Neurosurgery

NOTICE

Medicine is an ever-changing science. As new research and clinical experience broaden our knowledge, changes in treatment and drug therapy are required. The editors and the publisher of this work have checked with sources believed to be reliable in their efforts to provide information that is complete and generally in accord with the standards accepted at the time of publication. However, in view of the possibility of human error or changes in medical sciences, neither the editors nor the publisher nor any other party who has been involved in the preparation or publication of this work warrants that the information contained herein is in every respect accurate or complete, and they are not responsible for any errors or omissions or for the results obtained from use of such information. Readers are encouraged to confirm the information contained herein with other sources. For example and in particular, readers are advised to check the product information sheet included in the package of each drug they plan to administer to be certain that the information contained in this book is accurate and that changes have not been made in the recommended dose or in the contraindications for administration. This recommendation is of particular importance in connection with new or infrequently used drugs.

Neurosurgery

Second Edition
VOLUME II

Editors

Robert H. Wilkins, M.D.
Professor and Chief
Division of Neurosurgery
Duke University Medical Center
Durham, North Carolina

Setti S. Rengachary, M.D.
Professor of Neurosurgery
University of Minnesota Medical School
Minneapolis, Minnesota

McGRAW-HILL
Health Professions Division
New York St. Louis San Francisco Auckland Bogotá
Caracas Lisbon London Madrid Mexico City Milan Montreal
New Delhi San Juan Singapore Sydney Tokyo Toronto

McGraw-Hill
A Division of The **McGraw-Hill** *Companies*

Neurosurgery

123456780 DOW DOW 98765

ISBN 0-07-079991-1 (Set)
0-07-070313-2 (Volume I)
0-07-070314-0 (Volume II)
0-07-070315-9 (Volume III)

This book was set in Times Roman by York Graphic Services, Inc.
The editors were Martin J. Wonsiewicz and Mariapaz Ramos Englis;
the production supervisor was Clare Stanley; the cover designer was Karen Quigley.
The index was prepared by Alexandra Nickerson.
R. R. Donnelley and Sons, Inc., was printer and binder.

This book is printed on acid-free paper.

Library of Congress Cataloging-in-Publication Data

Neurosurgery / editors, Robert H. Wilkins, Setti S. Rengachary.—2d ed.
p. cm.
Includes bibliographical references and index.
ISBN 0-07-079991-1 (set : hard cover).—ISBN 0-07-070313-2 (v. 1 : hard cover).—ISBN 0-07-070314-0 (v. 2 : hard cover).—ISBN 0-07-070315-9 (v. 3 : hard cover)
1. Nervous system—Surgery. I. Wilkins, Robert H. II. Rengachary, Setti S.
[DNLM: 1. Nervous System Diseases—surgery. 2. Nervous System Diseases—diagnosis. 3. Neurosurgery—methods. WL 368 N4951 1996]
RD593.N417 1996
617.4′8—dc20
DNLM/DLC
for Library of Congress 95-35870

This book is dedicated to innovative neurosurgeons throughout the world

CONTENTS

Part V NEUROSURGICAL AND RELATED TECHNIQUES 515

Part VI NEURO-ONCOLOGY 653

Section A General Information

Section B Gliomas

Section C Metastatic Brain Tumors

Section D Meningiomas

Section E Epidermoid and Dermoid Tumors

Section F Tumors in the Region of the Pineal Gland

Section G Cerebellopontine Angle Tumors

VOLUME II

VOLUME III

Part X INFECTIONS 3267

Part XI DEVELOPMENTAL ANOMALIES AND NEUROSURGICAL DISORDERS OF CHILDHOOD 3409

CONTRIBUTORS

Numbers in brackets refer to the contributors' chapters.

Bizhan Aarabi, M.D.
Professor and Chairman, Division of Neurological Surgery, Shiraz University of Medical Sciences, Shiraz, Iran [279]

Rune Aaslid, Ph.D.
Research Associate Professor, Department of Neurological Surgery, University of Washington School of Medicine, Seattle, Washington [21]

Igor Z. Abolnik, M.D.
Assistant Professor, Department of Internal Medicine, University of Utah Health Sciences Center, Salt Lake City, Utah [331]

Jamshid Ahmadi, M.D.
Professor of Radiology and Neurological Surgery, University of Southern California School of Medicine, Los Angeles, California [263, 279]

Mark J. Alberts, M.D.
Assistant Professor, Division of Neurology, Duke University Medical Center, Durham, North Carolina [48]

Maurice Albin, M.D., M.S. (Anes.)
Professor and Vice Chairman Emeritus, Department of Anesthesiology, University of Texas Health Science Center at San Antonio, San Antonio, Texas [39]

A. Leland Albright, M.D.
Professor, Department of Neurological Surgery, University of Pittsburgh School of Medicine; and Chief, Department of Neurological Surgery, Children's Hospital of Pittsburgh, Pittsburgh, Pennsylvania [283]

E. Francois Aldrich, M.D., M.Med., F.C.S.
Associate Professor, Division of Neurological Surgery, University of Maryland Medical System, Baltimore, Maryland [134]

Eben Alexander, Jr., M.D.
Professor Emeritus, Department of Neurosurgery, The Bowman Gray School of Medicine, Winston-Salem, North Carolina [249, 397]

George S. Allen, M.D., Ph.D.
Professor and Chairman, Department of Neurological Surgery, Vanderbilt University Medical Center, Nashville, Tennessee [436]

Marshall B. Allen, Jr., M.D.
Professor Emeritus, Section of Neurosurgery, Medical College of Georgia, Augusta, Georgia [337]

Ossama Al-Mefty, M.D.
Professor and Chairman, Department of Neurosurgery, University of Arkansas for Medical Sciences, Little Rock, Arkansas [86, 94, 166]

Nayef Al-Rodhan, M.D., Ph.D.
Fellow, Department of Surgery (Neurosurgery), Harvard Medical School; and Molecular Neurogenetics Unit, Massachusetts General Hospital East, Charlestown, Massachusetts [222]

A. Loren Amacher, M.D., F.R.C.S.(C)
Neurosurgeon-in-Chief, Geisinger Medical Center, Danville, Pennsylvania [244]

Robert E. Anderson, B.S.
Department of Neurologic Surgery, Mayo Clinic, Rochester, Minnesota [191]

Edgardo J. C. Angtuaco, M.D.
Associate Professor, Department of Radiology, and Head of Neuroradiology and MRI, University of Arkansas for Medical Sciences, Little Rock, Arkansas [27, 216]

Mitchell S. Anscher, M.D.
Associate Professor, Department of Radiation Oncology, Duke University Medical Center, Durham, North Carolina [187]

Douglas C. Anthony, M.D., Ph.D.
Assistant Professor of Pathology, Harvard Medical School; and Director, Neuropathology, Children's Hospital, Boston, Massachusetts [173]

Ronald I. Apfelbaum, M.D.
Professor, Department of Neurological Surgery, University of Utah Health Sciences Center, Salt Lake City, Utah [293, 443]

Michael L.J. Apuzzo, M.D.
Edwin M. Todd/Trent H. Wells, Jr. Professor, Department of Neurological Surgery, University of Southern California School of Medicine, Los Angeles, California [73, 98, 188]

Arthur G. Arand, M.D.
Neurological Surgery, Cincinnati, Ohio [62]

Ehud Arbit, M.D.
Chief, Neurosurgery Service, Memorial Sloan-Kettering Cancer Center; and Professor of Surgery (Neurosurgery), Cornell University Medical College, New York, New York [83]

Simon J. Archibald, M.D.
Assistant Research Professor of Experimental Neurosurgery, Duke University Medical Center, Durham, North Carolina [315]

Joseph H. Arguelles, M.D.
Resident, Division of Neurosurgery, Oregon Health Sciences University, Portland, Oregon [318]

E. Joy Arpin, M.D.
Chief, Neurological Surgery, Cape Coral Hospital, Cape Coral, Florida [289]

Andrew W. Artenstein, M.D.
Assistant Professor of Medicine, Uniformed Services University of the Health Sciences, Bethesda, Maryland; and Division of Retrovirology, Walter Reed Army Institute of Research, Rockville, Maryland [329]

Sylvia L. Asa, M.D., Ph.D.
Associate Professor, Department of Pathology, University of Toronto and Mount Sinai Hospital, Toronto, Ontario, Canada [124]

David M. Asher, M.D.
Medical Officer, Laboratory of Central Nervous System Studies, National Institute of Neurological Disorders and Stroke, National Institutes of Health, Bethesda, Maryland [343]

James I. Ausman, M.D., Ph.D.
Professor and Head, Department of Neurosurgery, University of Illinois at Chicago, Chicago, Illinois [205]

Issam A. Awad, M.D., M.S.
Professor, Section of Neurological Surgery, and Head, Neurovascular Surgery Program, Yale University School of Medicine, New Haven, Connecticut [250]

Gregory J. Bailey, M.D., Ph.D.
Microsurgery and Brain Research Institute, P.C., St. Louis, Missouri [444]

Nevan G. Baldwin, M.D.
Assistant Professor, Division of Neurosurgery, The University of New Mexico School of Medicine, Albuquerque, New Mexico [23]

Marshall R. Ball, M.D.
Associate Professor, Department of Radiology, The Bowman Gray School of Medicine, Winston-Salem, North Carolina [197, 249]

H. Thomas Ballentine, Jr., M.D.
Clinical Professor of Surgery, Emeritus, Harvard Medical School; and Senior Neurosurgeon, Massachusetts General Hospital, Boston, Massachusetts [434]

Robert W. Baloh, M.D.
Professor of Neurology and Surgery (Head and Neck), University of California, Los Angeles School of Medicine, Los Angeles, California [11]

Peter N. Barboriak, M.D., Ph.D.
Director, Dementia Evaluation and Treatment Unit, Geropsychiatry Institute, John Umstead Hospital, Butner, North Carolina [132]

Gene H. Barnett, M.D.
Vice Chairman, Department of Neurosurgery, Cleveland Clinic Foundation, Cleveland, Ohio [386]

Daniel L Barrow, M.D.
Professor and Chairman, Department of Neurosurgery, Emory University School of Medicine, Atlanta, Georgia [227]

William J. Barwick, M.D.
Late Assistant Professor, Division of Plastic, Reconstructive, Maxillofacial, and Oral Surgery, Duke University Medical Center, Durham, North Carolina [269]

H. Hunt Batjer, M.D.
Marchese Professor and Chief, Division of Neurological Surgery, Northwestern University Medical School, Chicago, Illinois [221, 231, 240]

Janet W. Bay, M.D.
Clinical Associate Professor, Division of Neurosurgery, The Ohio State University College of Medicine, Columbus, Ohio [326]

William L. Bayer, M.D.
Director, Community Blood Center of Greater Kansas City, Kansas City, Missouri [38]

Donald P. Becker, M.D.
Eugene Stern Professor and Chief, Division of Neurosurgery, University of California, Los Angeles, School of Medicine, Los Angeles, California [265]

Myles Behrens, M.D.
Professor of Clinical Ophthalmology, College of Physicians & Surgeons of Columbia University; and Attending Ophthalmologist, Presbyterian Hospital, New York, New York [140]

Allan J. Belzberg, M.D., F.R.C.S.(C)
Assistant Professor, Department of Neurosurgery, The Johns Hopkins Medical Institutions, Baltimore, Maryland [319]

Gregory J. Bennett, M.D.
Assistant Professor, Department of Neurosurgery, School of Medicine and Biomedical Sciences, State University of New York at Buffalo, Buffalo, New York [300]

Edward C. Benzel, M.D.
Professor and Chief, Division of Neurosurgery, The University of New Mexico School of Medicine, Albuquerque, New Mexico [23, 282]

Mitchel S. Berger, M.D.
Associate Professor, Department of Neurological Surgery, and American Cancer Society Professor of Clinical Oncology, University of Washington Medical Center, Seattle, Washington [54]

Mark Bernstein, M.D., F.R.C.S.(C)
Associate Professor, Department of Surgery, University of Toronto; and Head, Division of Neurosurgery, The Toronto Hospital, Toronto, Ontario, Canada [169]

Darell D. Bigner, M.D., Ph.D.
Edwin L. Jones & Lucille Finch Jones Cancer Research Professor of Pathology, Duke University Medical Center, Durham, North Carolina [70, 75]

Sandra H. Bigner, M.D.
Professor, Department of Pathology, Duke University Medical Center, Durham, North Carolina [75]

Beverly M.K. Biller, M.D.
Assistant Professor of Medicine, Harvard Medical School; and Assistant in Medicine, Massachusetts General Hospital, Boston, Massachusetts [125]

José Biller, M.D.
Professor, Department of Neurology, Northwestern University Medical School, Chicago, Illinois [330]

Eugene F. Binet, M.D.
Warren Professor and Chairman, Department of Radiology, Medical College of Georgia, Augusta, Georgia [27, 216]

Keith L. Black, M.D.
Head, Neurosurgical Oncology, Division of Neurosurgery, School of Medicine and Medical Center, University of California, Los Angeles, Los Angeles, California [76]

Perry Black, M.D.
Professor, Department of Neurosurgery, Hahnemann University, Philadelphia, Pennsylvania [177]

Peter McL. Black, M.D., Ph.D.
Franc D. Ingraham Professor of Neurosurgery, Harvard Medical School; and Neurosurgeon-in-Chief, Brigham and Women's Hospital and Children's Hospital, Boston, Massachusetts [31, 129]

Jeffrey P. Blount, M.D.
Resident, Department of Neurosurgery, University of Minnesota School of Medicine, Minneapolis, Minnesota [119]

Bennett Blumenkopf, M.D.
Associate Professor, Department of Neurological Surgery, Vanderbilt University Medical Center, Nashville, Tennessee [421]

James E. Boggan, M.D.
Professor and Acting Chairman, Department of Neurological Surgery, School of Medicine, University of California, Davis, Sacramento, California [127, 328, 335]

Michael H. Bowman, M.D., Ph.D.
Attending Neurologist, Wake Medical Center, Raleigh, North Carolina [430]

Derald E. Brackmann, M.D.
Clinical Professor of Otolaryngology–Head and Neck Surgery, and Clinical Professor of Neurosurgery, University of Southern California School of Medicine, and President, House Ear Clinic, Los Angeles, California [163]

Charles L. Branch, Jr., M.D.
Associate Professor, Department of Neurosurgery, The Bowman Gray School of Medicine, Winston-Salem, North Carolina [312]

Jon Brillman, M.D.
Professor and Chairman, Department of Neurology, Allegheny Campus, Medical College of Pennsylvania, Pittsburgh, Pennsylvania [148]

Derek A. Bruce, M.B., Ch.B.
Clinical Professor of Neurosurgery, University of Texas Southwestern Medical Center; and Director, Center for Pediatric Neurosurgery, Children's Medical Center of Dallas, Dallas, Texas [115, 266, 270]

Jeffrey N. Bruce, M.D.
Assistant Professor, Departments of Neurological Surgery and Pathology, College of Physicians and Surgeons of Columbia University, New York, New York [102]

William A. Buchheit, M.D.
Professor, Department of Neurological Surgery, Jefferson Medical College, Philadelphia, Pennsylvania [107]

Dennis E. Bullard, M.D.
Raleigh Neurosurgical Clinic, Inc., Raleigh, North Carolina [74]

Elizabeth Bullitt, M.D.
Associate Professor of Surgery (Neurosurgery), University of North Carolina School of Medicine, Chapel Hill, North Carolina [344]

James L. Bundy, M.D.
Clinical Associate Professor of Neurosurgery and Radiology, State University of New York at Buffalo School of Medicine and Biomedical Sciences, Buffalo, New York [211]

Kim J. Burchiel, M.D.
John Raaf Professor and Head, Division of Neurosurgery, Oregon Health Sciences University, Portland, Oregon [318]

Peter C. Burger, M.D.
Professor of Pathology, The Johns Hopkins Medical Institutions, Baltimore, Maryland [77]

R. Stanley Burns, M.D.
Associate Professor, Department of Neurology, and Director, Vanderbilt Movement Disorders Clinic, Vanderbilt University Medical Center, Nashville, Tennessee [436]

Edward Byrd, M.D.
Assistant Clinical Professor of Neurological Surgery, George Washington School of Medicine and Health Sciences, Washington, District of Columbia [130]

J. Gregory Cairncross, M.D.
Professor, Departments of Clinical Neurological Sciences and Oncology, University of Western Ontario; and Attending Neurologist, London Regional Cancer Centre, London, Ontario, Canada [189]

James N. Campbell, M.D.
Professor, Department of Neurosurgery, The Johns Hopkins Medical Institutions, Baltimore, Maryland [319]

Peter W. Carmel, M.D., D.Med.Sc.
Professor and Chief, Section of Neurological Surgery, University of Medicine and Dentistry of New Jersey, New Jersey Medical School, Newark, New Jersey [136, 139]

Michael J. Caron, M.D.
Associate Medical Director, Chicago Institute of NeuroSurgery and NeuroResearch, Silver Cross Hospital, Joliet, Illinois [265]

Leonard J. Cerullo, M.D.
Medical Director, Chicago Institute of NeuroSurgery and NeuroResearch, Chicago, Illinois [61]

Venkata R. Challa, M.D.
Professor of Pathology, The Bowman Gray School of Medicine, Winston-Salem, North Carolina [87]

Fady T. Charbel, M.D.
Assistant Professor, Department of Neurosurgery, University of Illinois at Chicago, Chicago, Illinois [205]

Michael Chicoine, M.D.
Resident, Neurological Surgery, Washington University School of Medicine, St. Louis, Missouri [208]

Henry T. Ching, M.D.
Assistant Professor, Department of Radiology, The George Washington University Medical Center, Washington, District of Columbia [174]

Shelley N. Chou, M.D., Ph.D.
Professor Emeritus, Department of Neurosurgery, University of Minnesota Medical School, Minneapolis, Minnesota [398]

Ivan Ciric, M.D.
Bennett-Tarkington Chair in Neurosurgery, Northwestern University Medical School; and Head, Division of Neurosurgery, The Evanston Hospital, Evanston, Illinois [392]

Guy L. Clifton, M.D.
Professor and Chairman, Department of Neurosurgery, The University of Texas-Houston Health Science Center, Houston, Texas [44]

William Cobb, M.D.
Mount Sinai Medical School, New York, New York [131]

Alan R. Cohen, M.D.
Chief of Pediatric Neurosurgery, Rainbow Babies and Children's Hospital; and Associate Professor of Neurological Surgery and Pediatrics, Case Western Reserve University School of Medicine, Cleveland, Ohio [51]

Douglas S. Cohen, M.D.
Resident, Department of Neurological Surgery, Neurological Institute of New York, Columbia University, New York, New York [33]

R. E. Coleman, M.D.
Professor, Division of Nuclear Medicine, Duke University Medical Center, Durham, North Carolina [24]

Frances K. Conley, M.D.
Professor, Department of Neurosurgery, Stanford University School of Medicine, Stanford, California [97]

Edward S. Connolly, M.D.
Senior Neurosurgeon, Ochsner Medical Institution, Professor of Neurosurgery, Louisiana State University School of Medicine in New Orleans; and Clinical Professor of Neurosurgery, Tulane University School of Medicine, New Orleans, Louisiana [324, 395]

E. Sander Connolly, Jr., M.D.
Resident, Department of Neurological Surgery, Columbia-Presbyterian Medical Center and The Neurological Institute, New York, New York [136]

Shlomi Constantini, M.D., M.Sc.
Division of Pediatric Neurosurgery, Hadassah University Hospital, Jerusalem, Israel [60]

Wesley A. Cook, Jr., M.D.
Associate Professor, Division of Neurosurgery, Duke University Medical Center, Durham, North Carolina [296]

Paul R. Cooper, M.D.
Professor, Department of Neurosurgery, New York University Medical Center, New York, New York [276]

Bernard J. Cosman
Late Founder and Former President, Radionics, Inc., Burlington, Massachusetts [429]

Eric R. Cosman, Ph.D.
Professor of Physics, Emeritus, Massachusetts Institute of Technology, Cambridge; and President, Radionics, Inc., Burlington, Massachusetts [429]

William T. Couldwell, M.D., Ph.D.
Assistant Professor, Department of Neurosurgery, University of Southern California School of Medicine, Los Angeles, California [345]

Barbara J. Crain, M.D., Ph.D.
Associate Professor of Pathology and Neurology, The Johns Hopkins University School of Medicine, Baltimore, Maryland [167]

Kerry R. Crone, M.D.
Associate Professor, Department of Neurosurgery, University of Cincinnati College of Medicine, Cincinnati, Ohio [370, 377]

DeWitte Cross, M.D.
Assistant Professor of Radiology (Neuroradiology), Washington University School of Medicine, St. Louis, Missouri [208]

Robert M. Crowell, M.D.
Professor of Surgery (Neurosurgery), University of Massachusetts Medical Center, Worcester, Massachusetts; and Neurosurgeon, Berkshire Medical Center, Pittsfield, Massachusetts [202, 204]

C. J. Cummins, Ph.D.
Formerly of the National Institute of Neurological and Communicative Disorders and Stroke, National Institutes of Health, Bethesda, Maryland [72]

Ralph G. Dacey, Jr., M.D.
Professor and Chairman, Neurological Surgery, Washington University School of Medicine; and Neurosurgeon-in-Chief, Barnes Hospital, St. Louis, Missouri [208, 258]

Neil C. Davey, M.B., Ch.B., F.F.Rad.D.(S.A.)
Fellow and Associate in Neuroradiology, Department of Radiology, Duke University Medical Center, Durham, North Carolina [203]

Carlos A. David, M.D.
Resident, Department of Neurological Surgery, University of Miami School of Medicine, Miami, Florida [302, 303]

James N. Davis, M.D.
Professor and Chairman, Department of Neurology, State University of New York at Stony Brook, Stony Brook, New York [207]

Arthur L. Day, M.D.
James and Newton Eblen Scholar and Professor of Neurological Surgery, J. Hillis Miller Health Center and College of Medicine, University of Florida, Gainesville, Florida [223]

John H.N. Deck, M.D., F.R.C.P.(C)
Professor, Department of Pathology, University of Toronto, Toronto, Ontario, Canada [169]

George Robert DeLong, M.D.
Associate Professor, Department of Pediatrics, Duke University Medical Center, Durham, North Carolina [349]

R.A. de los Reyes, M.D.
Associate Professor of Neurosurgery and Director of Cerebral Vascular Surgery, Montefiore Medical Center, Bronx, New York [205]

Evandro DeOliveira, M.D.
Instituto Neurologico, São Paulo, Brazil [93]

Sylvie Destian, M.D.
Assistant Professor of Radiology, University of Southern California School of Medicine, Los Angeles, California [263]

Fernando G. Diaz, M.D., Ph.D.
Professor and Chairman, Department of Neurological Surgery, Wayne State University, Detroit, Michigan [205]

Curtis A. Dickman, M.D.
Associate Chief, Spine Section, Division of Neurological Surgery, Barrow Neurological Institute, Phoenix, Arizona [290]

Thomas S. Dina, M.D.
Director, Section of Neuroradiology, Department of Radiology and Radiological Sciences, Vanderbilt University and Medical Center, Nashville, Tennessee [174]

Jacques E. Dion, M.D., F.R.C.P.(C)
Associate Professor of Neuroradiology and Neurosurgery, and Head, Interventional Neuroradiology Section, University of Virginia Health Sciences Center, Charlottesville, Virginia [234]

Donald F. Dohn, M.D.
Department of Neurological Surgery (Ret.), Cleveland Clinic Foundation, Cleveland, Ohio [326]

George J. Dohrmann, M.D., Ph.D.
Associate Professor, Section of Neurosurgery, University of Chicago Medical Center, Chicago, Illinois [56, 117]

R.M. Peardon Donaghy, M.D.
Late Professor Emeritus, Division of Neurosurgery, College of Medicine, University of Vermont, Burlington, Vermont [4]

Charles G. Drake, M.D., O.C., F.R.C.S.(C)
Professor, Division of Neurosurgery, The University of Western Ontario, London, Ontario, Canada [229, 243]

Miles E. Drake, M.D.
Associate Professor of Neurology and Psychiatry, The Ohio State University College of Medicine, Columbus, Ohio [19]

Burton P. Drayer, M.D.
Radiologist-in-Chief, Barrow Neurological Institute, Phoenix, Arizona [25]

Thomas B. Ducker, M.D.
Annapolis, Maryland; Professor, Department of Neurosurgery, The Johns Hopkins Medical Institutions; and Clinical Professor, Division of Neurological Surgery, University of Maryland Medical System, Baltimore, Maryland [309]

Gary R. Duckwiler, M.D.
Endovascular Therapy Service, School of Medicine and Medical Center, University of California, Los Angeles, Los Angeles, California [65, 66]

Derek A. Duke, M.D.
Resident, Department of Neurologic Surgery, Mayo Clinic, Rochester, Minnesota [176]

David T. Durack, D.Phil.(Oxon), M.B., F.R.C.P., F.R.A.C.P.
Chairman, Department of Medicine, Health Care International, Ltd., Clydebank, Scotland [331]

Jonathan J. Dutton, M.D., Ph.D.
Professor, Department of Ophthalmology, Duke University Medical Center, Durham, North Carolina [322]

J. Donald Easton, M.D.
Professor and Chairman, Department of Clinical Neurosciences, Brown University School of Medicine; and Physician-in-Chief, Department of Neurology, Rhode Island Hospital, Providence, Rhode Island [201]

Michael J. Ebersold, M.D.
Associate Professor, Department of Neurologic Surgery, Mayo Clinic, Rochester, Minnesota [170]

Howard M. Eisenberg, M.D.
Professor and Head, Division of Neurological Surgery, University of Maryland Medical System, Baltimore, Maryland [134]

Magdy El-Kalliny, M.D.
Lecturer of Neurosurgery, Ain-Shams University, Cairo, Egypt [164]

Amr O. El-Naggar, M.D.
Neurosurgery, Somerset, Kentucky [422]

John D. England, M.D.
Associate Professor, Department of Neurology, Louisiana State University School of Medicine in New Orleans, New Orleans, Louisiana [325]

Fred J. Epstein, M.D.
Professor and Director, Division of Pediatric Neurosurgery, New York University Medical Center, New York, New York [60]

Joseph A. Epstein, M.D.
Clinical Professor of Neurological Surgery, Albert Einstein College of Medicine, Bronx; and Honorary Attending, Division of Neurosurgery, North Shore University Hospital, Manhasset, New York [391]

Mel H. Epstein, M.D.
Professor and Chairman, Department of Neurosciences, Brown University, Providence, Rhode Island [376]

Nancy E. Epstein, M.D.
Clinical Associate Professor of Surgery (Neurosurgery), Cornell University Medical College, New York; and Associate Attending, Division of Neurosurgery, North Shore University Hospital, Manhasset, New York [383, 391]

Andrea C. Erwin, B.A.
Technical Administrator, Clinical Neurophysiology Laboratory, Duke University Medical Center, Durham, North Carolina [19]

C. William Erwin, M.D.
Professor, Department of Psychiatry, and Associate Professor, Division of Neurology, Duke University Medical Center, Durham, North Carolina [19]

E. Fletcher Eyster, M.D.
West Florida Regional Medical Center, Pensacola, Florida [257]

Jacob I. Fabrikant, M.D., Ph.D.
Late Professor of Radiology, University of California, San Francisco and Berkeley; and Medical Scientist and Senior Scientist, Donner Pavilion and Donner Laboratory, Lawrence Berkeley Laboratory, University of California, Berkeley, Berkeley, California [184]

Joseph C. Farmer, M.D.
Professor, Division of Otolaryngology–Head and Neck Surgery, Duke University Medical Center, Durham, North Carolina [57]

Gary J. Felsberg, M.D.
Neuroradiologist, Magnetic Resonance Institutes, Boca Raton, Florida [26]

Richard G. Fessler, M.D., Ph.D.
Dunspaugh Dalton Chair of Brain and Spinal Surgery, Department of Neurological Surgery, University of Florida College of Medicine, Gainesville, Florida [298]

Michael R. Fetell, M.D.
Clinical Associate Professor, Department of Neurology, College of Physicians and Surgeons of Columbia University, New York, New York [102]

Paul J. Feustel, Ph.D.
Division of Neurosurgery, The Albany Medical College, Albany, New York [260]

Howard C. Filston, M.D.
Professor of Pediatric Surgery and Pediatrics, and Chief of Pediatric Surgery and Trauma, The University of Tennessee Graduate Medical Center at Knoxville, Knoxville, Tennessee [357]

John Fisher, M.D.
Section of Infectious Diseases, Medical College of Georgia, Augusta, Georgia [337]

Wink S. Fisher III, M.D.
Associate Professor, Division of Neurosurgery, University of Alabama at Birmingham, Birmingham, Alabama [238]

Robert D. Fitch, M.D.
Assistant Clinical Professor, Division of Orthopaedic Surgery, Duke University Medical Center, Durham, North Carolina [399]

Eugene S. Flamm, M.D.
Charles Harrison Frazier Professor and Chairman, Division of Neurosurgery, University of Pennsylvania, Philadelphia, Pennsylvania [224]

Ann Marie Flannery, M.D.
Associate Professor, Section of Neurosurgery, Medical College of Georgia, Augusta, Georgia [337]

J.F. Ross Fleming, M.D., F.R.C.S.(C)
Professor, Department of Surgery, University of Toronto, and Division of Neurosurgery, The Toronto Hospital, Toronto, Ontario, Canada [169]

Robert L. Flinner, M.D.
Resident, Department of Pathology, Latter Day Saints Hospital, Salt Lake City, Utah [130]

Eldon L. Foltz, M.D.
Professor Emeritus, Neurological Surgery, University of California Irvine Medical Center, Orange, California [369]

John A. Fox, M.D.
Fellow in Pediatric Orthopaedic Surgery, Texas Scottish Rite Hospital, Dallas, Texas [338]

Randal D. France, M.D.
Salt Lake City, Utah [402]

Arthur Frankel, M.D.
Associate Professor of Medicine, Medical University of South Carolina, Charleston, South Carolina [85]

Kenneth A. Frankel, Ph.D.
Assistant Adjunct Professor of Radiology, University of California, San Francisco; and Staff Scientist, Donner Pavilion and Donner Laboratory, Lawrence Berkeley Laboratory, University of California, Berkeley, Berkeley, California [184]

John G. Frazee, M.D.
Associate Clinical Professor, Division of Neurosurgery, University of California, Los Angeles, Los Angeles, California [233]

Glenn D. Frazer, Ph.D.
Assistant Professor, Department of Neurosurgery, Thomas Jefferson University Hospital, Philadelphia, Pennsylvania [198]

Arno H. Fried, M.D.
Associate Professor, Clinical Neurosciences (Neurosurgery) and Pediatrics, Brown University School of Medicine; and Chief, Section of Pediatric Neurosurgery, Rhode Island Hospital, Providence, Rhode Island [376]

Allan H. Friedman, M.D.
Professor, Division of Neurosurgery, Duke University Medical Center, Durham, North Carolina [25, 212, 218, 219, 226, 235, 344, 396, 411]

Herbert E. Fuchs, M.D., Ph.D.
Assistant Professor, Division of Neurosurgery, Duke University Medical Center, Durham, North Carolina [70, 75]

Gregory N. Fuller, M.D., Ph.D.
Assistant Professor of Pathology, Section of Neuropathology, The University of Texas M.D. Anderson Cancer Center, Houston, Texas [71, 77]

Eric M. Gabriel, M.D.
Resident, Division of Neurosurgery, Duke University Medical Center, Durham, North Carolina [268, 396]

Joseph H. Galicich, M.D.
Attending Surgeon, Neurosurgery Service, Memorial Sloan-Kettering Cancer Center; and Professor of Surgery (Neurosurgery), Cornell University Medical College, New York, New York [83]

Julio H. Garcia, M.D.
Professor of Pathology, Case Western Reserve University; and Head, Division of Neuropathology, Henry Ford Hospital, Detroit, Michigan [199]

H.D. Garretson, M.D., Ph.D.
Professor and Chairman, Department of Neurological Surgery, University of Louisville School of Medicine, Louisville, Kentucky [239]

Sarah J. Gaskill, M.D.
Pediatric Neurosurgery, San Antonio, Texas [52, 153]

Laurie E. Gaspar, M.D.
Assistant Professor, Department of Radiation Oncology, Wayne State University School of Medicine, Detroit, Michigan [187]

Emmanuel Gay, M.D.
Assistant de Neurochirurgie, Service de Neurochirurgie, Centre Hospitalier Universitaire de Grenoble, Grenoble, France [151]

Jack C. Geer, M.D.
Professor Emeritus, Department of Pathology, University of Alabama at Birmingham, Birmingham, Alabama [199]

Fred H. Geisler, M.D., Ph.D.
Director, Comprehensive Spine Care Center, Chicago Institute of NeuroSurgery and NeuroResearch Medical Group, S.C., Chicago, Illinois [271]

Thomas A. Gennarelli, M.D.
Professor and Chairman, Department of Neurosurgery, Center for Neurosciences, Medical College of Pennsylvania and Hahnemann University, Philadelphia, Pennsylvania [259]

Fred Gentili, M.D., M.Sc., F.R.C.S.(C)
Associate Professor, Division of Neurosurgery, University of Toronto and The Toronto Hospital, Toronto, Ontario, Canada [308]

Ralph P. George, M.D.
Clinical Professor of Internal Medicine, University of California, San Diego; and Vice-President, Medical Affairs, Mercy Health Care, San Diego, California [255]

Gregory S. Georgiade, M.D.
Associate Professor, Division of General Surgery, and Associate Professor, Division of Plastic, Reconstructive, Maxillofacial, and Oral Surgery, Duke University Medical Center, Durham, North Carolina [273]

Nicholas G. Georgiade, D.D.S., M.D.
Professor Emeritus, Division of Plastic, Reconstructive, Maxillofacial, and Oral Surgery, Duke University Medical Center, Durham, North Carolina [273]

Oded Gerber, M.D.
Assistant Professor, Department of Neurology, State University of New York at Stony Brook, Stony Brook, New York [207]

Christopher C. Getch, M.D.
Jefferson Hospital, Philadelphia, Pennsylvania [107]

George Giannakopoulos, M.D.
Hudson, Florida [177]

Steven L. Giannotta, M.D.
Professor, Department of Neurological Surgery, University of Southern California School of Medicine, Los Angeles, California [279]

Clarence J. Gibbs, Jr., Ph.D.
Deputy Chief, Laboratory of Central Nervous System Studies, National Institute of Neurological Disorders and Stroke, National Institutes of Health, Bethesda, Maryland [343]

Philip L. Gildenberg, M.D., Ph.D.
Director, Houston Stereotactic Center, Houston, Texas [431]

Lawrence E. Ginsberg, M.D.
Assistant Professor, Department of Diagnostic Radiology, University of Texas M.D. Anderson Cancer Center, Houston, Texas [88]

P. Langham Gleason, M.D.
Neurosurgical Service, Brigham and Women's Hospital and Children's Hospital, Boston, Massachusetts [31]

Larry B. Goldstein, M.D.
Assistant Professor, Division of Neurology, Duke University Medical Center, Durham, North Carolina [29, 43]

John P. Gorecki, M.D., F.R.C.S.(C)
Assistant Professor, Division of Neurosurgery, Duke University Medical Center, Durham, North Carolina [417, 419]

Liliana Goumnerova, M.D., F.R.C.S.(C)
Instructor in Surgery, Harvard Medical School; and Associate in Surgery, Childrens Hospital, Boston, Massachusetts [116]

Paul A. Grabb, M.D.
Assistant Professor, Division of Neurosurgery, The University of Alabama at Birmingham; and Section of Pediatric Neurosurgery, The Children's Hospital of Alabama, Birmingham, Alabama [283]

Carmelo Graffagnino, M.D.
Assistant Professor, Division of Neurology, Duke University Medical Center, Durham, North Carolina [48]

Brent Graham, M.D., F.R.C.S.(C)
Assistant Professor, Divisions of Orthopaedic Surgery and Plastic Surgery, University of Toronto, Toronto, Ontario, Canada [310]

Doyle G. Graham, M.D., Ph.D.
Professor and Chair, Department of Pathology, Vanderbilt University Medical Center, Nashville, Tennessee [172]

Linda Gray, M.D.
Assistant Professor, Department of Radiology, Duke University Medical Center, Durham, North Carolina [96, 105, 203]

Barth A. Green, M.D.
Professor and Chairman, Department of Neurological Surgery, and Clinical Professor, Department of Orthopaedic Surgery, University of Miami School of Medicine; and Director, Spinal Cord Injury Service, Jackson Memorial Medical Center, Miami, Florida [302, 303]

John R. Green, M.D.
Late Director, Barrow Neurological Institute, Phoenix, Arizona [1]

I.M. Greenberg, M.D.
Clinical Professor of Neurosurgery, State University of New York, Stonybrook, New York [59]

Samuel H. Greenblatt, M.A., M.D.
Associate Professor of Neurosurgery, Brown University, Providence, Rhode Island [6]

Daryl R. Gress, M.D.
Assistant Professor of Clinical Neurology, and Director, Neurovascular Service, University of California, San Francisco, San Francisco, California [202]

Oliver Woodhouse Grin, M.D.
Chief of Neurosurgery, Blodgett Memorial Medical Center, Grand Rapids, Michigan [438]

Peter Gruen, M.D.
Assistant Professor, Department of Neurological Surgery, University of Southern California School of Medicine, Los Angeles, California [98]

Abhijit Guha, M.D., M.Sc., F.R.C.S.(C)
Assistant Professor, Division of Neurosurgery, University of Toronto; and Scientist, Lunenfeld Research Institute, Mount Sinai Hospital, Toronto, Ontario, Canada [310]

Mary Kay Gumerlock, M.D.
Associate Professor, Department of Neurosurgery, The University of Oklahoma Health Sciences Center, Oklahoma City, Oklahoma [190]

Murali Guthikonda, M.D.
Assistant Professor and Chief of Skull Base Surgery, Department of Neurosurgery, Wayne State University, Detroit, Michigan [164]

A. Norman Guthkelch, M.Ch., F.R.C.S.
Formerly Professor of Neurosurgery, University of Pittsburgh, Pittsburgh, Pennsylvania [353]

Philip H. Gutin, M.D.
Professor and Chairman, Department of Neurological Surgery, School of Medicine, University of California, San Francisco, San Francisco, California [186]

Earl R. Hackett, M.D.
Neurologist, Springfield, Missouri [313]

Georges F. Haddad, M.D., F.R.C.S.(C)
Clinical Assistant Professor of Neurosurgery, American University of Beirut, Beirut, Lebanon [86, 94, 166]

Mark N. Hadley, M.D.
Associate Professor, Division of Neurosurgery, University of Alabama at Birmingham School of Medicine, Birmingham, Alabama [210, 288]

Stephen J. Haines, M.D.
Professor of Neurosurgery and Professor of Otolaryngology and Pediatrics, Department of Neurosurgery, University of Minnesota Medical School, Minneapolis, Minnesota [440]

F. Terry Hambrecht, M.D.
Head, Neural Prosthesis Program, Division of Fundamental Neurosciences, National Institute of Neurological Disorders and Stroke, National Institutes of Health, Bethesda, Maryland [435]

H. Bruce Hamilton, M.D.
Resident, Department of Neurosurgery, Louisiana State University School of Medicine in New Orleans, New Orleans, Louisiana [150]

William C. Hanigan, M.D., Ph.D.
Clinical Professor of Neurological Surgery, Department of Neuroscience, University of Illinois College of Medicine at Peoria, Peoria, Illinois [375]

William T. Hardaker, Jr., M.D.
Associate Professor, Division of Orthopaedic Surgery, Duke University Medical Center, Durham, North Carolina [286, 296, 297, 338]

Jules Hardy, O.C., C.Q., M.D., F.R.C.S.(C)
Professeur Titulaire, Université de Montréal; and Adjunct Professor, McGill University, Montreal, Quebec, Canada [137]

Russell W. Hardy, Jr., M.D.
Professor, Department of Neurological Surgery, Case Western Reserve University School of Medicine and University Hospitals of Cleveland, Cleveland, Ohio [305]

H. Louis Harkey, M.D.
Assistant Professor, Department of Neurosurgery, University of Mississippi Medical Center, Jackson, Mississippi [294]

Kristine D. Harper, M.D.
Assistant Professor, Division of Endocrinology, and Medical Director, Bone and Metabolism Clinic, Duke University Medical Center, Durham, North Carolina [380]

John M. Harrelson, M.D.
Associate Professor, Division of Orthopaedic Surgery, and Assistant Professor, Department of Pathology, Duke University Medical Center, Durham, North Carolina [178]

A. Basil Harris, M.D.
Professor, Department of Neurological Surgery, University of Washington School of Medicine, Seattle, Washington [420]

Steven J. Harrison, M.S., F.A.M.I.
Assistant Professor and Chairman, Department of Medical Illustration, Medical College of Georgia, Augusta, Georgia [161]

Griffith R. Harsh IV, M.D.
Associate Professor of Surgery, Harvard Medical School; and Visiting Associate Neurosurgeon, Massachusetts General Hospital, Boston, Massachusetts [90, 278]

B. Thomas Harter, Jr., M.D.
Clinical Associate Professor of Surgery, University of Louisville School of Medicine, Louisville, Kentucky [149]

Kathleen C. Harter, M.D.
Medical Director, Ford Louisville Assembly Plant, Louisville, Kentucky [149]

M. Peter Heilbrun, M.D.
Joseph J. Yager Professor and Chair, Department of Neurological Surgery, The University of Utah School of Medicine, Salt Lake City, Utah [426]

Carl B. Heilman, M.D.
Assistant Professor, Department of Neurosurgery, Tufts University School of Medicine and New England Medical Center Hospital, Boston, Massachusetts [146]

E. Ralph Heinz, M.D.
Professor, Department of Radiology, Duke University Medical Center, Durham, North Carolina [2]

David C. Hemmy, M.D.
Clinical Professor of Neurosurgery, Medical College of Wisconsin, Milwaukee, Wisconsin [180]

Nelson Hendler, M.D., M.S.
Assistant Professor of Neurosurgery, The Johns Hopkins Medical Institutions; and Associate Professor of Physiology, University of Maryland School of Dental Surgery, Baltimore; and Clinical Director, Mensana Clinic, Stevenson, Maryland [414]

Juha A. Hernesniemi, M.D.
Associate Professor, Department of Neurosurgery, University Hospital of Kuopio, Kuopio, Finland [229, 243]

Roberto C. Heros, M.D.
Professor and Co-Chairman, Department of Neurological Surgery, and Director, International Neurological Institute, University of Miami, Miami, Florida [225, 230]

Maie Kaarsoo Herrick, M.D.
Clinical Associate Professor of Pathology (Neuropathology) and Neurology, Stanford University, Santa Clara Valley Medical Center, San Jose, California [99]

Arnold M. Herskovic, M.D.
Professor, Department of Radiation Oncology, Wayne State University School of Medicine; and Medical Director, Department of Radiation Oncology, Oakwood Hospital, Dearborn, Michigan [182]

Lloyd A. Hey, M.D., M.S.
Assistant Professor, Division of Orthopaedic Surgery, Duke University Medical Center, Durham, North Carolina [384]

Alfred C. Higgins, M.D.
Wenatchee, Washington [421]

William E. Hitselberger, M.D.
Neurosurgeon, Los Angeles, California [109]

Charles J. Hodge, Jr., M.D.
Professor and Chairman, Department of Neurosurgery, State University of New York Health Science Center at Syracuse, Syracuse, New York [389]

Julian T. Hoff, M.D.
Professor and Head, Section of Neurosurgery, University of Michigan Medical Center, Ann Arbor, Michigan [381]

Harold J. Hoffman, M.D., B.Sc.(Med), F.R.C.S.(C)
Professor, Department of Surgery, University of Toronto; and Neurosurgeon-in-Chief, The Hospital for Sick Children, Toronto, Ontario, Canada [116, 372]

John M. Hoffman, M.D.
Associate Professor of Neurology and Radiology, Emory University School of Medicine, Atlanta, Georgia [24]

Rose Marie Holt, M.D.
Instructor, Department of Radiology, University of Washington School of Medicine, Seattle, Washington [79]

L.N. Hopkins, M.D.
Professor of Neurosurgery and Radiology, State University of New York at Buffalo School of Medicine and Biomedical Sciences, Buffalo, New York [211]

Eva Horvath, Ph.D.
Associate Professor, Department of Pathology, University of Toronto and St. Michael's Hospital, Toronto, Ontario, Canada [124]

William F. House, M.D.
Clinical Professor of Otolaryngology, University of Southern California School of Medicine, Newport Beach, California [109]

Edgar M. Housepian, M.D.
Professor of Clinical Neurological Surgery, College of Physicians & Surgeons of Columbia University; and Attending Neurological Surgeon, Presbyterian Hospital, New York, New York [140]

Frank P.K. Hsu, M.D., Ph.D.
Resident, Division of Neurosurgery, Oregon Health Sciences University, Portland, Oregon [247]

Alan R. Hudson, M.B., Ch.B., F.R.C.S.(C)
President and Chief Executive Officer, The Toronto Hospital; and Professor, Division of Neurosurgery, University of Toronto, Toronto, Ontario, Canada [308, 310]

Christine M. Hulette, M.D.
Assistant Professor of Neuropathology and Associate in Neurology, Duke University Medical Center, Durham, North Carolina [200]

Robin P. Humphreys, M.D., F.R.C.S.(C)
Professor, Department of Surgery, University of Toronto; and Associate Surgeon-In-Chief, Hospital for Sick Children, Toronto, Ontario, Canada [350]

Barrie J. Hurwitz, M.D.
Associate Professor, Division of Neurology, Duke University Medical Center, Durham, North Carolina [5]

Bermans J. Iskandar, M.D.
Chief Resident, Division of Neurosurgery, Duke University Medical Center, Durham, North Carolina [172, 213]

Ian T. Jackson, M.D., F.R.C.S., F.R.A.C.S.(Hon)
Director, Institute for Craniofacial Reconstructive Surgery, Providence Hospital, Southfield, Michigan [156]

Ivor M.D. Jackson, M.D.
Professor of Medicine and Director, Division of Endocrinology, Brown University; and Chief of Endocrinology, Rhode Island Hospital, Providence, Rhode Island [121]

Hector E. James, M.D.
Clinical Professor of Neurosurgery and Pediatrics, School of Medicine, University of California, San Diego, San Diego, California [22, 171]

Peter J. Jannetta, M.D.
Walter E. Dandy Professor and Chairman, Department of Neurological Surgery, University of Pittsburgh School of Medicine, Pittsburgh, Pennsylvania [321,409]

Ronald J. Jaszczak, Ph.D.
Professor, Department of Radiology and Department of Biomedical Engineering, Duke University Medical Center, Durham, North Carolina [25]

Iain H. Kalfas, M.D.
Head, Section of Spinal Surgery, Department of Neurosurgery, Cleveland Clinic Foundation, Cleveland, Ohio [386]

David F. Kallmes, M.D.
Instructor, Neuroradiology Section, University of Virginia Medical Center, Charlottesville, Virginia [96]

John E. Kalsbeck, M.D.
Professor of Surgery (Neurosurgery), Indiana University Medical Center; and James Whitcomb Riley Hospital for Children, Indianapolis, Indiana [142]

Uma P. Kalyan-Raman, M.D.
Department of Pathology, University of Illinois College of Medicine at Peoria, Peoria, Illinois [248]

John P. Kapp, M.D., Ph.D., J.D.
Kapp & Stewart Law Office, Winston-Salem, North Carolina [197, 213]

Howard H. Kaufman, M.D.
Professor and Chairman, Department of Neurosurgery, West Virginia University School of Medicine, Morgantown, West Virginia [28, 254, 284]

Mary Ann E. Keenan, M.D.
Chairman, Department of Orthopaedic Surgery, Albert Einstein Medical Center, Moss Rehabilitation Hospital, Philadelphia, Pennsylvania [42]

Diana B. Kelker, M.P.A.
Executive Director, THINK FIRST Foundation, Park Ridge, Illinois [257]

Jeffrey T. Keller, Ph.D.
Director of Education, Department of Neurosurgery, University of Cincinnati, Cincinnati, Ohio [164]

David L. Kelly, Jr., M.D.
Assistant Professor, Division of Neurosurgery, University of California, Los Angeles, School of Medicine and Harbor-UCLA Medical Center, Los Angeles, California [265]

David L. Kelly, Jr., M.D.
Professor and Chairman, Department of Neurosurgery, The Bowman Gray School of Medicine, Winston-Salem, North Carolina [312, 359]

Patrick J. Kelly, M.D.
Professor and Chairman, Department of Neurosurgery, New York University Medical Center, New York, New York [427]

Jerone D. Kennedy, M.D.
Resident, Department of Neurosurgery, University of Minnesota School of Medicine, Minneapolis, Minnesota [374]

John S. Kennerdell, M.D.
Professor and Chairman, Department of Ophthalmology, Allegheny Campus, Medical College of Pennsylvania, Pittsburgh, Pennsylvania [148]

John J. Kepes, M.D.
Professor Emeritus, Department of Pathology, University of Kansas Medical Center, Kansas City, Kansas [130]

Rashida A. Khakoo, M.D.
Professor, Department of Medicine, West Virginia University School of Medicine, Morgantown, West Virginia [28]

Jerome H. Kim, M.D.
Assistant Professor of Medicine, Uniformed Services University of the Health Sciences, Bethesda, Maryland; and Division of Retrovirology, Walter Reed Army Institute of Research, Rockville, Maryland [329]

Harold K. Kimelberg, Ph.D.
Division of Neurosurgery, The Albany Medical College, Albany, New York [260]

J. Philip Kistler, M.D.
Associate Professor of Neurology, Harvard Medical School; and Associate Neurologist and Director of the Stroke Service, Massachusetts General Hospital, Boston, Massachusetts [202]

Peter M. Klara, M.D., Ph.D.
Norfolk, Virginia; Associate Clinical Professor, Department of Orthopaedic Surgery, State University of New York, Syracuse, New York; and Assistant Clinical Professor, Department of Neurosurgery, F. Edward Herbert School of Medicine and Uniformed Services University of the Health Sciences, Bethesda, Maryland [301]

David G. Kline, M.D.
Professor and Head, Department of Neurosurgery, Louisiana State University School of Medicine in New Orleans, New Orleans, Louisiana [310, 311, 313]

Robin F. Koeleveld, M.D.
Raleigh Neurosurgical Clinic, Inc., Raleigh, North Carolina [74]

Thomas A. Kopitnik, Jr., M.D.
Associate Professor, Department of Neurological Surgery, University of Texas Southwestern Medical Center, Dallas, Texas [231]

Paul L. Kornblith, M.D.
Professor, Department of Neurosurgery, University of Pittsburgh School of Medicine, Pittsburgh, Pennsylvania [72]

Kalman Kovacs, M.D., Ph.D., D.Sc., F.R.C.P.(C), F.R.C. Path.
Professor, Department of Pathology, University of Toronto and St. Michael's Hospital, Toronto, Ontario, Canada [124]

John Krawchenko, M.D.
Watertown, New York [53]

George Krol, M.D.
Clinical Professor of Radiology, The New York Hospital-Cornell Medical Center; and Chief of Neuroradiology, Memorial Sloan-Kettering Cancer Center, New York, New York [179]

Walter Kucharczyk, M.D., F.R.C.P.(C)
Professor and Chairman, Department of Radiology, University of Toronto; and Director, TRI Hospital MRI, Division of Neuroradiology, The Toronto Hospital, Toronto, Ontario, Canada [123]

Ashok J. Kumar, M.D.
Professor, Department of Radiology, The University of Texas M.D. Anderson Cancer Center, Houston, Texas [168]

Howard J. Landy, M.D.
Associate Professor, Department of Neurological Surgery, University of Miami School of Medicine, Miami, Florida [303]

Lauren A. Langford, M.D.
Assistant Professor, Section of Neuropathology, The University of Texas M.D. Anderson Cancer Center, Houston, Texas [168]

Richard E. Latchaw, M.D.
Professor of Radiology and Neurosurgery, and Margaret and H.O. Peterson Chair of Neuroradiology, University of Minnesota, Minneapolis, Minnesota [147]

Edward R. Laws, Jr., M.D.
Professor, Department of Neurological Surgery, University of Virginia Health Sciences Center, Charlottesville, Virginia [128, 191]

Milam E. Leavens, M.D.
Professor, Department of Neurosurgery, The University of Texas M.D. Anderson Cancer Center, Houston, Texas [168]

Ronald J. Lemire, M.D.
Professor, Department of Pediatrics, University of Washington School of Medicine, Seattle, Washington [346]

Allan B. Levin, M.D.
Professor, Department of Neurological Surgery, University of Wisconsin, Madison, Wisconsin [40]

L. Scott Levin, M.D.
Assistant Professor, Division of Orthopaedic Surgery, and Assistant Professor, Division of Plastic, Reconstructive, Maxillofacial, and Oral Surgery, Duke University Medical Center, Durham, North Carolina [269]

Alice C. Levine, M.D.
Assistant Professor of Medicine, Division of Endocrinology, Mount Sinai Medical School, New York, New York [131]

Michael L. Levy, M.D.
Assistant Professor, Department of Neurological Surgery, University of Southern California School of Medicine, Los Angeles, California [73, 188, 279]

Richard P. Levy, M.D., Ph.D.
Department of Radiation Medicine, Loma Linda University Medical Center, Loma Linda, California [184]

Robert M. Levy, M.D., Ph.D.
Division of Neurological Surgery, Northwestern University Medical School, Chicago, Illinois [341]

Jeffrey D. Lewine, Ph.D.
Assistant Professor of Radiology and Psychology, The University of New Mexico School of Medicine, Albuquerque, New Mexico [23]

Adam I. Lewis, M.D.
Resident, Department of Neurosurgery, University of Cincinnati College of Medicine, Cincinnati, Ohio [251]

Christer Lindquist, M.D., Ph.D.
Associate Professor, Department of Neurosurgery, Karolinska Hospital; and Director, Karolinska Gamma Knife Center, Stockholm, Sweden [185]

John R. Little, M.D.
Spine and Neurologic Surgery Center, Naples, Florida [85]

John D. Loeser, M.D.
Professor, Departments of Neurological Surgery and Anesthesiology, and Director, Multidisciplinary Pain Center, University of Washington Medical Center, Seattle, Washington [413]

Christopher M. Loftus, M.D.
Professor, Division of Neurosurgery, The University of Iowa College of Medicine and The University of Iowa Hospitals and Clinics, Iowa City, Iowa [330]

Patrick E. Logue, Ph.D.
Associate Professor, Medical Psychology, Duke University Medical Center, Durham, North Carolina [7]

Don M. Long, M.D., Ph.D.
Harvey Cushing Professor of Neurosurgery, and Director, Department of Neurosurgery, The Johns Hopkins Medical Institutions, Baltimore, Maryland [155, 401, 439]

L. Dade Lunsford, M.D.
Professor and Chief, Department of Neurological Surgery, and Professor of Radiology and Radiation Oncology, University of Pittsburgh School of Medicine, Pittsburgh, Pennsylvania [246, 408]

W. David Lust, Ph.D.
Professor, Department of Neurological Surgery, Case Western Reserve University, Cleveland, Ohio [194, 196]

J. Scott Luther, M.D.
Medical Director, The Comprehensive Epilepsy Center, Southwest Texas Methodist Hospital, San Antonio, Texas [30]

George C. Lynch, C.M.I., F.A.M.I.
Emeritus Professor of Biomedical Communications, The Bowman Gray School of Medicine, Winston-Salem, North Carolina [312]

R. Loch Macdonald, M.D., Ph.D., F.R.C.S.(C)
Assistant Professor, Section of Neurosurgery, The University of Chicago, Chicago, Illinois [214, 237]

Robert J. Maciunas, M.D.
Associate Professor, Department of Neurological Surgery, Vanderbilt University Medical Center, Nashville, Tennessee [428, 436]

Roger D. Madison, Ph.D.
Associate Research Professor of Experimental Neurosurgery and Associate Medical Research Professor of Neurobiology, Duke University Medical Center, Durham, North Carolina [315]

Ghaus M. Malik, M.D.
Vice Chairman, Department of Neurological Surgery, Henry Ford Hospital, Detroit, Michigan [242]

Lloyd I. Maliner, M.D.
Fellow, Division of Neurosurgery, Penn State University, Hershey, Pennsylvania [41]

William J. Mallon, M.D.
Triangle Orthopaedic Associates, and Assistant Consulting Professor, Division of Orthopaedic Surgery, Duke University Medical Center, Durham, North Carolina [178]

John T. Manning, M.D.
Associate Professor, Section of Hematopathology, The University of Texas M.D. Anderson Cancer Center, Houston, Texas [168]

Kim J. Manwaring, M.D.
Director, Pediatric Neurosurgery, Phoenix Children's Hospital, Phoenix, Arizona [348]

Moshe H. Maor, M.D.
Professor, Department of Radiotherapy, The University of Texas M.D. Anderson Cancer Center, Houston, Texas [168]

Timothy B. Mapstone, M.D.
Associate Professor, Division of Neurological Surgery, University of Alabama at Birmingham School of Medicine, Birmingham, Alabama [15]

Kenneth R. Maravilla, M.D.
Professor of Radiology and Neurological Surgery, and Director of Neuroradiology, University of Washington School of Medicine, Seattle, Washington [79]

Stephen D. Mark, M.D.
Fellow, Reconstructive Urology and Urodynamics, Division of Urology, Duke University Medical Center, Durham, North Carolina [35]

Lawrence B. Marks, M.D.
Assistant Professor, Department of Radiation Oncology, Duke University Medical Center, Durham, North Carolina [187]

Joseph C. Maroon, M.D.
Professor and Chairman, Department of Surgery, Allegheny Campus, Medical College of Pennsylvania, Pittsburgh, Pennsylvania [148, 388]

Merlin D. Marquardt, M.D.
Former Assistant Professor, Department of Pathology, College of Physicians & Surgeons of Columbia University, New York, New York [140]

Lawrence F. Marshall, M.D.
Professor and Chief, Neurosurgical Services, University of California, San Diego, San Diego, California [267]

Sharon B. Marshall, B.S.N.
Assistant Clinical Professor, Division of Neurosurgery, University of California, San Diego, San Diego, California [267]

Neil A. Martin, M.D.
Associate Professor, Division of Neurosurgery, School of Medicine and Medical Center, University of California, Los Angeles, Los Angeles, California [66]

Robert J. Martin, M.D.
Assistant Professor, Department of Neurosurgery, State University of New York Health Science Center at Syracuse, Syracuse, New York [389]

Robert L. Martuza, M.D.
Professor and Chairman, Department of Neurosurgery, Georgetown University Medical Center, Washington, District of Columbia [68, 69]

John M. Mathis, M.D.
Associate Professor of Radiology and Head, Neuroradiology and Interventional Neuroradiology Sections, University of Maryland Medical System, Baltimore, Maryland [234]

Mitsunori Matsumae, M.D.
Department of Neurosurgery, Tokai University School of Medicine, Bohseidai, Isehara, Kanagawa, Japan [31]

Toshio Matsushima, M.D.
Assistant Professor, Department of Neurosurgery, Neurological Institute, Kyushu University, Fukuoka, Japan [113]

Dana Matthews, M.D.
Assistant Professor, Department of Radiology, University of Texas Southwestern Medical Center, Dallas, Texas [231]

Paul Kurt Maurer, M.D.
Assistant Professor, Division of Neurosurgery, University of Rochester Medical Center, Rochester, New York [292]

Robert E. Maxwell, M.D., Ph.D.
Professor and Head, Department of Neurosurgery, University of Minnesota Medical School, Minneapolis, Minnesota [404]

Mark May, M.D.
Clinical Professor, Department of Otolaryngology–Head and Neck Surgery, University of Pittsburgh Medical Center, Pittsburgh, Pennsylvania [111]

Marc R. Mayberg, M.D.
Associate Professor, Department of Neurological Surgery, University of Washington School of Medicine, Seattle, Washington [217]

J. Gordon McComb, M.D.
Professor, Department of Neurological Surgery, University of Southern California School of Medicine; and Head, Division of Pediatric Neurosurgery, Childrens Hospital, Los Angeles, California [358, 378]

Patrick W. McCormick, M.D.
Department of Neurosurgery, The Toledo Hospital, Toledo, Ohio [242]

Paul C. McCormick, M.D.
Assistant Professor, Department of Neurological Surgery, Columbia-Presbyterian Medical Center and The Neurological Institute, New York, New York [152, 175]

William F. McCormick, M.D.
Director, Forensic Pathology, James H. Quillen College of Medicine, Johnson City, Tennessee [261]

Michael W. McDermott, M.D., F.R.C.S.(C)
Assistant Professor and Co-Director, Radiosurgery Program, Department of Neurological Surgery, School of Medicine, University of California, San Francisco, San Francisco, California [186]

Dennis E. McDonnell, M.D.
Associate Professor and Acting Chief, Section of Neurosurgery, Medical College of Georgia, Augusta, Georgia [161]

John T. McElveen, Jr., M.D.
Head of Otology-Neurotology, Carolina Ear & Hearing Clinic, Raleigh, North Carolina [104, 109, 110, 323]

John E. McGillicuddy, M.D.
Professor, Section of Neurosurgery, University of Michigan Medical Center, Ann Arbor, Michigan [314]

Peter W. McLaughlin, M.D.
Associate Professor, Section of Hematology, The University of Texas M.D. Anderson Cancer Center, Houston, Texas [168]

Robert L. McLaurin, M.D., J.D.
Emeritus Professor, Department of Neurosurgery, University of Cincinnati College of Medicine, Cincinnati, Ohio [370, 377]

Roger E. McLendon, M.D.
Assistant Professor of Pathology and Associate Director of Neuropathology, Duke University Medical Center, Durham, North Carolina [95]

David G. McLone, M.D., Ph.D.
Professor of Surgery (Neurosurgery), Northwestern University Medical School; and Division Head, Pediatric Neurosurgery, Children's Memorial Medical Center, Chicago, Illinois [114]

Irvine G. McQuarrie, M.D., Ph.D.
Associate Professor, Department of Neurological Surgery, Case Western Reserve University School of Medicine; and Medical Investigator in Neurosurgery, Cleveland Veterans Affairs Medical Center, Cleveland, Ohio [316]

David F. Meaney, Ph.D.
Assistant Professor, Department of Bioengineering, School of Engineering and Applied Science, University of Pennsylvania, Philadelphia, Pennsylvania [259]

Arnold H. Menezes, M.D.
Professor and Vice Chairman, Division of Neurosurgery, The University of Iowa College of Medicine and The University of Iowa Hospitals and Clinics, Iowa City, Iowa [160, 336, 362]

Daniel M. Meyer, M.D., Ph.D.
Associate Professor, Division of Cardiothoracic Surgery, University of Texas Southwestern Medical Center, Dallas, Texas [231]

J. Parker Mickle, M.D.
L. D. Hupp Professor of Pediatric Neurological Surgery, Department of Neurological Surgery, University of Florida College of Medicine, Gainesville, Florida [245]

Rajiv Midha, M.D., M.Sc., F.R.C.S.(C)
Assistant Professor, Division of Neurosurgery, Sunnybrook Health Sciences Centre, University of Toronto, Toronto, Ontario, Canada [308]

Michael A. Mikhael, M.D., Ph.D.
Chicago Institute of NeuroSurgery and NeuroResearch, Chicago, Illinois [392]

Thomas H. Milhorat, M.D.
Professor and Chairman, Department of Neurosurgery, State University of New York Health Science Center at Brooklyn, Brooklyn, New York [365]

Michael E. Miner, M.D., Ph.D.
Professor and Director, Division of Neurosurgery, The Ohio State University College of Medicine, Columbus, Ohio [277]

Steven L. Mitchell, M.D.
Assistant Professor, Department of Radiology, University of Minnesota Medical School, Minneapolis, Minnesota [147]

Aage R. Møller, Ph.D.
Professor, Department of Neurological Surgery, University of Pittsburgh School of Medicine, Pittsburgh, Pennsylvania [55]

Lee H. Monsein, M.D., M.P.H.
Associate Professor of Radiology and Neurosurgery, The Johns Hopkins Medical Institutions, Baltimore, Maryland [247]

Walter Montanera, M.D., F.R.C.P.(C)
Assistant Professor, Department of Radiology, University of Toronto; and Division of Neuroradiology, The Toronto Hospital, Toronto, Ontario, Canada [123]

Thomas J. Montine, M.D., Ph.D.
Assistant Professor, Department of Pathology, Vanderbilt University Medical Center, Nashville, Tennessee [200]

Dixon M. Moody, M.D.
Professor of Radiology, The Bowman Gray School of Medicine, Winston-Salem, North Carolina [88]

Robert A. Morantz, M.D.
Clinical Associate Professor of Neurosurgery and Clinical Professor of Radiation Oncology, The University of Kansas School of Medicine, Kansas City, Kansas [81]

Richard B. Morawetz, M.D.
J. G. Galbraith Professor of Neurosurgery, and Director, Division of Neurosurgery, The University of Alabama at Birmingham, Birmingham, Alabama [342]

Joel C. Morgenlander, M.D.
Assistant Professor, Division of Neurology, Duke University Medical Center, Durham, North Carolina [17]

Karin M. Muraszko, M.D.
Chief of Pediatric Neurosurgery, Section of Neurosurgery, University of Michigan, Ann Arbor, Michigan [360]

Somnath Nair, M.D.
Associate Professor, Department of Neurosurgery, Hahnemann University, Philadelphia, Pennsylvania [177]

Blaine S. Nashold, Jr., M.D.
Emeritus Professor, Division of Neurosurgery, Duke University Medical Center, Durham, North Carolina [411, 421, 422]

James R.B. Nashold, M.D.
Chief Resident, Division of Neurosurgery, Duke University Medical Center, Durham, North Carolina [421]

Francis A. Neelon, M.D.
Associate Professor, Department of Medicine, Duke University Medical Center, Durham, North Carolina [132]

Edward A. Neuwelt, M.D.
Professor of Neurology and Associate Professor of Neurosurgery, The Oregon Health Sciences University, Portland, Oregon [190]

David W. Newell, M.D.
Associate Professor, Department of Neurological Surgery, University of Washington School of Medicine, Seattle, Washington [21]

Philippa Newfield, M.D.
Attending Anesthesiologist, California Pacific Medical Center, San Francisco, California [39]

Nancy M. Newman, M.D.
Department of Ophthalmology, Pacific Medical Center, San Francisco, California [10]

K. Thomas Noell, M.D.
Clinical Associate Professor, Department of Radiology, Louisiana State University School of Medicine in New Orleans; and Director, Romagosa Radiation Oncology Center, Lafayette, Louisiana [182]

G. Robert Nugent, M.D.
Professor, Department of Neurosurgery, West Virginia University School of Medicine, Morgantown, West Virginia [407]

Marc R. Nuwer, M.D., Ph.D.
Professor, Department of Neurology, University of California, Los Angeles School of Medicine, Los Angeles, California [46]

W. Jerry Oakes, M.D.
Professor, Division of Neurosurgery, The University of Alabama at Birmingham; and Chief of Pediatric Neurosurgery, The Children's Hospital of Alabama, Birmingham, Alabama [352, 363]

Christopher S. Ogilvy, M.D.
Assistant Professor of Surgery, Harvard Medical School; and Director, Cerebrovascular Surgery, Massachusetts General Hospital, Boston, Massachusetts [202, 204]

George A. Ojemann, M.D.
Professor, Department of Neurological Surgery, University of Washington School of Medicine, Seattle, Washington [433]

Robert G. Ojemann, M.D.
Professor of Surgery, Harvard Medical School; and Visiting Neurosurgeon, Massachusetts General Hospital, Boston, Massachusetts [89, 108, 204]

Edward H. Oldfield, M.D.
Chief, Surgical Neurology Branch, National Institute of Neurological Disorders and Stroke, National Institutes of Health, Bethesda, Maryland [252]

Ayub K. Ommaya, M.D., F.R.C.S.
Bethesda, Maryland [274]

Gary M. Onik, M.D.
Chairman, Department of Minimally Invasive Therapy, Princeton Hospital, Orlando, Florida [388]

Michio Ono, M.D.
Research Fellow, Department of Neurological Surgery, University of Florida College of Medicine, Gainesville, Florida [91]

Burton M. Onofrio, M.D.
Professor of Neurosurgery, Mayo Medical School, and Attending Neurosurgeon, Mayo Clinic, Rochester, Minnesota; and Senior Consultant for Pain Disorders, Neurosurgical Service, Massachusetts General Hospital, Boston, Massachusetts [410]

William W. Orrison, Jr., M.D.
Director, Magnetic Diagnostic Center, The New Mexico Regional Federal Medical Center, Albuquerque, New Mexico [23]

Richard K. Osenbach, M.D.
Assistant Professor of Surgery (Neurosurgery), Uniformed Services University of the Health Sciences, Bethesda, Maryland [330]

Jewell L. Osterholm, M.D.
Professor, Department of Neurosurgery, Thomas Jefferson University Hospital, Philadelphia, Pennsylvania [198]

Alan K. Osumi, M.D., Ph.D.
Staff Radiologist, Sierra Vista Community Hospital, Sierra Vista, Arizona [26]

Nelson M. Oyesiku, M.D., Ph.D.
Assistant Professor, Department of Neurosurgery, Emory University School of Medicine, Atlanta, Georgia [227]

Roger J. Packer, M.D.
Professor of Neurology and Pediatrics, George Washington University Medical Center; and Chairman, Department of Neurology, Children's National Medical Center, Washington, District of Columbia [78]

Robert B. Page, M.D.
Professor of Neurosurgery and of Neuroscience and Anatomy, Milton S. Hershey Medical Center of the Pennsylvania State University, Hershey, Pennsylvania [120]

Dachling Pang, M.D., F.R.C.S.(C)
Professor, Department of Neurological Surgery, and Chief, Pediatric Neurosurgery, University of California, Davis Medical Center, Sacramento, California [351, 356]

Manohar M. Panjabi, Ph.D.
Professor, Department of Orthopaedics and Rehabilitation, and Director of Biomechanics Laboratory, Yale University School of Medicine, New Haven, Connecticut [379]

Stephen M. Papadopoulos, M.D.
Associate Professor, Section of Neurosurgery, University of Michigan Medical Center, Ann Arbor, Michigan [381]

Christopher G. Paramore, M.D.
Assistant Professor, Division of Neurosurgery, The University of Alabama at Birmingham, Birmingham, Alabama [334]

Andrew D. Parent, M.D.
Professor and Chairman, Department of Neurosurgery, The University of Mississippi Medical Center, Jackson, Mississippi [133, 143]

Michael D. Partington, M.D.
Assistant Professor of Surgery (Neurosurgery), University of Colorado Health Sciences Center; and Attending Neurosurgeon, The Childrens Hospital, Denver, Colorado [114]

Roy A. Patchell, M.D.
Associate Professor of Surgery and Neurology, University of Kentucky Chandler Medical Center, Lexington, Kentucky [84]

Sunil J. Patel, M.D.
Associate Professor, Department of Neurosurgery, Medical University of South Carolina, Charleston, South Carolina [165]

Russel H. Patterson, Jr., M.D.
Professor and Chief, Division of Neurosurgery, The New York Hospital–Cornell Medical Center, New York, New York [138]

Troy D. Payner, M.D.
Indianapolis Neurosurgical Group, Inc., Indianapolis, Indiana [50, 220]

Warwick J. Peacock, M.D.
Professor, Division of Neurosurgery, University of California, Los Angeles School of Medicine, Los Angeles, California [46]

Sydney J. Peerless, M.D., F.R.C.S.(C)
Clinical Professor, Department of Neurological Surgery, University of Miami School of Medicine; and Director, Mercy Neuroscience Institute, Mercy Health System, Miami, Florida [229, 243]

Richard R. Pelker, M.D.
Professor, Department of Orthopaedics and Rehabilitation, Yale University School of Medicine, New Haven, Connecticut [379]

Richard D. Penn, M.D.
Professor of Neurosurgery, Rush Presbyterian-St. Luke's Medical Center, Chicago, Illinois [45, 47]

John R. Perfect, M.D.
Associate Professor, Division of Infectious Diseases, Duke University Medical Center, Durham, North Carolina [331]

Phanor L. Perot, Jr., M.D., Ph.D.
Professor and Chairman, Department of Neurosurgery, Medical University of South Carolina, Charleston, South Carolina [385]

Byron Cone Pevehouse, M.D., M.Sc.
Clinical Professor, Department of Neurological Surgery, University of Virginia Health Sciences Center, Charlottesville, Virginia [437]

Joseph H. Piatt, Jr., M.D.
Associate Professor of Surgery (Neurosurgery) and Pediatrics, Oregon Health Sciences University, Portland, Oregon [304, 366]

David G. Piepgras, M.D.
Professor and Chairman, Department of Neurosurgery, Mayo Graduate School of Medicine, Rochester, Minnesota [206, 222, 236]

Salvatore V. Pizzo, M.D., Ph.D.
Chairman, Department of Pathology, Duke University Medical Center, Durham, North Carolina [37]

Fred V. Plapp, M.D., Ph.D.
Medical Director, Department of Laboratory Medicine, Saint Luke's Hospital, Kansas City, Missouri [38]

Steven R. Plunkett, M.D.
Southeast Radiation Oncology Group, Charlotte; and Matthews Radiation Oncology Center, Matthews, North Carolina [183]

Larry B. Poe, M.D.
Attending Neuroradiologist, Department of Radiology, United Health Services Hospitals, Johnson City; and Clinical Assistant Professor, Department of Radiology, State University of New York Health Sciences Center at Syracuse, Syracuse, New York [112]

Michael Pollay, M.D.
Clinical Professor of Neurosurgery, Oklahoma University Health Sciences Center, Oklahoma City, Oklahoma [32]

A. John Popp, M.D.
Professor and Chairman, Department of Surgery, and Head, Division of Neurosurgery, The Albany Medical College, Albany, New York [260]

Randall W. Porter, M.D.
Resident, Division of Neurological Surgery, Barrow Neurological Institute, Phoenix, Arizona [257]

Elisabeth M. Post, M.D.
Attending Neurosurgeon, Rancocas Hospital, Willingboro, New Jersey [367]

Kalmon D. Post, M.D.
Professor and Chairman, Department of Neurosurgery, Mount Sinai Medical School, New York, New York [131, 152]

Stephen K. Powers, M.D.
Professor and Chief, Division of Neurosurgery, Milton S. Hershey Medical Center of Pennsylvania State University, Hershey, Pennsylvania [41]

Donald J. Prolo, M.D.
Clinical Associate Professor, Department of Neurosurgery, Stanford University School of Medicine; and Medical Director, Western Transplant Services, San Jose, California [275, 442]

Phillip D. Purdy, M.D.
Professor and Vice Chairman, Department of Radiology, University of Texas Southwestern Medical Center, Dallas, Texas [231]

Lynn M. Quast, R.N., B.S.N.
Department of Neurologic Surgery, Mayo Clinic, Rochester, Minnesota [170]

Donald O. Quest, M.D.
Professor of Clinical Neurological Surgery, Neurological Institute of New York, Columbia University, New York, New York [33]

Matthew R. Quigley, M.D.
Associate Professor of Surgery (Neurosurgery), Allegheny Campus, Medical College of Pennsylvania, Pittsburgh, Pennsylvania [388]

Ronald G. Quisling, M.D.
Professor, Department of Radiology, University of Florida College of Medicine, Gainesville, Florida [245]

Robert A. Ratcheson, M.D.
The Harvey Huntington Brown, Jr. Professor and Chairman, Department of Neurological Surgery, Case Western Reserve University and University Hospitals of Cleveland, Cleveland, Ohio [15, 194, 196]

Charles E. Rawlings III, M.D.
Forsyth Neurosurgical Associates, Winston-Salem, North Carolina [64, 390]

John B. Redford, M.D.
Distinguished Professor, Department of Rehabilitation Medicine, University of Kansas Medical Center, Kansas City, Kansas, and Chief, Rehabilitation Medicine Service, Veterans Affairs Medical Center, Kansas City, Missouri [382]

R. Lawrence Reed II, M.D.
Associate Professor of Surgery and Anesthesiology, and Director, Surgical Intensive Care Unit, Duke University Medical Center, Durham, North Carolina [264]

Andrew Reisner, M.D.
Assistant Professor, Department of Neurological Surgery, University of Louisville School of Medicine, Louisville, Kentucky [126]

Justin W. Renaudin, M.D.
Assistant Clinical Professor of Neurosurgery, University of California, San Diego; and Chief of Neurosurgery, Sharp Memorial Hospital, San Diego, California [255, 333]

Setti S. Rengachary, M.D.
Professor, Department of Neurosurgery, University of Minnesota Medical School, Minneapolis, Minnesota [8, 12, 13, 118, 119, 130, 176, 181, 209, 248, 256, 291, 295, 299, 306, 374, 382, 393]

Albert L. Rhoton, Jr., M.D.
R. D. Keene Family Professor and Chairman, Department of Neurological Surgery, University of Florida College of Medicine, Gainesville, Florida [91, 93, 106, 113, 122, 144, 145, 215]

Dan N. Richardson, M.D.
Neuroradiology Section, Austin Radiological Association, Austin, Texas [197]

Donald E Richardson, M.D.
Professor and Chairman, Department of Neurosurgery, Tulane University School of Medicine, New Orleans, Louisiana [419]

William J. Richardson, M.D.
Assistant Professor, Division of Orthopaedic Surgery, Duke University Medical Center, Durham, North Carolina [297, 338]

William J. Richtsmeier, M.D., Ph.D.
Professor and Chief, Division of Otolaryngology–Head and Neck Surgery, Duke University Medical Center, Durham, North Carolina [157, 159]

Ronald Riefkohl, M.D.
Associate Clinical Professor, Division of Plastic, Reconstructive, Maxillofacial, and Oral Surgery, Duke University Medical Center, Durham, North Carolina [273]

Rosario Maria S. Riel-Romero, M.D.
Resident, Department of Pediatrics, The Bowman Gray School of Medicine, Winston-Salem, North Carolina [349]

Daniele Rigamonti, M.D.
Associate Professor of Neurosurgery and Radiology, The Johns Hopkins Medical Institutions, Baltimore, Maryland [247]

Patricia C. Rinaldi, Ph.D.
Associate Professor, Department of Neurological Surgery, University of California Irvine Medical Center, Orange, California [424]

Edmond F. Ritter, M.D.
Assistant Professor, Division of Plastic, Reconstructive, Maxillofacial, and Oral Surgery, Duke University Medical Center, Durham, North Carolina [149]

Theodore S. Roberts, M.D.
Professor, Department of Neurological Surgery, University of Washington School of Medicine; and Chief, Division of Pediatric Neurosurgery, Children's Hospital & Medical Center, Seattle, Washington [361]

Richard L. Robertson, Jr., M.D.
Instructor of Radiology, Harvard Medical School; and Neuroradiologist, Boston Children's Hospital, Boston, Massachusetts [202]

James C. Robinson, M.D.
Department of Neurosurgery, The Bowman Gray School of Medicine, Winston-Salem, North Carolina [359]

Arthur E. Rosenbaum, M.D.
Professor, Department of Radiology, and Director, Neuroradiology Division, State University of New York Health Science Center at Syracuse, Syracuse, New York [112]

Michael Rosenberg, M.D.
Associate Professor, Department of Ophthalmology, Northwestern University Medical School, Chicago, Illinois [9]

William S. Rosenberg, M.D.
Assistant Professor, Department of Neurosurgery, and Director, Division of Neurotrauma and Critical Care, University of Cincinnati College of Medicine, Cincinnati, Ohio [278]

Shelley B. Rosenbloom, M.D.
Clinical Assistant Professor, Department of Radiology, University of Texas Southwestern Medical Center, Dallas, Texas [112]

Mark L. Rosenblum, M.D.
Professor, Department of Neurological Surgery, Case Western Reserve University, Cleveland, Ohio; and Chairman, Department of Neurosurgery, Henry Ford Health Sciences Center, Detroit, Michigan [339, 341]

Allen D. Roses, M.D.
Jefferson-Pilot Corporation Professor of Neurobiology and Neurology, and Chief, Division of Neurology, Duke University Medical Center, Durham, North Carolina [29, 48]

Richard A. Roski, M.D.
Quad City Neurosurgical Associates, P.C., Davenport, Iowa [228]

Hubert L. Rosomoff, M.D., D.Med.Sc.
Professor and Chairman Emeritus, Department of Neurological Surgery, and Medical Director, Comprehensive Pain and Rehabilitation Center, University of Miami School of Medicine, Miami, Florida [423]

Eugene Rossitch, Jr., M.D.
Late Assistant Professor of Surgery, Harvard Medical School; and Neurosurgeon, Brigham and Women's Hospital and Children's Hospital, Boston, Massachusetts [63, 373, 422]

William E. Rothfus, M.D.
Associate Professor of Radiologic Sciences, Medical College of Pennsylvania, Allegheny Campus; and Department of Diagnostic Radiology, Allegheny General Hospital, Pittsburgh, Pennsylvania [147]

Richard A. Rovit, M.D.
Professor of Neurosurgery, New York Medical College; and Chairman Emeritus, Department of Neurological Surgery, St. Vincent's Hospital and Medical Center, New York, New York [135]

Ranjan S. Roy, M.D., Ph.D.
Spine Fellow, Department of Neurological Surgery, University of Southern California School of Medicine, Los Angeles, California [285]

Marvin P. Rozear, M.D.
Associate Professor, Division of Neurology, Duke University Medical Center, Durham, North Carolina [340]

Jonathan M. Rubin, M.D., Ph.D.
Professor, Department of Radiology, University of Michigan Medical Center, Ann Arbor, Michigan [56]

Gregory L. Ruff, M.D.
Assistant Professor, Division of Plastic, Reconstructive, Maxillofacial, and Oral Surgery, Duke University Medical Center, Durham, North Carolina [273]

H. Earl Ruley, Ph.D.
Professor, Department of Microbiology and Immunology, Vanderbilt University School of Medicine, Nashville, Tennessee [67]

Kamran Sahrakan, M.D.
Resident, Department of Neurological Surgery, School of Medicine, University of California, Davis, Sacramento, California [328]

Ramesh Sajpaul, M.D.
Assistant Professor, Department of Clinical Neurological Sciences, University of Western Ontario; and Attending Neurosurgeon, University Hospital, London, Ontario, Canada [189]

Michael Salcman, M.D.
Towson, Maryland, and Clinical Professor of Neurosurgery, George Washington University Medical Center, Washington, District of Columbia [80]

Stephen P. Salloway, M.D., M.S.
Assistant Professor of Neurology, Brown University, Providence, Rhode Island [6]

John H. Sampson, M.D.
Resident, Division of Neurosurgery, Duke University Medical Center, Durham, North Carolina [68, 69, 154, 394, 421]

Duke S. Samson, M.D.
Clark Professor and Chairman, Department of Neurological Surgery, University of Texas Southwestern Medical Center, Dallas, Texas [221, 231, 232, 240]

Srinath Samudrala, M.D.
Resident, Department of Neurosurgery, New York University Medical Center, New York, New York [276]

Abhay Sanan, M.D.
Resident, Department of Neurosurgery, University of Minnesota Medical School, Minneapolis, Minnesota [256, 291, 295, 299]

James E. Saunders, M.D.
House Ear Institute, Los Angeles, California [104]

Raymond Sawaya, M.D.
Chairman, Department of Neurosurgery, The University of Texas M. D. Anderson Cancer Center, Houston, Texas [62]

Barry Schaitkin, M.D.
Clinical Assistant Professor, Department of Otolaryngology–Head and Neck Surgery, University of Pittsburgh Medical Center, Pittsburgh, Pennsylvania [111]

Richard L. Scher, M.D.
Assistant Professor, Division of Otolaryngology–Head and Neck Surgery, Duke University Medical Center, Durham, North Carolina [157, 159]

Wouter I. Schievink, M.D.
Resident, Department of Neurologic Surgery, Mayo Graduate School of Medicine, Rochester, Minnesota [236]

Henry H. Schmidek, M.D.
Marion, Massachusetts [101, 400]

Frederick A. Schmitt, Ph.D.
Associate Professor, Department of Neurology, University of Kentucky Medical Center, Lexington, Kentucky [7]

Sydney S. Schochet, Jr., M.D.
Professor, Departments of Pathology, Neurosurgery, and Neurology, West Virginia University School of Medicine, Morgantown, West Virginia [28]

S. Clifford Schold, Jr., M.D.
Cullum Professor and Chairman, Department of Neurology, The University of Texas Southwestern Medical Center at Dallas, Dallas, Texas [74, 189]

Luis Schut, M.D.
Professor of Neurosurgery and Pediatrics, University of Pennsylvania School of Medicine; and Chief, Neurosurgical Services, Children's Hospital of Philadelphia, Philadelphia, Pennsylvania [78, 115]

R. Michael Scott, M.D.
Professor of Surgery, Harvard Medical School; and Director, Section of Pediatric Neurosurgery, The Children's Hospital, Boston, Massachusetts [368]

Hervey D. Segall, M.D.
Professor of Radiology and Director of Neuroradiology, University of Southern California School of Medicine, Los Angeles, California [263]

Laligam N. Sekhar, M.D.
Professor and Chairman, Department of Neurological Surgery, George Washington University Medical Center, Washington, District of Columbia [151, 158, 162, 165]

Roy Selby, M.D.
Neurological Surgery, Texarkana, Texas [441]

Robert G. Selker, M.D.
Chairman, Department of Surgery, Chief, Division of Neurosurgery, and Director, Center for Neuro-Oncology, Western Pennsylvania Hospital, Pittsburgh, Pennsylvania [192]

Warren R. Selman, M.D.
Professor, Department of Neurological Surgery, Case Western Reserve University and University Hospitals of Cleveland, Cleveland, Ohio [194, 196]

Chandranath Sen, M.D.
Associate Professor of Neurosurgery and Otolaryngology, and Co-Director of Cranial Base Surgery, Mount Sinai Medical Center, New York, New York [92, 158, 179]

Donald Serafin, M.D.
Professor, Division of Plastic, Reconstructive, Maxillofacial, and Oral Surgery, Duke University Medical Center, Durham, North Carolina [149]

Daniel J. Sexton, M.D.
Associate Professor, Division of Infectious Diseases, and Assistant Professor, Department of Microbiology, Duke University Medical Center, Durham, North Carolina [338, 340]

Ehud Shalmon, M.D.
Neurotrauma Fellow, Division of Neurosurgery, University of California, Los Angeles, School of Medicine, Los Angeles, California [265]

Clough Shelton, M.D.
Associate Professor, Division of Otolaryngology–Head and Neck Surgery, University of Utah School of Medicine, Salt Lake City, Utah [109]

David G. Sherman, M.D.
Department of Medicine (Neurology), The University of Texas Health Science Center, San Antonio, Texas [201]

Jeffrey K. Shramek, M.D.
Director of Neuroradiology, Department of Radiology, St. Francis Hospital System, Greenville, South Carolina [105]

William A. Shucart, M.D.
Professor and Chairman, Department of Neurosurgery, Tufts University School of Medicine and New England Medical Center, Boston, Massachusetts [121, 146]

Joseph R. Siebert, Ph.D.
Research Associate Professor of Pathology, University of Washington School of Medicine, Seattle, Washington [346]

Jon M. Silver, M.D.
Mountain Neurological Center, P.A., Asheville, North Carolina [193]

Gerald D. Silverberg, M.D.
Professor, Department of Neurosurgery, Stanford University School of Medicine, Stanford, California [16]

Frederick A. Simeone, M.D.
Professor and Chairman, Department of Neurological Surgery, Jefferson Medical College; and Chief of Neurosurgery, Pennsylvania Hospital and Wills Neurosensory Institute, Philadelphia, Pennsylvania [387]

Marcia Sirotkin-Roses, M.A., L.P.T.
Carolina Sports Physical Therapy, Durham, North Carolina [415]

Frederick H. Sklar, M.D.
Clinical Associate Professor of Neurosurgery, University of Texas Southwestern Medical School, Dallas, Texas [34, 364]

Konstantin V. Slavin, M.D.
Research Fellow, Department of Neurosurgery, University of Illinois at Chicago, Chicago, Illinois [205]

Barry H. Smith, M.D., Ph.D.
Director, The Health Foundation, New York, New York [72]

Susan M. Snodgrass, M.D.
Assistant Professor, Department of Neurology, Case Western Reserve University, Cleveland, Ohio [74]

Robert A. Solomon, M.D.
Associate Professor, Department of Neurological Surgery, Columbia-Presbyterian Medical Center and The Neurological Institute, New York, New York [241]

Volker K. H. Sonntag, M.D.
Clinical Professor of Surgery (Neurosurgery), University of Arizona; and Vice Chairman and Chief of Spine Section, Division of Neurological Surgery, Barrow Neurological Institute, Phoenix, Arizona [288, 290]

Frederick S. Southwick, M.D.
Professor and Chief, Division of Infectious Diseases, University of Florida, Gainesville, Florida [332]

Robert F. Spetzler, M.D.
Director, Barrow Neurological Institute, Phoenix; and J. M. Harber Chairman of Neurological Surgery, University of Arizona, Tucson, Arizona [210, 228]

Constance A. Stanton, M.D.
Assistant Professor of Pathology, The Bowman Gray School of Medicine, Winston-Salem, North Carolina [87]

Loretta A. Staudt, M.S., P.T.
Division of Neurosurgery, University of California, Los Angeles School of Medicine, Los Angeles, California [46]

Hans Jacob Steiger, M.D.
Associate Professor, Department of Neurosurgery, Ludwig-Maximilians-University, Munich, Germany [50, 220]

Bennett M. Stein, M.D.
Byron Stookey Professor and Chairman, Department of Neurological Surgery, Columbia-Presbyterian Medical Center and The Neurological Institute, New York, New York [102, 175, 241]

Gary K. Steinberg, M.D., Ph.D.
Associate Professor, Department of Neurosurgery, Stanford University School of Medicine, Stanford, California [184]

Ladislau Steiner, M.D., Ph.D.
Alumni Professor of Neurological Surgery and Radiology, and Director, Lars Leksell Center for Gamma Knife Radiosurgery, University of Virginia Health Sciences Center, Charlottesville, Virginia [185]

John C. Stevenson, M.B. Ch.B., F.R.C.S.
Resident, Division of Neurosurgery, Duke University Medical Center, Durham, North Carolina [36, 286]

Donald H. Stewart, Jr., M.D.
Arlington, Virginia [53]

Charles B. Stillerman, M.D.
Assistant Professor and Director of Spine Surgery, Department of Neurological Surgery, University of Southern California School of Medicine, Los Angeles, California [285]

Warren J. Strittmatter, M.D.
Professor, Division of Neurology, Duke University Medical Center, Durham, North Carolina [48]

Michael Sturgill, M.D.
Department of Neurosurgery, Kaiser Permanente, Denver, Colorado [298]

Austin J. Sumner, M.D.
Professor and Head, Department of Neurology, Louisiana State University School of Medicine in New Orleans, New Orleans, Louisiana [313, 325]

Narayan Sundaresan, M.D.
Clinical Professor of Neurosurgery, Mount Sinai Medical Center; and Attending Surgeon, Lenox Hill Hospital, New York, New York [179]

Leslie N. Sutton, M.D.
Professor of Neurosurgery and Pediatrics, University of Pennsylvania School of Medicine; and Associate Neurosurgeon, Children's Hospital of Philadelphia, Philadelphia, Pennsylvania [78, 115]

Morton N. Swartz, M.D.
Professor of Medicine, Harvard Medical School; and Chief, James Jackson Firm, Medical Services, Massachusetts General Hospital, Boston, Massachusetts [332]

William H. Sweet, M.D., D.Sc.
Department of Neurosurgery, Massachusetts General Hospital, and Harvard Medical School, Boston, Massachusetts [406]

Patrick S. Swift, M.D.
Assistant Professor, Department of Radiation Oncology, University of California, San Francisco, San Francisco, California [187]

George W. Sypert, M.D.
Southwest Florida Neurosurgical Associates; and Chairman, Neurological Institute of Southwest Florida, Fort Myers, Florida [289]

Ronald R. Tasker, M.D., F.R.C.S.(C)
Professor, Division of Neurosurgery, University of Toronto and The Toronto Hospital, Toronto, Ontario, Canada [425]

Charles H. Tator, M.D., Ph.D., F.R.C.S.(C)
Professor and Chairman, Division of Neurosurgery, University of Toronto, Toronto, Ontario, Canada [281, 412]

Ethan Taub, M.D.
Fellow in Functional Neurosurgery, Division of Neurosurgery, University of Toronto, Toronto, Ontario, Canada [138]

John M. Tew, Jr., M.D.
Frank H. Mayfield Professor of Neurosurgery, and Chairman, Department of Neurosurgery, University of Cincinnati College of Medicine, Cincinnati, Ohio [50, 220, 251]

Kamal Thapar, M.D.
Resident, Division of Neurosurgery, University of Toronto, Toronto, Ontario, Canada [124]

Robert Tiel, M.D.
Assistant Professor, Department of Neurosurgery, Louisiana State University School of Medicine in New Orleans, New Orleans, Louisiana [339]

Robert D. Tien, M.D., M.P.H.
Associate Professor, Department of Radiology, and Section Head, Neuroradiology, Duke University Medical Center, Durham, North Carolina [26]

George T. Tindall, M.D.
Professor, Department of Neurosurgery, Emory University School of Medicine, Atlanta, Georgia [126]

Suzie C. Tindall, M.D.
Professor, Department of Neurosurgery, Emory University School of Medicine, Atlanta, Georgia [317, 320]

Tadanori Tomita, M.D.
Associate Professor of Surgery, Northwestern University School of Medicine; and Assistant Head, Division of Pediatric Neurosurgery, The Children's Memorial Hospital, Chicago, Illinois [272]

Thomas A. Tomsick, M.D.
Professor, Department of Radiology, and Director of Neuroradiology, University of Cincinnati College of Medicine, Cincinnati, Ohio [251]

Vincent C. Traynelis, M.D.
Assistant Professor, Division of Neurosurgery, University of Iowa College of Medicine and University of Iowa Hospitals and Clinics, Iowa City, Iowa [284]

J. Allan Tucker, M.D.
Associate Professor, Department of Pathology, and Director, Anatomic Pathology, University of South Alabama, Mobile, Alabama [173]

Noel B. Tulipan, M.D.
Associate Professor, Department of Neurological Surgery, Vanderbilt University Medical Center, Nashville, Tennessee [436]

Dennis A. Turner, M.D.
Associate Professor, Division of Neurosurgery, and Associate Professor, Department of Neurobiology, Duke University Medical Center, Durham, North Carolina [262, 268, 432]

Keisuke Ueki, M.D.
Fellow, Department of Neurosurgery, Mayo Graduate School of Medicine, Rochester, Minnesota [206]

Bruno J. Urban, M.D.
Professor, Department of Anesthesiology, Assistant Professor, Division of Neurosurgery, and Director, Pain Clinic, Duke University Medical Center, Durham, North Carolina [403, 416, 418]

John C. VanGilder, M.D.
Professor and Chairman, Division of Neurosurgery, University of Iowa College of Medicine and University of Iowa Hospitals and Clinics, Iowa City, Iowa [336, 362]

Kevan E. VanLandingham, M.D., Ph.D.
Assistant Professor, Division of Neurology, Duke University Medical Center, Durham, North Carolina [18]

Harry R. van Loveren, M.D.
Professor and Director, Division of Skull Base Surgery, Department of Neurosurgery, University of Cincinnati, Cincinnati, Ohio [164]

Fernando Viñuela, M.D.
Professor and Chief, Therapeutic Neuroradiology, Department of Radiological Sciences, School of Medicine and Medical Center, University of California, Los Angeles, Los Angeles, California [65, 234]

F. Stephen Vogel, M.D.
Executive Director, United States and Canadian Academy of Pathology, Inc., Augusta, Georgia [103]

Dennis G. Vollmer, M.D.
Assistant Professor, Neurological Surgery, Washington University School of Medicine, St. Louis, Missouri [258]

Rand M. Voorhies, M.D.
Assistant Clinical Professor, Department of Neurosurgery, Louisiana State University School of Medicine in New Orleans; and Department of Neurosurgery, Ochsner Clinic and Ochsner Foundation Hospital, New Orleans, Louisiana [150]

Brandy Walker, M.D.
Assistant Professor, Department of Radiology, University of Texas Southwestern Medical Center, Dallas, Texas [231]

Sidney Wallace, M.D.
Professor and Chairman, Department of Diagnostic Radiology, The University of Texas M.D. Anderson Cancer Center, Houston, Texas [168]

John W. Walsh, M.D., Ph.D.
Professor, Department of Neurosurgery, The University of Texas Medical School at Houston; and Hermann Neurosurgical Association, Houston, Texas [141]

David D. Weaver, M.D.
Professor and Director of Clinical Services, Department of Medical and Molecular Genetics, Indiana University School of Medicine, Indianapolis, Indiana [347]

George D. Webster, M.B., F.R.C.S.
Professor, Division of Urology, Duke University Medical Center, Durham, North Carolina [35]

Bryce Weir, M.Sc., M.D.C.M., F.R.C.S.(C), F.R.C.S.(Ed) Hon.
Maurice Goldblatt Distinguished Service Professor, Surgery and Neurology, Chief, Section of Neurosurgery, and Director, Brain Research Institute, The University of Chicago, Chicago, Illinois [214, 237]

Leonard Weiss, M.D.
Williamsville, New York, and Former Director, Department of Experimental Pathology, Roswell Park Memorial Institute, Buffalo, New York [82]

Martin H. Weiss, M.D.
Professor and Chairman, Department of Neurological Surgery, University of Southern California School of Medicine, Los Angeles, California [285]

Robert E. Wharen, Jr., M.D.
Associate Professor of Neurosurgery, Mayo Clinic, Jacksonville, Florida [191]

Augustus A. White III, M.D., Dr. Med. Sci.
Beth Israel Hospital, Boston Massachusetts [379]

Richard J. Whitley, M.D.
Loeb Eminent Scholar Chair in Pediatrics, and Professor of Pediatrics, Microbiology, and Medicine, The University of Alabama at Birmingham, Birmingham, Alabama [342]

Asa J. Wilbourn, M.D.
Associate Clinical Professor, Department of Neurology, Case Western Reserve University School of Medicine; and Director, EMG Laboratory, The Cleveland Clinic, Cleveland, Ohio [305]

Robert H. Wilkins, M.D.
Professor and Chief, Division of Neurosurgery, Duke University Medical Center, Durham, North Carolina [3, 49, 63, 64, 154, 193, 354, 355, 373, 390, 394, 405]

Harold A. Wilkinson, M.D., Ph.D.
Professor and Chairman, Division of Neurosurgery, and Professor, Anatomy/Cell Biology Program, University of Massachusetts Medical Center, Worcester, Massachusetts [327]

Charles B. Wilson, M.D.
Tong-Po Kan Professor, Department of Neurological Surgery, School of Medicine, University of California, San Francisco, San Francisco, California [90]

H. Richard Winn, M.D.
Professor and Chairman, Department of Neurological Surgery, University of Washington School of Medicine, Seattle, Washington [21]

Ken R. Winston, M.D.
Professor, Department of Surgery (Neurosurgery), The University of Colorado Health Sciences Center; and Director of Pediatric Neurosurgery, The Children's Hospital, Denver, Colorado [371]

Fremont P. Wirth, M.D.
Neurological Institute of Savannah, Savannah, Georgia [58]

Hugh S. Wisoff, M.D.
Associate Clinical Professor of Neurological Surgery, Albert Einstein College of Medicine; and Attending Neurosurgeon, Montefiore Medical Center, Bronx, New York [253]

Samuel M. Wolpert, M.D.
Professor, Department of Radiology, Tufts University School of Medicine; and Chief of Neuroradiology, New England Medical Center Hospital, Boston, Massachusetts [146]

James H. Wood, M.D.
Chief, Neurosurgical Section, West Paces Medical Center, Atlanta, Georgia [14]

Robert M. Worth, M.D., Ph.D.
Associate Professor, Section of Neurological Surgery, Indiana University School of Medicine, Indianapolis, Indiana [307]

Donald C. Wright, M.D.
Associate Professor and Vice Chairman, Department of Neurological Surgery, George Washington University Medical Center, Washington, District of Columbia [151, 158, 162]

Marek Wroński, M.D., Ph.D.
Research Fellow, Neurosurgery Service, Memorial Sloan-Kettering Cancer Center, New York, New York [83]

Isao Yamamoto, M.D.
Professor and Chairman, Department of Neurosurgery, School of Medicine, Yokohama City University, Yokohama, Japan [145]

Howard Yonas, M.D.
Associate Professor, Departments of Neurological Surgery and Radiology, University of Pittsburgh School of Medicine; and Chief of Neurosurgery, Montefiore Hospital, Pittsburgh, Pennsylvania [195]

Donald H. York, Ph.D.
Director, Department of Neuroscience, St. John's Mercy, St. Louis, Missouri [20]

Byron Young, M.D.
Johnston-Wright Chair of Surgery, University of Kentucky Chandler Medical Center, Lexington, Kentucky [84, 280]

Jacob N. Young, M.D.
Naval Medical Center, Portsmouth, Virginia [422]

Paul H. Young, M.D.
Associate Clinical Professor of Anatomy and Neurosurgery, St. Louis University School of Medicine, St. Louis, Missouri [444]

Ronald F. Young, M.D.
Director, Northwest Neurosciences Institute and Northwest Hospital Gamma Knife Center, Seattle, Washington; and Clinical Professor of Neurosurgery, University of California Irvine Medical Center, Orange, California [424]

Michael R. Zalutsky, Ph.D.
Professor, Department of Radiology, and Assistant Professor, Department of Pathology, Duke University Medical Center, Durham, North Carolina [75]

Chi Shing Zee, M.D.
Associate Professor of Radiology and Neuroradiology Education Coordinator, University of Southern California School of Medicine, Los Angeles, California [263, 345]

Nicholas T. Zervas, M.D.
Higgins Professor of Neurosurgery, Harvard Medical School; and Chief of the Neurosurgical Service, Massachusetts General Hospital, Boston, Massachusetts [125]

Robert A. Zimmerman, M.D.
Professor of Radiology, University of Pennsylvania School of Medicine; and Chief, Pediatric Neuroradiology and Pediatric MRI, Children's Hospital of Philadelphia, Philadelphia, Pennsylvania [100]

FOREWORD

The appearance of the second edition of "Wilkins and Rengachary" is a time for celebration by neurosurgeons. Containing 444 chapters with dozens of new and updated contributions, it is the most extensive compilation of neurosurgical knowledge ever assembled into one text for neurosurgeons. This product of hundreds of authors has been carefully edited to provide a concise but comprehensive and interlocking overview of the specialty.

As all of the contributors know, Dr. Wilkins and Dr. Rengachary bring great skill to the art of editing and crafting the world of neurosurgical knowledge into a practical and authoritative text. Based on their extensive service as editors of the leading journals and texts in the specialty and on their comprehensive review of the world's neurosurgical literature, they have carefully selected contributions from the authors and leaders in each facet of neurosurgery. The contributors received careful instructions about which data and figures were needed in order to ensure that their contributions are timely, thorough, and concise.

This work is for neurosurgeons and for those who aspire to be or to work with neurosurgeons. No neurosurgical text has ever tapped the wisdom and insights of so many neurosurgeons and other specialists and covered such a broad spectrum of topics. It deserves to be on the ready-access shelf and frequently in the hands of every neurosurgeon. Dr. Eben Alexander, Jr., in the foreword to the first edition, wrote "to have been asked to write this foreword is an honor, for this text is indeed an awesome compilation of neurosurgical knowledge," and I wholeheartedly agree.

Albert L. Rhoton, Jr., M.D.

PREFACE

"The only phenomenon that is constant in this universe is change."

How true is this statement with regard to clinical neurosciences! Rapid and explosive advances in all areas of neurosciences have overwhelmed most neurosurgical practioners, resulting in a tendency for choosing an area of focus and subspecialization. After the publication of the first edition of *Neurosurgery,* we tried to keep up with the advances by publication of *Updates I and II,* but it became evident to us that updates would no longer suffice; the entire book needed revision. This prompted a second edition of *Neurosurgery,* which is appearing now, a decade after the first edition.

We have made every attempt to incorporate virtually all of the advances that have occurred since the earlier edition. At the same time we have maintained the core subjects and the basic organization of the text, which have received enthusiastic response from readers worldwide. Particularly gratifying are the compliments from young neurosurgeons preparing for their board examinations, who found this book helpful as a single source of reference for the entire spectrum of neurosurgery. We have made every attempt to maintain the basic philosophy of the text in its first edition. The idea of blending basic science with clinical neurosciences has been maintained. The core subjects have been retained, such as clinical examination of the nervous system, techniques in basic neurosurgery, pathology of tumors, neuroanatomy, history of neurosurgery, etc. We have strived diligently to incorporate recent advances in neurosurgery that include ventriculoscopy, newer brain imaging methodologies, skull base approaches, frameless stereotactic surgery, radiosurgery, Lyme disease, dorsal rhizotomy for spasticity, and spinal instrumentation, to name a few.

We have incorporated most of the chapters from *Updates I and II,* and have added many new topics besides thoroughly revising and updating the chapters from the first edition. This has resulted in 444 chapters. We have strived to assemble a most comprehensive collection of neurosurgical information as of this date. We appreciate the comments from the various readers throughout the world and have made every attempt to incorporate their input into the second edition. We hope that this second edition will gain the popularity enjoyed by the earlier edition.

We thank all the contributors for their time and effort in sharing their expertise, without which this multiauthored text would have been impossible. We thank Mrs. Gloria K. Wilkins as managing editor and Ms. Mariapaz Ramos Englis and many others from McGraw-Hill for their help in compiling and editing this work. We also thank our family members for their forebearance and patience.

Robert H. Wilkins, M.D.
Setti S. Rengachary, M.D.

Neurosurgery

SECTION L

Tumors of the Scalp, Skull, Skull Base, and Upper Cervical Spine

149 Noninvasive Tumors of the Scalp

Edmond F. Ritter
B. Thomas Harter, Jr.
Kathleen C. Harter
Donald Serafin

Noninvasive tumors of the scalp are derived from structures commonly found in this region (Fig. 149-1). In addition to the epidermis and dermis, the most common structure found in this region is the hair follicle. Closely associated with the hair follicle are three different glandular structures: the sebaceous gland, the apocrine gland, and the eccrine sweat gland. All of these are of dermal origin.

The sebaceous gland continuously forms a complex lipoidal mixture, the sebum, which is excreted to the skin surface from the opening of the hair follicle. A common congenital tumor arising from rests of sebaceous cells is the nevus sebaceous of Jadassohn. Another benign neoplasm is the adenoma sebaceum.

The apocrine gland is a vestigial skin appendage of no known physiologic significance. It may be responsible for certain body odors when its milky secretion is acted upon by skin bacteria. Its greatest concentration is found in the axilla. Its secretion is also discharged from the orifice of the hair follicle. Although ectopic apocrine glands can be found in the scalp, this is unusual.

The eccrine sweat glands have a more uniform and generalized distribution pattern than do either sebaceous or apocrine glands. These glands are essential to thermal regulation, and discharge their secretion from a separate and distinct pore. The dermal eccrine cylindroma can be traced to rests of eccrine sweat glands.

Hair growth takes place as a holocrine process by the continuous formation of new cells, which move upward and gradually cornify. As indicated above, hair-bearing follicles are closely associated with sebaceous glands and are often referred to collectively as the pilosebaceous apparatus. A pilomatrixoma is thought to arise from a primitive cell which normally would differentiate into a hair matrix cell. Trichillemal cysts are thought to be derived from the trichillema, or external root sheath of the hair follicle.

Surgical Excision and Closure Techniques

Most noninvasive scalp tumors may be treated by simple excision and closure. The scalp is an unyielding structure lacking distensibility; therefore, if a large excision is required, it is not always possible to close the wound primarily. One method of organization of reconstructive methods is the reconstructive triangle as described by Mathes.[7] Techniques are catalogued by increasing complexity. The lowest rung on the reconstructive ladder is primary closure. Skin grafting is the next higher rung. Local tissue may be

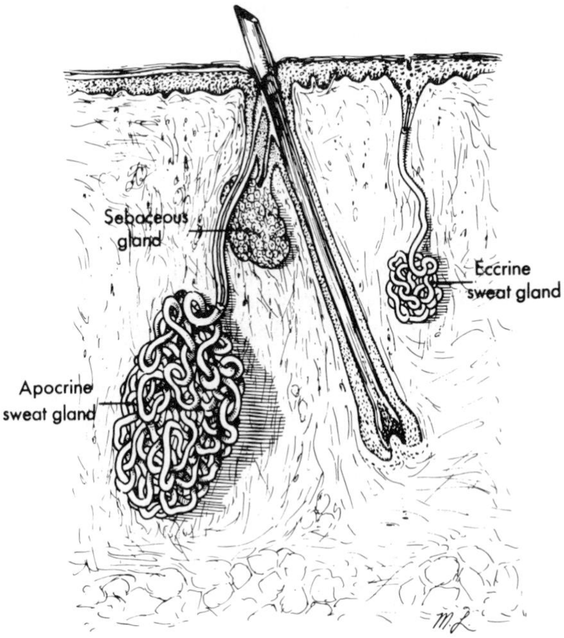

Figure 149-1 Illustration depicting a cross-section of hair-bearing skin.

advanced into the wound by the principle of rotation advancement with primary closure of the donor site or skin graft closure. A pedicled flap may be used to bring large amounts of tissue from a remote location. An example is the trapezius flap. Microsurgery provides a powerful method for transport of large amounts of healthy well-vascularized tissue to provide stable coverage of the calvarium. The latissimus muscle flap has become the work horse for scalp reconstruction, and when the microsurgical anastomoses are constructed meticulously to healthy vessels and attention is paid to the orientation and lie of the pedicle, this free flap may be transferred with a high degree of reliability. Usually the simplest method which will provide adequate qualitative and quantitative coverage is selected because more complex methods may be associated with a higher morbidity. The calvarium will accept a skin graft well when the periosteum is intact and healthy. If the periosteum has been disturbed, methods higher up on the reconstructive ladder must be selected. Large areas of skin graft often do not do well on the calvarium over a long term because they are subject to erosion.

Tissue expansion is a powerful technique which has come of age during the last decade. In this technique a silicone balloon-type device with fill ports is placed under a qualitatively adequate tissue and inflated serially. The overlying tissue is increased and may be advanced to close wounds. This technique is generally applicable as a secondary method of reconstruction when a wound has healed well. This technique is particularly worthwhile in the reconstruction of the scalp because it provides hair-bearing tissue. The scalp can be expanded by a factor of 2 in most patients, with an adequate aesthetic result. The technique of tissue expansion may be added to the surgeon's armamentarium when serial excision has failed to adequately remove a lesion due to the inadequate distensibility of the tissue.

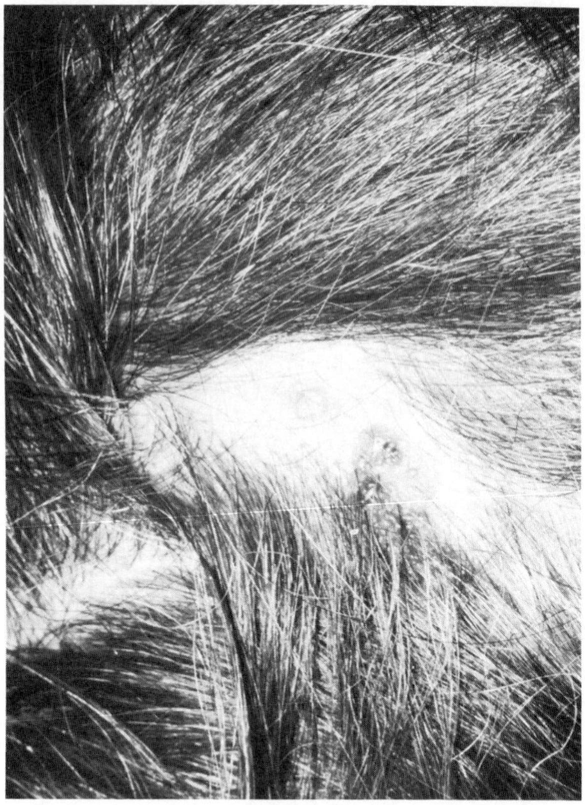

Figure 149-2 Photograph of a nevus sebaceous of Jadassohn. The lesion consists of a yellow or yellow-brown, slightly raised, waxy, hairless plaque. With advancing age, this tumor may undergo malignant change to a basal cell epithelioma.

Nevus Sebaceous

The nevus sebaceous was first described by Jadassohn in 1895 to characterize a lesion consisting of an excess of sebaceous glands. Its clinical course can be divided into three stages: childhood, puberty, and tumor development.

The nevus sebaceous is usually present at birth or in early childhood on the scalp or face. In childhood, the nevus usually appears as a yellow or yellow-brown, slightly raised, waxy, hairless plaque with a velvety texture. Histologically, it consists of underdeveloped sebaceous glands and hair roots.

Puberty ushers in the second phase of development, with the lesion becoming verrucose, and in some cases nodular. The surface is firm or rubbery, with either few or no hairs present. At this time there is enlargement of the lesion, which often achieves a linear rather than a circular form. Microscopically, this second phase is characterized by the proliferation of mature sebaceous glands in the dermis. Hair roots either completely disappear or remain small. In many cases apocrine glands become hyperplastic and cystic. The epidermis becomes more verrucose (Fig. 149-2).

The third phase is characterized by the development of neoplasms within the original nevus. In one series of 150 cases of nevus sebaceous where 52 tumors were found, 21 patients developed basal cell carcinomas and 8 developed papilliferous syringadenomas.[8]

Because of the natural course of this tumor, with proliferation during puberty and the possibility of later malignant change, it is advisable to perform excision during childhood.

Adenoma Sebaceum

Adenoma sebaceum was first described by Balzer and Ménétrier in 1885. It is an uncommon benign tumor which occurs most often in middle age on the nose, cheek, and scalp. Sebaceous adenomas appear clinically as discrete, small, flesh-colored or yellow nodules which may be several millimeters to several centimeters in size. The lesions are usually slow-growing and may have been present for a long time before the patient seeks treatment.

Microscopically, the tumors are arranged in lobules. Masses of small cells resembling basal cells line the periphery of the lobule. Larger cells containing fat vacuoles and cysts containing sebaceous material are found centrally. The adenoma is usually surrounded by a connective tissue layer.

Sebaceous adenomas should be excised (Fig. 149-3).

Pilomatrixoma (Calcifying Epithelioma of Malberle)

Pilomatrixoma usually occurs on the scalp, face, neck, and upper arms. It usually presents as an asymptomatic, solitary, firm nodule located in the dermis, although at times it may occur in the subcutaneous tissue. Varying in diameter from 0.5 to 5 cm, this lesion may develop at any age.

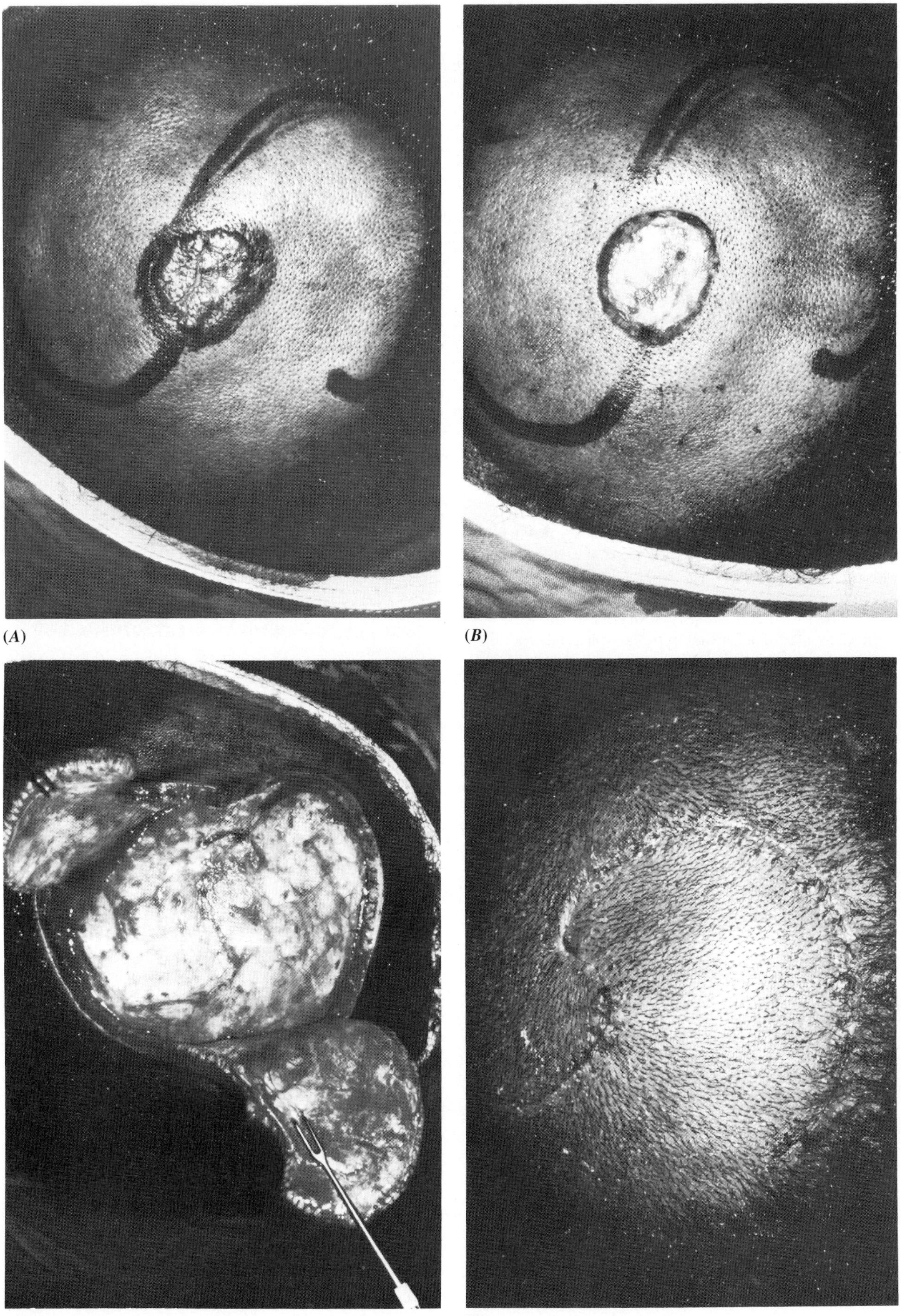

Figure 149-3 A sebaceous adenoma. *A.* Note that the large size of the lesion precludes simple excision and primary closure. *B.* Outline of rotation advancement flaps following tumor excision. *C.* Flaps elevated, exposing the periosteum of the cranium. *D.* Early postoperative result following successful wound closure.

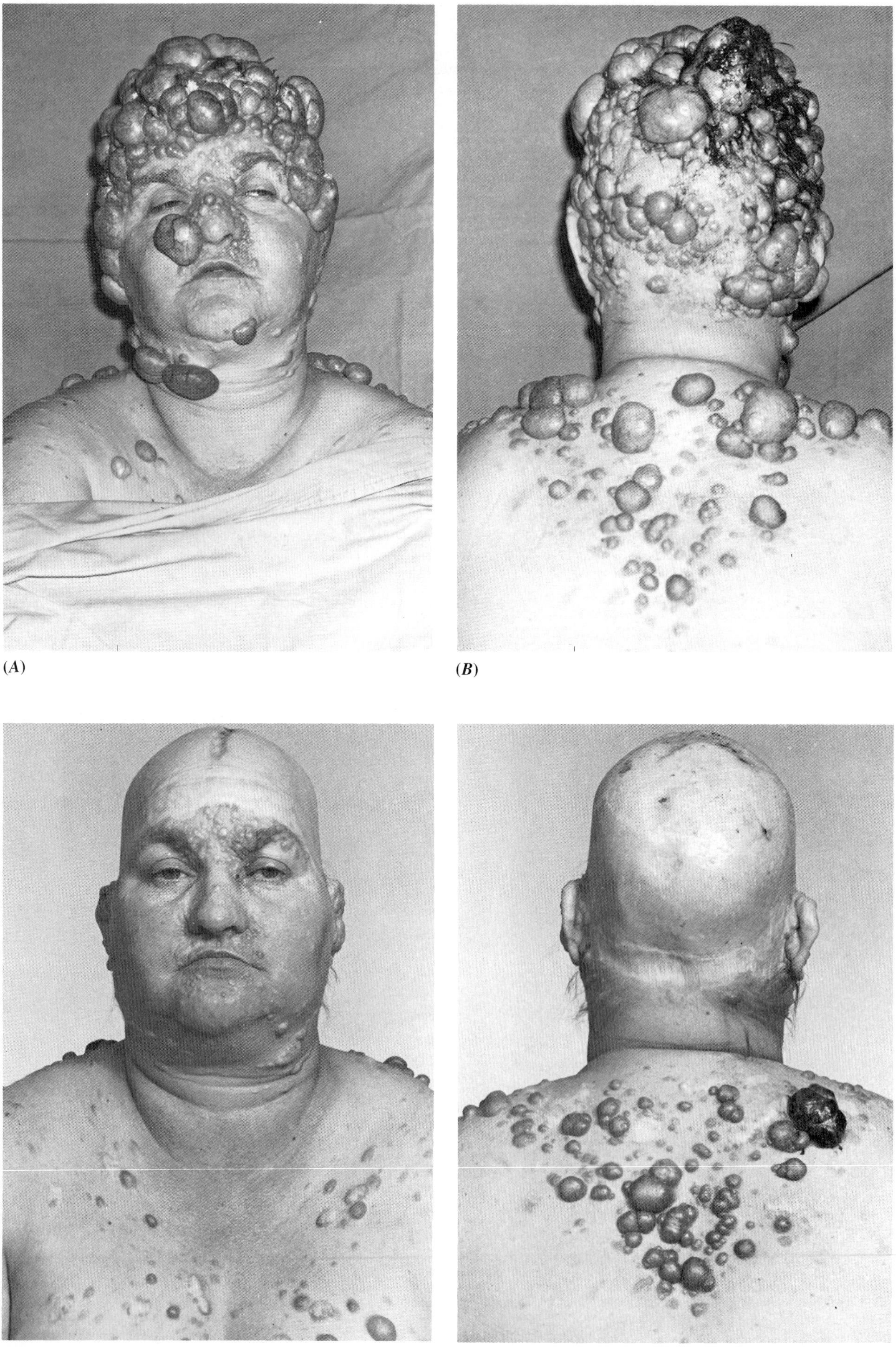

(*A*) (*B*) (*C*) (*D*)

Figure 149-4 *A, B.* Preoperative photographs of a patient with a dermal eccrine cylindroma. This tumor is commonly called a turban tumor. *C, D.* Postoperative photographs after excision of the entire scalp with application of a split-thickness skin graft.

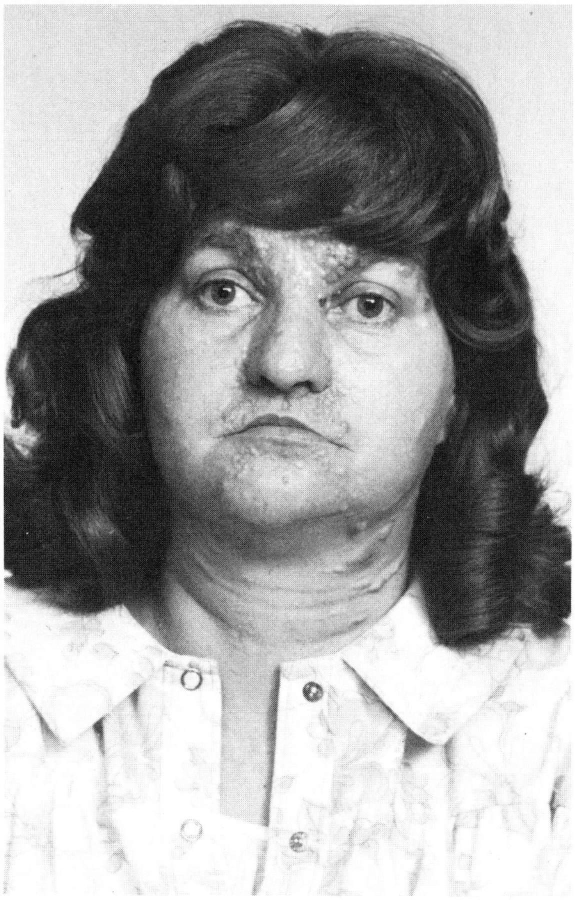

(*E*)

Figure 149-4 (*Continued*) *E.* Late postoperative result following completion of reconstruction, with the patient wearing an artificial hairpiece. (Photographs kindly supplied by Dr. Kenneth L. Pickrell.)

Microscopically, the tumor is encased by compressed collagen, and consists of folded sheets and bands of basophilic and shadow cells. The basal cells are small, with large, round, deeply basophilic nuclei and scanty cytoplasm. The cytoplasm of the shadow cells stains slightly, but the nucleus does not stain. The cells thus appear with an unstained ''shadow'' at the site of the nucleus, and hence their name, *shadow cells*. Basophilic cells develop into shadow cells, and older tumors usually show decreasing numbers of basophilic cells.[3]

It is postulated that this tumor arises from a primitive cell which is differentiating toward a hair matrix cell. Calcification is frequently seen in these tumors (84 percent in the study by Forbis and Helwig) and occurs in the areas of the shadow cells.[3]

Malignant change has not been shown to occur, and the pilomatrixoma is best removed by excision.

Dermal Eccrine Cylindroma

The dermal eccrine cylindroma has also been called Spiegler's tumor, cylindroma, and turban tumor since it was first described by Ancell in 1842. These tumors usually begin as small nodules in adolescence or early adulthood, and continue to grow slowly into mushroom-shaped rubbery masses measuring up to several centimeters. They are nonpainful, freely movable, and usually a red-blue or pink color.

The tumors most commonly appear on the scalp and face, and are usually multiple. They have been given the name *turban tumor* because they sometimes cover the entire scalp like a turban (Fig. 149-4).

The dermal eccrine cylindroma occurs more often in women than in men, and there is a positive family history in about 30 percent of the cases. These tumors usually do not bother the patient except as a cosmetic problem, and usually run a benign course.

Cylindromas of the scalp and facial trichoepitheliomas have been reported to occur as a single genetic entity with inheritance determined by an autosomal dominant gene with variable expression.[13] Another syndrome of trichoepitheliomas, milia, and cylindromas has also been reported.[11]

A dermal eccrine cylindroma originates from an eccrine sweat gland. It is usually unencapsulated and lies in the upper dermis. Microscopically, closely packed cords of basophilic round or oval cells are separated into lobules by strands of hyaline material. Cystic and ductlike spaces are also seen within the tumor.[2]

Biopsy is indicated to establish the diagnosis when a single lesion is present, and is often needed to differentiate multiple cylindromas from epidermal cysts.

These tumors usually require excision, and skin grafting is often needed if the area involved is large. It is not uncommon for these tumors to recur after excision in adjacent areas of uninvolved skin.

Keratoses

The keratoses represent localized hyperplastic changes in the epidermis. Both seborrheic and solar keratoses are commonly found on the scalp.

Seborrheic Keratoses

These lesions commonly develop during middle age and are most frequently found on the scalp, face, and trunk. They may occur singly or in large numbers, and appear as slightly raised, soft, greasy, brownish, circumscribed papules. Usually they measure only several millimeters, but may attain sizes up to several centimeters.

The epidermis is thickened in seborrheic keratoses. Cells resembling basal cells penetrate into the epidermis, forming a flat or irregular epithelial mass, or develop a reticular pattern with horn cysts or pseudocysts.[12]

The seborrheic keratosis may at times be difficult to distinguish from a solar keratosis or basal cell carcinoma. If the lesion is darkly pigmented, it may resemble a melanoma. In these cases, biopsy is needed to establish the diagnosis.

These lesions do not undergo malignant change and may be removed for cosmetic reasons by currettage, dermabrasion, or freezing with liquid nitrogen.

Solar Keratoses

Solar keratoses (also referred to as actinic keratoses) develop commonly on the sun-exposed areas of skin, most often in fair-complexioned individuals. These lesions usually occur in middle to old age as a function of the cumulative effect of solar radiation.

The lesions begin as dry, hard patches, usually less than 1 cm in diameter, which develop scales on an erythematous base. When the scales are removed, bleeding usually occurs, followed by further scale development.

Microscopically, the epidermis is parakeratotic and has lost its granular layer. The prickle cells have lost their orderly stratified arrangement and have become edematous. The basal layer no longer consists of small, darkly staining cells, but is now composed of cells resembling prickle cells. The dermoepidermal junctions may be flat and the epidermis thin, or the epidermis may be hyperplastic and acanthotic. The regular pattern of rete ridges and papillae is lost. The border of the keratosis is sharp and slants upward and away from the adjoining normal skin.[9]

Skin keratoses are considered premalignant lesions because they may undergo malignant degeneration. If induration or ulceration exists in a lesion, the diagnosis of squamous cell carcinoma must be entertained, and biopsy done to establish the diagnosis.

Removal of these lesions may be accomplished by curettage or liquid nitrogen. Recently, significant interest has developed in the use of the chemical peel for treatment of patients with multiple solar keratoses of the scalp. If many keratoses are present, 5-fluorouracil cream may be applied topically to the involved area.

Hemangiomas

Hemangiomas are benign vascular tumors and are the commonest tumors of childhood. They are subdivided by their histology into capillary hemangiomas and cavernous hemangiomas. Capillary hemangiomas are formed by aggregations of abnormal capillaries. Two types of capillary hemangiomas are found on the scalp—the port-wine stain and the strawberry mark.

Port-Wine Stain (Nevus Flammeus)

The port-wine stain is a flat, bright pinkish-red to bluish-purple lesion present at birth. It blanches with pressure, and refills when the pressure is released. The tumor is composed of masses of intradermal capillaries lined by mature endothelium. These vessels may follow a dermatomal distribution. When a port-wine stain located in a trigeminal ophthalmic distribution is associated with an intracranial collection of capillary blood vessels, the Sturge-Weber syndrome must be considered.

These lesions do not undergo spontaneous involution, nor do they grow; but their surface area increases with the growth of the area involved. Although some port-wine stains may fade slightly with time, small lesions may be treated by excision or by the use of cosmetic covering agents. Recently, the pulse dye laser has proved efficacious in the treatment of port-wine stains and has become the method of choice in most physicians' hands. The argon laser has been largely abandoned because of inferior cosmetic results.

Strawberry Mark

The strawberry mark is a bright red or purplish red, slightly raised lesion consisting of capillaries lined by embryonic endothelium. On palpation the strawberry mark feels firm and rubbery, and it blanches incompletely with pressure.

The hemangioma is usually not present at birth, but appears within a few weeks as a pink or red spot. It then begins a period of very active growth usually lasting about 6 months. Following a dormant period, the tumor begins to undergo a spontaneous involution during the next 6 to 12 months. With this involutional phase, small gray islets develop within the lesion. During the next 2 to 3 years, these islets increase and become confluent, and the hemangioma decreases in size. Eventually normal or atrophic skin remains in the area.[6]

The diagnosis of strawberry mark can usually be made by careful history and observation. In dealing with these hemangiomas, it is important to remember that 85 percent will undergo spontaneous resolution by the age of 5 years. Therefore, in most cases no treatment is necessary, and parents are best advised to wait until the involutional phase begins.

Surgical resection may be indicated in cases involving obstruction or loss of function of an organ, bleeding, or ulceration. The use of systemic steroids may also prove helpful in certain cases.

Scalp Cysts

Four types of cysts are found in the scalp: epidermoid inclusion cysts, trichilemmal cysts, dermoid cysts, and branchiogenic cysts. In the past the term *sebaceous cyst* was used to describe the common wen. However, studies have shown that these cysts are either epidermoid or trichilemmal cysts, and do not contain elements of the sebaceous gland. Hence, the term *sebaceous cyst* is not used in this discussion of scalp cysts.

Epidermoid Inclusion Cysts

Epidermoid cysts are slow-growing, rounded, subcutaneous masses. They lie in the dermis but are attached to the epidermis, and a central punctum may be seen on the overlying skin. The cysts vary in size from several millimeters to several centimeters. On palpation, the cyst may feel soft or firm, depending on its contents. Epidermoid cysts may undergo calcification or become inflamed and infected, leading to the development of an abcess.

These cysts commonly develop during adolescence and adulthood. Multiple epidermal cysts of the scalp and face are a component of Gardner's syndrome, which is also characterized by polyposis of the colon, fibromas, and lipomas of the skin.

Histologically, the wall of the cyst is composed of stratified squamous epithelium. It contains laminated keratin or an amorphous material with a high lipid content.[5] Pressure from these contents may cause flattening of the cyst wall.

These cysts are best handled by surgical excision, and the entire cyst must be removed to avoid recurrence. When the cyst is infected, incision and drainage may initially be undertaken, with excision planned at a later date after the inflammation has subsided.

Trichilemmal Cysts

Trichilemmal cysts occur most commonly on the scalp during the adult years and occur more frequently in females than in males. Cysts are often found within families, and inheritance is determined by an autosomal dominant gene.

These smooth, rounded cysts are located within the dermis.

They may occur as a single lesion, but usually are multiple and increase very slowly in size. About 50 percent of the affected individuals will develop increasing numbers of cysts with time, but it is unusual to find a large number of cysts on one person. In one study, only 10 percent of the patients had more than 10 cysts.[4] Multiple cysts usually appear all over the scalp and originate independently, but they may derive from one cyst or appear as recurrences following the removal of a cyst.

These cysts are derived from the trichilemma, or external root sheath of the hair follicle. The cyst wall consists of stratified epithelium and shows a characteristic lining of pale cells. These cells increase in vertical diameter as they lose their nuclei, and mature into keratin without the formation of a granular layer. The cyst is filled with keratin.[10]

Trichilemmal cysts show fewer inflammatory changes than do epidermoid cysts. These cysts usually are excised for cosmetic reasons.

Congenital Inclusion Dermoid Cysts

Displaced dermal cells along the lines of embryonic fusion may develop into dermoid cysts. In the scalp, they originate as the developing cranial bones grow toward each other. Dermal cells may become isolated from the overlying epithelium, creating the dermoid cyst.

Although these lesions are congenital, they usually enlarge later in life and may reach a diameter of several centimeters. The overlying skin is freely movable and the lesion feels cystic upon palpation. Stratified squamous epithelium lines the cyst wall and the cyst may contain a greasy keratinized material and hair.

Dermoid cysts occur frequently on the head and neck; only a small percentage appear on the scalp. In one study, the three dermoid cysts found on the scalp from among a total of 36 head and neck cases were located at the right parieto-occipital suture line, at the anterior fontanel, and at the bregma.[1]

These cysts are excised with careful attention to the possibility of a connection of the cyst wall to the underlying meninges, or of intracranial extension of the cyst.

Branchiogenic Cysts

Branchiogenic cysts and sinuses result from the failure of the branchial arches to close completely during embryonic development. The only branchiogenic cysts found in the scalp area involve lesions of the first branchial cleft, which appear anterior to the upper part of the external ear.

Although present at birth, these cysts may not become apparent until later in life, often in the third decade. They usually appear as smooth, painless lumps, slowly increasing in size.

The cyst is lined by stratified squamous or columnar epithelium, and contains caseous fluid. These cysts should be completely excised.

References

1. Colcock BP, Sass RE, Staudinger L. Dermoid cysts. *N Engl J Med* 1955; 252:373–379.
2. Crain RC, Helwig EB. Dermal cylindroma (dermal eccrine cylindroma). *Am J Clin Pathol* 1961; 35:504–515.
3. Forbis R Jr, Helwig EB. Pilomatrixoma (calcifying epithelioma). *Arch Dermatol* 1961; 83:606–618.
4. Leppard BJ, Sanderson KV. The natural history of trichilemmal cysts. *Br J Dermatol* 1976; 94:379–390.
5. Lund HZ. *Tumors of the Skin.* Washington: Armed Forces Institute of Pathology, 1957.
6. Margileth AM. Developmental vascular abnormalities. *Pediatr Clin North Am* 1971; 18:773–800.
7. Mathes SJ. Personal communication, December 1992.
8. Mehregan AH, Pinkus H. Life history of organoid nevi. *Arch Dermatol* 1965; 91:574–588.
9. Pinkus H. Keratosis senilis. *Am J Clin Pathol* 1958; 29:193–207.
10. Pinkus H. ''Sebaceous cysts'' are trichilemmal cysts. *Arch Dermatol* 1969; 99:544–555.
11. Rasmussen JE. A syndrome of trichoepitheliomas, milia, and cylindromas. *Arch Dermatol* 1975; 111:610–614.
12. Rook A, Dawber R. *Diseases of the Hair and Scalp.* Oxford: Blackwell, 1982.
13. Welch JP, Wells RS, Kerr CB. Ancell-Spiegler cylindromas (turban tumours) and Brooke-Fordyce trichoepitheliomas: evidence for a single genetic entity. *J Med Genet* 1968; 5:29–35.

150

Tumors of the Skull

H. Bruce Hamilton
Rand M. Voorhies

There have been two major developments in the treatment of skull tumors since the original chapter was written for the first edition of this textbook: magnetic resonance imaging (MRI) and the continued evolution of skull base surgery. The introduction of MRI has improved preoperative planning, and postoperative follow-up assessment. The capability of imaging in multiple planes and the absence of artifact at the skull base are important advantages of MRI over computed tomography (CT). Evaluation of flow void can also predict vascular involvement. However, despite the added benefits of MRI, definitive preoperative identification of tumor type has proved elusive in most cases. That is because most skull neoplasms share certain MRI characteristics, such as hypointensity on T1-weighted images, hyperintensity on T2-weighted images, and some degree of contrast enhancement.

Sometimes certain MRI patterns are suggestive of a particular diagnosis. Differentiation between nasopharyngeal carcinoma and a rare primary bone tumor at the skull base is often difficult. Nasopharyngeal carcinoma frequently causes destruction of the skull base, whereas a slowly growing primary bone tumor tends to cause erosion. Nasopharyngeal carcinoma has a strong tendency to spread via a perineural mechanism. Branches of the fifth cranial nerve are affected most often. This condition can be detected on coronal MR images well before CT scans show foraminal erosion. Fat-suppressed contrast-enhanced T1-weighted images can show perineural tumor involvement.[47]

On the other hand, a CT scan is better than MRI in actually mapping bone destruction. It is also more sensitive in picking up intratumoral calcification, which can sometimes be an important clue to the diagnosis. Authorities agree that MRI and CT are complementary in the preoperative evaluation of patients with skull tumors.[47,69,78,131]

Plain x-ray films of the skull are still important in the evaluation of calvarial neoplasms (Fig. 150-1). Occasionally a bone scan may be useful in providing preoperative localization of lesions which are poorly visualized on either skull films or CT scans (Fig. 150-2). Angiography may also be indicated in certain cases.

Even after extensive neuroradiologic evaluation, however, definitive preoperative diagnosis is rarely possible. Ashkenazi et al. suggest that preoperative fine needle aspiration should be considered in such cases, since knowledge of the tumor type will influence surgical decision making.[7] When metastatic tumor is diagnosed, the extent of disease may temper the surgeon's desire for a radical resection.

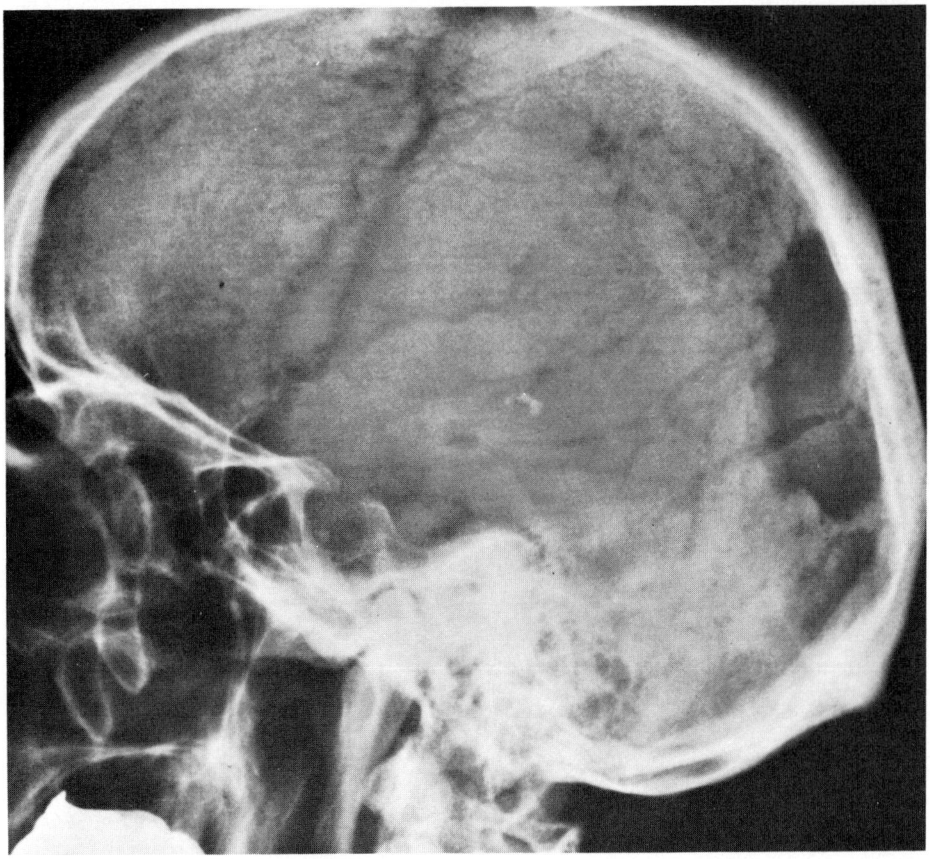

Figure 150-1 A lytic skull lesion with irregular, undermined edges. This appearance is suggestive of a malignant tumor.

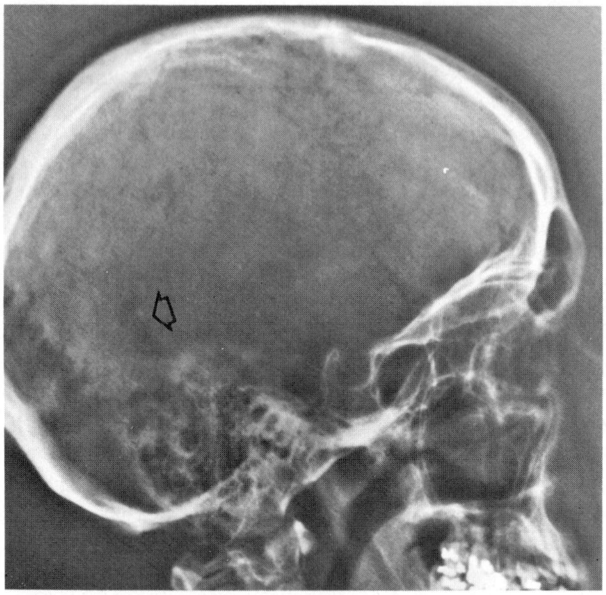
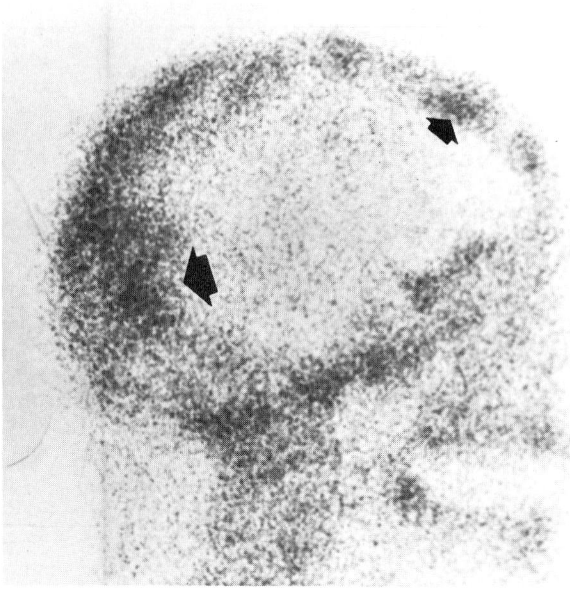

(*A*) (*B*)

Figure 150-2 *A*. A plain lateral roentgenogram showing minimal irregularity (*arrow*) that could not be demonstrated with bone windows on computed tomography. *B*. A radionuclide bone scan shows several areas of increased uptake (*arrows*). The biopsy site was selected by placing a scalp marker over the larger abnormal area. (Courtesy of Richard Benua, M.D.)

Until recently, many primary skull tumors were largely inaccessible, particularly when they were located at the skull base. Surgical intervention was often limited to biopsy. The development of new techniques in skull base surgery has resulted in a more aggressive approach to these lesions.[40,79,80,107–109,114] Knowledge of the expected clinical behavior of these tumors is now more than just of academic interest. Radical and potentially mutilating surgical procedures are not indicated when curettage will do, and vice versa. The surgical approaches to the skull base will be discussed elsewhere in this textbook.

This chapter attempts to catalogue the large number of tumors and tumor-like conditions which can arise primarily in the bones of the skull (Table 150-1). Many of these are quite rare, and the literature often consists of individual case reports. There is often controversy among the experts in bone pathology concerning the nomenclature and classification of some of these lesions. In many instances we have presented a simplified view. In addition there is a section on syndromes that can involve skull tumors (Table 150-2). Once again, we have employed a classification system that is modified from Huvos, and once again we lean very heavily on his book, now in its second edition.[59,60] For a more complete discussion, we encourage the reader to refer to this classic text, as well as to the original literature.

Bone-Forming Tumors—Benign

Osteoma

Osteomas are benign, slow-growing neoplasms composed of mature lamellar bone. They usually arise in bone formed by intramembranous ossification. There are two characteristic histologic types: the ivory osteoma and the spongy osteoma. The compact or ivory osteoma is the most frequently occurring variety. It consists of dense and compact mature lamellar bone with minimal marrow space (Fig. 150-3). On the other hand, the trabecular or spongy osteoma has a cancellous, trabecular architecture with a peripheral cortical bony margin.

Osteomas are the most common primary bone tumor found in the craniofacial skeleton. Most are not symptomatic and occur in as many as 0.43 percent of patients.[113] Osteomas develop in the paranasal sinuses, maxilla, mandible, mastoid sinus, external auditory canal, and cranial vault. The site of involvement determines the clinical manifestations. Tumors in the paranasal sinuses can present with frontal headache and recurrent sinusitis (Fig. 150-4). Smith and Calcaterra[113] recommend removal of asymptomatic osteomas that are located at the nasofrontal duct or that occupy more than 50 percent of the volume of the frontal sinus. Small and laterally located osteomas may be watched, provided the patient understands the potential for growth.

Intracranial extension is rare because osteomas of the vault tend to arise from the outer table and grow outward. However, large size and epidural compression can occur (Fig. 150-5). A giant osteoma with superior sagittal sinus compression has been reported.[34] Most present as a painless, slowly enlarging mass. Radiologic evaluation reveals a rounded sclerotic lesion that arises from one of the cortical tables of the skull (usually the outer table) without involvement of the diploe. Treatment of asymptomatic osteomas may be indicated for cosmetic reasons. Removal with a high-speed burr with sparing of the uninvolved inner table is generally sufficient.

In contrast to the ivory osteoma, the rarer spongy osteoma has been reported to be radiolucent and to present with localized headache and tenderness to palpation.[112] In this respect it is similar to osteoid osteoma.

The differential diagnosis of the ivory osteoma includes a solitary osteoblastic metastasis, for example from prostate carcinoma.

TABLE 150-1 Classification of Primary Tumors and Bone-Forming Conditions of the Skull

Bone-Forming Tumors—Benign
Osteoma
Ossifying fibroma
Osteoid osteoma
Osteoblastoma (giant osteoid osteoma)
Bone-Forming Conditions—Benign but Potentially Premalignant
Fibrous dysplasia
Paget's disease
Bone-Forming Tumors—Malignant
Osteogenic sarcoma
Secondary osteogenic sarcoma in association with Paget's disease, fibrous dysplasia, retinoblastoma, or radiation
Cartilage-Forming Tumors—Benign
Chondroma
Chondroblastoma (Codman's tumor)
Chrondromyxoid fibroma
Myxoma of the facial skeleton
Cartilage-Forming Tumors—Malignant
Chondrosarcoma
Connective Tissue Tumors—Benign
Desmoplastic fibroma
Connective Tissue Tumors—Malignant
Fibrosarcoma of bone
Histiocytic or Fibrohistiocytic Tumors—Benign
Giant cell "reparative" granuloma
Non-ossifying fibroma (benign fibrous histiocytoma)
Xanthoma of bone
Histiocytic or Fibrohistiocytic Tumors—Malignant
Ewing's sarcoma
Giant cell tumor of bone (osteoclastoma)
Malignant fibrous histiocytoma
Tumors of Blood or Blood Vessel Origin
Angiosarcoma of bone
Hemangiopericytoma
Malignant hemangioendothelioma
Eosinophilic granuloma of bone
Hemangioma of bone
Lymphangioma of bone
Lymphoma of bone
Plasmacytoma
Miscellaneous Tumors of Soft Tissue and Bone
Aneurysmal bone cyst
Benign nerve sheath tumor (schwannoma) of bone
Chordoma
Epidermoid and dermoid tumors of bone
Lipoma and liposarcoma of bone
Melanotic neuroectodermal tumor of bone
Intraosseous meningioma
Primary neuroendocrine (Merkle cell) carcinoma of bone
Primary tumors of bone with smooth muscle and skeletal muscle differentiation

Source: Adapted from Huvos.[59,60]

TABLE 150-2 Syndromes That Can Include Primary Tumors and Bone-Forming Conditions of the Skull

Gardner's syndrome
McCune-Albright syndrome
Nonthrombotic partial venous sinus occlusion near the torcular Herophili
Ollier's syndrome
Maffucci's syndrome

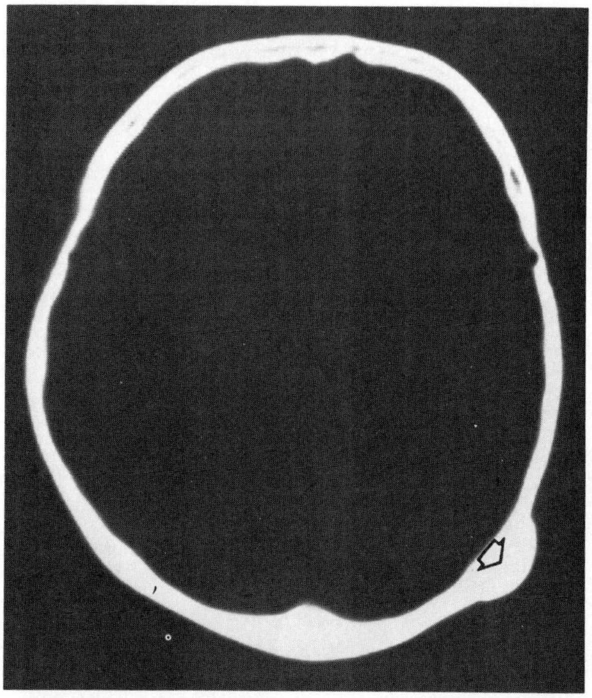

Figure 150-3 A CT scan with a skeletal window setting shows an osteoma arising from the outer table (*arrow*). The homogeneous dense appearance is characteristic.

The monostotic form of fibrous dysplasia can be purely sclerotic; but this is more common at the skull base and is composed of immature woven bone. Hyperostosis frontalis interna does not cross the midline, nor does it form over large cortical veins. Meningiomas are usually associated with increased vascular markings. For additional discussion on differential diagnosis the reader

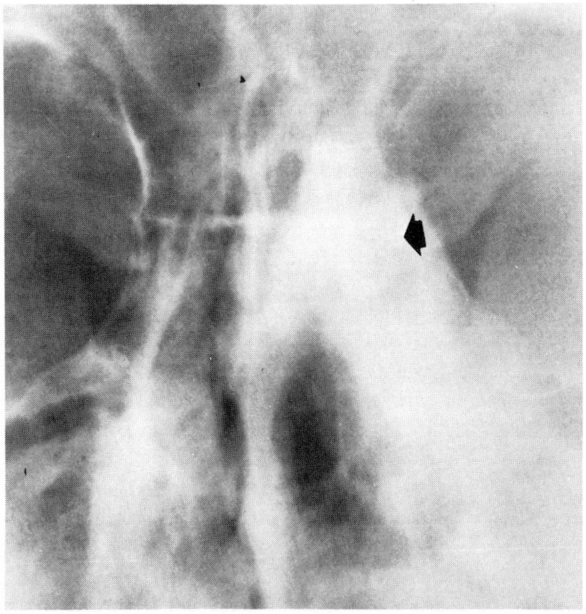

Figure 150-4 A skull film showing an osteoma of the paranasal sinuses (*arrow*). The radiographic differential diagnosis includes fibrous dysplasia and meningioma.

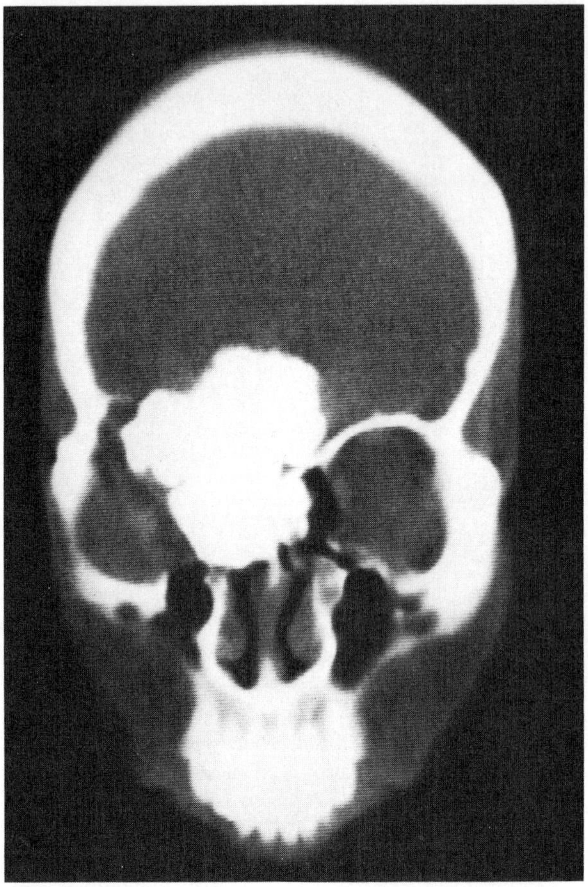

Figure 150-5 A CT scan in the coronal plane showing a large osteoma that originated in the frontal sinus but grew to involve the orbit and the maxillary and ethmoid sinuses. Note the marked extension into the anterior cranial fossa. Complete surgical resection required a craniofacial approach.

is referred to the other sections on benign bone tumors as well as the section on intraosseous meningioma.

Multiple osteomas should alert the clinician to the possibility of Gardner's syndrome. This dangerous condition carries an inevitable risk of cancer, most often occurring in the gastrointestinal tract. For additional discussion, see the section on Gardner's syndrome.

Ossifying Fibroma

Ossifying fibroma is a slow-growing sharply marginated benign tumor. It is composed of a fibrous stroma with varying amounts of woven bone, but has areas of mature lamellar bone at the periphery. It appears to represent part of the spectrum of fibro-osseous lesions that includes fibrous dysplasia. Some authorities believe that the only feature that separates ossifying fibroma from fibrous dysplasia is the presence of a ''capsule'' of lamellar bone that surrounds an ossifying fibroma. Others contend that they are distinct pathologic entities.[60]

Owing to the controversy surrounding the classification of these fibro-osseous lesions, the true incidence and most common location of this condition varies widely among reports. Ossifying fibroma is a very rare lesion, with no racial predilection; it may be more common in females. It appears in patients before the age of 40, with a peak incidence in the third and fourth decades. Ossifying fibroma most commonly occurs in the mandible and maxilla. The frontal and temporal bones are the most common sites in the calvaria. These lesions present as a slowly growing mass that is initially asymptomatic. Symptoms and signs are dependent on the location of the tumor.

Radiographically the lesions are radiolucent initially, but gradually acquire radiopaque, haphazardly arranged calcifications. Ossifying fibromas appear to expand the involved bone, usually with the preservation of a thin rim of cortex. Occasionally a densely sclerotic border is induced, creating a sharply defined radiopaque margin. In contrast, fibrous dysplasia has an indistinct margin with a ground-glass appearance. Skull films may show dilated vascular channels. CT images of ossifying fibroma reveal a well-delineated dense lesion. Angiography will occasionally reveal scalp and dural feeding vessels. Radionuclide ^{99m}Tc scans also may be positive.

Histologic examination reveals a uniformly cellular fibrous spindle cell growth arranged in a whorled or matted pattern. The bony fragments, which can be spherical, can be mistaken for meningioma psammoma bodies. Varying amounts of woven bone spicules are present, with lamellar bone development at the periphery. New bone formation normally occurs in stages, with woven bone appearing first and later maturing into lamellar bone. Lamellar bone has several distinguishing characteristics. Lamellar bone trabeculae polarize with widely spaced parallel birefringent lines. Furthermore, the trabeculae in lamellar bone are rimmed by osteoblasts and osteoclasts. Fibrous dysplasia, in which bone development is arrested in the woven bone stage, may be recognized by random birefringence when viewed under polarized light. Silver reticulin stains display tangled and disoriented fibers with no osteoblastic or osteoclastic activity present. Hemorrhage, inflammation, and giant cell reaction also can be present in fibrous dysplasia.[60]

The differential diagnosis of fibro-osseous lesions must include not only ossifying fibroma and fibrous dysplasia but also reactive bone formation. In reactive bone formation, spicules of bone appear along the lines of trauma with woven bone undergoing complete maturation to lamellar bone. Endochondral bone formation is also present.[60]

Juvenile ossifying fibroma is a rapidly growing destructive lesion of the maxilla occurring before the age of 15. Extension into the paranasal sinuses and orbit is common (Fig. 150-6). This lesion is identical histologically to the adult tumor, but its aggressive local invasiveness can be fatal.[123]

The preferred treatment of ossifying fibroma is complete surgical excision, which is easily accomplished when it occurs in the cranial vault.[141] In extremely large lesions and those of the skull base, subtotal removal has provided excellent results of more than ten years. Radiation therapy has been reported in therapy of these tumors, but malignant transformation limits this application.[60] Additional discussion is included in the section on fibrous dysplasia.

Osteoid Osteoma

Osteoid osteoma is a benign osteoblastic lesion consisting of a well-defined small osteolytic nidus surrounded by dense reactive cortical sclerosis. The nidus is characterized by a mixture of osteoid, bony trabeculae, and a vascular supportive tissue. Osteoid osteoma accounts for about 10 percent of all benign tumors and 2.6

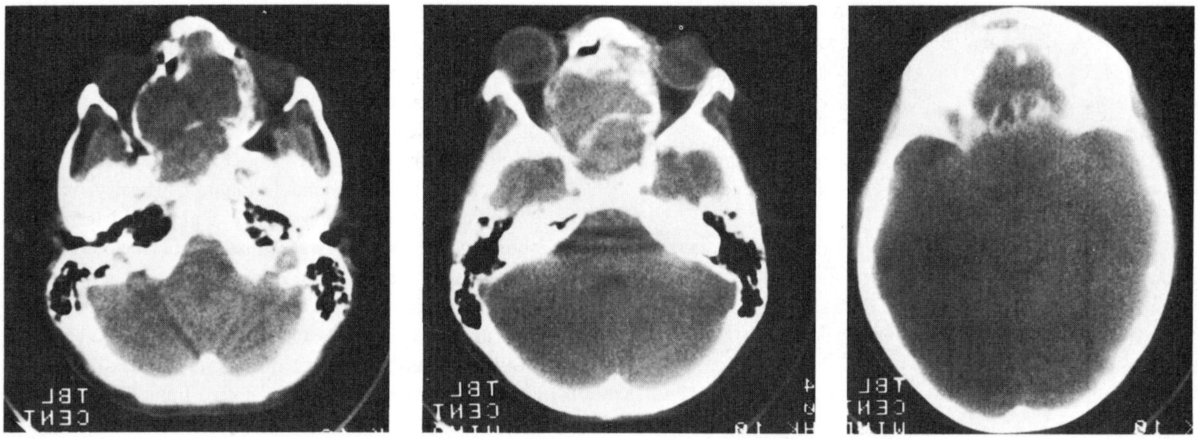

Figure 150-6 Serial CT scans in the axial plane showing a juvenile ossifying fibroma of the paranasal sinuses with early extension through the cribriform plate. (From Tomita et al.,[123] with permission.)

percent of excised primary bone tumors. It occurs predominantly between the ages of 10 and 25 and is twice as common in males.

These tumors occur throughout the skeleton, with some predilection for the bones of the legs. Location in the skull is extremely rare. Only a handful of cases involving the calvaria have been reported in the literature. Osteoid osteoma is characteristically accompanied by localized pain and tenderness, particularly at night. Classically this nocturnal pain is relieved by aspirin or other nonsteroidal anti-inflammatory agents. Sometimes these tumors are asymptomatic or may present as a vague discomfort or atypical head pain.

The nidus of osteoid osteoma is radiolucent, and has a surrounding zone of dense sclerosis. In cases when the cortical reaction of surrounding bone is very dense, the nidus can be obscured. Occasionally a lesion located in cortical bone will appear as a radiopaque center with a surrounding ringlike radiolucent band. Radionuclide bone scans have been shown to be effective in locating these lesions, even when roentgenograms of the skull and CT scans have been negative.[91] Angiography has been performed with variable success. Preoperative injection of tetracycline may allow for the more accurate identification of the nidus under ultraviolet light during resection.[60]

Histologically, the development of these lesions can be divided into three stages, although there is no correlation between these developmental stages and clinical symptoms. The initial stage is characterized by actively proliferating, densely packed, prominent osteoblasts within a highly vascular stroma. The intermediate phase, which is the most characteristic phase, exists when osteoid is deposited between the osteoblasts. The intercellular osteoid and trabeculae show varying degrees of calcification in the mature or osteoma stage. The osteoid eventually becomes well-calcified, compact trabeculae of atypical bone that is typically neither woven nor lamellar. Thickened cortical bone surrounds all three histologic stages.[60]

The differential diagnosis is mainly with osteoblastoma, which is histologically extremely similar to osteoid osteoma. The distinction is based on clinical features. Osteoblastoma also presents with pain, but does not share the classic occurrence at night or the response to aspirin. Osteoblastomas are also larger, and have potential for continued growth.

Treatment of osteoid osteoma is indicated to relieve pain. Surgical excision, either *en bloc* or by curettage of the nidus and adjacent sclerotic bone, is usually curative. Only transient symptom relief may result if the nidus is spared.[91] For additional discussion, the reader is referred to the following section on osteoblastoma.

Osteoblastoma

Osteoblastoma is a benign tumor of bone that is histologically very similar to osteoid osteoma; in the past it was sometimes known as giant osteoid osteoma. In fact, some authors consider size to be the most important discriminating criterion, and arbitrarily classify lesions larger than 1.5 cm as osteoblastomas.[71] Osteoblastomas are rare tumors, comprising about 1 percent of all primary bone tumors. Most arise in the second and third decades of life, with 90 percent occurring before the age of 30. Males are affected twice as often as females when the tumor occurs in extracranial locations.

Osteoblastomas occur most commonly in the vertebral column (34 percent), the long bones (30 percent), and the small bones of the hands and feet (13.5 percent).[60] Since back pain and scoliosis are common findings in patients with osteoblastoma of the spine (the most frequent localization), most cases are seen by orthopedic surgeons.[128] In a series of 98 osteoblastomas, only 3 were located in the bones of the skull.[71] One recent literature review found only 13 cases of calvarial involvement, while another found a total of 16 cases.[9,84] The average age at presentation was 27 years, with no sex predilection. The youngest reported patient was a 7-month-old female.[88] These tumors typically present with a localized, dull, aching pain, which in contrast to the pain of osteoid osteoma is not usually worse at night and is not relieved by aspirin.

Skull films typically show a well-demarcated lytic lesion with a smooth calcified rim. In that respect osteoblastomas resemble eosinophilic granulomas. However, some degree of mineralization is often present in the center of the lesion that gives it the appearance of a button sequestrum of the skull.[71] Angiography gives variable results. CT is helpful in demonstrating the thin surrounding sclerosis and subtle calcification within the tumor matrix. Most of these tumors enhance following the intravenous infusion of a contrast agent, but not always.[9] Radionuclide bone scans are always positive. On MRI the tumor is of low intensity on T1-weighted images and high intensity on T2-weighted images.[84]

Histologically these lesions possess fibrous stroma in which irregular osteoid deposition takes place. Highly vascularized tissue lies between the osseous trabecular network. Osteoblastoma can be confused with osteogenic sarcoma. However, in osteoblastoma the stromal cells are small and slender and do not resemble the sarcomatous spindle cells. Mitoses are rare, anaplastic cells are absent, there is no cartilage within the tumor, and the cells within the osteoid matrix are small and inconspicuous. When differentiating this tumor from osteoid osteoma, osteoblastoma is found to possess a more abundant fibrous stroma, many multinucleated giant cells, extravasated blood, and generally to be less osteoid. Size and symptoms help in the differential diagnosis. In many cases, aneurysmally dilated vascular spaces appear within these tumors, forming an associated aneurysmal bone cyst.

The main differential diagnosis includes the above-listed lesions: osteogenic sarcoma, osteoid osteoma, and aneurysmal bone cyst. Giant cell tumor of bone can be excluded because of the presence of calcification, osteoid, and bone formation.

Osteoblastoma is a benign lesion, but local recurrence has been reported following subtotal resection. Aggressive osteoblastomas have been reported, with multiple recurrences despite radiation.[1] The literature indicates a 10 percent recurrence rate.[128] Lesions of the cranial vault should generally be removed *en bloc*; however, curettage, even with residual tumor, has resulted in years of symptom-free existence. There is no agreement concerning the role of radiation therapy. Malignant transformation of osteoblastoma has been reported, both spontaneously as well as following radiation therapy.[60] For additional discussion, see the preceding section on osteoid osteoma.

Bone-Forming Conditions—Benign but Potentially Premalignant

Fibrous Dysplasia

Fibrous dysplasia is a nonheritable developmental anomaly of bone-forming mesenchyme. The normal evolutionary development of new bone formation from the woven bone stage to the lamellar bone stage does not occur. In addition, there is an overgrowth of a well vascularized fibrous stroma surrounding the haphazardly arranged bony trabeculae.[60]

Fibrous dysplasia has been divided into three categories: (1) the monostotic form, involving a single bony site; (2) the polyostotic form, involving multiple bony sites; and (3) the McCune-Albright syndrome. About 70 percent of afflicted patients have the monostotic form, 30 percent have the polysostotic form, and only about 3 percent have the McCune-Albright syndrome.[95,138]

Camilleri has provided an excellent discussion of the history and theories of causation of fibrous dysplasia.[22] Prior to 1937, cystic bone disease was attributed to parathyroid disease despite negative exploratory surgery. In that year the McCune-Albright syndrome was recognized. Lichtenstein first suggested the term "fibrous dysplasia" in 1938. The etiology of this condition is not clear and several theories have been proposed: (1) Lichtenstein and Jaffe (1942) believed there is a congenital defect of the bone-forming mesenchyme; (2) Schlumberger (1946) postulated that fibrous dysplasia is a reparative response to trauma; (3) Albright et al. in 1937 suggested some kind of primary endocrine dysfunction to explain the variant of fibrous dysplasia now known as McCune-Albright syndrome; (4) Changus in 1957 proposed that fibrous dysplasia represents a hyperplasia of osteoblasts in response to an unidentified stimulus; and (5) Shapiro believed that fibrous dysplasia results from a mutant gene whose protein product affects bone, pigment, and hormone metabolism. A genetic abnormality may indeed exist. There is no evidence, however, for a mendelian pattern of inheritance.[130]

Histologically, fibrous dysplasia is characterized by the presence of woven bone. New bone formation normally occurs in stages, with woven bone appearing first and later maturing into lamellar bone. Lamellar bone trabeculae, when viewed under polarized light, show widely spaced parallel birefringent lines. In addition, the trabeculae in lamellar bone are rimmed by osteoblasts and osteoclasts. Fibrous dysplasia, in which bone development is arrested in the woven bone stage, may be recognized by random birefringence when viewed under polarized light. The trabeculae are irregular and jumbled up like alphabet soup.[20] The anvil-shaped trabeculae of woven bone surrounded by swirls of abundant fibrous tissue are typical of fibrous dysplasia.[60] The osteocytic lacunae are large and have feathery margins. Silver reticulin stains display tangled and disoriented fibers, and there is little osteoblastic or osteoclastic activity. Hemorrhage, inflammation, and giant cell reaction can also be present in fibrous dysplasia.[60]

The radiographic appearance of fibrous dysplasia is divided into three presentations: (1) cystic, (2) sclerotic, and (3) mixed, or "pagetoid." The cystic type is seen in the vault; it affects mainly the outer table, which is thinned and bulged out. The inner table is slightly thickened, but usually preserved. The sclerotic form produces a diffuse, often symmetric, thickening of the floor of the anterior and middle cranial fossae (Figs. 150-7 and 150-8). The mixed form occurs in the vault and simulates the cystic variety. Intermixed with lucent areas are patches of increased density similar to those seen in Paget's disease, although they are more sharply defined.[8] The mixed form occurs in more than half the patients, most of whom are older than 30 years of age and have had symptoms for an average of 15 years. The sclerotic and cystlike patterns occurred in younger individuals (average age, 20 years) with less than 3 years of symptoms. This suggests that the pagetoid pattern may represent the natural progression of the sclerotic and cystlike

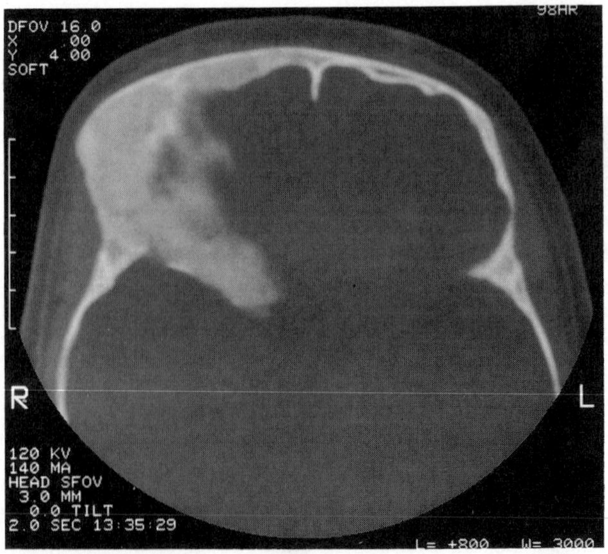

Figure 150-7 A CT scan in the axial plane showing fibrous dysplasia involving the floor of the right anterior cranial fossa. Thickening of the optic canal can result in loss of vision.

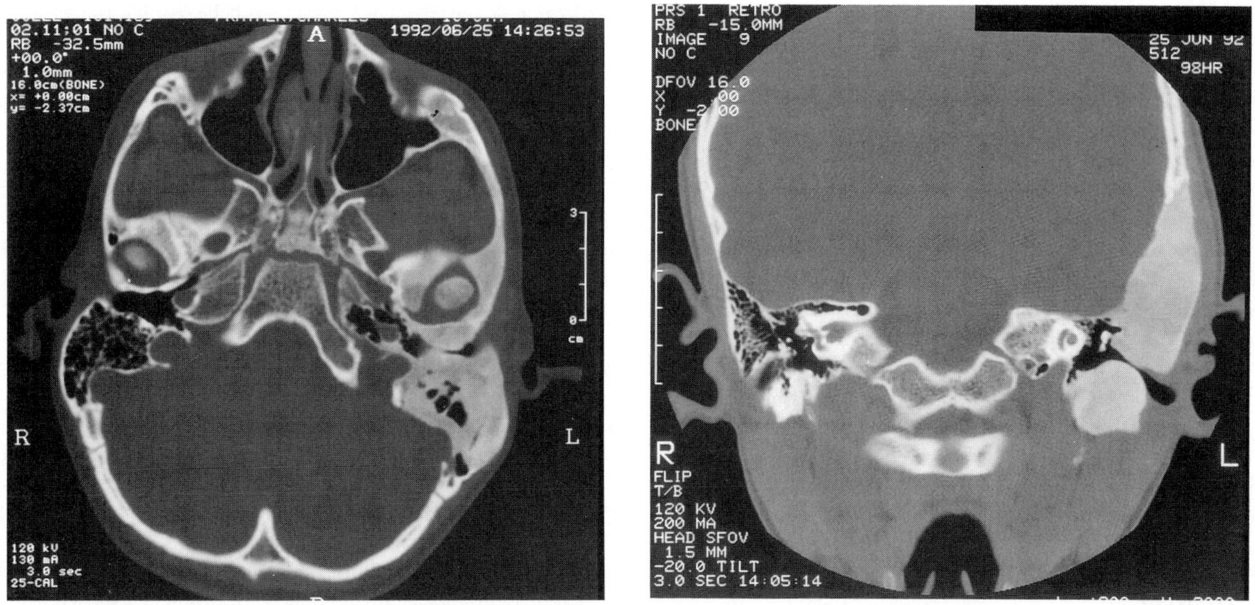

(*A*) (*B*)

Figure 150-8 *A*. A CT scan in the axial plane showing fibrous dysplasia involving the skull base. This is the sclerotic pattern, with expansion and replacement of the bone in the left middle cranial fossa. *B*. CT scan of the same patient in the coronal plane showing more clearly the compromise of the external auditory meatus. This patient presented with conductive hearing loss.

lesions.[22] Craniofacial fibrous dysplasia seems to ignore suture lines, so that in the majority of cases, more than one bone is involved at the time of presentation.[32] CT more clearly reveals an intradiploic, multilocular lesion separated by bony trabeculae. Angiography can show a faint tumor stain, but that is unusual.[97] Various types of radionuclide bone scans have been reported to aid in the assessment of the extent of bony involvement.[32,38,44,51,101]

The classic teaching is that the active phase of fibrous dysplasia occurs in the teenage years and that it becomes quiescent after adolescence. However, a recent report by Davies and MacPherson suggests that disease progression into adulthood, as well as initial presentation in adulthood, may be more common than previously thought.[36] The sex incidence in their series of 18 patients was equal. Fibrous dysplasia was most active during the teenage years, when there was a preponderance of male patients. Of the seven patients in whom there was evidence of progression in adulthood, all but one were female, as were six of the seven patients presenting in adulthood. Therefore, both disease progression into adulthood and initial presentation in adulthood seem much more common in females. Overall, 7 of 18 patients (38 percent) had their initial diagnosis as adults. Supporting this observation are case reports of a 49-year-old woman presenting with diplopia, and a 72-year-old woman suffering with trigeminal neuralgia-like pain, both secondary to fibrous dysplasia.[10,15]

Skull involvement occurs in 27 percent of monostotic and up to 50 percent of polyostotic patients. Surgical intervention is generally directed at the cosmetic facial deformities and cranial nerve compression. Chen and Noordhoff have divided the craniofacial skeleton into four zones in an attempt to develop principles of surgical treatment.[24] They recommend: total excision of dysplastic bone of fronto-orbital, zygomatic, and upper maxillary origin (zone 1) with bone reconstruction primarily; conservative excision of dysplastic skull in hair-bearing areas (zone 2), dysplastic bone in the central cranial base (zone 3), and dysplastic tooth-bearing bones (zone 4); and optic canal decompression for patients with orbital dysplasia and decreasing visual acuity. They found that radical excision of the dysplastic bone can cure the disease. However, when there was some residual disease, they found no invasion of the dysplasia into the reconstructed bones. The reconstructed bones retained their contour. This agrees with Camilleri's observation that autogenous bone grafts will successfully unite with remaining bone that still contains elements of fibrous dysplasia. Furthermore, resected dysplastic bone can be contoured, thinned, and replaced as a free graft to aid reconstruction, apparently without the risk of regrowth.[22]

The experience with optic nerve decompression is generally less impressive. Decreased vision after chronic compression usually cannot be reversed after decompression, and it is possible to damage the nerve further during the operation.[24,90] However, some authorities recommend prophylactic decompression for zone 3 growing lesions, particularly in children.[90] Nevertheless, on occasion optic nerve dysfunction is improved.[138] Munro[90] draws attention to the danger of another type of visual problem, which can occur as the result of corrective surgery. Sudden eye repositioning will cause diplopia. He states that most adults prefer to have just the forehead contour restored by burring and accept the downward displacement of the eye rather than risk permanent diplopia. In children and adolescents, the sudden elevation of the eye also will also produce diplopia, but this will usually disappear after several months.

Camilleri believes that traditional procrastination during the "active" phase in children is now increasingly considered unacceptable.[22] There is no indication that surgical procedures inhibit the growth rate of residual normal tissues. Furthermore, progression of disease can continue into adulthood.[36] A strategy based on an expected spontaneous regression in disease activity after adolescence may be ill-advised. Surgery is indicated at any age if important function is threatened, deformity becomes substantial, or complications develop. However, partial removal is associated with a 25 percent incidence of local recurrence.[22]

Radiation is not recommended because of the risk of malignant transformation.[89] Even in the absence of radiation, malignant tumors can develop. It is estimated that patients with fibrous dysplasia are about 400 times more likely than the general population to develop a malignant bone tumor.[24] The incidence of spontaneous malignant degeneration is about 0.5 percent, which is about one-fourth that of Paget's disease. Camilleri reported that the mean interval to the development of malignancy after the diagnosis of fibrous dysplasia is 12.5 years.[22] For additional discussion of fibrous dysplasia, the reader is referred to the sections on McCune-Albright syndrome, secondary osteogenic sarcoma, ossifying fibroma, and intraosseous meningioma.

Paget's Disease

Paget's disease is a benign but premalignant condition of unknown etiology. Both bone resorption and bone formation are increased. In progressively active Paget's disease, woven bone replaces cortical lamellar bone, and the haversian system is obliterated by bone of chaotic structure.[60] It usually occurs after the age of 55 years. The skull is the third most common site of involvement, following the lumbar vertebrae and sacrum.

The neurological symptoms and signs of advanced Paget's disease are caused by changes at the skull base. The thickened bone constricts neural foramina, producing cranial nerve deficits, particularly deafness. Basilar impression may develop, with cervicomedullary compromise.[20]

Malignant degeneration occurs in about 2 percent of afflicted patients.[60] Osteogenic sarcoma is the most commonly seen tumor, but others occur as well. For additional discussion, see the section on secondary osteogenic sarcoma.

Bone-Forming Tumors—Malignant

Osteogenic Sarcoma

The osteogenic sarcoma is the second most common primary malignant tumor of bone after multiple myeloma. It is twice as common as chondrosarcoma, three times more frequent than Ewing's sarcoma, and up to ten times more common than malignant fibrous hystiocytoma of bone.[60] There are 7400 new cases and 4200 deaths in the United States annually.[83] Osteogenic sarcoma can occur throughout all ages, but 61 percent of patients present during the first two decades of life and 85 percent before the age of 30.[49,60,129] In this age group the tumors most frequently arise in area of fastest bone growth, which is on either side of the knee in the distal femur or proximal tibia. A second and significantly smaller peak in incidence occurs in patients over the age of 60, accounting for approximately 10 percent of all osteogenic sarcomas. Craniofacial involvement is more common in older patients, with an average age of those presenting with calvarial tumors being 39.[129] Overall the craniofacial bones account for only 5 to 10 percent of osteogenic sarcomas, and most of these are located in the mandible and maxilla.[49] Less than 1 percent are found in the calvaria.[129]

Calvarial tumors usually present as a mass which may or may not be associated with pain, unlike the early pain found with tumors occurring in the long bones. As a general rule, the symptoms are subacute with a history only a few months in duration.

The radiographic features of osteogenic sarcoma reflect the bone production, destruction, and periosteal reaction. One series included eight patients with primary osteogenic sarcoma of the cranial bones; seven of these were osteolytic and one was osteoblastic.[76] All had soft-tissue extension, four (50 percent) contained calcification, and none had a periosteal reaction. Of the eight, five arose from the vault and three at the base. CT and plain films were found superior to MRI in detecting the matrix calcifications and bone destruction or reaction.[76] Extracortical soft tissue extension of tumor may display radiating striations giving the characteristic "sun-ray" appearance on tangential skull films, but this is not common (Fig. 150-9). Increased tracer uptake is usually demonstrated on bone scan.

The histologic diagnosis of osteogenic sarcoma depends on the identification of a malignant spindle cell stroma which directly produces osteoid or immature bone. There are three subtypes based on the predominant cell type forming the lesion. These are the fibroblastic, chondroblastic, and osteoblastic subtypes. In a series of primary osteogenic sarcomas of the calvarial bones, half were of the osteoblastic type, and half were fibroblastic. There were no chondroid variants in that group.[76] Lesions are also assigned a grade based on the relative anaplasia of the stromal element (grades 1 through 4). In general, there seems to be no significant prognostic difference among the subtypes or histologic grades. In most cases, a spindle cell malignant stroma is seen that may imitate fibrosarcoma, but production of osteoid directly by the tumor cells is pathognomonic. The secondary ossification and metaplastic bone formation of many chondrosarcomas may result in their erroneously being classified as osteogenic sarcomas. Differentiation is important because osteogenic sarcomas have a far poorer prognosis.

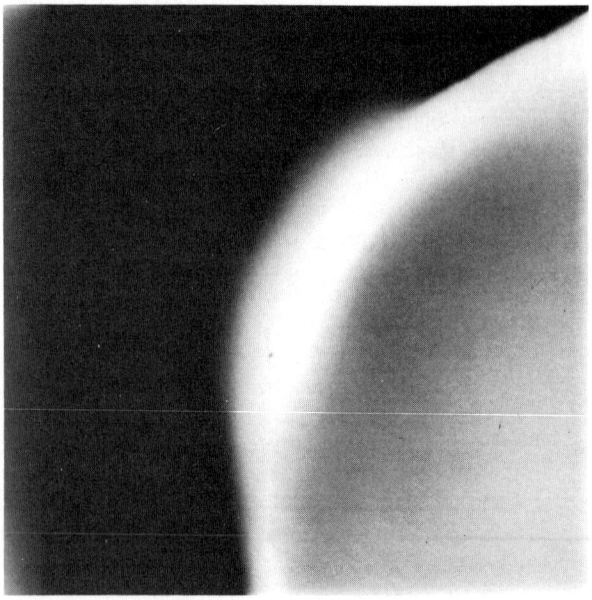

Figure 150-9 A tangential view of the skull showing an osteogenic sarcoma involving both tables with irregular new bone formation.

When osteogenic sarcoma occurs in the extremities, amputation is often performed. Despite radical surgery, the overall 5-year survival has been reported to be between 5 and 20 percent. Head and neck tumors have a much lower risk of distant metastasis than extremity tumors, but have a higher rate of local recurrence. This probably reflects the difficulty of obtaining wide surgical margins in this location. Surgery alone is clearly not the answer for these aggressive neoplasms. One report described a nonrandomized retrospective study of 18 patients.[83] Overall, 47 percent of the patients enjoyed a disease-free interval of 5 years or more. There were five patients who had surgery + radiation + chemotherapy as their initial treatment, and four (80 percent) were cured. The authors recommend multimodality treatment for osteogenic sarcoma of the head and neck.[83]

Secondary Osteogenic Sarcoma

Osteogenic sarcoma occurs with a higher frequency than that seen in the general population in patients with Paget's disease, fibrous dysplasia, or retinoblastoma, and in those who have been exposed to radiation therapy or thorium oxide (a radioactive scanning agent). In individuals younger than 21 years, 91 percent of osteogenic sarcomas arise in the absence of any risk factors. In older patients, 56 percent are secondary to one of these conditions.[60]

Sir James Paget reported five cases of osteitis deformans in 1877. Two of these (40 percent) eventually developed sarcomas.[86] The actual risk is much lower. The incidence of sarcomatous degeneration varies widely in the literature from 0.15 to 12 percent. The fairest estimate is probably that 2 percent of all patients with polyostotic Paget's disease will develop a secondary malignant bone tumor.[60] The most common sites of malignant transformation in Paget's disease include the femur, pelvis, humerus, and tibia. The most common tumor type is osteogenic sarcoma (Fig. 150-10), but fibrosarcomas, chondrosarcomas, and giant-cell tumors occur less frequently.[137] Paget's disease is a common entity in the western world. Prevalence is estimated to be about 5 percent of the population over 40 years of age. On the other hand, Paget's disease is apparently quite rare in India.[129] Osteosarcomas arising in Paget's disease account for between 20 and 30 percent of all osteosarcomas arising in patients over 40 years of age. Radionuclide bone scanning can be useful in diagnosing malignant degeneration and defining the extent of the tumor by increased uptake.[86]

The risk of spontaneous (without radiation) malignant transformation in fibrous dysplasia is about 0.5 percent, or about one-fourth that seen in Paget's disease. The true risk is actually lower because many patients with the monostotic form of fibrous dysplasia are asymptomatic and remain undetected.[116] In the monostotic form, the most common site for sarcomatous involvement are the facial bones and skull. However, in the polyostotic form the femur is the most frequent site.[25] The interval between diagnosis and malignant transformation can vary from 2 to 30 years. Pain, swelling, a significant alteration in radiographic appearance, and especially the development of a soft tissue mass indicate malignant change. The most common malignant tumor to develop in this setting is osteogenic sarcoma (53 percent), but fibrosarcoma (30 percent) and chondrosarcoma (16 percent) also occur. The literature indicates that about half of these tumors developed in the polyostotic form of fibrous dysplasia. Slightly less than half of the patients who developed osteogenic sarcoma had radiation therapy, usually in the setting of the polyostotic form. Most secondary chondrosarcomas and fibrosarcomas developed in fibrous dysplasia without prior irradiation.[89,116]

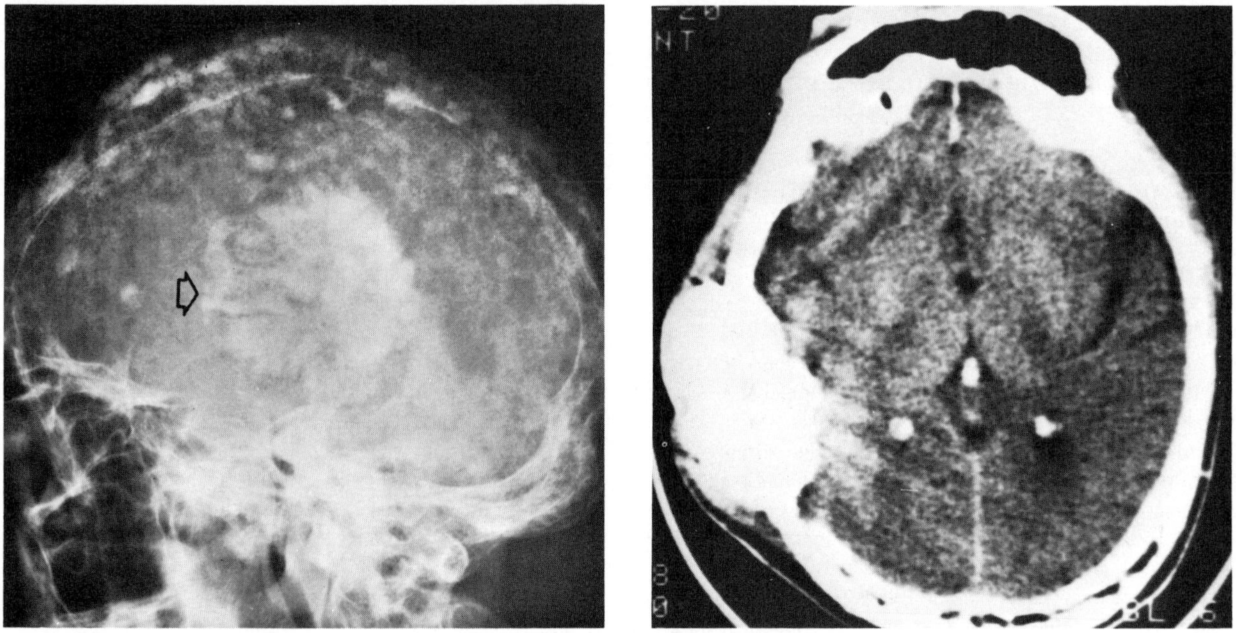

(A) ***(B)***

Figure 150-10 *A.* The sudden appearance of a rapidly growing skull mass in a patient with Paget's disease is classic for osteogenic sarcoma (*arrow*). *B.* A contrast-enhanced CT scan of an osteogenic sarcoma shows both intracranial extension and invasion of the soft tissues of the scalp. For complete surgical excision, wide resection of the scalp, skull, and dura with adequate margins is necessary.

Patients with retinoblastoma have an increased risk for developing osteogenic sarcoma independent of radiation exposure. Among patients with hereditary retinoblastoma, the incidence of osteogenic sarcoma is increased 500 times over the expected incidence.[83] Retinoblastoma seems to be related to genetic abnormalities. The first characterized tumor suppressor gene was the retinoblastoma gene. This is deleted or mutated not only in retinoblastomas but also in osteogenic sarcomas, small-cell lung carcinomas, breast cancers, and bladder cancers.[111]

Osteogenic sarcoma is known to arise after radiation treatment. The report by Lee et al. included 14 patients with postradiation osteosarcomas of the cranial-facial bones.[76] Patient ages ranged from 7 to 50, with a mean of 38. The latent period ranged from 4 years, 2 months, to 50 years, with a mean of 14 years. Information on radiation dose was available only on six patients, and ranged from 3500 to 6400 rad. Of the osteogenic sarcomas, 9 of 14 (64 percent) were osteolytic, 3 (21 percent) were osteoblastic, and 2 (14 percent) were mixed. All three subtypes were represented in the eight cases that were available for pathologic review: five were chondroblastic, one osteoblastic, and two were fibroblastic. The tumors tended to occur near the periphery of the radiation fields. In that zone the administered radiation was unable to destroy all viable cells but was able to induce malignant transformation. The authors concluded that it may be difficult to differentiate radiographically between postradiation osteosarcoma and simple radiation osteitis. Nevertheless, an associated soft-tissue extension strongly favors tumor and justifies a prompt tissue biopsy.[76] More recently, Sugita et al. reviewed the literature and found just eight cases, including their own, of postradiation osteogenic sarcomas involving the cranial vault. Five patients were less than 40 years old. The latent period varied from 3.5 to 21 years (mean, 9.1 years). The radiation dosage varied from 2052 to 11,000 rad (mean, 6122 rad). The radiographic appearance in this case was osteoblastic. Tangential x-ray films showed the typical ''sun-ray'' appearance.[115]

Cartilage-Forming Tumors—Benign

Chondroma

The chondroma is a benign tumor composed of mature hyaline cartilage. When a cartilaginous tumor arises in the peripheral skeleton, it is classified according to its relationship to the bony cortex. A tumor located within the medullary cavity is called an enchondroma. When one is found between the periosteum and cortex, it is a juxtacortical chondroma. An outward bony protrusion from the cortex with a cartilage-capped external surface is termed an osteochondroma. These distinctions lose their significance at the skull base, and these tumors are referred to simply as chondromas.

Chondromas are very rare tumors of the skull (comprising 0.1 to 0.2 percent of such tumors), are most common in the second through fifth decade, and have a female predominance.[4,70] These tumors arise in bone formed by endochondral ossification, and therefore are most commonly found at the basilar synchondroses and paranasal sinuses. The bones of the vault, which are formed by membranous ossification, are rarely involved. However, unusual locations have been reported, including the vault, choroid plexus, dura, arachnoid, and brain.[70] Chondromas are generally painless, slowly growing tumors whose symptoms and signs are dependent on their location.

Radiologically these tumors are well-circumscribed, with distinct areas of lucency caused by bone deformation and destruction at the skull base. The bony cortex may be expanded and thinned by the lesions. Many show varying degrees of degeneration and necrosis, with resulting calcification from granular to massive in amount. This calcification allows these tumors to be distinguished from metastasis or nasopharyngeal carcinoma. The tendency for intralesional calcification seems to be related to tumor location. The parasellar chondromas or chondrosarcomas (arising from the sphenopetrosal synchondrosis) show speckled areas of calcification, but tumors occurring in the posterior fossa (arising from the petro-occiptal synchondrosis) do not calcify.[21]

These tumors can occur as part of systemic disorders in Ollier's syndrome and Maffucci's syndrome. Malignant degeneration, particularly in the latter condition, is common. For additional discussion, the reader is referred to the section on chondrosarcoma, as well as the section on Ollier's syndrome and Maffucci's syndrome.

Chondroblastoma

Chondroblastoma is a rare, benign but locally aggressive tumor of bone consisting of immature cartilage cells. It was first recognized as a distinct entity by Codman in 1931. These tumors make up 1 to 2 percent of all primary bone tumors.[14] As with all cartilage tumors, they are usually found in bone formed by endochondral ossification. Classically, these occur at the epiphysis of long bones in patients younger than 25 years. Males are affected twice as often as females. This tumor involves the craniofacial bones about 7 percent of the time; when it does, it is usually in those older than 30.[11] Approximately 50 cases of chondroblastoma involving the skull have been reported, most occurring at the skull base, usually in the temporal bone.[5,11,14,57,73,118] Only two cases have been reported in the cranial vault.[11]

Symptoms and signs of this tumor are usually nonspecific. Pain and swelling can appear locally, with focal neurological findings dependent on tumor location. Radiologically the lesions are characterized by well-demarcated osteolytic areas, with varying degrees of central and peripheral calcification. These tumors may expand the cortex of bone, with about one-third of these cases possessing a periosteal reaction. CT scans show the presence of intralesional calcifications, which is important in differential diagnosis. Radionuclide bone scans show active uptake.

Histologically these lesions are composed of uniform, polyhedral, closely packed cells which may be difficult to distinguish from plasma cells. Chondroid differentiation and pericellular lattice-like calcifications arranged in a ''chicken wire'' pattern are the hallmarks of this lesion. Chondroblastomas must be differentiated from the more aggressive true giant-cell tumors and the nonneoplastic giant-cell ''reparative'' granulomas. If there is a lesion in the lateral portion of the temporal bone, the likelihood is that it is chondroblastoma. Giant-cell tumor is much less common in this location. On the other hand, giant-cell tumor should be definitely considered in the differential diagnosis for lesions of the body of the sphenoid. Giant-cell reparative granuloma can affect bones at the base of the skull, above the maxilla, but probably would not produce a circumscribed defect laterally in the temporal bone.[11]

When chondroblastoma is associated with aneurysmal bone cyst, some authors believe that there is a higher recurrence rate. This view is not shared universally.[14] An unusual histologic feature of cranial chondroblastoma is infiltration of tumor beyond the peripheral reactive rim of bone. This may account for the high rate of recurrence seen in cranial chondroblastoma treated with simple curettage. Dural invasion, and even temporal lobe involvement has been reported. Complete surgical excision is the preferred treatment.[57] There is no agreement concerning radiation therapy, because of the fear of irradiation-induced malignant transformation.

Chondromyxoid Fibroma

Chondromyxoid fibroma is a benign tumor of bone characterized by chondroid and myxoid differentiation with lobular growth. It was first described by Jaffe and Lichtenstein in 1948. It is a rare tumor, accounting for approximately 0.5 percent of all bone tumors. It appears slightly more commonly in males and presents most frequently in the second and third decades of life; 60 percent of patients reported are younger than 30.[60]

The most common site of involvement is the lower extremity, especially the proximal part of the tibia. Only 13 patients have been reported with tumors in the skull and facial bones. In case reports of the chondromyxoid fibroma of the skull, symptoms evolve slowly and insidiously. Calcification may be present on plain skull films. The basic histologic picture of chondromyxoid fibroma is one of lobulated areas of fibromyxomatous tissue, with a tendency toward chondroid differentiation, separated by fibrocellular bands. Histologic evidence of calcification is present in 75 percent.[67]

Chondromyxoid fibroma must be differentiated from chondrosarcoma and from chordoma. Chondrosarcoma contains, in addition to well-differentiated cartilage, pleomorphic and undifferentiated cells. Chordoma has the stellate and the physalipherous cell types. A third cell type identified by electron microscopy is the intermediate type, which is characteristic of the chordoma. Intracytoplasmic mucin or mitochondrial endoplasmic reticulum complexes are a prominent feature of the cells of a chordoma.[42]

Chondromyxoid fibroma is generally a benign and nonaggressive tumor, although malignant transformation has been reported. Subtotal resection by curettage results in a 10 to 15 percent recurrence rate, probably secondary to the remaining lobules which extend outside the resected area.[42,60] Therefore, total excision has been recommended.

Myxoma

Myxoma of the facial skeleton is a locally invasive neoplasm consisting of small, innocuous spindle-shaped cells in a mucoid myxoid stroma. Myxoma of the bone is extremely rare. Most reported cases are in the second and third decades, with a slight male predominance.

Myxomas occur in the mandible and maxilla, most commonly in the condylar region of the jaw and the zygomatic process. Pain may or may not be associated with an enlarging mass, while occasionally the symptoms are loose or displaced dentition.

Radiologically these lesions appear as a uniloculated or multiloculated radiolucent area divided by osseous trabeculation, giving it a "soap-bubble" appearance. Cortical thinning and expansion followed by destruction can be found. These tumors are often indistinguishable from ameloblastoma radiographically.

Histologically the lesion is quite acellular with a large amount of myxoid or mucoid intracellular substance. Stellate cells with long cytoplasmic processes are present.

Myxomas are locally aggressive lesions with a 25 percent recurrence rate following curettage. Irradiation seems to have no therapeutic effect.[60]

Cartilage-Forming Tumors—Malignant

Chondrosarcoma

Chondrosarcoma is a malignant tumor consisting of fully developed cartilage that does not directly form tumor osteoid. Secondary myxoid changes, calcification, and ossification may be present. It is the third most common malignant tumor of bone, following multiple myeloma and osteogenic sarcoma. Chondrosarcomas constitute approximately 11 percent of all malignant bone tumors, but only about 6.7 percent occur in the head and neck.[87] In one literature review, the authors found 40 cases of cranial chondrosarcoma.[92] Age at presentation varied from 9 to 68 years, with the incidence highest in the second decade. This contrasts with the average age of presentation of chondrosarcomas in extracranial locations, which is the fourth decade. There was no sex bias. Of these tumors, 32 (80 percent) were in the skull base, most commonly the middle cranial fossa; 6 (15 percent) were in the meninges of the vault; and 2 (5 percent) were located elsewhere.[92]

The criteria for malignancy in a cartilage-forming tumor include: the presence of an increased number of cartilage cells having plump nuclei, more than occasional binucleated cells, and mononuclear or multinucleated giant cartilage cells. Two or more cells within a cartilage lacuna in more than an occasional microscopic field characterizes a low-grade chondrosarcoma. There are two recognized subtypes of chondrosarcoma: myxochondrosarcoma and mesenchymal chondrosarcoma. The distinction has practical significance because, unlike the subtypes of osteogenic sarcoma, the subtypes of chondrosarcoma seem to have different biological behavior.

The presence of myxomatous changes and cystic degeneration correlates well with lower-grade lesions (myxochondrosarcoma). Absence of cartilage lobules and the presence of spindle-cell sarcomatous areas are characteristic of high-grade variants (mesenchymal chondrosarcoma). In one report, of the tumors that had recurred following surgical excision, 80 percent were the mesenchymal chondrosarcoma subtype.[53] Chondrosarcomas are also grouped into grades I, II, and III on the basis of nuclear size, cellularity, and mitotic rate. Among the cases reviewed by Oguro et al., the 10-year survival varied from 83 percent for grade I to 29 percent for grade III.[92] Some authorities believe that cranial chondrosarcomas are in general less aggressive than peripheral chondrosarcomas.[17]

Lytic and sclerotic changes may be present on plain x-ray films of the skull. In one report, 56 percent had calcification on either CT or plain films.[53] Tumors occurring at the petrous apex are generally of the myxochondrosarcoma subtype, and therefore are not calcified.[31] In the series reported by Hassounah et al., 80 percent of the mesenchymal chondrosarcoma subtypes showed hypervascularity on angiography, but the majority of chondrosarcomas were avascular.[53] There are no reliable radiologic characteristics that allow for accurate preoperative diagnosis. Meyers et al. concluded that: "In many cases, differentiation of these diagnostic entities that is based solely on MR imaging and CT characteristics may be impossible. However, a heterogeneously enhanced tumor located at the petrooccipital synchondrosis that has high signal intensity on long TR/TE images, contains chondroid mineralization, and is associated with erosive bone changes strongly favors the diagnosis of chondrosarcoma.''[87] When these tumors arise from the convexity dura or the falx, confusion with an atypical meningioma is possible (Fig. 150-11). However, the absence of hyperostosis and bone destruction as well as avascularity on angiography make chondrosarcoma more likely.[77]

Chondrosarcomas are bluish-white, pearly, translucent lesions that are frequently lobulated. Areas of calcification and ossification are represented by yellow or white areas of speckling. A mucoid, slimy character is seen when secondary myxomatous changes supervene. Slowly growing lesions elicit more reactive new bone formation. The histologic appearance has to be correlated with both the clinical and radiographic features in arriving at a diagnosis of a benign versus a malignant tumor. In the skull, chondrosarcoma must be distinguished from chondroblastic osteogenic sarcoma. Chondrosarcoma should not show direct osteoid or bone production by the sarcomatous stroma; careful examination of the entire specimen may be necessary. On occasion, an aggressive chondromyxofibroma may be mistaken for a chondrosarcoma. In addition, large locally aggressive benign mixed tumors of the salivary glands with prominent cartilaginous components may cause diagnostic difficulty if only a small biopsy sample is examined. The cartilage component in a benign mixed salivary gland tumor closely resembles well-differentiated hyaline cartilage with foci of myxochondroid growth streaks.

Bourgouin et al. have stated the importance of differentiating low-grade chondrosarcoma from chordoma, particularly if there is a significant myxoid tissue component.[17] In classic chordoma, large acidophilic cells with cytoplasmic vacuoles (physaliphorous cells) are observed in cohesive sheets, nestlike formations, and thick cords within a myxoid ground substance. Occasional cartilage foci may be present. In chondrosarcoma, the cells may have an acidophilic cytoplasm with intracytoplasmic vacuoles, but their growth pattern differs significantly from that of chordomas. The cells grow either individually in the myxoid ground substance or in uncohesive sheets and one-cell-thick strings. Cohesive sheets, nestlike formations, and thick cords are not identified. Immunocytochemical analysis also assists in differentiation. Chordoma is strongly immunopositive for epithelial markers (cytokeratin and epithelial membrane antigens) and the enzyme 5′-nucleotidase, but is immunonegative for vimentin. By comparison, in chondrosarcoma, vimentin is present but the epithelial markers and the enzyme 5′-nucleotidase are absent.[17] Most authorities believe that the term ''chondroid chordoma'' should be dropped and replaced with ''low-grade chondrosarcoma'' or myxochondrosarcoma. The distinction is important because the tumor grows much more slowly than chordoma.[19]

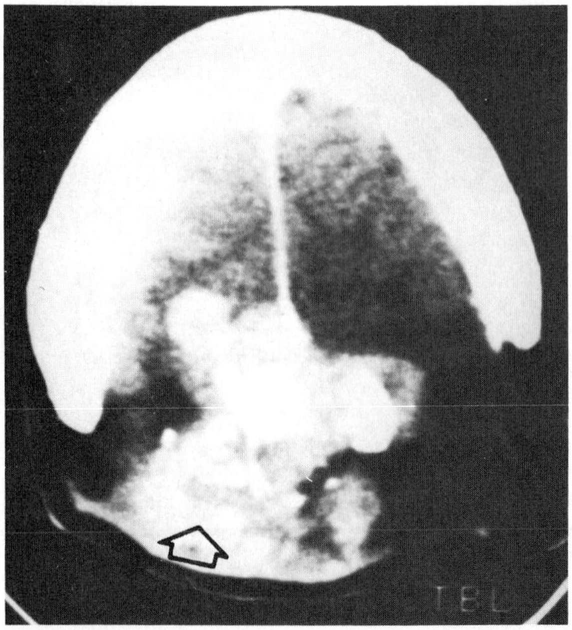

Figure 150-11 A CT scan of a mesenchymal chondrosarcoma involving the occipital bone, dura, and falx. Note the irregular, stippled calcifications (*arrow*).

Shen et al. found multiple gene rearrangements in a myxochondrosarcoma which may implicate a common molecular mechanism involved in tumor evolution.[111] Allele loss, rearrangement, or a small deletion involving chromosomes 10 and 22 have been demonstrated. Abnormalities involving chromosome 22 have been reported in various neuroectodermal tumors (e.g., meningioma, Ewing's sarcoma, peripheral neuroepithelioma, acoustic neuroma, and astrocytoma). Loss of chromosome 10 is also commonly found in high-grade gliomas and meningiomas.[111]

Chondrosarcoma may arise *de novo* or result from sarcomatous changes in a pre-existing chondroma. Malignant change can occur in patients afflicted with Ollier's syndrome and especially in those with Maffucci's syndrome. Previous radiation therapy, Paget's disease, or fibrous dysplasia can also predispose patients to develop these tumors.

Because of its local invasiveness and high rate of recurrence, radical resection is the treatment of choice for chondrosarcoma of the cranium. Because the majority of these arise from the skull base, complete resection presents a formidable challenge. New skull base techniques have increased exposure and allowed for gross total resection in some cases.[74] Adjunctive radiation therapy and chemotherapy have been reported, with occasional beneficial effect, but no consensus has been reached.[92] For additional discussion, refer to the sections on Ollier's syndrome and Maffucci's syndrome, secondary osteogenic sarcoma, and chondroma.

Connective Tissue Tumors—Benign

Desmoplastic Fibroma

Desmoplastic fibroma is a benign but locally aggressive intraosseous neoplasm that was first described in 1958 by Jaffe. It is a tumor of fibrous connective tissue origin marked by the formation of collagen. Sparse cellularity, lack of pleomorphism, and decreased mitotic activity characterize this tumor. Desmoplastic fibroma is very uncommon. It usually arises in the mandible, femur, or humerus. The peak incidence is during the second decade, and there is no sex predilection. Pain and/or swelling are the presenting symptoms in 80 percent. Involvement of the calvaria is extremely rare.[58,94]

Radiographically these tumors are well-defined lytic and expansile lesions with a soap-bubble appearance. Thinning of the overlying bony cortex in the absence of a periosteal reaction is common. Sclerotic reaction at the margins is mild to absent.[58]

Microscopically, the lesion is composed primarily of dense collagenous tissue. Scattered slender fibroblasts are haphazardly embedded in this matrix. No bone formation, mitotic activity, or necrosis is found. The fibroblasts may form obtuse bands or bundles, giving an appearance similar to, but not identical with, a ''herringbone'' pattern. However, the fibroblasts are relatively uniform in size and shape, and do not display much nuclear hyperchromatism or prominent mitotic figures.

Microscopically, the most important and often difficult differential diagnosis is primary low-grade fibrosarcoma of bone. Hypercellularity and the presence of mitotic activity and necrosis will help to establish a diagnosis of malignancy. Moderately well-differentiated fibrosarcomas are more cellular and present a herringbone arrangement of their spindle cells.

Both fibrous dysplasia and ossifying fibroma consist of varying amounts of an osseous component, which is absent in the desmoplastic fibroma. The presence of woven bone, the salient diagnostic feature of fibrous dysplasia, is noticeably absent in cases of desmoplastic fibroma.

Nonossifying fibroma (benign fibrous histiocytoma of bone) has rarely been reported in a cranial location. Osteoclastic giant cells and foamy macrophages, which may be predominant cellular elements of the nonossifying fibroma, are never found in desmoplastic fibroma. Furthermore, nonossifying fibroma is distinctively hypercellular when compared with desmoplastic fibroma. The fibroblasts form whorls and bundles, in contrast to the haphazard organization of desmoplastic fibroma.

Myxoma of the facial skeleton is characterized by polyhedral or stellate cells embedded in a mucinous matrix. The lack of such a myxoid stroma in desmoplastic fibroma removes the myxoma from consideration.

Desmoplastic fibroma is a locally aggressive tumor with a 20 to 30 percent recurrence rate reported; therefore, complete excision is recommended. Local excision and curettage with cryotherapy may be adequate for limited lesions and those inaccessible to complete resection. Radiation therapy is of no benefit in these tumors.[94]

Connective Tissue Tumors—Malignant

Fibrosarcoma of Bone

Fibrosarcoma of bone is a malignant fibroblastic tumor characterized by varying amounts of collagen production. There is a distinct absence of tumor bone, osteoid, or cartilage. Fibrosarcoma is one of the two least common primary malignant tumors of bone, and accounts for less than 5 percent of these lesions. Fibrosarcoma may arise *de novo* or secondary to fibrous dysplasia, Paget's disease, bone infarct, or osteomyelitis. Radiation-induced tumors have also been reported. Between 20 and 30 percent are secondary to these pre-existent lesions or follow irradiation.[60] There is a broad age distribution, with an average age of 38 years. Two distinct age peaks occur, during the third and fifth decades. There is a slight male predominance with this lesion. These tumors are classified as medullary or periosteal depending on the site of origin; the two types occur in a 2:1 ratio. The more common medullary tumors have a better prognosis.[60]

These tumors show a strong predilection for the long bones; however, between 11 and 15 percent arise from the craniofacial skeleton. The mandible and maxilla are most commonly involved, with rare occurrence in the skull. Medullary and periosteal lesions occur with equal frequency in the head and neck region.[60]

Most lesions present as a mass, which is associated with pain when the cortex and medullary cavity are involved. Pain, swelling, and loose teeth often accompany mandibular and maxillary involvement. The precise site of origin from scalp or bone may be impossible to determine. Intracranial extension is unusual; therefore, neurological sequelae are uncommon.[60]

Radiographically, fibrosarcomas are radiolucent lytic lesions of bone with thinning and widening of the overlying cortex (Fig. 150-12). Because of the absence of calcification and bone production, these lesions are extremely radiolucent. Very minimal periosteal reaction accompanies these tumors.

Fibrosarcoma of bone is histologically identical to that arising in the soft tissues. A low-grade, well-differentiated tumor exhibits ample intercellular collagen in a distinctive herringbone pattern, with rare mitoses in the fibroblasts. In secondary fibrosarcomas, focal areas of abundant collagen may be present in the absence of increased fibroblastic cellularity. Increased mitoses and pleomorphism usually suggest a higher grade malignancy. In the presence of numerous giant cells, malignant fibrous histiocytoma is an important consideration. Other entities which may mimic fibrosarcoma are the fibroblastic subtype of osteogenic sarcoma in which alkaline phosphatase activity is present, and the spindle cell variant of renal cell carcinoma which may present as a solitary skeletal lesion. Huvos states that many pathologists are tending to classify lesions as malignant fibrous histiocytomas that in the past they would have called fibrosarcomas.[60]

Fibrosarcoma of bone is a locally aggressive tumor with almost a 50 percent rate of metastasis, and wide excision is recommended. Preoperative and adjunctive chemotherapy may be of benefit in some patients, although results are not yet conclusive. Wide excision of the scalp, skull, and dura is advocated in lesions of the craniofacial bones. Despite radical surgery, a 30 and 11 percent recurrence rate is encountered in high-grade and well-differentiated tumors, respectively. Radiation therapy is of no benefit in

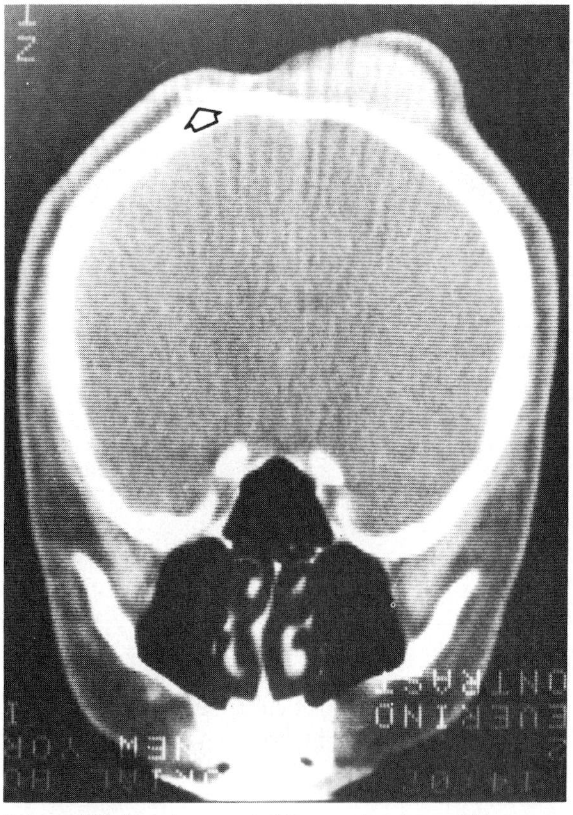

Figure 150-12 A coronal CT scan showing a fibrosarcoma involving the scalp and skull, with a satellite nodule (*arrow*).

these patients.[60] For additional discussion, refer to the sections on osteogenic sarcoma, secondary osteogenic sarcoma, desmoplastic fibroma, and malignant fibrous histiocytoma.

Histiocytic or Fibrohistiocytic Tumors—Benign

Giant Cell "Reparative" Granuloma

Giant cell "reparative" granuloma is a non-neoplastic lesion histologically very similar to the giant cell tumor of bone, and histologically indistinguishable from the "brown tumor" of hyperparathyroidism.[2,28,60] In 1953, Jaffe established this lesion as a distinct pathologic entity, and included the word reparative in the name to underscore his belief that it was a localized, reparative reaction to previous trauma. Many authorities now consider this etiology unlikely, and simply refer to this lesion as giant cell granuloma.[60]

This entity occurs most commonly in the mandible and maxilla. It has been reported in other bones, including the bones of the skull. The sphenoid, temporal, and ethmoid bones are the preferred sites in the calvaria. Just over 30 cases have been reported at the skull base. One case of vault involvement has been reported. Giant cell granuloma is a disorder of the young, with 75 percent occurring before 30 years of age. Females are affected twice as frequently as males.

Pain, swelling, and a rapidly growing mass are the most common initial complaints. Frontal headaches and diplopia are frequent symptoms with sphenoid involvement. Temporal bone involvement usually results in hearing problems and vertigo. These lesions are radiolucent, well-demarcated areas in plain films and may be multiloculated. Expansion and thinning of the bony cortex is common. Computed tomography reveals an isodense lesion which may erode the overlying cortical bone.

The histologic features of giant cell reparative granuloma consist of giant cells presenting in groups around hemorrhagic foci. Numerous spindle-shaped fibroblastic cells form the stroma. The giant cells have relatively few nuclei and seem to be generally smaller than those seen in the giant cell tumor of bone. Foci of osteoid and new bone formation are frequently present. In contrast, the giant cell tumor usually presents with quite a different histologic appearance. Giant cell tumor of bone is uniformly composed of oval undifferentiated mononuclear histiocytic or fibroblastic tumor cells with evenly dispersed, large multinucleated giant cells. There is a rich vascular network; fresh hemorrhage is slight to moderate; hemosiderin deposits are rare and small. The giant cells are generally larger and more rounded and have a greater number of nuclei. A key point in the differential diagnosis is that the stromal cells and giant cells resemble each other, particularly in regard to their nuclei, whereas in giant cell reparative granuloma the osteoclasts and the stromal cells of the fibroblastic type are distinctly different.[68]

Giant cell granuloma is a slowly growing lesion with frequent bone erosion. Malignant transformation and metastasis have not been reported. Curettage is the treatment of choice, but is still associated with a 12 to 16 percent recurrence rate. Some authorities believe that subtotal resection should be followed by radiation therapy.[28] For additional discussion, the reader is referred to the section on giant cell tumor.

Nonossifying Fibroma

Nonossifying fibroma is a benign lesion of bone characterized by a fibroblastic cellular proliferation with multinucleated giant cells and foamy xanthomatous cells. Fibrous cortical defects are seen in 30 to 40 percent of normal children past the age of 2, most between the age of 4 and 8 years. The cortex of the metaphysis of long bones is the usual site. When the lesion is larger and actively growing and involves the medullary cavity it is called a nonossifying fibroma. These lesions occur primarily in the long bones of the appendicular skeleton. There are a few reports of involvement of the mandible, clavicle, and vertebrae. Case reports involving the cranial vault are extremely rare.[3] These lesions are most common in the first two decades of life, and males are affected twice as often as females. Most patients are asymptomatic, although pain and swelling have been reported. Pathologic fracture can occur through these sites of involvement in the long bones. In the skull it has presented as a painless swelling.[3]

In the long bones the lesion is radiolucent, with sclerotic margins and interior bony trabeculae giving the appearance of soap bubbles or a bunch of grapes. A well-delineated thin sclerotic medullary border is usually present.

Spindly fibroblastic cells are arranged in matted whorls in a storiform pattern (*storea* means "rope mat" or "straw mat" in Latin). Some authors consider nonossifying fibroma and benign fibrous histiocytoma to be one and the same. Scattered giant cells and lipid-laden cells of the xanthoma variety are present. Xanthoma of bone is considered by some to be a subtype of nonossifying fibroma. The histologic appearance is similar to that of the stromal tissue of ossifying fibroma and fibrous dysplasia, but there is no bone formation in nonossifying fibroma. Desmoplastic fibroma is excluded by the presence of giant cells.

These benign lesions are asymptomatic in the vast majority of patients and are therefore not treated. Fracture or imminent fracture in tumors of the long bones is treated by curettage and fixation. Cranial lesions that become symptomatic can be cured by curettage or complete excision.

Xanthoma of Bone

The existence of pure xanthoma of bone is not universally established. Some authorities believe it to be a variant of nonossifying fibroma.[60] Others think it may be a "burnt-out" benign condition such as fibrous dysplasia or histiocytosis X.[12] Still others consider it to be a distinct pathologic entity.[62]

It occurs mainly in the flat bones of men, is small, and radiographically is lytic with surrounding sclerosis. Most patients are older than 20 years, and often present with local pain. These are benign conditions. Histologically they are characterized by cholesterol clefts, giant cells, foam cells, and fibrosis. In cases where foam cells predominate, it is important not to confuse the lesion with a metastatic clear cell hypernephroma.[12]

Xanthomata are usually associated with disorders of lipid metabolism which result in abnormally high circulating levels of cholesterol and lipids. Among the various hyperlipoproteinemia syndromes (types 1–5), xanthomata are especially common in electrophoresis pattern types IIA and IIB. They may also occur as secondary phenomena in other metabolic disorders, such as diabetes mellitus, hypothyroidism, and the nephrotic syndrome, and with biliary tract obstruction. In rare cases, disseminated xanthomata have occurred in patients who are normolipemic, presumably due to abberrant lipid storage.[62] Treatment includes reducing plasma lipids by dietary restriction and pharmacologic manipulation.

Histiocytic or Fibrohistiocytic Tumors—Malignant

Ewing's Sarcoma

Ewing's sarcoma is a malignant tumor that was first described by J. E. Ewing in 1921. It represents 6 to 9 percent of all primary malignant bone tumors, but is very rare in adulthood. It is the second most common bone tumor in children, with a peak incidence in the second decade of life. It is approximately twice as common in males as in females. Those of African and Chinese descent are very rarely affected. The common primary sites include the diaphyses of long bones, and the ribs, pelvis, and vertebrae. Primary involvement of the calvaria is extremely unusual.[30,35,132]

Histologically, Ewing's sarcoma is characterized by uniform, densely packed small cells with indistinct cytoplasmic borders and with round nuclei lacking prominent nucleoli. Many mitotic figures and occasional rosettes are seen. The initial differential diagnosis on clinical and histologic grounds includes neuroblastoma and malignant lymphoma. Periodic acid-Schiff (PAS) stains with and without diastase treatment show the intracellular glycogen and favors the diagnosis of Ewing's sarcoma rather than metastatic neuroblastoma. Metastatic neuroblastoma is also excluded by a normal 24-h urinary vanillylmandelic acid excretion. Embryonic rhabdomyosarcoma is the only other small cell tumor known to demonstrate intracellular glycogen.[35]

Pain and swelling are the most common symptoms of Ewing's sarcoma. Low-grade fever and general malaise are characteristic. The plain films typically show laminated periosteal changes (onion skin) with bone destruction and soft tissue extension. These pathognomonic clinical and radiographic features may be absent with cranial tumors.[35]

CT scans reveal an isodense mass, surrounded by a hypodense area and hyperostosis adjacent to the tumor. There is homogeneous enhancement with contrast administration. MRI shows a hypointense appearance on T1-weighted images and mixed intensity on T2-weighted images. There is contrast enhancement. Angiography shows a tumor stain.[132]

Only 11 cases of primary Ewing's sarcoma of the cranium have been reported. Fewer metastases and improved long-term survival are seen when these tumors affect the cranium as compared to all other primary sites.[132] The 5-year survival rate ranges from 39 to 65 percent. Multi-stage chemotherapy and radiation treatments are recommended.[35]

Giant Cell Tumor of Bone

Giant cell tumor of bone is an aggressive lesion characterized by well-vascularized tissue composed of plump, spindly, or ovoid stromal cells together with *uniformly dispersed* numerous large multinucleated giant cells. Because normal bone osteoclasts are multinucleated, this tumor is sometimes referred to as an osteoclastoma, particularly in the British literature. These tumors make up between 3 and 7 percent of all primary bone tumors.[39] There seems to be a slight female predominance. Giant cell tumors generally affect patients between 25 and 40 years of age and very rarely affect those under the age of 20.[28] More than 75 percent of these lesions are situated near the articular end of long bones, with more than half of all cases involving the long bones near the knee.[60] Origination in the skull is not frequent. When it occurs, the sphenoid bone is the most common site, followed by the nonsquamous portion of the temporal bone.[39,41,52,65,68,103,117,126,133,136] Even more rarely, some tumors are seen to involve bones derived from intramembranous ossification, such as the occipital bone.[54,110]

Physical findings relate to the site of involvement. Watkins et al. have offered a "typical" presentation for these tumors: a woman in her 20s or 30s having headaches, ocular palsy, and visual loss with erosion of the body of the sphenoid but with normal endocrine function.[133] However, pituitary involvement can occur.[65]

Radiographically, the most common finding is a mass in the region of the sphenoid bone and sinus with sellar erosion. CT scans usually reveal a tumor that is slightly increased in density before contrast administration, with intense and homogeneous enhancement after contrast administration (Fig. 150-13). Angiography often shows a faint tumor stain. MRI typically reveals that the signal intensity is not increased on T2-weighted images, unlike the usual appearance of many other intracranial neoplasms. Some other tumors also are known to remain with relatively low intensity on T2-weighted images. These include squamous and mucinous adenocarcinomas. Signal inhomogeneity within the mass, representing areas of necrosis, can sometimes be seen.[52]

The histologic differential diagnosis includes tumors in which giant cells are featured (Table 150-3). Giant cells may be found in osteogenic sarcomas, chondroblastomas, malignant fibrous histiocytomas, chondromyxoid fibromas, and eosinophilic granulomas.

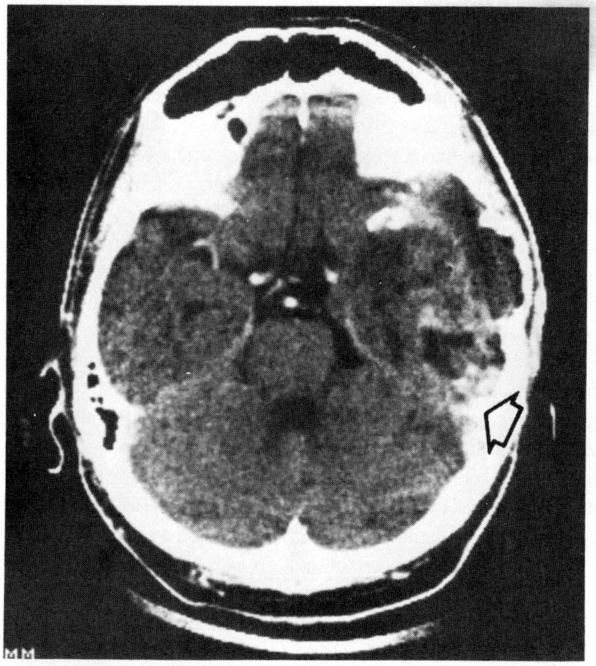

Figure 150-13 A CT scan with contrast enhancement, showing a giant cell tumor of the temporal bone with significant extension into the middle cranial fossa (*arrow*). (From Epstein et al.,[39] with permission.)

TABLE 150-3 Differential Diagnosis of Primary Tumors and Bone-Forming Conditions of the Skull That Contain Giant Cells

Lesion	Most Common Age Group	Radiologic Appearance	Sex (M:F) Distribution	Microscopic Features	
				Giant Cells	Stromal Cells
Giant cell tumor of bone	3d and 4th decades	Irregular expanded radiolucency	M < F	Abundant number uniformly distributed	Plump and polyhedral with abundant cytoplasm
Non-ossifying fibroma	1st decade	Oval defects	2:1	Focal in distribution; small with few nuclei	Slender and spindly with little cytoplasm
Aneurysmal bone cyst	1st and 2d decades	Irregular "soap-bubble" appearance	M = F	Focal around vascular channels	Large vascular channels; slender to plump cells with hemosiderin granules
Brown tumor of hyperparathyroidism	Any age	Absent lamina dura of teeth	M = F	Focal around hemosiderin pigment	Fibrous stroma with slender cells
Chondroblastoma	2d decade	Radiolucency with spotty opacities	M > F	Few and focal	Large, plump, and round with pericellular calcifications
Fibrous dysplasia	1st and 2d decades	"Ground-glass" appearance	M > F	Few and focal	Woven bone and fibrous tissue
Ossifying fibroma	2d and 3d decades	Radiopaque	M < F	Few and focal	Lamellar bony trabeculae in fibrous tissue
Osteogenic sarcoma	2d and 3d decades	Radiolucent	M > F	Focal distribution	Malignant spindle cells with direct osteoid formation
Chondromyxoid fibroma	2d and 3d decades	Eccentric with expanded cortex	M < F	Focal distribution	Chondroid and myxoid components
Osteoblastoma	2d and 3d decades	Radiolucent or dense	2:1	Focal distribution	Abundant osteoblasts between osteoid trabeculae

Source: Adapted from Huvos.[59,60]

An inflammatory cell background rich in eosinophils and the presence of Langerhans cells are typical of eosinophilic granuloma. Langerhans giant cells are identified with electron microscopy by the presence of Birbeck granules. These enigmatic cytoplasmic organelles are said to resemble tennis rackets.[20]

The main differential diagnostic challenge lies with giant cell reparative granuloma of bone and the "brown tumor" of hyperparathyroidism. Giant-cell reparative granuloma is thought to be a non-neoplastic lesion related to previous trauma and intraosseous hemorrhage. The age at onset is younger than that of giant cell tumor, usually in the 10- to 25-year range.[28] The histologic features consist of giant cells presenting in groups around hemorrhagic foci, and numerous spindle-shaped fibroblastic cells forming the stroma. The giant cells have relatively few nuclei and seem to be generally smaller than those seen in giant cell tumor. Foci of osteoid and new bone formation are frequently present. The giant-cell reparative granuloma has a benign course, presenting as a lytic lesion in bone and usually healing by new bone formation and sclerosis. In contrast, the giant cell tumor usually presents with a quite different histologic appearance. The tumor is uniformly composed of oval undifferentiated mononuclear histiocytic or fibroblastic tumor cells with evenly dispersed, large multinucleated giant cells. There is a rich vascular network; fresh hemorrhage is slight to moderate; hemosiderin deposits are rare and small. The giant cells are generally larger and more rounded and have a greater number of nuclei. A key point in the differential diagnosis is that the stromal cells and giant cells resemble each other, particularly in regard to their nuclei, whereas in giant-cell reparative granuloma the osteoclasts and the stromal cells of the fibroblastic type are distinctly different.[68] The brown tumor of hyperparathyroidism may preferentially affect the mandible or maxilla in its solitary form (Fig. 150-14). Histologically, it is identical to the giant cell reparative granuloma.[60] The diagnosis of brown tumor of hyperparathyroidism is based mainly on laboratory data such as serum and urinary levels of calcium, phosphates, and nephrogenous cAMP, radioimmunoassay for parathyroid hormone, phosphate clearance measurement, bone and serum alkaline phosphatase values, and evidence of hydroxyprolinuria. One has to bear in mind the later onset and frequent multiplicity of brown tumors.[2]

Giant cell tumor of bone is characterized by unpredictable, but often very aggressive, clinical behavior. Probably as a result of this unpredictability, there is considerable controversy concerning the management of these lesions. This is particularly true with regard to the role of radiation therapy. A literature review by Henderson and Whitwell revealed that after curettage alone the recurrence rate is 23 percent.[54] This falls to 7 percent after wide excision, but metastasis is reported to occur in 2 percent. Rengachary, in his comments on this report, stated that malignant degeneration occurs in 9 to 15 percent of cases, and that radiation not only is ineffective in preventing recurrences, but also triggers the onset of malignant degeneration.[54] Findlay et al. believe, on the other hand, that carefully planned and delivered supervoltage irradiation is safe and effective.[41] They believe that the poor results in the older literature reflect outmoded techniques of radiation therapy.[41] This pro-irradiation view is echoed in more recent papers.[126,133] For additional discussion, refer to the section on giant cell reparative granuloma.

Malignant Fibrous Histiocytoma

Malignant fibrous histiocytoma is a rare malignant tumor consisting of primitive mesenchymal cells which differentiate into two cell types: fibroblasts and histiocytes. Most of these tumors arise from soft tissues of the extremities but occasionally they may arise from bone. The long bones of the appendicular skeleton are involved in nearly 70 percent of these osseous lesions. Craniofacial

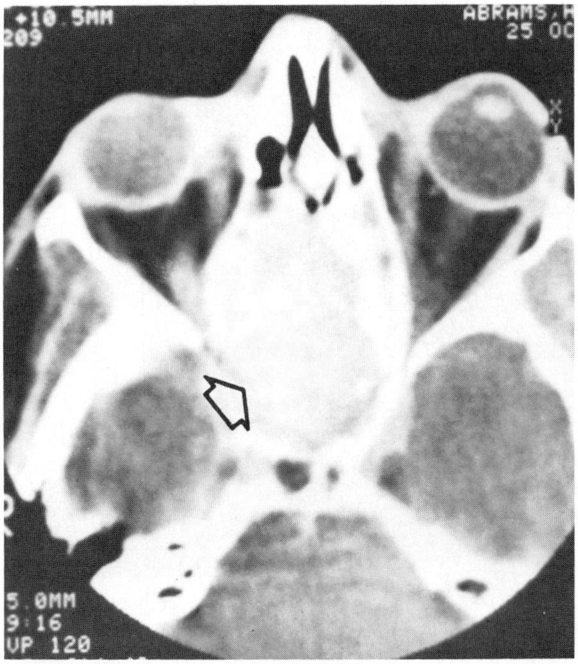

Figure 150-14 A patient with long-standing renal failure and known severe secondary hyperparathyroidism who had refused parathyroidectomy. A previous transnasal biopsy provided the diagnosis of brown tumor. The CT scan shows an expansile tumor of the ethmoid and sphenoid sinuses with destruction of the anteromedial border of the right middle cranial fossa (*arrow*).

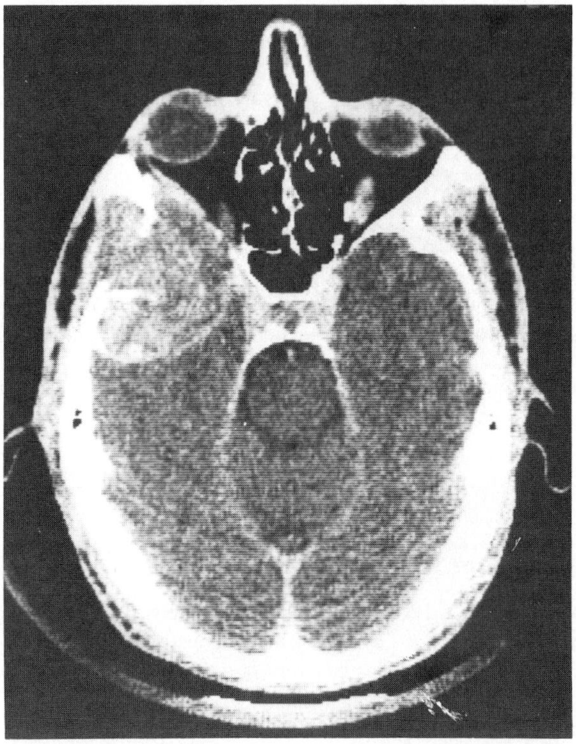

Figure 150-15 A CT scan shows a destructive tumor of the temporal bone with extradural extension along the floor of the middle cranial fossa. The pathologic diagnosis was malignant fibrous histiocytoma.

bones are the site of origin of 8.5 percent of the lesions, with the maxilla and mandible being the most commonly affected. Tumors of the skull are quite unusual. In general, malignant fibrous histiocytoma may affect persons of any age, but is more common in middle-aged and older adults, with a mean age of 40.5 years. Of these tumors, 70 percent arise as primary lesions whereas 30 percent arise from pre-existing conditions (such as Paget's disease) or following irradiation.[60] Primary disease reaches a peak incidence during the second and third decades of life; secondary tumors reach a peak incidence during the sixth and seventh decades. Males are affected more commonly than females. Pain and a palpable mass are the most common presenting complaints. Cranial lesions usually present as a painless mass. Intracranial extension of these tumors with brain invasion has been reported.[26,33,85]

Radiographically, these tumors appear as a poorly circumscribed osteolytic lesion with occasional areas of calcification. CT shows a destructive lesion expanding the inner and outer tables, with heterogeneous enhancement (Fig. 150-15).[85] A soft tissue mass is usually identifiable. Angiography may be positive.

Histologically, these neoplasms are extremely pleomorphic, exhibiting a definite ''storiform'' (rope-mat-like) pattern of growth, with spindle-shaped cells appearing in pinwheel configuration. They are predominantly fibrous with occasional tumor giant cells scattered throughout, while the histiocytic components incorporate lipid, hemosiderin, or erythrocytes, thereby manifesting phagocytic capacity. The histologic differential diagnosis includes malignant giant cell tumors, osteogenic sarcoma, histiocytic lymphoma, and metastatic carcinoma.[26]

The prognosis varies with tumor type. Atypical fibrous histiocytoma and epithelioid sarcoma have favorable 5- and 10-year survival rates, whereas survival rates for malignant histiocytoma are poor. Malignant fibrous histiocytoma is intermediate in prognosis, with two-thirds of the patients surviving 5 years and one-third surviving 10 years.[33] Radiation therapy and chemotherapy are recommended following surgical resection.[26,33,85]

Tumors of Blood or Blood Vessel Origin

Angiosarcoma of Bone

Angiosarcoma is a general term for malignant tumors of vascular origin. Included in this group of tumors is the hemangiopericytoma and malignant hemangioendothelioma.

Hemangiopericytoma

Hemangiopericytoma is an uncommon tumor of vascular origin. It is characterized by the proliferation of uniformly shaped pericytic cells arranged around irregular vascular spaces lined by a single layer of endothelial cells. Its occurrence in bone is very rare; however, a high proportion arise in the head and neck, with meningeal involvement most common.[48] Meningeal hemangiopericytoma corresponds to variant 1 of the angioblastic meningioma described by Cushing and Eisenhardt in 1938.[13] Very few cases arise from the skull. Patients from 16 to 83 years of age have been affected, and the sexes appear to be equally involved.

The most common complaints by patients are of a painful mass. Temporal lesions have been associated with hearing deficits and lower cranial nerve palsies.[13] Radiographically these lesions are destructive, with cortical erosion and reactive ossification. Some intralesional sclerosis is occasionally noted, with fine honeycombing striations.[60] Meningeal involvement is suggested by dual arterial supply, abundant corkscrew-like vessels (Fig. 150-16), dense tumor staining, and absent early venous drainage.[82] CT scans reveal heterogeneous enhancement with focal necrosis and a new, defined border.

Pericytes were described by Zimmerman in 1923, and are thought to represent immature smooth muscle cells derived from mesenchyme. They surround the vascular sheath of all vessels throughout the body and have the ability to contract. The extravascular location of the pericyte allows differentiation of hemangiopericytoma from hemangioendothelioma, in which the tumor cells are intraluminal.[13]

Wide local excision is the treatment of choice, giving an overall cure rate of 50 percent at all sites, and preoperative embolization is recommended. These tumors are largely resistant to radiation therapy and chemotherapy.

Malignant Hemangioendothelioma

Malignant hemangioendothelioma is composed of irregular vascular channels lined by one or more layers of atypical malignant endothelial cells. This is a very rare tumor, comprising less than 1 percent of primary malignant bone tumors. Calvarial involvement is most unusual. This lesion can occur at any age, with equal sex distribution. Patients most commonly present with a painful mass, often with associated swelling. Huvos states that the classification and grading of malignant vascular tumors is currently undergoing a thorough reassessment.[60] The small number of reported cases as well as the controversy among expert pathologists make detailed discussion of this entity here rather meaningless.

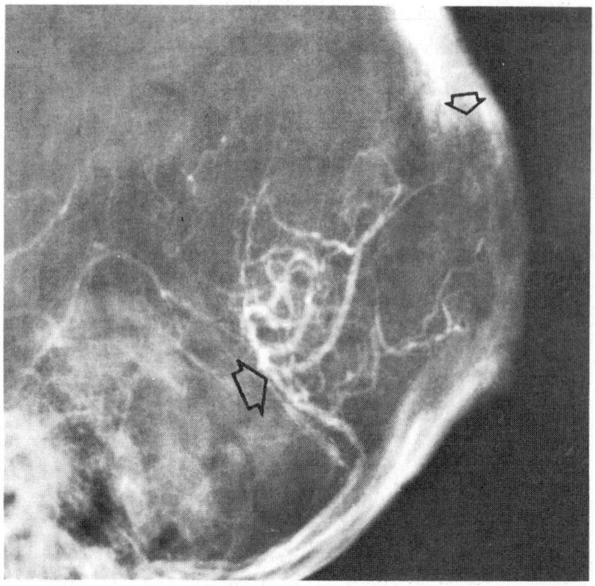

Figure 150-16 Angiogram of a malignant occipital bone tumor (*small arrow*) showing intracranial extension and neovascularity (*large arrow*). At operation a primary angiosarcoma of the occipital bone was resected.

Eosinophilic Granuloma of Bone

Solitary or multifocal eosinophilic granuloma of bone is a benign proliferative disease of Langerhans-type histiocytes. These lesions may affect almost any bone, with the skull being commonly affected. One-third of cases involving the temporal bone have been found to be bilateral. Solitary eosinophilic granuloma of bone is a disease of the young, with 34 percent younger than 4 years of age and 74 percent younger than 20 years of age. About half of the cases occur in the first decade of life. Males are twice as commonly affected by this disease as are females.[60]

Patients most commonly present with localized tenderness. One-third of those with Hand-Schüller-Christian disease develop the full triad of diabetes insipidus, exophthalmos, and bone lesions, which are usually in the skull.

The typical radiographic appearance is that of a radiolucent oval area which is well-demarcated without peripheral sclerosis, forming a ''punched-out'' defect. The ''button sequestrum'' calvarial doughnut-shaped lesion once thought to be diagnostic of eosinophilic granuloma of bone is also seen in a variety of other tumors.

These lesions are soft brownish masses that are often cystic and contain focal hemorrhagic areas. Histologically, mononuclear histiocytes are mixed with eosinophils, with areas of hemorrhage, necrosis, and associated multinucleated giant cells. The histiocytes stain for S-100 protein and on electron microscopic examination have Birbeck granules in their cytoplasm. These enigmatic cytoplasmic organelles are said to resemble tennis rackets.[20] This benign proliferative lesion is part of the spectrum of diseases known as histiocytosis X, which is discussed elsewhere in this textbook.

Hemangioma of Bone

Hemangioma is a benign lesion composed of capillary, cavernous, or venous blood vessels. Intraosseous hemangioma comprises 0.7 percent of all neoplasms of bone.[60] Most of these occur in the vertebral column.[55] The most common extravertebral location is the skull, particularly in the frontal or parietal bones.[56] Hemangioma was the second most common primary calvarial tumor (after osteoma) in two large series, comprising 10 percent of benign neoplasms of the skull.[120] The incidence of the lesions increases with age, but symptomatic lesions seem to appear in younger patients. A peak incidence occurs from the fourth to the sixth decades. Generally, females are affected two to four times more frequently than males, although a study of cases involving the skull found a twofold male predominance.[60]

Lesions involving the skull most commonly present as a small painless mass. Large size is unusual, but a 6 cm outwardly growing tumor has been reported in a newborn infant.[121] Significant intracranial extension is rare.[93] Hemangiomas can occur in the temporal bone near the internal auditory canal. In that location they behave more aggressively than acoustic neuromas of the same size, and hearing loss and facial paralysis are common.[45] Frontal bone involvement can cause proptosis.[56]

Calvarial hemangiomas occur in two forms: (1) The very rare globular variety, which arises from the skull base on a broad stalk, and acts like a space-occupying lesion; and (2) the more common sessile type, which causes expansion of the diploe of the vault. The sessile type is characterized by a well-defined lytic lesion. In a series of 333 patients with calvarial radiolucencies, 43 (13 percent) had hemangiomas.[120] Peripheral sclerosis occurs in one-third of lesions, in contrast to epidermoid cysts, where it is almost always seen. Intralesional bone remnants are visualized in 80 percent of hemangiomas, but in only 20 percent of epidermoids and 10 percent of histiocytomas. The well-known honeycomb or trabecular pattern occurs in about one-half of hemangiomas (Fig. 150-17), and the classic sunburst striations occur in only 10 to 15 percent. When present, the sunburst pattern of this lesion appears to radiate from a central point, while the sunburst observed with meningiomas has spicules arranged in parallel.[55,56,60] Furthermore, meningiomas often have associated enlarged vascular markings in the skull, a finding not usually found with hemangiomas. Outer table erosion with preservation of the inner table is frequently observed with hemangiomas. Bone scanning demonstrates increased activity. Computed tomography shows a lucent lesion with multiple trabeculae (Fig. 150-18). In magnetic resonance T1-weighted images the lesions appear isointense; they are hyperintense on T2-weighted images. Flow void is generally not found because the small size of the vascular channels causes slow flow.[100] Angiography shows an intraosseous hypervascular lesion with normally shaped but dilated vessels. Aneurysms have been observed on the feeding middle meningeal artery of an aggressive hemangioma.[93]

A brownish red lesion can be seen beneath the skull periosteum. Microscopically, hemangiomas are classified according to the size of the vessels, with capillary hemangiomas being rare in the skull. The vessels are usually of the cavernous type, being thin-walled without muscle or elastic tissue. A single layer of flattened endothelial cells is contained within the bony trabeculae. Aneurysmal bone cysts, which are also blood-filled spaces in bone, must be considered in the differential diagnosis. In contrast to hemangiomas, aneurysmal bone cyst cavities are lined by connective tissue, not endothelium. A similar honeycomb appearance may be present, but without radiation of spicules from a common center. Destruction of either cortex may occur, with new periosteal bone formation giving a sclerotic margin.[56]

Hemangiomas are benign lesions cured by *en bloc* resection. Occasionally, proximal vessel ligation may be necessary to minimize blood loss, especially for the rare globular hemangioma fouhd at the base of the skull. Radiation therapy has been used to arrest the growth of inaccessible lesions.[55]

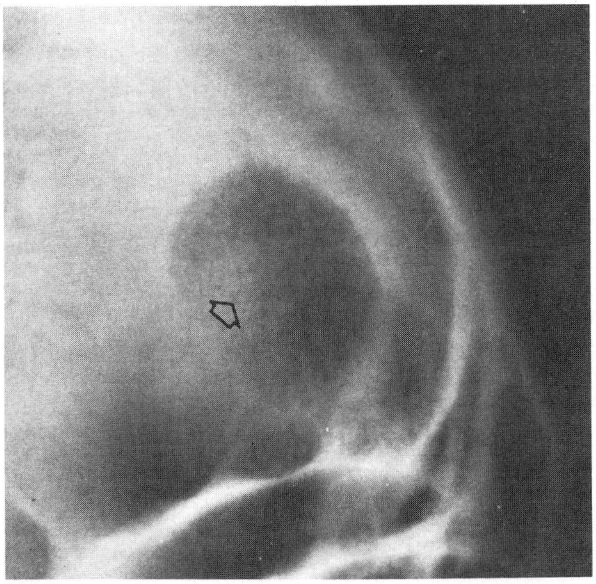

Figure 150-17 A skull film showing a well-demarcated, partially honeycombed (*arrow*) lytic lesion without significant marginal sclerosis. This appearance is classic for hemangioma.

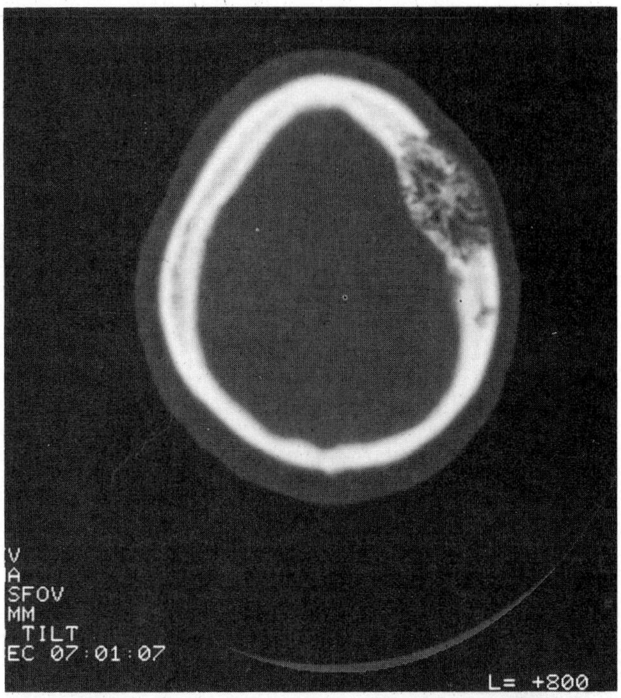

Figure 150-18 A CT scan (with a bone window setting) of a calvarial hemangioma in the axial plane reveals the expansion of both the inner and outer tables, with an intralesional honeycombed trabecular pattern.

Lymphangioma of Bone

Lymphangioma is an extremely rare benign lesion of bone composed of newly formed lymph vessels, usually in the form of dilated cystic spaces. Usually found in childhood and infancy, these lesions present as cystic defects in bone. Histologically the lesion consists of vascular channels filled with clear fluid. Lymphangiomas appear radiographically as lytic intramedullary lesions that are indistinguishable from hemangiomas on conventional x-ray examination. These need no treatment unless they become symptomatic, at which time resection will cure the condition.[60]

Lymphoma of Bone

Malignant lymphoma is a neoplastic proliferation of cells of the lymphoreticular system which can be divided into non-Hodgkin's and Hodgkin's types. Most commonly these types originate within lymph nodes. Extranodal involvement occurs most commonly with non-Hodgkin's lymphoma, with 5 to 25 percent of these tumors arising in extranodal sites.[60] Criteria that justify consideration of lymphoma as a primary tumor of bone have been variably applied. With best estimates, primary malignant lymphoma constitutes 2.5 percent of all bone tumors and 5 percent of all malignant bone tumors. Secondary bone involvement occurs in about 30 percent of malignant lymphomas.[60]

Practically all bones may give rise to these lesions, with almost half arising in the femur and pelvic bones. Primary lymphoma of the central nervous system (CNS) accounts for 0.5 to 3 percent of intracranial tumors. This number has increased rapidly among patients with acquired immunodeficiency syndrome, organ transplants, and bone marrow transplants. Primary non-Hodgkin's lymphoma (NHL) involving the cranial vault and the skull base is rare.[81,98,125] In the reported literature, primary NHL of bone can occur at any age but is most common after the second decade of life; it is quite rare in children. A peak incidence occurs in the fifth decade. Males are more frequently involved than are females.

Metastatic bone involvement in Hodgkin's disease occurs in 10 to 20 percent of patients clinically, and 34 to 78 percent of patients in autopsy studies. This is mostly by hematogenous dissemination or by direct extension, with primary Hodgkin's disease of bone being very rare and difficult to verify. The vertebral bodies are involved most commonly whereas the skull is involved very rarely.[119]

Patients with CNS lymphoma have 5-year survivals from 3 to 8 percent. Radiation is generally the treatment of choice, but there is an extremely high recurrence rate. Adjunctive chemotherapy in combination with irradiation and surgical resection have been used with variable results.

Plasmacytoma

Multiple myeloma is a malignant tumor of plasma cells which produces bone destruction. Multiple myeloma is the most common neoplasm of bone in adults, accounting for about one-half of all malignant bone tumors. The average age of patients at presentation is 60 years, with a range from the 20s to the 80s. Occurrence before 30 is rare. All bones may be involved with this disease, but the vertebral bodies, ribs, pelvic bones, and skull are most frequently involved.

Solitary plasmacytoma is an infrequent variant of multiple myeloma consisting of a solitary neoplastic mass of plasma cells without clinical or radiologic signs of systemic disease. Location in the skull is the least frequent (0.7 percent) within this group of tumors. Craniocerebral plasmacytomas are composed of two groups: (1) extramedullary plasmacytomas originating from the dura; and (2) plasmacytomas originating from the cranial vault. Only 16 cases of plasmacytoma originating from the calvaria have been reported.[37] The lesion is usually painless, and the overlying skin is normal except for enlarged scalp arteries. The tumor spreads subperiosteally, without invading the galea, and causes destruction of the bone. The tumor is extremely vascular, with the main blood supply derived from the scalp arteries. X-ray films of the skull reveal evidence of a lytic lesion involving both inner and outer tables and the diploe, with enlargement of the diploic veins. CT scans show the presence of an extradural, slightly hyperdense lesion with homogeneous enhancement after the intravenous injection of a contrast agent. There may be calcified areas inside the mass, representing bony inclusions. Carotid angiography shows a vascular lesion.

Miscellaneous Tumors of Soft Tissue and Bone

Aneurysmal Bone Cyst

Aneurysmal bone cyst (ABC) is regarded by some to be a secondary reactive bone lesion created when a primary lesion of bone develops an osseous arteriovenous fistula.[60] Others consider aneurysmal bone cyst to be a distinct pathologic entity. This benign lesion is composed of large vascular spaces separated by trabeculae of connective tissue and bone. It constitutes approximately 6 percent of tumors of bone. Aneurysmal bone cyst most commonly occurs in the long bones and the vertebrae, and is only rarely (3 to 6 percent) found in the skull.[29] Calvarial involvement has occurred most often in the frontal, occipital, and temporal bones.[18,23,29,61] Almost all patients are under 30 years of age, with 80 percent under 20. There appears to be an equal sex distribution.

Most of these lesions present as a painful swelling which is tender to palpation. Headache, proptosis, focal neurological signs, and signs of increased intracranial pressure have been reported. Aneurysmal bone cysts sometimes enlarge during pregnancy.[23]

Radiographically, aneurysmal bone cysts are well-demarcated lesions that arise in the diploe and expand both the inner and outer tables, which are usually thinned but intact. CT scans may show a multilocular lesion with regions of high and low density, the high-density lesions showing contrast enhancement. Multiple fluid levels are often present. The CT finding of a multiloculated expansile bone lesion is not specific for aneurysmal bone cyst. Other lesions share that characteristic, and include giant cell tumor, chondroblastoma, and fibrous dysplasia. However, fluid levels have only been found in ABCs and in osteogenic sarcomas with a large telangiectatic component, and their finding helps to lead to a more definitive diagnosis. Aneurysmal bone cysts, particularly in the long bones, vertebrae, and pelvis, are frequently highly vascular lesions. Marked vascularity is a less constant feature in ABC of the skull vault, and angiography is usually negative.[6,29]

After opening the thin wall of bone, a cystic lumen with unclotted blood and scant stringy tissue is encountered. Microscopically, the lesions are made up of numerous cavernous spaces that usually lack an endothelial lining. The walls consist of fibrous connective tissue and woven bone. Large accumulations of giant cells in relation to hemorrhage are seen in the septa. Aneurysmal bone cyst may coexist with other bone tumors, so it is important to give as much tissue to the pathologist as possible. Associated lesions are chondroblastoma, unicameral bone cyst, giant cell tumor, osteosarcoma, nonossifying fibroma, hemangioma, traumatic lesions, and fibrous dysplasia, among others.[60]

The recurrence rate of these benign lesions is as high as 50 percent following subtotal resection, and 20 to 30 percent following curettage. *En bloc* resection of a lesion involving the calvaria without dural involvement is usually curative. Radiation therapy results in local control comparable to that of curettage. However, it should be considered only in recurrent or unresectable lesions because of the danger of postradiation sarcoma formation.[18,60]

Benign Nerve Sheath Tumor (Schwannoma) of Bone

Schwannoma involving bone is a very rare tumor, comprising approximately 0.1 percent of all bone tumors. The most common intraosseous location is the mandible, probably because it contains a long segment of the mandibular nerve. The vertebrae and the sacrum are also reported sites. One case involving the skull has been reported.[106] Except in von Recklinghausen's disease, these are tumors of adults, with a peak incidence in the fifth and sixth decades. Benign schwannoma occurs slightly more frequently in females than in males. Lytic and dysplastic osseous lesions are associated with von Recklinghausen's disease, but it is uncertain whether these represent the known occurrence of nonossifying fibromas, or tumors of Schwann cell lineage.[60]

Radiographically, the reported lesion was well-circumscribed-lytic in nature with a sclerotic margin.[106] Histologically, the tissue was of the typical Antoni A type. Treatment is excision or curettage.

Chordoma

Chordoma is a malignant tumor arising from developmental remnants of the notochord in the axial skeleton; 35 percent of chordomas occur in the skull base. This entity is discussed in detail elsewhere in this textbook.

Epidermoid and Dermoid Tumors of Bone

Cranial epidermoid and dermoid cysts are benign congenital tumors which are derived from ectopic inclusions of epithelium. The incidence is approximately 1 percent. The most common locations of epidermoids are the cerebellopontine angle, parapituitary region, and calvaria. Dermoids tend to lie along the midline; when the skull is involved, it is usually at the anterior fontanelle. Epidermoid cysts most commonly involve males between the age of 20 and 50 years. Dermoids have no sex preference and arise most often in children.

Diploic lesions of the skull present as a painless swelling most commonly but may give rise to painless exophthalmos and headache. Osseous lesions rarely extend intracranially; therefore, neurological deficit is uncommon.[105] A malignant form of epidermoid can occur in the skull.[27]

Radiographically these lesions appear as a round lytic calvarial lesion with a dense sclerotic border. CT scans show a hypodense non-enhancing lesion with often irregular borders. Marginal enhancement and calcification may be present. MRI scans show inhomogeneous low-intensity lesions on T1-weighted images, and inhomogeneous high-intensity lesions on T2-weighted images.[96,99,105]

Epidermoid cysts have a thin capsule of stratified, keratinized squamous epithelium and are filled by desquamated epithelial cells and keratin. Dermoid cysts have, in addition, hair follicles and sebaceous and sweat glands.

Treatment is complete surgical resection with removal of the cyst wall. Complete removal is not associated with recurrence, whereas incomplete removal has a high recurrence rate. Intracranial dermoids and epidermoids are discussed elsewhere in this textbook.

Lipoma and Liposarcoma of Bone

Lipomas are extremely common benign tumors found primarily in the subcutaneous tissues, but they may occur in any location where fat is found. Despite the great amount of adipose tissue in marrow, intraosseous lipoma is extremely rare, accounting for approximately 100 reported cases. Six cases of skull lipoma have been reported in the literature.[122,139]

Radiographically these lesions appear as well-defined lytic areas without any periosteal reaction. Intralesional trabeculae are seen, which create a ground-glass appearance. CT shows an expanded high-density diploic lesion, with preservation of both tables on bone windows. All this may lead to a preoperative diagnosis of fibrous dysplasia.[122]

Benign lipomas are of little clinical significance except for their cosmetic effects and are unlikely to result in any neurological sequelae. It is also doubtful that liposarcomas ever arise from lipomas. Therefore, resection is needed only for cosmetic reasons.

Liposarcomas are clinically variable lesions, with the well-differentiated and myxoid forms being locally invasive and with a high recurrence rate following incomplete resection. Metastases are rare. Round cell and pleomorphic variants are highly aggressive, with widespread metastases and common local recurrence.[60]

Melanotic Neuroectodermal Tumor of Bone

Melanotic neuroectodermal tumor (MNET) of bone is rare and usually arises from the maxilla during the first year of life, although other sites have been reported. In a review of eight cases of MNET of the skull vault, seven arose from the anterior fontanel.[6,20] The tumor often presents as a rapidly growing soft tissue mass which may be associated with new bone formation. They arise from the neural crest cells and behave locally like malignant tures and frequent recurrence following surgical removal. Most of these lesions are cured by excision, but metastasis has occurred.[6,20]

Intraosseous Meningioma

Ectopic meningiomas have been reported in the finger, paravertebral areas, parotid gland, paranasal sinuses, face, neck, scalp, calvarial periosteum, and calvaria. In the calvaria, the majority of lesions are localized in the frontal and parietal region. They are thought to arise from the arachnoid cells within the sheath of the cranial nerves, and from arachnoid cell remnants that have been displaced during embryogenesis. They are believed to occur more frequently along the suture lines of the skull.[72]

Intraosseous meningioma can be mistaken for fibrous dysplasia.[16,43] Osteoma and osteoblastic metastasis are also in the differential diagnosis.[127] Kim et al. attempted to develop a classification system of the appearance of these lesions on CT with bone window settings.[66] In doing so, they hoped to differentiate among the hyperostotic patterns seen with meningioma *en plaque,* osteoma, and fibrous dysplasia. Only their "periosteal pattern" was found to be specific for meningioma, but this was seen only in two of nine cases. One feature which would exclude fibrous dysplasia is localized inward bulging of the inner table. The surface of the hyperostotic bone in intraosseous meningioma is usually irregular. Furthermore, intraosseous meningioma is often localized in the vicinity of the coronal suture. When fibrous dysplasia involves the convexity, the inner table is usually spared and the surface of the hyperostosis tends to be smooth. Differentiation from osteoma is based on the observations that osteoma usually arises from the outer table of the skull and rarely from the inner table. Another differential point is that osteomas do not extend across suture lines, whereas hyperostosis from meningiomas may cross suture lines.[66] Kim et al. did not find angiography to be useful in the diagnosis of intraosseous meningioma.[66] No cases demonstrated any tumor blush, and only one case showed enlargement of the middle meningeal artery. That finding is nonspecific, and can be seen with fibrous dysplasia.

These tumors are usually benign, but a primary intraosseous malignant meningioma of the skull has been reported.[75] For additional discussion, refer to the sections on fibrous dysplasia and osteoma.

Primary Neuroendocrine (Merkel Cell) Carcinoma of Bone

This is a malignant tumor of the skin. There is a slight female predominance, and the average age at presentation is 67.5 years. Of these neoplasms, 46 percent are located in the region of the head and neck, with only one case reported arising in the calvaria.[135]

Primary Tumors of Bone with Smooth Muscle and Skeletal Muscle Differentiation

These tumors are extremely rare tumors of bone, accounting for fewer than 50 cases in the literature. The smooth muscle tumors, leiomyoma and leiomyosarcoma, occur throughout all ages, with an average age of 47.7 years, but most commonly in the seventh and eighth decades of life. Males are affected slightly more often than females. Bones about the knee as well as the gnathic bones are most commonly affected.

Rhabdomyosarcoma (RMS) is the most frequent soft tissue sarcoma in children, having a predilection for the head and neck. Within the temporal bone it usually originates in the tympanic cavity, mastoid air cells, or external auditory canal, and clinical presentation includes hearing loss, otalgia, and hemorrhagic or purulent discharge from the external auditory canal, or evidence of a polypoid mass in the external ear. A case of primary RMS of the petrous ridge has been reported.[140] Rhabdomyosarcoma of the cranial vault in a 5-year-old girl has also been described.[6]

Syndromes That Can Include Primary Tumors and Bone-Forming Conditions of the Skull

Gardner's Syndrome

Gardner's syndrome was described in 1953. It is inherited as an autosomal dominant with complete penetrance and variable expression. It is considered by many authorities to be the same genetic entity as familial adenomatous polyposis (FAP). In addition to colonic polyposis there are multiple osteomas, cutaneous lesions, dental abnormalities, and desmoid tumors.

The osteomas can appear in the first decade of life. The ramus of the mandible and the frontal bone are the most common sites. The skin lesions include epidermoid cysts, fibromas, lipomas, leiomyomas, neurofibromas, and pigmented areas. Dental abnormalities include multiple unerupted permanent teeth, supernumary teeth, odontomes, and cemental lesions. Usually the skin and bony lesions predate the intestinal polyposis by as much as 10 years.[64]

Desmoid tumors contain mature fibroblasts and differ from most fibrous growths by their tendency to infiltrate into surrounding structures, causing intestinal obstruction when growing in the abdominal cavity. Subtotal resection of desmoid tumors is often followed by recurrence. Gallium-67 radionuclide scanning has been reported to be superior to CT as a follow-up examination, since scar tissue and residual desmoid tumor look the same on CT.[50]

The clinical importance of this condition lies in the pattern of inheritance and the universal development of cancer. Fifty percent of siblings of patients with FAP/Gardner's syndrome are affected. Therefore, the physician has a responsibility not only to the patient but to the patient's family as well. Unlike the hamartomatous polyps of Peutz-Jeghers syndrome, the colorectal polyps of the FAP/Gardner's syndrome have a 100 percent potential of becoming malignant. The malignant change occurs commonly in the 20- to 40-year age group. The upper gastrointestinal tract and biliary tree have also recently been recognized as having the potential for the development of malignancy. Patients who have more than 30 polyps or have evidence of dysplasia or malignant change in any polyp should undergo total colectomy and ileorectal anastomosis. Rectal preservation after colectomy carries a 25 percent risk of rectal carcinoma within 15 years, and frequent endoscopy is recommended.[64]

McCune-Albright Syndrome

The association of polyostotic fibrous dysplasia (POFD), hyperpigmented skin macules, and precocious puberty was first described in 1937 by McCune and Bruch and shortly thereafter by Albright. After sexual precocity, thyroid disorders are the second most common form of endocrinopathy associated with McCune-Albright syndrome. Pituitary adenoma has also been reported.[95] The McCune-Albright syndrome occurs in about 3 percent of patients with fibrous dysplasia. Ninety-five percent have been females.[101] All reported cases have been sporadic, with no known hereditary basis.[130]

The syndrome can begin in infancy with vaginal bleeding. The hyperpigmented skin lesions can cause confusion with neurofibromatosis. The hyperpigmented lesions in McCune-Albright syndrome are irregular, fewer in number, and much larger (sometimes regional or segmental) than those seen in von Recklinghausen's disease. Patients with extensive bone disease may present in early childhood with fractures and deformities of the long bones. Acromegaly, hyperparathyroidism, hyperthyroidism, and Cushing's syndrome have been found in association with the syndrome.[38,95] The serum alkaline phosphatase level is elevated in about 80 percent of patients, but does not predict the degree of bone involvement. Radionuclide bone scanning is recommended for determining the extent of bony disease.[38,101]

Nonthrombotic Partial Occlusion of the Venous Sinuses

Plant et al. have drawn attention to the fact that epidural nonthrombotic partial occlusion of the superior sagittal sinus is clinically very different from thrombotic occlusion.[102] With intraluminal thrombosis, there is usually associated cortical venous thrombosis, which results in infarcts and focal neurological deficits. As recovery ensues after the venous infarct, another draining vein on the opposite hemisphere may become thrombosed. This produces the rare but characteristic syndrome of *hemiplegia a bascule,* or alternating hemiplegia (bascule in French means "balance scale," which alludes to the alternating and reciprocal relationship of the two sides).

With epidural nonthrombotic partial occlusion, however, the

clinical presentation is that of raised intracranial pressure: papilledema with enlarged blindspots ultimately leading to optic atrophy and visual loss, sixth nerve palsies, etc. The most common metastatic neoplasm to cause this in the adult is myeloma, and in children and young adults, Ewing's sarcoma and neuroblastoma.[102] Epidural compression near the torcular Herophili has also been reported with primary calvarial tumors. Osteoma, eosinophilic granuloma, primary Hodgkin's disease of the skull, and epidermoid tumor have all been seen to cause this syndrome.[34,105,119,134]

Ollier's Syndrome and Maffucci's Syndrome

In 1899, when Ollier described the disease that bears his name, he characterized it as a dysplastic developmental anomaly in which cartilage fails to ossify and continues to proliferate.[104] The result is multiple rests and masses of hyperplastic cartilage found most commonly in the tubular bones of the hands and long bones of the extremities. These lesions are histologically identical to solitary enchondroma, which is a common benign tumor. Ollier's syndrome is an apparently noninheritable dysplasia of cartilage. It is generally not diagnosed until childhood, although occasionally a limb length discrepancy is noted at birth. Clinically, the disease is characterized by severe limb length discrepancies accompanied by gross bone deformities, such as genu valgum, cubitus varus, and multiple enchondromas. Histologically, the lesions consist of hyaline cartilage with irregularly arranged, variously sized cells with centers of ossification. Intracranial chondroma is a rare event in Ollier's syndrome.[46,124] Generally, Ollier's syndrome is not associated with tumors other than enchondromas. However, Rawlings et al. have discussed a patient with Ollier's syndrome who had two intracranial gliomas.[104]

The syndrome of multiple enchondromas combined with multiple soft-tissue hemangiomas were first described by Maffucci at the University of Naples in 1881.[63] The enchondromas and the dyschondroplasia in Maffucci's syndrome are the same as in Ollier's syndrome. The differences are the nonskeletal manifestations of Maffucci's syndrome, which consist primarily of simple or cavernous hemangiomas occurring in the subcutaneous tissues and occasionally involving the viscera. The subcutaneous bluish nodules are usually noted in infancy, involve the limbs, and vary greatly in size. In contrast to Ollier's syndrome, a generalized predisposition to neoplasia in adulthood has been well established in Maffucci's syndrome. Malignant transformation of enchondromas to chondrosarcomas has been noted in 15 to 20 percent of patients. Malignant degeneration of hemangiomas and lymphangiomas may also occur. Other tumors documented to be associated with this syndrome include fibrosarcoma, glioma, mesenchymal ovarian tumor, carcinoma of the pancreas, pituitary adenoma, uterine polyp, uterine fibroid, etc.[63] Bilateral chondrosarcomas in the cerebellopontine angle have been seen.[21] Overall, of the 98 cases of Maffucci's syndrome reported, only 8 had possible skull involvement. Although exact incidences are not available, authorities believe that skull involvement in Ollier's syndrome is even less common.[104]

References

1. Adler M, Hnatuk L, Mock D, Freeman JL. Aggressive osteoblastoma of the temporal bone: a case report. *J Otolaryngol* 1990; 19:307–310.
2. Alappat JP, Pillai AM, Prasanna D, Sambasivan M. Giant cell reparative granuloma of the craniofacial complex: case report and review of the literature. *Br J Neurosurg* 1992; 6:71–74.
3. Ando S, Tsuchida T, Hayakawa I. Diploic fibroma of the skull. *Surg Neurol* 1978; 10:108–109.
4. Angiari P, Torcia E, Botticelli RA, et al. Ossifying parasellar chondroma. Case report. *J Neurosurg Sci* 1987; 31:59–63.
5. Anim JT, Baraka ME. Chondroblastoma of temporal bone: unusual histologic features. *Ann Otol Rhinol Laryngol* 1986; 95:260–263.
6. Arthur RJ, Brunelle F. Computerised tomography in the evaluation of expansile lesions arising from the skull vault in childhood—a report of 5 cases. *Pediatr Radiol* 1988; 18:294–301.
7. Ashkenazi E, Constantini S, Oren R, et al. Fine needle aspiration biopsy for skull tumors: technical note and two demonstrative case reports. *Clin Neuropathol* 1992; 11:74–76.
8. Babu ML. Fibrous dysplasia skull (mixed type). *Semin Roentgenol* 1991; 26:3–4.
9. Banerjee AK, Kak VK. Benign osteoblastoma of the occipital bone. *Ear Nose Throat J* 1991; 70:215–216.
10. Barontini F, Maurri S, Sita D. Peripheral ophthalmoplegia as the only sign of late-onset fibrous dysplasia of the skull. *J Clin Neuroophthalmol* 1986; 6:109–112.
11. Bertoni F, Unni KK, Beabout JW, et al. Chondroblastoma of the skull and facial bones. *Am J Clin Pathol* 1987; 88:1–9.
12. Bertoni F, Unni KK, McLeod RA, Sim FH. Xanthoma of bone. *Am J Clin Pathol* 1988; 90:377–384.
13. Birzgalis AR, Ramsden RT, Lye RH, Richardson PL. Haemangiopericytoma of the temporal bone. *J Laryngol Otol* 1990; 104:998–1003.
14. Blaauw G, Prick JJ, Versteege C. Chondroblastoma of the temporal bone. *Neurosurgery* 1988; 22:1102–1107.
15. Bollen E, Vielvoye J, Van Dijk JG. Trigeminal neuralgia-like pain in an aged woman with fibrous dysplasia of the skull base. *Headache* 1990; 30:277–279.
16. Boon AP, Carey MP, Hockley A. Meningioma mimicking fibrous dysplasia of the skull. *J Neurol Neurosurg Psychiatry* 1990; 53:818 (letter; comment).
17. Bourgouin PM, Tampieri D, Robitaille Y, et al. Low-grade myxoid chondrosarcoma of the base of the skull: CT, MR, and histopathology. *J Comput Assist Tomogr* 1992; 16:268–273.
18. Branch CL Jr, Challa VR, Kelly DL Jr. Aneurysmal bone cyst with fibrous dysplasia of the parietal bone. Report of two cases. *J Neurosurg* 1986; 64:331–335.
19. Brooks JJ, LiVolsi VA, Trojanowski JQ. Does chondroid chordoma exist? *Acta Neuropathol (Berl)* 1987; 72:229–235.
20. Burger PC, Scheithauer BW, Vogel FS. *Surgical Pathology of the Nervous System and its Coverings*, 3d ed. New York: Churchill Livingstone, 1991.
21. Bushe KA, Naumann M, Warmuth-Metz M, et al. Maffucci's syndrome with bilateral cartilaginous tumors of the cerebellopontine angle. *Neurosurgery* 1990; 27:625–628.
22. Camilleri AF. Craniofacial fibrous dysplasia. *J Laryngol Otol* 1991; 105:662–666.
23. Cataltepe O, Inci S, Ozcan OE, et al. Aneurysmal bone cyst of the frontal bone. *Surg Neurol* 1990; 33:391–394.
24. Chen YR, Noordhoff MS. Treatment of craniomaxillofacial fibrous dysplasia: how early and how extensive? *Plast Reconstr Surg* 1990; 86:835–842.
25. Chetty R, Kalan MR, Kranold DH. Malignant transformation in fibrous dysplasia. A report of 3 cases. *S Afr J Surg* 1990; 28:80–82.
26. Chitale VS, Sundaresan N, Helson L, Huvos A. Malignant fibrous histiocytoma of the temporal bone with intracranial extension. *Acta Neurochir (Wien)* 1981; 59:239–246.
27. Ciappetta P, Artico M, Salvati M, et al. Intradiploic epidermoid cysts of the skull: report of 10 cases and review of the literature. *Acta Neurochir (Wien)* 1990; 102: 33–37.
28. Ciappetta P, Salvati M, Bernardi C, et al. Giant cell reparative granuloma of the skull base mimicking an intracranial tumor. Case report and review of the literature. *Surg Neurol* 1990; 33:52–56.

29. Clavier E, Thiebot J, Godlewski J, et al. Intracranial aneurysmal bone cyst: a rare CT appearance. *Neuroradiology* 1988; 30:269–271.
30. Colak A, Berker M, Ozcan OE, Erbengi A. CNS involvement in Ewing's sarcoma. A report of 12 cases. *Acta Neurochir (Wien)* 1991; 113:48–51.
31. Coltrera MD, Googe PB, Harrist TJ, et al. Chondrosarcoma of the temporal bone. Diagnosis and treatment of 13 cases and review of the literature. *Cancer* 1986; 58:2689–2696.
32. Conrad GR, Dean BL, Baumann RJ, Seabold JE. HMPAO scintigraphy, MRI, and CT of a vascular fibrous dysplasia of the craniofacial bones. *Clin Nucl Med* 1991; 16:743–746.
33. Cook BR, Vries JK, Martinez AJ. Malignant fibrous histiocytoma of the clivus: case report. *Neurosurgery* 1987; 20:632–635.
34. Corriero G, Maiuri F, Giamundo A, et al. Giant osteoma of the cranial vault with acromegaly and hydrocephalus. A case report. *J Neurosurg Sci* 1985; 29:331–334.
35. Davidson MJ. Ewing's sarcoma of the temporal bone. A case report. *Oral Surg Oral Med Oral Pathol* 1991; 72:534–536.
36. Davies ML, MacPherson P. Fibrous dysplasia of the skull: disease activity in relation to age. *Br J Radiol* 1991; 64:576–579.
37. Du Preez JH, Branca EP. Plasmacytoma of the skull: case reports. *Neurosurgery* 1991; 29:902–906.
38. Edeburn GF, Mortensson W. Value of bone scan in the McCune-Albright syndrome. Report of a case. *Acta Radiol Diagn (Stockh)* 1986; 27:719–721.
39. Epstein N, Whelan M, Reed D, Aleksic S. Giant cell tumor of the skull: a report of two cases. *Neurosurgery* 1982; 11:263–267.
40. Fagan PA, Bentivoglio PJ, Sheridan BF, et al. Surgical treatment of tumours of the skull base. *Med J Aust* 1992; 156:717–721.
41. Findlay JM, Chiasson D, Hudson AR, Chui M. Giant-cell tumor of the middle cranial fossa. Case report. *J Neurosurg* 1987; 66:924–928.
42. Frank E, Deruaz JP, de Tribolet N. Chondromyxoid fibroma of the petrous-sphenoid junction. *Surg Neurol* 1987; 27:182–186.
43. Frankel J, Ianotti F, Powell M, Schon F. Meningioma—an unrecognised complication of fibrous dysplasia of the skull? [letter] [see comments]. *J Neurol Neurosurg Psychiatry* 1989; 52:546–547.
44. Garzozi H, Garty I, Kaveh Z. Craniofacial fibrous dysplasia complicated by mucocele: the role of radionuclide scintigraphic methods in the diagnosis. *Ann Ophthalmol* 1989; 21:108–110.
45. Gavilan J, Nistal M, Gavilan C, Calvo M. Ossifying hemangioma of the temporal bone. *Arch Otolaryngol Head Neck Surg* 1990; 116:965–967.
46. Ghogawala Z, Moore M, Strand R, et al. Clival chondroma in a child with Ollier's disease. Case report. *Pediatr Neurosurg* 1991–1992; 17:53–56.
47. Ginsberg LE. Neoplastic diseases affecting the central skull base: CT and MR imaging. *Am J Roentgenol* 1992; 159:581–589.
48. Gudrun R. Haemangiopericytoma in otolaryngology. *J Laryngol Otol* 1979; 93:477–494.
49. Gupta D, Vishwakarma SK. Osteogenic sarcoma of the frontal sinus. *Ann Otol Rhinol Laryngol* 1990; 99:489–490.
50. Hardoff R, Ben Dov D, Front A. Gallium 67 scintigraphy in the evaluation of Gardner's syndrome. *Cancer* 1988; 61:2353–2358.
51. Hardoff R, Gips S. Radiographic and scintigraphic demonstration of mono-ostotic fibrous dysplasia of the skull. Advantage of SPECT imaging. *Clin Nucl Med* 1991; 16:869–871.
52. Harman SA, Pribram H. Case report 586: giant cell tumor of sphenoid bone. *Skeletal Radiol* 1990; 19:212–215.
53. Hassounah M, Al-Mefty O, Akhtar M, et al. Primary cranial and intracranial chondrosarcoma. A survey. *Acta Neurochir (Wien)* 1985; 78:123–132.
54. Henderson BT, Whitwell H. Giant cell tumor of the skull: case report. *Neurosurgery* 1988; 23:120–122.
55. Hoffman DF, Israel J. Intraosseous frontal hemangioma. *Head Neck* 1990; 12:160–163.
56. Hook SR, Font RL, McCrary JA, Harper RL. Intraosseous capillary hemangioma of the frontal bone. *Am J Ophthalmol* 1987; 103:824–827.
57. Horn KL, Hankinson H, Nagel B, Erasmus M. Surgical management of chondroblastoma of the temporal bone. *Otolaryngol Head Neck Surg* 1990; 102:264–269.
58. Hufnagel TJ, Artiles C, Piepmeier J, et al. Desmoplastic fibroma of parietal bone simulating eosinophilic granuloma. Case report. *J Neurosurg* 1987; 67:449–451.
59. Huvos AG. *Bone Tumors: Diagnosis, Treatment and Prognosis.* Philadelphia: Saunders, 1979.
60. Huvos AG. *Bone Tumors: Diagnosis, Treatment and Prognosis,* 2d ed. Philadelphia: Saunders, 1991.
61. Ikeda H, Niizuma H, Yoshimoto T. Aneurysmal bone cyst of the skull. *Surg Neurol* 1986; 25:145–148.
62. Jackler RK, Brackmann DE. Xanthoma of the temporal bone and skull base. *Am J Otol* 1987; 8:111–115.
63. Johnson TE, Nasr AM, Nalbandian RM, Cappelen SJ. Enchondromatosis and hemangioma (Maffucci's syndrome) with orbital involvement. *Am J Ophthalmol* 1990; 110:153–159.
64. Jones K, Korzcak P. The diagnostic significance and management of Gardner's syndrome. *Br J Oral Maxillofac Surg* 1990; 28:80–84.
65. Kemeny AA, Afshar F. Giant cell tumour of the sphenoid bone with coincidental galactorrhoea—a case report. *Br J Neurosurg* 1990; 4:343–346.
66. Kim KS, Rogers LF, Goldblatt D. CT features of hyperostosing meningioma en plaque. *Am J Roentgenol* 1987; 149:1017–1023.
67. Kitamura K, Nibu K, Asai M, et al. Chondromyxoid fibroma of the mastoid invading the occipital bone. *Arch Otolaryngol Head Neck Surg* 1989; 115:384–386.
68. Kiwit JC, Schober R, Nicola N, et al. Osteoclastomas of the petrous bone. *Surg Neurol* 1986; 26:59–62.
69. Kraus DH, Lanzieri CF, Wanamaker JR, et al. Complementary use of computed tomography and magnetic resonance imaging in assessing skull base lesions. *Laryngoscope* 1992; 102:623–629.
70. Krayenbühl H, Yasargil MG. Chondromas. *Prog Neurol Surg* 1975; 6:435–463.
71. Kroon HM, Schurmans J. Osteoblastoma: clinical and radiologic findings in 98 new cases. *Radiology* 1990; 175:783–790.
72. Kulali A, Ilcayto R, Rahmanli O. Primary calvarial ectopic meningiomas. *Neurochirurgia (Stuttg)* 1991; 34:174–177.
73. Kurt AM, Unni KK, Sim FH, McLeod RA. Chondroblastoma of bone. *Hum Pathol* 1989; 20:965–976.
74. Kveton JF, Brackmann DE, Glasscock ME III, et al. Chondrosarcoma of the skull base. *Otolaryngol Head Neck Surg* 1986; 94:23–32.
75. Lee WH, Tu YC, Liu MY. Primary intraosseous malignant meningioma of the skull: case report. *Neurosurgery* 1988; 23:505–508.
76. Lee YY, Van Tassel P, Nauert C, et al. Craniofacial osteosarcomas: plain film, CT, and MR findings in 46 cases. *Am J Roentgenol* 1988; 150:1397–1402.
77. Lee YY, Van Tassel P, Raymond AK. Intracranial dural chondrosarcoma. *Am J Neuroradiol* 1988; 9:1189–1193.
78. Leonetti JP. Preoperative evaluation of patients with advanced tumors of the skull base. *Ear Nose Throat J* 1991; 70:558–560.
79. Long DM, Holliday M, Zinreich SJ, Mattox DE. Uncommon tumors of the skull base and uncommon approaches to them. *Neurosurg Clin North Am* 1990; 1:225–242.
80. Long DM, Mattox DE. Tumors of the skull base. *Md Med J* 1990; 39:355–360.
81. Maiuri F, Corriero G, Giamundo A. Primary lymphoma of the cranial vault. *J Neurosurg Sci* 1987; 31:183–186.
82. Marc JA, Takei Y, Schechter MM, Hoffman JC. Intracranial haemangiopericytomas: angiography, pathology and differential diagnosis. *Am J Roentgenol* 1975; 125:823–832.
83. Mark RJ, Sercarz JA, Tran L, et al. Osteogenic sarcoma of the head and neck. The UCLA experience. *Arch Otolaryngol Head Neck Surg* 1991; 117:761–766.

84. Matsumoto K, Kakita K, Fukuma S. Large, benign osteoblastoma of the temporal bone—case report. *Neurol Med Chir (Tokyo)* 1989; 29:444–448.
85. Matsuura S, Takagi T, Tan EC, et al. Malignant fibrous histiocytoma of the occipital bone with intracranial extension—case report. *Neurol Med Chir (Tokyo)* 1991; 31:219–222.
86. Mehta RC, Wilson MA, Perlman SB. Osteosarcoma arising in Paget's disease of the calvarium. *J Nucl Med* 1988; 29:414–416.
87. Meyers SP, Hirsch WL Jr, Curtin HD, et al. Chondrosarcomas of the skull base: MR imaging features. *Radiology* 1992; 184:103–108.
88. Miyazaki S, Tsubokawa T, Katayama Y, et al. Benign osteoblastoma of the temporal bone of an infant. *Surg Neurol* 1987; 27:277–283.
89. Mortensen A, Bojsen-Moller M, Rasmussen P. Fibrous dysplasia of the skull with acromegaly and sarcomatous transformation. Two cases with a review of the literature. *J Neurooncol* 1989; 7:25–29.
90. Munro IR. Discussion of Chen YR, Noordhoff MS. Treatment of craniomaxillofacial fibrous dysplasia: how early and how extensive? *Plast Reconstr Surg* 1991; 87:799–800.
91. Neff S, Hansen K, Domanowski GF, Wu JL. Cryptic osteoid osteoma of the cranium: case report. *Neurosurgery* 1990; 27:820–821.
92. Oguro K, Nakahara N, Yamaguchi Y, et al. Chondrosarcoma of the posterior fossa—case report. *Neurol Med Chir (Tokyo)* 1989; 29:1030–1038.
93. Ohta H, Tanazawa T, Osuka K, et al. True aneurysms of the middle meningeal artery associated with cavernous hemangioma of the skull—case report. *Neurol Med Chir (Tokyo)* 1991; 31:203–205.
94. Okuno H, Yamamichi N, Watanabe I, Tokita N. Desmoplastic fibroma of the temporal bone. *J Otolaryngol* 1990; 19:311–314.
95. O'Laughlin RL, Selinger SE, Moriarty PE. Pituitary adenoma in McCune-Albright syndrome: MR demonstration. *J Comput Assist Tomogr* 1989; 13:685–688.
96. Olson JJ, Beck DW, Crawford SC, Menezes AH. Comparative evaluation of intracranial epidermoid tumors with computed tomography and magnetic resonance imaging. *Neurosurgery* 1987; 21:357–360.
97. Otsuka S, Nakatsu S, Matsumoto S, et al. Monostotic fibrous dysplasia of the left parietal bone—case report. *Neurol Med Chir (Tokyo)* 1989; 29:248–250.
98. Oyama H, Nagane M, Shibui S, et al. Skull base malignant lymphoma: a case report and review of the literature. *Jpn J Clin Oncol* 1992; 22:131–135.
99. Ozgen T, Oge HK, Erbengi A, Bertan V. Cranial dermoid and epidermoid cysts. *Neurochirurgia (Stuttg)* 1990; 33:16–19.
100. Peterson DL, Murk SE, Story JL. Multifocal cavernous hemangioma of the skull: report of a case and review of the literature. *Neurosurgery* 1992; 30:778–782.
101. Pfeffer S, Molina E, Feuillan P, Simon TR. McCune-Albright syndrome: the patterns of scintigraphic abnormalities. *J Nucl Med* 1990; 31:1474–1478.
102. Plant GT, Donald JJ, Jackowski A, et al. Partial, non-thrombotic, superior sagittal sinus occlusion due to occipital skull tumours. *J Neurol Neurosurg Psychiatry* 1991; 54:520–523.
103. Pradhan S, Datta NR, Krishnani N, et al. Giant cell tumour of the petrous bone. *Indian J Cancer* 1991; 28:177–180.
104. Rawlings CE III, Bullard DE, Burger PC, Friedman AH. A case of Ollier's disease associated with two intracranial gliomas. *Neurosurgery* 1987; 21:400–403.
105. Rubin G, Scienza R, Pasqualin A, et al. Craniocerebral epidermoids and dermoids. A review of 44 cases. *Acta Neurochir (Wien)* 1989; 97:1–16.
106. Schiffer J, Reif R, Lahat E, et al. Intraosseous neurilemmoma of skull—single case report. *Neurochirurgia (Stuttg)* 1991; 34:178–179.
107. Sekhar LN, Pomeranz S, Sen CN. Extradural petrous bone and petroclival neoplasms. *Acta Neurochir Suppl (Wien)* 1991; 53:183–192.
108. Sen CN, Sekhar LN, Schramm VL, Janecka IP. Chordoma and chondrosarcoma of the cranial base: an 8-year experience. *Neurosurgery* 1989; 25:931–940.
109. Shah JP, Kraus DH, Arbit E, et al. Craniofacial resection for tumors involving the anterior skull base. *Otolaryngol Head Neck Surg* 1992; 106:387–393.
110. Sharma V, Newton G. Osteoclastoma of occipital bone. *Yonsei Med J* 1991; 32:169–171.
111. Shen WP, Young RF, Walter BN, et al. Molecular analysis of a myxoid chondrosarcoma with rearrangements of chromosomes 10 and 22. *Cancer Genet Cytogenet* 1990; 45:207–215.
112. Shibata Y, Yoshii Y, Tsukada A, Nose T. Radiolucent osteoma of the skull: case report. *Neurosurgery* 1991; 29:776–778.
113. Smith ME, Calcaterra TC. Frontal sinus osteoma. *Ann Otol Rhinol Laryngol* 1989; 98:896–900.
114. Snyderman CH, Sekhar LN, Sen CN, Janecka IP. Malignant skull base tumors. *Neurosurg Clin North Am* 1990; 1:243–259.
115. Sugita Y, Shigemori M, Miyagi J, et al. Radiation-induced osteosarcoma of the calvaria—case report. *Neurol Med Chir (Tokyo)* 1992; 32:32–35.
116. Taconis WK. Osteosarcoma in fibrous dysplasia. *Skeletal Radiol* 1988; 17:163–170.
117. Tandon DA, Deka RC, Chaudhary C, Misra NK. Giant cell tumour of the temporosphenoidal region. *J Laryngol Otol* 1988; 102:449–451.
118. Tanohata K, Noda M, Katoh H, et al. Chondroblastoma of temporal bone. *Neuroradiology* 1986; 28:367–370.
119. Thomas CV, Kennedy BJ. Primary Hodgkin's disease of the skull following a 3-year history of pseudotumor cerebri. *Cancer* 1986; 58:318–320.
120. Thomas JE, Baker HL Jr. Assessment of roentgenographic lucencies of the skull: a systematic approach. *Neurology* 1975; 25:99–106.
121. Tokuda Y, Uozumi T, Sakoda K, et al. Giant congenital capillary hemangioma of pericranium—case report. *Neurol Med Chir (Tokyo)* 1990; 30:1029–1033.
122. Tomabechi M, Sako K, Daita G, Yonemasu Y. Lipoma involving the skull. Case report. *J Neurosurg* 1992; 76:312–314.
123. Tomita T, Huvos A, Shah J, Sundaresan N. Giant ossifying fibroma of the nasal cavity with intracranial extension. *Acta Neurochir (Wien)* 1981; 56:65–71.
124. Traflet RF, Babaria AR, Barolat G, et al. Intracranial chondroma in a patient with Ollier's disease. Case report. *J Neurosurg* 1989; 70:274–276.
125. Tucci DL, Lambert PR, Innes DJ Jr. Primary lymphoma of the temporal bone. *Arch Otolaryngol Head Neck Surg* 1992; 118:83–85.
126. Uttley D, Archer DJ. Giant cell tumour of the sphenoid sinus: an unusual skull base tumour. *J Laryngol Otol* 1991; 105:855–857.
127. Van Tassel P, Lee YY, Ayala A, et al. Case report 680. Intraosseous meningioma of the sphenoid bone. *Skeletal Radiol* 1991; 20:383–386.
128. Vara-Thorbeck R, Morales OI, Rosell J, Gomez M. Benign osteoblastoma of vertebral column and skull. Report of two cases. *Zentralbl Neurochir* 1990; 51:216–218.
129. Vege DS, Borges AM, Aggrawal K, et al. Osteosarcoma of the craniofacial bones. A clinico-pathological study. *J Craniomaxillofac Surg* 1991; 19:90–93.
130. Viljoen DL, Versfeld GA, Losken W, Beighton P. Polyostotic fibrous dysplasia with cranial hyperostosis: new entity or most severe form of polyostotic fibrous dysplasia? *Am J Med Genet* 1988; 29:661–667.
131. Volle E, Treisch J, Claussen C, Kaufmann HJ. Lesions of skull base observed on high resolution computed tomography. A comparison with magnetic resonance imaging. *Acta Radiol* 1989; 30:129–134.
132. Watanabe H, Tsubokawa T, Katayama Y, et al. Primary Ewing's sarcoma of the temporal bone. *Surg Neurol* 1992; 37:54–58.
133. Watkins LD, Uttley D, Archer DJ, et al. Giant cell tumors of the sphenoid bone. *Neurosurgery* 1992; 30:576–581.
134. Wightman H, Wheelock B. Eosinophilic granuloma of the occipital bone presenting as intracranial venous hypertension. *Can J Neurol Sci* 1991; 18:512–514.
135. Wojak JC, Murali R. Primary neuroendocrine (Merkel cell) carcinoma presenting in the calvarium: case report. *Neurosurgery* 1990; 26:137–139.

136. Wu KK, Ross PM, Mitchell DC, Sprague HH. Evolution of a case of multicentric giant cell tumor over a 23-year period. *Clin Orthop* 1986; 213:279–288.
137. Wu RK, Trumble TE, Ruwe PA. Familial incidence of Paget's disease and secondary osteogenic sarcoma. A report of three cases from a single family. *Clin Orthop* 1991; 265:306–309.
138. Yamaguchi K, Hayasaka S, Yamada T, et al. Orbitocranial fibrous dysplasia. A case report. *Ophthalmologica* 1986; 193:225–230.
139. Yasuda Y, Tsukada S, Okada T, Haseda Y. Intraosseous lipoma of the skull: a report of two cases. *Ann Plast Surg* 1987; 18:74–80.
140. Zampa V, Mascalchi M, Giodano GP, et al. Rhabdomyosarcoma of the petrous ridge. CT and MR imaging in an atypical case with multiple cranial nerve palsy. *Acta Radiol* 1992; 33:76–78.
141. Zappia JJ, LaRouere MJ, Telian SA. Massive ossifying fibroma of the temporal bone. *Otolaryngol Head Neck Surg* 1990; 103:480–483.

151

Chordomas and Chondrosarcomas of the Cranial Base

Laligam N. Sekhar
Emmanuel Gay
Donald C. Wright

Chordomas are a rare but difficult-to-manage group of neoplasms that have challenged neurosurgeons since their first description by Luschka in 1856.[45] Although pathologically distinct from chordomas, chondrosarcomas have similar biological behavior, radiologic features, location, and surgical treatment. Chordomas and chondrosarcomas are therefore considered together in this chapter.

Controversies exist regarding both the pathologic diagnosis and optimal treatment of these lesions. Much of this controversy stems from the fact that a number of these tumors grow slowly, yet have been difficult to cure. Modalities of therapy available at present in the treatment armamentarium include partial surgical removal followed by radiotherapy, extensive surgical removal with the aid of cranial base approaches, radiation with charged particles such as proton beams or helium ions, and radiosurgery. However, it has been difficult to conduct randomized studies of these various treatment options because of the small number of patients treated in most institutions, the variability of tumor size and extent, and the fact that at least a 10-year follow-up of patients treated by these methods is necessary.

Pathology

Chordoma

Chordomas develop from remnants of the notochord, an embryonic structure which is the forerunner of the axial skeleton. In the normal adult, remnants of the notochord are usually found only in the nucleus pulposus of the intervertebral discs. However, remnants may also be found in the clival bone marrow, and in the intradural clival area (''ecchordosis physaliphora'').[8,34,41,75]

Cranial base chordomas usually originate extradurally, although a primary intradural origin is possible in some patients. Dural invasion by extradural chordomas occurs late in their course, with very aggressive tumors, and in recurrent tumors when the dura was opened and not reconstructed during a previous operation.

Chordomas invade local and regional structures widely, and in an irregular fashion. However, they metastasize rarely, and late in their course. Of metastatic chordomas, only about 7 to 12 percent are from cranial base tumors.[12,20,41,72] Patients with cranial base chordomas usually die from the consequences of regional rather than metastatic disease.

Grossly, chordomas are grayish tumors, with foci of calcification and hemorrhage. They are firm to gelatinous in consistency. Their size is very variable. In a recent review of 60 tumors operated upon by the senior author's group, the tumors varied in volume from 1 cm^3 to 346 cm^3, with an average of 58 cm^3.[31]

Histologically, three features are typical of chordomas: large, vacuolated, mucus-containing cells called physaliphorous (physaliferous) cells; the lobular arrangement of these cells; and abundant extracellular mucoid tissue. A group of tumors with abundant cartilaginous matrices has been named ''chondroid chordoma'' by Heffelfinger. He and others have found a better survival with these tumors as compared to tumors without such features.[19,34,48,53–55,65,67] However, based on immunochemical features, other pathologists have considered these tumors to be low-grade chondrosarcomas.[7–9,25,51] Approximately 10 percent of chordomas show histologic features of malignancy such as nuclear pleomorphism, spindle-shaped elongated nuclei, and abundant mitoses. In our material, this was more commonly observed in patients who had undergone previous irradiation.

Immunochemistry is very useful for distinguishing chordomas from chondrosarcomas. Chordomas stain positively for epithelial markers such as cytokeratin, epithelial membrane antigen, and alpha fetoprotein. Some chordomas stain positively with vimentin antisera, reflecting mesenchymal differentiation.[8,73] Immunoreactivity with S-100 protein often occurs, but is not diagnostic.

Chondrosarcoma

Chrondrosarcomas have been classified into three categories: classic, mesenchymal, and dedifferentiated.[21,47] Classic chondrosarcomas contain many large cells with single or multiple nuclei, and an abundant cartilaginous matrix. Classic chondrosarcomas are divided into three grades, I–III. The distinction is based on mitotic rates, cellularity, the nuclear size of the cells, and the extent of the cartilaginous matrix.[28] Chondrosarcomas of a lower grade are less aggressive, and have minimal metastatic potential.[2,7,13,16,27,33,43] Low-grade chondrosarcomas may be difficult to distinguish from chordomas, but an accurate diagnosis can be made on the basis of immunochemistry, since both epithelial markers and oncofetal antigens are absent in chondrosarcomas.[8,9,71]

The dedifferentiated chondrosarcoma has features of anaplastic sarcoma. The mesenchymal chondrosarcoma has islands of undifferentiated mesenchymal cells, and islands of cartilage. Both dedifferentiated and mesenchymal chondrosarcomas are more aggressive than classic chondrosarcomas.[21]

Fortunately, most skull base chondrosarcomas are of the low-grade variety, which favors a good prognosis after surgical resection or after the combination of surgery and radiotherapy. Such tumors typically are paramedian in location, the most typical site of origin being the petrosphenoclival junction.

Incidence and Distribution

Chordomas occur most commonly in the sacrococcygeal region, second most frequently in the skull base area, and least commonly in other vertebrae. Approximately 40 percent of chordomas are intracranial, and 0.1 percent of all intracranial tumors are chordomas.[34,49,72]

Chondrosarcomas can occur anywhere in the skeletal system. Skull base chondrosarcomas also make up about 0.1 percent of all intracranial tumors.[14,41,43,75]

Chordomas occur in a wide range of ages, from childhood to old age. However, they are most common between the third and fifth decades of life. A male preponderance is found in some series,[2,20,34,39] but not in others.[41,48,49,69] In our series, a male:female ratio of 1.5:1 was observed.

Chondrosarcomas have a narrower age range than do chordomas (the age range in our series was 27 to 57 years), the most common age groups being the third and fourth decades of life. A strong male:female ratio is common,[27,33,37] being 3.7:1 in our series.

Tumor Location

We classify the cranial involvement of chordomas and chondrosarcomas as extradural, intradural, or extra- and intradural. Purely intradural lesions are rare, and are seen only with chordomas.

The tumor origin may involve the upper, middle, and lower clival regions, petrous apex and bone, cavernous sinus, foramen magnum, and sphenoethmoidal areas (Fig. 151-1). Each region has its distinct set of surgical problems. For instance, upper clival and sphenoidal lesions frequently involve the cavernous sinuses, and bilateral involvement may be seen. Lower clival and foramen magnum lesions may present with a significant retropharyngeal mass, and may also involve the occipital condyles and the extradural portions of the vertebral arteries. The greatest difficulty is experienced when an intradural tumor invades the brain stem or encases the basilar artery or its branches. Intra- and extradural tumors present the potential problem of cerebrospinal fluid communication to the exterior, once the tumor is excised.

Clinical Presentation

Despite the large size of these tumors, patients usually have minimal symptoms because of the slow growth of the tumor. Most patients present with headaches and diplopia (Table 151-1).[20,34,37,39,49,53,54] The most common finding on examination is abducens paresis or palsy. Less common symptoms include those referable to other cranial nerves such as hearing loss, dysphagia, dysarthria, and facial numbness, as well as symptoms of brain stem or cerebellar compression such as dysmetria, gait ataxia, motor weakness, and memory problems.

Patients may experience symptoms because of local tumor extension into the retropharyngeal area or nasal cavity (dysphagia or nasal obstruction). Patients with bilateral occipital condyle erosion by tumor may experience severe headaches and neck pain due to atlanto-occipital instability.

Radiologic Diagnosis and Evaluation

Plain skull films now are rarely used for diagnosis. However, if obtained incidentally, they may show areas of bone destruction and calcification.

Computed tomography (CT) scans without contrast enhancement reveal a lesion which is isodense with brain, with foci of calcification in 30 to 47 percent of cases. Bone-windowed CT shows areas of bone destruction and other important features of skull base anatomy. Contrast enhancement to a varying degree is always present.[7,37,39,46]

Magnetic resonance imaging (MRI) is most important for precise delineation of the extent of the tumor, the accompanying changes in the brain, and the involvement of blood vessels.[7,10,44,50,69] Chordomas are mostly isointense, and occasionally hypointense, on T1-weighted images. T2-weighted images show bright hyperintensity. The tumors enhance brightly with gadolinium. Fat suppression imaging is useful to distinguish chordomas from surrounding clival bone marrow.

Although a midline tumor is more likely to be a chordoma and a paramedian tumor is more likely to be a chondrosarcoma, the tumors cannot be clearly distinguished on the basis of radiologic

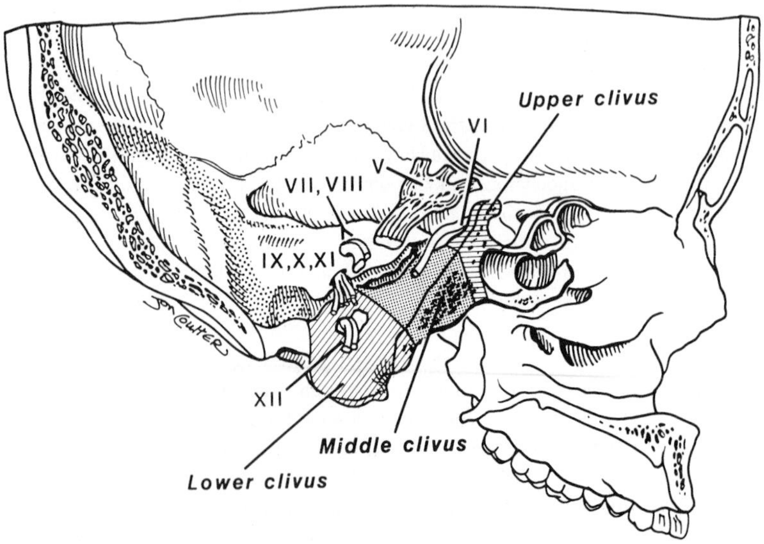

Figure 151-1 The anatomic division of the clivus into upper, middle, and lower legions is shown (From Sekhar et al.,[59] with permission).

TABLE 151-1 Presenting Symptoms and Signs in 64 Patients with Chordomas and Chondrosarcomas

Symptoms		Number (%)
Double vision		37 (58)
Headache		36 (56)
Hoarseness/Dysphagia		24 (38)
Facial numbness/Pain		20 (31)
Ptosis		11 (17)
Hearing loss/Vertigo		10 (16)
Facial paresis		9 (14)
Visual loss		8 (13)
General decline of functional status		7 (11)
Signs		**Number (%)**
Cranial nerve disorders:	VI	29 (45)
	V	19 (30)
	III	17 (27)
	IX–X	13 (20)
	XII	11 (17)
	VIII	10 (16)
	VII	9 (14)
	II	8 (13)
	Other CNs	<10%
Gait disturbance		11 (17)
Weakness, lower & upper limb		4 (6)

findings.[16] Lesions which are considered in the differential diagnosis include schwannoma, pituitary adenoma, adenoid cystic carcinoma, and other tumors arising from the basicranium such as chondromyxoma.[73]

Arteriography and Balloon Occlusion Test

If an operation is planned, cerebral angiography is important for large and giant-sized tumors to evaluate the status of the blood vessels and the collateral circulation. Balloon occlusion testing of the internal carotid artery (ICA) is important if the artery may need to be excised as part of the tumor resection.[24] For tumors near the jugular foramen or the clival area, evaluation of the vein of Labbé, and of the size and communication of the sigmoid sinuses is important.

Review of Natural History and Older Treatment Series

In the past, patients with nontreated chordomas had an average survival time of 0.6 to 2 years.[26,34,37] However, many of the lesions encountered in earlier years were already large at diagnosis; this must be taken into account in considering their poor natural history. Some patients may live for many years, even with growing tumors. For this reason, the quality of life of these patients is a very important consideration, in addition to disease-free survival.

In a series of 155 patients, Heffelfinger et al. demonstrated a 5.2-year average survival for chordoma patients treated by partial operative resection and radiotherapy, 4.8 years after radiotherapy alone, and 1.5 years after partial resection alone.[34] Other series have demonstrated poor survival rates of 51 percent at 5 years, and 35 percent at 10 years, after subtotal or partial tumor resection followed by radiotherapy.[19,29,34] Because recurrence of tumor is the major cause of death, "recurrence-free" survival is an important indicator of the efficacy of treatment.[27] When such "recurrence-free" survival is considered, 5- and 10-year survival rates fall to 33 and 20 percent, respectively.[29,30]

Classic chondrosarcomas have a better prognosis than do chordomas. Five-year survival rates are 90, 81, and 43 percent for grades I, II, and III lesions, respectively.[27] Mesenchymal and dedifferentiated chondrosarcomas have a poorer prognosis.

Treatment

Chemotherapy

Although some authors have reported the subjective improvement of patients with chordomas treated with a soft tissue sarcoma protocol or an osteogenic sarcoma protocol, effective chemotherapy is not yet available.[28,30] However, for patients who have failed both surgery and radiation therapy, and whose histologic findings reflect high mitotic rates and poor differentiation, chemotherapy can be tried as a last resort.

Radiotherapy

The efficacy of external beam irradiation on chordomas is questionable. The tumor is radiosensitive, but requires very high doses, in the range of 70 to 80 Gy. However, such high doses have a high risk of producing radiation necrosis.

A number of reports have been published regarding external beam radiotherapy for chordomas, but the results have generally been disappointing.[1,5,19,20,30,32,38,41,51,54,68] Doses in the range of 50 to 70 Gy have been administered. A recent report from the Mayo Clinic demonstrated, in a large series, that postoperative radiotherapy with external beam sources does not improve the survival time, but does significantly prolong disease-free survival.[29]

Because of this, several high-energy radiation sources have been tried in their treatment. Sources such as radioactive radon, iodine, and yttrium have been implanted stereotactically or microsurgically. However, because of the high incidence of local complications, these techniques have not become popular.[40,42,74]

Radiosurgery with the Leksell Gamma Knife or linear accelerator is an attractive way to treat small chordomas and chondrosarcomas.[40] When treated with the Gamma Knife, doses to the tumor and margins in the order of 20 Gy are typically administered. Long-term results are not yet available. However, because of the large size of the tumors, their irregular shape, and the poor delineation of tumor margins even with MRI, it is reasonable to assume that radiosurgery as the sole treatment is likely to fail. However, when small remnants remain after microsurgery, radiosurgery is an attractive adjuvant therapy because of the minimal effect on adjacent neural structures, and the short duration of treatment.

Proton beam radiotherapy uses charged particles which have a Bragg peak. This allows high radiation doses to be given to the tumor, with acceptable normal tissue doses. By fashioning a mold around the patient's head, the head is held in a fixed position during the treatment sessions. The total treatment is provided over several weeks, and the doses range from 50 to 75 cobalt Gy equivalents. Computerized three-dimensional planning has improved the results.[70] Applied after adequate debulking of tumor, this treatment leads to an overall local control rate of 76 percent at 5 years. Two hundred nine patients were treated at the Massachusetts General Hospital through December 1991, with a median follow-up of 48 months (range = 2 to 222 months). The results were better for chondrosarcomas (95 percent recurrence-free survival at 5 years), than for chordomas (63 percent recurrence-free survival at 5 years)[4,6,48] Tumor volume is a significant prognostic factor for local failure, so that adequate tumor debulking is important for success. A 34 percent complication rate has been described, consisting of endocrine, hearing, and visual problems, as well as brain injury, seizures, and radionecrosis.[48] High-energy irradiation with helium ions has also been used for these tumors, but long-term results are not available.[6] It must be kept in mind that since proton beam or helium ion radiotherapy is administered after surgical resection of tumor, several selection biases are introduced, and it is impossible to compare the results with purely surgical series. Many factors such as the size of the tumor, prior treatment, etc., introduce biases in this sort of comparison.

Chondrosarcomas are probably more radiosensitive than chordomas, even to external beam radiotherapy. Patients with skull base chondrosarcomas seem to have a consistently better survival than those with chordomas, following radiotherapy.

Surgical Resection

Because the tumors remain confined to the cranial base area for a long time and most recurrences are local, it is rational to assume that extensive surgical resection may provide long-term disease-free survival, and even a cure of these tumors. However, such resections have not been available in the past because the surgical techniques used to remove these tumors were in their infancy.

The majority of authors agree that surgical resection is important for a good outcome.[3,9,15,17,18,23,29,33,35,38,41,43,48,49,52,62,63,72] Some authors have reported success in removing the tumors totally, with disease-free control of tumor.[13,22,23,31,43,62]

Operative Approaches

Several operative approaches have been used to remove chordomas and chondrosarcomas (Table 151-2). To a large extent, the choice of the approach depends upon the location of the tumor and the experience and personal preference of the surgeon. The approaches may be broadly divided into three categories: anterior approaches, anterolateral approaches, and posterolateral approaches. These are summarized in Table 151-2.

In general, we have not preferred many of the anterior approaches because of the limited exposure achieved and the poor ability to reconstruct the skull base in the event of a large dural fistula at the end of the operation. However, we use the extended subfrontal approach frequently, and the extended maxillotomy approach is of value. The trans-sphenoidal and transethmoidal approaches are useful as adjuncts to other approaches or for diagnostic purposes. The transoral approach has a limited use for chordomas because of the limited lateral reach. However, palliative operations or conservative resections in older patients can be performed through this approach.

The *frontotemporal transcavernous approach* is necessary when the tumor involves the cavernous sinus extensively (Fig. 151-2). In some instances, the cavernous sinus is only compressed by the tumor; in other cases, the cavernous sinus is actually invaded, and the intracavernous portion of the ICA may be displaced or even encased by the tumor (Figs. 151-3 and 151-4). As the bony origin of such tumors still lies in the petrous bone or the sphenoid bone, the abnormal bone needs to be resected extensively in order to remove the tumor completely. During these operations, the tumor is exposed by a frontotemporal craniotomy combined with an orbitozygomatic osteotomy. Proximal control of the ICA is secured in the cervical segment. The cavernous sinus is opened at the most prominently bulging area, usually between cranial nerves (CNs) IV, V_1, V_2, and V_3, to remove the tumor. Extensive dissection of CN III is not necessary and is in fact avoided. Tumor removal from inside the cavernous sinus is easily performed. However, venous bleeding may obscure small islands of tumor (which frequently infiltrates venous spaces). The intracavernous ICA usually can be preserved by dissection from tumor. In our experience, vein graft replacement of the intracavernous ICA was necessary in only two patients (Fig. 151-5). After the removal of the tumor from the petrous bone and the sphenoid bone, the dead spaces need to be obliterated with autologous fat, and covered with vascularized tissue such as a pericranial flap or a temporalis muscle flap. The dural defect in the skull base area will have to be closed with a graft, which is secured with microsutures and with fibrin glue.

The *subtemporal, transpetrous apex, and transcavernous approach* is essential for tumors which arise from the region of the upper clivus (Fig. 151-6). Such tumors usually invade the clival dura, and one or both cavernous sinuses in their posterior regions. The brain stem is frequently compressed severely and may even be invaded. During the operation, a temporal craniotomy is combined with a zygomatic osteotomy (including the condylar fossa), and the roof of the bony ear canal is also removed, if necessary, to achieve a low exposure. The standard subtemporal exposure is enlarged by the opening of the posterior cavernous sinus and the intradural resection of the petrous apex area; these maneuvers get the surgeon as low as the abducens nerves. In this fashion, both the upper and lower poles of the tumor are exposed, and tumor resection is performed in the usual fashion. An extensive dural defect is frequently created after the resection of the tumor, and the dura must be reconstructed by means of a fascia lata graft. The advantage of this approach is that the brain stem, the vertebrobasilar vessels, and the cranial nerves can be seen and separated from the tumor under direct vision. The disadvantage is that if the sphenoclival bone is extremely involved by the tumor, it cannot be removed by this approach, but requires a separate, second operation via an extended subfrontal or trans-sphenoidal approach (Fig. 151-7).

The *extended subfrontal approach* is well suited for midline tumors that involve the sphenoethmoidal and upper and middle clival areas.[56,66] The dorsum sellae is a blind spot with this approach. Tumor extension into the medial aspects of the cavernous sinuses, into both petrous apices, and into the lower clivus (as low

TABLE 151-2 Operative Approaches to Chordomas and Chondrosarcomas

Anterior Approaches
Extended subfrontal (modified transbasal)
Transethmoidal
Maxillotomy and extended maxillotomy
Trans-sphenoidal and extended trans-sphenoidal
Transoral
Anterolateral Approaches
Frontotemporal, transcavernous
Subtemporal, transpetrous apex, and transcavernous
Subtemporal-infratemporal
Lateral and Posterolateral Approaches
Presigmoid petrosal, retrolabyrinthine or partial translabyrinthine
Extreme lateral, transcondylar

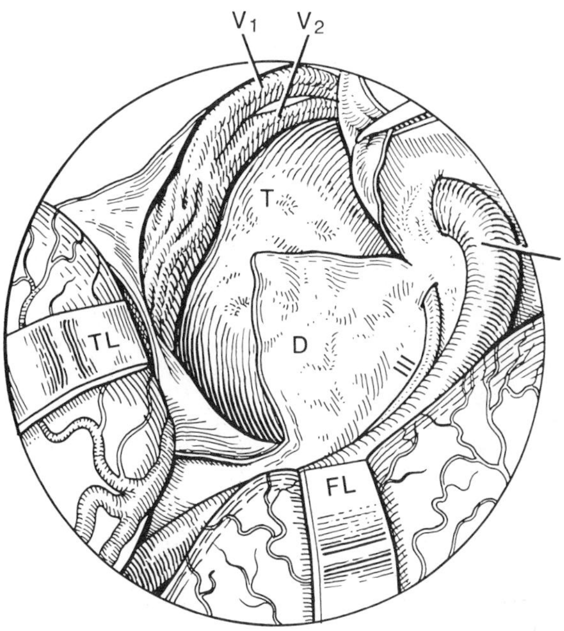

(*A*)

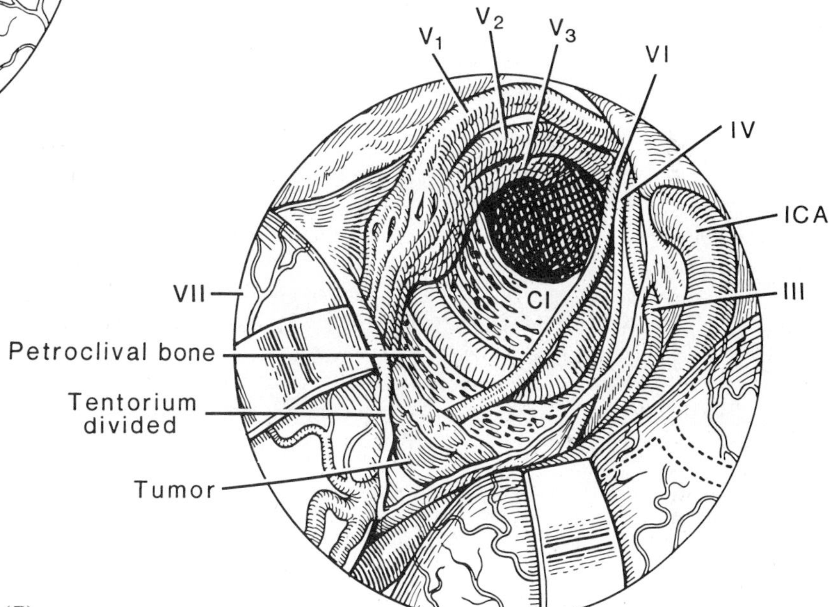

(*B*)

Figure 151-2 The frontotemporal transcavernous approach to an intracavernous chordoma or chondrosarcoma. *A*. The initial tumor exposure is shown. *B*. The appearance after tumor resection is demonstrated. Cl, clivus; D, dura mater; TL, temporal lobe; ICA, internal carotid artery; T, tumor; FL, frontal lobe; III, IV, V_1, V_2, V_3, VI, VII, cranial nerves. (From Sekhar et al.,[57] with permission).

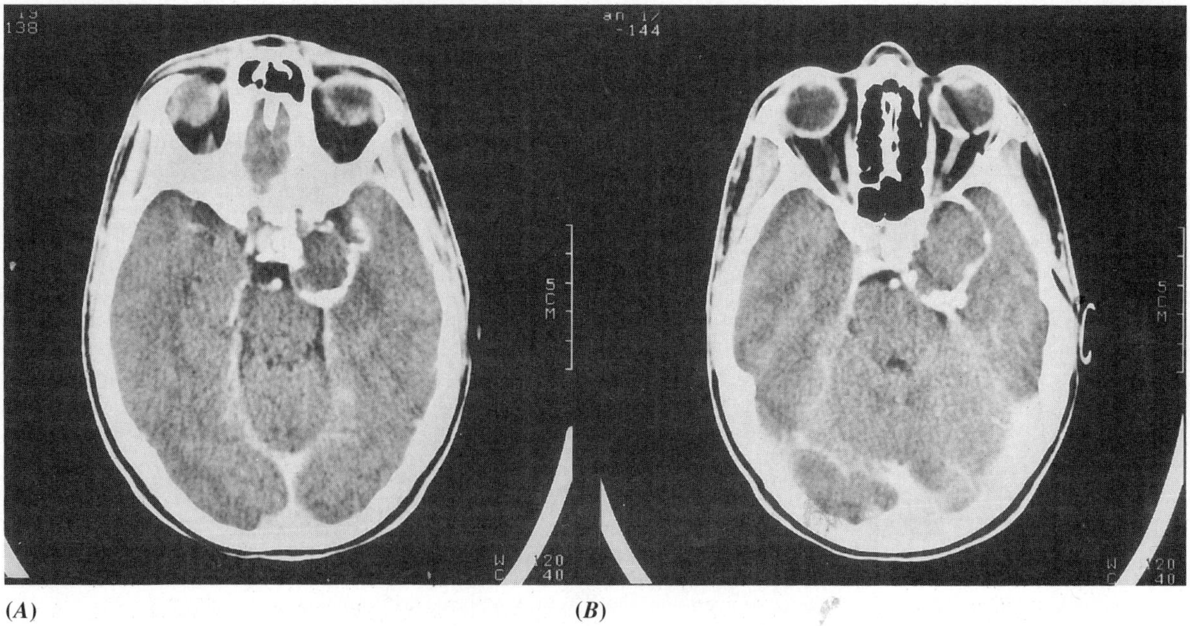

(*A*) (*B*)

Figure 151-3 Axial CT scans of a 38-year-old patient with a recurrent low-grade chondrosarcoma involving the left cavernous sinus and the sphenoid bone reveals multiple areas of calcification.

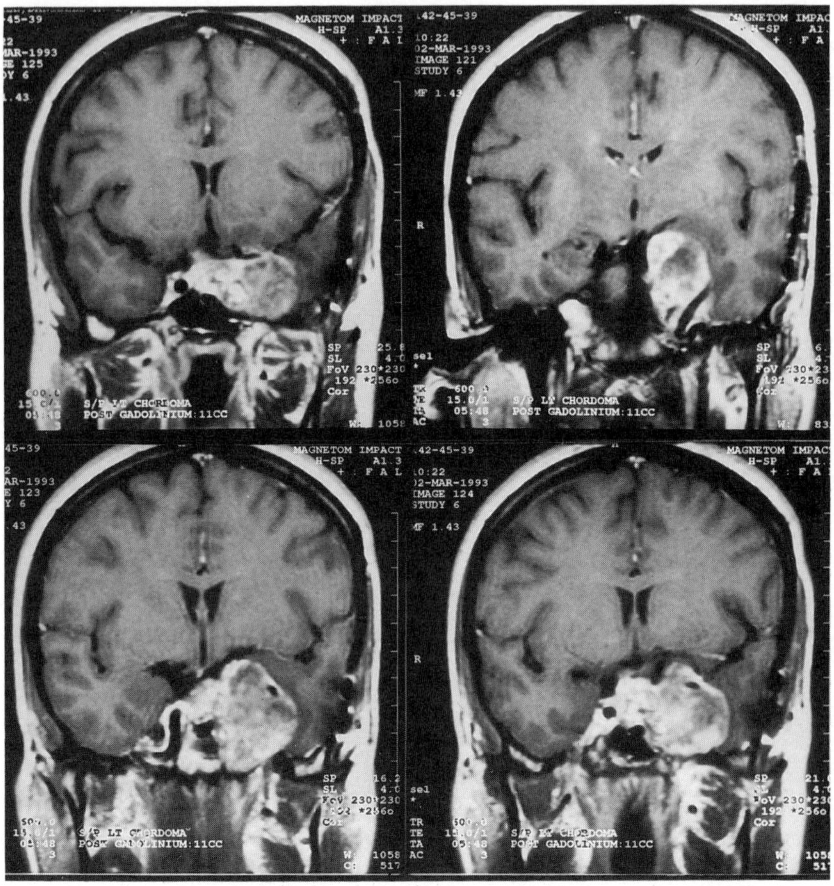

Figure 151-4 Coronal MRI views of the patient shown in Fig. 151-3 reveal a tumor arising from the sphenoid bone and the dorsum sellae and involving the ICA. The intracavernous portion of the ICA is encased and narrowed by the tumor.

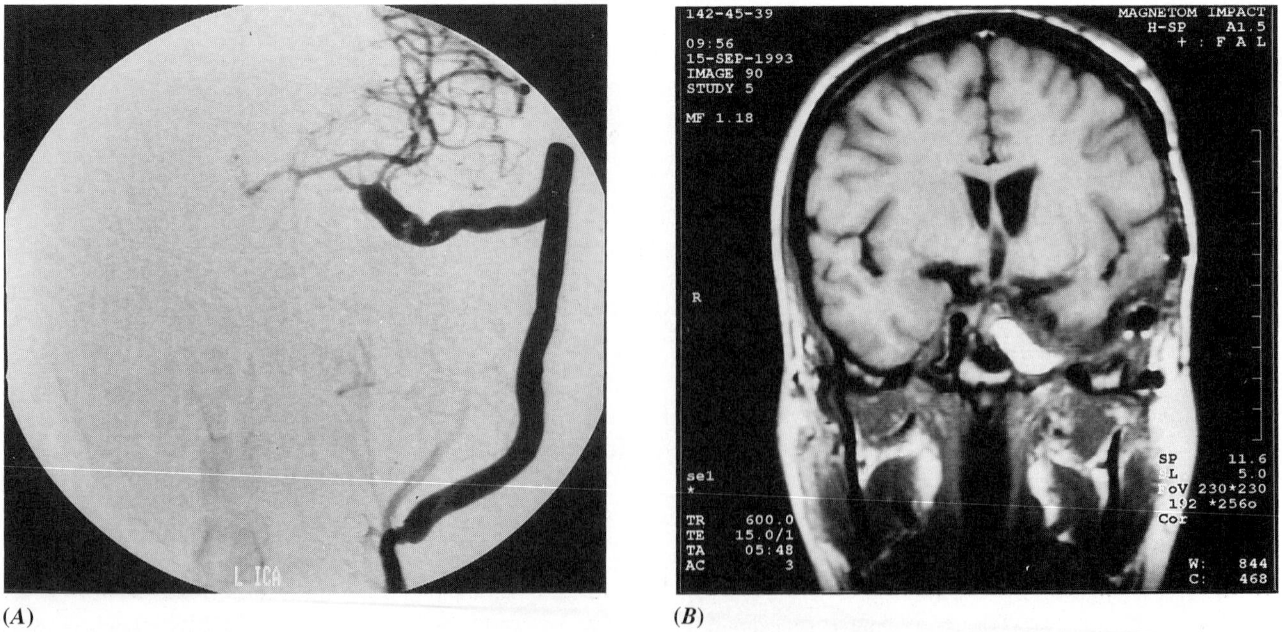

(*A*) (*B*)

Figure 151-5 This patient's tumor was removed in two stages. Because of the encasement of the intracavernous ICA and scar from the prior operation, the ICA was replaced with a vein graft from the cervical ICA to the middle cerebral artery, seen in the postoperative angiogram (*A*). The tumor was removed in a second operation via the frontotemporal transcavernous approach, as seen in the postoperative MRI scan (*B*). This coronal scan also demonstrates the fat and fascia used to reconstruct the cavernous sinus, after tumor resection.

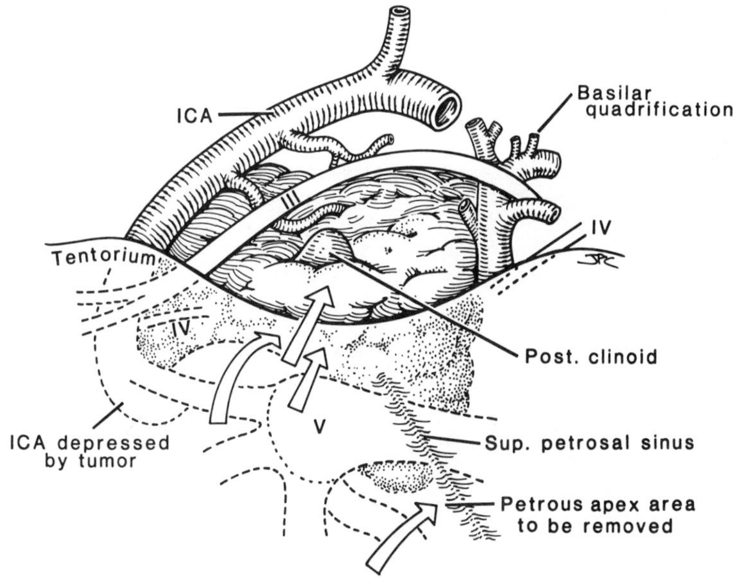

(*A*)

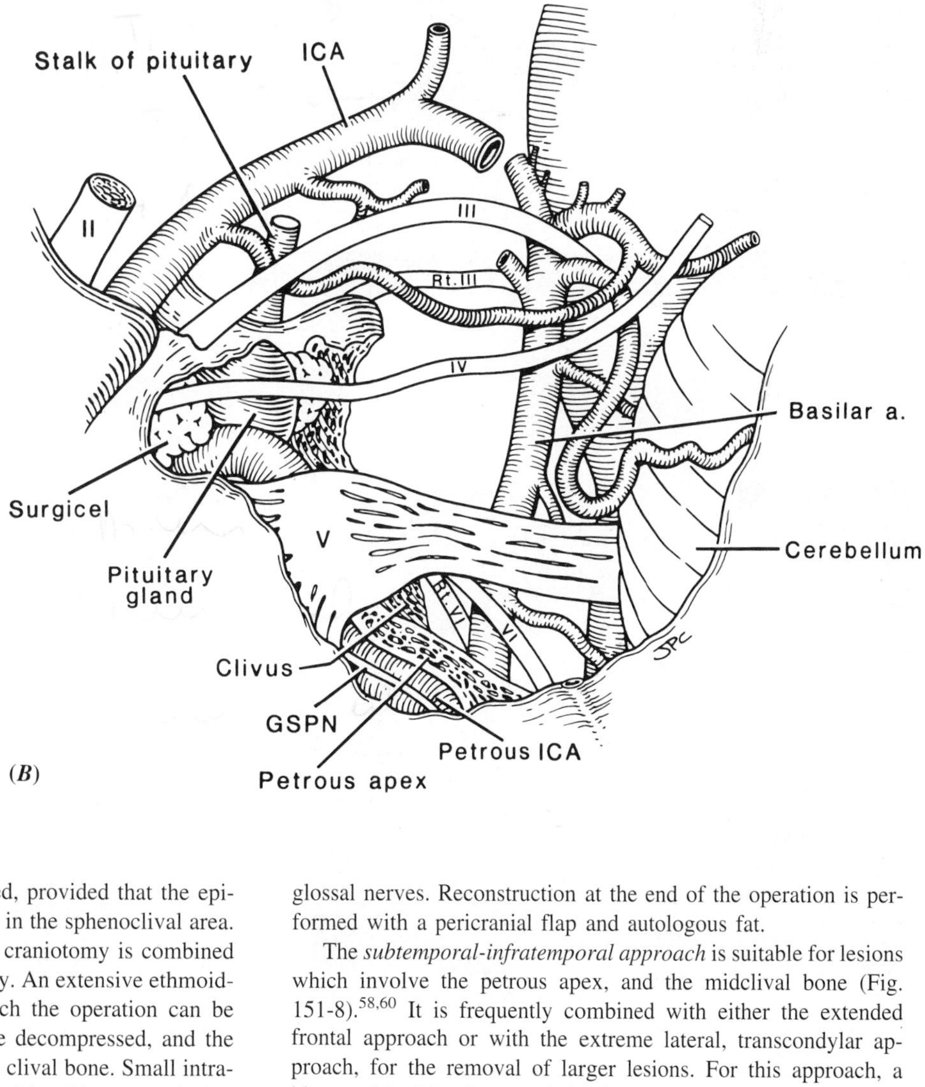

(*B*)

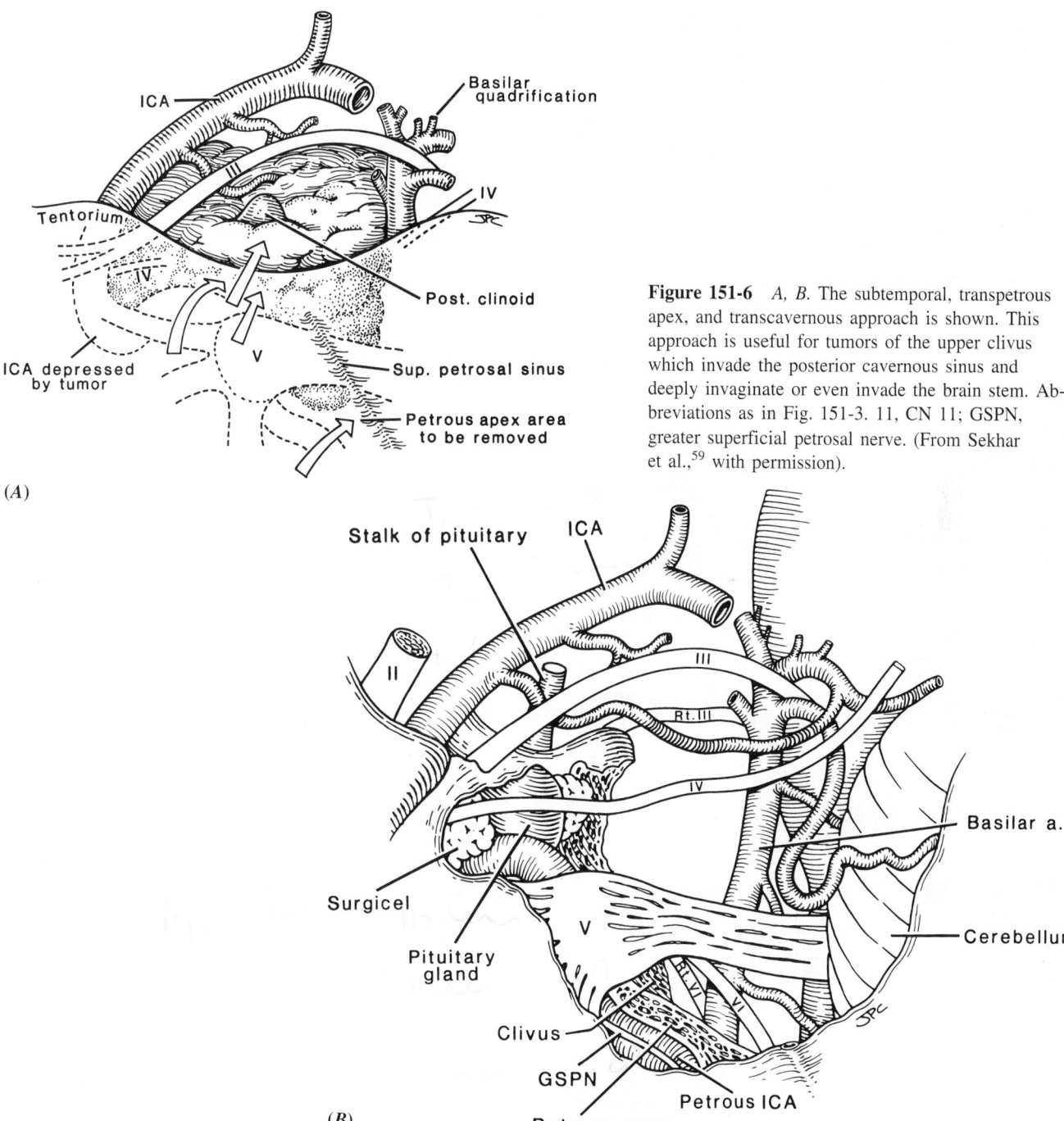

Figure 151-6 *A, B.* The subtemporal, transpetrous apex, and transcavernous approach is shown. This approach is useful for tumors of the upper clivus which invade the posterior cavernous sinus and deeply invaginate or even invade the brain stem. Abbreviations as in Fig. 151-3. 11, CN 11; GSPN, greater superficial petrosal nerve. (From Sekhar et al.,[59] with permission).

as the foramen magnum) can be removed, provided that the epicenter of the tumor is in the midline, and in the sphenoclival area. During this operation, a bilateral frontal craniotomy is combined with an orbitofrontal-ethmoidal osteotomy. An extensive ethmoidectomy enlarges the space through which the operation can be performed. One or both optic nerves are decompressed, and the tumor is dissected progressively from the clival bone. Small intradural extensions of tumor can be removed by this approach, but large intradural extensions cannot be removed safely. Dural defects are reconstructed by means of a fascia lata graft. By angling the microscope appropriately, and by rotating the patient's head or the patient from side to side, tumor removal can be performed laterally to the petrous apices, the abducens nerves, and the hypoglossal nerves. Reconstruction at the end of the operation is performed with a pericranial flap and autologous fat.

The *subtemporal-infratemporal approach* is suitable for lesions which involve the petrous apex, and the midclival bone (Fig. 151-8).[58,60] It is frequently combined with either the extended frontal approach or with the extreme lateral, transcondylar approach, for the removal of larger lesions. For this approach, a bicoronal incision is extended inferiorly into the preauricular region, and all the soft tissues in front of the ear—including the parotid gland, upper branches of the facial nerve, and the superficial temporal artery—are elevated from the masseter muscle. A temporal craniotomy is followed by a zygomatic osteotomy, including the condylar fossa. A subtemporal craniectomy is

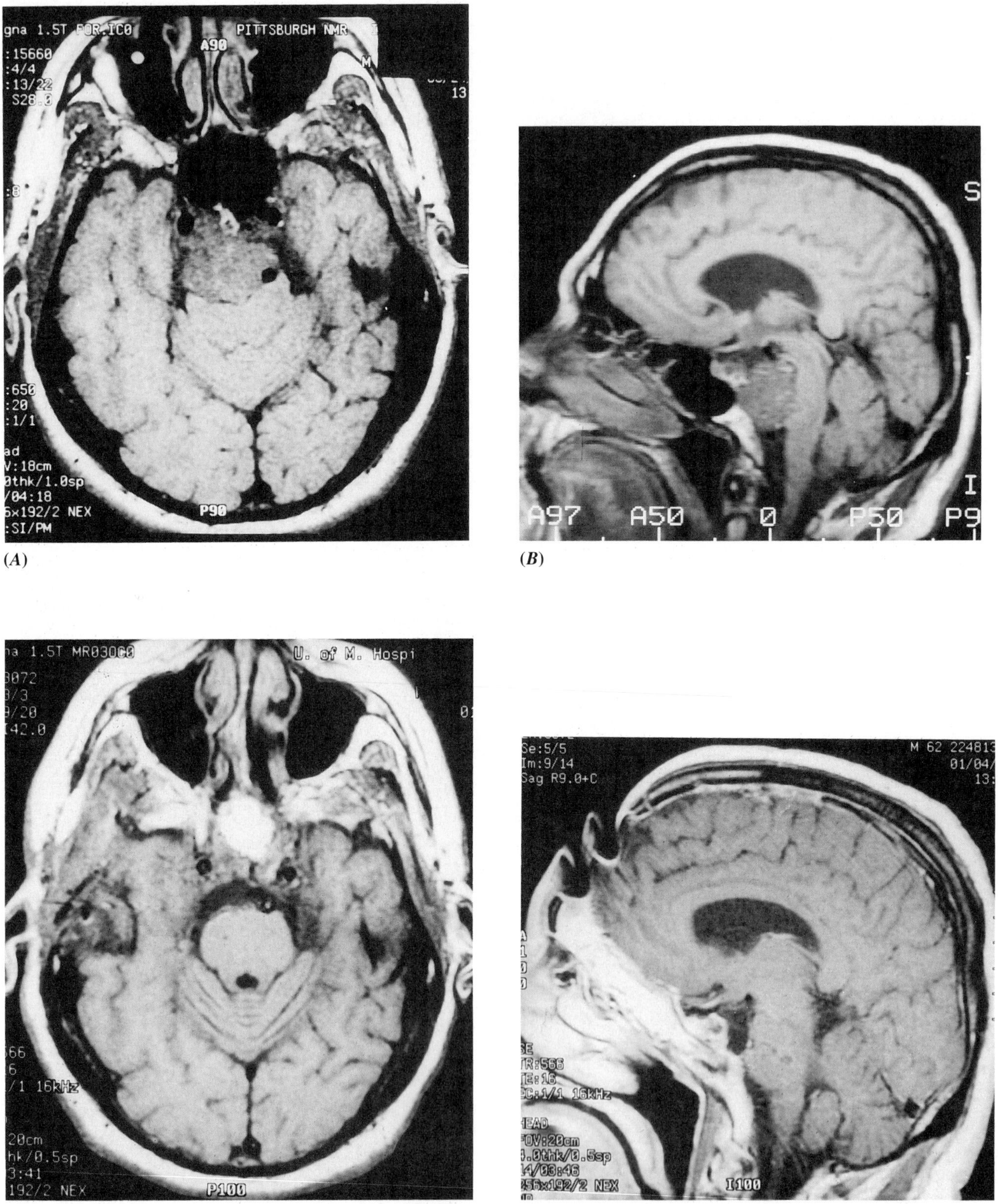

(*A*) (*B*) (*C*) (*D*)

Figure 151-7 Nonenhanced axial (*A*) and sagittal (*B*) MRI scans of a 62-year-old patient with a large upper clival chordoma with invasion of the cavernous sinus. He presented with abducens paresis. The tumor was removed via the extended frontal approach initially, followed by a subtemporal, transzygomatic, transpetrous apex, and transcavernous approach. The postoperative nonenhanced axial MRI scan (*C*) demonstrates fat and fascia in the tumor bed and sphenoid sinus. The enhanced sagittal MRI scan (*D*) shows the absence of tumor, and the enhancement due to the flaps.

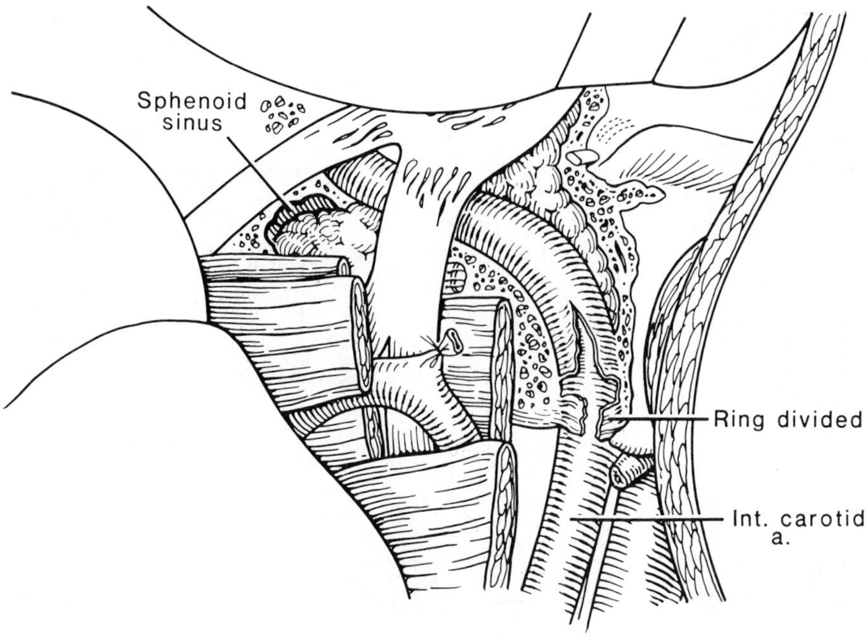

(*A*)

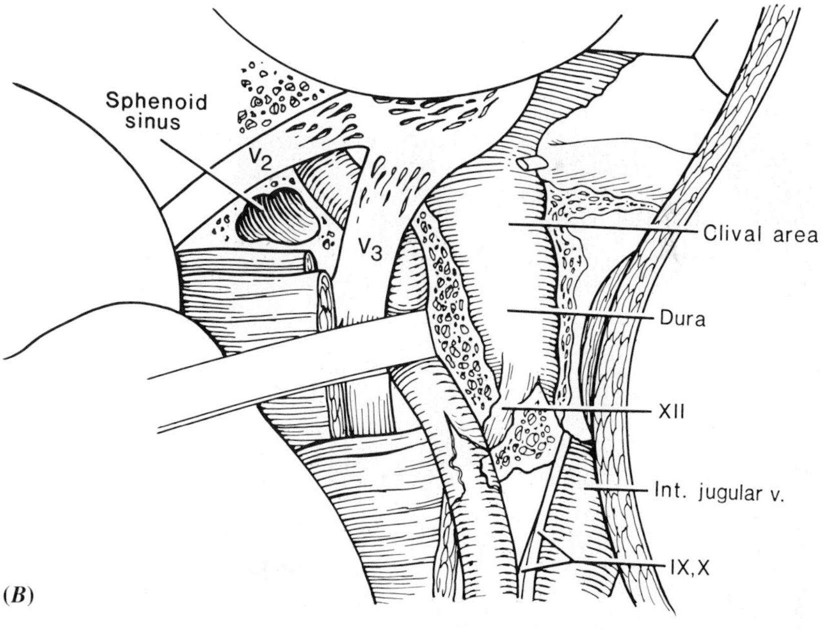

(*B*)

Figure 151-8 The subtemporal and infratemporal approach is shown in these figures. The exposure of the tumor is shown in *A* and the appearance after tumor resection is demonstrated in *B*. (From Sekhar et al.,[59] with permission).

performed, and is followed by unroofing the middle meningeal artery and the foramina ovale and rotundum. The greater superficial petrosal nerve is identified and sectioned. The petrous portion of the ICA is then completely unroofed from the upper cervical segment to the point where it enters the cavernous sinus, medial to the trigeminal ganglion. The eustachian tube has to be interrupted for this exposure, and its ends are closed with fat and sutures to prevent cerebrospinal fluid leakage. The petrous ICA is then mobilized forward from its canal, and the tumor which lies medial to the ICA is removed from the petroclival bone and the lateral aspect of the sphenoid bone. Reconstruction is done with autologous fat and a portion of the temporalis muscle (Fig. 151-9).

The *petrosal approach,* with or without partial labyrinthectomy, is rarely needed for chordomas or chondrosarcomas. However, tumors with considerable intradural extension, and with significant compression of the brain stem, will require this approach. For this operation, a mastoidectomy is performed, with unroofing of the labyrinth and the sigmoid sinus. A temporal craniotomy and a small retrosigmoid craniectomy are then performed. If more space is needed, the root of the zygoma and the bony roof of the external ear canal can be removed. The bony shell of the superior and posterior semicircular canals can be removed, with the preservation of hearing. The petrous apex bone can also be resected. All of these maneuvers increase the space available to work, while minimizing brain retraction. The presigmoid and temporal dura are opened, and the tentorium is divided, after ligation of the superior petrosal sinus. It is important to open the Meckel's cave in order to mobilize the trigeminal root. Tumor removal then proceeds with minimal retraction of the temporal lobe and cerebellum. At the end of the operation, dural closure is performed with a

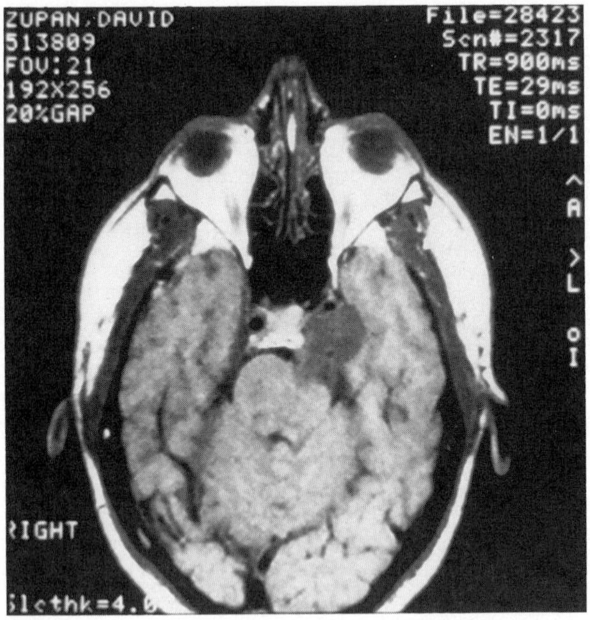

(*A*)

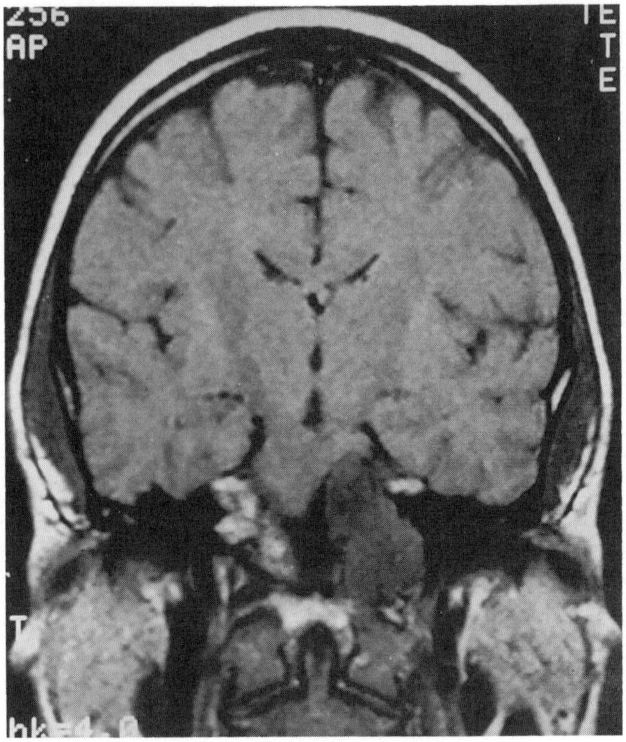

(*B*)

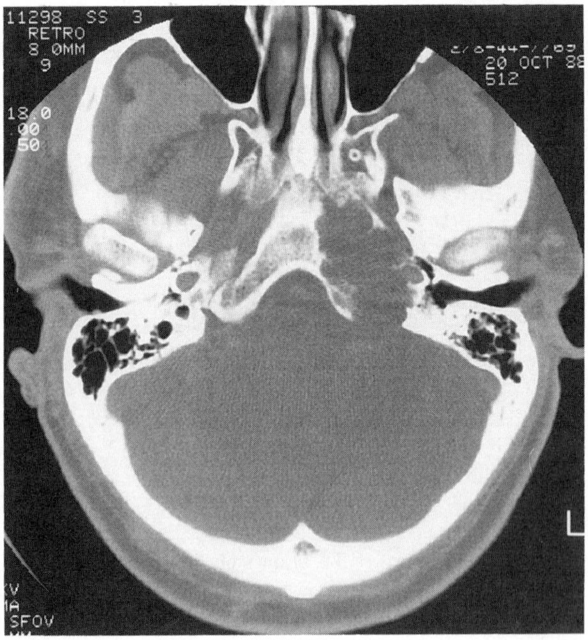

(*C*)

Figure 151-9 These axial (*A*) and coronal (*B*) MRI scans of a 33-year-old patient show a petroclival chondrosarcoma with extension into the posterior cavernous sinus. *C*. This bone windowed CT shows erosion of the petroclival bone. The tumor was resected completely via a subtemporal-infratemporal and transcavernous approach. No tumor regrowth was seen on follow-up for 4 years. (From Sekhar et al.[59] with permission).

fasica lata graft, and the mastoidectomy defect is obliterated with autologous fat. The middle ear is frequently packed gently with oxidized cellulose and fibrin glue, to provide a temporary seal against cerebrospinal fluid leakage.

The *extreme lateral, transcondylar approach* is suitable for lesions of the lower clivus, with extension into the occipital condyle, and even into the C1–C2 area.[61] This can be combined with an occiput to C1–C2 fusion, if complete resection of one or both condyles is necessary (Fig. 151-10). During this operation, the mastoid and retromastoid bone are exposed, and the lateral masses of C1 and C2 are exposed. The vertebral artery is exposed from the C2 transverse foramen to the dural entrance point. A mastoidectomy is performed, unroofing the sigmoid sinus and the posterior portion of the jugular bulb. A small retrosigmoid craniectomy, including the rim of the foramen magnum, is performed. The vertebral artery is displaced posteromedially after the C1 transverse foramen is opened. The dura mater is opened in the retrosigmoid area to permit inspection of the region medial to CNs IX–XII,

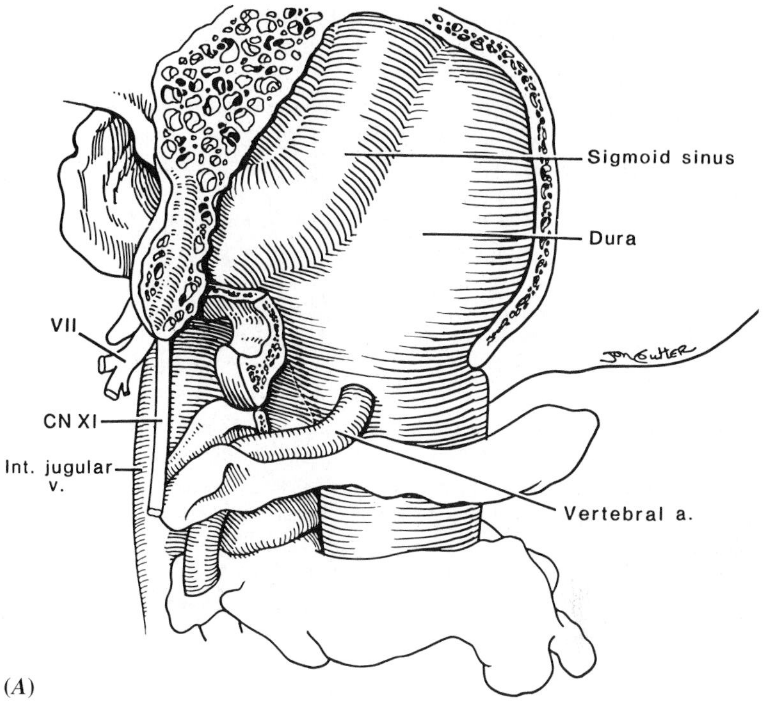

(*A*)

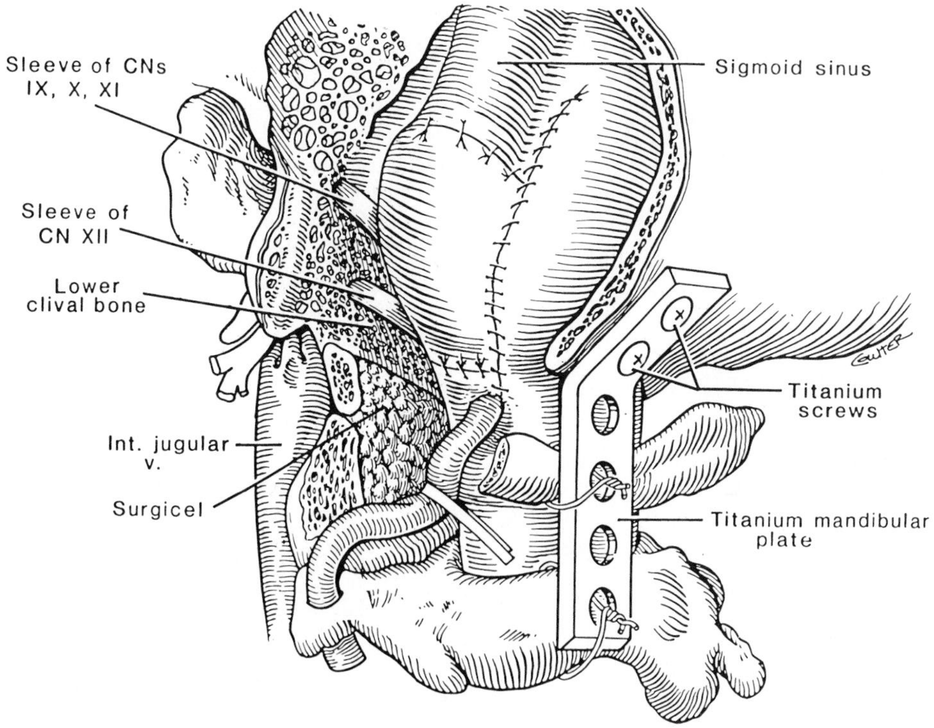

(*B*)

Figure 151-10 These figures illustrate the extreme lateral transcondylar approach. *A*. The vertebral artery has been exposed extradurally. A mastoidectomy and retrosigmoid craniectomy have been performed. *B*. The tumor has been removed after ligation of an invaded sigmoid sinus and the jugular bulb. The tumor-invaded occipital condyle has been resected and an occiput to C1, C2 fusion has been performed. (From Sekhar et al.,[59] with permission).

because tumor invasion may occur through this area. Extradural tumor resection is performed by working through the occipital condyle and the lateral mass of C1. If the sigmoid sinus is occluded, the surgeon can work through the occluded sinus and the jugular bulb, dissecting and carefully preserving CNs IX–XII. If both occipital condyles are involved by the tumor, tumor removal is performed in a staged fashion, after an occiput to C2–C3 fusion has been performed.

General Principles of Tumor Resection

The core of these tumors is generally easy to remove, since it is soft and cartilaginous or gelatinous. Occasionally, chondrosarcomas may be heavily calcified or even ossified. Such tumors may have to be removed piecemeal, with the use of rongeurs or even a high-speed drill. The use of a high-speed drill has made the removal of these tumors much easier, since the lesion can be removed with a light touch, which reduces the chances of the drill slipping and injuring critical structures.

After removal of the core of the tumor, the tumor-involved bony margins have to be removed until normal-looking bone marrow or venous channels in the bone are reached. These tumors appear to infiltrate the cancellous bone of the petroclival area well beyond the cortical clival bone. The hard bone of the otic capsule also seems to be resistant to tumor invasion. During surgery, it is difficult to be certain of the tumor margins, since frozen section of bone margins is not possible. At present, MRI is the most sensitive tool for revealing the extent of the tumor. However, the actual areas of tumor invasion may extend beyond the margins revealed by imaging.

In removing intradural tumor, the surgeon needs to be particularly careful with encased perforating arteries, the adherent veins of the brain stem, and the invaginated brain stem itself. The arachnoid plane of the brain stem may be invaded. In such patients, the surgeon removes only what comes easily, because attempts to remove every piece of tumor may result in brain stem injury or hematoma. Invasion of the dura mater is not a contraindication to complete tumor resection. In such patients, the invaded dura mater is excised and fascia lata reconstruction is performed.

Operation on recurrent or previously irradiated tumors is more difficult because of the scar tissue and the microangiopathy of surrounding tissues which makes postoperative healing difficult. Such patients are more prone to develop postoperative CSF leaks. This is especially true of patients operated on previously through anterior approaches, which destroy normal mucosal and submucosal tissues. In such patients, we have learned that vascularized tissue flaps are important for reconstruction; microvascular flaps such as the rectus abdominis flap and the radial forearm flap are very useful.[36,64] Patients who have undergone prior operations may also develop hydrocephalus postoperatively, which may require CSF shunting. Our philosophy has been to attempt complete tumor removal whenever possible, using staged operations and multiple approaches, if necessary.

Patient Series

Sixty-four patients with chordomas and chondrosarcomas were operated on over a 9-year period at the University of Pittsburgh Hospitals and at the George Washington University Medical Center. Sixty patients were followed for at least 1 year.

Forty-seven patients had chordomas and 17 had chondrosarcomas, mostly low-grade. Fifty percent of the patients had been operated on previously. The patients' symptoms and signs are listed in Table 151-1. The location of the tumors is shown in Table 151-3. Ten patients with chordomas (21 percent) had been given radiotherapy. Tumor sizes were defined as small (<1 cm^3), medium (1–14 cm^3), large (15–84 cm^3), and giant (≥ 85 cm^3). The majority of tumors were large (68 percent), the next common sizes being giant (16 percent) and medium (14 percent).

Multiple staged operations were performed in 52 percent of the cases, the average of surgical procedures per patient being 1.9. Total resection or near-total resection was accomplished in 65 percent of the patients. Subtotal resection was performed in 24 percent, and partial resection in 10 percent of the patients.

The most frequent postoperative complication was cranial nerve palsy or paresis, occurring in 48 patients. The most frequent nerve to be affected was the trigeminal nerve; the eighth, seventh, and sixth cranial nerves were affected less frequently. Many CN disorders improved or recovered during follow-up. One-third to one-half of the preoperative CN disorders also recovered during follow-up.

TABLE 151-3 Areas Invaded by Tumor in 64 Patients

Area Invaded	Number (%)
Cavernous sinus	48 (75)
Clivus	59 (92)
Foramen magnum extension	15 (23)
Sphenoid sinus invasion	22 (34)
Sellar and suprasellar extension	19 (30)
Cerebellopontine angle and petrous bone	39 (61)
Orbit	4 (6)
Nasal-ethmoidal area	6 (9)
Nasopharynx	19 (30)

The most important complication was CSF leakage, occurring in 19 patients (30 percent). Six of these patients developed meningitis, and 11 were reoperated on to repair the fistula. Four patients (6 percent) had small, nonoperated, postoperative hematomas. Wound infection occurred in 5 percent. Three patients died within 3 months after the operation, two from pulmonary embolism and one from probable myocardial infarction.

There was no statistical difference between the preoperative Karnofsky score (84 $\pm$ 11, with a range of 60 to 100), and the postoperative Karnofsky score (82 $\pm$ 15). However, the occurrence of CSF leakage had an adverse effect on patients' functional status. Sixty-seven percent of the patients who suffered postoperative CSF leakage had a permanent decrease in the postoperative Karnofsky score ($p < 0.05$).

Seven patients (11 percent) developed tumor recurrence during the follow-up period that ranged from 1 to 9 years (median, 3 years). Five patients died because of the recurrence. The mean time to recurrence after surgery for these patients was only 1.9 years. One additional patient died of unrelated causes. Two patients with chondrosarcomas died from side effects of radiotherapy—one from radiation necrosis of the brain stem, and another because of a radiation-induced malignant glioma of the brain stem.

Survival analysis revealed that the recurrence-free survival for all patients was 80 percent at 3 years, and at 76 percent at 5 years, respectively (Fig. 151-11*A*). The survival was worse for patients with chordoma (5-year recurrence-free survival of 65 percent) than for those with chondrosarcoma (5-year recurrence-free survival of 90 percent) (Fig. 151-11*B*). There was also a big difference between previously operated patients (5-year recurrence-free survival of 64 percent) and previously nonoperated patients (5-year recurrence-free survival of 93 percent) (Fig. 151-12). Patients with total or near-total resection had a better 5-year recurrence-free survival rate (84 percent) than did patients with partial or subtotal resection (64 percent) ($p < 0.05$) (Fig. 151-13).

Conclusion

Chordomas and chondrosarcomas are a rare group of tumors that are difficult to eradicate. A number of advances have occurred in our ability to treat these lesions in recent years, including surgical

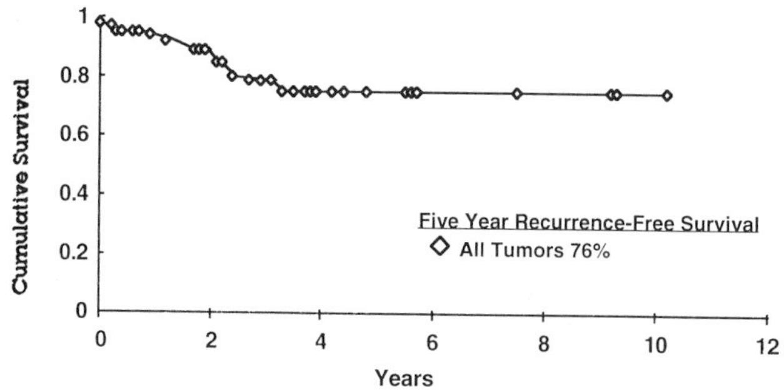

(*A*)

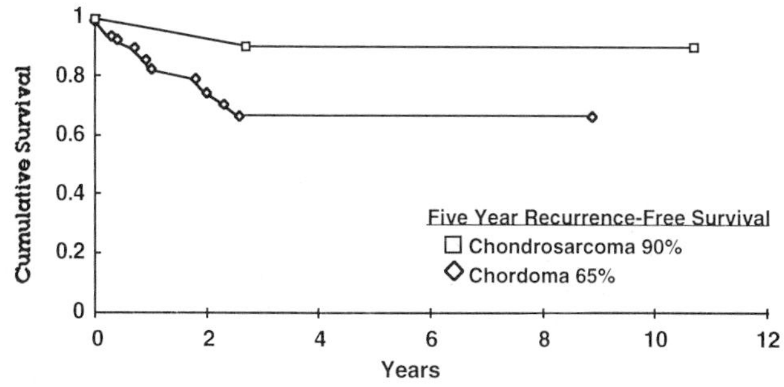

(*B*)

Figure 151-11 *A*. Five-year recurrence-free survival curve for all patients (all tumors) *B*. Five-year recurrence-free survival curves for patients with chondrosarcomas (90 percent) versus chordomas (65 percent).

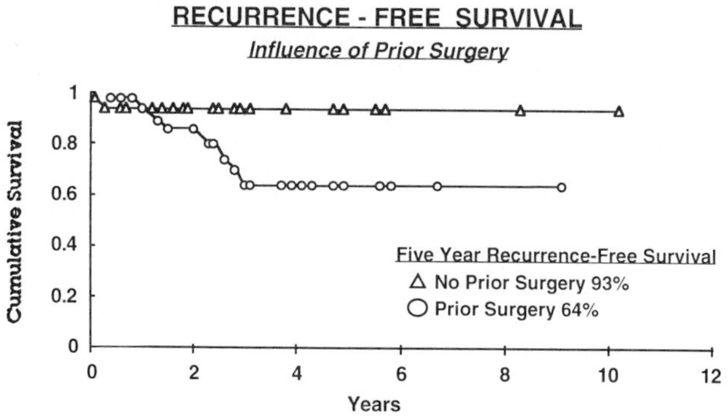

Figure 151-12 Five-year recurrence-free survival curves for patients who had undergone previous surgery (64 percent) and those who had not undergone previous surgery (93 percent).

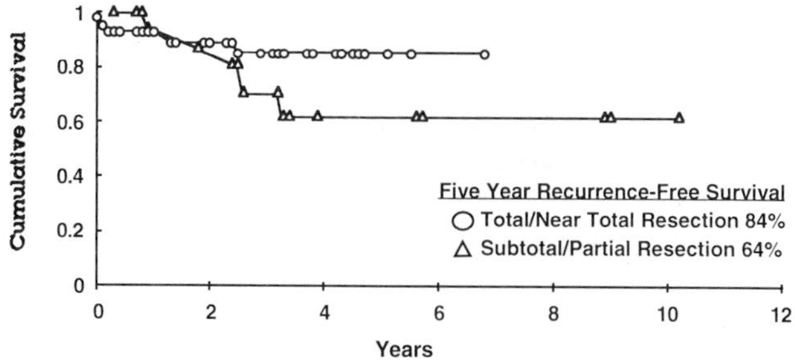

Figure 151-13 Five-year recurrence-free survival curves for patients who had underwent total or near-total resection (84 percent) and those who underwent subtotal or partial resection (64 percent).

advances that permit extensive tumor resection with minimal morbidity, and radiation therapy techniques that allow the delivery of high doses of radiation to the tumor, with minimal effects on surrounding brain. More extensive patient follow-up is necessary to determine whether these advances will produce improved long-term control of these tumors, or even cures. Further work in the molecular biology and genetics of these tumors is also necessary.[11,65]

References

1. Amendola BE, Amendola MA, Oliver E, McClatchey KD. Chordoma: role of radiation therapy. *Radiology* 1986; 158:839–843.
2. Ariel IM, Verdu C. Chordoma: an analysis of twenty cases treated over a twenty-year span. *J Surg Oncol* 1975; 7:27–44.
3. Arnold H, Herrmann HD. Skull base chordoma with cavernous sinus involvement. Partial or radical tumour-removal? *Acta Neurochir (Wien)* 1986; 83:31–37.
4. Austin-Seymour M, Munzenrider J, Goitein M, et al. Fractionated proton radiation therapy of chordoma and low-grade chondrosarcoma of the base of the skull. *J Neurosurg* 1989; 70:13–17.
5. Belza J. Double midline intracranial tumors of vestigial origin: contiguous intrasellar chordoma and suprasellar craniopharyngioma. Case report. *J Neurosurg* 1966; 25:199–204.
6. Berson AM, Castro JR, Petti P, et al. Charged particle irradiation of chordoma and chondrosarcoma of the base of skull and cervical spine: the Lawrence Berkeley Laboratory experience. *Int J Radiat Oncol Biol Phys* 1988; 15:559–565.
7. Bourgouin PM, Tampieri D, Robitaille Y, et al. Low-grade myxoid chondrosarcoma of the base of the skull: CT, MR, and histopathology. *J Comput Assist Tomogr* 1992; 16:268–273.
8. Bouropoulou V, Bosse A, Roessner A, et al. Immunohistochemical investigation of chordomas: histogenetic and differential diagnostic aspects. *Curr Top Pathol* 1989; 80:183–203.
9. Brooks JJ, LiVolsi VA, Trojanowski JQ. Does chondroid chordoma exist? *Acta Neuropathol (Berl)* 1987; 72:229–235.
10. Brown RV, Sage MR, Brophy BP. CT and MR findings in patients with chordomas of the petrous apex. *Am J Neuroradiol* 1990; 11:121–124.
11. Bushe KA, Naumann M, Warmuth-Metz M, et al. Maffuci's syndrome with bilateral cartilaginous tumors of the cerebellopontine angle. *Neurosurgery* 1990; 27:625–628.
12. Chambers PW, Schwinn CP. A clinicopathologic study of metastasis. *Am J Clin Pathol* 1979; 72:765–776.
13. Charabi S, Engel P, Bonding P. Myxoid tumours in the temporal bone. *J Laryngol Otol* 1989; 103:1206–1209.
14. Cianfriglia F, Ponpili A, Occhipinti E. Intracranial malignant cartilaginous tumours. Report of two cases and review of literature. *Acta Neurochir (Wien)* 1978; 45:163–175.
15. Cocke EW Jr, Robertson JH, Robertson JT, Crook JP. The extended maxillotomy and subtotal maxillectomy for excision of skull base tumors. *Arch Otolaryngol Head Neck Surg* 1990; 116:92–104.
16. Coltrera MD, Googe PB, Harrist TJ, et al. Chondrosarcoma of the temporal bone: diagnosis and treatment of 13 cases and review of the literature. *Cancer* 1986; 58:2689–2696.
17. Crockard HA. Transoral approach to intra/extradural tumors. In Sekhar LN, Janecka IP (eds): *Surgery of Cranial Base Tumors*. New York: Raven Press, 1993, pp 225–234.
18. Crockard HA. The transmaxillary approach to the clivus. In Sekhar LN, Janecka IP (eds): *Surgery of Cranial Base Tumors*. New York: Raven Press, 1993, pp 235–244.
19. Cummings BJ, Hodson DI, Bush RS. Chordoma: the results of megavoltage radiation therapy. *Int J Radiat Oncol Biol Phys* 1983; 9:633–642.

20. Dahlin DC, MacCarty CS. Chordoma: a study of fifty-nine cases. *Cancer* 1952; 5:1170–1178.
21. Dahlin DC, Unni KK. *Bone Tumors: General Aspects and Data on 8542 Cases,* 4th ed. Springfield, IL: Charles C Thomas, 1986, pp 244–267.
22. Derome P, Guiot G. Surgical approaches to the sphenoidal and clival areas. *Adv Tech Stand Neurosurg* 1979; 6:101–136.
23. Derome PJ, Visot A, Monteil JP, Maestro JL. Management of cranial chordomas. In Sekhar LN, Schramm VL Jr (eds): *Tumors of the Cranial Base: Diagnosis and Treatment.* Mount Kisco, NY: Futura 1987, pp 607–622.
24. Erba SM, Horton JA, Latchaw RE, et al. Balloon test occlusion of the internal carotid artery with stable xenon/CT cerebral blood flow imaging. *Am J Neuroradiol* 1988; 9:533–538.
25. Erbengi A, Tekkok IH, Acikgoz B. Posterior fossa chordomas—with special reference to transoral surgery. *Neurosurg Rev.* 1991; 14:23–28.
26. Eriksson B, Gunterberg B, Kindblom LG. Chordoma: a clinicopathologic and prognostic study of a Swedish national series. *Acta Orthop Scand* 1981; 52:49–58.
27. Evans HL, Ayala AG, Romsdahl MM. Prognostic factors in chondrosarcoma of bone. A clinicopathologic analysis with emphasis on histologic grading. *Cancer* 1977; 40:818–831.
28. Finn DG, Goepfert HG, Batsakis JG. Chondrosarcoma of the head and neck. *Laryngoscope* 1984; 94:1539–1544.
29. Forsyth PA, Cascino TL, Shaw EG, et al. Intracranial chordomas: a clinicopathological and prognostic study of 51 cases. *J Neurosurg* 1993; 78:741–747.
30. Fuller DB, Bloom JG. Radiotherapy for chordoma. *Int J Radiat Oncol Biol Phys* 1988; 15:331–339.
31. Gay E, Sekhar LN, Rubinstein E, et al. Chordomas and chondrosarcomas of the cranial base: results and follow-up of 60 patients. *Neurosurgery* 1995; 36:887–897.
32. Harwood AR, Krajbich JI, Fornasier VL. Radiotherapy of chondrosarcoma of bone. *Cancer* 1980; 45:2769–2777.
33. Hassounah M, Al-Mefty O, Akhtar M, et al. Primary cranial and intracranial chondrosarcoma. A survey. *Acta Neurochir (Wien)* 1985; 78:123–132.
34. Heffelfinger MJ, Dahlin DC, MacCarty CS, Beabout JW. Chordomas and cartilaginous tumors at the skull base. *Cancer* 1973; 32:410–420.
35. Janecka IP, Sen CN, Sekhar LN, Arriaga M. Facial translocation: a new approach to the cranial base. *Otolaryngol Head Neck Surg* 1990; 103:413–419.
36. Jones NF, Schramm VL, Sekhar LN. Reconstruction of the cranial base following tumour resection. *Br J Plast Surg* 1987; 40:155–162.
37. Kamrin RP, Potanos JN, Pool JL. An evaluation of the diagnosis and treatment of chordoma. *J Neurol Neurosurg Psychiatry* 1964; 27:157–165.
38. Keisch ME, Garcia DM, Shibuya RB. Retrospective long-term follow-up analysis in 21 patients with chordomas of various sites treated at a single institution. *J Neurosurg* 1991; 75:374–377.
39. Kendall BE. Cranial chordomas. *Br J Radiol* 1977; 50:687–698.
40. Kondziolka D, Lunsford LD, Flickinger JC. The role of radiosurgery in the management of chordoma and chondrosarcoma of the cranial base. *Neurosurgery* 1991; 29:38–46.
41. Krayenbühl H, Yaşargil MG. Cranial chordomas. *Progr Neurol Surg* 1975; 6:380–434.
42. Kumar PP, Good RR, Skultety FM, Leibrock LG. Local control of recurrent clival and sacral chordoma after interstitial irradiation with iodine-125: new techniques for treatment of recurrent or unresectable chordomas. *Neurosurgery* 1988; 22:479–483.
43. Kveton JF, Brackmann DE, Glasscock ME 3d, et al. Chondrosarcoma of the skull base. *Otolaryngol Head Neck Surg* 1986; 94:23–32.
44. Lee YY, Von Tassel P. Craniofacial chondrosarcomas: imaging findings in 15 untreated cases. *Am J Neuroradiol* 1989; 10:165–170.
45. Luschka H. Die Altersveranderungen der Zwischenwirbelknorpel. *Virchows Arch Pathol Anat Physiol Klin Med* 1856; 9:312–327.
46. Meyer JE, Oot RF, Lindfors KK. CT appearance of clival chordomas. *J Comput Assist Tomogr* 1986; 10:34–38.
47. Meyes SP, Hirsch WL Jr, Curtin HD, et al. Chondrosarcomas of the skull base: MR imaging features. *Radiology* 1992; 184:103–108.
48. Munzenrider JE. Proton beam radiation and chordomas and chondrosarcomas. Presented at the Third International Conference on Head and Neck Tumors. San Fransisco, CA, July 1992.
49. O'Neill P, Bell BA, Miller JD, et al. Fifty years of experience with chordomas in southeast Scotland. *Neurosurgery* 1985; 16:166–170.
50. Oot RF, Melville GE, New PF, et al. The role of MR and CT in evaluating clival chordomas and chondrosarcomas. *Am J Roentgenol* 1988; 151:567–575.
51. Pearlman AW, Friedman M. Radical and radiation therapy of chordoma. *Am J Roentgenol* 1970; 108:332–341.
52. Rabadan A, Conesa H. Transmaxillary-transnasal approach to the anterior clivus: a microsurgical anatomical model. *Neurosurgery* 1992; 30:473–482.
53. Raffel C, Wright DC, Gutin PH, Wilson CB. Cranial chordomas: clinical presentation and results of operative and radiation therapy in twenty-six patients. *Neurosurgery* 1985; 17:703–710.
54. Rich TA, Schiller A, Suit HD, Mankin HJ. Clinical and pathologic review of 48 cases of chordoma. *Cancer* 1985; 56:182–187.
55. Rupa V, Rajshekhar V, Bhanu TS, Chandi SM. Primary chondroid chordoma of the base of the petrous temporal bone. *J Laryngol Otol* 1989; 103:771–773.
56. Sekhar LN, Janecka IP, Jones NF. Subtemporal-infratemporal and basal subfrontal approach to extensive cranial base tumours. *Acta Neurochir (Wien)* 1988; 92:83–92.
57. Sekhar LN, Ross DA, Sen C. Cavernous sinus and sphenocavernous neoplasms: anatomy and surgery. In Sekhar LN, Janecka IP (eds): *Surgery of Cranial Base Tumors.* New York: Raven Press, 1993, pp 521–604.
58. Sekhar LN, Schramm VL, Jones NF. Subtemporal-preauricular infratemporal fossa approach to large lateral and posterior cranial base neoplasms. *J Neurosurg* 1987; 67:488–499.
59. Sekhar LN, Sen C, Synderman CH, Janecka IP. Anterior, anterolateral, and lateral approaches to extradural petroclival tumors. In Sekhar LN, Janecka IP (eds): *Surgery of Cranial Base Tumors.* New York: Raven Press, 1993, pp 157–223.
60. Sen CN, Sekhar LN. The subtemporal and preauricular infratemporal approach to intradural structures ventral to the brain stem. *J Neurosurg* 1990; 73:345–354.
61. Sen CN, Sekhar LN. An extreme lateral approach to intradural lesions of the cervical spine and foramen magnum. *Neurosurgery* 1990; 27:197–204.
62. Sen CN, Sekhar LN, Schramm VL, Janecka IP. Chordoma and chondrosarcoma of the cranial base: an 8-year experience. *Neurosurgery* 1989; 25:931–941.
63. Sindou M, Daher A, Vighetto A, Goutelle A. Chondrosarcome parasellaire: rapport d'un cas opéré par voie ptériono-temporale et revue de la littérature. *Neurochirurgie* 1989; 35:186–190.
64. Snyderman CH, Janecka IP, Sekhar LN, et al. Anterior cranial base reconstruction: role of galeal and pericranial flaps. *Laryngoscope* 1990; 100:607–614.
65. Spaar FW, Spaar U, Markakis E. DNA is chordomas of the clivus Blumenbachi. *Neurosurg Rev* 1990; 13:219–229.
66. Spetzler RF, Herman JM, Beals S, et al. Preservation of olfaction in anterior craniofacial approaches. *J Neurosurg* 1993; 79:48–52.
67. Spoden JE, Bumsted RM, Warner ED. Chondroid chordoma. Case report and literature review. *Ann Otol Rhinol Laryngol* 1980; 89:279–285.
68. Suit HD, Goitein M, Munzenrider J, et al. Definitive radiation therapy for chordoma and chondrosarcoma of base of skull and cervical spine. *J Neurosurg* 1982; 56:377–385.
69. Sze G, Uichanco LS 3d, Brant-Zawadzki MN, et al. Chordomas: MR imaging. *Radiology* 1988; 166:187–191.
70. Tatsuzaki H, Urie MM. Importance of precise positioning for proton beam therapy in the base of skull and cervical spine. *Int J Radiat Oncol Biol Phys* 1991; 21:757–765.
71. Tomlinson FH, Scheithauer BW, Forsythe PA, et al. Sarcomatous

transformation in cranial chordoma. *Neurosurgery* 1992; 31:13–18.
72. Volpe R, Mazabraud A. A clinicopathologic review of 25 cases of chordoma (a pleomorphic and metastasizing neoplasm). *Am J Surg Pathol* 1983; 7:161–170.
73. Walaas L, Kindblom LG. Fine-needle aspiration biopsy in the preoperative diagnosis of chordoma: a study of 17 cases with application of electron microscopic, histochemical, and immunocytochemical examination. *Hum Pathol* 1991; 22:22–28.
74. Zoltán L, Fényes I: Stereotactic diagnosis and radioactive treatment in a case of spheno-occipital chordoma. *J Neurosurg* 1960; 17:888–900.
75. Zülch KJ. *Brain Tumors. Their Biology and Pathology,* 3d ed. Berlin: Springer-Verlag, 1986, pp 476–482.

152 Trigeminal Neurinomas

Kalmon D. Post
Paul C. McCormick

Incidence and Classification

Neurinomas (schwannomas) arising from the intracranial portion of the trigeminal nerve are rare. They account for 0.07 to 0.36 percent of intracranial tumors and 0.8 to 8 percent of intracranial neurinomas.[1,4,9,11,13,15,18,21] These tumors are occasionally encountered in conjunction with multiple intracranial neurinomas as a manifestation of neurofibromatosis. In most of these cases, however, the trigeminal neurinoma does not represent the clinically significant pathology and is usually described as an incidental radiographic, operative, or postmortem finding.

Neurinomas can arise from the root, ganglion, or rarely, a proximal division of the trigeminal nerve. Since the intracranial course of the trigeminal nerve is closely applied to the skull base of both posterior and middle fossae, Jefferson classified trigeminal neurinomas into three types: (1) tumors mainly in the middle fossa, (2) predominantly posterior fossa tumors, and (3) tumors with significant components in both posterior and middle fossae.[8] This classification scheme has functional significance from a clinical, radiographic, and surgical perspective. A review of reported cases indicates that slightly more than 50 percent of trigeminal neurinomas arise within the middle fossa, with variable degrees of tumor extension into the posterior fossa. Approximately one-third are totally or predominantly confined to the posterior fossa, and less than 20 percent are dumbbell-shaped with significant tumor components in both middle and posterior fossae.

The data presented in this chapter reflect the experience at our institution with a series of 14 patients with trigeminal neurinoma managed operatively since 1970. To better define the clinical, radiographic, and pathologic aspects of these rare tumors, an additional 122 reported cases were analyzed.[11,15]

Surgical Anatomy and Pathology

The trigeminal root, consisting of a larger sensory root and a smaller medially situated motor root, arises from the lateral aspect of the rostral pons and courses in a lateral, anterior, and slightly superior direction through the anterior part of the cerebellopontine angle in the pontocerebellar cistern. The superior cerebellar artery usually passes above and the anterior inferior cerebellar artery below the root, but this relationship is not constant owing to the frequent anatomic variations and loops of these vessels. The petrosal vein lies lateral and posterior to the trigeminal root. The root passes under the trochlear nerve and free edge of the tentorium and enters the middle fossa through a dural cleft, the porus trigeminus, located just inferior to the lateral tentorial attachment and superior petrosal sinus. The root is then essentially extradural in location and terminates in the trigeminal ganglion.

The crescent-shaped trigeminal ganglion occupies a shallow bony recess on the anterior surface of the petrous apex known as Meckel's cave. Because the sensory root rotates anteriorly as it enters the trigeminal ganglion, the motor root becomes related to its inferior surface and passes under the ganglion before being incorporated into the mandibular nerve. Just anterior to Meckel's cave the connective tissue–filled foramen lacerum separates the distal part of the ganglion from the horizontal petrous segment of the internal carotid artery and the eustachian tube. The greater superficial petrosal nerve courses anteriorly beneath the trigeminal ganglion and is frequently injured during removal of neurinomas involving the ganglion. The dural covering of the trigeminal ganglion is continuous anteriorly with the posterolateral wall of the cavernous sinus.

The pathologic relationship of these tumors to the trigeminal root and ganglion is variable. The trigeminal ganglion is usually not visualized with tumors arising in Meckel's cave, although compressed remnants of ganglionic tissue may occasionally be identified after tumor removal. Although trigeminal nerve fibers may be seen on the surface of the tumor, in most cases, at least portions of the root appear to course through the tumor mass.

Microscopically, these tumors show the typical neurinoma appearance of bipolar elongated cells with fusiform darkly staining nuclei arranged in compact interlacing fascicles with a tendency toward palisade formation, the Antoni A pattern. A looser arrangement of cells, separated by a collagenous or hyalinized matrix, the Antoni B pattern, is less common. Thickened hyalinized blood vessels, occasionally thrombosed, and hemosiderin-laden macrophages (foam cells) are frequently present. Histologically malignant neurinomas and melanotic neurinomas are rare but have been described.[6,11]

Clinical Features

Among the cases we reviewed, the peak incidence occurred during the fourth decade of life, and the mean age at the time of diagnosis was 37 years (range, 1 to 67 years). The tumors were only slightly more common in women. The duration of symptoms preceding diagnosis ranged from 6 days to 16 years, with a mean of 39 months.

The initial symptom was recorded in 130 of the 136 cases. Subjective complaints of trigeminal nerve dysfunction were the initial symptoms in 55 percent (72 of 130) of the cases. These complaints included numbness (35 cases), pain (30 cases), and paresthesia (7 cases). Frequently, the complaint was initially localized to a portion of the sensory field in the distribution of one trigeminal division. In most cases, however, the entire trigeminal distribution was involved by the time of diagnosis. The remaining initial symptoms are listed in Table 152-1.

Eventual involvement of the trigeminal nerve was the general rule, so that, by the time of diagnosis, 86 percent (117 of 136) had either subjective or objective evidence of trigeminal nerve dysfunction. Varying degrees of hypesthesia, hypalgesia, and a diminished or absent corneal reflex were the most common findings

TABLE 152-1 Initial Symptom in 130 Patients with Trigeminal Neurinoma

Symptom	No. of Cases	Percent
Trigeminal nerve dysfunction	72	55
Numbness	35	27
Pain	30	23
Paresthesia	7	5
Headache	19	15
Diplopia	13	10
Hearing loss/tinnitus	10	8
Visual loss	7	5
Ear pain	4	3
Other*	10	8
Total	132	

*Other symptoms: Subarachnoid hemorrhage, vertigo, seizure, exophthalmos, gait difficulty, hemifacial spasm.

†Three patients presented with more than one initial complaint; one patient was asymptomatic.

(Table 152-2). Complete anesthesia was distinctly rare, and although one division of the trigeminal nerve was commonly more severely affected, there was usually diminished sensation in the entire trigeminal nerve distribution.

Weakness in the muscles of mastication was recorded in 53 (39 percent) patients. The paresis was generally mild, and atrophy of the masseter and temporalis muscles was noted only occasionally.

Facial pain was a prominent complaint on admission history in 52 (38 percent) patients. It was more common with tumors involving the trigeminal ganglion (52 percent) than with tumors arising from the trigeminal root (28 percent). The quality and intensity of the pain was variable, ranging from a dull ache to a severe burning pain. In most cases, the pain was constant and usually progressed in severity. Episodes of severe lancinating exacerbations of facial pain, suggestive of trigeminal neuralgia, were noted by one-third of these patients. True trigeminal neuralgia, characterized by trigger zones, prolonged pain-free periods, and the absence of objective trigeminal nerve deficits, however, was an initial symptom in only six patients. Three of these patients had tumors arising from the trigeminal root, and three patients had trigeminal ganglion tumors.

TABLE 152-2 Abnormal Findings on Admission Examination in 136 Patients with Trigeminal Neurinoma*

Neurological Abnormality	No. of Cases	Percent
Trigeminal nerve		
Decreased sensation	100	74
Diminished or absent corneal reflex	93	68
Motor weakness	53	39
Other cranial nerve deficits		
II	14	10
III	19	14
IV	9	7
VI	47	35
VII	31	23
VIII	44	32
IX, X	11	8
XI	2	1
XII	4	3
Cerebellar signs	31	23
Long tract signs	21	15
Exophthalmos	22	16
Papilledema	14	10

*Only 29 patients (21%) had abnormal findings limited to the trigeminal nerve.

Neurological deficits, other than trigeminal nerve abnormalities, were present in over 75 percent of patients by the time of diagnosis (Table 152-2). The majority of these deficits were in the form of cranial nerve palsies and were related to the location of the tumor. The abducens nerve was most commonly affected by ganglion tumors, probably as a result of the proximity of the intracavernous portion of the nerve to the medial aspect of the trigeminal ganglion. Posterior fossa tumors frequently caused deficits in the seventh and eighth cranial nerves. Large posterior fossa tumors were usually also associated with cerebellar and pyramidal tract signs.

A few patients with tumors located solely within the middle fossa were noted to have conductive hearing loss or facial weakness. The hearing loss was probably the result of compression of the eustachian tube as it passes under the cartilaginous floor of Meckel's cave. The facial paresis seen with middle fossa tumors is most likely due to traction on the greater superficial petrosal nerve.

Radiologic Investigation

Plain films of the skull, frequently with thin-section tomography, were obtained in 115 patients. Anteroposterior, base, and Stenver's views were the most useful projections in defining the bony changes associated with trigeminal neurinomas.

Erosion of the anteromedial portion of the petrous pyramid was the most common bony abnormality and was present in 67 cases. The defect was usually described as a sharply delineated amputation of the petrous apex with smooth, rarely sclerotic, margins (Fig. 152-1).[5,7,10,14,15] This finding was generally seen with Meckel's cave or dumbbell-shaped tumors.

Epidermoids, meningiomas, acoustic neurinomas, and primary bone tumors of the skull base, such as chordomas and osteochondromas, also have been reported to produce erosion of the petrous apex.[4,12,22] In most cases, however, associated bony abnormalities serve to distinguish these tumors from trigeminal neurinomas. Meningiomas frequently produce bone erosion with irregular margins or hyperostosis and may have visible intratumoral calcification. Acoustic neurinomas usually cause enlargement of the internal auditory meatus, a finding not seen with trigeminal neurinomas. Primary bone tumors of the skull base generally show more extensive destructive bony changes and are frequently calcified. Epidermoids, however, arising either in Meckel's cave or in the cerebellopontine angle, may produce bony changes identical to those seen with trigeminal neurinomas. Sclerosis at the margins of the bone defect, frequently seen with epidermoids, may help to distinguish between these tumors. Finally, aneurysms arising from the petrous, precavernous, or cavernous portions of the internal carotid artery may produce isolated erosion of the petrous apex.[12]

Additional bony abnormalities generally reflect a slowly expanding mass in the middle fossa. These findings include erosion of the floor of the middle fossa, enlargement of the basal foramina, and occasional erosion of the pterygoid plates. Medial and anterior tumor growth is associated with erosion of the lateral aspect of the sella turcica, dorsum sellae, anterior clinoid process, superior orbital fissure, and inferolateral aspect of the optic canal. The extradural location of these tumors in the middle fossa, growing under pressure exerted by the dura, may be responsible for the frequency and extent of bone erosion associated with these slow-growing benign tumors.

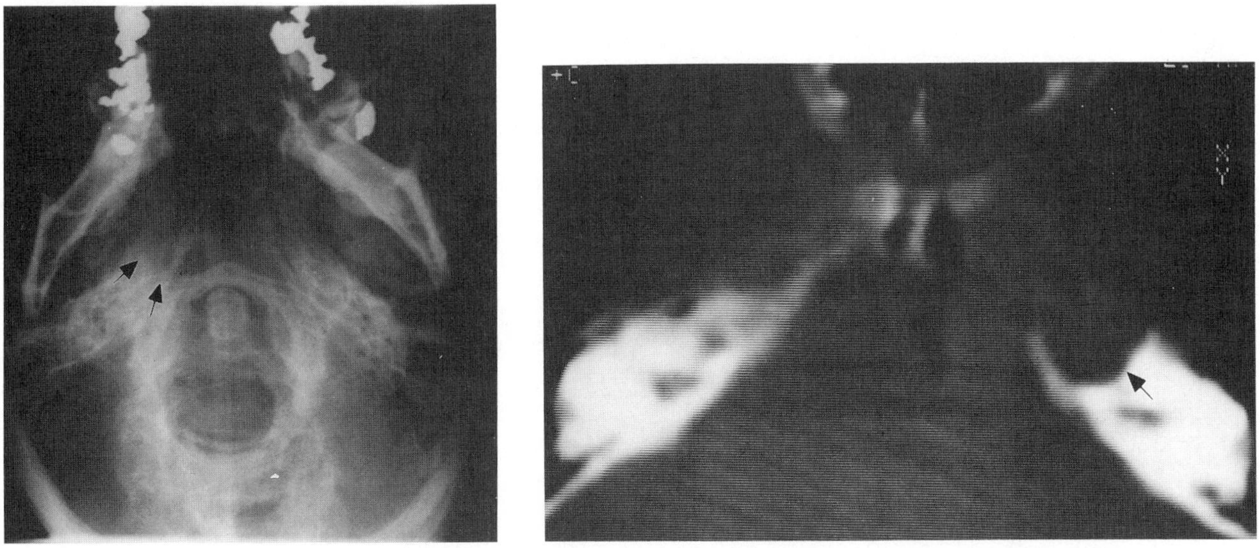

(*A*) (*B*)

Figure 152-1 *A.* A skull roentgenogram (base view) demonstrates amputation of the right petrous apex (*arrows*). *B.* An axial CT correlate on a different patient demonstrates similar erosion of the left petrous apex (*arrow*).

Bony changes are infrequently seen with trigeminal neurinomas in the posterior fossa. Although amputation of the petrous apex is occasionally seen, flattening of the posterior surface of the petrous apex is more common. This erosion may extend laterally to involve the anteromedial lip of the internal auditory meatus. Other bony abnormalities seen with posterior fossa neurinomas include erosion of the lateral aspect of the clivus and diffuse changes produced by increased intracranial pressure.

Cerebral angiography was performed in 63 patients. The results were reported as normal in 9 patients. All of these patients had small tumors arising either in Meckel's cave or from the trigeminal root. The remaining 54 patients exhibited abnormalities in the form of blood vessel displacement related to the location of the tumor.

Medial displacement of the initial extradural portion of the carotid siphon, the so-called ganglial or precavernous segment, was the most commonly reported abnormality associated with tumors originating in Meckel's cave (Fig. 152-2*A*). In most cases, there was associated anterior and inferior displacement of this portion of the siphon (Fig. 152-2*B*), but superior and posterior displacement, indicating tumor growth anterior to the ascending portion of the carotid siphon, was noted in some patients. Although displacement

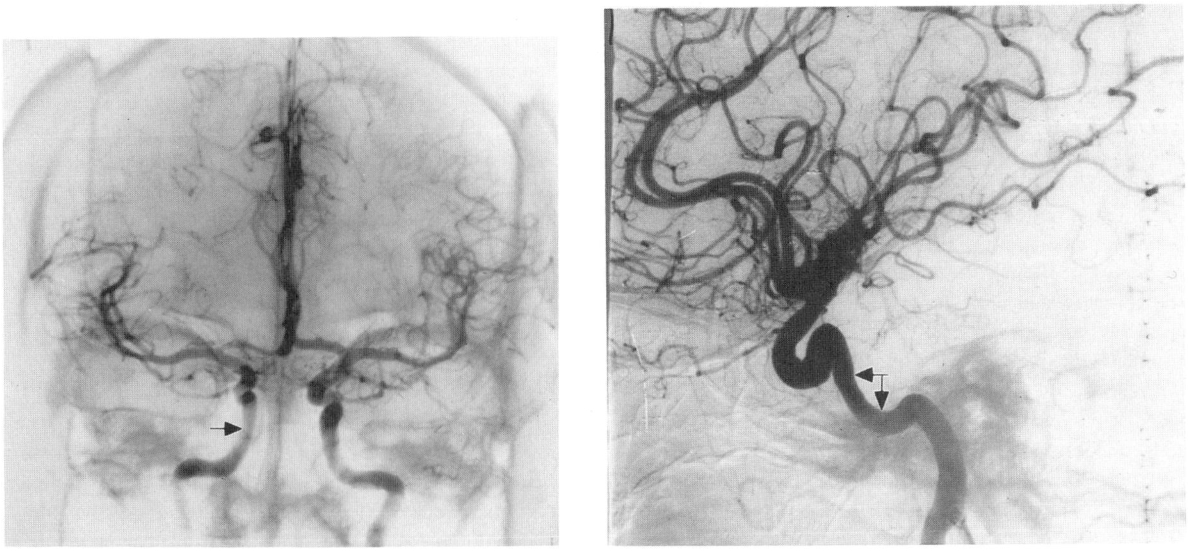

(*A*) (*B*)

Figure 152-2 *A.* Subtraction films from bilateral internal carotid artery angiograms (superimposed) show relative medial displacement of the precavernous segment of the right internal carotid artery (*arrow*). *B.* A lateral projection of an internal carotid angiogram shows anterior and inferior displacement of the precavernous (ganglial) segment of the internal carotid artery (*arrows*).

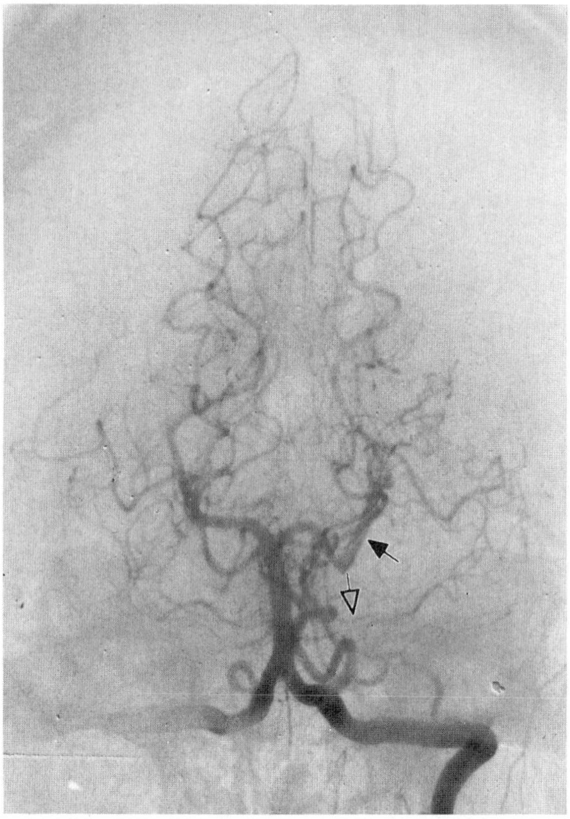

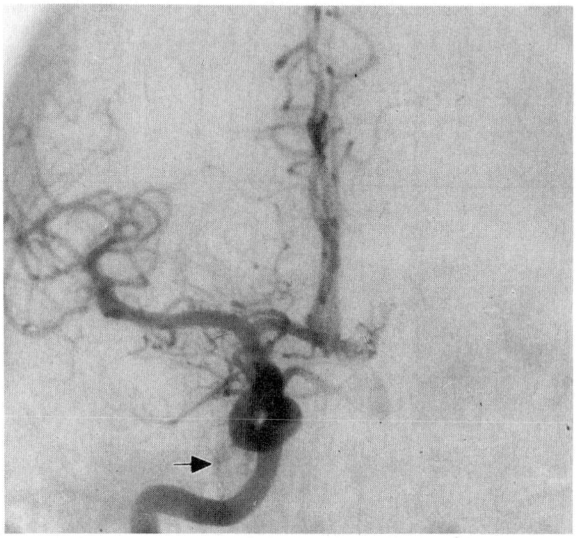

(*C*) (*D*)

Figure 152-2 (*Continued*). *C.* A subtraction angiogram of a left vertebral artery injection shows medial displacement of the proximal segments of the superior cerebellar and posterior cerebral arteries (*arrow*). The left anterior inferior cerebellar artery is displaced inferiorly (*open arrow*). *D.* A subtraction film (anteroposterior projection) from an internal carotid artery angiogram shows slight but definite neovascularity associated with a Meckel's cave neurinoma (*arrow*).

of the precavernous extradural segment of the carotid siphon may rarely be seen with large intra-axial masses arising in the temporal lobe, this finding is fairly specific for extracerebral, particularly extradural, masses arising from the skull base.[3,8]

Early posterior fossa extension through the porus trigeminus of a tumor arising in Meckel's cave was heralded by medial displacement of the proximal segments of the posterior cerebral and superior cerebellar arteries (Fig. 152-2*C*). Both of these vessels may also be elevated. Large posterior fossa trigeminal neurinomas, in addition, produce depression of the anterior inferior cerebellar artery and elevation or nonfilling of the petrosal vein. The basilar artery may be stretched and displaced contralaterally. Posterior displacement of the basilar artery may occasionally be seen and results from tumor growth ventral to the brain stem.

About 20 percent of trigeminal neurinomas demonstrate abnormal tumor vascularity consisting of enlarged feeding vessels or a tumor stain. The abnormal vessels are derived from the precavernous and cavernous segments of the carotid siphon or from branches of the external carotid artery (Fig. 152-2*D*).

Twenty-five of 30 patients[11,15] were studied preoperatively with CT. Typically, these tumors were isodense or slightly hyper- or hypodense with respect to surrounding brain on unenhanced scans. Most showed homogeneous enhancement after the intravenous administration of a contrast agent. Seven tumors showed areas of decreased attenuation after contrast administration, believed to represent either necrosis or cystic degeneration (Fig. 152-3). Axial and coronal sections of the skull base were particularly useful in identifying the extent of bone destruction in both middle and posterior fossae (Fig. 152-3*B*).

Although coronal CT sections provide important information in defining the relationship of the tumor to the cavernous sinus, tentorial notch, and extracranial tissues, magnetic resonance imaging (MRI) has thus far proved superior in these respects (Fig. 152-4). By MRI, the trigeminal neurinoma was typically a well-circumscribed mass that showed a decreased signal intensity on T1-weighted images and increased signal intensity on T2-weighted images when compared to surrounding brain.[15,17]

Differential Diagnosis

The differential diagnosis from a radiologic standpoint has been discussed. From a clinical perspective there is no distinct clinical syndrome produced by trigeminal neurinomas. Careful examination of the motor and sensory components of the trigeminal nerve will ultimately reveal deficits in the majority of patients harboring trigeminal neurinomas, but in about 10 percent of patients, no evidence of trigeminal nerve dysfunction will be found. Additional deficits are related to the location of the tumor. Neurinomas arising in Meckel's cave frequently produce various forms of a parasellar or paratrigeminal (Raeder's) syndrome.[16] Trigeminal neurinomas

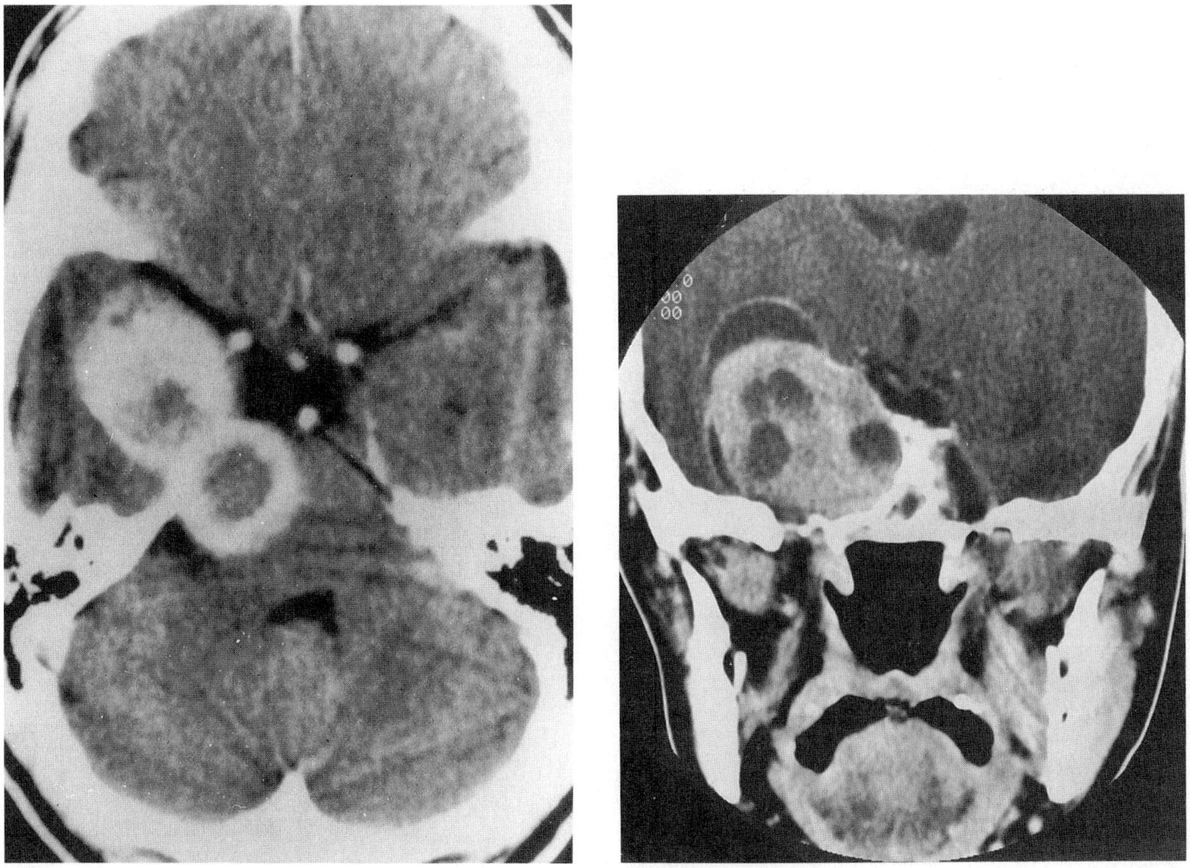

(*A*) (*B*)

Figure 152-3 *A*. A contrast-enhanced CT scan of a dumbbell-shaped tumor shows areas of decreased attenuation representing either necrosis or cystic degeneration. *B*. A contrast-enhanced coronal CT scan shows a large inhomogeneous mass in the right middle fossa with marked erosion of the dorsum sellae and upper clivus. Note the marked atrophy of the masseter and pterygoid muscles on the right side.

confined to the posterior fossa generally will produce some form of a cerebellopontine angle syndrome with facial paresis, hearing loss, and occasional long tract and cerebellar signs. Early involvement of the trigeminal nerve tends to distinguish these tumors from acoustic neurinomas, as will the early appearance of hearing loss generally seen with acoustic neurinomas. This distinction, however, may not always be possible since up to 10 percent of patients with acoustic neurinomas initially present with symptoms related to trigeminal nerve dysfunction. Conversely, hearing loss as an initial complaint was seen in 6 percent of patients with trigeminal neurinomas.

Although facial pain may occur early in the clinical course of the patient, its atypical nature is frequently misinterpreted as being caused by local processes such as tooth, temporomandibular joint, or paranasal sinus pathology. The acceptance that associated sensory deficits may be seen with trigeminal neuralgia further delays diagnosis, despite the fact that these patients respond poorly or not at all to medical treatment with carbamazepine or phenytoin.[2] Isolated paroxysms of facial pain are common, but the absence of trigger zones and the prolonged duration of these paroxysms, frequently lasting 30 min or longer, further differentiate the facial pain caused by tumors from true trigeminal neuralgia. It seems likely that minimal pressure on the trigeminal root or ganglion is capable of producing trigeminal neuralgia. With increasing pressure on either structure, the brief paroxysms of pain may give way to constant facial pain and the appearance of trigeminal nerve sensory deficits.

Surgical Techniques

The surgical approach to these tumors is dependent on their anatomic location. Accurate preoperative delineation of the tumor mass is essential in choosing the most appropriate surgical route. Much of this information can be obtained during the radiologic evaluation. Thin-section axial CT through the skull base, posterior fossa, and parasellar region, with and without bone windows, is the most useful study because it defines the relationship of the tumor to the skull base, quantifies the degree of bone erosion, and allows an accurate estimation of the size of the tumor in both middle and posterior fossae. Coronal sections, with either CT or MRI, more precisely define the relationship of the tumor to the cavernous sinus and will identify extracranial tumor extension into the pterygoid fossa or paranasal sinuses, which occurs in about 10 percent of patients with trigeminal neurinomas (Fig. 152-4*A*).

Cerebral angiography is routinely performed in the preoperative evaluation of patients with parasellar tumors, both to rule out a

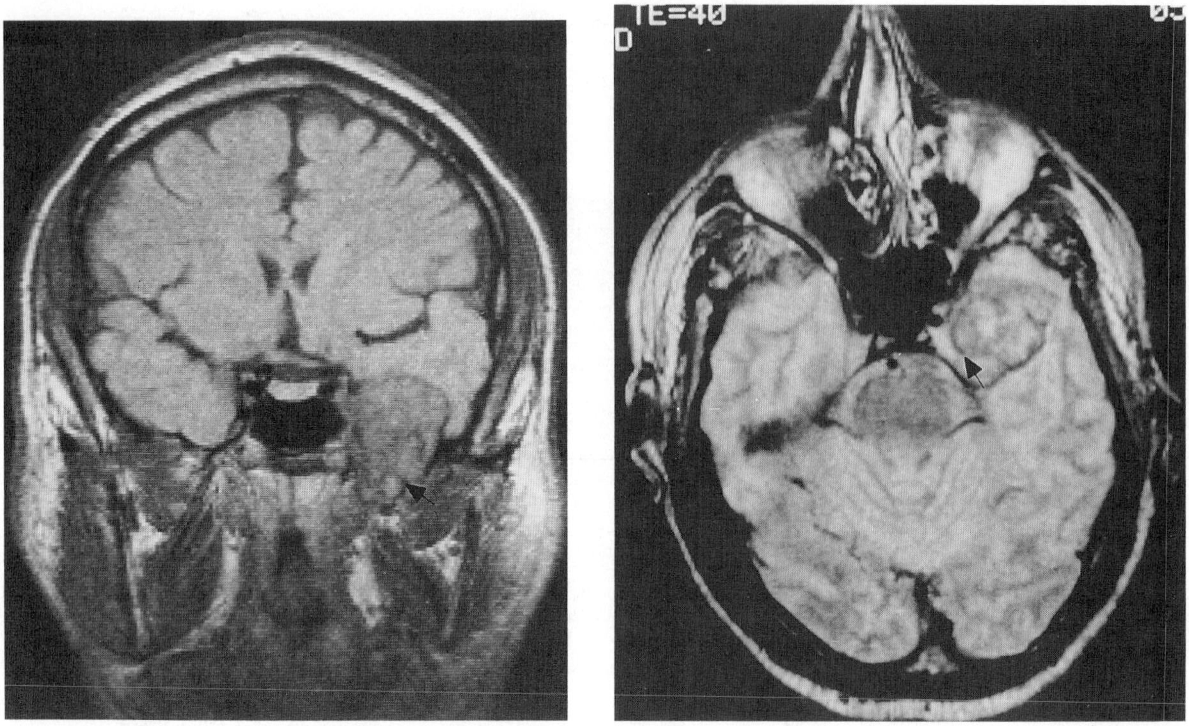

(*A*) (*B*)

Figure 152-4 *A.* A T1-weighted coronal MR image demonstrates an extra-axial mass eroding through the floor of the middle fossa into the pterygoid fossa (*arrow*). The tumor is inhomogeneous in signal intensity and somewhat hypointense with respect to the surrounding brain. Note the atrophy of the muscles of mastication on the side of the tumor. *B.* A T1-weighted axial MR image demonstrates the relationship of the tumor to the cavernous sinus. Note the integrity of the dura which clearly demarcates the tumor from the cavernous sinus (*arrow*).

petrous, precavernous, or cavernous carotid artery aneurysm, and to define the relationship of the tumor to these segments of the carotid artery. This second point is of particular importance, since there is frequently no intervening bone between the trigeminal ganglion and these segments of the carotid artery.

A balloon occlusion test of the ipsilateral internal carotid artery (ICA) with cerebral blood flow monitoring and neurological examination may be helpful to assess the adequacy of collateral circulation.[15,19] Temporary or permanent occlusion of the ICA may become necessary during surgery. In addition, intraoperative monitoring of brain stem auditory evoked potentials and somatosensory evoked potentials is extremely helpful and routinely utilized now.[15,19,20]

A subtemporal intradural approach is the preferred route in most cases, because it offers excellent exposure of the middle fossa floor and allows access into the posterior fossa. Alternatively, a predominantly extradural approach may be used, with removal of the superior rim and lateral wall of the orbit and the zygoma. This facilitates exposure of the cavernous sinus region and minimizes temporal lobe retraction while exposing the petrous apex region. Lumbar CSF drainage and the intravenous administration of mannitol are used to assist in temporal lobe retraction.

Access into the posterior fossa is obtained by incising the tentorium and ligating the superior petrosal sinus. The amount of tumor that can be removed from the posterior fossa through the subtemporal exposure depends largely on the degree of brain relaxation and the amount of erosion of the petrous apex. In most cases, significant tumor decompression can be obtained in the posterior fossa when the tumor is located primarily anteriorly in the cerebellopontine angle. Tumor extension ventral to the upper brain stem also may be removed through this exposure. Attempts to remove more caudally placed tumors below the seventh and eighth cranial nerves, especially if the tumor is closely applied to the lateral skull base (Fig. 152-5*A*) or ventral to the lower brain stem, will usually require an unacceptable amount of temporal lobe retraction. These portions of the tumor are more safely removed through a suboccipital route, performed either as part of a combined transtentorial approach or at a staged second operation.

Although a reasonable degree of access into the posterior fossa can be obtained via a subtemporal approach, only very limited access to the middle fossa can be obtained through a suboccipital approach. Thus, the suboccipital approach is appropriate only for those tumors either entirely limited to the posterior fossa or with minimal supratentorial extension (Fig. 152-5*B*).

The combined transtentorial approach is reserved for patients with posterior fossa tumors, the size or configuration of which prevents removal through a subtemporal approach, in which there is also tumor extension into the middle fossa (Fig. 152-5*A*). The position of the patient is supine with elevation of the ipsilateral shoulder and the head turned to the opposite side. The lateral sinus is not ligated when this approach is employed for tumor removal. Including the lateral sinus in the tentorial incision is a maneuver which essentially allows greater retraction of the brain stem, a situation usually already created by the tumor. However, if there is significant tumor extension ventral to the brain stem then ligation of the lateral sinus may be necessary.

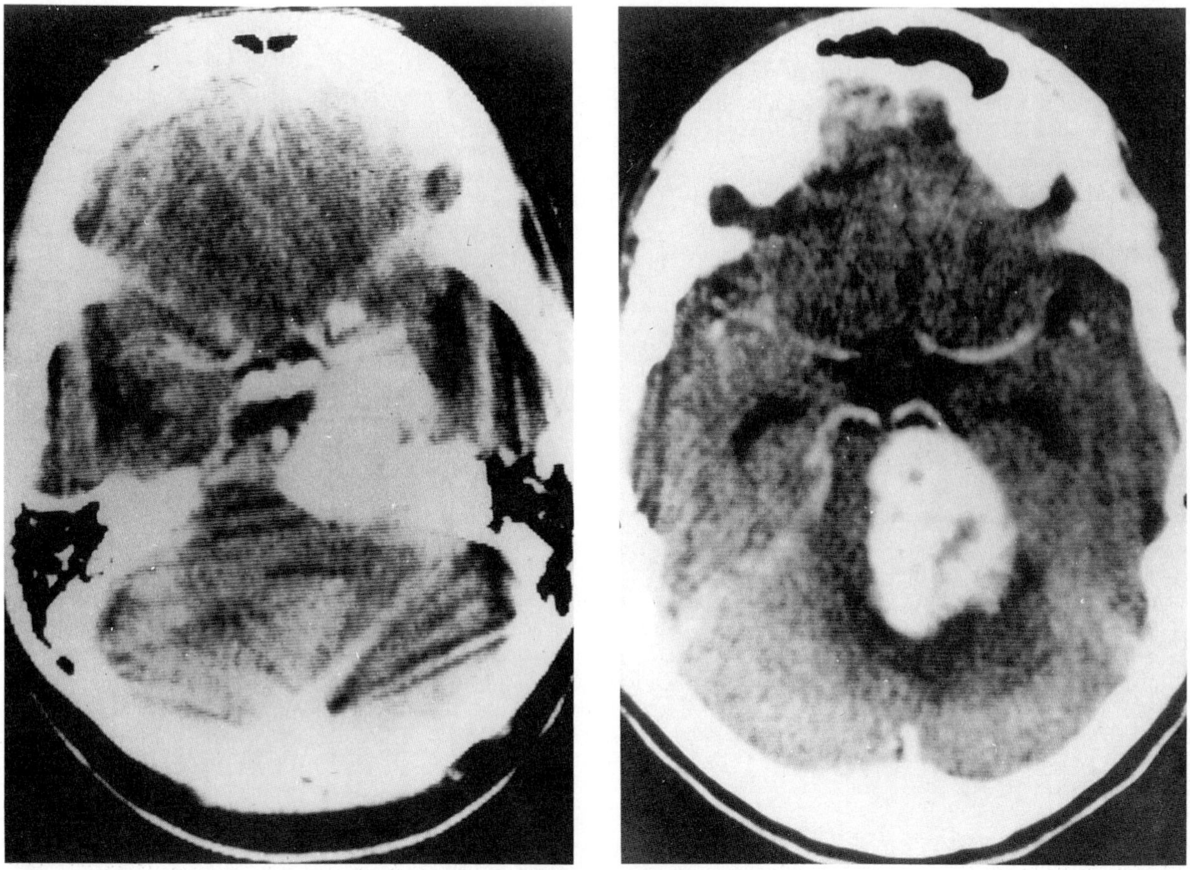

(*A*) (*B*)

Figure 152-5 *A*. An axial CT scan demonstrating a dumbbell-shaped tumor. Although the posterior fossa tumor component is not large, its wide-based apposition to the posterior aspect of the petrous pyramid makes it unlikely that this tumor can be removed safely through a subtemporal approach. *B*. An axial CT scan shows a large trigeminal root neurinoma totally confined to the posterior fossa.

The surgical techniques for tumor removal are similar to those employed for acoustic neurinomas. Adequate illumination and magnification with the operative microscope and adherence to microsurgical principles are essential prerequisites for successful removal of these tumors. An initial subcapsular decompression minimizes tumor manipulation and protects the third, fourth, sixth, seventh, and eighth cranial nerves, which are frequently adherent to the tumor capsule. The ultrasonic aspirator is useful in debulking the central portions of the tumor. Removal of the tumor capsule should be preceded by gentle dissection of the affected cranial nerves from the surface of the tumor. The altered anatomy of these cranial nerves depends on the size of the tumor. The trochlear nerve usually will be identified on the superior pole of the tumor, whereas the oculomotor nerve is frequently applied to the medial tumor surface. Large posterior fossa tumors will displace the seventh and eighth cranial nerves inferiorly or posteriorly. The abducens nerve may occasionally be exposed if medial extension of the extradural portion of the tumor elevates the dura from the petrous tip.

The obvious goal at operation is complete extirpation. This may not be possible, because the inferomedial portion of the tumor is frequently particularly adherent to the posterolateral wall of the cavernous sinus. Overly aggressive attempts to remove this part of the tumor pose a significant risk of injury to the cavernous sinus, carotid artery, and abducens nerve. However, in recent years, experience has grown with cavernous sinus surgery techniques. To achieve a complete removal, the tumor can be dissected from the ICA, the abducens nerve, and the lateral wall of the cavernous sinus with minimal morbidity.[19] A similar situation may exist in the posterior fossa, where part of the tumor capsule may be densely adherent to the brain stem. Rather than risking injury to these structures, the surgeon is probably better advised to accept a near-total removal in these cases. Long-term "tumor-free" intervals generally can be expected even when these portions of the tumor have been left behind. The removal of tumors that extend through the skull base into the pteryopalatine fossa and infratemporal fossa requires a surgical team consisting of a neurosurgeon and an otolaryngologist.

Postoperative Course

In the immediate postoperative period, the appearance of additional cranial nerve deficits is common but usually transient, resolving in 3 weeks to 4 months. Abnormalities of trigeminal nerve function, either of new onset or worsening of existing defects, are frequently seen and tend to be permanent. Improvement of preoperative deficits is also common. Among the cases we reviewed, diplopia resolved in 67 percent of patients, hearing returned to a functional level in 75 percent, and facial weakness improved in 67 percent of patients. Cerebellar and pyramidal tract signs resolved in all patients. Facial pain continued to be a problem in only one patient in our series.

Some degree of trigeminal sensory loss remains in most patients. Weakness in the muscles of mastication is evident in one-third of patients. All of these patients had at least partial resection of the trigeminal root, ganglion, or peripheral divisions at operation. Tarsorrhaphy for corneal ulceration secondary to neurotropic keratitis may be necessary.

CSF shunting may be required for hydrocephalus. CSF leakage and meningitis may be complications.

References

1. Arseni C, Dumitrescu L, Constantinescu A. Neurinomas of the trigeminal nerve. *Surg Neurol* 1975; 4:497–503.
2. Bullitt E, Tew JM, Boyd J. Intracranial tumors in patients with facial pain. *J Neurosurg* 1986; 64:865–871.
3. Chase NE, Taveras JM. Carotid angiography in the diagnosis of extradural parasellar tumors. *Acta Radiol (Diagn)* 1963; 1:214–224.
4. De Benedittis G, Bernasconi V, Ettorre G. Tumours of the fifth cranial nerve. *Acta Neurochir (Wien)* 1977; 38:37–64.
5. Gaal A: Zur Röntgendiagnose des Neurinoma trigemini. *Röntgenpraxis* 1935; 7:546–550.
6. Hedeman LS, Lewinsky BS, Lochridge GK, et al. Primary malignant schwannoma of the gasserian ganglion: report of two cases. *J Neurosurg* 1978; 48:279–283.
7. Holman CB, Olive I, Svien HJ. Roentgenologic features of neurofibromas involving the gasserian ganglion. *Am J Roentgenol* 1961; 86:148–153.
8. Jefferson G. The trigeminal neurinomas with some remarks on malignant invasion of the gasserian ganglion. *Clin Neurosurg* 1955; 1:11–54.
9. Krohm G, Marguth F. Zur Sympomatik der Trigeminus-neurinome. *Zentralbl Neurochir* 1964; 25:21–29.
10. Lindgren E: Das Röntgenbild bei Tumoren des Ganglion Gasseri. *Acta Chir Scand* 1941; 85:181–194.
11. McCormick PC, Bello JA, Post KD. Trigeminal schwannoma: surgical series of 14 patients and a review of the literature. *J Neurosurg* 1988; 69:850–860.
12. Mello LR, Tänzer A. Some aspects of trigeminal neurinomas. *Neuroradiology* 1972; 4:215–221.
13. Olive I, Svien HJ. Neurofibromas of the fifth cranial nerve. *J Neurosurg* 1957; 14:484–505.
14. Palacios E, MacGee EE. The radiographic diagnosis of trigeminal neurinomas. *J Neurosurg* 1972; 36:153–156.
15. Pollack IF, Sekhar LN, Jannetta PJ, Janecka IP. Neurilemomas of the trigeminal nerve. *J Neurosurg* 1989; 70:737–745.
16. Raeder JG. "Paratrigeminal" paralysis of the oculo-pupillary sympathetic. *Brain* 1924; 47:149–158.
17. Rigamonti D, Spetzler RF, Shetter A, et al. Magnetic resonance imaging and trigeminal schwannoma. *Surg Neurol* 1987; 28:67–70.
18. Schisano G, Olivecrona H. Neurinomas of the gasserian ganglion and trigeminal root. *J Neurosurg* 1960; 17:306–322.
19. Sekhar LN. Operative management of tumors involving the cavernous sinus. In Sekhar LN, Schramm VL Jr (eds): *Tumors of the Cranial Base: Diagnosis and Treatment.* Mt Kisco, NY: Futura Publishing, 1987, pp 393–419.
20. Takayasu M, Shibuya M, Suzuki Y, et al. Trigeminal sensory evoked potentials in patients with trigeminal neurinoma: report of two cases. *Neurosurgery* 1987; 20:453–456.
21. Tönnis W. Diagnostic der intrakraniellen Geschwülste. In Olivecrona H, Tönnis W (eds): *Handbuch der Neurochirurgie,* vol 4, pt 3. Berlin: Springer-Verlag, 1962, pp 68–72.
22. Westberg G. Angiographic changes in neurinoma of the trigeminal nerve. *Acta Radiol (Diagn)* 1963; 1:513–520.

153

Other Cranial Nerve Schwannomas

Sarah J. Gaskill

Schwannomas, which previously have been called neurinomas and neurilemomas in the literature, comprise less than 10 percent of all primary intracranial tumors.[42] Sensory nerves are preferentially affected, although the optic and olfactory nerves do not have a Schwann cell layer and therefore do not develop schwannomas. The acoustic and trigeminal nerves are the cranial nerves most often affected and are discussed in other chapters of this book. Schwannomas of the other cranial nerves are sufficiently rare that most have been reported as single case studies or small series based in part on previously published reports. This chapter presents a review of schwannomas arising from the nerves of ocular motility, the facial nerve, and the lower cranial nerves. The radiology of intracranial schwannomas is discussed elsewhere and will not be covered. Emphasis will be placed on the clinical presentation and management of these uncommon tumors.

Nerves of Ocular Motility

A 1992 survey of isolated schwannomas involving the oculomotor, trochlear, or abducens nerve reviewed 37 previously published cases and one of the authors' own.[4] Of these tumors, 22 (58 percent) involved the oculomotor nerve, 11 (29 percent) the trochlear nerve, and 5 (13 percent) the abducens nerve.

In contrast to schwannomas of the vestibular nerve, the tumors under discussion have been noted to have an origin distant from the glial-Schwann sheath junction. This junction is less than 4 mm from the neuraxis for the third nerve and about 1 mm from the neuraxis for the fourth and sixth nerves.[24] In their review, Celli et al. recommended that these tumors be classified by location as either cisternal, cisternocavernous, or cavernous.[4]

The clinical presentation of schwannomas of the nerves of ocular motility depends on the site of origin and the size of the tumor. In the patients reviewed by Celli et al.,[4] the mean age at presentation was 44 years, and there was a slight preponderance (60 percent) of females. The duration of symptoms was variable, with a tendency toward a shorter history for tumors involving the fourth or sixth nerves (2 years) and a somewhat longer history for tumors involving the third nerve (5 years).

In general, the most common presenting symptoms and signs reflect a disturbance of eye movements related to the involved nerve; there may also be evidence of brain stem compression. It should be noted, however, that despite the direct involvement of the nerves governing eye movements, one-third of patients present with no disturbance of ocular motility. The clinical presentation for schwannomas involving each of the individual nerves is discussed below.

Oculomotor nerve schwannomas most commonly present with a third nerve palsy, decreased visual acuity, gait ataxia, paresthesia in the distribution of the trigeminal nerve, and/or a hemiparesis. Trochlear nerve schwannomas are likely to present with an isolated third nerve palsy, gait ataxia, a contralateral hemiparesis, and/or a unilateral sensory disturbance. It is unusual for fourth nerve function to be affected by a trochlear nerve schwannoma. This fact has been explained by the observation that most trochlear nerve schwannomas are cisternal in location which allows displacement of the nerve with preservation of superior oblique function and results in a tendency for the tumor to present with symptoms and signs of brain stem compression. It should be noted that two reported cases of trochlear nerve schwannomas were initially misdiagnosed as brain stem lesions despite imaging with MRI or CT.[3,13] Abducens nerve schwannomas most commonly present with a sixth nerve palsy or symptoms of intracranial hypertension, most often headache. Given the rarity of abducens nerve schwannomas, it should be emphasized that paresis of the sixth nerve may be the first sign of a trigeminal schwannoma or some other intracranial process.

Surgical excision is currently the treatment of choice for these lesions. This approach allows for a correct tissue diagnosis as well providing decompression of vital structures, in particular the brain stem. The surgical approach depends on the location of the lesion. In most reported cases, tumor removal is total. Tumors in the region of the cavernous sinus can invade the sinus or adhere to the internal carotid or middle cerebral artery, precluding complete resection. In nearly all cases, a postoperative deficit involving the nerve of origin is to be expected. Often, complete resection mandates resection of a portion of the nerve. In other cases, the nerve is found to be disrupted by the tumor at the time of surgery. If possible, an anastomosis of the affected nerve should be performed at the time of the initial resection, as some reports of primary repair of the nerves governing eye movements have shown return of function.[15,20] Recurrence of these lesions, in particular when resection is subtotal, is a concern. However, follow-up on reported cases is usually limited to months or, in rare cases, 2 to 5 years. Vaquero et al. reported on the suprasellar recurrence of a completely resected oculomotor nerve schwannoma 13 years after the initial operation.[39]

Facial Nerve

The facial nerve is the third most common cranial nerve to be affected by schwannomas (after the acoustic and trigeminal nerves). These tumors can arise anywhere along the course of the facial nerve and are thought to arise from the sensory fibers of the nerve. Many originate in the region of the geniculate ganglion, a fact that has been attributed to the major structural reorganization that occurs in this portion of the facial nerve.[11] As these tumors are frequently intratemporal in location, they often fall in the venue of the otolaryngologist, and a significant number of cases have been reported in the otolaryngology literature[1,2,6,7,17,21,22,29,30,31,33,37]; in 1972, there was a comprehensive review of the subject by Pulec.[34] Some aspects of these cases are relevant to the neurosurgeon and are discussed below. Neurosurgical intervention is required when these tumors extend into the middle or posterior fossa. A smaller number of cases have been reported in the neurosurgical literature.[9,12,14,19,25,36]

The clinical presentation of facial nerve schwannomas depends on the site of origin and the size of the tumor. In a review by Lipkin et al.[26] of 238 facial nerve schwannomas reported in the world literature, the segment of nerve involved was found to be the tympanic segment in 58 percent, the vertical segment in 48 percent, and the labyrinthine/geniculate segment in 42 percent. These tumors can also be multicentric, with involvement of several branches or segments of the facial nerve, as occurred in 3 of 17 patients reported by Conley and Janecka.[7]

The most common presenting symptoms are hearing loss, facial paralysis, facial pain, hemifacial spasm, tinnitus, vertigo, otorrhea, and otalgia. As would be expected, the type of hearing loss is predictive of the location of the tumor. Sensorineural loss is most commonly caused by tumors within the internal auditory canal and the posterior fossa. Tumors in this location are often diagnosed preoperatively as acoustic tumors, with their actual origin from the facial nerve noted at surgery. Conductive hearing loss is typically seen with tumors involving the geniculate, horizontal, or vertical segments of the facial nerve.[29] Tumors that involve the distal facial nerve can present as a parotid mass.

Facial paralysis is noted in up to 45 percent of cases, although it is not always a presenting symptom or sign. Usually the weakness is of gradual onset, but an acute onset of facial weakness, similar to that of Bell's palsy, has been reported in up to 20 percent of cases.[11] In other cases, facial paralysis may be intermittent, with partial or complete recovery of function between episodes.

It is of note that schwannomas which present as a retrotympanic mass on otoscopic evaluation are typically confined to the geniculate, horizontal, or vertical segment of the nerve; in only 2 of 14 such cases did the tumor extend into the middle or posterior fossa.[29]

The surgical approach to facial nerve schwannomas depends on the location of the lesion. Tumors proximal to the geniculate ganglion but not extending significantly into the cerebellopontine angle can be approached in one of two ways, depending on the results of the patient's audiologic assessment. In cases where there is no hearing or poor cochlear reserve, a translabyrinthine approach is recommended.[23,26,34] If hearing is to be preserved, a middle fossa approach is recommended. A lateral suboccipital approach should be used for tumors in the cerebellopontine angle. In nearly all cases, a complete resection of the tumor can be accomplished; however, it usually necessitates removal of the involved segment of the facial nerve. Therefore, complete facial paralysis should be expected postoperatively. Symon et al. recommend restoration of facial nerve continuity at the time of tumor resection using an interposition graft of sural nerve or a facial-hypoglossal nerve anastomosis.[36] The latter technique is used in cases of nerve involvement close to the brain stem where there is an inadequate proximal stump. In some cases, the gap is sufficiently small to allow an end-to-end anastomosis. In this series, the most important determinant of facial nerve function was not the technique of anastomosis but, rather, the duration of preoperative facial paralysis. The poorest results were noted in the patients with the longest duration of facial paralysis. Follow-up in this series was from 3 to 80 months, with no recurrences noted.

Lower Cranial Nerves

The cranial nerves traversing the jugular foramen are the glossopharyngeal, vagus, and spinal accessory nerves. While the hypoglossal nerve does not leave the skull through the jugular foramen, it does pass from the brain stem in close proximity to the jugular foramen, and schwannomas of this nerve are therefore also discussed in this section.

Schwannomas identified as originating from a single lower cranial nerve are rare. I found in the literature reports of 37 schwannomas arising from a single lower cranial nerve. In eight of these cases, the tumor originated on the glossopharyngeal nerve (Fig. 153-1)[10]; these cases typically presented with hearing loss, palatal dysfunction, and hoarseness. In five cases, the tumor arose on the vagus nerve[10,28]; these cases typically presented with a jugular foramen syndrome (discussed below). In seven cases, the tumor arose from the spinal accessory nerve,[5,27] either in the jugular foramen or in the cistern, and presented with trapezius pain, dysesthesias in the upper extremity, and signs of brain stem compression. In one case, an accessory nerve schwannoma was thought preoperatively to be a pontomedullary glioma.[27] The most common lower cranial nerve to be affected by a schwannoma is the hypoglossal nerve, with 17 intracranial cases found.[8,38] These tumors presented with evidence of hypoglossal nerve dysfunction, other lower cranial nerve deficits, and brain stem compression.

In most cases, the exact site of origin of schwannomas of the lower cranial nerves cannot be determined. Such cases are grouped together as jugular foramen schwannomas (Fig. 153-2). Hakuba et al. have reviewed a total of 45 such lesions (including three of their own).[16] In nearly half the cases, the jugular foramen was noted to be enlarged (Fig. 153-3). Many of these patients presented with the jugular foramen syndrome, which includes a loss of taste in the posterior one-third of the tongue (nerve IX), paralysis of the vocal cords and palate (nerve X), and weakness of the trapezius and sternocleidomastoid muscles (nerve XI). However, the degree and type of nerve involvement can be highly variable with schwannomas in this region. Of the 45 cases reviewed by Hakuba et al., clinical involvement of the nerves was variable. Symptoms and signs of ninth nerve involvement were noted in 36 (80 percent), of tenth nerve involvement in 29 (64 percent), and of eleventh nerve involvement in 21 (47 percent). Thus, many jugular foramen schwannomas present with one of the allied syndromes of the jugular foramen (Schmidt's, Tapia's, Jackson's, Avellis's, Collet-Sicard's, or Villaret's syndrome), depending on the combination of nerves involved.[35]

The treatment of schwannomas of the jugular foramen is surgical excision. In many cases a total resection can be accomplished. However, significant morbidity is associated with the surgical removal of these lesions; there is a high incidence of postoperative deficits of lower cranial nerves resulting in dysphagia and potential respiratory compromise. Earlier authors even recommended preoperative tracheostomy, although with current operative techniques that may be somewhat aggressive.[18] Certainly a thorough assessment of postoperative swallowing function should be performed prior to any oral intake.

Treatment

As discussed in each section, the treatment of these lesions is surgical. The surgical approach depends on the tumor's location along

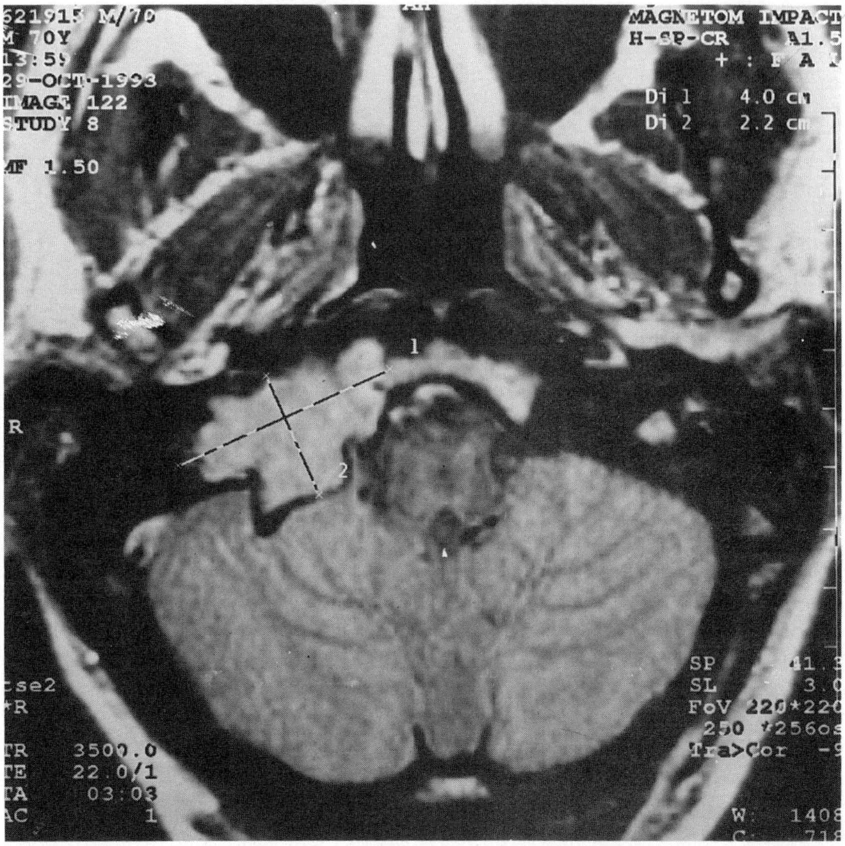

Figure 153-1 An axial MRI scan with gadolinium demonstrating a densely enhancing schwannoma in the region of the jugular foramen, which was found at surgery to arise from the glossopharyngeal nerve.

the nerve tract. Schwannomas in the cisterns can be approached by a subtemporal, transtentorial, frontotemporal, or suboccipital approach. With cisternal tumors, gross total resection is usually possible. Cavernous schwannomas can be approached frontotemporally, and those in a cisternocavernous location can be approached through a frontotemporal or subtemporal approach. If the region of the cavernous sinus is involved, resection is made difficult by tumor invasion of the cavernous sinus and adherence of the tumor to the internal carotid artery. In such cases, a subtotal resection is often the best that can be achieved. In most cases, the nerve

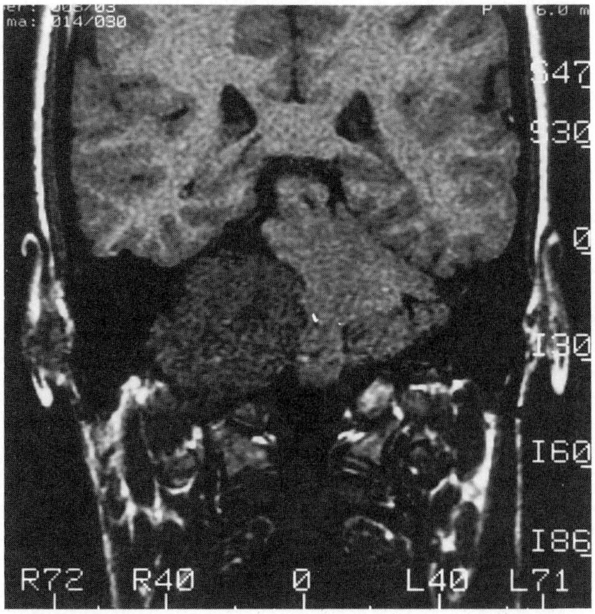

Figure 153-2 A coronal MRI scan without gadolinium demonstrating a large jugular foramen schwannoma with marked brain stem compression. The nerve of origin could not be determined at the time of surgery.

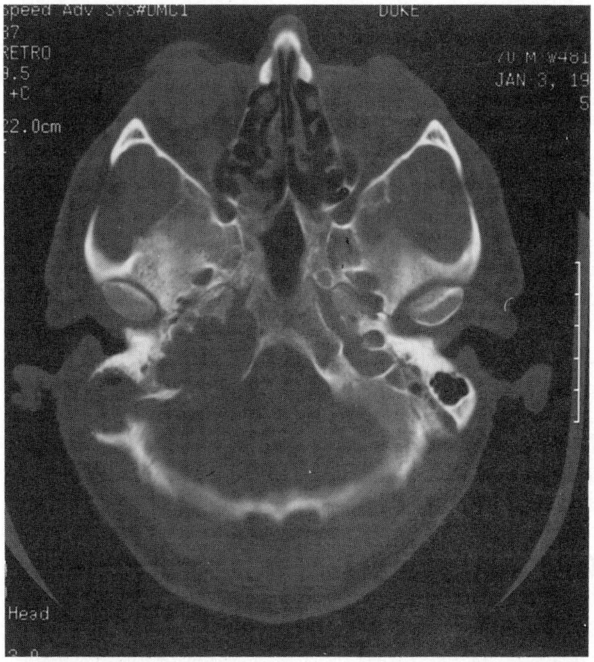

Figure 153-3 The bone window of this CT scan demonstrates the degree of jugular foramen erosion that can occur with tumors in the region of the jugular foramen.

involved with the tumor is not functional after resection of the schwannoma.

In addition to surgery, the use of radiation for nonacoustic schwannomas has been advocated by a number of authors.[32,40] In general, radiation is used as an adjunct to surgery when resection is incomplete. The rationale for using radiation to treat these lesions is based on reports that subtotally resected acoustic tumors treated with postoperative irradiation of greater than 45 Gy demonstrated a recurrence rate of 6 percent, as opposed to 46 percent for nonirradiated tumors.[41] In a series of 18 patients reported by Wallner et al.[40], with a follow-up ranging from 2 to 15 years, the following results were noted. A total resection was achieved in five cases. None of these patients was treated with radiation, and in none has the tumor recurred. Eight patients who had incomplete resection of non-eighth-nerve schwannomas were treated with postoperative megavoltage irradiation to a minimum tumor dose of 45 to 54 Gy. Of these, four developed recurrent tumors. Of four patients who underwent subtotal resection and were not treated with radiation, two developed recurrences. The outcome in one case is not clear. In all cases, the tumor recurred at the site of origin. Recently, a series of six trigeminal nerve and five jugular foramen schwannomas treated with gamma unit stereotactic radiosurgery has been reported.[32] Two of the six trigeminal nerve schwannomas in this study had been treated previously with surgery. Three of the six decreased in size and three showed no change. Of note, two of the six tumors showed a loss of central enhancement on CT scan, and two patients showed signs of clinical improvement (follow-up ranged from 7 to 35 months, with a mean of 21 months). Of the five jugular foramen schwannomas in this series, four had been treated previously with surgery. Over a follow-up period of 7 to 19 months (mean 10 months), one patient had a decrease in tumor size, two had no change, and one showed an increased cystic formation requiring surgery. One patient had no follow-up scan. With such limited information, it is difficult to determine precisely the role of irradiation in the treatment of nonacoustic schwannomas. Of concern is the fact that sensory nerves are particularly sensitive to radiation. We must await longer follow-up on patients treated with radiation to determine the role and efficacy of radiation in the treatment of these lesions.

Summary

Despite the benign pathologic nature of schwannomas of the "other" cranial nerves, their anatomic relationship to important structures, such as the brain stem and cavernous sinus, make prompt diagnosis and treatment important for avoiding serious neurological morbidity related to compression of vital structures.

References

1. Anand CS, Kumra PK, Anand T, Singh SK. Facial nerve schwannoma. *J Laryngol Otol* 1977; 91:1093–1099.
2. Bogdasarian RM. Neurinoma of the facial nerve. *Arch Otolargyngol* 1944; 40:291–294.
3. Broggi G, Franzini A. Value of serial stereotactic biopsies and impedance monitoring in the treatment of deep brain tumours. *J Neurol Neurosurg Psychiatry* 1981; 44:397–401.
4. Celli P, Ferrante L, Acqui M, et al. Neurinoma of the third, fourth, and sixth cranial nerves: a survey and report of a new fourth nerve case. *Surg Neurol* 1992; 38:216–224.
5. Christoferson LA, Leech RW, Grossman M. Intracranial neurilemoma of the spinal accessory nerve. *Surg Neurol* 1982; 18:18–20.
6. Collins EG, Thomson IS. Neurofibroma of the facial nerve: excision with nerve graft. *J Laryngol Otol* 1953; 67:48–50.
7. Conley J, Janecka I. Schwann cell tumors of the facial nerve. *Laryngoscope* 1974; 84:958–962.
8. Dolan EJ, Tucker WS, Rotenberg D, et al. Intracranial hypoglossal schwannoma as an unusual cause of facial nerve palsy. Case report. *J Neurosurg* 1982; 56:420–423.
9. Fagan PA, Misra SN, Doust B. Facial neuroma of the cerebellopontine angle and the internal auditory canal. *Laryngoscope* 1993; 103:442–446.
10. Fink LH, Early CB, Bryan RN. Glossopharyngeal schwannomas. *Surg Neurol* 1978; 9:239–245.
11. Fisch U, Rüttner J. Pathology of intratemporal tumors involving the facial nerve. In Fisch U (ed): *Facial Nerve Surgery*. Birmingham, AL: Aesculapius Publishing Company, 1977, pp 448–456.
12. Furlow LT. The neurosurgical aspects of seventh nerve neurilemmoma. *J Neurosurg* 1960; 17:721–735.
13. Garen PD, Harper CG, Teo C, et al. Cystic schwannoma of the trochlear nerve mimicking a brain-stem tumor: case report. *J Neurosurg* 1987; 67:928–930.
14. Gonzales-Pardo L, Brackett CE, Lansky LL. Facial nerve schwannoma in a 16-year old girl. *Child's Brain* 1980; 7:220–224.
15. Grimson BS, Ross MJ, Tyson G. Return of function after intracranial suture of the trochlear nerve. Case report. *J Neurosurg* 1984; 61:191–192.
16. Hakuba A, Hashi K, Fujitani K, et al. Jugular foramen neurinomas. *Surg Neurol* 1979; 11:83–94.
17. Hora JF, Brown AK. Neurilemmoma of the facial nerve. *Laryngoscope* 1964; 74:134–143.
18. Ignelzi RJ, Bucy PC. Intracranial hypoglossal neurofibroma: case report. *J Neurosurg* 1967; 26:352–356.
19. Isamat F, Bartumeus F, Miranda AM, et al. Neurinomas of the facial nerve. Report of three cases. *J Neurosurg* 1975; 43:608–613.
20. Iwabuchi T, Suzuki M, Nakaoka T, et al. Oculomotor nerve anastomosis. *Neurosurgery* 1982; 10:490–491.
21. Kettel K. Neurinoma of the facial nerve. *Arch Otolaryngol* 1946; 44:253–260.
22. Kettel K. Surgery of the facial nerve. *Arch Otolaryngol* 1963; 77:327–341.
23. King JS. Trochlear nerve sheath tumor. *J Neurosurg* 1976; 44:245–247.
24. Lang J. Über Bau, Länge und Gefassbeziehungen der "zentralen" und "peripheren" Strecken der intrazisternalen Hirnnerven. *Zentralbl Neurochir* 1982; 43:217–255.
25. Liliequist B, Thulin CA, Tovi D, et al. Neurinoma of the labyrinthine portion of the facial nerve: case report. *J Neurosurg* 1972; 37:105–109.
26. Lipkin AF, Coker NJ, Jenkins HA, et al. Intracranial and intratemporal facial neuroma. *Otolaryngol Head Neck Surg* 1987; 96:71–79.
27. Matsushima T, Fukui M, Matsunaga M, et al. Accessory nerve neurinoma mimicking a brain stem tumor on angiography: report of a case. *Neurosurgery* 1985; 16:839–842.
28. Mukherjee DK. Neurilemmoma of the vagus nerve. A case report. *J Laryngol Otol* 1979; 93:187–192.
29. O'Donoghue GMO, Brackmann DE, House JW, et al. Neuromas of the facial nerve. *Am J Otol* 1989; 10:49–54.
30. Parnes LS, Lee DH, Peerless SJ. Magnetic resonance imaging of facial nerve neuromas. *Laryngoscope* 1991; 101:31–35.
31. Pearman K, Welch AR. Schwannoma of the intratemporal facial nerve. Case report. *J Laryngol Otol* 1980; 94:779–784.
32. Pollock BE, Kondziolka D, Flickinger JC, et al. Preservation of cranial nerve function after radiosurgery for nonacoustic schwannomas. *Neurosurgery* 1993; 33:597–601.
33. Pulec JL. Facial nerve tumors. *Ann Otol Rhinol Laryngol* 1969; 78:962–982.

34. Pulec JL. Facial nerve neuroma. *Laryngoscope* 1972; 82:1160–1176.
35. Svien HJ, Baker HL, Rivers MH. Jugular foramen syndrome and allied syndromes. *Neurology* 1963; 13:797–809.
36. Symon L, Cheesman AD, Kawauchi M, et al. Neuromas of the facial nerve: a report of 12 cases. *Br J Neurosurg* 1993; 7:13–22.
37. Tremble GE, Penfield W. Operative exposure of the facial canal: with removal of a tumor of the greater superficial petrosal nerve. *Arch Otolaryngol* 1936; 23:573–579.
38. Ulso C, Sehested P, Overgaard J. Intracranial hypoglossal neurinoma: diagnosis and postoperative care. *Surg Neurol* 1981; 16:65–68.
39. Vaquero J, Martinez R, Salazar J. Suprasellar recurrence of third nerve neurinoma. *J Neurosurg* 1985; 62:317 (letter).
40. Wallner KE, Pitts LH, Davis RL, et al. Radiation therapy for the treatment of non-eighth nerve intracranial neurilemmoma. *Int J Radiat Oncol Biol Phys* 1988; 14:287–290.
41. Wallner KE, Sheline GE, Pitts LH, et al. Efficacy of irradiation for incompletely excised acoustic neurilemomas. *J Neurosurg* 1987; 67:858–863.
42. Zülch KJ. *Brain Tumors: Their Biology and Pathology,* 3d ed. Berlin: Springer-Verlag, 1986.

154

Paragangliomas of the Carotid Body and Temporal Bone

John H. Sampson
Robert H. Wilkins

Paragangliomas are neoplasms of the paraganglia. The paraganglia are small aggregates of cells derived from embryonic neuroepithelium that are distributed throughout the human body in close association with the autonomic nervous system. Historically, the paraganglia have been divided into chromaffin and nonchromaffin subtypes. The carotid bodies are the largest and best known of the nonchromaffin paraganglia, and, along with paraganglia of the temporal bone, are the most frequent source of paragangliomas encountered by the neurosurgeon.

Paragangliomas of the carotid body and temporal bone are slowly growing hypervascular tumors that originate at the carotid bifurcation and in the temporal bone, respectively. Patients with carotid body paragangliomas typically present with a painless mass at the angle of the jaw, while those with a temporal bone paraganglioma usually present with gradual hearing loss and unilateral pulsatile tinnitus. With larger lesions of either type, multiple lower cranial nerve palsies are common, and 1 to 3 percent of these tumors produce catecholamines that may give rise to additional symptoms. Although paragangliomas have a predominantly benign appearance histologically, they are invasive locally and, rarely, can metastasize. They can occur in multiple locations simultaneously, and at least some seem to be inherited. Multiplanar computed tomography (CT) or magnetic resonance imaging (MRI) is usually sufficient for making this diagnosis; therefore, angiography is usually reserved for outlining the blood supply to lesions that will be treated by embolization or surgical resection. Complete surgical excision is now possible for most carotid body and temporal bone paragangliomas and should be the goal for most patients. Radiation therapy, however, may be an appropriate and effective therapy for some patients.

Paraganglia: Structure and Function

Since their discovery, the structure and function of the carotid and temporal paraganglia have been debated. Naturally, this has led to an unfortunate proliferation of confusing synonyms being applied to these structures. More, recently, however, the role of these structures as chemoreceptors in a diffuse neuroendocrine system has been revealed. This system incorporates several organs that contain peptide-producing cells derived from neuroepithelium that are characterized by amine precursor uptake and decarboxylation (APUD).[23]

Anatomy

The carotid body is a vascular reddish brown structure, about the size of a grain of rice, located within the adventitia posteromedial to the bifurcation of the common carotid artery (CCA). Blood reaches the carotid body via a fibrovascular bundle, the ligament of Mayer, that runs from the posterior surface of the CCA to the inferior portion of the carotid body and supplies the normal carotid body with more blood by weight than the brain.

The carotid body is innervated by the intercarotid plexus and the carotid branch of the glossopharyngeal nerve, also called the carotid sinus nerve or the nerve of Hering.[32] Both receive contributions from the glossopharyngeal and vagus nerves and from the superior cervical sympathetic ganglion. Although the major innervation of the carotid body is sensory, efferent innervation for vasomotor tone control and inhibitory feedback mechanisms has also been proposed.

The temporal bone paraganglia are smaller ovoid masses located in various regions of the temporal bones. These bodies do not have a precise anatomic location but are always found in association with the nerves of Arnold and Jacobson. In 88 temporal bones from 44 patients, Guild found 248 temporal bone paraganglia.[9] Most temporal bones had at least one paraganglia while some had as many as 12. Most of the temporal bone paraganglia (135) were found along the course of the tympanic branch of the glossopharyngeal nerve (Jacobson's nerve) at its origin (14), in the adventitia of the jugular bulb (37), in the tympanic canaliculus (54), on the promontory (27), and distally along the lesser petrosal nerve (3). Fewer (113) were found in association with the auricular branch of the vagus nerve (Arnold's nerve) which runs a variable course. Most of the temporal bone paraganglia found along this nerve were located within the jugular fossa (81); the remainder were distributed distally along the mastoid canaliculi between the jugular fossa and the descending part of the facial canal (19), within the descending facial canal (7), or accompanying an aberrant branch of Arnold's nerve that passed external to the skull base between the jugular fossa and the stylomastoid foramen (6). The sex, race, or side studied appears to make no difference in the number or position of these bodies. The number of paraganglia seems to increase until the fourth decade of life and then to decline.

Both Arnold's and Jacobson's nerves are accompanied by branches of the inferior tympanic branch of the ascending pharyngeal artery. This vessel supplies blood to the normal temporal bone paraganglia. Neoplasms may recruit additional blood supply from a variety of other sources, however. The temporal bone paraganglia are innervated by Arnold's and Jacobson's nerves along with some branches from the superior cervical sympathetic ganglion.

Histology

The carotid and temporal paraganglia are indistinguishable histologically. Wide bands of cartilaginous connective tissue divide the parenchyma into lobules. Each lobule is nourished by a single arteriole and is divided into three to six cell nests. Each of these cell nests, called glomeruli or Zellballen, contains 20 to 40 cells of various types that are surrounded by a sinusoidal vascular network (Fig. 154-1).[32]

The parenchyma of the paraganglia consists of two primary cell types. These are best called type I and type II cells. Type I cells are more common and are typically round with indistinct cell borders. Type I cells may be further divided into light, dark, and pyknotic subtypes that may have different functions. The role of type I cells, however, remains unknown. Because they store a variety of biologically active amines, it is tempting to postulate that these substances are released in response to chemical changes in the blood. On the other hand, these chemicals could modulate other chemoreceptive nerve endings. Similarly, type I cells could act as interneurons. Type II cells are smaller and irregularly shaped. They are situated between the type I cells and the surrounding vascular sinusoids. These cells may act as glial-like sheaths for the type I cells.

Paragangliomas

Pathology

Operative specimens from carotid body or temporal bone paragangliomas are generally indistinguishable. Smaller tumors may be grooved by the carotid arteries while larger ones may have vessels imbedded in the sample. These tumors tend to be smooth and well circumscribed. They have a rubbery consistency, and the cut surface is usually homogeneous except for some occasional areas of necrosis, fibrosis, or hemorrhage.

Although paragangliomas of the carotid body and temporal bone are generally regarded as benign, they are histologically invasive and can metastasize.[4,33] Typically, rates of malignancy of 3 percent for temporal bone tumors and 12 percent for carotid body tumors are quoted, although some reports quote rates as high as 30 to 50 percent. The definition of malignancy for paragangliomas is difficult to establish, however. These tumors tend to develop spontaneously in multiple locations and to recur frequently. On the other hand, paragangliomas may grow very slowly and often lack histologic changes characteristic of other malignant tumors. Only relatively recently was a reduction in the proportion of type II cells and a poorer staining of type I cells for S-100 and glial fibrillary acidic protein (GFAP) reported to be correlated with an increased tumor grade.[16] Finally, although patients with metastatic paragangliomas may quickly succumb, their prognosis is completely unpredictable, and some patients with multiple metastatic lesions survive for several decades.

The nonchromaffin paragangliomas also have a familial tendency. An analysis of 15 pedigrees by van der Mey and colleagues found that paragangliomas were inherited in an autosomal dominant fashion but were transmitted almost exclusively by males.[29] For example, an affected father resulted in 28 percent (23/82) of descendants (11 males and 12 females) being affected, while in families with an affected mother, the disease was reported in only one descendant with a questionable diagnosis. This pattern of inheritance is best explained by a hypothesis of genomic imprinting by which a maternally derived mutant gene that leads to the development of a paraganglioma is inactivated during oogenesis only to be reactivated during spermatogenesis in a subsequent generation. Overall, half the patients in this series had a positive family history.

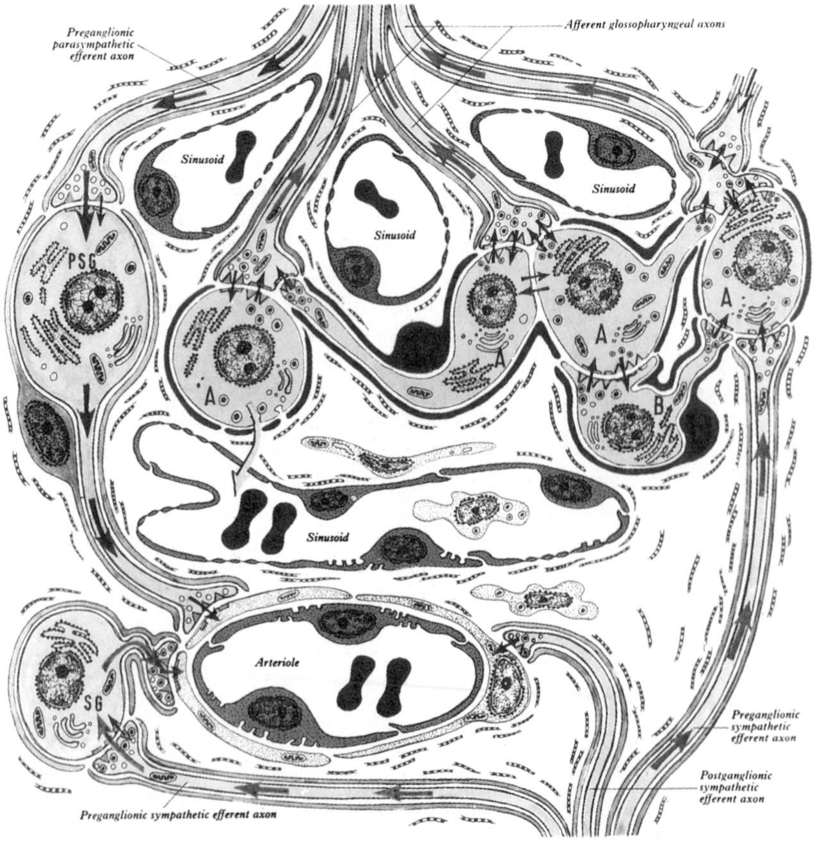

Figure 154-1 Diagram showing the microanatomic arrangement of the paraganglia. The type I (A) and type II (B) cells are shown within the vascular sinusoidal network. The innervation is also shown. (From Williams et al.,[32] with permission).

As could be expected, a positive family history also places a patient at increased risk for developing a second primary paraganglioma. In this circumstance, up to one-third of patients will have a second paraganglioma. Multicentric paragangliomas, however, are discovered in as many as 10 percent of patients without a significant family medical history. The onset of these multicentric tumors may be synchronous or delayed by several decades. Bilateral carotid body tumors are the most frequently encountered example. These are followed in frequency by the combination of a carotid body tumor and a temporal bone tumor and then other combinations. Plurifocal tumors can occur in 3 to 5 percent of patients.

Clinical Presentation

Carotid Body Paragangliomas

Carotid body tumors are the second most frequently encountered nonchromaffin paragangliomas after temporal bone paragangliomas. More than 1000 cases have now been reported in the literature.[33] These tumors usually present in patients in the fourth, fifth, or sixth decade of life, although reported cases range in age from 3 months to 89 years. An average tumor size is 4.5 × 3.5 × 3 cm, with the largest tumors exceeding 15 cm in diameter and weighing almost 200 g. There may be an increased incidence of these tumors in high-altitude dwellers, and although some reports show a female predominance greater than 5:1, carotid body tumors are less sex-specific than temporal bone paragangliomas.

Classically, carotid body tumors grow with progressive involvement of the internal and external carotid arteries, usually without constricting the arterial lumens. These lesions can extend into the base of the skull through a foramen or by bony erosion. Alternatively, they may grow medially or laterally and into the peripharyngeal space or inferiorly to invade the clavicle. The clinical manifestations of these tumors generally can be ascertained from these characteristic growth patterns. The widely accepted Shamblin classification system of carotid body tumors is primarily used for staging purposes, but also allows a comparison between different therapeutic modalities (Fig. 154-2).[10]

Patients with carotid body tumors typically present with a painless mass at the angle of the jaw that may be partially covered by the sternocleidomastoid muscle. Although many other possibilities exist in the differential diagnosis of such lesions (Table 154-1),[33] classically, the mass from a carotid body tumor is mobile laterally, but is restricted from vertical movement because of its attachment to the bifurcation of the CCA. These vascular tumors may transmit pulsations from the nearby carotid arteries or may be pulsatile inherently. The mass may shrink and reexpand spontaneously or with digital compression, and infrequently a bruit may also be heard over the mass. Larger tumors may produce a pharyngeal bulge that may displace or erode the tonsil, soft palate, or uvula. In these instances, patients may present with spontaneous oropharyngeal bleeding. Occasionally, however, these tumors are discovered incidentally at angiography, surgery, or autopsy.

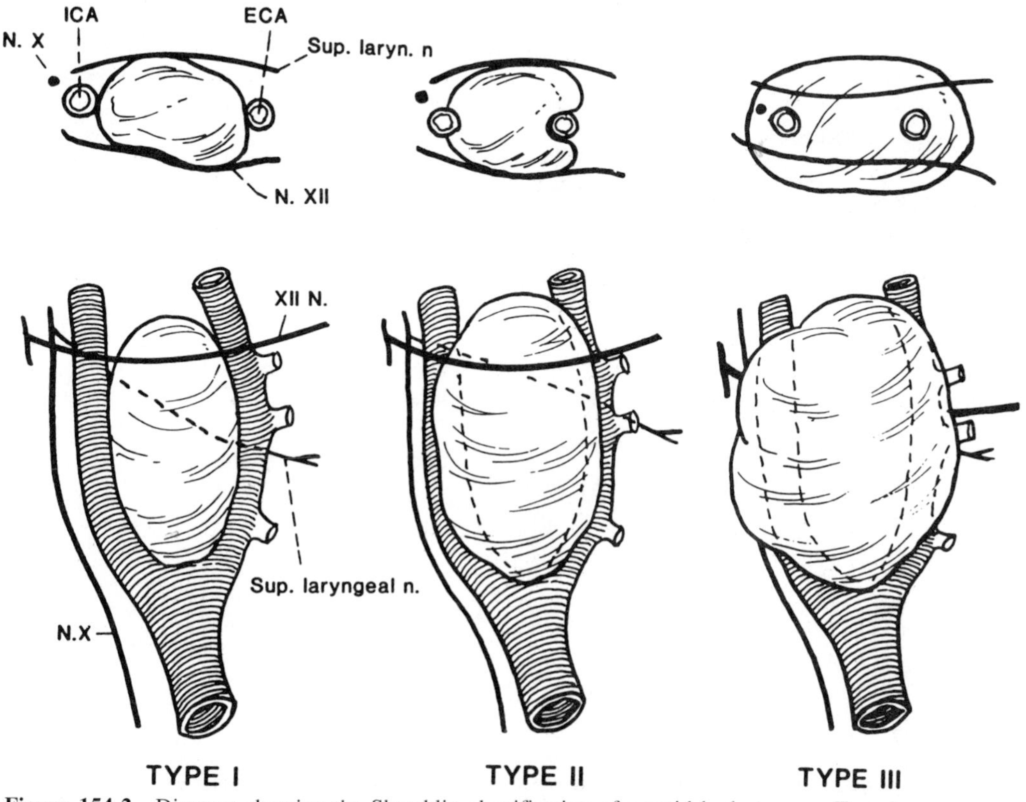

Figure 154-2 Diagram showing the Shamblin classification of carotid body tumors. Type I tumors are easily dissected from surrounding structures. Type II tumors partially surround the carotid arteries. Type III tumors encase the carotid arteries completely and are the most difficult to resect without vascular or neural injury. (From Hallett et al.,[10] with permission).

TABLE 154-1 Differential Diagnosis of Carotid Body Paragangliomas

Lymphadenitis	Fibroma, lipoma, hemangioma, dermoid, teratoma
Lympoma	Aneurysm
Branchial cleft cyst	Giant cell arteritis
Lymph node metastases	Hematoma
Lateral aberrant thyroid	Carotid stenosis with poststenotic dilatation
Vagal or sympathetic neurogenic tumors	Carotid calcification
Salivary gland tumors	

Source: Adapted from Zak and Lawson.[33]

An invasion of surrounding neural structures in the neck can result in a variety of additional sequelae. At the time of diagnosis, cranial nerve palsies are usually present in less than 10 percent of patients.[10,33] The vagus and hypoglossal nerves are most frequently involved, and this usually leads to dysphagia or hoarseness. Cranial nerves V and VII may also be involved, however. In addition, infiltration of the cervical or brachial plexus may result in the mass being painful or tender, while involvement of the cervical sympathetic chain can produce a Horner's syndrome.

The distant effects of these tumors are varied, and remain for the most part unexplained. Perhaps the best example of this phenomenon is the carotid sinus syndrome. This syndrome of bradycardia, hypotension, and a loss of consciousness may occur spontaneously or secondary to head movement or direct pressure on the tumor in some patients with carotid body paragangliomas. Additional reports of such systemic abnormalities that have resolved after tumor excision include alterations in gut motility with emesis on manipulation of the tumor, extensive skin alterations, constitutional symptoms such as weight loss and fever, and even one case of membranous glomerulonephritis.[33] Finally, while catecholamine production is exceedingly rare for extra-adrenal paragangliomas, a few patients with these tumors may present with a variety of symptoms or signs secondary to catecholamine production.[6,18,33] Norepinephrine is the usual product and hypertension is the most frequent finding. Although only a handful of such cases have been reported in the literature, being unaware of functional tumors can have disastrous consequences during embolization or surgery. Therefore, patients with suspicious findings should have free norepinephrine, epinephrine, and 3,4-dihydroxyphenylglycol measured in a 24-h urine collection.[5] If these tests confirm the presence of such a tumor then the patient should undergo an appropriate adrenergic blockade prior to embolization or surgery (Table 154-2).[6]

TABLE 154-2 Treatment Guidelines for Adrenergic Blockade

α-Adrenergic Blockade

At least 2 weeks before surgery, establish adequate blockade in all patients with norepinephrine- and epinephrine-secreting tumors.

Begin with phenoxybenzamine, 10 mg twice a day; increase by 10 mg/day at 3-day intervals; 10–20 mg 3 times a day usually suffices.

Maintain patient on generous salt diet to expand blood volume.

β-Adrenergic Blockade

Indicated in patients with a heart rate greater than 110 beats/min, history of arrhythmias or persistent ventricular extrasystoles, or predominantly epinephrine-secreting tumor; also in patients with pulse rate greater than 110 beats/min after initiation of phenoxybenzamine therapy.

For most patients, begin with propranolol, not to exceed 10 mg 3 times a day; 30–60 mg/day usually suffices. For patients with history of bronchospastic disease use low-dose metoprolol or equivalent cardioselective beta-blocker.

Do not initiate β-adrenergic blockade until α-adrenergic blockade is at least partially established.

Source: From Feldman,[6] with permission.

Temporal Bone Paragangliomas

Temporal bone paragangliomas are the most frequently encountered benign tumor of the temporal bone, and must be considered in the differential diagnosis of temporal bone lesions (Table 154-3).[33] Although frequent histologic misinterpretation, difficulties with nomenclature, and republication of cases make estimates of prevalence difficult, well over 1000 cases have been reported in the world literature.[33] These tumors usually present in patients in the fifth decade of life, although reported cases range in age from 22 months to 85 years of age. Females with temporal bone paragangliomas outnumber males approximately 3:1 in most large series and ratios of 10:1 have been reported. Larger studies also suggest a preference for the left side, especially in females.

Paragangliomas of the temporal bone are generally divided into those that originate within the middle ear, *glomus tympanicum tumors,* and those that originate within the jugular fossa, *glomus jugulare tumors.* This latter term, however, is often used to refer to large tumors where the origin is difficult to determine. The predominance of the paraganglia within the jugular fossa likely accounts for the increased frequency of tumors with this origin. Classification systems that have been developed for temporal bone paragangliomas are used for staging purposes, surgical planning, and comparison among different therapeutic modalities. The Glasscock-Jackson (Table 154-4)[12] and Fisch (Table 154-5)[7] classifications are the most widely employed.

The symptoms and signs that result from paraganglia of the temporal bone can be conveniently divided into otologic and neurological manifestations. Otologic symptoms usually predominate for both *glomus jugulare* and *glomus tympanicum* tumors. Unilateral hearing loss is the most frequent initial symptom and will be present in most patients. Typically it is gradual in onset, but an acute onset should not exclude the diagnosis. Although the hearing loss can be of the conductive type, sensorineural hearing loss is usually present at the time of diagnosis in most patients. This indicates involvement of the labyrinth or eighth cranial nerve and a

TABLE 154-3 Differential Diagnosis of Temporal Bone Paragangliomas

Otitis media	Meningioma
Otosclerosis	Metastasis
Chronic mastoiditis	Aneurysm
Cholesteatoma	Aberrant intrapetrous internal carotid artery
Cholesterol granuloma	Idiopathic hemotympanum
Eosinophilic granuloma	Arteriovenous malformation
Chordoma	Prominent jugular bulb
Vestibular schwannoma	Persistent stapedial artery

Source: Adapted from Zak and Lawson.[33]

TABLE 154-4 Glasscock-Jackson Classification of Temporal Bone Paragangliomas

Type I	Small tumor involving the jugular bulb, middle ear, and mastoid
Type II	Tumor extending under internal auditory canal; might have intracranial extension
Type III	Tumor extending into petrous apex; might have intracranial extension
Type IV	Tumor extending beyond petrous apex into clivus or infratemporal fossa; might have intracranial extension

Source: From Jackson et al.,[12] with permission.

poorer prognosis. Unilateral tinnitus, synchronous with the pulse, is the second most frequently reported symptom. Often, this is coincident with an audible bruit, and both can be reduced with neck turning or direct pressure on the tumor. Otoscopic examination may reveal a gray-red mass in the external auditory canal or a hypervascular or bulging tympanic membrane. This mass may not be pulsatile on first inspection, but pulsations usually can be demonstrated by increasing the pressure within the external auditory canal using a pneumatic otoscope. Examination with the otoscope can also confirm bleeding from the lesion or an associated chronic otitis media that may lead to otalgia, meningitis, or brain abscess.

Neurological symptoms and signs generally follow otologic symptoms by several years, but ultimately these tumors produce neurological symptoms or signs in one-third to two-thirds of patients. These neurological findings are very important in classifying the stage and extent of these tumors. Neurological manifestations of these lesions result from involvement of either the cranial nerves or the brain. Although temporal bone paragangliomas can lead to a palsy of any adjacent cranial nerve, the facial nerve is the most commonly involved. The facial nerve may be affected in the middle ear or by extension of the tumor into the mastoid or internal acoustic meatus. In a similar way, vertigo may be secondary to involvement of the labyrinth, or secondary to compression of the eighth nerve directly. The resultant nystagmus is usually horizontal, but vertical and rotatory nystagmus have been reported. The lower cranial nerves are also frequently involved. Patients with *glomus jugulare* tumors often present with a jugular foramen syndrome that includes palsies of the ninth, tenth, and eleventh cranial nerves. Greater cranial nerve involvement generally correlates with increased invasion of the nervous system and a worse prognosis.

Involvement of the central nervous system generally results from extension of the tumor into the middle or posterior cranial fossa, especially in the region of the cerebellopontine angle. Besides additional cranial nerve palsies, this can produce headache, increased intracranial pressure, cerebellar and long tract signs, or a Horner's syndrome. Seizures from temporal lobe penetration by a paraganglioma have been reported, and these tumors have been cited as the cause of cerebral ischemic events, congestive heart failure, and subarachnoid hemorrhage. A few patients with these tumors may also present with a variety of symptoms or signs secondary to catecholamine production as described above for carotid body tumors.[6,18,33]

TABLE 154-5 Fisch Classification of Temporal Bone Paragangliomas

Class A: Tumors limited to the middle ear cleft
Class B: Tumors limited to the tympanomastoid area without destruction of bone in the infralabyrinthine compartment
Class C: Tumors extending into and destroying bone of the infralabyrinthine and apical compartments of the temporal bone
- C_1: Tumors destroying the bone of the jugular foramen and jugular bulb with limited involvement of the vertical portion of the carotid canal
- C_2: Tumors destroying the infralabyrinthine compartment of the temporal bone and invading the vertical portion of the carotid canal
- C_3: Tumors involving the infralabyrinthine and apical compartments of the temporal bone with invasion of the horizontal portion of the carotid canal

Class D: Tumors with intracranial extension
- D_1: Tumors with intracranial extension up to 2 cm in diameter
- D_2: Tumors with an intracranial extension greater than 2 cm in diameter
- D_3: Tumors with inoperable intracranial extension

Note: For class D tumors, additional subscripts are used to further differentiate extradural (e) from intradural (i) intracranial extension of tumor.
Source: From Fisch et al.,[7] with permission.

Radiographic Evaluation

Patients suspected of having a carotid body or temporal bone paraganglioma should undergo a noninvasive radiographic study to exclude more common entities and to detect an additional unsuspected paraganglioma at another location. The initial radiographic investigation selected depends on the clinical impression. Patients with a temporal bone paraganglioma thought to be limited to the middle ear (*glomus tympanicum*) should undergo high-resolution, axial and direct coronal, bolus-enhanced CT of the temporal bone and surrounding structures.[27] A small glomus tympanicum tumor will appear as a contrast-enhancing soft tissue mass on the promontory within the middle ear cavity (Fig. 154-3). If the bony septum that separates the jugular bulb and carotid artery from the middle ear is intact, then several vascular abnormalities within the differential diagnosis can also be excluded. Furthermore, any tumor present can be considered limited to the middle ear. This has considerable importance in selecting the appropriate surgical approach.

Patients thought to have a carotid body paraganglioma or a temporal bone paraganglioma that extends beyond the middle ear or that originates next to the jugular bulb (*glomus jugulare*) should undergo multiplanar, thin-section, T1- and T2-weighted and gadolinium diethylenetriaminepenta-acetic acid (DTPA) enhanced MRI. Paragangliomas have an intermediate signal on T1-weighted and a high signal on T2-weighted images and enhance intensely (Fig. 154-4).[22] In addition, paragangliomas greater than 2 cm in size produce a characteristic salt-and-pepper appearance that results from the fast-flowing blood pools and large tumor vessels within these lesions. Although this appearance in the petromastoid region is almost pathognomonic for a temporal bone paraganglioma, renal and thyroid carcinoma metastases and hemangiomas can be confused with carotid body paragangliomas in the peripharyngeal space. Although MRI clearly proves involvement of the carotid arteries and jugular vein by these lesions, bony landmarks in the skull base are poorly defined by MR images, and parallel imaging with CT may be necessary.

Cerebral angiography remains the gold standard for the diagnosis of head and neck paragangliomas, but in practice, this study is reserved for patients who have larger tumors and who are scheduled for embolization or resection. The main goal of angiography in such patients is to delineate the vascular anatomy of the tumor.

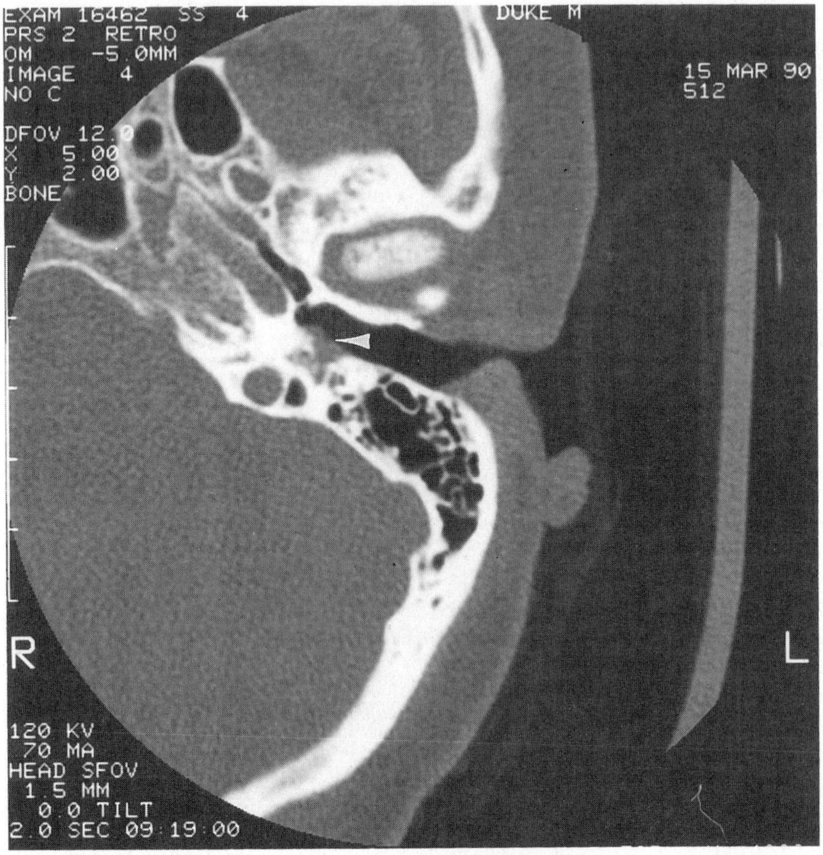

Figure 154-3 A high-resolution unenhanced axial computed tomogram of the left temporal bone with bone window processing demonstrates a *glomus tympanicum* temporal bone paraganglioma (*white arrowhead*).

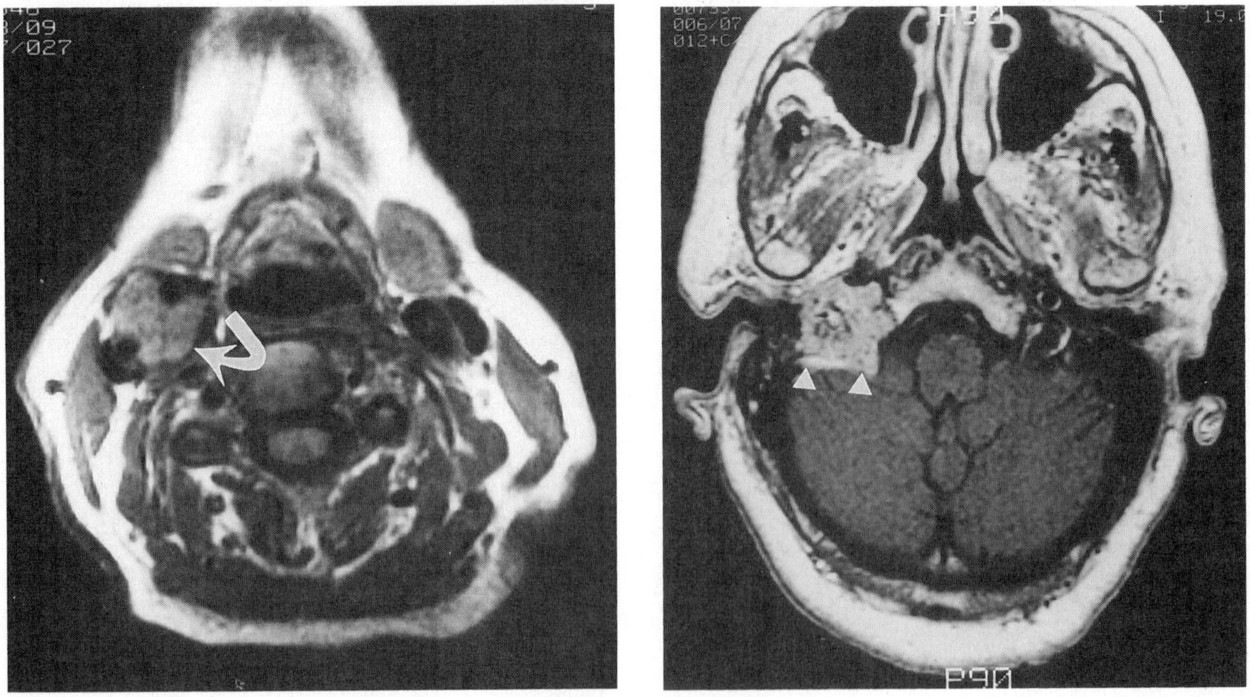

(*A*) (*B*)

Figure 154-4 Magnetic resonance images of carotid body and temporal bone paragangliomas. *A.* An axial T1-weighted image of a right carotid body paraganglioma (*curved white arrow*). The mass is well circumscribed and is located between the internal and external carotid arteries. *B.* An axial T1-weighted image of a temporal bone paraganglioma (*white arrowheads*) demonstrating the characteristic contrast enhancement. Note also the typical salt-and-pepper appearance of these tumors. (Courtesy of Dr. Gary J. Felsberg and Dr. Robert D. Tien)

However, it can also be used to determine the presence of internal carotid artery invasion and to evaluate for atherosclerotic disease, patency of the circle of Willis, and the patient's tolerance of balloon test occlusion. Both external carotid artery (ECA) and internal carotid artery (ICA) iodinated contrast injections are routinely employed. If intracranial extension is suspected, vertebrobasilar angiography will also be necessary.

Paragangliomas have an angiographic appearance midway between that of a meningioma and that of an arteriovenous malformation. Early phases show variably sized pathologic vessels around the tumor site. This is followed by an intense, occasionally inhomogeneous staining of the tumor. For temporal bone tumors such a tumor blush appears in the middle ear and may be obscured by the overlying temporal bone. Thus, subtraction techniques may be necessary. Other findings with temporal bone paragangliomas may include an increase in the number and size of branches passing from the ECA to the temporal bone and displacement of vessels within the middle or posterior cranial compartment. Besides the characteristic tumor blush in patients with a carotid body tumor, a characteristic distortion of the carotid bifurcation is also visible on angiography (Fig. 154-5). The ICA is generally pushed laterally and posteriorly while the ECA is displaced anteriorly.

Other diagnostic techniques may also be of value if applied under appropriate circumstances. For example, about half of all head and neck paragangliomas can be detected using iodine-123 metaiodobenzylguanidine (MIBG) scintigraphy.[30] Most nonchromaffin paragangliomas show low uptake of this tracer; therefore, single photon emission computed tomography (SPECT) images are needed to eliminate the interference created by the normal uptake of tracer in the parotid and submandibular glands. In addition, total body scintigraphy with ^{123}I-MIBG can be used as a screening tool to detect distant additional primary or metastatic lesions in patients or their near relatives. Although it is often speculated that such uptake, especially if intense, suggests a norepinephrine-producing tumor, the uptake of ^{123}I-MIBG can be independent of catecholamine secretory activity. In lesions that show tracer uptake, this technique can be used to document the results of therapy or to treat unresectable lesions by using radiotherapeutic doses of ^{131}I-MIBG.[15] Color Doppler ultrasound can also be used to demonstrate vascular lesions that disrupt the carotid bifurcation, but it will not reliably differentiate between carotid body tumors and other vascular lesions in the area.

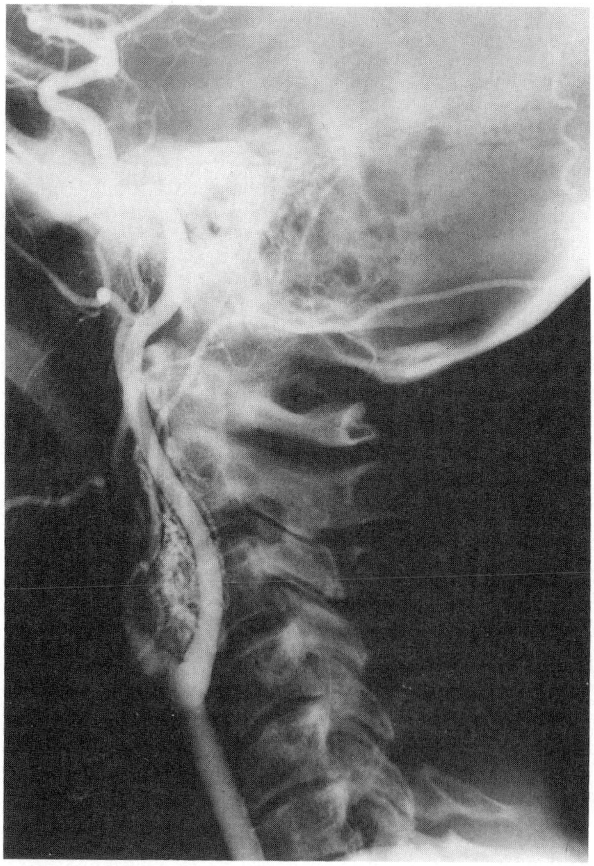

Figure 154-5 A lateral view of an angiogram demonstrating a carotid body paraganglioma. This hypervascular mass extends from the level of the bifurcation of the common carotid artery to the second cervical vertebra. Note the characteristic separation of the internal and external carotid arteries.

Treatment

There are four treatment options for patients with carotid body or temporal bone paragangliomas. These can be used alone or in various combinations. The ideal treatment for most patients is complete surgical excision of the tumor. Endovascular embolization can be used preoperatively to facilitate such a resection, but insufficient evidence exists to warrant its isolated use. In patients not suited for operative therapy, irradiation may be a useful measure for primary or metastatic disease. Chemotherapy, on the other hand, has been reserved for patients with systemic metastases and has no proven efficacy except for a few isolated case reports.[17]

Embolization

Endovascular embolization of carotid body or temporal bone tumors may reduce operative time and limit blood loss. This was shown in one representative work by Ward and colleagues who retrospectively compared six patients with carotid body tumors who underwent preoperative embolization to ten patients with 11 tumors who did not.[31] They found a reduction in average operative time from 4.24 h to 1.75 h. The blood loss was also reduced from 1250 ml to approximately 400 ml. Although these authors also observed a reduction in operative cranial nerve injuries in patients who underwent preoperative embolization, they provide no basis for comparison between the two groups for other important parameters such as tumor classification or size. Similarly, Murphy and Brackmann reported a series of patients with temporal bone tumors stratified according to the Fisch classification system.[21] Eighteen patients underwent preoperative embolization while 17 patients did not. When patients with tumors from all classifications were grouped together, embolized patients showed a significant reduction in operative blood loss from 2769 ml to 1122 ml ($p < 0.005$) and a reduction in operative time from 7.95 h to 7.04 h ($p < 0.005$). However, Murphy and Brackmann could not show a reduction in postoperative cranial nerve deficits with embolization. In both of the above studies, however, the embolized patients were always later in the series. Therefore, these conclusions are confounded by other variables such as an increase in the experience of the operative team. Although some authorities have not found preoperative embolization necessary, most now employ this technique for Shamblin type III carotid body tumors and Fisch type $C_{2,3}$ or D temporal bone tumors. Embolization usually takes place immediately following the diagnostic angiogram and is then followed soon after by surgery to prevent the recognized phenomena of collateral vessel formation and recanalization.

Temporal bone paragangliomas may be composed of up to four hemodynamically isolated compartments.[20,26] Each of these compartments is primarily supplied by different branches of the ECA. Therefore, superselective catheterization of specific branches of the ECA is necessary for complete embolization of a multicompartmental tumor. Blood supply from the internal carotid and vertebral arteries can be shown for some anteriorly located tumors that may be supplied by the caroticotympanic branch of the ICA. Large tumors with extradural intracranial extension may also be supplied by clival and cavernous branches of the ICA. The intradural component of Fisch type D_i tumors is always supplied by parenchymal branches from the vertebrobasilar system, usually the posterior inferior cerebellar artery at the level of the jugular foramen and the anterior inferior cerebellar artery in the cerebellopontine angle.

Complete devascularization of Fisch type C and at least partial devascularization of type D tumors can usually be achieved.[26] Tumors with an anterior component supplied by the caroticotympanic artery can be embolized completely only if this artery can be selectively catheterized and there is no evidence of contrast reflux into the ICA. Otherwise tumors with significant ICA blood supply can only be embolized by balloon occlusion of the petrous ICA provided the patient has tolerated temporary balloon occlusion and hypotensive testing before embolization. The intradural portion of type D tumors is supplied by the vertebrobasilar system and cannot be embolized safely.

Preoperative embolization of temporal bone paragangliomas is usually followed by a fever and transient ear pain.[26] This procedure may also be complicated by wound healing problems, cerebral ischemia, and lower cranial nerve palsies. Ischemic cerebral events are most likely to occur if arterial anastomoses exist between the branches of the ECA supplying the tumor and the ICA or vertebrobasilar arterial system. Such anastomoses, present in as many as one-third of patients, are not a contraindication to embolization, but special techniques such as temporary occlusion of the anastomotic artery or the use of embolic particles larger than the anastomotic artery must be employed. Similarly, permanent new cranial nerve palsies may develop if nonabsorbable embolization material is injected into the neuromeningeal branch of the ascending pharyngeal artery that supplies cranial nerves IX through XII or the stylomastoid and middle meningeal arteries that supply blood to cranial nerve VII. Absorbable materials such as Gelfoam (absorbable gelatin sponge; The Upjohn Company, Kalamazoo, MI) may still produce cranial nerve palsies, but these are usually transient.

Preoperative embolization of carotid body tumors follows the same basic principles as outlined above for temporal bone paragangliomas.[26] Most carotid body tumors are also multicompartmental, with the bulk of the blood supply coming from the ascending cervical artery and the musculospinal branch of the ascending pharyngeal artery. The tumor may also be supplied by the facial, lingual, thyroid, posterior auricular, occipital, and deep cervical arteries. The artery of the carotid body that also supplies these tumors cannot usually be identified on angiography, and therefore cannot be embolized.

Radiation Therapy

Opinions vary on the value of radiation therapy in the treatment of the paragangliomas of the carotid body and temporal bone. The debate centers on the radiosensitivity of these tumors. Histologically, radiation results in edema, fibrosis, hemosiderin pigmentation, and degeneration of the vessel walls with intimal proliferation leading to partial obliteration and thrombosis.[11,24] It seems not to affect the cellular elements of the paragangliomas, however, with most tumors retaining many areas that appear viable.

Unfortunately, there are no generally accepted criteria for successful radiation therapy of these lesions. While some authors claim that all patients treated with radiation therapy obtain symptomatic relief, few report significant regression of the tumor mass, and no evidence exists to show that local irradiation decreases the risk of developing metastases. To evaluate the results of radiation therapy for these lesions, Springate and colleagues reviewed the literature on the treatment of temporal body paragangliomas published from 1965 to 1988.[25] In this review, all patients without evidence of disease progression on clinical or radiographic examination were considered to have been treated successfully. Using this definition, they averaged the cases reported in the literature and found success rates of 86, 90, and 93 percent for surgery alone, irradiation with or without surgery, and irradiation alone, respectively. While such a comparison is used to advocate radiation therapy as a primary treatment for head and neck paragangliomas, it fails to recognize that the goal of surgical therapy, that is, eradication of disease, is different from the goal of radiation therapy, which is limitation of disease progression. As a result, no valid comparison between radiation and surgical therapy exists in the literature.

Despite these concerns, radiation therapy for patients with carotid body or temporal bone paragangliomas leads initially to symptomatic relief in most patients. Neurological deficits, however, are rarely relieved and may progress after irradiation. For example, Cummings and colleagues reported on a series of 45 patients who received radiation therapy for temporal bone paragangliomas.[3] In this group, most patients were relieved of tinnitus (30/38), pain (8/8), and vertigo (5/5), although this was sometimes delayed for several months. Furthermore, these symptoms recurred in only three patients during a follow-up period that ranged from 3 to 23 years. In contrast, only two patients had significant relief of cranial nerve deficits. Similarly, Valdagni and Amichetti reported on 13 carotid body tumors in seven patients followed from 1 to 19 years after irradiation.[28] While no patient in this series was considered to have progressive disease, only three tumors displayed regression and only seven patients had symptomatic relief.

Complications secondary to radiation therapy for temporal bone paragangliomas are generally more severe than those encountered during the treatment of carotid body tumors. The most serious sequelae from radiation of temporal bone paragangliomas include brain and temporal bone necrosis that may be life-threatening. This complication is reported in one or two patients in most series, for an average of slightly less than 4 percent.[2,25] These patients have almost always received more than the standard 3500–5000 rad megavoltage dose given via a homolateral wedge pair technique over 3 to 5 weeks in most centers. Other less severe complications associated with temporal body paraganglioma irradiation include protracted otorrhea or otitis, vertigo, ataxia, and external auditory canal stenosis. Although the complications associated with carotid body tumors are infrequent and generally trivial, radiation therapy may result in delayed hemiplegia, postradiation stricture of the larynx, and radionecrosis of the carotid artery and mandible.[33] Such radiation will also complicate subsequent surgery. Therefore, radiation therapy as a treatment should be limited to patients who are elderly and asymptomatic, who have undergone incomplete resection, who refuse surgery, or who develop recurrent or metastatic lesions. Patients who have bilateral paragangliomas with severe cranial nerve deficits, especially of the glossopharyngeal and vagus nerve on one side secondary to tumor progression or surgical excision, should also be considered for radiation therapy.

Experience is now accumulating with the radiosurgical treatment of temporal bone paragangliomas. Time will tell whether this approach is better than conventional radiotherapy.

Surgical Therapy: Carotid Body Paragangliomas

Complete surgical excision remains the preferred treatment for most patients with carotid body tumors. This is especially true for tumors that display aggressive or invasive growth locally. Small tumors, tumors that interfere with normal function, and tumors in young people should also undergo surgical removal. With advanced techniques, including intraoperative cerebral blood flow and electroencephalographic monitoring; ICA shunting, grafting, or reconstruction; and mobilization of the parotid gland; nearly all carotid body tumors can be resected completely with small risk of stroke or death. For example, among 30 cervical paragangliomas, mostly Shamblin type II carotid body tumors, resected between 1976 and 1986, Hallett and colleagues reported only one stroke and no deaths.[10]

Postoperative cranial nerve deficits and arterial injury, however, have remained a significant problem. While only 10 percent of patients in the above series were found to have cranial nerve deficits preoperatively, this number increased to 40 percent postoperatively.[10] Fortunately, these deficits were transient in one-half of these patients. The most frequently affected nerves were the hypoglossal nerve and the vagus nerve. The superior laryngeal nerve and the pharyngeal branches of the vagus nerve were especially at risk. Less frequently injured were the glossopharyngeal and spinal accessory nerves, the sympathetic chain, and the mandibular branch of the facial nerve. More than one of these nerves was injured in roughly one-third of these patients. In this same series, 33 percent of patients required ligation or resection of the ECA. The ICA required reconstruction in 25 percent and was directly repaired in an additional 9 percent. The carotid arteries were temporarily clamped in 9 percent. Patients in this series who underwent arterial repair required significantly more transfused blood (5.67 U versus 1.92 U) and had a higher complication rate.

Patients with larger tumors tend to have a higher incidence of cranial nerve and arterial injury. Other complications resulting from the surgical therapy of these lesions are infrequent but may include venous graft occlusion, hemorrhage, internal carotid artery spasm, and respiratory failure secondary to aspiration. Preoperative embolization, especially for larger tumors, may reduce these complications.[10,31]

The basic principle behind successful surgery for carotid body paragangliomas is preoperative preparation and early intraoperative identification of neural and vascular structures. This can be achieved by using a wide exposure, intraoperative monitoring of cerebral blood flow and electroencephalographic activity, periadventitial tumor dissection in an inferior to superior direction, appropriate grafting or shunting of the ICA, appropriate parotid gland mobilization, and meticulous hemostasis and microtechnique.

Our recommended surgical approach is that described by Meyer et al.[19] The patient is placed supine on the operating table and general anesthesia is induced. A nasoendotracheal tube is used to allow maximal upward displacement of the floor of the mouth. The operative field that extends from the clavicle to above the superior extension of the pinna of the ear is then prepared. Routinely, the ipsilateral lower extremity is also prepared for saphenous vein harvesting. Although for cosmetic considerations a high horizontal incision may be used for very small tumors, typically a vertical incision is used (Fig. 154-6*A*). Tumors that extend into the posterior fossa should be approached by a separate suboccipital craniectomy.

The initial goal of the operation is to identify specific neural and vascular structures (Fig. 154-6*B*). The distal ICA is isolated first. This requires mobilization of the parotid gland. Therefore, once the skin incision has been made, the superficial cervical fascia is opened and the posterior border of the parotid gland is elevated. The temporoparotid fascia between the parotid gland and the mastoid process is then incised and the main trunk of the facial nerve is identified. The lower division of the facial nerve and the marginal mandibular nerve are dissected free and the deep cervical fascia is divided. The parotid gland is then gently retracted superiorly. The digastric muscle, stylohyoid muscle, and stylomandibular ligament are then divided in turn to expose the distal ICA. The proximal CCA is then exposed and loose rubber tourniquets are placed around the ICA, ECA, and CCA. Some authorities recommend obtaining baseline preocclusion and occlusion ^{131}xenon cerebral blood flow measurements at this point in case rapid occlusion of the ICA is required later for hemostasis.[19] Next, the neural elements are identified. The submandibular dissection is continued and the course of the vagus nerve is identified (it may be incorporated within the tumor bed). The hypoglossal nerve, which is usually displaced posterosuperiorly, and the spinal accessory nerve are also identified proximal and distal to the tumor and are tagged (Fig. 154-6*C*).

Tumor dissection begins by outlining the superficial medial and lateral margins of the tumor. Major arterial and venous feeding and draining vessels are identified and occluded. A periadventitial tissue plane is developed near the bifurcation of the CCA at the lower end of the tumor. This allows coagulation of numerous vasa vasorum in this area that supply much of the blood supply of the tumor. Once the tumor has been at least partially devascularized, the superolateral portion of the tumor is mobilized away from the cranial nerves and the ICA under magnified vision. Finally, the posteromedial subadventitial attachment of the tumor is elevated and the superior laryngeal branch of the vagus nerve is dissected free. Great care must be taken in this region not to inadvertently enter the carotid artery. While temporary occlusion of the carotid artery or intravascular shunting is used routinely by some authors, it is usually not necessary. Once the tumor is removed, the arterial walls are inspected carefully, and cerebral blood flow may be measured again. The incision is then closed in anatomic layers, incorporating multiple closed suction drains.

Surgical Therapy: Temporal Bone Paragangliomas

The particular surgical approach used to resect temporal bone paragangliomas depends on the location and extent of the tumor. Paragangliomas originating from the promontory of the middle ear

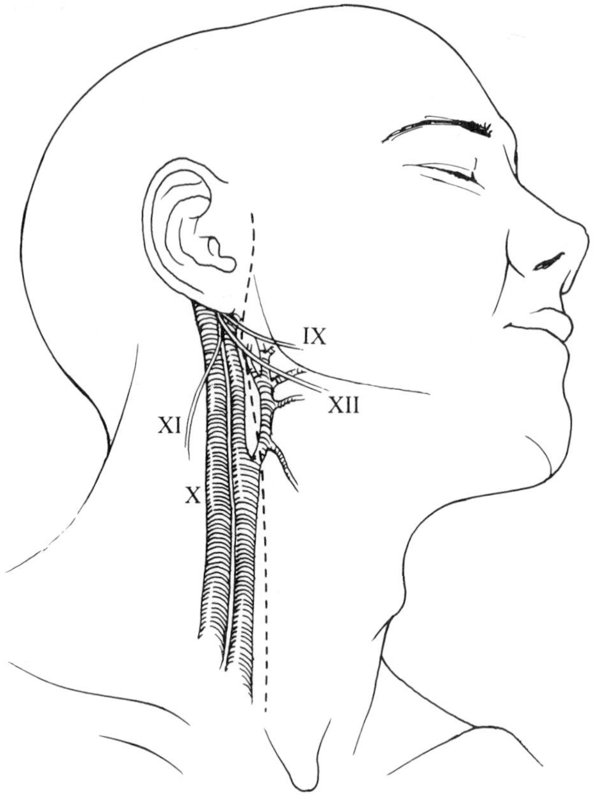

(*A*)

Figure 154-6 *A–C.* Diagrams demonstrating the surgical anatomy and technique for resection of carotid body tumors. See the text for details. Cranial nerves are identified by Roman numerals. A, artery; br, branch.

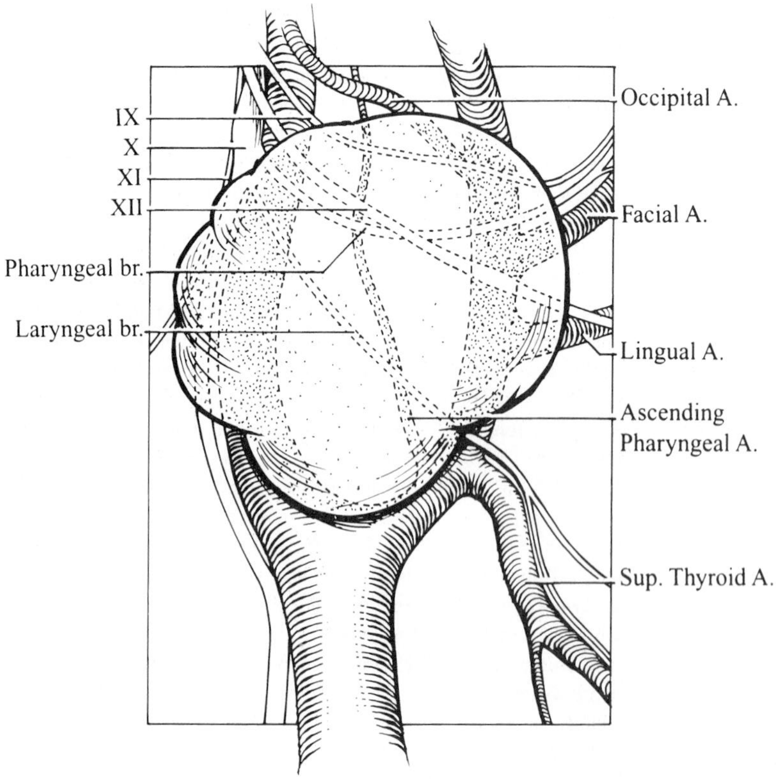

(*B*)

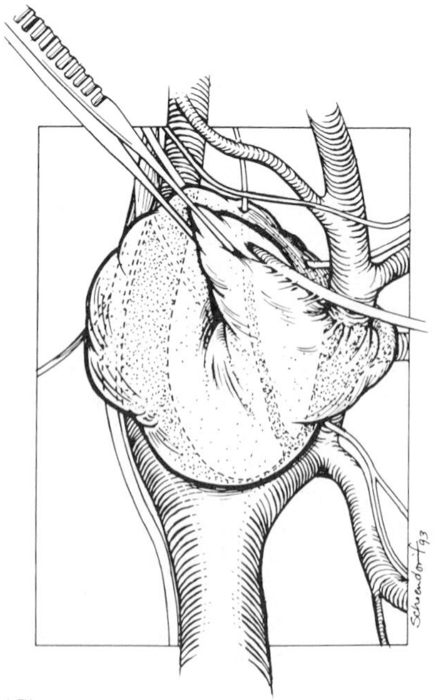

(*C*)

and isolated to the mesotympanum can be resected by elevating the tympanic membrane and removing the tumor using microdissection techniques. If the tumor extends into the hypotympanum or the mastoid, a tympanomastoidectomy is performed and the tumor resected.

Larger tumors that involve the jugular bulb or extend medial to the jugular bulb require more extensive dissection. Fortunately, with recent advances in the techniques of skull base surgery, extensive temporal bone paragangliomas can be resected completely by an experienced multidisciplinary team. For example, Jackson et al.[14] reported on the treatment of 49 patients with skull base tumors with intracranial extension of which 36 were paragangliomas originating in the temporal bone. In this series of formidable tumors, 76 percent of patients had gross total tumor resection, and most of those with incomplete removal were operated on early in the series. Now, according to these authors, tumors that involve the ICA or basilar artery, the foramen magnum, the cavernous sinus, or the clivus should no longer be considered unresectable.

Unfortunately, accurate data regarding the ability of surgery to cure these tumors are not available. Among those patients in the series referred to above with complete resection of a temporal bone paraganglioma, there were two recurrences after a mean follow-up of 5.1 years.[14] One patient with incomplete resection accounted for another recurrence. Another series reported a single recurrence among 17 patients with temporal bone paragangliomas, but the follow-up time was not clearly stated.[2] Still, these tumors usually grow slowly, and recurrent disease cannot be excluded for many years after surgical intervention. Therefore, meaningful results about the effects of aggressive modern surgical techniques on temporal bone paragangliomas will not be available for another decade or more.

Such aggressive resections in patients with larger tumors, however, are not without significant risk of complications (Table 154-6). For instance, in the series of Jackson et al., which is representative, 5 of the 49 patients died within 1 year of surgery.[14] Furthermore, only 24 percent of patients escaped cranial nerve deficit, with 47 percent of patients sustaining injury to the ninth and tenth cranial nerve complex. No patient in this series, however, required permanent tracheostomy or gastrostomy tube alimentation. Enhanced neural preservation can be achieved with smaller lesions, and this underscores the need for early diagnosis and treatment of these lesions. Irradiation prior to surgery may also curtail cranial nerve preservation.

A number of approaches to temporal bone paragangliomas have been described. Most of these are used to excise tumors without intracranial extension or as the first part of a two-stage operation where an intracranial tumor is removed through a separate suboccipital craniectomy.[7] More recently, a number of combined approaches have been developed that allow tumors with a large intracranial component to be resected by a multidisciplinary team during a single operation.[1,8]

After general anesthesia is induced, the patient is generally placed on the operating table in the supine position. The shoulder is then elevated to a variable degree depending on the location of the tumor or the preference of the surgeon. A more lateral position allows excellent exposure of the posterior fossa component of the tumor but compromises tumor removal from the neck and skull base. A nasoendotracheal tube is used to allow maximal upward displacement of the floor of the mouth. The pre- and postauricular areas and the neck are prepared from the clavicle to above the superior extension of the pinna of the ear. Routinely, the ipsilateral lower limb is also prepared for saphenous vein and fascia lata harvesting. The abdominal area is also prepared as a site for adipose tissue donation.

A postauricular curvilinear incision is then made as shown in Fig. 154-7*A*. This may be extended in either direction to improve exposure. As this flap is retracted, the external auditory canal is transected and closed as a blind sac. The attachment of the sternocleidomastoid muscle and the contents of the carotid sheath are then identified. The base of the skull that lies behind and lateral to the jugular foramen must then be exposed fully. This requires that the sternocleidomastoid muscle and the underlying splenius and suboccipital muscles be dissected off the base of the skull. Care must be taken in this step to avoid injury to the vertebral artery. The dissection is continued until it merges with one proceeding upward from the neck that has exposed the internal jugular vein, ICA, ECA, and the nerves of the jugular foramen (Fig. 154-7*B*).

TABLE 154-6 Representative Operative Complications and Outcome from Resection of Temporal Bone Tumors*[1,2,13,14]

	%	
Mortality	8	
Tumor recurrence	8	
Wound infection	11	
Cerebrospinal fluid leakage	20	
Meningitis	8	
Required treatments		
Vocal cord injection	23	
Tracheostomy	8	
Tarrsorrhaphy	19	
Cranial nerve deficits[2,13]		
	Preoperative (%)	**Postoperative (%)**
None	57	28
VII	13	42
VIII	15	15
IX	24	70
X	32	59
XI	15	46
XII	22	47

*The majority of the patients had intracranial tumor extension. Smaller tumors are associated with fewer complications.

Here the surgeon must avoid injury to the inferior petrosal sinus that may merge with the internal jugular vein after it exits the skull. Branches from the ECA that are supplying the tumor, usually the ascending pharyngeal, posterior auricular, and occipital arteries, are occluded, and vascular tapes are secured around the internal jugular vein, ICA, and ECA.

The second stage of the operation requires the use of a high-speed drill to perform an extensive mastoidectomy. First, the mastoid process is removed, and then the sigmoid sinus and the bony labyrinth are skeletonized. If the tumor extends along the ICA toward the petrous apex, the facial nerve is uncovered from the geniculate ganglion to the stylomastoid foramen and transposed anterosuperiorly out of the fallopian canal. A suboccipital craniotomy or craniectomy is then performed. The portion of the sigmoid sinus above the tumor is identified, and a ligature is passed through the dura and around the sinus in this location. A pair of similar ligatures are also placed around the internal jugular vein (below the tumor) and the vein is then transected between them. The lateral wall of the sigmoid sinus may be opened and any tumor invading this wall resected.

Attention is then turned to the ICA. It is followed up toward the skull base and into the petrous canal. This may require transection of the posterior belly of the digastric muscle and the stylohyoid muscle. Simultaneously, the lateral wall of the bony eustachian tube is drilled until the isthmus is identified, at which point the lumen is closed with bone wax and a fascial graft. The tumor is then mobilized progressively from various directions. As the superior pole of the tumor is drilled free, one must guard against opening into the basal turn of the cochlea or damaging the seventh and eighth cranial nerves. Finally, the jugular vein is lifted out of the neck and excised along with the lateral wall of the jugular bulb. Here the medial aspect of the tumor is carefully dissected from the cranial nerves. As this dissection proceeds, the inferior petrosal sinus with its multiple openings will be encountered and should be occluded. Finally, the extradural portion of the tumor is then divided from the intradural portion and removed.

The intradural portion of the tumor is then excised. First the dura is opened behind the sigmoid sinus. Meticulous hemostasis

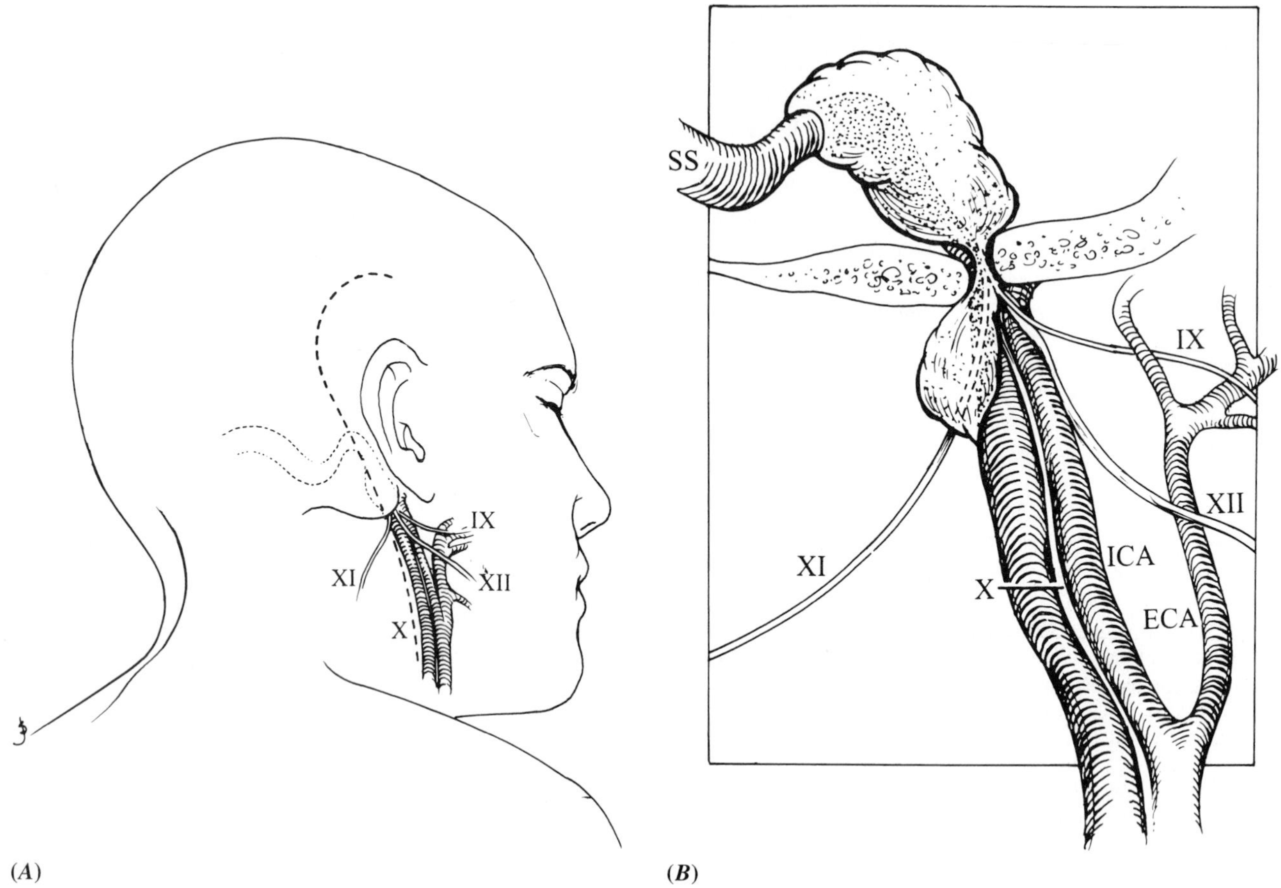

Figure 154-7 *A, B.* Diagrams demonstrating the surgical anatomy appropriate to the resection of temporal bone paragangliomas. Cranial nerves are identified by Roman numerals. ECA, external carotid artery; ICA, internal carotid artery; SS, sigmoid sinus.

must then be maintained as the tumor is separated from the parenchyma of the brain. If the tumor encroaches on the anterior compartment of the jugular foramen, the cranial nerves in this area may not withstand the manipulation required for complete tumor removal. Therefore, in this instance, the goal of complete tumor removal must be weighed against neurological deficit. The same situation occurs when one encounters tumor that extensively involves the ICA, basilar artery, clivus, foramen magnum, or cavernous sinus.

Once the intradural component of the tumor has been removed, the wound is closed. Fascia lata may be used as a dural graft. The cavity is then obliterated with adipose tissue. A vascularized temporalis muscle flap can be swung inferiorly and sutured to the operative margins. The skin is then closed in several anatomic layers incorporating several closed suction drains. Adjunctive procedures thought to be necessary such as the insertion of a parenteral feeding catheter, insertion of a lumbar cerebrospinal fluid drainage catheter, tracheostomy, or insertion of a feeding gastrostomy tube are then completed.

References

1. Bordi LT, Cheesman AD, Symon L. The surgical management of glomus jugulare tumours—description of a single-staged posterolateral combined otoneurosurgical approach. *Br J Neurosurg* 1989; 3:21–30.
2. Cece JA, Lawson W, Biller HF, et al. Complications in the management of large glomus jugulare tumors. *Laryngoscope* 1987; 97:152–157.
3. Cummings BJ, Beale FA, Garrett PG, et al. The treatment of glomus tumors in the temporal bone by megavoltage radiation. *Cancer* 1984; 53:2635–2640.
4. Dayal VS, Hinojosa R, Amenta CA III, et al. Surgical inferences from study of temporal bones with glomus jugulare tumor. *Otolaryngol Head Neck Surg* 1990; 102:690–697.
5. Duncan MW, Compton P, Lazarus L, et al. Measurement of norepinephrine and 3,4-dihydroxyphenylglycol in urine and plasma for the diagnosis of pheochromocytoma. *N Engl J Med* 1988; 319:136–142.
6. Feldman JM. Diagnosis and management of pheochromocytoma. *Hosp Pract (Off Ed)* 1989; 24:175–179, 182, 187–189.
7. Fisch U, Fagan P, Valavanis A. The infratemporal fossa approach for the lateral skull base. *Otolaryngol Clin North Am* 1984; 17:513–552.
8. Gardner G, Robertson JT, Robertson JH, et al. Glomus jugulare tumors—skull base surgery. In Schmidek HH, Sweet WH (eds): *Operative Neurosurgical Techniques. Indications, Methods and Results,* 2d ed. Orlando: Grune & Stratton, 1988, pp 739–752.
9. Guild SR. The glomus jugulare, a nonchromaffin paraganglion, in man. *Ann Otol Rhinol Laryngol* 1953; 62:1045–1071.
10. Hallett JW Jr, Nora JD, Hollier LH, et al. Trends in neurovascular complications of surgical management for carotid body and cervical paragangliomas: a fifty-year experience with 153 tumors. *J Vasc Surg* 1988; 7:284–291.
11. Hawthorne MR, Makek MS, Harris JP, et al. The histopathological and clinical features of irradiated and nonirradiated temporal paragangliomas. *Laryngoscope* 1988; 98:325–331.

12. Jackson CG, Cueva RA, Thedinger BA, et al. Conservation surgery for glomus jugulare tumors: the value of early diagnosis. *Laryngoscope* 1990; 100:1031–1036.
13. Jackson CG, Cueva RA, Thedinger BA, et al. Cranial nerve preservation in lesions of the jugular fossa. *Otolaryngol Head Neck Surg* 1991; 105:687–693.
14. Jackson CG, Glasscock ME III, McKennan KX, et al. The surgical treatment of skull-base tumors with intracranial extension. *Otolaryngol Head Neck Surg* 1987; 96:175–185.
15. Khafagi F, Egerton-Vernon J, van Doorn T, et al. Localization and treatment of familial malignant nonfunctional paraganglioma with ^{131}I-MIBG: report of two cases. *J Nucl Med* 1987; 28:528–531.
16. Kliewer KE, Wen D-R, Cancilla PA, et al. Paragangliomas: assessment of prognosis by histologic, immunohistochemical, and ultrastructural techniques. *Hum Pathol* 1989; 20:29–39.
17. Massey V, Wallner K. Treatment of metastatic chemodectoma. *Cancer* 1992; 69:790–792.
18. Matishak MZ, Symon L, Cheeseman A, et al. Catecholamine-secreting paragangliomas of the base of the skull: report of two cases. *J Neurosurg* 1987; 66:604–608.
19. Meyer FB, Sundt TM Jr, Pearson BW. Carotid body tumors: a subject review and suggested surgical approach. *J Neurosurg* 1986; 64:377–385.
20. Moret J, Picard L. Vascular architecture of tympanojugular glomus tumors. Its relevance in therapeutic angiography. *Semin Intervent Radiol* 1987; 4:291–308.
21. Murphy TP, Brackmann DE. Effects of preoperative embolization on glomus jugulare tumors. *Laryngoscope* 1989; 99:1244–1247.
22. Olsen WL, Dillon WP, Kelly WM, et al. MR imaging of paragangliomas. *Am J Roentgenol* 1987; 148:201–204.
23. Pearse AGE. The cytochemistry and ultrastructure of polypeptide hormone-producing cells of the APUD series and the embryologic, physiologic and pathologic implications of the concept. *J Histochem Cytochem* 1969; 17:303–313.
24. Spector GJ, Compagno J, Perez CA, et al. Glomus jugulare tumors: effects of radiotherapy. *Cancer* 1975; 35:1316–1321.
25. Springate SC, Haraf D, Weichselbaum RR. Temporal bone chemodectomas—comparing surgery and radiation therapy. *Oncology (Huntingt)* 1991; 5:131–137.
26. Valavanis A. Preoperative embolization of the head and neck: indications, patient selection, goals, and precautions. *Am J Neuroradiol* 1986; 7:943–952.
27. Valavanis A, Schubiger O, Oguz M. High-resolution CT investigation of nonchromaffin paragangliomas of the temporal bone. *Am J Neuroradiol* 1983; 4:516–519.
28. Valdagni R, Amichetti M. Radiation therapy of carotid body tumors. *Am J Clin Oncology* 1990; 13:45–48.
29. van der Mey AGL, Maaswinkel-Mooy PD, Cornelisse CJ, et al. Genomic imprinting in hereditary glomus tumours: evidence for new genetic theory. *Lancet* 1989; 2:1291–1294.
30. van Gils APG, van der Mey AGL, Hoogma RPLM, et al. Iodine-123-metaiodobenzylguanidine scintigraphy in patients with chemodectomas of the head and neck region. *J Nucl Med* 1990; 31:1147–1155.
31. Ward PH, Liu C, Vinuela F, et al. Embolization: an adjunctive measure for removal of carotid body tumors. *Laryngoscope* 1988; 98:1287–1291.
32. Williams PL, Warwick R, Dyson M, et al: *Gray's Anatomy,* 37th ed. London: Churchill Livingstone, 1989.
33. Zak FG, Lawson W: *The Paraganglionic Chemoreceptor System. Physiology, Pathology, and Clinical Medicine.* New York: Springer-Verlag, 1982.

155 Surgical Approaches to Tumors of the Skull Base: An Overview

Don M. Long

Tumors of the skull base have been terra incognita for neurosurgeons.[17] Most were approached by craniotomy for biopsy or unsatisfactory attempts at removal followed by irradiation.[18,61] The ones that are largely intracranial with a minor skull base component, such as the usual subfrontal or sphenoid wing meningioma, have been removed successfully.[23] Even with these tumors, however, the recurrence rate is high.[13] The only skull base tumors that are managed in a truly satisfactory fashion are pituitary and acoustic tumors.[53] There have been a few pioneers who have attempted to improve the approaches to both common and unusual tumors of the skull base. Fisch has been chief among these, writing for a decade about extracranial approaches to intracranial tumors.[19,27] A number of others have described individual approaches. In the recent past, there has been a considerable increase in the interest in these previously untreatable tumors.[42] A number of individual physicians and a few specialized centers interested in these tumors have appeared.[30,32,33,57]

This surgery is difficult and time-consuming and requires a number of skills that are not commonly taught in neurosurgical training. Most are in evolution. The anatomic considerations are now well understood. Technical advances have been such that radical removal of many tumors of the skull base is possible. What is still not clear are the indications for the various procedures and the degree to which radical removal should be undertaken. It is clear that now many of these tumors can be removed. We are not yet certain enough of the natural history of many, especially the meningiomas, to advocate either radical or conservative management for most tumors. We still must individualize and decide about the course of therapy after considering all the factors presented by any individual patient.[42]

Tumors of the Anterior Fossa

Midline Nasopharyngeal Tumors

The most common skull base lesions that require more than conventional craniotomy are malignancies of the paranasal sinuses and nasopharynx. These tumors can be approached by a combined operation in which the intracranial portion of the tumor is managed by craniotomy and the nasopharyngeal portion by the *en bloc* dissections of the head and neck surgeon. Current magnetic resonance (MR) and computed tomography (CT) imaging, particularly three-dimensional CT imaging, provide an accurate assessment of these tumors, their relationships, and their extent. Resectability can be determined in advance. At one time it was thought that any intracranial extension made these tumors inoperable. That is no longer the case, and wide resections including dura are possible for palliation and even cure.[17,34,55]

Operative Technique The neurosurgical portion of the operation is carried out with the patient in the supine position. Arrangements must be made for a bicoronal skin incision and bifrontal craniotomy to be followed by the head and neck procedure. The neurosurgical portion of the operation is done first. A standard coronal incision and bifrontal craniotomy carried as low as possible without regard for the frontal sinuses are the first steps. The pericranium must be preserved as a sheet for later reconstruction of the skull base. The pericranium must be lifted from the frontal bone without perforation and left attached to the supraorbital rim. If any perforation occurs, it must be closed at the time it is noticed, for it will be extremely difficult to find at the end of a long procedure. An extradural elevation of the frontal lobes is then performed. In most instances surgery is undertaken when there is no dural involvement. At one time it was thought that dural involvement precluded definitive operation. However, advances in technique now make it possible to widely excise the dura, lift the frontal lobe off the tumor mass, and then repair the dura with a graft after *en bloc* resection of the tumor from below. More commonly, the frontal lobes are elevated in an extradural fashion, and the dura remains intact to prevent a CSF leak. With the frontal fossa exposed, the location of the optic nerves is estimated, and a high speed drill or chisel used to cut through the frontal bone at the lateral margins of the ethmoid sinuses and the roof of the sphenoid sinus, leaving the orbits and optic canals intact. A cut is made through the cribriform plate anteriorly, and the entire mass is then freed from the intracranial contents. This allows the head and neck surgeon to carry out definitive resection from below and remove the skull base as a part of the tumor specimen. When the tumor is removed, the pericranial flap is then swung into the field and placed over the skull defect, and the frontal lobes allowed to return to their normal location. The double layer of pericranium and dura has been sufficient to prevent herniation of the brain through the bony defect. Reconstitution of the skull base with other materials has not been necessary. The results of this aggressive approach to these tumors are not yet documented by long-term follow-up, but it appears that cure is possible and may occur in 30 to 50 percent of cases.

Meningiomas and Other Tumors of the Sphenoid Bone, and Lateral and Posterior Orbit

The most common tumor to occur in the region of the sphenoid bone is the meningioma (Fig. 155-1).[15,31,39,45] Meningiomas of the optic sheath and sphenoid bone with major intracranial extensions are best managed by craniotomy. However, a significant number of these tumors arising within the sphenoid bone cause hyperostosis, restriction of eye mobility, pain, and, eventually, loss of vision.[15,31,35,39] These tumors may be approached by a standard craniotomy, but a lateral extradural approach is often better, as well as safer for the patient. That is the procedure of choice when there is

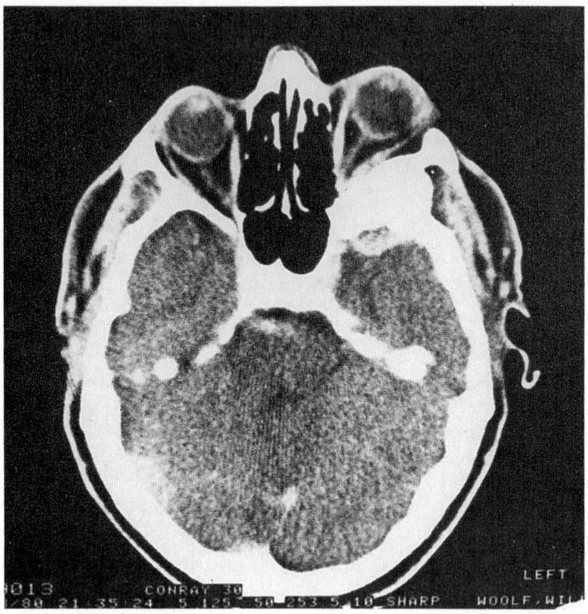

Figure 155-1 Hyperostosis of the sphenoid bone with a small tumor producing proptosis and mechanical limitation of vision. This tumor and bony abnormality are ideal for an extradural lateral approach.

little intracranial extension of the tumor.[21,62,66] A number of variations of the transtemporal transzygomatic approach have now been described. The operation is in common use to reach tumors of the gasserian ganglion and ones that principally involve the cavernous sinus. In combination with pterional craniotomy, it is the best procedure for meningiomas with both intracranial extension and intracavernous tumor. This extremely low approach is now appreciated for aneurysm surgery of the internal carotid artery in the cavernous sinus, ophthalmic artery aneurysms, and some aneurysms of the basilar apex.[22,52,58,66]

Operative Technique The operation is carried out with the patient under general anesthesia and prepared in the lateral position. A skin incision is made just behind the temporal hairline from above the level of insertion of the temporalis muscle down to the zygoma. It then turns posteriorly to parallel the zygoma to the tragus and then angles down behind the jaw in a convenient skin fold. If there is a large extension of the tumor into the pterygoid fossa, the incision can be carried down parallel to the anterior border of the sternocleidomastoid muscle. For tumors associated only with the orbit and sphenoid bone, that is not necessary. The temporalis muscle is cut from its attachments, leaving a small rim of muscle for resuturing, and is reflected down over the zygoma. If the tumor is large, it is probably wise to cut the zygoma at both extremities and then resuture it in place when the surgery is finished. The goal of surgery is to remove the abnormal tumor-bearing or hyperostotic sphenoid bone and the entire lateral orbit, most of its roof, and most of its floor in order to provide access to the posterior orbit and canal. This is done with a high speed drill. The drill is used to remove sphenoid bone medially until the anterior clinoid and orbital sheath are encountered. The clinoid can be removed and the orbital sheath skeletonized. It is possible to remove the orbital roof virtually to the midline. The floor can be removed extensively, and the entire sphenoid bone down to the superior orbital fissure is drilled away. When the tumor is exclusively in the sphenoid bone or when the problem is hyperostotic reaction to a small meningioma, the bony removal is all that is required. Small intracranial extensions are removed without opening the dura. The tumor is identified where it penetrates the dura and removed using standard techniques. If there is a sizable intracranial extension, it probably is wiser to open the dura, identify the mass, and be certain that there are no intimate connections with important structures before extradural removal is attempted. Tumors that penetrate the orbit usually leave the periorbita intact and can be removed as soon as the bone is drilled away. If the periorbita is penetrated, the tumor must be dissected free from the orbital contents. The major risks of the procedure are entering the carotid artery near the clinoid, entering the superior orbital fissure, and injuring the optic nerve near the orbital apex or in the canal.

Several factors mandate the use of a combined intradural-extradural approach for tumors of this location. If the mass appears to involve the chiasm, it is better to remove the portion that surrounds the intracranial optic apparatus directly and then continue the extradural dissection. If the carotid artery and cavernous sinus are involved, as they often are with these tumors, it is better to explore intracranially first to identify cranial nerves and the carotid artery. It is much easier to follow these structures into a tumor mass from their normal intracranial portions than to try to identify them in the cavernous sinus and posterior orbit in the tumor mass. These tumors often surround the cranial nerves and vessels, making it impossible to remove the tumor by way of the extracranial approach alone.

When the procedure is completed, the large bony defect that is left is filled with a fat graft harvested from the abdomen. Even if the dura is open, no closure is required.

The results of surgery of this kind are excellent. In 32 operations using various combinations of this intracranial-extracranial approach, there has been no mortality and no increased visual loss. The only morbidity has been the development of a sixth nerve palsy in two patients. Both palsies have been corrected, although one requires further revision of the muscle-shortening operation.

Tumors of the Medial Middle Fossa and Gasserian Ganglion

The Lateral Temporal Approach

The most common tumors that occur in the medial middle fossa and require more than a traditional craniotomy are meningiomas that have large extensions through the skull base into the pterygoid fossa, and schwannomas of the gasserian ganglion.[19] Both present with facial pain and sensory loss, trigeminal motor deficits, and abnormalities of extraocular function. Although the two tumors and the rare neurofibroma of the trigeminal system cannot be differentiated with certainty with imaging studies, it is possible to identify the anatomic configuration of the tumor and surrounding structures with accuracy.[40] Angiography should be employed if the tumor appears to involve the carotid artery. Schwannomas are usually circumscribed ovoid tumors, whereas meningiomas are more invasive and conform more to the anatomic configuration of the structures at the skull base. The approach to both is the same.[28,52,66]

Operative Technique The operation used is virtually identical to that for the lateral approach to the orbit. The procedure is performed under general anesthesia with the head and patient turned so that the zygoma is parallel with the floor. The same skin incision is made. The temporalis muscle is removed, and the zygoma is resected. If there is a significant pterygoid extension, it may be necessary to dislocate the mandible or to section it and reflect it forward. The squamous portion of the temporal bone and the base of the middle fossa are exposed by these maneuvers, and a high speed drill is used to drill away the floor of the middle fossa. It is not necessary to remove much bone over the lateral surface of the temporal lobe. The drilling is continued until the foramen ovale is skeletonized. The middle meningeal artery will be encountered and can be coagulated easily after the bone around it is totally removed. It must be divided. The drilling continues until the second division of the trigeminal nerve is also isolated. At that point it will be possible to palpate the tumor through the dura. If a schwannoma is expected, it will not be necessary to open into the subtemporal subarachnoid space. The junction of temporal dura with the dural covering of Meckel's cave is identified and opened. The tumor becomes immediately apparent. These tumors are soft and easily removable with an ultrasonic dissector or powerful suction. Often many fascicles of the trigeminal nerve can be saved. The same techniques that are employed for removal of large acoustic tumors will be satisfactory here. The capsule of the tumor is opened, its soft contents are evacuated, and then the capsule is gradually stripped from the surrounding dura and the remaining fascicles of the trigeminal nerve. Anteriorly and medially, the tumor will usually surround the carotid artery, and it may invade the cavernous sinus. However, the capsule is usually such that the cranial nerves in the cavernous sinus are simply adherent, and they can be dissected away. Venous bleeding can be packed with thrombin-soaked Gelfoam. If the tumor extends out along one of the branches or posteriorly into the canal, it may be necessary to extend the dural incisions appropriately.

If there is a significant mass of tumor in the posterior fossa, it is better to remove it through a more conventional dural opening. In such a situation, the tumor in the middle fossa is completely evacuated. The temporal lobe is allowed to return to normal position after hemostasis, and the temporal dura is opened at any convenient point along the base where it will be easy to close. The temporal lobe is then elevated to the free edge of the tentorium, and the tumor is identified. It can be removed using conventional intracranial techniques. The dural incision is then closed in a watertight fashion. It is not necessary to close the gasserian dura. Closure includes replacement of the zygoma, which is wired in place; reattachment of the temporalis muscle to bone; and routine skin closure.

For meningiomas, the techniques differ somewhat. In general, if the tumor is completely extradural, the approach can be as described. However, when the tumor is both intra- and extradural, it is necessary to add a standard craniotomy approach. This distinction can be very hard to make on imaging studies. Therefore, for a meningioma, the procedure should include a larger temporal craniectomy that will allow the lateral temporal dura to be opened and the temporal lobe elevated to expose the medial middle fossa and the region of the tumor. It is then possible to judge what can be done extradurally and what must be performed intradurally. It is usually easier to remove the intradural portion of the tumor first. Standard techniques are employed. There are some differences, however. It is possible to carry out radical tumor removal for extensions in the cavernous sinus. To do so, the cranial nerves entering the sinus should be isolated and followed until they enter the tumor. The tumor is then carefully peeled away, following the nerves through the sinus and only removing the tumor after the courses of all of the nerves are identified. Once the intracranial portion of the tumor is removed, the extracranial portion is then approached by the same technique described for trigeminal schwannomas. Meningiomas are much more difficult to deal with because they do not dissect as easily. The laser is an ideal tool in this location. It is easier to skeletonize the carotid artery from the extradural approach, but the surgeon may have to go back and forth between intradural and extradural exposures in order to verify the location of cranial nerves and the carotid artery to make tumor removal safe.

Meningiomas of the Cavernous Sinus

Most meningiomas of the cavernous sinus that require surgery have posterior fossa extensions with brain stem compression, or they compress the visual apparatus.[38,70] They are best approached by pterional craniotomy coupled with the transpterygoid approach. Once the tumor is exposed by these methods, the surgical techniques vary. It is usually better to remove the intradural soft portions before approaching the intra- and extradural portions in the sinus. This means dissecting the tumor free from the visual apparatus and removing all possible tumor in that location. Then the tumor compressing the brain stem is removed in the same way. The dissection of the visual apparatus, while delicate, is much easier than the removal of the posterior fossa tumor because lesions of this type that are under the tentorium virtually always involve the third, fourth, and sixth cranial nerves. The optic and trigeminal nerves, which are also involved, are larger structures and are easier to dissect. The tumor must be exposed so that its posterior and medial borders are seen as well as its superior surface. The cranial nerves should be identified before they enter the tumor. This is usually possible with the fourth and sometimes with the third nerve, but the sixth is almost always obscured by the tumor mass. A nerve-free segment of the tumor is thus identified, and the tumor is debulked using either ultrasonic dissection or a laser. The individual cranial nerves are then identified and dissected through the tumor mass. Additional tumor removal can continue only after the nerve has been dissected free. The small fourth and sixth nerves are extremely difficult to dissect through these invasive tumors. Sometimes it is simply impossible to do so. Fortunately, these nerves are usually redundant and can be sutured should they be divided during the dissection. The dissection can be carried into the sinus and tumor removed from within the sinus. There is usually enough medial reaction that venous bleeding is not a problem. However, if it should occur, packing with hemostatic agents, muscle, or fat will suffice to stop the bleeding. The risks of bleeding from the sinus have been overestimated, but lesions in this region can be approached only by those with a thorough understanding of the anatomy and techniques involved. The carotid artery also requires a delicate dissection. Sometimes the tumor has actually invaded the wall of the carotid. A preoperative angiogram that demonstrates compromise of the carotid lumen usually suggests direct invasion of the wall. Total removal is sometimes possible but may not be feasible without neurological deficit. In such situations, postoperative irradiation is used to reduce the risk of recurrence.

A major question with these tumors is whether the carotid artery needs to be resected and replaced by a graft. Two techniques have been described. One is a graft from the internal carotid artery in the neck to the intracranial internal carotid artery above the anterior clinoid. The other is a vein graft from the carotid in the petrous bone to the supraclinoid carotid. Both techniques have been described in detail and appear to be feasible, but the mortality/morbidity is currently high. Radical surgery with carotid grafting certainly could be indicated for malignant tumors that might be cured. Whether this radical step is indicated for meningiomas is not yet certain.[4]

The entire question of the radical removal of meningiomas from the cavernous sinus is still unsettled. We have found that these cavernous sinus meningiomas are very slow growing. Of the patients in our series, 75 percent showed no progression over an average period of three years; many of the follow-up periods were much longer. Nor is it certain that radical removal of these tumors means cure. Loss of extraocular muscular control is relatively common. It is going to require more patients with longer periods of evaluation to settle the issue of whether radical surgery is substantially better than the natural history for most patients with these meningiomas. On the other hand, there are meningiomas that grow rapidly and cannot be easily controlled by adjuvants. Certainly, the radical operation is indicated for these tumors.

At present, the risks of an aggressive approach in which the extraocular nerves are all dissected out of the tumor and the carotid artery is grafted are great enough that I believe it should only be employed when it is clear that the natural history of the particular tumor warrants it.[42,66,71]

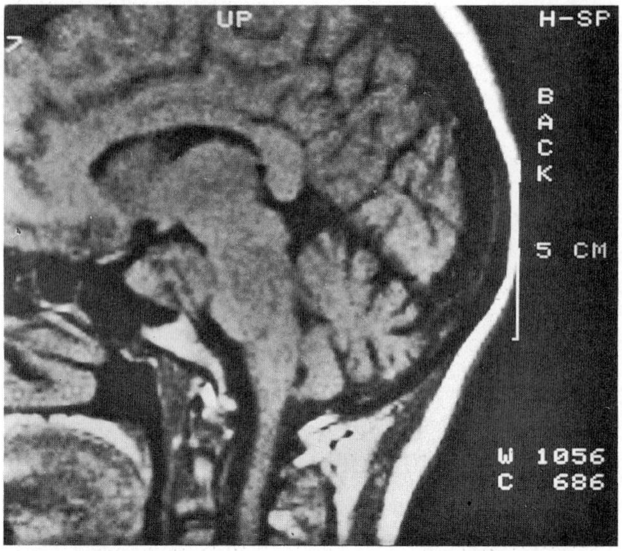

Figure 155-2 MRI reveals a small tumor in the upper clivus that encroaches on the brain stem and has a significant extension into the sphenoid sinus. The tumor can be approached via the pterional or trans-sphenoidal route.

Tumors of the Clivus

The most common tumor to involve the intracranial contents in the region of the clivus is the meningioma. The clivus itself is usually not involved, but the meningioma is located intracranially over the clivus and in front of the brain stem. In almost two-thirds of the 125 such patients in my personal series, the tumor occurred in the region of the posterior clinoid process, the petrous apex, and the upper third of the clivus. Radical surgery from one of several approaches was employed. The operative mortality was zero, but three patients were seriously disabled by the surgery and subsequently died. Permanent major neurological deficits did not occur in other patients, but cranial nerve palsies were common. The elderly fared as well as younger patients. Ninety-three percent of these patients continue to be functional individuals. Deterioration over time has occurred in only a small number. The tumors appear to be quite indolent. It appears that the surgical approaches, which were unusual only a few years ago, allow these tumors to be removed with safety.

Midline Tumors of the Upper Third of the Clivus

Tumors in the upper third of the clivus are usually chordomas. An occasional unusual pituitary tumor may present in this way, and meningiomas occur with enough frequency that they must be considered in the differential diagnosis.[11] All other tumors are exceedingly rare. The critical factor is whether the tumor has a significant intradural extension. This distinction can be difficult to make but is crucial. If the tumor has a large intradural extension, then a staged operation is required. In such a situation, the intracranial portion of the tumor is removed first and the dura reconstituted with a graft. Then one of the anterior midline approaches is employed.[12,34] If the tumor appears to be intraosseous and extradural, the midline approaches can be used[2,30,44] (Fig. 155-2).

Midline Approaches to the Upper Clivus

Trans-sphenoidal Approach

Tumors that involve only the clival bone and sphenoid sinus without major extensions can be approached by a simple trans-sphenoidal route, which may also be used to biopsy tumors. Large tumors of this type that are in the sinus can be easily biopsied by endoscopic techniques, so that a full-scale operation is rarely required for diagnosis alone. The trans-sphenoidal approach allows a tumor in the sinus to be removed, and a tumor that is in the upper third of the clivus but does not extend laterally or posteriorly can also be approached in this way.

Transpalatal Approach

Tumors that do not involve the sinus but are confined to the body of the clivus extending down as far as the upper cervical region may be approached by a simple transpalatal procedure. Significant lateral extensions cannot be easily removed, and large tumors require a greater exposure.

Again, the critical factor is intradural extension. MRI and three-dimensional CT scanning will usually settle this question. Angiography should be used if there is any suggestion that the basilar artery system may be involved.

Operative Technique These operations are carried out under general anesthesia with the patient in the supine position. Oral intubation is required, and a special tongue retractor which accommodates the tube is mandatory. The incision splits the uvula and soft palate. A portion of the hard palate can easily be removed without problem if necessary to get higher exposure on the clivus. The incision is then carried through the posterior pharyngeal wall, and the whole clivus, arch of C1, odontoid, and body of C2 can be exposed. The tumor is entered and debulked using standard techniques. Soft, gelatinous tumors such as chordomas can easily be removed entirely. Meningiomas are much more difficult to remove and could not be approached effectively before lasers and ultrasonic dissectors became available. It is very important not to enter the subarachnoid space. Leaks are very hard to control with this exposure and should be avoided.

The Transmandibular-Glossopharyngeal-Clival Approach

Large tumors involving the body of the clivus with extensive invasion of the skull base cannot be exposed adequately through the limited transpalatal approach. To deal with these tumors, it is necessary to split the mandible and divide the tongue and palate. This affords broad access to the entire skull base.[3,12,14,16] It is our practice for these procedures to be carried out by a team of surgeons. The otolaryngologist/head and neck surgeon is responsible for the approach; the neurosurgeon removes the tumor; and closure is carried out by the head and neck surgeon.[37]

Operative Technique The procedure is done under general anesthesia with a tracheostomy. The tracheostomy is carried out as the first step of the procedure. A midline incision is made through the lower lip, exposing the mandible in the midline. The mandible is divided with a small step to allow perfect reapproximation. Preformed bite blocks allow perfect occlusion at the end of the procedure but are not absolutely necessary. The tongue is split in the midline to and including its base. This step opens the entire pharyngeal area widely. The pharynx is opened in the midline after division of the soft palate. Much of the hard palate can be removed if necessary for exposure. The clival bone, C1, and C2 can be broadly exposed by this route. Many surgeons now use a bilateral maxillotomy instead of resecting the hard palate. This procedure essentially creates a maxillary fracture so that the maxilla is divided in the midline and the two halves of the maxillary bone are then swung laterally. This approach allows exposure of the entire skull base from the pituitary fossa down to C2.[3,12,14,16,37]

The tumors are removed in the conventional way. The ultrasonic dissector and laser are extremely important adjuncts. Chordomas, being soft, can usually be removed entirely, leaving the dura more or less intact. Other types of bony tumors of the clivus can usually be removed with an intact dura. Meningiomas are most likely to have involved the dura, and total removal may not be possible. The mass can be reduced in bulk to decompress the brain stem and make radiotherapy feasible. Tumors can be removed laterally. The principal limiting factors are the carotid and vertebral arteries and the twelfth nerves. A bilateral twelfth nerve paralysis is a catastrophe and must be avoided. Following tumor excision, the whole defect can be filled with fat taken from the abdomen. This provides a good CSF seal and eliminates the dead space that would otherwise exist in the bony defect. Reconstruction of the pharyngeal, glossal, and mandibular incisions is critical for a functional jaw. Restoration of proper occlusion is another important factor.

Midface Degloving

There are some tumors that are too widespread to be approached by simple trans-sphenoidal surgery but can be reached by the so-called midface degloving operation. The goal is a radical sphenoidectomy. Any clival tumor that has a major lateral extension on one or both sides can be managed by this approach.[55]

Operative Technique The operation is carried out under general anesthesia with the patient in the supine position. An oral endotracheal tube is used. The initial skin incision is made beneath the lip but is extended much more laterally than for transnasal trans-sphenoidal surgery. The skin of the face is then dissected up to the infraorbital nerves, and the skin of the nose lifted from the cartilaginous and bony nose. This allows the skin of the face to be elevated, exposing the entire anterior surface of the maxillary sinuses bilaterally to the level of the inferior rim of the orbit. One or both maxillary sinuses are entered and removed. Through the medial walls of one or both sinuses, the sphenoid sinus is opened and removed. The surgeon may work from either side. This approach gives a broad view of the upper clivus and allows far lateral dissection. It is most appropriate for tumors of the posterior sphenoid and clivus that have lateral extensions. It is particularly important not to enter the subarachnoid space from this approach because there is nothing left to use as packing to control a CSF fistula. This approach has been most useful for extraordinarily large pituitary tumors, asymmetric chordomas, and sinus carcinomas. Meningiomas may be palliated in this way, but total removal is unlikely.

Tumors Primarily in the Posterior Fossa

Petroclinoclival Meningiomas

Meningiomas that arise from the posterior clinoid and the petrous apex are particularly difficult surgical challenges.[41] They tend to grow to enormous size without causing symptoms (Figs. 155-3 and 155-4). They distort the brain stem and involve the basilar artery and its branches. They involve cranial nerves III through XII routinely, and they may extend anteriorly and involve the optic apparatus and pituitary as well.[67] Their total removal is a formidable

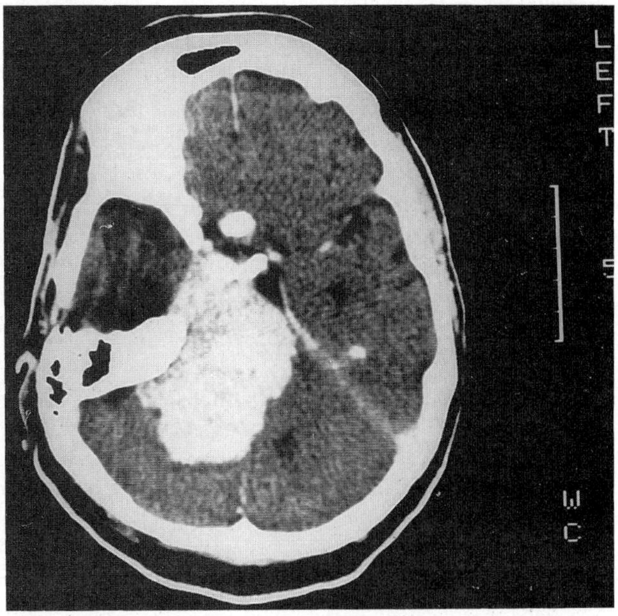

Figure 155-3 This enormous clival meningioma arises from the region of the posterior clinoid and upper clivus. It was approached through the posterior fossa and a total removal achieved.

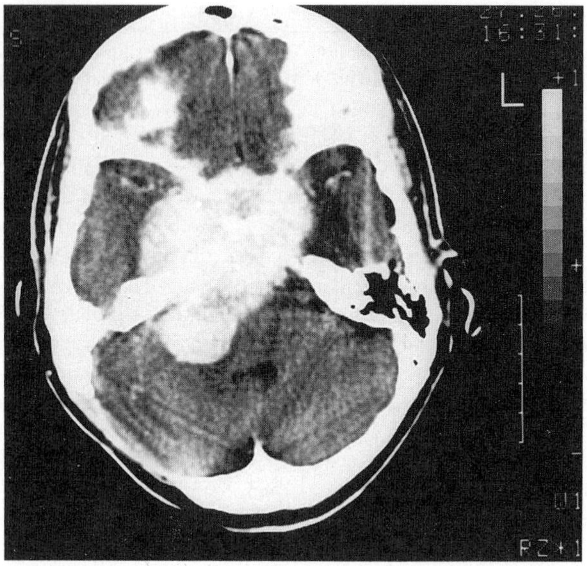

Figure 155-4 This enormous clival meningioma involves all four compartments. A lesion of this kind is beyond surgical cure at the moment. The patient was treated with removal of the posterior fossa component of the tumor that was causing brain stem compression. She has remained without neurological deficit, so no further treatment has been undertaken.

undertaking. Most of these tumors displace the neural and vascular structures and so are amenable to radical treatment. Another group, approximately 25 percent in our experience, so invest the blood vessels, particularly the basilar artery, that total removal is impossible. The bulk of these tumors can often be removed by the transoral route as long as there is no significant extension into the subarachnoid space. They can also be debulked by a more traditional subtemporal approach, as well as through the posterior fossa.[2]

The Posterior Fossa Approach to Petroclival Tumors

The traditional approach to petroclival tumors has been from beneath the temporal lobe.[29] However, the amount of brain retraction required puts the temporal lobe at risk, and the potential for cranial nerve injury is much greater than with an approach through the posterior fossa. This is now the favored route for partial or total removal of these tumors.[63]

Operative Technique The operations are done under general anesthesia with the patient in the lateral position with the head parallel to the floor. A unilateral posterior fossa incision suffices. Removal of one half of the occipital bone should be carried as far superiorly and laterally as possible without entering the venous sinuses. A rare tumor may require a combined supratentorial and infratentorial approach. Therefore, it is wise to prepare the occipitoparietal area for extension of the incision and a supratentorial craniotomy flap. The approach is identical to that used for large tumors of the cerebellopontine angle. CSF is drained from the cisterna magna until the cerebellum falls away; the operation can be carried out virtually without retraction once CSF is drained. The tumor itself displaces the brain stem posteriorly, and it is rarely necessary to put retractors on the brain stem until the final stages of removal of tumor from the basilar artery and its branches. The first step is to identify all the cranial nerves possible. It is not unusual for these tumors to involve cranial nerves II through XII. Access to the tumor will generally be between cranial nerve V and the VII-VIII complex or between VII-VIII and IX-X-XI. These structures should be identified first. As they are dissected from the posterior aspect of the tumor, a nerve-free area can be defined and entered. Internal debulking is the key to successful surgery. The ultrasonic aspirator or laser makes this task possible even with the extremely firm tumors that are so common in this location. Since these tumors share the twin characteristics of firmness and high vascularity, preoperative angiography and embolization can be an invaluable adjunct. As these tumors are debulked along the base, the cranial nerves become more obvious and the brain stem will begin to sag into the field. The portions adhering to the brain stem and basilar arteries should be removed last to minimize the need for brain stem retraction. The tumor should be allowed to do this work as long as possible. As the tumor shrinks, it should be possible to define cranial nerves IV and XII. The sixth cranial nerve is most likely to be lost during surgery because these tumors often arise from the area of Dorello's canal. Tumors of this type frequently enlarge the incisura of the tentorium so much that it is a simple matter to go up into the middle fossa and strip them from the carotid artery and even from the underside of the optic nerve and chiasm. The last step should be removal from the brain stem and dissection from the basilar artery. Sometimes the tumor is so adherent to the basilar artery that it is not safe to attempt removal.

The base of the tumor in bone is then vaporized with the laser, and any tumor-bearing bone is drilled away. Total removal even of extremely large tumors is frequently possible, and the outcome is excellent.

Combined Posterior and Middle Fossa Approaches to the Clivus

Some posterior fossa tumors are located both above and below the tentorium, and, while many of these can be approached by the suboccipital route alone, it is necessary to get more exposure for some that are in the incisura. The most common tumor in this location is meningioma. Epidermoids also occur here.

Preoperative Evaluation Before the decision for a combined posterior and middle fossa approach is made, the anatomy of the transverse sinuses has to be determined bilaterally. If the sinus is to be sacrificed, then it is essential that there is free communication to the opposite side. The location of the vein of Labbé is also important. Injury to this vein often produces catastrophic venous infarction and a hemiplegic patient. Embolization of these large tumors during angiography may be helpful, so the angiogram should be performed the day before surgery, with embolization planned if possible.

Operative Technique The suboccipital exposure is exactly as described. However, the incision is carried across the region of the sinus and then extended as a horseshoe flap or an elongated "S" above the ear. There is a tendency with these tumors to want to make the supratentorial flap too far posteriorly. The flap must allow subtemporal exposure up to the vein of Labbé at a minimum and as far as the sphenoid wing if the tumor extends to the visual apparatus. The usual flap is from the vein of Labbé toward the midline to allow the entire transverse sinus and the tentorium to be visualized.

There are two techniques for dealing with the part of the tumor that is above the tentorium. One is to simply elevate the parieto-occipital junction to expose the incisura, taking great care not to injure the vein of Labbé. The tentorium is cut behind the point where the fourth nerve begins to join the tentorial edge, but the sinus is left intact. This technique allows the whole area of the incisura to be widely opened and the tumor removed.

Even greater exposure is obtained if the sinus is divided. Once the cerebellum has been retracted and the brain elevated above, double ligatures can be passed around the sinus and the lumen obliterated. Then the sinus is divided, and the whole tentorium is cut into the incisura. This provides a dramatic exposure of the area, and tumor removal is much easier than if the sinus is intact. However, I personally do not like to divide the sinus unless absolutely necessary since it is my general rule to leave all normal anatomic structures in their natural state whenever possible.

Tumor removal is much as described above. The location of the tumor and its distortion of major vessels and cranial nerves must be determined, and the cranial nerves must be identified and dissected from the tumor. The position of blood vessels must be appreciated and the tumor removed from around them. Standard techniques employed for meningiomas everywhere suffice. The closure is equally straightforward. Both wounds are closed in the routine way.

There is one other point that must be considered. Some of these patients require pre- or postoperative shunting. When placing the shunt, it is important to remember where the approach to the tumor will be and to avoid putting a shunt in a place that will later be a problem for the exposure.

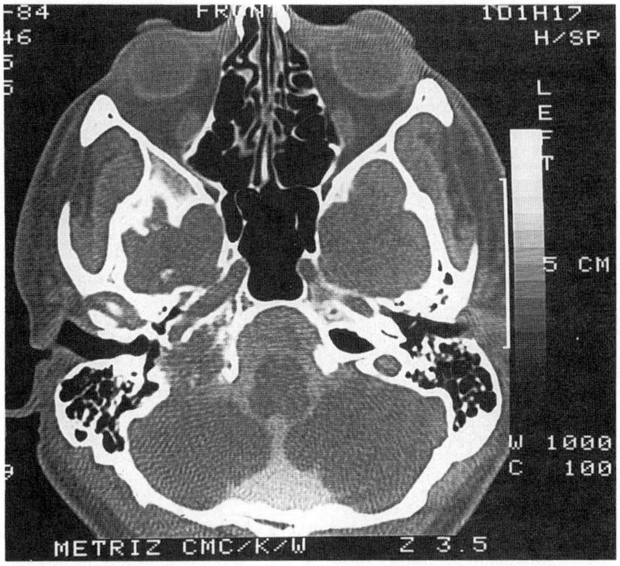

Figure 155-5 This glomus jugulare tumor has enlarged the jugular foramen and resulted in significant bone destruction. There is no intracranial extension. Such a tumor can be approached by either a one- or a two-stage procedure.

Lateral and Posterior Fossa Approaches to the Skull Base

Asymmetrical tumors involving the petrous bone and the skull base laterally around the exit foramina of the cranial nerves are best approached from a lateral exposure. The most common lesion in this location is the glomus tumor (Fig. 155-5).[8,9,25] Meningiomas are relatively common; chordomas occur in this location, as do chondromas and chondrosarcomas. Occasionally, a schwannoma or neurofibroma of a cranial nerve other than the eighth occurs here. Large cholesteatomas may also be encountered.

There are two ways to approach these lesions. One is by a single-stage operation designed for cure, and the other is by a two-stage operation for the same purpose.[5] There are no definitive data to indicate that one technique is superior to the other, so both will be described.[1]

Two-Stage Operation for Skull Base Tumors

The reason for a two-stage operation is to prevent a CSF fistula and to provide the greatest protection of the intracranial structures during surgery. When the two-stage operation is contemplated, the first approach is a standard unilateral suboccipital craniectomy carried out in the same fashion as for a large acoustic schwannoma. No attempt is made to remove glomus tumors on the first stage. However, other tumors may be debulked intracranially. The major goal is not to remove the tumor but to isolate cranial nerves and vessels from it. A dural graft is then interposed between these structures and the tumor. Fascia lata or the newer human dural substitutes may be used. Artificial substances are not effective in providing the desired CSF barrier. At a second stage, radical resection of the petrous bone and skull base from the lateral approach is undertaken, with the brain protected behind a thick layer of artificial dura. In our series of 13 patients treated with this procedure, no CSF leak has occurred.

The only differences from standard surgery relate to the skin incision. A curvilinear incision is made behind the ear. It is not carried down to the posterior cervical region but is swung forward toward the angle of the jaw so that it can be continued down into the neck to provide access to the major vessels. This is mandatory for glomus tumors, where control of both carotid artery and jugular vein must be achieved, and is desirable for all tumors in the skull base so that both carotid and jugular are under proximal control. This means that the cervical musculature is reflected medially off the occipital bone rather than being divided.

Single-Stage Operation for Petrous and Skull Base Tumors

The same operation can be carried out in a single stage. When the tumor involves principally the petrous bone and is extradural in location, there is no need to consider a two-stage procedure. In such circumstances, a curvilinear incision is made behind the ear, like that employed for an acoustic tumor but more laterally placed. The lower end of the incision curves to the angle of the jaw and is extended down the neck to expose the carotid artery and jugular vein. These structures are followed up to either the skull base or the tumor, whichever is encountered first. The cervical musculature is detached from the skull base and occipital bone. A drill is then used to drill away the structures of the bone of the skull base. This technique is not a usual neurosurgical skill. In our institution, these operations are shared between otolaryngology/head and neck surgery and neurosurgery. It is quite reasonable for neurosurgeons to do them, but it requires practice and anatomic knowledge not usually provided in neurosurgical training.[36] The surgeon must learn to spare the structures of the inner ear when necessary, to reroute the VIIth nerve, and to skeletonize the jugular bulb and sigmoid sinus. The extent of destruction of these structures relates entirely to the extent of the tumor. In most instances, hearing is already destroyed, so preservation of the inner ear is not important. However, the VIIth nerve must be preserved in all cases.

It is possible to go all the way to the petrous apex by this approach. The extent of the exposure can be from the petrous apex to the foramen magnum and below if indicated. Extensions upward into the middle fossa can be followed. This lateral posterior fossa approach is the most unfamiliar of all of the extracranial skull base approaches for the neurosurgeon. No one should undertake it without being thoroughly familiar with the techniques. A number of specialized publications are available for reference which detail the surgical procedures.

Tumors of the Inferior Third of the Clivus and Upper Cervical Area

The most common tumor in the inferior third of the clivus and the upper cervical area is meningioma.[11] Chordomas may occur here, and an occasional lymphoma of the bone is encountered. If no intradural extension is expected, the simple transoral route is the most effective way to remove these tumors.[46,49] Fusion undertaken through the mouth has a high incidence of infection, and, therefore, this approach can be used only when there is posterior stability so that fusion will not be necessary. If anterior fusion is contemplated, it is better to use the lateral superior cervical approach.[60]

Operative Technique The patient is intubated in the usual fashion in the supine position. The head is then turned to the side opposite the incision. It is easier for a right-handed surgeon to work on the left. A transverse incision is a convenient skin fold just below the mandible is made, and an approach anterior to the sternocleidomastoid similar to that employed for anterior cervical fusion at a lower level is performed. The jugular vein and carotid artery are reflected laterally with the sternomastoid. The digastric must be cut, and the laryngeal structures are reflected medially. It is usually necessary to cut some or all of the insertion of the sternocleidomastoid on the skull base. This should be done through the tendinous portion so it can be resutured upon closure. This approach brings the surgeon to the retropharyngeal space at the C1-C2 level. By dissecting upward it is possible to isolate the lower third of the clivus; C1, the odontoid, and the body of C2 are already exposed. Resection of the tumor is undertaken by standard techniques. A fibular or iliac graft is taken, molded to fit from the lower portion of the intact clivus into the body of C2, and firmly keyed into position. The patient should be stabilized in a halo postoperatively. It is critical not to enter the subarachnoid space by this route.

For tumors with large intradural extensions in this location, a modified lateral approach is preferred. The typical posterior fossa craniectomy is carried out, but the incision is extended farther down the neck to allow the arch of C1 and the spine and the lamina of C2 to be exposed. Cervical laminectomy is added to the craniectomy. The tumor usually has displaced the brain stem and upper cervical cord posteriorly, so that there is room to work in front of the cord and brain stem without retraction. The techniques for working between cranial and spinal nerves, debulking the tumor near the base, and gradually extracting the remaining capsule from beneath the brain stem and cord are the same for all clival tumors. The tumor can be devascularized by drilling away its bony base early in the course of the surgery. This requires careful preservation of the cranial nerves by skeletonizing the jugular foramen. The critical feature in total removal is likely to be the penetration of the tumor by the vertebral artery. The tumor must be dissected from the vertebral and posterior inferior cerebellar arteries. Skeletonization of the vertebral artery at the skull base in the tumor mass can be difficult.

The Posterior Fossa Approach to the Cerebellopontine Angle

Most tumors in the cerebellopontine angle are acoustic schwannomas (Fig. 155-6).[10,43,47,59] Meningiomas occur less commonly (Fig. 155-7), and other lesions such as cholesteatomas are unusual.[6,50,65,68] There are three basic approaches to these tumors: a posterior fossa craniectomy, a translabyrinthine approach, and middle fossa exposure. Much has been written about the utility of these approaches. My own preference is to use the posterior fossa approach whenever the tumor is large or hearing preservation is a goal. When the tumor is small—1.5 cm or less—and hearing preservation cannot be a goal, the translabyrinthine route is satisfactory and very safe for the patient. A translabyrinthine exposure for radical intracapsular removal of an exceptionally large tumor in an elderly or ill patient is also useful occasionally. We have virtually given up the middle fossa exposure. It has been advocated for small intracanalicular tumors where hearing preservation is a realistic goal.[48,51,56]

The Translabyrinthine Exposure

The translabyrinthine technique has been elaborated on at great length by a number of authors over the past 20 years. Those interested should consult the specialized articles that detail this operative approach.[32,33] The principal role of this approach in our practice is the treatment of small tumors that have already destroyed

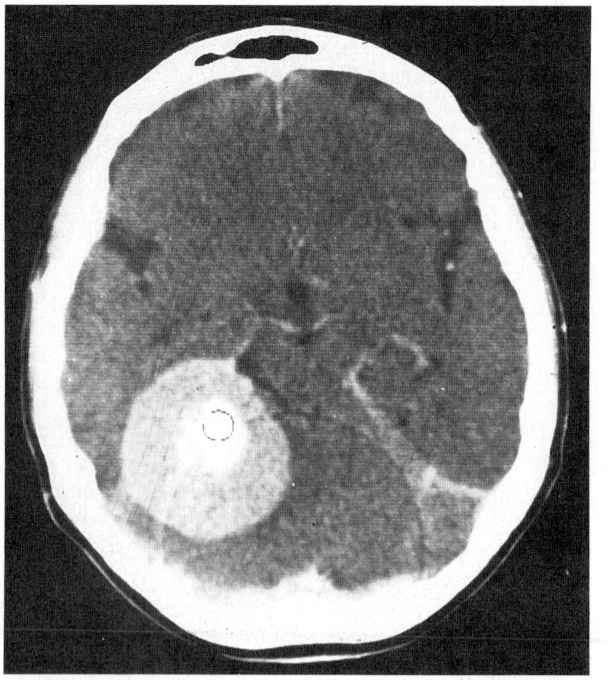

Figure 155-6 This is a typical giant vascular acoustic schwannoma. The tumor had recurred after two previous attempts at removal. Preoperative embolization followed by a radical posterior fossa approach resulted in total removal.

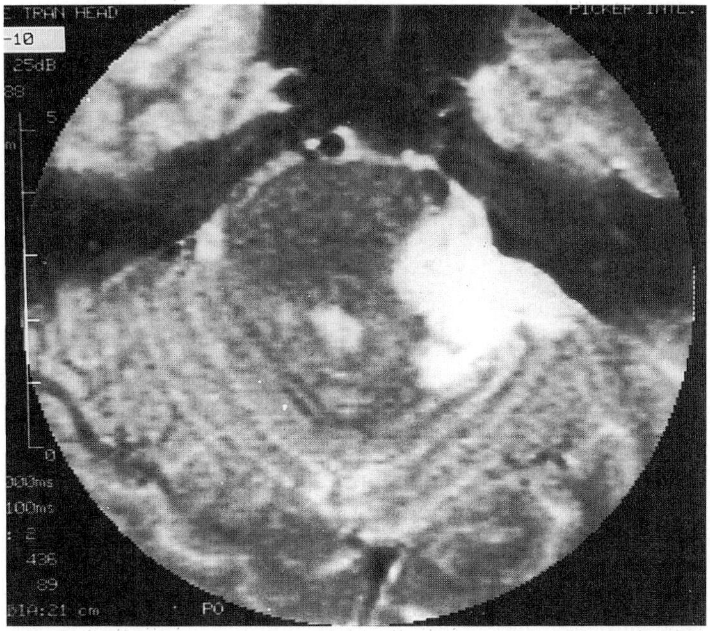

Figure 155-7 The typical features of a cerebellopontine angle meningioma are apparent. The tumor is irregular, broadly based, and highly vascular. Brain stem compression and the insinuation of tumor into the cerebellopontine angle are typical.

hearing. The translabyrinthine procedure, while it takes longer than direct intracranial exposure, does provide great safety and very small morbidity. It is also useful in elderly patients with large tumors. Sometimes total removal is not feasible because of the medical status of the patient. An intracapsular removal may decompress the brain stem and provide long-term palliation for such elderly patients, avoid the risk of facial nerve paralysis or other significant morbidity.[24]

The Posterior Fossa Approach

The standard neurosurgical approach to tumors of the cerebellopontine angle has also been described in great detail.[49] These approaches are familiar enough that they need little description. Most surgeons now use a lateral or supine position with the head turned and a unilateral retromastoid posterior fossa exposure. A limited craniectomy is carried out on the side of the tumor. The amount of bone removal will relate to the size of the lesion. Once the tumor is exposed, cranial nerves are dissected free, and the anterior inferior cerebellar artery and its branches are removed from the capsule.[54] Most surgeons employ an intracapsular removal to reduce the bulk of the tumor and then dissect the tumor capsule free from all surrounding vessels. At some point in the removal, the porus acusticus must be drilled open for 10 to 12 mm and the tumor then dissected free from all cranial nerves medially and laterally. Surgeons vary in their preference for lateral-to-medial or medial-to-lateral dissection to preserve the seventh nerve. Some monitor seventh nerve function, while others do not. The goal of the posterior fossa removal is cure of the tumor, and that is now accomplished routinely. Even the largest tumors can be treated at a single stage, and intracapsular removal is rarely indicated except in the most fragile of patients or for the most difficult of tumors.[26]

Current neurosurgical practice focuses on the preservation of hearing. How often that can be accomplished is not yet certain, but optimistic reports have appeared.[48,51,56]

Preservation of seventh nerve function is now routine.[64] A significant percentage of patients develop temporary paresis, but anatomic preservation of the nerve is accomplished most of the time, and virtually all of these patients have satisfactory recovery of function. Occasionally a seventh nerve is divided deliberately or accidentally. There is now good evidence that intracranial suturing with or without grafting provides recovery of function in most of these patients.[7,20]

The major questions with cerebellopontine angle tumors are no longer technical. Total removal is virtually always possible. The problems in management relate to decisions about what to do with certain kinds of patients.

The most frustrating of these patients are the ones that harbor bilateral tumors. It is the usual practice of most surgeons to allow the tumors to grow, retaining useful hearing as long as possible, and then to carry out tumor removal when hearing is lost. Patients are educated in sign language during the interval. As preservation of hearing becomes feasible, there is an increasing tendency to try to remove these tumors and preserve hearing in so doing. When this goal is achievable, a more aggressive approach to the bilateral tumor is indicated.

The very small tumor discovered almost accidentally is another management problem. Now that MRI is available, such tumors may be observed during repeat scanning on a regular basis. It is our practice to operate only when they begin to grow. However, there are some risks to this approach, as an occasional tumor will grow very rapidly. Strict monitoring with regular scans is required if these patients are not operated on.

Small tumors in elderly patients are a particular problem. It is our general practice not to operate on these tumors and to follow the patients until the tumors become symptomatic.

Huge tumors in elderly patients are another major problem. Some patients are simply not able to withstand the formidable operation required for total removal of these large tumors. In this situation, an intracapsular removal by the translabyrinthine route is a way to palliate the symptoms and provide a long period of functional survival for these elderly patients. Even repeat intracapsular removal is a reasonable way to maintain such patients. Another possibility is intracapsular removal followed by intracranial removal of a tumor that has been greatly reduced in bulk. Many elderly patients who could not have total tumor removal at one sitting can tolerate it well after the brain stem has returned to its normal position and hydrocephalus has come under control.

Preoperative Angiography and Embolization

Many skull base tumors are avascular. However, some, particularly meningiomas, angioneurofibromas, and an occasional schwannoma, may be very vascular (Fig. 155-6). The MRI and enhanced CT scan usually give a clue to vascularity. If the tumor appears to have an abundant blood supply, then preoperative angiography is useful. This should be coordinated with surgery so that the major feeding vessels of the tumor can be obliterated no more than 48 h before the operation. Occasionally, one of these tumors will swell after embolization, necessitating urgent surgery. It is our usual practice to perform the angiography and embolization the day before the proposed operation to maximize the reduction in blood flow. Adequate embolization will often so devascularize these tumors that they become necrotic, greatly aiding removal.

Conclusions

These extracranial and combined intracranial-extracranial approaches to paracranial tumors are unusual for neurosurgeons. They require a detailed understanding of the anatomy of the skull base. The surgeon must also understand the intracranial anatomy in the same detail and be able to visualize the intracranial anatomy with the dura intact. The surgeon must be skilled in the use of high speed surgical drills, capable of handling intracranial extensions, and prepared to repair transected cranial nerves and injured cerebral vessels. While there is no reason why one surgeon cannot manage all these factors as they relate to the orbit, petrous bone, clivus, and cranial contents, most current training programs do not provide the knowledge to do so. For this reason we have elected to approach these complex lesions through the use of a surgical team that includes neurosurgery, neuro-ophthalmology, and neuro-otology. The surgical duties are shared, with each surgeon responsible for the portion of the procedure in that specialty's domain. These lesions remain the most complex and surgically demanding of all three disciplines. The advances in skull base surgery over the past 10 years have been remarkable. Many more surgeons are involved from all of the surgical disciplines of the skull base. Dramatic improvements in mortality and morbidity have been achieved. Operations that were considered oddities a short time ago are now regularly described at meetings and are in common use by specialists in this area. Nevertheless, there are still major questions to be answered, and much improvement in technique is required. Disasters are still possible, and many tumors cannot be removed. Recurrence of meningiomas is still a problem. In the past 10 years, skepticism about the ability of surgeons to approach the skull base successfully has changed to general appreciation and some enthusiasm. Better evaluation of natural history and improved assessment of outcome remains important. These tumors require both skill and experience. Still, the outlook for patients with most of these tumors has improved dramatically in the recent past, and it is probable that improvements in outcome based upon greater experience and improved technique will continue. Advances are being made by all the disciplines involved with these patients, and the multi-disciplinary team continues to be the most popular option for their management.

References

1. Al-Mefty O, Fox JL, Rifai A, et al. A combined infratemporal and posterior fossa approach for the removal of giant glomus tumors and chondrosarcomas. *Surg Neurol* 1987; 28:423–431.
2. Al-Mefty O, Fox JL, Smith RR. Petrosal approach for petroclival meningiomas. *Neurosurgery* 1988; 22:510–517.
3. Arbit E, Patterson RH Jr. Combined transoral and median labiomandibular glossotomy approach to the upper cervical spine. *Neurosurgery* 1981; 8:672–674.
4. Arnold H, Herrmann HD. Skull base chordoma with cavernous sinus involvement. Partial or radical tumour-removal? *Acta Neurochir (Wien)* 1986; 83:31–37.
5. Bordi LT, Cheesman AD, Symon L. The surgical management of glomus jugulare tumours: description of a single-staged posterolateral combined otoneurosurgical approach. *Br J Neurosurg* 1989; 3:21–30.
6. Brackmann DE. A review of acoustic tumours: 1979–1982. *Am J Otol* 1984; 5:233–244.
7. Brackmann DE, Hitselberger WE, Robinson JV. Facial nerve repair in cerebellopontine angle surgery. *Ann Otol Rhinol Laryngol* 1978; 87:772–777.
8. Brammer RE, Graham MD, Kemink JL. Glomus tumours of the temporal bone: contemporary evaluation and therapy. *Otolaryngol Clin North Am* 1984; 17:499–512.
9. Britton BH. Glomus tympanicum and glomus jugulare tumors. *Radiol Clin North Am* 1974; 12:543–551.
10. Catz A, Reider-Groswasser I. Acoustic neurinoma and posterior fossa meningioma: clinical and CT radiologic findings. *Neuroradiology* 1986; 28:47–52.
11. Cherington M, Schneck SA. Clivus meningiomas. *Neurology* 1966; 16:86–92.
12. Cocke EW Jr, Robertson JH, Robertson JT, Crook JP Jr. The extended maxillotomy and subtotal maxillectomy for excision of skull base tumors. *Arch Otolaryngol Head Neck Surg* 1990; 116:92–104.
13. Cophignon J, Lucena J, Clay C, et al. Limits to radical treatment of spheno-orbital meningiomas. *Acta Neurochir (Wien)* 1979; 28(suppl):375–380.
14. Crockard HA. The transoral approach to the base of the brain and upper cervical cord. *Ann R Coll Surg Engl* 1985; 67:321–325.
15. Deen HG Jr, Scheithauer BW, Ebersold MJ. Clinical and pathological study of meningiomas of the first two decades of life. *J Neurosurg* 1982; 56:317–322.
16. Delgado TE, Garrido E, Harwick RD. Labiomandibular, transoral approach to chordomas in the clivus and upper cervical spine. *Neurosurgery* 1981; 8:675–679.
17. Derome PJ. Surgical management of tumours invading the skull base. *Can J Neurol Sci* 1985; 12:345–347.
18. Ferrara P, Cimino A, Tortorici M. Role of radiation therapy in glomus tumor. *Am J Otol* 1987; 8:390–395.
19. Fisch U. Infratemporal fossa approach for glomus tumors of the temporal bone. *Ann Otol Rhinol Laryngol* 1982; 91:474–479.
20. Fisch U, Dobie RA, Dmür A, et al. Intracranial facial nerve anastomosis. *Am J Otol* 1987; 8:23–29.
21. Fisch U, Pillsbury HC. Infratemporal fossa approach to lesions in the temporal bone and base of the skull. *Arch Otolaryngol* 1979; 105:99–107.
22. Fujitsu K, Kuwabara T. Zygomatic approach for lesions of the interpeduncular cistern. *J Neurosurg* 1985; 62:340–343.
23. Gagnon NB, Lavigne F, Mohr G, et al. Extracranial and intracranial meningiomas. *J Otolaryngol* 1986; 15:380–384.
24. Gardner G, Robertson JH, Clark WC. 105 patients operated upon for cerebellopontine angle tumors: experience using combined approach and CO_2 laser. *Laryngoscope* 1983; 93:1049–1055.

25. Glasscock ME III, Harris PF, Newsome G. Glomus tumors: diagnosis and treatment. *Laryngoscope* 1974; 84:2006–2032.
26. Glasscock ME III, Hays JW, Jackson CG, et al. A one-stage combined approach for the management of large cerebellopontine angle tumors. *Laryngoscope* 1978; 88:1563–1576.
27. Glasscock ME III, Miller GW, Drake FD, et al. Surgery of the skull base. *Laryngoscope* 1978; 88:905–923.
28. Goin DW. Surgical management of petrous apex meningioma. *Larygoscope* 1979; 89:204–213.
29. Grand W, Bakay L. Posterior fossa meningiomas: a report of 30 cases. *Acta Neurochir (Wien)* 1975; 32:219–233.
30. Hakuba A, Nishimura S. Total removal of clivus meningiomas and the operative results. *Neurol Med Chir (Tokyo)* 1981; 21:59–73.
31. Henderson JW, Campbell RJ. Primary intraorbital meningioma with intraocular extension. *Mayo Clin Proc* 1977; 52:504–508.
32. House WF, de la Cruz A, Hitselberger WE. Surgery of the skull base: transcochlear approach to the petrous apex and clivus. *Otolaryngology* 1978; 86:770–779.
33. House WF, Hitselberger WE. The transcochlear approach to the skull base. *Arch Otolaryngol* 1976; 102:334–342.
34. Janecka IP, Sen CN, Sekhar LN, Arriaga M. Facial translocation: a new approach to the cranial base. *Otolaryngol Head Neck Surg* 1990; 103:413–419.
35. Karp LA, Zimmerman LE, Borit A, et al. Primary intraorbital meningiomas. *Arch Ophthalmol* 1974; 91:24–28.
36. Kawase T, Toya S, Shiobara R, Mine T. Transpetrosal approach for aneurysms of the lower basilar artery. *J Neurosurg* 1985; 63:857–861.
37. Kennedy DW, Papel ID, Holliday N. Transpalatal approach to the skull base. *Ear Nose Throat J* 1986; 65:125, 127–133.
38. Leipzig B, English J. Sphenoid wing meningioma occurring as a lateral orbital mass. *Laryngoscope* 1984; 94:1091–1093.
39. Lloyd GAS. Primary orbital meningioma: a review of 41 patients investigated radiologically. *Clin Radiol* 1982; 33:181–187.
40. Lloyd GAS, Phelps PD. The investigation of petro-mastoid tumours by high resolution CT. *Br J Radiol* 1982; 55:483–491.
41. Mafee MF, Aimi K, Valvassori GE. Computed tomography in the diagnosis of primary tumors of the petrous bone. *Laryngoscope* 1984; 94:1423–1430.
42. Malis LI. Surgical resection of tumors of the skull base. In Wilkins RH, Rengachary SS (eds): *Neurosurgery*. New York: McGraw-Hill, 1985, pp 1011–1021.
43. Mawhinney RR, Buckley JH, Worthington BS. Magnetic resonance imaging of the cerebello-pontine angle. *Br J Radiol* 1986; 59:961–969.
44. Mayberg MR, Symon L. Meningiomas of the clivus and apical petrous bone: report of 35 cases. *J Neurosurg* 1986; 65:160–167.
45. McFadzean RM, Gowan ME. Orbital tumours: a review of 34 cases. *J R Coll Surg Edinb* 1983; 28:361–364.
46. Menezes AH, VanGilder JC, Graf CJ, McDonnell DE. Craniocervical abnormalities. A comprehensive surgical approach. *J Neurosurg* 1980; 53:444–455.
47. Morrison AW, King TT. Space-occupying lesions of the internal auditory meatus and cerebellopontine angle. *Adv Otorhinolaryngol* 1984; 34:121–142.
48. Nadol JB Jr, Levine R, Ojemann RG, et al. Preservation of hearing in surgical removal of acoustic neuromas of the internal auditory canal and cerebellar pontine angle. *Laryngoscope* 1987; 97:1287–1294.
49. Nedzelski JM, Tator CH. Surgical management of cerebellopontine angle tumors. *J Otolaryngol* 1980; 9:105–112.
50. Nedzelski J, Tator C. Other cerebellopontine angle (non-acoustic neuroma) tumors. *J Otolaryngol* 1982; 11:248–252.
51. Nedzelski JM, Tator CH. Hearing preservation: a realistic goal in surgical removal of cerebellopontine angle tumors. *J Otolaryngol* 1984; 13:355–360.
52. Neil-Dwyer G, Sharr M, Haskell R, et al. Zygomaticotemporal approach to the basis cranii and basilar artery. *Neurosurgery* 1988; 23:20–22.
53. Penzholz H. Development and present state of cerebellopontine angle surgery from the neuro- and otosurgical point of view. *Arch Otorhinolaryngol* 1984; 240:167–174.
54. Perneczky A, Perneczky G, Tschabitscher M, et al. The relationship between the caudolateral pontine syndrome and the anterior inferior cerebellar artery. *Acta Neurochir (Wien)* 1981; 58:245–257.
55. Price JC, Holliday MJ, Johns ME, et al. The versatile midface degloving approach. *Laryngoscope* 1988; 98:291–295.
56. Rosenberg RA, Cohen NL, Ransohoff J. Long-term hearing preservation after acoustic neuroma surgery. *Otolaryngol Head Neck Surg* 1987; 97:270–274.
57. Sekhar LN, Schramm VL Jr, Jones NF. Subtemporal-preauricular infratemporal fossa approach to large lateral and posterior cranial base neoplasms. *J Neurosurg* 1987; 67:488–499.
58. Sen CN, Sekhar LN. The subtemporal and preauricular infratemporal approach to intradural structures ventral to the brain stem. *J Neurosurg* 1990; 73:345–354.
59. Slooff JL. Pathological anatomical findings in the cerebellopontine angle. *Adv Otorhinolaryngol* 1984; 34:89–103.
60. Spetzler RF, Grahm TW. The far lateral approach to the inferior clivus and the upper cervical region. Technical note. *BNI Q* 1990; 6:35–38.
61. Stein BM. Operative approaches to midline tumors. *Acta Neurochir (Wien)* 1985; 35(Suppl):42–49.
62. Stern WE. Meningiomas in the cranio-orbital junction. *J Neurosurg* 1973; 38:428–437.
63. Susac JO, Smith JL, Walsh FB. The impossible meningioma. *Arch Neurol* 1977; 34:36–38.
64. Tator CH, Nedzelski JM. Facial nerve preservation in patients with large acoustic neuromas treated by a combined middle fossa transtentorial translabyrinthine approach. *J Neurosurg* 1982; 57:1–7.
65. Thomsen J. Cerebellopontine angle tumours, other than acoustic neuromas: a report on 34 cases; a presentation of 7 bilateral acoustic neuromas. *Acta Otolaryngol (Stockh)* 1976; 82:106–111.
66. Uttley D, Archer DJ, Marsh HT, Bell BA. Improved access to lesions of the central skull base by mobilization of the zygoma: experience with 54 cases. *Neurosurgery* 1991; 28:99–104.
67. Valavanis A, Schubiger O, Hayek J, et al. CT of meningiomas on the posterior surface of the petrous bone. *Neuroradiology* 1981; 22:111–121.
68. Valvassori GE. Benign tumors of the temporal bone. *Radiol Clin North Am* 1974; 12:533–542.
69. VanGilder JC, Menezes AH. Craniovertebral junction abnormalities. *Clin Neurosurg* 1983; 30:514–530.
70. Weisman PA. Meningioma of the sphenoid ridge: palliative surgery for facial involvement. *Panminerva Med* 1969; 11:117–122.
71. Yasargil MG, Mortara RW, Curcic M. Meningiomas of basal posterior cranial fossa. *Adv Tech Stand Neurosurg* 1980; 7:1–115.

156 Craniofacial Osteotomies to Facilitate the Resection of Tumors of the Skull Base

Ian T. Jackson

One of the main problems confronting those who, in the past, attempted to excise skull base tumors was exposure of the involved area. Without adequate exposure, *en bloc* resection is next to impossible, and when attempted can be highly dangerous. In an attempt to improve on this situation, structures were sacrificed, sometimes leading to adverse functional effects together with facial deformity. Experience in the correction of congenital craniofacial anomalies led to the development of "exposure osteotomies," methods of preventing infection (e.g., galeal frontalis myofascial flap[3]), and techniques of reconstruction (e.g., free cranial bone grafts[4,7] and vascularized cranial bone grafts[1,8]). Armed with these new developments, skull base tumor surgery has taken on a completely new look; exposure is usually adequate, and *en bloc* resection is frequent, with minimal complications.

Exposure Osteotomies

Exposure osteotomies have been described previously in a systematic fashion,[2–5] and these continue to be a convenient series of techniques to learn initially; however, after these techniques have been mastered, improvization is the key. The type of osteotomy performed is that which is necessary and possible to expose the tumor. Basically, anterior and lateral approaches are used.

The Anterior Approach

Under this heading, only upper face osteotomies will be discussed. The mandibular swing technique is used to resect infratemporal fossa tumors extending to the base of the middle cranial fossa; it is a good approach in selected cases, but it is unlikely that a neurosurgeon would ever choose to use it. By contrast, the upper face approaches, if studied on the skull or, better still, on the cadaver, could fall within the sphere of the neurosurgeon. This is not advocated. A team approach involving the head and neck surgeon is strongly advised. The surgery is accomplished more expeditiously and safely.

Supraorbital Osteotomy

For tumors lying in the superior or cranial segment of the orbit (Fig. 156-1), the approach should be a combined intra- and extracranial one, particularly if the lesions are malignant. There is nothing to recommend and everything to deprecate a subcranial approach through the upper lid. This approach virtually ensures inadequate resection with its inevitable consequences.

The orbit is exposed through a bicoronal flap. This should be raised using an incision from ear to ear. The older incision just within the hairline can cause an unacceptable and uncorrectable esthetic problem and should be abandoned. To claim that this allows better exposure is illogical. The frontal craniotomy should be that which gives adequate exposure and no more. This ensures that any problem such as infection will result in the loss of the smallest possible area of bone. If the tumor lies within the periorbitum, e.g., a neurilemoma, the periorbitum is elevated from the orbital walls medially, cranially, and laterally without disturbing the medial and lateral canthal ligaments. If the periorbitum of the orbital roof is involved, the uninvolved area only is dissected. The frontal lobe is elevated.

Using an air drill with a side cutting burr, or a saw (sagittal or reciprocal), the supraorbital rim is cut through vertically, medially, and laterally. If the periorbitum is intact, the orbital and cranial contents are protected with malleable retractors and the osteotomies are extended posteriorly through the roof near the orbital apex—usually a distance close to 4 cm. The cuts are joined and the osteotomy segments is removed.

When the periosteum is involved, the bony segment anterior to this area is removed. The involved posterior segment of the orbital roof will be removed *en bloc* with the orbital contents.

With this exposure, resection can be performed safely and accurately under direct vision. At the completion of the resection, the osteotomy is wired or miniplated back into position. If necessary, any orbital roof defect is reconstructed with a split cranial bone graft. This is also stabilized with wires or miniplates. If an orbital exenteration has been performed, the osteotomy is exposed in the orbit and must be covered with vascularized tissue. This is accomplished using the temporalis muscle taken through an ostectomy in the lateral orbital wall—the "letter box" technique. A split skin graft applied to the transposed temporalis muscle will give a very adequate socket.

Glabellar Osteotomy

Midline tumors that need only a limited bony exposure can be approached by midline trephination (Fig. 156-2). Associated skull base resection will result in a communication with the nasopharynx; infection was a problem in the past, and therefore removal of as little bone as possible is strongly advocated. The frontal lobes are elevated, and the contents of both orbits are dissected subperiosteally. This may have to be limited because of tumor extension into the periorbita.

Osteotomies are now made vertically from the edge of the trephine defect through the superior orbital rims into the orbits. Their cuts are taken back just in front of the crista galli and are then joined transversely. Anteriorly, the nasal mucoperiosteum is dissected off the undersurface of the nasal bones and medial orbital

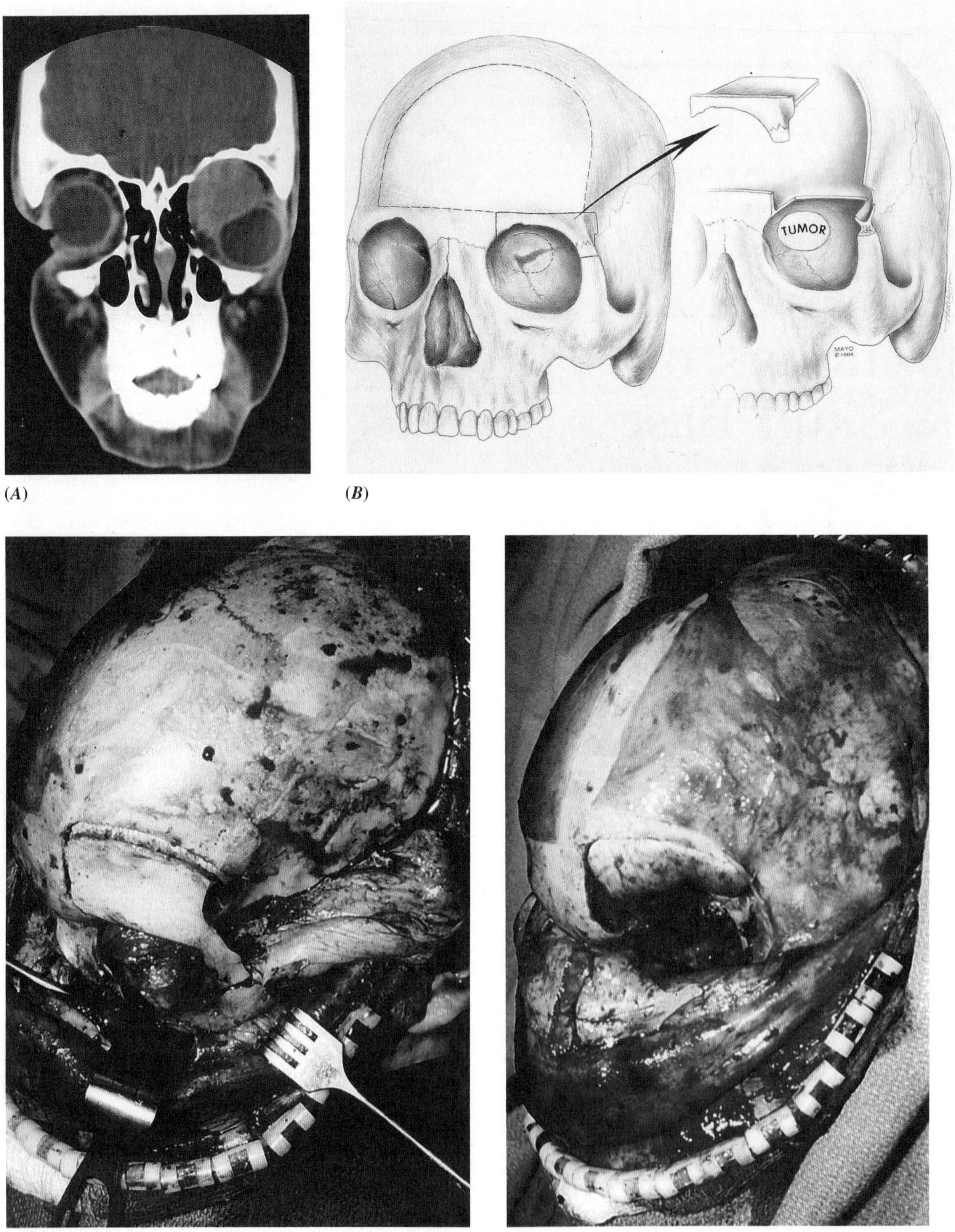

(*A*) (*B*)

(*C*) (*D*)

Figure 156-1 Supraorbital osteotomy. *A*. Coronal CT scan showing recurrent postradiotherapy rhabdomyosarcoma of the left orbit. *B*. Diagram illustrating the supraorbital exposure osteotomy. *C*. The osteotomy cuts have been outlined. *D*. The osteotomy has been removed for exposure. Following this, orbital exenteration in continuity with the roof of the orbit has been performed.

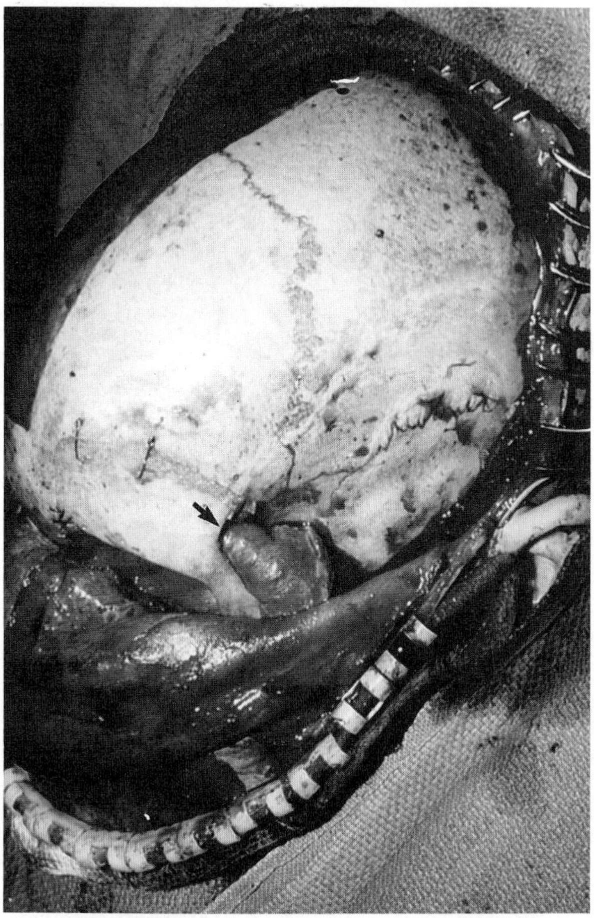

(*E*)

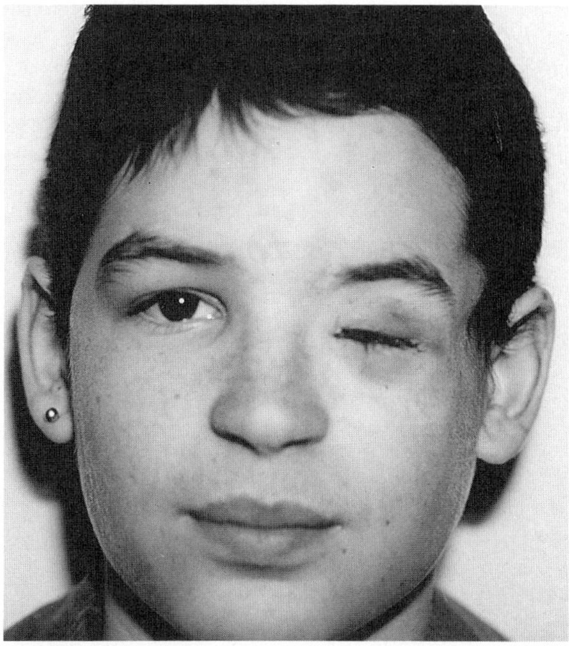

(*F*)

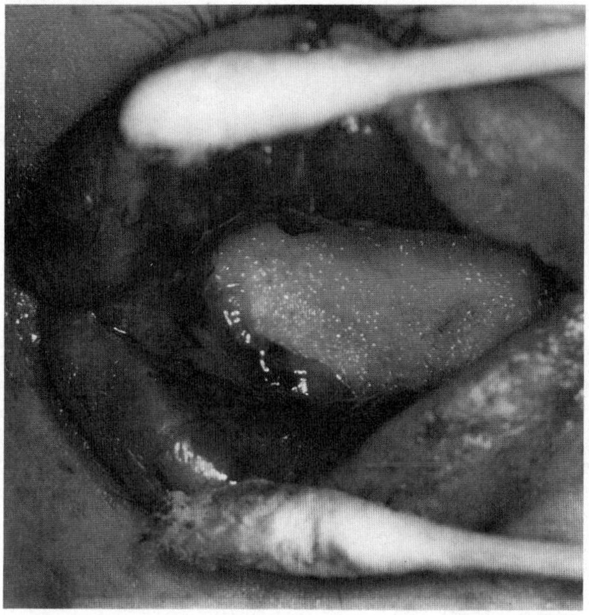

(*G*)

Figure 156-1 (*Continued*) *E.* Orbital roof bone has been grafted. The osteotomy has been wired back in position, and the temporalis muscle has been taken through a defect of the lateral orbital wall to line the socket (letter box technique; *arrow*). *F.* Result at 1 year. *G.* Split skin graft covering the transposed temporalis muscle.

walls. With the mucoperiosteum protected, cuts are made into the nose at the desired level and the glabellar and nasal bone block is removed.

This osteotomy gives excellent exposure, and it is possible to resect medial orbital walls, septum, ethmoid sinuses, cribriform plate, and sphenoid sinuses back to their posterior wall as a single block. At the completion of the procedure, holes are drilled through the edges of the anterior cranial base defect and a galeal frontalis myofascial flap is sutured carefully and securely to separate the anterior cranial fossa from the nasopharynx. It has not been found necessary to reconstruct the defect in the anterior cranial fossa floor; however, this can be done if it is needed for frontal lobe support. When the glabellar bone segment is reinserted, a portion is removed transversely from its lower end so that the pedicle of the flap is not constricted—the ''letter box'' technique. All replaced bone segments are stabilized with wires or miniplates. It is possible to carry out medial and orbital wall reconstruction with split cranial bone grafts. A second galeal frontalis myofascial flap may be necessary to cover these grafts, since otherwise they would be exposed into the nose.

Frontonasomaxillary Osteotomy

In a frontonasomaxillary osteotomy (Fig. 156-3), when midline lesions are positioned deep in the anterior cranial fossa and are extensive, a wider exposure may be necessary to ensure safety during the resection. The approach is again by the biocoronal flap, but on this occasion, a standard bifrontal cranial bone flap is removed. The approach to the face is greatly facilitated by a "face splitting" incision. This will usually result in a satisfactory scar. The orbital contents are dissected as completely as possible superiorly, medially, and inferiorly, depending on the tumor pathology and its extension. The frontal lobes and orbital contents are protected. Vertical osteotomies are taken through the medial third of the supraorbital rims into the orbits. These are taken back as far as possible in the orbital roof and are joined by a horizontal cut. The osteotomy is then taken down the medial wall of the orbit unilaterally or bilaterally; this continues into the floor of the orbit,

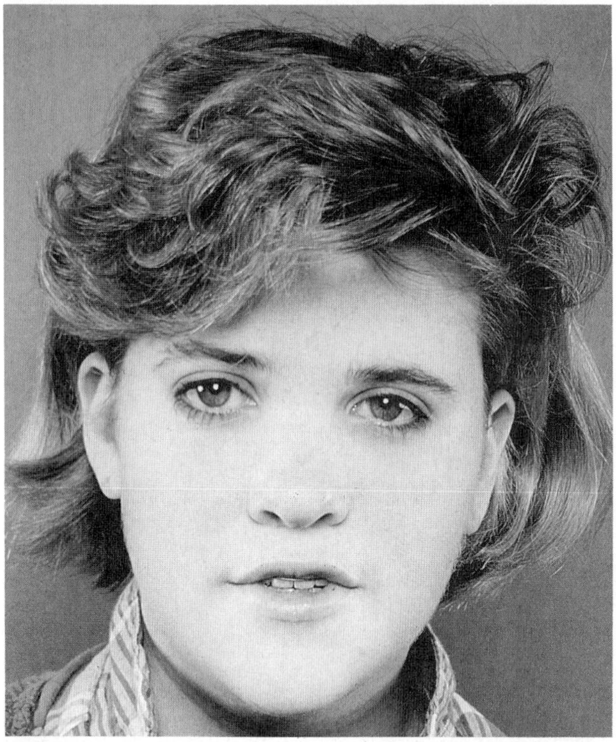
(*A*)

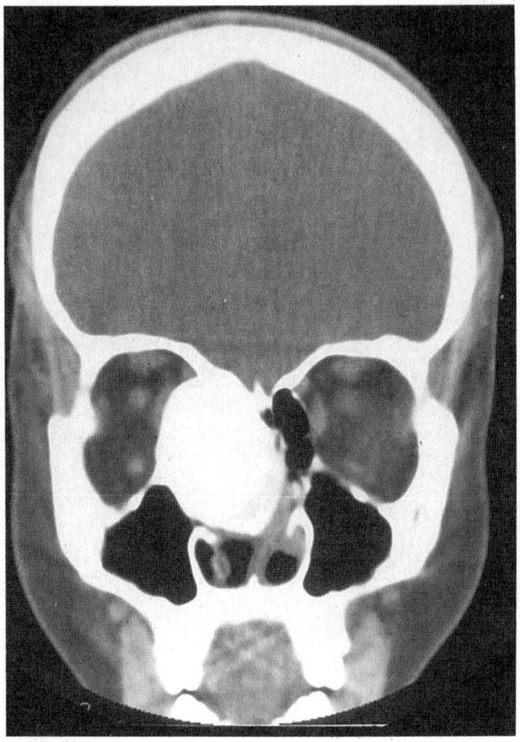
(*B*)

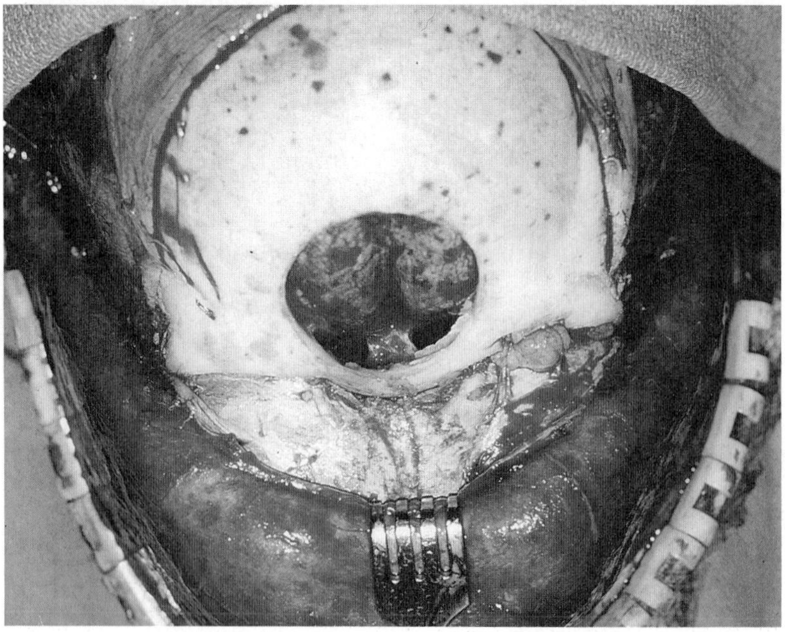
(*C*)

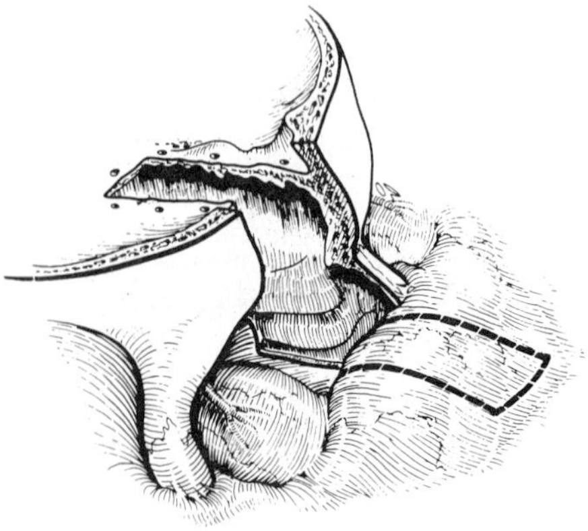
(*D*)

Figure 156-2 Glabellar exposure osteotomy. *A*, *B*. Patient with fibrous dysplasia involving the cribriform fossa, medial orbital wall, and nasal cavity. *C*. Trephine craniotomy. *D*. Diagram showing removal of glabellar region with resection of tumor. The galeal frontalis flap is shown.

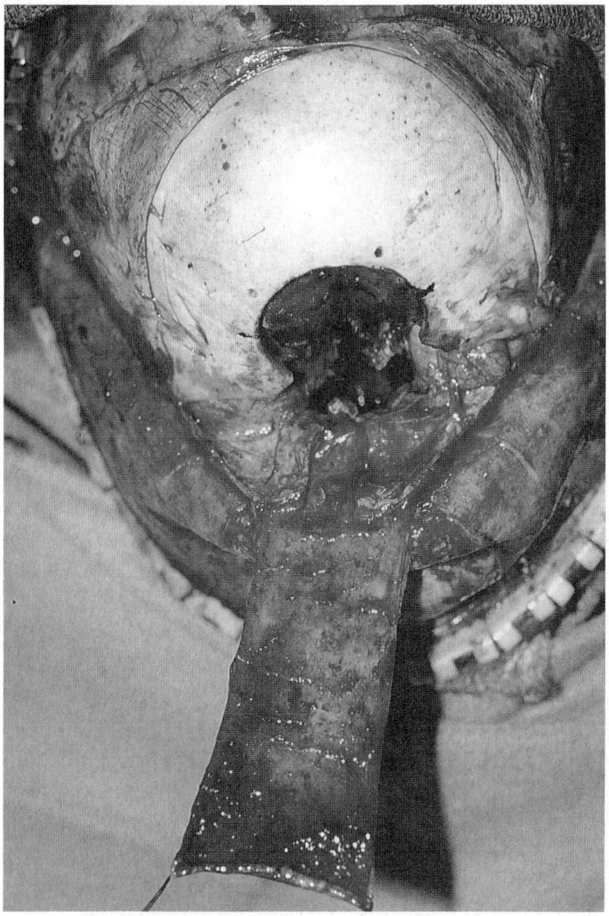

(*E*)

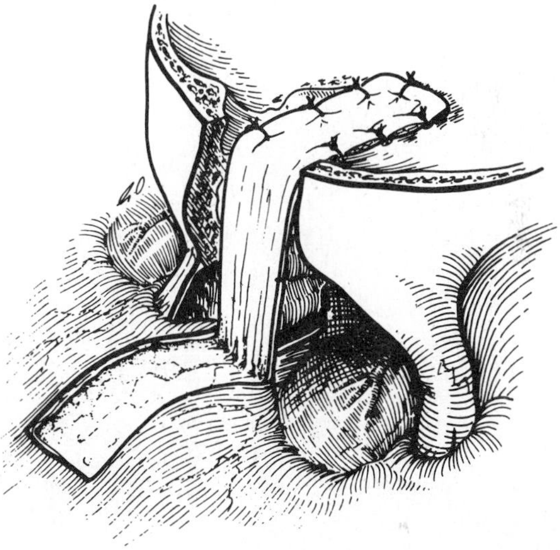

(*F*)

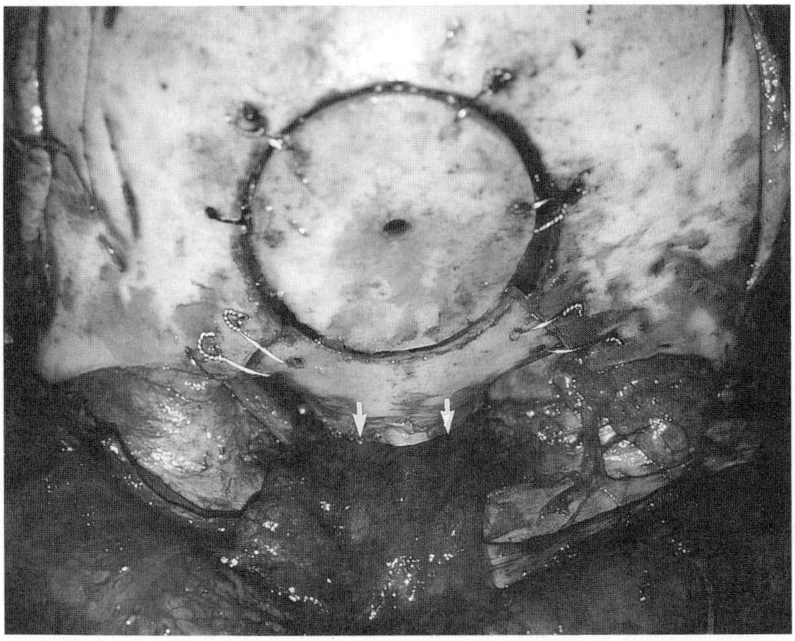

(*G*)

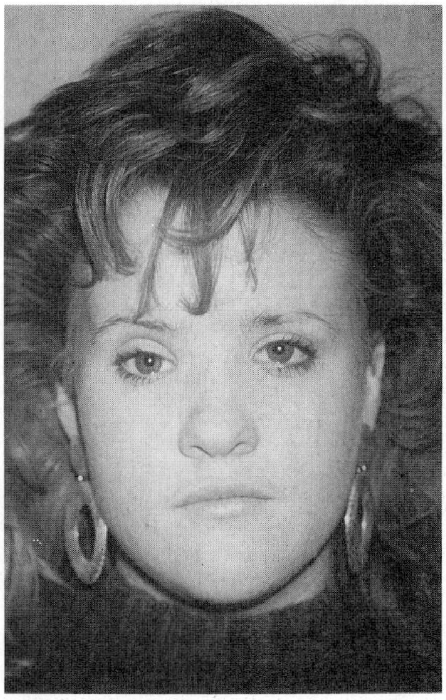

(*H*)

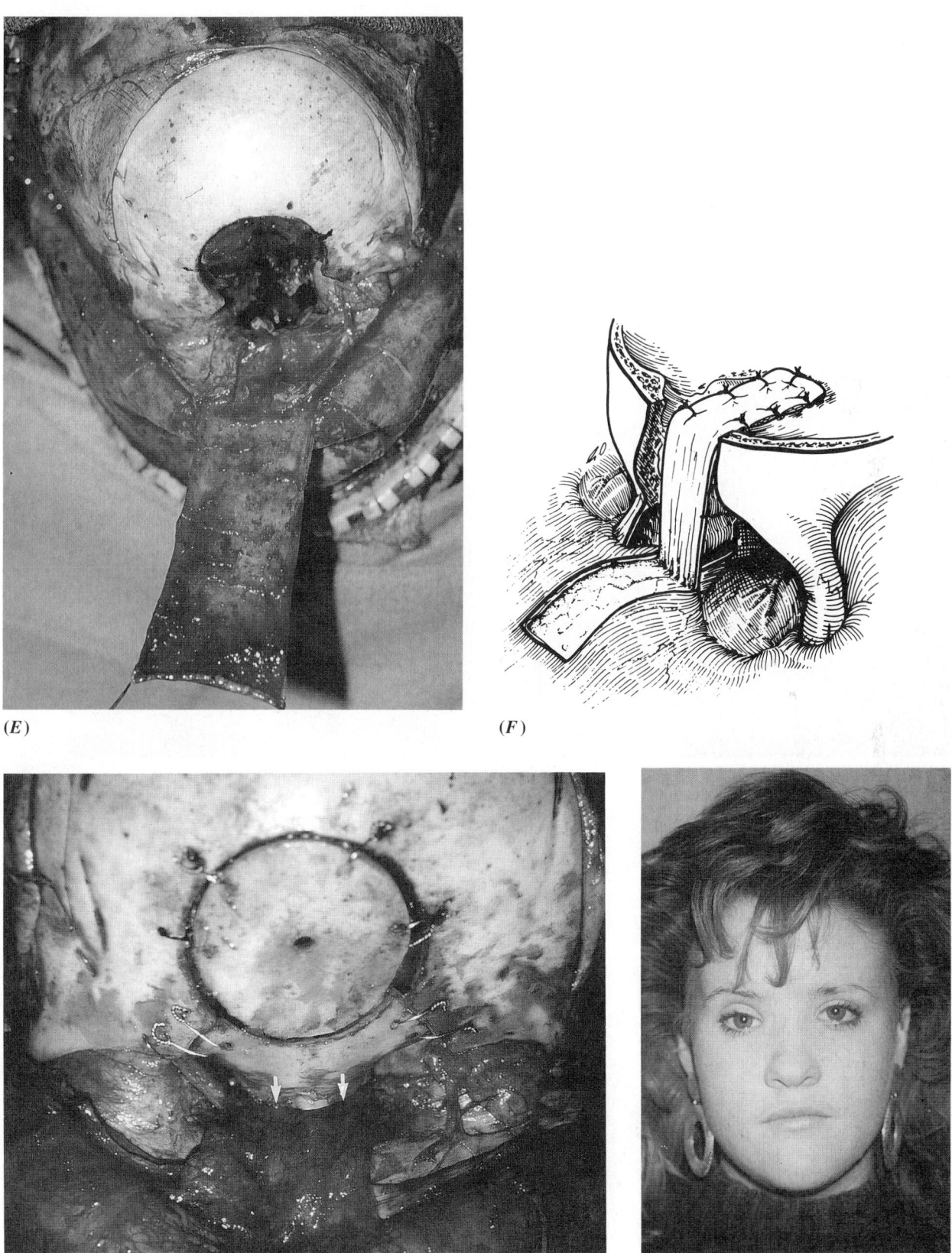

Figure 156-2 (*Continued*) *E*. Galeal frontalis flap ready to be inserted into the floor of the anterior cranial fossa. *F*. Diagram to show the galeal frontalis flap sutured in the anterior cranial fossa using the drill holes illustrated in *D*. *G*. Glabellar osteotomy and trephine craniotomy wired back in position. Note the galeal frontalis flap placed through the ''letter box'' under the glabellar osteotomy *(arrows)*. *H*. Result after 1 year.

stopping medial to the infraorbital nerve. The cut is then brought through the inferior orbital rim vertically down the maxilla to the same level as the pyriform aperture floor. It is then taken transversely to the lateral wall of the pyriform aperture. An osteotome introduced through the anterior cranial fossa osteotomy will, with gentle tapping, mobilize this whole bony segment and allow it to be removed without difficulty.

The tumor can now be removed safely under direct vision. If an orbit is involved in such a way that exenteration is judged to be necessary, this can be accomplished very easily in continuity with the central block. At the completion of the resection, the segment of osteotomized bone is replaced, and using the ''letter box'' technique, the connection between the extradural space and the nasopharynx is closed as described earlier. The interior of the replaced bone is covered by a contralateral galeal frontalis myofascial flap. In this way, resection can be readily accomplished without the complications which were so prone to occur in the past as a result of these procedures.

Le Fort I Osteotomy

The Le Fort I osteotomy (Fig. 156-4) is used to approach chordomas. It affords excellent exposure to the posterior aspect of the upper nasopharynx and central skull base (clivus) area.

Through an upper buccal sulcus incision extending between the first molars, the periosteum of the maxilla is elevated. This dissection is taken up to the infraorbital nerves. The mucoperiosteum of the pyriform aperture is elevated completely from anterior to posterior along the nasal floor and lateral walls. Laterally, the dissection is taken to the retrotuberosity area. A saw cut is made from the

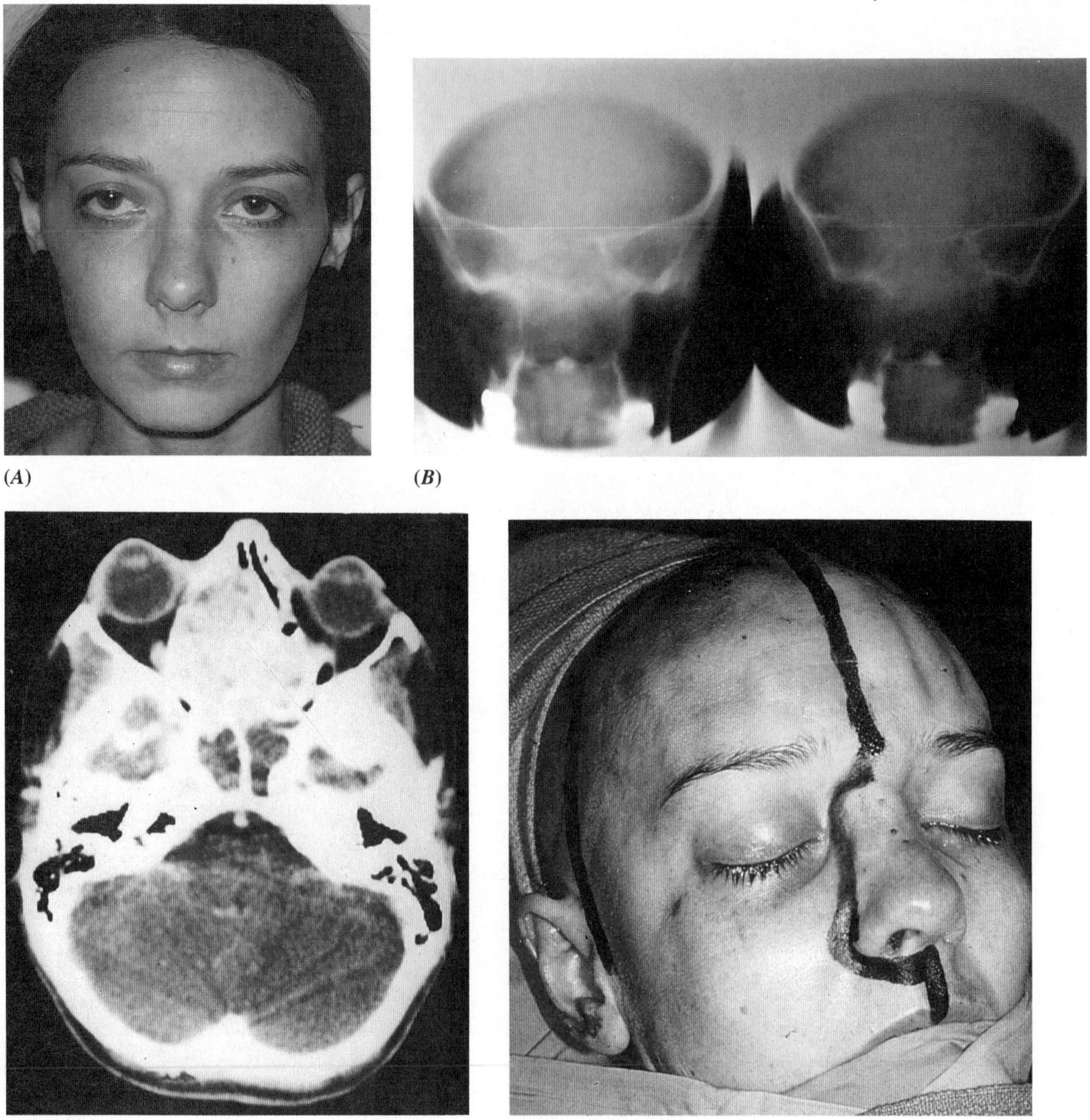

(*A*) (*B*) (*C*) (*D*)

Figure 156-3 Frontonasomaxillary osteotomy. *A, B.* Chondrosarcoma of the central anterior skull base. Its extent can be seen on tomography. *C.* Axial CT scan. *D.* Planned approach. Coronal flap and face splitting incision.

lateral margin of the pyriform aperture, with the mucoperiosteum protected, to the tuberosity and the pterygomaxillary groove. The lateral pyriform wall is cut completely from front to back, the cartilaginous septum is elevated from the vomerine ridge, and the vomer is cut with a notched osteotome.

A curved osteotome is placed in the pterygopalatine groove to separate the bony connection with the pterygoid plates. The maxillary fragment is now downfractured to gain posterior exposure.

When the resection has been completed, the maxilla is placed back in its correct position and held there with miniplates on the lateral margins of the pyriform fossa and the zygomaticomaxillary buttress. The patient is maintained on a soft diet for 1 month.

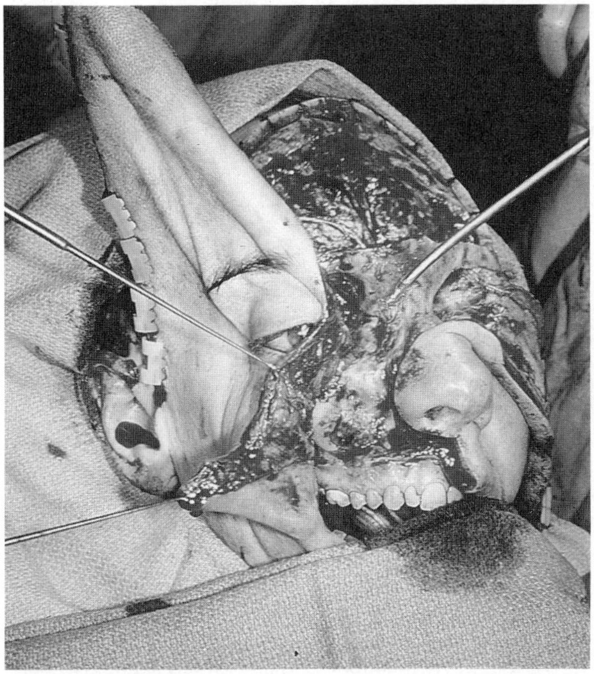

(*E*)

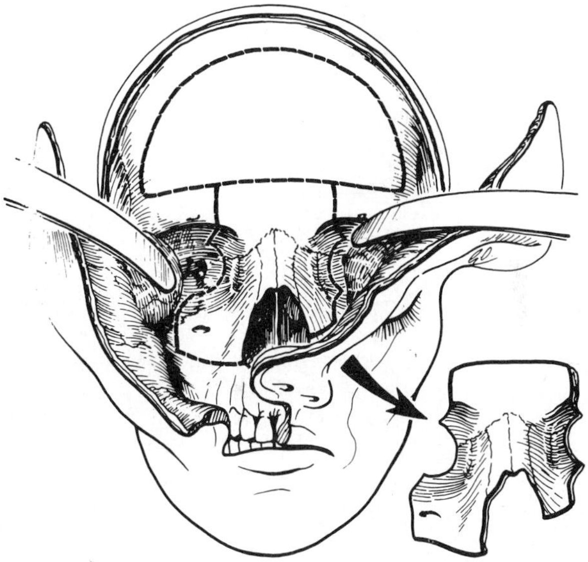

(*F*)

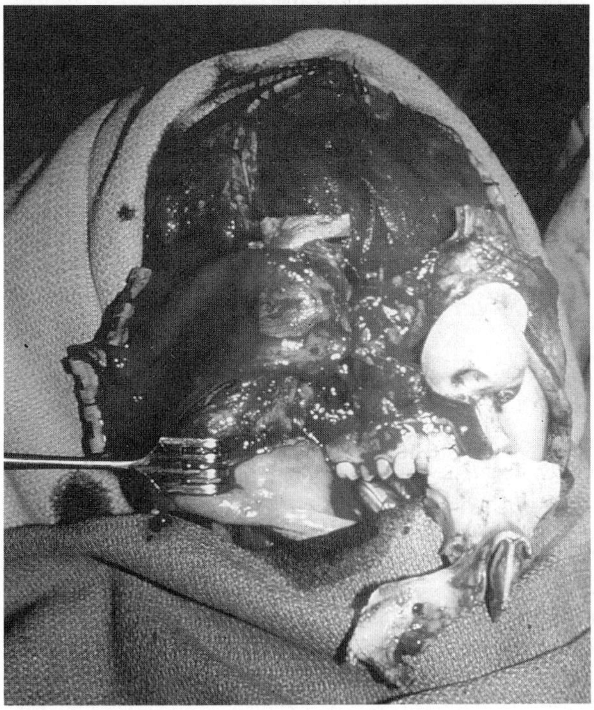

(*G*)

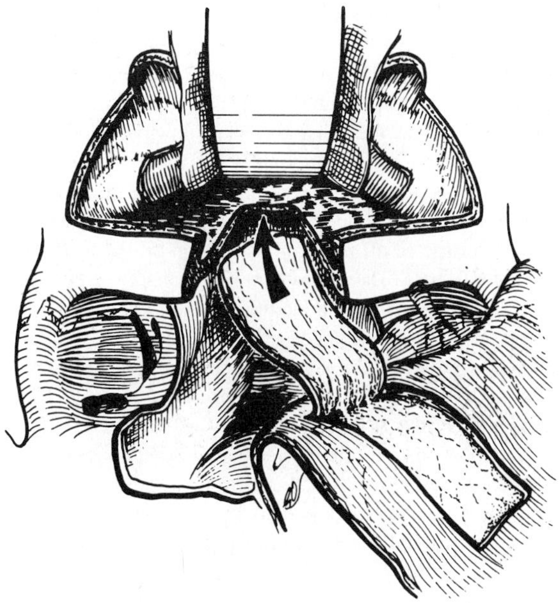

(*H*)

Figure 156-3 (*Continued*) *E*. Exposure of the nasomaxillary area through a face splitting incision and the anterior cranial fossa through a frontal craniotomy. *F*. Diagram of a frontomaxillary exposure osteotomy. *G*. The osteotomy has been completed to give good exposure of the tumor. *H*. Following resection, a galeal frontalis flap is used to separate the anterior cranial fossa from the nasopharynx.

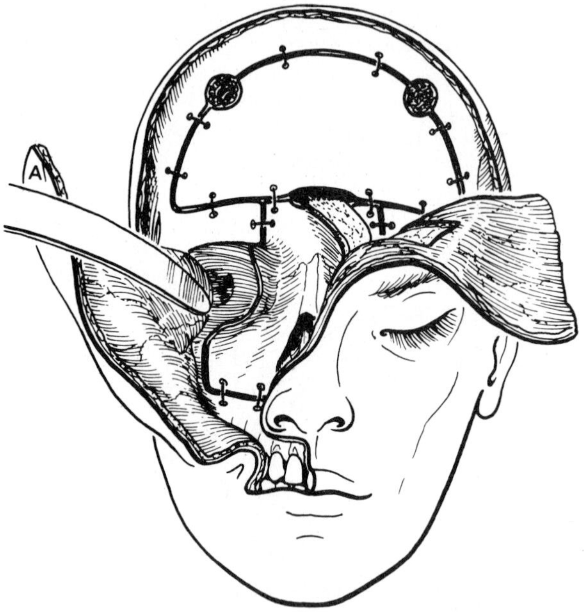

(*I*)

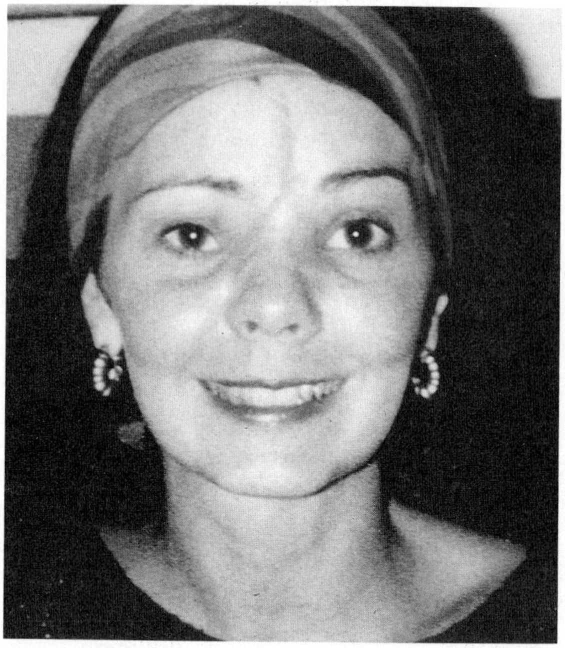

(*J*)

Figure 156-3 (*Continued*) *I.* The osteotomy is replaced and wired or plated in position. *J.* Patient 3 years after resection.

The Lateral Approach

Tumors involving the middle cranial fossa and the lateral orbit are exposed by a lateral approach.

Orbitozygomatic Osteotomy

The two lesions most commonly approached using the orbitozygomatic osteotomy (Fig. 156-5) have been sphenoid ridge meningiomas and fibrous dysplasia of that region. A coronal flap is again used, since this is most esthetically acceptable in terms of scarring. On the affected side, the incision is taken down to below the zygomatic arch. In the temporal area, the flap is elevated just above the deep temporal fascia to prevent damage to the frontal branch of the facial nerve. The temporalis muscle with the pericranium cranial to it is dissected off the skull and lateral orbital wall to expose the temporal fossa. The periosteum is elevated over the lateral orbital rim, the zygomatic arch, and the anterior surface of the maxilla. The periorbita is elevated superiorly, laterally, and inferiorly. A limited frontotemporal craniotomy is performed, and the frontal lobe is elevated. The supraorbital rim is cut through where indicated for exposure, as is the orbital roof with the periorbita protected. The most posterior part of the lateral orbital wall is cut vertically to the inferior orbital fissure. The osteotomy cuts are varied depending on how much maxilla and zygoma needs to be removed for exposure. The infraorbital rim is cut through onto the anterior aspect of the maxilla. From here a horizontal osteotomy is taken under the zygomatic arch; the arch is cut through. The bony segment is mobilized and removed. Any involved temporal and orbital bone is resected, as is the main lesion. During this procedure, the temporal lobe is protected. Since the exposure is good, an *en bloc* removal is possible on most occasions. The temporal bony defect is reconstructed with split bone grafts, and the exposure osteotomy is replaced. Stabilization is achieved with miniplates. The temporalis muscle is returned to its original position and is held in place using sutures through drill holes in the lateral orbital rim and temporal ridge.

Orbitozygomatic Mandibular Osteotomy

The orbitozygomatic mandibular osteotomy (Fig. 156-6) is used for infratemporal fossa lesions. These may be maxillary or intraoral tumors invading the skull base, or intracranial tumors escaping through a foramen into the infratemporal fossa.

The skin incision begins in the anterior temporal area and curves superiorly and posteriorly to then run down in the preauricular region into the neck where it is fashioned as a lazy S. After the skin and scalp have been elevated, as for a face-lift, the temporalis muscle is dissected up as described in the preceding section. A limited temporal craniotomy is used for access to the tumor to confirm resectability. A total parotidectomy with preservation of all branches of the facial nerve is performed. The zygomatic arch with or without a portion of the maxilla and lateral orbital wall is removed. If the mandible is involved by the tumor, the ascending ramus is sacrificed. If, however, this is not the case, an osteotomy is made through the angle after the periosteum has been elevated. The temporomandibular joint is disarticulated, and the ascending ramus is removed or, if possible, simply hinged forward on the masseter and/or pterygoid muscles.

A neck dissection with preservation of the sternomastoid muscle is usually performed. This allows identification of the jugular and carotid vessels, which makes for safer dissection in the skull base region. This specimen is then removed with an in-continuity resection of the infratemporal fossa contents and base of skull. On occasion, it may be necessary to include a portion of the maxilla with or without the orbital contents in the resected specimen.

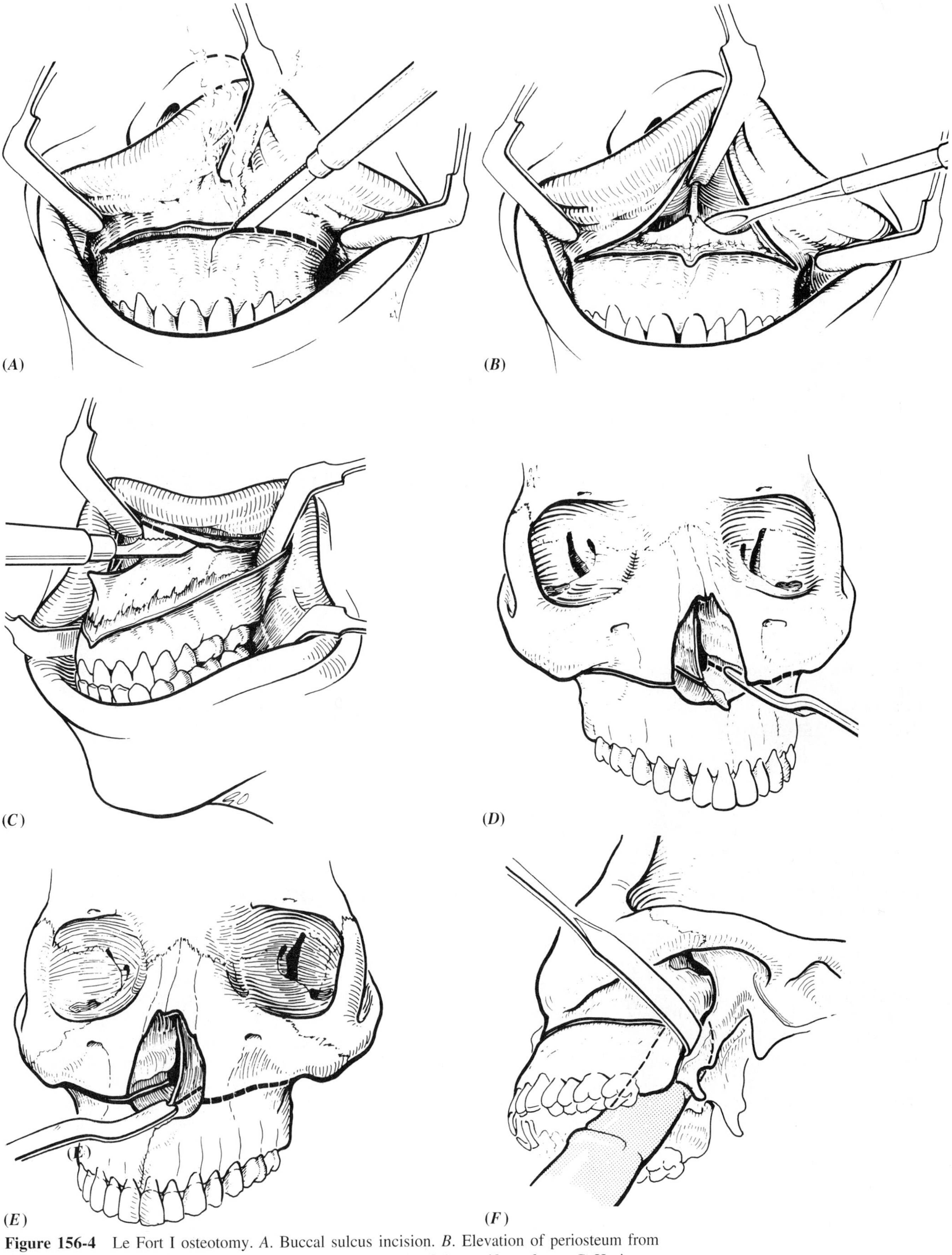

Figure 156-4 Le Fort I osteotomy. *A*. Buccal sulcus incision. *B*. Elevation of periosteum from the front of the maxilla and nasal floor, and the lateral wall of the pyriform fossa. *C*. Horizontal osteotomy of the maxilla using an oscillating saw. *D*. Division of the lateral wall of the pyriform fossa using a chisel. *E*. Notched osteotome to divide the vomer from the nasal septum. *F*. Curved osteotome to separate the maxillary segment from the pterygoid plates.

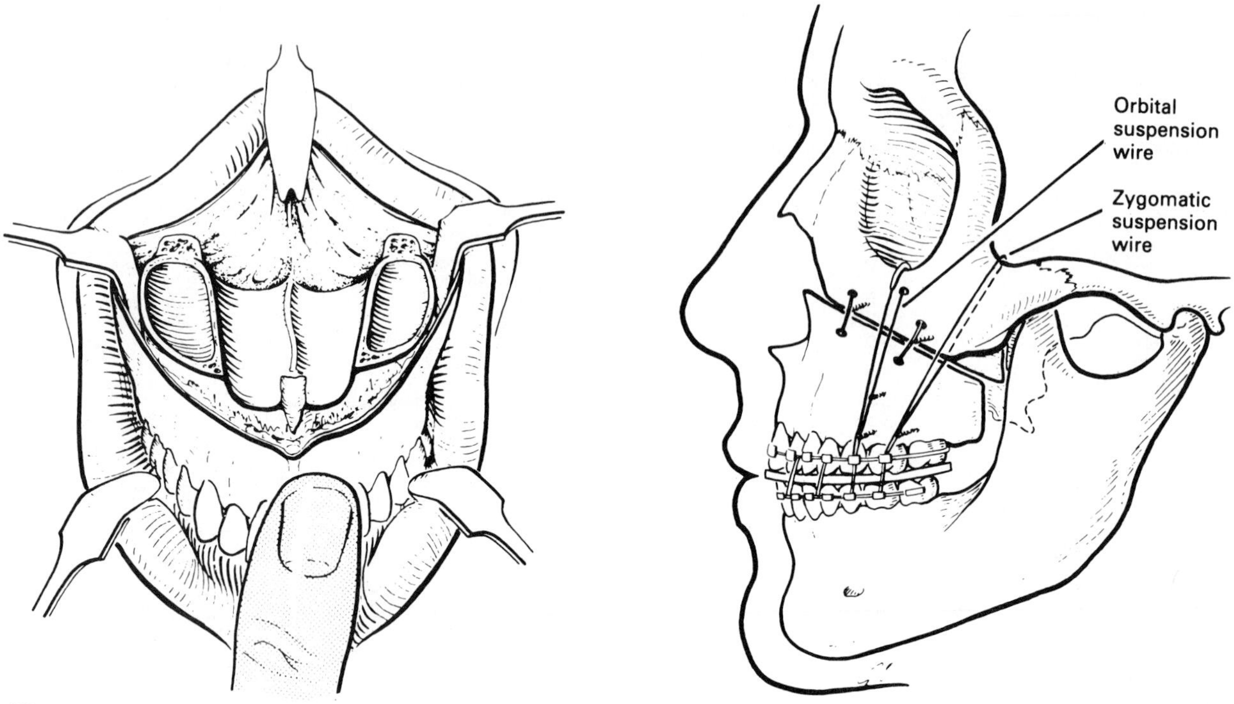

(*G*) (*H*)

Figure 156-4 (*Continued*) *G*. Downfracture of the maxilla to gain full mobility. *H*. Maxillary segments stabilized with wires; now, routinely, miniplates are used for rigid fixation.

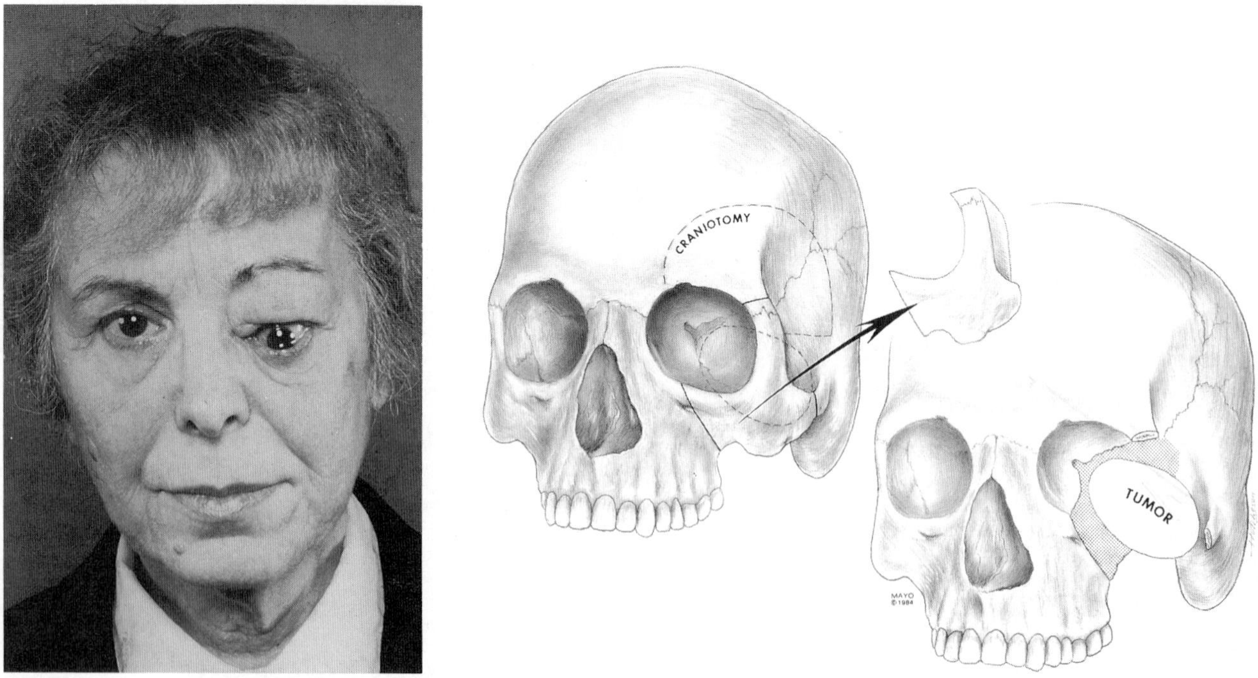

(*A*) (*B*)

Figure 156-5 Orbitozygomatic osteotomy. *A*. Patient with a left sphenoid wing meningioma invading the orbit. *B*. Diagram of an orbitozygomatic exposure osteotomy.

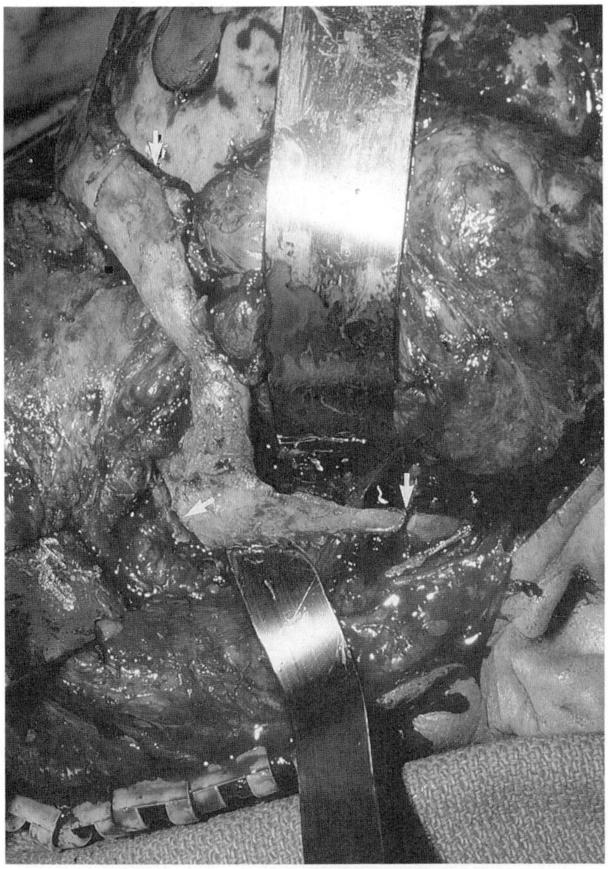

(C)

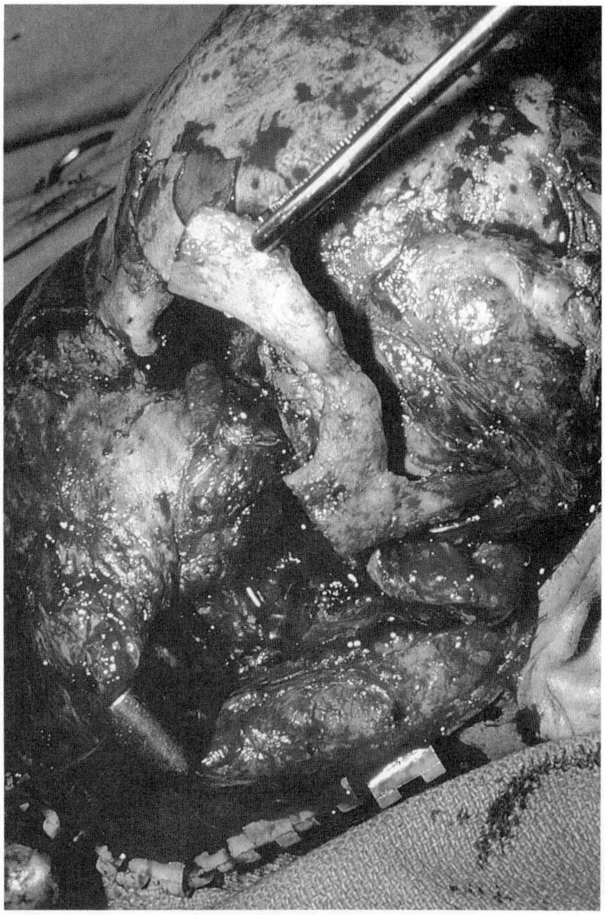

(D)

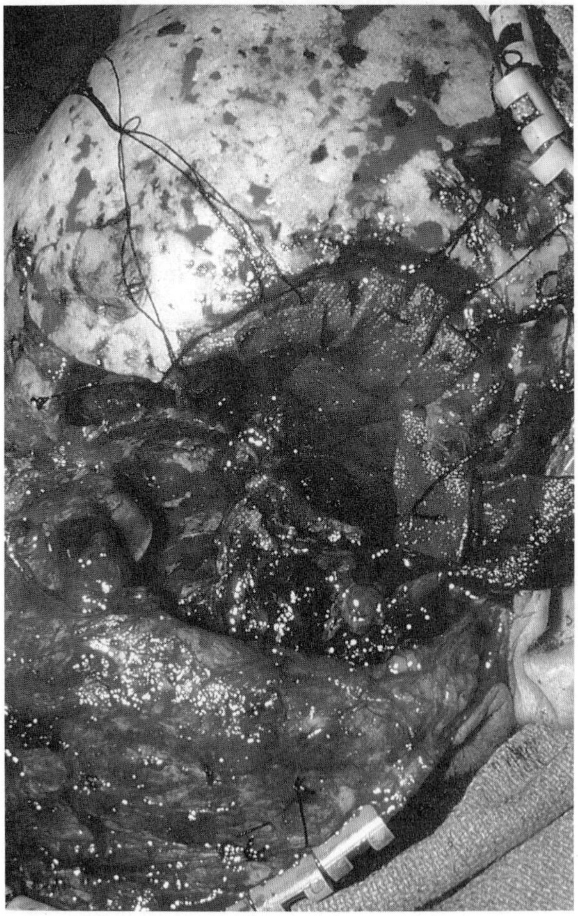

(E)

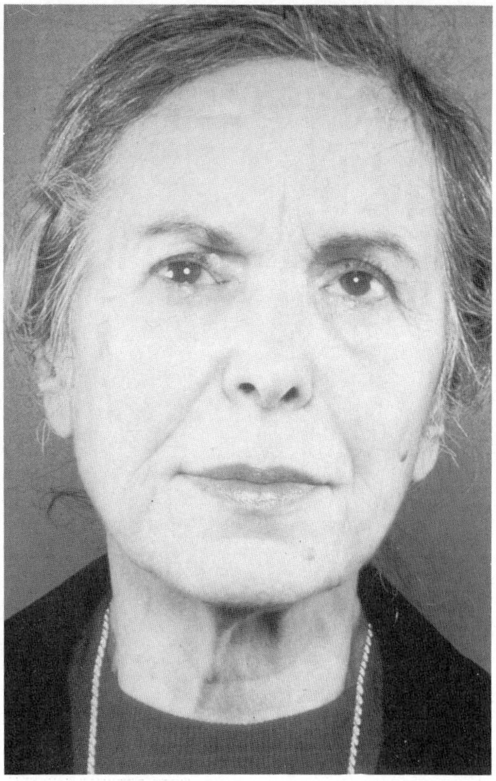

(F)

Figure 156-5 (*Continued*) *C*. The cuts for the osteotomy can be seen *(arrows)*. *D*. Osteotomized segments being removed. *E*. The meningioma has been excised completely. *F*. Result 2 years later.

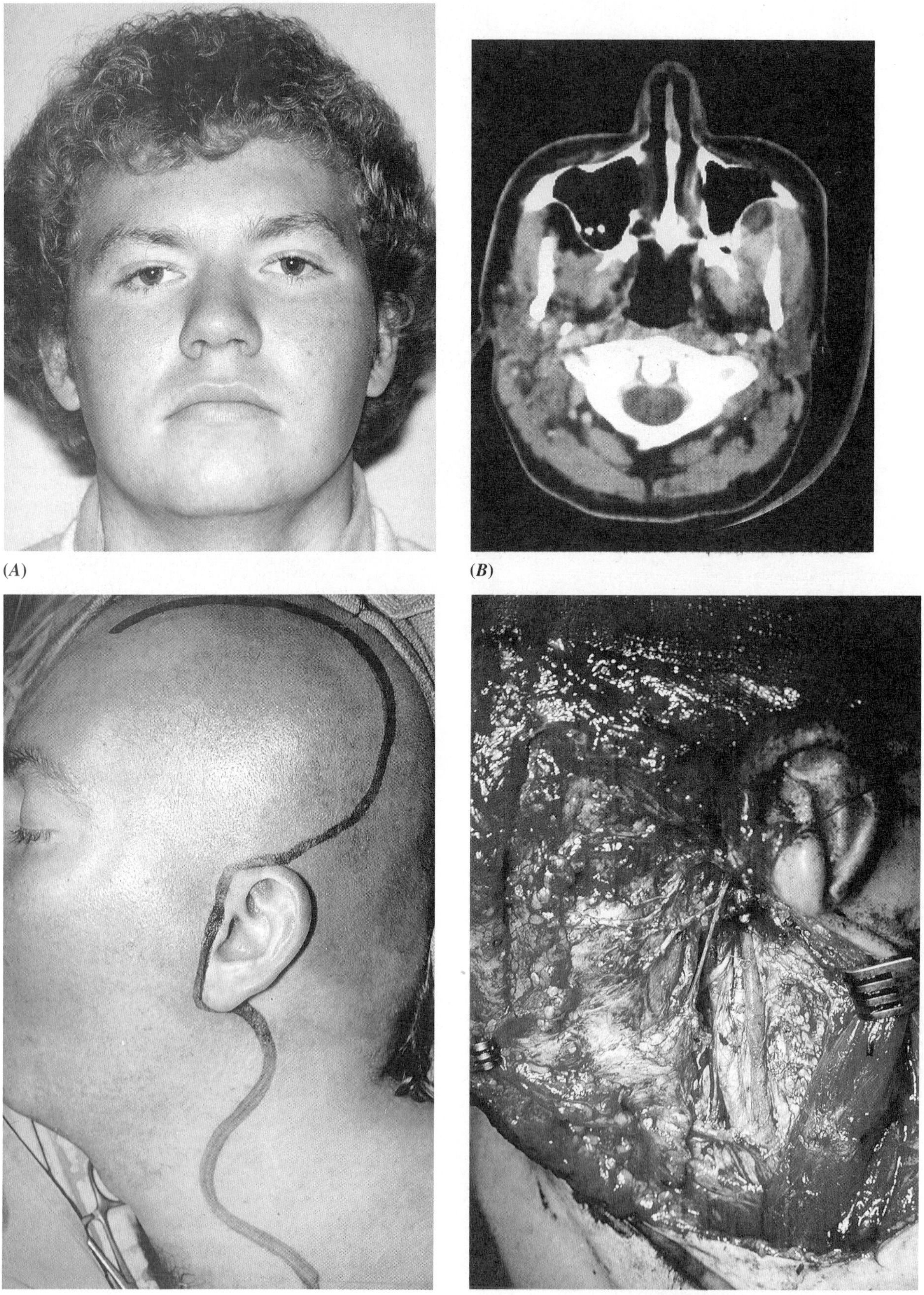

(*A*) (*B*) (*C*) (*D*)

Figure 156-6 Orbitozygomatic mandibular osteotomy. *A*, *B*. Patient with a left infratemporal fossa liposarcoma well seen on axial CT scan (*B*). *C*. Planned skin incision. *D*. Total parotidectomy with preservation of the facial nerve and all of its branches and modified radical neck dissection preserving the sternomastoid with good exposure of the internal carotid artery and external jugular vein.

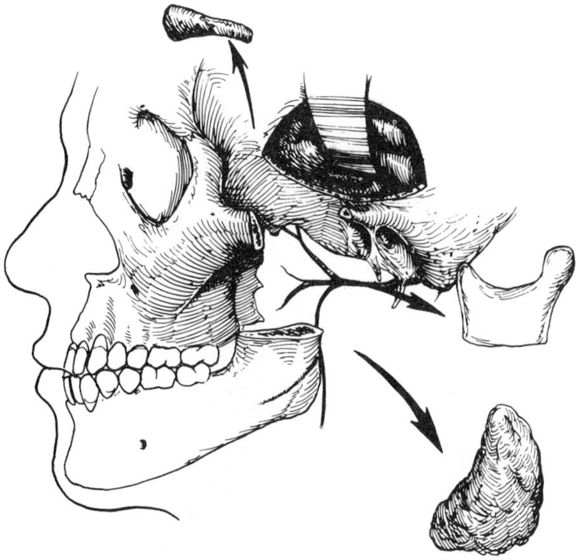

(*E*)

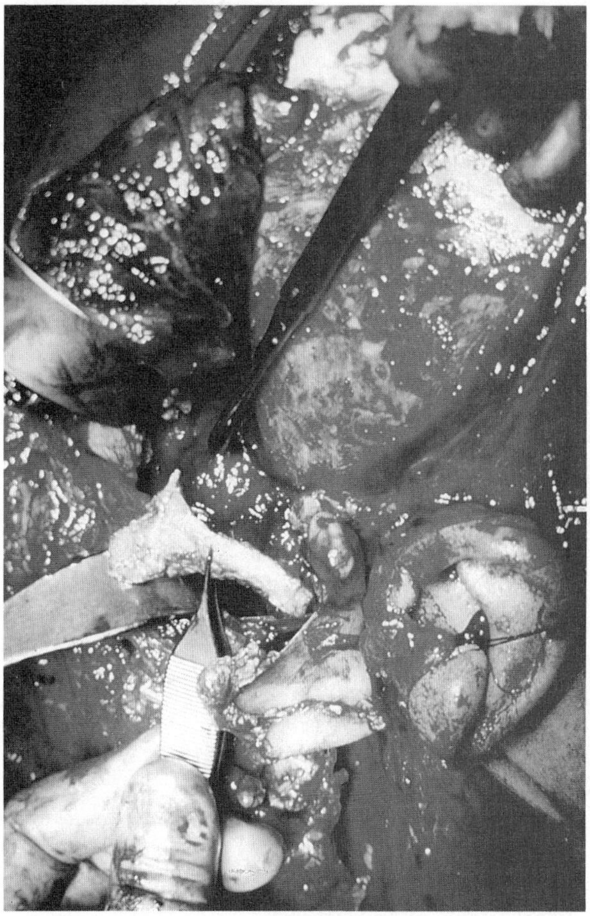

(*F*)

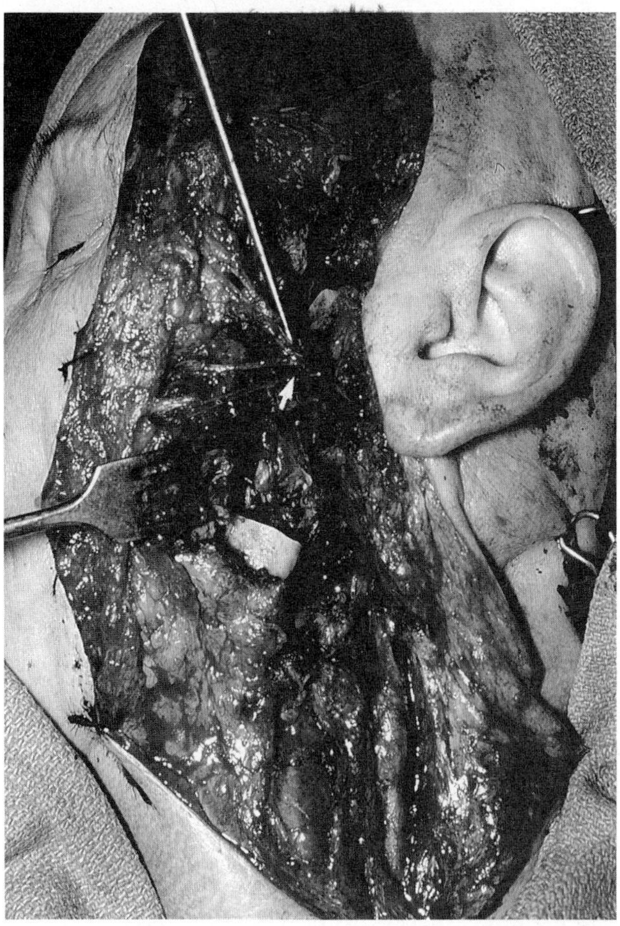

(*G*)

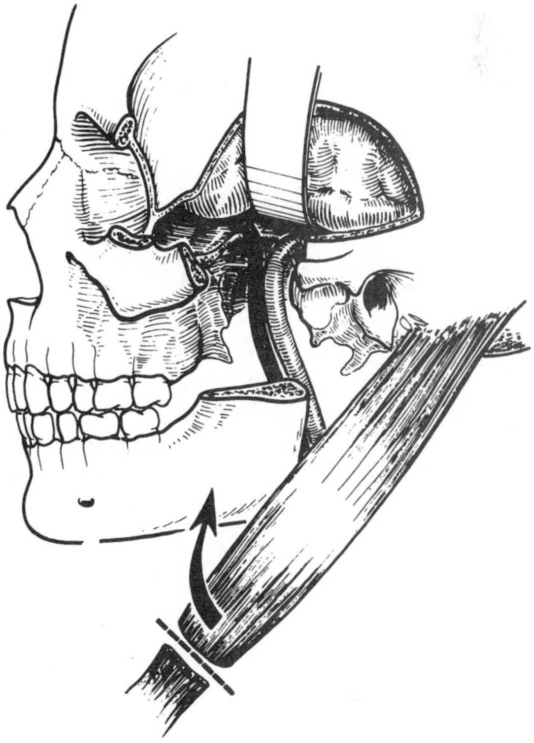

(*H*)

Figure 156-6 (*Continued*) *E*. Diagram of the orbitozygomatic mandibular exposure osteotomy with small temporal craniotomy. *F*. Zygomatic and maxillary segment being removed. *G*. Defect following resection of tumor involving the orbit and maxilla. The facial nerve is intact *(arrow)*. *H*. Sternomastoid muscle divided inferiorly to be swung up on its superior pedicle to fill up the infratemporal dead space.

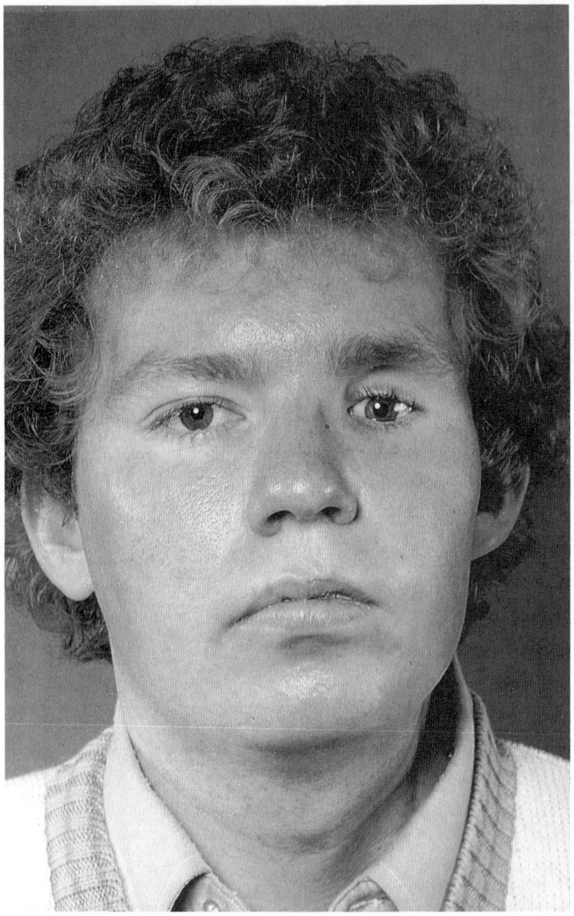

(*I*)

Figure 156-6 (*Continued*) *I.* Result 1 year later. The patient died 18 months postoperatively with spinal metastasis.

If necessary, the sternomastoid can be divided inferiorly and swung up on its superior vascular pedicle to fill any significant dead space in the infratemporal fossa. In selected cases, e.g., without prior radiotherapy, nonmalignant tumors, or less aggressive malignant tumors, the osteotomies can be replaced and stabilized with miniplates. The temporalis muscle is replaced as described in the previous section. The patient is kept on a soft diet for 1 month.

Multiple Osteotomies

For tumors situated in difficult anatomic areas (e.g., the cavernous sinus), it may be necessary to perform multiple osteotomies for adequate exposure. Portions of the facial skeleton may be removed for later replacement or swung aside, maintaining a soft tissue pedicle. This is well exemplified by the case presented in Fig. 156-7. In this case and in others, the concept of ''side table assembly''[6] has greatly decreased operating time. The fragments are assembled and plated by an assistant during the resection, using miniplates or microplates and screws, and the whole reconstruction is replaced very rapidly and stabilized with plates and screws at the end of the procedure.

Conclusion

These exposure osteotomies have made skull base surgery less complex and safer. In 272 cases in which malignant tumors outweighed nonmalignant by 2 to 1, there were no significant infections apart from one instance of meningitis, which responded to antibiotic therapy. There was one surgical death (i.e., within 24 h

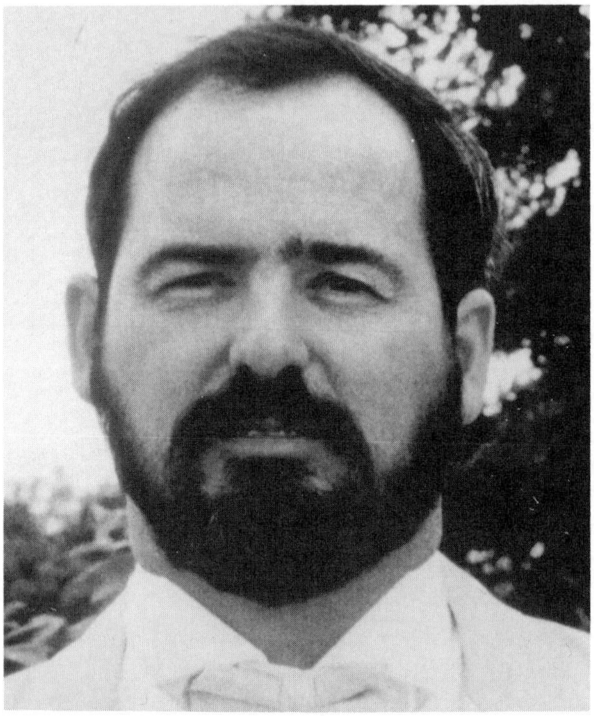

(*A*)

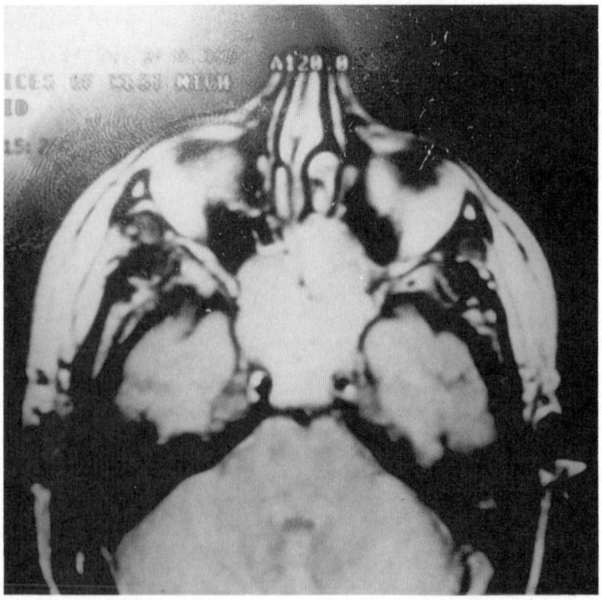

(*B*)

Figure 156-7 *A.* A 42-year-old male with an adenoid cystic carcinoma of the central skull base region. *B.* An axial CT scan showing the central skull base tumor position.

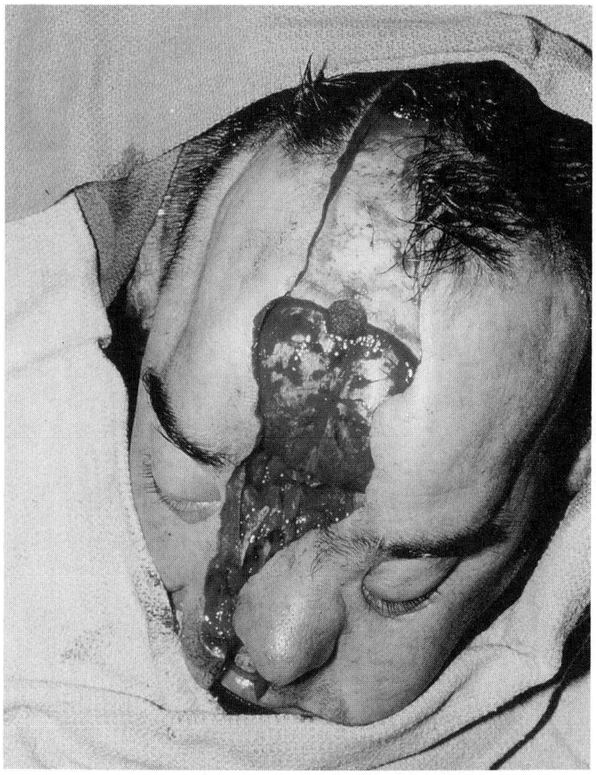
(*C*)

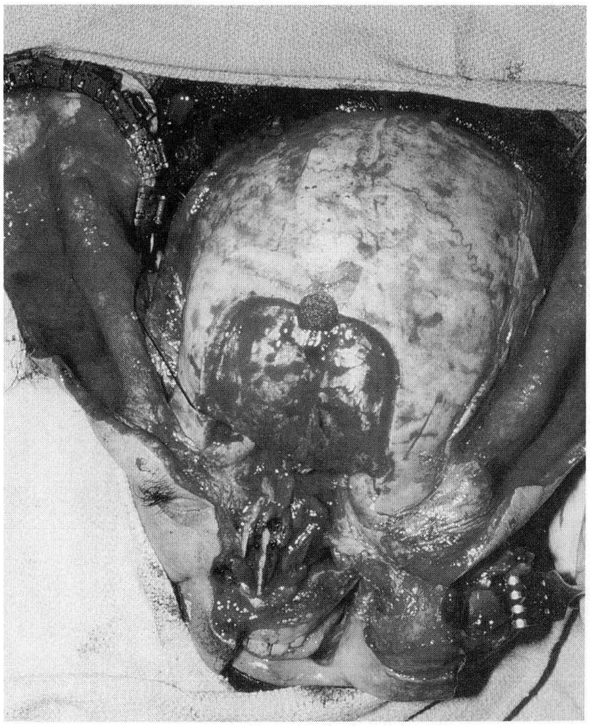
(*D*)

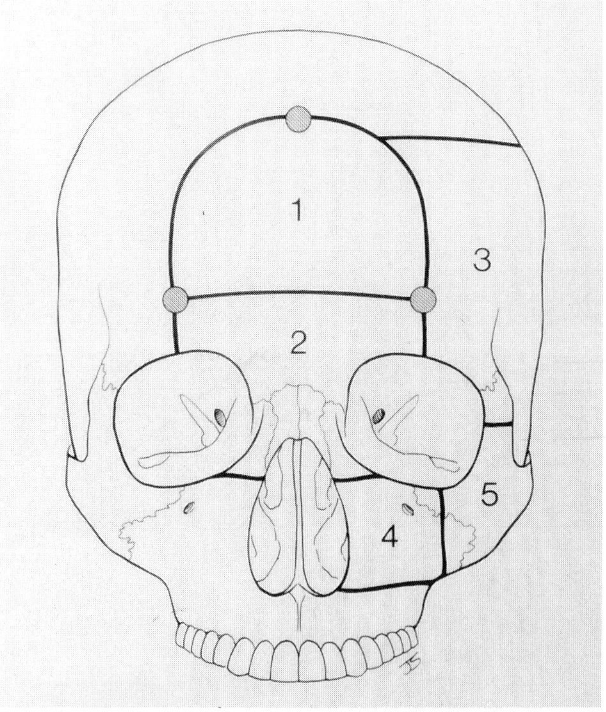

(*E*)

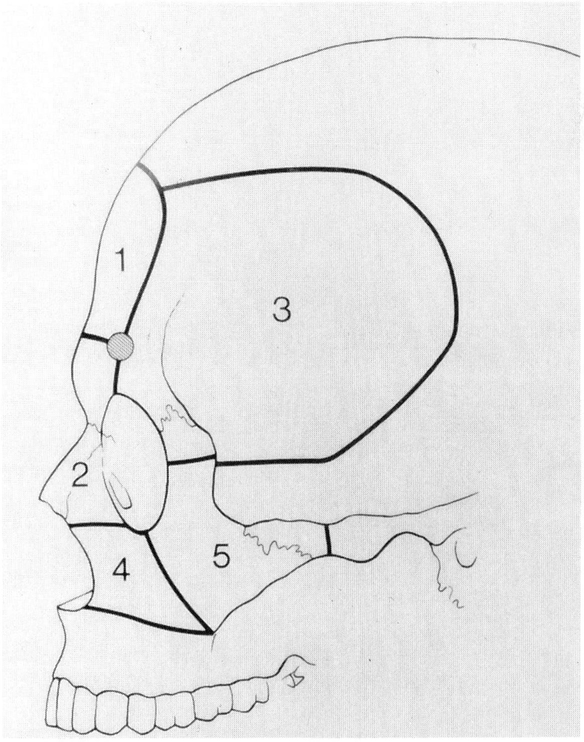

(*F*)

Figure 156-7 (*Continued*) *C*. Face-splitting approach with removal of bony, cartilaginous, and soft tissue nose on his left hemiface flap; frontal craniotomy. *D*. Exposure gained by the face-splitting incision and retraction of the left facial flap including the nose. *E, F*. Portions of facial bone removed.

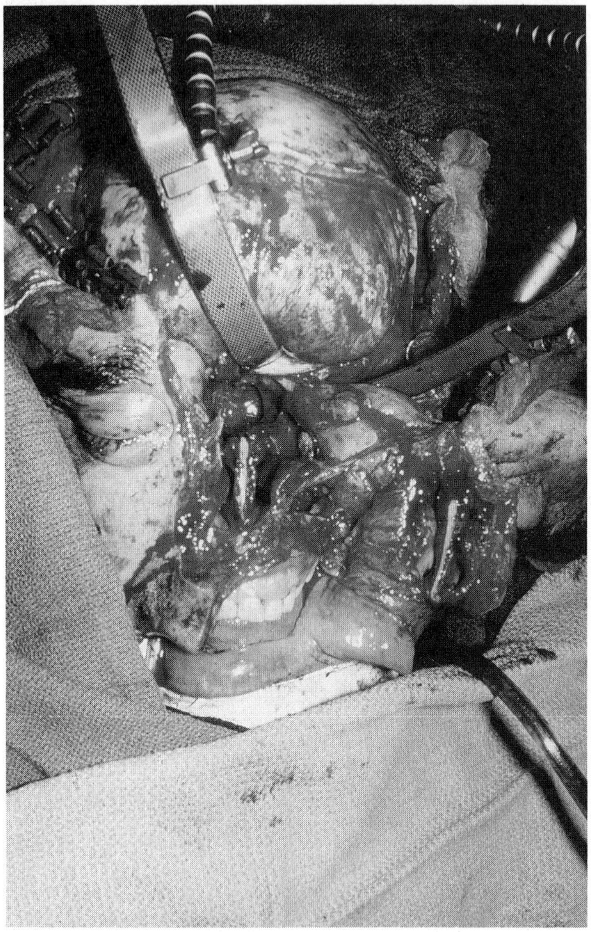

(*G*)

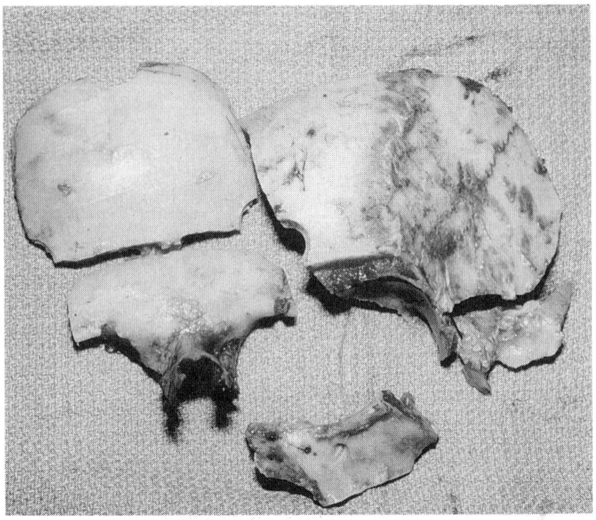

(*I*)

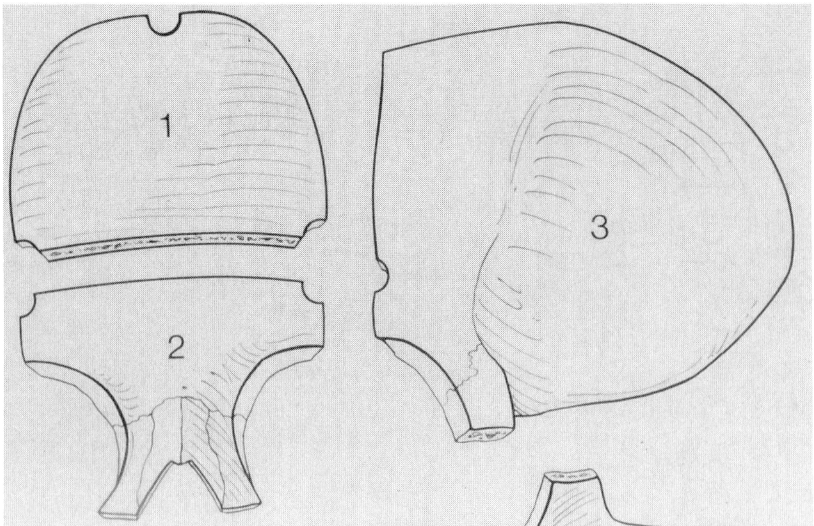

(*H*)

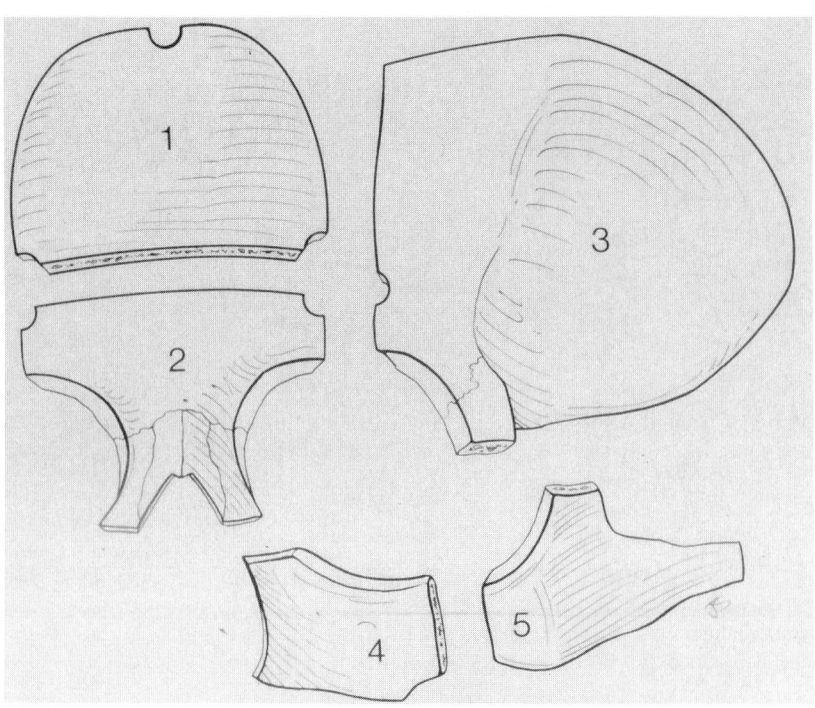

Figure 156-7 (*Continued*) *G*. Exposure to the tumor. Patient wished to retain his left eye. *H, I*. The portions of facial bones and skull removed for exposure.

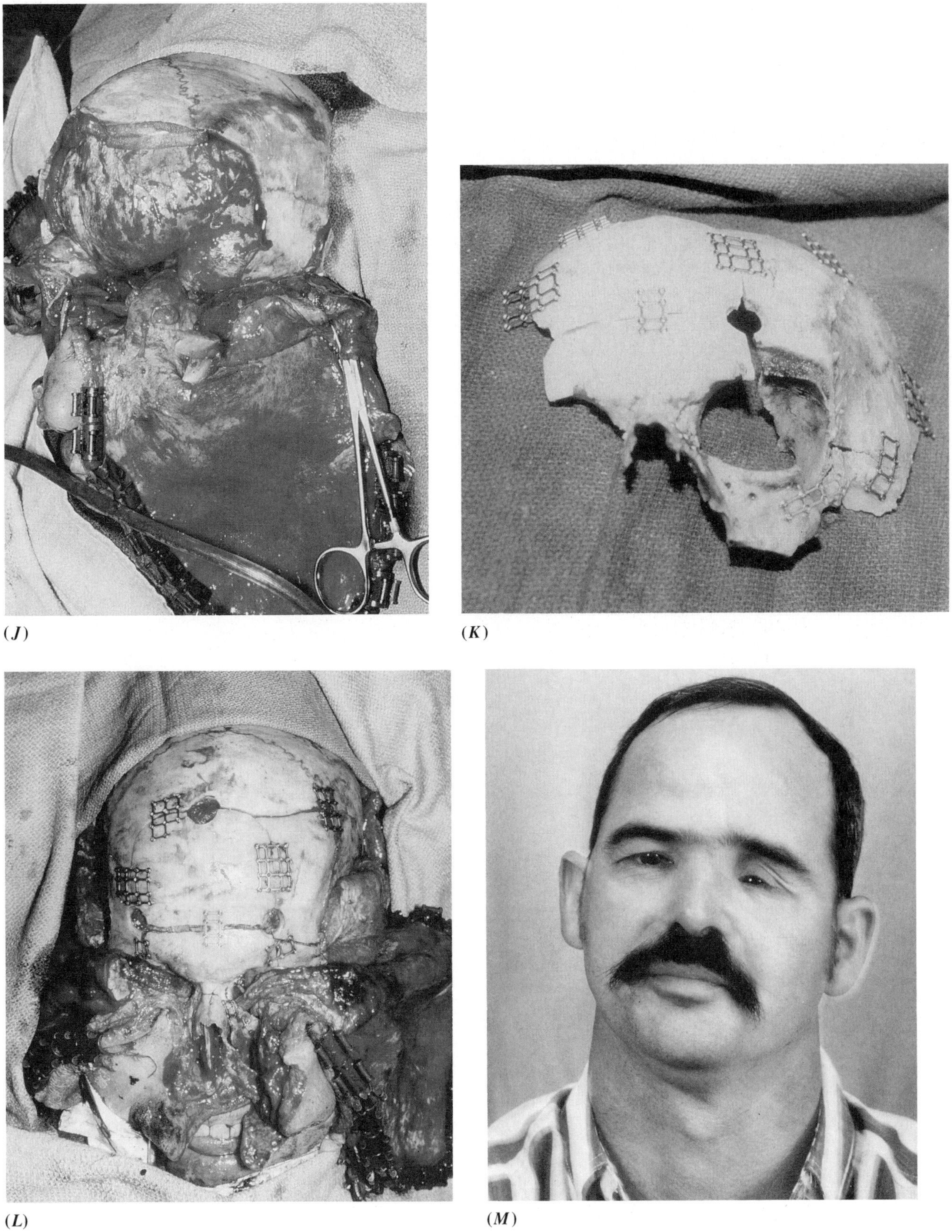

Figure 156-7 (*Continued*) *J*. Appearance following resection of tumor. The optic nerve can be clearly seen. *K*. Side table assembly of the resected bony parts. *L*. Facial skeleton plated back into position. *M*. Postoperative appearance with enophthalmos, which the patient did not wish to have corrected; 4-year follow-up.

after operation). What cannot be claimed at the moment is whether the improved exposure and consequently better resection will lead to an increase in survival rates. For 190 patients with malignant tumors of widely varying pathology, the majority of which were recurrent after surgery and radiotherapy, the 5-year survival rate was 48 percent. This is encouraging, but a larger number of cases with a longer follow-up need to be studied.

References

1. Bite U, Jackson IT, Wahner HW, et al. Vascularized skull bone grafts in craniofacial surgery. *Ann Plast Surg* 1987; 19:3–15.
2. Jackson IT. Craniofacial surgery for congenital deformities: its contribution to surgery of the skull. In: Chretien PB, Johns ME, Shedd DP, et al. (eds): *Head and Neck Cancer,* vol 1. St Louis: Mosby, 1985, pp 263–272.
3. Jackson IT, Adham MN, Marsh WR. Use of galeal frontalis myofascial flap in craniofacial surgery. *Plast Reconstr Surg* 1986; 77:905–910.
4. Jackson IT, Helden G, Marx R. Skull bone grafts in maxillofacial and craniofacial surgery. *J Oral Maxillofac Surg* 1986; 44:949–955.
5. Jackson IT, Marsh WR, Bite U, et al. Craniofacial osteotomies to facilitate skull base tumour resection. *Br J Plast Surg* 1986; 39:153–160.
6. Jackson IT, Ross JH, Fukuta K, et al. "Side table assembly"—an adjuvant to craniofacial reconstruction. *Br J Plast Surg* 1991; 44:348–350.
7. Tessier P. Autogenous bone grafts taken from the calvarium for facial and cranial applications. *Clin Plast Surg* 1982; 9:531–538.
8. van der Meulen JCH, Hauben DJ, Vaandrager JM, et al. The use of a temporal osteoperiosteal flap for the reconstruction of malar hypoplasia in Treacher Collins syndrome. *Plast Reconstr Surg* 1984; 74:687–693.

157

Craniofacial Resection of Anterior Skull Base Tumors

Richard L. Scher
William J. Richtsmeier

In 1943, Ray and McLean[13] ushered in the era of anterior skull base surgery with the report of a combined transcranial and transorbital resection of a retinoblastoma. Smith et al.[18] in 1954 followed this report with the description of a combined intracranial transfacial method for *en bloc* resection of extensive paranasal sinus cancers. The efficacy of this treatment for patients with paranasal sinus malignancies involving the skull base was demonstrated by Ketcham and colleagues in 1963.[6] Subsequent reports have detailed the effectiveness of the anterior craniofacial resection of malignant tumors that involve the superior nasal vault, ethmoid sinus complex, frontal sinus, and orbits, with extension to or through the floor of the anterior cranial fossa.[5,8,14,16,17,20]

Although it improved oncological outcome, anterior craniofacial resection was associated with significant morbidity. This morbidity was mainly the result of intracranial contamination due to communication with the sinonasal tract. Close cooperation between head and neck surgeons and neurosurgeons, combined with advances in perioperative care, surgical technique, and reconstructive methods, has helped reduce the incidence of significant morbidity following these major resections.[9,14] The 80 percent morbidity and 7 percent mortality rates associated with anterior craniofacial resection reported by Ketcham and associates in 1966[5] have been reduced to the much more acceptable rates of 30 to 40 percent morbidity and 0 to 2 percent mortality.[9,14] As a result, anterior craniofacial resection has been utilized not only for the treatment of malignant tumors but also for resection of certain benign neoplasms and infectious processes.

In this chapter, we discuss the following aspects of anterior craniofacial resection: indications, diagnostic evaluation, relevant anatomy, operative technique, postoperative care, outcome, and complications.

Indications for Anterior Craniofacial Resection

The anterior craniofacial resection is designed to provide complete resection of disease involving the anterior fossa skull base and contiguous paranasal structures. Virtually all disease processes that involve this area can be surgically treated by using this approach. Variations of this approach with extension laterally to include the orbit or posteriorly to involve additional regions of the skull base, such as middle fossa, cavernous sinus, nasopharynx, or infratemporal fossa, can also be designed. However, the anterior craniofacial resection proves to be ideal for the treatment of certain lesions. These include malignant tumors involving the nasal cavity, olfactory grooves, and paranasal sinuses, such as squamous cell carcinoma, adenocarcinoma, esthesioneuroblastoma, and chondrosarcoma. In addition, benign lesions present in these same regions, such as angiofibroma, meningioma, and inverting papilloma, can also be successfully treated by using this surgical technique. As stated above, extension of the approach to include resection of part or all of the orbital contents can also be utilized for the same and other diseases. Additionally, tumors that arise in the maxillary sinus and extend into the nasal cavity or ethmoid sinuses or tumors involving the facial skin with extension into the paranasal sinus region and skull base can also be encompassed by an anterior craniofacial approach.

Although the classic limitations to surgical resection of skull base tumors, such as involvement of the cavernous sinus and extensive involvement of dura, are no longer specific contraindications to surgical resection, there are still certain situations for which anterior craniofacial resection should probably not be utilized. Tumors that extend into the nasopharynx, cavernous sinus, middle cranial fossa, infratemporal fossa, and orbital apex are probably best managed by alternative approaches, such as combined anterolateral craniofacial resection or transtemporal approaches. Other contraindications to anterior craniofacial resection include extensive invasion of frontal lobe parenchyma by tumor; malignancies that carry an extremely poor prognosis, such as malignant melanoma or sinonasal undifferentiated carcinoma; and evidence of direct invasion of the internal carotid artery at the skull base. This last contraindication is not absolute, as newer techniques have allowed preoperative testing of cerebral vascular perfusion with the ability to isolate safely the intracranial segment of the carotid artery and include it with the resection specimen. Finally, patients with malignancy who present with evidence of distant metastases are probably best served by a palliative approach that has a lower morbidity than craniofacial resection. Patients with biopsy-proven evidence of malignant disease should therefore undergo preoperative evaluation to rule out distant metastases.

Preoperative Evaluation and Diagnosis

Anterior craniofacial resection is most commonly utilized in the treatment of neoplastic disease. Most patients with these diseases present with symptoms of nasal obstruction, epistaxis, anosmia, proptosis, diplopia, or headache, alone or in combination. Evaluation may reveal a nasal mass that is polypoid or appears friable and hemorrhagic. In patients with lesions arising from either the orbit or an intracranial location, physical examination may not reveal an obvious tumor mass. Transnasal endoscopy may be useful for surgical planning, as it allows evaluation of both the extent and the location of tumors.

Radiological imaging studies play a significant role in the evaluation of patients before anterior craniofacial resection.[11] Computed tomography (CT) scans are obtained with coronal and axial images, and they prove useful in determining both the extent and the location of a tumor. CT scanning is most helpful in evaluating bony invasion of the facial and skull base skeleton, especially in the area of the cribriform plate. Magnetic resonance imaging (MRI) is also an important adjunct preceding craniofacial resection (Fig. 157-1). T1- and T2-weighted images, without and with gadolinium enhancement, supplement the findings of CT scanning. MRI is better able to demonstrate the extent of disease in the soft tissue of the anterior skull base region, especially in assessing the relationship of the tumor to the cavernous sinus, petrous and cavernous portions of the internal carotid artery, dura and brain, and orbit. MRI is also useful in differentiating neoplasia from inflammatory mucosal disease of the paranasal sinuses.

Angiography can be helpful for patients in whom preoperative imaging studies seem to demonstrate that a tumor involves the cavernous or petrous carotid artery. Angiography can assist in determining whether the tumor invades the artery itself, and angiographically directed balloon occlusion testing can be useful in predicting neurological outcome, should carotid artery resection be necessary.

Once physical examination and radiographic evaluation have been accomplished, histological diagnosis of the lesion is necessary. Tumors in the paranasal sinus and nasal cavity are usually readily accessible for biopsy by a transnasal approach. This often can be accomplished in the office setting, but the surgeon should be prepared to control hemorrhage, as many of these tumors are quite vascular. In all cases, violation of overlying skin, mucosa, or bone should be avoided during biopsy of the tumor. This prevents tumor contamination of surrounding tissues before definitive resection and therapy. Tissue obtained at biopsy should be sent for pathologic analysis, with special immunohistochemical staining and electron microscopy performed as needed. These special studies may be necessary for tumors that appear poorly differentiated on routine histologic evaluation in order to rule out such neoplasms as lymphoma, rhabdomyosarcoma, or melanoma, which require therapy other than craniofacial resection. For certain tumors, such as meningioma, angiofibroma, and some of the fibro-osseous lesions, physical examination and radiographic imaging may be all that is necessary to provide a diagnosis, as the radiographic appearance of these lesions is quite characteristic.

When a diagnosis of malignant neoplasm is made, the patient should undergo an extensive workup to rule out metastatic disease. This may include CT scans of the chest and abdomen to rule out pulmonary and hepatic metastases. In addition, patients with malignant disease should be evaluated by a multidisciplinary team that includes radiation and medical oncologists. This approach allows for appropriate planning for adjuvant therapy with radiation or chemotherapeutic agents if they are indicated. For all patients for whom anterior craniofacial resection is planned, appropriate medical evaluation is necessary to ensure that any concomitant illnesses are adequately managed and to optimize the overall condition of the patient before surgery. Patients should undergo ophthalmological examination to establish baseline visual acuity and ocular movement and to assess for orbital invasion by tumor. Before surgical therapy, patients should be given the opportunity to donate autologous blood, should transfusion be necessary. Usually two or three units can be donated over a 2- to 3-week period.

Relevant Anatomy

The anterior craniofacial resection is designed to encompass the region of the ethmoidal labyrinth, including the cribriform plate,

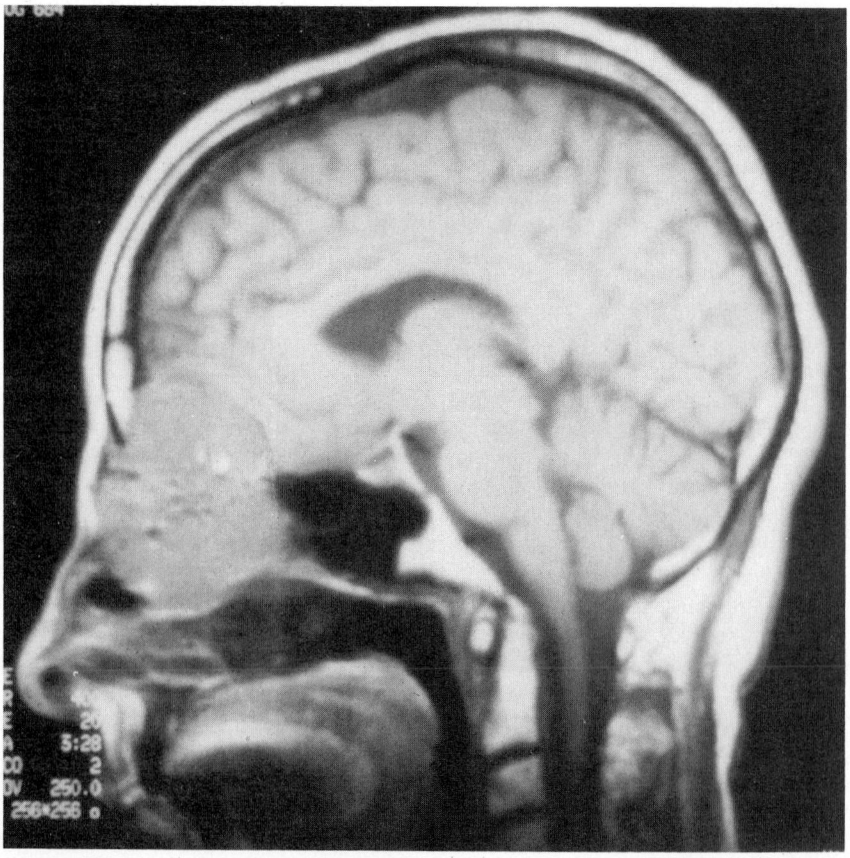

Figure 157-1 T1-weighted MRI demonstrating an esthesioneuroblastoma with extension through the anterior skull base, compressing the frontal lobes.

fovea ethmoidalis, ipsilateral lamina papyracea, and nasal septum. Depending upon the extent of the disease being resected, orbital exenteration, maxillectomy, or dural resection can be included in the operative approach. Access for craniofacial resection is usually accomplished through a bicoronal scalp incision along with either a lateral rhinotomy or midfacial degloving for the transfacial approach.

The intracranial anatomical considerations center on the region of the cribriform plate. In this area the dura is extremely adherent along each side of the midline crista galli. Dural extensions from the olfactory bulb pass through the cribriform plate along the olfactory nerves to reach the nasal cavity. Elevation of the dura from this region ordinarily results in multiple perforations, which must be repaired. Involvement of the dura by direct extension of tumor requires resection of the involved dura with reconstruction to prevent cerebrospinal fluid (CSF) leakage postoperatively. Resection of the olfactory nerves with craniofacial resection is almost always necessary and results in postoperative anosmia. The cribriform plates extend posteriorly to the region of the planum sphenoidale. In most cases, transection through the anterior sphenoid sinus is sufficient to encompass the tumor being resected. The relationship of the cavernous sinus along the lateral surface of the sphenoid must be kept in mind. Contained within this duplication of dura are the internal carotid artery and cranial nerves III, IV, V_1, and VI. The optic nerves cross from lateral to medial through the posterior ethmoidal cells toward the sphenoid sinus and optic chiasm. Resection should obviously remain anterior to the region of the optic chiasm. The intracavernous portion of the internal carotid artery along the lateral sphenoid sinus wall should also be recognized. The carotid artery often bulges into the sphenoid sinus to a variable extent and the bony covering can be dehiscent.

The lateral extent of the ethmoid bone, the lamina papyracea, often is involved with tumor. Resection of this region in continuity with the remainder of the specimen can include the periorbita if necessary. Periorbital reconstruction is possible, to provide adequate support to the orbital contents. The anterior and posterior ethmoidal arteries delineate the junction of the ethmoid and frontal bones. These arteries pass from lateral to medial through the orbit. The posterior ethmoidal artery is 3 to 7 mm anterior to the optic nerve. Anteriorly, the frontal sinus is connected through the ethmoidal labyrinth by the nasofrontal recesses. The most inferior extent of the posterior table of the frontal sinus is at the same level as the cribriform plate. Anterior to the ethmoid bone in the medial orbital wall is the lacrimal bone. Within the lacrimal crest are situated the nasolacrimal sac and nasolacrimal duct. The duct ends inferiorly lateral to the inferior turbinate in the inferior meatus. The nasolacrimal duct is transected during craniofacial resection. Drainage from the nasolacrimal system into the nasal cavity is usually adequate postoperatively without the need for dacryocystorhinostomy. The medial canthal tendon attaches to the lacrimal crest and must be reapproximated at the appropriate level to provide adequate cosmetic appearance to the eye and to prevent postoperative diplopia.

The anterior nasal septum is composed of the quadrilateral cartilage. This attaches anteriorly and caudally at the anterior nasal spine. Along the hard palate, the septum is held in place in the maxillary crest. The perpendicular plate of the ethmoid bone and the vomer constitute the posterior extent of the nasal septum, which is attached posteriorly to the anterior wall of the sphenoid sinus. The nasal bones join the frontal bone at the glabella. Attached to the nasal bones are the upper lateral cartilages. The lower lateral cartilages are joined laterally to the upper lateral cartilages and medially to the caudal end of the nasal septum. The lower lateral cartilages are separated from their attachments to the septum and upper lateral cartilages during a midfacial degloving approach. This provides adequate elevation of the nasofacial skin off the underlying nasal and facial skeleton during the resection.

The superficial layers of the scalp are composed of the skin and subcutaneous tissue closely adherent to the galea aponeurotica. This structure is continuous anteriorly with the frontalis muscle. Deep to the galea aponeurotica lies a layer of loose connective tissue that is continuous across the calvaria. Deep to this layer is the pericranium, continuous with the temporalis fascia overlying the temporalis muscle. The galea aponeurotica, pericranium, and temporalis muscle and fascia are all useful tissues for reconstruction of the anterior skull base defect following craniofacial resection. Vascular supply to this tissue is derived from branches of the frontal, supraorbital, and superficial temporal arteries and veins. An extensive anastomotic plexus is present both ipsilaterally and with the contralateral scalp.

Operative Technique

Patient Preparation

Craniofacial resection is performed by using a two-team approach involving a head and neck surgeon and a neurosurgeon. The patient is placed supine on the operative table. After the induction of anesthesia, the patient's head is supported on a head ring or Mayfield headrest. Before and after induction, appropriate intravenous catheters are inserted, along with an arterial line for arterial blood pressure measurement, a central venous catheter for central venous pressure measurement, and a urinary catheter. Prophylactic antibiotics are started, with broad spectrum coverage provided by a combination of cefotaxime and clindamycin, or chloramphenicol. The antibiotics are continued during the postoperative period until all nasal packing has been removed. A lumbar CSF drain or needles are placed in preparation for drainage of CSF during the intracranial portion of the resection. The patient's entire scalp and face are then prepared and draped sterilely, as are the lower quadrant of the abdomen and thigh, for possible harvesting of an abdominal adipose graft and split-thickness skin graft or fascia lata graft, respectively. A temporary tarsorrhaphy is placed in both eyes to provide corneal protection during the procedure. Anesthetic is administered through an orotracheal route. No need for tracheotomy exists in most cases.

Intracranial Resection

After patient preparation, the neurosurgical team begins the intracranial portion of the procedure. A bicoronal scalp incision is created, starting just above the pinna bilaterally and extending superiorly toward the vertex of the scalp. The scalp flap is developed deep to the galea aponeurotica and elevated anteriorly to the level of the supraorbital rims. Care must be taken to preserve the supraorbital and frontal vessels, as they provide the dominant blood supply both to the superficial layers of scalp and to the underlying pericranium. A pericranial flap is developed with an anteriorly based pedicle or a lateral pedicle based on the temporalis muscle (Fig. 157-2). This latter design can be used for larger anterior fossa defects that extend laterally toward the orbit.[15] A broad-based apron-shaped flap of pericranium is harvested and preserved in

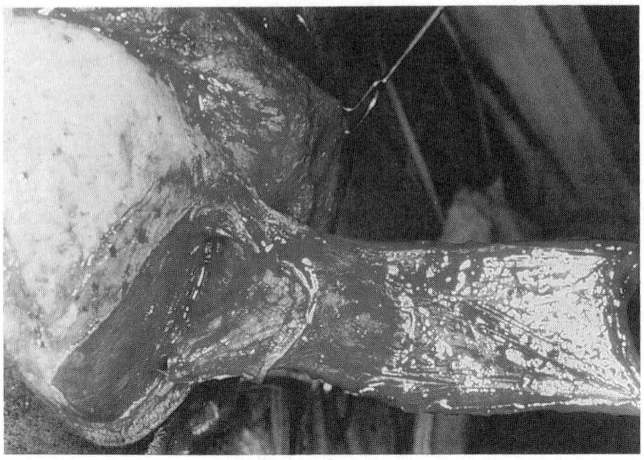

Figure 157-2 Development of a laterally based pericranial flap pedicled on the temporalis muscle after elevation from the calvaria. This design of pericranial flap allows reconstruction of more extensive anterior skull base defects than does an anteriorly based flap pedicled on the frontal and supraorbital vessels. (From Scher and Cantrell,[15] with permission.)

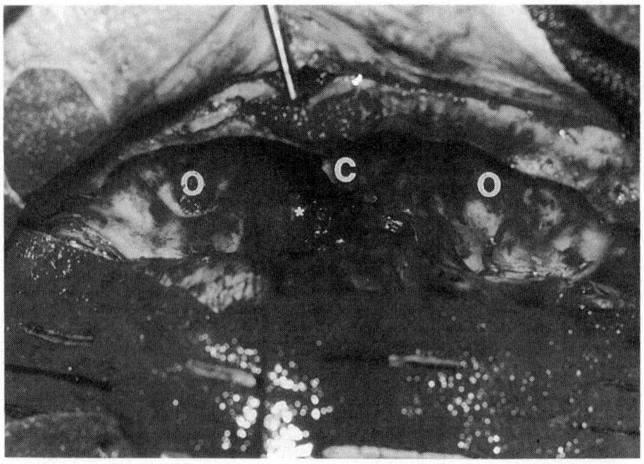

Figure 157-3 The anterior craniotomy has been completed and the frontal lobes have been allowed to retract posteriorly, with elevation of the dura from the anterior skull base and cribriform plate. Tumor is evident, eroding through the cribriform plate (*). The crista galli (C) is seen anterior to the tumor, and the orbital roofs (O) are noted laterally.

moist sponges until the completion of the procedure, when it is utilized for reconstruction.

After elevation of the scalp flap, a craniotomy is performed to provide access to the anterior fossa. A frontal craniotomy is usually done, although a supraorbital rim approach and an osteoplastic frontal sinus approach are alternatives, depending on the size of the lesion to be resected.[2,9] If a frontal sinus approach is chosen, the posterior table of the frontal sinus is removed and discarded, with the remaining frontal sinus mucosa removed in its entirety.

After removal of the bone flap, the frontal lobes are allowed to retract to provide exposure of the cribriform plate. Drainage of CSF from the lumbar drain assists in providing adequate retraction. Only enough CSF is removed to allow adequate exposure. Following retraction of the frontal lobes, the dura is elevated from the anterior fossa; the elevation begins laterally over the orbits. Once the region of the cribriform plate is reached, the dural extensions covering the olfactory nerves are cut to provide elevation of the frontal lobes and overlying dura from the skull base. The dura in this area is repaired immediately to prevent postoperative CSF leakage. If tumor invades the dura, an intradural dissection can be performed, allowing resection of the involved dura with later repair by a graft of pericranium, temporalis fascia, or fascia lata. The dura is elevated back to the planum sphenoidale, providing wide exposure of the anterior fossa skull base in the region of the cribriform plate (Fig. 157-3).

Intracranial osteotomies are then created around the ethmoidal complex. On the side ipsilateral to the tumor, the osteotomy is created lateral to the lamina papyracea through the roof of the orbit. On the contralateral side the osteotomy can be made through the fovea ethmoidalis unless tumor involves the lateral ethmoid extent. In the latter situation the osteotomy should be lateral to the lamina papyracea. The osteotomy can be extended laterally to include the orbit if the orbital contents are involved by tumor. The anterior osteotomies are created through the nasofrontal recess, whereas the posterior osteotomy is created through the sphenoid sinus anterior to the optic chiasm. In this way the anterior wall of the sphenoid will be included with the resected specimen. At this point the tumor has been freed from above in continuity with the cribriform plate, and the transfacial portion of the procedure can commence.

Transfacial Resection—Lateral Rhinotomy

The lateral rhinotomy approach has been used extensively for transfacial access during craniofacial resection.[1,8,16] The advantages of the lateral rhinotomy are wide exposure of the midfacial region and the ability to extend the incisions inferiorly through the lip for access to the palate or laterally through the inferior eyelid for access to the orbit. The lateral rhinotomy, although requiring facial incisions, nonetheless has an excellent cosmetic result. The disadvantages of the lateral rhinotomy approach include more difficult exposure of the contralateral side if it is involved with tumor as well as the possibility of an unsightly facial scar.

Before the lateral rhinotomy incision is made, the nasal cavity mucosa is vasoconstricted with topical and infiltrated vasoconstrictive agents. The proposed lateral rhinotomy incision is likewise injected with lidocaine, containing a solution of 1 : 100,000 epinephrine. The incision is created on the side of the tumor or on the side of the greater extent of disease. The incision begins just medial to the medial brow and is carried down along the nasofacial groove, halfway between the medial canthus and the nasal dorsum. The incision continues inferiorly around the alar rim and is carried into the nasal vestibule. If palatal resection is necessary, the lip can be split in the midline, although this is rarely needed. In addition, access to the orbit can be improved by lateral extension of the incision in a subciliary crease in the lower eyelid. It is not necessary to extend the incision across the root of the nose in most cases. Cheesman and colleagues[1] have reported an interesting variation of the lateral rhinotomy incision for access during craniofacial resection. The superior end of the lateral rhinotomy incision is extended vertically through the midportion of the forehead to provide access to the cranial cavity.

Following creation of the lateral rhinotomy incision, a lateral osteotomy is made through the ipsilateral frontal process of the maxilla. The periosteum is left attached to the nasal bone during performance of the osteotomy in order to preserve the blood supply to the underlying skeleton. The lateral osteotomy is then extended across the root of the nose in order to reflect the nasal skeleton and overlying soft tissue to the contralateral side (Fig. 157-4).

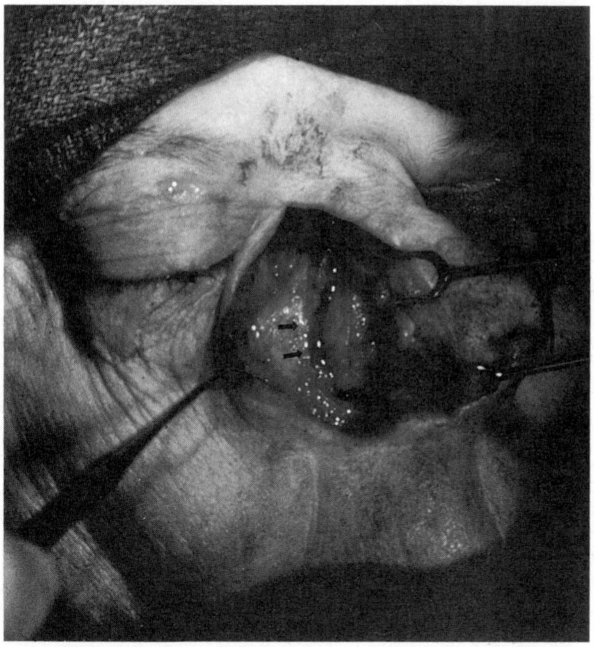

Figure 157-4 The lateral rhinotomy approach allows transfacial exposure for resection of nasal cavity and paranasal sinus tumors. The nasal structures are reflected to the contralateral side after creation of nasal osteotomies. In this patient the tumor is evident, protruding anteriorly beyond the piriform aperture (*arrows*).

The bony septum and posterior septal cartilage are separated dorsally from the nasal bones and external nasal structure. The medial canthal tendon is located and tagged for future identification. It is separated from the lacrimal crest and reflected laterally. The lacrimal duct is then transected to allow lateral displacement of the orbital contents. The periorbita is elevated from the medial and inferior surfaces of the orbit, the lamina papyracea and maxilla, respectively. If the periorbita is involved by tumor, it can be resected and included in the specimen. This portion of periorbita must be reconstructed with either a temporalis fascia or fascia lata graft to provide adequate support to the eye. The anterior and posterior ethmoidal arteries are identified, cauterized, and divided.

Osteotomies are created in order to perform medial maxillectomy and resection of the entire ethmoidal complex on the side of the tumor as well as part or all of the ethmoidal complex on the contralateral side if necessary. An osteotomy is created through the ipsilateral inferior meatus, extending anteriorly to posteriorly. A second osteotomy is created along the medial orbital floor, extending posteriorly and superiorly to the region of the frontoethmoid suture anterior to the optic foramen. This osteotomy encompasses the lamina papyracea on the side of the tumor. On the contralateral side the ethmoid is freed from the lamina papyracea unless there is tumor involvement of the lamina. In that case, osteotomies are created contralaterally to encompass the entire ethmoidal complex.

Once the osteotomies have been completed, the tumor specimen can be mobilized through both the transcranial and transfacial approaches. The remaining soft tissue attachments along the inferior nasal septum and posterolateral nasal walls are divided with Mayo scissors. The specimen is delivered through the facial incision *en bloc*. Packing is placed in the nasal cavity defect to control bleeding from the internal maxillary artery and its branches. After bleeding is controlled with cauterization and ligatures, any remaining tumor is removed. Frozen sections are taken from any suspicious areas at the margins of resection, with confirmation of clearance of tumor. Any remaining ethmoidal mucosa on the contralateral side is likewise removed.

Repair of the anterior fossa defect is performed, as described below. Reconstruction requires attention to cosmetic and functional detail. The medial canthal tendon is reapproximated to any residual lacrimal bone with a permanent suture. This ensures proper alignment of the medial canthus to the contralateral side to prevent a postoperative cosmetic defect and diplopia. The lateral rhinotomy incision is closed in layers, with antibiotic ointment placed over the incision.

Transfacial Resection—Midfacial Degloving

An alternative to the lateral rhinotomy approach for transfacial access is the midfacial degloving approach. In this approach the midfacial soft tissues are elevated superiorly from the underlying facial skeleton, providing wide access to the midface and anterior skull base.[10] The advantages of this approach include excellent cosmesis because no facial cutaneous incisions are created. Excellent bilateral exposure of the ethmoid and maxillary areas is provided, with ready access to the lateral maxillary regions and orbits. The disadvantages include somewhat limited exposure of the superior orbit and nasal root, possible nasal tip deformity and nasal vestibule stenosis, and facial paresthesias secondary to infraorbital nerve injury.

Before the incisions necessary for midfacial degloving are made, the nasal cavity mucosa and sublabial mucosa are vasoconstricted with topical and infiltrative agents containing epinephrine in a concentration of 1:100,000. Four incisions are necessary to elevate the midfacial structures off the underlying skeleton: (1) Bilateral sublabial incisions are created in the gingivolabial mucosa and carried down to the maxillary alveolus; (2) a complete intranasal transfixion incision is made between the columella and caudal end of the septum; (3) bilateral intercartilagenous incisions are created between the upper and lower lateral cartilages; (4) bilateral piriform aperture incisions are made and carried inferomedially to the vestibule of the nose. The intranasal incisions are connected to one another to allow separation of the nasal tip from the underlying nasal skeleton.

The soft tissue over the nasal bones and upper lateral cartilages is then elevated in a subcutaneous plane. Soft tissue is likewise elevated over the anterior wall of each maxilla to the level of the infraorbital rim. The infraorbital nerve should be preserved bilaterally if possible. Following complete elevation of the soft tissue, two wide Penrose drains are inserted through each nares and used to retract the midfacial soft tissue superiorly to the level of the glabella and orbits (Fig. 157-5).

Following complete elevation of the nasal soft tissues, osteotomies and soft tissue mobilization are performed. This is similar to the resection performed during the lateral rhinotomy approach described above. After resection and skull base reconstruction is performed, the nasal tip is returned to position. The columellar and intercartilagenous incisions are closed with interrupted 4-0 chromic catgut sutures. The sublabial incision is also closed with interrupted absorbable sutures. A nasal splint is placed over the nasal dorsum to provide immobilization and compression to prevent a postoperative hematoma.

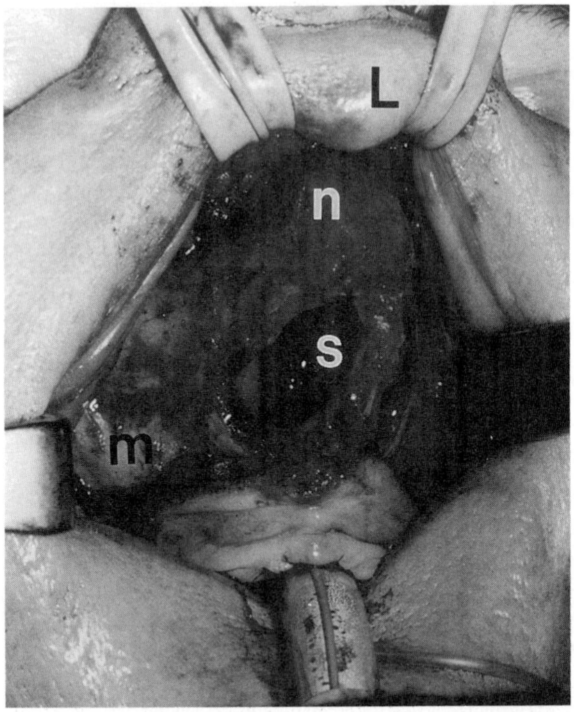

(*A*)

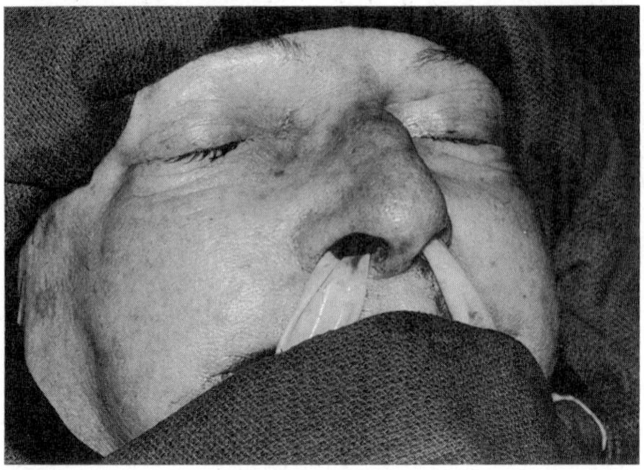

(*B*)

Figure 157-5 *A.* Midfacial degloving approach for transfacial access. The facial and nasal soft tissues have been elevated superiorly from the underlying maxilla (m) and the nasal skeleton (n). Access to the nasal cavity, septum (s), paranasal sinuses, and orbits is provided by this approach. The superior lip (L) can be elevated to the level of the glabella. *B.* The facial soft tissues have been redraped into position after the midfacial degloving. The Penrose drains placed through the nares are used to retract the soft tissue of the face superiorly during the resection.

Reconstruction of the Anterior Fossa Defect

Following complete resection of disease and control of hemorrhage, reconstruction of the anterior fossa defect can proceed. The pericranial flap that was developed during elevation of the scalp is rotated into the anterior fossa through the craniotomy. The pericranial flap can be based either anteriorly or laterally, depending upon the extent of the defect to be reconstructed. For lesions confined to the midportion of the anterior fossa, an anteriorly based pericranial flap provides adequate coverage.[3,19] Resections that include the orbit often require a laterally based pericranial flap to cover the defect adequately.[4,15] The pericranium is sutured to the margins of the dura as well as the margins of the bony resection. This provides support for the anterior fossa contents and separation of the nasal and intracranial cavities to prevent postoperative contamination.

A split-thickness skin graft, dermal graft, or fascia graft can be placed against the pericranium from the nasal surface. This graft is sutured in place to the margins of the bony defect. The graft is also held in position with antibiotic impregnated packing placed in the nasal cavity. This packing remains in place for 5 to 7 days postoperatively and is then removed.

In patients who previously underwent an operation and whose pericranium was resected, or in those with an extensive anterior cranial fossa defect following resection, a microvascular free flap of either rectus or latissimus muscle may be necessary for adequate closure and reconstruction.[4,14] Bone grafting with either microvascular compound osseous flaps or split calvarial grafts is rarely necessary for reconstruction of the anterior fossa floor defect; however, it may be necessary if there is resection of the anterior wall of the frontal sinus or other parts of the midfacial skeleton.

After the pericranial flap is secured over the anterior fossa defect, the frontal bone flap is re-placed into proper position. The bone flap is secured to the margins of the craniotomy by sutures placed through drill holes along the margins of the bone. The bone flap must be held in a position that prevents compression of the pericranial flap.

Postoperative Care

Before the patient leaves the operating room, the lumbar drain or drainage needles are removed. There is no reason to continue postoperative drainage of CSF, as this will only increase the likelihood of complications. The patient is observed in the intensive care unit for the first 24 to 48 h. During this time, the patient is maintained at bed rest in the supine position with the head slightly elevated to approximately 20 degrees.

Intravenous antibiotics are continued until the nasal packing is removed on the fifth to seventh postoperative day. Following removal of the nasal packing, the nasal cavity is cleaned and the anterior cranial fossa defect is inspected for any evidence of CSF leakage or breakdown of the pericranial flap. Postoperative radiotherapy, if it is to be administered, is not initiated for approximately 4 to 6 weeks to ensure adequate healing of the reconstruction.

Patient Outcome

Assessment of long-term survival following craniofacial resection is difficult because of the wide variety of tumors treated by this approach as well as the frequent use of combined modality therapy with radiatiotherapy and chemotherapy. Most authors have reported improvements in both local and regional disease control and overall survival when craniofacial resection is utilized for the treatment of benign or malignant disease.[1,8,14,16,17,20] Our experience supports the efficacy of anterior craniofacial resection.

In our series 32 patients have had craniofacial resection: 26 for

TABLE 157-1 Tumors Resected by Anterior Craniofacial Resection

Tumor	Number
Malignant	
Squamous cell carcinoma	9
Esthesioneuroblastoma	9
Adenoid cystic carcinoma	2
Small cell carcinoma	2
Sarcoma	2
Adenocarcinoma	1
Transitional cell carcinoma	1
Total	26
Benign	
Meningioma	2
Juvenile ossifying fibroma	1
Fibrous histiocytoma	1
Inverting papilloma	1
Osteoma	1
Total	6

treatment of malignant tumors and 6 for treatment of benign disease (Table 157-1).[14] In patients with malignant disease, 14 are alive with no evidence of disease at a mean follow-up of 28 months. In the 10 patients who died with disease, the mean survival before death was 22 months. Eight patients suffered local or regional recurrence with a mean follow-up time of 30.5 months. In all but one patient adjuvant therapy was used, with radiatiotherapy alone or in combination with chemotherapy.

The efficacy of craniofacial resection for management of certain malignant tumors, such as esthesioneuroblastoma, has been well documented. In one report, a survival rate of 37 percent for patients treated before the use of craniofacial resection was contrasted with a survival of 82 percent when craniofacial resection was performed.[8] Conversely, other tumors of the nasal cavity and paranasal sinus, such as sinonasal undifferentiated carcinoma, have such a poor prognosis that treatment approaches other than craniofacial resection should be considered.[7]

Dural invasion has been associated with a decreased survival rate.[21] In our experience, 5 of 11 patients with dural invasion who underwent craniofacial resection died of disease.[14] Periorbital invasion by tumor does not seem to carry the same grave prognosis. Resection of periorbita involved by tumor provides adequate tumor control as well as preservation and function of the eye.[12]

Complications

A procedure of the magnitude of anterior craniofacial resection is not without associated morbidity (Table 157-2). Recent advances in perioperative patient management have helped reduce the incidence of most of the severe complications; however, significant acute and long-term sequelae are still possible.[9,14] Minimizing trauma to the brain, dura, and orbits, and careful attention to wound closure with separation of the intracranial cavity from the nasal cavity are the operative strategies that help reduce postoperative complications.

In our experience, postoperative mortality has been low, with only one patient dying in the perioperative period.[14] In this previously neurologically intact patient, a fall occurring on the second postoperative day resulted in death. All other patients have survived the perioperative period, with an average hospital stay of 13 days.

TABLE 157-2 Potential Complications of Anterior Craniofacial Resection

Neurological
Pneumocephalus
Intracranial hemorrhage
Meningitis
CSF leakage
Cerebral edema
Cerebrovascular accident
Epidural abscess
Seizures
Diabetes insipidus
Depressed or altered mental status
Anosmia
Wound
Cellulitis
Infected cranial bone flap
Oronasal fistula
Necrosis of pericranial flap
Encephalocele
Crusting of nasal cavity
Orbital
Visual loss
Diplopia
Enophthalmos
Cosmetic
Facial scar
Burr hole depression
Ocular dystopia

The most significant postoperative complications have been neurological. Pneumocephalus, with resultant depression of mental status, has occurred in several patients. Acute management involves percutaneous aspiration of the air through an underlying burr hole, but direct evacuation of the air and revision of the anterior cranial base reconstruction may be required. Maneuvers that may help avoid this problem include placement of nasopharyngeal airways or tracheostomy to divert airflow from the upper airway. Patients with acute postoperative mental status changes should have an immediate CT scan to evaluate for pneumocephalus and associated cerebral compression (Fig. 157-6). CSF leakage and meningitis, although rare in our experience, are certainly possible.[5,9,14] Careful attention to the pericranial flap closure, dural reconstruction, and suture repair of dural defects helps prevent these complications. Epidural abscess, with resultant infection of the cranial bone flap, has occurred in two patients. This required removal of the bone flap and drainage of the abscess. Adequate separation of the nasal and cranial cavities and appropriate antibiotic coverage help avoid this problem. If loss of the bone flap occurs, secondary reconstruction of the frontal defect is necessary for adequate cosmesis.

Significant wound complications are uncommon. Infections of the facial and scalp incisions are treated with local wound care and antibiotic therapy. As stated above, infection of the cranial bone flap or facial skeleton is a significant complication, usually resulting from failure to separate adequately the intracranial cavity from the contaminated nasal surfaces. The pericranial flap has proved itself to be a hardy, well-vascularized reconstructive material. Necrosis of the flap has occurred in two of our patients following postoperative radiotherapy.[14] In both patients necrosis of the inferior frontal lobe was also present. This complication was managed

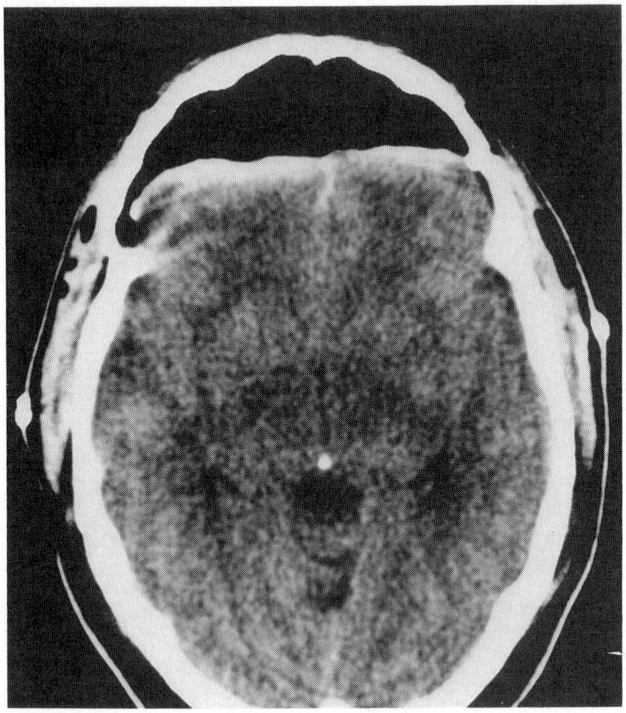

Figure 157-6 Postoperative CT scan demonstrates a large pneumocephalus.

by reconstruction of the floor of the cranial cavity with a myocutaneous free flap. Inadequate reconstruction of the anterior fossa floor can result in the development of an encephalocele. Defects that are too large to be reconstructed with a pericranial flap may require additional tissues, such as split calvarial bone grafts or free myocutaneous flaps.

Orbital sequelae following anterior craniofacial resection can include complete or partial loss of visual acuity, diplopia, and enophthalmos. Resection and retraction in the region of the orbital apex increase the risk of central retinal artery compression or optic nerve injury with resultant blindness. Similarly, adjuvant radiotherapy may increase the likelihood of blindness or altered visual acuity. Diplopia may result from restriction of the extraocular muscles or from injury to the ocular cranial nerves. Resection in the region of the cavernous sinus increases the incidence of this complication.[9] Extensive resections of the medial orbital wall with periorbita may result in enophthalmos. Reconstruction of the periorbita to provide adequate support helps alleviate this problem.

Postoperative cosmesis is usually acceptable to both patient and treating physician. Facial scarring is possible, especially when the lateral rhinotomy approach is utilized. However, the facial incisions are usually well camouflaged. Forehead depressions in the region of burr holes placed for the craniotomy can become problematic. Placement of the burr holes behind the hairline obviates the need for any type of reconstruction. Adequate alignment of the medial canthus and reconstruction of orbital support help prevent postoperative dystopia.

Summary

Anterior craniofacial resection has become a mainstay of surgical therapy for advanced lesions involving the nasal cavity, paranasal sinuses, and anterior skull base. Refinements in technique and perioperative management have reduced the morbidity and mortality associated with this procedure to levels that allow its application to a number of disease processes. A two-team approach combines the skill and expertise of neurosurgeons and head and neck surgeons, resulting in an improved outcome for the patient.

References

1. Cheesman AD, Lund VJ, Howard DJ. Craniofacial resection for tumors of the nasal cavity and paranasal sinuses. *Head Neck Surg* 1986; 8:429–435.
2. Jane JA, Park TS, Pobereskin LH, et al. The supraorbital approach: technical note. *Neurosurgery* 1982; 11:537–542.
3. Johns ME, Winn HR, McLean WC, Cantrell RW. Pericranial flap for the closure of defects of craniofacial resection. *Laryngoscope* 1981; 91:952–959.
4. Jones NF, Schramm VL, Sekhar LN. Reconstruction of the cranial base following tumour resection. *Br J Plast Surg* 1987; 40:155–162.
5. Ketcham AS, Hoye RC, Van Buren JM, et al. Complications of intracranial facial resection for tumors of the paranasal sinuses. *Am J Surg* 1966; 112:591–596.
6. Ketcham AS, Wilkins RH, Van Burean JM, Smith RR. A combined intracranial facial approach to the paranasal sinuses. *Am J Surg* 1963; 106:698–703.
7. Levine PA, Frierson HF Jr, Stewart FM, et al. Sinonasal undifferentiated carcinoma: a distinctive and highly aggressive neoplasm. *Laryngoscope* 1987; 97:905–908.
8. Levine PA, McLean WC, Cantrell RW. Esthesioneuroblastoma: the University of Virginia Experience 1960–1985. *Laryngoscope* 1986; 96:742–746.
9. Levine PA, Scher RL, Jane JA, et al. The craniofacial resection: eleven-year experience at the University of Virginia: problems and solutions. *Otolaryngol Head Neck Surg* 1989; 101:665–669.
10. Maniglia AJ. Indications and techniques of midfacial degloving: a 15-year experience. *Arch Otolaryngol Head Neck Surg* 1986; 112:750–752.
11. Paling MR, Black WC, Levine PA, Cantrell RW. Tumor invasion of the anterior skull base: a comparison of MR and CT studies. *J Compt Assist Tomogr* 1987; 11:824–830.
12. Perry C, Levine PA, Williamson BR, Cantrell RW. Preservation of the eye in paranasal sinus cancer surgery. *Arch Otolaryngol Head Neck Surg* 1988; 114:632–634.
13. Ray BS, McLean JM. Combined intracranial and orbital operation for retinoblastoma. *Arch Ophthalmol* 1943; 30:437–445.
14. Richtsmeier WJ, Briggs RJS, Koch WM, et al. Complications and early outcome of anterior craniofacial resection. *Arch Otolaryngol Head Neck Surg* 1992; 118:913–917.
15. Scher RL, Cantrell RW. Anterior skull base reconstruction with the pericranial flap after craniofacial resection. *Ear Nose Throat J* 1992; 71:210–217.
16. Schramm VL Jr, Myers EN, Maroon JC. Anterior skull base surgery for benign and malignant disease. *Laryngoscope* 1979; 89:1077–1091.
17. Shah JP, Sundaresan N, Galicich J, Strong EW. Craniofacial resections for tumors involving the base of the skull. *Am J Surg* 1987; 154:352–358.
18. Smith RR, Klopp CT, Williams JM. Surgical treatment of cancer of the frontal sinus and adjacent areas. *Cancer* 1954; 7:991–994.
19. Stiernberg CM, Bailey BJ, Weiner RL, et al. Reconstruction of the anterior skull base following craniofacial resection. *Arch Otolaryngol Head Neck Surg* 1987; 113:710–712.
20. Sundaresan N, Shah JP. Craniofacial resection for anterior skull base tumors. *Head Neck Surg* 1988; 10:219–224.
21. Van Tuyl R, Gussack GS. Prognostic factors in craniofacial surgery. *Laryngoscope* 1991; 101:240–244.

158

Extended Frontal Approach to Tumors and Aneurysms of the Cranial Base

Laligam N. Sekhar
Donald C. Wright
Chandranath Sen

The extended frontal approach is an extension of the subfrontal approach to the cranial base involving the addition of an orbital osteotomy or an orbitofrontoethmoidal osteotomy. The removal of the facial bones, with the optional removal of the ethmoid bone, greatly improves the exposure of cranial base structures while reducing frontal lobe retraction. Cosmesis is well preserved by the reattachment of the bones with titanium miniplates and the use of burr hole covers. The approach has applications to anterior fossa malignant tumors; sphenoclival neoplasms; olfactory groove, planum sphenoidale and optic canal meningiomas; large or giant anterior cerebral complex aneurysms; and complex traumatic lesions of the anterior cranial base.

Development of the Extended Frontal Approach

The concept of removing orbital rims to improve the exposure of the skull base was introduced by Frazier in 1913.[6] Derome et al. introduced the transbasal approach to the skull base in 1972.[5] The concept of using orbital osteotomies to approach cranial base lesions was developed by Tessier, Jane et al., Jackson et al., Sekhar et al., Al-Mefty and Smith, and a number of others.[1,2,7–11,13,16–19,21,22] A technique for olfactory preservation during the use of the extended frontal approach was described by Spetzler et al.[25]

A combined transcranial and transfacial approach to retinoblastoma was first described by Ray and McLean in 1943.[19] This combined approach to paranasal sinus malignancies was applied by Smith et al. in 1954,[23] Ketcham et al. in 1966,[14] and Van Buren et al. in 1968.[27] Several authors made contributions to resection of malignant lesions of the anterior cranial base.[3,16,20,26] The reconstruction of the cranial base by the use of pericranial, galeal, temporalis, and microvascular free flaps reduced the incidence of infection.[4,11,12,20,24]

Types of Lesions

Tumors

Tumors of the cranial base are of many pathologic varieties. *Meningiomas* originating from the basal meninges can be of two types. The first is the *en plaque* type, which spreads out over a wide area of the dura. This type is associated with hyperostosis of the underlying bone, which commonly manifests microscopic invasion by the tumor. Frequently, on the other side of the involved bone, tumor spreads into the air sinuses, the orbits, and the pterygoid and temporalis muscles. The second type, the *en masse* meningioma, is predominantly intracranial. En masse meningiomas include tumors of the olfactory groove, planum sphenoidale, and tuberculum sellae. Such tumors can extend inferiorly into the ethmoidal or sphenoidal sinuses with the destruction of the basal bony structures. Total removal of these tumors and their extensions, including the involved bone and dura, is essential to avoiding recurrence. Because the blood supply to these tumors enters from the cranial base, a very basal approach offers an excellent opportunity to interrupt the blood supply prior to the actual tumor removal.

Neoplasms that arise from the cranial bones and cartilage include chordomas, chondrosarcomas, chondromas, fibrous dysplasia of bone, ossifying fibromas, and osteogenic sarcomas. These tumors usually do not invade the dura unless they are aggressive or have recurred after prior transdural resection; however, the bony involvement can be much more extensive than is apparent on the preoperative magnetic resonance and computed tomographic images.

Tumors arising in the nasal cavity and the paranasal sinuses can extend superiorly to involve the cranial base and even the meninges of the brain. These include esthesioneuroblastomas, juvenile angiofibromas, squamous cell carcinomas, adenoid cystic carcinomas, inverted papillomas, and lymphomas. The removal of most of these tumors requires a wide excision with normal tissue margins.

Aneurysms

While many simpler *aneurysms of the anterior cerebral-communicating complex* can be operated on through traditional transsylvian or interhemispheric approaches, an extended subfrontal approach is quite useful for operations on large or giant aneurysms. During acute aneurysm surgery, the extended frontal approach can enable the operation to be performed even if the brain is tight.

Traumatic Lesions

The extended frontal approach can also be used for *complex traumatic lesions of the anterior cranial fossa* that require optic nerve decompression and dural and orbital repair.

Anatomy of the Anterior Cranial Base

The anterior cranial base consists of the frontal bone (including the frontal sinus) in front, the orbital roofs laterally, the ethmoid bones in the midline, and the lesser sphenoid wings posteriorly.[15] The foramen cecum lies immediately behind the frontal bone in the midline; the ethmoid bone forms the posterior and lateral boundaries of this foramen. The crista galli forms a bony ridge posterior to the foramen cecum. On either side of the crista lies the cribriform plate with the olfactory foramina, which transmit the anterior and posterior ethmoidal arteries and olfactory nerves, each of which carries a dural and arachnoidal sleeve. Behind the cribriform plate, the floor of the anterior cranial base is made up of the planum sphenoidale and the lesser wing of the sphenoid. The shape of the floor is important in understanding the mechanics of the approach. The cribriform plate and the planum sphenoidale are the lowest points of the floor. From there, the floor slopes upward and laterally over the orbits. Thus, removal of the orbital roofs along with the supraorbital rims and the downward retraction of the orbital contents allows a direct view with virtually no frontal lobe retraction.

The dura covering the orbitofrontal area is quite thick except in the region of the cribriform plates. There are usually several invaginations of the dura into the bone, posterior to the cribriform area, where tears can be produced during separation. The blood supply to this part of the dura comes from the ethmoidal, middle meningeal, and internal carotid arteries. The anterior falcial artery, a branch of the ethmoidal, supplies the anterior falx.

The frontal, ethmoidal, and sphenoidal paranasal sinuses make up the medial part of the anterior cranial base. They are pneumatized to a varying extent and are usually very thin-walled, permitting easy passage of tumors. It must be noted that, during surgery, either the drainage routes of these sinuses must be preserved or the mucosa must be denuded as thoroughly as possible to prevent the formation of a mucocele.

The orbit is an important neighbor of the anterior cranial base, and its relationships should be well understood for operative interventions in the anterior cranial fossa. The orbital process of the frontal bone, which is pneumatized to a variable degree, forms the orbital roofs. The lateral wall of the orbit is formed by the greater wing of the sphenoid bone and the zygomatic bone. This is the shortest wall of the orbit. Immediately beneath the greater wing is the base of the pterygoid plates. At the anterior end of the pterygoid plates is the foramen rotundum and the inferior orbital fissure. At the posterior end lies the foramen ovale. These structures frequently are involved by tumors arising from the nasopharynx and the sinuses. The medial wall of the orbit is composed of the lacrimal, ethmoid, and sphenoid bones. Important landmarks in this region are the ethmoidal foramina, usually two in number, which transmit the ethmoidal arteries. They are situated at the level of the frontoethmoidal suture and, in some cases, are on the frontal side of the suture. When approaching through the orbit, these foramina mark the floor of the medial part of the anterior cranial base. The posterior ethmoidal foramen is about 5 mm anterior to the orbital opening of the optic canal.

The optic foramen lies at the posterior limit of the anterior cranial base, from which the optic canal proceeds anteroinferolaterally at an angle of about 40 degrees to the sagittal plane. Extensions of the sphenoidal and ethmoidal sinuses can be found in the roof, floor, and medial wall of the canal.

Preoperative Evaluation

The exact extent of the lesion must be defined accurately to plan the operative approach and the limits of excision to be performed. Bony definition is obtained from axial and coronal computed tomography (CT) images, using bone algorithms. Opacification of the paranasal air sinuses, which is noted frequently, may be due to obstructive changes in the sinus or to actual tumor invasion. Magnetic resonance imaging (MRI) is an excellent way to make this distinction and to define the soft tissue extensions of the tumor. For both benign and malignant tumors, the plane of demarcation from the brain can be visualized preoperatively, and invasion of the parenchyma of the brain can be determined. The relationship of the optic nerves to the tumor, a very important piece of information, is readily determined from MRI. In most instances, the relation of vascular anatomy to the tumor can also be determined accurately with MRI. An arteriogram is obtained to determine the relationship of the major vessels to the tumor, the source of blood supply to the tumor, and the potential collateral channels (the anterior and posterior communicating arteries and the ophthalmic artery) available in the event of internal carotid artery (ICA) occlusion. If the tumor is very vascular, preoperative embolization can be performed to reduce intraoperative blood loss. If the internal carotid artery is displaced or encased by the tumor, a balloon occlusion test of the artery is performed. Both clinical evaluation and single photon emission tomography (SPECT) scanning are done with the balloon inflated in the upper cervical internal carotid artery to determine the circulatory reserve of the brain. We no longer perform excision of the ICA without vein graft replacement because of the unpredictable occurrence of stroke after ICA occlusion, even when the collateral circulation is excellent.

For complex aneurysms of the anterior communicating complex, the senior author has found that the use of rapid sequence CT imaging with three-dimensional imaging (CT-angiography) is very useful in addition to arteriography in planning the operation.

For traumatic lesions, CT scanning with soft tissue and bone algorithms and thin coronal bone windowed sections is adequate. If a vascular injury is suspected, arteriography is mandatory.

Operative Technique

Anesthesia

For most patients, a balanced anesthetic technique with muscle paralysis is used, after induction with intravenous sodium thiopental. If cranial nerve monitoring is anticipated, a nonparalytic technique should be employed. If the head position might be changed during the operation, it is wise to secure the endotracheal tube to the teeth with fine stainless steel wire passed interdentally, in addition to taping. Mild hypothermia (32° to 34°C) is used during tumor and vascular operations. During the operation, the anesthesiologist must be prepared to provide induced hypertension, as well as barbiturate coma to achieve burst-suppression on the electroencephalogram, to protect the brain in the event of temporary vascular occlusion. If excessive blood loss occurs during the operation, the anesthesiologist must monitor the patient's prothrombin time, partial thromboplastin time, and platelet count, and replace factors adequately *before* clinical manifestations of a dilutional coagulopathy. Indwelling arterial, central venous, and Foley catheters are routinely used during such operations. Good cooperation between the neurosurgeon and the anesthesiologist, and a good understanding of each other's work, are essential.

For extradural operations, a lumbar spinal drain is used. For intradural procedures, intravenous diuretics, cisternal drainage, and hyperventilation are adequate. If the brain is very tight during acute aneurysm surgery, lumbar spinal fluid drainage or ventriculostomy drainage can be used.

Neurophysiologic Monitoring

Monitoring of the electroencephalogram and the somatosensory evoked potentials is performed in most patients to detect evidence of cerebral ischemia caused by vascular compromise and to facilitate burst suppression in the event of vascular injury. In some patients, monitoring of the function of cranial nerves III and VI and of the brain stem evoked responses (BSER) may also be performed.

Patient Position and Incision

The patient is placed in the supine position, and the head is usually secured in a pin head holder, slightly elevated, extended, and turned 30 to 45 degrees away from the side of the approach. For midline lesions, the head is not turned. If the patient's head position may need to be changed during the operation as in a combined anterior and lateral approach, it is placed on a horse-shoe head rest and the endotracheal tube is secured to the teeth with stainless steel wire. For complex vascular cases, a radiolucent head holder is used to facilitate intraoperative angiography.

The incision is usually bicoronal, crossing the vertex about 15 cm above the nasion so that a pericranial flap will have an adequate length if used. If contralateral exposure is limited, the incision can be curved on the contralateral side toward the superior temporal hairline. The incision can be extended preauricularly if a lateral approach will be combined. If important to the patient, hair shaving can be limited to a strip around the incision, with careful preparation of the surrounding scalp and hair. In all patients, the thigh region is prepared for possible extraction of fat and fascia lata. The eyelids are taped or sewn shut. After infiltration with 2% xylocaine and 0.5% epinephrine, the incision is deepened to the bone and the scalp is elevated with the pericranium. As an alternative, the pericranium may be incised further posteriorly if a longer pericranial flap is desired for reconstruction. The superficial layer of the temporal fascia blends with the pericranium, and it is separated from the shiny deep layer of the temporal fascia and elevated along with the skin flap. The frontal branches of the facial nerve and the anterior branches of the superficial temporal artery are carefully preserved using this technique. The pericranium is densely attached to the rim of the orbit, and should be carefully separated. Although the supraorbital nerves and vessels usually lie inside a notch, they occasionally pass through a foramen that will have to be notched on either side of the neurovascular bundle to release it.

The periorbita is then carefully separated from the roof, lateral wall, and superomedial wall of the orbit (including the attachment of the trochlea), taking care to minimize injury to it and to avoid herniation of orbital contents. The separation should expose all of the orbital bone to be removed with the osteotomy. For an orbitofrontal-ethmoidal osteotomy, the periosteum will need to be separated carefully from the nasal bones, and the periorbita will have to be separated superomedially to the anterior ethmoidal arteries, which are cauterized and divided. If the periorbita is lacerated, it can be repaired with sutures after the orbitotomy. The temporalis muscle is elevated from the temporal fossa as needed, leaving a cuff of muscle and fascia for reattachment. After these initial steps, the procedure will be different for different lesions, and is described separately.

Malignant Anterior Cranial Lesions

Malignant anterior cranial lesions such as esthesioneuroblastomas and squamous cell carcinomas are usually removed by the combination of an extended frontal and a transfacial approach. However, malignant lesions restricted to the ethmoids and the anterior cranial fossa can be removed entirely via the extended frontal approach.[3]

A low bifrontal craniotomy is performed first. It is safer to perform a unilateral frontal craniotomy that extends to the midline, then separate the superior sagittal sinus from bone by tangential direct vision, and then perform a contralateral frontal craniotomy. After the relaxation of the brain with intravenous mannitol and the removal of spinal fluid, the frontal dura is separated from the roof of the orbit to the lesser wings of the sphenoid bone. The orbitotomy is then performed, including both orbital rims, the nasal bridge, and the roof of the orbit, but not including the tumor-involved ethmoid bone. Cuts through the orbital rims and the nasal bone are performed with a thin reciprocating saw, with protection of the dura and periorbita. Cuts through the roof of the orbit are completed using Midas Rex instrumentation (Midas Rex Instruments, Fort Worth, TX) with similar protection. The orbital osteotomy is further loosened with an osteotome and a mallet, and removed (Fig. 158-1). Further orbital roof bone is removed as necessary, with rongeurs, to achieve maximal exposure. The dura is excised circumferentially around the lesion. Tumor removal is effected in a piecemeal fashion for slow-growing malignancies but *en bloc* for fast-growing malignancies. *En bloc* tumor resection generally requires a transfacial approach via a lateral rhinostomy or a facial degloving incision.

Dural reconstruction is performed with fascia lata graft, followed by the development and application of an anteriorly based, well-vascularized pericranial flap to cover the defect. Bony reconstruction of the defect is not necessary. The pericranial flap is sutured to small holes in the posterior edges of the bony defect or to the dura of the planum sphenoidale area. The reconstruction may be reinforced with autologous fibrin glue. The osteotomy and bone plates are reattached with titanium miniplates, and burr hole covers are used. The incision is closed with gravity drainage. A head wrap is avoided, which appears to reduce the extent of periorbital edema. It is rarely necessary to employ postoperative spinal drainage.

Midline Sphenoclival Tumors

For midline sphenoclival tumors, which may extend into the medial aspect of the cavernous sinuses, the extended subfrontal ap-

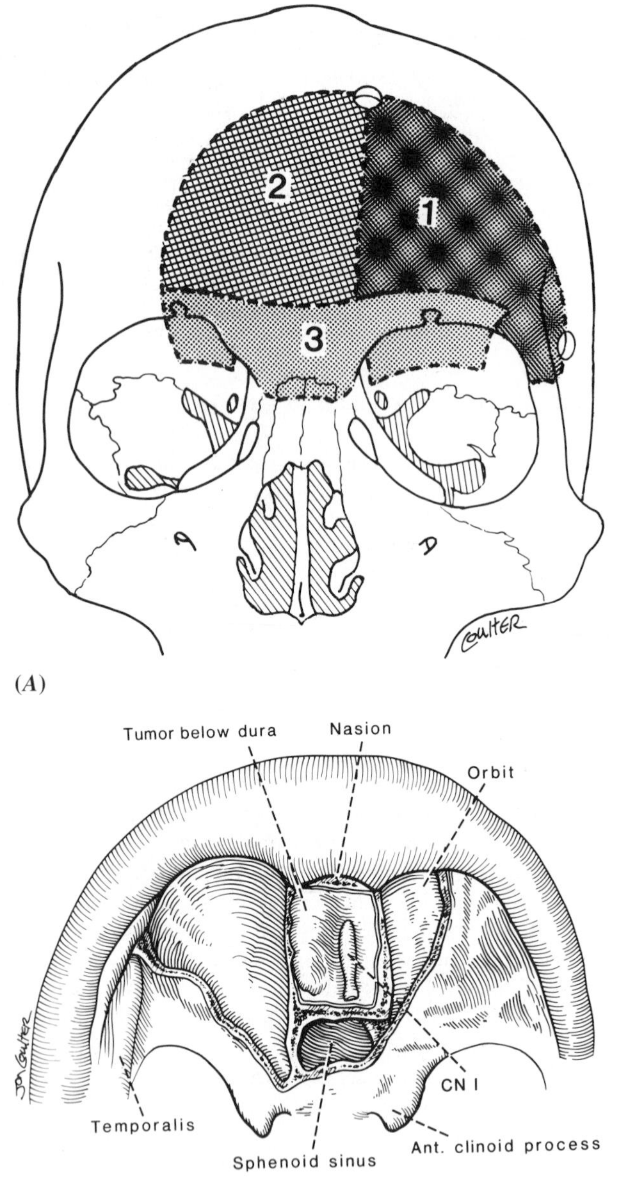

(*A*)

(*B*)

Figure 158-1 *A*. Craniotomy (areas 1 and 2) and orbital osteotomy (area 3) for an anterior cranial base malignant lesion. *B*. Superior view of the exposure of the anterior basal malignant lesion achieved after craniotomy and orbital osteotomy.

proach may be used in isolation. When extensive cavernous sinus invasion is present, a frontotemporal transcavernous approach is necessary. When the tumor extends extensively into the petrous apex, a subtemporal-extradural or subtemporal-infratemporal approach will need to be combined with the extended subfrontal approach. For tumors that have considerable invasion of the lower clivus or occipital condyles, the extreme lateral, transcondyle approach is essential.

For this approach, the olfactory nerves and the ethmoidal area dura are divided and elevated, and the dura is repaired. A bilateral orbitofrontoethmoidal osteotomy is then performed, as shown in Fig. 158-2. The posterior margin of the osteotomy must cross just behind the cribriform plate of the ethmoids and enter the sphenoid sinus to avoid injury to the optic nerves. The orbitofrontoethmoidal bone piece is then removed, and the ethmoidal mucosa is cauterized. One or both optic nerves are decompressed extradurally (Fig. 158-3). The sphenoid sinus is opened extensively, removing the bone of the planum and the sella. The posterior and middle ethmoidal cells are removed aggressively, which greatly expands the space available to work. The lateral walls of the body of the sphenoid bone (medial wall of the cavernous sinus) and the bone around the medial orbital apex are removed (Fig. 158-4). This step will expose the intracavernous ICA, which can be followed posteriorly to the petrous apices. The sphenodural bone and tumor can be removed aggressively, including uninvolved bony margins (Fig. 158-5). If the cavernous sinus is entered, venous bleeding can be controlled with small rolls of oxidized cellulose. Small dural defects that occur because of tumor invasion can be closed primarily. Larger dural defects are closed with fascia lata graft, microsutures, and fibrin glue. Reconstruction is completed with a pericranial flap, autologous fat, and fibrin glue (Fig. 158-3*C*). One must be careful to both obliterate the dead space and avoid overpacking the sinus. The osteotomy and craniotomy pieces are reattached as usual.

When the tumor is entirely extradural, the olfaction-preserving technique described by Spetzler[25] can be used. In this method, the cribriform plates are isolated by the osteotomy and lifted up with the frontal dura (Fig. 158-2*C*). They are reattached at the end of the operation with microplates. If a pericranial flap is used, it will have to be split in the midline to make an opening for the cribriform plates.

Olfactory Groove and Planum Meningiomas

Olfactory groove meningiomas (Fig. 158-6) and planum sphenoidale meningiomas are approached from the right side, unless vision is impaired in the left eye and not the right. The initial opening involves a right frontotemporal craniotomy with extension to the midline (Fig. 158-7). For larger tumors, a second frontal flap is removed, extending to the contralateral supraorbital notch. The orbital osteotomy is predominantly right-sided but extends just across the midline in front of the cribriform plate of the ethmoid bone. The remaining orbital roof of the right side is removed up to the optic canal and the anterior clinoid process, if doing so is feasible without excessive brain retraction.

The sylvian fissure is opened to obtain a lateral approach to the tumor and to visualize at least the ipsilateral optic nerve and anterior cerebral vessels. The dura and the periorbita are retracted together with sutures, enlarging the subfrontal space. Both olfactory tracts are dissected free of the frontal lobe. It is usually possible to spare the contralateral olfactory tract, but the ipsilateral one may have to be divided. The tumor is debulked toward its base and then removed. Dissection from the optic nerves, dorsum, and anterior cerebral vessels must be performed carefully. At times, the arteries may be encased by tumor.

For meningiomas of the planum and tuberculum sellae region, both optic nerves are usually decompressed inside the optic canal, and the dural sheath is opened. Tumor extensions in this area are common, even if they are not visualized in preoperative studies.

At the end of tumor resection, the involved dura and bone are resected in younger patients (<60 years old) and in patients with recurrent tumors. Reconstruction is performed with fascia lata, autologous fat, and a pericranial flap if the defect is large. The sphenoidal, ethmoidal, and frontal sinuses must be obliterated carefully.

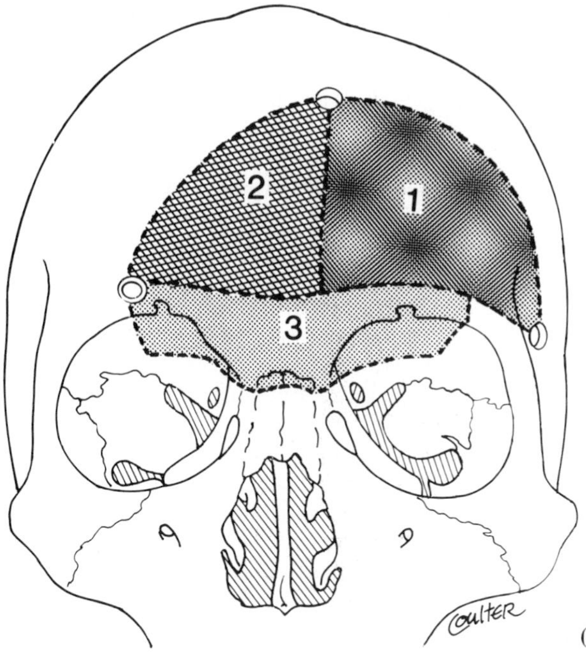

(*A*)

Figure 158-2 *A*. Craniotomy (areas 1 and 2) and orbitofronto-ethmoidal osteotomy (area 3) for a midline sphenocavernous tumor. *B*. Superior view of the orbitofrontoethmoidal osteotomy. The area of bone to be drilled away is also seen. *C*. The osteotomies that spare olfaction. The ethmoidal-cribriform area (2) is osteotomized and retracted upward with the olfactory mucosa.

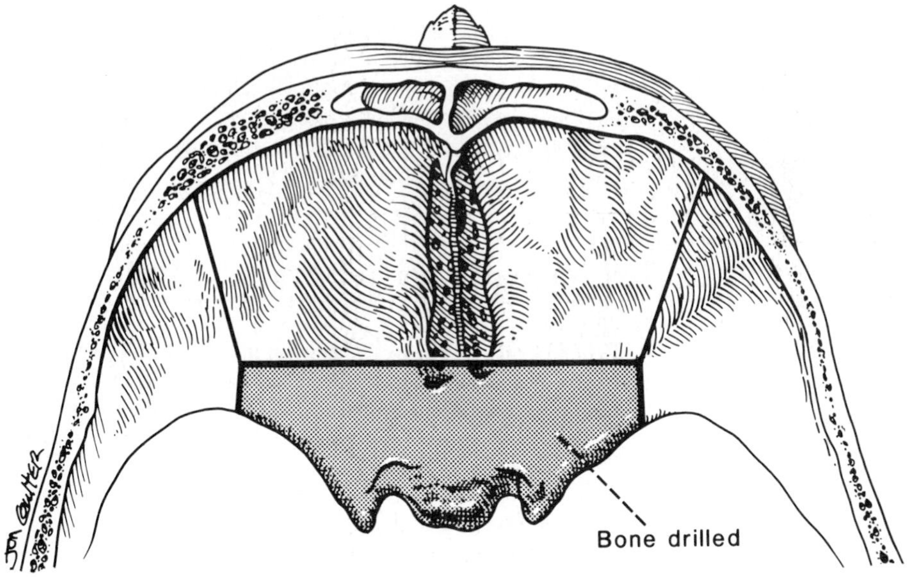

(*B*)

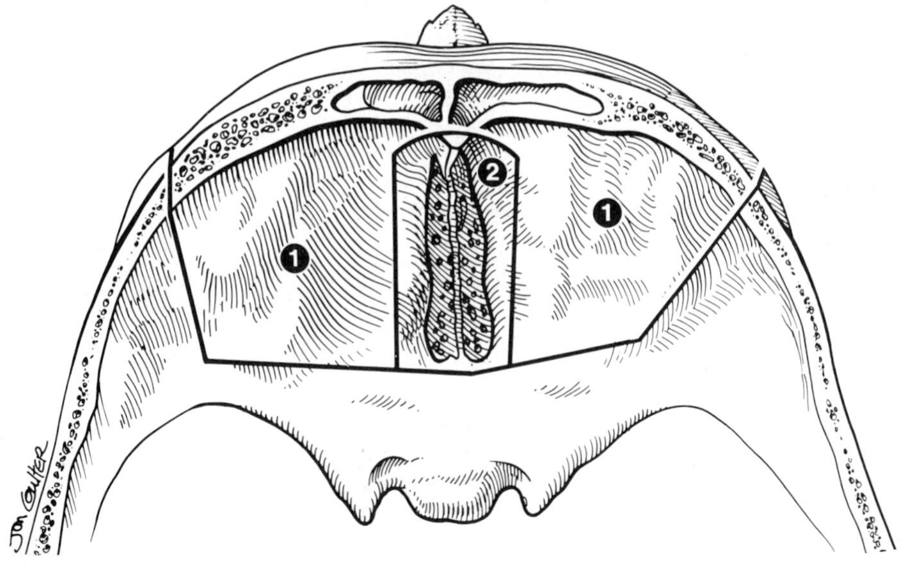

(*C*)

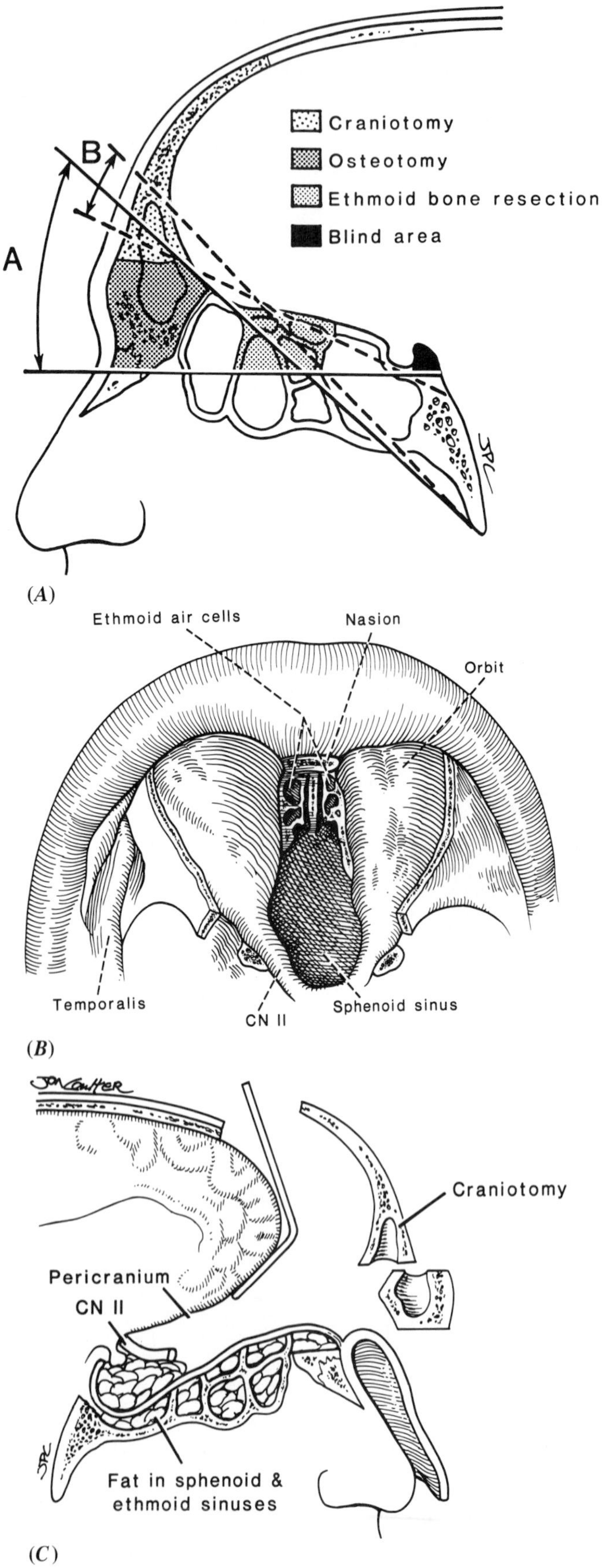

Figure 158-3 *A*. The exposure gained by the osteotomy. (From Sekhar et al.,[22] with permission.) *B*. The final exposure after orbital and optic nerve decompression. *C*. The reconstruction using a pericranial flap.

Other Benign Tumors

The extended frontal approach can be used for the removal of other benign neoplasms as well (Fig. 158-8; Table 158-1).

Anterior Communicating Artery Aneurysms

For large, giant, and complex anterior communicating complex aneurysms, and in the presence of a tight brain during early aneurysm surgery after subarachnoid hemorrhage, the extended subfrontal approach is very useful (Figs. 158-9 and 158-10). The patient is placed supine, with head extension and a 30 degree rotation to the contralateral side. A unilateral frontal craniotomy that extends to the midline and has a small temporal component is performed. A unilateral orbital osteotomy extending to the midline is then performed. Further removal of the orbital roof bone extends posteriorly to the optic nerve canal and anterior clinoid process and medially to the cribriform plate of the ethmoid bone. After the dura is opened, it is retracted inferiorly along with the orbital tissues by means of sutures. Occasionally, a retractor may also be placed on the orbital tissue.

The sylvian fissure is opened to release the frontal lobe and to identify the ipsilateral A_1 segment of the anterior cerebral artery. The ensuing approach to the aneurysm is subfrontal-transorbital, which is midway between the trans-sylvian and interhemispheric approaches. The approach can also be converted into an interhemispheric approach. With this approach, resection of gyrus rectus is minimal, brain retraction is reduced, and the angle of exposure is increased by 20 to 25 degrees.

Complications and Ways to Avoid Them

Cerebrospinal fluid leakage can occur in patients with a large dural resection and repair, especially if a transfacial resection of a malignant tumor has been performed. In such patients, the use of vascularized tissue such as a pericranial flap or radial forearm free flap is

TABLE 158-1 Lesions Operated on Using the Extended Frontal Approach

Type of Lesion	Number
Vascular lesions	
Anterior cerebral-communicating aneurysms	7
Neoplasms	
Benign	
Meningioma	13
Ossifying fibroma	3
Other lesions	5
Slow-growing malignancies	
Chordoma	16
Chondrosarcoma	4
Esthesioneuroblastoma	6
Adenoid cystic carcinoma	4
Pituitary adenoma	3
Other	3
Fast-growing malignancies	
Squamous cell carcinoma	7
Other	9
Cranial base defects	3
Total number	83

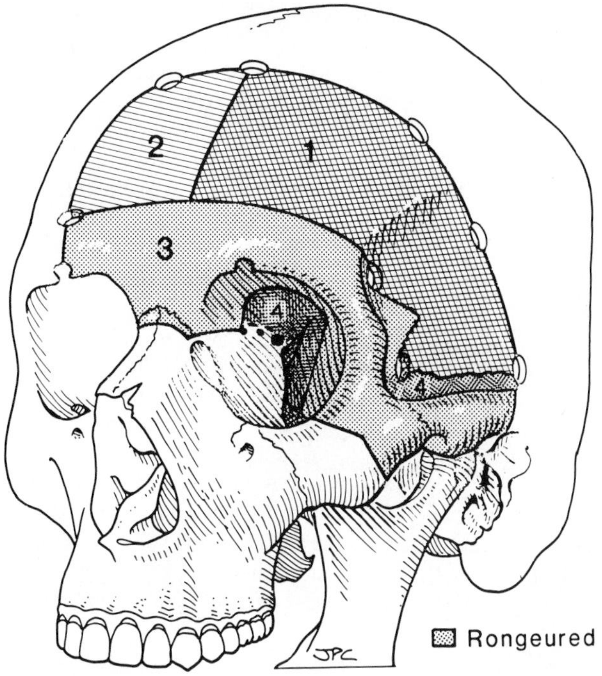

(*A*)

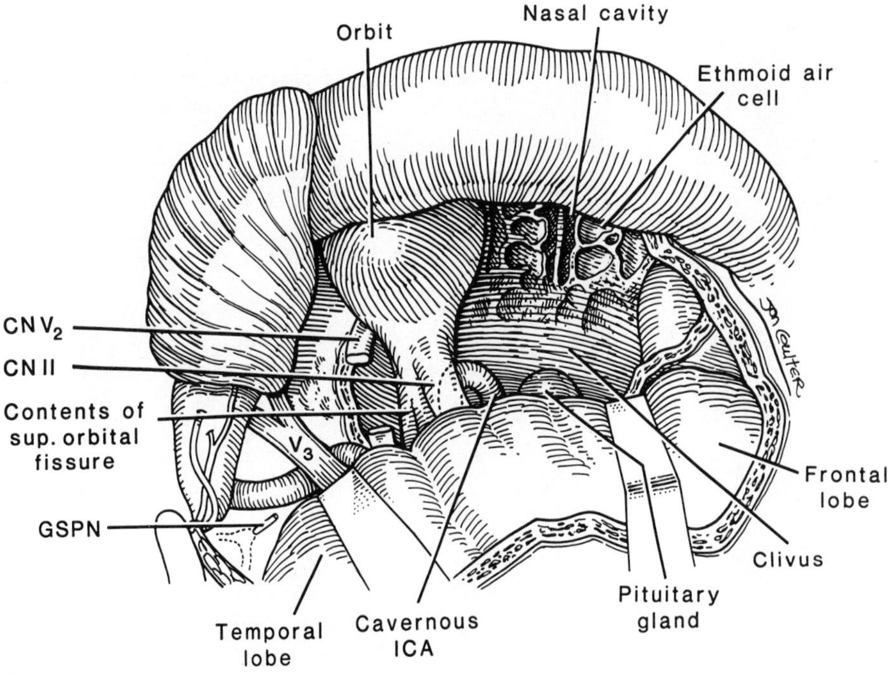

(*B*)

Figure 158-4 The combined anterior and lateral approach. *A*. The craniotomies (areas 1 and 2) and the orbitozygomatic osteotomy (area 3). *B*. The exposure obtained after tumor resection. (ICA, internal carotid artery; GSPN, greater superficial petrosal nerve). (*B* from Sekhar LN, Sen C, Snyderman CH, Janecka IP. Anterior, anterolateral, and lateral approaches to extradural petroclival tumors. In Sekhar LN, Janecka IP (eds): *Surgery of Cranial Base Tumors.* New York: Raven Press, 1993, pp 157–223, with permission.)

very important in addition to dural reconstruction. Such tissue flaps will have to be supported inferiorly by careful packing of the tumor resection cavity. Similarly, epidural infection occurs only in patients with a large cavity resulting from the resection of malignant tumors. If it does occur, the removal of the bone flap, drainage of the pus, and antibiotic treatment will be needed. It is generally not necessary to remove the orbital osteotomy segment because it is well vascularized.

As with all bifrontal operations, pneumocephalus and brain compression or shift can occur, especially if spinal fluid drainage is used. This can also lead to subsequent epidural infection. In older patients with a large volume of epidural space who have undergone the resection of a malignant nasoethmoidal tumor, if the brain is quite shrunken at the end of the operation, consideration is given to storing the bone flap in the abdominal soft tissue until the cranial base is well healed. The bone flap can be reimplanted during a subsequent, small operation.

Optic nerve injuries can occur during either the osteotomy or the tumor operation. The posterior osteotomy cut must be made just posterior to the cribriform plate of the ethmoid, with careful

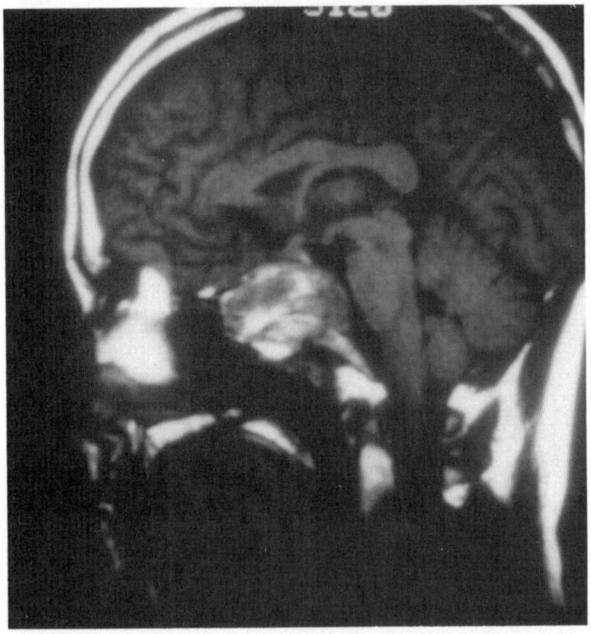

(*A*)

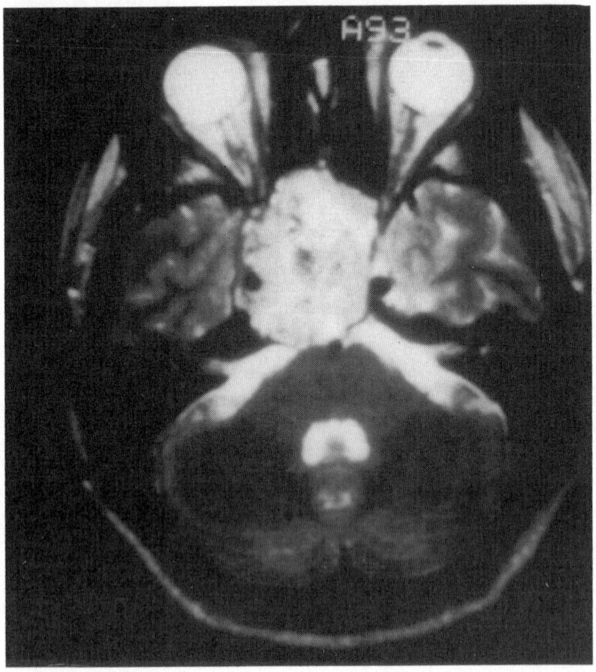

(*B*)

Figure 158-5 A clivus chordoma that was removed via the extended frontal approach. *A*. T1-weighted sagittal image. *B*. T2-weighted axial image. The lesion was resected totally.

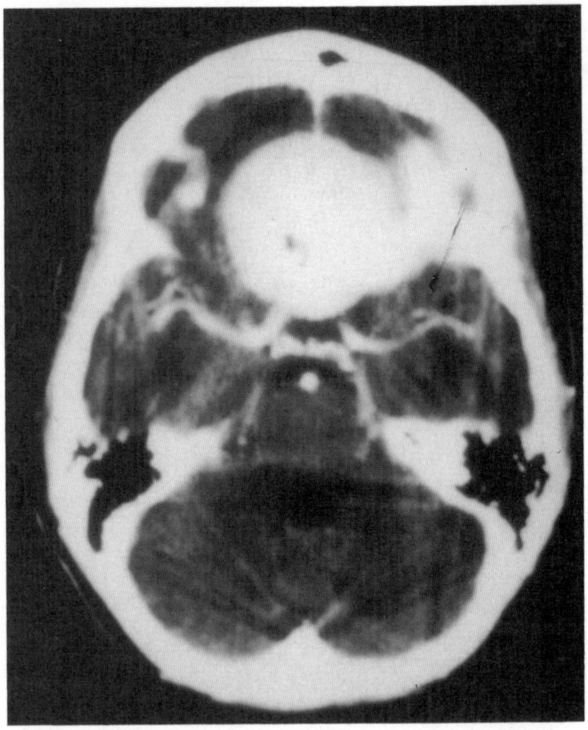

(*A*)

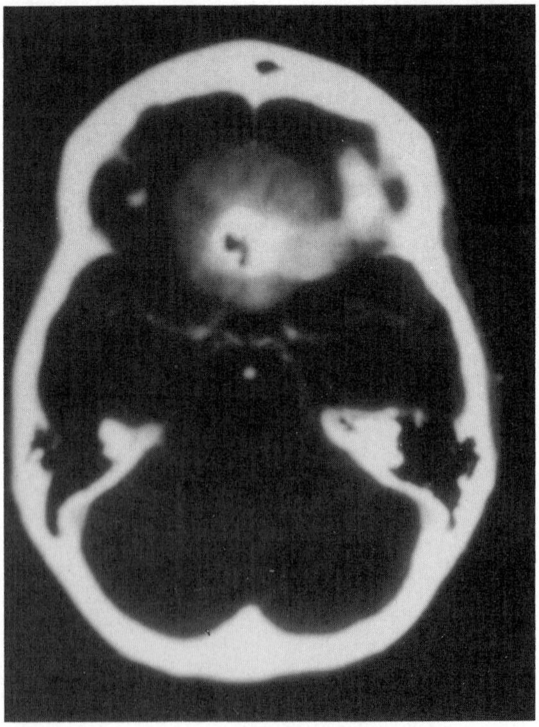

(*B*)

Figure 158-6 *A*. Olfactory groove meningioma that was removed via the extended frontal approach. *B*. Associated hyperostosis.

protection of the orbital tissue by means of a retractor. This approach will keep the bone cut in front of the optic canal. An osteotome should never be used in this area; a reciprocating saw or Midas Rex instrumentation is used. Optic nerve compression can be minimized by decompressing it carefully over a 270 degree circumference. Care must also be exercised during the reconstruction phase not to overpack the sphenoid sinus with fat, which can result in optic nerve compression (one patient in our series).

When the cavernous sinus is mostly patent, venous bleeding after tumor resection can be excessive. Overpacking with Surgicel must be avoided, since it can cause carotid artery stenosis. This occurred in two of our patients. In one it was recognized immediately because of the change in somatosensory evoked potentials, and was corrected. In the other, it was asymptomatic (recognized by MRI) and resolved with time. Injuries to cranial nerves VI and XII can occur where they cross the clival extradural space. Cranial nerve VI is particularly vulnerable near the petrous apex region.

Clinical Experience and Complications

The authors' clinical experience with the extended frontal approach for a variety of lesions is summarized in Table 158-1. Table 158-2 lists the location of the lesions and whether the extended frontal approach was used alone or in combination with other approaches. Table 158-3 lists the complications. The first series of patients were predominantly operated on at the University of Pittsburgh Hospitals, whereas the recent series were operated on mainly at the George Washington University Medical Center.

TABLE 158-2 Operative Approaches in Relation to the Location of the Lesion

	Location of Lesion*		
Operative Approach	**Anterior Base**	**Anterior and Middle Base**	**Middle and Posterior Base**
Extended frontal (EF)	9	14	4
EF + transfacial	16	12 (2)	0
EF + subtemporal-infratemporal or subtemporal-transzygomatic	0	9 (3)	18
EF + transcavernous	0	6 (2)	6 (5)
Totals	25	41	28

*Numbers in parentheses indicate the number of approaches which overlapped with other approaches.

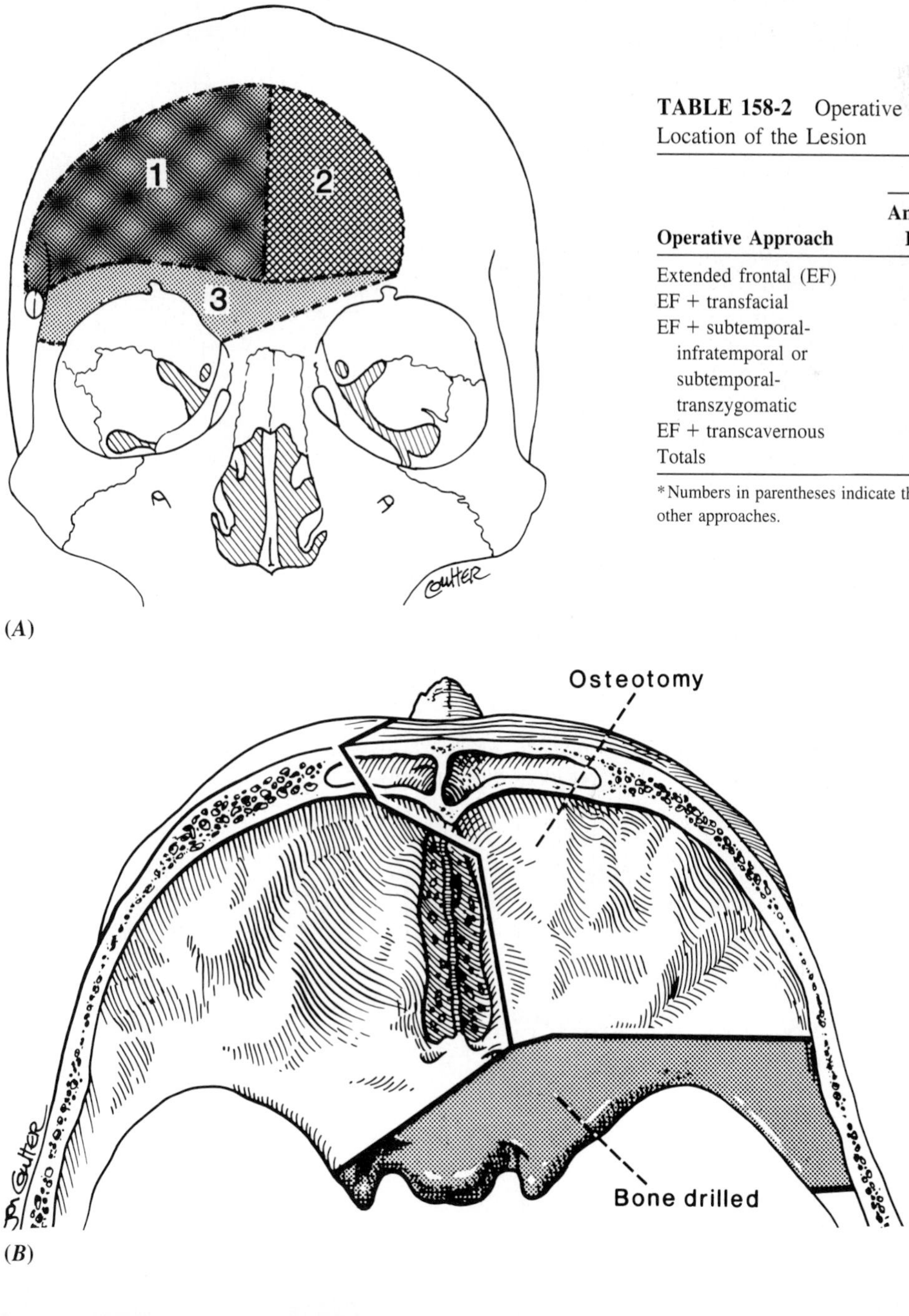

(*A*) (*B*)

Figure 158-7 *A, B.* Craniotomy and orbital osteotomy used for resecting a tumor involving the olfactory groove and planum sphenoidale region via the extended frontal approach. The olfactory groove bone may also need to be resected if involved pathologically.

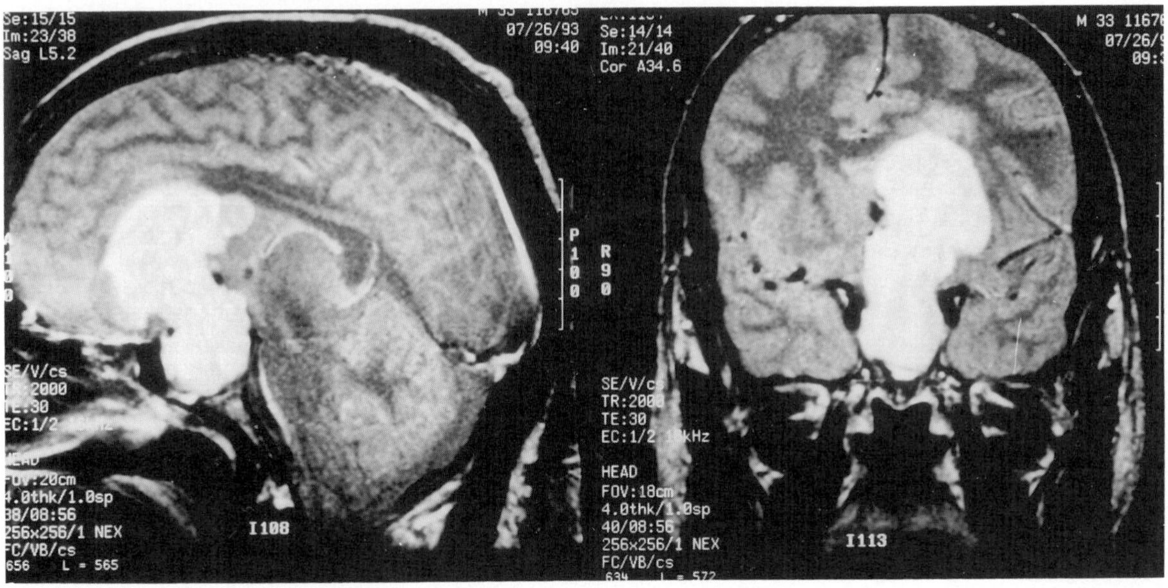

(*A*) (*B*)

Figure 158-8 *A, B.* Extensive pituitary adenoma (nonfunctioning) that was removed via a left frontotemporal and right frontal craniotomy combined with a left orbital osteotomy.

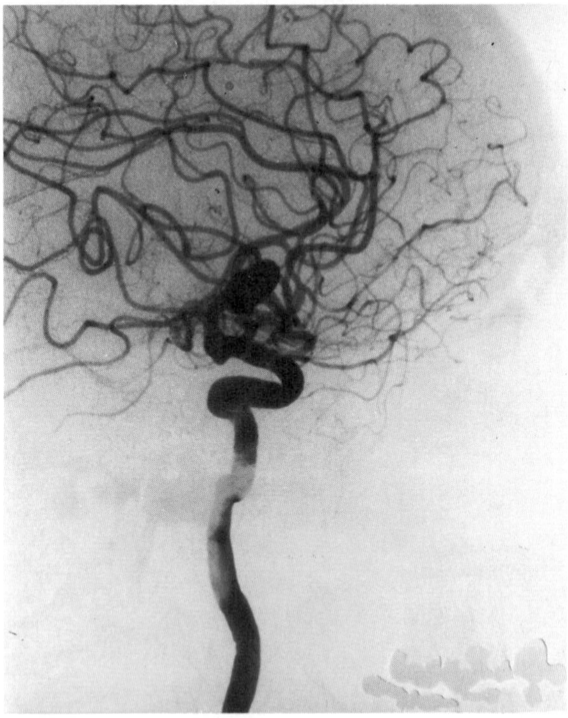

Figure 158-9 A large aneurysm of the anterior communicating artery complex treated via the extended frontal approach.

TABLE 158-3 Complications of Operations

Complication	Earlier Series (n = 49)	Recent Series (n = 34)
Death (superior mesenteric artery thrombosis)	1	—
Cerebrospinal fluid leak	2	1
Brain contusion or hematoma	4	—
Stroke due to hypotension	—	1†
Epidural abscess or infection	3	2
Transient neurological decline caused by excessive CSF drainage	2	—
Postoperative seizure	3	—
Cranial nerve palsy		
Nerve II	1*	3*
Nerves III, VI	1	1
Nerve V	1	2

*One patient in each group suffered delayed visual loss, in one case thought to be due to scar tissue and in the other to ischemic optic neuropathy.

†One patient with a tumor-occluded carotid artery suffered a stroke following significant intraoperative hypotension.

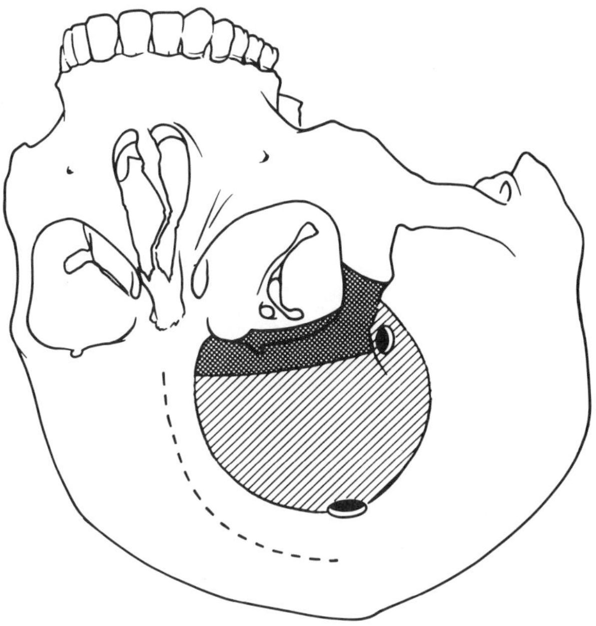

(A)

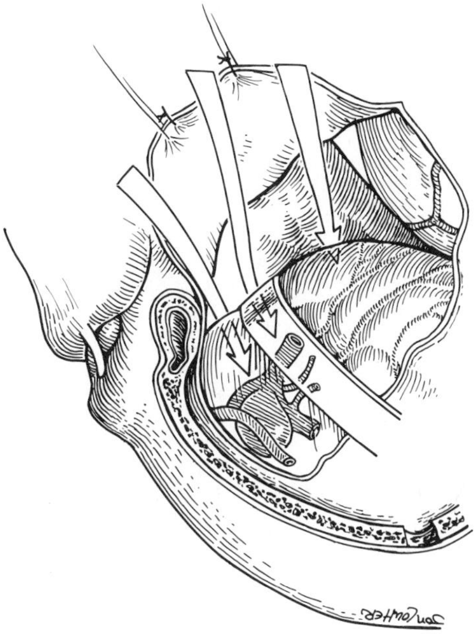

(B)

Figure 158-10 *A*. Craniotomy and orbital osteotomy for the patient shown in Fig. 158-9. *B*. Subfrontal, transorbital, and trans-sylvian approach. (From Sekhar LN, Kalia KK, Yonas H, et al. Cranial base approaches to intracranial aneurysms in the subarachnoid space. *Neurosurgery* 1994; 35:472–483, with permission.)

References

1. Alaywan M, Sindou M. Fronto-temporal approach with orbito-zygomatic removal. Surgical anatomy. *Acta Neurochir (Wien)* 1990; 104:79–83.
2. Al-Mefty O. Supraorbital-pterional approach to skull base lesions. *Neurosurgery* 1987; 21:474–477.
3. Blacklock JB, Weber RS, Lee YY, et al. Transcranial resection of tumors of the paranasal sinuses and nasal cavity. *J Neurosurg* 1989; 71:10–15.
4. Cocke EW Jr, Robertson JH, Robertson JT, et al. The extended maxillotomy and subtotal maxillectomy for excision of skull base tumors. *Arch Otolaryngol Head Neck Surg* 1990; 116:92–104.
5. Derome P. Les tumeurs spheno-ethmoïdales. Possibilités d'exérèse et de réparation chirurgicales. *Neurochirurgie* 1972; 18(Suppl 1):1–164.
6. Frazier CH. An approach to the hypophysis through the anterior cranial fossa. *Ann Surg* 1913; 57:145–150.
7. Hakuba A, Liu SS, Nishimura S. The orbitozygomatic infratemporal approach: a new surgical technique. *Surg Neurol* 1986; 26:271–276.
8. Jackson IT. Craniofacial osteotomies to facilitate the resection of tumors of the skull base. In Wilkins RH, Rengachary SS (eds): *Neurosurgery Update I.* New York: McGraw-Hill, 1990, pp 277–291.
9. Jackson IT, Marsh WR, Hide TA. Treatment of tumors involving the anterior cranial fossa. *Head Neck Surg* 1984; 6:901–913.
10. Jane JA, Park TS, Pobereskin LH, et al. The supraorbital approach: technical note. *Neurosurgery* 1982; 11:537–542.
11. Janecka IP, Sen CN, Sekhar LN, et al. Facial translocation: a new approach to the cranial base. *Otolaryngol Head Neck Surg* 1990; 103:413–419.
12. Jones NF, Schramm VL, Sekhar LN. Reconstruction of the cranial base following tumour resection. *Br J Plast Surg* 1987; 40:155–162.
13. Kawakami K, Yamanouchi Y, Kubota C, et al. An extensive transbasal approach to frontal skull-base tumors: technical note. *J Neurosurg* 1991; 74:1011–1013.
14. Ketcham AS, Hoye RC, Van Buren JM, et al. Complications of intracranial facial resection for tumors of the paranasal sinuses. *Am J Surg* 1966; 112:591–596.
15. Lang J. Anterior cranial base anatomy. In Sekhar LN, Schramm VL Jr (eds): *Tumors of the Cranial Base: Diagnosis and Treatment.* Mt Kisco, NY: Futura, 1987, pp 247–264.
16. Lesoin F, Pellerin P, Villette L, et al. Intérêt de la mobilisation du volet orbito-zygomatico-malaire. *Neurochirurgie* 1986; 32:90–93.
17. Persing JA, Jane JA, Levine PA, et al. The versatile frontal sinus approach to the floor of the anterior cranial fossa: technical note. *J Neurosurg* 1990; 72:513–516.
18. Raveh J, Vuillemin T. Advantages of an additional subcranial approach in the correction of craniofacial deformities. *J Craniomaxillofac Surg* 1988; 16:350–358.
19. Ray BS, McLean JM. Combined intracranial and orbital operation for retinoblastoma. *Arch Ophthalmol* 1943; 30:437–445.
20. Schramm VL Jr, Myers EN, Maroon JC. Anterior skull base surgery for benign and malignant disease. *Laryngoscope* 1979; 89:1077–1091.
21. Sekhar LN, Janecka IP, Jones NF. Subtemporal-infratemporal and basal subfrontal approach to extensive cranial base tumours. *Acta Neurochir (Wien)* 1988; 92:83–92.
22. Sekhar LN, Nanda A, Sen CN, et al. The extended frontal approach to tumors of the anterior, middle, and posterior skull base. *J Neurosurg* 1992; 76:198–206.
23. Smith RR, Klopp CT, Williams JM. Surgical treatment of cancer of the frontal sinus and adjacent areas. *Cancer* 1954; 7:991–994.
24. Snyderman CH, Janecka IP, Sekhar LN, et al. Anterior cranial base reconstruction: role of galeal and pericranial flaps. *Laryngoscope* 1990; 100:607–614.
25. Spetzler RF, Herman JM, Beals S, et al. Preservation of olfaction in anterior craniofacial approaches. *J Neurosurg* 1993; 79:48–52.
26. Sundaresan N, Shah JP. Craniofacial resection for anterior skull base tumors. *Head Neck Surg* 1988; 10:219–224.
27. Van Buren JM, Ommaya AK, Ketcham AS. Ten years' experience with radical combined craniofacial resection of malignant tumors of the paranasal sinuses. *J Neurosurg* 1968; 28:341–350.

159 Transfacial-Transmaxillary Approach to the Anterior Skull Base

William J. Richtsmeier
Richard L. Scher

History

Transmaxillary approaches have been employed for as long as anesthesia has been available to do them. Drommer in his review states that a horizontal osteotomy of the maxilla with successful postoperative healing was described well over 130 years ago by von Langbeck.[5] Kocher described the sagittal osteotomy in 1893 for exposure of the pituitary fossa. Simple maxillectomy is a tried and true, standard otolaryngologic procedure.

Indications

For the most part, the patients who require this approach are those with skull base tumors that extend to involve the skin of the face, orbit, or nasal complex or in which the area of involvement is so large that the operative exposure may need to be extended laterally or across the midline (Table 159-1). The most common transfacial surgical approach to this area involves the Weber-Fergusson incision, which is discussed in Chap. 157. The incision does not produce as good a result cosmetically as the facial degloving procedure or other approaches that do not incise the skin of the midface, but it provides excellent exposure of the maxillary and frontal sinuses, the orbit, and the entire nasal complex, and it can be extended laterally in the form of large cheek or temporal extensions. Tumors that begin in the maxillary-ethmoid complex and grow superiorly to involve the orbit or skull base or anteriorly to involve the skin benefit the most from this incision and approach.

Malignancies for which this approach is useful include esthesioneuroblastoma, minor salivary gland tumors, mucosal melanoma, squamous cell carcinoma, adenocarcinoma, chondrosarcoma, and osteosarcoma. Benign tumors include aggressive angiofibromas, fibrous dysplasia, small meningiomas, and inverted papillomas.

The transmaxillary approach provides good exposure to the sphenoid sinus and clivus. Patients who do not have a tumor in the sinuses or face may still need a translocation or resection of a portion of the maxilla to approach the middle skull base. If the resection is compromised by a surgical circumstance such as an inability to safely control the vasculature or to identify nerves, the following approaches are indicated. For patients who do not have a tumor in the sinuses or face but need an approach to the middle skull base through the maxilla, there are essentially two approaches. One can either perform a horizontal (Le Fort I) osteotomy,[9] mobilize the maxilla inferiorly, and approach the skull base through the opening created in the floor of the nose or alternatively, sagittally incise the hard palate, hingeing the maxilla medially on the mucosa, and approach the skull base through the maxillotomy.[3] The Le Fort I osteotomy described by Sasaki and colleagues differs from the facial degloving approach in not necessarily requiring a medial maxillectomy to give access to the posterior nose and in not requiring that the skin of the nose be lifted off of the cartilaginous pyramid.[9] However, all approaches require an understanding of the maxilla and its blood supply.

TABLE 159-1 Indications for the Transfacial-Transmaxillary Approach

Extradural (primarily) neoplasms involving the skull base and originating in the nose or sinuses
Meningoceles
Clival chordomas
Juvenile angiofibromas
Aneurysms of the mid-basilar region
Craniospinal malformations

Preoperative Evaluation

Preresection histologic evaluation of the tumor is important since the natural history of the disease and the radiosensitivity and biology of the tumor differ widely for different cell types.[2] Immunohistochemical evaluation is often needed to distinguish one tumor from another. Occasionally, electron microscopy is helpful, and material obtained at the time of biopsy should be set aside (in proper fixatives) for this study. An appropriate workup should be done to rule out lymphomas, which can involve this area but rarely if ever demand surgical intervention. In most circumstances, a transnasal biopsy can be performed so that neither the skin of the face nor the mucosa of the mouth is violated, thus avoiding a risk of tumor contamination and a potential site of recurrence. A few presentations, such as that of a clival chordoma, are either so characteristic that preresection biopsy is not necessary or lie behind bone so that it is not practicable.

Some malignant neoplasms originating in this location have a high propensity for metastases, such as osteosarcoma, melanoma, and undifferentiated carcinoma. Patients with these malignancies should have a metastatic workup, as metastatic disease can significantly shorten longevity. Despite a shortened survival with known metastasis, it should be kept in mind that many of these tumors cause severe pain due to involvement of the fifth cranial nerve or cause epistaxis or complete nasal obstruction. In these circumstances, obtaining a gross clear margin with a dry, healed cutaneous margin is a significant therapeutic triumph.

Preoperative consultation with prosthedontists is essential when one is considering a maxillary resection, so that impressions can be obtained. We have favored immediate placement of the prosthesis, although more simple obturators can be very effective. Nevertheless, full dental impressions need to be obtained prior to surgery if adequate reconstruction is to be achieved. Furthermore, the maxillary dentition should be evaluated preoperatively, especially if postoperative radiation therapy is considered, so as to avoid the possibility of osteoradionecrosis occurring around decayed teeth later.

Ophthalmologic consultation should be obtained prior to surgery in and around the ethmoid sinus, as tumors that impinge on the medial wall or floor of the orbit may require intervention that will defunctionalize the eye or may necessitate removal of the eye because of tumor involvement. If orbital exenteration is planned, it should be verified that vision in the contralateral eye is intact. The size of the defect should be estimated to indicate whether or not it will be possible to close the defect primarily, or whether it will require split-thickness skin graft or free flap coverage. Appropriate consultation should be obtained in the latter circumstance.

Most tumors present in such a way that there is ample time for the above consultation and testing. During this period, consideration should be given to autologous blood donation.

Relevant Anatomy and Physiology

The maxilla has both the structure and the physiology of a sinus, and this fact must be considered in choosing an approach to the skull base. One must appreciate the mucocillary transport pattern of the ethmoid and maxillary sinuses, in which mucus flow originates in the lateral inferior portion of the sinus, proceeds superiorly in all directions to the roof of the sinus, and then moves medially toward the natural ostia of the maxillary sinus.[6] Inferior meatal antrostomies do not change this pattern but can interrupt it by creating physical barriers. Incisions into the sinus should be planned so that normal mucocillary transport can continue after healing. If a medial maxillectomy is performed, it is important to include the natural ostia of the maxillary sinus, so that mucus is not trapped in the sinus by recirculation. Inferior turbinates are capable of swelling to enormous proportions after trauma, and adhesions to undesired parts of the nose are common if the swelling is not contained. It should be remembered that the lacrimal system traverses the anterior portion of the maxillary bone and exits under the inferior turbinate. An incision into the inferolateral portion of the nasal vestibule should be below the point of entry of the lacrimal duct if possible.

Blood is supplied to the posterior maxilla through the internal maxillary artery, which is the last branch of the external carotid artery before the superficial temporal artery (Fig. 159-1). This artery enters posteriorly and passes into the hard palate via the greater palatal foramen. There is considerable anastomosis via the facial and ascending pharyngeal artery systems. The maxilla can survive on the internal maxillary artery alone, but an atherosclerotic artery may not stay patent after being rotated through 90 degrees. The internal maxillary artery produces several important branches medially, including the middle meningeal and accessory meningeal arteries. In the pterygoid region, it passes upward and forward through the infratemporal fossa, sinking between the two heads of the external pterygoid muscle as it moves anteriorly into the pterygopalatine fossa. It sends branches to the masseteric, the temporal, the pterygoid, and the buccal muscles; the branches travel with the distribution of the maxillary nerve. The pterygopalatine portion of the internal maxillary artery provides major arteries to the maxilla and maxillary teeth, the nasal cavities, and the palate. It produces the posterior superior alveolar artery, the infraorbital artery, the descending palatine artery, the artery of the pterygoid canal, and the pharyngeal and sphenopalatine arteries. Again, each artery travels with a branch of the second division of the trigeminal nerve. It is the descending palatine (greater palatine) artery that passes through the greater palatine foramen and gives branches to the soft palate and the alveolar process of the maxilla.

The second division of the trigeminal nerve enters the posterior midface through the foramen rotundum. In the pterygopalatine

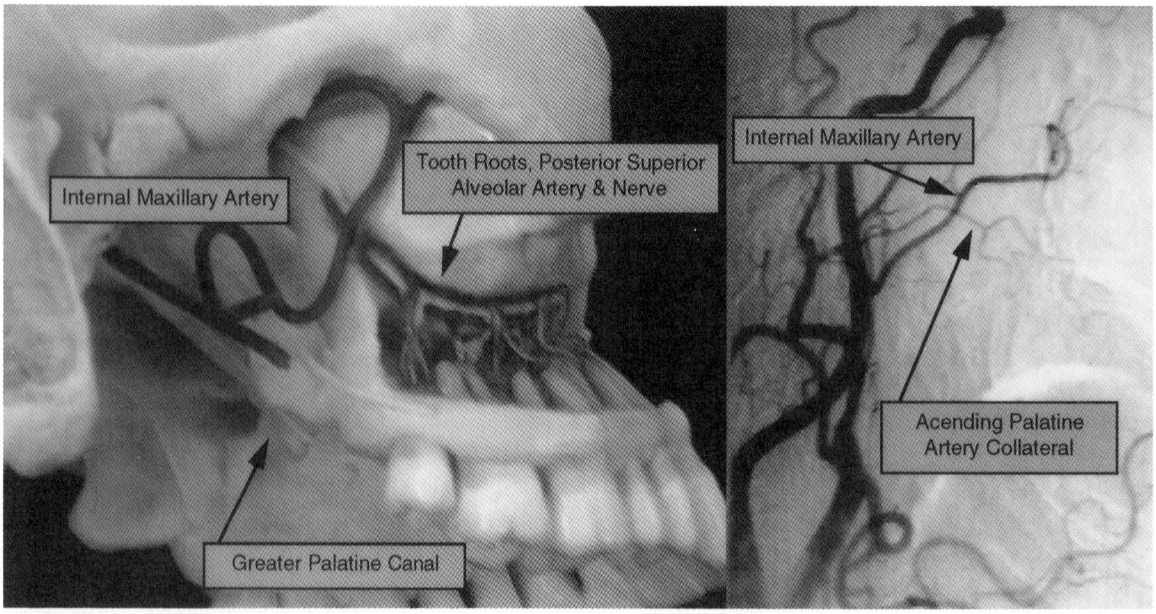

Figure 159-1 The relevant blood supply to the posterior, lower maxilla.

fossa it gives two major branches, one following the infraorbital groove and eventually giving sensation to the anterior cheek, upper lip, and dentition, and the other extending to the sphenopalatine ganglion and giving sensation to the posterior nose and palate.

Radiologic Workup

The radiologic assessment of patients with problems in this area routinely includes coronal and axial computed tomography (CT) scans. Coronal scans assess the relationship of the sinuses and nasal cavity to the skull base. Contrast enhancement is usually employed, but it does not always help to delineate tumors, as mucosal elements may show substantial contrast enhancement even under normal circumstances. In addition to the soft tissue films usually provided, bone windows are essential to evaluate tumor invasion of bone. Magnetic resonance imaging (MRI) makes it possible to differentiate between tumor and obstructed sinuses as well as routinely providing adequate identification of the vasculature. In addition, sagittal images can be obtained with this modality, which is not easy with CT. MRI also has the advantage of potentially detailing soft tissue intracranial penetration and identifying specific cranial nerve or cavernous sinus involvement. Angiography in one form or another may be helpful in determining whether tumor involves the artery itself or creates extravascular compression, and in many cases in which the posterior nasal vault is involved, preoperative balloon occlusion measurements with appropriate monitoring can identify whether or not the internal carotid artery can be sacrificed. Angiography is often helpful in evaluating basilar artery lesions[1] or situations where tumor involvement of the cavernous sinus may be unclear from CT or MRI.

Le Fort I (Horizontal) Osteotomy

Anesthesia

Patients requiring this surgery usually present no difficulty with craniocervical stabilization and can undergo a routine induction and endotracheal oral intubation. The oral tube will need to be removed to maximally displace the maxilla inferiorly, and therefore tracheostomy is often indicated after conventional induction. Routine monitoring and support for long operations should be employed, to minimize the chances of thrombophlebitis, measure urinary output, and assess the hemodynamics of the patient.

Room Setup

The anesthesia team is usually positioned inferiorly and to the patient's left, where they have access to an arm, giving the surgical team exposure from the left shoulder circumferentially around to the right chest. This arrangement allows the surgeon to stand either above the patient, working cephalad towards himself or herself, or on the patient's right side in the more traditional orientation. The retractors are routinely displaced more superiorly in their deep portions than at the nasal opening, and, therefore, a microscope with a built-in angle will help if the surgeon chooses to stand at the head of the operating table. Since the procedure is carried out through the mouth and nasal cavities, it is not realistic to achieve asepsis with any preparative material. Patients with unusually poor oral hygiene should have it attended to by a dental colleague prior to surgery.

Operative Technique

After the patient is properly positioned and draped, the nasal mucosa is decongested with pledgets soaked in oxymetazoline. The mucosa of the septum, floor, and lateral wall of the nose and the gingivobuccal sulcus are infiltrated with a solution containing 1:200,000 epinephrine, taking into account that there is a substantial surface area to be injected. The patients are given an infusion of agents to control organisms commonly encountered in the mouth and sinuses, which include *Pneumococcus, Staphylococcus aureus,* and anaerobes. We routinely use intravenous cefazolin and metronidazole.

An incision is then made in the gingivobuccal sulcus across the entire upper jaw, allowing 2 or 3 mm of free mucosa in the sulcus for suturing at closure.[9] The mucoperiosteum is elevated off the nasal floor and up over the canine fossa to the posterior aspect of the maxilla. An air-driven oscillating saw is then used to horizontally section the maxilla at the level shown in Fig. 159-2, taking care to avoid the lacrimal apparatus and the dental roots.

At this point, the maxilla is still stable because of its posterior attachments. Miniplates are applied across the saw cuts for postoperative stabilization, as shown in Fig. 159-3. As soon as they are placed, they are removed. The nasal septum is divided with a chisel to separate it from the maxillary spine and crest. The pterygoid plates are cut with a curved chisel, completing the Le Fort I osteotomy. At this point the maxilla can be down-fractured, exposing the mucosa of the nasal floor. The blood supply of the maxilla is provided by the greater palatine arteries and by smaller pharyngeal vessels, branches of the ascending pharyngeal arteries which arise from the faucial arches.

Primary exposure for the access to the nose is now complete, and the next step is an incision in the mucosa of the floor of the nose. The shape of this incision depends on whether the lesion is unilateral or bilateral and on whether it will be necessary to resect portions of the posterior aspect of the maxilla and/or septum. Where only an approach to the skull base is needed, the posterior portion of the septum can be excised and the anterior portion deflected laterally, with care being taken not to fracture the perpendicular plate of the ethmoid, which could cause an anterior cerebrospinal fluid (CSF) leak. The posterior aspects of the inferior turbinates may be removed with relative impunity to improve exposure. A transoral retractor is placed to provide adequate exposure; it can be either the Crockard retractor or a modified Dingman retractor. The Crockard retractor has the advantage of being able to place additional retracting arms circumferentially, whereas the Dingman only allows lateral retraction. Usually the smallest tongue blade is used, and it presses inferiorly on the maxilla. Every 30 min during the operation, the retractor is released for 2 min to compensate for any problems with circulation to the maxilla.

The posterior septum is followed to the face of the sphenoid and the upper portion of the clivus. The mucosal incision is extended, allowing for lateralization of the mucosal flaps, and lateral retractors are placed. The floor of the sphenoid sinus may be removed if necessary. In the posterior aspect of the sphenoid, indentations of the optic nerves and internal carotid arteries can often be observed; the bone over them may be dehiscent even under normal circumstances.

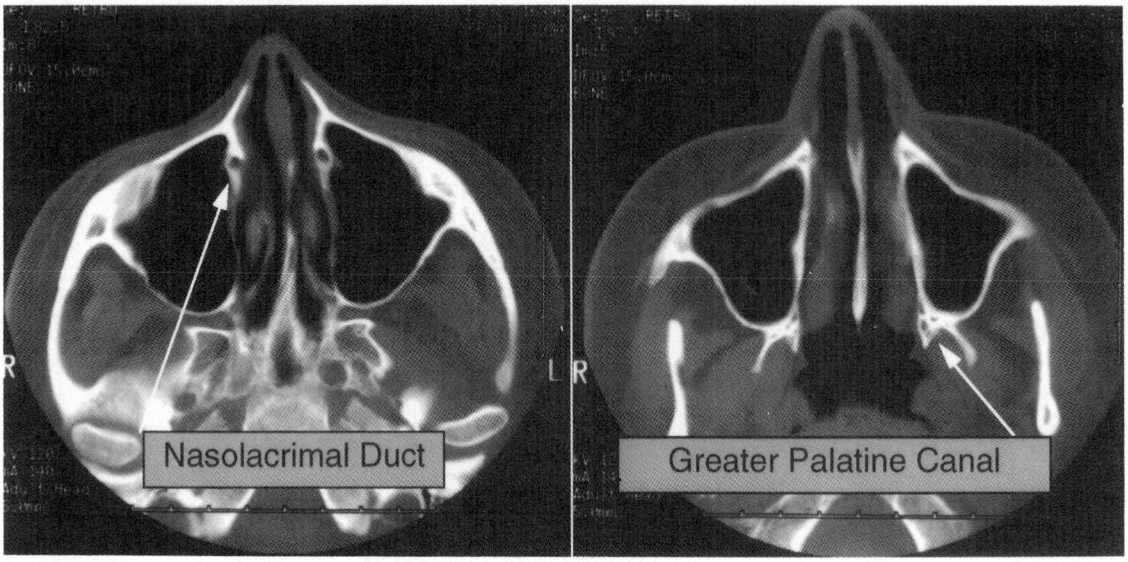

Figure 159-2 Axial CT scans through the level of the Le Fort I osteotomy (*right*) and the level immediately above the osteotomy (*left*).

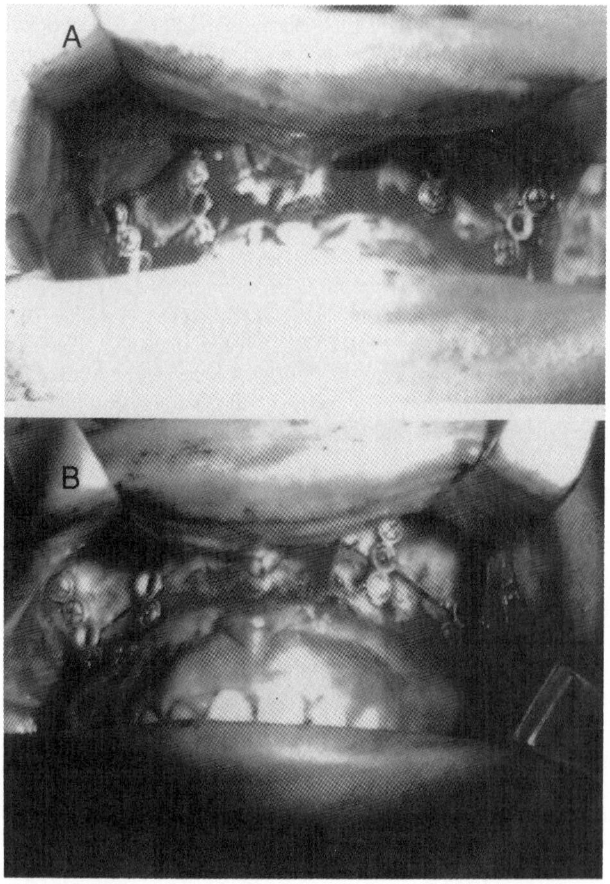

Figure 159-3 Two views of the anterior osteotomies and miniplate fixation of the Le Fort I osteotomy. *A*. View before completion of the osteotomy. *B*. View after completion of the resection and closure demonstrating the exact repair that ensures normal occlusion.

Crockard and Sen have proposed a midline split of the hard and soft palate to hinge each hemimaxilla laterally to increase the vertical dimension of the field.[4] The increased time required for exposure, a more challenging wound closure, and potential problems with soft palate function must be weighed against the advantage of a larger field.

A high-speed drill with a cutting burr is used to remove the bone of the clivus, which is often quite thick. Veins that communicate with the cavernous sinus may be encountered and need to be packed with bone wax or microfibrillar collagen. The clivus is drilled until cortical bone on its inner surface is identified. Bone across the entire surgical field is then thinned out until the width required for the surgical procedure is exposed. Finally, the inner cortical bone is thinned with a diamond burr, and the thin bone is gently removed with a dissector and Kerrison forceps. Significant bleeding may be encountered during final bone removal. Extradural tumors should be exposed by this point, care having been taken previously to identify the position of the carotid arteries and cranial nerves.

Dural integrity should be secured during closure, which may include the use of fascia, fat graft, microfibrillar collagen, or oxidized regenerated cellulose. Suturing in the traditional manner is difficult owing to the inaccessibility and thinness of the dura. The mucosal flaps are approximated with polyglactic acid sutures if possible, using a horizontal mattress stitch. A substance that can be packed over the mucosal closure and that will not adhere to it, such as Xeroform (bismuth tribromophenate; Sherwood Medical, St Louis, MO) petrolatum dressing is usually used. Subsequently, a traditional packing of either antibiotic-impregnated gauze or expandable sponge can be employed over the Xeroform petrolatum gauze to apply hemostatic pressure. Debris is evacuated from the rest of the surgical site, especially the maxillary sinuses. The hard palate is returned to its original position, and the titanium plates are reinserted to secure the upper jaw in its exact preoperative position. The oral mucosa is closed with interrupted absorbable sutures. The nasal septum is returned to its original position and sutured in place where appropriate, and the mucosa of the floor of the nose is packed into position anteriorly. As it is difficult to secure hemostasis in a nose with a nasogastric tube, an oral gastric tube is placed; initially it is used to evacuate the blood that may drain into the stomach, and then it is used for feeding once the period of nausea has passed.

Postoperative Management

As soon as the patient is awake and alert—at least by the second postoperative day—the tracheostomy tube can be changed to a noncuffed metal tube, which is easier to manage and allows speech. Many patients will prefer to breathe through the tracheostomy until their nasal packing is removed on the fifth postoperative day. Antibiotic coverage is continued until the nasal packs are removed, since the sinuses are often impacted with blood and provide a ready nutrient reservoir for any pathogen. Analgesia is initially provided with a pump, but oral medicines are substituted as soon as possible to allow for early ambulation in patients who can cooperate. Patients who are unable to ambulate wear sequential compression stockings.

Potential Complications

Potential complications for this procedure are listed in Table 159-2. Complications such as malocclusion, nonunion and late sinusitis can often be attributed to technical errors, and one way to minimize this problem is to use surgeons familiar with each area. Therefore, a surgical team composed of a neurosurgeon and an otolaryngologist–head and neck surgeon is often employed.

Bleeding may be encountered, particularly in and around the clivus, owing to the patient's anatomy. It is not uncommon for the mucosal incisions of the nose to lose a unit of blood, but rarely does this necessitate transfusion. The combined blood loss, however, may necessitate transfusion, and therefore in elective cases for nonmalignant tumors, autologous blood donation should be strongly considered. A compromised blood supply during surgery resulting in ischemic necrosis of the maxilla is uncommon,[8] but in patients who have been previously irradiated for malignancy, a late complication of osteoradionecrosis should be watched for and dealt with aggressively if there are signs such as exposed, nonhealing bone, persistent severe pain, or direct evidence of soft tissue necrosis. Cervical emphysema has been reported for Le Fort I osteotomy but should be minimal in a patient with a tracheostomy.

TABLE 159-2 Potential Complications of the Transfacial-Transmaxillary Approach

Malocclusion
Nonunion
Anosmia
Bleeding
Intraoperative (autologous blood should be obtained beforehand in patients with nonmalignant tumors)
Epistaxis
Chronic sinusitis
Infection
Loss of sinus mucocillary transport
Sinus ostia stenosis
Adhesions to turbinates
Nasal airway stenosis
Epiphora
Ischemic necrosis of maxilla
Compromised from retraction
Osteoradionecrosis
Incised tooth root
Insensate maxilla or teeth
Cervical emphysema
CSF leak—meningitis

Maxillotomy (Sagittal Osteotomy)

The maxillotomy procedure described by Cocke and colleagues,[3] and its management are very similar to those for the Le Fort I osteotomy, although the maxilla is retracted medially instead of inferiorly. An oral endotracheal tube can be used, although many surgeons prefer the safety and convenience of a tracheostomy. The room setup and patient preparation are similar to those for the Le Fort I osteotomy.

Procedure

In the case of large tumors, the approach to the more superior aspects of the maxilla is provided through either a modified Weber-Fergusson incision or a facial degloving. Small tumors can be approached through a sublabial incision, with extension as needed. Where extreme lateral exposure is required, the modified Weber-Fergusson incision is superior because its superior portion can be turned laterally into a subciliary incision to create a large, laterally based flap.

The maxillectomy, a standard otolaryngologic procedure,[7] is seldom the procedure of choice unless there is direct tumor involvement of the hard palate. Where appropriate, a vertical incision is made through the mucoperiosteum of the anterior maxilla. This incision is carried up to engage the nose and into the oral cavity, where it follows the alveolus laterally. Where the hemimaxilla is to be sacrificed, the incision should follow the gingiva around the teeth, maximizing the mucosa available for closure later. A similar lateral incision around the alveolus will allow primary closure of the palatal defect. If the maxilla is to be retraced inferomedially, then the palate incision is not used. Simple osteotomies through the lateral maxilla, posterior maxillary sinus ostia, and pterygoid plates will remove the hemimaxilla and give adequate exposure to the unilateral infratemporal fossa and nasal space. Additional exposure can be obtained by resecting portions of the zygomatic arch and/or attachments of the masseter muscle.

The sagittal maxillotomy technique is similar to that described above for the maxillectomy except that there are no hard palate mucosal incisions. A gingivobuccal incision is made so that the lateral maxilla can be incised. As in the horizontal maxillotomy, miniplates assure the return of the palate to the preoperative position at closure. The mucoperiosteum of the floor of the nose is elevated so that an oscillating saw cut can be made just lateral to the maxillary crest, with care taken not to cut the mucoperiosteum of the hard palate. The fibromuscular attachment of the soft palate to the pterygoid plates and hard palate is divided to expose the nasopharynx. A Gigli saw can be placed to make the posterior cut into the nasal cavity, thus allowing the maxilla to be removed from its osseous attachments and reflected contralaterally. This cut divides the descending and the posterior superior alveolar arteries, the terminal blood supply to the lower maxilla, which now relies on collateral flow through the mucosa of the hard palate. The exposure provided by the sagittal osteotomy is narrower than that obtained with the Le Fort I osteotomy, and it does not give bilateral access unless the septum is resected.

Closure is similar to that for the Le Fort I osteotomy, the palate being returned to its original position and secured with miniplates. Mucosal closure is performed with absorbable suture material such as chromic gut. If the hemimaxilla is removed and the mucosa is preserved up to the gingiva medially and laterally, a primary closure can usually be achieved, which makes the postoperative course for the patient less complicated and obviates the need for an obturator. Direct observation of the cavity is negated by primary closure, but flexible and telescopic examination of the nose and sinuses make this a less important issue today. The nose is packed as described for the Le Fort I osteotomy. Postoperative care is similar, keeping the patients on 6 weeks of liquid or soft diet.

Potential complications are similar to those for the horizontal maxillotomy, but the chance of losing an incisor tooth at the osteotomy site is greater.

References

1. Archer DJ, Young S, Uttley, D. Basilar aneurysms: a new transclival approach via maxillotomy. *J Neurosurg* 1987; 67:54–58.
2. Batsakis JG. *Tumors of the Head and Neck: Clinical and Pathological Considerations,* 2d ed. Baltimore: Williams & Wilkins, 1979.
3. Cocke EW Jr, Robertson JH, Robertson JT, Crook JP. The extended maxillotomy and subtotal maxillectomy for excision of skull base tumors. *Arch Otolaryngol Head Neck Surg* 1990; 116:92–104.
4. Crockard HA, Sen CN. The transoral approach for the management of intradural lesions at the craniovertebral junction: review of 7 cases. *Neurosurgery* 1991; 28:88–98.
5. Drommer RB. The history of the "Le Fort I osteotomy." *J Maxillofac Surg* 1986; 14:119–122.
6. Kennedy DW, Zeinrich SJ. The functional endoscopic approach to inflammatory sinus disease: current perspectives and technique modification. *Am J Rhinol* 1988; 2:89–96.
7. Loré JM Jr. Partial and radical Maxillectomy. *Otolaryngol Clin North Am* 1976; 9:255–267.
8. Nelson RL, Path MG, Ogle RG, et al. Quantitation of blood flow after Le Fort I osteotomy. *J Oral Surg* 1977; 35:10–16.
9. Sasaki CT, Lowlicht RA, Astrachan DI, et al. Le Fort I osteotomy approach to the skull base. *Laryngoscope* 1990; 100:1073–1076.

160 Transoral Approaches to the Clivus and Upper Cervical Spine

Arnold H. Menezes

The early pathologic descriptions of abnormalities affecting the clivus and upper cervical spine came from autopsy studies.[22] It was only after the radiographic studies of basilar invagination in 1939 by Chamberlain that the bony abnormalities affecting this region were considered as a clinical entity rather than pathologic and anatomic curiosities.[19] The surgical treatment of irreducible craniovertebral junction (CVJ) compressive pathology was posterior enlargement of foramen magnum and removal of the posterior arch of the atlas and axis. The postoperative mortality and morbidity associated with such treatment at the brain stem and upper cervical cord were high. In 1951, Scoville and Sherman stated that "the angulation of the medulla over an abnormally high odontoid process is the chief offender and causation of neurological signs and disability in platybasia. Future surgical advance lies in the development of successful removal of the odontoid, possibly through the mouth."[31] A transoral approach through the posterior pharyngeal wall had been used for drainage of retropharyngeal abscesses for many years. Although this route provided access to the CVJ, it had not gained its well-deserved place in the neurosurgical armamentarium because of initial reports of infection, limited exposure, cerebrospinal fluid (CSF) leakage, vertebral artery injury, and unacceptable patient morbidity and mortality. Fang and Ong, in 1962, reported their direct anterior approach to the upper cervical spine for the treatment of atlantoaxial instability and fusion, as well as tuberculous lesions.[8] Over the past three decades, the value of the anterior cervical approach to lesions of the ventral spinal canal has been defined in several disorders, including abnormalities of the clivus and the upper cervical spine with ventral compression of the brain stem and cervical cord.[18] Variations of the operation include combinations with lateral rhinotomy, the trans-sphenoidal operation, mandibular split with median glossotomy, and transpalatal approaches.[18,19] Despite the various approaches available, the adequate surgical exposure and successful removal with minimal postoperative morbidity of lesions that arise in the clivus and anterior upper cervical spine present a challenge (Fig. 160-1).[1,3,6,9,10,13–15,17,26,30,32,34,36,38]

In 1977, a surgical physiologic approach to correct pathology secondary to abnormality of the CVJ was presented formally by the author.[22] Using these guidelines, the high morbidity and mortality previously attendant with posterior decompression of ventrally placed lesions was not seen. The factors that influenced specific treatment were

1. the etiology of the lesion; whether it was bony or soft tissue, tumor or vascular;
2. the direction and mechanics of compression of the neural structures;
3. whether the bony abnormality could be reduced to its normal position; and
4. the associated neural abnormalities present.

The primary treatment of reducible lesions of the craniocervical junction (CCJ) is stabilization. Surgical decompression is required in patients with irreducible pathology causing compression of the cervicomedullary junction (CMJ), the transoral-transpalatopharyngeal approach being the procedure of choice for ventral decompression. This approach has been utilized in 263 individuals ranging in age from 4 to 82 years, 83 of whom were children.

Indications for Transoral Approaches

The primary indication for a transoral-transpalatopharyngeal approach to the clivus and upper cervical spine is ventral irreducible compression of the CMJ, a condition caused by a bony abnormality, a soft tissue epidural mass such as granulation tissue and tumor, and, rarely, an intradural ventral mass at the foramen magnum that defies treatment utilizing other surgical approaches.[1,3,5,20,24,27,29,37] Mere identification of a ventral abnormality at the CCJ, such as rheumatoid cranial settling, does not form an indication for a transoral operation. Except in the case of tumors, ventral operative decompression is of questionable value unless reduction of the lesion has been attempted by cervical traction. Of the 252 patients with rheumatoid basilar invagination and cranial settling in our surgical experience, only 53 required a ventral decompression. The remaining patients in this series had reduction with cervical traction and required only posterior stabilization.

Patients with a Chiari malformation and atlanto-occipital assimilation with basilar invagination require ventral decompression and subsequent dorsal decompression together with rerouting of CSF pathways to improve the CSF circulation. The primary approach to intra-arachnoid lesions should not be transoral unless other approaches have proven ineffective.[19] Numerous patients referred to our facility with clivus chordoma, meningioma, and schwannoma have undergone posterolateral procedures combined with middle and posterior fossa operations with complete surgical resection of the tumor (Fig. 160-1).[19,23,24,32,33]

The disadvantage of the transoral-transpalatopharyngeal approach is that access to the lateral extensions is limited by the position of the alveolar ridges of the maxilla.[3] This is especially true in distortion of the buccal cavity with severe craniofacial deformities. In such a situation, an extended maxillotomy that utilizes a transverse osteotomy at the LeFort I level accompanied by a midline sagittal split of both the maxilla and the soft palate allows for radical exposure of the base of the skull and upper cervical spine.[3,19] This has been utilized by the author, however in only four individuals who are not included in this series.

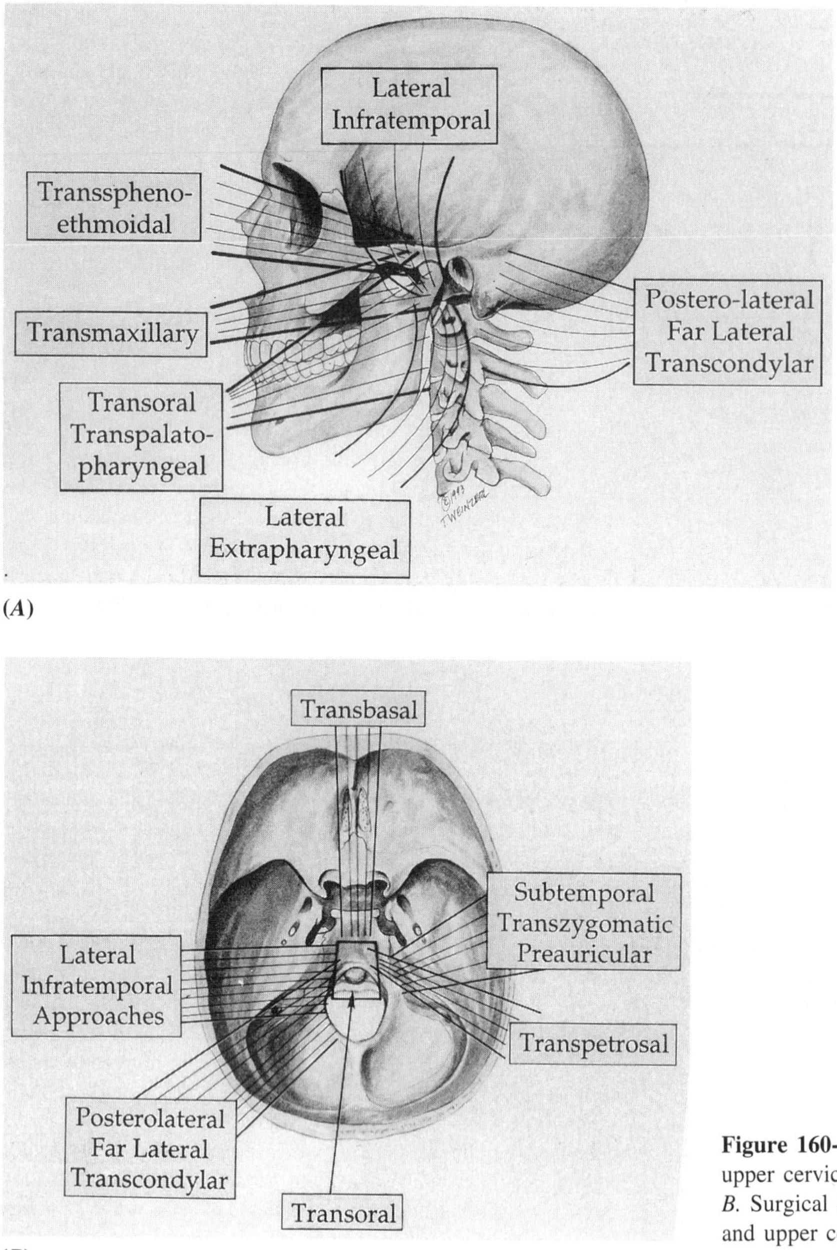

(*A*)

(*B*)

Figure 160-1 *A.* Surgical approaches to the clivus and upper cervical spine as seen on a lateral projection. *B.* Surgical approaches to the clivus, foramen magnum, and upper cervical spine as viewed from within the cranial base.

The term *median labial mandibular glossotomy* was coined in 1961 by Martin et al., who reintroduced the procedure for excision of midline lesions at the base of the tongue and posterior pharyngeal wall.[16] In 1980, Wood et al. described "median labial mandibular glossotomy, soft palate split, and hard palate resection" for selected congenital and acquired lesions of this area.[38] This author believes that the neurosurgical indications for this approach are extremely limited. The transoral-transpalatopharyngeal approach with an extended palatal incision serves the purpose in resection of lesions of the clivus, as well as those of the CVJ and the upper cervical spine. A median glossotomy extends the exposure to the C4 level, and when combined with a median mandibulotomy, usually in head and neck cancers, affords extensive lateral exposure.[1,5,11,25]

The transpalatal extension of the transoral-transpharyngeal approach adds significantly to the operative exposure; submucoparosteal dissection along the vomer allows a trans-sphenoidal or a transclival approach to midline skull base lesions, a technique especially useful in children because, unlike the standard sublabial trans-septal approach to the sphenoid and upper clivus, it does not disturb the forward growth of the face.

Investigative Studies

Modern neurodiagnostic techniques have enabled the accurate definition of the site and extension of lesions in the clivus and upper cervical spine, thereby opening this region to a number of new surgical approaches. The CCJ can be likened to a funnel that may be approached via various routes along its circumference in a rostral-caudal dimension. The neurodiagnostic procedures performed must complement each other and provide anatomic, pathologic, and biomechanical information for planning the surgical approach.

Plain roentgenograms of the skull and cervical spine are essential for recognition of the bony pathology, as well as for identification of oropharyngeal abnormalities that have a bearing on the surgical technique to be utilized. Paget's disease, osteogenesis imperfecta, platybasia, basilar invagination, Klippel–Feil syndrome, os odontoideum, and osseous tumors of the skull base are easily visualized on plain radiographs. In addition, instability of the CVJ and upper cervical spine is readily recognized by documenting reducibility with the flexed and extended positions. The neurodiagnostic procedure of choice is thin-section magnetic resonance imaging (MRI), accomplished in the coronal, sagittal and parasagittal, and axial planes to best identify neural, as well as osseous, abnormalities (Fig. 160-2*A*–*C*).[28] The flexed and extended positions must be viewed in the paracentral and midsagittal planes in both T1- and T2-weighted images. Suboptimal bone detail, the drawback of MRI, is best supplemented by dynamic pluridirectional tomography in the frontal and lateral planes, including the lateral flexed and extended positions (Fig. 160-2*D*–*G*).[19] When complemented by thin-section computed tomography (CT), these studies define the bony abnormalities in detail, as well as demonstrate abnormal biomechanical and translation forces, and the effect of cervical traction. In rheumatoid involvement of the CVJ, as well as with os odontoideum and atlantoaxial instability with associated ventral cervicomedullary compression, an MRI-compatible halo should be used to document the effects of cervical traction and the attempts to achieve reduction.

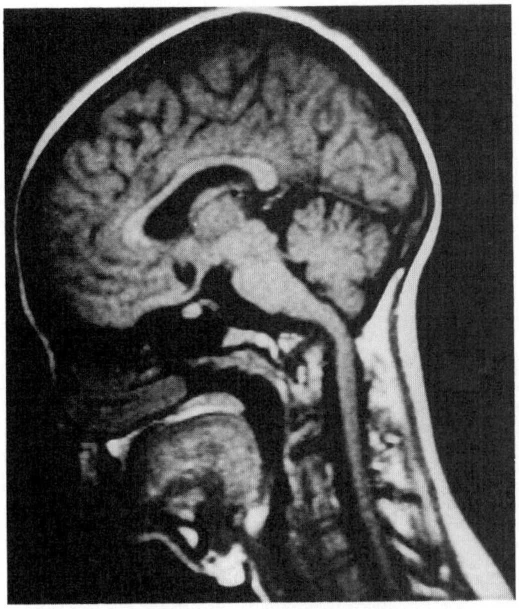
(A)

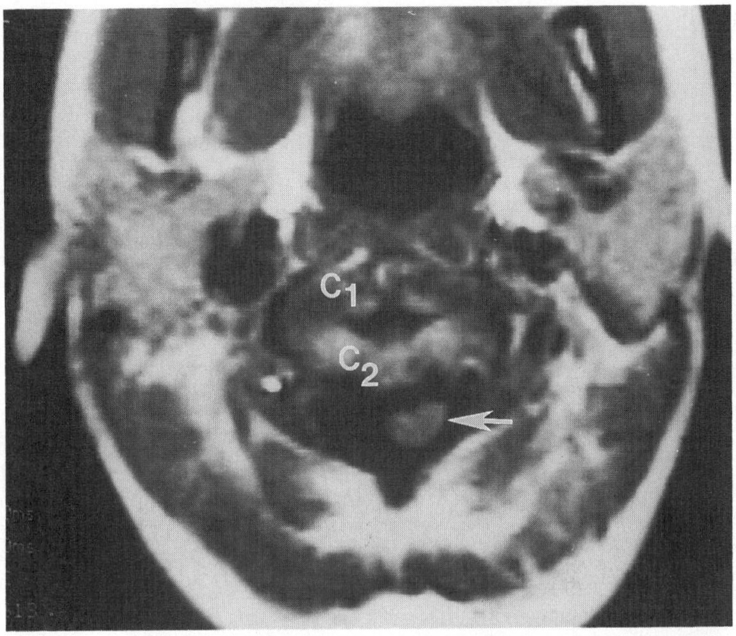

(B)

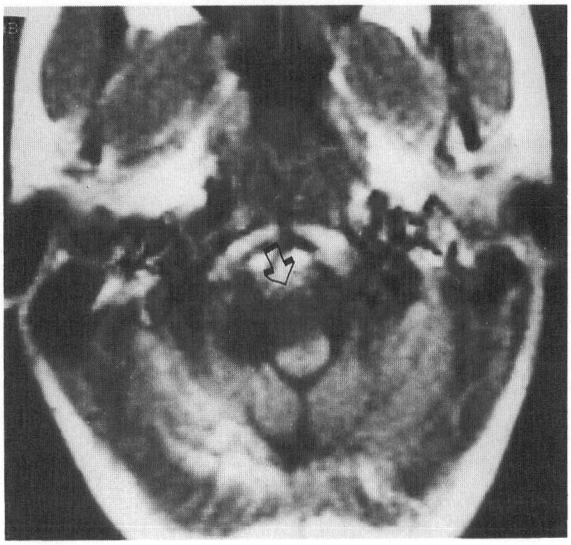
(C)

Figure 160-2 *A.* Midsagittal T1-weighted MRI scan of the head and neck. The patient presented with occipital headaches, mild quadriparesis, and speech and swallowing difficulties. Note the abnormal ventral CVJ with indentation of the ventral CMJ. *B.* Same patient. Axial T1-weighted MRI scan of the CVJ at the level of the foramen magnum. There is gross atlantoaxial luxation with dorsal displacement of the CMJ *(white arrow)*. *C.* Axial T1-weighted MRI scan of the CVJ, 15 mm above the level of the foramen magnum. Note the extradural bone and soft tissue mass *(open arrow)* indenting the lower medulla oblongata.

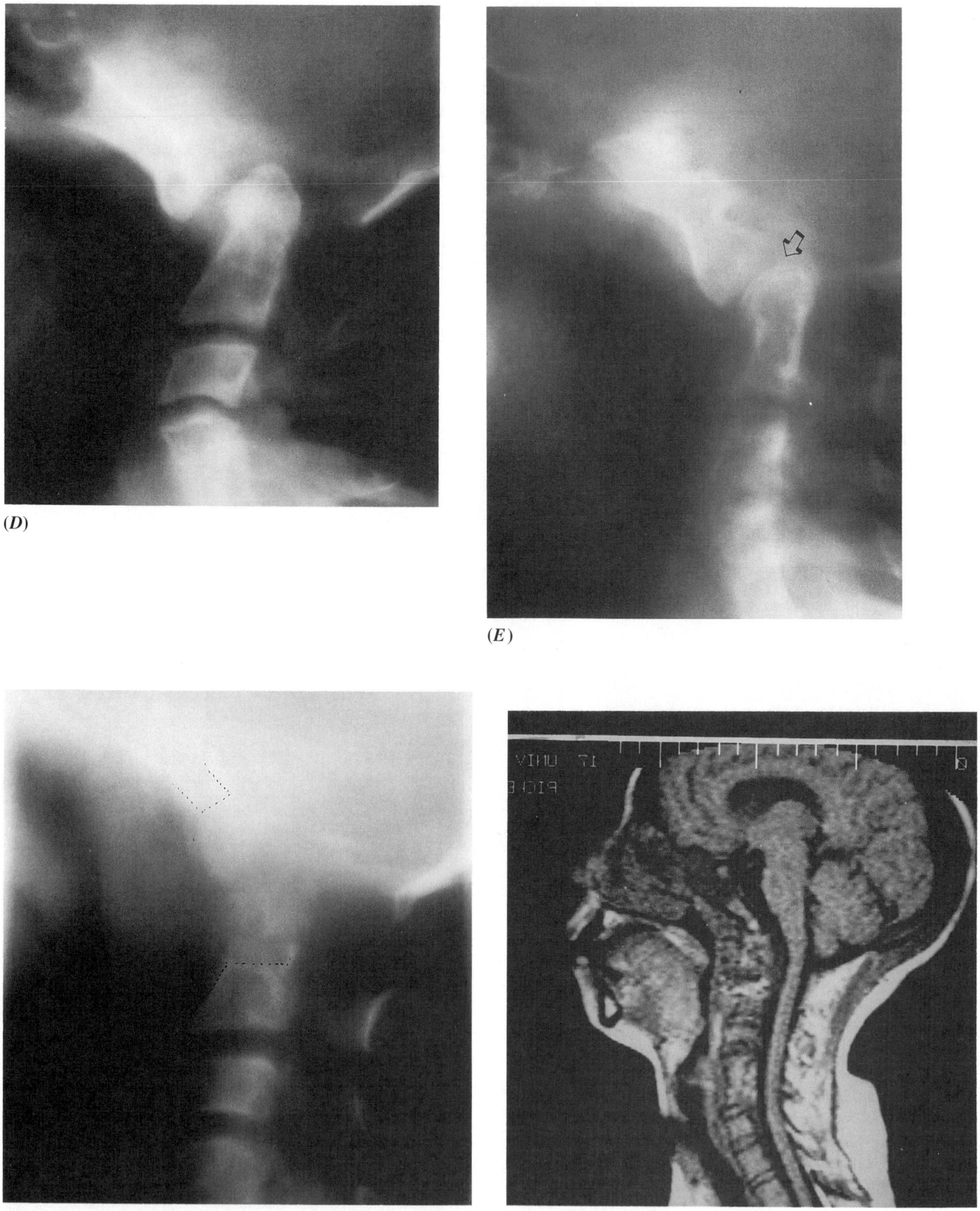

(*D*) (*E*) (*F*) (*G*)

Figure 160-2 (*Continued*) *D.* Midline lateral pluridirectional tomogram of the CVJ. There is complete atlas assimilation with basilar odontoid invagination into the posterior fossa, which was irreducible. *E.* Lateral paramedian tomogram of the CVJ demonstrates atlas assimilation. The superior facet of C2 articulates with the posterior aspect of the assimilated atlas lateral mass *(open arrow)*. *F.* Lateral midline tomogram of the CVJ made 6 days after transpalatopharyngeal resection of the assimilated atlas, anteriorly, and the odontoid process *(between dotted lines)*. *G.* T1-weighted MRI scan of the CVJ made 6 days after transpalatopharyngeal resection of the clivus-atlas and odontoid process. Note the decompressed CMJ.

Chordomas involving the clivus and cervical spine require complementary CT myelography of the CMJ.[19,20] This is essential to identify the precise location and nature of the invaginating mass and the sequestered bone. More importantly, intradural extension may be confirmed, providing the surgeon with additional information prior to the operative procedure.

Vertebral angiography has been a useful adjunct in evaluating selected cases where the symptomatology has been produced with abnormal head positions (such as with atlas assimilation and atlantoaxial instability) and in locating vessels when planning surgery in such cases as chordoma or severe Klippel–Feil abnormalities, in which preoperative MR angiography has proved unstatisfactory.

Relevant Anatomy

In order to understand CVJ abnormalities and their treatment, it is necessary to possess a knowledge of the embryology of this area, as well as its complex anatomy and biomechanics.

The occipitoatlantoaxial joints are approximated by multiple ligamentous structures that are responsible for its stability and complex movements. The ventral ligaments include the anterior atlanto-occipital membrane, which is the rostral extension of the anterior longitudinal ligament and its insertion on the anterior clivus. The principal stabilizer of the atlantoaxial joint is the transverse portion of the cruciate ligament, which inserts on the mesial aspect of the atlas and approximates the dens to the atlas. The atlas is connected to the occiput by the apical dens ligament, the cruciate ligament, the tectorial membrane, and the oblique alar ligaments. The posterior stabilizing tissues include the ligamentum flavum, the ligamentum nuchae, the posterior atlanto-occipital membrane, the supraspinous ligaments, and the paracervical musculature.

The occipitoatlantoaxial articulations are lined by synovial membrane, which is derived embryologically from the same unit. The lymphatic drainage of the occipitoatlantoaxial joints is into the retropharyngeal glands and then into the deep cervical chain.

Each hypoglossal nerve exits from the condylar foramen 1¾ to 2 cm from the midline, at the base of the skull. This limits the lateral extent of the exposure of the clivus in a transoral-transpalatal operative procedure. Likewise, the medial opening of the eustachian tubes at the upper level of the pharynx limits exposure at the CVJ to less than 1½ to 2 cm of either side of the midline. There is no posterior pharyngeal musculature over the clivus, and the posterior nasopharyngeal mucosa in this region is extremely thin. The circular sinus, also known as the marginal sinus, circumscribes the foramen magnum and thus is the first structure to be encountered behind the clivus at the foramen magnum. Opening this dural sinus requires cauterization of both its leaves or tamponade with hemostatic agents.

The angle of approach in a transoral operation is dependent on several factors:

1. The ability to open the oral cavity to its maximum, thus the integrity of the temporomandibular joints.
2. The presence of abnormal tonsillar and adenoid tissue.
3. Severe basilar invagination with platybasia, which can place the CVJ higher than the dorsum sellae.

The latter situation is not uncommon in conditions such as Paget's disease, osteogenesis imperfecta, and severe renal rickets.[3,19] This creates a narrow channel of approach that may require resection of a portion of the hard palate to gain access into this area. Alternately a LeForte I drop-down maxillotomy can be utilized. The inferior limit of a transoral-transpalatal operation is the C2–C3 junction.[36] Caudal exposure is obtained by midline splitting of the tongue or a combination of mandibular splitting and median glossotomy. An extensive midline surgical incision with preservation of neurovascular structures is possible in the tissues of the head and neck because these tissues, embryologically, develop bilaterally, resulting in midline fusion. This can result in a virtually bloodless midline field with minimal functional disability. Should an intradural operative procedure be envisioned through the transoral route, vertebral angiography is mandatory to identify the location of abnormal vascular structures and the vascularity of the tumor.

Operative Procedure

Nasopharyngeal cultures are obtained 3 days before the proposed surgery. If no pathologic flora are identified, 2,000,000 U penicillin G are administered 6 h before the operation, intraoperatively, and every 4 h for the first postoperative day.[2,20] Should a midline glossotomy and mandibulotomy be contemplated, it is essential that a panoramic radiographic view of the dentition be obtained and impressions of the upper and lower dentition made preoperatively for use in creating dental guards.

The patient is positioned supine and 5 to 7 lb of skeletal traction applied via an MRI-compatible halo ring. Fiberoptic awake oral endotracheal intubation is then accomplished and the patient repositioned and examined while awake to ensure no change in neurological status due to the intubation and positioning. General endotracheal and intravenous anesthesia is then administered.

Transoral-Transpalatopharyngeal Approach

An armored endotracheal tube, secured to the midline chin, is used for the operative procedure. Tracheostomy has been found to be unnecessary for this procedure and has not been used by this author for the past 5 years. The only circumstances in which a tracheostomy is performed are if the patient has severe brain stem dysfunction or in the situation where lower cranial nerves have been paralyzed preoperatively, as with chordoma. Another indication for tracheostomy is the performance of a median glossotomy and mandibulotomy. The nasopharyngeal passages are anesthetized with 5% cocaine and nasal packs placed so as to prevent drainage of nasal secretions into the high nasopharynx during the operation. Pharyngeal gauze packing is placed in the laryngopharynx to prevent fluid from going into the stomach. This allows free cleansing of the nasopharynx, the oropharynx, and laryngopharynx, as well as the oral cavity, with 10% povidone iodine solution. Hydrogen peroxide is then used to further cleanse the pharynx and a normal saline rinse completes the preparation. Previously made dental guards are placed over the upper and lower dentition and a self-retaining Dingman mouth retractor is positioned using the tongue blade for depression and incorporation of the endotracheal tube.

Should there be the concern of a dural violation, by tumor, bony masses, or attenuation of the dura, it is imperative that a lumbar subarachnoid drain be installed preoperatively (and opened only should a dural violation occur). Similarly, the anterior abdominal wall should be prepared for harvesting of fascia and fat for closure of a dural leak.

After the soft palate is infiltrated in the median raphe, an incision is made starting from either the right or the left of the base of the uvula to immediately attain the midline and ascend up the median raphe to the hard palate. Stay sutures are then placed in the soft palate and the leaves retracted to expose the nasopharynx.

In congenital and developmental osseous abnormalities of the CCJ, the author has found it necessary to carry the incision onto the hard palate for at least 2 to 3 cm along the midline. This requires appropriate preparation with infiltration of local anesthetic with epinephrine. The mucosa of the hard palate is then swept to either side and also along the nasal mucosa. If necessary, a portion of the hard palate 1 to 2 cm in length and 1 to 1½ cm to either side of the midline is removed, thus exposing the high nasopharynx and the sphenoid rostrum. The lateral exposure of the midline clivus is further facilitated by the development of the hard palate mucosal flaps on either side of the midline, which are then held apart with stay sutures. Retractor sets that assist in retracting the soft tissue are commercially available, however this author has no experience with them. Stay sutures are placed along the soft palate to allow its retraction over the springs of the Dingman mouth retractor. The operating microscope is then brought in to provide magnification and a concentrated light source.

The posterior pharyngeal mucosa is anesthetized with topical cocaine and the median raphe infiltrated with 0.5% lidocaine and 1/200,000 epinephrine. A midline incision in the posterior pharyngeal median raphe is carried through the mucosa, the constrictor muscles, and the pharyngeal fascia. The prevertebral fascia is swept away and retracted with stay sutures. Retracting the prevertebral fascia over the openings of the eustachian tubes protects them from damage. The longus colli muscles, as well as the longus capitis muscles, are separated from their ligamentous osseous attachments and retracted laterally for 1½ cm to either side of the midline, thus exposing the caudal half of the clivus and the axis and atlas as far laterally as the lateral atlantoaxial joints. The anterior longitudinal ligament and the occipital ligaments are cauterized with bipolar cautery and are sharply dissected free of the caudal clivus, the anterior arch of the atlas, and the ventral aspect of the axial body. Stay sutures help to maintain lateral retraction of the soft tissues. When necessary, the exposure can be carried as high up as the basisphenoid without any difficulty.

The caudal half of the clivus may be removed, if so indicated, with a high-speed air drill. The bone resection is then carried down to the anterior arch of the atlas, a 2½- to 3-cm wide portion which may be removed in the midline, to visualize the proximal odontoid process. Depending on the pathology, granulation tissue may be present behind the anterior arch of the atlas, preventing visualization of the proximal odontoid process. During resection of the caudal clivus, it is necessary to separate the dura from the posterior aspect to prevent bleeding from the marginal sinus. All soft tissue anterior to the odontoid process is then removed, and the odontoid process is resected in a rostral-caudal direction using a high-speed drill with a diamond burr. The shell of the odontoid process is finally removed with fine Kerrison rongeurs, and the additional granulation tissue is cauterized and subsequently removed far laterally toward the occipital condyles.[4,20,35] The extent of exposure is 3 cm in transverse dimension. It is only after resection of the tectorial membrane and additional granulation tissue that an adequate decompression is accomplished. The dura becomes pulsatile and occupies the decompression site. Rostral and caudal resection of the CVJ should be dictated by reference to the various diagnostic procedures (Fig. 160-3).

If an intradural exposure is planned, the lumbar subarachnoid drain is then opened. CSF is removed, relieving the turgidity of the ventral dura and allowing intradural exposure. A cruciate incision is then made in the dura caudal to the foramen magnum and extended vertically upward. Hemostatic clips are applied to the dura at the marginal sinus and sutures are used for self-retaining dural retraction for exposure of the intradural contents. The marginal sinus may be cauterized, if needed.

The intradural operative procedure must be carried out under highest-power magnification. Dural closure is performed with 4-0 polyglactin suture to be as complete as possible. The ideal closure is then completed by placing fascia, held in place with plasma glue, adjacent to the dural closure. Following this, a fat pad is used to reinforce the fascia. The longus colli muscles, the pharyngeal musculature, and the pharyngeal mucosa are then approximated in individual layers with dyed 3-0 polyglactin sutures. The soft palate is closed in two layers, the nasal mucosa of the soft palate being

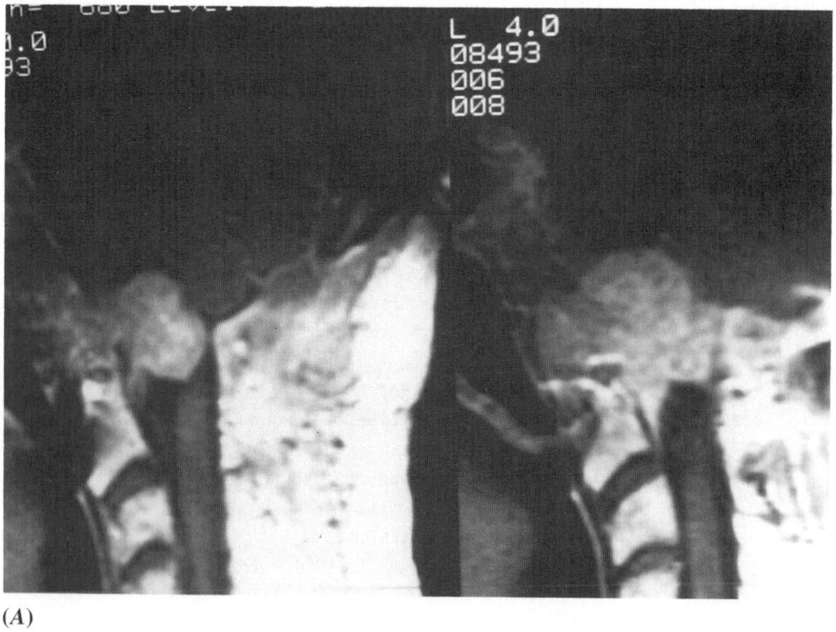

(*A*)

Figure 160-3 *A*. Composite of midsagittal (*left*) and parasagittal (*right*) T1-weighted gadolinium-enhanced MRI scans of the CVJ. The clivus, anterior arch of the atlas, and odontoid are replaced by recurrent chordoma.

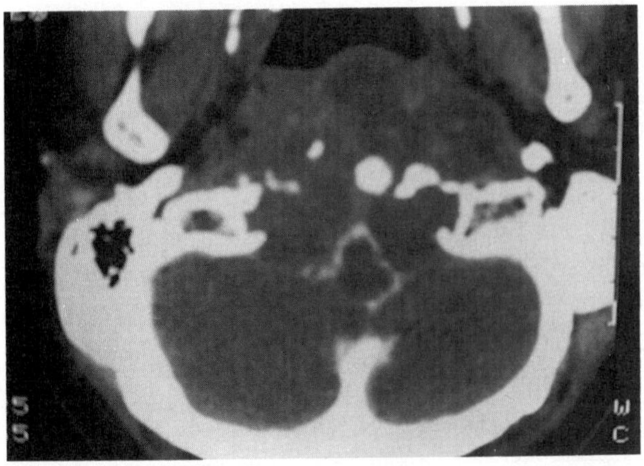

(*B*)

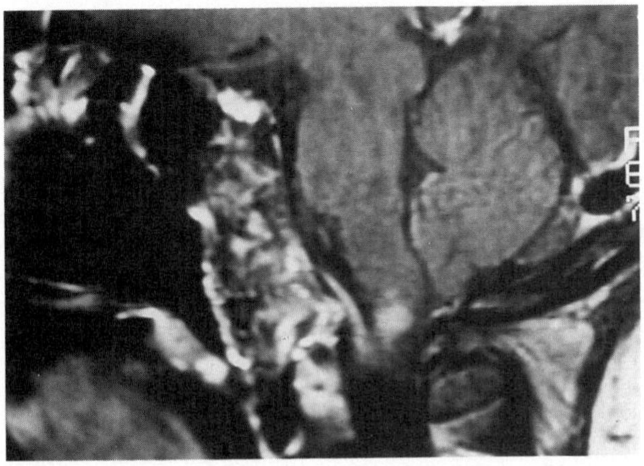

(*C*)

Figure 160-3 (*Continued*) *B.* Same patient. Axial CT myelogram made 2 cm above the level of the foramen magnum. Note the high retropharyngeal mass, extensive clivus destruction, and extradural medullary compression. *C.* Midsagittal T1-weighted gadolinium-enhanced MRI scan of the CVJ made 2 weeks after transoral-transpalatal resection of the recurrent CVJ chordoma. The clivus has been reconstructed with fascial graft. The posterolateral approach allowed removal of the remaining tumor and dorsal occipitocervical fusion.

approximated with interrupted sutures and the oral mucosa, together with the muscularis, brought together with horizontal mattress sutures.

In a series of 150 cases, intraoperative somatosensory responses and brain stem auditory evoked responses have proved to be ineffective in predicting neurological injury during the operation. Before closure of the posterior pharyngeal wall, aerobic and anaerobic cultures are obtained from the depths of the wound. Prior to closure of the soft palate, the throat pack is removed and a soft Kayo nasogastric feeding tube is passed via the nasal passages under direct vision into the stomach, its position confirmed by auscultation as air is instilled via the tube into the stomach. The tube is then anchored to the nostril with a transfixing suture.

At the termination of the transoral-transpalatopharyngeal portion of the procedure, the anesthesiologist replaces the armored oral endotracheal tube with a regular oral endotracheal tube using a tube exchanger. This tube is then secured to the angle of the mouth with a transfixing suture and is taped and secured into position. The latter maneuver is made to allow free movement of the tongue and to prevent prolonged postoperative lingual swelling. The patient is then nursed in a 25- to 30-degree head-up position with care taken to avoid pharyngeal suctioning. Nasogastric tube feedings are begun the day after the operative procedure. The skeletal traction may be discontinued, and a cervical Philadelphia collar is applied for postoperative stability. The oral endotracheal tube is removed once the laryngeal swelling has receded. Oral intake of clear fluids is permitted after the sixth postoperative day, and this is followed by gradually increased feedings to a regular diet by the end of the third week.

If the dura was opened and a fascial graft was used for repair, intravenous cefotaxime, metronidazole, and nafcillin are begun and continued for 5 days. If there is no CSF leakage and CSF cultures are normal, cefotaxime is discontinued and nafcillin and metronidazole are given for another 5 days, for a total of 10 days of antibiotic therapy. Prior to this, the spinal drainage is gradually reduced by elevation of the drainage container.[18,19] The spinal drain is then removed at the end of the 10th postoperative day and the patient is gradually ambulated. In our experience, a lumboperitoneal shunt has not been required.

Transpalatal-Transpharyngeal Approach

This is an extension of the previously described procedure. The soft palate incision is extended along the hard palate in the midline for a distance of 3 to 4 cm. The mucosa is swept laterally toward the alveolar margin, preserving the greater palatal vessels. The hard palate may be removed for a length of 2 to 3 cm, or even more; as required. The lateral extent of removal is 1½ cm to either side of the midline. The vomer is then identified and removed in its posterior aspect. Should the operative procedure only require exposure of the clivus, no further bone is removed and the remainder of the operation is carried out as previously described.

In children, tumors of the clivus, such as chordomas, may require opening of the sphenoid sinus (in the older child with an opacified sinus) in order to gain exposure of the basisphenoid (Fig. 160-3). In such circumstances, the primary incision is made just within the arch of the hard palate paralleling the upper dentition. This allows for the mucosa of the hard palate to be swept posteriorly and the hard palate to be removed in the midline. A subperiosteal exposure is then made along the vomer, which is swept to one side and traced up to the sphenoid rostrum, where the mucosa of the septum is separated to either side of the midline to allow for exposure of the sphenoid rostrum and thus its resection. The angle of approach then carries the surgeon from the planum sphenoidale to the pituitary fossa and posteriorly along the midline to the CVJ. Closure of this wound is easily made by approximating the mucosa of the septum and then approximating the posterior portion of the hard palate mucosa to the mucosa of the floor of the nasal cavity. This is facilitated by placing rubber finger stalls filled with triple antibiotic ointment-impregnated gauze tape into each nostril to serve as pressure packs in each nostril and to approximate the septal mucosa, as well as to reposition the nasal mucosa of the nasal passages. The oral aspect of the palatal mucosa is then approximated with interrupted sutures of 4-0 polyglycolic. The postoperative care is as described for the transoral operative procedure.

Median Glossotomy and Midline Mandibulotomy

A tracheostomy is performed at the start of the operative procedure, after general endotracheal anesthesia has been accomplished via fiberoptic oral endotracheal intubation. A midline incision from the lower lip to the hyoid bone is then made. This incision may be zig-zagged so as to result in a less cosmetically objectionable scar.[16,25] The periosteum at the mandibular symphysis is elevated in the midline. Step-like osteotomy of the midline mandible is accomplished with an air-powered microsagittal saw. We have not found it essential to remove the central incisor tooth.[1,5] Retention sutures are then placed on either side of the tip of the tongue and retracted superiorly. Using electrocautery, the tongue is incised along its median raphe to the midline epiglottic fold posteriorly. The incision is extended anteriorly through the floor of the mouth between the orifices of the submaxillary ducts and inferiorly to the hyoid bone. The mandibular-lingual halves are spread laterally and held in place with a self-retaining hinged scalp retractor. The exposure then can be carried down to the C5 vertebral body and pharyngeal exposure made in the midline, all utilizing a pharyngeal flap. The operation is then accomplished as described for the transoral procedure. An iliac crest bone graft, as with an anterior cervical fusion, has been utilized by some authors. Posterior pharyngeal closure is made in layers. The dorsum of the tongue is then sutured from posterior to anterior, utilizing 3-0 polyglycolic interrupted sutures. The intrinsic lingual musculature is approximated in a similar fashion with 2-0 polyglycolic interrupted sutures, and the ventral surface of the tongue and the floor of the mouth closed in this order. The mandibular osteotomy is repositioned and held in place with either figure-of-eight stainless-steel wire or miniplates. Application of arch bars and interdental wiring has been found to be unnecessary. The soft tissues of the lip, chin, and submental region are closed in a layered fashion and a Penrose drain is placed in the base of the tongue and brought out of the inferior end of the suture line. A cuffed tracheostomy tube is inserted and a bulky neck dressing applied.

Prophylactic antibiotic therapy is continued for 4 to 5 days and the Penrose drain is removed at the end of the third to fifth postoperative day. The tracheostomy cuff is usually deflated on the morning of the second postoperative day and left so unless intermittent positive-pressure respiratory therapy is necessary. A nasogastric feeding tube is placed at the time of surgery and feedings are begun at the end of 48 h. The tube feedings are maintained until the lingual edema is sufficiently reduced so that oral alimentation is possible. Tracheal decannulation is accomplished as soon as the upper airway is adequate using the sequential method of decreasing tracheostomy tube size and subsequent removal.

Evaluation of Postoperative Stability

Between the fifth and seventh days after the ventral operation, pluridirectional lateral tomography of the CVJ is done to visualize the resection and determine craniovertebral stability.[22] This is done both with and without traction in the flexed and extended positions. The tomography must visualize points of the facet joints to identify an offset at the lateral occipitoatlantoaxial articulations during flexion and extension. Excessive displacement of the cranial spinal axis with and without halo traction is indicative of instability. MRI of the CMJ is performed during this time before any other surgical intervention. If instability is identified, a posterior occipitocervical or atlantoaxial fusion is required.[7,20,22] In those individuals with bone fusion, occipitocervical immobilization is provided by a halo brace for 5 to 6 months. If a contoured loop instrumentation is made with bone fusion for stability, halo immobilization is necessary for only 3 months. Dorsal fixation is essential after a transoral clivus odontoid resection for abnormalities associated with atlas assimilation and segmentation failures of the upper cervical spine.[19] By definition, rheumatoid cranial settling is an unstable situation and all such patients will require occipitocervical fixation. Similarly, patients with dystopic os odontoideum require fixation.[21]

Discussion

The advantages of the transpalatopharyngeal approach to the CVJ over other operative approaches in treating irreducible ventral pathology are that (1) angulation of the brain stem is avoided during surgery through the use of the extended position, as opposed to the flexed position necessary for posterior or posterolateral approaches or the rotated angled position used in the lateral extrapharyngeal approach[33,34]; (2) the surgery is performed through the avascular pharyngeal median raphe and through the clivus; and (3) the impinging bony pathology and granulation tissue that is present with chronic instability is accessible via the ventral route alone.

The extent of lateral surgical exposure of the anterior CVJ is limited by the emergence of the hypoglossal nerves 1¾ to 2 cm lateral to the clivus midline, by the vertebral arteries, and by the eustachian tubes just below the base of the skull. However, these constraints do allow a total of 3 cm of transverse exposure, which is sufficient for removal of pathologic lesions from the clivus to the upper portion of the body of C3 (Fig. 160-4). Tumors, such as chordomas, provide the dissection; thus the exposure in such circumstances may extend as far as the jugular foramen on either side. Care is taken in such circumstances to avoid damage to the hypoglossal nerves. However, these are usually displaced laterally.

Because of the inherent possibility of infection through oral contamination, intra-arachnoid lesions should not be approached via the transoral route unless other avenues are ineffective. The lateral rhinotomy, combined with the transoral procedure, allows for midline anterior skull base resection, while the median labiomandibular glossotomy combined with the transoral approach adds exposure to lesions caudal to the C2 vertebral body. The importance of tracheostomy cannot be overemphasized in individuals who have severe respiratory insufficiency secondary to brain stem dysfunction.

The soft palate incision provides direct access to the lower clivus and the high CVJ. The technique of suture of the soft palate and retraction into the nasal cavity is advocated by some authors, but is not beneficial for exposure at the CVJ.

Experience with otolaryngologic procedures has shown that it is safe to conduct major operations in the upper airway and to use appropriate antibiotic coverage only when pathologic flora are identified. There appears to be an inherent host immunity of the nasopharyngeal structures to normal oral flora. However, the primary potential hazard is still infection, whether bacterial or fungal. Thus, it is important to have precise indications for the operation, as well as to limit the procedure to extradural compressive phenomena.

Injury to the vertebral arteries may be avoided by precise preoperative localization of the vertebrobasilar arterial vessels on the coronal and parasagittal MRI scans, and by limiting the lateral

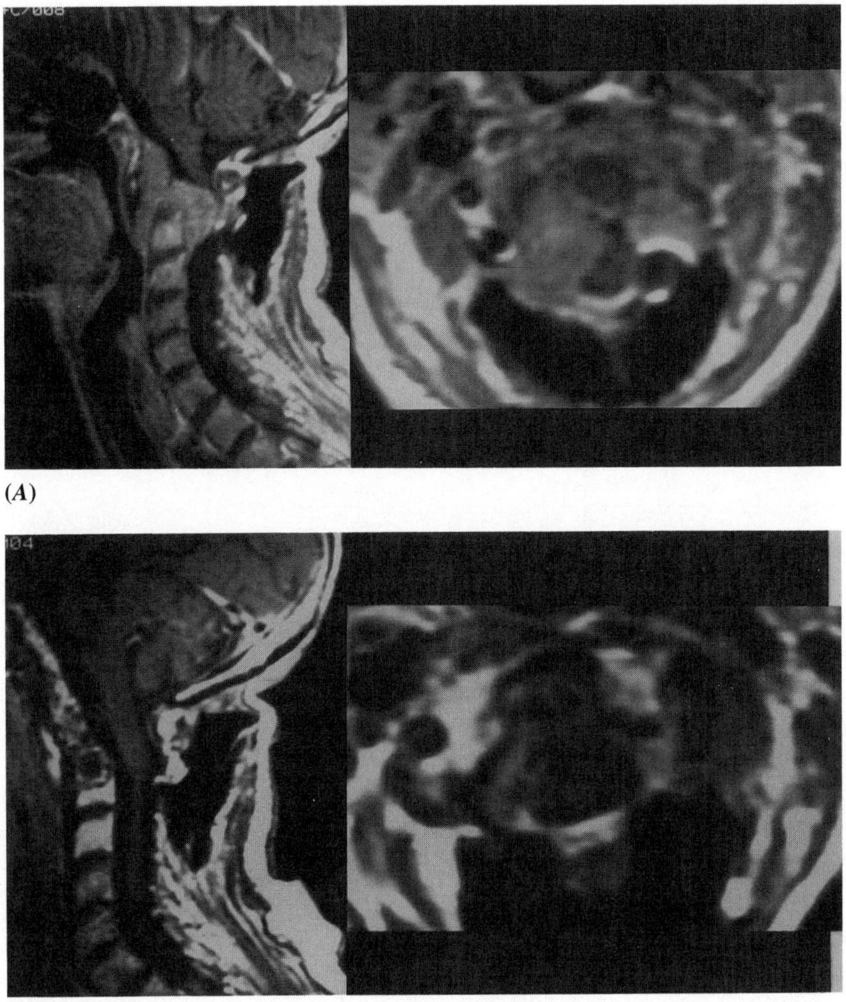

(A) *(B)*

Figure 160-4 *A.* Composite of T1-weighted MRI images of the CVJ in the midsagittal (*left*) and axial (*right*) planes at C1. Tumor, enhanced with gadolinium, is seen replacing the ventral atlas and axis, and circumscribing the CMJ (*right*). A dorsal C1-C2 Halifax fusion had been attempted previously. *B.* Composite of midsagittal (*left*) and axial (*right*) MRI scans, as in *A*, made 3 months after transoral resection of the solitary plasmacytoma replacing the atlas and axis. Note the cervicomedullary decompression.

dissection during the operation. Involvement of the vertebral arteries may occur if osteomyelitis develops secondary to an epidural retropharyngeal abscess. This is treated by immediate evacuation of the abscess and appropriate antibiotic coverage with adequate attention to the nutritional status of the patient.

Dehiscence of the pharyngeal closure is prevented by utilizing a pharyngeal flap,[12] and, at times, closure by secondary intention in the presence of infection. The key to wound healing during this time is adequate nutrition.[19] This can become difficult in rheumatoid patients who have been on corticosteroids over a long period.

Most patients do develop a serous otitis media and a transient sinusitis due to the supine position, which must be addressed as soon as possible. Failure to identify postoperative craniovertebral instability can be disastrous. It is thus imperative to investigate for postoperative stability by the end of the first week, and to recheck the postoperative stability at the end of 6 to 8 weeks, and subsequently at the end of 6 months. Most patients with brain stem dysfunction will require tube feedings to prevent aspiration. Recovery has been the rule.

Results

The youngest patient in the author's series was 4 years of age and the oldest was 82 years old. There were 83 children below the age of 16 years who underwent the ventral operation for primary basilar invagination, abnormal clivus–odontoid articulation, dystopic os odontoideum, malunion of occipitocervical dislocation, and clivus chordoma. The transverse portion of the cruciate ligament and the periosteum of the dens was not interrupted in 10 children below the age of 12. These children were immobilized in a halo brace or a sterno-occipitomandibular immobilizing brace for 3 months postoperatively. Four of these children later showed instability and required dorsal fixation.

A dural opening developed during transoral surgery in 33 individuals. This was seen in patients with a sequestered odontoid process that invaginated into the pons and medulla, in those with rheumatoid upward invagination of the odontoid process, as well as in patients with clivus chordoma who had undergone previous procedures.

Of the 263 patients who underwent a ventral transoral-transpalatal decompression of the CVJ, 225 required a dorsal fixation procedure (Table 160-1). In these individuals, postoperative immobilization was maintained for an average of 6 months.

Neurological recovery was the rule in all patients. Those individuals who were dependent on a ventilator before the operation (after either previous primary posterior decompression or trauma) had recovery of their neurological deficit during the immediate postoperative period.[20] Brain stem dysfunction, which was a prominent presenting feature in individuals with basilar invagination and Chiari malformation, regressed following the ventral decompression procedure.

TABLE 160-1 Pathology in 263 Patients Who Underwent Transoral-Transpalatopharyngeal Approach to the Clivus and Upper Cervical Spine (UIHC 1977–1993)

Primary basilar invagination and congenital anomalies	126
Rheumatoid irreducible cranial settling	53
Basilar invagination after malunion, O-C1 dislocation	12
Unfused C2 fracture (C1-C2 posterior fusion)	6
Dystophic os odontoideum complex	18
Granulation masses	6
Osteoblastoma	1
Clivus chordoma	19
Chondroma, clivus-C1	1
Plasmacytoma	3
Pseudogout	6
Miscellaneous (inflammatory ileitis, Goldenhar's syndrome, fetal warfarin, psoriasis, ankylosing spondylitis, osteogenesis imperfecta, osteomyelitis)	12
	263

Three patients died within the first month after operation. A 79-year-old rheumatoid male patient with cranial settling and basilar invagination had recovered neurological function, but died 4 weeks after operation from a myocardial infarction. A 52-year-old woman, admitted quadriplegic after a motor vehicle accident, died 3 weeks after the operation from *Escherichia coli* urinary sepsis that was existent at the time of her admission. She had recovered a great deal of her neurological deficit after the transoral operation. The third patient, a 73-year-old woman with extensive clivus chordoma, had undergone biopsy and conventional radiation of 6,000 rads at a referring facility. Progressive brain stem dysfunction and respiratory embarrassment prompted her referral at the end of her radiation therapy. She underwent ventral decompression, with recovery of her neurological dysfunction. Postoperatively, the dorsal posterolateral approach was utilized for the removal of the remaining tumor and relocation of the vertebral artery prior to entering the dura at foramen magnum. Postoperative occipitocervical fixation was performed. She had epistaxis at the end of the third week following the ventral operation, the source of which was unable to be detected. Bilateral vertebral angiography failed to reveal evidence of involvement of the vertebral arteries or branches, nor did carotid angiography identify the source of bleeding. This patient underwent an extrapharyngeal approach to the CVJ with placement of a sternomastoid vascularized pedicle graft into the area of ventral resection because no bleeding site was identified. She had a vertebral artery blow-out 4 weeks after the ventral operation, and at emergency surgery, the vertebral artery was found to have eroded at the site of tumor.

Two superficial wound dehiscences were treated with hyperalimentation and closed without any difficulty. The disturbing complication of velopalatal incompetence was seen, usually 4 to 6 months after the ventral transoral procedure. This occurred in seven young individuals, all of whom had brain stem dysfunction preoperatively. The velopalatal incompetence was successfully treated with a palatal prosthesis in four individuals, and in three others a pharyngeal flap was required.

Mandibular malunion is a possible complication of midline mandibulotomy. The possibility can be minimized by drilling the holes for the wires or screws prior to making the cuts in the mandible. Infection is likewise prevented by preserving the soft tissue adjacent to the mandibulotomy to allow for ample periosteal closure over the osteotomy. Retropharyngeal abscess is prevented by placement of a suction drain for 3 to 5 days.

References

1. Arbit E, Patterson RH Jr. Combined transoral and median labiomandibular glossotomy approach to the upper cervical spine. *Neurosurgery* 1981; 8:672–674.
2. Bartlett JG. Selective antibiotic therapy in surgery. Part 1. The normal flora. *J Surg Pract* 1977; July–August:12–16.
3. Crockard HA. Anterior approaches to the craniocervical junction. In Camins MB, O'Leary PF (eds): *Disorders of the Cervical Spine.* Baltimore: Williams & Wilkins, 1992, pp 381–389.
4. Crockard HA, Sett P, Geddes JF, et al. Damaged ligaments at the craniocervical junction presenting as an extradural tumour: a differential diagnosis in the elderly. *J Neurol Neurosurg Psychiatry* 1991; 54:817–821.
5. Delgado TE, Garrido E, Harwick RD. Labiomandibular, transoral approach to chordomas in the clivus and upper cervical spine. *Neurosurgery* 1981; 8(6):675–679.
6. Derome PJ. The transbasal approach to tumors invading the base of the skull. In Schmidek HH, Sweet WH (eds): *Current Techniques in Operative Neurosurgery.* New York: Grune & Stratton, 1977, pp 223–245.
7. Dickman CA, Locantro J, Fessler RG. The influence of transoral odontoid resection on stability of the craniovertebral junction. *J Neurosurg* 1992; 77:525–530.
8. Fang HSY, Ong GB. Direct anterior approach to the upper cervical spine. *J Bone Joint Surg [Am]* 1962; 44:1588–1604.
9. Fisch U, Pillsbury HC. Infratemporal fossa approach to lesions in the temporal bone and base of the skull. *Arch Otolaryngol* 1979; 105:99–107.
10. Gates GA. The lateral facial approach to the nasopharynx and infratemporal fossa. *Otolaryngol Head Neck Surg* 1988; 99:321–325.
11. Hall JE, Denis F, Murray J. Exposure of the upper cervical spine for spinal decompression by a mandible and tongue-splitting approach: case report. *J Bone Joint Surg [Am]* 1977; 59(1):121–123.
12. Hayakawa T, Kamikawa K, Ohnishi T, et al. Prevention of postoperative complications after a transoral transclival approach to basilar aneurysms: technical note. *J Neurosurg* 1981; 54:699–703.
13. Krespi YP, Har EG. Surgery of the clivus and anterior cervical spine. *Arch Otolaryngol Head Neck Surg* 1988; 114:73–78.
14. Lesoin F, Jomin M, Pellerin P, et al. Transclival transcervical approach to the upper cervical spine and clivus. *Acta Neurochir (Wein)* 1986; 80:100–104.
15. Levy ML, Chen TC, Weiss MH. Monostotic fibrous dysplasia of the clivus: case report. *J Neurosurg* 1991; 75:800–803.
16. Martin H, Tollefsen HR, Gerold FP. Median labiomandibular glossotomy: Trotter's median (anterior) translingual pharyngotomy. *Am J Surg* 1961; 102:753–759.
17. McAfee PC, Bohlman HH, Riley LH Jr, et al. The anterior retropharyngeal approach to the upper part of the cervical spine. *J Bone Joint Surg [Am]* 1987; 69:1371–1383.
18. Menezes AH. Anterior approaches to the craniocervical junction. *Clin Neurosurg* 1991; 37:756–769.
19. Menezes AH. Surgical approaches to the craniocervical junction. In Frymoyer JW (ed): *The Adult Spine: Principles and Practice.* New York: Raven Press, 1991, pp 967–986.
20. Menezes AH, VanGilder JC. Transoral-transpharyngeal approach to the anterior craniocervical junction. Ten-year experience with 72 patients. *J Neurosurg* 1988; 69:895–903.
21. Menezes AH, VanGilder JC, Clark CR, El-Khoury G. Odontoid upward migration in rheumatoid arthritis: an analysis of 45 patients with "cranial settling." *J Neurosurg* 1985; 63:500–509.
22. Menezes AH, VanGilder JC, Graf CJ, McDonnell DE. Craniocervical abnormalities: a comprehensive surgical approach. *J Neurosurg* 1980; 53:444–455.
23. Meyer FB, Ebersold MJ, Reese DF. Benign tumors of the foramen mangum. *J Neurosurg* 1984; 61:136–142.
24. Miller E, Crockard HA. Transoral transclival removal of anteriorly placed meningiomas at the foramen magnum. *Neurosurgery* 1987; 20:966–968.

25. Moore LJ, Schwartz HC. Median labiomandibular glossotomy for access to the cervical spine. *J Oral Maxillofac Surg* 1985; 43:909–912.
26. Mullan S, Naunton R, Hekmat-panah J, et al. The use of an anterior approach to ventrally placed tumors in the foramen magnum and vertebral column. *J Neurosurg* 1966; 24:536–543.
27. Ogata M, Ishikawa K, Ohira T. Cervical myelopathy in pseudogout: case report. *J Bone Joint Surg [Am]* 1984; 66(8):1301–1303.
28. Oot RF, Melville GE, New PFJ, et al. The role of MR and CT in evaluating clival chordomas and chondrosarcomas. *Am J Roentgenol* 1988; 151(3):567–575.
29. Resnick D, Pineda C. Vertebral involvement in calcium pyrophosphate dihydrate crystal deposition disease: radiographic-pathological correlation. *Radiology* 1984; 153(1):55–60.
30. Rosenfeld JV, Wallace D, Klug GL, et al. Transnasal stereotactic biopsy of a clivus tumor: technical note. *J Neurosurg* 1992; 76:878–879.
31. Scoville WB, Sherman IJ. Platybasia: report of ten cases with comments on familial tendency, a special diagnostic sign, and the end results of operation. *Ann Surg* 1951; 133:496–502.
32. Sekhar LN, Schram VL Jr, Jones NF. Subtemporal-preauricular infratemporal fossa approach to large lateral and posterior cranial base neoplasms. *J Neurosurg* 1987; 67:488–499.
33. Sen CN, Sekhar LN. An extreme lateral approach to intradural lesions of the cervical spine and foramen magnum. *Neurosurgery* 1990; 27(2):197–204.
34. Stevenson GC, Stoney RJ, Perkins RK, et al. A transcervical transclival approach to the ventral surface of the brain stem for removal of a clivus chordoma. *J Neurosurg* 1966; 24:544–551.
35. Sze G, Brandt-Zawadski MN, Wilson CR, et al. Pseudotumor of the craniovertebral junction associated with chronic subluxation: MR imaging studies. *Radiology* 1986; 161:391–394.
36. Uttley D, Moore A, Archer DJ. Surgical management of midline skull-base tumors: a new approach. *J Neurosurg* 1989; 71:705–710.
37. Wold LE, Laws ER Jr. Cranial chordomas in children and young adults. *J Neurosurg* 1983; 59:1043–1047.
38. Wood BG, Sadar ES, Levine HL, et al. Surgical problems of the base of the skull: an interdisciplinary approach. *Arch Otolaryngol Head Neck Surg* 1980; 106:1–5.

161

Anterolateral Cervical Approach to the Craniovertebral Junction

Dennis E. McDonnell
Steven J. Harrison

Patients suffering from encroachment on the ventral spinal canal at the craniovertebral junction have an element of basilar impression that causes a chronic and progressive myelopathy. The process may be developmental, neoplastic, inflammatory, or traumatic in origin. The resulting cervicomedullary mechanical distortion and compression may be further aggravated by the presence of any associated instability. Minor trauma may initiate symptoms when slow mechanical compression has been compensated for. Scoville and Sherman[38] reported spastic quadriparesis and nystagmus resulting from a combination of basilar impression ventrally, caused by platybasia and cranial settling, and the posterior cerebellar tonsillar compression of the Chiari I malformation with coexisting syringomyelia. Suboccipital craniectomy and tonsillar decompression was the treatment advocated. That treatment addressed the posterior compressive component, but ventral compression persisted owing to the cephalic migration of the odontoid process. Techniques for specifically addressing compressive lesions ventral to the spinal canal along the vertebral axis evolved as surgical and pathologic anatomy became better understood.[41]

It is now recognized that ventral surgical decompression, frequently followed by stabilization of the occiput to the cervical spine, is the accepted method of management for many of these problems.[7,29] The most popular approach is the transoral route, but it is hazardous because of the contaminated surgical field, particularly if the dura is opened and there is a cerebrospinal fluid (CSF) fistula. Exposure of vertebral segments caudal to C3 is limited. The transcervical approach offers a satisfactory alternative and avoids the hazards of a contaminated surgical field.

Historical Perspectives

Transoral Route

The oral cavity serves as a ready-made corridor to the anterior craniovertebral junction. The anterior tubercle of C1 is easily palpated through the posterior wall of the oral pharynx. Splitting the soft palate gives access to the nasopharynx, the anterior rim of the foramen magnum, and the caudal limit of the clivus.[2] Self-retaining retractors that engage the alveolar ridges and depress the tongue allow exposure. The operating microscope affords direct light and magnification. This route is direct, and the midsagittal plane is parallel to the surgeon's view so that the midline orientation is more easily maintained. Many surgeons have had success with this approach; so much so, that it has been well publicized and is the most popular approach to this region, particularly for extradural lesions.[12,16,28,42]

The mandible and tongue are barriers to immediate direct exposure of the upper cervical spine and clivus, resulting in a narrow, dark surgical field. These drawbacks have been partly overcome by innovative retraction devices, operative microscopes, and neurophysiologic monitoring.[16] The transoral approach has been modified and expanded to improve exposure by hemisection and rotation of the mandible and tongue.[4,17,49] Combining a midsagittal mandibular and glossal swing with the transcervical approach widens the exposure to the entire clivus and upper cervical spine, so that midline and lateral compartments of the skull base are available for surgical access.[1,22] These extensive midline sections and disarticulations are required to deal with lesions that extend beyond the midline compartment of the skull base. In selected cases, the transoral approach has been advocated for intradural lesions.[8] With the usual transoral approach, the lateral exposure is limited, and the access is deep and rather narrow. In addition, all of these transpharyngeal approaches take place through a field contaminated with bacteria. That creates a definite risk for infection, not only meningitis and CSF fistula formation but also infection in the cervical soft tissue planes. Palatal dysfunction, exposure limitations, anatomic complexity, and difficulty of vascular control and hemostasis, along with limited methods of dural closure, are obstacles that may not become evident until the surgeon is involved with the procedure.[13] The transcervical route offers an alternative that has fewer limitations of exposure and that minimizes the risks of CSF fistula formation and infection.

Anterolateral (Transcervical) Route

The transcervical route to the craniovertebral junction has evolved from the passage to the midcervical vertebral segments for intervertebral disc removal and fusion that was described in 1955 by Robinson and Smith.[36,40] Through either a transverse or a vertical anterior cervical incision, the sternocleidomastoid muscle and carotid sheath are dissected and retracted laterally, and the strap muscles, trachea, and esophagus are retracted medially to expose the retropharyngeal and prevertebral spaces from C3 to C7. This is now a standard procedure for treating lesions of the cervical vertebrae and ventral encroachments on the adjacent neuraxis. However, exposure of the *upper* cervical spine through soft tissue planes is more complex than for middle and lower segments. Therefore, the transoral route is more frequently used to approach the clival-atlantoaxial region.

In 1966, Stevenson et al. described the dissection of cervical soft tissues via a parapharyngeal approach to remove a clival chordoma through a combined transverse and vertical "T" incision; the microscope afforded light and magnification to assist the visualization required when using this approach.[43] Also in 1966, Whitesides and Kelly[47] described a lateral approach adapted from Henry's approach to the vertebral artery.[18] Through a lateral longitudinal incision, the sternocleidomastoid muscle is detached from the mastoid process and segmentally separated so as to be retracted posteriorly; the cervical spine up to C1 is then approached laterally behind the carotid sheath.[18,47] The lateral cervical approach was further detailed by Verbiest,[45] with special emphasis on the cervical course of the vertebral artery. De Andrade and MacNab, in 1969, described a method for exposing the atlanto-occipital condylar joint for fusion by using a vertical incision along the sternocleidomastoid muscle, dissecting the carotid sheath, transecting the omohyoid muscle, and dissecting bluntly to the occipitocervical articulation.[9] The complications for this procedure, which are also described, include retropharyngeal swelling, laryngeal nerve palsy, and the difficulty of achieving stability in the face of a previous cervical laminectomy. These complications attest to the difficulties inherent in surgical approaches to this region. In 1973, Riley described a procedure for exposing the entire anterior cervical spine from C1 to C7 via a posterior longitudinal incision, with transection of the sternocleidomastoid and omohyoid muscles, excision of the anterior scalenus muscle, ligation of external carotid artery branches, and mobilization of the vertebral artery.[35] Using the lateral approach through the ''hockey stick'' incision described in 1966, Whitesides and McDonald reported in 1978, their experience with ventral resection of a variety of lesions and with arthrodesis techniques for the basiocciput and C1-C2 lateral masses, along with the complications of such procedures.[48] In 1979, Nagashima et al. described success using Stevenson's approach in resecting a C2 vertebra destroyed by metastatic carcinoma; they attempted reconstruction using Kirschner wires from C4 through the anterior arch of C1 into the clivus and cementing the construct with acrylic polymer.[31] Lesoin et al. used a similar approach to treat atlantoaxial subluxation caused by rheumatoid arthritis, achieving stability with *in situ* acrylic from the clivus to C4 following multiple-vertebra resection and decompression.[24] They also reported this approach for treatment of C2 pedicle fractures with C2-C3 discectomy, interbody fusion, and fixation using a screw and plate construct.[25]

Recently, transarticular lateral mass fusion via the posterior approach has been advocated for managing atlantoaxial instability, and this procedure has been gaining popularity.[20] This lateral mass screw fixation has also been described by Lesoin et al. using the anterior transcervical approach.[23]

McAfee and associates have detailed and updated the results of Robinson and Southwick's modifications of the transcervical retropharyngeal approach to the upper cervical spine.[26] A transverse submandibular incision is used, with the option of an inferiorly directed vertical extension. Dissection of the cervical fascial planes is emphasized. The submandibular gland is excised. The digastric tendon is transected. The anterior border of the sternocleidomastoid muscle and the spinal accessory nerve are dissected. The carotid sheath is dissected and retracted laterally, so that the approach is made anteromedial to the carotid artery and jugular vein, as in the approaches described by Stevenson, Riley, and De Andrade but in contrast to the retrocarotid approaches described by Verbiest and Whitesides. The ''tethering'' branches of the external carotid artery, including the superior thyroid, lingual, ascending pharyngeal, and facial arteries and the accompanying veins, are ligated and transected to help mobilize the carotid sheath laterally. The superior laryngeal nerve is mobilized from its origin near the nodose ganglion of the vagus nerve to the larynx. Most of these authors advocate blunt dissection of the cervical fascia and adjacent structures, with ligation and transection of vessels and transection of muscles as well as excision of the submandibular gland. They also describe successful anterior fusion of the clivus to the upper cervical spine using a grooved iliac graft strut, which in their experience usually requires a supplemental posterior occipitocervical fusion.

This approach is relatively anterior in relation to neck structures, as is evident when it is compared to the most posterior and lateral approach to the distal internal carotid artery described by Batzdorf and Gregorius.[3] In that approach, the mandibular angle is mobilized by osteotomies through the superior ramus/coronoid process and by a second osteotomy through the body of the mandible. The masseter and pterygoid muscles are left attached to the freed mandibular angle, which can be mobilized out of the field to expose the origin of the stylohyoid muscle and posterior belly of the digastric muscle. The proximal hypoglossal nerve is dissected and mobilized and serves as a guide to the internal carotid artery. This approach allows enough access to repair the internal carotid artery. The exposure is well lateral to one giving access to the upper cervical spine. The carotid artery is not directly exposed in the approach proposed by the present authors. It remains posterolateral to this exposure and usually is not seen. However, it can be compromised by vigorous retraction or excessive skull base resection.

The basisphenoid, anterior foramen magnum, anterior C1 arch, odontoid, bodies of C2 and C3 and corresponding intervertebral discs, and superior epiphysis of C4 can be approached without the need to transect any of these structures. The approach stays well anterior to the carotid sheath, which therefore need not be dissected or mobilized. Wide dissection or cervical fascial planes allows adequate soft tissue release and achieves enough lateral exposure to show the lateral masses of the atlantoaxial articulation.[27] The surgeon must be familiar with the reflections of the cervical fascia and anatomy of the submandibular triangle, retromandibular fossa, and craniovertebral junction.

Anatomic Considerations

The surgical approach to the anterior craniovertebral junction should be tailored to the individual problem. The transcervical route to this region has the advantages over the transoral route of extensive exposure and relative safety from infection. The portal of passage is sequential methodical dissection of the superficial, middle, and deep layers of the cervical fascia. The superficial fascia is a continuous sheet extending from the head to the thorax and axillae. It takes origin from the mandible, inserts into fascia and skin over the upper chest, and contains the platysma muscle, which it separates from the subcutaneous fat. The middle and superficial layers of deep fascia fuse at the level of the hyoid bone, which forms a natural anatomic boundary between rostral and caudal pathways through the cervical viscera (thyroid gland, larynx, trachea, pharynx, esophagus, and adjacent neurovascular structures). The superficial layer of deep fascia is fused as it passes over and attaches to the hyoid bone and proceeds rostrally to envelop the structures of the submental and submaxillary divisions of the anterior triangle (collectively called the *submandibular space*). It fuses with the ventral sheath of the anterior belly of the digastric muscle; these two layers are separable. This deep fascial layer spreads laterally to fuse with the fascial sheaths of the posterior digastric belly and stylohyoideus muscles and splits to form the capsule of the submandibular gland. This fascial complex is a completely closed capsule that overlies the hyoglossus and superior constrictor muscles, which are in turn ensheathed in their own fascial capsule. The middle layer of the middle cervical fascia envelops structures caudal to the hyoid bone, which are not part of this exposure. The deepest division of the middle layer is the visceral fascia, which surrounds the trachea and esophagus. It extends rostrally to invest the thyroid cartilage and hyoid bone and extends to the skull base. It fuses posteriorly with the alar fascia and laterally with the carotid sheath. The alar fascia is the deepest layer of the deep fascia. It has two subdivisions: the alar and prevertebral fascia. The complete layer of fascia between the visceral and prevertebral fascia is the alar fascia, which is continuous laterally with the scalenus fascia and attaches to the tips of the transverse processes. It also fuses with the posterior layer of the carotid sheath. This combined alar fascia forms a midline prevertebral potential space that is continuous from the skull base to the coccyx. It forms the space of access for the transcervical parapharyngeal approach to the craniovertebral junction. These fascial structures and relationships were elaborately described by Grodinsky and Holyoke in 1938.[14] The anatomic structures and fascial reflections are beautifully illustrated in Pernkopf's anatomy atlas.[33]

The perspective of the bony landmarks is almost the same as that of the transoral approach except that the condyle-atlantis articulation is rotated on the axis, so that the ipsilateral articulation is more prominent and is forward of the one on the contralateral side. This fact must be kept in mind throughout the procedure to maintain proper orientation. The rostral limit for this exposure is the pharyngeal tubercle at the junction of the basisphenoid and basiocciput, which forms the attachment site of the superior pharyngeal constrictor muscle to the skull base. Rock et al. have determined measurements of key structures in reference to the midsagittal plane.[37] The vertebral artery in the foramen transversarium averages only 1.54 cm from the midline. The hypoglossal foramina were found to be on average 1.43 cm superolateral to the medial tip of the occipital condyle; this relationship should be appreciated when bone resection is extended to the condylar-C1 lateral mass articulation. These perspectives and measurements hold true for the transcervical approach. The risk for neural and vascular injury is the same for the transcervical and transoral routes.

Clinical Indications and Patient Selection

Neuraxis Compression

Pathologic conditions that require the procedure under discussion are uncommon but are potentially life-threatening when they occur. The pathology is primarily in the midline and includes such conditions as nonunion unstable odontoid or C2 fracture, rheumatoid dissolution of C1-C2 with cranial settling, congenital platybasia, neoplasms (both primary and metastatic) with pathologic fracture and spinal instability, osteomyelitis with vertebral destruction, and neuraxis compression. Any lesion (extradural or intradural) from the midclivus caudally that is amenable to the transoral approach can be handled by the transcervical approach.

Cervicomedullary compression from lesions at the craniovertebral junction is often chronic and progressive and is frequently misdiagnosed. Patients may become severely impaired and quadriparetic with compromised respiration and nutrition; their symptoms often are ignored or treated inadequately.[19] The most common complaint is suboccipital neck pain, often in the C2 nerve root distribution. The pain is frequently aggravated by head and neck movement. Patients may hold the head and neck stiffly and resist movement because of severe pain. Paresthesias and sensory disturbances are the next most common symptom and may involve upper or lower extremities. Gait disturbance, hyperreflexia, and extensor plantar responses are the most common neurological findings. Cervicomedullary compressive lesions are often misdiagnosed as demyelinating disease, degenerative spondylosis, or carpal tunnel syndrome.[30] When the cervicomedullary compression lesion is properly diagnosed, its management must be individually planned, and often is staged to achieve the best possible outcome. The risks of infection and CSF fistula should be considered when deciding which surgical approach to use. Many patients who suffer from lesions that cause dorsal compression, such as Chiari malformation, syringomyelia, and dural fibrous ring, may be helped by anterior decompression. However, this holds true only if the major deformity is ventral; otherwise, posterior decompressive measures are preferable.[11,21] Metastatic tumors in this location may not require decompression because neurological deficit is uncommon but pain is intractable. These patients may be adequately palliated by posterior stabilization followed by radiation therapy.[34]

Diagnostic and imaging techniques, such as thin-section computed tomography (CT) and magnetic resonance imaging (MRI), allow precise visualization of these pathologic processes and the characteristics of the neural compression. That is invaluable for planning treatment strategy. The degree of basilar impression no longer needs to be analyzed by lines drawn through the skull base because the lesions and their relationship to the neuraxis can be viewed directly. Wackenheim's clivus canal line is an exception; it is a helpful radiographic guide in assessing ventral cervicomedullary compression. A line is drawn along the inner surface of the clivus and along the floor of the cervical spinal canal; the intersection of the two lines forms Wackenheim's angle. The tip of the odontoid should not intersect the tangent of the line, and the angle should be greater than 150 degrees.[44,46]

Craniovertebral Instability

Instability with abnormal movement and displacement that occurs with normal head and neck motion can aggravate neuraxis compression and worsen neurologic function. It may result primarily from the local destructive changes caused by the pathologic entity, as when rheumatoid dissolution of the dens and transverse ligament leads to craniovertebral settling and subluxation. Instability may also result directly from surgical decompression or trauma. Anterior resection of the dens, anterior C1 arch, and lower clivus does not fully destabilize the spine; however, subclinical pathologic instability may be activated by the procedure. Delayed instability may occur. One study reported that 8 of 27 patients (30 percent) remained stable without requiring fusion after transoral resection of the odontoid over a 14-month follow-up period.[10] Surgically induced instability must be assessed and managed from the outset and may require temporary skull traction or placement of a halo-vest orthosis. At times, cranial settling and subluxation can be reduced by traction, which effects adequate decompression and precludes the need for a ventral surgical decompression procedure, so that all that is required is a posterior arthrodesis.[28] Attempts at anterior strut graft fusion of the clivus to the upper cervical spine after ventral resection have resulted in graft dislodgment, which required posterior occipital fusion.[26] In the author's (D.E.M.) experience, cranial torso bracing with a halo orthotic device has *not* been adequate for stabilizing a craniovertebral junction that is surgically destabilized by ventral decompression in the absence of an occipital cervical fusion construct. Such patients may become quadriparetic and go into respiratory arrest owing to a craniocervical flexion subluxation that causes cervicomedullary compression, even in the face of ventral "decompression." Such patients do best when they are nursed supine in continuous skull traction until they subsequently undergo an occipital cervical fusion as a staged procedure. Therefore, assessing postoperative decompression stability is critical to the overall management of these patients.

Menezes' classification of cervicomedullary junction lesions into *reducible* and *nonreducible* pathology has been a valuable framework for approaching patients with problems in this region, which are almost always complex.[29] *Reducible* means that the normal anatomic relationships of the craniovertebral junction can be restored. At times, simple analysis of the radiographs with flexion and extension views of CT with coronal and sagittal reconstruction, and of MR images of the lesion can indicate which category the patient falls in. Other patients must be observed during bed rest in extension or skull tong traction to determine if the lesion is reducible. Nonreducible lesions must be further analyzed to determine if either anterior or posterior decompression is required. If anterior decompression is necessary, then the transoral or transcervical approach is chosen. Often this choice depends on the experience and preference of the surgeon. If the lesion requires exposure of the lateral masses, is caudal to the mid-clivus, requires vertebral resection caudal to C2, or requires opening of the dura, then the transcervical approach may be preferable.

Anterolateral (Transcervical) Route

The anterolateral route runs through the platysma muscle to the submandibular trigone, beneath the submandibular gland, inferior to the digastric muscle, inferior to the hypoglossal nerve, superior to the greater cornu of the hyoid bone, and posteriorly past the lateral aspect of the superior pharyngeal constrictor muscle to the retropharyngeal space and precervical fascia. A series of 13 patients who had symptomatic cervicomedullary compression underwent ventral decompression by this procedure. All suffered chronic progressive myelopathy caused by ventral compression at the cervicomedullary junction. They underwent planned multistaged treatment, which included transcervical ventral resection of the compressive elements.

Sequential wide dissection of the cervical fascial planes is the key to exposing this region. Anatomic landmarks serve as guides along the way. Transection of tendons, muscles, and arteries is not required for the exposure.

Surgical Preparation

Preliminary Preemptive Procedures

Nutrition

Adequate nutrition is critical for the recovery of any stressed patient. Nutritional insufficiency is aggravated by a debilitated state. The pharyngeal and upper airway edema that result from this procedure impair swallowing for several days. Aggravation of a nutritional catabolic state can be avoided by preoperative placement of a gastrostomy/jejunostomy. Optimal nutritional support helps to prevent sepsis; it also facilitates ambulation and rehabilitation.

Respiration

Upper airway obstruction from soft tissue swelling is a major postoperative challenge with this procedure, and is particularly a concern with myelopathic and debilitated patients. Even patients who are neurologically intact may require preemptive tracheostomy to avoid ventilatory obstruction. Endotracheal intubation is needed for several days to insure an adequate airway. Pneumonitis from either aspiration or atelectasis must be continually fought off in the immediate postoperative period. Positive end-expiratory pressure (PEEP) of 5 to 10 cmH_2O on the ventilator is prophylactic for atelectasis. A rotokinetic bed assists pulmonary drainage. A feeding jejunostomy may prevent aspiration.

Skeletal Traction

Skeletal traction is often necessary to maintain position in spinal instability. The head can hang over an extra-thick pad or short mattress to allow neck extension. The head position to be used during the operation is tried before induction of anesthesia to verify that it is tolerated neurologically by the patient. Skull tongs can be applied after anesthesia has been induced.

CSF Diversion

An external lumbar subarachnoid drain is placed before starting the procedure if a dural opening is planned. If the dura is inadvertently opened, the lumber drain can be placed after completing the procedure. The lumbar catheter is tunneled subcutaneously for several centimeters before being externalized and attached to the drainage reservoir. CSF drainage will reduce hydrostatic pressure and avoid a CSF fistula.

Anesthesia

Nasotracheal airway intubation under topical and local anesthesia using a fiberoptic bronchoscope may avoid overmanipulation of a patient compromised by craniovertebral compression. Adequate venous access is necessary for cardiovascular monitoring and intravenous fluid balancing.

Operative Positioning

The operating table can be prepared for fluoroscopy oriented for the lateral projection. Fluoroscopic control of the operative field is very helpful for maintaining orientation in the sagittal plane. The patient's head is supported on a sponge doughnut or horseshoe headrest, rotated 30 degrees to the contralateral side, and placed into extension so as to raise the mandible up and away from the surgeon's line of sight to the field (Fig. 161-1). The head can also be maintained in a halo traction system.

Side of Approach

The side of approach depends on the pathology of the lesion. If there is unilateral lower cranial nerve impairment, the approach should be made from the side of impairment to avoid additional cranial nerve deficit. The surgeon's perspective will be at approximately a 20 degree angle from the midsagittal plane and a 30

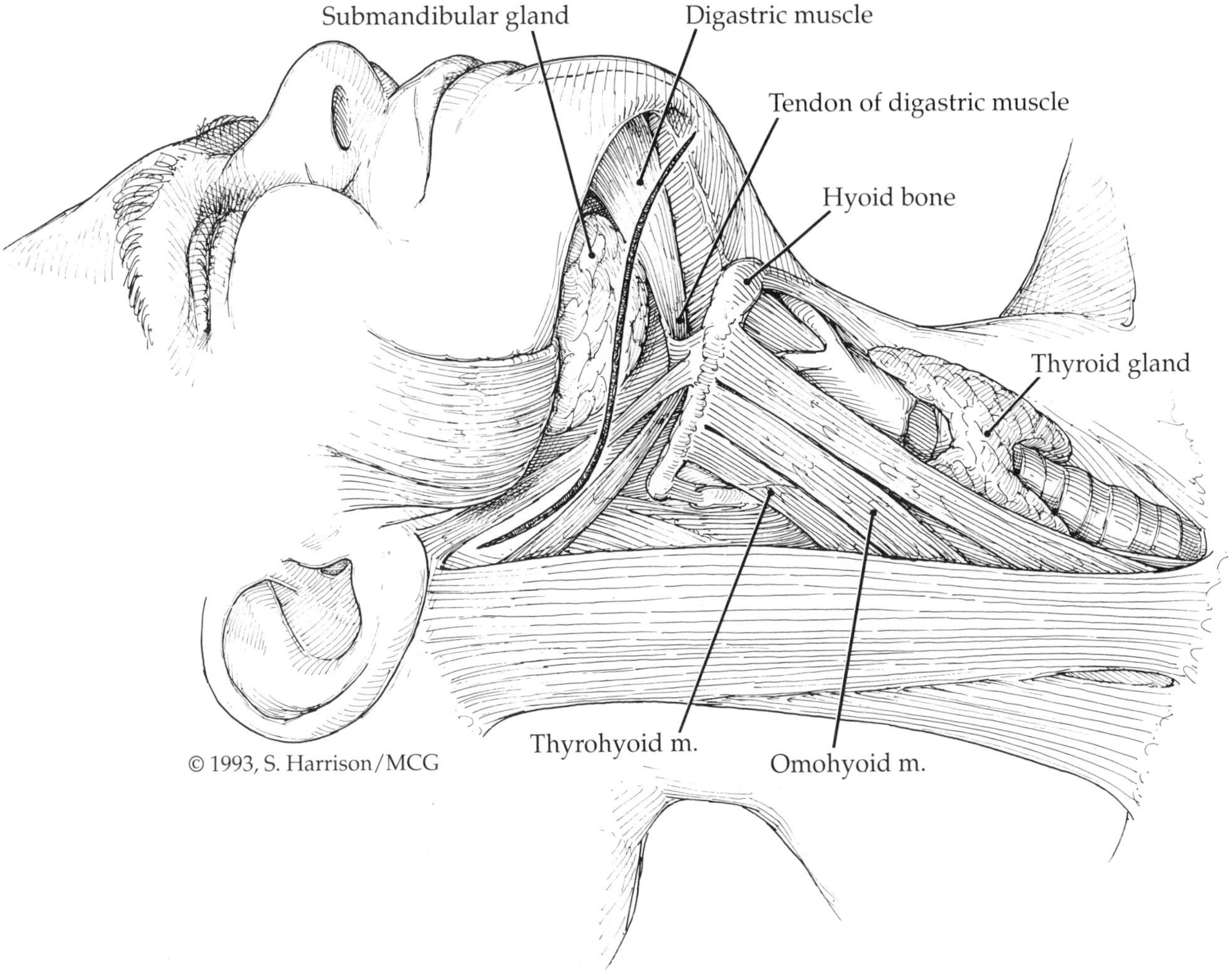

Figure 161-1 The patient is positioned with the head extended and rotated contralaterally to the side of the approach. The curvilinear incision is 2 to 3 cm below and parallel to the edge of the mandible.

degree angle from the transverse/horizontal plane; this perspective gives a good view of deep structures contralateral to the side of approach. Choosing the side of approach is important in preoperative planning, particularly with lesions eccentric from the midline. When dealing with midline pathology, the side of approach is usually that of the surgeon's preference.

Operative Approach

Skin Incision

The choice of incision depends on the craniovertebral exposure required. The transverse incision is used routinely. The key to adequate exposure for this approach is wide dissection of the cervical fascial planes. The incision parallels the mandible 2 cm below the lower edge. It extends from the angle of the mandible to the base of the mental protuberance beyond the midline (Fig. 161-1). Care is taken to avoid the marginal mandibular branch of the facial nerve that supplies the mental muscles of the lower lip.

General Plan of Dissection

The key to adequate exposure is wide sharp dissection of each layer or plane of the cervical fascia, beginning with the development of a wide subcutaneous flap on either side of the incision superficial to the platysma muscle (Fig. 161-2). Anatomic landmarks identify each plane and guide the way. Each landmark is dissected free of its fascial investment and is preserved both anatomically and functionally. Keeping the fascia taut with countertraction on the fascia as the dissection progresses helps to define the fascial plane being dissected. When lifted and opened, the areolar fibrous texture of the fascia is revealed. Its transparency allows a view of the structures it contains. Wide opening of each fascial layer in a sequential, methodical manner will ensure adequate exposure of the deeper structures while preserving the intervening structures. The dissection can be compared to the one performed on a cadaver in the anatomy laboratory for anatomic presentation. Therefore, this procedure requires a ''cadaveric'' dissection of the cervical fascia and its enclosed structures.

The previously dissected skin edges and subcutaneous flaps are retracted, thus exposing the superficial surface of the platysma muscle.

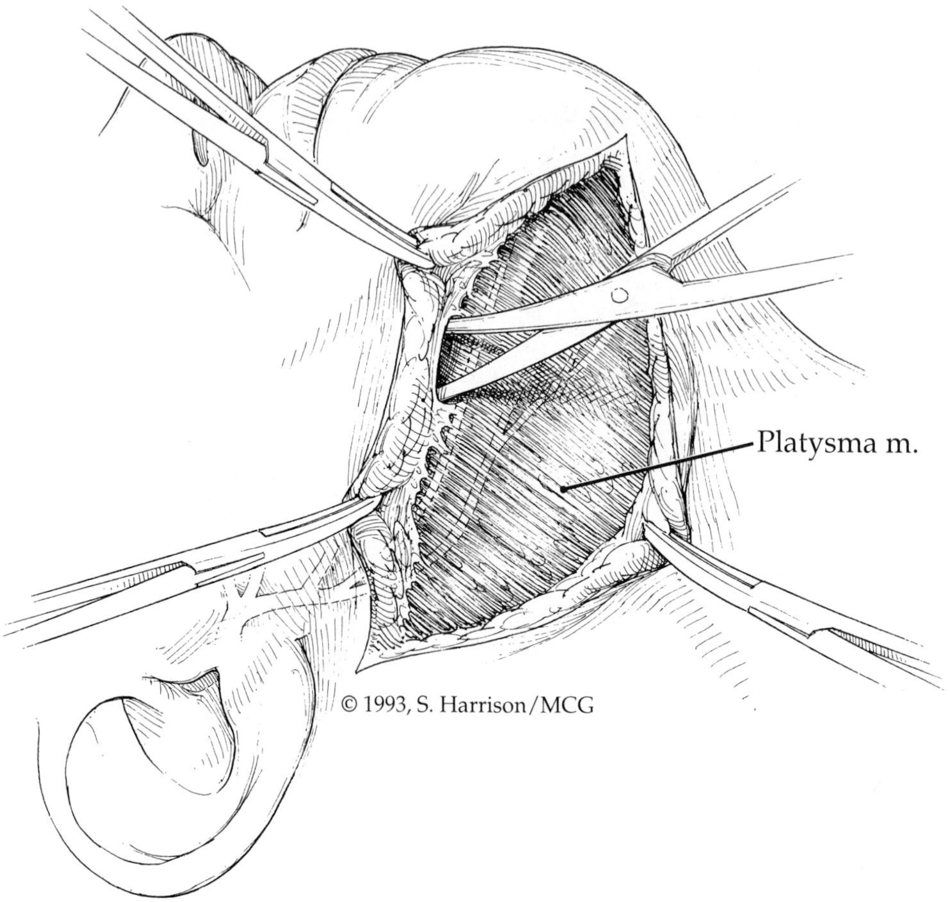

Figure 161-2 Wide dissection of the subcutaneous layer opens the most superficial layer of the cervical fascia, exposing the outer surface of the platysma muscle. Care is taken to avoid injuring the mental branch of the facial nerve, which can cause a droop of the ipsilateral lower lip.

Platysma Muscle

The medial edge of the platysma is grasped in the midline, and a hole is cut in the medial fascial raphe to gain entrance to the next fascial layer. Vertical dissection undermines this fascial layer in the midline in a cephalocaudal direction. The fascial sheet thus formed is then cut vertically in the midline for a length of 6 cm from the mandibular symphysis to the median notch of the thyroid cartilage (Fig. 161-3). This cut defines the medial edge of the platysma muscle and initiates vertical access, to allow freer retraction. The medial edge of the platysma is elevated. The platysma undersurface is then dissected and freed. The platysma is then transected across its fibers in line with the primary incision. The platysma edges are undermined to form flaps to be retracted.

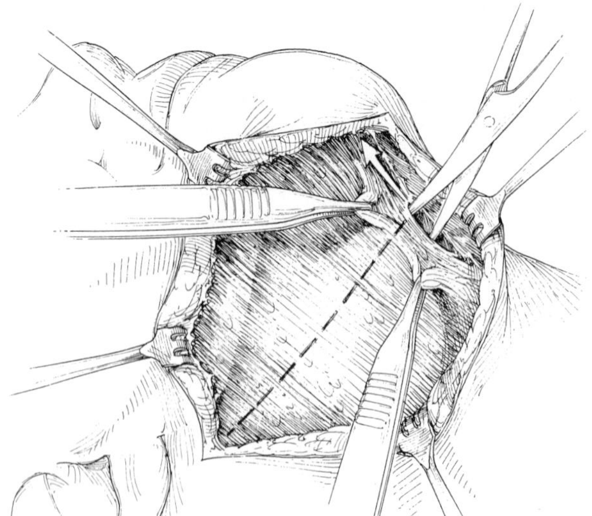

Figure 161-3 The medial border of the platysma muscle is found at the midline and split vertically from the mental symphysis to the superior notch of the thyroid cartilage; this step opens access to the next layer of cervical fascia.

Submandibular Gland

The next fascial layer is identified by the submandibular gland, which bulges beneath it (Fig. 161-4). The *inferior* edge of the gland is grasped and elevated. The fascia is opened, undermined, and dissected in line with the incision. The facial artery and vein are encountered crossing the field of dissection posterolateral to the submandibular gland. They are then dissected along their course. This maneuver further opens the submandibular fascial plane. The facial vein is transected. The facial artery is preserved (Fig. 161-4). Dissection of the facial artery proximally leads to the carotid sheath, the lateral limit of the exposure. When the facial

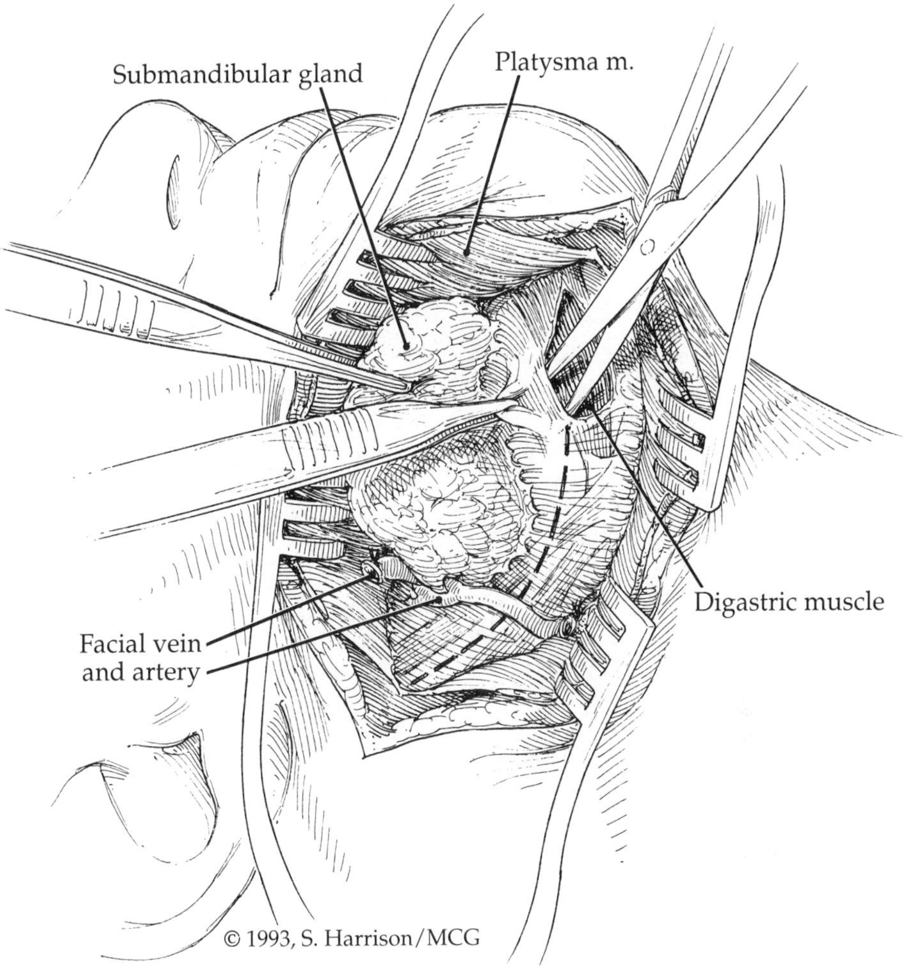

Figure 161-4 The platysma muscle is transected; lifting the tissues with grasping forceps and applying countertraction assists with the dissection. This step exposes the next fascial layer. Retraction of the platysma exposes the submandibular gland and the facial artery and vein. Dissection of these structures opens the next layer of cervical fascia. The anterior belly of the digastric muscle is exposed when the facial vein is transected and the submandibular gland is elevated and retracted superiorly.

artery is dissected, it can be retracted and not cut, as it assists orientation. Retracting the submandibular gland superiorly exposes the next landmark, the digastric tendon.

Digastric Muscle and Tendon

The tendon of the digastric muscle is identified as a glistening white cord running parallel to the incision beneath the inferior edge of the submandibular gland (Fig. 161-4). It leads to the next fascial layer. The fascial sling of the digastric tendon attached to the greater wing of the hyoid bone is transected along the course of the tendon. This frees the tendon so that it can be retracted rostrally toward the mandible. This retraction is facilitated by freeing the undersurface of the anterior and posterior digastric muscle bellies. When the digastric tendon is retracted toward the mandible, the next fascial layer becomes visible. The hypoglossal nerve comes into view, coursing just deep, slightly inferior, and parallel to the digastric tendon.

Hypoglossal Nerve

The hypoglossal nerve is gently dissected along its course and carefully preserved (Fig. 161-5). Posterolaterally the dissection is carried along the nerve trunk toward the descending hypoglossal ramus, which is another guide to the region of the carotid artery. Again, it is not necessary to dissect along the medial border of the carotid sheath unless segments caudal to C4 are to be exposed. Thus freed, the hypoglossal nerve is retracted superiorly, exposing the hypoglossus muscle. The greater cornu of the hyoid bone now comes into view.

Hyoid Bone

The greater cornu of the hyoid bone can now be seen and palpated. The fascia overlying it is opened along the course of the hyoid bone to the carotid sheath (Fig. 161-5). The carotid artery is easily palpated and is the lateralmost limit of the dissection. It is retracted laterally by a right-angled retractor blade. This maneuver opens the retropharyngeal space. It is not necessary to cut any muscles, nerves, or vessels. At this point, it is important to avoid compromising the superior laryngeal nerve (SLN). The SLN courses deep to the internal carotid artery along the middle pharyngeal constrictor muscle toward the superior cornu of the thyroid cartilage. The SLN is therefore caudal and lateral to the route of the exposure described here. Entrance to the retropharyngeal space by this procedure is along the greater cornu of the hyoid bone and adjacent to the superior pharyngeal constrictor muscle. Although the SLN is not seen in the dissection of this approach, it is vulnerable to stretch injury from retraction. Wide dissection of the fascial

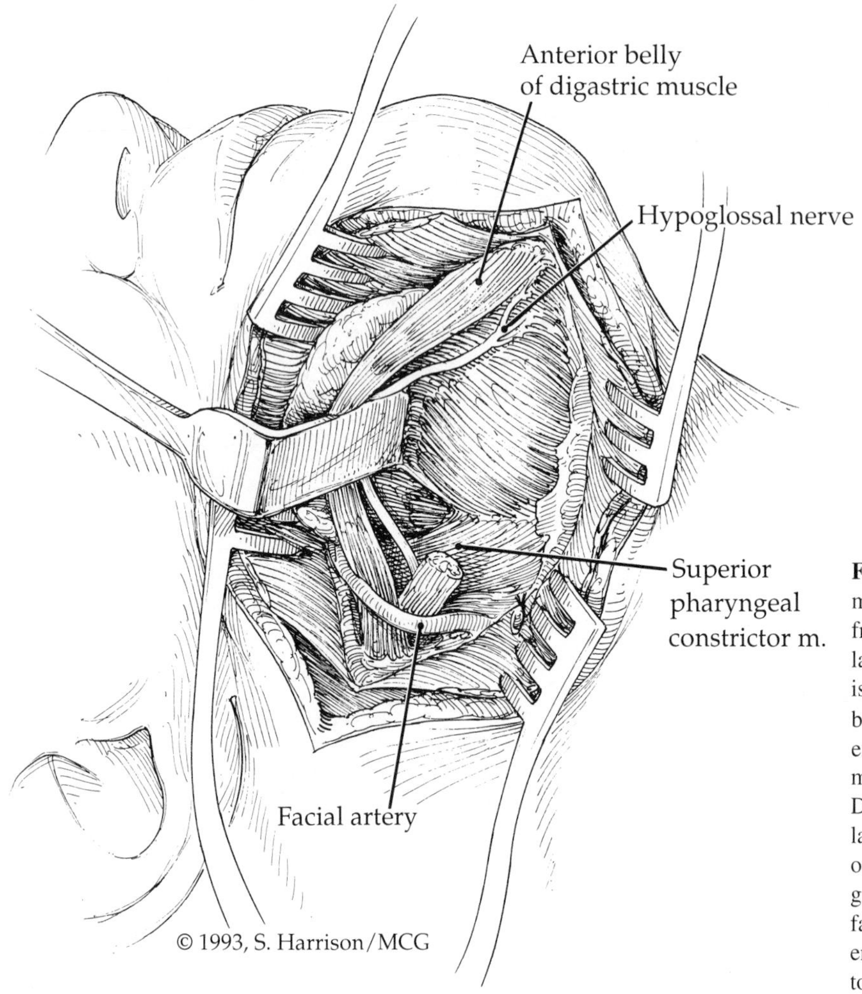

Figure 161-5 Transecting the fascial investment of the digastric muscle exposes and frees the next landmark and opens the next layer of cervical fascia. The digastric tendon is separated from its fascial sling at the hyoid bone and is retracted superiorly. This step exposes the hypoglossal nerve, the next landmark, and the next layer of cervical fascia. Dissection of the hypoglossal nerve opens this layer of cervical fascia and allows retraction of the nerve to expose the next landmark, the greater cornu of the hyoid bone. Opening the fascia along the hyoid bone exposes the lateral wall of the superior pharyngeal constrictor muscle.

planes, as described here, should tend to protect the SLN from retraction injury, as less force is required to separate the tissues that are freed by the fascial dissection. The SLN is not involved in the soft tissues retracted superiorly for this exposure. It is vulnerable to injury if the deep cervical fascia is opened inferiorly in the more lateral extent of this exposure. If access to C4 or lower cervical segments is needed by this route, the SLN is identified and preserved.

The pharyngeal constrictor muscles are retracted medially by a deep right-angled retractor. The retropharyngeal areolar tissue is opened with scissors. The anterior surface of the cervical spine is easily palpated. The prominence of the anterior tubercle of C1 is palpated and offers the surgeon rostral orientation. The midline of the cervical spine indicates the midsagittal plane, which is further identified between the longus colli and longus capitis muscles (Fig. 161-6).

Longus Colli Muscles

The converging medial borders of the longus colli muscles are cauterized and elevated from the anterolateral surfaces of C2 and C3 by sharp dissection. The retractor blade engaged along the dissected border is used to separate the longus colli muscles. This preliminary soft tissue retraction initiates access to deep structures. The microscope with CO_2 laser attached is adjusted to the field. Laser dissection facilitates the exposure of the anterior arch of C1 and the atlas and axis lateral mass articulations. It allows muscle separation up to the pharyngeal tubercle of the basiocciput. Viewing these most rostral structures requires vertical retraction using a deep, narrow, right-angled retractor blade (See Fig. 161-8). This retraction is critical for exposure and access. The medial one-half of the C1 and C2 lateral masses as well as the anterior rim of the foramen magnum and adjacent basiocciput (structures rostral to the anterior arch of C1) should be in view before proceeding.

C1 Anterior Arch Median Tubercle

The C1 anterior tubercle is a guide that helps the surgeon stay in orientation with the midsagittal plane (Fig. 161-6). The perspective to structures of interest is upward and angled at 45 degrees. The C1 arch, base of the dens, preodontoid space, and lateral mass articulations are seen. Laser removal of overlying soft tissue helps to clear the view. The dens, body of C2, and atlantotransverse ligament can be removed, leaving the anterior arch of C1 intact, if so desired. The transverse ligament is a tough, rather thick, well-defined, pale-yellow ligamentous band behind the dens. This ligament comes into view after the dens has been resected. It serves as a guide after the C1 arch and odontoid have been removed, but may be obscured by destructive changes of disease.

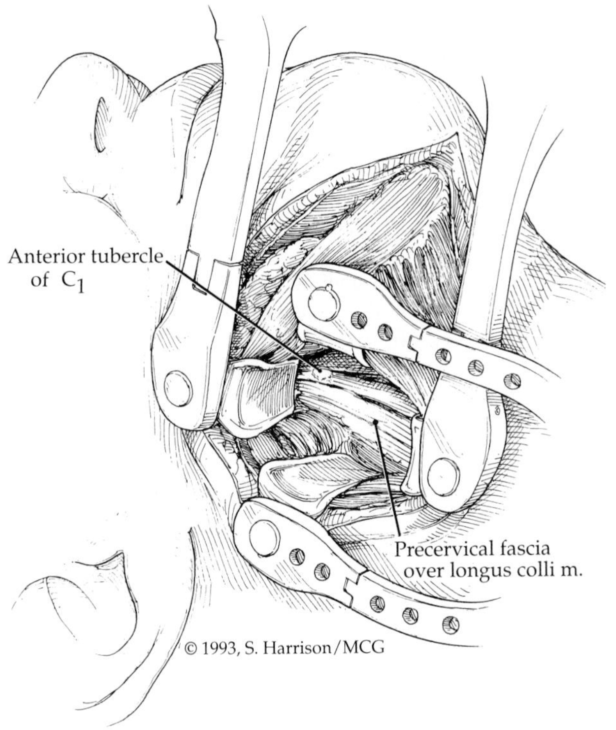

Figure 161-6 Retraction of the superior pharyngeal constrictor opens the retropharyngeal space and exposes the precervical fascia and longus colli muscles. The anterior tubercle of C1 identifies the midline. The longus colli muscles are dissected from the anterior arch of C1 and the anterior surface of C2 and C3 using a CO_2 laser.

Foramen Magnum Anterior Rim

The anterior rim of the foramen magnum is the next landmark just above the C1 arch. The basiocciput can be palpated and seen between the attachments of the longus colli and longus capitis muscles. It can be drilled away if entrance into the ventral aspect of the posterior fossa is needed. The pharyngeal tubercle is the rostral-most landmark and superior limit to this approach.

Resection

A high-speed drill with cutting burr is used to resect the bone. Usually, the anterior arch of C1 can be removed to give a full view of the dens and adjacent articulations. The dens should be resected from the apex caudally, keeping its base intact (Fig. 161-7). It should be thinned out like an eggshell. The diamond burr is used at this point to avoid inadvertent tearing of the adjacent soft tissues. The medial wall of the lateral masses can be removed to widen the ventral exposure; this is necessary if the lesion is intradural. The transverse ligament is identified to verify the orientation (Fig. 161-7). This ligament, along with the apical bursa, cruciform, and tectorial ligaments, must be separated from the dura and removed. The CO_2 laser, slightly defocused at 5 to 10 W, allows ''no touch'' removal of these structures. These ligaments and pannus can be thick, resilient, and difficult to remove when there has been long-standing instability at C1-C2. The anterior rim of the foramen magnum can now be drilled away.

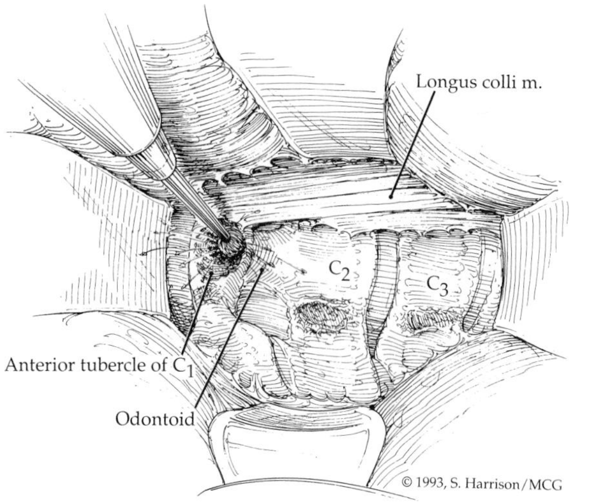

Figure 161-7 The anterior arch of C1 is being removed, which exposes the dens. The dens is best drilled away from its apex to its base. The transverse ligament is the next landmark. Along with the posterior longitudinal ligament, it must be removed to adequately decompress the neuraxis.

The ventral aspect of the dural sac must bulge and pulsate into the resection site to ensure adequate decompression of the neuraxis (Fig. 161-8). The dura may be transparent enough to reveal the pial vessels of the underlying spinal cord.

The dura is opened longitudinally. Traction sutures on the dural edge help to widen the exposure. For neoplasms, the laser is indispensable for atraumatic removal and compensates for the long reach required by this approach. The laser is particularly effective for tumor removal and is also amenable to the transoral approach.[32] Bleeding from venous sinuses and epidural veins in this region can be challenging. Micro bipolar coagulation, bone wax, topical microfibrillar collagen, and gentle suction compression are used for hemostasis.

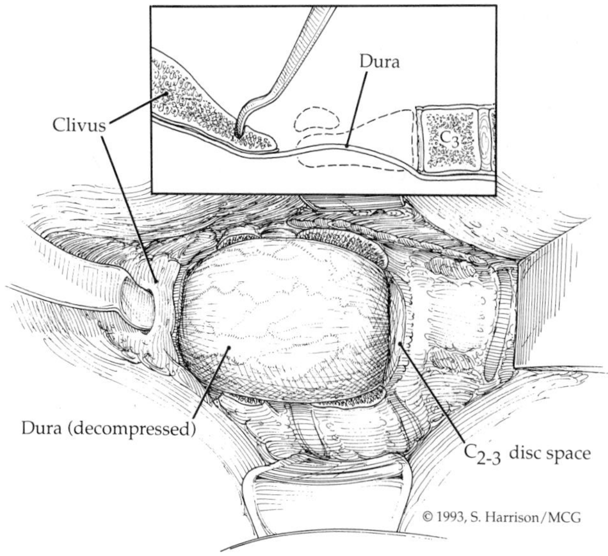

Figure 161-8 Bulging of the dura into the resection site ensures adequate decompression. Note the position of the retractor, which was inserted into the clivus *(inset)*.

Closure Techniques

Dural Closure

The dura cannot be closed primarily here. An autograft or allograft fascia tacked on all four sides at several places or held by a running stitch can also be used for dural closure. The milliwatt CO_2 laser can be used to ''weld'' the edges. The most effective dural closure supplement is fibrin glue.[15,39] Cryoprecipitate can be applied topically over the graft, which is then sprayed with thrombin, giving a thick layer of coagulum that helps to seal the dural closure. Composite baffles of fascia lata and small bone plate have also been successful in closing the defect transorally by wedging the bone plate behind the cranial base defect.[5]

CSF Drainage

A catheter placed percutaneously into the lumbar subarachnoid space at the beginning of the procedure and brought to continuous drainage will usually be effective in preventing an external CSF cutaneous fistula. It can be left in place for 7 to 12 days, provided it has been tunneled under the skin for a few centimeters. Excessive drainage can lead to intracranial hypotension and headache. CSF drainage should be monitored closely to avoid complications.

Spinal Stabilization

Spinal stabilization is important in preoperative planning. Skull tongs are placed before starting, and light traction (5 to 10 lb) is maintained throughout the procedure. Traction can be maintained as a temporizing measure postoperatively until final stabilization is accomplished. Osseous fusion *in situ* is an option. The C1-C2 lateral masses are available for interarticular arthrodesis via this approach. An intact C1 anterior arch can be used as a graft purchase. These alternatives assume a stable atlanto-occipital articulation, which must be verified.

An external orthosis (halo brace) is rarely adequate as the sole source for stability after this procedure. However, it often supplements surgical arthrodesis of the craniovertebral junction and is continued for several months. Occipitocervical arthrodesis is performed subsequently in the face of craniovertebral instability, and the patient is kept in skull traction until it is accomplished.

Suture Closure

Absorbable suture material is preferred for wound closure. The platysma muscle is closed as a separate layer. Interrupted horizontal mattress sutures placed separately in the subcutaneous layer gives strength to the closure. A continuous subcuticular stitch skin edge approximation will provide a cosmetically pleasing scar, particularly if the transverse incision has been used.

Specialized Instruments

Retractors

Adequate retraction is essential for this procedure because of the deep access and angle of approach. A narrow, 90 degree angle, 8-cm blade can be used to lift soft tissues rostrally for initial precervical dissection of the superior corner at C1 and the clivus. The deep blades of the Cloward or Caspar self-retaining retraction systems are adequate for ongoing retraction after dissection of the longus colli muscles. However, their purchase on the tissues is not secure, and they can migrate out of position. Adequate soft tissue dissection prior to retraction facilitates safe exposure of the approach. The author uses a bent, reversed-hook, narrow, long-bladed retractor that is inserted into a drill hole in the outer cortex of the basiocciput and then pulled rostrally by rubber bands and secured to the drapes at the patient's vertex. This arrangement pushes the soft tissues rostrally and allows good visualization of the midline compartment of the craniovertebral junction (Fig. 161-8).

Laser

The microsurgical CO_2 laser facilitates dissection of paraspinal muscles, resection of ligaments, and excision of pannus or tumor. Complete removal of offending lesions is possible even in hard-to-reach areas. Mechanical trauma is also avoided, thus improving the safety of the procedure.

Sutures

A small, strong, cutting, semicircular needle is needed for suturing in this cramped space. The P-2 Ethicon (Ethicon, Somerville, NJ) needle works well here. The suture material is 5-0 polydioxanone; it can be used for dural traction, dural patch repair, or dural graft closure. An alternate needle and suture for this purpose is 5-0 Dexon Plus on the PR-1 needle by Davis + Geck (Davis + Geck, Inc., Manati, PR).

Clinical Series

The first author's personal experience over a 9-year period with 13 patients is summarized in Table 161-1. The patients ranged from 14 to 66 years old, and the sex ratio was even. Six patients were quadriparetic. All patients had neck pain severe enough to interfere with overall comfort and life-style, and all were pain-free after recovering from the procedures. Six patients had neoplasms, each of a different histologic type. All patients underwent a fusion procedure. Two underwent anterior fusion during the initial transcervical ventral decompression—in one case, by an iliac wedge graft supplemented by a screw plate and halo brace, which fused (patient MS in Table 161-1); in the other case, by an iliac wedge graft from the C2 body to the C1 arch, which failed and necessitated subsequent posterior occipital cervical fusion (patient AS).

Complications

All patients experienced ipsilateral hypoglossal nerve paresis with hemiglossal atrophy, which improved but remained evident on examination even after long-term follow-up. This deficit was always well compensated for functionally, and no patient complained of glossal dysfunction. Five patients developed a CSF leak that formed a neck swelling which transilluminated light and/or was evident on postoperative MRI scans. These patients all were treated initially with continuous percutaneous lumbar subarachnoid catheter external drainage. Three ultimately required internalization of the shunt. In two of these three patients, the shunt was

TABLE 161-1 Clinical Series of Patients Who Underwent Transcervical Resection of Craniovertebral Junction Lesions

Clinical Series*										
Patient and Date of Operation	Sex	Age	Diagnosis	Preoperative Function	Duration	Pathology	Complications	Posterior Fusion	Neurofunctional Status, Time Course	
DB 8/20/85	M	42	Chordoma, C1-C2 dissolution	Neck pain	6 wk	Chordoma clivus, C1, C2	None	9/3/85	Left IX, X palsy; recurrence	Died 5 yr after operation
WR 10/18/85	F	60	Angled fx. C2 AP diam. 7 mm	Quadriparetic	9 mo	Thick fibrosis, nonunion fx.	CSF fistula	10/31/85	Independent	6 mo
DD 2/3/86	M	31	Os odontoideum, basilar impression	Quadriparetic	4 yr	Odontoid loose, unstable fibrosis	SIADH	2/11/86	Spastic gait, self care	6 mo
JS 11/12/86	M	43	Os odontoideum, basilar impression	Quadriparetic	3 yr	Odontoid loose, unstable fibrosis	None	11/25/86	Neurologically intact, back to work	3 mo
TS 11/24/87	M	16	Neurofibromas, ventral canal C2-C7	Quadriparetic	3 mo	Mult. neurofib. cervical roots	CSF fistula	12/11/87	Mild spasticity, carpenter work	1 yr
JD 3/1/88	F	66	Rheumatoid pannus, odontoid	Quadriparetic	2 yr	Rheumatoid pannus	Bronchial spasm	3/9/88	Neurologically intact, independent	2 yr
MS 11/10/89	F	63	Ca breast metastasis, path. fx. C2	Neck pain	3 mo	Path. compression fx. C2	Airway obstruction	Anterior fusion	Neurologically intact, independent	6 mo Died 1 yr after operation
AR 1/26/90	F	36	Hangman's fx. C2, HNP C2-C3	Neck pain	2 wk	Unstable fx. C2, HNP C2-C3	None	Anterior fusion	Neurologically intact, independent	2 mo
DY 6/15/90	M	64	Rheumatoid sublux. C1-C2	Quadriparetic	8 mo	Anterior subluxation C1-C2	CSF fistula	6/26/90	Died of cardiac arrest, coagulopathy	6/27/90
VS 6/18/90	F	45	Meningioma ventral foramen mag. C1	Mild myelopathy	1 yr	Meningioma with ventral compression	CSF fistula	6/29/90	Neurologically intact, independent	3 mo
AS 5/5/91	M	42	Type II odontoid fx., unstable nonunion	Mild myelopathy	8 yr	Odontoid, loose scar	Dysphagia	5/15/91	Neurologically intact, independent	3 mo
AR 6/29/92	F	14	Plexiform neurofibroma, C1-C2	Neck pain	1 yr	Neurofibroma	CSF fistula	7/10/92	Neurologically intact, independent	6 mo
EF 4/19/93	M	21	Ewing sarcoma, C1-C2	Neck pain	8 mo	Ewing sarcoma	None	5/3/93	Neurologically intact, independent	2 mo Positron rad.

*Ca, cancer; CSF, cerebrospinal fluid; diam., diameter; fx., fracture; HNP, herniated nucleus pulposus; mag., magnum; Mult., multiple; neurofib., neurofibromas; path., pathological; rad., radiation; SIADH, syndrome of inappropriate antidiuretic hormone secretion; sublux., subluxation.

closed with a clip under local anesthesia; one of these patients (TS) developed a CSF ascites syndrome, which resolved after shunt occlusion, and the other (AR) had persistent headache, presumably from low intracranial pressure. The retropharyngeal pseudomeningocoeles have not recurred in these patients. Two patients suffered from troubling dysphagia that persisted for several months and gradually subsided. The mechanism of dysphagia is unclear, but it was not due to pharyngeal swelling, as it persisted after the swelling had resolved. Voice hoarseness was noted in four patients and resolved in all but one (MS). It was due to superior laryngeal nerve dysfunction. This approach is well above the recurrent laryngeal nerve.[6] The sole death in the series, of patient DY, was caused primarily by a coagulopathy that developed after occipitocervical fusion; the patient was a 64-year-old woman who was bedridden with chronic rheumatoid arthritis and myelopathy from a C1-C2 subluxation.

Conclusion

The transcervical approach to the craniovertebral junction is an effective alternative to the transoral approach. A lesion caudal to the pharyngeal tubercle of the clivus and amenable to the transoral approach can be exposed via the transcervical approach. Dural leakage of CSF is more safely managed with this approach. Instrumentation and implantation can be placed with relatively safety. Anatomical fascial dissection need not restrict exposure or involve structural transection, if landmarks are followed.

The results can be improved and complications reduced by the following steps:

1. Careful selection of a treatment plan based on an algorithm that considers reduction of malalignment and specific imaged anatomy of neural compression
2. Pre-emptive and elective tracheostomy and feeding gastrostomy/jejunostomy tube placement
3. Hydrodynamic control of CSF with external lumbar subarachnoid drain placement and tunneling of the catheter under the skin; permanent CSF peritoneal shunt placement if required
4. Wide anatomic dissection of fascial planes
5. Microsurgical technique under fluoroscopic control
6. Nursing on a rotokinetic bed with skull traction

References

1. Ammirati M, Ma J, Cheatham ML, et al. The mandibular swing-transcervical approach to the skull base: anatomical study. Technical note. *J Neurosurg* 1993; 78:673–681.
2. Apuzzo MLJ, Wise MH, Heiden JS. Transoral exposure of the atlantoaxial region. *Neurosurgery* 1978; 3:201–207.
3. Batzdorf U, Gregorius FK. Surgical exposure of the high cervical carotid artery: experimental study and review. *Neurosurgery* 1983; 6:657–661.
4. Biller HF, Shugar JMA, Krespi YP. A new technique for wide-field exposure of the base of the skull. *Arch Otolaryngol* 1981; 107:698–702.
5. Bonkowski JA, Gibson RD, Snape L. Foramen magnum meningioma: transoral resection with a bone baffle to prevent CSF leakage. *J Neurosurg* 1990; 72:493–496.
6. Bulger RF, Rejowski JE, Beatty RA. Vocal cord paralysis associated with anterior cervical fusion: considerations for prevention and treatment. *J Neurosurg* 1985; 62:657–661.
7. Crockard HA, Pozo JL, Ransford AO, et al. Transoral decompression and posterior fusion for rheumatoid atlanto-axial subluxation. *J Bone Joint Surg [Br]* 1986; 68:350–356.
8. Crockard HA, Sen CN. The transoral approach for the management of intradural lesions at the craniovertebral junction: review of 7 cases. *Neurosurgery* 1991; 28:88–98.
9. De Andrade JR, MacNab I. Anterior occipito-cervical fusion using an extrapharyngeal exposure. *J Bone Joint Surg [Am]* 1969; 51:1621–1626.
10. Dickman CA, Locantro J, Fessler RG. The influence of transoral odontoid resection on stability of the craniovertebral junction. *J Neurosurg* 1992; 77:525–530.
11. Di Lorenzo N, Fortuna A, Guidetti B. Craniovertebral junction malformations. Clinico-radiological findings, long-term results, and surgical indications in 63 cases. *J Neurosurg* 1982; 57:603–608.
12. Fang D, Leong JCY, Fang HSY. Tuberculosis of the upper cervical spine. *J Bone Joint Surg [Br]* 1983; 65:47–50.
13. Goel A. Transoral approach for removal of intradural lesions at the craniocervical junction. *Neurosurgery* 1991; 29:155–156. Letter.
14. Grodinsky M, Holyoke EA. The fasciae and fascial spaces of the head, neck, and adjacent regions. *Am J Anat* 1938; 63:367–408.
15. Hadley MN, Martin NA, Spetzler RF, et al. Comparative transoral dural closure techniques: a canine model. *Neurosurgery* 1988; 22:392–397.
16. Hadley MN, Spetzler RF, Sonntag VKH. The transoral approach to the superior cervical spine. A review of 53 cases of extradural cervicomedullary compression. *J Neurosurg* 1989; 71:16–23.
17. Hall JE, Denis F, Murray J. Exposure of the upper cervical spine for spinal decompression by a mandible and tongue-splitting approach: case report. *J Bone Joint Surg [Am]* 1977; 59A:121–123.
18. Henry AK. *Extensile Exposure.* London: Livingstone, 1962, pp 58–72.
19. Howe JR, Taren JA. Foramen magnum tumors: pitfalls in diagnosis. *JAMA* 1973; 225:1061–1066.
20. Jeanneret B, Magerl F. Primary posterior fusion C1/2 in odontoid fractures: Indications, technique, and results of transarticular screw fixation. *J Spinal Disord* 1992; 5:464–475.
21. Kohno K, Sakaki S, Shiraishi T, et al. Successful treatment of adult Arnold-Chiari malformation associated with basilar impression and syringomyelia by the transoral anterior approach. *Surg Neurol* 1990; 33:284–287.
22. Krespi YP, Har-EL G. Surgery of the clivus and anterior cervical spine. *Arch Otolaryngol Head Neck Surg* 1988; 114:73–78.
23. Lesoin F, Autricque A, Franz K, et al. Transcervical approach and screw fixation for upper cervical spine pathology. *Surg Neurol* 1987; 27:459–465.
24. Lesoin F, Pellerin P, Thomas CE III, et al. Acrylic reconstruction of an arthritic cervical spine using the transcervical-transclival approach. *Surg Neurol* 1984; 22:329–334.
25. Lesoin F, Pellerin P, Villette L, et al. Anterior approach and osteosynthesis for recent fractures of the pedicles of the axis. *Neurosurgery* 1986; 19:374–377.
26. McAfee PC, Bohlman HH, Riley LJ Jr, et al. The anterior retropharyngeal approach to the upper part of the cervical spine. *J Bone Joint Surg [Am]* 1987; 69A:1371–1383.
27. McDonnell DE. Anterolateral cervical approach to the craniovertebral junction. In Rengachary SS, Wilkins RH (eds): *Neurosurgical Operative Atlas,* vol 1. Baltimore: Williams & Wilkins, 1991, pp 147–164.
28. Menezes AH, VanGilder JC. Transoral-transpharyngeal approach to the anterior craniocervical junction. Ten-year experience with 72 patients. *J Neurosurg* 1988; 69:895–903.
29. Menezes AH, VanGilder JC, Graf CJ, et al. Craniocervical abnormalities. A comprehensive surgical approach. *J Neurosurg* 1980; 53:444–455.
30. Meyer FB, Ebersold MJ, Reese DF. Benign tumors of the foramen magnum. *J Neurosurg* 1984; 61:136–142.
31. Nagashima C, Iwasaki T, Okada K, et al. Reconstruction of the atlas and axia with wire and acrylic after metastatic destruction. Case report. *J Neurosurg* 1979; 50:668–673.

32. Panje WR, Scher N, Karnell M. Transoral carbon dioxide laser ablation for cancer, tumors, and other diseases. *Arch Otolaryngol Head Neck Surg* 1989; 115:681–688.
33. Pernkopf E. *Atlas of Topographical and Applied Human Anatomy.* Monsen H (trans). Philadelphia: Saunders, 1963, pp 237–280.
34. Phillips E, Levine AM. Metastatic lesions of the upper cervical spine. *Spine* 1989; 14:1071–1077.
35. Riley LH Jr. Surgical approaches to the anterior structures of the cervical spine. *Clin Orthop* 1973; 91:16–20.
36. Robinson RA, Smith GW. Anterolateral cervical disc removal and interbody fusion for cervical disc syndrome. *Bull Johns Hopkins Hosp* 1955; 96:223–224 (abstr).
37. Rock JP, Tomecek FJ, Ross L. Transoral surgery: an anatomic study. *Skull Base Surg* 1993; 3:109–116.
38. Scoville WB, Sherman IJ. Platybasia: report of ten cases with comments on familial tendency, a special diagnostic sign, and the end results of operation. *Ann Surg* 1951; 133:496–502.
39. Shaffrey CI, Spotnitz WD, Shaffrey ME, et al. Neurosurgical applications of fibrin glue: augmentation of dural closure in 134 patients. *Neurosurgery* 1990; 26:207–210.
40. Smith GW, Robinson RA. The treatment of certain cervical-spine disorders by anterior removal of the intervertebral disc and interbody fusion. *J Bone Joint Surg [Am]* 1958; 40:607–624.
41. Southwick WO, Robinson RA. Surgical approaches to the vertebral bodies in the cervical and lumbar regions. *J Bone Joint Surg [Am]* 1957; 39:631–644.
42. Spetzler RF, Selman WR, Nash CL Jr, et al. Transoral microsurgical odontoid resection and spinal cord monitoring. *Spine* 1979; 4:506–510.
43. Stevenson GC, Stoney RJ, Perkins RK, et al. A transcervical transclival approach to the ventral surface of the brain stem for removal of a clivus chordoma. *J Neurosurg* 1966; 24:544–551.
44. VanGilder JC, Menezes AH, Dolan KD: *The Craniovertebral Junction and Its Abnormalities.* Mount Kisco, New York: Futura, 1987, pp 43–118.
45. Verbiest H. A lateral approach to the cervical spine: technique and indications. *J Neurosurg* 1968; 28:191–203.
46. Wackenheim A. Radiologic diagnosis of congenital forms, intermittent forms and progressive forms of stenosis of the spinal canal at the level of the atlas. *Acta Radiol Diagn (Stockh)* 1969; 9:759–768.
47. Whitesides TE, Kelly RP. Lateral approach to the upper cervical spine for anterior fusion. *South Med J* 1966; 59:879–883.
48. Whitesides TE, McDonald AP. Lateral retropharyngeal approach to the upper cervical spine. *Orthop Clin North Am* 1978; 9:1115–1127.
49. Wood BG, Sadar ES, Levine HL, et al. Surgical problems of the base of the skull: an interdisciplinary approach. *Arch Otolaryngol* 1980; 106:1–5.

162 Preauricular Subtemporal-Infratemporal and Combined Approaches to the Cranial Base

Laligam N. Sekhar
Donald C. Wright

Among the various new approaches to the cranial base area, the preauricular subtemporal-infratemporal (ST-IT) approach has an important place, providing ready access to the middle clival, petrous apex, and other areas, with the loss of the eustachian tube as its only disadvantage. This approach was developed by Sekhar and colleagues as a modification of the infratemporal approaches developed by Ugo Fisch.[2,7] Since its initial description, further technical refinements have been added, and its reach has been extended by combining it with other approaches. As with all "new" operative approaches, we have been able to define the limitations and potential complications of this approach, as well as their management.

Regions Accessed by This Approach

The ST-IT approach accesses the cranial base from an anterolateral direction, taking advantage of a subtemporal, extradural, transzygomatic, and transfacial exposure. The key element of this approach is the exposure and mobilization of the petrous segment of the internal carotid artery (ICA), and the extradural dissection of the trigeminal nerve and ganglion. From a lateral to a medial direction, the accessed areas include the temporal and infratemporal fossae, the petrous apex, the midclival area (especially the ipsilateral half), the inferior half of the cavernous sinus, and the lateral orbit. Lesions in this area may be neoplasms, aneurysms of the petrous or posterior intracavernous ICA, developmental anomalies, and other conditions such as cavernous hemangioma and cholesterol granuloma.

Preoperative Evaluation

For most lesions of this area, preoperative imaging studies include magnetic resonance imaging (MRI) scans, computed tomography (CT) scans using 3-mm slices and bone windows, and, if necessary, cerebral arteriography using the intra-arterial digital subtraction technique. Although in the past we used carotid occlusion testing routinely, we now use it selectively, only for lesions that encase the ICA. Because of our present policy of vein graft (or direct) reconstruction of all injured ICAs, the only current value of a preoperative carotid occlusion test is to know the patient's tolerance for temporary ICA occlusion.

A preoperative audiogram is important. If the patient has preoperative deficits of ocular, facial, or other neurological functions, they must be documented adequately.

Operative Technique

A general operative technique is presented here, with further discussion of an extended and an abbreviated version of the method. Later sections describe its combination with other approaches.

For extradural lesions, a lumbar spinal drain is used. A balanced anesthetic technique is employed, with short-acting muscle relaxants, to allow for intraoperative monitoring of facial nerve function. Since excessive blood loss may occasionally occur during surgery, the patient's coagulation parameters must be monitored every 2 h. Appropriate replacement with red blood cells, fresh frozen plasma or cryoprecipitate, and platelets is indicated to prevent a coagulopathy.

Intraoperative neurophysiological monitoring includes electroencephalography and measurement of somatosensory evoked potentials and facial nerve electromyographic activity. If there is concern about hearing preservation, brain stem evoked responses may also be monitored. In the event of injury to the carotid artery, the patient is placed under electroencephalographic burst suppression, induced by barbiturates and etomidate, and the blood pressure is raised about 30 to 40 mmHg while the artery is repaired primarily or replaced with a vein graft.

The patient is placed in the supine position, with the head turned approximately 60 degrees away from the side of the lesion, with a roll under the shoulder. For most lesions not requiring a vein graft, we shave only a strip of hair along the marked incision, with extensive cleansing of the scalp, hair, ear, and neck. A bicoronal or hemicoronal incision is made and extended preauricularly, sharply curved in a V-shape for better cosmesis (Fig. 162-1). The scalp flap includes the pericranium and the superficial layer of the temporal fascia, which blends with the periosteum over the zygomatic arch and with the deep fascia over the masseter muscle. The upper branches of the facial nerve lie superficial to this fascia, in the subcutaneous tissue. Extending this dissection plane over the zygomatic arch into the face allows the parotid gland, the superficial temporal artery, and the upper branches of the facial nerve to be elevated from the deeper tissues in a degloving fashion. The attachment of the deep temporal fascia to the zygomatic arch is then divided, and the entire temporalis muscle is separated and elevated from the temporal fossa. The masseter muscle is also detached from the zygomatic arch.

After administration of intravenous mannitol, hyperventilation, and gradual withdrawal of about 50 ml of cerebrospinal fluid (CSF) from the lumbar drain, a temporal craniotomy is performed,

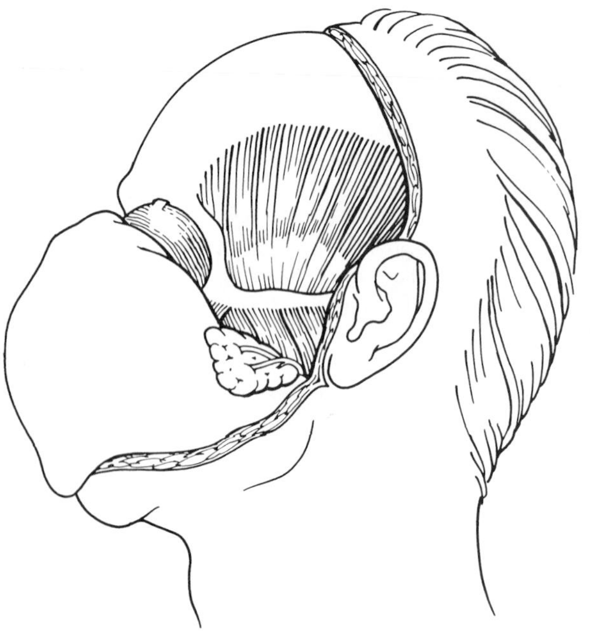

(*A*)

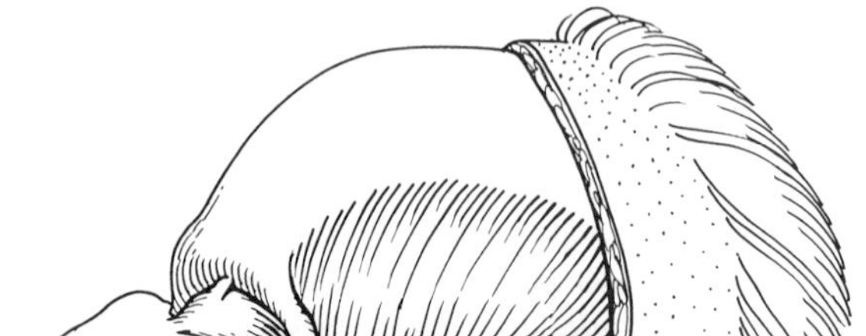

(*B*)

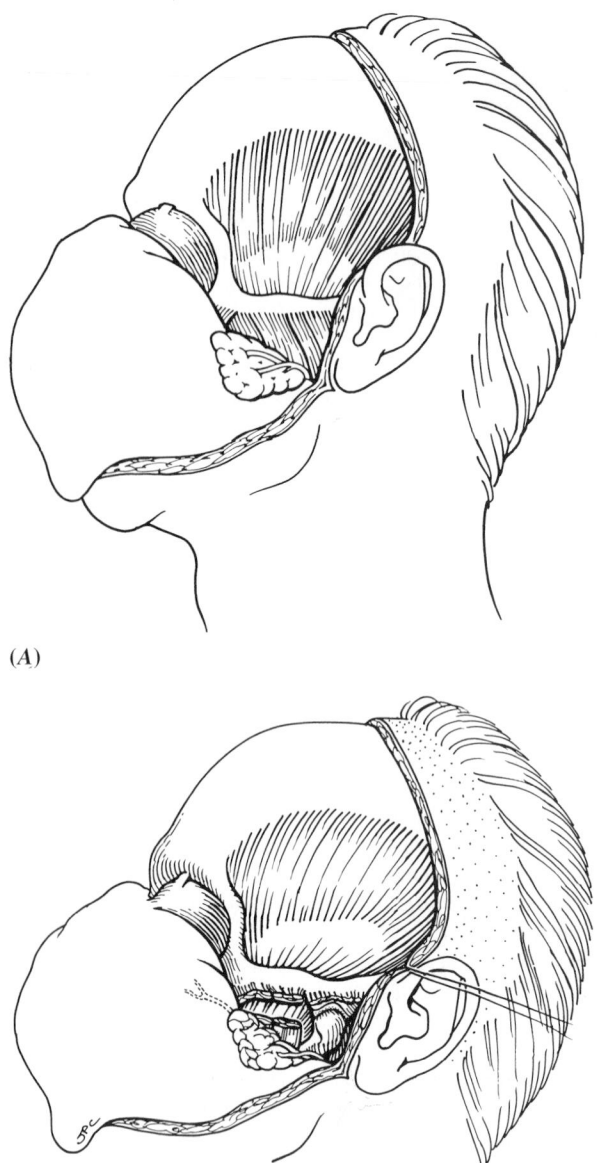

Figure 162-1 Subtemporal-infratemporal approach, bicoronal incision. *A.* Initial exposure after reflection of the scalp and facial tissues. *B.* The masseter muscle has been separated from the zygomatic arch, and the temporomandibular joint has been opened. (From Sekhar et al.,[8] with permission.)

extending anteriorly to the limits of the middle fossa and posteriorly over the base of the mastoid process. Dural tack-up sutures are placed. A subsequent step is the zygomatic osteotomy, which includes the condylar fossa but preserves the mandibular condyle and the meniscus of the temporomandibular (TM) joint. Removal of the zygomatic arch as a separate piece is preferred because of the danger of including the condylar fossa, and the fact that, in the event of epidural infection, the zygomatic arch can be left in situ even if the bone flap has to be removed (Fig. 162-2).

The capsule of the TM joint is opened sharply, and the meniscus and the mandibular condyle are dissected from the temporal bone and depressed. Under the magnification of the surgical microscope, the temporal dura is dissected away from the floor of the middle cranial fossa to expose the middle meningeal artery, the maxillary nerve and foramen rotundum, the mandibular nerve and foramen ovale, the roof of the TM junction, and the arcuate eminence. The latter structure can be found deep, at the level of the external ear canal, as a ridge that runs almost perpendicular to the long axis of the petrous temporal bone. The greater superficial petrosal nerve (GSPN) exits from a foramen anteromedial to the arcuate eminence and runs toward the foramen ovale. Its identity can be confirmed by stimulating it near the foramen with a 1 mA current. Because of retrograde spread of current, facial muscle contractions will be observed. A structure that may be confused with this is the lesser superficial petrosal nerve, which exits lateral to the GSPN and runs forward to the foramen spinosum (Fig. 162-3).

The zygomatic osteotomy is then performed, using a reciprocating saw or Midas Rex (Midas Rex Instruments, Fort Worth, TX) instrumentation. The anterior cut is made in a >-shaped fashion, near the zygomaticomaxillary suture. The posterior cut may include the bony roof of the external ear canal or be just anterior to it, and is made in a V-shaped fashion, just medial to the limits of the roof of the condylar fossa. The zygomatic piece is loosened with a chisel and then removed.

The foramina ovale and rotundum are unroofed, under magnification provided by the surgical microscope. The middle meningeal artery is cauterized and divided, and the foramen spinosum is unroofed. To further elevate the temporal dura and expose the petrous apex area, the outer dural layer over the mandibular and maxillary nerves is opened, and the dura of the middle fossa is peeled away from the trigeminal roof in Meckel's cave. This maneuver also allows the surgeon to access the basal aspect of the cavernous sinus.

By this time, the tumor in the petrous apex area, as well as the horizontal segment of the petrous ICA, may be exposed. The horizontal segment of the petrous ICA lies inferior to the GSPN. The GSPN usually has to be divided, close to its exit from its foramen, to allow the petrous ICA to be mobilized. Now, the tympanic and petrous temporal bone lateral to the petrous ICA is gradually removed using a high-speed drill. Both the tensor tympani muscle and the eustachian tube, which lie lateral to the genu of the petrous ICA, will have to be divided. The posterior (bony) end of the eustachian tube will need to be packed with muscle or fat to close it. The cartilaginous segment of the eustachian tube is divided just medial to V_3, packed with fat, and sutured shut, to occlude the communication with the nasopharynx. As bone is being removed, care must be taken in the area posteromedial to the genu of the petrous ICA, wherein lies the cochlea. As the entrance to the bony carotid canal is unroofed, a fibrocartilaginous ring which surrounds the entrance of the petrous ICA comes into view. This ring, which is fused to the periosteal layer around the petrous ICA, will have to be divided and partially excised to allow mobilization of the petrous ICA. The cervical ICA passes medial to the styloid process before it enters the carotid canal, and it usually makes a posteromedial curve as it enters the bony canal. The jugular bulb and the pars nervosa of the jugular foramen lie just posterior to the upper cervical ICA and the vertical segment of the petrous ICA (Fig. 162-4).

All the bone between the petrous ICA, V_3, and V_2 is now resected. The petrous ICA is then gradually separated from the remainder of the bony canal, along with its periosteal sheath, and mobilized anteriorly. If the periosteal sheath is invaded by tumor, it can be opened. Inside this sheath, around the carotid artery, lie a venous plexus and the sympathetic nerves. When the artery is mobilized forward, it is held with a stitch through the periosteal layer, without any kinks. It is important to remove bone medial to V_3 in order to prevent sharp compression of the artery (Fig. 162-5).

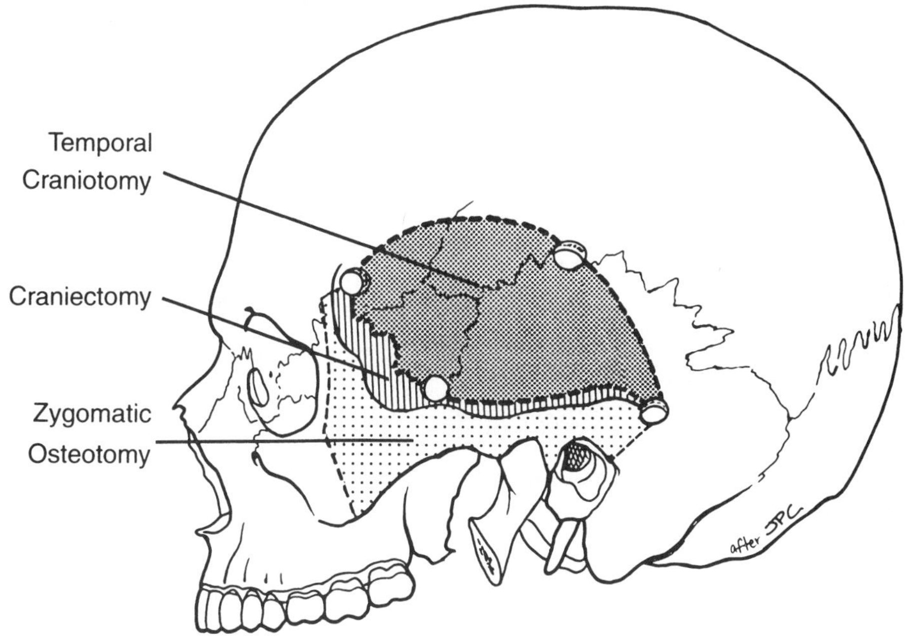

Figure 162-2 A temporal craniotomy, a craniectomy, and a zygomatic osteotomy are performed. The osteotomy includes the condylar fossa and the roof of the external ear canal.

The tumor that lies in the petroclival epidural area is now well exposed. It is removed in a piecemeal fashion. In the case of epidermoid cysts and cholesterol granulomas, it is important to remove the capsule. In the case of chondrosarcomas and chordomas, it is important to drill away surrounding bone until healthy, bleeding bone is reached. In these cases, the petroclival dura will be exposed at the end of the tumor resection. The endoscope can be used to examine hard-to-reach corners. If the jugular bulb is invaded by tumor, it can be opened to remove the tumor and packed with Gelfoam (absorbable gelatin sponge; The Upjohn Company, Kalamazoo, MI) to seal the opening. The hypoglossal canal lies in the clival bone posteromedial to the vertical segment of the petrous ICA. The anterior end of the cavernous sinus can be further accessed by unroofing the posterior end of the orbit and peeling the middle fossa dura in a posterior direction starting from the superior orbital fissure. The lateral aspect of the sphenoid sinus is often entered by this approach.

In order to extend the reach further toward the contralateral side, V_3 can be divided at or below its exit from the cavernous sinus (Fig. 162-6). This allows the temporal lobe and the ipsilateral cavernous sinus structures to be elevated, with access into the sphenoid sinus and the contralateral half of the clivus. The mandibular nerve is resutured at the end of the operation. However, patients seem to experience the recovery of sensation only, and not the motor function of the nerve. Because of this, we prefer to combine the ST-IT approach with the extended frontal approach in such cases, rather than divide V_3.

For intradural lesions of the midclival area, the dura is opened to expose the lesion.[10] This approach can be used for midbasilar or vertebrobasilar junction aneurysms (Fig. 162-7), when the brain stem is swollen, or when the lesion is inadequately exposed by the presigmoid petrosal approach.[5] Unless the intradural tumor is a small extension of the extradural lesion, we do not prefer this approach.

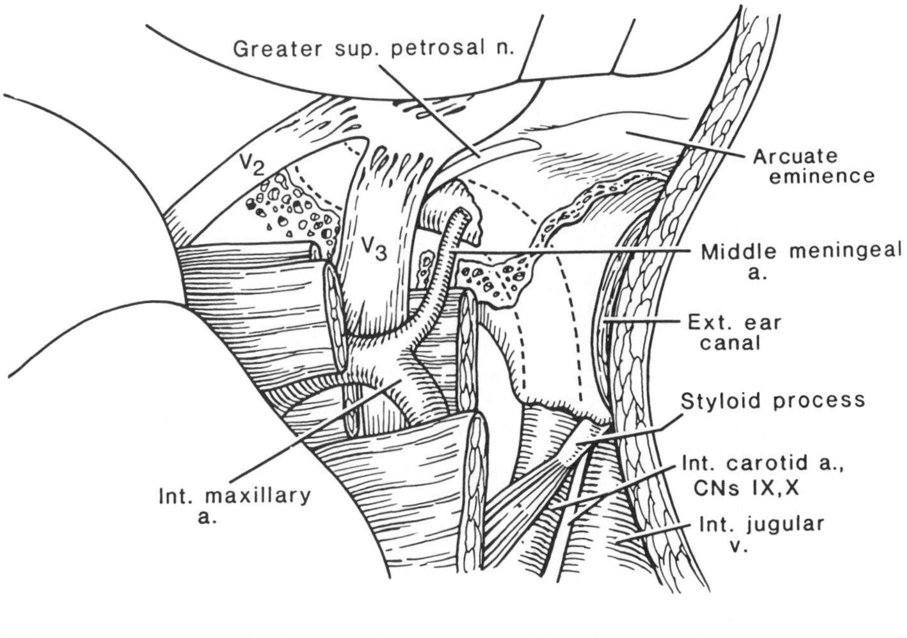

Figure 162-3 Key landmarks in the middle cranial fossa used in the subtemporal-infratemporal approach. (From Sekhar et al.,[8] with permission.)

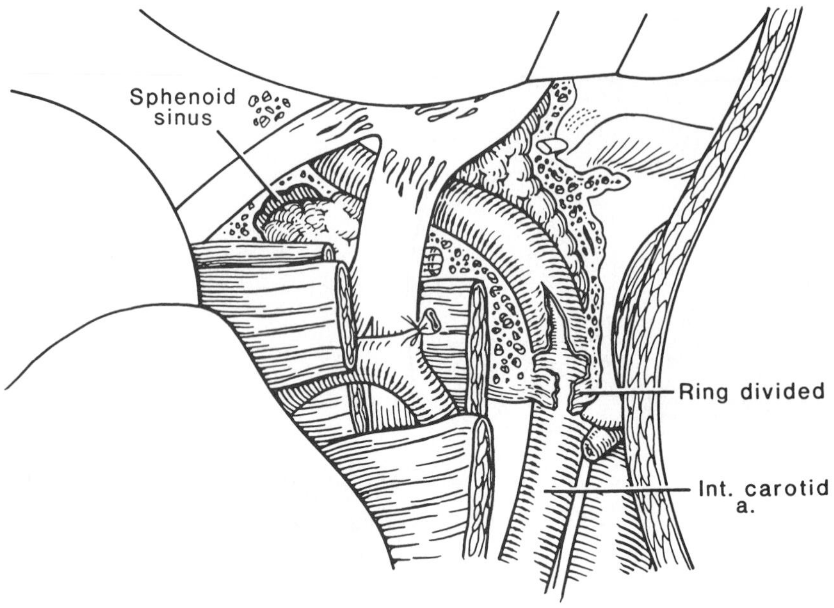

Figure 162-4 The exposure of the petrous ICA and a tumor in the petroclival area. (From Sekhar et al.,[8] with permission.)

Combination with Other Approaches

There are a number of areas of the cranial base that are inadequately exposed by the ST-IT approach. In these situations, combination with other approaches in the same or a second operation is necessary.[8] When the tumor extends into the sphenoethmoidal sinuses, the medial aspect of the cavernous sinus, and the mid- and upper clivus, the extended subfrontal approach is used.[4,6] This approach provides an excellent exposure at the price (in most patients) of permanent anosmia. If the tumor extends laterally into the petrous bone, a combination of the two approaches is essential (Fig. 162-8). When the tumor has extensively invaded the middle cranial fossa or the cavernous sinus, an intradural frontotemporal approach is necessary.

If the tumor reaches extensively into the petrous bone in the labyrinthine, retrolabyrinthine, or infralabyrinthine area (jugular bulb), a retroauricular T incision is made, and a transmastoid transpetrosal approach is combined with the ST-IT approach (Fig.

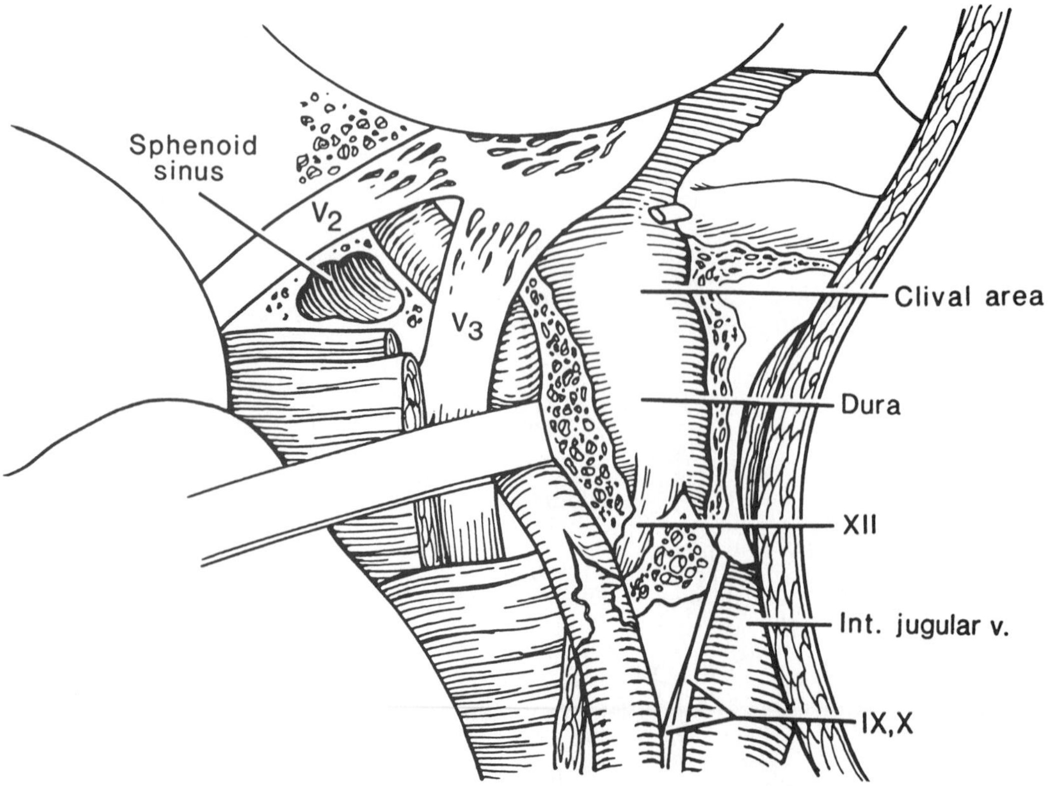

Figure 162-5 The petrous ICA has been displaced forward, and tumor has been resected. (From Sekhar et al.,[8] with permission.)

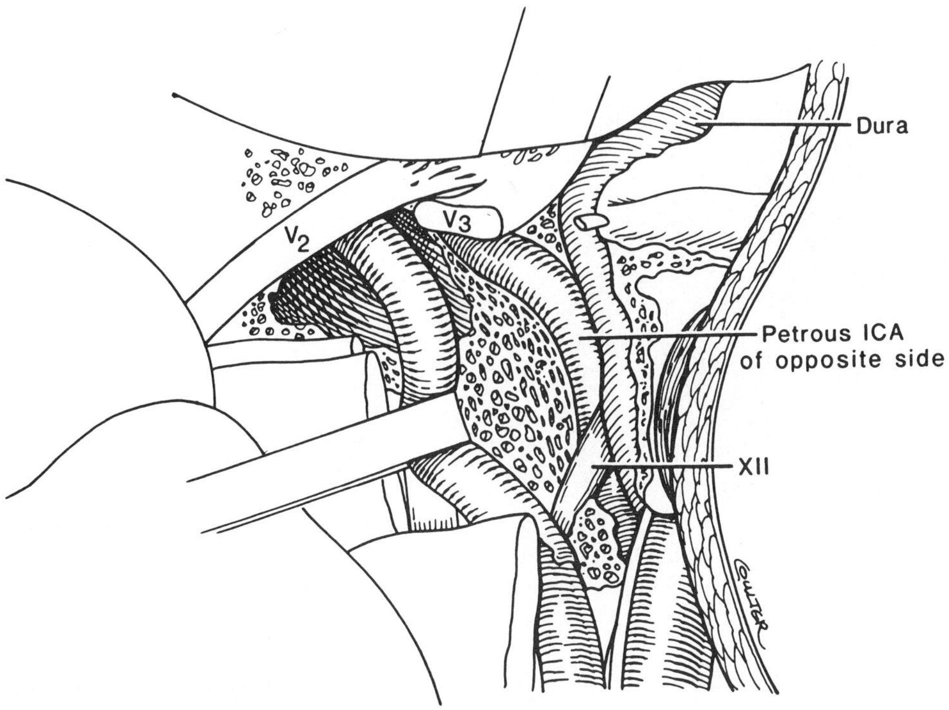

Figure 162-6 The division of the mandibular nerve to access the contralateral side of the clivus and the petrous ICA. (From Sekhar et al.,[8] with permission.)

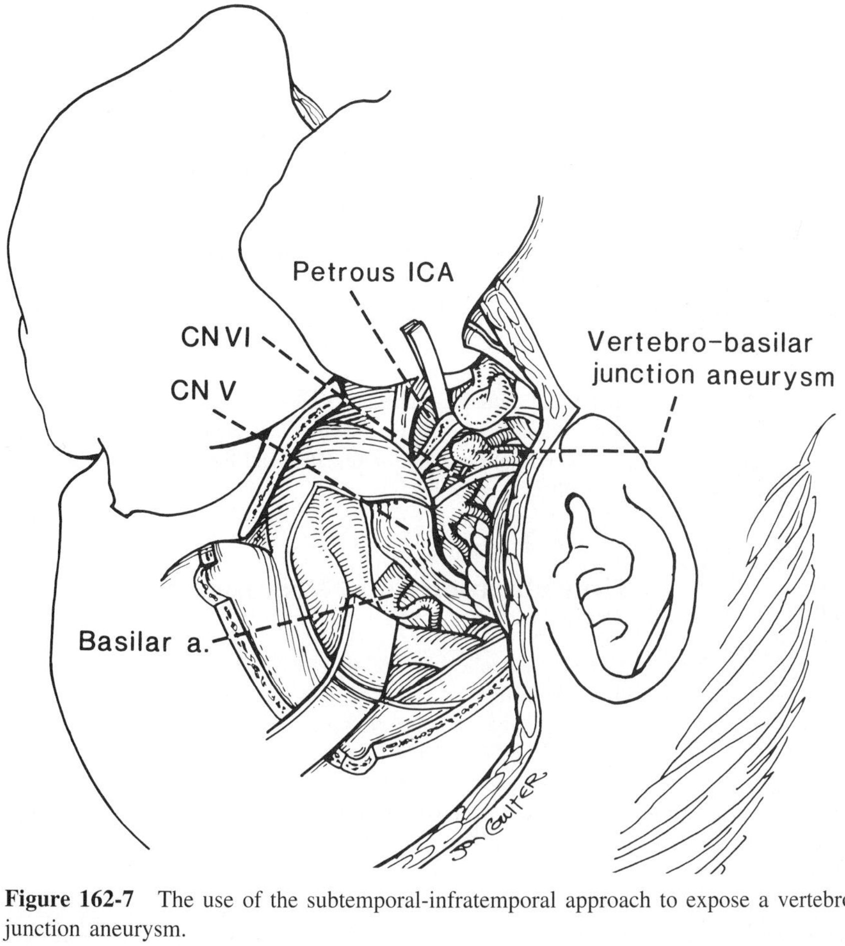

Figure 162-7 The use of the subtemporal-infratemporal approach to expose a vertebrobasilar junction aneurysm.

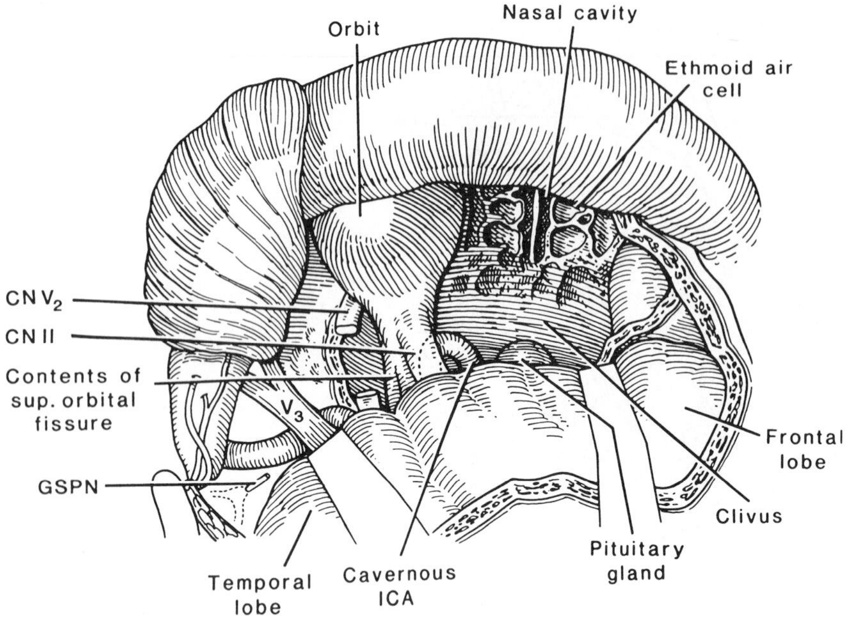

Figure 162-8 The combination of the extended subfrontal and the subfrontal-infratemporal approach. (From Sekhar et al.,[8] with permission.)

162-9). This can be done with the preservation of excellent hearing and normal facial function, unless the inner ear structures are involved.

When the foramen magnum, occipital condyle, and C1 areas are involved by the tumor, the extreme lateral, transcondylar approach is combined (Fig. 162-9). Chordomas and chondrosarcomas frequently involve one or both occipital condyles. In such cases, the entire occipital condyle is resected and an occiput-to-cervical fusion is performed with rods and bone chips.[1,9]

Malignant Tumors and Upper Cervical Extension

In the case of highly malignant tumors, a more extensive exposure is often needed. In such patients, an upper cervical incision is combined with a preauricular incision and the facial nerve is exposed from the stylomastoid foramen to its branches in the face. The mandibular condyle is resected to its neck, and the parts of the tumor medial to the mandibular condyle and at the entrance to the cranial base are well exposed.

For fast-growing malignancies such as squamous cell carcinomas, a wider exposure is necessary to achieve an *en bloc* resection, if possible. If the ICA is involved by such a tumor, it must be replaced by a vein graft from the cervical ICA to the intracranial ICA or the middle cerebral artery (MCA), running retroauricularly, about 2 to 3 weeks before the tumor operation. This prevents rupture of the carotid artery from exposure to pharyngeal contents, since such tumors frequently extend into the nasopharynx.

Tumors Lateral to the Petrous ICA

For excision of benign or malignant tumors that occupy the extradural temporal area or the infratemporal space lateral to the petrous ICA and the petrous bone, a much simpler exposure is performed with a zygomatic osteotomy anterior to the condylar fossa. The resection of such a tumor (e.g., a trigeminal schwannoma) is quite easy.

Reconstruction

After tumor resection, any dural defect is closed with a fascia lata or pericranial graft, with circumferential sutures and fibrin glue. Watertight closure is not usually possible. The dead space created by tumor removal is filled with autologous fat and then covered with a vascularized flap derived from the temporalis muscle. Depending on the size of the defect, either the entire muscle or the posterior half is used, taking care to preserve its vascularity (Fig. 162-10).

When the defect is very large, for example after resection of a cancerous lesion, or if the temporalis muscle has poor vascularity, a free flap transfer is indicated.[3] This procedure is performed by a plastic surgeon. A rectus abdominis muscle flap or a radial forearm flap is attached by microvascular anastomosis to an artery and vein in the neck, and the transplanted tissue is used to fill the dead space (Fig. 162-11). The zygomatic arch and the craniotomy piece are reattached with titanium miniplates, and the remaining closure is performed as usual.

Complications and Prevention

Potential complications of the ST-IT approach include petrous ICA injury, facial palsy, hearing loss, and CSF leakage. Infections and hematomas are also possible.

Petrous ICA injuries are the most serious complication. They may occur during drilling, mobilization of the artery from the bony canal, or dissection from a tumor or of an aneurysm. Many of these injuries result from an unfamiliarity with the anatomy, or are related to some local pathology of the vessel wall. Before performing this operative approach, surgeons must learn the anatomy by repeated dissection of cadavers. If the surgeon is inexperienced, or

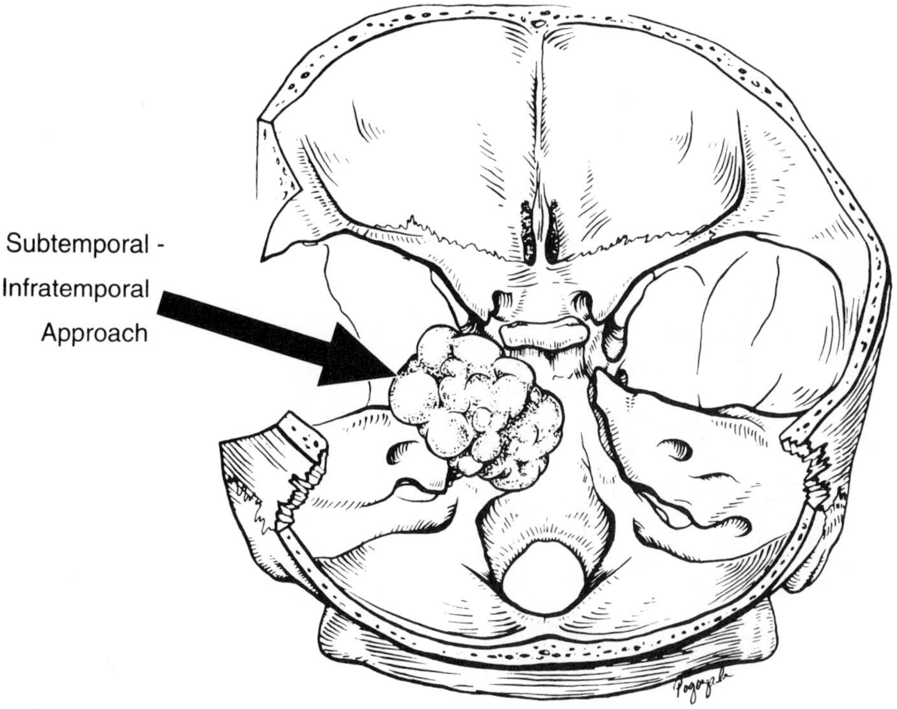

(A)

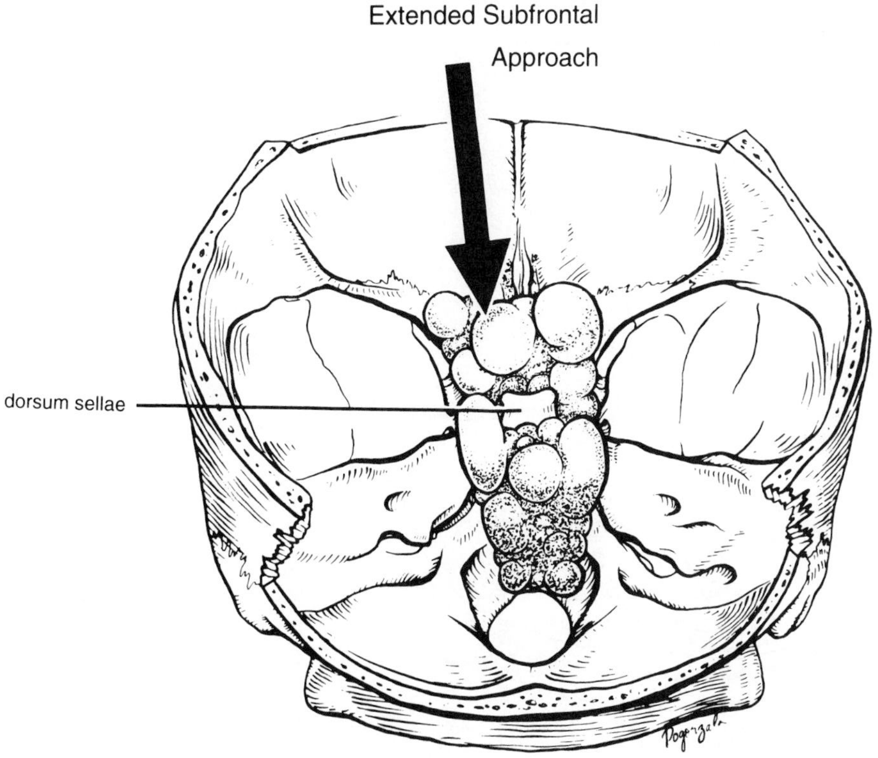

(B)

Figure 162-9 These figures show the areas of the cranial base exposed by the subtemporal-infratemporal approach *(A)*, the extended subfrontal approach *(B)*,

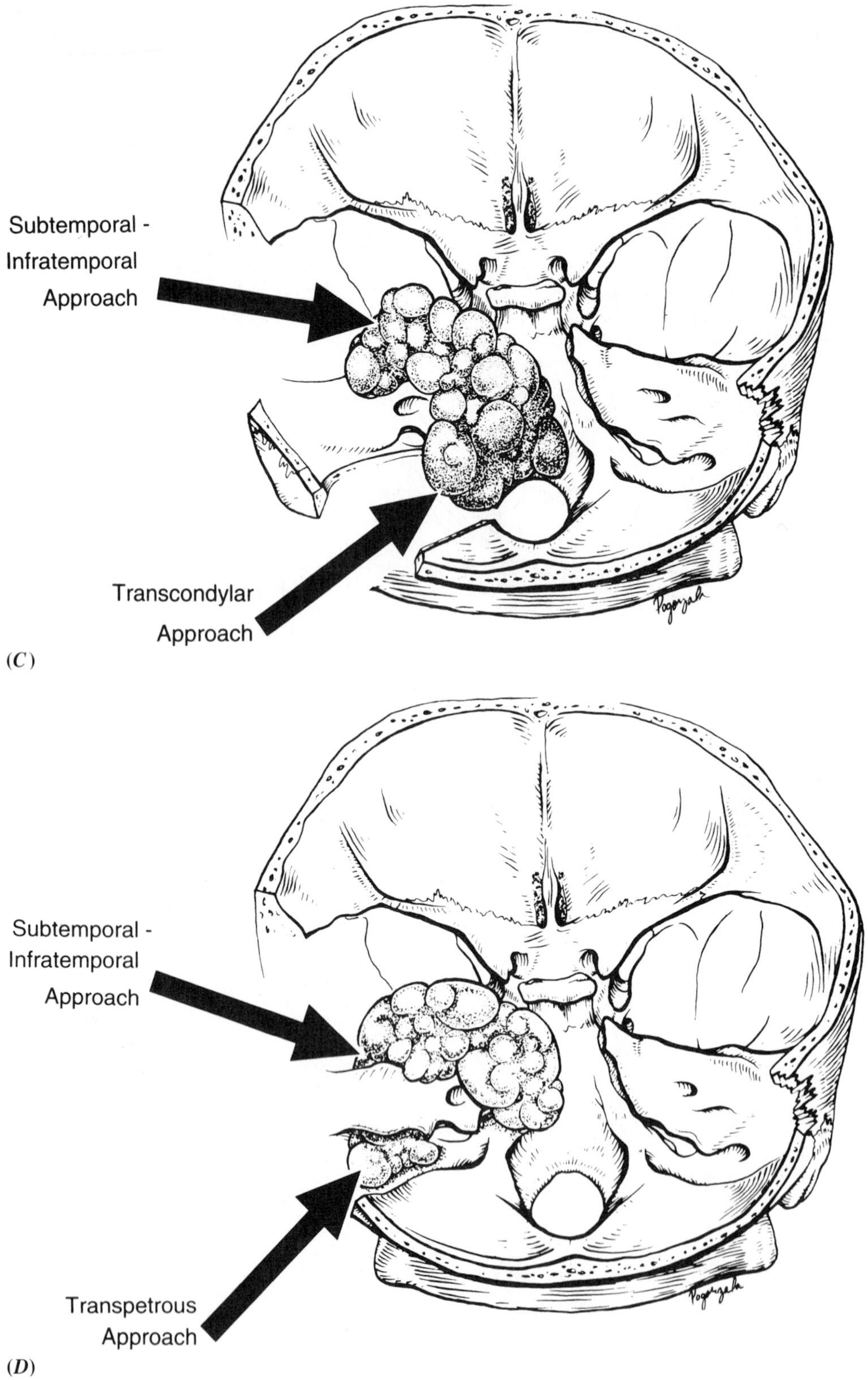

Figure 162-9 (*Continued*) the combination of the subtemporal-infratemporal and transcondylar approaches *(C)*, and the combination of the subtemporal-infratemporal approach with the transpetrous approach *(D)*.

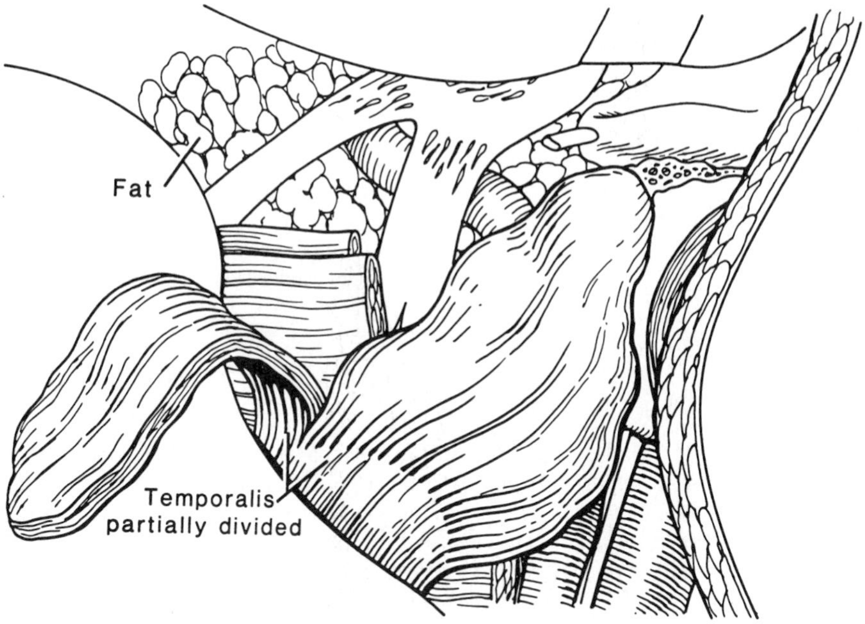

Figure 162-10 The use of the temporalis muscle flap and abdominal fat graft reconstruction after the subtemporal-infratemporal approach. (From Sekhar et al.,[8] with permission.)

if severe vascular pathology is present, proximal control of the cervical ICA is recommended before exposing the petrous ICA. It is best to expose the segment of the petrous ICA (vertical segment, genu, or horizontal segment) that is uninvolved by the lesion, and to trace it to the abnormal area. When the exposure of an area is inadequate, the surgeon must enlarge it (rather than work in a narrow space). The use of a high-speed drill, especially combined with a low torque, allows the use of a "feather touch" that can prevent injuries caused by excessive pressure on the bone. If ICA injury occurs, bleeding is controlled with cotton patties and gentle pressure, and a temporary clip is applied to the ICA proximally. Distal exposure and control are then obtained, and the injured area is repaired by a direct suture vein patch or an interposition vein graft. Rarely, the injured (and pathologic) segment is so abnormal that a saphenous vein bypass graft from the cervical ICA to the intracranial ICA or MCA is needed. During the period of ICA occlusion, the patient's blood pressure is raised 30 to 40 mmHg, 2000 units of heparin are given intravenously, and the patient is placed in a barbiturate- or etomidate-induced coma to achieve burst suppression on the electroencephalogram. Intraoperative or postoperative angiography must be performed to confirm patency of the ICA or graft.

Injuries to the facial nerve may be caused near the geniculate ganglion or in the facial area by traction, direct trauma, or devascularization. The use of facial nerve monitoring is very helpful in preventing injuries, but it is not foolproof.

Hearing loss may occur because of inadvertent injury to the cochlea or dislocation of the middle ear ossicles. Familiarity with the general anatomy of the approach, and with the specific anatomy of the patient as shown by thin-section, bone-windowed CT head scans, can help prevent such injuries.

Leakage of CSF can occur when the dura was opened, and either the middle ear or the eustachian tube was inadequately closed or not closed at all. Hydrocephalus due to poor spinal fluid absorption may also be responsible for CSF leakage.

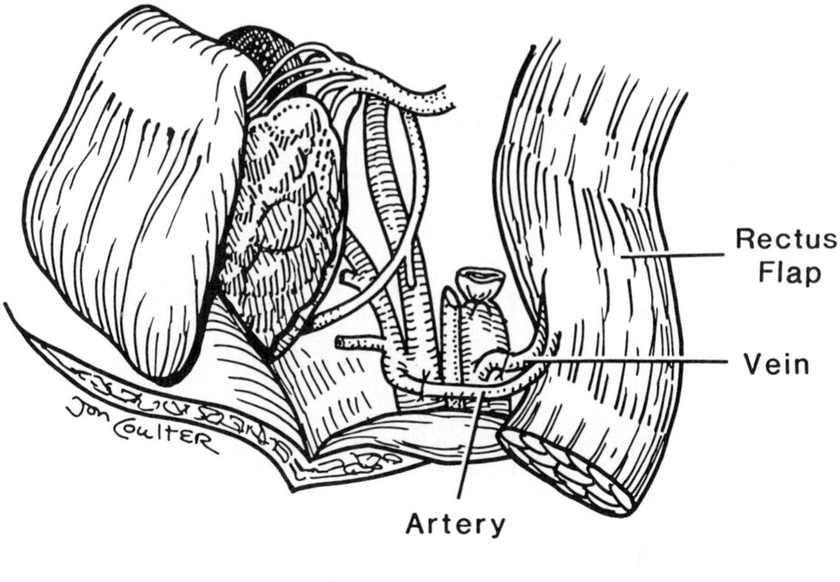

Figure 162-11 The use of a rectus abdominis microvascular free flap for reconstruction. (From Sekhar et al.,[8] with permission.)

Infections and hematomas (temporal lobe, epidural, or subdural) are rare and are managed in the usual fashion. Complications such as vascular injuries and CSF leaks are more common in previously operated or previously irradiated patients.

Illustrative Cases

Cholesterol Granuloma (Patient BA)

This 38-year-old woman underwent the transsphenoidal drainage of a cholesterol granuloma one year previously. She presented with facial twitching and numbness and progressive regrowth of the lesion. In MRI scans, the lesion was seen to occupy the extradural petroclival and jugular bulb areas on the left (Fig. 162-12). A subtemporal-infratemporal approach was carried out. The capsule of the lesion had inflamed and eroded the wall of the petrous ICA on the left, and, during exposure, the vertical segment of the petrous ICA was lacerated. The abnormal area of the ICA was excised and the artery was repaired primarily. The cyst contained a mixture of solid and liquid materials, and the capsule was thick. It was excised completely. An intraoperative arteriogram showed a 50 percent stenosis of the ICA. On postoperative MR angiography a few months later, the vessel was normal. MRI revealed complete tumor resection. After placement of a tympanostomy tube, the patient had no neurological deficits.

Extensive Clivus Chordoma (Patient AH)

This 53-year-old man presented with a 13-year history of lateral rectus muscle palsy and the recent onset of neck and trigeminal pain, dysphagia, dysarthria, and weight loss. Neurological examination revealed palsies of the left sixth and twelfth cranial nerves and of both ninth and tenth cranial nerves. Computed tomography and MRI scans (Fig. 162-13) revealed a giant petroclival-sphenoidal chordoma extending down to C1, with severe brain stem compression. The tumor was resected by petrosal, subtemporal-infratemporal, and transcondylar approaches, in two operations. An occiputto-C1-C2 fusion with titanium rods and bone chips was also necessary. The patient required a postoperative tracheostomy and gastrostomy, and his gait worsened transiently. He recovered well after rehabilitation, and was able to return to normal life. Postoperative MRI scans revealed a small tumor residue. The patient elected to be followed with serial imaging studies, without further treatment.

Patient Series and Complications

The ST-IT approach was used on approximately 80 patients, from 1984 through 1993, at the University of Pittsburgh Medical Center (UPMC). It was used subsequently on 22 patients at George Washington University Medical Center (GWUMC), from April 1993 through November 1994, and this experience is described briefly. This patient group was a subset of 237 patients with cranial base tumors operated on during the same period. The ST-IT approach was not used for any aneurysm cases at GWUMC, but it was used for one such case at UPMC.

The tumors accessed by the approach are shown in Table 162-1. They include meningiomas, chordomas, a chondrosarcoma, paragangliomas (glomus jugulare), cholesterol granulomas, carcinomas of different types, and a malignant fibrous histiocytoma. Total or near-total resection was accomplished in 17 patients, subtotal resection in 4, and partial resection in 1 (Table 162-2). The subtemporal-infratemporal approach was used by itself in only seven patients, and in the remainder it was combined with other approaches (Table 162-3). Complications of surgery are listed in Table 162-4, including their management and outcome. One patient with a recurrent chordoma suffered multiple postoperative hematomas secondary to a coagulopathy that was not recognized

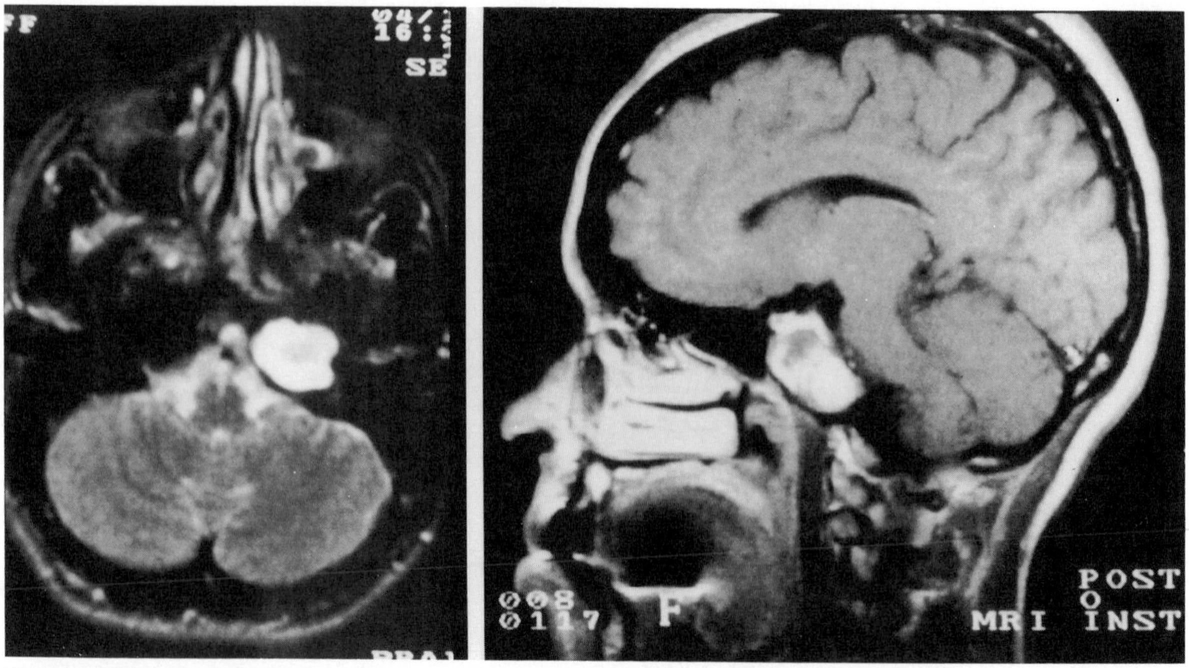

Figure 162-12 T2-weighted axial, and T1-weighted sagittal MRI scans of patient BA, showing a cholesterol granuloma.

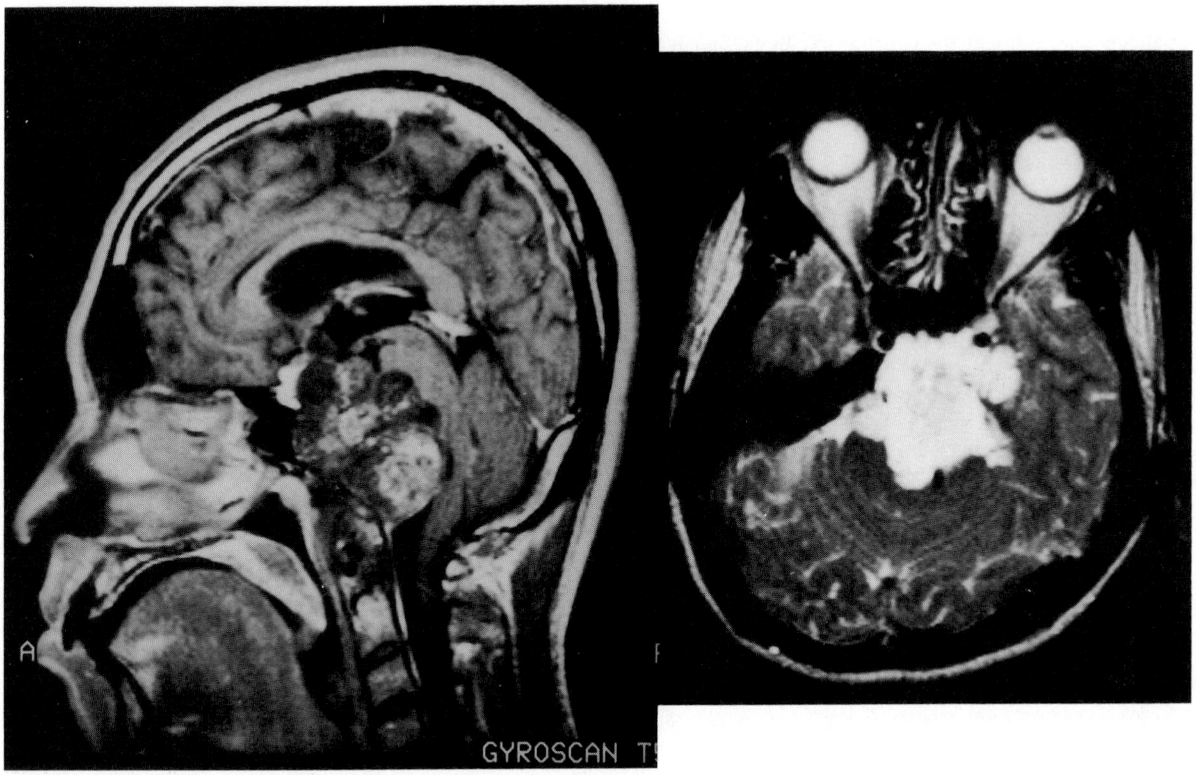

Figure 162-13 Enhanced sagittal and T2-weighted axial MRI scans of patient AH showing a giant sphenopetroclival and cervical chordoma.

TABLE 162-1 Tumors Resected by the Subtemporal-Infratemporal Approach, 1993–1994

Type of Tumor	No. Patients Operated on by ST-IT Approach
Benign tumors	8
Meningioma	4
Paraganglioma	2
Cholesterol granuloma	2
Malignant, slow-growing	11
Chordoma, first operation	2
Chordoma, recurrent	6
Chondrosarcoma	1
Malignant fibrous histiocytoma	1
Adenoid cystic carcinoma	1
Malignant, fast-growing	3
Adenocarcinoma	1
Undifferentiated carcinoma	1
Synovial carcinoma	1
Total	22

TABLE 162-2 Extent of Tumor Resection

Extent of Resection	Number
Total or near-total	17
Subtotal	4
Partial	1

TABLE 162-3 Approaches Used in the Series of 22 Patients

Approach Used	Number
ST-IT only	7
ST-IT + subtemporal, intradural	1
ST-IT + petrosal, intradural	3
ST-IT + frontotemporal, transcavernous	3
ST-IT + extended subfrontal	4
ST-IT + transpetrous, extradural	1
ST-IT + transcondylar, transjugular	5
ST-IT + transmaxillary	1
Total	25*

*Three patients had two of the above approaches.

TABLE 162-4 Complications: Management and Outcome

Complication	Number	Management	Outcome
Multiple hematomas, uncorrectable coagulopathy	1	Evacuation, factor & platelet transfusions	Death
Petrous ICA injury (tumor invasion)	3	Direct repair—1 Vein grafts—2	Excellent
Cerebrospinal fluid leak	2	Free flap repair—1 Intradural repair—1	Excellent
Facial palsy	1	Expectant	Recovered to House grade III
Abducens palsy	1	—	No recovery

preoperatively. She died despite eventual correction of the problem. Three patients sustained petrous ICA injuries; all had tumor invasion of the vessel wall. One patient, detailed above, had a direct repair, and the other two underwent vein grafts. Four additional patients underwent vein graft replacement of the ICA electively, before the planned operation, because of radiographic evidence of tumor invasion or inability to preserve the ICA. None of these patients sustained cerebral infarction.

Conclusions

The subtemporal-infratemporal approach is an essential element in the cranial base surgeon's armamentarium. Before using this approach, the surgeon must master the microsurgical anatomy of this area through cadaver dissections, and must observe experienced surgeons performing such operations.

References

1. Babu RP, Sekhar LN, Wright DC. Extreme lateral transcondylar approach: technical improvements and lessons learned. *J Neurosurg* 1994; 81:49–59.
2. Fisch U, Pillsbury HC. Infratemporal fossa approach to lesions in the temporal bone and base of the skull. *Arch Otolaryngol* 1979; 105:99–107.
3. Jones NF, Schramm VL, Sekhar LN. Reconstruction of the cranial base following tumour resection. *Br J Plast Surg* 1987; 40:155–162.
4. Sekhar LN, Janecka IP, Jones NF. Subtemporal-infratemporal and basal subfrontal approach to extensive cranial base tumours. *Acta Neurochir (Wien)* 1988; 92:83–92.
5. Sekhar LN, Kalia KK, Yonas H, et al. Cranial base approaches to aneurysms in the subarachnoid space. *Neurosurgery* 1994; 35:472–481.
6. Sekhar LN, Nanda A, Sen CN, et al. Extended frontal approach to tumors of the anterior, middle, and posterior skull base. *J Neurosurg* 1992; 76:198–206.
7. Sekhar LN, Schramm VL Jr, Jones NF. Subtemporal-preauricular infratemporal fossa approach to large lateral and posterior cranial base neoplasms. *J Neurosurg* 1987; 67:488–499.
8. Sekhar LN, Sen C, Snyderman CH, Janecka IP. Anterior, anterolateral, and lateral approaches to extradural petroclival tumors. In Sekhar LN, Janecka IP (eds): *Surgery of Cranial Base Tumors.* New York: Raven Press, 1993, pp 157–223.
9. Sen CN, Sekhar LN. An extreme lateral approach to intradural lesions of the cervical spine and foramen magnum. *Neurosurgery* 1990; 27:197–204.
10. Sen CN, Sekhar LN. The subtemporal and preauricular infratemporal approach to intradural structures ventral to the brain stem. *J Neurosurg* 1990; 73:345–354.

163

Postauricular Infratemporal Fossa Approach to Tumors Involving the Skull Base

Derald E. Brackmann

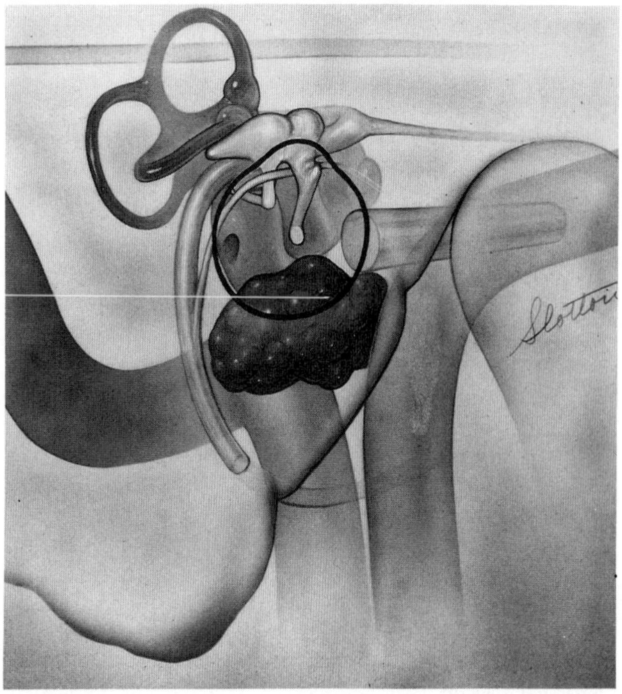

Figure 163-1 Diagram of a glomus jugulare tumor contacting the internal carotid artery. The overlying tympanic ring and facial nerve prevent adequate exposure of the tumor and carotid artery.

Treatment of lesions of the skull base presents a formidable challenge. They occupy areas that are relatively inaccessible and dangerous to approach because of important surrounding neural and vascular structures. Until recently many of these lesions were considered inoperable. Development of computed cranial tomography and magnetic resonance imaging makes accurate delineation of the extent of these tumors possible. The development of microsurgical techniques has allowed removal of tumors heretofore considered inoperable.

One of the most significant advances in our ability to treat skull base lesions is the posterior lateral infratemporal fossa approach developed by Fisch et al.[3,4] This approach allows access to the entire intratemporal course of the internal carotid artery and to cranial nerves V through XII. It offers a possibility of complete removal of even large posterior-medially situated tumors with acceptable morbidity and preservation of a good quality of life. In this chapter, I describe the types of infratemporal fossa approaches, discuss the indications for surgery and patient selection, and then report on the difficulties with this approach and the results in a series of patients.

Relevant Anatomy

Lesions of the skull base are in close proximity to the internal carotid artery, the major venous sinuses, and cranial nerves III through XII. The facial nerve blocks direct access to the area (Fig. 163-1). The tumors frequently extend into the posterior or middle fossa. The primary advantage of the infratemporal fossa approach is to allow direct lateral access to the internal carotid artery throughout its course from the carotid foramen to the cavernous sinus. In order to accomplish this access, the facial nerve is permanently transposed arteriorly, and this requires removal of the external auditory canal, tympanic membrane, and malleus and incus, with a resultant permanent conductive hearing impairment (Fig. 163-2). This is an acceptable morbidity for treatment of these difficult problems.

Surgical Techniques

Type A Approach

The type A approach is primarily used for glomus tumors of the temporal bone. The following is a description of the surgical procedure for that lesion.

Hair is removed from approximately 6 cm about the ear, and an incision is made approximately 2 cm posterior to the postauricular sulcus. The incision is stopped at the mastoid tip at this point in the dissection. A simple mastoidectomy is completed, and the facial recess is opened. The incudostapedial joint is disarticulated to protect inner ear function. The external auditory canal is transected at the level of the bony-cartilaginous junction. The skin of the meatus is everted and closed with 5-0 nylon sutures. The periosteum of the postauricular area is sutured behind the opening in the meatus to further reinforce the closure. The skin of the external auditory canal is removed along with the tympanic membrane, malleus, and incus. The bony external auditory canal is then removed. Following this, the facial nerve is freed of bone from the geniculate ganglion through the stylomastoid foramen.

Fisch originally described exposure of the facial nerve through the stylomastoid foramen into the parotid with permanent anterior transposition of the facial nerve.[3] In my experience, this always produced a temporary facial paralysis and sometimes a minor permanent residual facial weakness. I have modified this approach as follows.[1]

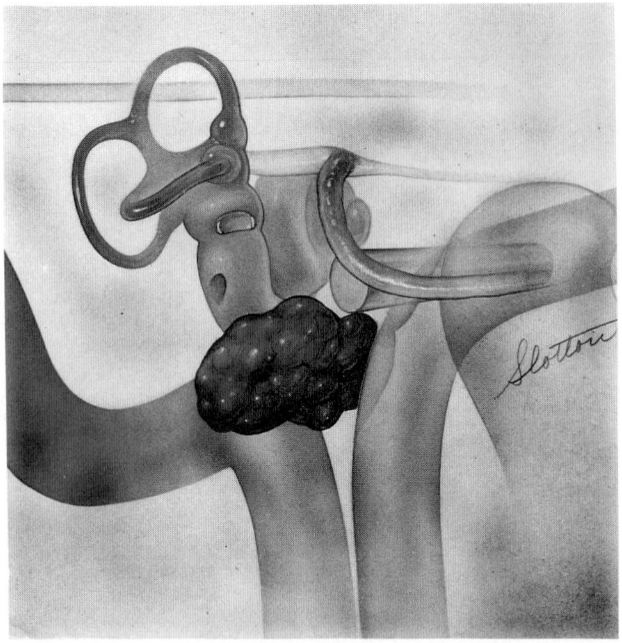

Figure 163-2 Diagram of infratemporal fossa exposure. The tumor and carotid artery are exposed by removal of the tympanic ring and anterior rerouting of the facial nerve.

The postauricular incision is now extended into the neck along the anterior border of the sternocleidomastoid muscle. Rather than exposing the facial nerve into the parotid as Fisch described, I elevate the entire tail of the parotid along with the periosteum of the stylomastoid foramen and the nerve. The facial nerve is then carefully freed from the fallopian canal with sharp dissection. There are multiple fibrous connections that are sharply incised in the descending portion of the nerve. In the tympanic portion of the nerve, there are no adhesions, and this section elevates readily. The entire tail of the parotid with the contained facial nerve is then elevated lateral to the mandibular ramus. A large silk suture is placed through the periosteum of the stylomastoid foramen and attached to the soft tissue in the area of the root of the zygoma. This elevates the facial nerve and prevents its being stretched when the retractors are placed.

For the past 6.5 years, I have been using continuous monitoring of facial nerve activity during this dissection. EMG electrodes are placed into the facial muscles and the activity of the muscles is monitored continuously. Even minor manipulation of the facial nerve produces activity in the facial muscles. This technique has significantly improved postoperative facial nerve function.[5]

After the facial nerve and parotid gland are elevated, I place a large Perkins retractor beneath the angle of the mandible and retract the entire mandible forward. I have not had to resect the mandibular condyle, even in large tumors extending far into the infratemporal fossa.

Transposition of the facial nerve allows exposure of the skull base in the area of the jugular foramen and carotid artery (Fig. 163-3). The internal carotid artery is followed through the skull base to its intratemporal course. The ninth, tenth, and eleventh cranial nerves are identified in the neck and followed into the jugular foramen. The twelfth cranial nerve is also identified and followed to its foramen.

The sigmoid sinus is double ligated with silk sutures. The jugular vein is elevated and the tumor freed inferiorly. The tumor is then freed from the carotid artery anteriorly. Bleeding corticotympanic vessels are controlled with bipolar cautery. If the tumor is adherent to the internal carotid artery it is best to leave a portion of it on the artery at this point and remove the bulk of the tumor. Removal of the last bit of the tumor from the artery is then saved for the conclusion of the procedure. The tumor is freed superiorly and posteriorly and then medially, and total removal of the tumor is thus accomplished.

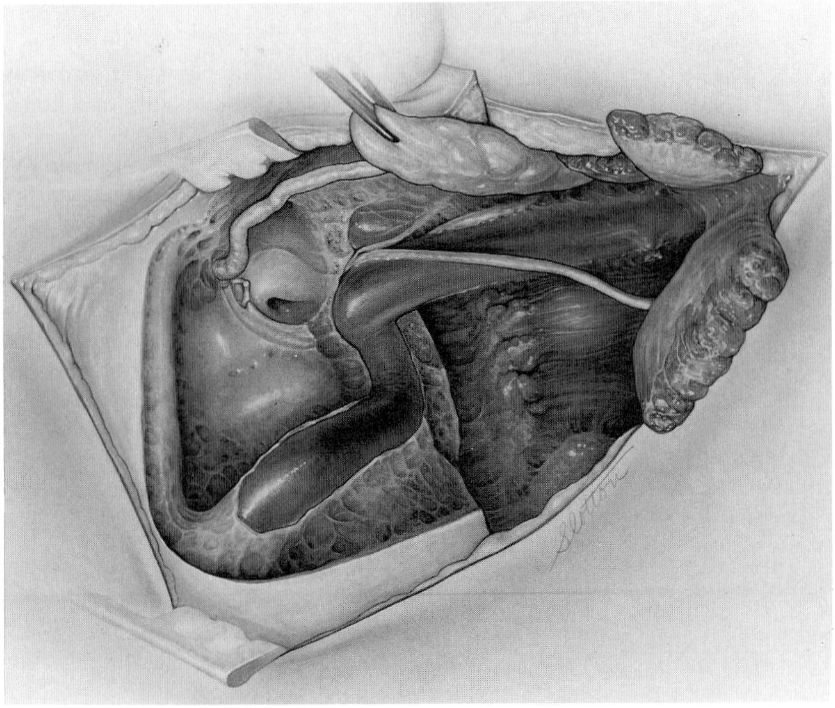

Figure 163-3 Infratemporal fossa exposure. See text for details.

If there is intracranial extension of the tumor, a decision must be made at this point whether to attempt a total removal of the tumor. We base this decision upon the amount of blood loss to this point. If the blood loss has been limited to less than 3000 ml, we proceed with the removal of the intracranial extension of the tumor. All glomus jugulare tumors now receive preoperative embolization with polyvinyl alcohol sponge (Ivalon). Since utilizing this technique, blood loss is greatly reduced and we are almost always able to accomplish a total removal of tumors even with large intracranial extensions.[6] If there has been greater than 3000 ml of blood loss, one may encounter problems with bleeding despite the replenishment of the clotting factors with fresh frozen plasma and platelet packs. In such a case we prefer a two-stage procedure with removal of the intracranial portion of the tumor approximately 6 months after the primary surgery.

The removal of the intracranial portion of the tumor is often easier than the removal of that within the temporal bone. By the time one is ready for the removal of the intracranial extension, the blood supply has often been controlled. The blood supply to the intracranial portion of the tumor is usually discrete and can be controlled with bipolar cautery as with other cerebellopontine-angle tumors. If tumor has been left along the internal carotid artery, this is now removed. Closure is accomplished by obliterating the mastoid defect with strips of abdominal fat. If the CSF space has been entered, continuous lumbar drainage is used for approximately 5 days until the wound is sealed.

Type B Approach

The most common skull base tumor requiring this approach is the clival chordoma. The description which follows describes that procedure. The incision is as for the type A approach except that it extends more forward superiorly. The external auditory canal is transected and closed and the flap anteriorly is undermined widely. The facial nerve is identified in the retromandibular fossa, and the superior branches are dissected peripherally to allow freeing and inferior displacement of the frontal ramus.

Holes that will later be used to rewire the zygoma are drilled in the arch, which is then divided between them. Posteriorly, the zygomatic arch is sectioned at the area of the temporomandibular joint. The zygomatic arch with the attached masseter muscle and freed temporalis muscle are displaced inferiorly and folded over the inferiorly displaced frontal ramus of the facial nerve to protect it. The external auditory canal and tympanic bone are then removed as described for the type A approach. The bone of the glenoid fossa is removed and the temporomandibular joint is disarticulated and retracted inferiorly with an infratemporal fossa retractor. The internal carotid artery is then exposed throughout its course to the foramen lacerum. This requires detachment of the medial cartilaginous portion of the eustachian tube.

When it is necessary to reach the anterior part of the clivus, the middle meningeal artery and the third division of the trigeminal nerve are coagulated and divided. To reach the anterior clivus, the tensor veli palatini muscle, cartilaginous eustachian tube, and pterygoid processes are displaced inferiorly.

After tumor exposure, the soft portions of the tumor are removed with suction and curettes. Diamond burrs are used until firm bone or dura is encountered. Care must be taken not to injure the contralateral internal carotid artery.

Closure is accomplished by packing with abdominal fat after the zygomatic arch has been wired in place anteriorly.

Type C Approach

The most frequent indication for the type C approach is nasopharyngeal carcinoma (failing radiotherapy) and advanced juvenile nasopharyngeal angiofibroma.

The dissection as described for the type B approach is first accomplished. After the displacement of the mandibular condyle inferiorly, the middle meningeal artery and the mandibular division of the trigeminal nerve are divided. Both pterygoid plates are removed, and the internal carotid artery is exposed from the middle ear to the foramen lacerum. The lateral wall of the nasopharynx covered by the palatal and pterygoid muscles can then be removed *en bloc* with the infiltrating tumor. Juvenile nasopharyngeal angiofibromas are dissected bluntly along their capsule. Extensions into the sphenopalatine fossa, sphenoid sinus, or nasal cavity are reached after complete removal of the pterygoid processes and division of the maxillary division of the trigeminal nerve at the foramen rotundum.

Closure is accomplished by obliteration of the anterior operative cavity with a pedicle of the temporalis muscle. Posteriorly, the mastoid cavity is obliterated with abdominal fat and the zygomatic arch is wired into its original position.

Indications

A variety of skull base lesions may be treated by the infratemporal fossa approach. Tables 163-1, 163-2, and 163-3 list the most common tumors treated by the different approaches.

Contraindications

An absolute contraindication to the infratemporal fossa approach is a malignant tumor extending across the skull base. However, Fisch et al. have stated that even in extensive carcinomas, surgery may be worthwhile for relief of trigeminal pain and general palliation.[4]

Involvement of one internal carotid artery is not a contraindication to surgery. Balloon occlusion studies are performed with continuous EEG monitoring. Xenon blood flow studies or technetium scans are also performed. If these studies indicate that sacrifice of the internal carotid artery would not be tolerated, plans must be made either for extracranial-intracranial bypass grafting or saphenous vein grafting of the resected internal carotid artery.

Relative contraindications to surgery include poor general health. These procedures are extensive, and the patient's general health must be carefully assessed before recommending the procedure.

TABLE 163-1 Type A Infratemporal Fossa Approach

Glomus tumor
Temporal bone carcinoma
Primary cholesteatoma
Jugular foramen neuroma
Meningioma
Sarcoma

TABLE 163-2 Type B Infratemporal Fossa Approach

Chordoma
Chondrosarcoma
Squamous cell carcinoma
Dermoid and primary cholesteatoma
Meningioma

In general, I do not recommend surgery for glomus tumors of the temporal bone in elderly patients. In my experience, radiation therapy is a better modality for treating the elderly person with a glomus tumor.[2]

Advantages and Limitations of the Infratemporal Fossa Approach

The advantage of the infratemporal fossa approach is the wide exposure of lesions of the skull base. Total exposure and protection of the carotid artery is a major advantage. With this technique the facial nerve is mobilized and preserved. Exposure of cranial nerves V through XII is possible and allows protection and preservation of these nerves when they are not involved by the tumor.

One disadvantage of the approach is the permanent conductive hearing impairment which results from blind sac closure of the external auditory canal and removal of the conductive hearing mechanism. Sensorineural hearing function is preserved in the majority of patients unless the tumor invades the labyrinthine capsule. In such cases, complete tumor removal requires sacrifice of sensorineural hearing function.

A temporary facial paralysis may result from mobilization of the facial nerve in the type A approach. In the types B and C approaches, weakness of the musculature innervated by the frontal branch is common. As discussed previously, intraoperative monitoring of facial nerve function and not exposing the nerve at the stylomastoid foramen have greatly decreased the incidence of facial paralysis. Hypesthesia in the distribution of the second and third divisions of the fifth cranial nerve accompany the types B and C infratemporal fossa approaches.

Hoarseness of the voice and aspiration to a variable degree occur with sacrifice of the ninth and tenth cranial nerves. I do not do a preoperative tracheotomy or gastrostomy even when I know that these nerves will be sacrificed. Most patients will tolerate these deficits in the immediate postoperative period. Early Teflon (E.I. duPont de Nemours & Co., Wilmington, DE) injection of the vocal cord is performed. Cricopharyngeal myotomy is also beneficial to enhance swallowing and decrease aspiration. Shoulder discomfort is common with sacrifice of the eleventh cranial nerve. Exercises are beneficial for this problem.[7]

TABLE 163-3 Type C Infratemporal Fossa Approach

Nasopharyngeal carcinoma
Juvenile nasopharyngeal angiofibroma
Adenoid cystic carcinoma
Meningioma
Sarcoma
Ameloblastoma

When tumors extend intracranially, a CSF leak is a potential problem. When the CSF space has been entered, a lumbar subarachnoid drain is routinely placed and remains until the wound is well sealed, which is usually about 5 days. Meningitis is an infrequent complication. Intra- and perioperative antibiotics are not used routinely.

Tumors with large intracranial extensions may involve the posterior fossa circulation, making total tumor removal impossible. Surgery in these cases may still be beneficial by decreasing the blood supply to the tumor with removal of its main bulk.

Results

As of October 1992, I had performed 116 infratemporal fossa approaches for various tumors of the skull base. The results with these cases are summarized in Table 163-4. The most common tumor that I have treated is the glomus jugulare tumor, although a variety of other lesions have also been operated upon. Total removal of the tumor was accomplished in most cases. Incomplete removal was performed on several early cases with large intracranial extensions. Second-stage procedures were planned, but follow-up has shown no growth of the tumor so they are currently being observed. Removal of the intracranial portion of the tumor will be accomplished if growth is demonstrated. Extensive involvement of the cavernous sinus has been a second indication for partial removal in three cases. These patients are also being monitored carefully, and if aggressive tumor growth is demonstrated, further surgery or focused beam irradiation will be recommended.

Only one patient in the series has died from the disease. This patient had a very large meningioma of the skull base which had previously been operated upon. It extended to the cavernous sinus. We thought that a total removal had been accomplished, but recurrent disease developed. She had further surgery elsewhere but had rapid regrowth of tumor following that and died of intracranial extension of the disease. Two patients have died of other disease without evidence of residual tumor in the temporal bone or infratemporal fossa.

A number of patients have been given postoperative x-ray therapy. In general, I do not recommend this for glomus tumors unless residual tumor is left and this demonstrates growth. In that case, a relatively small dose of therapy is recommended to decrease the blood supply to the tumor.[2] Postoperative x-ray therapy of chordoma and chondrosarcoma is somewhat controversial but has been employed in three of the four patients in this series. The patient with the recurrent papillary adenoma with intracranial extension also received postoperative x-ray therapy.

The quality of life in these patients has been excellent. All have returned to full activity without the need for tracheotomy or gastrostomy, even though these measures were employed immediately postoperatively in a number of patients.

Conclusion

The postauricular infratemporal fossa approach is a significant advance in our ability to treat extensive skull base lesions. Total removal of even large tumors is usually possible, with preservation of good quality of life.

TABLE 163-4 Summary of Results (N = 116)

Tumor Type	Primary Surgery	Surgery for Recurrence	Total Removal	Partial Removal	Alive without Disease	Alive with Disease	Died of Disease	Died of Other Disease	Postoperative Irradiation
Meningioma, $N = 11$	9	2	10	1	10		1		1
Jugular fossa neuroma, $N = 8$	8		8		8				
Glomus jugulare tumor, $N = 80$	73	7	73	7	72	7		1	6
Glomus vagale tumor, $N = 5$	4	1	4	1	4	1			1
Chordoma, $N = 2$	2		2		1			1	2
Chondrosarcoma, $N = 5$	4	1	4	1	4	1			1
Cholesteatoma, $N = 3$	2	1	3		3				
Papillary adenoma, $N = 2$	1	1	2		2				1

References

1. Brackmann DE. The facial nerve in the infratemporal approach. *Otolaryngol Head Neck Surg* 1987; 97:15–17.
2. Brackmann DE, House WF, Terry R, et al. Glomus jugulare tumors: effect of irradiation. *Trans Am Acad Opththalmol Otolaryngol* 1972; 76:1423–1431.
3. Fisch U. Infratemporal fossa approach for glomus tumors of the temporal bone. *Ann Otol Rhinol Laryngol* 1982; 91:474–479.
4. Fisch U, Fagan P, Valavanis A. The infratemporal fossa approach for the lateral skull base. *Otolaryngol Clin North Am* 1984; 17(3):513–552.
5. Leonetti JP, Brackmann DE, Prass RC. Improved preservation of facial nerve function in the infratemporal approach to the skull base. *Otolaryngol Head Neck Surg* 1989; 101:74–78.
6. Murphy TP, Brackmann DE. Effect of preoperative embolization on glomus jugulare tumors. *Laryngoscope* 1989; 99:1244–1247.
7. Saunders WH, Johnson EW. Rehabilitation of the shoulder after radical neck dissection. *Ann Otol Rhinol Laryngol* 1975; 84:812–816.

164

Surgical Anatomy of the Cavernous Sinus

Harry R. van Loveren
Murali Guthikonda
Magdy El-Kalliny
Jeffrey T. Keller

The cavernous sinus is a paired structure consisting of a plexus of variously sized veins located on either side of the body of the sphenoid bone and interconnected by venous channels. Anteriorly the cavernous sinus extends from the superior orbital fissure, which is formed by the greater and lesser wings of the sphenoid bone. Posteriorly it extends to the apex of the petrous temporal bone. It averages 2 cm in length and 1 cm in width.

Surgery of the cavernous sinus has become possible since this anatomy has been unraveled. The demystification of the cavernous sinus begins with its name; the cavernous sinus is neither cavernous nor a sinus. Embryologically, it is formed from a secondary venous plexus derived from the head vein.[27] Bedford[2] and Harris and Rhoton[10] believe that the sinus is largely an unbroken trabeculated venous channel. More appropriately, the cavernous sinus may be considered an epidural venous plexus in continuity with the basilar epidural venous plexus. In this context, the cranial nerves are considered to be extradural as they leave the intradural space at their respective dural foramina (i.e., the oculomotor foramen and Dorello's canal) rather than at the superior orbital fissure where they actually become extracranial.

The enthusiasm that surrounded Parkinson's first venture into the cavernous sinus to repair a carotid-cavernous fistula was short-lived owing to the perceived need for circulatory arrest. Interest was later revived by other investigators, including Hakuba et al.[8] and Dolenc,[4] who not only described the anatomy of this region but also demonstrated its safe and effective application in human surgery.

In this chapter, we describe the anatomy of the cavernous sinus and its relation to the structures in and adjacent to it. Specific topics include the osseous, dural, neural, and vascular relationships of the sinus. This anatomic information serves as a framework for the surgical approaches to the region, thus amounting to "surgical" as well as "cadaveric" anatomy.

Osseous Relationships

Bony landmarks relevant to the cavernous sinus include the body of the sphenoid, the greater wing (alisphenoid), the lesser wing (orbitosphenoid), the anterior and posterior clinoid processes, the carotid clinoid foramen, and the interclinoid osseous bridge. Occasionally a prominent middle clinoid process is seen on the lateral surface of the sphenoid body.

The cavernous sinus is a paired structure of considerable size, extending approximately 2 cm along the lateral aspects of the body of the sphenoid bone from the superior orbital fissure anteriorly to the petrous apex posteriorly. The body of the sphenoid bone is cubelike and consists of two parts, the anterior presphenoid and the posterior basisphenoid, which are imperceptibly fused. The lateral surfaces of the body are united with the greater wings (alisphenoids) and the medial pterygoid plates. Above the attachment of each wing is the broad carotid sulcus (groove) for the internal carotid artery (ICA). The carotid sulcus is deepest at its posterior end, where it is overhung medially by the petrosal process and is limited laterally by a sharp margin called the lingula, which projects posteriorly into the foramen lacerum.[27] The lesser wings of the sphenoid bone extend medially, forming the optic canal roof, and fuse in the midline, forming the jugum sphenoidale.

The anterior clinoid process, a triangular projection superior and lateral to the optic foramen, is a medial and posterior extension of the lesser wing. In a study of 135 dry skulls and 25 cadaveric dissections performed in our laboratory, the length of the anterior clinoid process ranged from 3 to 18 mm (average 7 mm) and its width ranged from 2 to 4 mm (average 3 mm). On its inferomedial aspect, the anterior clinoid process is connected to the sphenoid body via the optic strut, which forms the inferolateral boundary of the optic foramen. The anterior clinoid process is composed of a thin shell of outer cortical bone surrounding inner cancellous bone. Occasionally the anterior clinoid process is pneumatized, communicating with the sphenoid sinus.

The posterior clinoid processes are the cephalad projections of the dorsum sellae and may be pneumatized with the sphenoid sinus. The posterior fossa dura bridging the gap between the posterior clinoid process and the petrous apex forms the posterior limit of the cavernous sinus.

The middle clinoid process is a bony projection from the lateral surface of the body of the sphenoid. It varies in shape from a small spicule to a prominent projection that fuses with the anterior clinoid process.

Carotid Clinoid Foramen

Complete bony fusion between the anterior and middle clinoid processes forms a carotid-clinoid foramen; this fusion was identified in 13 percent of the 135 specimens examined (Fig. 164-1) and was present bilaterally twice as often as unilaterally. In an additional 24 percent of the specimens, incomplete bony fusion resulted in a pseudoforamen that was closed by a connection of thickened fibrous tissue called the carotid-clinoid ligament. The ICA traverses the carotid-clinoid foramen in coursing from the cavernous to the clinoidal to the intradural ophthalmic segments. The distal dural ring lies just beyond this foramen.

Interclinoid Osseous Bridge

In 6 percent of our specimens, a bony connection called the interclinoid osseous bridge was noted between the anterior and posterior clinoid processes. In this study, an interclinoid osseous bridge was always associated with a carotid-clinoid foramen. Thus, whenever an interclinoid osseous bridge was present, two foramina

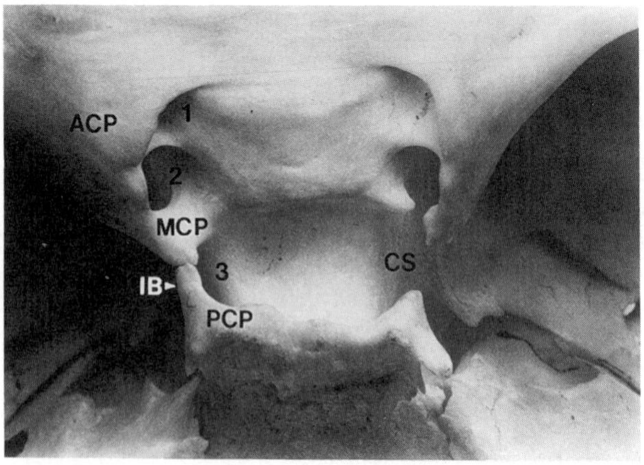

Figure 164-1 Variations in the anatomy of the sphenoid bone. ACP, anterior clinoid process; MCP, middle clinoid process; PCP, posterior clinoid process; IB, interclinoid bridge; CS, carotid sulcus; 1, optic foramen; 2, carotid-clinoid foramen; 3, posterior interclinoid foramen.

were formed: a carotid-clinoid foramen and a posterior-interclinoid foramen. In specimens lacking an osseous interclinoid bridge, a thick fibrous band, or interclinoid ligament, connects the anterior and posterior clinoid processes.

Clinical Significance

In surgically exploring the cavernous sinus, an initial step is to "unlock" the contents of the sinus from their bony confines. This step includes unroofing and mobilizing the optic nerve, and then removing the anterior clinoid process (Fig. 164-2). This phase of the operation can be performed in an extradural or intradural fashion.

During an extradural anterior clinoidectomy, the lesser wing of the sphenoid bone and the posterior orbital roof are removed. The optic canal is unroofed from the optic foramen to its junction with the periorbita. The anterior clinoid process is cored by drilling within its cancellous center using a diamond burr and is subsequently disconnected from the optic strut. If resistance is encountered during removal, a significant connection may exist between the anterior clinoid process and the middle or posterior clinoid process; final removal should then be done intradurally after visualizing the intracranial structures. Generous irrigation and drilling with diamond burrs should be used along with magnification for this part of the operative procedure.

Dural Relationships

Surfaces and Folds

The cavernous sinus has four surfaces: a superior surface, which is covered by the dura mater; an inferior surface, which is covered by the periosteum floor; and lateral and medial surfaces. The tentorium cerebelli contributes significantly to the cavernous sinus roof, and the dural propria of the middle cranial fossa contributes to the lateral wall of the cavernous sinus.

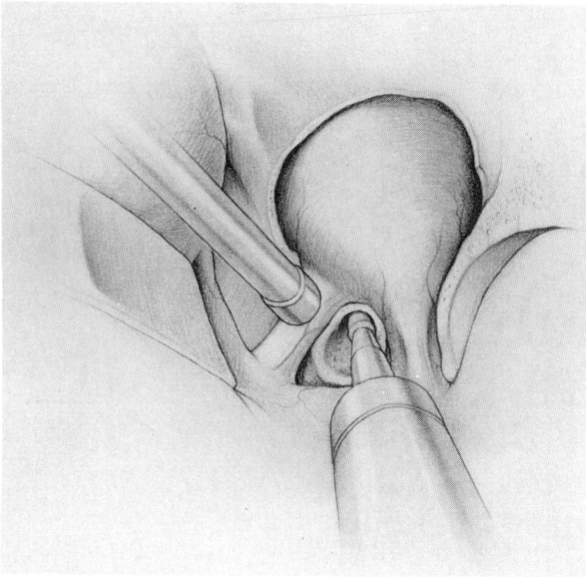

Figure 164-2 Technique of right extradural clinoidectomy. A posterior orbitotomy has been completed, and the dura overlying the superior orbital fissure has been exposed. The suction tip indicates the optic nerve unroofed in the optic canal with its dural sheath intact. A diamond burr cores out the anterior clinoid process. (From Tew JM Jr, van Loveren HR. *Atlas of Operative Microneurosurgery,* vol 1. *Aneurysms and Arteriovenous Malformations.* Philadelphia: Saunders, 1994, p 87, with permission.)

The superior surface or the cavernous sinus roof is formed by the anterior extension of the tentorium cerebelli and the lateral extension of the diaphragma sellae. As the tentorium curves anteromedially, it gives rise to two dural folds: first, the anterior clinoid fold extending anteriorly to the anterior clinoid process; and, second, the posterior clinoid fold extending to the posterior clinoid process. An interclinoid fold connects the anterior and posterior clinoid processes. These three folds form the boundaries of the oculomotor trigone, which constitutes the posterior two thirds of the roof of the cavernous sinus and, in essence, the lateral extension of the diaphragma sellae. The oculomotor nerve penetrates the oculomotor trigone. Although this portion of the roof is accessible by direct intradural exploration, the anterior one third is hidden by the anterior clinoid process, which must be removed to gain access to this region.

The anterior clinoid fold splits into two layers which enclose the anterior clinoid process: a superficial layer that extends on its superior surface and onto the tuberculum sellae, and a deeper layer on its undersurface. This deeper layer encircles the ICA proximal to the ophthalmic artery to form the distal dural ring (Fig. 164-3). The periosteal layer encircles the internal carotid artery as it emerges from the cavernous sinus to form the proximal ring and extends laterally to the third cranial nerve as the carotid-oculomotor membrane.

The lateral wall of the cavernous sinus is formed by the superficial dura propria of the middle fossa and a deeper reticular layer (or inner membranous layer).[25] This deeper layer is actually formed by the epineurium of the cranial nerves traversing the lateral wall of the cavernous sinus. The medial wall is formed by the dura propria and the endosteum of the sella turcica's lateral wall. The floor is formed by the endosteum of the sphenoid body.

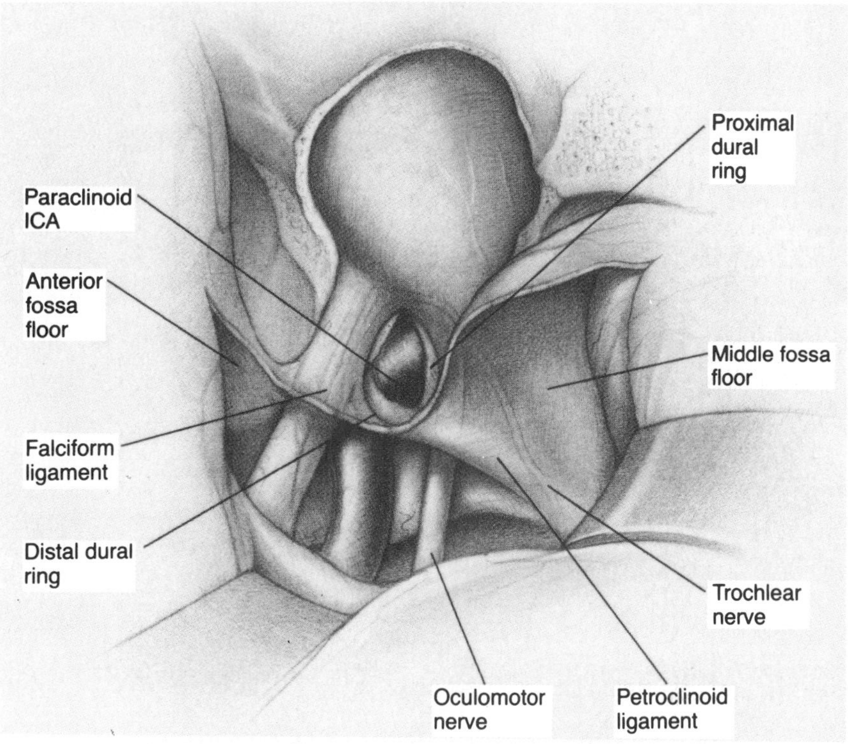

Figure 164-3 The proximal and distal dural rings after right anterior clinoidectomy and dural opening. (From Tew JM Jr, van Loveren HR. *Atlas of Operative Microneurosurgery,* vol 1. *Aneurysms and Arteriovenous Malformations.* Philadelphia: Saunders, 1994, p 89, with permission.)

Clinical Significance

The anterior loop of the ICA can be mobilized after anterior clinoidectomy and circumferential division of the distal ring. This mobilization allows the surgeon to manage aneurysms of the anterior loop and clinoidal segment of the ICA. Sectioning the proximal ring allows mobilization of the entire anterior loop and entry into the anterior cavernous sinus. The limiting factor is the ophthalmic artery, which can be safely sacrificed in most patients without causing visual loss, owing to retrograde filling of the ophthalmic artery and its central retinal arterial branch.

Lesions of the cavernous sinus can be divided by location into those that are contained within the cavernous sinus, those that are located in the lateral wall of the cavernous sinus between the dura propria and inner membranous layers (Fig 164-4), and those that invade these layers, thus disrupting the normal anatomy of the lateral wall.

Because there is a distinct cleavage plane between the dura propria and the inner membranous layer, tumors of the lateral wall, such as epidermoid tumors and some trigeminal neuromas, can be exposed without entering the cavernous sinus proper.[5] Tumors within the cavernous sinus are generally approached by mobilizing the dura propria and are followed by exploring the sinus through various defined triangles bordered by the cranial nerves that traverse it (Fig. 164-5). Lesions that invade the lateral wall, such as sphenoid wing meningiomas, also can invade neurovascular structures within the cavernous sinus. The total resection of these lesions remains both challenging and controversial.

Neural Relationships

Cranial nerves III through VI are closely associated with the cavernous sinus (Fig. 164-6). The oculomotor nerve courses above the posterior petroclinoid fold lateral to the posterior clinoid process and enters the cavernous sinus via the oculomotor foramen in the oculomotor trigone. Cranial nerve III travels along the lateral wall of the cavernous sinus where its epineurium interweaves with the epineurium of the trochlear nerve and V_1; this interweaving forms the inner layer of the cavernous sinus. Cranial nerve III courses anteriorly along the inferolateral surface of the anterior clinoid process and enters the superior orbital fissure. The carotid-oculomotor membrane stretches between the anterior loop of the ICA and the third nerve as it crosses the artery, giving rise to the proximal dural ring. The oculomotor nerve enters the superior orbital fissure between the two heads of the lateral rectus muscle within

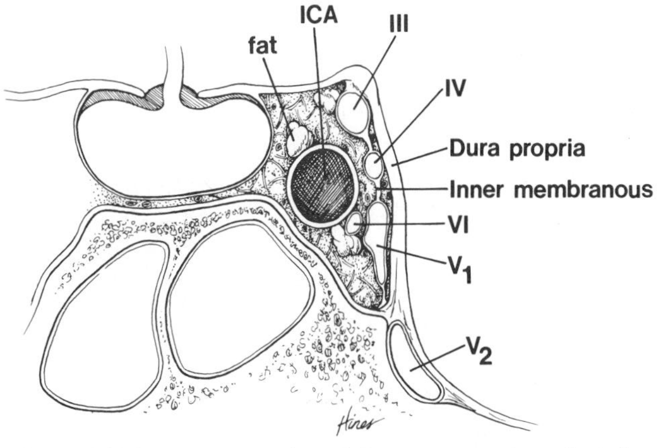

Figure 164-4 A cross-section of the cavernous sinus depicting the dura propria of the lateral wall, the inner membranous layer, and the neurovascular relationships of the internal carotid artery (ICA), cranial nerves III, IV, V_1, V_2, and VI, and the veins between the lateral wall and inner membranous layer and within the cavernous sinus.

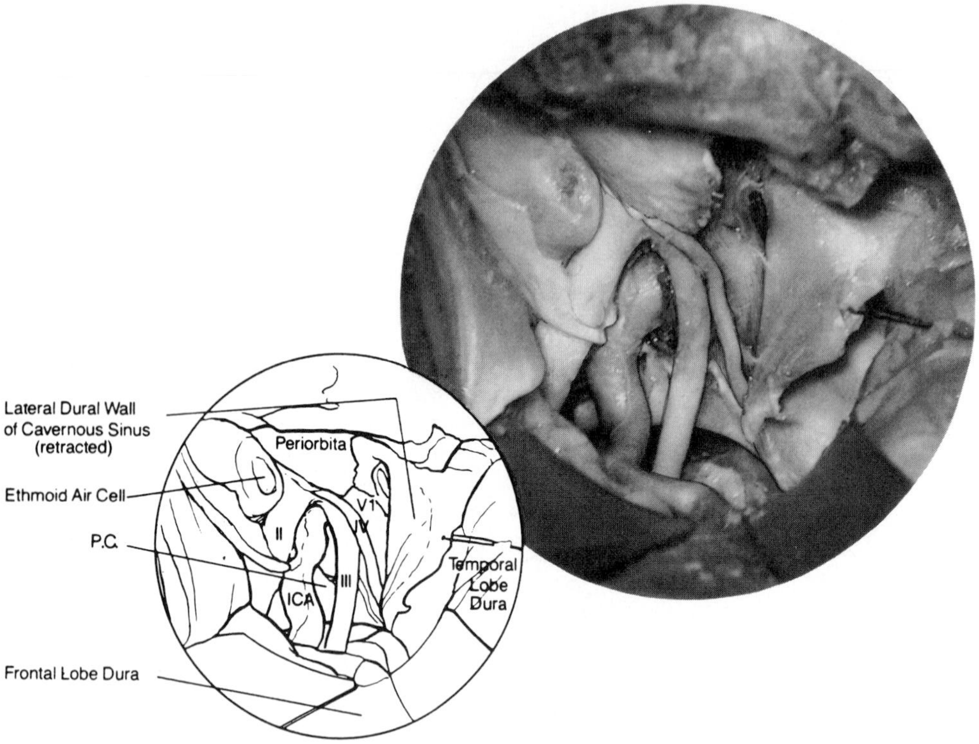

Figure 164-5 Mobilization of the lateral wall (dura propria) of the cavernous sinus. PC, posterior clinoid process; ICA, internal carotid artery. (From van Loveren HR et al.,[26] with permission.)

the annulus of Zinn; there it divides into superior and inferior divisions. The superior division innervates the levator palpebrae superioris and the superior rectus. The inferior division innervates the medial and inferior recti and the inferior oblique.

The trochlear nerve penetrates the margin of the tentorium posterolateral to the posterior clinoid process between its diverging anterior and posterior petroclinoid folds. This nerve travels along the tentorium for a few millimeters before entering the lateral wall of the cavernous sinus. In the lateral wall, it travels anteriorly below and lateral to the oculomotor nerve, deep to the dura propria and suspended within the inner membranous layer. Cranial nerve IV crosses over the third nerve before entering the superior orbital fissure; it is located outside the annulus of Zinn. Here, the nerve passes between the levator palpebrae superioris and the periorbita to enter the orbital surface of the superior oblique muscle.

The ophthalmic division (V_1) of the trigeminal nerve enters the lateral wall of the cavernous sinus at its most posterior end. V_1 courses below and lateral to the trochlear nerve in the lateral wall

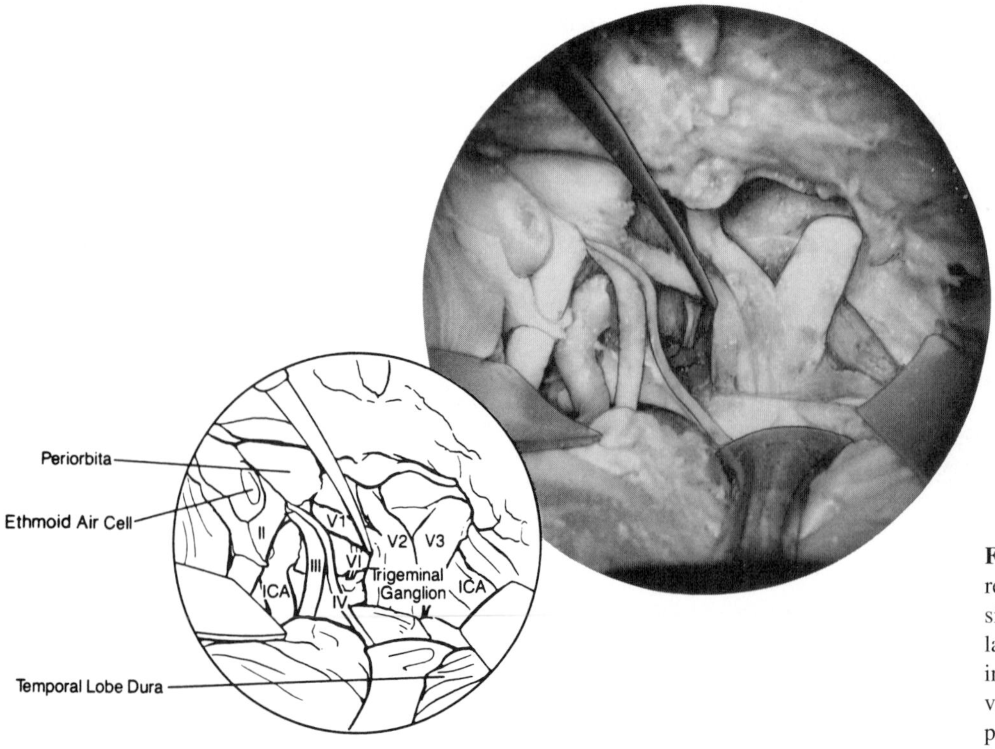

Figure 164-6 Neurovascular relationships of the cavernous sinus after mobilization of the lateral wall (dura propria). ICA, internal carotid artery. (From van Loveren HR et al.,[26] with permission.)

and lateral to it in the superior orbital fissure. In the superior orbital fissure, V_1 divides into three branches. The large frontal branch courses with the trochlear nerve and the small lacrimal branch travels in the lateralmost part of the fissure; both these branches are outside the annulus of Zinn. The intermediate nasociliary branch enters the orbit through the anulus between the two heads of the lateral rectus muscle. The dura of the cavernous sinus is innervated by the ophthalmic and maxillary branches of the trigeminal nerve.

The abducens nerve penetrates the clival dura and ascends toward Dorello's canal, which is the space between the petrous apex and the posterior clinoid process. Dorello's canal is bridged by a ligamentous or osseous petroclinoid ligament. After passing through Dorello's canal, the nerve penetrates the posterior cavernous sinus and drapes over the lateral surface of the ICA. The abducens nerve is branched, either in duplicate or triplicate. The sympathetic fibers from the carotid plexus join the sixth nerve in its intracavernous course.

The arterial supply of cranial nerves is frequently overlooked. Because a disregard for cranial nerve vascularization can lead to loss of neurological function, understanding this supply is important. The portions of cranial nerves III, IV, VI, V_1, and V_2 associated with the cavernous sinus receive vascular supply from multiple sources.[14–16] Before entering the cavernous sinus, cranial nerves III, IV, and VI receive branches from the vertebrobasilar system. Cranial nerves IV and VI are each supplied by arteries that arise separately, whereas the arteries supplying cranial nerve III may arise from a common trunk close to the posterior perforated substance or from a branch of the posterior cerebral artery. The proximal portion of the trigeminal nerve receives arterial supply from a branch of the basilar trunk, a vestige of the trigeminal artery. Within the cavernous sinus, the inferolateral trunk, a cavernous branch of the ICA, largely supplies all the cranial nerves coursing through the sinus.[14–16] The inferolateral trunk divides into four branches: a superior or tentorial branch supplying cranial nerves III and IV; an anteromedial branch supplying cranial nerves III, IV, VI, and V_1; a lateral branch supplying cranial nerve V_2; an anterior lateral branch supplying cranial nerve V_2; and a posterior branch supplying cranial nerve V_3.

Clinical Significance

Cranial nerve palsy is the most common manifestation of pathologic processes involving the cavernous sinus. Diplopia is often the presenting symptom; in one study, multiple cranial neuropathies occurred in 82 percent of patients.[7] Primary aberrant regeneration of the third cranial nerve without a previous history of acute paralysis has been reported.[20] A sixth cranial nerve palsy with postganglionic Horner's syndrome suggests a cavernous sinus lesion.[12] Sensory symptoms in the distribution of V_1 and occasionally V_2 are also common presenting symptoms of cavernous sinus lesions. Impaired visual acuity is less often a presenting symptom than double vision.[7]

Most cavernous sinus explorations are for benign disease with the goal of preserving and improving cranial nerve function.[22,23] Exploration of the cavernous sinus usually follows mobilization of the lateral wall and entry through one or more of the various triangles formed by these cranial nerves and dural folds.

Anatomic Triangles

The cranial nerves in conjunction with dural folds and some osseous structures of the skull base tend to form a pattern of nine triangles[26] (Table 164-1; Fig. 164-7). A thorough knowledge of the anatomic layout of these triangles is essential before undertaking any exploration in this area.

TABLE 164-1 Anatomic Triangles of the Cavernous Sinus

	Boundaries			
Triangle	**Medial**	**Lateral**	**Base**	**Contents**
Anteromedial	CN II	CN III	Anterior petroclinoid fold	Anterior clinoid process, carotid rings, anterior loop, distal horizontal ICA
Paramedial	CN III	CN IV	Anterior petroclinoid fold	Horizontal ICA, inferolateral trunk
Parkinson's	CN IV	V_1	Anterior petroclinoid fold	Medial loop, horizontal ICA (distal), CN VI
Anterolateral (Mullen's)	V_1	V_2	Superior orbital fissure to foramen rotundum	Horizontal ICA, CN VI
Lateral	V_2	V_3	Foramen rotundum to foramen ovale	Lateral loop of ICA
Posterolateral (Glasscock's)	Greater superficial petrosal nerve	Arcuate eminence to foramen spinosum	V_3 lateral margin	Posterior and lateral loops of ICA, tensor tympani, lateral loop of eustachian tube
Posteromedial (Kawase's)	V_3, gasserian ganglion	Greater superficial petrosal nerve	Petrous apex	Posterior surface of medial loop, petrous apex with Meckel's cave, posterior fossa dura

Abbreviations: CN, cranial nerve; ICA, internal carotid artery; V_1, V_2, V_3, the ophthalmic, maxillary, and mandibular divisions of the trigeminal nerve.

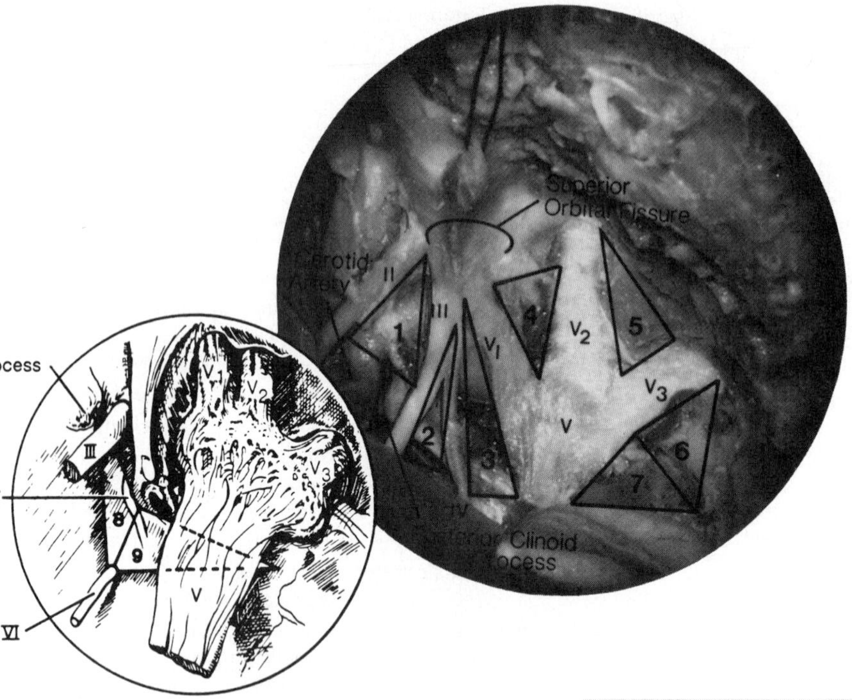

Figure 164-7 Anatomic triangles of the cavernous sinus: 1, anteromedial (Dolenc); 2, paramedial; 3, Parkinson's; 4, anterolateral (Mullen's); 5, lateral; 6, posterolateral (Glasscock's); 7, posteromedial (Kawase's); 8, inferomedial; 9, inferolateral. Photo enhanced. (From van Loveren HR et al.,[26] with permission.)

Vascular Relationships

Arterial

The ICA begins at the common carotid artery and extends rostrally as the cervical portion (C1) of the ICA to the external orifice of the carotid canal (Fig. 164-8*A*).[6] It enters the base of the skull via the carotid foramen anterior to the jugular foramen. The ICA runs vertically at first and becomes horizontal through the petrous temporal bone, thus forming the posterior loop (Fig. 164-8*B*). The artery crosses over the foramen lacerum under the trigeminal ganglion and ascends toward the cavernous sinus, thus forming the lateral loop. These two segments of the artery are relatively fixed to the skull base. After penetrating the posterior inferior cavernous sinus, the ICA ascends toward the posterior clinoid process, where it becomes nearly horizontal, forming the medial loop. After traversing the sinus as the horizontal segment, the ICA reverses its course and exits from the sinus; this course forms the vertical clinoid and almost horizontal supraclinoid segments, thereby forming the anterior loop. The medial loop and the intracavernous segments are very mobile. However, the anterior loop, oriented at 30 degrees to the horizontal plane, is firmly fixed to the skull base by the distal dural ring. The segment of the artery between the proximal and the distal rings is extracavernous, infraclinoid, and extradural.[13]

The intracavernous ICA gives rise to three branches[24]: the meningohypophyseal trunk, the inferolateral trunk, and McConnel's capsular artery. The meningohypophyseal trunk, which is the most

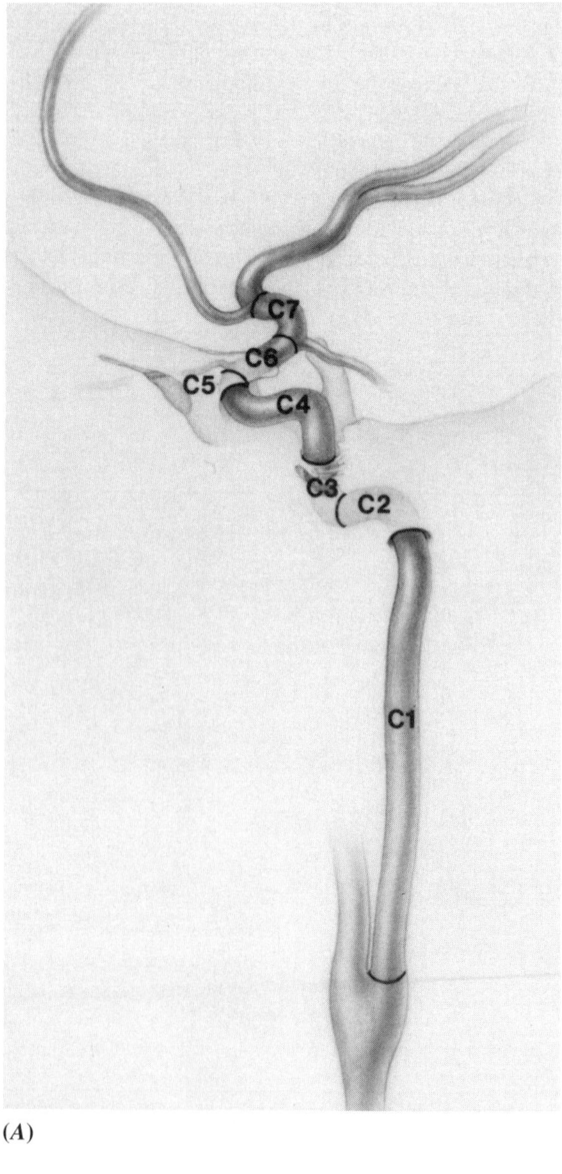

(*A*)

Figure 164-8 Segments and loops of the internal carotid artery. *A*. Modified Fischer classification according to A Bouthillier, HR van Loveren, and JT Keller (personal communication). Segments are C1, cervical; C2, petrous; C3, lacerum; C4, cavernous; C5, paraclinoid; C6, ophthalmic; C7, communicating.

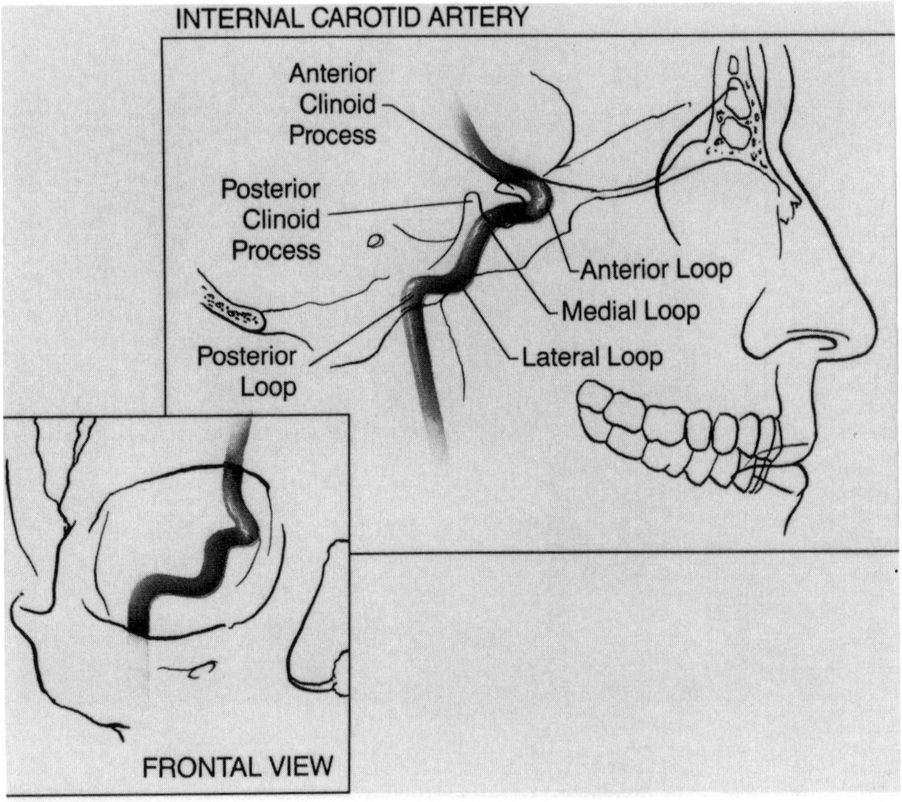

Figure 164-8 (*Continued*) *B.* Loops of the cranial internal carotid artery. (*B* from van Loveren HR et al.,[26] with permission.)

(*B*)

consistently present of these branches (seen in 100 percent of our specimens), arises from the medial loop and divides into three branches: the inferior hypophyseal, tentorial (artery of Bernasconi and Cassinari), and clival (dorsal meningeal) branches. The inferolateral trunk, also called the inferior cavernous sinus branch, which was present in 84 percent of our specimens, arises from the lateral surface of the horizontal segment and supplies the sixth nerve. The capsular artery of McConnell, seen in 28 percent of our specimens, arises from the medial surface of the horizontal segment and is often paired. The ophthalmic artery arose from the intracavernous segment of the carotid artery in 8 percent of our specimens. A persistent trigeminal artery can arise from the medial loop near the meningohypophyseal trunk. This trigeminal artery enters the posterior fossa lateral to Dorello's canal, adjacent to the trigeminal ganglion.[19]

Venous

Multiple tributaries drain into and away from the cavernous sinus (Fig. 164-9). Veins entering the cavernous sinus include, anteriorly, the superior ophthalmic vein, which enters via the superior orbital fissure; the sphenoparietal sinus located under the lesser wing of the sphenoid; and the sylvian and temporal lobe draining veins. Posterosuperiorly, the superior petrosal sinus connects the cavernous sinus to the transverse-sigmoid junction. Posteroinferiorly, the inferior petrosal sinus located in the petroclival fissure connects the cavernous sinus with the jugular bulb. Posteriorly, the basilar plexus connects the cavernous sinus to the vertebral epidural venous plexus. Laterally, multiple emissary veins connect the sinus to the pterygoid plexus. The right and left cavernous sinuses are interconnected by the anterior and posterior intracavernous sinuses across the diaphragma sellae and by a plexus in the dura of the sellar floor.

Clinical Significance

Lesions of surgical importance affecting the cavernous carotid artery range from aneurysms[17] to spontaneous and traumatic arteriovenous (carotid-cavernous) fistulae.[1] Aneurysms arising from the anterior loop can project into the subarachnoid space and therefore can present with subarachnoid hemorrhage if they rupture. Mobilization of the anterior loop after sectioning the distal dural ring allows clipping of the aneurysm neck, which is often hidden by the anterior clinoid process. Truly intracavernous aneurysms tend to present with cranial nerve palsies and retro-orbital pain. These aneurysms can reach significant size and are often bilateral. Indications and modalities for treating them remain controversial. Treatment ranges from simple observation to balloon occlusion and trapping of the segment with or without a vascular bypass. The bypass can extend from the cervical or petrous carotid artery to the supraclinoid carotid artery or the M2 segment of the middle cerebral artery. The bypass uses a venous or arterial graft or an anastomosis of the superficial temporal artery to the inferior trunk (M2 segment) of the middle cerebral artery.

The relatively fixed paraclinoid segment between the proximal and distal rings is susceptible to developing traumatic aneurysms upon fracturing of the sphenoid bone.[4] These traumatic aneurysms can manifest with epistaxis.

Patients with carotid-cavernous fistulae present with chemosis, proptosis, and pulsatile exophthalmos when drainage is predomi-

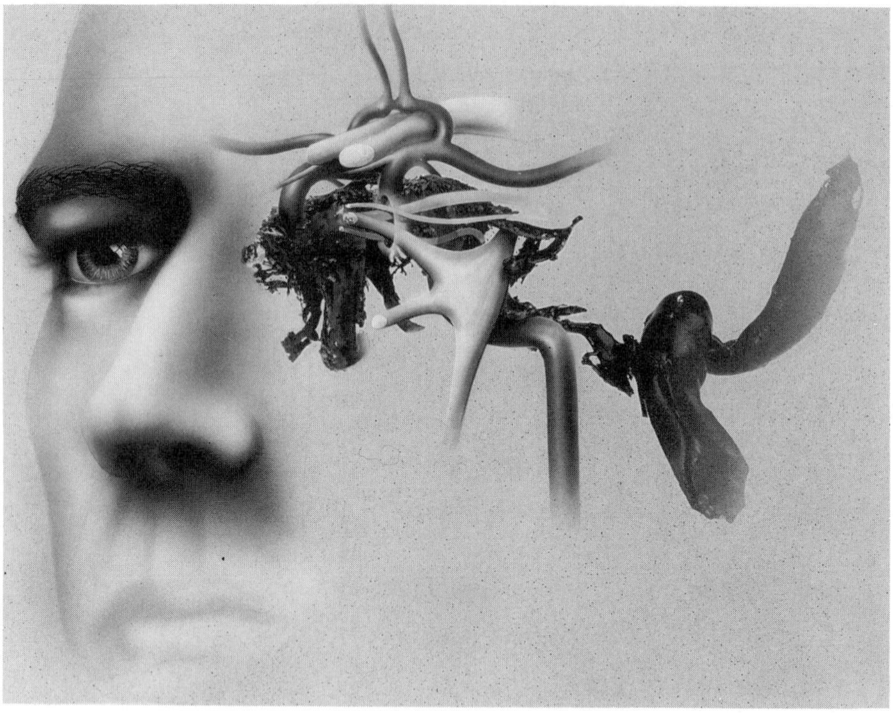

Figure 164-9 Venous anatomy of the cavernous sinus. An artist's rendering of the internal carotid artery and cranial nerves II through VI superimposed onto a photograph of a plastic cast of the cavernous sinus produced by Dr. Oscar Batson of the University of Cincinnati circa 1929. (From van Loveren HR et al.,[26] with permission.)

nantly anterior toward the superior ophthalmic vein. Progressive visual loss is ascribed to a combination of reduced arterial perfusion, orbital venous hypertension, and accompanying glaucoma.[1]

Approaches to Lesions in the Cavernous Sinus Region

There are essentially three directions of entry into the cavernous sinus: a superior approach, a lateral approach, and a combination of both.[9,11,18,21]

Superior Approach

After the removal of the anterior clinoid process and mobilization of the anterior loop of the ICA, the cavernous sinus can be entered medial or lateral to the artery. The dural incision is extended along the sinus roof posteriorly toward the posterior clinoid process. The anterior petroclinoid fold and the third cranial nerve are retracted laterally, making it possible to explore regions medial and lateral to the cavernous carotid artery. The medial limiting structures with this approach are the optic nerve and hypophysis. The abducens nerve is at risk for injury during dissection lateral to the ICA. The capsular artery medially and the inferior cavernous artery laterally may be sacrificed to further mobilize the ICA within the sinus. Sacrifice of the ophthalmic artery may be necessary for additional mobilization of the anterior loop and can be tolerated in most cases without visual compromise. Aneurysms of the anterior loop and pituitary tumors with lateral extension can be dealt with by the superior approach.

Lateral Approach

Limited access to the cavernous sinus can be achieved through Parkinson's triangle, which forms a relatively fixed landmark. The incision is made about 4 mm below the point where the third cranial nerve disappears in the oculomotor trigone; the incision extends approximately 1 cm anteriorly and posteriorly, parallel to the free edge of the tentorium. This incision is bisected at its midpoint by a 1-cm vertical incision.[11] The medial loop of the ICA and the sixth nerve are identified through this triangle.

Mobilization of the lateral wall (dura propria) as described by Dolenc[3] allows exploration of the entire venous space lateral to the ICA. The dura propria is reflected as a flap from the inner membranous layer of the lateral wall of the cavernous sinus and the trigeminal ganglion. This flap is made by incising along the oculomotor nerve and then reflecting the dura propria at the superior orbital fissure. Exploration of the sinus is done between the oculomotor and trochlear nerves (medial triangle), between the trochlear nerve and V_1 (Parkinson's triangle), and between V_1 and V_2 (Mullen's triangle).

Combined Approach

Surgery for infiltrative lesions of the cavernous sinus may require both superior and lateral approaches.

Conclusions

The essential prerequisites for surgical exploration of the cavernous sinus are, first, a thorough understanding of its anatomy; second, sufficient surgical skill to mobilize the lateral dura propria and explore the cavernous sinus without increasing the neurological deficit; and third, sound surgical judgment that will reflect the first principal of the task, "first do no harm." We have a limited understanding of the natural history of benign disease of the cavernous sinus, which may often progress only to diplopia. For this reason, we must be ever critical of our results while trying to improve them.

References

1. Barrow DL, Fiandaca MS. Carotid cavernous sinus fistulas: anatomical considerations, diagnosis and management. Part 1. *Contemp Neurosurg* 1988; 10:No 11.
2. Bedford MA. The "cavernous sinus." *Br J Ophthalmol* 1966; 50:41–46.
3. Dolenc V. Direct microsurgical repair of intracavernous vascular lesions. *J Neurosurg* 1983; 58:824–831.
4. Dolenc VV. *Anatomy and Surgery of the Cavernous Sinus.* New York: Springer-Verlag, 1989.
5. El-Kalliny M, van Loveren H, Keller JT, et al. Tumors of the lateral wall of the cavernous sinus. *J Neurosurg* 1992; 77:508–514.
6. Gibo H, Lenkey C, Rhoton AL Jr. Microsurgical anatomy of the supraclinoid portion of the internal carotid artery. *J Neurosurg* 1981; 55:560–574.
7. Golnick KC, Miller NR. Meningiomas of the anterior visual system. *Neurosurg Q* 1991; 1:79–96.
8. Hakuba A, Nishimura S, Shirakata S, et al. Surgical approaches to the cavernous sinus. Report of 19 cases. *Neurol Med Chir (Tokyo)* 1982; 22:295–308.
9. Hakuba A, Tanaka K, Suzuki T, et al. A combined orbitozygomatic infratemporal epidural and subdural approach for lesions involving the entire cavernous sinus. *J Neurosurg* 1989; 71:699–704.
10. Harris FS, Rhoton AL Jr. Anatomy of the cavernous sinus: a microsurgical study. *J Neurosurg* 1976; 45:169–180.
11. Inoue T, Rhoton AL Jr, Theele D, et al. Surgical approaches to the cavernous sinus: a microsurgical study. *Neurosurgery* 1990; 26:903–932.
12. Johnston JA, Parkinson D. Intracranial sympathetic pathways associated with the sixth cranial nerve. *J Neurosurg* 1974; 40:236–243.
13. Knosp E, Muller G, Perneczky A. The paraclinoid carotid artery: anatomical aspects of a microneurosurgical approach. *Neurosurgery* 1988; 22:896–901.
14. Lapresle J, Lasjaunias P. Cranial nerve ischaemic arterial syndromes: a review. *Brain* 1986; 109:207–216.
15. Lasjaunias PL, Berenstein A. *Craniofacial and Upper Cervical Arteries: Functional, Clinical, and Angiographic Aspects.* Baltimore: Williams & Wilkins, 1981.
16. Lasjaunias P, Moret J, Mink J. The anatomy of the inferolateral trunk (ILT) of the internal carotid artery. *Neuroradiology* 1977; 13:215–220.
17. Linskey ME, Sekhar LN, Hirsch WL Jr, et al. Aneurysms of the intracavernous carotid artery: natural history and indications for treatment. *Neurosurgery* 1990; 26:933–938.
18. Parkinson D. A surgical approach to the cavernous portion of the carotid artery. Anatomical studies and case report. *J Neurosurg* 1965; 23:474–483.
19. Parkinson D, Shields CB. Persistent trigeminal artery: its relationship to the normal branches of the cavernous carotid. *J Neurosurg* 1974; 40:244–248.
20. Schatz NJ, Savino PJ, Corbett JJ. Primary aberrant regeneration: a sign of intracavernous meningioma. *Arch Neurol* 1977; 34:29–32.
21. Sekhar LN, Burgess J, Akin O. Anatomical study of the cavernous sinus emphasizing operative approaches and related vascular and neural reconstruction. *Neurosurgery* 1987; 21:806–816.
22. Sekhar LN, Moller AR. Operative management of tumors involving the cavernous sinus. *J Neurosurg* 1986; 64:879–889.
23. Sekhar LN, Sen CN, Jho HD, et al. Surgical treatment of intracavernous neoplasms. A four-year experience. *Neurosurgery* 1989; 24:18–30.
24. Tran-Dinh H. Cavernous branches of the internal carotid artery: anatomy and nomenclature. *Neurosurgery* 1987; 20:205–210.
25. Umansky F, Nathan H. The lateral wall of the cavernous sinus: with special reference to the nerves related to it. *J Neurosurg* 1982; 56:228–234.
26. van Loveren HR, Keller JT, El-Kalliny M, et al. The Dolenc technique for cavernous sinus exploration (cadaveric prosection): technical note. *J Neurosurg* 1991; 74:837–844.
27. Warwick R, Williams PL. *Gray's Anatomy,* 35th British ed. Philadelphia: Saunders, 1973.

165

Surgical Treatment of Tumors Involving the Cavernous Sinus

Sunil J. Patel
Laligam N. Sekhar

Recent advances in imaging methods and surgical techniques have made it possible to use direct surgery for tumors involving the cavernous sinus (CS).[1,3,9,10] The basic requirements for learning surgery in this region include facility with contemporary microsurgical techniques and a thorough knowledge of the anatomy of and approaches to the CS. Performance of cadaveric dissections and observation of experienced surgeons working in this region are also essential. Of equal importance is the surgeon's ability to recognize preoperatively the various factors that should be considered to avoid complications. Involvement of the air sinuses, encasement or invasion of the internal carotid artery (ICA), the patient's age and general condition, the size and extent of the tumor, and the patient's ability to tolerate ICA occlusion are a few of the factors that should be assessed carefully.

Anatomic Overview

Several references are available that give a detailed account of the relevant anatomy,[4,6] and only a general overview is provided here (Fig. 165-1).

The lateral wall of the CS consists of two dural layers, an outer thick layer continuous with the dura and an inner thin layer continuous with the periosteum. The ICA, the sixth cranial nerve (CN), and sympathetic nerves lie within the CS, while the third and fourth CNs and the first and second divisions of the fifth CN lie between the layers of the lateral wall.

Intracavernous branches of the ICA include the constant meningohypophyseal and inferolateral trunks, the less frequent capsular artery of McConnell, and, occasionally, the ophthalmic artery and other small unnamed vessels. Fibrous rings invest the ICA at its entrance into (periosteal) and exit from (dural) the CS. At its exit, there are two rings that fuse medial to the ICA and are separated by the anterior clinoid process laterally. The "clinoid space," exposed by removing the anterior clinoid process, quite often contains extensions of the cavernous venous plexus, thus making this space part of the CS.

Classification of Cavernous Sinus Tumors

Besides classifying these tumors by pathology and biological behavior (malignant vs. benign), a rational classification is necessary to assess degrees of CS involvement and ICA encasement, since these factors relate directly to the technical difficulty of resection. This assessment would also allow reasonable methods for comparing surgical results. Table 165-1 shows a classification based on features noted on magnetic resonance imaging (MRI). Generally, tumors of grades I and II are easier to resect, while tumors of grades III through V may require CS-ICA resection and vein graft reconstruction. Another method of classifying tumors of the CS, which is surgically relevant and more often useful for benign tumors such as meningiomas, is to specify whether they are *confined* to the CS or *extensive*. Confined tumors are defined as small tumors that arise from the CS itself or its immediate surroundings and that involve Meckel's cave, the medial middle fossa, and/or the sella turcica in addition to the CS. Extensive CS tumors can also involve distant areas such as the orbit, anterior fossa, infratemporal fossa, contralateral CS, posterior fossa, and/or petroclival regions.[8,12]

Preoperative Imaging and Assessment

Although MRI with contrast enhancement provides a superior way to screen for suspected CS lesions and clearly defines dural extension and ICA involvement, computed tomography (CT) with bone windows is important in defining the bony anatomy and tumor involvement, the knowledge of which is essential in planning surgery.

The importance of preoperative assessment with angiography cannot be overstated. In addition to revealing tumor vascularity and allowing for embolization when feasible, angiography can also better define surgically relevant contralateral ICA disease and any other vascular pathology. In order to better prepare for temporary or permanent ICA occlusion during CS surgery, the surgeon should perform preoperative balloon test occlusion (BTO) of the ICA and ICA-occluded cerebral blood flow (CBF) studies. Patients who clinically tolerate a 15-min BTO and show CBF > 35 ml/min per 100 g on xenon-CT during ICA occlusion are considered to have a low risk for a subsequent stroke should the ICA

TABLE 165-1 Radiologic Classification of Intracavernous Neoplasms

Grade	Cavernous Sinus Involvement	ICA Encasement	ICA Narrowing
I	One area	None	None
II	Two or more	Partial	None
III	All	Total	None
IV	All	Total	Stenosis or occlusion
V	Bilateral	+/−	+/−

Source: Adapted from Sekhar et al.[10]

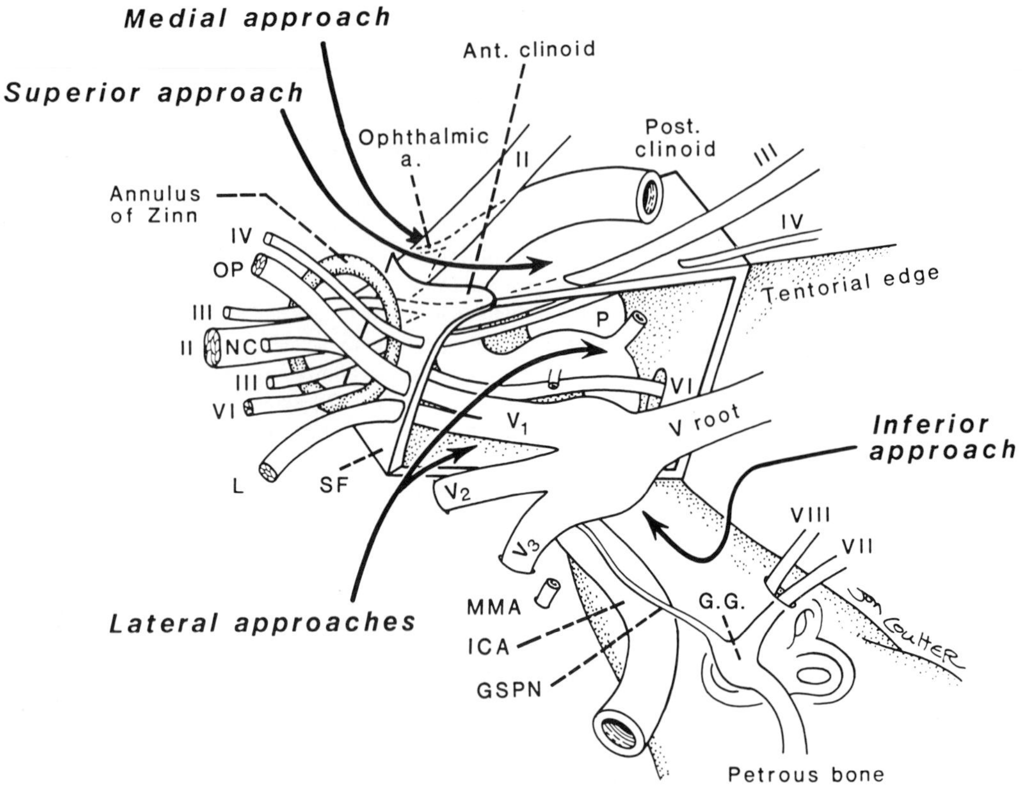

Figure 165-1 Schematic view of the anatomy of the cavernous sinus and the routes of cavernous sinus entry. MMA, middle meningeal artery; ICA, internal carotid artery; GSPN, greater superficial petrosal nerve; GG, geniculate ganglion; OP, ophthalmic branch of CN V; NC, nasociliary branch; L, lacrimal branch; SF, superior orbital fissure; P, pituitary gland. (From Sekhar et al.,[10] with permission.)

be permanently occluded (75 percent of patients fall in this category). Those with BTO tolerance but CBF < 35 ml/min per 100 g are considered at moderate risk, while those who do not tolerate BTO are at high risk for a stroke after permanent ICA occlusion. At present, the philosophy of the senior author is to reconstruct the ICA with a vein graft whenever it is totally encased. In our experience, the risk of stroke after ICA occlusion is not completely eliminated even in patients who tolerated the balloon occlusion test without reduction of CBF. The risk of vein graft occlusion has been greatly reduced—indeed, practically eliminated—with the use of intraoperative angiography.

Indications for Surgery

Generally, for meningiomas involving the CS, symptom progression and/or tumor growth on serial imaging are indications for resection of the tumor from the CS. We tend to be more conservative in managing patients with grade III and IV tumors as compared to those with grade I and II tumors. Grade V tumors are treated even more conservatively, and only the symptomatic side is operated on. For patients who have asymptomatic, extensive tumors and/or are elderly, only extracavernous resection is performed, with the intention of treating the remnant tumor in the CS with radiosurgery. In general, the CS portion is often easier to remove for meningiomas than neurilemomas, cavernous hemangiomas, juvenile angiofibromas, craniopharyngiomas, pituitary adenomas, chordomas, and chondrosarcomas. Operations can thus be performed for these tumors with the intention of completely resecting them from the CS.

Surgery for fast-growing malignant lesions (e.g., squamous cell carcinomas) in this region is controversial. *En bloc* resection of the entire CS with the ICA and cranial nerves is justifiable only if complete extracavernous resection is feasible. Bilateral CS involvement is a contraindication for any surgery.

Operative Technique

As with any prolonged operation, adequate positioning is essential and preparations should be made to deal with heavy blood loss, to prevent deep venous thrombosis, and to detect venous air embolism. Appropriate anesthesia is administered for electromyographic (EMG) monitoring of cranial nerves and neurophysiologic monitoring of cerebral hemispheric function (Fig. 165-2). Antibiotic prophylaxis and high-dose steroid administration are recommended. During temporary ICA occlusion, whenever necessary, measures should be taken to protect the brain (hypothermia to 32 to 34°C, barbiturate coma to electroencephalography (EEG) burst suppression levels, and induced hypertension).

Craniotomy and Osteotomy

The basic surgical principles are a low basal approach to minimize brain retraction, provide adequate exposure, and gain control of the

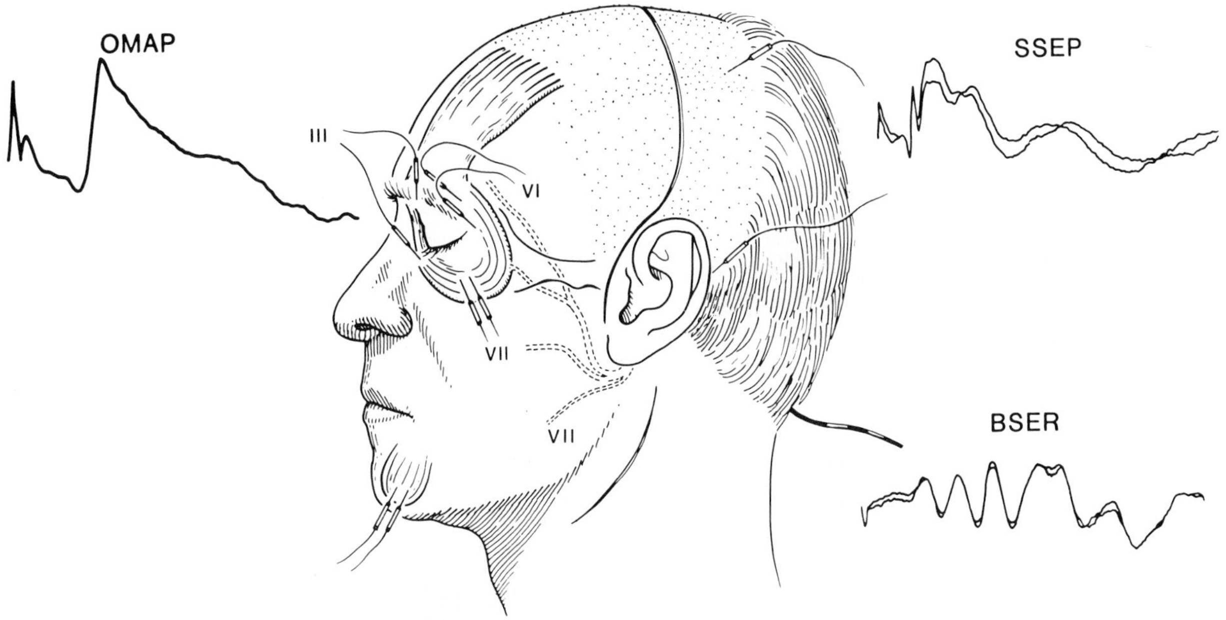

Figure 165-2 The monitoring modalities and typical incision used in cavernous sinus surgery. (From Sekhar et al.,[10] with permission.)

ICA and, finally, proper closure to prevent CSF leakage and provide a cosmetically good result. For unilateral lesions, a frontotemporal-orbitozygomatic approach is used. A bicoronal or curvilinear incision is made, extending below the zygomatic arch and just anterior to the tragus, thus preserving facial nerve branches and the superficial temporal artery. The scalp flap is elevated subperiosteally with the superficial temporalis muscle fascia and is brought forward to expose the orbital rim and the entire zygoma. Dissecting between the superficial and deep layers of the temporalis muscle fascia and staying deep to the parotid gland avoids injury to the facial nerve. The temporalis muscle is completely mobilized and the periosteum elevated from the orbital roof and lateral wall, up to the inferior orbital fissure. A frontotemporal craniotomy is performed, and any remaining pterional and squamous temporal bone is removed (Fig. 165-3*A*). Dura is then elevated subfrontally and subtemporally to expose the roof of the condylar fossa. Brain relaxation, essential for this procedure, is achieved with diuretics and/or lumbar cerebrospinal fluid (CSF) drainage.

An orbitozygomatic osteotomy is performed using a reciprocating saw so that the rim, roof, and lateral wall of the orbit and the zygomatic arch are removed as a single piece (Fig. 165-3*B*). The anterior zygomatic osteotomy is directed laterally from the inferior orbital fissure to avoid entering the maxillary sinus. After temporomandibular disarticulation and separation of the meniscus from the condylar fossa, the posterior zygomatic osteotomy is made through the condylar fossa, staying within its confines to avoid the middle ear and ICA. Removing the condylar fossa in this manner allows for better restoration of the temporomandibular joint. When vein graft reconstruction of the ICA is not planned, as with grade I or II tumors, the zygomatic osteotomy can be made without involving the condylar fossa.

Proximal (ICA) Exposure

Exposure of the ICA in the neck is necessary only when its petrous portion is short or encased by tumor or hyperostosis or when a long vein bypass graft is planned. Usually, however, petrous ICA exposure is sufficient. After the orbitozygomatic osteotomy, the subtemporal dura is further elevated in the lateral-to-medial and posterior-to-anterior directions, and the following landmarks are identified: the tegman tympani, the arcuate eminence, the lesser superficial petrosal nerve (LSPN), the greater superficial petrosal nerve (GSPN), the middle meningeal artery, and the mandibular nerve (V_3). The horizontal segment of the petrous ICA is usually visible without a bony covering just medial and inferior to the GSPN. Removal of bone over and around the ICA should not be carried too far inferolaterally or posterolaterally, to avoid the eustachian tube and cochlea, respectively. If the eustachian tube is opened, it must be closed with autologous fat and suture ligation to prevent a CSF leak, and a tympanostomy may be required postoperatively. The hiatus fallopii (exit foramen of the GSPN from the petrous bone) marks the location of the underlying inferomedial cochlea. The bony anatomy of the floor of the middle fossa, the location of the cochlea, foramen spinosum (middle meningeal artery), and foramen ovale (V_3) should be well studied on preoperative CT bone window scans to discover any anatomic variations. Exposure of the petrous ICA is carried out from its posterior genu proximally to the cavernous sinus distally. The periosteum of the carotid canal can be left intact unless ICA reconstruction is planned (Fig. 165-4). One drawback of exposing the petrous ICA is the need for transecting the GSPN, which results in dryness of the eye. This sequela is especially a problem in patients who also have corneal anesthesia. If corneal denervation is expected to result from the operation, we prefer to perform cervical rather than petrous ICA exposure.

Approaches to the Cavernous Sinus for Resecting Tumor

The surgeon must be knowledgeable about the various intra- and extradural approaches that have been described for resecting tumors of the CS. Usually one approach alone does not suffice, and a combination has to be used. The inferior subtemporal-

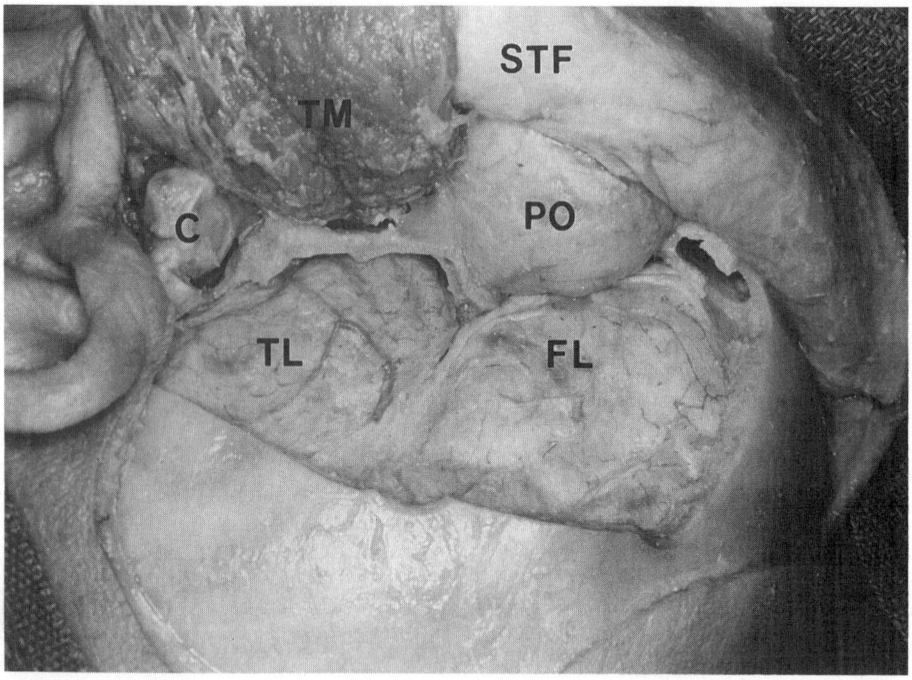

(*A*)

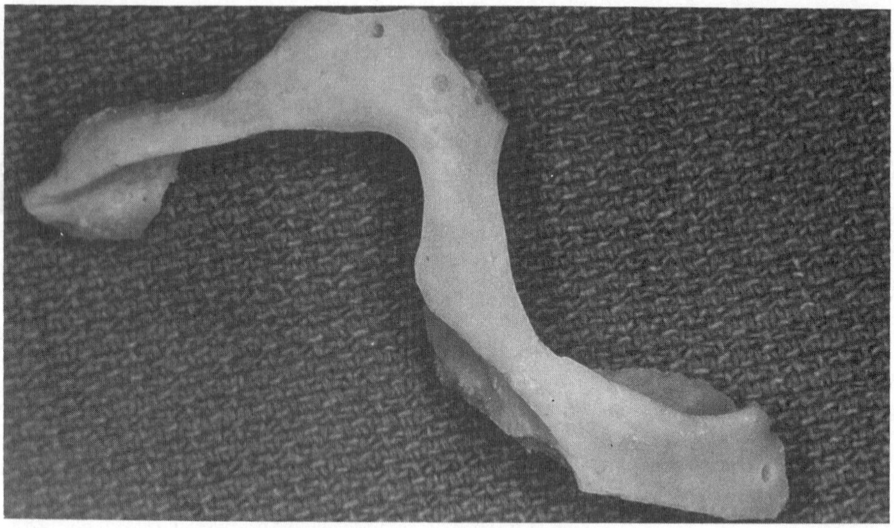

(*B*)

Figure 165-3 *A.* A cadaver dissection showing the initial exposure after a frontotemporal craniotomy and orbitozygomatic osteotomy. STF, superficial temporalis fascia, PO, periorbita, TM, temporalis muscle, TL, temporal lobe, FL, frontal lobe, C, meniscus of temporo-mandibular joint. *B.* Single-piece removal of the orbitozygomatic bone, including the condylar fossa.

infratemporal extradural approach can be used to remove tumors that invade V_3 or extend infratemporally. The medial approach (extradural) is useful only for chordomas, craniopharyngiomas, pituitary adenomas, and meningiomas with limited contralateral tumor involvement. For tumors that are intracavernous and extradural-extracavernous, the anterolateral-extradural approach between V_1 and V_2 and/or V_2 and V_3 may be useful. These tumors may include juvenile angiofibromas, adenoid cystic carcinomas, and trigeminal neurilemomas.

Generally, extradural approaches are inadequate for complete resection of meningiomas involving this region. All CS meningiomas require an intradural approach for complete tumor resection (Figs. 165-5 through 165-10). After dural opening, trans-sylvian dissection allows improved exposure through independent manipulation of the frontal and temporal lobes and facilitates exposure of the supraclinoid ICA and proximal branches of the middle cerebral artery (MCA). Subdural tumor (in the anterior or middle fossa and tentorial notch region) is first resected in the usual fashion; for some extensive tumors, a small temporal lobectomy may also be necessary.

Tumor extending into the orbital apex is removed after the optic canal is unroofed, the anterior clinoid process drilled, and the dura propria of the optic nerve opened. The latter procedure is usually done intradurally to avoid injuring the ICA at its exit from the CS.

Intradural Cavernous Sinus Dissection

The intradural superior approach exposes the regions superior and medial to the horizontal portion of the cavernous ICA and the anterior genu and vertical segments of the cavernous ICA. The clinoidal ICA is exposed by anterior clinoid process removal, the optic canal is unroofed, and the dura propria is opened to

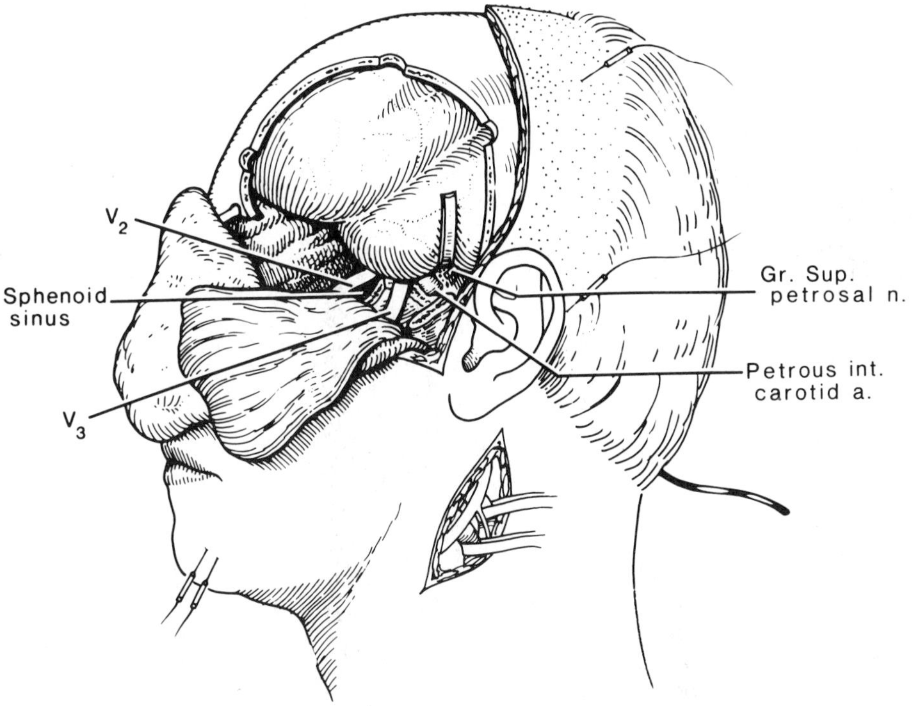

Figure 165-4 A subtemporal, extradural exposure of the petrous internal carotid artery, middle meningeal artery, greater superficial petrosal nerve, mandibular nerve, maxillary nerve, and orbital tissue. (From Sekhar et al.,[10] with permission.)

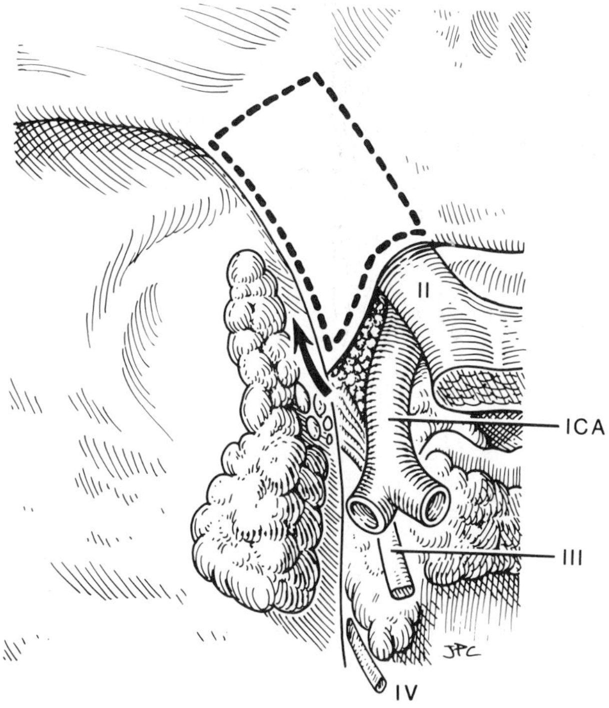

Figure 165-5 The first step in the resection of a cavernous sinus meningioma (the subsequent steps are shown in Figs. 165-6 through 165-10). The sylvian fissure has been opened and the subdural tumor exposed. The dura around the optic canal and the anterior clinoid process is removed in preparation for intradural removal of the anterior clinoid process and the bony roof of the optic canal. (From Sekhar et al.,[10] with permission.)

decompress the optic nerve. The distal intracavernous ICA is mobilized by opening the two dural rings around the ICA in this area. The superior wall of the CS is incised from the clinoid space toward the posterior clinoid, and the edge of the tentorium is retracted laterally—cautiously, since the ICA may be adherent to the dura. Care is taken during this opening procedure, since the oculomotor nerve lies just inferolateral to the clinoid space. The posterior vertical segment and bend of the ICA and CNs VI, V_2, and V_3 are not always well seen by this approach alone, so that a complete dissection of the lateral wall is necessary, especially for meningiomas.[6] The dura at the point where CN III enters the CS is opened slightly to decompress the often deformed nerve. The outer dural layer of the lateral wall is dissected away from the sphenoparietal sinus anteriorly, from the second and third divisions of the trigeminal nerve inferiorly, from the tentorial edge superiorly, and from the region of the superior petrosal sinus posteriorly. Cranial nerves III, IV, and V_1 can be positively identified from their segments in the extracavernous subarachnoid space and Meckel's cave, respectively. Electrical stimulation, although useful, should not be relied on alone. The dura around CNs III and IV is left to the end to protect the nerves from damage during dissection.

Tumor removal then proceeds through the spaces between the identified CNs of the lateral wall. The intracavernous portion of CN VI, which is most susceptible to injury, can be located and traced either forward from its posterior fossa (extracavernous) segment behind Dorello's canal by removing the petrous apex, or backward from the CS apex just inferior to V_1. The sympathetic nerves should be preserved if possible. During dissection of tumor from the ICA, lacerations of the artery should be repaired primarily, with temporary trapping of the artery if necessary. Arterial hemorrhage from the intracavernous branches of the ICA, such as the often enlarged inferolateral trunk, can be stopped by bipolar cautery. With meningiomas of grades III and IV, which usually cannot be entirely dissected from the ICA, the vessel should be excised after a vein graft bypass is established. Venous bleeding, encountered most often at the completion of tumor removal, is

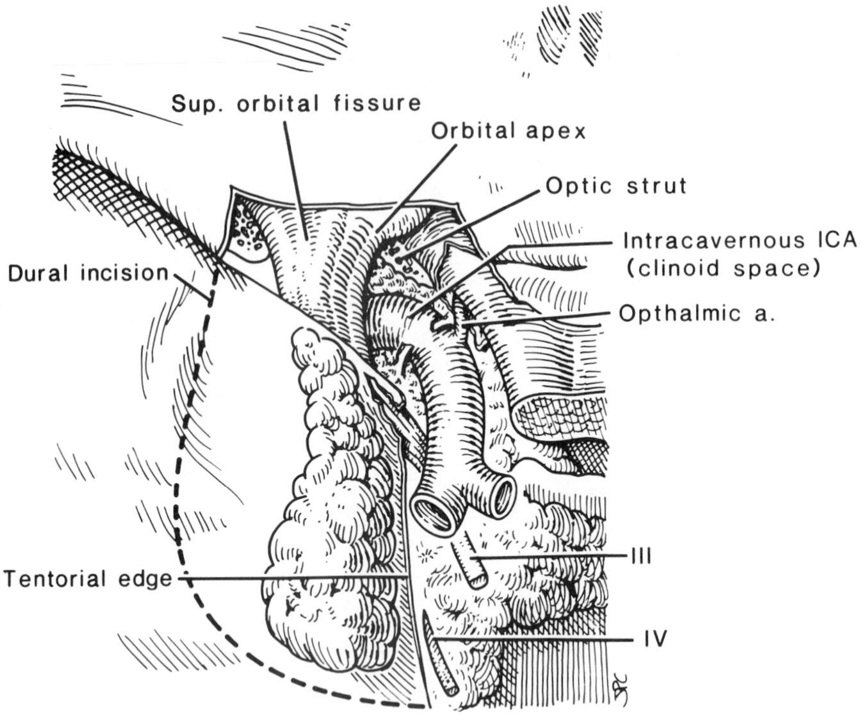

Figure 165-6 The extradural portion of the optic nerve, the clinoid space, and the superior orbital fissure have been unroofed. (From Sekhar et al.,[10] with permission.)

controlled by gentle packing with Surgical (oxidized regenerated cellulose, Johnson & Johnson Medical, Inc., Arlington, TX). Slight head elevation may be useful in controlling venous bleeding; however, it increases the risk of air embolism.

Resection of Nonmeningeal Tumors

Tumors such as neurilemomas, pituitary adenomas, cavernous hemangiomas, chordomas, and chondrosarcomas can usually be removed without extensive dissection of CNs III and IV, thus minimizing postoperative morbidity. In such cases, the CS is opened through the area of most prominent expansion, usually between CNs IV, V_1, and V_2. Removal of chordomas and chondrosarcomas should also entail extensive bone drilling, since these tumors infiltrate the bone (Figs. 165-11 and 165-12).

Transcavernous Tumor Removal

Tumor located medial to the gasserian ganglion and the trigeminal root (medial to Meckel's cave) can be removed by splitting the trigeminal root and ganglion between V_2 and V_3 and occasionally between V_1 and V_2. For meningiomas of grades III through V, the

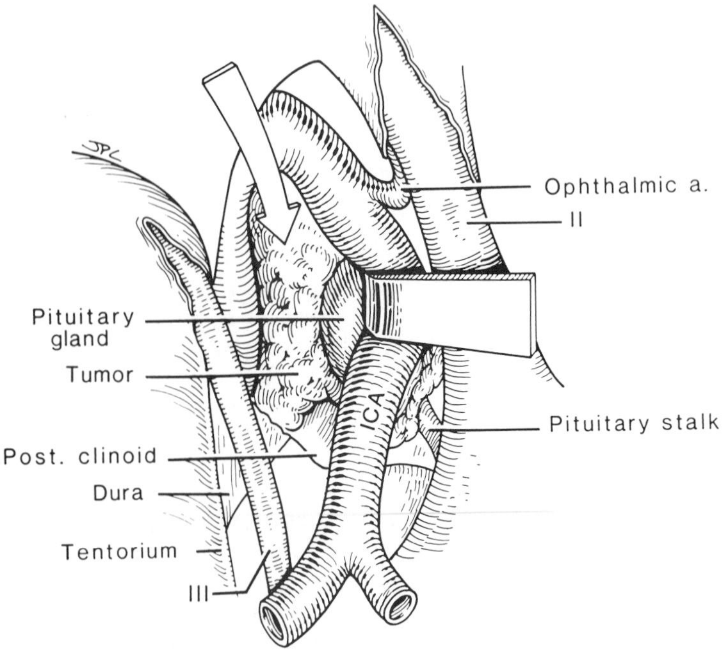

Figure 165-7 The distal dural ring around the exit of the ICA from the clinoid space has been opened. The cavernous sinus has been opened by a superior approach to remove tumor. (From Sekhar et al.,[10] with permission.)

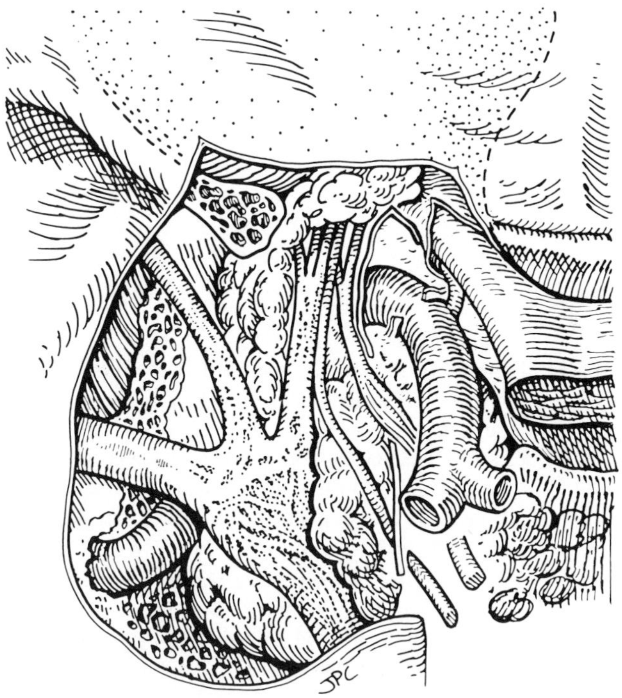

Figure 165-8 The lateral wall of the CS has been peeled away to expose CNs III, IV, and V, which are imbedded in the lateral wall. (From Sekhar et al.,[10] with permission.)

medial and inferior dural walls of the sella turcica are often invaded and should be removed, which often allows inspection of the contralateral CS. Upper clival dura should also be resected in these cases. All resections of intracavernous meningiomas should also include transcavernous intradural rongeuring and drilling of the petrous apex and dorsum sellae.

ICA Vein Graft Reconstruction

A cavernous ICA vein graft bypass is considered in patients in whom the vessel is encased by the tumor, with or without vascular narrowing.[11,13] Younger patients and those who may have contralateral tumor growth, aneurysm, or occlusive disease are also candidates for a bypass. Patients who are determined preoperatively to be at a high risk for stroke after ICA occlusion are not candidates for such a direct ICA-to-ICA bypass, and subtotal resection is a better option. If ICA resection is considered mandatory in such patients, a vein graft bypass from the external carotid artery (ECA) to the M_2 segment of the MCA can be performed with subsequent gradual ICA occlusion.

Whenever ICA reconstruction is planned, the proximal saphenous vein (8 to 10 cm) is exposed at the beginning of the procedure and is harvested just before actual reconstruction. Methylprednisolone sodium succinate (1 g) is administered systemically prior to vein harvesting, and the patient is mildly heparinized (1500 to 2000 U) during the grafting procedure. Measures to protect the brain (hypothermia, induced hypertension, and barbiturate or etomidate coma) are instituted before blood flow is interrupted. For short vein graft bypasses, first the distal anastomosis (end-to-end or end-to-side) is performed with 8-0 nylon suture (proximal to the posterior communicating artery), and then the proximal anastomosis to the petrous ICA (end-to-end) is performed using interrupted stitches with 7-0 or 8-0 monofilament suture. Twisting or tension on the graft is avoided, to allow for its retraction during tumor removal. A long vein graft from the cervical ICA or ECA to the M2 segment of the MCA is also an option for bypass. In these cases, cerebral ischemia can be limited to 45 min, that is, only the time of the MCA occlusion.

In all cases of vein graft bypass, intraoperative angiography should be done so that any vessel occlusion will be recognized and immediately corrected. At present, the senior author prefers the long vein graft over the short one, not only because it reduces the duration of ischemia but also because it makes it possible to avoid sectioning of the greater superficial petrosal nerve and the resulting "dry eye."

Cranial Nerve Reconstruction

Primary repair or grafting of cranial nerves should be undertaken for injured nerves, since good results can be expected.[2,5] The function of CN III recovered partially in two patients after primary reapproximation, and in one of two patients after nerve grafting.

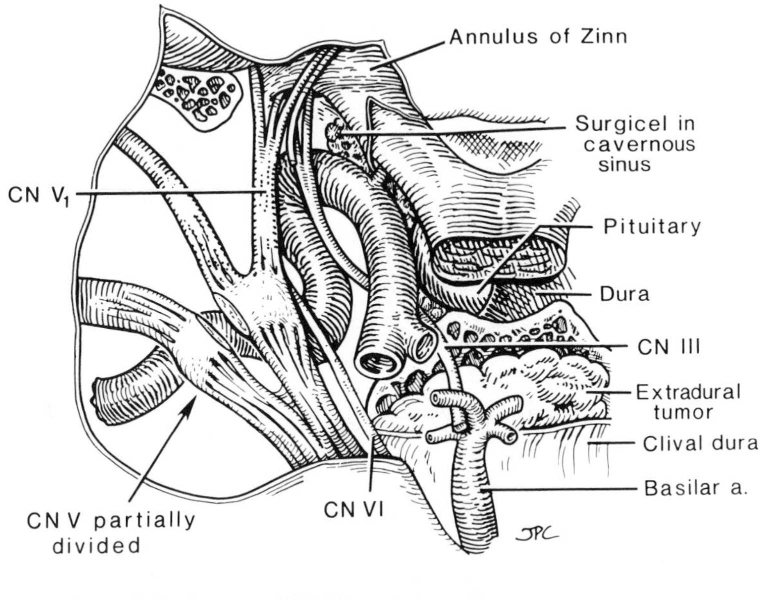

Figure 165-9 Tumor has been removed from inside the CS, with preservation of the ICA and CN VI. The trigeminal nerve and ganglion have been split between V_2 and V_3 to gain access medial to them. (From Sekhar et al.,[10] with permission.)

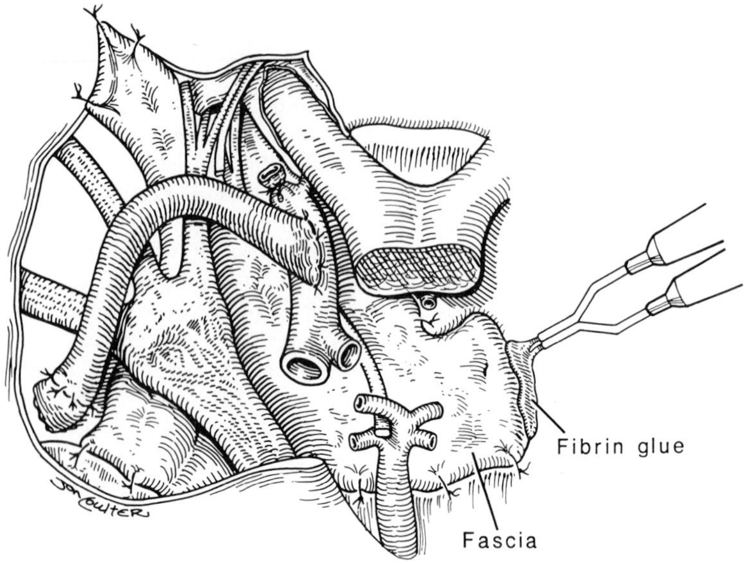

Figure 165-10 The cavernous ICA could not be preserved in this patient and had to be resected with the tumor. A petrous-to-supraclinoid-ICA vein graft bypass was created. Tumor involving the sphenoid bone was removed, and the sphenoid sinus was closed with fat, fascia lata, and a pericranial flap. (From Sekhar et al.,[10] with permission.)

CN VI recovered function in five patients after it was reconstructed. CN IV is usually not reconstructed. Grafts can be obtained from the greater auricular or sural nerve.

Closure

To prevent CSF leakage, opened air sinuses must be adequately stripped of mucosa, lined with a pedicled pericranial flap, and packed with autologous fat, and the dura must be reconstructed over them as well as possible with a free fascia lata or pericranial graft sutured circumferentially and held with fibrin glue. Large defects of the infratemporal fossa and sphenoid sinus are filled with bulkier vascularized tissue, such as temporalis muscle or a revascularized rectus abdominis muscle flap. The dura is closed completely using fat, pericranium, and/or fascia lata where primary closure is not possible. The orbitozygomatic bone piece is replaced and secured, and the remaining craniotomy closure is done in the usual fashion.

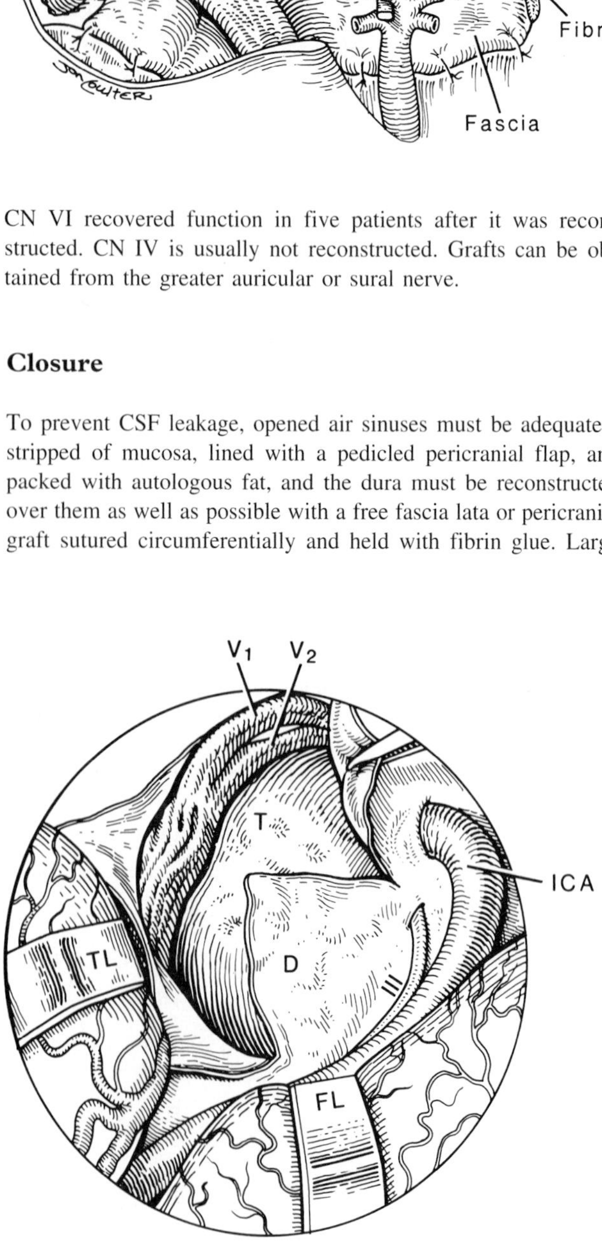

Figure 165-11 When the tumor is not a meningioma, as here, extensive dissection of the cranial nerves is usually not necessary, which results in a better functional outcome. Here, the dura is being peeled away over the most prominent aspect of the tumor, to gain entry between CNs IV and V_1 and/or between V_1 and V_2. (From Sekhar et al.,[10] with permission.)

Combined or Staged Procedures

Large petroclival meningiomas that extend into the CS require a separate staged procedure for complete resection. A subtemporal-transpetrosal (with partial labyrinthectomy), presigmoid approach is employed in these cases.[8] For tumors that involve the petroclival or sphenoid bone in the midline, such as chordomas and chondrosarcomas, the frontotemporal-orbitozygomatic approach is combined with the extended frontal approach.[7,12] The bicoronal scalp incision used in these cases also provides a long galeopericranial flap that is sufficient to cover the opened sphenoid sinus during closure.

In patients with extensive tumors that have air sinus involvement and in whom ICA reconstruction has been planned, staged procedures are recommended. First, the major intradural tumor is resected (without entering the CS or the air sinus) and a vein graft bypass of the ICA is performed. After a few weeks' healing, the resection of tumor from the sinuses is completed as a second stage. This approach minimizes the risk of infection and subsequent graft ''blow-out.''

Combined extended frontal and subtemporal-infratemporal approaches may be required for extensive clival chordomas and chondrosarcomas that extend into the CS, especially when the ICA is involved and the tumor extends lateral to it.

Postoperative Care

Usually, postoperative care involves observation in the intensive care unit for 2 days followed by another week's hospital stay. An especially careful watch is kept for CSF leakage in cases in which

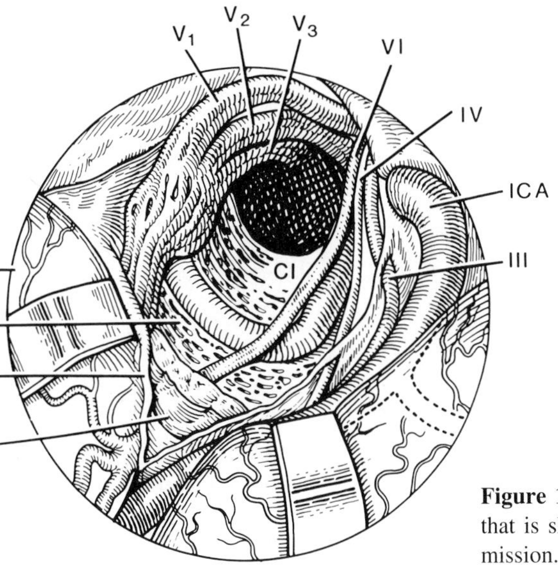

Figure 165-12 The removal of a tumor through the exposure that is shown in Fig. 165-11. (From Sekhar et al.,[10] with permission.)

an air sinus was entered or the eustachian tube violated. A leak is usually managed with lumbar drainage (50 ml per 8 hour shift) for 3 to 5 days, but if the leak persists, then open repair is performed. CT scans of the head are routinely obtained on the first postoperative day to observe for any contusion, hemorrhage, or edema. In patients with partial third nerve paralysis, an eye patch is applied and other corneal precautions instituted. An ophthalmologist should be consulted so that protracted ocular muscle palsies can be managed with botulinum toxin, eye muscle surgery, or other conventional measures. A dry eye should be treated with frequent application of a viscous lubricant; if the condition proves bothersome, punctal occlusion may be considered. All patients in whom the ICA was reconstructed or extensively manipulated should undergo an angiogram postoperatively. Owing to manipulation of the pituitary gland itself or to deprivation of its blood supply during CS surgery, pituitary dysfunction is to be expected in the immediate postoperative period. Routine electrolyte checks and an adequate record of urinary output are mandatory. Both diabetes insipidus and the syndrome of inappropriate secretion of antidiuretic hormone (SIADH) are common but usually transient. Before discontinuing steroid coverage postoperatively, an adequate endocrine evaluation should be done.

Clinical Series

Between 1983 and 1993, 252 patients with cavernous sinus tumors underwent surgery, and in 228 of them an attempt was made to resect tumor from the cavernous sinus. The operations were performed by the senior author (LNS), in collaboration with Dr. Donald Wright and Dr. Chandranath Sen, at the University of Pittsburgh. Of these lesions, 159 were benign and 69 were malignant (Tables 165-2 and 165-3). Most of the benign tumors were meningiomas (114 patients), while chordomas and chondrosarcomas (both considered slow-growing malignancies) were the most frequent malignant tumors that were treated with CS surgery.

The results of CS surgery and its complications are presented separately for malignant and benign tumors, owing to the obviously dissimilar oncologic goals and neural conservation principles applied to these lesions at the time of surgery. For the same reasons, chordomas, chondrosarcomas, and adenoid cystic carcinomas should be considered separately, since they are slow-growing in comparison to the other malignancies (e.g., squamous cell carcinoma).

TABLE 165-2 Benign Cavernous Sinus Tumors Operated upon from 1983 to 1993 (n = 159): Degrees of Resection and Recurrence or Regrowth in All Areas*

	Total Resection		Partial Resection	
Tumor	**No. (%)**	**No. with Recurrence (%)**	**No.**	**No. with Regrowth**
Meningioma (n = 114)	83 (73)	4 (5)	31	6
Others (n = 45)	34 (76)	1 (3)	11	4
Subtotals (n = 159)	117 (74)	5 (3)	42	10

*Unpublished data

TABLE 165-3 Malignant Cavernous Sinus Tumors Operated upon from 1983 to 1993 (n = 69): Degrees of Resection, Recurrence, and Regrowth

Tumor	**Total**	**Total Resections (Recurrence)**	**Partial Resections (Regrowth)**
Slow-growing			
Chordoma	24	13 (2)	11 (7)
Chondrosarcoma	13	7 (−)	6 (−)
Adenoid cystic carcinoma	11	4 (2)	7 (2)
Others	3	2 (1)	1 (1)
Subtotals	51	26 (5)	25 (10)
Fast-growing			
Squamous cell carcinoma	5	2 (2)	3 (2)
Malignant meningioma	4	2 (1)	2 (1)
Others	9	5 (1)	4 (1)
Subtotals	18	9 (4)	9 (4)

Results

Not only are malignant tumors less often completely resected than benign tumors, but as expected, their rates of recurrence and regrowth are higher (Table 165-3). Among the malignant group, fast-growing tumors recurred more often than slow-growing ones. Also, in the malignant group, residual tumor was often left outside the CS.

Complete resection was more often achieved with benign tumors (74 percent) (Table 165-2). All four patients with a hemangioma had total resection with no recurrence (at a follow-up ranging from 1 to 4.5 years). Neurilemomas were the next most resectable tumor (87 percent with total resection), followed by meningiomas (73 percent). Tumors that were extensive or had scar formation related to prior operations and/or irradiation were least likely to be resected totally. Of the 42 patients with benign tumors that were not totally resected, 37 had extensive tumors and/or prior irradiation or surgery. Of the remaining five patients, four were not candidates for vein graft reconstruction and had meningiomas that encased the cavernous ICA. The remaining patient had an epidermoid cyst, and remnants of cyst wall were left adhering to the brain stem. Of the patients who underwent total resection of benign CS tumors, 3 percent (5 of 117) had recurrence. In one of these patients, the tumor was an angiofibroma and recurred far from the CS. Four patients had meningiomas that recurred adjacent to either the CS or the resection site. Tables 165-4 and 165-5 relate the size (extent) and CS grade of the benign tumors with the degree of resection achieved. Tumors that were confined or of grade I or II had higher complete resection rates, although the grade IV tumors in this series also had a relatively high total resection rate. The latter statistic is due to the fact that vein graft reconstruction of the cavernous ICA has allowed for more complete resection of high-grade tumors since 1987.[11] In 18 patients with benign CS tumors, a bypass was performed to make it possible to resect the encased cavernous ICA and achieve total tumor resection.

Complications

Tables 165-6 and 165-7 show the complications that were encountered in the series. None of the patients died intraoperatively. One patient in the benign group who had undergone near-total resection of an extensive meningioma died from pulmonary embolism one day after discharge. Two patients died in the immediate postoperative period (less than one month after surgery): One, who had had a recurrent malignant meningioma and whose treatment included a vein graft bypass of the ICA, died of a massive stroke from ICA dissection and occlusion; the other died from progresison of an extensive carcinoma. Two patients who had undergone resection of a meningioma died 11 and 33 months postoperatively, both in a vegetative state after suffering fulminant meningitis; one of them also had an intracerebral hematoma.

Six patients with benign CS tumors developed cerebral infarctions after tumor resection. In three of these patients, the infarction was due either to ICA injury or to vein graft occlusion, and in one of them the eventual outcome was severe disability (Karnofsky score of 40). One patient, who was already disabled preoperatively, had a small infarction but experienced no significant change in her condition. The remaining three patients had strokes unrelated to cavernous ICA manipulation, two owing to injury to vessels during dissection of scar, and one from vasospasm. Two of these patients fortunately recovered to a level of fairly independent living, although they are not able to work, and one recovered to the point of self-care, but then died from a pulmonary embolism.

Cerebrospinal fluid leakage is the most common complication of this operation, especially in patients who have had previous surgery and/or radiation therapy or whose air sinuses were opened

TABLE 165-4 Cavernous Sinus Surgery (Benign Tumors): Relation of Tumor Size (Extent) to Degree of Resection and Recurrence or Regrowth

	Total Resection (from Ipsilateral Side)		Partial Resection	
Tumor Type	No. (%)	No. with Recurrence	No. (%)	No. with Regrowth
Confined (n = 48)	39 (81)	2	9 (19)	1
Extensive (n = 111)	78 (70)	3	33 (30)	9
Totals (n = 159)	117 (74)	5	42 (26)	10

TABLE 165-5 Cavernous Sinus Surgery (Benign Tumors): Relation of CS Grade to Degree of Resection and Recurrence or Regrowth

	Total Resection (from Ipsilateral Side)		Partial Resection	
CS Grade	No. (%)	No. with Recurrence	No.	No. with Regrowth
I (n = 22)	19 (86)	1	3	1
II (n = 35)	32 (91)	1	3	1
III (n = 38)	24 (63)	3	14	2
IV (n = 39)	30 (77)	0	9	3
V (n = 25)	12 (48)	0	13	3
Totals (n = 159)	117 (74)	5	42	10

TABLE 165-6 Cavernous Sinus Surgery for Benign Tumors (n = 159): Complications

Complication	No.
Cerebral infarction	6 (4%)
Cerebral edema	2
Hematoma	11 (1 evacuated) (7%)
CSF leaks from the:	27 (17%)
Sphenoid sinus	13 (11 required operation)
Incision	5 (4 required reclosure)
Eustachian tube	3 (2 required operation)
Ear canal	3 (2 required operation)
Frontal sinus	2 (1 required operation)
Maxillary sinus	1
Infections	
Meningitis—following CSF leak	7 (7%)
Meningitis—without CSF leak	5
Pneumonia	15
Pituitary dysfunction	
Diabetes insipidus	17 (1 permanent)
SIADH, transient	14
Pulmonary embolism	4
Outcome of complications	
Death	1 (0.7%)
Disablement (dependent)	8 (5%)
(Mild/moderate)	6
(Severe)	2

TABLE 165-7 Cavernous Sinus Surgery for Malignant Tumors (n = 69): Complications

Complication	No. with Slow-Growing Tumors	No. with Fast-Growing Tumors
Cerebral infarction	3	1
Cerebral edema	0	0
Hematoma	0	0
CSF leaks from the:		
Sphenoid sinus	3 (1 repaired)	1
Eustachian tube	5 (3 repaired)	0
Nose	2 (1 repaired)	0
Incision	1 (repaired)	0
Infections		
Meningitis—with CSF leak	7	0
Meningitis—no CSF leak	0	0
Pneumonia	5	1
Pituitary dysfunction		
Diabetes insipidus, transient	3	3
SIADH, transient	5	1
Pulmonary embolism	3	1
Outcome of complications		
Death	1	1
Disabled (dependent)	5	0

during surgery. Most of these patients had extensive tumors. CSF leakage was also slightly more frequent in patients who had resections of malignant tumors (26 percent) than benign tumors (17 percent). For persistent leakage, free flaps (vascularized) were used in two cases, although these may be too bulky to permit closure of the sinus.

Meningitis occurred in 12 patients, 7 of whom had a CSF leak. Intravenous antibiotics and prompt treatment of the leak usually sufficed. A poor outcome occurred in two patients mentioned earlier. Postoperative pituitary dysfunction was almost always transient. Diabetes insipidus and SIADH were almost equal in frequency (10 percent and 9 percent for benign tumors), and only one patient required permanent hormone replacement. Diabetes insipidus usually occurred in patients who had undergone dissection of tumor from the sella or resection of the ICA, probably owing to interruption of arterial supply to the pituitary gland or to direct injury of the gland.

Ophthalmoparesis, a common sequela of CS surgery, is often temporary if the nerves are well preserved. The functional outcome for the extraocular muscles is assessed using a grading scale for binocular vision (Table 165-8). Table 165-9 shows the preoperative and final follow-up results for binocular vision in the first 97 of the 159 patients who underwent CS surgery for benign tumors. These patients were followed for an average of 30 months. In only slightly over half of them (57 percent) does the grade of function stay the same or improve between these points. Surgeons should

TABLE 165-8 Grading System for Binocular Vision (Ocular Motility)

Excellent: Singular binocular vision in primary gaze and the reading position; extends 20 degrees in right, left, up, and down gaze.
Good: Singular binocular vision in primary gaze and the reading position, but diplopia out of these gaze positions. Partial ptosis.
Fair: Diplopia in primary gaze or reading position, but patient has singular binocular vision with a head posture.
Poor: Moderate to severe ptosis. Nearly total opthalmoparesis.
Not applicable: No useful vision in one eye.

TABLE 165-9 Preoperative and Postoperative (Follow-up ≥12 months) Binocular Vision in the First 97 Patients Operated on for Benign Intracavernous Tumors*

Preoperative Function	Excellent 47	Good 24	Fair 5	Poor 12	N/A 9
Postoperative Function in Corresponding Patients					
Excellent (n = 31)	24	5	0	1	1
Good (n = 25)	15	7	1	1	1
Fair (n = 11)	4	4	2	1	0
Poor (n = 16)	1	7	2	4	2
N/A (n = 14)	3	1	0	5	5

*Grading system as given in Table 165-8.

therefore avoid operating on patients whose tumors are benign and not changing in size radiographically and who are either assymptomatic or have nonprogressive symptoms.

Appropriate precautions should be taken to avoid neurotrophic keratitis in patients who have corneal anesthesia and/or reduced tearing postoperatively. Routine application of eye lubricants will suffice, although a temporary tarsorrhaphy is occasionally required. Frequent follow-up with an ophthalmologist is strongly advised, especially for patients who may require corrective surgery for permanent ophthalmoplegia.

The overall functional outcome in these patients is assessed using the Karnofsky performance score. For instance, of the first 97 patients with benign tumors in this series (all followed for more than a year), 90 (93 percent) were able to care for themselves, and 79 (81 percent) were working.

Follow-Up

Protracted follow-up MRI studies are often necessary to distinguish residual tumor from surgical changes. ICA vein grafts are followed by yearly MR angiograms. Focused radiation therapy is usually offered as adjuvant therapy for residual benign tumors that are either unresectable or were left intentionally. Stereotactic radiosurgery is the preferred modality of therapy in such cases. For small tumors that meet the size criteria for stereotactic radiosurgery, the primary modality of treatment is still often debated, although in such cases, histologic diagnosis should be sought before instituting any therapy. In addition, prior radiation therapy often makes resection more difficult and increases the risks of CSF leakage and infection. External beam radiation therapy is not recommended if it can be avoided.

References

1. Al-Mefty O, Smith RR. Surgery of tumors invading the cavernous sinus. *Surg Neurol* 1988; 30:370–381.

2. Grimson BS, Ross MJ, Tyson G. Return of function after intracranial suture of the trochlear nerve. *J Neurosurg* 1984; 61:191–192.
3. Hakuba A, Tanaka K, Suzuki T, Nishimura S. A combined orbitozygomatic infratemporal epidural and subdural approach for lesions involving the entire cavernous sinus. *J Neurosurg* 1989; 71:699–704.
4. Parkinson D. Surgical anatomy of the lateral sellar compartment (cavernous sinus). *Clin Neurosurg* 1990; 36:219–239.
5. Samii M. Reconstruction of the trigeminal nerve. In Samii M, Jannetta PJ (eds): *The Cranial Nerves.* New York: Springer-Verlag, 1981, pp 352–358.
6. Sekhar LN, Burgess J, Akin O. Anatomical study of the cavernous sinus emphasizing operative approaches and related vascular and neural reconstruction. *Neurosurgery* 1987; 21:806–816.
7. Sekhar LN, Janecka IP, Jones NF. Subtemporal-infratemporal and basal subfrontal approach to extensive cranial base tumours. *Acta Neurochir (Wien)* 1988; 92:83–92.
8. Sekhar LN, Javed T, Jannetta PJ. Petroclival meningiomas. In Sekhar LN, Janecka IP (eds): *Surgery of Cranial Base Tumors.* New York: Raven Press, 1993, pp 605–659.
9. Sekhar LN, Møller AR. Operative management of tumors involving the cavernous sinus. *J Neurosurg* 1986; 64:879–889.
10. Sekhar LN, Ross DA, Sen C. Cavernous sinus and sphenocavernous neoplasms. Anatomy and surgery. In Sekhar LN, Janecka IP (eds): *Surgery of Cranial Base Tumors.* New York: Raven Press, 1993, pp 521–604.
11. Sekhar LN, Sen CN, Jho HD. Saphenous vein graft bypass of the cavernous internal carotid artery. *J Neurosurg* 1990; 72:35–41.
12. Sekhar LN, Sen C, Snyderman CH, et al. Anterior, anterolateral, and lateral approaches to extradural petroclival tumors. In Sekhar LN, Janecka IP (eds): *Surgery of Cranial Base Tumors.* New York: Raven Press, 1993, pp 157–223.
13. Spetzler RF, Fukushima T, Martin N, Zabramski J. Petrous carotid-to-intradural carotid saphenous vein graft for intracavernous giant aneurysm, tumor, and occlusive cerebrovascular disease. *J Neurosurg* 1990; 73:496–501.

166

Approaches to Petroclival Tumors

Georges F. Haddad
Ossama Al-Mefty

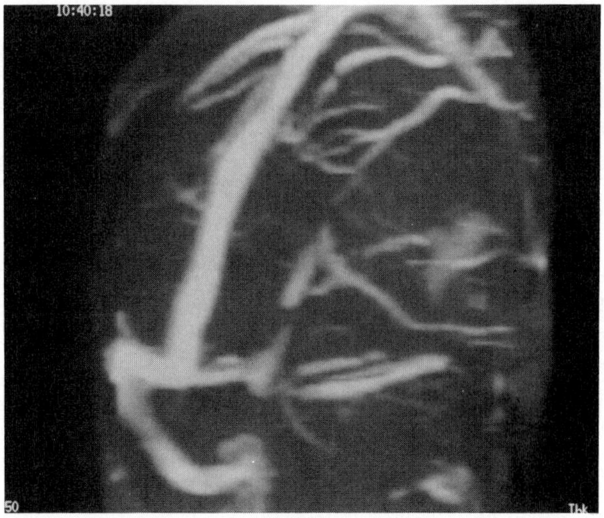

Figure 166-1 Magnetic resonance angiogram showing the cerebral venous system. The torcular Herophili is well visualized. The left sigmoid sinus is obliterated. This fact was confirmed by multiple MRA views (not shown).

Surgical access to the clivus and petrous apex remains a formidable challenge. Despite numerous approaches designed to reach lesions at this deep-seated and vital location, there are still many disappointments and shortcomings; the perfect approach has yet to be developed. Detailed preoperative radiologic studies are crucial for surgical planning. Computed tomography (CT) and magnetic resonance imaging (MRI) not only reveal the presence of a lesion in this area but also depict the exact location of the mass, its extension, and, frequently, its nature. Coronal and sagittal imaging enhances the information obtained by these studies. The authors still perform angiography to identify vascular lesions, depict tumor blood supply, demonstrate the location and displacement of cerebral arteries, and determine the anatomy and patency of the dural venous sinuses. However, magnetic resonance angiography (MRA) is rapidly replacing conventional angiography in this regard (Fig. 166-1).

Approach Selection

Approaches to the posterior cranial base can be grouped into three main categories: anterior extradural, conventional intradural, and lateral (Fig. 166-2). The various anterior extradural approaches are detailed in other chapters of this book. This chapter will briefly discuss approach selection for petroclival tumors and describe the approaches for intradural tumors.

The most fitting approach to a particular tumor depends on its location (intradural, extradural, or both), extension (upper, lower, or entire clivus), nature (benign, invasive, or malignant), and size.

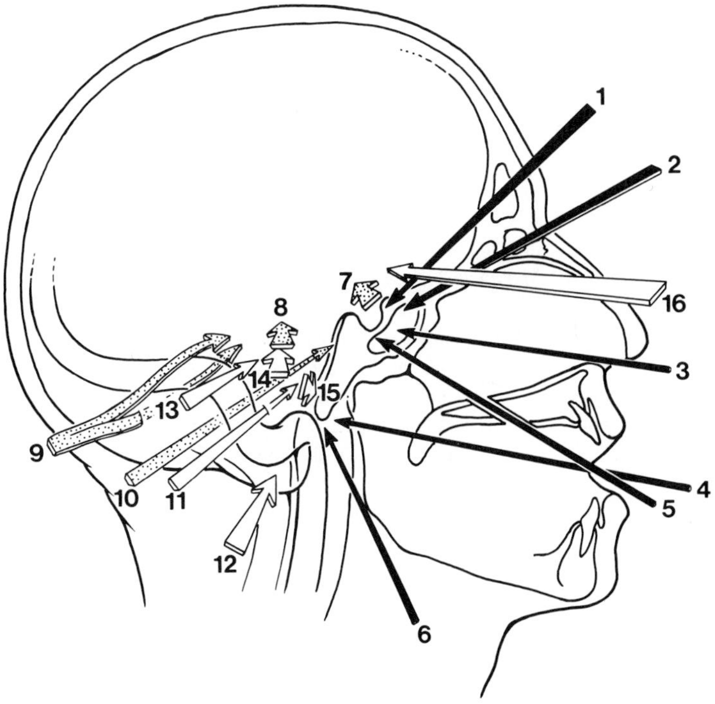

Figure 166-2 Approaches to the skull base: Anterior approaches (*black arrows*): 1, transbasal; 2, transethmoidal; 3, trans-sphenoidal; 4, transoral; 5, transmaxillary; 6, transcervical. Conventional approaches (*stippled arrows*): 7, pterional; 8, subtemporal; 9, combined subtemporal and suboccipital; 10, suboccipital. Skull base approaches (*white arrows*): 11, translabyrinthine-transcochlear; 12, transcondylar; 13, petrosal; 14, extended middle fossa; 15, infratemporal; 16, cranio-orbital zygomatic.

The transoral, transpalatal, and trans-sphenoidal approaches are used for midline extradural tumors.

Intradural tumors are divided into three categories involving three distinct areas. The first area comprises the dorsum sellae, the posterior wall of the sphenoid sinus, and the petrous apex down to a horizontal line joining the acoustic meati. The second area extends from the spheno-occipital synchondrosis to the level of the jugular foramina. The third area comprises the rest of the clivus down to the anterior rim of the foramen magnum. For tumors involving the first area, a cranio-orbital zygomatic or an extended middle fossa approach is preferable. Tumors in the midclival area are best handled through a petrosal or transtemporal approach, depending on the preoperative hearing status. The best approach to the lower clivus is a transcondylar approach (Table 166-1). Even though this conceptualization is helpful in choosing the surgical avenue, most tumors do involve more than one compartment and other structures such as the cavernous sinus and the internal acoustic meatus. Thus, choosing the best approach to petroclival meningiomas is, in fact, a matter of choosing the best compromise, keeping in mind that combined approaches and two-step operations are valid options. Large extra- and intradural tumors are reached through a combined infratemporal approach with a suboccipital craniectomy.

Anterior Extradural Approaches

Anterior extradural approaches include the transoral (with or without glossotomy and mandibulotomy), transpalatal, transcervical, trans-sphenoidal, transethmoidal, transmaxillary, and transbasal approaches. An anterior extradural approach allows direct exposure of a lesion situated ventral to the brain stem, and obviates brain retraction or resection; also, the access to the lesion is not blocked by neural structures. Major disadvantages of these approaches are as follows: (1) Septic sequelae may result from transgressing the contaminated oral and nasal pharynx (transcervical is an exception), (2) the surgeon must work at considerable depth, (3) the exposure is restricted to the midline (transmaxillary is an exception), (4) the lateral extension of a tumor cannot be visualized or dissected, (5) vascular control is not reliable, (6) obtaining a good dural repair is difficult, and (7) neurovascular structures in the posterior fossa are not visualized during the major portion of the dissection. Although these approaches have been used or suggested for intradural tumors, they are most suitable for extradural tumors.

Conventional Intradural Approaches

Several conventional and combined intradural approaches have been used to reach petroclival tumors. These include the frontotemporal, subtemporal transtentorial, occipital transtentorial, suboccipital, and combined subtemporal and suboccipital approaches.[4,6,13,16,17] The intradural approaches allow visualization of the neurovascular anatomy and its relation to the tumor. However, they have several disadvantages: (1) they require varying degrees of brain retraction, (2) the field is deep, (3) exposure of the ventrally located clival tumor is limited, (4) exposure of neural and vascular structures around the brain stem is inadequate, and (5) the surgeon must work between cranial nerves and vessels in the posterior fossa and at the tentorial hiatus.

TABLE 166-1 Approaches to Intradural Clival Tumors

Tumor Location	Additional Factors	Approach
Upper clivus	Involves cavernous sinus	Cranio-orbitozygomatic
	No involvement of cavernous sinus	Extended middle fossa approach
Mid-clivus	Hearing preserved	Petrosal
	No hearing	Transtemporal
Lower clivus		Transcondylar

The *frontotemporal* approach, as it is used for clival and petroclival meningiomas, has been elegantly described and illustrated by Yaşargil and colleagues.[17] Their results for these meningiomas are most impressive. Most neurosurgeons are familiar with the approach, the splitting of the sylvian fissure, and the clear exposure of the upper clivus. This approach is limited, however, to the upper clival area; dissection behind the dorsum sellae is carried out in an extremely narrow space between the carotid artery and the third nerve or the carotid artery and the optic nerve. In our practice, this approach is replaced by the cranio-orbital zygomatic approach described below.

The *subtemporal* approach has been used frequently to remove tumors in the petroclival area. Opening the tentorium allows the surgeon to reach a tumor extending caudally into the posterior fossa. The temporal lobe is retracted, and the tentorium is incised parallel to the petrous ridge, from the free edge of the tentorium to the lateral sinus. The approach may be anterior or posterior, according to the part of the temporal lobe to be elevated. The subtemporal approach has several advantages: (1) Surgeons are familiar with the anatomy; (2) the superior pole of the tumor is clearly exposed; (3) the third and fourth cranial nerves are directly visualized upon exposure of the tentorial hiatus; and (4) the fifth, seventh, and eighth cranial nerves, which are displaced superiorly or anteriorly, are visualized early. The major disadvantage is the need for temporal lobe retraction, which often results in temporal lobe swelling. This occurs more often with a posterior subtemporal than with the anterior approach and is particularly devastating on the dominant hemisphere. There is considerable difficulty in reaching and exposing the inferior pole of the tumor when the tumor has a deep extension. Since the upper cranial nerves (III, IV) are prominent in the field, their injury is a potential risk. In our practice, we have replaced this approach with the zygomatic-extended middle fossa approach described below.

The *suboccipital* approach is also a standard in neurosurgery that is more suitable for a tumor located in the cerebellopontine angle (CPA) than for those that extend to the petrous apex or upper clivus.[15,17] The exposure requires some cerebellar retraction. However, it provides access to the lower part of the clivus down to the foramen magnum. A larger tumor can be removed through this approach. The approach, which is posterior, provides poor access to a ventrally located lesion; a further hindrance is the requirement of working between the cranial nerves.

The *combined subtemporal and suboccipital* approach has also been used for many years to remove petroclival and tentorial tumors. In 1939, Bailey described an approach through a unilateral osteoplastic flap incorporating bone over the occipital lobe as well as over the posterior fossa.[3] The occipital lobe was retracted superiorly and the tentorium was split after ligation of the transverse sinus. After tumor removal the sinus ends were reunited. Bailey believed that a well-developed sinus on the contralateral side was a prerequisite for this operation. Several authors have used a modification of this approach. Malis extended the posterior fossa craniectomy with a lateral mastoidectomy.[13] He emphasized ligation of the transverse sinus with preservation of the vein of Labbé drainage through the opposite transverse sinus. This combined approach provides better exposure to clival and petroclival tumors that extend into the tentorial hiatus and the posterior fossa. However, excessive retraction of the temporal lobe and the cerebellum may still be required. Before the undertaking of this approach, radiologic confirmation of the patency of both sigmoid sinuses, and the connection of both through the torcular herophili, is mandatory. Although many authors have stated that the sigmoid sinus can be ligated safely, there have been reports of complications due to sinus ligation. Sacrifice of the sinus is not necessary.

Lateral Approaches

The lateral approaches evolved from the translabyrinthine approach. As early as 1904, Fraenkel and Hunt described an operation consisting of a wide suboccipital craniectomy with extension over the sigmoid sinus down to the point where the sinus enters the jugular bulb.[8] These authors believed that this was a more direct approach to the CPA and that the cerebellum incurred less pressure from retraction. In 1905, Borchardt reported a similar exposure.[5] He extended the bone removal over the lateral sinus and forward through the labyrinth, divided the sigmoid sinus, and exposed the CPA. House and colleagues refined and popularized a similar exposure and further modified it to include the cochlea,[11] whereas Fisch and Pillsbury have advocated the infratemporal approach, preserving the cochlea and the labyrinth with anterior transposition of the facial nerve.[7] Other modifications and combinations have been used by other authors.

A lateral approach shortens the distance to the clivus, provides excellent exposure of the middle and lower clivus with excellent visualization of the ipsilateral brain stem, and requires no brain retraction. Major septic spaces are not transgressed, and, with good closure and obliteration of the eustachian tube, the risk of cerebrospinal fluid (CSF) leakage is minimal. Disadvantages of a lateral approach are hearing loss, either conductive or total; temporary paralysis of the seventh nerve after its mobilization or anterior transposition; poor exposure of the contralateral surface of the brain stem; and the sacrifice of the sigmoid sinus. A lateral approach can be tailored to suit the size and location of the lesion. The extent of the exposure can vary from a limited retrolabyrinthine space to a wide transtemporal exposure. These approaches are suitable for tumors with extension on the lower half of the clivus, as well as for tumors that extend both intra- and extradurally (large jugular foramen neuromas and giant glomus jugulare tumors). A subtemporal approach may also be added, with or without violation of the labyrinth.[2,10,14]

Skull Base Approaches

Petroclival tumors can be reached from three main directions: anterior (cranio-orbital zygomatic approach), lateral (extended middle fossa, petrosal, and transtemporal approaches), and posterolateral (transcondylar approach) (Fig. 166-3).[1,2] Following are descriptions of the five approaches used for intradural tumors along the clivus.

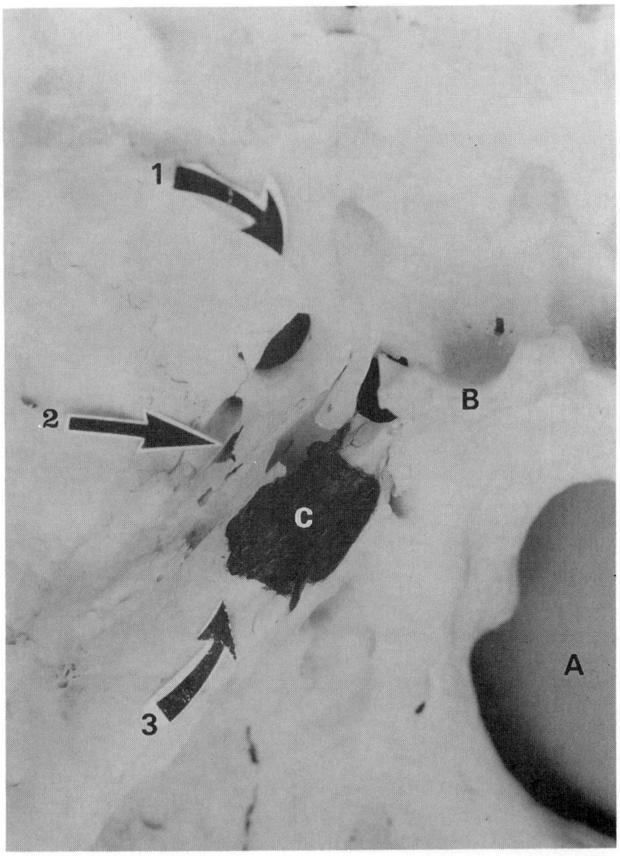

Figure 166-3 The petrous apex can be drilled through different approaches to allow access to the petroclival area: A, foramen magnum; B, dorsum sellae; C, petrous apex. 1, cranio-orbital zygomatic approach; 2, extended middle fossa approach; 3, petrosal approach.

Cranio-Orbital Zygomatic Approach

The cranio-orbital zygomatic approach is best suited for tumors of the interpeduncular fossa and upper clivus, especially if the tumor extends into the cavernous sinus and the parasellar area (Fig. 166-4*A*, *B*). For this approach the patient is placed supine, and the head rotated 30 to 40 degrees to the opposite side, dropped toward the floor and tilted 20 to 40 degrees. The axis of visualization is changed by turning the table from side to side.

A bicoronal incision is made behind the hairline, extending from the zygomatic arch on the side of the lesion to the superior temporal line on the opposite side. The scalp is incised, with care taken to preserve the superficial temporal artery. The plane of dissection, between the galea and the pericranium, is carried as far posteriorly as possible. The two layers of the temporalis fascia are cut along a line extending from the keyhole to the zygomatic root. The frontal branches of the facial nerve run within the space bounded by the two fascial layers anterior to the incision described above. The deep fascia is dissected from the muscle layer and reflected anteriorly with the skin, thus preserving the frontal branches of the facial nerve.

With the cautery, the pericranium is cut as far posteriorly as possible and along both superior temporal lines. The pericranium is dissected free from the skull; its intact base is dissected free

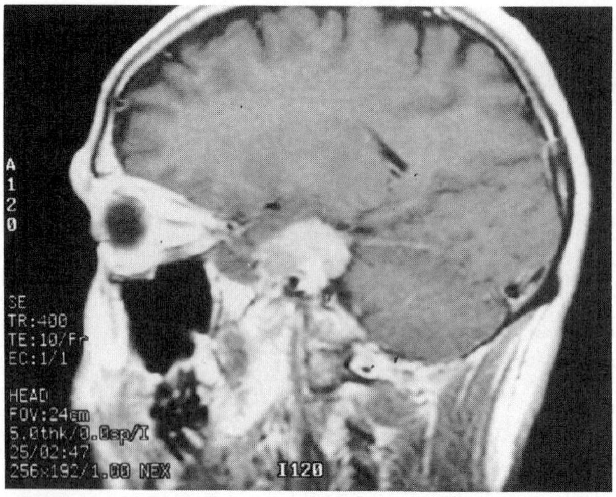

(*A*)

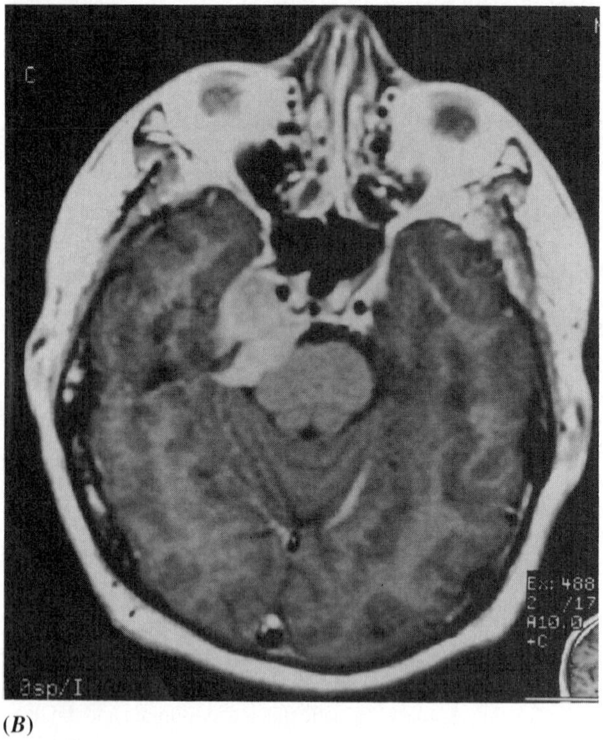

(*B*)

Figure 166-4 A preoperative T1-weighted MRI scan with gadolinium (*A*, sagittal view; *B*, axial view) of a patient with a tumor involving the right cavernous sinus and the right petroclival area. The cranio-orbital-zygomatic approach is best for this tumor.

from the roof and lateral wall of the orbit. This vascularized pericranial flap is crucial for repair of the floor of the frontal fossa and and to cover the frontal and ethmoid sinuses to avoid leakage of CSF. It may be necessary to use a high-speed air drill around the supraorbital notch to free the supraorbital nerve.

The periorbita is sharply dissected from the roof and lateral wall of the orbit, care being taken not to injure the periorbita. The zygomatic arch is dissected in subperiosteal fashion and is incised at its most anterior and posterior ends. The cuts are made obliquely so that the zygomatic arch can be anchored during reattachment. The temporalis muscle passes inferior to the zygoma and attaches to the coronoid process of the mandible, whereas the masseter muscle is attached to the underside of the zygoma. After sectioning, the zygoma is displaced downward with its masseter attachment. The temporalis muscle is detached from its insertion, then retracted posteriorly and inferiorly.

Three holes are placed initially. The first, MacCarty's keyhole, is made in the temporal fossa at the frontosphenoidal junction (Fig. 166-5). This keyhole lies at the level of the frontozygomatic point (the junction of the zygomatic process of both the frontal and zygomatic bones). The upper portion of MacCarty's keyhole opens into the frontal fossa, while its lower half opens into the orbit. The two halves of the burr hole are separated by the roof of the orbit. The second burr hole is drilled posteriorly at the level of the floor of the middle fossa. The third hole is placed in a frontal paramedian position above the nasion. To keep it as small as possible, this hole is made with a high-speed drill. In adults this hole will invariably pass through the anterior and posterior walls of the frontal sinus. If the dura is not dissected easily from the overlying bone, an extra burr hole can be placed.

The keyhole and temporal burr holes are connected with a craniotome. The bony cut should follow the floor of the middle fossa; the sphenoid ridge may have to be removed with a drill. The temporal and frontal holes are joined with a craniotome. This cut passes through the frontal bone about 4 cm above the superior orbital rim. With a fine-bit high-speed air drill, a groove is made from the frontal hole through the medial part of the superior orbital rim, preserving the trochlea. This groove must include both the anterior and posterior walls of the frontal sinus. The contents of the orbit are protected with a brain spatula while the lateral orbital rim is sectioned. This cut is carried to the keyhole. The orbital roof may be cut with a high-speed drill, a chisel, or a Gigli saw. The removed craniotomy flap thus includes the superior orbital rim and the upper half of the lateral orbital rim, the anterior portion of the orbital roof, and portions of the frontal and temporal bones. The air drill is used to remove a small bone flap from the roof of the orbit. In doing this, care should be taken not to enter the superior orbital fissure. Later this bone flap will be wired to the craniotomy flap. This reconstruction reduces the likelihood of both postoperative pulsating exophthalmos and enophthalmos. If necessary, the superior orbital fissure is exposed and anterior clinoid process is removed under the microscope.

The dura is opened in a crescent and tented. The sylvian fissure is split. The temporal lobe is mobilized outward and upward, and the frontal and temporal lobes supported with malleable retractors. The cavernous sinus and parasellar areas are reached readily through this approach. The interpeduncular fossa is reached by splitting Liliequist's membrane, which runs upward from the dorsum sellae and posterior clinoid processes toward the mammillary bodies of the hypothalamus. This membrane spreads between both oculomotor nerves and separates the inferior part of the carotid and chiasmatic cisterns from the superior part of the interpeduncular cistern. Tumor dissection can be performed in the space between the carotid artery and the optic nerve, as well as lateral to the carotid artery between the artery and the oculomotor nerve (Fig. 166-6). Wide splitting of the sylvian fissure allows exposure along the incisura, making the third nerve the center of the exposure. The prominent posterior clinoid process is drilled away with a fine diamond bit. Further exposure can be obtained by incising the tentorium posterior to the entry of the fourth nerve.

The preoperative angiogram should be studied carefully to determine the adequacy of the anastomotic blood flow in the circle of

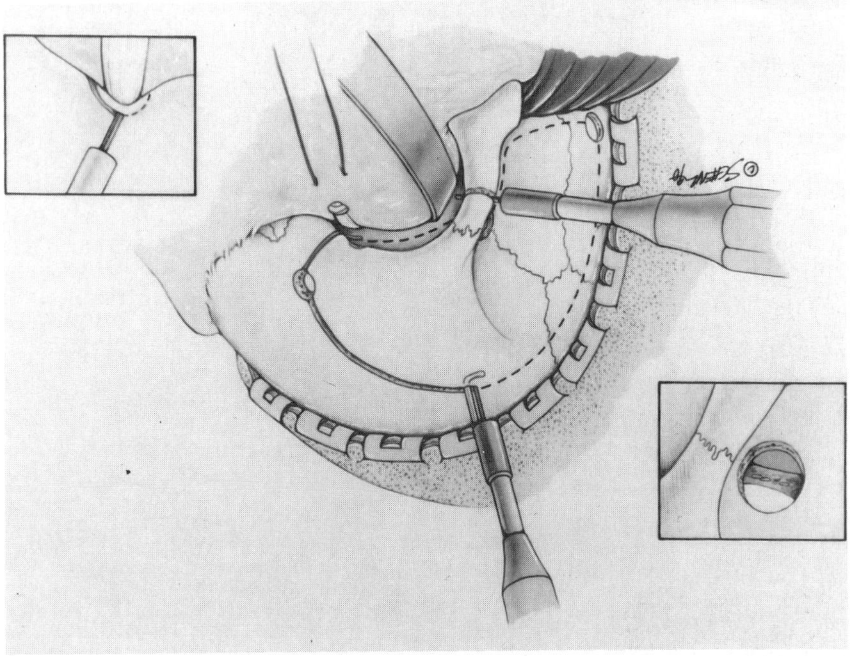

Figure 166-5 Cranio-orbital-zygomatic craniotomy. The orbital contents are gently retracted with a malleable retractor. The *insets* show the freeing of the supraorbital nerve and the placement of MacCarty's keyhole at the level of the fronto-zygomatic suture.

Willis. The presence of any large, dominant superficial middle cerebral vein emptying into the sphenoparietal sinus should be noted. The surgeon may be unable to sacrifice such a vein safely; this restriction prevents wide splitting of the sylvian fissure and greatly limits surgical access to the interpeduncular fossa. Temporary clipping of the sylvian vein is recommended before sacrifice. The temporal lobe should be observed for any signs of ischemia, and the evoked potentials should be monitored closely during temporary clipping.

Zygomatic Extended Middle Fossa Approach

If the tumor involves the upper clivus only or extends into Meckel's cave, a zygomatic extended middle fossa approach is chosen (Fig. 166-7*A*, *B*). The patient is supine with a roll placed under the ipsilateral shoulder, and the head is rotated to keep the zygoma near horizontal. A preauricular curvilinear incision is made. The zygoma is sectioned as described above. The coronoid process is cut and reflected superiorly along with the temporalis muscle. A limited craniotomy abutting the floor of the middle fossa is performed, and the temporal lobe and dura are supported with a malleable retractor (Fig. 166-8). The first landmark to be encountered is the middle meningeal artery leading to the foramen spinosum. This artery is coagulated and cut. The foramen ovale and the greater superficial petrosal nerve (GSPN) running in the sphenopetrosal groove are then identified. The lesser superficial petrosal nerve (LSPN) may be seen lateral to the GSPN. The GSPN is sharply divided to avoid traction injury to the facial nerve. The petrous carotid runs in the carotid canal deep to the GSPN. The petrous apex is then drilled to allow easy access to the posterior fossa. The drilled area will be limited by the following structures: trigeminal ganglion anteriorly, carotid canal laterally, and internal auditory canal and cochlea posteriorly. Whereas the petrous apex is easy to drill, the cochlea is encased in hard, compact bone. The change in bone texture will alert the surgeon to stop drilling (Fig. 166-9). The temporal dura is then opened, and the superior petrosal sinus coagulated and transected. The tentorium is divided up to the tentorial hiatus. Care must be taken to visualize the trochlear nerve and cut the tentorium behind the point where the nerve pierces it. The space provided by drilling the petrous apex (about 1 × 2 cm) allows the surgeon a better avenue to the upper clivus.[12]

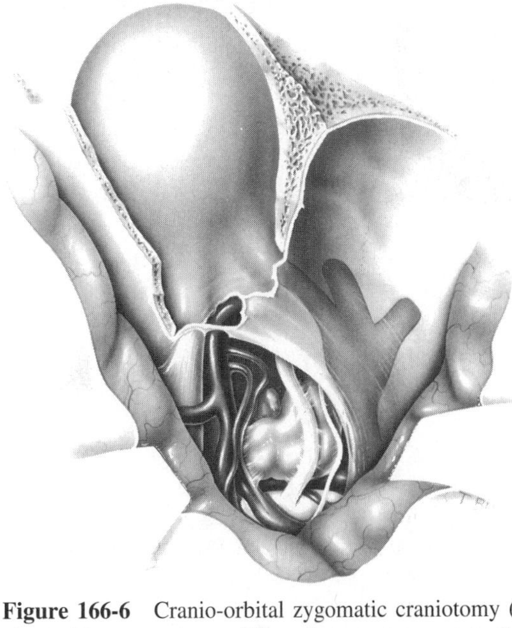

Figure 166-6 Cranio-orbital zygomatic craniotomy (surgeon's view). The tumor is straddling the superior aspect of the clivus. The frontal and temporal lobes are gently supported with malleable retractors. The third and fourth cranial nerves are splayed by the tumor. The trigeminal nerve and the contents of the cavernous sinus are shadowed.

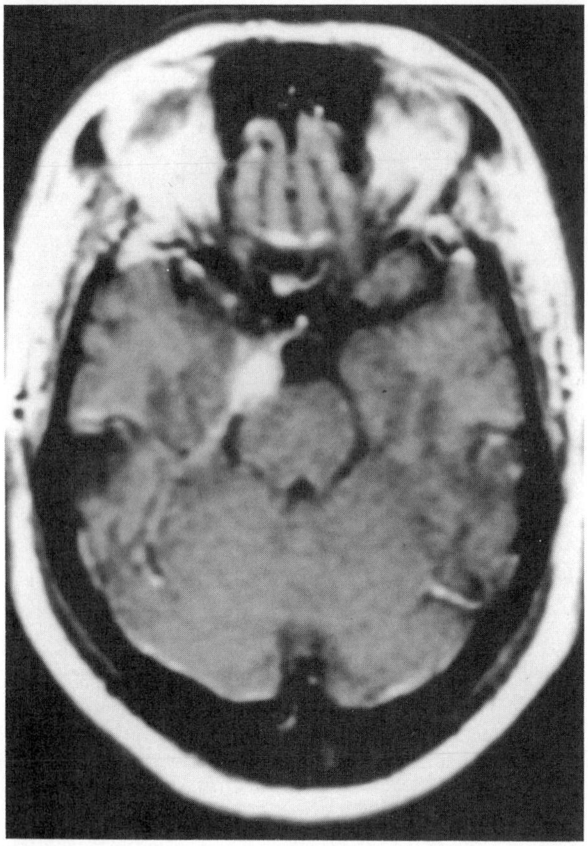

(A)

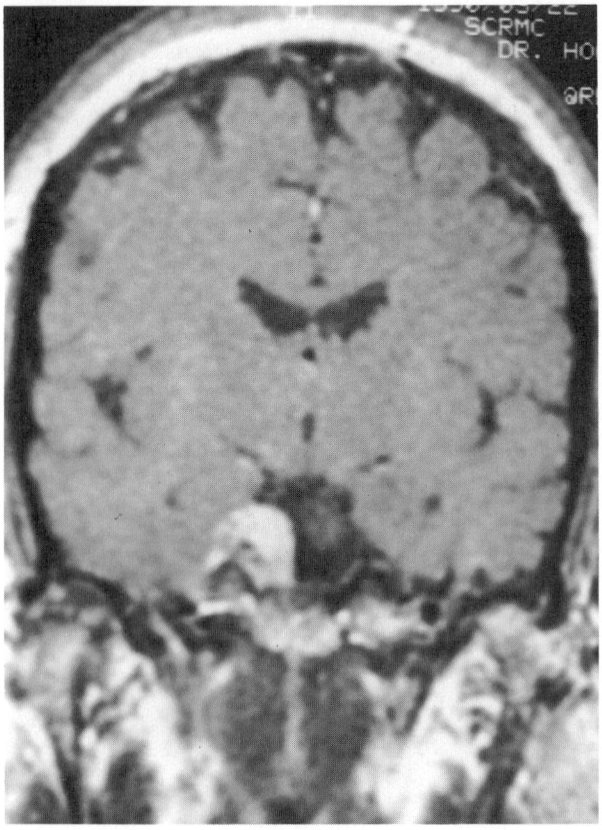

(B)

Figure 166-7 Preoperative T1-weighted MRI scan with gadolinium (*A*, axial view; *B*, coronal view) of a patient with a tumor involving the right petroclival area. The tumor does not involve the cavernous sinus. The extended middle fossa approach is best suited for this tumor.

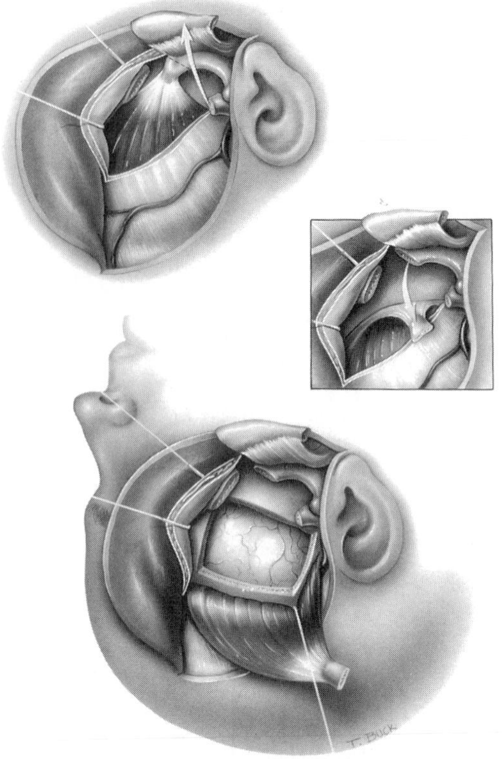

Figure 166-8 Extended middle fossa approach. The temporalis fascia is retracted anteriorly with the skin flap. The zygoma is resected. The coronoid process is sectioned and the temporalis muscle elevated. A middle fossa craniotomy then is performed. (From Haddad GF, Al-Mefty O. The road less traveled: transtemporal access to the CPA. *Clin Neurosurg* 1994; 41:150–167, with permission.)

Petrosal Approach

The petrosal approach is chosen for petroclival tumors involving the middle third of the clivus (Figs. 166-10*A*, *B* and 166-11*A*, *B*). This approach is best suited to patients with intact hearing on the side of surgery. This approach is centered on the petrous bone, creating several advantages: (1) The cerebellar and temporal lobes are retracted minimally; (2) the operative distance to the clivus is shortened by 3 cm as compared to a standard subtemporal approach; (3) the surgeon has a direct line of sight to the lesion and the anterior and lateral aspects of the brain stem; (4) the neural and otologic structures, including the cochlea, labyrinth, and facial nerve, are preserved; (5) the transverse and sigmoid sinuses, as well as the vein of Labbé and the basal veins, are preserved; (6) the tumor's vascular supply is interrupted early in the procedure; and (7) multiple axes for dissection are provided.

For this approach, the patient is placed supine with the ipsilateral shoulder slightly elevated. The head is turned away from the side of the tumor, inclined toward the floor, and tilted toward the opposite side, making the petrous base the highest point of the operative field. The head is fixed in a three-point Mayfield headrest. During the operation, the surgeon's line of sight can be altered by rotating the table from side to side or up and down.

A reverse question-mark incision is made, starting at the zygoma in front of the ear, circling above the ear, and descending 1 cm behind the mastoid process. The skin flap is elevated and retracted anteriorly and inferiorly. Care is taken not to injure the temporalis fascia. This fascia is cut anteriorly and superiorly and dissected from the underlying muscle. The fascia is kept in continuity with the periosteum and the fascia of the sternocleidomastoid muscle. After the insertion of the sternocleidomastoid is detached, the temporalis fascia, periosteum, and sternomastoid muscle and

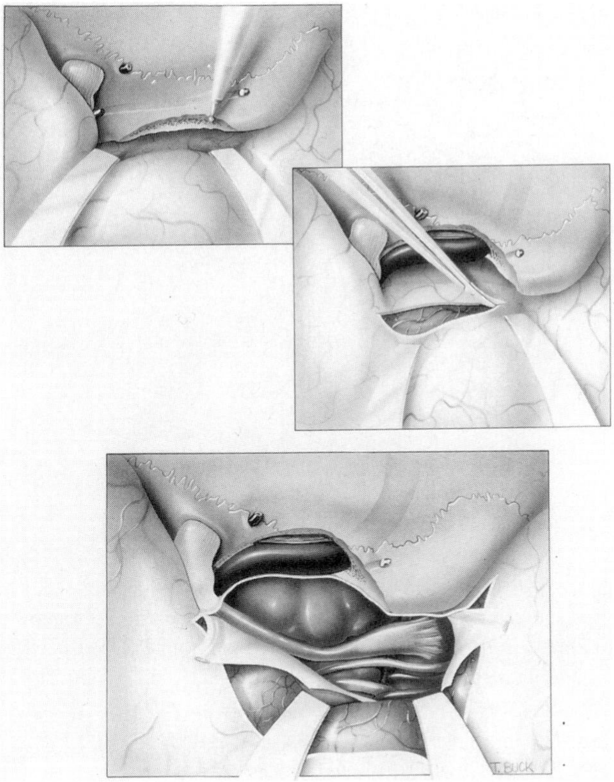

Figure 166-9 Extended middle fossa approach. The temporal lobe is gently supported by self-retaining retractors. The middle meningeal artery has been coagulated and cut. The greater superficial petrosal nerve has been cut. The carotid canal is drilled with a diamond burr. The dura is opened parallel to the petrous ridge, and the tentorium incised. The tumor is identified stretching the trigeminal nerve. The occulomotor and trochlear nerves are identified. The basilar artery and its terminal branches are also seen. (From Haddad GF, Al-Mefty O. The road less traveled: transtemporal access to the CPA. *Clin Neurosurg* 1994; 41:150–167, with permission.)

fascia are reflected as one unit inferiorly and posteriorly. The temporalis muscle then is detached from its insertion, using the cautery. The muscle is reflected anteriorly. The bony surface of the temporal fossa, the mastoid, and the lateral posterior fossa are thus exposed.

Four burr holes are made, two on each side of the transverse sinus (Fig. 166-12). A hole made just medial and inferior to the asterion opens into the posterior fossa below the transverse-sigmoid sinus junction, whereas a hole located at the squamal and mastoid junction of the temporal bone, along the projection of the superior temporal line, opens into the supratentorial compartment. The burr hole at each of these points will flank the sigmoid sinus. The other two burr holes are placed slightly more medial than the first two and closer together, flanking the transverse sinus. The temporal bone and a portion of the parietal bone above the tentorium, as well as the occipital bone below the tentorium, are incised between burr holes with the foot attachment of the Midas Rex drill (Midas Rex Pneumatic Tools, Inc, Fort Worth, TX). The foot attachment is not used to cross over the sinus. The burr holes flanking the transverse sinus are then connected using a thin rongeur or the Midas Rex drill. Special care should be taken to avoid tearing the wall of the venous sinus. The bone may be very adherent to the dura where the sigmoid and transverse sinuses meet. The craniotomy flap is then elevated.

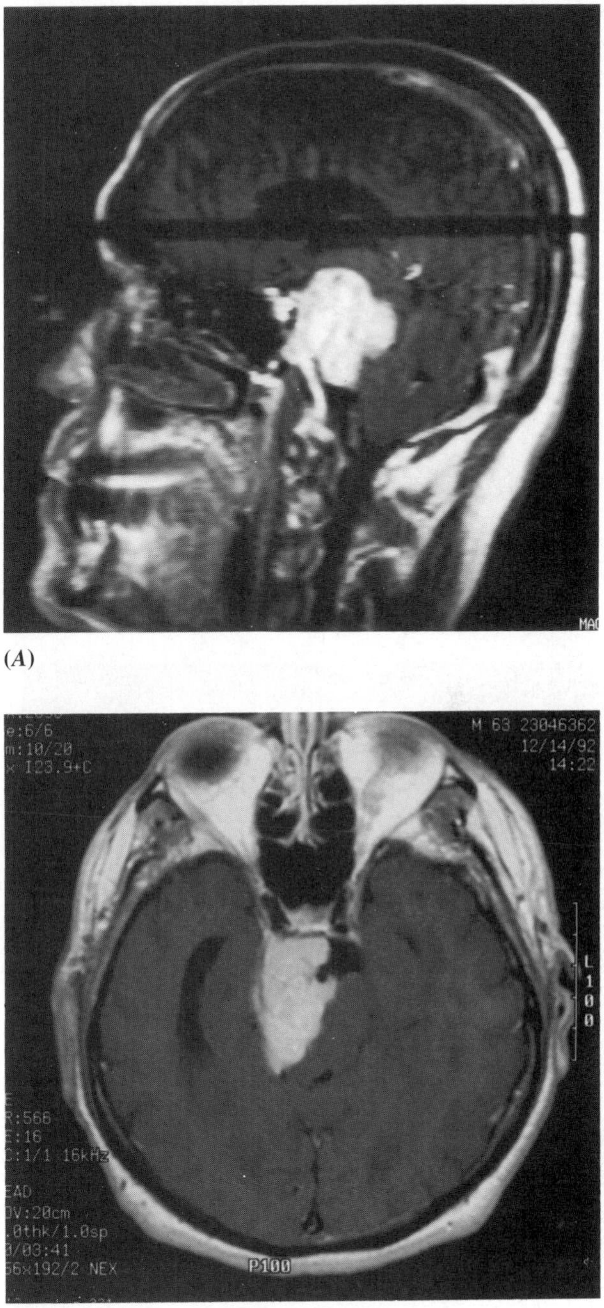

(*A*)

(*B*)

Figure 166-10 Preoperative T1-weighted MRI scan with gadolinium (*A*, sagittal view; *B*, axial view) of a patient with a meningioma involving the middle part of the clivus. The tumor was operated upon through a petrosal approach.

Drilling of the temporal bone requires a thorough knowledge of the anatomy of the petrous bone and surrounding structures. The orifice of the external acoustic meatus lies below the posterior root of the zygomatic arch. Along the superior wall of the external acoustic meatus is the suprameatal spine. Above this spine lies the temporal line, which extends posteriorly from the zygomatic root. The area between these two lines is the suprameatal triangle, which is used as a guide in locating the mastoid antrum 1.5 cm medially within the bone. The facial (fallopian) canal and the inner ear structures, including the semicircular canals, lie deep and anterior to the antrum. The first level of mastoidectomy can be

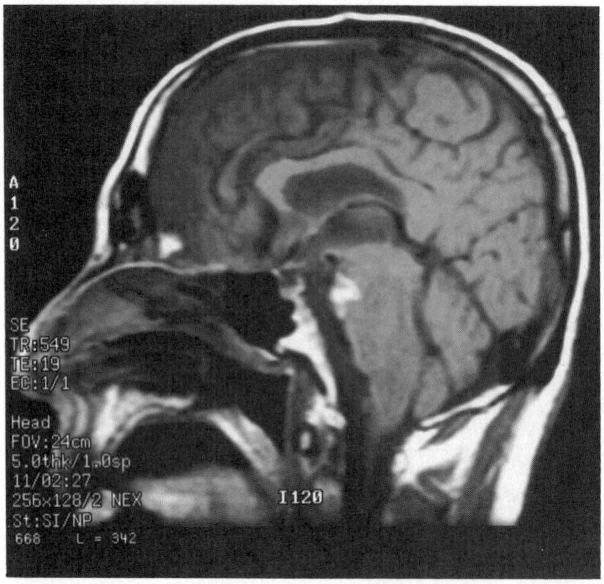

(*A*)

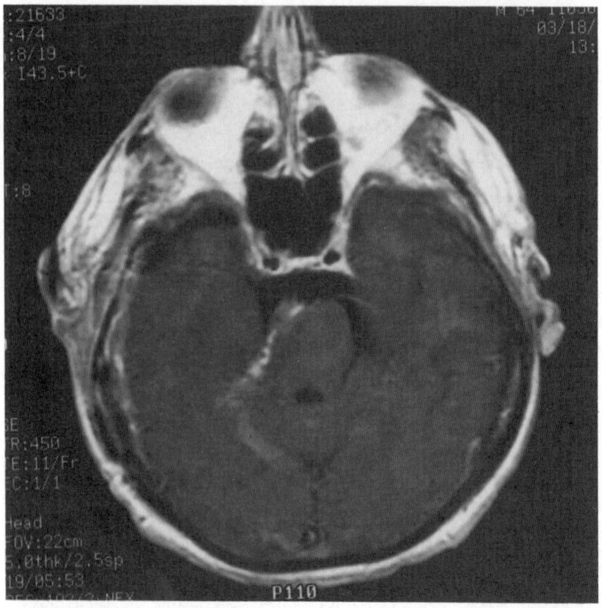

(*B*)

Figure 166-11 Postoperative films of the patient depicted in Figure 166-10 (same MRI sequences, similar cuts). Total tumor resection has been achieved. The hyperintense area seen on the sagittal film represents absorbable gelatin sponge.

performed quickly with a cutting drill. The mastoid cortex overlying the antrum is first drilled. Once the antrum is identified, the drilling is confined in a posterior direction. At this stage, the two structures that must be preserved are the sigmoid sinus posteriorly and the facial nerve inferiorly as it emerges from the stylomastoid foramen, medial to the digastric notch. The rest of the mastoidectomy is performed with a diamond drill under the microscope.

The solid angle is identified just medial to the antrum. It is characterized by a noticeable increase in bone density and houses the three semicircular canals. The facial canal is exposed and identified just below this solid angle. The sigmoid sinus is skeletonized

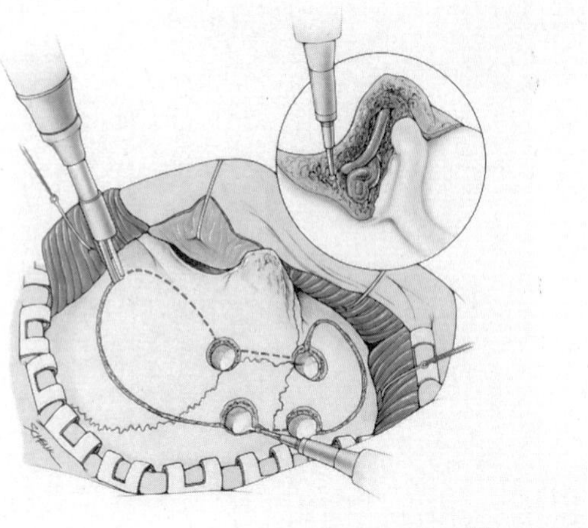

Figure 166-12 Petrosal approach. Placement of the four burr holes and craniotomy. *Insert* shows details of mastoidectomy. [Modified from Al-Mefty O, Schenk MP, Smith RR. Petroclival meningiomas. In Rengachary SS, Wilkins RH (eds): *Neurosurgical Operative Atlas*, vol 1. Park Ridge, IL: American Association of Neurological Surgeons, 1991, pp 339–350, with permission.]

down to the jugular bulb. Opened air cells are obliterated with bone wax.

The posterior fossa dura anterior to the sigmoid sinus is opened along the anterior margin of the sinus. The incision is then extended upward toward a supratentorial dural incision made along the floor of the middle fossa. The sinodural (Citelli's) angle, which identifies the position of the superior petrosal sinus, is thus exposed. The vein of Labbé is preserved. The superior petrosal sinus is clipped or coagulated and transected; the incision is continued on the tentorium, parallel to the pyramid, and extended through the incisura. During this maneuver the surgeon should preserve the trochlear nerve by keeping the incision through the tentorial notch behind the area where the fourth nerve enters the tentorial dural fold. By opening the tentorium one gains excellent exposure of the upper pole of the tumor and the anterior and lateral aspects of the brain stem. A retractor is placed to support the temporal lobe with the posterior part of the tentorium; another retractor holds medially the sigmoid sinus and the cerebellum (Fig. 166-13).

When the lesion is large and extends significantly into both supra- and infratentorial compartments, the dura of the posterior fossa is opened along both sides of the sigmoid sinus. The sigmoid sinus need not be transected; exposure may be obtained by alternating the visualized field above and below the tentorium.

Further relaxation is obtained by opening the arachnoid of the cerebellopontine cistern and draining CSF. The tumor is devascularized by coagulating its insertion on the pyramid and its meningeal feeders over the tentorium. When the tumor is small or moderate in size, the seventh and eighth cranial nerves usually are stretched posteriorly and thus are easily identified. When the tumor reaches a large size, however, it may well engulf these nerves. A suitable area on the tumor is selected, and the arachnoid over the tumor is opened. The tumor then is debulked—with extreme caution, because the seventh and eighth nerves, as well as

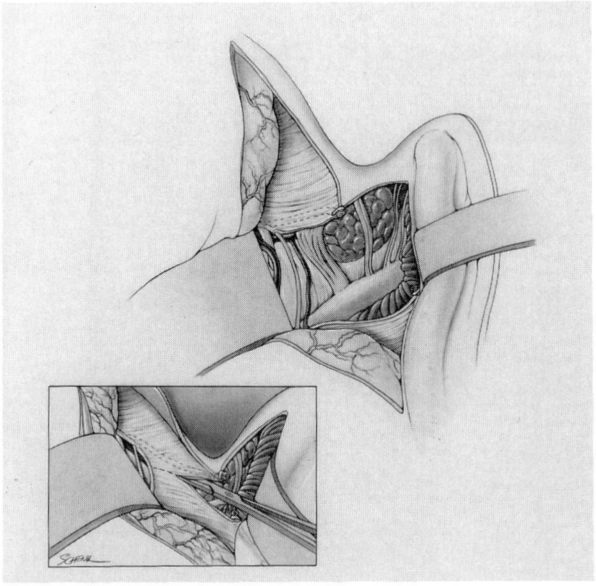

Figure 166-13 Petrosal approach. The dura is opened along the floor of the middle fossa and the anterior border of the sigmoid sinus. The superior petrosal sinus is clipped and cut. The tentorium is opened behind the entry point of the trochlear nerve. The tumor splays the fifth, seventh, eighth, ninth, and tenth cranial nerves. [Modified from Al-Mefty O, Schenk MP, Smith RR. Petroclival meningiomas. In Rengachary SS, Wilkins RH (eds): *Neurosurgical Operative Atlas*, vol 1. Park Ridge, IL: American Association of Neurological Surgeons, 1991, pp 339–350, with permission.]

the posterior inferior cerebellar artery (PICA) and anterior inferior cerebellar artery (AICA), may be embedded in it. The trigeminal nerve rootlets are found under the tentorium, frequently stretched and separated by the tumor.

The tumor capsule then is dissected free from the surrounding structures. It is crucial that one keep dissection within the arachnoidal planes, to preserve the vital neural and vascular structures. No cut edge of the tumor should be allowed to slip away, lest the plane of cleavage be lost. The lower cranial nerves are dissected off the inferior pole of the tumor through the infratentorial avenue. Gentle dissection is required to avoid hypotension and bradycardia from vagal stimulation. The basilar artery, if it is not embedded in the tumor, usually is displaced to the opposite side. The need to preserve the main and small branches of the basilar artery cannot be overemphasized. If the tumor has extended into the internal auditory meatus, the meatus wall is drilled and the tumor removed. Because the petrous apex contains no vital structures, it can easily be drilled away, exposing tumor attachments and easing dissection of the fifth and sixth cranial nerves. The area removed extends from the internal auditory meatus to Meckel's cave and medial to the petrous carotid artery.

The dura is closed watertight. A fascia lata graft is used if necessary. The mastoidectomy cavity is filled with fat taken from the thigh. The temporal muscle is then rotated over the defect and sutured to the sternocleidomastoid muscle, and the temporalis fascia flap is brought back to its original position and sutured into place. The soft tissues are closed in layers.

The need for a preoperative angiogram is obvious. The position and displacement of the arteries should be studied. Particular attention should also be paid to the venous pattern, because venous infarction of the temporal lobe has grave sequelae. How big is the vein of Labbé? Is it the dominant venous drainage of the temporal lobe? Are there other basal temporal veins that may be equally vital? Does the patient have two transverse sinuses, and do these sinuses connect at the torcular Herophili?

Transtemporal Approach

A transtemporal approach is appropriate for tumors involving the middle portion of the clivus in a patient who has completely lost hearing before surgery. This approach is the same as the petrosal approach except for the amount of drilling of the temporal bone. The external auditory meatus is transected and the skin edges are inverted and closed watertight as a blind sac. The tympanic membrane and the middle ear ossicles are removed and the eustachian tube is obliterated. Drilling in this case continues to incorporate the translabyrinthine and transcochlear exposures. The lateral and posterior semicircular canals are removed. The facial nerve lies anterior to this plane. The facial nerve is skeletonized from the genu to the stylomastoid foramen. If necessary, the facial nerve is then mobilized. Further exposure can be achieved by removing the cochlea with a diamond drill and skeletonizing the carotid artery anteriorly. The entire petrous apex then is removed, allowing superb access to the tumor (Fig. 166-14).

Transcondylar Approach

The transcondylar approach is selected for tumors involving the lower third of the clivus and the anterior lip of the foramen magnum (Figs. 166-15*A*, *B* and 166-16*A*, *B*). This approach allows removal of both caudal extensions in the cervical canal and cephalad extensions in the posterior fossa. The axis of visualization is lateral, providing direct visualization and dissection of the lesion from the ventral surface of the medulla and spinal cord. The vertebral artery is exposed for proximal and distal control, and the contaminated nasopharyngeal cavity is not transgressed. This

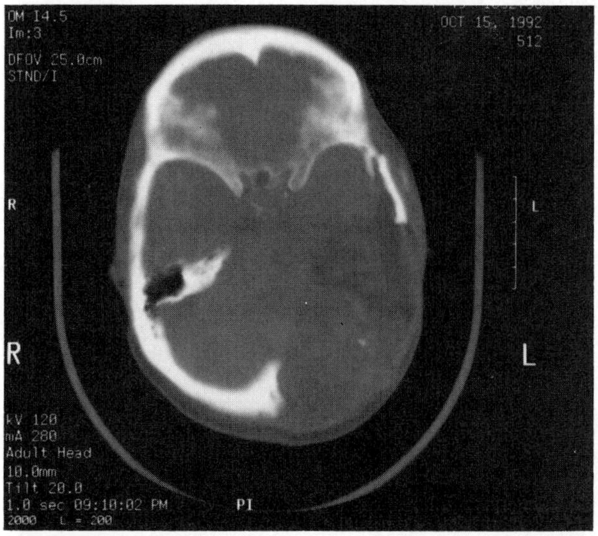

Figure 166-14 Transtemporal approach. Postoperative CT scan (bone window settings). Note the amount of bone removal on the left side.

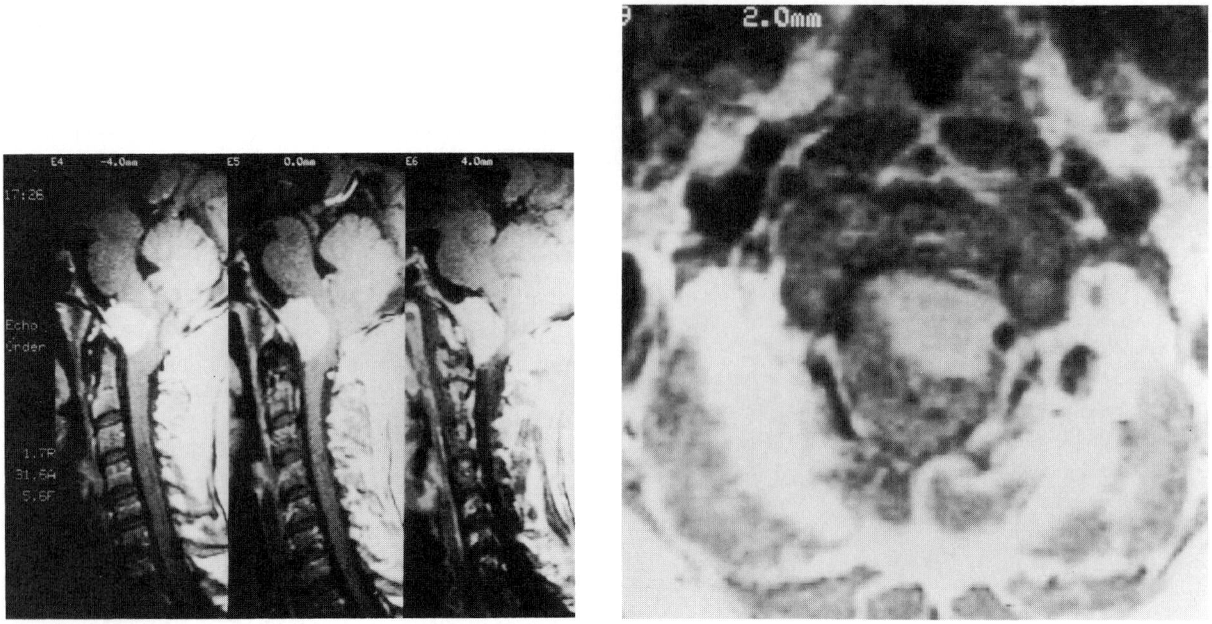

(*A*) (*B*)

Figure 166-15 Preoperative T1-weighted MRI scan with gadolinium (*A*, sagittal view; *B*, axial view) of a patient with a meningioma involving the lower clivus and foramen magnum.

approach combines the principles of the extreme suboccipital craniectomy and the high lateral cervical exposure.[9]

For the transcondylar approach, the patient is placed in the lateral decubitus position with the axis of the body lying at 45 degrees from the horizontal. A neutral craniospinal axis is maintained. The ipsilateral shoulder may be gently pulled down and secured. The axis of visualization is changed by turning the table from side to side.

An open C-shaped incision is made extending downward along the edge of the sternocleidomastoid muscle, which is detached from its mastoid insertion and retracted inferiorly and medially. Bleeding from the mastoid emissary vein is controlled with bone wax. Special care must be taken to avoid injury to the eleventh cranial nerve during this maneuver.

The retromastoid muscles are arranged in three layers. The muscles of the upper two layers are detached in succession. The

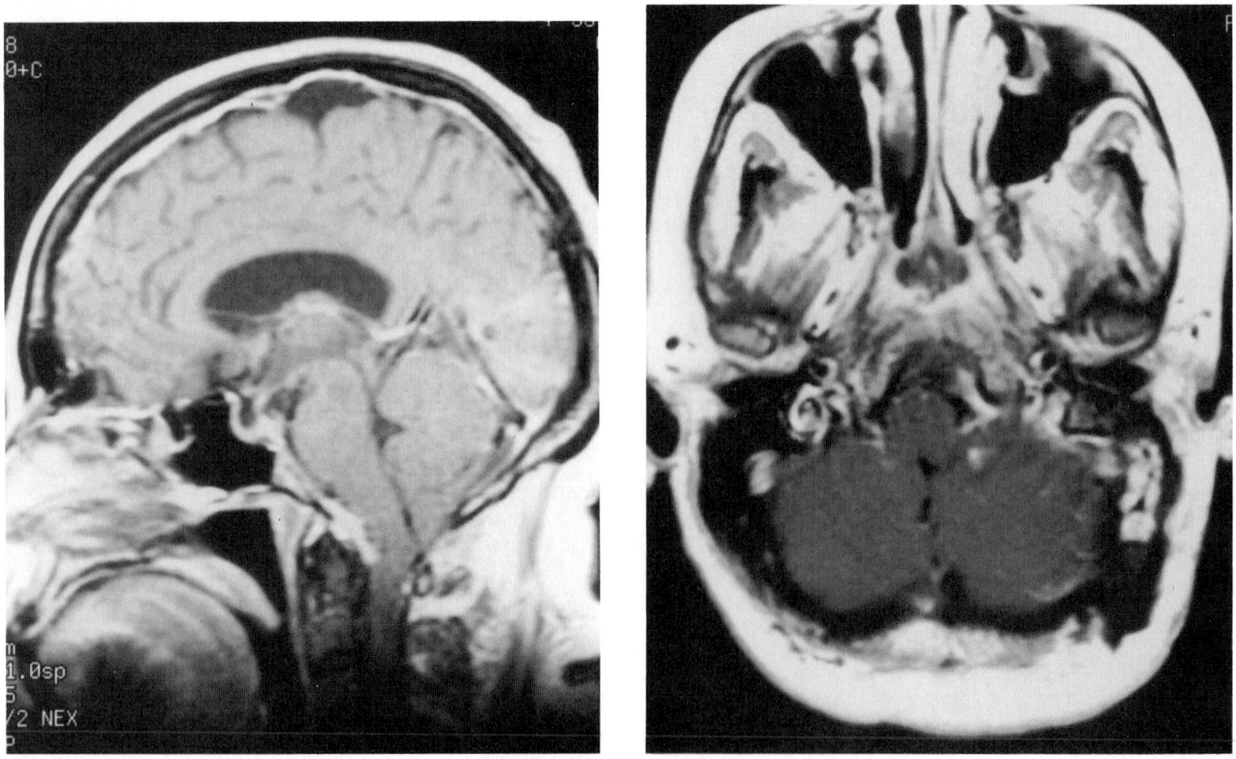

(*A*) (*B*)

Figure 166-16 Postoperative MRI scan of the patient depicted in Fig. 166-15. Same sequences, similar cuts (*A*, sagittal view; *B*, axial view). The tumor was totally removed.

most superficial muscle is the sternocleidomastoid, which inserts on the mastoid process and partially covers the splenius capitis. The splenius capitis itself inserts on the mastoid process and in the lateral end of the superior nuchal line. These two muscles constitute the first layer. The second layer consists of the semispinalis and longissimus capitis muscles. The longissimus capitis inserts onto the mastoid process deep to the splenius capitis. The semispinalis inserts onto the occipital bone between the superior and inferior nuchal lines. These two layers are detached and reflected posteriorly to expose the suboccipital triangle. The boundaries of this triangle comprise the third muscular layer. The recti (major and minor) form the medial border, while the superior oblique capitis forms the lateral border. The inferior oblique arises from the spine of the axis and inserts on the transverse process of the atlas, thus constituting the inferior border of the suboccipital triangle (Fig. 166-17).

The lateral mass of the first cervical vertebra is easily palpable. The muscles are detached in a subperiosteal fashion from their insertions in the first and second vertebrae. As the inferior oblique muscle is detached, the dorsal ramus of the first spinal root is identified and followed, exposing the vertebral artery between the arch of C1 and the occiput. The artery is surrounded by a venous plexus in this area, which might be a source of bleeding if severed. Once the vertebral artery is identified, its course is followed by both cephalad, as it pierces the dura, and caudally into the foramina transversaria of the first and second vertebrae. The foramen transversarium of C1 is opened and the vertebral artery is freed and mobilized medially.

A burr hole is made in the lower lateral aspect of the posterior fossa. A small, lateral posterior fossa craniectomy is carried out with a rongeur. The sigmoid sinus and the jugular bulb are skeletonized using a drill. Care is taken not to injure the facial nerve in the fallopian tube. Drilling is continued to remove the laminae of the first and second cervical vertebrae if necessary.

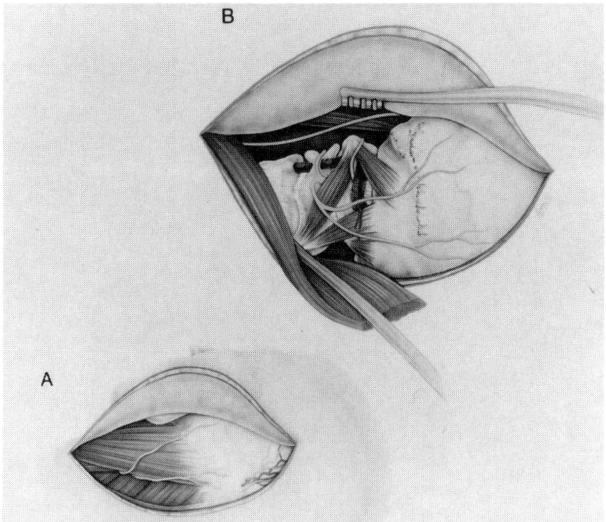

Figure 166-17 Transcondylar approach. *A.* C-shaped retromastoid skin incision. Note the greater auricular and lesser occipital nerves. *B.* Suboccipital triangle delineated by major and minor recti (medial border), inferior oblique (inferior border), and superior oblique (lateral border).

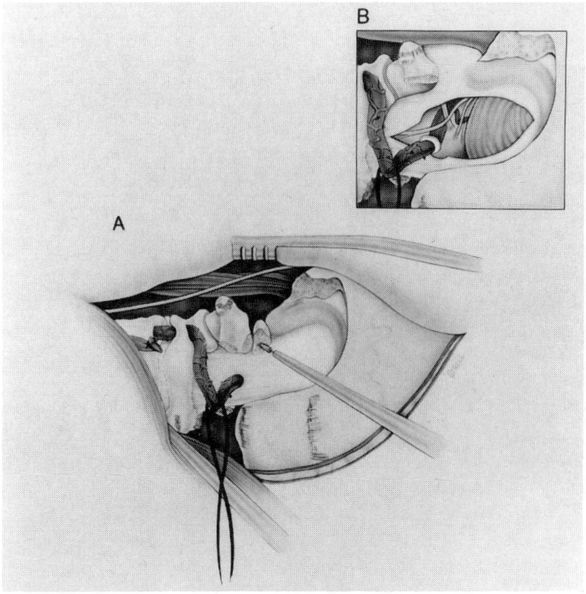

Figure 166-18 Transcondylar approach. *A.* C1 laminectomy has been performed. The vertebral artery has been mobilized. A suboccipital craniectomy has been performed. Drilling of the lateral mass of C1 and the occipital condyle is under way. *B.* Dural opening. Note cranial nerves IX to XII.

The lateral mass of the first vertebra and the occipital condyle are then drilled in their posterior and lateral portions. The anterior halves of these articular surfaces usually can be spared to ensure structural stability. If it became necessary to drill more than half of the condyle, then stabilization with fusion is needed. Lesions with a sizable component in the posterior fossa may require a larger suboccipital craniectomy. The dura mater is opened starting from behind the sigmoid sinus, extending downward across the foramen magnum and down to the area of entry of the vertebral artery. The incision extends longitudinally in the lateral aspect of the upper cervical dural sac. The dural ring around the vertebral artery is opened fully, thus mobilizing the vertebral artery (Fig. 166-18). The spinal cord is usually displaced posteriorly and to the opposite side. This dural opening exposes the tumor directly without the threat of cord herniation. The spinal portion of the spinal accessory nerve, as well as the upper cervical roots, are displaced laterally and draped over the tumor. The arachnoid over the tumor is opened between the spinal roots, and the tumor is debulked. Every effort is made to preserve the radicular arteries and the PICA. Once the tumor is debulked, a plane of arachnoidal membrane allows careful dissection of the tumor from the ventral surface of the cord and the medulla. In recurrent tumors, however, this plane is lost, making dissection more difficult and hazardous. The tumor's extension into the posterior fossa is dissected from the lower cranial nerves and cerebellar vessels.

Conclusion

We have reviewed five skull base approaches to the petroclival area. The approach selection depends on the size, location, and extent of the tumor. Other factors, such as vascular anatomy and the presence or absence of hearing, also come into consideration in choosing the optimal approach.

References

1. Al-Mefty O. *Surgery of the Cranial Base*. Boston: Kluwer Academic Publishers, 1989, pp 239–258.
2. Al-Mefty O, Fox JL, Smith PR. Petrosal approach for petroclival meningiomas. *Neurosurgery* 1988; 22:510–517.
3. Bailey P. Concerning the technic of operation for acoustic neurinoma. *Zentralbl Neurochir* 1939; 4:1–5.
4. Bonnal J, Louis R, Combalbert A. L'abord temporal transtentoriel de l'angle ponto-cérébelleux et du clivus. *Neurochirurgie* 1964; 10:3–12.
5. Borchardt M. Zur operation der tumoren des Kleinhirn-Brückenwinkels. *Berl Klin Wochenschr* 1905; 42:1033–1035.
6. Cushing HW, Eisenhardt L. *Meningiomas: Their Classification, Regional Behavior, Like History, and Surgical End Results*. Springfield: Charles C Thomas, 1938, pp 169–223.
7. Fisch U, Pillsbury HC. Infratemporal fossa approach to lesions in the temporal bone and base of the skull. *Arch Otolaryngol Head Neck Surg* 1979; 105:99–107.
8. Fraenkel J, Hunt JR. Contribution to the surgery of neurofibroma of the acoustic nerve. *Ann Surg* 1904; 40:293–319.
9. George B, Dematans C, Cophignon J. Lateral approach to the anterior portion of the foramen magnum. *Surg Neurol* 1988; 29:484–490.
10. Hakuba A, Nishimura S, Tanaka K, et al. Clivus meningioma: six cases of total removal. *Neurol Med Chir (Tokyo)* 1977; 17:63–77.
11. House WF, Hitselberger WE, Horn KL. The middle fossa transpetrous approach to the anterior-superior cerebellopontine angle. *Am J Otol* 1986; 7:1–4.
12. Kawase T, Ryuzo S, Shigeo T. Anterior transpetrosal-transtentorial approach for sphenopetroclival meningiomas: surgical method and results in 10 patients. *Neurosurgery* 1991; 28:869–876.
13. Malis LI. Surgical resection of tumors of the skull base. In Wilkins RH, Rengachary SS (eds): *Neurosurgery*. New York: McGraw-Hill, 1985, pp 1011–1021.
14. Morrison AW, King TT. Experiences with a translabyrinthine-transtentorial approach to the cerebellopontine angle: technical note. *J Neurosurg* 1973; 38:382–390.
15. Ojemann RG. Meningiomas: clinical features and surgical management. In Wilkins RH, Rengachary SS (eds): *Neurosurgery*. New York: McGraw-Hill, 1985, pp 635–654.
16. Symon L. Surgical approaches to the tentorial hiatus. *Adv Tech Stand Neurosurg* 1982; 9:69–112.
17. Yaşargil MG, Mortara RW, Curcic M. Meningiomas of basal posterior cranial fossa. *Adv Tech Stand Neurosurg* 1980; 7:1–115.

SECTION M

Miscellaneous Neoplasms and Non-neoplastic Tumors

167 Primitive Neuroectodermal Tumors

Barbara J. Crain

The term *primitive neuroectodermal tumor* (PNET) refers to a group of highly malignant tumors that usually occur in young children. The spectrum of lesions within this category includes the medulloblastoma, cerebral neuroblastoma, spongioblastoma, ependymoblastoma, and other tumors characterized by predominantly undifferentiated small round cells with scant cytoplasm. Whether these tumors should be categorized according to their location and their differentiation, however focal, or whether they should be considered as variations of a single lesion has been debated. Proponents of both points of view have used neuroembryologic data to justify their classification systems.[23,25,26] The purpose of this chapter, therefore, is to review the concept of the PNET from the point of view of classic and modern neuroembryology. After a review of the early development of the nervous system, the controversy over nosology will be outlined. Finally, the problems and conclusions of clinical studies of patients with PNETs will be summarized.

Early Development of the Nervous System

During the third week after fertilization, a specialized region of ectoderm appears on the dorsal surface of the human embryo.[15,21] This single layer of columnar epithelial cells is known as the neural plate. It will eventually give rise to the cells of the brain and spinal cord, including neurons, astrocytes, oligodendroglia, and ependymal cells. Immediately adjacent to the neural plate is another region of specialized neuroepithelium, the neural crest. Neural crest derivatives will include the dorsal root ganglia, autonomic ganglia, melanocytes, Schwann cells, and the bones and musculature of the face.

Soon after the appearance of the neural plate, the neural tube is formed by a process known as neurulation. The lateral borders of the neural plate rise as the neural folds and fuse dorsally, beginning in the future cervical region. Fusion then extends rostrally and caudally. At about 4 weeks, the newly formed neural tube sinks below the surface of the embryo. At this point, the neural tube consists of a single layer of pseudostratified columnar neuroepithelium surrounding the neural canal (future ventricular system).

Once neurulation is complete, neural tube cells begin to proliferate. The nuclei within the columnar cells migrate back and forth centrally and peripherally in a rhythmic to-and-fro manner; mitoses occur when the nuclei are adjacent to the lumen of the neural canal.[15,21] Eventually, one daughter cell may become postmitotic. The postmitotic "neuroblast," more properly termed a young neuron since it will never again divide, migrates away from the future ventricular region. Some glioblasts also migrate away from the ventricular zone; these will continue to divide in their new locations. Eventually, the epithelium of the ventricular zone ceases production of neurons and glia and differentiates terminally into ependymal cells.

There are two exceptions to the general rule that cell division is limited to the ventricular zone.[15,21] First, some proliferating cells arise from the ependymal or ventricular layer of the rhombic lip and migrate beneath the pia as the external granule cells of the cerebellum. They eventually develop into the granule cells, stellate cells, and basket cells of the cerebellum.[15,21,28] Whether the external granular layer also produces glial cells has been a matter of much debate. With the development of ^{3}H-thymidine autoradiographic techniques for labeling dividing cells, the consensus finally seemed to be that the external granular layer produces glial cells surrounding Purkinje cells.[15,21] However, a subsequent autoradiographic study using correlative light and electron microscopy found no labeled glial cells in the molecular layer.[28] Whether the Purkinje cell layer was included in the analysis was unclear. In addition, the possibility that glial cells had been labeled, but had undergone multiple mitoses with subsequent dilution of the signal to undetectable levels, was not considered. Nonetheless, this study is often cited as definitive evidence against glial cell production by the external granular layer.

The second exception to the rule that cell division is limited to the ventricular zone occurs in the mammalian forebrain. Owing to the vast number of cells required to develop the forebrain, not all the cells can be produced from the columnar neuroepithelial cells in this relatively small area. Thus, some actively proliferating cells migrate a short distance from the ventricular zone to the immediately adjacent subventricular zone (Fig. 167-1) and continue to divide.[15,18,21] Both the ventricular and the subventricular zones contribute neurons and glia to the forebrain. The subventricular zone persists as the germinal matrix adjacent to the ependyma of the lateral ventricles throughout the third trimester and into the early months of postnatal life, when it gives rise solely to glia.[15]

As a population, the neuroepithelial cells of the ventricular and subventricular zones clearly give rise to neurons, glia, and ependymal cells.[15,21] However, whether there are individual stem cells which can give rise to more than one cell type and, if there are such stem cells, when and where they exist remain major unanswered questions in neuroembryology.

The lack of definitive data has not been paralleled by a lack of theories. Over the last hundred years, numerous hypotheses about the histogenesis of the nervous system have been proposed; these have been reviewed in detail elsewhere.[8,15,18,21] In 1889, His described two types of cells in what is now called the ventricular zone (Fig. 167-1). He proposed that the rounded "germinal cell" and the columnar "spongioblast" are precursors to neurons and glia, respectively. Later, Schaper (in 1897) and Sauer (in 1935) correctly observed that His's "germinal cell" and "spongioblast" actually represent a single cell type in different phases of the mitotic cycle. Schaper therefore hypothesized that all the cells of the ventricular zone are stem cells not yet committed along either neuronal or glial lines. In his model, the undifferentiated ventricular cells give rise to cells which migrate away from the ventricle and then either differentiate into neurons or undergo further mitoses and later differentiate into both neurons and glia.[15,18,21]

Like Schaper and Sauer, Fujita (in 1963) emphasized the homogeneity of the ventricular zone.[15,18,21] Using ^{3}H-thymidine autoradiography to label dividing cells, Fujita concluded that a homogeneous population of dividing stem cells in the ventricular zone gives rise first to neurons and later to glia (and eventually to ependyma).[15,21] However, the ^{3}H-thymidine technique has two limitations.[18] First, labeling of all the ventricular cells with ^{3}H-thymidine only indicates that all the cells are synthesizing DNA during the period of injection. It does not necessarily imply that the dividing cells are a homogeneous population. Second, embryonic glial cells undergo repeated cell divisions after the label is incorporated, resulting in dilution of the signal to undetectable levels. Thus, the ^{3}H-thymidine technique cannot determine the onset of glial differentiation.

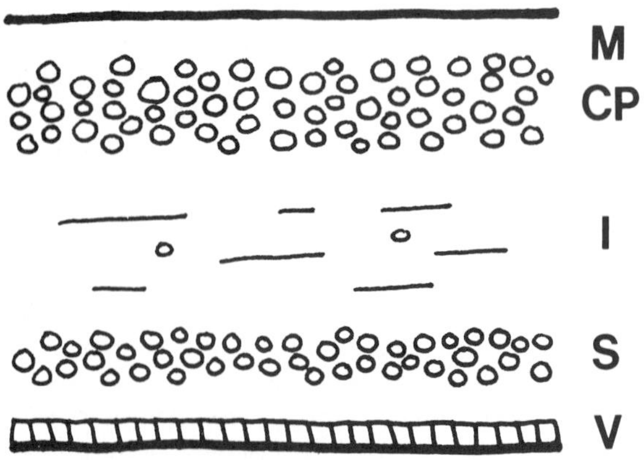

Figure 167-1 A diagrammatic cross-section through the developing neocortex shows the ventricular zone (V) lining the ventricle below. Remnants of this zone will form the ependyma. The subventricular zone (S) is immediately adjacent to the ventricular zone. Postmitotic neuroblasts and dividing glioblasts leaving the ventricular and subventricular zones migrate through the intermediate zone (I) or future white matter, to the cortical plate (CP) which will give rise to cortical layers 2 to 6. Layer 1 of the neocortex will form in the marginal zone (M) adjacent to the pia. (Terminology according to the Boulder Committee.[15])

The first indication that separate proliferating neuronal and glial cell lines might coexist during development was provided by Rakic and his coworkers. They described the radial glial cells which provide guides for migrating young neurons during the development of the neocortex and cerebellum.[15,18,21] Because radial glial cells are present and increase in number prior to and during the peak of neurogenesis, the precursors for these two cell types must be present concomitantly, not sequentially as postulated by earlier authors. Using immunocytochemical studies of glial fibrillary acidic protein (GFAP), Levitt et al. demonstrated that GFAP-positive and GFAP-negative mitotic cells coexist in the ventricular zone during the peak period of neurogenesis in the monkey.[18] They concluded that there were at least two populations of ventricular cells: labeled ones already showing glial differentiation and unlabeled ones which were presumably neuronal precursors. Since neurons and differentiated radial glial cells coexist very early in the development of the cerebral wall, neuronal and glial lines may be separate from the time that neurogenesis begins. However, this study could not answer two questions. First, does a common stem cell give rise to both the glial and neuronal precursor types? Second, are the unlabeled cells a uniform neuronal precursor pool or do they include multiple cell classes including some "indifferent" cells?[18]

Although true multipotential stem cells have not yet been isolated from the developing brain, recent tissue culture studies do suggest that they may exist. In the peripheral nervous system, individual neural crest cells placed in vitro can proliferate and either differentiate into several types of neurons, nonneuronal cells, and melanocytes, or remain actively dividing multipotential stem cells.[3,27] Even more remarkably, postmitotic cells isolated from the striatum of adult mice can reenter the mitotic cycle and produce either neurons or glia, depending on culture conditions.[22] Whether single cells are capable of such feats, and therefore classifiable as true stem cells, has not yet been determined. However, the dividing striatal cells do express nestin,[22] an intermediate filament characteristic of primitive neuroepithelium. Interestingly, many PNETs (and normal blood vessels) also express nestin.[29] Whether similar cells exist in the human brain, and where they might be along the neuraxis, is still unknown.

Neuropathology: Controversies Regarding Nosology

The issue of the existence of a common precursor for neurons, astrocytes, oligodendroglia, and ependymal cells continues to haunt not only neuroembryologists but also physicians seeking to understand the neoplasms encompassed by the term *primitive neuroectodermal tumors*. Both the advocates of lumping all these tumors into the PNET group and the advocates of splitting them into distinct categories assume that differences (or lack of differences) in microscopic appearances of tumors reflect differences in tumor histogenesis. They therefore use neuroembryologic data to justify their classifications. The purpose of this section is to describe the two major classification schemes and to discuss the assumptions each makes about cell lineage and neurohistogenesis.

The Traditional Classification Scheme

The traditional classification scheme for the primitive brain tumors of childhood is derived largely from the histogenetic scheme of Bailey and Cushing and has been described in detail by Rubinstein.[25,26] Under this system, six intracranial tumors can be recognized. First, the sharply demarcated *medulloepithelioma* is characterized by papillary and tubular collections of columnar cells closely resembling the structure of the primitive neural tube itself. Divergent differentiation along neuronal, ependymal, astrocytic, and oligodendroglial cell lines may be present and the stroma may be prominent. Both meningeal and distant metastases have been reported. The *cerebral neuroblastoma* is also well defined grossly and often contains cystic foci. Microscopically the tumor is very cellular and may be composed either of compact sheets of closely packed cells or cells arranged in small clumps, short trabeculae, or irregular syncytial groups. Poorly formed neuroblastic rosettes may be identified but differentiation into clearly identifiable ganglion cells is rare. Again, a mesenchymal stromal reaction may be prominent. The postulated cell of origin is a replicating neuroepithelial cell already committed to neuronal differentiation. The *polar spongioblastoma* is also well demarcated and prone to metastasize widely in the meninges. The histologic picture is very characteristic, with poorly differentiated cells aligned in parallel compact bands or palisades. Occasionally, more advanced astrocytic and oligodendroglial differentiation may be seen. As the name suggests, the migrating polar spongioblast is the putative cell of origin. That the polar spongioblast is a common precursor for astrocytes and oligodendroglial cells is assumed. The *ependymoblastoma* is a highly malignant primitive tumor with clear areas of ependymomatous differentiation which spreads widely through the CSF. Primitive neuroepithelial cells committed to ependymal differentiation are the hypothetical cell of origin. Origin from a "polar ependymoglioblast" would explain the occasional ependymoblastoma with focal features of polar spongioblastoma. The *pineoblastoma* is a primitive tumor arising in the pineal gland. It has a marked tendency to spread through CSF pathway and appears microscopically as a primitive embryonal glioma with poorly formed neuroblastic rosettes. Occasional examples show photoreceptor differentiation which mimics the transient photoreceptor differentiation in the normal embryonic pineal gland. The *medulloblastoma* is a relatively discrete lesion which spreads through CSF pathways (Fig. 167-2). A highly cellular, primitive tumor, it may nevertheless have multiple microscopic appearances. Although it often shows neither neuronal nor glial differentiation, either or both may be present. In the desmoplastic medulloblastoma, a stromal reaction may be prominent. The histogenesis of the medulloblastoma is uncertain but is generally attributed to either of two main sources. The first is the external granular cell layer of the cerebellum or its remnants, and the second is the neuroepithelial lining of the fourth ventricle.

In addition to the intracranial tumors just described, the *retinoblastoma* is a primitive ocular tumor which may show either neuroblastic or photosensory receptor (cone) differentiation. Because of its primitive histology and its ability to show neuronal differentiation, it may be classed with the PNETs.[4,6,26] However, its autosomal dominant inheritance pattern and extracranial site are distinctive. The primitive neuroepithelial cell of the optic cup (an outpouching from the diencephalon) is the proposed cell of origin.

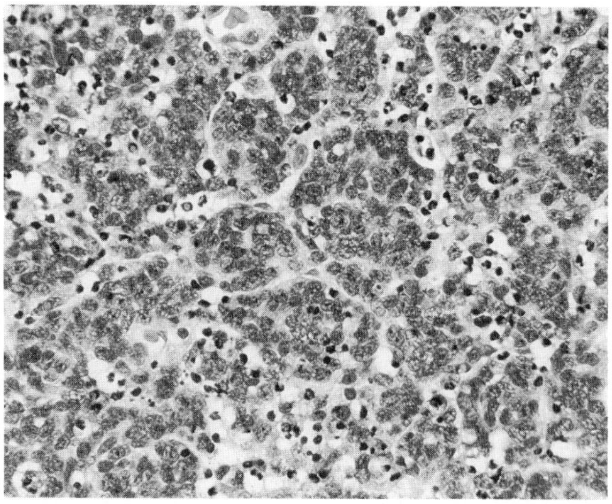

Figure 167-2 Sheets of small tumor cells with angular, hyperchromatic nuclei and scant cytoplasm characterize the undifferentiated areas of both the medulloblastomas (the diagnosis in this cerebellar tumor) and other tumors in the PNET group. (Hematoxylin and eosin, ×293.)

What assumptions about normal histogenesis does this tumor classification scheme make? First, by assigning the cells of the neural tube as the cells of origin of the medulloepithelioma, it assumes that one very primitive neuroepithelial cell can produce not only abortive neural tubes but all the derivatives of the neural tube—neurons, glia, and ependyma. Thus, the neural tube must include at least some precursor or stem cells capable of producing all these cell lines. This is certainly a plausible view, but there is no direct experimental evidence that it is true. On the contrary, some brain stem neurons are already postmitotic at the neural plate stage, before the neural tube has even formed,[8,15,18] and some cells in both the ventricular and subventricular zones are GFAP-positive.[18] Nonetheless, other cells may still be uncommitted. The second assumption is that regional specificity is important in the development of the nervous system. This hypothesis is amply justified. Ablation studies, in which part of the neural plate is destroyed and the animal's brain is analyzed later in development, allow creation of "fate maps" indicating regional specification even before neurulation occurs.[15] The third assumption is that morphologic similarities between normal embryonic cells and tumor cells indicate a cell of origin. In a sense this is an untestable hypothesis, though it underlies much of current oncology. The embryonic central nervous system (CNS) tumors listed above have each been given a putative cell of origin often indicated by the name of the tumor. That neural tube epithelial cells, neuroblasts, polar spongioblasts, ependymoblasts, and pineoblasts all exist at some time during embryogenesis is generally accepted. Whether the tumors with corresponding names actually arise from these cells is unknown. No true medulloblast exists. At the tissue level, the primitive neuroepithelium of the fourth ventricle can differentiate along both neuronal and glial lines,[15,21] but the assumption that individual cells in this region can give rise to both neurons and glia is untested. The assumption that the external granular layer also gives rise to both neurons and glia, thus accounting for glial differentiation in medulloblastomas, is less secure. Some authors claim that only neurons are produced in this layer,[28] a point of view Rubinstein incorporated into later versions of his model.[26]

The First Description of PNET

Although Rubinstein's classification can account for up to 90 percent of the primitive tumors of childhood,[26] Hart and Earle have emphasized that there is a group of largely undifferentiated cerebral neoplasms that do not fit any of the categories outlined by Rubinstein.[13] They thought that these largely undifferentiated brain tumors share enough biological and pathologic properties to justify classifying them as a single entity, the *primitive neuroectodermal tumor* (PNET). Clinically, the cases noted by Hart and Earle were characterized by their predominance in early life, with a mean age of onset of 8 years, and by their aggressive behavior, with death usually occurring in less than 1 year. The lesions occurred deep in the cerebrum and were often grossly cystic and hemorrhagic, with sharp borders. Microscopically, the tumors were malignant and predominantly (90 to 95 percent) undifferentiated, with evidence of focal glial, neuronal, or ependymal differentiation in some cases. Nuclear pleomorphism, hyperplasia, high mitotic rates, and necrosis were all common. Because this study antedated the use of immunocytochemistry, only routine light microscopic techniques, relying strongly on paraffin sections stained by hematoxylin and eosin, were used to identify areas of differentiation.

Hart and Earle thought the cell of origin of the PNET was a primitive neuroepithelial cell whose location was not specified.[13] Thus, they assumed the existence of a single stem cell capable of producing daughter cells with neuronal, glial, and ependymal differentiation. As discussed above, this hypothesis was proposed first by His[8] and later by Fujita,[15,21] but it has never been proved or disproved.

A Broader View of the PNET

The term *primitive neuroectodermal tumor* as used by Hart and Earle[13] was a tumor type described in addition to those described by Rubinstein.[25,26] In contrast, Rorke took a dramatically different approach to the problem of the primitive neuroectodermal tumor.[23] She thought that, with the exception of the medulloepithelioma, all the embryonal tumors in this general category, including the medulloblastoma, represent a continuum in both morphology and behavior, with no clear criteria separating them into unique classes. She therefore proposed that CNS tumors composed primarily of undifferentiated round neuroepithelial cells be termed "primitive neuroectodermal tumors" with the additional terminology "with glial, ependymal, neuronal, or multi- or bipotential differentiation" being given strictly on a descriptive basis. To these were added the terms "medulloblastoma" if the tumor was located in the cerebellum and "pineal parenchymal tumor" if the tumor was located in the pineal body. Pineal parenchymal tumor was retained because of the specialization of the normal pineal gland. Medulloblastoma was retained because of the tumor's frequent occurrence and the term's deep entrenchment in the medical literature. However, Rorke rejected the concept of the medulloblastoma as a separate entity for two reasons. First, histologically identical tumors may arise above the tentorium. Second, she believed that the external granular layer produces only neurons[28] and therefore cannot be the source of medulloblastomas, which may show glial differentiation. Instead, she proposed that the cell of origin for PNETs at all levels of the neuraxis is the germinal matrix cell in the subventricular zone.

There are three underlying assumptions about neurohistogenesis in this view of the PNET. The first assumption is that the subventricular zone actually exists at all levels of the neuraxis. However, this is not the case. The subventricular zone is limited to the forebrain.[15,21] Thus, the medulloblastoma cannot originate from the subventricular zone of the fourth ventricle because no such zone exists. A localized portion of the ventricular ("ependymal") zone surrounding the fourth ventricle is the source of Purkinje cells, Golgi II neurons, the neurons of the deep cerebellar nuclei, the proliferating cells of the external granular layer, and some glial cells.[15,21] Ventricular cells are present at all levels of the neuraxis, but they were not considered as possible cells of origin for the PNETs in this model.

The second assumption, very closely related to the first, is that there are no regional differences within the subventricular zone. Strictly speaking, this is not true. Since the anterior-posterior and medial-lateral axes of the nervous system are already determined at the neural plate stage, as shown by grafting experiments,[15] regional differences must also be present at subsequent stages of development. Indeed, the prosencephalon (future forebrain), mesencephalon (future midbrain), rhombencephalon (future hindbrain), and optic cups (future retina) are distinguishable grossly by the end of neurulation. However, positional information available to the subventricular germinal cells about the exact numbers and types of neurons to be produced at various levels of the forebrain may not be relevant to the issue of the cell of origin of the PNET.

The third assumption, the one that is key for the forebrain, is that the subventricular zone is a uniform population of cells, each with the potential to differentiate into neurons, astrocytes, oligodendroglia, and ependymal cells. Whether any of the cells in the subventricular zone ever reenter the ependymal epithelium is unknown. As noted above, many neural plate cells, as well as ventricular and subventricular cells, already represent glial or neuronal precursors,[8,15,18,21] but the possibility of common stem cells remains.[3,22,27] Whether astrocytes and oligodendrocytes share a common precursor is also unknown. However, the observation of apparent transitional forms and the observation that astrocyte precursor cells may develop into oligodendroglial cells under appropriate tissue culture conditions support this hypothesis.[8]

Modifications of the PNET Hypothesis

Rorke's original model of the PNET[23] has been modified by many authors. Becker and Hinton divided this group of tumors into two general categories.[4] First were PNETs with no differentiation, a category in which they included the PNET of the cerebrum and the medulloblastoma. Their second general category was PNET with differentiation, which could be along the lines of the neural tube (medulloepithelioma), neuron (neuroblastoma), astrocyte (polar spongioblastoma), ependyma (ependymoblastoma), pineal gland (pineoblastoma), retina (retinoblastoma), olfactory receptor cell (olfactory neuroblastoma), melanocyte (melanotic medulloblastoma), muscle (myomedulloblastoma), oligodendroglia, Schwann cell, or other lines. They thus implied a one-to-one correspondence between Rubinstein's classic terminology (cerebral neuroblastoma, ependymoblastoma, etc.) and the PNET terminology (PNET with neuronal differentiation, PNET with ependymal differentiation, etc.). They favored the PNET terminology because they thought it did not necessarily imply a cell of origin.

A similar approach was adopted by Dehner.[6] Like Becker and Hinton,[4] he used the term PNET as an inclusive designation for a group of childhood tumors. For CNS tumors with differentiation, he too used terms such as PNET with ependymal differentiation (ependymoblastoma). Importantly, Dehner extended the concept of the PNET to include not only tumors in the central nervous system but tumors of the peripheral nervous system as well. The latter may be neural crest derivatives. His paper is recommended as a critical review of the concept of PNETs.[6] He emphasized that phenotypic similarities between tumors do not necessarily imply a common histogenesis.

Rorke and associates have also modified the PNET terminology.[24] Their revised classification provides more detailed morphologic criteria for the diagnosis of PNETs than any of the earlier models. The use of special stains and immunohistochemistry is laid out in detail. In this system, ''primitive'' neuroectodermal tumors (''P''NET) fall into three major categories. The first category is the ''P''NET tumor, not otherwise specified, which occurs most commonly in the cerebellum but may be located anywhere in the CNS including the pineal gland. These tumors tend to spread widely through CSF pathways and may rarely metastasize outside the CNS, most commonly to bone. Histologically, the tumors are composed of poorly differentiated neuroepithelial cells; neuroblastic rosettes may be present. The second category is ''P''NET with astrocytes, oligodendroglia, ependymal cells, neuronal cells, other cells (melanocytes, mesenchymal cells), or mixed cellular elements. Such terms as ''astrocytic differentiation'' are eliminated because of their histogenetic connotations. The third category is medulloepithelioma. Tumors in this category may or may not contain astrocytes, oligodendroglia, ependymal cells, neuronal cells, other cell types, or mixed cellular elements. ''P''NET (pineoblastoma) is listed separately under ''pineal cell tumors'' because it is thought to arise from the neuroepithelial anlage of the pineal. Its histologic features are identical to the ''P''NETs, with the additional possibility of retinoblastomatous differentiation.

The modified scheme of Rorke et al. specifically avoided assumptions about the cell of origin of the ''P''NET and explicitly stated that its histogenesis is unknown. Instead, they outlined the unresolved questions: ''(1) Is the cell of origin unique to the region of the nervous system in which the tumor arises, e.g., external granule cell in cerebellum, pineoblast in pineal gland, etc., or does it arise from a primitive or undifferentiated cell common to all portions of the nervous system, including the pineal gland; or (2) Do the tumors arise from a single primitive multipotential neuroepithelial cell or, alternatively, do the tumors originate from a clone of cells, some of which are already committed to become astrocytes or neurons or simply to remain as undifferentiated neoplastic cells; or (3) The possibility also exists that these tumors do not arise from 'primitive' neuroepithelial cells; rather, the apparently undifferentiated or 'primitive' cell is a previously mature transformed neoplastic cell. Until such time as there is incontrovertible scientific evidence in support of one view, the nosologic problem will persist.''[24]

Finally, it should be noted that all these classification systems assume that undifferentiated cells comprise a significant proportion of the tumor mass. This assumption is based on a combination of conventional light microscopy and immunohistochemistry on paraffin-embedded material. However, one study using snap-frozen sections of 22 PNETs found immunohistochemical evidence of both neuroendocrine and glial differentiation in 21 cases, including 17 medulloblastomas, 1 ependymoblastoma, 2 neuroblastomas, 1 anaplastic astrocytoma, and 1 unclassified anaplastic tumor. Furthermore, double- and triple-labeling studies confirmed that individual ''primitive'' cells could express both neuronal and glial antigens, as well as various intermediate filament markers.[12] Such an unusual labeling pattern might in itself be a reason to group these lesions.

Problems in Clinical Studies of PNETs

As is evident from the foregoing discussion, the nosology of tumors in the PNET category is confusing and controversial. The underlying uncertainty over the pathologic definition of PNET undermines the clinical studies of cases reported as PNET. Because different authors have used the term in different ways, and have seldom defined their pathologic criteria very clearly, there is no way to ascertain the comparability of neoplasms in different series. In all likelihood they are very different. The situation is further complicated by the fact that, excluding the medulloblastomas, PNETs (however defined) are rare tumors, accounting for only 3 to 7 percent of primary brain tumors of children.[4,20] Thus, most studies are either small (fewer than half a dozen cases) or include retrospective reviews of previous cases which often had incomplete records. The few large reviews[2] of PNETs include previously published series of ''cerebral neuroblastomas'' and ''supratentorial gliomas'' of childhood and discuss them all as a single uniform entity, the PNET, which was not always the original authors' intent.

In spite of these significant problems in nosology and case identification, certain generalities about PNETs become apparent. Most occur in infants or young children and produce nonspecific symptoms and signs (irritability, nausea, vomiting, and papilledema), although focal findings are present in some cases.[1,2,5,13,16,17,20] Computed tomography[9,13] and magnetic resonance imaging[9] studies of PNETs describe large, enhancing tumors that are often calcified, with cystic or necrotic areas. The transition between tumor and brain is often abrupt, with surprisingly little edema. Hemorrhage is common.

Nowhere are the limitations of the clinical studies of PNETs more apparent than in the reports of surgical and adjunctive therapy. There have been no large, prospective, randomized studies comparing the efficacies of various treatment modalities. Rather, individual series with only a few patients with poorly described tumors and with different treatments have been compared across institutions and across time. Most frequently these have not indicated how or by whom the histologic diagnoses were established. The result is that undoubtedly heterogeneous groups of patients have been given heterogeneous treatments. Nonetheless, some authors have reviewed the literature and their own experience and made suggestions about patient management.[10,14,30]

Most patients have received some form of surgery. Although complete resection of PNETs is recommended by some,[10,14] most of these large lesions are subtotally excised. The extent of the resections in different series is unclear. Some form of radiation therapy is generally administered as well. Although the radiation protocols vary, the doses are usually in the range of 3600 to 4000 rad to the cranium or craniospinal axis with 1500 rad as a local boost to the tumor site.[10,14,20] Higher doses have also been used.[30] There is some evidence that surgery plus radiation prolongs survival compared with surgery alone.[1,2,10,14,20]

Although some authors advocate aggressive chemotherapy,[30] its usefulness in the treatment of PNETs remains unproved.[2,6,10] Chemotherapeutic protocols have been varied and not always described in detail. No single regimen has been given to more than a few patients.

The prognosis for patients with a PNET (diagnosed by any criteria) or for patients with one of the embryonal tumors described by Rubinstein[25,26] is generally poor. Most patients develop local recurrence; leptomeningeal dissemination[19] or systemic metastasis occurs in some cases. In spite of surgery, radiation therapy, and aggressive chemotherapy, most patients survive less than 24 months.[2,7,10,11,13,17] Nonetheless, many of the same studies also report a few long-term survivors (5 to 17 years) whose prolonged courses could not be predicted on clinical grounds. No studies have assessed the prognostic significance of the amount and type of histologic differentiation or the location of the tumor (cerebrum, pineal, cerebellum, brain stem, spinal cord). Such prognostic information would promote the development of more effective treatments for tumors in the PNET category and would also help support or refute the hypothesis that the PNETs are truly a single tumor type.

Conclusions

The PNET is not a well-defined pathologic entity. Some authors have used the term as a synonym for a group of embryonal tumors without specifying a cell of origin.[4,6] This usage emphasizes the histologic similarities of many of these tumors without completely obscuring potential differences among them. Others have used PNET as a specific diagnosis, implying that all such tumors are a single entity with a cell of origin in the subventricular zone of the developing nervous system.[24] The danger in this approach is the very real possibility of obscuring distinct clinicopathologic entities that might respond to specific treatments. Careful, well-documented pathologic diagnoses and prospective, randomized treatment protocols involving large numbers of patients will be necessary to test the PNET hypothesis.

References

1. Altman N, Fitz CR, Chuang S, et al. Radiologic characteristics of primitive neuroectodermal tumors in children. *Am J Neuroradiol* 1985; 6:15–18.
2. Ashwal S, Hinshaw DB Jr, Bedros A. CNS primitive neuroectodermal tumors of childhood. *Med Pediatr Oncol* 1984; 12:180–188.
3. Baroffio A, Dupin E, Le Douarin NM. Clone-forming ability and differentiation potential of migratory neural crest cells. *Proc Natl Acad Sci USA* 1988; 85:5325–5329.
4. Becker LE, Hinton D. Primitive neuroectodermal tumors of the central nervous system. *Hum Pathol* 1983; 14:538–550.
5. Dehner LP. Primitive neuroectodermal tumors of the central nervous system in childhood: retrospective and overview. In Humphrey GB, Dehner LP, Grindey GB, et al (eds): *Pediatric Oncology 1.* Hague: Martinus Nijhoff, 1981, pp 277–288.
6. Dehner LP. Peripheral and central primitive neuroectodermal tumors: a nosologic concept seeking a consensus. *Arch Pathol Lab Med* 1986; 110:997–1005.
7. Duffner PK, Cohen ME, Heffner RR, et al. Primitive neuroectodermal tumors of childhood: an approach to therapy. *J Neurosurg* 1981; 55:376–381.
8. Fedoroff S. Macroglial cell lineages. In Edelman GM, Gall WE, Cowan WM (eds): *Molecular Bases of Neural Development.* New York: Wiley, 1985, pp 91–117.
9. Figeroa RE, el Gammal T, Brooks BS, et al. MR findings on primitive neuroectodermal tumors. *J Comput Assist Tomogr* 1989; 13:773–778.
10. Gaffney CC, Sloan JP, Bradley NJ, et al. Primitive neuroectodermal tumours of the cerebrum: pathology and treatment. *J Neurooncol* 1985; 3:23–33.
11. Ganti SR, Silver AJ, Diefenbach P, et al. Computed tomography of primitive neuroectodermal tumors. *Am J Neuroradiol* 1983; 4:819–821.
12. Gould VE, Jansson DS, Molenaar WM, et al. Primitive neuroectodermal tumors of the central nervous system. Patterns of expression of neuroendocrine markers, and all classes of intermediate filament proteins. *Lab Invest* 1990; 62:498–509.
13. Hart MN, Earle KM. Primitive neuroectodermal tumors of the brain in children. *Cancer* 1973; 32:890–897.
14. Humphrey GB, Dehner LP, Kaplan RJ, et al. Overview on the management of primitive neuroectodermal tumors. In Humphrey GB, Dehner LP, Grindey GB, et al (eds): *Pediatric Oncology 1.* Hague: Martinus Nijhoff, 1981, pp 289–294.
15. Jacobson M. *Developmental Neurobiology,* 2d ed. New York: Plenum Press, 1978.
16. Kingsley DPE, Harwood-Nash DCF. Radiological features of the neuroectodermal tumours of childhood. *Neuroradiology* 1984; 26:463–467.
17. Kosnik EJ, Boesel CP, Bay J, et al. Primitive neuroectodermal tumors of the central nervous system in children. *J Neurosurg* 1978; 48:741–746.
18. Levitt P, Cooper ML, Rakic P. Coexistence of neuronal and glial precursor cells in the cerebral ventricular zone of the fetal monkey: an ultrastructural immunoperoxidase analysis. *J Neurosci* 1981; 1:27–39.
19. Packer RJ, Siegel KR, Sutton LN, et al. Leptomeningeal dissemination of primary central nervous system tumors of childhood. *Ann Neurol* 1985; 18:217–221.
20. Parker JC Jr, Mortara RH, McCloskey JJ. Biologic behavior of the primitive neuroectodermal tumors: significant supratentorial childhood gliomas. *Surg Neurol* 1975; 4:383–388.
21. Purves D, Lichtman JW. *Principles of Neural Development.* Sunderland, MA: Sinauer Associates, Inc., 1985.
22. Reynolds BA, Weiss S. Generation of neurons and astrocytes from isolated cells of the adult mammalian central nervous system. *Science* 1992; 255:1707–1710.
23. Rorke LB. The cerebellar medulloblastoma and its relationship to primitive neuroectodermal tumors. *J Neuropathol Exp Neurol* 1983; 42:1–15.
24. Rorke LB, Gilles FH, Davis RL, et al. Revision of the World Health Organization classification of brain tumors for childhood brain tumors. *Cancer* 1985; 56:1869–1886.
25. Rubinstein LJ. Cytogenesis and differentiation of primitive central neuroepithelial tumors. *J Neuropathol Exp Neurol* 1972; 31:7–26.
26. Rubinstein LJ. Embryonal central neuroepithelial tumors and their differentiating potential: a cytogenetic view of a complex neuro-oncological problem. *J Neurosurg* 1985; 62:795–805.
27. Stemple DL, Anderson DJ. Isolation of a stem cell for neurons and glia from the mammalian neural crest. *Cell* 1992; 71:973–985.
28. Swarz JR, Del Cerro M. Lack of evidence for glial cells originating from the external granular layer in mouse cerebellum. *J Neurocytol* 1977; 6:241–250.
29. Tohyama T, Lee VM-Y, Rorke LB, et al. Nestin expression in human neuroepithelium and in human neuroepithelial tumor cells. *Lab Invest* 1992; 66:303–313.
30. Tomita T, McLone DG, Yasue M. Cerebral primitive neuroectodermal tumors in childhood. *J Neurooncol* 1988; 6:233–243.

168

Primary Central Nervous System Lymphomas

Milam E. Leavens
John T. Manning
Lauren A. Langford
Ashok J. Kumar
Moshe H. Maor
Peter McLaughlin
Sidney Wallace

Primary central nervous system lymphoma (PCNSL) is a malignant neoplasm of lymphocytic derivation that is localized to the CNS, at least on initial presentation. The possibility of systemic lymphoma must be excluded by clinical staging or by autopsy. The synonyms that have been used to denote PCNSL include malignant lymphoma, non-Hodgkin's lymphoma, reticulum cell sarcoma, microgliomatosis, microglioma, reticulum cell sarcoma–microgliomatosis, perithelial sarcoma, perivascular sarcoma, reticuloendothelial cell sarcoma, malignant reticulosis, malignant reticuloendotheliosis, histiocytic lymphoma, immunoblastic sarcoma, and granulomatous encephalitis.

Incidence

PCNSL is occurring with increasing frequency. In a review of the pathologic material obtained from 8,070 patients with brain tumors, Kernohan and Uihlein, in 1962, found that only 40 (0.5 percent) of the patients had reticulum cell sarcoma or lymphoma of the brain.[44] Freeman et al. reported that 23 (0.18 percent) of 12,447 lymphoma patients had primary lymphoma in the CNS, and Henry et al. reported 83 (0.7 percent) similar patients among 11,712 lymphoma patients in the Armed Forces Institute of Pathology files.[22,35] CNS lymphoma was primary in 8 (7.6 percent) of 105 patients with non-Hodgkin's CNS lymphoma reported by Mackintosh et al.[51] Remick and coworkers[68] (and personal communication, Richard Selik, M.D., 1989) state that 0.4 percent of 28,920 AIDS patients reported to the Centers for Disease Control had PCNSL at the time of diagnosis of AIDS. This is an underestimation, since AIDS patients who subsequently developed PCNSL were not reported. Hochberg and coworkers[36] stated that PCNSL occurs probably in 2.5 percent of AIDS patients. An increase in the incidence of PCNSL in immunocompetent patients was noted by DeAngelis and coworkers.[13,15,16] The incidence increased from 2.7 cases per 10 million population in 1973 to 7.25 cases per 10 million in 1984.[18] The risk of transplant patients developing PCNSL is 100 times greater.[36]

Location and Gross Pathology

PCNSL may involve numerous regions, including the brain parenchyma, the meninges, the intradural spinal cord, and the vitreous and retina of the eye.[36] The brain lesions tend to be invasive with poorly defined margins. PCNSL can occur in all areas of the brain[11,47,74]; however, primary lymphomas of the spinal cord are extremely rare.[10,42,57,74,87] The cerebral hemispheres are the most commonly involved sites, especially in the periventricular area; but the basal ganglia, thalamus, brain stem, and cerebellum are all sites of occurrence. A solitary mass was the most common lesion in some series,[11,47] whereas a high incidence of multifocal (about 50 percent of patients) or diffuse involvement has been emphasized by others.[6,50,87] A predilection toward involvement of the corpus callosum has been found by some.[6,39,74] "Butterfly tumors," involving the corpus callosum and extending symmetrically and bilaterally into the perivascular and deep white matter of the cerebral hemispheres, have been frequent in some series.[17,39]

A common gross appearance is a gray-pink, homogeneous, circumscribed mass that is firmer than the surrounding brain parenchyma. The appearance and texture will be more heterogeneous if necrosis, hemorrhage, or cavitation is present. This pattern of brain involvement produces a mass lesion effect with increased intracranial pressure, midline displacement, and herniation of brain structures.[11,45] A less common gross appearance is an ill-defined area that looks swollen but lacks a distinct tumor mass.[1,6,87] Peritumor edema is often absent, in contrast to that seen in metastatic brain tumors.[13]

Microscopic Pathology

The central part of the tumor mass is characterized by high cellularity. Necrosis may be present. Diffuse infiltration of the parenchyma for some distance beyond the grossly evident tumor has often been emphasized.[6,20,35,69] The infiltrating tumor cells at the advancing edge often have a strikingly perivascular orientation. Infiltration and distention of perivascular (Virchow-Robin) spaces is a highly characteristic feature, usually seen most easily near the tumor border (Fig. 168-1). Perivascular cuffing of lymphoma cells is associated with an increase of reticulin, which appears as concentric rings in reticulin stained sections.[35,69] Some investigators have interpreted this as evidence of the perivascular origin of the tumors and refer to these neoplasms as *perithelial* or *perivascular sarcomas*.[4,35] While it is a helpful diagnostic feature, vascular and perivascular infiltration is not specific for lymphoma; granulocytic sarcoma (myeloblastoma), and even metastatic carcinoma, can infiltrate in exactly the same manner.

Besides perivascular extension, diffuse parenchymal, leptomeningeal, and subpial spread are characteristic, and the choroid plexus may be involved.[35,69,74] Reactive gliosis may be prominent either at the periphery or in the center of the tumor.

The majority of PCNSL are classifiable as diffuse, large cell lymphomas and are essentially indistinguishable from lymphomas

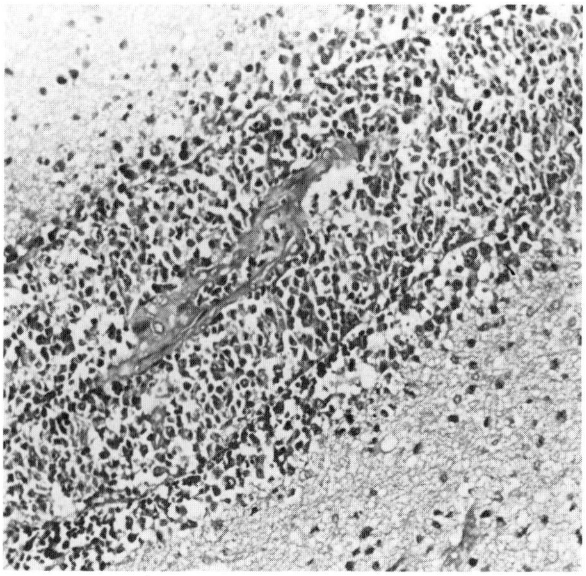

Figure 168-1 Tumor cells infiltrate the perivascular (Virchow-Robin) space at the periphery of the lesion (H & E, ×150).

of the same type arising in lymph nodes or extranodal sites outside the CNS (Fig. 168-2). There are, however, several notable differences between the relative occurrence rates of lymphomas of histologic types originating within, and types originating outside, the CNS. A larger percentage of lymphomas arising in the CNS, particularly those arising in association with primary or acquired immunodeficiency, appear to be B-cell immunoblastic sarcomas.[23,54,61,80] Another difference is the absence in the CNS of nodular (follicular) lymphoma, a type of non-Hodgkin's lymphoma that is common outside the CNS.[33,42,47,80] And third, examples of Hodgkin's disease restricted to the CNS are rare or nonexistent.[42,47,80] Although such cases were reported in earlier series with some frequency, most, if not all, were probably B-cell immunoblastic sarcomas.[47,77,80]

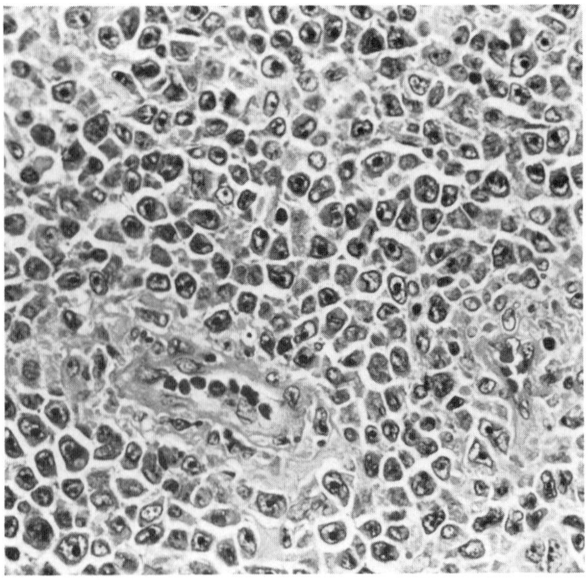

Figure 168-2 Same case as Fig. 168-1. Diffuse, large cell lymphoma (B-immunoblastic sarcoma) of the brain, with high cellularity in the central area of the left posterior frontal lobe mass. The plasmacytoid features of the tumor cells are apparent (H & E, ×380).

Lymphomas having the histologic features of undifferentiated Burkitt's lymphoma or lymphoblastic (convoluted cell) lymphoma have been reported.[26,33,42,80]

Terminology and Origin

A semantic disagreement over terminology existed for a number of years, and even today there is considerable lack of uniformity in the reporting of cases. Bailey provided perhaps the earliest description of these tumors and regarded them as perivascular sarcomas and perithelial sarcomas, for reasons mentioned above.[4] Yuile considered them to be indistinguishable from reticulum cell sarcomas originating outside the CNS, and preferred that term.[86] Kinney and Adams also preferred that term and thought that such tumors originated from primitive reticulum cells.[45] Russell and other British pathologists were impressed by the affinity of tumor cells for the silver carbonate stain, which they regarded as being specific for microglia. They argued that *reticulum cell sarcoma* was not appropriate, since the primitive reticulum cell should not show affinity for the silver carbonate stain, and thought *microgliomatosis* to be a more accurate name.[71] Burstein and coworkers concluded that the dispute was basically a semantical one caused by different interpretations of the term *reticulum cell*, since both sides agreed that the tumors were derived from brain histiocytes. They therefore proposed *reticuloendothelial cell sarcoma* as a name denoting the basic histiocytic nature of the tumors.[11] Rubinstein preferred the term *reticulum cell sarcoma–microglioma* as a better compromise.[69]

An assumption made by workers on both sides of the dispute was that these tumors derived from the reticular component of the reticuloendothelial (lymphoreticular) system and not from lymphocytes, since only the former were intrinsic to the CNS. In the light of modern knowledge it is now apparent that this assumption was incorrect. Virtually all lymphomas, including those restricted to the CNS, derive from lymphocytes. Intracytoplasmic immunoglobulin has been demonstrated in a high percentage of PCNSLs by immunoperoxidase staining of tissue sections for light and heavy chains, and primary lymphoma cell suspensions and cell cultures have shown B-lymphocyte membrane markers.[4,39,58] Electron microscopy has shown them to have the ultrastructural features of immunoblasts.[82]

So the terms *reticulum cell sarcoma, microglioma*, and *microgliomatosis* are all inappropriate in view of current knowledge. *Histiocytic lymphoma*, a term still in wide usage among experienced hemopathologists, is also misleading, since very few of these lymphomas are of histiocytic derivation.[83] To this date, lymphocyte marker studies of primary intracranial lymphomas have not shown any to be T-cell lymphomas.[58]

PCNSL occurs in patients who are immunoincompetent for various reasons, and in patients who are immunocompetent.[14,27,37] The high reported incidence of CNS lymphomas in AIDS patients, renal transplant recipients, and patients with primary immunodeficiency diseases—and also with other primary malignancies—has generated considerable interest in the cause of these tumors.[5,23,34,59,65,75] It has been proposed that the various lymphoproliferative disorders occurring in persons with primary and acquired immunodeficiency are caused by proliferation of

B lymphocytes infected by Epstein-Barr virus (EBV).[67,72] EBV, the B-lymphocytotrophic herpes virus, is the cause of infectious mononucleosis (IM). During acute EBV infection the B-lymphocytic proliferation is controlled by, and EBV forced into latency in large part by, the cell-mediated (T-lymphocyte) immune system, as well as by specific antibodies to viral-related antigens and possibly by natural killer cell activity.[71,72] Viral genomes remain present in the B-lymphocytes of asymptomatic seropositive individuals, and immortal lymphoblastoid cell lines can be readily established from the blood of such individuals.[25,72] There is now substantial evidence that the lymphoproliferative disorders (fatal IM and malignant lymphoma) occurring after renal transplantation in patients with X-linked lymphoproliferative syndrome and in other diverse types of immunodeficiency are caused by EBV infection (either primary infection or reactivation).[32,37,52,60,67,72] Following renal transplantation, patients develop high antibody titers to EBV and shed large numbers of virus particles in their oropharyngeal secretions. Tumor biopsy specimens from renal transplant recipients contain lymphoma cells with Epstein-Barr nuclear antigen and EBV genomes.[32] Similarly, the tissues of patients with X-linked lymphoproliferative syndrome (an affliction of young males who are unable to mount an immune response to EBV and who usually die at an early age from a lymphoproliferative process such as IM or immunoblastic sarcoma), as well as the tissues of patients with various other primary immunodeficiency states, contain significant numbers of EBV genomes in their cells.[72] Lymphomas arising in X-linked lymphoproliferative syndrome, in Wiskott-Aldrich syndrome, and in renal transplant recipients all have similar features with regard to histology and type of presentation. Most are B-cell immunoblastic sarcomas, and they frequently have localized extranodal presentations. There is a high rate of CNS involvement, and the occurrence of PCNSL in association with these immunodeficiency states has been reported in a number of instances.[5,23,32,34,54,59,65,67,72,75] Its occurrence has also been reported in association with other abnormal immune states, such as Waldenström's macroglobulinemia and immunoglobulin A (IgA) deficiency, and in immunosuppressed patients with immunoinflammatory diseases such as necrotizing vasculitis.[28,29,41] Thus, the primary difference between lymphomas in non-immunocompromised and immunocompromised persons is that EBV is only rarely present in the PCNSLs of non-immunocompromised persons.[52] Not only do patients with AIDS have an increased risk of developing CNS lymphoma, but these tumors represent a major source of morbidity and mortality in the HIV-infected population. In these patients most PCNSLs are associated with EBV, in contrast to AIDS-related systemic lymphomas, of which only 30 to 50 percent are associated with EBV.[30,52] Two lymphoma morphologies commonly seen in AIDS patients are diffuse, frequently immunoblastic, large cell tumors and diffuse, Burkitt-like, small noncleaved cell tumors. Large cell tumors resemble those associated with organ transplantation and are more often associated with EBV than the small non-cleaved cell tumors, which are usually negative for the EBV genome.[30] The association with EBV suggests that large cell tumors may have a different pathogenesis from that of the small cell, or Burkitt-type, lymphoma.

The high rate of CNS occurrence of lymphomas associated with immunodeficiency may be related to the fact that the brain is an immunologically privileged site where the cell-mediated immune response is weaker than in other tissues. Such lymphomas may well arise in the systemic tissues but favor growth in the CNS.[19,25] This may also help to explain how lymphomas arise in an organ that contains no lymphatics or lymphoid tissue.

Clinical Characteristics

The clinical presentations of 193 patients with PCNSL reported in the literature,[11,20,31,35,39,48,73,74] as well as those of 4 of our patients, are reviewed.

Age and Sex Incidence

The patients studied included 121 males and 76 females. Their ages at the time of diagnosis ranged from 2 months to 90 years. The greatest incidence was in the fourth through sixth decades of life, with a mean age of about 55 years; there was a separate early peak incidence in the first decade.[6,11,20,35,47,74]

Considerable variation in the duration of symptoms prior to diagnosis was detected in these patients. The symptom duration in the majority was 2 to 7 months. Four had symptoms for only 1 to 2 weeks prior to diagnosis. Seven had symptoms ranging from 1 to 20 years. One patient had intermittent depression and diplopia for 20 years before exhibiting progressive neurological symptoms and signs. Still another patient had intermittent neurological complaints over an 8-year period before a definitive diagnosis was made.

Clinical Presentation

The clinical presentations of patients with primary lymphoma in the brain differ because of variations in tumor involvement of the brain and meninges and because of variations in the biological behavior of these tumors. The various clinical presentations seen in such patients may be catalogued as follows: (1) symptoms and signs of a rapidly expanding intracranial mass lesion, (2) a clinical course suggesting encephalitis, (3) a course suggesting a demyelinating disease, (4) symptoms suggesting cerebrovascular disease, and (5) symptoms and signs indicating meningeal involvement by tumor.

An estimated 60 percent of the patients with primary lymphoma of the brain present clinically with a rapidly growing mass lesion in the brain similar to that seen in patients with glioblastoma multiforme or metastatic carcinoma.[73] Such patients usually have a circumscribed lymphoma in the brain surrounded by some edema; the disease is fatal and its course is relatively rapid.[20] Symptoms and signs indicate raised intracranial pressure, and focal symptoms and signs indicate specific site involvement in the brain. Usually, the symptoms and signs are such that a diagnosis of an expanding lesion above or below the tentorium can be made and lateralized correctly.[31]

Approximately 25 percent of the patients with primary lymphoma in the brain have a clinical course that suggests an erroneous diagnosis of either a viral encephalitis or a demyelinating disease. Seven reported patients had a clinical course suggesting influenza or encephalitis.[11,73] Each patient had several of the following symptoms and signs: fever, chills, vertigo, insomnia, fatigue, malaise, anorexia, sore throat, dizziness, somnolence, lethargy, headache, vomiting, diarrhea, and neck stiffness. Early in the course of the disease, some patients underwent carotid arteriography and pneumoencephalography. Neither of these procedures revealed evidence of an intracranial mass lesion. Spinal fluid pressures were normal, CSF total protein content was elevated, the glucose level was low, there was CSF lymphocytosis, and cultures were negative. Late in the disease some patients developed specific neurological deficits or symptoms and signs of increased intracranial pressure, which led to a diagnosis of a space-occupying intracranial lesion. The duration of symptoms prior to diagnosis varied from 2 weeks to 9 months (mean, 3.4 months). The tumor location varied (temporal lobe, thalamus, frontal and parietal lobes, bilateral frontal lobes and corpus callosum, and cerebellum). In some patients the tumor was diffuse or multicentric. Two patients had multiple brain lesions.

A few patients, including one of our patients who had primary lymphoma of the brain, had exacerbations and remissions of neurological symptoms for 8 to 20 years, resulting in the initial diagnosis of a demyelinating disease.[73,74] These patients, 1 to 2 years prior to being diagnosed as having lymphoma in the brain, developed progressive neurological symptoms and signs. One patient had diffuse lymphoma in the brain stem, thalamus, and cerebellar vermis and peduncle. Another patient had a frontal lobe lymphoma.

PCNSL, as well as toxoplasmosis, bacterial abscess, and viral infections of the brain, should be included in the differential diagnosis of brain lesions in the setting of AIDS.

The clinical course of lymphoma of the brain may simulate cerebrovascular disease in approximately 7 percent of patients.[73] One such patient was 70 years old when she developed aphasia and a right homonymous hemianopsia.[73] Angiography was negative for a mass or abnormal vascularity. Postmortem examination revealed diffuse lymphoma in both frontal lobes, the corpus callosum, the basal ganglia, and the frontal horn of the lateral ventricle.

Primary lymphoma may occur in the meninges and may be manifested by a clinical course similar to that seen in patients with meningeal carcinomatosis or gliomatosis.[74] Patients with such a condition have a clinical course of 4 to 7 months during which they may develop headache, nausea, neck stiffness, multiple cranial nerve palsies, and spinal root and/or spinal cord involvement.

There are a few reports in the literature of the duration of life after appearance of the first symptom in patients with primary lymphoma of the brain who had only supportive care or no treatment at all. Twenty-four patients who did not undergo definitive treatment had symptoms 3 weeks to 21 months (mean, 5.6 months) prior to death.[11,73,74] Fifteen similar patients had symptoms an average of 3.3 months prior to death.[35]

Clinical Diagnosis and Staging

From the above, it is evident that the symptoms and neurological findings are not specific for PCNSL but are shared by other pathologic disorders of the CNS. PCNSL should be on the differential diagnosis list in a patient suspected of having a brain tumor, vascular lesion in the brain, encephalitis, spinal cord lesion, or leptomeningeal disease in the absence of symptoms or physical findings outside the CNS. PCNSL in the leptomeninges, vitreous, and retina may not be symptomatic; CSF and eye examination may be required to establish the diagnosis.

Patients recommended for PCNSL staging include three high risk groups: transplant recipients, congenitally immunodeficient persons, and AIDS patients.[36] Others are immunocompetent or have a past history of a malignant tumor.[13,36]

PCNSL staging recommended by Hochberg and coworkers[36] includes:

1. CT or MRI scan of the brain, without and with contrast.
2. Slit lamp examination of the eye.
3. CSF examination by lumbar puncture (in the absence of significant intracranial mass effect) for tumor lymphocytes bearing B-cell monoclonal immunocytologic markers.
4. Determination of HIV status.
5. Routine chest and abdomen CT and bone marrow examination have little value, since fewer than 5 percent of PCNSL patients have systemic lymphoma at the time of diagnosis.

DeAngelis and coworkers[15] staged 32 PCNSL patients and found that 19 percent had ocular involvement and 69 percent had definite or probable leptomeningeal lymphoma. The diagnosis may be established in some patients by CSF examination or aspiration of the vitreous. In many PCNSL patients, CT or MRI examination of the brain reveals parenchymal abnormalities that indicate the possibility of PCNSL. The diagnosis in those patients is established by brain biopsy.

Radiologic Features

Primary lymphoma of the brain can be solitary or multiple. Focal intracranial masses are the common initial presentation. Even though it is not always possible to distinguish lymphoma of the brain from glioblastoma or metastasis, these tumors have distinct imaging characteristics.

Primary lymphoma of the brain is commonly located in the basal ganglia, thalamus, corpus callosum, and periventricular white matter (Fig. 168-3*A*, *B*). The vermis and cerebellar hemispheres are less commonly involved. The supratentorial structures are involved in 75 to 85 percent of patients at initial presentation.[37] Up to 75 percent of lymphomatous masses are seen in contact with ependyma, meninges, or both.[40]

Magnetic Resonance Imaging

Advantages

MRI scanning of the brain has proved to be the imaging modality of choice for evaluation of intracranial pathology, especially because of its ability to localize and characterize intracranial neoplasms. With the use of an intravenous contrast agent—namely, gadolinium-DTPA—MRI has clearly claimed its superiority over CT. While CT is still useful in the evaluation of intracranial neoplasms, MRI has distinct advantages, such as (1) multiplanar capability; (2) more precise anatomic location of lesions; (3) lack of radiation; (4) ability to discern differences in tissue by variation in signal intensity; (5) ability to distinguish tumor necrosis from cyst; (6) ability to detect old blood not visible on CT; (7) sensitivity in the detection of subtle enhancement of tumors where CT fails to show enhancement, particularly in subtle leptomeningeal metastasis; and (8) usefulness in the differentiation of peritumoral edema from tumor, including the ability to detect vascular enhancement by tumor. More recently, three-dimensional MRI techniques have enabled the surgeon to plan an operative approach to intracranial masses and the radiation oncologist to plan radiotherapy. Also, MR angiography has proved a valuable replacement for the invasive routine cerebral angiography in the differentiation of vascular tumors from nonvascular tumors.

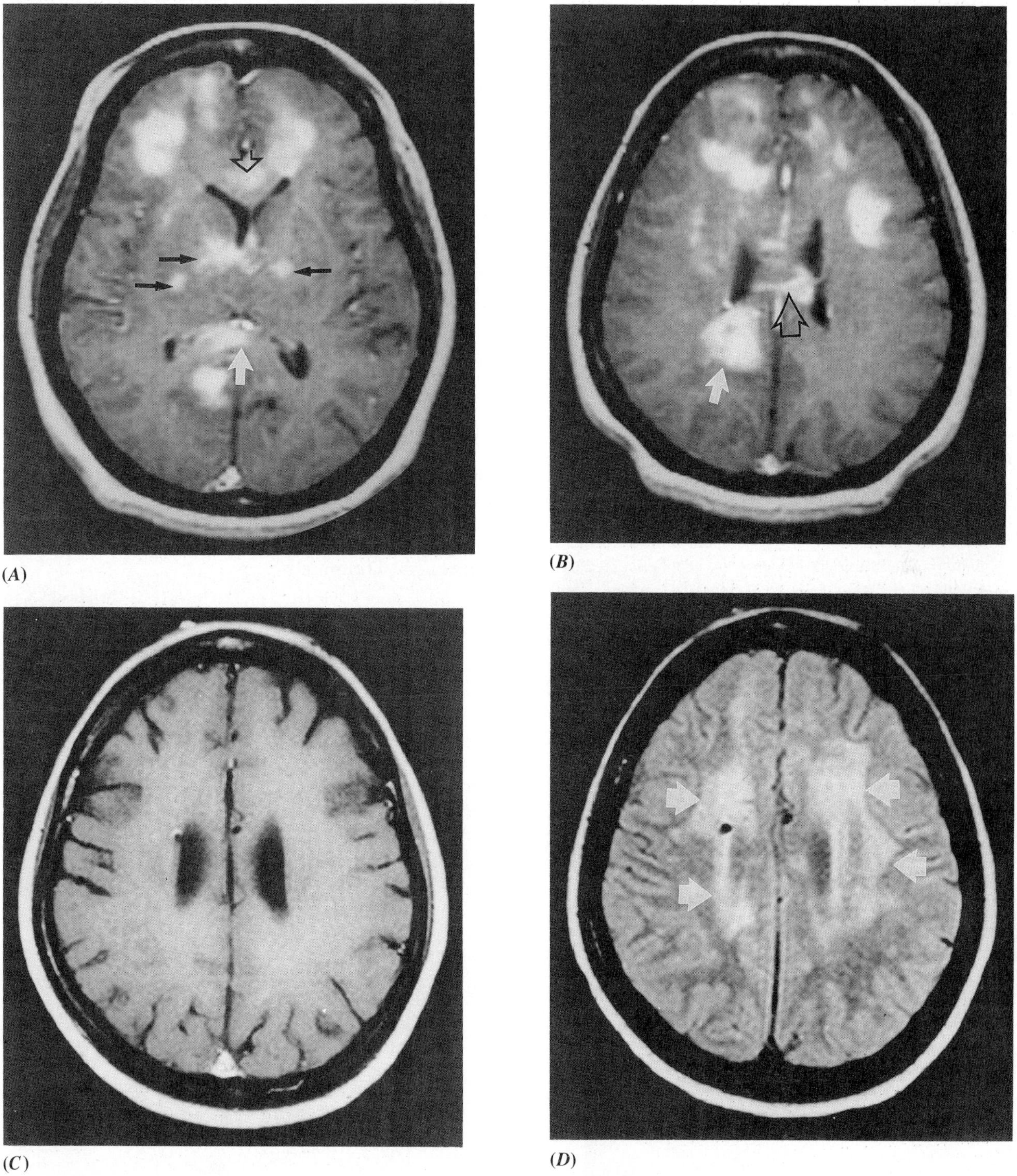

(*A*) (*B*) (*C*) (*D*)

Figure 168-3 Multicentric primary lymphoma of the brain seen on postcontrast MRI scans of the brain. *A*. T1-weighted image showing a section at the level of the frontal horns. Multiple enhancing masses of varying sizes are seen involving both frontal lobes, genu of the corpus callosum (*open arrow*), basal ganglia (*black arrows*), and splenium of the corpus callosum (*white arrow*). *B*. T1-weighted image showing a section at the level of the lateral ventricles. In addition to lymphomatous involvement of both frontoparietal lobes, the body of the corpus callosum (*open arrow*) and deep parietal periventricular white matter (*white arrow*) are seen to be involved. *C*. Follow-up postcontrast MRI scan at 3 months posttherapy (T1-weighted image). A section of the brain comparable to that seen in *B*. All lesions within the brain have disappeared completely. Mild hydrocephalus is present. *D*. Another follow-up scan at 3 months posttherapy (T2-weighted image). Radiation-induced periventricular leukoencephalopathy (*arrows*) is clearly visible in this sequence.

Signal Intensity

Lymphomatous masses are isointense to gray matter in all sequences, because of hypercellularity, but can be hyperintense in a T2-weighted pulse sequence.[3]

Pattern of Enhancement

Intense homogeneous enhancement is a common feature; however, heterogeneous enhancement with a central area of necrosis can be seen. Ring-like peripheral enhancement of tumor also can be seen.

Edema

The degree of edema is less than that seen with glioblastoma and metastatic lesions.[13]

Leptomeningeal Metastasis

Contrast MRI is directly superior to contrast CT in detecting leptomeningeal metastasis. However, MRI is less sensitive in detecting leptomeningeal metastasis from lymphoma or leukemia in patients with proven cytologic evidence of neoplastic seeding, compared with other causes of leptomeningeal metastasis. This discrepancy may be due to the lack of macroscopic invasion of the meninges by lymphoma.[85]

Computed Tomography

On noncontrast CT scan the lymphoma is seen as an area of increased density (Fig. 168-4*A*). Calcification and hemorrhage within the tumor are not features of lymphomas. Intravenously enhanced CT scanning can reveal intense enhancement of the tumor (Fig. 168-4*B*). The enhancement pattern of the tumor is usually homogeneous but can be heterogeneous with areas of necrosis (Fig. 168-5).

Diagnostic Patterns

Primary Lymphoma in AIDS Patients

In these patients lymphomas tend to be multifocal with ring enhancement and can have pronounced edema.

Secondary CNS Lymphoma

Involvement of dura (Fig. 168-6) and skull is more commonly seen in secondary lymphomas than in PCNSL.

Differential Diagnosis

The CT and MRI scan patterns of some PCNSLs can be confused with those of glioblastoma, metastasis, toxoplasmosis, and multi-

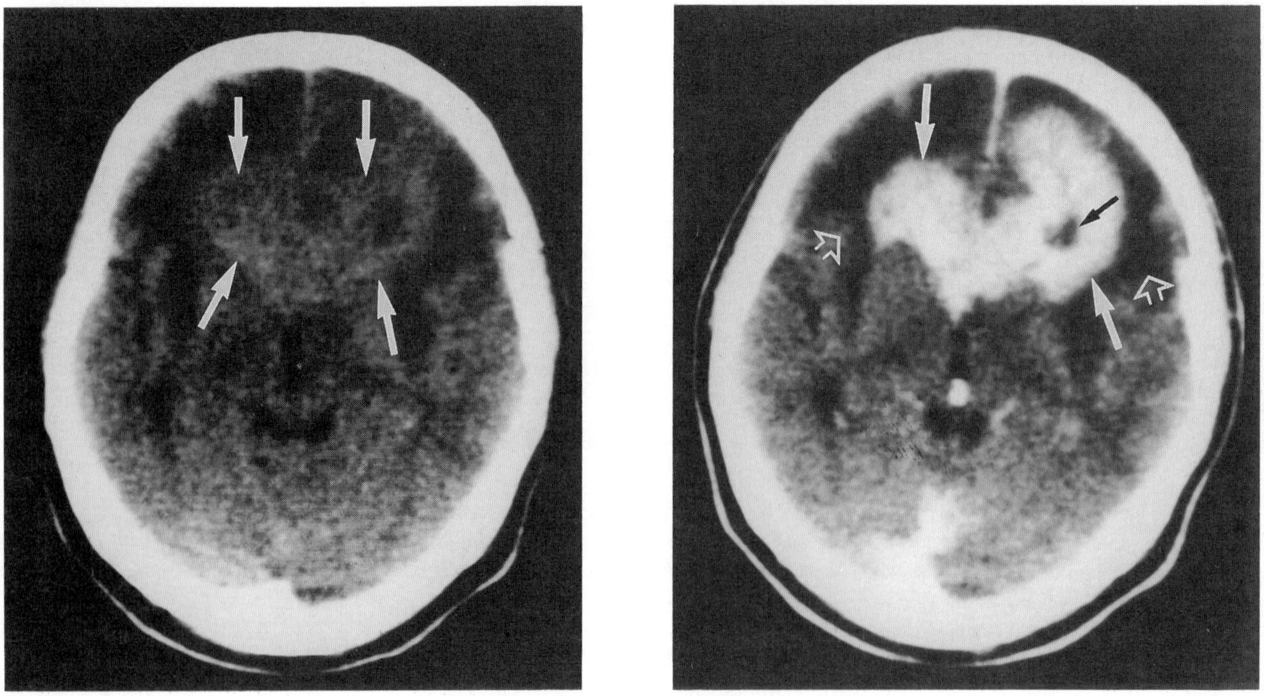

(*A*) (*B*)

Figure 168-4 Primary lymphoma involving both frontal lobes, spreading across the genu of the corpus callosum. *A*. Noncontrast CT. The tumor is slightly dense (*arrows*). *B*. Contrast CT. The tumor intensity enhances with contrast (*arrows*) except for small focal areas of cystic degeneration (*black arrow*). There is relatively less edema (*open arrows*) for the large size of the tumor. Glioblastoma can give rise to a similar appearance.

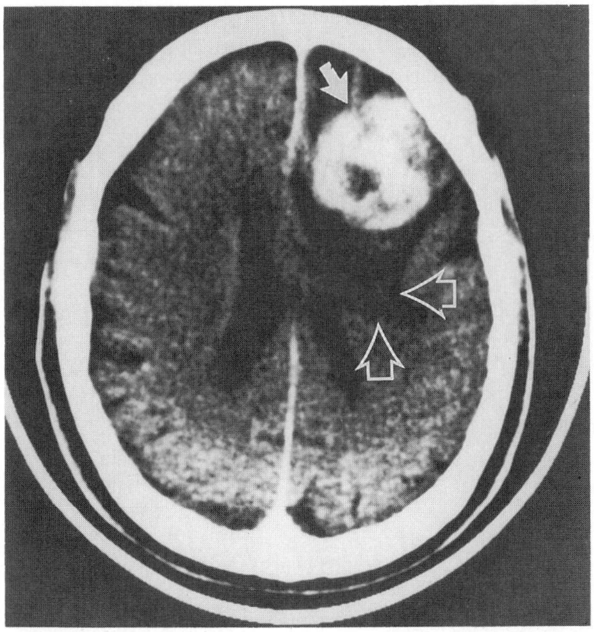

(*A*)

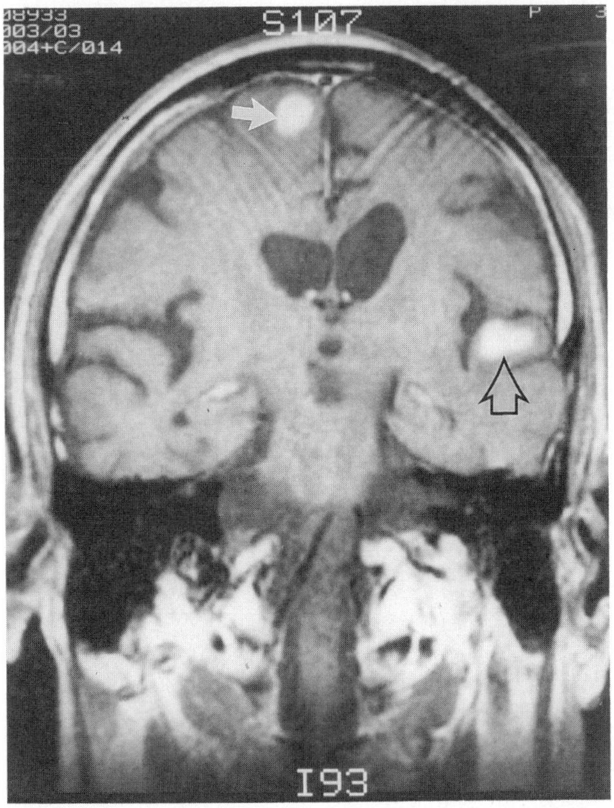

(*B*)

Figure 168-5 Lymphoma resembling metastasis. *A*. Enhanced CT. A solitary well-defined enhancing mass (*arrow*) with central necrosis is seen within the left frontal lobe, with a moderate degree of edema (*open arrows*). *B*. Postcontrast coronal MRI taken 15 months later, after therapy. The original lesion has disappeared. Two new enhancing lesions have appeared in the right parietal lobe (*arrow*) and left temporal lobe (*open arrow*).

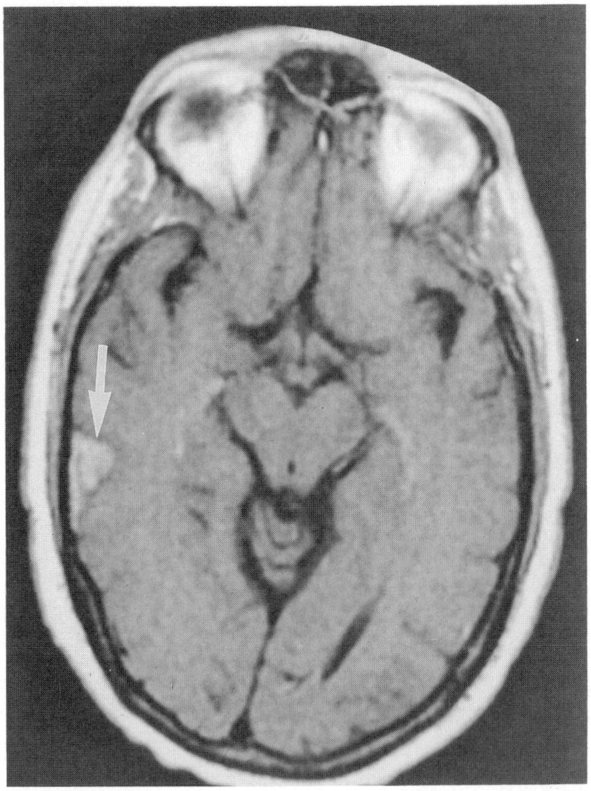

Figure 168-6 Durally based secondary lymphoma of the brain mimicking meningioma, seen on a postcontrast axial T1-weighted MRI scan. A dural-based enhancing mass is seen involving the right temporal lobe (*arrow*). Meningioma was excluded on the basis of lack of hyperostosis of adjacent bone and relatively lesser degree of enhancement of tumor.

ple sclerosis. Dural-based lymphomas can mimic meningiomas. However, if one sees one or multiple intensely enhancing masses along the periventricular location with relatively little edema, the diagnosis of lymphoma should be entertained and a stereotactic biopsy should be recommended.

Glioblastoma and metastasis tend to have moderate-to-severe edema with mass effect on adjacent structures. Toxoplasmosis lesions are not dense on noncontrast CT scan and they exhibit peripheral ring enhancement. Unlike lymphoma, subependymal spread and ventricular capping are not seen in toxoplasmosis nor in multiple sclerosis. MRI is also useful in evaluating the response to therapy (Figs. 168-3*C* and *D*, 168-5*B*).

The Neurosurgeon's Role in the Management of PCNSL

Hochberg and coworkers[36] use corticosteroids in PCNSL patients to reduce morbidity and tumor burden. These tumors are steroid-sensitive. Commonly, 24 mg of dexamethasone is given daily. Within hours the brain lesions may be reduced or may disappear as tumor cells are killed. Eighty percent of patients benefit within 5 days of treatment. The benefits of steroids tend to disappear within 6 months of treatment but may last longer. The tumor will reappear within 1 week after the corticosteroids are discontinued.[36,38,70,76,81,84]

Steroids may be so effective against these tumors that their use prior to brain biopsy may eliminate the possibility of establishing the diagnosis with certainty. DeAngelis and coworkers[16] recommend withholding corticosteroids prior to biopsy in a patient suspected of having PCNSL, unless herniation is imminent.

The results of treating patients who have primary lymphoma in the brain by surgery alone are available in a few reports in the literature.[11,20,35,74] The postoperative survival of 12 patients was between 1 day and 9 months (mean, 1.4 months).[11,20,74] In another report, the mean postoperative survival of 28 patients was 4.6 months.[35] The results are poor and substantiate the opinion that patients with primary lymphoma in the brain require additional postoperative treatment for improved tumor control.

The main role of the surgeon in patients suspected of having PCNSL is in establishing the diagnosis by CT, MRI, or ultrasound-guided brain biopsy. Total removal of PCNSL is not possible, because of the invasive nature and deep locations of these tumors. Attempts at total removal increase the risk of permanent postoperative neurological deficit.[16,48] Subtotal removal does not add to survival; it should be considered only in patients with imminent herniation and in selected patients who do not respond to, or have recurrent tumor following, chemotherapy and radiotherapy. The placement of a frontal Ommaya reservoir[46] to administer methotrexate into the ventricles is recommended as part of the management of PCNSL by DeAngelis and coworkers.[16]

Radiotherapy

Primary brain lymphoma responds quickly and effectively to external radiation. Complete responses, based on follow-up CT scanning, were found in 80 percent of patients treated in a prospective protocol by the Radiation Therapy Oncology Group.[62] Yet this tumor behaves differently from other extranodal lymphomas, in that recurrence within the radiation field is the rule rather than the exception. Patterns of failure were reviewed for 254 patients reported in 11 publications.[62] Local failure in the brain occurred in 79 percent, and only 7 percent had failure outside the CNS. Isolated failure in the spinal cord or spinal fluid happened in 4 percent of patients. The high local failure rate led to early death and resulted in a median survival of 1 to 2 years in most patients. Prognosis was shown to be better for patients under age 60 and for patients with higher performance levels.[56,62,66] A total radiation dose of more than 50 Gy was also found to improve survival.[53]

The optimal volume to be irradiated depends on the nature of the tumor and the tolerance of the critical normal tissue. Primary brain lymphoma has a tendency to multicentricity, deep paraventricular invasion, and involvement of meninges. For these reasons, whole brain radiation including the base of the skull and all cranial meninges is required. The eyes are included in this field only if they are found to be involved on ophthalmologic examination.[53,56] Elective irradiation of the spinal cord and meninges is not justified, because of the low recurrence rate there as compared to the high recurrence rate at the primary site. Furthermore, the bone marrow toxicity inherent in total spine irradiation significantly lowers the tolerance for chemotherapy. The recommended dose to the whole brain is 40 to 45 Gy, at 1.8 to 2 Gy per fraction. A boost to the volume of the initial tumor is added, to achieve a total tumor dose of 55 to 60 Gy. When required by involvement, the eyes and the spine are treated to doses of 40 Gy.

The ever-growing subgroup of patients with AIDS and primary brain lymphoma deserves special attention. Their prognosis is significantly worse than that of patients with brain lymphoma without AIDS, and their results have to be reported separately. The lymphoma of AIDS patients also responds well to radiation therapy both clinically and radiologically.[7,21,27] Nevertheless, mean survival was only 2.5 months or 5.5 months.[21,27] In spite of this short-term palliation, patients who had no radiation did much worse.[7] Autopsy findings showed that patients who did not receive radiation died of tumor progression, whereas those who completed radiation died of opportunistic infections.

The same guidelines for radiation therapy apply also to AIDS patients with brain lymphomas. Hypofractionation, with abbreviation of the total treatment time, should be considered in poor-prognosis AIDS patients.

At present, the treatment of primary brain lymphoma with radiation alone remains disappointing. Radiation treatment in this disease is generally insufficient to achieve long-term local control of the tumor.

Chemotherapy

Because of the generally poor long-term results with radiotherapy (XRT) only,[15,24,63] and the high rate of local failure, considerable attention has been focused recently on the role of systemic chemotherapy in the treatment of PCNSL. Several reports have suggested improved survival when chemotherapy is added to XRT. Areas of ongoing research include the impact of the blood-brain barrier (BBB), the consequent choice of active chemotherapeutic agents, the possible long-term sequelae of combined chemotherapy-XRT, and the daunting problem of devising effective and tolerable therapy for patients with PCNSL in the setting of AIDS.

The BBB is disrupted in the presence of active CNS neoplasm, but fairly quickly becomes intact once initial tumor control occurs.[64] Hence, regimens known to be effective against systemic lymphoma, such as CHOP (cyclophosphamide, doxorubicin, vincristine, and prednisone), have been found to be effective in PCNSL. But partly because of concerns about reestablishment of the BBB, reliance on chemotherapy alone has been infrequent; most regimens for PCNSL that start with chemotherapy make an early crossover to XRT.

One approach that has focused on the independent role of the chemotherapy is that of Neuwelt and coworkers. They have disrupted the BBB with intra-arterial mannitol, and delivered intravenous cyclophosphamide, intra-arterial high-dose methotrexate (HD-MTX), and oral procarbazine and dexamethasone on a monthly basis for 12 courses to a group of 30 patients with PCNSL.[63] Thirteen of the patients had received prior XRT; for the other 17, chemotherapy alone was used and XRT was reserved for cases of incomplete response or progression. Of the 30, there were 2 early deaths from sepsis and 1 early withdrawal by patient choice. The remaining 27 had a complete remission (CR) rate of 70 percent, and the others achieved partial remission. While the majority of patients who had chemotherapy alone have relapsed and subsequently received XRT, 5 patients have remained in remission following BBB-disruption chemotherapy alone. Moreover, the medial survival of the 17 patients treated with primary chemotherapy was 44 months, an apparent improvement over XRT approaches. BBB disruption and intra-arterial chemotherapy may be effective, but it is not used by others, because it is believed to be cumbersome and may be associated with significant toxicity. Another objection is that therapy is delivered only within the disrupted BBB arterial territory.[16]

The more common and technically simpler chemotherapy approach has been to employ regimens based on agents that can cross the BBB. Hochberg and coworkers have recently updated their experience with HD-MTX prior to XRT.[36] Of 22 patients treated, two-thirds were found to achieve CR before XRT, and the remainder responded partially. With a median follow-up of over 2 years, the median survival is greater than 37 months. Similarly, DeAngelis and coworkers have updated the Memorial Sloan-Kettering experience with 31 patients treated with intravenous and intraventricular MTX and dexamethasone prior to XRT, followed by high-dose cytosine arabinoside (ara C) after XRT, which has resulted in a median survival of 42 months. Intraventricular MTX is given to deliver adequate chemotherapy to the CSF in all patients whether or not they have proven leptomeningeal disease.[15] Other, smaller, series have also reported encouraging results with regimens based on drugs that cross the BBB. McLaughlin and coworkers, at the M.D. Anderson Cancer Center, reported a high response rate with the DHAP (dexamethasone, high-dose ara C, and cisplatin) regimen in 10 patients with parenchymal brain lymphoma, 4 of whom had PCNSL.[55] Of these 4 patients, 2 remain in continuous CR for over 5 years, including one who was managed with primary chemotherapy alone (Fig. 168-7). The PCV (procarbazine, CCNU, and vincristine) regimen has been used as adjuvant therapy following XRT, and apparent prolongation of remission has been noted.[12]

When MTX follows CNS XRT in children, there is a well-established risk of leukoencephalopathy; the addition of intrathecal MTX increases this risk.[8] CNS toxicity has similarly been observed in patients with PCNSL following XRT and MTX.[9,51] When HD-MTX is used without XRT, the risk of leukoencephalopathy is probably quite low, but close spacing of doses and sustained CNS MTX levels may increase the risk.[2] Largely because of these concerns, the most common current use of MTX is prior to XRT; a finite number of doses are employed (usually two or three). With this sequence the risk of leukoencephalopathy is believed to be quite low, but long-term follow-up is limited.

The inclusion of chemotherapy for patients with AIDS-related PCNSL is problematic. Among AIDS patients with systemic lymphoma, intensive chemotherapy can be employed without excessive toxicity in some patients,[49] but the morbidity and mortality of therapy is significantly higher in patients with poor performance status, a prior history of opportunistic infections, and low CD4 cell counts.[43] Since the majority of patients with AIDS-related PCNSL have poor performance status and often have had AIDS-defining opportunistic infections before their lymphoma,[68] the experience with chemotherapy in AIDS-related PCNSL has been limited and predictably bad. Directions for the future include improvements in supportive care, such as the integration of colony stimulating factors, the development of therapies that are less immunosuppressive (such as targeted therapies), and, of course, advances in the therapy of the underlying AIDS.

Most patients with PCNSL have parenchymal brain disease, but some present with meningeal disease, making intrathecal chemotherapy a major consideration. Meningeal disease as the only manifestation of PCNSL is rare but has been well described. The frequency of meningeal involvement along with parenchymal brain disease is somewhat difficult to estimate, since in many series CSF analysis is avoided because of concern about increased intracranial pressure. For those series in which CSF analysis is done, the reported rate of positive cytology ranges from rare[37] to as high as 60 to 77 percent,[9] so a conservative estimate of about 30 percent is reasonable. When present, meningeal lymphoma is most commonly managed with intraventricular therapy via an Ommaya reservoir. A common practice is to instill MTX 12 to 15 mg twice weekly until the CSF is clear, then weekly for 1 month, then

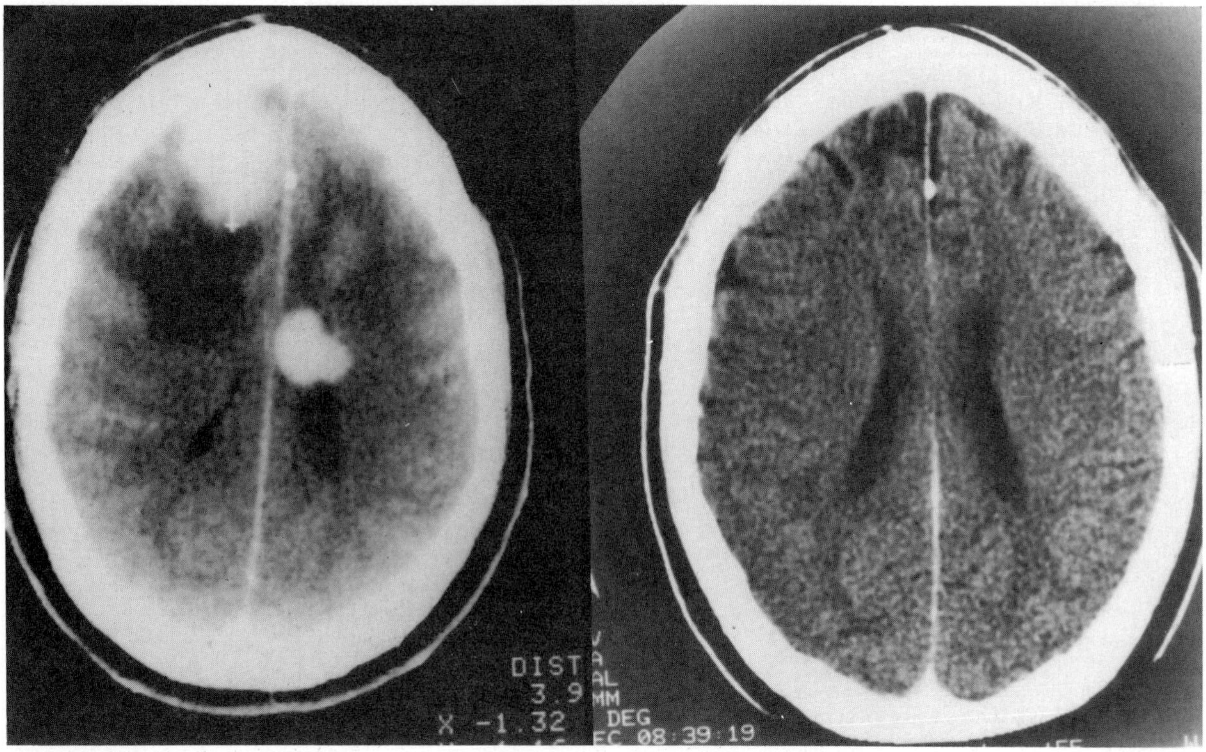

Figure 168-7 CT of the brain before therapy (*left panel*) and after two cycles of DHAP (*right panel*). This patient has been in continuous remission for 5 years. (From McLaughlin et al.,[55] with permission.)

monthly for 1 to 2 years. On the basis of pediatric experience with meningeal leukemia, it may be preferable to use a three-drug combination of MTX, cytosine arabinoside, and hydrocortisone.[79] For adults, intraventricular doses of MTX 15 mg, cytosine arabinoside 75 mg, and hydrocortisone 15 mg have been used in combination.[78]

DeAngelis and coworkers suggest that if chemotherapy can be improved substantially, PCNSL may become the first primary malignant brain tumor to be cured by chemotherapy alone.[16]

References

1. Adams JH. The classification of microgliomatosis with particular reference to diffuse microgliomatosis. *Acta Neuropathol (Berl) [Suppl].* 1975; 6:119–123.
2. Allen JC, Rosen G, Mehta BM, Horten B. Leukoencephalopathy following high-dose IV methotrexate chemotherapy with leucovorin rescue. *Cancer Treat Rep* 1980; 64:1261–1273.
3. Atlas SW. Intraaxial brain tumors. In Atlas SW (ed): *Magnetic Resonance Imaging of the Brain and Spine.* New York: Raven Press, 1991, pp 223–326.
4. Bailey P. Intracranial sarcomatous tumors of leptomeningeal origin. *Arch Surg* 1929; 18:1359–1402.
5. Bale JF Jr, Wilson JF, Hill HR. Fatal histiocytic lymphoma of the brain associated with hyperimmunoglobulinemia-E and recurrent infections. *Cancer* 1977; 39:2386–2390.
6. Barnard RO, Scott T. Patterns of proliferation in cerebral lymphoreticular tumours. *Acta Neuropathol (Berl) [Suppl]* 1975; 6:125–130.
7. Baumgartner JE, Rachlin JR, Beckstead JH, et al. Primary central nervous system lymphomas: natural history and response to radiation therapy in 55 patients with acquired immunodeficiency syndrome. *J Neurosurg* 1990; 73(2):206–211.
8. Bleyer WA. The clinical pharmacology of methotrexate: new applications of an old drug. *Cancer* 1978; 41:36–51.
9. Bogdahn U, Bogdahn S, Mertens HG, et al. Primary non-Hodgkin's lymphomas of the CNS. *Acta Neurol Scand* 1986; 73:602–614.
10. Bruni J, Bilbao JM, Gray T. Primary intramedullary malignant lymphoma of the spinal cord. *Neurology (Minneap)* 1977; 27:896–898.
11. Burstein SD, Kernohan JW, Uihlein A. Neoplasms of the reticuloendothelial system of the brain. *Cancer* 1963; 16:289–305.
12. Chamberlain MC, Levin VA. Adjuvant chemotherapy for primary lymphoma of the central nervous system. *Arch Neurol* 1990; 47:1113–1116.
13. DeAngelis LM. Primary central nervous system lymphoma: a new clinical challenge. *Neurology* 1991; 41:619–621.
14. DeAngelis LM. Primary central nervous system lymphoma as a secondary malignancy. *Cancer* 1991; 67:1431–1435.
15. DeAngelis LM, Yahalom J, Heinemann MH, et al. Primary CNS lymphoma: Combined treatment with chemotherapy and radiotherapy. *Neurology* 1990; 40:80–86.
16. DeAngelis LM, Yahalom J, Thaler HT, Kher U. Combined modality therapy for primary CNS lymphoma. *J Clin Oncol* 1992; 10(4):635–643.
17. Ebels EJ. Reticulosarcomas of the brain presenting as butterfly tumors: possible implications for treatment. *Eur Neurol* 1972; 8:333–338.
18. Eby NL, Grufferman S, Flannelly CM, et al. Increasing incidence of primary brain lymphoma in the U.S. *Cancer* 1988; 62:2461–2465.
19. Epstein AL, Herman MM, Kim H, Dorfman RF, Kaplan HS. Biology of the human malignant lymphomas: III. Intracranial heterotransplantation in the nude, athymic mouse. *Cancer* 1976; 37:2158–2176.
20. Foncin JF, Faucher JN. Primary and borderline brain lymphosarcoma: a neuropathological review of nine cases. *Acta Neuropathol (Berl) [Suppl]* 1975; 6:107–113.
21. Formenti SC, Gill PS, Lean E, et al. Primary central nervous system lymphoma in AIDS. Results of radiation therapy. *Cancer* 1989; 63(6):1101–1107.
22. Freeman C, Berg JW, Cutler SJ. Occurrence and prognosis of extranodal lymphomas. *Cancer* 1972; 29:252–260.
23. Frizzera G, Rosai J, Dehner LP, et al. Lymphoreticular disorders in primary immunodeficiencies: new findings based on an up-to-date histologic classification of 35 cases. *Cancer* 1980; 46:692–699.
24. Gabbai AA, Hochberg FH, Lingood R, et al. High-dose methotrexate for non-AIDS primary central nervous system lymphoma: report of 13 cases. *J Neurosurg* 1989; 70:190–194.
25. Giovanella B, Nilsson K, Zech L, et al. Growth of diploid, Epstein-Barr virus–carrying human lymphoblastoid cell lines heterotransplanted into nude mice under immunologically privileged conditions. *Int J Cancer* 1979; 24:103–113.
26. Giromini D, Peiffer J, Tzonos T. Occurrence of a primary Burkitt-type lymphoma of the central nervous system in an astrocytoma patient. *Acta Neuropathol (Berl)* 1981; 54:165–167.
27. Goldstein JD, Dickson DW, Moser FG, et al. Primary central nervous system lymphoma in acquired immune deficiency syndrome: a clinical and pathologic study with results of treatment with radiation. *Cancer* 1991; 67:2756–2765.
28. Gregory MC, Hughes JT. Intracranial reticulum cell sarcoma associated with immunoglobulin A deficiency. *J Neurol Neurosurg Psychiatry* 1973; 36:769–776.
29. Gunderson CH, Henry J, Malamud N. Plasma globulin determinations in patients with microglioma: report of five cases. *J Neurosurg* 1971; 35:406–415.
30. Hamilton-Dutoit SJ, Pallesen G, Franzmann MB, et al. AIDS-related lymphoma: histopathology, immunophenotype, and association with Epstein-Barr virus as demonstrated by in situ nucleic acid hybridization. *Am J Pathol* 1991; 138:149–163.
31. Hanbery JW, Dugger GS. Perithelial sarcoma of the brain: a clinicopathological study of thirteen cases. *Arch Neurol Psychiatry* 1954; 71:732–761.
32. Hanto DW, Frizzera G, Purtilo DT, et al. Clinical spectrum of lymphoproliferative disorders in renal transplant recipients and evidence for the role of Epstein-Barr virus. *Cancer Res* 1981; 41:4253–4261.
33. Hassoun J, Andrac L, Gambarelli D, Toga M. Lymphomes malins primitifs du systeme nerveux central: etude anatomoclinique, ultrastructurale et immunocytochimique. A propos de 23 cas. *Ann Pathol* 1981; 1:193–203.
34. Heidelberger KP, LeGolvan DP. Wiskott-Aldrich syndrome and cerebral neoplasia: report of a case with localized reticulum cell sarcoma. *Cancer* 1974; 33:280–284.
35. Henry JM, Heffner RR Jr, Dillard SH, et al. Primary malignant lymphomas of the central nervous system. *Cancer* 1974; 34:1293–1302.
36. Hochberg FH, Loeffler JS, Prados M. The therapy of primary brain lymphoma. *J Neurooncol* 1991; 10:191–201.
37. Hochberg FH, Miller DC. Primary central nervous system lymphoma. *J Neurosurg* 1988; 68:835–853.
38. Homo-Delarche F. Glucocorticoid receptors and steroid sensitivity in normal and neoplastic human lymphoid tissues: a review. *Cancer Res* 1984; 44:431–437.
39. Houthoff HJ, Poppema S, Ebels EJ, Elema JD. Intracranial malignant lymphomas: a morphologic and immunocytologic study of twenty cases. *Acta Neuropathol (Berl)* 1978; 44:203–210.
40. Jack CR Jr, O'Neill BP, Banks PM, Reese DF. Central nervous system lymphoma: histologic types and CT appearance. *Radiology* 1988; 167:211–215.
41. Jellinger K, Kothbauer P, Weiss R, Sunder-Plassmann E. Primary malignant lymphoma of the CNS and polyneuropathy in a patient with necrotizing vasculitis treated with immunosuppression. *J Neurol* 1979; 220:259–268.
42. Jellinger K, Radaskiewicz TH, Slowik F. Primary malignant lymphomas of the central nervous system in man. *Acta Neuropathol (Berl)* [Suppl] 1975; 6:95–102.
43. Kaplan LD, Abrams DI, Feigal E, et al. AIDS-associated non-Hodgkin's lymphoma in San Francisco. *JAMA* 1989; 261:719–724.

44. Kernohan JW, Uihlein A. *Sarcomas of the Brain.* Springfield, IL: Charles C Thomas, 1962.
45. Kinney TD, Adams RD. Reticulum cell sarcoma of the brain. *Arch Neurol Psychiatry* 1943; 50:552–564.
46. Leavens ME, Aldama-Luebert A. Ommaya reservoir placement: technical note. *Neurosurgery* 1979; 5:264–266.
47. Letendre L, Banks PM, Reese DF, et al. Primary lymphoma of the central nervous system. *Cancer* 1982; 49:939–943.
48. Littman P, Wang CC. Reticulum cell sarcoma of the brain. *Cancer* 1975; 35:1412–1420.
49. Lopez TM, Hagemeister FB, McLaughlin P, et al. Small noncleaved cell lymphoma in adults: superior results for stages I–III disease. *J Clin Oncol* 1990; 8:615–622.
50. Lukin R, Tomsick TA, Chambers AA. Lymphoma and leukemia of the central nervous system. *Semin Roentgenol* 1980; 15:246–250.
51. Mackintosh FR, Colby TV, Podolsky WJ, et al. Central nervous system involvement in non-Hodgkin's lymphoma: an analysis of 105 cases. *Cancer* 1982; 49:586–595.
52. MacMahon EME, Glass JD, Hayward SD, et al. Epstein-Barr virus in AIDS-related primary central nervous system lymphoma. *Lancet* 1991; 338:969–973.
53. Maiuri F. Visual involvement in primary non-Hodgkins's lymphomas. *Clin Neurol Neurosurg* 1990; 92(2):119–124.
54. Matas AJ, Hertel BF, Rosai J, et al. Post-transplant malignant lymphoma. *Am J Med* 1976; 61:716–720.
55. McLaughlin P, Velasquez WS, Redman JR, et al. Chemotherapy, with dexamethasone, high-dose cytarabine, and cisplatin for parenchymal brain lymphoma. *J Natl Cancer Inst* 1988; 80:1408–1412.
56. Michalski JM, Garcia DM, Kase E, et al. Primary central nervous system lymphoma: analysis of prognostic variables and patterns of treatment failure. *Radiology* 1990; 176:855–860.
57. Mitsumoto H, Breuer AC, Lederman RJ. Malignant lymphoma of the central nervous system: a case of primary spinal intramedullary involvement. *Cancer* 1980; 46:1258–1262.
58. Miyoshi I, Kubonishi I, Yoshimoto S, et al. Characteristics of a brain lymphoma cell line derived from primary intracranial lymphoma. *Cancer* 1982; 49:456–459.
59. Model LM. Primary reticulum cell sarcoma of the brain in Wiskott-Aldrich syndrome: report of a case. *Arch Neurol* 1977; 34:633–635.
60. Morgello S. Epstein-Barr and human immunodeficiency viruses in acquired immunodeficiency syndrome-related primary central nervous system lymphoma. *Am J Pathol* 1992; 141:441–450.
61. Nakhleh RE, Manivel JC, Hurd D, Sung JH. Central nervous system lymphomas. Immunohistochemical and clinicopathologic study of 26 autopsy cases. *Arch Pathol Lab Med* 1988; 113:1050–1056.
62. Nelson DF, Martz KL, Bonner H, et al. Non-Hodgkin's lymphoma of the brain: can high dose, large volume radiation therapy improve survival? Report on a prospective trial by the radiation therapy oncology group (RTOG): RTOG 8315. *Int J Radiat Oncol Biol Phys* 1992; 23:9–17.
63. Neuwelt EA, Goldman DL, Dahlberg SA, et al. Primary CNS lymphoma treated with osmotic blood-brain barrier disruption: prolonged survival and preservation of cognitive function. *J Clin Oncol* 1991; 9:1580–1590.
64. Ott RJ, Brada M, Flower MA, et al. Measurements of blood-brain barrier permeability in patients undergoing radiotherapy and chemotherapy for primary cerebral lymphoma. *Eur J Cancer* 1991; 27:1356–1361.
65. Pattengale PK, Taylor CR, Panke T, et al. Selective immunodeficiency and malignant lymphoma of the central nervous system. *Acta Neuropathol (Berl)* 1979; 48:165–169.
66. Pollack IF, Lunsford DL, Flickinger JC, Dameshek HL. Prognostic factors in the diagnosis and treatment of primary central nervous system lymphoma. *Cancer* 1989; 63:939–947.
67. Purtilo DT. Epstein-Barr-virus–induced oncogenesis in immune-deficient individuals. *Lancet* 1980; 1:300–303.
68. Remick SC, Diamond C, Migliozzi JA, et al. Primary central nervous system lymphoma in patients with and without the acquired immune deficiency syndrome: a retrospective analysis and review of the literature. *Medicine (Baltimore)* 1990; 69:345–360.
69. Rubinstein LJ. *Tumors of the Central Nervous System.* Washington, D.C.: Armed Forces Institute of Pathology, 1972, pp 215–234.
70. Ruff RL, Petito CK, Rawlinson DG. Primary cerebral lymphoma mimicking multiple sclerosis. *Arch Neurol* 1979; 36:598.
71. Russell DS, Marshall AHE, Smith FB. Microgliomatosis: a form of reticulosis affecting the brain. *Brain* 1948; 71:1–15.
72. Saemundsen AK, Purtilo DT, Sakamoto K, et al. Documentation of Epstein-Barr virus infection in immunodeficient patients with life-threatening lymphoproliferative diseases by Epstein-Barr virus complementary RNA/DNA and viral DNA/DNA hybridization. *Cancer Res* 1981; 41:4237–4242.
73. Samuelsson SM, Werner I, Ponten J, et al. Reticuloendothelial (perivascular) sarcoma of the brain. *Acta Neurol Scand* 1966; 42:567–580.
74. Schaumburg HH, Plank CR, Adams RD. The reticulum cell sarcoma–microglioma group of brain tumours: a consideration of their clinical features and therapy. *Brain* 1972; 95:199–212.
75. Schneck SA, Penn I. De-novo brain tumours in renal-transplant recipients. *Lancet* 1971; 1:983–986.
76. Singh A, Strobos RJ, Singh BM, et al. Steroid-induced remissions in CNS lymphoma. *Neurology* 1982; 32:1267–1271.
77. Sparling HJ Jr, Adams RD. Primary Hodgkin's sarcoma of the brain. *Arch Pathol* 1946; 42:338–344.
78. Stewart DJ, Maroun JA, Hugenholtz H, et al. Combined intraommaya methotrexate, cytosine arabinoside, hydrocortisone and thio-TEPA for meningeal involvement by malignancies. *J Neurooncol* 1987; 5:315–322.
79. Sullivan MP, Moon TE, Trueworthy R, et al. Combination intrathecal therapy for meningeal leukemia: two versus three drugs. *Blood* 1977; 50:471–479.
80. Taylor CR, Russell R, Lukes RJ, Davis RL. An immunohistological study of immunoglobulin content of primary central nervous system lymphomas. *Cancer* 1978; 41:2197–2205.
81. Vaguero J, Martinez R, Rossi E, et al. Primary cerebral lymphoma: the "ghost tumor." case report. *J Neurosurg* 1984; 60:174–176.
82. Varadachari C, Palutke M, Climie ARW, et al. Immunoblastic sarcoma (histiocytic lymphoma) of the brain with B cell markers: case report. *J Neurosurg* 1978; 49:887–892.
83. Warnke R, Miller R, Grogan T, et al. Immunologic phenotype in 30 patients with diffuse large-cell lymphoma. *N Engl J Med* 1980; 303:293–300.
84. Williams RS, Crowell RM, Fisher CM, et al. Clinical and radiologic remission in reticulum cell sarcoma of the brain. *Arch Neurol* 1979; 36:206–210
85. Yousem DM, Patrone PM, Grossman RI. Leptomeningeal metastases: MR evaluation. *J Comput Assist Tomogr* 1990; 14:255–261.
86. Yuile CL. Case of primary reticulum cell sarcoma of the brain. Relationship of microglia cells to histiocytes. *Arch Pathol* 1938; 26:1036–1044.
87. Zimmerman HM. Malignant lymphomas of the nervous system. *Acta Neuropathol (Berl) [Suppl]* 1975; 6:69–74.

169

Intracranial Sarcomas

Mark Bernstein
John H. N. Deck
J. F. Ross Fleming

Intracranial sarcomas are uncommon, representing only 1 to 2 percent of all intracranial neoplasms. Because this group of tumors is so rare, and because the pathologic description of sarcomas in the brain and at other sites seems to be changing,[13] their nature has not been well understood. Early classifications were somewhat confusing and included several tumors no longer considered to be sarcomas.

The most common intracranial sarcoma that a neurosurgeon is likely to encounter is gliosarcoma, which is a sarcoma arising in continuity with a malignant glioma and occuring in up to 8 percent of malignant gliomas.[17] Other intracranial sarcomas include sarcoma arising in meningioma, sarcoma induced by ionizing radiation, and primary sarcoma arising *de novo* in the brain and meninges; this last sarcoma is exceedingly rare, and occurs most commonly in infants and children.[7,24] In this chapter we present a simple working classification of intracranial sarcomas and review their pathologic features. The clinical features and management will be reviewed briefly, although most of the clinical features of intracranial sarcomas are shared by other more common malignant neoplasms and are not particularly distinctive.

Classification

Intracranial sarcomas may be classified according to their site of origin as (1) sarcomas arising in the brain, meninges, and cranial nerves; (2) primary sarcomas of the skull; or (3) metastatic sarcomas of the brain, secondary to primary sarcomas elsewhere in the body. Only sarcomas arising in the brain and meninges will be considered in this chapter.

Sarcomas of the brain and meninges are those malignant tumors that arise from the mesenchymal tissues present within the cranial cavity, that is, from dura mater, from pia-arachnoid, from blood vessels of the subarachnoid space and brain, and from the tela choroidea. They can be classified into four groups.

1. Primary sarcoma of the brain and meninges arising *de novo*
2. Sarcoma arising in continuity with malignant glioma (gliosarcoma)
3. Sarcoma arising in meningioma
4. Sarcoma arising after cranial irradiation.

Sarcomas arising from the skull and presenting as intracranial tumors are discussed separately in another chapter. Also excluded from this chapter are the rare sarcomas that are metastatic to the brain; these tumors have few clinical features to distinguish them from other metastatic tumors and they are discussed elsewhere. Primary lymphoma of the central nervous system, formerly referred to as reticulum cell sarcoma, is a highly distinctive tumor which shares few features with the nonlymphoreticular sarcomas; it is therefore excluded from this chapter and is discussed in another chapter. Also excluded are the rare examples of malignant tumors arising from cranial nerves, such as malignant schwannomas and neurofibrosarcomas.

There are, in addition, some highly undifferentiated tumors that in the past were classified as sarcomas by some pathologists, but for which alternative designations are now widely preferred. These tumors include the ''circumscribed sarcoma of the cerebellum'' and ''monstrocellular sarcoma.'' The circumscribed sarcoma of the cerebellum was classified as a sarcoma because of its prominent reticulin formation; however, it is now generally accepted as a subtype of medulloblastoma that has stimulated leptomeningeal proliferation or desmoplasia. The monstrocellular sarcoma was so-called because of the prominence of reticulin and of vascular structures. The nature of its giant cells was quite uncertain until their glial nature was demonstrated by stains for glial fibrillary acidic protein (GFAP); this tumor is now widely accepted as a giant cell variant of glioblastoma multiforme. The use of GFAP as a glial cell marker has resulted in the reclassification of yet another tumor, ''meningeal fibrous xanthosarcoma,'' which has proved to be a pleomorphic xanthoastrocytoma and not a sarcoma.

Primary Sarcoma of the Brain and Meninges

Primary sarcomas arising *de novo* in the meninges or brain constitute fewer than 1 percent of all intracranial tumors; Paulus et al. reported the incidence as only 0.1 percent based on a retrospective review of 25,000 brain tumor biopsies.[18] These tumors tend to occur more frequently in children and are extremely rare in adults. The more histologically malignant tumors tend to occur in younger patients. They affect males and females with equal frequency.

These sarcomas form a spectrum of tumors in which the degree of malignancy varies widely. Christensen and Lara divided them into three histologic subgroups of increasing malignancy: fibrosarcoma, spindle cell sarcoma, and polymorphic cell sarcoma.[5] Fibrosarcoma represents a low-grade malignancy, and survival of patients with fibrosarcoma in Christensen and Lara's series averaged 74 months, with occasional very long term survival. Survival of patients with spindle cell sarcoma averaged 27 months, and with polymorphic cell sarcoma it was less than 1 year.

The description of sarcoma subtypes put forward by Christensen and Lara is supported by the observations of Russell and Rubinstein,[20] but is different from that of Paulus et al. who reported on 19 primary intracranial sarcomas in adults collected over 25 years from three institutions in Europe.[18] They diagnosed the tumors according to current pathologic criteria for soft tissue sarcomas[8]; the most common tumor type in their series was malignant fibrous histiocytoma (6 of 19 cases) with only one tumor being designated as a fibrosarcoma. Another recent case report draws attention to this entity.[12] It is likely that many tumors previously reported as fibrosarcoma would today be designated malignant fibrous histiocytoma and that this diagnosis will be made more frequently in the future.

Gross and Microscopic Features

A sarcoma usually appears as a discrete mass involving the meninges and compressing and invading the underlying brain. Occasionally, a sarcoma may lie entirely within the brain parenchyma, presumably arising from perivascular pia-arachnoid sheaths or cells of blood vessels. A rare form of sarcoma that occurs exclusively in infants is meningeal sarcomatosis, in which an extensive sheet of highly anaplastic tumor extends widely over the intracranial and spinal dura.

Sarcomas tend to be large, clearly demarcated masses. The fibrosarcomas, especially, may be sufficiently clearly delineated to make gross total surgical removal possible. The production of collagen may give fibrosarcomas a relatively firm texture, whereas the more cellular sarcomas tend to be soft and friable. They are usually homogeneous and pale, and foci of necrosis occur, since vascular stroma is sparse.

The presence of reticulin and a characteristic pattern of infiltration into adjacent brain tissue typify these sarcomas. Fibrosarcomas have abundant reticulin and collagen and are moderately cellular with mostly spindle-shaped tumor cells. Spindle cell sarcomas (Fig. 169-1) are more densely cellular, and reticulin is easily demonstrated, but there is less collagen; the cells tend to be arranged in parallel bundles, and microscopic areas of necrosis and pseudopalisades may be seen. Polymorphic cell sarcomas (Fig. 169-2) are the least differentiated and most malignant variant, with highly variable, large, irregularly shaped cells and little stroma; reticulin stroma may be fine or absent, and the tumor is usually very soft and extensively necrotic. On immunohistochemical study, sarcomas of the brain and meninges are uniformly GFAP-negative and vimentin-positive.[18]

Sarcomas infiltrate the brain in a characteristic way. Tongues of tumor penetrate irregularly into adjacent parenchyma, and collars of sarcoma cells surround blood vessels; the advancing tumor encompasses distinct islands of neuroglia. Adjacent astrogliosis may be quite marked.

Histologic Variants

Rare examples of primary sarcoma of the brain and meninges showing different histologic patterns of differentiation have been reported. Such tumors include angiosarcoma,[16] leiomyosarcoma,[18] rhabdomyosarcoma,[6] osteosarcoma,[19] chondrosarcoma,[11] mesenchymal chondrosarcoma,[21] and Ewing's sarcoma.[18] Rarely, mixed patterns of differentiation suggest an origin from incompletely differentiated mesenchymal cells, giving rise to the mixed malignant mesenchymoma.[18] One recent cytogenetic study has documented monosomy 22 in cerebral rhabdomyosarcoma.[4]

Sarcomas of the brain and meninges often give rise to conspicuous reactive gliosis in adjacent brain tissue. A number of cases have been reported in which the view has been taken that the reactive gliosis has progressed to glial neoplasia.[14] The development of such a ''sarcoglioma'' must be an extremely rare event. Such a development is very difficult to distinguish from the relatively common and widely accepted development of sarcoma secondary to glioma, termed *gliosarcoma*, which is discussed below.

Management

The principles for treatment of patients with intracranial sarcomas are the same as those for patients with any malignant intracranial tumor. The preoperative differential diagnosis based on neuroimaging includes metastasis, glioma, and meningioma (Fig. 169-3). Once the diagnosis is suspected on frozen section at craniotomy (or stereotactic biopsy), the goal is surgical removal of all, or as much as is safely possible, of the tumor; gross total removal may be achieved in some cases of fibrosarcoma. Little but temporary palliation can be achieved in patients with the highly malignant polymorphic cell sarcoma, and meningeal sarcomatosis will run its rapid course in spite of all endeavors to arrest it. There is no definite evidence that radiation therapy or chemotherapy, either alone or in combination, will affect the survival time of patients with intracranial sarcomas, although these treatment measures should be offered to patients with a good quality of life (i.e., a good performance status) following surgery.

Sarcoma Arising in Continuity with Malignant Glioma (Gliosarcoma)

One of the cardinal features of glioblastoma multiforme is the presence of hyperplasia of tumor blood vessels with proliferation of both endothelial and adventitial cells, forming glomeruloid structures. Such vascular hyperplasia is believed to reflect the production of angiogenic factors by the tumor, and although it is not unique to glioblastoma multiforme, vascular hyperplasia is more

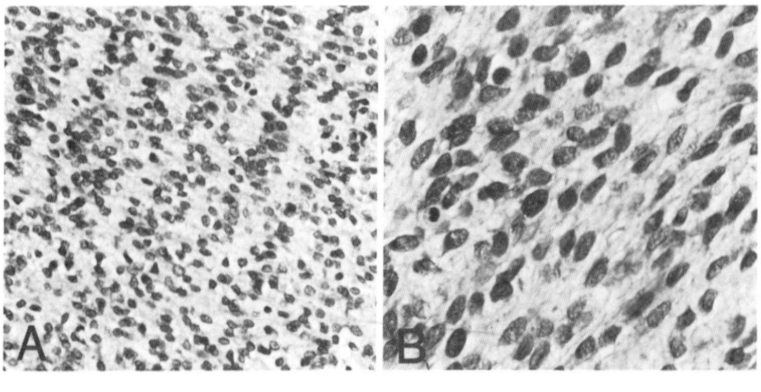

Figure 169-1 Spindle cell sarcoma. Tumor cells are elongated with oval nuclei. Note the streaming pattern and the tendency to palisading of nuclei. Mitotic figures are numerous and stroma is scant. (H & E; original magnifications: *A*, ×10; *B*, ×25.)

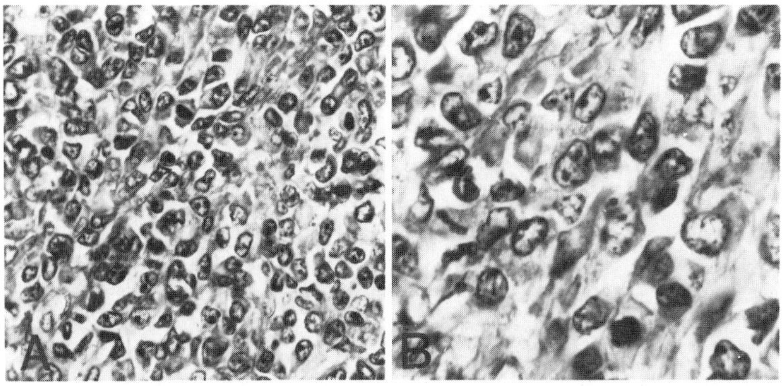

Figure 169-2 Polymorphic cell sarcoma. Tumor cells with scant cytoplasm have highly variable nuclei with a coarse pattern of nuclear chromatin. Mitotic figures are numerous; stroma is scant. Extensive necrosis was present but is not shown in these views. (H & E; original magnifications: *A*, ×25; *B*, ×40.)

prominent in this than in any other brain tumor. A recent study of this vascular hyperplasia has shown that the great majority of hyperplastic cells are positive for smooth muscle–specific α-actin and are therefore smooth muscle cells.[9] Hyperplastic vascular proliferation may progress to neoplasia, and the mesenchymal proliferation acquires both the cellular atypia and the aggressive growth characteristic of sarcomatous malignancy.[22] This progression is supported by the observation that in gliosarcomas the sarcomatous cells are also positive for smooth muscle–specific α-actin.[10] The entity of gliosarcoma is now generally accepted, and although earlier reports suggested that sarcoma was an uncommon development in glioblastoma, with increased awareness of the process, it is now reported in as many as 8 percent of glioblastomas.[17] Since glioblastoma multiforme is the most common primary brain tumor and the incidence of sarcoma secondary to it is substantial, sarcomas of the brain occurring in this way represent the great majority of intracranial sarcomas.

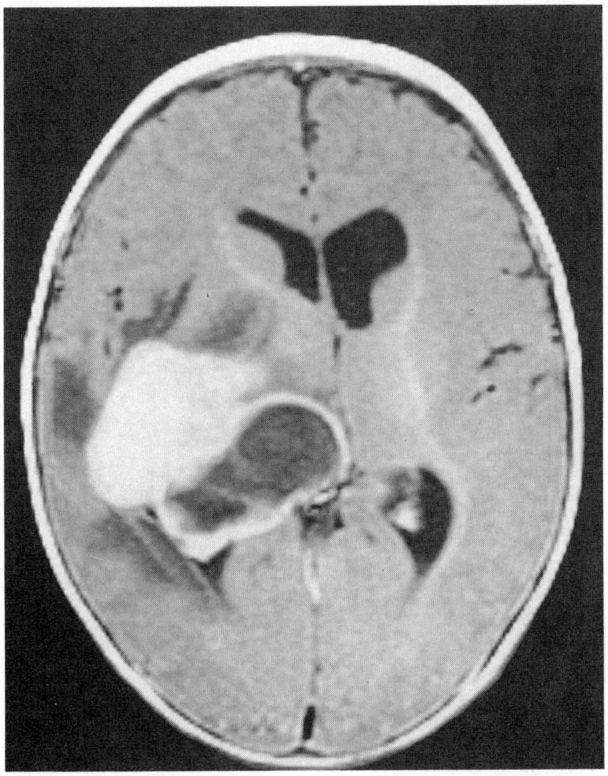

Figure 169-3 Gadolinium-enhanced axial T1-weighted magnetic resonance image of a 4-month-old child with a 2-week history of a bulging fontanel and left hemiparesis. A gross total resection of the tumor was performed. At surgery, the tumor was noted to be firm, avascular, and clearly demarcated from brain. Pathologic examination revealed an undifferentiated (i.e., polymorphic cell) sarcoma. (MRI courtesy of Dr. J. Drake and Dr. J. Rutka, Hospital for Sick Children, Toronto.)

Histology

The sarcomatous areas of gliosarcoma usually exhibit a pattern of spindle-shaped cells with reticulin formation, and glial cells are lacking. Two distinct but intermingled tumor patterns are thus produced (Fig. 169-4), a gliomatous pattern and a sarcomatous pattern. The gliomatous component consists of astrocytes which are readily identified by GFAP stains and by the absence of reticulin and collagen. The sarcomatous component is rich in reticulin and collagen but is devoid of GFAP-positive cells. Cellular atypia and mitotic figures are prominent in both areas, since both are malignant tumor patterns (Fig. 169-5). Occasionally, the intimate admixture of glioma and sarcoma produces such a confusing histologic picture that the gliomatous tumor may be completely overlooked. The amount of collagen in the sarcoma is variable but is usually sufficient to produce a tumor of quite firm consistency. The sarcoma may become the dominant tumor and overgrow the glioma, so that the pre-existing glioma may become obscured. Gliosarcoma is more prone to metastasize to extracranial sites (such as the liver and lung) than glioblastoma.[26] The metastases may contain either the gliomatous or the sarcomatous elements or both.

Variants

The majority of sarcomas arising in continuity with gliomas exhibit no specialized differentiation and can be described as spindle cell sarcomas or fibrosarcomas. However, smooth muscle differentiation is frequently present, and myofibrils in the cytoplasm that stain positively with phosphotungstic acid hematoxylin (PTAH) may easily be mistaken for glial fibrils, which also stain positively with PTAH; this error in interpretation was almost unavoidable prior to the advent of GFAP stains.

The development of chondroid or osteoid differentiation within the sarcoma is much less common.[23] Here, the cartilage and bone

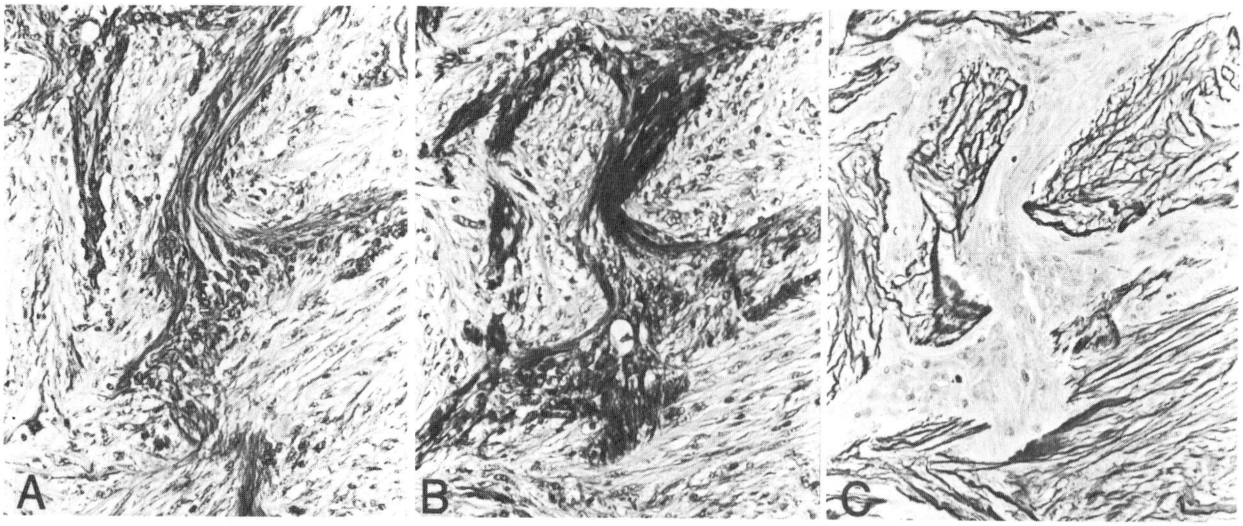

Figure 169-4 Gliosarcoma. Identical fields from three serial sections of the tumor are stained as follows: *A*, PTAH; *B*, GFAP; *C*, reticulin. Dark-staining areas are composed of astrocytes rich in glial fibrils which are PTAH positive (*A*) and GFAP positive (*B*). *C*. The astrocytic areas are pale, since they are devoid of reticulin. (Original ×10.)

exhibit the malignant features of chondrosarcoma and osteosarcoma and are thought to represent a type of metaplasia of the sarcomatous cells (Fig. 169-6).

Clinical Features

The clinical features of gliosarcoma are similar to those of malignant astrocytoma or glioblastoma multiforme. As with glioblastoma there is a slight male predominance; among 24 patients with gliosarcoma reviewed by Morantz et al. there were 14 men and 10 women ranging in age from 37 to 68 years.[17] Gliosarcomas occur more often in the temporal lobe than in any other part of the brain; in 10 of the 24 patients, the tumor was confined to the temporal lobe, and in another four a substantial portion was in the temporal lobe; six tumors were parietal and four were frontal. This temporal predominance is confirmed in other published series, and is not seen in glioblastoma.

The diagnosis of gliosarcoma was first made at the time of a repeat craniotomy done for the removal of a tumor recurrence in several of our own cases; in these cases, the diagnosis at the initial operation had been glioblastoma multiforme. Upon review of some cases, however, sarcomatous features could be found in the tissue that had been removed at the initial operation. In other cases, it is possible that the sarcomatous change had not yet occurred at the time of the first operation, or that the tissue biopsied was remote from the sarcomatous area of the tumor. With increasing awareness of its features, the diagnosis of gliosarcoma is now being made more frequently.

Gliosarcomas are usually firm or even hard, and are often well-circumscribed. They commonly present at the surface of the brain, and may be firmly attached to the dura. The outer surface may be lobulated, and the tumor may be dissected fairly readily from the surrounding brain substance. Because of these features, a gliosarcoma may be mistaken for a meningioma at the time of operation. A superficially located gliosarcoma may have a rich external carotid blood supply, so that its angiographic appearance also resembles that of a meningioma. The tumor center is often necrotic, and the gross features may be quite variable and include those commonly seen in glioblastoma multiforme.

Survival time is similar to that of patients with glioblastoma multiforme. The median survival time in the 24 patients reported by Morantz et al. was approximately 4 months after surgery.[17]

Only 13 of the 24 patients reported by Morantz et al. lived long enough to complete a radiation therapy dose of 50 to 60 Gy; in this selected group, the survival rate was somewhat longer, being 37

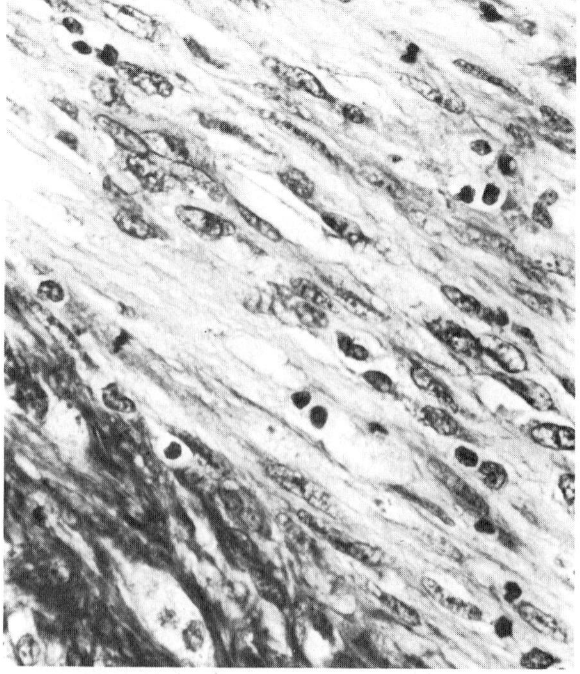

Figure 169-5 Gliosarcoma. High-power view of sarcoma showing streaming pattern of somewhat pleomorphic spindle-shaped cells and numerous mitotic figures. (H & E, original ×25.)

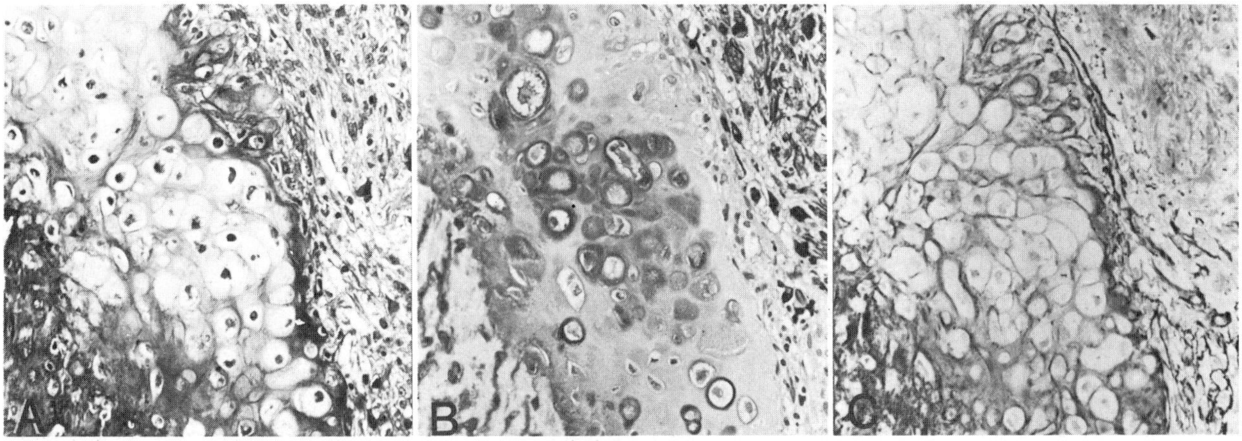

Figure 169-6 Gliosarcoma showing chondroid and osteoid differentiation. The astrocytic component of the tumor is on the right in each picture. Identical fields from three serial sections of the tumor are stained as follows: *A*, Masson's trichrome; *B*, GFAP; *C*, reticulin. *B*. Astrocytes in the upper right stain darkly for GFAP. The dark staining of bone and cartilage is due to the hematoxylin counterstain. *C*. The absence of reticulin in the astrocytic tumor is noted at the upper right. (Original ×10.)

weeks from the onset of symptoms and 33 weeks after surgery. Chemotherapy in addition to radiation made no significant difference in survival rate. However, these treatment groups were biased by the selection of only patients who had survived at least 5 weeks postoperatively. There is, as yet, no statistical evidence to show that either radiation therapy or chemotherapy confers any benefit or prolongs the survival time in patients with gliosarcoma, but based on randomized studies demonstrating the benefit of radiation for patients with malignant astrocytoma and glioblastoma, it is recommended to administer conventional fractionated radiation to patients with gliosarcoma following surgery.

Thus, with our present knowledge, the principles of management of patients with gliosarcoma are exactly the same as for those with glioblastoma multiforme. In addition, it must be remembered that gliosarcomas not uncommonly metastasize to extracranial sites.

Sarcoma Arising in Meningioma

Malignancy in meningiomas is uncommon, but on rare occasions a benign meningioma may change into a tumor which has features of malignancy or even of frank sarcoma. Meningiomas are subclassified on the basis of histologic appearance, but these categories do not reflect differences in behavior except in the case of angioblastic meningiomas. Almost all angioblastic meningiomas are now recognized to be histologically identical to hemangiopericytomas; they have a tendency to aggressive growth characteristic of the hemangiopericytoma, but are not generally regarded as sarcomas.

There are, however, meningiomas that deserve the designation of malignant meningioma. These tumors are not sharply distinguished from their benign counterparts; in fact, there may over time be a gradual evolution from a picture that appears entirely benign to one which, while retaining the general histologic picture of meningioma, has additional features of malignancy. This malignant change is characterized by a pattern of infiltration into brain tissue, frequent mitoses (Fig. 169-7), and the development of a distinctive papillary epithelioid pattern rarely if ever seen in benign meningiomas (Fig. 169-8). The malignant meningioma provokes a marked hyperplastic astroglial reaction in the invaded brain tissue, unlike the very limited astroglial reaction in the compressed brain adjacent to a benign meningioma. Cytogenic analysis reveals that the cells of a malignant meningioma are likely to be tetraploid and demonstrate a 4C peak on fluoresence cytometry.[1] As well, there is evidence that the quantity of argyrophilic nucleolar organizer region proteins may correlate with the level of malignancy in meningioma.[15]

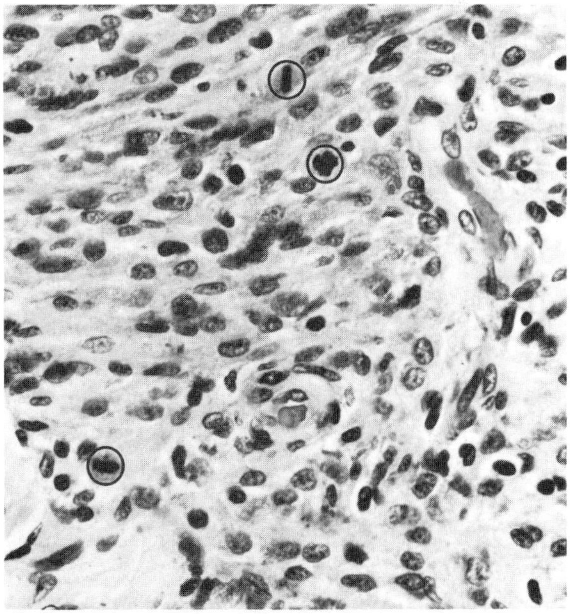

Figure 169-7 A portion of a meningothelial meningioma undergoing malignant change. As many as six mitotic figures were seen per high-power field. The three mitotic figures in this field are indicated by circles. (H & E, original ×25.)

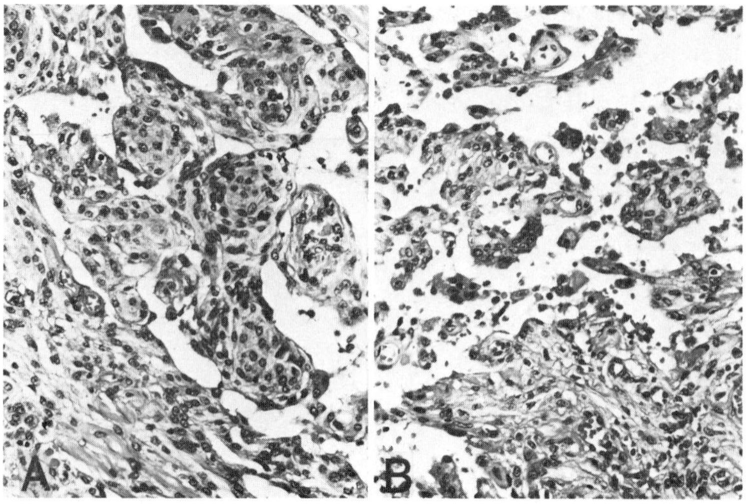

Figure 169-8 Malignant meningioma. *A* and *B* are from the same case. Note the typical whorling pattern (*A*), interrupted by cleftlike spaces to produce a papillary pattern, more developed in *B*. (H & E, ×10.)

The process of malignant evolution of a meningioma progresses on rare occasions to a frankly sarcomatous appearance in which all histologic evidence of the pre-existing meningioma is lost. The tumor is then difficult to distinguish from a primary meningeal sarcoma. Neuroimaging studies may suggest a benign meningioma, although frequently the images look atypical (e.g., irregular, invasive-looking tumor margin) and are predictive of a more aggressive histologic picture (Fig. 169-9).

Treatment of the sarcomatous meningioma consists of radical surgical removal of the initial tumor and of any and all recurrences, as long as it is feasible to do so. While there is some evidence that radiation therapy may retard the growth rate of benign meningiomas, no information is available as to the benefit of radiation therapy in patients with malignant meningiomas. However, conventional radiation is to be strongly recommended after the initial surgery for a frankly malignant meningioma, and, in fact, high-dose focused radiation (i.e., radiosurgery) may be considered if the anatomy of residual or recurrent tumor is appropriate for this modality. However, in spite of radical surgery and radiation, these tumors may behave in a most aggressive fashion (Fig. 169-10).

Sarcoma Arising after Cranial Irradiation

The development of sarcoma many years after radiation therapy is uncommon but well-recognized, and has been reported in a number of different tissues of the body. Intracranial sarcomas have occurred following radiation of a variety of intracranial tumors, but most commonly following radiation of pituitary tumors. Postradiation sarcomas are usually fibrosarcomas, although other types, including osteogenic sarcoma and chondrosarcoma,[3] have occurred.

Sarcomas that develop following radiation therapy of pituitary tumors arise in the field of radiation in or near the sella, where the dose was maximal, but are not necessarily contiguous with the radiated tumor. Waltz and Brownell reviewed 10 such cases from the literature, and described three more cases of their own.[25] The time interval between radiation and the diagnosis of sarcoma ranged from 2.5 to 20 years, with a mean of 10.1 years; this latent interval is similar to that encountered in the development of sarcomas at the site of radiation elsewhere in the body. In an extensive review of radiation-induced intracranial tumors by Bernstein and Laperriere,[2] the minimum radiation dose which was followed by subsequent sarcoma development was 20 Gy, the mean latency interval was 10.5 years, and multiple courses of radiation increased the risk of developing sarcoma. As more successful treatment regimens produce longer survival for brain tumor patients, especially

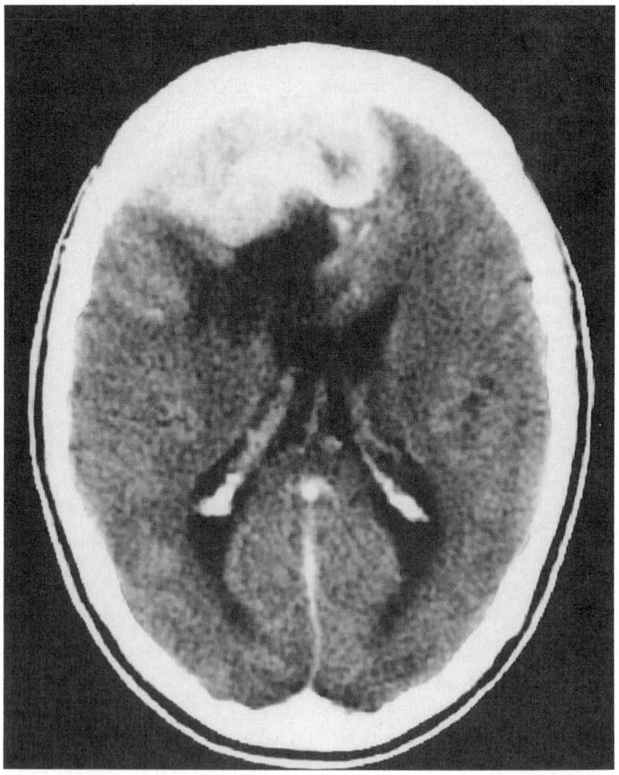

Figure 169-9 An enhanced axial CT scan of a 78-year-old woman with a 2-month history of frontal headaches, confusion, and a mild left hemiparesis. The preoperative differential diagnosis based on neuroimaging included malignant glioma and malignant meningioma. At surgery a rather ill-defined plane between tumor and brain was encountered, but a gross total resection was achieved. Pathologic examination revealed a frankly malignant meningioma with cellular pleomorphism, numerous mitotic figures, and widespread areas of necrosis producing a pseudopapillary appearance.

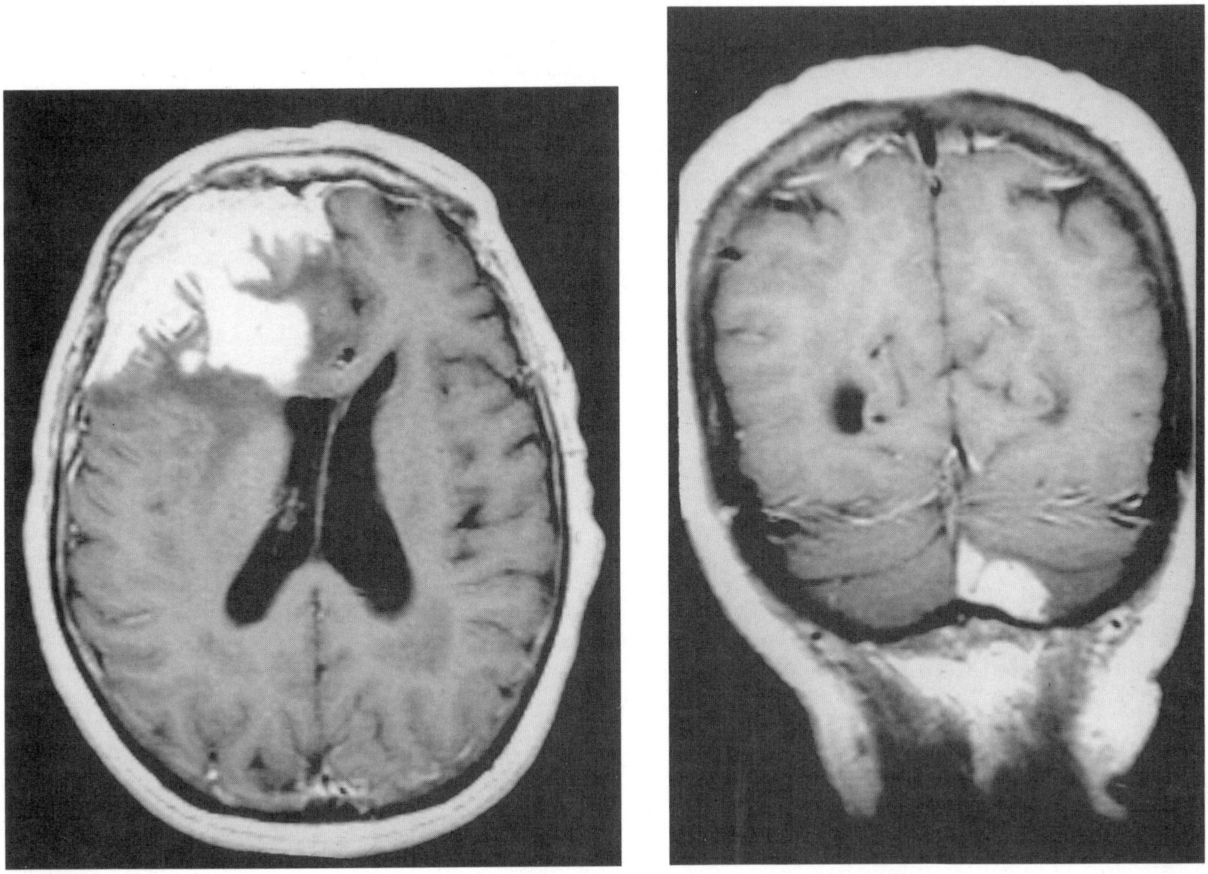

(*A*) (*B*)

Figure 169-10 Gadolinium-enhanced MRI study from the same patient shown in Figure 169-9, 9 months following gross total resection and conventional fractionated radiation for malignant meningioma. The patient has tumor recurrence in the right frontal region (*A*), as well as at distant dural-based sites including the posterior fossa (*B*).

children, the clinician must maintain a high index of suspicion for the development of a second, radiation-induced tumor later in the patient's life.

The clinical features of postradiation sarcomas are similar to those of other intracranial sarcomas and will not be detailed here. Surgical removal of the sarcoma, if possible, is the treatment of choice, followed by some form of focused radiation (i.e., radiosurgery or brachytherapy) if the anatomy of the lesion is appropriate, so that the brain is not exposed to a second, potentially damaging course of conventional fractionated external beam therapy.

References

1. Ahyai A, Spaar FW. DNA and prognosis of meningiomas: a comparative cytological and fluorescence-cytophotometrical study of 71 tumours. *Acta Neurochir (Wien)* 1987; 87:119–128.
2. Bernstein M, Laperriere N. Radiation-induced tumors of the nervous system. In Gutin PH, Leibel SA, Sheline GE (eds): *Radiation Injury to the Nervous System.* New York: Raven Press, 1991, pp 455–472.
3. Bernstein M, Perrin RG, Platts ME, Simpson WJ. Radiation-induced cerebellar chondrosarcoma. Case report. *J Neurosurg* 1984; 61:174–177.
4. Biegel JA, Rorke LB, Packer RJ, Emmanuel BS. Monosomy 22 in rhabdoid or atypical tumors of the brain. *J Neurosurg* 1990; 73:710–714.
5. Christensen E, Lara DE. Intracranial sarcomas. *J Neuropathol Exp Neurol* 1953; 12:41–56.
6. Dropcho EJ, Allen JC. Primary intracranial rhabdomyosarcoma: case report and review of the literature. *J Neurooncol* 1987; 5:139–150.
7. Ellams ID, Hildebrandt G, Vuia O, Kaufmann U. Intracranial sarcoma in childhood. *Childs Nerv Syst* 1985; 1:169–171.
8. Enzinger FM, Weiss SW. *Soft Tissue Tumors,* 2d ed. St. Louis: Mosby, 1988.
9. Haddad SF, Moore SA, Schelper RL, Goeken JA. Vascular smooth muscle hyperplasia underlies the formation of glomeruloid vascular structures of glioblastoma multiforme. *J Neuropathol Exp Neurol* 1992; 51:488–492.
10. Haddad SF, Moore SA, Schelper RL, Goeken JA. Smooth muscle can comprise the sarcomatous component of gliosarcomas. *J Neuropathol Exp Neurol* 1992; 51:493–498.
11. Hassounah M, Al-Mefty O, Akhtar M, et al. Primary cranial and intracranial chondrosarcoma. A survey. *Acta Neurochir (Wien)* 1985; 78:123–132.
12. Ho YS, Wei CH, Tsai MD, Wai Y. Intracerebral malignant fibrous histiocytoma: case report and review of the literature. *Neurosurgery* 1992; 31:567–571.
13. Ironside JW. Classification of primary intracranial sarcomas and other central nervous system neoplasms. *Histopathology* 1991; 18:483–486.
14. Lalitha VS, Rubinstein LJ. Reactive glioma in intracranial sarcoma: a form of mixed sarcoma and glioma (''sarcoglioma''). Report of eight cases. *Cancer* 1979; 43:246–257.
15. Maier H, Ofner D, Hittmair A, et al. Classic, atypical, and anaplastic meningioma: three histopathological subtypes of clinical relevance. *J Neurosurg* 1992; 77:616–623.

16. Mena H, Ribas JL, Enzinger FM, Parisi JE. Primary angiosarcoma of the central nervous system. Study of eight cases and review of the literature. *J Neurosurg* 1991; 75:73–76.
17. Morantz RA, Feigin I, Ransohoff J. Clinical and pathological study of 24 cases of gliosarcoma. *J Neurosurg* 1976; 45:398–408.
18. Paulus W, Slowik F, Jellinger K. Primary intracranial sarcomas: histopathological features of 19 cases. *Histopathology* 1991; 18:395–402.
19. Reznik M, Lenelle J. Primary intracerebral osteosarcoma. *Cancer* 1991; 68:793–797.
20. Russell DS, Rubinstein LJ. *Pathology of Tumours of the Nervous System,* 5th ed. Baltimore: Williams & Wilkins, 1989.
21. Scheithauer BW, Rubinstein LJ. Meningeal mesenchymal chondrosarcoma. Report of 8 cases with review of the literature. *Cancer* 1978; 42:2744–2752.
22. Slowik F, Jellinger K, Gaszo L, Fischer J. Gliosarcomas: histological, immunohistochemical, ultrastructural, and tissue cultural studies. *Acta Neuropathol (Berl)* 1985; 67:201–210.
23. Tada T, Katsuyama T, Aoki T, et al. Mixed glioblastoma and sarcoma with osteoid-chondral tissue. *Clin Neuropathol* 1987; 6:160–163.
24. Tomita T, Gonzalez-Crussi F. Intracranial primary nonlymphomatous sarcomas in children: experience with eight cases and review of the literature. *Neurosurgery* 1984; 14:529–540.
25. Waltz TA, Brownell B. Sarcoma: a possible late result of effective radiation therapy for pituitary adenoma. Report of two cases. *J Neurosurg* 1966; 24:901–907.
26. Weaver D, Vandenberg S, Park TS, Jane JA. Selective peripancreatic sarcoma metastases from primary gliosarcoma. Case report. *J Neurosurg* 1984; 61:599–601.

170 Meningeal Hemangiopericytomas

Michael J. Ebersold
Lynn M. Quast

Meningeal hemangiopericytoma (M-HPC) is a rare neoplasm arising from perivascular pericytes.[3] The M-HPC is similar in phenotype to peripheral soft tissue HPC. Other tumors with an HPC-like pattern include synovial sarcomas, malignant schwannomas, leiomyosarcomas, liposarcomas, and malignant fibrous histiocytomas.[32]

The first description of hemangiopericytoma was of a tumor outside the central nervous system (CNS). These tumors frequently involve the soft tissues of the thigh, buttock, and retroperitoneum. Stout and Murrary developed the concept of hemangiopericytoma, a vascular tumor featuring Zimmerman's pericytes; only one of Stout's 25 subsequently reported cases was stated to involve the meninges.[39] A review of the literature, however, reveals that Bailey and co-workers had already described three "angioblastic meningiomas" in 1928.[2] Although strong opinions have been expressed as to whether they represent separate entities, many now consider the angioblastic meningioma and the hemangiopericytoma to be identical, an opinion with which we concur.[15] The clinicopathologic features of these morphologically identical tumors have been confused not only because authors have long referred to them as distinct lesions but also because some have reported the existence of tumors with intermediate features.[34] It is nonetheless probable that most reports and reviews of angioblastic meningiomas refer to a tumor synonymous with hemangiopericytoma of the CNS.[9] There are a number of excellent clinicopathologic reviews of meningeal hemangiopericytomas.[10,11,14,30,33,35,40] Much of our present understanding and the views expressed herein are based on these reviews, on other sources,[20,22,25] and on a review of 44 patients with meningeal hemangiopericytoma seen at our institution. Since our review of these 44 patients, we have seen 12 additional patients who have undergone surgery for M-HPC. During this same 6-year period, 405 patients have undergone surgery for meningiomas. All of these patients had the presumptive preoperative diagnosis of meningioma. Even with modern computed tomography scanning, angiography, and magnetic resonance imaging (MRI), the diagnosis depends on pathologic confirmation.

Incidence and Behavior

In spite of the radiographic similarities between meningioma and M-HPC (or angioblastic meningioma), it is important to recognize that the latter is distinct from ordinary meningiomas. Grossly, both have a similar topographic distribution, arising preferentially from the falx, tentorium, dural sinuses, and skull base. In addition, both meningioma and hemangiopericytoma are dural-based, compress rather than invade the brain, and are frequently found to be very vascular at the time of surgery. In many instances, these tumors seem to involve the leptomeninges, making it difficult to maintain an avascular surgical plane. Total resection may also be complicated by the tendency of both types of tumors to be irregular at their interface with adjoining tissue.

A review of our own data based on 2381 patients who underwent surgery for meningioma between 1960 and 1992 revealed 56 hemangiopericytomas; the incidence of this lesion was therefore 2.4 percent of the incidence of meningiomas. This value agrees with the ones given by other authors, who have found the incidence to be less than 4 percent that of meningiomas[5,11,17,19,30,33,37,42] and approximately 0.5 percent that of all tumors of the CNS. Hemangiopericytoma in tissue outside the brain is a well-established entity; several large series have been reported.[10,27]

These publications stress frequent recurrence and rates of metastasis approaching 50 percent. Long-term follow-up is mandatory, because recurrence or metastasis may be delayed for years. A recent analysis of published series demonstrated a 90 percent 9-year actuarial risk for local recurrence following surgical resection alone. Only 33 percent of these recurrences were noted in the first 5 years.[3] In a previously published series of 26 patients from this institution, it was found that the aggressive nature of the hemangiopericytoma resulted in a recurrence rate of 80 percent and a rate of metastasis of 23 percent.[14] More recently, we had the opportunity of enlarging the study group and extended the duration of follow-up; it was observed that the patients who had undergone surgery between the years 1938 and 1987 experienced 1-, 5-, and 10-year recurrence rates of 15, 65, and 76 percent, respectively, and that the rate of metastasis at 10 and 15 years was 33 percent and 64 percent, respectively.[15]

Meningiomas are much less likely to recur following surgical removal, and metastases are very rare. For patients whose tumors were treated with gross total removal, Simpson found the recurrence rate to be only 9 percent.[37] Simpson reported a 19 percent recurrence rate for meningiomas that were totally removed but for which cauterization of the dural attachment site was required.

Pathology

Light Microscopy

Light microscopy shows a hemangiopericytoma to consist of plump to spindle-shaped cells (Fig. 170-1). Occasional zones of hypocellularity are found, but microcysts are uncommon. Mitotic figures are frequent; in the 1978 review, these ranged from 1 to 5 per 10 high-power fields,[14] and in our subsequent review, they averaged 7 per 20 high-power fields.[15]

Nuclei are generally delicate and round to fusiform, and demonstrate neither coarse chromatin nor nucleolar prominence. Binucleation or multinucleation of tumor cells is very infrequent; however, cellularity is generally high and may be either dense and patternless or show some fibrogenesis. Vascularity is quite variable, with some of these tumors demonstrating abundant thin-walled vascular networks that have a staghorn-like arrangement and are lined with flat inconspicuous endothelial cells. Some cells

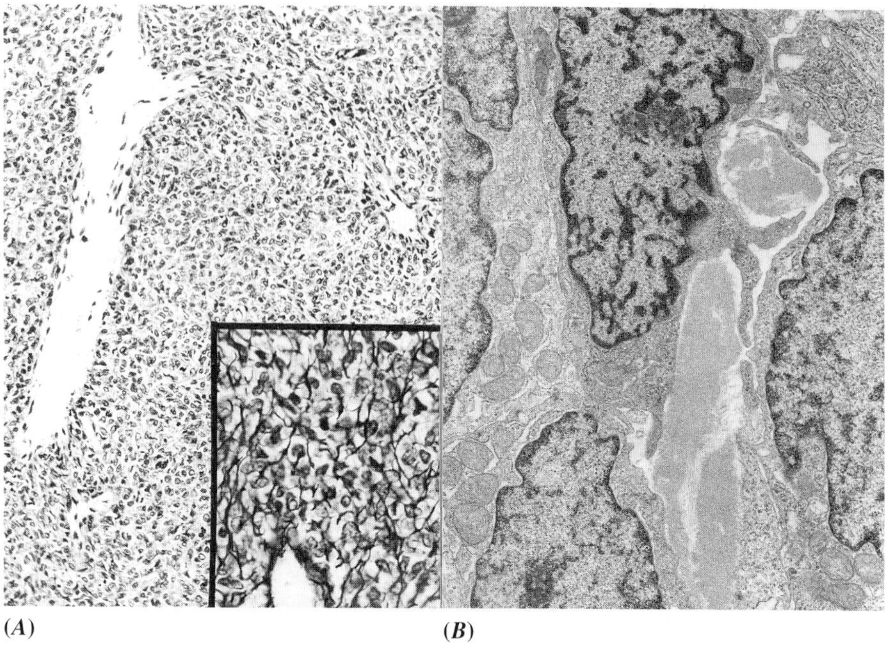

Figure 170-1 Microscopic appearance of a hemangiopericytoma. *A.* The typical light microscopic appearance of a hemangiopericytoma, composed of small ovoid to elongated cells associated with staghorn vascular channels. (Hematoxylin and eosin stain, ×160.) *Inset:* A reticulin stain demonstrating a dense intercellular reticulin pattern (×400). *B.* An electron micrograph demonstrating cohesion of elongated tumor cells with scant processes; note the lack of frequent intercellular junctions, a feature prominent in meningiomas. Note the intercellular basement membrane-like material, the basis of the reticulin reaction (×9000).

or groups of cells are surrounded by fine reticulin-staining fibers. The reticulin stain often, but not invariably, shows a typical pattern of fine fibers surrounding individual tumor cells or small groups of tumor cells.

Interestingly, no significant tendency to increasing anaplasia was demonstrated when recurrent or metastatic lesions were compared to the original or primary tumor.[15] Nevertheless, 3 of 11 cases in the 1978 review demonstrated "dedifferentiation," with plumper cells, more prominent nucleoli, and less reticulin among tumor cells in later specimens.[14]

Immunocytology

Winek and colleagues,[43] in a study of immunohistochemical characteristics of 9 peripheral and 13 CNS hemangiopericytomas as well as 40 ordinary meningiomas, noted similar immunoprofiles for the hemangiopericytoma regardless of site (positive for vimentin; negative for epithelial membrane antigen). In contrast, reactivity to both epithelial membrane antigen and vimentin was observed in all ordinary meningiomas studied. These results support the concept that hemangiopericytoma and meningioma are distinct neoplasms. Iwaki and colleagues also have presented immunohistochemical data that support the concept that the meningeal hemangiopericytoma is composed of poorly differentiated cells that originate from a perivascular mesenchymal cell of the meninges but not from the arachnoidal cap cells.[16] Morphologic, ultrastructural, and immunochemical data indicate that meningeal hemangiopericytoma represents the intracranial counterpart of soft tissue hemangiopericytomas. The existence of meningiomas with hemangiopericytoma-like growth patterns is another reason for much of the confusion.[8] The immunostaining pattern of M-HPC is nonspecific; however, the use of markers for soft tissue tumors can help exclude other diagnoses.[32]

Electron Microscopy

Electron microscopic studies of ordinary meningiomas have demonstrated their ultrastructural similarity to normal arachnoid membrane. The cells are cohesive, show intricate interdigitation of the cell membrane with those of adjoining cells, demonstrate numerous intercellular desmosomes, and have no pericellular basement membrane. The cytoplasm contains varying numbers of intermediate filaments, the basis of the vimentin reaction noted above. In contrast, the cells in a hemangiopericytoma are often less cohesive, show few and structurally simpler intercellular junctions, and contain fewer as well as less dispersed cytoplasmic microfilaments. The intercellular space often contains deposits of basement-membrane-like material, which is apparent on reticulin stains (Fig. 170-1).[9] Nevertheless, the interpretation of ultrastructural findings is complicated by the paucity of readily recognizable ultrastructural features in pericytes.[32] The pericytes in HPC do show smooth muscle-like features but do not express α-smooth muscle actin, the differentiation marker of smooth muscle tumors that is present in glomus tumors.[9,28,36]

Location

Although hemangiopericytomas have been reported to arise at both extra- and intracranial sites, those involving the CNS often, but not invariably, originate in the meninges. In general, these tumors do not originate intraparenchymally. However, a hemangiopericytoma originating in the choroid plexus has been reported.[26] Some authors have reported that 10 to 30 percent of CNS lesions involve the spinal cord.[33,35] A recent review at our institution demonstrated that only 2 of 56 tumors were primary spinal hemangiopericytomas, although one tumor did produce a spinal metastasis.[15] The intracranial distribution of hemangiopericytomas is similar to that reported for ordinary meningiomas. Of our 56 patients, 37 (66 percent) presented with supratentorial tumors, the favored locations of which included the parasagittal region, tentorium, and sphenoid wing.

Clinical Presentation

In contrast to patients with meningiomas, of whom two-thirds are female, 55 to 70 percent of hemangiopericytomas occur in males.[5,7,19,30] In addition, hemangiopericytomas occur in a slightly younger age group, averaging 38 to 42 years old,[17,33,35] unlike patients with meningiomas, who have a mean age in the early fifties.[5,19,30,38] Although M-HPC is generally considered a tumor of adults, an orbital-anterior fossa HPC and a giant meningeal HPC have been reported in newborns.[1,18] There have also been several other reports of M-HPC in children.[4,31] As reported by others, we confirmed the finding that patients with a hemangiopericytoma are often symptomatic for less than a year before diagnosis.[11,33,35,40] This contrasts to similar reviews of meningiomas, wherein most patients exhibit symptoms for 1 to 2 years.[30] In our series, the average symptomatic interval for hemangiopericytoma was approximately 14 months during the computed tomography (CT) era.[15]

Not surprisingly, the clinical presentation of hemangiopericytomas reflects the location of the tumor. Of our 56 patients, 57 percent presented with headaches and 14 percent with seizures. Patients with posterior fossa lesions were most likely to have gait disturbance and dysequilibrium.[15]

Radiographic Diagnosis

Plain x-ray films are generally not revealing. At present, the diagnosis will almost always be established before there is radiographic evidence of increased intracranial pressure. Although ordinary meningiomas may at times be associated with hyperostosis, this sign has not been reported with a hemangiopericytoma. One of our 56 patients with hemangiopericytoma showed a lytic lesion on skull films.

The CT and MRI appearances of a hemangiopericytoma are usually indistinguishable from those of an ordinary meningioma (Fig. 170-2). Indeed, a diagnosis of meningioma is most often rendered. The finding of calcium within a tumor, however, is strong evidence against the diagnosis of hemangiopericytoma.

The angiographic appearance of a hemangiopericytoma likewise resembles that of a meningioma. Of the 25 most recent angiograms in our patients with hemangiopericytoma, 15 showed vascular lesions with the typical tumor blush and 11 demonstrated avascular masses. The blood supply may be from the brain parenchyma, from an extradural source, or from a combination of both. In patients that have an extremely vascular tumor where the blood supply is primarily from an extraparenchymal source, embolization may be considered in an effort to decrease the blood loss at the time of surgery (Fig. 170-3).

Surgical Treatment

The surgical treatment of a hemangiopericytoma is essentially that of a meningioma. Preoperative embolization may be considered for the small proportion of tumors that are highly vascular and also derive their major blood supply from vessels appropriate for embolization. Because of the significant tendency of these tumors to recur locally and to eventually metastasize, aggressive and thorough resection is the goal.

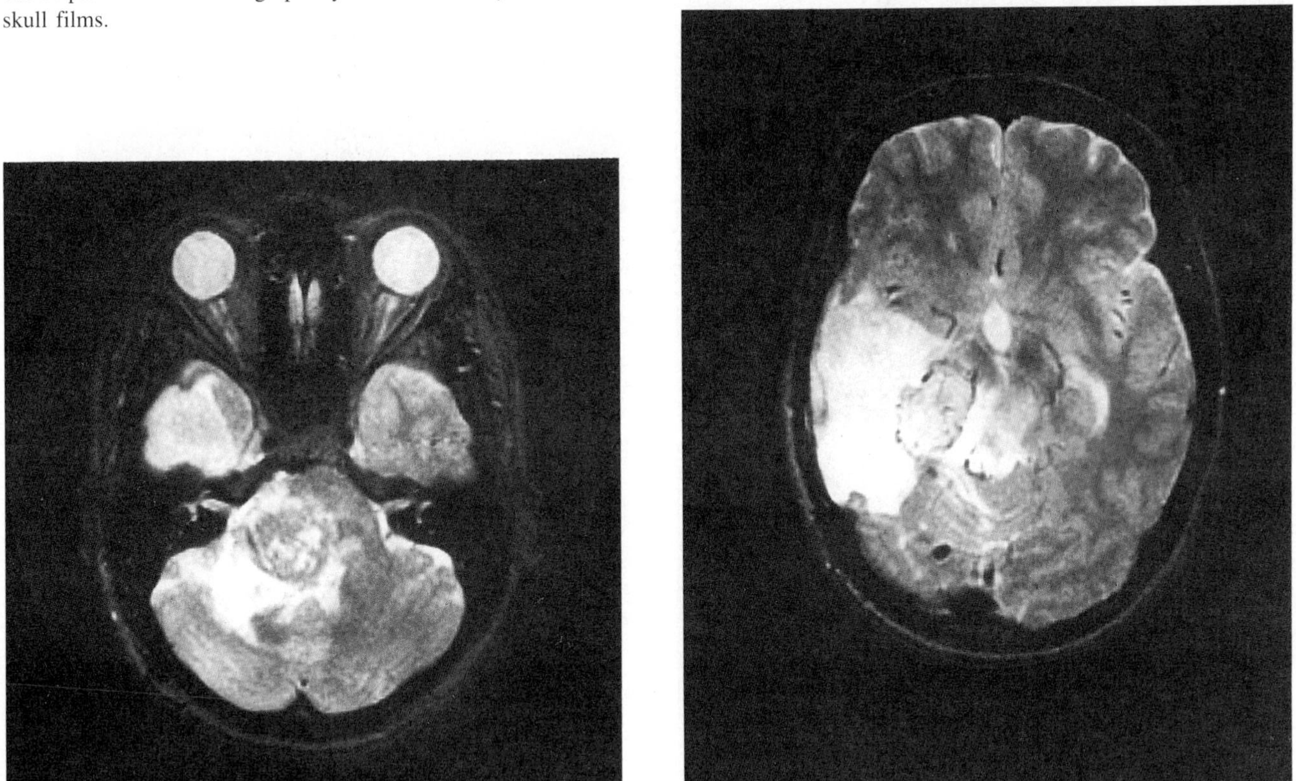

(*A*) (*B*)

Figure 170-2 *A*. A T2-weighted axial MR image through the posterior fossa demonstrates a lobulated tumor mass with mixed signal intensities in the right cerebellopontine angle. Note the marked displacement of the brain stem and the surrounding edema in the cerebellum. *B*. A T2-weighted axial image at a higher level demonstrates the mass extending through the tentorial notch. The high-intensity area in the middle cranial fossa is secondary to previous surgery.

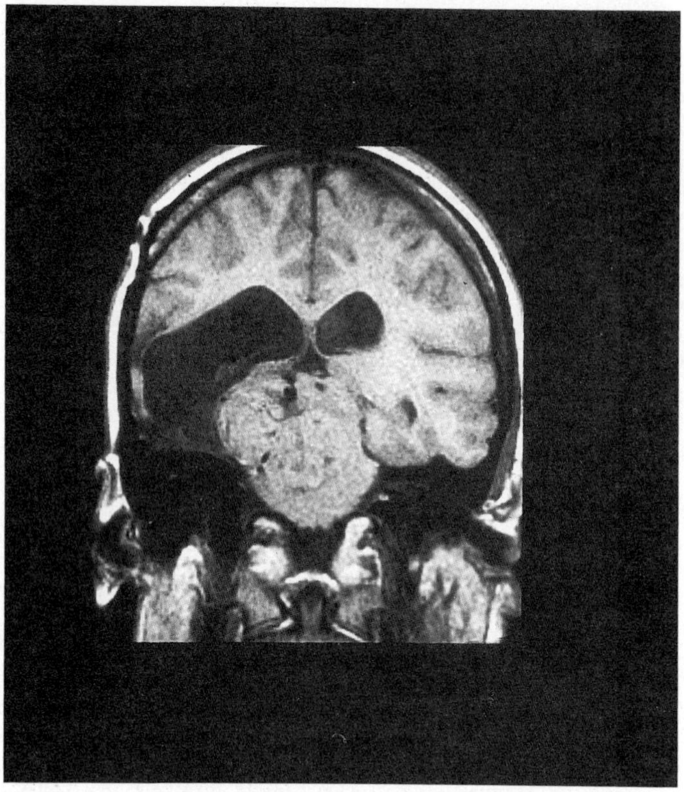

(*C*)

Figure 170-2 (*Continued*) *C.* A T1-weighted coronal image shows the predominantly isointense mass, with focal areas of hypointensity consistent with cyst formation or areas of necrosis, involving the posterior and middle cranial fossae. Note the marked indentation and displacement of the brain stem.

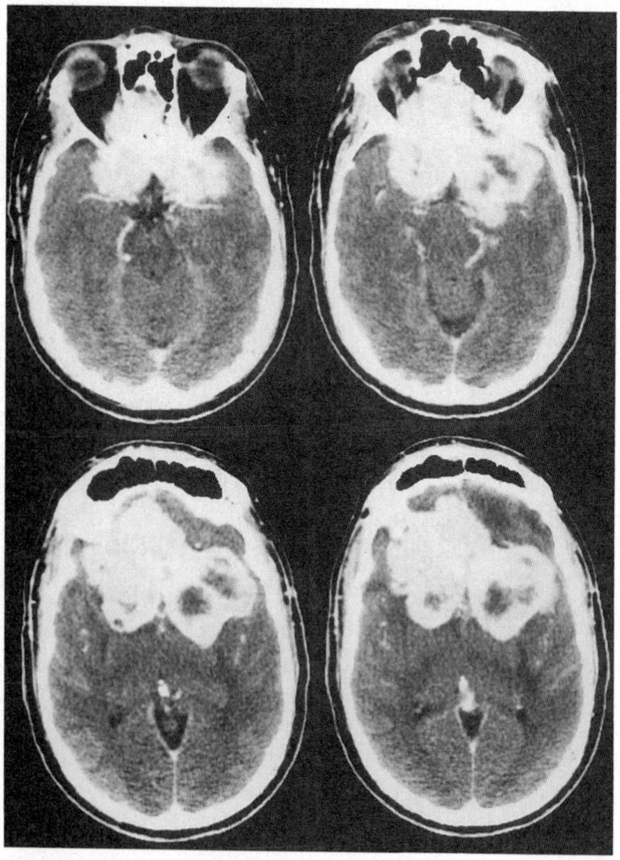

(*A*)

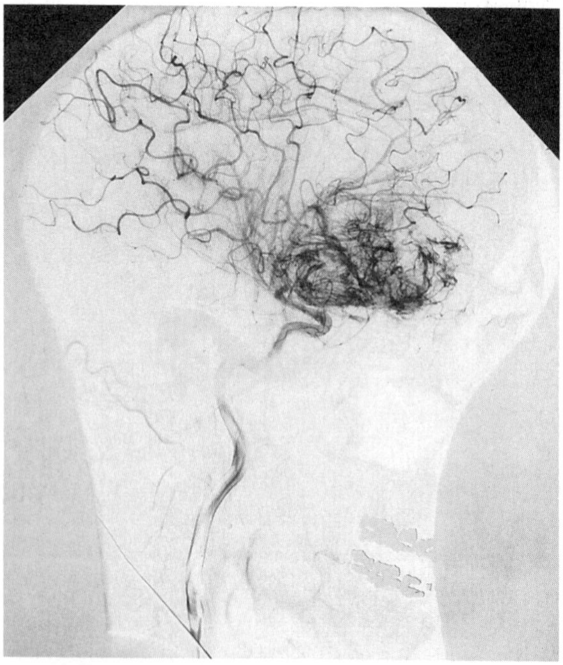

(*B*)

Figure 170-3 *A.* A CT scan of a 38-year-old man who had progressive lethargy and memory loss. *B.* This angiogram shows a very vascular tumor with an obviously large internal carotid supply. There was also a very significant supply from the meningeal vessels, with extensive shunting of blood from the meningeal supply to the tumor mass. Because of this, embolization of the meningeal source was performed.

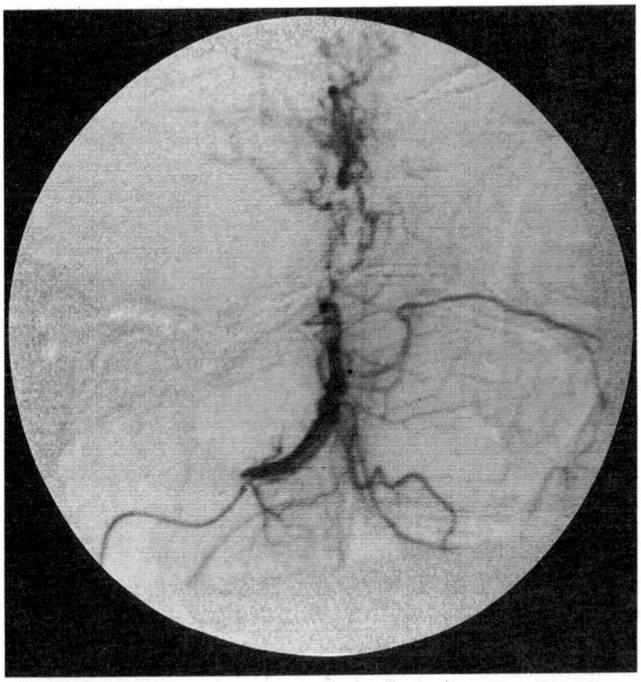

(*C*)

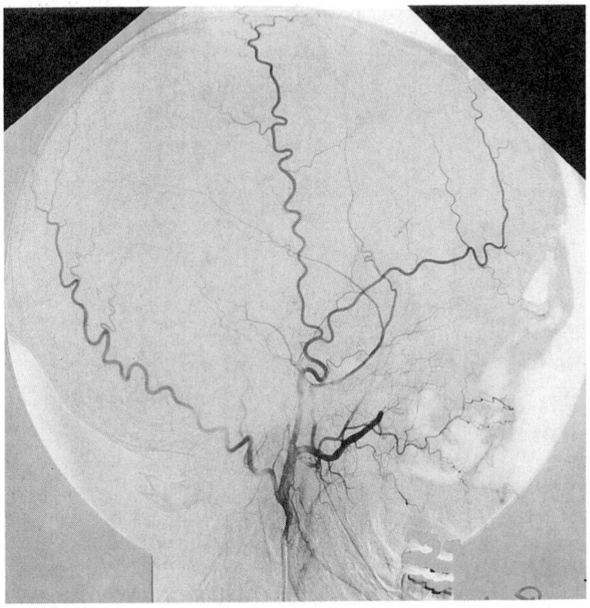

(*D*)

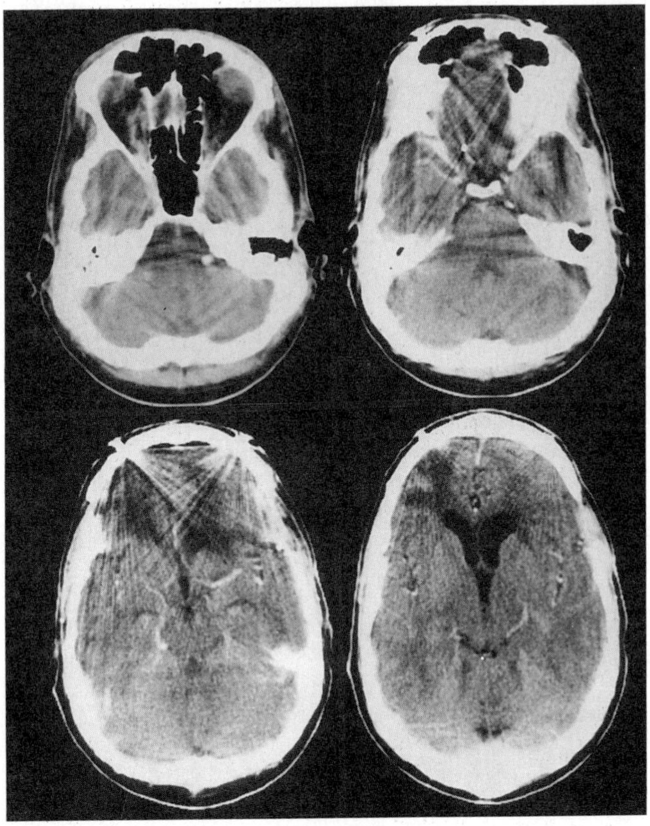

(*E*)

Figure 170-3 (*Continued*) *C.* Preoperatively, the patient underwent embolization of the right and the left external carotid artery supply to this subfrontal lesion. Even though there remained a significant supply from the ophthalmic ethmoidal perforating arteries bilaterally, it was thought that this measure markedly decreased the blood loss at the time of surgery. *D.* The result after embolization shows obliteration of the blood supply to the tumor from the external carotid system. After this embolization procedure, the patient underwent a bifrontal craniotomy with removal of the tumor. *E.* The blood supply from the internal carotid system was very meticulously eliminated as the plane was developed between the tumor and the brain. Anything that can be done to decrease the blood flow from the external carotid system to the tumor enhances this dissection.

Despite efforts at achieving complete removal whenever possible, local recurrence and, to a lesser extent, metastasis are all too common. Among the last 36 patients who had their initial operation at our institution, slightly over half (19) developed local recurrence at an average of 43 months after the initial operation. Eleven of the 36 also developed at least one metastasis by 8 months to 20 years after the initial operation (lung, four; bone, four; soft tissue, one; liver, one; retroperitoneum, one; diffuse in meninges, one). Multiple metastases were noted in two cases.

The frequency of recurrence reflects the fact that it is often impossible to be sure that complete removal has been accomplished. In our own review, the mean survival of the patients who had gross total tumor removal was just under 8 years, whereas subtotal removal was associated with an average survival of 5.5 years. For technical reasons, it seems to be particularly difficult to achieve gross total removal in cases wherein the posterior fossa and tentorium are involved; our own data support this conclusion and highlight the surgical challenge. In addition to the technical difficulties encountered in resecting posterior fossa tumors, patients do not tolerate posterior fossa tumor recurrence as well as supratentorial recurrence. The difficulties and limitations inherent in repeat posterior fossa surgery no doubt worsen the survival statistics. In a previous review of 44 patients, for instance, the average survival of patients undergoing gross total removal of tentorial or posterior fossa tumors and that of patients undergoing subtotal removal were 76 and 53 months, respectively, whereas patients with similarly treated supratentorial tumors survived 110 and 75 months, respectively.[15] The operative mortality rate in our most recent review of 56 patients was 7.1 percent, but there have been no surgical deaths in the last 21 years.

Postoperative Radiation Therapy

The impressive recurrence rate of hemangiopericytoma coupled with its potential for metastasis despite apparent total removal make it clear that surgery alone cannot be considered the solution to the treatment of hemangiopericytoma. As early as 1949, Stout reported a reduction in tumor volume with radiation therapy in an 11-year-old girl with a rectal hemangiopericytoma.[39] The response of peripheral hemangiopericytoma to radiation therapy has also been reported by others.[10–12] In addition, several authors have suggested that radiation is beneficial in the treatment of meningeal hemangiopericytomas.[13,14,21,23,24,29,42] For instance, Fukui and colleagues documented the reduction in size of meningeal hemangiopericytomas 6 months after irradiation with 4000 to 6000 cGy.[13]

Our own review of the effects of radiation therapy on hemangiopericytomas showed definite benefits. Even though we were more likely to recommend radiation therapy in cases wherein incomplete tumor removal was likely, patients receiving radiation therapy did better than those treated by surgery alone. Several years ago we reviewed 32 patients, 17 of whom underwent radiation therapy and 15 of whom did not. In this heterogeneous group, radiation therapy increased the recurrence-free interval from 34 months to 75 months ($p < 0.05$). It was our observation that doses in excess of 4500 cGy, especially doses above 5100 cGy, were more likely to prevent local recurrence.[15] The three patients who received 5130, 5200, and 5600 cGy, respectively, had no recurrence. In addition, we noted that patients who received radiation therapy after their first operation survived an average of 2.5 years longer than those who did not. This observation, however, was not statistically significant because of the small number of such patients.[15]

Despite the beneficial effects of radiation therapy, it is of interest that all intracranial recurrences after radiation lay within the treatment field. It is our opinion, therefore, that little is to be gained from whole brain or spinal axis irradiation.

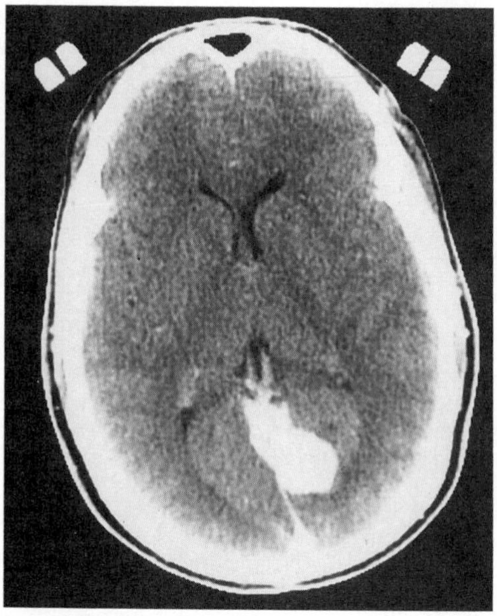

(*A*)

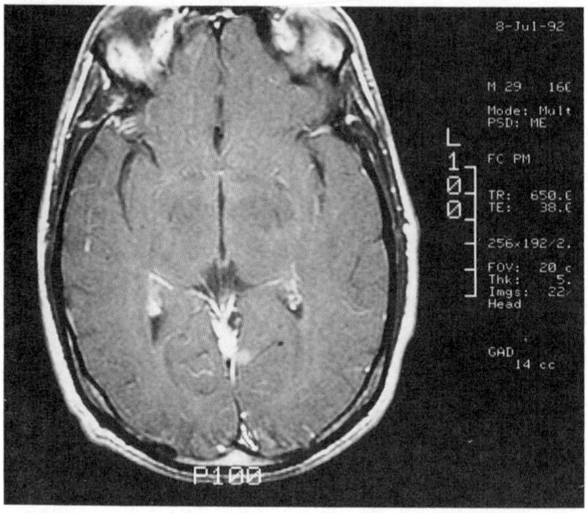

(*B*)

Figure 170-4 *A*. A stereotactic contrast-enhanced CT scan of a recurrent falx-tentorial junction hemangiopericytoma prior to radiosurgical treatment. *B*. An MRI scan through essentially the same level of the brain showing a nice response to Gamma Knife therapy. The follow-up MRI one year after the Gamma Knife treatment did not show any evidence of tumor recurrence.

Stereotactic Radiosurgery

The use of stereotactic radiosurgical procedures provide another treatment option, especially for the patient whose hemangiopericytoma is already histologically proven. Radiosurgery appears to cause a dramatic early reduction in the size of small and medium-sized hemangiopericytomas that have recurred or developed after previous surgery and/or radiation therapy (Fig. 170-4). A recent review of this subject by Coffey and coworkers at our institution discusses the treatment of five patients with eleven meningeal lesions.[6] Radiosurgical techniques allow for the delivery of additional high-dose focal irradiation in patients who have already undergone radiation therapy. All of the patients treated in this series responded to radiosurgical treatment. It would seem that previously unirradiated patients with multiple recurrent tumors and extensive dural tumor involvement should be considered as candidates for fractionated radiation therapy and follow-up MRI. If the patient has persistent or progressive tumor within the external beam radiation ports, then radiosurgical treatment might be expected to result in further tumor shrinkage and help to achieve local tumor control. It would seem that these tumors are more amenable to radiosurgical treatment than the more commonly encountered varieties of meningioma. At our institution, the Gamma Knife has been used to treat seven patients with hemangiopericytomas. Three of these patients had recurrent lesions. Although six patients did have regression in tumor size with Gamma Knife treatment, tumor recurrence or spread outside the field of treatment occurred in two patients, necessitating additional treatment. One of these patients who had an additional treatment with Gamma Knife radiation, however, died of the lesion 17 months after the treatment.

Conclusions

The meningeal hemangiopericytoma is a rare and aggressive lesion which is considered synonymous with angioblastic meningioma. Unlike the classic meningiomas, which are more common in females, hemangiopericytomas are more common in males. Typically, meningeal hemangiopericytomas occur in a somewhat younger age group than do meningiomas. In our patients, such factors as tumor cellularity, cytologic atypia, and mitotic activity were of little or no prognostic significance. The same was true of patient sex and age at the time of diagnosis.

Recurrence and, to a lesser extent, metastasis are common and mandate an aggressive approach with complete surgical removal if possible. Postoperative radiation treatment to the operative site should be seriously considered for tentorial or posterior fossa tumors as well as in instances in which gross total removal could not be achieved. Doses in the range of 5400 to 5700 cGy directed to the primary tumor bed and surrounding margin are suggested by our recent review.[15] Postoperative radiation therapy has been recommended even in cases of complete tumor removal.[41] Other reviews also suggest that these tumors are relatively radiosensitive and that radiotherapy substantially reduces the risk of local recurrence and prolongs survival.[3] The role of chemotherapy remains investigational; however, some patients with metastatic hemangiopericytoma seem to benefit from adriamycin-based regimens.[3] Long-term follow-up, at least to 15 years, is necessary, in that late recurrence and late metastases to lung, bone, and soft tissue are not uncommon.

References

1. Aouad N, Vital C, Rivel J, et al. Giant supratentorial meningeal haemangiopericytoma in a newborn. *Acta Neurochir (Wien)* 1991; 112:154–156.
2. Bailey P, Cushing H, Eisenhardt L. Angioblastic meningiomas. *Arch Pathol Lab Med* 1928; 6:953–990.
3. Bastin KT, Mehta MP. Meningeal hemangiopericytoma: defining the role for radiation therapy. *J Neurooncol* 1992; 14:227–287.
4. Blank W, Spring A, Giesen H, et al. Intracranial haemangiopericytoma in a child. *Klin Padiatr* 1988; 200:422–425.
5. Chan RC, Thompson GB. Morbidity, mortality, and quality of life following surgery for intracranial meningiomas: a retrospective study in 257 cases. *J Neurosurg* 1984; 60:52–60.
6. Coffey RJ, Cascino TL, Shaw EG. Radiosurgical treatment of recurrent hemangiopericytomas of the meninges: preliminary results. *J Neurosurg* 1993; 78:903–908.
7. Cushing H, Eisenhardt L. *Meningiomas: Their Classification, Regional Behaviour, Life History and Surgical End Results.* Springfield, IL: Charles C Thomas, 1938.
8. D'Amore ESG, Manivel JC, Sung JH. Soft-tissue and meningeal hemangiopericytomas: an immunohistochemical and ultrastructural study. *Hum Pathol* 1990; 21:414–423.
9. Dardick I, Hammar SP, Scheithauer BW. Ultrastructural spectrum of hemangiopericytoma: a comparative study of fetal, adult, and neoplastic pericytes. *Ultrastruct Pathol* 1989; 13:111–154.
10. Enzinger FM, Smith BH. Hemangiopericytoma: an analysis of 106 cases. *Hum Pathol* 1976; 7:61–82.
11. Fabiani A, Favero M, Trebini F. On the primary meningeal tumors with special concern to the hemangiopericytoma pathology and biology. *Zentralbl Neurochir* 1980; 41:273–284.
12. Friedman M, Egan JW. Irradiation of hemangiopericytoma of Stout. *Radiology* 1960; 74:721–730.
13. Fukui M, Kitamura K, Nakagaki H, et al. Irradiated meningiomas: a clinical evaluation. *Acta Neurochir (Wien)* 1980; 54:33–43.
14. Goellner JR, Laws ER Jr, Soule EH, et al. Hemangiopericytoma of the meninges: Mayo Clinic experience. *Am J Clin Pathol* 1978; 70:375–380.
15. Guthrie BL, Ebersold MJ, Scheithauer BW, et al. Meningeal hemangiopericytoma: histopathological features, treatment, and long-term follow-up of 44 cases. *Neurosurgery* 1989; 25:514–522.
16. Iwaki T, Fukui M, Takeshita I, et al. Hemangiopericytoma of the meninges: a clinicopathologic and immunohistochemical study. *Clin Neuropathol* 1988; 7:93–99.
17. Jääskeläinen J, Servo A, Haltia M, et al. Intracranial hemangiopericytoma: radiology, surgery, radiotherapy, and outcome in 21 patients. *Surg Neurol* 1985; 23:227–236.
18. Jellinger K, Machacek E. Rare intracranial tumours in infancy and childhood. In Voth D, Gutjahr P, Langmaid C (eds): *Tumours of the Central Nervous System in Infancy and Childhood.* Berlin: Springer, 1982, pp 44–52.
19. Jellinger K, Slowik F. Histological subtypes and prognostic problems in meningiomas. *J Neurol* 1975; 208:279–298.
20. Kernohan JW, Uihlein A. *Sarcomas of the Brain.* Springfield, IL: Charles C Thomas, 1962.
21. King DL, Chang CH, Pool JL. Radiotherapy in the management of meningiomas. *Acta Radiol Ther Phys Biol* 1966; 5:26–33.
22. Kochanek S, Schröder R, Firsching R. Hemangiopericytoma of meninges. I. Histopathological variability and differential diagnosis. *Zentralbl Neurochir* 1986; 47:183–190.
23. Lal H, Sanyal B, Pant GC, et al. Hemangiopericytoma: report of three cases regarding role of radiation therapy. *Am J Roentgenol* 1976; 126:887–891.
24. Lesoin F, Bouchez B, Krivosic I, et al. Hemangiopericytic meningioma of the pineal region: case report. *Eur Neurol* 1984; 23:274–277.
25. Lolova I, Kamenova M. Hemangiopericytoma of the brain: histological and histochemical study of four cases. *J Neurosurg* 1973; 39:636–641.
26. McDonald JV, Terry R. Hemangiopericytoma of the brain. *Neurology* 1961; 11:497–502.
27. McMaster MJ, Soule EH, Ivins JC. Hemangiopericytoma: a clinicopathologic study and long-term follow-up of 60 patients. *Cancer* 1975; 36:2232–2244.
28. Miettinen M. Antibody specific to muscle actins in the diagnosis and classification of soft tissue tumors. *Am J Pathol* 1988; 130:205–215.
29. Mira JG, Chu FCH, Fortner JG. The role of radiotherapy in the management of malignant hemangiopericytoma: report of eleven new cases and review of the literature. *Cancer* 1977; 39:1254–1259.
30. Mirimannoff RO, Dosoretz DE, Linggood RM, et al. Meningioma: analysis of recurrence and progression following neurosurgical resection. *J Neurosurg* 1985; 62:18–24.
31. Nakamura Y, Becker LE. Meningeal tumors of infancy and childhood. *Pediatr Pathol* 1985; 3:341–358.
32. Nemes Z. Differentiation markers in hemangiopericytoma. *Cancer* 1992; 69:133–140.

33. Pitkethly DT, Hardman JM, Kempe LG, et al. Angioblastic meningiomas: clinicopathologic study of 81 cases. *J Neurosurg* 1970; 32:539–544.
34. Russell DS, Rubeinstein LJ. *Pathology of Tumours of the Nervous System,* 4th ed. Baltimore: Williams & Wilkins, 1977, pp 74–79.
35. Schröder R. Firsching R, Kochanek S. Hemangiopericytoma of meninges. II. General and clinical data. *Zentralbl Neurochir* 1986; 47:191–199.
36. Schurch W, Skalli O, Lagace R, et al. Intermediate filament proteins and actin isoforms as markers for soft-tissue tumor differentiation and origin. III. Hemangiopericytomas and glomus tumors. *Am J Pathol* 1990; 136:771–786.
37. Simpson D. The recurrence of intracranial meningiomas after surgical treatment. *J Neurol Neurosurg Psychiatry* 1957; 20:22–39.
38. Skullerud K, Löken AC. The prognosis in meningiomas. *Acta Neuropathol (Berl)* 1974; 29:337–344.
39. Stout AP. Hemangiopericytoma: a study of twenty-five new cases. *Cancer* 1949; 2:1027–1035.
40. Thomas HG, Dolman CL, Berry K. Malignant meningioma: clinical and pathologic features. *J Neurosurg* 1981; 55:929–934.
41. Uemura S, Kuratsu J, Hamada J, et al. Effect of radiation therapy against intracranial hemangiopericytoma. *Neurol Med Chir (Tokyo)* 1992; 32:328–332.
42. Wara WM, Sheline GE, Newman H, et al. Radiation therapy of meningiomas. *Am J Roentgenol* 1980; 123:453–458.
43. Winek RR, Scheithauer BW, Wick MR. Meningioma, meningeal hemangiopericytoma (angioblastic meningioma), peripheral hemangiopericytoma and acoustic schwannoma: a comparative immunohistochemical study. *Am J Surg Pathol* 1989; 13:251–261.

171

Choroid Plexus Papillomas

Hector E. James

Choroid plexus papillomas are benign neoplastic growths that arise from the ventricular choroid plexus and can be considered of ependymal origin.[8] They are slow-growing. They remain asymptomatic for considerable periods, are commonly associated with hydrocephalus, and are liable to hemorrhage spontaneously.[8,9]

Incidence

Considering adults and children together, choroid plexus papillomas are rare, constituting less than 1 percent of all primary intracranial tumors. Although they occur at any age, the majority occur in the first decade; thus in children they constitute 1.8 to 3 percent of intracranial neoplasms.[4,5] Forty-eight percent of those reported in the literature were in children under 10 years of age and 20 percent in infants under 1 year of age.[5] They are among the more frequent tumors in children under the age of 3 years.[4,5]

The tumor affects both sexes equally. Genetic factors do not seem to play a role.

Pathology

In adults, the choroid plexus papilloma is most often located in the fourth ventricle, whereas in children it usually arises in the lateral ventricles.[2,4,5,8,9] The third ventricle is seldom involved.[4,10]

To gross examination the tumor is a dark pink or red meaty mass with an irregular papillary surface. In the lateral ventricle it is accompanied by a considerable enlargement of the ventricle. If it is located in the lateral recess of the fourth ventricle, it can significantly distort surrounding structures. It is characteristically easy to separate from the surrounding brain. Small foci of hemorrhage may be present in its interior.[8,9]

Typical of the choroid plexus papilloma in microscopic examination is its resemblance to the normal choroid plexus. Resting on a slender vascular connective tissue stroma is a delicate arrangement of papillary formations, usually of single layers of cuboidal or columnar epithelium (Fig. 171-1). Cilia and blepharoplasts are found in some infantile tumors.[8] Malignant changes indicate that the tumor is the rare choroid plexus carcinoma, representing an entirely different clinical condition than the choroid plexus papilloma.[2,4,5,8,9]

On occasion, gross and microscopic spread in the leptomeninges of a benign choroid plexus papilloma is seen at postmortem examination. In these cases there are no malignant histologic changes, and such lesions do not cause clinical symptoms.[8]

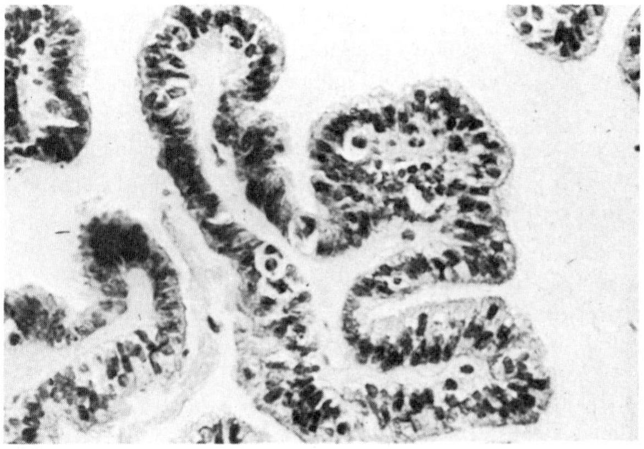

Figure 171-1 Microscopic appearance of a choroid plexus papilloma. Note the delicate papillary structures formed by a single layer of epithelium on a fine connective tissue stroma. Hematoxylin-eosin stain. (Courtesy of Dr. Luis Schut.)

In the differential histologic diagnosis, papillary ependymoma and xanthogranuloma of the choroid plexus must be considered. In the former the cells are usually piled up in multiple layers and the stromal support is neuroglial, not connective tissue. The latter consists of small lesions, yellowish and firm, with deposition of cholesterol in their stroma; they are often bilateral.[8]

Pathogenesis of Hydrocephalus

Ventricular enlargement is seen in association with most but not all choroid plexus papillomas. This may be due to a combination of factors: overproduction of CSF, obstruction of CSF pathways by the tumor mass, or subarachnoid scarring due to recurrent bleeding from the tumor.

In those tumors located in the fourth and third ventricles the tumor may reach a size that can obstruct CSF flow. In these cases removal of the tumor mass may resolve the hydrocephalus.

Recurrent occult bleeding is a known complication of these tumors. The subarachnoid obstruction due to basal meningitis and fibrosis may then lead to hydrocephalus, thus accounting for the lack of resolution of the hydrocephalus despite tumor removal in some cases.[9]

Overproduction of CSF by the tumor mass has long been suspected and was thought to be documented in two patients.[1,6] In one of these, measurement of CSF production by ventriculolumbar perfusion revealed a formation rate of 1.05 ml/min prior to surgical removal of the tumor; 8 weeks after surgery it was measured at 0.2 ml/min.[6] This may explain the resolution of hydrocephalus in some cases after the removal of a choroid plexus papilloma from the lateral ventricle.[2,4,5,7]

In a series of 23 patients with choroid plexus tumors, 18 had hydrocephalus at the time of presentation. Thirteen of these went on to require a CSF diversionary procedure.[4]

Clinical Features

Clinical Presentation

Choroid plexus papillomas may present with overt intracranial hypertension with or without focal neurological signs, with progressively increasing head size, or with insidious hydrocephalus.

As indicated above, obstruction to CSF flow by the tumor mass, subarachnoid fibrosis, or overproduction of CSF will create hydrocephalus. As volume increases, intracranial hypertension follows. Thus, except for headaches, irritability, vomiting, and malaise, there may be no symptoms and a paucity of findings. In the tumor situated in the lateral ventricle, hemiparesis and corticospinal tract findings may be present.

In infancy a common referral is for macrocephaly, and the tumor may then be detected as part of a hydrocephalus workup. In 16 of 23 children in Matson's series,[5] progressive enlargement of the head was one of the important findings. Papilledema was present in over half the patients.[5]

The hydrocephalus may have a slow and progressive course in the adult patient, leading to an insidious presentation. In these cases difficulty with mentation and occasional headaches may be the only symptoms.

In children, irritability and malaise may be seen in 33 percent, headaches in 18 percent, and visual difficulties in 18 percent.[2] Seizures, as a form of early presentation, may be seen in 18 percent.[2]

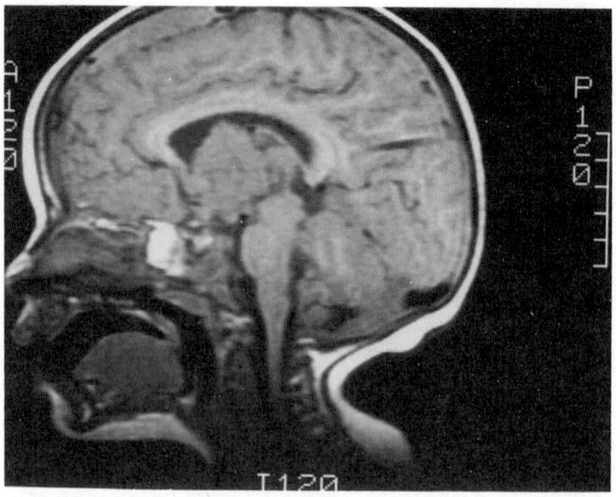

Figure 171-2 Cranial MRI of a 1-year-old infant with a choroid plexus papilloma of the III ventricle. Note the enlargement of the III ventricle by the mass.

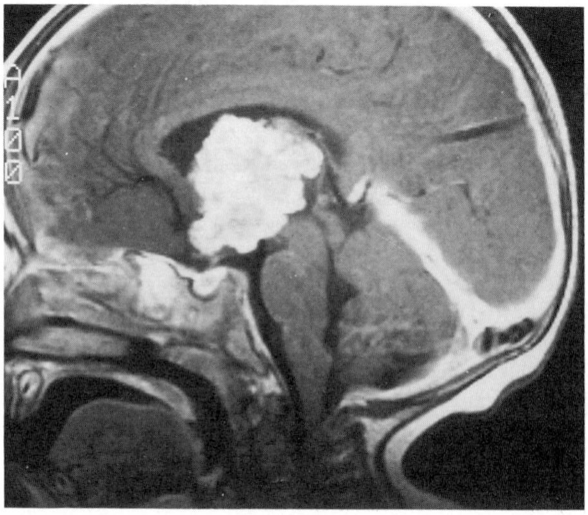

Figure 171-3 Cranial MRI of the patient shown in Fig. 171-2, following the administration of gadolinium. Note the uniform increase in signal throughout the tumor.

CSF Findings

Elevation of CSF protein values is characteristic in choroid plexus papillomas and is found in over two-thirds of patients.[5] In 50 percent of patients there is some degree of xanthochromia, but frank blood is uncommon.[5] When measured, the lumbar CSF pressure has nearly always been elevated.[5]

Radiologic Findings

Plain skull roentgenograms will reveal nonspecific changes of elevated intracranial pressure, such as separation of sutures, craniofacial disproportion, and the ''beaten silver'' appearance of the calvarium.[3] In children, tumor calcification has been reported in 21 percent.[3]

On noncontrast CT scanning the tumor is noted to be similar in density to brain tissue, but there is dramatic enhancement with intravenous injection of a contrast agent.[3] CT provides detail about the outline, extent, and size of the tumor and demonstrates the degree of hydrocephalus.[3] On MRI the tumor may have a signal similar to that of the surrounding brain, and following gadolinium infusion, a strong increase in the signal is noted (Figs. 171-2 and 171-3).

Cerebral angiography reveals the vascular supply of the tumor, which can aid in surgical planning.[2,3] The tumor is fed by the corresponding choroidal arteries and shows a diffuse blush in the capillary phase. In choroid plexus carcinomas and in ependymomas, the irregular vessels and early venous shunting seen may aid in the differential diagnosis.[2,3]

Surgical Therapy

The treatment of choroid plexus papilloma is total surgical excision with minimal damage to the surrounding neural elements. Subtotal removal and radiation therapy play no role.[2,4,10]

Tumor in the fourth ventricle location is reached through a midline suboccipital approach. Interruption of the vascular plexus coming from the choroid supply aids in removal of the tumor. Those tumors in the fourth ventricle are commonly quite free and easy to remove. Those in the cerebellopontine angle and foramen of Luschka are best treated by piecemeal removal through both the angle and the fourth ventricle.[7]

The rare third ventricle tumors are best approached through a transcallosal incision, although a transfrontal cortical incision and access through an enlargement of the foramen of Monro has been described.[5,10]

Tumors in the lateral ventricle are most commonly located in the trigone. Two approaches have been advocated for choroid papillomas in this location. One is via a temporoparietal craniotomy, with a linear cortical incision in a convenient thinned gyrus overlying the tumor if the ventricles are enlarged or through an opening of a cone of cerebral tissue to the ventricle if the ventricles are small.[4,5] Another approach to the trigone is through a linear incision in the superior temporal gyrus which allows access to the choroid supply under the tumor, rather than approaching it superiorly.[4,6] In both approaches, emphasis is placed on interrupting the vascular supply early in the operation, since this can reduce the tumor size dramatically and minimize bleeding from the highly vascular neoplasm.

Total surgical removal of the neoplasm not only cures the tumor but may lead to complete resolution of the hydrocephalus.[2,5,7] However, in 50 percent of cases the hydrocephalus will not resolve and a shunt will be needed.[2,5,7] It is imperative, therefore, to follow these patients in the postoperative period and assess the size of their ventricles.

Results and Complications

Total surgical removal of a choroid plexus papilloma cures the disease, and no recurrence following such a procedure has been noted.[2,4,5,7] Although a mortality of 22 percent was noted by Matson,[5] the death of 5 of the 23 patients was not due to the operative intervention itself in 2, and 2 others were moribund upon admission. Present-day anesthesia, microneurosurgery, and pediatric intensive care support should allow for an operative and perioperative mortality of less than 1 percent.[2,4,10]

Neurological handicaps vary according to the size of the tumor and the location and degree of transcortical surgery. Postoperative epilepsy can occur in those patients with supratentorial neoplasms. However, overall the surgeon can expect a good outcome in these patients.[2,4,10]

References

1. Eisenberg HM, McComb JG, Lorenzo AV. Cerebrospinal fluid overproduction and hydrocephalus associated with choroid plexus papilloma. *J Neurosurg* 1974; 40:381–385.
2. Ellenbogen RG, Winston KR, Kupsky WJ. Tumors of the choroid plexus in children. *Neurosurgery* 1989; 25:327–335.
3. Harwood-Nash DC, Fitz CR. *Neuroradiology in Infants and Children.* St Louis: Mosby, 1976, pp 751–754.
4. Humphreys RP, Nemoto S, Hendrick EB, Hoffman HJ. Childhood choroid plexus tumors. In Marlin AE (ed): *Concepts in Pediatric Neurosurgery,* vol 7. Basel: Karger, 1987, pp 1–18.
5. Matson DD. *Neurosurgery of Infancy and Childhood,* 2d ed. Springfield, IL: Charles C Thomas, 1969, pp 581–595.
6. Milhorat TH. *Pediatric Neurosurgery* (Contemporary Neurology Series, vol 16). Philadelphia: Davis, 1978, pp 95–99.
7. Raimondi AJ, Gutierrez FA. Diagnosis and surgical treatment of choroid plexus papillomas. *Childs Brain* 1975; 1:81–115.
8. Rubinstein LJ. *Tumors of the Central Nervous System* (Atlas of Tumor Pathology, 2d ser, fasc. 6). Washington: Armed Forces Institute of Pathology, 1972, pp 257–262.
9. Russell DS, Rubinstein LJ. *Pathology of Tumours of the Nervous System,* 3d ed. Baltimore: Williams & Wilkins, 1971, pp 163–166.
10. Schijman E, Monges J, Raimondi AJ, Tomita T. Choroid plexus papillomas of the III ventricle in childhood. *Childs Nerv Syst* 1990; 6:331–334.

172

Intracranial Lipomas

Bermans J. Iskandar
Doyle G. Graham

Incidence and Location

Although lipomas are common in the rest of the body, intracranial lipomas are usually found incidentally at autopsy (0.08 to 0.2 percent of all autopsies) or on radiographic studies (0.06 to 0.3 percent of all computed tomography scans),[10] and constitute fewer than 0.1 percent of intracranial tumors. Owing to their embryologic origin from the meninx primitiva (see below), lipomas occur in the cerebrospinal fluid cisterns of the brain. Nearly 50 percent of reported cases are located in the pericallosal cistern (commonly called lipomas of the corpus callosum); 20 percent in the ambient, quadrigeminal plate, and chiasmatic cisterns combined; 12 percent in the cerebellopontine angle and/or the internal auditory meatus; and 7 percent in the brain convexities, most commonly around the sylvian fissure.[10] A larger percentage of lipomas in children occur in the pericallosal cisterns; otherwise, there appear to be no age differences, and, with one minor exception (the preponderance of cerebellopontine angle lipoma in males),[38] there are no sex differences.[10,11,17,23,30,49]

Although Rokitansky first described the corpus callosum lipoma in 1856, the first mention of an intracranial lipoma in the literature was as early as 1818, when Meckel described a chiasmatic lesion; these tumors were observed incidentally at autopsy until 1939, when Sosman described their appearance using plain skull radiography and pneumoencephalography.[43,46] Nearly 200 cases have been reported since, especially after the advent of computed tomography (CT) and magnetic resonance imaging (MRI).

Pathologic Findings

Intracranial lipomas are deep yellow lesions, which vary from less than a millimeter to several centimeters in dimension (Fig. 172-1). They are composed of adult fat cells with peripheral, sometimes indented, nuclei. The mass of fat cells is surrounded by a collagenous capsule, which may be intimately bound to surrounding structures. The capsule and surrounding parenchyma frequently contain calcifications, which are sometimes associated with bone formation. Bone formation is one of the few features that differentiate these lipomas from lipomas outside the central nervous system.[6,12,26] The lesions have a spectrum of vascularity, ranging from the minimally vascularized lipoma to the "angiolipoma," which is a mixture of adipose and hemopoietic tissues.[26,31,44,48] Finally, large vessels and nerves course through the lipoma undisturbed. Common examples include the anterior cerebral artery in the case of the pericallosal lipoma and the trochlear nerve in ambient cistern lipomas.

Histogenesis

The term *lipoma,* which implies that the biology of the lesion is that of an enlarging neoplasm, is a misnomer. In a brilliant analysis of the hypotheses that had previously been proposed to explain the embryogenesis of intracranial lipomas, Truwit and Barkovich[46] gave persuasive evidence that these lipomas are congenital lesions. They are thought to result from "abnormal persistence and maldifferentiation of the meninx primitiva during the development of the subarachnoid space."[46] The meninx primitiva,[32] the anlage of the meninges, is a mesenchymal derivative of the neural crest, which, starting at 32 to 44 days of gestation, dissolves to form the subarachnoid spaces. In some cases, "a persistent, therefore abnormal focus of meninx primitiva is somehow induced into adipose tissue and matures into a lipoma."[46]

The dissolution of the meninx occurs in an orderly fashion, starting ventral to the brain stem (forming the prepontomedullary cisterns), then extending dorsally (forming the peri- and dorsomesencephalic cisterns) and later cephalad (supratentorial cisterns). The last meninx to resorb is in the area of the lamina terminalis. This order is found to correspond inversely to the frequency of lipoma formation in the cisterns. Thus, pericallosal lipomas, which have the most time to form, are more common than quadrigeminal plate lipomas, which are in turn more common than interpeduncular ones. In addition, areas of flexure in the neural tube, such as the pontomedullary junction, are sites of redundant meninx primitiva and are thus more likely to develop lipomas. Finally, because the lipoma is "a maldifferentiated subarachnoid space, whatever courses through the cisterns (vessels, nerves) can course through the lipoma" without being compressed or displaced.[46]

Other theories of the formation of intracranial lipomas have included (1) hypertrophy of fatty tissues that are already present in the meninges, (2) formation of a lipomatous glioma from brain parenchyma, (3) metaplasia of meningeal connective tissue into fat, (4) inclusion of mesodermal tissue in the lips of a closing neural tube, and others. None of these postulates, however, can explain the fact that vessels and cranial nerves run undisturbed in their course. In addition, the first three hypotheses cannot explain the concomitant formation of neighboring neural defects (the reader is referred to the excellent paper by Truwit and Barkovich[46] for a more thorough analysis.) Finally, one may argue that there is never fat in the CNS. However, both the meninx primitiva and early precapillary parenchyma have been proposed as cells from which fat could differentiate.[26] In fact, in certain species of fish, fat cells are normal constituents of the meninges.[2]

Clinical Manifestations

One-third of patients with intracranial lipomas reported to date have been asymptomatic. In the remaining two-thirds of cases, certain symptoms and signs have been found to be associated with these lesions irrespective of their location intracranially.[10] However, because of the malformational, noncompressive, and nongrowing nature of the lipomas, most of these symptoms and signs

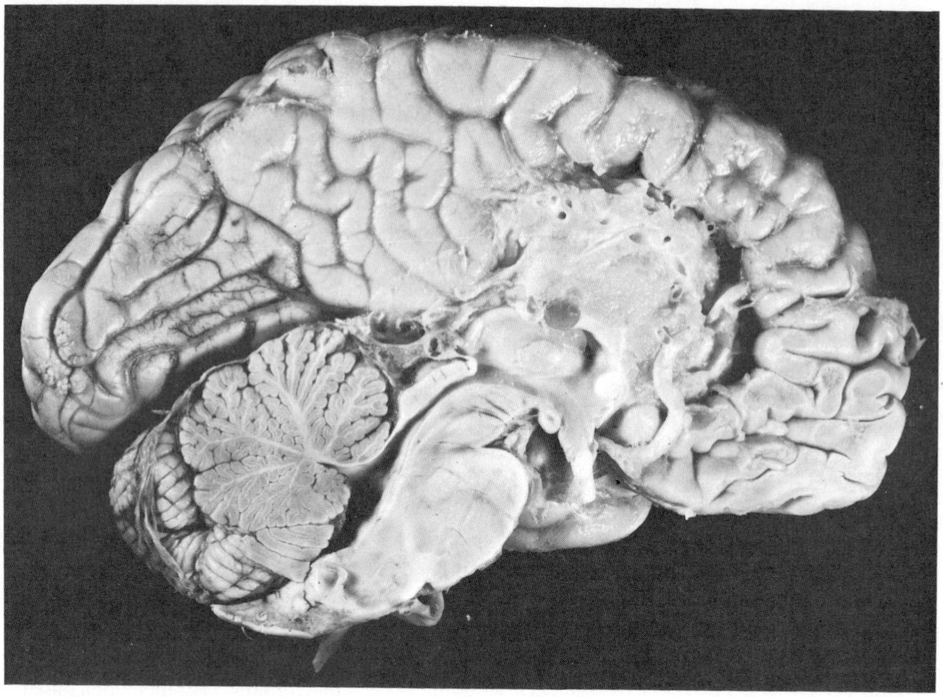

Figure 172-1 The brain of a 56-year-old man who died of renal cell carcinoma contained this asymptomatic lipoma in the region of a congenitally absent corpus callosum. The lesion was canary yellow except for the unusual nodule of cartilage seen just superior to the massa intermedia. (From Burger PC, Vogel FS. *Surgical Pathology of the Nervous System and Its Coverings,* 2d ed. New York: Wiley, 1982, p 109, with permission.)

are unlikely to be directly caused by the lipoma; instead, they are thought to be due to other associated, usually neighboring, stable brain malformations. In general, 30 percent of lipoma patients have a seizure disorder, which is often severe, is focal or generalized, and has an average onset age of 15 years. Recurrent headaches are a presenting symptom in 25 percent, and, last, 10 to 15 percent have behavioral disturbances and/or mental retardation.[10] Other less commonly reported features include fainting spells, vomiting, episodic leg weakness, blurred vision, sleepwalking, diencephalic disturbances such as adiposogenital dystrophy and hypothermia, and even transient ischemic attacks.[10,11] Patients with infratentorial lesions occasionally present with hydrocephalus, cerebellar ataxia, motor weakness, or sleep apnea[17,23,30,43]; there are also rare reports of ocular motor apraxia[41] and cranial nerve symptoms and signs such as hemifacial spasm,[39] vertigo, and hearing loss. Symptoms characteristic of lipomas at specific locations will be discussed under the appropriate subheadings below.

Associated Anomalies

Just as agenesis of the corpus callosum is associated with virtually half of pericallosal lipomas,[49] hypogenesis of neural structures adjacent to lipomas at other locations may also occur. A typical example is the occasional hypogenesis of the mamillary bodies with a lipoma along the mamillary-infundibular axis. The lack of resorption of the meninx primitiva presumably interferes with the development of neighboring brain tissue, thus resulting in local structural malformations (Fig. 172-2), most commonly hypogenesis. Because the meninx of the lamina terminalis is the last to be resorbed, it is the one with the most chance to maldevelop. Therefore, anterior interhemispheric (i.e., pericallosal) lipomas, hypogenesis of the corpus callosum, and malformations of the frontal brain and skull are the anomalies most likely to occur (Table 172-1).[10,45,46]

Intracranial lipomas also occur as part of specific syndromes. These include the Bannayan syndrome,[21] encephalocraniocutaneous lipomatosis,[3,15] Goldenhar-Gorlin syndrome,[1,5] neurifibromatosis variants,[36] and frontonasal dysplasia.[33] The importance of diagnosing these syndromes remains unclear, with the exception of the Bannayan syndrome. The latter is an autosomal dominant disorder in which early diagnosis provides the possibility of genetic counseling.[21]

Neuroradiologic Findings

Plain Radiographs

The larger lipomas of the corpus callosum are occasionally recognized on plain x-ray films as radiolucent zones in the midline of the frontal region, best demonstrated on the lateral view. The lesion is surrounded by curvilinear calcifications (Fig. 172-3), which may be punctate in the capsular region and may rarely resemble tumor calcification. Associated findings may be asymmetry of the skull or midline skull defects.[10,11,23]

Carotid Angiography

Carotid angiography may reveal enlarged and tortuous neighboring of feeding arteries. In the case of pericallosal lipomas, for instance, dilated, tortuous anterior cerebral arteries may be found, with occasionally only a single pericallosal artery, and even pericallosal aneurysms.[13] Rarely, pathologic neovascularity has been seen.

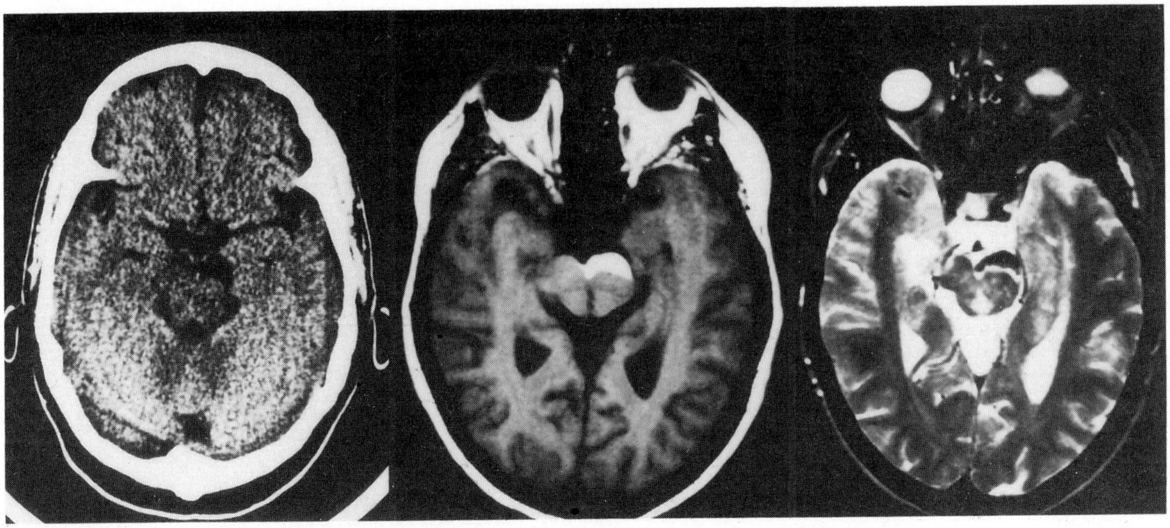

Figure 172-2 Cerebral peduncle lipoma in a neurologically intact patient. *A.* hypodensity on unenhanced brain CT scan; *B.* high signal intensity on T1-weighted axial MR image *C.* low signal intensity on T2-weighted axial MR image, with a prominent chemical shift artifact. Note the malformed cerebral peduncle. (MR images courtesy of Linda Gray, M.D.)

Computed Tomography

CT is a very accurate method for the diagnosis of intracranial lipomas, for two main reasons: (1) its ability to delineate calcification and (2) the low attenuation values of fat (−40 to −100 Hounsfield units) (Fig. 172-2). However, very small lesions that do not occupy one whole CT slice may show higher attenuation owing to the "partial volume" effect of the lipoma and surrounding tissue. This may cloud the diagnosis, making the lipoma look like a dermoid or epidermoid tumor. In addition, lipomas do not enhance with contrast and do not cause peritumoral edema.[10,23,30]

TABLE 172-1 Anomalies Associated with Intracranial Lipomas

Neural (Intracranial)
Agenesis/hypogenesis of neighboring neural tissue (e.g., corpus callosum)
Frontal encephalocele
Heterotopia
Chiari type I malformation
Hydrocephalus
Absent septum pellucidum
Other intracranial lipomas at different sites
Neighboring Soft Tissue and Bone
Frontal bone defect
Facial dysplasia/hypoplasia
Neighboring soft tissue lipoma
Neighboring Blood Vessels
Tortuous and dilated vasculature
Pericallosal artery aneurysm
Azygous anterior cerebral artery
Absent vessel
Neighboring Cranial Nerves
Absence (e.g., of trochlear nerve)
Duplication
Unusual branching patterns
Other Body Parts (Incidental?)
Webbed toes
Funnel chest
Spina bifida
Myelomeningocele
Other sporadic anomalies

Source: (See specific syndromes mentioned in text)

Data from Tart and Quisling[45] and Zettner and Netsky.[49]

Magnetic Resonance Imaging

MRI is the study of choice for detecting intracranial lipomas. First, it is the best modality available for the detection of associated brain anomalies; second, it provides sagittal and coronal images, making reconstruction unnecessary; and, third, it allows the visualization of cranial nerves and vessels, which either penetrate or surround the lipoma. Lipomas are homogeneous structures (in contrast to dermoids, epidermoids, and teratomas) with high signal intensity on T1-weighted images, hypo- to isointensity (compared to brain) on T2-weighted images, and no enhancement with gadolinium diethylaminetriaminepentaacetic acid (DTPA) (unlike other tumors typical of the same locations). Flow voids within vessels, and, less commonly, calcifications, may show up as signal voids within the lipomas. In doubtful cases, fat suppression techniques yield the diagnosis; and, finally, a chemical shift artifact, if present, is pathognomonic (Fig. 172-2).[4,18,37,42]

Special Features

Pericallosal Lipomas

Comprising about 50 percent of intracranial lipomas, lipomas of the corpus callosum are asymptomatic 42 percent of the time, with the most common presenting complaint being seizures, followed by motor dysfunction, then headaches.[10] Pericallosal lipomas were recently divided into two important types[45,46]: tubulonodular lipo-

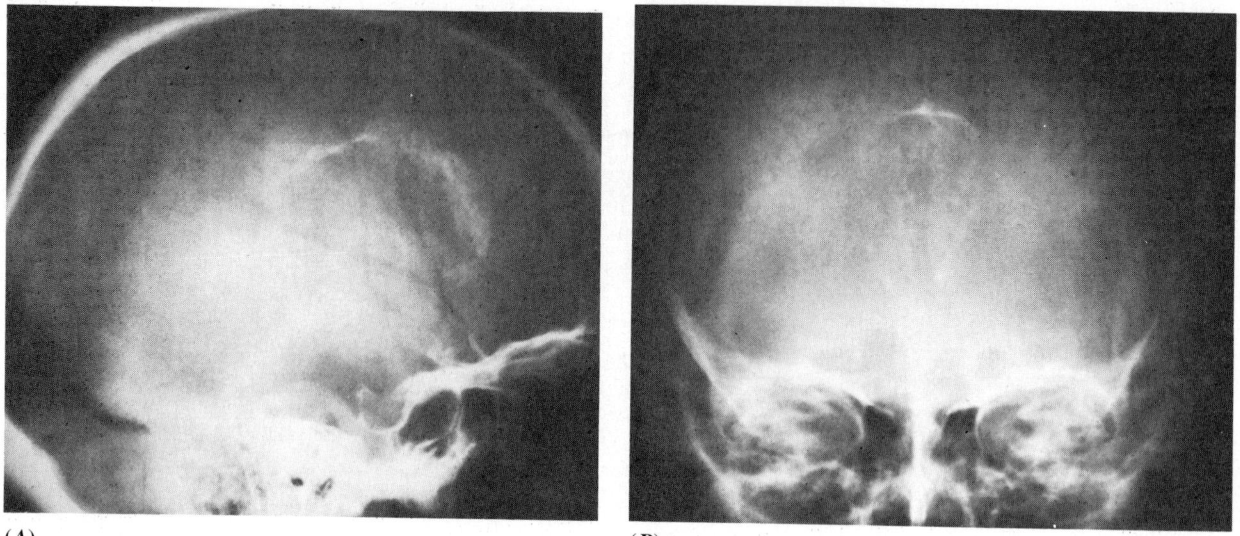

(*A*) (*B*)

Figure 172-3 Lateral (*A*) and anteroposterior (*B*) skull films showing a rim of calcification in the periphery of a lipoma of the corpus callosum.

mas and curvilinear lipomas. The former are usually large (greater than 2 centimeters in diameter), are round or cylindrical, and occur over the anterior aspect of the corpus callosum. These lesions are frequently associated with severe frontal anomalies. Conversely, the curvilinear lipomas are thin, ''ribbon-like'' structures that occur over the posterior aspect of the corpus callosum, curving around the splenium. They are more likely to be asymptomatic and have a much lower incidence of associated anomalies; moreover, even when other anomalies occur, they are usually less severe.[46] Truwit and Barkovich again gave convincing explanations for these observations. The anterior corpus callosum develops earlier than its posterior counterpart. Therefore, an early problem in the meninx of the lamina terminalis would cause complete agenesis of the corpus callosum, as opposed to a later problem, which may only cause hypogenesis of the more posterior part. In addition, the posterior corpus callosum develops after closure of the anterior neuropore, and thus a late abnormality is less likely to be associated with frontal brain malformations. Finally, earlier lesions cause bigger lipomas, presumably because more meninx is still available early on.[45,46]

Lipomas of the Cerebellopontine Angle and Internal Auditory Canal

Lipomas of the cerebellopontine (CP) angle are relatively common in the literature, and are usually divided into small lesions that are limited to the internal auditory canal (IAC), and others that occur elsewhere in the CP angle, with or without extension into the IAC. They are twice as common in males as in females, and are usually not associated with other obvious brain malformations. They often involve surrounding cranial nerves, with the eighth nerve being involved in most cases. This involvement is usually very intimate, with no intervening capsule, making surgery extremely hazardous. CP angle lipomas represent 0.14 percent of CP angle tumors and are distinguished from the others by MRI characteristics. Schwannomas, meningiomas, epidermoid tumors, and metastatic growths, unlike fatty lesions, show low signal intensity on T1-weighted images, and usually enhance with gadolinium-DTPA. Lipomas that are limited to the IAC are only rarely visible on CT.[8,34,35,38,40] Symptoms include tinnitus, vertigo, otalgia, and trigeminal neuralgia. However, hearing loss is the most common symptom, occurring in most cases, and in all of the reported cases of lipomas invading the IAC. The occurrence of symptoms attributed to vestibulocochlear nerve dysfunction is somewhat puzzling, considering that patients with lipomas involving other cranial nerves are usually not symptomatic (see lipomas of the ambient and quadrigeminal plate cisterns below). Anatomic malformations of cranial nerves have, however, been reported (e.g., trochlear nerve duplication or branching). The occasional case report of CP angle lipomas causing new or progressive symptoms[38] makes the controversy even more interesting, since lipomas are not expected to grow, and therefore should not be causing symptoms to progress. More thorough evaluations using serial MRI scans, audiograms, and evoked potentials are needed to help clarify the pathophysiology underlying these symptoms.

Surgery is usually not indicated for two reasons: first, because there is no evidence that the symptoms are directly related to the lipoma; and second, because it is very difficult to save the involved cranial nerves, especially the facial and vestibulocochlear nerves, during these procedures. However, a nonaggressive debulking procedure using a translabyrinthine approach has been suggested in some patients with progressive symptomatology (such as recent-onset vertigo),[38] with the goal of decompressing the area with minimal injury to the facial nerve. It would be interesting to find out if the occasional symptomatic improvement reported after this procedure is actually due to sectioning of the vestibulocochlear nerve rather than resection of the lipoma. Hearing conservation with various surgical approaches has, in general, not been successful.[23,25,38]

Sylvian Lipomas

Located in the sylvian fissure, these lipomas usually enclose the middle cerebral artery and its branches, but without any compression or displacement of the vessels. Half of the patients reported had seizures with late onset, including at least one case of uncinate fits. Surgical resection of the lipoma is dangerous and is ineffective in treating the seizures. Instead, medical control of the seizure disorder has been successful in most cases.[27,28]

Lipomas of the Ambient and Quadrigeminal Plate Cisterns

Lipomas of the mesencephalic cisterns usually enclose one or both trochlear nerves without damaging or compressing them. Nevertheless, the nerve itself may be duplicated, branched, or absent, most probably owing to a separate developmental error that is associated in some way with the lipoma formation.[22] Hydrocephalus[19,29] is not rare and is probably due to an aqueductal malformation, or, less likely, to compression of the cerebral aqueduct by the fatty tissue.[20,23] Symptoms and signs are very rare; if present, they may include ataxia, hemiparesis, paralysis of upgaze, and intellectual deterioration associated with the hydrocephalus. Complete extirpation of the lipoma would be dangerous because of its frequent infiltration of the brain stem and/or the superior medullary velum. Ventricular shunting is necessary, however, to treat the hydrocephalus.

Lipomas of the Medullary Cisterns

Lipomas in the region of the medulla usually enclose several of the lower cranial nerves, and may cause nuchal pain as well as truncal and appendicular ataxia. No symptoms attributable to cranial nerve dysfunction have been reported to date. Careful partial resection may cause improvement of symptoms (according to a case report), but complete removal of the lesion would again be dangerous and of little, if any, use.[7]

Lipomas of the Tuber Cinereum and Infundibulum

These lipomas are very consistent in physical characteristics and location along the infundibular-mamilary axis. They are almost always situated in the midline, attached to the tuber cinereum or the anterior aspect of the mamillary bodies. They are usually pea-sized and nearly perfectly spherical, and contain a highly organized bone spherule; hence the name osteolipoma. They have a dense collagenous capsule that blends with the surrounding leptomeninges, with lobules of adipose tissue infiltrating the nervous tissue.[16] These lesions are usually asymptomatic, except for rare reports of endocrinologic problems.[14] They are difficult to recognize radiographically because of their size, and virtually impossible to resect entirely because of their adherence to surrounding structures.[14,16,23]

Choroid Plexus Lipomas

Lipomas of the choroid plexus of the lateral ventricles very frequently are extensions of corpus callosum lipomas through the choroidal fissures and are occasionally associated with hydrocephalus.[23,46] Again, treatment of the hydrocephalus is the recommended form of therapy.

Lipomas at Other Locations

Other rare reports of asymptomatic or minimally symptomatic lesions have included lipomas of the interpeduncular cisterns (Fig. 172-2), septum pellucidum,[24,47] and pineal region.

Treatment

It is generally accepted that radical surgical extirpation is contraindicated[17,27,28,43] for the following two reasons: first, because the frequently severe vascularity of the lipoma and its adherence to surrounding neural tissue, especially cranial nerves, makes resection technically difficult and hazardous; and second, because the lesion does not grow or compress brain tissue, which makes surgery unimportant in the setting of stable or no symptomatology (that is, in most cases). This is notwithstanding the fact that most symptoms are likely to be due to the associated stable malformations (for instance, a frontal skull defect), not directly to the lipoma. Even seizures are thought to be caused not by compression from the lipoma but by an associated neural malformation, which may suggest that infiltration by the lipoma capsule is present and causes an irritative focus.[17]

Therapy[9,31] for intracranial lipomas follows three major guidelines: placement of a ventricular shunt if there is hydrocephalus; medical management of the seizure disorder; and repair of the cosmetic deformities that may be caused by a large frontal lipoma or the associated bone and soft tissue malformations. The etiology of symptoms associated with intracranial lipomas is still not well understood. As a result, the usefulness of surgical interventions aimed at the relief of specific, medically intractable symptoms (such as vertigo or trigeminal neuralgia), remains inconclusive.

References

1. Aleksic S, Budzilovich G, Greco MA, et al. Intracranial lipomas, hydrocephalus and other CNS anomalies in oculoauriculo-vertebral dysplasia (Goldenhar-Gorlin syndrome). *Child's Brain* 1984; 11:285–297.
2. Bailey P, Bucy PC. The origin and nature of meningeal tumors. *Am J Cancer* 1931; 15:15–54.
3. Bamforth JSG, Riccardi VM, Thisen P, et al. Encephalocraniocutaneous lipomatosis. Report of two cases and a review of the literature. *Neurofibromatosis* 1989; 2:166–173.
4. Barkovich AJ. Brain development: normal and abnormal. In Atlas SW (ed): *Magnetic Resonance Imaging of the Brain and Spine.* New York: Raven Press, 1991, pp 129–173.
5. Beltinger C, Saule H. Imaging of lipoma of the corpus callosum and intracranial dermoids in the Goldenhar syndrome. *Pediatr Radiol* 1988; 18:72–73.
6. Budka H. Intracranial lipomatous hamartomas (intracranial "lipomas"): a study of 13 cases including combinations with medulloblastoma, colloid and epidermoid cysts, angiomatosis and other malformations. *Acta Neuropathol (Berl)* 1974; 28:205–222.
7. Cho DY, Wang YC, Li CS, Chang SM. Intracranial lipoma of the medulla oblongata. *Surg Neurol* 1991; 36:384–387.
8. Christensen WN, Long DM, Epstein JI. Cerebellopontine angle lipoma. *Hum Pathol* 1986; 17:739–743.
9. Clarici G, Heppner F. The operative approach to lipomas of the corpus callosum. *Neurochirurgia (Stuttg)* 1979; 22:77–81.
10. Donati F, Vassella F, Kaiser G, Blumberg A. Intracranial lipomas. *Neuropediatrics* 1992; 23:32–38.

11. Eghwrudjakpor PO, Kurisaka M, Fukuoka M, Mori K. Intracranial lipomas: current perspectives in their diagnosis and treatment. *Br J Neurosurg* 1992; 6:139–144.
12. Ehni GJ, Adson AW. Lipoma of the brain. Report of cases. *Arch Neurol Psychiatry* 1945; 53:299–304.
13. Eldevik OP, Gabrielsen TO. Fusiform aneurysmal dilatation of pericallosal artery: a sign of lipoma of corpus callosum. *Acta Radiol [Suppl]* 1975; 347:71–76.
14. Esposito S, Nardi P. Lipoma of the infundibulum. Case report. *J Neurosurg* 1987; 67:304–306.
15. Fishman MA. Encephalocraniocutaneous lipomatosis. *J Child Neurol* 1987; 2:186–193.
16. Friede RL. Osteolipomas of the tuber cinereum. *Arch Pathol Lab Med* 1977; 101:369–372.
17. Gastaut H, Regis H, Gastaut JL, et al. Lipomas of the corpus callosum and epilepsy. *Neurology* 1980; 30:132–138.
18. Goldberg HI. Extraaxial brain tumors. In Atlas SW (ed): *Magnetic Resonance Imaging of the Brain and Spine.* New York: Raven Press, 1991, pp 327–378.
19. Halmagyi GM, Evans WA. Lipoma of the quadrigeminal plate causing progressive obstructive hydrocephalus. Case report. *J Neurosurg* 1978; 49:453–456.
20. Hara M, Kawachi S, Hirano A. Lipoma of the superior medullary velum with schwann cells. Report of a case and review of the literature. *Acta Pathol Jpn* 1981; 31:825–833.
21. Higginbottom MC, Schultz P. The Bannayan syndrome: an autosomal dominant disorder consisting of macrocephaly, lipomas, hemangiomas, and risk for intracranial tumors. *Pediatrics* 1982; 69:632–634.
22. Hori A. Lipoma of the quadrigeminal region with evidence of congenital origin. *Arch Pathol Lab Med* 1986; 110:850–851.
23. Kazner E, Stochdorph O, Wende S, Grumme T. Intracranial lipoma: diagnostic and therapeutic considerations. *J Neurosurg* 1980; 52:234–245.
24. Kobayashi H, Hayashi M, Kawano H, et al. Lipoma of the cerebral peduncle. Case report. *Zentralbl Neurochir* 1989; 50:166–167.
25. Lalwani AK. Meningiomas, epidermoids, and other nonacoustic tumors of the cerebellopontine angle. *Otolaryngol Clin North Am* 1992; 25:707–728.
26. List CF, Holt JF, Everett M. Lipoma of the corpus callosum. A clinicopathologic study. *Am J Roentgenol* 1946; 55:125–134.
27. Maiuri F, Cirillo S, Simonetti L, et al. Intracranial lipomas: diagnostic and therapeutic considerations. *J Neurosurg Sci* 1988; 32:161–167.
28. Maiuri F, Cirillo S, Simonetti L. Lipoma of the sylvian region. *Clin Neurol Neurosurg* 1989; 91:321–323.
29. Maiuri F, Corriero G, Gallicchio B, Simonetti L. Lipoma of the ambient cistern causing obstructive hydrocephalus. *J Neurosurg Sci* 1987; 31:53–58.
30. Nabawi P, Dobben GD, Mafee M, Espinosa GA: Diagnosis of lipoma of the corpus callosum by CT in five cases. *Neuroradiology* 1981; 21:159–162.
31. Nalesnik MA, Martinez AJ, Heros RC. Intracranial lipoma with hematopoietic elements (myelolipoma). Report of a case with successful surgical resection. *Cancer* 1982; 50:295–299.
32. O'Rahilly R, Müller F. The meninges in human development. *J Neuropathol Exp Neurol* 1986; 45:588–608.
33. Pascual-Castroviejo I, Pascual-Pascual SI, Pérez-Higueras A. Frontonasal dysplasia and lipoma of the corpus callosum. *Eur J Pediatr* 1985; 144:66–71.
34. Pensak ML, Glasscock ME III, Gulya AJ, et al. Cerebellopontine angle lipomas. *Arch Otolaryngol Head Neck Surg* 1986; 112:99–101.
35. Rosenbloom SB, Carson BS, Wang H, et al. Cerebellopontine angle lipoma. *Surg Neurol* 1985; 23:134–138.
36. Ross GW, Miller JQ, Persing JA, Urich H. Hemimegalencephaly, hemifacial hypertrophy and intracranial lipoma: a variant of neurofibromatosis. *Neurofibromatosis* 1989; 2:69–77.
37. Rubio G, Garcia Guijo C, Mallada, JJ. MR and CT diagnosis of intracranial lipoma. *Am J Roentgenol* 1991; 157:887–888.
38. Saunders JE, Kwartler JA, Wolf HK, et al. Lipomas of the internal auditory canal. *Laryngoscope* 1991; 101:1031–1037.
39. Sprik C, Wirtschafter JD. Hemifacial spasm due to intracranial tumor. An international survey of botulinum toxin investigators. *Ophthalmology* 1988; 95:1042–1045.
40. Steimlé R, Pageaut G, Jacquet G, et al. Lipoma in the cerebellopontine angle. *Surg Neurol* 1985; 24:73–76.
41. Summers CG, MacDonald JT, Wirtschafter JD. Ocular motor apraxia associated with intracranial lipoma. *J Pediatr Ophthalmol Strabismus* 1987; 24(5):267–269.
42. Suzuki M, Takashima T, Kadoya M, et al. Pericallosal lipomas: MR features. *J Comput Assist Tomogr* 1991; 15:207–209.
43. Tahmouresie A, Kroll G, Shucart W. Lipoma of the corpus callosum. *Surg Neurol* 1979; 11:31–34.
44. Takeuchi J, Handa H, Keyaki A, et al. Intracranial angiolipoma. *Surg Neurol* 1981; 15:110–113.
45. Tart RP, Quisling RG. Curvilinear and tubulonodular varieties of lipoma of the corpus callosum: an MR and CT study. *J Comput Assist Tomogr* 1991; 15:805–810.
46. Truwit CL, Barkovich AJ. Pathogenesis of intracranial lipoma: an MR study in 42 patients. *Am J Neuroradiol* 1990; 11:665–674.
47. Wilberger JE Jr, Abla A, Rothfus W. Lipoma of the septum pellucidum: case report. *J Comput Assist Tomogr* 1987; 11:79–82.
48. Wilkins PR, Hoddinott C, Hourihan MD, et al. Intracranial angiolipoma. *J Neurol Neurosurg Psychiatry* 1987; 50:1057–1059.
49. Zettner A, Netsky MG. Lipoma of the corpus callosum. *J Neuropathol Exp Neurol* 1960; 19:305–319.

173

Langerhans Cell Histiocytosis (Histiocytosis X)

Douglas C. Anthony
J. Allan Tucker

Langerhans cell histiocytosis is a term that encompasses a spectrum of clinical conditions, ranging from a single, sometimes self-limited osteolytic bone lesion to a fulminant, disseminated process that may be fatal. The etiology of this disorder, or disorders, is unknown, and there is no consensus on how to classify these patients. What is now recognized, however, is that the lesions in these patients share a common feature: a clonal proliferation of a histiocytic cell type known as the Langerhans cell.

Historically, three clinical entities were described that were considered subtypes of Langerhans cell histiocytosis. Hand-Schüller-Christian disease, presenting in its classic form with a triad of calvarial defects, exophthalmos, and diabetes insipidus, was reported independently by Hand, Schüller, and Christian between 1893 and 1920. Letterer-Siwe disease, a fulminant progressive proliferative disease of infancy which clinically resembles a malignancy, was reported in 1924 and 1933. Eosinophilic granuloma, as a solitary osteolytic lesion of bone, was described in 1940. Farber recognized a histologic similarity among these disparate conditions,[10] and Lichtenstein suggested that although certain differences existed between groups of patients, a reliable distinction could not be made in individual cases on the basis of histopathology alone.[21] In 1953, Lichtenstein introduced the term *histiocytosis X* to denote a proliferation of histiocytes, with "X" to convey the uncertain histogenesis of the disease. The subsequent demonstration that all of these lesions feature a proliferation of Langerhans cells supports the concept of grouping them under the term *Langerhans cell histiocytosis.* Interestingly, it now appears that each type of Langerhans cell histiocytosis involves the proliferation of a clone of Langerhans cells,[39] suggesting that the disease may be a neoplastic disorder with a variable clinical course.

The Langerhans cell is a distinct member of the mononuclear phagocytic system,[36] a system that includes tissue histiocytes and macrophages. The Langerhans cell is derived from the bone marrow and is a normal resident of the skin, buccal lining, lymph nodes, and other sites. Like macrophages, the Langerhans cell expresses Fc and C_3 surface receptors and is thought to function in presenting antigen to lymphocytes. It has several unique features among the mononuclear phagocytic system, however, which allow its identification: It expresses CD1 (T6) and CD4 (T4) surface antigens, has a high adenosine triphosphatase (ATPase) activity, has a nuclear and membrane affinity for peanut agglutinin, contains a high cytoplasmic content of S-100 protein,[11] and possesses a characteristic cytoplasmic membranous structure known as the Birbeck, or Langerhans cell, granule. Also unlike macrophages, the Langerhans cell does not contain significant amounts of lysozyme or α_1-antitrypsin, and it is much less phagocytic.

Histopathology of Langerhans Cell Histiocytosis

The lesions of Langerhans cell histiocytosis are composed of a polymorphous cellular infiltrate (Fig. 173-1*A*). Large histiocytic cells are present, sometimes including foamy or multinucleated forms, and are mixed with inflammatory cells, which may include eosinophils, neutrophils, lymphocytes, and occasional plasma cells.[4] The mixture of inflammatory cells is extremely variable from case to case and may be related to the chronicity of the process. The inflammatory infiltrate sometimes features a prominent number of eosinophils, which may provide a clue to the nature of the lesion. The key to diagnosis, however, is recognizing that many or all of the histiocytic cells are Langerhans cells.

On routine hematoxylin and eosin stained sections, Langerhans cells contain an abundant eosinophilic homogeneous cytoplasm and often have well-defined cytoplasmic borders. The nuclei are large, with vesicular chromatin and occasional small nucleoli. The most important feature in recognizing these cells as Langerhans histiocytes by light microscopy is a characteristic nuclear shape. The nuclei are typically sharply grooved or indented along one surface, much like an open clam (Fig. 173-1*B*). In perpendicular sections, the nuclei are reniform, and, when viewed *en face,* they resemble a coffee bean with a midline linear groove. Ploidy analysis most often reveals a lack of a significant aneuploid population.[29,30]

The phenotypic properties of the normal Langerhans cell are often useful in the identification of Langerhans cell histiocytosis. The most important and practical of these is that the cells have a high cytoplasmic content of S-100 protein. Immunoperoxidase stains for S-100 protein can be performed on routinely fixed, paraffin-embedded tissue, so that essentially any biopsy in which Langerhans cell histiocytosis is suspected can be studied with this technique. Langerhans cells also express CD1 (T6) and CD4 (T4) surface membrane antigens.[11] Detection of these antigens requires frozen tissue or preservation in an immunofixative. Less commonly used is the affinity of the nuclear membrane of these cells for peanut agglutinin.

Electron microscopy is of great value in the diagnosis of Langerhans cell histiocytosis. Ultrastructurally, Langerhans cell nuclei have a characteristic contorted and often deeply indented contour (Fig. 173-1*B*). The cytoplasm contains unique cytoplasmic structures called Birbeck, or Langerhans cell, granules, whose function remains unknown (Fig. 173-1*C–D*). These granules are disc-shaped with a central paracrystalline lattice, so that in cross section they appear as rod-shaped profiles with the central lattice producing a line or a zipper-like structure. The disc may also have a marginal vesicular swelling; a cross section through the disc including the vesicular area then produces a profile with the shape of a tennis racket. The membranes of a Birbeck granule are sometimes continuous with the plasma membrane, suggesting that these granules arise as invaginations of the plasma membrane. The granules are found only in Langerhans cells, so electron microscopy can be used for the definitive identification of Langerhans cells. However, since Langerhans cells occur normally in some sites, identification of a Langerhans cell does not necessarily indicate a

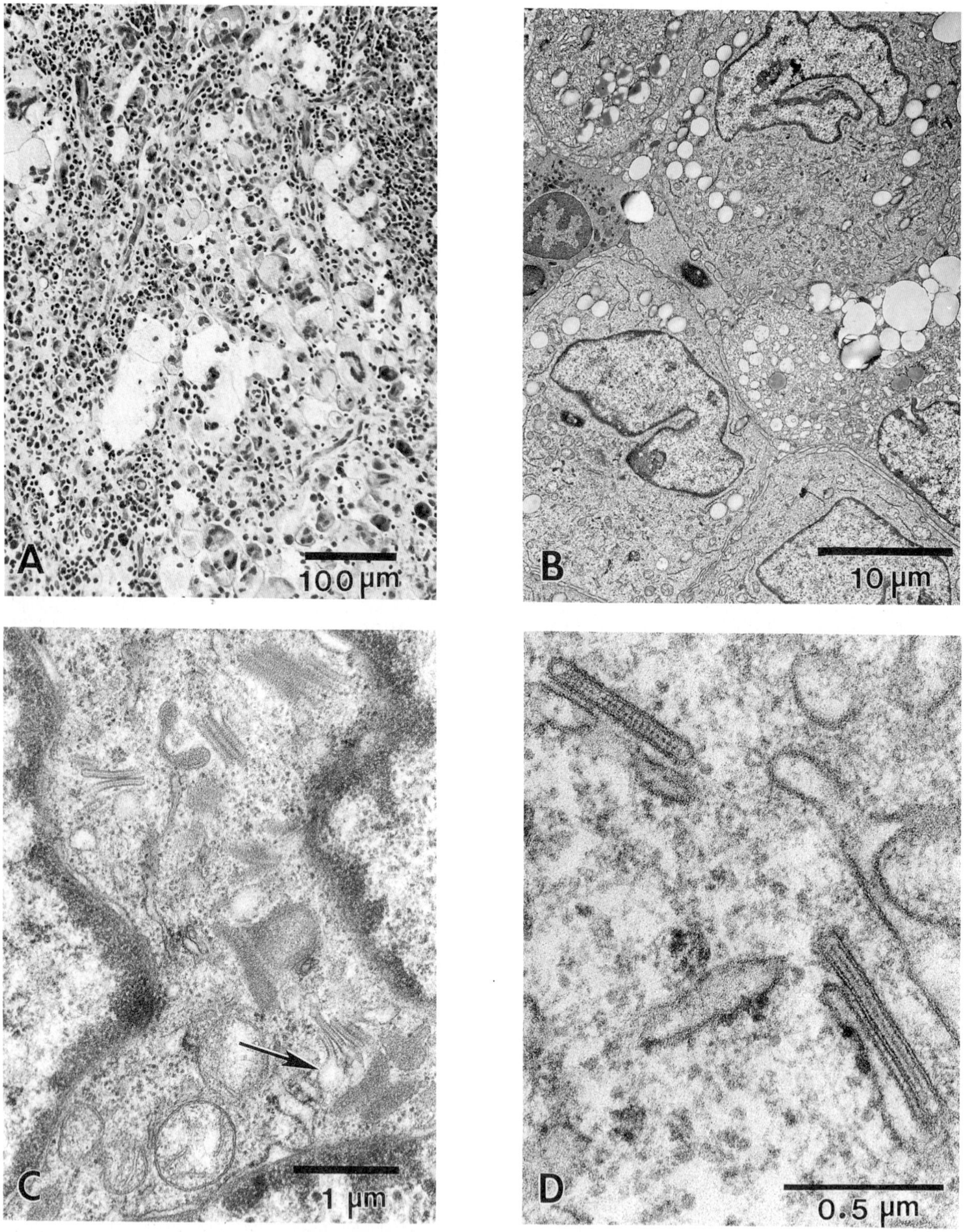

Figure 173-1 Histologically, Langerhans cell histiocytosis features a mixed cellular infiltrate *(A)*, with lymphocytes, neutrophils, and plasma cells amid a background population of histiocytes, some of which have foamy cytoplasm and are multinucleated. Electron microscopy reveals the typical appearance of a sharp groove in the histiocytic nuclei *(B)*, a finding which is characteristic of Langerhans cell histiocytosis. The definitive morphologic finding is the presence of Birbeck granules in the cytoplasm *(C)*. These granules may include a vesicular component resulting in a tennis-racket appearance (arrow). The Birbeck granule is pentalaminar *(D)*, with a central lattice that shows a periodicity, or zipper, configuration.

diagnosis of Langerhans cell histiocytosis. Therefore, these specialized diagnostic techniques should be employed only to further evaluate a lesion that is suggestive of Langerhans cell histiocytosis by light microscopy and clinical findings.

Although there is a consensus on the histologic diagnosis of Langerhans cell histiocytosis, there is much more controversy on the topic of histologic subclassification. Some authors contend that abundant foam cells and multinucleated giant cells are seen more often in the clinical setting of multiple skull lesions with diabetes insipidus (Hand-Schüller-Christian disease), whereas others argue that this characteristic reflects chronicity and may be seen in any of the disparate clinical situations.[28] Certain histologic features, including large numbers of noncohesive Langerhans cells, few giant cells, paucity of necrosis, and a brisk mitotic rate, have been suggested as indicating a more aggressive clinical course, although such a correlation is not a consistent observation among different institutions.[32] Thus, there is no uniform set of criteria for histologic subclassification.

On the other hand, specific recommendations have been made for recognizing Langerhans cell histiocytosis and the distinguishing it from other lesions that can have similar morphology. There are a number of conditions from which Langerhans cell histiocytosis must be distinguished, and the precise differentiation depends on the clinical features and histological appearance. An osseous lesion of Langerhans cell histiocytosis with giant cells must be distinguished from an infectious granulomatous process, fibrous dysplasia, osteomyelitis, malignant histiocytosis, and primary bone tumors with a giant cell (osteoclast) component. In the case of a skin lesion, the differential diagnosis includes juvenile xanthogranuloma and reticulohistiocytoma. In the case of a disseminated process in early childhood, storage diseases and leukemia or lymphoma may also need consideration. It is a matter of opinion and some debate as to when a diagnosis of Langerhans cell histiocytosis is established. Using a three-tier system for the histologic diagnosis,[40] a ''presumptive diagnosis'' is based on typical light microscopic findings; a ''diagnosis'' requires additional studies, including S-100 immunolocalization, cytoplasmic ATPase demonstration, peanut agglutinin studies, or CD4 surface markers; and a ''definitive diagnosis'' is secure only with CD1 (T6) surface marker studies or ultrastructural documentation of Birbeck granules. Although these suggestions have merit for investigational studies, they may be somewhat stringent for widespread clinical application and would deny a ''definitive diagnosis'' of Langerhans cell histiocytes in much of the available literature. In practice, each of the markers of Langerhans cells is recognized to have some diagnostic value, but they cannot be demonstrated in all cases of Langerhans cell histiocytosis.[2,41]

Occurrence and Distribution of Langerhans Cell Histiocytosis in the Central Nervous System and Its Coverings

The breadth of the spectrum of Langerhans cell histiocytosis is reflected in the very different clinical situations as they were originally recognized. The mildest form of Langerhans cell histiocytosis is a single osteolytic lesion of bone known as an eosinophilic granuloma. This monostotic form can occur in almost any bone, but preferred sites are the calvaria, the vertebral bodies, the ribs, and the long bones of the limbs. The Hand-Schüller-Christian triad consists of osteolytic skull defects, exophthalmos, and diabetes insipidus. Hand-Schüller-Christian disease has been viewed as a chronic progressive form of Langerhans cell histiocytosis, often with a remitting and relapsing clinical course, and may be associated with cutaneous and pulmonary lesions. Letterer-Siwe disease is characterized by an acutely progressive course, often with fever, pancytopenia, hepatomegaly, diffuse pulmonary infiltrates, and a cutaneous eruption.

Although this historical classification has been used to subclassify patients with Langerhans cell histiocytosis, many authors have raised the objection that patients often do not fit well into these categories, leaving issues of prognosis and therapy unresolved. In general, most of the proposed classification schemes include distribution of disease (e.g., hepatomegaly), dysfunction of organs (e.g., elevated liver function tests), and/or age of the patient. With differing emphasis on particular features, the schemes arrive at a score, or stage, of disease and provide an estimate of prognosis.

Overall, it appears that patients in whom the disease is limited to bony sites have a good prognosis, and these patients should be viewed separately from those with a disseminated form of the disease.[40] If the disease is limited to a single bone lesion, the prognosis is excellent, and the well-established terms *eosinophilic granuloma* and *monostotic eosinophilic granuloma* are acceptable. If more than one site is involved, but the lesions are limited to bone, again the prognosis is good, and the terms *polyostotic eosinophilic granuloma* and *multifocal eosinophilic granuloma* have been applied.[6] For patients with multifocal disease including extraskeletal involvement, the process is best viewed as disseminated Langerhans cell histiocytosis, and the prognosis depends on the patient's age and the extent and magnitude of the extraskeletal involvement. Finally, there are examples of isolated extraosseous Langerhans cell histiocytosis, but the rarity of these cases precludes a definitive statement concerning prognosis. For the remainder of this discussion, only four forms of Langerhans cell histiocytosis will be considered: monostotic, polyostotic, disseminated, and unifocal extraskeletal.

Monostotic eosinophilic granuloma is the most common form of Langerhans cell histiocytosis. It occurs predominantly in children, with 75 percent of cases occurring before the age of 20. The most common sites of involvement are the skull (usually the vault rather than the base), rib, femur, jaw, humerus, and vertebral body. It has been estimated that the overall incidence of Langerhans cell histiocytosis is 0.6 case per million children less than 15 years old,[11] and most of these cases involve monostotic eosinophilic granuloma. A slight male predominance has been noted for monostotic eosinophilic granuloma, and it rarely progresses to a disseminated form of disease.

Polyostotic eosinophilic granuloma occurs in a similar age group and carries only a slightly worse prognosis.[6] This process exhibits a greater predilection for the skull, and multiple skull lesions are often discovered at once. The local effects of the osseous lesions, such as diabetes insipidus, do not worsen the prognosis[28]; however, any evidence of extraskeletal involvement should be viewed as an expression of a disseminated process. Thus, the presence of calvarial defects with diabetes insipidus, which would be considered by some to represent Hand-Schüller-Christian disease, is compatible with polyostotic eosinophilic granuloma; however, the presence of hepatic or cutaneous involvement warrants a designation of disseminated Langerhans cell histiocytosis.

Disseminated Langerhans cell histiocytosis may follow a chronic, relapsing course or an acute fulminant course, and some authors subclassify the disseminated disease along these lines. As prognosis is related to age and extent of involvement, however, it would appear best to concentrate on determining the location of the disease and whether there is compromise of organ function. After bone, the sites most frequently involved are the skin, liver, spleen, lymph nodes, bone marrow, and lungs. The disseminated form occurs in infants and young children, with approximately 50 percent of cases occurring before the age of 2.

Unifocal extraskeletal Langerhans cell histiocytosis is uncommon. It may occur in many sites, including the lung, where it is usually referred to as eosinophilic granuloma of the lung, and as a process confined to the skin, where it may be self-limited.[23] Involvement of the central nervous system, although not rare in disseminated Langerhans cell histiocytosis, is quite uncommon as an isolated extraskeletal lesion. The most common intracerebral location is the hypothalamus, where histologic features suggestive of Langerhans cell histiocytosis have been referred to as Gagel's granuloma, granuloma infiltrans of the hypothalamus, and Ayala's disease.[16] Although cases of isolated Langerhans cell histiocytosis of the central nervous system have been identified primarily by means of routine histologic methods without confirmatory studies such as electron microscopy, there are a number of reasons for suspecting that some of these cases represent a cerebral form of Langerhans cell histiocytosis.[16] In addition, some of these lesions have been documented to contain Birbeck granules, satisfying the criteria for a "definitive diagnosis" as outlined by the Histiocyte Society.[40] Other, less frequent, unifocal forms affecting the nervous system include intracerebral masses,[15] posterior fossa masses, spinal cord tumors,[1] and isolated lesions of the cranial or spinal meninges and cauda equina. A somewhat distinctive histologic feature of Langerhans cell histiocytosis in the central nervous system as compared to the features of extracranial forms is higher phagocytic activity, including phagocytosis of inflammatory cells, especially plasma cells.[16]

Clinical Presentation of Langerhans Cell Histiocytosis

The clinical features of Langerhans cell histiocytosis depend on the form of the disease. Monostotic eosinophilic granuloma usually presents as local tenderness or a small mass lesion in a child, although it is not restricted to this age group. Occasionally, the lesion may reveal its presence through the pathologic fracture of a long bone, while in other cases it may be completely asymptomatic, discovered only as an incidental finding on an x-ray film obtained for other reasons. Vertebral involvement is frequently manifested as localized back pain. Polyostotic eosinophilic granuloma may present with pain or mass lesions of the scalp, or with local effects at the base of the skull. These include diabetes insipidus, proptosis, or recurrent otitis media, where the diagnosis of Langerhans cell histiocytosis can be suspected from the additional finding of osteolytic skull lesions. Other signs of pituitary-hypothalamic involvement may occur, such as growth retardation or amenorrhea, and these functional disturbances occasionally precede detectable osseous involvement.

Disseminated Langerhans cell histiocytosis is extremely variable in clinical presentation, and the diagnosis may be elusive. In the more indolent forms, multiple skin macules and papules with osteolytic bone lesions, reticulonodular pulmonary infiltrates, or hepatomegaly may be present. The more aggressive forms may commence with fever, hepatosplenomegaly, anemia, leukopenia, thrombocytopenia, purpura, and lymphadenopathy, raising a suspicion of leukemia. In any of the disseminated forms, localized lesions of the central nervous system may occur as a component and bring the patient to the neurosurgeon for evaluation.

The isolated cerebral form of Langerhans cell histiocytosis presents with localizing symptoms and a mass effect, and Langerhans cell histiocytosis is frequently suspected only after biopsy. The only exception is the hypothalamic location, where the location and radiographic appearance may suggest the diagnosis.

Radiologic Features of Langerhans Cell Histiocytosis

In bone, whether as a localized eosinophilic granuloma or as part of a disseminated process, the lesions of Langerhans cell histiocytosis are osteolytic, usually with complete absence of bony trabeculae and without a sclerotic rim. This "punched out" appearance is characteristic and, in the appropriate clinical setting, may be quite suggestive of Langerhans cell histiocytosis (Fig. 173-2).

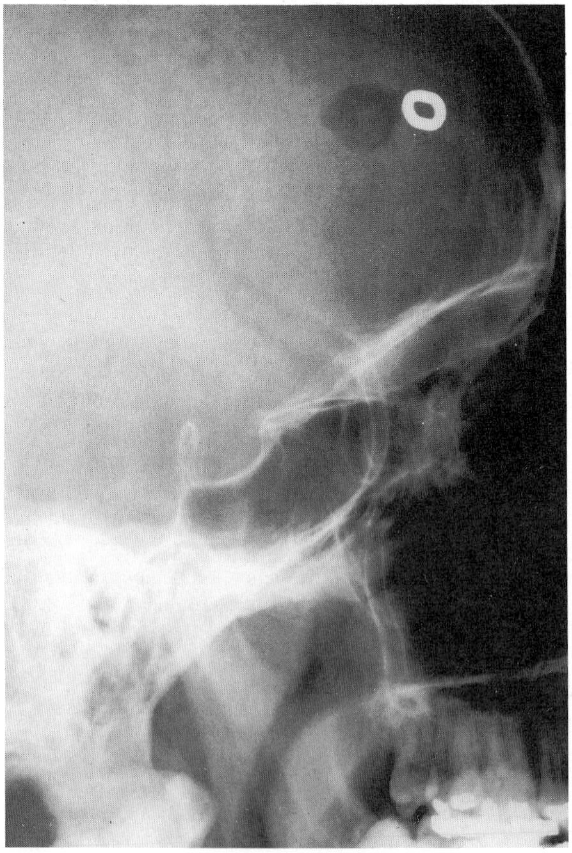

Figure 173-2 A single osteolytic calvarial lesion was discovered in this 23-year-old man who presented with frontal headaches and an area of tenderness in the left frontal region. The radiographic appearance of osteolysis without a sclerotic rim is characteristic of Langerhans cell histiocytosis. A radiopaque marker has been placed over the symptomatic area and aids in the intraoperative localization of the osseous lesion for biopsy.

Metastatic carcinoma, metastatic neuroblastoma, or primary Ewing's sarcoma may give a similar radiologic appearance, and these cancers may enter into the differential diagnosis in some patients. Computed tomography (CT) similarly reveals the osteolytic lesions and provides information concerning intracranial extension or bilateral involvement.[8]

Langerhans cell histiocytosis of the lung, as an isolated lesion or as part of a disseminated process, usually is identified on chest x-ray films as a reticulonodular pattern. With progression, a honeycomb appearance may develop, at times complicated by a pneumothorax.

The best radiologic demonstration of Langerhans cell histiocytosis in the central nervous system has been attained with CT, and, more recently, with magnetic resonance imaging (MRI). Most intracerebral lesions show a low-density lesion on CT, usually with a moderate degree of enhancement. Intracranial involvement may be suspected in a patient with this radiographic appearance and an established diagnosis of Langerhans cell histiocytosis; however, in the case of an isolated cerebral lesion, the preoperative suspicion is of a glioma or an encephalitic process. MRI shows prolonged T1 and T2 values in the lesion, with surrounding vasogenic edema. In some instances, MRI may be more sensitive than CT for detecting hypothalamic involvement.[12]

Management and Prognosis

The first step in management is to establish the diagnosis of Langerhans cell histiocytosis, which is done by biopsy. Skull lesions tend to involve the full thickness of the skull, and lesions of the calvaria are a readily accessible site for biopsy. There is usually some elevation of the galea, and the lesion is soft and frequently tan or yellow on biopsy. The pathologist should be alerted to the suspicion of Langerhans cell histiocytosis at the time of biopsy so that extra steps can be taken to establish the diagnosis. Unstained frozen sections may be prepared at this time and stored for immunocytochemical localization of surface markers. In addition, small, noncrushed tissue fragments may be preserved in glutaraldehyde to optimize the electron microscopic search for Birbeck granules. When clinical, radiologic, and histopathologic features are typical of Langerhans cell histiocytosis, these immunodiagnostic and ultrastructural studies may be unnecessary; however, it is best to prepare for them should diagnostic difficulties arise.

Once a diagnosis of Langerhans cell histiocytosis has been established, investigation should be directed to determining whether the process is localized. Although lesions of Langerhans cell histiocytosis occur in virtually any location, a limited number of features have been associated with prognosis,[17,20,27,31] and clinical attention should be directed to these. Evidence of skin lesions should be sought, and a distinction should be made between seborrheic involvement and a maculopapular rash. Pulmonary involvement may be symptomatic, including dyspnea, tachypnea, coughing, pneumothorax, or pleural effusion; this symptomatology carries a worse prognosis than an asymptomatic abnormality on chest films.[17] Similarly, hepatic dysfunction (total protein <5.5 g/dl, albumin <2.5 g/dl, total bilirubin >1.5 mg/dl, edema, or ascites) is a significant feature that should be evaluated.[17] A radiographic skeletal survey or bone scan will usually reveal any additional bony lesions. Bone marrow dysfunction is indicated by anemia (<10 g/dl hemoglobin), leukopenia (<4000 white cells/mm^3), neutropenia (<1500 neutrophils/mm^3), or thrombocytopenia ($<100{,}000$ platelets/mm^3).[17] The presence of lymphadenopathy and splenomegaly is the usual clinical indication of involvement at these sites. Most studies have also shown that age at diagnosis is associated with the ultimate outcome, with those greater than 2 years of age faring better than those under 2.[27] On the basis of relatively few additional studies, a stage for a disseminated process can then be established that will provide an estimate of the patient's prognosis.

One of the earliest and most widely used systems is the Lahey score, which assigns one point for each of eight features: skin involvement, hepatic dysfunction, splenomegaly, respiratory symptoms, bone involvement, pituitary involvement, anemia or leukopenia, and thrombocytopenia or purpura.[20] As the Lahey score approaches 7 or 8, the 2-year mortality without treatment approaches 100 percent. The prognostic groups defined by the Southwest Oncology Group are "good risk" for patients older than 2 years without organ dysfunction, "intermediate risk" for patients under 2 years without organ dysfunction, and "poor risk" for patients with organ dysfunction, regardless of age.[17] The 5-year survival rates in these groups were found to be approximately 90, 66 and 47 percent, respectively.[17]

The therapy for Langerhans cell histiocytosis is extremely variable and ranges from observation only to systemic multiagent chemotherapy. A solitary eosinophilic granuloma is almost always a localized process when it occurs in older children and adults, and the disease may resolve spontaneously. Therapeutic recommendations for a solitary lesion reflect these features and may consist of curettage, resection, or the intralesional injection of methylprednisolone[7]; the patient is then followed with observation. Radiation therapy should be reserved for patients with clear progression, when lesions have such a location and size that waiting may have serious consequences (e.g., vertebral lesions in which the possibility of spinal cord injury is substantial), or when symptomatic lesions require treatment.[8,34] Radiation has also been used with some success in the treatment of diabetes insipidus.[26] A course of radiation therapy, when used for bone lesions, is generally 450 to 1000 rad in 200-rad daily fractions.[5] In general, however, monostotic disease may be managed conservatively.

Numerous studies have been performed to evaluate therapy for disseminated Langerhans cell histiocytosis, and a variety of chemotherapeutic agents have been reported to have efficacy in this setting. Agents including chlorambucil, vincristine, vinblastine, 6-mercaptopurine, cyclophosphamide, and methotrexate alone or with prednisone have been advocated in the treatment of disseminated disease, all with comparable response rates of 30 to 65 percent.[35] More recently, treatment has been reported with α-interferon,[14,33] cyclosporine,[22] bone marrow transplantation,[13,37] and etoposide[3,24,38]; etoposide has shown particular promise.[18,19] That the mortality rate from disseminated Langerhans cell histiocytosis seems to have declined over the last 20 years suggests that these therapeutic interventions have been of benefit. This potential response rate must be weighed against the complications of therapy,[25] which may include short-term immunosuppression, and, rarely, the later induction of a malignancy.

The management of polyostotic disease is more controversial, although in some cases the process may be self-limited without therapy. If a single symptomatic lesion requires treatment, surgical and/or radiation therapy may be beneficial.[5] In younger children, there is a greater risk of developing a disseminated process, and chemotherapy may be warranted.[35] Unifocal lesions of the brain or spinal cord have been treated with surgical resection, either alone or with subsequent radiotherapy or chemotherapy.[1,9,15]

References

1. Al-Rodhan NRF, Al-Mefty O, Goodwin JT, et al. Histiocytosis-X of the spinal cord: a case report. *Neurosurgery* 1986; 19:837–840.
2. Azumi N, Sheibani K, Swartz WG, et al. Antigenic phenotype of Langerhans cell histiocytosis: an immunohistochemical study demonstrating the value of LN-2, LN-3, and vimentin. *Hum Pathol* 1988; 19:1376–1382.
3. Broadbent V, Pritchard J, Yeomans E, Etoposide (VP16) in the treatment of multisystem Langerhans cell histiocytosis (histiocytosis X). *Med Pediatr Oncol* 1989; 17:97–100.
4. Burger PC, Scheithauer BW, Vogel FS. *Surgical Pathology of the Nervous System and Its Coverings,* 3d ed. New York: Churchill Livingstone, 1991, pp 6–10.
5. Cassady JR. Current role of radiation therapy in the management of histiocytosis-X. *Hematol Oncol Clin North Am* 1987; 1:123–129.
6. Chase DC, Eversole LR, Hall HD. Histiocytosis X with jaw involvement. *J Oral Surg* 1974; 32:494–502.
7. Cohen M, Zornoza J, Cangir A, et al. Direct injection of methylprednisolone sodium succinate in the treatment of solitary eosinophilic granuloma of bone: a report of 9 cases. *Radiology* 1980; 136:289–293.
8. Cunningham MJ, Curtin HD, Butkiewicz BL. Histiocytosis X of the temporal bone: CT findings. *J Comput Assist Tomogr* 1988; 12:70–74.
9. Eriksen B, Janinis J, Variakojis D, et al. Primary histiocytosis X of the parieto-occipital lobe. *Hum Pathol* 1988; 19:611–614.
10. Farber S. The nature of "solitary or eosinophilic granuloma" of bone. *Am J Pathol* 1941; 17:625–629.
11. Favara BE, McCarthy RC, Mierau GW. Histiocytosis X. *Hum Pathol* 1983; 14:663–676.
12. Graif M, Pennock JM. MR imaging of histiocytosis X in the central nervous system. *Am J Neuroradiol* 1986; 7:21–23.
13. Greinix HT, Storb R, Sanders JE, et al. Marrow transplantation for treatment of multisystem progressive Langerhans cell histiocytosis. *Bone Marrow Transplant* 1992; 10:39–44.
14. Halton J, Whitton A, Wiernikowski J, et al. Disseminated Langerhans cell histiocytosis in identical twins unresponsive to recombinant human alpha-interferon and total body irradiation. *Am J Pediatr Hematol Oncol* 1992; 14:269–272.
15. Hammar S, Weaver RA, Keranen VJ. Left temporal lobe cerebral cortex mass in a 19-year-old male. *Ultrastruct Pathol* 1986; 10:583–591.
16. Kepes JJ, Kepes M. Predominantly cerebral forms of histiocytosis X: a reappraisal of "Gagel's hypothalamic granuloma," "granuloma infiltrans of the hypothalamus" and "Ayala's disease" with a report of four cases. *Acta Neuropathol (Berl)* 1969; 14:77–98.
17. Komp DM, Herson J, Starling KA, et al. A staging system for histiocytosis X: a Southwest Oncology Group study. *Cancer* 1981; 47:798–800.
18. Ladisch S, Gadner H. Treatment of Langerhans cell histiocytosis. Evolution and current approaches. *Br J Cancer (Suppl)* 1994; 23:S41–S46.
19. Ladisch S, Gadner H, Arico M, et al. LCH-I: a randomized trial of etoposide vs. vinblastine in disseminated Langerhans cell histiocytosis. *Med Pediatr Oncol* 1994; 23:107–110.
20. Lahey ME. Prognosis in reticuloendotheliosis in children. *J Pediatr* 1962; 60:664–671.
21. Lichtenstein L. Histiocytosis X: integration of esosinophilic granuloma of bone, "Letterer-Siwe disease," and "Schuller-Christian disease" as related manifestations of a single nosologic entity. *Arch Pathol Lab Med* 1953; 56:84–102.
22. Mahmoud HH, Wang WC, Murphy SB. Cyclosporine therapy for advanced Langerhans cell histiocytosis. *Blood* 1991; 77:721–725.
23. Marsh WL Jr, Lew SW, Heath VC, et al. Congenital self-healing histiocytosis X. *Am J Pediatr Hematol Oncol* 1983; 5:227–233.
24. Mayou SC, Chu AC, Munro DD, et al. Langerhans-cell histiocytosis—excellent response to etoposide. *Clin Exp Dermatol* 1991; 16:292–294.
25. McLelland J, Broadbent V, Yeomans E, et al. Langerhans cell histiocytosis: the case for conservative treatment. *Arch Dis Child* 1990; 65:301–303.
26. Minehan KJ, Chen MG, Zimmerman D, et al. Radiation therapy for diabetes insipidus caused by Langerhans cell histiocytosis. *Int J Radiat Oncol Biol Phys* 1992; 23:519–524.
27. Nezelof C, Frileux-Herbet F, Cronier-Sachot J. Disseminated histiocytosis X: analysis of prognostic factors based on a retrospective study of 50 cases. *Cancer* 1979; 44:1824–1838
28. Oberman HA. Idiopathic histiocytosis: a clinicopathologic study of 40 cases and review of the literature on eosinophilic granuloma of bone, Hand-Schüller-Christian disease and Letterer-Siwe disease. *Pediatrics* 1961; 28:307–327.
29. Ornvold K, Carstensen H, Larsen JK, et al. Flow cytometric DNA analysis of lesions from 18 children with Langerhans cell histiocytosis (histiocytosis X). *Am J Pathol* 1990; 136:1301–1307.
30. Rabkin MS, Wittwer CT, Kjeldsberg CR, et al. Flow-cytometric DNA content of histiocytosis X (Langerhans cell histiocytosis). *Am J Pathol* 1988; 131:283–289.
31. Raney RB Jr, D'Angio GJ. Langerhans' cell histiocytosis (histiocytosis X): experience at the Children's Hospital of Philadelphia, 1970–1984. *Med Pediatr Oncol* 1989; 17:20–28.
32. Risdali LJ, Dehner LP, Duray P, et al. Histiocytosis X (Langerhans' cell histiocytosis): prognostic role of histopathology. *Arch Pathol Lab Med* 1983; 107:59–63.
33. Sato Y, Ikeda Y, Ito E, et al. Histiocytosis X: successful treatment with recombinant interferon-alpha A. *Acta Paediatr Jpn* 1990; 32:151–154.
34. Selch MT, Parker RG. Radiation therapy in the management of Langerhans cell histiocytosis. *Med Pediatr Oncol* 1990; 18:97–102.
35. Starling KA. Chemotherapy of histiocytosis-X. *Hematol Oncol Clin North Am* 1987; 1:119–122.
36. Steinman RM. The dendritic cell system and its role in immunogenicity. *Annu Rev Immunol* 1991; 9:271–296.
37. Stoll M, Freund M. Schmid H, et al. Allogeneic bone marrow transplantation for Langerhans' cell histiocytosis. *Cancer* 1990; 66:284–288.
38. Viana MB, Oliveira BM, Silva CM, et al. Etoposide in the treatment of six children with Langerhans cell histiocytosis (histiocytosis X). *Med Pediatr Oncol* 1991; 19:289–294.
39. Willman CL, Busque L, Griffith BB, et al. Langerhans-cell histiocytosis (histiocytosis X)—a clonal proliferative disease. *N Engl J Med* 1994; 331:154–160.
40. Writing Group of the Histiocyte Society. Histiocytosis syndromes in children. *Lancet* 1987; 1:208–209.
41. Ye F, Huang SW, Dong HJ. Histiocytosis X. S-100 protein, peanut agglutinin, and transmission electron microscopy study. *Am J Clin Pathol* 1990; 94:627–631.

SECTION N

Spinal Tumors

174 Imaging of Spinal Tumors

Thomas S. Dina
Henry T. Ching

The selection of the appropriate diagnostic imaging procedure has become considerably more complex since the advent of magnetic resonance imaging (MRI). Formerly there were few options beyond the usually non-enlightening plain film radiograph. Myelography in any form, as well as computed tomography (CT), contrast-enhanced CT (CECT), and CT myelography (CTM), are anatomic-site directed; that is, a specific level or segment of the spine is studied. Imaging technique is little influenced by the suspected compartment or level of the abnormality. For example, there are only minor variations in imaging technique, if any, when using CTM to study intramedullary, intradural, or extradural lesions. Options to maximize soft tissue contrast and spatial resolution are relatively few and limited in capability. With CT, multiplanar imaging is provided indirectly by computerized reformation of axial images. MRI has become the neuroimaging modality of choice for most disorders of the spine and spinal canal, providing information sufficient for definitive patient management, including operative intervention.

Neuroimaging Procedures

MRI

MRI variables offer an almost infinite number of options from which must be selected the sequences most likely to solve the diagnostic problem. The specifics of a clinical problem, in addition to the anatomic site of concern, have taken on greater importance. The advantages of MRI are well known. They include the lack of ionizing radiation, multiplanar imaging, superior soft tissue contrast, and high lesion detection sensitivity.

Some patients are unable to undergo MRI examination, because of their inability to cooperate, a need for sedation or anesthesia with monitoring, uncontrollable claustrophobia, or a medical contraindication. Such medical contraindications include cardiac pacemakers, many types of aneurysm clips, stapes and penile prostheses, and ferromagnetic foreign bodies, especially in or near the eye. Orthopedic devices, including metal plates, rods, and screws, are usually safe but interfere with magnetic resonance by deleting information from the immediately adjacent area.

Detailed MRI of the spine requires the use of surface coils. Dedicated surface coils greatly improve signal-to-noise ratios (SNR), affording greater soft tissue contrast resolution, thinner slices, and volume acquisitions, which provide greater spatial resolution. Surface coils have size limitations that require repositioning of the patient or coil in order to cover the entire spine. Specially designed coils with multiple independent arrays, which can be activated independently, provide electronic movement of the coil or simultaneous study of two adjacent segments of the spine.

Patient movement, even physiologic movement (e.g., respiration and cardiovascular pulsations), degrades the image. In the cervical spine, swallowing can produce significant artifacts; and in the thoracic and lumbar areas, pulsation artifacts from the heart and great vessels are a problem. Particularly menacing to spine imaging are CSF pulsations, which can result in either a false increase or a false decrease in signal intensity; both can obscure lesions and mimic mass lesions and vascular malformations. There are several methods to decrease artifact created by CSF pulsations. One involves gating the imaging sequence in synchrony with the cardiac cycle, using the ECG or peripheral pulse as the trigger. A more common method uses specific gradient pulses that correct for proton movement during the imaging sequence. These are known as *gradient-moment nulling* or *flow compensation.* In the axial plane, artifact arising from major vessel pulsations can be directed transversely across the image, anterior to the spine and away from the area of interest. In the sagittal plane, saturation pulses can eliminate all signal from such arteries and thus greatly reduce artifact generated by their pulsations.

Still, many artifacts are inherent to MRI. Common examples include magnetic-susceptibility artifacts, chemical-shift artifact, and truncation artifact. Each can be minimized by the selection of appropriate imaging parameters and by a simple awareness of their appearance.

The sagittal plane provides most diagnostic information and will detect the majority of abnormalities. The axial plane, and less often the coronal plane, adds anatomic information, characterizing lesion extent more fully. For most spinal imaging, both T1-weighted and T2-weighted images are obtained. T1-weighted images are used for sagittal imaging; they are short-TR (repetition time), short-TE (echo time) sequences. On T1-weighted images, CSF has decreased signal intensity relative to the spinal cord. The size and shape of the cord is well defined and cystic cavities may be demonstrated. T1-weighted sequences provide good definition of the vertebrae and are sensitive to marrow replacement lesions. In combination with T2-weighted images, they may confirm the presence of hemorrhage.

T2-weighted images, which are long-TR, long-TE sequences, are necessary to obtain maximum soft tissue contrast and optimize intramedullary lesion detection. T2-weighted images display CSF with high signal intensity, creating a myelographic effect. Spinal intramedullary lesions will be detected in the presence of a normal-sized cord. T2-weighted images can be acquired with either conventional long TR/TE spin echo (SE) sequences; single slice, multiplanar, or volume-acquired T2* sequences; or fast spin echo sequences (FSE). Conventional SE long TR/TE sequences have long imaging times and are most susceptible to CSF pulsation artifact. Gradient-recalled-echo (GRE) pulse sequences are short TR/TE sequences with a partial flip angle. A flip angle of 20 degrees or less achieves a T2-like effect with excellent contrast. These T2* images depend on the T2 properties of protons in the tissue imaged but are also susceptible to signal decay from static field inhomogeneity and magnetic susceptibility. Properly used, GRE T2* images afford detection of intramedullary lesions equal, or nearly so, to that of conventional T2, images particularly with high-field-strength magnets. FSE sequences provide true T2 decay information, not T2*, with a time saving of 2 to 16 times that of conventional SE. This time saving allows longer TRs, which increase SNR, improve T2 contrast, and allow larger matrices for increased resolution.

Spatial resolution depends on image slice thickness and pixel size, which is determined by the field of view (FOV). When slice thickness and FOV are decreased to increase spatial resolution, the inherent loss in SNR must be compensated for. To obtain images less than 3.0 mm thick (e.g., for evaluation of cervivical neuroforamina, or to allow multiplanar reformation) a volume acquisition is used to maintain adequate SNR. One must be aware that osseous margins are exaggerated, because of magnetic susceptibility effects, and spinal cord dimensions may be misrepresented unless proper window width and level settings are used.

Contrast enhancement is essential for intraspinal extraosseous tumor detection. Intravenously administered paramagnetic ions, such as gadolinium, reduce T1 relaxation times. The delivery method and chelating agent to which the ion is bound determine the site of activity. Several gadolinium compounds are available that remain intravascular in intact tissue but provide enhancement of tumors and other lesions due primarily to blood-brain barrier breakdown. Since the action of paramagnetic ions is to shorten T1 relaxation times of surrounding protons, increased signal intensity is seen on T1-weighted images obtained shortly after contrast material administration. In general, lesions are detected that are not seen on conventional SE images or are obscured by surrounding edema, tumor margins are better defined, solid components are differentiated from cystic components, and detection of pial metastases is greatly improved.

CT and CECT

High-resolution CT developed to advanced levels, and the application of CT to diseases of the spine became well established, long before MRI reached its current level of utility and availability. CT remains a valuable diagnostic tool for patients in whom MRI is contraindicated or unavailable. CT is used as a focal diagnostic procedure. While an entire spinal segment (lumbar, cervical, or upper or lower thoracic) may be screened with CT, a focal area of interest is usually first determined by clinical findings, conventional radiography, radionuclide scanning, or myelography.

High-resolution CT is achieved with thin slices and a small field of view, approximately 17 cm. The scanning plane should parallel that of the intervertebral disk for study of disk, endplate, or single body lesions; it should be angled perpendicularly to the spinal canal for study of multilevel or intraspinal abnormalities. Slice thicknesses no greater than 5 mm are used in the lumbar spine, spaced at 4- or 5-mm intervals, but contiguous 3-mm-thick slices will improve resolution. The smaller size of cervical vertebrae and disks demands thinner slices. Continuous spiral scanning techniques allow the acquisition of 1 scan slice per second for up to 30 to 60 slices. Interleaved or overlapping scans can then be reconstructed from the raw scan data without further radiation for 3D or multiplanar reformations. CT scans are imaged with both wide and narrow windows to allow assessment of both the bony and soft-tissue components of a lesion. Primary bone lesions and fractures are acquired by means of a bone algorithm technique.

CT scanning after the administration of intravenous (IV) contrast material (CECT) may provide additional information. One should first be well informed on the use of iodinated contrast material, including the risk of side effects, as well as on the choices to be made regarding specific contrast agents, concentration, dose, rate and timing of administration, and patient premedication, if appropriate. IV contrast may aid in the localization of extradural lesions and in the delineation of the extent of intradural, including intramedullary, tumors—thus helping to differentiate cystic from solid components.[8]

Myelography (and CT Myelography)

Conventional myelography has assumed a lesser role in the diagnosis of spinal tumors. Myelography is now an outpatient procedure. The use of small-gauge spinal needles (22 to 26g) and nonionic, low-osmolar, water-soluble contrast material has significantly lowered the side effects and complication rate. The role of myelography is to localize lesions, both to level and to compartment (extra- or intradural, extra- or intramedullary). It remains nonspecific as to etiology. Lesion characterization is greatly aided by CT scanning following the myelogram while contrast material remains within the thecal sac.[21] When studying a focal lesion or area, one may forgo conventional myelogram radiographs. The simple intrathecal injection of a small volume of isotonic nonionic contrast material through a small-gauge needle, followed by CT, minimizes discomfort and morbidity while at the same time providing more information. Not only are the intrathecal contents imaged, but so are the adjacent bone and paraspinous soft tissues. Imaging parameters are similar to those for standard CT. The detection of intradural extramedullary nodules, root thickening, and arachnoiditis has been notoriously difficult with myelography, unenhanced CT, and unenhanced MRI. CT myelography (CTM) in those patients who cannot undergo MRI remains the most sensitive imaging modality. Contrast-enhanced MRI, however, remains equal or superior to CTM in the detection of such lesions.

Spinal Tumors

Intramedullary Tumors

Astrocytoma and Ependymoma

MRI with non-enhanced T1- and T2-weighted images will detect the great majority of intramedullary tumors. MRI, although a highly sensitive imaging procedure, is nonspecific in distinguishing astrocytoma from ependymoma and other primary spinal cord tumors.[2] Both astrocytomas and ependymomas have low to intermediate signal intensity on T1-weighted images and produce fusiform swelling of the spinal cord, usually over several segments. Inhomogeneity of signal intensity may be due to hemorrhage breakdown products or cystic components (Fig. 174-1). Since both tumor and surrounding edema have prolonged T2 relaxation times, on T2-weighted images both ependymomas and astrocytomas appear to infiltrate adjacent cord tissue and thereby appear ill defined and larger than they actually are.[12] Ependymomas in the cauda equina or filum terminale may be obscured by the high signal intensity of CFS on T2-weighted images.

Focal markedly hypointense areas are occasionally seen, at the superior and inferior margins of tumors, that appear to correspond to a relatively firm pseudocapsule—which likely developed secondarily to old hematomas at the tumor–normal-cord interface (Fig. 174-2). This finding has been seen more frequently in ependymomas and is suggestive, although not pathognomonic, of ependymoma.[11] Occasionally there is also evidence of prior intratumoral hemorrhage seen as low-signal foci of hemosiderin.

The vast majority of tumors will exhibit enhancement on enhanced MR. Ependymomas tend to enhance more markedly, more homogeneously, and with sharper margins than do astrocytomas. Ependymomas tend to occupy the whole width of the spinal cord, whereas astrocytomas tend to be eccentrically positioned and in some instances exophytic.[12] While patchy, less-marked enhancement is more common in astrocytomas, there is considerable overlap between the two groups. In general, enhancement of intramedullary lesions may be increased on delayed images. This increase is usually mild enough that immediate post-contrast imaging should suffice to depict most lesions.[18]

Tumor cysts appear either as intratumoral cavities of neoplastic origin or as rostral or caudal cystic cavities that delineate the superior or inferior extent of the tumor but are not of tumorous origin.[6] Intratumoral cavity detection depends on the cavity's contents. The more CSF-like its contents, the more likely it is to be detected on T1-weighted images. Necrosis and highly proteinaceous material may appear isointense to the tumor and therefore be obscured on non-enhanced MRI. Cystic cavities capping the rostral or caudal poles of intramedullary tumors are usually readily identified as cavities with low signal intensity on T1-weighted images and high signal intensity on T2-weighted images. Enhanced MRI is especially important when the adjacent cyst has proteinaceous contents that image isointense to tumor. In such cases, enhanced MRI will usually differentiate tumor margin from adjacent cyst.[4,16] Lack of enhancement surrounding a cyst extending inferiorly or superiorly from the tumor suggests that the cyst formed as a reactive response to the neoplasm, rather than as a part of it.[19]

Spinal cord expansion due to syringohydromyelia unassociated with tumor is apparent on nonenhanced MRI when the cavity has distinct margins, uniform signal intensity, and isointensity to CSF. Enhanced MRI is especially important in those cysts in which a high protein concentration produces nonuniform signal intensity or ill-defined margins.[22] Cyst inhomogeneity may also be due to pulsatile flow of CSF which produces a focal area of signal loss [the CSF flow void sign (CFVS)]. This sign has been reported in 40 percent of syrinx cavities. This sign may be present in rostral or caudal tumor cysts, but not in intratumoral cysts.[15]

Hemangioblastoma

On nonenhanced MR, hemangioblastomas are seen as areas of irregular and diffuse widening of the spinal cord. Heterogeneous signal intensity reflects cavities alternating with areas of cord thickening. Although long TR/TE images will show the signal intensity within the cavity to be greater than that of the tumor nidus, enhanced MRI will more distinctly differentiate the highly vascular tumor nidus from areas of cystic change.[12] A uniformly enhancing nodule associated with a well-defined cyst strongly suggests hemangioblastoma. Enhanced MRI may also reveal additional small, unsuspected, solid tumor nodules in the spinal cord or posterior fossa.[14]

Myelography and CTM (the latter especially) detect intramedullary spinal cord tumors by virtue of cord swelling or expansion. CT also demonstrates vertebral body scalloping (remodeling) and pedicle and lamina thinning indicative of long-standing or slowly progressive cord expansion. Although delayed rescanning approximately 6 h following CTM may reveal opacification of a cavity, simple syringomyelia cannot reliably be differentiated from syringomyelia associated with tumor on the basis of cyst opacification. The opacified cavity must account fully for the cord expansion.[7] Intravenous CECT may also demonstrate the extent of the tumor and help separate solid and cystic components. Hemangioblastomas most consistently enhance, often densely.[8]

Metastases

Intramedullary metastases are nonspecific in their appearance. MRI is most sensitive in demonstrating cord widening, increased signal intensity with T2 weighting (even in the absence of cord widening), and contrast enhancement of the lesion (Fig. 174-3). Furthermore, MRI allows screening of the entire spine even in the presence of a myelographic block. The diagnosis is suspected in the setting of multiple lesions, often associated with brain lesions, in a patient with known primary malignancy.[13]

Intradural/Extramedullary Tumors

Nerve Sheath Tumors

Schwannomas and neurofibromas have similar appearances on MRI. They tend to be smoothly rounded and well marginated, isointense or slightly hypointense to the cord on T1-weighted images, and to have increased signal intensity (often markedly so) on T2-weighted images. They consistently enhance, usually intensely. Neurofibromas occasionally exhibit a low-signal area within the mass, representing dense areas of collagenous stroma.[3] Heterogeneous enhancement has been described in schwannomas, occasionally with peripheral enhancement around cystic areas.[5] Nerve sheath tumors may grow through and expand neural foramina, resulting in a ''dumbbell'' shape (Fig. 174-4). They deviate and compress the spinal cord and widen the subarachnoid space, as

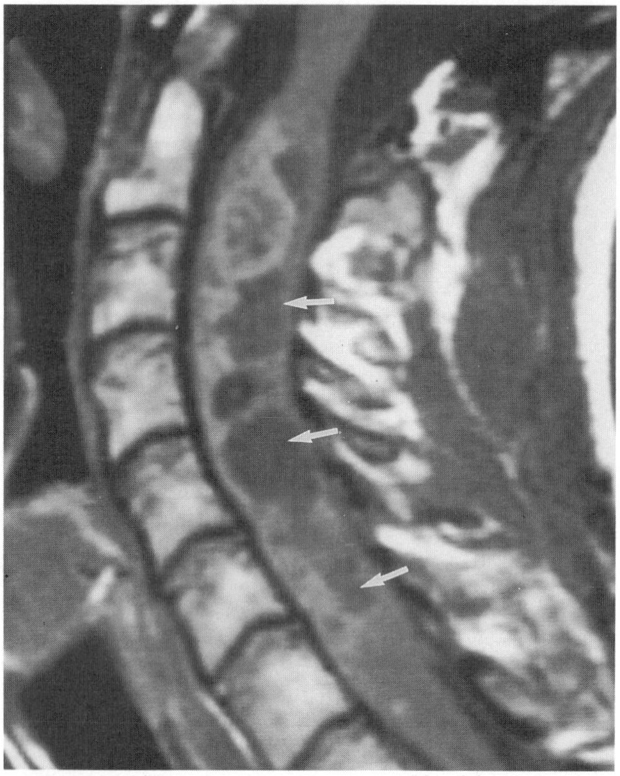

(*A*)

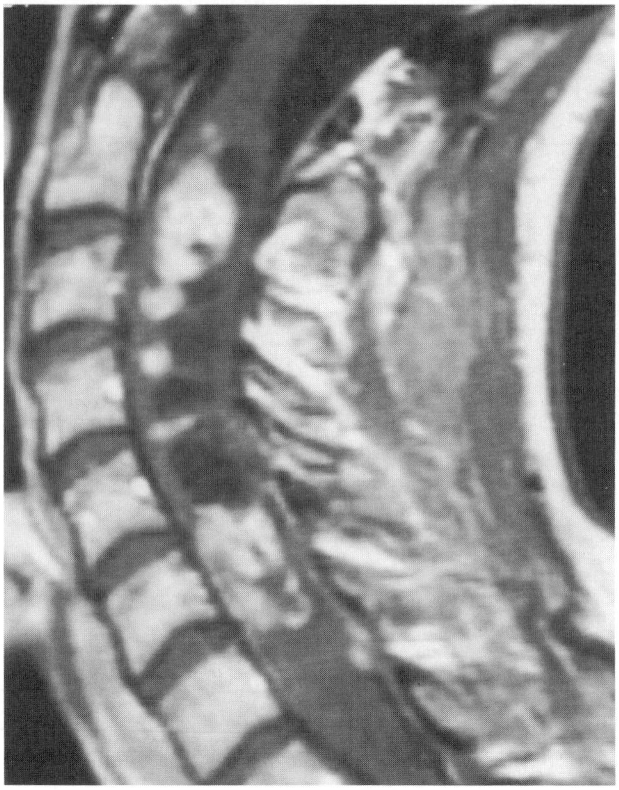

(*C*)

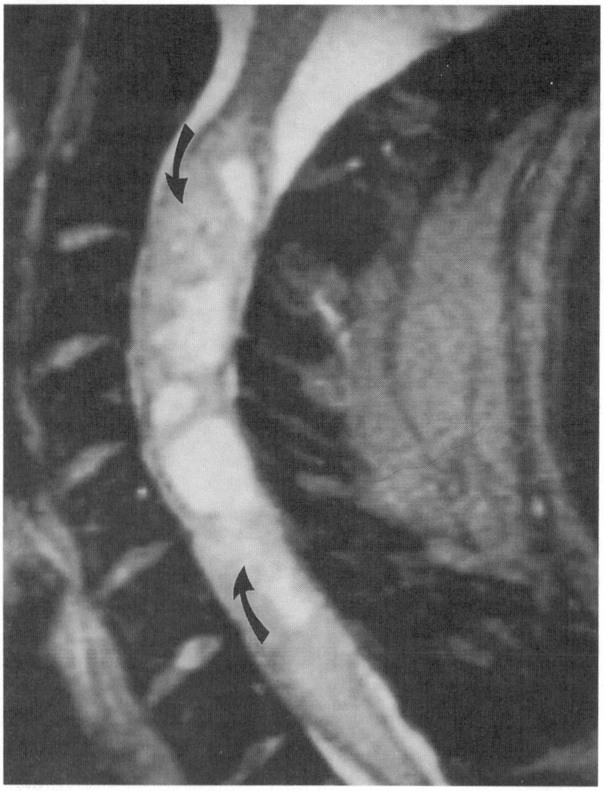

(*B*)

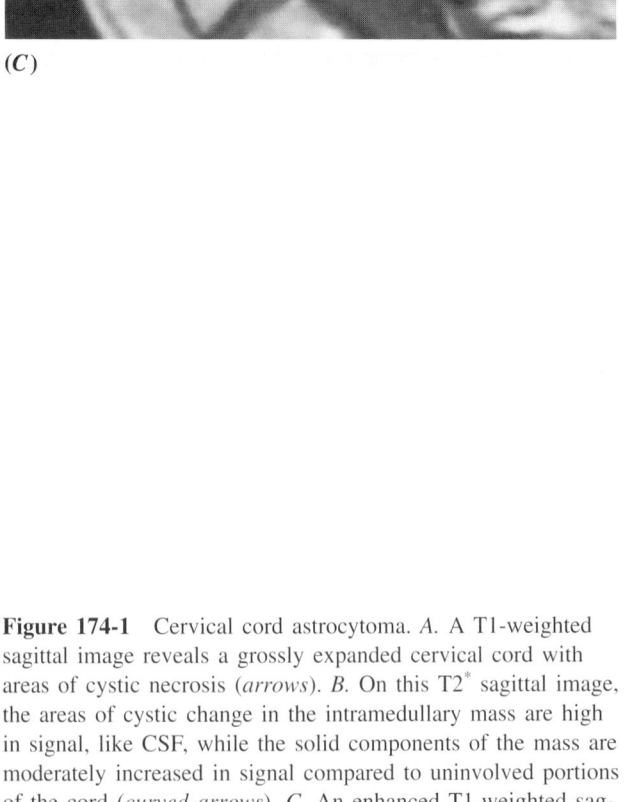

Figure 174-1 Cervical cord astrocytoma. *A*. A T1-weighted sagittal image reveals a grossly expanded cervical cord with areas of cystic necrosis (*arrows*). *B*. On this T2* sagittal image, the areas of cystic change in the intramedullary mass are high in signal, like CSF, while the solid components of the mass are moderately increased in signal compared to uninvolved portions of the cord (*curved arrows*). *C*. An enhanced T1-weighted sagittal image demonstrates marked enhancement of solid portions of the tumor. Necrotic areas within the tumor do not enhance and are therefore better delineated.

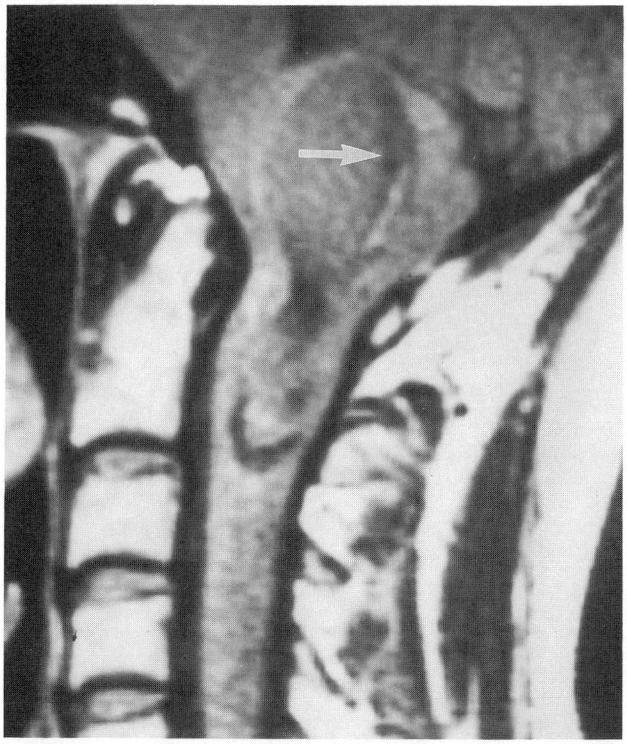

(*A*)

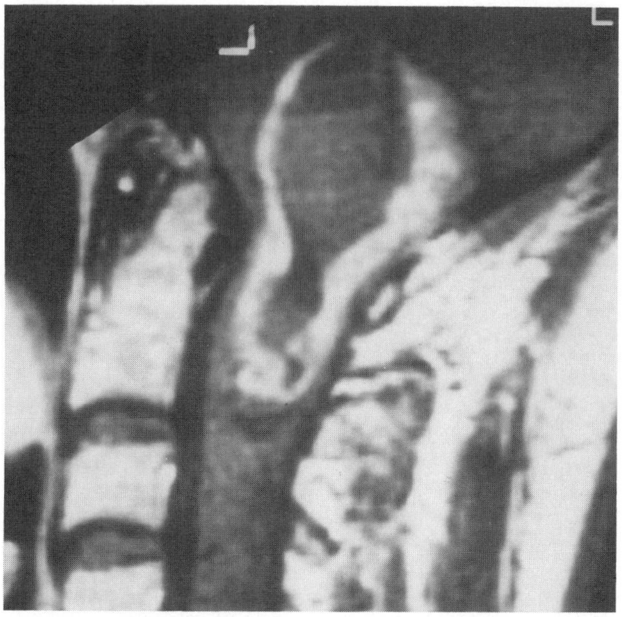

(*C*)

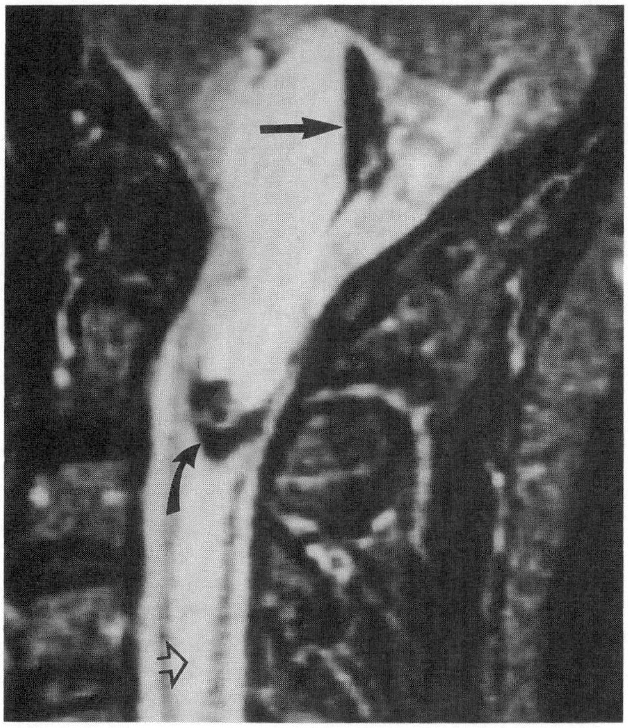

(*B*)

Figure 174-2 Intramedullary ependymoma. *A.* A T1-weighted sagittal image reveals marked expansion and deformity of the medulla and upper cervical cord by an intramedullary mass that has central areas of low-signal necrosis. The solid portion of the mass is isointense to cord. The fluid-fluid level present in the posterior aspect of the region of necrosis (*arrow*) is due to intratumoral hemorrhage. *B.* On the T2* sagittal image the entire mass is increased in signal, especially the necrotic portions. The fluid-fluid level is better seen (*arrow*). The more posterior, dependent fluid component contains the more cellular, proteinaceous blood products and is therefore low in signal; the less dependent portion is more serous in nature and therefore higher in signal. The ''cap'' of low signal at the inferior aspect of the ependymoma (*curved arrow*) is likely related to old hemorrhage with consequent hemosiderin deposition, which is lower in signal on T2-weighted images compared to T1- or proton-weighted images. Note the increased signal within the cord caudad to the tumor, due to peritumoral edema (*open arrow*). *C.* This enhanced sagittal image demonstrates enhancement of the non-necrotic periphery of the mass and therefore better defines the mass. Note, however, that there may still be tumor cells located outside the area of enhancement.

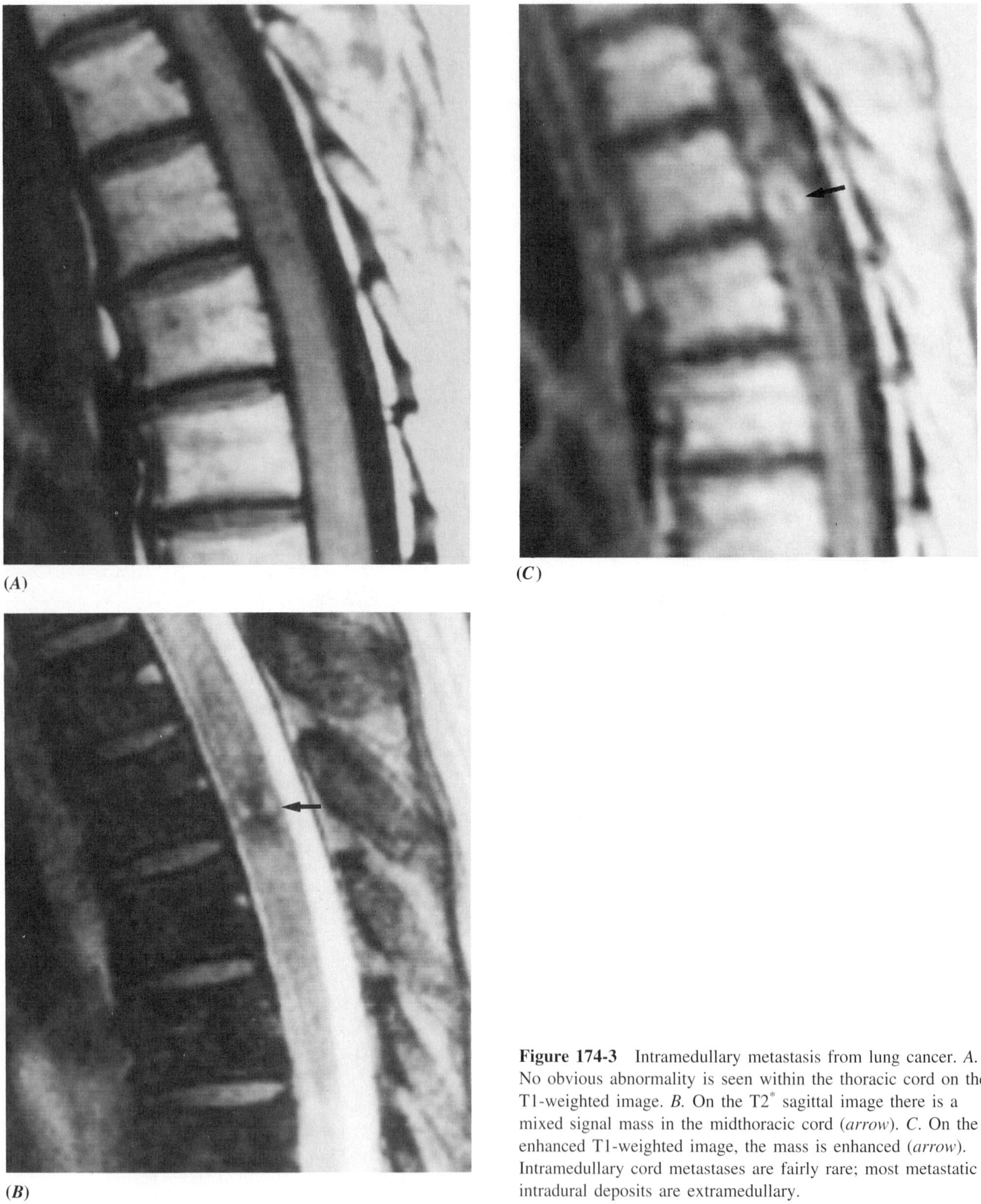

Figure 174-3 Intramedullary metastasis from lung cancer. *A*. No obvious abnormality is seen within the thoracic cord on the T1-weighted image. *B*. On the T2* sagittal image there is a mixed signal mass in the midthoracic cord (*arrow*). *C*. On the enhanced T1-weighted image, the mass is enhanced (*arrow*). Intramedullary cord metastases are fairly rare; most metastatic intradural deposits are extramedullary.

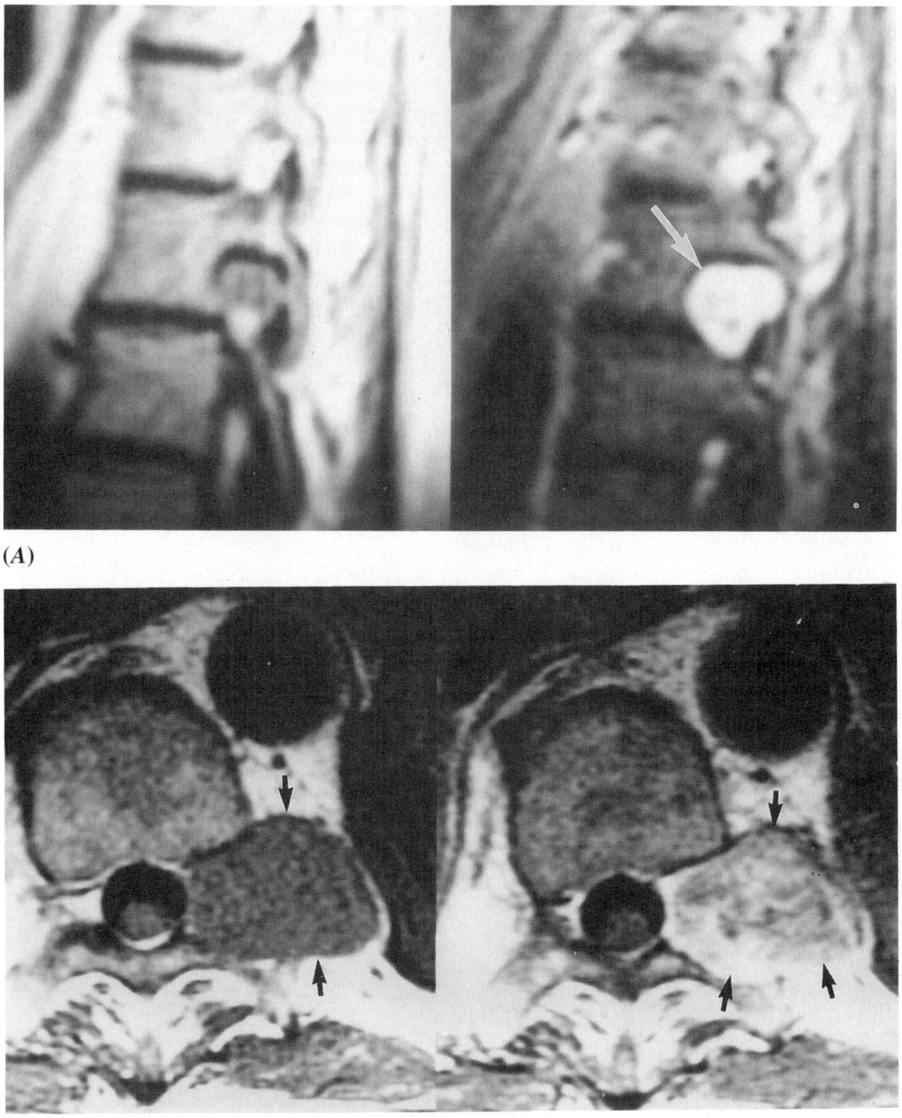

(*A*)

(*B*)

Figure 174-4 Neurofibroma. *A.* Proton density (*left*) and T2-weighted (*right*) parasagittal images of the thoracic spine demonstrate obliteration of the epidural fat in the neural foramen by a mass that is isointense on the proton density image and hyperintense on the T2-weighted image (*arrow*). The neural foramen is enlarged. *B.* T1-weighted (*left*) and enhanced T1-weighted (*right*) images show a large oval soft tissue mass partly within the spinal canal and extending through the neural foramen into the left paraspinal space (*arrows*). The mass is low-to-intermediate in signal on the T1-weighted image and heterogeneously enhancing on the enhanced T1-weighted image. These are the most typical signal characteristics and enhancement patterns of neurofibromas.

does any intradural extramedullary mass. In the cauda equina, they may be attached to a nerve root, free from the dura (Fig. 174-5).

Meningiomas

Meningiomas also usually appear as rounded, sharply marginated masses displacing and compressing the spinal cord. They are most often isointense to the spinal cord on T1-weighted images and isointense, or slightly hyperintense, on T2-weighted images. Since meningiomas are highly vascular extra-axial lesions with no blood-brain barrier, immediate and uniform—and usually intense—enhancement occurs. Calcification may result in irregular enhancement and signal void.

Nerve sheath tumors and meningiomas may appear similar on MRI or any other kind of imaging study. Nerve sheath tumors tend to be anterolateral in the spinal canal, occasionally are multiple, may extend through a neural foramen, may have a central focus of decreased signal, and may be attached to a nerve root free from dura. Meningiomas tend to be posterolateral (except in the cervical area), usually are solitary, are dural based, and only on rare occasion extend through a neural foramen.

Myelography readily demonstrates larger lesions with cord displacement and asymmetric widening of the subarachnoid space. An intradural location is usually evident, with capping of the rounded margin of the mass. CTM may identify the extraforaminal component of a "dumbbell" mass.

Metastases

Intradural extramedullary metastases of sufficient size are demonstrated on unenhanced MRI with the aid of secondary findings of cord displacement or compression and an asymmetric subarachnoid space. Lesions may be obscured, especially below the conus, on T2-weighted images, since the MR relaxation characteristics of these lesions may approach those of surrounding CSF—especially if the CSF is abnormally proteinaceous. Myelography will demonstrate larger nodules and CTM will aid in the demonstration of smaller nodules, especially cord cloaking nodules and those attached to nerve roots[17] (Fig. 174-6). Enhanced MRI, however, is the most sensitive modality for detection of intradural metastases and is the only means of demonstrating tiny nodules and thin sheets of pial metastases[10] (Fig. 174-7).

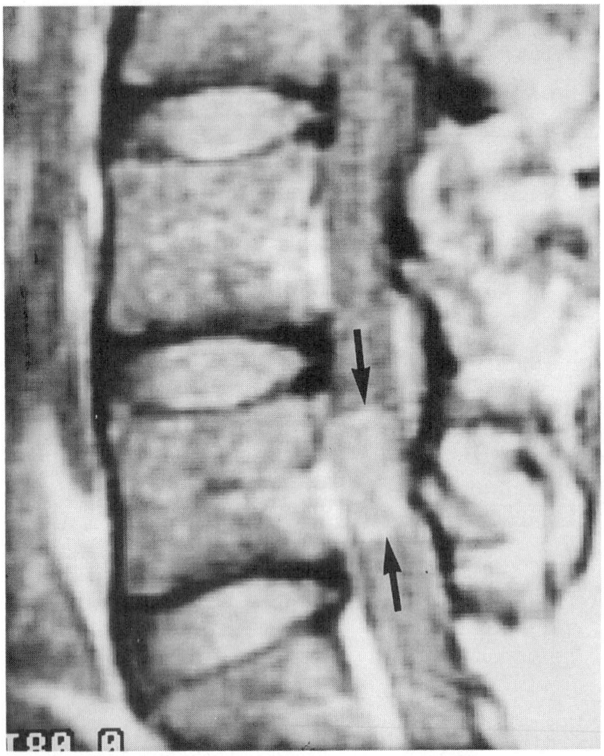

(*A*)

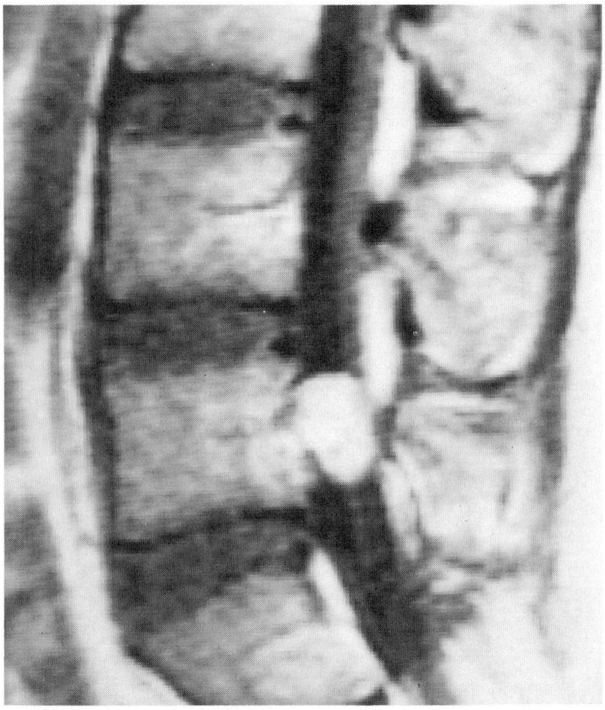

(*C*)

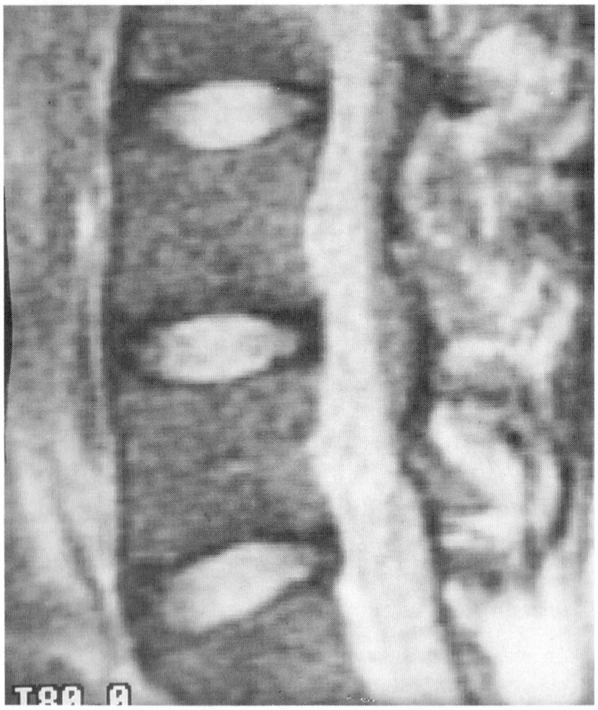

(*B*)

Figure 174-5 Neurofibroma. *A*. The intradural, extramedullary rounded soft tissue mass is hyperintense to CSF on the proton density sagittal image (*arrows*). *B*. It is isointense to CSF and obscured by CSF on the T2-weighted image. *C*. It is strongly enhancing on the enhanced T1-weighted image.

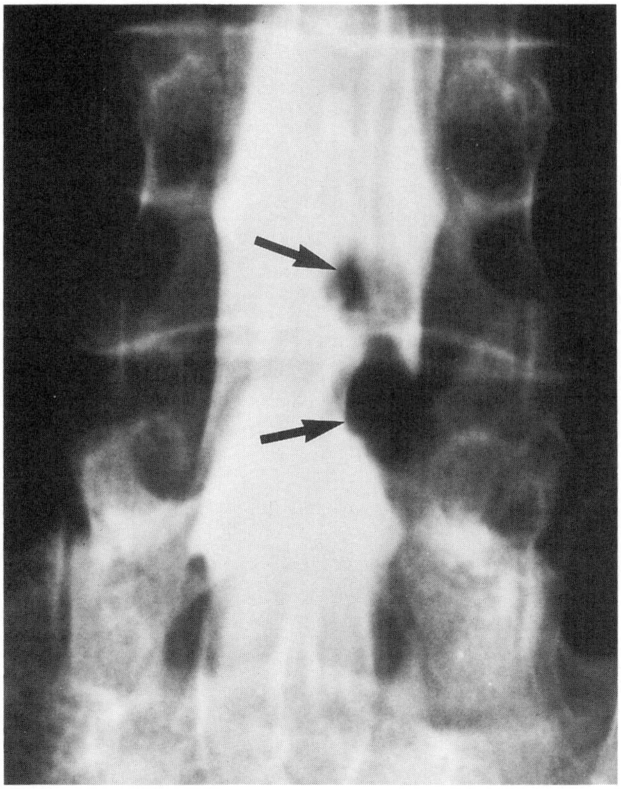

(*A*)

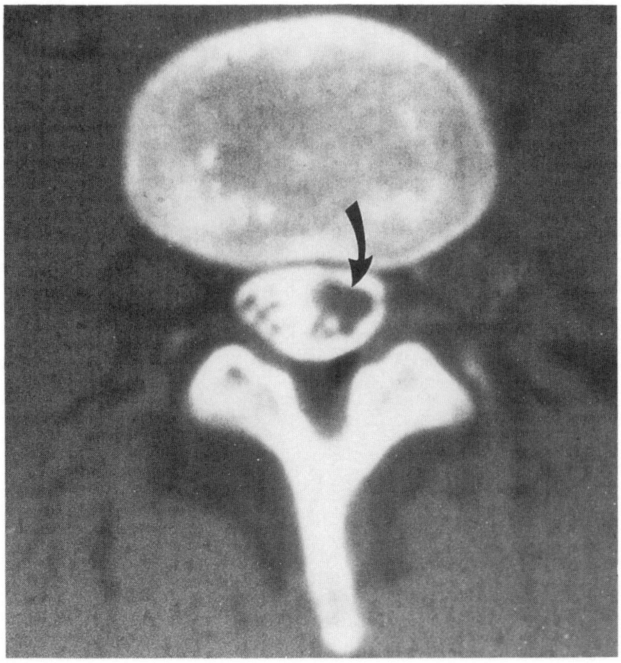

(*B*)

Figure 174-6 Drop metastasis from lung cancer metastatic to the cerebellum. *A.* Lumbar myelography, frontal projection, using water-soluble contrast material, shows a 1-cm by 2-cm lobulated intradural filling defect on the left at the L4-L5 level (*arrows*). *B.* Post-myelographic CT (CTM) confirms the intradural location of the mass, as well as its attachment to intrathecal nerve roots (*curved arrow*).

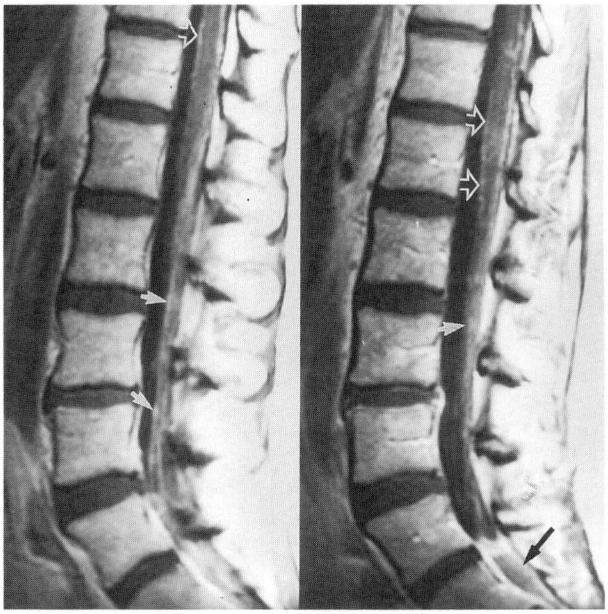

Figure 174-7 Drop metastases from pituitary carcinoma. Enhanced T1-weighted sagittal images show involvement of the lower thoracic cord and conus by drop metastases (*open arrows*). There is nodular enhancement along nerve roots (*white arrows*) and a larger mass filling the caudal end of the thecal sac (*black arrow*). MRI surpasses myelography in the detection of drop metastases of this nature. The fine coating of the cord surface by tumor would not likely be detected by myelography.

Extradural Tumors

Unenhanced MRI is generally excellent for the detection of spinal osseous lesions. MRI has greater sensitivity than either plain films or radionuclide bone scans for metastatic disease in the spine. The high signal intensity of marrow fat usually outlines marrow-replacing lesions. Increased T2 signal intensity will be more obvious with fat-suppression imaging techniques. MRI has the advantage of detecting the osseous component, epidural extension, and thecal sac compression. Few lesions have characteristic imaging properties.

Vertebral Hemangioma

Vertebral hemangioma is one of the few primary neoplasms that exhibit a distinctive imaging appearance (Fig. 174-8). Increased signal intensity on T1-weighted MR images reflects the fatty component; the increased signal intensity on T2-weighted images is more difficult to explain, but probably is related to the more cellular component. Some appear isointense to marrow on T2-weighted images. The "thickened trabeculae" and vertically striated appearance (also seen on plain films and CT) are characteristic. More aggressive hemangiomas have less fat content and, therefore, less-marked signal intensity on T1-weighted images.[9] Enhanced MRI aids in the delineation of extraosseous, especially epidural, extension.

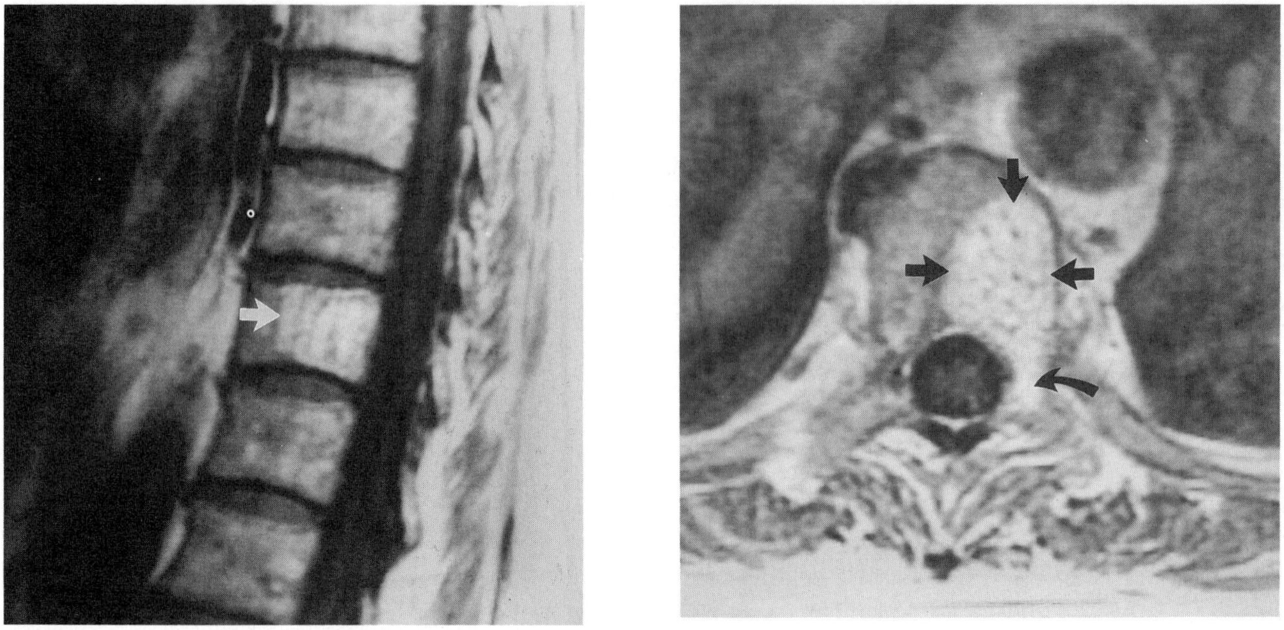

(*A*) (*B*)

Figure 174-8 Vertebral body hemangioma. *A.* A T1-weighted sagittal image shows the classic appearance of a vertebral body hemangioma (*arrow*). It is hyperintense in signal because of fatty elements within the benign tumor. Vertical low-signal striations are due to osseous trabeculations. Hemangiomas are variable in signal on long-TR images, but are usually isointense or mildly increased in signal. *B.* An enhanced T1-weighted axial image shows enhancement of the hemangioma (*arrows*), which extends posteriorly into the left pedicle (*curved arrow*).

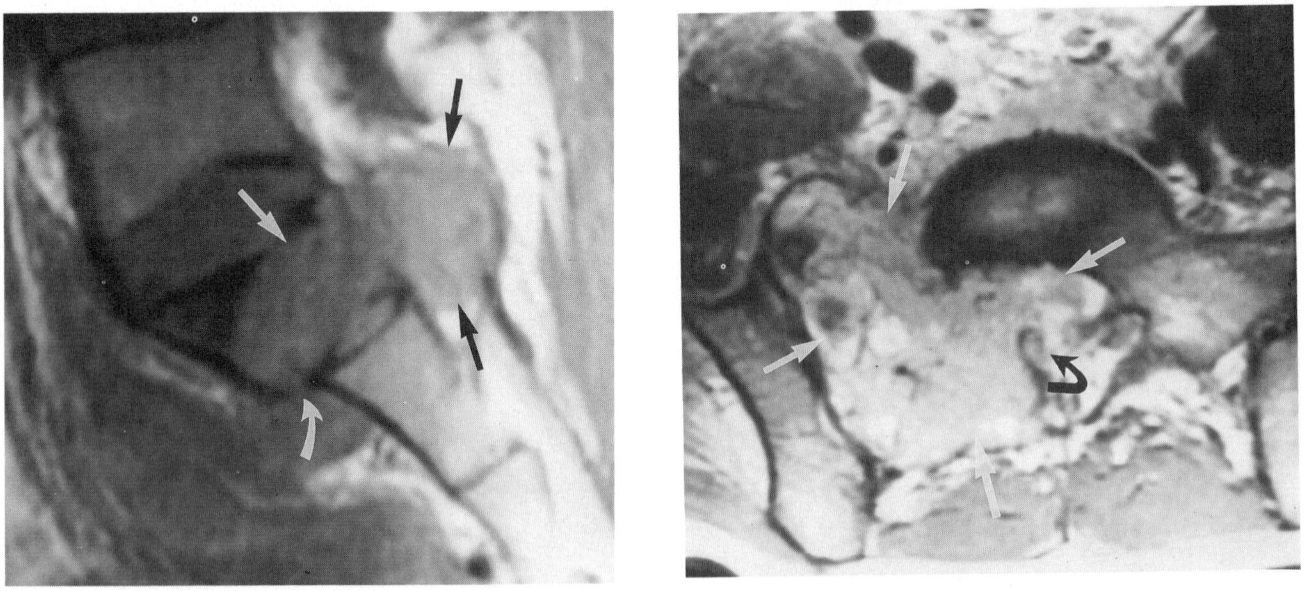

(*A*) (*B*)

Figure 174-9 Giant cell tumor of the sacrum. *A.* A T1-weighted sagittal image demonstrates a destructive soft tissue mass of intermediate signal intensity (*arrows*) in the upper sacrum, with pathologic fracture through the S1 vertebral body (*curved arrow*). *B.* A proton density axial image shows a heterogeneous generally hyperintense expansile mass involving the right side of the sacrum (*arrows*) with extension into the spinal canal and encroachment on neural foramina (*curved arrow*). The differential diagnosis includes chordoma, aneurysmal bone cyst, metastatic disease, and sarcoma.

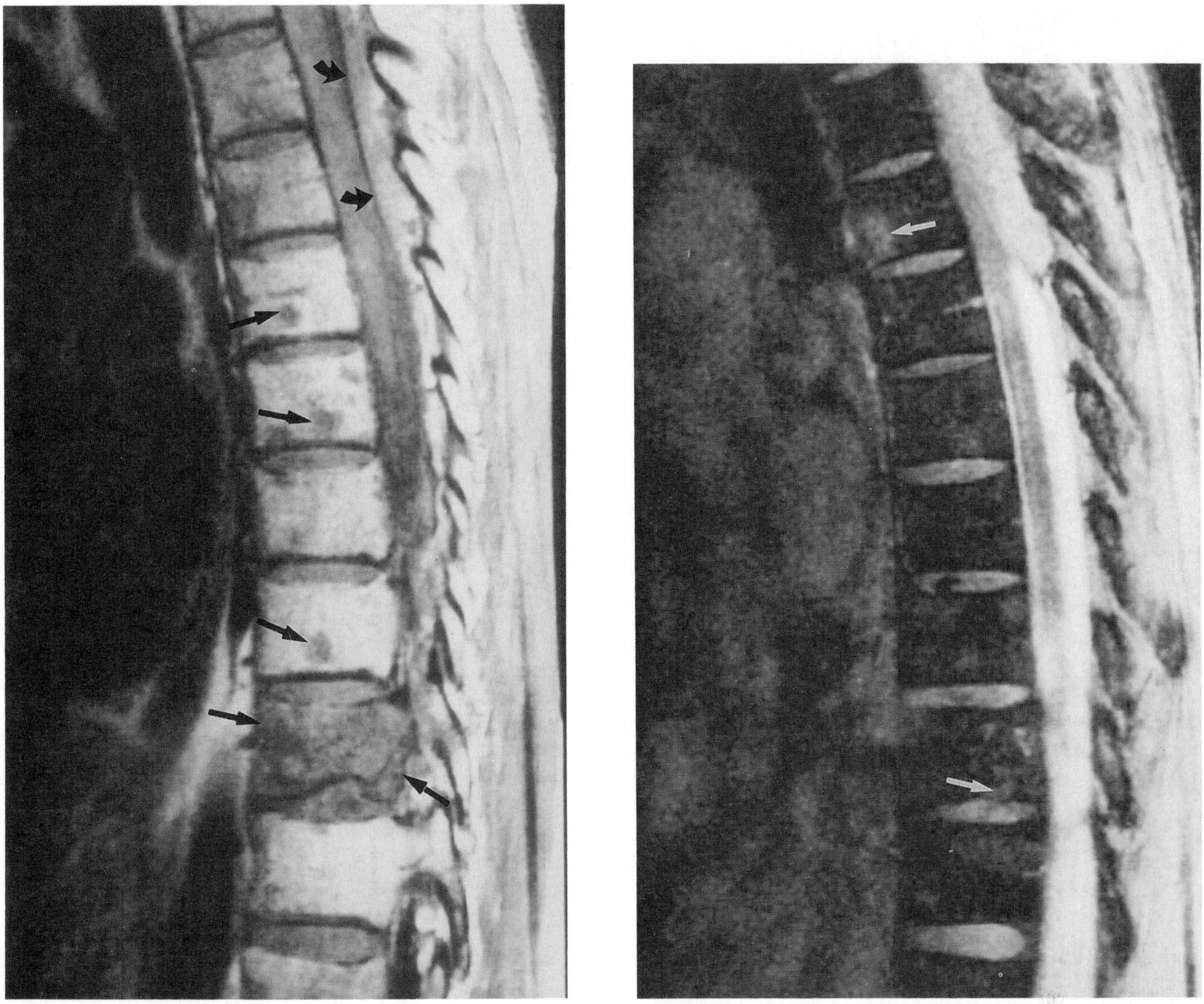

(*A*) (*B*)

Figure 174-10 Extradural metastases of lymphoma. *A.* A T1-weighted sagittal image demonstrates multiple areas of abnormal low signal within several vertebral bodies, representing bone marrow replacement by lymphoma (*arrows*). There is an isointense lymphomatous mass within the epidural space posterior to the spinal cord in the upper thoracic region (*curved arrows*). *B.* A T2*-weighted sagittal image reveals hyperintense metastatic foci within the vertebral bodies (*arrows*) and intermediate signal intensity of the epidural soft tissue mass. Not all lesions present on the T1-weighted image are seen on the T2* image; this shows the increased sensitivity of T1-weighted images compared to T2* images in identifying marrow-replacing metastatic bone disease.

Other Primary Tumors

Most primary spine neoplasms are neoplasms of bone and will be detected on plain radiographs and well defined on CT. MRI has the added advantage of defining soft tissue limits and degree of spinal canal compromise. Specific diagnoses are suggested by a constellation of imaging properties and by lesion location.

Osteochondromas are confined to the posterior elements and contain a cartilaginous cap. Most osteoid osteomas involve the posterior elements and contain an often-calcified characteristic nidus, which enhances intensely. The more expansile osseous lesions, of which osteoblastoma, aneurysmal bone cyst, and giant cell tumor are a partial list, have many imaging similarities—as do their malignant counterparts (Fig. 174-9). CT better defines cortical bone destruction and calcified tumor matrix, while MRI is superior in defining spinal canal invasion and paraspinous soft tissue extension.[1]

Metastases

Spinal metastases are usually apparent on T1-weighted images, because of fatty marrow replacement. The degree of increased signal intensity on T2-weighted images is variable. Enhanced MRI greatly aids in the delineation of epidural as well as paraspinous spread.[20] Enhanced lesions may be isointense to marrow fat; therefore, unenhanced T1-weighted images are necessary to detect both enhancing and non-enhancing lesions. Conspicuity is increased with fat-suppressed enhanced images (Fig. 174-10). Although CTM is also sensitive in demonstrating osseous destruction, thecal

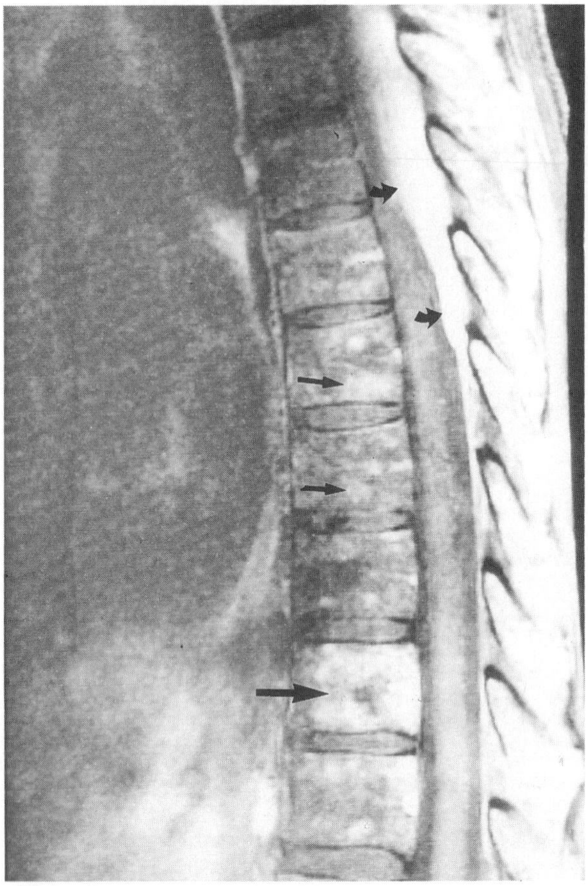

(C)

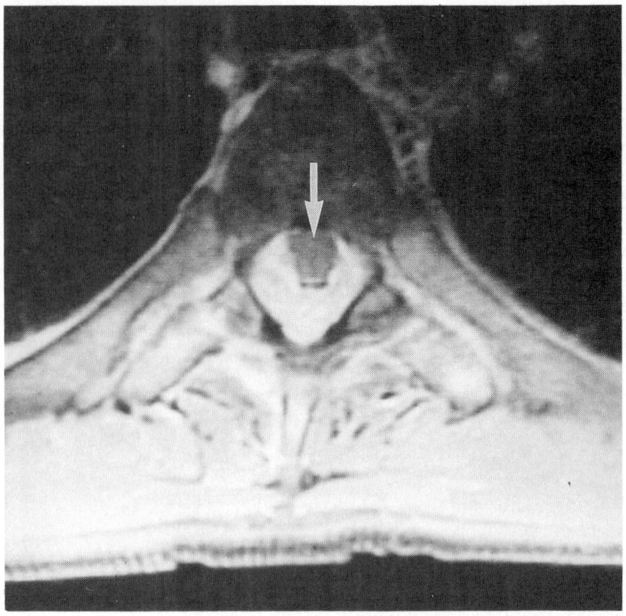

(D)

Figure 174-10 (*Continued*) *C.* Fat-suppressed enhanced T1-weighted sagittal image demonstrates enhancement of the osseous metastases (*arrows pointing to a few of the many lesions*) and the epidural tumor (*curved arrows*). *D.* This enhanced T1-weighted axial image best demonstrates transverse compression of the spinal cord (*arrow*).

sac compression, and paraspinous extension, MRI is superior and has the added advantage of allowing screening the entire spine.

References

1. Beltran J, Noto AM, Chakeres DW, et al. Tumors of the osseous spine: staging with MR imaging versus CT. *Radiology* 1987; 162:565–569.
2. Brotchi J, Dewitte O, Levivier M, et al. A survey of 65 tumors within the spinal cord: surgical results and the importance of preoperative magnetic resonance imaging. *Neurosurgery* 1991; 29(5):651–657.
3. Burk DL Jr, Brunberg JA, Kanal E, et al. Spinal and paraspinal neurofibromatosis: surface coil MR imaging at 1.5 T. *Radiology* 1987; 162:797–801.
4. Dillon WP, Norman D, Newton TH, et al. Intradural spinal cord lesions: Gd-DTPA-enhanced MR imaging. *Radiology* 1989; 170:229–237.
5. Friedman DP, Tartaglino LM, Flanders AE. Intradural schwannomas of the spine: MR findings with emphasis on contrast-enhancement characteristics. *Am J Neuroradiol* 1992; 158:1347–1350.
6. Goy AMC, Pinto RS, Raghavendra BN, et al. Intramedullary spinal cord tumors: MR imaging, with emphasis on associated cysts. *Radiology* 1986; 161:381–386.
7. Kan S, Fox AJ, Viñuela F, et al. Delayed CT metrizamide enhancement of syringomyelia secondary to tumor. *Am J Neuroradiol* 1983; 4:73–78.
8. Lapointe JS, Graeb DA, Nugent RA, et al. Value of intravenous contrast enhancement in the CT evaluation of intraspinal tumors. *Am J Neuroradiol* 1985; 6:939–943.
9. Laredo JD, Assouline E, Gelbert F, et al. Vertebral hemangiomas: fat content as a sign of aggressiveness. *Radiology* 1990; 177:467–472.
10. Lim V, Sobel DF, Zyroff J. Spinal cord pial metastases: MR imaging with gadopentetate dimeglumine. *Am J Neuroradiol* 1990; 11:975–982.
11. Nemoto Y, Inoue Y, Tashiro T, et al. Intramedullary spinal cord tumors: significance of associated hemorrhage at MR imaging. *Radiology* 1992; 182:793–796.
12. Parizel PM, Balériaux D, Rodesch G, et al. Gd-DTPA-enhanced MR imaging of spinal tumors. *Am J Neuroradiol* 1989; 10:249–258.
13. Post MJD, Quencer RM, Green BA, et al. Intramedullary spinal cord metastases, mainly of nonneurogenic origin. *Am J Neuroradiol* 1987; 8:339–346.
14. Rothwell CI, Jaspan T, Worthington BS, et al. Gadolinium-enhanced magnetic resonance imaging of spinal tumours. *Br J Radiol* 1989; 62:1067–1074.
15. Sherman JL, Barkovich AJ, Citrin CM. The MR appearance of syringomyelia: new observations. *Am J Neuroradiol* 1986; 7:985–995.
16. Slasky BS, Bydder GM, Niendorf HP, et al. MR imaging with gadolinium-DTPA in the differentiation of tumor, syrinx, and cyst of the spinal cord. *J Comput Assist Tomogr* 1987; 11(5):845–850.
17. Stanley P, Senac MO Jr, Segall HD. Intraspinal seeding from intracranial tumors in children. *Am J Roentgenol* 1985; 144:157–161.
18. Sze G, Bravo S, Krol G. Spinal lesions: quantitative and qualitative temporal evolution of gadopentetate dimeglumine enhancement in MR imaging. *Radiology* 1989; 170:849–856.
19. Sze G, Krol G, Zimmerman RD, et al. Intramedullary disease of the spine: diagnosis using gadolinium-DTPA-enhanced MR imaging. *Am J Neuroradiol* 1988; 9:847–858.
20. Sze G, Krol G, Zimmerman RD, et al. Malignant extradural spinal tumors: MR imaging with Gd-DTPA. *Radiology* 1988; 167:217–223.
21. Tadmor R, Cacayorin ED, Kieffer SA. Advantages of supplementary CT in myelography of intraspinal masses. *Am J Neuroradiol* 1983; 4:618–621.
22. Williams AL, Haughton VM, Pojunas KW, et al. Differentiation of intramedullary neoplasms and cysts by MR. *Am J Neuroradiol* 1987; 8:527–532.

175 Spinal Intradural Tumors

Bennett M. Stein
Paul C. McCormick

Victor Horsley is credited with the first successful removal of a spinal cord tumor.[11] The tumor was intradural and extramedullary, and was typed as a fibromyxoma. The condition had been diagnosed by William Gowers; Horsley proceeded with the surgery with a great deal of trepidation because at that time (1887) even the successful performance of a laminectomy was rare. The patient was a captain in the British army who suffered relentless progression of the disease to a paraplegia. The operation was performed under ether anesthesia with the patient in a semiprone position. The patient subsequently made excellent progress and became ambulatory. Horsley's conclusion about spinal cord tumors was "there is but one treatment, viz. removal of the source of pressure by operation."

Although Cushing[5] is given credit for the first successful removal of an intramedullary ependymoma, the technique of intramedullary spinal cord tumor surgery as well as the diagnosis and treatment of all spinal tumors is epitomized by Elsberg's 1925 masterpiece on this subject.[7] He pointed out, "Not so many years ago 'chronic myelitis' and 'transverse myelitis' were considered diseases of frequent occurrence; we now know that, excluding the secondary and traumatic forms, they are rare." Symptoms and findings leading to these erroneous diagnoses were due to tumors of the spinal cord. Elsberg underscored the tremendous advance from Gowers and Horsley's first diagnosis and successful removal of a spinal cord tumor in 1887 to his review in 1924.

In spite of the remarkable progress in spinal tumor surgery during the 37 years cited by Elsberg, it is notable and ironic that little progress[16] was made in the treatment of intramedullary tumors for 43 years after Elsberg's pioneering work, until Greenwood reported on a large series of patients who underwent the successful removal of intramedullary tumors.[12,13] Since then, the rapidly increasing sophistication of imaging and microsurgical techniques has allowed surgery to evolve into the definitive treatment modality for most intradural tumors.

Incidence

Intradural spinal cord tumors are categorized as intra- or extramedullary. They are uncommon (approximately 20 percent as common as cerebral tumors), with an incidence of from 3 to 10 per 100,000 population.[19,38] The ratio of intradural to extradural tumors is approximately 3 to 2. This discussion is primarily related to intradural tumors, including extramedullary and intramedullary tumors. The ratio of intramedullary to extramedullary tumors is somewhat higher in children (about 50 percent) than in adults (about 30 percent).[6,8,34] These tumors occur predominantly in the middle decades, and except for the unusually high incidence of meningiomas in females, the sex ratio is about equal. Because of the relative proportions of cord substance, the most common location is the thoracic region; the cervical region is the next most likely location, and the lumbosacral region the least likely. The ependymoma, besides being intramedullary, has a predilection for occurrence at the conus medullaris, where it may be both intra- and extramedullary, with an ectophytic component extending into the cauda equina. Dermoids, epidermoids, and teratomas are found in intra- and extramedullary locations.

The most common extramedullary-intradural tumors are the nerve sheath tumors, which constitute approximately 30 percent of spinal tumors, and the meningiomas, which constitute approximately 25 percent of tumors.[38] The most common intramedullary tumors, having about equal incidence, are the astrocytomas and ependymomas. A variety of other intramedullary tumors, including hemangioblastomas, dermoids, epidermoids, and mixed tumors, are common.

Ninety percent of all intradural spinal cord tumors are benign and potentially resectable.[31,36] Therefore, the outlook after surgical therapy is excellent. Similarly, severe defects due to spinal cord compression in relatively young individuals can be reversed by removing these tumors, with the expectation of improvement of neurological function.

Clinical Symptoms and Signs

In interpreting symptoms, the surgeon must consider certain factors, including (1) anatomic discrepancies between segmental levels of the spinal cord and of the vertebral bodies; (2) variations produced by a blood supply flowing predominantly to specific regions of the spinal cord, producing a watershed effect that may result in relative ischemia in other areas of the spinal cord distant from the primary lesion; (3) an anchoring of the spinal cord to its adjacent structures, which may produce unpredictable stresses within the cord structure, perhaps at some distance from the tumor; and (4) known anatomic features, such as the two- to three-level crossing of the anterolateral spinothalamic tract.

The spinal cord is shorter than the vertebral canal, which causes a discrepancy between spinal cord segments and their analogous vertebral bodies. This discrepancy increases caudally. For example, the C8 spinal cord level lies between vertebral bodies C6 and C7. The fourth thoracic segment of the spinal cord is opposite the third thoracic vertebra. The twelfth thoracic cord segment is opposite the T10–11 interspace, and the L5–S1 spinal cord segment lies opposite the L1 vertebral body. In searching for appropriate changes in the bone structure, the surgeon must consider these discrepancies.

The arterial blood supply to the spinal cord derives from different sources at different levels.[20] The anterior spinal artery is supplied predominantly by branches of the intracranial portions of the vertebral arteries, and it nourishes the upper cervical spinal cord, assisted by a major radicular artery at C6. In the thoracic region the major arterial supply is at T7, and in the lower spinal cord segments, the predominant supply is via the artery of Adamkiewicz, which may enter the cord anywhere from T9 to L2. Therefore, the intermediate areas of the spinal cord have a watershed blood supply; if the predominant arterial supply related to this watershed is compromised by tumor, the watershed area at some distance from the primary lesion will be the first to suffer. These vascular relationships may explain the necrosis of central areas of the spinal cord in the lower cervical region at some distance from tumors of the high cervical area.

The spinal cord is anchored to some extent by the dentate ligaments and the dorsal and ventral roots. Masses displacing the spinal cord produce stresses within the interior of the spinal cord that may be altered by these tethering structures.[17]

Fibers of the pain pathway mediated by the anterolateral spinothalamic tract take from two to three segments to cross before they enter the ascending tract. This has significance for neurological localization.

Irrespective of the location of tumors, symptoms precede the discovery of the tumor by an average of 2 years. Pain is an early symptom, regardless of whether the tumor is extra- or intramedullary.[21,22,27,28,30] The clinical syndrome depends primarily on the longitudinal rather than the coronal location of the tumor, that is, on whether the tumor is intra- or extramedullary, although there are a few classic discrepancies. In general, extramedullary tumors tend to be eccentric, lying to the side of the spinal cord either dorsally or ventrally. Therefore, the compressive effect is asymmetrical. This results in a higher incidence of a Brown-Sequard syndrome, in which the corticospinal tract and dorsal column functions are affected ipsilateral to the lesion while involvement of the ipsilateral spinothalamic tract, which contains crossed fibers, produces contralateral abnormalities of pain and temperature sensation. Conversely, because of the topographic arrangement of the spinothalamic tract, intramedullary tumors are associated with a relative sparing of the lumbosacral pain- and temperature-conducting fibers, which are located more externally. This is a theoretical consideration, and although sacral sparing would be expected with intramedullary tumors, this is not always the case.

Most spinal cord tumors produce symptoms and signs with a combination of local or segmental and distant features. Segmental involvement of the dorsal root entry zone or the anterior horn cells and roots results in specific sensory and lower motor neuron defects. Distant features are related to involvement of the longitudinally oriented ascending and descending tracts, which interrupt function below the level of the tumor. In the corticospinal tract, this results in upper motor neuron defects; in the spinothalamic tract, a decrease in pain and temperature sensation; and in the dorsal columns, a decrease in position and vibratory sensation. Involvement of the descending autonomic pathways, which are located between the corticospinal and spinothalamic tracts, results in both sympathetic and parasympathetic disturbances below the level of the lesion. This is most important when the lesion affects function bilaterally and thereby impairs respiratory, bowel, bladder, and sexual function. The volume of the tumor in longitudinal and transverse orientation dictates, to some extent, the degree of involvement of these systems. However, the clinical presentation can be variable and seemingly inconsistent. Theoretically, other factors, such as age, vascular distribution, relative size of the spinal column, and tethering structures, may modify the clinical course. The surgeon is always amazed to find large tumors, either intrinsic or extrinsic, with severe spinal cord compression that produce very few abnormalities.

Specific syndromes related to the rostrocaudal site of the tumor can be identified. Lesions of the upper cervical spine or foramen magnum region produce a unique syndrome characterized by (1) a disproportionate loss of position and vibration sense in the upper, compared with the lower, extremities, and (2) atrophy of the intrinsic muscles of the hands.[42] This finding has been a topic of speculation. It has been suggested that compromise of the arterial blood supply to the spinal cord results in central necrosis of the anterior gray matter at C8–T1. This suggestion is inconsistent with the pattern of blood supply to the cervical spinal cord. Similarly, pressure on the central canal at the high cervical level has been incriminated, and the hypothesis has been forwarded that a central hydromyelia or cystic degeneration is created at lower levels. Perhaps the most attractive hypothesis is the interruption of the venous channels by the high cervical lesion, with venous infarction and central necrosis at lower levels.[44] Involvement of the dorsal roots of C2 results in both pain and sensory loss over the occipital region. Nystagmus has been attributed to pressure on the sulcomarginal fibers, which are an extension of the medial longitudinal fasciculus. Involvement of the other pathways of the spinal cord eventually leads to a host of neurological abnormalities below the level of the lesion.

Involvement of the middle and lower cervical regions by intramedullary tumors produces a suspended, capelike sensory loss with pain that involves the upper extremities, most often the shoulders or fingers. Horner's syndrome may be seen unilaterally or bilaterally, depending on the degree of involvement of the sympathetic system.

Involvement of the upper thoracic region evokes pain in a girdle-type distribution, sometimes mistaken for angina pectoris, coronary thrombosis, or pleurisy. Similarly, in the middle and lower thoracic regions, pain may wrongly suggest an abdominal lesion.

Tumors at the lumbosacral or conus medullaris regions of the spinal cord affect the parasympathetic innervation of the bladder, bowel, and sexual organs. The ensuing symptoms and signs, including enuresis and disturbances in sexual capacity, may precede other overt neurological abnormalities by many months or years. These are often misdiagnosed as psychological problems, as cystocele in women of child-bearing age, and as prostatic disease in men. Involvement of the lumbosacral interface may lead to the fascinating neurological picture of upper motor neuron deficits in the sacral myotomes and lower motor neuron deficits in the affected lumbar myotomes.

Tumors of the cauda equina may selectively impair the function of a single dorsal root for many months. This leads to persistent, discrete dermatomal appreciation of pain, which may be mistaken for disc prolapse or psychological symptoms.

Although it may seem reasonable to assume that intramedullary and extramedullary tumors produce different syndromes in practical experience it is often difficult to differentiate these two conditions on clinical grounds alone.

In the adolescent child the clinical syndromes are often similar to those of the adult. In the younger child, tumors frequently present as extremity weakness or growth deformities and are first recognized by the orthopedic surgeon who sees the child for kyphoscoliosis. This is especially common with extensive intramedullary astrocytomas. Beside deformities of the spine, gait abnormalities or deformities of the feet, such as talipes equinovarus or pes cavus, may be witnessed in the young child. Enuresis in the previously toilet-trained child is another symptom of a caudal tumor.[6,34] Although rare, congenital tumors, such as the teratomas, dermoids, and epidermoids, have a higher incidence in children than in adults; there may be associated abnormalities, such as a sinus tract or a hairy or pigmented cutaneous lesion.

Pathology

Nerve sheath tumors usually arise from the dorsal roots at the various segmental levels of the spinal cord. They are relatively avascular, globoid, and without calcification. The nerve root is intimately involved in the tumor's matrix and can rarely be spared in the surgical removal of the tumor (Fig. 175-1). When associated with von Recklinghausen's disease, the tumors are multiple, occurring at numerous levels of the spinal canal in various stages of growth (Fig. 175-2). The protein content of the spinal fluid is often elevated beyond a range ascribable to CSF block. In the region of the cauda equina, these tumors may have some degree of mobility because of the elasticity of the parent nerve root. Only when these tumors have a dumbbell configuration, following the nerve root through the dural sleeve into the extradural space, do they have an attachment to and blood supply from the dura. In the dumbbell nerve sheath tumor, the size of the extradural mass may exceed that of the intradural mass. This may result in a large soft tissue mass visible on chest or abdominal x-ray films or a mass palpable in the cervical region.

Rare instances have been described of a wholly intramedullary nerve sheath tumor, presumably arising from aberrant nerve roots, with growth predominantly into the spinal cord.[24] These tend to be museum cases; however, it is important to recognize their possibility because they are eminently resectable, unlike some of the other intramedullary tumors.

Seventy-five to 85 percent of meningiomas occur in women, and about 80 percent are thoracic.[21,27] They may arise in any age group, but most occur between the 5th and 7th decades of life. They presumably arise from arachnoid cluster cells and therefore are located at the exit zones of nerve roots or the entry zones of arteries into the spinal canal. They are often lateral or ventrolateral (uncommonly dorsal) to the spinal cord (Fig. 175-3). The growth of a foramen magnum meningioma is intimate to the entry of the vertebral artery into the subarachnoid space. Meningiomas caudal to the level of the conus medullaris are rare. In spite of their relationship to root entry and exit zones, they can often be separated from the nerve roots and do not have the same intimate relationship to these roots that nerve sheath tumors have.

Nearly one-half of all central nervous system (CNS) ependymomas arise within the spinal canal.[38] Most are intramedullary,

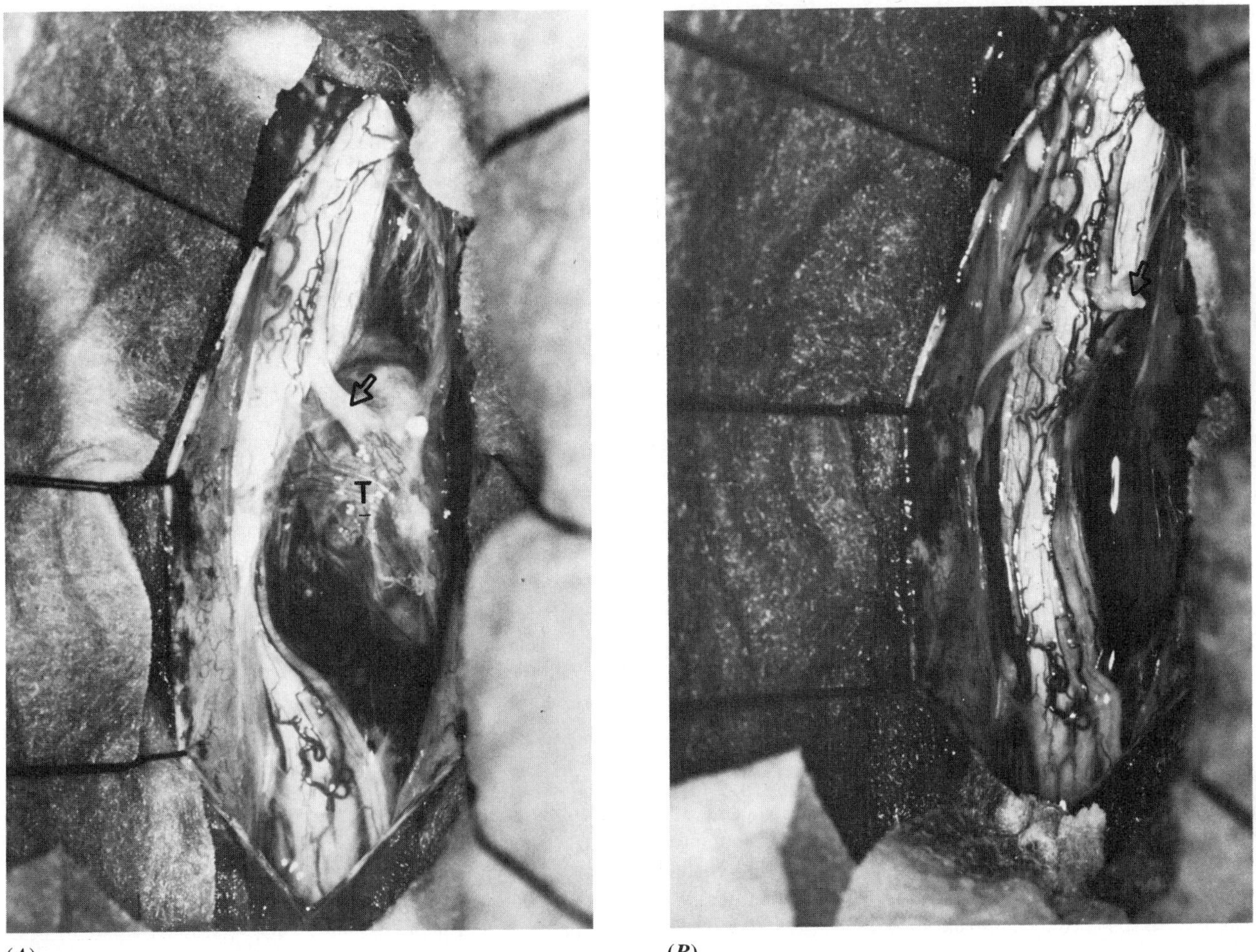

(*A*) (*B*)

Figure 175-1 *A.* Operative photograph showing a discrete neurofibroma (T) lateral to the thoracic cord. The parent nerve root is indicated by an arrow. *B.* Operative photograph after removal of the neurofibroma showing the cut end of the sacrificed nerve root (*arrow*).

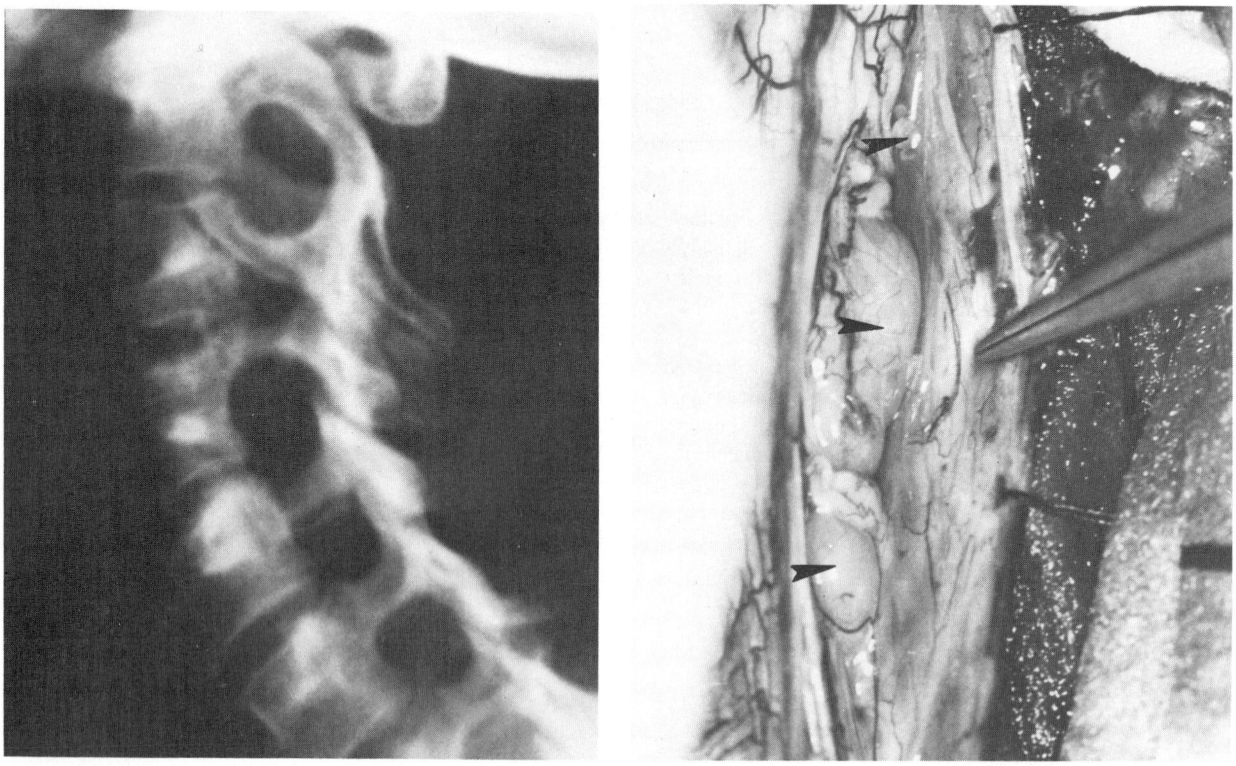

(*A*) (*B*)

Figure 175-2 *A.* Lateral x-ray film of the cervical spine showing multiple enlargements of the neural foramina. *B.* Operative photograph showing multiple neurofibromas (*arrowheads*) in a case of von Recklinghausen's disease.

but about 40 percent arise from the filum terminale. They occur throughout the spinal cord, although most series report a cervical or cervicothoracic predominance.[9,30] In the conus region, the tumor may be partially intramedullary and partially exophytic. Rarely, an intramedullary ependymoma may extend through a root entry zone to present with an exophytic component. These tumors are rarely malignant and are often associated with intramedullary cysts containing fluid of high protein content. Rarely, when the tumor is malignant, it may seed throughout the spinal and cranial axes. In cases of exophytic components of this tumor, the protein content of the CSF is disproportionately elevated and has been associated with papilledema.[2] These tumors are well circumscribed and relatively avascular. When involving the filum terminale—presumably arising from the ependyma of the central canal—they may be mobile and change position during surgery (Fig. 175-4). This accentuated mobility may make differentiation from a nerve sheath tumor difficult. Grossly at operation it may also be hard to distinguish a nerve sheath tumor attached to a nerve root of the cauda equina from a globoid ependymoma attached to a thin filum.

The astrocytoma is invariably intramedullary, relatively avascular, usually distinguishable from neural tissue in color and contour, and soft without calcification. In adults, approximately 50 percent of astrocytomas have a well-defined plane between tumor and neural tissue and often are associated with cysts; accordingly, they can be resected.[28] In other instances, the plane between the tumor and the spinal cord may be indistinguishable around most of the tumor; however, the characteristic features of the tumor may allow it to be gutted without injuring the surrounding spinal cord. This is frequently feasible in the case of benign intramedullary astrocytoma of childhood.[8] About 20 percent of intramedullary astrocytomas are malignant—grades III or IV. Their growth is rapid, the color and contour differences between neural tissue and tumor are absent, and the tumor has a propensity for seeding the spinal and sometimes the intracranial subarachnoid spaces.[4] Interestingly, the low-grade astrocytomas, although extensive, do not often violate the junction between the spinal cord and the brain stem. The sister tumor within the cerebral hemisphere is similar in growth, histologic features, and anatomical division between tumor and neural tissue.

Uncommon intradural tumors include the dermoids, epidermoids, lipomas, and teratomas. The rare teratomas are intramedullary. The dermoid and epidermoid tumors occur both in an intramedullary location and in the region of the cauda equina. In the latter instances, an epidermoid tumor has been attributed to one or more preceding lumbar punctures presumably carrying cutaneous tissue into the spinal canal. The capsule of these tumors creates a reaction in the surrounding neural tissue that may thwart total removal of the capsule and contents. Nevertheless, these tumors are slow-growing, avascular, encapsulated, and usually resectable. Experience indicates that residual diaphanous portions of the capsule apparently remain static or grow at such a slow rate that cures have been recorded for a decade or more. Lipomas are not true neoplasms but probably arise from inclusion of normal mesenchymal tissue.[23,45] These lesions generally enlarge and produce symptoms in early and middle adult years through increased fat deposition in these metabolically normal fat cells. Total removal of these subpial lesions are not possible because their margins are densely adherent to the surrounding functional spinal cord tissue. In general, a longitudinal pial incision over the extent of the lesion and conservative subtotal internal decompression are sufficient to provide long-term symptom control.

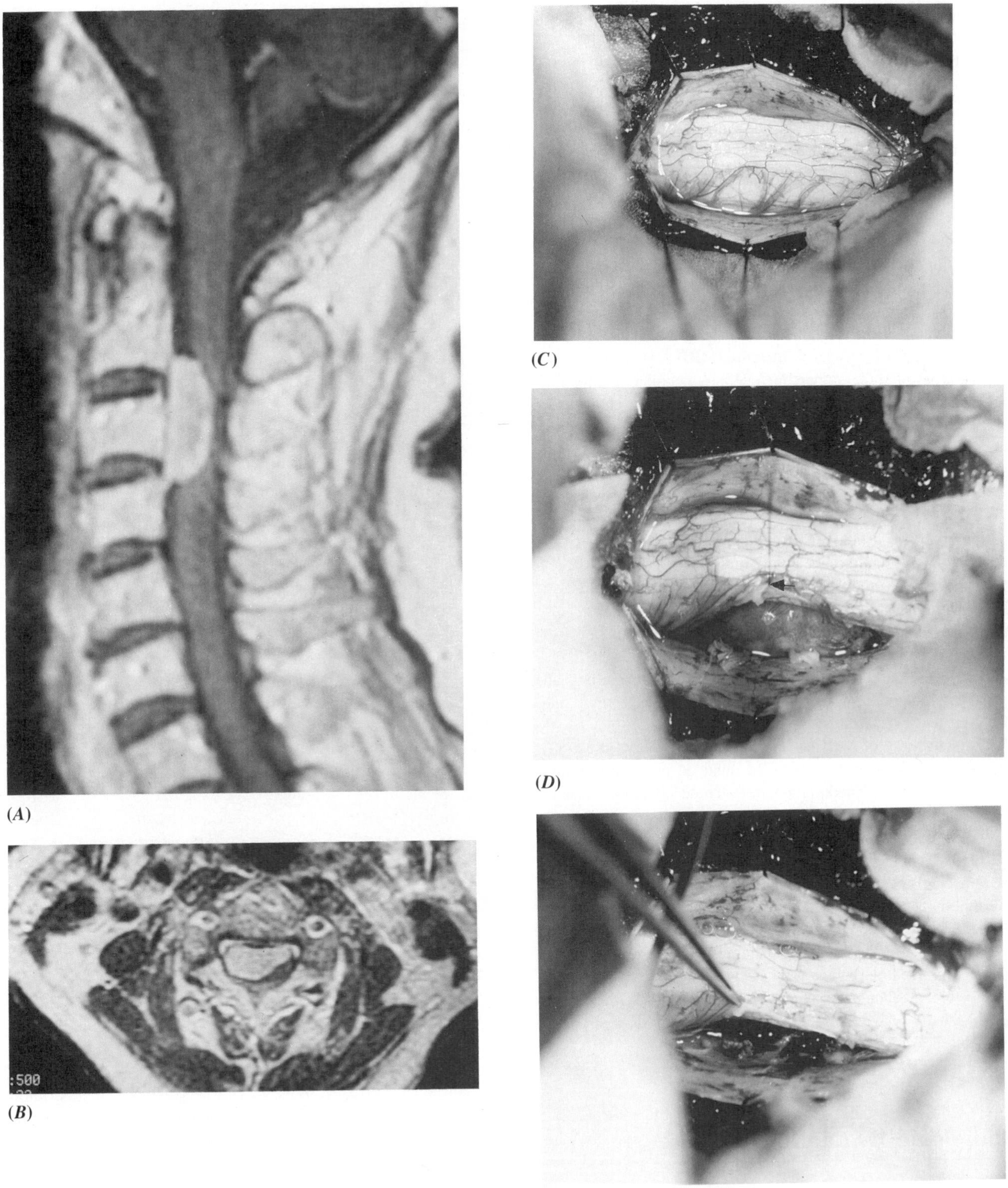

(E)

Figure 175-3 T1-weighted gadolinium-enhanced sagittal (*A*) and axial (*B*) MRI demonstrates a uniformly enhancing broad-based ventral meningioma of the upper cervical spine. *C.* The tumor is not visible following initial exposure via laminectomy. The spinal cord is splayed over the ventral mass. *D.* The ventral tumor is now visualized following dorsal root division. Suture retraction on a divided dentate ligament (*arrow*) further assists visualization of the ventral tumor. *E.* Operative photograph following gross total tumor removal.

Hemangioblastomas may occur as solitary tumors or as part of the broader spectrum of the von Hippel-Lindau syndrome.[3,14,32] They most commonly involve the cervical or thoracic region. Their vascularity varies; however, they are the most vascular variety of intradural tumor. They may be wholly intramedullary, but most frequently they gain the dorsal surface of the spinal cord and are visible upon initial exposure of the involved area (Fig. 175-5). They are discrete and well circumscribed, and they rarely involve more than one or two segments of the spinal cord. They are often associated with cysts that may extend some distance from the body of the tumor. These tumors are benign and are amenable to surgical resection. In several cases, we have witnessed an unexplained widening of the spinal cord below the level of the lesion without an associated cyst or another hemangioblastoma.[39] Following the total removal of the tumor, this widening regressed, as shown on follow-up magnetic resonance imaging (MRI).

Rare types of spinal tumors include intramedullary carcinomatous metastases, mixed tumors that include malignant elements of a variety of tumors, and neurenteric cysts, which often compress the cord from a symmetrical ventral location and mimic an intramedullary tumor upon initial exploration of the spinal cord.[1,29,43] These latter tumors are very rare and are discussed elsewhere in this textbook.

Nontumorous pathology should also be included in the differential diagnosis of an intramedullary mass lesion. Vascular pathology, such as a cavernous malformation or venous aneurysm associated with an arteriovenous malformation, may occasionally present as an intramedullary mass.[26] Although inflammatory or infectious spinal cord involvement generally produces acute transverse myelitis, certain conditions, such as an intramedullary abscess, tuberculoma, sarcoidosis, or parasitic involvement, may rarely present as a mass lesion.[29]

The sensitivity of MRI has allowed inflammatory, infectious, and paraneoplastic syndromes to be included in the differential diagnosis of an intramedullary tumor. These conditions usually produce an acute transverse myelitis that progresses rapidly over several hours to a few days. MRI exquisitely images these lesions, and the surgeon often is asked to evaluate for biopsy. The MRI appearance of these lesions can be variable and ranges from focal uniform enhancement to patchy irregular enhancement over long segments of the cord (Fig. 175-6). There is minimal, if any, spinal cord enlargement, which further distinguishes these lesions from a surgical intramedullary mass. In these patients, operative intervention for biopsy should be undertaken with caution, since biopsy results usually reveal nonspecific information that does not assist in diagnosis or treatment.

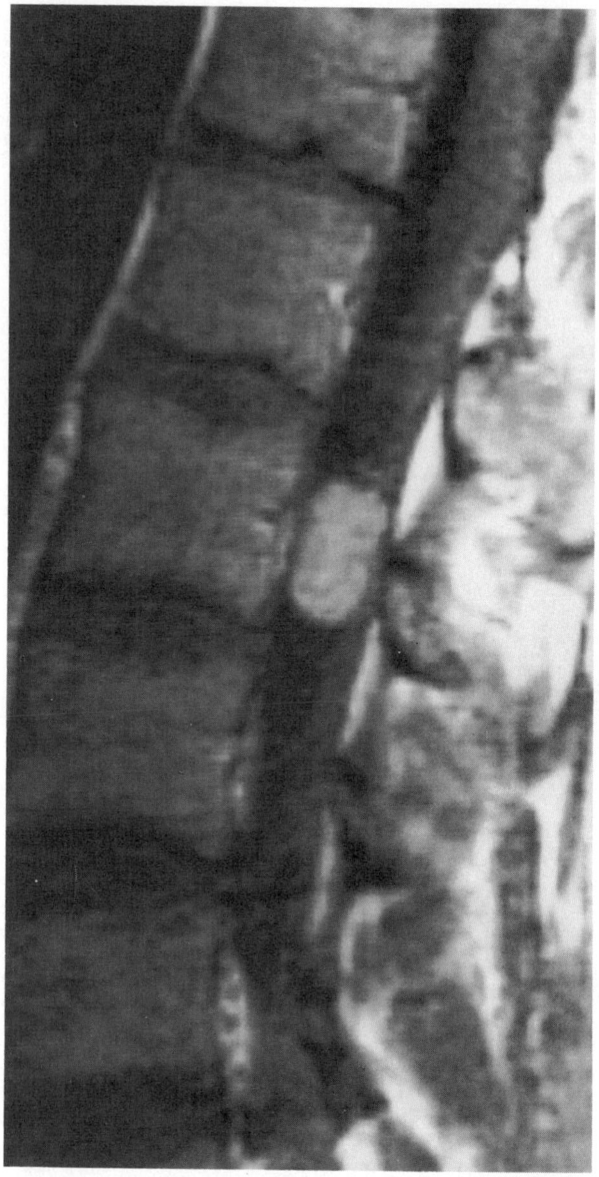

(*A*)

Figure 175-4 *A.* T1-weighted gadolinium-enhanced sagittal MRI demonstrates a well-circumscribed, homogeneously enhancing mass at the level of the filum terminale and cauda equina.

Radiologic Evaluation

The radiologic evaluation of nearly all intradural lesions is performed with MRI. Gadolinium-enhanced images sensitively identify even small intradural mass lesions. Most intradural tumors are isointense or slightly hypointense with respect to the spinal cord and cauda equina or T1-weighted images. Intramedullary lesions can be easily overlooked on noncontrasted T1-weighted images if only subtle spinal cord widening is present. Most intradural tumors exhibit some degree of contrast enhancement (Fig. 175-7). Meningiomas and ependymomas usually demonstrate uniform contrast enhancement, but heterogeneous enhancement can be seen with some frequency, especially with ependymomas. Heterogenous enhancement is frequently seen with nerve sheath tumors. Intramedullary cysts are commonly seen as polar cysts in association with intramedullary tumors and may extend over several cord segments (Fig. 175-7*C*). In the absence of an associated Chiari malformation or previous history of trauma, an underlying tumor should be suspected when an isolated syrinx is identified on a noncontrasted MRI. In these cases, a gadolinium-enhanced study of the entire spinal cord is indicated. Postoperative MRI also allows sensitive periodic surveillance of tumor recurrence. This provides an objective parameter by which to gauge efficacy of treatment, which is particularly important in defining operative treatment of intramedullary astrocytomas.

Myelography and postmyelographic computed tomography (CT) is rarely utilized in the evaluation of intradural pathology. Nevertheless, spatial resolution of postmyelography CT remains superior to MRI, and this study may provide useful information in

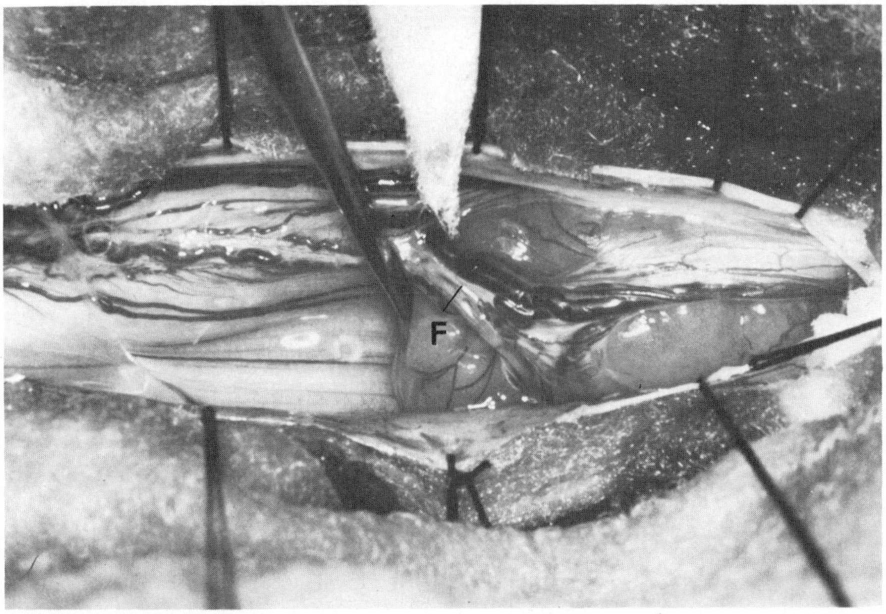

(*B*)

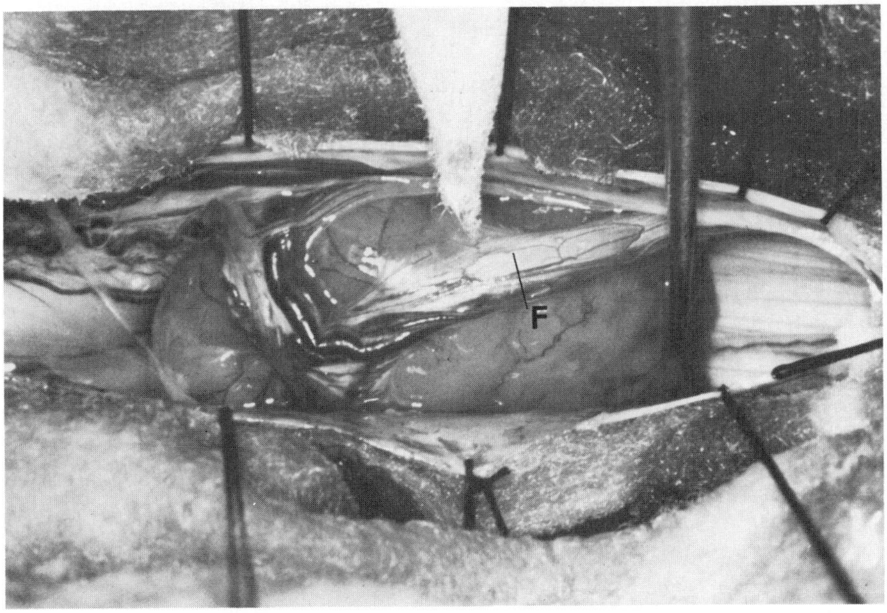

(*C*)

Figure 175-4 (*Continued*) *B.* and *C.* Operative photographs showing an ependymoma of the filum (F). The white cottonoid marker remains static in position, demonstrating the mobility of this tumor. *B.* Tumor displaced caudally. *C.* Tumor displaced rostrally.

some cases. Questionable intradural involvement of a paraspinal tumor is one such instance. An unnecessary intradural exploration would be avoided if postmyelography CT reveals no intradural extension.

Surgical Considerations

Although the clinical picture is important in suggesting a spinal tumor and assisting in the localization of the process, the radiographic diagnosis is the key to preparing for surgery. Armed with clinical and radiographic information, the surgeon can design exposures that minimize the removal of bone and maximize the potential for removal of the benign tumors afflicting the spinal cord. Generally, the earlier the recognition of the problem at a time of minor neurological deficit, the better are the prognosis and surgical result. Patients who are neurologically devastated—especially older people—are unlikely to experience satisfactory resolution of neurological defects.

The patient is prepared for surgery by steroid medication and by a medical evaluation to identify any coagulation deficiencies or pulmonary problems, especially in association with cervical tumors, which may cause additional respiratory problems postoperatively. Many of these patients have taken aspirin or other platelet-inhibiting medications to relieve their pain and do not inform the

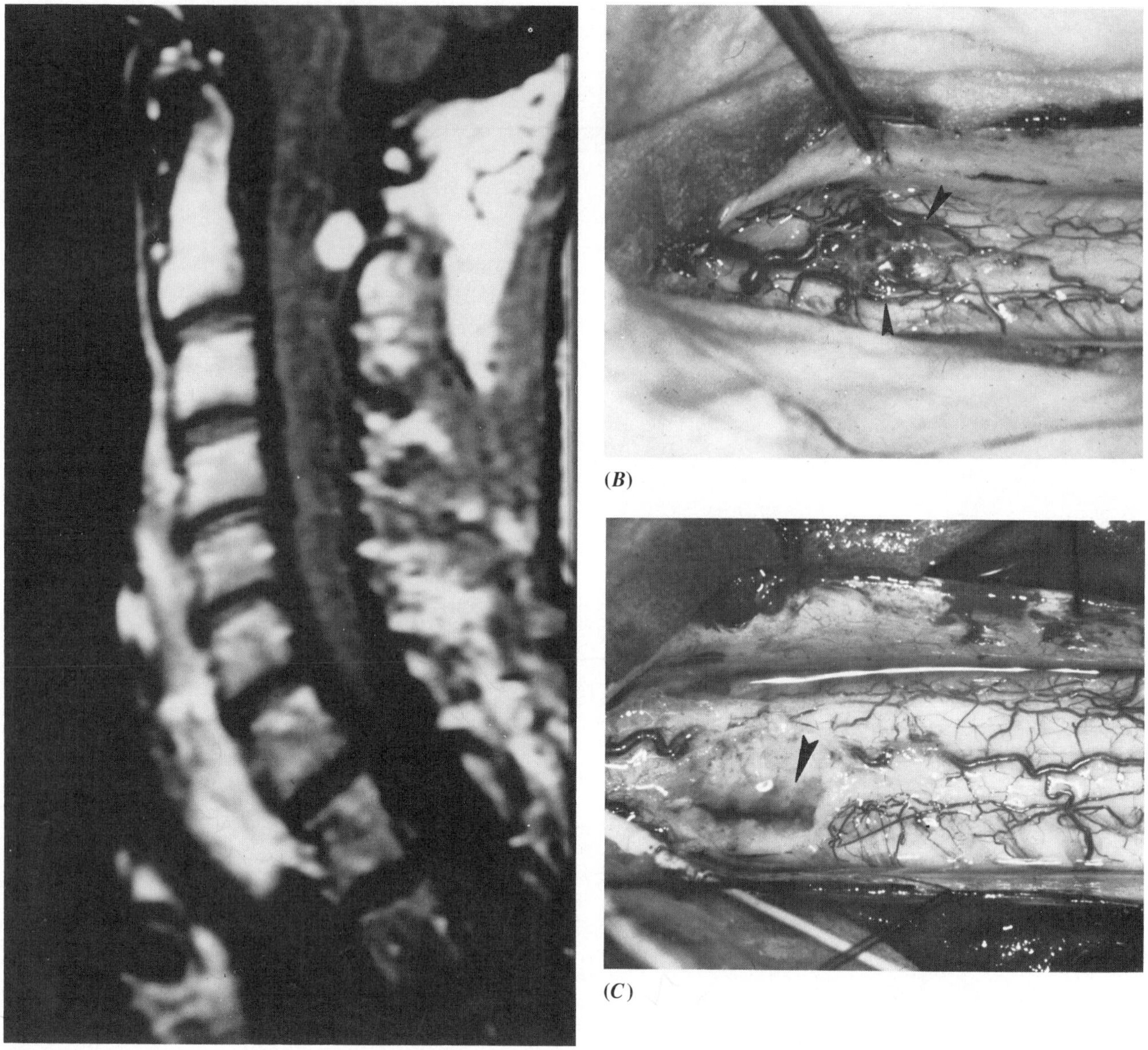

(*B*)

(*C*)

(*A*)

Figure 175-5 *A.* T1-weighted gadolinium-enhanced sagittal MRI shows a small, intensely enhancing intramedullary hemangioblastoma located in the spinal cord at the C2 level. Note the significant spinal cord enlargement above and below the small tumor mass. *B.* Operative photograph showing a cervical hemangioblastoma (*arrowheads*), intramedullary but with a portion reaching the surface. *C.* Operative photograph following tumor removal. A small cyst is marked by an arrowhead. The widening of the cervical cord below the level of the tumor remains unexplained.

physician of these circumstances before the operation. Such medications may create problems with hemostasis.

The surgeon discusses the operation in detail with the patient and family, emphasizing that these tumors often occupy a high percentage of the spinal space, severely compressing spinal cord tissue, and that the patient's symptoms and signs may not truly reflect the huge extent of the tumor. The implication is that any additional injury or compression to the spinal cord may lead to a neurological disaster during or immediately after the operation. Patients with cervical tumors should be warned that it may be necessary to maintain intubation for 24 to 48 h postoperatively to ensure an adequate airway. Furthermore, because flexion of the head on the cervical spine is necessary for operations involving the cervical region, a preoperative test should be done with the patient awake to see if the flexion is tolerated. The area to be operated on is kept relatively high above the heart to maximize venous drainage and prevent any congestion around the area of the surgery. A free abdomen or chest and excellent ventilation are absolutely essential. A midline incision is utilized, and a relatively wide laminectomy sparing the intervertebral articulations is carried out.

Because of the confined nature of the spinal canal and the size of tumors relative to the diameter of the spinal cord, the use of the operating microscope is advisable. The prone position is preferred because it maximizes the use of the surgical assistant working, via the binocular sidearm of the microscope, face to face with the operating surgeon. Some surgeons prefer the sitting position for tumors located in the cervical or upper thoracic region; however, this position makes it almost impossible to use the assistant effectively. The spinal exposure should encompass the area of the pathologic process, leaving a modest amount of space at the rostral and caudal margins to prepare for mobilization of the tumor. In children, laminoplasty may reduce the incidence of postoperative deformity.[33] Spinal stability is always an important consideration in operations on these tumors, especially those that are more extensive in the rostrocaudal dimension. In adults, laminotomy is not a practical consideration and laminectomy is always performed. If the tumor is intradural but extramedullary, the laminectomy must be wide on the ipsilateral side and may include the joint facets and the intervertebral foramen, especially in the case of a dumbbell nerve sheath tumor. While bone and ligaments are preserved whenever possible, nerve roots and radicular arteries must also be preserved when feasible in the removal of even the largest tumors. The dorsal roots, which often are impediments to tumor removal, may be sacrificed over a number of segments in the thoracic

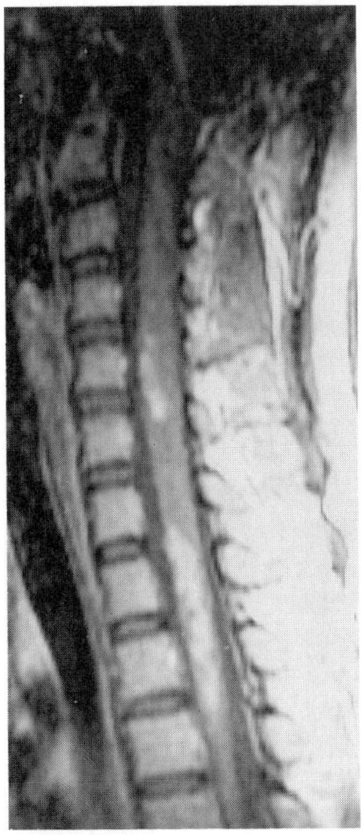

(*A*)

Figure 175-6 T1-weighted gadolinium-enhanced sagittal MRI in a woman with the acute onset of back pain and rapidly progressive neurological deficit shows irregular patchy enhancement over several spinal cord segments. The acute clinical onset and lack of significant spinal cord enlargement establish this as a transverse myelitis rather than a surgical lesion.

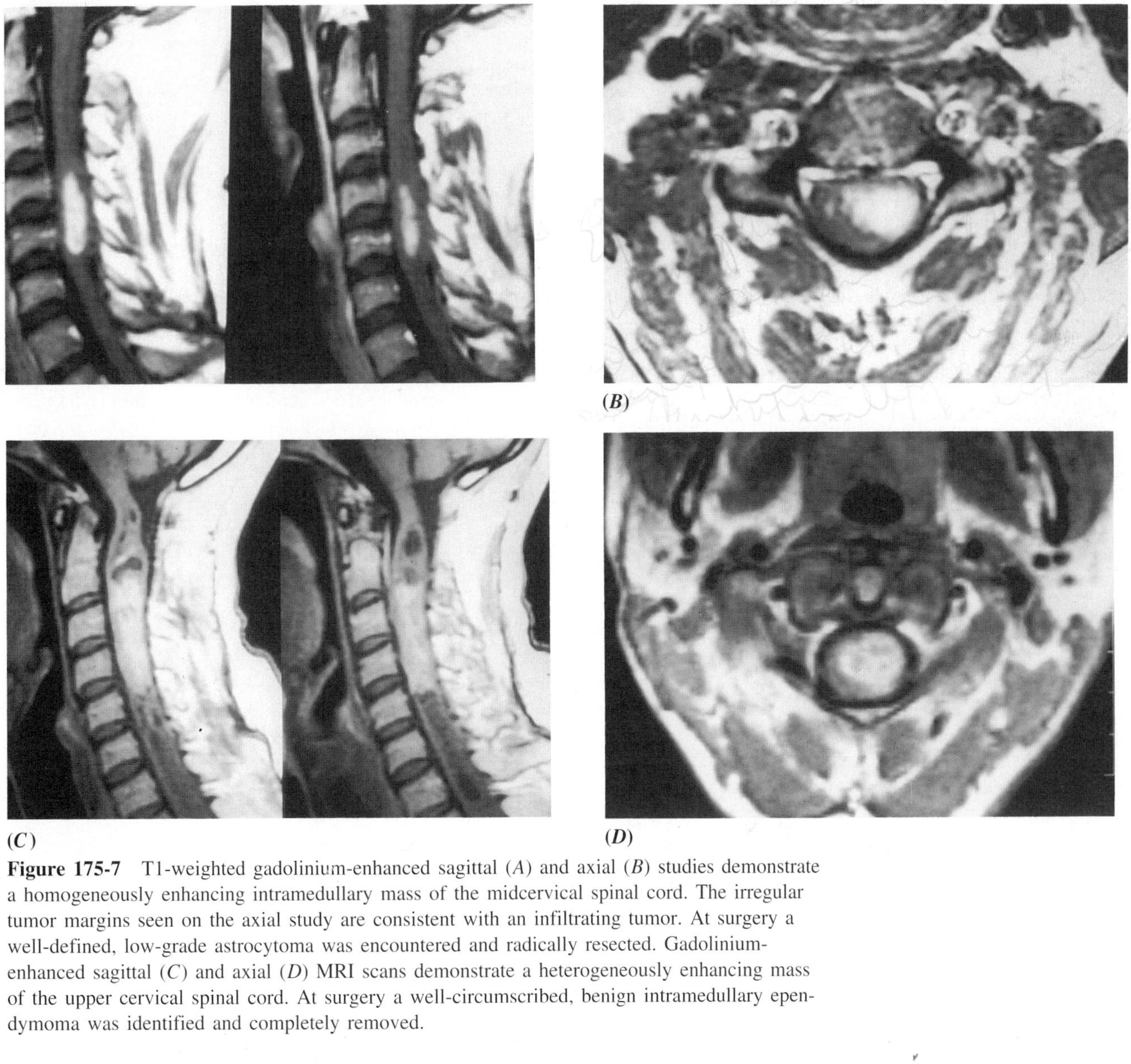

(*B*)

(*C*) (*D*)

Figure 175-7 T1-weighted gadolinium-enhanced sagittal (*A*) and axial (*B*) studies demonstrate a homogeneously enhancing intramedullary mass of the midcervical spinal cord. The irregular tumor margins seen on the axial study are consistent with an infiltrating tumor. At surgery a well-defined, low-grade astrocytoma was encountered and radically resected. Gadolinium-enhanced sagittal (*C*) and axial (*D*) MRI scans demonstrate a heterogeneously enhancing mass of the upper cervical spinal cord. At surgery a well-circumscribed, benign intramedullary ependymoma was identified and completely removed.

region; however, the surgeon should attempt to preserve the dorsal roots in the midcervical region whenever possible.

In the case of extramedullary-intradural tumors, surgical principles employed elsewhere for benign tumors also apply to the spinal region. One should create traction only on the lesion, not on the neural tissue. In larger tumors this may be accomplished by an intracapsular decompression before the tumor is removed, to spare nerve roots and other vital structures. For these tumors a CUSA unit (Cavitron ultrasonic surgical aspirator; Cooper Medical, Stamford, CT) is most beneficial because it creates a rapid debulking without displacing neural or tumor tissue. The surgeon is advised to seek out the vascular supply, no matter how minimal, before debulking or finally removing the tumor to keep the operative field relatively free of blood. This assists in the removal of the tumor because the anatomic and color planes between the tumor and neural tissue are maintained in a virgin state, without staining of the tissues by blood.

In extramedullary tumors located ventral or ventrolateral to the spinal cord, a wide laminectomy with transverse cutting of the dura facilitates undercutting and debulking of the tumor and permits the surgeon to maneuver it out from under the critical ventral area of the spinal cord. In most instances, meningiomas and nerve sheath tumors receive little blood from the spinal cord and are attached by few adhesions to the spinal cord. The foramen magnum meningioma often encases or envelopes the vertebral artery; great care must be taken not to injure this structure. When the tumor extends above the foramen magnum, it often incorporates the 12th cranial nerve, and it may be impossible to remove the tumor without sacrificing this nerve.

In surgery for conus medullaris and cauda equina tumors—especially ependymomas, which occur both in and out of the spinal cord—first the exophytic portion of the tumor is removed, and then the intramedullary portion may be separable from the conus medullaris region. The tumor often is situated like a cork in a bottle, coming away from a cystic extension within the conus medullaris region of the spinal cord with relative ease. In removing an ependymoma of the filum terminale, it is often necessary to remove the latter as well (without consequent neurological deficit). A nerve sheath tumor of the cauda equina is easily removed, usually with sacrifice of a single dorsal root (with no consequence).

Dermoid and epidermoid tumors in the cauda equina region present a unique problem. The surgeon must be careful not to spill the noxious contents of these tumors into the subarachnoid space because this will cause arachnoiditis and adhesions around the conus, leading to distressing postoperative pain and neurological deficits. Therefore, these tumors must be carefully debulked, and a persistent, careful attempt made to remove the capsule from the surrounding nerve roots. This may present difficulties, and it may be necessary to leave diaphanous portions of the capsule adherent to the roots so as not to sacrifice them. The result should be good.

Dumbbell tumors with significant extension into the paraspinal region may require complex spinal exposure. Although two-stage operations may be performed to manage separately the intraspinal and paraspinal tumor components, a single-stage procedure is preferable. For cervical tumors, the vertebral artery is an additional consideration. Most cervical dumbbell tumors can be adequately accessed through a standard laminectomy and complete unilateral facetectomy. This allows for paraspinal access up to 3 cm from the lateral dural margin. A second-stage anterior procedure may be required if further tumor extension is present. The vertebral artery is displaced anteromedially by these tumors, and an intervening layer of periosteum and venous plexus serves as an effective dissection plane and protects the artery from injury. Contralateral facet fusion prevents delayed instability. In the thoracic and lumbar spine, the lateral extracavitary approach provides extensive intraspinal exposure through a single "hockey stick" incision.[25] The peritoneal and pleural cavity are avoided, which diminishes the risk of a CSF fistula.

The removal of intramedullary tumors has evolved over many decades (Fig. 175-8).[8–10,15,23,40,41] These tumors tend to be avascular and in a majority of instances can be totally removed, resulting in a cure. The exposure must encompass the entire extent of the intramedullary process, whether it be cystic or solid. In most instances the tumor spans a number of segments. The dura will be tense because of underlying compression by the tumor and should be opened at either end of the tumor. At the caudal end, the surgeon is more apt to encounter dilated veins, therefore, it may be safer to open the dura from the rostral end. Once the entire area of spinal cord widening has been exposed, the surgeon must select a site for myelotomy. In a minority of instances, the intramedullary tumor will be visible through the translucent dorsal or dorsolateral portion of the spinal cord. However, in most instances, the tumor lies beneath the surface so that it is not readily visible.

A myelotomy should be carried out as close to the midline as possible. The incision must be straight and parallel to the longitudinal plane of the spinal cord. With the ladder-like arrangement of arteries and veins that occurs over the dorsal surface of the spinal cord, it will be necessary to interrupt a number of small vascular channels. This is accomplished with a bipolar cautery set at low level and used under irrigation; the myelotomy is then made by a sharp dissection. The myelotomy should be carried over the entire extent of widening of the spinal cord, so that any planes between the tumor and the spinal cord are not missed. Once this has been performed, the pial margins are held back with fine sutures under tension, to open the cord as one would open a book. If the myelotomy has been extensive, a plane between the tumor and the spinal cord is readily visible. This is further developed by gentle use of dissectors, bipolar cautery, and cottonoids. If the surgeon is fortunate enough to encounter a cyst at one or both ends of the tumor, this significantly facilitates the removal of the tumor. It often may not be necessary to debulk the interior of the tumor to effect a total removal. In debulking the tumor's interior, care must be taken not to allow any bleeding, which spills over and obscures the plane between the external surface of the tumor and the spinal cord. It is essential that this area be kept dry, so that the surgeon can carefully follow the contour and coloration provided by the margin of a resectable tumor. Combining these maneuvers allows the surgeon to remove the tumor expeditiously.

In the astrocytoma there may be a plane that encompasses most of the tumor but in some places tends to face into the surrounding spinal cord. The surgeon must use judgment to define where this plane is or should be, and removal is carried out radically. Removal should continue as long as the surgeon can clearly differentiate the tumor from the surrounding spinal cord. Because a clear correlation between radical removal and clinical tumor control has not been established for benign astrocytomas, preservation of neurological function is the treatment priority for these frequently indolent tumors.

For intramedullary dermoid tumors, it may be impossible to remove every filament of the fine tumor capsule; the surgeon should attempt the most radical removal possible without injuring the surrounding spinal cord tissue. Recently we used sensory evoked potential monitoring during radical tumor removal. The potentials are recorded from the spinal cord above the site of operation and from the cortex. The usefulness of this procedure is yet to be determined. It appears to signal when cord function is

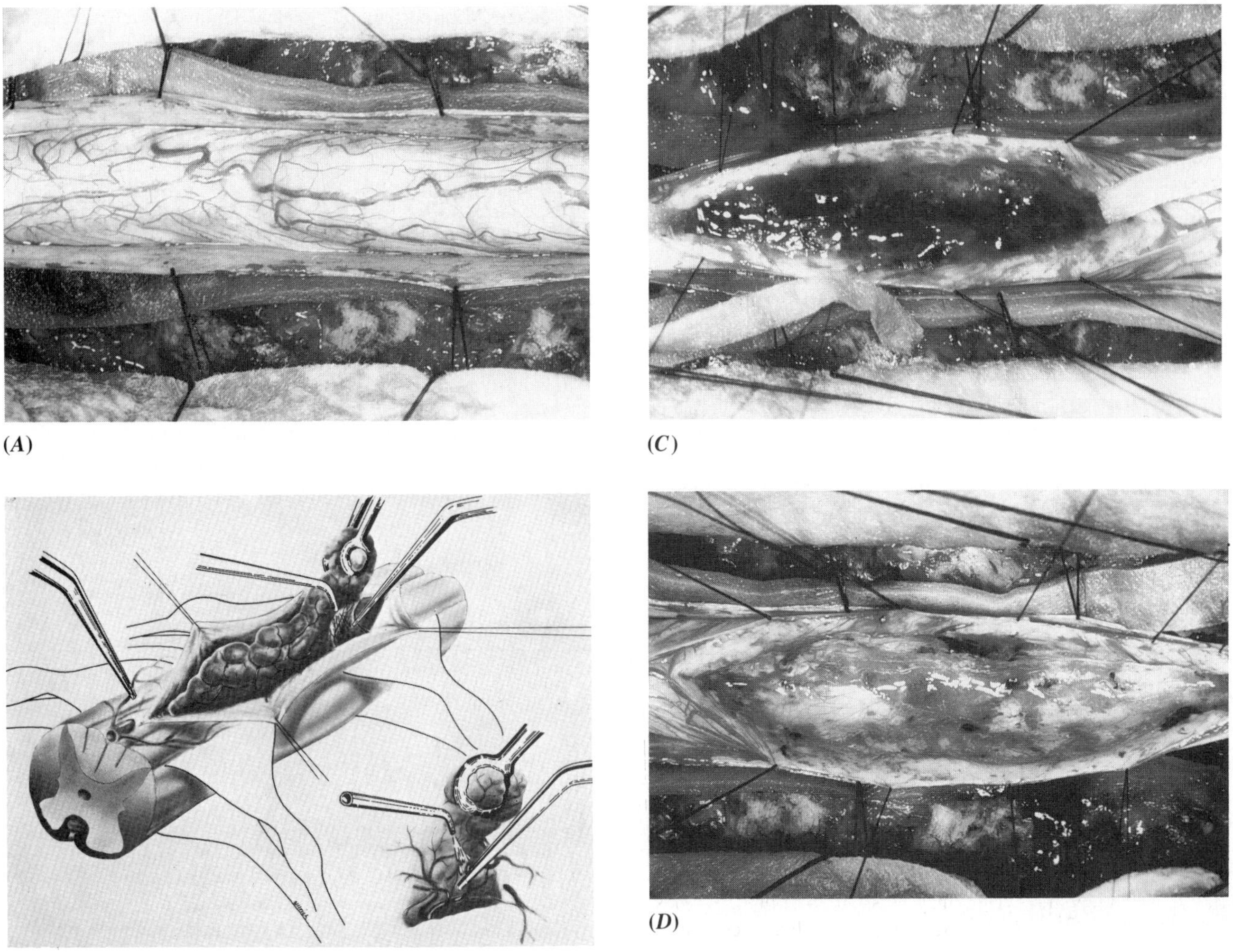

(*A*) (*C*) (*D*) (*B*)

Figure 175-8 *A*. Operative photograph of a widened cervical cord caused by an intramedullary ependymoma. *B*. A drawing showing the steps in the removal of an intramedullary tumor, including bipolar cautery under irrigation. *C*. Intraoperative photograph following midline myelotomy with initial exposure of the dorsal tumor surface. Note the glistening tumor surface and clear demarcation from the surrounding spinal cord, which are typical of an intramedullary ependymoma. *D*. Operative photograph of the resection bed following complete tumor removal.

affected during removal of the tumor. However, if the surgeon is carefully dissecting with the microscope, it may be necessary to give up at this point because the loss of potentials appears to be occasionally reversible.

For an intramedullary hemangioblastoma, the tumor area is exposed by appropriate laminectomy and dural opening; care is taken not to injure any of the vasculature. The arterial supply to the tumor, which is easily recognized, is interrupted first; this is similar to the technique used to remove an arteriovenous malformation from either the spinal cord or the brain. After a myelotomy directed rostrally and caudally in the midline a short distance from the tumor, a bipolar cautery is used to caress the margin of the tumor, around which a circumscribing incision is made. Gradually the vascular adhesions to the tumor are interrupted, preserving a large, easily visible draining vein until the final removal of the tumor, which is swung out on this venous pedicle that is then cauterized and divided between clips. Any associated cysts are drained in the process.

At the completion of the removal of an intramedullary tumor, we have found no need to appose the pial margins of the opened spinal cord. They are released and tend to collapse together. We have not observed the development of cysts under tension within the spinal cord following these resections.

After a spinal tumor is removed, the dura is closed or a dural substitute (preferably autologous fascia) is used to close the opening. In patients who have been previously operated on and given radiation, the surgeon is doubly concerned about the integrity and watertightness of the closure. Any leakage from the area of operation may lead to a disastrous infection, or at least to a nagging inflammatory reaction in the surrounding tissues and agony for both the surgeon and the patient in the postoperative period. If a laminotomy has been done, then these fragments are wired or sewn back into position, and the muscles and fascia are closed in meticulous fashion. The muscle layers are carefully approximated, and the surgeon takes care that these heavy sutures are not placed too close to the dorsal surface of the cord, which might lead to a guillotine-like compression of the spinal cord when the spine moves.

For high cervical lesions, whether intra- or extramedullary, it is often advisable to leave the endotracheal tube in position until the surgeon is assured of normal respiratory function. A 24- to 48-h interval of careful monitoring of respiratory function may be needed before the endotracheal tube can be removed. Also, special care must be given to bladder function in the postoperative period. Extensive tumors (whether intra- or extramedullary) above the lumbosacral region, especially cervical and high thoracic tumors, may lead to sympathetic denervation and therefore to postural hypotension as the patient is mobilized postoperatively.

The use of radiotherapy to treat intramedullary tumors is controversial.[28,30,46] Optimistic reports of the effect of radiation on intramedullary tumors, such as ependymomas and low-grade astrocytomas, appear to be without foundation. An analysis of these reports reveals that the follow-up period is purely clinical and is too short relative to the normal evolution of these tumors.[37,47] The beneficial results attributed to such treatment may be related more to the decompressive laminectomy. Unfortunately, follow-up MRI has not been performed in the vast majority of these cases to indicate resolution or involution of the tumor following radiation therapy. Orthopedists have also reported that radiotherapy in childhood has a deleterious effect on growth of the spine.[18] In many instances, we observed deleterious effects of radiotherapy of the central areas of the spinal cord adjacent to the tumor when patients were operated upon some time after a course of radiotherapy.[40,41] Lacking definitive evidence of a beneficial effect of radiation upon benign intramedullary tumors, we rarely recommend such treatment for benign pathology. Rather we prefer to observe these patients and consider a second operation, should the clinical and radiographic situation so dictate.

Prognosis and Results

The immediate results and future prognoses in the common extramedullary-intradural tumors, including meningiomas and nerve sheath tumors, have been well established: These tumors are benign, and if they are carefully and thoroughly removed, the patients should be cured, with excellent prognosis. Even in patients who have been devastated neurologically by the growth of these tumors before surgical intervention, there is some hope—especially in young individuals—that many of the neurological abnormalities may resolve slowly in the postoperative period. It may take 18 months to 2 years to maximize the resolution of these neurological deficits, and some patients have improved progressively beyond this time.

Most intramedullary tumors are benign and resectable, provided that the tumor is clearly demarcated from the surrounding spinal cord. Long-time tumor control or cure can be achieved when a discrete benign intramedullary tumor has been removed totally.[28,35] In our series of 155 intramedullary tumors, there has been only one operative mortality. Postoperative morbidity is most closely related to the preoperative neurological condition of the patient. Individuals who have maximal neurological deficits before the operation have made no significant functional recovery after successful tumor removal. In individuals with mild or modest neurological deficits, excellent functional recovery may be expected when the tumor has totally been removed. This underscores the importance of early diagnosis and aggressive initial surgical treatment before a significant neurological deficit develops, When only a portion of the tumor has been removed, the subsequent course depends upon the growth pattern of the tumor. If the tumor is static or indolent, neurological deficits may diminish or remain chronic. Malignant tumors are associated with significant operative morbidity and carry a poor prognosis. Surgical manipulation may result in tumor seeding via the CSF. The results of radiotherapy have been similarly disappointing for a primary malignancy of the spinal cord.

Long-term follow-up of our published series of 23 patients who underwent gross total removal of benign intramedullary ependymomas reveals only one radiographic tumor recurrence. It occurred 6 years after total removal and was completely removed at a second operation. Three other patients from an accumulated series of 70 intramedullary ependymomas have had small linear areas of contrast enhancement without mass effect on follow-up MRI and are being monitored with a serial MRI. A repeat MRI is done biyearly in the remainder of patients. The recurrence rate following varying degrees of removal of benign intramedullary astrocytomas is about 25 to 30 percent at 5 years. Age, rather than the degree of resection, seems to be the most important prognostic factor.

References

1. Agnoli AL, Laun A, Schonmayr R. Enterogenous intraspinal cysts. *J Neurosurg* 1984; 61:834–840.
2. Arseni C, Maretsis M. Tumors of the lower spinal cord associated with increased intracranial pressure and papilledema. *J Neurosurg* 1967; 27:105–110.
3. Christoferson LA, Gustafson MB, Petersen AG. von Hippel-Lindau's disease. *JAMA* 1961; 178:280–282.
4. Cohen AR, Wisoff JH, Allen JC, et al. Malignant astrocytomas of the spinal cord. *J Neurosurg* 1989; 70:50–54.
5. Cushing H. The special field of neurological surgery. *Bull Hopkins Hosp* 1905; 16:77–87.
6. DeSousa AL, Kalsbeck JE, Mealey J Jr, et al. Intraspinal tumors in children: a review of 81 cases. *J Neurosurg* 1979; 51:437–445.
7. Elsberg CA. *Tumors of the Spinal Cord and the Symptoms of Irritation and Compression of the Spinal Cord and Nerve Roots: Pathology, Symptomatology, Diagnosis, and Treatment.* New York: Paul B. Hoeber, 1925.
8. Epstein F, Epstein N. Surgical treatment of spinal cord astrocytomas of childhood: a series of 19 patients. *J Neurosurg* 1982; 57:685–689.
9. Fischer G, Mansuy L. Total removal of intramedullary ependymomas: follow-up study of 16 cases. *Surg Neurol* 1980; 14:243–249.
10. Garrido E, Stein BM. Microsurgical removal of intramedullary spinal cord tumors. *Surg Neurol* 1979; 7:215–219.
11. Gowers WR, Horsley V. A case of tumour of the spinal cord. Removal; recovery. *Med-Chir Trans* 1888; 2nd s 53:377–428.
12. Greenwood J Jr. Intramedullary tumors of spinal cord: a follow-up study after total surgical removal. *J Neurosurg* 1963; 20:665–668.
13. Greenwood J Jr. Surgical removal of intramedullary tumors. *J Neurosurg* 1967; 26:276–282.
14. Guidetti B, Fortuna A. Surgical treatment of intramedullary hemangioblastoma of the spinal cord. Report of 6 cases. *J Neurosurg* 1967; 27:530–540.
15. Herrmann HD, Neuss M, Winkler D. Intramedullary spinal cord tumors resected with CO_2 laser microsurgical technique: recent experience in fifteen patients. *Neurosurgery* 1988; 22:518–522.
16. Horrax G, Henderson DG. Encapsulated intramedullary tumor involving the whole spinal cord from medulla to conus: complete enucleation with recovery. *Surg Gynecol Obstet* 1939; 68:814–819.
17. Kahn EA. The role of the dentate ligaments in spinal cord compression and the syndrome of lateral sclerosis. *J Neurosurg* 1947; 4:191–199.
18. Katzman H, Waugh T, Berdon W. Skeletal changes following irradiation of childhood tumors. *J Bone Joint Surg (Am)* 1969; 51A:825–842.

19. Kurland LT. Frequency of intracranial and intraspinal neoplasms in the resident population of Rochester, Minnesota. *J Neurosurg* 1958; 15:627–641.
20. Lazorthes G, Gouaze A, Zadeh JO, et al. Arterial vascularization of the spinal cord: recent studies of the anastomotic substitution pathways. *J Neurosurg* 1971; 35:253–262.
21. Levy WJ Jr, Bay J, Dohn D. Spinal cord meningioma. *J Neurosurg* 1982; 57:804–812.
22. Levy WJ Jr, Latchaw J, Hahn JF, et al. Spinal neurofibromas: a report of 66 cases and a comparison with meningiomas. *Neurosurgery* 1986; 18:331–334.
23. Malis LI. Intramedullary spinal cord tumors. *Clin Neurosurg* 1978; 25:512–540.
24. Mason TH, Keigher HA. Intramedullary spinal neurilemmoma: case report. *J Neurosurg* 1968; 29:414–416.
25. McCormick PC. The lateral extracavitary approach to the thoracic and lumbar spine. In Holtzman RNN, McCormick PC, Farcy JPC (eds): *Spinal Instability*. New York: Springer-Verlag, 1993, pp 335–348.
26. McCormick PC, Michelsen WJ, Post KD, et al. Cavernous malformations of the spinal cord. *Neurosurgery* 1988; 23:459–463.
27. McCormick PC, Post KD, Stein BM. Intradural extramedullary tumors in adults. *Neurosurg Clin North Am* 1990; 1:591–608.
28. McCormick PC, Stein BM. Intramedullary tumors in adults. *Neurosurg Clin North Am* 1990; 1:609–630.
29. McCormick PC, Stein BM. Miscellaneous intradural pathology. *Neurosurg Clin North Am* 1990; 1:687–699.
30. McCormick PC, Torres R, Post KD, et al. Intramedullary ependymoma of the spinal cord. *J Neurosurg* 1990; 72:523–532.
31. Mork SJ, Loken AC. Ependymoma. A follow-up study of 101 cases. *Cancer* 1977; 40:907–915.
32. Neumann HPH, Eggert HR, Weigel K, et al. Hemangioblastomas of the central nervous system: a 10-year study with special reference to von Hippel-Lindau syndrome. *J Neurosurg* 1989; 70:24–30.
33. Raimondi AJ, Gutierrez FA, di Rocco C. Laminotomy and total reconstruction of the posterior spinal arch for spinal canal surgery in childhood. *J Neurosurg* 1976; 45:555–560.
34. Rand RW, Rand CW. *Intraspinal Tumors of Childhood.* Springfield, IL: Charles C Thomas, 1960.
35. Rawlings CE III, Giangaspero F, Burger PC, et al. Ependymomas: a clinicopathologic study. *Surg Neurol* 1988; 29:271–281.
36. Russell DS, Rubinstein LJ. *Pathology of Tumours of the Nervous System,* 5th ed. Baltimore: Williams & Wilkins, 1989.
37. Schwade JG, Wara WM, Sheline GE, et al. Management of primary spinal cord tumors. *Int J Radiat Oncol Biol Phys* 1978; 4:389–393.
38. Sloof JL, Kernohan JW, MacCarthy CS. *Primary Intramedullary Tumors of the Spinal Cord and Filum Terminale.* Philadelphia: Saunders, 1964.
39. Solomon RA, Stein BM. Unusual spinal cord enlargement related to intramedullary hemangioblastoma. *J Neurosurg* 1988; 68:550–553.
40. Stein BM. Surgery of intramedullary spinal cord tumors. *Clin Neurosurg* 1979; 26:529–542.
41. Stein BM. Management of intramedullary spinal cord lesions. *Neurol Neurosurg Update Ser* 1983; 4:1–12.
42. Stein BM, Leeds NE, Taveras JM, et al. Meningiomas of the foramen magnum. *J Neurosurg* 1963; 20:740–751.
43. Stein BM, Richardson EP Jr. Spinal-cord disorder in a 19-year-old man. *N Engl J Med* 1975; 293:33–38.
44. Taylor AR, Byrnes DP. Foramen magnum and high cervical cord compression. *Brain* 1974; 97:473–480.
45. Thomas JE, Miller RH. Lipomatous tumors of the spinal canal: a study of their clinical range. *Mayo Clin Proc* 1973; 48:393–400.
46. Whitaker SJ, Bessell EM, Ashley SE, et al. Postoperative radiotherapy in the management of spinal cord ependymoma. *J Neurosurg* 1991; 74:720–728.
47. Wood EH, Berne AS, Taveras JM. The value of radiation therapy in the management of intrinsic tumors of the spinal cord. *Radiology* 1954; 63:11–24.

176

Paragangliomas of the Cauda Equina

Setti S. Rengachary
Derek A. Duke

Paraganglia and Tumors of the Paraganglion System

A brief overview of the paraganglion system and the tumors arising from it is necessary for a logical understanding of a paraganglioma arising from a specific site such as the cauda equina region. Most paraganglia are small spherical bodies measuring 2 to 4 mm in diameter. They represent collections or aggregates of neuroepithelial cells containing neurosecretory vesicles; the latter are best demonstrated by electron microscopy. The neurosecretory vesicles contain varying proportions of biogenic amines (catecholamines and serotonin) and peptides (somatostatin).[32]

The term paraganglia derives from the fact that most of these bodies are located in intimate relationship to the abdominal sympathetic ganglia. Although they may be located within the sympathetic ganglia, the majority are located just outside the ganglia. The adrenal medulla represents the largest member of the paraganglion system in the adult; it is thus customary to subdivide the paraganglion system into adrenal and extra-adrenal paraganglion systems. Some members of the paraganglion system such as the glomus jugulare, glomus tympanicum, carotid body, and aortic body are not intimately related to the autonomic ganglia, yet the term paraganglion is customarily applied to them, and justifiably so. Their structure and organization are no different from those of paraganglia elsewhere. A prominent member of the paraganglion system in the fetus is the organ of Zuckerkandl, a large paraganglion located within the mesenteric sympathetic plexus just below the origin of the inferior mesenteric artery. The paraganglia are widely distributed in the head, neck, and trunk. The distribution of paraganglia in the fetus is depicted in Fig. 176-1 and summarized in Table 176-1.

The functions of the paraganglion system, except for certain of its members, such as the carotid and aortic bodies and the adrenal medulla, are unknown. The paraganglia reach their maximal size between the fifth and eighth months of intrauterine life and start to regress thereafter. In the adult, most are recognizable by microscopic examination only. They probably have an important function during fetal development, but the exact role they play is unknown.

The tumors arising from the paraganglia resemble normal paraganglia in their histology and are generically termed paragangliomas. The most common site of origin of paragangliomas are the adrenal medulla, the carotid body, and the glomus jugulare; tumors arising from the rest of the paraganglion system are rare. Exceptionally, paragangliomas may arise in certain locations where paraganglia do not normally exist, for example, sellar and parasellar regions,[2] the cavernous sinus,[13] the pineal area,[39] the petrous apex,[21] the duodenum,[36] and the cauda equina.[1,3,6,8,10,11,14,15,17–19,22,23,25–28,30,33,37,38,40–45] It is estimated that about 10 percent of the paragangliomas are malignant. The tumors may be familial[12] or multicentric[35] or may be associated with other neuroectodermally derived tumors such as neurofibromas.[9]

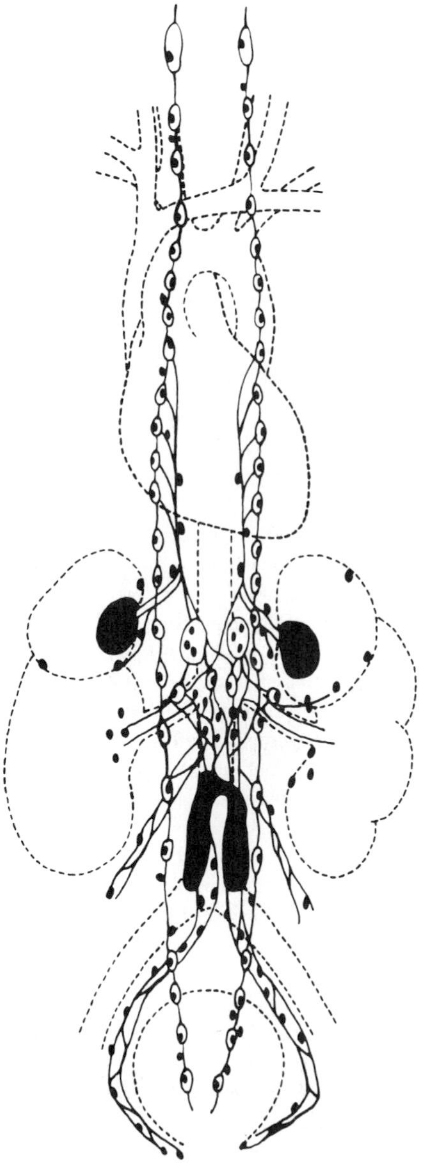

Figure 176-1 The distribution of paraganglia in the fetus. (Redrawn from Coupland RE. *The Natural History of the Chromaffin Cell.* Boston: Longmans, 1965, p 194, Fig. 64.) The chains of clear ovals represent the sympathetic ganglia. The dark dots represent the paraganglia. The adrenal medulla is the largest member of the paraganglion system. The horseshoe-shaped paraganglion just above the aortic bifurcation is the organ of Zuckerkandl. Some components of the paraganglion system such as the carotid and aortic bodies, glomus jugulare, and glomus tympanicum are not represented in this drawing. Most of the paraganglia involute in the adult human.

TABLE 176-1 Paraganglion System and Paragangliomas

Location of Paraganglia	Special Nomenclature, if Any, for the Corresponding Paraganglioma, with Synonyms
Head	
Orbit	—
Petrous bone in the middle fossa	—
Nasal mucosa	—
In the adventitia of the jugular bulb In the jugular ganglion of the vagus nerve Along the tympanic branch of the glossopharyngeal nerve Along the auricular branch of the vagus nerve	Glomus jugulare tumor; glomus tympanicum tumor; pheochromocytoma of the glomus jugulare (functional paraganglioma arising from the glomus jugulare); chromaffin and nonchromaffin paragangliomas of the glomus jugulare
Neck	
Carotid body	Carotid body tumor, chemodectoma
Larynx	—
Vagus nerve	—
Chest	
Aortic arch	—
Subclavian artery	—
Lung	—
Mediastinum	—
Heart	—
Abdomen	
Adrenal gland	Pheochromocytoma
Retroperitoneal, para-aortic sympathetic ganglia	—
Sympathetic plexus (organ of Zuckerkandl)	—
Mesentery	—
Urogenital tract (kidney, bladder, testis, ovary)	—
Gallbladder	—
Gastrointestinal tract	—
Liver	—

The paragangliomas arising from the adrenal medulla are generally called pheochromocytomas (from the Greek root *pheo,* meaning brown) because of the brown discoloration of the tumor with stains containing chromium salts (see the discussion of the chromaffin reaction in the next paragraph). The tumors arising from the aortic and carotid bodies are called chemodectomas, but histologically they are no different from paragangliomas elsewhere. Certain paragangliomas are designated by their anatomic site (e.g., the glomus jugulare tumor). In addition, paragangliomas have been divided into chromaffin and nonchromaffin types, but this classification is of historic interest only.

Historically, the earliest observation that led to the use of chromaffin staining to demonstrate catecholamines within tissues was an empirical observation by Henle that a dark brown color appeared in adrenal medullary tissue when it was exposed to chromic acid or potassium dichromate. Following the identification and synthesis of epinephrine in 1900, it became apparent that the hormone can be oxidized easily and that oxidized epinephrine is brown in color. Also, it was noted that a brown color can be produced by combining epinephrine with powerful oxidizing agents other than chromium compounds. A chromaffin reaction, then, is a nonspecific oxidation reaction that stains catecholamine-containing tissue a brown color. Pathologists over the years have found that this is an undependable, capricious, and insensitive method to detect the presence of a catecholamine in tissue. "Nonchromaffin" paraganglionic tissues and tumors have been shown to contain various catecholamines by sensitive biochemical assay techniques and formaldehyde-induced fluorescence. Indeed, by definition, all paraganglia and tumors arising from them should contain neurosecretory vesicles, which in turn contain catecholamines. In a small fraction of such tumors, the secretions get into the blood stream (most notably in tumors arising from the adrenal medulla, carotid body, and glomus jugulare) and cause a hypersecretion syndrome. In the modern context, it is more logical to classify paragangliomas as functional or nonfunctional rather than as chromaffin or nonchromaffin tumors.

The paraganglion system, with certain exceptions, is embryologically derived from the neural crest. The primordial cells are represented by a mass of undifferentiated sympathochromaffin cells. At a later stage these cells differentiate into small sympathoblasts, giving rise to sympathetic nerve cells, and large chromaffin cells, giving rise to paraganglion cells. This common origin from the neural crest explains several observed phenomena: (1) the close association of the paraganglion system with the autonomic nervous system, (2) the synchronous occurrence of neurofibromas and paragangliomas in the same individual, and (3) the multicentric occurrence of paraganglion tumors.

The embryologic origin of the carotid and aortic bodies is not entirely clear. They are probably not of direct neural crest origin. The carotid body, for instance, is thought to arise from the wall of the third branchial cleft, closely related to the development of a branch of the glossopharyngeal nerve.

Paragangliomas of the Cauda Equina Region

Clinical Features

Paraganglioma of the cauda equina is a disease of adults. It usually manifests in midlife, most commonly in the fifth decade, although it has been reported in individuals 13 to 71 years old. It is extremely rare under the age of 20. It is seen one and a half to two times more frequently in men than in women. There does not seem to be an ethnic or geographic preference.

In most instances, the tumor originates at a nearly constant locus opposite the L2-L3 interspace, approximately 5 cm caudal to the tip of the conus medullaris, and grows slowly and insidiously. As the tumor grows, it expands in all directions, encroaching on the lumbar and sacral roots in the caudal direction, the conus medullaris in the cephalic direction, and the vertebral bodies, the retroperitoneal space, and the laminae in anterior and posterior directions. The clinical features parallel this scheme of origin and growth. Because the lumbar spinal canal is capacious, the cauda equina roots can tolerate considerable pressure, and the growth of the tumor is slow, the symptoms and signs, at least in the early stages, are surprisingly minimal with respect to the size of the tumor. The initial symptom is a vague and poorly localized back pain. There is no characteristic distinguishing clinical feature that suggests a specific diagnosis of paraganglioma of the cauda equina at any stage of the disease. Symptoms of catecholamine excess such as paroxysmal hypertension, anxiety attacks, sweating, and facial flushing might be expected to be helpful but none of the authentic paragangliomas of the cauda equina has been a functional tumor. (One of the patients reported by Boker et al.[4] had long-standing flushing episodes and had high levels of norepinephrine in the urine, but the histology of the resected tumor was indeterminate.) In fact, the early clinical features of the tumor are indistinguishable from those of degenerative disc disease. A diagnosis of paraganglioma is not suspected until diagnostic imaging studies are completed, if then.

Some patients may give a history of trauma such as a work-related accident, a fall, or a sudden snap after lifting a heavy object, but a retrospective analysis will not prove a causal relationship to the tumor. The most commonly involved root is either L3 or L4. Thus, the patient complains of pain radiating to the anterior thigh. On examination, there may be weakness or atrophy of the quadriceps, sensory loss over the anterior thigh, loss of the patellar reflex, and a positive femoral stretch test. As the tumor grows, additional roots of the cauda equina are involved. The back pain worsens, which may be aggravated by activity or Valsalva's maneuver. In the terminal stages, the back pain may be intense, may be present at rest, and may be aggravated by the slightest motion. When this occurs, there is considerable paraspinal muscle spasm and rigidity. As more caudal lumbar and sacral roots are involved, the pain radiates to the posterior thigh, the anterior or posterior aspects of the leg, or the ankle and foot on one or both sides. Tingling and paresthesias may be present in this distribution instead of pain. The signs at this stage are those of a typical cauda equina syndrome consisting of bilateral but asymmetrical involvement of multiple lumbar and sacral roots, with corresponding multiroot motor atrophy, weakness, sensory loss, and hyporeflexia. The straight leg raising test may be positive. Sphincter disturbances occur late in the course of the disease and may reflect involvement of the sacral roots of the cauda equina or the conus medullaris. A mixed conus-cauda syndrome consisting of flexor spasms of the hip, patellar clonus, absent ankle reflexes, and sphincter disturbance is rare.

Diagnostic Imaging

Roentgenograms of the lumbar spine are nearly always normal. Rarely, in very advanced stages, erosive changes may be present in the vertebral bodies (posterior aspects), pedicles, and laminae. Lumbar myelography shows a smooth, rounded, crescentic intradural defect with varying degrees of block, in both the anteroposterior and lateral views (Fig. 176-2). The cauda equina roots are seen

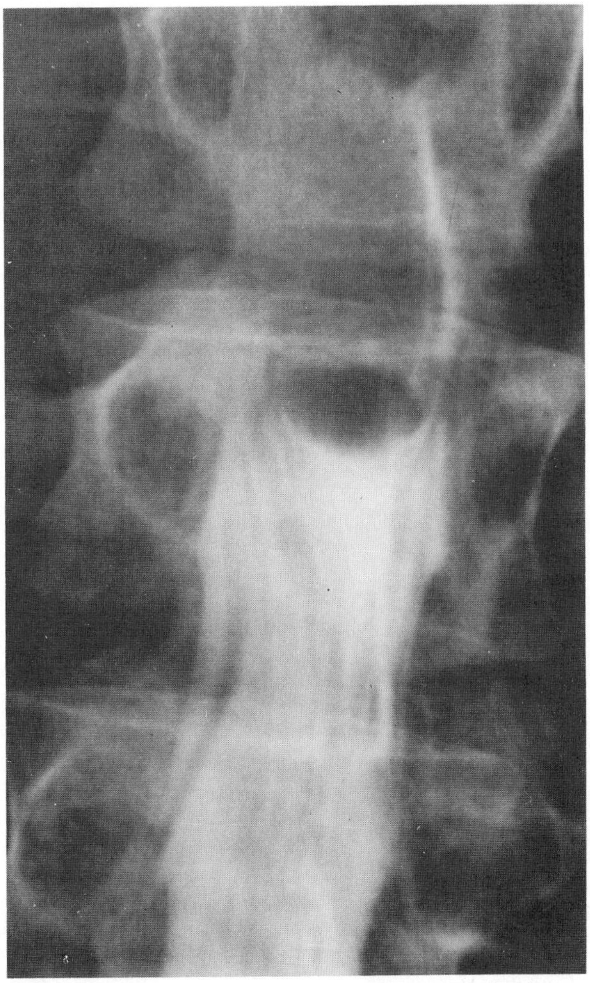

Figure 176-2 Lumbar myelogram with a water-soluble contrast agent showing a smooth, rounded, intradural filling defect near the L2, L3 interspace. The cauda equina roots are seen splayed around the mass.

to be splayed around the mass. Serpentine filling defects representing dilated vascular channels feeding the neoplasm may be seen rostral to the lesion. The spinal fluid protein value is invariably elevated, considerably so in patients with a complete myelographic block. Spinal angiography confirms the rich vascular supply to the tumor. Computed tomography done after the intrathecal administration of a contrast agent confirms the presence of an intradural mass. MRI shows a discrete hyperintense intradural mass in T1-weighted images and an isointense lesion in the proton density-weighted images (Fig. 176-3). The tumor enhances with intravenous contrast injection.[16,29,31,32]

Of interest is the use of radioactive metaiodobenzyl-guanidine (MIBG) in the imaging and treatment of paragangliomas.[5,20] This compound is a physiologic analogue of norepinephrine. It is an "aralkylguanidine which combines the benzyl portion of bretylium with the guanidino group of guanethidine, making it resistant to catabolism by catechol-*o*-methyltransferase and monoamine oxidase, respectively."[20] It is taken up in vivo through the sodium-dependent neuron 1 uptake system and stored in the neurosecretory vesicles, much like norepinephrine. It may be labeled with ^{123}I or ^{131}I, but the former is said to provide superior images. This radioactive compound was used originally to image pheochromocytomas arising from the adrenal medulla, but more recently, related

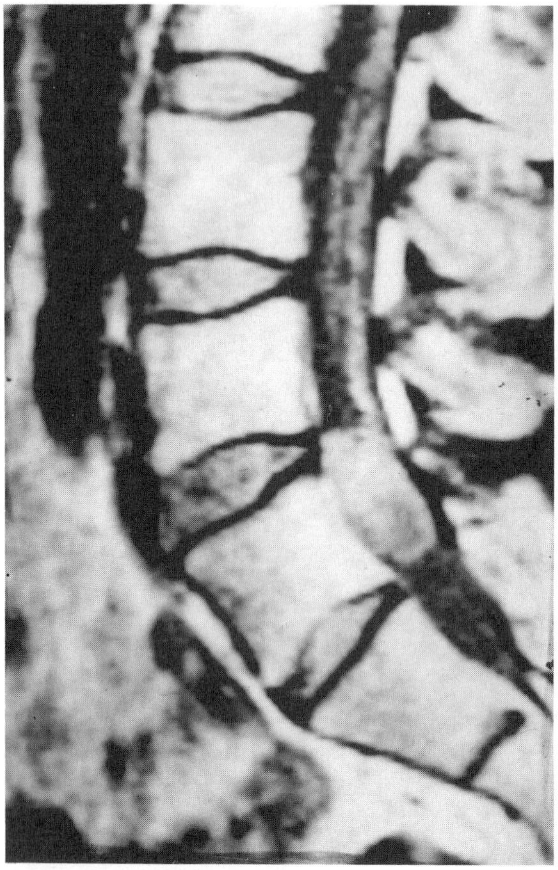

Figure 176-3 MRI appearance of a paraganglioma of the cauda equina.

tumors containing neurosecretory granules such as extra-adrenal paragangliomas and neuroblastomas have been imaged successfully. Although there is no good correlation between the functional activity of the tumor and the ^{123}I MIBG uptake, there seems to be a linear relationship between the amount of stored granules and the ^{123}I MIBG uptake. It is a potentially useful test, having the following advantages: (1) it helps to differentiate paragangliomas from ependymomas and neurilemomas, the two most common tumors of the cauda equina, because the latter do not contain neurosecretory vesicles; (2) the imaging is done of the entire paraganglion system and therefore, multicentric tumors can be detected; and (3) metastatic spread of a malignant paraganglioma can be detected.

Surgical Therapy

Ideally, the patient should be placed in the knee-chest position. Induced hypotension is not necessary except in patients with an invasive tumor that has spread beyond the confines of the dura. Long-acting paralyzing agents are avoided at the induction of anesthesia should electrical stimulation of cauda equina roots be necessary intraoperatively. A total laminectomy is done, centered on the tumor as based on the myelographic findings. The dura is usually tense and the mass may be palpated through the dura.

The tumor is intradural and intra-arachnoid, and is not attached to either of these structures. Typically, the mass is dark purplish red in color and appears extremely vascular (Fig. 176-4). The intraspinal site of attachment varies. Usually the tumor is suspended by a single large feeding artery and its accompanying vein at the cephalic pole of the tumor. Occlusion of these vessels generally renders the tumor virtually avascular. In other instances, the tumor may be attached to the filum terminale. The roots of the cauda equina are splayed by the tumor. It is not uncommon for one or two roots of the cauda to be loosely attached to the surface of the tumor. These can be separated easily. If a root courses entirely through the center of the tumor, it may have to be sacrificed. Piecemeal removal or diagnostic biopsy is not recommended as these maneuvers induce troublesome bleeding. For the same reason, the use of an ultrasonic aspirator is contraindicated. Every attempt should be made to remove the tumor in a single piece after ligating or clipping the vascular pedicle and dissecting it off the cauda equina. Extensive tumors may require tedious dissection from the cauda equina, the conus medullaris, the dura, and even the vertebral bodies. In such instances, resection may be less than complete.

Pathology

The tumor consists of nests or clusters (''Zellballen'') of large uniform polygonal cells with pale eosinophilic granular cytoplasm (Fig. 176-5). The cell nests are sharply circumscribed by a fibrovascular stroma best appreciated with Gomori and phosphotungstic acid hematoxylin (PTAH) stains. Mitotic figures

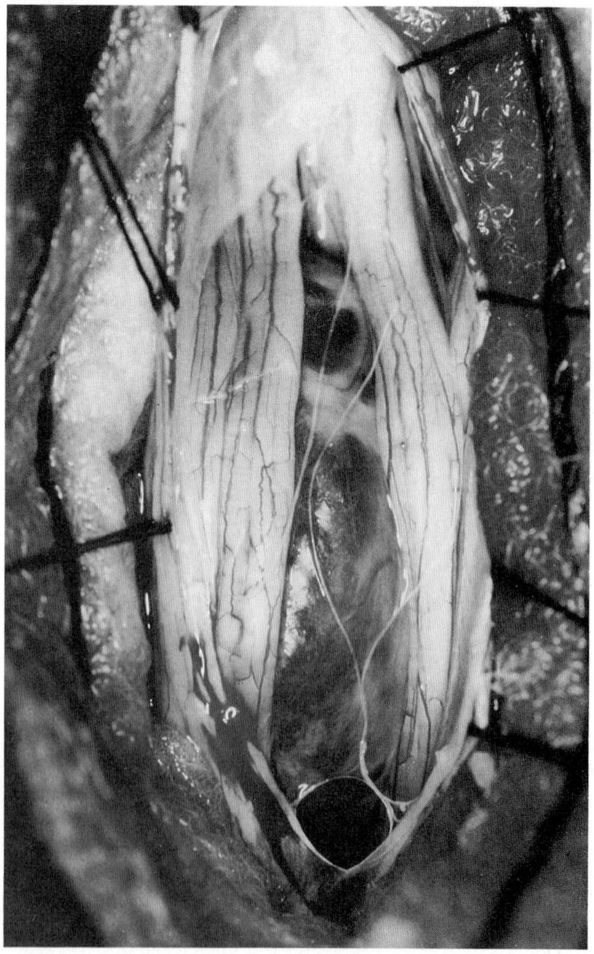

Figure 176-4 Operative exposure of a paraganglioma of the cauda equina. The tumor is intra-arachnoid and is highly vascular. The roots of the cauda equina are splayed around the mass and are clearly separate from it.

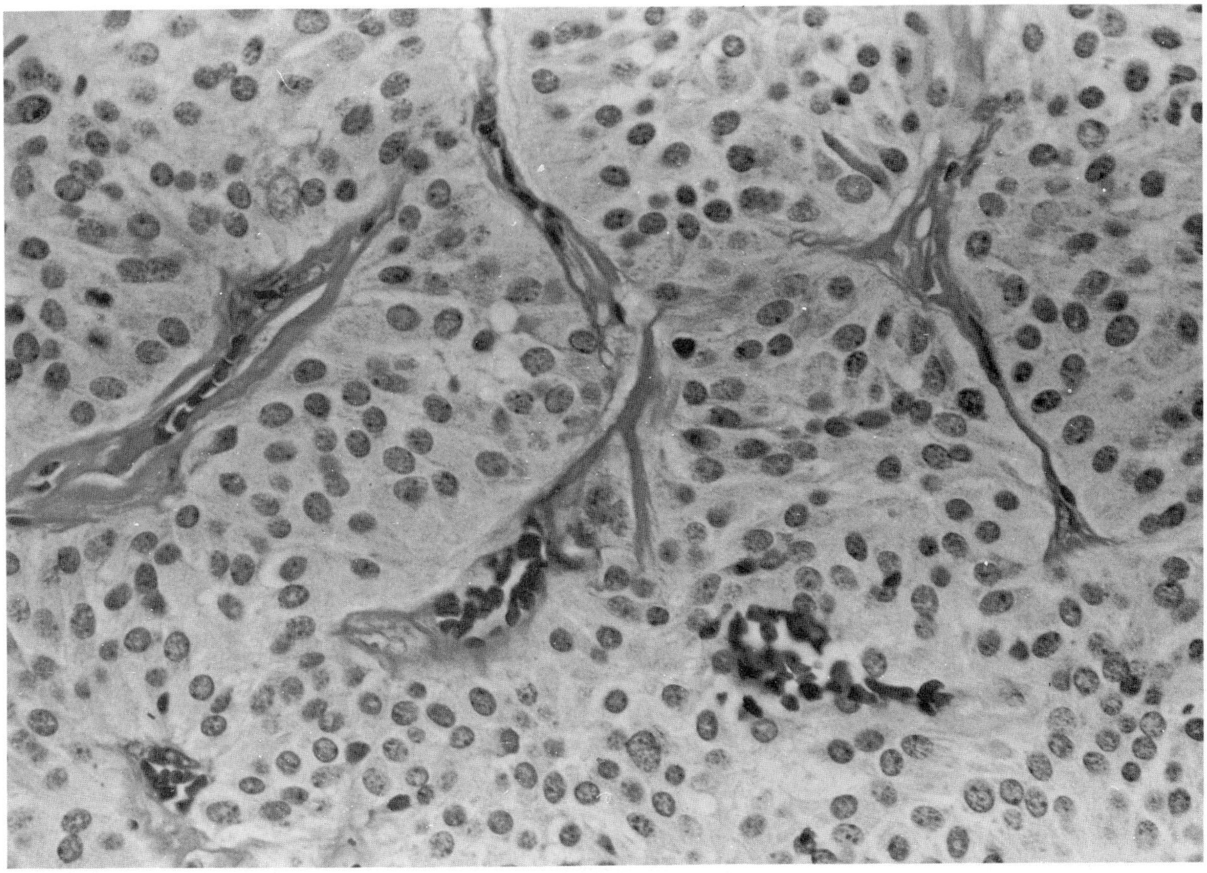

Figure 176-5 Light microscopic appearance of a paraganglioma showing the characteristic "Zellballen" pattern with nests or lobules of polyhedral cells separated by a network of capillaries. (Hematoxylin and eosin, ×250.)

are rarely observed. Occasional pseudopapillary structures may cause a misleading resemblance to ependymoma, but the immunostain for glial fibrillary acidic protein (GFAP) is negative. However, tumors with authentic ependymal and paraganglionic differentiation have been reported.[7] In about 50 percent of the tumors, mature neurons are scattered among the tumor cells—the gangliocytic variant of paraganglioma (Fig. 176-6). The Grimelius stain is usually positive, demonstrating argyrophilic granules. A positive immunostain for synaptophysin confirms the presence of neurosecretory granules within the tumor and is thought to be more specific than neuron-specific enolase or protein gene product 9.5 (PGP 9.5).[31,34] Electron microscopy shows variable numbers of dense core vesicles measuring 80 to 300 nm in diameter (Fig. 176-7). Cytoplasmic filaments of the intermediate type may be demonstrated.

Benign and malignant paragangliomas look alike histologically. The diagnosis of malignancy is made more on the basis of biological behavior, such as involvement of lymph nodes or distant metastases at sites where paraganglion cells are not normally present. One study has shown a definite relationship between the expression of certain neuropeptides [such as (Leu^5)-enkephalin, (Met^5)-encephalin, somatostatin, pancreatic polypeptide, vasoactive intestinal polypeptide, substance P, adrenocorticotropic hormone, calcitonin, bombesin, and neurotensin] and the biological behavior of paragangliomas.[24]

Prognosis and Adjunctive Therapy

The prognosis of paragangliomas of the cauda equina is generally excellent. There have been no reports of recurrence of tumor when gross total removal has been accomplished. Ordinarily, the postoperative neurological deficit is limited to one or two roots, if any. However, involvement of the conus medullaris or extradural invasion adversely affects the prognosis. To this date, all of the reported cases of intradural paraganglioma of the cauda equina have been benign. No patient has ever died of the disease, even in recurrent cases. "Recurrence" has been noted after a tumor has been incompletely resected, because of either extensive disease or a mistaken histologic diagnosis. Such an event is better designated as regrowth rather than recurrence.

Because these tumors are inherently benign, have very slow growth characteristics, and are uncommon, it is difficult to assess the role of radiation therapy in their management. Radiation therapy is clearly unwarranted in an uncomplicated case of intradural paraganglioma of the cauda equina. In fact, if the radiation therapy had been initiated with a mistaken diagnosis of ependymoma or metastatic carcinoma, the therapy should be interrupted immediately as soon as a definitive diagnosis of paraganglioma is made. In the case of an incompletely resected tumor, it may be better to attempt a second operation to achieve a total resection and surgical cure before resorting to palliative radiation therapy.

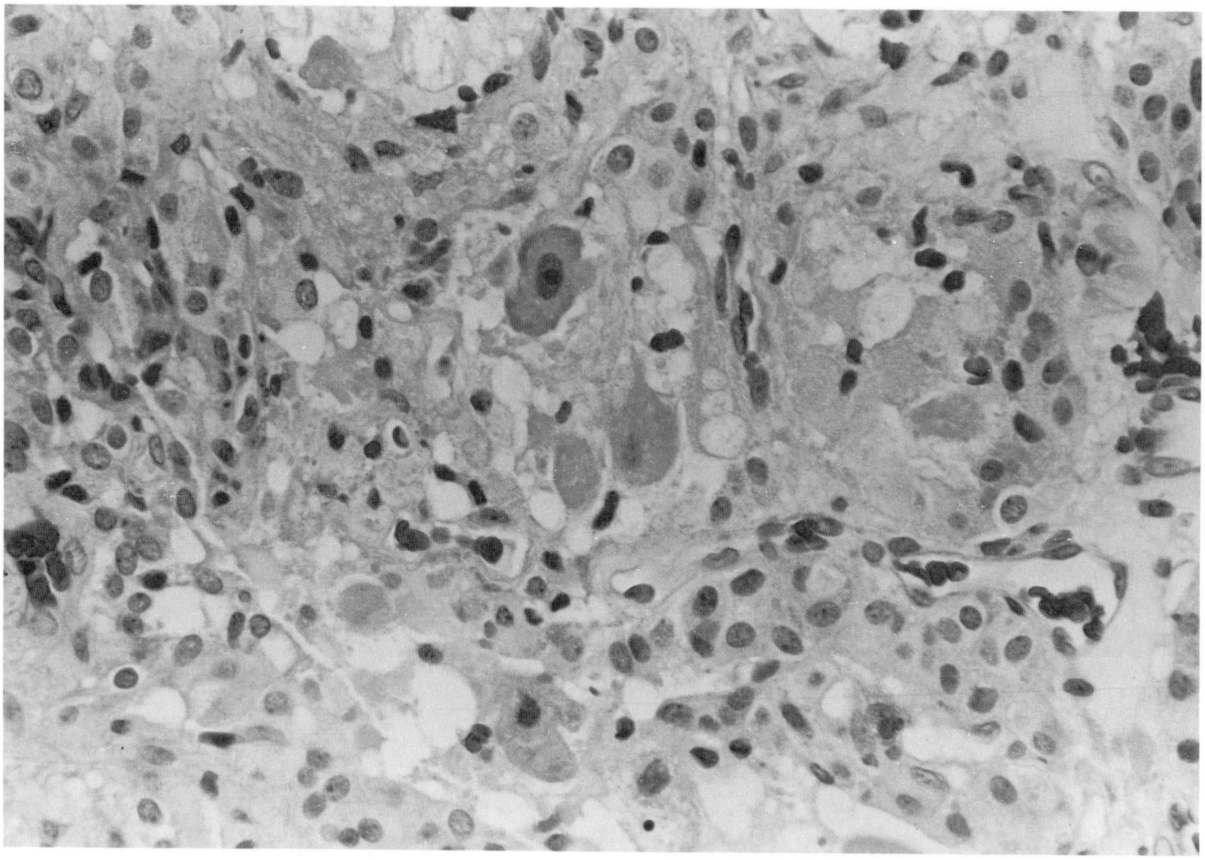

Figure 176-6 An area of a paraganglioma showing gangliocytic differentiation. (Hematoxylin and eosin, ×250.)

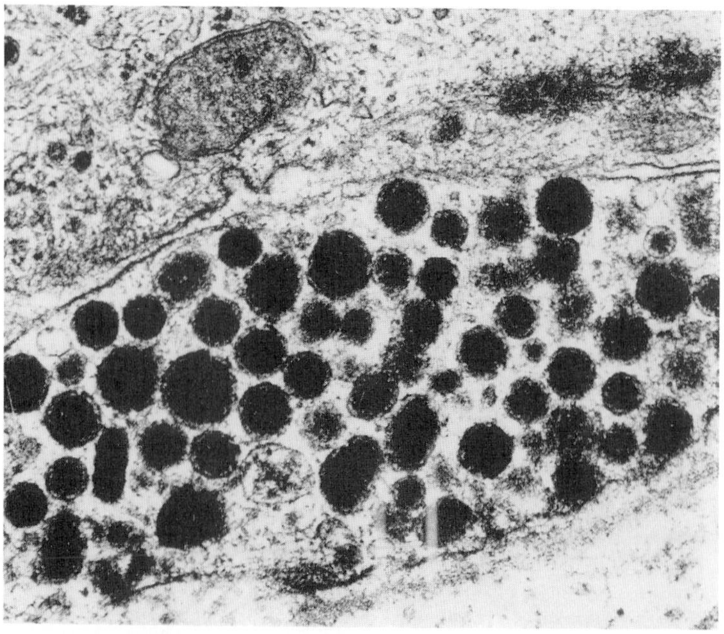

Figure 176-7 An electron micrograph showing dense core vesicles (×54,000).

References

1. Anderson JR, Gullan RW. Paraganglioma of the cauda equina: a case report. *J Neurol Neurosurg Psychiatry* 1987; 50:100–103.
2. Bilbao JM, Horvath E, Kovacs K, et al. Intrasellar paraganglioma associated with hypopituitarism. *Arch Pathol Lab Med* 1978; 102:95–98.
3. Binkley W, Vakili ST, Worth R. Paraganglioma of the cauda equina: case report. *J Neurosurg* 1982; 56:275–279.
4. Boker DK, Wassmann H, Solymosi L. Paragangliomas of the spinal canal. *Surg Neurol* 1983; 19:461–468.
5. Bomanji J, Levison DA, Flatman WD, et al. Uptake of iodine-123 MIBG by pheochromocytomas, paragangliomas, and neuroblastomas: a histopathological comparison. *J Nucl Med* 1987; 28:973–978.
6. Cabello A, Ricoy JR. Paraganglioma of the cauda equina. *Cancer* 1983; 52:751–754.
7. Caccamo DV, Ho KL, Garcia JH. Cauda equina tumor with ependymal and paraganglionic differentiation. *Hum Pathol* 1992; 23:835–838.
8. Cole G, Varma T, Hourihan M, et al. Paraganglioma of the cauda equina. *J Neurol Neurosurg Psychiatry* 1987; 51:1558 (letter).
9. DeAngelis IM, Kelleher MB, Post KD, et al. Multiple paragangliomas in neurofibromatosis: a new neuroendocrine neoplasia. *Neurology* 1987; 37:129–133.
10. Djindjian M, Ayache P, Brugieres P, et al. Giant gangliocytic paraganglioma of the filum terminale: case report. *J Neurosurg* 1990; 73:459–461.
11. Gaffney EF, Doorly T, Dinn JJ. Aggressive oncocytic neuroendocrine tumour ('oncocytic paraganglioma') of the cauda equina. *Histopathology* 1986; 10:311–319.
12. Grufferman S, Gillman MW, Pasternak LR, et al. Familial carotid body tumors: case report and epidemiologic review. *Cancer* 1980; 46:2116–2122.
13. Ho KC, Meyer G, Garancis J, et al. Chemodectoma involving the cavernous sinus and semilunar ganglion. *Hum Pathol* 1982; 13:942–943.
14. Horoupian DS, Kerson LA, Sainotz H, Valsamis M. Paraganglioma of cauda equina: clinicopathologic and ultrastructural studies of an unusual case. *Cancer* 1974; 33:1337–1348.
15. Ilgren EB, Teddy PJ. Chemodectoma of the cauda equina: case report. *Clin Neuropathol* 1984; 3:148–152.
16. Iliya AR, Davis RP, Seidman RJ. Paraganglioma of the cauda equina: case report with magnetic resonance imaging description. *Surg Neurol* 1991; 35:366–367.
17. Ironside JW. Paraganglioma of the cauda equina. *J Neurol Neurosurg Psychiatry* 1988; 51:740 (letter).
18. Ironside JW, Royds JA, Taylor CB, et al. Paraganglioma of the cauda equina: a histological, ultrastructural and immunocytochemical study of two cases with a review of the literature. *J Pathol* 1985; 145:195–201.
19. Kamalian N, Abbassioun K, Amirjamshidi A, Mohammed S. Paraganglioma of the filum terminale internum. Report of a case and review of the literature. *J Neurol* 1987; 235:56–59.
20. Khafagi F, Egerton-Vernon J, Van Doorn T, et al. Localization and treatment of familial malignant nonfunctional paraganglioma with iodine-131 MIBG: report of two cases. *J Nucl Med* 1987; 28:528–531.
21. Kruse F Jr. Petrous ridge chemodectoma (non-chromaffin paraganglioma) simulating meningioma: case report. *J Neurosurg* 1960; 17:1108–1111.
22. Lagace R, Delage C, Gagne F. Paraganglioma of the filum terminale. *Can J Neurol Sci* 1978; 5:257–260.
23. Lerman RI, Kaplan ES, Daman L. Ganglioneuroma-paraganglioma of the intradural filum terminale. Case report. *J Neurosurg* 1972; 36:652–658.
24. Linnoila RI, Lack EE, Steinberg SM, et al. Decreased expression of neuropeptides in malignant paragangliomas: an immunohistochemical study. *Hum Pathol* 1988; 19:41–50.
25. Lipper S, Decker RE. Paraganglioma of the cauda equina. A histologic, immunohistochemical, and ultrastructural study and review of the literature. *Surg Neurol* 1984; 22:415–420.
26. Llena JF, Hirano A, Rubin RC. Paraganglioma in the cauda equina region. *Acta Neuropathol (Berl)* 1979; 46:235–237.
27. Llena JF, Wisoff HS, Hirano A. Gangliocytic paraganglioma in cauda equina region, with biochemical and neuropathologic studies: case report. *J Neurosurg* 1982; 56:280–282.
28. Miller CA, Torack RM. Secretory ependymoma of the filum terminale. *Acta Neuropathol (Berl)* 1970; 15:240–250.
29. Olsen WL, Dillon WP, Kelly WM, et al. MR imaging of paragangliomas. *Am J Roentgenol* 1987; 148:201–204.
30. O'Sullivan MG, Keohane C, Buckley TF. Paraganglioma of the cauda equina: a case report and review of the literature. *Br J Neurosurg* 1990; 4:63–67.
31. Pigott TJ, Lowe JS, Morrell K, et al. Paraganglioma of the cauda equina: report of three cases. *J Neurosurg* 1990; 73:455–458.
32. Raftopoulos C, Flament-Durand J, Brucher JM, et al. Paraganglioma of the cauda equina: report of 2 cases and review of 59 cases from the literature. *Clin Neurol Neurosurg* 1990; 92:263–270.
33. Reyes MG, Torres H. Intrathecal paraganglioma of the cauda equina. *Neurosurgery* 1984; 15:578–582.
34. Rode J, Dhillon AP, Doran JF, et al. PGP 9.5, a new marker for human neuroendocrine tumours. *Histopathology* 1985; 9:147–158.
35. Sato T, Saito H, Yoshinaga K, et al. Concurrence of carotid body tumor and pheochromocytoma. *Cancer* 1974; 34:1787–1795.
36. Scheithauer BW, Nora FE, LeChago J, et al. Duodenal gangliocytic paraganglioma: clinicopathologic and immunocytochemical study of 11 cases. *Am J Clin Pathol* 1986; 86:559–565.
37. Schmitt HP, Wurster K, Bauer M, et al. Mixed chemodectoma-ganglioneuroma of the conus medullaris region. *Acta Neuropathol (Berl)* 1982; 57:275–281.
38. Shuangshoti S, Suwanwela N, Suwanwela C. Combined paraganglioma and glioma of conus medullaris and cauda equina. *J Surg Oncol* 1984; 25:162–167.
39. Smith WT, Hughes B, Ermocilla R. Chemodectoma of the pineal region, with observations on the pineal body and chemoreceptor tissue. *J Pathol* 1966; 92:69–76.
40. Soffer D, Pittaluga S, Caine Y, Feinsod M. Paraganglioma of the cauda equina. A report of case and review of the literature. *Cancer* 1983; 51:1907–1910.
41. Sonneland PRL, Scheithauer BW, LeChago J, et al. Paraganglioma of the cauda equina region: clinicopathologic study of 31 cases with special reference to immunocytology and ultrastructure. *Cancer* 1986; 58:1720–1735.
42. Steinberg GK, Rowan LM, White JE, Krist DA. An unusual neoplasm of the cauda equina with gangliomatous and ependymomatous elements. *Surg Neurol* 1984; 22:164–166.
43. Taxy JB. Paraganglioma of the cauda equina. Report of a rare tumour. *Cancer* 1983; 51:1904–1906.
44. Tsao M-S, Bilbao J, Richardson P, Finlayson M. Cauda equina paraganglioma. *Can J Neurol Sci* 1983; 10:266–269.
45. Van Alphen HA, Bellot SM, Stam FC. Paraganglioma of cauda equina. *Clin Neurol Neurosurg* 1977; 79:316–322.

177

Spinal Epidural Tumors

Perry Black
Somnath Nair
George Giannakopoulos

Incidence

Metastatic lesions of the spine represent the large majority of spinal epidural tumors. Approximately 5 percent of cancer patients with solid neoplasms—both adults[4] and children[33]—develop spinal epidural tumor deposits, although not all of these become clinically evident. Spinal metastasis as a clinical problem is likely to increase in the future as the life expectancy of cancer patients is prolonged with advances in therapy.

Benign tumors such as neurilemomas (schwannomas), neurofibromas, and meningiomas are generally intradural but occasionally have an extradural component or may be limited to the extradural space (Figs. 177-1 to 177-3).

Pathology

Origin of the Metastatic Lesion

In adults, the common primary sources are lung, breast, prostate, and kidney tumors, and lymphoma. In almost one-tenth of cases, the patient is not known to have cancer, and the spinal cord compression is the initial symptom of malignancy; half of these are subsequently found to have lung cancer.[49] In an additional one-tenth of cases, the primary lesion cannot be identified, even after diagnostic study.[23]

Latent Interval

The time between the original diagnosis of cancer and the occurrence of spinal metastasis varies widely. In one series the range was 0 to 19 years, with the longest interval occurring in patients with breast carcinoma.[23]

Sex and Age Distribution

Metastatic Tumors

There is a slight preponderance of metastatic tumors in males (60 percent) compared with females[23,52]; this sex difference may reflect the incidence of primary breast versus prostate tumors in a given series.[16] All ages may be affected, but the period of highest incidence coincides with the relatively high cancer risk period of 40 to 65 years of age.

Benign Tumors

Males and females are equally affected by neurilemomas; these tumors occur predominantly from 30 to 50 years of age. Eighty percent of spinal meningiomas occur in females in the age range of 40 to 70 years.[46]

Route of Metastatic Spread to the Spinal Canal

Extraspinal malignant tumors are believed to metastasize to the spine and extradural space mainly by hematogenous spread either (1) through the arterial system to the bone marrow of the vertebral body and then into the anterior or posterior epidural space via venous channels,[3] or (2) retrogradely through Batson's paravertebral and extradural venous plexus, which is devoid of valves.[5] Tumors may also gain entry to the spinal extradural space by bone erosion or by direct extension through a neural foramen; invasion of the spinal canal through a foramen is a characteristic pathway for lymphoma,[25,52,57] and for spinal metastases in children.[33]

Distribution of Spinal Tumors

Metastatic Tumors

Metastatic deposits may occur in any portion of the spinal canal. For each portion of the canal, the incidence of involvement corresponds roughly to the proportion of that part to the total length of the spine; thus the thoracic spine is involved in about 60 percent of the cases. A majority of the tumors are localized to one or two adjacent vertebral segments; 17 to 30 percent of patients, however, show evidence of compression of the spinal cord or cauda equina at two or more noncontiguous sites[23,42,54] (Figs. 177-4 and 177-5). Unexpected epidural lesions are commonly asymptomatic clinically. Multiple noncontiguous levels of spinal involvement occur particularly in breast[29] and prostate metastasis,[40] and in multiple myeloma.[4] *The possibility of multiple separate levels of involvement points to the desirability of diagnostic imaging of the entire spinal canal in patients suspected of having spinal metastasis.*

Metastasis to the vertebral column may involve any portion of one or more vertebral elements, including the vertebral body, pedicle, lamina, and spinous process. Although the vertebral body may be destroyed, the intervertebral disc is maintained because it is resistant to invasion by tumor; this feature is a useful radiographic diagnostic aid in distinguishing neoplastic destruction of a vertebral body from infection (vertebral osteomyelitis), in which case the disc is often destroyed along with the vertebral body.

When a metastasis invades the spinal canal, it is usually restricted to the extradural space. Experimentally, the expanding mass causes breakdown of the blood–spinal cord barrier and vasogenic edema.[18,53] Autopsy studies in humans have shown vascular congestion, hemorrhage, and edema at the site of cord compression.[4] The dura mater is a barrier to penetration of tumor cells into the subdural or subarachnoid space; for this reason surgeons are generally reluctant to open the dura when resecting an epidural metastasis. Within the epidural space there is variable tumor

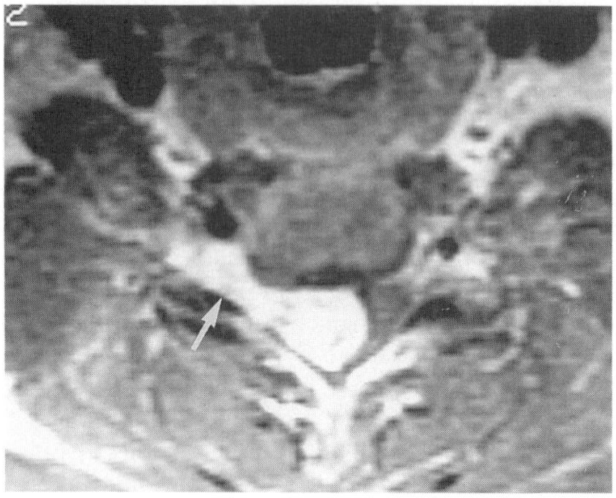

(*A*)

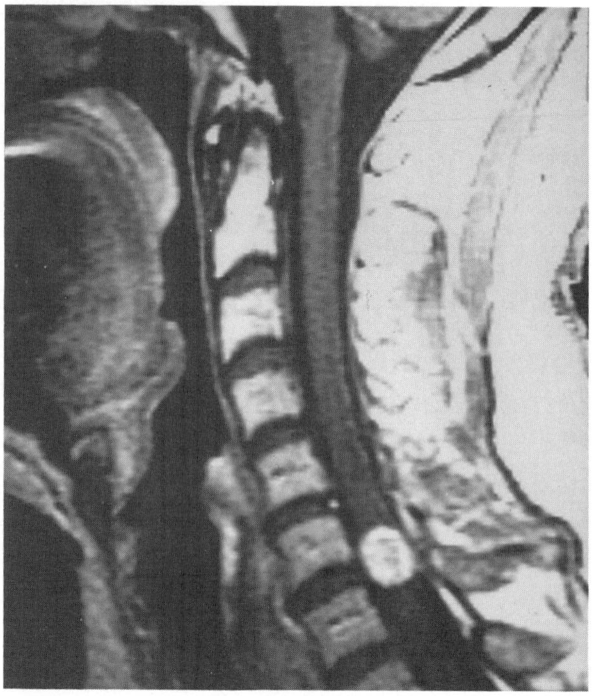

(*B*)

Figure 177-1 Recurrent cervical neurilemoma in a 45-year-old man who presented with a 3-month history of progressive pain and weakness in the right upper extremity, and asymmetrical myelopathy (Brown-Sequard's syndrome). *A.* T1-weighted contrast-enhanced axial MRI scan demonstrating a dumbbell-shaped neurilemoma extending through the right neural foramen *(arrow). B.* T1-weighted contrast-enhanced midline sagittal MRI scan demonstrating a densely enhancing intradural extramedullary neurilemoma at C6–7. Microsurgical technique via a hemilaminectomy was used to excise the lesion, which extended through an enlarged neural foramen. The pain and weakness improved, but dysesthesias in the upper extremity persisted. (Courtesy of Thomas McCormack, M.D.)

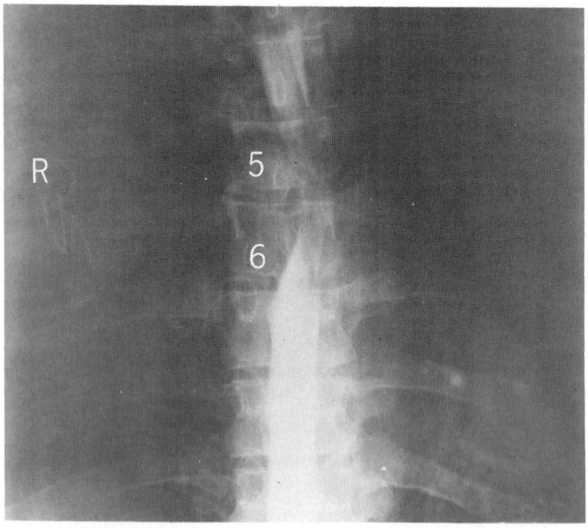

Figure 177-2 Epidural neurilemoma at T5–T6 in a 34-year-old man with a 1-year history of pain in the midthoracic and upper lumbar regions and progressive weakness and sensory impairment in the lower extremities. He also had difficulty with micturition. The myelogram showed a subtotal block at T5–T6, suggestive of an extradural mass lesion. Although MRI is preferred for imaging in such cases, myelography with subsequent CT is a suitable alternative. Microsurgical excision of the lesion was carried out, and rapid postoperative recovery of neurological function ensued.

involvement of the anterior (ventral) compartment, the lateral gutters, and the posterior compartment (or any combination of these sites). The location of the extradural metastatic lesion has important surgical implications in that a metastatic tumor mass in the posterior extradural compartment is easily accessible to the surgeon by a laminectomy, whereas it is preferable to approach a ventral mass by an anterior or anterolateral route.

Intradural extramedullary metastasis is uncommon, with a reported incidence of 1 to 4 percent.[13,34,57] Invasion of the spinal cord parenchyma is even less common; in one series, intramedullary metastasis accounted for 2 percent of the spinal metastases.[13]

Benign Tumors

Neurilemomas (schwannomas) and neurofibromas are both intradural and extramedullary in approximately 70 percent of cases, and the remaining 30 percent are equally divided between a strictly extradural location and a dumbbell or hourglass configuration (involving the intradural and/or extradural compartment with extension into the paraspinal space) (Fig. 177-1); 1 percent is intramedullary.[36] Half of all neurilemomas and neurofibromas are located in the thoracic spine (Fig. 177-2); the next most frequent site is the cervical region (Fig. 177-1), and the least frequent is the lumbar area (Fig. 177-3).

Meningiomas are generally intradural and extramedullary, but 15 percent are extradural. They are often attached to the insertion of the dentate ligaments and may be seen as multiple lesions in von Recklinghausen's disease. Meningiomas may be located in any

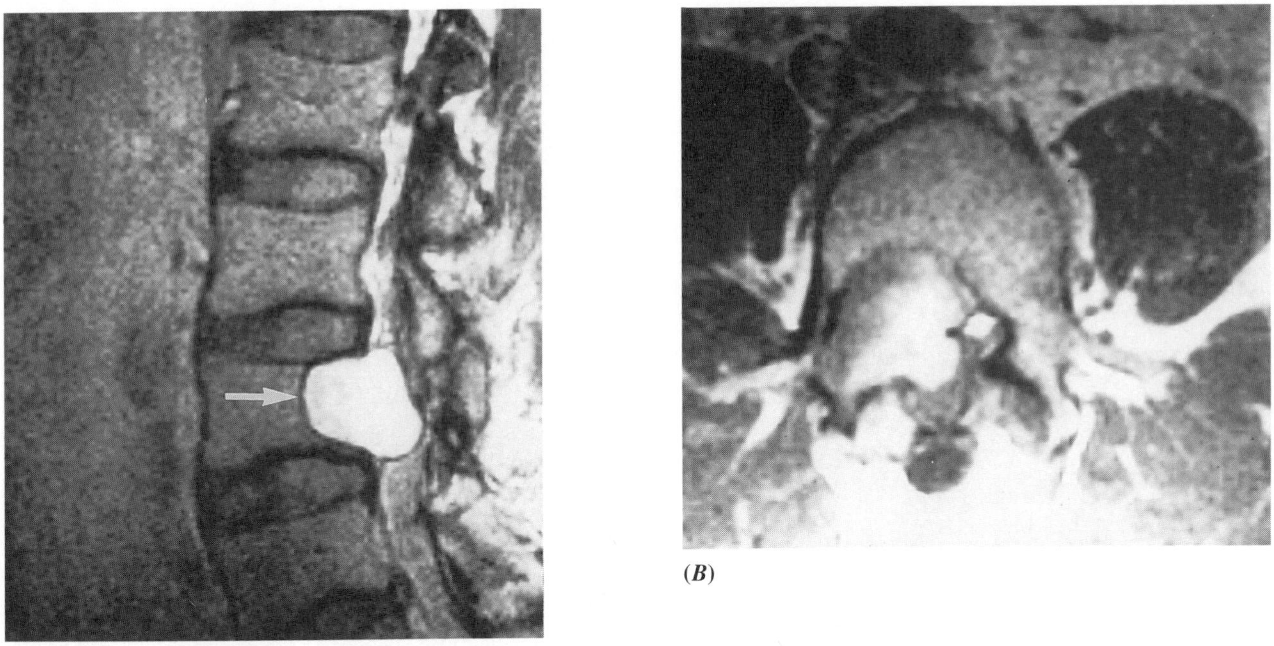

(*A*) (*B*)

Figure 177-3 Recurrent neurilemoma in a 50-year-old man who had undergone removal of the tumor at the same site 15 years earlier. He now presented with low back pain, right sciatica, and weakness at the right ankle. *A.* T1-weighted contrast-enhanced sagittal MRI scan to the right of the midline showing an intra- and extradural neurilemoma with scalloping *(arrow)* of the posterior L4 vertebral body and encroachment upon the cauda equina. *B.* Corresponding axial image. Microsurgical excision via a laminectomy was carried out, yielding relief of pain, but weakness of the right ankle extensors persisted.

portion of the spinal canal, but two-thirds are found in the thoracic region.

Symptoms and Signs

Metastatic Tumors

The onset of symptoms of spinal cord or nerve root compression may be acute or insidious. The duration of symptoms before diagnosis varies from 5 days to 2 years (with a median of 2 months).[23] Pain is usually the initial symptom (in 96 percent of cases), preceding other symptoms by 5 days to 2 years (with a median of 7 weeks).[23] Local pain in the vertebral column is generally located close to the site of the lesion. Radicular pain, less common than local spinal pain, is also of localizing value, as it radiates in the dermatomal distribution of the compressed or tumor-infiltrated nerve roots.

Weakness, usually in the lower extremities, rarely occurs as a first symptom, but is common (76 percent of cases) by the time the diagnosis is made.[23] Despite an antecedent history of spinal or radicular pain, some 15 percent of patients present with paraplegia[23]; this underlines the importance of placing a high index of suspicion of spinal or radicular pain in following patients with known cancer.

More than half the patients with spinal cord compression secondary to metastatic disease have bladder and bowel dysfunction at the time of diagnosis. Sphincter dysfunction is usually associated with motor and sensory loss, although a few patients with compression limited to the conus medullaris do not have weakness or sensory impairment of the lower limbs.

Sensory symptoms such as numbness or paresthesias in the extremities or trunk do not generally occur as initial symptoms but are present in about half the patients at the time of diagnosis.[23]

In the presence of paraplegia, a presumptive diagnosis of spinal cord compression is readily made. There is flaccid paralysis of the lower limbs and a distended bladder; the level of motor or sensory loss approximates the site of spinal cord compression. The deficit may be more subtle, however, in cases of early spinal cord compression. Anterior (ventral) cord compression is suspected when there is weakness in the extremities and loss of spinothalamic tract function (pain and temperature sense) below the level of the lesion, with preservation of dorsal column sensation (touch, position, vibration).[6] The loss of dorsal column sensation with preservation of other sensory or motor functions suggests pressure on the posterior spinal cord.

The level of motor loss, except in thoracic cord involvement, is a somewhat more reliable indicator of the spinal cord segment involved than is the level of sensory loss. The sensory level on the chest or abdomen is the most useful localizing sign in thoracic spinal cord compression. The abdominal reflexes may also help in localization because their innervation originates from segments T8–12. The motor and sensory deficits are generally symmetrical, but occasionally asymmetrical compression of the spinal cord or interference with its blood supply produces Brown-Sequard's syndrome.

The lumbar and sacral nerve roots of the cauda equina are loosely arranged in the spinal canal. Compression of the cauda equina is, therefore, often irregular, giving rise to patchy and

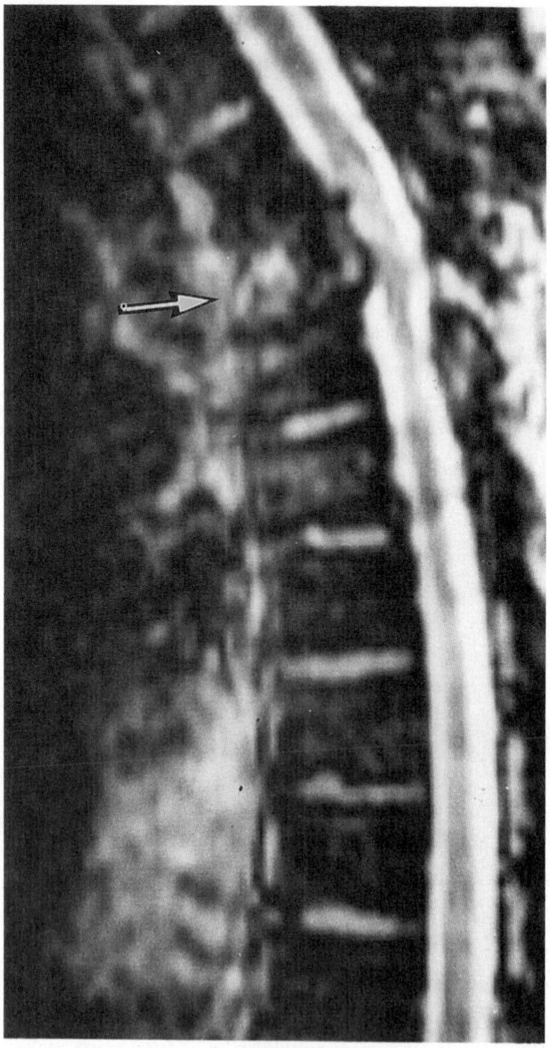

(*A*)

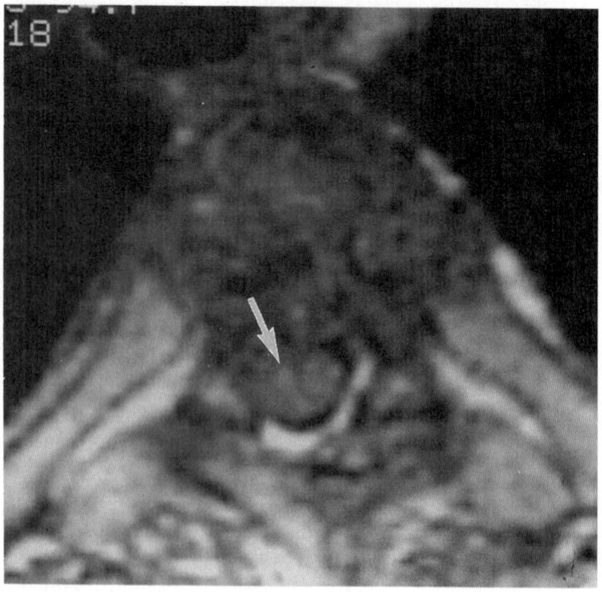

(*B*)

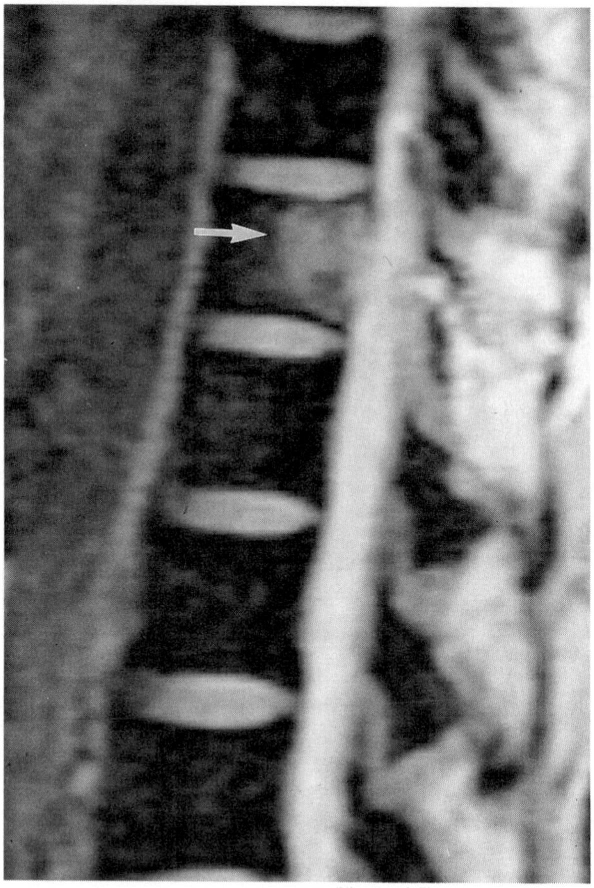

(*C*)

Figure 177-4 Spinal epidural lymphoma in a 40-year-old man presenting with a 2-week history of upper thoracic spinal pain and paraparesis progressing rapidly to paraplegia. *A.* Relatively T2-weighted gradient sagittal MRI scan of the thoracic spine showing a high-signal-intensity lesion of the T3 vertebral body *(arrow)* with retropulsion into the ventral epidural space. At surgery, the lesion proved to be a lymphoma, which more typically involves the epidural space without bony involvement. *B.* Corresponding axial T1-weighted spin-echo MRI scan through the T3 vertebral level showing destruction of the vertebral body and extension of tumor into the ventral epidural space and anterior paravertebral region. Note the anterolateral cord compression *(arrow)*, which, as shown here, is better evaluated with axial, rather than sagittal, imaging sequences. *C.* Relatively T2-weighted gradient sagittal MRI scan of the lower thoracic/upper lumbar spine in the same patient showing a high-signal-intensity tumor *(arrow)* involving the T12 vertebral body. This lesion was clinically ''silent.'' Noncontiguous multilevel metastases occur in up to 30 percent of cases, necessitating imaging of the entire spinal axis. A posterolateral thoracotomy was carried out for resection of the T3 vertebral body with decompression of the ventral and lateral epidural space. Bone struts fashioned from the resected rib were placed in the corpectomy site to reconstruct the vertebral body. The patient received postoperative radiotherapy, but failed to recover power or sensation in the lower extremities.

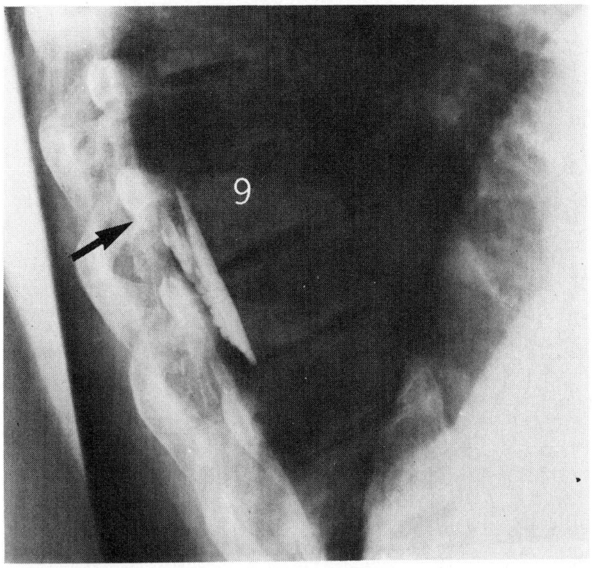

Figure 177-5 A case illustrating the desirability of *complete* MRI or myelographic visualization of the spinal canal prior to radiotherapy or surgery. This patient was a 65-year-old man with a history of prostatic carcinoma who presented with low back pain and mild weakness in the legs. Plain x-ray films showed multiple osteolytic lesions of the midlumbar region for which he received a course of radiotherapy, but without a prior MRI scan or myelogram. Lumbar pain was relieved, but 3 weeks after completion of radiotherapy he was referred to the neurosurgical service with a 1-week history of rapid development of paraparesis. This myelogram showed a complete block at T8–T9 *(arrow)*, several segments above the uppermost limit of the radiotherapy exposure. If the patient had had the myelogram prior to radiotherapy, the T8–T9 metastatic lesion would probably have been identified and the radiation ports would have been extended to include the thoracic metastatic deposit. Radiotherapy to the thoracic region was now out of the question, because the radiotherapy port would be adjacent to an area of the cord that had already been maximally exposed to radiation. Consequently, surgical decompression was carried out, giving only slight improvement in the paraparesis. MRI or myelography to visualize the entire spinal canal, and not restricted to the area of obvious clinical concern, is recommended, in order to identify multiple tumor deposits that may have a bearing on management by radiotherapy or surgical decompression.

asymmetrical motor and sensory loss in the lower limbs. By comparison, compression of the lower spinal cord (conus medullaris) may be identified by a more complete and symmetrical distribution of neurological signs. Compression of the conus or cauda equina characteristically produces saddle anesthesia and loss of sphincter control.

On examination of the spine, the patient's characteristic pain is commonly reproduced by spinal movement or by palpation or gentle fist percussion over the vertebral spinous processes at the affected level.

When there is some question regarding bladder dysfunction, the situation can be clarified by having the patient void, then introducing a urinary catheter to measure the volume of residual urine (''postvoid residual''). A neurogenic bladder may be assumed to be present if the residual urine volume is more than 150 ml.

Benign Tumors

When located in the epidural space, a benign tumor (neurilemoma, neurofibroma, or meningioma) is likely to cause nerve root irritation with associated radicular pain or dysesthesia (Figs. 177-1 to 177-3). As the tumor enlarges and produces spinal cord compression, segmental sensory or motor disturbances develop. Brown–Sequard's syndrome is more apt to occur in benign tumors than in epidural metastatic tumors because benign tumors are more commonly confined to one side. Besides their absence of a history of malignant disease, patients with benign epidural tumors are likely to have symptoms of longer duration—months to years—than patients with metastatic tumors.

Diagnostic Studies

Diagnostic imaging of spinal tumors is presented in Chapter 174. However, some general principles concerning selection of diagnostic studies, of particular relevance to epidural tumors, are discussed here.

Spinal Roentgenography

A minimum of 50 percent local bone destruction must occur in order for a lesion to be detected on plain x-ray films[14]; roentgenography may therefore miss early metastatic lesions. In one study, 15 percent of patients with a complete high-grade epidural block had no bony involvement on roentgenograms.[23] Metastatic spinal involvement may appear as osteolytic or osteoblastic lesions (Fig. 177-6*A*); there may be associated vertebral body collapse, but the disc space is generally preserved. Plain films of the suspected portion of the vertebral column show evidence of metastatic involvement in about 60 percent of patients who are subsequently shown to have spinal cord or nerve root compression.[52] Plain films are normal in two-thirds of cases with spinal involvement secondary to lymphoma.[25] The radiographic lesion corresponds approximately to the level of spinal cord or nerve root compression, although epidural tumor may be present without radiographic evidence of vertebral involvement.

In view of its relatively unpredictable diagnostic yield, we do not recommend roentgenography for routine screening in patients suspected of harboring one or more spinal metastases. Roentgenography is of value, however, in identifying areas of bone destruction and malalignment in planning surgical intervention. Portenoy et al.[37] attempted to develop criteria to select patients for definitive imaging on the basis of patients' symptoms (focal pain or neurological dysfunction), plain films, and radioisotope scans. In their study, 86 percent of symptomatic patients with abnormal roentgenograms were subsequently found to have epidural disease compared with 8 percent of similar patients with normal roentgenograms. Vertebral collapse on plain films was highly predictive of an epidural lesion. The combination of an abnormal roentgenogram and an abnormal isotope bone scan was even more predictive.

Despite such criteria for selecting patients for additional imaging studies, we are of the opinion that plain films do not have sufficient diagnostic yield to warrant their use for routine screening of patients with suspected spinal metastasis. In view of the importance of *early* treatment, the clinician needs to identify not only metastatic epidural lesions but also those metastases limited

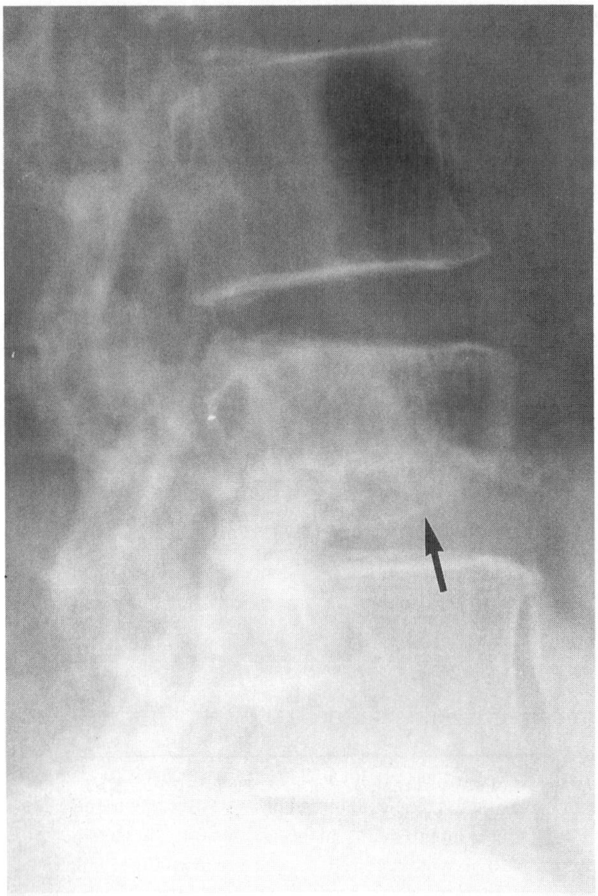

(*A*)

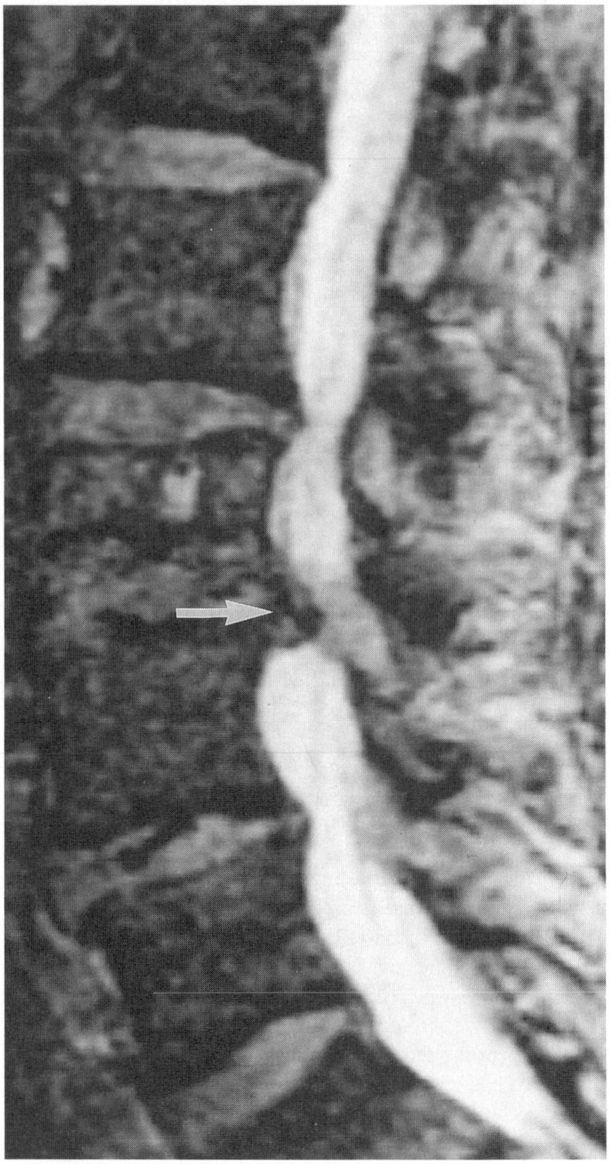

(*B*)

Figure 177-6 Metastatic breast carcinoma in a 70-year-old woman who presented with a several-week history of low back pain, paraparesis, and difficulty with micturition. *A.* Lateral plain film of the lumbar spine showing osteolytic metastatic disruption *(arrow)* of the L3 vertebral body with a pathologic compression fracture. *B.* Sagittal T2-weighted MRI scan showing posterior epidural extension of tumor and possibly retropulsed bone fragments with compression of the thecal sac. When radiotherapy failed to control the pain, and in view of the progressive paraparesis, a decompressive laminectomy was carried out with removal of the ventral epidural compression and stabilization by means of posterior rods and pedicular screws.

to bone. To minimize the risk of delaying diagnosis with nondefinitive studies, the cost and time of roentgenography (and isotope bone scans) can be avoided; resources are better directed to expeditious spinal neuroimaging [magnetic resonance imaging (MRI), myelography, or computed tomography (CT)–myelography].

Radioisotope Bone Scanning

Abnormal uptake of an isotope may ''light up'' a metastatic deposit in the spine before it becomes radiographically evident.[14] The resolution of such scans is not adequate, however, to clearly define the anatomy of a lesion; other imaging studies are therefore necessary to aid in diagnosis and management. An advantage of a skeletal isotope survey is the early identification of extraspinal bony and soft tissue (e.g., liver, brain) metastasis.[14] In a study of the predictive value of isotope scans in identifying patients with epidural disease, it was found that 69 percent of symptomatic patients with abnormal scans had epidural disease, compared with 0 percent of those with normal scans.[37] Isotope scanning has been shown to be a more sensitive, but less specific, indicator of epidural disease than spine roentgenography.

Magnetic Resonance Imaging

Magnetic resonance imaging is emerging as the best screening study for evaluating patients with suspected spinal metastasis. Because of the relatively high incidence (17 to 33 percent)[23,42,54] of multiple separate metastases, it is desirable to image the *entire* spine, even though there may be no clinical evidence of spinal involvement in a particular area (Figs. 177-4*C* and 177-5); some lesions may be clinically ''silent.'' MRI is superior to myelography in revealing paravertebral masses. However, CT is superior to MRI in detecting cortical bone destruction because the MRI signal

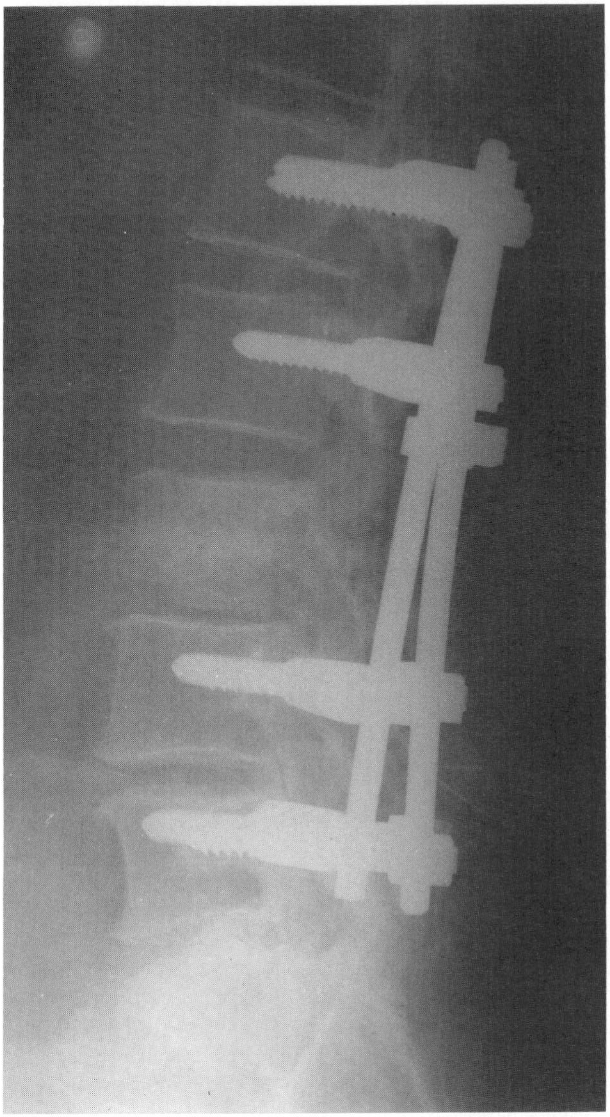

(*C*)

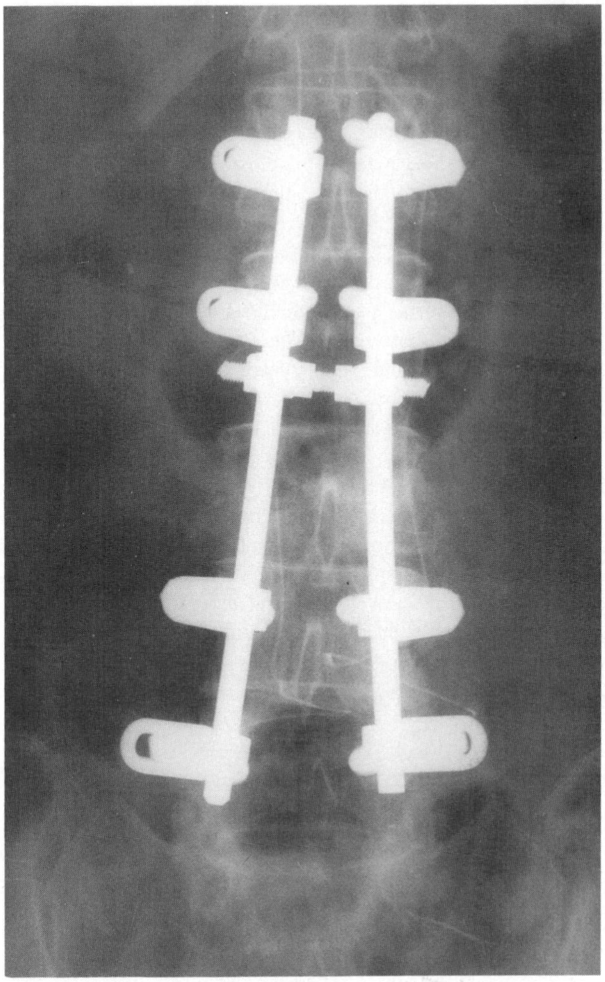

(*D*)

Figure 177-6 (*Continued*) Lateral (*C*) and anteroposterior (*D*) plain films of the lumbar spine show the instrumentation. Postoperatively, the pain and weakness improved but the bladder symptoms persisted.

from cortical bone is relatively poor.[55] MRI is comparable to myelography in detecting large epidural masses compressing the cord,[47] but smaller epidural lesions causing radiculopathy are better identified with myelography.[26] Gadolinium enhancement has further increased the value of MRI.[51] Epidural tumors show patchy enhancement and the contrast may also differentiate epidural tumor from disc herniation because disc material does not enhance. Bone metastases successfully treated with radiation do not enhance, whereas unresponsive metastases continue to show enhancement.

The cost of spinal MRI is comparable to the combined cost of a myelogram followed by postcontrast CT; MRI has the advantage of being noninvasive. Movement artifact can degrade the MRI, however, so this modality may not be useful in an uncooperative patient; claustrophobia and the presence of ferrous-metal implants represent other limitations.

Myelography

In situations where MRI is not available or not feasible (e.g., in uncooperative or claustrophobic patients and in those with ferrous-metal implants), myelography is a suitable alternative for identifying an epidural mass lesion. Myelography is superior to MRI for detecting small epidural lesions.[26] Myelography and MRI are equivalent in detecting clinically significant (large) epidural lesions.[47] As in the case of MRI, it is desirable to visualize the *entire* spinal axis in search of multiple lesions. ''Blind'' radiotherapy or ''blind'' surgical decompression, relying on clinical examination and limited visualization of the spinal axis, risks missing multiple tumor deposits at different levels (Figs. 177-4 and 177-5). Although an extradural tumor deposit is usually limited to one or two adjacent vertebral segments, clinically unsuspected multiple separate tumor deposits occur in different portions of the spinal canal in 17 to 30 percent of cases.[23,42,54]

In the presence of a complete myelographic block, it is important to visualize the upper limit of the block. If the contrast agent (generally a water-soluble agent) does not flow spontaneously around the block to reach the upper end, tilting the patient on the fluoroscopy table with the head inclined downward and injecting a few milliliters of air from below will slightly increase the pressure in the subarachnoid space and thereby force a small quantity of the contrast medium past the obstruction. If this measure fails to identify the upper end of the block, contrast medium can be injected into the spinal subarachnoid space laterally between C1 and C2 or posteriorly in the midline into the cisterna magna. The advantage of a separate injection from above is its ability to reveal the upper end of the lesion as well as to visualize the remainder of the spinal canal above the block. Alternatively, the cephalad limit of the metastasis may be defined by a postmyelogram spinal CT scan; in most cases, sufficient contrast medium leaks around the mass to show the upper end of the block on the CT scan.[8] A disadvantage of the latter technique is that the spinal canal above the block is not fully visualized. Regardless, however, whether a separate injection of contrast medium is made above the level of the block, postcontrast CT through the abnormal areas shown on the myelogram is a useful adjunct in revealing greater detail of the relationship between the tumor, the neural elements, and bone.

An acute increase in neurological deficit may occur after myelography, generally thought to be the result of downward herniation of the spinal cord induced by the reduction of cerebrospinal fluid (CSF) pressure below the lesion. This has been reported in 14 percent of cases following lumbar myelography.[31] In the latter study, however, myelography carried out by C1–2 puncture was not associated with postmyelographic deterioration, and the authors therefore recommended C1–2 puncture as a safe and effective alternative for myelography in patients suspected of having spinal epidural metastasis.

Computed Tomography Scanning

Computed tomography is more sensitive and specific than plain roentgenography or radionuclide scanning in identifying spinal metastases[10] or benign tumors. It is best used, however, following myelography or as an adjunct to MRI. As an aid in planning surgical intervention, CT with bone windows is useful for defining the anatomy of bone destruction.[17] CT is limited in identifying cortical disruption in cases of severe osteoporosis; cortical margins may also appear indistinct in cases with osteoblastic metastases (such as those arising from prostate cancer).

Ancillary Diagnostic Studies

Routine chest roentgenography and, depending on circumstances, studies such as prostatic-specific antigen (PSA), mammography, and abdominal and chest CT may identify a primary neoplasm. Fluoroscopic or CT-guided biopsy of the paraspinal tumor mass by the open or percutaneous needle technique may reveal the diagnosis in patients in whom surgical decompression of the mass is not feasible. Lumbar puncture for examination of CSF is generally not necessary except in instances where CSF cytopathology may be needed in patients suspected of having leptomeningeal carcinomatosis or an infection (such as an abscess in the extradural or subdural space).

Management

Metastatic Epidural Cancer

Complexity of the Problem

Because cure is usually beyond expectation, palliation is a reasonable goal in the management of patients with spinal metastasis. Preservation or restoration of neurological function—ambulation and bladder control—is the criterion of successful therapy. Pain relief is also an important, but secondary, goal that may often be achieved by treatment of the metastatic tumor. When the decision is not to treat the metastatic tumor, control of pain becomes the primary concern.

Radiotherapy and surgical decompression are the keystones of management. Despite long experience with both therapeutic modalities, individually and in combination, the relative merits of each for spinal metastases have not yet been clarified. Much of the difficulty in analysis relates to sorting out the influence of factors such as the biological activity, radiosensitivity, and systemic spread of the primary tumor; the rate of progression and degree of neurological deficit; and the associated involvement of the vertebral column. This multiplicity of factors is compounded by the fact that to date there have not been any large, prospective, controlled series comparing radiotherapy and surgery; a small prospective clinical trial was inconclusive.[58]

Radiotherapy

Radiotherapy to the area of the spine involved by metastatic tumor produced significant neurological improvement (over pretreatment status) in 13 to 45 percent of patients in different studies.[7,16,23,58] The results are somewhat better for radiosensitive tumors, such as Hodgkin's and non-Hodgkin's lymphoma, multiple myeloma, seminoma, and neuroblastoma, with an improvement rate of about 50 percent.[7] The outlook is less favorable for tumors less sensitive to radiotherapy, including the carcinomas, melanomas, and soft tissue sarcomas.[23]

There has been concern that radiation therapy may result in neurological deterioration, presumably by inducing radiation edema in the tumor and/or spinal cord. This concern has been an important factor prompting the use of decompressive surgery before starting the patient on a course of radiotherapy. Experimental studies, however, do not support the concept of radiation edema. It has been postulated that the increase in tumor volume following small daily radiation doses is caused by the inadequacy of such doses to slow tumor growth rather than by radiation edema.[41]

The usual radiotherapy dose is approximately 3000 to 4000 cGy for treatment of spinal metastasis.[2,28,43] To minimize the risk of radiation myelopathy, fractionation schedules of 2000 cGy in 5 fractions or 3000 cGy in 10 fractions have been recommended as safe regimens for the thoracic spinal cord.[56]

Surgical Decompression Alone (without Radiotherapy)

Neurosurgeons' attitudes regarding surgery for metastatic tumor compression of the spinal cord or cauda equina have varied widely over the years. The proportion of patients significantly benefited by traditional decompressive laminectomy alone was 17 percent in one large series[16] and 20 percent in another.[48] (The more recently introduced *anterior* approaches to the spine, generally combined with radiotherapy, are discussed in the next section of this chapter.)

The operative mortality—death within the first month after laminectomy—has ranged from 3 to 14 percent in various series, with an average mortality of 9 percent.[7] Worsening of neurological status was reported in various studies, with an overall mean of 12 percent.[7] Surgical morbidity following laminectomy (independent of neurological deterioration) included wound infection, CSF leakage, and instability with subluxation of the spine, with a mean of 11 percent.[7] In summary, the hazards of laminectomy consist of an estimated 9 percent risk of death, 12 percent risk of neurological worsening, and 11 percent risk of other complications.

Prior to the past decade, surgical decompression for spinal metastasis almost always implied a wide laminectomy in the region of the tumor mass. In some cases, the decompression was limited to a laminectomy or hemilaminectomy, without any tumor resection; spinal stabilization (except in the cervical region[15]) was usually not carried out. An unknown proportion of the laminectomy cases probably had ventral cord compression by tumor and/or vertebral body collapse. This factor may account for the relatively low rate of improvement (17 to 20 percent), because decompressive laminectomy limits the neurosurgeon's ability to remove tumors other than those located in the posterior portion of the epidural space. In a series of 118 patients with spinal metastasis, Hall and Mackay[27] reported that posterior decompression (laminectomy) improved 39 percent of the patients when the tumor was posterior, 35 percent when the lesion was lateral, 25 percent when the tumor was circumferential, and only 9 percent when the lesion was in the anterior epidural space. This suggests that, because laminectomy is effective primarily for posteriorly and laterally placed tumors, an anterior or lateral surgical approach to the spine is needed when the tumor or bone mass is located ventrally. In this regard, the majority of epidural tumors are believed to arise in a vertebral body.[3,4,52]

Combined Therapy: Surgical Decompression Plus Radiotherapy

In various reported series of combined therapy in which *laminectomy* was the surgical technique employed, pooled data revealed a mean improvement rate of 44 percent.[7,16,48] In two of the large retrospective series, the combination of laminectomy plus radiotherapy resulted in improved neurological status in a mean of 36 percent of patients, compared with 26 percent of those treated with radiotherapy alone and 18 percent with surgery alone.[16,48] A prospective study of 29 patients comparing the combination of laminectomy plus radiotherapy versus radiotherapy alone revealed improvement in 16 percent of the patients in both groups.[58] For tumors of the lymphoma type, the results after combined therapy were considerably better, with a pooled improvement rate of 68 percent.[7]

In the above series of combined therapy in which *laminectomy* was the surgical technique employed, no indication was given by the authors as to the proportion of cases that had *anterior* compression of the cord and/or vertebral body collapse. Surgical decompression by laminectomy in those situations where the tumor mass lies anterior to the cord is not likely to achieve the maximum potential of surgical intervention.

In the early 1980s, reports began to appear concerning an anterior approach to the spine for metastatic epidural cord or cauda equina compression. The technique consists of vertebral body resection and stabilization in the cervical, thoracic, or lumbar spine.[17,28,44,50] Significant improvement in ambulation was reported in 51 to 87 percent of cases, even in some patients who were paraplegic; a high percentage of patients also experienced pain relief and, in two of the series,[28,50] almost half to three-quarters of patients with nerve-root deficit showed neurological improvement. Mortality ranged from 0 to 7 percent, neurological worsening, 0 to 6 percent; and other morbidity, 10 to 15 percent.[17,28,44,50]

Although the average mortality and operative morbidity are roughly comparable for both the anterior and posterior (laminectomy) approaches, the anterior approach *seems* to be superior with respect to the prospect for neurological improvement and the lower chance of neurological worsening. However, direct comparison of the relative merits of the anterior versus the posterior approach is unwarranted, because previous reports of laminectomy probably included cases with *anterior* cord compression and instability. The apparently less-favorable outcome of laminectomy may well reflect, to some degree, the inappropriate use of the posterior approach.

As surgical experience has evolved, some authors have recommended a ''blend'' of the posterior laminectomy or hemilaminectomy approach, modified with the addition of pedicle resection to permit safe access to the ventral aspect of the spinal canal.[32,43] Results in terms of ambulation, mortality, and morbidity are comparable to those of the anterior approach.[17,28,44,50] There is thus a place for the respective anterior and posterior (laminectomy) approaches, each with its own indications and limitations. The neurosurgeon has a range of options, the selection of approach being based on analysis of the neurological and neuroimaging factors in each case.

Regardless of the approach, the mortality/morbidity risk must be weighed against the potential benefit in the individual patient and needs to be taken into account when comparing surgical intervention with other forms of therapy.

Surgical decompression—by laminectomy or by an anterior approach—is carried out initially to effect prompt relief of cord compression. An internal stabilization procedure (with methyl methacrylate and/or bone graft, metal rods, wire, or plates) is added when spinal stability needs to be restored.[15,28,44,50] Postoperative radiotherapy is intended to eradicate or suppress the regrowth of residual tumor tissue. Reduction of the ''tumor burden'' by surgical resection is also thought to enhance the effectiveness of radiotherapy.[11,28] Methyl methacrylate and metal instrumentation provide immediate spinal stability (so that postoperative orthoses are not necessary) and do not interfere with subsequent radiotherapy. Radiation, however, may compromise fusion with bone so that, in such cases, the total dose of radiation may need to be reduced[28]; there is also concern that tumor may grow into the bone graft. Some authors, however, report the use of bone grafts without mention of their being affected by subsequent radiotherapy.[15,44,50]

Recommended Guidelines for Management

The following guidelines are proposed as tentative criteria for management, to be modified with the further evolution of clinical experience and research.

Radiotherapy may be viewed as the primary or basic mode of treatment for the management of metastatic disease of the spine in the absence of neurological deficit; or where pain is the main symptom. It is most clearly indicated for radiosensitive tumors, such as the lymphomas and myeloma; its advantages are less clear-cut for radioresistant neoplasms. When there is a known diagnosis of extraspinal lymphoma, a trial of local spinal irradiation would be reasonable without the need for tissue biopsy of the spinal lesion or surgical decompression.[1] When there is radiographic evidence of bony involvement only, without encroachment on the spinal canal, radiotherapy can be expected to provide satisfactory pain relief.[16,28] It has been suggested that ''curative resection'' may be considered when the metastasis is limited to the vertebral body.[50] If spinal stability is preserved, additional support and pain relief may be provided by an external brace. When there is a question regarding stability, internal fixation by fusion and instrumentation, followed by postoperative irradiation, should be considered.

Indications for Surgical Intervention

The following six indications are presented as relative rather than absolute criteria for surgery because a number of other considerations must be taken into account, including general medical condition, histology of the primary tumor, extent of metastatic disease elsewhere, and the patient's attitude concerning aggressive treatment. Minimum life expectancy of 3 to 4 months appears reasonable.[17]

1. *Spinal instability or compression by bone.* When spinal instability endangers spinal cord or nerve root function, or when a pathologic fracture produces direct compression of the neural structures, surgical decompression and possible fusion and instrumentation should be strongly considered.
2. *Failure to respond to radiotherapy.* In the case of relatively radiosensitive tumors, further decline in neurological function or failure to improve during the course of radiotherapy should prompt early consideration of surgical decompression.
3. *Known radioresistance of the tumor.* When the tumor is known to be radioresistant, decompressive surgery might be considered as the primary mode of therapy, supplemented by postoperative radiation in the hope that it might retard tumor regrowth.
4. *Previous radiation exposure of the spinal cord.* Surgical decompression may have to be considered when the patient has had a previous course of radiotherapy to the spine such that further radiotherapy might exceed the spinal cord tolerance for radiation. This applies even in the case of highly radiosensitive tumors.
5. *Diagnosis in doubt.* Surgical decompression is advisable to establish a tissue diagnosis when the nature of the intraspinal lesion is in doubt. Surgery in these cases should generally be followed by radiotherapy. When there is a paraspinal mass, it may be feasible to obtain a percutaneous needle biopsy under fluoroscopic or CT guidance.
6. *Repeat surgical decompression for recurrent tumor.* When radiotherapy cannot be used, reoperation for removal of recurrent tumor is warranted for relapse occurring months or years after previous spinal decompression for metastatic tumor.

Surgical Technique

It is important to individualize the approach to the spine on the basis of the location of the tumor mass or bony compression in the spinal canal. Consideration also must be given to the necessity to maintain or restore spinal stability. Irrespective of the surgical approach employed in a given case, a measure of safety is added by intraoperative neurophysiological monitoring with somatosensory or motor-evoked potentials.

Posterior and Posterolateral Approaches (Laminectomy) Lesions situated in the posterior compartment of the spinal canal are approached through a standard, wide multilevel laminectomy, extending longitudinally one level above and below the area of dural compression. After resection (debulking) of the epidural tumor, a rubber catheter is passed cephalad and caudad in the extradural space to detect any additional lesions.

In the case of a circumferential epidural mass lesion without bone involvement and without a history of cancer, a laminectomy for diagnosis and decompression is a reasonable approach. In the absence of vertebral involvement, lymphoma is a diagnostic consideration.

When a decompressive laminectomy is carried out in the presence of vertebral body collapse, there is considerable risk that the removal of the laminar arch may increase the instability and result in further cord and/or nerve root compression.[22,28,50] In such instances, the surgical plan may include laminectomy (or hemilaminectomy) and posterior stabilization, or combined anterior and posterior decompression with stabilization.[32,43] In the lumbar area, in view of the greater mobility of the cauda equina (below the level of L2), it is often possible to achieve satisfactory decompression by a posterior (laminectomy) approach even when the mass is located ventral to the dural sac (Fig. 177-6). To approach a ventral mass or vertebral body in the thoracic or lumbar spine, it may be necessary to remove the facets and pedicle, at least on one side. When there is associated instability in the cervical, thoracic, or lumbar area, posterior fusion and instrumentation is carried out during the same operation (Fig. 177-6). Simultaneous posterior and anterior stabilization may be desirable when both the posterior and anterior elements are disrupted.[32]

Anterior and Lateral Approaches Metastatic lesions involving the vertebral body are best managed by an anterior or lateral decompression and stabilization.[15,17,28,44,50] An outline of anterior and lateral approaches to the cervical, thoracic, and lumbar spine is shown in Table 177-1.

In the cervical region and down to the level of T1–2, the standard anterior approach is used with a transverse incision on either the right or left side for a one-level exposure; an oblique incision (parallel to the sternocleidomastoid muscle) is used for a multilevel cervical corpectomy. For cervical decompression by either the anterior or posterior route, awake endotracheal intubation minimizes excessive neck manipulation in the process of intubation and positioning the patient. Gardner–Wells tongs for intraoperative traction provide stability,[15] although this may not be essential.[28]

To approach the thoracic spine (T3–11), a posterolateral thoracotomy or costotransversectomy approach is used. The exposure may be from either side, depending on the site of bony involvement; for the upper thoracic spine (T1–4), a right-sided thoracic exposure avoids the aortic arch. (T1 and T2 may also be reached by the standard anterior cervical route.) The skin incision for the

TABLE 177-1 Anterior and Lateral Approaches to the Spine

Cervical	
C1–C2	Anterior cervical/retropharyngeal, or transmandibular median glossotomy
C3–C7	Anterior cervical (transverse or oblique incision)
Thoracic	
T1–T2	Anterior cervical/transsternal, or posterolateral thoracotomy
T3–T11	Posterolateral thoracotomy or costotransversectomy
Thoracolumbar	
T11–L2	Posterolateral thoracotomy/retroperitoneal (flank incision)
Lumbar	
L2–L5	Retroperitoneal (flank incision)
L5–S1	Transabdominal (laparotomy)

Source: Modified from Sundaresan et al.[50]

transthoracic approach is made in the intercostal space corresponding to the level above the involved vertebral body, and the rib is resected.[28] Segmental vessels are ligated one segment above and one segment below the target vertebra to avoid tearing these vessels when the vertebral space is expanded with a spreader.[28]

A combined posterolateral thoracotomy/retroperitoneal approach is used for lesions in the region of the thoracolumbar junction (T11–L2). A left-sided skin incision is preferred and is centered two intercostal interspaces above the target vertebra. The posterolateral corner of the diaphragm can be detached to facilitate the exposure.[9]

The lower lumbar vertebrae can be approached through a retroperitoneal flank incision (preferably on the left side), but a transabdominal laparatomy approach may provide better exposure at the L5–S1 level.[50]

Having reached the appropriate spinal level, a corpectomy is carried out at the involved vertebral body, including the adjacent discs. The posterior cortex of the vertebral body and the posterior longitudinal ligament need to be removed in order to decompress the anterior and anterolateral extradural space.[15,44]

Stabilization is achieved with bone and/or methyl methacrylate,[44] with Steinman pins[50] or distraction rods and hooks[28] incorporated in the acrylic. A modification of the technique for vertebral reconstruction involves bridging the vertebral defect with Silastic tubing that is then filled with methyl methacrylate; the Silastic tube, the ends of which are fitted into a trough in the vertebrae above and below the defect, prevents dislodgement of the acrylic.[20] Another option is the application of metal plates and screws to the anterolateral aspect of the adjacent vertebral bodies.

Posterolateral decompression and stabilization has been recommended as an alternative to the anterior approach for thoracic or lumbar metastases.[32,43] The technique, similar to that recommended by Erickson et al.[19] for thoracolumbar fractures, entails a midline posterior incision. In the thoracic region, the approach is similar to a costotransversectomy but includes a hemilaminectomy and resection of the facet and pedicle so as to gain exposure to the lateral portion of the vertebral body. Another variation is a lateral parascapular extrapleural approach to the upper thoracic spine.[21] These various techniques permit decompression of both the posterior and anterior aspects of the cord or cauda equina in one stage. Stabilization is then carried out posteriorly with Harrington distraction rods or Luque–Drummond instrumentation with sublaminar wiring, or other fixation methods.[43] The approach also permits partial or complete vertebrectomy (corpectomy) followed by anterior stabilization with a high-density polyethylene prosthesis or with methyl methacrylate bone cement.[32] Physiologically, an advantage of the posterolateral approach is the avoidance of the thoracic and abdominal cavities.

Spinal Metastases in Children

Similar to the incidence in adults, 5 percent of children with solid malignant tumors develop spinal epidural metastases with cord compression.[33] In contrast to adults, the common primary neoplasms are Ewing's sarcoma, neuroblastoma, osteogenic sarcoma, rhabdomyosarcoma, Hodgkin's disease, soft tissue sarcoma, and germ cell tumor. In a series of children with cord compression from metastatic sarcoma (Ewing's sarcoma, soft tissue sarcoma, osteogenic sarcoma, and rhabdomyosarcoma), over 50 percent (depending on degree of paraparesis) were significantly improved with decompressive laminectomy.[33] In another study, radiotherapy alone was effective for radiosensitive tumors in patients who were neurologically intact (dosage 2,000 to 5,000 cGy)[39]; however, those with severe cord compression benefited significantly from a combination of decompressive laminectomy for tumor removal followed by adjuvant therapy.

Tumors in the pediatric age group invade the spinal canal via the neural foramen and compress the cord circumferentially so that decompressive laminectomy is an effective surgical approach.[33]

Steroids

Dexamethasone has been shown experimentally in animals to have a dose-related beneficial effect on spinal cord function associated with improvement of blood–spinal cord barrier breakdown and a reduction of edema in the compressed cord.[18] In view of this experimental evidence of the benefit of high-dose steroids in animals, a trial of high-dose steroids combined with radiotherapy was undertaken in humans[24]; dexamethasone 100 mg was given on day 1, then 96 mg daily in four divided doses, then tapered to 0 by day 14. Pain was improved in most patients, but there was no neurological improvement in patients who were paraplegic. Another study with similar high doses of dexamethasone plus radiotherapy for epidural metastasis likewise showed no benefit in ambulation; however, serious complications, thought to be secondary to high-dose steroids, occurred in 14 percent of the patients.[30] The complications included one fatal ulcer hemorrhage, rectal bleeding, and gastrointestinal perforation. The high-dose regimen was abandoned in favor of a more standard dosage (16 mg daily, reduced to 0 in 14 days); this was associated with several complications, none serious.

It has been reported that steroids (dexamethasone, 16 mg daily) may have an oncolytic effect on spinal epidural metastases[38]; in four patients, the epidural tumor was noted to shrink or disappear on myelography, but the tumor subsequently recurred in all cases.

In current practice, corticosteroids in standard dosage are recommended for their protective effect on the spinal cord and nerve roots, and serve as a supplement to radiotherapy or surgical decompression.

Other Adjuvant Therapeutic Modalities

Chemotherapy has not been shown to be of benefit for spinal metastatic carcinoma but may be useful, when combined with radiotherapy, in cord compression secondary to lymphoma,[35] Hodgkin's disease,[45] seminoma,[38] and Ewing's sarcoma.[38]

Nonambulatory patients are prone to deep venous thrombosis and pulmonary embolism, for which prophylactic subcutaneous heparin may be considered. Other preventive measures are antiembolism stockings and pneumatic intermittent compression boots, particularly in the perioperative period. Simple elevation of the lower extremities (easily accomplished by elevating the foot-end of the mattress about 15 degrees) helps to diminish venous stasis by promoting venous return.

External spinal bracing helps to maintain spinal stability and reduce pain. Urinary retention and urinary tract infection may be prevented by intermittent catheterization or, if necessary, with an indwelling Foley catheter. Stool softeners are used to prevent constipation and a regular schedule of enemas may be needed. For patients who are bedridden, skin-care precautions are taken to prevent decubitus ulcers.

No Active Treatment Warranted

When a patient is terminally ill with widely disseminated cancer, there seems to be little value in aggressive management with

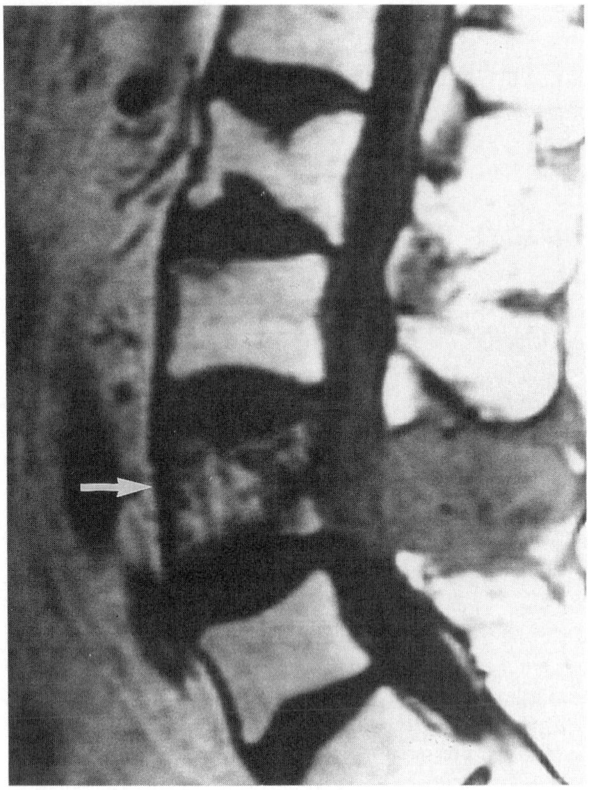

(*A*)

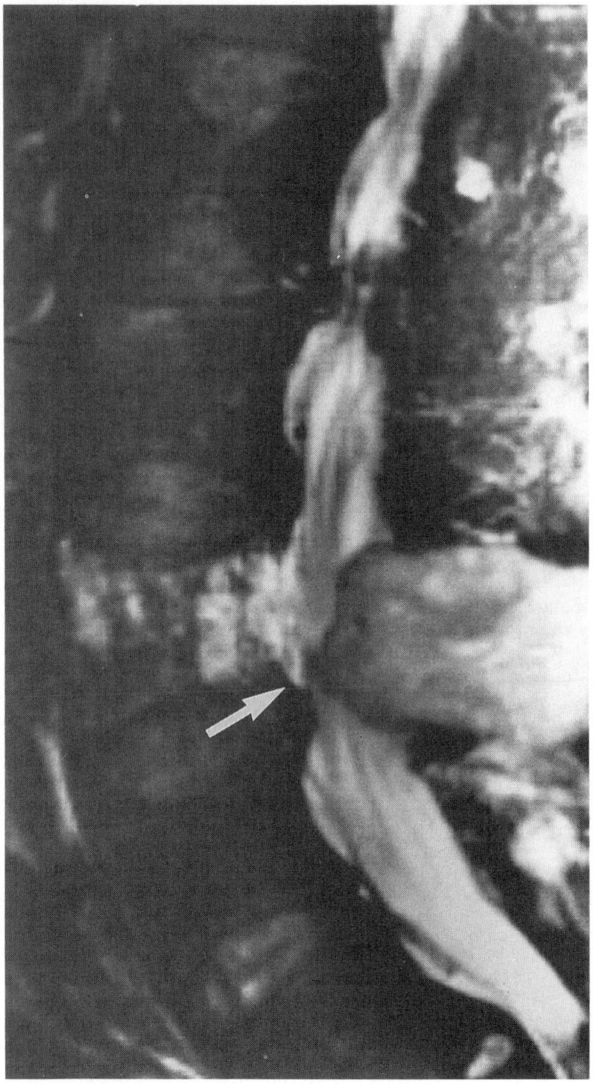

(*B*)

Figure 177-7 Metastatic renal carcinoma in a 66-year-old man with a 2-month history of low back pain, bilateral sciatica, and mild paraparesis with bladder involvement. He was given a course of radiotherapy, which afforded moderate relief of pain but no improvement in the paraparesis. *A*. Following completion of the radiotherapy, the sagittal T1-weighted MRI scan showed metastatic destruction of L4 vertebral body *(arrow)* with associated expansile tumor involvement of the posterior elements. Note the incidental effect of prior radiotherapy with complete fatty marrow replacement, and also benign (degenerative) loss of stature of the L2 vertebral body. *B*. Corresponding T2-weighted sagittal MRI scan shows that the low-signal-intensity tumor in *A* becomes relatively hyperintense with evidence of epidural tumor extension *(arrow)*. A radionuclide bone scan showed widespread metastatic tumor deposits, including in the liver. Life expectancy was less than 3 to 4 months. Nonsurgical palliative hospice care was undertaken.

radiotherapy or surgery. Despite the probability, however, that life expectancy in such patients is limited to a matter of weeks or a few months, radiotherapy may be of value if spinal pain is a problem (Fig. 177-7). An alternative for pain management in such patients is the use of the spinal morphine pump or a similar device, which is usually effective for control of cancer pain. Hospice care is often helpful in these terminal situations.

Benign Epidural Tumors

The treatment of neurilemomas, neurofibromas, and meningiomas is surgical excision, and this can generally be achieved completely. Microsurgical technique contributes considerably to the safety of their removal (Figs. 177-1 to 177-3). Occasionally, meningiomas with a broad attachment and dumbbell neurilemomas or neurofibromas cannot be removed completely. Radiotherapy is not indicated for these benign tumors.

Prognosis

The patient with spinal metastasis is in double jeopardy: from the primary neoplastic disease with its systemic manifestations and the superimposed hazard of spinal cord or cauda equina compromise. Regardless of the nature of treatment, the histology of the primary neoplasm has an important bearing on both survival and the potential for recovery of neurological function. After radiotherapy, the median survival in patients with a lung primary is 1.5 months and for patients with breast primary, the median survival is 9.2 months.[48]

For both benign and malignant epidural tumors, rapid onset and progression of neurological deterioration are associated with a worse prognosis than a gradual onset and slow progression. There is a positive correlation between pretreatment motor status and functional outcome; 60 percent of patients who can walk at the time of diagnosis retain that ability after treatment, whereas only 35 percent of those who are initially paraparetic (mild to moderate weakness) become ambulatory.[12] For patients who present with paraplegia, the outlook for regaining the ability to walk is highly variable; in general, the prognosis is relatively poor if the paraplegia came on abruptly and has been present longer than 24 h; only 0 to 25 percent (in different series) who present with paraplegia recover ambulation,[23,27,34,57] although some authors report a better outlook for such patients.[28,33,43,50]

Conclusions

The majority of patients with spinal metastatic disease present with prodromal symptoms of spinal or radicular pain. In patients with a history of cancer, such symptoms should signal a high index of suspicion of spinal metastasis. Early treatment may avert catastrophic loss of spinal cord or cauda equina function. Therefore, such patients who present with the classical prodromal symptoms—and certainly those who already have myelopathy or radiculopathy—should proceed promptly with definitive neuroimaging. Plain cervical spine films are not a reliable guide to identify those patients who need specialized spinal imaging. MRI has emerged as the most useful imaging modality for spinal metastatic disease; however, when MRI is not feasible or unavailable, myelography with a water-soluble contrast agent (and followed by CT of abnormal areas) is a suitable alternative. Because two or more separate epidural lesions may be present—and may be clinically "silent"—it is necessary to image the entire spinal axis to aid in planning radiotherapy or surgery. The radionuclide scan is a useful adjunct in identifying metastatic disease elsewhere in the body.

The ideal treatment for spinal metastatic disease has not been established. The current mainstay of treatment is radiotherapy alone for radiosensitive tumors (with or without neurological compromise), and in combination with surgical decompression/stabilization for radioresistant tumors. Regardless of the radiosensitivity of the tumor, surgery is considered when the compression is due to retropulsed bone or disc fragments or secondary to spinal malalignment. Surgery is also warranted in situations where the histology of the spinal lesion is unknown. The selection of surgical approach is predicated on the location of the mass lesion in the spinal canal (anterior versus posterior) and the need to maintain or restore spinal stability. The wide range of surgical options for decompression and stabilization offer the patient with metastatic spinal disease an improved outlook for maintenance or recovery of neurological function.

References

1. Aabo K, Walbom-Jorgensen S. Central nervous system complications by malignant lymphomas: radiation schedule and treatment results. *Int J Radiat Oncol Biol Phys* 1986; 12:197–202.
2. Ampil FL. Epidural compression from metastatic tumor with resultant paralysis. *J Neurooncol* 1989; 7:129–136.
3. Arguello F, Baggs RB, Duerst RE, et al. Pathogenesis of vertebral metastasis and epidural spinal cord compression. *Cancer* 1990; 65:98–106.
4. Barron KD, Hirano A, Araki S, Terry RD. Experiences with metastatic neoplasms involving the spinal cord. *Neurology* 1959; 9:91–106.
5. Batson OV. The function of the vertebral veins and their role in the spread of metastases. *Ann Surg* 1940; 112:138–149.
6. Black P. Injuries of the vertebral column and spinal cord: mechanisms and management in the acute phase. In Zuidema GD, Rutherford RB, Ballinger WF II (eds): *The Management of Trauma,* 3d ed. Philadelphia: Saunders, 1979, pp 226–253.
7. Black P. Spinal metastasis: current status and recommended guidelines for management. *Neurosurgery* 1979; 5:726–746.
8. Boesen J, Johnsen A, Helweg-Lersen S, Soelberg Sorensen P. Diagnostic value of spinal computer tomography in patients with intraspinal metastases causing complete block on myelography. *Acta Radiol* 1991; 32:1–2.
9. Bradford DS, Winter RB, Lonstein JE, Moe JH. Techniques of anterior spinal surgery for the management of kyphosis. *Clin Orthop* 1977; 128:129–139.
10. Braunstein EM, Kuhns LR. Computed tomographic demonstration of spinal metastases. *Spine* 1983; 8:912–915.
11. Brice J, McKissock W. Surgical treatment of malignant extradural spinal tumours. *Br Med J* 1965; 1:1341–1344.
12. Bruckman JE, Bloomer WD. Management of spinal cord compression. *Semin Oncol* 1978; 5:135–140.
13. Chade HO. Metastatic tumours of the spine and spinal cord. In Vinken PJ, Bruyn GW (eds): *Handbook of Clinical Neurology,* vol 20. Amsterdam: North-Holland, 1976, pp 415–433.
14. Charkes ND, Sklaroff DM, Young I. A critical analysis of strontium bone scanning for detection of metastatic cancer. *Am J Roentgenol* 1966; 96:647–656.
15. Conley FK, Britt RH, Hanbery JW, Silverberg GD. Anterior fibular strut graft in neoplastic disease of the cervical spine. *J Neurosurg* 1979; 51:677–684.
16. Constans JP, de Divitiis E, Donzelli R, et al. Spinal metastases with neurological manifestations. Review of 600 cases. *J Neurosurg* 1983; 59:111–118.
17. Cooper PR, Errico TJ, Martin R, et al. A systematic approach to spinal reconstruction after anterior decompression for neoplastic disease of the thoracic and lumbar spine. *Neurosurgery* 1993; 32:1–8.
18. Delattre JY, Arbit E, Thaler HT, et al. A dose–response study of dexamethasone in a model of spinal cord compression caused by epidural tumor. *J Neurosurg* 1989; 70:920–925.
19. Erickson DL, Leider LL Jr, Brown WB. One-stage decompression-stabilization for thoracolumbar fractures. *Spine* 1977; 2:53–56.
20. Errico TJ, Cooper PR. A new method of thoracic and lumbar body replacement for spinal tumors: technical note. *Neurosurgery* 1993; 32:678–681.
21. Fessler RG, Dietze DD Jr, Millan MM, Peace D. Lateral parascapular extrapleural approach to the upper thoracic spine. *J Neurosurg* 1991; 75:349–355.
22. Findlay GFG. The role of vertebral body collapse in the management of malignant spinal cord compression. *J Neurol Neurosurg Psychiatry* 1987; 50:151–154.
23. Gilbert RW, Kim JH, Posner JB. Epidural spinal cord compression from metastatic tumor: diagnosis and treatment. *Ann Neurol* 1978; 3:40–51.
24. Greenberg HS, Kim JH, Posner JB. Epidural spinal cord compression from metastatic tumor: results with a new treatment protocol. *Ann Neurol* 1980; 8:361–366.
25. Haddad P, Thaell JF, Kiely JM, et al. Lymphoma of the spinal extradural space. *Cancer* 1976; 38:1862–1866.
26. Hagenau C, Grosh W, Currie M, Wiley RG. Comparison of spinal magnetic resonance imaging and myelography in cancer patients. *J Clin Oncol* 1987; 5:1663–1669.
27. Hall AJ, Mackay NNS. The results of laminectomy for compression of the cord or cauda equina by extradural malignant tumour. *J Bone Joint Surg [Br]* 1973; 55:497–505.
28. Harrington KD. Anterior cord decompression and spinal stabilization for patients with metastatic lesions of the spine. *J Neurosurg* 1984; 61:107–117.
29. Harrison KM, Muss HB, Ball MR, et al. Spinal cord compression in breast cancer. *Cancer* 1985; 55:2839–2844.

30. Heimdal K, Hirschberg H, Slettebo H, et al. High incidence of serious side effects of high-dose dexamethasone treatment in patients with epidural spinal cord compression. *J Neurooncol* 1992; 12:141–144.
31. Hollis PH, Malis LI, Zappulla RA. Neurological deterioration after lumbar puncture below complete spinal subarachnoid block. *J Neurosurg* 1986; 64:253–256.
32. Johnston FG, Uttley D, Marsh HT. Synchronous vertebral decompression and posterior stabilization in the treatment of spinal malignancy. *Neurosurgery* 1989; 25:872–876.
33. Klein SL, Sanford RA, Muhlbauer MS. Pediatric spinal epidural metastases. *J Neurosurg* 1991; 74:70–75.
34. Livingston KE, Perrin RG. The neurosurgical management of spinal metastases causing cord and cauda equina compression. *J Neurosurg* 1978; 49:839–843.
35. Murphy WT, Bilge N. Compression of the spinal cord in patients with malignant lymphoma. *Radiology* 1964; 82:495–501.
36. Nittner K. Spinal meningiomas, neurinomas and neurofibromas and hourglass tumors. In Vinken PJ, Bruyn BW (eds): *Handbook of Clinical Neurology*, vol 20. Amsterdam: North-Holland, 1976, pp 177–322.
37. Portenoy RK, Galer BS, Salamon O, et al. Identification of epidural neoplasm. Radiography and bone scintigraphy in the symptomatic and asymptomatic spine. *Cancer* 1989; 64:2207–2213.
38. Posner JB, Howieson J, Cvitkovic E. "Disappearing" spinal cord compression: oncolytic effect of glucocorticoids (and other chemotherapeutic agents) on epidural metastases. *Ann Neurol* 1977; 2:409–413.
39. Raffel C, Neave VCD, Lavine S, McComb JG. Treatment of spinal cord compression by epidural malignancy in childhood. *Neurosurgery* 1991; 28:349–352.
40. Rubin H, Lome LG, Presman D. Neurological manifestation of metastatic prostatic carcinoma. *J Urol* 1974; 111:799–802.
41. Rubin P. Extradural spinal cord compression by tumor: Part I. Experimental production and treatment trials. *Radiology* 1969; 93:1243–1248.
42. Ruff RL, Lanska DJ. Epidural metastases in prospectively evaluated veterans with cancer and back pain. *Cancer* 1989; 63:2234–2241.
43. Shaw B, Mansfield FL, Borges L. One-stage posterolateral decompression and stabilization for primary and metastatic vertebral tumors in the thoracic and lumbar spine. *J Neurosurg* 1989; 70:405–410.
44. Siegal T, Siegal T, Robin G, et al. Anterior decompression of the spine for metastatic epidural cord compression: a promising avenue of therapy? *Ann Neurol* 1982; 11:28–34.
45. Silverberg IJ, Jacobs EM. Treatment of spinal cord compression in Hodgkin's disease. *Cancer* 1971; 27:308–313.
46. Slooff JL, Kernahan JW, McCarty CS. *Primary Intramedullary Tumors of the Spinal Cord and Filum Terminale*. Philadelphia: Saunders, 1964.
47. Smoker WRK, Godersky JC, Knutzon RK, et al. The role of MR imaging in evaluating metastatic spinal disease. *Am J Roentgenol* 1987; 149:1241–1248.
48. Sorensen PS, Borgesen SE, Rohde K, et al. Metastatic epidural spinal cord compression. Results of treatment and survival. *Cancer* 1990; 65:1502–1508.
49. Stark RJ, Henson RA, Evans SJ. Spinal metastasis: a retrospective survey from a general hospital. *Brain* 1982; 105:189–213.
50. Sundaresan N, Galicich JH, Lane JM, et al. Treatment of neoplastic epidural cord compression by vertebral body resection and stabilization. *J Neurosurg* 1985; 63:676–684.
51. Sze G, Krol G, Zimmerman RD, Deck MDF. Malignant extradural spinal tumors: MR imaging with Gd-DTPA. *Radiology* 1988; 167:217–223.
52. Törmä T. Malignant tumours of the spine and the spinal extradural space: a study based on 250 histologically verified cases. *Acta Chir Scand [Suppl]* 1957; 225:1–176.
53. Ushio Y, Posner R, Posner JB, Shapiro WR. Experimental spinal cord compression by epidural neoplasms. *Neurology* 1977; 27:422–429.
54. van der Sande JJ, Kroger R, Boogerd W. Multiple spinal epidural metastases: an unexpectedly frequent finding. *J Neurol Neurosurg Psychiatry* 1990; 53:1001–1003.
55. von Einsiedel HG, Stepan R. Magnetic resonance imaging of spinal cord syndromes. *Eur J Radiol* 1985; 5:127–132.
56. Wara WM, Phillips TL, Sheline GE, Schwade JC. Radiation tolerance of the spinal cord. *Cancer* 1975; 35:1558–1562.
57. Wright RL. Malignant tumors in the spinal extradural space: results of surgical treatment. *Ann Surg* 1963; 157:227–231.
58. Young RF, Post EM, King GA. Treatment of spinal epidural metastases. Randomized prospective comparison of laminectomy and radiotherapy. *J Neurosurg* 1980; 53:741–748.

178 Primary Neoplasms of the Spine

William J. Mallon
John M. Harrelson

Although the spine is the most common site of metastasis to bone from a distant primary malignant neoplasm, we will be considering here only those skeletal tumors which arise primarily in the vertebral column. Chordoma, which arises from rests of embryonic notochordal tissue and usually affects either the sacrum or the cervico-occipital region, will not be considered.

Primary tumors of the spine are rare entities. In several large series published by Dahlin and Unni,[12] Enneking,[15] and Schajowicz,[38] primary skeletal tumors arose in the spine in only 11 percent of cases. Because of this rarity, the possibility of a primary tumor in the spine is often overlooked. The symptoms from a spinal tumor will often mimic those of a herniated disc. Unless there is obvious radiographic evidence of a tumor, the physician will often not search any further. Because of the potential morbidity and mortality from bone tumors, they should always be excluded as a diagnosis when dealing with patients with back or neck pain.

Biological and Anatomic Factors

A skeletal tumor tends to grow outward from its site of origin and to stimulate a response from the adjacent normal tissue at its margins. In bone, osteoid is the reactive tissue that attempts to encapsulate the tumor. Slow-growing benign and malignant tumors will usually be surrounded by a well-developed pseudocapsule. With increasing aggressiveness of the lesion, the capsule is less well developed and transgression by the tumor is common.

Certain anatomic structures may serve as barriers to tumor growth. Typically, cartilage, cortical bone, and major fascial planes constitute such barriers and tissue bounded by these structures constitutes an anatomic compartment. In the vertebral column, the anatomic compartments are bounded by cortical bone, the intervertebral discs, the anterior and posterior longitudinal ligaments, the interspinous and intertransverse process ligaments, and, posteriorly, the juxtaspinal musculature.

Clinical Evaluation

In patients with primary spinal tumors, the most common presenting complaint is pain.[19,31] One of the difficulties with diagnosis is the similarity in symptoms and signs between spinal tumors and herniated discs.[44] Pain associated with spinal tumors can be distinguished because it rarely improves with rest, and it is often worse at night and when lying supine.[19]

The patient's age is of importance because different skeletal lesions appear in characteristic age groups.[19,31] Primary spinal tumors in children tend to be benign, whereas in adults they tend to be malignant.[6,48] Spinal column lesions appearing during the patient's fifth decade or beyond are most likely multiple myeloma or metastatic carcinoma.[31]

Laboratory evaluation to assess the causes of back pain should include a complete blood count, erythrocyte sedimentation rate, urinalysis, and serum and urine protein electrophoresis. The white blood cell count and sedimentation rate will suggest or help rule out an infectious process. Multiple myeloma is suggested by the combination of anemia and an elevated sedimentation rate; protein electrophoresis will usually confirm or rule out this diagnosis. Measurement of levels of prostate-specific antigen (PSA) (for suspected metastatic prostate carcinoma), urinary hydroxyproline (for suspected Paget's disease), or even urinary vanillylmandelic acid (for a child with suspected metastatic neuroblastoma[31]) may also be helpful.

Diagnosis of a primary tumor of the spine requires radiologic imaging. The single imaging modality most likely to establish the diagnosis of a skeletal tumor is conventional high-quality radiography.[31] However, it should be remembered that 60 percent of bone must be replaced by tumor for the lesion to be visible on plain radiographs.[13] These films should be obtained in any patient with persistent back pain or an appropriate neurological deficit, and in any child presenting with back pain.[48] Magnetic resonance imaging (MRI) and computed tomography (CT) are required to evaluate the exact extent of the tumor. CT has been proved to be more sensitive in the evaluation of cortical bone, whereas MRI is the most accurate and sensitive indicator of medullary and soft tissue involvement. Technetium bone scans are of great importance in evaluating primary bone tumors. Increased uptake in the primary lesion indicates that the lesion is either producing bone, destroying bone, or eliciting a response from the host bone. If multiple ''hot'' lesions are found on the bone scan, metastatic disease is by far the most likely diagnosis. It is important to remember that multiple myeloma will often be ''cold'' (decreased uptake) or negative (normal uptake) on radionuclide bone scanning.

Staging of Benign and Malignant Tumors

Staging is the process whereby radiographic, histologic, and anatomic data are used to categorize tumors. Staging has prognostic implications and provides a rationale for treatment decisions. Where skeletal tumors are concerned, the staging system devised by Enneking et al.[16] has proved to be the most useful. Benign lesions are graded primarily by radiographic appearance, but this is influenced to some degree by histology and knowledge of the natural history of the lesion. Stage 1 lesions are static or tend to heal spontaneously. Stage 2 lesions show a more aggressive appearance

TABLE 178-1 Staging of Benign Tumors

Stage	Behavioral Characteristics
1	Latent, heal spontaneously
2	Active, progressive growth
3	Locally aggressive

Source: From Enneking,[15] with permission.

TABLE 178-2 Staging of Malignant Tumors

Stage	Grade	Site	Metastasis
IA	Low	Intracompartmental	None
IB	Low	Extracompartmental	None
IIA	High	Intracompartmental	None
IIB	High	Extracompartmental	None
III	Any	Any	Present

Source: From Enneking,[15] with permission.

radiographically, are less mature histologically, and show evidence of continued growth. Stage 3 lesions are locally aggressive and histologically immature and demonstrate progressive growth not limited by natural barriers. Anatomic location and size are not factors in the staging of benign tumors (Table 178-1).

Sarcomas of bone are graded primarily by histologic appearance into low-grade (designated I and corresponding to Broders' grades 1 and 2) and high-grade (designated II and corresponding to Broders' grades 3 and 4).[7] Anatomic location is specified as intracompartmental (designated A) or extracompartmental (designated B). Malignant bone tumors are thus classified as IA, IB, IIA, or IIB. Lesions which demonstrate distant or regional metastasis are designated as stage III regardless of grade or anatomic location and carry the worst prognosis (Table 178-2). From a prognostic point of view, a tumor of high grade or extracompartmental location carries a more ominous prognosis. From a treatment point of view, high-grade and extracompartmental tumors generally require more aggressive surgery.

By this staging system, adequate extirpation of a IA or IB malignant bone tumor requires the complete removal of the tumor along with a cuff of normal tissue, termed a wide excision. In IIA lesions, adequate treatment is considered to be complete removal of the compartment containing the tumor. It is thought that IIB lesions require radical amputation above above the lesion, i.e., an amputation high enough to remove all of the compartments involved by the tumor. Such an approach to bone sarcomas works better in the extremities than in the spine. Because of the proximity of the spinal cord and the need to maintain stability of the spinal column, the tumor surgeon must often settle for less than a complete excision, as defined above, often an intralesional or marginal resection. This will be dealt with further below.

Biopsy

Technically, the biopsy is part of the staging procedure but it is sufficiently important to deserve separate consideration. All malignant and many benign tumors can be implanted by surgical manipulation. Implantation can occur either by direct transfer of tumor tissue to extralesional sites or by the dissection of a hematoma from the biopsy along adjacent fascial planes and structures. Thus, the surgical approach for the biopsy must be planned with some thought about the malignant potential or possible implantability of the lesion in question. Failure to consider these factors may result in extension of the influence of the tumor, convert an intracompartmental lesion into an extracompartmental one, and potentially sacrifice structures which might otherwise have been saved. Second, a surgical plan for definitive treatment should be formulated before biopsy for the various possible stages of the lesions. Such planning allows the biopsy incision to be resectable as a part of the specimen if wider excision is necessary.

For biopsy of lesions of the posterior elements of the spine, a longitudinal posterior midline incision will suffice in almost all cases and still allow resection of the biopsy tract at a later stage. It is almost impossible to biopsy lesions of the vertebral body without contaminating multiple compartments which are not easily sacrificed. These lesions may be biopsied under fluoroscopic or CT guidance by a needle placed through a posterior approach.[40] However, this will provide less material for pathologic diagnosis and, in some ways, is more demanding and more hazardous than the open procedure.[19] It is cautioned that such an approach should be performed only by a practitioner with experience and only if the pathologist feels comfortable making diagnoses from such specimens.[18]

Treatment Modalities

General Considerations

Excision of a primary bone tumor in the spine is very difficult because of the proximity of the neural structures as well as the possibility of creating an unstable spine. The goal of the surgery is to completely remove the tumor and retain stability of the spine.[33] Occasionally, the surgeon must settle for less than the recommended margins in order to preserve the patient's quality of life.[27]

Reconstruction of the spine in order to avoid instability is usually performed using bone grafts, including both strut grafts anteriorly (from either a fibula, iliac crest, or rib) and cancellous bone posteriorly (usually obtained from an iliac crest). In addition, instrumentation must be used for support and stability until fusion occurs.[13] Currently popular techniques used for the instrumentation of scoliotic and degenerative spines can be used to provide immediate stability. As a rule, combined anterior and posterior stabilization is recommended for the reconstruction of a spine which is unstable due to neoplastic destruction.[27,30] Spinal cord monitoring of evoked potentials is useful during these procedures to help avoid catastrophic neurological complications.[33]

In cases of metastatic lesions, there have been many reports of the use of methyl methacrylate to provide even stronger immediate stability.[9,14,20,30] This is rarely indicated in the treatment of primary bone tumors of the spine. Methacrylate provides excellent short-term stability but undergoes fatigue failure quickly in the spinal column; over the long term, collapse and instability often occur.[30] Currently, such a construct is only recommended to improve the quality of life when the patient will have an expected survival of less than a year.

Surgical Reconstruction of the Cervical Spine

Primary bone tumors in the cervical spine are rare. Needle biopsy under radiographic control is the preferred technique for initial diagnosis according to Enneking,[15] but Bohlman et al.[6]

recommended an open biopsy. For open biopsy, incisions should be oriented vertically, both anteriorly and posteriorly.

In patients with a radiographic lesion in the cervical spine, the age of the patient is highly prognostic. Younger patients generally have benign tumors and survive without symptoms after appropriate treatment, whereas older patients more frequently have malignant lesions with a more guarded prognosis.[6]

Benign stage 2 lesions of the cervical spine usually require *en bloc* excision of a vertebral body to obtain a marginal excision. Reconstruction can be with a strut graft between the contiguous vertebral bodies. If more than one vertebral body must be excised, a preliminary posterior fusion from one level above to one level below the excised segments is indicated.[15]

Stage 3 benign and grade I malignant lesions in the cervical spine are fortunately quite rare. About 50 percent of such lesions of the bodies will have microscopic extensions into the pedicles, precluding all but an intracapsular excision. Adjuvant radiotherapy or chemotherapy should be considered in these cases. If this is expected, minimal stripping of the posterior soft tissues should be done to lessen the risk of transverse myelitis from radiation. As with stage 2 lesions, prophylactic posterior stabilization and fusion may be necessary.[15]

Surgical Reconstruction of the Thoracic Spine

The thoracic spine is very unforgiving in that the canal is narrow and the risk of irreversible myelopathy from neurological encroachment is high. However, the ribs provide a stabilizing effect which allows wider margins than in the cervical spine. Preliminary studies are important. Roentgenograms are seldom definitive because of the overlap of the ribs, and computed tomography is probably necessary in all cases. Arteriography may have its greatest use in the thoracic spine because it localizes the critical intraspinal vasculature to the cord in the critical area between T7 and T10.[15]

Needle biopsy can be performed in this area[40] by practitioners who are skilled in the technique. Open biopsy is probably performed more commonly. Lesions of the body can be approached through a midline longitudinal incision posteriorly. The lesion is then biopsied through a pedicle. Very anterior lesions are probably better handled through a costotransversectomy incision, although this will make complete excision of the biopsy tract virtually impossible. However, because of the proximity of the aorta and vena cava it may be the only choice.

Lesions in the body will usually be contained by the barrier of the pedicles except in stage II tumors. Marginal or wide excisions can thus be obtained for stages 1, 2, 3, or I lesions by *en bloc* vertebral body excision. Reconstruction is performed by the use of a strut graft, from either a fibula, iliac crest, or rib. Although the ribs do provide stability, a posterior fusion, either secondarily or prophylactically, is usually necessary if the entire body is excised.

Surgical Reconstruction of the Lumbar Spine

Lesions in the lumbar spine are quite accessible and are less dangerous with regard to neurological problems because of the wider canal and the transition of the spinal cord to the cauda equina. However, because of the lack of ribs and the great mechanical stress on this region, reconstruction must be more aggressive in order to achieve stability.[15] Needle biopsy can be performed in the lumbar spine,[15,40] although it has been best studied with metastatic carcinoma and marrow-cell lesions. Open biopsy can be performed easily either anteriorly or posteriorly, depending on the location of the lesion.

Lesions in the posterior elements can be marginally or widely excised with segmental posterior reconstruction and fusion. Anteriorly, lesions of the body can be excised by removal of the entire vertebral body with fusion by the use of a strut graft (fibula, iliac crest, or rib). Fusion is augmented by the use of cancellous bone packed about the strut. Internal stabilization until fusion occurs can be anterior or posterior. Multiple systems of internal fixation are available and can be chosen according to the surgeon's preference.

Surgical Reconstruction of the Sacrum

Primary bone tumors of the sacrum are quite rare and most of the lesions will be either chordomas, giant cell tumors, or aneurysmal bone cysts. Presentation is commonly with low back pain and the diagnosis is often overlooked for some time because of the difficulty of visualizing the sacrum on standard pelvic x-ray films. Neurological symptoms commonly will include urinary incontinence. A less common but distinctive presenting sign is an external rotation contracture of the ipsilateral hip in lesions of the sacral wing, presumably because of pain from the overlying psoas muscle.[15]

Because of the difficulty imaging the sacrum by standard radiographic techniques, CT or MRI is a necessity. Lesions can be biopsied through a midline posterior approach, either open or by needle biopsy. As both a staging study and for preoperative planning, arteriography is helpful. Because sacral lesions can cause massive intraoperative bleeding, preoperative embolization during the arteriogram may be helpful if the study demonstrates large feeding vessels.

In large lesions, wide excision can often not be performed without the sacrifice of several nerve roots. In such cases, intralesional curettage with adjuvant radiotherapy, cryotherapy, or methacrylate packing may be preferable.[15] Radiation has a significant morbidity and methacrylate packing is technically difficult in the sacrum.[15] Methacrylate packing also risks thermal damage to the sacral nerve roots. Bilateral sacrifice of the S3, S4, and S5 nerve roots will cause no loss of urogenital sphincter function but will cause perianal numbness. Preservation of one S2 root will allow for adequate urinary and anal continence in about one-half of the patients. The other half will be incontinent.[15]

Benign lesions totally contained within the sacrum can usually be fully excised through a transverse posterior approach as described by Localio et al.[26] Lesions with anterior extension will lie near the major vessels and the colon, and a combined anterior and posterior approach with the help of a general surgeon is necessary. Reconstruction after sacral excision is usually not required. Even complete removal of the sacrum usually will allow spontaneous fusion of L5 to the iliac wings, although prolonged recumbency will be required.[15] The available reconstructive options are minimal because of the presence of the multiple nerve roots.

Primary Skeletal Neoplasms

It is convenient to categorize primary skeletal tumors by their cell of origin.[39] Both benign and malignant neoplasms may evolve from the osseous, cartilaginous, and fibrous elements of the skeleton (Table 178-3). Tumors of marrow origin are invariably malignant and are often an expression of systemic disease. It should be

TABLE 178-3 Primary Skeletal Neoplasms

Cell of Origin	Benign Neoplasms	Malignant Neoplasms
Osseous	Osteoid osteoma* Osteoblastoma*	Osteosarcoma* (and variants)
Cartilaginous	Osteochondroma* Enchondroma Chondroblastoma Chondromyxoid-fibroma	Chondrosarcoma* primary/secondary)
Fibrous	Fibroma	Fibrosarcoma Malignant fibrous histiocytoma
Marrow	None	Ewing's sarcoma* Multiple myeloma* Lymphoma* Metastasis
Other	Giant cell tumor* Hemangioma* Related lesions: Eosinophilic granuloma* Aneurysmal bone cyst*	

* Indicates occurrence in the spine with some frequency; these lesions are discussed in the text.
Source: Adapted from Schajowicz.[39]

emphasized again that primary tumors of the spine are rare lesions. Although virtually all known skeletal tumors have been described in the spine, we will deal in detail only with those that occur with any frequency.

Benign Lesions

Osteoid Osteomas

Osteoid osteomas are benign lesions seen predominantly in children or young adults from 10 to 25 years of age. They have a strong predilection for the posterior elements of the vertebra, with the lamina and pedicle being the most frequent sites of involvement.[1,22] Within the spinal column they are slightly more common in the lumbar area, followed by the cervical, thoracic, and sacral regions.[22]

Virtually all patients will present with back pain. The classic history is that the pain is not relieved by rest, is worse at night and with recumbency, and is frequently relieved by aspirin.[22] The incidence of neurological deficit reported in the literature is between 0 and 25 percent.[25,28] More commonly, the patients will present with scoliosis.[24,25] Osteoid osteoma is the most frequent cause of painful scoliosis in adolescents.[1,24,35] In addition, Keim and Reina reported a rapid onset of scoliosis.[24] Typically, the tumor will be located near the apex of the curve on the concave side.[24,25,28] Sabanas et al. studied the natural history of osteoid osteoma of the spine and suggested that the natural course is self-limiting in 4 to 8 years.[37] However, persistence of symptoms or progressive spinal deformity usually will necessitate surgical intervention.

Osteoid osteoma is often diagnosed late, with the delay reported in several series being between 18 and 72 months.[1,22,24,25,35] Radiologically, the lesion is characterized by a radiolucent area with a central nidus and surrounding sclerosis (Fig. 178-1). In addition, to differentiate an osteoid osteoma from its large twin, the osteoblastoma, the lesion must arbitrarily be less than 1.5 cm in diameter. Early in its course, plain roentgenograms will often be normal.[35] Because back pain in the presenting age group is rather uncommon, any back pain of greater than 6 weeks' duration in children and young adults should be studied by a technetium bone scan when plain x-ray films are negative. The bone scan will show increased radionuclide uptake at the site of the lesion, but the central nidus will often be visible, as it will be relatively "cold" compared with the "hot" image shown by the area of surrounding sclerosis.

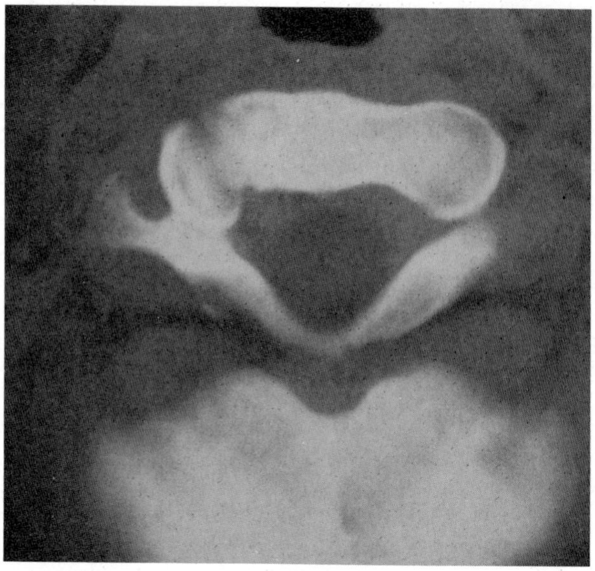

Figure 178-1 An axial CT scan showing an osteoid osteoma in the anterior body of the C2 vertebra.

Preoperative planning should include a CT scan to exactly localize the area of the tumor. The gross pathology of an osteoid osteoma is not significantly different from that of the surrounding normal bone. Thus it can be difficult to know when the entire tumor is removed. This problem can be obviated by labeling the lesion with radioactive technetium. This is usually injected on the morning of the operation. Intraoperatively, a sterilized radioactive counter can be used to localize the lesion precisely. When the lesion has been fully removed, the surrounding bone will no longer be "hot" to the counter.

When lesions involve the posterior elements, they can usually be completely removed through a posterior approach. Spinal fusion is rarely needed, even if one articular process has been violated.[1,24] Whether to proceed with instrumentation and fusion for scoliosis depends on the duration of the symptoms. If the symptoms have been present for 15 months or less, the deformity will most likely decrease or correct completely.[25,35] Symptoms of longer duration imply a structural deformity which will probably require instrumentation and fusion to avoid further progression even after removal of the osteoid osteoma.

Complications from surgery for osteoid osteoma are rare. If the lesion has been completely removed, recurrence is unlikely. Pain after removal usually implies incomplete removal of the lesion.

Osteoblastomas

Osteoblastoma is an aggressive benign tumor which commonly occurs in the spine. More than 40 percent of the reported cases involved the spine and more than half of these were associated with scoliosis.[1] Although osteoblastomas occur in a slightly older age group than do osteoid osteomas, 80 percent of the patients are under 30 years of age. Osteoblastomas also have a predilection for the posterior spinal elements.[19] Although they occasionally occur in the vertebral body, this is rare without concurrent involvement of the pedicle. Janin et al. reported an almost equal distribution among cervical, thoracic, and lumbar sites of origin.[22]

Histologically, osteoblastoma is indistinguishable from osteoid osteoma. The division between the two lesions has been arbitrarily defined as a diameter of 1.5 cm. In contrast to osteoid osteoma, night pain and dramatic relief of pain by aspirin is less common in osteoblastoma.[19] Neurological deficit is more likely in patients with osteoblastoma owing to the larger size of the tumor and the extension of the tumor toward the spinal cord.[22] As with osteoid osteoma, the presenting problem is often a painful scoliosis.[25]

Radiologically, osteoblastomas demonstrate less abundant sclerosis than do osteoid osteomas. However, they may show expansion and cystic changes and may occasionally mimic the radiographic appearance of an aneurysmal bone cyst.[3]

The nature and natural history of the spinal deformity associated with osteoblastoma are similar to those of osteoid osteoma.[1] Surgical excision of an osteoblastoma is desirable, although cure has been reported with incomplete excision.[29] For posterior lesions, excision through a posterior approach is usually adequate. Because of the large size of these lesions, excision may require destabilization of the spine, necessitating stabilization with fusion and instrumentation. Since these patients will often be slightly older than those with osteoid osteoma, the scoliosis may become structural after only 6 to 9 months of symptoms, requiring earlier instrumentation and fusion.

Osteoblastomas recur more frequently than do osteoid osteomas. Recurrence of an osteoblastoma may be related to its larger size which makes complete excision more difficult, or to its aggressive behavior with recurrence even after seemingly complete excision.

Osteochondromas

Osteochondromas are the most common of bone tumors. They are benign lesions which can occur in a single or multiple form. They will occasionally degenerate into malignant chondrosarcomas, and this is much more common (about 10 percent) in patients with multiple lesions. An osteochondroma is a cartilage-capped bony protuberance that is thought to develop from an adjacent physis or a cartilaginous remnant of the physis.

Osteochondromas usually occur in the posterior elements, especially the spinous process. More than one spinous process may be involved by the tumor.[32] They rarely arise in the vertebral body.[34] Osteochondromas are not inherently painful but cause symptoms from pressure on adjacent neurological structures, from formation of a painful bursa over the cartilage cap, or from malignant degeneration. Sumptoms can be relieved by excision of the lesion.

Giant Cell Tumors

Giant cell tumors are benign lesions of unknown cell origin. Histologically they are composed of multiple giant cells with a fibrous stroma. They most commonly affect the metaphysis or epiphysis in young adults.[19] In the spine, giant cell tumors have a predilection for the vertebral body and they are most commonly found in the thoracic area (Fig. 178-2).[10] Radiographically they appear as a cystlike lesion, which should be differentiated from an

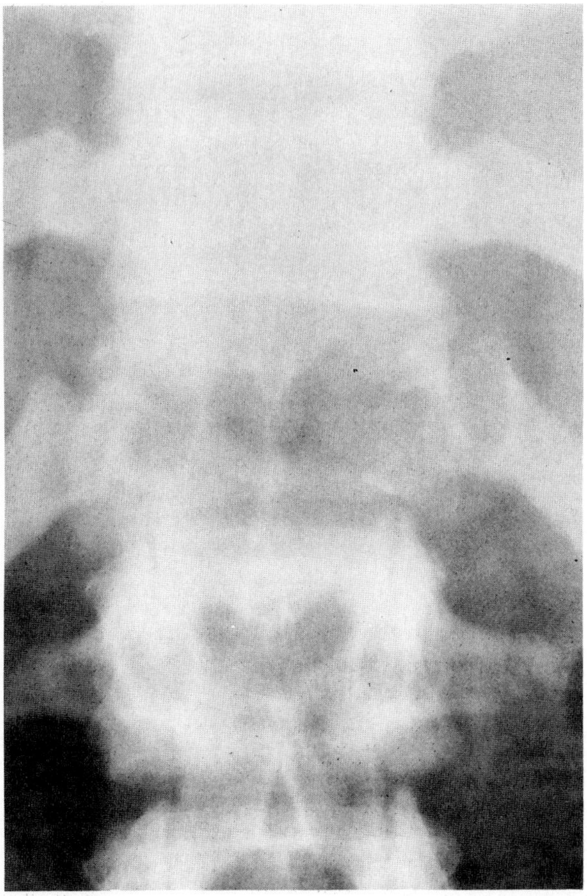

Figure 178-2 Erosion of the pedicle and expansion of the lateral aspect of the body secondary to a giant cell tumor involving the T11 vertebra.

aneurysmal bone cyst and an osteoblastoma.[10] In Dahlin's series, he noted a very young age of occurrence (the first and second decades) and he suggested that giant cell tumors of vertebrae may be basically different from giant cell tumors found elsewhere.[10]

Although benign, giant cell tumors have a tendency to recur and can even metastasize.[12] In the spine, the recurrence rate has been reported to be as high as 50 percent; metastases occur in 15 percent.[10,19,47] Thus, treatment must involve an attempt to surgically extirpate the entire lesion, preferably with a wide margin of normal tissue. As discussed above, this can be difficult to achieve. In lesions which cannot be completely excised, consideration may be given to postoperative radiotherapy.[19]

Aneurysmal Bone Cysts

Aneurysmal bone cysts are benign lesions which arise in the spine between 11 and 20 percent of the time.[8,21] They are more frequent in the second and third decades of life.[23] Hay et al. reported that 60 percent of these lesions occur in the posterior elements.[21] Capanna et al. stated that none of their patients had involvement of the vertebral body alone without involvement of the pedicle.[8] Aneurysmal bone cysts are slightly more common in the lumbar spine.[8,21,23] Patients will commonly present with back pain. A neurological deficit is relatively common, being reported in 55 percent of cases by Capanna et al.[8] and by Akbarnia.[2] As with osteoid osteoma and osteoblastoma, an aneurysmal bone cyst can cause a painful scoliosis.[3]

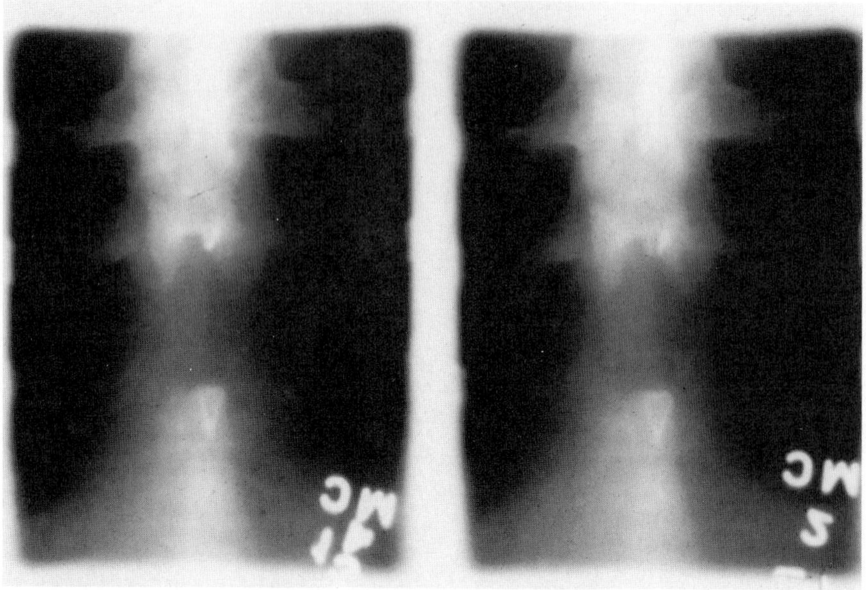

Figure 178-3 Tomographic images demonstrating marked thinning and expansion of the C7 posterior arch secondary to an aneurysmal bone cyst.

Radiographically, an aneurysmal bone cyst has the features of a cystic lesion (Fig. 178-3). Rarely, they may cross a joint or extend to an adjacent rib. Many aneurysmal bone cysts will have a soft tissue component.[2,8,46] The radionuclide bone scan will usually show increased uptake, but it may occasionally be normal. Histologically, aneurysmal bone cysts contain many fluid-filled spaces separated by fibrous septae. Aneurysmal bone cysts may be either primary or secondary to another bony lesion. Secondary cysts will show histologic evidence of the original lesion.

A definitive diagnosis by roentgenograms is rarely possible. Needle biopsy of a suspected aneurysmal bone cyst of the spine should be discouraged because extradural bleeding following such a needle biopsy has been reported to cause neurological deficits.[21] An open biopsy is thus recommended and should be done by the most appropriate approach, depending on the location of the lesion. Treatment consists of complete excision, if possible. Unfortunately, in the spine this can rarely be achieved because these lesions usually are quite large by the time the patient presents. Hay et al. reported a 25 percent recurrence rate when biopsy and incomplete excision were performed.[21] Capanna et al., however, reported no recurrences if the lesion was treated surgically (with or without complete excision) or by surgery and radiation combined.[8] Karparov and Kitov also reported good results with incomplete excision.[23] Although radiation to the spine presents many risks, including myelopathy, scoliosis, growth arrest, and possible sarcomatous degeneration, it can be used as adjuvant therapy in cases where complete excision is not possible.

Eosinophilic Granulomas

Eosinophilic granuloma is a benign tumor-like condition of bone characterized histologically by numerous histiocytes and eosinophils. In one study it was found to be the most common benign spinal tumor occurring in the first two decades of life.[45] The lesion may be solitary or may occur as part of systemic involvement. Letterer-Siwe and Hand-Schüller-Christian disease represent the acute and chronic forms of the systemic disease, respectively.[32]

Eosinophilic granuloma usually occurs in the first or second decade, with a peak incidence between 5 and 10 years of age. In the spine, the lesion more commonly affects adolescents and presents with an acute onset of back pain. It occurs most commonly in the thoracic area and the classic presentation is that of a symmetrically flattened vertebral body (vertebral plana). It can also present as a lytic lesion in the body without collapse (Fig. 178-4). Although vertebral plana is classically associated with eosinophilic granuloma, it can occur with other lesions, and needle biopsy is indicated.

The systemic forms of eosinophilic granuloma are treated with various chemotherapeutic regimens. Solitary eosinophilic granuloma is a self-limited disease and treatment in the spine can consist solely of a body cast or orthosis to maintain alignment of the spine and relieve pain during the actual episode.[41]

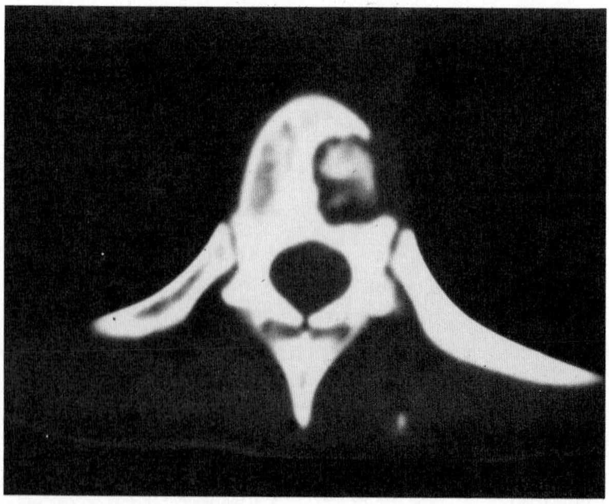

Figure 178-4 An axial CT scan showing an area of lytic destruction with a central radiodensity secondary to eosinophilic granuloma. In this case, the central density is residual bone. The lesion is too large for an osteoid osteoma.

Hemangiomas

A hemangioma is a benign tumor of vascular origin. Hemangiomas are probably the most common benign tumor in the spine but they rarely cause clinical problems and are often found incidentally at autopsy.[19] When found during life, the patients are usually over 40 years old.

More than 50 percent of hemangiomas occur in the spine and skull.[32] They commonly occur in either the thoracolumnbar or lumbar spine. Radiographically, they present with a classic appearance with coarse vertical striations (Fig. 178-5). This is because the horizontal trabeculae are commonly destroyed by the tumor and the vertical traberculae undergo compensatory hypertrophy and are easily seen on the x-ray films.

Most hemangiomas become symptomatic only after vertebral collapse or pathologic fracture. Most of these can be treated by radiation therapy. External bracing may also help in alleviating discomfort.[19] Surgery is reserved for instances in which cord compromise occurs. In those cases, the possibility of severe hemorrhage must be kept in mind and preoperative embolization of the tumor may be helpful.

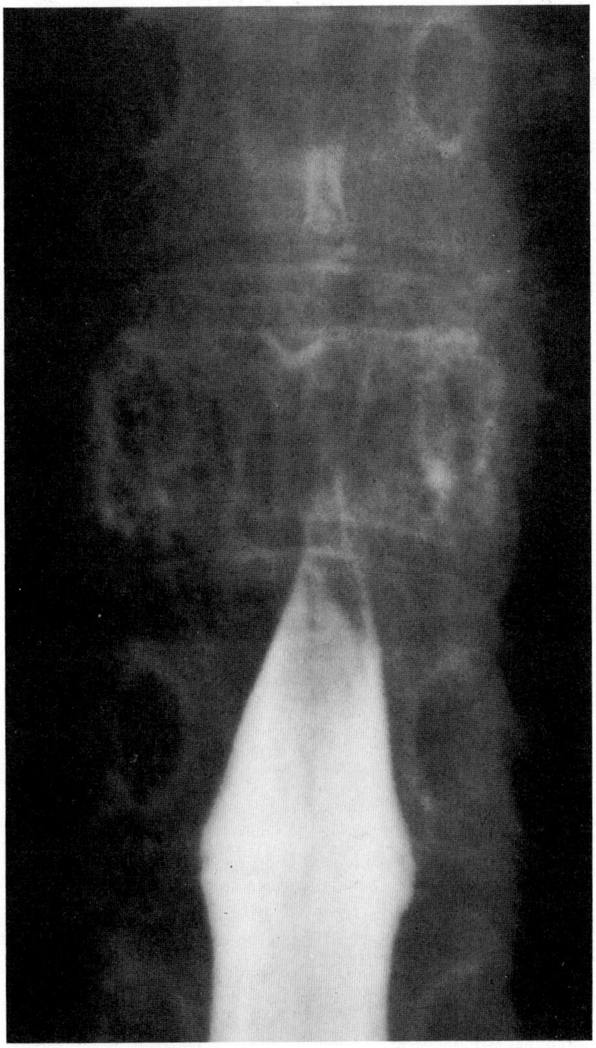

Figure 178-5 The vertebral body immediately above the myelographic contrast column shows the vertical striations characteristic of a hemangioma of the vertebral body.

Malignant Lesions

Osteosarcomas

Primary osteosarcoma of the spine is very rare.[42] When osteosarcoma does occur in the spine, it more commonly is as a metastasis from an extremity primary, or secondary to either radiation or Paget's disease.[17,19] Primary osteosarcoma of the spine occurs in a slightly older age group than does that of the extremities.[42] Radiographically, spinal osteosarcoma typically demonstrates a combined lytic and blastic destruction of the vertebral body or posterior elements (Fig. 178-6).[19,42]

Extremity osteosarcoma should be treated by radical resection or limb salvage after adjuvant chemotherapy. Neither approach is possible in the spine. Total extirpation cannot be accomplished without jeopardizing the integrity of the spinal column and spinal cord. Neoadjuvant chemotherapy for this disease commonly includes intra-arterial chemotherapy in the extremities, but in the spine this is hazardous because of the risk of jeopardizing the blood supply to the spinal cord.

When there are signs of cord compression or the structural integrity of the spine is jeopardized, patients may require debulking of the lesion, decompression of the spinal cord, and reconstruction of the vertebral column.[4] Patients with unresectable lesions or with multiple involvement are treated with local irradiation and chemotherapy. Cordotomy may be considered in terminal patients who suffer from intractable pain.[4] The overall prognosis of osteosarcoma of the spine is dismal. In the series of Shives et al., only 1 of 30 patients was alive without disease at 12 years, and only 4 patients survived more than 3 years.[42]

Chondrosarcomas

Although chondrosarcoma commonly occurs in the long bones and the pelvis, vertebral column involvement is not unusual.[4] This tumor commonly presents in the fourth to the seventh decade[5] and may occur either as a primary lesion or secondary to malignant degeneration of a pre-existing enchondroma or osteochondroma. Chondrosarcomas exhibit a wide spectrum of biological activity

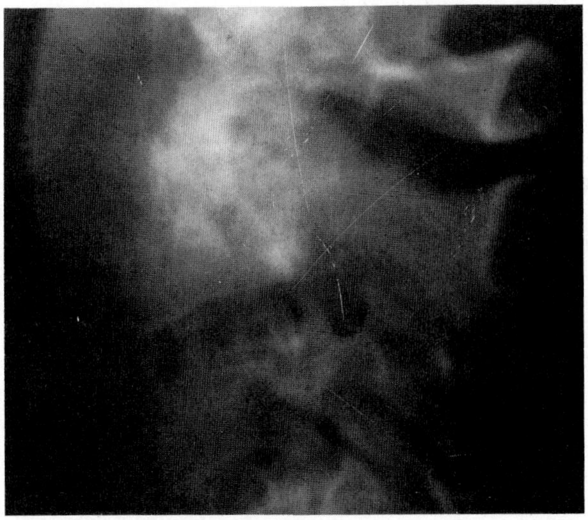

Figure 178-6 This lateral radiographic view of C2 shows dense blastic new bone in the body and erosion of the anterior cortex secondary to osteosarcoma.

from indolent slow growth to aggressive metastatic disease. Unfortunately, prediction of this behavior based on histologic appearance has been unreliable.[19] Dahlin and Henderson reported that the closer the tumor is to the axial skeleton, the more likely it is to be malignant, which forebodes poorly for patients with spinal lesions.[11]

Chondrosarcoma should be treated by wide resection when possible. As with osteosarcoma, this can rarely be achieved in the spine. Neither radiation therapy nor chemotherapy has been shown to be of much benefit in chondrosarcoma, but these may be used for adjuvant therapy in the event of less-than-complete tumor resection.[43] Chondrosarcoma of the pelvis and spine, including the sacrum, has the poorest prognosis because of the difficulty in achieving complete ablation.

Ewing's Sarcoma

Ewing's sarcoma is a malignant small cell tumor of bone whose cell of origin is unclear. It presents in children and adolescents and rarely involves the spine as a primary lesion, although metastasis to the spine is not uncommon. In general, the prognosis for survival with Ewing's sarcoma is considered less favorable for lesions in the trunk than for those in the extremities.[36] Thommesen and Poulsen reported it to be the most common malignant tumor found in the spine in the first two decades of life.[45] Many patients with Ewing's sarcoma will present with low-grade fever, anemia, leukocytosis, and an elevated erythrocyte sedimentation rate, which can cause confusion with osteomyelitis.[19]

Classically, surgery has had little role in the treatment of Ewing's sarcoma; chemotherapy and radiotherapy have been the recommended treatments. Recently, surgical excision of the primary lesion has been done as a supplement, with good results. However, in the spine, surgery is considered to have little role except for spinal cord decompression and vertebral reconstruction.[19] A combination of chemotherapy and radiotherapy has provided better long-term results in the spine to date.[4]

Multiple Myeloma

Multiple myeloma is the most common malignant neoplasm of bone in adults.[19] It usually affects patients over the age of 50.[19] It is a malignant tumor of plasma cells and, as a result of widespread bone marrow involvement, most patients will present with normocytic and normochromic anemia. They will also usually have an elevated erythrocyte sedimentation rate.[4,19] A definitive diagnosis requires bone marrow aspiration or open biopsy. In addition, the abnormal proliferation of plasma cells will cause a change in the normal electrophoretic pattern of protein seen in the serum and urine.

Radiographically, the tumor is usually identified by lytic lesions which often have a moth-eaten appearance and rarely show a bony capsule about the lesion (Fig. 178-7). Lesions in multiple myeloma may often be "cold" or negative on radionuclide bone scanning, and that study is not a useful screening device. Should the diagnosis of multiple myeloma be made, the patient should undergo a skeletal survey with plain roentgenograms to detect any occult lesions which may place bones at risk for fracture.

Chemotherapy is the primary treatment of multiple myeloma. Radiotherapy can be used locally for single painful lesions.[19] Surgery for lesions in the spine is reserved for those instances where acute neurological compromise occurs or where collapse from

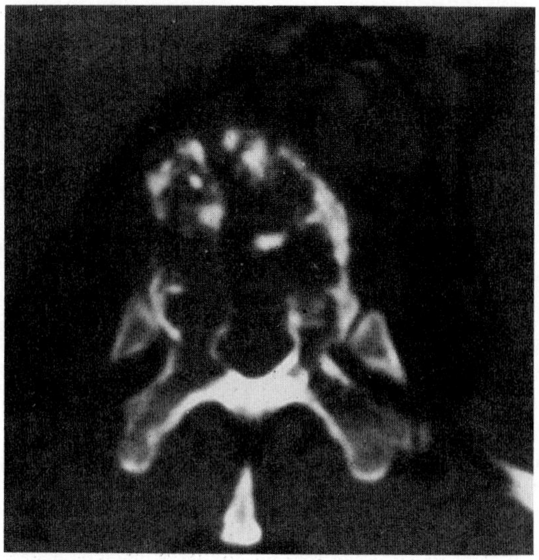

Figure 178-7 An axial CT scan showing marked destruction of the vertebral body and portions of the posterior elements secondary to myeloma.

a lesion is causing structural instability. In those cases, decompression and reconstruction should be considered. In advanced cases, external bracing of the spine with local irradiation can be considered.

Lymphomas

Lymphoma of bone is histologically similar to any lymphoma occurring in the lymph nodes or other soft tissues. It is most common in young adults and is much more likely to involve the peripheral skeleton.[19] In the spine, it usually involves the vertebral body.[4] It appears radiographically as an ill-defined lytic lesion which may eventually break through the cortex. A definitive diagnosis cannot be made radiographically but requires either open or needle biopsy. Surgery is rarely used for lymphomas of the spinal column. Irradiation is the treatment of choice for solitary lesions. A combination of radiotherapy and chemotherapy may improve the overall prognosis.[4]

References

1. Akbarnia BA. Osteoid osteoma and osteoblastoma of the spine. *Spine: State of the Art Reviews* 1988; 2:249–263.
2. Akbarnia BA. Aneurysmal bone cysts of the spine. *Spine: State of the Art Reviews* 1988; 2:265–274.
3. Akbarnia BA, Rooholamini SA. Scoliosis caused by benign osteoblastoma of the thoracic or lumbar spine. *J Bone Joint Surg* [*Am*] 1981; 63A:1146–1155.
4. Aprin H. Primary malignant tumors of the spine. *Spine: State of the Art Reviews* 1988; 2:289–299.
5. Blaylock RL, Kempe LG. Chondrosarcoma of the cervical spine: case report. *J Neurosurg* 1976; 44:500–503.
6. Bohlman HH, Sachs BL, Carter JR. Primary neoplasms of the cervical spine: diagnosis and treatment of twenty-three patients. *J Bone Joint Surg* [*Am*] 1986; 68A:483–494.
7. Broders AC, Hargrave R, Meyerding HW. Pathological features of soft

tissue fibrosarcoma: with special reference to the grading of its malignancy. *Surg Gynecol Obstet* 1939; 69:267–280.
8. Capanna R, Albisinni U, Picci P, et al. Aneurysmal bone cyst of the spine. *J Bone Joint Surg [Am]* 1985; 67A:527–531.
9. Clark CR, Keggi KJ, Panjabi MM. Methylmethacrylate stabilization of the cervical spine. *J Bone Joint Surg [Am]* 1984; 66A:40–46.
10. Dahlin DC. Giant-cell tumor of the vertebrae above the sacrum: a review of 31 cases. *Cancer* 1977; 39:1350–1356.
11. Dahlin DC, Henderson ED. Chondrosarcoma, a surgical and pathological problem: review of 212 cases. *J Bone Joint Surg [Am]* 1956; 38A:1025–1038.
12. Dahlin DC, Unni KK. *Bone Tumors,* 4th ed. Springfield, IL: Charles C Thomas, 1986.
13. Delamarter RB, Sachs BL, Thompson GH, et al. Primary neoplasms of the thoracic and lumbar spine: an analysis of 29 consecutive cases. *Clinical Orthop* 1990; 256:87–100.
14. Dunn EJ. The role of methyl methacrylate in the stabilization and replacement of tumors of the cervical spine: a project of the Cervical Spine Research Society. *Spine* 1977; 2:15–24.
15. Enneking WF. *Musculoskeletal Tumor Surgery.* New York: Churchill Livingstone, 1983.
16. Enneking WF, Spanier SS, Goodman MA. A system for the surgical staging of musculoskeletal sarcoma. *Clin Orthop* 1980; 153:106–120.
17. Fielding JW, Fietti VG Jr, Hughes JEO, et al. Primary osteogenic sarcoma of the cervical spine: a case report. *J Bone Joint Surg [Am]* 1976; 58A:892–894.
18. Frager DH, Goldman MJ, Seimon LP, et al. Computed tomography guidance for skeletal biopsy. *Skel Radiol* 1987; 16:644–646.
19. Friedlaender GE, Southwick WO. Tumors of the spine. In Rothman RH, Simeone FA (eds): *The Spine.* Philadelphia: Saunders, 1982, pp 1022–1040.
20. Harrington KD. The use of methylmethacrylate for vertebral-body replacement and anterior stabilization of pathological fracture-dislocations of the spine due to metastatic malignant disease. *J Bone Joint Surg [Am]* 1981; 63A:36–46.
21. Hay MC, Paterson D, Taylor TKF. Aneurysmal bone cysts of the spine. *J Bone Joint Surg [Br]* 1978; 60B:406–411.
22. Janin Y, Epstein JA, Carras, R, et al. Osteoid osteomas and osteoblastomas of the spine. *Neurosurgery* 1981; 8:31–38.
23. Karparov M, Kitov D. Aneurysmal bone cyst of the spine. *Acta Neurochir (Wien)* 1977; 39:101–113.
24. Keim HA, Reina EG. Osteoid-osteoma as a cause of scoliosis. *J Bone Joint Surg [Am]* 1975; 57A:159–163.
25. Kirwan EO'G, Hutton PAN. Pozo JL, et al. Osteoid osteoma and benign osteoblastoma of the spine: clinical presentation and treatment. *J Bone Joint Surg [Br]* 1984; 66B:21–26.
26. Localio SA, Francis KC, Rossano PG. Abdominosacral resection of sacrococcygeal chordoma. *Ann Surg* 1967; 166:394–402.
27. Lonstein JE. Spinal stability after tumor resection by laminectomy. *Spine: State of the Art Reviews* 1988; 2:363–373.
28. Maclellan DI, Wilson FC Jr. Osteoid osteoma of the spine: a review of the literature and report of six new cases. *J Bone Joint Surg [Am]* 1967; 49A:111–121.
29. Marsh BW, Bonfiglio M, Brady LP, et al. Benign osteoblastoma: range of manifestations. *J Bone Joint Surg [Am]* 1975; 57A:1–9.
30. McAfee PC, Bohlman HH, Ducker T, et al. Failure of stabilization of the spine with methylmethacrylate. *J Bone Joint Surg [Am]* 1986; 68A:1145–1157.
31. McGuire MH. Evaluation of patients with spinal column tumors. *Spine: State of the Art Reviews* 1988; 2:183–194.
32. Merenda JT. Other primary benign tumors and tumor-like lesions of the spine. *Spine: State of the Art Reviews* 1988; 2:275–287.
33. Morley TR. The management of spinal tumours. *J Bone Joint Surg [Br]* 1991; 73B:158.
34. Novick GS, Pavlov H, Bullough PG. Osteochondroma of cervical spine: report of two cases in preadolescent males. *Skel Radiol* 1982; 8:13–15.
35. Pettine KA, Klassen RA. Osteoid-osteoma and osteoblastoma of the spine. *J Bone Joint Surg [Am]* 1986; 68A:354–361.
36. Russin LA, Robinson MJ, Engle HA, et al. Ewing's sarcoma of the lumbar spine: a case report of long-term survival. *Clin Orthop* 1982; 164:126–129.
37. Sabanas AO, Bickel WH, Moe JH. Natural history of osteoid osteoma of the spine: review of the literature and report of three cases. *Am J Surg* 1956; 91:880–889.
38. Schajowicz F. *Tumors and Tumor-Like Lesions of Bones and Joints.* Berlin: Springer-Verlag, 1982.
39. Schajowicz F. Classification of tumors and tumor-like lesions of the spine. *Spine: State of the Art Reviews* 1988; 2:169–181.
40. Schajowicz F. Results of needle biopsy in spinal tumors. *Spine: State of the Art Reviews* 1988; 2:239–247.
41. Seimon LP. Eosinophil granuloma of the spine. *J Pediatr Orthop* 1981; 1:371–376.
42. Shives TC, Dahlin DC, Sim FH, et al. Osteosarcoma of the spine. *J Bone Joint Surg [Am]* 1986; 68A:660–668.
43. Shives TC, McLeod RA, Unni KK, et al. Chondrosarcoma of the spine. *J Bone Joint Surg [Am]* 1989; 71A:1158–1165.
44. Sim FH, Dahlin DC, Stauffer RN, et al. Primary bone tumors simulating lumbar disc syndrome. *Spine* 1977; 2:65–74.
45. Thommesen P, Poulsen JO. Primary tumours in the spine and pelvis in adolescents: clinical and radiological features. *Acta Orthop Scand* 1976; 47:170–174.
46. Tillman BP, Dahlin DC, Lipscomb PR, et al. Aneurysmal bone cyst: an analysis of ninety-five cases. *Mayo Clin Proc* 1968; 43:478–495.
47. Verbiest H. Giant-cell tumours and aneurysmal bone cysts of the spine: with special reference to the problems related to the removal of a vertebral body. *J Bone Joint Surg [Br]* 1965; 47B:699–713.
48. Weinstein JN, McLain RF. Primary tumors of the spine. *Spine* 1987; 12:843–851.

179 Spinal Chordomas

Narayan Sundaresan
George Krol
Chandranath Sen

Chordomas are rare primary malignant tumors arising predominantly from the axial skeleton.[78] They have traditionally been considered slow-growing, locally invasive neoplasms and have constituted between 1 and 4 percent of malignant bone tumors in several large series.[16,29,61,84] Although more than 1000 cases have been reported to date, the only true epidemiologic data were provided by two studies published in the Scandinavian literature. In the Swedish Registry, Eriksson and co-workers noted an annual incidence of 0.5 percent per million population, with chordomas accounting for 17.5 percent of all primary malignant tumors of bone.[37] Over a 12-year period (1958 to 1970), 979 tumors were registered, of which 290 were malignant tumors arising from the axial skeleton. Of these, chordomas accounted for close to 20 percent. A similar incidence in Finland was noted by Paavolainen and Teppo.[92] Approximately 50 percent of all chordomas arise in the sacrococcygeal region, 35 percent in the sphenoid and occipital bones in the region of the clivus, and 15 percent in the true vertebrae above the sacrum (the mobile spine).[13,14,20,118,138] In addition, there have been reports of "ectopic" chordomas arising outside the skeletal axis, within the maxilla, sinuses, larynx, and other soft tissues.[9,11,17,51,108,126]

The site of origin of chordomas is presumed to be the embryonic notochord.[53,56,57,75,102] Among animals of the phylum Chordata, the notochord is the first skeletal structure to be formed. It gives way to the axial skeleton in the subphylum Vertebrata. Portions of notochord persist in the trunk and tail of fish, but only vestiges remain in modern reptiles, birds, and mammals. Embryologically, the notochord itself is seen in the somite stage, that is, from the 20th to the 30th day of human development. It originates as a group of cells that pass laterally from the primitive streak to form the intraembryonic mesoderm. As the intraembryonic mesoderm develops, the ectoderm thickens at one end to form Hensen's node, or the primitive knot. A cord of cells migrates forward from Hensen's node between the endoderm and ectoderm, forming the *head process.* As development proceeds, the notochordal process fuses with and is intercalated in the embryonic endoderm, ultimately forming a flattened plate of columnar cells termed the *notochordal plate.* The notochord itself develops as the notochordal plate folds longitudinally and separates from the endoderm. This separation proceeds in a cranial–caudal direction, leaving rests of notochordal cells closely associated with the developing pharynx.

During the development of the axial skeleton, the vertebral bodies themselves are formed from loose mesenchymal cells that collect segmentally from the para-axial mesoderm as sclerotomes. The sclerotomes give rise to all skeletal elements, connective tissue and cartilage, as well as bone. The organization of the sclerotomes into segmental levels results in the development of a cranial portion that is less condensed and a caudal portion that is more condensed. Fusion of the adjacent segments traps the notochord within the disc; thus the nucleus pulposus is the only remaining derivative of the notochord in the adult. Three-dimensional reconstruction experiments performed on serial sections of human embryos have shown complex interrelationships at the rostral and caudal ends of the embryo. Forking of the ends was observed; this may explain the sites and presumed origin of the vestigial rests when the notochord regresses. The distribution of these rests would also explain the observed skeletal distribution of chordomas.[102] In the animal kingdom, chordomas are commonly seen in ferrets.[35]

Luschka is credited with the earliest description (in 1856) of jelly-like excresences of tissue around the clivus.[61] A year later, Virchow named the unique jelly-like excresences "ecchondrosis physalifora," believing them to be of cartilaginous origin.[130] In 1858, Muller was the first to postulate that they were persisting notochordal relics, naming them "ecchordosis physalifora." His view did not gain support until 1894, when Ribbert, and later Congdon, produced experimental lesions in rabbits by perforating the anterior intervertebral ligaments with a needle and noting that the resulting proliferating lesion resembled chordoma.[24,99] Willis noted that embryonic rests around the clivus are found in 0.5 to 2.0 percent of autopsies; it has been suggested that chordoma arises from aberrant vestiges such as these.[139] Electron microscopy and tissue culture studies also suggest a histologic similarity between chordoma and disc tissue. It is curious, however, that chordomas arise from the vertebral body and the sacrum and have not been associated with the one structure traditionally associated with the notochord, that is, the nucleus pulposus. Ulich and Mirra have reported finding a microscopic ectopic remnant of notochord and hyaline cartilage within the vertebral body and postulate that these remnants may be the origin of chordomas developing in the spine.[129]

Anatomic Distribution and Clinical Features

Chordomas represented approximately 5 percent of all primary bone tumors in the Mayo Clinic series, and 1 percent of tumors in the series reported by Huvos.[29,61] It is important to recognize, however, that they represent a primary diagnostic consideration whenever a neoplasm of the sacrum or skull base is encountered.[15,31,33,85,118,122,131] In the mobile spine, the prevalent tumor by far is metastatic disease; thus both metastatic cancer and chordoma should be in the differential diagnosis whenever a neoplasm of the spine is seen. Although chordomas are tumors of bone, they have also been reported at extraosseous sites, predominantly in the parapharyngeal area. In addition, chordomas along the central nervous system axis without either bone or dural attachment may also be seen.[108,128,136] Chordomas may be multicentric or arise as a second neoplasm.[3,134]

Chordomas occur in almost all age groups,[22,142] although they are predominantly tumors of the fifth through seventh decades of life. Over a 36-year period (1949 to 1985), a total of 88 patients with histologically verified spinal chordomas were treated at the Memorial Sloan-Kettering Cancer Center.[55,119,120] Of these, 54 patients were treated in the earlier 27 years, and the more recent 34 patients were treated within the latter 7 years. In the entire series, there were 60 males and 28 females. Fifty-six lesions were located in the sacrococcygeal region, and 30 involved the vertebral column at a higher level (i.e., the true vertebrae). There were two tumors involving the clivus and skull base. The youngest patient was 2½ years old, and the oldest was 74 years old. The mean age of the sacrococcygeal group was approximately 56 years, whereas tumors originating in the true vertebrae (vertebral chordomas) occurred in a younger age group (mean 47 years). In the literature, chordoma has been reported as a congenital tumor presenting with hydrocephalus, and we have recently encountered such a patient in the ninth decade of life.[96] In a large series of patients encountered at the Mayo Clinic, approximately 50 percent had tumors in the sacrococcygeal region and 40 percent had skull base tumors. Approximately 15 percent of tumors arose in the true vertebrae. This anatomic distribution is not always seen in medical centers because of the skewed referral of patients. The male/female ratio in most series reflects a preponderance of males, with a ratio of slightly larger than 2:1.

In the previously mentioned series of 88 patients, the clinical symptoms and signs varied with the location and extent of the tumor.[119] In general, symptoms associated with sacrococcygeal tumors were present 6 months to a year before diagnosis. The most frequent symptom was pain, located either in the low back or in the sacrum or coccyx, which was reported in 75 percent of our patients. Occasionally, patients complained of pain in the buttocks or perineum. There were no specific characteristics of the pain, which was described variously as dull, sharp, continuous, or intermittent. Because these early symptoms were insidious and nonspecific, they were frequently ignored by the patient or the physician. Fifteen percent of the patients related the pain to a prior history of trauma to the lower back. Rectal dysfunction (change in bowel habits, tenesmus, or rectal bleeding) was noted as an additional symptom in approximately 20 percent of the patients. Occasionally, patients reported urinary incontinence, a symptom less common than in the past because diagnosis is established by computed tomography (CT) or magnetic resonance imaging (MRI) at an earlier stage of the disease.

Twelve patients in the early series noted a mass over the coccyx, and on several occasions this mass was presumed to be a pilonidal cyst. In addition, radicular pain in the sciatic distribution, sensory loss, and other neurological deficits were present in 10 patients. Frequently, pain was referred along the corresponding dermatome; thus, patients with L1–2 lesions generally complained of pain in the hip, knee, groin, or sacroiliac region. Many of these patients were treated for degenerative arthritis, disc disease, coccydynia, or hemorrhoids for several months before the true diagnosis was established. In every sacral tumor patient examined, there was a palpable presacral mass that did not involve the rectal mucosa. The longest time to clinical detection in our more recent series of 34 patients involved an asymptomatic lytic lesion of the sacrum that had been followed for more than 10 years prior to clinical growth and onset of symptoms.[120] There appeared to be no tendency toward earlier clinical detection in the recent group of 34 patients when compared with the previous group of 54 patients.

Patients with chordomas generally present with a shorter duration of symptoms; although radicular pain and neurological deficits are common, the prevertebral mass may frequently become symptomatic, especially in the cervical and nasopharyngeal regions.[9,17,38,51,89] Thus, dysphagia or nasal obstruction may lead to the erroneous diagnosis of a nonosseous retropharyngeal tumor. Although chordomas are rare in the thoracic region, they may present as a posterior mediastinal mass resembling a neurogenic tumor or lymphoma.[2,18,25] Two of the lumbar chordomas in our previous series presented as intra-abdominal masses for which exploratory laparotomies were performed without the spinal origin of the tumor being recognized. Fortunately, it is now rare that a patient is completely paralyzed secondary to spinal cord compression, because most spinal tumors are now diagnosed earlier with MRI.

Although this chapter reviews the presentation and management of spinal tumors, the clinical features of clival lesions may overlap those of lesions of the most cephalad portion of the spinal axis.[72,97,110,112,131,137] Sometimes, it may be impossible to discern the exact site of origin. Clival tumors present with ocular symptoms (either diplopia or visual impairment) in half the cases. Headache and an insidious onset of sixth nerve palsy are the most common presenting features of both chordomas and chondrosarcomas arising at the skull base. A normal neurological examination is almost invariably seen in chordoma patients, whereas visual loss, facial numbness, and multiple cranial neuropathies are more common in patients with chondrosarcoma.

Radiologic Features

Several papers have analyzed both the plain radiographic and CT features of spinal chordomas.[30,34,40,49,70,113,135] The most consistent radiologic finding in sacral chordomas is destruction of several segments of the sacrum associated with a soft tissue tumor mass anterior to it (Figs. 179-1 and 179-2). The degree of calcification in the tumor may vary from 40 to 80 percent, depending on whether this is sought on plain radiographs or CT scans. We agree with Smith et al. that these calcifications are more likely to represent bone debris because calcification is not generally seen in histologic sections.[113] The soft tissue mass is disproportionately larger than the area of bone destruction, and frequently the soft

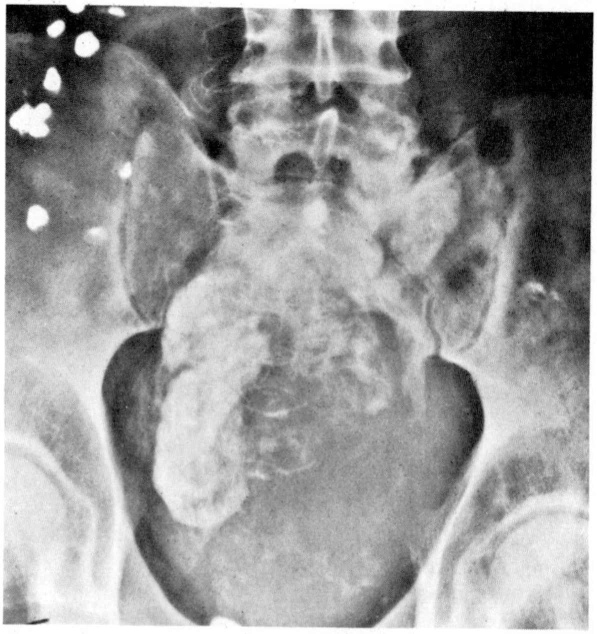

Figure 179-1 Plain x-ray film showing destruction of the sacrum over several segments.

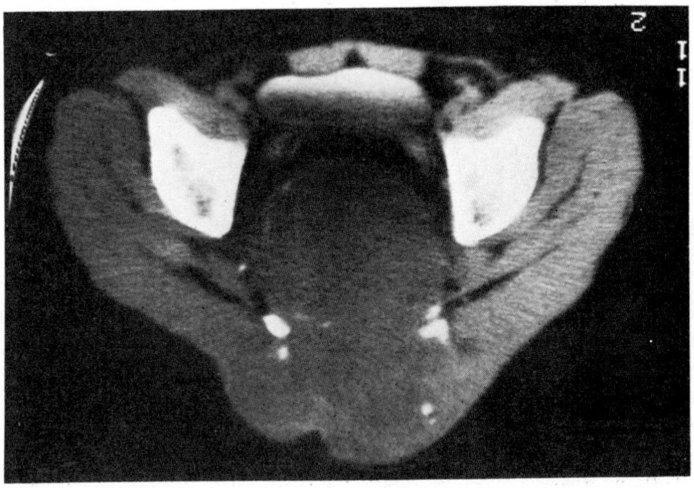

Figure 179-2 CT scan demonstrating a presacral mass displacing the rectum, with destruction of the sacrum and amorphous peripheral calcification.

tissue limits of the mass may be well beyond the level of bone involvement. Generally, the calcification is amorphous and peripheral in location. Tumors involving the true vertebral body are lytic (Fig. 179-3), with surrounding reactive sclerosis. Involvement of adjacent vertebral bodies with sparing of the intervertebral disc is a common feature of chordomas. An anterolateral paraspinal mass is seen in all these patients, and in a few, the intraosseous extension may be barely perceptible. In our more recent patients, the actual amount of bone destruction visualized on plain radiography was minimal.

CT-myelography will reveal epidural extension of tumor in more than 90 percent of patients with tumors involving the true vertebrae; however, it is rarely indicated if high-quality MRI is available. We reserve myelography (in conjunction with CT) for patients who have had extensive spinal instrumentation.

Radionuclide bone scans rarely show positive uptake in the tumor. Spinal angiography is performed in some patients, often to determine whether the tumor is vascular. In the majority, the tumor is relatively avascular, but selective angiography frequently reveals a focal tumor blush.

Although traditional radiographic methods of tumor staging include pyelography, barium studies, and even angiography and venography, it is clear that both CT and MRI are capable of disclosing the total extent of the tumor mass without the need for additional studies. No enhancement is seen with the administration of an intravenous contrast agent during CT examination, which is therefore not recommended for patients with spinal lesions.

The introduction of MRI has added another useful radiodiagnostic tool. MRI is superior to CT because it allows tumor evaluation in the axial, sagittal, and coronal planes. A variety of recent papers have dealt with the MR features of both skull base and spinal chordomas in an effort to distinguish them from other tumors of the bone, such as chondrosarcomas.[34,47,52,59,67,73,74,83,101,115,123,143] On short TR/short TE images, chordomas have a low to intermediate signal intensity. After gadolinium-DTPA administration, all chordomas demonstrate some degree of contrast enhancement. On long TR/long TE images, chordomas generally have a very high, heterogenous signal intensity. Skull base lesions frequently show encasement of intracranial vessels, and tumor extension into structures such as the cavernous sinus, sella, nasopharynx, and hypoglossal canal. The distinction between chordoma and chondrosarcoma may be very difficult on conventional sequences. Chordomas tend to be more lobulated, have peripheral enhancement on administration of a contrast agent, and show markedly low signal intensity on inverson recovery sequences.[124] Recently, Rosenthal and colleagues have shown that MRI provides superior contrast to CT because of the prolonged T1 and T2 times of the tumors.[101] The soft tissue tumor masses are especially well shown by long TR and TE (T2-weighted) MRI scans. Invasion of the rectum—a site that is rarely involved by these tumors—is easily visualized. MRI cannot detect the effects of radiation or the small polyp-like extension of tumor into the surrounding pseudocapsule described by Hudson and Galceran.[59] In our experience, recurrent tumors of the spinal axis tend to spread along the perineurium and sometimes extend into the subarachnoid space. The radiologic findings, that is, the presence of a soft tissue extension with bone involvement, are so characteristic that there should rarely be difficulty in making the radiologic diagnosis. Although these tumors grow strictly in the midline, diagnostic confusion may occasionally result if the tumor grows eccentrically and presents as a pelvic mass with minimal or no apparent intraosseous involvement.

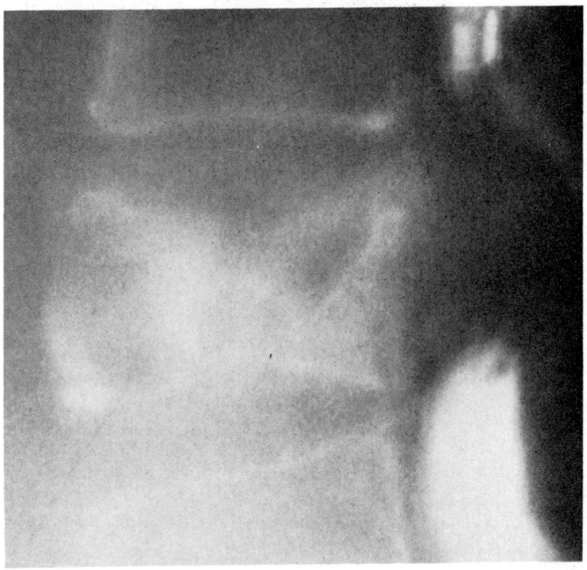

Figure 179-3 Tomogram of a lumbar chordoma showing the combination of lytic destruction, collapse, and epidural extension of tumor.

To facilitate MRI evaluation after tumor resection, titanium implants should be used in spinal instrumentation whenever feasible. If rods and heavy cables are used for reconstruction, removal of these implants once fusion has occurred will allow periodic MRI to evaluate tumor recurrence.

Pathology

Grossly, chordomas are lobulated, gray, partially translucent, glistening, cystic or solid masses that resemble cartilage tumors or occasionally a mucin-producing carcinoma. Their consistency varies from firm and focally ossified or calcified, to extremely soft, myxoid, gelatinous, or even semifluid. These tumors appear to be well circumscribed owing to pseudocapsule formation within soft tissue, but this is not evident within bone. In all sacral tumors, intact and elevated periosteum anteriorly forms the pseudocapsule of the tumor. In the bone itself, the tumor appears to be multifocal, invading between trabeculae without a clear margin of reactive bone.

Microscopically, the tumors are characterized by a distinct, lobular architecture that is formed by the physaliphorous (''soap bubble'') cells with ample vacuolated cytoplasm, as well as by the presence of ''signet ring''-type cells (Fig. 179-4). A dense, often incomplete layer of fibrous tissue is usually seen secondary to soft tissue compression; this layer may be invaded by infiltrating tumor cells. The intracytoplasmic mucus droplets vary greatly in size, and they stain positively for both glycogen and mucin. The smaller, better preserved tumor nodules often have polygonal cells in close proximity to each other similar to carcinoma cells with mucin production. In addition, larger tumor lobules have ample extracellular mucin with only a few stellate cells scattered about, especially in the peripheral areas. Volpe and Mazabrund have stressed that chordoma is a pleomorphic tumor, containing ghost cells, large epithelial cells with acidophilic cytoplasm, small round

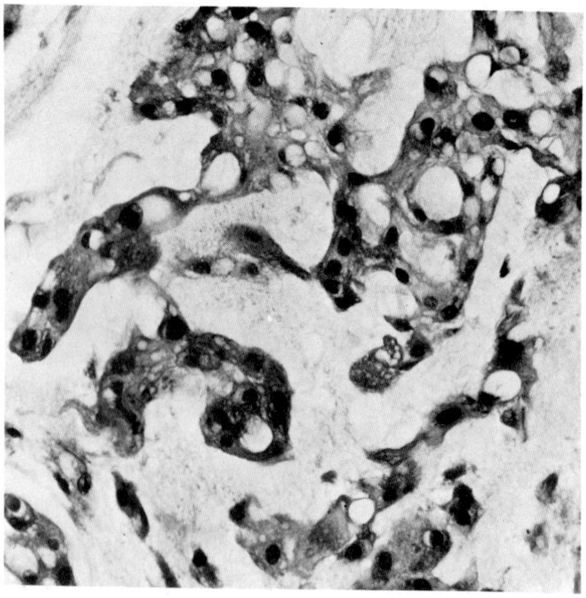

Figure 179-4 Tumor cells arranged in sheets and cords, with individual cells showing marked vacuolation (physaliphorous cells). (Hematoxylin-eosin, ×280; courtesy of Andrew G. Huvos, M.D.)

compact cells, and occasional binucleate forms and multinucleated giant cells in some cases.[132] Although mitotic figures are rare, cellular anaplasia and increased mitotic activity do not seem to correlate with a more virulent clinical course. Histologically, it has previously been accepted that the only prognostic finding is the presence of chondroid differentiation.[54,86,141]

Chondroid chordomas are particularly common in the skull base. Such chondroid differentiation is associated with a median survival of 10 years according to data from a Mayo Clinic study.[54] In a more recent study, Bjornsson et al.[14] analyzed the clinicopathologic features of 40 patients with spinal chordomas, and reviewed several different features from ''classic'' chordoma. These included chondroid differentiation, tumor necrosis, spindle cell transformation, cellular atypia, and areas of compact epithelioid growth. Although the number of patients with these specific features was small, the authors could not correlate biological behavior with histologic features.

Several recent reports suggest that ''dedifferentiated'' chordoma, which resembles a spindle cell sarcoma, may arise de novo even in the absence of prior irradiation. In a recent review of 52 patients with skull base chordoma, two tumors (4 percent) showed anaplastic features, both de novo without evidence of prior irradiation.[127] This was associated with loss of reactivity for keratin and epithelial membrane antigen. Huvos suggests that the term *dedifferentation* is inaccurate because the spindle cell component generally denotes the emergence of a novel phenotype arising from stem cells of mesodermal origin, rather than retrograde differentiation of more mature cellular elements.[61] In some patients, the spindle cell component appears after solitary or several local recurrences. Clearly, the prognosis for chordomas with high-grade spindle cell sarcomatous change is much worse than that for the conventional classic chordoma. These tumors have the highest propensity to disseminate widely by hematogenous metastasis.

At the present time, the most important differential diagnosis in spinal tumors is chondrosarcoma and mucin-producing adenocarcinomas. The availability of small biopsy specimens from percutaneous techniques may pose a technical challenge for the histopathologist. The recent introduction of immunohistochemical methods has greatly facilitated the diagnosis.[1,39,81,82,86,95,133,141] When confronted with a small biopsy showing a small cellular myxoid or mucinous tumor, the differential diagnosis includes mucinous adenocarcinoma, renal cell carcinoma, and myxopapillary ependymoma.[21,87] Using an array of immunohistochemical tests, it has been established that all chordomas are immunoreactive for vimentin and cytokeratin, and approximately 89 percent stain for epithelial membrane antigen and S100 protein.[1,21,81] Myxopapillary ependymomas are distinguished by immunoreactivity for vimentin and glial fibrillary acid protein in all cases; approximately 50 percent react with S100 protein. Most colon cancers are positive for cytokeratin, epithelial membrane antigen, and carcinoembryonic antigen, while renal cancers are uniformly reactive for epithelial membrane antigen and cytokeratin, nonreactive for carcinoembryonic antigen, and variably reactive for S100 protein and vimentin.[141] Although all classic chordomas stain for cytokeratin, less than one-third of chondroid chordomas stain with epithelial markers. A recent study by Mitchell et al. attempted to use immunohistochemical methods to determine prognosis.[86] They noted that regardless of tumor subtype, age was the most important variable in determining survival. There were no significant survival differences in patients with cartilage-containing tumors that were either cytokeratin positive or negative. With increasing dedifferentiation and transformation into spindle cell sarcoma, immunoreactivity to cytokeratin may be lost.[82]

Cytogenetic analysis of two sacral chordomas was reported by Persons et al.[94] These studies showed clonal chromosomal abnormalities, including numerical and structural aberrations. With flow-cytometric studies, aneuploid chromosome numbers were observed in both tumors, and the involvement of the same chromosome band 21q22 suggests that this band may contain genes important in the development of chordoma. Two human proto-oncogenes, ERL and ETS2, have been mapped to this region. Further studies are obviously indicated to confirm these observations.

Frequently, the histologic distinction between chondrosarcoma and chordoma may be difficult, especially in the clival region. The tendency for both intra- and extracellular mucin production helps to distinguish chordomas from cartilaginous tumors. Cartilage lesions have a positive staining reaction with phosphotungstic acid hematoxylin (PTAH), while chordomas are mostly negative for PTAH. Chordomas contain readily-impregnated (by silver-staining) reticulin fibers that support the tumor cells.[26] With the widespread availability of immunohistochemical techniques, however, these special stains are rarely required.

Ultrastructural studies of the tumor have been carried out by several authorities. These show the presence of two cell types: the stellate and the physaliphorous cells, with many transitional forms. The small, compactly arranged stellate cells appear to be the primary cell type, with elongated indented nuclei and sparse cytoplasmic organelles, including agranular endoplasmic reticulum, occasional profiles of rough endoplasmic reticulum, and mitochondria. The physaliphorous cells are identified by the abundant cytoplasm containing vesicles or vacuoles of different types. It has been suggested that the stellate cell is the primary neoplastic cell, which subsequently evolves into the physaliphorous cell and accounts for the autonomous growth of the tumor. The evolution of the stellate cell into the physaliphorous cell supposedly occurs through a process of cisternal dilatation and internal secretion, a process that has been observed in the developing notochord.

Metastases

Whereas the tendency of chordomas to recur locally is well known, the propensity for these tumors to metastasize may not be. Chordoma should be considered a malignant neoplasm even though the clinical behavior is relatively indolent in most patients. Currently, we estimate that between 5 and 10 percent of chordomas may behave as high-grade sarcomas at initial presentation, while 10 to 30 percent metastasize to multiple sites following attempts at resection.[10,23,41,50,58,88,90,132] The final evolutionary stage is the development of a malignant fibrous histiocytoma, an event that is usually but not invariably linked to radiotherapy.[10]

In our earlier series, 11 of 18 vertebral chordoma patients and 10 of 36 sacral chordoma patients were found to have disseminated metastases. The difference in incidence between the two groups was statistically significant. Metastases appeared uniformly throughout the course of therapy and were discovered as early as 1 year and as late as 10 years after tissue diagnosis, and therefore did not merely reflect a long follow-up period. There was no obvious correlation between the incidence of metastases and the mode of treatment of the primary tumor. Sites of metastases included soft tissues, lymph nodes, lung, bone, liver, and other intra-abdominal viscera. Occasionally, widely disseminated metastases to organs including the heart, pleura, and brain were found. In our more recent experience, 30 percent of the patients developed metastases, similar to what has been reported in several different series.

Chambers and Schwinn found an incidence of 30 percent in 27 cases, but curiously the metastases in their study were predominantly to skin and bone.[19] In two of three patients with dermal metastases, the lesions in the skin were diagnosed even prior to the primary tumor. In their study, the histologic appearance of the tumor—anaplasia and the degree of mitosis—did appear to correlate with the presence of metastases. In a more recent study, Su et al. reported on a series of 19 patients with skin involvement from chordoma.[116] These represented local recurrence or metastases in 12, direct extension in 6, and distant metastases in 1. In seven patients, cutaneous lesions were detected when the diagnosis of primary chordoma was made. Metastatic lesions in chordoma have little impact on overall survival because death frequently results from complications of local treatment failure.

The presence of metastatic disease has offered the opportunity to study the biological doubling time of chordoma. In patients with primary tumors, Cummings and coworkers estimated a doubling time of the primary lesion of approximately 6 months.[27] Metastatic tumor nodules, on the other hand, may have much shorter doubling times, ranging from 9 to 36 days; in another report, metastatic nodules in the lung had average doubling times of 3.3 months.

Treatment

There is general agreement that complete surgical resection is the treatment of choice in chordomas, but this type of surgery may not always be technically feasible in advanced cases or in patients with medical contraindications.[5,8] The last decade has witnessed a virtual explosion of the development of surgical approaches aimed at "gross total resection" of chordomas of the skull base, and it is now accepted that more than two-thirds of skull base or craniocervical chordomas can be resected.[4,31,36,42,44,69,72,106,109–112,137] Although there is a tendency to pool patients with chordomas at various sites in many surgical and radiotherapy series, this approach does not allow accurate comparison of the various treatment modalities currently available, and should be avoided. Most skull base and upper cervical spine chordomas are generally removed piecemeal by intralesional curettage, whereas virtually all sacral tumors are potentially amenable to curative en bloc resection by sacrectomy. In the early years, the majority of patients with sacrococcygeal tumors presented with involvement of the first sacral segment, which was considered a contraindication to curative resection. This was based on the assumption that an intact first sacral segment was necessary for maintenance of pelvic strength and stability. Further, complete functional loss of the second through fourth sacral segments leads to complete irreversible loss of bladder and bowel function, often considered unacceptable in a seemingly benign tumor.

The evolution of sacral surgery for chordoma began with the pioneering work of MacCarty and colleagues at the Mayo Clinic,[79] and this surgical approach (posterior sacretomy) is still valid for tumors below the third sacral segment. Removal of sacral tumors is currently carried out using a strictly posterior or a combined anterior–posterior approach.[45,63,76,100,103,121]

The posterior approach is performed with the patient in the Kraske position. A midline incision is made over the sacrum and coccyx, with skin flaps fashioned. Both the midline skin and a portion of the subcutaneous tissue may have to be resected with the sacrum if the tumor extends posteriorly. The gluteal muscles and piriformis muscles are divided to reach the sacroiliac joint. With a perianal skin incision and perineal dissection, the rectum and pelvic organs are mobilized to protect them during later sacral resection. The sacrum and ilium are then osteotomized, usually at the S2–3 level, unless the tumor extends more proximally. The sacral resection should be carried above the tumor in order to avoid contaminating the wound with tumor cells. The proximal nerve roots, including the pudendal nerve and sacral nerves, are carefully identified and preserved. The sacrum is removed, leaving a large space into which suction drains are placed. The coccyx is removed with the specimen. If the caudal sac of the spinal cord is cut, this is carefully repaired. The gluteal muscles may be rotated to fill in the defect.

Of the 50 patients in the Mayo Clinic series who underwent excision of the tumor using this approach, 25 patients had wide local excision without the tumor being entered, while the remainder had inadvertent incision of tumor during resection.[62] For those patients with violation of tumor, the recurrence rate was 64 percent; for those patients in whom the tumor was removed en bloc, the recurrence rate was 28 percent. Complciations related to surgical treatment consisted of bladder dysfunction in 40 percent, which in most cleared spontaneously. Fecal incontinence was noted in 20 percent, but all had gradual clinical improvement. Wound-related complications occurred in another 8 percent. In the overall series of 63 patients, 25 percent were continuously free of disease.

In a more recent series, Samson et al. reported their experience with the posterior approach in 21 patients over a 20-year period (1972 to 1992).[103] They used this approach even for tumors involving the higher levels (S1 segment). In 5 patients (24 percent), the operation was preceded by a colostomy. They used a midline incision with excision of the biopsy scar. The incision was extended either cephalad or caudad in the shape of a hockey stick or an inverted Y, or was carried along the posterior iliac wing. The sacretomy was carried out after mobilizing the sacrum from the rectum and musculoligamentous attachments. They made efforts to preserve as many sacral roots as possible, even if this meant that the tumor pseudocapsule was violated. A wide excision was possible in 10 patients, 3 patients had a marginal excision, and in 7 patients only intralesional curettage was performed. Seven patients (33 percent) had problems with the sacral wound, and 4 underwent additional procedures for wound complications. More than 75 percent of patients received radiotherapy: 5 before and after the operation, and 8 only before the operation; the remaining 3 patients received postoperative radiotherapy. Four patients (19 percent) had evidence of local recurrence, and 3 died of metastatic disease. Their actuarial 5-year survival was 77 percent and 10-year survival was 50 percent. They noted that local recurrences occurred principally in the first 3 years, but metastases appeared late in the clinical course.

With regard to functional results, half the patients who had both second sacral roots spared had normal bowel and bladder function. The surgeons' philosophy was that while the tumor should be removed, as many nerve roots as possible should be spared to preserve normal bladder, bowel, and sexual function.

Although the posterior approach may lead to a lower incidence of complications, we currently believe that chordomas that extend to the second sacral segment can best be managed by a combined anterior–posterior procedure, as originally described by Localio et al. and subsequently modified by others.[12,15,60,63,64,76,77]

An oblique incision is made from the left iliac crest and costal margin; the left colon is mobilized along with the rectum and is displaced anteriorly and to the patient's right. The left ureter is identified. The iliac vessels are also mobilized and are held by tapes for temporary occlusion. The middle sacral vessels and lateral sacral veins are suture ligated. Posteriorly, a transverse incision is made over the sacrum and skin flaps are developed. The gluteal muscles are dissected free from their iliac attachments. The anococcygeal ligaments are incised and the presacral space is entered to join the abdominal dissection. Surgery proceeds with sectioning of the sacroiliac, sacrotuberous, and sacrospinous ligaments. The piriformis muscles are cut. To mobilize the sacrum, osteotomies have to be performed through the sacroiliac articulations and the sacrum. Nerve roots below the level of the sacral osteotomy are included in the resection. The tumor specimen is then completely mobilized. The wounds are then closed over suction drains. Maintenance of the suction drains for prolonged periods will lessen the possibility of serous effusions that may lead to secondary wound infections, which are very common after this type of surgery.

Profuse blood loss may accompany such procedures, and therefore the use of hypotensive anesthesia or a cell saver is recommended. In Localio's series of five patients, there were four long-term survivors. In view of the propensity for blood loss, a preliminary laparotomy during which time both internal iliac vessels are secured and ligated has been recommended. During the initial exploration, the tumor itself is completely mobilized and freed from the rectum, and the middle sacral vessels are ligated. The abdominal incision is then closed, and the patient undergoes posterior sacral resection after being placed in a prone position. In our view, ligation of the internal iliac vessels does not reduce bleeding from the sacral osteotomies, which are the major cause of blood loss during operation.

For much larger tumors, the approach described by Stener and Gunterberg should be used.[114] At least one vertebra proximal to the radiologic limit of the tumor should be removed to ensure tumor-free margins. In younger patients, the argument that preservation of bladder and bowel function is important does not take into account the fact that the majority of recurrent tumors will cause an irreversible loss of bladder and bowel function, with death resulting from local tumor. Stener has shown that if all sacral nerves are sacrificed on one side, there may be little clinical impairment of urogenital and anorectal function. Furthermore, transection of the sacrum above the level of pelvic stability and strength is compatible with ambulation in the upright posture. In Stener's series of eight patients with chordoma, five have remained free of tumor for more than 5 years. We have rarely encountered patients in whom the osteotomy has to be carried through at the lumbosacral junction for a chordoma.

For chordomas arising in the vertebral body, accurate radiologic assessment of tumor extent by a combination of MRI and CT should be performed. Even if the tumors are hypovascular, superselective angiography and embolization to minimize intraoperative blood loss should be considered. In the past, laminectomy and tumor resection from a posterior approach was useful in relieving cord compression, but the majority developed local recurrences within the first 3 years despite postoperative radiation. Currently, successful total resection of the tumor requires that all gross disease be removed by a combined anterior–posterior or staged approach.[48] Removal of the entire vertebra (spondylectomy) and all involved soft tissue may require vertebrectomy at more than one level, and simultaneous exposure of the posterior elements. Following tumor resection, reconstruction of the vertebral body anteriorly with bone grafts and instrumentation, as well as posteriorly by instrumentation, is feasible with minimal morbidity. Although purely intraosseous tumor may be removed by en bloc techniques, intralesional curettage or drilling may be required for bone adjacent to the dura. Carefuly packing and isolation of the operative site should minimize the possibility of surgical contamination.

With these techniques, we have achieved disease-free 5-year survival rates exceeding 67 percent for tumors involving the true vertebrae.[121] Careful repeat evaluation by serial CT is required to detect early recurrences.

Chordomas of the cervical spine may involve one or both vertebral arteries, which can be an impediment to radical tumor resection.[110] Although tumor extensions into the posterior elements can be adequately addressed through the posterior appraoch, the standard anterior approach is insufficient for the anterior tumor. Several authors have advocated the transoral and extended transmandibular approaches for lesions of the upper cervical spine.[4,106,111,140] In addition to the limitations of access to the lateral aspect of the tumor, anterior strut grafting to provide axial support to the spine is not advisable through the contaminated transpharyngeal route. It is recommended that for tumors below C2 an anterolateral approach (posterior to the carotid sheath) be performed as an initial step.[46] This allows isolation and dissection of the vertebral artery and also delineation of the nerve roots and thecal sac from the lateral border of the tumor. At this point the surgeon goes anterior to the carotid sheath as in a Cloward-type anterior approach and completes the vertebrectomy and stabilization with bone grafts and titanium locking plates and screws. Preoperative testing in these patients must include bilateral vertebral arteriography, and in certain situations, if the artery cannot be dissected from the tumor, it can be reconstructed with a saphenous vein graft. A posterior approach is subsequently used at the same or separate operation to resect the involved posterior elements and stabilize the spine with facet plates and screws and bone grafts. In dealing with tumors of the upper two cervical vertebrae, the lateral extrapharyngeal approach is preferred.[111] This approach allows the surgeon to deal with the lower cranial nerves, the vertebral artery, the occipital condyle, and lateral mass of C1 on one side. Anterior instrumentation is usually not possible in such high lesions and impacting a bone graft between the clivus and spine may have to suffice along with posterior instrumentation. Involvement of the opposite side may require the use of a lateral approach from the other side at a later operation. Posterior instrumentation should include the occiput (occipitocervical stabilization) in order to provide long-term stability and alignment of the spine. Sequential postoperative imaging is important in these patients and if possible, titanium devices should be used. If stainless steel rods are used, we recommend that these implants be removed after fusion is complete to allow radiologic monitoring. With these approaches, our current disease-free survival at 5 years exceeds 67 percent.

Because a substantial portion of chordomas recur, repeat surgery to remove localized recurrences is indicated. In some instances, cryosurgery may be used to obtain local control of sacral recurrences in lieu of the need for additional sacral bone resection and loss of stability.[32] Multiple procedures for removal of recurrent chordoma is the norm in most patients with spinal tumors, and morbidity can be minimized if patients do not receive irradiation to the spine.

Radiotherapy

Although it is currently possible to achieve gross total resection in the majority of patients with spinal chordomas, most patients are referred for radiation following either biopsy or subtotal resection.[80,98] Although chordomas are not very responsive to radiation, there may still be a role for this modality as a palliative rather than potentially curative treatment of pain and neurological deficit. In an extensive review of the literature, Cummings and co-workers found no difference in survival between those who had undergone prior biopsy only and those who had subtotal resection prior to radiotherapy.[27] Because chordomas exhibit a wide range of growth rates, the potential impact of any treatment cannot be measured easily. In general, the rate of response of the tumor to irradiation is slow, as can be expected from the relatively acellular and slowly proliferating tumor cells. Even though the predominant effect of the irradiation is on the cellular portion, small reductions in tumor volume may result in symptomatic pain relief and improvement in neurological deficits. In the series of Cummings et al., the 5-year survival rate of 24 patients was 65 percent and the 10-year survival rate was 28 percent.[28] Pearlman and Friedman concluded that chordomas would not respond to doses less than 5000 cGy, but would respond to doses above 6000 to 8000 cGy.[93] It is therefore considered traditional to treat sacrococcygeal chordomas with doses ranging from 6000 to 7000 cGy for curative intent, and to use lesser doses of 4000 to 5000 cGy for palliation. In another review, Cummings et al. found that a 5-year symptomatic response was just as likely at doses of 3500 to 4500 cGy (in 6 of 9 patients) as at doses of 6500 to 8500 cGy (in 4 of 10 patients).[27,28] They did not find a significant dose–response curve in the 3500- to 8500-cGy range. As a result, the tendency had been for most radiotherapists to recommend doses in excess of 5000 cGy for sacral lesions. However, no dose–response relationship was found by Cummings et al. in the recent radiotherapy literature, and the value for such high doses of radiation must be balanced against the potential for delayed radiation effects and complications from subsequent surgery, as well as the small possibility of a radiation-related sarcoma. Unfortunately, there are no good data on the actual impact of external-beam radiation following subtotal resection, although several retrospective studies seem to suggest a small survival advantage.[43,65,84,97,105,125]

Physicians at some institutions have used preoperative irradiation to allow surgery to be carried out closer to the tumor plane (marginal) or directly through it; however, it is clear that prior irradiation has a major impact on wound healing and all patients who have undergone irradiation have a substantially higher incidence of complications following surgery.[103] Additional risks of irradiation include potential injury to the brain stem and spinal cord, as well as the possibility of soft tissue necrosis in the pelvis. Radiation itself has been implicated in the malignant transformation of chordoma into sarcoma, as well as the potential development of a second neoplasm within the surrounding bone.

Currently, with conventional radiotherapy alone, local control is achieved in approximately 35 percent at 3 years. In view of the failure of conventional radiotherapy to produce significant cure rates, or even to alter the median time to tumor relapse, several different techniques have been used to deliver focused high-beam therapy with reduced doses to the surrounding critical tissues. These include the use of wedge filter techniques, rotational beam therapy, and radiosurgery, as well as the use of permanent ^{125}I seeds or removable ^{192}Ir implants.[66,68,71,120]

For this reason, Suit and Castro have pioneered the use of high-dose charged-particle radiation.[6,7,91,104,107,117] At the Lawrence Berkeley Laboratory, the charged-particle beams include helium and neon with energies of 232 to 934 MeV per nucleon. The goal of treatment is to deliver a dose of at least 65 to 70 Gy-equivalents to the longest volume while keeping the dose to the center of the load to 45 Gy-equivalents. In a recent report, 24 patients (12 with chordoma and 12 with chondrosarcoma) with tumors involving the cervical, thoracic, and lumbar spine were treated. The majority had undergone subtotal resection. The 3-year local control rates were

83 percent for chondrosarcoma and 33 percent for chordoma. They noted that chordoma patients tended to have bulkier tumors (>150 cc), which contributed to the poorer local control. In addition, local control was significantly influenced not only by volume but also whether treatment was for recurrent or initial disease. In a similar series of patients with sacral tumors, the 5-year local control rate was 55 percent.[107]

Suit et al. have used proton-beam irradiation at the Harvard Cyclotron Laboratory to treat chordomas and chondrosarcomas of the skull base and cervical spine. In the overall series, local control was achieved in 111 of 141 patients. The complex treatment plan included a prescribed target does of 70 Cobalt Gy-equivalents to gross disease, and 45 Cobalt Gy-equivalents to areas of microscopic disease. Of the 26 failures, 10 involved tumors of the cervical spine. The authors attributed this to the larger size of residual tumors (120 cc) for tumors in this location. However, although the 3-year local control rates are high, there is a tendency for the incidence of local failure to increase over time. Chordomas are prone to recur many years after initial treatment.[75] At present, the actuarial local control rate at 5 years for chordomas in the cervical spine is 67 percent (Hug et al. Personal communication, 1993).

Chemotherapy

There has been no concerted effort to treat patients with chordomas using chemotherapy regimens because they are generally considered to be resistant to chemotherapy. The majority of patients are referred for treatment only after maximum radiotherapy has been given or for treatment of metastatic disease. Reports in the literature have suggested occasional subjective and objective responses to chemotherapy. A small number of patients with metastatic disease have been given either single agents or combination chemotherapy, with poor results. In our initial series, 14 patients received single-agent or combination therapy, and only short-term subjective relief of pain was seen in two patients. In our more recent series, seven patients were treated with sarcoma regimens (incorporating doxorubicin), but no major response was noted. Fleming et al. have recently reported complete remissions to chemotherapy in two patients with dedifferentiated chordoma.[41] In one patient a six-drug regimen was used; in the other, high-dose ifosfamide was used. We have also observed chemotherapy responses in high-grade sarcomatous variants of chordoma using doxorubicin, platinum, or ifosfamide combinations. In patients having chordomas with spindle cell features suggesting malignancy, early chemotherapy in conjunction with radiotherapy might be warranted.

Results of Treatment

In view of the slow-growing nature of the tumor, the actual impact of newer treatment modalities is difficult to assess. Some authorities have concluded that the natural history of disease is only marginally affected by treatment, but we believe that this pessimistic view is not justified in view of the remarkable technical advances in surgery that have occurred within the past few years. The median survival time reported in the literature is approximately 5 years for sacral lesions and survival varies from 20 to 40 percent at the 10-year level. However, only 10 to 30 percent of patients were rendered disease-free by treatment.[119,120] More recently, however, surgical resection alone can be expected to produce disease-free survival rates of 67 to 75 percent at 5 years, a figure that is also similar to data available from centers using particle-beam therapy.[44]

The role of radiotherapy following curative total resection is still unclear. Although particle-beam irradiation has been advocated as being superior to conventional photon-beam therapy, the major determinant affecting local control still remains residual tumor volume following surgery. Because chordomas tend to recur many years after treatment, 5-year survival statistics may be misleading.

Despite the vast surgical literature, very little is known about this tumor at the molecular level, knowledge of which is crucial to improving results in the future.

With the sophisticated technique of radiologic imaging with MRI, earlier and smaller tumors, as well as their extension into various anatomic compartments, can be visualized. This should clearly result in better disease-free survival both for skull base and spinal chordomas. Unfortunately, attempts at resection are often being made by surgeons with little experience in the management of these complex tumors. Because prior surgery and irradiation negatively impact on a subsequent surgical attempt at cure, we believe that the initial curative surgery should be attempted only at centers that offer the best possibilities for cure.

References

1. Abenoza P, Sibley RK. Chordoma—an immunohistologic study. *Hum Pathol* 1986; 17:744–747.
2. Ahrendt MN, Wesselhoeft CW. Chordoma presenting as a posterior mediastinal mass in a pediatric patient. *J Pediatr Surg* 1992; 27:1515–1518.
3. Anderson WB, Meyers HI. Multicentric chordoma—report of a case. *Cancer* 1968; 21:126–128.
4. Arbit E, Patterson RH Jr. Combined transoral and median labromandibular glossotomy approach to the upper cervical spine. *Neurosurgery* 1981; 8:672–674.
5. Ariel IM, Verdu C. Chordoma: An analysis of twenty cases treated over a twenty-year span. *J Surg Oncol* 1975; 7:27–44.
6. Austin JP, Urie MM, Cardenosa G, Munzenrider JE. Probable causes of recurrence in patients with chordoma and chondrosarcoma of the base of skull and cervical spine. *Int J Radiat Oncol Biol Phys* 1993; 25:439–444.
7. Austin-Seymour M, Munzenrider J, Goitein M, et al. Fractionated proton radiation therapy of chordoma and low-grade chondrosarcoma of the base of the skull. *J Neurosurg* 1989; 70:13–17.
8. Azzarelli A, Quagliuolo V, Cerasoli S, et al. Chordoma: natural history and treatment results in 33 cases. *J Surg Oncol* 1988; 37:185–191.
9. Batsakis JG, Kittleson AC. Chordomas: otorhinolaryngolocic presentation and diagnosis. *Arch Otolaryngol* 1963; 78:168–175.
10. Belza MG, Urich H. Chordoma and malignant fibrous histiocytoma: Evidence for transformation. *Cancer* 1986; 58:1082–1087.
11. Berryhill BH, Armstrong BW. Extracranial presentation of craniocervical chordoma. *Laryngoscope* 1984; 94:1063–1065.
12. Bethke KP, Neifeld JP, Lawrence W Jr. Diagnosis and management of sacrococcygeal chordoma. *J Surg Oncol* 1991; 48:232–238.
13. Birrell JHW. Chordomata: A review of nineteen cases of chordomata including five vertebral cases. *Aust NZ J Surg* 1953; 22:258–267.
14. Bjornsson J, Wold LE, Ebersold MJ, Laws ER. Chordoma of the mobile spine. A clinicopathologic analysis of 40 patients. *Cancer* 1993; 71:735–740.
15. Bohm B, Milsom JW, Fazio VW, et al. Our approach to the

management of congenital presacral tumors in adults. *Int J Colorectal Dis* 1993; 8:134–138.
16. Brondi LA, Podrecca S, Cataldo I. Chordoma: study of 245 cases verified at the Instituto Nazionale dei Tumori de Milano. *Rev Paul Med* 1980; 95:71–73.
17. Campbell WM, McDonald TJ, Unni KK, et al. Nasal and paranasal presentations of chordomas. *Laryngoscope* 1980; 90:612–618.
18. Castellano GC, Johnston HW. Intrathoracic chordoma presenting as a posterior mediastinal tumor. *South Med J* 1975; 68:109–112.
19. Chambers PW, Schwinn CP. Chordoma: A clinicopathologic study of metastasis. *Am J Clin Pathol* 1979; 72:765–776.
20. Chetty R, Levin CV, Kalan MR. Chordoma: A 20-year clinicopathologic review of the experience at Groote Schuur Hospital, Cape Town. *J Surg Oncol* 1991; 46:261–264.
21. Coffin CM, Swanson PE, Wick MR, Dehner LP. An immunohistochemical comparison of chordoma with renal cell carcinoma, colorectal adenocarcinoma, and myxopapillary ependymoma: a potential diagnostic dilemma in the diminutive biopsy. *Mod Pathol* 1993; 6:531–538.
22. Coffin CM, Swanson PE, Wick MR, Dehner LP. Chordoma in childhood and adolescence. A clinicopathologic analysis of 12 cases. *Arch Pathol Lab Med* 1993; 117:927–933.
23. Congdon CC. Benign and malignant chordomas. A clinico-anatomical study of twenty-two cases. *Am J Pathol.* 1952; 28:793–821.
24. Congdon CC. Proliferative lesions resembling chordoma following puncture of the nucleus pulposus in rabbits. *J Nat Cancer Inst* 1952; 12:893–907.
25. Cotler HB, Cotler JM, Cohn HE, et al. Intrathoracic chordoma presenting as a posterior superior mediastinal tumor. *Spine* 1983; 8:781–786.
26. Crawford T. The staining reactions of chordoma. *J Clin Pathol* 1958; 11:110–113.
27. Cummings BJ, Esses S, Harwood ARI. The treatment of chordoma. *Cancer Treat Rev* 1982; 9:299–311.
28. Cummings BJ, Hodson DI, Bush RS. Chordoma: the results of megavoltage radiation therapy. *Int J Radiat Oncol Biol Phys* 1983; 9:633–642.
29. Dahlin DC, Unni KK. *Bone Tumors: General Aspects and Data on 8542 Cases,* 4th ed. Springfield, IL: Charles C Thomas, 1986, pp 379–393.
30. De Bruine FT, Kroon HM. Spinal chordoma: radiologic features in 14 cases. *Am J Roentgenol* 1988; 150:861–863.
31. Derome PJ, Visot A, Monteil JP, et al. Management of cranial chordomas. In Sekhar LN, Schramm VL (eds): *Tumors of the Cranial Base: Diagnosis and Treatment.* New York: Futura, 1987, pp 607–622.
32. De Vries J, Oldhoff J, Hadders HN. Cryosurgical treatment of sacrococcygeal chordoma. Report of four cases. *Cancer* 1986; 58:2348–2354.
33. Di Lorenzo N, Delfini R, Ciappetta P, et al. Primary tumors of the cervical spine: surgical experience with 38 cases. *Surg Neurol* 1992; 38:12–18.
34. Ducou le Point H, Brugieres P, Chevalier X, et al. Imaging of chordomas of the mobile spine. *J Neuroradiol* 1991; 18:267–276.
35. Dunn DG, Harris RK, Meis JM, Sweet DE. A histomorphologic and immunohistochemical study of chordoma in twenty ferrets (*mustela putorius furo*). *Vet Pathol* 1991; 28:467–473.
36. Erba SM, Horton JA, Latchaw RE, Yonas H. Balloon test occlusion of the internal carotid artery with stable xenon/CT cerebral blood flow imaging. *Am J Neuroradiol* 1988; 9:533–538.
37. Eriksson B, Guterberg B, Kindblom LG. Chordoma: A clinicopathologic and prognostic study of a Swedish national series. *Acta Orthop Scand* 1981; 52:49–58.
38. Fernandez Liesa R, Fraile Rodrigo J, Rivares Esteban J, Perez OJ. Chordoma cervical. *Acta Otorbinolaryingol Esp* 1991; 42:121–124.
39. Finley JL, Silverman JF, Dabbs DJ, et al. Chordoma: diagnosis by fine-needle aspiration biopsy with histologic immunocytochemical, and ultrastructural confirmation. *Diagn Cytopathol* 1986; 2:330–337.
40. Firooznia H, Pinto RS, Lin JP, et al. Chordoma: radiologic evaluation of twenty cases. *Am J Roentgenol* 1976; 127:797–805.
41. Fleming GF, Heimann PS, Stephens JK, et al. Dedifferentiated chordoma. Response to aggressive chemotherapy in two cases. *Cancer* 1993; 72:714–718.
42. Forsyth PA, Cascino TL, Shaw EG, et al. Intracranial chordomas: a clinicopathological and prognostic study of 51 cases. *J Neurosurg* 1993; 78:741–747.
43. Fuller DB, Bloom JG. Radiotherapy for chordoma. *Int J Radiat Oncol Biol Phys* 1988; 15:331–339.
44. Gay E, Sekhar LN, Rubinstein E, et al. Chordomas and chondrosarcomas of the cranial base: results and follow-up of 60 patients. Presented at the 62nd Annual Meeting of the American Association of Neurological Surgeons, San Diego, California, April 11, 1994.
45. Gennari L, Azzarelli A, Quagliuolo V. A posterior approach for the excision of sacral chordoma. *J Bone Joint Surg [Br]* 1987; 69B:565–568.
46. George B, Zerah M, Lot G, Hurth M. Oblique transcorporeal approach to anteriorly located lesions in the cervical spinal canal. *Acta Neurochir (Wien)* 1993; 121:187–190.
47. Golfieri R, Baddeley H, Pringle JS, et al. Primary bone tumors. MR morphologic appearance correlated with pathologic examinations. *Acta Radiol* 1991; 32:290–298.
48. Gregorius FK, Batzdorf U. Removal of thoracic chordoma by staged laminectomy and thoracotomy: a case report. *Am Surg* 1977; 45:535–537.
49. Hagenlocher HU, Ciba K. Radiologische Aspekte des zervikalen Chordoms. *ROFO Fortschr Geb Rontgenstr Nuklearmed* 1976; 125:228–232.
50. Halpern J, Kopolovic J, Catane R. Malignant fibrous histiocytoma developing in irradiated sacral chordoma. *Cancer* 1984; 53:2661–2662.
51. Hampal S, Flood LM, Jones RA. Chordoma of the parapharyngeal space. *J Laryngol Otol* 1992; 106:549–552.
52. Hardie RC. Magnetic resonance appearance of a rare intradural chordoma. *Wis Med J* 1992; 91:627–628.
53. Heaton JM, Turner DR. Reflections on notochordal differentiation arising from a study of chordomas. *Histopathology* 1985; 9:543–550.
54. Heffelfinger MJ, Dahlin DC, MacCarty CS, Beabout JW. Chordomas and cartilaginous tumors at the skull base. *Cancer* 1973; 23:410–420.
55. Higinbotham NL, Phillips RF, Farr HW, et al. Chordoma: thirty-five year study at Memorial Hospital. *Cancer* 1967; 20:1841–1850.
56. Horowitz T. Chordal ectopia and its possible relationship to chordoma. *Arch Pathol* 1941; 31:354–362.
57. Horowitz T. *The Human Notochord. A Study of its Development and Regression, Variations, and Pathologic Derivative, Chordoma.* Indianapolis: Limited Private Printing, 1977.
58. Hruban RH, Traganos F, Reuter VE, Huvos AG. Chordomas with malignant spindle cell components: a DNA flow cytometric and immunohistochemical study with histogenic implications. *Am J Pathol* 1990; 137:435–447.
59. Hudson TM, Galceran M. Radiology of sacrococcygeal chordoma: difficulties in detecting soft tissue extension. *Clin Orthop* 1983; 175:237–242.
60. Huth JF, Dawson EG, Eilber FR. Abdominosacral resection for malignant tumors of the sacrum. *Am J Surg* 1984; 48:157–161.
61. Huvos AG. *Bone Tumors: Diagnosis, Treatment, and Prognosis.* Philadelphia: Saunders, 1979, pp 373–391.
62. Kaiser TE, Pritchard DJ, Unni KK. Clinicopathologic study of sacrococcygeal chordoma. *Cancer* 1984; 53:2574–2578.
63. Karakousis CP. Sacral resection with preservation of continence. *Surg Gynecol Obstet* 1986; 163:270–273.
64. Karakousis CP, Park JJ, Fleminger R, Friedman M. Chordomas: diagnosis and management. *Am Surg* 1981; 47:497–501.
65. Keisch ME, Garcia DM, Shibuya RB. Retrospective long-term follow-up analysis in 21 patients with chordomas of various sites treated at a single institution. *J Neurosurg* 1991; 75:374–377.
66. Kelley CD, Reid A, Simpson LD, et al. The Proimos device: a gravity

oriented blocking system for use in external radiation therapy. *Clin Bull* 1976; 6:107–113.
67. Kollias SS, Barkovich AJ, Edwards MS. Magnetic resonance analysis of suprasellular tumors of childhood. *Pediatr Neurosurg* 1991; 17:284–303.
68. Kondziolka D, Lunsford LD, Flickinger JC. The role of radiosurgery in the management of chordoma and chondrosarcoma of the cranial base. *Neurosurgery* 1991; 29:38–46.
69. Kratimenos GP, Crockard HA. The far lateral approach for ventrally placed foramen magnum and upper cervical spine tumours. *Br J Neurosurg* 1993; 7:129–140.
70. Krol G, Sundaresan N, Deck M. Computerized tomography in axial chordomas. *J Comput Assist Tomogr* 1983; 7:286–289.
71. Kumar PP, Good RR, Skultety FM, et al. Local control of recurrent clival and sacral chordoma after interstitial irradiation with iodine-125: new techniques for treatment of recurrent or unresectable chordomas. *Neurosurgery* 1988; 22:479–483.
72. Lanzino G, Hirsch WL, Pomonis S, et al. Cavernous sinus tumors: neuroradiologic and neurosurgical considerations on one hundred and fifty operated cases. *J Neurosurg Sci* 1992; 36:183–196.
73. Larson TC III, Houser OW, Laws ER Jr. Imaging of cranial chordomas. *Mayo Clin Proc* 1987; 62:886–893.
74. Leproux F, De Toffol B, Aesch B, Cotty P. MRI of cranial chordomas: the value of gadolinium. *Neuroradiology* 1993; 35:543–545.
75. Lewis NDC. A contribution to the study of tumors from the primitive notochord. *Arch Intern Med* 1921; 28:434–452.
76. Localio SA, Eng K, Ranson JH. Abdominosacral approach for retrorectal tumors. *Ann Surg* 1980; 191:555–560.
77. Localio SA, Francis KC, Rossano PG. Abdominosacral resection of sacrococcygeal chordoma. *Ann Surg* 1967; 166:394–402.
78. Mabrey RE. Chordoma: a study of 150 cases. *Am J Cancer* 1935; 25:501–517.
79. MacCarty CS, Waugh JM, Mayo CW, Conventry MB. The surgical treatment of presacral tumor: a combined problem. *Proc Staff Meet Mayo Clin* 1952; 27:73–84.
80. Magrini SM, Papi MG, Marletta F, et al. Chordoma—natural history, treatment, and prognosis: the Florence Radiotherapy Department experience (1956–1990) and a critical review of the literature. *Acta Oncol* 1992; 31:847–851.
81. Meis JM, Giraldo AA. Chordoma—An immuno-histochemical study of twenty cases. *Arch Pathol Lab Med* 1988; 112:553–558.
82. Meis JM, Raymond AK, Evans HL, et al. "Dedifferentiated" chordoma: a clinicopathologic and immunohistochemical study of three cases. *Am J Surg Pathol* 1987; 11:516–525.
83. Meyers SP, Hirsch WL Jr, Curtin HD, et al. Chordomas of the skull base: MR features. *Am J Neuroradiol* 1992; 13:1627–1636.
84. Mindell ER. Chordoma. *J Bone Joint Surg [Am]* 1981; 63A:501–505.
85. Mirra JM. *Bone Tumors: Clinical, Radiologic, and Pathologic Correlations.* Philadelphia: Lea & Febiger, 1989.
86. Mitchell A, Scheithauer BW, Unni KK, et al. Chordoma and chondroid neoplasms of the spheno-occiput. An immunohistochemical study of 41 cases with prognostic and nosologic implications. *Cancer* 1993; 72:2943–2949.
87. Moelleken SM, Seeger LL, Eckardt JJ, Batzdorf U. Myxopapillary ependymoma with extensive sacral destruction: CT and MR findings. *J Comput Assist Tomogr* 1992; 16:164–166.
88. Morris AA, Rabinovitch R. Malignant chordoma of the lumbar region; report of a case with autopsy; comment on usual metastases to the brain, lungs, pancreas, sacrum and axillary and iliac lymph nodes. *Arch Neurol Psychiatry* 1947; 57:547–564.
89. Murali R, Rovit RL, Benjamin MV. Chordoma of the cervical spine. *Neurosurgery* 1981; 9:253–256.
90. Nanda A, Hirsch LF, Antoiniades K. Malignant fibrous histiocytoma in a recurrent thoracic chordoma: case report and literature review. *Neurosurgery* 1991; 28:588–592.
91. Nowakowski VA, Castro JR, Petti PL, et al. Charged particle radiotherapy of paraspinal tumors. *Int J Radiat Oncol Biol Phys* 1992; 22:295–303.
92. Paavolainen P, Teppo L. Chordoma in Finland. *Acta Orthop Scand* 1976; 47:46–51.
93. Pearlman AW, Friedman M. Radical radiation therapy of chordoma. *Am J Roentgenol Radiat Ther Nucl Med* 1970; 108:333–341.
94. Persons DL, Bridge JA, Neff JR. Cytogenic analysis of two sacral chordomas. *Cancer Genet Cytogenet* 1991; 56:197–201.
95. Plate KH, Bittinger A. Value of immunocytochemistry in aspiration cytology of sacrococcygeal chordoma: a report of two cases. *Acta Cytol* 1992; 36:87–90.
96. Probst EN, Zanella FE, Vortmeyer AO. Congenital clivus chordoma. *Am J Neuroradiol* 1993; 14:537–539.
97. Raffel C, Wright DC, Gutin PH, Wilson CB. Cranial chordomas: clinical presentation and results of operative and radiation therapy in twenty-six patients. *Neurosurgery* 1985; 17:703–710.
98. Reddy EK, Mansfield CM, Hartman CV. Chordoma. *Int J Radiat Oncol Biol Phys* 1981; 7:1709–1711.
99. Ribbert H. Ueber die Ecchondrosis physalifora sphenooccipitalis. *Zentralbl Allg Pathol* 1894; 5:457–461.
100. Rich TA, Schiller A, Suit HD, Mankin HJ. Clinical and pathologic review of 48 cases of chordoma. *Cancer* 1985; 56:182–187.
101. Rosenthal DI, Scott JA, Mankin HJ, et al. Sacrococcygeal chordoma: magnetic resonance imaging and computed tomography. *Am J Roentgenol* 1985; 145:143–147.
102. Salisbury JR, Deverall MH, Cookson MJ, Whimster WF. Three-dimensional reconstruction of human embryonic notochords: clue to the pathogenesis of chordoma. *J Pathol* 1993; 171:59–62.
103. Samson IR, Springfield DS, Suit HD, Mankin HJ. Operative treatment of sacrococcygeal chordoma. A review of twenty-one cases. *J Bone Joint Surg [Am]* 1993; 75A:1476–1484.
104. Saunders WM, Chen GTY, Austin-Seymour M, et al. Precision, high dose radiotherapy. II. Helium ion treatment of tumors adjacent to critical central nervous system structures. *Int J Radiat Oncol Biol Phys* 1985; 11:1339–1347.
105. Saxton JP. Chordoma. *Int J Radiat Oncol Biol Phys* 1981; 7:913–915.
106. Scamoni C, Marra A, Dario A, et al. Surgical approaches to the clivus and upper cervical spine. *J Neurosurg Sci* 1991; 35:123–129.
107. Schoenthaler R, Castro JR, Petti PL, et al. Charged particle irradiation of sacral chordomas. *Int J Radiat Oncol Biol Phys* 1993; 26:291–298.
108. Sebag G, Dubois J, Beniaminovitz A, et al. Extraosseous spinal chordoma: radiographic appearance. *Am J Neuroradiol* 1993; 14:205–207.
109. Sekhar LN, Janecka IP, Jones NF. Subtemporal-infratemporal and basal subfrontal approach to extensive cranial base tumours. *Acta Neurochir (Wien)* 1988; 92:83–92.
110. Sen C, Eisenberg M, Casden AM, et al. Management of the vertebral artery in excision of extradural tumors of the cervical spine. *Neurosurgery* 1995; 36:106–116.
111. Sen CN, Sekhar LN. Surgical management of anteriorly placed lesions at the craniocervical junction—an alternative approach. *Acta Neurochir (Wien)* 1991; 108:70–77.
112. Sen CN, Sekhar LN, Schramm VL, Janecka IP. Chordoma and chondrosarcoma of the cranial base: an 8-year experience. *Neurosurgery* 1989; 25:931–941.
113. Smith J, Ludwig RL, Marcove RC. Sacrococcygeal chordoma. A clinicoradiological study of 60 patients. *Skeletal Radiol* 1987; 16:37–44.
114. Stener B, Gunterberg B. High amputation of the sacrum for extirpation of tumors: principles and technique. *Spine* 1978; 3:351–366.
115. Stephens GC, Schwartz HS. Lumbosacral chordoma resection: image integration and surgical planning. *J Surg Oncol* 1993; 54:226–232.
116. Su WP, Louback JB, Gagne EJ, Scheithauer BW. Chordoma cutis: a report of nineteen patients with cutaneous involvement of chordoma. *J Am Acad Dermatol* 1993; 29:63–66.
117. Suit HD, Goitein M, Munzenrider J, et al. Definitive radiation therapy for chordoma and chondrosarcoma of the base of the skull and cervical spine. *J Neurosurg* 1982; 56:377–385.
118. Sundaresan N. Chordomas. *Clin Orthop* 1986; 204:135–142.

119. Sundaresan N, Galicich JH, Chu FCH, Huvos AG. Spinal chordomas. *J Neurosurg* 1979; 50:312–319.
120. Sundaresan N, Huvos AG, Krol G, Brennan MB. Surgical treatment of spinal chordomas. *Arch Surg* 1987; 122:1479–1482.
121. Sundaresan N, Krol G, Sachdev VP. Chordomas of the spine: an 8-year experience with radical resection. Presented at the 60th Annual Meeting of the American Association of Neurological Surgeons, San Francisco, California, April 13, 1992.
122. Sundaresan N, Schmidek HH, Schiller AL, Rosenthal DI. *Tumors of the Spine: Diagnosis and Clinical Management.* Philadelphia: Saunders, 1990.
123. Sze G, Uichanco LS, Brant-Zawadzki MN, et al. Chordomas: MR imaging. *Radiology* 1988; 166:187–191.
124. Tashiro T, Inoue Y, Nemoto Y, et al. Magnetic resonance (MR) imaging of chordoma and chondroma in the skull base—differential diagnosis by IR sequence. *Nippon Igaku Hoshasen Gakkai Zasshi* 1992; 52:589–593.
125. Tewfik HH, McGinnis WL, Nordstrom DG, Latourette HB. Chordoma: evaluation of clinical behavior and treatment modalities. *Int J Radiat Oncol Biol Phys* 1977; 2:959–962.
126. Thakar A, Tandon DA, Bahadur S, Yijayaraghavan M. Extranotochordal chordoma presenting as multiple neck masses: report of a case. *J Laryngol Otol* 1993; 107:942–945.
127. Tomlinson FH, Scheithauer BW, Forsythe PA, et al. Sarcomatous transformation in cranial chordoma. *Neurosurgery* 1992; 31:13–18.
128. Tomlinson FH, Scheithauer BW, Miller GM, Onofrio BM. Extraosseous spinal chordoma: case report. *J Neurosurg* 1991; 75:980–984.
129. Ulich TR, Mirra JM. Ecchordosis physaliphora vertebralis. *Clin Orthop* 1982; 163:282–289.
130. Virchow R. *Untersuchungen uber die Entwickelung des Schadelgrundes im gesunden und krankhaften Zustande und uber den Einfluss der selben auf Schadelform, Gesichtsbildung und Gehirnbau.* Berlin: G. Reimer, 1857, p 128.
131. Volpe NJ, Liebsch NJ, Munzenrider JE, Lessel S. Neuro-ophthalmologic findings in chordoma and chondrosarcoma of the skull base. *Am J Opthalmol* 1993; 115:97–104.
132. Volpe R, Mazabrund A. A clinicopathologic review of 25 cases of chordoma (a pleomorphic and metastasizing neoplasm). *Am J Surg Pathol* 1983; 7:161–170.
133. Walaas L, Kindblom LG. Fine-needle aspiration biopsy in the preoperative diagnosis of chordoma: a study of 17 cases with application of electron microscopic, histochemical, and immunocytochemical examination. *Hum Pathol* 1991; 22:22–28.
134. Walsh TM, Mayer PJ. Chordoma of the thoracic spine presenting as a second primary malignant lesion. A case report. *Spine* 1992; 17:1524–1528.
135. Wang AM, Joachim CL, Shillito J Jr, et al. Cervical chordoma presenting with intervertebral foramen enlargement mimicking neurofibroma: CT findings. *J Comput Assist Tomogr* 1984; 8:529–532.
136. Warnick RE, Raisanen J, Kaczmar T Jr, et al. Intradural chordoma of the tentorium cerebelli. Case report. *J Neurosurg* 1991; 74:508–511.
137. Watkins L, Khudados ES, Kaleoglu M, et al. Skull base chordomas: a review of thirty-eight patients, 1958–1988. *Br J Neurosurg* 1993; 7:241–248.
138. Wellinger CL. Le chordome rachidien—revue de la littérature depuis 1960. *Rev Rhum Mal Osteoartic* 1975; 42:109–116.
139. Willis RA. *Pathology of Tumours,* 4th ed. London: Butterworth 1967, p 937.
140. Windle-Taylor PC. Cervical chordoma: report of a case and the technique of transoral removal. *Br J Surg* 1977; 64:438–441.
141. Wojno KJ, Hruban RH, Garin-Chesa P, Huvos AG. Chondroid chordomas and low-grade chondrosarcomas of the craniospinal axis. An immunohistochemical analysis of 17 cases. *Am J Surg Pathol* 1992; 16:1144–1152.
142. Wold LE, Laws ER Jr. Cranial chordomas in children and young adults. *J Neurosurg* 1983; 59:1043–1047.
143. Yuh WT, Flickinger FW, Barloon TJ, et al. MR imaging of unusual chordomas. *J Comput Assist Tomogr* 1988; 12:30–35.

180 Vertebral Hemangiomas

David C. Hemmy

Incidence

Vertebral hemangioma is the most commonly encountered tumor of the vertebral column. Its incidence has been noted variously from 2 to 12 percent in routine autopsy material. It occurs slightly more commonly in females than males. It is also a disease of advancing age, encountered only infrequently in children and most commonly beyond the fourth decade of life in adults. The hemangioma may involve any portion of the spine, including the sacrum, but occurs most often in the thoracic spine and next most often in the lumbar spine. It rarely occurs in the cervical spine, but cases have been described in which the tumor has caused cord compression or radicular symptoms.

In slightly less than two-thirds of the cases, a single vertebral body is involved. Two to five lesions are encountered in approximately one-third of the cases. Involvement of more than five vertebral bodies is extremely rare.

Pathology

Vertebral hemangiomas can be either cavernous or capillary. More common is the cavernous form, which consists of large, irregular spaces filled with blood and lined by a single layer of endothelial cells. The capillary hemangioma consists of small blood vessels lined by a single layer of cuboidal cells.

The blood supply to the lesion consists of small branches of the intercostal or lumbar arteries which arise proximal to the radicular branches. The lesion is functionally an arteriovenous shunt.

Clinical and Radiologic Features

Most often, a vertebral hemangioma is an asymptomatic, incidental finding. For those that do produce symptoms, the clinical presentation is often insidious. The patient may note local pain, radicular symptoms, or a slowly progressive paraparesis.

Frequently, but not always, changes on plain x-ray films are pathognomonic of the lesion. Vertical trabeculae buttressed by new bone produce axial sclerotic strands between areas of rarefaction (Fig. 180-1). Such areas represent the tumor tissue, which is sometimes mingled with fat. The tumor most often involves a vertebral body but may extend into the pedicles, laminae, and transverse and spinous processes. Vertebral end plates are usually preserved, but extension into disc spaces and neighboring ribs has been described. Simulation of destruction by metastasis may appear radiographically if the pedicles are involved and ill-defined.

Extraspinal contiguous extension of the tumor may produce a paravertebral soft tissue shadow that suggests tuberculosis. In hemangioma, however, the disc space usually remains intact. The presence of a paravertebral mass without bone changes usually suggests an inflammatory or neoplastic process. However, hemangioma may present in a similar fashion. Similarities to Paget's disease will be observed when a hemangioma presents with coarse trabeculation that is accentuated at the periphery of a vertebral body. Furthermore, expansion of the vertebral body may occur, as in Paget's disease. The presence of a high alkaline phosphatase value and involvement of other bones will serve to differentiate Paget's disease.

Plain-film examination of the spine will usually show, in addition to the characteristic features of vertebral hemangioma, loss of vertebral height suggesting recent collapse of the vertebra (Fig. 180-1). Computed tomography (CT) should be employed to best determine the degree of bone destruction that has occurred (Fig. 180-2). The occasional annular constriction of the spinal canal because of involvement of the pedicles, laminae, and vertebral body is also best shown by CT studies.

Unlike most osseous lesions, vertebral hemangiomas display an increased signal on T1- and T2-weighted magnetic resonance imaging (MRI), serving to distinguish them from other osseous lesions. This characteristic is due to the fact that adipose tissue is contained in these lesions. It has been suggested that the fat content of the lesion may be inversely proportional to the aggressiveness of the lesion. Thus, high MRI T1 and T2 signal intensity and decreased opacification on contrast-enhanced CT may represent less active vertebral hemangiomas, whereas less T1 and T2 signal intensity and increased opacification on enhanced CT may represent a more active vascular lesion.[4]

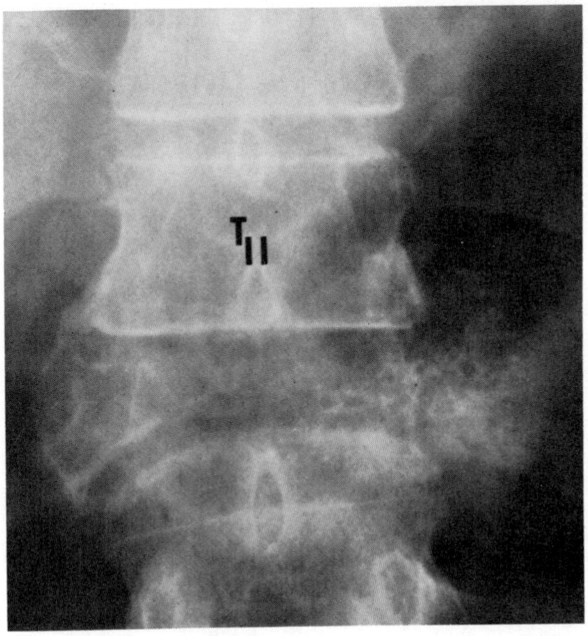

Figure 180-1 Characteristic appearance of a vertebral hemangioma. There is a coarse vertical trabeculation and loss of vertebral height with preservation of the interspaces. (From Hemmy et al.,[3] with permission.)

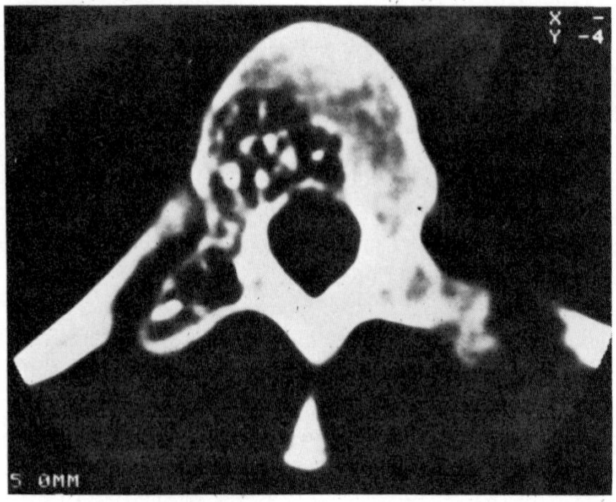

Figure 180-2 A CT section through a vertebral hemangioma, showing involvement of the vertebral body and transverse process.

In the past, I preferred to use either gas myelography with sagittal polytomography (Fig. 180-3) or CT-myelography to determine the extent of tumor involvement of the spinal canal and the relationship of the tumor to the spinal cord. Now MRI with axial and sagittal views is the preferred modality.

Angiography is most valuable in defining the nature and the blood supply of the tumor. Enlarged intercostal arteries will be noted. Furthermore, contrast medium tends to opacify the vertebral body because of the large blood sinuses within the bone (Fig. 180-4).

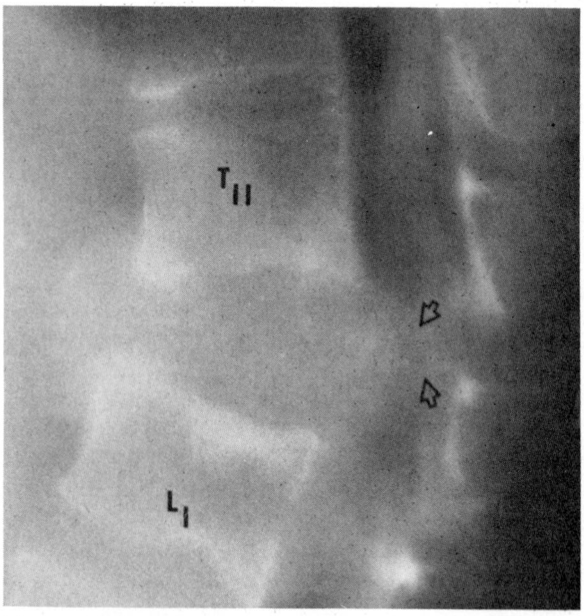

Figure 180-3 Gas myelogram with a sagittal polytomographic section. There is a complete spinal subarachnoid block with cord compression by the tumor (*arrows*). Kyphosis has developed at the site of the lesion. (From Hemmy et al.,[3] with permission.)

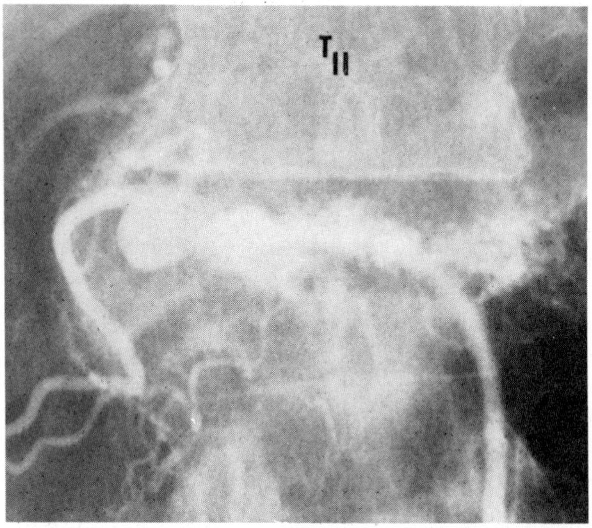

Figure 180-4 Selective spinal arteriography showing rich perfusion. The lesion is supplied by the intercostal vessels. (From Hemmy et al.,[3] with permission.)

Therapy

Several methods of treatment have been employed when hemangioma causes neurological dysfunction. Surgical therapy alone is quite hazardous and is not to be recommended because of the threat of exsanguination. Furthermore, laminectomy is not recommended except in those cases of annular constriction with hypertrophy of the laminae alone. Most frequently the lesion lies anterior to the spinal cord and proper anatomic reconstruction of the spinal canal cannot be performed through a posterior approach. Because of the hazards of surgery, alternative modes of therapy have been proposed, including radiotherapy and embolization of the mass. Radiotherapy is said to offer arrest of the progression of myelopathy, but generally it has not resulted in significant improvement. Furthermore, radiation treatment offers the added risk of radiation myelopathy.

Embolization of the tumor through selective arterial catheterization has been employed as a method of treatment.[1] Although improvement has been demonstrated with the use of this method, I believe that this improvement is due to the collapse of angiomatous vessels that lie within the epidural space rather than to any effect on the involved vertebral body.

Because most symptomatic patients have collapsed vertebral bodies, significant kyphosis, and encroachment upon the vertebral canal, surgical therapy should be directed toward relief of spinal angulation and restoration of the anatomic continuity of the spinal canal. Because the vertebral body is usually the major offending structure, the surgical approach will be anterior or anterolateral to the spinal canal. I find the lateral extrapleural or lateral extraperitoneal approach preferable because of the paravertebral mass frequently associated with the tumor, which may have an intimate relationship to major thoracic or lumbar vessels. This approach permits subtotal resection of the vertebral body, allowing the surgeon to visualize the dura prior to resecting the tumor, and it permits the anterior portions of the vertebral body, which, as indicated, may be intimately related to great vessels, to remain behind (Fig. 180-5). This approach must, however, be preceded by preoperative embolization of the tumor mass. Embolization should be

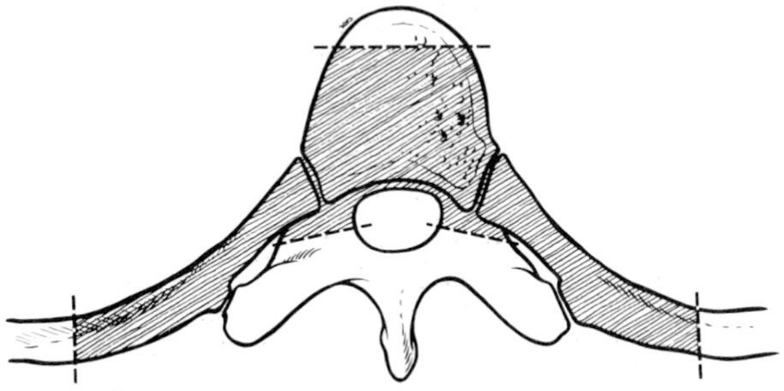

Figure 180-5 Bone to be resected through the lateral extracavitary approach. (From Hemmy et al.,[3] with permission.)

performed on the day prior to surgery. It is best performed via a transfemoral approach utilizing a nontapered French catheter. The largest catheter that can be completely wedged into the lumen of the proper arterial branch should be selected. This will prevent retrograde reflux of emboli. Complete wedging of the catheter prior to embolization should be confirmed by fluoroscopy.

Because surgery is to follow, embolization with Gelfoam (absorbable gelatin sponge; The Upjohn Company, Kalamazoo, MI) emboli can be used. The chief disadvantage of Gelfoam embolization is that later recanalization of the lesion may occur. This usually occurs months after the initial embolization; nonetheless, I think that a rapid angiographic assessment of the site of the lesion should be made on the day of surgery to confirm the continued obliteration of the lesion by the emboli (Fig. 180-6). The 24-h delay between embolization and surgery is to confirm that the lesion has remained obliterated over this period.

I suggest that the artery of Adamkiewicz be identified at the time of angiography. However, it is unlikely that the artery of Adamkiewicz will arise from the intercostal branches serving the

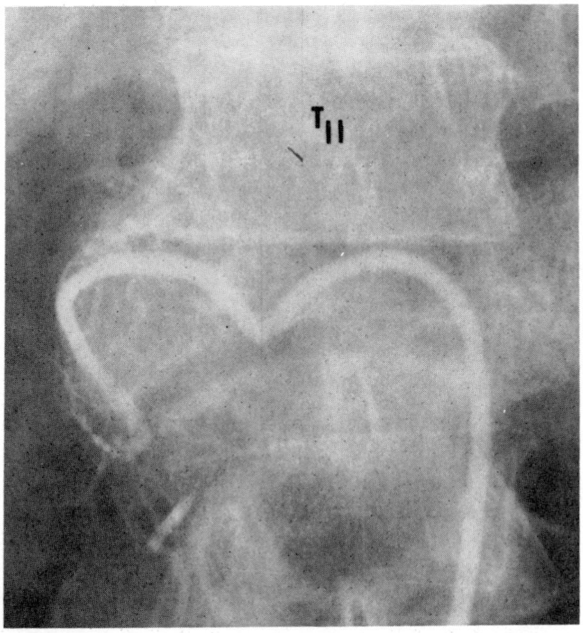

Figure 180-6 Preoperative angiography showing complete obliteration of the blood supply to a hemangioma following embolization. (From Hemmy et al.,[3] with permission.)

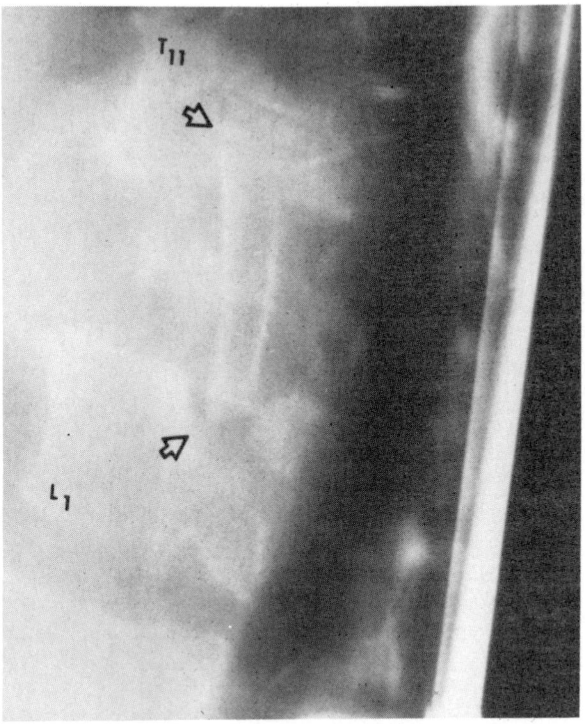

Figure 180-7 Polytomogram showing the extent of the tumor resection, correction of angulation, and placement of the bone graft (*arrows*). (From Hemmy et al.,[3] with permission.)

angioma because of its fistulous nature. Following successful embolization, excision of the tumor is quite easy because of the friability of the tumor, and minimal blood loss should be encountered.[3]

Because many of these patients have angular deformities of the spine, application of spinal instrumentation such as Harrington or Luque rods or Weiss springs (Zimmer, Inc., Warsaw, IN) will serve to correct the angulation and stabilize the spine. Finally, spinal fusion should be performed between the vertebral bodies adjacent to the tumor, utilizing iliac crest donor bone (Fig. 180-7). This technique will permit significant improvement in myelopathy and, in most cases, early ambulation. It remains the procedure of choice.[2]

In those few cases that are due to angiomatous hypertrophy of the posterior elements, laminectomy following embolization is the preferred form of treatment.

References

1. Benati A, DaPian R, Mazza C, et al. Preoperative embolization of a vertebral hemangioma compressing the spinal cord. *Neuroradiology* 1974; 7:181–183.
2. Djindjian M, Nguyen JP, Gaston A, et al. Multiple vertebral hemangiomas with neurological signs: case report. *J Neurosurg* 1992; 76:1025–1028.
3. Hemmy DC, McGee DM, Armbrust FH, Larson SJ. Resection of a vertebral hemangioma after preoperative embolization: case report. *J Neurosurg* 1977; 47:282–285.
4. Laredo JD, Assouline E, Gelbert F, et al. Vertebral hemangiomas: fat content as a sign of agressiveness. *Radiology* 1990; 177:467–472.

181 Masses of the Sacrum

Setti S. Rengachary

Masses occurring in the sacrococcygeal region often present problems that overlap many medical fields, including pediatrics, teratology, neurosurgery, colorectal surgery, orthopedics, gynecology, and genitourinary surgery. The neurosurgeon's role is twofold—first, to diagnose and treat developmental or neoplastic neurogenic lesions occurring in this area; and second, to assist surgeons in other fields in the resection of non-neurogenic lesions, with special emphasis on preserving neural elements within the sacrum.

Clinical Features

The symptoms and signs due to a sacral mass are generally disproportionately mild with respect to the size of the mass. This results from insidious growth of the tumor into the capacious sacral canal, with chronic pressure erosion of the sacral vertebral bodies and further extension into the potentially large retrorectal space. The sacral nerves tend to withstand chronic pressure well, with minimal manifestation of neurological deficit.

The symptoms frequently start with vague, nondescript low back pain or pelvic pressure. The pain may radiate to the buttock and the back of the thigh but radiation below the knee is somewhat uncommon. A persistent sensation of fullness in the perineum or pelvis may occur. In malignant infiltrative lesions, the low back pain may be relentlessly persistent. Rectal symptoms may be due either to direct pressure by the mass on the rectum or to neural impairment. Chronic constipation results from the former and incontinence from the latter.

There may be no visible or palpable external mass, but if one is noted it may be in the subcutaneous area behind the sacrum, in the intergluteal cleft, in the buttock, or in the perineum (Fig. 181-1). Proctoscopy and digital examination of the rectum may reveal a retrorectal mass, as evidenced by the ability to glide the rectal mucosa over the mass. The rectal sphincter may be patulous if the S2 and S3 roots are involved. Rarely, a presacral mass may grow large enough to be palpable through the anterior abdominal wall.

Motor weakness and atrophy may be manifest in the gluteal, hamstring, or gastrocnemius-soleus groups. Sensory impairment may be detected in the perianal or saddle area. The ankle reflex(es) may be impaired or absent.

Investigation

Changes in the plain radiographs of the sacrum may be missed unless special attention is paid. Fecal material and bowel gas frequently overlie and obscure the sacrum, particularly when the sacral nerves are compromised. The curvilinear shape of the sacrum makes it difficult to evaluate on standard anteroposterior projections. A modified sacral projection with the x-ray beam angled 15 to 30 degrees cephalad and with the patient's hips flexed can greatly facilitate detection of a bony abnormality. A lateral projection will often yield more useful information than the frontal projection (Fig. 181-2). In contemporary practice, one rarely depends upon plain radiographs alone to make definitive diagnosis of any sacral lesion.

Bone scanning with bone-seeking radionuclides gives nonspecific positive information when there is bone destruction, bone repair, or increased blood flow in the sacral area. The principal advantage of bone scanning is to determine whether the pathologic process is confined to the sacral area or is disseminated or multifocal.

Lumbar myelography with a water-soluble contrast agent is especially helpful when the lesion communicates with the subarachnoid space (e.g., a meningocele) (Fig. 181-3). In other lesions, the distal thecal sac may show nonspecific displacement (Fig. 181-4).

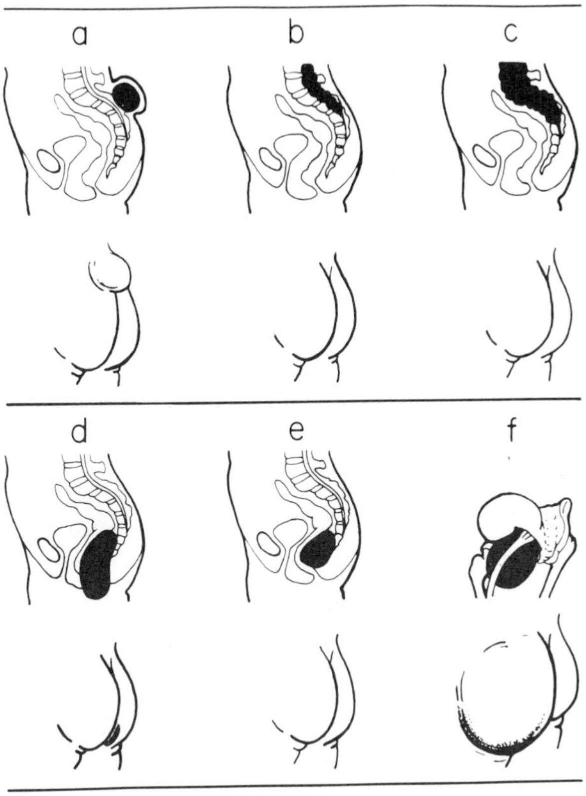

Figure 181-1 Principal anatomic spaces in the sacrococcygeal region where mass lesions occur. *a*. Subcutaneous space behind the sacrum (lipoma, meningocele, ectopic ependymoma, hemangioma). *b*. Neural canal of the sacrum (ependymoma, neurilemoma). *c*. Osseous elements of the sacrum (chordoma, giant cell tumor, osteogenic sarcoma, chondrosarcoma, aneurysmal bone cyst). *d, e*. Presacral space, with and without presentation of a mass in the perineum (teratoma, dermoid, ganglioneuroma, neurilemoma). *f*. Buttock. Unilateral buttock enlargement can be caused by a presacral teratoma, with extension of the mass into the buttock through the greater sciatic notch.

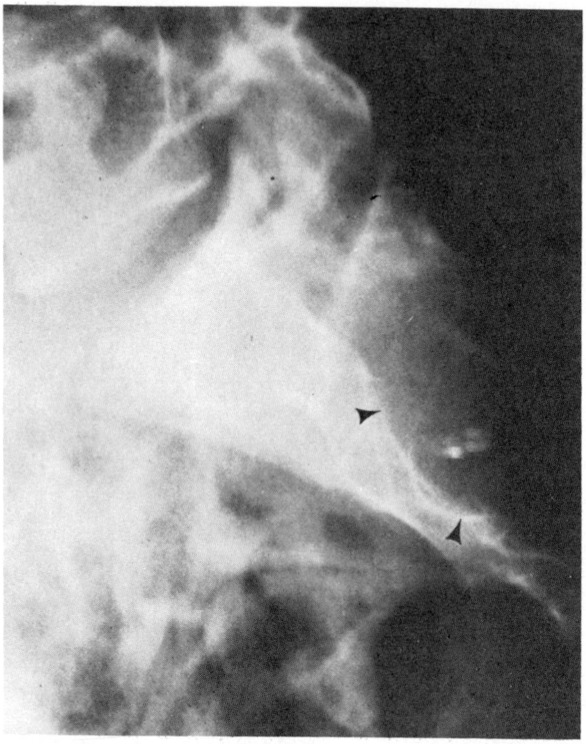

Figure 181-2 Roentgenogram of the sacrum in the lateral projection, showing bony erosion with sclerotic margins (*arrowheads*) caused by an intrasacral cyst.

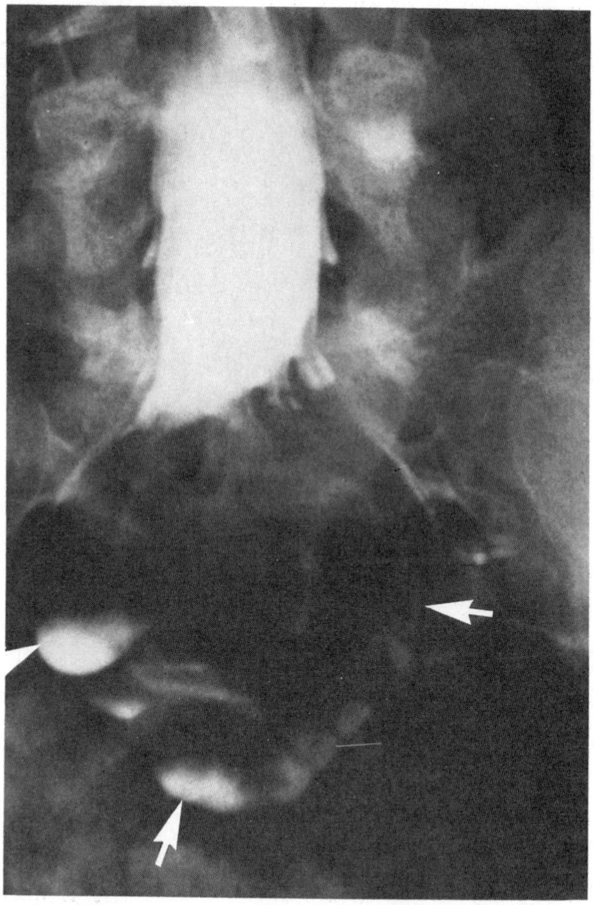

Figure 181-3 Anteroposterior view of a metrizamide lumbar myelogram showing a large multiloculated cyst within the sacrum (*arrows*).

High-resolution computed tomography (CT) is a very useful noninvasive diagnostic test; it may be advantageously performed in conjunction with metrizamide myelography. The principal advantage of computed tomography is its ability to distinguish between a far wider spectrum of radiologic densities than can conventional radiographs. Thus, soft tissue masses and their relationships to neighboring structures are delineated better by CT (Figs. 181-5 and 181-6). Calcifications not visible on plain radiographs are often clearly visible on CT. Image manipulation with various window width settings optimally demonstrates either the soft tissue component or the bony margin of a tumor. As a general rule, smooth sclerotic margins around a mass tend to denote a longstanding and benign process, whereas irregular destructive margins suggest a malignant lesion.

Arteriography seldom adds any useful information in diagnosing sacrococcygeal lesions. However, arteriography is necessary if preoperative embolization of a vascular sacral neoplasm is considered.

Magnetic resonance imaging (Fig. 181-7) has proved to be extremely useful in the diagnosis of sacral lesions. It is particularly useful in the diagnosis of tethered cord syndrome, lipoma, meningoceles (posterior, intrasacral, and anterior sacral), and neoplasms of various types. In most situations, MRI alone may provide all the information desired. Destructive or erosive bony changes, however, are better appreciated on CT.

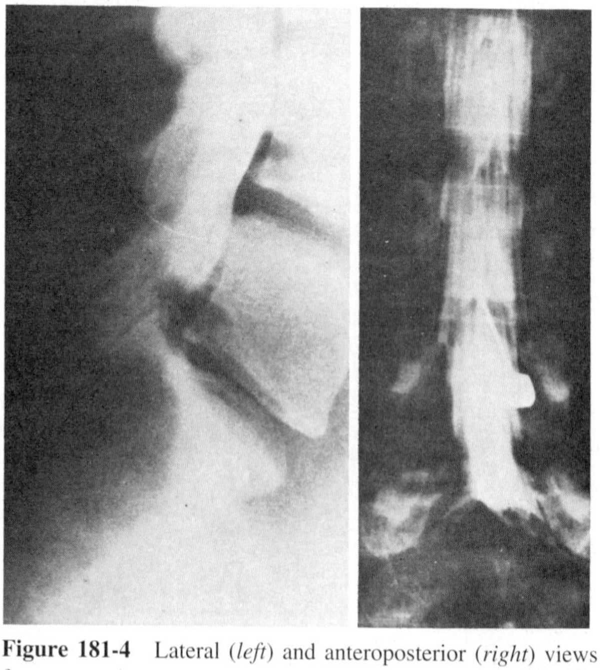

Figure 181-4 Lateral (*left*) and anteroposterior (*right*) views from a metrizamide lumbar myelogram showing a complete block at the lower border of L5, with displacement of the dural sac to the patient's right by a large intrasacral schwannoma. Erosion of the posterior surface of the sacral vertebral bodies is evident in the lateral view.

Differential Diagnosis of Sacral Masses

A vast array of mass lesions of different etiologies occur in the sacrococcygeal area (Table 181-1). When confronted with a

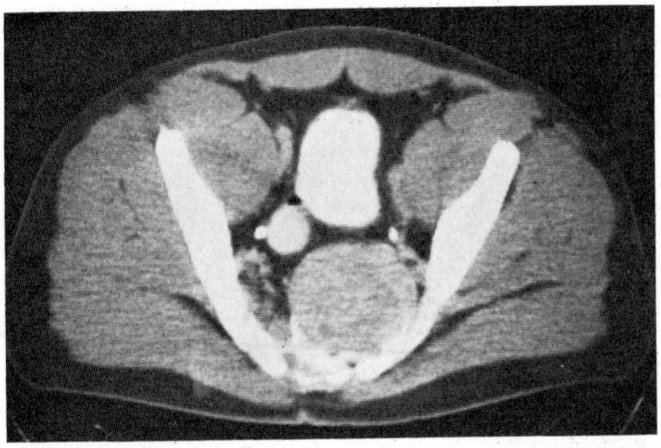

Figure 181-5 Computed tomogram of the lower sacral area shows extension into the presacral space by a large neurilemoma arising from the neural canal of the sacrum. The mass has a smooth, globular outline.

patient with a sacrococcygeal mass, critical and methodical analysis of certain factors is likely to lead to a logical diagnosis.[3,11]

Precise Anatomic Location

There are five principal anatomic spaces in the sacrococcygeal region where masses may occur (Fig. 181-1). They are (1) the subcutaneous space behind the sacrum, (2) the buttocks, (3) the osseous elements of the sacrum, (4) the sacral canal, and (5) the presacral or retrorectal space.

A mass occurring in the subcutaneous area behind the sacrum may represent a lipoma, meningocele, ectopic ependymoma, pilonidal cyst, or hemangioma. Unilateral buttock enlargement is commonly seen in infants with a presacral teratoma that extends into the buttock through the greater sciatic notch. In adults, a sarcoma arising from the ilium may produce unilateral buttock enlargement. A primary tumor arising from the osseous elements of the sacrum, such as a giant cell tumor, osteogenic sarcoma, chondrosarcoma, osteoma, or aneurysmal bone cyst, may produce a palpable bony mass. Chordoma, thought to arise from notochordal remnants (ecchordosis physaliphora) in the osseous element of the sacrum, is discussed in detail elsewhere in this textbook. Metastatic tumors to the sacrum, such as those from the prostate, seldom produce a mass lesion or offer any diagnostic difficulty. Neurogenic tumors (ependymoma, neurilemoma) most commonly occur in the sacral canal. The presacral space or retrorectal area is a potential space bounded anteriorly by the posterior wall of the rectum, posteriorly by the sacrum and coccyx, superiorly by the peritoneal reflection, and inferiorly by the levator ani and coccygeus muscles of the pelvic floor; the iliac vessels and ureters define the lateral margins. Lesions such as dermoid cyst, teratoma, ectopic kidney, ectopic ependymoma, neurilemoma, ganglioneuroma, or anterior sacral meningocele occur in this area.

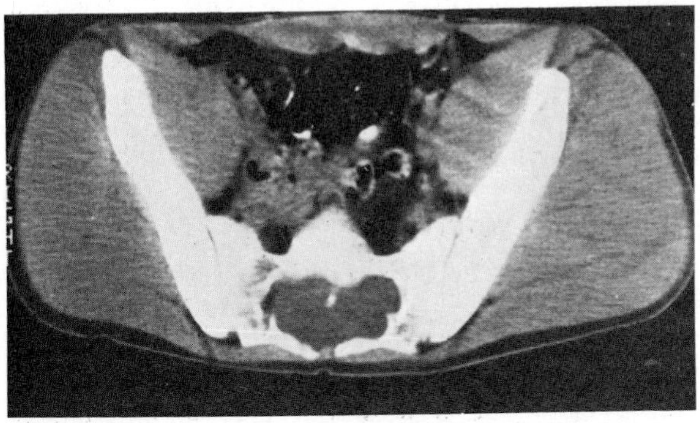

Figure 181-6 Computed tomogram of the sacrum, showing an intrasacral cyst.

Cystic or Solid Form

A purely cystic lesion in this area generally implies a developmental lesion, such as a meningocele, or an inclusion cyst, such as an epidermoid or dermoid cyst. Solid or nodular lesions are usually neoplastic in nature.

Communication of a Cystic Mass with the Subarachnoid Space

This can be determined in an infant by palpating the mass both when the infant is quiet, especially immediately after a feeding or during sleep, and when it is crying. An increase in tension in the cyst during straining suggests communication with the subarachnoid space. CT will show the cyst to have attenuation values for water, and myelography will demonstrate the communication (Figs. 181-3 and 181-6). MRI may demonstrate direct continuity of the spinal subarachnoid space with a meningocele (Fig. 181-7).

Age of Patient

Teratoma, meningocele, and lipoma are the most common sacrococcygeal lesions in the neonate. Anterior sacral meningoceles may not be detected until late in adulthood. It is noteworthy that teratomas manifest in the newborn tend to be benign, whereas those occurring after 3 months of age tend to be malignant. Chordomas, although thought to arise from notochordal remnants, are rarely seen in childhood. Ependymomas and neurilemomas occur in young to middle-aged adults.

Presence of Neurological Impairment

Neurological impairment is most commonly observed with ependymomas and neurilemmomas. Benign sacrococcygeal teratomas, even when they assume enormous size, seldom produce neurological impairment. Chordomas and osseous neoplasms may produce neurological impairment late in the course of the disease. Meningoceles, because of their low location, produce minimal or no neurological deficit.

Presence of Bone Destruction or Pressure Erosion

Typically, destructive or invasive lesions are malignant neoplasms, whereas a lesion with smooth sclerotic margins is a developmental process or a benign tumor.

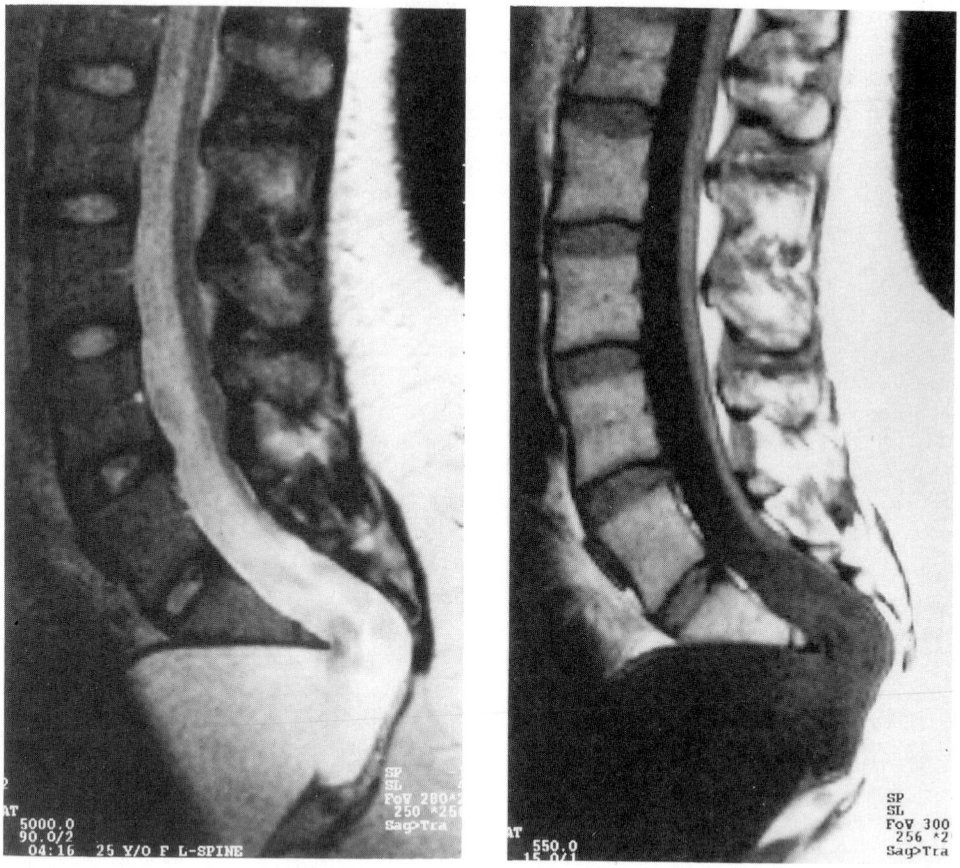

(*A*) (*B*)

Figure 181-7 Sagittal T2-weighted (*A*) and T1-weighted (*B*) MRI views, showing a large anterior sacral meningocele communicating with the spinal subarachnoid space.

Dissemination of Lesion

A disseminated or multifocal lesion generally implies a metastatic or multifocal neoplastic process such as plasmacytoma.

Certain Sacral Lesions of Neurosurgical Interest

Intrasacral Extradural Arachnoid Cyst

Synonyms include intrasacral cyst, occult intrasacral meningocele, expansion of subarachnoid space in the lumbosacral region, and intraspinal meningocele.[2,10] This is discussed in detail elsewhere in this textbook.

Neurogenic Tumors

The two most common tumors occurring in the cauda equina are neurilemoma[1] and ependymoma.[8] Most commonly these tumors occur in the lumbar region, but rarely they may occur in the sacral area. An intradural ependymoma occurring low in the lumbar thecal sac, if highly invasive, may extend into the sacral canal and may present in part as an intrasacral tumor.[12]

Less than 5 percent of all spinal ependymomas occur extradurally in the sacrococcygeal region.[7] The age at onset may range from 3 months to 65 years, with a mean of 26 years. Extradural ependymomas occur in three characteristic locations in the sacrococcygeal area: (1) in the subcutaneous soft tissue posterior to the sacrum. When occurring in this location, the tumor presents as a slow-growing mass in the intergluteal fold; (2) within the sacral canal but lying extradurally. In late stages the tumor may infiltrate and erode the sacrum either anteriorly or posteriorly, with extension into the presacral space or retrosacral tissue, respectively; (3) in the retrorectal (presacral) space. In this location the tumor is usually quite large on initial discovery, since it may attain enormous size without impingement upon any structure that will produce symptoms.

The origin of extradural ependymomas in the sacrococcygeal region has been the subject of debate. No unitary hypothesis would explain all cases. Heterotopic ependymal cell rests may be the source of tumor in some cases, especially those occurring in the subcutaneous tissue. Some authorities have suggested an origin from the coccygeal medullary vestige, which is an ependymal-lined cavity remaining in the caudal portion of the neural tube beneath the skin of the postanal pit. A few have theorized that persistent remnants of the notochordal canal give rise to ependymomas.

Neurilemomas occasionally occur in the sacral canal; they may attain enormous size before symptoms occur (Fig. 181-5).[1] Unlike ependymomas, these are benign tumors and thus cause smooth pressure erosion rather than invasion or destruction of bone.[9]

TABLE 181-1 Sacral and Presacral Masses

Congenital Masses
Anterior sacral meningocele
Chordoma
Dermoid cyst
Ectopic kidney
Epidermoid cyst
Intrasacral meningocele
Teratoma
Neurogenic masses
Ependymoma (intraspinal and ectopic)
Ganglioneuroma
Metastatic neuroblastoma
Neurofibroma
Neurilemoma
Osseous masses
Aneurysmal bone cyst
Chondroma
Chondrosarcoma
Ewing's sarcoma
Giant cell tumor
Osteogenic sarcoma
Osteoma
Miscellaneous tumors
Fibrosarcoma
Hemangioendothelioma
Leiomyosarcoma
Liposarcoma
Metastatic carcinoma
Myeloma
Rhabdomyosarcoma
Inflammatory conditions
Abscess
Granuloma

Surgical Approach to Sacrococcygeal Masses

The surgical approach to the sacrococcygeal lesion will depend greatly upon the exact anatomic site and the nature of the lesion.[4,5] Subcutaneous masses behind the sacrum are amenable to wide local excision. Neurilemomas and ependymomas in the sacral canal may be excised after the posterior wall of the sacrum is removed. Chordomas require an attempt at radical resection.[6] In regard to preservation of sacral roots, it is useful to remember that the critical roots are S2 and S3, which subserve sphincter function; saving these roots only on one side will maintain sufficient visceral function. The S1 root subserves significant motor function in the lower extremity and should be preserved. Purely presacral lesions are best approached through the abdomen.

References

1. Abernathy CD, Onofrio BM. Sacral neurilemmoma. In Doty JR, Rengachary SS (eds): *Surgical Disorders of the Sacrum.* New York: Thieme, 1994, pp 184–196.
2. Doty JR. Benign sacral meningeal cysts. In Doty JR, Rengachary SS (eds): *Surgical Disorders of the Sacrum.* New York: Thieme, 1994, pp 124–132.
3. Luken MG III, Michelsen WJ, Whelan MA, Andrews DL. The diagnosis of sacral lesions. *Surg Neurol* 1981; 15:377–383.
4. MacCarty CS, Waugh JM, Coventry MB, Cope WF Jr. Surgical treatment of sacral and presacral tumors other than sacrococcygeal chordoma. *J Neurosurg* 1965; 22:458–464.
5. McCormick PC, Post KD. Surgical approaches to the sacrum. In Doty JR, Rengachary SS (eds): *Surgical Disorders of the Sacrum.* New York: Thieme, 1994, pp 257–265.
6. Mindell ER. Current concepts review: chordoma. *J Bone Joint Surg* 1981; 63A:501–505.
7. Morantz RA, Kepes JJ, Batnitzky S, Masterson BJ. Extraspinal ependymomas: report of three cases. *J Neurosurg* 1979; 51:383–391.
8. Post KD, McCormick PC. Intrasacral ependymoma. In Doty JR, Rengachary SS (eds): *Surgical Disorders of the Sacrum.* New York: Thieme, 1994, pp 181–183.
9. Rengachary SS, O'Boynick P, Batnitzky S, Kepes JJ. Giant intrasacral schwannoma: case report. *Neurosurgery* 1981; 9:573–577.
10. Rengachary SS, O'Boynick P, Karlin CA, et al. Intrasacral extradural communicating arachnoid cyst: case report. *Neurosurgery* 1981; 8:236–240.
11. Turner ML, Mulhern CB, Dalinka MK. Lesions of the sacrum: differential diagnosis and radiological evaluation. *JAMA* 1981; 245:275–277.
12. Vara-Thorbeck R, Sanz-Esponera J. Intrasacral ependymoma: case report. *J Neurosurg* 1970; 32:589–592.

SECTION O

Adjunctive Therapy of Central Nervous System Tumors

182 Principles of Radiotherapy of Central Nervous System Tumors

K. Thomas Noell
Arnold M. Herskovic

Put simply, all modes of therapeutic irradiation inject energy into biochemical systems such as cellular nuclei. The addition of energy into a previously stable biochemical unit, like heating a strip of bacon, causes rapid and often permanent alteration.

The mutual intent of radiotherapy and chemotherapy is to eradicate by nonextirpative means the aberrant cells that form a tumor. If effective, both treatment methods cause a fatal derangement of cellular functions. All chemotherapeutic agents are subject to common pharmacologic considerations, such as binding to plasma proteins, diffusibility, membrane transport, biochemical activation, and excretion, as is any medication. Once within neoplastic cells, these drugs, or their derivatives, may have the intended deranging and lethal effect. Ionizing radiation, which is composed of packets of energy, reaches the cellular targets without pharmacologic processing. The deposited energy causes the creation of new biochemical moieties within the cell. At the level of the therapeutic target, then, radiotherapy and chemotherapy may be roughly comparable. Methods of application and intermediate (processing) steps are very different, however, as are results.

The Nature of Ionizing Radiation

Ionizing radiation deposits energy in absorbing materials such as tissue. Energized electrons are freed from their irradiated atoms; ions are thus formed. Electromagnetic radiation has the physical properties of both waves and subatomic particles (photons). Such radiation may be x-rays or gamma rays; both are photons. The former are produced by extranuclear events; the sudden deceleration of a stream of electrons in the metallic target of an x-ray tube produces x-rays and heat as the result of the law of conservation of energy. Gamma rays are identical to x-rays except for their source; they are the result of intranuclear rearrangements to a lower, more stable energy state, with the residual energy discharged as gamma rays.[16,19] Therapeutic sources of gamma rays are cobalt machines, and radioactive elements used for implants.

In an irradiated medium, energy absorption occurs by processes known as *photoelectric absorption, Compton absorption,* and *pair production,* or by combinations thereof, depending on the energy spectrum of the incident photons.[16,18]

Photoelectric absorption predominates at low incident photon energies (40 to 125 keV). A tightly bound electron is escalated to an energized orbit more distant from the atomic nucleus; when this energized electron then falls back to a closer, less energized orbit, its excess energy is released as a stream of photons, which may be in the form of detectable light. Photoelectric absorption varies directly with the cube of the absorbing materials' electron content (atomic number, or Z). Thus, tissues composed of atoms with high atomic numbers distinctly attenuate the radiation beam. This yields the visible contrast between iodinated contrast agent, bone, and soft tissue in diagnostic roentgenograms (high, medium, and lower Z, respectively).

In Compton interactions, the collision of photons is with outer orbital, or less strongly bound, electrons of the atom, so that the x-rays are mainly scattered rather than absorbed. In contrast to photoelectric absorption, the probability of Compton absorption depends not on the atomic number, but rather on the electron density. Soft tissue, composed mostly of elements of lower atomic number, has a high electron density.

Pair production requires higher energies than do the other processes described. At photon energies of more than 1.02 MeV, absorption of a photon yields simultaneous production of an electron and its oppositely charged equivalent, the positron; energy has thus been converted into matter. The resultant species then dissipate their remaining energy within the absorbing medium.

X-ray sources, including linear accelerators, produce a continuous spectrum of x-ray energies up to a maximum, or peak, energy. A 250-kV peak (250,000 V peak) x-ray unit, for example, produces a spectrum of x-rays with energies ranging from just above 0 to 250,000 eV. Six million electron volts (6 MeV) in the linear accelerator produces a spectrum also, up to a maximum x-ray energy of 6 MeV. The average energy of emitted x-rays is about one-third of the maximum, as a rough generalization. At 50 keV and below, photoelectric absorption predominates in the target material; from 50 to 200 keV, both photoelectric and Compton absorption occur; from 200 keV to 1 MeV, Compton absorption predominates; and with yet higher x-ray, or gamma ray, energy, pair production increasingly occurs.

As their energy increases, photon beams can be thought of as more penetrating: a greater proportion of their incident energy reaches a specific tissue depth. X-ray units yielding up to 125 keV are considered to give superficial irradiation. Orthovoltage radiations with peak energies in the 200- to 400-keV range were used for the "deep x-ray therapy" of the 1930 to 1950 era. Megavoltage, or supervoltage, radiations (greater than 1 MeV) have since become dominant. Megavoltage irradiation has several important advantages over orthovoltage, including greater penetrability and skin sparing in addition to a relatively lower dose in denser materials, especially bone.

Skin sparing results when the energized electrons are scattered away from the atmosphere–tissue interface. The electron scatter is deeper, with reference to the path of the x-rays from their origin. Hence less energy is deposited in the epidermis, and the epidermal reaction is less.

Equilibrium dose is the point in the absorbing medium at which the number of energized electrons arriving is matched by the number of scattered electrons leaving. This is the point of maximum energy dose. In isodose distributions the maximum dose (D_{max}) is normalized at 100 percent, and dosages at greater depth are described as percentages of D_{max}. For cobalt 60 machines, D_{max} is 0.5 cm below the skin surface; for 4-MeV linear accelerators, 1 cm; and for higher-beam energies, yet deeper. The reviled radiation burns caused by orthovoltage x-rays essentially disappeared as megavoltage therapy became increasingly available in the 1970s.

The International Commission on Radiation Units and Measurements first defined the Roentgen (R) as the unit of radiation. Roentgens are a measure of exposure in air, not the absorbed dose. The rad was the first unit for energy absorbed; 1 rad equals 100 ergs per gram. The gray (Gy) recently replaced the rad; one Gy equals one joule of energy absorbed per kilogram, or 100 rad. One centigray (cGy) equals 1 rad.

Particle irradiation uses a beam of accelerated particles such as neutrons, nuclei of helium or other atoms, protons, or pions. Usually produced in cyclotrons, these are considered in another chapter. Brachytherapy, in which a radiation source is placed within or next to the tumor by interstitial or intracavitary means, is also discussed in another chapter.

Teletherapy Machines

Teletherapy is treatment with the radiation source at a distance from the patient. *Brachytherapy* refers to the replacement of radiation sources within the patient, and generally within the tumor itself. Only megavoltage teletherapy units will be discussed in this chapter. Prior to the 1950s, some machines utilizing radium were used for teletherapy, but in fact, it was only in the 1950s that megavoltage therapy became a practical reality. In 1952, Johns and coworkers reported the use of the first cobalt teletherapy machine, which was made possible by the activation of cobalt 59 to cobalt 60 by neutron bombardment in a nuclear reactor.[18] The radioactive cobalt is encapsulated in stainless steel, and is surrounded by heavy shielding except for a window in the treatment direction. During treatment, the cobalt 60 source is positioned over this window in the shield, exposing the patient to the gamma rays, which reach the patient after passing a series of beam-shaping collimators. The relatively large size of the source (2 to 3 cm) results in an indistinct beam edge, or *penumbra,* which becomes more pronounced as the distance from the source increases. As the source-to-target distance increases, the dose per unit time decreases because of the inverse-square law, which states that dose decreases inversely with the square of the distance from the source. Another disadvantage of cobalt units is the relatively large amount of shielding required in the head of the machine, because the radiation source can never be turned off, but just shielded (Fig. 182-1). Because cobalt 60 has a half-life of 5.25 years, the source must be replaced at approximately 5-year intervals. However, cobalt 60 machines still have the advantages of electrical simplicity, operational dependability, and beam uniformity (1.25 MeV).

Historically, other types of teletherapy units have been outmoded by linear accelerators, for a variety of practical reasons. These include Cesium 137 units, Van de Graaf generators, and betatrons.

Since the 1970s, the linear accelerator (Fig. 182-2) has become the principal external-beam irradiation machine. These are compact and relatively stable machines that can be rotated around the patient. Available at multiple x-ray and electron beam energies, these machines contain an electron gun, which injects electrons

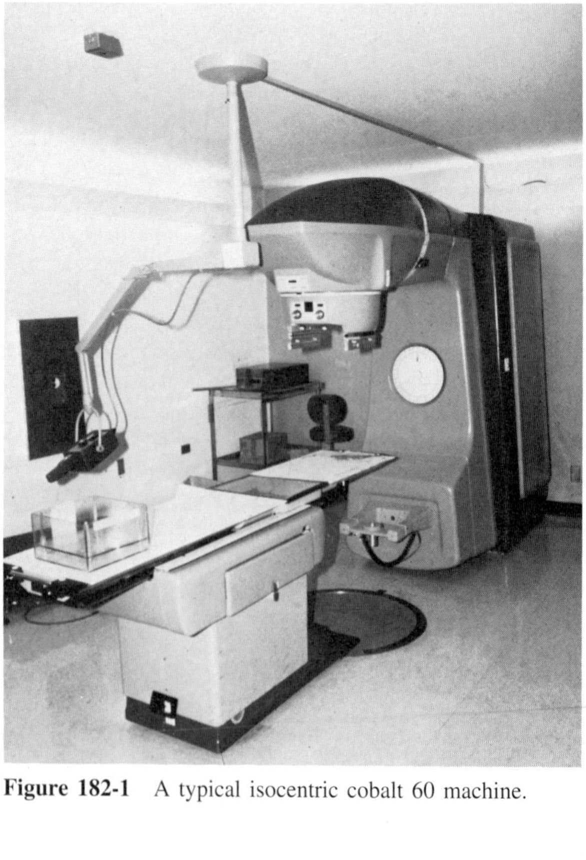

Figure 182-1 A typical isocentric cobalt 60 machine.

into a straight (linear) wave guide. The electrons accelerated through the wave guide hit a metallic foil target and produce x-rays by a process known as *Bremsstrahlung*. If the metallic foil is moved out of the path of the electron beam, the electrons themselves emerge from the unit. Linear accelerators provide irradiation pulses of 1 to 5 μs repeated some 5 to 500 times per second.

The linear accelerator has made use of electron beams practical in most major facilities. The critical property that makes use of electrons appealing is their rapid falloff, or decrease in dose, beyond D_{max}. This confines the therapeutic dose predictably to a thickness of superficial tissue, proportional to electron-beam energy. The deposited energy may have an effective range of from about 2 cm for a 6-MeV beam to 5 cm for 20 MeV. As the electron-beam energy increases, the falloff becomes more gradual and clinically less useful. In contrast to photons (x-rays), skin sparing decreases as electron-beam energy increases.

A 1990 census of radiotherapy in the United States showed that 492,120 new patients were treated at 1321 facilities with 2397 treatment machines (1893 accelerators and 504 cobalt units).[27]

The dose distribution of a radiation beam can be described by diagramming a vertical cross section at the central axis (Fig. 182-3). The dose of a representative orthovoltage beam decreases rather rapidly from the maximum at the surface to 50 percent at a depth of about 6 cm; it is the maximum dose at the skin surface that limits the patient's tolerance to treatment. For the cobalt 60 beam there is a buildup zone of 5 mm, and a 50 percent dose at about 10 cm. Isodose distributions will show comparable off-axis doses. The beam edges, or penumbras, are relatively wide in cobalt and orthovoltage irradiation, whereas the penumbra is narrow for linear accelerator photon beams, which also feature a significant buildup zone and greater penetration. In comparison, electron-beam isodose distributions show a rapid falloff of dose beyond the maximal, and a wider curve, or sideward bulge, near the surface (Fig. 182-4*A*).

Radiation beams have to be carefully measured; this is usually done in water-filled phantoms with ionization chambers. Other means of measurement are thermoluminescent dosimetry and photographic film densitometry. The beams themselves can be altered by placing various field-shaping blocks, wedges, or compensators in their paths.

Treatment Planning and Simulation

Increasingly, computed tomography (CT) through the tumor is performed with the patient in the treatment position to improve treatment accuracy. Tissue densities and dimensions are measured.

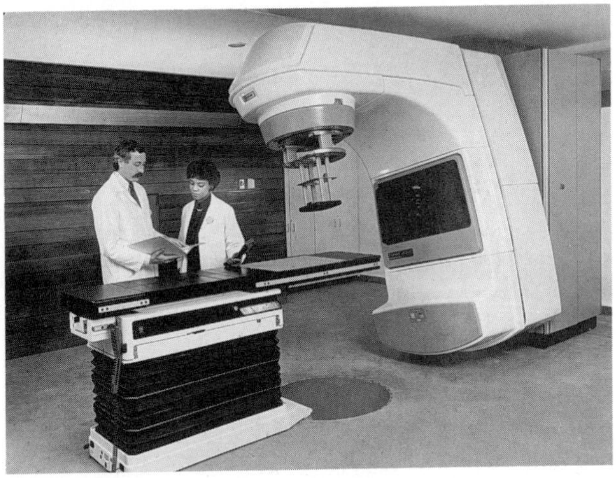

(*A*)

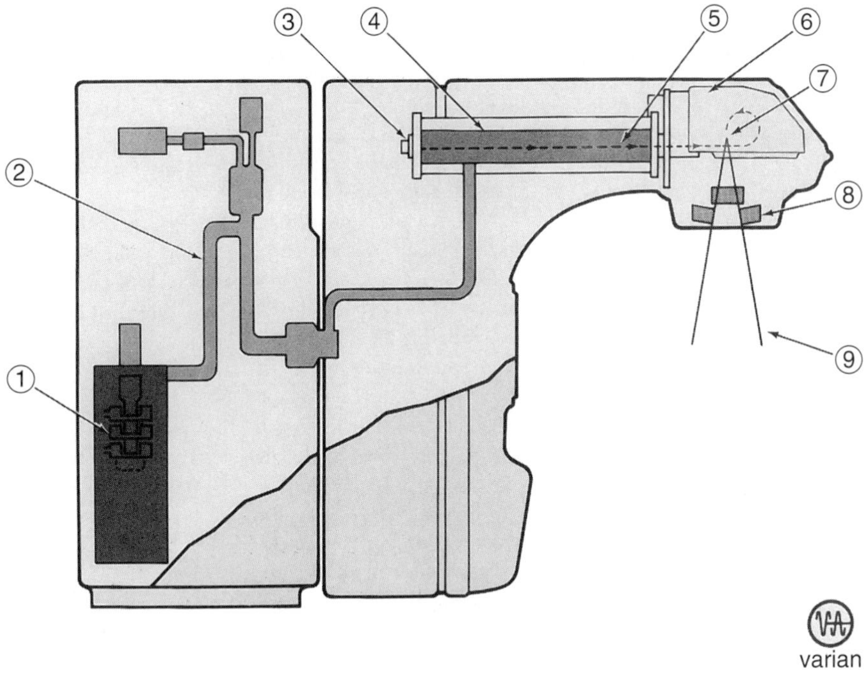

(*B*)

Figure 182-2 *A*. A high-energy linear accelerator. (Courtesy of Varian Associates, Inc., Palo Alto, CA.) *B*. Schematic of a high-energy linear accelerator. (1) Klystron tube generates high-power microwaves used to accelerate electrons in the accelerator guide; (2) wave guide carries microwave power from Klystron to accelerator guide; (3) electron gun injects electrons into accelerator; (4) accelerator guide has special inner structure so that microwave power accelerates electrons in a straight (linear) path to the correct energy; (5) beam of electrons accelerated to near the speed of light; (6) magnet causes electron beam to turn 270°; (7) electron beam hits metal target producing high-energy x-rays. Target also can be removed from beam path to permit treatment with electrons; (8) movable collimators shape the x-ray beam; (9) x-ray beam is directed to treatment area in patient. (Courtesy of Varian Associates, Inc., Palo Alto, CA.).

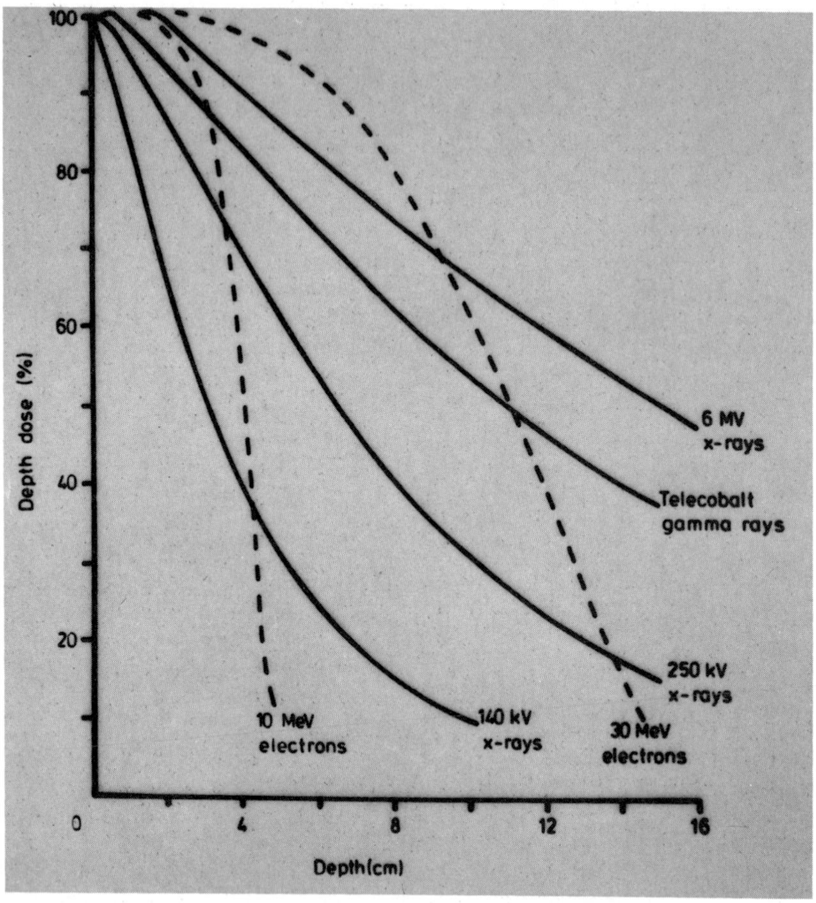

Figure 182-3 Comparison of dose profiles along the central axis. The beam is positioned on the left with the skin at depth = 0. Typical orthovoltage curves are shown for 140-kV and 250-kV x-ray machines; note the relatively high dose at the surface and low dose at depth. Two megavoltage beams, cobalt 60 and 6 MV, are represented. They give a lower dose at the surface (with skin sparing) and a higher dose at depth. Electrons have a rapid falloff. Note that the 10-MeV electrons are almost perfect for treating at a depth of 4 cm and limiting the dose to deeper structures. The higher-energy electrons (e.g., the 30 MeV) fall off more gradually.

Next, the cross-sectional skin contour, critical dose-limiting normal structures, and treatment volume (tumor volume plus appropriate margins) are digitized into the dedicated treatment-planning computer. This computer has files of the measured isodose data for the radiation beam energy or energies specific to the linear accelerator that will treat the lesion. A variety of beam energies, beam directions, and beam modifiers (such as wedge filters) are then modelled on the computer, and the best combination of parameters is selected as the treatment plan. Software for three-dimensional reconstruction of tumor and specific normal tissue volumes are in development but not generally commercially available yet.

The treatment plan is next transferred to the patient using a simulator, a device that mimics the treatment machine's geometry, generates diagnostic-quality radiographs, and usually has an image intensifier for fluoroscopy.

Simulation precedes computed dosimetry when the beam direction(s) does not require modelling, to better define the volumes to be irradiated and spared (e.g., a posterior field to cover the T7 to T11 vertebrae with a right T9 paraspinous mass), and simulator films are used in making customized field-shaping blocks. After satisfactory simulation, the patient can be marked with small skin tattoos to identify each field; this is very useful for future reference.

The axis about which a rotational therapy unit moves is called an *isocenter*. In multifield techniques, placement of the isocenter in the volume of interest means that any beam from that machine will pass through the treatment volume. This is thought to decrease the chance and significance of error in the clinical setup of patients.

Optimal treatment requires reproducible execution of the treatment plan with respect to field size, beam-modifying devices, beam direction, patient position, and immobilization. Variations in any parameter may adversely affect the outcome of the treatments. Verification films are prudently taken during treatment for quality assurance. Laser optical pointers mounted on the walls of the treatment room, or on the treatment machine, are aligned with marks on the center and both sides of the patient. This places the patient in the same position for each treatment at the same isocenter. Wedge filters and tissue compensators improve dose distribution in the treatment volume by partial attenuation of the radiation beam. Quality-assurance measures during a course of radiotherapy include periodic field verification films, independent dose calculation review by a second person, and microdosimetry to compare the dose measured with that calculated as given.

Radiation Fields

The best biological effects are achieved if *all* fields directed to one treatment volume are treated every treatment day.[39]

Single Field

This is the simplest form of radiotherapy, in which the beam is directly aimed at the tumor. The radiation oncologist accepts a dose gradient as the beam traverses the treatment volume (Fig.

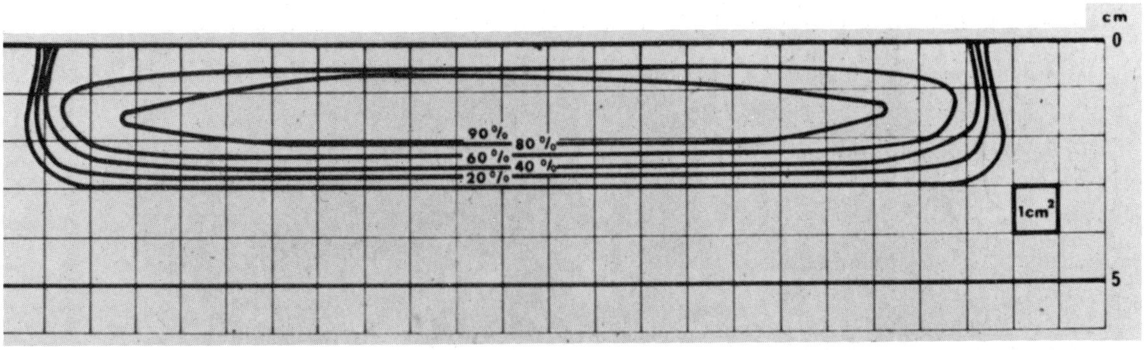

(*A*)

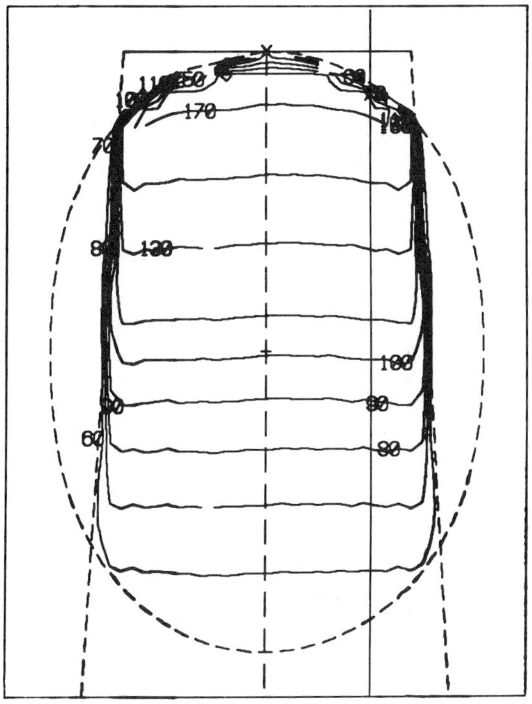

(*B*)

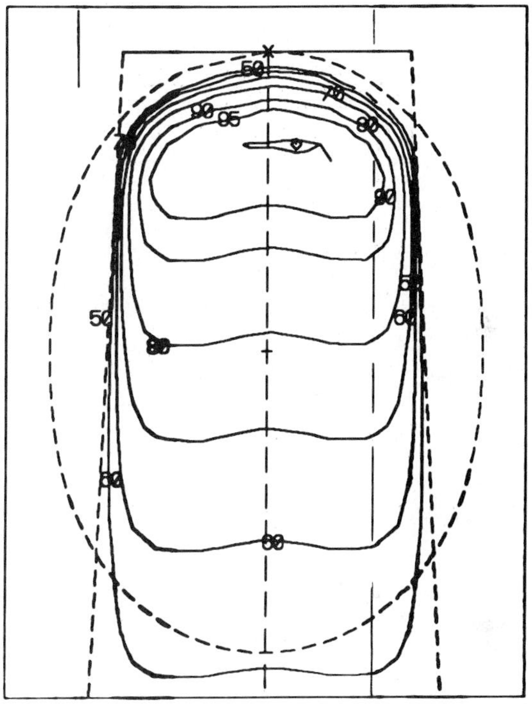

(*C*)

Figure 182-4 *A.* A typical electron beam isodose curve; note the rapid falloff at depth. *B.* A typical cobalt 60 beam isodose profile; note the relatively wide beam edge or penumbra and 50 percent isodose at 10 cm depth. *C.* A typical high-energy linear accelerator 15-MeV x-ray beam isodose profile; note the sharper beam edge and greater penetration.

182-4). The gradient would be used in treating tumor volume that is closer to a beam's entry point than to its exit, for example, the spinal cord. The clinician accepts a dosage gradient, from the D_{max} point just under the skin through the defined tumor depth, and actually irradiates tissues on the far side of the treatment volume with a lower dose. The dose gradient depends on the energy of the treatment beam; for example, a 6-MeV photon beam has less of a dose gradient than does a cobalt beam. The most frequent application of single fields in the central nervous system (CNS) is in treatment of the spinal cord or spine. However, it should be noted that the lumbosacral vertebrae are often almost midline in the sagittal plane, and parallel opposed anterior and posterior fields may be used as an alternative treatment to yield a more homogeneous dose.

Parallel Opposed Fields

This is the most frequently used field arrangement because it produces a relatively homogeneous dose distribution throughout the treatment volume (Fig. 182-5). Such homogeneity is dependent on the distance of separation of the fields and on beam parameters such as energy and source-to-skin or source-to-axis distances. Parallel opposed fields yield relatively uniform doses if field separation is less than twice the depth of the 50 percent dose. There is a dose variation at the edges of the field, the amount depending chiefly on the ''flatness'' characteristic of the beam. A flattening filter can be used for compensation. An anomaly of the flattening filter is that the beam for the linear accelerator tends to be corrected to flatness for 10 cm depth, and that there is an increased

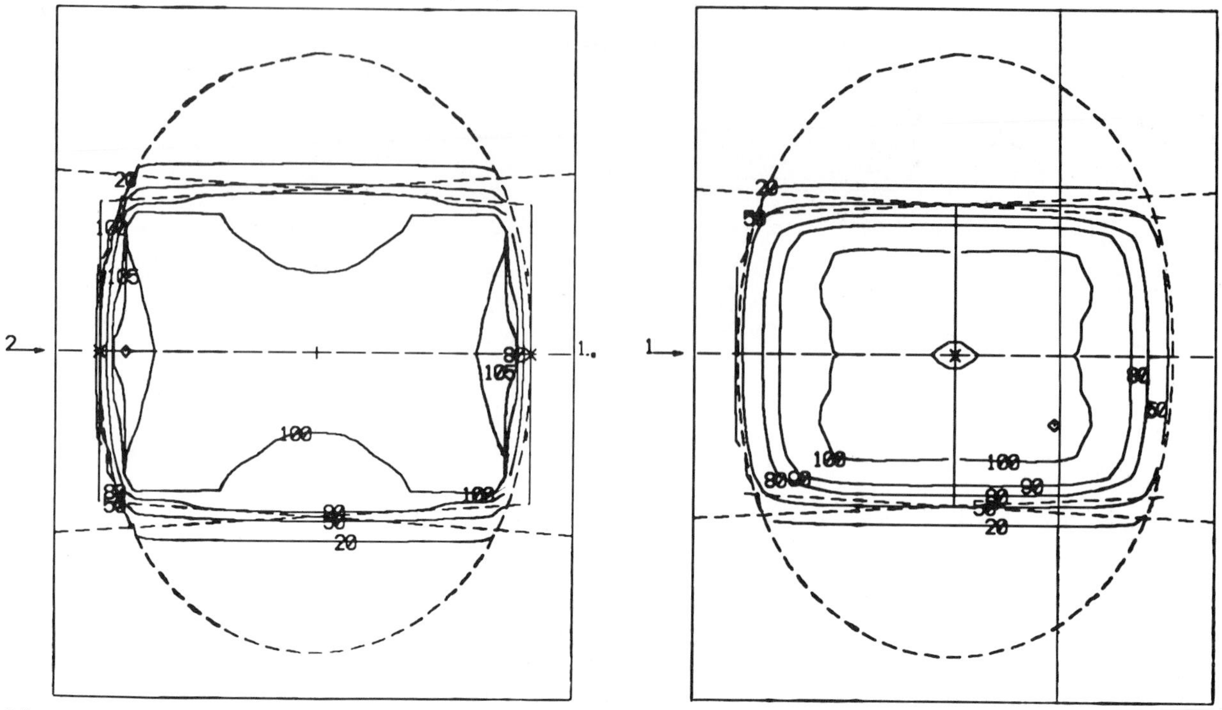

(*A*) (*B*)

Figure 182-5 Comparison of the isodose curves of parallel opposing lateral (partial brain) fields: *A.* Cobalt 60; note the higher dose (105 percent) at entrance and exit and narrowed isodose area at mid-depth compared to *B. B.* The curves produced by a 15-MeV x-ray beam.

dose nearer the surface at the edges of the treatment field. Occasionally one side is treated more heavily than the other, for lateralized lesions. As this ''differential loading'' produces a higher surface dose on the more heavily irradiated side, it is not frequently used. The parallel opposed technique is used for most patients who have whole-brain treatment for metastatic foci.

Wedge filters are frequently used to form slanted isodose lines. A pair of wedge fields, for example, an anterior brain field and a lateral brain field, can be combined to treat one frontal lobe. The two wedge fields together deposit energy homogeneously within a limited volume and subject the contralateral frontal lobe and ipsilateral posterior parts of the brain to lower exit doses. These lower doses to normal tissue should translate into lower morbidity and therefore a greater therapeutic ratio (Fig. 182-6).

Adjacent Fields

Spinal cord injury is probably the number one cause of radiotherapy malpractice suits, as the morbidity is severe and permanent and may occur in patients who have a long life expectancy. Most frequently it is related to the use of adjacent, abutting fields without accurate determination of the appropriate gap on the skin between adjacent fields, which is needed because radiation beams diverge. Because this is extremely critical, it may be advisable to move the junctions between fields during treatment so that no single small area receives an unacceptably high dose as a result of beam overlap.

Arc Rotational Therapy

An isocentric treatment machine lends itself well to arc rotational therapy, in which the arc (or the entire 360-degree rotation) of the machine is used to concentrate the dose in the required treatment volume; the lowered dose to interposed normal tissue reduces treatment morbidity. Such techniques can be modified to become fairly sophisticated, with the placement of wedges, blocks, or compensators in the beam. The arc rotational technique is frequently employed for tumors that have a well-defined, central location, for example, pituitary lesions (Fig. 182-7). Multiple arcs in different planes through the same isocenter are the basis of ''linac scalpel'' radiosurgery.

Multifield Technique

Numerous fields can be used to summate the radiation dose at a specified volume: pituitary treatment using a three-field technique with bilateral wedges can be used with essentially the same result as the arc rotational technique. Computer-aided treatment planning is the most efficient method for combining isodose curves; these computers add the doses to multiple points and can take into consideration variations in tumor volume and beam attenuation (Fig. 182-8).

Tissue Compensators

The intention of tissue compensators is to produce beam attenuation proportional to differences in the thickness of tissues interposed between the radiation source and the tumor that would otherwise cause undesirable variation in doses. If the compensator is placed near the radiation source (not near the patient), skin-sparing effects can be preserved.

Clinical use of compensators has been limited because of practical inefficiencies in measuring surface irregularities, and in manufacturing these topographically irregular, highly customized

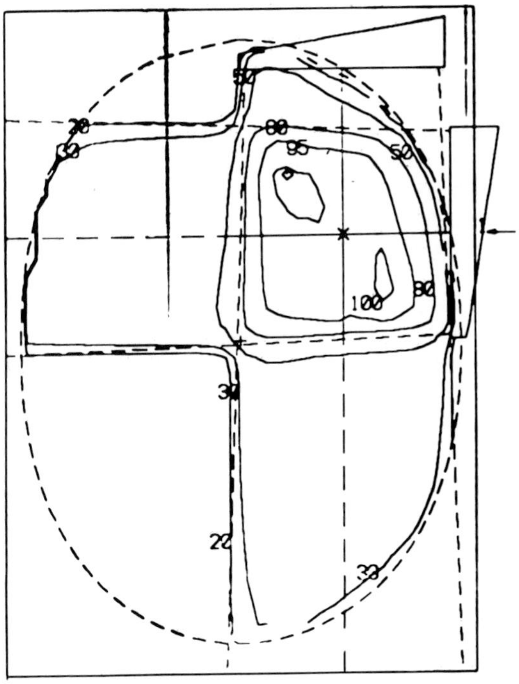

Figure 182-6 A plan that uses lateral and anterior wedged fields. A fairly homogeneous distribution results, with limited irradiation of other brain areas.

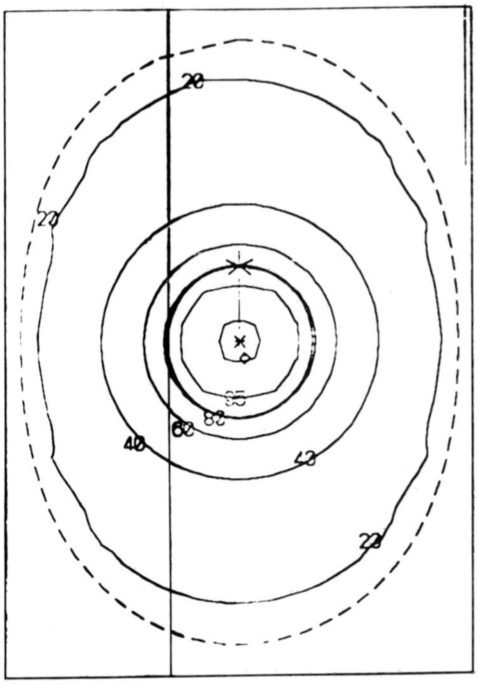

Figure 182-7 Rotational field as for a pituitary tumor. The plan uses a 5 × 5 cm field and 15-MeV x-rays.

beam modifiers. Compensator production systems using specific software in personal computers, and milling machines, have recently become commercially available, and clinical use of compensators is expected to increase.

Radiobiological Considerations

The exact mechanism of radiation kill remains unknown but is obviously extremely efficient, as the energy equivalent to raise the temperature of the human body only 0.0012°C, or 500 cGy of total body irradiation, is lethal. Ionizing radiation produces ionic and nonionic free radicals. Free radicals are chemically very reactive. Radiolysis of water is fundamental; the resulting hydroxyl and hydrogen-free radicals react with oxygen to form hydrogen peroxide. Organic molecules react with these radiolytic products, and are thus "damaged."[25]

Available evidence points to DNA as the critical cellular target for radiation lethality in mammalian cells. In clonogenic assays, cells that cannot multiply are considered dead even though they may be metabolically and morphologically viable. Cell survival curves are semilog plots of surviving clonogenic fraction versus radiation dose; the dose reducing the surviving fraction to 37 percent of the original number of cells is D_0, which is related to the slope of the curve (Fig. 182-9). The survival curve will initially show an area of reduced dose efficiency, a shoulder of nonlinear slope; this is thought to represent sublethal damage, repair of which is overcome by increasing the dose. Cells defective in DNA repair functions are more radiosensitive.

Elkind and Sutton divided the dose of irradiation and determined that when the radiation doses are given a few hours apart, the shoulder of nonlinear slope is reproduced.[7] The difference between these two doses represents the effect of repair, which is probably complete in 3 h in most tissue. With multiple treatments there is interference by many factors, such as partial cell cycle synchronization, changes in cellular oxygenation, tumor repopulation and revascularization, and probably selection of clones of different responsiveness to irradiation. As the dose rate of irradiation

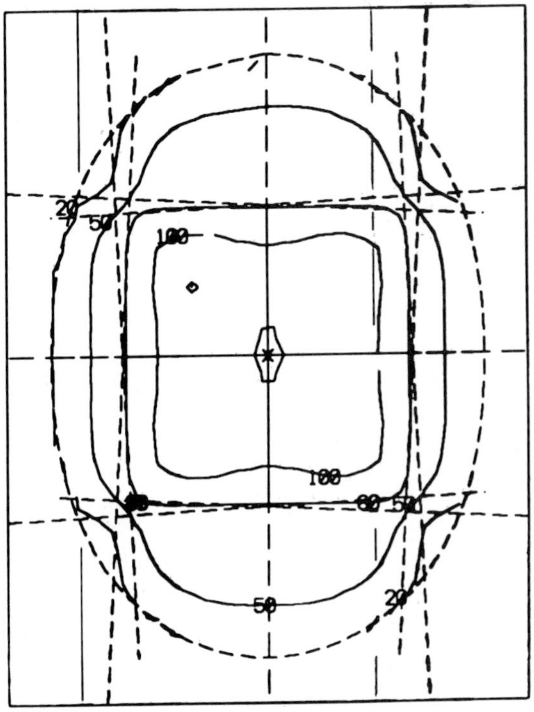

Figure 182-8 A four-field 15-MeV x-ray plan to limit the dose to the areas outside the target volume.

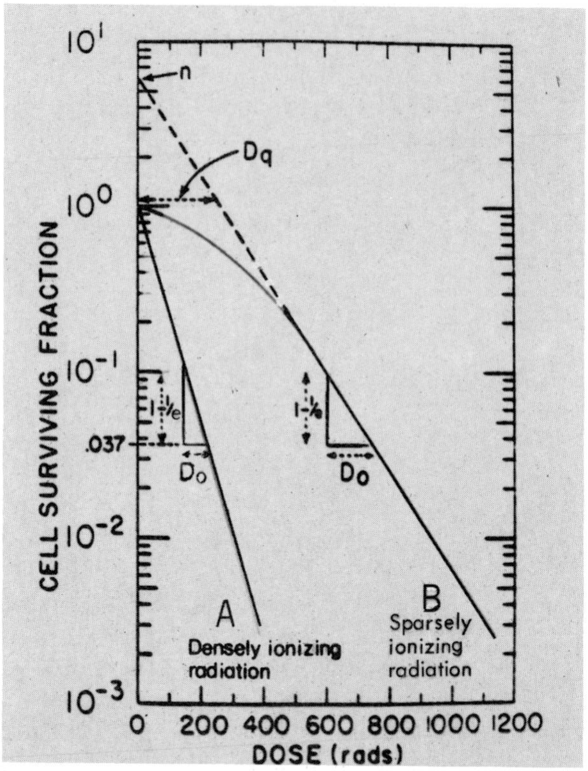

Figure 182-9 Cell survival curves (see text). Conventional irradiation is represented by Line *B*. High-LET irradiation (e.g., neutrons) is better described by Line *A*.

decreases, the efficiency of cell kill per rad (cGy) also decreases. This is thought to be due to the repair of sublethal injury, which is believed to be maximal at a dose rate of about 100 rad per hour or less (common in brachytherapy) and minimal above 100 rad per minute (as in external-beam teletherapy). A second form of cellular injury is termed *potentially lethal damage.* This occurs in cells not actively proliferating. Such damage is enhanced by conditions that increase progression through the cell cycle to mitosis. Recovery from this damage is enhanced by conditions that slow the normal progression through the cycle, such as hypothermia.

The most important modifier of irradiation effect is thought to be oxygen. In 1952, Read demonstrated the need for a greater radiation dose in a hypoxic environment than in an oxic one.[29] The oxygen enhancement ratio (OER) describes the ratio of cell kill in oxic versus hypoxic environments. The exact mechanism is uncertain but the clinical influence is undeniable. The oxygen effect is most significant when x rays (photons) are used (OER $\cong$ 3), and less with subatomic particle beams such as helium nuclei (alpha particles) or neutrons (OER = 1–2). Thomlinson and Grey predicted that the diffusion range of oxygen tension was limited to 150 μm from a capillary.[34] It appears that reoxygenation occurs mostly in cells at 100 to 150 μm from capillaries, as cells beyond that distance are essentially anoxic or necrotic. Importantly, anoxia and severe hypoxia occur in tumors, not normal tissue. Several clinical studies have defined a benefit from the use of hyperbaric oxygen with small numbers of radiation treatments, but the technique was found to be cumbersome and difficult for the patient and treatment staff, prohibiting careful beam definition and beam modification and occasionally being hazardous.[37] The use of sensitizers for hypoxic cells is conceptually more attractive and has been explored. These compounds may actually reach more areas of the tumor than does hyperbaric oxygen.[28]

Of the four phases of the cell cycle, G2 and M are most sensitive, but late G1 and S phases are relatively radiation resistant. In the laboratory, mitotic delay induced by radiation may synchronize the cells so that the next dose fraction may come when cells are in their most resistant phase. However, tumor cells usually tend to desynchronize and redistribute themselves within the cell cycle. Chemotherapeutic agents of different toxicities may be combined with irradiation. The combination of multiple-drug chemotherapy and irradiation may produce a clinical response that is additive, synergistic, or even antagonistic. Obviously, the therapeutic ratio is the critical criterion in determining the clinical usefulness of such combinations.

Relative biological effectiveness (RBE) is the ratio of doses of different radiation types that produce the same biological effect; this is important in comparing particle beams to conventional radiation beams. RBE varies only modestly for clinical photon-beam energies.[25]

Unfortunately, cell survival curve characteristics do not allow the differentiation of normal from malignant cells or sensitive from resistant cells.[38] Dose–response curves can be generated experimentally by implanting tumor cells, allowing the tumor to become palpable, and then testing the effects of different doses of a therapeutic agent. Thus the classic sigmoid curve can be produced, with a relatively constant slope in the middle of the curve; control increases dramatically with dose. Hellman states that the dose necessary to increase the likelihood of tumor control from 10 percent to 90 percent is 3 times the D_0 dose.[15] If tumor cells are relatively radioresistant, the radiation survival curve will become shallow. Then the dose–tumor control curve will be shallow also.

As a generalization, larger tumors have a smaller portion of their cell population proceeding through the cell cycle to division (the *growth fraction*) than smaller tumors, presumably due to chronic metabolic deficiencies that result from an inadequate microvasculature. Interference with a tumor's ability to produce tumor angiogenesis factor may limit tumor growth, as described by Folkman.[10]

Those tissues made of cells that do not divide, particularly neural and muscular tissue, have long been regarded as relatively resistant to irradiation; however, they are supported by vascular and connective tissue cells that do divide, and that may ultimately determine the response (in the CNS, necrosis and gliosis) to radiation.[31] Filler et al. describe a D_q (shoulder) of 340 cGy and D_0 of 170 cGy, with N = 7 for these endothelial cells, which are similar to epithelial cells.[9]

Total-body irradiation in the range of 10,000 rad (cGy) produces rapid death; this occurs within hours and is characterized by vomiting, diarrhea, nausea, sweating, fever, headache, rapidly evolving to obtundation, seizures, and coma. In the range of 500 to 1000 cGy, death occurs within several days from gastrointestinal mucosal damage that results in profuse diarrhea, hemorrhage, sepsis, and dehydration. At doses of 100 to 500 cGy, hematopoietic failure occurs, with death 2 to 4 weeks later because of the differential survival of end-product cells in the marrow and peripheral blood. The number of lymphocytes falls first, the number of platelets and granulocytes in about 5 to 6 days, and the number of red blood cells last.

Radiation has definite effects on the immune response; for example, following whole-body irradiation, most of the lymphocytes die immediately. Anderson and Warner reached the following conclusions: B lymphocytes and T-lymphocyte precursor cells are sensitive to irradiation; the homing potential of immunocompetent cells may be altered; resting cells just having been stimulated are less sensitive; and effects of whole-body irradiation are different from those of localized irradiation.[1]

Localized radiotherapy will produce a lymphopenia of both T and B cells in humans. However, established immunity recovers quickly. Claims that patients treated with radiation to the chest wall and regional lymph nodes after mastectomy have an increased mortality due to immunosuppression have been repudiated.[21]

Normal Tissue Consequences of Therapeutic Irradiation

Radiation carcinogenesis is a subject of considerable concern. After the exposure of a population to irradiation, there is a gradual increase in tumor incidence with time until a plateau is reached, as evidenced by studies of atomic bomb survivors in Japan and of patients irradiated for benign diseases.[4,11,14,33] The tumor induction period can range from 3 to 5 years for leukemia to 10 to 15 years or longer for solid tumors. Patients treated for benign diseases with modest radiation doses (1000 cGy or less) to the pelvis have a higher incidence of secondary malignancies than do patients treated with tumoricidal higher doses to the same volume.[2] Radiation is both teratogenic and carcinogenic for in utero exposure and is also an abortifacient.

The basic principle of fractionation of radiotherapy was described by Coutard, who observed a relationship between acute reaction and late effects and established the importance of multiple daily doses, or *fractionation.*[5] The rationale of fractionation is that normal cells recover better from sublethal radiation damage than do neoplastic cells, and that this recovery takes place between successive treatment sessions. In addition, partial reoxygenation of hypoxic tumor cells probably takes place gradually as multiple radiation doses are administered.

Normal tissue radiation responses are either early reacting (e.g., skin, mucosa, bone marrow) or late reacting (e.g., brain, spinal cord). The late reactions are the responses of nonproliferating tissue or slowly proliferating vascular and connective tissue. Clinical radiation dose prescriptions attempt to predict the tolerance of early- and late-reacting normal tissues, and the late effects are generally dose limiting (e.g., brain necrosis). Differing radiation time–dose–fractionation (TDF) schedules that yield identical tissue effects are termed *isoeffective.* Strandqvist established this concept in 1944. Subsequent developments of the isoeffect concept include the nominal standard dose (NSD) of Ellis[8] in 1965, and the TDF factors of Orton and Ellis[26] in 1973.

The usefulness of NSD and TDF proved to be limited, and in the 1980s became replaced by the linear quadratic model:

$$S = e^{-E} \text{ and } E = D(\alpha + \beta d) \text{ and } D = nd$$

where S is the surviving cell fraction, D is the total dose, n is the number of fractions, d is the dose per fraction, and alpha and beta are constants.[12] Mathematically, the equations can be solved for the alpha/beta ratio but not the individual constants. Alpha/beta ratios can be calculated from experimental and clinical data. Basically, rapidly multiplying (early-reacting) tissues have high alpha/beta ratios, generally above 10; slowly proliferating (late-reacting) tissues have low ratios, usually 2 to 5. Tolerance to irradiation is also related to the anatomic location of the treatment volume, which must be considered in the patient's overall treatment plan.

In certain situations irradiation and surgery are most useful when combined, because irradiation is usually very effective in the (oxygenated) periphery of the tumors, whereas surgery can fail in those areas, particularly when vital or resection-limiting structures are involved. The disadvantages of using preoperative radiotherapy are (1) the surgical definition of tumor extent is not known, (2) it is difficult to evaluate the histologic specimen obtained at operation for the viability of any remaining tumor cells, and (3) there may be some delay in healing after surgery. If 4000 to 5000 cGy are given to a potential operative site, a 4- to 6-week delay prior to surgery is necessary while capillary dilatation subsides. If higher doses are given, even greater healing problems may be evident. A major problem is the combined toxicity of irradiation and surgery; particularly evident is increased fibrosis in the area of scars, which may lead to damage to underlying vessels, muscles, or nerves.

It is probably best that radiation-related cerebral edema be anticipated clinically, because it may be prevented by surgical decompression, medical means, or a combination of both. The clinician does occasionally see patients whose symptoms and signs, such as headache, obtundation, nausea, and vomiting are increased when brain irradiation begins. In the past it has been common to begin with low individual radiation doses and gradually increase the daily dose, but that approach has largely been abandoned with the advent of steroid medication. If patients are irradiated postoperatively, this should be delayed until the wound is healed (usually 7 to 14 days).

It is difficult to determine if necrosis in irradiated brain is related to tumor, treatment, or a combination of the two. Brain tolerance is probably in the range of 6000 photon cGy given in 30 to 35 treatments over 6 to 7 weeks. Frequently brain necrosis is seen in patients after radiotherapy for recurrent disease, an anticipated complication that may be justified because of a desperate situation. The physician is occasionally able to effect a reasonable remission in these patients. There also seems to be a greater incidence of brain necrosis in patients treated with a higher dose per fraction. A third parameter, treatment volume, is seldom mentioned when considering the incidence of brain necrosis but clearly has a major effect (Fig. 182-10).

In 1992, Kleinberg and associates reported the performance status of 30 adults who were disease free more than 1 year after cranial irradiation for gliomas at Memorial Sloan-Kettering Cancer Center.[20] Twenty-five patients had anaplastic gliomas or glioblastomas, and median follow-up was 3.5 years. Treatment volume was partial brain, or whole brain with partial-brain boost; total dose was 5400 to 6600 cGy at 170 to 200 cGy per fraction. These patients' rather high Karnofsky performance status (mean, 84 preradiation) generally remained stable (mean, 84 at last follow-up), with no change in 80 percent. Sixty-eight percent returned to work in capacities similar to premorbid work, with 90 percent of these working 1 year later, and 85 percent working at last follow-up. These authors conclude that long-term glioma survivors with relatively good preradiation performance did not experience declines in cognitive function after radiotherapy.

A common delayed reaction of irradiation to the whole brain is a somnolence syndrome, first described in 1929 in patients irradiated for ringworm of the scalp. Its onset is about 6 to 8 weeks following radiotherapy, and it persists for about 2 weeks. More recently, symptoms have been reported recurring in children several months after completion of treatment for acute leukemia.[13] The symptoms were nonfocal and transient; all of the children had spontaneous complete recovery. Late delayed effects can occur within a range of 4 months to 12 years. They tend to peak in 1 to 3 years and are characterized by insidiously progressive deterioration, focal neurological signs, dementia, and seizures. Differentiation from recurrence of the brain tumor is difficult at times because

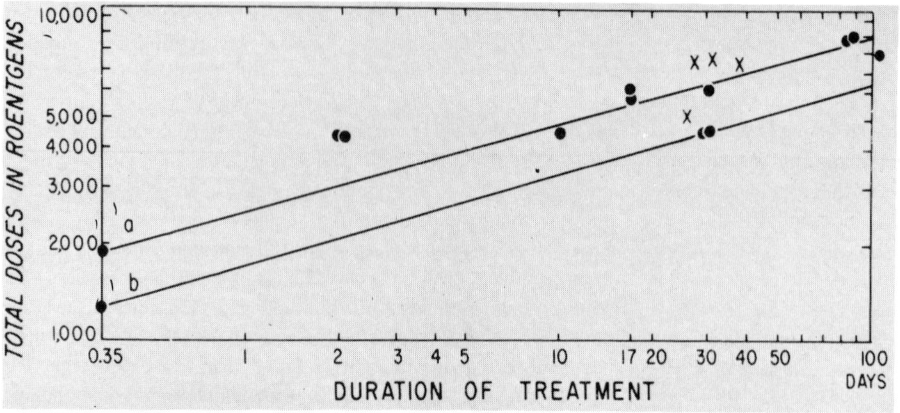

Figure 182-10 Modified Strandqvist diagram. The dose above Line *a* involves great risk of cerebral necrosis. Line *b* represents the lowest dose level producing cerebral necrosis. The slope of both lines is 0.26. (From Rubin and Casarett,[31] with permission.)

both may produce increased spinal fluid protein levels, increased uptake in a radioisotope scan, focal electroencephalographic dysfunction, and CT and MRI scan changes. This is usually due to progressive changes in white matter caused by vasculopathy involving small and large blood vessels (Fig. 182-11).

Investigators involved with pediatric patients in recent years have been concerned about the long-term effects of brain irradiation and chemotherapy. In combined group studies of 108 patients there was no evident decrease in verbal performance IQs found in irradiated children, but several intellectual limitations have been recognized. Other pediatric studies involving patients with brain tumors showed that irradiation resulted in a disproportionate number of patients who were severely disabled mentally. For example, Hirsch et al. compared the IQs of children with medulloblastoma with those of children with cerebellar astrocytoma; the latter were presumed to have a lower chance of having a significant increase in intracranial pressure. There was a striking difference between these two populations, with a higher IQ in those patients who had cerebellar astrocytoma.[17] A study done at Roswell Park Memorial Institute noted deterioration of full-scale IQ of at least 25 points in each of four children who had intelligence testing before and after treatment. CT scans after brain irradiation may show leukoencephalopathy as evidenced by large ventricles, widened sulci, hypodense areas, and calcifications. The implication of these studies is that brain irradiation in childhood has definite adverse effects that are probably worse in children treated with higher doses.

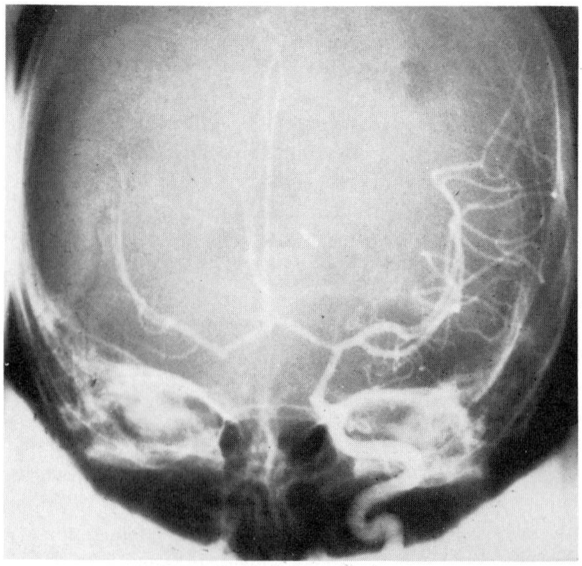

Figure 182-11 Left carotid arteriogram of a child with medulloblastoma treated with external irradiation and intrathecal radioactive gold colloid. Note the narrowing of the intracranial segment of the left internal carotid artery and of the left anterior cerebral artery.

Endocrine dysfunction (a decrease in growth hormone release) was noted in children treated prophylactically to prevent CNS leukemia, but normal follicle-stimulating hormone, luteinizing hormone, cortisol, and testosterone levels were noted.[13,36] Tumoricidal radiotherapy for cancer of the nasopharynx can slowly cause broad reductions in hypothalamic–pituitary function, although the exact incidence is unknown.[32] Thyroid dysfunction and neoplasia resulting from irradiation of the thyroid gland has been well documented.[23,24]

Irradiation of the spinal axis in children can produce a decrease in sitting height in adulthood, with or without scoliosis. The basic rule for tumoricidal radiotherapy in children is that immature tissues within the radiation beam are at risk for hypoplasia.

Transverse myelopathy caused by irradiation is usually irreversible. It develops 6 months to 5 years after treatment, and no effective treatment is known. The likelihood of myelopathy tends to increase with the length of spinal cord irradiated, and if doses over 5000 cGy are given at 180 to 200 cGy per treatment, 5 days per week; if higher doses per treatment are used, spinal cord injury may follow total doses less than 5000 cGy. Spinal cord irradiation is particularly a problem at field junctions, where there is a risk of overlapping beams; the upper thoracic spinal cord is most susceptible.[31]

Lhermitte's sign occurs occasionally 1 to 3 months after spinal doses of 3500 to 4000 cGy. It does not precede radiation myelopathy and resolves in several weeks. Its precise pathogenesis is unclear because tissue for pathological study has not been available.

Other potential adverse effects of radiotherapy range from otitis media (if a middle ear is irradiated) to seizures (presumably due to focal gliosis) and cataracts (if a lens is irradiated). These adverse effects can be minimized by careful treatment planning, daily treatment precision, and due consideration of tolerance doses, but are not completely eliminated, unless tumor treatment is seriously compromised.

Radiation Sensitizers

A true radiosensitizer will increase radiation cell kill without inherent cytotoxic effects. Despite a great deal of work, the radiosensitizers have to date not yielded improved clinical results. Desirable features of a radiosensitizer include a lack of cell-cycle specificity, no intrinsic cytotoxicity, easy diffusibility, and for hypoxic cell sensitizers, high electron affinity. The nitroimidazoles, particularly metronidazole and misonidazole, have been used in numerous clinical trials as hypoxic cell radiosensitizers, showing little advantage despite significant toxicity. Peripheral and central neuropathies occur with some frequency.[3,6,30]

Other classes of potential radiosensitizers include the halogenated pyrimidines BUdR (bromodeoxyuridine) and IUdR[22] (iododeoxyuridine); perfluorocarbons, which improve oxygen transport to hypoxic cells; and drugs that bind with, or reduce synthesis of, intracellular glutathione, because glutathione and other thiols are radioprotectors.[3,30]

Oxygen is still the best radiosensitizer of hypoxic cells.[25]

Radioprotectors

At the cellular level, repair by reduction competes with fixation of damage by oxidation. Promising radioprotective compounds tend to have a sulfhydryl and an aminopropyl group.[25] Interestingly, the protection is greater in the oxygenated than in the hypoxic cell population. WR2721, an aminopropylthioic acid, has these groups.[35] It is the most promising of a series of possible radioprotectors developed under the auspices of the U.S. Army. Its intracellular concentrations are greater in normal than in tumor tissue. Primary toxicity is vomiting and hypotension. Unfortunately, the drug is not lipophilic and therefore is poorly concentrated in central nervous tissue, making its role unlikely in neuro-oncology. It affords greater protection for bone marrow, mucosa, skin, and renal and hepatic tissues.[3,25]

References

1. Anderson RE, Warner NL. Ionizing radiation and the immune response. *Adv Immunol* 1976; 24:215–335.
2. Boice JD, Hutchinson GB. Leukemia in women following radiotherapy for cervical cancer: ten year follow-up of an international study. *J Nat Cancer Inst* 1980; 65:115–129.
3. Brown JM, Bigalow JE, Hall EJ, et al. Sensitizers and protectors to radiation and chemotherapeutic drugs. *Cancer Treat Symp* 1984, 1:85–101.
4. Brown WM, Doll R. Mortality from cancer and other causes after radiotherapy for ankylosing spondylitis. *Br Med J* 1965; 2:1327–1332.
5. Coutard H. Roentgen therapy of epitheliomas of the tonsillar region, hypopharynx and larynx from 1920–1926. *Am J Roentgenol* 1932; 28:313–331.
6. Dische S. Chemical sensitizers for hypoxic cells: a decade of experience in clinical radiotherapy. *Radiother Oncol* 1985; 3:97–115.
7. Elkind MM, Sutton H. Radiation response of mammalian cells grown in culture. 1: Repair of x-ray damage in surviving Chinese hamster cells. *Radiat Res* 1960; 13:556–593.
8. Ellis F. The relationship of biological effect to dose-time-fractionation factors in radiotherapy. *Cur Top Radiat Res* 1965; 4:357–397.
9. Filler RM, Tefft M, Vawter GF. Hepatic lobectomy in childhood: effects of x-ray and chemotherapy. *J Pediatr Surg* 1969; 4:31–41.
10. Folkman J. Tumor angiogenesis: a possible control point in tumor growth. *Ann Intern Med* 1975; 82:96–100.
11. Folley JH, Borges W, Yamawaki T. Incidence of leukemia in survivors of atomic bomb in Hiroshima and Nagasaki, Japan. *Am J Med* 1952; 13:311–321.
12. Fowler JF. The linear-quadratic formula and progress in fractionated radiotherapy, *Br J Radiol* 1989; 62:679–694.
13. Freeman JE, Johnston PGB, Voke JM. Somnolence after prophylactic cranial irradiation in children with acute lymphoblastic leukemia. *Br Med J* 1973; 4:523–525.
14. Gray LH. Radiation biology and cancer. In *Symposium on Fundamental Cancer Research; Cellular Radiation Biology*. Baltimore: Williams & Wilkins, 1965; pp 7–25.
15. Hellman S. Principles of radiation therapy. In DeVita VT Jr, Hellman S, Rosenberg SA (eds): *Cancer—Principles and Practice of Oncology*. Philadelphia: Lippincott, 1993, p 264.
16. Hendee WR. *Radiation Therapy Physics*. Chicago: Year Book, 1981, pp 1–19, 56–78, 83–114.
17. Hirsch JF, Renier D, Czernichow P, et al. Medulloblastoma in childhood: survival and functional results. *Acta Neurochir (Wien)* 1979; 48:1–15.
18. Johns HE, Bates LM, Watson TA. 1000 Curie cobalt units for radiation therapy: I. Saskatchewan cobalt 60 unit. *Br J Radiol* 1952; 25:296–302.
19. Johns HE, Cunningham JR. *The Physics of Radiology*, 3d ed. Springfield, IL: Charles C Thomas, 1969.
20. Kleinberg L, Malkin M, Wallner K. Performance status of long term disease free survivors of intracranial gliomas. *Int J Radiat Oncol Biol Phys* 1992; 24(Suppl 1): 302 (abstr).
21. Levitt SH, McHugh RB. Early breast cancer and postoperative irradiation. *Lancet* 1975; 2:1258–1259.
22. McGinn CJ, Kinsella TJ. The experimental and clinical rationale for the use of S-phase-specific radiosensitizers to overcome tumor cell repopulation. *Semin Oncol* 1992; 19(Suppl 11): 21–28.
23. National Council on Radiation Protection and Measurements. Induction of thyroid cancer by ionizing radiation. NCRP Report No. 80. Bethesda, MD: The Council, 1985.
24. Nelson DF, Reddy KV, O'Mara RE, et al. Thyroid abnormalities following neck irradiation for Hodgkin's disease. *Cancer* 1978; 42:2553–2562.
25. Nias AHW. *An Introduction to Radiobiology*. New York: John Wiley, 1990, pp 53–60, 112–114, 164–183, 271–275.
26. Orton CG, Ellis F. A simplification in the use of the NSD concept in practical radiotherapy. *Br J Radiol* 1973; 46:529–537.
27. Owen JB, Coia LR, Hanks GE. Recent patterns of growth in radiation therapy facilities in the United States: a patterns of care study report. *Int J Radiat Oncol Biol Phys* 1992; 24:983–986.
28. Phillips TL. Radiation sensitizers and protectors. In DeVita VT Jr, Hellman S, Rosenberg SA (eds): *Cancer—Principles and Practice of Oncology*. Philadelphia: Lippincott, 1982, pp 1822–1836.
29. Read J. The effect of ionizing radiations on the broad beam group: Part X. The dependence of the x-ray sensitivity on dissolved oxygen. *Br J Radiol* 1952; 25:89–99.
30. Rockwell S. Use of hypoxia-directed drugs in the therapy of solid tumors. *Semin Oncol* 1992; 19(Suppl 11), 29–40.
31. Rubin P, Casarett GW. *Clinical Radiation Pathology*. Philadelphia: Saunders, 1968, p 651.
32. Samaan NA, Maor M, Sampiere VA, et al. Hypopituitarism after external irradiation of nasopharyngeal cancer. In Linfood JA (ed): *Recent Advances in the Diagnosis and Treatment of Pituitary Tumors*. New York: Raven Press, 1979, pp 315–330.
33. Smith PG, Doll R. Late effects of x irradiation in patients treated for metropathia haemorrhagica. *Br J Radiol* 1976; 49:224–232.
34. Thomlinson RH, Grey LH. The histological structure of some human

lung cancers and the possible implications for radiotherapy. *Br J Cancer* 1955; 9:539–549.

35. Turrisi AT, Glover DV, Hurwitz S, et al. Final report of the Phase I trial of single-dose WR-2721 [S-2-(3-aminopropylamino)ethylphosphorothioic acid]. *Cancer Treat Rep* 1986; 70:1389–1393.
36. Voorhees M, Brecher ML, MacGillivray M, et al. Effect of different forms of central nervous system (CNS) prophylaxis on pituitary function of children with acute lymphocytic leukemia (ALL). *Proc Am Soc Clin Oncol* 1981; 22:396 (abstr).
37. Watson ER, Halnan KE, Dische S, et al. Hyperbaric oxygen and radiotherapy: a Medical Research Council trial in carcinoma of the cervix. *Br J Radiol* 1978; 51:879–887.
38. Weichselbaum RR, Nove J, Little JB. X-ray sensitivity of human tumor cells in vitro. *Int J Radiat Oncol Biol Phys* 1980; 6:437–440.
39. Wilson CS, Hall EJ. On the advisability of treating all fields at each radiotherapy session. *Radiology* 1971; 98:419–424.

183

Conventional Radiotherapy of Specific Central Nervous System Tumors

Steven R. Plunkett

Radiation therapy is a well-established tool in the treatment of many CNS neoplasms. Various modalities of irradiation have been used for many years in efforts to improve local control and prevent regional spread, as well as to improve both quality and length of survival. Recent advancements in the development of linear accelerators, along with improvements in computer-assisted treatment planning and dosimetry, have increased the effectiveness of radiation therapy in treating CNS tumors.

Conformal radiotherapy, using three-dimensional computer-assisted tomography, is currently being used in many centers. This technique should allow the radiation oncologist to more clearly define tumor volume and allow higher doses of radiation to be administered with fewer adverse effects on normal tissue.

Many recent studies more clearly define the role of radiation therapy in the management of a broad spectrum of brain and spinal cord neoplasms.

Malignant Gliomas

External beam irradiation has been used in the treatment of high-grade gliomas for a number of years. There have previously been uncertainties as to the optimum dose, field size, and fractionation scheme which should be used in managing these aggressive neoplasms. Fortunately, several excellent studies have more clearly defined the use of radiotherapy in the treatment of these tumors.

The most comprehensive study relating to the role of radiotherapy in the treatment of these tumors was conducted by the Brain Tumor Study Group (BTSG).[49] In this study, a group of 222 patients with histologically confirmed anaplastic gliomas were studied in a prospective, randomized fashion. The patient population was divided into four groups. The first group received no postoperative radiotherapy or chemotherapy but received the best conventional care; the second group received 1,3-bis(2-chloroethyl)-1-nitrosourea (BCNU) postoperatively; the third group received radiotherapy following surgical resection; and the fourth group received a combination of BCNU and radiotherapy postoperatively. The patient groups were broken down into those who received any amount of therapy (the Valid Study Group, VSG) and those who were deemed to have been adequately treated (the Adequately Treated Group, ATG). The ATG included patients in all four of the treatment arms. Patients who received radiotherapy and/or BCNU were included in the ATG if they received at least 5000 cGy of radiotherapy, received at least 2 courses of chemotherapy, and survived a minimum of 8 weeks after treatment.

There were no differences among the four groups in patient age or sex, diagnosis, characteristics and location of tumor, or the amount of corticosteroids used. The results were broken down into median survival times for patients in the VSG and for those in the ATG. Median survival times of patients in the VSG were as follows: best conventional care, 14 weeks; BCNU, 18 weeks; radiotherapy, 35 weeks; and radiotherapy plus BCNU, 34.5 weeks. Median survival times of patients in the ATG were: best conventional care, 17 weeks; BCNU, 25 weeks; radiotherapy, 37.5 weeks; and radiotherapy plus BCNU, 40.5 weeks. Clearly, radiotherapy was found to have a favorable prognostic effect in this study. The median survival time in those patients who received radiotherapy was increased by approximately 150 percent. Although BCNU did not alter the median survival times in either of the patient groups in which it was used, a significantly greater fraction of surviving patients was noted at 18 months in the group that received a combination of BCNU and radiotherapy.

The technique of radiotherapy was delineated rather specifically in the BTSG studies, and this needs to be emphasized. Patients were treated with a dose of 6000 cGy over 6 to 7 weeks, using 5 fractions per week. Large parallel opposing lateral fields were used, and the entire cranial contents were encompassed within the irradiated area. The daily fraction size was 170 to 200 cGy and the dose was calculated at the midplane of the patient's brain.

The importance of radiotherapy dose in regard to patient survival was emphasized in another study involving a much larger patient population within the Brain Tumor Study Group.[50] This study demonstrated that patient survival increases as the dose of radiotherapy is increased. Six hundred twenty-one patients were analyzed for the median survival times relative to the doses of radiotherapy which were given (Table 183-1). Those patients who received 4500 cGy or less had a median survival of 13.5 weeks; 5000 cGy, 28 weeks; 5500 cGy, 36 weeks; and 6000 cGy, 42 weeks. Those patients who received 4500 cGy or less comprised a heterogeneous group of patients, and this group as a whole is difficult to analyze. However, the use of radiotherapy at a dose of 6000 cGy increased the patients' median life span by 2.3 times as compared to those patients who received no radiotherapy. A 5000-cGy dose resulted in an increased life expectancy of 1.6 times, and life expectancy was doubled with a 5500-cGy dose. In this study, the difference in toxicity between a dose of 5000 cGy and one of 6000 cGy was not thought to be clinically significant.

The need for relatively large radiation fields in treating the malignant gliomas was emphasized over 30 years ago.[7] The extent of supratentorial gliomas was analyzed by autopsy studies in 30 patients who expired shortly after admission to the hospital for radiotherapy. The investigators consistently found that the tumor was larger and more extensive than had been anticipated on the basis of clinical and radiographic examinations. Those patients who were treated with large fields had a much greater chance of having the entire tumor volume encompassed within the treated field. This study demonstrated that there is no place for small- or medium-sized treatment volumes in the radiotherapeutic management of malignant gliomas. Indeed, the number of patients in

TABLE 183-1 Median Survival of Patients in Each Therapeutic Subgroup*

Nominal Dose (cGy)	Number Entered	Percentage Failed	Median Survival (weeks)	Wilcoxon Test†			
0	194	98	18.0	†			
≤ 4500	61	97	13.5	0.346	†		
5000	56	91	28.0	0.001	0.003	†	
5500	33	97	36.0	0.001	0.001	0.174	†
6000	270	89	42.0	0.001	0.001	0.004	0.110

*Results of the Brain Tumor Study Group analysis of median survival relative to the total dose of whole brain irradiation for malignant glioma.

†The Wilcoxon test was applied between the survival time indicated on each line by a dagger and each succeeding survival time below the dagger.

Source: From Walker et al.,[50] with permission.

whom, had they survived, tumors would have been missed was greatest in those patients who were being treated with small- or medium-sized fields.

Advancements in treatment planning utilizing better imaging studies [e.g., computed tomography (CT) and magnetic resonance imaging (MRI)] and computer-assisted dosimetry have made it possible to more clearly define tumor volumes, thus allowing the radiation oncologist to spare more normal brain tissue from unnecessary radiation. In general, radiation therapy is administered to a volume which encompasses the area of tumor and surrounding edema with a margin of 2 to 4 cm. Some protocols call for a decrease in this volume after a dose of 4500 to 5000 cGy to a volume which includes the primary tumor plus a 2 to 3 cm margin.

The use of radiotherapy in doses greater than those conventionally used has been studied by Salazar et al.[41] All patients underwent surgical resection and were then treated with megavoltage equipment. This retrospective analysis included a group of patients considered to have received very high dose treatment. These patients received 5000 to 6000 cGy of whole brain irradiation followed by an additional dose to a smaller volume encompassing the primary lesion. The total dose to the primary region was between 7000 and 8000 cGy. Patients in the medium high dose group received 6000 cGy of whole brain irradiation. Patients in the conventional dose group received between 5000 and 5500 cGy. The patients were analyzed in separate groups, according to the histologic grade of their tumors. In those patients who had grade IV lesions, there was statistically significant improvement in median survival in those patients who received the very high doses compared to those who received conventional doses. However, the difference was not maintained after 2 years from the beginning of treatment. Patients with grade III lesions were found to have statistically significant differences in their median survival between each group. These differences were maintained for 4 years after the initiation of treatment. The patients who received the higher doses of irradiation tolerated their treatments fairly well. There were no documented cases of brain tissue necrosis. It is important to realize that the higher doses did not alter the long-term survival of patients. In addition, the patients who received very high (7500 to 8000 cGy) doses to the primary region still did not have tumor sterilization.

Alterations in dose rate and fraction size have been attempted in many clinical trials. One of the more common approaches has been to study the results of external beam radiotherapy utilizing multiple fractions per day. These trials, usually using twice daily or three times daily treatments, have not shown any consistent survival benefit.[15,16]

The technique used in delivering radiotherapy can make a great difference in terms of patient tolerance, patient compliance, and side effects. The use of high-energy x-rays, sometimes in combination with lower-energy sources, is often of benefit. It is essential to use CT scans and MRI scans as well as computerized dose distributions in order to concentrate the dose of irradiation to a specific region of the tumor and reduce the dose to the surrounding soft tissues and normal brain substance. The use of compensating filters and specially cut blocks for each patient can enhance hair growth, even out the dose distribution, and rèduce undesirable side effects (Fig. 183-1). In general, since the treatment of malignant gliomas requires whole brain irradiation, the use of high-energy sources with equal loading on each portal results in an adequate dose distribution while minimizing the risk of complications. Certainly as the dose of irradiation is increased, the number of complications to both the cerebral tissue and the overlying soft tissue is increased as well. It is for this reason that some prefer treating a larger area with a dose of approximately 4500 to 5000 cGy, followed by higher doses to a reduced volume encompassing the area of the primary lesion. In making a decision about the dose to be used in treating these patients, the physician must weigh the possibility of improved tumor control against the greater risk of complications at the higher dose levels. Other techniques for treating these neoplasms include concomitant chemotherapy, stereotactic radiosurgery, and brachytherapy. The use of these modalities is discussed elsewhere in this text.

Low-Grade Astrocytomas

The role of postoperative radiotherapy in the low-grade astrocytomas is not as clear-cut as in the case of the malignant gliomas. It has been said that low-grade astrocytomas (grades I and II) are radioresistant and that radiotherapy is not useful in their treatment. There are several convincing retrospective studies, however, which indicate that radiotherapy can be effective against these tumors. These studies suggest that postoperative irradiation of incompletely resected low-grade astrocytomas results in prolonged survival. Many of the studies lack a control arm and the radiation doses are often inconsistent. A 5-year survival of 49 percent was reported for a patient population which was studied by Bouchard and Peirce.[5] These patients were described as having received adequate irradiation for their astrocytomas. However, it is unclear exactly how the patients who received postoperative irradiation were selected.

A convincing retrospective analysis which involved 147 patients seen over a 25-year period was reported by Leibel et al.[27] In this study, the patient population consisted of 80 males and 67

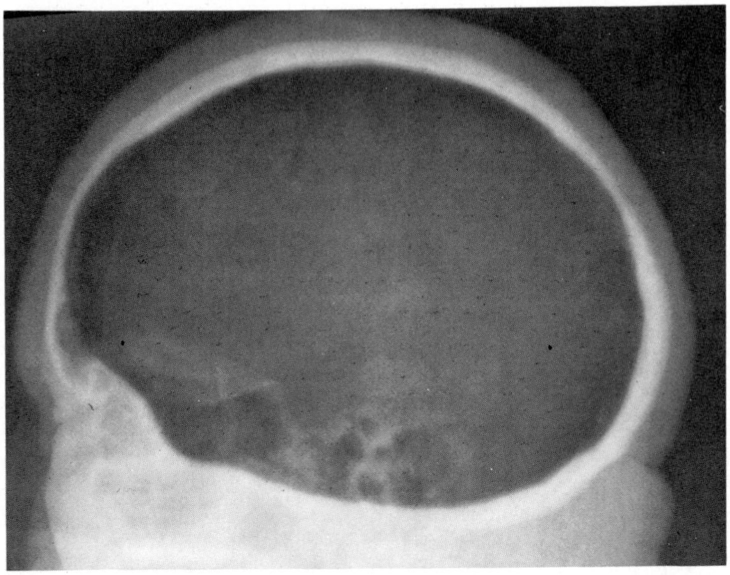

Figure 183-1 Port film of a patient with a malignant glioma who is receiving whole brain irradiation. Specially cut blocks of Cerrobend (Cerro Sales Corp, New York, NY) made for each patient can reduce the dose of irradiation to surrounding soft tissues and decrease the incidence of undesirable side effects.

females over a wide age range. All patients had histologic confirmation of a grade I or grade II astrocytoma, and all patients underwent surgical resection of the primary lesion. Only 14 of these 147 patients were thought by the surgeon to have had complete resection of the tumor. These 14 patients were treated by surgery alone and all survived 5 years or longer. Some of the patients in whom the lesion was considered to be incompletely resected were referred for postoperative irradiation. In reviewing the patient population, the authors did not think that there was any bias regarding which patients were referred for irradiation. During the latter portion of the study, however, a larger percentage of patients were referred for postoperative irradiation. Of the 147 patients, 25 were eliminated because of early postoperative death. These patients did not have the opportunity to receive radiotherapy and were excluded from the analysis. Of the remaining 122 patients, 108 had incompletely resected tumors. Thirty-seven of these patients were treated with surgery alone and the remainder received postoperative radiotherapy. Treatment was administered to fields which included the area of known disease and a margin of several centimeters around the tumor to allow for the possibility of additional tumor extent. No patients received whole brain irradiation. The tumor dose varied from less than 3500 to 5500 cGy. Only four patients received radiotherapy in doses of less than 3500 cGy, and none of these patients survived 5 years. However, there was no difference in survival between those patients who received 3500 to 4500 cGy and those who received doses greater than 4500 cGy. Overall, patients who received postoperative irradiation for incompletely excised tumors had a longer survival time than those who did not receive treatment (Table 183-2). This was true for both grade I and grade II lesions, but patients with grade I astrocytomas experienced a greater survival rate. In the group as a whole, the 5-year survival rate for those patients who did not receive postoperative irradiation after incomplete resection was 19 percent. When irradiation was given, the 5-year survival rate increased to 46 percent. The authors found no evidence of complications induced by the radiotherapy. The 10- and 20-year survival rates without irradiation were 11 percent and 0 percent, compared to rates of 35 percent and 23 percent, respectively, in the irradiated group.

Recent retrospective studies confirm that surgery followed by radiotherapy offers the best chance for long-term survival. Patients more recently diagnosed with low-grade astrocytomas, treated with surgery and radiation therapy, have better survival than patients studied in prior retrospective studies. This is probably due to the widespread use of CT scanning, which results in earlier diagnosis of these lesions. A recent retrospective review demonstrated a median survival of 7¼ years in a group of adults with supratentorial low-grade astrocytomas who were treated with surgery and postoperative radiation therapy. A 10-year median survival was demonstrated in the subset of patients with cerebral hemisphere tumors.[30]

It would thus appear that postoperative radiotherapy does play

TABLE 183-2 Survival Rates According to Therapy*

		Surgery Alone		Surgery + Irradiation
Interval (years)	**All Cases**†	**Total Resection**	**Incomplete Resection**	**Incomplete Resection**
1	65% (33/51)	100% (14/14)	51% (19/37)	80% (57/71)
3	47% (24/51)	100% (14/14)	27% (10/37)	59% (42/71)
5	41% (21/51)	100% (14/14)	19% (7/37)	46% (33/71)
10	33% (16/49)	100% (12/12)	11% (4/37)	35% (19/54)
15	24% (9/37)	89% (8/9)	4% (1/28)	25% (8/32)
20	26% (7/27)	88% (7/8)	0% (0/19)	23% (6/26)

* Survival rates in patients with low-grade astrocytoma, according to the therapy received.
† Includes two patients lost to follow-up and considered dead of disease.
Source: From Leibel et al.,[27] with permission.

a role in the incompletely resected low-grade astrocytoma. Although the optimum dose has not been fully determined, most radiation oncologists would recommend treating these patients with a dose of 5000 to 5500 cGy.

The benefits of postoperative irradiation may not be identified in short-term survival rates. A survival advantage is more likely to appear in survival rates after several years. In particular, patients who receive postoperative irradiation do seem to have an improved survival rate at the 5-, 10-, and 20-year marks.

Oligodendrogliomas

These rare tumors of glial cell origin are similar in many ways to the gliomas which have already been discussed. In particular, complete surgical resection is often difficult, and there are good data in the literature documenting the effectiveness of postoperative irradiation in prolonging survival and improving the quality of the patient's life. As for many CNS neoplasms, the advent of CT scanning has improved survival rates. A recent meta-analysis confirmed that a survival advantage exists in patients receiving surgery and radiation therapy as compared to patients treated with surgery alone.[46]

The various treatment modalities utilized in a group of 54 patients have been reported.[6] Follow-up data on 35 of these patients were available for 5-year survival analysis. Eleven patients received surgery only and 24 received postoperative irradiation. The 5-year survival rate for the surgery group was 82 percent, and for the radiotherapy group, 100 percent. Tumor doses varied from 5300 to 7000 cGy given over a total elapsed time of 49 to 66 days. The surgical procedure included complete tumor excision combined with electroencephalography to indicate if any abnormal areas of tissue remained. If an abnormal corticogram was noted, an additional attempt was made to remove the remaining neoplastic tissue. Thus, the patients had fairly radical surgical excision, but in spite of this the group receiving postoperative irradiation responded more favorably.

Similar data are available in a retrospective review of 37 patients with a histologically confirmed diagnosis of oligodendroglioma.[45] The neurosurgeon made an attempt in each case to remove as much of the tumor as possible. However, complete tumor excision was not thought to have been achieved in any of these patients. Since five patients died within 2 weeks of their operation, they were excluded from the analysis. The 32 remaining patients were divided equally between those who received postoperative irradiation and those who did not. One patient in each group was lost to follow-up. The 5- and 10-year survival rates for the patients who underwent surgical resection only were 31 and 25 percent, respectively. Those patients who received postoperative irradiation had a 5-year survival rate of 85 percent and a 10-year survival rate of 55 percent. Analysis revealed that the difference between the 5-year survival rates was statistically significant.

Since complete tumor excision is very difficult in the patient with an oligodendroglioma, postoperative irradiation is indicated. The recommended tumor dose ranges from 5000 to 6000 cGy. Some radiation oncologists recommend whole brain irradiation, while others think that irradiation to the tumor-bearing volume, with adequate margins, is sufficient. The actual technique of irradiation may vary depending on the location and size of the tumor. Although there are no data relating to the optimum time over which irradiation should be given, it is recommended that treatments be initiated when the patient has recovered from surgery sufficiently and the surgical incision site has healed satisfactorily.

Metastatic Disease

The value of radiotherapy in the treatment of tumors metastatic to the brain has been known for many years. There have been numerous studies documenting the effectiveness of radiotherapy in providing symptomatic improvement in these patients, and a number of different fractionation schemes have been used. Some authors report that a prolonged course of treatment with high doses is the most effective both in symptomatic control of the disease and in prolongation of survival. Others think that a more rapid fractionation scheme is just as effective.

The most extensive clinical trials of irradiation in the treatment of brain metastases were conducted by the Radiation Therapy Oncology Group (RTOG).[26] In the first trial, different doses of whole brain irradiation were delivered with different fractionation schedules. There was also a treatment arm which utilized a single high dose of irradiation to the whole brain. Patient assessment was done on the basis of improvement in the patient's neurological status and overall condition. Only 12 percent of the total patient population in this study had undergone a prior surgical procedure. This group included those patients who had gross removal of the tumor as well as those who underwent biopsy only.

The dose of whole brain irradiation varied from 1000 cGy in a single treatment (optional in this study) to 4000 cGy in 4 weeks given at 200 cGy per day; patients could be treated with 4000 cGy in 3 weeks, 3000 cGy in 3 weeks, or 3000 cGy in 2 weeks. At the completion of the study, the most favorable treatment arms were found to be those in which 4000 cGy were given in 3 weeks and 3000 cGy were given in 2 weeks. No significant difference existed between these two arms in terms of patients' general performance or neurological function. Thus, 3000 cGy given to the whole brain in 2 weeks (300 cGy per fraction) seems to be an optimum dosage schedule. This is not only as effective as the higher-dose treatment, but it also allows the patient to be treated over a shorter time interval and thus could be a factor in improving the quality of the patient's life.

Although the use of corticosteroids was not a controlled factor in the RTOG study, it was considered in the analysis of the results. As a general rule, the patients who had more significant symptoms were given corticosteroids. These patients had a more rapid improvement in their neurological function than did patients who did not receive corticosteroids. However, this improvement was not noted after the fourth week. The patients who received steroids did not have an improved median survival time. Thus, it seems that steroids are effective in alleviating the initial symptoms, but it appears that they have no significant antitumor effect. However, they are useful when used in combination with radiotherapy. It is interesting to note that in 40 percent of the patients analyzed, their ultimate deaths did not appear to be related to the brain metastases.

In another prospective randomized trial, a dose of 3000 cGy given in 2 weeks was compared to a dose of 1000 cGy in a single fraction.[18] All patients received whole brain irradiation with two parallel opposed fields. The dose was calculated at the midline. Of the 101 patients eligible for analysis, there was no significant difference in median survival time between the two groups. A slightly higher percentage of patients in the single-dose group had acute complications of nausea, vomiting, headache, or increased neurological deficit (40 percent, vs. 27 percent in the fractionated group). Overall, there was no significant difference in frequency of response, degree of response, or complication rate. Although overall survival rates did not differ significantly between the two groups, the curve delineating probability of survival did appear to slightly favor the group receiving 3000 cGy in 10 fractions.

The patient with a solitary metastatic deposit poses an additional therapeutic challenge. Certain tumors with a potentially long course do have a propensity for solitary metastatic lesions, and patients with these tumors are sometimes treated with a surgical approach. In particular, malignant melanoma and carcinomas of the colon and uterus sometimes present with solitary metastases and can be managed surgically. In other situations, surgery is the initial treatment because the metastasis may be the only known manifestation of disease before the primary lesion has been found. In cases where a solitary metastatic deposit has been removed surgically, many radiation oncologists would recommend a course of whole brain irradiation following the surgical procedure in order to decrease the incidence of clinical manifestations from micrometastases which may already have been present in other areas of the brain. Depending on the operative findings, a boost to the tumor bed may also be considered.

It is sometimes of beneficial to retreat the patient who has previously undergone a course of external beam irradiation for cerebral metastases.[8] In general, the results of reirradiation are not as favorable as those of the initial treatment. However, if the patient has had a relatively long interval of symptomatic improvement after the initial course of treatments, it may be of benefit to attempt another trial of whole brain irradiation. The patients are sometimes treated with slightly lower doses and over a slightly longer period of time in order to decrease the chance of radiation complications in the reirradiated brain.

Meningeal Carcinomatosis

Malignant disease involving the meninges is a perplexing and difficult problem. Numerous treatment techniques for meningeal carcinomatosis have been used, and the results of treatment have generally been less than encouraging. Despite appropriate treatment, meningeal carcinomatosis often progresses rapidly and results in death of the patient within a fairly short period.

CNS irradiation has been utilized in the treatment of this disorder with varying success. It was probably first used in the treatment of meningeal leukemia. (The meninges were frequently found to be a site of relapse in patients who otherwise had no evidence of disease.) The most encouraging results in the treatment of meningeal carcinomatosis in patients with solid tumors appeared in a group with carcinoma of the breast.[54] In this study, 40 patients with meningeal carcinomatosis underwent treatment with whole brain irradiation combined with intrathecal and intraventricular methotrexate with citrovorum factor rescue. The patients were diagnosed as having meningeal involvement on the basis of the presence of malignant cells in the CSF and the absence of mass lesions on either radionuclide brain scans or CT. Patients received whole brain irradiation consisting of 3000 cGy given over a 2-week period. They also received 16 mg of dexamethasone per day and continued with dexamethasone for 1 week after the completion of treatment. Patients also received intrathecal methotrexate, 20 mg, with citrovorum factor rescue. At the completion of whole brain irradiation, an Ommaya reservoir was inserted for the instillation of intraventricular methotrexate. This was done in 36 of the 40 patients who were in systemic remission or who were thought likely to have a survival time of greater than 8 weeks. In patients who had a complete response, malignant cells disappeared from the CSF. In addition, the CSF protein, glucose, and carcinoembryonic antigen (CEA) levels returned to normal. Patients also had clinical improvement of their neurological function. Patients defined as having a partial response had complete disappearance of tumor cells from the CSF, but there was not complete normalization of CSF or significant improvement in the patients' functional status. Twenty-six of the 40 patients had complete responses and 1 had a partial response. Thus, the overall response rate was an encouraging 67 percent. In patients who responded, the survival time was 23 weeks. This compared favorably to a median survival time of 4 weeks in the patients who did not respond. There did not appear to be a relationship between a patient's response and the initial degree of neurological dysfunction. However, patients who had neurological symptoms for more than 4 weeks were found to have a shorter median survival time (7 weeks) and a lower response rate (47 percent) than those patients who had neurological symptoms for less than 4 weeks; the latter group had response rates greater than 75 percent and survival times longer than 18 weeks.

Comparable results have been obtained in patients with carcinomatous meningitis from primary malignancies other than breast carcinoma.[43] In this study, an Ommaya reservoir was used to treat 67 patients. Thirty of these patients had solid tumors, seven had lymphoma, and 30 had leukemia. Fifty-eight percent of the patients with solid tumors improved, while 100 percent of the leukemic patients improved from a clinical standpoint, and ninety percent of the leukemic patients improved from the standpoint of normalization of CSF. It is interesting that in the solid tumor group, patients with breast carcinoma and patients with lymphoma showed the greatest amounts of improvement. All but four of the patients with solid tumors received CNS irradiation, and half of the patients with leukemia received this treatment. Thus, comparable response rates can be obtained in patients who have neoplasms other than carcinoma of the breast.

The actual benefit of whole brain irradiation in patients with meningeal carcinomatosis is difficult to assess, since the vast majority of patients were treated with a combination of radiotherapy and chemotherapy. Because the approach to management of meningeal carcinomatosis has not been consistent in most centers and early diagnosis has been difficult, it has been difficult to assess the actual role of the specific modalities used in treating this disorder. However, there are now reports in the literature that show some encouraging results, and whole brain irradiation with a dose of approximately 3000 cGy in 10 to 12 fractions combined with intrathecal and/or intraventricular chemotherapy can lead to improved control of this condition.

Meningiomas

The meningiomas are typically considered to be rather slow-growing, benign lesions which are well circumscribed and can often be completely resected. Recurrence after complete tumor removal has been reported and is found to occur in 10 to 15 percent of cases. The recurrence rate after incomplete resection is significantly higher.[53]

The role of radiotherapy in the treatment of meningiomas, primarily to prevent recurrence, is controversial, although many studies do indicate a beneficial effect in subtotally resected meningiomas.[23] In 1946, McWhirter indicated that roughly 43 percent of meningiomas are radiosensitive.[31] Since these tumors tend to be slow-growing, patients generally have a long survival time and therefore survival time per se may not be an accurate indication of the value of postoperative irradiation. This problem was circumvented in a report from King et al., who studied the interval between initial treatment and subsequent recurrence (the recurrence interval).[23] Forty-eight of the 79 patients studied were treated with surgery and radiotherapy. Twenty-five patients had surgery alone and 6 received radiotherapy alone. The tumors were histologically divided into meningiomas, angioblastic meningiomas, and malignant or sarcomatous meningiomas. The mean interval to recurrence for all meningiomas was analyzed; those treated with surgery alone had a recurrence interval of 44.5 months and those treated with a combination of surgery and radiotherapy had a recurrence interval of 54.5 months. The difference was not statistically significant. However, when the angioblastic meningiomas were analyzed separately, the average recurrence interval after surgery alone was 39 months as compared to 72 months after treatment with the combined approach. Patients with sarcomatous meningiomas had a 10-month average recurrence interval following surgery alone and an 83-month recurrence interval following surgery and radiotherapy. Thus, the authors suggest that these two subtypes of meningioma do respond to radiotherapy and that radiotherapy is indicated in treating these lesions. However, there were fairly small numbers of patients in both of the histologic subtypes. These authors did not find radiotherapy alone to be of benefit as the primary mode of treatment.

Another study involving a fairly large number of patients indicated that histologic subtypes did not have a bearing on the response of meningiomas to irradiation.[52] In this study, 188 patients were treated by surgery with or without irradiation. If the patients were thought to have had complete removal of their tumors, no further treatment was given. Forty-four percent of the patients were thought to have had total surgical removal; there was no recurrence in this group of patients. Fifty-eight of the remaining 104 patients who had subtotal removal of tumor did not receive postoperative irradiation. In this patient group the recurrence rate was 74 percent. Ninety-four patients had subtotal resection and had immediate postoperative irradiation. The recurrence rate in this group was 29 percent. There was an additional group of 12 patients who had tumors which were initially not thought to be totally resectable. These patients underwent either limited partial resection or biopsy only, followed by radiotherapy. Patients in this group were scheduled for reoperation about 6 months after completion of the radiation therapy. In this group, eight patients underwent total resection following the course of radiotherapy. Seven of these patients were alive and well with no recurrence at an interval of between 4 and 13 years after surgery.

A more recent study provides additional evidence for the benefits of radiation therapy in subtotally resected meningiomas. Patients with subtotally resected tumors who did not receive postoperative radiotherapy had a progression-free survival rate of 48 percent at 8 years whereas the 17 patients whose tumors were irradiated had a progression-free survival rate of 88 percent. In the group of patients who had an incomplete resection at the time of first recurrence, 11 percent of the surgery-only group were progression free, as compared to 78 percent in the group receiving radiation therapy postoperatively (Fig. 183-2).[32]

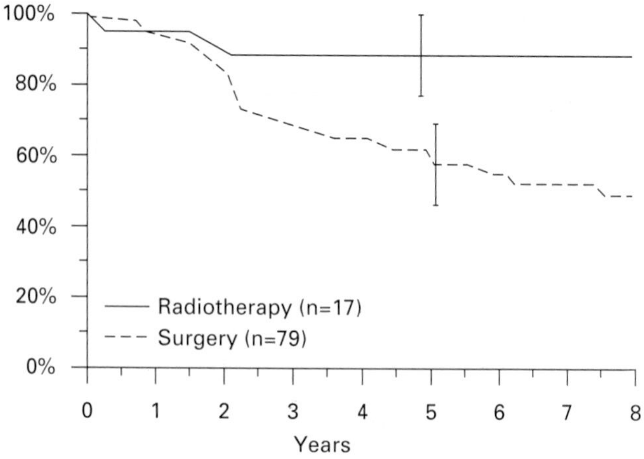

(*A*)

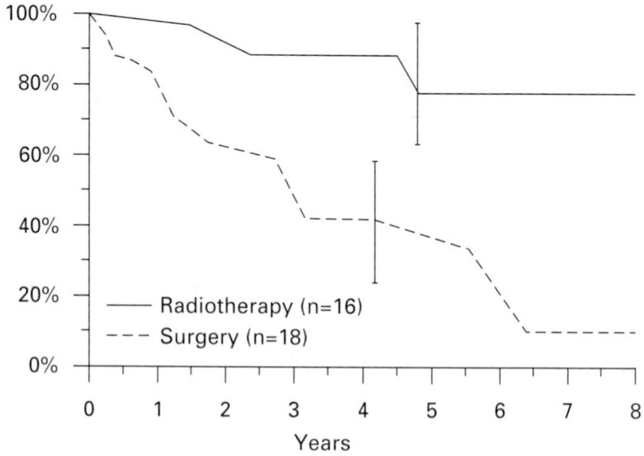

(*B*)

Figure 183-2 Progression-free survival rates in patients with subtotally resected meningioma with or without postoperative irradiation. *A*. After primary subtotal excision. *B*. After first salvage subtotal excision. (From Miralbell et al.,[32] with permission.)

It would thus appear that complete surgical removal is the preferred treatment in the patient with a meningioma. However, in those cases where the neoplasm cannot be completely resected, radiotherapy may well be effective in either totally preventing or delaying the onset of recurrence. There is some controversy as to whether the histologic subtype of the meningioma is related to its sensitivity to irradiation. There has been some indication that the meningiomas which are very vascular may respond favorably to irradiation, and that the resectability of these tumors may be improved with a course of preoperative radiotherapy. The patient with a meningioma should be treated through fields which encompass the known area of disease, with adequate margins around the primary lesion. High-energy equipment should be utilized in the vast majority of cases. The dose should be 5000 to 5500 cGy at a rate of 170 to 200 cGy/day. If a recurrent meningioma which has not been previously irradiated is not amenable to further surgical resection, radiotherapy may play a very effective role in controlling this tumor for a prolonged period.

Pineal Tumors

Neoplasms in this region are rather uncommon. MRI, CT, and microneurosurgical techniques have greatly facilitated the diagnosis and management of these neoplasms. However, because of their anatomic location, surgical excision is often not possible and radiotherapy plays a primary role in their management. There continue to be questions regarding the optimum field size and dose to use in these tumors, and the question of neuraxis irradiation for the germinomas occurring in this region remains to be clearly answered. In cases where imaging studies document spinal metastases, or if the CSF cytology is positive, craniospinal irradiation is indicated.

For those patients in whom neuraxis irradiation is not deemed necessary, the question still remains as to what are the optimum field size and dose for tumor control. In one study, 22 patients with a clinical diagnosis of tumor in the pineal region were treated with radiotherapy.[40] The patients were thought to have pineal-region tumors when they presented with a combination of increased intracranial pressure and altered pupillary function and upward-gaze paralysis. Air studies and CT scans were obtained and demonstrated a defect in the posterior third ventricle, with associated hydrocephalus. Patients with ectopic tumors generally had diabetes insipidus, visual disturbances, and some amount of hypopituitarism. Radiologic studies showed a defect in the anterior third ventricle, with or without hydrocephalus. These 22 patients received irradiation with megavoltage equipment. Patients received a daily dose of 150 to 180 cGy given 5 times per week. Twelve patients received whole brain irradiation and 10 received less than whole brain treatment. Five of these patients were treated with fields which included the entire ventricular system, and the other five patients had smaller portals which were limited to the primary tumor with an adequate margin.

A review of the results of treatment indicated that the patients who received whole brain irradiation or who received maximum doses greater than 5000 cGy had a longer survival time than did those patients who received lower doses or less extensive treatment portals. Three of five patients who were treated with whole brain irradiation had no evidence of disease 10 years after diagnosis, whereas only one of eight patients who were treated with partial brain fields was alive at 10 years.

The authors included a review of the literature in an attempt to further document the effectiveness of irradiation. Adequate radiotherapy data were available for 67 patients. The favorable prognosis in this tumor is reflected by the fact that the median survival time in this patient population was 10 years. Sixty-two percent of the patients had no evidence of disease at 5 years, and 60 percent of all failures had occurred by 4 years after diagnosis. Patients who were treated with fields that included the whole brain had better survival rates than did those patients who received less than whole brain treatment. The difference between those patients receiving whole brain irradiation and those receiving partial brain treatment was maintained for up to 10 years from the date of diagnosis. In the patient group that received treatment with fields that included the entire ventricular system, the survival rate was better for 3 years as compared to that in patients who received treatment to smaller portals. The failure rates were comparable for patients with ectopic tumors and those with pineal-area tumors. There was no difference in failure rates between the patients who were under 12 years old and those who were over 12 years old at diagnosis.

Since the surgical procedure in these patients may be limited to a shunting procedure to relieve intracranial pressure, radiotherapy remains the primary treatment modality. It appears that doses in excess of 5000 cGy given at conventional fractionation are indicated, and large treatment fields seem to improve the survival. As a minimum, patients should receive treatment to the entire ventricular system, and many radiation oncologists would advocate whole brain irradiation. This can be adequately achieved with opposing bilateral fields. In some institutions, the whole brain is treated with a moderate dose, and then the fields are reduced to bring the dose to the area of tumor volume up to the 5000- to 5500-cGy level. Some authorities have suggested that a reduction in total dose by approximately 20 percent should be considered in children who are under 3 years of age. There is evidence that the cerebral tissue of young children is more sensitive to the damaging effects of irradiation than that of older patients.

The question of neuraxis irradiation is a controversial one. Certainly there are documented instances of spinal cord seeding from primary tumors of this type, and after seeding has occurred, the disease is difficult to control with irradiation. If malignant cells are found in the CSF, neuraxis irradiation is indicated. The recommended dose to the spinal cord may vary depending on the clinical, radiographic, and pathologic findings. There have been some instances where a patient has been found to have an elevated alpha-fetoprotein level or an elevated human chorionic gonadotropin level in the CSF studies. The question of whether to treat the neuraxis in the face of positive markers and in the absence of malignant cells is also controversial. The benefit of neuraxis irradiation in patients with positive markers in the CSF has yet to be proven. In the young child, radiotherapy to the neuraxis can result in significant long-term sequelae. These include the arrest of bone growth, as well as the possibility of long-term growth abnormalities in the soft tissues and vasculature within the irradiated field. If the physician thinks that inclusion of the entire subarachnoid space is necessary, the treatment field must be extended to the level of S2. Treatment to this inferior border could result in radiation damage to the gonads as well.

In a study by the Childrens Cancer Study Group, the incidence of spinal cord metastases was 8 percent (9 of 118 patients).[51] Two of these nine patients had primary recurrences as well. None of the patients received spinal irradiation. It was not thought that the 8 percent incidence of metastasis warranted prophylactic neuraxis irradiation. It is interesting to note, however, that of the patients who had biopsy-proven germinomas, 14 percent developed spinal metastases, in contrast to a 1.7 percent incidence of metastases in the group that did not receive biopsies.

Cerebellar Astrocytomas

Cerebellar astrocytomas are found in the pediatric age group in the vast majority of cases. These lesions generally have a good prognosis, possibly because the symptoms occur early in neoplasms in this location. In addition, these tumors are commonly low-grade and cystic, and tend to be relatively noninvasive. These characteristics permit complete surgical removal of the lesion in the majority of patients. These tumors, like the low-grade astrocytomas of the optic nerve, carry a favorable prognosis.

Because of the characteristics of these tumors, there is some controversy as to the specific role of radiotherapy in their management. If the tumor is completely removed, 5-year survival rates as high as 80 percent or better are reported. One study included 14

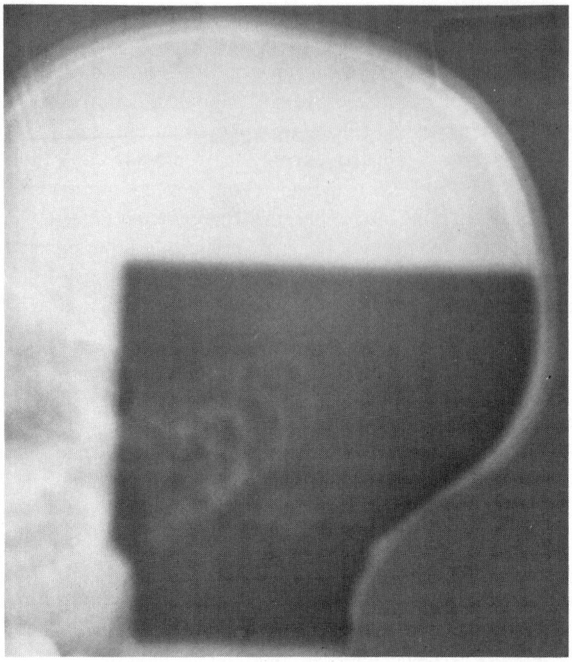

Figure 183-3 Port film indicating the treatment field in a patient with a cerebellar astrocytoma. An individually made Cerrobend block was used to treat the specific area of risk.

patients who received postoperative irradiation for cerebellar astrocytoma.[4] In this series, 12 patients survived from 5 to 22 years. Only one patient was physically impaired and this was because of an unsteady gait.

There seems to be no role for radiotherapy in cases where the lesion has been completely excised. However, radiotherapy is indicated if the tumor has been incompletely excised. Treatment can be delivered either through bilateral opposed fields or through three fields consisting of a posterior field in conjunction with two lateral fields. The dose should be in the range of 5500 cGy, with some consideration for reduction of the total dosage if the patient is under 2 years of age. The solid astrocytoma that is subtotally removed is more likely to recur than a solid tumor that is totally removed or a cystic tumor that is subtotally removed. Although long-term radiation-induced complications in these patients have been difficult to document, utilization of small fields which adequately encompass the tumor volume, along with appropriate fractionation schemes, should reduce treatment-related morbidity (Fig. 183-3).

Medulloblastomas

This relatively uncommon neoplasm, which primarily affects children, is routinely treated with a combination of surgical resection and postoperative irradiation. It has long been known that surgery alone is ineffective in the management of these patients, resulting in a survival time which averages from 6 to 12 months. Radiation therapy has been used in the management of these neoplasms for over 60 years.[10,34] Many studies have documented the vital role of irradiation in managing these neoplasms.

Appropriate irradiation includes treatment to the entire craniospinal axis. It has been known for approximately 40 years that radiotherapy to this volume is necessary, and recent data indicate that survival can be improved in this patient population if postoperative irradiation is administered to the appropriate fields and in appropriate doses. A large study looked retrospectively at 122 patients with histologic confirmation of medulloblastoma who received radiotherapy postoperatively.[2] Since the review covered 21 years, various doses and treatment techniques were utilized, but some interesting conclusions can be drawn. In this patient population, 36 percent were thought to have had macroscopically complete tumor resection, while 54 percent had subtotal removal, and 10 percent had biopsy only. Most of the patients were treated with cobalt 60, but early in the study, some patients received treatment with kilovoltage irradiation only. In the entire patient group, the median dose to the whole brain was 3500 cGy. The posterior fossa received a boost, and median dose to this region was 5000 cGy. Patients received a median spinal cord dose of 3500 cGy. Survival rates from the date of surgery were 56 percent of the entire group at 5 years and 43 percent at 10 years. The relapse-free rates were 49 and 38 percent, respectively. The amount of tumor resection had a bearing on survival rates in that 64 percent of the patients who had what were thought to be total resections survived 5 years, while 33 percent of those patients who received biopsy only survived 5 years. The survival rate for subtotal resection was 56 percent at 5 years. When the dose of irradiation to the posterior fossa was analyzed, no statistical difference was found in survival rates relative to the dose received. Yet there did seem to be a trend of increasing survival when higher doses were given to the posterior fossa (Fig. 183-4). However, the posterior fossa was the site of first relapse in 46 percent of the patients, and there was a relationship between the dose to the posterior fossa and recurrence in this

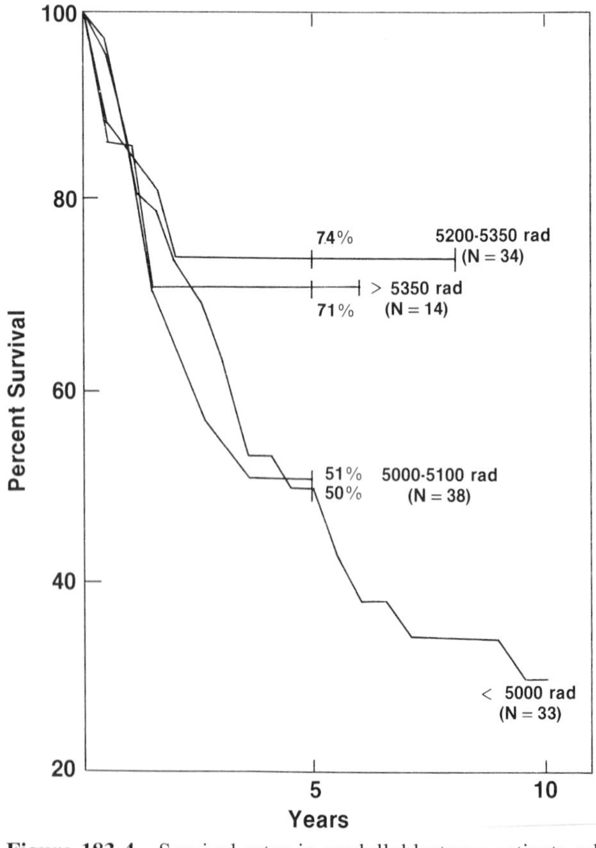

Figure 183-4 Survival rates in medulloblastoma patients relative to the dose of irradiation which was given to the posterior fossa. (From Berry et al.,[2] with permission.)

area. The relapse-free rate was 79 percent in patients who received more than 5350 cGy, 82 percent in those who received between 5200 and 5350 cGy, 74 percent in those who received 5000 to 5100 cGy, and only 42 percent in those who received less than 5000 cGy. There did not appear to be any difference in survival between the patients for whom radiotherapy was initiated within 10 days of surgical treatment and those patients for whom the initiation of treatment was delayed because of postoperative complications.

Further data indicating a relationship between the dose to the posterior fossa and control of the tumor come from a retrospective study involving 33 children under the age of 20.[9] During the later portion of this study, patients received a dose of 4500 cGy to the whole brain, with an additional 1000-cGy boost to the posterior fossa. The spinal cord received 4500 cGy. Treatments were given at 180 cGy per fraction to the brain and 160 cGy per fraction to the spinal cord. In those children who were under 3 years of age, the total dose to each area was decreased by 1000 cGy. In those patients who received posterior fossa doses of 5500 cGy, the local control rate was 86 percent (six of seven patients) while local control was achieved in only 17 percent (two of 12 patients) when the posterior fossa doses were less than 5000 cGy. Although the incidence of recurrence might be highest in the first 2 to 3 years after treatment, two patients in this series had recurrences at 47 and 62 months. A similar correlation of dose and response was noted in the spinal cord. In those patients who received cord doses of 4000 cGy the 5-year control rate was 62 percent (eight of 13 patients), whereas in those who received less than 3500 cGy the 5-year local control rate was 33 percent (two of six patients).

Various techniques have been developed for irradiating the whole brain and spinal cord. In an acceptable technique, the patient is placed in a prone position, with treatment of the brain and upper cervical cord via lateral opposed portals. The spine is treated through a direct posterior field, which can be done in either one or two segments, depending on the length of the patient's spine. In order to avoid a dose overlap between abutting fields, the field junctions are moved at regular intervals during the course of treatment (Fig. 183-5). The posterior fossa can be boosted with an additional dose with lateral fields after the completion of the whole brain irradiation.

Since this patient population tends to be fairly young and the radiotherapy is rather extensive, complications can be significant. These patients receive treatment to at least 20 percent of the functioning marrow, and neutropenia and/or thrombocytopenia can sometimes be a problem. In all patients treated, a moderate depression of the blood counts is expected. If the white blood cell count drops to less than 1000 or the platelet count decreases to significantly below 100,000, some radiation oncologists would consider interrupting treatment until the counts have recovered. Long-range complications include endocrine disturbances caused by irradiation of the hypothalamopituitary axis, impairment of bone growth, and hypoplasia of some of the soft tissue structures which may have been included in the irradiated field. Many radiation oncologists think that a lower dose is justified in patients under 3 years of age because of the decreased myelinization present within the CNS of patients in this age range. For children under the age of 3, chemotherapy should be considered, and radiation therapy withheld until the child is older.

It thus appears that patients with medulloblastoma should be treated first with surgical resection of as much tumor as is reasonably possible without causing significant morbidity. This should be followed by external beam megavoltage irradiation to the entire neuraxis. The posterior fossa should receive a boost to a higher dose. This higher dose appears to be effective in decreasing local recurrences. Since the posterior fossa is a common site of initial relapse, by controlling the disease in this area, the physician might decrease the incidence of disease in other areas. If imaging studies demonstrate focal areas of CSF spread, additional radiation therapy to these regions is often recommended. Patient tolerance to irradiation is generally good, but the patient should be monitored closely during the course of treatment with frequent blood counts. The technique used to deliver treatment is extremely important; it is essential to avoid overlapping fields that increase the risk of spinal cord myelitis due to overdosage to a segment of the cord.

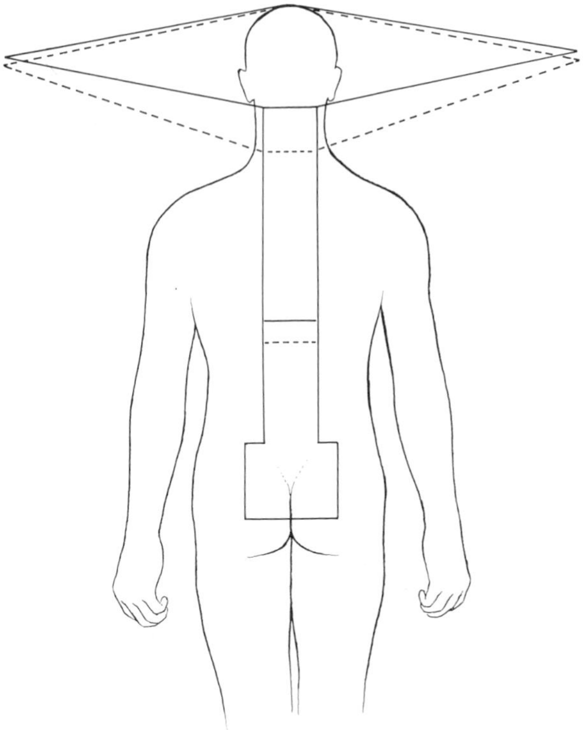

Figure 183-5 Field arrangement utilized in treating the craniospinal axis in patients with medulloblastoma. The brain and upper cervical cord are treated via lateral portals, and the spine is treated posteriorly. Field junctions are moved at regular intervals to avoid overdosing the cord. Solid and dashed lines indicate field arrangements on alternating days.

Brain Stem Gliomas

Brain stem gliomas are often diagnosed on radiologic and clinical grounds, since these tumors are not often surgically accessible. Because of their critical location, the vast majority of these neoplasms have been treated primarily with radiotherapy. Analysis of treatment results relating to brain stem tumors is sometimes difficult because tumors of various anatomic locations are included within this group. Some series include tumors of the thalamus, midbrain, and fourth ventricle, while others are limited to the area of the medulla oblongata and pons. In addition, since biopsy is often not possible, the specific histologic subtype is often not known. These tumors occur in patients of a wide age range, and the results of treatment will vary depending on the ages of the patients in the study group. Certainly those studies which include a large proportion of pediatric patients may report a more favorable prognosis than do studies dealing only with adults.

One retrospective review reported the results of radiotherapy in treating patients with primary brain stem tumors.[22] Approximately half of these patients were under 20 years of age. In 45 patients the primary lesion was located in the pons, in 11 in the medulla oblongata, and in 18 the exact location was not known. Histologically, 54 percent of the patients had low-grade astrocytomas and 38 percent had higher-grade gliomas.

The patients were treated with megavoltage equipment, using fields to the posterior fossa and upper cervical cord. Of the 63 patients who received full courses of radiotherapy, 44 received doses of over 5000 cGy. The survival rate for those patients who received over 5000 cGy was better, and all of the survivors of 5 years or more received doses of at least 5000 cGy. There was a correlation between survival rate and response to treatment. Those patients who were poor responders had a poor survival rate, while the long-term survivors all exhibited a good initial response to the radiotherapy.

External beam irradiation remains the mainstay of treatment in patients with brain stem gliomas. Localized fields that include the posterior fossa and upper cervical cord are generally recommended. The dose should be in the range of 5000 to 6000 cGy, at a daily dose rate of between 160 and 200 cGy per fraction. Various field arrangements have been used in treating these patients, including bilateral opposed fields as well as rotational and three-field techniques. A clear-cut advantage of one treatment plan over another has not been demonstrated. In the younger patient, the physician should consider decreasing the total dose because some think that the developing nervous system in children under the age of 3 is more sensitive to the damaging effects of irradiation.

The dose-response relationship in pediatric brain stem gliomas has also been demonstrated in a more recent study. The most important predictor of survival was the response to initial radiotherapy. Higher doses of radiation seem to increase the response rate, but normal tissue tolerance is the limiting factor. Hyperfractionated radiation has not been clearly shown to provide improved disease control in these neoplasms.[17]

Ependymomas

Neoplasms of ependymal cell origin are relatively rare. Because of this, it has not been possible to look at the role of radiotherapy in a prospective fashion. However, there are a number of retrospective reports which indicate a clear role for radiotherapy in treating these neoplasms.

In one study, the role of radiotherapy was analyzed in 31 patients who survived 2 months after subtotal surgical removal of ependymomas.[36] Twenty-eight of these patients received radiotherapy. Twenty-five received postoperative irradiation, and three were treated preoperatively. Ten patients either received radiation doses of less than 3500 cGy or did not receive any irradiation at all. Only one of these 10 patients was a 5-year survivor. In the patient group receiving 4500 cGy or more, 13 of 15 were 5-year survivors. The difference between the 5-year survival rates of patients receiving less than 3500 cGy and those receiving more than 4500 cGy was statistically significant. The overall 5-year survival rate in the entire patient population was 40 percent. The 5-year survival rate was 56 percent for those patients who survived surgery and 87 percent for the patients who were thought to have adequate radiotherapy, consisting of a dose of at least 4500 cGy.

The same study addressed the question of spinal seeding within the subarachnoid space. This is a controversial subject, and there have been conflicting data regarding the need for prophylactic irradiation to the entire neuraxis. The authors of this study found that the incidence of clinically significant subarachnoid seeding was very low, and it was thought that irradiation of the cerebrospinal axis was not indicated. Although some autopsy studies have indicated that the incidence of microscopic subarachnoid seeding is somewhat higher, the low incidence of clinically significant subarachnoid seeding would seem to justify this treatment approach. In some instances, however, neuraxis irradiation may be indicated. In those patients who have very poorly differentiated ependymoma involving the posterior fossa, the incidence of spinal cord seeding might be significantly higher, and neuraxis irradiation should be seriously considered in these situations. As in many other CNS neoplasms, the grade of the primary tumor has an impact on survival, with higher grade neoplasms yielding a poorer prognosis.[20]

The site of origin of the ependymoma within the CNS may have a direct influence on the clinical characteristics of the tumor.[29] In a series of 61 patients with ependymomas located in various areas within the CNS, the subgroup of patients with infratentorial lesions was noted to have improved local control with increasing biologically effective doses of irradiation.[29] No such correlation could be demonstrated in patients with tumors in other locations. The incidence of spinal cord seeding was found to be 11 percent in pathologic specimens, but it was clinically evident in only 4 percent of these patients. Of the five patients who had pathologically documented spinal metastases, four had infratentorial primary tumors and in one the lesion was located supratentorially. Eight patients in this study had also received intrathecal gold 198 as a part of their therapy. Three of these eight patients developed a radiation myelopathy and/or cauda equina syndrome, from 3.5 to 17 years after treatment.

On the basis of a number of retrospective analyses, it appears that postoperative irradiation has a clear-cut role in the treatment of ependymomas. The actual treatment approach will vary depending on the location and histology of the tumor. In general, the more distally located lesions have more favorable prognoses. That is, lesions of the cauda equina have the most favorable prognosis, whereas supratentorial lesions have the least favorable prognosis. Tumors of the infratentorium and spinal cord have an intermediate prognosis.

The optimum treatment for most ependymomas is surgical removal of as much tumor as is possible without inducing significant morbidity, followed by radiotherapy. The radiotherapy should be given with a generous margin around the primary tumor. Doses in the range of 5000 to 5500 cGy at conventional fractionation are appropriate. In some cases, the whole brain can be treated with 4500 to 5000 cGy, followed by an additional 500 cGy to a reduced volume encompassing the primary lesion. Parallel opposed portals are sufficient for most patients. Whole neuraxis irradiation should be considered in those patients who have cytologic or radiologic evidence of spinal cord seeding. The dose to the spinal cord should be in the range of 3000 to 3500 cGy at conventional fractionation. This dose is well tolerated and carries a minimal risk of myelopathy.

Pituitary Tumors

Most tumors of the pituitary are histologically benign. However, they are often malignant in their behavior due to their critical ana-

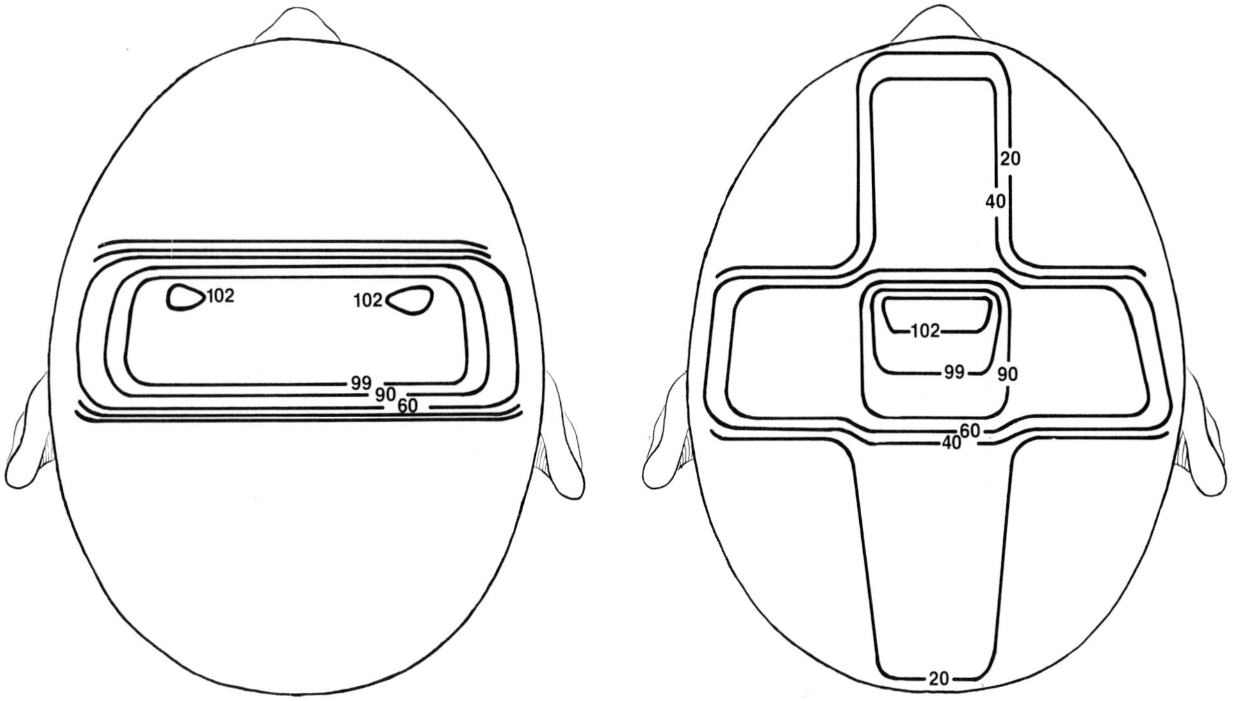

(*A*) (*B*)

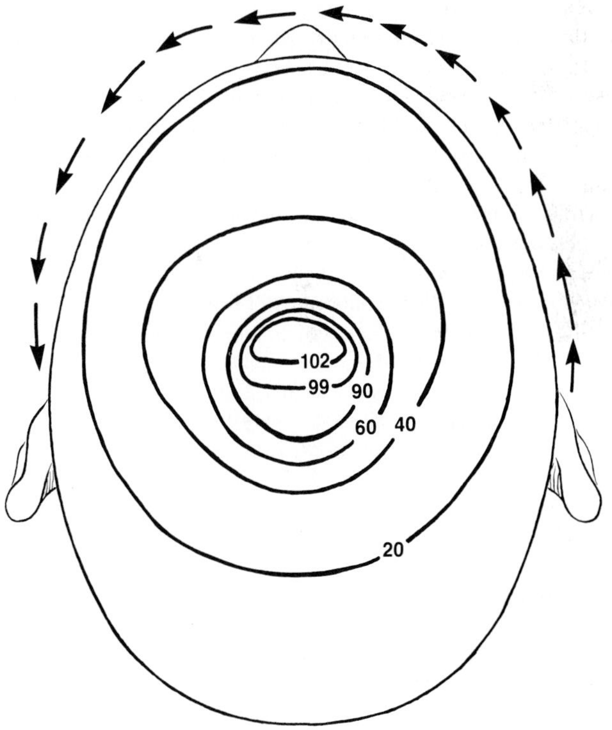

(*C*)

Figure 183-6 Isodose distributions for various techniques used in the treatment of pituitary tumors. *A.* Bilateral opposed portals. *B.* Three-field technique utilizing two lateral ports and a single anterior port. *C.* Arc rotational therapy.

tomic location. It has been reported that normal pituitary tissue is relatively resistant to the effects of ionizing irradiation, and that doses in the usual therapeutic range do not produce significant signs of hypopituitarism.[5] However, it may take many years for the pituitary gland to display any evidence of damage induced by irradiation, and long-term endocrinologic follow-up of these patients is often lacking.

External beam irradiation has long been recognized as an effective therapeutic modality in the treatment of pituitary adenomas. A number of different techniques have been utilized in treating these lesions, including the use of two parallel opposed fields, three-field techniques, and arc rotational therapy (Fig. 183-6). These lesions require moderate doses for control, generally in the range of 4500 to 5000 cGy at conventional fractionation (180 to 200 cGy/day). It has been clearly shown that the combination of surgery followed by postoperative irradiation is effective in controlling the chromophobe adenomas. In a study involving 107 patients, Sheline analyzed the determinant control rate in patients treated with surgery alone compared with those who received both surgery and radiotherapy.[44] At 5 years, the control rate with surgery only was 38 percent (9 of 24 patients) versus a control rate of 96 percent (65 of 68 patients) in the group which received surgery plus postoperative irradiation. At 10 years, the control rates were 14 and 83 percent, respectively.

External beam irradiation has also been shown to be a very effective technique for treating acromegaly.[13] A group of 47 patients with documented acromegaly comprised the study group. The patients received between 4000 and 5000 cGy of external beam irradiation and were followed for up to 10 years. This treatment approach was found to be quite effective, but it should be emphasized that the decline in growth hormone levels took place quite gradually, over 5 to 10 years after completion of treatment. In 81 percent of the patients, plasma growth hormone values were less than 10 ng/ml. As the growth hormone level declined, the objective changes induced by growth hormone (GH) excess improved as well. Although the decline was gradual, conventional irradiation was found to produce the same fall in the GH level as do other forms of treatment for acromegaly. (The incidence of hypopituitarism was also noted to increase throughout the follow-up period.) The authors therefore thought that conventional external beam irradiation had fewer serious side effects than do the surgical techniques which are normally employed for the treatment of acromegaly.

Surgical removal of prolactinomas has been found to be an effective method of reducing an elevated prolactin level to normal. In those patients who have persistently elevated prolactin levels postoperatively, radiotherapy can be effective in further reducing the serum level.[24] In addition, it has been shown that radiotherapy alone can result in normalization of the serum prolactin level.[12] A group of six women with evidence of prolactin-secreting pituitary adenomas were treated with a course of external beam irradiation consisting of 5000 cGy given over 5.5 weeks. Half of these patients had normalization of their serum prolactin levels and two of the patients had normal pregnancies. In the third patient, a normal menstrual cycle was re-established. The fall in the prolactin level was fairly rapid, with five of the six patients having a substantial reduction in the serum prolactin level after a brief period. It is important to realize that after radiotherapy these patients were given maintenance bromocriptine treatments. In the remaining three patients, radiotherapy did not appear to have beneficial effects. All six of the patients in this study had been previously treated with various medications, and the drugs had not been effective in controlling their prolactin-secreting tumors.

In 1932, Dr. Harvey Cushing introduced the use of x-irradiation for a syndrome which he attributed to a basophilic adenoma. Since that time, a number of investigators have documented the beneficial effects of radiotherapy in treating Cushing's disease. As diagnosis of this disease became more specific and advances were made in radiotherapy, there were a number of treatment plans used in the management of this disease. An attempt to establish some correlation between time-dose factors and control of the primary lesion was made in a study of 45 patients with Cushing's disease.[1] This study was limited to patients with hypercortisolism which was caused by excessive pituitary ACTH secretion. These patients were treated with megavoltage equipment, using either a three-field technique (one anterior and two lateral portals), parallel opposed portals, or rotational therapy. Three patients were treated with five to seven isocentric stationary fields. Patients were considered to have been cured of their disease if urinary hydrocortisone excretion was less than 7 mg/g creatinine and the plasma hydrocortisone level was either normal or subnormal. In 39 patients, follow-up observations of from 2 to 15 years were available. Twenty-five percent of the patients were considered cured. An additional 28 percent were found to have improved to the point that they either required aminoglutethimide or no further therapy. Nineteen patients failed and subsequently underwent adrenalectomy or hypophysectomy. Complications developed in three patients (necrosis of the brain stem in one, progressive blindness in another, and blindness of one eye in the third patient).

When the time-dose factors were reviewed, it was found that treatment with less than 4000 cGy was not satisfactory. At doses between 4500 and 5000 cGy the maximum benefits of radiotherapy were noted. It appears that the complication rate increased as the dose exceeded 4500 cGy. There were no clear relationships between the field size or the technique used and the development of complications. In particular, patients who received treatment via opposed lateral fields were not found to have a higher incidence of complications.

Thus, using conventional fractionation and megavoltage equipment and a dose of approximately 4500 cGy in 5 weeks (treating 5 times per week), Cushing's disease can be controlled in approximately 50 percent of the patients. Since the tumor tends to occupy a fairly small volume, small treatment fields can be utilized. It is difficult to assess the advantage of one particular treatment technique over another. Certainly bilateral opposed fields are technically simpler to reproduce, but some radiation oncologists think that the dose distribution is somewhat better when three fields are used. Bilateral opposed fields will result in an increased dose to the temporal lobes, and may increase the likelihood of subsequent temporal lobe necrosis. Other authorities prefer the arc rotational technique. Each technique is effective, and no advantage of one treatment method over another has been demonstrated. An additional technique uses proton beams, and this treatment modality is discussed elsewhere in this text.

Although Cushing's disease is uncommon in childhood, the use of conventional radiotherapy in this patient population has also been studied.[21] Fifteen patients were diagnosed as having Cushing's disease, and all underwent radiotherapy with an 8 MeV linear accelerator, using doses from 3500 to 5000 cGy at a daily fractionation of 150 to 200 cGy. Most of the patients were treated with opposed lateral fields. Within 11 to 18 months after the initiation of irradiation, 12 of the 15 patients were thought to be cured. The three patients who failed subsequently underwent bilateral adrenalectomies. Sexual development was normal in all 15 patients, and growth resumed in 12 of the 15 patients treated. Pituitary irradiation was thought to be a safe and effective therapy for Cushing's disease in the pediatric patient population.

Craniopharyngiomas

These histologically benign tumors are malignant by virtue of their location and their locally invasive characteristics. They can produce considerable morbidity. A significant proportion of patients will eventually succumb to their disease process.

The clinical course of the patient with a craniopharyngioma can vary considerably, depending on the size and characteristics of the tumor. This fact has led to some controversy regarding the optimum management of these neoplasms. Some have advocated a radical surgical approach only, while others think that limited surgical excision followed by postoperative irradiation is the treatment of choice. Most of the reports involving limited surgical procedures followed by irradiation indicate that control rates are quite good and treatment complications are less.

One report analyzed 35 patients with craniopharyngioma who were classified into three separate treatment groups.[28] Nineteen patients had surgery alone and 11 were treated with limited surgery followed by irradiation. Eleven were treated for recurrent disease; four of these were from the group which had originally received surgery only. The minimum follow-up was 3 years in the 35 patients suitable for analysis. Twelve of these patients were older than 18 years and 23 were 18 or younger.

In the group receiving surgery only, three of eight patients who were thought to have had total resection had recurrences. Five of the nine who had partial removal of their tumor had recurrences. Therefore, a 47 percent recurrence rate was noted in these groups. The group receiving both surgery and radiotherapy had a rate of local recurrence of 20 percent (two of 10 patients). It is interesting to note that one of these recurrences occurred in a patient who had received an inadequate dose of radiation (3450 cGy). There were no recurrences in eight patients who had fairly small tumors and to whom adequate doses of postoperative irradiation were given.

In the group of 11 patients who had recurrent disease, 7 received irradiation with or without limited resection and 4 received surgery only. Five patients from the irradiated group were alive and four showed no evidence of disease within the minimum follow-up of 3 years. In contrast, only one patient from the group that received surgery alone remained alive without evidence of recurrence. Only three patients from the reirradiated group were thought to have a good initial result following their retreatment. Overall, the complications of treatment were fewer in the group of patients who received both limited surgical resection and postoperative irradiation.

The findings of this study confirmed other reports which indicated that irradiation after surgical decompression is the treatment of choice for patients with craniopharyngioma. The radiotherapy should be given with megavoltage equipment and using field sizes which correspond to the area of tumor volume, with an adequate margin. Communication between the surgeon and the radiation oncologist is extremely important in localizing the tumor, and radiologic imaging techniques are very helpful as well. The dose to the tumor volume should be between 5000 and 6000 cGy, delivered in 5 treatments per week in fractions of from 160 to 200 cGy. Some have advocated using lateral opposed portals, while others think that a three-field technique using lateral wedged portals and an anterior field is optimum. There have not been any studies which show a significant advantage of one type of field arrangement over another.

Optic Nerve Gliomas

The majority of these tumors are slow-growing astrocytomas, and a number of different therapeutic approaches have been successful in their management. Suggestions for appropriate treatment have included complete excision, inspection and biopsy only, and partial removal followed by radiotherapy. Indeed, there have been cases of long-term control after only incomplete excision. Thus, the optimum management of the optic nerve glioma remains somewhat controversial. Most treatment reports have been retrospective analyses, and have included patients whose gliomas were confined to the optic nerve as well as those whose tumors extended to involve the chiasm or hypothalamus. Certainly those patients with chiasmal and/or hypothalamic involvement have a less favorable prognosis than do those patients with involvement of the optic nerve only.

One analysis involved 18 children with optic nerve gliomas who underwent treatment with external beam irradiation.[11] All of these patients had rather extensive disease in that none of them had neoplasms limited to a single optic nerve. Eight patients were noted to have chiasmal lesions; 10 had neoplasms which involved the hypothalamus and chiasm, and of these 10, six had hydrocephalus as well. Of the entire group of 18 patients, seven had partial resection, seven had biopsy, two had surgical inspection without biopsy, and two had the diagnosis made on neuroradiologic findings. All the patients received treatment with megavoltage equipment, and received doses of 5000 to 6000 cGy. Sixteen of the 18 patients underwent their radiotherapy when the initial diagnosis was made. The other two patients underwent treatment after they developed signs of disease progression. This occurred 1.5 years after the initial diagnosis had been made.

Five-year survival statistics were available for 12 of the 18 patients. In this group, the 5-year survival rate was 83 percent (10 of 12 patients). The 10-year survival rate was 73 percent (eight of 11 patients). Of the five patients with chiasmal lesions, all survived 5 years, and four of the five survived 10 years. The seven patients who had involvement of the hypothalamus or third ventricle had a 5-year survival rate of 71 percent and a 10-year survival rate of 66 percent. Of the total group, 14 of the 18 patients were thought to have improvement or maintenance of their visual status. The remaining four patients had decreased vision after completion of treatment.

The primary goal in treating the optic nerve glioma is to achieve long-range survival. Above this, it is hoped to either preserve or improve the patient's vision. If optic nerve gliomas are asymptomatic, close follow-up without any therapeutic intervention is reasonable. There are certain clinical situations where total surgical removal of the tumor is not possible, i.e., for those tumors that extend to the chiasm or involve the hypothalamus and/or third ventricle. Thus, there is a patient population that would benefit from postoperative irradiation. When there is a question of preserving the patient's vision, a biopsy followed by irradiation may be the most appropriate treatment approach.

A number of different techniques have been used in the treatment of optic nerve gliomas, including bilateral opposed fields, arc rotational therapy, and a three-field technique. The optimum tumor dose should be in the range of 5000 to 6000 cGy at conventional fractionation. Some radiation oncologists have recommended that children under the age of 2 be treated with lower doses, in the range of 4500 cGy, at slightly lower daily dose fractions. For the low-grade gliomas, treatment fields should include the extent of known tumor, with adequate margins. Precise localization of the tumor, using both radiologic and surgical findings, can be extremely important in limiting the total volume of the irradiated field. In those unusual instances where the patient may have a higher-grade glioma, more generous fields should be utilized. In cases where an adult presents with an optic nerve glioma, some radiation oncologists have recommended increasing the tumor dose to the range of 6500 cGy. The efficacy of this higher-dose range has not been shown conclusively.

Chordomas

These rare tumors have traditionally been considered to be radioresistant. There is evidence, however, to indicate that they do respond to irradiation. Because of the difficulty of completely resecting these tumors, radiotherapy is often utilized in their management. The malignancy of these tumors is caused primarily by their locally aggressive nature, high recurrence rate, and critical anatomic location. Although these neoplasms do metastasize, it is the local tissue damage and high recurrence rate that generally lead to the death of the patient.

Although it has been reported that these tumors vary in their sensitivity to irradiation, the consensus is that the chordomas require radical doses for control. The primary limiting factor in treating these tumors is the tolerance of the normal surrounding structures. Recent advances both in image localization of these tumors and in use of high-energy photon and proton beams have resulted in some encouraging results.

The clinical histories of 46 patients with chordoma who were evaluated over a 35-year period were reviewed by Higinbotham et al.[19] Thirty of the patients in this series had chordomas that were of sacral origin. This incidence is somewhat higher than that reported by others, in which approximately 50 percent of the chordomas are located in the sacrococcygeal area. It is interesting as well that in this series 43 percent of the patients had documented metastases. This is significantly higher than the usually described metastatic rate of approximately 15 percent. Eighteen of the thirty cases with sacrococcygeal chordoma underwent radiotherapy. The authors noted that both the symptomatic relief and the objective tumor response increased as the dose of radiation was increased. In the eight cases where an objective response was noted, the minimum tumor dose which produced this response was 3900 cGy. In addition, five other patients were found to have had significant relief of symptoms. The authors thought that a tumor dose of up to 7000 cGy can result in significant benefit for those patients in whom the tumor is incompletely resected.

In an attempt to more clearly define the optimal dosage of radiation required to control these tumors, a scatter diagram of control rates was constructed.[35] The patients were divided into a group whose tumors were destroyed or who were free of regrowth for 5 years or longer and a group whose tumors persisted after treatment or in whom regrowth occurred, usually within 2 years. Tumor doses of less than 4000 cGy were of little benefit in controlling the tumors. Doses of 8000 cGy or more were found to be most likely to be successful. Eight of 11 patients were thought to have successful treatment with doses in this range. An increasing local control rate was seen with increasing doses (Table 183-3). This particular analysis did not consider the size or location of the tumor. Certainly with doses of 7000 cGy and higher, there is a significant risk of damaging normal tissues, and doses in this range make considerations of reirradiation very difficult. The risk of serious radiation sequelae limits the use of these doses to those anatomic regions which are not surrounded by vital structures, in particular the sacrococcygeal area.

Some promising results have been obtained with the use of proton beam irradiation in these tumors.[47] This series of 10 patients included six with chordoma, three with chondrosarcoma, and one with neurofibrosarcoma. The patients were treated with a combination of photons and 160 MeV proton beams. All tumors were located in the base of the skull and/or upper cervical spine region. The proton beam used in treating these patients allowed a higher dose to be given to a very specific area of the tumor volume. Therefore, the patient's tumor was localized very carefully in each case. Overall doses ranged from a dose equivalent to 6500 cGy to as high as 7620 cGy. In all 10 patients, local control was achieved for follow-up periods of up to 6 years. One patient was thought to have a marginal failure because of an error in calculating the actual extent of disease. An additional advantage of the proton beam is that it allows for a fairly rapid falloff of the dose outside of the designated treatment volume, thus sparing much of the surrounding normal tissue.

The relative radioresistance of the chordoma, the increasing risk of complications at higher doses, and frequent presence of critical anatomic structures within the area of the tumor mass make therapeutic considerations in these patients quite difficult. Because of the slow-growing nature of the tumor, the response of the tumor to radiation is often slow. Patients who present with pain or discomfort caused by their tumors may not have achieved much relief of their symptoms at the completion of treatments. However, over the next few weeks or months the patients may notice decreased pain, and an objective response in terms of tumor regression may be noted as well. This regression may continue for several months after the completion of treatment. Although radiation in and of itself has not been shown to be a curative modality in these tumors, it often presents the possibility of substantial palliation and either regression or stabilization of the tumor. Most studies indicate that the most effective treatment approach in these tumors is surgical resection of as much tumor as is reasonably possible, with postoperative irradiation in doses which approach normal tissue tolerance.

Primary Lymphomas of the Brain

A malignant lymphoma originating in the CNS and without systemic manifestations is an uncommon condition which comprises only 1 to 2 percent of all of the extranodal lymphomas. However, with the recent increase in AIDS, as well as the use of immunosuppressive drugs for organ transplantation, the incidence of primary CNS lymphoma is increasing.

Primary CNS lymphoma has traditionally had a poor response to treatment. The median survival in these patients has generally been from 4 to 6 months. These lesions have been called by a number of different names, including reticulum cell sarcoma, microglioma, and reticuloendothelial sarcoma. Pathologic studies have documented that the histologic findings of primary CNS lymphoma are similar to those of malignant lymphomas that originate in the reticuloendothelial system of other organs. More recently, CNS lymphomas have been designated according to the more common terminology utilized for the non-Hodgkin's lymphomas which arise outside the central nervous system.

A report documenting 24 histologically confirmed cases of intracranial lymphoma indicates that there may be a time-dose factor involved in controlling this disease.[39] Twenty-one of these 24 patients primarily had involvement of intra-axial structures, and three were found to have extradural and meningeal involvement. Every patient in the study had surgical exploration. Some patients underwent subtotal tumor removal, while others had only biopsy. Four patients died postoperatively and did not receive radiotherapy. The other 20 patients received postoperative irradiation and 18 were available for evaluation. In this patient group, there were six who received a tumor dose of less than 3000 cGy. The tumor was not controlled locally in any of these patients. The 12 remaining patients received tumor doses in excess of 3000 cGy, and local control was achieved in 50 percent. The authors thought that failure to

TABLE 183-3 Radical Radiotherapy of Chordoma*

Tumor Dose (cGy)	Failure		Significant Palliation		Success	
	Number	Percentage	Number	Percentage	Number	Percentage
To 4000	47	85	5	9	3	6
4001–6000	18	60	6	20	6	20
6001–8000	8	43	5	31	4	26
Over 8000	2		1		8	80

*Dose-response rates in patients receiving radiotherapy for chordoma.
Source: From Pearlman and Friedman,[35] with permission.

control the disease could have been caused by inadequate tumor dose or by failure to recognize the actual extent of disease. In addition, the presence of multiple involved sites within the CNS sometimes led to use of an inadequate field size. Thus, it was concluded that whole brain irradiation would be the most appropriate treatment and that a minimum dose of 3500 cGy delivered with conventional fractionation was indicated. More recently, 5000 cGy has been recommended as the optimum dose for these lesions.[48]

A recent RTOG study utilized treatment to the 6000 cGy level. In this study, patients were treated to a dose of 4000 cGy to the whole brain, and a local boost of 2000 cGy was administered to the area of known disease. Forty-eight percent of the patients were alive at 1 year, and 28 percent at 2 years.[33]

Some patients treated for intracranial disease subsequently develop lymphoma involving the spinal canal. Although this suggests that primary irradiation to the entire neuraxis might be indicated, studies have shown that spinal cord involvement from primary intracranial lymphoma is not a common occurrence, and most radiation oncologists would not recommend neuraxis irradiation. However, in situations where symptoms or radiologic studies indicate that disease involves the spinal canal, the indications for larger fields, possibly including the entire neuraxis, are more clear-cut.

Results of irradiation to the entire neuraxis have been reported.[38] Twelve patients with primary CNS lymphoma were studied. Four patients received neuraxis irradiation consisting of 4000 to 4500 cGy to the whole brain and 3000 to 3300 cGy to the spinal cord. All four patients who received neuraxis irradiation survived for more than 1 year. One patient had no evidence of disease at 3 years, one patient was alive with possible disease at 35 months, and two patients survived for 13 and 16 months. The patients who received whole neuraxis irradiation were thought to have primary lymphoma in an "unfavorable" condition, meaning that the disease was diffuse or multifocal, was located in the vital structures around the brain stem, or had positive CSF cytology.

Even in those patients who do not have a significant prolongation of survival after treatment with irradiation, the symptomatic response to treatment is often good and there is very little morbidity associated with treatment. In most of the reported cases, patients noted an improvement in both neurological symptoms and general physical status. It would thus appear that radiotherapy for primary CNS lymphoma is important not only as a possible modality for prolonging survival, but also for improving the quality of the patient's life.

Spinal Cord Tumors

Primary neoplasms of the spinal cord are relatively rare and there are few published reports involving large series of patients. Thus, the specific role of radiotherapy for the various intramedullary neoplasms is difficult to assess.

A retrospective review of 34 patients who received radiotherapy for primary spinal cord neoplasms indicates that postoperative irradiation is of benefit in many of these patients.[42] The initial diagnoses included 12 patients with ependymoma, seven with astrocytoma, and two with chordoma. Of the 12 patients with ependymoma, four received only biopsies, seven had incomplete resection, and one was thought by the surgeon to have had total resection of the tumor. With a minimum follow-up of 2.5 years, all patients with ependymoma were alive. One patient who was alive 16 years after treatment developed a severe neurological deficit and became paraplegic. Three of the seven patients with astrocytoma had subtotal resections and the other four had biopsy only. Four of these seven patients were alive and without evidence of disease at a follow-up time of 4 to 11 years.

It is difficult to delineate a dose-response curve for primary astrocytoma of the spinal cord.[25] In contrast, a dose-response relationship has been noted in patients with primary ependymoma of the spinal cord. This retrospective analysis converted the dose of irradiation and the time over which it was given into a factor termed the time, dose, and fractionation factor (TDF). By doing so, the investigators hoped to determine an optimum dosage for response of these tumors. In this patient population, local control was achieved in five of the seven patients who were treated with irradiation alone. In addition, local control was maintained in one patient who underwent subtotal resection plus irradiation. None of the patients in this study had complete removal of their astrocytoma at operation. Since the intramedullary astrocytomas did not exhibit any significant correlation of control and TDF, it must be assumed that they vary in their sensitivity to irradiation. It is important to remember that this study dealt with a fairly small series of patients. In the ependymoma group, a dose-response relationship was established. In seven of eight ependymoma patients who received irradiation after subtotal resection, tumor control was achieved. The actuarial 5-year survival rates were 100 percent for ependymoma and 58 percent for astrocytoma. At 10 years, actuarial survival figures for ependymoma and astrocytoma were 73 and 23 percent, respectively (Fig. 183-7). On the basis of the findings

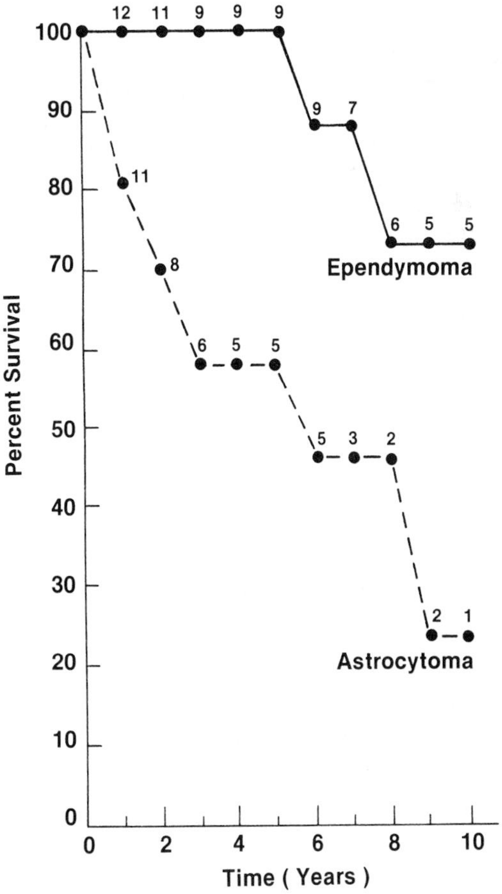

Figure 183-7 Actuarial survival rates for spinal cord ependymoma and astrocytoma. (From Kopelson et al.,[25] with permission.)

of this study, a dose of 4000 to 4500 cGy given in fractions of 180 to 200 cGy per treatment was recommended. The authors of this study also analyzed the functional results in the patient population. In the 19 irradiated patients, there were 45 deficits present prior to the initiation of treatments. Thirty-four of these 45 deficits resolved completely and eight of the deficits improved. The implication is that a minimal surgical procedure is indicated for histologic confirmation of tumor type, followed by definitive irradiation. Others would argue that surgical removal of as much tumor as is functionally possible should be done and then postoperative irradiation should be given.

The use of neuraxis irradiation for primary ependymomas of the spinal cord is controversial. The question is difficult to answer because CSF cytologic studies are generally not obtained in these patients. It appears that the incidence of intracranial recurrence is fairly low. Many radiation oncologists prefer to irradiate only the area of known disease, with a 2 to 3 cm margin around the tumor. Others recommend neuraxis irradiation with a dose of 3500 cGy, followed by additional treatment to the area of known tumor. This seems a reasonable approach in patients in whom positive CSF cytology has been demonstrated. Of course, the presence of other abnormal neuroradiologic findings during the initial evaluation of the patient with a primary spinal cord tumor would have an additional bearing on the decision to give neuraxis irradiation.

Primary tumors of the spinal cord are treated mainly through direct posterior portals, with the dose generally calculated at the spinal cord. The depth of different segments of the cord varies from 3 to 5 cm in most patients, and the particular segment being irradiated needs to be considered when calculating the depth at which the dose of irradiation is to be given. For the astrocytomas, most radiation oncologists would recommend tumor doses in the range of 4500 to 5000 cGy. Many would recommend a similar dose for the ependymomas, but others think that ependymomas might be slightly more sensitive to irradiation, and would prefer a dose in the range of 4000 to 4500 cGy. Both of these doses should be fairly well tolerated, and the risk of radiation myelitis at these doses should be minimal. However, if a large segment of the spinal cord is being treated or high daily doses are being utilized, the incidence of myelitis might be considerably higher. Reirradiation of these lesions after documented recurrence has been attempted on several occasions, but the number of patients is too small for meaningful analysis.

Metastatic Epidural Tumors

Metastatic disease involving the epidural space and causing neurological compromise is a fairly common problem. There has been some controversy regarding the optimum management of these patients, and certainly no single treatment approach is optimum for all patients. As the life expectancy of cancer patients increases and their clinical course becomes longer, the incidence of epidural metastases may increase as well. Indeed, metastatic disease is the most common neoplasm which occurs in the spinal canal.

Radiotherapy has been used in the management of metastatic epidural lesions for some time. It has been shown to be effective, resulting in improvement of significant neurological symptoms in one-third to one-half of the patients.[3] In addition, patients who are treated with external beam therapy usually receive significant relief of painful symptoms. There are some data to support the concept that patients with tumors which are more radioresponsive (e.g., lymphomas) have a higher rate of neurological improvement than those patients with tumors which are generally considered relatively radioresistant. The most important predictor of outcome in this patient population is the degree of motor function at presentation.[14]

There are no firmly established data regarding the optimum radiation schedule to be used in this patient population. Comparable results have been obtained using various dose and fractionation schedules. Some radiation oncologists advocate using higher doses for the first three treatments, followed by continuation of therapy at more conventional fractionation for the remaining course of treatment. In general, most think that multiple fractions, resulting in a tumor dose of 3000 to 4000 cGy, are more effective than a single high-dose treatment. A common schedule is to deliver 300 to 400 cGy daily for 3 days, followed by continuation of treatment at reduced fractionation. Others argue that patients can be treated equally as well with treatment given in 2 to 5 fractions.[37] The field should include the area of known extradural defect, with an adequate margin. Often, the field is extended to include other areas of bony involvement or other potential extradural defects.

Patients are often treated with dexamethasone concomitantly, and the question of radiotherapy causing edema has often been raised. In experimental models, radiation-induced edema has not been shown to be a problem, and, in fact, higher doses of radiation cause more tumor regression without the induction of significant edema. Dexamethasone should still be used to minimize the edema which may result from the metastatic deposit.

The diagnosis of spinal cord compression in its early stages requires a high index of suspicion. Once the diagnosis has been made, treatment should be initiated immediately using a combination of steroids and external beam irradiation. In selected cases, laminectomy is done prior to the initiation of treatment, and most radiation oncologists would recommend giving postoperative irradiation when the patient has recovered sufficiently from the surgical procedure.

References

1. Aristizabal S, Caldwell WL, Avila J, Mayer EG. Relationship of time dose factors to tumor control and complications in the treatment of Cushing's disease by irradiation. *Int J Radiat Oncol Biol Phys* 1977; 2:47–54.
2. Berry MP, Jenkin RDT, Keen CW, et al. Radiation treatment for medulloblastoma: a 21-year review. *J Neurosurg* 1981; 55:43–51.
3. Black P. Spinal metastasis: current status and recommended guidelines for management. *Neurosurgery* 1979; 5:726–746.
4. Bouchard J. *Radiation Therapy of Tumors and Diseases of the Nervous System.* Philadelphia: Lea & Febiger, 1966.
5. Bouchard J, Peirce CB. Radiation therapy in the management of neoplasms of the central nervous system, with a special note in regard to children: twenty years' experience, 1939–1958. *Am J Roentgenol* 1960; 84:610–628.
6. Chin HW, Hazel JJ, Kim TH, Webster JH. Oligodendrogliomas: I. A clinical study of cerebral oligodendrogliomas. *Cancer* 1980; 45:1458–1466.
7. Concannon JP, Kramer S, Berry R. The extent of intracranial gliomata at autopsy and its relationship to techniques used in radiation therapy of brain tumors. *Am J Roentgenol* 1960; 84:99–107.
8. Cooper JS, Steinfeld AD, Lerch IA. Cerebral metastases: value of reirradiation in selected patients. *Radiology* 1990; 174:883–885.
9. Cumberlin RL, Luk KH, Wara WM, et al. Medulloblastoma: treatment results and effect on normal tissues. *Cancer* 1979; 43:1014–1020.
10. Cushing H. Experiences with the cerebellar medulloblastomas: a critical review. *Acta Pathol Microbiol Scand* 1930; 7:1–86.

11. Danoff BF, Kramer S, Thompson N. The radiotherapeutic management of optic nerve gliomas in children. *Int J Radiat Oncol Biol Phys* 1980; 6:45–50.
12. De Schryver A, VandeKerckhove D, Debruyne G. Prolactin-secreting pituitary adenoma: observations in irradiated patients. *Acta Radiol Oncol Radiat Phys Biol* 1980; 19:169–175.
13. Eastman RC, Gorden P, Roth J. Conventional supervoltage irradiation is an effective treatment for acromegaly. *J Clin Endocrinol Metab* 1979; 48:931–940.
14. Findlay GF. Adverse effects of the management of malignant spinal cord compression. *J Neurol Neurosurg Psychiatry* 1984; 47:761–768.
15. Fulton DS, Urtasun RC, Scott-Brown I, et al. Increasing radiation dose intensity using hyperfractionation in patients with malignant glioma: final report of a prospective phase I-II dose response study. *J Neurooncol* 1992; 14:63–72.
16. Halperin EC. Multiple-fraction-per-day external beam radiotherapy for adults with supratentorial malignant gliomas. *J Neurooncol* 1992; 14:255–262.
17. Halperin EC, Wehn SM, Scott JW, et al. Selection of a management strategy for pediatric brainstem tumors. *Med Pediatr Oncol* 1989; 17:116–126.
18. Harwood AR, Simpson WJ. Radiation therapy of cerebral metastases: a randomized prospective clinical trial. *Int J Radiat Oncol Biol Phys* 1977; 2:1091–1094.
19. Higinbotham NL, Phillips RF, Farr HW, Hustu HO. Chordoma: thirty-five-year study at Memorial Hospital. *Cancer* 1967; 20:1841–1850.
20. Imhof HG, Hany M, Wiestler OD, Glanzmann CH. Long-term follow-up in 39 patients with an ependymoma after surgery and irradiation. *Strahlenther Onkol* 1992; 168:513–519.
21. Jennings AS, Liddle GW, Orth DN. Results of treating childhood Cushing's disease with pituitary irradiation. *N Engl J Med* 1977; 297:958–962.
22. Kim TH, Chin HW, Pollan S, et al. Radiotherapy of primary brain stem tumors. *Int J Radiat Oncol Biol Phys* 1980; 6:51–57.
23. King DL, Chang CH, Pool JL. Radiotherapy in the management of meningiomas. *Acta Radiol Oncol Radiat Phys Biol* 1966; 5:26–33.
24. Kleinberg DL, Noel GL, Frantz AG. Galactorrhea: a study of 235 cases, including 48 with pituitary tumors. *N Engl J Med* 1977; 296:589–600.
25. Kopelson G, Linggood RM, Kleinman GM, et al. Management of intramedullary spinal cord tumors. *Radiology* 1980; 135:473–479.
26. Kramer S, Hendrickson F, Zelen M, Schotz W. Therapeutic trials in the management of metastatic brain tumors by different time/dose fraction schemes of radiation therapy. *Natl Cancer Inst Monogr* 1977; 46:213–221.
27. Leibel SA, Sheline GE, Wara WM, et al. The role of radiation therapy in the treatment of astrocytomas. *Cancer* 1975; 35:1551–1557.
28. Lichter AS, Wara WM, Sheline GE, et al. The treatment of craniopharyngiomas. *Int J Radiat Oncol Biol Phys* 1977; 2:675–683.
29. Marks JE, Adler SJ. A comparative study of ependymomas by site of origin. *Int J Radiat Oncol Biol Phys* 1982; 8:37–43.
30. McCormack BM, Miller DC, Budzilovich GN, et al. Treatment and survival of low-grade astrocytoma in adults—1977–1988. *Neurosurgery* 1992; 31:636–642.
31. McWhirter R. Radiation treatment of cerebral tumors. *Proc R Soc Med* 1946; 39:673–679.
32. Miralbell R, Linggood RM, de la Monte S, et al The role of radiotherapy in the treatment of subtotally resected benign meningiomas. *J Neurooncol* 1992; 13:157–164.
33. Nelson DF, Martz KL, Bonner H, et al. Non-Hodgkin's lymphoma of the brain: can high dose, large volume radiation therapy improve survival? Report on a prospective trial by the Radiation Therapy Oncology Group (RTOG): RTOG 8315. *Int J Radiat Oncol Biol Phys* 1992; 23:9–17.
34. Paterson E, Farr RF. Cerebellar medulloblastoma: treatment by irradiation of the whole central nervous system. *Acta Radiol* 1953; 39:323–336.
35. Pearlman AW, Friedman M. Radical radiation therapy of chordoma. *Am J Roentgenol* 1970; 108:333–341.
36. Phillips TL, Sheline GE, Boldrey E. Therapeutic considerations in tumors affecting the central nervous system: ependymomas. *Radiology* 1964; 83:98–105.
37. Podd TJ, Carpenter DS, Baughan CA, et al. Spinal cord compression: prognosis and implications for treatment fractionation. *Clin Oncol (R Coll Radiol)* 1992; 4:341–344.
38. Rampen FHJ, van Andel JG, Sizoo W, van Unnik JAM. Radiation therapy in primary non-Hodgkin's lymphomas of the CNS. *Eur J Cancer* 1980; 16:177–184.
39. Sagerman RH, Cassady JR, Chang CH. Radiation therapy for intracranial lymphoma. *Radiology* 1967; 88:552–554.
40. Salazar OM, Castro-Vita H, Bakos RS, et al. Radiation therapy for tumors of the pineal region. *Int J Radiat Oncol Biol Phys* 1979; 5:491–499.
41. Salazar OM, Rubin P, Feldstein ML, Pizzutiello R. High dose radiation therapy in the treatment of malignant gliomas: final report. *Int J Radiat Oncol Biol Phys* 1979; 5:1733–1740.
42. Schwade JG, Wara WM, Sheline GE, et al. Management of primary spinal cord tumors. *Int J Radiat Oncol Biol Phys* 1978; 4:389–393.
43. Shapiro WR, Posner JB, Ushio Y, et al. Treatment of meningeal neoplasms. *Cancer Treat Rep* 1977; 61:733–743.
44. Sheline GE. Treatment of nonfunctioning chromophobe adenomas of the pituitary. *Am J Roentgenol* 1974; 120:553–561.
45. Sheline GE, Boldrey E, Karlsberg P, Phillips TL. Therapeutic considerations in tumors affecting the central nervous system: oligodendrogliomas. *Radiology* 1964; 82:84–89,.
46. Shimizu KT, Tran LM, Mark RJ, Selch MT. Management of oligodendrogliomas. *Radiology* 1993; 186:569–572.
47. Suit HD, Goitein M, Munzenrider J, et al. Definitive radiation therapy for chordoma and chondrosarcoma of base of skull and cervical spine. *J Neurosurg* 1982; 56:377–385.
48. Uematsu M, Kondo M, Dokiya T, et al. Primary non-AIDS related brain lymphoma: patterns of failure following radiotherapy. *Acta Oncologica* 1992; 31:551–554.
49. Walker MD, Alexander E Jr, Hunt WE, et al. Evaluation of BCNU and/or radiotherapy in the treatment of anaplastic gliomas: a cooperative clinical trial. *J Neurosurg* 1978; 49:333–343.
50. Walker MD, Strike TA, Sheline GE. An analysis of dose-effect relationship in the radiotherapy of malignant gliomas. *Int J Radiat Oncol Biol Phys* 1979; 5:1725–1731.
51. Wara WM, Jenkin RDT, Evans A, et al. Tumors of the pineal and suprasellar region: Childrens Cancer Study Group treatment results 1960–1975. A report from Childrens Cancer Study Group. *Cancer* 1979; 43:698–701.
52. Wara WM, Sheline GE, Newman H, et al. Radiation therapy of meningiomas. *Am J Roentgenol* 1975; 123:453–458.
53. Yamashita J, Handa H, Iwaki K, Abe M. Recurrence of intracranial meningiomas, with special reference to radiotherapy. *Surg Neurol* 1980; 14:33–40.
54. Yap HY, Yap BS, Rasmussen S, et al. Treatment for meningeal carcinomatosis in breast cancer. *Cancer* 1982; 50:219–222.

184 Charged-Particle Irradiation of Intracranial Lesions

Richard P. Levy
Jacob I. Fabrikant
Gary K. Steinberg
Kenneth A. Frankel

Charged-particle irradiation of intracranial lesions has been the subject of biomedical research and clinical development since 1946, when Wilson[76] proposed the therapeutic use of charged-particle beams, based on the unique physical characteristics of alpha-emitting radionuclides first observed by Bragg in 1904.[4] After completion of the 184-inch synchrocyclotron at the University of California at Berkeley–Lawrence Berkeley Laboratory (UCB–LBL) in 1947,[5] Tobias and Lawrence and their colleagues[72–74] began the study of the biological effects of beams of protons, deuterons, and helium ions, with particular emphasis on reaction to radiation injury in the brain.

Since 1954, more than 7000 patients worldwide with intracranial and juxtaspinal lesions have been treated with charged-particle irradiation. (Only charged particles of proton mass or greater are considered in this chapter.) The majority of these patients have been treated at UCB–LBL,[7,16,39,66] the Harvard Cyclotron Laboratory–Massachusetts General Hospital (HCL–MGH),[24,25,27,69] the Institute for Theoretical and Experimental Physics in Moscow (ITEP),[58,61] and the Institute of Nuclear Physics in St. Petersburg (INPh).[28] Most patients have been treated with single-dose irradiation or with a few large-dose fractions (i.e., a *stereotactic radiosurgical* approach), but several hundred patients with primary malignant tumors have been treated using conventional fractionation schedules.[6–8,69]

Clinical applications were constrained initially by the limitations of neuroradiologic techniques for treatment planning, stereotactic localization, and dose distribution.[39] Early clinical trials, therefore, were restricted to pituitary-ablation treatment, in which high-dose radiation was used to induce selective destruction of small, well-defined intracranial target volumes. The first stereotactic irradiation procedures utilizing charged particles in clinical patients were performed by Lawrence and colleagues[30] at UCB–LBL in 1954 for pituitary-hormone suppression in the treatment of metastatic breast carcinoma. Shortly thereafter, charged-particle radiosurgery was applied to the pituitary-ablation treatment of patients with proliferative diabetic retinopathy[35,36] and to the treatment of pituitary adenomas.[27,34,45] During these early years, limited numbers of patients were also treated for other conditions, including certain functional disorders and malignant brain tumors.[34] With the development of improved techniques of stereotaxis and cerebral angiography, the charged-particle radiosurgical approach, using Bragg-peak protons, was applied to the treatment of arteriovenous malformations (AVMs) at HCL–MGH by Kjellberg et al.[24] in 1965. More recently, the advent of high-resolution computed x-ray tomography (CT) and magnetic resonance imaging (MRI) has made it possible for reliable stereotactic localization and irradiation techniques to be applied to the treatment of a diverse collection of disorders.[37] The expanded application of charged-particle irradiation for intracranial lesions is an important development in neurosurgery and radiation oncology, which promises new and innovative approaches that will influence therapeutic strategies, not only in the brain but elsewhere in the central nervous system and at other sites within the body. In the past few years, advances in neurological imaging have been accompanied by technologic advances and by computer software dedicated to charged-particle treatment planning and dose delivery. During the past 5 years, especially, all these factors have contributed to increased numbers of institutions worldwide building and/or planning charged-particle treatment facilities.[39]

Our objectives in this chapter are to present the rationale for the use of charged-particle irradiation as a neurosurgical and/or radiotherapeutic procedure and to describe the spectrum of human research studies thus far carried out in the development of charged-particle irradiation for intracranial lesions. A comprehensive review of these topics is beyond the scope of this chapter. Selected historically significant or representative studies and reviews, therefore, have been summarized and/or cited for further reference.

Physical Properties of Charged-Particle Beams

Ionizing radiations used for external-beam irradiation may be classified as high-energy photons (e.g., x-rays or gamma rays) or accelerated charged particles (e.g., protons or helium ions). As photons traverse and interact with tissue, their ionization events attenuate with depth in tissue (Fig. 184-1); satisfactory dose distributions in deep-seated lesions are achieved, at the cost of a relatively high integral dose to the patient, by using beams from many different angles or intersecting dynamic arcs. Charged-particle beams manifest very different physical properties that can be exploited to place a high dose of radiation preferentially within the boundaries of a deeply located target volume.[19,39,64] These properties include (1) a well-defined *range* that can be adjusted precisely so that the beam *stops* at the distal edge of the target and deep within the tissue, resulting in little or no exit dose; (2) an initial region of low dose (the *plateau*) as the beam penetrates through tissue, followed by a region of high dose (the *Bragg ionization peak*) at the end of the range of the beam that can be adjusted to conform to the location and dimensions of the target, so that the entrance dose can be kept to a minimum; and (3) very sharp lateral edges that can be shaped by metal apertures to conform to the projected cross-sectional contour of the target, so that negligible dose is absorbed by the adjacent normal tissues (Figs. 184-1 to 184-4).

Each charged-particle beam can be directed to place individually shaped three-dimensional high-dose regions precisely within the brain by using an appropriately shaped aperture, spreading the Bragg peak and adjusting the beam range (Fig. 184-3). For irregularly shaped lesions and to accommodate skull curvature, tissue-equivalent compensators positioned in the beam path are used to match the distal edge of the spread-out Bragg peak (across the transverse profile of the beam) to the distal surface of the target volume.[19,39] Several entry angles and beam ports (typically, four) are directed stereotactically so that the high-dose regions of the individual beams intersect within the target volume, with a much lower dose to immediately adjacent and intervening normal brain tissues.[16,19,38,39]

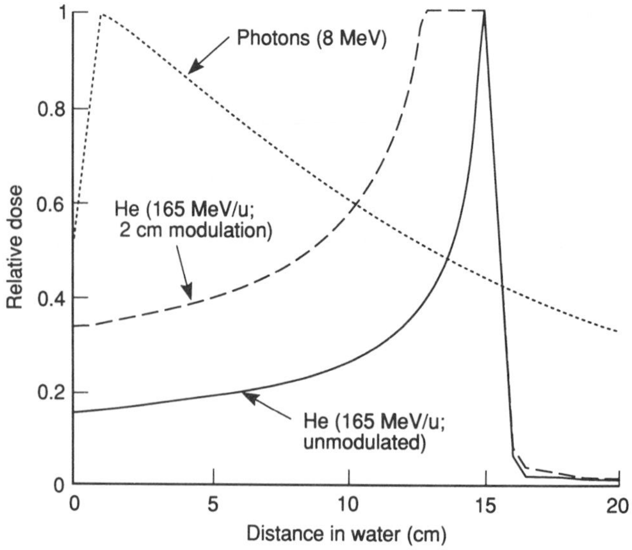

Figure 184-1 Relative dose in water as a function of depth is shown for 8-MeV photons (*dotted line*), an *unmodulated* helium-ion (165 MeV/U) beam (*solid line*), and a helium-ion beam with a spread-out Bragg peak (SOBP) *modulated* to 2-cm width (*dashed line*) by interposing variable-thickness absorbers in the beam path. The unmodulated Bragg peak produces a narrow beam with high energy deposition at the end of the range, suitable for producing small intracranial lesions. For most radiosurgical applications, it is necessary to spread out the width of the Bragg peak to ensure optimum dose distribution throughout the lesion. (From Levy et al.,[39] with permission.)

Treatment Planning and Dose Delivery*

The application of charged-particle irradiation to the treatment of intracranial lesions presents a number of problems not encountered in conventional radiotherapy.[10,19,75] Treatment planning and dose delivery consist of sequential neuroradiologic imaging studies, computer-assisted image correlation and calculation of dose distribution, positioning of the patient and target volume within a three-dimensional frame of reference, and delivery to the target of carefully monitored charged-particle beams.[16,19,53,63] In this section, we consider briefly the methods of treatment planning and dose delivery that have been developed at UCB–LBL for stereotactic radiosurgery for Bragg-peak and plateau-beam irradiation of vascular and other disorders; similar techniques in principle are employed at other charged-particle facilities and are applicable as well to extended-fractionation delivery of charged-particle irradiation. The reader is referred to Frankel et al.[19] for a more-detailed review.

*Portions of this section are adapted, with permission, from Frankel et al.[19]

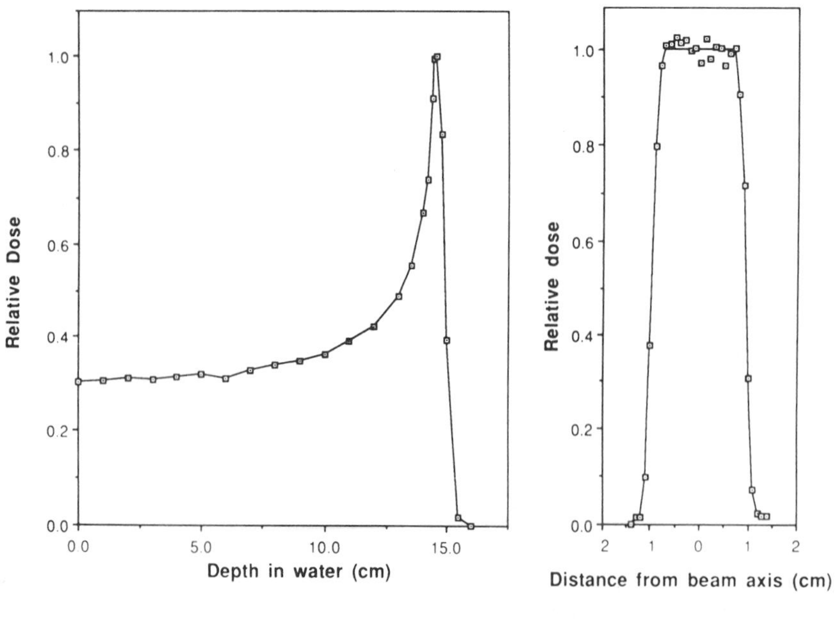

Figure 184-2 The Bragg ionization curve and its transverse profile for the 165-MeV/U helium-ion beam at the UCB–LBL Bevatron. *Left,* the Bragg-peak-to-plateau dose ratio is approximately three, and the relative biological effectiveness in the peak is estimated to be about 1.3; thus, the biological effect in the peak is about 4 times that in the plateau region. Dose fall-off from 90 percent to 10 percent occurs within 2 to 3 mm distal to the Bragg peak. *Right,* the transverse profile of the Bragg peak demonstrates sharp edges; the lateral dose fall-off from 90 percent to 10 percent occurs within 2.5 mm. This profile was measured 1 cm proximal to the distal edge of a beam with a 7-cm residual range and with the Bragg peak spread 2 cm. Distal and lateral dose fall-off are negligibly affected by spreading the Bragg peak. (From Fabrikant et al.,[16] with permission.)

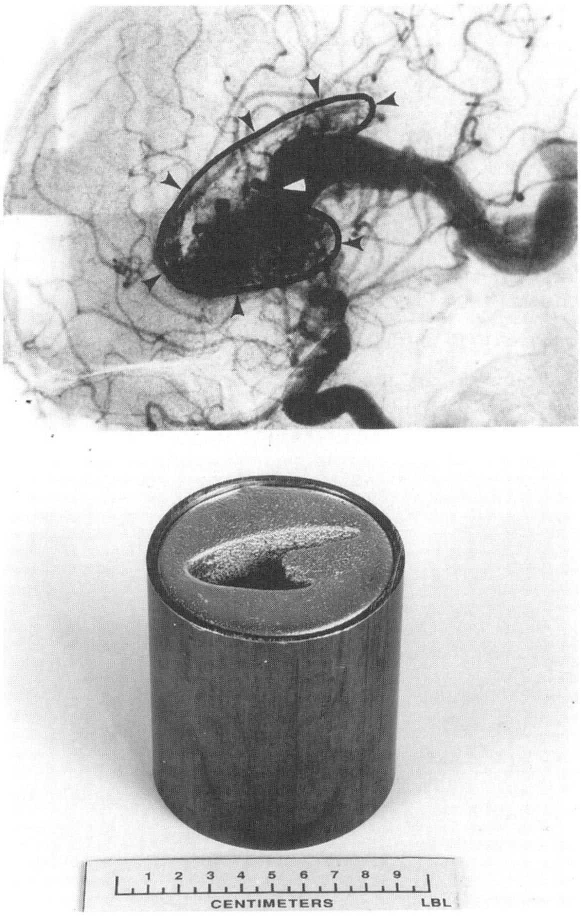

Figure 184-3 Charged-particle beams can be readily contoured by metal apertures shaped to conform to the cross-sectional size and shape of the target volume in any projection. *Top,* a lateral projection view of a stereotactic cerebral angiogram (left internal carotid artery injection) demonstrates a large AVM occupying the genu and body of the corpus callosum. The composite radiosurgical target, selected after evaluation of the multivessel cerebral angiogram study, has been outlined (*arrowheads*). *Bottom,* an individually tailored brass and Cerrobend (a low-melting-temperature dense alloy) aperture has been fabricated from computer-defined contours derived from the cerebral angiogram to conform to the radiosurgical target. The aperture is inserted into the beam line for appropriate shaping of the lateral beams during radiosurgery (cf. Fig. 184-5). (From Levy et al.,[39] with permission.)

Stereotactic Localization

A transportable stereotactic frame-mask system, consisting of an individualized thermoplastic immobilizing head mask and stereotactic frame with fiducial markers, has been developed to permit accurate and reproducible positioning of the patient's head for neuroradiologic procedures, including target definition and localization, treatment planning, and radiosurgical treatment (Fig. 184-5).[53] The stereotactic frame can be attached to neuroradiologic couches and to the stereotactic positioning couch—the Irradiation Stereotactic Apparatus for Humans (ISAH) (Fig. 184-4).[52,53] This system has proved to be safe and reliable in more than 1300 patients.[39]

Neuroradiologic Evaluation and Image Correlation

Methods for correlation of stereotactic MRI and CT images have been developed for target definition and localization for neoplastic disorders and angiographically occult vascular malformations (AOVMs).[16,19,42] In the patient whose brain-stem lesion is illustrated in Figure 184-6, radiosurgical target contours are delineated on stereotactic MRI and CT images. The MRI-derived target contours are transferred to CT for comparison with CT-derived contours, and a final set of target contours is then defined on the noncontrast CT images. For each CT slice, the inner and outer tables of the skull are digitized, along with selected other bony landmarks, such as the pituitary sella, frontal plates, and anterior and posterior protuberances. A computerized digitization program then generates CT-derived treatment-localization overlays (alignment aids), based on the final target contours and the digitized bony landmarks.[63] The CT data are also used to determine the coordinates required to position the patient on ISAH. The radiosurgical treatment of pituitary adenomas represents a special situation for which the localization procedure is greatly simplified, because the sella turcica can usually be readily identified and localized on plain orthogonal radiographs.[19]

For AVMs, stereotactic cerebral angiography is the most precise imaging method for determining the shape and location of the lesion. (MR and CT imaging, however, are useful for demonstrating relationships of the AVM to adjacent anatomic structures.) The contours of the AVM target, derived from selected orthogonal angiographic films and transferred to the CT images, form the basis for the stereotactic treatment-planning procedure.[16,19,63] Via geometric optics, the digitization program uses the positions of the fiducial markers of the stereotactic frame as they appear on the radiographs, in conjunction with their known positions on the frame, to calculate radiographic magnification factors and the coordinates of the target volume within the frame. The digitized angiographic data are also used to calculate the initial translational coordinates of the patient-positioning couch and to generate overlays of the stereotactic-frame fiducial markers, angiographically derived target contours, and midplane bony landmarks of the skull for lateral and anteroposterior localization radiographs (Fig. 184-7).

The digitization program also models the angiographically derived AVM target volume as a series of ellipses on corresponding axial CT slices. The CT data and derived target contours for each axial CT slice are reformatted to generate relevant views in coronal and sagittal planes. The reformatted target contours, which are corrected for parallax and magnification, then have approximately the same shape and location as the AVM target delineated on the orthogonal angiographic films.[63] In the case of irregularly shaped AVMs, MR and CT image information may be used to modify the target contours.[19]

Computer-Assisted Treatment Planning

For homogeneous tissues, the task of positioning the Bragg peak at a specified depth is quite straightforward. For the heterogeneous tissues of the skull and brain, however, this procedure is more complex.[10,75] Generally, denser bone tissue slows the incident stream of charged particles more per unit length of tissue than does less-dense parenchymal tissue. Thus, a beam traversing denser tissue will have its Bragg-peak region displaced proximally to a greater extent than a beam traversing less-dense tissue. Knowledge

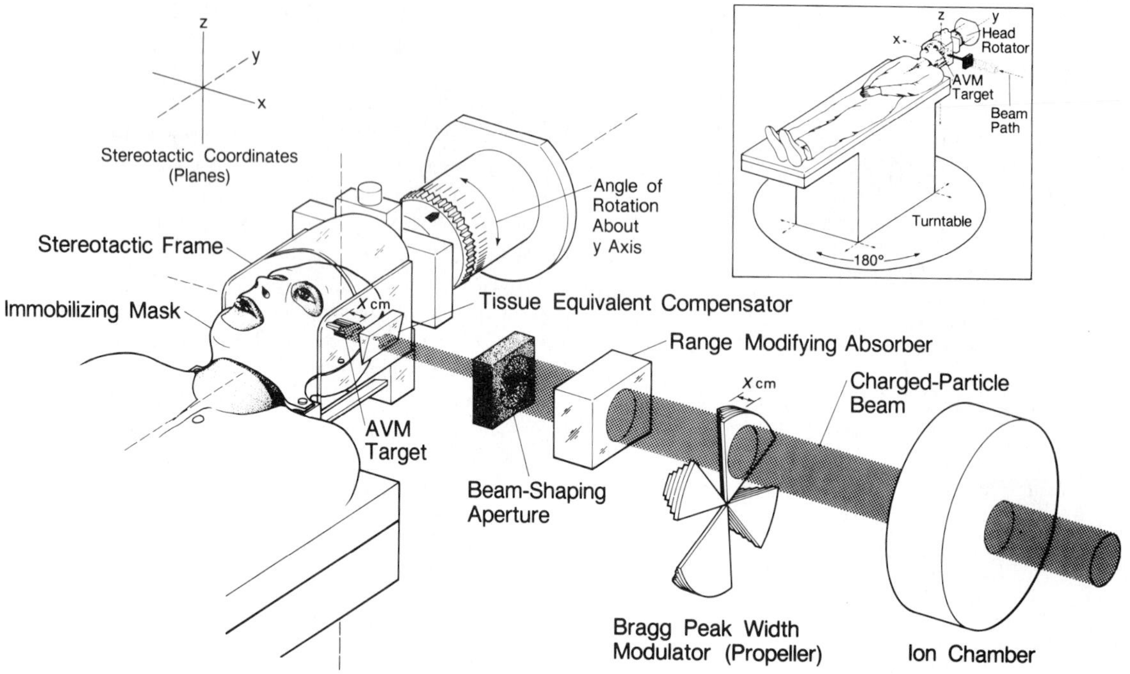

Figure 184-4 Schematic diagram of charged-particle-beam delivery system at UCB–LBL for stereotactic radiosurgery of intracranial tumors and vascular disorders. The stereotactic patient-positioning system (ISAH) allows translation along three orthogonal axes (x,y,z) and rotation about the y and z axes, thereby providing precise patient immobilization and positioning for stereotactically directed charged-particle-beam therapy. The width of the high-dose Bragg ionization peak within the brain can be spread to the prescribed size by interposing a modulating filter of comparable maximum thickness (x cm) in the beam path, schematically shown here as a variable-thickness propeller. The range in tissue of the Bragg-peak region is determined by a range-modifying absorber. At the Bevatron accelerator, the range and modulation of the Bragg peak are controlled by use of a variable-position water-column absorber. An individually designed aperture, specifically tailored to the size and configuration of the intracranial lesion, shapes the beam in cross-section. Tissue-equivalent compensators further improve the precision placement of the high-dose Bragg-peak region by adjusting for irregular target contours, skull curvature, and tissue inhomogeneities. Ion chambers monitor the dose delivered in each beam. (From Levy et al.,[38] with permission.)

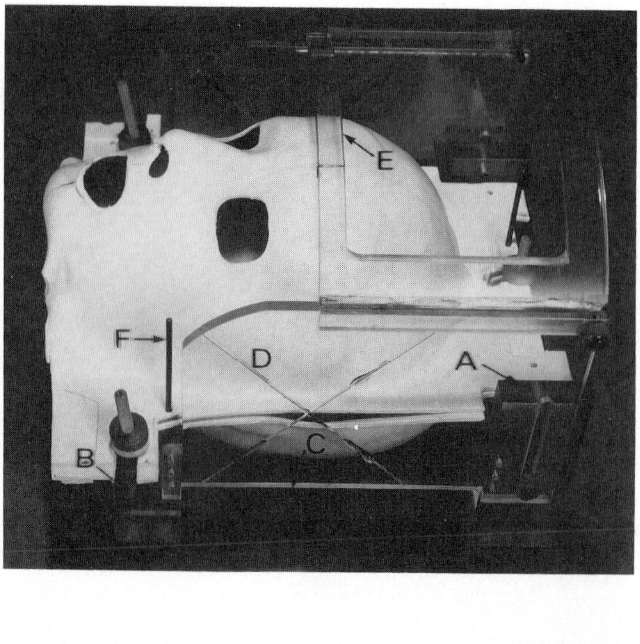

Figure 184-5 Stereotactic frame and patient mask system (cf. Fig. 184-4). The head-immobilization mask is formed of thermoplastic material, and it is molded individually for each patient's head. Letters denote components of the stereotactic frame: A, Top cross member. B, Yoke. C, Graphite support bar with fiducial marker. An identical bar is present on the other side of the frame. D, Sideplates with fiducial markers. The clear Lucite sideplates have two grooves machined at right angles. Fine copper wires cemented into the grooves are imaged on lateral radiographs and serve as markers for angiograms and CT. For MRI, fine tubes filled with olive oil are substituted into the grooves. E, Arch with fiducial markers. The arch supports two copper wire markers (or oil-tube markers for MRI) that are imaged on anteroposterior radiographs. F, Positioning pins. (From Lyman et al.,[53] with permission.)

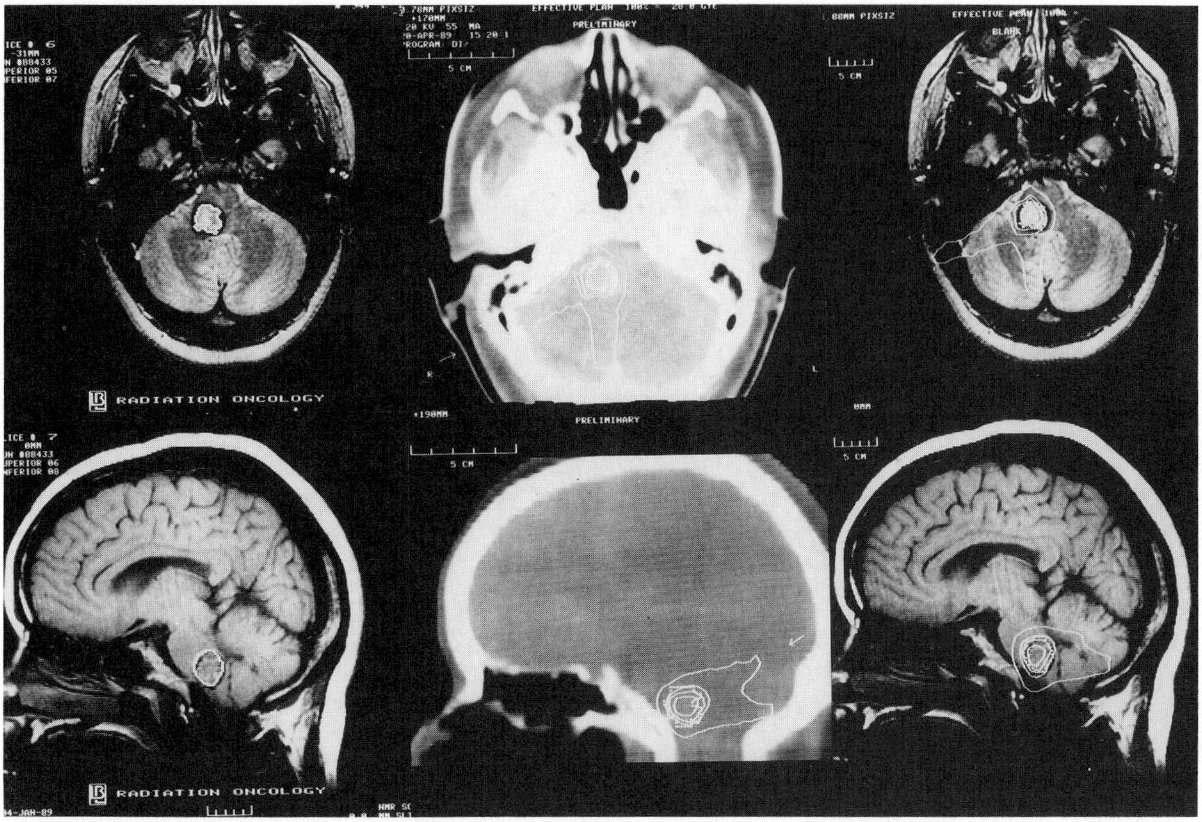

Figure 184-6 Stereotactic helium-ion Bragg-peak radiosurgery treatment plan for a 29-year-old woman with a symptomatic angiographically occult vascular malformation in the pons. *Left* (*upper* and *lower*), diagnostic stereotactic MRI scans in the axial and sagittal planes are used to define the target volume (*ring of white dots*) for stereotactic radiosurgery. *Middle* (*upper* and *lower*), the target contour data are then transferred to corresponding stereotactic CT images for treatment planning and calculation of isodose contours for display. *Right* (*upper* and *lower*), the isodose-contour information is then transferred back to the original MRI scans to permit the explicit demonstration (and modification, where required) of isodose-contour distributions in all desired anatomic planes. Isodose contours displayed here in the axial and sagittal planes are calculated for 10, 50, 70, and 90 percent of the maximum central dose. (From Fabrikant et al.,[16] with permission.)

of the physical characteristics of each volume element of tissue along the beam path on a pixel-by-pixel basis is necessary for precise determination of dose distribution and for calculating the depth of penetration of the beam. Noncontrast-CT data provide electron-density information (x-ray absorption coefficients), which is converted to charged-particle energy loss by established calibration functions.[10] Dose-absorbing filters of appropriate thickness are placed in the beam path to adjust the range in tissue precisely to the desired value (Fig. 184-4).

A computer-assisted treatment-planning program is used to calculate dose distributions and to generate isodose curves.[10] Figures 184-8 and 184-9 are representative examples of the isodose-contour displays of treatment plans for small and large AVMs, respectively. The size, shape, and location of the lesion, and the dose to the target volume and adjacent brain structures are interrelated factors that affect the choice of beam ports, entry angles, and dose-configuration patterns. The final treatment plan is selected after iterative refinement of a number of preliminary treatment plans.

Target Localization and Treatment Procedure

The radiosurgical procedure requires that the target volume be localized precisely at the intersection of the charged-particle beam and the isocenter of ISAH.[52] ISAH has three degrees of freedom for translation, two degrees of freedom for rotation (the third degree of rotational freedom is effected by rotation of the beam-shaping aperture) and a mechanical precision of 0.1 mm and 0.1 degree. (Based on the limits of resolution of imaging data and correlation and the intrinsic uncertainties in patient positioning, the overall localization and alignment system is reproducible in repeated diagnostic and therapeutic sessions to approximately 1.5 mm and 1.5 degrees in each translational and rotational degree of freedom, respectively.[53,63]

At treatment, the patient is positioned on ISAH in the stereotactic frame-mask system, and orthogonal localization radiographs are obtained. Final alignment of the patient is verified by comparing the localization radiographs and port films exposed immediately prior to treatment to the computer-generated treatment-

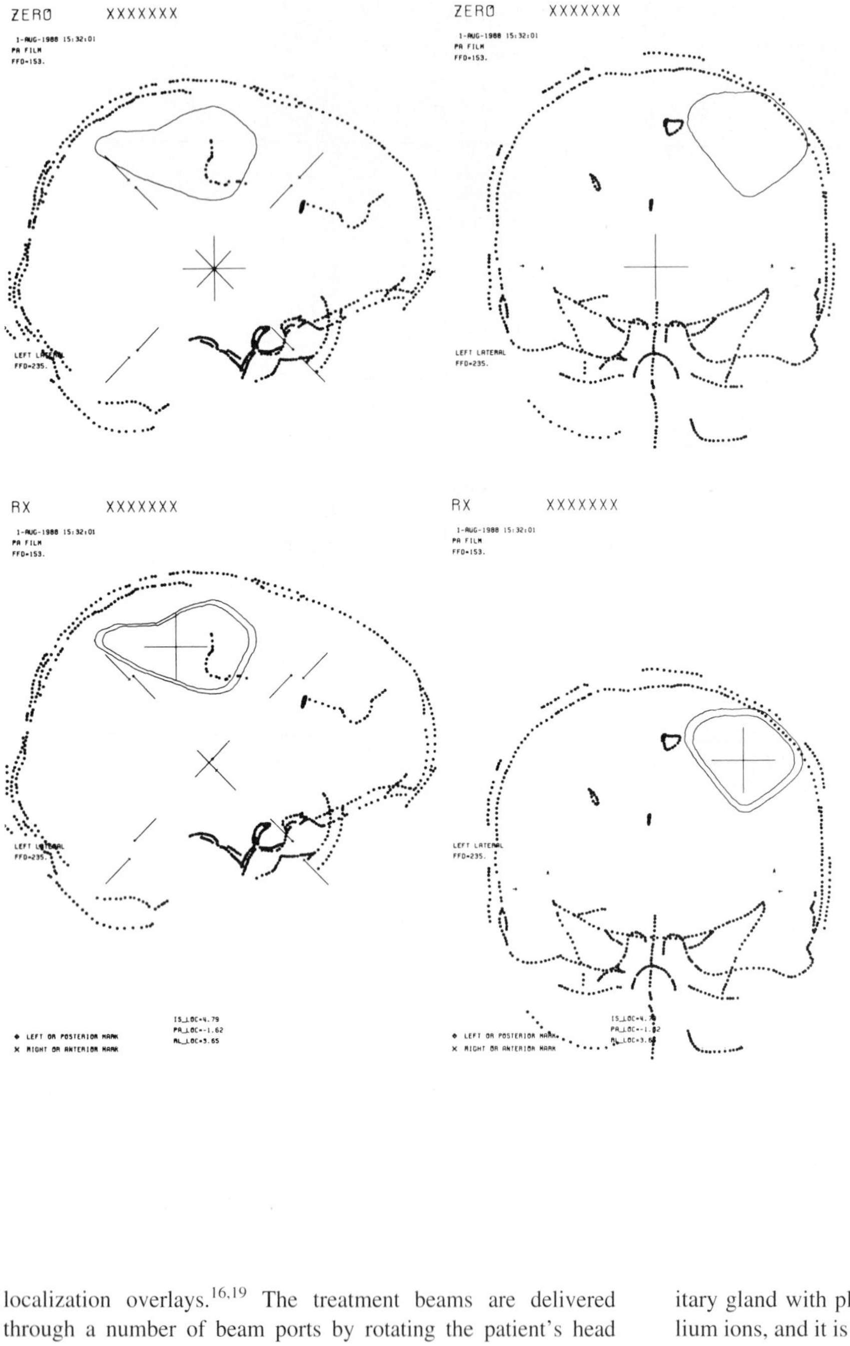

Figure 184-7 Computer-reformatted overlay of digitized angiographic films for treatment-planning procedures, used to transfer the three-dimensional target volume for dose localization and to align the patient for the radiosurgical procedure. The overlay maps target contours, midplane bony landmarks, fiducial markers from the stereotactic frame, and the isocenter of the patient positioner (denoted by the *cross*). *Upper,* lateral and anteroposterior views demonstrate the relative orientation of these elements when the stereotactic frame center is located at the isocenter of ISAH (*upper left*). *Lower,* corresponding views demonstrate the relative orientation when the patient has been moved so as to place the center of the lesion at the isocenter of the immobilization system (''treatment position''). The two concentric target contours reflect the angiographically derived target contour magnified to match the localization radiograph (outer contour) and the actual size of the AVM (inner contour), respectively. (From Phillips et al.,[63] with permission.)

localization overlays.[16,19] The treatment beams are delivered through a number of beam ports by rotating the patient's head and/or treatment couch sequentially to predetermined fixed positions. Each beam port requires 10 to 15 min for patient positioning, aperture adjustment, and compensator placement and 1 to 3 min for beam exposure. The entire treatment procedure typically requires about 30 to 60 min.

Plateau-Beam Stereotactic Irradiation

When a charged-particle beam of sufficiently high energy, and hence greater depth of penetration, is available, radiosurgery can be performed with the plateau-ionization portion of the beam. In this treatment configuration, the beam passes completely through the head, depositing plateau-region radiation in the brain; the Bragg-peak dose is absorbed in the wall of the treatment room opposite the beam line. This method was developed by Lawrence and colleagues[30,31,70,73] at UCB–LBL for irradiation of the pituitary gland with plateau beams of protons and (subsequently) helium ions, and it is currently applied to radiosurgery of small intracranial target volumes at several proton-irradiation centers in Russia.[28,60,61]

With the plateau-beam-irradiation technique, consideration of the tissue inhomogeneity normally encountered in the head is not important, but accurate stereotactic localization of the intracranial target volume and precise isocentric technique are essential. The plateau-beam radiosurgical system developed at UCB–LBL uses a stereotactic positioning table and head holder in combination with individually fabricated plastic head masks for immobilization (Fig. 184-10). Following delineation of the target volume, the charged-particle beam is centered on the sella turcica by means of orthogonal localization radiographs and port films, and the beam contour is shaped by a brass aperture. During irradiation, the head is turned in pendulum motion around a horizontal axis while the patient is positioned sequentially at 12 discrete angles around a vertical axis (Fig. 184-10). The irradiation arcs are directed such that the dose fall-off is very rapid in the anteroposterior direction and toward the

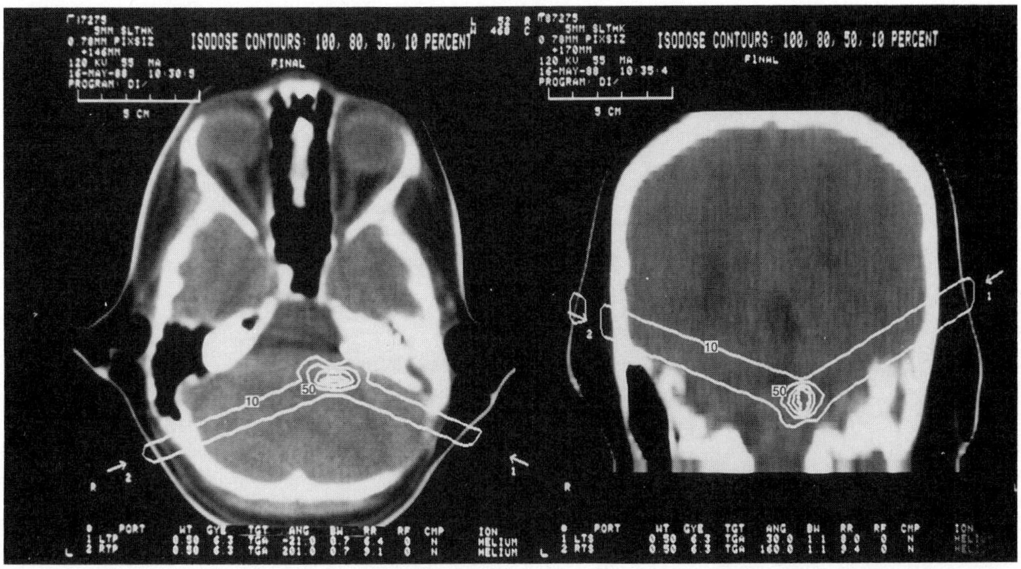

Figure 184-8 Stereotactic helium-ion Bragg-peak radiosurgery treatment plan for a 12-year-old girl with an AVM of the brain stem (*inner ring of white dots*). Isodose contours have been calculated at 10, 50, 80, and 100 percent of the maximum dose in the axial (*left*) and coronal (*right*) planes. The 100 percent contour conforms precisely to the periphery of the lesion. There is a very rapid fall-off in dose outside the AVM target volume. Because four noncoplanar beams are used, very little normal brain tissue receives even as much as 10 percent of the dose to the AVM and most of the brain receives no radiation at all. There is virtually complete sparing and protection of midbrain and pontine structures. The helium-ion beam was collimated by an elliptical brass aperture measuring 8.5 × 11.5 mm; treatment was performed using four ports in 1 day, to a volume of 0.3 cc (dose, 25 GyE). (From Levy et al.,[38] with permission.)

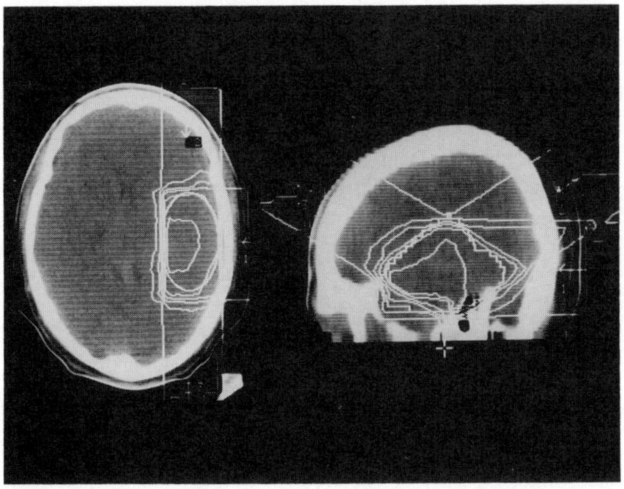

Figure 184-9 Stereotactic helium-ion Bragg-peak radiosurgery treatment plan for a large (54 cc) left temporal and deep central AVM in a 39-year-old man. *Left,* axial plane; *right,* sagittal plane. The helium-ion beam was collimated by 61- × 50-mm and 55- × 42-mm individually shaped brass and Cerrobend apertures; 27 GyE was delivered in 3 days to the lesion (defined by the *ring of white dots*) using four noncoplanar beams. Isodose contours have been calculated for 10, 30, 50, 70, 90, and 99 percent of the maximum dose. The 90 percent isodose contour borders precisely on the periphery of the lesion. There is rapid dose fall-off to the 70 percent level, and the 10 percent isodose contour completely spares irradiation of the contralateral hemisphere. (From Fabrikant et al.,[16] with permission.)

optic chiasm; the dose fall-off decreases more slowly laterally toward the temporal lobes (Fig. 184-11). With this method, the optic chiasm, hypothalamus, and outer portions of the sphenoid sinus receive less than 10 percent of the central-axis pituitary dose.[70] Plateau-beam radiosurgery can also be used for treatment of disorders other than pituitary adenomas. For these applications, however, it is necessary to incorporate the more-general methods of stereotactic target localization described previously.[19]

The dose distributions that result from the use of isocentrically directed arcs of plateau-beam irradiation are quite comparable to those produced with stereotactic radiosurgical systems using x-rays or gamma rays. Their application, therefore, is similarly limited primarily to the treatment of lesions less than 2- to 3-cm diameter.[64]

Clinical Applications*

Four decades have now passed since the first patient was treated with charged-particle irradiation of the brain. Clinical experience has been obtained in the following categories: pituitary hormone suppression, pituitary adenomas, malignant gliomas, vascular malformations, juxtaspinal tumors, and ocular melanomas. In this section, we review selected aspects of the worldwide clinical experience with charged-particle irradiation of intracranial and

*Portions of this section are adapted, with permission, from Fabrikant et al.,[16] Levy et al.,[39] and Steinberg et al.[66,68]

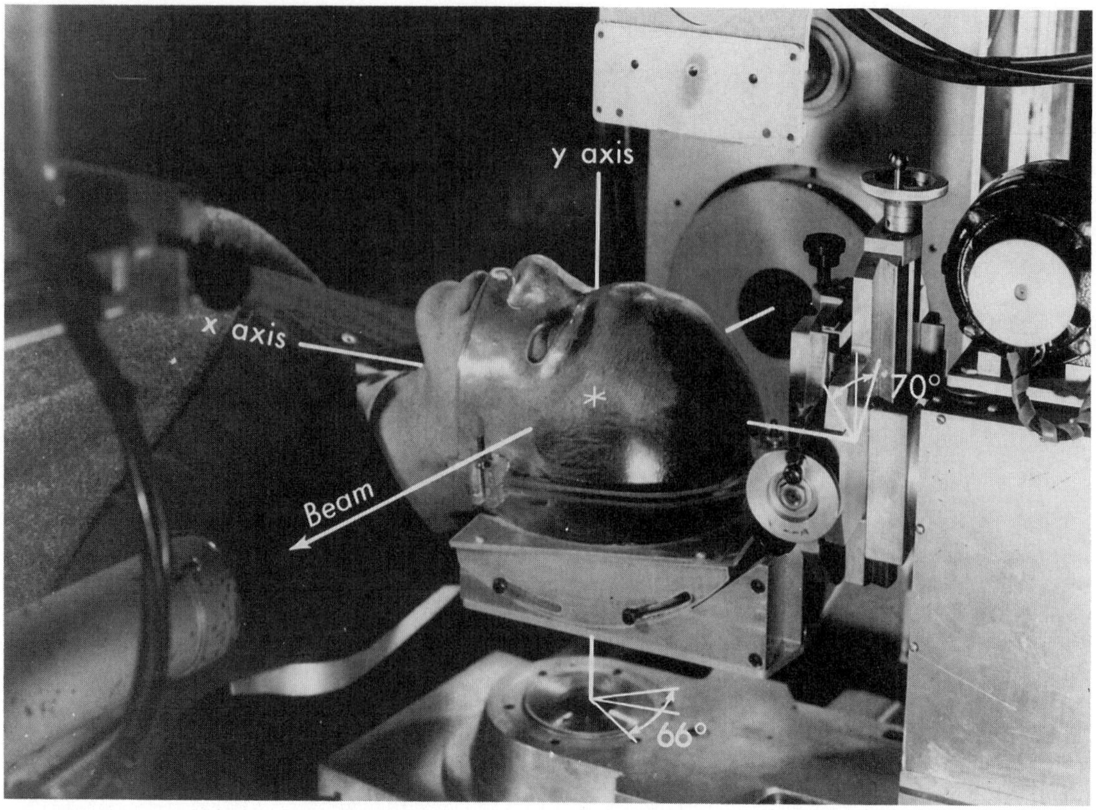

Figure 184-10 Stereotactic positioning table and head holder for the plateau-beam helium-ion pituitary-irradiation system developed at the UCB-LBL 184-inch synchrocyclotron. The mask is a rigid transparent polystyrene unit that is tailored for each patient. During irradiation, the patient is positioned sequentially at 12 discrete angles, covering a 66-degree arc around the vertical (y) axis; at each position, the patient's head is turned in pendulum motion through a 70° arc around the horizontal (x) axis. (From Levy et al.,[39] with permission.)

juxtaspinal lesions; for more-detailed information, the reader is referred to several reviews.[14,16,37,39] The relative emphasis here on helium-ion irradiation reflects the authors' experience at UCB–LBL and at Stanford University Medical Center (SUMC); this experience has been paralleled by extensive experience with proton-beam therapy elsewhere.

Pituitary Hormone Suppression

Charged-particle irradiation of the pituitary gland has been shown in more than 1300 patients to be very effective for inducing suppression of normal pituitary function with minimal associated risk of inducing injury in adjacent neural structures.[39,65] The primary applications of charged-particle hypophysectomy have been to control the metastatic spread of selected hormone-responsive carcinomas (e.g., breast and prostate cancer)[11,28,30,32,34,35,48,58,61,62,73] and to induce regression of proliferative diabetic retinopathy.[26,28,35,36,44,58,61]

In North America, pituitary-ablation treatment is no longer in common use. In the case of metastatic breast carcinoma, for example, modern antiestrogenic drugs are now available for selective use, guided, in part, by reliable estrogen-receptor classification of tumors. In the case of diabetic retinopathy, pituitary-ablation treatment has also fallen out of favor. Nonetheless, the extensive clinical experience accrued has served to provide considerable information about radiation tolerance of the pituitary gland, parasellar tissues, cranial nerves, and temporal lobes.[65]

Hormone-Dependent Metastatic Carcinoma

Between 1954 and 1972 at UCB–LBL, stereotactically directed plateau beams of protons (initial 26 cases) or helium ions (157 cases) were used for pituitary-ablation treatment in 183 patients with metastatic breast carcinoma.[34] Patients received 180 to 220 Gy stereotactic plateau-beam helium-ion irradiation to the pituitary gland, in order to control the metastatic spread of carcinoma by effecting hormonal suppression through induction of hypopituitarism. The total dose was given in six to eight fractions over 2 to 3 weeks in the early years of the clinical program and in three or four fractions over 5 days in later years. Each dose fraction consisted of 30 to 50 Gy. Many patients experienced long-term remissions. Eight cases of focal radiation necrosis limited to the adjacent portion of the temporal lobe occurred; all were from an earlier group of patients who had received higher doses to suppress pituitary function as rapidly as possible.[56] Clinical manifestations of temporal lobe injury and transient cranial nerve involvement occurred in only four of these patients.

Minakova et al.[48,62] have reported excellent results following stereotactic plateau-beam proton radiosurgery at ITEP in a series of 489 patients with metastatic breast carcinoma and in a series of 92 patients with metastatic prostate carcinoma (Minakova YeI: Personal communication). Konnov et al.[28] have also reported excellent clinical results in breast carcinoma patients treated with 120 to 180 Gy plateau-beam proton radiosurgery at INPh. In a series of 91 patients with bone metastases, 93 percent had relief of pain following treatment. Of 45 patients treated for metastatic disease

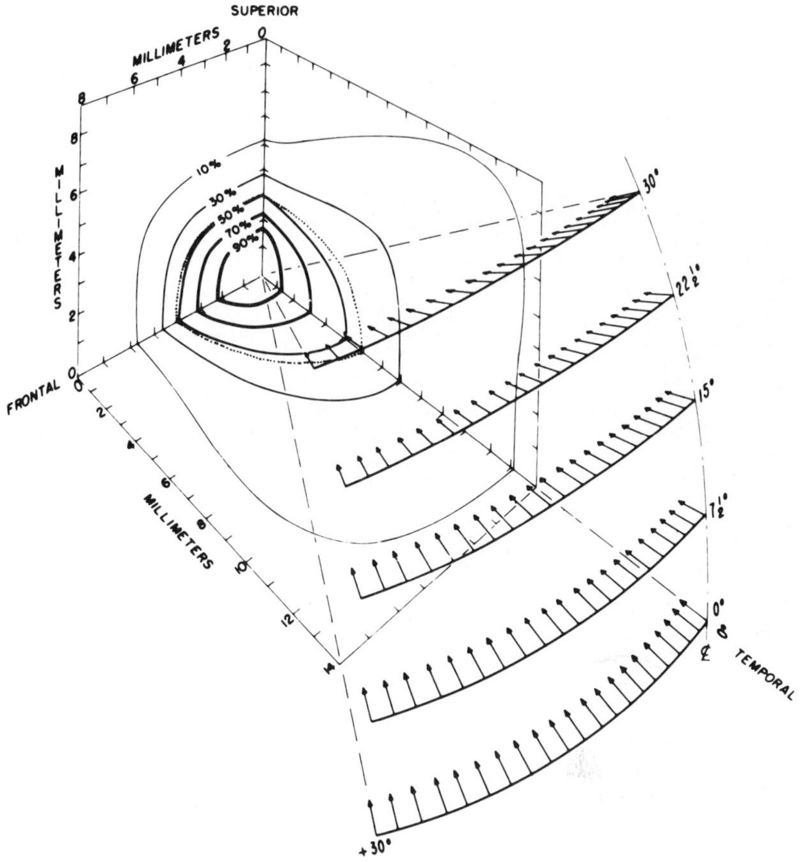

Figure 184-11 Three-dimensional isodose contours for one octant of the radiation field used to treat pituitary adenomas at the UCB-LBL 184-inch synchrocyclotron. Stereotactic irradiation is performed with the plateau-ionization portion of the 230-MeV/U helium-ion beam. The dose fall-off from 90 percent to 10 percent occurs in less than 4 mm in the frontal plane. The technique produces very favorable dose distributions for the treatment of small intracranial lesions.

with combined medical therapy and proton-beam hypophysectomy, 20 had no signs of recurrence or metastases after a follow-up period of 2 to 6 years. Kjellberg et al. have used Bragg-peak proton-beam therapy of the pituitary to treat 31 patients with metastatic breast cancer at HCL–MGH (Kjellberg RN: Personal communication).

Diabetic Retinopathy

Between 1958 and 1969 at UCB–LBL, 169 patients with proliferative diabetic retinopathy received stereotactic plateau-beam helium-ion pituitary irradiation. This procedure was performed to evaluate the effects of pituitary hormonal suppression on proliferative diabetic retinopathy. [Earlier reports had suggested that surgical hypophysectomy resulted in regression of proliferative retinopathy in many diabetic patients, a phenomenon suspected to be related to decreased insulin requirements and lowered growth hormone (GH) levels.[50]] The first 30 patients in this cohort were treated with 160 to 320 Gy delivered in six to eight fractions (27 to 50 Gy per fraction) over 11 days to effect total pituitary ablation; the subsequent 139 patients underwent subtotal pituitary ablation with 80 to 150 Gy. Most patients had a 15 to 50 percent decrease in insulin requirements; this result occurred sooner in patients receiving higher doses, but ultimately both patient groups had comparable insulin requirements. Fasting GH levels and reserves were lowered within several months after irradiation. Moderate to good vision was preserved in at least one eye in 59 of 114 patients at 5 years after pituitary irradiation (Lawrence JH: Unpublished). Of 169 patients treated, 69 patients (41 percent) ultimately required thyroid replacement and 46 patients (27 percent) required adrenal hormone replacement. There were four deaths from complications of hypopituitarism. Focal temporal lobe injury was limited to an early group of patients that had received at least 230 Gy to effect rapid pituitary ablation in advanced disease; four patients in this high-dose group developed extraocular palsies. Neurological injury was rare in those patients receiving doses less than 230 Gy (Lawrence JH: Unpublished data).

In a series of 25 patients treated with 100 to 120 Gy plateau-beam proton radiosurgery, Konnov et al.[28] found that those with higher visual acuity and without proliferative changes in the fundus had stabilization and regression of retinopathy after treatment; microaneurysms were decreased and visual acuity was stabilized or improved. However, patients with poor visual acuity and progressive proliferative retinopathy responded less favorably. A reduction in insulin requirements was observed in all patients. Kjellberg et al.[26] reported comparable results following stereotactic Bragg-peak proton radiosurgery in 183 patients.

Histopathologic Studies

Histopathologic observations on autopsies from early patients, who had received helium-ion pituitary irradiation for hormonal suppression of metastatic breast carcinoma, confirmed that more than 95 percent of pituitary cells were destroyed and replaced with connective tissue in a period of several months with doses of 180 to 220 Gy delivered in 2 or 3 weeks total time (Fig. 184-12).[56,77] At lower doses, the magnitude of the histologic effect depended on the dose at the periphery of the pituitary gland, where viable hormone-secreting cells were usually found.

Woodruff et al.[77] performed autopsies on 15 patients who had been treated with stereotactic plateau-beam helium-ion irradiation of the pituitary gland at UCB–LBL. Ten of these patients had been

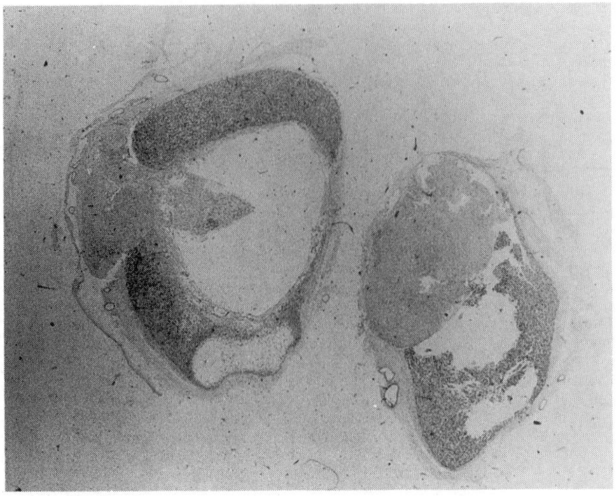

Figure 184-12 Autopsy specimen of the pituitary gland of a patient with metastatic breast carcinoma 14 years after stereotactic helium-ion radiosurgery performed for hormonal suppression. The central coagulative necrosis and the sharply defined peripheral rim of functioning pituitary gland are seen. (From Fabrikant et al.,[15] with permission.)

treated for progressive diabetic retinopathy with average doses of 116 Gy delivered in six fractions. All cases demonstrated pituitary fibrosis without radiation changes in the surrounding brain tissue or cranial nerves.

Pituitary Adenomas

Since 1958, more than 2000 patients worldwide with pituitary adenomas have been treated with charged-particle irradiation of the pituitary gland as a primary noninvasive treatment, as adjunctive radiotherapy for incomplete operative resection and/or medical therapy, and as treatment for late recurrences after surgery.[25,27,28,33,43,45,51,60] Charged-particle radiosurgery has been applied to the treatment of acromegaly, Cushing's disease, Nelson's syndrome, and prolactin-secreting tumors, as well as to the treatment of nonfunctioning and selected other adenomas.

Prior to the introduction of transsphenoidal microsurgery, surgical hypophysectomy was often associated with high morbidity and mortality, and charged-particle radiosurgery was considered to be an excellent alternative treatment. With the development of safe and effective transsphenoidal techniques, the extensive clinical use of primary radiosurgical treatment, concentrated for many years in the UCB–LBL and HCL–MGH programs, has decreased significantly. Currently, primary radiosurgery for treatment of microadenomas is most often limited to patients who are considered to be poor surgical candidates or who have refused surgery. Proton-beam radiosurgery, however, remains as a primary therapeutic procedure for treatment of pituitary tumors in Russia.[28,37,51,59,60] The charged-particle radiosurgical approach is now being applied mostly as adjunctive therapy in combination with microsurgery, where complete removal of large adenomas is not possible, or for recurrences of tumor growth.

The therapeutic goals in the primary radiosurgical treatment of pituitary adenomas are control of tumor growth and hormonal hypersecretion, with acceptably low hormonal and neurological complications. These goals have been met with remarkable success over the past 35 years, especially considering the limitations of the available neuroradiologic imaging methods during the early years of these investigations. (The great majority of patients were treated before the advent of CT and MRI, and adenoma assessment and target-volume determination, therefore, relied on relatively crude neuroradiologic procedures such as polytomography and pneumoencephalography.) The clinical and metabolic follow-up data describing the response of pituitary adenomas to charged-particle radiosurgery have been reported extensively; the reader is referred to the work of Fabrikant and Levy[14] and Levy et al.[39] for more-detailed reviews. In this section, the emphasis is limited to selected clinical studies and complications of treatment.

Acromegaly

At UCB–LBL, stereotactic helium-ion plateau-beam radiosurgery has proved to be very effective for the treatment of acromegaly in 318 patients.[31,33,43] The maximum dose to the pituitary tumor ranged from 30 to 50 Gy, most often delivered in four fractions over 5 days. The choice of dose varied according to the extent of disease and the corresponding size of the target volume. Maximum pituitary doses were selected so that the cortex of the temporal lobes received no more than 15 Gy. As the dose fell off rapidly from the central axis, the dose to the periphery of larger tumors was considerably less than the peripheral dose to smaller ones. A sustained decrease in serum GH secretion was observed in most patients; the mean serum GH level in a cohort of 234 of these patients decreased nearly 70 percent within 1 year and continued to decrease thereafter (Fig. 184-13). Normal levels were sustained during more than 10 years of follow-up. Comparable long-term results were observed in a cohort of 65 patients who were irradiated with helium ions because of residual or recurrent metabolic abnormalities persisting after surgical hypophysectomy. Serial GH levels were examined before and after helium-ion irradiation as a function of neurosurgical grade. Statistically significant differences ($P < 0.01$) in fasting GH existed only between the microadenoma patients with normal sellar volumes (Hardy's grade I[21]) and patients with macroadenomas (grades II through IV).[43] Grade I patients had lower initial GH levels, responded more rapidly to treatment, and had a good prognosis for cure; a lower incidence of post-treatment hypopituitarism was also observed in these patients. The more-invasive tumors were slower to respond, but by 4 years after irradiation they were associated with GH levels not statistically different from levels found in patients with grade I tumors. Clinical and metabolic improvement (e.g., improved glucose tolerance, normalization of serum phosphorus levels) was observed in most patients within the first year, even before a significant fall in serum GH level was noted.

Treatment failures following helium-ion irradiation generally resulted from failure to assess accurately the degree of extrasellar tumor extension.[33,43] With recent advances in MRI and CT scanning, the radiosurgical target can now be better delineated, which in turn should lead to improved rates of tumor cure and control. These same imaging improvements also make possible more reliable determination of tissue inhomogeneities in the brain and adjacent tissues and correspondingly more precise positioning of the Bragg ionization peak within the target volume.[19,39]

Kjellberg et al.[25,27] have treated about 600 patients with acromegaly using Bragg-peak proton irradiation at HCL–MGH. Using a nomogram based on lesion size and complication rate in a large number of treated patients, doses selected are inversely related to the beam diameter; intrasellar tumors typically receive maximal

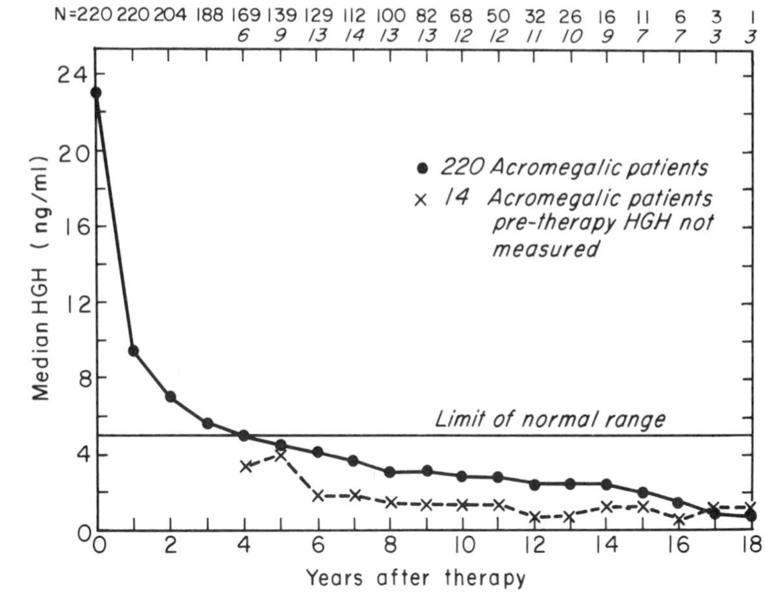

Figure 184-13 Median plasma human growth hormone (hGH; HGH) levels in 234 patients with acromegaly treated with stereotactic plateau-beam helium-ion radiosurgery. The numbers of patients used to calculate the median plasma levels before radiosurgery and for each time interval thereafter are shown at the top of the graph. Fourteen patients did not have pretreatment hGH measurements, but their hGH levels measured 4 to 18 years after radiosurgery were comparable with those of the other 220 patients. The 20 patients in the series who subsequently underwent pituitary surgery or additional pituitary irradiation were included until the time of the second procedure.

central doses of 60 to 120 Gy. Selected adenomas with extrasellar extension are treated using a "beam-within-a-beam" technique; here, a subnecrotizing dose (e.g., 10 Gy) is given to the larger overall target volume, and an additional necrotizing dose (e.g., 35 Gy) is given to the smaller infraclinoid volume. Therapy has resulted in objective clinical improvement in about 90 percent of a cohort of 145 patients 24 months after irradiation. By this time, 60 percent of patients were in remission (GH level ≤10 ng/ml); after 48 months, 80 percent were in remission. About 10 percent of patients failed to enter remission or to improve, and they required additional treatment (usually transsphenoidal hypophysectomy).

Another approach under consideration for the charged-particle-irradiation treatment of invasive macroadenomas is the use of more extended fractionation schedules. Historically, stereotactic irradiation regimens have not been designed to exploit the differential response between normal cells and tumor cells that is the biological basis for the use of fractionated external-beam irradiation.[41] With the development of stereotactic immobilization systems capable of reliable serial repositioning, this approach offers the potential for improved treatment outcome by combining the excellent dose-localization and dose-distribution characteristics of charged-particle irradiation with the favorable radiobiological properties of fractionated irradiation.

In the Russian experience, plateau-beam proton radiosurgery has also proved successful for treatment of acromegalic tumors. Minakova et al.[60] reported excellent results in 93 patients with acromegaly treated at ITEP. Konnov et al.[28] observed partial or total remission in 89 percent of 145 patients treated with doses of 100 to 120 Gy at the INPh.

Cushing's Disease

Cushing's disease has been treated successfully at UCB–LBL using stereotactic helium-ion plateau-beam irradiation.[33,43,45] In 83 patients (aged 17 to 78 years) treated, mean basal cortisol levels in a cohort of 44 patients and urinary fluorogenic corticosteroids in a cohort of 37 patients returned to normal values within 1 year after treatment, and these indices remained normal during more than 10 years of follow-up (Fig. 184-14). All five teenage patients were

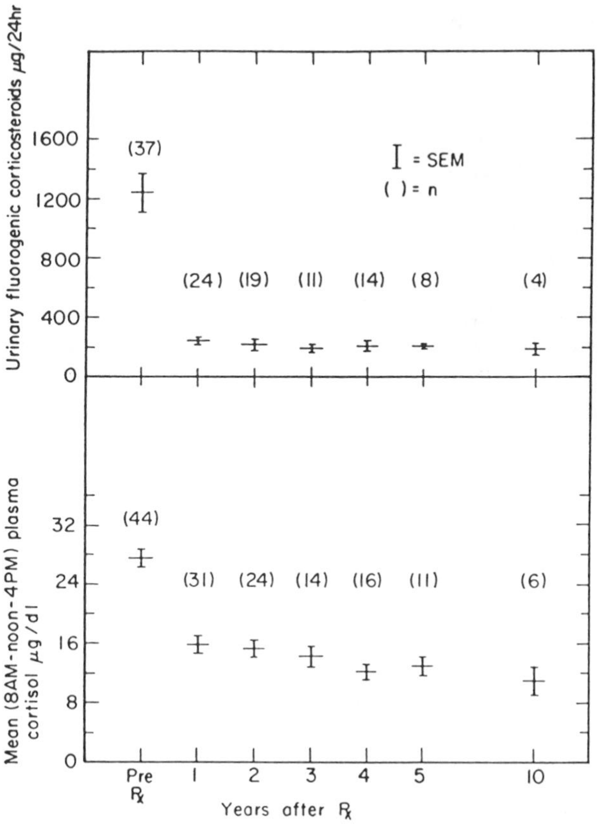

Figure 184-14 Pre- and post-treatment levels (mean ±SEM) of urinary fluorogenic corticosteroids (*top*) and plasma cortisol (*bottom*) are shown for Cushing's disease patients treated with helium-ion radiosurgery. Normal levels of plasma and urinary cortisols were achieved 1 year after treatment and these levels were maintained for at least 10 years follow-up. The number of patients studied at each time is shown in parentheses. (From Linfoot,[43] with permission.)

cured by doses of 60 to 120 Gy without concomitant hypopituitarism or neurological sequelae; however, 9 of 59 older patients subsequently underwent bilateral adrenalectomy or surgical hypophysectomy because of relapse or failure to respond to treatment. Of the nine treatment failures, seven occurred in the earlier group of 22 patients treated with 60 to 150 Gy in six alternate-day fractions; when the same total doses were given in three or four daily fractions, 40 of 42 patients were cured.[43]

Kjellberg et al. have treated more than 175 Cushing's disease patients with Bragg-peak proton-beam irradiation at HCL–MGH.[25] Doses are inversely related to the beam diameter selected (typically, 60 to 120 Gy). Complete remission with restoration of normal clinical and laboratory findings has occurred in about 65 percent of a cohort of patients followed-up for 24 months; another 20 percent were improved to the extent that no further treatment was considered necessary.

Minakova et al.[58,60] have reported excellent results in 224 Cushing's disease patients treated with plateau-beam proton radiosurgery at ITEP. Konnov et al.[28] have reported that plateau-beam proton radiosurgery (doses, 100 to 120 Gy) has induced partial or total remission in 34 of 37 patients who were followed 6 to 15 months after treatment.

Nelson's Syndrome

Plateau-beam helium-ion radiosurgery has been used at UCB–LBL in 17 patients with Nelson's syndrome.[33,43] Treatment doses and fractionation schedules were comparable to those for the Cushing's disease group, i.e., 50 to 150 Gy in four fractions. Six patients had prior pituitary surgery, but persistent tumor or elevated serum-ACTH levels indicated that further treatment was required. All patients in the Nelson's syndrome group had marked decreases in ACTH levels, but rarely to normal levels. All but one patient, however, had neuroradiologic evidence of local tumor control.

Kjellberg and Kliman[25] reported similar findings in patients treated with Bragg-peak proton irradiation. Of a cohort of 19 patients treated, 12 of 14 patients experienced some depigmentation following treatment; headache was reduced or eliminated in 8 of 11 patients. ACTH levels were decreased in all four patients for whom data were available, but levels became normal in only one patient.

Prolactin-Secreting Adenomas

Twenty-nine patients with prolactin-secreting pituitary tumors were treated at UCB–LBL using stereotactic plateau-beam helium-ion radiosurgery.[31,43] Treatment dose and fractionation were comparable to those used for the Cushing's disease and Nelson's syndrome groups, i.e., 50 to 150 Gy in four fractions. Helium-ion irradiation was the sole treatment in 17 patients; the remaining patients were irradiated after surgical hypophysectomy had failed to provide complete or permanent improvement. Of 20 patients followed 1 year after irradiation, 19 had a marked fall in prolactin level (12 to normal levels) (Fig. 184-15). Amenorrhea and galactorrhea often resolved before prolactin levels returned to normal.[43] Two patients became pregnant after treatment.

Konnov et al.[28] have reported partial or total remission in about 85 percent of patients with prolactin-secreting tumors treated with plateau-beam proton radiosurgery (doses, 100 to 120 Gy) at INPh. Excellent clinical results have also been reported in 75 patients treated with plateau-beam proton radiosurgery at ITEP (Minakova YeI: Personal communication), and in 132 patients treated with Bragg-peak proton therapy at the HCL–MGH (Kjellberg RN: Personal communication).

Complications

Variable degrees of hypopituitarism developed as sequelae of attempts at subtotal destruction of pituitary function in about one-third of the patients following stereotactic helium-ion plateau-beam radiosurgery, although endocrine deficiencies were rapidly corrected in most cases with appropriate hormonal replacement therapy.[43,65] Retrospectively, it seems likely that, in many cases, larger portions of the pituitary gland had to be designated for radiosurgical treatment to ensure sufficient dose to the adenoma than would now be indicated based on current MRI and CT techniques. Diabetes insipidus has not been observed in any pituitary patient treated with helium-ion irradiation.[43] Other than hormonal insufficiency, complications in the pituitary tumor patients treated with helium-ion plateau radiosurgery were relatively few and limited most frequently to those patients who had received prior photon

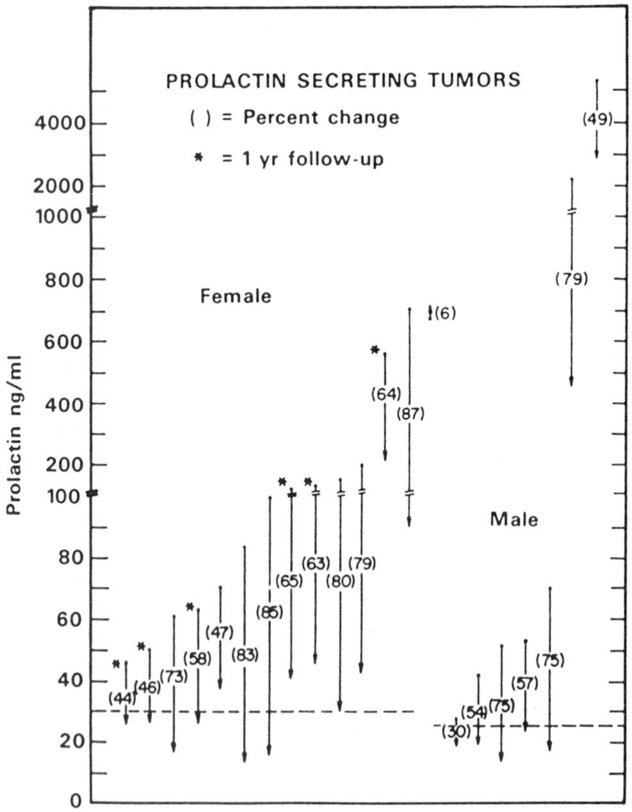

Figure 184-15 Fasting plasma prolactin levels are shown before treatment and 1 year following helium-ion radiosurgery for females (*left*) and males (*right*) with prolactin-secreting tumors. A marked decrease in prolactin, usually to normal levels (*dashed line*), was observed in many patients at 1 year (*) post-treatment. Percent change is shown in parentheses. (From Linfoot,[43] with permission.)

irradiation. These sequelae included mild or transient extraocular nerve palsies, partial visual field deficits, and seizures due to limited temporal lobe injury.[43,56,65] There were very few significant complications after the initial high-dose group of patients. After appropriate adjustments of dose schedules based on this early experience, focal temporal lobe necrosis and transient cranial nerve injury have been rare sequelae, in the range of 1 percent or less, and no other permanent therapeutic sequelae have occurred. A very low incidence of significant adverse sequelae has also been reported in patients treated with Bragg-peak proton irradiation at HCL–MGH and ITEP and with plateau-beam proton irradiation at INPh.[25,28]

Other Benign Tumors

Charged-particle irradiation has been applied to the treatment of a variety of benign intracranial tumors, including meningiomas, acoustic neuromas, and craniopharyngiomas.[39] Selection criteria, treatment parameters, and long-term clinical results in most cases have not yet been clearly defined. More-detailed follow-up evaluation is available for selected cohorts of patients with meningiomas.

Luchin et al.[49] used proton-beam irradiation (two to four fractions; plateau-beam or Bragg-peak method) to treat 52 patients with cavernous sinus meningiomas. Maximum central doses of 50 to 70 Gy were used. With mean follow-up of 40.6 months (range, 13 to 77 months), local control was obtained in 84 percent of patients; five patients with inadequate dose distribution in the tumor volume exhibited continued tumor growth.

Excellent local control has also been reported in patients treated with conventionally fractionated helium-ion irradiation for sphenoid ridge meningioma, where the optic nerves and/or chiasm were considered critical dose-limiting tissues. Tumor doses ranged from 53 to 80 gray-equivalents (GyE) (mean, 63.5 GyE) (Castro JR: Personal communication). The local control rate (minimum follow-up of 2 years) in a series of 24 patients was 88 percent; the 3-year Kaplan-Meier actuarial survival was 87 percent. This series includes patients with partially unresectable lesions or gross recurrences. While the range of follow-up extends to more than 8 years in some patients, the only failures occurred within 36 months of therapy in several early patients accepted for treatment with massive recurrent lesions. Treatment tolerance has been excellent.

Malignant Gliomas

Malignant gliomas are among the human tumors that respond relatively poorly to conventional megavoltage irradiation. Treatment failures in resistant tumors can often be attributed, at least in part, to two factors: (1) tumor-dose limitations imposed by tolerance of adjacent normal tissues; and (2) intrinsic radioresistance of the tumor. Neon-ion irradiation has been proposed as a solution to both problems.[46,71] Neon-ion beams have the favorable dose-distribution characteristics of lighter charged-particle beams (see the section on "Physical Properties of Charged-Particle Beams"), as well as the increased relative biological effectiveness (RBE) associated with high linear energy transfer (LET). High-LET radiations include neutrons, pions, and heavier-charged particles (e.g., neon ions). The dense ionization in tissue associated with these particles gives rise to several radiobiological properties of potential value for the treatment of selected malignancies resistant to low-LET irradiation with protons and photons.[3,8,65,71] These properties include (1) improved oxygen enhancement ratio, i.e., reduction of the radioresistance typical of hypoxic tumor cells; (2) decreased variation in the cell-cycle-specific radiosensitivity of tumor cells; (3) reduced ability of irradiated cells to repair potentially lethal and sublethal damage; and (4) diminished radioresistance attributable to cell-density or cell-contact effects. The increased RBE of high-LET radiation has been demonstrated by decreased cell survival in cultured mammalian cells and by reduced repair of radiation damage in vitro and in vivo.

The role of neon-ion irradiation in the treatment of malignant glioma is as yet undefined, and outcomes have thus far not been better than those obtained with conventional irradiation. Preliminary studies have been limited to 16 patients treated with fractionated Bragg-peak neon-ion irradiation at the UCB–LBL Bevatron.[8,46] Because of limited availability of the neon-ion beam, most patients received mixed-beam treatments combining neon, helium, and photon irradiation to bring total tumor doses to prescribed levels. Doses were calculated as gray-equivalent (GyE), using experimentally derived RBE factors that accounted for fraction size, type of tissue irradiated, beam energy, Bragg-peak width, and biological endpoint chosen.[46] In this formulation, neon RBE values ranged from 2.0 to 3.5, and helium RBE values ranged from 1.2 to 1.4.

Nine patients with glioblastoma (GBM) and seven with anaplastic astrocytoma (AA) received total equivalent doses ranging from 48.0 to 69.0 GyE (median, 49.3 GyE), with neon physical doses ranging from 13.8 to 25.0 Gy (median, 18.6 Gy).[46] Follow-up ranged from 3 to 77 months. Local control was obtained in only one patient (with GBM), who died 31 months after treatment. The only patient surviving at the time of analysis had developed local recurrence of AA 25 months following treatment. Two patients treated solely with neon for GBM developed fatal radiation necrosis. One had received 54.4 GyE (assumed RBE, 2.43); the other patient died from combined local failure and brain necrosis (48.0 GyE; assumed RBE, 2.98). Although the acute skin reaction in each case was consistent with these assumed RBE values, the RBE for late brain necrosis was revised upward to a range of 4.0 to 4.5. It remains uncertain whether the potential benefits of high-LET irradiation for malignant gliomas will be realized.

Vascular Malformations and Carotid-Cavernous Fistulae

More than 2000 patients worldwide since 1965 have been treated with charged-particle radiosurgery for vascular malformations of the brain, primarily at UCB–LBL,[16–18,38,42,66–68] HCL–MGH,[22–24] ITEP,[58,59,61] and INPh.[28,29,57] Between 1980 and 1992, we treated 426 patients with intracranial vascular malformations using helium-ion beams, initially at the UCB–LBL 184-inch synchrocyclotron and subsequently at the UCB–LBL Bevatron. This total includes 379 patients with angiographically demonstrable AVMs and 47 patients with AOVMs. The therapeutic goals of radiosurgery for the treatment of AVMs are to achieve (1) reduction or elimination of intracranial hemorrhage; (2) stabilization or reversal of progressive neurological dysfunction; (3) lower frequency of seizures; and (4) improvement in frequency and intensity of headaches. In this section, we describe the methods of patient selection and evaluation, and clinical and neuroradiologic outcome and complications in a cohort of 86 consecutive patients with angiographically demonstrable AVMs, who were treated between 1983 and 1988 through the collaborative LBL–SUMC radiosurgery program.[66] The results of other programs using proton radiosurgery for treatment of AVMs and carotid-cavernous fistulae are then discussed briefly, as is our experience with the helium-ion treatment of AOVMs.

Arteriovenous Malformations: Berkeley–Stanford Series

Patient Selection In the LBL–SUMC patient series,[66] there were 47 females and 39 males, ranging in age at the time of treatment from 9 to 69 years (mean, 33 years). Many patients presented with more than one symptom; 60 had experienced hemorrhage, 11 had neurological deficits unassociated with hemorrhage, 35 had seizures, and 40 had headaches. Sixty patients (70 percent) were graded clinically (using the Drake[13] neurosurgical scale) as *excellent* before radiosurgery, 24 (28 percent) as *good,* and two (2 percent) as *poor.* Prior to radiosurgery, 17 patients had undergone partial resection of their AVMs, 7 had had flow-directed embolization, and 5 had had both embolization and surgery. Nearly half of these patients (44 percent) had AVMs located in the brain stem, corpus callosum, thalamus, or basal ganglia, and most of the remainder had large malformations in critical areas of the cerebrum—the sensory, motor, language, or visual areas of the cortex. Using *angiographic-volume* criteria (the volume of the parallelepiped enclosing the AVM target volume delineated on orthogonal stereotactic cerebral angiograms), the preradiosurgical volumes of the malformations were 0.33 to 288 cc; 25 percent of AVMs were larger than 25 cc.

Clinical Follow-Up and Outcome Clinical evaluation, performed 24 to 72 months (mean, 38 months) after radiosurgery, found that 63 percent of patients presenting with seizures and 68 percent of patients presenting with headaches had improvement of these symptoms.[66] Of 11 patients presenting with progressive neurological deficits unrelated to hemorrhage, there was improvement in 3 patients and stabilization of neurological status in 6 patients. The mechanisms underlying the observed improvements in seizure activity and headache syndromes and the stabilization or improvement of progressive nonhemorrhagic neurological dysfunction following radiosurgery are poorly understood. These changes seem to be associated, in large measure, however, with improved regional cerebral blood flow, stabilization of hemodynamic imbalance, and reversal of vascular steal associated with progressive thrombosis of the malformation.[16,66] Table 184-1 shows the distribution of clinical grades for patients before radiosurgery and at most recent follow-up. Clinical outcome was *excellent* in 58 percent and *good* in 36 percent of all patients in the series.

Neuroradiologic Response Cerebral angiography was performed at yearly intervals to evaluate postradiosurgical changes. In general, the observed patterns of response can be summarized as follows: (1) after a variable latency period, the likelihood of achieving complete AVM obliteration increases progressively over a period of about 3 years; (2) the probabilities of eventual AVM obliteration and adverse treatment sequelae both increase as the radiation dose increases; (3) the entire AVM must be thrombosed to achieve an optimal clinical outcome; and (4) favorable response is achieved more readily with smaller lesions. The first hemodynamic changes observed include a decrease in blood flow through the AVM, probably due to progressive obliteration of the small shunting vessels, with a decrease in size of the feeding arteries and draining veins. This stage is followed by a progressive decrease in the AVM volume until stabilization or complete obliteration of the AVM occurs. Many uncertainties remain regarding optimal radiosurgical treatment parameters for malformations of various sizes and locations in the brain[16,66] and the evolving role of embolization and/or microsurgery in combination with charged-particle radiosurgery.[55,68]

The angiographic results 2 years after radiosurgery (Table 184-2) indicate that complete obliteration of the AVM occurred in 70 percent, partial obliteration (10 to 99 percent obliteration) in 23 percent, and no change in 7 percent. By 3 years after treatment, 90 percent of patients had complete AVM obliteration, 6 percent had partial obliteration, and 4 percent had no change. The rate and extent of obliteration appear to be threshold phenomena directly related to the AVM volume and the radiation dose. Smaller AVMs

TABLE 184-1 Clinical Outcome in 86 Patients with Arteriovenous Malformations after Stereotactic Radiosurgery

	Before Treatment		After Treatment	
Overall Outcome	**n**	**(%)**	**n**	**(%)**
*Grade**				
Excellent	60	(70)	50	(58)
Good	24	(28)	31	(36)
Poor	2	(2)	2	(2)
Dead			3	(3)

Source: Adapted from Steinberg et al.[66]
*Drake[13] neurosurgical scale.

TABLE 184-2 Number of Patients with Angiographically Detectable Obliteration of Their Arteriovenous Malformations after Stereotactic Radiosurgery, According to Volume of AVM before Treatment

	Degree of Obliteration						
	Complete		Partial†		No Change		Total
Volume (cc)*	**n**	**(%)**	**n**	**(%)**	**n**	**(%)**	**n**
After 1 year (11–13 months)							
<4	9	(53)	7	(41)	1	(6)	17
4–25	7	(29)	12	(50)	5	(21)	24
>25	1	(6)	15	(83)	2	(11)	18
All	17	(29)	34	(58)	8	(13)	59
After 2 years (24–27 months)							
<4	17	(94)	1	(6)	0		18
4–25	15	(75)	3	(15)	2	(10)	20
>25	8	(42)	9	(47)	2	(11)	19
All	40	(70)	13	(23)	4	(7)	57
After >3 years (>36 months)							
<4	18	(100)	0		0		18
4–25	19	(95)	0		1	(5)	20
>25	11	(73)	3	(20)	1	(7)	15
All	48	(90)	3	(6)	2	(4)	53

Source: Adapted from Steinberg et al.[66]
*A 4-cc volume equals a sphere approximately 2.0 cm in diameter; a 25-cc volume equals a sphere approximately 3.7 cm in diameter.
†Denotes a 10 to 99 percent reduction in volume as detected angiographically.

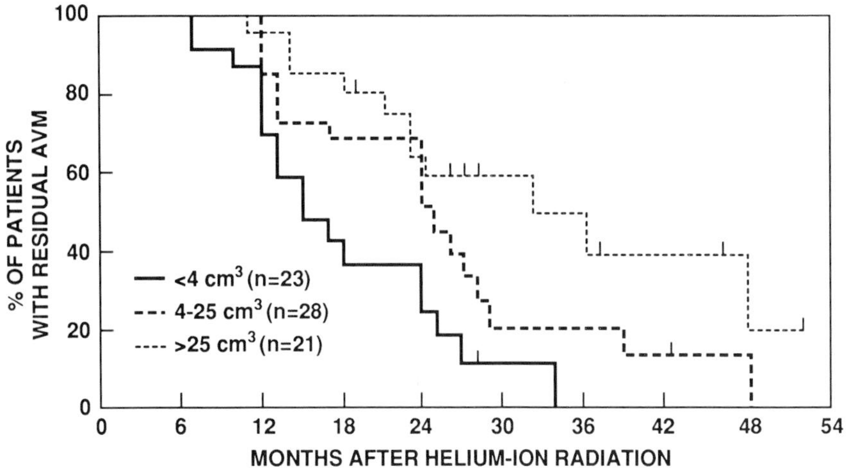

Figure 184-16 Kaplan–Meier cumulative plots illustrate the temporal pattern of complete AVM obliteration as a function of AVM size prior to helium-ion radiosurgery in 71 patients with angiographic follow-up. *Solid line,* pretreatment angiographic volumes <4 cc (23 patients); *dashed line,* volumes 4 to 25 cc (28 patients); *dotted line,* volumes >25 cc (20 patients). *Vertical lines* represent patients with residual AVM. The smallest lesions obliterate most frequently and with the shortest latency intervals. (From Steinberg et al.,[68] with permission.)

had higher rates of obliteration than larger ones ($P < 0.005$ after 1 and 2 years, Mann–Whitney test). AVMs smaller than 4 cc thrombosed more rapidly and more completely than larger lesions ($P < 0.05$ for the comparison with AVMs 4 to 25 cc in volume and $P < 0.001$ for the comparison with those >25 cc, Cox test) (Fig. 184-16). Intermediate-sized AVMs were obliterated more rapidly and more completely than large AVMs ($P < 0.05$, Cox test).

Complete obliteration occurred more frequently in malformations treated with higher doses (30 to 45 GyE) ($P < 0.05$ after 1 and 2 years, Mann–Whitney test) (Table 184-3). AVMs treated with intermediate doses (24 to 28 GyE) also responded well at 2 and 3 years. Preliminary results with the lowest-dose group (11.5 to 20 GyE) were encouraging after 3 years follow-up, but thus far the number of patients in this group is too small to permit firm conclusions.

TABLE 184-3 Number of Patients with Angiographically Detectable Obliteration of Their Arteriovenous Malformations after Stereotactic Radiosurgery, According to Treatment Dose

	Degree of Obliteration						
	Complete		Partial†		No Change		Total
Dose (GyE)*	n	(%)	n	(%)	n	(%)	n
After 1 year (11–13 months)							
11.5–20	3	(17)	10	(56)	5	(27)	18
24–28	5	(20)	18	(72)	2	(8)	25
30–45	9	(56)	6	(38)	1	(6)	16
After 2 years (24–27 months)							
11.5–20	6	(50)	4	(33)	2	(17)	12
24–28	18	(67)	8	(29)	1	(4)	27
30–45	16	(89)	1	(6)	1	(6)	18
After >3 years (>36 months)							
11.5–20	8	(100)	0		0		8
24–28	20	(87)	2	(9)	1	(4)	23
30–45	20	(95)	0		1	(5)	21

Source: Adapted from Steinberg et al.[66]
* 1 GyE equals physical dose in Gy (100 rad) multiplied by a relative biological effectiveness of 1.3 for the Bragg ionization peak of helium ions.
† Denotes a 10 to 99 percent reduction in volume as detected angiographically.

Post-Treatment Hemorrhage Ten of 86 patients (12 percent) have experienced hemorrhage from residual angiographically demonstrable AVMs after radiosurgery, 7 patients during the first year and 3 thereafter.[66] Hemorrhage resulted in permanent new neurological deficits in 3 patients and death in 2 patients; the other 5 patients recovered fully. AVMs in 7 of these 10 patients had bled before treatment. No patients with angiographic evidence of complete obliteration of the malformation experienced hemorrhage subsequently. Until complete obliteration occurs, patients remain at risk; one patient with 95 percent AVM obliteration had a hemorrhage 34 months after treatment.

Complications and Sequelae Serious early sequelae have been negligible following radiosurgery.[16,38,40,66] A few patients with a prior history of seizures had transiently increased seizure activity that was readily controlled by adjustment of anticonvulsant medications. A few patients who presented initially with severe headaches required increased doses of oral analgesics for a few days following treatment. No patients experienced nausea, vomiting, or hyperpyrexia. No deaths have occurred from the irradiation procedure.

Several categories of delayed radiation injury have been observed.[38,40,54,65] On the basis of MRI, CT, angiography, and clinical evaluation, the treatment-associated sequelae can be classified as white matter changes or vasculopathy and include vasogenic edema, occlusion of functional vasculature, and radiation necrosis. The manifestations and incidence of clinical sequelae depend, in part, on the region of the brain involved, the volume of normal and abnormal brain tissue affected, the radiation dose, the presence of prior tissue injury from spontaneous hemorrhage or previous interventional procedures, and the timing and nature of therapeutic measures.

Clinical complications following radiosurgery were most common in patients with AVMs in the brain stem, thalamus, or basal ganglia. About 20 percent of patients (17 of 86) experienced complications between 3 and 38 months after treatment (mean, 13.4 months). Seven patients had minor complications, such as visual field deficit, diplopia, unilateral hearing impairment, slight gait ataxia, or mild paresis; three of them recovered completely and four partially. Ten patients (12 percent) had major complications, including hemiparesis, gait ataxia, cranial nerve palsies, partial aphasia, or hypothalamic syndrome; two recovered fully, seven recovered partially, and one remained unchanged. Some patients had more than one complication. Hemiparesis was the most common major complication and visual field deficit was the most common minor complication.

In about half of all the patients (33 of 65) examined after radiosurgery with MRI and CT, deep-white-matter changes occurred between 4 and 26 months after treatment (mean, 15.3 months); 20 of these patients were asymptomatic. In the 13 patients who were clinically symptomatic, the white-matter changes had MRI and CT patterns consistent with those described following radiation-induced brain injury, viz., abnormal signals on MRI or low attenuation on CT scans. These findings usually were associated with an appreciable amount of cerebral edema. A biopsy of the involved white matter in one patient revealed areas of tissue necrosis. Of 13 symptomatic patients, changes observed on MRI and CT resolved partially in 11 patients, and completely in 2 patients. Radiation-induced vasculopathy occurred in 3 patients and was characterized by arterial stenosis or thrombosis on cerebral angiograms and by MRI and CT changes consistent with cerebral ischemia. Doses ranged from 25 to 45 GyE, delivered to *angiographic volumes* of 0.85 to 40 cc.

Complications were more prevalent with higher doses and larger volumes of treated brain tissue (Fig. 184-17). Among the 20 patients who received doses above 25 GyE and whose angiographic volumes of treated tissue were more than 13 cc, 10 experienced major or minor complications; these represented almost 60 percent of all clinical complications. Complications were limited to the initial 46 patients treated in the higher-dose phase of the dose-searching protocol. None of the 40 patients in the series treated with lower doses in the later phases of the protocol experienced any complications during this last 5-year period since 1986.

Additional Therapy In selected patients in whom radiosurgery has not achieved complete AVM obliteration within 3 years, we have carried out additional treatment with microsurgery, embolization, or both.[55] In three patients who underwent open surgery for residual AVM several years after radiosurgery, we found the AVM to be markedly less vascular and more easily resected than expected had the patient not received radiosurgery. In another patient whose AVM was not obliterated 3 years following radiosurgical treatment, we were able to achieve complete thrombosis of the AVM using endovascular embolization alone. It appears that the small-vessel component of the AVM had likely been obliterated by the radiosurgical treatment, and that embolization-induced occlusion of the limited number of residual fistulae was able to obliterate fully the remaining AVM shunts. Although our experience with helium-ion radiosurgery prior to open microsurgery and embolization is limited, this approach may prove useful in the multistage management of some unusually large and complex AVMs in which complete obliteration has not occurred by 3 years or more.

Partial-Volume Radiosurgery Certain sequelae of the treatment procedure may arise from the hemodynamic alterations of the AVM as it undergoes obliteration.[40] The creation of high-flow shunting within the AVM may increase the probability of intracranial hemorrhage.[47] This is a potential hazard of any incomplete treatment. Undesirable shunts can be created acutely, by subtotal surgical excision or embolization, or subacutely, by limited focal irradiation (*partial-volume radiosurgery*). During the initial phase of our clinical protocol, a selected number of patients with large hemispheric AVMs were treated with stereotactic focal irradiation limited to the earliest-filling component of the arterial phase, that is, the so-called *nidus* of the AVM, rather than the entire angiographic arterial phase, that is, the complete AVM *core*. In many cases, this approach resulted in obliteration of the target volume,

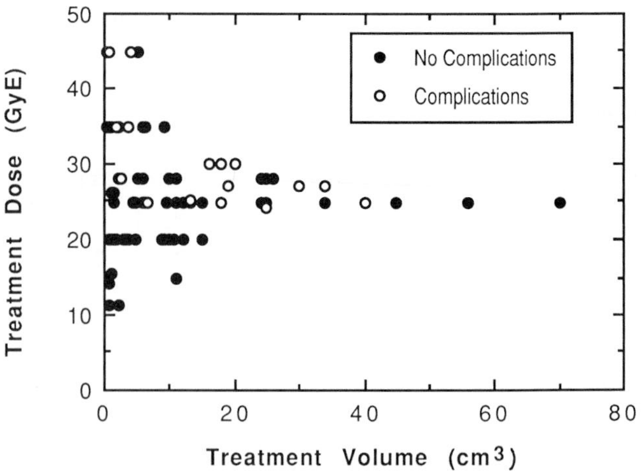

Figure 184-17 The frequency of clinical complications (major and minor) following helium-ion radiosurgery in relation to treatment dose and volume of treated AVM in 86 patients. The maximum doses (*ordinate*) and treatment volumes (*abscissa*) are given; the 90 percent isodose surface was contoured to the periphery of the target volume. Open circles, patients with complications; solid circles, patients with no complications. (Adapted from Steinberg et al.[66])

but the periphery of the malformation was left intact, thereby creating an undesirable shunt with attendant risks of hemorrhage. We no longer consider it acceptable to treat an AVM without encompassing its entire arterial phase with a homogeneous dose distribution. Those patients whose initial radiosurgical treatment failed to meet these criteria are re-evaluated and given additional treatment if residual AVM shunts persist.

Arteriovenous Malformations: Other Series

Kjellberg and associates[22–24] have used single-fraction Bragg-peak proton (160 MeV) therapy at HCL–MGH to treat more than 1300 patients with vascular malformations of the brain (Kjellberg RN: Personal communication). Irradiation generally is delivered with parallel opposed treatment fields. Doses (typically, 10 to 50 Gy) are selected according to diameter of the AVM, using a nomogram based on lesion size and complication rate in a large number of treated patients.[24] Findings of follow-up evaluation in 1000 patients with AVMs, 2 to 24 years after treatment with proton-beam therapy, have been reported.[23] In 104 patients, the clinical outcome was unrelated to hemorrhage or proton-beam therapy. Of the remaining 896 patients, 818 (91.3 percent) were the same or improved as compared to their neurological status at the time of treatment; 27 (3 percent) had moderate deficits from hemorrhage or proton-beam therapy but functioned independently at pretreatment levels; seven (0.8 percent) had severe deficits and were dependent to varying degrees; two (0.2 percent) were vegetative; 39 (4.4 percent) were dead (37 from hemorrhage and two from treatment complications); three (0.3 percent) were lost to follow-up after surviving hemorrhage.[23] Analysis by actuarial life-table methods showed 98.4 percent 24-year survival for patients with AVMs $\leq$3 cm in diameter and 93 percent 24-year survival for all patients[23]; these data were contrasted to a 24-year survival of 77 percent reported for an untreated historical control group. Of the 37 patients who died from hemorrhage, 22 died within the first 2 years after treatment; 33 lethal hemorrhages occurred in patients with AVMs >3 cm in diameter. An additional 101 patients survived hemorrhage, including the three above-mentioned patients who were lost to follow-up. Complications of treatment occurred in 17 patients (6 months to 6.5 years after treatment), but only seven were in the last 925 patients following downward adjustments in treatment doses. In general, treatment doses used in this patient series were significantly lower than those used in the LBL–SUMC series described above.

Minakova and colleagues[58,59,61] have used Bragg-peak proton radiosurgery at ITEP in 66 patients with AVMs (Minakova YeI: Personal communication). The Bragg-peak is spread to a width of 15 to 25 mm as required; seven or eight beam ports are used. Single-fraction maximum doses of 30 to 50 Gy are used, depending on the size and location of the AVM; the periphery of the lesion is treated to the 50 percent isodose. Of 28 patients followed-up angiographically for 2 years after treatment, 71 percent demonstrated total or partial obliteration. Two patients sustained hemorrhage within the first year after treatment. Two patients experienced neurological sequelae with corresponding CT findings of edema, the onset occurring in one patient at 22 months, and in the other, 18 months after radiosurgery (dose, 50 Gy; beam diameter, 20 mm). Both patients responded well to brief courses of high-dose steroids.

Konnov and co-workers[28,57] have used plateau-beam proton radiosurgery at INPh to treat 187 patients with AVMs and 6 patients with arterial aneurysms (Konnov BA: Personal communication). Of the first 148 AVM patients treated, embolization and partial surgical excision were performed in 18 patients and 16 patients, respectively. Using isocentrically directed converging irradiation arcs, maximal doses of 40 to 80 Gy were delivered to diameters of 5 to 10 mm; the irradiated-field size was defined by the extent of the 50 percent isodose contour.[28] Larger AVMs were treated with two isocenters. Five patients died from recurrent hemorrhage during the first year. Angiographic follow-up 1 to 8 years after treatment was obtained in 109 patients. Complete AVM obliteration was achieved in 23 of 36 patients (64 percent) with angiographically determined AVM volumes ≤2.0 cc, in 7 of 20 patients (35 percent) with 2.1- to 4.0-cc AVMs, in 3 of 10 (30 percent) with 4.1- to 6.0-cc AVMs, and in 1 of 43 (2 percent) with AVMs >6.0 cc.[57] Nearly all cases of complete AVM obliteration occurred within the first 3 years after treatment. AVM obliteration and volume decrease were positively correlated with both average absorbed dose and dose to the margin of the treatment volume.[57]

Carotid-Cavernous Fistulae

Stereotactic radiosurgery with plateau-beam proton irradiation has been used by Minakova and colleagues[29,58,59,61] to treat 24 patients with carotid-cavernous fistulae (Minakova YeI: Personal communication). Patients were treated with 40 to 60 Gy in one or two fractions, using 10- to 12-mm beams. Thus far, all patients have had regression of ocular symptoms and headaches, usually between 4 and 8 months after treatment. In four of eight patients examined, complete obliteration of the fistulae was observed on follow-up angiograms; three other patients had partial fistulae obliteration. No patient experienced adverse sequelae.

Angiographically Occult Vascular Malformations

Stereotactic radiosurgery of AOVMs presents complex problems in diagnosis, patient selection criteria, treatment planning, choice of dose, and criteria for clinical and neuroradiologic follow-up evaluation.[39,42,67] Since 1983 we have treated 47 patients with symptomatic AOVMs with stereotactic heavy-charged-particle Bragg-peak radiosurgery (dose range, 8 to 45 GyE), using the helium-ion beams at the UCB–LBL 184-inch synchrocyclotron and Bevatron. There were 25 males and 22 females, ranging in age at the time of treatment from 13 to 64 years. Twenty-eight AOVMs (60 percent) were located in the brain stem, 15 (32 percent) in the thalamus, internal capsule, or basal ganglia, 3 (6 percent) in the motor or language cortex, and 1 (2 percent) in the cerebellopontine angle. AOVMs measured between 0.1 and 15.2 cc. Twenty-two patients (47 percent) were in *excellent* grade prior to treatment, 20 (43 percent) in *good* grade, and 5 (10 percent) in *poor* grade. There was clinical and radiologic evidence of hemorrhage in all patients; most had experienced repeated hemorrhage.

Clinical follow-up grade was *excellent* in 47 percent of patients, *good* in 34 percent, and *poor* in 9 percent; five patients (10 percent) died. Thirty-seven patients in *excellent* or *good* condition prior to treatment remained stable or improved neurologically. Two patients initially in *poor* condition, who had previously received conventional large-field radiotherapy (approximately 50 Gy) and chemotherapy for presumed brain stem glioma, died of disease progression 9 and 14 months after radiosurgical treatment; a third patient with a large hypothalamic AOVM who was initially in *good* condition deteriorated from recurrent hemorrhage 26 months after treatment and died 4 months later. These three patients had been treated with radiosurgical doses ≤10 GyE. A fourth patient initially in *poor* condition deteriorated markedly as a result of hemorrhage 13 months following treatment, and died with severe brain-stem dysfunction 3 years later; she had been treated with a dose of 20 GyE. Another patient in *poor* condition prior to radiosurgery died 7 years after treatment (dose, 25 GyE) from recurrent hemorrhage.

Eight other patients had transient or permanent neurological deterioration due to recurrent AOVM hemorrhage 2 months to 5 years after treatment (five within 13 months). Five of these patients recovered fully to their previous condition, including three following microsurgical resection of their AOVMs 20 months, 3 years, and 5 years, respectively, after radiosurgery; histologic examination confirmed that these AOVMs were partially thrombosed.[67] The other three patients had permanent neurological worsening following hemorrhage.

Seven of 47 patients (15 percent) with AOVMs had possible or probable treatment-associated sequelae 3 to 12 months after helium-ion radiosurgery; six of these patients had findings of enhanced signal on T2-weighted MRI. Two patients recovered fully without surgical treatment, three recovered to their baseline neurological status following microsurgical resection of their AOVMs, and two patients had permanent worsening. Undetected recurrent hemorrhage or spontaneous thrombosis of adjacent vessels may have also contributed to neurological deterioration in some of these patients.

Most patients demonstrated little change on sequential MRI scans over time, other than what could be explained by partial resorption or evolution of pre-existing hemorrhage.[42] No AOVM had associated radiologic findings comparable to those seen following radiosurgery for angiographically demonstrable AVMs (i.e., MRI findings typically associated with obliteration of abnormal vascular structures were not seen).[38] Follow-up CT scanning has been of limited value, other than for diagnosing acute recurrent hemorrhage where clinically suspected.[42]

The clinical results following helium-ion radiosurgery for AOVMs are not as favorable as the results of high-flow

AVMs.[16,42,67] Considerable clinical research is required to define more precisely the selection criteria for stereotactic radiosurgery in patients with AOVMs. The optimal treatment dose and radiosurgical target volume must be determined for the treatment of AOVMs in various locations within the brain. Neuroradiologic imaging methods are presently not able to demonstrate the vascular structures in most AOVMs or obliterative changes in response to radiosurgery. We have concluded that microsurgical resection should be the primary treatment for surgically accessible, symptomatic AOVMs. The potential value of helium-ion radiosurgery for surgically inaccessible AOVMs remains uncertain.

Juxtaspinal Tumors

The management of juxtaspinal and skull base tumors (e.g., chordomas and chondrosarcomas) is a complex problem in neurosurgery and radiation oncology.[2,7] Complete surgical resection is uncommon, and most patients require postoperative irradiation. The proximity of these tumors to the spinal cord or brain stem, however, limits the radiation dose that can be delivered safely to the tumor with conventional radiotherapy techniques. Charged-particle radiotherapy delivered with conventional fractionation (60 to 75 GyE tumor dose, approximately 2 GyE per fraction) has been used with excellent results.

From 1978 through 1991, 85 patients with chordoma or chondrosarcoma of the cranial base or cervical spine were treated at LBL with helium-ion irradiation, most following subtotal surgical resection.[2,6] A minority of patients had received the first part of their radiation treatment with photons and were referred for helium-ion "boost" treatment; another group of patients was referred because of recurrent disease. Total helium-ion doses ranged from 36 to 80 GyE (mean, 67 GyE). Local control was obtained in 59 of 85 patients (70 percent) with a follow-up period ranging from 2 to 163 months (median, 34 months). The projected 5-year Kaplan–Meier actuarial survival was 67 percent; the actuarial survival and local control for these patients at 3 years were 70 and 68 percent, respectively. Patients treated for primary disease had a 78 percent actuarial local control rate at 2 years, whereas the rate for patients with recurrent disease was 33 percent.[2] Those patients with smaller tumor volumes ($<$20 cc) had a significantly better local control rate than patients with larger tumor volumes (80 versus 33 percent actuarial rate at 5 years), as did patients whose radiation treatment was solely with charged particles. Local control was better for chondrosarcoma than for chordoma, and in the skull base than in the cervical spine. Serious complications included three patients with unilateral vision loss, two who became blind, and four with radiation injury to the brain stem.

Fractionated proton therapy has also proven successful for treatment of chordoma and chondrosarcoma of the skull base; 5-year actuarial local control rates of about 80 percent have been reported.[1,69] By contrast, the local recurrence rate for these tumors following conventional photon irradiation is 64 percent.[69]

Ocular Melanomas

Several thousand patients in the United States and Europe have been treated for ocular melanoma using Bragg-peak irradiation with protons or helium ions (50 to 80 Gy) typically delivered in five fractions over 7 to 12 days.[9,12,20,78] In these clinical series, local control exceeding 95 percent has been achieved in selected patient groups, but distant metastases occurred in about 20 percent of patients. A large proportion of patients have maintained useful vision in the treated eye; however, enucleation due to complications has been required in 7 to 12 percent of patients.

Summary

Charged-particle beams manifest unique physical properties that offer advantages for neurosurgery and radiation oncology. These properties include a finite range in tissue, a Bragg ionization peak, and very sharp lateral edges. Charged-particle irradiation can be applied effectively using either the Bragg-peak method, where the charged particles *stop* within the target volume, or the plateau-beam method, where the charged particles pass completely through the patient's head. In either case, the target volume must be defined and located precisely within a reproducible three-dimensional frame of reference, the physical properties of the materials to be traversed by the beam must be determined accurately, and the patient must be positioned exactly with respect to the beam. Treatment planning consists of sequential stereotactic neuroradiologic imaging studies, computer-assisted correlations among the different types of imaging information, and calculations of dose distribution.

Since 1954, more than 7000 patients worldwide have been treated with charged-particle irradiation for various intracranial and juxtaspinal lesions. Most patients have been treated with single-dose irradiation or with a few large-dose fractions, but several hundred patients have been treated using conventional fractionation schedules. Therapeutic efficacy has been clearly demonstrated for the treatment of selected lesions and sites, e.g., pituitary adenomas, AVMs, juxtaspinal tumors, and ocular melanomas. Optimal treatment parameters (dose, fractionation, and choice of charged-particle species) have yet to be determined for lesions of varying histology, size, and location. Improved three-dimensional treatment planning and beam delivery can be expected to improve cure rates and minimize adverse sequelae of treatment, especially for large or irregularly shaped lesions.

References

1. Austin-Seymour M, Munzenrider J, Goiten M, et al. Fractionated proton radiation therapy of chordoma and low-grade chondrosarcoma of the base of the skull. *J Neurosurg* 1989; 70:13–17.
2. Berson AM, Castro JR, Petti P, et al. Charged particle irradiation of chordoma and chondrosarcoma of the base of skull and cervical spine: the Lawrence Berkeley Laboratory experience. *Int J Radiat Oncol Biol Phys* 1988; 15:559–565.
3. Blakely EA, Ngo FQH, Curtis SB, et al. Heavy-ion radiobiology: cellular studies. In Lett JT (ed): *Advances in Radiation Biology,* vol 11. New York: Academic Press, 1984, pp 295–389.
4. Bragg WH, Kleeman RD. On the ionization curves of radium. *Philosoph Mag* 1904; 8:726–738.
5. Brobeck WM, Lawrence EO, MacKenzie KR, et al. Initial performance of the 184-inch cyclotron of the University of California. *Physics Rev* 1947; 71:449–450.
6. Castro JR. High-LET charged particle radiotherapy. In Dewey WC, Edington M, Fry RJM, et al. (eds): *Proceedings of the 9th International Congress of Radiation Research,* vol 2. New York: Academic Press, 1992, pp 635–640.

7. Castro JR, Collier JM, Petti PL, et al. Charged particle radiotherapy for lesions encircling the brain stem or spinal cord. *Int J Radiat Oncol Biol Phys* 1989; 17:477–484.
8. Castro JR, Saunders WM, Austin-Seymour MM, et al. A phase I–II trial of heavy charged particle irradiation of malignant glioma of the brain: a Northern California Oncology Group study. *Int J Radiat Oncol Biol Phys* 1985; 11:1795–1800.
9. Char DH, Castro JR, Kroll SM, et al. Five-year follow-up of helium ion therapy for uveal melanoma. *Arch Ophthalmol* 1990; 108:209–214.
10. Chen GTY, Singh RP, Castro JR, et al. Treatment planning for heavy ion radiotherapy. *Int J Radiat Oncol Biol Phys* 1979; 5:1809–1819.
11. Constable JD, Lawrence JH, Born JL, et al. Effect of alpha particle hypophysectomy on disseminated cancer of male breast. *JAMA* 1960; 174:1720–1723.
12. Decker M, Castro JR, Linstadt DE, et al. Ciliary body melanoma treated with helium particle irradiation. *Int J Radiat Oncol Biol Phys* 1990; 19:243–247.
13. Drake CG. Cerebral arteriovenous malformations: considerations for and experience with surgical treatment in 166 cases. *Clin Neurosurg* 1979; 26:145–208.
14. Fabrikant JI, Levy RP. Radiation therapy of pituitary tumors. In Barrow DL, Selman WR (eds): *Neuroendocrinology.* Baltimore: Williams & Wilkins 1992, pp 367–393.
15. Fabrikant JI, Levy RP, Phillips MH, et al. Neurosurgical applications of ion beams. *Nucl Instrum Methods Phys Res B* 1989; 40/41:1376–1384.
16. Fabrikant JI, Levy RP, Steinberg GK, et al. Charged-particle radiosurgery for intracranial vascular malformations. *Neurosurg Clin North Am* 1992; 3:99–139.
17. Fabrikant JI, Lyman JT, Frankel KA. Heavy charged-particle Bragg peak radiosurgery for intracranial vascular disorders. *Radiat Res* (Suppl) 1985; 104:S244–S258.
18. Fabrikant JI, Lyman JT, Hosobuchi Y. Stereotactic heavy-ion Bragg peak radiosurgery for intra-cranial vascular disorders: method for treatment of deep arteriovenous malformations. *Br J Radiol* 1984; 57:479–490.
19. Frankel KA, Levy RP, Fabrikant JI, et al. Heavy-charged-particle radiosurgery: rationale and method. In Alexander E 3d, Loeffler JS, Lunsford LD (eds): *Stereotactic Radiosurgery.* New York: McGraw-Hill 1993, pp 87–103.
20. Gragoudas ES, Seddon JM, Egan K, et al. Long-term results of proton beam irradiated uveal melanomas. *Ophthalmology* 1987; 94:349–353.
21. Hardy J. Transsphenoidal microsurgical treatment of pituitary tumors. In Linfoot JA (ed): *Recent Advances in the Diagnosis and Treatment of Pituitary Tumors.* New York: Raven Press, 1979, pp 375–388.
22. Kjellberg RN. Stereotactic Bragg peak proton beam radiosurgery for cerebral arteriovenous malformations. *Ann Clin Res* 1986; 18 (Suppl 47):17–19.
23. Kjellberg RN, Candia GJ. Stereotactic proton beam therapy for cerebral AVMs. *Harvard Radiosurgery Update.* Chestnut Hill, MA, 1990 (abstr).
24. Kjellberg RN, Hanamura T, Davis KR, et al. Bragg peak proton-beam therapy for arteriovenous malformations of the brain. *N Engl J Med* 1983; 309:269–274.
25. Kjellberg RN, Kliman B. Lifetime effectiveness—a system of therapy for pituitary adenomas, emphasizing Bragg peak proton hypophysectomy. In Linfoot JA (ed): *Recent Advances in the Diagnosis and Treatment of Pituitary Tumors.* New York: Raven Press, 1979, pp 269–288.
26. Kjellberg RN, McMeel JW, McManus N, Koehler AM. Pituitary suppression in diabetic retinopathy by proton beam in surgically "unfit" patients. In Goldberg MF, Fine SL (eds): *Symposium on the Treatment of Diabetic Retinopathy.* Arlington, VA: U.S. Public Health Service (Publication No. 1890), 1968, pp 249–276.
27. Kjellberg RN, Shintani A, Frantz AG, et al. Proton-beam therapy in acromegaly. *N Engl J Med* 1968; 278:689–695.
28. Konnov B, Melnikov L, Zargarova O, et al. Narrow proton beam therapy for intracranial lesions. In Heikkinen E, Kiviniitty K (eds): *International Workshop on Proton and Narrow Photon Beam Therapy.* Oulu, Finland: University of Oulu, 1989, pp 48–55.
29. Krymsky VA, Serbinenko FA, Minakova YeI, et al. Proton beam irradiation of spontaneous arteriosinusal anastomoses of the cavernous sinus area. *Med Radiol (Mosk)* 1987; 32(8):57–61 (in Russian).
30. Lawrence JH. Proton irradiation of the pituitary. *Cancer* 1957; 10:795–798.
31. Lawrence JH. Heavy particle irradiation of intracranial lesions. In Wilkins RH, Rengachary SS (eds): *Neurosurgery.* New York: McGraw-Hill, 1985, pp 1113–1132.
32. Lawrence JH, Born JL, Tobias CA, et al. Clinical and metabolic studies in patients after alpha particle subtotal or total hypophysectomy. In *Medicine in Japan in 1959. Proceedings of the 15th General Assembly of the Japan Medical Congress,* vol 5. Tokyo, 1959, pp 859–862.
33. Lawrence JH, Linfoot JA. Treatment of acromegaly, Cushing disease and Nelson syndrome. *West J Med* 1980; 133:197–202.
34. Lawrence JH, Tobias CA, Born JL, et al. Heavy-particle irradiation in neoplastic and neurologic disease. *J Neurosurg* 1962; 19:717–722.
35. Lawrence JH, Tobias CA, Born JL, et al. Heavy particles in experimental medicine and therapy. *JAMA* 1966; 196:166–170.
36. Lawrence JH, Tobias CA, Linfoot JA, et al. Heavy particles, the Bragg curve and suppression of pituitary function in diabetic retinopathy. *Diabetes* 1963; 12:490–501.
37. Levy RP, Fabrikant JI. Clinical applications of stereotactic radiosurgery. In Phillips MH (ed): *Physical Aspects of Stereotactic Radiosurgery.* New York: Plenum, 1993, pp 239–278.
38. Levy RP, Fabrikant JI, Frankel KA, et al. Stereotactic heavy-charged-particle Bragg peak radiosurgery for the treatment of intracranial arteriovenous malformations in childhood and adolescence. *Neurosurgery* 1989; 24:841–852.
39. Levy RP, Fabrikant JI, Frankel KA, et al. Charged-particle radiosurgery of the brain. *Neurosurg Clin North Am* 1990; 1:955–990.
40. Levy RP, Fabrikant JI, Frankel KA, et al. Clinical-radiological evaluation of sequelae of stereotactic radiosurgery for intracranial arteriovenous malformations. In Steiner L (ed): *Radiosurgery: Baselines and Trends.* New York: Raven Press, 1992, pp 209–220.
41. Levy RP, Lo EH, Fabrikant JI. Biologic basis for stereotactic radiosurgery. In Phillips MH (ed): *Physical Aspects of Stereotactic Radiosurgery.* New York: Plenum, 1993, pp 189–238.
42. Levy RP, Steinberg GK, Fabrikant JI, et al. Stereotactic heavy-charged-particle radiosurgery for angiographically occult vascular malformations. In Lunsford LD (ed): *Stereotactic Radiosurgery Update.* New York: Elsevier, 1992, pp 177–183.
43. Linfoot JA. Heavy ion therapy: alpha particle therapy of pituitary tumors. In Linfoot JA (ed): *Recent Advances in the Diagnosis and Treatment of Pituitary Tumors.* New York: Raven Press, 1979, pp 245–267.
44. Linfoot JA, Born JL, Garcia JF, et al. Metabolic and ophthalmological observations following heavy particle pituitary suppressive therapy in diabetic retinopathy. In Goldberg MF, Fine SL (eds): *Symposium on the Treatment of Diabetic Retinopathy.* Arlington, VA: U.S. Public Health Service (Publication No. 1890), 1968, pp 277–289.
45. Linfoot JA, Lawrence JH, Born JL, et al. The alpha particle or proton beam in radiosurgery of the pituitary gland for Cushing's disease. *N Engl J Med* 1963; 269:597–601.
46. Linstadt DE, Castro JR, Phillips TL. Neon ion radiotherapy: results of phase I/II clinical trial. *Int J Radiat Oncol Biol Phys* 1991; 20:761–769.
47. Lo EH, Fabrikant JI, Levy RP, et al. An experimental compartmental flow model for assessing the hemodynamic response of intracranial arteriovenous malformations to stereotactic radiosurgery. *Neurosurgery* 1991; 28:251–259.
48. Lopatkin NA, Khazanov VG, Minakova YeI, et al. Proton irradiation of the hypophysis in the combined antiandrogenical treatment of cancer of the prostate. *Khirurgiia (Sofiia)* 1988; 3:1–3 (in Bulgarian).
49. Luchin YI, Minakova YeI, Krymsky VA. Proton beam irradiation of cavernous sinus meningiomas. In Heikkinen E, Kiviniitty K (eds): *International Workshop on Proton and Narrow Photon Beam Therapy.* Oulu, Finland: University of Oulu, 1989, pp 99–100.

50. Luft R. The use of hypophysectomy in juvenile diabetes mellitus with vascular complications. *Diabetes* 1962; 11:461–462.
51. Lyass FM, Minakova YeI, Rayevskaya SA, et al. The role of radiotherapy in the treatment of pituitary adenomas. *Med Radiol (Mosk)* 1989; 34(8):12–24 (in Russian).
52. Lyman JT, Chong CY. ISAH: a versatile treatment positioner for external radiation therapy. *Cancer* 1974; 34:12–16.
53. Lyman JT, Phillips MH, Frankel KA, et al. Stereotactic frame for neuroradiology and charged particle Bragg peak radiosurgery of intracranial disorders. *Int J Radiat Oncol Biol Phys* 1989; 16:1615–1621.
54. Marks MP, DeLaPaz RL, Fabrikant JI, et al. Intracranial vascular malformations: imaging of charged-particle radiosurgery. Part II. Complications. *Radiology* 1988; 168:457–462.
55. Marks MP, Lane B, Steinberg GK, et al. Endovascular treatment of cerebral arteriovenous malformations following radiosurgery. *Am J Neuroradiol* 1993; 14:297–305.
56. McDonald LW, Lawrence JH, Born JL, et al. Delayed radionecrosis of the central nervous system. In Lawrence JH (ed): *Semiannual Report. Biology and Medicine. Donner Laboratory and Donner Pavilion. Fall 1967.* Berkeley: Regents of the University of California, Report UCRL-18066, 1967, pp 173–192.
57. Melnikov LA, Konnov BA, Yalynych NN. Radiosurgery of cerebral AVM. In Heikkinen E, Kiviniitty K (eds): *International Workshop on Proton and Narrow Photon Beam Therapy.* Oulu, Finland: University of Oulu, 1989, pp 92–98.
58. Minakova YeI. Review of twenty years proton therapy clinical experience in Moscow. In *Proceedings of the Second International Charged Particle Workshop.* Loma Linda, CA, 1987, pp 1–23.
59. Minakova YeI. Twenty years clinical experience of narrow proton beam therapy in Moscow. In *Proceedings of the International Heavy Particle Therapy Workshop.* Paul Scherrer Institute, Villigen, Switzerland, 1990, pp 158–162.
60. Minakova YeI, Kirpatovskaya LYe, Lyass FM, et al. Proton therapy of pituitary adenomas. *Med Radiol (Mosk)* 1983; 28(10):7–13 (in Russian).
61. Minakova YeI, Krymsky VA, Luchin YeI, et al. Proton beam therapy in neurosurgical clinical practice. *Med Radiol (Mosk)* 1987; 32 (8):36–42 (in Russian).
62. Minakova YeI, Vasil'eva NN, Svyatukhina OV. Irradiation of the hypophysis with single large dose of high energy protons for advanced breast carcinoma. *Med Radiol (Mosk)* 1977; 22 (1):33–39 (in Russian).
63. Phillips MH, Frankel KA, Lyman JT, et al. Heavy charged-particle stereotactic radiosurgery: cerebral angiography and CT in the treatment of intracranial vascular malformations. *Int J Radiat Oncol Biol Phys* 1989; 17:419–426.
64. Phillips MH, Frankel KA, Lyman JT, et al. Comparison of different radiation types and irradiation geometries in stereotactic radiosurgery. *Int J Radiat Oncol Biol Phys* 1990; 18:211–220.
65. Rodriguez A, Levy RP, Fabrikant JI. Experimental central nervous system injury after charged-particle irradiation. In Gutin PH, Leibel SA, Sheline GE (eds): *Radiation Injury to the Nervous System.* New York: Raven Press, 1991, pp 149–182.
66. Steinberg GK, Fabrikant JI, Marks MP, et al. Stereotactic heavy-charged-particle Bragg-peak radiation for intracranial arteriovenous malformations. *N Engl J Med* 1990; 323:96–101.
67. Steinberg GK, Levy RP, Fabrikant JI, et al. Stereotactic helium ion Bragg peak radiosurgery for angiographically occult intracranial vascular malformations. *Stereotact Funct Neurosurg* 1991; 57:64–71.
68. Steinberg GK, Levy RP, Marks MP, et al. Charged-particle radiosurgery. In Alexander E III, Loeffler JS, Lunsford LD (eds): *Stereotactic Radiosurgery.* New York: McGraw-Hill, 1993; pp 122–135.
69. Suit HD, Goitein M, Munzenrider J, et al. Definitive radiation therapy for chordoma and chondrosarcoma of base of skull and cervical spine. *J Neurosurg* 1982; 56:377–385.
70. Tobias CA. Pituitary radiation: radiation physics and biology. In Linfoot JA (ed): *Recent Advances in the Diagnosis and Treatment of Pituitary Tumors.* New York: Raven Press, 1979, pp 221–243.
71. Tobias CA, Alpen EL, Blakely EA, et al. Radiobiological basis for heavy-ion therapy. In Abe M, Sakamoto K, Phillips TL (eds): *Treatment of Radioresistant Cancers.* Amsterdam: Elsevier, 1979, pp 159–183.
72. Tobias CA, Anger HO, Lawrence JH. Radiologic use of high energy deuterons and alpha particles. *Am J Roentgenol* 1952; 67:1–27.
73. Tobias CA, Lawrence JH, Born JL, et al. Pituitary irradiation with high-energy proton beams: a preliminary report. *Cancer Res* 1958; 18:121–134.
74. Tobias CA, Roberts JE, Lawrence JH, et al. Irradiation hypophysectomy and related studies using 340-MeV protons and 190-MeV deuterons. In *Proceedings of the International Conference on the Peaceful Uses of Atomic Energy,* vol 10. New York: United Nations Publications, 1956, pp 95–106.
75. Verhey L, Goitein M. Problems of inhomogeneities in particle beam therapy. In Skarsgard LD (ed): *Pion and Heavy-Ion Radiotherapy. Pre-Clinical and Clinical Studies.* New York: Elsevier, 1983, pp 159–168.
76. Wilson RR. Radiological use of fast protons. *Radiology* 1946; 47:487–491.
77. Woodruff KH, Lyman JT, Lawrence JH, et al. Delayed sequelae of pituitary irradiation. *Hum Pathol* 1984; 15:48–54.
78. Zografos L, Bercher L, Egger E, et al. Le traitement des tûmeurs oculaires par faisceau de protons accélérés. *Klin Mbl Augenheilk* 1992; 200:431–435.

185 Radiosurgery for Tumors

Christer Lindquist
Ladislau Steiner

The term *radiosurgery*, introduced by the late Lars Leksell as early as 1951, describes the procedure wherein ionizing radiation is used, as is any neurosurgical tool, to destroy circumscribed volumes of tissue in a single session. This is made possible by focusing the radiation from multiple sources using stereotactic techniques. The dose gradient at the periphery of the target volume is very sharp and therefore surrounding normal tissue is spared the untoward effects of the ionizing beams. Tumors diffusely infiltrating surrounding eloquent tissue are therefore theoretically not suitable targets for this treatment modality. The ideal targets among tumors are those that are well circumscribed and growing in noninfiltrating fashion. With the success of radiosurgery has followed modifications of radiotherapy, i.e., delivery of ionizing radiation in a fractionated form, which also includes adaptation of stereotactic techniques. This specialized form of radiotherapy is now emerging under the name *stereotactic radiotherapy* (SRT) and should be distinguished from *stereotactic radiosurgery*. Whereas radiosurgery utilizes only the physical properties of the technique to deliver deadly radiation doses to tumors, the radiotherapeutic techniques benefit from the differences in radiobiological properties between normal and pathologic tissue. The development of stereotactic radiotherapy is still in its early infancy and little information on its efficacy exists. The adaptation of stereotactic techniques in radiotherapy will probably lower treatment morbidity and possibly improve treatment results in the management of infiltrating brain tumors. SRT belongs to the domains of radiotherapy and is beyond the scope of this chapter.

The traditional management of circumscribed tumors includes microsurgical removal and, in case of metastatic tumors or partially removed benign tumors, sometimes postoperative radiotherapy. Microsurgical results are constantly improving and it is against this management technique that the results of radiosurgery should be weighed. Total removal of a benign tumor usually means a permanent cure even if the number of recurrences following so-called gross total removal of skull base tumors is not insignificant. The surgeon's own intraoperative evaluation and/or modern postoperative imaging is most often a good predictor of the final outcome. Following radiosurgery, on the other hand, a modest decrease of tumor volume or even a tumor volume remaining unchanged for many years may be the only available objective evidence of disease control. With radiosurgery the definition of cure must be redefined. In this predicament it has been a slow process for radiosurgery to become an accepted treatment alternative. However, 25 years of work with the gamma knife has yielded enough results to secure radiosurgery a place in the management of tumors. The total number of patients now treated is around 20,000. The first acoustic neuroma and the first pituitary microadenoma were radiated with the gamma knife in 1969, the first meningioma in 1975, and the first metastatic brain tumor also in 1975. Long-term clinical and radiologic follow-up results are now becoming available. We are, however, still searching for a method by which the biological effects of the radiation could be monitored objectively at an earlier stage. Positron emission tomography (PET) and magnetic resonance spectroscopy may satisfy this need in the future.

Radiosurgical Techniques

Radiosurgery is performed by crossfiring of the target volume with photons or heavy particles, such as protons or helium, from an external source of radiation or by utilizing the so-called Bragg peak of heavy particle radiation. Photons are delivered from cobalt 60 (^{60}Co) and from linear accelerators. Heavy particle irradiation requires larger and more expensive accelerators available at only a few sites worldwide. The longest and quantitatively most important experience has been accumulated with the gamma knife, which utilizes 201 ^{60}Co sources to deliver gamma rays. It is considered the gold standard of radiosurgical equipment against which emerging techniques are compared. Radiosurgical linear accelerators are usually common radiotherapy machines modified to improve accuracy and precision to meet the needs of steep dose gradients. There is ongoing debate regarding the preferred technique. Experienced linear accelerator users seem to agree that linear accelerators dedicated to radiosurgery rather than machines also used for conventional radiotherapy are needed to meet demands on quality and safety of the treatment. The reader is referred to other publications for more elaborate presentations of radiosurgical techniques.[88]

Some neurosurgeons consider treatment with radiation from implanted radioactive isotopes a form of radiosurgery.[82] However, interstitial stereotactic radiosurgery or interstitial brachytherapy differs in important aspects from linac, heavy particle, and gamma knife radiosurgery. The interstitial technique implies implantation of radioactive isotopes (most commonly iodine125) by an open stereotactic technique and it is thus an open surgical procedure. The gamma radiation is delivered at a much slower rate—approximately 10 cGy/h as compared to 100 to 400 cGy/min for the gamma knife. This difference in dose rate probably has significant implications for the biological effect. The protracted radiation is thus, in this respect, more akin to radiotherapy. Stereotactic interstitial brachytherapy has mainly been applied to treatment of gliomas[3,14,23,31,82,98] but also to metastatic tumors[57] and skull base tumors.[7,30,58] Compared with brachytherapy, radiosurgery has the advantage of lower initial morbidity, reduced hospital stay, reduced radiation exposure to personnel, and lower costs.[26] In this chapter, only brief and incomplete reference is given to results obtained with this treatment technique.

Radiosurgery is a three-part procedure consisting of stereotactic imaging, dose-planning, and the radiation exposure. The crucial part for the outcome is the dose-planning. The planning determines the risks and the chances for success. The distribution of the radiation is modified to avoid damaging doses to neighboring normal structures such as cranial nerves and eloquent brain. The volume and shape of the radiation may be modified a number of ways: (1) beam collimation; (2) blocking individual beams; (3) multiple isocenters (i.e., utilizing several target points within the tumor); and (4) "weighting" between multiple isocenters (i.e., allowing different treatment times of the targets within the tumor). Optimization of the dose plan is achieved by interactively working with the dose-planning computer using these four options in various combinations. A prerequisite for a successful dose plan is the same as that for microsurgery—a thorough knowledge of surgical anatomy. The dexterity required for microsurgery is supplanted by experience and knowledge of radiobiology.

Radiosurgical Considerations

Optimizing a dose plan involves selection of the proper minimal tumor-killing dose and configuration of the dose distribution to the tumor volume. Although the radiotherapy literature is extensive and the knowledge of the reaction of the tumor tissue to radiation is profound, there is surprisingly little information on how brain tumors and normal human brain react to the single high doses of radiation used in radiosurgery. The current dose recommendations and radiosurgical treatment strategies are mainly based on experiences accumulated at our gamma knife centers. Obviously, tumors of different kinds may require different doses of radiation and various structures of the CNS differ in their tolerance of radiation. Nevertheless, a few simple generally applicable statements can be made.

Cellular Effects

The primary target in the cell for the radiation effect is the deoxyribonucleic acid (DNA) molecule. Depending on the dose absorbed, the injury can be lethal or repairable. In radiosurgery of tumors the idea is to give a lethal dose in a single session. The dose delivery must therefore be very precise in order to avoid damage to normal cells. In fractionated radiotherapy, on the other hand, doses low enough to incur lethal damage to only some cells is given in each fraction, but the surrounding tissue is also damaged to some extent. The thought is that normal tissue has a higher potential for repair between radiation fractionations and thus the net result of the fractionation scheme is more damage to the tumor than to normal tissue. Cell death may require one or more cell generations to occur and in clinical practice the time from the radiosurgical treatment to a visible effect on the tumor is therefore dependent on the inherent growth rate of the tumor, as well as on the dose given. In normal brain, the most rapidly proliferating cell populations are the endothelial cells of the blood vessels, the glial cells, and the stem cells of the subependymal plate. The endothelial cell population may be, even in some slow-growing benign tumors, the most rapidly proliferating cells. It is therefore quite possible, but not yet shown, that vascular thrombosis and ischemia secondary to radiation-induced endothelial damage may also be responsible for or at least contribute to tumor death.

Dose–Effect Relationships

In optimizing the dose plan for tumor radiosurgery, dose homogeneity and dose–volume relationships must also be considered. In traditional radiotherapy a homogeneous distribution of the radiation dose has always been considered optimal. In radiosurgery the core dose delivered to a tumor is often considerably higher than that to the tumor surface. Because normal nervous tissue usually abuts the tumor surface, the minimal dose and the steepest isodose gradient should be delivered there. When discussing radiosurgical doses, we usually refer to the tumor surface dose and the treatment dose. However, for two reasons it may also be important to deliver a high dose to the tumor core. The first reason is that the center of a tumor may be less well oxygenated, which predisposes to a lesser biological effect of the radiation. Second, a high central tumor dose increases the chances for tumor cell kill without increasing the risks of undue effects outside the tumor. In fact, dose–volume relationships are such that a given dose to a population of cells is more damaging when neighboring cells receive a higher dose of radiation.[117] The limits of radiosurgery are set by the tolerance of the normal CNS structures. The tolerance dose is related to the total dose, the dose rate, and the volume receiving the dose. The dose rate delivered by available radiosurgery equipment varies within ranges with similar biological responses. The biological effects of variations in radiated volume and doses are considerable, not well known, and related to the pathology treated. Treatment with acceptable risk is probably restricted to maximum tumor volumes of approximately 25 cc but meningiomas of several times this volume have been treated. Many benign tumors treated by radiosurgery are located at the central skull base adherent or adjacent to vessels of the circle of Willis or to cranial nerves. Information on the radiosensitivity of these structures is therefore crucial but available to a very limited extent.

Vascular Effects

There are occasional reports in the literature on stroke secondary to radiation damage of the carotid artery.[9,15,76,119] In rabbits, extensive atheromatous plaques were found in the carotids after doses as low as 5 Gy.[59] On the other hand, no changes were found in the basilar or middle cerebral arteries in normal and hypercholesterolemic rabbits 2 to 24 months following gamma knife irradiation with an 8-mm collimator in doses of 10 to 100 Gy. These findings were in contrast to the fact that brain radionecrosis was seen within 9 to 18 months in all animals exposed to 50 or 100 Gy.[49] A reasonable assumption is that endothelial damage occurring in vessels with a large lumen in most situations does not result in thrombosis but is quickly repaired. In our clinical experience of several hundred patients in whom major cerebral vessels have been exposed to radiation doses of 15 to 25 Gy we have seen stenosis or occlusion of a major arterial vessel in less than 1 percent and in only one case resulting in a clinical deficit (quadrantanopia). In clinical practice the major vessels therefore never set the limit on the radiation dose prescribed for radiosurgery of a tumor.

Cranial Nerve Sensitivity

Radiation injury of cranial nerves is probably secondary to damage of small vessels and protective Schwann cells or oligodendroglia. The relative vulnerability of the cranial nerves differs. This is not surprising in view of their differences in morphology as well as in function. Thus the optic as well as the statoacoustic nerves are actually fiber tracts of the CNS and carriers of much more complex information than the simple sensory and motor cranial nerves. The clinical experience suggests that these specialized sensory nerves are more susceptible to radiation injury and do not seem to have any capacity for restoration of function once a clinical deficit has occurred. Although desirable, it is not possible to state a "tolerance" dose for a particular nerve. For obvious reasons it has not been possible to work out dose–response curves for normal human cranial nerves, and animal data, even if it would be available, probably cannot be transferred directly to humans as the dose–volume relationships are quite different. In a treatment situation the problem is even more complex because the nerves in jeopardy may also be exposed to secondary influences from the tumor to be treated. Thus the facial nerve on the surface of an acoustic neuroma is subjected to mechanical stress in addition to the radiation exposure. Currently, reports on which doses cranial nerves have tolerated in connection with treatment of various tumors must suffice.

The largest experience on cranial nerve radiation tolerance involves the trigeminal and facial nerve roots. In 15 patients with trigeminal neuralgia 50 to 100 mm^3 of the root at its exit from the brain stem were exposed to a minimum dose of 60 to 80 Gy. Only one patient received 80 Gy and this dose resulted in a modest hypesthesia and a small volume of gadolinium enhancement visible on magnetic resonance imaging (MRI) of the nerve root. Consequently, it could be stated that the trigeminal nerve root tolerates a single exposure of 60 to 70 Gy. However, 19 percent of 254 patients radiated for small acoustic neuromas experience "trigeminal neuropathy" as a sequela from doses in the range 10 to 25 Gy.[79] This apparent difference in tolerance could be due to the added effect of mechanical stress on the nerve root in the tumor cases, but with small tumors this should not be an important factor. It is more likely that a difference in volume of nerve root exposed explains the difference. In the same group of acoustic neuroma patients the facial nerve was injured in 17 percent of the patients, but always with a subsequent improvement of function.[79] Also the facial nerve root has a considerably higher tolerance when small volumes of the root are exposed. Thus we have seen acoustic neuroma patients receive 50 Gy to small volumes of the nerve root without undue effects. In an attempt to analyze the risk factors for the trigeminal and facial nerves, Linskey, Flickinger, and Lunsford found that within a minimum tumor dose range of 12 to 20 Gy, the incidence of delayed trigeminal or facial neuropathy depended more on the estimated length of nerve irradiated than the tumor dose or tumor volume.[65]

In our practice, nerves of the cavernous sinus have often received 20 to 25 Gy in the course of treatment for cavernous sinus meningiomas or dural arteriovenous malformations. The maximum doses delivered to nerves in the cavernous sinus were recently related to clinical deficit in 29 patients following linac and in 33 patients following gamma knife radiosurgery. Over the 3- to 41-month observation period there were new neuropathies in 12 patients but they all seemed unrelated to the maximum dose received in the interval 10 to 40 Gy. The conclusion from this study was that it is "relatively" safe to give doses of up to 40 Gy to cranial nerves (III to VI) in the cavernous sinus.[109] In the same 62 patients, 17 received a maximum dose of more than 8 Gy to the optic system and 4 of them developed radiation-related visual complications. In 35 patients receiving less than 8 Gy to the optic system there were no visual complications. The recommendation of these authors of limiting the dose to 8 Gy is in line with our current practice. In the past probably more than 100 patients with pituitary and parasellar tumors had small parts of their optic apparatus exposed with impunity to 10 to 15 Gy. There are even reports of visual improvement following doses of 12 to 15 Gy to the optic apparatus in patients in whom treatment with the gamma knife relieved compression on the optic pathways from parasellar meningiomas.[85] Again there is the question of how big is the volume exposed to radiation and which are the secondary effects of tumor compression.[101]

Vestibular Schwannomas (Acoustic Neuromas)

The first vestibular schwannoma or acoustic neuroma was treated by Leksell, Steiner, and Greitz with the gamma knife in 1969 at the Karolinska Institute.[61] Today more than 500 patients have been treated at this institution alone and in recent years several hundred more have been treated at other radiosurgical centers. By far, the largest number of patients have been treated with the gamma knife. The largest series of linac-treated patients numbers 32 and the follow-up over 4 to 59 months was recently reported.[73] The learning curve of radiosurgery for these tumors has been retarded by the nonelucidation effect of the treatment on the tumor, the effect often being no further growth or slight diminution of tumor volume, which should be compared to the often very slow or erratic growth of untreated tumors. The time course of the development of undue effects also required considerable time to be established. Not until now are we, therefore, in a position to evaluate the role of radiosurgery in the treatment of vestibular schwannomas.

Indications for Radiosurgery

Among the community of neurosurgeons the opinions regarding the indications for radiosurgery of vestibular schwannomas have changed with the results of long-term follow-up, as have our own management strategies. Currently there is consensus that a tumor volume that is causing mass effect on the brain stem with clinical deficit is a contraindication for radiosurgery. Many neurosurgeons now agree that patients with tumors with a maximal intracisternal diameter of 3 cm or less should be given the option of gamma knife surgery. Within this group of patients the decision-making becomes more intricate and should be made in light of the consistently improving results of both microsurgery and gamma knife surgery. The yardstick by which to measure radiosurgical results should be the results of the best available microsurgery. In elderly patients no treatment may be the best choice, especially if there is useful hearing remaining on the affected side. In younger patients the pivotal point for selecting the treatment modality is probably hearing preservation. With the current dose prescription, hearing preservation following gamma knife surgery is probably superior to that of microsurgery, but it is still too early to evaluate tumor control in these dose ranges. When hearing is already lost, gamma knife surgery as well as first-class microsurgery offer excellent results with very low morbidity. Gamma knife surgery is a better treatment strategy than leaving a tumor remnant.[38] It is the opinion of the authors that if a neurosurgeon with extensive experience in acoustic neuroma surgery, with proven excellent results, is available, small tumors in young patients as well as tumors larger than 3 cm should be removed by microsurgery.[102] However, Norén contends that with the improved dose-planning systems now available for gamma knife surgery, even large tumors can be safely treated by radiosurgery.

Results

Changes in the follow-up computed tomography (CT) scans or MR images were seen 6 to 12 months after treatment in 70 percent of 254 tumors followed at the Karolinska Institute for a minimum of 12 months. The changes included loss of contrast or gadolinium enhancement, particularly in the center of the tumors. There was a decrease of tumor volume in 55 percent, no volume change in 33 percent, and an increase in 12 percent of the unilateral tumors. In patients with documented neurofibromatosis, type 2 (NF2), the corresponding numbers were 33 percent, 43 percent, and 24 percent.[79] Similar short-term experience has been reported from other radiosurgical centers.[53,66,73,103] In 49 cases Steiner treated with gamma knife surgery and with a follow-up ranging from 6 months to 7 years, a decrease in size was observed in 73 percent (Figs. 185-2 and 185-3), no change in 21 percent, and increase in 6 percent of the tumors. The review of 47 cases in which tumor residuals have been treated using the gamma knife following microsurgery is not yet complete. It is of practical importance to know that the initial loss of contrast enhancement is often followed by a period when the tumor may appear increased in volume and again densely enhancing. This finding should not be of concern because it is usually followed by shrinkage of the tumor (Figs. 185-1 and 185-2).

Understandably, critics of this treatment modality have pointed out the relatively low percentage of tumors actually decreased in volume 1 to 2 years after treatment and have called for much longer follow-up periods. Recently, Norén analyzed the radiologic and clinical follow-up results on patients treated for unilateral tumors at the Karolinska Institute during the period 1969 to 1980. Forty-one of the 46 patients treated during this time can now be considered to have received treatment with a proper dose plan. The average follow-up time in this patient cohort was 12.3 years (range 4 to 22 years, median 12.1 years). Only four of the patients did not respond to a proper treatment, but two of them responded after a second treatment, whereas two tumors were removed. In this long-term follow-up, the growth control rate (shrinkage or unchanged size) is thus 90 percent to the initial treatment and 95 percent if the two patients treated twice are included. The fact is that with time, the number of tumors showing a decreased volume increases: at 2 years to 40 percent, at 4 years to 64 percent, and at 10 years to 91 percent. Recurrences usually become apparent within 2 to 3 years and always within 5 years after the gamma knife procedure.[81] A similar analysis of 18 patients with NF2 and 24 patients with vestibular schwannomas found a growth-control rate following a single treatment of 73 percent and if a second treatment was included, 86 percent. The average observation time in this series was 6.7 years (median 6.5 years, range 0.6 to 17.3 years). In addition to a poorer response of tumors in NF2 patients there were also signs of recurrence appearing as late as 10 years after treatment. Thus NF2 patients should probably have life-long annual follow-up after radiosurgery treatment, whereas in other patients annual follow-up for 5 years is sufficient, and then only if clinical deterioration occurs.

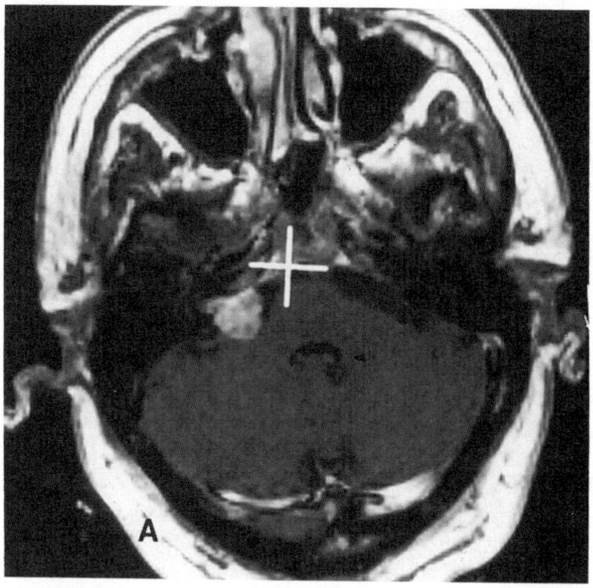

(*A*)

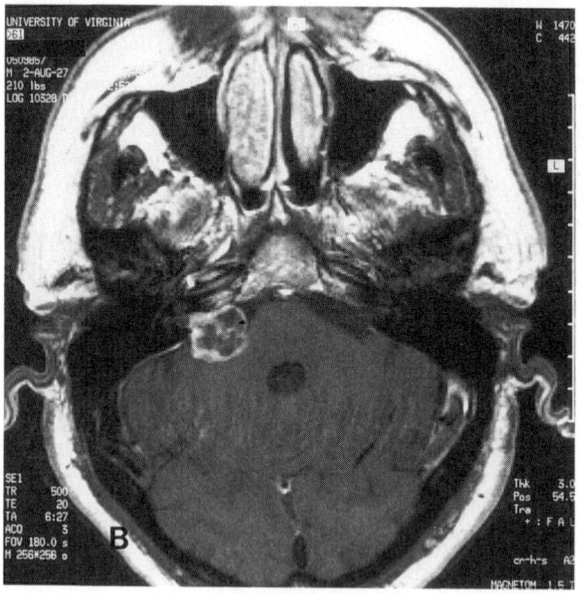

(*B*)

Figure 185-1 Gadolinium-enhanced magnetic resonance imaging (MRI) scan of a right 18 × 17 × 15-mm vestibular schwannoma in a 65-year-old man. An MRI study before (*A*) and 6 months after gamma knife surgery with loss of contrast enhancement in the central part of the tumor (*B*). The tumor is slightly increased in size. This changing pattern of contrast enhancement and its time course is typical for 70 percent of vestibular schwannomas following gamma knife surgery.

Complications

To make a correct evaluation of the gamma knife surgery, an account also needs to be made for the undue effects. Although cerebellar and/or brain stem edema occurs in 5 percent of patients 6 to 12 months after treatment, this rarely causes disturbing vertigo and/or ataxia. Thus edema has always been transient and is not practically important. Of more concern is the relatively high number of disturbances of facial and trigeminal nerve function. In the initial Karolinska series of 254 patients, facial nerve function was disturbed in 17 percent of the patients, but there was always recovery. The early experience from the University of Pittsburgh and Tokyo University Gamma Knife centers gave an even higher number of transient facial nerve problems,[66] but in 96 patients treated at the University of Virginia, there was only one case of facial weakness lasting for only 6 weeks and six transitory trigeminal neuropathies.[103]

Analysis of the causes for the facial weakness as well as the problems of trigeminal neuropathy indicated that they were related to the dose of radiation[70,80] and to the length of nerve exposed to radiation.[65] Consequently, in some radiosurgical centers the marginal tumor dose has been decreased and the incidence of facial and trigeminal dysfunction decreased to approximately 1 to 2 percent. Improvements in three-dimensional dose-planning and the

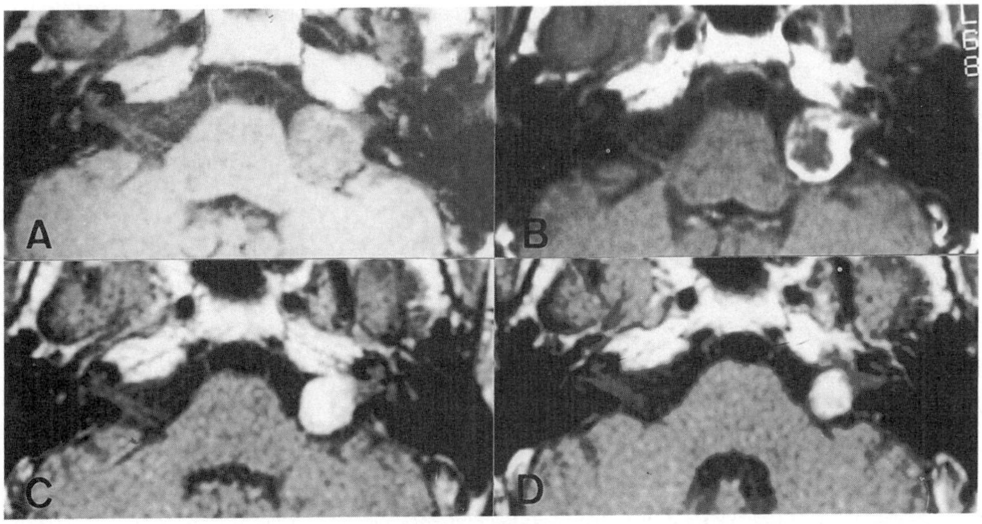

Figure 185-2 T1-weighted (*A–D*) gadolinium-enhanced (*B–D*) MRI scans of a 19-mm diameter left vestibular schwannoma before (*A*) and 5 months (*B*), 12 months (*C*), and 25 months (*D*) after gamma knife surgery. Loss of contrast enhancement is first seen in the central part of the tumor (*B*). Contrast enhancement is then regained (*C*) while a continuing decrease of the tumor volume occurs to an intracranial diameter of 14 mm (*D*). The peripheral dose was in this case 13 Gy and the maximum dose 19 Gy. (Courtesy of Georg Norén, M.D., Karolinska Institute, Stockholm, Sweden.)

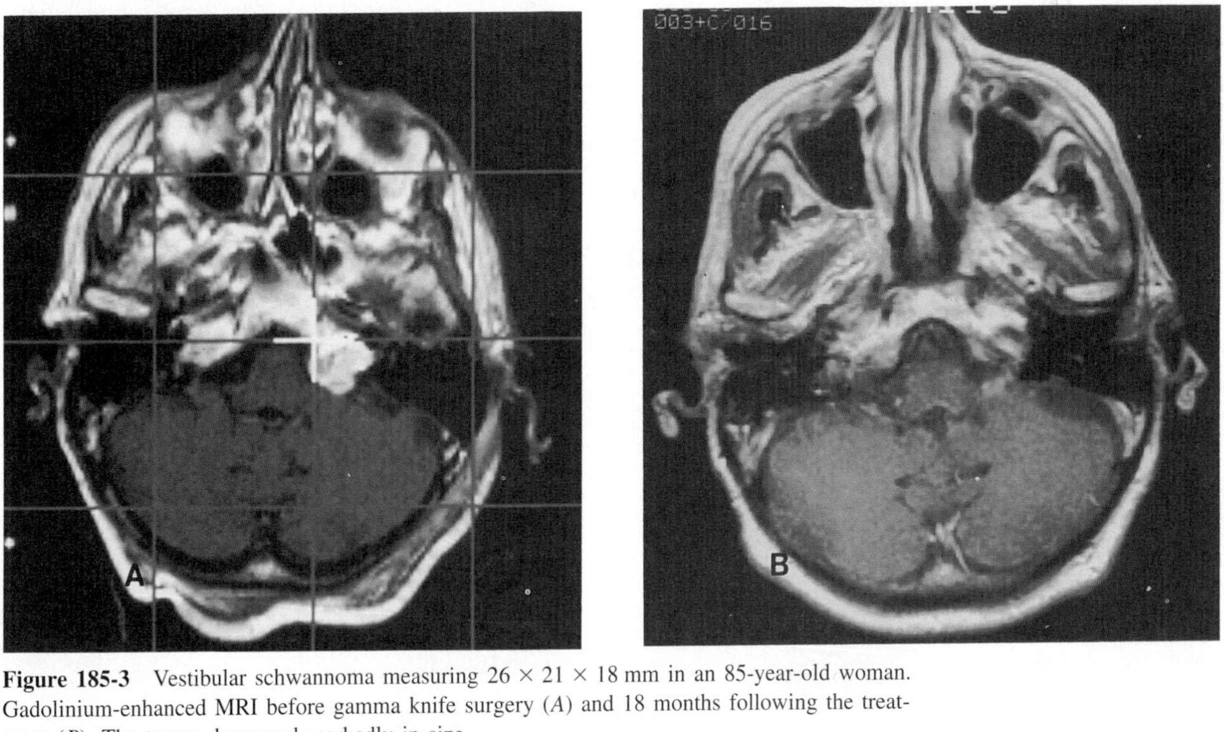

Figure 185-3 Vestibular schwannoma measuring 26 × 21 × 18 mm in an 85-year-old woman. Gadolinium-enhanced MRI before gamma knife surgery (*A*) and 18 months following the treatment (*B*). The tumor decreased markedly in size.

use of multiplanar MRI for tumor localization are certainly also important contributions to superior results. Currently, these centers recommend marginal doses for small tumors of 14 Gy; for medium-sized tumors, 12 Gy; and for large tumors, 10 Gy.[80] The experience with this dose prescription has involved 150 patients over 3 years. Despite the insignificant morbidity, the tumor control rate is still around 90 percent.

Hearing Preservation

Hearing preservation has become the major goal of vestibular schwannoma management following reduction of the facial nerve problems to negligible levels. There are only two reports in peer-reviewed journals addressing hearing preservation after gamma knife surgery, the combined experience of which was some hearing preservation in 8 of 12 patients.[66,77] There is a report by Norén et al. of the Karolinska experience with 54 patients with unilateral schwannoma and 10 patients with schwannomas and NF2. In these patients preserved hearing, which was defined as a maximum post-treatment loss of 20 dB pure tone average, occurred in 56 percent at 1 year; in 54 percent at 2 years; but in only 28 percent at 6 years.[78] These results were all in patients treated before 1987 before magnetic resonance imaging (MRI) localization was available and when comparatively high doses were prescribed with an inferior dose-planning system. With the dose-planning techniques and strategies available for the last 3 years, long-term hearing preservation may be possible in up to 70 percent of patients. If these results hold up, contentions that radiosurgery should be used as a primary treatment modality for small and medium-sized vestibular schwannomas will probably be more insistent. We believe that even with such a development, microsurgery, in the best hands, in young patients, may be preferable. If the best hands are not available, radiosurgery should not be easily discarded.

Pituitary Adenomas

Heavy particle irradiation of pituitary tumors was already being performed during the 1950s in a large number of patients in Boston,[52] Berkeley,[63] St. Petersburg, and Moscow. Since 1954, 840 patients have been treated at the Lawrence Berkeley Laboratory with stereotactic charged particle radiosurgery of the pituitary gland. In the great majority of the 475 patients treated for pituitary tumors, marked and sustained biochemical and clinical improvement was observed. Variable degrees of hypopituitarism developed in about one-third of patients treated with radiosurgery only.[63] However, these treatments were not performed under strict stereotactic conditions and they involved three or four fractions. They were, therefore, not, in the original definition of the word, true radiosurgical treatments.

However, the results, particularly on growth hormone (GH) secretion in acromegaly, definitely inspired Leksell to initiate a program of gamma knife surgery for pituitary adenomas. At the time satisfactory treatment for hormone-secreting microadenomas was lacking. Pituitary gamma knife irradiation had been performed in patients with hormone-dependent malignancies, and it had been shown in post-mortem studies that very well circumscribed lesions could be made in the pituitary gland with the gamma knife.[5] The stereotactic localization techniques available in the early era were stereotactic pneumoencephalography and, later, CT-cisternography. Direct visualization of the tumor mass was not possible with these techniques. Nevertheless, the results were encouraging, particularly in suppressing adrenocorticotropic hormone (ACTH) secretion in Cushing's disease. The availability of stereotactic MRI has opened the possibility of direct tumor visualization, which should improve results and decrease the number of pituitary insufficiencies. However, available MRI techniques still often fail to clearly visualize adenomatous tissue and radiosurgery remains a second-line treatment modality in all but special patients. Petrosal venous sampling of hormones may be helpful but in postoperative situations, interpretation of the findings may be ambiguous. Today, the best indication for radiosurgery is probably as an adjuvant to microsurgery, particularly in dealing with tumors invading the cavernous sinus.

Follow-up of patients treated for pituitary adenomas should today include not only ophthalmologic and neurological examinations, but also MRI and careful hormonal evaluation. Particularly in regard to the latter in hormone-secreting tumors, there are differences in the definition of cure that must be kept in mind when comparing different patient materials.

Nonsecreting Adenomas

For treatment of nonsecreting pituitary adenomas the gamma knife has been used after failure of total resection and for recurrences after conventional treatment by surgery and postoperative irradiation. Also linac-radiosurgery performed for the same purpose has been reported, but it is unclear how many of these patients had nonsecreting tumors.[20,112] Clinical and radiologic results have been reported on 35 patients from seven Gamma Knife centers. There is consensus on the safety of the procedure. No neuro-ophthalmologic complications have been reported, and only one case of postirradiation panhypopituitarism. In at least 15 of the 35 patients there was a significant decrease of tumor volume, and no further growth or minor volume decrease was noted in the others.

The dose requirements for treatment of nonsecreting tumors seem to be lower than those for secreting tumors. This is beneficial as it makes treatment of larger tumors feasible without jeopardizing the function of the optic system. Doses to the chiasm and optic nerves should be kept at or below 8 Gy. Edge doses to the tumors of 10 to 15 Gy seem to be effective.

As reports of larger series of patients treated and long-term follow-up become available, radiosurgery can already be recommended as an adjuvant therapy in cases in which microsurgery followed by conventional irradiation has failed.

GH-Producing Tumors

GH-producing tumors not infrequently pose a surgical problem by parasellar growth. Whereas conventional orthovoltage radiation is of definite value for these patients, it takes 15 years for 90 percent of treated patients to reach GH-levels below 5 ng/ml and in patients with initial values above 100 ng/ml it may fail altogether. Panhypopituitarism is also an expected sequela.[22,28]

Results

GH-producing pituitary adenomas have been treated with the gamma knife at the Karolinska Institute in 60 patients with acromegaly. The majority of patients were surgical failures with tumor extension into the cavernous sinus. The dose plan has always been aimed at cure from the first treatment. Doses to the tumor margin have been 20 to 40 Gy (maximum dose 40 to 70 Gy). In general, the dose limitation has been set by the inevitable dose to the optic apparatus, keeping it below 15 Gy and in recent years, below 8 Gy. Adjustments of the dose have been made for previous radiotherapy. Retreatments were performed once in eight patients, twice in one patient, and three times in one patient.

The first 21 patients treated have been the subjects of a report. Fourteen of them had previous surgery and eight had additional radiotherapy. Radiosurgery was the initial treatment for seven patients. The patients were observed during a period of 1 to 21 years from the first radiosurgical session. Two young patients had a clinical remission with a substantial decline of GH levels to near normal serum profiles. Another eight patients obtained reduction of GH levels and clinical activity. More than half of the patients (11 of 21) had minor or no effect from the treatment. The only complication in the 13 patients who had not been previously irradiated was pituitary insufficiency in two.[108] More encouraging are the follow-up of GH serum levels in nine consecutive patients who were selected for gamma knife surgery based on previous treatment failure and visibility of the tumor on MRI. In three of these patients, GH serum levels fell below 4.5 ng/ml. The time to cure was 6, 9, and 30 months, respectively. The other six patients all have reduced GH values.

Reports on 38 patients with acromegaly treated at seven other Gamma Knife centers are also available. In general, these Centers report better results. At the University of Virginia[66] and at Brown University, four of nine patients had normalized GH values within 1 year of a single gamma knife treatment. In Fig. 185-4, the decrease in the size of a tumor treated by Steiner is illustrated. The Gamma Knife center at Kyung-Hee University in Korea reports "reduced hormone hypersecretion" within 2 to 12 months in 25 of 27 patients treated for secreting adenomas (GH-, ACTH-, and prolactin-secreting tumors).[60] The improvement in results must be ascribed to better tumor localization using multiplanar MRI and to developments in three-dimensional dose-planning.

ACTH-Producing Tumors

ACTH-producing tumors are often microadenomas and therefore attractive targets for radiosurgery. The initial results of gamma knife surgery at the Karolinska Institute built the hopes that an elegant cure for Cushing's disease had been found.[90] However, radiosurgery was hampered by the poor tumor localization techniques available, which not infrequently caused initial treatment failures and a need for repeated treatments. The latency to cure was therefore often long and when the results of transsphenoidal surgery improved, gamma knife radiosurgery for Cushing's disease was pushed back to the secondary armamentarium. It remains an attractive treatment option for the 10 to 20 percent of patients failing or experiencing tumor recurrence after surgery in whom reoperation has a high failure rate and high incidence of pituitary insufficiency.[92]

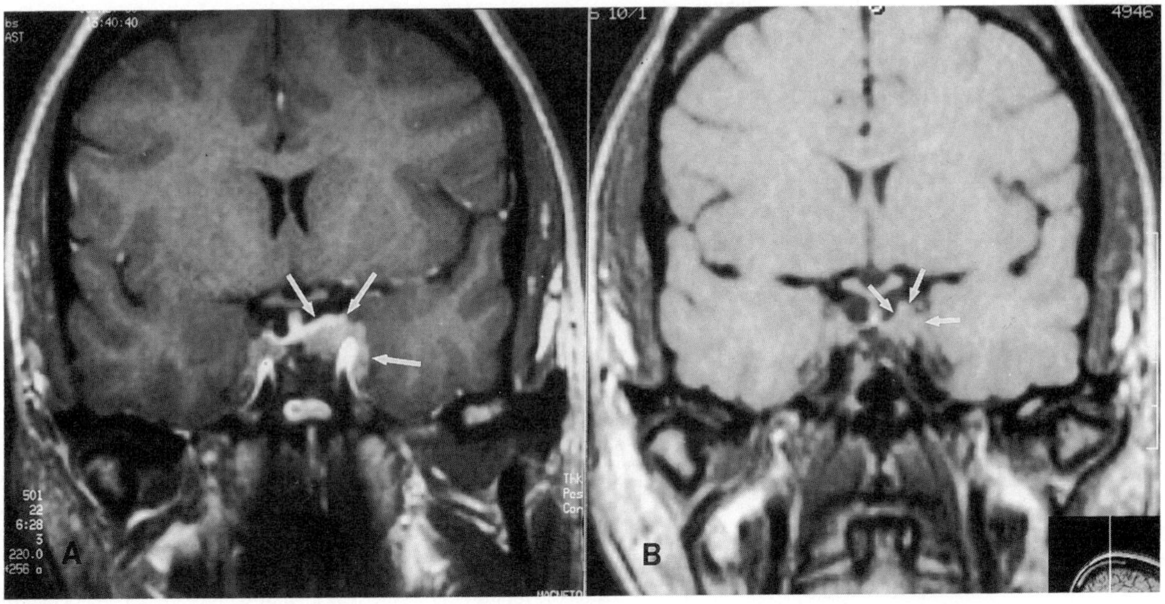

(*A*) (*B*)

Figure 185-4 MRI studies with coronal cuts before and after gamma knife surgery for a growth hormone-secreting pituitary adenoma. The patient, a 45-year-old woman with acromegaly, had trans-sphenoidal microsurgery. Following recurrence of the tumor, gamma knife surgery was carried out in November 1989. *A.* The pretreatment MRI shows the central and left laterally located recurrent tumor measuring 18 × 12 × 9 mm (*arrows*). *B.* A follow-up MRI in May 1994 reveals a small amount of residual tumor to the left of the sella that measures 8 × 9 × 8 mm (*arrows*).

Results

To date, 112 patients with pituitary-dependent Cushing's disease have been treated at the Karolinska Gamma Knife Center since 1974. Fourteen patients have been retreated once; eight patients, twice; four patients, three times; and one patient has been treated four times. The doses prescribed have, as with the GH-producing tumors, mainly been limited by the assumed tolerance dose of the optic apparatus. Because the vast majority of tumors have been intrasellar microadenomas, the assumed edge doses to the tumors have been higher [35 to 50 Gy (maximum doses 70 to 100 Gy)] than for the GH-producing tumors. The initial experience comprising 35 patients has been reported. This report includes only cases treated before stereotactic MRI and petrosal vein hormone sampling was available. In 29 patients the observation time was 3 to 9 years and sufficient for a more detailed scrutiny of the results. In 14 (18 percent) there was clinical remission and normal urinary cortisol output after a single treatment. Eight patients were in remission after two to four radiosurgery treatments. In total, there was a complete remission in 22 of the 29 patients (76 percent). Normalized hormone values were obtained within 1 year in 12 patients and within 3 years in another 10 patients. In contrast to the results of microsurgery, there have been no single late recurrences even now, 8 years after publication of this report. Pituitary insufficiency with follicle-stimulating hormone, thyroid-stimulating hormone, or ACTH failure was demonstrated in 12 of 22 patients in remission. These failures were documented 4 months to 7 years after the first irradiation. In a more recent series of 11 consecutive patients in whom the tumor was localized for gamma knife surgery by stereotactic MRI, the results were better. Seven were in remission with an average latency of 7.5 months. There was improvement to the point that the hormone output could be normalized by medication in two patients. One patient is scheduled for retreatment, and adrenalectomy had to be performed in one patient before remission because of a serious catabolic state.

Other gamma knife centers have reported a total of 34 Cushing patients treated so far. Although the rate of remission after a single treatment has not surpassed the initial Karolinska experience, there is still enthusiasm because of the virtual absence of morbidity in the cases treated. The impact of modern imaging techniques and corollary improvement of targeting seems to have been that of shortening the response latency. There are frequent reports of drop in hormonal values already after 2 to 3 months in some cases.

Prolactinomas

Prolactinomas are well managed by bromocriptine or surgery and rarely need to be considered for radiosurgery. The assembled experience is therefore low. Fifteen patients were treated by us: six in Stockholm; six at the University of Virginia; and three in Providence. In the Stockholm (Karolinska) series the follow-up time is 1 to 11 years. One patient died of unrelated causes 2 years after treatment with a prolactin level that was still elevated. The hormonal values were normalized in the other five patients but in two, bromocriptine was required. Tumors in three of the six cases treated at the University of Virginia decreased in size; the prolactin level returned to normal in two patients and decreased in four.[103]

Craniopharyngiomas

Controversy still prevails regarding the best management for craniopharyngiomas. The controversy centers around how aggressive surgery should be; what the role of postoperative conventional radiation is; and to what extent stereotactic techniques such as cyst aspiration, intracavitary radiation, and radiosurgery should be used.

Conventional Treatment

Excellent surgical results in a series of 144 patients, with total removal in 90 percent and recurrence only in 7 percent of the patients, have been reported by Yasargil et al.[120] Symon et al. reported three recurrences (6 percent) in 50 cases of total tumor excision.[105] From The Children's Hospital in Toronto, Hoffman et al. reported total excision in 45 of 50 patients operated on, but there were recurrences in 17 of the children after a mean time of 33 months.[37] In other series including patients operated on with modern microsurgical techniques, total excision has been possible in 50 to 80 percent of the cases,[4,41,43,110,115] with a 0 to 20 percent recurrence rate.[116] Attempt at total excision still carries an operative mortality of a few percent.[37,43,105] Surgical morbidity varies with the size and location of the tumor and is higher after repeat surgery. Unfortunately, it is also higher after more radical attempts at removal.[10]

Late-occurring recurrences after presumed total excisions and significant surgical morbidity have prompted many neurosurgeons to take a more conservative attitude, particularly in treating children. Long-term results are now available.

Nineteen children were followed for a median of 21 years (range, 8 to 28 years) following surgery and postoperative radiation. Five of 19 (26 percent) developed recurrence following radiation. The overall 20-year survival was 62 percent.[94]

The Joint Center for Radiation Therapy in Boston reported treatment results in 61 children after a median of 10 years (range, 2 to 20.5 years). All nine of the children treated only with radiation therapy are alive; none have had a recurrence. Nine of the 15 children treated with surgery alone have had a recurrence; seven of the 37 patients treated with surgery plus radiotherapy have had a recurrence. The 10-year actuarial freedom from progression for the surgery group was 31 percent compared with 100 percent for patients treated with radiation therapy only, and 86 percent for patients treated with surgery plus radiotherapy at diagnosis. There were two treatment-related deaths, but in the surgery plus radiotherapy group. A higher incidence of visual loss and diabetes insipidus was associated with the use of aggressive surgery. Patients treated with surgery alone had a significantly higher incidence of progression when compared to patients treated with surgery and radiation therapy or radiation therapy only.[35]

Between 1950 and 1986, 173 patients with craniopharyngioma were treated at the Royal Marsden Hospital in London with radiotherapy only or following surgery. Survival and progression-free survival were not influenced by the extent of surgical excision. Visual field defects improved after radiotherapy in 38 of 106 patients (36 percent), and visual acuity in 27 of 91 (30 percent).[91]

Proponents of aggressive surgery emphasize the long-term risks of radiotherapy and especially the risks of retardation of intellectual development in children. It is also rightly pointed out that the significant improvements in microsurgical techniques and postoperative intensive care have considerably lowered morbidity, making comparisons with older material invalid. From all surgical reports it can be concluded that the results are much better following the first operation and that the morbidity is higher with surgery of large tumors. It seems reasonable to reserve postoperative radiotherapy for partially resected tumors and for tumors recurring after "total excision." The results of radiotherapy at recurrence are similar to those of conservative surgery and radiotherapy at the time of presentation.[40]

The Stereotactic Approach

A third way of attacking craniopharyngiomas is by a combination of stereotactic techniques. In an autopsy study it was found that approximately 70 percent of these tumors were predominantly cystic.[86] In surgical specimens 34 percent were predominantly cystic and 43 percent mixed.[106] Already in the 1950s Leksell proposed treatment of cystic tumors with intracavitary radioactive isotopes.[62] His pupil, Backlund, then developed and advocated this technique for the management of cystic craniopharyngiomas. Solid tumor parts were left alone, operated on and given radiotherapy, or treated by gamma knife surgery. Of 42 consecutively treated patients, 31 were alive and available for follow-up after 10 to 23 years. There was no perioperative mortality. The patients were "socially well adapted with a high rate of full-time work and a low rate of intercurrent disease." Most patients had panhypopituitarism.[96]

Radiosurgery

Gamma knife surgery has been part of the stereotactic management strategy for craniopharyngiomas at the Karolinska Institute since 1968, when the first patient was treated with the gamma knife. Altogether 51 patients have been treated. In a small minority of patients the gamma knife surgery has been the primary treatment modality. Most patients were first operated on and then often treated by instillation of yttrium 90 (^{90}y) in cystic parts of the tumor. Solid portions were then treated by radiosurgery. Hence, it is very difficult to single out the contribution of radiosurgery to the outcome in these patients. The peripheral dose to the target tumor has been limited by the proximity of the optic apparatus. Peripheral doses of 10 to 20 Gy were prescribed. In many cases there has been considerable shrinkage of tumor volume 6 to 12 months following the treatment (Fig. 185-5). In other tumors of equal size no further growth has occurred. A possible explanation for the differential effect is tumor histology, as it has been shown that the squamous cell variety of craniopharyngioma is more radiosensitive than the adamantinomatous type.[39] There also seems to be a higher risk of recurrence after conventional treatment for the adamantinomatous craniopharyngioma.[106] Differences in histology should in the future be taken into account when selecting treatment and evaluating treatment results.

Nine patients have been treated at the University of Virginia by gamma knife surgery with peripheral doses of 10 to 15 Gy (maximum dose 20 to 50 Gy) following one or two conventional operations. In three cases the radiosurgery was combined with intracavitary radiation of a cystic component using phosphorus[32] (^{32}P) and one patient had previously received intracavitary treatment with ^{90}Y. Eight patients were available for follow-up. In five of those, the tumor volume had decreased, in one it was unchanged, and in one patient there had been continued tumor growth. Clinical improvement was seen in six of the eight cases.[103]

Ten patients (five children and five adults) were treated by gamma knife surgery following partial removal (seven cases), stereotactic biopsy and cyst drainage (two cases), or radiologic diagnosis (one case) at the Komaki City Hospital in Japan. The mean volume of these tumors was ~6 cc and the mean marginal dose around 14 Gy. All tumors responded with volume reduction during the observation period, which was 4 to 29 months. In seven cases the volume reduction was marked.[54]

It is premature to define the role of radiosurgery in the current management of craniopharyngioma. It seems a reasonable prediction that it could supplant postoperative conventional radiotherapy when the remaining tumor is of reasonable size. In selected cases of small tumors it could possibly be used as the only treatment modality. Microsurgery aiming at total excision remains the first treatment option for the majority of patients.

Meningiomas

The primary treatment modality for meningiomas is definitely microsurgical removal. Most patients can be cured by removal of the tumor, but this fact does not justify radical surgical attempts carrying the risk of leaving the patient with a poor quality of life. Undoubtedly there has been considerable progress in skull base surgical techniques and tumors can now sometimes be completely removed even from these difficult locations. The good results reported from a few excellent neurosurgical centers have inspired less well-trained neurosurgeons to attack meningiomas in the central skull base and cavernous sinus. Many patients therefore present for adjuvant therapy with neurological deficits actually created by the neurosurgeon.[69] In view of this fact, partial resection of central skull base meningiomas or even leaving them alone should be considered.

A recent review of the hospital records of 325 patients with skull base meningiomas managed at the Karolinska Institute between 1947 and 1982 and followed for an average of 18 years (range, 10 to 36 years) gave some perspectives on this issue and on the requirements that should be set for studies concerning therapy of meningiomas. As expected with radical removal (Simpson grade 1), without adjuvant therapy the recurrence rate at 5 years was low (3.5 percent), continued to be low at 10 years (7 percent), and at 25 years was 13 percent. The corresponding numbers for subtotal removal was 5 years, 25 percent; 10 years, 39 percent; and 25 years, 76 percent. Of particular interest were the 38 patients with tumors remaining in the cavernous sinus who were followed for more than 10 years or until their death. Twenty-nine patients died from their tumor within 10 years, six were alive with progressive symptoms at 10 to 15 years, and only three were alive and asymptomatic at 10 to 15 years (Mathiesen T, Kihlström L, Lindquist C, et al.: Unpublished data.) These figures strongly suggest that a "wait and see" attitude should not be adopted for central skull base meningiomas, except maybe for very old patients.

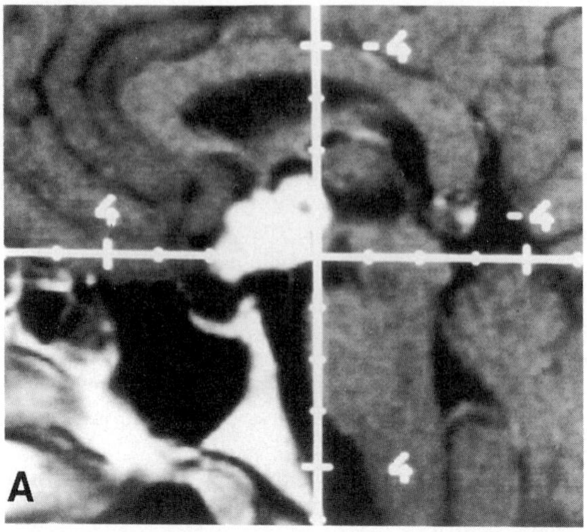

(*A*)

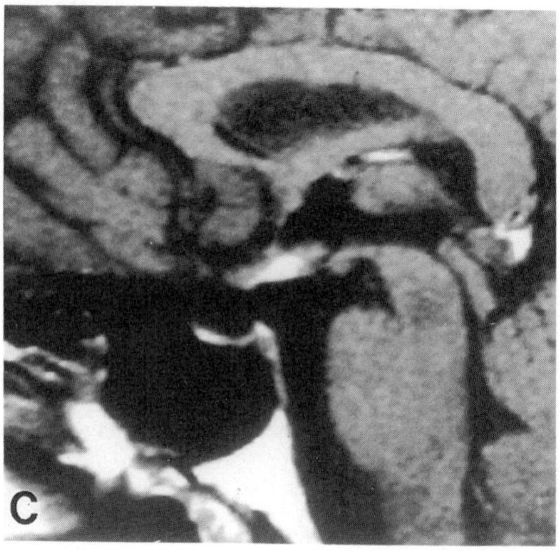

(*C*)

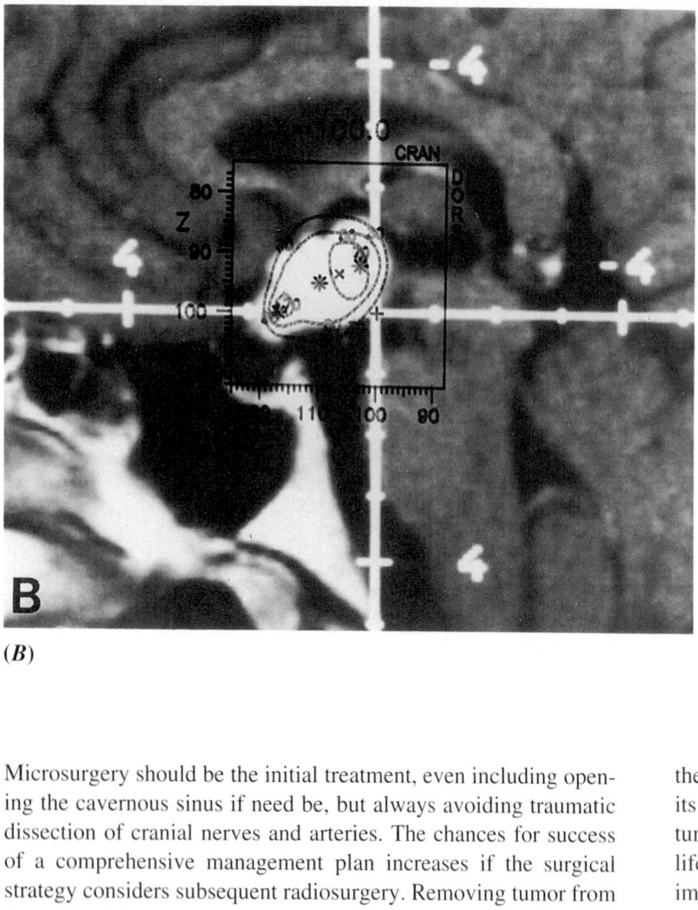

(*B*)

Figure 185-5 T1-weighted gadolinium-enhanced MRI scans of a 45-year-old man with a craniopharyngioma recurrence after microsurgery. Before (*A*), at the time of the gamma knife surgery (*B*), and 5 months after the treatment (*C*).

Microsurgery should be the initial treatment, even including opening the cavernous sinus if need be, but always avoiding traumatic dissection of cranial nerves and arteries. The chances for success of a comprehensive management plan increases if the surgical strategy considers subsequent radiosurgery. Removing tumor from the optic chiasm and nerves and minimizing the tumor volume facilitates dose-planning. Ideally the microsurgery and the radiosurgery are performed by the same person.

Rationale for Radiosurgery

There is now compelling evidence that postoperative radiation therapy of residual meningioma prolongs progression-free survival of the patient.[6,12,29,74,87,107] The rationale for using radiosurgery as the specific radiation adjuvant is that this technology is unique in its accuracy and precision and thus minimizes risks. Furthermore, tumors actually shrink following treatment; therefore, the use of life-table statistics is not the only means of data analysis. More importantly, no undue effects such as dementia or neoplasia have been seen after 26 years of using the gamma knife. Last, but not least, the single-session treatment is convenient for the patient.

Localization for Radiosurgery

Tumor localization for radiosurgery should now be made with stereotactic MRI, without and with gadolinium enhancement. This imaging modality gives an excellent display of the tumor but also visualizes the optic apparatus and sometimes the other cranial nerves in proximity to skull base meningiomas. Again in the treatment of parasellar meningiomas we are careful not to overdose the optic pathways and therefore keep the dose to these structures at or below 8 Gy. The nerves in the cavernous sinus are more resistant and usually do not limit the marginal dose to the tumor, which is 12 to 20 Gy depending on tumor volume.

Long-Term Results

Benign meningiomas are slowly growing tumors and recurrences may develop very late. We have seen recurrences in two patients who had negative CT scans at 15 and 17 years following surgery, respectively. Very long follow-up is therefore required to prove the effectiveness of any treatment modality. Over such prolonged observation periods treatment techniques improve, which further complicates the comparison of results.

A number of reports consider the efficacy of radiosurgery for meningioma growth control in the short-term perspective. These studies and our own experience indicate that the whole tumor should be included in an optimal radiosurgical treatment plan. When we started to treat meningiomas at the Karolinska Gamma Knife Center in 1976, stereotactic MRI was not available and CT was of poor quality. The treatment strategy was therefore often to cover the vascular supply of the tumor and/or part of the "tumor blush" seen on a stereotactic angiogram. We recently examined the results of patients treated by this partial tumor irradiation. Of the 30 consecutive cases, 21 were available for a minimum follow-up of 10 years. The tumors were located in the cavernous sinus and parasellar area in 11 of these patients; in the petroclival area in three; and in the cerebellopontine angle in seven. The first patient treated, a man in his thirties, is still alive without clinical symptoms 18 years after treatment of his cavernous sinus meningioma. In total, there is no sign of further growth or a decrease of tumor size in 15 of the 21 patients. Two patients had partial surgical removal of their tumors because of continued growth, two patients died related to their tumor (one from a seizure), and two patients died of unrelated causes. The cranial nerve function improved in five patients and deteriorated over the observation time in four patients. Deterioration of cranial nerve function was ascribed to the treatment in two cases and to further tumor growth in two cases. Obviously the results of this suboptimal radiosurgical treatment compare favorably with the natural or postoperative course of the disease. The treatment morbidity also appears to be less than that from microsurgery, although reports detailed enough to make just comparisons are not available.

Short-Term Results

In a short-term perspective, the Pittsburgh group has reported on 81 meningioma patients treated by gamma knife surgery since 1987, of whom 73 had a minimum follow-up of 6 months. Nineteen (26 percent) showed a reduction in tumor volume, while in 46 (63 percent) tumors did not show further growth. Five patients had delayed tumor growth and three patients underwent surgery. Clinical improvement was seen in nine cases. The results of treatment of meningiomas in the cavernous sinus was the subject of a special report from the same group. No patient of the 34 treated had signs of further growth during the median follow-up of 26 months. Tumor regression was observed in 19 cases (56 percent). Eight patients (24 percent) improved clinically, two developed a permanent new cranial nerve deficit, and two a transient new cranial nerve deficit. No patient developed an endocrinopathy or new extraocular muscle paresis.[21]

Among the 160 meningioma patients treated by Steiner, 139 had previous surgery (emphasizing our treatment policy) and 120 were available for follow-up from 4 months to 13 years (9 patients). More than 5 years of follow-up was available in 58 cases. Fifty-two of these tumors remained unchanged and 61 decreased in size. Seven lesions have increased. Clinical improvement was seen in nine patients, and deterioration in two. The meningioma was located in the cavernous sinus in 86 of the patients. Follow-up was available in 62 of them. Decrease in size was observed in 30 (48.3 percent), 29 (46.8 percent) were unchanged, and the tumor increased in volume in three patients.[103] In Fig. 185-6 a meningioma treated by Lindquist is illustrated.

Short-term results of another 93 meningiomas treated by three additional gamma knife centers were recently reported (at the Sixth Leksell Gamma Knife Society meeting in Kyoto, Japan in 1994). Two groups reported 50 percent of the tumors to be decreasing and the third group saw 26 percent of tumors decreasing over an average observation time of 9.5 months.

Metastases

Malignant primary tumors of the brain are in general not well suited for radiosurgery because of their infiltrating character. Secondary malignancies are, on the other hand, usually well circumscribed and therefore well suited for this therapy. It is estimated that approximately 20 to 30 percent of all patients harboring malignant disease develop metastases to the brain.[8,11,118] In lung cancer patients the probability of developing cerebral metastases is estimated to be 30 to 40 percent; in breast cancer, 15 to 50 percent; in melanoma, 10 to 65 percent; and in renal cancer, 4 to 10 percent.[46,55,84,97,111,118] It is not infrequent that metastasis to the brain is the first evidence of spread,[2,51] and untreated patients are likely to die from the cerebral metastases regardless of the nature of the primary tumor.[11]

Based on CT scan evaluations, it was found that almost half (49 percent) of the patients had a single metastasis,[19] which corresponds well with findings from an autopsy series in which the frequency was 42 percent.[111] Assuming that half of the patients with a single metastasis are suitable for a craniotomy, at least 25 patients per million inhabitants would profit from neurosurgical care.[121]

Established Therapy

Presently the prevailing therapy for the treatment of cerebral metastases is craniotomy followed by whole-brain radiation therapy (WBRT). There is profound evidence that surgical extirpation of a single metastasis prolongs survival and improves quality of life.[11] In retrospective studies, it was shown that the addition of postoperative WBRT prolonged the interval to tumor relapse in the brain and reduced the number of patients dying from neurological disease.[18,33,100] In a randomized prospective study by Patchell et al.,

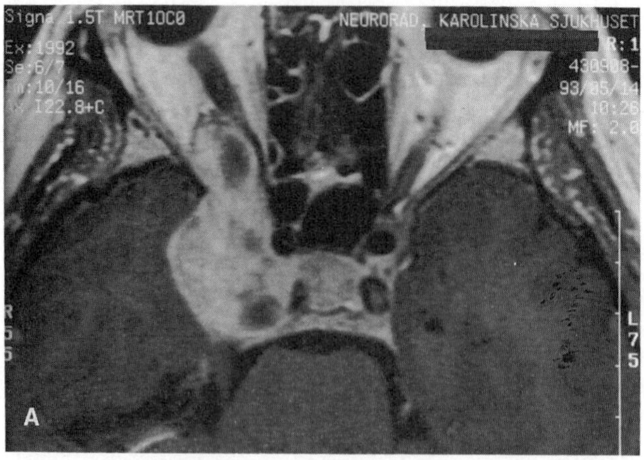

(*A*)

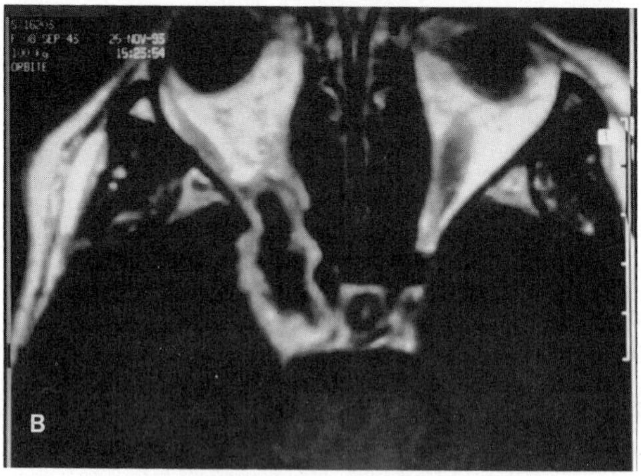

(*B*)

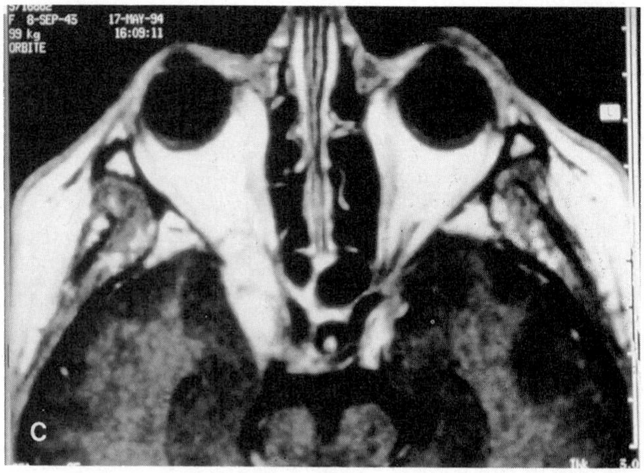

(*C*)

Figure 185-6 Meningioma extending from the left cavernous sinus into the middle cranial fossa and involving the optic canal, in a 50-year-old woman with transitory third-nerve weakness in the right eye in 1980. Microsurgery was carried out in 1989 and the diagnosis was established. Following surgery there was complete blindness in the right eye. Because of growth of the residual tumor, gamma knife surgery was performed in 1992. *A*. MRI before gamma knife treatment. *B*. Six months after the treatment there is no central enhancement and irregular circumferential enhancement. *C*. One year after the treatment the size of the tumor is 28 × 12 mm in the axial plane as compared to the measurements of 44 × 23 at the time of the gamma knife procedure.

surgery alone and surgery followed by WBRT for a single metastasis were compared.[83] Length of survival as well as quality of life were superior in the group treated with operation plus WBRT, and the number of local recurrences was lower.

Rationale for and Results of Radiosurgery

Although of definite value, WBRT separates the patient from the family for a significant time. The short- and long-term side effects may also be a significant problem. In one study, 11 percent of patients surviving for more than 1 year developed dementia.[17] These facts prompted us to start gamma knife surgery for metastases in 1975. There are now two different radiosurgical treatment strategies. In both strategies radiosurgery has taken the place of craniotomy. In one strategy radiosurgery is used as a local boost in combination with WBRT. This strategy is based on the assumption that undetected tumors and potential tumor deposits outside the imaging-defined tumor margin will be affected by the general radiation. The radiosurgical dose has been approximately 20 Gy in combination with about 35 Gy of fractionated WBRT. Good local control and stabilization or improvement of neurological symptoms have been reported with this technique for a single metastasis.[1,13,68,104] The other strategy is to use radiosurgery exclusively for single or multiple metastases. The minimum dose given to the tumor in these treatments has been somewhat higher, or 25 to 30 Gy, depending on volume. This is the strategy currently used in our institutions, and the results have been reported.[46–48,64] At a recent follow-up of 200 patients, half of the tumors were no longer visible (Fig. 185-9), one-third had significantly decreased in size, 5 percent were unchanged, and 10 percent had increased in size. Increase in tumor volume could be shown to be due to radionecrosis in half of the cases and to local recurrence in one-fourth (Figs. 185-7 and 185-8).[42] Defining successful treatment as arrest of tumor growth or decrease in tumor size yields a success rate of up to 90 percent (Figs. 185-7 to 185-9).

A number of factors influence the outcome of treatment for brain metastases. Obviously, the general condition of the patient at the time of treatment is very important, as is the nature of the underlying primary malignancy. Before the advent of radiosurgery, neurosurgical treatment was more or less reserved for patients with a single metastasis and others were treated by WBRT or steroids only. The convenience of radiosurgery has encouraged a more liberal attitude toward treatment, and patients late in the course of their malignancies are now being managed by radiosurgery.

To prove the superior efficacy of radiosurgery, randomized prospective studies are still desirable but available data give a good indication of the outcome to be expected from such trials. The best efficacy indicator is probably the rate of recurrences at the treatment site. Of 375 gamma knife procedures performed at the Karolinska Institute there were recurrences in 27 cases (7 percent). In a multi-institutional trial of gamma knife surgery for a single metastasis there were 17 local recurrences in 116 patients treated (15 percent).[25] These figures should be compared to the 20 percent local recurrence rate after surgery and WBRT, and to the 50 percent recurrence rate for WBRT as the sole treatment modality.[83] It can be argued that the local recurrence rate is related to the time the patient survives after treatment, but this parameter also indicates the superiority of gamma knife surgery. In the Karolinska group of patients with a single metastasis, the mean survival following treatment was 46 weeks, which is similar to the 11 months reported from the multi-institutional trial,[25] a little longer than the 10 months reported for patients treated by surgical removal followed by WBRT, and significantly longer than the 15 weeks that was the outcome for patients randomized to WBRT alone.[83] Local control after radiosurgery thus seems to be as effective with radiosurgery alone as in combination with WBRT but the question of whether WBRT gives protection against metastases appearing elsewhere in the brain remains. Among 191 patients with a single metastasis, 47 (26 percent) had distant recurrences following gamma knife surgery only. It is not known whether the addition of WBRT would lower this incidence.

It is hoped that randomized trials now under way will resolve this issue. The short survival of patients with a single metastasis treated by WBRT does, however, not favor WBRT. Our preliminary observations indicate that a single metastasis appearing distant to the original treatment site is treated equally well by radiosurgery and therefore makes this an attractive treatment option. It must be realized that WBRT only has a chance to kill tumor cells present in the brain at the time of therapy and does not prevent later seeding.

Indications for Radiosurgery

Granted the efficacy and convenience of radiosurgery for brain metastases, the indications for the treatment must be addressed. Stringent rules cannot be given. Although effective, it must be realized that radiosurgery at best can only kill intracranial tumor cells. Suffering should not be prolonged by treatment of terminal patients.

Which tumors should be treated? Any secondary tumor responds to radiosurgery, even such less radiosensitive tumors as melanomas and renal cell cancers. In fact, the longest mean survival following treatment in the Karolinska series has been seen in melanoma patients. The best local control in another series of patients was achieved in melanoma and renal cell cancer patients.[25]

How many tumors can and should be treated? Again, assessments for the individual patient must be made. However, we have observed that the risk for distant recurrences is double (50 percent) in patients treated for more than three metastases as compared to patients with a single metastasis (25 percent). The nature of the primary tumor is also of importance in these assessments. In melanoma patients and in patients with renal cell cancer we have seen prolongation of a good quality of life even in patients treated for multiple metastases. On the other hand, patients with lung cancer have a shorter life expectancy than most other patients with brain metastases (in 103 patients the average time to death after treatment was 25 weeks).

Radiosurgery is recommended as the primary treatment modality for brain metastasis (except for tumors large enough to threaten the patient's life by mass effect). Histologic confirmation should be obtained prior to treatment unless circumstantial evidence for a specific diagnosis is very strong. Stereotactic biopsy is the method of choice, but we and others[95] have seen spread of tumor in the trajectory of the biopsy needle. We therefore usually perform the stereotactic biopsy immediately after the gamma knife surgery with the stereotactic frame in the same position to prevent seeding of untreated tumor cells.

Follow-Up

Concomitant edema often subsides following treatment or can be treated by steroids. Tumor shrinkage is usually visible within 1 to 2 months. Follow-up by MRI or CT should be made bimonthly. If increase of tumor size is seen after treatment, radionecrosis can be differentiated from tumor progression by positron emission tomography (PET) studies with fluoride 18-deoxyglucose (FDG) or by multiple stereotactic biopsies.[75]

Gliomas

Tumors of neuroepithelial tissue and (perhaps) in particular the astrocytoma series are difficult to classify. The expected natural course is dependent on the grade of tumor and consequently a marginal impact of any new therapy is difficult to elucidate. Histologic diagnosis is mandatory even in the age of high-resolution neuroimaging techniques.[56] Because of their infiltrating growth, it is difficult to outline these tumors and to give a tumoricidal dose without jeopardizing the function of surrounding normal brain. The experience of radiosurgery for gliomas is very limited and few publications are available. In our review we distinguish pilocytic astrocytomas, including optic gliomas, grade I according to the World Health Organization (WHO); low-grade astrocytomas, WHO grade II; malignant gliomas and anaplastic astrocytomas, WHO grade III; and glioblastomas, WHO grade IV. Gliomas are commonly too voluminous for safe radiosurgery and most treatments have been made following surgical debulking and/or conventional radiotherapy.

Pilocytic Astrocytoma (Astrocytoma I)

Pilocytic astrocytomas tend to occur in younger patients, are circumscribed, and are amenable to cure with gross total resection. There is no role for the routine use of postoperative radiotherapy in these patients.[99] We concur with this statement and add that the well-defined borders of these tumors make them well suited for radiosurgery also. Contrast enhancement on CT or MRI defines the tumor volume and should be used for stereotactic localization. These benign lesions are often located in the thalamus, hypothalamus, or basal ganglia. In these locations resection is still possible with reasonable safety with the aid of stereotactic microsurgery.[44]

Results

There are no publications on results after radiosurgical treatment of pilocytic astrocytomas but a fairly extensive experience on

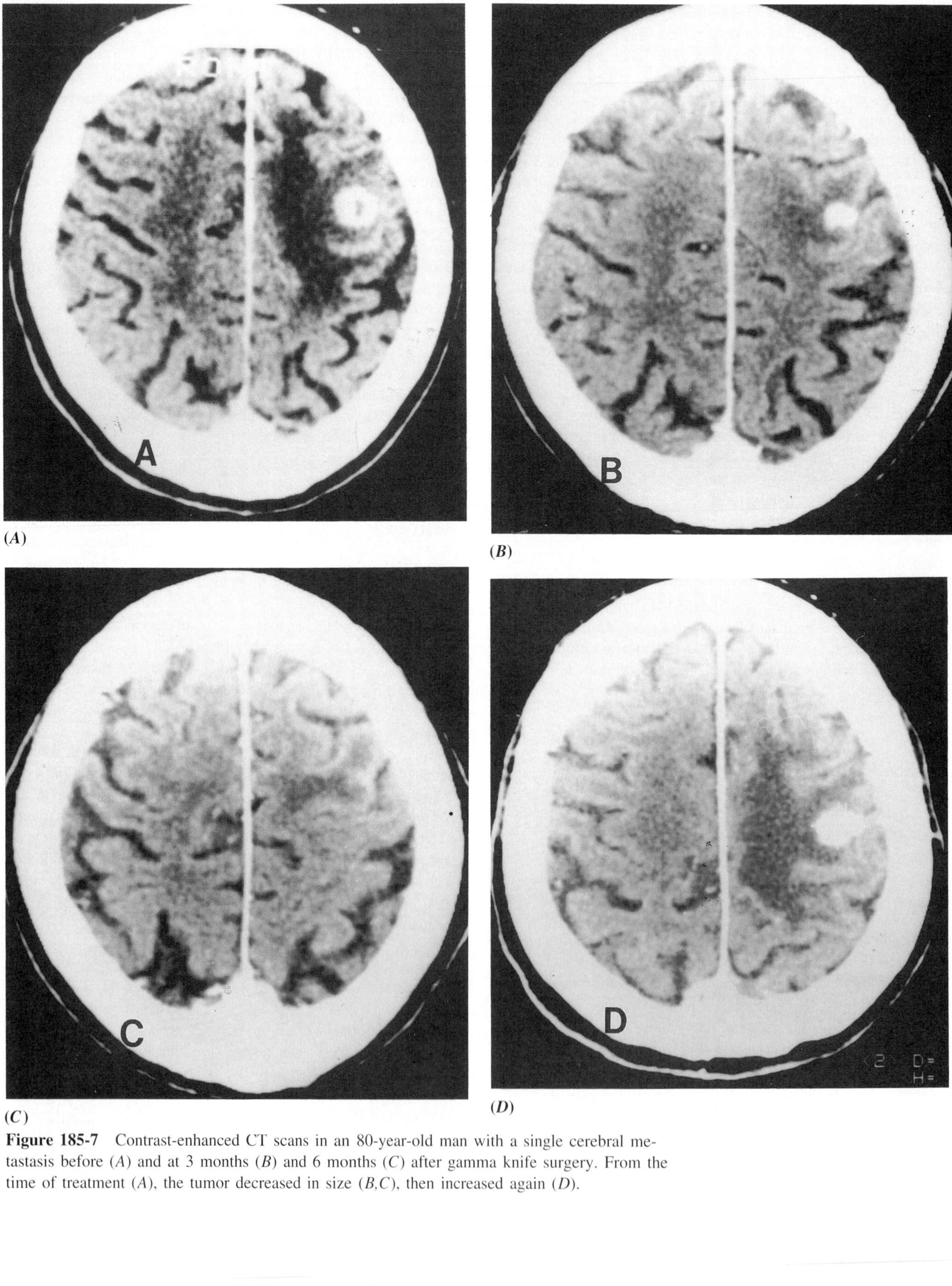

(*A*) (*B*) (*C*) (*D*)

Figure 185-7 Contrast-enhanced CT scans in an 80-year-old man with a single cerebral metastasis before (*A*) and at 3 months (*B*) and 6 months (*C*) after gamma knife surgery. From the time of treatment (*A*), the tumor decreased in size (*B,C*), then increased again (*D*).

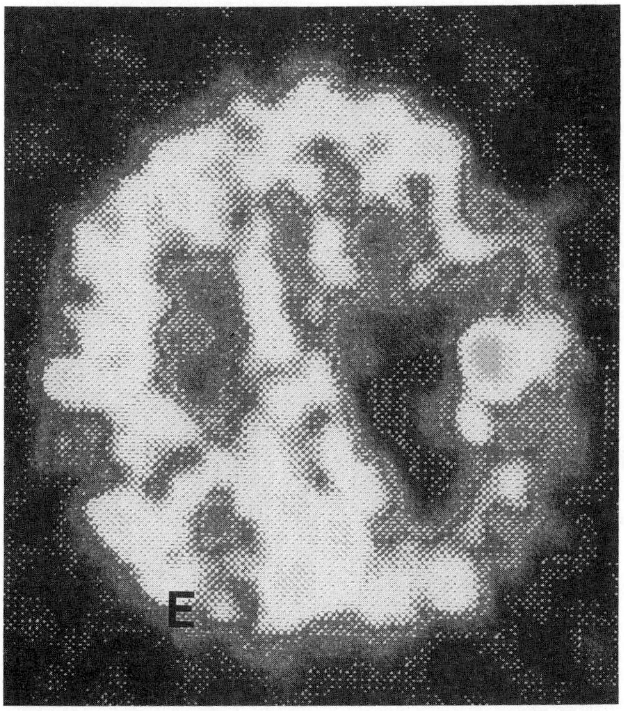

(*E*)

Figure 185-7 (*Continued*) To differentiate between tumor growth and radiation-induced swelling, PET with [^{18}F] FDG was performed. The PET scan revealed higher metabolism than surrounding brain in the tumor area (*E*)—evidence of living tumor.

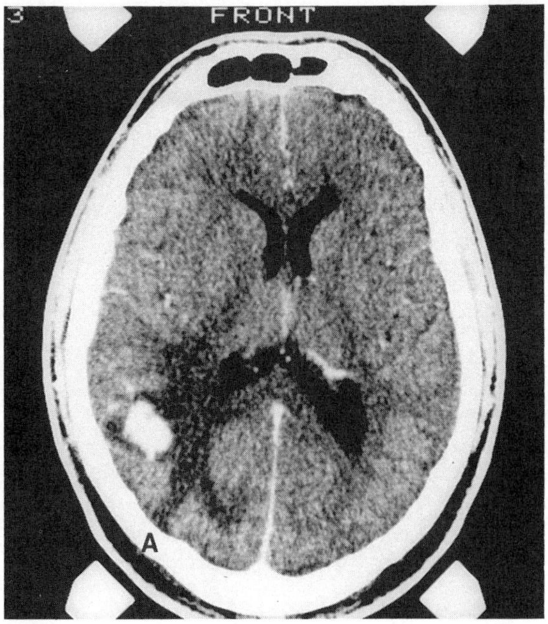

(*A*)

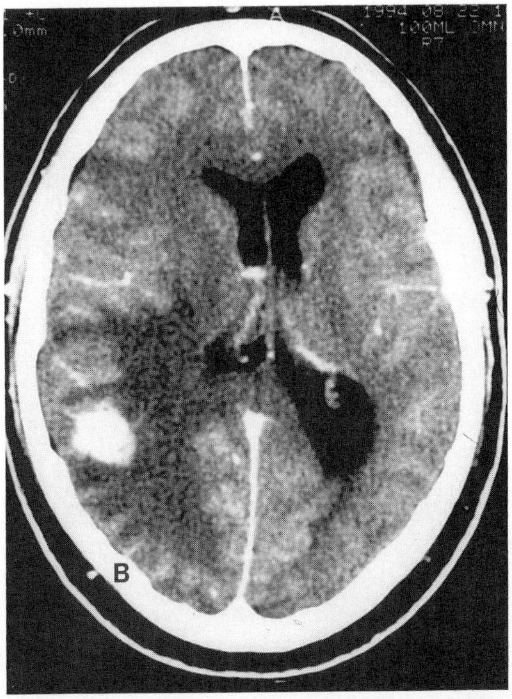

(*B*)

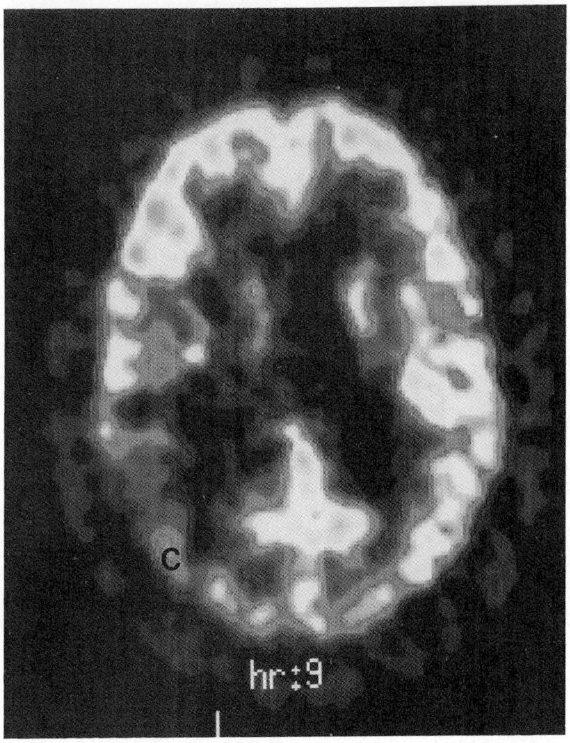

(*C*)

Figure 185-8 Contrast-enhanced CT scans (*A,B*) in a 45-year-old man with a single cerebral metastasis before (*A*) and 2 months after (*B*) gamma knife surgery. The tumor volume at 2 months is a bit larger than before. In this case PET with [^{18}F] FDG shows lower metabolism in the tumor area in comparison to the surrounding normal brain (*C*). This indicates that the increased tumor volume is due to swelling secondary to radiation-induced necrosis rather than to an increased number of tumor cells.

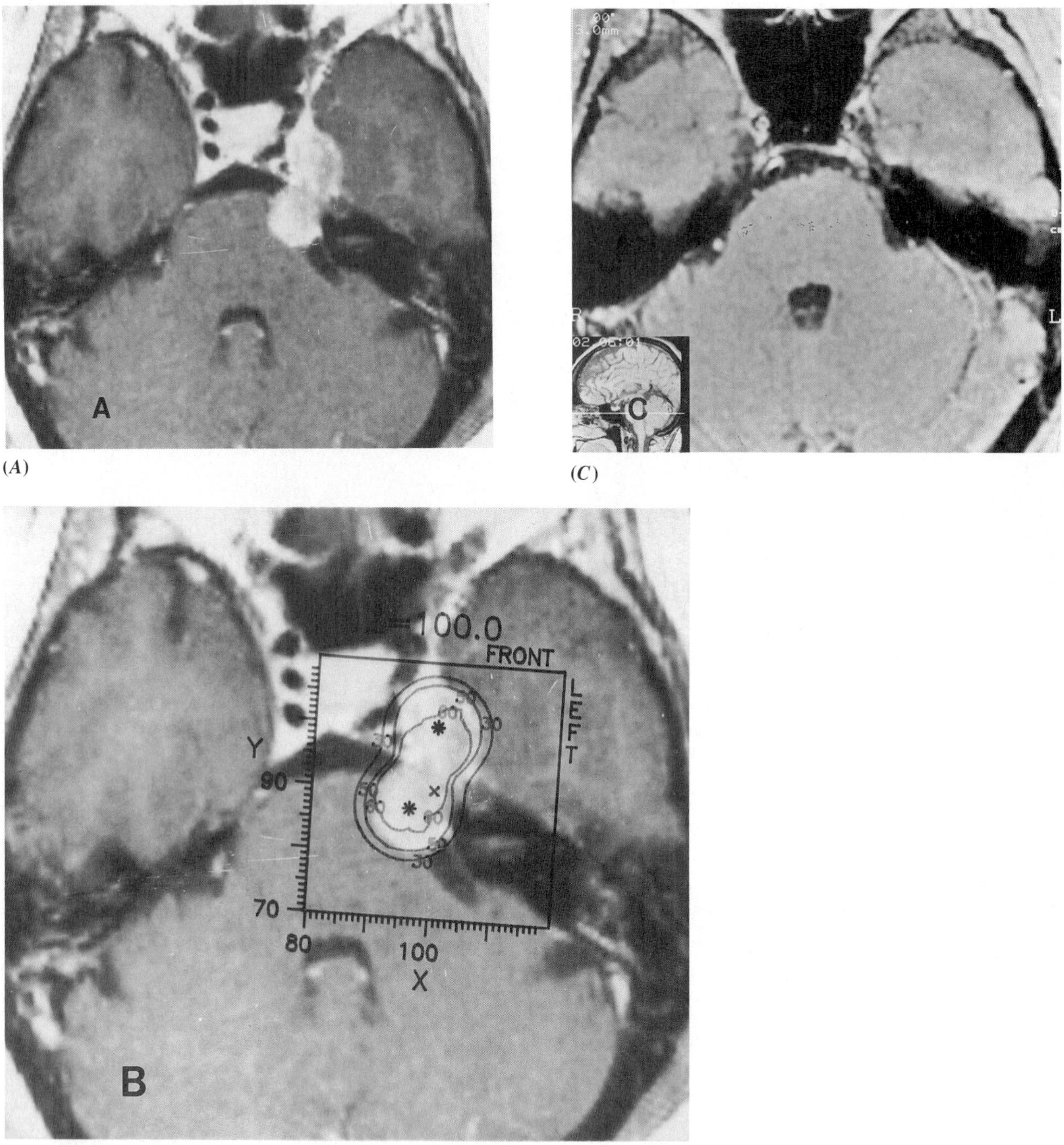

(*A*) (*C*) (*B*)

Figure 185-9 A 50-year-old woman with a metastatic tumor from breast carcinoma at the level of Meckel's cave and the gasserian ganglion. Contrast-enhanced T1-weighted MR images before (*A*), at the time of gamma knife surgery (*B*), and 6 months after the treatment (*C*). Regression of the tumor.

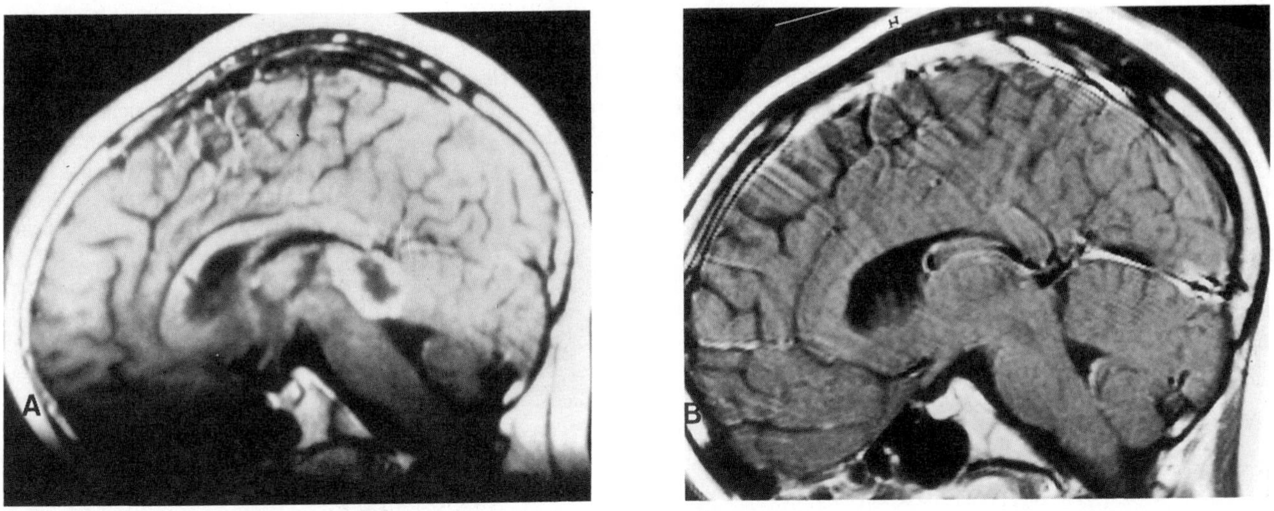

(*A*) (*B*)

Figure 185-10 *A*. Sagittal T2-weighted MR image in a 9-year-old girl revealing a tumor within the tectum of the midbrain. The diagnosis of a low-grade astrocytoma was secured by a stereotactic biopsy. Gamma knife surgery was carried out in August 1989. Following the treatment the tumor progressively decreased in size and finally disappeared. The girl remains in excellent condition and serial MRI studies, the most recent in April 1994, revealed no recurrence (*B*).

treatment of pilocytic astrocytomas of the optic pathways in children by ''interstitial stereotactic radiosurgery'' has been reported from the University of Freiburg. Treatment was given with ^{125}I seeds temporarily implanted into the tumor. At 10 cGy/h, 5000 to 8000 cGy were given to 115 children. Tumor response could be detected by a decrease of tumor volume on CT in 71 percent of the children, clinical improvement occurred in 58 percent, and in those with ophthalmologic symptoms, improvement occurred in 86 percent. The 5-year survival rate was 86 percent and the treatment morbidity only 2 percent.[114] We have used gamma knife surgery for eight patients with pilocytic astrocytomas; following subtotal stereotactic microsurgical resection from the deep ganglia and as a primary modality for tumor in the brain stem. Tumor volume decrease or no further growth has been seen in this small number of patients (Fig. 185-10).

Low-Grade Astrocytoma (Astrocytoma II)

Radiosurgery faces the same problem with low-grade astrocytomas as open surgery, i.e., tumor destruction without injuring surrounding brain. The infiltration of the tumor margin into surrounding brain makes this difficult in eloquent areas of the brain. Postoperative radiotherapy appears to improve survival, particularly in adults.[99] In some situations, deferring treatment may be the best option.[93] Several ongoing clinical trials are addressing two issues: observation versus radiotherapy and low-dose versus high-dose radiotherapy in patients with ordinary astrocytomas, oligoastrocytomas, and mixed oligoastrocytomas.[99]

Colombo and his group were the first to publish results on radiosurgery of low-grade gliomas. The target volume was defined with CT performed under stereotactic conditions. A total dose of 16 to 50 Gy was administered in either one fraction or two fractions 8 days apart. Patients were followed up for 11 to 48 months. Twelve of 14 patients had a partial or complete response to treatment, as demonstrated by CT.[89]

At the University of Virginia, we treated 30 low-grade glioma patients and follow-up was obtained in all after 3 to 44 months. The tumor disappeared in 4 cases, decreased in 15, increased in 7, and was unchanged in 4. Two patients ultimately succumbed to their illness as a result of tumor progression.

In Stockholm seven patients with low-grade gliomas in the tectum presenting with ophthalmologic problems or hydrocephalus were treated by the gamma knife from 1979 to 1991. The patients have been followed for an average of 6 years (range, 2 to 15 years). In five cases the tumor had shrunk after treatment. In one patient the cystic tumor was too large to be completely covered by an effective radiation dose and the tumor had to be removed 3 years after treatment. There have been no other cases of tumor progression or cases of dedifferentiating tumor. All patients were treated using one isocenter and the 14-mm collimator but with different peripheral tumor doses. In the first two cases the dose prescription was based on previous experience from treatment of arteriovenous malformations (peripheral dose, 25 to 30 Gy). These doses resulted in severe radiation-induced neurological complications and subsequently lower doses were prescribed. This is a good example of the fact that not only the volume of the target but also its biological nature is of importance in dose selection. Currently the recommended peripheral dose to a low-grade glioma is 10 to 14 Gy. At the latest follow-up one patient had improved after treatment, no change was noted in two, and one patient had aggravated symptoms secondary to radiation injury.[50] Encouraging results have also been seen in the treatment of patients with partial complex epilepsy and medial temporal lobe low-grade gliomas.

Malignant Glioma (Anaplastic Astrocytoma, Glioblastoma)

Rationale

Even anaplastic astrocytomas and glioblastomas are generally localized. Only 3 percent of glioblastomas are multifocal.[71] In a study of patients with glioblastoma it was found at autopsy that the tumor in 29 of 35 patients did not extend beyond the abnormalities on CT scan in the living patient.[36] The T2-weighted MR image correlates even better with the extension of the infiltrating tumor as shown in a study correlating such images with serial biopsies obtained by a stereotactic technique.[16,45] Thus, covering the tumor volume, as visualized by a T2-weighted MR image with a generous margin, with a tumoricidal dose should have a chance of curing the patient. Unfortunately, a tumoricidal dose appears to be beyond the limits that can be tolerated by the normal brain. In an often-quoted study, Walker et al. showed that the median survival time for glioblastoma patients increased with the median dose of WBRT administered, reaching 56 weeks with 75 Gy delivered in fractions.[113] This dose is beyond the 54 to 55 Gy that can be delivered in a 6-week fractionation scheme without risking radionecrosis.[72] The attraction of radiosurgery is that it can deliver precise radiation to the target volume and thus limit the risks of necrotizing surrounding normal brain. However, despite surgical debulking the volumes needed to be treated remain large and the dose requirement high.[24] A major impact of radiosurgery in the management of malignant infiltrating brain tumors should therefore not be expected.

Results

Radiosurgery has usually been used as an adjunct when conventional therapy fails or as a first-line treatment as part of a comprehensive management protocol. The largest experience has probably been accumulated at the Joint Center for Radiation Therapy in Boston. A report of their initial experience using linac radiosurgery has been published. They treated 23 patients with glioblastoma and 14 patients with anaplastic astrocytoma. All patients received conventional radiotherapy (5910 cGy in 33 fractions) to the tumor area with a 3- to 4-cm margin following surgical debulking (20 patients) or biopsy (17 patients). Thirty-seven patients underwent radiosurgery according to the protocol and were assessable for survival and complications of treatment. Radiosurgery was delivered 2 to 4 weeks after completion of the conventional radiotherapy to a median tumor volume of 4.8 cc (range, 1.2 to 77 cc) with a minimum dose of 1250 to 2000 cGy. Adjuvant chemotherapy was not given. After a median follow-up of 19 months, only 9 of 37 (24 percent) patients had died. Six patients (all with glioblastoma multiforme) died of recurrent tumor, whereas death was attributable to complications of treatment in two cases and intercurrent disease in one case. The authors conclude that "radiosurgery is a useful adjunct to other modalities in the initial management of patients with small, radiographically well-defined malignant gliomas."[67]

Gamma knife centers have also reported preliminary experiences. In 55 consecutive cases of "inoperable" malignant glioma (15 astrocytoma III and 10 astrocytoma IV) treated in Chicago, a median survival of 13.1 months after treatment was observed.[34] Of particular interest is a report from the University of California, San Francisco, a center leading the development of interstitial brachytherapy for brain tumors. They reported results of gamma knife treatment of 26 patients with malignant gliomas of volumes up to 29 cc with minimal doses of 14 to 22 Gy. The treatment was used as a boost to conventional radiotherapy or as treatment for recurrences. Twenty-two of the 26 patients have shown either a reduction in tumor volume or disease stability 4 to 12 months or longer after radiosurgery. The overall "response rate" was 85 percent.[32]

Our personal experience in radiosurgery for malignant gliomas is limited to some 30 patients. We have rarely used radiosurgery as a primary treatment modality. In 12 patients gamma knife radiosurgery with 40 Gy to the gadolinium-enhancing margin was used in combination with cisplatin as a radiosensitizer following surgery and conventional radiotherapy. Twenty grays were delivered 1 to 1.5 cm around this volume. The very high doses given were based on published work on the in vitro sensitivity of malignant glioma cells.[72] In all patients there were transient radiation-induced neurological symptoms during the first 72 h, but at 3 to 6 months only three patients required steroids.

It must be concluded that radiosurgery has, so far, not had a major impact on the management of malignant gliomas. Dose requirements and treatment schedules are still being investigated and it is possible that radiosurgery will have a place as an adjuvant to other treatment modalities.

References

1. Adler JR, Cox RS, Kaplan I, Martin DP. Stereotactic radiosurgical treatment of brain metastases. *J Neurosurg* 1992; 76:444–449.
2. Akslen LA, Hove LM, Hartveit F. Metastatic distribution in malignant melanoma. A 30-year autopsy study. *Invasion Metast* 1987; 7:253–263.
3. Alexander E III, Loeffler JS, Wen P, Black PM. Results of stereotactic brachytherapy used in the initial management of patients with glioblastoma. *J Neurosurg* 1991; 74:344A (abstr).
4. Amendola BE, Gebarski SS, Bermudez AG. Analysis of treatment results in craniopharyngioma. *J Clin Oncol* 1985; 3:252–258.
5. Backlund EO, Rähn T, Sarby B, et al. Closed stereotaxic hypophysectomy by means of ^{60}Co gamma radiation. *Acta Radiol Ther Phys Biol* 1972; 11:545–555.
6. Barbaro NM, Gutin PH, Wilson CB, et al. Radiation therapy in the treatment of partially resected meningiomas. *Neurosurgery* 1987; 20:525–528.
7. Bernstein M, Gutin PH. Interstitial irradiation of skull base tumours. *Can J Neurol Sci* 1985; 12:366–370.
8. Black P. Brain metastases: current status and recommended guidelines for management. *Neurosurgery* 1979; 5:617–631.
9. Bowen J, Paulsen CA. Stroke after pituitary irradiation. *Stroke* 1992; 23:908–911.
10. Bucci MN, Chin LS, Hoff JT. Perioperative morbidity associated with operative resection of craniopharyngioma: a review of ten years experience. *Neurochirurgia (Stuttg)* 1987; 30:135–138.
11. Cairncross JG, Posner JB. The management of brain metastases. In Walker MD (ed): *Oncology of the Nervous System.* Boston: Martinus Nijhoff, 1983, pp 341–377.
12. Carella RJ, Ransohoff J, Newall J. Role of radiation therapy in the management of meningiomas. *Neurosurgery* 1982; 10:332–339.
13. Coffey RJ, Flickinger JC, Bissonette DJ, Lunsford LD. Radiosurgery for solitary brain metastases using the cobalt-60 gamma unit: methods and results in 24 patients. *Int J Radiat Oncol Biol Phys* 1991; 20:1287–1295.
14. Coffey RJ, Friedman WA. Interstitial brachytherapy of malignant brain tumors using computed tomography-guided stereotaxis and available imaging software: technical report. *Neurosurgery* 1987; 20:4–7.
15. Conomy JP, Kellermeyer RW. Delayed cerebrovascular consequences of therapeutic radiation: a clinicopathologic study of a stroke associated with radiation-related carotid arteriopathy. *Cancer* 1975; 36:1702–1708.
16. Daumas-Duport C, Scheithauer BW, Kelly PJ. A histologic and cytologic method for the spatial definition of gliomas. *Mayo Clin Proc* 1987; 62:435–449.
17. DeAngelis LM, Delattre JY, Posner JB. Radiation-induced dementia in patients cured of brain metastases. *Neurology* 1989; 39:789–796.
18. DeAngelis LM, Mandell LR, Thaler HT, et al. The role of postoperative radiotherapy after resection of single brain metastases. *Neurosurgery* 1989; 24:798–805.
19. Delattre JY, Krol G, Thaler HT, Posner JB. Distribution of brain metastases. *Arch Neurol* 1988; 45:741–744.
20. DeSalles AA, Bajada CL, Goetsch S, et al. Radiosurgery of cavernous sinus tumors. *Acta Neurochir Suppl (Wien)* 1993; 58:101–103.
21. Duma CM, Lunsford LD, Kondziolka D, et al. Stereotactic radiosurgery of cavernous sinus meningiomas as an addition or alternative to microsurgery. *Neurosurgery* 1993; 32:699–705.
22. Eastman RC, Gorden P, Glatstein E, Roth J. Radiation therapy of acromegaly. *Endocrinol Metab Clin North Am* 1992; 21:693–712.
23. Etou A, Mundinger F, Mohadjer M, Birg W. Stereotactic interstitial irradiation of diencephalic tumors with Iridium 192 and Iodine 125: 10 years follow-up and comparison with other treatments. *Childs Nerv Syst* 1989; 5:140–143.
24. Fischer H, Hartmann GH, Sturm V, et al. In vitro model for the response to irradiation of different types of human intracranial tumours. *Acta Neurochir (Wien)* 1987; 85:46–49.
25. Flickinger JC, Kondziolka D, Lunsford LD, et al. A multi-institutional experience with stereotactic radiosurgery for solitary brain metastasis. *Int J Radiat Oncol Biol Phys* 1994; 28:797–802 (see comments).
26. Flickinger JC, Loeffler JS, Larson DA. Stereotactic radiosurgery for intracranial malignancies. *Oncology (Huntingt)* 1994; 8:81–86.
27. Gay PC, Litchy WJ, Cascino TL. Brain metastasis in hypernephroma. *J Neurooncol* 1987; 5:51–56.
28. Goffman TE, Dewan R, Arakaki R, et al. Persistent or recurrent acromegaly. Long-term endocrinologic efficacy and neurologic safety of postsurgical radiation therapy. *Cancer* 1992; 69:271–275.
29. Goldsmith BJ, Wara WM, Wilson CB, Larson D. Postoperative irradiation for subtotally resected meningiomas. *J Neurosurg* 1994; 80:195–201.
30. Gutin PH, Leibel SA, Hosobuchi Y, et al. Brachytherapy of recurrent tumors of the skull base and spine with iodine-125 sources. *Neurosurgery* 1987; 20:938–945.
31. Gutin PH, Prados MD, Phillips TL, Lamborn K. Stereotactic interstitial ^{125}I "boost" in the initial management of malignant gliomas. *J Neurosurg* 1991; 74:353A (abstr).
32. Gutin PH, Torres R, Harsh GR, et al. Gamma knife radiosurgery of malignant gliomas. *Acta Neurochir (Wien)* 1993; 122:152 (abstr).
33. Hagen NA, Cirrincione C, Thaler HT, et al. The role of radiation therapy following resection of single brain metastasis from melanoma. *Neurology* 1990; 40:158–160.
34. Helenowski TK, Clark SK, Grutsch J, et al. Survival of high grade astrocytoma patients following gamma knife radiosurgery. *Acta Neurochir (Wien)* 1993; 122:151–152 (abstr).
35. Hetelekidis S, Barnes PD, Tao ML, et al. 20-year experience in childhood craniopharyngioma. *Int J Radiat Oncol Biol Phy* 1993; 27:189–195 (see comments).
36. Hochberg FH, Pruitt A. Assumptions in the radiotherapy of glioblastoma. *Neurology* 1980; 30:907–1011.
37. Hoffman HJ, De Silva M, Humphreys RP, et al. Aggressive surgical management of craniopharyngiomas in children. *J Neurosurg* 1992; 76:47–52.
38. Hudgins WR. Patients' attitude about outcomes and the role of gamma knife radiosurgery in the treatment of vestibular schwannomas. *Neurosurgery* 1994; 34:459–465.
39. Inoue HK, Nakamura M, Ono N, et al. Radiosensitive squamous cell craniopharyngioma: clinical and pathological comparison with the adamantinomatous type. *Noshuyo Byori* 1993; 10:27–31.
40. Jose CC, Rajan B, Ashley S, et al. Radiotherapy for the treatment of recurrent craniopharyngioma. *Clin Oncol (R Coll Radiol)* 1992; 4:287–289.
41. Kang JK, Song JU. Results of the management of craniopharyngioma in children. An endocrinological approach to the treatment. *Childs Nerv Syst* 1988; 4:135–138.
42. Karlsson B, Kihlström L, Lindquist C. Medical controversy: is gamma knife the treatment of choice for cerebral metastases—the neurosurgeons' opinion. *Trends Exp Clin Med* 1994; 4:396–402.
43. Kawano N, Ohwada T, Yada K. Radical removal of craniopharyngioma: a long-term follow-up. *Neurol Med Chir (Tokyo)* 1993; 33:543–546.
44. Kelly PJ. *Tumor Stereotaxis.* Philadelphia: Saunders; 1991, p 409.
45. Kelly PJ, Daumas-Duport C, Kispert D, et al. Image-based stereotaxic serial biopsies in untreated intracranial glial neoplasms. *J Neurosurg* 1987; 66:865–874.
46. Kihlström L, Karlsson B, Lindquist C. Gamma knife surgery in brain metastases. In Lunsford LD (ed): *Stereotactic Radiosurgery Update.* New York: Elsevier, 1992, pp 429–434.
47. Kihlström L, Karlsson B, Lindquist C. Gamma knife surgery for cerebral metastases. Implications for survival based on 16 years experience. *Stereotact Funct Neurosurg* 1993; 61(Suppl 1):45–50.
48. Kihlström L, Karlsson B, Lindquist C, et al. Gamma knife surgery for cerebral metastasis. *Acta Neurochir Suppl (Wien)* 1991; 52:87–89
49. Kihlström L, Lindquist C, Adler J, et al Histological studies of gamma knife lesions in normal and hypercholesterolemic rabbits. In

Steiner L, Lindquist C, Forster D, et al (eds): *Radiosurgery: Baseline and Trends.* New York: Raven Press, 1992, pp 111–119.
50. Kihlström L, Lindquist C, Lindguist M, Karlsson B. Stereotactic radiosurgery for tectal low-grade gliomas. *Acta Neurochir* 1994; Suppl 62:55–57.
51. Kiricuta IC, Kolbl O, Willner J, Bohndorf W. Central nervous system metastases in breast cancer. *J Cancer Res Clin Oncol* 1992; 118:542–546.
52. Kjellberg RN, Shintani A, Frantz AG, Kliman B. Proton-beam therapy in acromegaly. *N Engl J Med* 1968; 278:689–695.
53. Kobayashi T, Tanaka T, Kida Y. The early effects of gamma knife on 40 cases of acoustic neuroma. In Lindquist C (ed): *1st Congress of the International Stereotactic Radiosurgery Society.* Stockholm, Sweden. Berlin: Springer-Verlag, 1993, pp 135–184.
54. Kobayashi T, Tanaka T, Kida Y. Stereotactic gamma radiosurgery of craniopharyngioma. In Ganz J (ed): *6th Annual Leksell Gamma Knife Society Meeting, Kyoto, Japan.* Basel: S Karger, 1994.
55. Komaki R, Cox JD, Stark R. Frequency of brain metastasis in adenocarcinoma and large cell carcinoma of the lung: correlation with survival. *Int J Radiat Oncol Biol Phys* 1983; 9:1467–1470.
56. Kondziolka D, Lunsford LD, Martinez AJ. Unreliability of contemporary neurodiagnostic imaging in evaluating suspected adult supratentorial (low-grade) astrocytoma. *J Neurosurg* 1993; 79:533–536.
57. Kreth FW, Warnke PC, Ostertag CB. Interstitial implant radiosurgery for cerebral metastases. *Acta Neurochir Suppl (Wien)* 1993; 58:112–114.
58. Kumar PP, Patil AA, Syh HW, et al. Role of brachytherapy in the management of the skull base meningioma. Treatment of skull base meningiomas. *Cancer* 1993; 71:3726–3731.
59. Lamberts HB, de Boer WGRM. Contributions to the study of immediate and early X-ray reactions with regard to chemoprotection: VII. X-ray-induced atheromatous lesions in the arterial wall of hypercholesterolemic rabbits. *Int J Radiat Biol* 1963; 6:343–350.
60. Leem W, Yj L. Gamma knife radiosurgery in pituitary adenoma. In Ganz J (ed): *6th Annual Leksell Gamma Knife Society Meeting, Kyoto, Japan.* Basel: S Karger, 1994.
61. Leksell L. A note on the treatment of acoustic tumours. *Acta Chir Scand* 1971; 137:763–765.
62. Leksell L, Lidén K. A therapeutic trial with radioactive isotopes in cystic brain tumour. In Ministry of Supply. *Radioisotope Techniques Vol I. Medical and Physiological Applications.* London: Her Majesty's Stationery Office, 1953, pp 76–78.
63. Levy RP, Fabrikant JI, Frankel KA, et al. Heavy-charged-particle radiosurgery of the pituitary gland: clinical results of 840 patients. *Stereotact Funct Neurosurg* 1991; 57:22–35.
64. Lindquist C. Gamma knife surgery for recurrent solitary metastasis of a cerebral hypernephroma: case report. *Neurosurgery* 1989; 25:802–804.
65. Linskey ME, Flickinger JC, Lunsford LD, et al. Cranial nerves length predicts the risk of delayed facial and trigeminal neuropathies after acoustic tumor stereotactic radiosurgery. *Int J Radiat Oncol Biol Phys* 1993; 25:227–233.
66. Linskey ME, Lunsford DL, Flickinger JC. Radiosurgery for acoustic neurinomas: early experience. *Neurosurgery* 1990; 25:736–745.
67. Loeffler JS, Alexander E III, Shea WM, et al. Radiosurgery as part of the initial management of patients with malignant gliomas. *J Clin Oncol* 1992; 10:1379–1385 (see comments).
68. Loeffler JS, Kooy HM, Wen PY, et al. The treatment of recurrent brain metastases with stereotactic radiosurgery. *J Clin Oncol* 1990; 8:576–582 (see comments).
69. Lunsford LD. Contemporary management of meningiomas: radiation therapy as an adjuvant and radiosurgery as an alternative to surgical removal? *J Neurosurg* 1994; 80:187–190 (editorial).
70. Lunsford L, Kondziolka D, Ogunrinde O, Flickinger J. The evolution of technique in stereotactic radiosurgery of acoustic tumours. In Lindquist C (ed): *1st Congress of the International Stereotactic Radiosurgery Society, Stockholm, Sweden.* Berlin: Springer-Verlag, 1993, p 164.
71. Marks JE. Ionizing radiation. In Salcman M (ed): *Neurobiology of Brain Tumors.* Baltimore: Williams & Wilkins, 1991, pp 299–320.
72. Marks JE, Baglan RJ, Prassad SC, et al. Cerebral radionecrosis: incidence and risk in relation to dose, time, fractionation, and volume. *Int J Radiat Oncol Biol Phys* 1981; 7:243–252.
73. Mendenhall WM, Friedman WA, Bova JF. Linear accelerator-based stereotactic radiosurgery for acoustic schwannomas. *Int J Radiat Oncol Biol Phys* 1994; 28(4):803–810 (see comments).
74. Mirimanoff RO, Dosoretz DE, Lingood RM, et al. Meningioma: analysis of recurrence and progression following neurosurgical resection. *J Neurosurg* 1985; 62:18–24.
75. Mogard J, Kihlström L, Ericson K, et al. Recurrent tumor vs radiation effects after gamma knife radiosurgery of intracerebral metastases: diagnosis with PET-FDG. *J Comput Assist Tomogr* 1994; 18:177–181.
76. Murros KE, Toole JF. The effect of radiation on carotid arteries. A review article. *Arch Neurol* 1989; 46:449–455.
77. Norén G, Arndt J, Hindmarsh T. Stereotactic radiosurgery in cases of acoustic neurinoma: further experiences. *Neurosurgery* 1983; 13:12–22.
78. Norén G, Arndt J, Hindmarsh T, Hirsch A. Stereotactic radiosurgical treatment of acoustic neurinomas. In Lunsford LD (ed): *Modern Stereotactic Neurosurgery.* Boston: Martinus Nijhoff, 1988, pp 481–429.
79. Norén G, Greitz D, Hirsch A, Lax I. Gamma knife surgery in acoustic tumours. *Acta Neurochir Suppl (Wien)* 1993; 58:104–107.
80. Norén G, Lax I. Dosimetry in gamma knife radiosurgery of vestibular schwannomas. In Lindquist C (ed): *1st Congress of the International Stereotactic Radiosurgery Society, Stockholm, Sweden.* Berlin: Springer-Verlag, 1993, pp 165–166.
81. Norén G, Mosskin M, Hirsch A, Lax I. Long-term follow-up results after gamma knife radiosurgery of acoustic neuromas. Presented at the 61st Annual Meeting of the American Association of Neurological Surgeons, Boston, April 27, 1993.
82. Ostertag CB. Brachytherapy—interstitial implant radiosurgery. *Acta Neurochir Suppl (Wien)* 1993; 58:79–84.
83. Patchell RA, Tibbs PA, Walsh JW, et al. A randomized trial of surgery in the treatment of single metastases to the brain. *N Engl J Med* 1990; 322:494–500 (see comments).
84. Pechova-Peterova V, Kalvach P. CT findings in cerebral metastases. *Neuroradiology* 1986; 28:254–258.
85. Pendl G, Schrottner O, Friehs G. Stereotactic radiosurgery of skull base meningiomas. In Ganz J (ed): *6th Annual Leksell Gamma Knife Society Meeting, Kyoto, Japan.* Basel: S Karger, 1994.
86. Petito CK, DeGirolami U, Earle KM. Craniopharyngiomas: a clinical and pathological review. *Cancer* 1976; 37:1944–1952.
87. Petty AM, Kun LE, Meyer GA. Radiation therapy for incompletely resected meningiomas. *J Neurosurg* 1985; 62:502–507.
88. Phillips MH, *Physical Aspects of Stereotactic Radiosurgery.* New York: Plenum, 1993.
89. Pozza F, Colombo F, Chierego G, et al. Low-grade astrocytomas: treatment with unconventionally fractionated external beam stereotactic radiation therapy. *Radiology* 1989; 171:565–569.
90. Rähn T, Thoren M, Hall K, et al. Stereotactic radiosurgery in the treatment of MB Cushing. In Szilka G (ed): *Stereotactic Cerebral Irradiation.* Amsterdam: Elsevier, 1979, pp 207–211.
91. Rajan B, Ashley S, Gorman C, et al. Craniopharyngioma—long-term results following limited surgery and radiotherapy. *Radiother Oncol* 1993; 26:1–10.
92. Ram Z, Nieman LK, Cutler GB Jr, et al. Early repeat surgery for persistent Cushing's disease. *J Neurosurg* 1994; 80:37–45.
93. Recht LD, Lew R, Smith TW. Suspected low-grade glioma: is deferring treatment safe? *Ann Neurol* 1992; 31(4):431–436 (see comments).
94. Regine WF, Kramer S. Pediatric craniopharyngiomas: long-term results of combined treatment with surgery and radiation. *Int J Radiat Oncol Biol Phys* 1992; 24:611–617.
95. Rosenfeld JV, Murphy MA, Chow CW. Implantation metastasis of

96. Sääf M, Thoren M, Bergstrand CG, et al. Treatment of craniopharyn-pineoblastoma after stereotactic biopsy: case report. *J Neurosurg* 1990; 73:287–290.
giomas—the stereotactic approach in a ten to twenty-three years' perspective. II. Psychosocial situation and pituitary function. *Acta Neurochir (Wien)* 1989; 99:97–103.
97. Saitoh H, Shimbo T, Tasaka T, et al. Brain metastasis of renal adenocarcinoma. *Tokai J Exp Clin Med* 1982; 7:337–343.
98. Salcman M, Sewchand W, Amin PP, Bellis EH. Technique and preliminary results of interstitial irradiation for primary brain tumors. *J Neurooncol* 1986; 4:141–149.
99. Shaw EG, Scheithauer BW, O'Fallon JR. Management of supratentorial low-grade gliomas. *Oncolory (Huntingt)* 1993; 7:97–104.
100. Smalley SR, Schray MF, Laws EJ, O'Fallon JR. Adjuvant radiation therapy after surgical resection of solitary brain metastasis: association with pattern of failure and survival. *Int J Radiat Oncol Biol Phys* 1987; 13:1611–1616.
101. Steiner L, Lindquist C, Steiner M. Meningioma and gamma knife radiosurgery. In Al-Mefty O (ed): *Meningiomas.* New York: Raven Press, 1991, pp 263–272.
102. Steiner L, Lindquist C, Steiner M. Radiosurgery. *Adv Tech Stand Neurosurg* 1992; 19:19–102.
103. Steiner L, Prasad D, Lindquist C, et al. Gamma knife surgery in cerebral vascular lesions and tumors. In Schmidek HH, Sweet WH (eds): *Operative Neurosurgical Techniques: Indications, Methods, and Results,* 3d ed. Philadelphia: Saunders, 1995, pp 667–694.
104. Sturm V, Kober B, Hover KH, et al. Stereotactic percutaneous single dose irradiation of brain metastases with a linear accelerator. *Int J Radiat Oncol Biol Phys* 1987; 13:279–282.
105. Symon L, Pell MF, Habib AH. Radical Excision of craniopharyngioma by the temporal route: a review of 50 patients. *Br J Neurosurg* 1991; 5:539–549.
106. Szeifert GT, Sipos L, Horvath M, et al. Pathological characteristics of surgically removed craniopharyngiomas: analysis of 131 cases. *Acta Neurochir (Wien)* 1993; 124:139–143.
107. Taylor BW Jr, Marcus RB Jr, Friedman WA, et al. The meningioma controversy: postoperative radiation therapy. *Int J Radiat Oncol Biol Phys* 1988; 15:299–304.
108. Thoren M, Rähn T, Guo WY, Werner S. Stereotactic radiosurgery with the cobalt 60 gamma unit in the treatment of growth hormone-producing pituitary tumors. *Neurosurgery* 1991; 29:663–668.
109. Tishler RB, Loeffler JS, Lunsford LD, et al. Tolerance of cranial nerves of the cavernous sinus to radiosurgery. *Int J Radiat Oncol Biol Phys* 1993; 27(2):215–221 (see comments).
110. Tomita T, McLone DG. Radical resections of childhood craniopharyngiomas. *Pediatr Neurosurg* 1993; 19:6–14.
111. Tsukada Y, Fouad A, Pickren JW, et al. Central nervous system metastasis from breast carcinoma. Autopsy study. *Cancer* 1983; 52:2349–2354.
112. Valentino V. Postoperative radiosurgery of pituitary adenomas. *J Neurosurg Sci* 1991; 35:207–211.
113. Walker MD, Strike TA, Sheline GE. An analysis of dose-effect relationship in the radiotherapy of malignant gliomas. *Int J Radiat Oncol Biol Phys* 1979; 5:1725–1731.
114. Warnke P, Kreth F, Ostertag C. Interstitial stereotactic radiosurgery of gliomas of the optic pathway. *Acta Neurochir (Wien)* 1993; 122:152 (abstr).
115. Wen BC, Hussey DH, Staples J, et al. A comparison of the roles of surgery and radiation therapy in the management of craniopharyngiomas. *Int J Radiat Oncol Biol Phys* 1989; 16:17–24.
116. Wen DY, Seljeskog EL, Haines SJ. Microsurgical management of craniopharyngiomas. *Br J Neurosurg* 1992; 6:467–474.
117. Withers HR, Taylor JM. Volume effect in spinal cord. *Br J Radiol* 1988; 61:973–975.
118. Wright D. Metastatic brain tumors. In Tindall GT (ed): *Contemporary Neurosurgery*, vol 12, no 6. Baltimore: Williams & Wilkins, 1990, pp 1–6.
119. Wright TL, Bresnan MJ. Radiation-induced cerebrovascular disease in children. *Neurology* 1976; 26:540–543.
120. Yasargil MG, Curcic M, Kis M, et al. Total removal of craniopharyngiomas. Approaches and long-term results in 144 patients. *J Neurosurg* 1990; 73:3–11.
121. Young B, Patchell RA. Surgery for a single brain metastasis. In Wilkins RH, Rengachary SS (eds): *Neurosurgery Update I.* New York: McGraw-Hill, 1990, pp 473–476.

186

Interstitial Brachytherapy of Primary Brain Tumors

Michael W. McDermott
Philip H. Gutin

The practice of brain tumor brachytherapy began with Frazer, who, in 1914, implanted radium into the tumor bed of a malignant glioma at the time of craniotomy.[68] Radium implants continued to be used until the late 1930s, when the necessity of shielding from radiation became apparent and the development of high-energy teletherapy machines offered another way to deliver radiation safely and effectively. The development in the late 1940s and early 1950s of new radioisotopes, including gold 198 (^{198}Au) and iridium 192 (^{192}Ir), coupled with the development of frame-based stereotactic systems by Leksell, brought about a renewed interest in interstitial brachytherapy for treating brain tumors. The early experience in European centers was with permanent implants for inoperable low-grade tumors.[63,80] More recently, brachytherapy using iodine 125 (^{125}I) and ^{192}Ir has been investigated in selected patients for the treatment of primary malignant supratentorial gliomas.[6,8,9,13,15,16,21,24,28-33,39,41,43,45,47,53,54,57,61,62,64-66,69,70,72,79,81,87-89] Our clinical experience to date indicates that brachytherapy can prolong survival in patients with glioblastoma multiforme (GM), when used in the initial phases of treatment, and in selected patients with recurrent malignant GM and nonglioblastoma malignant glioma (NGMG).[33,69,72]

Radiation therapy is experimentally and clinically the single most effective form of therapy for malignant gliomas. In 1978, the Brain Tumor Study Group confirmed this with a controlled, prospective, randomized trial evaluating the use of carmustine (BCNU) and radiation therapy in patients with malignant gliomas.[83] The median survival for patients who received BCNU alone was 25 weeks, compared to 37.5 and 40.5 weeks for patients who received radiation or a combination of radiation and BCNU. A later study that analyzed the results for patients in three successive Brain Tumor Study Group trials showed that a higher dose of radiation improved survival without increasing toxicity. The median survival was 28 weeks for patients who received 50 Gy and 42 weeks for those who received 60 Gy ($P = 0.004$).[84]

Modifications of the total dose and fractionation schedule, and the use of radiation sensitizers and particle-beam therapy have failed to significantly improve survival for patients with malignant glioma.[12,18,55,71,75] Interstitial brachytherapy attempts to improve the therapeutic ratio by using a radiation modality that has radiobiologic advantages over high-dose-rate systems and permits high doses of radiation therapy to be delivered to localized volumes, without causing significant irradiation to the surrounding normal brain.

Questions have been raised about the use of a focal form of therapy in tumors that are clearly infiltrating.[37] Pathologic studies indicate that isolated tumor cells exist at a distance beyond the contrast-enhancing margin of tumor seen on computed tomography (CT) scans or magnetic resonance (MR) images, yet clinical studies indicate that the most common pattern of failure is within 2 cm of the primary tumor site.[40] In a postmortem study of glioblastomas, the maximum thickness of infiltrating cells from the border of solid tumor tissue varied from 4 to 33 mm and constituted only 25 percent of the total tumor volume.[10] Even in untreated lesions, isolated tumor cells were not found beyond 3 cm from the periphery of necrotic areas at postmortem examination.[11] Comparison of CT and MR imaging findings with the results of stereotactic biopsy showed that isolated tumor cells could be identified on CT in the low-density area of brain outside of the contrast-enhancing area, and as areas of increased signal intensity on T2-weighted MR images.[42] These pathologic and radiologic characteristics of infiltrating gliomas seem to contradict what is known about patterns of failure in patients who receive whole-brain irradiation with or without an additional dose (''boost'') using coned-down radiation fields. In several studies between 1980 and 1992, local recurrence within 2 cm of the primary tumor site was the most common pattern of failure in 72 to 100 percent of the cases treated.[3,14,27,40,49,60,85] Therapeutic failures due to metastasis to distant sites within the brain occurred in 0 to 10 percent of patients; systemic metastasis occurred in 0 to less than 1 percent. Thus, the local control rate with conventional external-beam radiation therapy alone remains poor. This is the problem interstitial brachytherapy attempts to address.

Radiobiology

Interstitial brachytherapy increases the therapeutic ratio in cases of malignant brain tumors because it permits the placement of radioactive sources within the tumor volume, thereby localizing the dose. The stereotactic intratumoral placement of radioactive sources protects surrounding normal brain from potentially toxic cumulative doses of radiation that may occur after conventional external-beam radiation therapy. The dose rate falls off quickly at greater distances from the radioactive source, although not precisely according to the inverse square law. Within the first centimeter or so from the radioactive source, there is a build-up of radiation from scattered secondary photons,[73] and beyond this distance, the radiation dose distribution depends on the number of radioactive sources within the implanted volume, their spatial relationship to one another, the density or radiation permeability of surrounding tissue, and the energy of the radiation emitted. The use of modern computer-based stereotactic planning systems permits isodose distributions to be conformed to the margins of the contrast-enhancing tumor with surprising ease, allowing the dose to the normal brain to be kept to a minimum.

The dose rate is an important determinant of the biological effect of any radiation dose on tissue, but, in general, the lower the dose rate, the smaller the biological effect of a particular dose.[7,26] The effect of the dose rate is observable particularly between 0.01

and 1.0 Gy/min. Dose rates from interstitial brachytherapy sources are commonly on the order of 0.4 to 0.6 Gy/h, compared to 1.8 to 2.0 Gy/min with conventional linear accelerators. Continuous low-dose-rate irradiation has a therapeutic advantage because of the differences in the repair of sublethal damage between tumor and normal tissue, the redistribution of proliferating cells into the more radiation-sensitive phases of the cell cycle, the reduced importance of oxygen enhancement on radiation damage, and the inhibition of repopulation because of the total radiation dose delivered to tumor cells during their cell cycle.

The repair of sublethal damage (SLD) is largely responsible for the dose rate phenomenon.[7,34-36,59] The time required for repair of SLD is normally 1 to 1.5 h; normal tissues repair radiation damage more effectively than do tumor cells. Continuous low-dose-rate irradiation allows for an accumulation of SLD, which prevents cell proliferation and ultimately leads to cell death. As radiation-sensitive cells are destroyed, other tumor cells in the nonproliferating pool and those in the resistant phases of the cell cycle will eventually enter the more radiation-sensitive phases (G_2 and M phases). Thus, as proliferation takes place in a malignant tumor, the cells are continually subjected to irradiation, and, in a typical interstitial implant, the center of a tumor, which contains the most resistant cells, usually gets a radiation dose two to three times greater than the dose at the margin. Hypoxic cells, traditionally regarded as being resistant to conventional radiation therapy, are relatively more sensitive to the effects of continuous low-dose-rate irradiation.[51] Repopulation of tumor cells is less likely to be an issue with interstitial brachytherapy because, during a standard course of clinical treatment, at least one cell cycle is irradiated with at least two to three times the dose necessary to inhibit mitoses. The total dose per cell cycle necessary to inhibit mitosis has been estimated to be 720 to 900 cGy.[30] Assuming a dose rate of 0.4 to 0.6 Gy/h, a cell-cycle time for malignant gliomas of anywhere between 24 and 120 h, and a total implant duration of 4 to 6 days, the total dose delivered per cell cycle will be well above the critical amount necessary to inhibit mitosis.

Recently, a linear quadratic model has been used to assess the radiation dosages that are most effective in sparing surrounding normal tissue in the stereotactic irradiation of brain tumors, using either radioactive interstitial implants or radiosurgical techniques.[50] A figure of merit, which was used to assess the two irradiation modalities, was defined as a ratio of tumor to normal tissue biological effective dose, expressed as a ratio of early to late radiation effects. A radiobiological advantage was demonstrated for temporary ^{125}I versus permanent ^{125}I implants or fractionated radiosurgical techniques. Permanent lead implants (palladium 103), which have a higher dose rate than ^{125}I, but retain the same radiation safety advantages, had nearly equivalent figures of merit for tumors with long doubling times. Permanent ^{125}I implants were effective for those tumors with doubling times greater than 10 to 15 days, because of the low-dose-rate irradiation, which permitted a larger total dose to be given, while preferentially sparing normal tissue. An evaluation of the biologically effective dose in tissues with a very short half-life of repair of SLD showed that pulsed brachytherapy at 3 Gy/h resulted in a greater biological effect than continuous low-dose-rate treatment at 0.5 Gy/h.[23] While there may be theoretical advantages to pulsed brachytherapy, temporary implants that deliver radiation therapy continuously over 5 to 7 days achieve some balance between theoretical radiobiological advantages and practical issues of time and personnel availability related to treating patients.

In vitro results with boron-neutron-capture enhancement of californium 252 (^{252}Cf) brachytherapy may be a promising development, as both the absorbed dose and the frequency of high linear energy-transfer events at 3 to 5 cm from the sources are increased. The absorbed dose enhancement is roughly 23 percent at a distance of 3 cm from the californium sources and over 50 percent at a distance of 5 cm.

Isotopes

Several isotopes have been used for brain tumor brachytherapy, including ^{198}Au, ^{192}Ir, ^{252}Cf, and ^{125}I.[4,7,46,67] ^{125}I has become the preferred isotope for temporary implants and is provided by the manufacturer as standard low-activity (0.5 mCi) and high-activity (10 to 50 mCi) sources. High-activity sources have been used mainly to treat primary brain tumors at the University of California, San Francisco (UCSF); low-activity sources are reserved for permanent implantation in skull base neoplasms.[31-33]

The ^{125}I high-activity seed is a titanium capsule approximately 4 mm in length and 0.8 mm in diameter. The 0.05-mm-thick titanium capsule surrounds the radioactive isotope, which is absorbed on resin balls within this shell. ^{125}I decays by electron capture and emits gamma rays, x-rays, and electrons. The electrons and L-characteristic x-rays are completely absorbed by the titanium jacket and only the gamma and K-characteristic x-rays are important for therapeutic effect.[44,73] The energy of the ^{125}I photons is in the range of 27 to 35 keV, as compared to 300 to 610 keV for ^{192}Ir. This lower energy range results in higher tissue attenuation and less irradiation of normal brain surrounding the tumor for a similar volume than is true for ^{192}Ir, and also provides improved radiation safety.[7] The relative biological effectiveness of ^{125}I is slightly better than that of ^{192}Ir and cesium-137 in both plant and animal models.[7,17,25,58,59] Photoelectric absorption of these low-energy photons is also relative to the atomic number of the interposed tissues.[44] Therefore, the absorption in a tissue such as bone will be four to five times that of soft tissue, a fact that contributes to the improved radiation safety of ^{125}I over ^{192}Ir.

Ultimately, isotope selection depends on a number of factors. We use the ^{125}I high-activity seeds because of their ease of handling, relative safety, and reusability. Calibration and dosimetry are problems, however, because of the low energy of x-rays emitted. Also, the anisotropy of radiation fields surrounding the seeds that result from the titanium end-welds on the capsule must be taken into account. This is particularly important when calculating dosimetry of multiple linear arrays of seeds and catheters. We are currently involved in a trial combining interstitial brachytherapy with the radiation sensitizer iododeoxyuridine (IUdR). Goodman et al.[29] have proposed samarium-145 sources for implantation when using IUdR. This isotope releases low-energy 38- to 61-keV photons and has a long half-life of 340 days.

Case Selection

The selection criteria for patients suitable for interstitial brachytherapy have evolved over time and relate to both patient and tumor factors (Table 186-1). Generally, patients must be in good neurological condition with a Karnofsky performance status (KPS)

TABLE 186-1 Selection Criteria

Patient	
Karnofsky performance status ≥70	
Informed consent	
Life expectancy >3 months	
Available for follow-up	
Tumor	
Size	
<6 cm maximum one dimension	
Type	
Newly diagnosed glioblastoma multiforme	
Recurrent glioblastoma multiforme or nonglioblastoma malignant glioma	
Clearly seen on contrast-enhanced computed tomography	
Location	
Supratentorial	
Cortical/subcortical	
Unifocal	
No spread to corpus callosum or ependyma	

≥70. They must be able to understand the issues related to the potential benefits and risks of interstitial brachytherapy, be available for the interval of follow-up review recommended, and have a life expectancy of greater than 3 months.

The size, location, radiographic appearance, and histologic type of the tumor also determine whether the patient is a suitable candidate for implantation. The largest acceptable tumor size for implantation is 6 cm in diameter. Patients with purely cystic tumors are considered less-than-ideal candidates because of the risk of fluid draining from the tumor cavity during implantation, which would change the final dose distribution. Patients with diffuse tumors that appear to be multicentered or that involve the corpus callosum or ependymal lining of the ventricles are not considered appropriate candidates, nor are patients with infratentorial tumors, because of the fear of brain stem injury. Because of the current software system that relies on CT-based stereotactic imaging studies to generate a treatment plan and determine dose distributions, only those patients with contrast-enhancing tumors can be implanted.

Our experience suggests that all patients with recurrent GM or anaplastic astrocytoma may benefit from interstitial brachytherapy.[33,47,69,72] Only patients with GM had a survival benefit from "boost" brachytherapy after external-beam irradiation, according to the Northern California Oncology Group (NCOG) trial 6G-82-2, which included patients newly diagnosed with brain tumors between January 1982 and January 1990, including 34 patients with glioblastoma and 29 with anaplastic gliomas other than glioblastoma.[33] Therefore, only patients newly diagnosed with glioblastoma are considered appropriate candidates for brachytherapy. The implantation is performed after external-beam radiation therapy is completed, and a postirradiation CT scan is obtained.

The influence of selection bias on the survival of patients deemed appropriate for brachytherapy in an analysis of consecutive, conventionally treated adults with newly diagnosed supratentorial tumors has been evaluated.[22] On the basis of imaging studies and KPS, patients were designated as eligible or ineligible for brachytherapy. Of 101 consecutive patients, only 32 were considered eligible. These patients were younger and had higher KPS scores and larger surgical resections. Forty percent of the patients with glioblastoma were eligible. Their median survival time was 13.9 months versus 5.8 months for the ineligible group. The improved outcome after adjunctive brachytherapy for malignant glioma was thought to be due partly to the criteria by which patients were selected.

Implantation Procedure

Pretreatment Planning

At UCSF, patients who are appropriate for implantation are brought to the postanesthetic care recovery room on the morning of the procedure. Under local anesthesia in adults and under general anesthesia in children, the Brown-Robert-Wells (BRW) stereotactic base ring is fixed to the patient's skull. The patient is then transferred to the neuroradiology department, where the BRW graphite-rod localizing system is attached to the base ring, a dose of intravenous contrast agent is administered, and a CT scan is performed using 3-mm slices in the axial plane to cover the entire tumor volume. A magnetic tape containing the digital information from the stereotactic CT scan is then transferred to the department of radiation oncology, where the information is transferred to a Vax 4000 computer. CT scan slices can then be viewed on a computer monitor by using the BRAIN software interface developed at UCSF and in use since 1986.[86]

The target volume is outlined on axial slices at the outer rim of enhancement on the CT image by the radiation oncologist and neurosurgeon. A series of catheters and ^{125}I sources are positioned empirically on reconstructed images by the radiation physicist to derive a plan that covers the entire target volume, keeps the number of catheters to a minimum, and delivers a smooth dose distribution to the margin of the tumor. Multiple iterations are performed until a final treatment plan is derived. The program does not require that individual catheters be parallel to one another, and we attempt to maintain a catheter orientation that is perpendicular to the outer table of skull. Catheter positions are specified by catheter tip and trajectory. The catheter tip is defined as a target point in the BRAIN program and anteroposterior (AP), lateral, and vertical coordinates are generated that will be placed into the phantom base at the time of surgery. The catheter trajectory is defined by the BRW frame angles alpha, beta, delta, and gamma.

An inventory program lists the seeds currently available, from which appropriate ^{125}I sources are selected. Seeds are placed at intervals along the catheters beginning at the catheter end, along with some combination of intervening plastic spacers. Two to four catheters are commonly used, with one to five seeds placed in each catheter. From the positions and activities of the seeds, the computer calculates and superimposes any desired dose-rate line (40 to 60 cGy/h) over the target volume. The dose-rate distributions are then reviewed in the sagittal, coronal, and axial planes. The final treatment plan is reviewed by the radiation oncologist and neurosurgeon and a hard copy of catheter target values and BRW frame angles is produced. A thermal color-printer copy of the computer screen, with the catheters numbered, is used by the surgeon for reference during the implantation procedure. The entire treatment planning process takes approximately 1 to 1½ h.

In a recent review of 307 adult patients who received interstitial brachytherapy for glioma between December 1979 and June 1990, the mean number of catheters placed in each patient was 2.7, the mean number of sources was 6.5, and the median total activity was

132 mCi. The median prescription dose rate for the target volume was 40 cGy/h with a median duration of 138 h. The median dose delivered during the implant time for all tumors implanted was 56 Gy at the tumor margin.[72]

Surgical Technique

In order to improve the therapeutic ratio for brachytherapy, a defined dose of radiation should be selectively delivered to the tumor volume while sparing the surrounding normal brain. For that reason, our implantation technique strives to encompass the tumor volume with a specific isodose surface (40 to 60 cGy/h). This technique results in a smooth dose distribution at the margin of the tumor, giving less importance to dose inhomogeneity within the tumor volume. Several implantation systems have been described that use a rigid template by which catheters are placed in a fixed spatial pattern in an attempt to produce a homogeneous dose distribution within the target volume.[5,56] Such a system requires placement of more catheters than ours, which aims only for a smooth dose distribution at the margin of the tumor.

The patient is transferred to the operating room and the BRW base ring is attached to the table with a Mayfield apparatus. The area of implantation on the overlying scalp is then shaved of hair and prepared with povidone scrub and iodine solution. The remaining hair on the scalp is then wetted and taped out of the field with 3-inch paper tape. The skin overlying the implantation site is covered with an adhesive plastic drape. One gram of vancomycin is given intravenously before the procedure begins. The AP, lateral, and vertical coordinates for a catheter tip or target point are entered into the phantom-base ring. The corresponding alpha, beta, delta, and gamma arc settings for the trajectory of the same catheter are entered into the arc-ring system, which is placed on the phantom-base ring. A metal stylet is directed along the guide tube to confirm the accuracy of the coordinates. The arc-ring system is then transferred to the patient-base ring and a 3.4-mm twist drill is advanced to the level of the skin. The skin is anesthetized with lidocaine with epinephrine and the plastic drape is removed. The skin is then incised with a no. 15 blade down to the bone and a twist-drill hole is fashioned. The dura is then perforated with successively larger sizes of Kirschner wires and enlarged with a blunt dilator, and a trial pass is made on a metal stylet with an outer Silastic catheter (1.57 mm inside diameter, 2.16 mm outside diameter) that has been lubricated with mineral oil (Fig. 186-1). The arc-ring system is returned to the phantom base and a single half-sheet is placed around the patient to drape out a sterile field. A 2-0 braided nylon suture is then placed in a purse-string fashion around the site of the twist-drill hole. The ends of the suture are taped to the plastic drape with a sterile adhesive strip.

Next, the surgeon returns to the arc ring on the phantom base, and, with the Silastic catheter on a metal stylet with a plastic stop apparatus at its end, sets the length of the catheter required by placing the tip of the metal stylet at the pointer tip of the phantom-base ring. This target point defines the catheter tip on the treatment plan. After the catheter length is determined, the arc-ring system is then returned to the patient-base ring. The outer Silastic catheter is then advanced through a Silastic collar button through the dura to the target point. The position of the Silastic catheter relative to the top of the Silastic collar button is marked on the Silastic catheter with an indelible marking pen (Fig. 186-2). Should the position of the outer catheter relative to the collar button change, it will be noted by malalignment of these marks. Cyanoacrylate glue is immediately placed at the junction of the collar button opening and the outer catheter, fixing the two together. The inner stylet is removed and the redundant catheter is cut with straight scissors. The arc-ring system is then returned back to the phantom base, and, again, a small sterile sheet is used to drape out the area. The Silastic collar button is marked with the appropriate number for the catheter and then sutured to the skin with a 4-0 nylon suture. In a similar fashion, the remaining outer Silastic catheters are placed. As most of the patients undergoing this procedure have previously undergone an open operation and/or radiation therapy, the brain surface is usually scarred under the center of the flap; bleeding from cortical arteries or veins is rare.

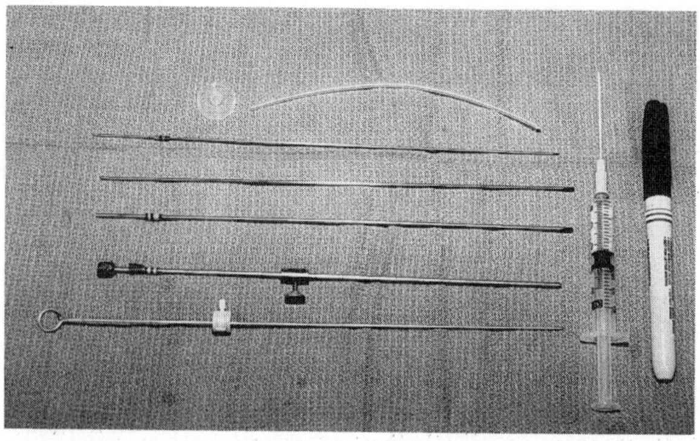

Figure 186-1 Equipment for ^{125}I implantation. Top to bottom are: Silastic collar button and outer Silastic catheter; three Kirschner wires of increasing size for perforating the dura; blunt cannula with metal stop for dilating the dural opening; metal stylet, over the top of which an outer Silastic catheter is placed for directing to the target point. (*Right*) 3-ml syringe with glue and plastic angiocatheter attached and indelible marking pen.

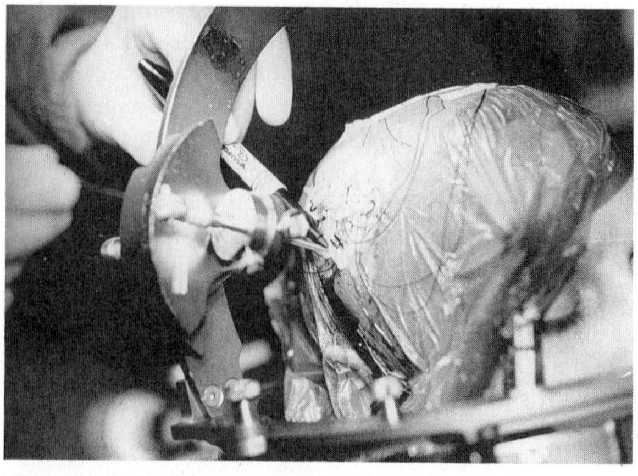

Figure 186-2 Surgeon marking the position of the outer catheter relative to the Silastic collar button. Should movement of the outer catheter occur, it will be detected by malalignment of these marks and corrected before the end of the procedure.

While the surgeon places the outer Silastic catheters, the radiation physicist prepares the inner nylon catheters (1.04 mm inside diameter, 1.47 mm outside diameter) with the ^{125}I seeds and the plastic spacers. The loaded catheters are then marked with tape at their ends with the appropriate catheter number and are transported to the operating room in a lead-lined metal container. The entire container is then sterilized in a routine fashion by using an autoclave system and is brought into the operating room. All operating-room personnel are required to wear lead aprons and radiation exposure badges. The surgeon handling the sources must also wear leaded glasses, a thyroid shield, leaded vinyl-rubber gloves, and a radiation exposure ring. Only after adequate protection has been ensured for everyone in the operating room does the afterloading technique begin. The inner nylon catheters containing radioactive sources are dipped in mineral oil to facilitate passage down the center of the implanted Silastic outer catheters. Long-handled forceps are used to handle the radioactive catheters. The surgeon double-checks that the inner catheter is seated to its deepest position by the feedback of firm resistance at the end of the Silastic outer catheter. After all the nylon catheters have been loaded into their corresponding outer Silastic catheters, the inner and outer catheters are secured with a single hemostatic clip. A surgical gauze is held in place with long-handled forceps and the sterile dressings and tape are removed from the patient's head. Metered readings of radiation output are obtained by the radiation technologist in the operating room before and after a lead-lined cap is placed on the patient's head. After these measures have been taken, AP and lateral orthogonal roentgenograms are taken with a fiducial box that mounts to the patient-base ring. The resulting films are used to check the accuracy of the seed location and to derive a postimplantation plan. An analysis of the accuracy of seed placement in 50 patients has revealed an average difference of 3.8 mm $\pm$ 3.3 mm between calculated and actual seed positions.[86] These differences usually result from the deflection of the catheter at bone edges by wire sutures holding the bone flap in place, or by gliotic brain, or deflection where the catheters may on occasion abut the floor of the middle or anterior cranial fossa. Should any large discrepancy between the pretreatment plan and the final position of the seeds be discovered, the inner catheter can be removed and reloaded with the necessary modifications to improve the dose plan. A day and time for seed removal are determined and entered into the patient's treatment plan record.

After the orthogonal roentgenograms have been taken, the BRW base ring is removed from the patient and small bandages are applied to the pin sites. Wearing a lead-lined cap, the patient is taken to a private room on the neurosurgery ward. At the end of the calculated treatment time, the catheters are removed at the bedside using sterile technique and local anesthesia. The twist-drill holes are closed with a figure-eight of 4-0 nylon sutures, which are left in place for 2 weeks.

Radiation Safety

Despite the low-energy radiation emitted using ^{125}I, radiation shielding is an important consideration through all phases of the preparation, transport, implantation, and postoperative care of patients. Federal and state regulations require that the maximum exposure for hospital personnel be no more than 100 mrem/week for 50 weeks a year. When preparing the inner nylon catheters into which the ^{125}I seeds are loaded, the radiation physicist wears leaded-vinyl rubber gloves and a leaded glass eye shield. The prepared catheters are transported to the operating room by the radiation technologist and oncologist in a lead-lined stainless steel tray. The radiation precautions taken by the surgeon and operating room staff during the process of afterloading the catheters have already been described. After the inner catheters have been loaded, a soft cloth cap with compartments that accept 0.5-mm-thick lead panels is placed over the patient's head. Readings are taken in the operating room at a distance of 1 m from all four sides of the patient's head, before and after the lead-lined cap is placed. These readings are recorded in the chart and on a sheet placed on the door of the patient's room (Fig. 186-3). Nurses and visitors must wear lead-lined aprons when visiting the patient and no children or pregnant visitors are allowed in the room. Visitors are required to sit at least 1 m away from the side opposite the implant. Although no radiation precautions are required for human waste, utensils used for meals are disposable, as are linens, and garbage is monitored daily before disposal by the radiation oncology department. A radiation counter, a small surgical tray for sutures, long-handled forceps, and a lead container to hold removed seeds are kept in the room at all times. Metered readings from the implantation side of the patient, taken when the lead-lined cap is in place, are usually zero, and in such cases, the patient is allowed to walk around the neurosurgery floor.

Follow-Up

After patients are discharged from the hospital, their dose of dexamethasone is slowly tapered if their clinical symptoms are stable. Neurological examinations and follow-up CT scans or MR images are obtained at 2-month intervals. At each visit, clinical symptoms, dexamethasone dose, neurological status, KPS score, and results of imaging studies are all recorded. Changes in any of these characteristics are noted, and, when there is a question of tumor recurrence or radiation necrosis, the case is reviewed at a multidisciplinary tumor board meeting. Nuclear-medicine imaging studies with either positron emission tomography (PET) or single-photon emission computed tomography (SPECT) are used in attempts to differentiate radiation necrosis from recurrent tumor. Reoperation is considered after brachytherapy when neurological deterioration occurs in a patient with a recurrent tumor confirmed by PET, or in a patient with an expanding contrast-enhancing mass when symptoms cannot be controlled by increasing doses of steroids, the lesion is surgically accessible, and the patient's general medical condition and KPS permit.

Responses to Treatment

Newly Diagnosed Gliomas

Between January 1982 and January 1990, 107 patients newly diagnosed with malignant glioma were entered into NCOG trial 6G-82-2 using brachytherapy after external-beam irradiation as part of initial therapy.[33] Thirty-four of the initial 64 patients with GM and 29 of the initial 37 patients with NGMG completed the prescribed course of treatment, which consisted of hydroxyurea (300 mg/m^2 PO) every other day during external-beam irradiation (60 Gy).

DO NOT DISCARD THIS FORM

Patient Radiation Survey Form

Name________________________ Room ______ Unit No________

Type of Implant________________________ Removable/Permanent

Post-implant Survey: Date______________ Time__________

Survey instrument: Mfgr & model______________ S/N________

Dose rate at 1 m______________ mR/hr Initials__________

Area survey without patient present: Reading above bkgnd? Y N

If Y, resolution________________________________

Radioactive-alert wrist tag attached? ☐

Room Survey - readings at indicated points X in mR/hr

Date______________ Time__________

Survey meter:
Mfgr:__________
Model__________
S/N__________

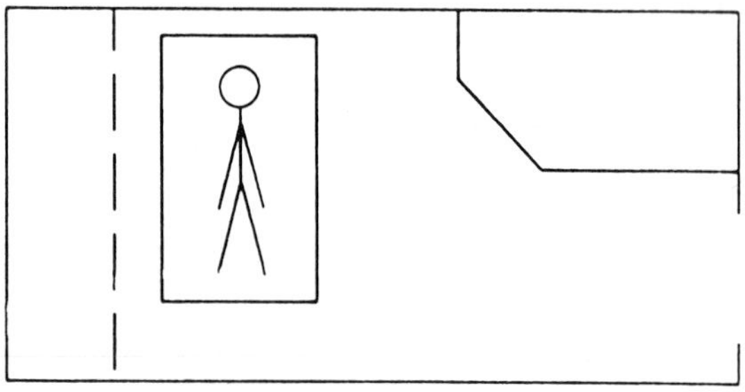

Safety instructions: Time spent near patient not to exceed:

______________ hrs/week at 1 meter from implant

______________ hrs/week behind shields

Additional instructions________________________________

____

Signature: ______________ **6-4811, 6-1208**Radiation Oncology***

Post-removal Survey: Date______________ Time__________

Survey instrument: Mfgr & model______________ S/N________

Dose rate at 1 m______________ mR/hr Initials__________

Reading in room above bkgnd? Y N

If Y, resolution________________________________

DO NOT DISCARD THIS FORM

Figure 186-3 Radiation safety sheet placed on the door of the patient's room detailing patient and room radiation survey readings during brachytherapy and after removal of the sources.

Within 3 weeks, a temporary ^{125}I seed implantation was performed, providing a median dose of 5193 cGy in the GM group and 5500 cGy in the NGMG group. Two weeks after brachytherapy, patients received a combination of lomustine (CCNU), procarbazine, and vincristine (PCV). The doses were CCNU 110 mg/m^2 orally on day 1, procarbazine 60 mg/m^2 orally on days 8 to 21, and vincristine 1.4 mg/m^2 intravenously on days 8 and 29. Chemotherapy was repeated every 6 to 8 weeks for 1 year or until tumor progression. The median survival times were 88 weeks for the 34 GM patients and 157 weeks for the 29 NGMG patients (Fig. 186-4). Forty-four percent of the GM group required reoperation at a median time of 46 weeks after their implantation. The median survival after diagnosis in patients who underwent reoperation was 108 weeks, as compared to 77 weeks for patients who did not have reoperation (Fig. 186-5), and their survival rates were significantly different ($P = 0.047$). Fifty-two percent of the NGMG patients had reoperation at a median time of 41 weeks after their implantation; their median survival was 165 weeks, as compared to 105 weeks for patients who did not have reoperation, and their survival rates were not significantly different ($P = 0.43$).

The quality of survival in patients who received brachytherapy appears to be acceptable. Whereas our selection criteria required an initial KPS $\geq$ 70, the mean KPS of patients with GM was 86 at 1 month and 75 at 24 months after brachytherapy. Similarly, for NGMG patients, the mean KPS was 91 at 1 month and 78 at 30 months after brachytherapy. Most patients were placed on stable doses of steroids after surgery; 6 to 30 months after implantation, 13 to 33 percent required increased doses.

The NCOG trial 6G-61 combining external irradiation with hydroxyurea followed by PCV resulted in median survival times of 50.4 weeks for the GM group and 157.1 weeks for the NGMG group.[48] Brachytherapy used as part of the initial treatment plan (''upfront'' brachytherapy) was considered to be valuable only in prolonging survival for patients with GM. A comparison of the survival times for patients receiving ''upfront'' brachytherapy with those in NCOG trial 6G-61 indicates to us that ''upfront'' brachytherapy is valuable in prolonging survival in patients with GM, not those with NGMG.

In patients newly diagnosed with malignant glioma who were treated in a similar fashion to the NCOG trial, Prados et al.[69] found

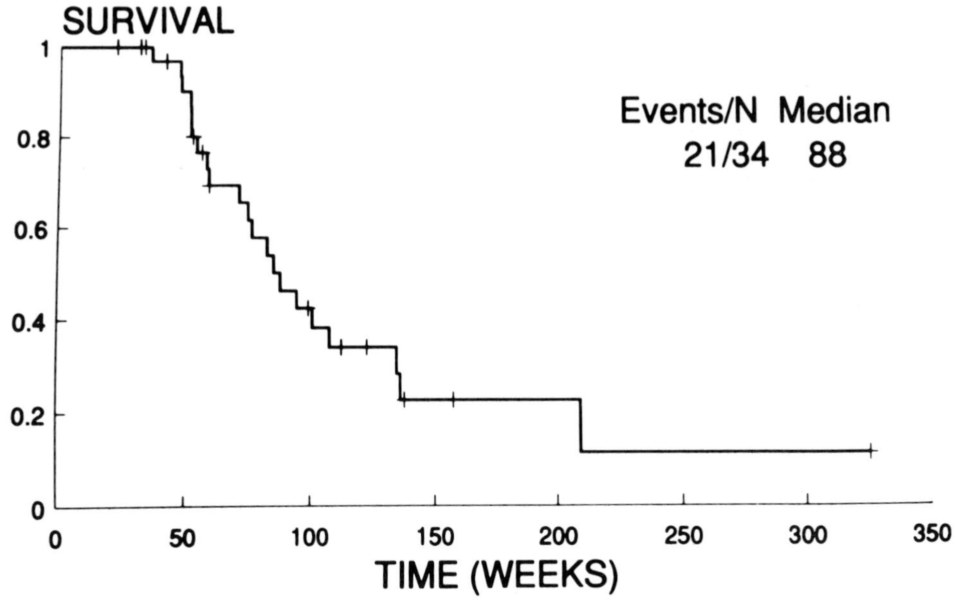

Figure 186-4 Kaplan-Meier representation of the probability of survival for patients newly diagnosed with glioblastoma multiforme treated with "boost" brachytherapy on the NCOG 6G-82-2 protocol. (From Gutin et al.,[33] with permission.)

that 59 percent of the 56 GM patients and 75 percent of the 32 NGMG patients received chemotherapy after their implantation. The median survival was 87 weeks for GM patients and 160 weeks for NGMG patients. Fourteen percent of GM and 32 percent of NGMG patients lived 3 years or longer. Forty-six percent of GM and 56 percent of NGMG patients required reoperation. This study suggested that for selected patients with GM, brachytherapy prolonged survival, but that for patients with NGMG, the toxicity associated with treatment outweighed its advantages.

Scharfen et al.[72] found median survival times that were similar to those reported by Prados et al.[69] and the NCOG study. The median survival times were 88 weeks for 106 patients with GM, 142 weeks for 52 patients with NGMG, and 226 weeks for 16 patients with low-grade NGMG. There was no difference in survival between patients who were on or off a protocol study at UCSF, and no difference between patients who received postimplantation chemotherapy and those who did not. As a consequence of this study, we no longer use adjuvant chemotherapy after brachytherapy for patients newly diagnosed with GM. Of the 307 patients in the study by Scharfen et al.[72] who received brachytherapy, 40 percent required a reoperation; there was no association between the reoperation rate and the total activity of the implant or implant volume. Of the 124 patients who had reoperations, 5 percent had necrosis only, 29 percent had tumor only, and 66 percent had both tumor and necrosis. Median survival after reoperation did not differ among patients in whom necrosis only, tumor only, or both was found. The total acute complication rate for the 307 patients was 7.8 percent and the mortality rate was 0.7 percent. Two patients died within 30 days of their implantation, but neither death was related to an intracranial event; one had sepsis and the other had a pulmonary embolism.

Two prospective randomized trials are currently underway to evaluate "boost" brachytherapy in the initial management of patients with malignant gliomas. These are the Brain Tumor

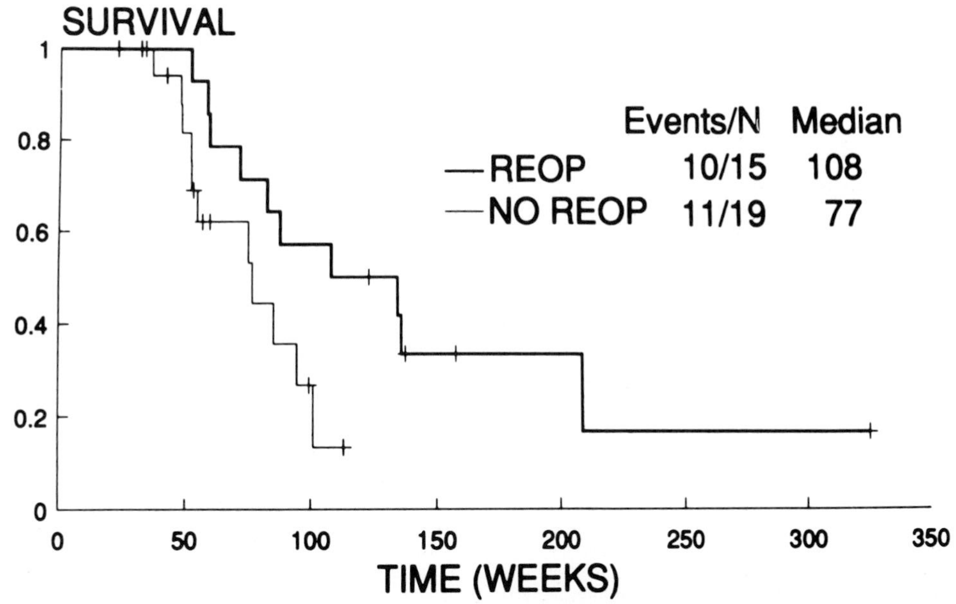

Figure 186-5 Kaplan-Meier representation of the probability of survival for patients with glioblastoma who did or did not have reoperation after brachytherapy ($P = 0.047$). (From Gutin et al.,[33] with permission.)

Cooperative Group study 87-01 and the University of Toronto brachytherapy trial.

Table 186-2 lists the results of published series for patients newly diagnosed with malignant glioma who were treated with brachytherapy using either temporary or permanent implants.

Recurrent Gliomas

The results of interstitial brachytherapy for recurrent malignant gliomas at UCSF have been reported.[32,47,72] In the most recent report,[72] the median survival from the date of implantation was 49 weeks for patients with recurrent glioblastoma (n = 66), 52 weeks for patients with recurrent NGMG (n = 45), and 81 weeks for those with recurrent low-grade NGMG (n = 22) (Fig. 186-6). The 1- and 3-year survival rates were 50 and 15 percent for the recurrent glioblastoma group, 49 and 24 percent for the recurrent NGMG group, and 68 and 30 percent for the recurrent low-grade NGMG group. Reoperation significantly prolonged median survival after implantation (90 weeks versus 37 weeks; $P = 0.0052$). The reoperation rate was 38 percent for recurrent GM, 47 percent for recurrent NGMG, and 36 percent for recurrent low-grade NGMG.

The KPS did not deteriorate significantly during follow-up for long-term survivors with recurrent malignant glioma who were treated with interstitial brachytherapy.[47] The mean and median KPS were 79 and 80 for the patients who survived 18 months and 76 and 80 for those who survived for 36 months. Long-term steroid dependency was a problem; 67 percent of the 18-month and 53 percent of the 36-month survivors were steroid dependent. Other reports also document the efficacy of interstitial brachytherapy in prolonging the survival of patients with recurrent malignant glioma.[8,38,54,87,89]

An interesting observation in patients who have a reoperation after interstitial brachytherapy is that apparently viable tumor cells, seen along with necrotic material in histologic preparations, do not appear to have the proliferative potential of anaplastic astrocytes outside the heavily radiated area, as evidenced by the lack of disease progression after reoperation alone and no other treatment.[47,72] Arbit et al.[2] recently reported on the viability and clonogenic potential of cells retrieved from eight patients after brachytherapy and four patients both before and after interstitial brachytherapy. All unirradiated samples grew well in primary culture, whereas those from tumors subjected to brachytherapy only formed small colonies of 50 to 100 cells, and these degenerated within 14 to 21 days. All specimens from within 3 cm of the

TABLE 186-2 Results of Brachytherapy for Patients Newly Diagnosed with Malignant Glioma

Author (Year)	Isotope (Temporary/ Permanent)	Tumor Type (Number)	Survival (Median)
Drake et al.[20] (1963)	^{192}Ir* (temp)	MG† (6)	10.5 months
	^{137}Cs* (temp)	MG (3)	6 months
Mundinger and Ostertag[62] (1978)	^{192}Ir* (temp)	GM (59)	10.9 months (mean)
Rougier et al.[70] (1984)	^{192}Ir‡ (temp)	GM (13)	7 months
		AA (12)	5 years
Szikla et al.[79] (1984)	^{192}Ir*‡ (3/4)	Grade 3 (7)	55%—5 years
	^{192}Ir*‡ (4/5)	Grade 4 (9)	44%—1 year
Patchell et al.[67] (1988)	^{252}Cf‡ (temp)	MG (56)	10 months
Willis et al.[87] (1988)	^{125}I‡ (temp)	GM (5)	21.3 months
Chun et al.[15] (1989)	^{192}Ir‡ (temp)	GM (20)	14.5 months
		AA (9)	15.5 months
Etou et al.[21] (1989)	^{125}I* (perm)	Grade 3 (6)	17%—3 years
Kumar et al.[45] (1989)	^{60}Co‡ (temp)	GM (30)	7 months
Bernstein et al.[8] (1990)	^{125}I‡ (temp)	MG (23)	60 weeks
Goodman et al.[29] (1990)	^{192}Ir‡ (temp)	MG (13)	64%—2 years
Loeffler et al.[53] (1990)	^{125}I‡ (temp)	GM (35)	40%—2 years
Gutin et al.[33] (1991)	^{125}I‡ (temp)	GM (34)	88 weeks
		NGMG (29)	157 weeks
Lucas et al.[54] (1991)	^{192}Ir‡ (temp)	GM (6)	10 months
		AA (20)	23 months
Hitchon et al.[39] (1992)	^{125}I‡ (temp)	GM (13)	100 weeks
		AA (7)	100 weeks
Malkin[57] (1992)	^{125}I‡ (temp)	GM (20)	22 months
Ostertag and Kreth[66] (1992)	^{125}I* (73% perm)	GM (34)	6 months
	(79% perm)	AA (75)	8 months
Prados et al.[69] (1992)	^{125}I‡ (temp)	GM (56)	87 weeks
		NGMG (32)	160 weeks
Scharfen et al.[72] (1992)	^{125}I‡ (temp)	GM (106)	88 weeks
		NGMG (52)	142 weeks
Zamorano et al.[89] (1992)	^{125}I‡ (temp)	MG (25)	60.4 weeks
	(perm)	(37)	90%—1 year

*Brachytherapy as the only source of radiation therapy.

†MG, malignant glioma; GM, glioblastoma multiforme; NGMG, nonglioblastoma malignant glioma; AA, anaplastic astrocytoma.

‡Brachytherapy boost after conventional external-beam irradiation.

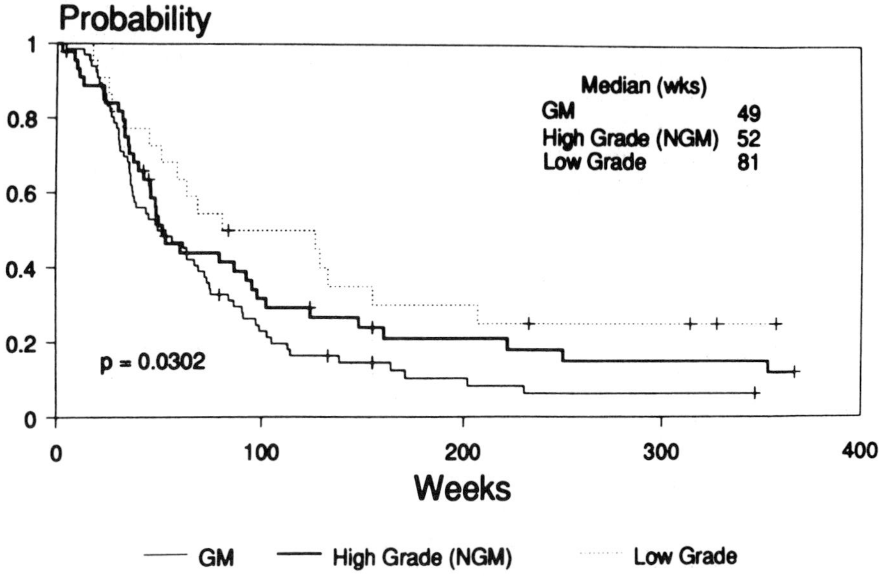

Figure 186-6 Kaplan-Meier representations of the probability of survival for patients with recurrent gliomas treated with implant alone. (From Scharfen et al.,[72] with permission.)

plantation site failed to grow as a monolayer in culture and all cell growth stopped within 8 weeks. A viable cell line grew in only one sample, which was obtained from 2 to 4 cm away from the implantation site. Sensitivity to external-beam radiation therapy persisted in cell lines after brachytherapy, which implies that local failure may have resulted from undertreatment.

Recurrence after Brachytherapy

Several studies have confirmed the initial report of Hochberg and Pruitt[40] on the pattern of recurrence after external-beam radiation therapy, which found that local recurrence (less than 2 cm from the rim of contrast enhancement) was the predominant pattern of treatment failure in over 80 percent of the patients after external-beam irradiation alone. Gaspar et al.[27] recently examined treatment failure patterns in the whole brain and in areas treated with a local "boost" of external-beam irradiation. The original enhancing tumor was entirely within the irradiated field in only 57 percent of patients. In 53 patients who had a recurrence during the follow-up period, recurrence was within the irradiated field in 72 percent, partly outside the field in 23 percent, outside the field but within the brain in 2 percent, in the field and in the spinal cord in 2 percent and in the spinal cord alone in 2%. All recurrences were found within 4 cm of the enhancing tumor as defined by the preoperative CT scan. Recurrences outside the volume that received the "boost" were more common when the "boost" margins were inadequate, the tumor was located in the temporal lobe, the "boost" volumes were small, or when the wedge-pair technique was used. In a study of 12 patients who had a second recurrence after external irradiation,[60] most recurrences (66%) occurred within 2 cm of the contrast-enhancing margin of the first recurrence after external-beam irradiation.

The reported patterns of recurrence after interstitial brachytherapy vary. In 22 patients who underwent ^{125}I brachytherapy, the recurrence was more than 2 cm from the original tumor margin in 82 percent, less than 2 cm from the margin in 18 percent, 2 to 5 cm from the tumor margin in 36 percent, and greater than 5 cm from the margin in 46 percent.[52] In contrast, another study found that among 24 patients who had a recurrence after ^{125}I brachytherapy, 72 percent of recurrences were within 2 cm of the original margin.[1] Recurrence separate from the pretreatment margin occurred in 6 percent, cerebrospinal fluid metastases in 2.4 percent, and systemic metastases in 4.3 percent. In NCOG trial 6G-82-2, of the recurrences that developed in 22 patients, 77 percent were less than 2 cm from the original site, 17 percent were 2 to 5 cm from the original site, and 5 percent were systemic metastases.[76] Local control again remains the primary problem for patients with malignant gliomas, even after "boost" brachytherapy.

Recurrent tumor and radiation necrosis are indistinguishable by CT or MR imaging. We prefer to use PET scanning to make this distinction during follow-up review of patients who undergo brachytherapy. The predictions of PET scanning correlated with pathologic findings in 84 percent of 34 patients who underwent reoperation for an increasing contrast-enhancing mass or recurrent tumor.[82] The PET scan was performed with rubidium 82 to assess the integrity of the blood–brain barrier and fluoro-18-fluordeoxyglucose to assess metabolic activity. Schwartz et al.[74] have reported on the use of SPECT thallium 201 (^{201}Th) and technetium-99m-hexamethylpropyleneamine oxime (^{99m}Tc-HMPAO) scanning. Fourteen of 15 patients were treated with conventional irradiation, nine received brachytherapy, two underwent stereotactic radiosurgery, and one underwent two implantations without prior external-beam treatment. All patients with high ^{201}Th uptake in their treated tumor beds had local tumor recurrence and all those with low uptake had radiation necrosis alone at biopsy or reoperation. An intermediate level of ^{201}Th uptake and preserved ^{99m}Tc-HMPAO perfusion were indicative of recurrent tumor and decreased perfusion was indicative of radiation necrosis. The dual-isotope SPECT scanning correlated with pathologic findings in 93 percent of cases.

Hyperthermia

In an attempt to improve the effects of brachytherapy alone, the combination of interstitial hyperthermia before and after brachytherapy has been evaluated. The rationale for combining these two modalities is that they may act both independently and synergistically. By itself, heat above 41 to 42°C kills tumor cells as a function of time and temperature, can impair the recovery of cells from radiation-induced SLD, and is effective against the relatively radiation-resistant S-phase and hypoxic cells.[19]

Previous clinical trials have suggested that hyperthermia improves tumor control and response rates. Sneed et al.[77] reported on 48 patients who underwent thermoradiotherapy using interstitially implanted microwave antennas, including thermometry probes within the same implant volume. The tumors were heated before and after brachytherapy. The number of catheters required for this combined treatment ranged from 3 to 11; these catheters permitted us to place between 1 and 8 antennas and 1 and 3 thermometry probes. The protocol attempted to heat as much tumor as possible to 42.5°C for 30 min. The actuarial median survival after hyperthermia was 47 weeks for patients with recurrent GM and had not been reached for recurrent NGMG; 65 percent of the NGMG patients were alive 18 months after treatment. Acute complications occurred in 27 percent of patients; the most common problem (19 percent) was seizures during the heat treatments. Progression-free median survival times were similar for the GM and NGMG groups (19 and 25 weeks, respectively).

One of the difficulties with hyperthermia is the inability to adequately heat the tumor volume to its edge without increasing the thermal conduction and convection to normal brain. One measure of the effectiveness of heating the tumor volume is the T90, i.e., the temperature exceeded by 90 percent of the measured intratumoral temperatures. Sneed et al.[77] achieved values of T90 that were greater than or equal to 41.5°C for the first 15 patients treated and in 19 of the next 34 patients. Only T90 value and minimum tumor temperature significantly influenced the probability of freedom from recurrence. However, another study found no correlation between T90 values and survival in 28 patients treated with ^{192}Ir brachytherapy and ferromagnetic implants for hyperthermia.[78] A prospective, randomized, phase 2 trial has begun in which newly diagnosed GM patients will be randomized to receive "boost" brachytherapy, with or without heat, after undergoing conventional radiation therapy.

References

1. Agbi CB, Bernstein M, Laperriere N, et al. Patterns of recurrence of malignant astrocytoma following stereotactic interstitial brachytherapy with iodine-125 implants. *Int J Radiat Oncol Biol Phys* 1992; 23:321–326.
2. Arbit E, Shapiro JR, Fiola M, et al. The significance of morphologically viable glioma cells found at the time of operation after interstitial brachytherapy. *Neurosurgery* 1993; 32:105–110.
3. Bashir R, Hochberg F, Oot R. Regrowth patterns of glioblastoma multiforme related to planning of interstitial brachytherapy radiation fields. *Neurosurgery* 1988; 23:27–30.
4. Beach JL, Schroy CB, Ashtari M, et al. Boron neutron capture enhancement of ^{252}Cf brachytherapy. *Int J Radiat Oncol Biol Phys* 1990; 18:1421–1427.
5. Beach L, Young AB, Patchell RA. A template for rigid stereotaxic afterloading brachytherapy of the brain. *Int J Radiat Oncol Biol Phys* 1993; 26:347–351.
6. Benabid AL, Chirossel JP, Mercier C, et al. Removable, adjustable and reusable implants for stereotactic interstitial radiosurgery of brain tumors. *Appl Neurophysiol* 1987; 50:278–280.
7. Bernstein M, Gutin PH. Interstitial irradiation of brain tumors: a review. *Neurosurgery* 1981; 9:741–750.
8. Bernstein M, Laperriere N, Leung P, et al. Interstitial brachytherapy for malignant brain tumors: preliminary results. *Neurosurgery* 1990; 26:371–380.
9. Bouzaglou A, Dyck P, Solt-Bohman LG, et al. Stereotactic interstitial implantation of brain tumors. *Endocurietherap Hypertherm Oncol* 1985; 1:9–112.
10. Burger PC. Pathologic anatomy and CT correlations in the glioblastoma multiforme. *Appl Neurophysiol* 1983; 46:180–187.
11. Burger PC, Dubois PJ, Schold SC Jr, et al. Computerized tomographic and pathologic studies of the untreated, quiescent, and recurrent glioblastoma multiforme. *J Neurosurg* 1983; 58:159–169.
12. Castro JR, Saunders WM, Austin-Seymour MM, et al. A phase I-II trial of heavy charged particle irradiation of malignant glioma of the brain: a Northern California Oncology Group Study. *Int J Radiat Oncol Biol Phys* 1985; 11:1795–1800.
13. Chin HW, Fruin AH, Estes T Jr, et al. Brain brachytherapy for malignant gliomas at Creighton University. *Nebr Med J* 1990; 75:258–262.
14. Choucair AK, Levin VA, Gutin PH, et al. Development of multiple lesions during radiation therapy and chemotherapy in patients with gliomas. *J Neurosurg* 1986; 65:654–658.
15. Chun M, McKeough P, Wu A, et al. Interstitial iridium-192 implantation for malignant brain tumours: Part II. Clinical experience. *Br J Radiol* 1989; 62:158–162.
16. Coffey RJ, Friedman WA. Interstitial brachytherapy of malignant brain tumors using computed tomography-guided stereotaxis and available imaging software: technical report. *Neurosurgery* 1987; 20:4–7.
17. Da Silva VF, Gutin PH, Deen DF, et al. Relative biological effectiveness of ^{125}I sources in a murine brachytherapy model. *Int J Radiat Oncol Biol Phys* 1984; 10:2109–2111.
18. Deutsch M, Green SB, Strike TA, et al. Results of a randomized trial comparing BCNU plus radiotherapy, streptozotocin plus radiotherapy, BCNU plus hyperfractionated radiotherapy, and BCNU following misonidazole plus radiotherapy in the postoperative treatment of malignant glioma. *Int J Radiat Oncol Biol Phys* 1989; 16:1389–1396.
19. Dewey WC, Freeman ML, Raaphorst GP, et al. Cell biology of hyperthermia and radiation. In Meyn RE, Withers HR (eds): *Radiation Biology in Cancer Research.* New York: Raven Press, 1980, pp 589–621.
20. Drake CG, Pfalzner PM, Linell EA. Intracavitary irradiation of malignant brain tumours. *J Neurosurg* 1963; 20:428–434.
21. Etou A, Mundinger F, Mohadjer M, et al. Stereotactic interstitial irradiation of diencephalic tumors with iridium 192 and iodine 125: 10 years follow-up and comparison with other treatments. *Childs Nerv Syst* 1989; 5:140–143.
22. Florell RC, MacDonald DR, Irish WD, et al. Selection bias, survival, and brachytherapy for glioma. *J Neurosurg* 1992; 76:179–183.
23. Fowler JF. Why shorter half-times of repair lead to greater damage in pulsed brachytherapy. *Int J Radiat Oncol Biol Phys* 1993; 26:353–356.
24. Frank F, Fabrizi AP, Gaist G, et al. Late considerations in the treatment of low-grade malignancy cerebral tumors with iodine-125 brachytherapy. *Appl Neurophysiol* 1987; 50:302–309.
25. Freeman ML, Goldhagen P, Sierra E, et al. Studies with encapsulated ^{125}I sources: II. Determination of the relative biological effectiveness using cultured mammalian cells. *Int J Radiat Oncol Biol Phys* 1982; 8:1355–1361.
26. Fu KK, Phillips TL, Kane LJ, et al. Tumor and normal tissue response to irradiation in vivo: variation with decreasing dose rates. *Radiology* 1975; 114:709–716.
27. Gaspar LE, Fisher BJ, MacDonald DR, et al. Supratentorial malignant glioma: patterns of recurrence and implications for external beam local treatment. *Int J Radiat Oncol Biol Phys* 1992; 24:55–57.
28. Godano U, Frank F, Fabrizi AP, et al. Stereotactic surgery in the management of deep intracranial lesions in infants and adolescents. *Childs Nerv Syst* 1987; 3:85–88.
29. Goodman JH, Gahbauer RA, Kanellitsas C, et al. Theoretical basis and clinical methodology for stereotactic interstitial brain tumor irradiation using iododeoxyuridine as a radiation sensitizer and ^{145}Sm as a brachytherapy source. *Stereotact Funct Neurosurg* 1990; 54–55:531–534.

30. Gutin PH, Bernstein M, Sano Y, et al. Combination therapy with 1,3-bis(2-chloroethyl)-1-nitrosourea and low dose rate radiation in the 9L rat brain tumor and spheroid models: implications for brain tumor brachytherapy. *Neurosurgery* 1984; 15:781–786.
31. Gutin PH, Leibel SA, Hosobuchi Y, et al. Brachytherapy of recurrent tumors of the skull base and spine with iodine-125 sources. *Neurosurgery* 1987; 20:938–945.
32. Gutin PH, Philips TL, Wara WM, et al. Brachytherapy of recurrent malignant brain tumors with removable high-activity iodine-125 sources. *J Neurosurg* 1984; 60:61–68.
33. Gutin PH, Prados MD, Phillips TL, et al. External irradiation followed by an interstitial high activity iodine-125 implant "boost" in the initial treatment of malignant gliomas: NCOG study 6G-82-2. *Int J Radiat Oncol Biol Phys* 1991; 21:601–606.
34. Hall EJ. Radiation dose-rate: a factor of importance in radiobiology and radiotherapy. *Br J Radiol* 1972; 45:81–97.
35. Hall EJ. The promise of low dose rate: has it been realized? *Int J Radiat Oncol Biol Phys* 1978; 4:749–750.
36. Hall EJ. The biological basis of endocurietherapy. *Endocurietherap Hypertherm Oncol* 1985; 1:141–152.
37. Halperin EC, Burger PC, Bullard DE. The fallacy of the localized supratentorial malignant glioma. *Int J Radiat Oncol Biol Phys* 1988; 15:505–509.
38. Hitchon PW, Jani SK, VanGilder JC, et al. Interstitial radiation in recurrent malignant gliomas. *Appl Neurophysiol* 1987; 50:292–294.
39. Hitchon PW, VanGilder JC, Wen BC, et al. Brachytherapy for malignant recurrent and untreated gliomas. *Stereotact Funct Neurosurg* 1992; 59:174–178.
40. Hochberg FH, Pruitt A. Assumptions in the radiotherapy of glioblastoma. *Neurology* 1980; 30:907–911.
41. Hosobuchi Y, Phillips TL, Stupar TA, et al. Interstitial brachytherapy of primary brain tumors: preliminary report. *J Neurosurg* 1980; 53:613–617.
42. Kelly PJ, Daumas-Duport C, Scheithauer BW, et al. Stereotactic histologic correlations of computed tomography and magnetic resonance imaging-defined abnormalities in patients with glial neoplasms. *Mayo Clin Proc* 1987; 62:450–459.
43. Kelly PJ, Olson MH, Wright AE. Stereotactic implantation of iridium-192 into CNS neoplasms. *Surg Neurol* 1978; 10:349–354.
44. Krishnaswamy V. Dose distribution around a ^{125}I seed source in tissue. *Radiology* 1978; 126:489–491.
45. Kumar PP, Good RR, Jones EO, et al. Survival of patients with glioblastoma multiforme treated by intraoperative high-activity cobalt 60 endocurietherapy. *Cancer* 1989; 64:1409–1413.
46. Larson GL, Wilbanks JH, Dennis WS, et al. Interstitial radiogold implantation for the treatment of recurrent high-grade gliomas. *Cancer* 1990; 66:27–29.
47. Leibel SA, Gutin PH, Wara WM, et al. Survival and quality of life after interstitial implantation of removable high-activity iodine-125 sources for the treatment of patients with recurrent malignant gliomas. *Int J Radiat Oncol Biol Phys* 1989; 17:1129–1139.
48. Levin VA, Silver P, Hannigan J, et al. Superiority of post-radiotherapy adjuvant chemotherapy with CCNU, procarbazine, and vincristine (PCV) over BCNU for anaplastic gliomas: NCOG 6G61 final report. *Int J Radiat Oncol Biol Phys* 1990; 18:321–324.
49. Liang BC, Thornton AF Jr, Sandler HM, et al. Malignant astrocytomas: focal tumor recurrence after focal external beam radiation therapy. *J Neurosurg* 1991; 75:559–563.
50. Ling CC, Chui CS. Stereotactic treatment of brain tumors with radioactive implants or external photon beams: radiobiophysical aspects. *Radiother Oncol* 1993; 26:11–18.
51. Ling CC, Spiro IJ, Mitchell J, et al. The variation of OER with dose rate. *Int J Radiat Oncol Biol Phys* 1985; 11:1367–1373.
52. Loeffler JS, Alexander E III, Hochberg FH, et al. Clinical patterns of failure following stereotactic interstitial irradiation for malignant gliomas. *Int J Radiat Oncol Biol Phys* 1990; 19:1455–1462.
53. Loeffler JS, Alexander E III, Wen PY, et al. Results of stereotactic brachytherapy used in the initial management of patients with glioblastoma. *J Natl Cancer Inst* 1990; 82:1918–1921.
54. Lucas GL, Luxton G, Cohen D, et al. Treatment results of stereotactic interstitial brachytherapy for primary and metastatic brain tumors. *Int J Radiat Oncol Biol Phys* 1991; 21:715–721.
55. Ludgate CM, Douglas BG, Dixon PF, et al. Superfractionated radiotherapy in grade III, IV intracranial gliomas. *Int J Radiat Oncol Biol Phys* 1988; 15:1091–1095.
56. Lulu BA, Lutz W, Stea B, et al. Treatment planning of template-guided stereotaxic brain implants. *Int J Radiat Oncol Biol Phys* 1990; 18:951–955.
57. Malkin MG. Interstitial irradiation of malignant gliomas. *Rev Neurol (Paris)* 1992; 148:448–453.
58. Marchese MJ, Goldhagen PE, Zaider M, et al. The relative biological effectiveness of photon radiation from encapsulated iodine-125, assessed in cells of human origin: 1. Normal diploid fibroblasts. *Int J Radiat Oncol Biol Phys* 1990; 18:1407–1413.
59. Marchese MJ, Hall EJ, Hilaris BS. Clinical, physical and radiobiological aspects of encapsulated iodine-125 in radiation oncology. *Endocurietherap Hypertherm Oncol* 1985; 1:67–82.
60. Massey V, Wallner KE. Patterns of second recurrence of malignant astrocytomas. *Int J Radiat Oncol Biol Phys* 1990; 18:395–398.
61. Mundinger F, Braus DF, Krauss JK, et al. Long-term outcome of 89 low-grade brain-stem gliomas after interstitial radiation therapy. *J Neurosurg* 1991; 75:740–746.
62. Mundinger F, Ostertag C. Post-operative stereotactic Curie-therapy using the iridium-192 GammaMed contact irradiation apparatus combined with radio-sensitizers in treating multiform glioblastomas. *Acta Neurochir (Wein)* 1978; 42:73–77.
63. Mundinger F, Riechert T. Stereotaxic irradiation-procedure of brain tumors and pituitary adenomas by means of radio-isotopes and its results. *Confin Neurol* 1962; 22:190–203.
64. Mundinger F, Weigel K. Indication and results of stereotactic curietherapy with iridium-192 and iodine-125 for non-resectable tumours of the hypothalamic region. *Acta Neurochir Suppl (Wien)* 1984; 33:323–330.
65. Mundinger F, Weigel K. Long-term results of stereotactic interstitial curietherapy. *Acta Neurochir Suppl (Wien)* 1984; 33:367–371.
66. Ostertag CB, Kreth FW. Iodine-125 interstitial irradiation for cerebral gliomas. *Acta Neurochir (Wien)* 1992; 119:53–61.
67. Patchell RA, Maruyama Y, Tibbs PA, et al. Neutron interstitial brachytherapy for malignant gliomas: a pilot study. *J Neurosurg* 1988; 68:67–72.
68. Pierquin B, Wilson JF, Chassagne D. *Modern Brachytherapy.* New York: Masson, 1987, pp 1–6.
69. Prados MD, Gutin PH, Phillips TL, et al. Interstitial brachytherapy for newly diagnosed patients with malignant gliomas: the UCSF experience. *Int J Radiat Oncol Biol Phys* 1992; 24:593–597.
70. Rougier A, Pigneux J, Cohadon F. Combined interstitial and external irradiation of gliomas. *Acta Neurochir Suppl (Wien)* 1984; 33:345–353.
71. Saroja KR, Mansell J, Hendrickson FR, et al. Failure of accelerated neutron therapy to control high grade astrocytomas. *Int J Radiat Oncol Biol Phys* 1989; 17:1295–1297.
72. Scharfen CO, Sneed PK, Wara WM, et al. High activity iodine-125 interstitial implant for gliomas. *Int J Radiat Oncol Biol Phys* 1992; 24:583–591.
73. Schultz RJ, Chandra P, Nath R. Determination of the exposure rate constant for ^{125}I using a scintillation detector. *Med Phys* 1980; 7:355–361.
74. Schwartz RB, Carvalho PA, Alexander E III, et al. Radiation necrosis vs high-grade recurrent glioma: differentiation by using dual-isotope SPECT with ^{201}Tl and ^{99m}Tc-HMPAO. *Am J Neuroradiol* 1991; 12:1187–1192.
75. Shapiro WR, Green SB, Burger PC, et al. Randomized trial of three chemotherapy regimens and two radiotherapy regimens in postoperative treatment of malignant glioma. Brain Tumor Cooperative Group Trial 8001. *J Neurosurg* 1989; 71:1–9.

76. Sneed PK, Gutin PH, Prados MD, et al. Patterns of recurrence of glioblastoma multiforme after external irradiation followed by implant boost. *Int J Radiat Oncol Biol Phys* 1993; 27(Suppl 1):177 (abstr).
77. Sneed PK, Gutin PH, Stauffer PR, et al. Thermoradiotherapy of recurrent malignant brain tumors. *Int J Radiat Oncol Biol Phys* 1992; 23:853–861.
78. Stea B, Kittelson J, Cassady JR, et al. Treatment of malignant gliomas with interstitial irradiation and hyperthermia. *Int J Radiat Oncol Biol Phys* 1992; 24:657–667.
79. Szikla G, Schlienger M, Blond S, et al. Interstitial and combined interstitial and external irradiation of supratentorial gliomas. Results in 61 cases treated 1973–1981. *Acta Neurochir Suppl (Wien)* 1984; 33:355–362.
80. Talairach J, Ruggiero G, Aboulker J, et al. A new method of treatment of inoperable brain tumours by stereotaxic implantation of radioactive gold—a preliminary report. *Br J Radiol* 1955; 28:62–74.
81. Thomson ES, Afshar F, Plowman PN. Paediatric brachytherapy. *Br J Radiol* 1989; 62:223–229.
82. Valk PE, Budinger TF, Levin VA, et al. PET of malignant cerebral tumors after interstitial brachytherapy: demonstration of metabolic activity and correlation with clinical outcome. *J Neurosurg* 1988; 69:830–838.
83. Walker MD, Alexander E Jr, Hunt WE, et al. Evaluation of BCNU and/or radiotherapy in the treatment of anaplastic gliomas. A cooperative clinical trial. *J Neurosurg* 1978; 49:333–343.
84. Walker MD, Strike TA, Sheline GE. An analysis of dose-effect relationship in the radiotherapy of malignant gliomas. *Int J Radiat Oncol Biol Phys* 1979; 5:1725–1731.
85. Wallner KE, Galicich JH, Krol G, et al. Patterns of failure following treatment for glioblastoma multiforme and anaplastic astrocytoma. *Int J Radiat Oncol Biol Phys* 1989; 16:1405–1409.
86. Weaver K, Smith V, Lewis JD, et al. A CT-based computerized treatment planning system for I-125 stereotactic brain implants. *Int J Radiat Oncol Biol Phys* 1990; 18:445–454.
87. Willis BK, Heilbrun MP, Sapozink MD, et al. Stereotactic interstitial brachytherapy of malignant astrocytomas with remarks on postimplantation computed tomographic appearance. *Neurosurgery* 1988; 23:348–354.
88. Wu A, Chun M, Kadson D, et al. Interstitial iridium-192 implantation for malignant brain tumours: Part I. Techniques of dosimetry planning. *Br J Radiol* 1989; 62:154–157.
89. Zamorano L, Yakar D, Dujovny M, et al. Permanent iodine-125 implant and external beam radiation therapy for the treatment of malignant brain tumors. *Stereotact Funct Neurosurg* 1992; 59:183–192.

187

Radiation Injury of the Brain and Spinal Cord

Mitchell S. Anscher
Patrick S. Swift
Laurie E. Gaspar
Lawrence B. Marks

The ill effects of ionizing radiation on the central nervous system (CNS) have been studied extensively. In this chapter we will review the common forms of radiation injury of the brain and spinal cord, the radiobiological factors that influence injury, and clinical strategies for dealing with injury.

Radiobiology

The Concept of Tolerance

The dose of radiation that can be delivered to a tumor will often be limited by the tolerance to irradiation of the surrounding normal tissues. The concept of minimal and maximal tissue tolerance dose (TTD) was developed in an attempt to provide useful guidelines for the tolerance to irradiation of normal tissues and organs.[177] The minimal tissue tolerance dose ($TTD_{5/5}$) is defined as the dose associated with a 5 percent rate of complications occurring within 5 years of treatment. The maximal tissue tolerance dose ($TTD_{50/5}$) is the dose associated with a 50 percent complication rate over the same time span. $TTD_{5/5}$ and $TTD_{50/5}$ values for normal tissues have been published.[178] These values assume a standard set of treatment conditions: (1) megavoltage irradiation (1 to 10 MeV); (2) a dose-delivery schedule of 2.0 Gy/day, 5 fractions per week (10 Gy/week) with 2-day rest intervals; and (3) completion of treatment in 6 to 8 weeks. Some of the published values represent best estimates based on indirect data or a consensus of clinical experience where experimental documentation is lacking.

The Relationship of Dose per Fraction to Radiation Injury

The radiobiologist defines cell death as a loss of reproductive integrity—that is, a loss of the capacity for sustained proliferation. In this sense, the term *cell death* is used in the same sense as in microbiology: cell death means clonogenic death. The in vitro cell-survival curve describes the relationship between absorbed doses of radiation and the surviving fraction of irradiated cells.

A typical survival curve for a mammalian cell line is shown in Fig. 187-1. The dose of radiation is plotted on a linear scale, and the surviving fraction on a logarithmic scale. For sparsely ionizing radiation such as therapeutic x-rays, the survival curve has an initial shoulder followed by an almost straight portion. This curve may be expressed by a linear dose coefficient (α) and a coefficient (β) for the square of the dose. The effect of irradiation is proportional to αD plus βD^2, where D equals dose of radiation.[200]

The linear-quadratic formula can be used to fit a continuously bending curve to cell-survival data: $SF = e^{-(\alpha D+\beta D^2)}$. The linear component of the dose–survival relationship, αD, dominates the response at low doses of radiation. With radiotherapy delivered at the conventional doses per fraction, on the order of 2 Gy, the α component is of major significance. It is thought that this α component is the result of single-hit radiation killing of cells.[200]

The dose range over which the linear component dominates in a linear-quadratic survival curve relationship depends on the relative values of α and β. The higher the relative value of α, the more linear the response at low doses and the less sensitive one would expect a cell line to be to fractionation of radiation dose. If, on the other hand, α is low relative to β, the survival curve will be "curvier." A low α/β ratio will indicate more bending down of the curve after a relatively small initial linear region. There will therefore be a marked effect of dose fractionation. As another way to state this observation, a high α/β ratio implies little fractionation effect at low doses of radiation. Conversely, a low α/β ratio indicates that dose fractionation will have a marked sparing effect on the survival of cell populations.

Current measurements of the values for α and β indicate that early-responding tissues tend to have a high α/β ratio. For example, tissues that respond in an acute way to irradiation, such as bowel mucosa, the oropharyngeal epithelium, and spermatic cells, have an α/β ratio ranging from 7 to 13. On the other hand, tissues responding late to irradiation, such as the brain and spinal cord, have low α/β ratios, on the order of 1.6 to 5.[212]

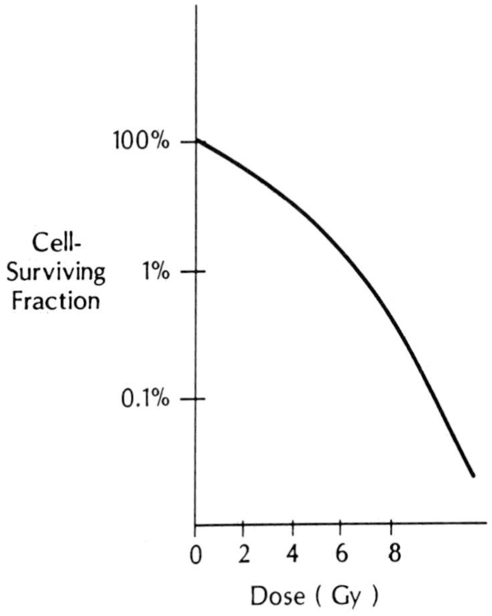

Figure 187-1 A schematic radiation cell-survival curve following single doses of x-rays.

Over recent years, it has become clear that there is a consistent difference between early- and late-responding tissues in their response to radiotherapy fractionation. When large dose fractions are given, the late effects of irradition are more severe than if low doses per fraction are given. Many of the ill effects of irradiation on the CNS are attributable to the use of high-dose-per-fraction irradiation.

The effects of fractionation on normal tissue toxicity may be expressed with "isoeffect curves." Such curves show the change in the total dose of a course of radiation that can be administered, as the dose per fraction is changed, to achieve an equal biological effect (isoeffect). In Fig. 187-2, we show the increase in the total isoeffective dose with the decrease in size of each fraction of radiation for multifraction animal experimentation. In the spinal cord, it can be seen that there is a marked decrease in the total dose of radiation that can be administered as the dose per fraction increases. This effect is less marked in an acute-reacting tissue such as the jejunum. Such experimental evidence confirms the findings of α/β ratio mathematical models. That is, high doses per fraction are much more likely to produce ill effects in late-responding tissues than low doses per fraction.

Review of data from patients who have developed necrosis of the brain or spinal cord following irradiation confirms that the dose per fraction is the most important factor in determining CNS tissue tolerance in humans.[164] As the dose per fraction increases above 2.0 Gy, the total dose that may be delivered safely to the CNS decreases rapidly. There are some suggestions in the literature that as the dose per fraction decreases below 2.0 Gy, tolerance of CNS tissue may increase very slowly.

Earlier experimental work with irradiation of the rat spinal cord suggests that there is no further increase in tolerance below doses of 2.0 Gy/fraction.[5] However, more recent evidence suggests that there is sparing of the spinal cord at doses below 2.0 Gy/fraction. There appears to be little change in the ED_{50} (the radiation dose producing paralysis in 50 percent of experimental animals). However, there is a suggestion that the threshold dose for the induction of radiation myelitis may be increased with lower doses per fraction. The sparing of the spinal cord occurs to a lesser extent than that predicted by the linear-quadratic model, suggesting that the spinal cord repairs sublethal radiation damage less rapidly or less completely after small doses than was predicted based on clinical experience with larger doses per fraction.[101,207]

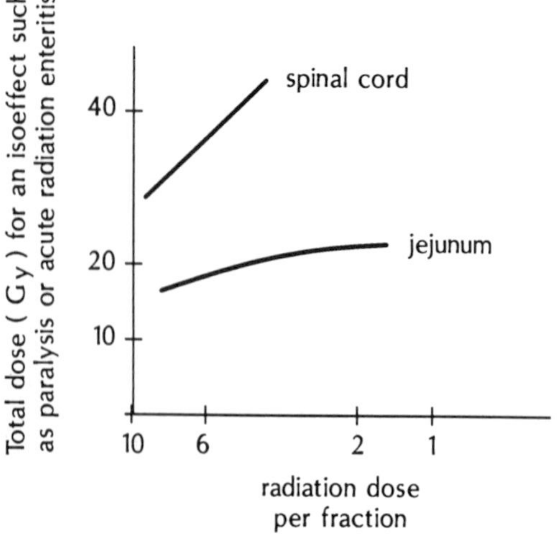

Figure 187-2 An isoeffect curve, based on animal experiments, showing the difference in fractionation effect on an acute-reacting tissue (jejunum) compared to a late-reacting CNS tissue (spinal cord). (Modified, with permission, from Withers HR. Biologic basis for altered fractionation schemes. *Cancer* 1985, 55:2086–2095.)

Recent studies suggest that the tolerance of the brain also increases as the dose decreases below 2.0 Gy/fraction. The Pediatric Oncology Group performed a series of dose-escalation studies in the treatment of brain stem tumors in children. They found no increase in late radiation injury when doses of 66 Gy in 1.1-Gy fractions twice daily were used, as compared to expected complication rates when using 1.8- to 2.0-Gy fractions once daily to 55 Gy (standard therapy).[55,56] Similar findings were noted when 70.2 Gy was delivered in 1.17-Gy fractions twice daily. In the first study, 4 to 6 h of time elapsed between fractions, and in the second study a 6-h time interval between fractions was mandated. Similar findings were noted using doses up to 78 Gy in 1.0-Gy fractions given twice daily at the University of California at San Francisco (UCSF).[114]

Clinical Aspects of Radiation Injury

The Acute Forms

Acute radiation necrosis refers to the acute destruction of irradiated tissue within hours or days of exposure. This response usually requires an extremely high dose of radiation (≥100 Gy) delivered in a short period of time. Severe nausea and vomiting develop, usually within minutes. These are followed by disorientation, loss of muscular coordination, respiratory distress, diarrhea, seizures, coma, and eventually death.[72] Such exposures may be administered in animal experiments but should only occur in human radiation therapy under the controlled circumstances of stereotactic radiosurgery. Exposures of this magnitude may occur in atomic accidents.

It has been claimed that edema resulting in increased intracranial pressure or spinal cord compression may occur after a single dose of 2.0 Gy to the brain or spinal cord. However, there is no good evidence that any acute reaction occurs in normal CNS tissue at clinically used radiotherapeutic dose levels.[94]

The Subacute Forms

Subacute effects appear a few weeks to several months after irradiation. These subacute effects may be the result of irradiation-induced demyelination.[13]

Lhermitte's sign, characterized by numbness, tingling, or electrical sensations in the upper and/or lower extremities, has been observed after irradiation of the spinal cord. These symptoms may be present continuously and exacerbated by flexion of the head and neck. More commonly, patients are asymptomatic except when they flex the head and neck, which causes an immediate onset of numbness, tingling, or an electrical sensation radiating into the back or extremities. This syndrome is thought to result from transient demyelinization of the posterior columns, the lateral spinothalamic tracts, or both. Lhermitte's sign usually appears 1 to 3 months following completion of irradiation and lasts from 1 to 9 months, with an average duration of 3 to 4 months. The paresthesia usually subsides gradually, leaving no sequelae. Rarely, Lhermitte's sign has been reported to herald the onset of permanent myelopathy.[94] This sign has been reported to occur with doses to the spinal cord as low as 26.3 Gy, and it will occur in 10 to 15 percent of patients with Hodgkin's disease receiving 30 to 40 Gy to a mantle field.[81]

Irradiation of the brain can result in the somnolence syndrome. This syndrome was first described by Druckmann in 1929.[38] He noted a period of marked somnolence that appeared in a small percentage of children treated with radiation for ringworm of the scalp. The somnolence persisted up to 14 days and then resolved spontaneously. The syndrome may consist of somnolence, anorexia, low-grade fevers, apathy, headaches, dizziness, nausea, occasional vomiting, and, rarely, cranial nerve palsies. The onset usually occurs 4 to 8 weeks after completion of irradiation. This syndrome has been reported to occur in most children with acute lymphoblastic leukemia (ALL) receiving prophylactic cranial irradiation to doses as low as 18 Gy.[117] The role of systemic and intrathecal chemotherapy in the production of this syndrome in these children is not well defined. This syndrome also occurs in a small proportion of adult patients receiving partial- or whole-brain irradiation.[184] These symptoms are transient, usually resolving spontaneously in 4 to 14 days. However, persistent electroencephalographic abnormalities, learning disabilities, and clinical seizure disorders have been reported to be more frequent in children with ALL who developed the somnolence syndrome.[19]

Watne et al.[209] have described a syndrome occurring in 5 percent of patients receiving radiation therapy and chemotherapy for low-grade astrocytomas. In its mild form, the syndrome consisted of mild fatigue or somnolence beginning 2 to 3 months after irradiation. Computed tomography (CT) demonstrated marked edema in the irradiated volume without contrast enhancement. CT changes usually normalized within 3 months, and the symptoms regressed. In the severe form of this syndrome, patients manifested exacerbations of their presenting clinical signs, beginning 3 to 8 months after irradiation. CT demonstrated marked edema with areas of contrast enhancement mimicking recurrent tumor. Both the mild and the severe forms of the syndrome responded to corticosteroid therapy. Thus, in this setting, a trial of steroids may be warranted prior to surgical intervention. Similar findings have been reported by others as well.[13,170]

A vary rare, severe subacute effect consisting of rapidly progressive ataxia, focal motor signs, cranial neuropathies, and nystagmus has been reported. This sequela occurred 6 to 13 weeks after the completion of radiotherapy. Although recovery in 6 to 8 weeks occurred in two patients, two other reported patients had progressive deficits resulting in death. Punched-out areas of demyelination with a predilection for subependymal regions in the lower pons and upper medulla were seen pathologically. These patients had received doses of 50 to 57 Gy over approximately 1 month.[99,170]

The pathogenesis of subacute radiation injury appears to be a temporary interruption of myelin synthesis resulting from injury to the oligodendroglial cells. The latency in recovery time from subacute radiation injury corresponds to the turnover time of myelin.[42,78,81]

The Late Forms

Late effects of irradiation-induced damage to CNS tissue may occur from 6 months to many years after irradiation, peaking between 1 and 3 years. Late effects rarely appear for the first time more than 4 to 5 years after the completion of irradiation, with the exception of the development of second malignancies.[95]

Delayed radiation necrosis is characterized by (1) partial tissue necrosis after therapeutic doses of radiation (40 to 70 Gy over 2 to 7 weeks); (2) a clinically silent interval between the irradiation and the necrosis; and (3) characteristic histopathologic changes. Widely accepted values of $TTD_{5/5}$ for brain necrosis are 60 Gy for irradiation of the whole brain and 70 Gy for irradiation of 25 percent or less of the brain.[178] Review of the literature has yielded only 25 reported cases of brain necrosis following single courses of irradiation to doses < 72.5 to 75 Gy at 2.0 Gy/fraction.[184] The actual incidence of brain necrosis is difficult to determine because reports in the literature are anecdotal. The determination of these values is further complicated by the fact that it is often difficult to differentiate radiation necrosis from recurrent brain tumor except by postmortem examination.

Reagan and colleagues identified three specific categories of late radiation myelopathy: acute complete paraplegia/quadriplegia, lower motor neuron disease, and chronic progressive radiation myelitis.[167] Acute complete paraplegia/quadriplegia involves a dramatic progression, over a span of hours to days, from an intact neurological state to one of a complete neurological deficit. The lower motor neuron syndrome involves the development of lower motor neuron signs, including muscle atrophy, loss of deep tendon reflexes, and fasciculations.[62]

Chronic progressive radiation myelitis is perhaps the most dreaded of all late complications of radiotherapy. Symptoms typically present within 9 to 15 months after treatment in the form of paresthesia and inability to perceive pain and temperature. Subsquently, a steady progression usually follows over the next 6 months, involving loss of all cord functions.[98]

The widely accepted value of tolerance for necrosis of the spinal cord is 45 Gy for the thoracic spinal cord and 50 Gy for the cervical and lumbar spinal cord.[8,95,164,178] Review of the literature suggests that the risk of necrosis at doses of 45 to 50 Gy, given at 1.8 to 2.0 Gy/fraction, 5 fractions per week, approaches 0 percent. As total dose increases above 50 Gy, the risk of necrosis increases in a sigmoid fashion. The incidence of spinal cord necrosis is difficult to determine because reports in the literature are anecdotal. If long segments of the spinal cord ($>$10 cm) are irradiated, the tolerance may be decreased.[73,164]

Tolerance data suggests that the thoracic spinal cord is more sensitive than the cervical or lumbar spinal cord. It has been proposed that such a difference could be related, at least in part, to a more vulnerable vascular supply in the "watershed area" of the upper thoracic spinal cord.[61] There is little evidence to support this argument.

An intrinsic difference in tolerance to irradiation between the brain and spinal cord is suggested by the above tolerance values. There is little evidence documenting such a difference. This apparent difference may be a result of (1) functional deficits that may not be clinically apparent if necrosis occurs in "silent" areas of the brain; and (2) the unwillingness of clinicians to accept any incidence of spinal cord necrosis because of the devastating functional deficits that result.

Previous damage to CNS tissue may decrease its tolerance to irradiation. In patients with brain tumors who receive whole-brain irradiation to doses of 50 to 60 Gy at 1.7 to 2.0 Gy/fraction, a strong predilection for necrosis in the white matter adjacent to the neoplasm has been found, suggesting that these areas may be more susceptible to irradiation-induced injury.[15]

The use of systemic and/or intrathecal chemotherapy may also significantly decrease the tolerance of CNS tissue to irradiation. This is strongly suggested by studies in children with leukemia and patients with small cell carcinoma of the lung and brain tumors, all of whom received CNS irradiation and systemic and/or intrathecal chemotherapy. These patients all appear to be at increased risk for necrosis as well as functional deficits.

Age appears to be an importat factor in the tolerance of CNS tissues to irradiation. Children less than 3 to 5 years old have an increased risk of developing functional deficits when treated with cranial irradiation.

Pathology of Late Radiation Injury

In terms of gross morphology, the advanced stages of delayed radiation necrosis of the brain are manifested by a tissue defect. The cortex of the brain is shriveled and shrunken. This is an indication of cavitation of the underlying white matter. Telangiectasias and focal hemorrhage may be encountered. Delayed radiation necrosis of the spinal cord is generally characterized by a narrowing of the cord. On cross section, the gray columns of the spinal cord have a washed-out appearance, and the area occupied by the white tracts is reduced in size.

The histopathology of delayed radiation necrosis is characterized by large areas of confluent, coagulative necrosis of the white matter and the deepest layers of the cortex, atypia or absence of endothelial cells of the vessels, vascular thickening, telangiectasia formation, and vascular proliferation. The vascular degenerative changes are seen in almost every case.[73,214]

When the lesions of delayed radiation necrosis are distant from an intracranial neoplasm, their identity is readily established if the appropriate histologic findings are present. It is, however, quite frequent that the lesions of delayed radiation necrosis occur adjacent to a neoplasm. In this setting, delayed radiation necrosis must be distinguished from therapeutic necrosis of the tumor or spontaneous necrosis. The astrogliosis that can occur at the edge of delayed radiation necrosis can be difficult to distinguish from a glioma. The vascular lesions, however, can be identified and allow one to make the diagnosis.[73]

Because radiation necrosis can occur adjacent to a neoplasm, one must be cautious in interpreting the effects of new chemotherapeutic agents on "tumors" whose recurrence is documented only by imaging studies. Some of these "recurrences" may actually represent delayed radiation necrosis. The responses of brain tumors to drugs may not be the response of tumor to treatment but, rather, the natural history of radiation necrosis, that is, shrinkage of the involved area.[73]

Lyman, Kupalov, and Scholz made a major contribution to our understanding of the pathogenesis of delayed radiation necrosis with their 1933 report of experimentally induced "Roentgen ray" CNS damage.[130] At a Leningrad laboratory, four adult dogs were given large doses of x-rays to the occipital lobes of the brain. During the second to twelfth week following irradiation, the conditioned reflexes (measured in Professor I.P. Pavlov's laboratory) were always below the normal range. One dog was allowed to live for 6 months after irradiation. In the fifth month there were signs of cortical and subcortical damage. At autopsy, there were marked hyalin degeneration and obliterating sclerosis of the arterioles, with numerous areas of complete and incomplete necrosis. Lyman and colleagues postulated that x-rays did not exert their primary CNS effects on the cells of the cerebral cortex. Rather, these effects were secondary to vascular changes, which brought "the appearance of necrosis in their wake." For over 50 years, this vascular mechanism has been most often cited for delayed radiation necrosis. This postulated mechanism is consistent with the almost uniform finding of vascular lesions in cases of delayed necrosis.

All aspects of the morphology of delayed radiation necrosis, however, are not explicable by the vascular hypothesis. Demyelination may precede the observation of vascular damage. Delayed radiation necrosis is primarily a white matter lesion, whereas circulatory insufficiency is usually thought to be more injurious to gray matter. As an alternative to the vascular insufficiency hypothesis, Zeman and Samorajski suggested a radiobiological theory based on clonogenic death of glial cells.[214] The radiation-induced reproductive death of slowly reproducing oligodendrocytes, they postulated, shifts oxidative enzyme activity to the astrocytes. This may result in demyelination. Radiation-induced endothelial cell death, the hypothesis continues, will also promote necrosis.

A third hypothesis, offered as an alternative to both the vascular and the primary cell death hypotheses, is that of an allergic origin of delayed radiation necrosis. In some cases, the lesions of delayed radiation necrosis consist of disseminated plaques of demyelination with central necrosis and occasional petechial hemorrhage. Patent blood vessels are present, and there is perivascular cuffing with lymphocytes and plasma cells. An autoimmune pathogenesis of this disseminated radiation-induced sclerosis has been proposed. The postulated mechanism is that an antigenic substance is produced by the reaction of x-rays with the oligodendromyelin complex and its enzyme systems. These antigens then stimulate the accumulation of inflammatory cells.[27,99]

It is likely that no one hypothesis explains the origin of delayed radiation necrosis. The pathogenesis, in any individual case, may be explicable by some combination of these three proposed mechanisms.

Imaging of Late Radiation Injury

Changes due to radionecrosis are seen on CT scanning of the brain either as regions of low density without a mass effect or contrast enhancement, as a localized, low-density, contrast-enhancing mass, or as diffuse lesions of varying density without a mass effect but with occasional enhancement.[142,143] The lesions appear from 9 to 28 months following irradiation. They appear sooner with higher doses. Enhancement may be central or peripheral, and may be seen even if the original tumor did not enhance.[142] None of these findings is specific, and one cannot distinguish recurrent tumor from radiation necrosis by CT alone. Correlating the CT changes with the high-dose regions on the patient's radiation isodose reconstruction maps may be helpful, but is still not diagnostic of radiation necrosis. Histologic confirmation should be obtained whenever possible.[143]

Radiation myelopathy may appear on CT at the time of diagnosis as a widening of the cord, which returns to near normal size several months later.[204] Changes on CT are not diagnostic, but CT can be used to rule out tumor recurrence or metastases and may help lead to the diagnosis of radiation myelopathy if the rest of the clinical picture fits the diagnosis.

Postradiation changes seen on magnetic resonance imaging (MRI) of the brain are also nonspecific. Radiation injury to the brain results in an increase in tissue water content, producing prolonged T1 and T2 relaxation times. Increased signal intensity compared to normal white matter is seen on T2-weighted and proton density images. Decreased signal intensity relative to normal white matter is seen on T1-weighted images. The changes seen on MRI correspond to abnormalities on CT[105] but cannot be used to distinguish recurrent tumor from necrosis.[36,103]

Zweig and Russell[215] have recently described the findings of radiation myelitis on MRI. They found abnormally increased signal intensity on proton density and T2-weighted images corresponding to the site of injury. Precontrast T1-weighted images were normal; however, postcontrast (gadopentetate dimeglumine) T1-weighted images showed focal enhancement corresponding to the area of abnormality on T2-weighted images. These findings are not specific, however, for radiation myelitis.

Positron emission tomography (PET) may be able to distinguish tumor recurrence from necrosis in selected situations.[35,37] Using rubidium 82 (^{82}Rb) to define regions in which the blood-brain barrier (BBB) was absent or altered and [^{18}F]2-fluoro-2-deoxy-D-glucose([^{18}F]FDG) to evaluate the metabolic state of these regions, Doyle and colleagues were able to distinguish radiation necrosis from tumor recurrence in nine of nine patients with high-grade gliomas.[37] These authors noted that the recurrent tumors appeared more metabolically active than adjacent tissues. Areas of necrosis demonstrated less metabolic activity than adjacent regions. Histologic confirmation of the PET scan diagnosis was obtained in seven of nine patients. However, Di Chiro and colleagues noted that the [^{18}F]FDG results demonstrated increased metabolic activity in only 4 of 40 patients with low-grade gliomas.[34,35]

PET scanning with the combination of ^{18}F[FDG] and L-methyl-^{11}C-methionine (^{11}C-Met) may be useful in distinguishing radiation injury from recurrent tumor. Ogawa and colleagues[155] demonstrated that ^{11}C-Met uptake in patients with radiation injury was similar to that of normal cortical tissue. Recurrent brain tumor, however, appeared as focal areas of increased accumulation of ^{11}C-Met. In this study, PET scanning with ^{18}F[FDG] demonstrated hypometabolism in all patients with radiation injury but also in one patient with recurrent malignant glioma. Thus, the combination of hypometabolism on ^{18}F[FDG] PET scanning and normal uptake on ^{11}C-Met PET scanning is strongly suggestive of radionecrosis. These data, however, are based on a small number of patients and deserve further study.

Dual-isotope single photon emission computed tomography (SPECT) with thallium 201 (^{201}Tl) in the perfusion agent technetium-99m-hexamethylpropyleneamine oxime (^{99m}Tc-HMPAO) may also prove to be useful in differentiating tumor growth from radiation changes. Schwartz and colleagues[181] studied 15 patients with high-grade gliomas who developed worsening symptoms after radiation therapy. All patients with high ^{201}Tl uptake in the area in question had local tumor recurrence. All patients with low ^{201}Tl uptake showed only radiation changes. In patients with intermediate ^{201}Tl uptake, the addition of ^{99m}Tc-HMPAO scanning allowed a tumor recurence to be distinguished from radiation change in seven of eight cases. This technique is promising and deserves further study.

Therapy of Late Radiation Injury

Histologic confirmation is usually required to differentiate radionecrosis from recurrent tumor. Surgical resection of the lesion may result in marked improvement or complete recovery if the lesion is focal and in a favorable location[109] or if symptomatic increased intracranial pressure is present. Diffuse lesions or lesions involving the brain stem or optic nerves are not amenable to resection. If the lesion can be resected, then surgery is the treatment of choice.

In lesions not amenable to surgery, corticosteroids may be effective in producing improvement or even complete resolution of all clinical and radiographic abnormalities. Lee and colleagues noted that complete disappearance of all symptoms and CT scan findings (lasting at least 6 months after steroids have been discontinued) occurred in 14 (19.4 percent) of 72 patients treated with dexamethasone for radionecrosis.[102] An additional 11 patients (15.3 percent) had complete disappearance of symptoms and greater than 50 percent reduction in the size of the CT scan abnormalities. No responders had experienced a relapse. These authors recommended using 12 to 16 mg/day of dexamethasone for 4 to 6 weeks, then tapering slowly over 4 months.

Hyperbaric oxygen (HBO) administration may be useful in the treatment of radiation injury of the CNS. Six patients were treated by Hart and Mainous for radionecrosis of the brain (one patient) or spinal cord (five patients) with HBO.[74] Improvement was noted in the patient suffering injury to the brain. All five patients with myelitis demonstrated improved sensory function following HBO, but there was no significant improvement in motor function.

Two patients with progressive symptomatic radionecrosis in spite of surgery and corticosteroids have been reported to show evidence of improvement both clinically and on CT scanning after treatment with heparin followed by warfarin. This improvement persisted after the warfarin was discontinued.[171]

Other Manifestations of Late Radiation Injury

Damage to the Retina, Optic Nerve, and Optic Chiasm Radiation retinopathy may develop when > 50 Gy is delivered to the retina.[162] Chemotherapy may lower the dose threshold.[162] Radiation retinopathy presents 1.5 to 6 years after irradiation as a painless, progressive loss of vision in the treated eye.[109,162] On examination, the retinal changes resemble those of diabetic retinopathy. There are capillary microaneurysms, flame hemorrhages, and cotton-wool and hard exudates. Neovascularization, retinal detachment, and vitreous hemorrhage may also be seen. Fluorescein angiography demonstrates leakage of plasma from damaged vessels, obliteration of small retinal vessels, ischemia, edema, and neovascularization.[162] Neovascularization may also be seen in the iris (rubeosis iridis), leading to angle closure glaucoma. This form of glaucoma is not responsive to medical therapy.[162] As in diabetic retinopathy, treatment with laser photocoagulation may be helpful.[162]

The manifestations of radiation damage to the optic nerve depend on the region of the nerve that has been damaged. Injury to the head of the optic nerve produces ischemic optic neuropathy secondary to injury to the posterior ciliary arteries. This is characterized by the gradual onset of progressive visual loss beginning 2 to 4 years after irradiation.[162] Physical examination reveals papilledema, pallor of the optic disc, and splinter hemorrhages on or near the disc. In contrast, injury to the proximal portion of the optic nerve produces retrobulbar optic neuropathy from small-vessel injury. This presents as the sudden onset of partial or total visual loss, which may be associated with pain. Clinical symptoms and signs may occur 1 to 9 years after irradiation. The risk of both forms of optic nerve injury is related to the total radiation dose and the daily fraction size.[162] Doses of ≤ 5000 Gy at 1.8 to 2 Gy/fraction should prevent the occurrence of optic nerve damage.[109,162] Every effort should be made to prevent radiation optic nerve damage, because no effective therapy exists.

Damage to the Hypothalamic-Pituitary Axis Many endocrinologic abnormalities have been described following cranial irradiation for tumors remote from the hypothalamic–pituitary axis. The incidence of hypothalamic–pituitary dysfunction as a function of dose is unknown. The lowest dose of radiation capable of causing hypothalamic–pituitary dysfunction is not precisely known, but a steep dose-tolerance curve may exist, with the threshold lying somewhere in the range of 15 to 25 Gy.[82,116,183] In the absence of a sellar or suprasellar tumor, no evidence of direct hypothalamic–pituitary deficiency was reported following 10 to 13.2 Gy to the whole brain in 3 to 5 days.[116] However, higher doses of 27 to 29 Gy have been associated with endocrine deficiency in 40 to 80 percent of patients followed for 2 years or more.[82,183] Radiation treatment in the dose range used for benign or malignant brain tumors (>45 Gy) will result in almost certain dysfunction of the hypothalamic–pituitary axis.[97,183,203] Conventional external-beam fields for treatment of sellar or suprasellar tumors frequently encompass the hypothalamus, pituitary stalk, and pituitary fossa.[115,139] Radiosurgery with avoidance of the suprasellar region may result in a reduced risk of radiation-induced endocrine deficiency, although this has yet to be demonstrated conclusively.[201] The incidence of direct radiation injury to the posterior lobe of the pituitary has not been studied thoroughly.

Surgical disruption or manipulation of the sellar–suprasellar region increases the subsequent risk of endocrine dysfunction; however, it is always difficult to exclude direct tumor effects.[41,139] Chemotherapy may also increase the risk of hypothalamic–pituitary dysfunction, although specific agents have not been identified.[82]

The risk of hypothalamic–pituitary radiation injury clearly increases with time, occurring as early as 3 months after irradiation.[82,97,115,116] Growth hormone (GH) deficiency and prolactin hypersecretion will usually manifest within 2 years of treatment, while other hormones must be observed for more than 5 years. Using life table analysis, Littley and colleagues[115] demonstrated the difference in radiation sensitivity of the anterior pituitary hormones. By 5 years, 100 percent of patients were GH deficient, 91 percent were gonadotropin deficient, 77 percent were corticotropin deficient, and 42 percent thyrotropin deficient. GH deficiency commonly develops first, followed by deficiencies in gonadotropin, corticotropin, and thyrotropin, although other sequences may occur.[97,115]

The incidence of hypothalamic–pituitary dysfunction reported will also depend on the diagnostic tests and criteria applied. Evaluation of GH and corticosteroid levels following insulin or glucagon stimulation, in conjunction with thyrotropin and gonadotropin releasing hormone tests and basal estimations of prolactin, thyroid hormones, and testosterone or estradiol, will uncover clinical and subclinical hormonal dysfunction.

Although the pituitary itself may be damaged by radiation, the actual site of injury in most cases is probably the hypothalamus.[26,141] There are several observations that suggest that radiation-induced hypothalamic dysfunction occurs early and with a higher frequency than pituitary dysfunction. In a large series of children with primary brain tumors, pituitary–hypothalamic injury was observed most frequently after the use of radiation techniques that could not allow for shielding of the hypothalamus, suggesting that the hypothalamus is the primary site of injury, leading to secondary pituitary insufficiency.[82] A delayed pituitary response to hypothalamic releasing hormone stimulation tests is often demonstrated, suggesting that the hypothalamus is the primary site of radiation-induced damage.[97,116] In addition, prolactin hypersecretion, reflecting hypothalamic damage, occurs often within 1 year of radiation therapy.[203] Destruction of dopaminergic neurons or disruption of the hypothalamic–pituitary vascular communication may be responsible for the hypothalamic injury.

The most common abnormality is a deficiency in GH. Growth abnormalities due to GH deficiency (i.e., a growth rate of less than 4 cm/year in children < 4 years old, or any decrease in growth rate in younger children) occur in 40 percent of children following radiation therapy for primary brain tumors.[41,82,183] This may be detected as early as 3 months after irradiation. Most patients destined to become GH deficient do so within the first year after irradiation.[41,182]

Although not a clinical problem in adults, GH deficiency may result in short stature in children. Studies in children with ALL have demonstrated abnormal GH release responses to insulin and arginine stimulation following doses of 24 Gy to the whole brain. However, no clear-cut relationship has been found between the blunting of the GH response to stimulation tests and clinically significant linear growth delay. In addition, functional recovery of the hypothalamic–pituitary axis in these children has been found 6 to 12 months after completion of treatment. In contrast, most children with brain tumors receiving higher doses of radiation have an abnormal GH response to stimulation tests and decreased linear growth.[40]

Even children who are not GH deficient after cranial irradiation may demonstrate a diminished growth rate. Growth in the irradiated child is influenced by multiple factors: spinal irradiation, nutrition, GH level, chemotherapy, and recurrent tumor. All children receiving cranial irradiation, even those receiving low doses,[41] should have their growth rate plotted over time. Careful longitudinal follow-up is required to detect an age-inappropriate decline in growth rate, indicating the need for a complete endocrine workup. Treatment with GH replacement may be indicated if GH deficiency is documented,[41,182] depending on the age and projected height of the child. Several studies have documented the safety and effectiveness of recombinant GH replacement in children; there is no apparent association between GH replacement and tumor recurrence or persistence. Normal growth and even "catch-up" growth will occur if hormonal replacement is initiated at the proper time.[41,82] Furthermore, the success of GH replacement is independent of the gender, the sites irradiated, and the use of chemotherapy. GH replacement must be started when abnormal growth rate is detected, prior to the closure of the epiphyses. Appropriate thyroid, corticoid, and gonadotropin replacement also will be necessary for normal growth and development.

As previously noted, irradiation of the hypothalamic–pituitary axis may also cause hypothyroidism and hyperprolactinemia.[26] Both of these entities occur significantly more often following doses > 55 Gy.[26] There is a long latent period, amounting to about 58 months for hyperprolactinemia and 22 to 55 months for hypothyroidism. The clinical spectrum ranges from asymptomatic elevations of prolactin and thyroid stimulating hormone (TSH) values to amenorrhea and/or diminished libido due to elevated prolactin levels and frank hypothyroidism accompanied by diminished levels of thyroxine (T_4). Therapy of hypothyroidism consists of thyroid replacement. Hyperprolactinemia may respond to bromocriptine.

Other uncommon endocrine abnormalities that have been described include gonadotropin deficiency[208] and panhypopituitarism.[28] Depending on the age of onset, problems range from failure to enter puberty or loss of secondary sexual characteristics to infertility resulting from gonadotropin deficiency. Panhypopituitarism results in all of the deficiencies noted above, plus diabetes insipidus (DI) and glucocorticoid deficiency. DI is treated with D-amino-D-arginine vasopressin, and glucocorticoid deficiency may be corrected with corticosteroid administration. Because corticotropin deficiency may occur prior to other hormone deficiencies, steroid coverage under periods of stress should be considered if results of basal or stimulation studies are not available. Gonadotropin deficiency is the most difficult problem to correct. If fertility is not desired, men may be treated with testosterone replacement and women with cyclic estrogen and progesterone. If fertility is desired, treatment requires the use of human gonadotropins. In prepubertal males, testosterone replacement requires a balanced hormonal environment to be effective, especially adequate GH levels. The subsequent fertility following hormone replacement of patients who were rendered gonadotropin-deficient or whose gonadotropin releasing sequence was disturbed, has not been evaluated.

Endocrinologic evaluation at least yearly, with a baseline evaluation prior to radiation therapy, is recommended if irradiation of the hypothalamic–pituitary region is required. Stimulation studies may not always be a part of the endocrinologic evaluation but should be done if growth or sexual maturation is abnormal, despite normal basal hormone levels. Somatomedin-C is a useful laboratory screen for GH deficiency, although normal thyroid function must be present for accurate results.[82] Children with midline tumors should have a complete baseline endocrine workup. Other children should have, as baseline, T_4 and TSH testing and a review of prior growth curves. Growth curves should be watched closely, and thyroid function should be checked every 6 months for 3 years.[41] The development of puberty should be monitored in prepubertal children. If the growth rate declines inappropriately or thyroid abnormalities are detected, a full endocrine workup should be undertaken.

Prior to cranial radiotherapy, adults should have baseline thyroid studies. A full endocrine workup should be considered for those with midline brain tumors. In the follow-up period, thyroid function should be monitored. A full endocrine workup should follow the detection of an abnormality. Other endocrine abnormalities are rare (with the exception of hyperprolactinemia) and are unlikely to present without detectable defects in GH or thyroid function. Routine biochemical monitoring is not warranted. One should, however, inquire about amenorrhea, loss of libido, impotence, and other symptoms that may indicate the need for an endocrinologic evaluation.

Intellectual Deficits Intellectual deficits have been noted to develop in both adults and children following cranial irradiation. With improvements in survival following treatment of primary or metastatic brain tumors, there is increasing concern about the neuropsychological sequelae and quality of life of long-term survivors.[18,31,96,104,132,145,161,176,189] Radiation-induced deficits can be difficult to distinguish from direct tumor effects or the side effects of other treatments, such as surgery and chemotherapy. Other factors are even more difficult to control for (i.e., CNS paraneoplastic effects, or the changes in educational/social environment that occur following the diagnosis of malignancy). However, several series have documented progressive intellectual decline in patients with controlled malignancy, suggeting that irradiation is at least partly responsible.[20,31,39,44,96,132,161,175]

In adults, intellectual deficits have been most frequently associated with prophylactic cranial irradiation (PCI) for small cell lung cancer, and they may be seen in up to 45 percent of long-term survivors.[75] They also occur following irradiation for primary brain tumors.[132]

In children, radiation therapy, surgery, chemotherapy, the tumor and its location, increased intracranial pressure, stress, time lost from school, parental education level, and rehabilitation all contribute to intellectual development. The radiation-associated decline in intelligence quotient (IQ) is generally in the area of performance, especially visual-motor and spatial integration, although a decline in verbal IQ has also been noted.[43,77,189] As in adults, previously acquired knowledge is not lost, but there is a decline in the rate at which new skills are acquired.[147] These deficits may progress with time, stabilize, or improve.[146] A greater decline may be seen in children whose IQs are high before treatment.[140] Because myelinization is not complete until the age of 2 to 3 years, young children are at greater risk.[28]

A prospective study using standardized intelligence tests demonstrated a significant intellectual decline after whole-brain irradiation only in children treated before age 9.[44] Children less than 5 years old had a larger intelligence quotient (IQ) decline than children 7 to 8 years old, suggesting that the younger the child, the larger the deficit to be anticipated. In a similar study of children with intracranial tumors not involving the cortical or subcortical regions, a drop in overall intelligence was measured 2 years following 24 to 36 Gy whole-brain radiation, usually with a posterior fossa boost.[161] Children less than 7 years of age at the time of radiation had a mean decline in full-scale IQ of 25 points.[161] A comparison of cognitive function between children who received prophylactic cranial irradiation for ALL and their siblings demonstrated a significant difference in IQ, an average difference of 10.5 points on standard IQ tests.[80] The difference was greatest for children irradiated at 7 years of age or less.

The influence of extent of radiation (whole-brain versus partial-brain) on subsequent neuropsychological deficits has not been thoroughly evaluated. Most studies in children pertain almost exclusively to whole-brain irradiation because this is the conventional technique for many common pediatric malignancies such as acute leukemia or medulloblastoma. Partial-brain irradiation in children may cause less subsequent intellectual deficit.[44] Cognitive deficits have been reported in adults treated with partial-brain radiation, although the relationship between intellectual deficits and radiation field size or site has not been investigated rigorously.[104,132]

In view of studies showing cognitive deficits following cranial irradiation, and the suspicion that the incidence and severity of these deficits is higher with larger doses of radiation, attempts have been made to omit radiation or lower its dose.[71,153,175,176] A cranial radiation dose reduction from 24 Gy to 18 Gy in children with ALL treated at UCSF resulted in smaller declines in IQ and academic performance, evident 6 years or longer after treatment.[71] Unfortunately, other studies using 18 Gy whole-brain irradiation have documented late cognitive deficits, suggesting that even these low doses have potential negative consequences.[175,176] Cranial irradiation may be omitted in appropriate groups of children with low-risk ALL, decreasing the neuropsychological consequences. However, the long-term toxicity of intrathecal or parenteral methotrexate requires further study in view of the electroencephalographic and radiologic changes reported.

The poor prognosis after treatment for primary malignant adult brain tumors has made it difficult to assess the true incidence of cognitive impairment. Studies in adults have documented progressive intellectual deterioration starting as early as 5 months after completion of treatment.[31,132] In the absence of clinical or radiologic evidence of tumor recurrence or progression, overall intellectual function may remain in the normal range, but the ability to conceptualize, reason, analyze, and synthesize new information is impaired.[6,104,132] Other reports are more alarming. Data from the Memorial Sloan-Kettering Cancer Center (MSKCC) yield an estimate that 1.9 to 5.1 percent of patients receiving radiation therapy for brain metastases will suffer severe dementia within 5 to 36 months (median, 14 months).[31] Assuming a 10 percent survival at 1 year, the risk of developing radiation-induced dementia would have been 19 percent in the MSKCC experience. Rapid fractionation schemes commonly used for palliation of metastases (i.e., 3 to

6 Gy/fraction) have been implicated because the total doses of 25 to 39 Gy would not otherwise have been expected to cause such serious problems. Cooperative groups in North America (Radiation Therapy Oncology Group, Southwestern Oncology Group) are conducting a prospective study, randomizing patients with resected solitary brain metastases to either immediate cranial irradiation or close observation only. Such a study is needed to determine the efficacy and neurotoxicity of prophylactic irradiation. Controversy also surrounds the projected risk : benefit ratio of prophylactic cranial irradiation for small cell lung cancer following reports of extensive neurological and radiologic deficits in treated patients.[100] Extensive neuropsychological tests have not always been performed, making it difficult to interpret studies that otherwise demonstrate little long-term deficit.[17]

Compared with children receiving PCI for ALL, more severe deficits have been found in children with brain tumors receiving higher doses (40 to 55 Gy). The intensity of other CNS treatment influences the likelihood of a child's developing intellectual deficits. This is most readily apparent in PCI for ALL, where the incidence of intellectual dysfunction ranges from 2 to 10 percent for PCI plus intrathecal methotrexate to upward of 45 percent with PCI, intrathecal methotrexate, and high-dose systemic methotrexate.[77,109]

The correlation between gender and risk of radiation-induced cognitive problems is not known, but there are studies suggesting that females at all ages are at increased risk.[80,104] Other studies have looked for but have not found such a correlation.[175]

Environmental factors clearly play an important role in intellectual development. Whitt and colleagues, using a multivariant analysis to compare children with ALL treated with intrathecal chemotherapy alone or in combination with 24 Gy PCI, demonstrated that the most significant predictor of the cognitive and academic abilities of these children was the education level of their parents.[210] Factors that do not appear to influence intellectual development following cranial irradiation include hydrocephalus[28] and the extent of surgical resection of the tumor.[44]

Necrotizing leukoencephalopathy has been observed primarily in children with ALL treated with concurrent intravenous methotrexate and/or intrathecal methotrexate and cranial irradiation.[172] Symptoms may include developmental regression, dementia, spasticity, ataxia, seizures, hemiplegia, and pseudobulbar paresis, and may progress to obtundation and coma in the latter stages of the syndrome. These symptoms can present at various times after completion of radiotherapy, though most patients have been observed to develop deficits 4 to 12 months after treatment. Pathologically one sees multiple areas of necrotic white matter. The overlying gray matter is preserved. CT scans demonstrate hypodensity of the white matter corresponding to the areas of severe destruction.[169] MRI usually demonstrates a diffuse increase in signal intensity throughout the white matter on T2-weighted images, particularly around the ventricles. Necrotizing leukoencephalopathy may stabilize, but often progresses to coma and death.

Mineralizing microangiopathy is another distinct clinicopathologic syndrome occurring in children with ALL treated with combined methotrexate and cranial irradiation. In contrast to necrotizing leukoencephalopathy, the clinical symptoms are usually mild and transient or temporary in nature. Pathologically, an accumulation of calcium in the walls of vessels has been described. This has been noted in up to 17 percent of autopsy specimens in children with ALL treated as noted above.[166] The lesion typically involves small vessels in the gray matter, particularly the region of the lenticular nucleus, with or without involvement of the cerebral cortex. Radiation increases the risk of leukoencephalopathy and mineralizing microangiopathy if given before or concurrent with methotrexate, by reducing the BBB and allowing increased drug delivery and toxicity.[163,166,168] While mineralizing microangiopathy is most widely described in ALL, similar dystrophic calcifications occur after cranial irradiation for other malignancies.[106]

All children should undergo detailed neuropsychological evaluation before beginning radiation and/or chemotherapy to the brain. Children should be followed closely for signs of decline in school performance, at which time the evaluation should be repeated to identify specific deficits. Advocates of early testing to reveal intellectual deficits believe in the ability of special educational programs to maximize potential.[96,132,146] Although medical treatments such as anticoagulation, steroids, or barbiturates have been proposed to treat or prevent radiation brain necrosis, studies have yet to demonstrate the impact of early medical management on the prevention or reversal of radiation-induced dementia.[38,39,58,157] Ventriculoperitoneal shunting has infrequently been of benefit in patients with radiologic evidence of nonobstructive hydrocephalus.[7,31] Unfortunately, the treatment of radiation-induced cognitive impairment is primarily in the area of prevention (i.e., avoidance, delay, or minimization of radiation).

All adults should receive preradiotherapy neuropsychological evaluation. Special psychological and educational assistance, as well as an early return to work, may be of benefit.[132] Further study is needed regarding the role of neuropsychological support.

Carcinogenesis The development of second malignancies is well documented in irradiated patients who survive their primary tumor. An increased incidence of meningiomas as well as other benign and malignant neoplasms of the head and neck area has been seen in children irradiated for tinea capitis.[144] The dose of radiation delivered to the brain was estimated at 1.4 Gy. An interval of 22 to 45 years between irradiation and the development of meningiomas was noted in these patients. Gliomas, as well as meningiomas, have been reported to develop following higher-dose irradiation of CNS tissue in the treatment of other benign or malignant lesions. These lesions have developed between 3.75 and 25 years from the time of initial irradiation.[23,138] The risk of developing second CNS malignancies and its relationship to dose, age of patient, and other treatment such as chemotherapy is poorly understood and requires further study.

Radiosurgery

Complications Following Radiosurgery

Radiosurgery is the delivery of a large dose of radiation, usually in a single fraction, to a small volume in the brain. While conventional fractionated therapy is usually delivered over many days, with a small dose of radiation given each day, radiosurgery is generally delivered in a single treatment.[200]

In spite of the evidence presented earlier in this chapter suggesting that higher doses per fraction increase the risk of injury to the CNS, it is possible to perform radiosurgery safely because the volume of brain irradiated to a high dose is small. This is achieved by delivering the radiation to the target from multiple directions (Fig. 187-3). When the tumor is irradiated with two opposed beams (e.g., right and left lateral portals), all of the brain in the path of the beams receives a dose very similar to that received by the target. The situation improves markedly when three or four fields are used, as shown. As the number of fields increases further, the shape of the irradiated volume conforms closer to the

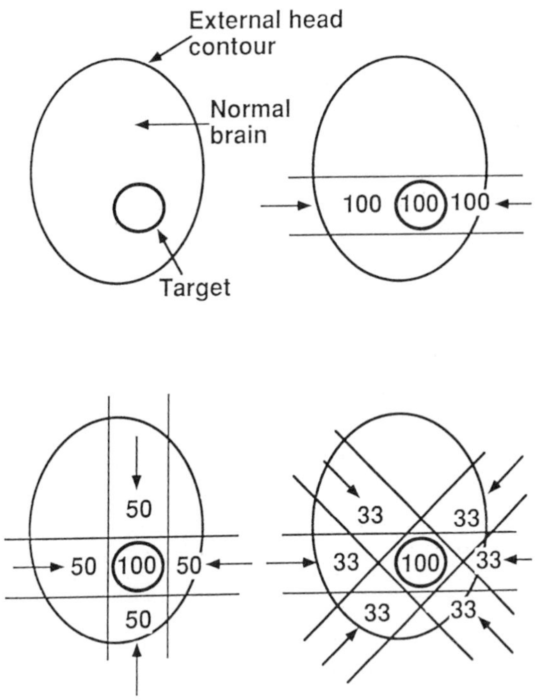

Figure 187-3 Schematic diagram illustrating the dose delivered to the surrounding normal brain when the target lesion is irradiated with different beam arrangements. As the number of beams increases, the volume of normal brain receiving the same dose as the tumor decreases, while the volume of normal brain receiving any dose of radiation increases.

shape of the target, and the volume of normal brain receiving a high dose of radiation is further reduced. However, with each successive increase in the number of fields, the volume of brain receiving *any* dose of radiation increases. The surrounding normal brain generally can tolerate the low doses of radiation that they receive with this technique.

Thus, the physical advantages of radiosurgery, which provides a tight dose distribution around the target, offset the biological disadvantages of not fractionating. Nevertheless, there is growing interest in the use of fractionated radiosurgery (often termed *stereotactic radiation therapy*) to take advantage of both the biological advantages of fractionation and physical advantages of radiosurgery.

Risk Factors for Radiation Injury After Radiosurgery

Several factors play a central role in determining the risk of developing CNS injury from radiosurgery.

Irradiated Volume The risk of brain injury increases with irradiated volume. The data from several series demonstrating this point are summarized in Tables 187-1 to 187-4. No complications have been observed among patients with arteriovenous malformations (AVMs) < 15 mm[51,52] (Table 187-1), primary brain tumors < 20 mm[152] (Table 187-4), or meningiomas < 20 mm[92] (Table 187-4). Most of the reported complications were in patients with larger lesions. Therefore, lesions ≥ 3 to 4 cm are not considered appropriate for radiosurgery. A similar finding has been reported in experimental animals.[9]

TABLE 187-1 Complications Following Radiosurgery for Arteriovenous Malformations

Center	Number of Patients	Months of Follow-Up (Median)	Minimum Dose (Gy)	Lesion Diameter (mm)[a] (Average)	Radiographic Complication Rate (%)*	Clinical Complication Rate (%)*	Months Between Treatment and Complication	Temporary/ Permanent	Mild/ Severe	Reference
Pittsburgh	72	12–35 (23)	15–27	7–30	31[b]	14[b]	5–18 (12 median)	4//5		51, 52
	18	7–19	17.5–25	7–29 (17)		5 (1/18)	4	0//1		4
Pittsburgh[c]	24		16–20	≤15		0				
				>15		36 (4/11)				
Berkeley[d]	24		18–40.5			28 (7/24)	4–28		2//5	137
	86	24–72 (38)	7.9–31	10–50	51 (33/65)	20 (17/86)	3–33 (13 median)	5//15	7//10	191
				≤35		0				47
				>30		50 (10/20)				
Univ. Florida	47	1–27 (13.5)	10–25	10–35 (23)		4 (2/47)	10, 12	0//2	2//0	57
Joint Center	16		15–25			12 (2/16)	6, 7	2//0	2//0	122
Mass. Genl. Hosp.	74	24–192	10–100	7–50		11 (8/74)				89
	636					0.3–0.5			2//0	87, 88
Vicenza[†]	97	1–49 (17)	15–30	4–40		3 (3/97)		1//2	0//3	24, 25
Karolinska	26		50	8, 14		0				194
	20		75–125	8, 14		20 (4/20)				194
	135		30–125	≈20–30		3 (4/135)	3–11	1//3	1//3	192
	300					2 (5/300)		1//4	1//4	193
	247					4 (9/247)				195
McGill	33	1–32 (16)	<25–50	8–25		6 (2/33)	6, 9	1//1	0//2	188
Sheffield	50	>12	25			0				83
	160	>24	25			4 (6/160)	9–17	3//3		198
Buenos Aires	52			<12–60		4 (2/52)	6, 9	2//0	0//0	12
Heidelberg	55	Mean 23	8–28	10–54 (31)		13 (7/55)	6–12	6//1		45

[a]When the lesion volume is known, this is the diameter of a sphere with the equivalent volume. Irradiated volumes are not necessarily spherical
[b]Two year actuarial risks
[c]Data for angiographically occult vascular malformations
[d]Doses are given in helium gray, and therefore the photon equivalent dose is approximately 30% higher. The prescribed doses were given in 1–3 fractions.
*Complication rates are crude unless otherwise noted. The values listed in the table are frequently approximates, as exact data are not always available in the publications.
[†]Doses given in 1–2 sessions

TABLE 187-2 Complications Following Radiosurgery for Acoustic Neuromas

	Pittsburgh[50,113]	Karolinska[76,154]	Vicenza[24]
Patient number	135	110	8
Minimum dose (Gy)	12–20	18–25	18–25
Hearing			
Any hearing loss	65%	72%	
Total hearing loss	29%	20%	
Onset (months)	0–12 (median 6)		
Facial Nerve Function			
Any reduction in function	29% (4 yr actuarial risk)	15%	
Onset (months)	0–16 (median 5)	4–15	
Trigeminal Nerve Function			
Reduction in function	33% (4 yr actuarial risk)	18%	75%
Onset (months)		6–9	6–18
Other Toxicities			
Imbalance	31%		
Worsening vertigo	4%		
Persistent nausea	3%		
Persistent headache	5%		

Radiation Dose The dose of radiation delivered in a single fraction during radiosurgery is an extremely important determinant of the risk of radiation injury. This has been shown in animal and clinical studies (see Tables 187-1 to 187-4). It is often very difficult to separate the effects of dose and volume and, therefore, one needs to consider both of these factors quite carefully.

Location Just as it is possible to surgically resect portions of the brain without causing severe disability, it is possible to irradiate some portions of the brain without causing significant injury. Injury to critical structures such as the brain stem are much more likely to cause clinical symptoms than are injuries to the anterior portions of the frontal or temporal lobes, which are relatively ''silent'' regions. In a series of patients treated at Berkeley for AVMs, complications were more frequent among patients with lesions in the brain stem, thalamus, or basal ganglia.[191] Several of the cranial nerves are very sensitive to large single doses of radiation. In particular, the optic nerves appear to be very sensitive. In a recent report from the University of Pittsburgh and the Joint Center for Radiation Therapy, 3 of 19 patients (16 percent) who received 8 Gy to the optic structures developed permanent visual complications, compared to none of 36 patients who received a lesser dose. Injuries to cranial nerves (CN) III, IV, VI, and VII have been reported, though these nerves do not seem to be as sensitive as the optic nerves.[202] Radiosurgery to a volume including CN VIII is associated with a high rate of hearing dysfunction.[50,154]

Number of Isocenters Nedzi and colleagues,[152] from the Joint Center for Radiation Therapy, reported that complications were more common in patients irradiated with multiple isocenters. It is likely that dose heterogeneity, rather than the fact that multiple isocenters were used, is responsible for this finding. Furthermore, it is possible that patients with larger tumors were treated with multiple isocenters. In contrast, the group at the University of Pittsburgh reached the opposite conclusion. They have noted a lower complication rate among patients treated with multiple isocenters, and have attributed this to the fact that the therapy was more conformal and, therefore, included less normal brain when multiple isocenters were used. This issue requires further study.

Type of Intracranial Lesion Radiosurgery for brain metastases is generally not associated with a high rate of complication. This may be due to the fact that brain metastases displace surrounding normal brain tissue rather than infiltrating it. In the review from the Joint Center for Radiation Therapy, the complication rates among patients with brain metastases was clearly lower than for other intracranial lesions. In contrast to brain metastases, primary gliomas diffusely infiltrate the surrounding brain. Radiosurgery for these lesions has been associated with a higher risk of complication (Table 187-4).

Prescription Isodose Line The prescription isodose line is an indirect indication of the dose heterogeneity within the target volume. If a dose of 20 Gy is delivered to the 50 percent isodose line,

TABLE 187-3 Complications Following Radiosurgery for Pituitary Adenomas

Center	Patient Number	Dose (Gy)	Neural Complications	Hypopituitarism	References
Berkeley	283	30–50*	2/283	33%	110
	83	30–150	3/83		
	183†	180–320	4/183		
Karolinska	35	70–100	0	50%	33
Mass. Genl. Hosp.	571		≈4%	10–15%	85–88

*Dose given in up to four to eight fractions. Doses are in helium Gy and therefore the photon equivalent dose is ≈30% higher.
†Patients had pituitary ablation therapy.

TABLE 187-4 Complications Following Radiosurgery for Metastatic and Primary Brain Tumors

Center	Lesion Type	Patient Number	Minimum Dose (Gy)[a] (Average)	Lesion Diameter (mm)(Avg)[a,b]	Clinical Complication Rate (%)[a]$	Months Between Treatment and Complication (Average)	Prior XRT (%)[a,c]	Prior XRT Dose (Gy) (Avg)[a]	References
Joint Center	Metastasis	65	9–25 (17)	10–37.5	6 (4/65)	7–20	94	30–60 (36)	120, 124
Pittsburgh	Metastasis	24	16–20	≤30	0		96	30–42.5	21, 22
Heidelberg	Metastasis	37	10–40		14 (5/37)	0–6	24	50	45
McGill	Metastasis	9	20	10–30	0		88	18–50 (30)	16
Joint Center	Primary CNS tumor	30		13–44 (26)	47 (14/30)	0–7 (3)	58	35–60	3
				≤20	0 (0/5)				152
				≥20	65 (13/20)				
	Primary CNS tumor	22	10–25	20–37	14 (3/22)		91		125
	Glioma	17	10–20	20–40	35 (6/17)	2–7		54–72 (59)	2
	Glioma	37	10–20 (12)	10–50	46[d]	1–14 (5)		59	121
Pittsburgh	Meningioma	65			7@2 yr[e]	3.5–12			92
			15–20	≤20	0 (0/14)				
			15–20	>20	23 (3/13)				
Heidelberg	Meningioma	17		18–52 (40)	35 (6/17)	5–18			46

[a]The numbers listed are approximates, as the exact data are not always supplied.
[b]The lesion diameter is not always given. If the volume was stated, the diameter of the sphere with an equivalent volume is shown.
[c]Percent of patients that received prior external beam radiotherapy.
[d]46% of the patients evaluable at 1 year required continued steroids (14/30). Nearly all patients required steroids at some time; seven (19%) required reoperation.
[e]2 year actuarial rate.
$Complication rates are crude rates, unless otherwise noted.
XRT, external beam radiotherapy; CNS, central nervous system.

then the volume of brain included within the 100 percent isodose line receives 40 Gy. For a solid metastatic lesion, this higher dose within the tumor may not be relevant; however, for an infiltrating glioma, this high dose region may include normal brain. On the other hand, if the same 20 Gy is delivered to the 80 percent line, then the maximum dose (at the 100 percent line) within the tumor will be 25 Gy. The prescription isodose line also determines what dose is delivered to regions of the brain away from the lesion but included in the lower isodose lines. The prescription isodose line used depends on the size, shape, and orientation of the radiation beams.

Prior Radiation Therapy Many patients who are treated with radiosurgery have received prior fractionated external-beam radiation therapy. The data suggest that patients who have received such prior therapy are at an increased risk of developing complications following radiosurgery.[110] Among patients previously irradiated for gliomas, up to 20 to 50 percent require steroids and/or reoperation following subsequent radiosurgery (Table 187-4). This is not as frequent a problem in patients with brain metastasis. First, the dose of external-beam radiation previously received for metastases is usually lower than for gliomas (30 Gy versus 60 Gy). Second, less normal brain is usually included in radiosurgery for metastases because metastatic lesions tend to displace surrounding brain while gliomas usually infiltrate normal structures.

Treatment Era and Duration of Follow-Up Some of the early studies from pioneering institutions reported fairly high complication rates. A 20 percent, 28 percent, and 11 percent complication rate was reported following radiosurgery for AVMs at the Karolinska Institute, in Berkeley, and at the Massachusetts General Hospital, respectively.[89,111,112,137,194] Three institutions have since reported far lower complication rates, resulting from improved techniques, reduced doses, and better patient selection.

As shown in the tables, complications may become clinically apparent months to years after radiosurgery. Therefore, reports that include patients with very short follow-up likely underestimate the risks. Actuarial calculations are usually not done. A good example of this potential problem is shown in the Pittsburgh data for AVMs. A report from 1989 noted a 5 percent crude complication rate. A later report, with additional follow-up, noted a 14 percent 2-year actuarial complication rate. Similarly, an early report from Sheffield noted no complications among 50 patients. A later report, with additional follow-up, noted a 4 percent complication rate.

Treatment Equipment There are no convincing data to suggest that the use of the Gamma Knife, modified linear accelerator, or charged particles is more or less likely to cause complications[156] (Tables 187-1 to 187-4). This is not surprising, as the radiation dose distribution provided by each technique is very similar.[165] This is especially true for "spherical" lesions. For larger lesions with more complex geometries, a more uniform dose distribution may be achievable with charged particles.

Predicting the Risk of CNS Injury from Radiosurgery

When planning radiosurgery, it would be helpful if we were able to predict the risk of injury based on the dose, volume, and location of the therapy. Pioneering work in this area was performed by Kjellberg. Based on clinical and laboratory data, he generated the lines that are reproduced in Fig. 187-4. The 1 percent line was meant to denote the dose that could be delivered to a particular volume of normal brain and produce a 1 percent risk of brain necrosis. Even in his very early work, he noted that structures such as the optic nerves were more sensitive than the remainder of the brain. A review of clinical data performed by Marks and Spencer[136] suggests that this 1 percent necrosis line initially proposed by Kjellberg underestimates the clinically observed risk of brain injury. Based on their calculations, they estimate that this 1 percent necrosis corresponds to a 3 to 8 percent risk of

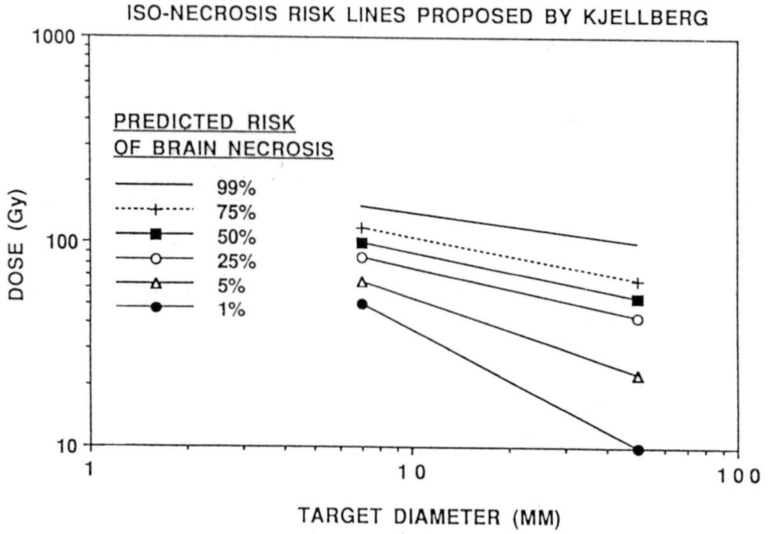

Figure 187-4 These idealized lines were proposed by Kjellberg and were meant to predict the risk of necrosis based on the dose and volume irradiated. The 1 percent risk line has been used to select radiation doses during radiosurgery (see text). (Modified from Kjellberg and Abe.[88])

developing any clinically significant radiation reaction.[135,136] It is important to recognize that not all toxicities are necessarily due to necrosis, and that not all instances of necrosis necessarily result in clinical symptoms. Flickinger et al. have performed theoretical calculations using the integrated logistic model, and suggest that Kjellberg's proposed 1 percent line corresponds to the 3 percent risk line.[54]

Regardless of the mathematical model, it is clear that the risk of complication increases with both dose and volume. Therefore, extreme care should be taken to minimize the volume of normal brain irradiated during radiosurgery. This requires close cooperation among the radiologists, neurosurgeons, and radiation oncologists so that the target volume can be appropriately delineated. Furthermore, the physicists and physicians must work closely together to develop radiation treatment plans that minimize unnecessary irradiation of neighboring brain. To this end, techniques of optimization of radiation treatment beams are being developed.[127]

Clinical Aspects

Acute Syndromes

While radiosurgery appears to be useful in the treatment of many intracranial lesions, the complication rates that are accepted for radiosurgery are higher than those reported for conventional fractionated radiotherapy (Tables 187-1 to 187-4). Similar to conventional fractionated radiotherapy, radiation injury after stereotactic radiosurgery can be divided into acute and late syndromes.

Immediately following radiosurgery, patients may develop transient headache.[47,128] Acute nausea and vomiting occur in approximately 10 to 20 percent of patients and generally last less than 1 day. Premedication with steroids may reduce this risk.[2,3,113,128] The risk of developing nausea appears to be related to incidental irradiation of the area postrema in the brain stem.[125] Patients with a pre-existing seizure disorder may experience increased seizure activity. Pre- and postirradiation treatment with anticonvulsants and steroids seems to reduce this risk.[89,128,129]

Late Syndromes

Significant radiation injury to the brain usually becomes apparent months to years following radiosurgery. The reported late complication rates following radiosurgery for various intracranial lesions are shown in Tables 187-1 to 187-4. In general, the rates shown are those of clinically significant reactions that may be transient or permanent. These reactions may be due to necrosis, vascular insufficiency, or severe edema.[118] The doses of radiation used in recent years are lower than those used in the past. In general, this has resulted in a reduction of the complication rates, especially when care is taken to minimize the volume of normal brain treated.

Complication Rates for Specific Disease Entities

Arteriovenous Malformations

The reported incidences of complications following radiosurgery for AVMs are shown in Table 187-1. As for other intracranial lesions, there is a distinct difference between the incidence of finding radiological evidence of radiation injury and clinical complication rates. In the study from the University of Pittsburgh,[52] the 2-year actuarial risk of developing radiological or clinical abnormalities consistent with radiation injury was 31 percent and 14 percent respectively. Radiological abnormalities present in the deep structures (midbrain and brain stem) were almost always associated with symptoms. Serial scans revealed that the vast majority of radiological abnormalities resolved spontaneously, and the projected actuarial rate of resolution of these imaging changes was 88 percent.[52] The median time of onset of the radiological abnormalities was 12 months (range, 5 to 18 months). The risk of developing a radiological abnormality was higher in the patients irradiated to larger volumes. Following radiosurgery for AVMs, toxicity referable to cerebrovascular insufficiency has been reported. This may be secondary to the obliteration of blood vessels supplying normal portions of the brain and may occur in approximately 1 to 3 percent of patients.[47,87,88,191,195,196] The limited data from Pittsburgh suggest that complications are more common following radiosurgery for angiographically occult vascular malformations than for AVMs.[93]

Acoustic Neuromas

Radiosurgery for acoustic neuromas is associated with a fairly high risk of cranial nerve dysfunction (Table 187-2). Complete preservation of hearing at pretreatment levels was achieved in approximately one-third patients treated at the University of Pittsburgh.[53] Similarly, at the Karolinska Institute, only one-quarter of patients had preservation of hearing. A slight decrease in hearing was observed in approximately one-half of patients, and severe hearing loss in the remaining one-quarter. In addition to CN VIII injury, injury to CNs V and VII is frequently seen following radiosurgery for acoustic neuromas. In the series from Pittsburgh, the actuarial incidence of facial and trigeminal neuropathy was approximately 29 and 33 percent at 4 years, respectively. While only 10 to 20 percent of these neuropathies totally resolve, > 50 percent of patients have some degree of improvement. Delayed transient trigeminal and facial nerve dysfunction was reported in 18 and 15 percent of patients, respectively, in the Karolinska series.

Injury to CNs V and VII occur more commonly in patients with larger tumors. This is a recurring theme, as patients with larger tumors are generally treated to larger volumes, with a corresponding increase in the volume of normal tissue irradiated. Lesions were generally < 30 mm in diameter in all three of the series listed. Interestingly, in the Pittsburgh series, the risk of cranial nerve injury was less in patients who were treated with a larger number of isocenters. They attribute this to the fact that, in general, the use of multiple isocenters allows them to better conform the irradiated volume to the target. This finding is different from that reported from the Joint Center for Radiation Therapy, where a higher rate of complications was seen with multiple-isocenter treatments.[152] Cranial nerve injury is also dose related, as no patient receiving a maximum dose < 27 Gy developed a facial nerve injury in the Karolinska experience.

Patients can also develop problems with balance, nausea, headache, and dizziness.[113,154] This may be due to peritumoral edema or impairment of circulation to the posterior fossa.[113,154] Communicating hydrocephalus, thought to be due to protein release from the tumor, can occur months to years following radiation.[113,154]

Pituitary Tumors

The data from several series in which radiosurgery was used to treat pituitary adenomas are summarized in Table 187-3. Hypopituitarism occurs in 10 to 50 percent of patients. Neuronal complications, including visual, oculomotor, and temporal lobe injury, occur in approximately 0 to 4 percent of patients. These cranial nerve injuries can occur years after irradiation and may be transient.[110] The risks are highest in patients who have been previously irradiated with conventional external-beam radiotherapy.[110,197]

Primary and Metastatic Brain Tumors

The reported complication rates following radiosurgery for various malignant brain lesions are shown in Table 187-4. The complication rates are generally higher than what is seen in patients with AVMs. In general, many of the patients with malignant tumors have received prior radiotherapy and/or chemotherapy. These lesions also may be larger than the AVMs. Both of these factors probably contribute to the relatively high complication rate. Complications are less common in patients with metastatic lesions compared to primary lesions.

Interstitial Brachytherapy

Focal radionecrosis of brain tissue in the high-dose region of a stereotactic brain implant is a common result of interstitial brachytherapy (the implantation of radioactive sources directly into the brain) as it is currently employed in the management of primary or recurrent CNS malignancies.[1,10,11,48,49,65–70,123,180,213] The extent of radionecrosis is linked to the isotope used,[63,84,160,199] the volume implanted, and the total dose delivered,[106,108,109,133,134,159,160,179,213] as well as to the dose rate at which it is delivered.[106] The symptomatology associated with the insult is dependent on the volume of injured tissue, the anatomic location, the extent of surrounding edema with associated mass effect, and the underlying defect due to the original tumor. As greater experience has been gained with the procedure, more information regarding the relative contribution of these factors has been accumulated.

Animal Studies

Temporary Implants with Iodine 125

Fike et al. temporarily implanted 35-mCi ^{125}I sources in the white matter of canine brains to deliver doses ranging from 10 to 100 Gy at a dose rate of 30 to 40 cGy/h to a reference point 10 mm from the source.[48,49] Serial CT scans were obtained in the weeks to months after explantation to compare the changes on CT scan with the various dose regions of each implant. Three regions of interest were identified on CT scan. First, a central region of hypodensity occurred in the high-dose region and gradually increased in volume over time. This area of hypodensity on CT was found, on histologic examination, to be a region of coagulative necrosis. The minimum dose necessary to produce necrosis averaged 180 to 200 Gy. A second region of contrast enhancement surrounded the low-density center and corresponded to the region that received 60 to 190 Gy. Contrast enhancement gradually disappeared by 6 months after the delivery of reference doses of 10 Gy. Pathologically, this region was found to contain lipid-laden macrophages, gliosis, and diffuse vascular changes, including endothelial cell proliferation, fibrinoid necrosis, perivascular cuffing with lymphocytes, and minute hemorrhages. A third region, characterized histologically by axonal swelling, partial demyelination, and edema, surrounded the contrast-enhancing region. On CT, generalized low-density changes were noted in the remaining implanted hemisphere, most notably in the white matter. After 4 weeks, the hypodense lesion began to decrease in size, with increasing contrast enhancement seen in the low-density region.[205]

Interstitial irradiation was also found to alter regional cerebral blood flow (CBF) and vascular volume. Gobbel and colleagues implanted single ^{125}I sources temporarily in the frontal white matter of beagles.[60] These sources delivered 20 Gy at 45 cGy/h to a reference point 0.75 cm from each source. Drops in regional CBF and vascular volume were recorded in the immediate 3 weeks after explantation. From 3 to 6 weeks regional CBF markedly increased although transit time remained depressed, suggesting a strong neovascular response in the necrotic region. Simultaneously, CT scans revealed increasing contrast enhancement within the central low-density region. Reduction in CBF was also consistently found in regions outside the necrotic mass associated with cerebral edema.

Permanent Implants with Iodine 125 and Iridium 192

Ostertag and colleagues investigated the serial effects of low-dose-rate ^{125}I seeds permanently implanted in canine brains.[160] They delivered doses ranging from 79 Gy in 24 days to 320 Gy in 368 days to reference volumes 5 mm from the source. A zone of central calcified necrosis was found immediately surrounding the implanted seeds as early as 25 days after implant. This zone reached its maximum size by day 70. An astrocytic reaction was confined to a narrow region surrounding the necrotic zone. In gray matter, morphologic changes were confined to a very narrow margin (<0.2 mm) surrounding the central necrosis, whereas changes in white matter were more extensive and consisted of marked gliosis. Breakdown of the BBB was consistently present in a narrow zone within millimeters of the central necrotic region.[63] This developed as early as 7 days postimplantation[63] and remained relatively constant for the first year, then gradually returned toward normal by 2 years after explantation. Necrosis appeared to correspond to regions that received ≥ 270 Gy via low-dose-rate permanent implant. The BBB was relatively unimpaired at calculated doses ≤ 135 Gy.

Permanently implanted ^{192}Ir seeds produced a different pattern of histologic change from that seen with ^{125}I.[160] Following permanent ^{192}Ir implants, calcified necrosis changed to liquefactive necrosis after 70 days. The zone of transition from necrosis to normal brain tissue was more poorly demarcated because of the greater depth of penetration of the higher-energy gamma radiation of ^{192}Ir (300 to 610 keV versus 35 keV for ^{125}I). Vasogenic edema in the white matter was more extensive than that seen with ^{125}I.

Clinical Studies

Autopsy Series

Autopsy studies of patient treated with permanent or temporary ^{125}I implantation for CNS malignancies have revealed three zones of damage.[30,84] Central coagulative necrosis was constant in regions that received doses ≥ 200 Gy, but has been seen to extend into zones of lower doses, even as low as 20 Gy.[30,84] A second zone, which received 40 to 150 Gy, was characterized by significant demyelination with a variable inflammatory and vascular response. Vasculature was preserved in this region but was markedly altered, corresponding to the contrast-enhanced regions noted on the CT scan. A third zone of cerebral edema and gliosis was present after 20 to 40 Gy. There was significant variability in the extent of these changes, owing to the presence or absence of residual tumor and preimplant therapy (i.e., prior radiation or chemotherapy).

Temporary Iodine 125 Implants: Acute Complications

Early complications following temporary interstitial implantation of ^{125}I have been reported to occur in up to 23 percent of patients. Most of these early side effects are correctable. Many of them do not involve injury to the brain, but are a result of the operative procedure. Several series have recently been published that report early complication rates after brachytherapy. From 1979 through June 1990, 392 patients underwent high-activity ^{125}I implantation at UCSF. Of these, 307 were adults being treated for primary or recurrent intracerebral gliomas. Implants were part of the initial therapy in 174, whereas 133 received implants at the time of recurrence. Forty-two additional patients received hyperthermia in conjunction with their implants, of whom 26 were children and 17 were patients treated for metastases. Acute complications were relatively uncommon. Of the 307 patients reported by Scharfen and colleagues,[180] 6 percent (19 patients) developed grade 3 complications, defined as severe but non-life-threatening, including four seizures, four cases of infection, three hemorrhages, one non-life-threatening pulmonary embolus, and seven cases in which nontransient neurological deterioration occurred. There were three (10 percent) separate life-threatening complications: one case of temporary brain stem dysfunction, one case of sepsis, and one severe pulmonary embolus. Only two deaths were attributable to the implant: one fatal pulmonary embolus and one fatal episode of sepsis.

In 35 patients with glioblastoma multiforme (GBM) treated from 1987 to 1990 at the Joint Center for Radiation Therapy with external-beam radiation therapy (59.40 Gy) followed by ^{125}I implantation for an additional 48 to 54 Gy, only six acute complications were reported: four scalp infections, one brain abscess, and one hemorrhage.[123] Twenty-three patients underwent implantation with ^{125}I at Toronto for newly diagnosed malignant astrocytomas.[1] The acute complication rate was 21.7 percent. Other smaller studies show acute complication rates ranging from 14 to 23 percent.[1,20,123,126,211]

In an earlier report on 95 UCSF patients treated for recurrent gliomas,[107] all patients had unifocal disease measuring ≤ 6 cm in maximum dimension, not crossing the mid-line or involving the corpus callosum. These patients had all previously been treated with a median dose of 60 Gy (66 patients had received whole-brain irradiation, while 29 had received partial-brain irradiation). Minimum tumor dose from the brachytherapy was a mean of 74.44 Gy, with a range of 52.70 to 150 Gy. A mild increase in cerebral edema was commonly seen immediately after implantation. Complications included one major increase in cerebral edema, one abscess in the tumor bed, one case of bacterial meningitis (these last two prior to the institution of routine intraoperative antibiotics), two wound dehiscences requiring graft placement, one intracranial hemorrhage, and two mild increases in hemiparesis.

Delayed Effects

Late complications after brachytherapy are a result of necrosis and edema producing neurological deterioration. Reoperation is frequently necessary for those patients who develop worsening neurological symptoms in conjunction with CT evidence of an enlarging mass effect due to necrosis, tumor regrowth, or both. Of 307 patients implanted at UCSF, 40 percent of patients required reoperation for relief of symptoms at a median of 33 weeks after implantation.[180] The avascular central necrotic zone was easily distinguished from surrounding viable brain tissue.[106] Of the reoperated patients, 95 percent had residual evidence of tumor, 5 percent had necrosis only, 29 percent had tumor only with no evidence of necrosis, and 66 percent had a combination of tumor and necrosis. The presence of tumor cells in the necrotic region is probably of little significance, as cells in the high-dose necrotic region have little or no clonogenicity.[29,119] Viable tumor cells in the periphery of the necrotic zone, however, correlate more closely with tumor recurrence.[29,106,119]

The addition of adjuvant therapies, such as radiosensitizers or chemotherapy, does not seem to increase the need for subsequent reoperation. In NCOG 6G-82-2, patients with anaplastic glioma or GBM received concomitant external-beam radiation therapy (60 Gy) and hydroxyurea, followed by 50 to 60 Gy by ^{125}I implant.[70] Patients then received 1 year of chemotherapy with procarbazine, lomustine, and vincristine. A total of 107 patients were entered into this trial from 1982 to 1990, of whom 66 successfully underwent implantation. Forty-four percent of the GBM cases required reoperation, as did 52 percent of the non-GBM cases.

Reoperation rates are similar for patients implanted at the time of recurrence and for those who receive an implant as part of their initial therapy. Among patients with recurrent glioma treated with implants at UCSF, 56 percent of those with anaplastic astrocytoma and 42 percent of those with GBM underwent reoperation at a median time of 29 weeks.[70] In a separate series of 18 patients who received implants at the time of recurrence of malignant astrocytoma, using a dose of 70 Gy, 28 percent required reoperation, with 11 of 12 having mixed necrosis and tumor, and 1 of 12 having pure necrosis only.[10] Reoperation rates of 25 to 47 percent have been reported in other series.[1,20,67,106,211]

As a result of the high reoperation rate after brachytherapy, the issue of quality of life following this procedure has been raised. Liebel and colleagues have attempted to address this issue in a series of 98 patients with recurrent gliomas who underwent implantation.[107] Median survival was inversely related to total dose delivered: 95 weeks for those who received $\leq$ 70 Gy, 79 weeks for 71 to 100 Gy, and 69 weeks for $>$ 100 Gy. The mean pretreatment KPS for these patients was 90. After implantation the mean KPS declined slightly over 6 months to 80, and remained stable at 79 by 18 months. Patients who survived to 36 months had a mean KPS of 76. Steroid dependence was also analyzed as an assessment of quality of life. Of 33 patients who survived 18 months or longer, all but one of whom were steroid-dependent prior to implantation, 67 percent remained steroid-dependent at 18 months. Similarly, of those patients alive at 36 months after implantation, 53 percent remained steroid dependent.

Temporary Iridium 192 Implants

It is difficult to compare complication rates in patients treated with ^{192}Ir versus those treated with ^{125}I because fewer patients have been implanted with ^{192}Ir sources. Twenty-nine patients underwent ^{192}Ir implantation at Tufts University after 6000 cGy external-beam radiation therapy to boost malignant astrocytomas to a total dose of 12,000 to 16,000 cGy. A complication rate of 23 percent was seen, including two cases of meningitis in those patients treated before the routine use of intraoperative antibiotics. Twenty-five percent of patients required reoperation.

Willis and colleagues reported a group of 39 patients with primary or recurrent malignant gliomas or metastatic disease implanted with ^{192}Ir and receiving doses ranging from 27 to 62 Gy (mean, 48 Gy) after external-beam doses of 29 to 94 Gy (mean total dose of 101 Gy).[211] An acute complication rate of 12 percent was reported, and only 9 percent of patients required reoperation because of the development of a mass effect.

Temporary ^{192}Ir implants were given either as the sole treatment (50 Gy over 4 to 7 days for lesions $<$ 3 cm in size) or in conjunction with 25 Gy external-beam radiation (35 Gy for larger lesions) in 61 patients.[106,199] Acute complication and reoperation rates were not discussed. After an initial period of improvement in neurological symptoms, ''late brain swelling'' was noted at 6 to 16 months, often requiring steroid intervention. This late effect was associated with an enlarging area of contrast enhancement on CT scan corresponding to the high-dose region of the implant. Deterioration proceeded over 3 months, followed by spontaneous stabilization of clinical symptoms and improvement of CT findings.

Permanent Implantation with Iodine 125 or Iridium 192

Permanent implantation of low- and high-grade astrocytomas that were unresectable because of location in the diencephalon, pineal gland, pituitary gland, or brain stem has been accomplished in over 1200 cases using ^{192}Ir (1965 to 1979) and ^{125}I (1979 to the present) in Freiburg, Germany.[148,151] Only survival information has been reported, with no details of complication rates.

Radiographic Evaluation of Postimplant Changes

As is the case following external-beam irradiation, the characteristic CT findings of a central low-density region surrounded by a limited region of contrast enhancement with more extensive low-density changes beyond the ring of enhancement cannot distinguish between tumor regrowth and radionecrosis.[106] The finding of new areas of contrast enhancement beyond the implanted tissue, on the other hand, is strongly suggestive of new tumor. Stereotaxic biopsy data reveal that the central zone invariably shows radionecrosis, commonly intermingled with tumor cells of questionable clonogenicity.[106] Tumor cells are frequently found in the ring-enhancing region and beyond in regions appearing normal on CT. Similarly, MRI scans are also poor differentiators of radiation injury and progressive disease in the high-dose region of implants.[11,32,36,59,158,206] Autopsy review after MRI scans reveals that MRI significantly underestimates the extent of radiation injury after interstitial brachytherapy.[158]

PET with ^{82}Rb to demonstrate breakdown in the BBB and with [^{18}F]FDG to illustrate the glucose metabolic state has had greater success than MRI or CT in differentiating between necrosis and persistent tumor.[206] An increase or equivalent amount of [^{18}F]FDG uptake in the region of interest compared to surrounding normal tissue is interpreted as evidence of recurrent disease. Lesser uptake in the area of concern, however, provides little helpful information. Valk and colleagues retrospectively studied 34 patients with malignant gliomas who had interstitial implants as part of their therapy and underwent PET scanning prior to clinical (16 of 34) or surgical (18 of 34) assessment of tumor status.[206] The overall accuracy of PET for differentiating between radionecrosis and tumor regrowth was 84 percent. A sensitivity of 88 percent for regrowth and a specificity of 81 percent was reported.

Thermoradiotherapy

Hyperthermia has been investigated as a modality to improve the chance of local tumor control in patients with malignant gliomas undergoing interstitial brachytherapy.[64,90,91,131,173,174,185,187,190] One goal of this approach would be to allow for the reduction in radiation dose required with a subsequent reduction in the risk and extent of radiation necrosis.[185] Heat-induced damage to normal tissue is dependent on the maximum tissue temperature achieved and the duration that the temperature is maintained.[185,187] In the ideal, hyperthermia techniques produce therapeutic temperatures (42.5 to 45°C) in tumor tissue while maintaining normal tissues at temperatures below 42.5°C.[185] Technical difficulties combined with physiologic conditions make it impossible to attain uniform desired temperatures throughout the entire tumor without exceeding tolerance levels of surrounding and intermingled normal tissue. Conversely, maintaining all normal tissues at acceptable level results in a portion of the tumor being heated to subtherapeutic temperatures.

Sneed and colleagues, using interstitially implanted microwave antennae operating at frequencies of 915 and 2450 MHz in a canine brain, maintained a temperature of 43 to 44°C at a reference point 0.5 cm from the microwave antennal junction for 30 min in five animals.[186] All dogs developed some degree of hemiparesis immediately after treatment, but it promptly resolved in four of five dogs within 24 h. The fifth dog had persistent mild stable hemiparesis. Minor tissue damage was noted in the overlying scalp muscle due to overheating in one dog. Thermal lesions were characterized by CT scanning and pathologic examination; a region of focal low density developed by the first week in the tissue treated to ≥ 44°C for 30 min, corresponding pathologically to an area of coagulative necrosis. This region was surrounded by a ring of contrast enhancement in the area heated to 43 to 44°C for 30 min, which demonstrated damaged but viable tissue with intense neovascular proliferation on microscopic examination. Beyond this region of vascular change, CT revealed diffuse edema that histopathologically consisted of variable degrees of vacuolization, demyelination, and edema. By 4 weeks the contrast enhancement had resolved, and by 16 weeks the previously hypodense necrotic region had consolidated to a hyperdense compact stable lesion consisting of fibrosis and neovascular proliferation. Other experimental animal studies have indicated a range of normal brain tolerance ranging from 42 to 42.5°C for 50 to 70 min or 42.7 to 43°C for 30 min.[14,79,84]

A microwave system was used to deliver heat in conjunction with interstitial brachytherapy in 48 patients with recurrent malignant gliomas or solitary brain metastases at UCSF from 1987 to 1990.[185] Three to eleven catheters were implanted for use with microwave antennae, fiberoptic thermometry probes, and ^{125}I seeds. Eighty-nine treatments were delivered, with a treatment goal of attaining a temperature of 42.5°C throughout as much of the tumor as possible for 30 min. Normal tissue temperatures were held at or below 42.5°C. Maximum tumor temperatures were maintained below 50°C. Complications included 13 patients with quickly reversible neurological changes, 8 cases of transient seizures, 1 prolonged focal seizure, 3 minor infections of a bone flap or wound, 1 case of meningitis, 1 pulmonary embolus, and 1 scalp burn. The requirement for reoperation was 47 percent, similar to that seen for patients treated with interstitial brachytherapy without hyperthermia. Similarly, mean KPS gradually decreased from 82 (preimplant) to 79 at 12 months.

Stea and colleagues at the University of Arizona used ferromagnetic seeds to deliver hyperthermia in conjunction with ^{192}Ir brachytherapy to treat 14 patients with primary or recurrent malignant gliomas.[190] Intratumoral target temperatures of 42.5 to 45°C were maintained for 60 min. Two patients did not complete the heat session because of temporary seizures without prolonged sequelae. In 19 attempted heating sessions, four minor (three seizures, one transient increase in brain edema) and two major complications occurred. The first major complication seen was the development of hydrocephalus immediately after implantation of the catheters before heating could be started. The second major complication was irreversible brain edema and coma in a patient whose tumor volume was in excess of 100 cc. All minor complications resolved within 24 h with no prolonged sequelae.

One unique study used scanned focused ultrasound to deliver hyperthermia to involved brain after removal of a bone flap in 15 patients who were being treated with external-beam radiation but no brachytherapy.[64] The heat treatments were scheduled on a weekly basis during external-beam therapy, and required placement of catheters stereotactically within the tumor for use with thermometry probes. Nine of the 15 underwent four treatments each; the remainder had fewer than four treatments for a variety of reasons. Four patients developed intracranial hemorrhages at the time of catheter insertion during 41 total treatments. Acute complications included two thermal scalp blisters and two temporary CSF leaks, in addition to the hemorrhages noted above. The five patients who went on to autopsy were all found to have hyperthermia-induced necrosis in conjunction with persistent disease.

Several other smaller studies have been reported using various technologies to deliver brain hyperthermia and interstitial brachytherapy for malignant gliomas.[64,90,91,173,174,185,187,190] Patients generally tolerated hyperthermia well, and morbidity was only marginally increased over that seen with interstitial brachytherapy alone.

References

1. Agbi CB, Bernstein M, Laperriere N, et al. Patterns of recurrence of malignant astrocytoma following stereotactic interstitial brachytherapy with iodine-125 implants. *Int J Radiat Oncol Biol Phys* 1992; 23:321–326.
2. Alexander E III, Kooy HM, Nedzi L, Loeffler JS. Linear accelerator radiosurgery for metastatic tumors. Presented at *Radiosurgery Update,* Boston, 1990, pp 1–4.
3. Alexander E III, Loeffler JS. Radiosurgery using a modified linear accelerator. *Neurosurg Clin North Am* 1992; 3:167–190.
4. Altschuler EM, Lunsford LD, Coffey RJ, et al. Gamma knife radiosurgery for intracranial arteriovenous malformations in childhood and adolescence. *Pediatr Neurosci* 1989; 15:53–61.
5. Ang KK, van der Kogel AJ, van der Schueren E. Lack of evidence for increased tolerance of rat spinal cord with decreasing fraction doses below 2 Gy. *Int J Radiat Oncol Biol Phys* 1985; 11:105–110.
6. Archibald YM, Lunn D, MacDonald DR, et al. Cognitive functioning in treated long-term survivors with high grade primary brain tumors—a prospective study. Presented at the 20th Annual Meeting of the International Neuropsychological Society, San Diego, February, 1992.
7. Asai A, Matsutani M, Kohno T, et al. Subacute brain atrophy after radiation therapy for malignant brain tumor. *Cancer* 1989; 63:1962–1974.
8. Atkins HL, Tretter P. Time-dose considerations in radiation myelopathy. *Acta Radiol (Ther)* 1966; 5:79–94.
9. Berg NO, Lindgren M. Relation between field size and tolerance of rabbit's brain to roentgen irradiation (200 kV) via a slit-shaped field. *Acta Radiol Ther Phys Biol* 1963; 1:147–168.
10. Bernstein M, Laperriere N, Leung P, McKenzie S. Interstitial brachytherapy for malignant brain tumors: preliminary results. *Neurosurgery* 1990; 26:371–379.
11. Bernstein M, Marotta T, Stewart P, et al. Brain damage from I-125 brachytherapy evaluated by MR imaging, a blood brain-barrier tracer, and light and electron microscopy in a rat model. *J Neurosurg* 1990; 73:585–593.
12. Betti OO, Munari C, Rosler R. Stereotactic radiosurgery with linear accelerator: treatment of arteriovenous malformations. *Neurosurgery* 1989; 24:311–321.
13. Boldrey E, Sheline G. Delayed transitory clinical manifestations after radiation treatment of intracranial tumors. *Acta Radiol (Ther)* 1966; 5:5–10.
14. Britt RH, Pounds DW, Lyons BE. Feasibility of treating malignant brain tumors with focussed ultrasound. *Prog Exp Tumor Res* 1984; 28:232–245.
15. Burger PC, Mahaley MS Jr, Dudka L, et al. The morphologic effects of radiation administered therapeutically for intracranial gliomas: a postmortem study of 25 cases. *Cancer* 1979; 44:1256–1272.
16. Caron J-L, Souhami L, Podgorsak EB. Dynamic stereotactic radiosurgery in the palliative treatment of cerebral metastatic tumors. *J Neurooncol* 1992; 12:173–179.
17. Catane R, Schwade JG, Yarr I, et al. Follow-up neurological evalua

tion in patients with small cell lung carcinoma treated with prophylactic cranial irradiation and chemotherapy. *Int J Radiat Oncol Biol Phys* 1981; 7:105–109.
18. Ch'ien L, Mauer A, Simone J. Comparison of neurospychologic functioning and clinical indicators of neurotoxicity in long-term survivors of childhood leukemia given cranial radiation or parenteral methotrexate: a prospective study. *J Clin Oncol* 1991; 9:145–151.
19. Ch'ien LT, Aur RJ, Stagner S, et al. Long-term neurological implications of somnolence syndrome in children with acute lymphoblastic leukemia. *Ann Neurol* 1980: 8:273–277.
20. Chun M, McKeough P, Wu A, et al. Interstitial iridium-192 implantation for malignant brain tumours: Part II. Clinical experience. *Br J Radiol* 1989; 62:158–162.
21. Coffey RJ, Flickinger JC, Bissonette DJ, Lunsford LD. Radiosurgery for solitary brain metastases using the cobalt-60 gamma unit: methods and results in 24 patients. *Int J Radiat Oncol Biol Phys* 1991; 20:1287–1295.
22. Coffey RJ, Flickinger JL, Lunsford LD. Boost radiosurgery for solitary brain metastases: results in 23 consecutive patients. *Int J Radiat Oncol Biol Phys* 1990; 19(Suppl 1): 148(abstr).
23. Cohen ME, Duffner PK. *Brain Tumors in Children: Principles of Diagnosis and Treatment*. New York: Raven Press, 1984, pp 308–327.
24. Colombo F. Linear accelerator radiosurgery: a clinical experience. *J Neurosurg Sci* 1989; 33:123–125.
25. Colombo F, Benedetti A, Pozza F, et al. Linear accelerator radiosurgery of cerebral arteriovenous malformations. *Neurosurgery* 1989; 24:833–840.
26. Constine LS, Rubin P, Woolf PD, et al. Hyperprolactinemia and hypothyroidism following cytotoxic therapy for central nervous system malignancies. *J Clin Oncol* 1987; 5:1841–1851.
27. Crompton MR, Layton DD. Delayed radionecrosis of the brain following therapeutic x-radiation of the pituitary. *Brain* 1961; 84:85–101.
28. Danoff BF, Cowchock FS, Marquette C, et al. Assessment of the long-term effects of primary radiation therapy for brain tumors in children. *Cancer* 1982; 49:1580–1586.
29. Daumas-Duport C, Blond S, Vedrenne C, Szikla G. Radiolesion versus recurrence: bioptic data in 39 gliomas after interstitial, or combined interstitial and external radiation treatment. *Acta Neurochir [Suppl] (Wien)* 1984; 33:291–299.
30. Davis RL, Barger GR, Gutin PH, Phillips TL. Response of human malignant gliomas and CNS tissue to I-125 brachytherapy: a study of seven autopsy cases. *Acta Neurochir Suppl (Wien)* 1984; 33:301–305.
31. DeAngelis LM, Delattre JY, Posner JB. Radiation-induced dementia in patients cured of brain metastases. *Neurology* 1989; 39:789–796.
32. Deck MDF. Imaging techniques in the diagnosis of radiation damage to the central nervous system. In Gilbert HA, Kagan AR (eds): *Radiation Damage to the Central Nervous System: A Delayed Therapeutic Hazard*. New York: Raven Press, 1980, pp 107–127.
33. Degerblad M, Rahn T, Bergstrand G, Thoren M. Long-term results of stereotactic radiosurgery to the pituitary gland in Cushing's disease. *Acta Endocrinol (Copenh)* 1986; 112:310–314.
34. Di Chiro G, DeLa Paz RL, Brooks RA, et al. Glucose utilization of cerebral gliomas measured by [^{18}F] fluorodeoxyglucose and positron emission tomography. *Neurology* 1982; 32:1323–1329.
35. Di Chiro G, Oldfield E, Wright DC, et al. Cerebral necrosis after radiotherapy and/or intraarterial chemotherapy for brain tumors: PET and neuropathologic studies. *Am J Roentgenol* 1988; 150:189–197.
36. Dooms GC, Hecht S, Brant-Zawadzki M, et al. Brain radiation lesions: MR imaging. *Radiology* 1986; 158:149–155.
37. Doyle WK, Budinger TF, Valk RE, et al. Differentiation of cerebral radiation necrosis from tumor recurrence by [^{18}F]FDG and ^{82}Rb positron emission tomography. *J Comput Assist Tomogr* 1987; 11:563–570.
38. Druckmann A. Schlafsucht als Folge der Röntgenbestrahlung: Beitrag zur Strahlenempfindlichkeit des Gehirns. *Strahlenther Onkol* 1929; 33:382–384.
39. Duffner PK, Cohen ME, Parker MS. Prospective intellectual testing in children with brain tumors. *Ann Neurol* 1988; 23:575–579.
40. Duffner PK, Cohen ME, Thomas PR, et al. The long-term effects of cranial irradiation on the central nervous system. *Cancer* 1985; 56:1841–1846.
41. Duffner PK, Cohen ME, Voorhees ML, et al. Long-term effects of cranial irradiation on endocrine function in children with brain tumors: a prospective study. *Cancer* 1985; 56:2189–2193.
42. Edwards MS, Wilson CB. Treatment of radiation necrosis. In Gilbert HA, Kagan AR (eds): *Radiation Damage to the Nervous System. A Delayed Therapeutic Hazard*. New York: Raven Press, 1980, pp 129–143.
43. Eiser C. Intellectual abilities among survivors of childhood leukaemia as a function of CNS irradiation. *Arch Dis Child* 1978; 53:391–395.
44. Ellenberg L, McComb JG, Siegel SE, Stowe S. Factors affecting intellectual outcome in pediatric brain tumor patients. *Neurosurgery* 1987; 21:638–644.
45. Engenhart R, Kimmig B, Sturm V. Stereotactically guided convergent beam irradiation of solitary brain metastases and cerebral arteriovenous malformations. In Dyck P, Bouzaglou A (eds): *Neurosurgery: State of the Art Reviews*, vol 4. Philadelphia: Hanley & Belfus, 1989, pp 119–132.
46. Engenhart R, Kimmig BN, Hover K-H, et al. Stereotactic single high dose radiation therapy of benign intracranial meningiomas. *Int J Radiat Oncol Biol Phys* 1990; 19:1021–1026.
47. Fabrikant JI, Levy RP, Steinberg GK, et al. Charged-particle radiosurgery for intracranial vascular malformations. *Neurosurg Clin North Am* 1992; 3:99–139.
48. Fike JR, Cann CE, Gutin PH, et al. Radiation damage to normal canine brain induced by radiation from interstitially-implanted I-125 sources. *Acta Neurochir [Suppl] (Wien)* 1984; 33:307–309.
49. Fike JR, Cann CE, Phillips TL, et al. Radiation brain damage induced by interstitial I-125 sources: a canine model evaluated by quantitative computed tomography. *Neurosurgery* 1985; 16:530–537.
50. Flickinger JC, Lunsford LD, Coffey RJ, et al. Radiosurgery of acoustic neurinomas. *Cancer* 1991; 67:345–353.
51. Flickinger JC, Lunsford LD, Kondziolka D. Dose prescription and dose-volume effects in radiosurgery. *Neurosurg Clin North Am* 1992; 3:51–59.
52. Flickinger JC, Lunsford LD, Kondziolka D, et al. Radiosurgery and brain tolerance: an analysis of neurodiagnostic imaging changes after gamma knife radiosurgery for arteriovenous malformations. *Int J Radiat Oncol Biol Phys* 1992; 23:19–26.
53. Flickinger JC, Lunsford LD, Linskey ME, et al. Gamma knife radiosurgery for acoustic tumors: four year results and multivariate analysis of treatment technique. *Int J Radiat Oncol Biol Phys* 1992; 24(Suppl 1): 128 (abstr).
54. Flickinger JC, Schell MC, Larson DA. Estimation of complications for linear accelerator radiosurgery with the integrated logistic formula. *Int J Radiat Oncol Biol Phys* 1990; 19:143–148.
55. Freeman CR, Krisher J, Sanford RA, et al. Hyperfractionated radiotherapy in brain stem tumors: results of a Pediatric Oncology Group study. *Int J Radiat Oncol Biol Phys* 1988; 15:311–318.
56. Freeman CR, Krisher JP, Sanford RA, et al. Hyperfractionated radiation therapy in brain stem tumors. Results of treatment at the 7020 cGy dose level of Pediatric Oncology Group Study #8495. *Cancer* 1991; 68:474–481.
57. Friedman WA, Bova FJ, Spiegelmann R. Linear accelerator radiosurgery at the University of Florida. *Neurosurg Clin North Am* 1992; 3:141–166.
58. Glantz MJ. Treatment of cerebral radiation necrosis (CRN) and radiation plexopathy (RP) with anticoagulation (AC). *Neurology* 1990; 40(Suppl 1): 398 (abstr).
59. Glantz MJ, Hoffman JM, Coleman RE, et al. Identification of early recurrence of primary central nervous system tumors by

[18F]fluorodeoxyglucose positron emission tomography. *Ann Neurol* 1991; 29:347–355 (see comments).
60. Gobbel GT, Seilhan TM, Fike JR. Cerebrovascular response after interstitial irradiation. *Radiat Res* 1992; 130:236–240.
61. Goldwein JW. Radiation myelopathy: a review. *Med Pediatr Oncol* 1987; 15:89–95.
62. Greenfield MM, Stark FM. Post-irradiation neuropathy. *Am J Roentgenol* 1948; 60:617–622.
63. Groothuis DR, Wright DC, Ostertag CB. The effect of I-125 interstitial radiotherapy on blood-brain barrier function in normal canine brain. *J Neurosurg* 1987; 67:895–902.
64. Guthkelch AN, Carter LP, Cassady JR, et al. Treatment of malignant brain tumors with focused ultrasound hyperthermia and radiation: results of a phase I trial. *J Neurooncol* 1991; 10:271–284.
65. Gutin PH, Bernstein M. Stereotactic interstitial brachytherapy for malignant brain tumors. *Prog Exp Tumor Res* 1984; 28:166–182.
66. Gutin PH, Leibel SA. Stereotaxic interstitial irradiation of malignant brain tumors. *Neurol Clin* 1985; 3:883–893.
67. Gutin PH, Leibel SA, Wara WM, et al. Recurrent malignant gliomas: survival following interstitial brachytherapy with high-activity iodine-125 sources. *J Neurosurg* 1987; 67:864–873.
68. Gutin PH, Phillips TL, Hosobuchi Y, et al. Permanent and removable implants for the brachytherapy of brain tumors. *Int J Radiat Oncol Biol Phys* 1981; 7:1371–1381.
69. Gutin PH, Phillips TL, Wara WM, et al. Brachytherapy of recurrent malignant brain tumors with removable high-activity iodine-125 sources. *J Neurosurg* 1984; 60:61–68.
70. Gutin PH, Prados MD, Phillips TL, et al. External irradiation followed by an interstitial high-activity iodine-125 implant "boost" in the initial treatment of malignant gliomas: NCOG study 6G-82-2. *Int J Radiat Oncol Biol Phys* 1991; 21:601–606.
71. Halberg FE, Kramer JH, Moore IM, et al. Prophylactic cranial irradiation dose effects on late cognitive function in children treated for acute lymphoblastic leukemia. *Int J Radiat Oncol Biol Phys* 1991; 22:13–16.
72. Hall E. *Radiobiology for the Radiologist,* 3d ed. Philadelphia: Lippincott, 1988, pp 367–368.
73. Halperin EC, Burger PC. Conventional external beam radiotherapy for central nervous system malignancies. *Neurol Clin* 1985; 3:867–882.
74. Hart GB, Mainous EG. The treatment of radiation necrosis with hyperbaric oxygen (OHP). *Cancer* 1976; 37:2580–2585.
75. Herskovic AM, Orton CG. Elective brain irradiation for small cell anaplastic lung cancer. *Int J Radiat Oncol Biol Phys* 1986; 12:427–429.
76. Hirsch A, Norén G. Audiological findings after stereotactic radiosurgery in acoustic neurinomas. *Acta Otolaryngol (Stockh)* 1988; 106:244–251.
77. Hirsch JF, Renier D, Czernichow P, et al. Medulloblastoma in childhood: survival and functional results. *Acta Neurochir (Wien)* 1979; 48:1–15.
78. Hoffman WF, Levin VA, Wilson CB. Evaluation of malignant glioma patients during the postirradiation period. *J Neurosurg* 1979; 50:624–628.
79. Hoopes PJ, Roberts DW, Ryan TP, et al. Assessment of interstitial microwave hyperthermia in dog brain: a time-temperature study. Unpublished manuscript.
80. Jannoun L. Are cognitive and educational development affected by age at which prophylactic therapy is given in acute lymphoblastic leukaemia? *Arch Dis Child* 1983; 58:953–958.
81. Jones A. Transient radiation myelopathy: with reference to Lhermitte's sign of electrical paresthesia. *Br J Radiol* 1964; 37:727–744.
82. Kanev PM, Lefebvre JF, Mauseth RS, Berger MS. Growth hormone deficiency following radiation therapy of primary brain tumors in children. *J Neurosurg* 1991; 74:743–748.
83. Kemeny AA, Dias PS, Forster DM. Results of stereotactic radiosurgery of arteriovenous malformations: an analysis of 52 cases. *J Neurol Neurosurg Psychiatry* 1989; 52:554–558.
84. Kiessling M, Kleihues P, Gessaga E, et al. Morphology of intracranial tumours and adjacent brain structures following interstitial iodine-125 radiotherapy. *Acta Neurochir [Suppl] (Wien)* 1984; 33:281–289.
85. Kjellberg RN. Isoeffective dose parameters for brain necrosis in relation to proton radiosurgical dosimetry. In Szikla G (ed): *Stereotactic Cerebral Irradiation: INSERM Symposium No. 12.* Amsterdam: Elsevier, 1979, pp 157–166.
86. Kjellberg RN. Stereotactic Bragg peak proton radiosurgery results. In Szikla G (ed): *Stereotactic Cerebral Irradiation: INSERM Symposium No. 12.* Amsterdam: Elsevier, 1979, pp 233–240.
87. Kjellberg RN. Proton beam therapy for arteriovenous malformations of the brain. In Schmidek HH, Sweek WH (eds): *Operative Neurosurgical Techniques.* New York: Grune & Stratton, 1988, pp 911–915.
88. Kjellberg RN, Abe M. Stereotactic Bragg peak proton beam therapy. In Lunsford LD (ed): *Modern Stereotactic Neurosurgery.* Boston: Martinus Nijhoff, 1988, pp 463–470.
89. Kjellberg RN, Hanamura T, Davis KR, et al. Bragg-peak proton-beam therapy for arteriovenous malformations of the brain. *N Engl J Med* 1983; 309:269–274.
90. Kobayashi T, Kida Y. Interstitial hyperthermia of brain tumors by stereotactically implanted heating system. *Stereotact Funct Neurosurg* 1990; 54-55:514–518.
91. Kobayashi T, Kida Y, Tanaka T, et al. Interstitial hyperthermia of malignant brain tumors by implant heating system: clinical experience. *J Neurooncol* 1991; 10:153–163.
92. Kondziolka D, Lunsford LD. Radiosurgery of meningiomas. *Neurosurg Clin North Am* 1992; 3:219–230.
93. Kondziolka D, Lunsford LD, Coffey RJ, et al. Stereotactic radiosurgery of angiographically occult vascular malformations: indications and preliminary experience. *Neurosurgery* 1990; 27:892–900.
94. Kramer S, Lee KF. Complications of radiation therapy: the central nervous system. *Semin Roentgenol* 1974; 9:75–83.
95. Kramer S, Southard ME, Mansfield CM. Radiation effect and tolerance of the central nervous system. *Front Radiat Ther Oncol* 1972; 6:332–334.
96. Kun LE, Mulhern RK Jr. Neuropsychologic function in children with brain tumors: II. Serial studies of intellect and time after treatment. *Am J Clin Oncol* 1983; 6:651–656.
97. Lam KSL, Tse VKC, Wang C, et al. Effects of cranial irradiation on hypothalamic-pituitary function—a 5-year longitudinal study in patients with nasopharyngeal carcinoma. *Q J Med* 1991; 78:165–176.
98. Lambert PM. Radiation myelopathy of the thoracic spinal cord in long term survivors treated with radical radiotherapy using conventional fractionation. *Cancer* 1978; 41:1751–1760.
99. Lampert PW, Davis RL. Delayed effects of radiation on the human central nervous system. *Neurology* 1964; 14:912–917.
100. Laukkanen E, Klonoff H, Allan B, et al. The role of prophylactic brain irradiation in limited stage small cell lung cancer: clinical neuropsychologic, and CT sequelae. *Int J Radiat Oncol Biol Phys* 1988; 14:1109–1117.
101. Lavey RS, Johnstone AK, Taylor JMG, McBride WH. The effect of hyperfractionation on spinal cord response to radiation. *Int J Radiat Oncol Biol Phys* 1992; 24:681–686.
102. Lee AW, Ng SH, Ho JHC, et al. Clinical diagnosis of late temporal lobe necrosis following radiation therapy for nasopharyngeal carcinoma. *Cancer* 1988; 61:1535–1542.
103. Lee AWM, Cheng LOC, Ng SH, et al. Magnetic resonance imaging in the clinical diagnosis of late temporal lobe necrosis following radiotherapy for nasopharyngeal carcinoma. *Clin Radiol* 1990; 42:24–31.
104. Lee PWH, Hung BKM, Woo EKW, et al. Effects of radiation therapy on neuropsychological functioning in patients with nasopharyngeal carcinoma. *J Neurol Neurosurg Psychiatry* 1989; 52:488–492.
105. Lee YY, Glass JP, Van Eys J, Wallace S. Medulloblastoma in infants and children: computed tomographic follow-up after treatment. *Radiology* 1985; 154:677–682.
106. Liebel SA, Gutin PH, Davis RL. Factors affecting radiation injury after interstitial brachytherapy for brain tumors. In Gutin PH, Leibel

SA, Sheline GE (eds): *Radiation Injury to the Nervous System*. New York: Raven Press, 1991, pp 257–270.

107. Leibel SA, Gutin PH, Wara WM, et al. Survival and quality of life after interstitial implantation of removable high-activity iodine-125 sources for the treatment of patients with recurrent malignant gliomas. *Int J Radiat Oncol Biol Phys* 1989; 17:1129–1139.
108. Leibel SA, Sheline GE. Radiation therapy for neoplasmas of the brain. *J Neurosurg* 1987; 66:1–22.
109. Leibel SA, Sheline GE. Tolerance of the central and peripheral nervous system to therapeutic irradiation. In Lett JT, Altman KI (eds): *Advances in Radiation Biology:* Vol 12. *Relative Radiation Sensitivities of Human Organ Systems*. Orlando: Academic 1987, pp 257–288.
110. Levy RP, Fabrikant JI, Frankel KA, et al. Heavy-charged-particle radiosurgery of the pituitary gland: clinical results of 840 patients. In Marin P, Mandrillon P (eds): *European Particle Accelerator Conference,* Nice, France, June 1990. Gif-sur-yvette, France: Editions Frontihres.
111. Lindquist C, Steiner L. Stereotactic radiosurgical treatment of arteriovenous malformations. In Lunsford LD (ed): *Modern Stereotactic Neurosurgery*. Boston: Martinus Nijhoff, 1988, pp 491–505.
112. Lindqvist M, Steiner L, Blomgren H, et al. Stereotactic radiation therapy of intracranial arteriovenous malformations. *Acta Radiol [Suppl]* 1986; 369:610–613.
113. Linskey ME, Lunsford LD, Flickinger JC, et al. Stereotactic radiosurgery for acoustic tumors. *Neurosurg Clin North Am* 1992; 3:191–205.
114. Linstadt DE, Edwards MSB, Prados M, et al. Hyperfractionated irradiation for adults with brainstem gliomas. *Int J Radiat Oncol Biol Phys* 1991; 20:757–760.
115. Littley MD, Shalet SM, Beardwell CG, et al. Hypopituitarism following external radiotherapy for pituitary tumours in adults. *Q J Med* 1989; 70:145–160.
116. Littley MD, Shalet SM, Morgenstern GR, Deakin DP. Endocrine and reproductive dysfunction following fractionated total body irradiation in adults. *Q J Med* 1991; 78:265–274.
117. Littman P, Rosenstock J, Gale G, et al. The somnolence syndrome in leukemic children following reduced daily dose fractions of cranial radiation. *Int J Radiat Oncol Biol Phys* 1984; 10:1851–1853.
118. Lo EH, Frankel KA, Steinberg GK, et al. High-dose single-fraction brain irradiation: MRI, cerebral blood flow, electrophysiological, and histological studies. *Int J Radiat Oncol Biol Phys* 1992; 22:47–55.
119. Loeffler JS, Alexander E III, Hochberg FH, et al. Clinical patterns of failure following stereotactic interstitial irradiation for malignant gliomas. *Int J Radiat Oncol Biol Phys* 1990; 19:1455–1462.
120. Loeffler JS, Alexander E III, Kooy HM, et al. Radiosurgery for brain metastases. In DeVita VT, Hellman S, Rosenberg SA (eds): *Cancer: Principles & Practice of Oncology, PPO Updates,* vol 5. Philadelphia: Lippincott, 1991, pp 1–12.
121. Loeffler JS, Alexander E III, Shea WM, et al. Radiosurgery as part of the initial management of patients with malignant gliomas. *J Clin Oncol* 1992; 10:1379–1385.
122. Loeffler JS, Alexander E III, Siddon RL, et al. Stereotactic radiosurgery for intracranial arteriovenous malformations using a standard linear accelerator. *Int J Radiat Oncol Biol Phys* 1989; 17:673–677.
123. Loeffler JS, Alexander E III, Wen PY, et al. Results of stereotactic brachytherapy used in the initial management of patients with glioblastoma. *J Natl Cancer Inst* 1990; 82:1918–1921.
124. Loeffler JS, Kooy HM, Wen PY, et al. The treatment of recurrent brain metastases with stereotactic radiosurgery. *J Clin Oncol* 1990; 8:576–582.
125. Loeffler JS, Siddon RL, Wen PY, Alexander E III. Stereotactic radiosurgery of the brain using a standard linear accelerator. A study of early and late effects. *Radiother Oncol* 1990; 17:311–321.
126. Lucas GL, Luxton G, Cohen D, et al. Treatment results of stereotactic interstitial brachytherapy for primary and metastatic brain tumors. *Int J Radiat Oncol Biol Phys* 1991; 21:715–721.
127. Lulu BA. Stereotaxic radiosurgery optimal dose normalization and isocenter separation for multi-isocenter treatments: a dose-volume histogram approach. *Int J Radiat Oncol Biol Phys* 1992; 24(Suppl 1): 232–233 (abstr).
128. Lunsford LD, Kondziolka D, Bissonette DJ, et al. Stereotactic radiosurgery of brain vascular malformations. *Neurosurg Clin North Am* 1992; 3:79–98.
129. Lunsford LD, Kondziolka D, Flickinger JC, et al. Stereotactic radiosurgery for ateriovenous malformations of the brain. *J Neurosurg* 1991; 75:512–524.
130. Lyman RS, Kupalov PS, Scholz W. Effect of roentgen rays on the central nervous system: results of large doses on the brains of adult dogs. *Arch Neurol Psychiatry* 1933; 29:56–87.
131. Lyons BE, Britt RH, Strohbehn JW. Localized hyperthermia in the treatment of malignant brain tumors using an interstitial microwave array. *IEEE Trans Biomed Eng* 1984; 31:53–62.
132. Maire JP, Coudin B, Guérin J, Caudry M. Neuropsychologic impairment in adults with brain tumors. *Am J Clin Oncol* 1987; 10:156–162.
133. Marks JE, Baglan RJ, Prassad SC, Blank WF. Cerebral radionecrosis: incidence and risk in relation to dose, time, fractionation and volume. *Int J Radiat Oncol Biol Phys* 1981; 7:243–252.
134. Marks JE, Wong J. The risk of cerebral radionecrosis in relation to dose, time and fractionation. A follow-up study. *Prog Exp Tumor Res* 1985; 29:210–218.
135. Marks LB. Conventional fractionated radiation therapy vs. radiosurgery for arteriovenous malformations (AVMs) and other intracranial lesions. In Lunsford LD (ed): *Stereotactic Radiosurgery Update*. Amsterdam: Elsevier, 1992, pp 307–310.
136. Marks LB, Spencer DP. The influence of volume on the tolerance of the brain to radiosurgery. *J Neurosurg* 1991; 75:177–180.
137. Marks MP, Delapaz RL, Fabrikant JI, et al. Intracranial vascular malformations: imaging of charged-particle radiosurgery. Part II. Complications. *Radiology* 1988; 168:457–462.
138. Marus G, Levin V, Rutherfoord GS. Malignant glioma following radiotherapy for unrelated primary tumors. *Cancer* 1986; 58:886–894.
139. McCollough WM, Marcus RB Jr, Rhoton Jr., AL, et al. Long-term follow-up of radiotherapy for pituitary adenoma: the absence of late recurrence after $\geq$ 4500 cGy. *Int J Radiat Oncol Biol Phys* 1991; 21:607–614.
140. Meadows AT, Gordon J, Massari DJ, et al. Declines in IQ scores and cognitive dysfunctions in children with acute lymphocytic leukemia treated with cranial irradiation. *Lancet* 1981; 2:1015–1018.
141. Mechanick JI, Hochberg FH, LaRocque A. Hypothalamic dysfunction following whole brain irradiation. *J Neurosurg* 1986; 65:490–494.
142. Mikhael MA. Radiation necrosis of the brain: correlation between computed tomography, pathology, and dose distribution. *J Comput Assist Tomogr* 1978; 2:71–80.
143. Mikhael MA. Radiation necrosis of the brain: correlation between patterns on computed tomography and dose of radiation. *J Comput Assist Tomogr* 1979; 3:241–249.
144. Modan B, Baidatz D, Mart H, et al. Radiation-induced head and neck tumours. *Lancet* 1974; 1:277–279.
145. Moore BD III, Ater J, Copeland DR. Improved neuropsychological outcome in children with brain tumors diagnosed during infancy and treated without cranial irradiation. *J Child Neurol* 1992; 7:281–290.
146. Mulhern RK, Kun LE. Neuropsychologic function in children with brain tumors: III. Interval changes in the six months following treatment. *Med Pediatr Oncol* 1985; 13:318–324.
147. Mulhern RK, Wasserman AL Fairclough D, et al. Memory function in disease-free survivors of childhood acute lymphocytic leukemia given CNS prophylaxis with or without 1,800 cGy cranial irradiation. *J Clin Oncol* 1988; 6:315–320.
148. Mundinger F. CT-guided stereotactic biopsy and interstitial curietherapy with Ir-192 and I-125 of non-resectable midline and brain stem gliomas. In Samii M (ed): *Surgery in and around the Brainstem and the Third Ventricle*. New York: Springer-Verlag, 1986, pp 509–517.
149. Mundinger F. Stereotactic biopsy and technique of implantation

(instillation) of radionuclids. In Jellinger K (ed): *Therapy of Malignant Brain Tumors*. New York: Springer-Verlag, 1987, pp 134–194.
150. Mundinger F, Braus DF, Krauss JK, Birg W. Long-term outcome of 89 low-grade brain-stem gliomas after interstitial radiation therapy. *J Neurosurg* 1991; 75:740–746.
151. Mundinger F, Weigel K. Long-term results of stereotactic interstitial curietherapy. *Acta Neurochirur [Suppl] (Wien)* 1984; 33:367–371.
152. Nedzi LA, Kooy H, Alexander E III, et ai. Variables associated with the development of complications from radiosurgery of intracranial tumors. *Int J Radiat Oncol Biol Phys* 1991; 21:591–599.
153. Nesbit ME Jr, Sather HN, Robinson LL, et al. Presymptomatic central nervous system therapy in previous untreated childhood acute lymphoblastic leukaemia: comparison of 1800 rad and 2400 rad: a report for children's cancer study group. *Lancet* 1981; 1:461–466.
154. Noren G, Arndt J, Hindmarsh T, Hirsch A. Stereotactic radiosurgical treatment of acoustic neurinomas. In Lunsford LD (ed): *Modern Stereotactic Neurosurgery*. Boston: Martinus Nijhoff, 1988, pp 481–489.
155. Ogawa T, Kanno I, Shishido F, et al. Clinical value of PET with ^{18}F-fluorodeoxyglucose and L-methyl-^{11}C-methionine for diagnosis of recurrent brain tumor and radiation injury. *Acta Radiol* 1991; 32:197–202.
156. Ogilvy CS. Radiation therapy for arterial venous malformations: a review. *Neurosurgery* 1990; 6:725–735.
157. Oldfield EH, Friedman R, Kinsella T, et al. Reduction in radiation-induced brain injury by use of pentobarbital or lidocaine protection. *J Neurosurg* 1990; 72:737–744.
158. Oppenheimer JH, Levy ML, Sinha U, et al. Radionecrosis secondary to interstitial brachytherapy: correlation of magnetic resonance imaging and histopathology. *Neurosurgery* 1992; 31:336–343.
159. Ostertag CB. Stereotactic interstitial radiotherapy for brain tumors. *J Neurosurg Sci* 1989; 33:83–89.
160. Ostertag CB, Groothuis D, Kleihues P. Experimental data on early and late morphologic effects of permanently implanted gamma and beta sources (Iridium-192, Iodine-125 and Yttrium-90) in the brain. *Acta Neurochir [Suppl] (Wien)* 1984; 33:271–280.
161. Packer RJ, Sutton LN, Atkins TE, et al. A prospective study of cognitive function in children receiving whole-brain radiotherapy and chemotherapy: 2-year results. *J Neurosurg* 1989; 70:707–713.
162. Parsons JT, Fitzgerald CR, Hood CI, et al. The effects of irradiation on the eye and optic nerve. *Int J Radiat Oncol Biol Phys* 1983; 9:609–622.
163. Phillips PC. Methotrexate neurotoxicity. In Rottenberg DA (ed): *Neurological Complications of Cancer Treatment*. Boston: Butterworth-Hienemann, 1991, pp 115–130.
164. Phillips TL, Buschke F. Radiation tolerance of the thoracic spinal cord. *Am J Roentgenol* 1969; 105:659–664.
165. Podgorsak EB, Pike GB, Olivier A, et al. Radiosurgery with high energy photon beams: a comparison among techniques. *Int J Radiat Oncol Biol Phys* 1989; 16:857–865.
166. Price RA, Birdwell DA. The central nervous system in childhood leukemia. III. Mineralizing microangiopathy and dystrophic calcification. *Cancer* 1978; 42:717–728.
167. Reagan TJ, Thomas JE, Colby MY Jr. Chronic progressive radiation myelopathy: its clinical aspects and differential diagnosis. *JAMA* 1968; 203:128–132.
168. Reinhold HS, Calvo W, Hopewell JW, Van Den Berg AP. Development of blood vessel-related radiation damage in the fimbria of the central nervous system. *Int J Radiat Oncol Biol Phys* 1990; 18:37–42.
169. Riccardi R, Brouwers P, Di Chiro G, Poplack DG. Abnormal computed tomography brain scans in children with acute lymphoblastic leukemia: serial long-term follow-up. *J Clin Oncol* 1985; 3:12–18.
170. Rider WD. Radiation damage to the brain: a new syndrome. *J Can Assoc Radiol* 1963; 14:67–69.
171. Rizzoli HV, Pagnanelli DM. Treatment of delayed radiation necrosis of the brain: a clinical observation. *J Neurosurg* 1984: 60:589–594.
172. Robain O, Dulac O, Dommergues JP, et al. Necrotising leukoencephalopathy complicating treatment of childhood leukaemia. *J Neurol Neurosurg Psychiatry* 1984; 47:65–72.
173. Roberts DW, Coughlin CT, Wong TZ, et al. Interstitial hyperthermia and iridium brachytherapy in treatment of malignant glioma. A phase I clinical trial. *J Neurosurg* 1986; 64:581–587.
174. Roberts DW, Strohbehn JW, Coughlin CT, et al. Iridium-192 brachytherapy in combination with interstitial microwave-induced hyperthermia for malignant glioma. *Appl Neurophysiol* 1987; 50:287–291.
175. Rowland JH, Glidewell OJ, Sibley RF, et al. Effects of different forms of central nervous system prophylaxis on neuropsychologic function in childhood leukemia. *J Clin Oncol* 1984; 2:1327–1335.
176. Rubenstein CL, Varni JW, Katz ER. Cognitive functioning in long-term survivors of childhood leukemia: a prospective analysis. *J Dev Behav Pediatr* 1990; 11:301–305.
177. Rubin P, Casarett G. A direction for clinical radiation pathology: the tolerance dose. *Front Radiat Ther Oncol* 1972; 6:1–15.
178. Rubin P, Cooper RA Jr, Phillips TL. The dose limiting organs in radiation oncology. In Cooper RA Jr, Phillips TL (eds): *Radiation Biology and Radiation Pathology Syllabus*. Chicago: American College of Radiology, 1975.
179. Safdari H, Fuentes JM, Dubois JB, et al. Radiation necrosis of the brain: time of onset and incidence: related to total dose and fractionation of radiation. *Neuroroadiology* 1985; 27:44–47.
180. Scharfen CO, Sneed PK, Wara WM, et al. High activity Iodine-125 interstitial implant for gliomas. *Int J Radiat Oncol Biol Phys,* 1992; 24:583–591.
181. Schwartz RB, Carvalho PA, Alexander E III, et al. Radiation necrosis versus high grade recurrent glioma: differentiation by using dual-isotope SPECT with ^{201}Tl in ^{99m}Tc-HMPAO. *Am J Neuroradiol* 1991; 12:1187–1192.
182. Shalet SM. Growth and hormonal status of children treated for brain tumors. *Childs Brain* 1982; 9:284–293.
183. Shalet SM, Beardwell CG, Pearson D, Morris Jones PH. The effect of varying doses of cerebral irradiation on growth hormone production in childhood. *Clin Endocrinol (Oxf)* 1976; 5:287–290.
184. Sheline GE, Wara WM, Smith V. Therapeutic irradiation and brain injury. *Int J Radiat Oncol Biol Phys* 1980; 6:1215–1228.
185. Sneed PK, Gutin PH, Stauffer PR, et al. Thermoradiotherapy of recurrent malignant brain tumors. *Int J Radiat Oncol Biol Phys* 1992; 23:853–861.
186. Sneed PK, Matsumoto K, Stauffer PR, et al. Interstitial microwave hyperthermia in a canine brain model. *Int J Radiat Oncol Biol Phys* 1986; 12:1887–1897.
187. Sneed PK, Stauffer PR, Gutin PH, et al. Interstitial irradiation and hyperthermia for the treatment of recurrent malignant brain tumors. *Neurosurgery* 1991; 28:206–215.
188. Souhami L, Olivier A, Podgorsak EB, et al. Radiosurgery of cerebral arteriovenous malformations with the dynamic stereotactic irradiation. *Int J Radiat Oncol Biol Phys* 1990; 19:775–782.
189. Spunberg JJ, Chang CH, Goldman M, et al. Quality of long-term survival following irradiation for intracranial tumors in children under the age of two. *Int J Radiat Oncol Biol Phys* 1981; 7:727–736.
190. Stea B, Cetas TC, Cassady JR, et al. Interstitial thermoradiotherapy of brain tumors: preliminary results of a phase I clinical trial. *Int J Radiat Oncol Biol Phys* 1990; 19:1463–1471.
191. Steinberg GK, Fabrikant JI, Marks MP, et al. Stereotactic heavy-charged-particle Bragg-peak radiation for intracranial arteriovenous malformations. *N Engl J Med* 1990; 323:96–101.
192. Steiner L. Treatment of arteriovenous malformations by radiosurgery. In Wilson CB, Stein BM (eds): *Intracranial Arteriovenous Malformations*. Baltimore: Williams & Wilkins, 1984, pp 295–313.
193. Steiner L. Radiosurgery in cerebral arteriovenous malformations. In Fein JM, Flamm ES (eds): *Cerebrovascular Surgery,* vol 4. New York: Springer-Verlag, 1985, pp 1161–1215.
194. Steiner L, Grietz T, Backlund E-O, et al. Radiosurgery in arteriovenous malformations of the brain. Undue effects. In Szikla G (ed): *Stereotactic Cerebral Irradiation. INSERM Symposium No. 12*. Amsterdam: Elsevier, 1979, pp 257–269.

195. Steiner L, Lindquist C, Adler JR, et al. Clinical outcome of radiosurgery for cerebral arteriovenous malformations. *J Neurosurg* 1992; 77:1–8.
196. Stelzer K, Griffin B, Eskridge J, et al. Results of neutron radiosurgery for inoperable arteriovenous malformations of the brain. *Med Dosim* 1991; 16:137–141.
197. Stephanian E, Lunsford LD, Coffey RJ, et al. Gamma knife surgery for sellar and suprasellar tumors. *Neurosurg Clin North Am* 1992; 3:207–218.
198. Sutcliffe JC, Forster DMC, Walton L, et al. Untoward clinical effects after stereotactic radiosurgery for intracranial arteriovenous malformations. *Br J Neurosurg* 1992; 6:177–185.
199. Szikla G, Schlienger M, Blond S, et al. Interstitial and combined interstitial and external irradiation of supratentorial gliomas. Results of 61 cases treated 1973–1981. *Acta Neurochir [Suppl] (Wien)* 1984; 33:355–362.
200. Thames HD, Hendry JH. *Fractionation in Radiotherapy*. London: Taylor & Francis, 1987.
201. Thoren M, Rahn T, Guo WY, Werner S. Stereotactic radiosurgery with the cobalt-60 gamma unit in the treatment of growth hormone-producing pituitary tumors. *Neurosurgery* 1991; 29:663–668.
202. Tishler RB, Duma C, Loeffler JS, et al. Cranial neuropathies following radiosurgery for cavernous sinus lesions: Joint Center for Radiation Therapy and University of Pittsburgh experience. *Int J Radiat Oncol Biol Phys* 1992; 24(Suppl 1): 128–129 (abstr).
203. Trampe EA, Lundell G, Lax I, Werner S. External irradiation of growth hormone producing pituitary adenomas: prolactin as a marker of hypothalamic and pituitary effects. *Int J Radiat Oncol Biol Phys* 1991; 20:655–660.
204. Tugendhaft P, Baleriaux D, Gerard JM, et al. Sequential CT scanning in radiation myelopathy. *J Neurooncol* 1984; 2:249–252.
205. Turowski K, Fike JR, Cann CE, et al. Normal brain iodine-125 radiation damage: effect of dose and irradiated volume in a canine model. *Radiology* 1986; 158:833–838.
206. Valk PE, Budinger TF, Levin VA, et al. PET of malignant cerebral tumors after interstitial brachytherapy. Demonstration of metabolic activity and correlation with clinical outcome. *J Neurosurg* 1988; 69:830–838.
207. Van der Schueren E, Landuyt W, Ang KK, Van der Kogel AJ. From 2 Gy to 1 Gy per fraction: sparing effect in rat spinal cord? *Int J Radiat Oncol Biol Phys* 1988; 14:297–300.
208. Wara WM, Richards GE, Grumbach MM, et al. Hypopituitarism after irradiation in children. *Int J Radiat Oncol Biol Phys* 1977; 2:549–552.
209. Watne K, Hager B, Heier M, Hirshberg H. Reversible oedema and necrosis after irradiation of the brain. Diagnostic procedures and clinical manifestations. *Acta Oncol* 1990; 29:891–895.
210. Whitt JK, Wells RJ, Lauria MM, et al. Cranial radiation in childhood acute lymphocytic leukemia: neuropsychologic sequelae. *Am J Dis Child* 1984; 138:730–736.
211. Willis BK, Heilbrun MP, Sapozink MD, McDonald PR. Stereotactic interstitial brachytherapy of malignant astrocytomas with remarks on postimplantation computed tomographic appearance. *Neurosurgery* 1988; 23:348–354.
212. Withers HR, Biologic basis of radiation therapy. In Perez CA, Brady LW (eds): *Principles and Practice of Radiation Oncology*. Philadelphia: Lippincott, 1987, pp 67–98.
213. Wowra B, Schmitt HP, Sturm V. Incidence of late radiation necrosis with transient mass effect after interstitial low dose rate radiotherapy for cerebral gliomas. *Acta Neurochir (Wien)* 1989; 99:104–108.
214. Zeman W, Samorajski T. Effects of irradiation on the nervous system. In Berdjis CC (ed): *Pathology of Irradiation*. Baltimore: Williams & Wilkins, 1971, pp 213–277.
215. Zweig G, Russell EJ. Radiation myelopathy of the cervical spinal cord: MR findings. *Am J Neuroradiol* 1990; 11:1188–1190.

188

Immunotherapy of Human Gliomas

Michael L. Levy
Michael L. J. Apuzzo

Since the early part of this century, when the rejection of transplanted tumors in animals was observed and the existence of tumor antigens and immune responses postulated, there has been periodic enthusiasm for immunotherapy as a mode of cancer treatment. During the past two decades, as basic mechanisms have increasingly been the focus of research, animal tumor systems have been employed to demonstrate that this approach is feasible. In general, animal studies have taken two major forms: (1) immunoprophylactic experiments in which immunotherapy is applied before neoplastic cell challenge or oncogenic virus inoculation, with a subsequent lower incidence of tumors, and (2) tumor implantation or induction, with subsequent immunotherapy on various schedules in relation to concurrent application of the more common forms of cytoreductive therapy. In these systems it has become apparent that tumor masses of less than 10^6 cells are more responsive to immunotherapy than are larger ones. Thus, cytoreductive measures may be an adjuvant to immunotherapy in reducing the critical neoplastic mass. In addition, unlike surgery, radiotherapy, or chemotherapy, which have limiting toxic side effects on normal tissues, immunotherapy is inherently more specific in its selective killing of tumor cells. In view of our current comprehension of immune mechanisms,[6] the primary objectives of immunotherapy should include (1) activation of cell-mediated cytotoxic responses, (2) activation of humorally mediated cytoxic responses, and (3) mitigation of the emergence of blocking factors and suppressor mechanisms.

In a variety of animal models, various immunotherapeutic modalities have shown promise. A number of these have been applied to glioma-bearing human patients. Such endeavors have been prompted by discovery of the following properties of malignant glial tumors: (1) moderate tumor-associated antigenicity or soluble tumor antigen, (2) humoral responses that are tumor-associated and capable of initiating complement-mediated cytotoxic responses, (3) depression of cell-mediated immune responses, (4) the presence of blocking factors in serum components, (5) antigen-antibody complexes, and (6) nonspecific suppressor humoral substances released by the tumor.

Many of the immunotherapeutic studies in glioma patients have used no controls, performed no assays of specific immune impact, and employed no external pathologic review, and were undertaken in individuals with excessive tumor burden; therefore, their data are difficult to evaluate. To date, immunotherapy of gliomas has remained largely within classic categories that relate to techniques of immunization,[86] namely, active nonspecific, active specific, adoptive, passive, and immunorestorative. With the exception of passive immunotherapy, all have been or are being evaluated for use in the treatment of glioma.

It should be noted that despite many immune responses to primary brain tumors, normal astrocytes are somewhat free from immune interaction, owing to the presence of the blood-brain barrier and the absence of a central nervous system (CNS) lymphatic system. Furthermore, brain cells do not express major histocompatibility complex (MHC) antigens, which are necessary for the initiation of an immune response.[120]

Active Immunotherapy

Active immunotherapy techniques attempt to stimulate the intrinsic immune response to the neoplasm. The method may involve a specific or nonspecific mode or a combination of the two.

Active Specific Immunotherapy

Active specific immunotherapy is based on specifically immunizing the host with neoplastic cells, cell products, or cross-reacting viral or bacterial antigens. Attempts have been made to alter tumor cells to enhance their generally weak natural immunogenicity by adding haptenic groups or by treating them with neuraminidase to remove the sialic acid coating (thus revealing membrane antigens). It has been suggested that the glycoprotein oligosaccharide components of glial cell membranes may be antigenic with regard to identification and destruction by natural killer (NK) cells. Thus, treating tumor cells with neuraminidase should enhance their destruction. Treatment with neuraminidase increased the sensitivity to NK lysis of grades I through III glioma cells, but did not influence the sensitivity of grade IV gliomas.[67] Miyatake and colleagues found similar results, with increased susceptibility to cytolysis following acid pretreatment in the glioma-derived GI-1 cell line. Acid pretreatment also decreased the expression of class I human leukocyte antigen (HLA) on tumor cells. On the other hand, Miyatake and colleagues reported that treatment with interferon-γ (IFN-γ) decreased the susceptibility of GI-1 cells to lymphokine-activated killer (LAK) cell cytolysis and increased expression of class I HLA antigen. Natural killer ($CD16^+$) cells had high cytotoxic activity against untreated cells but low activity against IFN-γ-treated cells in both the precursor and effector phases.[90] Butanol extracts have likewise been employed for this purpose. Tumor cells killed by either x-rays or chemical agents such as mitomycin-C have also been used to prepare cell-free antigen extracts.

Active specific immunotherapy, like active immunization for infectious disease, has a promise of emerging as a reliable form of immunotherapy since it elicits memory T cells that permit long-term recognition of offending antigens. However, this form of therapy may also cause the emergence of tumor-specific suppressor elements and thus enhance tumor progression. Also, in glioma-bearing patients, the treatment carries the risk of inducing experimental allergic encephalomyelitis (EAE) due to cross-reacting antigenic components shared with brain and brain-derived neoplastic tissues.

Bloom and colleagues reported tumor growth at 10 of 12 sites following subcutaneous autologous injection in a single patient with glioma. At autopsy the patient had no evidence of immune response peripherally or in the brain.[17] In a comparable study, Grace and colleagues observed evidence of immune rejection at the peripheral graft site in two of six cases without apparent evidence of alteration in the patient's course.[34] A randomized prospective trial was reported by Bloom and colleagues in 1973.[16] All patients had surgery and radiotherapy, and approximately half of them had concomitant specific immunotherapy. The immunotherapy group (27 patients) received various numbers of injections of irradiated autologous tumor cells. No positive therapeutic response was observed. One case of EAE was detected on external pathologic review.

Most recently, investigators have been interested in the immunogenicity of transplantable gliomas in animal models. Experiments using two transplantable rat gliomas, F98 and D74, found no in vivo protection in animals immunized and cross-challenged with either.[141]

Active Nonspecific Immunotherapy

Active nonspecific immunotherapy, which is the type most used so far, employs compounds or materials that have no antigenic similarity to the tumor but that enhance the immune capacity of the host. These include microorganisms such as bacillus Calmette-Guerin (BCG) and *Corynebacterium parvum*,[8,88] as well as newer chemical agents such as glucan, pyran, fluorenone derivative, and certain interferon inducers such as polyadenylic-uradilic acid (poly AU) and polyinosinic-cytidilic acid (poly IC). In the laboratory these agents can reduce tumor growth and abort the growth of small established tumors. These materials fundamentally act on macrophages, activating them to be cytotoxic and to act as T-cell stimulators. They also boost both cell-mediated and humoral immune responsiveness.

In addition to their inherent toxicity, these substances likewise enhance mechanisms of suppression. The apparent effects of any nonspecific modulator represent the net effect of its activities on the effector and suppressor arms of the immunoregulatory system. Suppressor macrophages that act via prostaglandins are particularly problematic, as they impede the emergence of cytotoxic T cells.[110] Use of *C. parvum* therapy was reported in six patients with intrinsic glial tumors; intracranial pressure was increased with administration, and no alteration in survival time was apparent.[125] Intradermal BCG was employed in 45 patients who were purified protein derivative (PPD)-negative.[85] Increased survival time was reported in those who converted to PPD-positive, but no external pathologic review was described.

An increasing array of biological response modifiers are emerging as potential agents in the immunotherapeutic management of patients with glial neoplasms. Lymphokines such as the interferons have been advocated in this regard as agents that might stimulate the immune system to respond to tumor antigenicity.

Combination Immunotherapy

Combinations of specific extracts and potentiating nonspecific adjuvants may be used in immunotherapy. The presence of adjuvants significantly increases the risk of EAE. To date, the most elaborate study in this regard is that of Trouillas.[137] The immunotherapy consisted of weekly injections of autologous tumor extracts emulsified with complete Freund's adjuvant. Sixty-five patients were randomized after surgery into four groups, for which treatment consisted of immunotherapy (10 patients), immunotherapy and radiotherapy (18 patients), radiotherapy (20 patients), or no postoperative treatment (7 patients). A moderate but significant increase in survival time was observed in the immunotherapy groups, and there were signs of strong antiglioma immunization. Four of six tumors evaluated showed increased round cell responses. One case of EAE was observed. Bigner and colleagues think that the threat of EAE induction and the potential difficulty of detecting it in a disabled glioma patient receiving active specific or nonspecific immunotherapy warrant subjecting immunizing CNS material to screening in experimental animals before administering it to patients.[12]

Clinical combination therapies for malignant glioma patients involving adjuvant irradiation, chemotherapy, and interferon have been reported. Treatment combined with IFN resulted in an increase in helper T cells and a reduction in suppressor T cells.[106] It has also been demonstrated that brain tumor-specific cytotoxic T lymphocytes (CTLs) could be produced by priming in vivo followed by secondary stimulation with brain tumor cells in vitro using either RT2 (an astrocytoma) or 9L (a gliosarcoma) and *C. parvum*.[39]

Adachi and colleagues have reported that recombinant tumor necrosis factor-α (rTNF-α) increases the density of epidermal growth factor receptor (EGF-R) in glioma cell lines in culture as determined by anti-EGF-R monoclonal antibody (mAb) 425. Given the ability of ^{125}I-labeled mAb 425 to lyse glioma cells in culture, the authors propose treating glioma patients with a combination of ^{125}I-labeled mAb 425 and rTNF-α.[1] Nagai[95] has reported on radioimmunotherapy as a potential therapeutic option. Specifically, human CLN-IgG was labeled with ^{131}I and administered into the tumor. Incorporation was confirmed by gamma-scintigraphy. Concurrent administration of interferon enhanced the efficacy of the therapy.

The combination of different modes of immunotherapy holds promise for future trials. Examples include a combination of adoptive immunotherapy with cytolytic monoclonal antibodies or adoptive immunotherapy with cytokines such as TNF or IFN-γ, which synergize with interleukin-2 (IL-2).[2,3] Biological response modification is currently of particular interest in the approach to immunotherapy. Other combinations of lymphokines, such as TNF with IFN-γ, exert synergistic antitumor effects in vivo in mice. To date none of these combinations has been tried in the treatment of human glioma; controlled trials have yet to establish their efficacy in vivo.

Adoptive Immunotherapy

The potential role of adoptive immunotherapy, specifically that involving lymphokine-activated killer cells (LAKs) and tumor-infiltrating lymphocytes (TILs), in the treatment of malignant glioma is being evaluated at the basic science and clinical levels. Adoptive immunotherapy is the transfer of immunity by means of lymphoid cells or subcellular information. Initially, it was accomplished by transferring histocompatible lymphocytes from one patient to another, and now it involves the transfer of autologous peripheral blood lymphocytes. These carefully matched lymphocytes have prevented tumor growth in experimental systems. Sensitized cellular components or fractions thereof may be transferred from one host to another or from the peripheral blood to a tumor site. Takakura and colleagues have transferred histocompatible adult marrow into children with a variety of tumors, with no controls.[132] In addition, the same group infused white cells into tumor beds postoperatively.[133] Long survival times were reported anecdotally. Once again, the tumor population was mixed, and no control data were presented. Seventeen patients who had failed conventional therapy for glioblastoma were treated by Young and colleagues with intratumoral infusions of autologous lymphocytes.[155] These autologous lymphocytes were isolated from peripheral blood and placed in direct contact with the tumor cells in an attempt to induce in vitro sensitization. Eight of the patients demonstrated unequivocal clinical improvement and were alive as long as 17 months later. There was no indication of EAE on clinical or pathologic assays.

In vitro techniques have improved since those efforts.[85] The ability to clone T cells and preserve their helper or cytotoxic function is due to the identification of T-cell growth factor (IL-2). The use of autologous sensitized cells circumvents the ethical issue of donor sensitization and the serious problem of graft-versus-host responses, which may be initiated by recognition of minor histocompatibility antigens. Autologous lymphocytes from tumor-bearing patients may be assayed for their in vitro reactivity and then restimulated in vitro by incubation with killer tumor cells. Clonal selection and/or expansion is a potential strategy.

Other promising modes of adoptive therapy involve the use of lymphokines, monokines (from a macrophage source), and various other well-characterized lymphocytic factors. Interleukin-1 (a monokine) and interleukin-2 (a lymphokine) are discrete biological entities that can be isolated and administered. These substances afford the ability to transfer homogeneous defined materials and to activate lymphocytes and macrophages in vivo. It has also been reported that the incubation of lymphocytes in IL-2 resulted in the generation of activated lymphoid cells capable of lysing fresh autologous, syngeneic, or allogenic tumor cells but not fresh normal cells.[156]

Studies suggest that IFN-γ may influence tumor cell susceptibility to CTL-mediated cytolysis differently than IFN-β. In addition, the mechanisms for recognizing target tumor cells likely differ between CTLs and LAK cells.[91] It has also been demonstrated that limiting dilution analysis (LDA) microcultures can be used as a powerful tool to differentiate tumor-reactive CTLs from other effector cell populations.[140] A new method for the sterile sorting of NK cells by negative selection using FITC-labeled monoclonal antibodies has also been described.[51] It is believed that the activation of the secretory function of tumor-specific CTLs is antigen-specific. Soluble factors in the secretory granules are likely to be associated with the mechanism of target cell lysis. Iwasaki and coworkers analyzed the ultrastructure of the tumor-lymphocyte interaction and found that CTLs increased in size following stimulation by the glioma-derived cell line GI-1 and that the intracytoplasmic secretory granules increased in number and size.[43]

Takamura has provided evidence that B-cell-line cells can enhance the nonspecific cytotoxic activity of human mononuclear leukocytes by increasing IL-2 production. He suggests that such lines should be studied as potential effective biological response modifiers in cancer immunotherapy.[134] Expression of the variable region of the T-cell receptor (Vα) has been reported in tumor-infiltrating lymphocytes invading malignant glial tumors. It was concluded that these TILs could be isolated, expanded, and used therapeutically for the treatment of malignant brain tumors.[101]

Cytofluorometric studies on glial cell lines indicate that sensitivity to destruction by NK cells may reflect the growth fraction of the target. Tumors with a higher proportion of cycling cells are more susceptible to lysis by NK cells. The potential effectiveness of NK cells against tumors with a low proliferative rate is being explored.[94]

Lymphokine-Activated Killer Cells

LAK cells differ phenotypically from cytotoxic T lymphocytes. Most LAK cell precursors have the surface markers Leu 4-11$^+$ 15$^+$.[126] LAK cells have been reported to kill fresh tumor cells that are unaffected by NK cells in an MHC-unrestricted fashion. The killing of glioma cells by LAK cells in vitro has been reported by Jacobs and colleagues.[45] A phase-1 clinical trial in which nine patients with malignant glioma were treated with IL-2 or LAK cells[46] failed to show any signs of systemic or neural toxicity following treatment.

Given the large number of peripheral blood leukocytes (PBLs) that have to be obtained by leukapheresis for LAK therapy, in addition to the difficulty of obtaining large numbers in children or elderly patients, methods to increase the yield of these CD4$^+$ helper/killer T cells have been explored. Anti-CD3 antibody has been found to increase the number of LAK cells for therapy.[53,99,100] Unfortunately, these LAK cells showed weaker killing activity than cells stimulated with recombinant IL-2 (rIL-2) alone. Their surface phenotypes were more sensitive to CD3 and FACS analysis. TILs generated using recombinant IL-2 and an anti-CD3 antibody were also found by others to be less cytotoxic than LAK cells against 10 glioma specimens in a standard 4-h ^{51}Cr release assay.[54] Another technique that generates large numbers of autologous cytolytic T cells with nonrestricted antitumor activity involves PBLs activated with phytohemagglutinin-P and recombinant human IL-2, and then proliferated in vitro for up to 5 months with IL-2.[149]

The supernatant of certain glioma cell lines has been found to suppress the functional response of IL-2-activated lymphocytes. Also, concurrent administration of steroids, which are frequently used in glioma patients, limits the potential yield of LAK cells.[108] This is a concern when one considers the environment in which LAK cells must function to respond to tumor cells. LAK cells obtained from patients with glioma had a level of cytotoxicity similar to that of LAK cells from normal subjects.[18] Yet other investigators have reported a marked reduction in the number of circulating mononuclear cells in patients with glioma. These findings are consistent with the compromised status of cellular immunity in glioma patients. Thus, while LAK cells derived from patients with glioma are highly cytotoxic, the low yield of LAK cells from these patients is a major limitation in their efficacy.

Multicellular tumor spheroid models of a human malignant glioma cell line have allowed for ultrastructural investigation of the infiltrative and cytotoxic cell-to-cell interactions between LAK cells and tumor cells. It was demonstrated that LAK cells infiltrated toward the inner areas of the tumor spheres and caused a progressive tumor destruction, with the number of viable tumor cells in the spheroids decreasing in direct relation to the increase in number of LAK cells.[41] Iwasaki et al. found that the infiltrating LAK cells were composed of heterogeneous subpopulations of T-like cells as well as large granular lymphocyte-like cells that were tightly adherent to the tumor cells.[42] Of interest is the finding in tumor spheroid models that LAK cells release membrane-damaging agents that potentially remain active outside the target area.[44]

Maleci and colleagues demonstrated that phorbol ester pretreatment of a LAK cell-sensitive glioma cell line decreased the susceptibility of glial cells to LAK cell-mediated lysis.[75] Protein kinase C (PKC) inhibitors failed to block this phenomenon. Tzeng and colleagues[139] indicated that curative, adoptive immunotherapy of an intracerebral F98 rat glioma by means of purified adherent lymphokine-activated killer (A-LAK) cells and interleukin-2 is impossible. Though the A-LAK cells demonstrated greater activity against F98 tumor cells than conventional LAK cells on chromium release assays, there was no evidence of therapeutic efficacy (Winn assay).

Kruse and colleagues[60] evaluated response to adoptive immunotherapy using recombinant interleukin-2 and various effector cells in the Fischer strain 9L rat gliosarcoma model. Improved survival was shown for groups treated with nonadherent or adherent LAK cells or syngeneic or allogeneic CTLs using Mantel-Haenzel nonparametric log-rank equations. Only allogeneic CTLs prevented tumor take. The killer activity of thymocytes has been found to be superior to that of splenocytes following incubation with IL-2 in tumor models. Thus, it is likely that the precursors of LAK cells are not NK cells.[78]

Therapy using LAK cells and rIL-2 has not proved to be effective in preliminary clinical trials. We continue to have a poor understanding of the interactions between LAK cells and tumor target cells, and specifically of the events that lead to tumor destruction. This prevents us from mounting an effective therapeutic regimen to date. Other clinical studies have failed to find any therapeutic difference in the in vitro antitumor cytolytic activity of IL-2-activated glioma-infiltrating lymphocytes separated from tumor tissue versus IL-2-activated peripheral blood lymphocytes.[119]

Merchant and colleagues[83] reported on a series of 23 patients with recurrent glioblastoma and 1 patient with a high-grade oligodendroglioma treated with recombinant IL-2 and LAK cells. An initial intraparenchymal injection of LAK cells with rIL-2 into the tissue surrounding the tumor cavity was followed by daily injections of rIL-2 into the tumor cavity for three days. On the 10th postoperative day, the patients received an additional course of intracavitary LAK and rIL-2. The median time for tumor recurrence was 22 months. Twelve patients had local recurrence or progression visible on follow-up radiographic imaging. Ten patients died without evidence of tumor recurrence or with tumor recurrence at distant sites. Only two patients were without recurrence on long-term follow-up. Thus, this therapy did no better than conventional treatment.

The clinical use of LAK cells treated with bispecific antibody is currently being investigated in the treatment of glial tumors. Nitta and colleagues reported on targeting therapy using LAK cells treated with an anti-CD3 mAb conjugated to an anti-glioma mAb in 10 patients with malignant glioma. A second group of 10 patients were treated with untreated LAK cells. Of those receiving targeting therapy, four showed tumor regression, and four appeared to have postsurgical tumor eradication, as indicated by computed tomography (CT) and histology. No recurrence was detected in the 10 to 18 months of follow-up. Nine patients receiving untreated LAK cells had recurrences within 1 year. Eight patients died within 4 years.[104]

The Denver Brain Tumor Research Group has reported on clinical trials using autologous human rIL-2-activated lymphocytes to treat 20 patients with recurrent high-grade gliomas. Surgical resection was followed by intracavitary implantation of LAK cells and autologous stimulated lymphocytes (ASLs) along with rIL-2 in a plasma clot. One month later, stimulated lymphocytes and rIL-2 were infused through a Rickham reservoir attached to a catheter directed into the tumor bed. No significant difference in survival was found between patients who received this therapy and those who did not. The use of steroids or prior chemotherapy did not influence the in vitro generation of ASLs or LAK cells.[66] Conversely, Merchant and colleagues have found that dexamethasone used to control cerebral edema may depress the antitumor activity of rIL-2 by depressing the capacity of lymphocytes to develop normal LAK activity.[82] In clinical trials, rIL-2 has been found to be safe, even though cerebral edema around the site of treatment has been a consistent finding.

The experience at our institution with stereotactic methods has allowed us to develop special catheters for the delivery of LAK cells and/or cytokines as part of immunotherapeutic protocols. The catheters are flanged and are compatible with standard Luer-Lok syringe systems to allow for serial injections. Predetermined points at or beyond the tumor margins are stereotactically defined using CT or magnetic resonance imaging (MRI) with catheter placement under local anesthesia. The catheters can then be removed at the bedside after treatment. Thus, with the use of CT or MRI, we can deliver immunotherapeutic regimens to specifically defined regions. This represents a marked improvement over conventional open methods in terms of patient morbidity and the ability to incorporate the leading edge of the tumor.

Restorative Therapy

Restorative therapy consists in direct or indirect attempts to restore deficient immune function by any means except direct adoptive transfer of cells. Restoration of depressed cell-mediated immunity may be selectively attempted by the administration of agents such as levamisole. This agent can convert T-cell precursors, including some null cells, into functional T cells. In a rigidly designed and well-controlled study, Mahaley et al. evaluated levamisole therapy in a group of 85 patients with anaplastic glioma who had undergone surgical resection and who were also treated with radiotherapy and chemotherapy.[73] No significant differences in survival time were observed between the treated and nontreated groups, nor did assays of cellular or humoral immunity show significant differences between the two groups. The same group of investigators reported that BCG in combination with levamisole was effective in an animal model and proposed future pilot studies.

Thymic hormones are currently under investigation as agents that, in various fractions, selectively alter depressed T-cell function to restore T-cell populations to normal levels and restore physiologic mechanisms related to this group of cells.[20] Thymosin in particular has been fractionated and found to cause differentiation of precursors into specific T-cell subfractions in mice. It may soon be possible to selectively augment various components of the T-cell compartment. Other substances, such as cyclophosphamide, have the ability to inhibit suppressor cells, thereby enhancing overall immune system activity. To date there is no substantial clinical evidence for the efficacy of this therapy against glioma.

Passive Immunotherapy

The transfer of antibodies from immunized individuals to tumor-bearing recipients constitutes passive immunotherapy. Not only does the method carry the theoretical danger of tumor enhancement, but antibodies are short-lived and in general are less important in tumor rejection than is cell-mediated immunity. In addition, technical problems in screening sera of donors and ethical restraints against immunization of individuals have made this form of therapy one of the most restrictive and least desirable approaches. No significant report relating to this form of therapy for malignant gliomas has appeared. However, the development of hybridoma techniques and the production of monoclonal antibodies have given new impetus to consideration of this method.[89]

Biological Response Modification

What has been called *immunotherapy* might more aptly be called *biological response modification* or *biomodulation.*[15] All therapeutic approaches to neoplastic disorders that attempt to modify the antigenic structure or growth characteristics of the tumor and thus influence the host-neoplasm interaction may be considered to fall in this province. An agent may be considered a biomodulator if it accomplishes one or more of the following actions:

1. Altering characteristics of the cell membrane or tumor so as to increase antigenicity or increase susceptibility to cytotoxic drugs or immune mechanisms.
2. Enhancing the host's ability to tolerate injury by cytotoxic modalities, as by increasing the number of leukocyte precursors in bone marrow.
3. Enhancing the host's defenses by being an effector or mediator.
4. Inhibiting suppressor mechanisms.
5. Directly enhancing the host's response by stimulating an increase in the amount of effector cells or soluble mediators, such as T-cell lymphokines or macrophage monokines.
6. Preventing or reversing transformation or increased maturation of the primitive tumor cells.

Biomodulation based on precise comprehension of immune neoplastic mechanisms emerges as a logical province for investigative enterprise in relation to the enigmatic issue of malignant glioma therapy.

Future Perspectives and Approaches to Immunotherapy

The progression of malignancy can be thought of as resulting from a lack of immune response to the neoplasm. This lack most likely results from the poor antigenicity of the neoplasm. Therefore, the isolation and identification of tumor-specific antigens is of the utmost importance. The current hybridoma models and the mAbs produced using them are facilitating the search. The development of mAbs that could inactivate suppressor proteins produced by glial tumors is another avenue of current interest.[55]

A rational approach to mobilizing immune mechanisms in the treatment of glial tumors requires a sophisticated understanding of the immune system. This is one of the main reasons why attempts at adjunctive immunotherapy have had so little success. As our understanding of the immune system develops, more precise modes of intervention and manipulation will emerge.

Some of the newer concepts of immunotherapy have been detailed previously. In addition, specific removal of blocking antibodies and circulating immune complexes appears to be a logical approach to restoring effective immunity and ultimately improving control of malignant disease. There is interest in the therapeutic use of immunoabsorption for this purpose.[135] Blocking antibodies may compete with cytotoxic antibodies for antigenic loci on tumor cells. Immune complexes ultimately stimulate the emergence of suppressor predominance in T-cell and macrophage populations. The end result of these events is a globally reduced effector immune response in tumor-bearing patients.

Immunoabsorption can be performed by perfusing the patient's blood through an absorptive column containing antigen and antibody bound to immobilized charcoal. Immune substances complementary to the bound reagent are removed by the column, and the filtered plasma is returned to the patient. The method has been effective in the laboratory and has shown promising results in a small number of patients with carcinoma of the breast.

Ways to antagonize suppressor responses are another area of interest.[86] Cyclophosphamide in low doses can specifically inhibit precursors of suppressor T cells, thereby augmenting cytotoxic effector function. In addition, antagonists of prostaglandin synthetase, such as indomethacin, inhibit the effects of suppressor macrophages, which are mediated through prostaglandin E. Combining these agents with the immunoabsorption technique could be an interesting strategy.

The hybridoma technique is a potent tool for identifying antigenic determinants and producing antibodies against them. By employing sensitized B cells and a myeloma tumor cell line, large quantities of monoclonal antibodies specific for cellular determinants can be obtained. Thus is it likely that our understanding of tumor antigens will increase and also that antibodies specific to individual neoplasms will become available for passive immunotherapy. Specific immunization is conceivable.

The retinoid derivatives of vitamin A have been effective in redirecting the maturation of metaplastic cells back toward normalcy. When administered with carcinogens, retinoids may prevent and occasionally reverse progression of malignant transformation. Extensive epidemiologic evidence supports the protective role of these agents in high-risk cancer populations. These agents can augment the immune response by increasing antibody production and cell-mediated cytotoxicity. In brief, these agents have both direct and indirect effects on transformed cells.

The interferons, a family of inducible secretory glycoproteins, need evaluation in glioma management and will be discussed below. These agents exert a number of potential therapeutic effects on neoplastic processes, including (1) antiviral impact, (2) inhibition of cellular proliferation, (3) alteration of membrane antigenicity and structure, (4) enhancement of lymphocytic cytotoxic responses, (5) augmentation of natural killer cell and macrophage cytotoxicity, and (6) augmentation of antibody-dependent cell-mediated responses. Because of issues related to blood-brain barrier permeability, alternative administration modes and delivery systems are being evaluated in glioma cases. In addition, a number of interferon inducers such as poly IC, poly AU, and pyran require further study.

Tumor-Specific Antigens, Monoclonal Antibodies, and Cytokines: Current Modalities and Potential Therapeutic Implications

Cell Lines and Antigenicity

As we learn more about tumor-related antigens, we need antigenic cell lines to allow us to elucidate the mechanisms of tumor destruction. One such human glioma-derived cell line expresses glial fibrillary acidic protein (GFAP) and glutamine synthetase (GS) in addition to cell-surface gangliosides recognized by the A2B5 monoclonal antibody.[56] Another cell line that expresses GFAP is the SRB.10A glial line. Three new human medulloblastoma cell lines expressed vimentin, neurofilament proteins, and the synaptic vesicle membrane glycoprotein synaptophysin.[38]

Bilzer and colleagues have reported marked variability in the surface antigens in glial-derived cell lines. They found differential expression of glial fibrillary acidic protein, S-100 protein, Leu-7, and GAA as defined by mAbs. In primary tumors, epidermal growth factor receptors and nerve growth factor receptors were found mostly in short-term cultures. They concluded that this may represent the control by effector molecules of the growth of malignant glioma.[13] Westphal and colleagues emphasize that only rigidly standardized culture conditions will assure that comparisons of data from primary cultures are valid.[144]

Immunostains and Cell Growth

The proliferative potential of gliomas has been a problematic factor in determining the most appropriate approach to therapy, especially in the instance of low-grade lesions. Brain tumor growth results from the relative proportions of cells in three populations: (1) cycling/proliferative; (2) quiescent (G0)/static, and (3) terminally differentiated/dying. The cytokinetic analyses of gliomas is based on markers of cell proliferation ([^{3}H]thymidine and BuDR) and the detection of growth-dependent proteins (proliferating cell nuclear antigen, Ki-67). Disadvantages of these methods include the necessity of administering the label before surgical resection.

Numerous markers have been defined and used in the evaluation of glial tumors. Kaluza and Adamek have proposed that the determination of GFAP antigenicity can assist in evaluating both the differentiation and the heterogeneity of tumors.[49] High-grade gliomas contain more tumor cells rich in epidermal growth factor receptor (EGFR) than do low-grade gliomas. Reactive astrocytes also have been found to express EGFR, whereas small neurons and normal glial cells do not.[136] Detta and Hitchcock have reported a method for estimating the proliferating/labeling indices of brain tumors using bromodeoxyuridine.[27] Other studies have also suggested that qualitative and quantitative differences in antigenic heterogeneity may identify stages in glial tumor progression.[47]

Ki-67 was initially raised against Reed Sternberg cells.[33] The nuclear antigen it recognizes is present only in the G_1, S, G_2, and M phases of the cell cycle. Zuber and colleagues,[157] studying frozen glioma specimens, demonstrated that the Ki-67 index of proliferating cells correlated with the histologic classification of these tumors. Most notable is the ability of Ki-67 to distinguish between anaplastic and low-grade gliomas. Tsanaclis and colleagues reported on the Ki-67 labeling index in 48 human brain tumors.[138] The Ki-67 index increases with increasing histologic grade and also appears to be a useful indicator of the active tumor volume and margin.[107] A nonlinear relationship between the mitotic index and the Ki-67 labeling index has been reported in glioma.[123] Immunostaining with DNA polymerase α has also been reported to more accurately predict the cellular proliferation rate of brain tumors than the mAb Ki-67.[61]

Proliferating cell nuclear antigen (PCNA) is a protein that accumulates in the nucleus during the S phase of the cell cycle. The labeling indices (LIs) of PCNA and Ki-67 were both found to increase with increasing tumor grade in glial tumors.[70] PCNA is a cell-cycle-regulated protein. Allegranza and colleagues have demonstrated a significant correlation between the PCNA labeling index, the histologic grade of the tumor, and the labeling indices for thymidine, BrdU, and Ki-67.[5] Recently the mAb S-44 has been found to identify a nuclear protein, statin, expressed only in nonproliferating cells. Statin may be useful in the evaluation of the cytotoxic effects of anticancer drugs used to treat gliomas.[121]

Using a cDNA probe, Quackenbush and colleagues have characterized the expression of CD44 in several normal and malignant cell types. High levels were expressed in astrocytoma lines. The CD44 complex is related to the ability of cells to adhere to matrix proteins and endothelium. Thus, high levels of CD44 could be associated with an increased capacity for invasiveness and metastasis.[111] Immunohistologic stains of human brain tumors, brain metastases, and normal brain demonstrated strong expression of CD44 in high-grade gliomas and weak expression in meningiomas, medulloblastomas, and normal brain.[63]

Anti-Leu-M1 reactivity was reported in 10 of 24 astrocytomas, 4 of 22 oligodendrogliomas, and 9 of 15 ependymomas studied. This finding suggests that neoplastically transformed gliocytes are no longer capable of expressing lacto-*N*-fucopentose III. Anti-Leu-M1 reactivity has proved to be helpful in distinguishing between benign and malignant CNS neoplasms.[128]

S-100 β immunoreactivity in immunostaining has been reported to decrease in parallel with the degree of malignancy. Hayashi and colleagues suggest that immunostaining for S-100 α and S-100 β proteins might become a useful diagnostic procedure in the evaluation of brain tumors.[37]

Tumor-Specific Antigens

As mentioned previously, the identification of tumor-specific antigens is essential to the development of antitumor antibodies to facilitate the cell-mediated killing of glioma cells. Although the use of tumor-specific mAbs has been shown to be effective in murine models, it does carry the danger of creating antigen-antibody complexes and attendant enhancement of tumor growth. The conjugation of mAbs with cytotoxic chemicals or radionuclides are other potential uses for mAbs.

Monoclonal antibodies produced by the hybridoma technique initially established by Kohler and Milstein in 1975[57] have made it possible to produce large quantities of antibodies that will react with a specific antigenic determinant. Such antibodies make it possible to identify and characterize antigens present on human neoplastic cells. This technique has been used to show that glial tumors have numerous antigens that are not present in normal brain. These antigens include oncofetal antigens of neuroectodermal origin,[152] major histocompatibility antigens (both class I and class II), and the products of oncogenes residing in the epidermal growth factor receptor.

As stated above, a good deal of evidence supports the existence of tumor-associated antigens in gliomas. Tumor-specific antigens have remained an elusive goal. Gliomas are known to express over a hundred antigens. To date, no specific antigen unique to glioma cells has been isolated; however, several glioma antigens have been recognized, often with primary representation on glioma cells but with minor representation on other cellular constituents.[25] To further complicate the issue, cells of brain tumors have a constantly varying multiprobable antigenicity[26]; cellular antigen expression varies with cell age, attempted therapy, and the heterogeneity of the original cell clonogene. Antigenic components of tumor cells include biochemically defined proteins, extracellular matrix antigens, muscle antigens, melanoma antigens, cellular proliferation antigens, specificities shared by nervous system-lymphoid cells, oncoembryonic-oncofetal determinants, and tumor-restricted or glial antigens. Cellular proliferation antigens will become increasingly important in predicting the prognosis of gliomas. Our understanding of tumor-associated antigens and the subsequent development of mAbs has been fostered by the benefits of hybridoma technology. Simply, most vertebrate cells will perish after a limited number of divisions in culture, whereas hybridoma cell lines are immortal and grow rapidly and to high densities in culture. The supernatants of these hybridoma lines of glioma tissue can then be screened. It is important to note that cells in culture may diverge phenotypically (and in some cases genotypically) from their predecessors. One example is the downregulation of MHC class I antigen in the B16 melanoma cell line.

The production of mAbs specific for glioma-associated antigens has assisted in their identification and characterization. In addition, panels of mAbs used in the immunohistochemical evaluation of frozen tumor tissue has revealed the heterogeneity of antigen expression among tumors. Such heterogeneity may have profound clinical ramifications. We will discuss the applications of mAbs in the immunohistochemical and immunocytologic evaluation of tumor tissue, the localization of radiolabeled mAbs in experimental and clinical models, and the mechanisms of antibody transport and interaction with antigenic molecules (including the transport of immunotoxins[129]). Preclinical studies involving intravenous or intracarotid injection of mAbs found them to accumulate specifically in tumor, although in amounts insufficient for therapeutic use. This low accumulation may result from the failure of some cell populations to express given tumor-associated antigens, from low affinity for the antigen, or from the presence of the blood-brain barrier. In the near future, the clinical use of mAbs as carrier molecules in the immunotherapeutic management of glial neoplasms will become a reality.

Central to this discussion is the concept of mesenchymal drift and its relationship to tumor antigenicity. Mesenchymal drift is the tendency of gliomas to progressively lose glial and gain mesenchymal features, as represented by the generation of multiple cell types with differing antigenic expression. Although the source of these cells is unknown, it is likely that endothelial proliferation results in the rapid growth of fibronectin-positive mesenchymal cells, which subsequently overgrow GFAP-positive cells. Unfortunately, this phenomenon does not occur in culture. Precursor glial cells may initiate mesenchymal drift by altering gene expression. Glial cells that express the antigenicity of multiple cell lines also may initiate mesenchymal drift by altering gene expression. Studies now suggest that cultured gliomas may alter the phenotypic expression of their genes, resulting in mesenchymal drift.[81]

Monoclonal Antibodies

Monoclonal antibodies have made it possible to identify neuroectodermal and neurohemopoietic antigens on the cell surface as well as glial cytoplasmic antigens such as glial fibrillary acidic protein.[80,150] Neural differentiation antigens, such as neuroectodermal-oncofetal and neurohemopoietic-shared antigens, have also been isolated with mAbs. Yoshida and colleagues evaluated the sera from 27 patients with malignant glioma for antibodies to surface antigens of cultured human glioma cells. They were able to define specific associated antigens as well as common antigens present on both cultured normal and malignant cells.[154]

Kokunai and colleagues report on a human mAb (CLN-IgG), produced from a human-human hybridoma derived from lymphocytes of a patient with cervical carcinoma, that reacted with various human glioma cells but not with normal or fetal brain. They believe that the CLN mAb recognizes an antigen related to cell proliferation in malignant gliomas.[58]

Yakabayashi and colleagues[147] identified an mAb (G-22) that recognizes a 67-kDa neuroectodermal antigen expressed on the surface of glioma, melanoma, and pulmonary adenocarcinoma. The antigen is expressed on normal fetal brain but is not expressed by nongliomatous adult brain. The recognition of this antigen by enzyme-linked immunosorbent assay (ELISA) in CSF or adult brain tumor tissue could be used to differentiate glioma from nongliomatous tumor tissue. Schrappe and colleagues have found a correlation between the expression of a proteoglycan synthesized by glioblastoma and capillary brain endothelial cells in culture (recognized by mAb 9.2.27.) and the malignant phenotype of astroglial cells.[122]

Mouse myeloma cells were fused with spleen cells from mice that had been immunized with a human ependymoma-derived cell line, KMS II. Hybridomas producing mAbs derived from a human ependymoma cell line recognized a cell-surface membrane antigen. There was no cross-reactivity with normal adult or fetal brain. This antigen defined by the mAb (Ep-C4) is specific for ependymoma cells.[84] B-cell hybridomas from mice immunized with human glioma extracts were cloned and subcloned by limiting dilution, yielding six mAbs that were entirely specific, a polypeptide pattern possibly related to human GFAP.[77] Fetal antigen 2 was found around vessels, pia, and arachnoid in normal brain and glial tumors, whereas in gliosarcoma it was distributed diffusely in the sarcoma region.[112]

Takahashi and colleagues produced two mAbs in mice immunized with cultured human malignant glioma cells. Both bound strongly to cultured glioma cells and led to their destruction by human peripheral blood lymphocytes, and thus are candidates for the immunotherapy of human malignant gliomas. Both mAbs bound more strongly to sections of frozen gliomas than to normal brain. Carcinomas of various histologic types were completely unreactive.[130] Takahashi and colleagues also reported that a neutralizing mouse monoclonal antibody (against fibroblast growth factor, FGF) inhibited the growth of two human glioblastoma cell lines that expressed both the basic FGF and the FGF receptor genes. The subcutaneous administration of this antibody suppressed tumor growth in nude mice.[131] Antihuman transferrin receptor monoclonal antibody–ricin A-chain conjugate (anti-TfR-A) immunotoxins were found to be potent in vitro cytotoxins for human glioma cell lines expressing human transferrin receptor, as assessed by flow cytometry.[113]

Monoclonal antibody 425 has been reported to bind to the epidermal growth factor receptor with a specificity for human glioma but not normal brain. mAb 425 has been found to inhibit the growth of subcutaneous glioma xenografts in nude mice. Although the mechanism of this inhibition remains unknown, it may be mediated by murine macrophages or may be related to the capacity of the mAb to antagonize growth.[9]

Nitta and colleagues[102] tested a bifunctional antibody that simultaneously recognized the CD3 complex on T cells and glioma-associated antigens, thus cross-linking effector and target cells. Of a group of human glioma patients in whom this antibody was tested, one showed disappearance of the tumor as judged by CT.

A patient receiving only LAK therapy had recurrence one year after LAK treatment. The authors suggest that this bifunctional antibody may be useful in anti-glioma immunotherapy.[103]

Radiolabeled Monoclonal Antibodies

The rationale behind using radiolabeled monoclonal antibodies in the treatment of malignant gliomas is that they will deliver an effective radiation dose to the tumor while sparing normal tissues. Monoclonal antibody G-22 is directed against a human glioma-associated surface antigen.[151] Using radiolabeled monoclonal and polyclonal antibodies, Williams and colleagues have assessed tumor targeting in nude mice bearing human glioma xenografts. Monoclonal P96.5 specifically binds the U-251 human glioma. They concluded that common cell surface antigens among neuroectoderm-derived neoplasms may provide a basis for human glioma radioimmunotherapy.[146]

It has become apparent that the specific uptake of the radiolabeled antibody by tumor (as opposed to normal tissue) will have to be increased if radioimmunotherapy is to be effective. A new method has been proposed to increase tumor uptake and the tumor-to-normal tissue uptake ratio. Tenascin is an antigen expressed by the stroma of malignant gliomas. The ATE method [labeling the IgG2b glioma-reactive antitenascin monoclonal antibody 81C6 with ^{131}I using *N*-succinimidyl-3-(tri-*n*-butylstannyl)benzoate] may significantly improve the therapeutic efficacy of radioiodinated monoclonal antibodies.[124] 3H9 is a murine mAb with activity against human malignant glial cell lines. Radiolabeled 3H9 can detect human brain tumor xenografts in nude mice in vivo.[65] Riva and colleagues stereotactically injected an anti-tenascin mAb (BC-2) radiolabeled with ^{131}I into a series of 10 patients in whom glioblastoma had recurred despite surgery, radiotherapy, or chemotherapy. They reported an initial complete remission in one patient with relapse after 11 months. Of the other patients, four showed no response, three had no progression, and two had partial remission.[115]

Other groups have also reported that the use of mAbs as carrier molecules for the administration of ^{131}I or drug conjugates can depress glioma cell proliferation in vitro and in vivo.[127] Bergh and colleagues defined a mAb (MUC 2-63) raised against a neuroectodermal antigen expressed on human malignant gliomas, neuroblastomas, and melanomas. Seven patients with brain tumors received radiolabeled MUC 2-63, and six showed an uptake of 0.01 to 0.04 percent of the injected dose at the site of the tumor.[11] Brady and colleagues, in a pilot phase I/II project, administered ^{125}I-labeled anti-epidermal growth factor receptor-425 via the internal carotid artery in patients with recurrent glioblastoma. Of the 15 patients, 1 had a complete response, 2 had a partial response, and 5 had stable disease.[19]

Mel-14 is an mAb reactive with the chondroitin sulfate proteoglycan antigen of gliomas. Colapinto and colleagues reported that a prior intravenous injection of ^{131}I-labeled Mel-14 resulted in prolonged survival in athymic mice transplanted intracerebrally with human glioma xenografts.[21] Another mAb currently being evaluated is P96.5, which specifically binds to U-251 human glioma. Radiolabeled P96.5 has been reported to specifically target U-251 human glioma xenografts in a murine model, in addition to causing tumor regression.[145]

Potential Problems

One potential problem with regard to the specificity of mAbs is that human mAbs derived from patients with astrocytic tumors might recognize subtle antigenic specificities that differ from those recognized by murine systems. Thus, hybridoma models should incorporate human myeloma cell lines. In a recent study, four of a total of five human monoclonal antibodies produced from the fusion of a human myeloma-like cell line with peripheral blood lymphocytes from four patients with astrocytic tumors were directed to cell-surface glycolipids.[24] An immunohistochemical evaluation of antigen expression in primary human glioblastomas and in the tumors from first and second recurrences confirmed that the phenotypic variability of tumor cells makes it difficult to identify the origin of cells in human glioblastomas on the basis of their antigenicity.[14]

Jones and colleagues identified epidermal growth factor receptor immunohistochemically in 62 of 110 malignant gliomas. They also noted that there is a potential for error in the use of mAbs to study the EGFR because there is cross-reactivity with blood group A antigen in certain cell lines.[48] An evaluation of the immunoreactivities of 35 different mAbs that were specific for intermediate filaments in cryostat sections of 14 human gliomas and normal brain found marked heterogeneity.[30]

Cytokines

The interferons (IFNs) can be subdivided into those that are virally induced (α), fibroblast-derived (β), and immune-derived (γ). In vitro, recombinant IFN-β has been reported to inhibit the replication of human glioma cells.[59,71] While some clinical studies have reported a response to the intrathecal or intratumoral administration of IFN-β,[96] others have failed to replicate these findings.[28] IFN-α also has been reported to inhibit the replication of human glioma cells in vitro.[97] Mahaley and colleagues reported a response in 7 of 17 patients treated with intravenous or intramuscular IFN-α.[74] They were unable to replicate this response in a series of 14 patients treated with IFN-γ.[72] In addition, the administration of IFN-γ was associated with hypotension during infusion as well as chills, fever, nausea, vomiting, and elevated liver enzyme levels. Interferons or TNF may be injected into the carotid artery to achieve high local concentrations in the tumor vasculature while minimizing systemic toxicity. Because large amounts of these recombinant lymphokines can be produced, immunologic reactions can be manipulated in vivo in ways not previously possible.[116]

There has been little success in the development of immunotherapy with IFN-β1 and even less with adoptive immunotherapy using LAK cells plus IL-2. It is known that the lysis of tumor cell requires the recognition of specific antigens in association with the presentation of MHC class I or II antigen. Certain cytokines are believed to enhance class I and class II antigen expression in certain mouse glioma cell lines in vitro. Current studies are evaluating the impact of MHC upregulation on the response of brain tumors to immunotherapy.[4]

Interleukin-4 has the ability to generate LAK cells and is synergistic with IL-2 in the generation of LAK cells in mice. IL-4 also helps promote the growth and differentiation of T cells exclusive of its effects on LAK cell generation. Pollack and colleagues concluded that in four low-passage human malignant glioma lines, PDGF may function as a mitogen to enhance DNA synthesis and autocrine stimulation.[109] IFN-γ has been found to induce the expression of MHC class I and class II antigens in gliomas. Glial neoplasms also have been reported to secrete the lymphokines IL-1, IL-3, and IL-6 in addition to factors that depress the immune response, including transforming growth factor-β2 (TGF-β2) and prostaglandin E_2 (PgE_2). Glioma cells are known to secrete

TGF-β2 and PgE_2, which may in part be responsible for this lack of immune response. The depression of the host immune response is strong enough to suppress any response on the part of the host to the tumor-associated antigenicity (resulting from the presence of tumor-associated antigens along with the expression of MHC) in an environment not protected by the blood-brain barrier.

The combination of systemic IL-2 and lymphocytes activated by IL-2 has been reported to result in the regression of pulmonary tumors in a murine model.[79] Given that the immunomodulatory effects of IL-2, at least in vitro, depend on the dose of the lymphokine to which peripheral blood lymphocytes are exposed, attempts at defining dosage regimens are of the utmost importance. Mitchell and colleagues[87] have demonstrated that LAK cells may be generated in humans after the administration of minimally toxic doses of IL-2. Dose-limiting toxicity of intravenous IL-2 has been reported by Lotze and colleagues.[69] This toxicity was manifested by fever, malaise, anorexia, gastrointestinal symptoms, and weight gain. Kedar and colleagues[52] reported that high-dose IL-2 may elicit immunosuppression mediated by lymphokine-activated killer cells and nonspecific suppressor cells.

The cooperative study on using IFN-β as therapy for glioblastoma and malignant astrocytoma reported response rates of 24.0 percent in low-grade glioma and 20.0 percent in medulloblastoma. Overall, a response rate of 19.2 percent was reported for 120 cases. When IFN-β therapy was combined with chemotherapy (using ACNU) and radiotherapy, the response rate was 41.2 percent, as opposed to 19.6 percent for patients treated with ACNU and radiation alone. Interferon-β is also being evaluated as maintenance therapy for malignant glial tumors.[95] Rosenblum and colleagues assessed the antiproliferative effects of human recombinant IFN-α and IFN-β in vitro against seven human glioma cell lines. They suggest that while these cell lines bound both IFN-α and IFN-β, the biological response may be due to only certain IFN subtypes.[118]

Nezu and colleagues have reported that IFN-γ activates a receptor-mediated calcium influx via the second messenger protein kinase C with subsequent induction of HLA class II expression on glioblastoma cell lines.[98] Wen and colleagues corroborated this finding by reporting that IFN-γ increased class I MHC expression in 9L cells in vitro. Intratumor injections of IFN-γ led to increased numbers of inflammatory cells in the tumor and class II^+ mononuclear phagocytes at its periphery, and increased MHC class I or II expression by endothelial and ependymal cells.[143]

Adhesion Molecules

Adhesion molecules may play a role in the homing of immune cells to tumors and in the regulation of tumor invasion. A more complete understanding of adhesion molecule expression on immune cells and/or gliomas may one day permit us to modulate this expression to enhance tumor kill by the immune system. In addition, manipulation of molecules involved in the adhesion of tumor cells to the extracellular matrix or to endothelial cells may increase our ability to limit local invasion.[22] Adhesion molecules have been found to be expressed on glioma cells, tumor-infiltrating lymphocytes, and endothelial cells in tumors.

With regard to the involvement of glial cells in the immune response, it has been found that the synthesis of inducible proteins such as intercellular adhesion molecule-1 (ICAM-1) was required for glial cells to assist in the induction of anti-CD3 antibody-mediated proliferation of T cells.[148] Immunohistochemical evaluation of frozen tissue sections has demonstrated that glioblastoma cells and intratumoral vessel cells express ICAM-1, CD44, and lymphocyte function-associated antigen-3 (LFA-3). Antibodies to LFA-1α, LFA-1β, and ICAM-1 were found to block the binding of LAK cells or TILs to human glioblastoma cells. Thus it is likely that these molecules play a role in the binding and subsequent migration of lymphocytes into brain tumor tissue.[62]

An anti-GD2 mAb (DMAb-20) was shown to be specific for 16 of 20 (80 percent) malignant gliomas and for 5 of 5 medulloblastoma cell lines. DMAb-20 levels were also higher in the glioma and medulloblastoma cell lines than in normal brain. Longee and colleagues conclude that DMAb-20 will be useful in determining the functional role of GD2 in cell-cell interaction, adhesion, and invasion in in vitro models.[68]

ICAM-1 has recently been identified as one of the ligands for LFA-1. Kuppner and colleagues have demonstrated ICAM-1 expression on human glioblastoma cells and neovascular endothelial cells. In addition, the expression of ICAM-1 in glioblastoma cells was similar to the expression of MHC class II. Incubation of tumor with IL-1β, TNF-α, and IFN-γ increased the surface expression of ICAM-1.[64] Suramin, a polysulfonated naphthylurea, has been found to inhibit astrocytoma proliferation. This inhibition was caused by an accumulation of the neural cell adhesion molecule at the cell surface.[36]

Genetic Manipulation

Progress toward Gene Therapy and Molecular Neurosurgery

One of the most exciting areas of molecular biology is the potential for gene therapy, in which a disease would be corrected by either modifying the expression of a mutant gene or introducing new genetic information into defective tissue in vivo. Means exist to alter the coding sequence of a gene or its regulatory regions so as to change either the functional properties of the protein product or the amount of product produced. The result of the genetic modification can be analyzed by inserting the gene into an expression vector. In addition, engineered genes can be inserted permanently into the germ line of mice, producing transgenic animals that display the effect of the modified or aberrantly expressed gene. Transgenic animals have provided important information on the regulation of mammalian genes and on oncogenes. For example, transgenic mice with tissue cells expressing either the *myc* or the H-*ras* oncogene have cells that grow at an increased rate; a few of the cells may develop into neural tumors.

Direct gene replacement can also now be achieved. Advances in the understanding of molecular biology and human disease have made gene therapy a realizable goal. The replacement or correction of a gene at its normal site in the genome is just beginning to be developed and refined experimentally. More practical are approaches for modifying the effects of mutant genes in defective cells by introducing normal genes (i.e., gene augmentation). One method is the introduction of genetic information at nontargeted sites to provide a functional gene product without the removal or correction of the endogenous mutant gene.

Retroviruses have been proved useful for many in vitro studies. Retroviruses can infect a broad range of species and tissue types, integrate efficiently into the host genome, and, in general, do not injure their host cells. Unfortunately their usefulness in vivo is limited by the fact that high viral titers are needed for the transduction and expression of modified DNA sequences in nonreplicating or fully differentiated postmitotic cells such as neurons. Because of these difficulties, neurotropic vectors such as herpesviruses have become interesting for the delivery of modified genetic information to neurons throughout the CNS. Over the past 10 years, various immunotherapeutic regimens have been reported to result in tumor regression in a subset of patients with advanced metastatic disease. Attempts have been made to use gene therapy to augment these regimens.

Moses and colleagues have mapped an IFN-γ-responsive element upstream of the DRA promoter in a glioblastoma multiforme line. This region of the HLA-DRA gene is necessary for IFN-γ inducibility.[93] In an interesting study, four glioma cell lines that did not express HLA-DR or HLA-DQ did so after transfection with genes encoding HLA-DR and DQ. Most important, the tumor cells then elicited an enhanced immune response (as judged by the mixed leukocyte reaction).[153]

Transfection of the human glioblastoma multiforme cell line GBM-18 with an expression-vector plasmid containing the human multidrug resistance gene pHaMDR1/A has been used to study the effect of drug resistance on the response to recombinant IFN-β and IFN-γ.[114] Miyatake and colleagues have suggested that the transfection of cytotoxic T lymphocytes with the IFN-γ gene could serve as a means to improve the efficacy of adoptive immunotherapy against cancer.[92]

In a more recent study, the expression of T-cell receptor (TCR) genes in tumor infiltrating lymphocytes in human malignant brain tumors was examined. Certain specific TCR genes were preferentially expressed. It was concluded that TILs with such expression could be isolated, propagated, and used therapeutically for the treatment of malignant brain tumors.[101]

Nitta and colleagues have described a method for incorporating surrogate receptors into effector cells, thereby enhancing the toxicity of the killer cells by directing them specifically to the desired target glioma cells. In studies, these cells showed more lytic potential than did ordinary, antibody-dependent cellular cytotoxicity.[105] Clinical applications are being pursued.

Humphrey and colleagues have indicated that it is possible to generate site-specific antipeptide antibodies that are highly selective for mutant proteins in human tumors.[40] Specifically, human gliomas have been described that amplify and rearrange the epidermal growth factor receptor gene. Site-specific antipeptide antibodies have been developed that react selectively to the glioma deletion mutant.

Gene expression of products resultant from the introduction of foreign genes into eukaryotic hosts is the basis for success in gene therapy. Certain lymphocytic populations can be safely labeled and followed in vivo.[50,117] A gene coding for neomycin phosphotransferase was introduced into tumor-infiltrating lymphocytes with murine leukemia retrovirus.[10] Neomycin phosphotransferase confers resistance to the antibiotic neomycin, thus allowing adoptively transferred TILs to be distinguished from host lymphocytes. Southern blotting and the polymerase chain reaction indicated that one copy of the viral genome was present in each recipient TIL.

Given the obvious safety and efficacy of retroviral-mediated gene transduction and the observation that TILs accumulated at tumor sites, attempts were made to enhance the cytotoxicity of these cells for specific tumors.[29,35] A gene for the cytokine TNF-α was introduced into TILs by means of a murine leukemia retrovirus. Clinical trials are in progress using TNF gene-modified TILs in patients with advanced cancer. In addition, studies evaluating the insertion of other cytokines, including IL-2, IL-4, and IFN-γ, as well as class 1 major MHC antigen, into TILs are under way.[7,31,32,142]

In cell culture, a thymidine kinase-negative mutant of herpes simplex virus-1 was able to eradicate both long- and short-term human glioma cell lines. Intraneoplastic administration of this mutant virus inhibited tumor growth in nude mice with implanted subcutaneous and subrenal human gliomas and prolonged survival in mice with intracranial U87 gliomas.[76]

The in situ administration of genetic material into rapidly proliferating tumors in an environment of nondividing neural tissue has been evaluated as a potential therapeutic option. Murine fibroblasts underwent the insertion of a herpes simplex thymidine kinase (HS-tk) gene that allowed for the production of a retroviral vector. Rats with a cerebral glioma received stereotactic injection of HS-tk in this model. Following the transduction of the glioma cells, the rats were treated with the anti-herpes drug ganciclovir with subsequent complete tumor regression.[23]

References

1. Adachi K, Belser P, Bender H, et al. Enhancement of epidermal growth factor receptor expression on glioma cells by recombinant tumor necrosis factor alpha. *Cancer Immunol Immunother* 1992; 34:370–376.
2. Agah R, Malloy B, Sherrod A, et al. Therapy of disseminated Nk-resistant tumor by the synergistic effects of recombinant interleukin-2 and tumor necrosis factor. *J Biol Response Mod* 1988; 7:140–151.
3. Agah R, Malloy B, Sherrod A, Mazumder A. Successful therapy of natural killer-resistant pulmonary metastases by the synergism of gamma-interferon with tumor necrosis factor and interleukin-2 in mice. *Cancer Res* 1988; 48:2245–2248.
4. Akbasak A, Oldfield EH, Saris SC. Expression and modulation of major histocompatibility antigens on murine primary brain tumor in vitro. *J Neurosurg* 1991; 75:922–929.
5. Allegranza A, Girlando S, Arrigoni GL, et al. Proliferating cell nuclear antigen expression in central nervous system neoplasms. *Virchows Arch [A]* 1991; 419:417–423.
6. Apuzzo MLJ, Mitchell MS. Immunological aspects of intrinsic glial tumors. *J Neurosurg* 1981; 55:1–18.
7. Asher AL, Mule JJ, Kasid A, et al. Murine tumor cells transduced with the gene for tumor necrosis factor-alpha. Evidence for paracrine immune effects of tumor necrosis factor against tumors. *J Immunol* 1991; 146:3227–3234.
8. Band PR, Jao-King C, Urtasun RC, Haraphongse M. Phase I study of *Corynebacterium parvum* in patients with solid tumors. *Cancer Chemother Rep* 1975; 59:1139–1145.
9. Bender H, Takahashi H, Adachi K, et al. Immunotherapy of human glioma xenografts with unlabeled, ^{131}I-, or ^{125}I-labeled monoclonal antibody 425 to epidermal growth factor receptor. *Cancer Res* 1992; 52:121–126.
10. Bender MA, Palmer TD, Gelinas RE, et al. Evidence that the packaging signal of Moloney murine leukemia virus extends into the *gag* region. *J Virol* 1987; 61:1639–1646.
11. Bergh J, Nilsson S, Liljedahl C, et al. Radioimaging of human malignant gliomas using indium-labelled monoclonal antibodies. *Nucl Med Commun* 1990; 11:437–444.
12. Bigner DD, Pitts OM, Wikstrand CJ. Induction of lethal experimental allergic encephalomyelitis in nonhuman primates and guinea pigs with human glioblastoma multiforme tissue. *J Neurosurg* 1981; 55:32–42.
13. Bilzer T, Stavrou D, Dahme E, et al. Morphological, immunocytochemical and growth characteristics of three human glioblastomas established in vitro. *Virchows Arch [A]* 1991; 418:281–293.
14. Bilzer T, Stavrou D, Wechsler W, et al. Antigen variation in a human glioblastoma: from the primary tumor to the second recurrence, permanent cell line and xenotransplantation tumors. *Anticancer Res* 1991; 11:547–553.

15. Biological Response Modifiers: Subcommittee Report. *Natl Cancer Inst* 1983; Monograph 63.
16. Bloom HJG, Peckham MJ, Richardson AE, et al. Glioblastoma multiforme: a controlled trial to assess the value of specific active immunotherapy in patients treated by radical surgery and radiotherapy. *Br J Cancer* 1973; 27:253–267.
17. Bloom WH, Carstairs KC, Crompton MR, McKissock W. Autologous glioma transplantation. *Lancet* 1960; 2:77–78.
18. Bosnes V, Hirschberg H. Comparison of in vitro glioma cell cytotoxicity of LAK cells from glioma patients and healthy subjects. *J Neurosurg* 1988; 69:234–238.
19. Brady LW, Markoe AM, Woo DV, et al. Iodine-125 labeled anti-epidermal growth factor receptor-425 in the treatment of malignant astrocytomas. A pilot study. *J Neurosurg Sci* 1990; 34:243–249.
20. Cohen MH, Chretien PB, Ihde DC, et al. Thymosin fraction V and intensive combination chemotherapy: prolonging the survival of patients with small-cell lung cancer. *JAMA* 1979; 241:1813–1815.
21. Colapinto EV, Zalutsky MR, Archer GE, et al. Radioimmunotherapy of intracerebral human glioma xenografts with ^{131}I-labeled F(ab′)2 fragments of monoclonal antibody Mel-14. *Cancer Res* 1990; 50:1822–1827.
22. Couldwell WT, de Tribolet N, Antel JP, et al. Adhesion molecules and malignant gliomas: implications for tumorigenesis. *J Neurosurg* 1992; 76:782–791.
23. Culver KW, Ram Z, Wallbridge S, Ishii H. In vivo gene transfer with retroviral vector-producer cells for treatment of experimental brain tumors. *Science* 1992; 256:1-150–1152.
24. Dan MD, Schlachta CM, Guy J, et al. Human antiglioma monoclonal antibodies from patients with astrocytic tumors. *J Neurosurg* 1992; 76:660–669.
25. de Muralt B, de Tribolet N, Diserens AC, et al. Reactivity of antiglioma monoclonal antibodies for a large panel of cultured gliomas and other neuroectoderm derived tumors. *Anticancer Res* 1983; 3:1–6.
26. de Tribolet N, Frank E, Mach JP. Monoclonal antibodies: their application in the diagnosis and management of CNS tumors. *Clin Neurosurg* 1988; 34:446–456.
27. Detta A, Hitchcock E. Rapid estimation of the proliferating index of brain tumours. *J Neurooncol* 1990; 8:245–253.
28. Duff TA, Borden E, Bay J, et al. Phase II trial of interferon-Beta for treatment of recurrent glioblastoma multiforme. *J Neurosurg* 1986; 64:408–413,
29. Fisher B, Packard BS, Read EJ, et al. Tumor localization of adoptively transferred indium-111 labeled tumor infiltrating lymphocytes in patients with metastatic melanoma. *J Clin Oncol* 1989; 7:250–261.
30. Franke FE, Schachenmayr W, Osborn M, Altmannsberger M. Unexpected immunoreactivities of intermediate filament antibodies in human brain and brain tumors. *Am J Pathol* 1991; 139:67–79.
31. Gansbacher B, Bannerji R, Daniels B, et al. Retroviral vector-mediated gamma-interferon gene transfer into tumor cells generates potent and long lasting antitumor immunity. *Cancer Res* 1990; 50:7820–7825.
32. Gansbacher B, Zier K, Daniels B, et al. Interleukin 2 gene transfer into tumor cells abrogates tumorigenicity and induces protective immunity. *J Exp Med* 1990; 172:1217–1224.
33. Gerdes J, Schwab U, Lemke H, Stein H. Production of a mouse monoclonal antibody reactive with a human nuclear antigen associated with cell proliferation. *Int J Cancer* 1983; 31:13–20.
34. Grace JT Jr, Perese DM, Metzgar RS, et al. Tumor autograft responses in patients with glioblastoma multiforme. *J Neurosurg* 1961; 18:159–167.
35. Griffith KD, Read EJ, Carrasquillo JA, et al. In vivo distribution of adoptively transferred indium-111-labeled tumor infiltrating lymphocytes and peripheral blood lymphocytes in patients with metastatic melanoma. *J Natl Cancer Inst* 1989; 81:1709–1717.
36. Guo XJ, Fantini J, Roubin R, et al. Evaluation of the effect of suramin on neural cell growth and N-CAM expression. *Cancer Res* 1990; 50:5164–5170.
37. Hayashi K, Hoshida Y, Horie Y, et al. Immunohistochemical study on the distribution of alpha and beta subunits of S-100 protein in brain tumors. *Acta Neuropathol (Berl)* 1991; 81:657–663.
38. He XM, Wikstrand CJ, Friedman HS, et al. Differentiation characteristics of newly established medulloblastoma cell lines (D384 Med, D425 Med, and D458 Med) and their transplantable xenografts. *Lab Invest* 1991; 6:833–843.
39. Holladay FP, Lopez G, De M, et al. Generation of cytotoxic immune responses against a rat glioma by in vivo priming and secondary in vitro stimulation with tumor cells. *Neurosurgery* 1992; 30:499–505.
40. Humphrey PA, Wong AJ, Vogelstein B, et al. Anti-synthetic peptide antibody reacting at the fusion junction of deletion-mutant epidermal growth factor receptors in human glioblastoma. *Proc Natl Acad Sci USA* 1990; 87:4207–4211.
41. Iwasaki K. Infiltrative and cytolytic activities of lymphokine-activated killer (LAK) cells against a human glioma mass: ultrastructural analysis using a three-dimensional multicellular spheroid model. *Nippon Geka Hokan* 1990; 59:39–54.
42. Iwasaki K, Kikuchi H, Miyatake S, et al. Infiltrative and cytolytic activities of lymphokine-activated killer cells against a human glioma spheroid model. *Cancer Res* 1990; 50:2429–2436.
43. Iwasaki K, Kikuchi H, Miyatake S, et al. Clonal analysis in the ultrastructure of cell-to-cell interaction between a human glioma cell line and autologous tumor-specific cytotoxic T lymphocytes. *Cell Immunol* 1990; 126:164–175.
44. Jaaskelainen J, Lehtonen E, Heikkila P, et al. Damage to multicellular human H-2 glioma spheroids incubated with LAK cells: an ultrastructural study. *J Natl Cancer Inst* 1990; 82:497–501.
45. Jacobs SK, Wilson DJ, Kornblith PL, Grimm EA. In vitro killing of human glioblastoma by interleukin-2-activated autologous lymphocytes. *J Neurosurg* 1986; 64:114–117.
46. Jacobs SK, Wilson DJ, Kornblith PL, Grimm EA. Interleukin-2 and autologous lymphokine-activated killer cells in the treatment of malignant glioma: preliminary report. *J Neurosurg* 1986; 64:743–749.
47. Jennings MT, Asadourian LL, Jennings VD, et al. Factor analysis of the immunophenotypes of astrocytomas and malignant gliomas: correlations with tumor grade and patient survival. *J Neurooncol* 1990; 9:265–273.
48. Jones NR, Rossi ML, Gregoriou M, Hughes JT. Investigation of the expression of epidermal growth factor receptor and blood group A antigen in 110 human gliomas. *Neuropathol Appl Neurobiol* 1990; 16:185–192.
49. Kaluza J, Adamek D. Expression of GFAP (glial fibrillary acidic protein) antigenicity and differentiation of glioma tumor cells of astrocytic origin. *Folia Histochem Cytobiol* 1990; 28:155–159.
50. Kasid A, Morecki S, Aebersold P, et al. Human gene transfer: characterization of human tumor-infiltrating lymphocytes as vehicles for retroviral-mediated gene transfer in man. *Proc Natl Acad Sci USA* 1990; 87:473–477.
51. Kawamoto K, Fujiwara H, Numa Y, Matsumura H. Antineoplastic effects of natural killer cells sorted with flow cytometry on brain tumors. *Hum Cell* 1991; 4:157–164.
52. Kedar E, Rezai AR, Giorgi JV, et al. Immunomodulating effects in vitro of interleukin-2 and interferon-gamma on human blood and bone marrow mononuclear cells. *Nat Immun Cell Growth Regul* 1988; 7:13–30.
53. Kikuchi T, Sakai H, Nakamura N, et al. Analysis of cytolytic activity and cell surface phenotypes of lymphokine activated killer cells stimulated with R-IL-2 and an anti-CD3 antibody. *No To Shinkei* 1990; 42:575–580.
54. Kikuchi T, Watanabe M, Ohno T. Cytological characteristics of human glioma-infiltrating lymphocytes stimulated with recombinant interleukin 2 and an anti-CD3 antibody. *Jpn J Cancer Res* 1991; 82:339–345.
55. Kim B, Warnaker P, Iverson M, Imbembo AL. Immunotherapy of pulmonary metastases using monoclonal antibody to T-cell suppressor factor and interleukin-2. *Arch Surg* 1987; 122:1455–1459.
56. Knott JC, Pilkington GJ. A2B5 surface ganglioside binding distinguishes between two GFAP-positive clones from a human glioma-derived cell line. *Neurosci Lett* 1990; 118:52–56.

57. Kohler G, Milstein C. Continuous cultures of fused cells secreting antibody of predefined specificity. *Nature* 1975; 256:495–497.
58. Kokunai T, Tamaki N, Matsumoto S. Antigen related to cell proliferation in malignant gliomas recognized by a human monoclonal antibody. *J Neurosurg* 1990; 73:901–908.
59. Korosue K, Takeshita I, Mannoji H, Fukui M. Interferon effects on multiplication, cytoplasmic protein and GFAP content, and morphology in human glioma cells. *J Neurooncol* 1983; 1:69–76.
60. Kruse CA, Lillehei KO, Mitchell DH, et al. Analysis of interleukin 2 and various effector cell populations in adoptive immunotherapy of 9L rat gliosarcoma: allogeneic cytotoxic T lymphocytes prevent tumor take. *Proc Natl Acad Sci USA* 1990; 87:9577–9581.
61. Kunishio K, Mishima N, Matsuhisa T, et al. Immunohistochemical demonstration of DNA polymerase alpha in human brain-tumor cells. *J Neurosurg* 1990; 72:268–272.
62. Kuppner MC, Hamou MF, de Tribolet N. Activation and adhesion molecule expression on lymphoid infiltrates in human glioblastomas. *J Neuroimmunol* 1990; 29:229–238.
63. Kuppner MC, van Meir E, Gauthier T, et al. Differential expression of the CD44 molecule in human brain tumours. *Int J Cancer* 1992; 4:572–577.
64. Kuppner MC, van Meir E, Hamou MF, de Tribolet N. Cytokine regulation of intercellular adhesion molecule-1 (ICAM-1) expression on human glioblastoma cells. *Clin Exp Immunol* 1991; 81:142–148.
65. Lee WH, Yeh MY, Tu YC. Tumor localization of human brain malignant glioma xenograft in nude mice with a radiolabeled monoclonal antibody. *Neurosurgery* 1990; 26:381–390.
66. Lillehei KO, Mitchell DH, Johnson SD, et al. Long-term follow-up of patients with recurrent malignant gliomas treated with adjuvant adoptive immunotherapy. *Neurosurgery* 1991; 28:16–23.
67. Lisianyi KI, Markova OV, Romodanov SA. Sensitivity of human glial tumor cells of different grade of anaplasia to lysis due to natural killers depending on some characteristics of the glycoprotein structure of tumor cell membranes. *Biull Eksp Biol Med* 1991; 112:190–191.
68. Longee DC, Wikstrand CJ, Mansson JE, et al. Disialoganglioside GD2 in human neuroectodermal tumor cell lines and gliomas. *Acta Neuropathol (Berl)* 1991; 82:45–54.
69. Lotze MT, Matory YL, Ettinghausen SE, et al. In vivo administration of purified human interleukin 2. II: Half life, immunologic effects, and expansion of peripheral lymphoid cells in vivo with recombinant IL 2. *J Immunol* 1985; 135:2865–2875.
70. Louis DN, Edgerton S, Thor AD, et al. Proliferating cell nuclear antigen and Ki-67 immunohistochemistry in brain tumors: a comparative study. *Acta Neuropathol (Berl)* 1991; 81:675–679.
71. Lundblad D, Lundgren E. Block of glioma cell line in S by interferon. *Int J Cancer* 1981; 27:749–754.
72. Mahaley MS Jr, Bertsch L, Cush S, Gillespie GY. Systemic gamma-interferon therapy for recurrent gliomas. *J Neurosurg* 1988; 69:826–829.
73. Mahaley MS Jr, Steinbok P, Aronin P, et al. Immunobiology of primary intracranial tumors. *J Neurosurg* 1981; 54:220–227.
74. Mahaley MS Jr, Urso MB, Whaley RA, Blue M. Immunobiology of primary intracranial tumors. Part 10: Therapeutic efficacy of interferon in the treatment of recurrent gliomas. *J Neurosurg* 1985; 63:719–725.
75. Maleci A, Alterman RL, Sundstrom D, et al. Effect of phorbol esters on the susceptibility of a glioma cell line to lymphokine-activated killer cell activity. *J Neurosurg* 1990; 73:91–97.
76. Martuza RL, Malick A, Markert JM, et al. Experimental therapy of human glioma by means of a genetically engineered virus mutant. *Science* 1991; 252:854–856.
77. Matsuda M, Fischer DK, Narayan RK, Atassi MZ. Preparation and characterization of antisera and of murine monoclonal antibodies to human glioma-associated antigen(s). *Adv Exp Med Biol* 1991; 303:271–283.
78. Matsuura H, Imaya H. Comparison of lymphokine-activated killer activities between thymocytes and splenocytes in rats with brain tumors. *Cancer Immunol Immunother* 1991; 33:50–53.
79. Mazumder A, Rosenberg SA. Successful immunotherapy of natural killer-resistant established pulmonary melanoma metastases by the intravenous adoptive transfer of syngenic lymphocytes activated in vitro by interleukin 2. *J Exp Med* 1984; 159:495–507.
80. McComb RD, Bigner DD. The biology of malignant gliomas: a comprehensive survey. *Clin Neuropathol* 1984; 3:93–106.
81. McKeever PE, Davenport RD, Shakui P. Patterns of antigenic expression of human glioma cells. *Crit Rev Neurobiol* 1991; 6:119–147.
82. Merchant RE, Ellison MD, Young HF. Immunotherapy for malignant glioma using human recombinant interleukin-2 and activated autologous lymphocytes. A review of pre-clinical and clinical investigations. *J Neurooncol* 1990; 8:173–188.
83. Merchant RE, McVicar DW, Merchant LH, Young HF. Long-term follow-up of patients with recurrent malignant glioma treated with intraparenchymal injections of lymphokine-activated killer cells and recombinant interleukin-2. Presented at the 57th Annual Meeting of the American Association of Neurological Surgeons, Washington, DC, April 3, 1989.
84. Mihara Y, Matsukado Y, Goto S, et al. Monoclonal antibody against ependymoma-derived cell line. *J Neurooncol* 1992; 12:1–11.
85. Miki Y, Sano K, Takakura K, Mizutani H. Adjuvant immunotherapy with BCG for malignant brain tumors. *Neurol Med Chir (Tokyo)* 1976; 16:357–364.
86. Mitchell MS. Principles of tumor immunology and their application to the biomodulation of cancer. In Calabresi P, Schein PS (eds): *Medical Oncology,* 2d ed. New York: McGraw-Hill, 1993, pp 323–344.
87. Mitchell MS, Kempf RA, Harel W, et al. Effectiveness and tolerability of low-dose cyclophosphamide and low-dose intravenous interleukin-2 in disseminated melanoma. *J Clin Oncol* 1988; 6:409–424.
88. Mitchell MS, Murahata RI. Modulation of immunity by bacillus Calmette-Guerin (BCG). *Pharmacol Ther* 1979; 4:329–353.
89. Mitchell MS, Oettgen HF (eds). *Hybridomas in Cancer Diagnosis and Treatment.* (*Progress in Cancer Research and Therapy,* vol 21). New York: Raven Press, 1982.
90. Miyatake S, Kikuchi H, Oda Y, et al. Decreased susceptibility of lined human gliosarcoma cells to lymphokine-activated killer cell cytolysis by gamma-interferon treatment. *Cancer Res* 1990; 50:596–600.
91. Miyatake S, Kondou S, Aoki T, et al. Immunomodulatory effects of interferons on target human gliosarcoma cells in the tumor-specific CTL- and LAK-mediated cytolysis. *No Shinkei Geka* 1991; 19:1053–1059.
92. Miyatake S, Nishihara K, Kikuchi H, et al. Efficient tumor suppression by glioma-specific murine cytotoxic T lymphocytes transfected with interferon-gamma gene. *J Natl Cancer Inst* 1990; 82:217–220.
93. Moses H, Sasaki A, Ting JP. Identification of an interferon-gamma-responsive element of a class II major histocompatibility gene in rat type 1 astrocytes. *J Neuroimmunol* 1991; 31:273–278.
94. Myers RL, Whisler RL, Stephens RE, et al. Sensitivity of human glioma and brain cells to natural killer cell lysis. Effects of serum concentration, epidermal growth factor, and time in culture. *J Neurosurg* 1992; 76:986–990.
95. Nagai M. Advances of BRM therapy of malignant brain tumors. *Gan To Kagaku Ryoho* 1991; 18:188–194.
96. Nagai M, Arai T. Clinical effect of interferon in malignant brain tumours. *Neurosurg Rev* 1984; 7:55–64.
97. Nederman T, Benediktsson G. Effects of interferon on the growth rate and radiation sensitivity of cultured, human glioma cells. *Acta Radiol Oncol* 1982; 21:231–234.
98. Nezu N, Ryu K, Koide Y, Yoshida TO. Regulation of HLA class II molecule expressions by IFN-gamma. The signal transduction mechanism in glioblastoma cell lines. *J Immunol* 1990; 145:3126–3135.
99. Nishimura T, Nakamura Y, Takeuchi Y, et al. Bispecific antibody-directed antitumor activity of human CD4+ helper/killer T cells induced by anti-CD3 monoclonal antibody plus interleukin 2. *Jpn J Cancer Res* 1991; 82:1207–1210.
100. Nishimura T, Nakamura Y, Takeuchi Y, et al. Generation, propagation, and targeting of human CD4+ helper/killer T cells induced by anti-CD3 monoclonal antibody plus recombinant IL 2. An efficient

strategy for adoptive tumor immunotherapy. *J Immunol* 1992; 148:285–291.
101. Nitta T, Ikeda M, Cogen P, et al. T cell receptor repertoire in tumor infiltrating lymphocytes within malignant brain tumors. *No Shinkei Geka* 1992; 20:559–566.
102. Nitta T, Ishizawa A, Ito M, et al. Induction of cytotoxicity from human lymphocytes coated with bispecific antibody against human glioma cells. *No Shinkei Geka* 1990; 18:1001–1006.
103. Nitta T, Sato K, Okumura K, Ishii S. Induction of cytotoxicity in human T cells coated with anti-glioma × anti-CD3 bispecific antibody against human glioma cells. *J Neurosurg* 1990; 72:476–481.
104. Nitta T, Sato K, Yagita H, et al. Preliminary trial of specific targeting therapy against malignant glioma. *Lancet* 1990; 335:368–371.
105. Nitta T, Yagita H, Sato K, Okumura K. Surrogate receptor-mediated cellular cytotoxicity against malignant human glioma cells. *Neurosurgery* 1991; 280:394–399.
106. Numa Y, Kawamoto K, Matsumura H. Multidisciplinary therapy using interferon and immunological evaluation for glioma patients: two-color analysis of T cell subsets. *No Shinkei Geka* 1991; 19:121–128.
107. Parkins CS, Darling JL, Gill SS, et al. Cell proliferation in serial biopsies through human malignant brain tumours: measurement using Ki67 antibody labelling. *Br J Neurosurg* 1991; 5:289–298.
108. Parrillo JE, Fauci AS. Mechanisms of corticosteroid action on lymphocyte subpopulations. III: Differential effects of dexamethasone administration on subpopulations of effector cells mediating cellular cytotoxicity in man. *Clin Exp Immunol* 1978; 31:116–125.
109. Pollack IF, Randall MS, Kristofik MP, et al. Response of low-passage human malignant gliomas in vitro to stimulation and selective inhibition of growth factor-mediated pathways. *J Neurosurg* 1991; 75:284–293.
110. Powles TJ, Bockman RS, Honn KV, Ramwell P (eds). *Prostaglandins and Cancer: First International Conference,* vol 2. New York: Alan R Liss, 1982.
111. Quackenbush EJ, Vera S, Greaves A, Letarte M. Confirmation by peptide sequence and coexpression on various cell types of the identity of CD44 and P85 glycoprotein. *Mol Immunol* 1990; 27:947–955.
112. Rasmussen HB, Teisner B, Schroder HD, et al. Fetal antigen 2 in primary and secondary brain tumors. *Tumour Biol* 1991; 12:330–338.
113. Recht LD, Griffin TW, Raso V, Salimi AR. Potent cytotoxicity of an antihuman transferrin receptor-ricin A-chain immunotoxin on human glioma cells in vitro. *Cancer Res* 1990; 50:6696–6700.
114. Reddy PG, Graham GM, Datta S, et al. Effect of recombinant fibroblast interferon and recombinant immune interferon on growth and the antigenic phenotype of multidrug-resistant human glioblastoma multiforme cells. *J Natl Cancer Inst* 1991; 83:1307–1315.
115. Riva P, Arista A, Sturiale C, et al. Treatment of intracranial human glioblastoma by direct intratumoral administration of ^{131}I-labelled anti-tenascin monoclonal antibody BC-2. *Int J Cancer* 1992; 51:7–13.
116. Rosenberg SA. Immunotherapy of cancer using interleukin-2: current status and future prospects. *Immunol Today* 1988; 9:58–62.
117. Rosenberg SA, Aebersold P, Cornetta K, et al. Gene transfer into humans: immunotherapy of patients with advanced melanoma, using tumor-infiltrating lymphocytes modified by retroviral gene transduction. *N Engl J Med* 1990; 323:570–578.
118. Rosenblum MG, Yung WK, Kelleher PJ, et al. Growth inhibitory effects of interferon-beta but not interferon-alpha on human glioma cells: correlation of receptor binding, 2′,5′-oligoadenylate synthetase and protein kinase activity. *J Interferon Res* 1990; 10:141–151.
119. Sawamura Y. Isolation and expansion of glioma-infiltrating lymphocytes in vitro: an analysis of their surface phenotypes and antitumor activities. Hokkaido Igaku Zasshi 1991; 66:868–878.
120. Sawamura Y, de Tribolet N. Immunobiology of brain tumors. *Adv Tech Stand Neurosurg* 1990; 17:3–64.
121. Schipper HM, Skalski V, Panasci LC, Wang E. Statin expression in the untreated and SarCNU-exposed human glioma cell line, SK-MG-1. *Cancer Chemother Pharmacol* 1990; 26:383–386.
122. Schrappe M, Klier FG, Spiro RC, et al. Correlation of chondroitin sulfate proteoglycan expression on proliferating brain capillary endothelial cells with the malignant phenotype of astroglial cells. *Cancer Res* 1991; 51:4986–4993.
123. Schroeder R, Bien K, Kott R, et al. The relationship between Ki-67 labeling and mitotic index in gliomas and meningiomas: demonstration of the variability of the intermitotic cycle time. *Acta Neuropathol (Berl)* 1991; 82:389–394.
124. Schuster JM, Garg PK, Bigner DD, Zalutsky MR. Improved therapeutic efficacy of a monoclonal antibody radioiodinated using N-succinimidyl-3-(tri-n-butylstannyl)benzoate. *Cancer Res* 1991; 51:4164–4169.
125. Selker RG, Wolmark N, Fisher B, Moore P. Preliminary observations on the use of *Corynebacterium parvum* in patients with primary intracranial tumors: effect on intracranial pressure. *J Surg Oncol* 1978; 10:299–303.
126. Shau H, Gray JD, Mitchell MS. Studies on the relationship of human natural killer and lymphokine-activated killer cells with lysosomal staining and analysis of surface marker phenotypes. *Cell Immunol* 1988; 115:13–23.
127. Stavrou D. Monoclonal antibodies in neuro-oncology. *Neurosurg Rev* 1990; 13:7–18.
128. Szymas J, Hossmann KA, Weber F, Oschlies U. Detection of Leu-M1 immunoreactivity in brain tissue and brain tumors. *Zentralbl Allg Pathol* 1990; 136:171–179.
129. Tada M, Aida T, Hosokawa M, et al. Antiproliferative effect of trapidil on PDGF-associated growth of human glioma cell lines in vitro. *Neurol Med Chir (Tokyo)* 1991; 31:313–317.
130. Takahashi H, Belser PH, Atkinson BF, et al. Monoclonal antibody-dependent, cell-mediated cytotoxicity against human malignant gliomas. *Neurosurgery* 1990; 27:97–102.
131. Takahashi JA, Fukumoto M, Kozai Y, et al. Inhibition of cell growth and tumorigenesis of human glioblastoma cells by a neutralizing antibody against human basic fibroblast growth factor. *FEBS Lett* 1991; 288:65–71.
132. Takakura K, Miki Y, Kubo O. Adjuvant immunotherapy for malignant brain tumors in infants and children. *Childs Brain* 1975; 1:141–147.
133. Takakura K, Miki Y, Kubo O, et al. Adjuvant immunotherapy for malignant brain tumors. *Jpn J Clin Oncol* 1972; 2:109–120.
134. Takamura S. Enhancement of mononuclear leukocyte-mediated antitumoral activity by cells of the B cell-line. *Gan No Rinsho* 1990; 36:457–477.
135. Terman DS, Young JB, Shearer WT, et al. Preliminary observations of the effects on breast adenocarcinoma of plasma perfused over immobilized protein A. *N Engl J Med* 1981; 305:1195–1200.
136. Torp SH, Helseth E, Dalen A, Unsgaard G. Epidermal growth factor receptor expression in human gliomas. *Cancer Immunol Immunother* 1991; 33:61–64.
137. Trouillas P. Immunologie et immunothérapie des tumeurs cérébrales: état actuel. *Rev Neurol (Paris)* 1973; 128:23–38.
138. Tsanaclis AM, Robert F, Michaud J, Brem S. The cycling pool of cells within human brain tumors: in situ cytokinetics using the monoclonal antibody Ki-67. *Can J Neurol Sci* 1991; 18:12–17.
139. Tzeng JJ, Barth RF, Clendenon NR, Gordon WA. Adoptive immunotherapy of a rat glioma using lymphokine-activated killer cells and interleukin 2. *Cancer Res* 1990; 50:4338–4343.
140. Tzeng JJ, Barth RF, Orosz CG. Quantitation of glioma-reactive cytolytic T lymphocyte precursors by means of limiting dilution analysis. *J Immunol Methods* 1992; 146:177–184.
141. Tzeng JJ, Barth RF, Orosz CG, James SM. Phenotype and functional activity of tumor-infiltrating lymphocytes isolated from immunogenic and nonimmunogenic rat brain tumors. *Cancer Res* 1991; 51:2373–2378.
142. Weber JS, Rosenberg SA. Effects of murine tumor MHC class 1 expression on the antitumor activity of tumor infiltrating lymphocytes. *J Natl Cancer Inst* 1990; 82:755–761.
143. Wen PY, Lampson MA, Lampson LA. Effects of gamma-interferon on major histocompatibility complex antigen expression and

lymphocytic infiltration in the 9L gliosarcoma brain tumor model: implications for strategies of immunotherapy. *J Neuroimmunol* 1992; 36:57–68.
144. Westphal M, Nausch H, Herrmann HD. Antigenic staining patterns of human glioma cultures: primary cultures, long-term cultures and cell lines. *J Neurocytol* 1990; 19:466–477.
145. Williams JA, Wessels BW, Edwards JA, et al. Targeting and therapy of human glioma xenografts in vivo utilizing radiolabeled antibodies. *Cancer Res* 1990; 50(Suppl):974–979.
146. Williams JA, Wessels BW, Wharam MD, et al. Targeting of human glioma xenografts in vivo utilizing radiolabeled antibodies. *Int J Radiat Oncol Biol Phys* 1990; 18:1367–1375.
147. Yakabayashi T, Yoshida J, Seo H, et al. Characterization of neuroectodermal antigen by a monoclonal antibody and its application in CSF diagnosis of human glioma. *J Neurosurg* 1988; 68:449–455.
148. Yamada M, Kakimoto K, Shinbori T, et al. Accessory function of human glioma cells for the induction of CD3-mediated T cell proliferation: a potential role of glial cells in T cell activation in the central nervous system. *J Neuroimmunol* 1992; 38:263–273.
149. Yamamoto RS, Coss J, Vayuvegula B, et al. Generation of stimulated, lymphokine activated T killer (T-LAK) cells from the peripheral blood of normal donors and adult patients with recurrent glioblastoma. *J Immunol Methods* 1991; 137:225–235.
150. Yoshida J, Kagayama N, Ueda R, Takahashi T. Human glioma associated and related antigens, identified by monoclonal antibodies. *Neurosurg Rev* 1984; 7:23–28.
151. Yoshida J, Mizuno M, Inoue I, et al. Radioimaging of human glioma xenografts with ^{123}I labeled monoclonal antibody G-22 against glioma-associated antigen. *J Neurooncol* 1990; 8:221–229.
152. Yoshida J, Wakabayashi T, Kito A, et al. Clinical application of monoclonal antibodies against glioma-associated antigens. *Prog Exp Tumor Res* 1987; 30:44–56.
153. Yoshida S, Takahashi H, Tanaka R. Expression of MHC class II antigens on human glioma cells modulated by transfection with genes encoding these antigens. *Neurol Med Chir (Tokyo)* 1991; 31:623–628.
154. Yoshida S, Tanaka R, Ono K. Serological analysis of tumor antigens in malignant glioma patients. *Neurol Med Chir (Tokyo)* 1991; 31:559–562.
155. Young H, Kaplan A, Regelson W. Immunotherapy with autologous white cell infusions (''lymphocytes'') in the treatment of recurrent glioblastoma multiform. *Cancer* 1977; 40:1037–1044.
156. Yron I, Wood TA Jr, Spiess PJ, Rosenberg SA. In vitro growth of murine T cells. V: The isolation and growth of lymphoid cells infiltrating syngeneic solid tumors. *J Immunol* 1980; 125:238–245.
157. Zuber P, Hamou M-F, de Tribolet N. Identification of proliferating cells in human gliomas using the monoclonal antibody Ki-67. *Neurosurgery* 1988; 22:364–368.

189

Chemotherapy of Primary Brain Tumors

S. Clifford Schold, Jr.
J. Gregory Cairncross
Ramesh Sajpaul

Standard forms of treatment for patients afflicted with primary malignant brain tumors have had only limited success. Surgery and radiotherapy prolong survival, but cures are rare. These limitations and the success chemotherapy has achieved in other types of cancer led to an assessment of the value of antineoplastic drug therapy in patients with malignant brain tumors. Although major advances in treatment have been limited, there has been progress in several areas of clinical importance. Prognostic factors that influence outcome have been identified; the science of prospective controlled clinical trials has been refined; unequivocal antineoplastic activity has been documented in some patients using some forms of chemotherapy; and these initial steps have stimulated detailed investigations of basic aspects of brain tumor chemotherapy. Studies of the blood-brain barrier and its manipulation, of blood flow and metabolic activity in normal and neoplastic brain, and of the molecular basis of drug resistance, as well as the development of chemosensitivity testing of human brain tumors, represent active areas of research with potential for clinical impact.

History and Basic Principles

History

The history of brain tumor chemotherapy begins shortly after the introduction of the first antineoplastic chemicals in the late 1940s and early 1950s. Pioneer neurosurgeons such as B. Woodhall, G. Odom, G. Owens, C. Wilson, J. French, and M. S. Mahaley, among others, used agents such as nitrogen mustard, vincristine, and mithramycin to treat patients with anaplastic gliomas. This early work, which was necessarily based on limited experimental data, demonstrated the technical feasibility of intracarotid drug administration, the potential brain and eye toxicity of some of these agents, and the limited efficacy of even highly aggressive approaches.[26] However, there were a few apparent responses, and these investigators can be credited with laying the foundation for the modern era of brain tumor chemotherapy.

In 1962 the nitrosoureas were introduced. These drugs were of special importance to those interested in nervous system tumors because of their impressive efficacy in experimental intracranial tumors. 1,3-bis(2-chloroethyl)-1-nitrosourea (carmustine or BCNU), the most active nitrosourea experimentally, also showed activity in patients with recurrent gliomas, and it was introduced into large-scale clinical trials. The use of the nitrosoureas and the introduction of the randomized clinical trial permanently changed the management of patients with anaplastic brain tumors. A new chemotherapeutic agent is now usually compared to a nitrosourea in carefully controlled trials.

Basic Principles of Cancer Chemotherapy

In the design and interpretation of chemotherapeutic trials, a number of basic principles must be considered (Table 189-1). First, the greater the tumor burden, the less effective are therapeutic maneuvers and the worse is the prognosis. This principle, which is intuitively obvious and which has now been demonstrated repeatedly in experimental systems, is especially important to the neurosurgeon dealing with primary brain tumors. Surgical decompression of a tumor is important not only to relieve symptoms and to establish a diagnosis, but also because it allows other forms of therapy to begin under more favorable circumstances. This will become increasingly important as more active drugs are introduced.

Second, there is often a steep dose-response curve with any chemotherapeutic agent.[14] The practical consequence of this principle is that antineoplastic agents should be given in the highest tolerated dose. Bone marrow toxicity is often the dose-limiting factor with anticancer drugs, and a certain degree of hematologic toxicity and risk should be accepted to be certain that as much of the drug as possible is being given. Circumventing the primary site of toxicity, such as by reinfusion of autologous bone marrow, allows use of higher doses and could improve therapeutic effects.

Third, it is now clear that, with few exceptions, curative cancer chemotherapy requires drug combinations.[8] There are many explanations for this, including tumor cell heterogeneity and acquired drug resistance, but if two or more drugs are available for the treatment of a particular tumor, their use in combination is likely to be more effective than using one drug alone. When used in combination, drugs again should be given at the maximum tolerated dose. While doses must be modified because of overlapping toxicity, often almost a full dose of each agent can be given without a significant increase in toxicity. Again, the importance of drug combinations in brain tumor chemotherapy will increase as more effective agents are introduced.

Fourth, scheduling of combined-modality therapy can influence results. When surgery, radiotherapy, and multiple-agent (or multiple-route) chemotherapy are considered, the permutations of treatment order are staggering, and it would be impractical to test all of them. Even when drugs alone are considered, certain agents, such as methotrexate, are much more effective in multiple lower

TABLE 189-1 Important Basic Principles of Cancer Chemotherapy

Therapeutic success is inversely related to tumor volume.
Dose-response curves are steep.
Drug combinations improve responses.
Therapeutic scheduling affects outcome.
Drugs must be delivered adequately.
Response must be carefully defined.

doses than in a single high dose; others, such as the alkylating agents, appear to be more effective in a single large dose. The order and timing of single doses of different agents can be important both because of "priming" of the tumor (by altering its kinetics) by one drug and because overlapping toxicity can be avoided.

Fifth, to be effective, an antineoplastic agent must be delivered appropriately to the tumor cells. The problem of adequate drug delivery is especially complex in tumors of the nervous system because of the variable preservation of the blood-brain barrier in these tumors. To the extent that the barrier is preserved in anaplastic brain tumors, efforts to either disrupt or circumvent it are important in delivering certain chemotherapeutic agents.

Finally, the problem of the evaluation of response to a drug must be addressed very carefully. "Response," "treatment failure," and similar terms must be defined precisely in any study or useful information may be lost. This again is especially difficult in brain tumor therapy because clinical deficits may persist even though the tumor mass is reduced and because neuroimaging may not always give an accurate representation of tumor burden.

Even though the introduction of active agents in brain tumor chemotherapy has been painfully slow, many basic principles of combined-modality cancer therapy are now understood. As new agents are introduced and alternate delivery routes refined, an appreciation of these basic principles will permit their optimal implementation in the brain tumor patient.

Development of New Drugs

Preclinical Evaluation of Potential Agents

The National Cancer Institute screens over 10,000 compounds annually for anticancer activity. Substances come from various sources, ranging from folk remedies to research laboratories. The screening system has changed from a purely in vivo system to a stem cell assay.[36] Agents that show activity in this system are then used to treat experimental tumors, including mouse leukemias P388 and L1210, the Lewis lung tumor, B16 melanoma, and human tumor xenografts. Drugs that are active in these systems are then advanced to more detailed testing.

The standard tumor cell lines used for screening potential brain tumor drugs are the intracranial L1210 leukemia and the mouse ependymoblastoma. Both tumor lines were initiated in the 1940s by the application of a carcinogen, and both are sensitive to nitrosoureas. They have the advantages of highly reproducible growth and an established experimental track record. However, both lines have limitations as models for human brain tumors. The L1210 line is a leukemia or lymphoma and biologically has little resemblance to tumors of the nervous system. Treatment of the intracranial L1210 addresses the drug delivery problem, but it does not necessarily reflect what is likely to be the cellular sensitivity of human brain neoplasms. The mouse ependymoblastoma is a primary brain neoplasm, but it is histologically dissimilar to the most common human brain tumors, and its relation to the human tumor is uncertain. Other experimental brain tumor lines, such as the 9L gliosarcoma and the avian sarcoma virus–induced astrocytoma, have also been used to evaluate therapeutic approaches. The use of human brain tumors growing in athymic mice offers significant theoretical advantages over animal tumor lines, but this is a much more expensive model and its value in comparison to the standard screens remains to be demonstrated.

Clinical Evaluation of New Agents

Once drugs show activity in standard experimental tumors and their toxicity in large animals has been assessed, they may be introduced into clinical trials. Clinical protocols for new agents are commonly divided into phase I, II, and III studies.

Phase I studies are designed to assess toxicity. Standard practice is to begin phase I studies of new drugs in specialized cancer centers, treating patients with extensive disease whose disease has progressed on conventional agents. Drug dosages are increased until significant toxicity develops, and the highest tolerated doses are then used in phase II studies. Information about therapeutic efficacy is collected, but it is recognized that drug activity will be underestimated in patients with advanced disease in phase I studies.

Phase II protocols are designed to test efficacy. Drugs are given to patients with measurable disease, using a schedule and dose based on phase I results. Criteria for response are carefully defined, and both the percentage of patients responding and the duration of the responses are compared to those achieved with currently available therapy. Phase II studies may of course involve drug combinations as well as single agents. If the new agent compares favorably with conventional drugs, phase III trials may be initiated.

In phase III trials the new therapeutic regimen is compared in carefully controlled fashion to the best available conventional treatment. Patient selection and therapeutic schedule are controlled, and usually alternative therapies are chosen by randomization. Relative efficacy is then compared, using a standard measure such as time to tumor recurrence or survival time. Occasionally phase III studies are conducted using historical controls, but this approach is risky.

Human Brain Tumor Chemotherapy

Drug Delivery in Brain Tumor Chemotherapy

Successful cancer chemotherapy requires that tumor cells be properly exposed to cytotoxic agents to which they are sensitive. Intrinsic cellular susceptibility is poorly understood and currently impossible to predict. Consequently, in the last decade attempts to improve therapeutic results using standard agents have emphasized improving drug delivery.

Drug delivery in its broadest sense encompasses basic pharmacologic properties such as absorption, protein binding, metabolism, and excretion. These properties are important in the treatment of any neoplasm in any location, but the blood-brain barrier (BBB) adds unique complexity to the chemotherapy of central nervous system tumors. Molecules that are small, lipid-soluble, and nonionized are best suited to cross the intact barrier, and these characteristics have been considered essential in the design of agents for the treatment of CNS neoplasms.[28] Yet several lines of evidence show that the BBB is disrupted in anaplastic brain tumors. Both radiographic evidence of abnormal vascular permeability and elevation of CSF protein concentration are crude but definite measures of loss of barrier integrity in patients with brain tumors. More detailed observations using quantitative autoradiographic methods in a rat brain tumor model indicate marked variability of barrier function both within individual tumors and among different tumors.[17] Similar methods applied in patients with brain tumors could, in theory, permit individualization of therapy on the basis of the degree of preservation of the barrier.

The other critical variable in drug delivery to central nervous system tumors is blood flow. Quantitative autoradiographic measurements of blood flow in tumor-bearing rat brain demonstrate marked regional variability in large tumors.[17] Flow is markedly diminished in the necrotic center of a tumor and increases toward normal levels at the periphery. In very small cerebral tumors, blood flow is normal or minimally reduced. These findings support the clinicopathologic impression that central necrosis in rapidly expanding cerebral neoplasms reflects relative ischemia. Direct measurement of blood flow in human cerebral neoplasms is now being obtained; findings of regional variability and diminished blood flow would have major implications for chemotherapeutic approaches to these tumors. As a result of blood flow alterations, tumor cells may escape cytotoxic drugs or be exposed to sublethal concentrations, the latter a factor that may be important in the emergence of drug resistance. At the same time, tumor cells may survive and proliferate under these relatively ischemic conditions.

Direct intra-arterial administration of chemotherapeutic agents theoretically could improve the therapeutic index of these treatments by exposing the tumor to higher concentrations of drug and by reducing systemic toxicity. It has been demonstrated in animals that higher intracerebral levels of BCNU can be achieved by intracarotid than by intravenous administration of the drug. However, significant ocular and brain toxicity offset any potential benefits of intra-arterial BCNU[35] and possibly of intra-arterial nitrosoureas in general.[39] Favorable response rates and less significant local toxicity with intracarotid cisplatin[25] suggest that this agent warrants further study.

Improved drug delivery by direct infusion into the ventricles, tumor, or tumor cavities or by transient BBB disruption has also been attempted. Implantation of drug-impregnated biodegradable polymers at the tumor site in an attempt to allow prolonged local exposure with minimal systemic exposure has been studied with BCNU-impregnated wafers, and it appears that this form of treatment is well tolerated.[3] A placebo-controlled randomized clinical trial is currently being analyzed to evaluate the efficacy of this relatively new treatment modality.

Assessment of the effectiveness of chemotherapy for malignant gliomas is based on clinical and radiographic criteria. One must be certain that the apparent effectiveness of a particular chemotherapy regimen is not due to factors known to mimic treatment effects, including delayed CT scan improvement following radiotherapy, steroid-induced clinical and CT scan improvements,[5] and spontaneous resolution of postoperative CT scan changes.[6] Many older series described patients treated in the pre-CT era. In others, the response criteria were loosely defined, thus possibly overestimating the effectiveness of chemotherapy. More recent series have adhered to rigid response criteria and have provided a more accurate assessment of the response to chemotherapy.

Pharmacology of Specific Chemotherapeutic Agents

Antineoplastic agents may be classified according to their presumed mechanism of action. Traditionally, cytotoxic agents fall into one of two major groups: drugs that act during specific phases of the cell cycle (cell cycle specific, CCS), including the folate antagonists, pyrimidine analogues, purine analogues, and vinca alkaloids; and those whose activity does not depend on the cell cycle phase (cell cycle nonspecific, CCNS), including the alkylating agents, many antitumor antibiotics, and a variety of miscellaneous compounds. CCS drugs arrest proliferating cells by interfering with crucial functions such as DNA replication, protein synthesis, or mitotic spindle formation. CCNS agents are equally toxic to both resting and proliferating cells. Theoretically, cell cycle-specific agents are ideally suited to the treatment of CNS neoplasms since tumor cells represent the only actively proliferating cells in the target tissue. However, single-agent chemotherapy using CCS drugs has been disappointing. The most effective drugs to date have been the CCNS drugs, including the nitrosoureas (especially BCNU), procarbazine, and cisplatin. The failure of CCS chemotherapeutic agents has been attributed to the low proportion of tumor cells that are actively dividing (i.e., low growth fraction) in many CNS neoplasms. Nevertheless, selected CCS drugs (e.g., hydroxyurea, VM-26, vincristine) may prove useful when administered in combination with the alkylating agents. Table 189-2 lists typical dosage schedules and common toxic effects of some drugs used in brain tumor chemotherapy.

TABLE 189-2 Characteristics of Drugs Commonly Used in Human Brain Tumor Chemotherapy

Drug	Usual Dosage and Route of Administration	Common Toxic Effects
Nitrosoureas		Bone marrow toxicity is delayed and cumulative. BCNU is associated with pulmonary fibrosis in total doses exceeding 1400 mg/m^2.
BCNU	200 mg/m^2 IV q 6–8 weeks	
CCNU	130 mg/m^2 PO q 6 weeks	
meCCNU	125–200 mg/m^2 PO q 6 weeks	
Procarbazine	100 mg/m^2 PO daily for 14 days	Bone marrow suppression. Allergic rash occurs in 10 percent of patients.
Cisplatin	50–100 mg/m^2 IV q 4 weeks	Nausea may be severe. Kidney damage can be prevented with hydration. Peripheral neuropathy is uncommon.
Vincristine	0.5–1.5 mg/m^2 IV weekly	Polyneuropathy is the dose-limiting toxic effect. Bone marrow suppression is mild.
Carboplatin	400 mg/m^2 IV q 4 weeks	Myelosuppression (usually reversible). Nausea and vomiting (may be severe).
VP-16	45 mg/m^2 IV daily ×7, or 86 mg/m^2 IV twice weekly, or 290 mg/m^2 IV once weekly. Oral preparation available	Leukopenia; mild nausea and vomiting; severe peripheral neuropathy if previously treated with vincristine.

Nitrosoureas

The chloroethylnitrosoureas are small, highly lipid-soluble CCNS alkylating agents with clinical activity against a variety of neoplasms. Many derivatives incorporating this basic structure have been synthesized (including BCNU, CCNU, methyl-CCNU, PCNU, ACNU, streptozotocin, chlorozotocin, and clomesome). Decomposition of these agents in aqueous solution yields two reactive intermediates, a chloroethyldiazohydroxide and an isocyanate group. The former alkylates DNA, producing strand breaks and cross-links. The latter has been related to the drugs' toxicity rather than to their antitumor effect. Parent compounds disappear rapidly from plasma after absorption or intravenous infusion. These agents readily cross the intact blood-brain barrier, which may partially explain their efficacy against CNS neoplasms. Myelosuppression, which is both delayed and cumulative, is their most notable and consistent toxic effect. Prolonged administration has also been associated with pulmonary fibrosis.

Procarbazine

Procarbazine (PCB) is a water-soluble agent with a molecular weight of 258. It has monoamine oxidase–inhibiting activity, but its antineoplastic action is produced by DNA alkylation. The drug requires metabolic activation, yielding an end product with alkylating activity. Procarbazine is readily absorbed from the gastrointestinal tract, disappears rapidly from plasma, and readily crosses the intact blood-brain barrier. Cerebrospinal fluid levels are in equilibrium with plasma within minutes of intravenous administration. Nausea and anorexia may be dose-limiting, myelosuppression is mild to moderate in degree, and clinically significant neurotoxicity is very uncommon. An allergic rash appears in fewer than 10 percent of the patients taking the drug.

Cis-diamminedichloroplatinum (II)

Cis-platinum (cisplatin, CDP) is a water-soluble CCNS agent with a molecular weight of 300. It is the first heavy metal to be used as an anticancer agent. It appears to act through interstrand and intrastrand cross-linking of DNA. After intravenous administration, most of the drug is protein-bound and inactive, and drug not bound to tissues or plasma proteins is excreted in the urine. Cisplatin penetrates poorly into the central nervous system; the ratio of drug concentration in plasma to CSF is 25:1 or greater. The major dose-limiting effect is renal toxicity. This is minimized by vigorous hydration in conjunction with a mannitol-induced diuresis, but dosage should be reduced in the presence of impaired renal function. Severe nausea and vomiting occur frequently, although this can now be effectively controlled with newer antiemetics. Ototoxicity and peripheral neuropathy may also complicate cisplatin therapy. Myelosuppression is usually mild, which can be an advantage in patients who are receiving or who have received myelotoxic drugs.

Hydroxyurea

Hydroxyurea (HU) is a water-soluble CCS drug with a molecular weight of 76. It interferes with DNA synthesis by inhibiting the enzyme ribonucleoside diphosphate reductase. This enzyme catalyzes the conversion of ribonucleotides to deoxyribonucleotides, a process which is necessary for DNA synthesis. In experimental systems, hydroxyurea has been shown to potentiate radiation damage. It readily crosses the blood-brain barrier and is excreted in the urine. Myelosuppression is its major dose-limiting toxic effect.

Vincristine

Vincristine (VCR) is a water-soluble CCS agent with a molecular weight of 923. It acts as a mitotic spindle poison, resulting in metaphase arrest. Vincristine is administered intravenously, metabolized in the liver, and excreted via the biliary and gastrointestinal tracts. Under normal circumstances the drug does not cross the blood-brain barrier to any significant extent. Sensory-motor and autonomic neuropathies are usually the dose-limiting toxic effects of vincristine, and the bone marrow is relatively spared.

Carboplatin

Carboplatin (Paraplatin) has biochemical properties similar to those of cisplatin, thus producing predominantly interstrand DNA cross-links. Approximately 87 percent of carboplatin is protein-bound within 24 h of administration. Drug excretion is primarily in the urine, and so pre-existing severe renal impairment is a contraindication to its use. The major dose-limiting toxicity is myelosuppression (unlike cisplatin) which is usually reversible and not cumulative. Nausea and vomiting occur frequently and are often severe without aggressive antiemetic therapy. Neurological adverse effects include a low incidence of peripheral neuropathy and ototoxicity, similar to cisplatin. Allergic reactions are similar to those with cisplatin.

VP-16

VP-16 is a synthetic glycosidic derivative of podophyllotoxin that binds to tubulin and inhibits microtubule assembly. Despite its high lipid solubility, VP-16 penetrates poorly into CSF. At least 30 percent of the administered VP-16 dose is excreted unchanged. An oral ampule preparation is available but because of decreased bioavailability, at least a twofold increase in dose is required if the drug is given orally. The dose-limiting toxicity is leukopenia. Although gastrointestinal side effects such as nausea and vomiting are uncommon with the intravenous preparations, they occur in approximately one-half of patients receiving oral VP-16. A mild peripheral neuropathy (usually paresthesia or reduced tendon reflexes) is seen in fewer than one-half of the patients receiving VP-16. High dose VP-16 has been administered with autologous bone marrow reinfusion but produces severe mucositis and leukopenia.

Chemotherapy of Anaplastic Gliomas

Anaplastic gliomas are a heterogeneous group of primary malignant brain neoplasms, variously referred to as anaplastic astrocytomas, malignant astrocytomas, astrocytomas grades 3 and 4, and glioblastoma multiforme.[15] Also included under this designation are the less common anaplastic oligodendrogliomas, mixed anaplastic gliomas, and gliosarcomas. These are predominantly supratentorial tumors of adults, with a peak incidence in the fifth or sixth decade of life and a slight preponderance in males.

The natural history of the malignant gliomas is remarkably

uniform, yet variables independent of treatment significantly influence prognosis. One of the major contributions of the Brain Tumor Study Group (BTSG) of the National Cancer Institute has been the identification of these prognostic variables. Age, duration of symptoms prior to diagnosis, histopathologic type, and pretreatment performance status are the most important clinical characteristics influencing outcome. Considering these variables, Walker et al. have identified a favorable-prognosis group in which the expected median survival exceeds 40 months.[41] The design of clinical trials must account for the impact of these factors on results and conclusions.

A partial list of studies of the chemotherapeutic response rates of recurrent malignant gliomas is found in Tables 189-3 and 189-4. Relatively recent studies and studies involving large numbers of patients have been emphasized. In certain instances the results have been edited to permit concentration on anaplastic gliomas, and individual reports should be consulted for details. A number of drugs and drug combinations have produced objective response rates exceeding 20 percent.[10,31,34] These include BCNU, intra-arterial BCNU, high-dose BCNU with autologous bone marrow rescue, CCNU, PCB, CDP, VM-26, diaziquone (AZQ), cyclophosphamide, BCNU plus VCR, BCNU plus PCB, BCNU plus 5-fluorouracil, BCNU plus dianhydrogalactitol (DAG), CCNU plus VM-26, DAG plus VP-16, CCNU plus PCB plus VCR, and others. In general, response durations rarely exceed 9 months; response rates have been lower in patients previously exposed to chemotherapeutic agents; and studies in which strict response criteria, especially with respect to corticosteroid use, have been defined report lower rates of response. Surprisingly, many commonly available chemotherapeutic agents have not been examined carefully for activity against anaplastic glial tumors.

In contrast to most malignant glial tumors, malignant oligodendrogliomas seem to be uniquely chemosensitive tumors. Encouraging results have been achieved with nitrosourea-based regimens for pure and mixed anaplastic oligodendrogliomas, with response rates up to 79 percent and long-term tumor control.[4]

Encouraging results from response studies have led to an analysis of the role of adjuvant chemotherapy in the treatment of patients with anaplastic gliomas. The results of several major studies of adjuvant chemotherapy are summarized in Table 189-5. In most, survival was the therapeutic end point, concurrent randomized controls were used, and at least 5000 rad were administered to the tumor bed. However, details vary, and the individual reports should be reviewed.

A landmark study was reported by the BTSG in 1978, in which patients were randomized after surgery into one of four arms: no further therapy, BCNU alone, radiotherapy (RT) alone, or RT plus BCNU.[40] These data established unequivocally the benefit of RT

TABLE 189-3 Selected Studies of the Response of Recurrent Anaplastic Gliomas to Single-Agent Chemotherapy

Drug*	No. of Patients†	% Responding†	Response Criteria	Comment‡	Reference§
AZQ	25	24	Clinical and CT improvement	7 patients with SD	Feun, 1984
AZQ	15	40	Clinical and CT improvement		Schold, 1984
AZQ	33	6	Clinical and CT improvement	13 SD	EORTC, 1985
AZQ	34	3	CT improvement only	17 patients with SD	Chamberlain, 1985
AZQ	23	35	Clinical and CT improvement	1 CR	Maral, 1985
AZQ	51	6	Clinical and CT improvement		Taylor, 1985
BCNU	19	37	Clinical improvement	Includes only patients who received at least 2 chemotherapy courses	Wilson, 1970
BCNU high dose & marrow rescue	20	55	Clinical and CT improvement	Significant visceral toxicity	Takvorian, 1983
BCNU high dose & marrow rescue	27	44	Clinical and CT improvement	Significant toxicity	Philips, 1986
Cisplatin	31	13	Clinical and CT improvement	3 SD	Stewart, 1983
Cisplatin	14	29	Clinical and CT improvement		Spence[37]
Cisplatin	15	7			Grunberg, 1987
Carboplatin	29	14	Clinical and CT improvement	No prior chemotherapy	Yung[42]
Melphalan	14 (GBM) 13 (AA)	0 8	Improvement in CT or MRI after 1 cycle		Chamberlain, 1988
MTX, high dose & citrovorum factor rescue	9	78	Clinical and/or CT improvement	(1) Steroids not mentioned (2) Intracarotid injections in 3 patients	Djerassi, 1985
Procarbazine	83	6 (GBM) 8 (A. glioma)	CT or MRI improvement	No CRs	Rodriguez, 1989
Trimetrexate	14	0	Clinically stable or improved and >50% reduction in tumor size on CT		Cairncross, 1990
VP 16	18	17	Clinical and CT improvement		Tirelli, 1984

*AZQ, diaziquone; MTX, methotrexate.
†GBM, glioblastoma multiforme; AA, anaplastic astrocytoma; A. glioma, anaplastic glioma.
‡SD, stable disease; CR, complete response.
§All references before 1991 are listed in Mahaley.[24]

TABLE 189-4 Selected Studies of the Response of Recurrent Anaplastic Gliomas to Multiple-Agent Chemotherapy

Drug*	No. of Patients†	% Responding	Response Criteria	Comment‡	Reference§
BCNU, PCB	45	29	Clinical & brain scan improvement with stable or decreasing corticosteroids		Levin, 1976
BCNU, 5-FU	29	31	Improvement in 2 of: clinical, CT, and brain scan	Includes only patients completing two courses of therapy; 15 SD	Levin, 1978
DFMO, BCNU	10 (GBM) 21 (AA)	0 10	Clinical and CT improvement		Prados, 1989
BCNU, 5-FU, HU, 6-MP	29 (GBM) 45 (A. glioma)	17 31	Clinical and brain scan improvement with stable or decreasing corticosteroids		Levin, 1986
AZQ, BCNU	32 (GBM) 10 (AA)	22 30	Clinical and CT improvement		Schold, 1987
AZQ, BCNU	8 (GBM) 10 (AA)	15 10	Improvement in 2 of: clinical, CT, and performance status		Yung, 1989
AZQ, PCB	42 (GBM) 19 (AA)	12 47	CT and clinical improvement		Schold, 1987
VCR, CPA	16	50	Clinical and CT improvement		Longee, 1990
Cisplatin, Ara C	25	40	CT improvement	2 CR	Stewart, 1984
VP-16, Carboplatin	38	21	CT improvement; clinically stable or improvement		Jeremic[19]
DAG, VP-16	15	40	Clinical and CT improvement; stable or decreasing steroids	Median age = 35	Eagan, 1981
meCCNU, PCB, VCR	28	32	Clinical and either CT or brain scan improvement off corticosteroids	No prior RT	Avellanosa, 1979
"Eight-in-One"	10	50			Rozenthal, 1989

*PCB, procarbazine; 5-FU, 5-fluorouracil; DFMO, difluoromethylornithine; HU, hydroxyurea; 6-MP, 6-mercaptopurine; VCR, vincristine; CPA, cyclophosphamide; DAG, dianhydrogalactitol.
†GMB, glioblastoma multiforme; AA, anaplastic astrocytoma; A. glioma, anaplastic glioma.
‡SD, stable disease; CR, complete response; RT, radiation therapy.
§All references before 1991 are listed in Mahaley.[24]

in this disease. They also suggested the additional value of BCNU chemotherapy, since the percentage of survivors at 18 months was significantly greater in the group treated with combination therapy than in the group treated with RT alone. Since then, surgery plus RT and BCNU has been considered the standard form of treatment against which new forms of therapy must be compared. Other important observations made in adjuvant chemotherapy studies include the activity of PCB,[16] the apparent radiosensitizing effect of HU in patients with glioblastoma,[23] and the curious observation that patients in whom CCNU chemotherapy was delayed until the time of clinical recurrence did at least as well as those in whom drug treatment was instituted immediately after diagnosis.[11]

These adjuvant studies are difficult to compare because of different eligibility criteria and because of differences in other forms of therapy, notably radiotherapy. The variable results in the control arms of different studies emphasize this point. Furthermore, many of the earlier studies are difficult to interpret because of the small numbers of patients in each treatment arm and because the importance of non-treatment-related prognostic variables was not appreciated. Clinical trials are now more tightly controlled and their outcomes more rigorously analyzed. Nevertheless, results of these prospective controlled clinical trials support the use of BCNU, CCNU, or PCB in the management of patients with anaplastic glioma.

The value of combination chemotherapy using cytotoxic agents that were judged to be effective as single agents in previous adjuvant or response studies has been addressed in several trials.[21] Many of these reports describe a substantial advantage for the multi-drug regimen over (usually historical) control series using BCNU alone, with reported response rates of up to 60 percent. However, a significant selection bias exists in most of these trials in that patients eligible for the trials tended to have more favorable prognostic variables and thus such optimistic results using combination chemotherapy are not equivalent to improved survival in phase III studies utilizing a concurrent control group. In a study by Levin et al.,[22] multi-drug regimens did not prove superior to BCNU alone in terms of prolonging survival, but there was a suggestion that for anaplastic tumors (i.e., not glioblastomas), PCV was superior to BCNU. Still others think that chemotherapy (BCNU) plus radiotherapy affords a small increase in survival over radiotherapy alone only in younger patients (40–60 years old).[7]

Among the anaplastic gliomas are the malignant brain stem gliomas and the anaplastic ependymomas. An evaluation of chemotherapy in the treatment of these predominantly pediatric tumors is hampered by the small number of patients in any one center and by the absence of a tissue diagnosis in many patients with intrinsic brain stem neoplasms. A variety of single agents and combinations of agents have been used in conjunction with

TABLE 189-5 Selected Studies of the Adjuvant Chemotherapy of Anaplastic Gliomas

Treatment*	No. of Patients	Median Survival	Comment†	Reference‡
No further treatment	31	14 wks	RT vs. no further treatment, $p = 0.001$	Walker, 1978
RT	68	36 wks		
BCNU	51	19 wks	RT v. RT, BCNU—no significant difference in median survival but more long-term survivors in RT, BCNU arm ($p < 0.01$).	
RT, BCNU	72	35 wks		
RT, BCNU	124	50 wks	Survival figures are for VSG. BCNU, PCB arms both significantly better than methylprednisolone alone.	Green[16]
RT, methylprednisolone	141	40 wks		
RT, PCB	128	47 wks		
RT, BCNU, methylprednisolone	134	41 wks		
RT	55	31 wks	Figures indicate time to tumor progression. No significant difference.	EORTC, 1981
RT, CCNU, VM-26	61	39 wks		
RT	94	36 wks	Survival figures are for VSG. RT, BCNU not significantly better than RT alone. meCCNU alone significantly worse than other arms.	Walker[41]
meCCNU	81	24 wks		
RT, BCNU	92	51 wks		
RT, BCNU (GBM)	26	31 wks	Differences significant for GBM but not for MG, $p = 0.002$	Levin, 1979
RT, BCNU, HU (GBM)	36	49 wks		
RT, BCNU (MG)	20	73 wks		
RT, BCNU, HU (MG)	17	50 wks		
RT, CCNU	42	43 wks	Favorable prognosis patients only. Survival at least as good if CCNU held until recurrence, $p = 0.07$.	EORTC, 1978
RT, delayed CCNU	39	62 wks		
RT	32	11 mos	RT, CCNU significantly better than RT alone ($p < 0.03$).	Solero, 1979
RT, BCNU	34	12 mos		
RT, BCNU	36	16 mos		
RT	20	35 wks	RT, DAG significantly better than RT alone ($p = 0.002$).	Eagan, 1979
RT, DAG	22	67 wks		
RT	30	40 wks	RT alone worse than RT, DBD ($p = 0.02$) or RT, DBD, CCNU ($p = 0.0015$). CCNU provides only marginally better survival but more long-term survivors.	Afra, 1983
RT, DBD	26	57 wks		
RT, DBD, CCNU	28	60 wks		
RT, CCNU	56	55 wks	No significant difference.	Eyre, 1983
RT, CCNU, PCB	59	50 wks		
RT, BCNU	114	54 wks	No significant difference.	Nelson, 1983
RT, BCNU, misonidazole	112	46 wks		
RT	148	10 mos	No significant difference. Significant toxicity with CCNU, DTIC. Small beneficial effect on survival of RT, BCNU in 40–60 y group	Chang, 1983
RT & 1000 rad. boost	105	8 mos		
RT BCNU	165	10 mos		
RT methyl CCNU, DTIC	136	10 mos		
RT	58	43 wks	No significant differences.	Hatleroll, 1985
RT, CCNU	60	43 wks		
RT, misonidazole	60	43 wks		
RT, CCNU, misonidazole	66	43 wks		
RT, BCNU	82	45 wks	No significant differences. Response rate better in PCB and DTIC arms.	Eyre, 1986
RT, PCB	83	31 wks		
RT, DTIC	78	39 wks		
RT	104	45 wks	No significant difference.	Trojanowski, 1989
RT, CCNU	94	52 wks		
RT	69	49 wks	No significant difference.	Peszyrski, 1988
RT, CCNU	68	49 wks		
RT, BCNU	166	13 mos	No significant differences.	Shapiro, 1989
RT, CCNU, PCB	176	11 mos		
RT, BCNU, HU/PCB, VM-26	168	14 mos		
RT, BCNU	140	10 mos	No significant differences.	Deutsh, 1989
RT, streptozocin	136	11 mos		
Hypperfrac. RT, BCNU	142	10 mos		
RT, misonidazole, BCNU	139	9 mos		
RT	125	52 wks	No significant difference.	EORTC[12]
RT, cisplatin	121	46 wks		
RT, BCNU	—	48 wks	No significant difference; 346 total patients.	Dinapoli[9]
RT, PCNU	—	48 wks		
RT, AZQ	121	46 wks	No significant difference; survival is from randomization, which occurred after RT.	Schold[33]
RT, BCNU	128	54 wks		

*Abbreviations as in Tables 189-3 and 189-4. MG, malignant glioma; DBD, dibromodulcitol; DTIC, dacarbazine.

†VSG, valid study group.

‡All references before 1991 are listed in Mahaley.[24]

radiotherapy or at the time of tumor progression, and although occasional responses have been described, the role of chemotherapy remains uncertain. Radiotherapy is unquestionably of benefit in the treatment of patients with anaplastic ependymomas, and the tendency for this tumor to seed the subarachnoid space has led to whole neuraxis irradiation following surgical removal in some patients. There is no defined role for chemotherapy in the management of patients with anaplastic ependymomas, although there have been several documented responses of recurrent ependymal tumors to cisplatin-based regimens.

Chemotherapy of Other Primary Brain Tumors

Perhaps one-third of all primary glial tumors of adults and children are histologically benign. Treatment of these lesions varies among centers but usually includes surgical removal followed by cranial irradiation. The role of chemotherapy in the treatment of these diseases has not been addressed. Since patients with low-grade gliomas may live for many years following conventional treatment, the toxicity and potential long-range complications of cytotoxic agents weigh heavily against their use.

Medulloblastoma is the most common primary malignant CNS tumor of childhood. Conventional treatment includes surgical resection followed by whole neuraxis irradiation. The latter is recommended because of the propensity for this tumor to spread throughout the subarachnoid space. Using this approach, prolonged control of the disease is accomplished in approximately 40 percent of patients. Relapse usually occurs at the primary site, although occasionally leptomeningeal or systemic metastases are the first indication of tumor recurrence. Until recently, chemotherapy has been reserved for patients with evidence of recurrent or progressive disease. In this setting, response rates of over 50 percent have been achieved for varying periods of time in small series of patients (median duration of response: 6 to 18 months). A number of cytotoxic agents have been used, alone or in combination, including procarbazine, CCNU, vincristine, cisplatin, and methotrexate. Methotrexate has been administered intravenously or into the subarachnoid space via either the lumbar or intraventricular routes.

There have been two large independent multi-institution randomized trials [International Society of Pediatric Oncology (SIOP); Children's Cancer Study Group (CCSG)] to determine the benefit of chemotherapy when used after radiotherapy for children with medulloblastoma or primitive neuroectodermal tumor (MB/PNET). According to Packer,[27] these studies are flawed by today's standards because of the unavailability of CT in some institutions and incomplete postoperative staging of other patients for residual primary site disease; however, they did demonstrate, for the first time, benefit of the addition of chemotherapy in some children with MB/PNET. In the SIOP trial, children with brain stem involvement at diagnosis who were treated with radiation and chemotherapy (CCNU, vincristine) had a significantly higher ($p < 0.003$) 5-year event-free survival rate than did children treated with radiation alone.[38] In the CCSG study there was no significant difference in either the estimated 5-year event-free survival probability between children treated with radiation alone or radiation plus chemotherapy (CCNU, vincristine, prednisone); however, in a small number of patients with extensive tumor, those receiving chemotherapy had significantly better metastatic event-free survival and overall survival.[13] In another study of children with poor-risk MB/PNET,[27] those treated with weekly vincristine during radiotherapy and cisplatin, CCNU, and vincristine after radiotherapy had a significantly better survival when compared to matched poor-risk historical controls receiving radiotherapy alone or radiotherapy plus chemotherapy with CCNU and vincristine.

Although flawed, these studies suggest that although chemotherapy does not benefit patients with low-grade MB/PNET, it probably improves the short-term survival for children with poor-risk MB/PNET when compared to radiotherapy alone. Recently reported survival figures for poor-risk MB/PNET children treated with radiotherapy and chemotherapy suggest that these patients may survive at a rate equal to or greater than average-risk children treated with radiotherapy alone.

Another potential benefit of chemotherapy for MB/PNET is that it may be useful as a partial replacement for radiation therapy in very young children who might otherwise be severely damaged by therapeutic cranial irradiation. To this end, very young children with MB/PNET have been treated with MOPP chemotherapy (mechlorethamine, vincristine, procarbazine, and prednisone) with encouraging results at M.D. Anderson Hospital in an attempt to obviate or delay the need for radiation.

Various drug combinations have been utilized in the adjuvant treatment of MB/PNET but none has been shown to result in a significantly better overall response rate when compared to single agents, although there is a somewhat longer median time to recurrence with multi-agent chemotherapy (so-called eight-drugs-in-one-day therapy) and although initial results were encouraging with tolerable toxicity, the long-term therapeutic advantage remains to be proved.

The pineal region tumors are a heterogeneous group of neoplasms that are often indistinguishable from one another on clinical grounds and that may be difficult to biopsy or remove. Astrocytomas, germinomas, and teratomas are the most common pineal region neoplasms; true neoplasms of pineal cells are rare. At times, these tumors can be distinguished on the basis of CSF tumor markers or CSF cytology. Although pineal region tumors may seed the subarachnoid space, the necessity for whole neuraxis radiation is debated because of the risk of bone marrow suppression, growth arrest of the spine, and radiation effects on the ovaries or testes, which attend this form of treatment. The incidence of spinal metastasis is uncertain, with estimates ranging from 15 to 57 percent, and its incidence varies with the tumor type. At the present time, adjuvant chemotherapy in patients with pineal region tumors of unknown histologic type cannot be recommended. Rational chemotherapeutic approaches to the treatment of recurrent tumors of known histology are possible, however. CNS germinomas should respond to agents such as cisplatin that are active against gonadal cell tumors. There is good evidence that cisplatin-based chemotherapy is useful in the management of primary CNS germ cell tumors of all types, with excellent reported response rates and early indications of improved long-term survival.[1] Prospective trials evaluating the routine incorporation of cisplatin-based chemotherapy into the management of primary CNS germ cell tumors are underway.

Other primary malignant CNS neoplasms such as meningeal sarcomas and malignant meningiomas are sufficiently rare that guidelines with respect to the chemotherapy of recurrent disease are wanting.

Therapeutic Sensitivity Testing

One of the major problems in the chemotherapy of human cancer is our limited ability to design treatments for individual patients. Sensitivity testing of individual tumors is in its infancy, so for the most part therapeutic decisions are based on results in large-scale clinical trials. However, neoplasms of similar origin and histologic type are often heterogeneous in their therapeutic sensitivity, and it would be very desirable to choose agents based on a tumor's measured drug sensitivity profile. Since currently available antineoplastic agents appear to inhibit the growth of only a minority of anaplastic brain tumors, a rational method of choosing a particular drug for a particular patient and tumor would be a major advance.

In Vitro Chemosensitivity

There has been considerable interest in the development of an in vitro assay of therapeutic sensitivity of individual tumors.[18] These assays are based on the presumption that the clonogenic or stem cells that grow in soft agar represent the proliferative cells of a neoplasm and that their sensitivity to agents in vitro will parallel the clinical response of the parent tumor. The assays have largely been used for drug screening, but some promising studies of their direct clinical application have been reported.[30] As indicated earlier, these assays have now been incorporated into the drug screening process of the National Cancer Institute. The studies are limited by the extremely low clonogenicity of most human tumors and by the difficulty of transferring in vitro pharmacologic data into an in vivo setting.

Little information in this regard is available for human brain tumors. Both Rosenblum et al.[29] and Kornblith et al.[20] have developed in vitro chemosensitivity assays using glioma cells, and they have found a correlation between the in vitro response (or lack of response) to BCNU and the response of the tumor in situ to the same agent. Although this observation is important, clonogenicity is less than 1 percent, even with the most anaplastic tumors, and the assays are subject to a number of technical factors. Their general applicability is therefore uncertain. Although this work may be important for an appreciation of the biological basis of drug sensitivity and resistance in these tumors, neither group of investigators has used the assays to design therapy for individual patients.

Human Tumor Xenografts

A number of laboratories have now reported successful transplantation of human neoplasms into congenitally or artificially immunosuppressed animals. Anaplastic brain tumors grow especially well after heterotransplantation into congenitally athymic mice, and a number of these transplanted tumor lines have been used for therapeutic studies.[32] In general, drugs that show some clinical activity against human brain tumors show efficacy against the transplanted tumors, and such tumor lines are now being used to evaluate new agents in the preclinical stage of development. In this manner, an athymic mouse system can be used as a secondary screen for possible new agents.[2] However, xenografted brain tumors usually require many months before therapy can be evaluated, and so far this prolonged latency has limited any attempts to use these animals to design therapy for individual patients.

Biochemical Markers of Drug Resistance

In addition to direct sensitivity testing of tumor cells, it may be possible to predict sensitivity of a tumor based on its biochemical phenotype. For example, high O6-alkylguanine-DNA alkyltransferase activity in glioma xenografts correlates with resistance to alkylating agents, whereas low activity predicts sensitivity. Similarly, the multi-drug-resistant (MDR) phenotype predicts sensitivity to large, naturally occurring antineoplastic agents, such as adriamycin, vincristine, and taxol. These and other markers of drug resistance might aid in the prediction of a tumor's sensitivity.

Drug Toxicity and Patient Acceptance

Most chemotherapeutic agents are potent cell poisons that produce toxic effects on normal tissues. In general, toxicity is most prominent in rapidly proliferating tissues, such as gut and bone marrow, but some agents produce distinctive organ toxicity. The neuropathy of the vinca alkaloids, the nephropathy from cisplatin, and pulmonary fibrosis from BCNU are notable examples among the agents used in brain tumor chemotherapy. These complications are usually preventable and may be reversible, and given the overall circumstances, the potential benefits outweigh the risks. However, in patients treated for longer periods, unexpected side effects may appear and must be monitored. Finally, other considerations being equal, patient acceptance is improved by oral rather than parenteral medications and by infrequent treatments. Acceptance of any treatment program will also be enhanced by an open explanation of therapeutic options and expectations, as well as of possible adverse effects.

References

1. Allen JC, Kim JH, Packer RJ. Neoadjuvant chemotherapy for newly diagnosed germ-cell tumors of the central nervous system. *J Neurosurg* 1987; 67:65–70.
2. Bellet RE, Danna V, Mastrangelo MJ, Berd D. Evaluation of a "nude" mouse-human tumor panel as a predictive secondary screen for cancer chemotherapeutic agents. *J Natl Cancer Inst* 1979; 63:1185–1188.
3. Brem H, Mahaley MS Jr, Vick NA, et al. Interstitial chemotherapy with drug polymer implants for the treatment of recurrent gliomas. *J Neurosurg* 1991; 74:441–446.
4. Cairncross JG, Macdonald DR. Successful chemotherapy for recurrent malignant oligodendroglioma. *Ann Neurol* 1988; 23:360–364.
5. Cairncross JG, Macdonald DR, Pexman JHW, Ives FJ. Steroid-induced CT changes in patients with recurrent malignant glioma. *Neurology* 1988; 38:724–726.
6. Cairncross JG, Pexman JHW, Rathbone MP. Post-surgical contrast enhancement mimicking residual brain tumor. *Can J Neurol Sci* 1985; 12:75.
7. Chang CH, Horton J, Schoenfeld D, et al. Comparison of postoperative radiotherapy and combined postoperative radiotherapy and chemotherapy in the multidisciplinary management of malignant gliomas. *Cancer* 1983; 52:997–1007.
8. DeVita VT, Schein PS. The use of drugs in combination for the treatment of cancer: rationale and results. *N Engl J Med* 1973; 288:998–1006.
9. Dinapoli RP, Brown L, Buckner J, et al. Phase III comparative evaluation of PCNU and BCNU combined with radiation therapy (RT) for high-grade glioma: a collaborative trial of North Central Treatment Group and Mayo Clinic. *Neurology* 1991; 41(Suppl 1):382 (abstr).
10. Edwards MS, Levin VA, Wilson CB. Brain tumor chemotherapy: an evaluation of agents in current use for phase II and III trials. *Cancer Treat Rev* 1980; 64:1179–1205.
11. European Organization for Research on Treatment of Cancer (EORTC) Brain Tumor Group. Evaluation of CCNU, VM-26 plus CCNU, and procarbazine in supratentorial brain gliomas: final evaluation of a randomized study. *J Neurosurg* 1981; 55:27–31.
12. EORTC Brain Tumor Group: cisplatin does not enhance the effect of radiation therapy in malignant gliomas. *Eur J Cancer* 1991; 27:568–571.
13. Evans AE, Jenkin RDT, Sposto R, et al. The treatment of medulloblas-

toma: results of a prospective randomized trial of radiation therapy with and without CCNU, vincristine, and prednisone. *J Neurosurg* 1990; 72:572–582.

14. Frei E III, Canellos GP. Dose: a critical factor in cancer chemotherapy. *Am J Med* 1980; 69:585–594.
15. Fuller GN, Burger PC. Gliomas: Pathology. Chapter 77, this textbook.
16. Green SB, Byar DP, Walker MD, et al. Comparison of carmustine, procarbazine, and high-dose methylprednisolone as additions to surgery and radiotherapy for the treatment of malignant glioma. *Cancer Treat Rev* 1983; 67:121–132.
17. Groothuis DR, Molnar P, Blasberg RG. Regional blood flow and blood-to-tissue transport in five brain tumor models: implications for chemotherapy. In Rosenblum M, Wilson CB (eds): *Progress in Experimental Brain Tumor Research*. New York: Karger, 1984, pp 132–153.
18. Hamburger AW, Salmon SE. Primary bioassay of human tumor stem cells. *Science* 1977; 197:461–463.
19. Jeremic B, Grujicic D, Jevremovic S, et al. Carboplatin and etoposide chemotherapy regimen for recurrent malignant glioma: a phase II study. *J Clin Oncol* 1992; 10:1074–1077.
20. Kornblith PL, Smith BH, Leonard LA. Response of cultured human brain tumors to nitrosoureas: correlation with clinical data. *Cancer* 1981; 47:255–265.
21. Kornblith PL, Walter M. Chemotherapy for malignant gliomas. *J Neurosurg* 1988; 68:1–17.
22. Levin VA, Silver P, Hannigan J, et al. Superiority of post-radiotherapy adjuvant chemotherapy with CCNU, procarbazine, and vincristine (PCV) over BCNU for anaplastic gliomas: NCOG 6G61 final report. *Int J Radiat Oncol Biol Phys* 1989; 18:321–324.
23. Levin VA, Wilson CB, Davis R, et al. A phase III comparison of BCNU, hydroxyurea, and radiation therapy to BCNU and radiation therapy for the treatment of primary malignant gliomas. *J Neurosurg* 1979; 51:526–532.
24. Mahaley MS Jr. Neuro-oncology index and review (adult primary brain tumors): radiotherapy, chemotherapy, immunotherapy, photodynamic therapy. *J Neurooncol* 1991; 11:85–147.
25. Mahaley MS Jr, Hipp SW, Dropcho EJ, et al. Intracarotid cisplatin chemotherapy for recurrent gliomas. *J Neurosurg* 1989; 70:371–378.
26. Owens G. Intraarterial chemotherapy of primary brain tumors. *Ann NY Acad Sci* 1969; 159:603–607.
27. Packer RJ. Chemotherapy for medulloblastoma/primitive neuroectodermal tumors of the posterior fossa. *Ann Neurol* 1990; 28:823–828.
28. Rall DP, Zubrod CG: Mechanisms of drug absorption and excretion: passage of drugs in and out of the central nervous system. *Annu Rev Pharmacol Toxicol* 1962; 2:109–128.
29. Rosenblum ML, Gerosa MA, Wilson CB, et al. Stem cell studies of human malignant brain tumors. Part 1: Development of the stem cell assay and its potential. *J Neurosurg* 1983; 58:170–176.
30. Salmon SE, Hamburger AW, Soehnlen B, et al. Quantitation of differential sensitivity of human-tumor stem cells to anticancer drugs. *N Engl J Med* 1978; 298:1321–1327.
31. Schold SC Jr. Chemotherapy of primary central nervous system neoplasms. *Semin Neurol* 1981; 1:189–201.
32. Schold SC Jr, Bullard DE, Bigner SH, et al. Growth, morphology, and serial transplantation of anaplastic human gliomas in athymic mice. *J Neurooncol* 1983; 1:5–14.
33. Schold SC Jr, Herndon JE, Burger PC, Halperin EC, et al. Randomized comparison of diaziquone and carmustine in the treatment of adults with anaplastic glioma. *J Clin Oncol* 1993; 11:77–83.
34. Shapiro WR. Treatment of neuroectodermal brain tumors. *Ann Neurol* 1982; 12:231–237.
35. Shapiro WR, Green SB, Burger PC, et al. A randomized comparison of intra-arterial versus intravenous BCNU, with or without intravenous 5-fluorouracil, for newly diagnosed patients with malignant glioma. *J Neurosurg* 1992; 76:772–781.
36. Shoemaker RH. New approaches to antitumor drug screening: the human tumor colony-forming assay. *Cancer Treat Rev* 1986; 70:9–12.
37. Spence AM, Berger MS, Livingston RB, et al. Phase II evaluation of high-dose intravenous cisplatin for treatment of adult malignant gliomas recurrent after chloroethylnitrosourea failure. *J Neurooncol* 1992; 12:187–191.
38. Tait DM, Thorton-Jones H, Bloom HJG, et al. Adjuvant chemotherapy for medulloblastoma: the first multi-centre control trial of the International Society of Paediatric Oncology (SIOP I). *Eur J Cancer* 1990; 26:464–469.
39. Tonn JC, Roosen K, Schachenmayr W. Brain necroses after intra-arterial chemotherapy and irradiation of malignant gliomas—a complication of both ACNU and BCNU? *J Neurooncol* 1991; 11:241–242.
40. Walker MD, Alexander E Jr, Hunt WE, et al. Evaluation of BCNU and/or radiotherapy in the treatment of anaplastic gliomas: a cooperative clinical trial. *J Neurosurg* 1978; 49:333–343.
41. Walker MD, Green SB, Byar DP, et al. Randomized comparisons of radiotherapy and nitrosoureas for the treatment of malignant glioma after surgery. *N Engl J Med* 1980; 303:1323–1329.
42. Yung WKA, Mechtler L, Gleason MJ. Intravenous carboplatin for recurrent malignant glioma: a phase II study. *J Clin Oncol* 1991; 9:860–864.

190

Blood-Brain Barrier Modification in the Delivery of Antitumor Agents

Mary Kay Gumerlock
Edward A. Neuwelt

Perhaps the most unique anatomic aspect of brain tumors from the chemotherapeutic point of view is the presence of the blood-brain barrier (BBB), a morphologic entity based on the brain capillary endothelial cell tight junctions.[38] This structural barrier serves both protective and regulatory functions by constraining diffusion across capillaries in relation to lipid solubility and molecular weight. Brain tumor vascularity and the integrity of the blood-tumor barrier have long been debated. Suffice it to say that while the permeability of the barrier may vary from one tumor nodule to another, from the chemotherapeutic point of view, the state of the blood-brain and blood-tumor barriers must be factored into each drug delivery equation.[18]

The *selectivity* of the BBB is defined as its ability to limit the penetration of substances into the CNS on the basis of their size, molecular weight, charge, and lipid solubility. In conjunction with the continuous production of CSF, this selective exclusion leads to the concept of the "sink action" of the cerebrospinal fluid (CSF).[20] Because the CSF circulates, it acts as a sump for solutes that cross the blood-brain barrier. Thus, low drug concentrations in brain parenchyma are the result not only of slow penetration through the blood-brain barrier but also of the efficient sink action of the CSF, where active removal by CSF bulk flow into venous blood prevents a diffusional equilibrium from being established.

Tumor pharmacology must also be taken into consideration. Tumor blood flow varies, so drug delivery to a tumor with or without a blood-tumor barrier will be variable. Blood flow and capillary permeability are often low in brain tumors, and the intercapillary distance is usually increased, which further compromises diffusion of administered drugs. Because there is also a decrease in the diffusion of oxygen and nutrients, tumor cells often become quiescent and thus unable to take up drugs.[14] The rate of CNS drug uptake also depends on local CBF differences, capillary surface area, and capillary permeability. These three factors are known to vary considerably from region to region and also from time to time, in response to the general physiologic state of the patient and probably also to neurotransmitter changes.

As described above, the CSF and normal brain surrounding a tumor may act as a diffusional sink for any drug that enters the tumor. CNS drug uptake will vary depending on the proximity of parenchymal tissue to the CSF. Thus, the increased availability of drug to tumor afforded by increased local permeability is rapidly reduced by diffusion. In addition, brain tumors appear to have an efficient perivascular drainage system. Thus the important factor in effective drug delivery, that of *sufficient concentration over a sufficient time,* may not be realized to any therapeutic advantage using most current methods of brain tumor chemotherapy.

Modes of Drug Administration to Circumvent the BBB

Intra-Arterial Administration

The purpose of intra-arterial (IA) chemotherapy infusion is to increase the ratio of peak concentration to infusion time. This route of administration offers an advantage over the conventional intravenous (IV) route only during the first pass; thereafter IA concentrations are similar to IV levels.[13,35] If rates of biotransformation, metabolism, and excretion during the first pass are high, the IA route delivers more drug to the brain for a given degree of systemic toxicity. Recently, a number of agents have been evaluated for this route of administration, including methotrexate, vincristine, vinblastine, mechlorethamine, melphalan, BCNU, cisplatin, etoposide, and tenoposide.[23]

Intra-arterial chemotherapy with the currently available drugs has the potential for significant local toxicity. Balloon catheterization with superselective arterial drug delivery increases the selective drug delivery but carries risk of thromboembolic complications and cerebral ischemia.[41,45,46] It is therefore important to determine which drugs can be used without significant local toxicity but with a diminution in systemic toxicity. Several methods for further direct arterial catheterization are under investigation.

Intrathecal Administration

The intrathecal method of chemotherapeutic administration has developed as an attempt to deliver high-molecular-weight or polar drugs past the BBB. Drug distribution in the CSF is influenced by a number of factors, including bulk CSF flow, diffusion through the extracellular spaces of the brain and spinal cord, transport across the choroid plexus, removal by CSF absorption, and diffusion from the extracellular space into the capillaries of the CNS.[37] Drugs administered intrathecally have short half-lives, necessitating repeat administration. Lipid-based formulations of encapsulated cytarabine or methotrexate (MTX) have been developed; the CSF half-life for encapsulated MTX is 5.4 days, as compared to 0.3 days for unencapsulated MTX.[7]

Administration by CSF Perfusion

The CSF perfusion method of drug therapy has the theoretical advantage of exposing the CSF to prolonged high levels of drug with supposedly less systemic absorption and thus less systemic toxicity. Investigators have attempted to prolong infusion of various agents directly into the CSF.[2,39] While these techniques do result in an increased parenchymal drug concentration, the effect is limited to approximately 3 mm beneath the subarachnoid space, even after long perfusion. Direct intraventricular perfusion also produces a 10-fold concentration difference between the ventricular and surface subarachnoid tissue.[20] It is thus well to remember that CSF levels of a drug have no correlation with parenchymal or tumor drug concentrations. This route has limited usefulness, except perhaps in the case of pure carcinomatous meningitis. Even in this situation, though, the plugging of the Virchow-Robin spaces with cancer cells will result in poor drug penetration in these subarachnoid channels. This fact may account for the short duration of response to intrathecal treatment in carcinomatous meningitis.

Direct Instillation into the Tumor Bed or Tumor Cyst

Another method for bypassing the BBB is direct instillation of chemotherapeutic agents into the tumor bed and/or into associated tumor cysts.[4,23,24] Use of the Ommaya reservoir, an adapted tumor cyst device, or multiple microcatheters allows for direct instillation of several chemotherapeutic agents. If a cyst is part of the tumor complex, access to tumor fluid and ongoing biochemical analysis is available. Kinetic drug studies can also be performed. The more recent development of the Ommaya tumor cyst device allows the tumor bed cavity to persist. The use of intracystic/intratumoral drugs presupposes a focal disease process and is therefore of somewhat limited usefulness for most primary brain tumors.

Packaging in Liposomes

Another way to achieve an adequate drug concentration over a sufficient period is to use liposomes as drug carriers.[16] This technique first requires that the antimitotic drugs be incorporated into liposomes. Liposomes are phospholipid vesicles formed by the dispersion of bilayer lipid lamellae. These micelles can be inverted so that the polar region is inside and the nonpolar phospholipid tails are outside, thus rendering them more lipid-soluble and able to penetrate membranes. Such drug-containing liposomes can then act as a depot for slow drug release. While this method of CNS chemotherapy may be limited by the amount of drug packageable, it represents a unique approach both to penetrating the BBB and to maintaining prolonged tissue concentrations.

Packaging in Biodegradable Polymers

Biodegradable polymers are frequently composed of polyanhydrides that have a labile linkage and thus undergo surface degradation. When these polymers are mixed with a given concentration of chemotherapeutic agent, the rate of drug release is proportional to the polymer erosion rate. Kubo and colleagues first described the treatment of malignant brain tumors with such polymer composites.[26] Brem and coworkers reported on the surgical implantation of drug-impregnated polymers and subsequent chemical analysis after reoperation.[5] This interesting new technology allows for prolonged maintenance of a high drug level in surrounding brain tissue (1-cm radius).[5,19] Clinical trials are in progress.

Blood-Brain Barrier Disruption Chemotherapy

Background

As detailed above, several methods for increasing the amount of drug delivered to CNS tumors have been developed, each having particular toxicities and effects. Also, as mentioned above, one of the unique aspects of tumors in the CNS is the presence of the BBB, an anatomic and physiologic barrier to substances in the bloodstream. A unique though quite rational approach to the problem of chemotherapeutic drug delivery therefore has been to transiently disrupt the BBB while the drug is being administered.

In the 1940s, Broman and Olsson showed that the BBB opens reversibly in response to iodinated contrast agents that are hyperosmolar.[6] This observation largely lay dormant until Rapoport began his elaborate studies on rats, rabbits, and monkeys detailing the physicochemical parameters of the BBB and its role in the passage of substances from the blood to the CNS extracellular space.[38] He described methods for using hyperosmolar mannitol, urea, or arabinose to reversibly open the BBB by temporarily opening the tight junctions, thus permitting transient unregulated entry of circulating substances into the CNS. Neuwelt subsequently applied these observations and techniques to the clinically relevant problem of chemotherapeutic drug delivery in animals and then patients with primary and metastatic CNS tumors.[31]

How do the basic principles outlined above apply to this modality? First, the existence and character of the BBB in tumors has been debated and studied from various angles. Suffice it to say that the state of the BBB in tumors differs anatomically and physicochemically to various degrees from one tumor nodule to another, from one type of tumor to another, and within any given single focus of tumor. The state of the BBB in tumors, though, becomes a moot point because substances diffuse from areas of high concentration to areas of lower concentration to the point of equilibrium. Therefore, even if a tumor has no BBB, the fact that the barrier remains intact in the surrounding brain parenchyma (thus inhibiting drug delivery in the CNS tissue) means that a drug that is initially delivered in higher concentration to the tumor will rapidly diffuse out to equilibrate with the rest of the CNS (the sink effect). Thus, any concentration advantage is lost too quickly to be effective.

The technique of blood-brain barrier disruption (BBBD) evades this problem by providing a higher and more uniform delivery of drug to the whole CNS, thus decreasing the rate at which the drug diffuses away from the tumor and causing the tumor to be exposed to a higher concentration of drug for a longer period.[28] As this method also exposes the normal CNS to much higher concentrations of anticancer agents, one must be alert to potential increased toxicity. This problem may limit the number of drugs for which BBBD and chemotherapy can be used.

The technique of reversible osmotic BBBD involves opening the BBB in the distribution of one artery (a carotid or vertebral artery). The exact distribution of disruption depends on the flow as determined by these vessels and the circle of Willis. One selects the left carotid, right carotid, or vertebral artery on the basis of tumor location. For tumors in a border zone, two disruptions may be performed sequentially over two days. No attempt at three sequential disruptions has been described, but all three circulations have been used in two-day pairwise disruptions, which have been repeated at monthly intervals.

To cause reversible disruption of the BBB, a hyperosmolar saturated solution of 25% mannitol (lower concentrations are inadequate) is injected at a sufficient rate and volume to essentially replace blood flow for a period of 30 s. Because the degree and extent of barrier disruption vary, the disruption must be measured. This can be done with either nonionic iodinated contrast and CT scanning or radionuclide brain scanning.[21,40] The procedure carries the attendant risks of thromboembolic ischemia or infarction, which are symptomatic in less than 0.6 percent of procedures. Blood-brain barrier disruption allows nonselective entry of substances into the CNS and tumor for a period of approximately 30 min. It is important to be aware of the potential toxicities of any other medications that are present in the patient's bloodstream and are normally excluded by the BBB, as they too will enter the brain parenchyma during the period of disruption.

Chemotherapy with BBBD is not yet in widespread clinical use, but several centers are beginning to report their experience.[21] While the protocols at different institutions vary in terms of mannitol infusion time, determination of BBBD, and chemotherapeutic agents used, these data emphasize the clinical feasibility of the approach and suggest that it is associated with a significant improvement in the median survival of patients with certain brain tumors.

Malignant Gliomas

The published series of brain tumor patients treated with BBBD and chemotherapy include 176 patients with malignant gliomas.[3,9,15,21,25,27–30,33,42,43,47] For 78 percent (138/176 patients), follow-up data are available. Of the latter patients, 53 percent (73 patients) showed clinical and radiographic improvement, 32 patients had stabilization of their disease, and 33 patients had tumor progression.

It has been standard practice to treat malignant brain tumors with radiation immediately after surgical diagnosis, saving chemotherapy for use thereafter. However, 4 of the 16 patients in the series of Fauchon and colleagues[15] received BBBD and chemotherapy prior to radiation treatment, as did 4 of 16 patients in the series of Miyagami and colleagues.[30,42,43] While the practice of preradiation chemotherapy has been gaining popularity in the treatment of pediatric CNS malignancy, its use in adults with glioblastoma has been less common. Three of four patients in the Japanese series remained alive at 24 to 44 months after diagnosis. Our own series of approximately 25 patients receiving BBBD and chemotherapy before radiotherapy demonstrates tumor response to BBBD and chemotherapy as measured by CT scan. The question of whether chemotherapy before radiation will offer improved survival and/or decreased toxicity is being evaluated.

In summary, the treatment of patients with high-grade malignant gliomas using adjuvant chemotherapy administered in conjunction with osmotic blood-brain barrier disruption affords a significant chance for improved survival (18 to 22 months median survival for malignant glioma) and a stable Karnofsky performance score.[21,33] The intra-arterial infusion of mannitol prior to the administration of chemotherapeutic agents is not associated with additional risks beyond those of standard intra-arterial chemotherapy. This route of drug administration has advantages over standard intravenous, intra-arterial, intrathecal, and intra-tumoral methods with respect to both the length of time a therapeutic level is achieved in the tumor and the ability to treat tumor cells that have infiltrated beyond the defined tumor edge into normal brain tissue. Full quantitation of the advantage of BBBD and chemotherapy over more conventional brain tumor chemotherapy awaits further assessment.

Cerebral Lymphoma

The results of BBBD and chemotherapy in the treatment of primary cerebral lymphoma are impressive, and serve to emphasize the fact that increasing the delivery of drugs to malignant brain tumors improves survival, particularly when the tumors are sensitive to the chemotherapeutic agents used.[22] Although combination chemotherapy for systemic non-Hodgkin's lymphoma results in long-term remission for most patients, it has had only modest efficacy in the treatment of CNS lymphoma. The best results have been with high-dose MTX protocols, which result in transient responses. These protocols attempt to overcome the BBB through sheer high intravenous dosage. However, because MTX penetrates the CNS poorly, tumor drug levels are still subtherapeutic, especially in the case of infiltrative brain tumors such as lymphoma. Intraventricular and intrathecal MTX infusion also fails to produce therapeutic levels except in the superficial CNS parenchyma.[2] Ott and colleagues have measured BBB permeability in three patients with primary CNS lymphoma treated with chemotherapy before radiation treatment.[36] They clearly demonstrated a marked decrease in blood-brain barrier permeability between week 1 and week 4 of treatment. They concluded that such early reestablishment of the BBB after one course of chemotherapy may preclude the entry of further drugs into the CNS, thus perhaps protecting any remaining malignant cells in the brain parenchyma.

Clinical studies have documented the efficacy of chemotherapy in conjunction with osmotic BBBD for patients with primary cerebral lymphoma. The most recent report extends observations to include 30 consecutive patients with CNS lymphoma treated with BBBD and chemotherapy using methotrexate, cyclophosphamide, procarbazine, and dexamethasone.[32] The patients in group 1 ($n = 13$) were initially treated with cranial radiation and subsequently received BBBD and chemotherapy for persistent or recurrent tumor. Patients in group 2 ($n = 17$) received initial BBBD and chemotherapy and underwent radiation only for persistent or recurrent tumor.

Survival differences between these two groups were assessed using the Fisher Exact Test and the log-rank statistic applied to the Kaplan-Meier survival curves. The difference in median survival after diagnosis, 17.8 months for group 1 and 44.5 months for group 2, is statistically significant ($p < 0.04$). One patient in group 1 and eight in group 2 remain alive and disease-free at a follow-up ranging from 15 to 98 months. Morbidity and mortality in these 30 patients undergoing 471 BBBD/chemotherapy procedures include three deaths within 30 days of the last procedure (two from sepsis and one from disease progression), two cerebral infarctions, three episodes of prolonged obtundation, and a periprocedural seizure incidence of 7 percent. Neuropsychological testing at one year shows stable or improved function in most of the patients tested.[10,11]

Enzyme and Monoclonal Antibody Delivery Across the Blood-Brain Barrier

The penetration of monoclonal antibodies (mAbs) into brain tumors has been notably poor, raising the question of whether BBBD might improve mAb delivery to tumor. Three patients with malignant melanoma metastatic to the CNS have received a ^{131}I-mAb specific for a melanoma-associated cell-surface proteoglycan.[34] A radionuclide brain scan following BBBD and mAb administration demonstrated increased uptake in the affected cerebral hemisphere, but additional tumor-specific binding could not be detected with this imaging modality. However, in the single patient with malignant cells in the CSF, tumor-specific binding was documented by immunohistochemistry.[31,34]

Another new application of monoclonal antibody techniques is the conjugation of the antibody to an enzyme (alkaline phosphatase) to form a relatively high-molecular-weight molecule.[44] Osmotic disruption can be used to deliver conjugate across the BBB into the brain, where it binds to a brain tumor surface antigen; the barrier then returns to its predisrupted state. A low-molecular-weight phosphorylated prodrug which can be activated to the cytotoxic agent by the antibody-bound enzyme is subsequently given, resulting in localized drug therapy. Preliminary studies of this technique are encouraging.

Other Barrier-Opening Techniques

Black and colleagues have pioneered the use of leukotrienes to enhance drug delivery to CNS tumors. They have demonstrated that intracarotid infusion of leukotrienes selectively increases the transfer constant for permeability within tumors without altering drug permeability in normal brain.[8] While this method of blood-tumor barrier opening has the advantage of minimizing the exposure of normal brain to antitumor agents, it may not prevent rapid diffusion of the drug away from the critical tumor area. Phase I clinical trials are in progress to evaluate the feasibility of this chemotherapeutic regimen.

The permeation of peptides across the BBB has been controversial. It is now recognized that they do penetrate the CNS either unidirectionally or bidirectionally not only via saturable transport mechanisms, but also via nonsaturable transmembrane and paracellular diffusion pathways.[1] Further study of the principles of peptide permeability is allowing the development of therapeutically useful peptide analogs.

Along similar lines, peptides such as bradykinin, histamine, and other receptor-mediated "membrane permeabilizers" may usefully be combined with drugs to increase chemotherapeutic delivery to the CNS. Larger molecules such as nerve growth factor (NGF) can cross the BBB when conjugated to a transferrin receptor antibody.[17]

Conclusion

Given that we have some 40 years of experience in general antineoplastic chemotherapy and some 30 years of experience with brain neoplasia, where does the neuroclinician stand? We have accumulated a substantial amount of data on malignant cell cycles and tumor cell kinetics using tight experimental constructs, and these data must now be extrapolated to in vivo malignancy. For CNS tumors, the methodology must account for the BBB and the CSF circulation. The general anatomic parameters of infiltrative primary brain tumors and multifocal metastatic disease have been defined, and we have recognized their importance in treatment protocols. Perhaps the most dramatic illustration of this importance is the phenomenon, observed separately by Neuwelt and Stewart, of tumor that regressed in a circulatory zone where it was treated while simultaneously progressing in an adjacent untreated region.[31,45]

As safe, adequate, and rational chemotherapy develops, the role of radiation treatment (prominent only by default) will come up for risk-benefit analysis. Advances in molecular biology have established the role of monoclonal antibodies in the diagnosis and treatment of brain neoplasia. The role of oncogenes in CNS tumorigenesis suggests making more prominent use of such agents as cytarabine and dactinomycin (inhibitors of reverse transcriptase) in progressive chemotherapy.

Emphasis on the role of the BBB in defining adequate drug delivery has resulted in a clinically feasible new approach to brain tumor chemotherapy. Current results with the technique of disrupting the BBB osmotically just before administering multiagent chemotherapy establishes this treatment regimen as an alternative to other drug protocols. The use of a regimen of etoposide and carboplatin in combination with osmotic BBB disruption is now under study and will add significantly to the therapeutic regimen, as these drugs are more effective against primary CNS tumors.

As experience is gained in treating malignant tumors with BBB disruption and chemotherapy, such methods may offer improved treatment of other less malignant CNS diseases. Techniques that increase the concentration of a drug in the brain parenchyma and techniques that target drugs to specific cells or brain regions are applicable to many CNS problems, such as enzyme deficiencies, multiple sclerosis, and Alzheimer's disease.

References

1. Banks WA, Audus KL, Davis TP. Permeability of the blood-brain barrier to peptides: an approach to the development of therapeutically useful analogs. *Peptides* 1992; 13:1289–1294.
2. Blasberg RG, Patlak C, Fenstermacher JD. Intrathecal chemotherapy: brain tissue profiles after ventriculocisternal perfusion. *J Pharmacol Exp Ther* 1975; 195:73–83.
3. Bonstelle CT, Kori SH, Rekate H. Intracarotid chemotherapy of glioblastoma after induced blood-brain barrier disruption. *Am J Neuroradiol* 1983; 4:810–812.
4. Bouvier G, Penn RD, Kroin JS, et al. Direct delivery of medication into a brain tumor through multiple chronically implanted catheters. *Neurosurgery* 1987; 20:286–291.
5. Brem H, Mahaley MS Jr, Vick NA, et al. Interstitial chemotherapy with drug polymer implants for the treatment of recurrent gliomas. *J Neurosurg* 1991; 74:441–446.
6. Broman T, Olsson O. Experimental study of contrast media for cerebral angiography with reference to possible injurious effects on the cerebral blood vessels. *Acta Radiol* 1949; 31:321–334.
7. Chatelut E, Kim T, Kim S. A slow-release methotrexate formulation for intrathecal chemotherapy. *Cancer Chemother Pharmacol* 1993; 32:179–182.
8. Chio CC, Baba T, Black KL. Selective blood-tumor barrier disruption by leukotrienes. *J Neurosurg* 1992; 77:407–410.
9. Chiras J, Dormont D, Fauchon F, et al. Intra-arterial chemotherapy of malignant gliomas. *J Neuroradiol* 1988; 15:31–48.
10. Crossen JR, Garwood D, Glatstein E, Neuwelt EA. Neurobehavioral sequelae of cranial irradiation in adults: review of radiation-induced encephalopathy. *J Clin Oncol* 1994; 12:627–642.
11. Crossen JR, Goldman DL, Dahlborg SA, Neuwelt EA. Neuropsychological assessment outcomes of nonacquired immunodeficiency syndrome patients with primary central nervous system lymphoma before and after blood-brain barrier disruption chemotherapy. *Neurosurgery* 1992; 30:23–29.

12. DeAngelis LM, Yahalom J, Thaler HT, et al. Combined modality therapy for primary CNS lymphoma. *J Clin Oncol* 1992; 10:635–643.
13. Dedrick RL, Oldfield EH, Collins JM. Arterial drug infusion with extracorporeal removal. I. Theoretic basis with particular reference to the brain. *Cancer Treat Res* 1984; 68:373–380.
14. DeVita VT Jr. The relationship between tumor mass and resistance to chemotherapy: implications for surgical adjuvant treatment of cancer. *Cancer* 1983; 51:1209–1220.
15. Fauchon F, Chiras J, Poisson M, et al. Intra-arterial chemotherapy by cisplatin and cytarabine after temporary disruption of the blood-brain barrier for the treatment of malignant gliomas in adults. *J Neuroradiol* 1986; 13:151–162.
16. Firth G, Oliver AS, McKeran RO. Studies on the use of antimitotic drugs entrapped within liposomes and of their action on a human glioma cell line. *J Neurol Sci* 1984; 63:153–165.
17. Friden PM, Walus LR, Watson P, et al. Blood-brain barrier penetration and in vivo activity of an NGF conjugate. *Science* 1993; 259:373–377.
18. Groothuis DR, Molnar P, Blasberg RG. Regional blood flow and blood-to-tissue transport in five brain tumor models: implications for chemotherapy. *Prog Exp Tumor Res* 1984; 27:132–153.
19. Grossman SA, Reinhard C, Colvin OM, et al. The intracerebral distribution of BCNU delivered by surgically implanted biodegradable polymers. *J Neurosurg* 1992; 76:640–647.
20. Gumerlock MK. Blood-brain barrier and its manipulation: implications for neutron capture therapy. In Allen BJ, Moore DE, Harrington BV (eds): *Progress in Neutron Capture Therapy for Cancer.* New York: Plenum, 1992, pp 531–536.
21. Gumerlock MK, Belshe BD, Madsen R, Watts C. Osmotic blood-brain barrier disruption and chemotherapy in the treatment of high grade malignant glioma: patient series and literature review. *J Neurooncol* 1992; 12:33–46.
22. Gumerlock MK, Neuwelt EA. Primary cerebral lymphoma. *Cancer Treat Res* 1993; 66:111–126.
23. Gumerlock MK, Neuwelt EA. Chemotherapy of brain tumors: innovative approaches. In Morantz RA, Walsh JW (eds): *Brain Tumors, A Comprehensive Text.* New York: Marcel Dekker, 1994, pp 763–778.
24. Harbaugh RE. Novel CNS-directed drug delivery systems in Alzheimer's disease and other neurological disorders. *Neurobiol Aging* 1989; 10:623–629.
25. Heimberger K, Samec P, Podreka I, et al. Reversible Blut-Hirn-Schrankenöffnung in der Chemotherapie Maligner Gliome. *Wien Klin Wochenschr* 1987; 99:385–388.
26. Kubo O, Himuro H, Inoue N, et al. Treatment of malignant brain tumors with slowly releasing anticancer drug-polymer composites [Japanese]. *No Skinkei Geka* 1986; 10:1189–1195.
27. Li V, Levin AB, Turski P. Intra-arterial chemotherapy following blood-brain barrier disruption in patients with recurrent high grade astrocytomas. Presented at the 56th Annual Meeting of the American Association of Neurological Surgeons, Toronto, April 24–28, 1988 (poster).
28. Markowsky SJ, Zimmerman CL, Tholl D, et al. Methotrexate disposition following disruption of the blood-brain barrier. *Ther Drug Monit* 1991; 13:24–31.
29. Miyagami M, Kagawa Y, Tsubokawa T. ACNU delivery to malignant glioma tissue by osmotic blood brain barrier modification with intracarotid infusion of hyperosmolar mannitol [Japanese]. *No Shinkei Geka* 1985; 13:955–963.
30. Miyagami M, Tsubokawa T, Tazoe M, Kagawa Y. Intra-arterial ACNU chemotherapy employing 20% mannitol osmotic blood-brain barrier disruption for malignant brain tumors. *Neurol Med Chir (Tokyo)* 1990; 30:582–590.
31. Neuwelt EA, Dahlborg SA. Blood-brain barrier disruption in the treatment of brain tumors: clinical implications. In Neuwelt EA (ed): *Implications of the Blood-Brain Barrier and Its Manipulation*, vol 2. New York: Plenum, 1989, pp 195–261.
32. Neuwelt EA, Goldman DL, Dahlborg SA, et al. Primary CNS lymphoma treated with osmotic blood-brain barrier disruption: prolonged survival and preservation of cognitive function. *J Clin Oncol* 1991; 9:1580–1590.
33. Neuwelt EA, Howieson J, Frenkel EP, et al. Therapeutic efficacy of multiagent chemotherapy with drug delivery enhancement by blood-brain barrier modification in glioblastoma. *Neurosurgery* 1986; 19:573–582.
34. Neuwelt EA, Specht HD, Barnett PA, et al. Increased delivery of tumor-specific monoclonal antibodies to brain after osmotic blood-brain barrier modification in patients with melanoma metastatic to the central nervous system. *Neurosurgery* 1987; 20:885–895.
35. Oldfield EH, Dedrick RL, Chatterji DC, et al. Arterial drug infusion with extracorporeal removal. II. Internal carotid carmustine in the rhesus monkey. *Cancer Treat Res* 1985; 69:293–303.
36. Ott RJ, Brada M, Flower MA, et al. Measurements of blood-brain barrier permeability in patients undergoing radiotherapy and chemotherapy for primary cerebral lymphoma. *Eur J Cancer* 1991; 27:1356–1361.
37. Poplack DG, Bleyer WA, Horowitz ME. Pharmacology of antineoplastic agents in cerebrospinal fluid. In Wood JH (ed): *Neurobiology of Cerebrospinal Fluid. I.* New York: Plenum, 1980, pp 561–578.
38. Rapoport SI. *Blood-Brain Barrier in Physiology and Medicine.* New York: Raven Press, 1976.
39. Riccardi R, Bleyer WA, Poplack DG. Enhancement of delivery of antineoplastic drugs into cerebrospinal fluid. In Wood JH (ed): *Neurobiology of Cerebrospinal Fluid. II.* New York: Plenum, 1983, pp 453–466.
40. Roman-Goldstein S, Clunie DA, Stevens J, et al. Osmotic blood-brain barrier disruption: CT and radionuclide imaging. *Am J Neuroradiol* 1994; 15:581–590.
41. Saris SC, Wright DC, Oldfield EH, Blasberg RG. Intravascular streaming and variable delivery to brain following carotid artery infusions in the Sprague-Dawley rat. *J Cereb Blood Flow Metab* 1988; 8:116–120.
42. Sato S, Toya S, Otani M. Blood-brain barrier opening microcirculation in human brain tumor [Japanese]. *No To Shinkei* 1985; 37:109–113.
43. Sato S, Yoshinori A, Kodama R, et al. Blood-brain barrier opening CT [Japanese]. *CT Kenkyu* 1985; 7:43–48.
44. Senter PD. Activation of prodrugs by antibody-enzyme conjugates: a new approach to cancer therapy. *FASEB J* 1990; 4:188–193.
45. Stewart DJ. Novel modes of chemotherapy administration. *Prog Exp Tumor Res* 1984; 28:32–50.
46. Stewart DJ, Grahovac Z, Maroun J, et al. Intraarterial (IA) chemotherapy (CT) for brain tumors (BT). *Proc Am Soc Clin Oncol* 1985; 4:132 (abstr).
47. Yamada K, Takahama H, Nakai O, et al. Intra-arterial chemotherapy for malignant glioma after osmotic blood-brain barrier disruption [Japanese]. *Gan To Kagaku Ryoho* 1985; 16:2692–2696.

191

Photoradiation Therapy for Malignant Gliomas

Edward R. Laws, Jr.
Robert E. Wharen, Jr.
Robert E. Anderson

The concept of photoradiation therapy (PRT) is based upon the ability of certain substances known as photosensitizers to concentrate preferentially in malignant tissue. These photosensitizers then have the capability for the selective destruction of malignant tissue when activated by light of the appropriate wavelength and intensity in the presence of oxygen. Phototherapy, photodynamic therapy, and photochemotherapy are all terms for this phenomenon of photoradiation therapy.

The action of a photosensitizer is produced by the absorption of photons of a wavelength sufficient to promote electrons within the sensitizer to an excited triplet state. This excited molecule may then interact either directly with substrates within a cell or indirectly with those substrates through the production of singlet oxygen ($^1O_2$). The various photochemical reactions that are excited by light are subsequently capable of killing cells through multiple interactions with the cell membrane, cytoplasm, nuclear membrane, and nucleus.

An ideal photosensitizer should (1) be nontoxic to normal tissues, (2) be selectively absorbed or retained by all neoplastic or dysplastic cells, (3) have some characteristic such as fluorescence that makes it easily detectable, and (4) be efficient in killing malignant tissue following the application of light at a wavelength capable of significant tissue penetration.

The search for an ideal photosensitizer is currently being pursued. Although far from ideal, the photosensitizer which has received the most extensive investigation both in the laboratory and clinically is hematoporphyrin derivative (HpD).

History of Photoradiation Therapy

The first application of HpD to the management of brain tumors took place in the 1950s at The Johns Hopkins Hospital.[35,42] At that time, a series of experiments were performed to evaluate HpD fluorescence in the detection of brain tumors at the time of surgery. These experiments demonstrated that detectable levels of HpD would concentrate in brain tumors and that HpD was effectively excluded by an intact blood-brain barrier.

The first studies that suggested that photoactivation of HpD might by cytotoxic to brain tumors were performed in 1975.[17] In a tumor model system, cell death was produced by exposure of the tumor containing HpD to light. Interest in this phenomenon was rekindled in Italy,[31–33] Australia,[15,19] and the United States[23] in 1980–1981 when several groups reported the initial results of photodynamic therapy (PDT) directed toward brain tumors in humans.

The application of PRT in neurosurgery was initially very encouraging. A number of investigators have reported the capability of HpD to kill glioma cells both in vitro and in vivo.[2,4–7,13,16,37,41] More recent reports have described additional attempts at the use of PRT for the treatment of malignant brain tumors,[11,12,19,22,24–30,33,34,38–40] and although the results are equivocal, it is evident that despite major differences in the protocols by various investigators, HpD phototherapy is capable of tumor cell destruction in humans. Hematoporphyrin is not entirely contained within neoplastic tissue, and some HpD accumulates in brain tissue. This small amount of HpD within normal brain tissue can produce significant morbidity and mortality in experimental animals upon application of a sufficient dose of light.[8]

Efforts to quantitate the uptake of hematoporphyrin within tumors and normal tissue have been performed,[14,20,30,36] and Wharen et al. have quantitated the amount of HpD achieved in human gliomas and normal brain tissue 24 to 48 h after the administration of 5 mg/kg HpD.[37] The uniformity of brain tumor uptake was assessed by Boggan et al.,[6] who found considerable heterogeneity of uptake in their tumor model and attributed cell death in such tumors as much to an effect on the vasculature[3] as to direct toxicity to tumor cells.

Current efforts are being directed toward an understanding of the fundamental principles and the scientific application of this modality of PRT. This has been stimulated by the desire to develop a treatment which may open new possibilities for therapy of malignant tumors where surgery, radiotherapy, and chemotherapy are inadequate.

Current Status of Photoradiation Therapy

Analysis of the Photoactive Drug

In parallel with our initial clinical investigations,[23] a number of laboratory experiments were performed. These utilized cell culture models of human and experimental brain tumors and an animal model of malignant ethylnitrosourea (ENU)-induced brain tumors in rats.[37,42] These experiments have confirmed HpD photodynamic cytotoxicity for brain tumor cells at practical concentrations of HpD and achievable doses of light. They also provided information relative to the time course and quantitative aspects of HpD concentration within the tumor cells. Several aspects of PDT were elucidated by these studies. First, a dose of 5 mg/kg of HpD seemed adequate. Second, a delay of 4 to 24 h resulted in satisfactory concentrations of HpD in the tumor cells and optimal tumor/brain ratios. Third, the exclusion of HpD by an intact blood-brain barrier was again confirmed. Fourth, the superiority of violet light (405 nm) activation to red light activation was confirmed. Fifth, the superiority of red light (633 nm) to violet light penetration of brain and brain tumor was confirmed. Subsequent experiments have suggested that the postulated cytotoxic mechanisms are dependent upon production of singlet oxygen in these experimental brain tumors.[12,18]

The optimum time to administer photoradiation therapy after drug administration would be when the HpD concentration in tumor is maximum, as compared to normal brain, provided that the absolute amount in normal brain is low enough to be nontoxic. Although Wharen et al. noted a ratio approximately twofold higher at 4 h compared to 24 h after drug administration,[37] Boggan et al. found maximal ratios at 24 h.[4] This ratio will also be dependent upon the HpD preparation, and further development is necessary before the timing of photoradiation therapy after drug administration can be optimized. Efforts to use subfractions of HpD (Hp, porphyrin C) or other photoactive compounds such as phthalocyanines, are also being investigated.

The toxicity of HpD in clinical applications has thus far been limited primarily to skin sensitization. Patients must remain out of bright sunlight for approximately 4 weeks after drug administration. McCulloch et al. have also reported one patient who developed cerebral edema following the administration of 150 J/cm^2 of red light 48 h after the injection of 5 mg/kg of HpD.[26] As suggested by El-Far and Pimstone[14] and Dougherty,[12] the use of a more pure preparation of HpD or a different porphyrin such as uroporphyrin-I may limit or eventually eliminate skin toxicity.

Analysis of the Drug-Light Interaction

The action mechanism in PRT and in dye-sensitized photo-oxidation reactions for both in vitro and in vivo systems has been an area of avid research from which some understanding of the basic processes involved has developed.

With few exceptions, photosensitized oxidations proceed by way of a triplet sensitizer. The excited triplet state (^{3}S) of the sensitizer (S) is produced by the absorption of a photon of light with an energy sufficient to raise the sensitizer to an excited singlet state (^{1}S). Subsequent intersystem crossing results in the transformation of an excited singlet state (^{1}S) to an excited triplet state (^{3}S), because the direct excitation of the triplet state (^{3}S) from the ground state (S) is a forbidden process.

The excited triplet state (^{3}S) can then react with biological substrates by two major mechanisms: either directly with the substrate (type I) by electron or hydrogen-ion transfer, or indirectly with the substrate (type II) through the production of single molecular oxygen.

The efficiency of each path is dependent upon the relative concentrations of oxygen (O_2) and substrate available for the sensitizer (^{3}S) to react, and the relative rate constants for each reaction (K_{O_2} and K_S) and for the rate of triplet decay (K_d). The overall process is limited by the quantum yield of triplet sensitizer formation. The rate constants will be dependent upon such factors as the chemical structure of the sensitizer (^{3}S), the aggregation state of the prophyrin, and the nature of the reaction medium.

The transfer of energy from the excited triplet state of the sensitizer (^{3}S) to oxygen proceeds by a process of electronic or resonance energy transfer, which is a diffusion-controlled process. The $^1O_2$-producing ability of photoexcited porphyrins and hence their photosensitizing efficiency is directly related to the lifetime or the decay rate of the porphyrin triplet state.

Dougherty et al. proposed in 1976 that singlet oxygen ($^1O_2$) was the cytotoxic agent responsible for the in vitro inactivation of TA-3 mouse mammary carcinoma cells exposed to HpD photoradiation using red light therapy.[13] $^1O_2$ was produced by the transfer of energy from an excited triplet state of hematoporphyrin to oxygen with a quantum yield for $^1O_2$ of 0.16 within the TA-3 cells. Further work has demonstrated that although most porphyrin-sensitized reactions occur via a type II mechanism involving $^1O_2$, other type I mechanisms involving electron transfer may be important. It has been documented that HpD (photofrin I and II) which consists of porphyrin aggregates produces $^1O_2$ with significantly smaller yields than Hp. Thus, although the use of $^1O_2$ quenchers such as β-carotene, ascorbic acid, and N_3 along with the enhancing effect of D_2O on the production of $^1O_2$ have clearly demonstrated the participation of $^1O_2$ in reactions in vivo, no photodynamic action so far investigated in vivo is solely explained by the $^1O_2$ mechanism.

The mechanisms responsible for the loss of cell viability in photoradiation therapy are difficult to characterize because of the multiplicity of damaging reactions that occur. Photoradiation of porphyrin-loaded cells results in inhibition of membrane transport functions and membrane damage; effects which may occur from photodynamic cross-linking of membrane proteins. Photodynamic damage to DNA and to lysosomes also occurs.[18]

Proteins, nucleic acids, unsaturated lipids, NADH, NADPH, hyaluronic acid, and other biomolecules are photo-oxidized with porphyrins as sensitizers. The predominant susceptible sites on proteins are the unprotonated thiol group of cysteine, the unprotonated imidazole ring of histidine, the thio-ether group of methionine, the indole ring of tryptophan, and the phenolate anion of tyrosine. Photo-oxidation of these sites on proteins results in the loss of enzymatic and hormonal activity, loss of toxic properties of snake venoms and bacterial toxins, loss of antigenic properties, and loss of antibody reactivity. Unsaturated lipids and cholesterol are converted to hydroperoxides. Nucleic acids are photo-oxidized by porphyrins predominately at guanine residues, and both single and double strand breaks can be produced in DNA.

Inactivation of cells by photoradiation can be classified into three major modes of action. First the porphyrin remains either outside the cell or within the cell membrane. In this case, the cell membrane would be expected to be the major site of photodamage. Membrane damage would result from the photo-oxidation of membrane lipids, structural proteins, and enzymes with resultant inhibition of transport processes, alterations of receptors, changes in permeability, or cross-linking of proteins in the membrane. Second, the porphyrin penetrates into the cytoplasm, resulting in damage to mitochondria, lysosomes, ribosomes, and proteins. Cell death would then occur from uncoupling or inhibition of oxidative phosphorylation, leaking of hydrolases from lysosomes into the cytoplasm, and inhibition of microsomal activity. Third, the prophyrin penetrates the nucleus to sensitize the nucleic acids and chromosomes, with resulting chromosomal breaks. As yet, no chromosomal breaks have been demonstrated in mammalian cells. Currently, the modes of action of porphyrin photosensitized reactions are considered to be multifactorial involving predominately the cell membrane and cytoplasm.

Optimization of the parameters of photoradiation therapy involves not only considerations of the uptake, distribution, and action mechanisms of the dye but also considerations of the wavelength, quantity, and energy density of light necessary to achieve cell kill. The action spectrum for porphyrin-sensitized cytotoxicity corresponds closely to the absorption spectrum of the porphyrin. Kinsey et al. found that the cytotoxic action of HpD was directly proportional to the number of light quanta absorbed by HpD in the cell.[21] For thin layers of cells, the Soret band at 405 nm had 12 to 30 times the cytotoxicity of red light.

Anderson et al. investigated the effect of optical spectrum, power density, HpD concentration, and HpD preparation on the HpD tumor cell killing efficiency of MEWO cells in culture.[2] Using a trypan blue exclusion assay, cell survival curves were obtained following irradiation with violet (405 nm), red (630 nm), and white (340 to 680 nm) light at energies of 0 to 320 J and at power densities of 20 to 160 mW/cm^2 for cells exposed for 6 h to HpD concentrations of 0 to 25 μg/ml.

Not only the wavelength and power density but also the type of light appears to affect the cellular killing efficiency of HpD-photoradiation therapy. Cowled et al. observed no difference in the HpD cell killing efficiency of a continuous-wave argon-pumped dye laser using rhodamine B with a wavelength of 625 to 635 nm when compared to a pulsed-wave gold vapor laser at a pulse frequency of 10 to 14 kHz having a wavelength of 627.8 nm.[9] Wharen et al. found a markedly decreased cellular killing efficiency for pulsed red light (625 to 645 nm) produced from a tunable flash-pumped dye laser at a repetition rate of one to six per second compared to continuous-wave red light (625 to 635 nm) from a filtered xenon arc lamp.[39] In addition, it has been reported that pulsed light from a nitrogen laser with a wavelength of 332 nm and a repetition rate of 30 Hz had a HpD cellular killing efficiency greater than that of a continuous light from an argon ion laser with a wavelength of 334 nm. This was attributed to a mechanism of two-photon absorption and production of cytotoxic radicals of HpD. It appears that not only the wavelength of light but also the form of the light (pulsed versus continuous) and the repetition rate, pulse width, and peak pulse power are all important variables in need of further study.

After all the drug and light parameters have been maximized in HpD photoradiation therapy, the limiting factor in its clinical application may remain the penetration of light through brain and tumor tissue. Light penetration into tissue is determined by the optical characteristics of the tissue, the wavelength of the light, and the concentration of the photosensitizer that has been used. Photons are either absorbed or scattered, and the ultimate penetration of light is both wavelength- and tissue-dependent in an exponential manner.

The relative penetration of light through in vivo cat brain as a function of wavelength has been measured and demonstrates the significantly greater depth of penetration of red light (630 nm) compared to violet light (405 nm). Dougherty, however, has stated that the useful penetration of visible light in adult brain at 630 nm is on the order of 1 to 1.5 mm.[12] If that is the case, then the depth of penetration of light at 630 nm represents a significant limiting factor for the use of photoradiation therapy for brain tumors. It is known, however, that the penetration of light through tissue continues to improve by several orders of magnitude as the wavelength increases from approximately 600 nm to 1.1 m. Thus, the possibility exists that photoradiation therapy at these wavelengths might provide a more effective depth of tissue penetration.

Clinical Studies

Clinical experience (Table 191-1) has expanded slowly. The majority of patients have had recurrent malignant tumors and have failed prior attempts at therapy. The mean survival for those patients who died after surgery was 11.6 months.

At present, a number of modalities of PDT for malignant brain tumors are suggested. For inoperable deep tumors, the stereotactic implantation of one or more quartz fibers to provide argon-dye laser photoradiation (500 to 1000 J) has been utilized, in conjunction with prior intravenous administration of HpD. For recurrent tumors which can be resected, PDT of the tumor bed has been utilized after intravenous and, in some cases, additional topical administration of HpD. The light delivery system has consisted of a filtered high-intensity xenon-arc lamp and a fiberoptic cable with a Lucite tip. The latter is inserted into a diffusion medium (0.1% Liposol in saline) which fills the tumor bed and also may be used to cool the operative field. A dose of 150 to 200 J is employed. A third mechanism of PDT is employed for cystic or cavitary lesions. After intravenous and/or topical administration of HpD, the cyst or cavity is filled with a diffusion medium and illuminated either with the laser-quartz fiber system or the high-intensity xenon-arc lamp fiberoptic system.

The technical aspects of these clinical trials in brain tumor patients have been quite satisfactory. There have been no adverse effects related to either intravenous or topical administration of HpD.

The light delivery systems have functioned well, but the importance of temperature monitoring should be emphasized. Power densities greater than 200 mW of red light through a 0.6-mm quartz fiber will produce significant heating of tissue. There is less significant heating when light is delivered through a large diameter (>5.0-mm) fiberoptic system. Because hyperthermia has its own cytotoxic effects, and because heat interferes with the photodynamic effect, it is essential to monitor this parameter and to avoid any significant thermal effects while delivering photoradiation.

If tissue heating is avoided, we have not recognized any significant degree of post-therapy cerebral edema in any of these patients, all of whom had CT scans within 48 h of treatment. Two patients had new neurological signs related to either surgery or PDT, but they were transient in both. All patients were managed with pre- and postoperative corticosteroid therapy. Two patients developed postoperative wound infections, which is not surprising in light of the extensive prior therapy both had received. Both responded to antibiotic therapy. One patient died postoperatively of disseminated intravascular coagulopathy (DIC), and one late death occurred at 4 months from a pulmonary embolus. Two patients developed symptoms and signs of cutaneous photosensitivity as a result of disregarding advice to protect themselves from direct sunlight.

As mentioned earlier, the analysis of this series of brain tumor patients treated by PDT with HpD does not yet permit any conclusions as to the effectiveness of the method. The results, however, are encouraging for several reasons. The theoretical basis of PDT for brain tumors still appears to be sound. The administration of effective amounts of HpD is relatively well tolerated by these patients. The light delivery systems are practical in use. At least some of these patients appear to have derived some benefit from PDT. These conclusions have been supported by the work of others.[33]

As basic knowledge with regard to PDT and malignant brain tumors increases and further laboratory work in cell culture and animal model systems progresses, it should be possible to improve the efficiency and the efficacy of PDT. Clinical indications may expand as well, to include the treatment of nonmalignant but invasive brain tumors such as meningiomas, pituitary adenomas, and craniopharyngiomas and the treatment of some forms of brain abscesses or parasitic infestations. Other prospects for the future include the following: new light-drug combinations[1] of higher efficiency, less toxicity, and deeper penetrations of tumor tissue; new light delivery systems, such as multiple fiber lasers, for more complete photoradiation of tumor tissue; the development of methods (systemic or topical) to improve dye uptake by tumor cells; the use of metabolic enhancers of the cytotoxic effect in tumor tissue[10] and quenchers of the photodynamic effect in normal tissue; and

TABLE 191-1 Brain Tumor Patients Treated by HpD-Photodynamic Therapy

Tumor	Location	HpD	Light	Result
Malignant astrocytoma	Right frontal	5 mg/kg IV, 48 h	Laser—630 nm	Alive, 6 months
Malignant astrocytoma	Left frontal	5 mg/kg IV, 72 h	Laser—630 nm	Dead, 5 months
Malignant astrocytoma, cystic	Left temporal	5 mg/kg IV, 48 h	Laser—630 nm	Dead, 37 months
Malignant astrocytoma	Right frontal	5 mg/kg IV, 48 h	Laser—630 nm	Dead, 4 months
Malignant astrocytoma	Left temporal	5 mg/kg IV, 36 h	Postresection, xenon lamp—450 + 630 nm	Dead, 7 months
Malignant astrocytoma	Left parietal	5 mg/kg IV, 24 h	Postresection, xenon lamp—white	Dead, 9 months
Malignant astrocytoma	Right frontal	5 mg/kg IV, 24 h	Postresection, xenon arc—white	Dead, 26 months
Malignant astrocytoma	Right thalamus	5 mg/kg IV, 24 h	Postresection, xenon arc—white	Alive, 33 months
Malignant astrocytoma	Right thalamus	5 mg/kg IV, 6 h	Postresection, xenon arc—630 nm	No follow-up
Malignant astrocytoma	Left frontal	5 mg/kg IV, 6 h	Postresection, xenon arc—630 nm, diffusion medium	Dead, 2 months
Malignant astrocytoma	Left frontal	5 mg/kg IV, 8 h	Postresection, xenon arc—630 nm, diffusion medium	Dead, 2 months
Malignant astrocytoma	Left frontal	5 mg/kg IV, 8 h	Postresection, xenon arc—630 nm, diffusion medium	Alive, with recurrence, 13 months
Malignant oligodendroglioma	Right frontal	5 mg/kg IV, 48 h	Postresection, xenon arc—405 + 630 nm	Dead, 3 months
Malignant small cell neoplasm (probably metastatic)	Right frontal	5 mg/kg IV, 48 h	Laser 630 nm	Dead, 1 month, infection
Malignant small cell neoplasm (probably metastatic)	Right frontal	5 mg/kg IV, 48 h	Laser—630 nm	Alive, 6 months
Medulloblastoma	Cerebellum	5 mg/kg IV, 6 h	Postresection, xenon arc—white	Alive, 31 months
Medulloblastoma	Cerebellum	5 mg/kg IV, 6 h	Postresection, xenon arc—630 nm, diffusion medium	Alive, 13 months
Ependymoma	Cerebellum	5 mg/kg IV, 4 h	Postresection, xenon arc—405 nm	Dead, postoperative, DIC
Ependymoma	Cerebellum	5 mg/kg IV, + topical, 6 h	Postresection, xenon arc—630 nm, diffusion medium	Alive, 8 months
Metastatic carcinoma (pulmonary)	Left parietal	5 mg/kg IV, 6 h	Postresection, xenon arc—630 nm, diffusion medium	Alive, with recurrence, 11 months
Metastatic melanoma	Left frontal	5 mg/kg IV, 10 h	Postresection, xenon arc—620 nm, diffusion medium	Alive, 9 months
Rhabdomyosarcoma	Left orbit	5 mg/kg IV, 24–72 h	Xenon arc—405 + 630 nm	Dead, 2 months
Craniopharyngioma	Sella turcica	Topical 5 mg/ml, 15 min	Xenon arc—630 nm	Dead, pulmonary embolus, 4 months

Source: Adapted from Laws et al.[25]

combination of PDT with other methods (stereotactic CO_2 laser resection, interstitial and conventional chemotherapy, radiation therapy,[22] hyperthermia, immunotherapy) in an effort to achieve ultimate control of these devastating tumors.

References

1. Abernathey CD, Anderson RE, Kooistra KL, et al. Activity of phthalocyanine photosensitizers against human glioblastoma in vitro. *Neurosurgery* 1987; 21:468–473.
2. Anderson RE, Wharen RE Jr, Jones CA, et al. Parameters of hematoporphyrin derivative tumor cell killing efficiency: decomposition of hematoporphyrin derivative at high power densities. In Doiron DR, Gomer CJ (eds): *Porphyrin Localization and Treatment of Tumors.* New York: Liss, 1984, pp 483–500.
3. Berenbaum MC, Hall GW, Hoyes AD. Cerebral photosensitization by haematoporphyrin derivative: evidence for an endothelial site of action. *Br J Cancer* 1986; 53:81–89.
4. Boggan JE, Berns M, Edwards M. Uptake, distribution, and retention of hematoporphyrin derivative in metastic and intrinsic rat tumor models. Presented at the Clayton Foundation Symposium on Porphyrin Localization and Treatment of Tumors, Santa Barbara, California, 1983.

5. Boggan JE, Bolger C, Edwards MSB. Effect of hematoporphyrin derivative photoradiation therapy on survival in the rat 9L gliosarcoma brain-tumor model. *J Neurosurg* 1985; 63:917–921.
6. Boggan JE, Walter R, Edwards MSB, et al. Distribution of hematoporphyrin derivative in the rat 9L gliosarcoma brain tumor analyzed by digital video fluorescence microscopy. *J Neurosurg* 1984; 61:1113–1119.
7. Boisvert DP, McKean JD, Tulip J, et al. Penetration of hematoporphyrin derivative into rat brain and intracerebral 9L glioma tissue. *J Neurooncol* 1985; 3:113–118.
8. Cheng MK, McKean J, Boisvert D, et al. Effects of photoradiation therapy on normal rat brain. *Neurosurgery* 1984; 15:804–810.
9. Cowled PA, Grace JR, Forbes IJ. Comparison of the efficacy of pulsed and continuous-wave red laser light in induction of phototoxicity by hematoporphyrin derivative. *Photochem Photobiol* 1984; 39:115–117.
10. Cowled PA, MacKenzie L, Forbes IJ. Potentiation of photodynamic therapy with haematoporphyrin derivatives by glucocorticoids. *Cancer Lett* 1985; 29:107–114.
11. Diamond I, Granelli SG, McDonagh AF, et al. Photodynamic therapy of malignant tumors. *Lancet* 1987; 2:1175–1177.
12. Dougherty TJ. Photodynamic therapy (PDT) of malignant tumors. *CRC Crit Rev Oncol Hematol* 1984; 2:83–116.
13. Dougherty TJ, Gomer CJ, Weishaupt KR. Energetics and efficiency of photoinactivation of murine tumor cells containing hematoporphyrin. *Cancer Res* 1976; 36:2330–2333.
14. El-Far MA, Pimstone NR. Selective in vivo tumor localization of uroporphyrin isomer I in mouse mammary carcinoma: superiority over other porphyrins in a comparative study. *Cancer Res* 1986; 46:4390–4394.
15. Forbes IJ, Cowled PA, Leong AS, et al. Phototherapy of human tumours using haematoporphyrin derivative. *Med J Aust* 1980; 2:489–493.
16. Gomer CJ, Doiron DR, Bucker N, et al. Examination of action spectrum, dose rate and mutagenic properties of haematoporphyrin derivative photoradiation therapy. In Doiron DR, Gomer CJ (eds): *Porphyrin Localization and Treatment of Tumors.* New York: Liss, 1984, pp 459–469.
17. Granelli SG, Diamond I, McDonagh AF, et al. Photochemotherapy of glioma cells by visible light and hematoporphyrin. *Cancer Res* 1975; 35:2567–2570.
18. Grossweiner LI, Patel AS, Grossweiner JB. Type I and type II mechanisms in the photosensitized lysis of phosphatidylcholine liposomes by hematoporphyrin. *Photochem Photobiol* 1982; 36:159–167.
19. Kaye AH, Morstyn G, Brownbill D. Adjuvant high-dose photoradiation therapy in the treatment of cerebral glioma: a phase 1-2 study. *J Neurosurg* 1987; 67:500–505.
20. Kessel D. Components of hematoporphyrin derivatives and their tumor-localizing capacity. *Cancer Res* 1982; 42:1703–1706.
21. Kinsey JH, Cortese DA, Moses HL, et al. Photodynamic effect of hematoporphyrin derivative as a function of optical spectrum and incident energy density. *Cancer Res* 1981; 41:5020–5026.
22. Kostron H, Weiser G, Fritsch E, et al. Photodynamic therapy of malignant brain tumors: clinical and neuropathological results. *Photochem Photobiol* 1987; 46:937–943.
23. Laws ER Jr, Cortese DA, Kinsey JH, et al. Photoradiation therapy in the treatment of malignant brain tumors: a phase I (feasibility) study. *Neurosurgery* 1981; 9:672–678.
24. Laws ER Jr, Wharen RE, Anderson RE. Photodynamic therapy of brain tumors. In Jori G, Perria C (eds): *Photodynamic Therapy of Tumors and Other Diseases.* Padova: Libreria Progetto, 1985, pp 311–316.
25. Laws ER Jr, Wharen RE Jr, Anderson RE. The treatment of brain tumors by photoradiation. In Pluchino F, Broggi G (eds): *Advanced Technology in Neurosurgery.* Berlin: Springer-Verlag, 1988, pp 46–60.
26. McCulloch GAJ, Forbes IJ, See KL, et al. Phototherapy in malignant brain tumors. In Doiron DR, Gomer CJ (eds): *Porphyrin Localization and Treatment of Tumors.* New York: Liss, 1984, pp 709–717.
27. Muller PJ, Wilson BC. Photodynamic therapy of malignant primary brain tumors: clinical effects, postoperative ICP, and light penetration of the brain. *Photochem Photobiol* 1987; 46:929–935.
28. Muller PJ, Wilson BC. Photodynamic therapy of malignant brain tumours. *Can J Neurol Sci* 1990; 17:193–198.
29. Origitano TC, Karesh SM, Henkin RE et al. Photodynamic therapy for intracranial neoplasms: investigations of photosensitizers uptake and distribution using indium-III photofrin-II single photon emission computed tomography scans in humans with intracranial neoplasms. *Neurosurgery* 1993; 32:357–364.
30. Origitano TC, Karesh SM, Reichman OH et al. Indium-III photofrin-II scintillation scan. *Neurosurgery* 1989; 24:547–556.
31. Perria C. Photodynamic therapy of human gliomas by hematoporphyrin and He-Ne laser. *IRCS Med Sci (Cancer)* 1981; 9:57–58.
32. Perria C, Capuzzo T, Cavagnaro G, et al. First attempts at the photodynamic treatment of human gliomas. *J Neurosurg Sci* 1980; 24:119–129.
33. Perria C, Carai M, Falzoi A, et al. Photodynamic therapy of malignant brain tumors: clinical results of, difficulties with, questions about, and future prospects for the neurosurgical applications. *Neurosurgery* 1988; 23:557–563.
34. Powers SK, Cush SS, Walstad DL, et al. Stereotactic intratumoral photodynamic therapy for recurrent malignant brain tumors. *Neurosurgery* 1991; 29:688–696.
35. Rasmussen-Taxdal DS, Ward GE, Figge FHJ. Fluorescence of human lymphatic and cancer tissues following high doses of intravenous hematoporphyrin. *Cancer* 1955; 8:78–81.
36. Rounds DE, Jacques S, Shelden CH, et al. Development of a protocol for photoradiation therapy of malignant brain tumors: Part I. Photosensitization of normal brain tissue with hematoporphyrin derivative. *Neurosurgery* 1982; 11:500–505.
37. Wharen RE Jr, Anderson RE, Laws ER Jr. Quantitation of hematoporphyrin derivative in human gliomas, experimental central nervous system tumors, and normal tissues. *Neurosurgery* 1983; 12:446–450.
38. Wharen RE Jr, Anderson RE, Laws ER Jr. Photoradiation therapy with hematoporphyrin derivative in the management of brain tumors. In Fasano VA (ed): *Advanced Intraoperative Technologies in Neurosurgery* Vienna: Springer-Verlag, 1987, pp 211–227.
39. Wharen RE Jr, Anderson RE, Laws ER Jr. Photoradiation therapy of malignant brain tumors. In Cerullo LJ (ed): *Application of Lasers in Neurosurgery.* Chicago: Year Book Medical Publishers, 1988, pp 156–171.
40. Wharen RE Jr, Anderson RE, Laws ER Jr. Photoradiation therapy of brain tumors. In Salcman M (ed): *Neurobiology of Brain Tumors.* Baltimore: Williams & Wilkins, 1991, pp 341–357.
41. Wharen RE Jr, So S, Anderson RE, et al. Hematoporhyrin derivative photocytotoxicity of human glioblastoma in cell culture. *Neurosurgery* 1986; 19:495–501.
42. Wise BL, Taxdal DR. Studies of the blood-brain barrier utilizing hematoporphyrin. *Brain Res* 1957; 4:387–389.

192 Hyperthermia in the Treatment of Intracranial Tumors

Robert G. Selker

The current "best accepted" therapy for glioblastoma provides a median survival period of approximately 55 weeks.[23] Attempts to increase survival time by expanding the limits of current therapy (surgery, radiation, chemotherapy) result in an increase in morbidity and a decrease in overall quality of life. Clearly, one cannot resect the thalamus, the brain stem, the corpus callosum, or the majority of the dominant hemisphere and expect a reasonably functional result. Similarly, radiation dose levels above 6500 rad may result in damage of normal tissue, especially when given as a total head dose. If radiation is confined to the tumor bed plus a 2-cm border (the area of recurrence), viability of surrounding normal tissue still remains an important consideration.[5] Whereas, experimentally, cell kill rates may be increased with increasing levels of chemotherapy, systemic toxicity precludes that level of use in the human. Immunotherapy, be it active or passive, specific or nonspecific, cannot control (at least at present) large tumor burdens. Hence, the need for a modality to enhance the effectiveness of currently employed agents, hopefully utilizing inherent biological differences between normal and abnormal tissue to control tumor growth and increase the quality of survival. Such a modality may be hyperthermia.

Before the turn of the century, Coley published a report on the use of a toxin derived from a strain of Streptococcus, which, when injected directly into malignancies of the head and neck, produced fever, chills, suppuration, and a remarkable reduction in tumor size.[2] Why this occurred remains a subject of much debate. Was the remission, in fact, related to the degree of body temperature elevation? Possibly; patients not experiencing a febrile response seemed destined not to demonstrate a tumor response. Was the beneficial effect of the toxin related to a nonspecific immune response on the part of the host, with invasion of the area by lymphocytes and macrophages? Or, in fact, did this local effect on malignant cells represent suppuration with subsequent cell destruction?

In vitro experiments and some clinical data suggest that the febrile response is important, as evidenced by the relationship of cell kill rates to the degree of temperature elevation and the length of time of application; and that these factors are inversely proportional (i.e., the higher the temperature, the less time required to achieve cell kill) (Fig. 192-1). Furthermore, experimental evidence[19] suggests a synergistic effect when heat is combined with radiation therapy, yielding a therapeutic enhancement ratio (TER), where TER = rad dose/rad dose + heat. The enhancement is most pronounced when both modalities are delivered simultaneously.

If, then, this combined modality synergism can be demonstrated to occur in tumor tissue, it is proper to inquire as to the effect on surrounding normal tissue. Would, for instance, a differential effect on normal versus abnormal tissue therapeutic gain factor (TGF), where TGF = TER of tumor/TER of normal tissue, subsequently accrue? In point of fact, it would appear that if two modalities (heat and radiation) are delivered simultaneously, a major therapeutic enhancement does occur, but without a normal tissue differential. Hence, the modalities may need to be separated temporally, unless a defined volume is delineated and targeted for destruction. Hence, the case for local defined application. Which modality (in the case of radiation and heat) is best delivered first remains a matter of conjecture, although most investigators favor a preheating radiation dosage schedule. It must be concluded, then,

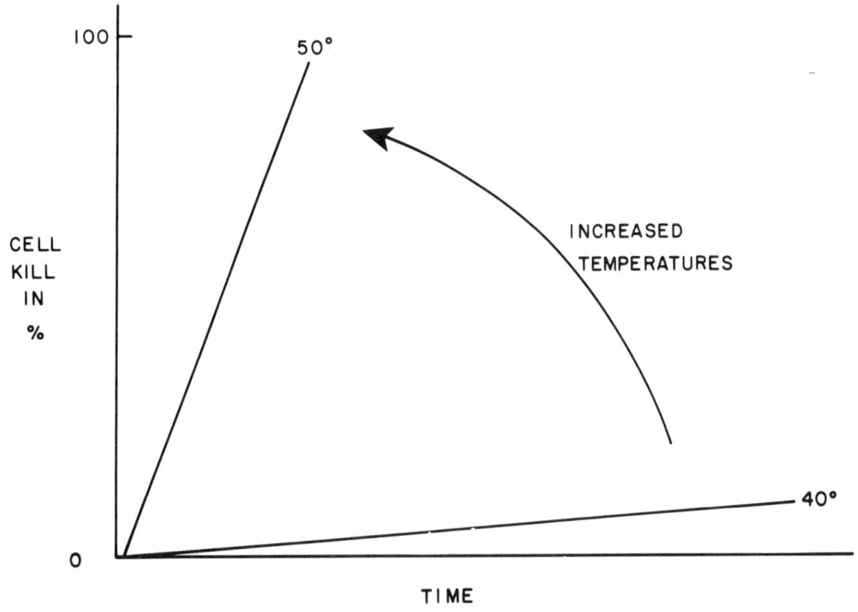

Figure 192-1 Relationship of time and temperature to cell kill rate.

that an increase in the TER when modalities are globally employed simultaneously may be achieved at the expense of the TGF (Fig. 192-2). The higher the TGF, the less damage to normal tissue there will be, presumably with less tumor effect as well. The key to success lies in the differential rates of metabolism and DNA repair in normal versus tumor cells.

A similar enhancement effect has been demonstrated in rats when elevated body temperatures are employed with 1, 3-bis (2-chloroethyl)-1-nitrosourea (BCNU), bleomycin, adriamycin, 5-fluorouracil, and methotrexate.[4,5,13] These reports support a therapeutic enhancement ratio of approximately 2, perhaps mandating up to a 50 percent reduction in drug dosage to avoid untoward systemic toxicity. Our own clinical experience, using 75 percent of the usual calculated dose per square meter of body surface and greater than 450°/min of total-body heat, confirms this previously published experimental expectation.[13] (See later explanation of degree/minutes.)

The laboratory evidence is now sufficient to allow the clinical introduction of hyperthermia as an adjuvant to existing treatment modalities. But how should this tool be applied? How can its possible toxicity be controlled and its potential enhanced? Should it be applied locally, regionally, or as a total body effort? What standard units of dosimetry are applicable? How can these modalities be combined in a hospital setting? Does repeated heating of tumor cells create thermal tolerance and/or resistant mutants in humans? These and other perplexing questions remain only partially answered, creating a technologic and biological dilemma.

Methodology

Local Intratumoral Hyperthermia

In many ways the brain tumor lends itself admirably to the application of local intratumoral heating. The glioblastoma is, in most instances, a local infiltrating disease supplied by a well-defined vascular perfusion bed which can be diagnostically imaged by a number of methods. Blood flow within the tumor is, as a rule, slower than in surrounding normal tissue, thereby creating a ''heat sink'' of poorly dissipated energy. By employing newly developed microwave, ultrasound, conductive, and radio-frequency techniques (some requiring indwelling antennae), temperatures in the range of 45° to 50°C can be produced and monitored by specifically designed thermocouples which do not participate in the created energy field.[12,14,15,20-22] Computer-controlled heat energy distribution within the mass strives to maintain uniform temperatures within the target volume. In effect, the physician is committed to heating a geometric volume of tissue which may contain normal and abnormal tissue as well as varying degrees of necrotic central tissue (making uniform intratumoral heating difficult) and yet may not contain an extension of tumor tissue beyond the volume of heating. Some recent work indicates the possibility of differing effects on normal and abnormal tissue within a heated geometric volume, depending upon the energy sources.[17,21] If this is the case, a major advance in local heating technology will have been made.

Methods of applying local heat energy to the exact confines of the tumor disclosed on computed tomographic (CT) or magnetic resonance (MR) images are currently undergoing study. Since a border area is also to be treated, a moderate amount of normal tissue and, more importantly, perhaps, deeper, functionally vital areas may still remain within the treatment field. Implantation of antennae or catheters (or other invasive devices), required for some local heat-generation techniques, faces a similar problem in that the surgeon can little afford to thread devices into the brain stem, thalamus, or similar sensitive areas, let alone destroy that volume of tissue. Further, the combination of modalities (interstitial heating and interstitial radiotherapy) may require separate implant systems (thermoseed vs. conductive devices vs. antennae) to effect simultaneous delivery. However, the introduction of a single catheter system for both interstitial radiation and interstitial hyperthermia (Cook, Inc., Bloomington, IN) may at last permit simultaneous application of these modalities.

From a practical point of view, many of the tumors encountered by neurologists and neurosurgeons are metastatic. Once the tumor is palliated by surgery and radiation, the usual cause of death is

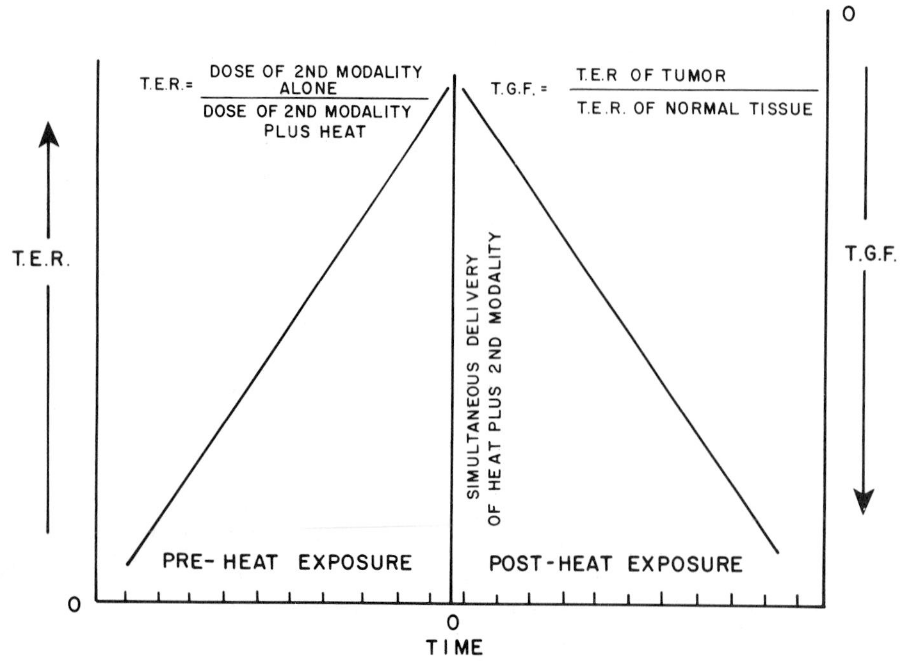

Figure 192-2 Enhancement of a second modality when employed with heat. Presumed effects on therapeutic enhancement ratio (TER) and therapeutic gain factor (TGF).

systemic dissemination and not the intracranial problem. Can a local heating technique be expected to heat all metastatic deposits in bone, brain, lung, marrow, etc.? With the current state-of-the-art equipment, it seems unlikely. However, local intracranial-intratumoral heating is an attractive technique because it (1) has the ability to achieve intratumoral temperatures much higher than can be tolerated by the human organism as a whole, (2) has the ability to locally enhance the effect of systemic or regionally delivered chemotherapy, (3) in some cases utilizes technology which can be employed without hospitalization or anesthesia, (4) can be repeated on frequent occasions within a short time span, (5) provides the ability to retreat an area at the time of recurrence without concern for cumulative total body toxicity, (6) can easily be imaged by CT or MRI, and (7) allows for preheating dosimetry planning and stereotactic or CT-guided implantation.

Regional Hyperthermia

Regional hyperthermia for melanoma of the limb, utilizing a closed-circuit system and extracorporeal circulator, has achieved acknowledged success.[7,18] Its application to a similar isolated perfusion area, the brain and/or head and neck, has not been as successful.[16] All perfusion methods involving the intracranial circulation suffer from the inability to restrict the circulatory ''leak'' of chemotherapeutic agents and from the rapid dissipation of heat from the region as a result of the rapid blood flow perfusing the intra- and extracranial tissue. Total body temperature elevation may occur before any significant intracranial temperature gradient can be achieved. Current work with energy sources in the 13.7 MHz range as used for regional heating elsewhere may show an advantage, but again, blood flow rates and the effect of total brain heating may outweigh the usefulness of the technique.[17]

Thermal Gradient

Popovic and Masironi reported dramatic observations of tumor regression in the experimental animal when tumor tissue was maintained at normothermic or hyperthermic levels while remaining body tissues were cooled to 30°C utilizing systemic hypothermia.[10] Their findings indicate cell kill rates to be dependent upon the length of time the gradient is applied and the span of the gradient between normal and abnormal tissue temperatures. When combined with a systemic chemotherapeutic agent, the advantage of the gradient is obvious. In attempting to apply this principle to the glioblastoma, the physician is immediately confronted with the same restrictions as outlined for local intracranial-intratumoral heating: the need for an implanted heating device, the volume of tissue to be heated, the inability to be certain of thermic homogeneity, and the uncertainty of cellular infiltration surrounding the target volume. Although it is a method not to be discarded for use in intracranial tumors, a thermal gradient would be technically difficult to effect, control, and monitor.

Total Body Hyperthermia

This form of hyperthermia uniformly heats (±0.05° to 0.10°C at equilibration) and affects all organ systems of the body. That feature of the procedure is a double-edged sword. On the one hand, the effects of heating and its enhancing capability when combined with other modalities are equally distributed throughout the body (an advantage in metastatic disease). On the other hand, human organ systems cannot withstand total body temperatures much beyond 42°C (a level needed to effect a major cell kill rate when heat is used alone), nor can they withstand heating's potential toxicity when it is employed with simultaneously administered systemic chemotherapy and/or large-volume irradiation. Although much of the literature on total body hyperthermia is concerned with efforts directed to a single agent (heating), most authors now believe a combined-modality approach to be the most beneficial; that is, radiotherapy, immunotherapy, chemotherapy, and heat in some combination and time relationship. As an adjuvant, the concept of total body heating is based on the assumption that inherent biological differences exist between normal and abnormal cells in pH, oxygen consumption, sugar metabolism, blood flow, and rates of DNA replication and repair. In the glioblastoma, for instance (and in some other solid tumor systems), the inherent phenomenon of anerobic metabolism can be capitalized upon by deliberately creating systemic nonketotic hyperglycemia, resulting in increased levels of intratumoral lactate production and a further decrease in an already lower intratumoral pH, thereby contributing to the differential effect of treatment.[3] Continuous intracranial pressure monitoring and previous cytoreductive efforts are mandatory when using this technique. The application of total body heating to the glioblastoma patient now has assumed a secondary (if any) role when one considers the local heating technologies available.

The procedure for total body hyperthermia is technically simple in comparison to the use of electronic instrumentation for local heating. Its potential effects on the organism, however, creates the need for multiparameter physiologic monitoring during the procedure. Considering the fine line of normal tissue (brain and liver) temperature tolerance at about 42°C, multisite temperature surveillance must be accurate to within less than 0.1°C, standardized to a recognized international reference probe. Rectal, esophageal, and bladder temperatures have been described[8,9] by various authors; however, our own experience indicates the pulmonary artery temperature, as measured by a Swan-Ganz thermocouple, to be the most predictive of core and brain temperature at equilibration.

The current methods of induction of total body hyperthermia include (1) molten wax immersion,[9] (2) use of an extracorporeal heat exchanger,[8] (3) use of a radiant oven,[11] (4) use of standard hyperthermia blankets,[6] (5) use of converted space suits or respirator-like devices with hot-air convection heating,[1] and (6) water bath immersion. Some of these methods require general anesthesia; all are inpatient procedures; and all cause changes in basal metabolic rate, cardiovascular physiology, fluid and electrolyte balance, colloid osmotic pressure, peripheral resistance, intracranial pressure, oxygen consumption, liver metabolism, and platelet function. All effects become extremely critical when dealing with intracranial mass effect and increased intracranial pressure.

As with local hyperthermia, dosimetry becomes important in estimation of therapeutic effect. The exact amount of heating required (in time and temperature) to create a response in the glioblastoma is largely unknown. It is assumed to be at least similar to that required in other solid tumor systems and to follow the outlines of previously enumerated time and temperature parameters (Figs. 192-1 and 192-2). Our own experiments indicate glioma cells to be resistant to 2 h of 40.5°C heating when in a sugar-containing tissue culture medium. However, when glioma cells are heated in a non-sugar-containing medium, they cannot be replated and are ultimately determined to be nonviable. At temperatures above 42° to 43°C, cell metabolic rates seem to preclude survival regardless of the sugar content of the medium.

In general, the term *degree/minutes* is used to rate or standardize total body heating dosage. In their simplest form, degree/minutes are calculated by multiplying the number of degrees of body temperature elevation above 40°C by the time that the temperature is maintained at that level. It is, in effect, an expression of the area beneath the described temperature curve. The limit for human tolerance has been quoted as 300°/min, with the highest achieved central temperature being somewhat less than 42°C.[9] Our own experience indicates tolerance to 450°/min when combined with midheating chemotherapy (BCNU) at 50 percent of the usual dose per square meter of body surface. There can be reversible toxicity in the form of platelet loss (<15,000), elevated prothrombin times (>20/10), and major changes in hepatic enzymes. In three patients treated with heat at 450°/min and 75 percent of the usual dose per square meter of body surface, proximal myopathy (and/or a Guillain-Barré–like syndrome) has occurred, although some investigators claim to have used a sustained temperature of 41.5°C for as long as 30 h, apparently without major clinical effect or damage to normal tissue.

Our clinical experience with total body hyperthermia has been exclusively with the use of a water bath immersion technique. It is simple, inexpensive, and easily controlled, does not require anticoagulation (an important feature with intracranial lesions), and reduces insensible fluid loss to a minimum. We have had experience with a number of primary and metastatic lesions to the brain, selecting where possible a target and a control lesion (Fig. 192-3). The target lesion is subjected to preheating sensitizing radiation (500 to 750 rad and a presumed TER of 2), thereby making it the object of a three-modality protocol (i.e., midheating chemotherapy, preheating irradiation, and heat), while the control lesion receives only midheating chemotherapy and heat. Our experience thus far in a series of terminal patients, not all of whom could tolerate a planned monthly treatment protocol, seems to indicate that three modalities are in fact required in order to control tumor growth. If this is true, this requirement could be satisfied with a half-body single-fraction low-dose radiation schedule, lending application to patients with widespread dissemination who also harbor an intracranial lesion. Our experience also indicates the need to reduce increased intracranial pressure to normal (or near-normal) levels by some surgical means prior to total body heating. In our hands, this has taken the form of repeat cytoreductive surgery and/or some external ventricular drainage (EVD) device. The same need may be present when local intracranial-intratumoral heating is employed, depending upon the degree of enhanced blood flow and tissue swelling, and the volume to be heated. In patients with an intracranial mass who are undergoing total body heating, vasodilatation and intracranial suffusion have caused recorded pressures as high as 40 torr, necessitating aborting the procedure or controlling the rise by venting CSF through a previously placed reservoir or EVD.

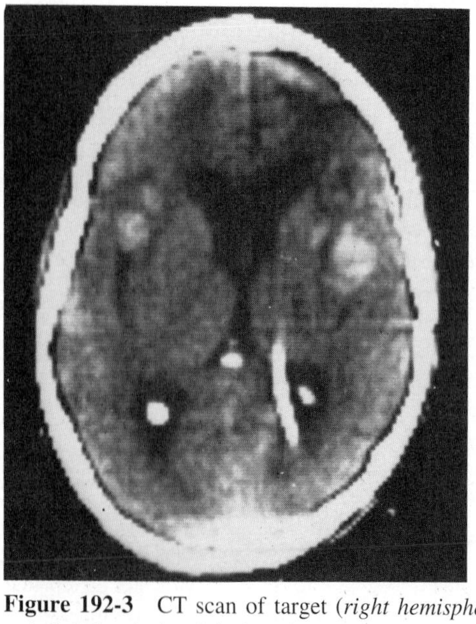

Figure 192-3 CT scan of target (*right hemisphere*) and control (*left hemisphere*) lesions in a patient with metastatic malignant melanoma.

Hyperthermia in Combination with Newer Modalities of Radiation and Drug Delivery

In previous paragraphs the use of heat combined with chemotherapy and external radiation has been described. In the glioblastoma, BCNU remains the drug of choice; the effects of BCNU are fortunately (or unfortunately) enhanced by heat. Whether to give the drug before, during, or after the hyperthermia remains a matter of conjecture. Still to be determined is the effect of a single intracarotid injection of the drug during heating versus sustained release throughout the period of heating. However, considering the overall morbidity of an intracarotid injection of BCNU in the unheated patient (about 15 percent), this route of delivery may be beyond the realm of experimental tolerance. Still, locally applied intratumoral hyperthermia combined with the systemic administration of a chemotherapeutic agent may be productive of an increased cell kill rate.

The use of local hyperthermia along with external beam radiation in nonintracranial lesions is acknowledged to have some advantage, is currently employed in many centers, and has resulted in a dramatic reduction of local tumor burden and mass effect. New radiation treatment planners coupled to the computed tomography scanner and stereotactic radiosurgery, may promote a greater effect on glioblastoma regardless of the type of local heating employed, but may in some cases present a major logistical problem. The effect of local hyperthermia on the glioblastoma may be further enhanced with the use of interstitial irradiation. Radiation sources implanted stereotactically (by "afterloading" or "hot loading") can provide a constant simultaneous source of therapy to a local area and permit continuous simultaneous or intermittent enhancement by multiple heatings, yet confine the main effect to a local intracranial volume. Although complex in its dosimetry requirements, the advantages of using this combination may overcome the labor-intensive cost requirements. Again, as with any procedure requiring local implants, tumors in functionally sensitive areas of the brain may be beyond the scope of this procedure.

References

1. Bull JM, Lees D, Schuete W, et al. Whole body hyperthermia: a phase-I trial of a potential adjuvant to chemotherapy. *Ann Intern Med* 1979; 90:317–323.
2. Coley WB. The treatment of malignant tumors by repeated inoculations of erysipelas: with a report of 10 original cases. *Am J Med Sci* 1893; 105:487–511.

3. Duggins EL. Effects of insulin and glucose on the interstitial pH differential between normal and tumor tissues during normo and hyperthermia. Unpublished manuscript.
4. Hahn GM, Braun J, Har-Kedar I. Thermochemotherapy: synergism between hyperthermia (42-43°) and adriamycin (or bleomycin) in mammalian cell inactivation. *Proc Natl Acad Sci USA* 1975; 72:937–940.
5. Hochberg FH, Pruitt A. Assumptions in the radiotherapy of glioblastoma. *Neurology (NY)* 1980; 30:907–911.
6. Larkin JM, Edwards WS, Smith DE, Clark PJ. Systemic thermotherapy: description of a method and physiologic tolerance in clinical subjects. *Cancer* 1977; 40:3155–3159.
7. Martin H, Oldhoff J, Koops HS. Hyperthermic regional perfusion with melphalan and a combination of melphalan and actinomycin D in the treatment of locally metastasized malignant melanomas of the extremities. *J Surg Oncol* 1982; 20:9–13.
8. Parks LC, Minaberry D, Smith DP, Neely WA. Treatment of far-advanced bronchogenic carcinoma by extracorporeally induced systemic hyperthermia. *J Thorac Cardiovasc Surg* 1979; 78:883–892.
9. Pettigrew RT, Galt JM, Ludgate CM, Smith AN. Clinical effects of whole-body hyperthermia in advanced malignancy. *Br Med J* 1974; 4:679–682.
10. Popovic VP, Masironi R. Disappearance of normothermic tumors in shallow (30°C) hypothermia. *Cancer Res* 1966; 26:863–864.
11. Robbins HI. Clinical use of a radiant head device (RHD) for whole-body hyperthermia (WBH). Presented at a meeting of the International Clinical Hyperthermia Society, London, June 1982.
12. Salcman M, Samaras GM. Hyperthermia for brain tumors: biophysical rationale. *Neurosurgery* 1981; 9:327–335.
13. Selker RG, Bova E, Kristofik M, et al. Effect of total body temperature on toxicity of 1,3-bis(2-chloroethyl)-1-nitrosourea (BCNU). *Neurosurgery* 1979; 4:157–161.
14. Selker RG, Wolfson SK Jr. The creation of thermal gradients in primates in the treatment of brain tumors. *J Med Primatol* 1975; 4:351.
15. Selker RG, Wolfson SK Jr, Medal R, Miller M. Creation of a chemothermal gradient in treatment of brain tumors. *Surg Forum* 1973; 24:461–463.
16. Shingleton WW, Bryan FA Jr, O'Quinn WL, Krueger LC. Selective heating and cooling of tissue in cancer chemotherapy. *Ann Surg* 1962; 156:408–416.
17. Silberman AW, Morgan DF, Storm FK, et al. Localized magnetic-loop induction hyperthermia of the rabbit brain. *J Surg Oncol* 1982; 20:174–178.
18. Stehlin JS Jr, Greeff P, Giovanella BC, Williams LJ Jr. Dramatic response of cancer to localized hyperthermia. *NY State J Med* 1980; 80:70–72.
19. Stewart FA, Denekamp J. Combined x-ray and heating: is there a therapeutic gain? In Streffer C, van Beuningen D, Dietzel F, et al. (eds): *Cancer Therapy by Hyperthermia and Radiation Therapy. Proceedings of Second International Symposium, Essen, June 2–4, 1977.* Baltimore: Urban & Schwarzenberg, 1978, pp 249–250.
20. Sutton CH, Carroll FB. Experimental studies on the use of temperature gradients to increase blood flow in malignant gliomas. Presented at a meeting of the European Association of Neurological Societies, September 1975.
21. Tanaka R. Radiofrequency hyperthermia therapy of experimental brain tumors. Presented at the Brain Tumor Meeting, Nikko, Japan, October 1981.
22. Thackray P, Meiskin ZH, Wolfson SK, Selker RG. Indirect heating source for treatment of malignant brain tumors. *Electrocomp Sci Technol* 1974; 1:91–96.
23. Walker MD, Green SB, Byar DP, et al. Randomized comparison of radiotherapy and nitrosoureas for the treatment of malignant glioma after surgery. *N Engl J Med* 1980; 303:1323–1329.

Part VII

Vascular Diseases of the Nervous System

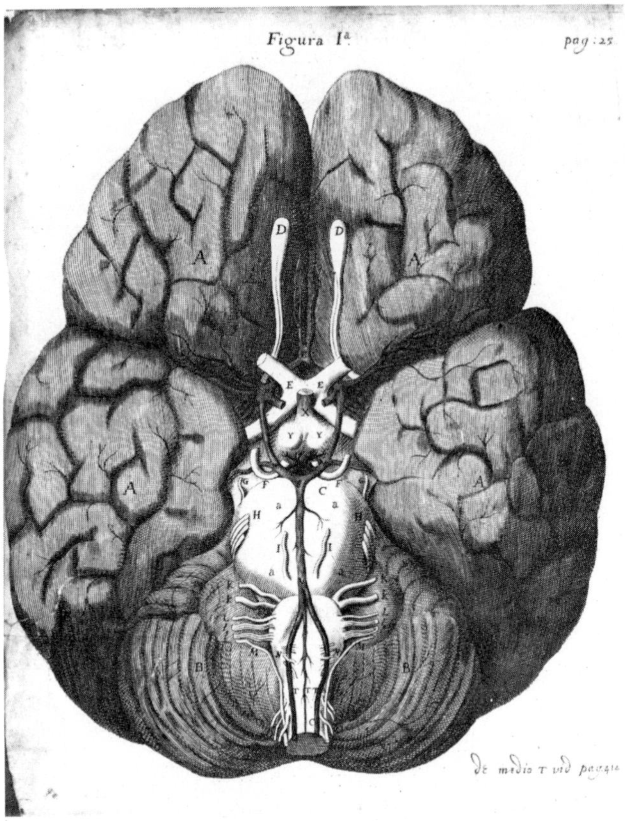

Willis T. *Cerebri Anatome.* London: Martyn & Allestry, 1664. An engraving of the base of the brain by Christopher Wren, illustrating the circle of Willis.

SECTION A

General Information

193

Persistent Embryonic Intracranial and Extracranial Vessels

Jon M. Silver
Robert H. Wilkins

Variations in the normal cerebrovascular anatomy, particularly with respect to persistent embryonic vessels, are of primary interest to individuals studying the central nervous system. Those involved in the treatment of diseases of the head and neck need to be aware of these deviations from the normal anatomy in order to plan neurodiagnostic as well as surgical strategies. Pathologic conditions associated with these abnormalities, including aneurysms, arteriovenous fistulae, and cranial nerve syndromes need also be considered.

The primary focus of this chapter will be variations in what is thought to be the standard vascular anatomy. The anatomy and clinical significance of these persistent embryonic vessels will be addressed. A brief review of the embryologic development of the arteries and veins of the head and neck will be provided first, as a basis for understanding abnormal persistent vessels.

Embryologic Development of the Cerebral Circulation

Arterial Embryology

Much of our current understanding of the normal embryology of the cranial arterial system is derived from the contributions of Dorcas Padget. Her monumental work concerning the development of the cranial arteries involved the study of embryos at various stages.[26]

At approximately 3-mm crown-rump length, specific cranial vessels first become apparent. The internal carotid arteries form as branches of the first aortic arches. By 4 mm, the internal carotids extend rostrally from the paired dorsal aortae. At this time the first and second aortic arches regress and the internal carotids become continuous with the third aortic arches, which serve as their roots. Also at this time, a pair of vessels called the longitudinal neural arteries develop at the base of the hindbrain, dorsal and parallel to the internal carotids.

As this 4-mm stage progresses, many changes take place in the structure of the internal carotid arteries. Each advances rostrally and, at the level of the optic vesicle, divides into cranial and caudal branches. The cranial branch will provide the anterior choroidal, middle cerebral, and primitive olfactory arteries, as well as the anterior cerebral artery at its terminal end. The caudal branch gives off the diencephalic, mesencephalic, and posterior choroidal branches. It will later join with the ipsilateral longitudinal neural artery (see below). By this stage, the formation of three additional arteries has taken place; these arise from the internal carotid artery to supply the longitudinal neural artery. They are called the trigeminal, otic, and hypoglossal arteries as determined by their relationship with the trigeminal ganglion, otic vesicle, and hypoglossal nerve. At the caudal end of the longitudinal neural artery, a branch from the dorsal aorta called the proatlantal intersegmental artery forms to provide blood supply here. Also at this stage, a remnant of the second aortic arch called the hyoid artery can be found.

At the 5- to 6-mm stage, the caudal branch of the internal carotid artery communicates with the ipsilateral longitudinal neural artery. With blood flow via this communication as well as via the proatlantal intersegmental artery, the three primitive arteries mentioned above regress—first the otic artery, followed by the hypoglossal artery, and finally the trigeminal artery. The connection from the caudal branch of the internal carotid artery to the longitudinal neural artery becomes the posterior communicating artery. A second pair of longitudinal channels, dorsal to the longitudinal neural arteries, are formed; they are called the primitive lateral basilovertebral anastomoses. These join the proatlantal intersegmental arteries and also communicate with the longitudinal neural arteries by transverse channels. They form anastomoses between the vertebral and basilar arteries and give rise to each posterior inferior cerebellar artery (PICA). During this stage, two other changes occur; the ventral pharyngeal artery, the precursor of the external carotid artery, arises from the aortic sac, and the hyoid artery, near its origin, gives off a branch called the stapedial artery.

By 7- to 12-mm crown-rump length, several changes take place in the posterior circulation. The longitudinal neural arteries fuse to form the basilar artery. The intersegmental arteries that arise from the dorsal aortae to supply the cervical somites fuse at their dorsal ends in a rostrocaudal fashion. As this occurs, all communications to each dorsal aorta regress except that from the sixth intersegmental artery. This dorsal channel becomes the vertebral artery, and the sixth intersegmental artery contributes to the subclavian artery. The cranial portion of the internal carotid artery also undergoes further change, giving rise to the anterior choroidal and middle cerebral arteries and terminating in the anterior cerebral and primitive olfactory arteries.

During the next phase of development (12- to 15-mm crown-rump length), the stapedial artery bifurcates into a dorsal branch that continues on to supply the middle meningeal artery and the supraorbital region, and a ventral or maxillomandibular branch. This latter artery divides into the maxillary and mandibular arteries. Following this, at approximately 15- to 17-mm crown-rump length, a branch of the external carotid artery called the internal maxillary artery joins the maxillomandibular artery. At this point, the anatomy is such that the middle meningeal, supraorbital, maxillary, and mandibular arteries are supplied by both the internal carotid artery and the developing external carotid artery. This relationship becomes important when persistent anastomoses between the internal and external carotid arteries are encountered. Also during this stage, the major branches of the internal carotid and basilar arteries develop further. From the former, the anterior cerebral arteries, with their plexiform anterior communicating channel, and the middle cerebral arteries become major branches. The stem of the ophthalmic artery is also seen. From the basilar artery, the superior cerebellar (SCA) and anterior inferior cerebellar artery (AICA) on each side become prominent.

Further development continues at 20- to 24-mm crown-rump length: the anterior communicating artery is now a single channel, thus completing the circle of Willis. Significant changes also take place with respect to the stapedial artery. The proximal portion of the stapedial artery begins to regress, and the hyoid artery becomes a small remnant called the caroticotympanic artery. The remaining, distal remnant of the stapedial artery is now known as the superior tympanic artery. The supraorbital branch becomes a minor branch called the anterior middle meningeal artery, and the middle meningeal artery remains. The branches of the maxillomandibular artery, the maxillary and the mandibular, become the infraorbital and the inferior alveolar arteries, respectively. Therefore, at this point, the middle meningeal artery and the maxillomandibular artery are branches of the external carotid artery via the internal maxillary artery.

Finally, at approximately 40 mm, the major arterial supply of the head has approached its adult configuration. The ophthalmic artery; anterior, middle, and posterior cerebral arteries; and the cerebellar arteries are comparable to those in the adult, and further changes principally involve further growth.[19]

Venous Embryology

An understanding of the embryologic development of the cranial venous system has been greatly advanced with the notable contributions of Mall,[22] Evans,[8] Streeter,[35] and Padget[27,28] in their studies of the human embryo. A basic knowledge of the evolution of the veins of the head and neck is essential before any discussion of venous anomalies that persist into adult life. The material presented below is derived mainly from the works of Streeter[35] and Padget.[27,28]

At the earliest stage of venous development, approximately 4-mm crown-rump length, a chain of angioblasts extends from the dorsal aortae as a plexus to the forebrain and midbrain. Shortly thereafter, bilateral longitudinal channels form at the ventrolateral margins of the hindbrain which communicate anteriorly with this primary plexus and caudally with the anterior cardinal vein. Active proliferation of this endothelial meshwork continues in all directions, and from this meshwork, a more lateral and superficial channel forms called the primary head vein. This has also been termed the primary head sinus by Padget[28] because of its dural location. The primary plexus divides into deep and superficial portions, the former being a capillary sheet investing the brain wall and the latter forming larger channels for the dura. These are connected by intermediate channels. Three main tributaries from the superficial plexus that drain into the primary head vein are formed, and these are referred to as the anterior, middle, and posterior dural plexuses. The anterior plexus drains the forebrain and midbrain and enters the primary head vein in front of the semilunar ganglion, the middle plexus drains the cerebellum and enters between the semilunar and acousticofacial complex, and the posterior plexus drains the medullary region and enters caudal to the otic capsule. Ventrally, two major drainage channels are formed, serving the optic vesicle and the mandibular and hyoid regions; these are termed the maxillary and ventral pharyngeal veins, respectively. These changes take place during the stage from 5- to 8-mm crown-rump length.

At approximately 8 to 12 mm, further changes take place due, in part, to the development of the dura and pia-arachnoid. This begins at the base and extends toward the vertex.[35] As this occurs, there is a decrease in the number of intermediate channels joining the superficial and deep plexuses, with only major communications remaining. These channels persist such that each of the five divisions of the brain has a major drainage channel; for example, first the diencephalic veins and then the telencephalic veins drain into the anterior dural plexus. The primary head vein migrates lateral to the facial and vagus complexes while remaining medial to the trigeminal ganglion, and its medial remnant becomes the myelencephalic vein. During this stage a primitive marginal sinus surrounding the developing cerebral hemispheres arises from the anterior dural plexus, and the posterior dural plexus migrates caudally to become directly continuous with a portion of the anterior cardinal vein that will later become the internal jugular vein.

By 14 mm, a second tributary draining the optic region is formed called the supraorbital vein. It joins with the primary head sinus or the anterior dural plexus and eventually becomes the superior orbital vein. At this point, only one or two veins drain each of the five major divisions of the brain as the small tributaries undergo compression with growth of the hemispheres. In the neck, the cervical intersegmental veins join, forming the vertebral vein. Also at this point, the dorsal portions of the anterior and middle dural plexuses advance toward the midline to form the early sagittal plexus, which will later become the superior and inferior sagittal sinuses. Anteriorly, this plexus dips between the cerebral hemispheres; however, it is not easily distinguished from the remainder of the superficial plexus.

Following this, from about 17- to 20-mm crown-rump length, major changes take place in the primary head vein. With growth of the otic capsule, the middle portion of the primary head vein becomes crowded laterally, and drainage between the middle and posterior plexuses takes place dorsally via an intrachondrocranial channel, the future sigmoid sinus. The dwindling middle plexus and middle portion of the primary head vein will later contribute to the superior petrosal sinus. Anastomotic channels between the anterior and middle dural plexuses actually increase. Also, the ventral pharyngeal vein becomes the linguofacial vein and anastomoses with the maxillary vein. To summarize up to this point, the primary head vein is now divided into three portions: an anterior portion (or trigeminal portion) that will later become the cavernous sinus; a middle portion lateral to the otic capsule; and a cervical portion, now called the internal jugular vein. These relationships are outlined in Fig. 193-1.

By 20- to 21-mm crown-rump length, the cavernous sinus has become better defined and drains the ophthalmic and maxillary veins as well as large cerebral veins from the lateral wall of the diencephalon. These latter veins eventually become the middle cerebral veins. The cavernous sinus is now one of the few remaining portions of the primary head vein. It drains into the forming transverse sinus via the superior petrosal sinus that has formed from the stem of the middle dural plexus and the middle portion of the primary head vein. The transverse sinus is situated dorsal to the dwindling primary head vein and arises from the stems of the anterior and middle dural plexuses. The tentorium has also begun to take shape between the caudal pole of the cerebral hemispheres and the cerebellum. Imbedded in this loose tissue is the tentorial plexus, a meshwork of the anterior and middle dural plexuses. At this stage, the posterior dural plexus undergoes far fewer changes. It will eventually form the occipital sinus as well as the marginal sinus of the foramen magnum.

During the period from 20 to 24 mm, changes occur in many areas of the developing venous system. The falx cerebri begins to take shape, and the sagittal plexus can now be located in its dorsal margin. The plexus contains fewer channels now, one of which will become the superior sagittal sinus. The straight sinus also forms at the lower part of the developing falx cerebri and receives the internal cerebral veins that have formed along the roof of the diencephalon. With cardiac enlargement and the formation of the sinus venosus, a detour to flow on the left side is established such that the majority of cerebral venous flow through the superior sagittal and straight sinuses is to the right. In the facial region, the maxillary vein anastomoses with the developing anterior facial vein and its stem dwindles. The supraorbital vein no longer drains into the anterior stem, as it has regressed, but now drains into the remnant of the middle dural stem, called the pro-otic sinus.[28] The tentorial sinus (not to be confused with the tentorial plexus, above) forms from the anterior dural plexus and receives the middle cerebral veins as well as the ventral diencephalic vein. The pairs of large veins that initially drained each of the five major regions now have become single stems. The tentorial plexus, with the growth of the cerebral and cerebellar hemispheres, changes shape and migrates caudally to eventually become the torcular. Finally, the external jugular system becomes apparent from a cranial tributary of the jugulocephalic vein. This system begins to annex the common facial (linguofacial) vein, which at this point still partly drains into the internal jugular system.

By 40-mm crown-rump length, the venous system starts to resemble its adult configuration. The great cerebral vein of Galen has formed, draining into the straight sinus. It receives the internal cerebral veins that represent a continuation of the developing superior choroidal veins. In this region, the septal and thalamostriate veins later become apparent. Draining the choroidal masses ventrally are the inferior choroidal veins. They are tributaries of the ventral diencephalic veins and will become important as the basal cerebral veins develop. The superficial middle cerebral veins continue into the tentorial sinus and subsequently into the transverse sinus. Anastomoses form between these middle cerebral veins and the superior cerebral veins, remnants of the anterior dural plexus, which represent primitive anastomotic veins of Trolard. The primitive middle meningeal sinus joins the pro-otic sinus to drain membranous bone. One of the five regional veins, the myelencephalic vein, contributes to the forming inferior petrosal sinus that joins the cavernous sinus. The midportion of the transverse sinus is transferred caudally with growth of the cerebral and cerebellar hemispheres. The tentorial sinus begins to elongate and curves around the ventral margin of the temporal lobe, and the dorsal diencephalic and mesencephalic veins pass through this region to continue with the transverse sinus. In the orbital region, a permanent stem of all orbital veins is formed from the stem of the maxillary vein. Primitive emissary veins are being formed and join the external jugular system. Significant emissaries exist in the temporal region, draining the temporoparietal ossification and, in the frontal region, joining the primitive supraorbital vein with the anterior facial vein. Also at this point, the superficial temporal vein forms to join the external jugular system.

Between 60- and 80-mm crown-rump length, the venous system undergoes many of the final changes that bring it to the

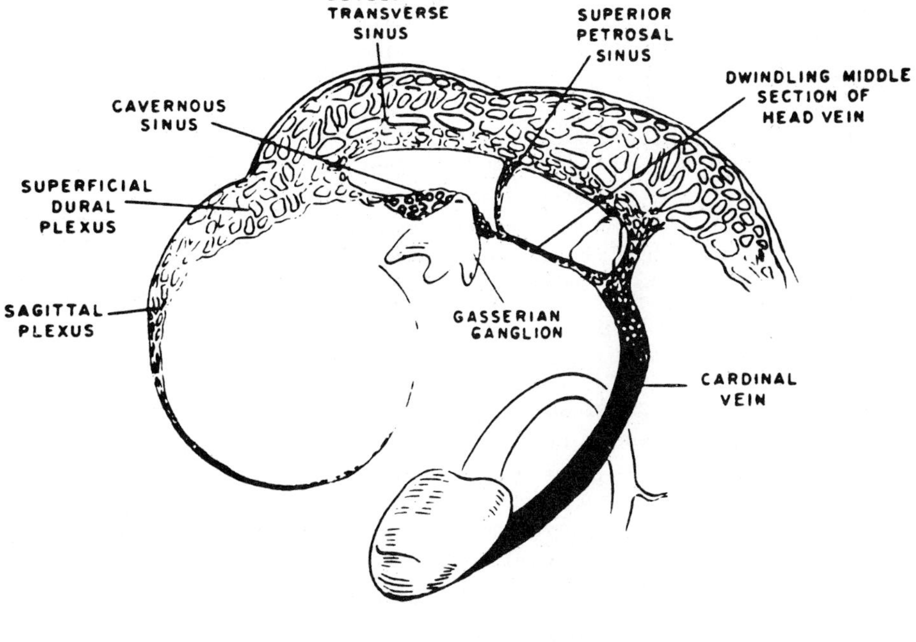

Figure 193-1 Lateral drawing of venous anatomy at 17 to 20 mm. Note the regression of the middle section of the primary head vein with the majority of flow via the transverse and sigmoid sinuses. (From Browder and Kaplan,[4] with permission.)

postnatal state; the cranial portion of the superior sagittal sinus ecomes a single channel either by selection of a single channel with compression of all others or by fusion of several channels into one.[35] The caudal portion is still more plexiform in nature. The transverse sinus is complete and assumes its adult position with a caudal swing into the sigmoid sinus. The tentorial plexus is reduced in size with continued growth of the hemispheres, and it marks the junction of the transverse, superior sagittal, and straight sinuses—the confluens of sinuses. At the junction of the sigmoid and transverse sinuses, the tentorial sinus enters, receiving the superficial cerebral veins. This sinus elongates and becomes somewhat attenuated with further growth. Its remnant is referred to as the sphenotemporal sinus.[28] The orbital veins now primarily drain via the inferior petrosal and cavernous sinuses, although there is still some drainage via the pro-otic sinus. The pro-otic sinus itself is carried cranially with expansion of the otic capsule. Its major function now becomes related to the drainage of the diploic system, and the middle meningeal sinus draining into it enlarges with continued bone growth. A portion of the pro-otic sinus will become the petrosquamosal sinus.[28]

Significant changes also occur with respect to the cerebral and cerebellar veins. The basal cerebral vein (of Rosenthal) forms as a channel from the primary veins draining the five regions of the brain, with the telencephalic, diencephalic, and mesencephalic veins becoming the primary tributaries. The lateral mesencephalic vein becomes a significant outlet of the basal cerebral vein into the superior petrosal sinus by way of the anterior cerebellar vein, the former metencephalic vein. This channel is one of the primary drainage channels of the cerebellum.

At this point, the venous system closely resembles that of the adult. Continued growth of the skull and brain results in final minor changes in the configuration of these vessels.

Congenital Anomalies of Arterial Anatomy

A review of the embryology of the intracranial arterial circulation reveals that many channels exist between future normal adult vessels, and these usually regress during development. These channels may, however, persist into adult life, often related to the failure of development of the normal arterial structures. These persistent embryonic vessels are of importance to the anatomist, to the radiologist in planning and interpreting cerebrovascular studies, to the clinician in evaluating various pathologic conditions, and to the surgeon in planning surgical strategies.

The various communications between the carotid-basilar, carotid-vertebral, internal-external carotid, and internal-internal carotid arterial systems will be discussed. In addition, a brief description of congenital abnormalities of the carotid system will be offered because these may be of significance in determining persistent embryonic channels.

Persistent Carotid-Basilar and Carotid-Vertebral Anastomoses

The blood supply to the hindbrain in the developing embryo is via a series of channels from the developing carotid arteries to the longitudinal neural arteries (Fig. 193-2). At approximately 4-mm

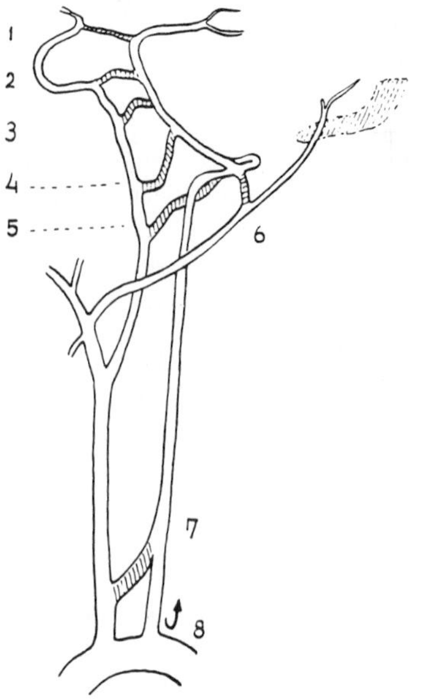

Figure 193-2 Various anastomotic channels between the carotid and vertebrobasilar systems, lateral view: (1) posterior communicating artery, (2) trigeminal artery, (3) otic artery, (4) hypoglossal artery, (5) proatlantal intersegmental artery, (6) vertebral-occipital anastomosis, (7) persistent cervical intersegmental artery, (8) retrograde filling. (From Lie,[19] with permission.)

crown-rump length, the trigeminal artery seems to serve this function and, soon after, the hypoglossal and otic arteries appear. These are known as the presegmental arteries. At the caudal end, the proatlantal intersegmental artery is responsible for the blood supply. With the formation of the posterior communicating artery cranially and the vertebrobasilar system caudally, the presegmental and the proatlantal intersegmental arteries regress, and this is usually completed by the 14-mm stage. The otic is the first to disappear, and this is then followed by the hypoglossal and then the trigeminal.

The *primitive trigeminal artery* (PTA) is the vessel most frequently observed to persist into adult life. Richard Quain has been credited with the first anatomic description of this vessel in 1844,[19] the first angiographic description was given by Sutton in 1950.[36] The incidence of the PTA on angiographic studies has been found to be 0.1 to 0.6 percent.[11,19] There have also been reports of bilateral PTAs.[2] The reason for its relatively high incidence is related to the fact that it is the major anastomotic channel of the presegmental arteries and also the last to disappear. The artery originates just before or at the point where the internal carotid artery enters the cavernous sinus. It then continues in one of two courses, each occurring in about half of the cases[20]; in the first, it travels extradurally between the trigeminal sensory root and the lateral portion of the sella and then under the petroclinoid ligament to join the basilar artery between the superior and anterior inferior cerebellar arteries; in the second, the artery travels in a groove in the dorsum sellae and perforates the dura near the clivus to join the basilar artery.

On angiography, an abnormal vessel between the cavernous carotid artery and the basilar artery can be demonstrated (Fig. 193-3). Saltzman has described three angiographic conditions related to a PTA: in type I, the distal basilar, superior cerebellar, and posterior cerebral arteries fill via the trigeminal, and the posterior

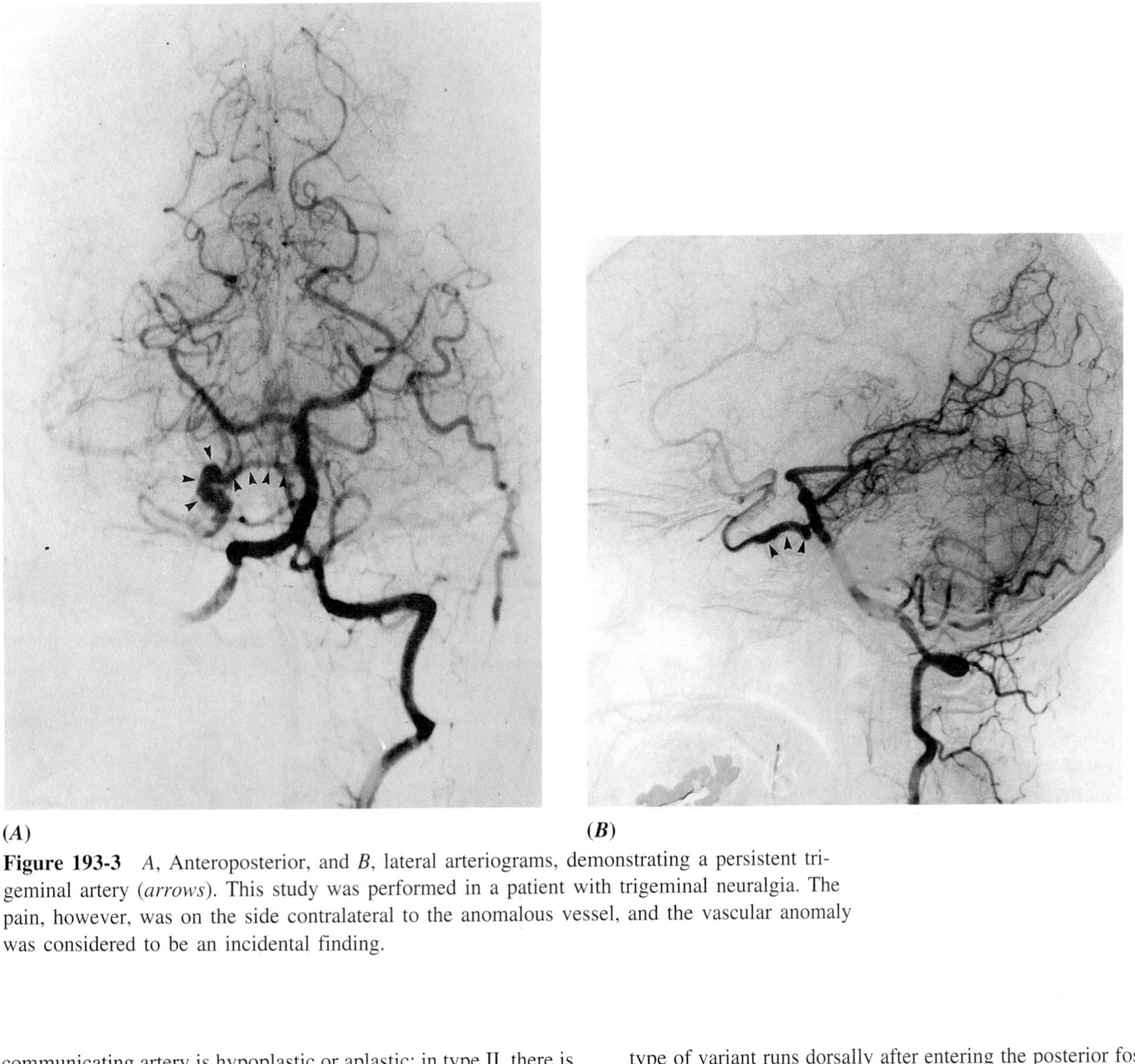

(*A*) (*B*)

Figure 193-3 *A*, Anteroposterior, and *B*, lateral arteriograms, demonstrating a persistent trigeminal artery (*arrows*). This study was performed in a patient with trigeminal neuralgia. The pain, however, was on the side contralateral to the anomalous vessel, and the vascular anomaly was considered to be an incidental finding.

communicating artery is hypoplastic or aplastic; in type II, there is similar filling except that the ipsilateral posterior cerebral artery is filled by the internal carotid artery via the posterior communicating artery; and in type III, there is poor filling of the distal basilar and superior cerebellar arteries, with each posterior cerebral artery filled by its respective posterior communicating artery.[32] In general, the basilar artery is hypoplastic, as is one or both of the vertebral arteries.

The relationship between the trigeminal artery and the cranial nerves in the cavernous sinus is depicted in Fig. 193-4. As the artery leaves the carotid, it travels below the third and fourth cranial nerves and medial to the first division of the trigeminal nerve. It often runs with the sensory root of the trigeminal and then passes below the abducens nerve before turning medially to join with the basilar artery. The importance of these relationships will become apparent when cranial nerve syndromes related to a PTA are discussed below.

Apart from the normal PTA, a variant of this artery has also been described, termed the primitive trigeminal artery variant (PTAV).[6,12,37] In this variation, one of the cerebellar arteries, usually AICA or SCA, is supplied by the internal carotid artery. This is thought to arise when there is a persistent trigeminal artery along with incomplete fusion of the longitudinal neural arteries.[12] This type of variant runs dorsally after entering the posterior fossa and is in close proximity to the root entry zone of the fifth nerve. This will be discussed below when considering facial pain from persistent vessels.

Although the PTA is usually an incidental finding on angiography, several clinical entities have been associated with its existence. Intracranial aneurysms have been described in association with a PTA, as have the rarer instances of aneurysms of the PTA itself.[10,11,20] George et al. stated that there is a 13.8 percent incidence of an intracranial aneurysm when a PTA is found to exist.[11] Some authors have suggested that structural defects in the walls of these abnormal vessels could make them more prone to develop an aneurysm and that subarachnoid hemorrhage without an identifiable lesion could be due to bleeding from this abnormal vessel.[11,20] Aneurysms of the PTA itself have been treated conservatively for the most part because the PTA may afford significant blood supply to the posterior circulation. Two cases of surgical treatment have been described, one with surgical ligation of the PTA and one with ligation of the cervical internal carotid artery.[10] In this latter case, a carotid-cavernous fistula resulted that was treated successfully.

Trigeminal neuralgia has also been attributed to the PTA[14,20,23] as well as to the PTAV.[24] Kempe and Smith reported a case of typical trigeminal neuralgia in a patient with a PTA discovered on

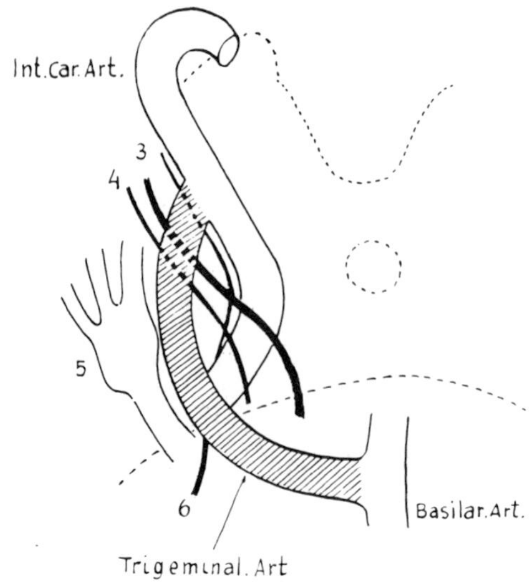

Figure 193-4 The relationship of the cranial nerves and the trigeminal artery. (From Lie,[19] with permission.)

angiography.[14] A retrogasserian nerve root section was performed, and the PTA was dissected from the nerve root. Merry and Jamieson described a patient with typical facial pain and diplopia who demonstrated a PTA and a hypoplastic ipsilateral vertebral artery.[23] A supra- and infratentorial approach was used to dissect a thick membrane that had encased the fifth and sixth cranial nerves, anchoring them to the PTA. This was divided, and a piece of absorbable gelatin sponge (Gelfoam) was placed, yielding good relief of pain and resolution of diplopia. Morita et al. described eight cases of trigeminal neuralgia associated with persistent embryonic arteries.[24] One patient demonstrated compression of the fifth nerve by a PTA and also by the superior and anterior inferior cerebellar arteries. The nerve was decompressed at all three sites with good relief of pain. The remaining seven cases were thought to be due to a PTAV compressing the trigeminal root. Again, microvascular decompression was performed via a retromastoid approach with excellent relief of pain. These authors thought that the PTAV is more likely to cause typical trigeminal neuralgia because it runs dorsally near the nerve root entry zone, whereas the PTA courses more medially and joins the basilar artery just after entering the posterior fossa.

Carotid-cavernous fistulae from the PTA itself,[15] from a presumed congenital PTA aneurysm,[7] and from a traumatic PTA aneurysm[9] have all been reported. Balloon embolization was used to successfully treat the first and third cases described, and excellent results were obtained by cervical carotid ligation in the second case.

In addition to the syndromes just discussed, other conditions that have been associated with a PTA include transient ischemic attacks involving the brain stem caused by microemboli originating in the carotid artery and being carried to the posterior circulation through a PTA,[40] and moyamoya disease in two patients with PTA found on angiographic study.[17]

A persistent *primitive otic artery* (POA) is extremely rare. Of the presegmental arteries, it is the least important for blood supply and also the first to disappear, thus leading to its low incidence. The POA, according to Lie, should originate from the carotid canal, run through the internal auditory meatus, and join the basilar at a caudal point.[19] Kempe and Smith reported a case of a POA found at autopsy in a patient who presented with hemifacial spasm and who died soon after of unrelated causes; the ipsilateral vertebral artery was also noted to be hypoplastic.[14] Reynolds et al. demonstrated a POA in a patient who underwent angiography for a right frontal lesion.[31] Here the ipsilateral vertebral artery could not be identified, and the contralateral vertebral artery was hypoplastic. A third case reported by Krayenbühl and Yasargil is thought to be only speculative by some authors because it was only demonstrated on angiography with a lateral projection.[19]

It is also rare for the *primitive hypoglossal artery* (PHA) to persist. The incidence of a PHA found on arteriography has been estimated to be approximately 0.02 to 0.03 percent.[20] The anomalous vessel originates from the cervical portion of the internal carotid artery at the level of C1 to C3 and runs dorsally, lateral to the hypoglossal nerve, to enter the hypoglossal canal. It then joins the caudal basilar artery. The vertebral arteries are usually hypoplastic bilaterally or hypoplastic contralateral to the PHA and aplastic ipsilateral to the PHA. Often the posterior communicating arteries are absent bilaterally. As is the case with the PTAV, a variant of the PHA has also been demonstrated which gives rise to the PICA.[38] The development of this variant can be explained by examining the embryologic development of the hypoglossal artery. The artery itself is composed of three parts: the first, near the origin of the internal carotid; the second, which is derived from the lateral anastomotic channels (lateral basilovertebral anastomosis) which also give rise to the posterior inferior cerebellar artery; and the third, which is composed of the transverse anastomotic channels that join the lateral anastomotic channels to the paired longitudinal neural arteries. In the PHA variant, this third part fails to develop normally and the PICA is supplied by the PHA.[38]

Aneurysms of the anterior cerebral artery,[19] anterior communicating artery,[16] internal carotid artery bifurcation,[19] superior cerebellar artery,[34] and basilar artery[1] have been described in association with a PHA, as have aneurysms of the hypoglossal artery itself.[16,20] With a limited number of reported cases of PHA associated with an intracranial aneurysm, it is difficult to determine if there is a true association or if the PHA is purely an incidental finding. As is the case with aneurysms of the PTA, great care must be taken if surgical ligation is considered, because the PHA may be the major source of blood to the basilar artery.

A second clinical syndrome related to a PHA has been reported by Kempe and Smith,[14] their patient presented with pain in the tonsillar fossa and in the posterior portion of the tongue. At operation, a close association of the ninth, tenth, and eleventh cranial nerves with a PHA was discovered. Sectioning of the ninth nerve and upper portions of the tenth nerve was performed, but no mention is made regarding the outcome of surgery.

The proatlantal intersegmental artery and the cervical intersegmental arteries are the major channels that join the carotid and vertebral arteries. Recall from their embryologic development that after normal regression of the hypoglossal artery on each side, the caudal portion of the longitudinal neural artery on each side is supplied by the ipsilateral proatlantal intersegmental artery. These proatlantal arteries arise from the paired dorsal aortae and travel between the last occipital and first cervical somites. The cervical intersegmental arteries also arise from the dorsal aortae, fuse dorsally, and then regress to form the vertebral artery on each side. The sixth intersegmental artery, however, remains to form the subclavian artery.

Persistence of the *proatlantal intersegmental artery* is rare, with fewer than 20 cases reported in the literature,[20,33] including 1 case of bilateral persistent arteries.[21] Their low incidence is quite surprising as they are a major source of blood to the hindbrain along with the trigeminal artery. The artery is a fairly large vessel that usually arises from the internal carotid artery at the C2 level, joins the horizontal portion of the vertebral artery suboccipitally, and then continues intracranially in the same course as the vertebral. The ipsilateral vertebral artery is absent and the contralateral vertebral may be normal, hypoplastic, or aplastic.[19] Occasionally, the proatlantal intersegmental artery arises from the external carotid artery, probably via an anastomosis between the occipital artery and a vertebral artery that is maldeveloped proximally.[20] There are no clinical syndromes attributed to persistent proatlantal intersegmental arteries, but it is important, of course, to realize their existence should embolization or ligation of feeding vessels to a vascular malformation or tumor be considered. Bour et al., for example, reported a case of a patient with a persistent proatlantal artery who had a tight stenosis of the ipsilateral carotid artery that required balloon angioplasty.[3] Because of the carotid's essential contribution to the blood supply to the posterior circulation territory, dilatations were performed in two separate sessions at a six-month interval. In a similar case in which endarterectomy might be planned, insertion of a temporary shunt would seem critical.

A persistent *cervical intersegmental artery* is seen as an abnormal origin of the vertebral artery either from the aortic arch or from the common carotid artery. Vertebral arteries with two or three roots can also be seen due to failure of regression of all except the sixth cervical intersegmental artery.[19]

Parkinson et al. have reported a case of an additional anastomosis between the cervical carotid and vertebral arteries.[29] In a patient undergoing arteriography for an anterior communicating artery aneurysm, the internal carotid was found to fill from a vertebral injection only and not from a common carotid injection. An anastomotic channel was demonstrated at the C2-C3 level.

Anomalous Anastomoses between the Internal and External Carotid Arteries

Occlusion of the internal carotid artery dictates the need for alternative channels to supply the brain. This collateral circulation may be through the circle of Willis or via an external-internal carotid artery anastomosis. A number of internal carotid–external carotid collaterals exist and usually involve the ophthalmic artery and various branches of the external carotid including the facial, superficial temporal, and internal maxillary arteries.[25] Aside from these normal channels, a number of potential congenital anastomoses are formed by persistent embryonic vessels.

The stapedial artery is one such vessel that is important in internal to external carotid anastomoses. To briefly review, the stapedial artery is a branch of the hyoid artery, which originates from the internal carotid. It has two major branches, a cranial branch that supplies the future middle meningeal artery and the supraorbital artery, which later becomes the anterior middle meningeal artery, and a caudal branch that gives rise to the maxillary and mandibular arteries. The internal maxillary artery joins this caudal trunk, and the stapedial artery then normally regresses, resulting in a middle meningeal artery arising from the external carotid. With failure of regression, the stapedial artery provides an anastomotic channel between the internal and external carotid arteries. Its persistence also results in the middle meningeal artery being supplied by the internal carotid. Anatomically, the stapedial artery originates at the hyoid branch of the internal carotid, penetrates the floor of the middle ear cavity, and travels to the posterior part of the promontorium. It then enters a bony canal and runs up and back between the crura of the stapes. It enters the facial canal, joins the facial nerve, and then exits, coursing along the floor of the middle fossa to join the middle meningeal artery.[41]

Persistence of the supraorbital branch of the stapedial artery also provides a channel for communication between the internal and external carotid systems. Normally the supraorbital branch involutes and becomes the minor anterior middle meningeal branch. It can, however, become a major anastomosis between the ophthalmic and the middle meningeal arteries. It enters the superior orbital fissure and connects with the lacrimal artery. It can therefore supply the orbit in cases of occlusion of the more proximal ophthalmic artery[19] and can also provide blood to the middle meningeal territory by reversal of flow into this vessel.[20]

In a discussion of internal carotid–external carotid anastomoses, the rete mirabile caroticum deserves some mention. This structure, which exists mainly in animals, is a network of small anastomosing vessels proximal to the circle of Willis that is found both intra- and extracranially. These retia are believed to assist in pituitary hormone exchange because they are close to the hypophysis; they may also offer a ''counter-current'' mechanism to prevent congestion in the heads of animals that normally graze.[19] The supply to the rete usually involves the internal maxillary, ascending pharyngeal, and occipital arteries or may be from the internal carotid artery. The afferents to the retia are the arteria anastomoticus, which enters via the orbital fissure, and the ramus anastomoticus, which enters through the foramen ovale. The distal end of the rete is a single trunk into the circle of Willis.

In man, such retia have been observed on rare occasions to develop in individuals with absent or hypoplastic carotid arteries.[19,25] The accessory meningeal artery, arising from the internal maxillary or middle meningeal artery and entering the foramen ovale, is thought to represent the ramus anastomoticus. It forms an anastomosis with the cavernous portion of the internal carotid artery. Meningeal branches of the ascending pharyngeal artery that pass through the foramen lacerum supply the petrous portion of the internal carotid artery. Finally, anastomosing arteries similar to the arteria anastomotica may pass through the superior orbital fissure to connect the internal maxillary artery to the cavernous portion of the carotid.[19]

Intercarotid Anastomoses

Under usual circumstances, when there is aplasia of one internal carotid artery, that side of the brain is supplied via collaterals through the circle of Willis, either through the anterior communicating artery or the posterior communicating artery. There have, however, been rare reports of an anastomotic channel between the intracavernous portions of the internal carotid arteries.[20,39] In all of these cases, there has been absence of the proximal internal carotid artery and of the A1 segment of the ipsilateral anterior cerebral artery.[39] This unusual anastomosis has been seen to cross either at the base of the dorsum sellae or through the floor of the sella. Lie had originally suggested that this anastomosis might be the result of fused bilateral persistent trigeminal arteries.[19] It is currently believed that the anterior anastomosis may be bilateral inferior hypophyseal arteries joined in the midline, these being the adult remnants of the primitive maxillary arteries, and that the posterior anastomosis may be the dorsal meningeal arteries fused in a similar fashion. Persistence of these channels is important to note if a procedure involving the contralateral carotid artery or if trans-sphenoidal surgery is anticipated.

Congenital Anomalies of Venous Anatomy

The cranial veins can basically be grouped into three systems: the outer system draining the scalp, frontal and occipital musculature, and galea; the middle system draining the skull, diploe, and dura mater; and the inner system draining the brain itself. Variations in each of these systems occur, and although they are usually not of pathologic significance, an appreciation of their existence is of importance to surgeons of the head and neck.

There are few channels that join the outer and middle systems. When present, they are usually situated in the superior midline.[35] Often with thrombotic or occlusive lesions of the transverse or superior saggital sinus, enlargement of the diploic and scalp veins can be seen.[4] In addition, Browder and Kaplan have described a 10 percent incidence of a channel that passes through the occipital protuberance, joining the confluens with the diploic system and subsequently the occipital veins.[4]

There are many variations that occur in the dural or middle system and in the inner system. These are of primary importance to the neurosurgeon because surgical strategies are often planned with the anatomy of the dural sinuses and superficial cerebral veins in mind.

The superior sagittal sinus courses through the dorsal margin of the falx cerebri to join the confluens of sinuses (torcular Herophili) at the level of the tentorium. Although the rostral portion of the superior sagittal sinus is usually a uniform, single channel, large vascular networks are not infrequently observed in the dura around the middle third of the superior sagittal sinus and near the confluens of sinuses. This meshwork may even be of sufficient size to compromise the sinus lumen. It is thought to represent persistence of the embryonic meshwork from which these dural sinuses arise. This "lacunar system" of vessels has been observed in 20 percent of specimens in some series and in up to 90 percent in others.[4] It has been speculated that this system may play a part in outflow regulation through the sinuses, but this idea has been challenged.[4] In addition to being present in the dura of the superior sagittal sinus, these channels have been found in 10 percent of falx cerebri specimens and may join the superior and inferior sagittal sinuses at their caudal margins.[4] They are less often observed in the rostral portion of the superior sagittal sinus in small children.

Variations also exist in the superior sagittal sinus itself. Approximately 20 percent of specimens have been found to have a horizontal membrane dividing the sinus in two.[4] This usually occurs between the rostral and middle third of the sinus and has been found to be as large as 6 cm in length. The transverse sinus may enter one of these divisions and exit rostral to the torcular. In addition, orifices of the superficial cerebral veins can be seen in just one portion, usually the ventral division.[4]

Variations also occur in the anatomic configuration of the venous system at the base of the cerebral hemispheres. The tentorium is surrounded by major venous structures. Within it, the straight sinus normally travels posteriorly and fuses with the transverse sinuses at the torcular Herophili. Rostrolaterally, the tentorium is bordered by the superior petrosal sinuses. A small venous channel is also found at the middle, rostral border of the tentorium. Although these comprise the major venous circulation around the tentorium, substantial channels also course within the tentorium itself.[4] Recall that in early embryonic stages there exists a large tentorial plexus that regresses with continued growth of the cerebral and cerebellar hemispheres. Modifications of this plexus contribute to many of the channels surrounding the tentorium, described above. Persistence of these embryonic channels may join the straight and transverse sinuses rostral to the confluens of sinuses and may join the transverse sinus with its ipsilateral superior petrosal sinus. These channels are usually found in the posterior half of the tentorium.

The straight sinus, which is a tributary of the inferior sagittal sinus and the vein of Galen, may have multiple openings into the confluens of sinuses. This, again, is due to the meshwork-like nature of the embryonic straight sinus.[4] Rarely, the straight sinus may be absent. In these cases, drainage may occur via persistent channels joining the caudal inferior sagittal sinus with the superior sagittal sinus or the transverse sinus.[4] The vein of Galen and its major tributaries, the internal cerebral and basal veins, also may demonstrate variability. With occlusion of the great cerebral vein, deep cerebral drainage can occur through the sigmoid sinus via the basal and mesencephalic veins and the superior petrosal sinus.[28] Recall also from the prior discussion of embryology that the great anterior cerebellar vein (prior metencephalic vein) that drains into the superior petrosal sinus may provide significant outflow for the basal cerebral vein.[28]

It has been suggested that the vein of Galen aneurysm exhibits retention of a normally transient venous channel rather than an "hypertrophied vein of Galen," this structure being a persistent median porencephalic vein.[30] This vessel is also referred to by Padget as the primitive internal cerebral vein which initially drains the choroid regions.[28] This theory is supported by Lasjaunias et al., who suggest that vein of Galen aneurysms form early in embryonic development, at or near the end of the second month.[18]

Neurosurgeons performing posterior fossa surgery are all too familiar with a venous plexus involving the dura overlying the posterior aspects of the cerebellar hemispheres and the falx cerebelli. As with the other networks described above, these probably result from a failure of regression of the primitive embryonic meshwork. Approximately 25 percent of all infants and children have significant venous channels in this region.[5] This network joins the confluens with the marginal sinus and is quite important in venous outflow in children. Although it normally dwindles with continued growth, 2 percent of adults have these large channels in addition to an enlarged occipital sinus that represents the major drainage channel from the superior sagittal and straight sinuses.[4] The occipital sinus itself, normally a small channel in the falx cerebelli, may be doubled or tripled in approximately 20 percent of all specimens.[4] These networks are often seen in association with atresia of the transverse sinus.[13] Surgeons performing posterior fossa operations need to be aware of these significant channels.

Finally, in addition to anomalies of each of the major sinuses themselves, variations may be seen at their junction, the confluens of sinuses or torcular Herophili. One-third of specimens show a superior sagittal sinus to the right, continuing as the right transverse sinus, 8 percent demonstrate the same relationship to the left, and 16 percent show a split superior sagittal sinus with subsequent absence of a true confluens.[4] The transverse sinus itself may have multiple openings into the confluens of sinuses or, as mentioned above, there may be atresia of one of the transverse sinuses. Occasionally, a persistent embryonic mesh may narrow the lumen of the transverse sinus.[13] The straight sinus may join the confluens via multiple channels,[4] and some of these may even join the superior sagittal or occipital sinuses directly. In the most extreme cases, the torcular itself may be absent and the four major sinuses may join in a circular pattern.[4] A working knowledge of these variations is important for cranial surgery as well as for radical neck surgery if ligation of the jugular system is anticipated. Descriptions of additional variations of the torcular have been given elsewhere.[4,13,42]

References

1. Anderson M. Persistent primitive hypoglossal artery with basilar aneurysm. *J Neurol* 1976; 213:377–381.
2. Binet EF, Young RF. Bilateral persistent trigeminal arteries: case report. *J Neurosurg* 1977; 47:619–622.
3. Bour P, Bracard S, Frisch N, et al. Persistent proatlantal artery associated with carotid artery stenosis treatment by percutaneous transluminal balloon angioplasty. *Ann Vasc Surg* 1991; 5:38–40.
4. Browder J, Kaplan HA. *Cerebral Dural Sinuses and Their Tributaries.* Springfield, IL: Charles C Thomas, 1976.
5. Browder J, Kaplan HA, Krieger AJ. Venous lakes in the suboccipital dura mater and falx cerebelli of infants: surgical significance. *Surg Neurol* 1975; 4:53–55.
6. Cobb SR, Hieshima GB, Mehringer CM, et al. Persistent trigeminal artery variant: carotid-anterior inferior cerebellar artery anastomosis. *Surg Neurol* 1983; 19:263–266.
7. Enomoto T, Sato A, Maki Y. Carotid-cavernous sinus fistula caused by rupture of a primitive trigeminal artery aneurysm. *J Neurosurg* 1977; 46:373–376.
8. Evans HM. Development of the vascular system. In Keibel F, Mall FP (eds): *Manual of Human Embryology.* Philadelphia: Lippincott, 1912, pp 570–709.
9. Flandroy P, Lacour P, Marsault C, et al. The intravascular treatment of a cavernous fistula caused by rupture of a traumatic carotid trigeminal aneurysm. *Neuroradiology* 1987; 29:308–311.
10. Freitas PE, Aquini MG, Chemale I. Persistent primitive trigeminal artery aneurysm. *Surg Neurol* 1986; 26:373–374.
11. George AE, Lin JP, Morantz RA. Intracranial aneurysm on a persistent primitive trigeminal artery: case report. *J Neurosurg* 1971; 35:601–604.
12. Haughton VM, Rosenbaum AE, Pearce J. Internal carotid artery origins of the inferior cerebellar arteries. *Am J Roentgenol* 1978; 130:1191–1192.
13. Kaplan HA, Browder J, Knightly JJ, et al. Variations of the cerebral dural sinuses at the torcular Herophili: importance in radical neck dissection. *Am J Surg* 1972; 124:456–461.
14. Kempe LG, Smith DR. Trigeminal neuralgia, facial spasm, intermedius and glossopharyngeal neuralgia with persistent carotid basilar anastomosis. *J Neurosurg* 1969; 31:445–451.
15. Kerber CW, Manke W. Trigeminal artery to cavernous sinus fistula treated by balloon occlusion: case report. *J Neurosurg* 1983; 58:611–613.
16. Kodama N, Ohara H, Suzuki J. Persistent hypoglossal artery associated with aneurysms: report of two cases. *J Neurosurg* 1976; 45:449–451.
17. Kwak R, Kadoya S. Moyamoya disease associated with persistent primitive trigeminal artery: report of two cases. *J Neurosurg* 1983; 59:166–171.
18. Lasjaunias P, Garcia-Monaco R, Rodesch G, et al. Deep venous drainage in great cerebral vein (vein of Galen) absence and malformations. *Neuroradiology* 1991; 33:234–238.
19. Lie TA. *Congenital Anomalies of the Carotid Arteries.* Amsterdam: Excerpta Medica Foundation, 1968.
20. Lie TA. Variations in cerebrovascular anatomy. In Fox JL (ed): *Intracranial Aneurysms,* vol 1. New York: Springer-Verlag, 1983, pp 432–489.
21. Lui CC, Liu YH, Wai YY, et al. Persistence of both proatlantal arteries with absence of vertebral arteries. *Neuroradiology* 1987; 29:304–305.
22. Mall FP. On the development of the blood-vessels of the brain in the human embryo. *Am J Anat* 1905; 4:1–18.
23. Merry GS, Jamieson KG. Operative approach to persistent trigeminal artery producing facial pain and diplopia: case report. *J Neurosurg* 1977; 47:613–618.
24. Morita A, Fukushima T, Miyazaki S, et al. Tic douloureux caused by primitive trigeminal artery or its variant. *J Neurosurg* 1989; 70:415–419.
25. Mount LA, Taveras JM. Arteriographic demonstration of the collateral circulation of the cerebral hemispheres. *Arch Neurol Psychiatry* 1957; 78:235–253.
26. Padget DH. The development of the cranial arteries in the human embryo. *Contrib Embryol* 1948; 32:205–262.
27. Padget DH. The cranial venous system in man in reference to development, adult configuration, and relation to the arteries. *Am J Anat* 1956; 98:307–355.
28. Padget DH. The development of the cranial venous system in man, from the viewpoint of comparative anatomy. *Contrib Embryol* 1957; 36:81–140.
29. Parkinson D, Reddy V, Ross RT. Congenital anastomosis between the vertebral artery and internal carotid artery in the neck: case report. *J Neurosurg* 1979; 51:697–699.
30. Raybaud CA, Strother CM. Persisting abnormal embryonic vessels in intracranial arteriovenous malformations. *Acta Radiol (Suppl) [Stockh]* 1986; 369:136–138.
31. Reynolds AF Jr, Stovring J, Turner PT. Persistent otic artery. *Surg Neurol* 1980; 13:115–117.
32. Saltzman GF. Patent primitive trigeminal artery studied by cerebral angiography. *Acta Radiol* 1959; 51:329–336.
33. Sato H, Fujiwara S, Otabe K, et al. A case of persistent primitive proatlantal intersegmental artery (proatlantal artery I) with an aneurysm: case report. *Neurol Surg (Tokyo)* 1985; 13:117–121.
34. Springer TD, Fishbone G, Shapiro R. Persistent hypoglossal artery associated with superior cerebellar artery aneurysm: case report. *J Neurosurg* 1974; 40:397–399.
35. Streeter GL. The developmental alterations in the vascular system of the brain of the human embryo. *Contrib Embryol* 1918; 8:7–38.
36. Sutton D. Anomalous carotid-basilar anastomosis. *Br J Radiol* 1950; 23:617–619.
37. Teal JS, Rumbaugh CL, Bergeron RT, et al. Persistent carotid-superior cerebellar artery anastomosis: a variant of persistent trigeminal artery. *Radiology* 1972; 103:335–341.
38. Teal JS, Rumbaugh CL, Segall HD, et al. Anomalous branches of the internal carotid artery. *Radiology* 1973; 106:567–573.
39. Tracy PT. Unusual intercarotid anastomosis associated with anterior communicating artery aneurysm: case report. *J Neurosurg* 1987; 67:765–767.
40. Waller FT, Simons RL, Kerber C, et al. Trigeminal artery and microemboli to the brain stem: report of two cases. *J Neurosurg* 1977; 46:104–106.
41. Willinsky R, Lasjaunias P, Berenstein A. Intracavernous branches of the internal carotid artery (ICA): comprehensive review of their variations. *Surg Radiol Anat* 1987; 9:201–215.
42. Woodhall B. Variations of the cranial venous sinuses in the region of the torcular Herophili. *Arch Surg* 1936; 33:297–314.

194

Cerebral Blood Flow

Warren R. Selman
W. David Lust
Robert A. Ratcheson

Our understanding of the relationship between cerebral circulation and cerebral function has evolved through refinements in the delineation of cerebral anatomy and physiology.[39] The relationship was known to exist by at least the sixth century B.C., when Pythagoras characterized the brain as the organ of reasoning. His student, Alcmeon of Croton, recognized that blood ebbs and flows in the veins and that this blood flow is important to proper cerebral function. Diogenes of Apollonia emphasized the importance of air, or pneuma, which was distributed by the heart through the vascular system, to proper functioning of the brain.[81]

Ischemic injury may be a final common pathway in many types of cerebral insults. During cerebrovascular procedures, ischemic injury may result from an unanticipated complication of planned permanent or temporary vessel occlusion. An understanding of the physiologic controls of normal cerebral blood flow and the pathophysiology of ischemic injury is necessary for planning effective strategies to minimize the consequences of cerebral ischemia.

The effects of an interruption of cerebral circulation on brain function have also been recognized for centuries. Leonardo da Vinci described the vessels of the neck and recognized that cervical compression would produce unconsciousness.[12] A more modern demonstration and quantification of this relationship (from a technological if not an ethical viewpoint) was offered by Rossen and coworkers.[67] Pneumatic compression of the neck in normal volunteers revealed that a loss of consciousness followed interruption of cerebral blood flow within 10 s.

In this chapter we review the blood flow requirements of the normal brain, the mechanisms that control cerebral blood flow, and the relation of cerebral blood flow thresholds to neuronal function and viability.

Normal Cerebrovascular Control

The brain is unique in that it is supplied by four major arteries that join in an equalizing manifold, the circle of Willis. The carotid arteries each supply approximately 40 percent of the total perfusion requirements of the brain.

The traditional view of the cerebral circulation saw the arterial supply as being functionally and morphologically separated into two distinct categories: the *extracerebral vessels,* including the major arteries at the base of the brain and the pial vessels, and the *intracerebral vessels,* or the penetrating arteries. Subsequent morphologic and functional studies have not confirmed this assumption, and these two groups of vessels are in fact similar.[14]

Four major, interdependent mechanisms are involved in the control of cerebral blood flow: metabolic coupling; neural control, involving both extrinsic and intrinsic neural pathways; P_{CO_2}; and autoregulation. Although this division may be somewhat artificial and these control mechanisms probably operate in concert, it is useful to consider each separately.

Metabolic Control

Local cerebral blood flow (CBF) is regionally heterogenous. The varied pattern of CBF is neither random nor related to the anatomic organization of the cerebral vasculature or to known differences in the innervation patterns of the cerebral vessels. Neuronal activity is the principal energy-consuming process in the brain. Local cerebral blood flow adjusts to the level of energy generation; therefore, it is the activity in the neuronal circuits that is the major determinant of variations and regional patterns of cerebral blood flow.[14]

Normally there is exquisite coupling between the regional cerebral metabolic demand for oxygen and glucose generated by local neuronal activity and the volume of blood flowing through that tissue[25,45] (Fig. 194-1). This coupling, termed *metabolic regulation,* was first demonstrated by simultaneous measurements of regional glucose metabolism and local blood flow in 1975,[83] although indirect evidence supporting this mechanism had existed for many years.[14,42,61,68,82] From their classic experiments in 1890, Roy and Sherrington noted that "the chemical products of cerebral metabolism contained in the lymph which bathes the wall of the arterioles of the brain can cause variations of the caliber of the cerebral vessels. In this reaction the brain possesses an intrinsic mechanism by which its vascular supply can be varied locally in correspondence with local variations of functional activity."[68] While this doctrine was undisputed for nearly a century, the precise mechanisms responsible for this coupling have remained elusive.[82] Alterations in the concentrations of local metabolites may lead to changes in regional CBF. Several chemical species capable of altering local vascular tone generated during periods of enhanced neuronal or glial activity have been considered as mediators of the coupling between flow and metabolism[14] (Fig. 194-2).

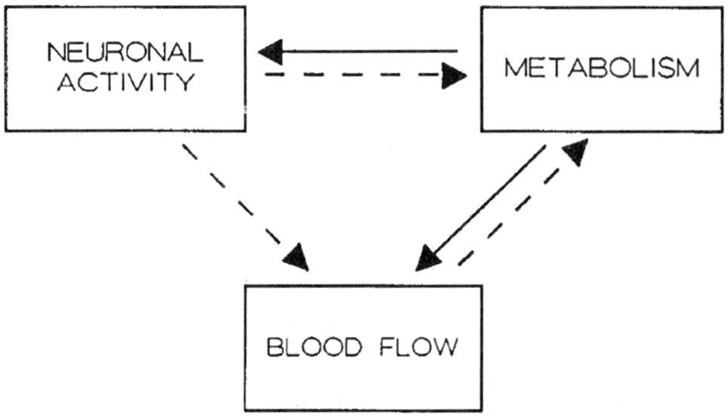

Figure 194-1 Interrelationship of neuronal activity, metabolism, and blood flow in the central nervous system. The solid arrows represent known control mechanisms, and the dashed arrows indicate putative physiologic regulatory interactions that may also be evoked during pathologic conditions in the brain. (From Selman et al.,[74] with permission.)

YEAR	PROPOSED FACTOR
1890	Chemical products of cerebral metabolism
1945	Oxygen (O_2)
1959	Carbon dioxide (CO_2)
1965	Hydrogen ion (H^+)
1972	Potassium
1975	Adenosine
1985	Glycolytic intermediates

Figure 194-2 Putative neurochemical mediators of blood flow and metabolism coupling. (Modified from Edvinsson et al.,[14] with permission.)

These include extracellular pH, P_{CO_2}, adenosine, glycolytic intermediates, and extracellular potassium (indirectly, through its role in neuronal and smooth muscle cell membrane function, even though it is not directly involved in energy metabolism).

Silver has shown that local blood flow increases as soon as 1 s after neuronal excitation and that the zone of increase is limited to 250 μm around the site of the increased activity.[80] These results indicate that flow can be adjusted very rapidly at the microvascular level according to metabolic demands in discrete functional subunits. While each of the species cited in Fig. 194-2 may be involved in the control of blood flow, none demonstrates precisely the correct time profile for the relation between their appearance in the extravascular space and acute alterations of local flow patterns. Furthermore, there are a number of examples of increases in flow that are disproportionate compared to metabolism during activation. Such overcompensation has been demonstrated at both cellular and macroscopic levels.[17,80]

A review of the information cited above indicates that (1) the metabolic hypothesis of Roy and Sherrington does not fully explain the phenomenon of metabolic coupling, since CBF may increase out of proportion to metabolic demands; (2) to date, none of the candidates suggested as mediating this coupling demonstrates the necessary temporal profile between its accumulation in the perivascular space and the flow increase; and, finally, (3) these metabolites may be involved in the maintenance of flow and metabolism levels after this relationship has been set at a different level by a yet undetermined rapid initiator, such as a neurogenic stimulus.[14]

Neurogenic Control

The association of metabolism and flow does not prove that metabolism determines flow. The two variables may be governed by a common third factor. The perivascular innervation is a candidate for playing such a role. The possible arrangements between neuronal systems and the cerebral vasculature are depicted in Fig. 194-3. It is important to consider not only the extrinsic nerve supply from the cranial ganglia to the cerebral arteries, arterioles, and veins, but also the role of intracerebral neurons serving the intracerebral vasculature. A dense plexus of nerve fibers in the walls of cerebral vessels, forming a "minibrain" or regulatory center, has been

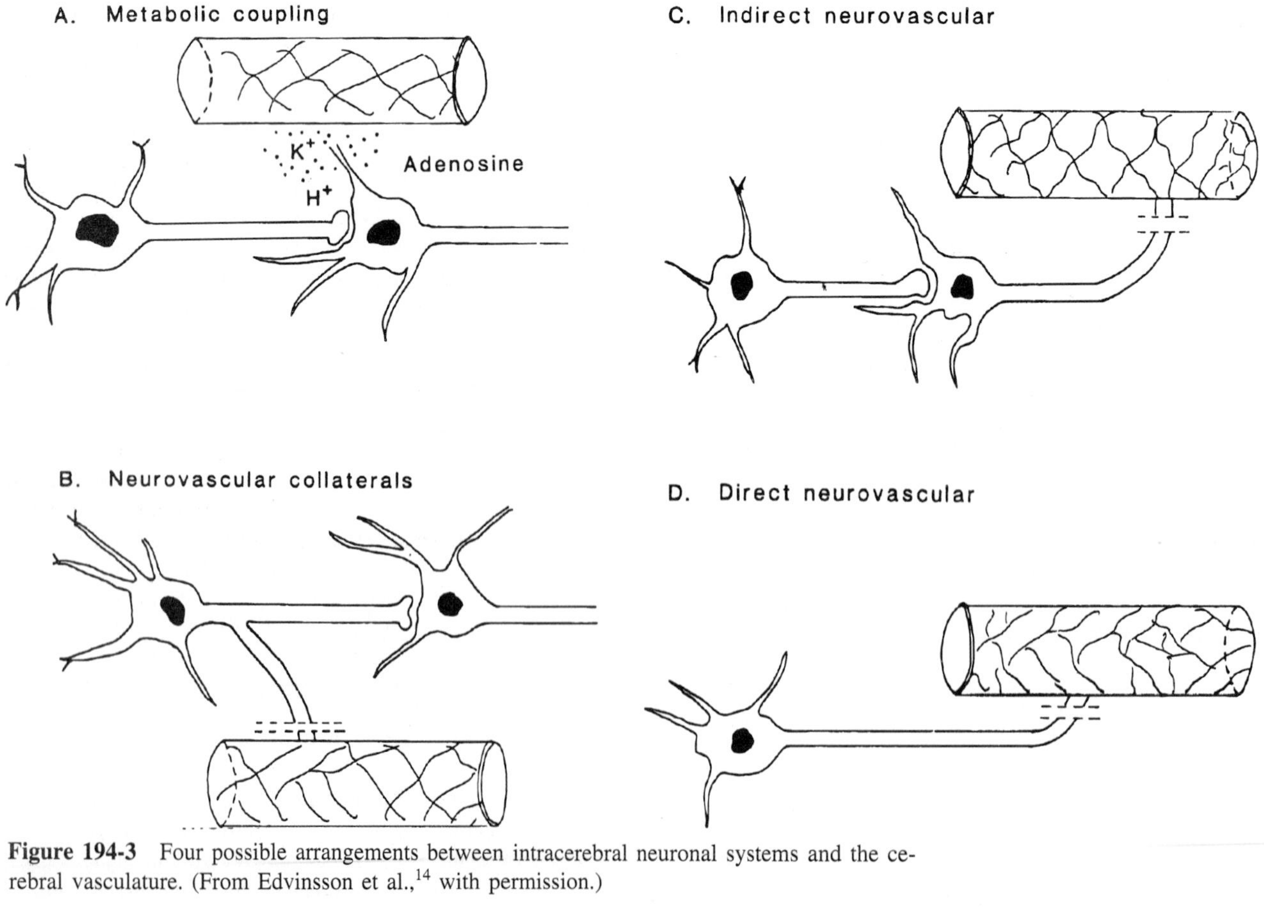

Figure 194-3 Four possible arrangements between intracerebral neuronal systems and the cerebral vasculature. (From Edvinsson et al.,[14] with permission.)

documented (Fig. 194-4).[14] Given this arrangement, neurons could form the coupling mechanism between metabolism and flow. Although systemic administration of various neurotransmitter agonists and antagonists may not produce dramatic effects on cerebral blood flow, in experiments where the blood-brain barrier has been circumvented, marked changes are seen, again suggesting a more prominent role for neurotransmitter action from nerves that synapse directly on the cerebral vasculature.[14] Extrinsic nerves, intrinsic nerves, and intrinsic brain regions all may bring their influence to bear on the cerebral vessels.

Theories of neurogenic control of the cerebral vasculature have focused on the role of efferent nerves that follow large arteries to innervate the cerebral vessels. Three types of extrinsic nerve systems, with distinct origins and neurotransmitters, have been identified. One consists of sympathetic neurons arising principally from the superior cervical ganglion. These neurons contain norepinephrine (NE) and neuropeptide-Y (NPY), which are both vasoconstrictors.[90] A second system consists of parasympathetic neurons in the sphenopalatine and otic ganglia, which contain acetylcholine (ACh) and often coexpress vasoactive intestinal peptide (VIP).[7,75] The third consists of sensory fibers originating in the trigeminal ganglion. These contain substance P (SP) and calcitonin gene-related peptide (CGRP), both of which are vasodilators.[14]

Most of the neuron fibers investing the cerebral vasculature are sympathetic. They appear to function by reducing CBF under conditions where it has been increased by metabolic demand, and they may raise the threshold for the breakthrough of autoregulation that occurs with arterial hypertension.[30] Attempts to manipulate CBF by either stimulation or ablation of sympathetic innervation have been largely unsuccessful. The parasympathetic nerves do not appear to play an important role in the tonic control of flow, but they may have some effect in pain-mediated vasodilatory responses.[23]

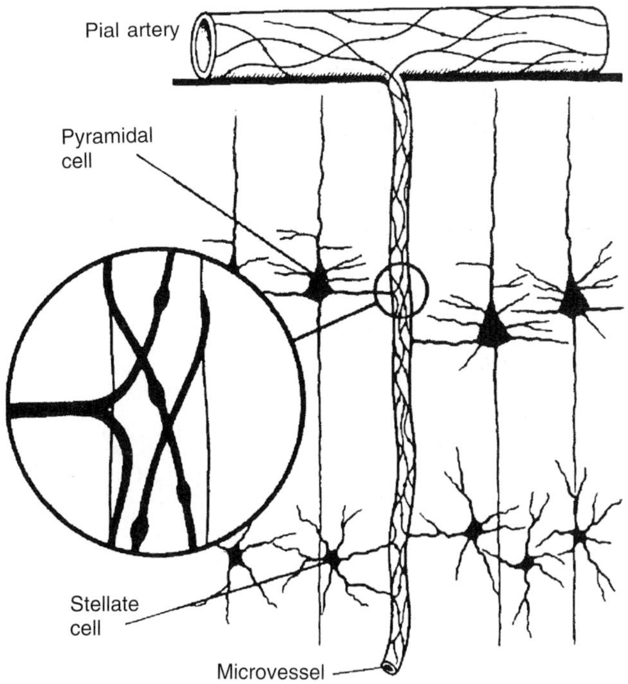

Figure 194-4 Hypothetical collateral innervation of a microvessel in a collateral column with neuronal ''minibrain.'' (From Edvinsson et al.,[14] with permission.)

Trigeminal nerves appear to become important only under special circumstances, such as hypertension and seizures, when their stimulation can effect a substantial increase in CBF.[69] Despite the abundance of these nerve fibers, CBF appears to be primarily regulated by local metabolism with only minor modulation by extrinsic nerves. It is unclear how these peripheral neurons may contribute to the moment-by-moment governance of the cerebral circulation during normal activity.

The possibility that the brain could regulate its own blood flow was recognized by several early researchers in the field, though for many years most investigators did not consider this to be a significant regulatory mechanism.[72,84,91] With the advent of both autoradiographic methods for the determination of regional CBF and positron emission tomography (PET) studies of cerebral circulation and metabolism in humans, as well as an explosion of techniques and knowledge in biochemical neuroanatomy, a growing body of evidence supports the concept that the brain can regulate its own blood flow through intrinsic neural networks.[63,65,75] Cerebrovascular control may in part be regulated by intrinsic neural systems within the medulla oblongata and may not (as traditionally believed), depend entirely on responses by vessel walls and/or endothelium.[64]

Carbon Dioxide (CO_2)

It has been well established that alterations in Pa_{CO_2} result in marked vasodilation.[60] There is an exponential relationship between Pa_{CO_2} and CBF within a Pa_{CO_2} range of 25 to 60 mmHg, with a CBF change of approximately 4 percent per millimeter of mercury.[52]

Flow changes induced by alterations in Pa_{CO_2} occur within 2 min and reach a new plateau within 12 min.[62] This regulatory mechanism has been shown to be a function of changes in the perivascular pH in the vicinity of the vascular smooth muscle cells, rather than a direct effect of CO_2 per se.[92] In addition to the direct effects of hydrogen ions on the vascular smooth muscle, local changes in pH can modulate the vasomotor responses to other agents that affect vessel caliber, such as norepinephrine.[11] Since changes in systemic Pa_{CO_2} are detected by carotid artery chemoreceptors, this regulatory mechanism can be effected by reflex pathways. In support of this, it has been observed that a lesion of the tegmental reticular formation diminishes the cerebrovascular response to alterations in Pa_{CO_2}.[76] Recent investigation has suggested that the powerful effects of CO_2 on the cerebral circulation are mediated by endothelium-derived relaxing factor.[35]

Prolonged alterations in Pa_{CO_2} result in chronic adaptation, and after approximately 36 h the blood flow changes tend to return to prealteration levels. At Pa_{CO_2} levels of 70 mmHg, maximal vasodilation has occurred, and CBF does not increase as Pa_{CO_2} increases further. Similarly, Pa_{CO_2} levels less than 20 mmHg cause no further decrease in CBF. These low Pa_{CO_2} levels should be avoided in the clinical setting, since the ensuing blood flow reductions can lead to tissue ischemia.

Autoregulation

Autoregulation is defined as the physiologic maintenance of a constant flow over a moderate range of perfusion pressures.[44] This restricted use of the term *autoregulation,* in contrast to the broader meaning of the term—the capacity of an organ to regulate its blood supply in accordance with its underlying functional or metabolic needs—avoids confusion with other mechanisms involved in cerebrovascular regulation, such as metabolic coupling (see above).[48]

According to the general equation of flow, CBF can be described by the relationship between cerebral perfusion pressure (CPP) and cerebrovascular resistance (CVR):

$$CBF = CPP/CVR$$

Cerebral perfusion pressure is equal to mean arterial blood pressure (MABP) [where MABP = ⅓(systolic pressure − diastolic pressure) + diastolic pressure] minus intracranial pressure and sagittal sinus pressure. In the absence of pathologic conditions, intracranial pressure and sagittal sinus pressure are negligible compared to systemic arterial pressure, and CPP is roughly equivalent to MABP. According to the previous equation, autoregulation must be mediated by changes in CVR. The *Hagen-Poiseuille* equation, which describes the flow of Newtonian fluids in rigid tubes, offers an approximation of the factors that govern CVR and suggests that resistance is inversely proportional to blood viscosity and proportional to the fourth power of the radius of the vessel.[93] Thus, changes in the radius of cerebral blood vessels can produce marked alterations of CVR. A decrease in CPP produces dilation of the precapillary resistance vessels, whereas an increase produces constriction. Largely by variation in the degree of constriction of the cerebral resistance vessels, average hemispheric CBF is maintained at a fairly constant level, near 50 ml/100 g per minute in the adult human brain at rest.

Although myogenic, neurogenic, and metabolic mechanisms have been postulated, the precise control of the autoregulatory response remains unknown.[14] Pioneering work done by Bayliss on the myogenic basis of autoregulation showed that reflex changes in the tone of arteriolar smooth muscle are elicited by changes in transmural pressure.[3] According to this hypothesis, an increase in the transluminal pressure leads to stretching of smooth muscle within the vessel wall. Reflex contraction of radial fibers then results in constriction of vessel diameter, and an opposite effect is seen with a decrease in transluminal pressure.

A growing body of evidence suggests that endothelium-dependent mechanisms function as the primary mediating factor of vascular tone, and they are now considered as a facet of the myogenic hypothesis of autoregulation. The endothelium acts as a transducer of hemodynamic forces that lead to the release of vasoactive substances.[43] Synthesis of the endothelium-derived relaxing factor, either nitric oxide (EDRF/NO) or a closely related molecule derived from the amino acid L-arginine, appears to affect vascular tone, both under basal conditions and in response to the application of specific agonists.[15,16,18,19,47,66] The proposed mechanism for this effect is that stimulation of soluble guanylate cyclase by EDRF/NO raises the level of cyclic guanosine monophosphate (cGMP) in vascular smooth muscle and results in vascular relaxation.[49] Dilation of large cerebral arteries and pial arterioles in response to the application of acetylcholine in vivo is dependent on the formation of NO by nitric oxide synthase and can be blocked by a competitive antagonist of that enzyme, *N*-monomethyl-L-arginine (L-NMMA).[16] Intravenous administration of a similar NO synthase antagonist in rats caused a 40 percent increase in MABP and a 60 percent reduction in the lumen diameter of pial arteries.[57] This L-arginine/NO/cGMP pathway appears to be critical in the control of vascular tone and is increasingly accepted as the dominant mediator of the autoregulatory response.[21,40,41,57]

In the brain, autoregulation is manifest as the lack of major fluctuation in CBF despite changes in mean arterial blood pressure between 60 and 150 mmHg.[28,44,85] Cerebral autoregulation may be thought of as a homeostatic mechanism that is superimposed on the baroceptive reflexes.[14] It is important to stress that both the upper and the lower limits of autoregulation can be affected by many factors, including sympathetic nerve activity, Pa_{CO_2}, and pharmacologic agents (Fig. 194-5). The most important factor that can affect autoregulation is chronic arterial hypertension. As a result of thickening of the cerebral arteries, the upper and lower limits of autoregulation are both displaced to higher levels in patients with chronic hypertension.[85] The consequence of these alterations is that symptoms of cerebral hypoperfusion can occur at higher values of mean arterial pressure in patients with chronic hypertension than in normotensive individuals (Fig. 194-6).

A knowledge of the cerebrovascular status of the patient with respect to hypertension may also be a consideration in the planning of temporary vessel occlusion during cerebrovascular surgery. Some experimental evidence suggests that intermittent temporary occlusion is less damaging than a single sustained episode.[24] Other experimental work directed specifically at determining the response in both normotensive and hypertensive animals demonstrates that in the latter group, intermittent occlusion was associated with a greater degree of ischemic injury.[73]

Cerebral Blood Flow and Ischemic Thresholds

The unique metabolic requirements of the brain form the central basis for understanding the relationship between blood flow and ischemic tolerance. Although the brain represents only 2 percent of the total body weight, it receives 18 percent of the cardiac output and uses 20 percent of the oxygen supply. Its high metabolic demand and lack of appreciable energy reserves render the central nervous system uniquely susceptible to alterations of blood supply. The use of PET has greatly enhanced our understanding of the pathophysiologic alterations that occur in focal cerebral ischemia in humans. The simultaneous measurement of regional CBF, oxygen metabolism (CMR_{O_2}), oxygen extraction fraction (OEF, or amount of oxygen extracted from the blood as it travels from artery to vein), and cerebral blood volume (CBV, or the volume of blood

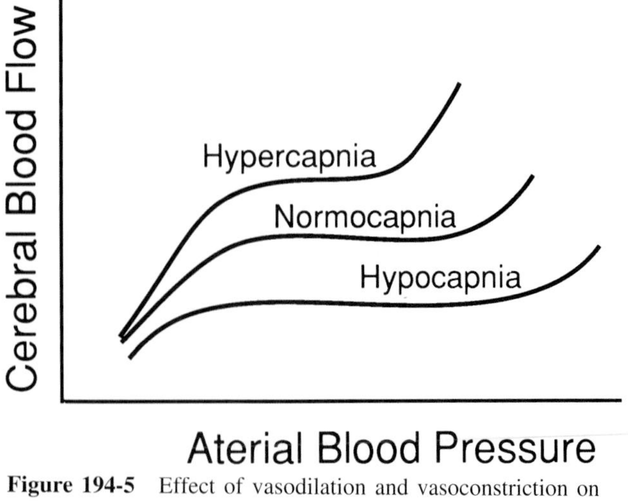

Figure 194-5 Effect of vasodilation and vasoconstriction on autoregulatory control. (From Edvinsson et al.,[14] with permission.)

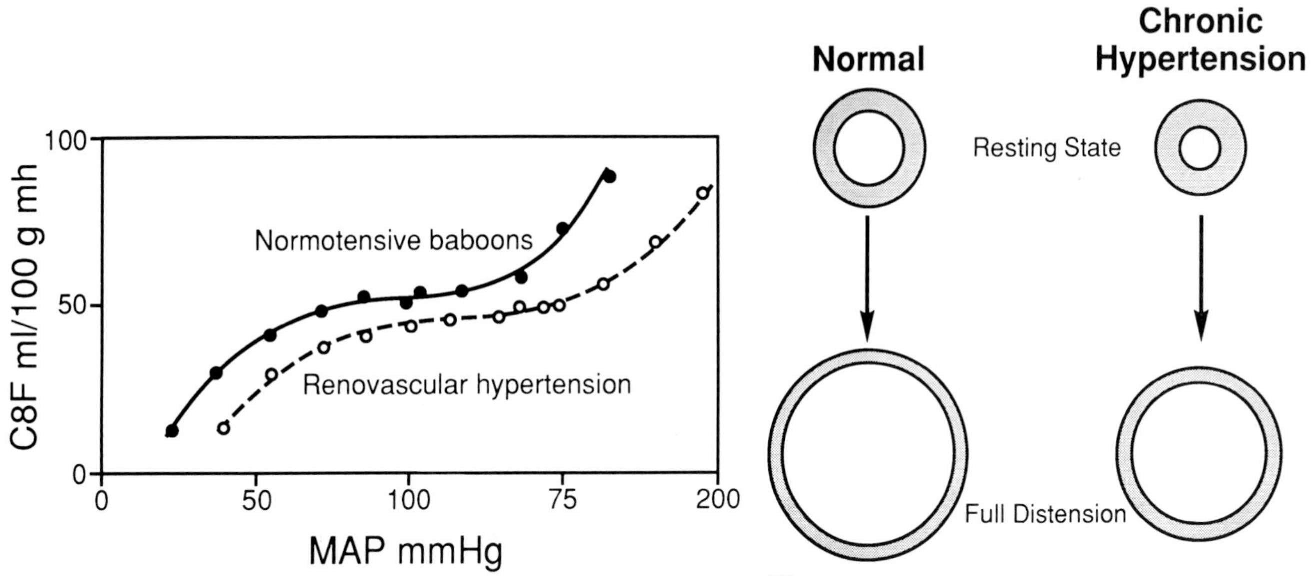

(*A*) (*B*)

Figure 194-6 *A.* Change in autoregulatory curve in response to hypertension. *B.* Vessel alterations associated with change in autoregulatory response from hypertension. (From Edvinsson et al.,[14] with permission.)

in the cerebral parenchyma) has permitted the identification of three successive stages of severity in an ischemic injury to the brain (Fig. 194-7).[13,22,54,55,56,86] As CPP initially falls, autoregulation occurs and vasodilation of precapillary resistance vessels causes an increase in CBV while maintaining both CBF and CMR_{O_2}. At the lower limit of autoregulation, maximal compensatory dilation of cerebral resistance vessels has occurred. Further reductions in CPP lead to a fall in CBF. The oxygen extraction fraction (OEF) then increases to maintain CMR_{O_2}. If CBF reduction is modest, the increased extraction of oxygen and glucose by the brain from remaining blood flow can maintain normal brain metabolism and function. A leftward shift of the oxygen-hemoglobin affinity curve, which is produced by the decreased local pH, results in an increased transfer of oxygen from blood to tissue and is largely responsible for the increased OEF. When the OEF reaches its maximum (approximately 90 percent), no further compensation can occur. As CBF falls further, the metabolic demands of the brain can no longer be satisfied, and CMR_{O_2} decreases. The metabolic alterations that occur during cerebral ischemia are detailed in a subsequent chapter.

The alterations of cerebral function that occur as these compensatory systems become overwhelmed in the face of increasingly severe ischemia may be best understood in the context of ischemic thresholds and the ischemic cascade.

Flow Thresholds

Modern electrophysiologic techniques and accurate cerebral blood flow determinations have refined our understanding of the relationship between neuronal function, tissue viability, and critical levels of regional cerebral blood flow.

Experimental studies of middle cerebral artery occlusion in various species have demonstrated a blood flow gradient from normal

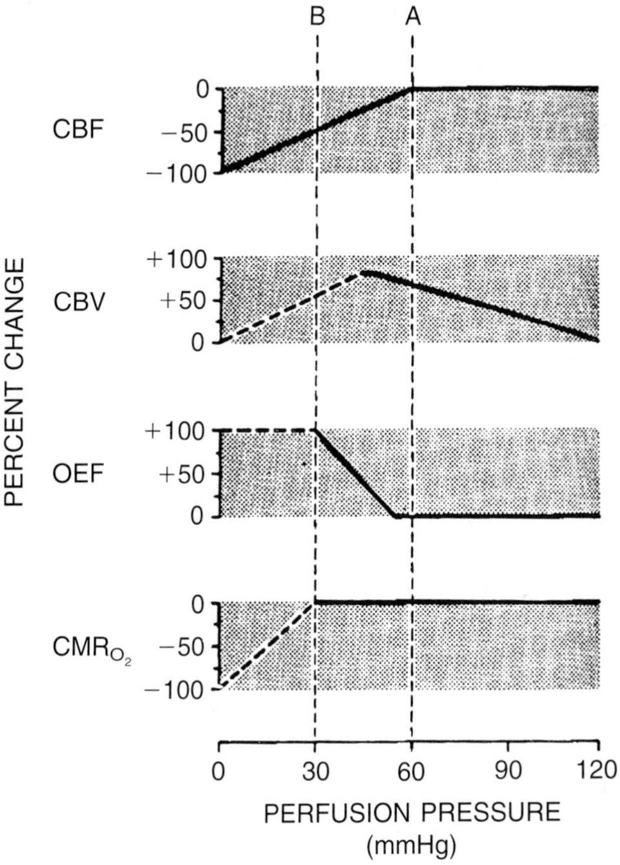

Figure 194-7 PET characterization of stages of blood flow reduction to the brain and compensatory mechanisms. See text for description. (From Powers,[54] with permission.)

flow in areas outside the affected territory, to modest decreases in the adjacent perifocal region, to a profound drop in the ischemic core.[50,51,87] The slope of this gradient depends on the extent and functional capacity of collateral blood supply. While some authors have attempted to make a distinction between the events occurring in the ischemic core and those that occur in tissue affected by a global ischemic insult, on a biochemical basis it is difficult to clearly dissociate the events occurring in these two environments. The tissue in the border zone between normal perfusion and the ischemic core—the perifocal region—may be subjected to unique challenges to its homeostatic mechanisms, however.[77,78]

Different cellular functions, which require specific minimum levels of blood flow, are affected in these regions depending on the level of blood flow reduction. Certain functional perturbations occur once blood flow decreases below these thresholds (Fig. 194-8). Critical values for loss of synaptic transmission, corresponding to loss of neuronal function, are between 15 and 18 ml/100 g per minute.[6,29] The threshold for membrane pump failure, and thus for loss of cellular integrity, is approximately 10 ml/100 g per minute.[2,5] The level of blood flow reduction for ion pump failure appears to be similar to that for energy failure. The presence of these two distinct thresholds implies that some regions in the perifocal area contain cells that are electrophysiologically quiescent but nonetheless viable. These regions constitute the ischemic penumbra, defined by Astrup, Siesjö, and Symon as areas with EEG quiescence and low extracellular K^+.[1] These thresholds were determined in experimental models using both primates and other higher vertebrates. Similar values have been reported in humans.[77,78] While absolute values may vary somewhat depending on the species and anesthetic factors, the percent reduction from normal flow to these thresholds appears to be uniform and constant.

Flow reduction is one component that determines the severity of an ischemic insult, but the duration of flow reduction is also of paramount importance (Fig. 194-9). Jones and coworkers demonstrated that the threshold for infarction in monkeys was approximately 12 ml/100 g per minute, but that the *duration* as well as the *degree* of blood flow reduction was important, since infarction developed only if blood flow was reduced to below 12 ml/100 g per minute for periods lasting 2 h or longer.[37,50] Since the time course for irreversible damage in complete global ischemia models is much shorter—approximately 10 min[36,40,58,59]—it is reasonable to suspect that areas with more profound blood flow reduction in focal ischemia have a shorter tolerance than areas with higher levels of blood flow.

The existence of two distinct thresholds suggests that some areas in the perifocal region contain cells that are electrically silent but nonetheless viable. These cells are the likely targets for prevention of ischemic injury, since they should be the most susceptible to therapeutic rescue. The ability to maintain a low extracellular potassium concentration in the perifocal region implies that sufficient energy stores remain to maintain near-normal electrochemical gradients, but the neuronal paralysis and reduced blood flow suggest that the penumbra is clearly at risk for further damage. Siesjö has applied a pragmatic definition to this region by defining a *reperfusion penumbra* and a *pharmacologic penumbra,* which represent the tissue that would inevitably become infarcted without the timely institution of either reperfusion or pharmacologic intervention.[77,78]

Therapeutic Manipulation of Residual Flow and Alteration of Flow Thresholds

The Role of Blood Viscosity

The importance of blood viscosity in the routine regulation of CBF remains controversial.[20,26,31,33,46,71,88,93] Several studies suggest that in normal brain the effect of blood viscosity on cerebral perfusion is nonexistent or minimal.[8,9,27] Under ischemic conditions, however, even small alterations in the rheologic properties of blood may have significant functional relevance.[26,38,53,70,88]

This selective contribution of viscosity to the regulation of CBF under impaired flow conditions can be explained by the inconstant nature of blood viscosity, which results from erythrocyte deformability and aggregation.[93] Therefore, the relationship between blood flow and viscosity is imprecisely described by the Hagen-Poiseuille equation, especially at low flow rates. In low-flow states, perfusion pressure is reduced and compensatory vasodilation of the microcirculation occurs. Under these conditions, blood flow is further reduced by an increase in viscosity. Thus, under ischemic conditions an intricate relationship exists between vasomotor compensatory mechanisms and blood viscosity, and even small alterations in the rheologic properties of blood have significant functional relevance.

Blood viscosity is determined by several factors, hematocrit

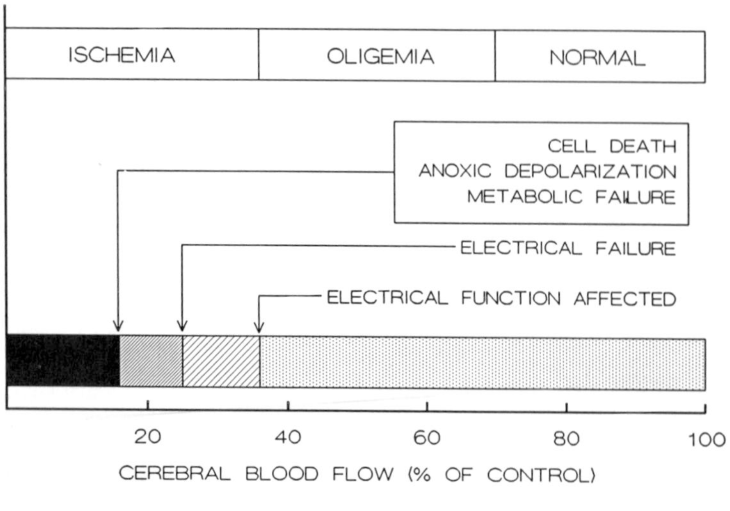

Figure 194-8 Relationship of relative cerebral blood flow to changes in cellular function and viability. (From Bhatti et al.,[4] with permission.)

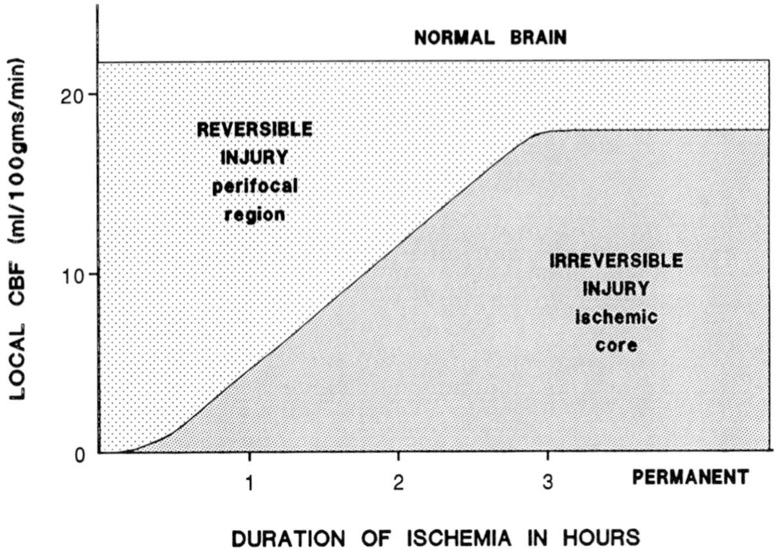

Figure 194-9 Relationship of time and severity of ischemia to the development of ischemic injury following focal cerebral ischemia. (Modified from Jones et al.,[37] with permission.)

being the most important, especially when shear rates are low. The steep portion of the hematocrit–viscosity curve falls in the physiologic range of hematocrit. Reductions in hematocrit within the physiologic range significantly reduce blood viscosity, and this effect is most marked at the low shear rates seen in focal cerebral ischemia.

Experimental studies have shown augmentation of diminished CBF following the acute reduction of hematocrit.[89,94] Although reduction of hematocrit (and thus hemoglobin content) reduces the oxygen content of blood, relative oxygen transport capacity has been calculated to increase owing to improved CBF with hematocrit reductions to approximately 30 percent.[93] Below this hematocrit level, the decrease in blood oxygen content outweighs the beneficial effect of decreased viscosity on CBF in the microcirculation. This finding is consistent with reports that indicate that a hematocrit range of 30 to 32 percent is optimal for tissue oxygen delivery.[32,34,93]

The Role of Reperfusion

The results of experimental work with reperfusion suggest that there is a definite time limit after which such restoration of flow will not be beneficial. Whether such treatment is in fact harmful is a matter of some debate. That reperfusion can lead to aggravation of edema and hemorrhagic transformation has been clearly documented. On a cellular and pathophysiologic level, it has also been shown that ''reperfusion injury'' occurs in some organs. This type of injury is speculated to occur in the brain, but definitive evidence is lacking.[77,78] It has nevertheless been shown that reperfusion achieved by the endovascular route in the early evolution of ischemic damage in the clinical setting does improve neurological outcome and offers a promise of revolutionizing the treatment of stroke.[10]

The Role of Calcium Homeostasis

While there are many promising areas of investigation into the pharmacologic control of the cerebral circulation, including adrenergic mechanisms and the roles of dopamine, serotonin, acetylcholine, histamine, prostaglandins, neuropeptides, and glutamate, few have generated as much interest among neurosurgeons as the possible uses of calcium antagonists.[14]

The role of calcium in the control of both cerebrovascular smooth muscle function and intracellular homeostasis offers opportunities for the treatment of ischemia and ischemia-producing disorders. The pharmacologic effects exerted by calcium entry blockers on vascular reactivity through an effect on excitation-contraction coupling involve three main processes: the influx of extracellular calcium or release of calcium from intracellular stores, the transport of calcium out of the cells and uptake into various cell organelles, and the processes that are regulated by the intracellular concentration of free calcium and that affect the activity of contractile proteins themselves or other cellular processes.[14]

The final common pathway for initiating contraction in vascular smooth muscle cells is believed to be an increase in the concentration of free ionized calcium within the cell. The current concept is that vasoconstrictor agents cause a depolarization of smooth muscle cells that in turn increases their spike frequency and ultimately leads to vascular contraction.[14] Of great therapeutic interest is the ability of some pharmacologic agents to induce contraction independent of any change in membrane potential (pharmacomechanical coupling).[14] These effects on smooth muscle function have resulted in the use of calcium antagonists as therapeutic agents in the treatment of cerebral vasospasm. Their precise role in this setting needs further clarification, since it is unclear whether the reported beneficial effects are due to changes in blood flow at the microcirculatory level or are directly related to ischemic cell protection, since dramatic changes in angiographic spasm are not seen with these agents.

Loss of Ca^{2+} homeostasis leading to an elevated level of intracellular Ca_i^{2+} has been implicated as a cause of irreversible cell injury in ischemia.[79] Both voltage-sensitive and agonist-operated calcium channels control the movement of calcium into the cell, and the latter are predominantly involved in the initiation of the pathologic processes resulting from ischemia (Fig. 194-10). Since Ca^{2+} plays an important role as an intracellular messenger, the rise in Ca_i^{2+} may disrupt several intracellular processes and thus compromise the cell's ability to recover from the insult.

The importance of Ca^{2+} as an intracellular messenger can be appreciated by the number of different mechanisms employed by

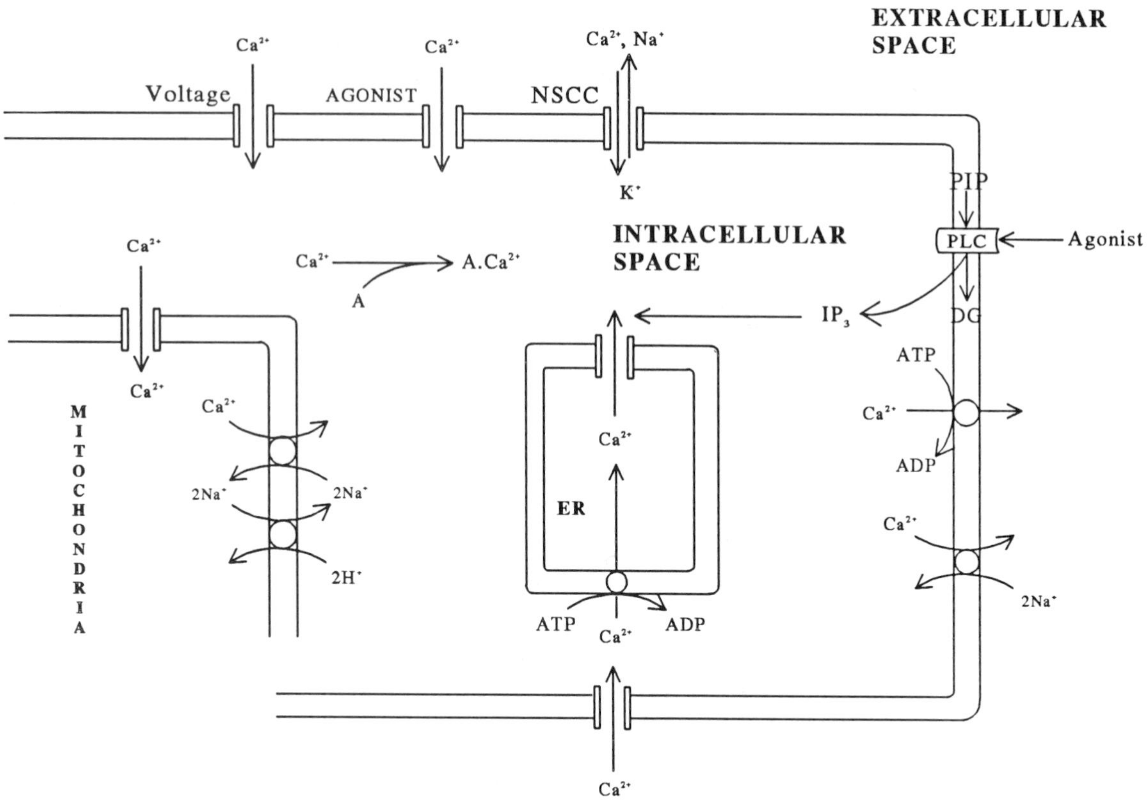

Figure 194-10 Schematic diagram illustrating mechanisms that play a role in calcium homeostasis. NSCC, nonspecific calcium channel; PIP, polyphospsoinositides; PLC, phospholipase C; IP_3, inositol triphosphate; DG, diglycerides; A^-, calcium binding proteins; ER, endoplasmic reticulum. (Modified from Siesjö and Bengtsson,[79] with permission.)

the cells to maintain Ca^{2+} homeostasis (Fig. 194-10). Intracellular Ca^{2+} concentration is maintained around 10^{-7} *M*, while extracellular concentration is in the range of 10^{-3} *M*. This large concentration gradient together with the electrical gradient exerts large inward force on Ca^{2+} ions. This gradient takes energy to maintain, requiring the active extrusion of Ca^{2+} from the cell either by a Ca^{2+}-activated ATPase or by electrogenic (3:1) Na^+/Ca^{2+} exchange, which uses the membrane Na^+ gradient as the energy source. Regulation of intracellular Ca^{2+} over the short term can be achieved by the binding or sequestration of calcium. Virtually all of the intracellular Ca^{2+} is bound to calcium-binding proteins or other molecules. Sequestration of Ca^{2+} also is energy-dependent, and it occurs primarily in the endoplasmic reticulum and mitochondria.

There is substantial evidence that a massive influx of calcium occurs during ischemia. The excessive rise in Ca_i^{2+} that results from an ischemia-induced failure of these homeostatic mechanisms represents a nonphysiologic stimulus that activates a wide array of intracellular receptors, membrane channels, and phosphorylases, which lead to compromise of the cell's functional and structural integrity.

Summary and Conclusions

Although the precise mechanisms remain to be elucidated, it can be appreciated from the material discussed that cerebral blood flow is strictly maintained and controlled. Pathologic conditions, induced by either disease or therapeutic intervention, can disrupt the regulation of blood flow and metabolism, and the neurosurgeon must be aware of these alterations to avoid untoward sequelae.

References

1. Astrup J, Siesjö BK, Symon L. Thresholds in cerebral ischemia—the ischemic penumbra. *Stroke* 1981; 12:723–725.
2. Astrup J, Symon L, Branston NM, et al. Cortical evoked potential and extracellular K^+ and H^+ at critical levels of brain ischemia. *Stroke* 1977; 8:51–57.
3. Bayliss WM. On the local reactions of the arterial wall to changes of internal pressure. *J Physiol (Lond)* 1902; 28:220–231.
4. Bhatti SU, Selman WR, Lust WD, et al. Techniques of neuroprotection. *Neurosurg Q,* 1991; 1:197–213.
5. Branston NM, Hope DT, Symon L. Barbiturates in focal ischemia of primate cortex: effects on blood flow distribution, evoked potential and extracellular potassium. *Stroke* 1979; 10:647–653.
6. Branston NM, Symon L, Crockard HA, et al. Relationship between the cortical evoked potential and the local cortical blood flow following acute middle cerebral artery occlusion in the baboon. *Exp Neurol* 1974; 45:195–208.
7. Brayden JE, Bevan JA. Acetylcholine and vasoactive intestinal polypeptide in the cerebral circulation: histochemical and biochemical indices of innervation. In Owman C, Hardebo JE (eds): *Neural Regulation of Brain Circulation.* Amsterdam: Elsevier, 1986, pp 371–381.

8. Brown MM, Marshall J. Regulation of cerebral blood flow in response to changes in blood viscosity. *Lancet* 1985; 1:604–609.
9. Brown MM, Pickles H. Effect of epoprostenol (prostacyclin, PGI2) on cerebral blood flow in man. *J Neurol Neurosurg Psychiatry* 1982; 45:1033–1036.
10. Camarata PJ, Heros RC, Latchaw RE. "Brain attack": the rationale for treating stroke as a medical emergency. *Neurosurgery* 1994; 34:144–158.
11. Dacey RG Jr, Duling BR. Effect of norepinephrine on penetrating arterioles of rat cerebral cortex. *Am J Physiol* 1984; 246:H380–H385.
12. daVinci L. *The Notebooks.* Translated by Edward MacCurdy. New York: Empire State Book, 1923.
13. Donnan GA, D'Alton JG, Chang JY, et al. Alterations in cerebral blood flow (CBF) and metabolism (CMR_{O_2}) after transient ischemic attacks. *Neurology* 1983; 33(Suppl 2):115 (abstr).
14. Edvinsson L, Mackenzie ET, McCulloch J. *Cerebral Blood Flow and Metabolism.* New York: Raven Press, 1993, pp 40, 92, 116, 122, 161, 163, 168, 169, 183, 355, 378, 483, 565–570.
15. Faraci FM. Role of nitric oxide in regulation of basilar artery tone *in vivo. Am J Physiol* 1990; 259:H1216–H1221.
16. Faraci FM. Role of endothelium-derived relaxing factor in cerebral circulation: large arteries vs. microcirculation. *Am J Physiol* 1991; 261:H1038–H1042.
17. Fox PT, Raichle ME. Focal physiological uncoupling of cerebral blood flow and oxidative metabolism during somatosensory stimulation in human subjects. *Proc Natl Acad Sci USA* 1986; 83:1140–1144.
18. Furchgott RF. Role of endothelium in responses of vascular smooth muscle. *Circ Res* 1983; 53:557–573.
19. Furchgott RF, Zawadzki JC. The obligatory role of endothelial cells in the relaxation of arterial smooth muscle by acetylcholine. *Nature* 1980; 288:373–376.
20. Gaehtgens P, Marx P. Hemorheological aspects of the pathophysiology of cerebral ischemia. *J Cereb Blood Flow Metab* 1987; 7:259–265.
21. Gardiner SM, Compton AM, Bennett T, et al. Control of regional blood flow by endothelium-derived nitric oxide. *Hypertension* 1990; 15:486–492.
22. Gibbs JM, Wise RJS, Leeders KL, et al. Factors associated with hydrocephalus after subarachnoid hemorrhage: a report of the Cooperative Aneurysm Study. *Arch Neurol* 1989; 46:744–752.
23. Goadsby PJ, Lance JW. Brain stem effects on intra- and extracerebral circulations. Relation to migraine and cluster headache. In Olesen J, Edvinsson L (eds): *Basic Mechanisms of Headache.* Amsterdam: Elsevier, 1988, pp 413–427.
24. Goldman MS, Anderson RE, Meyer FB. Effects of intermittent reperfusion during temporary focal ischemia. *J Neurosurg* 1992; 77:911–916.
25. Greenberg J, Hand P, Sylvestro A, et al. Localized metabolic-flow couple during functional activity. *Acta Neurol Scand* 1979; 72:12–13.
26. Grotta J, Ackerman R, Correia J, et al. Whole blood viscosity parameters and cerebral blood flow. *Stroke* 1982; 13:296–301.
27. Häggendal E, Norbäck B. Effect of viscosity on cerebral blood flow. *Acta Chir Scand [Suppl]* 1966; 364:3–12.
28. Harper AM. Autoregulation of cerebral blood flow: influence of the arterial blood pressure on the flow through the cerebral cortex. *J Neurol Neurosurg Psychiatry* 1966; 29:398–403.
29. Heiss WD, Hayakawa T, Waltz AG. Cortical neuronal function during ischemia: effects of occlusion of one middle cerebral artery on single-unit activity in cats. *Arch Neurol* 1976; 33:813–820.
30. Heistad DD, Kontos HA. Cerebral circulation. In Shephard JT, Abboud FM (eds): *Handbook of Physiology.* Section 2: *The Cardiovascular System,* vol 3. Bethesda, MD: American Physiological Society, 1983, pp 137–182.
31. Henriksen L, Paulson OB, Smith RJ. Cerebral blood flow following normovolemic hemodilution in patients with high hematocrit. *Ann Neurol* 1981; 9:454–457.
32. Hint H. The pharmacology of dextran and the physiological background for the clinical use of Rheomacrodex and Macrodex. *Acta Anaesthesiol Belg* 1968; 19:119–138.
33. Humphrey PRD, DuBoulay GH, Marshall J, et al. Cerebral blood-flow and viscosity in relative polycythaemia. *Lancet* 1979; 2:873–878.
34. Hunt WE, Hess RM. Surgical risk as related to time of intervention in the repair of intracranial aneurysms. *J Neurosurg* 1968; 28:14–20.
35. Iadecola C. Does nitric oxide mediate the increases in cerebral blood flow elicited by hypercapnia? *Proc Natl Acad Sci USA* 1992; 89:3913–3916.
36. Ito U, Spatz M, Walker JT Jr, et al. Experimental cerebral ischemia in mongolian gerbils. I. Light microscopic observations. *Acta Neuropathol (Berl)* 1975; 32:209–223.
37. Jones TH, Morawetz RB, Crowell RM, et al. Thresholds of focal cerebral ischemia in awake monkeys. *J Neurosurg* 1981; 54:773–782.
38. Kee DB Jr, Wood JH. Blood viscosity and cerebral blood flow. In Plum F, Pulsinelli WA (eds): *Cerebrovascular Disease: 14th Research (Princeton-Williamsburg) Conference.* New York: Raven Press, 1985, pp 107–117.
39. Kety SS. The cerebral circulation. In Fishman AP, Richards DW (eds): *Circulation of the Blood: Men and Ideas.* New York: Oxford University Press, 1964, pp 703–742.
40. Kirino T. Delayed neuronal death in the gerbil hippocampus following ischemia. *Brain Res* 1982; 239:57–69.
41. Kozniewska E, Oseka M, Stys T. Effects of endothelium-derived nitric oxide on cerebral circulation during normoxia and hypoxia in the rat. *J Cereb Blood Flow Metab* 1992; 12:311–317.
42. Kuschinsky W, Wahl M. Local chemical and neuronic regulation of cerebral vascular resistance. *Physiol Rev* 1978; 58:656–689.
43. Lansman JB. Endothelial mechanosensors; going with the flow. *Nature* 1988; 331:481–482.
44. Lassen NA. Cerebral blood flow and oxygen consumption in man. *Physiol Rev* 1959; 39:183–238.
45. Lebrun-Grandie P, Baron JC, Soussaline F, et al. Coupling between regional blood flow and oxygen utilization in the normal human brain: a study with positron tomography and oxygen 15. *Arch Neurol* 1983; 40:230–236.
46. Marshall J. The viscosity factor in cerebral ischemia. *J Cereb Blood Flow Metab* 1982; 2(Suppl 1): S47–S49.
47. Marshall JJ, Kontos HA. Endothelium-derived relaxing factors: a perspective from in vivo data. *Hypertension* 1990; 16:371–386.
48. McDowall DG. Drugs and cerebral autoregulation. *Eur J Clin Invest* 1982; 12:377–378.
49. Moncada S, Palmer RMJ, Higgs EA. The discovery of nitric oxide as the endogenous nitrovasodilator. *Hypertension* 1988; 12:365–372.
50. Morawetz RB, Crowell RH, DeGirolami U, et al. Regional cerebral blood flow thresholds during cerebral ischemia. *Fed Proc* 1979; 38:2493–2494.
51. Morawetz RB, DeGirolami U, Ojemann RG, et al. Cerebral blood flow determined by hydrogen clearance during middle cerebral artery occlusion in unanesthetized monkeys. *Stroke* 1978; 9:143–149.
52. Olesen J. Quantitative evaluation of normal and pathologic cerebral blood flow regulation to perfusion pressure: changes in man. *Arch Neurol* 1973; 143–149.
53. Ott EO, Ladurner G, Lechner H. Relationship between disturbed rheological properties and cerebral hemodynamics in recent cerebral infarction. *Prog Biochem Pharmacol* 1977; 13:349–352.
54. Powers WJ. Cerebral hemodynamics in ischemic cerebrovascular disease. *Ann Neurol* 1991; 39:231–240.
55. Powers WJ, Grubb RL Jr, Baker RP, et al. Regional cerebral blood flow and metabolism in reversible ischemia due to vasospasm: determination by positron emission tomography. *J Neurosurg* 1985; 62:539–546.
56. Powers WJ, Raichle ME, Grubb RL Jr. Positron emission tomography to assess cerebral perfusion. *Lancet* 1985; 1:102–103.
57. Prado R, Watson BD, Kuluz J, et al. Endothelium-derived nitric oxide synthase inhibition: effects on cerebral blood flow, pial artery diameter, and vascular morphology in rats. *Stroke* 1992; 23:1118–1124.
58. Pulsinelli WA, Brierley JB. A new model of bilateral hemispheric ischemia in the unanesthetized rat. *Stroke* 1979; 10:267–272.

59. Pulsinelli WA, Brierley JB, Plum F. Temporal profile of neuronal damage in a model of transient forebrain ischemia. *Ann Neurol* 1982; 11:491–498.

60. Purves MJ. *The Physiology of the Cerebral Circulation.* Cambridge: Cambridge University Press, 1972.

61. Raichle ME, Grubb RL Jr, Gado MH, et al. Correlation between regional cerebral blood flow and oxidative metabolism. In vivo studies in man. *Arch Neurol* 1976; 33:523–526.

62. Raper AJ, Kontos HA, Patterson JL Jr. Response of pial precapillary vessels to changes in arterial carbon dioxide tension. *Circ Res* 1971; 28:518–523.

63. Reis DJ. Central neural control of cerebral circulation and metabolism. In Mackenzie ET, Seylaz J, B-es A (eds): *Neurotransmitters and the Cerebral Circulation.* New York: Raven Press, 1984, pp 91–119.

64. Reis DJ, Iadecola C. Central neuronic regulation of cerebral blood flow. In Seylaz J, Sercombe R (eds): *Neurotransmission and Cerebrovascular Function II.* (Excerpta Medica International Congress Series, nos 869–870.) Amsterdam: Elsevier, 1989, pp 369–390.

65. Reis DJ, Iadecola C, Nakai M. Control of cerebral blood flow and metabolism by intrinsic neural systems in brain. In Plum F, Pulsinelli WA (eds): *Cerebrovascular Diseases: 14th Research (Princeton-Williamsburg) Conference.* New York: Raven Press, 1985, pp 1–22.

66. Rosenblum WI, Nishimura H, Nelson GH. Endothelium-dependent L-Arg- and L-NMMA-sensitive mechanisms regulate tone of brain microvessels. *Am J Physiol* 1990; 259:H1396-H1401.

67. Rossen R, Kabat H, Anderson JP. Acute arrest of cerebral circulation in man. *Arch Neurol Psychiatry* 1943; 50:510–528.

68. Roy CS, Sherrington CS. On the regulation of the blood-supply of the brain. *J Physiol (Lond)* 1890; 11:85–108.

69. Sakas DE, Moskowitz MA, Buzzi MG, et al. Trigeminovascular fibers increase blood flow in cortical gray matter by axon reflex-like mechanisms. *J Cereb Blood Flow Metab* 1989; 9:S31.

70. Sakuta S. Blood filtrability in cerebrovascular disorders, with special reference to erythrocyte deformability and ATP content. *Stroke* 1981; 12:824–828.

71. Schmid-Schonbein H. Macrorheology and microrheology of blood in cerebrovascular insufficiency. *Eur Neurol* 1983; 22 (Suppl 1):2–22.

72. Schmidt CF, Pierson JC. The intrinsic regulation of the blood vessels of the medulla oblongata. *Am J Physiol* 1934; 108:241–263.

73. Selman WR, Bhatti SU, Rosenstein CC, et al. Temporary vessel occlusion in spontaneously hypertensive and normotensive rats: effects of single and multiple episodes on tissue metabolism and volume of infarction. *J Neurosurg* 1994; 80:1085–1090.

74. Selman WR, LaManna JC, Ratcheson RA, Lust WD. Metabolic correlates of focal ischemia. In Bazan NG, Braquet P, Ginsberg MD (eds): *Neurochemical Correlates of Cerebral Ischemia.* (Advances in Neurochemistry, vol 7.) New York: Plenum, 1992, pp 9–39.

75. Seylaz J, Hara H, Pinard E, et al. Effect of stimulation of the sphenopalatine ganglion on cortical blood flow in the rat. *J Cereb Blood Flow Metab* 1988; 8:875–878.

76. Shalit MN, Reinmuth OM, Shimojyo S, Scheinberg P. Carbon dioxide and cerebral circulatory control. 3. The effects of brain stem lesions. *Arch Neurol* 1967; 17:342–353.

77. Siesjö BK. Pathophysiology and treatment of focal cerebral ischemia. Part I: Pathophysiology. *J Neurosurg* 1992; 77:169–184.

78. Siesjö BK. Pathophysiology and treatment of focal cerebral ischemia. Part II. Mechanisms of damage and treatment. *J Neurosurg* 1992; 77:337–354.

79. Siesjö BK, Bengtsson F. Calcium fluxes, calcium antagonists, and calcium-related pathology in brain ischemia, hypoglycemia and spreading depression. A unifying hypothesis. *J Cereb Blood Flow Metab* 1989; 9:127–140.

80. Silver IA. Cellular microenvironment in relation to local blood flow. *Ciba Found Symp* 1978; 56:49–67.

81. Singer CJ. *A Short History of Anatomy from the Greeks to Harvey: The Evolution of Anatomy,* 2d ed. New York: Dover, 1957.

82. Sokoloff L. Relationships among local functional activity, energy metabolism, and blood flow on the central nervous system. *Fed Proc* 1981; 40:2311–2316.

83. Sokoloff L, Reivich M, Kennedy C, et al. The [^{14}C]-deoxyglucose method for the measurement of local cerebral glucose utilization: theory, procedure, and normal values in the conscious and anesthetized albino rat. *J Neurochem* 1977; 28:897–916.

84. Stavraky GW. Response of cerebral blood vessels to electric stimulation of the thalamus and hypothalamic regions. *Arch Neurol Psychiatry* 1936; 35:1002–1028.

85. Strandgaard S, Olesen J, Skinhoj E, et al. Autoregulation of brain circulation in severe arterial hypertension. *Br Med J* 1973; 1:507–510.

86. Sutton LN, McLaughlin AC, Dante S, et al. Cerebral venous oxygen content as a measure of brain energy metabolism with increased intracranial pressure and hyperventilation. *J Neurosurg* 1990; 73:927–932.

87. Symon L, Pasztor E, Branston NM. The distribution and density of reduced cerebral blood flow following acute middle cerebral artery occlusion: an experimental study by the technique of hydrogen clearance in baboons. *Stroke* 1974; 5:355–364.

88. Thomas DJ, Marshall J, Russell RW, et al. Effect of haematocrit on cerebral blood-flow in man. *Lancet* 1977; 2:941–943.

89. Tu YK, Heros RC, Karacostas D, et al. Isovolemic hemodilution in experimental focal cerebral ischemia. 2. Effects on regional cerebral blood flow and size of infarction. *J Neurosurg* 1988; 69:82–91.

90. Tuor UI, Kelly PAT, Tatemoto K, et al. Neuropeptide Y and the cerebral circulation. In Owman C, Hardebo JE (eds): *Neural Regulation of Brain Circulation* Amsterdam: Elsevier, 1986, pp 333–354.

91. von Sāntha K, Cipriani A. Focal alterations in subcortical circulation resulting from stimulation of the cerebral cortex: an experimental demonstration of cortico-subcortical connections. *Res Publ Assoc Res Nerv Ment Dis* 1937; 18:346–362.

92. Wahl M, Deetjen P, Thurau K, et al. Micropuncture evaluation of the importance of perivascular pH for the arteriolar diameter on the brain surface. *Pfleugers Arch* 1970; 316:152–163.

93. Wood JH, Kee DB Jr. Hemorheology of the cerebral circulation in stroke. *Stroke* 1985; 16:765–772.

94. Wood JH, Simeone FA, Fink, EA, et al. Hypervolemic hemodilution in experimental focal cerebral ischemia: elevation of cardiac output, regional cortical blood flow, and ICP after intravascular volume expansion with low molecular weight dextran. *J Neurosurg* 1983; 59:500–509.

195 Measurement of Cerebral Blood Flow

Howard Yonas

An early attempt at the understanding of the nature of cerebral blood flow (CBF) was made in the late 1770s when Monro proposed that the quantity of blood flow within the head must be the same or nearly so at all times. He believed that because the brain is enclosed in bone and it is incompressible, the volume of blood within the cranium also has to be constant. Although this is basically correct, a false assumption was also made: that the vasculature is passive and incapable of actively changing its diameter. The later work of Roy and Sherrington in the late 1800s established an active role for the vasculature following observations of the pial vasculature through cranial window preparations.

A major step toward quantitation of cerebral blood flow was made in the 1920s with the capability of obtaining jugular bulb blood samples, which in turn made possible a measure of the arterial to jugular venous O_2 difference. This approach subsequently laid a solid scientific foundation for our current understanding of cerebral blood flow physiology and established the dominant role of CO_2 as a regulator of cerebral blood flow.

In 1945 Kety and Schmidt described a method of quantifying cerebral blood flow in humans, based on the Fick principle, that utilized nitrous oxide, a metabolically inert and highly lipid-soluble gas, as the tracer of blood flow.[7] The Fick principle had stated that the quantity of a gas taken up by a tissue per unit of time (Q_i) is equal to the quantity entering it via the arterial blood minus the quantity leaving in the venous blood: $dQ_i/dt = F_i(C_a - C_v)$, where F_i is equal to blood flow and C_a and C_v are equal to the arterial and venous gas concentrations, respectively. Knowing the time course of the changes in the inert gas concentration in the arterial blood flowing into the brain and the venous blood leaving it, as well as the blood/brain partition coefficient, enables one to calculate the average cerebral blood flow. The governing relationship as characterized by Kety and Schmidt for a single tissue compartment, i, is

$$C_i(T) = \lambda_i k_i C_a(\mu) e^{-k_i(T-\mu)} d\mu$$

where flow is $F_i = \lambda_i k_i$. The input functions for this equation are the partition coefficient (λ_i), the flow rate constant (k_i), the time-dependent tracer concentration in the arterial blood $C_a(\mu)$, and the time-dependent tracer concentration in the venous blood. For this relationship the tissue concentration ($C_i T$) is assumed to be equal to the venous blood content divided by λ. This equation is then valid for saturation or desaturation studies depending on the boundary conditions that are set. This measurement of global cerebral blood flow with nitrous oxide required the following assumptions: (1) blood flow is in a steady state during the period of study and is not affected by the tracer, (2) the venous blood from the superior internal jugular vein is representative of the mixed cerebral venous blood with no contamination from extracerebral blood, (3) the period of measurement is long enough to allow equilibration of gas in the brain with the cerebral venous blood, (4) no significant arterial-venous shunts are present in the brain, and (5) the value of the partition coefficient of the inert gas is representative of the entire brain. The initial studies with nitrous oxide demonstrated that blood flow studies with this tracer did meet the above assumptions under most situations, the exception being in a region of disturbed physiology, where arteriovenous shunting may be significant and where the partition coefficient is likely to be altered.

A major advance toward the broad clinical application of cerebral blood flow measurement came with the substitution of radiolabeled ^{85}Kr for nitrous oxide and scintillation counting as the direct measure of tracer movement within the tissue, the latter measure being substituted for the difference of the arterial and venous concentrations of the tracer. This approach provided a regionality of blood flow determination that was lacking in the global blood flow measures provided by nitrous oxide, but this was significantly hampered by a weak signal and contamination from extracranial emissions. Initially this was dealt with experimentally by the injection of ^{85}Kr directly into the internal carotid artery and by scintillation counting over the cortex. Subsequently with the substitution of the gamma emitter, ^{133}Xe, for ^{85}Kr, higher and more adequate counting rates were obtained through the skull. The application of this technique with internal carotid artery injection then became widely utilized, both clinically and experimentally, as a means of obtaining regional CBF measurements. Because this approach requires an internal carotid artery catheter, its application has generally remained limited to situations where patients were undergoing angiography.

A broader approach became possible, however, with the work of Obrist, who, utilizing a multicompartmental analysis of the Kety-Schmidt equation, was able to divide the washout curve into three components, with the extracranial contamination appearing as a well-defined, late washout (Table 195-1). If this contamination is subtracted from the remaining fast (gray matter) and slow (white matter) curves, an analysis of flow can then be done, with an additional correction being made for the recirculation of gas. The later measure was made by a separate recording of the end tidal ^{133}Xe concentration as an indirect measure of the capillary (and therefore arterial) concentration of the gas. As a "noninvasive" inhalation study, ^{133}Xe inhalation flow determinations have been shown to maintain the numerical reliability of the intracarotid injection method.[10] In recent years most centers have turned to intravenous bolus introduction of ^{133}Xe as a simpler means of delivering the tracer. Refinements have permitted a relatively short period of data acquisition (10 min) during the clearance phase in which only the fast "gray matter" flows are extracted, again without significant loss of validity against the intracarotid technique. Commercially available units utilizing this methodology commonly incorporate about 16 to 32 NaI scintillation counters, which are placed about both hemispheres so that each is perpendicular to the surface of the brain. The ultimate in collimation was developed in Lassen's laboratory, where 254 independent collimators were made into a unilateral array (Fig. 195-1).[8] Elegant studies of regional flow disturbance in disease and during activation studies of

TABLE 195-1 Methods of Measuring Cerebral Blood Flow

	Quality					
Technique	**Quantitative Flow**	**Qualitative Flow**	**Local Flow**	**Repeatable <1 h**	**Accessibility**	**Metabolism**
^{133}Xe	X			X	X	
^{133}Xe SPECT	X		X	X	X	
Xe/CT	X		X	X	X	
PET	X		X	X		X
HmPAO SPECT		X	X		X	
MRI		X*	X	X		X
TCD		X		X	X	
CT Transit		X		X	X	
^{99m}Tc Transit		X		X	X	

*Can record absence of perfusion.

physiologic stimulation have been demonstrated with this technique. Portable ^{133}Xe cerebral blood flow units utilizing four to five probes over each hemisphere are now available, permitting studies to be performed at the bedside.

The ^{133}Xe methodology, however, suffers from a number of significant limitations. Counts arising from extracranial tissues still provide a signal contamination, as do emissions arising from the opposite hemisphere. This technique is dependent on the use of ''normal'' partition coefficients, which in diseased states can alter flow values by as much as 50 percent. Although a careful analytic approach to data analysis with this technique has been able to positively identify the side of a cerebral infarction in 80 percent of the cases in which a stroke was evident on computed tomography, regions of no flow may be totally missed.[5] This technique may detect raised or normal flow in a region of no flow because counts from the hyperemic rim can overshadow the area of low or no flow just below it. As a major limitation of this technique, this ''look-through'' phenomenon has prompted the development of a single photon emission computed tomography (SPECT) imaging system for ^{133}Xe.[8] Due to Compton scatter and a weaker signal from central regions, ^{133}Xe SPECT still suffers from poor resolution, especially centrally within the brain. This technology is also limited because of a dependence on ''normal'' partition coefficient values (λ). Tomographic CBF measurements with ^{133}Xe are best acquired with dedicated multi-head rotating cameras. A single rotating gamma camera can be utilized with ^{133}Xe, but the time for adequate data acquisition may be over 1 h compared with 20 to 30 min for multi-head units.

Other quantitative and regionally specific techniques for blood flow determination include positron emission tomography (PET)[2] and stable xenon-enhanced tomography (Xe/CT).[12] The major advantage of PET is its ability to measure not only flow, but also a

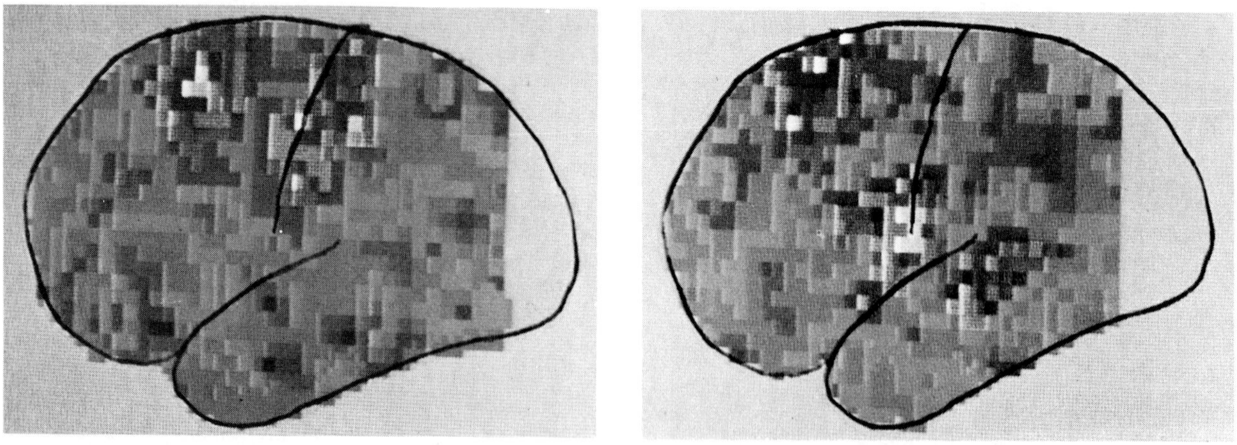

(*A*) (*B*)

Figure 195-1 These are cerebral blood flow studies utilizing ^{133}Xe introduced by intracarotid injection with imaging through an array of 254 externally placed scintillation detectors. Each detector is collimated to scan approximately 1 cm^2 of the brain surface. Lightest shades of gray indicate rates of flow up to 20 percent above baseline; the darkest shades indicate 20 percent below baseline. *A*. This study demonstrates an enhanced focal pattern which accompanies hand movements of the opposite side. *B*. This study demonstrates the flow pattern that accompanies counting out loud. Note enhanced flow values not only in the area of the cortex thought to cause mouth motions, but also in the supplemental motor area and the auditory cortex. (Courtesy of Drs. N. A. Lassen, D. H. Ingvar, and E. Skinhøj, Bispebjerg Hospital, Copenhagen, Denmark, and University Hospital, Lund, Sweden.)

theoretically limitless list of other potentially vital parameters at the same time (refer to Chap. 24 for further discussion). The relatively high cost of acquisition and its requirement for short-lived isotopes make PET a demanding technology requiring a team of individuals, thus limiting its potential for wide availability. Interpretation of PET-derived physiologic data is also limited due to a lack of direct anatomic correlation, and quantitative reliability is weakened by a dependence on numerous physiologic assumptions which do not necessarily pertain in disease states.

Another tomographic approach for acquiring cerebral blood flow information involves the inhalation of 26 to 33 percent stable xenon, an inert radiodense gas which is highly lipid-soluble, as a marker of flow combined with transmission computed tomography (Fig. 195-2).[6] For this technique, CT scans obtained before and during approximately 4.5 min of xenon-oxygen inhalation are utilized to record the movement of this lipid-soluble and radiodense gas into the brain substance. Because the relatively slow process of diffusion of this agent is being characterized, scans obtained at 1-min intervals provide the required data. Rapid scanning techniques with incremental table movements permit data acquisition at three or more additional levels during each inhalation sequence. The end tidal xenon concentration as measured by a thermoconductivity analyzer is utilized to indirectly record the arterial concentration during the buildup and/or washout of xenon. This information, plus the degree of image enhancement, is then used to derive λ and the local cerebral blood flow by multivariable analysis. Concurrent studies using radiolabeled microspheres, iodoantipyrine, and ^{133}Xe have shown excellent correlation with Xe/CT CBF. Anatomic resolution is high, approaching the resolution of the CT scanners, with equal quantitative accuracy within the center and on the surface of the brain. Clinical studies suggest that this method has the potential for broad application as a noninvasive, repeatable means of obtaining clinically useful CBF information. Although it has been shown that xenon moderately alters cerebral blood flow and may alter the sensorium of 10 to 15 percent of individuals, moderate flow activation does not significantly alter flow values, although sensorial effects can at times make it difficult to obtain studies without motion.

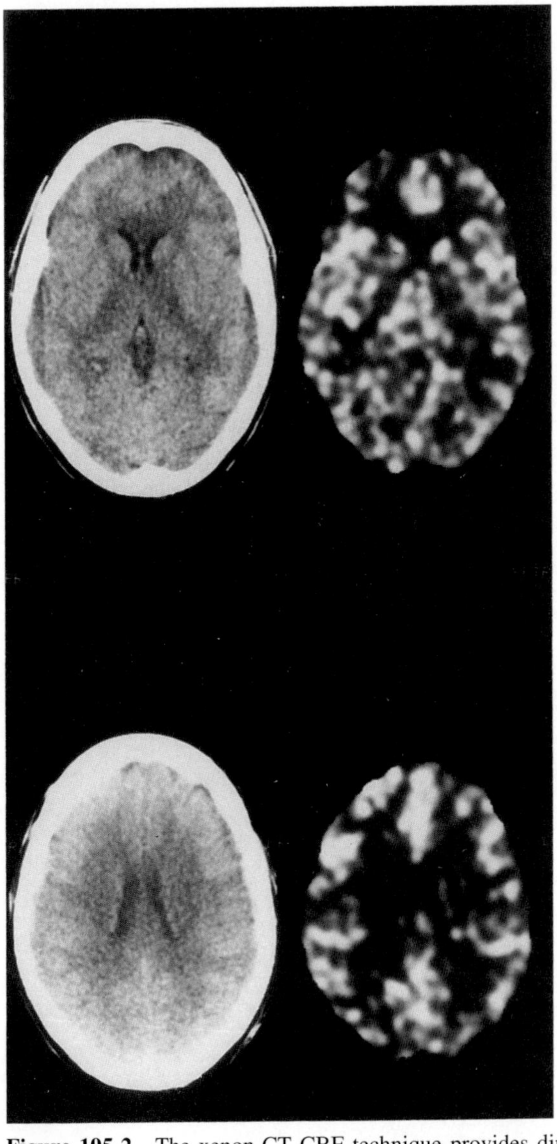

Figure 195-2 The xenon-CT CBF technique provides direct correlation between CT and high resolution, quantitative CBF data. (Reprinted from Yonas et al.,[12] with permission.)

Qualitative information about cerebral blood flow is also being provided by two older and four newer approaches. Clearance curves of ^{99m}Tc-labeled technetium pertechnetate combined with rapid data acquisition on a single-crystal Anger camera has been utilized for a decade to provide information about the movement of blood within comparative blood pools. The absence of supratentorial flow by this technique has become a standard test for brain death. The same type of data, but with better localization, is also being provided by rapid CT scanning following an intravenous iodine bolus. Studies at the level of the middle cerebral arteries or at the level of the brain stem have been shown to provide a readily accessible means of evaluating regional asymmetries of movement within blood pools. Because of the broad availability of this technology and the possible importance of flow asymmetry, this technique has a broad potential application for the assessment of regional blood flow.

New radiopharmaceuticals combined with SPECT imaging have received much attention of late.[3,9] SPECT CBF derived with radiolabeled isotopes that behave as biological microspheres today provide relatively high-resolution three-dimensional qualitative CBF imaging. While rotating angle cameras provide information for the entire intracranial volume, such studies require prolonged acquisition times (>40 to 60 min). Newer dedicated multihead SPECT units provide more rapid acquisition and higher resolution. Normally, repeat studies are performed at 24-h intervals, allowing tracer clearance. Repeat studies at briefer intervals can be performed using the fractional dosing of a single study. Quantitative data can be obtained if a reference arterial blood curve for tracer activity is acquired.

Diffusion imaging with magnetic resonance imaging provides information concerning the presence or absence of blood movement. The combination of excellent anatomic imaging and the ability to identify the absence of flow should have direct clinical utility, especially if linked to MR spectroscopy. At this time, MRI is unable to differentiate gradients of flow unless diffusible tracers of CBF such as fluorocarbons are combined with imaging.

Direct monitoring of cortical blood flow is available today utilizing either thermal dilution or laser Doppler technologies. Both techniques are able to record flow changes repeatedly and provide information from a very focused region of only the outer few millimeters of the cerebral cortex. Both are limited by the inability to maintain fixation with the cortical surface, so that the interpretation of variations in flow may be complicated by uncertainty as to whether the probe has remained in position.

Transcranial Doppler (TCD) velocity measurement of intracranial vessels in and directly about the circle of Willis is now widely available.[1,4] This relatively simple and low-cost bedside measurement can be made frequently or continuously. Although a single velocity measurement is not tightly linked to CBF, the change of velocity induced by a physiologic challenge is related to a proportional CBF change. This provides a valuable means of assessing the response to diagnostic and therapeutic efforts. TCD has also been very useful for recording the occurrence of cerebral emboli.

Three additional approaches to cerebral blood flow measurement are applicable only in the laboratory. These are autoradiography with iodo[^{14}C]antipyrine,[11] sequential injections of different radiolabeled isotope microspheres, and hydrogen clearance techniques.[12]

Autoradiography utilizing iodo[^{14}C]antipyrine as a diffusible indicator of flow has proved to be a highly quantitative means of obtaining data concerning flow with a high degree of spatial resolution. For this study the animal needs to be sacrificed shortly after the intravenous injection of iodo[^{14}C]antipyrine. The brain is then removed and frozen to $-70°$, followed by thin sectioning and application of tissue slices to radiographic plates for 5 to 6 days. Multiple sequential arterial blood samples are used to provide the arterial input function. The emission densities on the photographic plates are then interpretable as measures of blood flow which contain a high degree of spatial resolution. The major limitation of this approach is that it permits a measure of flow at only one point in time, although some work has suggested that two isotopes with differential counting can be used to record flow at two points in time.

Radiolabeled microspheres measuring 6 to 8 μm in diameter provide a nondiffusible means of measuring flow. Microspheres of this size are extracted into the microcirculation at a rate of over 90 percent for a single pass through the cerebral circulation. By recording the rate of extraction of radiolabeled isotopes from the arterial circulation and then directly counting the number of counts in each tissue volume, blood flow data are obtained. Currently up to five independent isotope injections (^{141}Ce, ^{133}Sn, ^{85}Sr, ^{95}Nb, ^{46}Sc) and therefore blood flow determinations can be made after isotope separation utilizing a matrix algebra approach for the solution of simultaneous equations. The major disadvantage of this approach in a laboratory is that a volume of $8 \times 8 \times 8$ mm is typically required to obtain adequate counts for reliable statistical determinations.

The third approach involves measuring the clearance of hydrogen gas from about a reference platinum-iridium probe previously placed within the brain substance. Fine probe diameters (0.01 in) with exposure of only the terminal 2 mm are commonly being utilized. An array of as many as six simultaneous probes are currently being used, and this approach has been shown to provide a highly reproducible and locally specific means of repeatedly determining local cerebral blood flow. This technique has the advantage of repeatability with the opportunity to make flow calculations every 10 to 15 min for days or even weeks. A critical review of this topic has suggested that the tissue volume of study may be $5 \times 5 \times 5$ mm.[13] The only major limitation to this approach is that the data acquisition is limited to only the immediate region about the tip of the probe, which does require disturbance of the tissue to be studied by its placement.

Blood flow is an important monitor of cerebral function and impaired blood flow is often the pathway through which cerebral injury occurs. Many technologies, each having advantages and disadvantages, have become available for the measurement of CBF. Choosing the most appropriate CBF tool will depend on the particular study subject and the specific question to be answered.

References

1. Aaslid R, Markwalder TM, Norues H. Noninvasive transcranial Doppler ultrasound recording of flow velocity in basal cerebral arteries. *J Neurosurg* 1982; 57:769–774.
2. Ackerman RH, Subramanyam R, Correia JA, et al. Positron imaging of cerebral blood flow during continuous inhalation of $C^{15}O_2$. *Stroke* 1980; 11:45–49.
3. DeRoo M, Mortelmans L, Devos P, et al. Clinical experience with Tc-99m HM-PAO high resolution SPECT of the brain in patients with cerebrovascular accidents. *Eur J Nucl Med* 1989; 15:9–15.
4. Grosset DG, Straiton J, duTrevou M, Bullock R. Prediction of symptomatic vasospasm after subarachnoid hemorrhage by rapidly increasing transcranial Doppler velocity and cerebral blood flow changes. *Stroke* 1992; 23:674–679.
5. Halsey JH Jr, Nakai K, Wariyar B. Sensitivity of rCBF to focal lesions. *Stroke* 1981; 12:631–635.
6. Johnson DW, Stringer WA, Marks MP, et al. Stable Xenon/CT: cerebral blood flow imaging: rationale for and role in clinical decision making. *Am J Neuroradiol* 1991; 12:201–213.
7. Kety SS, Schmidt CF. The determination of cerebral blood flow in man by the use of nitrous oxide in low concentrations. *Am J Physiol* 1945; 143:53–66.
8. Lassen NA, Henriksen L, Paulson O: Regional cerebral blood flow in stroke by ^{133}xenon inhalation and emission tomography. *Stroke* 1981; 12:284–288.
9. Nakano S, Kinoshita K, Jinnouchi S, et al. Comparative study of regional cerebral blood flow images by SPECT using xenon-133, iodine-123 imp, and technetium -99 m HM-PAO. *J Nucl Med* 1989; 30:157–164.
10. Obrist WD, Thompson HK Jr, King CH, Wang HS. Determination of regional cerebral blood flow by inhalation of 133-Xenon. *Circ Res* 1967; 20:124–135.
11. Sakurada O, Kennedy C, Jehle J, et al. Measurement of local cerebral blood flow with iodo[^{14}C]antipyrine. *Am J Physiol* 1978; 234:H59–H66.
12. Yonas H, Darby JM, Marks EC, et al. CBF measured by Xe-CT: approach to analysis and normal values. *J Cereb Blood Flow Metab* 1991; 11:716–725.
13. Young W: H_2 clearance measurement of blood flow: a review of technique and polarographic principles. *Stroke* 1980; 11:552–564.

196

Normal Cerebral Energy Metabolism

Robert A. Ratcheson
Warren R. Selman
W. David Lust

The brain is a fastidious organ, requiring a continuous supply of nutrients to feed its tens of billions of cells. It performs many activities, from processing and storing information to controlling vital functions in the organism. Maintaining the structure and function of this complex tissue requires a disproportionately large amount of energy as compared to other organs. This is clear from the fact that the brain constitutes about 2 percent of total body mass but accounts for about 20 percent of the total basal O_2 consumption and receives approximately 15 percent of the resting cardiac output.

This chapter gives an overview of cerebral energy metabolism and its tight coupling to the maintenance of the brain's function and structure. The brain derives its energy from the oxidation of glucose (Fig. 196-1). The equation for the oxidative catabolism of glucose is

$$C_6H_{12}O_6 + 6\,O_2 \longrightarrow \text{energy} + 6\,CO_2 + 6\,H_2O$$

The oxidation of glucose can be considered in three stages: glycolysis, the tricarboxylic acid (TCA) cycle, and electron transport coupled with oxidative phosphorylation. Each glucose molecule is reduced to two molecules of pyruvate through the glycolytic pathway, with a yield of two molecules each of adenosine triphosphate (ATP) and NADH. Pyruvate is oxidized by pyruvate dehydrogenase to yield acetyl-CoA, which enters the TCA cycle. The oxidation of acetyl-CoA produces both reduced pyridine nucleotides (NADH) and reduced flavin mononucleotides ($FADH_2$). The NADH and $FADH_2$ serve as substrates for the respiratory chain, and the proton gradient generated across the inner mitochondrial membrane drives the phosphorylation of adenosine diphosphate (ADP) (oxidative phosphorylation). Each NADH contains enough usable energy to phosphorylate three ADPs, whereas each $FADH_2$ produces only two ATP molecules. Through these three pathways, 36 ATPs are produced from each glucose moiety, with most of the energy production occurring during electron transport and oxidative phosphorylation. Subsequent sections will describe the specific pathways in the oxidation of glucose.

The standard free energy yield (ΔG) for the oxidation of glucose to carbon dioxide and water at 25°C and pH 7 is approximately −686 kcal/mole (note the negative standard free energy, which favors the forward reaction). Given that the brain cannot use thermal or mechanical energy, chemical energy is produced in the form of ATP. The energy for most of the active processes in the brain comes from the hydrolysis of ATP in coupled reactions, where either the adenylate or phosphate moiety is first covalently bound to an enzyme or a substrate molecule and then one of the moieties is released in the form of either free ADP or P_i. The free-energy change in the brain from the hydrolysis of ATP has been estimated to be −7.46 kcal/mole, as determined by the following equation:

$$\Delta G = \Delta G^{\circ\prime} + RT \ln\,[\mathrm{ADP}][\mathrm{P_i}]/[\mathrm{ATP}]$$

where ΔG is the free-energy change, $\Delta G^{\circ\prime}$ is the standard free-energy change, R is the gas constant, T is temperature in degrees Kelvin, [ADP] is the concentration of adenosine diphosphate, [ATP] is the concentration of adenosine triphosphate, and [P_i] is the concentration of inorganic phosphate in the brain. The actual free-energy change may be as much as −14.1 kcal/mole based on the observation that free ADP in the cytosol is actually about 5 percent of the total tissue concentration (i.e., 30 μmol/g).[76,77] The higher free-energy change would increase the efficiency of energy conservation in the brain, which has been estimated to be approximately 20 percent.[72] ATP can be hydrolyzed to other products, such as adenosine monophosphate (AMP) and inorganic pyrophosphate, but these energy-yielding reactions are less common in the cell. Thus, the oxidation of glucose provides cellular energy in the form of ATP, which upon hydrolysis serves most of the active processes in the brain. For the interested reader, a more extensive description of the various aspects of cerebral energy metabolism can be found in books and review articles by Erecinska and Silver,[16] Lehninger et al.,[38] Siegal et al.,[62] and Siesjo.[63]

Relationship of Cerebral Energy Metabolism to Cerebral Blood Flow

The endogenous reserves of glucose, oxygen, and high-energy phosphates in the brain are minimal.[41,47] The only storage form of high-energy phosphate besides ATP is phosphocreatine, which, given the high metabolic rate of the brain, would be rapidly depleted if the supply of glucose or oxygen were cut off. There is no storage form for oxygen in the brain, and the concentration of glycogen, a storage form of glucose, is relatively low.[41] Table 196-1 shows the energy reserves of the brain as determined experimentally. The high-energy phosphate equivalents (HEPEs) for each of the reserves in an ischemic brain can be estimated from the following equation, derived by Lowry and colleagues[40,41]:

$$\text{HEPE} = \text{phosphocreatine} + 2\ \text{ATP} + \text{ADP} + 2\ \text{glucose} + 2.9\ \text{glycogen}$$

If the total reserves are equal to 27.7 μmol/g of brain and the HEPE utilization rate in normal brain is between 20 and 25 μmol/g per minute, then the energy available for active processes would be lost in less than 2 min after the onset of ischemia. Clearly, the margin of safety in the brain is scant when blood flow fails. The susceptibility of the human brain to nutrient deprivation has been confirmed experimentally in volunteers by Rossen and coworkers. They demonstrated that a complete loss of blood flow to the brain produced by inflation of a pneumatic cuff around the neck caused a loss of consciousness within 10 s.[58]

While total ischemia represents the extreme in nutrient deprivation for the brain, other conditions where nutrients become limiting also cause marked changes in brain function. Siesjö and

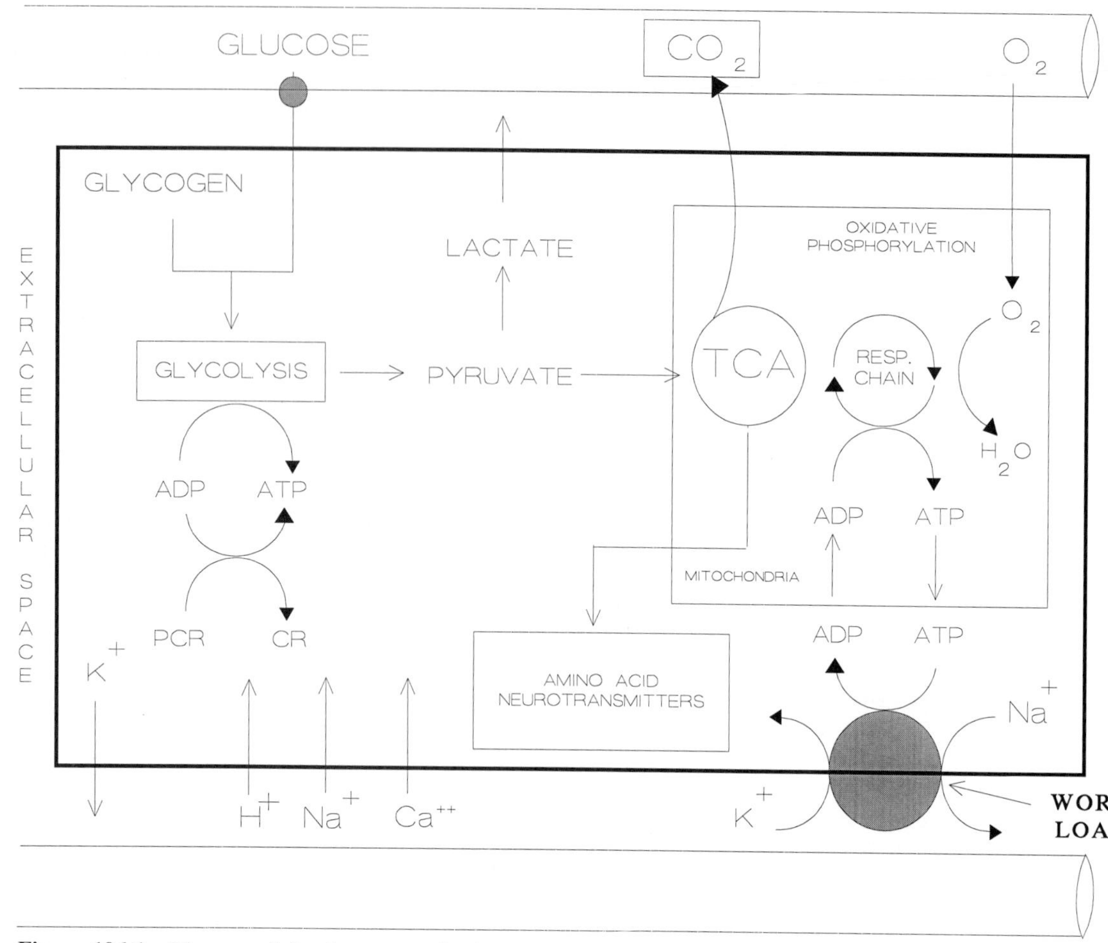

Figure 196-1 Diagram of the three stages in the oxidation of glucose to CO_2 and H_2O in the brain. The pathways in the oxidative metabolism of glucose are glycolysis (cytosolic), the TCA cycle, and electron transport with oxidative phosphorylation, the last two pathways both being in the mitochondria. Glucose from the vessels enters the brain through a glucose transporter and is metabolized to pyruvate by glycolysis. Pyruvate is metabolized to acetyl-CoA, which is then oxidized by the TCA cycle, yielding reduced pyridine nucleotides. The NADH serves as a substrate for the respiratory chain and, through a series of membrane-bound oxidoreductases, a proton gradient is generated. Passage of the protons down their electrochemical gradient provides energy for the phosphorylation of ADP. The energy produced in the form of ATP, whether by glycolysis or oxidative phosphorylation, is used for both biosynthetic and osmotic work, the latter predominantly by Na^+/K^+-ATPase to maintain the electrochemical gradients. There is some emerging evidence that the Na^+/K^+-pump may be coupled to the production of cytosolic ATP.[2]

coworkers have demonstrated that a number of physiologic processes are affected by increasing degrees of hypoxia.[70] Decreasing the percent of O_2 in inspired air from 20 percent to 17 percent causes a delay in dark adaption, and a decrease to 13 percent has an effect on short-term memory. At 8 percent O_2, consciousness is lost, even though cerebral blood flow (CBF) has increased by 70 percent to compensate for the low oxygen tension. Hypoglycemia also affects neuronal function by altering cerebral metabolism.[57] A 50 percent reduction in blood glucose can cause lethargy and coma, and further reductions can cause convulsions and death.[33]

Thus, there is an interdependency of CBF, metabolism, and function in the CNS. This relationship is of prime importance to the neurosurgeon, who routinely deals with conditions or procedures that compromise cerebral blood flow. Just how much the CBF can be manipulated before causing brain damage can be estimated by comparing the metabolic rate of the brain to the amounts of nutrients delivered by the blood. Sokoloff has reported that the CBF of the human brain is approximately 57 ml/100 g per minute and that the rates of oxygen and glucose consumption are 156 and 31 μmol/100 g per minute, respectively.[71] Knowing that the normal arterial oxygen pressure is approximately 100 mmHg and the normal arterial glucose level is about 4.4 m*M*, it is possible to estimate the quantity of nutrients removed from the blood under conditions of normal flow. In arterial blood, the availability of glucose is approximately 250 μmol/100 g per minute, and the brain consumes only about 12 percent of this amount. This fact suggests that glucose would be ample even with a marked reduction of CBF. It should be noted that 25 percent of the glucose is initially extracted from the blood, but half of that amount is returned to the blood, suggesting that the flux of glucose across the blood-brain barrier (BBB) is bidirectional (see below). Assuming that both hemoglobin and plasma are saturated at a value of

TABLE 196-1 Concentrations of Metabolites in the Rat Brain and the Amount of High-Energy Phosphate Equivalents Produced from Each Metabolite in the Absence of Blood Flow to the Brain

Metabolites	Cortical Concentrations (μmol/g wet weight)	High-Energy Phosphate Equivalents (μmol/g)
Phosphocreatine	4.50[a]	4.50
ATP	2.92[a]	5.84
ADP	0.29[a]	0.29
Glucose	4.53[a]	9.06
Glycogen	2.76[b]	8.00
		TOTAL = 27.7

Source: Average values for the various metabolites in rodent brains were taken from (*a*) Ponten et al.,[55] and (*b*) Veech.[76] The high-energy phosphate equivalents were calculated from the equation shown in the text (Lowry et al.[40,41]).

100 mmHg for arterial oxygen, the total available oxygen in arterial blood is approximately 430 μmol/100 g per minute, and approximately 36 percent of this amount is consumed by brain metabolism. From the amounts of oxygen and glucose extracted from the blood in a single pass through the brain, it would seem logical that CBF could be reduced by more than 50 percent and still provide the brain with enough substrates for normal metabolism. It has been shown experimentally that neuronal function remains essentially intact until the CBF is reduced to 15 to 18 ml/100 g per minute, or about 25 percent of control blood flow.[8,25] In complete ischemia, however, the residual blood oxygen and glucose would be exhausted within seconds, since blood volume is only about 4 percent of the weight of the brain. Oxidative metabolism of glucose would cease immediately in the absence of oxygen, and the endogenous glucosyl units (from endogenous glucose and glycogen catabolism) would be consumed through anaerobic glycolysis. Under these conditions the critical factors to be considered by a neurosurgeon are the duration of the insult, how long the brain will survive in the absence of nutrients before the onset of irreversible brain damage, and what measures can be taken to reduce the energy demands of the brain during a period of compromised blood flow.

Brain Work

What processes in the brain account for its inordinate energy consumption? While the rate of energy use in muscle (i.e., thermodynamic work) can be readily measured in terms of mechanical work and loss of heat, this measurement is not easy to make in the brain. Nevertheless, it is important to comprehend what "brain work" amounts to, and to do this we must look at the energy-requiring processes of the brain.

For the sake of simplicity, brain work has been arbitrarily divided into two categories: biosynthetic work and osmotic work.[48] Most of the biosynthetic work in the brain consists of the production of polysaccharides, lipids, proteins, and nucleic acids, and the processes are generally similar to those in other tissues. There are some processes that are largely unique to the brain, however, such as the synthesis, release, and uptake of neurotransmitters; axonal transport; certain protein phosphorylation reactions; and the active transport of certain nonelectrolytes across membranes.

Osmotic work is related to the specialized function of the brain and is involved in the reception, transmission, and storage of information by neurons. The normal functioning of neurons is supported by two other populations of cells, the glia and the endothelium, which optimize the external milieu for neuronal activity. Ion transport in all cells of the CNS, as well as axonal transport, accounts energetically for most of the specialized osmotic work of the brain (Fig. 196-2). Passive movement of ions across membranes can occur by two processes (1) a slow leakage of the ions across the membrane, which is exacerbated by the large surface-to-volume ratio of the cells and their processes in the brain, and (2) an active receptor-mediated flux through ion-specific channels. For example, calcium enters the cell through voltage-dependent channels following glutamate activation of the *N*-methyl-D-aspartate (NMDA) receptor. It has been estimated that biosynthetic requirements may be responsible for as much as half of the normal resting brain energy production, leaving the remaining energy for osmotic work.[3,44]

A major portion of the energy produced by the brain is used to counter passive ion movements, thereby maintaining ionic gradients and the electrical potential difference across the neuronal membrane.[80] When an action potential is generated in a neuron, there is a net efflux of potassium ions and a net influx of sodium ions. Since the ability of the neuron to generate action potentials depends on the maintenance of ionic disequilibrium across the neuronal membrane, the electrochemical gradients must be reestablished as action potentials dissipate them. The concentration of ions in neurons is continuously restored by a membrane-bound sodium/potassium-dependent ATPase, which couples the hydrolysis of one molecule of ATP with the extrusion of three Na^+ ions and the uptake of two K^+ ions across the neuronal membrane (site 1 in Fig. 196-2). While it is difficult to assess directly the total amount of energy consumed by the Na^+/K^+-ATPase in the brain, Astrup and coworkers have shown that ouabain, an inhibitor of the Na^+/K^+-ATPase, reduces brain metabolism by 20 to 25 percent, indicating that one-fourth of the brain's energy is used for the transport of sodium and potassium.[3] The other ion distributions that are altered during neuronal activity, especially those of calcium and hydrogen ions, also ultimately depend on metabolism, either directly through ATP-powered pumps or indirectly through the energy derived from the sodium gradient (sites 2 through 4 in Fig. 196-2). This list of active transport processes is incomplete, since there is often great redundancy in the homeostasis of these important cations. For example, the intracellular calcium concentration is kept low not only by the calcium pump and Na^+/Ca^{2+} cotransporter on the plasma membrane but also by active transport into mitochondria and the endoplasmic reticulum and by binding to proteins such as calmodulin.[69] The consumption of energy for these other energy-dependent cation transporters has been estimated to be minor compared to that for Na^+/K^+-ATPase.[16] Nevertheless, excess accumulation of intracellular calcium or prolonged acidification can be as devastating to function as disruption in the sodium and potassium gradients. Thus, there is a close coupling of neuronal activity, neuronal energy metabolism, and glucose use. An uncorrected disruption of the electrochemical gradients will at first cause loss of function and eventually cause the cell to swell and burst owing to the influx of sodium, chloride, and osmotic water. Therefore, the brain must have powerful homeostatic mechanisms to restore and maintain ion gradients. In terms of total brain work, this component of energy consumption is continual, and generally any change in activity causes a proportional change in the metabolic rate. Even when the activity of the brain is reduced, its energy demands remain high. For instance, during sleep the rate of energy use by the brain decreases by only about 25 percent.[32]

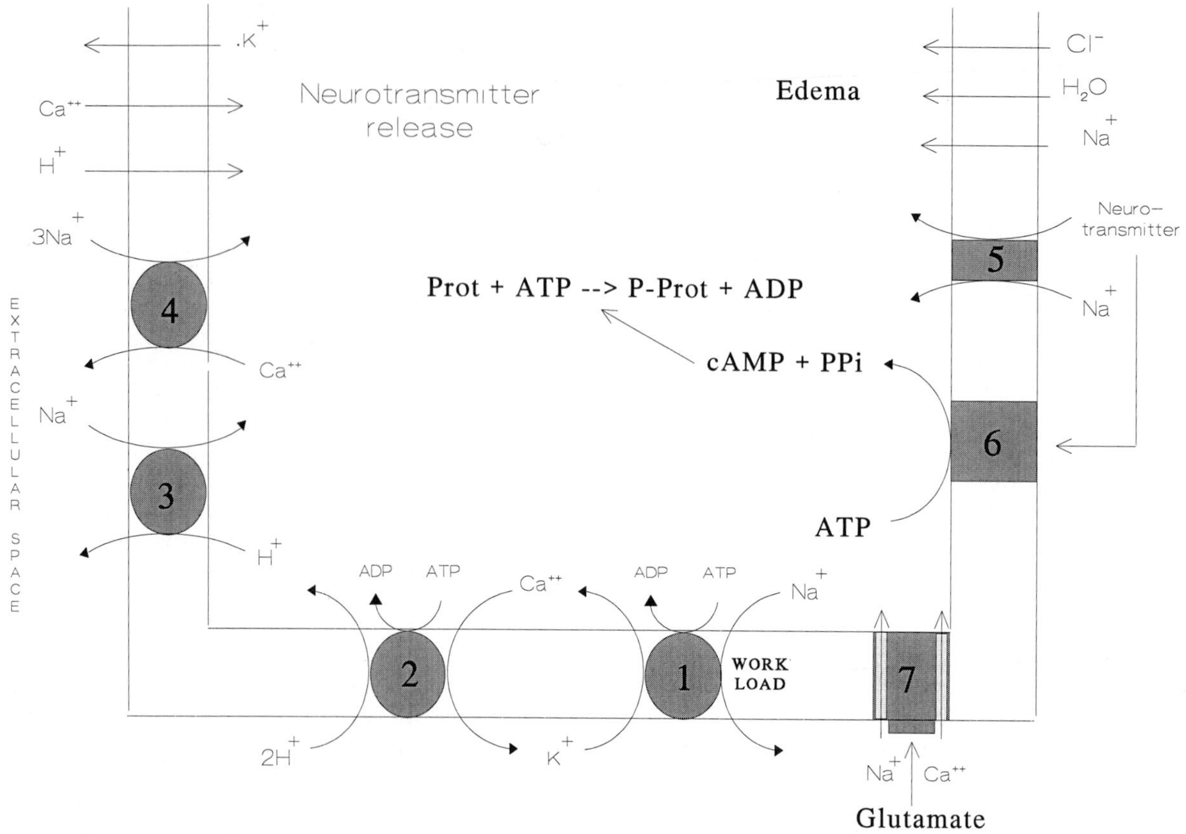

Figure 196-2 Diagram of the various homeostatic processes of the brain. There are both passive and active fluxes of cations within the CNS, and if the compartmentation of the ions is not maintained, CNS function will cease. The numbers indicate the following active homeostatic processes in the brain: (1) ATP-dependent Na^+/K^+ pump; (2) ATP-dependent calcium pump; (3) Na^+/H^+ cotransporter; and (4) Na^+/Ca^{2+} cotransporter. The other numbers indicate representative energy dependent processes in the brain: (5) sodium-dependent neurotransmitter uptake system; (6) adenylate cyclase; and (7) NMDA receptor, which when activated opens gated ion channels. Sodium and potassium gradients are maintained primarily by the Na^+/K^+-ATPase transport system. Regulation of intracellular acid-base balance is, in part, controlled by the Na^+/H^+ cotransporter (3), while the low levels of intracellular calcium are regulated by Na^+/Ca^{2+} cotransporter (4) and the ATP-dependent Ca^{2+} transporter (2). Passive fluxes of cations and chloride are shown at the top of the diagram, and a representative of receptor-mediated influx of cations is shown at the bottom (7). Inactivation of certain neurotransmitters is indicated by (5), where the uptake of the neurotransmitter is driven by the sodium gradient. Energy is also consumed by activation of certain receptors (6), where ATP is used for both the synthesis of cyclic AMP and for the phosphorylation of proteins by the various protein kinases in the brain.

Unlike most tissues, the brain consumes primarily glucose, even though other metabolic substrates can produce energy in the brain. The brain is also more isolated from the circulation than most other tissues, owing to the BBB. These unique aspects of the brain and their importance to energy metabolism will be considered in the following sections.

Substrates for Energy Metabolism

Although in vitro brain preparations can be supported by a number of metabolic substrates, the major substrate of the living brain is glucose. Under normal physiologic conditions the only substrates in the adult brain to exhibit a positive steady-state arteriovenous difference, indicating net uptake and use, are glucose and oxygen.[71] The total daily consumption of oxygen and glucose in an adult brain is 74 liters and 115 g, respectively, which corresponds to a daily energy requirement in the range of 250 kcal for a 1500-g brain. A number of factors, including age, gender, and dementia have been shown by positron emission tomography to affect these nutrient requirements.[13,19,35,83]

Too great a fall in blood glucose causes confusion and even coma.[33] Attempts to reverse these symptoms by administering other substrates have been unsuccessful; only glucose will work. Additional evidence for the primacy of glucose in the brain is provided by the brain's respiratory quotient (that is, the ratio of the rates at which O_2 is consumed and CO_2 produced), which is close to 1.0, indicating that energy is produced almost solely through the oxidation of glucose.

Under normal physiologic conditions, the arteriovenous differences for the ketone bodies produced from fatty acid catabolism (e.g., 3-hydroxybutyrate and acetoacetate) are minimal, even though D-β-hydroxybutyrate dehydrogenase, β-ketoacyl-CoA transferase, and thiolase—the enzymes for converting ketone bodies to acetyl-CoA—are present in the brain. However, Owen et al. showed that when the supply of glucose to the brain was limited, oxidation of ketone bodies could provide up to 50 percent of the total cerebral energy supply.[50] Ketone bodies alone, however, cannot maintain or restore normal cerebral function in the absence of glucose, suggesting an obligatory need for glucose, which is most likely related to a need for glycolysis. Since ketone bodies can be metabolized in brain tissue in vivo when glucose availability is limited, the relatively low consumption of this alternative substrate in the CNS has been attributed to the limited supply of ketone bodies in blood. If blood glucose is limiting or ketone body levels increase, as is the case during starvation or diabetes, then conditions are more favorable for them to pass the BBB and be metabolized.[24]

While ketone body metabolism may serve as a survival mechanism in adults, significant use of ketone bodies by the brain is normal in human fetuses,[1] infants,[60] and children.[54] Neonates tend to be hypoglycemic and to become ketotic owing to the high fat content of human milk. Ketosis and ketone body metabolism decrease when the infant is weaned onto a carbohydrate diet.

Several reports have also indicated that lactate is an important neonatal brain substrate.[26,39,43] Studies on the brains of neonatal dogs and rats have shown that radioactive lactate has a positive arteriovenous difference and is taken up and converted to CO_2 in the presence of negligible gluconeogenesis. The latter finding suggests that the lactate is oxidized through the tricarboxylic acid cycle to produce ATP. Furthermore, these studies indicated that lactate may be the primary metabolic fuel for the brain in the early neonatal period. Medina found that newborn rats respired as much as 65 percent of their endogenous lactate stores in the first 2 h of life.[43]

Parenthetically, many of the alternative substrates that have been shown to support energy metabolism in the brain in vitro (for example, glutamate[85]) probably cannot be used as effectively in vivo because they do not cross the BBB well or because the concentrations never reach levels sufficient to fuel the metabolic pathways.

Transport of Substrates from Blood to Brain

The capillary endothelial cells of the blood-brain barrier mediate substrate delivery to the brain. Since glucose, lactate, and ketone bodies are not gaseous or lipid-soluble, a transport mechanism to carry them across the BBB is required. Specific transport systems have been identified for glucose, amino acids, monocarboxylic acids, and other nutrients. Many transporters operate by means of facilitated diffusion and therefore are saturable, stereospecific, and subject to inhibition by competitive agents.[52]

The issue of how the brain is supplied with glucose obviously is important. Experimentally, it has been shown that the passage of small organic molecules into the brain is slow and that the BBB prevents the passage of certain small molecules, like glutamate, which could adversely affect function. Glucose does cross the BBB at a low rate by simple diffusion, but this means of entry is probably inadequate to meet the glucose demands of the brain. The pioneering work of Crone in 1965 described a facilitated transfer of glucose into the brain by a process which, together with simple diffusion, ensured that the glucose supply of the brain would be adequate despite fluctuations in blood glucose level.[12] The presence of facilitated diffusion was indicated by the fact that the fraction of glucose extracted from blood decreases with increasing blood glucose levels and that the extraction of fructose is always less than that of glucose.

Many advances have been made in understanding the glucose transporter in the brain, and for the most part they support the conclusions that the BBB carries out facilitated diffusion of glucose and that the site of glucose transport is at the level of the capillaries (for review, see Pelligrino et al.[53]) The glucose transporter has been shown to be nonconcentrative, saturable, subject to competition by other hexoses and to inhibition by phloretin, phlorizin, and cytochalasin B, and apparently independent of sodium and insulin. Of the five known glucose transporters, only GLUT1 (glucose transporter 1) and GLUT3 are found in the brain. The GLUT1 transporter is found on both the luminal and abluminal sides of endothelial cells. This observation agrees with the finding that there is exchange diffusion of glucose in the brain, such that a portion of the extracted glucose is not metabolized but is returned to the blood. A number of pathophysiologic conditions, such as hypoglycemia, hyperglycemia, hypometabolism, hypermetabolism, and Alzheimer's disease, apparently affect the density and/or affinity of the glucose transporter on the endothelium.[14,22,30] The mechanism by which the density of the glucose transporter is altered remains to be determined.

During early postnatal life, the BBB is not fully functional, and substrate delivery can occur by simple diffusion.[56] Studies of the kinetics of carrier-mediated transport across the BBB in young suckling rats[10] indicate that the rate of transport of ketone bodies and lactate is, respectively, 3 and 10 times higher than in adult rats. Transport of glucose, on the other hand, is twofold higher in adult than in suckling rats. Changes in the transport mechanisms for the various substrates during growth explain in part why glucose becomes the substrate of preference in the adult brain.[11]

Energy Production

As was indicated previously, the coupled hydrolysis of ATP is the principal source of energy in brain cells, and its production depends on the metabolism of glucose. The overall equation for the production of ATP through the oxidation of glucose is

$$C_6H_{12}O_6 + 6\,O_2 + 36\,\text{ADP} + 36\,P_i \longrightarrow 6\,CO_2 + 42\,H_2O + 36\,\text{ATP}$$

Inherent in this equation and critical to the formation of ATP is the transfer of electrons from glucose to intermediates through redox reactions. The final acceptor of the electrons in this system is oxygen, which has a high affinity for electrons. The process uses electron carriers that can be readily oxidized and reduced by certain intermediates in the metabolism of glucose. Nicotine adenine dinucleotide (NAD^+) and flavin adenine dinucleotide (FAD) are two such electron carriers that are critical to the oxidation of glucose. The reduced forms of these carriers (NADH and $FADH_2$) are generated by a number of dehydrogenases found both in the mitochondria and cytosol. For instance,

$$NAD^+ + 2\,e^- + 2\,H^+ \longrightarrow NADH + H^+$$

where e^- is the electron and H^+ is the hydrogen ion donated by the reduced substrate of the dehydrogenase reaction. The NAD^+

diffuses passively to the cytochrome chain in the inner mitochondrial membrane, and in the oxidized form to the various dehydrogenases of the mitochondrial matrix. In the following sections, the three stages in the oxidation of glucose will be examined in greater detail, showing how the redox reactions lead to the production of usable energy in the form of ATP.

Metabolic Pathways

Aerobic Glycolysis

Glycolysis is the main metabolic pathway for glucose and consists of 10 enzymic reactions that occur in the cytosol. Glycolysis converts one molecule of glucose into two molecules of pyruvate with the production of two ATP and two NADH molecules from their precursors ADP and NAD^+, respectively. Under aerobic conditions, the end-product of glycolysis, pyruvate, is transported into the mitochondrial matrix, where it is decarboxylated to form acetyl-CoA.

There are a number of sites in glycolysis at which the flux through the pathway is controlled by either allosteric interactions or substrate concentration (for a review, see Beitner[5]). The major regulatory site for entry of glucose into the glycolytic pathway is phosphofructokinase-1 (PFK-1), an enzyme that catalyzes the addition of a phosphate group to fructose-6-phosphate in the third step of glycolysis. PFK activity is pH-dependent, decreasing as pH falls.[74] PFK is also allosterically regulated by ATP and Mg^{2+}, which decrease its affinity for substrate. Conversely, allosteric regulation by 5′-AMP, ADP, cyclic AMP, P_i, K^+, NH_4^+, ribose-1,5-diphosphate, and fructose-2,6-bisphosphate increase its affinity for substrate in the brain.[40,49,51] Therefore, when the energy supply is low, the flux through glycolysis increases until ATP levels are returned to normal. The other two enzymes thought to regulate glycolytic rate are hexokinase and pyruvate kinase. Hexokinase, the first enzyme of the pathway, effectively traps glucose in cells by phosphorylating it to glucose-6-phosphate. Hexokinase may be either bound to mitochondria or free in the cytosol, and the activity of bound hexokinase is higher than that of the cytosolic (unbound) enzyme.[36,37,75,78] Recent evidence also suggests that bound hexokinase is more responsive to mitochondrial adenylates than is cytosolic hexokinase.[6] Pyruvate kinase, the final enzyme in the pathway, regulates the exit of glucose-derived compounds from glycolysis.[23,40] Experimental evidence indicates that these key enzymes can be regulated by hormones as well as by acute allosteric regulators.[34]

Anaerobic Glycolysis

Under normal circumstances, the end-product of glycolysis, pyruvate, is further oxidized in the TCA cycle. However, when oxygen becomes rate-limiting, as during ischemia or hypoxia, certain glycolytic adaptations occur. One major change is the reversal of the Pasteur effect. The Pasteur effect normally inhibits glucose consumption and production of lactate by approximately 90 percent in the presence of oxygen, and it is apparently mediated by an alteration in PFK activity. During hypoxia or anoxia, ADP increases and ATP decreases owing to the inability of the mitochondria to rephosphorylate ADP. Two mitochondrial intermediates, citrate and isocitrate, also decrease in concentration. Since both ATP and citrate are inhibitors of PFK, their reduction tends to disinhibit PFK. At the same time, the elevation of ADP stimulates PFK, so the result is an increase in the glycolytic flux. A high rate of glycolysis in the absence of oxygen could in theory maintain the energy status of the tissue, although at low efficiency. However, there is another problem, involving the glycolytic enzyme glyceraldehyde phosphate dehydrogenase (GPDH), which catalyzes the following reaction:

$$\text{D-3-phosphoglyceraldehyde} + NAD^+ + P_i \xrightleftharpoons{\text{GPDH}} \text{D-3-phosphoglyceroyl phosphate} + NADH + H^+$$

The activity of this enzyme clearly depends on the availability of cytosolic NAD^+. Under aerobic conditions, the NADH produced by the reaction is efficiently reoxidized to NAD^+ by the mitochondrial respiratory chain, and the supply of NAD^+ is not limiting. In the absence of oxygen, the available NAD^+ is rapidly consumed, which effectively would turn off glycolysis. However, NADH is reoxidized to NAD^+ in the absence of oxygen by the lactate dehydrogenase (LDH) reaction:

$$\text{Pyruvate} + NADH + H^+ \xrightleftharpoons{\text{LDH}} \text{lactate} + NAD^+$$

Anaerobic glycolysis allows the production of some ATP during periods of hypoxia or anoxia.

Anaerobic glycolysis alone, however, will not maintain the metabolic viability of the brain over a sustained period, since the brain's energy demands are so high and the production of ATP by glycolysis so low. In addition, the accumulation of lactate causes tissue acidification, which impairs CNS function and can contribute to the evolution of brain damage.[27]

Tricarboxylic Acid Cycle

The two-carbon fragment acetyl-CoA is converted to CO_2 in a series of nine reactions within the mitochondrial matrix called the tricarboxylic acid cycle or Krebs cycle (Fig. 196-3). Acetyl-CoA is produced by the catabolism of proteins and lipids as well as of carbohydrates. Unlike the glycolytic pathway, the TCA cycle is cyclical, with one of the substrates for the first reaction (oxaloacetic acid) also being the product of the cycle. Before pyruvate can enter the TCA cycle, it must be oxidized to acetyl-CoA. This step is catalyzed by the enzyme complex pyruvate dehydrogenase (PDH). The reaction involves three enzymes, pyruvate dehydrogenase, lipoate acetyltransferase, and lipoamide dehydrogenase, and requires the coenzymes thiamine pyrophosphate, lipoic acid, CoA, and flavin. The overall reaction for pyruvate dehydrogenase is

$$\text{Pyruvate} + \text{CoA} + NAD^+ \xrightarrow{\text{PDH}} \text{acetyl-CoA} + CO_2 + NADH + H^+$$

The phosphorylated form of PDH is inactive, and the dephosphorylated form is active. In addition, NADH, ATP, and acetyl-CoA are allosteric inhibitors of the PDH reaction. Because the enzyme is highly regulated, it is thought to be a major determinant of TCA cycle activity.

The initial step in the TCA cycle is the condensation of oxaloacetate with acetyl CoA to form citrate, which is catalyzed by citrate synthase. The dehydration of citrate, catalyzed by aconitase, produces *cis*-aconitate, which is then hydrated to isocitrate. Isocitrate dehydrogenase converts isocitrate to α-ketoglutarate, producing one molecule each of NADH and CO_2. The enzyme α-ketoglutarate dehydrogenase converts α-ketoglutarate to succinyl-CoA, NADH, and CO_2, and succinyl-CoA synthase in the presence of guanosine diphosphate converts the succinyl-CoA to succinate and guanosine triphosphate. In the lone reaction using FAD in the TCA cycle, succinate is converted by succinate dehydrogenase to fumarate, which in turn is hydrated by fumarase to yield malate. Malate dehydrogenase dehydrates malate to oxaloacetate, yielding another molecule of NADH. Therefore, each turn of the TCA cycle processes one acetyl-CoA molecule and produces two molecules of CO_2, three molecules of NADH, and one molecule of $FADH_2$. There is no net gain or loss of carbon fragments in the TCA cycle, since the two carbon fragments contributed by each acetyl-CoA are lost in the two molecules of CO_2 produced.

Although the TCA cycle is the major catabolic pathway in the production of ATP, it is also central to a number of anabolic processes, providing biosynthetic precursors for protein and lipid synthesis. TCA cycle intermediates drawn off for anabolism are replaced by a series of anaplerotic reactions, being replenished ultimately through either pyruvate carboxylase or transaminase reactions.

Electron Transport

The respiratory chain and oxidative phosphorylation are the processes in which the electrons carried by NADH and $FADH_2$ are transferred to O_2 (producing H_2O), and the resulting release of energy is used to power the synthesis of ATP. The flow of electrons down the electron transport chain takes place in the inner mitochondrial membrane and drives the formation of a proton electrochemical gradient across the inner membrane, which in turn powers the synthesis of ATP. At three electron transfer points along the respiratory chain, there is a sufficient drop in energy to drive the transport of hydrogen ions from the mitochondrial matrix to the intermembrane space. The flow of protons from the intermembrane space back into the matrix is coupled to ATP production by the membrane-bound enzyme ATP synthase (Fig. 196-3).

The overall equation for respiration shown above indicates that one molecule of glucose produces 36 equivalents of ATP under normal oxidative conditions. Production of ATP by the citric acid cycle, respiratory chain, and oxidative phosphorylation requires a constant source of oxygen to regenerate NAD^+ and FAD and to provide an acceptor for the continuous flow of electrons. Under conditions of high energy demand or anoxia, the brain reverts to anaerobic glycolysis for ATP production, which is far less efficient

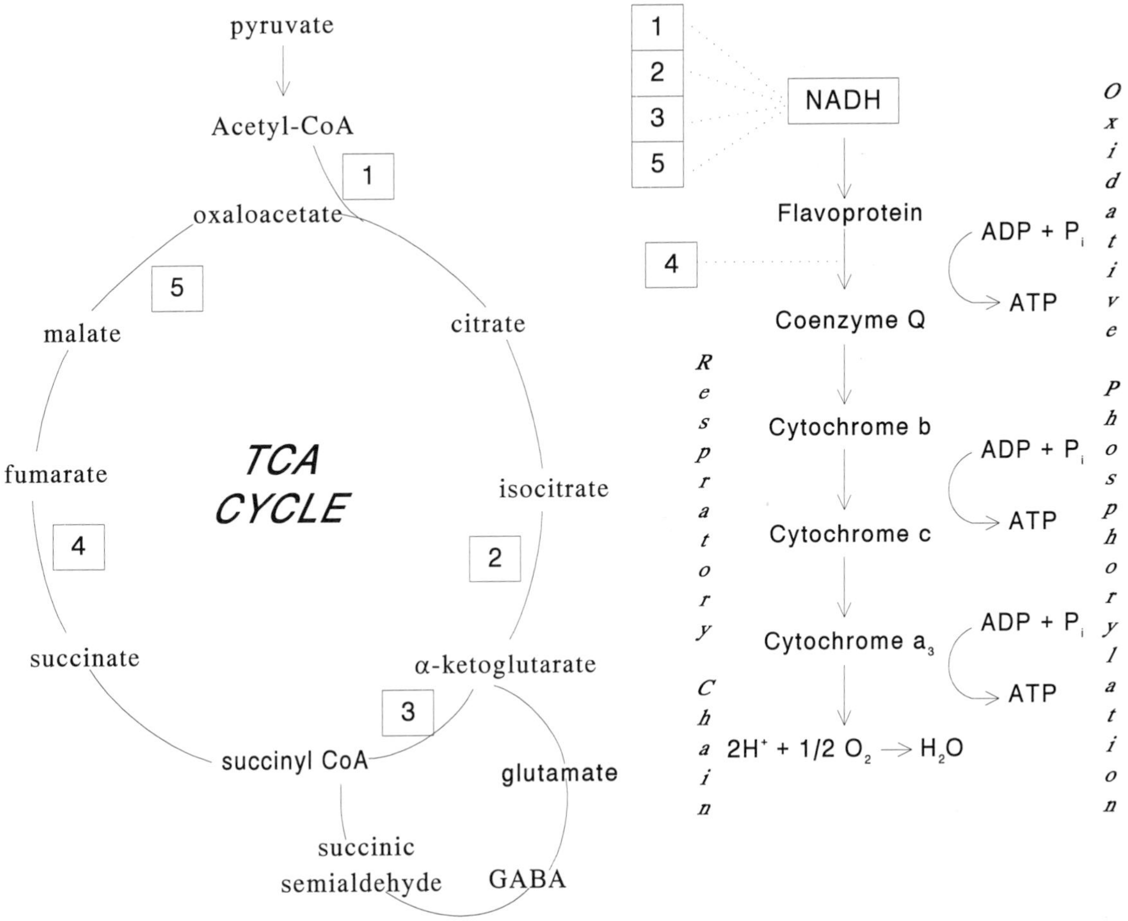

Figure 196-3 Diagram of the tricarboxylic acid cycle, respiratory chain, and oxidative phosphorylation. Oxidation of acetyl-CoA yields four molecules of NADH (at sites 1, 2, 3, and 5) and one molecule of $FADH_2$ (left side of schema), and the reduced pyridine nucleotides serve as substrates for the respiratory chain (right side of schema). As the electrons from NADH are passed along the respiratory chain, the energy created by the proton gradient serves to phosphorylate ADP at three different sites.

than oxidative metabolism and supplies only two ATP molecules per glucosyl unit.

Peripheral Metabolic Pathways in Glucose Oxidation

Glycogen is a macromolecule composed of glucosyl units and is the major storage form of glucose in the CNS. The level of glycogen is highly regulated through its biosynthetic and degradative enzymes, glycogen synthase and glycogen phosphorylase.[21] The degradation of glycogen is tightly regulated by a cascade of enzymes, including adenylate cyclase, cyclic AMP-dependent protein kinase, phosphorylase kinase *b* (active and inactive), phosphorylase *b*, and phosphorylase *a* (active). A signal for glycogenolysis will be rapidly amplified by this enzyme cascade, resulting in the production of substrates for glycolysis. Normally, only 20 percent of the phosphorylase activity in the brain is in the active form, phosphorylase *a*, indicating that the degradation of glycogen could be increased by almost fivefold.[42] Despite the exquisite control of glycogen levels in the CNS, the importance of this pathway has yet to be determined. Given the relatively low glycogen content of the brain, it seems unlikely that the only role of the glycogen cycle would be to supply glucosyl units.

The pentose pathway converts glucose-6-phosphate through a series of reactions to D-ribose-5-phosphate and two molecules of NADPH. Reducing equivalents in the form of NADPH, in contrast to those in the form of NADH, are used for the synthesis of lipids and steroids and not directly for the production of ATP.

Another important secondary pathway of cerebral metabolism is the gamma-aminobutyric acid (GABA) shunt, which is important primarily because it can supply both inhibitory (GABA) and excitatory (glutamate) neurotransmitters (Fig. 196-3). Glucose oxidation is closely linked to the synthesis of a number of neurotransmitters, and it is possible that perturbations in cerebral energy metabolism could affect function by altering the steady-state levels of neurotransmitters. Glutamate is the most abundant amino acid in the brain, and it can be converted to GABA by a single enzyme, glutamic acid decarboxylase. Glutamate is formed from the TCA intermediate α-ketoglutarate by glutamate dehydrogenase or from glutamine by glutaminase. In addition, glutamic acid can also be formed from α-ketoglutarate by a number of reversible transaminases, such as alanine transaminase (ALAase) and aspartate transaminase (ASPase):

$$\alpha\text{-Ketoglutarate} + \text{asparate} \xrightleftharpoons{\text{ASPase}} \text{glutamate} + \text{oxaloacetate}$$

$$\alpha\text{-Ketoglutarate} + \text{alanine} \xrightleftharpoons{\text{ALAase}} \text{glutamate} + \text{pyruvate}$$

The metabolic consequences of the GABA-glutamate cycle stem from the fact that it bypasses two steps in the citric acid cycle. GABA is synthesized by the decarboxylation of glutamate, and it can be converted to succinate via several enzymatic steps to reenter the citric acid cycle. The second of these reactions is catalyzed by succinic semialdehyde dehydrogenase, which generates NADPH rather than NADP. Although the GABA-shunt version of the TCA cycle yields two fewer ATPs per turn than the full TCA cycle (because it bypasses the substrate-level phosphorylation catalyzed by succinyl CoA synthase, with the production of $FADH_2$), the GABA shunt allows glutamate to act as a substrate in energy metabolism. Cultured astrocytes have been shown to use glutamate as an energy substrate in the presence of glucose.[85]

The glutamate-glutamine cycle plays a prominent role in the regulation of neurotransmitters by astrocytes and neurons. Both neurons and astrocytes participate in the uptake of glutamate, although most glutamate accumulates in astrocytes.[84] The uptake and hydrolysis of glutamate to glutamine by astrocytes terminates transmitter activity at the synapse and results in a compound that can be shuttled safely between astrocytes and neurons. Once in neurons, glutamine can be converted back to glutamate.[86] It has been estimated that as much as 10 percent of the carbon oxidized in the CNS passes through the GABA shunt.[61]

Heterogeneity of Cerebral Metabolism

Having established the major metabolic pathways in the CNS, it is necessary to ask whether the metabolic machinery is distributed evenly throughout the brain and whether some areas of the brain are more active than others. The regional energy metabolism and glucose use in the brain have been shown to be highly heterogeneous. Glucose use in rats can be 1.5-fold to 7-fold higher in gray matter than in white matter.[80] The rate of glucose use has been quantitatively related to the rate and intensity of the stimuli,[81,82] indicating a close relationship between local functional activity and glucose use.

The deoxyglucose method of Sokoloff has allowed the measurement of local energy metabolism in neuronal tissue.[73] It was assumed that metabolic activity would be higher in the neuronal cell body, since that was the traditional location for recording of action potentials. Experimental evidence, however, suggests that energy metabolism is higher in the synaptic region than in the cell body.[29,31,59,73] Kadekaro and coworkers measured the effect of stimulation on the dorsal root ganglion, where the cell bodies are clearly separated from the synapses.[29] While stimulation caused no significant changes in the rate of glucose use in the cell body region of the ganglion, there was a quantitative relationship between stimulation frequency and rate of glucose use in the terminal zones of the pathway. These findings, obtained with the 2-deoxyglucose method, are supported by other studies that found high levels of Na^+/K^+-ATPase[4,20] and cytochrome c oxidase activity[79] and large numbers of mitochondria[46] in the synaptic area. In another study, Borowsky and Collins compared the distributions of lactate dehydrogenase (a glycolytic enzyme) and cytochrome oxidase (a mitochondrial enzyme complex) in the hippocampus and olfactory bulb.[7] They found a negative correlation between the two enzyme distributions, with cytochrome oxidase most abundant in the synaptic regions, which also had the highest capillary density and rate of glucose use. While there seemed to be some overlap in the distributions of these two enzyme activities, the findings provide additional evidence that synaptic activity may require a higher capacity for energy production than that found in the cell bodies.

The lack of a significant increase in glucose metabolism with functional stimulation in the neuronal cell body presents an apparent paradox. Given that the work performed by the Na^+/K^+-ATPase is responsible for a considerable portion of a neuron's energy expenditure, how does the action potential traverse the cell body from the dendrites to the axon without raising glucose use in the cell body? The low level of voltage-dependent sodium channels in the cell body suggests that the transmission of the action potential in this region could be electrotonic. Essentially, the larger diameter of the cell body provides a low resistance to electrical flow and, therefore, voltage transients pass through it quickly and need not be regenerated because they suffer little loss of signal amplitude (signal amplitude representing simply ion redistribution). Thus, the energy cost of maintaining electrochemical gradients in the face of impulse transmission could be greater in cellular processes than in the cell body.[72]

While the coupling mechanisms between function, metabolism, and blood supply are only partially understood,[63,64] certain regulatory sites have been well established. The delivery of glucose and oxygen and the removal of carbon dioxide depend on the tissue blood supply. The use of positron emission tomography, which allows quantitative measurements of regional cerebral glucose utilization, has shown that regional blood flow dynamically reflects regional metabolism in the brain.[17,28] A logical mechanism would be that neuronal activity directly stimulates metabolism, and that increased metabolism directly leads to increased blood flow. However, there is some evidence that primary changes in blood flow result in changes in metabolism by limiting substrate availability independent of neuronal activity. Thus, one can imagine that there is reciprocal regulation of brain blood flow and brain metabolism.

Energy Metabolism and the Neurosurgeon

It should be clear that CNS function is absolutely dependent on a continuous supply of glucose and oxygen from the blood. While inborn errors of metabolism can affect cerebral metabolism,[15] more critical to the neurosurgeon are vascular events that affect the brain's energy metabolism. If the blood supply to the brain is severely perturbed, energy failure will occur within a matter of minutes, and the host of secondary events shown in Fig. 196-4 will be triggered. There is a disruption of the electrochemical gradients,

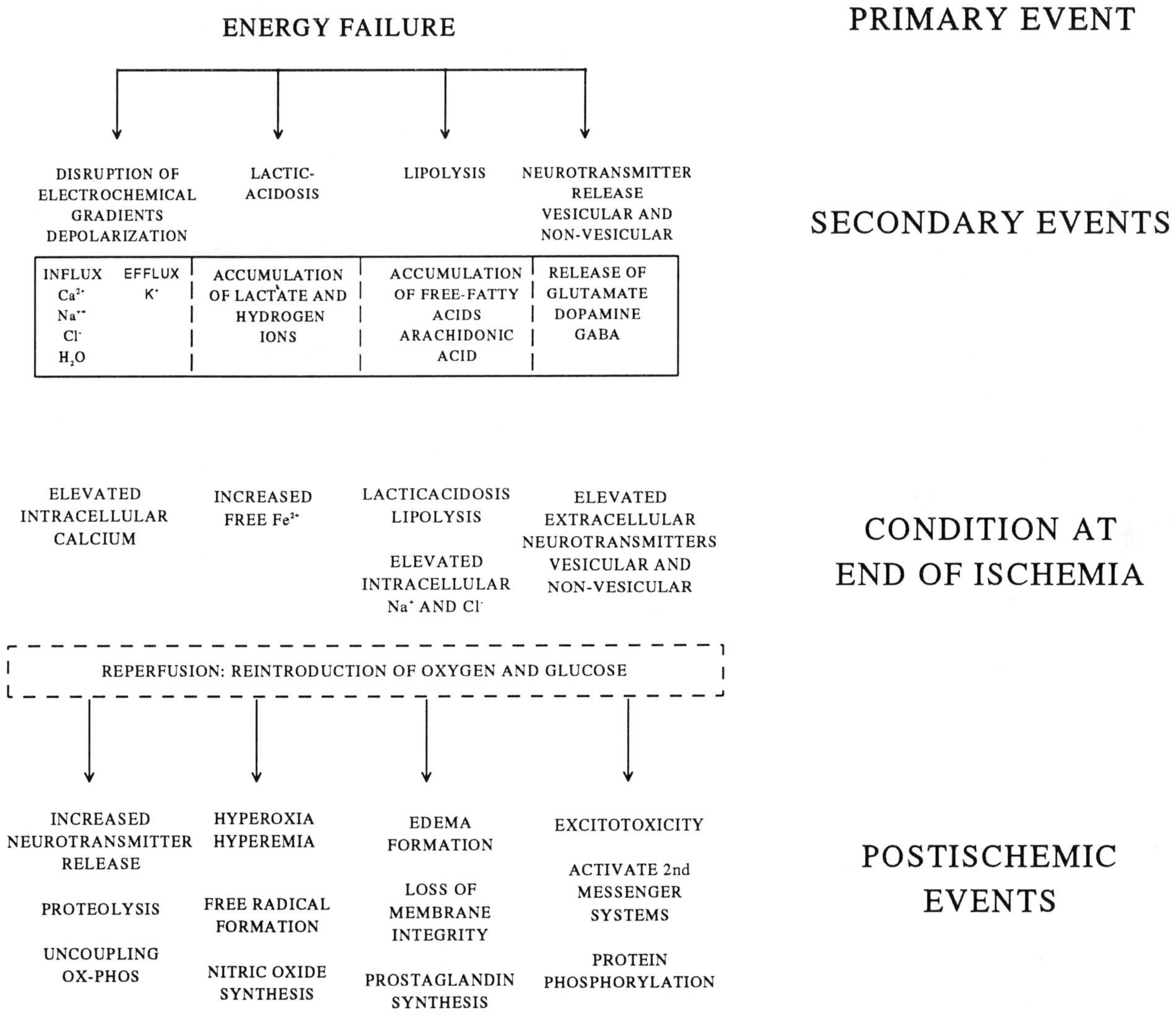

Figure 196-4 Cascade of effects following ischemia and reperfusion. The pervasive effects of energy failure include, for example, the disruption of electrochemical gradients, lactic acidosis, lipolysis, and excessive neurotransmitter release. The magnitude of the response depends on the duration of energy failure, and the perturbations within the cellular milieu are greater with increasing periods of ischemia. The combination of the restoration of energy metabolism with reperfusion and the pathologic condition of the brain creates an abnormal situation, which results in a number of unique postischemic events. Free-radical formation, edema formation, hyperoxia, and so forth could contribute to the onset of irreversible damage of the brain following ischemia.

including an excessive influx of calcium, as well as lactic acidosis, loss of membrane integrity, and an increased release of most neurotransmitters.[18,65,67,68] Restoration of blood flow sets off another set of unique pathologic events which could cause damage, including free radical formation, hyperemia, leukocyte adhesion, edema formation, and a burst of prostaglandin synthesis.[45,67] While energy failure alone does not cause irreversible brain damage, function in the affected region will immediately cease. If the ischemia persists, however, brain damage will ensue; in general, the severity of injury is a function of the duration of the episode and degree of CBF reduction.

What can the neurosurgeon do to counteract the cascade of events caused by loss of normal cerebral energy metabolism? When it is necessary to occlude a vessel to the brain, it is of primary importance to minimize the duration of ischemia. If the procedure necessitates prolonged occlusion, then there are other ways to minimize the impact on cerebral energy metabolism. Because the energy status of the brain reflects a balance between energy production and energy use, reducing the workload of the brain should delay the onset of energy failure. For example, this might be accomplished either by inducing hypothermia or by pharmacologically reducing the electrical activity of the brain prior to the occlusion. While these interventions will not prevent energy failure, they may delay its onset and thus provide the neurosurgeon with additional time before damage occurs. Alternatively, if it were possible to improve the efficiency of energy production or to increase the necessary nutrients, this too would retard the onset of energy failure. While increasing blood glucose does delay the onset of anoxic depolarization and thus should be protective, this effect is offset by the deleterious effects of a greater lactic acidosis, which negates the advantages of hyperglycemia. As the mystery of the pathophysiology of stroke is unraveled, it becomes increasingly evident that there are a number of potential targets for novel therapies other than energy failure.[9,66] It may be ultimately feasible to intervene directly in the evolution of the pathogenic events caused by energy failure and thus to increase the margin of safety for the neurosurgical patient.

References

1. Adam PAJ, Raiha N, Rahiala E-L, Kekomaki M. Oxidation of glucose and D-B-OH-butyrate by the early human fetal brain. *Acta Paediatr Scand* 1975; 64:17–24.
2. Andersen BJ, Marmarou A. Functional compartmentalization of energy production in neural tissue. *Brain Res* 1992; 585:190–195.
3. Astrup J, Sørensen PM, Sørensen HR. Oxygen and glucose consumption related to Na^+,K^+ transport in canine brain. *Stroke* 1981; 12:726–730.
4. Atterwill CK, Cunningham VJ, Balazs R. Characterization of Na^+, K^+-ATPase in cultured and separated neuronal and glial cells from rat cerebellum. *J Neurochem* 1984; 43:8–18.
5. Beitner R. *Regulation of Carbohydrate Metabolism,* vols 1 and 2. Boca Raton, FL: CRC Press, 1985.
6. Beltran del Rio H, Wilson JE. Hexokinase of rat brain mitochondria: relative importance of adenylate kinase and oxidative phosphorylation as sources of substrate ATP, and interaction with intramitochondrial compartments of ATP and ADP. *Arch Biochem Biophys* 1991; 286:183–194.
7. Borowsky IW, Collins RC. Metabolic anatomy of brain: a comparison of regional capillary density, glucose metabolism, and enzyme activities. *J Comp Neurol* 1989; 288:401–413.
8. Branston NM, Symon L, Crockard HA, Pasztor E. Relationship between the cortical evoked potential and local cortical blood flow following acute middle cerebral artery occlusion in the baboon. *Exp Neurol* 1974; 45:195–208.
9. Choi DW. Cerebral hypoxia: some new approaches and unanswered questions. *J Neurosci* 1990: 10:2493–2501.
10. Cremer JE. Measurement of brain substrate utilization in adult and infant rats using various ^{14}C-labeled precursors. In Passonneau JV, Hawkins RA, Lust WD, Welsh FA (eds): *Cerebral Metabolism and Neural Function.* Baltimore: Williams & Wilkins, 1980, pp 300–308.
11. Cremer JE. Nutrients for the brain: problems in supply. *Early Hum Dev* 1981; 5:117–132.
12. Crone C. Facilitated transfer of glucose from blood into brain tissue. *J Physiol (Lond)* 1965; 181:103–113.
13. de Leon MJ, George AE, Ferris SH, et al. Positron emission tomography and computed tomography assessments of the aging human brain. *J Comput Assist Tomogr* 1984; 8:88–94.
14. Duckrow RB, Bryan RM Jr. Regional cerebral glucose utilization during hyperglycemia. *J Neurochem* 1987; 48:989–993.
15. Eadie MJ, Tyrer JH. *Biochemical Neurology.* New York: Alan R. Liss, 1983.
16. Erecinska M, Silver IA. ATP and brain function. *J Cereb Blood Flow Metab* 1989; 9:2–19.
17. General discussion: Brain energy metabolism: cell body or synapse? In *Exploring Brain Functional Anatomy with Positron Tomography. Ciba Found Symp* 1991; 163:43–51.
18. Globus MY-T, Busto R, Dietrich WD, et al. Effect of ischemia on the in vivo release of striatal dopamine, glutamate and gamma-aminobutyric acid studied by intracerebral microdialysis. *J Neurochem* 1988; 51:1455–1464.
19. Goldstein S, Reivich M. Cerebral blood flow and metabolism in aging and dementia. *Clin Neuropharmacol* 1991; 14(Suppl 1):S34–S44.
20. Grisar T, Frere J-M, Franck G. Effect of K^+ ions on kinetic properties of the (Na^+,K^+)-ATPase (EC 3.6.1.3) of bulk isolated glial cells, perikarya and synaptosomes from rabbit brain cortex. *Brain Res* 1979; 165:87–103.
21. Gutman A. Regulation of glycogen metabolism. In Beitner R (ed): *Regulation of Carbohydrate Metabolism.* vol 2. Boca Raton, FL: CRC Press, 1985, pp 33–52.
22. Harik SI, LaManna JC. Vascular perfusion and blood-brain glucose transport in acute and chronic hyperglycemia. *J Neurochem* 1988; 51:1924–1929.
23. Hawkins RA, Mans AW. Intermediary metabolism of carbohydrates and other fuels. In Lajtha A (ed): *Handbook of Neurochemistry,* vol 3. New York: Plenum, 1983, pp 259–294.
24. Hawkins RA, Mans AW, Davis DW. Regional ketone body utilization by rat brain in starvation and diabetes. *Am J Physiol* 1986; 250:E169–E178.
25. Heiss WD, Hayakawa T, Waltz AG. Cortical neuronal function during ischemia. Effects of occlusion of one middle cerebral artery on single-unit activity in cats. *Arch Neurol* 1976; 33:813–820.
26. Hernandez MJ, Vannucci RC, Salcedo A, Brennan RW. Cerebral blood flow and metabolism during hypoglycemia in newborn dogs. *J Neurochem* 1980; 35:622–628.
27. Hochachka PW, Mommsen TP. Protons and anaerobiosis. *Science* 1983; 219:1391–1397.
28. Ingvar DH, Philipson L. Distribution of cerebral blood flow in the dominant hemisphere during motor ideation and motor performance. *Ann Neurol* 1977; 2:230–237.
29. Kadekaro M, Crane AM, Sokoloff L. Differential effects of electrical stimulation of sciatic nerve on metabolic activity in spinal cord and dorsal root ganglion in the rat. *Proc Natl Acad Sci USA* 1985; 82:6010–6013.
30. Kalaria RN. The blood-brain barrier and cerebral microcirculation in Alzheimer disease. *Cerebrovasc Brain Metab Rev* 1992; 4:226–260.
31. Kennedy C, DesRosiers MH, Sakurada O, et al. Metabolic mapping of the primary visual system of the monkey by means of the autoradiographic [^{14}C]deoxyglucose technique. *Proc Natl Acad Sci USA* 1976; 73:4230–4234.
32. Kennedy C, Gillin JC, Mendelson W, et al. Local cerebral glucose

utilization in non-rapid eye movement sleep. *Nature* 1982; 297:325–327.
33. Kety SS, Woodford RB, Harmel MH, et al. Cerebral blood flow and metabolism in schizophrenia. The effects of barbiturate semi-narcosis, insulin coma and electroshock. *Am J Psychiatry* 1948; 104:765–770.
34. Kostanyan A, Nazaryan K. Rat brain glycolysis regulation by estradiol-17β. *Biochim Biophys Acta* 1992; 1133:301–306.
35. Kuhl DE, Metter EJ, Riege WH, Phelps ME. Effects of human aging on patterns of local cerebral glucose utilization determined by the [^{18}F] fluorodeoxyglucose method. *J Cereb Blood Flow Metab* 1982; 2:163–171.
36. Lai JCK, Blass JP. Differences in the responses of brain cytosolic and mitochondrial hexokinases to three essential divalent metal ions. *Comp Biochem Physiol [C]* 1985; 80:285–290.
37. Land JM, Booth RFG, Berger R, Clark JB. Development of mitochondrial energy metabolism in rat brain. *Biochem J* 1977; 164:339–348.
38. Lehninger AL, Nelson DL, Cox MM: *Principles of Biochemistry,* 2d ed. New York: Worth, 1993.
39. Levitsky LL, Fisher DE, Paton JB, Delannoy CW. Fasting plasma levels of glucose, acetoacetate, D-β-hydroxybutyrate, glycerol, and lactate in the baboon infant: correlation with cerebral uptake of substrates and oxygen. *Pediatr Res* 1977; 11:298–302.
40. Lowry OH, Passonneau JV. The relationships between substrates and enzymes of glycolysis in brain. *J Biol Chem* 1964; 239:31–42.
41. Lowry OH, Passonneau JV, Hasselberger FX, Schulz DW. Effect of ischemia on known substrates and cofactors of the glycolytic pathway in brain. *J Biol Chem* 1964; 239:18–30.
42. Lust WD, Passonneau JV, Veech RL. Cyclic adenosine monophosphate, metabolites, and phosphorylase in neural tissue: a comparison of methods of fixation. *Science* 1973; 181:280–282.
43. Medina JM. The role of lactate as an energy substrate for the brain during the early neonatal period. *Biol Neonate* 1985; 48:237–244.
44. Michenfelder JD. The interdependency of cerebral functional and metabolic effects following massive doses of thiopental in the dog. *Anesthesiology* 1974; 41:231–236.
45. Mori E, del Zoppo GJ, Chambers JD, et al. Inhibition of polymorphonuclear leukocyte adherence suppresses no-reflow after focal cerebral ischemia in baboons. *Stroke* 1992; 23:712–718.
46. Nafstad HJ, Blackstad TW. Distribution of mitochondria in pyramidal cells and boutons in hippocampal cortex. *Z Zellforsch Mikrosk Anat* 1966; 73:234–245.
47. Nioka S, Chance B, Hilberman M, et al. Relationship between intracellular pH and energy metabolism in dog brain as measured by ^{31}P-NMR. *J Appl Physiol* 1987; 62:2094–2102.
48. Nordstrom CH, Rehncrona S, Siesjö BK. Cerebral metabolism. In Youmans JR (ed): *Neurological Surgery.* Philadelphia: Saunders, 1990, pp 623–651.
49. Ogush S, Lawson JWR, Dobson GP, et al. A new transient activator of phosphofructokinase during initiation of rapid glycolysis in brain. *J Biol Chem* 1990; 265:10943–10949.
50. Owen OE, Morgan AP, Kemp HG, et al. Brain metabolism during fasting. *J Clin Invest* 1967; 46:1589–1595.
51. Pardridge WM, Oldendorf WH. Transport of metabolic substrates through the blood-brain barrier. *J Neurochem* 1977; 28:5–12.
52. Passonneau JV, Lowry OH. Phosphofructokinase and the Pasteur effect. *Biochem Biophys Res Commun* 1962; 7:10–15.
53. Pelligrino DA, LaManna JC, Duckrow RB, et al. Hyperglycemia and blood-brain barrier glucose transport. *J Cereb Blood Flow Metab* 1992; 12:887–899.
54. Persson B, Settergren G, Dahlquist G. Cerebral arterio-venous difference of acetoacetate D-β-hydroxybutyrate in children. *Acta Paediatr Scand* 1972; 61:273–278.
55. Ponten U, Ratcheson RA, Salford LG, Siesjö BK. Optimal freezing conditions for cerebral metabolites in rats. *J Neurochem* 1973; 21:1127–1138.
56. Quadbeck G. Enzymology of energetics and ionic movement. 4: Inhibition and activation of sodium transport across the blood-brain barrier. *Acta Neurol Scand [Suppl]* 1962; 1:5 (abstr).
57. Ratcheson RA, Blank AC, Ferrendelli JA. Regionally selective metabolic effects of hypoglycemia in brain. *J Neurochem* 1981; 36:1952–1958.
58. Rossen R, Kabat H, Anderson JP. Acute arrest of cerebral circulation in man. *Arch Neurol Psychiatry* 1943; 50:510–528.
59. Schwartz WJ, Smith CB, Davidsen L, et al. Metabolic mapping of functional activity in the hypothalamo-neurohypophysial system of the rat. *Science* 1979; 205:723–725.
60. Settergren G, Lindblad BS, Persson B. Cerebral blood flow and exchange of oxygen, glucose ketone bodies, lactate, pyruvate and amino acids in infants. *Acta Paediatr Scand* 1976; 65:343–353.
61. Shank RP, Aprison MH. Glutamate as a neurotransmitter. In Kvamme E (ed): *Glutamine and Glutamate in Mammals.* Boca Raton, FL: CRC Press, 1988, pp 3–19.
62. Siegal GJ, Agranoff BW, Albers RW, Nolinoff P. *Basic Neurochemistry: Molecular, Cellular, and Medical Aspects,* 5th ed. New York: Raven Press, 1994.
63. Siesjö BK. *Brain Energy Metabolism.* Chichester, UK: Wiley, 1978.
64. Siesjö BK. Cerebral circulation and metabolism. *J Neurosurg* 1984; 60:883–908.
65. Siesjö BK. Acidosis and ischemic brain damage. *Neurochem Pathol* 1988; 9:31–88.
66. Siesjö BK. Pathophysiology and treatment of focal cerebral ischemia. Part II: Mechanisms of damage and treatment. *J Neurosurg* 1992; 77:337–354.
67. Siesjö BK, Agardh CD, Bengtsson F. Free radicals and brain damage. *Cerebrovasc Brain Metab Rev* 1989; 1:165–211.
68. Siesjö BK, Bendek G, Koide T, et al. Influence of acidosis in lipid peroxidation in brain tissue in vitro. *J Cereb Blood Flow Metab* 1985; 5:253–258.
69. Siesjö BK, Bengtsson F. Calcium fluxes, calcium antagonists, and calcium-related pathology in brain ischemia, hypoglycemia, and spreading depression: a unifying hypothesis. *J Cereb Blood Flow Metab* 1989; 9:127–140.
70. Siesjö BK, Johannsson H, Ljunggren B, Norberg K. Brain dysfunction in cerebral hypoxia and ischemia. *Res Publ Assoc Res Nerv Ment Dis* 1974; 53:75–112.
71. Sokoloff L. Metabolism of the central nervous system in vivo. In Field J, Magoun HW, Hall VE (eds): *Handbook of Physiology.* Section 1: *Neurophysiology,* vol 3. Washington, DC: American Physiological Society, 1960, pp 1843–1864.
72. Sokoloff L. The brain as a chemical machine. *Prog Brain Res* 1992; 94:19–33.
73. Sokoloff L, Reivich M, Kennedy C, et al. The [^{14}C]-deoxyglucose method for measurement of local cerebral glucose utilization: theory, procedure, and normal values in the conscious and anesthetized albino rat. *J Neurochem* 1977; 28:897–916.
74. Trivedi B, Danforth WH. Effect of pH on the kinetics of frog muscle phosphofructokinase. *J Biol Chem* 1966; 241:4110–4112.
75. Uyeda K. Interactions of glycolytic enzymes with cellular membranes. *Curr Top Cell Regul* 1992; 33:31–46.
76. Veech RL. Freeze-blowing of brain and interpretation of the meaning of certain metabolite levels. In Passonneau JV, Hawkins RA, Lust WD, Welsh FA (eds): *Cerebral Metabolism and Neural Function.* Baltimore: Williams & Wilkins, 1980, pp 34–41.
77. Veech RL, Lawson JW, Cornell NW, Krebs HA. Cytosolic phosphorylation potential. *J Biol Chem* 1979; 254:6538–6547.
78. Wilson JE. Regulation of mammalian hexokinase activity. In Beitner R (ed): *Regulation of Carbohydrate Metabolism,* vol 1. Boca Raton, FL: CRC Press, 1985, pp 45–85.
79. Wong-Riley M. Changes in the visual system of monocularly sutured or enucleated cats demonstrable with cytochrome oxidase histochemistry. *Brain Res* 1979; 171:11–28.
80. Yarowsky PJ, Ingvar DH. Neuronal activity and energy metabolism. *Fed Proc* 1981; 40:2353–2362.
81. Yarowsky P, Jehle J, Ingvar DH, Sokoloff L. Relationship between functional activity and glucose utilization in the rat superior cervical ganglion in vivo. *Soc Neurosci Abstr* 1979; 5:421.
82. Yarowsky P, Kadekaro M, Sokoloff L. Frequency-dependent activation of glucose utilization in the superior cervical ganglion by electri-

cal stimulation of cervical sympathetic trunk. *Proc Natl Acad Sci USA* 1983; 80:4179–4183.

83. Yoshii F, Barker WW, Chang JY, et al. Sensitivity of cerebral glucose metabolism to age, gender, brain volume, brain atrophy, and cerebrovascular risk factors. *J Cereb Blood Flow Metab* 1988; 8:654–661.
84. Yu ACH, Hertz L. Uptake of glutamate, GABA, and glutamaine into predominantly GABAergic and a predominantly glutamatergic nerve cell population in culture. *J Neurosci Res* 1982; 7:23–35.
85. Yu ACH, Lee YL, Eng LF. Glutamate as an energy substrate for neuronal-astrocytic interactions. *Prog Brain Res* 1992; 94:251–259.
86. Yudkoff M, Pleasure D, Cregar L, et al. Glutathione turnover in cultured astrocytes; studies with [^{15}N]glutamate. *J Neurochem* 1990; 55:137–145.

197

The Cerebral Venous System

Marshall R. Ball
John P. Kapp
Dan N. Richardson

Developments in radiology during the past decade have truly revolutionized the clinician's ability to identify disorders of the venous system of the brain. Yet this ability has only emphasized how functional and trouble-free the elegant, simple, and fragile structures which drain blood from the brain really are. Although cerebral venous disease remains rare, heightened awareness of the cerebral venous system has stimulated interest in its anatomy and physiology, as well as in the development of operative techniques applicable to it.

Gross Anatomy*

Using a classification suggested by Kaplan, the cerebral venous drainage comprises three segments: an outer or superficial segment that drains the scalp, underlying muscle, and tendons and that is subserved by the scalp veins; an intermediate segment for the skull, diploe, and dura mater, consisting of the diploic veins, emissary veins, meningeal veins, and dural venous sinuses; and a cerebral segment which consists of the veins that drain the brain.[28]

Blood normally drains from the scalp into the extracranial venous system and to a lesser extent into the intracranial venous sinuses through the emissary veins. Reversal of flow in these veins has been noted in patients with raised intracranial pressure. In these instances, blood flows from the intracranial sinuses into the scalp veins. This flow may then increase the size of the emissary and scalp veins.

The veins of the scalp accompany the arteries and have multiple connections with the diploic veins and with the dural venous sinuses. The diploic veins are located between the tables of the skull and drain into the superior sagittal, transverse, or sphenoparietal sinus, or the torcular. In the child, the calvarium consists of a single layer in which the veins grow and communicate with each other. Marrow then develops and with its ingrowth comes the formation of an outer and inner table of the skull and of the diploic layer. While the cranial bones are separated from one another, these veins are confined to particular bones; later, when the sutures are obliterated, the veins unite, increase in size, and communicate with the scalp veins, meningeal veins, and dural venous sinuses.

The diploic veins and the scalp veins function as collateral pathways for the venous outflow from intracranial structures if the outflow of the superior sagittal sinus is obstructed.[21] The scalp veins are rarely visualized on cerebral angiograms and therefore, when seen, indicate either an excessive amount of contrast agent or the presence of a vascular anomaly, a tumor of the scalp or skull, or occlusion of the superior sagittal sinus.

The meningeal veins are located between the skull and the dura mater and parallel the course of the meningeal arteries. These veins communicate with the emissary, diploic, and cerebral veins and empty into the major dural venous sinuses. The small meningeal veins of the falx cerebri drain into the superior sagittal sinus, and the veins of the tentorium join the superior sagittal and transverse sinuses.

The dural venous sinuses surround the brain, receive contributions from the brain, the meninges, and the diploe, and communicate through emissary channels with the veins outside the skull. The posterosuperior group of dural sinuses includes the superior sagittal sinus, inferior sagittal sinus, straight sinus, two transverse sinuses, sigmoid sinus, and occipital sinus; and the anteroinferior group includes the cavernous sinuses, superior petrosal sinus, and basilar plexus. Most of the blood in these sinuses either flows posteriorly to empty through the sigmoid sinuses into the internal jugular veins or is directed to the cavernous sinuses, the internal jugular veins, the veins of the orbit, and the vertebral venous plexus (Fig. 197-1*A*).

The veins of the brain are subdivided into superficial and deep cerebral veins. The superficial cerebral veins arise in brain substance, cross the subarachnoid and subdural spaces, and drain toward the superior sagittal or transverse sinuses. The superficial veins include the major anastomotic veins of Labbé and Trolard and the superficial veins on the cortex, of which the rolandic vein is the largest; the rolandic vein drains the precentral and postcentral gyri and empties into the dural sinuses. The vein of Trolard unites the superior and inferior groups of veins, and the vein of Labbé unites the sylvian vein with the superior petrosal sinus, where it joins the lateral sinus. Veins from the tentorial aspect of the brain empty into the transverse and superior petrosal sinuses. Large cortical areas, especially on the inferior and medial surfaces, are drained into the vein of Galen. These anastomotic veins connect the superficial and deep venous systems and include the occipital vein, the basal vein of Rosenthal, and the posterior callosal vein.

The deep cerebral veins of importance are the internal cerebral veins, the thalamostriate veins, the anterior septal veins, and the vein of Galen. The internal cerebral veins are formed at the level of the interventricular septum by the union of the anterior septal and the thalamostriate veins. These veins enter the tela choroidea of the third ventricle and pass through the velum interpositum to the level of the splenium of the corpus callosum. The internal cerebral veins receive veins that drain the roof of the lateral ventricles, veins from the occipital horns, thalamic veins, and superior choroidal veins. The thalamostriate vein drains the caudate nucleus, internal capsule, and deep white matter of the posterior frontal and anterior parietal lobes. The anterior part of the thalamostriate vein passes through the interventricular foramen. The anterior septal vein drains the white matter of the anterior portion of the frontal lobe and passes lateral to the columns of the fornix to join the ipsilateral thalamostriate vein to form the internal cerebral vein.

*This section is reprinted, with permission, from Schmidek HH, Auer LM, Kapp JP. The cerebral venous system. *Neurosurgery* 1985; 17:663–678.

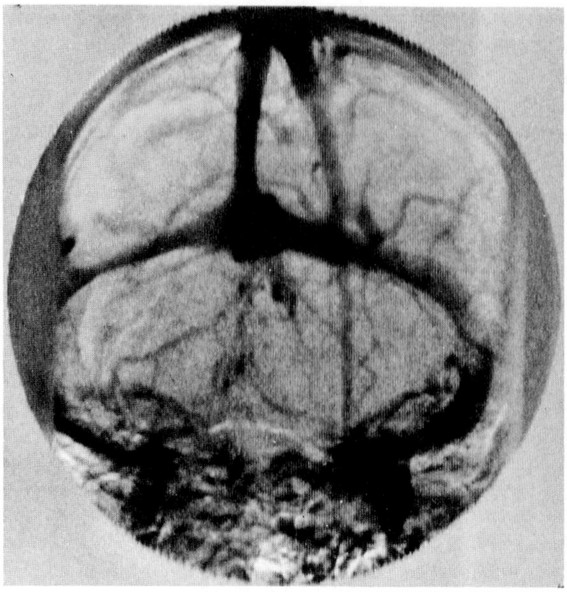

(*A*)

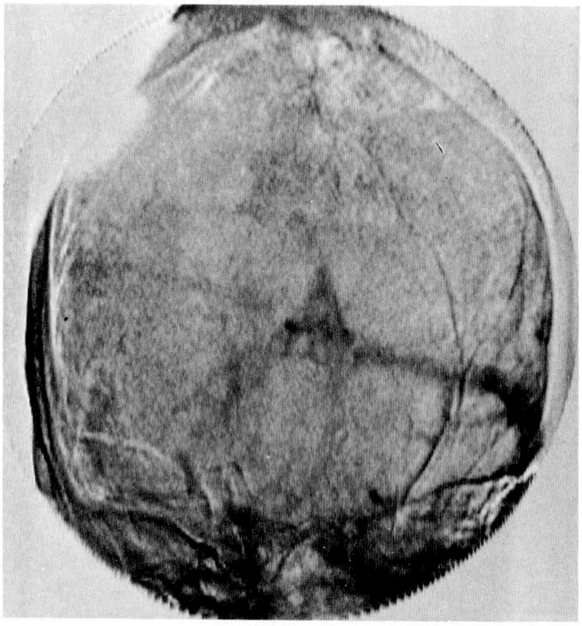

(*B*)

Figure 197-1 *A*. A normal digital subtraction angiogram from an aortic injection, 15 degree oblique posteroanterior projection, demonstrates filling of all of the major dural sinuses. *B*. Digital subtraction angiography from an aortic injection, venous phase. The superior sagittal sinus, the right transverse sinus, the right sigmoid sinus, and the right jugular vein do not fill in this patient with dural sinus thrombosis.

The vein of Galen originates beneath the splenium of the corpus callosum by the union of the two internal cerebral veins. It passes through the upper portion of the quadrigeminal cistern to join the inferior sagittal sinus and form the straight sinus. The vein of Galen receives the two basal veins and the posterior pericallosal, internal occipital, posterior mesencephalic, precentral, and superior vermian or superior cerebellar veins, thereby providing venous drainage for the medial areas of the diencephalon, the basal ganglia, the midbrain, the medial aspect of the cerebral hemisphere, and the corpus callosum.

The cerebellum has a surface network of veins that drain predominantly into the adjacent venous sinuses. These veins are grouped into the superior, anterior, and posterior cerebellar veins. The superior cerebellar veins pass from the rostral part of the vermis to terminate in the vein of Galen or in the straight sinus. The anterior cerebellar vein (or petrosal vein) receives tributaries from the brain stem and the anterior cerebellar hemisphere, and then runs into the superior petrosal sinus. The posterior cerebellar veins divide into medial and lateral branches and empty into the straight sinus and the straight or transverse sinus, respectively.

Functional Anatomy

The general design of the cerebral venous system appears to be geared to the maintenance of patency in the face of negative pressure. Thus, the major venous sinuses split the leaves of the dura, so that they are triangulated and relatively noncollapsible. Bridging veins enter the sinuses opposite the direction of sinus blood flow, perhaps minimizing collapse of bridging veins in the upright position.

The dural sinuses are noncontractile. Cerebral veins less than 200 μm in diameter rarely contain smooth muscle cells in their walls.[48,56] Their walls consist of a continuous endothelial cell layer surrounded by a perithelial cell layer reinforced by dense collagen bundles. The function of the perithelial cell layer is poorly understood. Contractile elements are visible in endothelial cells and perithelial cells. The perivascular collagen bundles are probably responsible for the rigidity of the venous walls.[48] The innervation of the cerebral venules is controversial, although the walls of both the intracerebral and the meningeal veins contain noradrenergic and peptidergic fibers.[8,9,19]

Physiology

Of the three major intracranial components, cerebral blood volume can change most rapidly, although its proportionate share of the total intracranial volume is small, compared to tissue volumes. Because 70 to 80 percent of cerebral blood volume is located in the venous system,[39] a study of regulatory mechanisms for cerebral blood volume must focus on cerebral veins.

Pressure in the confluens sinuum has been measured in anesthetized patients in a variety of surgical positions. In adults, the pressure was 9.8 $\pm$ 2.8 cmH_2O with the upper half of the body at a -10 degrees inclination. Pressure decreased almost linearly when the upper half of the body was raised to a mean low of -12.7 ± 3.0 cmH_2O at 90 degrees, i.e., in the sitting position. When the confluens sinuum was 15 degrees higher than the level of the right atrium, the pressure was usually 0 or slightly positive. Negative pressures in the confluens sinuum were not recorded in young children. Positive pressure respiration had a negligible effect on sinus pressure. Sinus pressure was promptly elevated by jugular compression and retroflexion of the neck.[25] With the patient in the supine position, sinus pressure was consistently increased by rotation of the head to the right. Rotation of the head to the left was followed by reduction in sinus pressure in 60 percent of cases, and an increase of lesser magnitude in the remaining 40 percent.[26]

Transmural pressure in cerebral veins, i.e., the difference between intravascular and perivascular pressure, rarely exceeds a few millimeters of mercury. An increase in intracranial pressure (ICP) is followed by a parallel increase in pressure in cortical veins, bridging veins, and lateral lacunae.[12,41] Pressure within the superior sagittal sinus does not always parallel a rising ICP. Some investigators have suggested that a sudden pressure drop between cortical veins and sagittal sinus may be related to "cuffing" of bridging veins secondary to increased cerebrospinal fluid (CSF) pressure.[41] Compression of veins against the skull and dura mater or overcoming arteries might also account for venous compression and congestion at extremely high intracranial pressures.

In animal experiments, electrical stimulation of the cervical sympathetic nerve causes significant constriction of pial veins as small as 50 μm.[3,4,7,23] The degree of vasoconstriction is greater than that of arterial constriction, especially in vessels larger than 100 μm. Venous constriction rapidly follows sympathetic stimulation, suggesting an active constrictive mechanism rather than passive collapse of veins as a response to arterial constriction.[9] Topical application of norepinephrine to pial veins has been reported to cause significant venous constriction.[8,20,57] Studies with blocking agents suggest that the sympathoadrenergic mechanism is mediated by α-receptors.[9] Sympathetic nerve stimulation significantly reduces intracranial pressure.[6,8,9] In mice, cerebral blood volume can be raised by sympathectomy and lowered by sympathetic stimulation.[20]

When intracranial pressure is elevated, sympathetic stimulation still induces venous constriction and a reduction in ICP. An increase in spontaneous cervical sympathetic activity can be recorded.[62] However, studies in cats suggest that only an 8 to 20 percent reduction in ICP follows cervical sympathetic stimulation at elevated ICP.[50]

Systemic barbiturate administration is associated with venous constriction.[50] Substance P and vasoactive intestinal peptide, when applied topically to cerebral veins, are mild dilators.[20,21] Topically applied 5-hydroxytryptamine dilates small cerebral veins and constricts larger veins.[2,5,36] Potassium and pH do not seem to have any influence on venous diameter.[38] Variations of arterial perfusion pressure do not usually induce a response within the venous side of the circulation.[50]

The effect of hypercapnia is complex. Increasing cerebral blood flow associated with hypercapnia is associated with increased sensitivity of the cerebral venous system to sympathetic stimulation.[11,32] The effects vary with vessel size and level of CO_2. Constriction of pial arteries in response to sympathetic stimulation decreases as Pa_{CO_2} increases, reaching zero at a Pa_{CO_2} of 60 mmHg. At a Pa_{CO_2} of 60 mmHg, small pial veins (below 50 μm in resting diameter) constrict significantly more than larger veins, whereas under resting conditions the reverse is true. The net result is that the sympathetic system exerts significant control over cerebral blood volume, even under hypercapnic conditions.

Acute elevations of arterial pressure may be transmitted to the venous system through the capillary bed. The breakdown in autoregulation results in foci of extremely elevated flow. Within the foci of elevated flow, venous pressure may exceed intracranial pressure, leading to venous distention and protein extravasation primarily in the postcapillary venular bed.[2]

Increasing intracranial pressure results in a complex series of pathologic circumstances. The pressure in cortical and bridging veins parallels the ICP over a wide range of pressure. Sagittal sinus pressure may remain low despite high ICP. Elevated cortical venous pressure drops suddenly in the lateral lacunae.

At high intracranial pressures, compression of veins against solid structures or even arteries may create focal geometric distortions and irregularities so that flow in them no longer conforms to conventional physical principles. Sympathetic tone rises with ICP, constricting cerebral veins, reducing cerebral blood volume, and consequently tending to lower ICP.[50]

CSF Absorption

The traditional concept holds that cerebrospinal fluid (CSF) is secreted by the choroid plexus, circulates through the ventricular outflow pathways to the basal cisterns, and then to the subarachnoid spaces over the cerebral hemispheres in bulk, where it is absorbed through arachnoid villi into the venous sinuses. Investigations during the past two decades have revealed this concept to be an oversimplification. CSF is a mixture of several components, and appearance curves for various components at different sites have shown that different components are absorbed primarily at different rates by different structures. Thus, tritiated water injected into the cisterna magna is equilibrated almost immediately with intravascular water. Radioactive sodium appears in highest concentration in convexity veins, and labeled albumin absorption is predominantly into the sagittal sinus.[45] Movement of radioactive sodium into brain tissue is accelerated by circulatory arrest, a finding which suggests that the cerebrospinal fluid compartment is maintained by an energy-consuming process.[31]

The evidence is compelling that the extracellular compartment of the brain is directly continuous with the ventricular and subarachnoid cerebrospinal fluid compartments.[46] Bidirectional diffusion of various substances from CSF into brain tissue occurs. Penetration of various CSF components (e.g., potassium ion into brain tissue) may occur at different rates from the ventricular compartment and the subarachnoid space.[44] Clearance of metabolites from the brain parenchyma underlying the highly vascular subarachnoid space occurs rapidly, whereas there may be little or no clearance from the brain parenchyma abutting the ventricular system.[61] The tight junctions between the endothelial cells of the cerebral microvasculature not only restrict passage of various substances from blood to brain, but may operate to restrict or regulate flow in the opposite direction as well.[16] Carrier-mediated transport mechanisms which control movement across this barrier have been identified for a number of metabolites, including various amino acids, nucleic acid precursors, and choline.[13,22,33,34]

Absorption of cerebrospinal fluid into the venous system through the arachnoid villi appears to be driven by a differential in pressure between the subarachnoid space and the intraluminal pressure of the dural sinuses. If sinus pressure is greater than the pressure in the subarachnoid space, the villus endothelium has no intracellular vacuolization and no major surface bulges. As the pressure gradient across the villus is increased, large vacuoles within the cytoplasm of the endothelial cells develop, with overlying bulges on the surface of the cell. Direct communication between the vacuole and the subarachnoid space or the lumen of the sinus can be seen, and occasionally the same intracytoplasmic vacuole may communicate with both the subarachnoid space and the lumen of the sinus, giving rise to a transcellular channel. The intra-endothelial cell junctions are not disturbed regardless of the pressure differential, and other structural communications between the subarachnoid space and the venous system within the arachnoid villus have not been identified.[46] The arachnoid villi function to clear particulate material and large molecules from the CSF by a process of bulk flow. The flow across the villus is unidirectional and a pressure differential between the subarachnoid space and the lumen of the sinus is required for flow.

Cerebral Venous Thrombosis

Spontaneous thrombosis of cerebral veins and dural venous sinuses occurs most frequently in association with infections involving the face, cranial air sinuses and air cells, and meninges. Three significantly different clinical syndromes of dural sinus thrombosis can be identified, which depend on the sinus involved—the cavernous sinus, lateral sinus, or sagittal sinus. Southwick et al. summarized cases reported between 1940 and 1984, and have added all cases seen at the Massachusetts General Hospital between 1948 and 1984.[54]

The cavernous sinus is most frequently involved by septic thrombosis. In the preantibiotic era, the common sites of primary infection were the medial face, orbits, tonsils, and soft palate. In recent years, infections involving the sphenoid and ethmoid sinuses, often misdiagnosed, have become the more common primary sites of infection. The common organisms are *Staphylococcus aureus, Streptococcus, Pneumococcus,* and gram-negative bacilli. The usual clinical presentation begins with fever and periorbital edema followed by headache, ptosis, and ocular muscle palsies. Less frequently, dilated or sluggishly reactive pupils and fifth nerve sensory deficits have been described. Papilledema or dilated tortuous retinal veins and decreased visual acuity may be present. Visual impairment, due to corneal ulceration from failure of lid closure; occlusion of the central retinal artery due to pressure at the orbital apex, emboli, or intracavernous internal carotid arteritis; or elevated intraocular pressure may progress to blindness. The diagnosis is usually made on clinical grounds. Radiographic examination of the sphenoid and ethmoid sinuses is mandatory in cases of suspected cavernous sinus thrombosis. Computed tomography (CT) after the intravenous injection of a contrast agent has not proved sensitive in demonstrating occlusion of the cavernous sinus. Carotid angiography shows narrowing or occlusion of the intracavernous segment of the carotid artery in the majority of cases. Orbital venography may be supplanted by high-resolution surface coil magnetic resonance imaging (MRI) as the definitive diagnostic test. Treatment consists of eradication of the primary source of infection and the administration of antibiotics and anticoagulants. Infected sinuses should be drained on an emergency basis. High-dose broad spectrum antibiotic coverage should be directed at *Staphylococcus,* other gram-positve organisms, and anaerobes. Review of reported cases suggests that the mortality is significantly lower in patients who receive heparin, 14 percent versus 36 percent. Since the introduction of antibiotics, the mortality in cases of septic cavernous sinus thrombosis has dropped from between 88 and 100 percent to 30 percent.

Septic lateral sinus thrombosis is almost uniformly associated with acute or chronic otitis media and mastoiditis. The organisms involved reflect the bacteriology of otitis media—*Proteus* species, *Staphylococcus aureus, Escherichia coli,* and anaerobes. Earache usually precedes headache by several weeks. Nausea, vomiting, and diplopia are also common complaints. Less common symptoms are photophobia and vertigo. Lateral sinus thrombosis is usually a subacute illness, and symptoms frequently have been present for several weeks before the patient is hospitalized. Physical findings include purulent drainage from a ruptured tympanic membrane (or, less commonly, an unruptured but dull erythematous tympanic membrane), postauricular swelling (Griesinger's sign), bilateral papilledema, and sixth cranial nerve palsy. Other focal neurological signs are usually absent. The diagnosis may be suggested by CT findings of mastoiditis or MRI findings of mastoiditis and an abnormality of blood flow in the lateral sinus, and is usually confirmed by digitial subtraction angiography. Initial therapy consists of antibiotics directed at likely pathogens, and mastoidectomy in some cases to eradicate the focus of infection. Anticoagulation is not recommended. If increased intracranial pressure results in visual loss, a lumbar subarachnoid-peritoneal shunt may be inserted if the cerebrospinal fluid is sterile and CT shows no intracranial mass. In rare patients who have inadequate collateral venous drainage from the brain on a long-term basis, from either hypoplasia of the opposite lateral sinus or bilateral lateral sinus thrombosis, bypass grafting from a patent segment of sinus to a cervical vein may afford relief.[52] The reported mortality has fallen from 20 to 30 percent in the preantibiotic era to 12 percent.

Septic thrombosis of the superior sagittal sinus is most frequently associated with meningitis. Less frequently, infections in the ethmoid, maxillary, and frontal sinuses may involve the sagittal sinus, either by spread through the epidural space or via ethmoidal veins. Common bacterial pathogens are *Streptococcus pneumoniae* (40 percent), *Staphylococcus aureus, Streptococcus,* and gram-negative organisms. The initial symptom is usually severe headache, followed by nausea, seizures, vomiting, and confusion which progresses rapidly to coma. Physical examination may reveal hemi- or quadriparesis in addition to an abnormal mental status, neck stiffness, and high fever. Abnormalities shown by CT may be pathognomonic in some instances or may suggest the diagnosis in others. The extent of thrombosis can be precisely delineated by digital subtraction angiography (Fig. 197-1*B*). Treatment consists of the intravenous administration of appropriate antibiotics, and surgical drainage of infected air sinuses and the epidural space. Craniotomy has frequently been followed by rapid clinical deterioration, however, and should be avoided unless a definite abscess has been demonstrated. Anticoagulants are contraindicated because of the frequent occurrence of venous hemorrhagic infarcts. Mannitol and corticosteroids in theory have both advantages and disadvantages. The limited reported experience with the use of these drugs has not been encouraging. Mortality in the antibiotic era remains high (78 percent).

Radiographic Signs of Venous Disease

Newer neuroradiologic techniques have revolutionized the diagnosis of cerebrosinovenous occlusive disease. Adequate visualization of the venous phase of angiography has been available since the advent of rapid sequence filming and photographic subtraction techniques. With major dural sinus occlusion, the cerebral circulation time may be prolonged and delayed filming may be required. Intraluminal filling defects may be due to unopacified blood entering the dural sinuses from vessels not injected when selective arteriography has been performed.[29]

Digital subtraction angiography from the arterial route rather than the intravenous route has become the main confirming diagnostic test of occlusive disease of the major dural sinuses. The arterial route requires much lower doses of contrast, has less patient motion with better subtraction, and has a lower incidence of contrast reaction. Selectivity is not desirable when studying the venous system. An aortic root injection of 25 ml of a 60 percent iodinated contrast medium delivered at 15 ml/s will adequately opacify all the veins of the central venous system simultaneously. Real-time digital subtraction allows one to continue the study until optimal venous visualization is accomplished. Turning the head 15 degrees off vertical in the posteroanterior position allows for adequate demonstration of the anterior and posterior aspects of the dural sinuses, including the lateral sinuses and both jugular bulbs. Figure 197-1*A* demonstrates normal filling of the superficial and deep systems. Nonfilling of a segment of the dural sinuses is highly suggestive of sinovenous occlusive disease (Fig. 197-1*B*). (Rarely, the anterior third of the superior sagittal sinus or one of the lateral sinuses may fail to develop.)

The initial suggestion of sinovenous occlusive disease is often based on computed tomography because of the universal application of CT to patients with neurological disease. However, normal CT scans do not exclude the diagnosis because 10 percent of proven cases have normal scans. Rarely, a positive delta sign is seen in acute thrombosis (Fig. 197-2). Both uninfused and infused CT scans should be performed: the uninfused scan demonstrates hemorrhages and the infused scan is necessary to demonstrate the negative delta or empty triangle of subacute thrombosis (Fig. 197-3), gyral enhancement, tentorial enhancement, and enlarged intramedullary veins.[59] When the infused CT scan is perpendicular to the sinus, the leaves of the dura are enhanced and an empty low-density center filled with thrombus rather than contrast-enhanced flowing blood creates the empty triangle or negative delta sign[17,18,47,58] in 35 percent of cases. Multiple bilateral parasagittal hemorrhages are noted in 20 percent of reported cases and are nonspecific but highly suggestive of sagittal sinus thrombosis (Fig. 197-4). Gyral enhancement is seen in 32 percent of patients. Tentorial enhancement due to venous engorgement has been reported. Direct visualization of an occluded vein, the "cord sign," is highly diagnostic of cortical venous thrombosis but was seen in only 2 of 32 cases reported by Rao et al.[47]

Magnetic resonance imaging is now clinically useful in the diagnosis of cerebral sinovenous occlusive disease. MRI signs of cerebral sinovenous occlusive disease parallel those of CT [e.g., parasagittal hemorrhages, venous infarctions, and gyral enhancement with gadolinium diethylenetriamine pentaacetic acid (Gd-DTPA)]. Special characteristics of flow in MR imaging allow a unique way of imaging thrombosed sinuses. Figure 197-5 demonstrates a spin-echo MR sequence in sagittal sinus occlusion. The occluded sinus gives a high signal in this T2-weighted image while the adjacent cortical veins and arteries demonstrate signal voids of flowing blood. Thrombosis usually presents as increased signal in all the usual multislice spin echo sequences; however, breakdown products within an intraluminal clot may produce signal loss on T2-weighted images due to paramagnetic effects, which will mimic the signal void of flow.[35]

Although flowing blood usually creates a loss of signal within vessels during spin echo MR sequences, several circumstances will produce increased signal within vessel lumina which may be mistaken for thrombus. These include slow or stagnant flow,[10] chance synchronization of TR and the pulse rate to produce pseudogating,[14] flow-related enhancement,[15] and even echo rephasing.[14] Several MR techniques have been suggested to help differentiate intraluminal thrombus and flow-related effects. These include phase imaging techniques,[60] nonselective 90-degree and 180-degree pulses for spin echo sequences,[55,59] and flow-sensitive gradient recalled echo sequences.[42]

To overcome these artifacts, when dural sinus thrombosis is suspected by history or on preliminary review of MR images, a

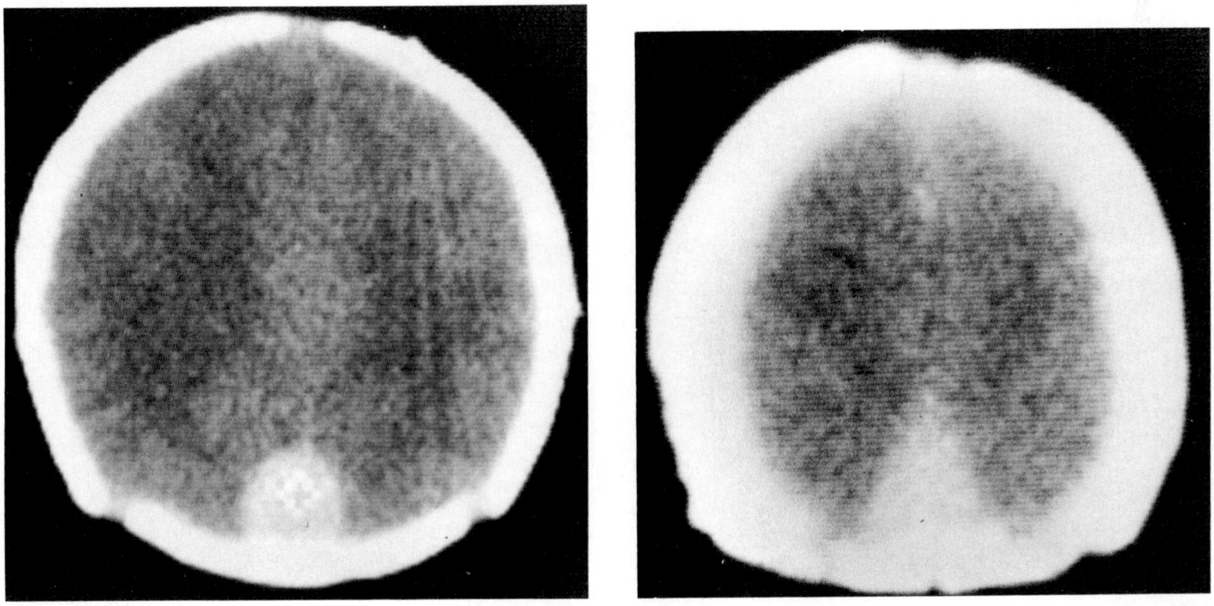

(*A*) **(*B*)**

Figure 197-2 Middle (*A*) and high (*B*) convexity CT of an infant with acute sagittal sinus thrombosis. Note the bulging dense thrombosed superior sagittal sinus posteriorly in these uninfused slices. (Courtesy of Dr. T. Hans Newton, San Francisco, CA.)

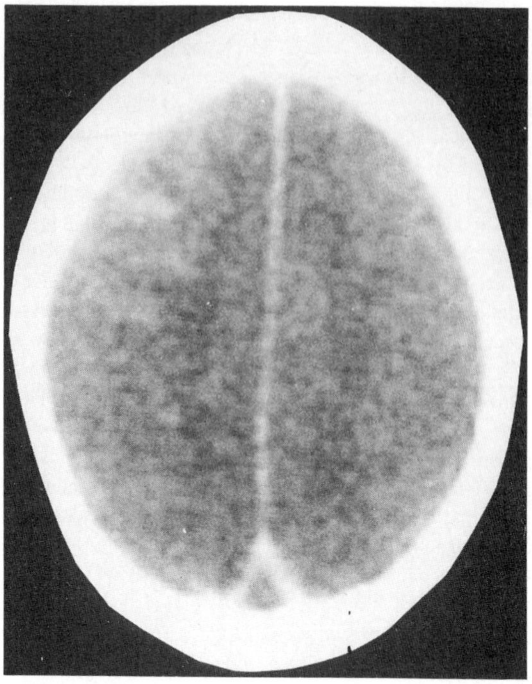

Figure 197-3 An axial infused CT at the centrum semiovale level. Note the posterior empty triangle or negative delta sign pathognomonic of sagittal sinus occlusion. Right frontal gyral enhancement, a nonspecific sign, is also seen.

special imaging sequence should be considered. Figure 197-6 demonstrates a single slice gradient refocused echo technique which confirms the absence of flow in the isointense occluded right sigmoid sinus compared to the bright patent left sinus.

MR angiography is still in the developmental stage and is fraught with artifacts but portends a great diagnostic future. In current examinations, if MR angiography is normal, significant vascular pathology is probably excluded. If abnormal, the finding may be real or artifactual. Magnetic susceptibility at the skull base, turbulent flow, partially thrombosed vessels, inadequate spatial resolution, and patient motion cause major interpretive problems for MR angiography as they do for conventional MR imaging.[49]

Surgery of Cerebral Veins and Dural Venous Sinuses

Surgical management of lesions of cerebral veins and dural sinuses follows established principles of vascular surgery. Adequate proximal and distal exposure of the lesion is required except for certain endovascular approaches. Most lesions are best managed by venous ligation unless reconstruction can be more readily accomplished. Autogenous veins have proven to be satisfactory graft materials for venous reconstruction. The suture techniques borrowed from vascular surgery are applicable to dural venous sinus reconstruction, and adequate patency rates may be expected.[30]

The question of which cerebral veins and venous sinuses can be safely ligated must be answered without a large amount of factual data. The sparse literature has been summarized by Kaplan[27] and by Smith and Sanford.[53] Briefly summarized, it seems that a significant risk of neurological deficit or death accompanies occlusion of the dominant vein of Labbé, the rolandic vein, the superior sagittal sinus posterior to the entrance of the rolandic vein, or a transverse sinus if its counterpart on the opposite side is hypoplastic. Ligation of the internal cerebral vein, the vein of Galen, and the straight sinus may be hazardous, although the precise degree of risk is unknown.[53]

A major development has been the transvenous approach to lesions such as vein of Galen aneurysms and their occlusion with occluding spring emboli (''Gianturco coils''). This procedure is accomplished by percutaneous puncture of the torcular Herophili in neonates or via a small craniectomy over the torcular in older

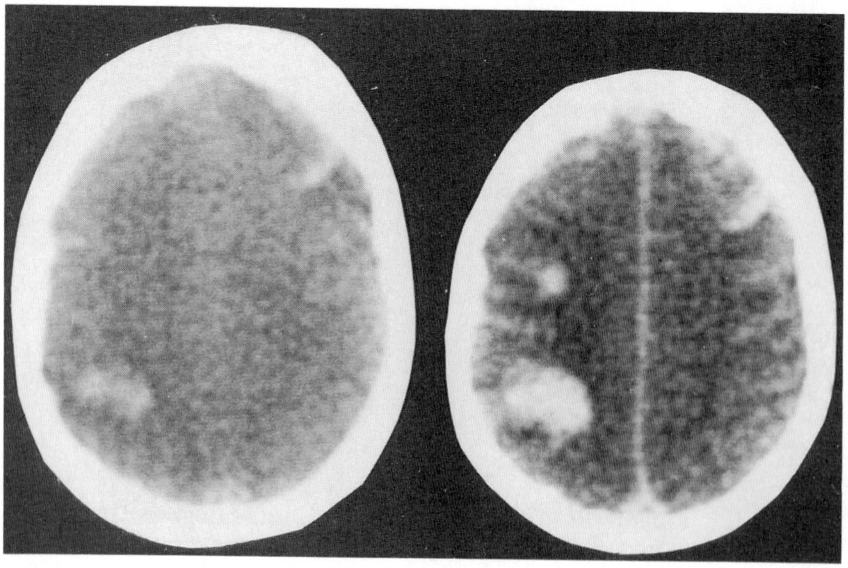

Figure 197-4 Uninfused (*left*) and infused (*right*) CT in sagittal sinus thrombosis. The uninfused scan demonstrates bilateral hemorrhages in unusual locations. After contrast infusion, gyral enhancement and an empty triangle sign confirm the diagnosis of sagittal sinus thrombosis.

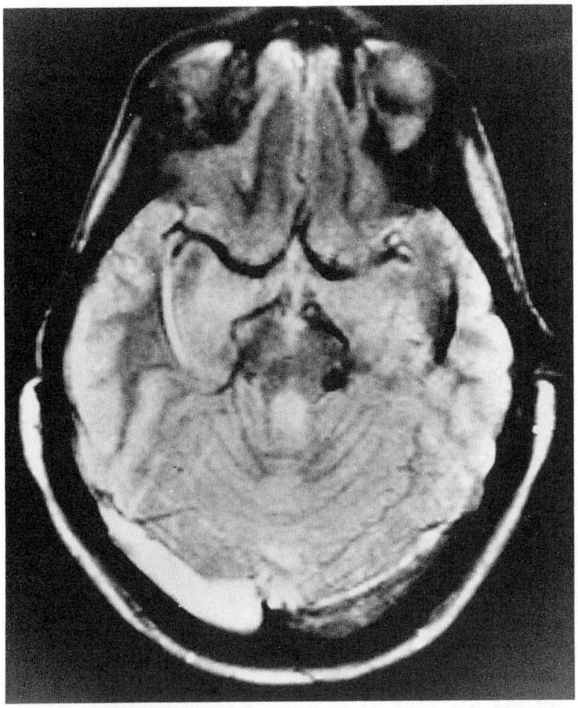

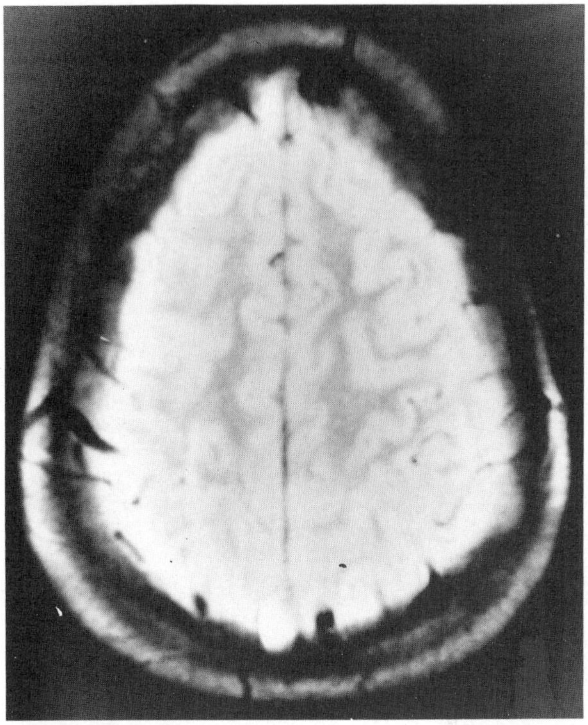

(*A*) (*B*)

Figure 197-5 *A.* An MR spin echo image (TR = 2000 ms, TE = 80 ms) demonstrates a high signal in the occluded right transverse sinus. Note flow voids in this 17-year-old woman with headaches and papilledema. *B.* While multiple cortical veins demonstrate flow voids, the occluded sagittal sinus shows increased signal. (Courtesy of Dr. Ron Cowley, Greenville, SC.)

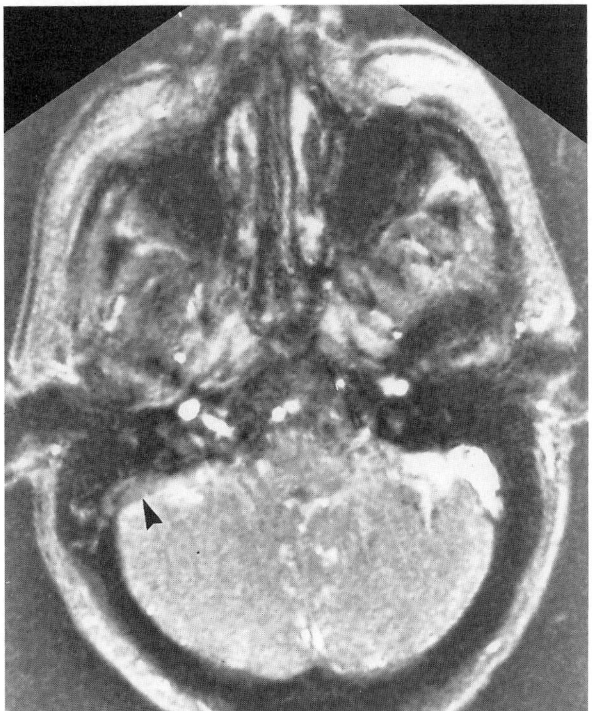

Figure 197-6 An MR single-slice gradient refocused echo technique confirms absent flow in an isointense occluded right sigmoid sinus (*arrowhead*). In this special pulse sequence, the patent left sigmoid sinus demonstrates an increased signal (TR = 50 ms, TE = 10 ms, flip angle = 60 degrees).

patients. A guide wire is positioned in the aneurysm under fluoroscopic control, and a standard 8- to 10-cm angiography introducer is threaded over the wire into the center of the aneurysm. Four to eight 15-cm Gianturco coils are inserted into the aneurysm, using a special tethering plunger system which allows retrieval of a misplaced coil. The goal of the first stage of the procedure is to reduce flow through the aneurysm by about 50 percent. The procedure is repeated in 3 to 21 days, at which time the goal is to completely eliminate flow through the aneurysm. To date, the results of treatment of six patients have been published; there has been one death.[37,40,43] (An unusual case of spontaneous thrombosis of a vein of Galen aneurysm is shown in Fig. 197-7.)

Additional experience has been gained with saphenous vein bypass grafting of an occluded transverse sinus. The technique, first described by Sindou et al., involves placement of a saphenous vein graft between the distal transverse sinus and a large neck vein.[52] Indications include surgical ligation of a sinus, thrombosis, hypoplasia, jugular vein stenosis, and congenital anomalies. To date, the procedure has been performed on 10 patients; the postoperative patency rate is 80 percent in this series.[24]

Surgical removal of neoplasms from the cavernous sinus has been shown to be feasible in two series of patients. Al-Mefty and Smith have provided a detailed description of the surgical anatomy and operative approach.[1] The cavernous sinus is a plexus of veins rather than a large venous space with multiple trabeculations. The lateral wall of the cavernous sinus consists of two layers. The deep layer is separable from the superficial layer and is formed by the sheaths of the third and fourth cranial nerves and the first and second divisions of the fifth cranial nerve connected by a reticular membrane. This membrane has a gap between the third and fourth nerves above, and the fifth below. Because the venous plexus is

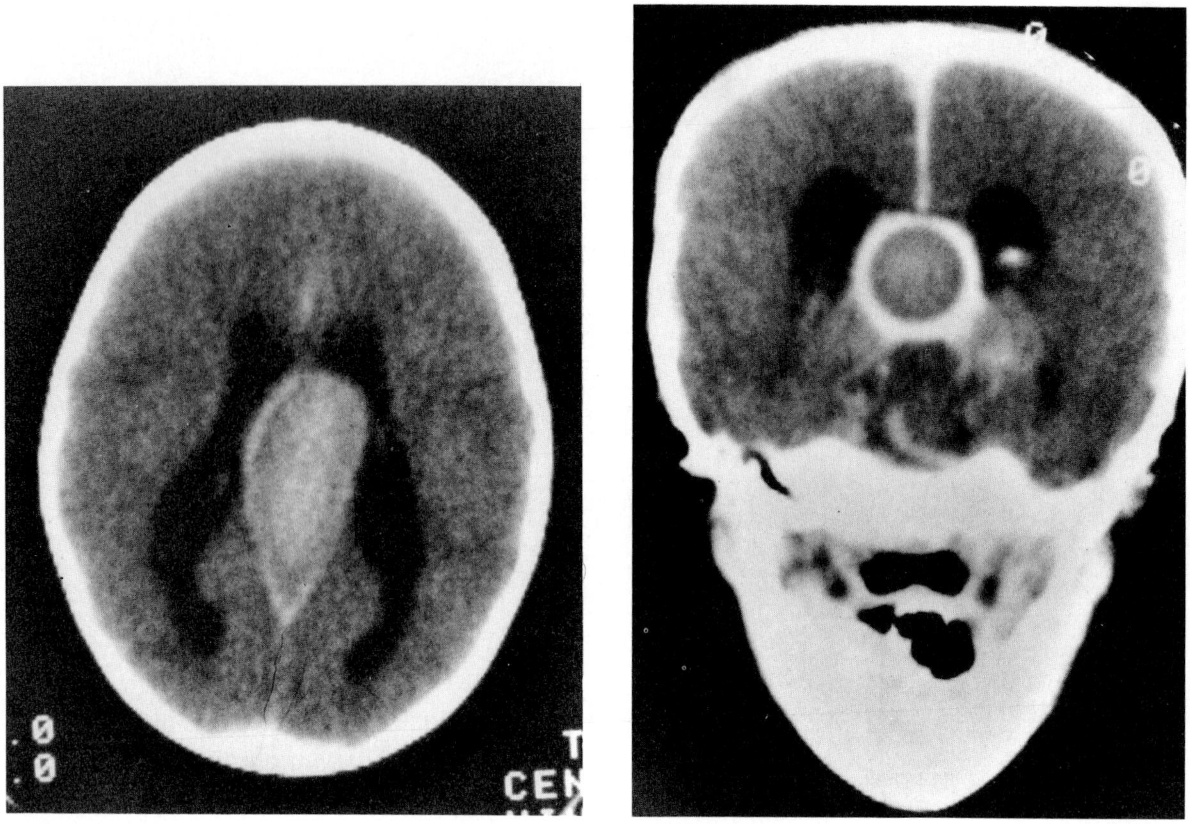

(*A*) (*B*)

Figure 197-7 Axial (*A*) and coronal (*B*) infused CT in a 4-year-old patient presenting with spontaneous thrombosis of a vein of Galen aneurysm. Similar but iatrogenic-induced thrombosis is the goal of percutaneous transvenous embolization with occluding spring coils.

compressed by the tumor, venous bleeding usually does not occur until the later stages of tumor removal. This bleeding can usually be controlled by packing and head elevation. Separation of the tumor from the carotid artery may or may not be easily accomplished. Preoperative carotid occlusion testing, using balloons and cerebral blood flow measurements, is recommended. The surgeon should be prepared to repair a laceration in the carotid artery, or to resect a segment of artery invaded by tumor and replace it with a vein graft or perform an extracranial-intracranial (EC-IC) anastomosis if preoperative testing suggests that the patient will not tolerate carotid occlusion.

Subsequently, Sekhar et al. reported a series of 42 patients who underwent surgical removal of neoplasms involving the cavernous sinus.[51] These authors described intradural-extradural approaches to the cavernous sinus from the superior and lateral aspect, and from inferior, anterolateral, and medial approaches; both the cervical internal carotid artery and the petrous segment of the internal carotid artery were exposed. Preoperative balloon occlusion of the carotid artery with cerebral blood flow measurement was done. One carotid artery was resected and replaced with a vein graft, and three carotid arteries were excised without replacement. There were no operative deaths.[51]

The emerging frontier in surgery of the cerebral venous system appears to be the reconstruction of the medium-size veins. Significant technical problems, which in the past have confronted the surgeon attempting such procedures, may have been solved by Kirsch, who has developed a nonpenetrating edge everting microclip system for such anastomoses.[63] A novel applicator permits clip placement in a rapid and facile manner in confined spaces. The method can be used for end-to-end, end-to-side, vessel caliber and wall thickness mismatch, and prosthetic anastomosis. Values for long- and short-term patency, blood flow velocity, intimal repair, and burst and tensile strength have been reported to be equivalent to or superior to those obtainable with conventional microsuture techniques. The system with three different size clips has been extended to vessels as small as 400 μm in diameter, with a wall thickness of 100 μm.

References

1. Al-Mefty O, Smith RR. Surgery of tumors invading the cavernous sinus. *Surg Neurol* 1988; 30:370–381.
2. Auer LM. The pathogenesis of hypertensive encephalopathy: experimental data and their clinical relevance with special reference to neurosurgical patients. *Acta Neurochir (Wien) [Suppl]* 1978; 27:1–111.
3. Auer LM. Cerebrovascular activity of the calcium antagonist nimodipine. In Reivich M, Hurtig HI (eds): *Cerebrovascular Diseases: Thirteenth Research (Princeton) Conference.* New York: Raven Press, 1983, 13, pp 375–386.
4. Auer LM, Edvinsson L, Johansson BB. Effect of sympathetic nerve stimulation and adrenoceptor blockade on pial arterial and venous calibre and on intracranial pressure in the cat. *Acta Physiol Scand* 1983; 119:213–217.

5. Auer L, Haydn F. Multichannel videoangiometry for continuous measurement of pial microvessels. *Acta Neurol Scand [Suppl]* 1979; 72:208–209.
6. Auer LM, Johansson BB. Pial venous constriction during cervical sympathetic stimulation in the cat. *Acta Physiol Scand* 1980; 110:203–205.
7. Auer LM, Johansson BB. Cervical sympathetic nerve stimulation decreases intracranial pressure in the cat. *Acta Physiol Scand* 1981; 113:565–566.
8. Auer LM, Johansson BB, Lund S. Reaction of pial arteries and veins to sympathetic stimulation in the cat. *Stroke* 1981; 12:528–531.
9. Auer LM, Kuschinsky W, Johansson BB, et al. Sympathoadrenergic influence on pial veins and arteries in the cat. In Heistad DD, Marcus ML (eds): *Cerebral Blood Flow: Effect of Nerves and Neurotransmitters.* New York: Elsevier/North Holland, 1982, pp 291–300.
10. Axel L. Blood flow effects in magnetic resonance imaging. *Am J Roentgenol* 1984; 143:1157–1166.
11. Bar T. The vascular system of the cerebral cortex. *Adv Anat Embryol Cell Biol* 1980; 59:1–62.
12. Benabid AL, Persat JC, deRougemont J, et al. Intracranial pressure: IV. Relationships with postcapillary vascular pressures. *J Physiol* 1978; 74:369–378.
13. Betz AL, Goldstein GW. Polarity of the blood-brain barrier: neutral amino acid transport into isolated brain capillaries. *Science* 1978; 202:225–227.
14. Bradley WG Jr,Waluch V. Blood flow: magnetic resonance imaging. *Radiology* 1985; 154:443–450.
15. Bradley WG Jr, Waluch V, Lai KS, et al. The appearance of rapidly flowing blood on magnetic resonance images. *Am J Roentgenol* 1984; 143:1167–1174.
16. Brightman MW, Reese TS. Junctions between intimately apposed cell membranes in the vertebrate brain. *J Cell Biol* 1969; 40:648–677.
17. Buonanno FS, Moody DM, Ball MR. CT scan findings in cerebral sinovenous occlusion. *Neurology* 1979; 29:1433–1434 (letter).
18. Buonanno FS, Moody DM, Ball MR, et al. Computed cranial tomographic findings in cerebral sinovenous occlusion. *J Comput Assist Tomogr* 1978; 2:281–290.
19. Edvinsson L, Högestätt ED, Uddman R, et al. Cerebral veins: fluorescence histochemistry, electron microscopy, and in vitro reactivity. *J Cereb Blood Flow Metab* 1983; 3:266–230.
20. Edvinsson L, McCulloch J, Uddman R. Feline cerebral veins and arteries: comparison of autonomic innervation and vasomotor responses. *J Physiol (Lond)* 1982; 325:161–173.
21. Edvinsson L, McCulloch J, Uddman R. Noradrenaline-, substance P-, and vasoactive intestinal polypeptide-containing nerve fibers and vasomotor responses of cerebral arteries and veins. In Heistad DD, Marcus ML (eds): *Cerebral Blood Flow: Effects of Nerves and Neurotransmitters.* New York: Elsevier/North Holland, 1982, pp 219–222.
22. Fenstermacher JD, Davson H. Distribution of two model amino acids from cerebrospinal fluid to brain and blood. *Am J Physiol* 1982; 242:F171–F180.
23. Forbes HS, Cobb SS. Vasomotor control of cerebral vessels. *Brain* 1938; 61:221–233.
24. George B, Sainte-Rose C, Sindou M, et al. Lateral sinus reconstructive surgery: treatment of intracranial hypertension by venous anastomosis. *Neurol Res* 1984; 6:203–206.
25. Iwabuchi T, Sobata E, Suzuki M, et al. Dural sinus pressure as related to neurosurgical positions. *Neurosurgery* 1983; 12:203–207.
26. Iwabuchi T, Tsubakisaka H. Letter to the Editor. *Neurosurgery* 1983; 13:473.
27. Kaplan HA. Results of obliteration of specific cerebral veins and dural venous sinuses: animal and human studies. In Kapp JP, Schmidek HH (eds): *The Cerebral Venous System and Its Disorders.* New York: Grune & Stratton, 1984, pp 275–282.
28. Kaplan HA, Browder J. Neurological consideration of some features of the cerebral dural sinuses and their tributaries. *Clin Neurosurg* 1976; 23:155–169.
29. Kapp JP. Nonseptic venous occlusive disease. In Wilkins RH, Rengachary SS (eds): *Neurosurgery.* New York: McGraw-Hill, 1985, pp 1300–1307.
30. Kapp JP, Gielchinsky I, Deardourff SL. Operative techniques for management of lesions involving the dural venous sinuses. *Surg Neurol* 1977; 7:339–342.
31. Kapp J, Paulson G. The nature of the cerebrospinal fluid-brain barrier and its response to circulatory arrest: I. The effect of circulatory arrest on the movement of cerebrospinal sodium into brain. *Neurology* 1967; 17:720–723.
32. Kapp JP, Schmidek HH (eds). *The Cerebral Venous System and Its Disorders.* New York: Grune & Stratton, 1984.
33. Lajtha A, Toth J. The brain barrier system: III. The efflux of intracerebrally administered amino acids from the brain. *J Neurochem* 1962; 9:199–212.
34. Levin E, Sepulveda FV, Yudilevich DL. Pial vessel transport of substances from cerebrospinal fluid to blood. *Nature* 1974; 249:266–267.
35. Macchi PJ, Grossman RI, Gomori JM, et al. High field MR imaging of cerebral venous thrombosis. *J Comput Assist Tomogr* 1986; 10:10–15.
36. MacKenzie ET, Young AR, Stewart M, et al. Effect of serotonin on cerebral function, metabolism and circulation. *Acta Neurol Scand [Suppl]* 1977; 64:76–77.
37. McCord FB, Shields MD, McNeil A, et al. Cerebral arteriovenous malformation in a neonate: treatment by embolisation. *Arch Dis Child* 1987; 62:1273–1275.
38. McCulloch J, Edvinsson L, Watt P. Comparison of the effects of potassium and pH on the calibre of cerebral veins and arteries. *Pflugers Arch* 1982; 393:95–98.
39. Mellander S, Johansson B. Control of resistance, exchange, and capacitance functions in the peripheral circulation. *Pharmacol Rev* 1968; 20:117–196.
40. Mickle JP, Quisling RG. The transtorcular embolization of vein of Galen aneurysms. *J Neurosurg* 1986; 64:731–735.
41. Nakagawa Y, Tsuru M, Yada K. Site and mechanism for compression of the venous system during experimental intracranial hypertension. *J Neurosurg* 1974; 41:427–434.
42. Needell WM, Maravilla KR. MR flow imaging in vascular malformations using gradient recalled acquisition. *Am J Neuroradiol* 1988; 9:637–642.
43. Nelson M, Dickinson DF, Wilson N. Transtorcular coil embolisation of malformations of the vein of Galen: rapid resolution of heart failure in neonates. *Int J Cardiol* 1988; 18:437–441.
44. Pape LG, Katzman R. ^{42}K distribution in brain during simultaneous ventriculocisternal and subarachnoid perfusion. *Brain Res* 1972; 38:49–69.
45. Paulson G, Kapp JP. Movement of sodium-22, radioiodinated protein, and tritiated water from the cisterna magna into the cerebrovascular circulation. *J Neurosurg* 1967; 27:138–141.
46. Povlishock JT, Levine JE. Cerebrospinal fluid absorption. In Kapp JP, Schmidek HH (eds): *The Cerebral Venous System and Its Disorders.* New York: Grune & Stratton, 1984, pp 251–274.
47. Rao KCVG, Knipp HC, Wagner EJ. Computed tomographic findings in cerebral sinus and venous thrombosis. *Radiology* 1981; 140:391–398.
48. Roggendorf W, Cervós-Navarro J, Lazaro-Lacalle MD. Ultrastructure of venules in the cat brain. *Cell Tissue Res* 1978; 192:461–474.
49. Ross JS, Masaryk TJ, Haucke EM, et al. MR angiography furnishes detailed vascular images. *Diagn Imaging* 1988; 10:96–103.
50. Schmidek HH, Auer LM, Kapp JP. The cerebral venous system. *Neurosurgery* 1985; 17:663–678.
51. Sekhar LN, Sen CN, Jho HD, et al. Surgical treatment of intracavernous neoplasms: a four-year experience. *Neurosurgery* 1989; 24:18–30.
52. Sindou M, Mercier P, Bokor J, et al. Bilateral thrombosis of the transverse sinuses: microsurgical revascularization with venous bypass. *Surg Neurol* 1980; 13:215–220.
53. Smith RR, Sanford RA. Disorders of the deep cerebral veins. In Kapp JP, Schmidek HH (eds): *The Cerebral Venous System and Its Disorders.* New York: Grune & Stratton, 1984, pp 547–555.

54. Southwick FS, Richardson EP Jr, Swartz MN. Septic thrombosis of the dural venous sinuses. *Medicine (Baltimore)* 1986; 65:82–106.
55. Sze G, Simmons B, Krol G, et al. Dural sinus thrombosis: verification with spin-echo techniques. *Am J Neuroradiol* 1988; 9:679–686.
56. Takahashi M. Electron microscopic study of the intracranial veins of rats. *Kaibogaku Zasshi* 1968; 43:238–254.
57. Ulrich K, Auer LM, Kuschinsky W. Cat pial venoconstriction by topical microapplication of norepinephrine. *J Cereb Blood Flow Metab* 1982; 2:109–111.
58. Virapongse C, Cazenave C, Quisling R, et al. The empty delta sign: frequency and significance in 76 cases of dural sinus thrombosis. *Radiology* 1987; 162:779–785.
59. Wehrli FW, Shimakawa A, MacFall JR, et al. MR imaging of venous and arterial flow by a selective saturation-recovery spin echo (SSRSE) method. *J Comput Asssist Tomogr* 1985; 9:537–545.
60. White EM, Edelman RR, Wedeen VJ, et al. Intravascular signal in MR imaging: use of phase display for differentiation of blood-flow signal from intraluminal disease. *Radiology* 1986; 161:245–249.
61. Wolfson LI, Katzman R, Escriva A. Clearance of amine metabolites from the cerebrospinal fluid: the brain as a ''sink.'' *Neurology* 1974; 24:772–779.
62. Yamato S, Higashi S, Fujii H. Vasomotor response in acute increased intracranial pressure. Presented at the Fifth International Symposium on Intracranial Pressure. Tokyo, 1982.
63. Zhu YH, Kirsch WM, Cushman R, et al. Comparison of suture and clip for microvascular anastomoses. *Surg Forum* 1985; 36:492–495.

SECTION B

Occlusive Cerebrovascular Disease

198

Pathophysiologic Consequences of Brain Ischemia

Jewell L. Osterholm
Glenn D. Frazer

A number of diseases may result in ischemia of the brain. Although stroke is usually first to come to mind, other emergency clinical syndromes such as cardiac arrest, severe shock, cerebral or subarachnoid hemorrhage, cerebral trauma, and elevated intracranial pressure due to a neoplasm may all result to some degree in cerebral ischemia. Common to all of these clinical abnormalities is a reduction of cerebral blood flow below levels that are sufficient to maintain normal cerebral metabolic function.[12]

In the conditions mentioned above, the ischemia may affect blood flow to the whole brain, and therefore is called *global ischemia,* or it may affect blood flow to a localized area, in which case it is termed *focal ischemia.* In addition, the ischemic insult may be characterized by the degree to which blood flow to the brain is reduced. For example, in incomplete ischemia the brain circulation is not totally abolished, resulting in a hypoxic state, whereas complete ischemia implies a total absence of cerebral circulation, resulting in an anoxic state. Another important factor is the duration of ischemia. Short periods of global ischemia may affect only the most vulnerable neurons; as the ischemia is prolonged greater numbers of cells and cell types will be damaged.[25,26] It is important to recognize that the duration of ischemia, the degree of reduced blood flow, and the magnitude of the area of the brain affected are all pertinent variables in this discussion of altered metabolic responses following the insult of cerebral ischemia.

The final outcome of ischemic insult is often unpredictable.[31] There are certain neurophysiological changes, however, that have been found to regularly occur following decreases in cerebral blood flow.[17] The normal cerebral blood flow ranges from 45 to 60 ml/100 g per minute. The blood flow may be reduced to a threshold level of 20 to 25 ml/100 g per minute without affecting EEG activity in a normothermic, lightly anesthetized individual. Below that threshold level, the EEG activity gradually disappears, and at a blood flow of 15 ml/100 g per minute, the evoked electrical cortical response disappears. At cerebral flow rates of approximately 10 to 12 ml/100 g per minute, ion homeostasis is lost. There is a sudden and complete neuronal depolarization with loss of potassium from the cell and an influx of sodium and calcium. This is followed by osmotically driven water uptake and cell swelling.[10]

From several experimental observations there may be two pathophysiologic or thresholds in response to ischemia.[2] Ischemia at the first threshold, which is generally reversible, induces inhibition of synaptic transmission as a result of neurotransmitter depletion. In order to restore the transmitter materials into the synaptic granules, adenosine triphosphate (ATP) is required. Energy depletion therefore results in reuptake failure and synaptic arrest. The second threshold of ischemia is associated with loss of ionic homeostasis leading to structural changes in the neuron such as microtubule and microfilament disassembly and degradation of membrane phospholipids.[30] This results from a lack of high energy phosphates for synthesis, and activation of degradative processes by elevated intracellular calcium and acidosis.[36] This has been viewed as an irreversible state.

Under conditions of rapid circulatory arrest, the brain is more susceptible to injury than other organs because the brain has a high energy requirement, and a relatively low store of high-energy phosphates and oxygen. With a sudden loss of blood flow to the brain, the cellular store of oxygen is depleted and there is an immediate cessation of oxidative phosphorylation, resulting in a rapid decrease in tissue levels of phosphocreatine and adenosine triphosphate.[5] The $NADH^+/NAD$ ratio increases, adenosine diphosphate (ADP), adenosine monophosphate (AMP) and cyclic AMP (cAMP) contents rise, and there is an attendant loss of the cellular energy charge. At this point phosphocreatinine levels fall toward zero as do ATP levels.[16,17,35]

The next metabolic response to ischemia is an activation of cerebral glycolysis, and the available stores of glucose are rapidly utilized. Increased glucose utilization appears to occur even before overt anaerobic metabolism can be detected following mild ischemia. The metabolic trigger for glycolysis, which may reach levels greater than tenfold, is an elevated activity of phosphofructokinase, because this enzyme is upregulated by accumulating levels of ADP. With increases in cerebral norepinephrine levels, as governed by the locus ceruleus, there is a rise in cyclic AMP, which stimulates glycogenolysis. Glycogen is rapidly broken down, as are the available stores of pyruvate NADH [reduced form of nicotinamide-adenine dinucleotide (NAD)], ketone bodies, and α-ketoglutarate.

Lactate accumulates as a consequence of primarily anaerobic metabolism. An increased intracellular hydrogen ion concentration ensues due to the excessive lactate presence. All available glucose, glycogen, and other suitable materials are metabolized to lactate. The actual degree of glycolysis under different ischemic conditions has been related to pathologic, metabolic, and structural reactions.

Experimental animals that were rendered hyperglycemic prior to stroke production did not fare as well as their normoglycemic mates.[32,34] In the high glucose group, the intracellular pH dropped to 6.1 as compared with 6.6 for the other group. The pH difference between the two groups was associated with a disparity in recovery of the EEG, which was substantially delayed in the hyperglycemic group. In a similar study that examined neurological recovery following global ischemia, all hyperglycemic animals died acutely whereas all normoglycemic animals lived. Hypoglycemic animals in the same study also fared badly but did have some survivals.[33] These results have recently been found in a focal model of cerebral ischemia.[40]

A destructive effect has been noted if tissue concentrations of lactate exceed 25 μg/g of tissue. Animals that had cerebral cortex lactate of either 15 or 35 mm/liter were studied. In animals with lower lactate levels, there was considerable recovery of the cellular energy state and electrical activity during recirculation after ischemia. The animals with higher lactate levels, however, had persistent energy failure with no return of electrical activity. The low lactate specimens had minor structural alterations, but the high lactate group had extensive and severe tissue damage. As a result, there is considerable evidence to implicate the degree of tissue lactic acidosis as a prime feature associated with not only the progressively worsening cellular effects but also the development of irreversible ischemic nerve cell injury.[27]

The relationship between pH changes and structural damage requires discussion. Ultrastructural and metabolic changes following total ischemia are less severe than those that occur under conditions of partial blood flow.[24] This apparent contradiction has been explained by the fact that the pH fall is abrupt but not sustained after the tissue glucose pool is exhausted in global ischemia. Partial ischemia, however, provides some glucose trickle so that there is continued accumulation of lactate and hydrogen ions, which reach levels that can be incompatible with cellular survival.[22]

Another sequence of events that occurs with severe ischemia is loss of membrane integrity. Membranes are disturbed both at the intracellular and axonal level. Under normal circumstances, a large amount of total brain energy production is consumed in re-establishing ionic gradients of Na^+ and K^+ after axonal depolarization. ATP is required to pump the ions against a gradient under the influence of the membrane-bound Na^+,K^+-ATPase. The rapid decline of ATP following ischemia makes it impossible to maintain normal ionic movements and gradients.[3] Extracellular K^+ rises from 3.0 mm to 28.5 mm after 4 min of ischemia, and to 48.1 mm in 8 min.[38] Extracellular acidosis is evident at both time points. As potassium leaves the cell, calcium, sodium, and water enter. The glia are also involved in this pathophysiologic process because it has been found that glial nuclei are significantly depleted of potassium as early as 15 s after an ischemic insult.[14] This change is associated with a concomitant and significant drop in high-energy substrates in the glial nuclei as well as the total brain. These observations have important implications in terms of glial swelling, which is commonly associated with postischemic states.

In terms of irreversible cell damage in ischemia, the loss of calcium homeostasis is extremely important. Intracellular calcium is normally highly regulated between 10^{-5} and 10^{-7} mol/liter, and functions as a controller of many cell processes such as enzyme activation and synaptic vesicle release. The intracellular calcium level is regulated by exchange with extracellular sodium (sodium gradient dependent), sequestered by endoplasmic reticulum (ATP dependent) or calmodulin, or taken up by the mitochondria in exchange for H^+, (thus competing with ATP synthesis for respiratory energy). Loss of oxidative metabolism and the subsequent depletion of high energy metabolites and membrane depolarization lead to influx of extracellular calcium and to disabling of normal calcium storage mechanisms, thus elevating intracellular calcium levels. Recovery of ATP synthesis upon restoration of oxygen supply to the tissue is therefore impaired by reuptake of calcium into the mitochondria, which takes precedence over ATP synthesis.[37]

Elevated levels of intracellular calcium can produce damage to the cell membranes because calcium activates phospholipases and stimulates release of free fatty acids (FFAs).[9] The extensive surface area of excitable and intracellular membranes contains a wide variety and quantity of phospholipids. It has been found that immediately after interrupting the blood supply to the brain, a strikingly rapid increase of FFAs takes place.[4] The rate of production of the cerebral FFAs is the same as that observed in adipose tissue under maximal lipolytic hormonal stimulation. It has been postulated that the cascade regulatory process of producing FFAs is mediated by membrane-bound phospholipase A_2. This enzyme is responsible for producing arachidonic acid, docosahexanoic acid, and other unsaturated fatty acids. Also elaborated under this stress are palmitic, stearic, and oleic acids. In the course of experiments using electroshock, FFAs are produced in the brain in a fashion similar to that observed attending ischemia. These data suggest that membrane lipids in the CNS actively deacylate and reacylate long-chain unsaturated fatty acids. An analysis of myelin and mitochondrial lipids from ischemic brain showed a decrease in fatty acid content. The components of decreased fatty acids fractions corresponded well with the types and amounts of FFAs accumulating in the ischemic brain. An important consequence of the increased FFA production is an impairment of cerebral energy functions.[19] These materials play an important role in uncoupling oxidative phosphorylation at the respiratory chain. Active ionic transport across plasma membranes is severely affected by the FFAs. The addition of FFAs, glycerol, glycerol phospholipids, and deoxycholate in low concentrations inhibits calcium accumulation in the mitochondria.[39] The accumulation of calcium ions in the brain mitochondria is decreased by 35 percent after ischemia. Thus, increased FFAs impair brain function by (1) disturbing ionic transport across plasma membranes, and (2) by uncoupling oxidative phosphorylation at the respiratory chain level.

The main FFA believed to have toxic properties is arachidonic acid. Increased arachidonic acid leads to increased production of prostaglandins E_2 and $F_{2\alpha}$. Prostaglandin formation via cyclooxygenase requires a precursor fatty acid to be in free form and is substrate limited. Prostaglandin synthesis leads to the generation of free radicals and endoperoxides that can initiate lipid peroxidation.[18]

During normal electron transport various partial oxidation productions possessing single unpaired electrons, termed *free radicals,* are formed through the action of molecular oxygen on membrane proteins.[31] A constant level of free radical oxidation reactions, or peroxidation, is normally maintained in the cell through a delicate balance of activators to inhibitors of these reactions. A major peroxidation activator is molecular oxygen, but the partially reduced superoxide, perhydroxyradicals also contribute to peroxidation, as do the partially degraded fatty acid moieties. Endogenous peroxidation inhibitors include certain intracellular enzymes, such as catalase and superoxide dismutase as well as antioxidants such as ubiquinone, ascorbic acid, α-tocopherol, and glutathione. A change in the relationship of the optimum ratio of catalyst to inhibitors leads to development of pathologic changes. An example of this would be a marked decrease in antioxidant tissue ability, since this would cause an accumulation of free radicals and specific degradation products of peroxidation that constitute disruptive influences.

Associated with ischemia is an alteration in the proteins of the electron transport chain, producing a state of excessive reduced membrane proteins capable of reacting pathologically with residual tissue oxygen to produce additional free radicals. Membrane disruption also follows as the pathological free radicals react with the unsaturated fatty acid moieties of the phospholipids which comprise the major portions of the cellular membranes, particularly those of the cellular organelles such as mitochondria. Disruptions of the membrane phospholipids may sufficiently damage the physiochemical state so as to alter ion selectivity and disturb functional capability of the membrane itself. An end result of this pathologic chain reaction is an irreversible injury of the inner membrane of mitochondria. With pH decreased because of increases in acidic metabolites and the breakdown of functional proteins, ATP net synthesis is no longer possible.

Ischemia also causes substantial disruption of amino acid metabolism.[20,28] During the first minute of ischemia there is an accelerated α-ketoglutarate consumption, and a marked increase in γ-aminobutyric acid (GABA) levels. Within 4 min pyruvate levels are decreased, which subsequently affects the glutamate and alanine levels. Glutamate is remarkably increased during anoxia. This accumulation can be explained in the following way:

1. The utilization of glutamate as an oxidative substrate may be inhibited during ischemia.
2. Nucleotides may stimulate the synthesis of glutamate using the increased levels of ammonia available.
3. Glutamate content may be increased as a result of enhanced glutamine decay.
4. Glutamate release from presynaptic stores is enhanced by elevated intracellular calcium levels.
5. Neural and glial reuptake mechanisms which are energy dependent are impaired.

The elevation in extracellular glutamate then activates postsynaptic receptors that enhance calcium influx into the postsynaptic neuron. This is the basic mechanism for enhanced vulnerability to ischemia in those cells with high densities of glutamate receptors, such as the CA1 cells of the hippocampus and Purkinje's cells of the cerebellum.[29]

There is a late accumulation of cystine, proline, methionine, cystidine, tryptophan, and tyrosine while lysine and phenylalanine decline. A hallmark chemical change in ischemia is an increased ammonia production in cerebral tissue. The ammonia may originate from glutamine, nucleotide, or protein amide groups. It is theorized that a decrease in the amount of glutamine early in ischemia is caused by a deamidation of this product.

Regional protein synthesis was measured at intervals of up to 48 h after cerebral ischemia of 10 or 30 min duration.[8] One hour following the 10-min ischemia period protein synthesis, as measured by incorporation of [^{14}C]valine into protein, was inhibited by 67 percent. However, protein synthesis at normal rates was achieved within 4 h of recirculation. In animals subjected to longer ischemic periods, protein synthesis was inhibited by 83 percent during the first hour. Thereafter protein synthesis recovery was slow and required 25 to 48 h for restitution. ^{14}C autoradiography revealed that pyramidal neurons and neurons in the hippocampus and caudate nucleus failed to recover normal protein synthesis rates even after 48 h of recovery.[7]

In addition to the excitatory amino acid transmitters glutamate and asparate, other neurotransmitters are affected by ischemia and may play roles in the pathophysiology of cerebral ischemia. Serotonin (5-hydroxytryptamine) is implicated in cerebral edema, as shall be discussed below. Dopamine and norepinephrine have been reported to have an increased turnover during the first 2 h following ischemia.[6] Norepinephrine probably activates adenyl cyclase to elevate cyclic AMP, resulting in early metabolic changes in ischemia. It has been found that electrical stimulation of the locus ceruleus triggers an induction of cyclic AMP throughout the ipsilateral hemisphere.[11] One important function of cyclic AMP under these conditions is to stimulate glycogen breakdown and hence initiate improved glycolysis as the first line of metabolic defense against ischemia. Dopamine fibers have been found to be most sensitive to ischemia and are damaged by mild degrees of ischemia that are well tolerated by other cells.

A major pathophysiologic change that occurs after ischemia is tissue edema.[1] Cerebral edema has been categorized into cytotoxic and vasogenic types, and is defined by an abnormal water accumulation associated with increase in brain tissue volume.[15] Cytotoxic edema involves primarily the parenchymal structural elements that are affected directly by noxious chemical factors, resulting in intracellular swelling, whereas vasogenic edema causes an increase mainly in extracellular water content. Early in the course of ischemia the predominant edema type is almost purely cytotoxic. Cytotoxic edema is associated with sodium entering the cell and potassium escaping into the extracellular compartment. Water follows the intracellular movement of sodium, resulting in tissue edema. Vasogenic edema becomes prominent at a later stage of cerebral ischemia and coincides primarily with the reflow period. During restoration of the cerebral blood flow there is an accelerated leakage of plasma constituents from the blood due to damage of the blood-brain barrier. After short periods of ischemia a prompt restoration of cerebral blood flow drastically reduces the degree of brain edema. Following longer periods of ischemia, however, the return of cerebral blood flow enhances greatly the degree of vasogenic cerebral edema.

A better understanding of the mechanism of cerebral edema that occurs after ischemic insult has been obtained through biochemical investigations.[21] For example, the liberation of FFAs from nervous tissue has been linked with tissue edema in postischemic states.[4] Experimental studies involving intracerebral injection of various polyunsaturated fatty acids indicate that these substances are capable of producing tissue edema. When injected into the brain, arachidonic acid, which has been identified in the brain after ischemia, can result in severe edema similar to that seen after stroke. This is most likely due to free radical production in the cerebral vessels. Superoxide, a free radical product of either cyclooxygenase or xanthine oxidase has been detected in endothelial and smooth muscle cells of cerebral arterioles following ischemia. It is associated with leakage of serum albumin into the tissue.

Blockage of the permeability defect can be achieved by pretreatment with enzymes that remove superoxide, namely superoxide dismutase and catalase. Chelation of iron also reduces vascular permeability increases after ischemia thus indicating a role for the hydroxyl radical in the process.[23]

A complex cascade of pathophysiologic events attending cerebral ischemia has been described. During the initial ischemia stages glycolysis is preserved through the breakdown of glycogen to glucose under the influence of catecholamines and cyclic AMP. Ketone bodies may also be utilized during this period. Under these anaerobic conditions the end metabolic product is lactate. The prolongation of glycolytic anaerobic metabolism is detrimental due to the formation of lactate. The high tissue lactate level lowers intracellular pH and may contribute to irreversible cerebral injury following an ischemic insult. The continued progress of glycolysis obtained during incomplete ischemia is more harmful to the cerebral tissues than is complete circulatory arrest. In the latter conditions all the metabolites are utilized quickly, thereby preventing the accumulation of the excessive lactate and the decline of intracellular pH. After cellular energy stores are exhausted, ionic membrane pumps fail, with an attendant dislocation of ionic components and the production of cytotoxic edema. After activation of phospholipases by elevated intracellular calcium, fatty acids accumulate as degradation materials from the phospholipid membrane walls. In the presence of large quantities of fatty acids the pathologic changes that occur include the formation of vasogenic edema, increased synthesis of the prostaglandins, and disturbances of the mitochondrial membranes. There are also changes in the physical state of the proteins themselves. Free-radical induced lipid peroxidation can, under some circumstances, be initiated, and the consequences of this reaction have been discussed. The central issue of reversibility versus irreversibility probably hangs on a complex number of factors. The most important factors are the degree of intracellular acidosis, the elevation in intracellular calcium, the presence or absence of continued anaerobic metabolism, and the relative integrity of the mitochondrial and cellular membranes.

At this time there is extensive experimental evidence to support the contention that neurons can survive ischemia for extended periods under very specific conditions. Resuscitation has been obtained in vivo after global ischemia of 1-h duration.[13] We found that in brain slices in vitro following ischemia, the brain slices would reinitiate uptake of glucose and norepinephrine after as long as 4 h of ischemia when they were resupplied with glucose and oxygen. Stroke therapy will be improved when methods are designed to effectively control intracellular pH levels, to resupply the neurons within their limits of ischemia tolerance, and to reextablish the blood supply.

References

1. Abe K, Abe T, Klatzo I, Spatz M. Effect of endogenous central nervous system depressants in ischemic cerebral edema of gerbils. *Adv Neurol* 1980; 28:429–441.
2. Astrup J. Energy-requiring cell functions in the ischemic brain: their critical supply and possible inhibition in protective therapy. *J Neurosurg* 1982; 56:482–497.
3. Astrup J, Rehncrona S, Siesjö BK. The increase in extracellular potassium concentration in the ischemic brain in relation to the preischemic functional activity and cerebral metabolic rate. *Brain Res* 1980; 199:161–174.
4. Bazan NG, Rodriguez de Turco EB. Membrane lipids in the pathogenesis of brain edema: phospholipids and arachidonic acid, the earliest membrane components changed at the onset of ischemia. *Adv Neurol* 1980; 28:197–205.
5. Benzi G, Dagani F, Arrigoni E. Acute model for the estimation of the cerebral energy state during or after hypoxia and complete or incomplete ischaemia. *Eur Neurol* 1978; 17 (Suppl I):87–96.
6. Bralet J, Beley P, Bralet AM, Beley A. Catecholamine levels and turnover during brain ischemia in the rat. *J Neural Transm* 1980; 48:143–155.
7. Diemer NH, Siemkowicz E. Increased 2-deoxyglucose uptake in hippocampus, globus pallidus and substantia nigra after cerebral ischemia. *Acta Neurol Scand* 1980; 61:56–63.
8. Dienel GA, Pulsinelli WA, Duffy TE. Regional protein synthesis in rat brain following acute hemispheric ischemia. *J Neurochem* 1980; 35:1216–1226.
9. Edgar AD, Strosznajder J, Horrocks LA. Activation of ethanolamine phospholipase Az in brain during ischemia. *J Neurochem* 1982; 39:1111–1116.
10. Hansen AJ. Effect of anoxia on ion distribution in the brain. *Physiol Rev* 1985; 65:101–148.
11. Harik SI, Busto R, Martinez E. Norepinephrine regulation of cerebral glycogen utilization during seizures and ischemia. *J Neurosci* 1982; 2:409–414.
12. Heiss WD. Experimental evidence of ischemic thresholds and functional recovery. *Stroke* 1992; 23:1668–1672.
13. Hossmann KA, Sato K. Recovery of neuronal function after prolonged cerebral ischemia. *Science* 1970; 168:375–376.
14. Ignelzi RJ. Sodium, potassium, and metabolic studies of glial, liver, and kidney nuclei under anoxic-ischemic conditions. *Neurol Res* 1980; 2:35–46.
15. Ito U, Ohno K, Nakamura R, et al. Brain edema during ischemia and after restoration of blood flow: measurement of water, sodium, potassium content and plasma protein permeability. *Stroke* 1979; 10:542–547.
16. Keykhah MM, Welsh FA, Miller AS, et al. Cerebral energy metabolite levels and survival following exposure to low inspired oxygen concentration. *Crit Care Med* 1978; 6:330–334.
17. Kogure K, Scheinberg P, Utsunomiya Y, et al. Sequential cerebral biochemical and physiological events in controlled hypoxemia. *Ann Neurol* 1977; 2:304–310.
18. Kontos HA, Wei EP, Povlishock JT, et al. Cerebral arteriolar damage by arachidonic acid and prostaglandin G2. *Science* 1980; 209:1242–1245.
19. Kuwashima J, Nakamura K, Fujitani B, et al. Relationship between cerebral energy failure and free fatty acid accumulation following prolonged brain ischemia. *Jpn J Pharmacol* 1978; 28:277–287.
20. Melitauri NN, Chikvaidze VN, Nikolaishvili LN. Change in the content of free amino acids in the brain of rabbits under circulatory hypoxia (ischemia). *Neuropatol Pol* 1979; 3:379–389.
21. Mršulja BB, Djuričić BM, Cvejić V, et al. Biochemistry of experimental ischemic brain edema. *Adv Neurol* 1980; 28:217–230.
22. Nakai H, Yamamoto YL, Diksic M, et al. Triple-tracer autoradiography demonstrates effects of hyperglycemia on cerebral blood flow, pH, and glucose utilization in cerebral ischemia of rats. *Stroke* 1988; 19:764–772.
23. Nelson CW, Wei EP, Povlishock JT, et al. Oxygen radicals in cerebral ischemia. *Am J Physiol* 1992; 263:H1356–H1362.
24. Nordstrom C, Siesjö B. Influence of phenobarbital on changes in the metabolites of the energy reserve of the cerebral cortex following complete ischemia. *Acta Physiol Scand* 1978; 104:271–280.
25. Pulsinelli WA. Selective neuronal vulnerability: morphological and molecular characteristics. *Prog Brain Res* 1985; 63:29–37.
26. Pulsinelli WA, Brierley JB, Plum F. Temporal profile of neuronal damage in a model of transient forebrain ischemia. *Ann Neurol* 1982; 11:491–498.
27. Rehncrona S, Rosen I, Siesjö BK. Excessive cellular acidosis: an important mechanism of neuronal damage in the brain? *Acta Physiol Scand* 1980; 110:435–437.
28. Rossowska M, Zalewska T. Effect of hypoxia and ischemia on the

distribution of protein in brain cellular fractions. *Neurochem Res* 1979; 4:15–23.
29. Rothman SM, Olney JW. Glutamate and the pathophysiology of hypoxic-ischemic brain damage. *Ann Neurol* 1986; 19:105–111.
30. Schlaepfer WW, Zimmerman UJ. Mechanisms underlying the neuronal response to ischemic injury: calcium-activated proteolysis of neurofilaments. *Prog Brain Res* 1985; 63:185–196.
31. Shaller CA, Jacques S, Shelden CH. The pathophysiology of stroke: a review with molecular considerations. *Surg Neurol* 1980; 14:433–443.
32. Siemkowicz E, Gjedde A. Post-ischemic coma in rat: effect of different pre-ischemic blood glucose levels on cerebral metabolic recovery after ischemia. *Acta Physiol Scand* 1980; 110:225–232.
33. Siemkowicz E, Hansen AJ. Clinical restitution following cerebral ischemia in hypo-, normo- and hyperglycemic rats. *Acta Neurol Scand* 1978; 58:1–8.
34. Siemkowicz E, Hansen AJ. Brain extracellular ion composition and EEG activity following 10 minutes ischemia in normo- and hyperglycemic rats. *Stroke* 1981; 12:236–240.
35. Siesjö BK. *Brain Energy Metabolism.* New York, Wiley, 1978.
36. Siesjö BK. Pathophysiology and treatment of focal cerebral ischemia. Part 1. Pathophysiology. *J Neurosurg* 1992; 77:169–184.
37. Siesjö BK, Wieloch T. Molecular mechanisms of ischemic brain damage: Ca^{2+}-related events. In Plum F, Pulsinelli WA (eds): *Cerebrovascular Diseases,* Fourteenth Research (Princeton-Williamsburg) Conference. New York: Raven Press, 1985, pp 187–200.
38. Silver IA. Changes in PO_2 and ion fluxes in cerebral hypoxia-ischemia. *Adv Exp Med Biol* 1977; 78:299–312.
39. Strosznajder J. Role of phospholipids in calcium accumulation in brain mitchondria from adult rat after ischemic anoxia and hypoxic hypoxia. *Bull Acad Pol Sci [Biol]* 1980; 27:683–692.
40. Yip PK, He YY, Hsu CY, et al. Effect of plasma glucose on infarct size in focal cerebral ischemia-reperfusion. *Neurology* 1991; 41:899–905.

199 Atherosclerosis

Julio H. Garcia
Jack C. Geer

Definition of the Problem

Transient malfunction of the central nervous system or cell necrosis therein, associated with vascular lesions may involve any of a growing number of vascular diseases, atherosclerosis is the most common one. A precise diagnosis of the probable causative vascular lesion is essential before therapeutic or preventive interventions can be attempted. Vascular lesions affecting the brain can be localized to one or more of four anatomic locations: carotid arteries, vertebral arteries, intracranial arteries, and microvessels. The lesions of atherosclerosis are primarily found in the large and medium-size vessels: carotids, vertebrals, and medium-size intracranial arteries. In contrast, intraparenchymal vessels (small arteries and arterioles) are most commonly affected by a degenerative process of the tunica muscularis, generally known as arteriolosclerosis.[14]

Natural History of Cerebral Atherosclerosis

The clinically significant lesion of atherosclerosis evolves over a period of decades at a specific site in the arterial wall: the inner coat or tunica intima.[17,34] Small lipid deposits, predominantly cholesteryl esters, are seen in the aorta early in the first decade of life. These lesions, which appear as grossly visible yellow streaks or dots, are called *fatty streaks.* The extent of aortic fatty streaks increases with age. Coronary artery fatty streaks appear early in the second decade of life and also increase in size and number with age. Fatty streaks are considered incapable of producing symptoms.

The *plaque lesions* of atherosclerosis appear in the middle of the third decade of life in both the aorta and coronary arteries. With age, plaque lesions increase variably in number and size in the aorta, and coronary, carotid, vertebral, cerebral, and femoral arteries. The variability depends on genetic and risk factors. The plaque lesions are significant because they may cause disease by giving rise to critical stenosis, local thrombosis, embolism, or weakening the wall of the artery with aneurysm formation. Atheromatous plaques consist of a core of lipid-rich debris (atheroma) covered on the luminal side by a layer of collagen and collagen-producing smooth muscle cells.[7,12] Plaques often become ''complicated'' with the passage of time. Complications of atherosclerosis include calcification; vascularization originating from the tunica adventitia (vasa vasorum)[1,4]; hemorrhage from the vasa vasorum; ulceration of the endothelium and underlying collagen wall, causing hemorrhage into the plaque; and thrombosis secondary to plaque ulceration. Diseases attributed to atherosclerosis are thought to be associated with plaques causing critical lumen stenosis, complete arterial occlusion due to thrombosis, or distal embolism of either fibrin thrombi or atheromatous material.

The lesions of atherosclerosis begin their evolution in the carotid, vertebral, and intracranial arteries later in life than do the morphologically identical lesions in the aorta and coronary arteries. Fatty streaks and plaques first appear in the cranial arteries in the fourth decade of life. The rate of progression for fatty streaks and plaques is much slower in the vertebral and intracranial arteries than in the carotid arteries. Each arterial bed has predictable sites of plaque development. In the internal carotid artery those sites are the bulb and siphon. In the vertebral arteries it is the portion of the vessel adjacent to the arches of the vertebral bodies. The branching points in the circle of Willis and the entire length of the basilar artery are the sites where atheromatous plaques most frequently appear in the intracranial arteries.

Risk Factors

Certain characteristics of persons with symptomatic atherosclerosis tend to distinguish them from others of similar age and gender who do not have atherosclerotic disease. The natural history of the atherosclerotic lesions, presented briefly above, tells us that those with and those without disease have atherosclerotic arteries. What distinguishes persons with disease from those without it is the extent of the plaque lesions, the location of the lesions, the degree of arterial occlusion, and the types of plaque complications. The personal characteristics associated with symptomatic atherosclerosis are referred to as *risk factors.* For atherosclerosis (carotid or otherwise) these risk factors include advanced age, family history, male gender, arterial hypertension, diabetes mellitus, cigarette smoking, low levels of high-density serum lipoprotein, and high levels of serum cholesterol (low-density lipoprotein), uric acid, fibrinogen, and factor VIII. Obesity and hypertriglyceridemia are more controversial risk factors for complicated atherosclerosis.

Risk factors are primarily general conditions affecting the body as a whole, yet the arterial beds are selectively affected. Within each bed there are sites of increased susceptibility to the atherosclerotic process.[30] Thus, local differences at these arterial sites must be responsible for the increased susceptibility. The nature of these differences is unknown. Some authors have attempted to relate certain risk factors to specific arterial sites. Arterial hypertension, cigarette smoking, and high serum fibrinogen levels tend to be more common with symptomatic carotid atherosclerosis than with atherosclerosis in other arteries.[35,37] However, the predictive power of this tendency is insufficient to be useful in diagnosis.

Although there are discrepancies in the extent of atherosclerosis between two separate vascular beds, there are also some close correlations. Symptomatic carotid atherosclerosis correlates well with coronary atherosclerosis; if the carotid lesions are either extensive or advanced, those in the coronary arteries are likely to be so.[8,20,21,31] Some recent publications report a reciprocal relationship: The extent and severity of coronary atherosclerosis predict the extent and severity of carotid artery lesions. This information is useful only in guiding interventional therapy; persons with extensive and occluding carotid plaques are likely to have similar lesions in the coronary arteries, and vice versa.

Significant Carotid Artery Plaques

Carotid artery plaques can be surgically removed by endarterectomy, a procedure that has low morbidity and mortality. The important challenge is to identify carotid lesions whose surgical removal will prevent either transient ischemic attacks or ischemic stroke.[2,3,9,33] The first consideration is the condition of the arteries distal to the carotid bulb lesion. Given arterial patency distal to the site of the internal carotid artery plaque, what characteristics of the lesion predict clinical significance? The most logical possibility is the degree of luminal occlusion.[3,9,13] Narrower arteries are more likely to cause clinical disease. Three double-blind prospective studies compared medical and surgical treatments; they concluded that for selected patients with symptoms of retinal or cerebral ischemic injury in the distribution of high-grade (>80 percent narrowing) internal carotid artery stenosis, carotid endarterectomy can effectively reduce the risk of subsequent ipsilateral cerebral ischemic events.[11,24,28]

A prospective study of 242 asymptomatic persons who did not undergo operation (selected because of a carotid bruit or other risk factor) studied by B-mode ultrasonography over a mean of 27.4 months revealed that the annual "stroke rate" correlates with high-grade stenosis (>80 percent); the progression of carotid atherosclerosis correlates well with the number of transient ischemic attacks and ischemic stroke, but these events almost uniformly occur on the contralateral side and develop abruptly and independently of changes in the carotid artery lesion.[5]

Some morphologic studies of carotid endarterectomy specimens suggested that plaque characteristics such as ulceration and intraplaque hemorrhage with or without thrombus formation could be the determinant factors in causing symptoms.[2,33] Angiography has been demonstrated to be an unreliable tool for determining carotid artery ulceration,[10,32] whereas B-mode ultrasonography detects plaque hemorrhage and ulceration with considerable accuracy. However, neither characteristic has been a powerful predictor of clinical significance.[3,6,23] The problem that appears so simple, mainly occlusion reducing distal blood flow to a critical level or plaque ulceration causing embolization or occlusive thrombus formation, may be far more complex. In recent reports, elevated serum fibrinogen and interleukin-6 levels have been associated with ischemic stroke; this finding suggests that changes in the microvasculature distal to the site of the atheromatous plaques may play a role in the pathogenesis of ischemic necrosis. The challenge is to determine whether the observed increase in fibrinogen and interleukin-6 is an effect or a cause of the ischemic stroke. Further studies are needed to assess the role of risk factors and coagulation factors in carotid narrowing, plaque ulceration, and plaque composition to identify a sufficiently powerful predictor of disease to warrant interventional therapy.

Vertebral and Intracranial Artery Lesions

The pathogenesis of lesions in these arteries has been studied far less often than that of lesions in the carotid bulb. There is a strong association between intracranial artery atherosclerosis and systemic hypertension. Early recognition and effective therapy of arterial hypertension might retard or prevent the development of plaques in the intracranial arteries. The widespread treatment of arterial hypertension, started several years ago, may explain the reduction in stroke incidence observed over the past 2 decades.[22]

There is no reason to believe that the pathogenesis of a brain infarct associated with a vertebral or intracranial artery plaque lesion differs from that associated with a carotid plaque; however, there is no evidence that carotid and vertebral forms of atherosclerosis follow an identical course. The former statement seems logical, as did narrowing and plaque ulceration for carotid lesions; yet it appears to explain the phenomenon only partially or to be simply untrue.

Atherogenesis

Atherogenesis is characterized by intimal thickening with focal deposition of lipid derived from the blood plasma, smooth muscle cell proliferation, influx of blood monocytes, and connective tissue formation.[12] Two theories attempt to account for the phenomenon.

The *thrombogenic hypothesis* states that thrombi form on the vascular surface, presumably in response to endothelial injury.[29] Subsequently, these thrombi become incorporated into the intima by endothelial overgrowth. The thrombotic material degenerates in the intima, releasing bound lipids and lipid from lipoproteins, thereby yielding the lipid component of the lesion.[7] Smooth muscle cells in the adjacent intima or media proliferate and synthesize connective tissues (collagen and glycosaminoglycans), which are characteristic of the organization (scarring) process. Cholesterol is the predominant lipid constituent of atherosclerotic lesions at all stages of development. If organizing thrombi are the common pathogenetic pathway, it must be assumed that the phospholipids and triglycerides derived from cellular or lipoprotein degeneration are catabolized by smooth muscle cells or blood monocytes that have migrated into the developing lesion. Cholesterol cannot be catabolized by smooth muscle cells and monocytes; thus cholesterol becomes a "foreign body" that must be either removed from the tissue or sequestered.[15] Most students of atherosclerosis do not believe that mural thrombosis and organization represent a common or major mechanism for the fatty streak lesions of atherosclerosis. However, few question that this mechanism commonly increases the mass of atheromatous plaques.

The dominant theory for the initiation and progression of early atherosclerotic lesions is the *filtration* or *insudation hypothesis*. It states that blood plasma constituents traverse the endothelium into the intima, wherein they stimulate cellular proliferative and connective tissue responses that characterize the lesions.

Diffuse Intimal Thickening

Compositional-structural changes in the arterial intima may be a prerequisite to the deposition of blood plasma constituents that are the supposed stimuli for lesion formation. The intima of human arteries progressively thickens with age, up to the fourth decade of life. The components of the thickened intima are smooth muscle cells, glycosaminoglycans, collagens, and elastin. One or more of these components may trap blood plasma constituents that eventually produce the atheromatous core of the lesion and stimulate the cellular and connective tissue reaction. Intimal thickening (commonly referred to as diffuse intimal thickening) has been observed in all human populations.[25] If intimal thickening is necessary for the development of atherosclerosis, we can conclude that all population and racial groups are susceptible to atherosclerosis and will develop the disease if the necessary etiologic factors are imposed. This hypothesis is supported by epidemiologic observations: a population or racial group that migrates from an area or environment with a low incidence of atherosclerotic diseases to one with a high incidence subsequently manifests an increased incidence of atherosclerotic diseases. Evidence indicates that all human populations exposed to the known risk factors for atherosclerosis will develop plaque lesions and atherosclerotic diseases; however, any population shows wide individual variability of the extent to which such lesions develop. We believe that this variability is both genetically and environmentally determined.

Plasma Lipids

Cholesterol is the predominant lipid constituent of the lesions and is derived almost exclusively from the blood plasma.[26] Thus, the amount of cholesterol in the blood may be an etiologic factor for atherogenesis. Plasma cholesterol level correlates positively with atherosclerotic disease on many epidemiologic studies. This correlation has stimulated extensive research on lipoprotein metabolism and diet, which indicates that low-density lipoprotein cholesterol level and dietary cholesterol and saturated fat are significant etiologic factors for atherogenesis. High-density lipoprotein (HDL), particularly HDL-2, appears to have a negative correlation, affording some measure of protection against atherosclerosis. The mechanism for HDL protection remains to be elucidated and proved. HDL may play a role in the removal of cholesterol from tissue, which is necessary because the smooth muscle cells cannot catabolize cholesterol.[18]

Critics of the hypothesis that hypercholesterolemia causes atherogenesis cite the large number of persons with atherosclerotic diseases who do not have hypercholesterolemia or hyperlipidemia of any recognized type. However, commonly used methods of assaying lipoproteins do not detect remnant or variant lipoproteins that are atherogenic and commonly found in serum. These lipoproteins include remnant chylomicrons; partially delipidated, very low density lipoprotein; and heavy low-density lipoprotein. Low levels of the putative protective high-density lipoprotein also could be an atherogenic factor among subjects whose plasma levels of total cholesterol are in the normal range. Current research should clarify the role of remnant or variant lipoproteins in atherogenesis as well as their possible relation to established risk factors for atherosclerosis: diet, smoking, arterial hypertension, diabetes mellitus, and obesity.

Endothelium

The filtration hypothesis requires movement of plasma constituents from the blood compartment across the endothelium and into the intimal compartment. Endothelial injury causing increased permeability may contribute to atherogenesis by increasing influx into the intima of plasma constituents, which in turn stimulate the cellular and connective tissue responses. Most attention has been directed to lipid influx because of the large amount of lipid that accumulates in the lesions. Other plasma constituents that may also contribute to the intimal cellular and connective reaction include albumin, fibrinogen, apolipoproteins, and globulins.

The mechanism by which plasma constituents are transported across the endothelium remains unelucidated. Endothelial injury and the resultant increased permeability could have several causes, among which are hemodynamic stress and vasoactive substances. The injury could alter the endothelial glycocalyx and cause platelet adhesion. Platelets may then aggregate and release vasoactive substances, such as thromboxane A_2, serotonin, or cationic protein, that increase endothelial permeability. Endothelial cell injury also could decrease prostacyclin formation, which would permit platelet adhesion and aggregation.[27] These mechanisms are speculative and must be substantiated. A curious phenomenon occurs in an experimental model in which the vascular endothelium is removed by balloon catheter; in the presence of induced hyperlipidemia, arterial intimal lipid deposition occurs only after the endothelium regenerates.

Infectious-immune causes of endothelial or intimal cellular reactive changes have been suggested.[19] Chickens with Marek virus infection develop arterial lesions. Hyperlipidemic rabbits with serum sickness develop arterial plaques that closely resemble those of human beings. Vasectomized monkeys develop more arterial lesions than do normal monkeys. Transplanted hearts are more likely to develop atherosclerosis than are normal hearts. These observations suggest the possibilities of virus-induced cellular change and immune complex injury. Immune complexes may fix complement on the endothelium, thereby causing increased cell permeability or cell death. That infectious-immune mechanisms are major and common etiologic factors for atherogenesis is difficult to reconcile with available epidemiologic data for atherosclerosis, unless infection susceptibility and immune responses can be related to diet, hypertension, and other established risk factors for atherosclerosis.

Smooth Muscle Cells

Smooth muscle cells, monocyte-derived macrophages, and mast cells are found in atherosclerotic lesions. Smooth muscle cells are predominant in most human lesions, whereas mast cells are present in small number. The role of mast cells in atherogenesis is unknown. Smooth muscle cells in diffuse intimal thickening, fatty streaks, and plaques are thought to be derived from medial smooth muscle cells that migrate into the intima. Smooth muscle cells in the intima increase in number by mitotic division. Intimal smooth muscle cells accumulate cytoplasmic lipid and synthesize connective tissues.

Stimuli for smooth muscle cell proliferation in vitro include a platelet-derived growth factor and low-density lipoprotein. Whether these substances react similarly in vivo remains to be determined. Yet-unidentified plasma- and cell-derived mitogenic substances may be involved.

Smooth muscle cells in atherosclerotic lesions perform at least two functions: storage of intracellular lipid and synthesis of connective tissue. Smooth muscle cells may acquire numbers of cytoplasmic lipid inclusions that presumably contain cholesteryl esters. Cellular and extracellular lipid accumulation suggests the possibility of abnormal lipid metabolism in the arterial wall as an etiologic or pathogenic factor for atherogenesis. Esterification of cholesterol appears to be a normal or protective reaction by cells in the artery wall; nonesterified cholesterol, which is potentially membrane-damaging, is changed to biologically inert cholesteryl esters.[16] Lipid composition studies of atherosclerotic lesions provide little support for the abnormal metabolism hypothesis. However, future studies may reveal effects on cellular integrity and function by lysosomal enzymes, hydroxy fatty acids, prostaglandins, oxidant injury, or leukotrienes.

Monocyte-Macrophage Foam Cell

The role of the monocyte-macrophage in atherogenesis has received recent attention.[15] Foam cells (cells laden with cholesteryl esters) have long been recognized in atherosclerotic lesions. The foam cell is derived from blood monocytes that migrate into the intima and are activated by unknown mechanisms to become macrophages. The identity of the foam cell as a monocyte-macrophage has been established by the demonstration of C3 and Fc membrane receptors, which smooth muscle cells do not possess. The macrophage probably plays a major role in atherogenesis and regression of lesions.[15,16,19] The stimulus for its migration from the blood into the intima is unknown. The activated monocyte (macrophage) has, in addition to its phagocytic property, the capacity to synthesize a wide range of substances, including collagenase, elastase, and platelet-activating factor; many of these are likely involved in atherogenesis. The number of foam cells in experimental lesions induced by diet hyperlipidemia is markedly reduced in lesions that have been allowed to regress by removing the diet stimulus to hyperlipidemia. Normalization of blood lipid level is associated with a marked reduction in the number of intimal foam cells and a sharp reduction in the cholesteryl ester content of the lesion. It is assumed that foam cells migrate from the intima into the blood.

Connective Tissues

Smooth muscle cell–derived connective tissues are major constituents of atherosclerotic lesions. These tissues, particularly collagens, are scar tissue presumably stimulated by intimal deposition of plasma constituents. Connective tissues probably are also involved in binding plasma constituents in the intima. Lipid deposition in the intima could result from increased endothelial permeability (increased load) or impaired transport through the intima. As stated previously, glycosaminoglycans and elastin bind lipoproteins. Binding (trapping) of lipid or other plasma constituents may be a major causative factor for the cellular reactions in the intima. This hypothesis differs in no substantial way from that proposed by Virchow over 100 years ago. The probable role of remnant or variant lipoproteins may be related to connective tissue binding. Future studies of binding of lipoproteins, molecular structure of connective tissues, and cellular reactions to bound lipoproteins should materially advance our knowledge of atherogenesis. Presently developed methods of cell culture, lipoprotein isolation, and connective tissue isolation methods make such studies feasible.

Fibrous Plaques

Causes of and mechanisms by which fatty streaks transform into plaques remain unknown. Indeed, some believe that fatty streaks are not the precursors of plaques. We believe that some fatty streaks progress to plaque lesions, whereas others either remain static or regress. Structural and biochemical studies of fatty streaks have disclosed no differences between fatty streaks from various anatomic locations or population groups that might explain differences in potential. The basic question is: What are the stimuli for plaque formation and increase in plaque mass once the lesion is formed? Previous considerations of atherogenesis all obtain to some degree, but which are the most and least important is unknown.

A hypothetical stimulus for plaque formation is necrosis of lipid-laden intimal cells, releasing lipid and other cellular contents into the interstitial space and thus forming the atheroma that somehow stimulates smooth muscle cell proliferation and connective tissue synthesis in the adjacent tissue. Cellular necrosis can be demonstrated in human lesions, but its role in plaque formation is conjectural. Another hypothesis is smooth muscle transformation, that is, monoclonal proliferation. Studies of glucose-6-phosphate dehydrogenase isozymes in human plaques have shown a single isozyme in the lesions, suggesting monoclonal proliferation, a neoplastic transformation.[36] This interpretation has been questioned and an alternative explanation proposed, that of selective growth potential. Selective growth potential means that cells with one isozyme are more likely to proliferate and thus survive than those with the other isozyme; thus the monoclonicity is apparent but not real.

Once formed, the plaque can increase its volume by several mechanisms. One mechanism is connective tissue synthesis; plaques may be composed largely of collagen with little or no apparent atheroma. Whether such a plaque is primarily due to connective tissue synthesis or represents a lesion in which the atheromatous debris has been removed by macrophages is unknown. Mural thrombosis and organization are observed frequently in plaque lesions, and unquestionably they represent a common mechanism for increasing plaque volume. The causes of the injury that stimulates thrombus formation are unknown. Hemodynamic stresses on the endothelium produced by the mass lesion protruding into the lumen may cause the injury. Lipid accumulation from the blood plasma is another mechanism for plaque growth. Foam cells are observed frequently in the fibrous cap of a plaque lesion, suggesting lipid deposition. Alternatively, these foam cells could reflect lipid transport from the lesions to the blood. There is currently no way to know which role these cells play, and indeed, both processes could operate simultaneously. Lipid composition studies demonstrate clearly that the apparently inert atheroma lipid is turning over. Another mechanism by which plaques may increase in volume is hemorrhage into the lesion. Hemorrhage may be due to focal rupture (ulceration, fissure) of the fibrous cap of the lesion (Fig. 199-1) or rupture of the vasa vasorum, which are small blood vessels that proliferate through the tunica media into the base of the lesion. It is not yet possible to identify which of the above mechanisms is more common. Observation of human lesions suggests that mural thrombosis and lipid accumulation are the most common mechanisms of plaque growth.

Total thrombotic occlusion of an artery associated with atherosclerosis is almost invariably associated with rupture of a plaque. Atheroma material is a strong procoagulant. For a totally occlusive thrombus to form, it is necessary that, in addition to plaque rupture and procoagulant activation of the coagulation system, blood flow be slowed. Evidence for the previous statement is indirect but substantial. Endarterectomy, balloon angioplasty, or experimental balloon de-endothelialization results in minimal thrombus formation if blood flow is rapid. Reduced blood flow in arteries with ruptured plaques may be due to distal occlusive atheromatous plaques or vasospasm.

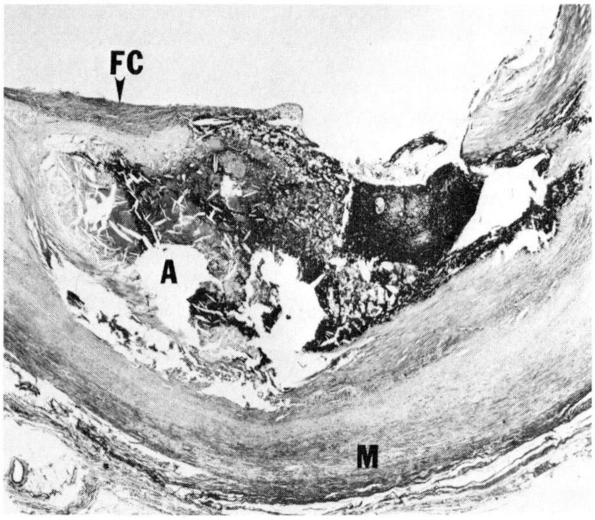

Figure 199-1 Histologic section of the distal portion of the carotid bulb of a 72-year-old man dying with extensive neoplasm and pulmonary embolism. He had no clinical symptomatology related to the central nervous system, and no embolic lesions were found at autopsy. Shown is an ulcerated atheromatous plaque that had caused an approximately 40 percent stenosis of the lumen. Rupture of the fibrous cap (FC) is evident to the right of center, with hemorrhage into the atheroma (A). There is no evidence of thrombus formation. M, media.

Summary

The lesions of atherosclerosis evolve over many years. They are apparent earliest in the aorta, next in the coronary arteries, and later in the arteries supplying the brain. With age, the extent of atherosclerotic lesions increases in predictable anatomic locations; their severity varies greatly among individuals. In general, plaques are found about a decade after fatty streaks develop. Both lesions increase in extent and size with age, but the rate of this increase is variable among individuals. The increasing severity of atherosclerosis correlates with most of the risk factors previously mentioned, but the exact effect of any risk factor on the pathogenesis of the lesions is unknown. Risk factors that reliably predict atherosclerosis in the brain arteries include arterial hypertension, cigarette smoking, and raised serum levels of fibrinogen and factor VIII.

Atherosclerosis in the carotid siphon, vertebral arteries, and intracranial arteries is a neglected subject. This subject appears to deserve more attention, especially the evaluation of carotid bulb lesions in aged persons, particularly those in the eighth decade and older. Plaques in the carotid bulb have been the subject of many studies, primarily to ascertain the lesion characteristics that predict future transient ischemic attacks and stroke. None of the studied characteristics has clearly correlated with clinical significance. It is possible, therefore, that changes in the distal intraparenchymal vasculature secondary to protracted low flow and aging play a key role in the development of symptomatic ischemic events. If this is true, it is possible that a long time passes between the development of a large and complicated carotid bulb atherosclerotic plaque and the onset of clinical disease.

References

1. Alpern-Elran H, Morog N, Robert F, et al. Angiogenic activity of the atherosclerotic carotid artery plaque. *J Neurosurg* 1989; 70:942–945.
2. Avril G, Batt M, Guidoin R, et al. Carotid endarterectomy plaques: correlations of clinical and anatomic findings. *Ann Vasc Surg* 1991; 5:50–54.
3. Bassiouny HS, Davis H, Massawa N, et al. Critical carotid stenoses: morphologic and chemical similarity between symptomatic and asymptomatic plaques. *J Vasc Surg* 1989; 9:202–212.
4. Bo WJ, McKinney WM, Bowden RL. The origin and distribution of vasa vasorum at the bifurcation of the common carotid artery with atherosclerosis. *Stroke* 1989; 20:1484–1487.
5. Bock RW, Gray-Weale AC, Mock PA, et al. The natural history of asymptomatic carotid artery disease. *J Vasc Surg* 1993; 17:160–171.
6. Bornstein NM, Krajewski A, Lewis AJ, et al. Clinical significance of carotid plaque hemorrhage. *Arch Neurol* 1990; 47:958–959.
7. Cornwell DG, Geer JC, Panganamala RV. Development of atheroma and the lipid composition of the deposit. In Masoro EJ (ed): *Pharmacology of Lipid Transport and Atherosclerotic Processes.* Oxford: Pergamon, 1975, pp 445–483.
8. Craven TE, Ryu JE, Espeland MA, et al. Evaluation of the associations between carotid artery atherosclerosis and coronary artery stenosis: a case-control study. *Circulation* 1990; 82:1230–1242.
9. Dempsey RJ, Diana AL, Moore RW. Thickness of carotid artery atherosclerotic plaque and ischemic risk. *Neurosurgery* 1990; 27:343–348.
10. Estol C, Claasen D, Hirsch W, et al. Correlative angiographic and pathologic findings in the diagnosis of ulcerated plaques in the carotid artery. *Arch Neurol* 1991; 48:692–694.
11. European Carotid Surgery Trialists' Collaborative Group. MRC European Carotid Surgery Trial: interim results for symptomatic patients with severe (70–99%) or with mild (0–29%) carotid stenosis. *Lancet* 1991; 337:1235–1243.
12. Feeley TM, Leen EJ, Colgan MP, et al. Histologic characteristics of carotid artery plaque. *J Vasc Surg* 1991; 13:719–724.
13. Fisher M, Fieman S. Geometric factors of the bifurcation in carotid atherogenesis. *Stroke* 1990; 21:267–271.
14. Garcia JH, Ho K-L. Pathology of hypertensive arteriopathy. *Neurosurg Clin North Am* 1992; 3:497–507.
15. Gerrity RG. The role of the monocyte in atherogenesis: I. Transition of blood-borne monocytes into foam cells in fatty lesions. *Am J Pathol* 1981; 103:181–190.
16. Goldstein JL, Hoff HF, Ho YK, et al. Stimulation of cholesteryl ester synthesis in macrophages by extracts of atherosclerotic human aortas and complexes of albumin/cholesteryl esters. *Arteriosclerosis* 1981; 1:210–226.
17. Haust MD. The morphogenesis and fate of potential and early atherosclerotic lesions in man. *Hum Pathol* 1971; 2:1–29.
18. Hollander W, Paddock J, Colombo M. Lipoproteins in human atherosclerotic vessels: 1. Biochemical properties of arterial low density lipoproteins, very low density lipoproteins, and high density lipoproteins. *Exp Mol Pathol* 1979; 30:144–171.
19. Holm J, Hansson G. Cellular and immunologic features of carotid artery disease in man and experimental animal models. *Eur J Vasc Surg* 1990; 4:49–55.
20. Howard G, Ryu JE, Evans GW, et al. Extracranial carotid atherosclerosis in patients with and without transient ischemic attacks and coronary artery disease. *Arteriosclerosis* 1990; 10:714–719.
21. Keys A. Coronary heart disease: the global picture. *Atherosclerosis* 1975; 22:149–192.
22. Klag MJ, Whelton PK, Seidler AJ. Decline in US stroke mortality: demographic trends and antihypertensive treatment. *Stroke* 1989; 20:14–21.

23. Leen EJ, Feeley TM, Colgan MP, et al. "Haemorrhagic" carotid plaque does not contain haemorrhage. *Eur J Vasc Surg* 1990; 4:123–128.
24. Mayberg MR, Wilson SE, Yatsu F, et al. Carotid endarterectomy and prevention of cerebral ischemia in symptomatic carotid stenosis. *JAMA* 1991; 266:3289–3294.
25. McGill HC (ed). *The Geographic Pathology of Atherosclerosis.* Baltimore: Williams & Wilkins, 1968.
26. McGill HC Jr. The relationship of dietary cholesterol to serum cholesterol concentration and to atherosclerosis in man. *Am J Clin Nutr* 1979; 32:2664–2702.
27. Moncada S. Prostacyclin and arterial wall biology. *Arteriosclerosis* 1982; 2:193–207.
28. North American Symptomatic Carotid Endarterectomy Trial Collaborators. Beneficial effect of carotid endarterectomy in symptomatic patients with high-grade carotid stenosis. *N Engl J Med* 1991; 325:445–453.
29. Ross R, Glomset JA. The pathogenesis of atherosclerosis. *N Engl J Med* 1976; 295:369–377, 420–425.
30. Schneidau A, Harrison MJ, Hurst C, et al. Arterial disease risk factors and angiographic evidence of atheroma of the carotid artery. *Stroke* 1989; 20:1466–1471.
31. Segrest JP, Chung BH, Cone JT, et al. Coronary heart disease risk: assessment by plasma lipoprotein profiles. *Ala J Med Sci* 1983; 20:76–83.
32. Senkowsky J, Bell WH III, Kerstein MD. Normal angiograms and carotid pathology. *Am Surg* 1990; 5:726–729.
33. Sterpetti AV, Hunter WJ, Schultz RD. Importance of ulceration of carotid plaque in determining symptoms of cerebral ischemia. *J Cardiovasc Surg* 1991; 32:154–158.
34. Strong JP. Atherosclerotic lesions: natural history, risk factors, and topography. *Arch Pathol Lab Med* 1992; 116:1268–1275.
35. Tell GS, Howard G, Evans GW, et al. Cigarette smoking and extracranial carotid atherosclerosis. *Adv Exp Med Biol* 1990; 273:39–49.
36. Thomas WA, Reiner JM, Janakidevi K, et al. Population dynamics of arterial cells during atherogenesis: X. Study of monotypism in atherosclerotic lesions of black women heterozygous for glucose-6-phosphate dehydrogenase (G-6-PD). *Exp Mol Pathol* 1979; 31:367–386.
37. Whisnant JP, Homer D, Ingall TJ, et al. Duration of cigarette smoking is the strongest predictor of severe extracranial carotid artery atherosclerosis. *Stroke* 1990; 21:707–714.

200 Pathology of Ischemic Cerebrovascular Disease

Thomas J. Montine
Christine M. Hulette

Ischemia in the central nervous system (CNS) is a function of several variables. These include etiologic factors, efficiency of anastomotic connections, anatomic idiosyncrasies of the circle of Willis, and the patient's age. The major causes of CNS ischemia may be broadly categorized according to the component of the cerebral vasculature that is affected: arterial, arteriolar, capillary, venous, or general failure of the systemic circulation. Regional ischemic injury may result from occlusive diseases of arteries and arterioles, e.g., atherosclerosis, thromboembolism, vasospasm, malformation, vasculitis, dissection, and hypertension, or as a complication of diseases that do not primarily damage vessels, e.g., blood dyscrasias and hypercoagulability. In contrast, global ischemic damage may be produced by profound reductions in cerebral perfusion pressure.

Aside from being regional or global, the consequences of ischemia assume one of three general forms depending on the severity of the insult: necrosis of all tissue elements (complete infarction), selective necrosis of neurons with reactive astrogliosis (incomplete infarction), and functional derangement without permanent tissue damage. This chapter will present the basic patterns of tissue damage that can be observed following CNS ischemia.[1–9]

Regional Ischemic Injury

Arteries

Complete Infarct

The extra- and intracranial arteries that perfuse the brain are common sites of cerebrovascular occlusion. Thrombosis complicating atherosclerosis is a frequent means of occlusion of the larger of these arteries, while lodgment of emboli is the predominant mechanism of occlusion in the major branches of the circle of Willis, especially at the trifurcation of the middle cerebral artery. As a general rule, thrombotic infarcts are anemic or bland, while embolic infarcts are hemorrhagic (Fig. 200-1). Regardless of the cause, arterial infarcts share a common evolution of coagulative

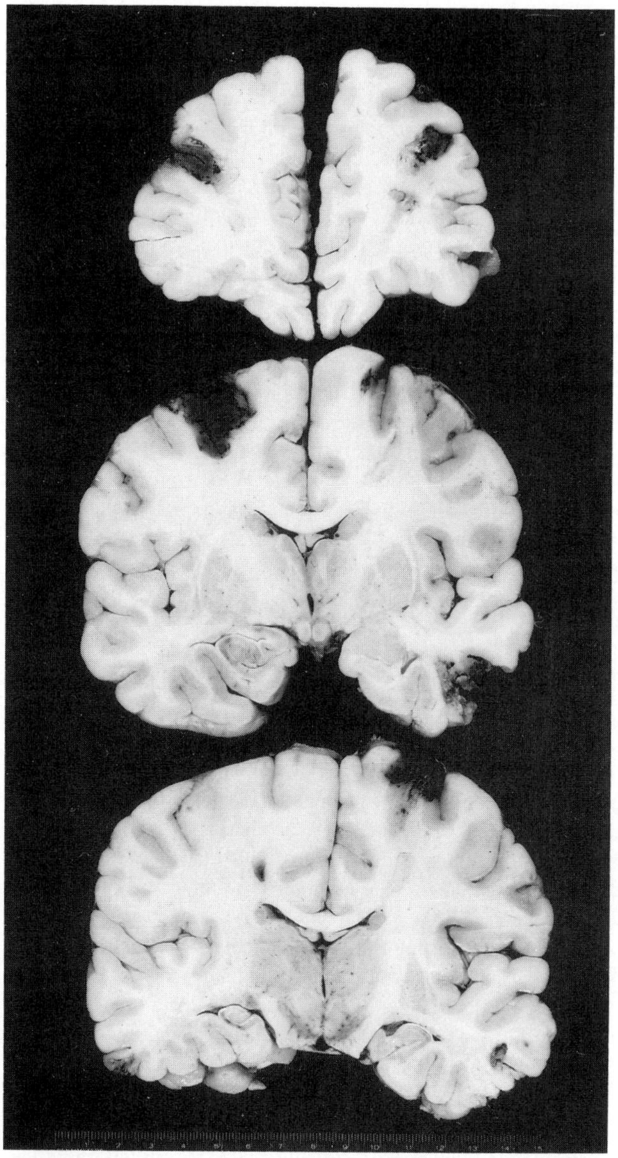

Figure 200-1 Hemorrhagic infarcts. Multiple hemorrhagic infarcts (about 1 week) that followed embolization from a left ventricular mural thrombus.

necrosis leading to liquefaction that culminates in cavity formation. Microscopically, the quintessential feature of an infarct is, at least at its core, destruction of all tissue elements.

Although death occurs in CNS tissue within minutes of arterial occlusion, the earliest sign of damage is not apparent until 12 to 24 h following the ictus when it takes the form of coagulative necrosis of neurons, or "red neuron" formation. The histologic hallmarks of this process are neuronal karyolysis and cytoplasmic hypereosinophilia. Infarcts become macroscopically apparent 24 to 36 h after onset. At this time, the lesion is tumorous, distending the normal surface contour, and is poorly delineated, soft, and boggy. Anatomical landmarks within the affected tissue, e.g., the gray-white junction, are obscured in the edematous tissue. In addition to neuronal coagulative necrosis, microscopic changes now include marked tissue edema, myelin pallor, diapedesis of erythrocytes, margination of neutrophils, and conspicuously swollen axons.

Approximately 2 days after infarction, the devitalized tissue develops a more distinct demarcation from the surrounding brain, a feature that allows identification of the vascular territory of the occluded artery. Histologically, this phase of infarct evolution is characterized by disintegration of necrotic neurons, capillary prominence, endothelial cell hypertrophy, and a short-lived influx of neutrophils that are rapidly replaced by macrophages.

Once recruited, the activity of macrophages defines both the gross and microscopic appearances of an infarct. Initially, macrophages may be difficult to discern in the inflamed and necrotic tissue, but within several days they accumulate to very high density and become enlarged with phagocytized material; this is the phase of liquefaction (Fig. 200-2). These debris-laden macrophages, also called "gitter cells" or "compound granular corpuscles," ultimately return to the bloodstream. When their task is completed, the solid mass of necrotic and expansile tissue that characterized the acute infarct has been transformed into a contracted, fluid-filled cavity that is traversed by a fine mesh of atretic vessels and that may harbor a few residual macrophages for many years (Fig. 200-3). Usually, the cavitated infarct is surrounded by a narrow zone of astrogliosis and neuron loss that abuts with histologically normal brain parenchyma. Distal degeneration of fiber tracts is also a late manifestation of cerebral cortical infarction (Fig. 200-4).

Incomplete Infarct

Under some circumstances, arterial ischemia may damage some cells without leading to necrosis of all tissue elements. Neurons and, to a lesser degree, oligodendroglia are more vulnerable to ischemia than other cells, and they can undergo coagulative necrosis and disintegration following an insult that does not destroy other tissue elements. There is minimal inflammatory infiltration with this type of lesion, and the liquefactive and cavitation phases that are typical of a complete infarct do not develop. The ultimate tissue manifestation of an incomplete infarct resembles the edge of a complete infarct; that is, neuronal and oligodendroglial depopulation, myelin pallor, astrogliosis, and capillary prominence.

Edema

All infarcts initially are edematous; however, in large infarcts the edema can be pronounced, and it may take on features of a

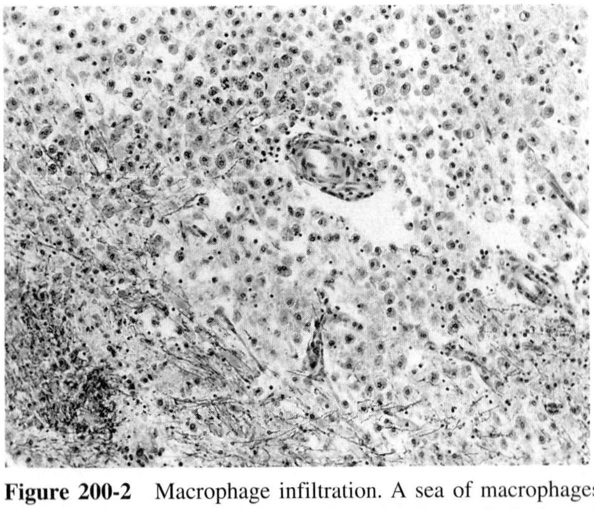

Figure 200-2 Macrophage infiltration. A sea of macrophages, phagocytizing devitalized tissue, abuts the shore of gliotic and demyelinated parenchyma in a 10-day-old cerebral infarct (hematoxylin and eosin, Luxol fast blue, ×130).

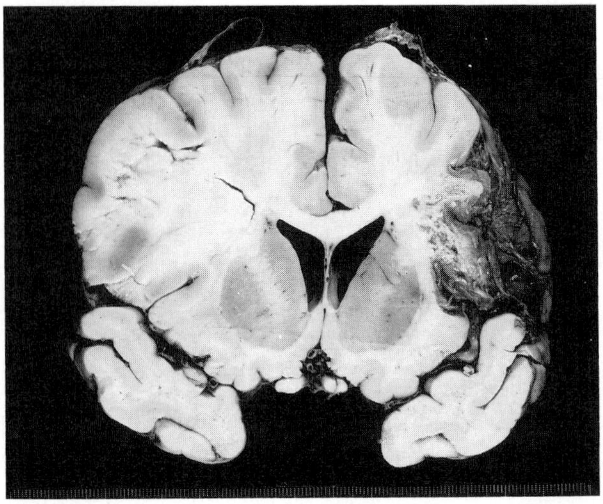

Figure 200-3 Cerebral infarcts of different ages. A 65-year-old woman was incapacitated by right hemiplegia and expressive dysphasia following a stroke 8 months prior to death. Two days before her death, she experienced the sudden onset of left arm weakness that progressed over minutes to include the left leg and culminated in unresponsiveness. This coronal section of the brain displays an old cavitated infarct in the left cerebral hemisphere. A recent infarct also is present in the distribution of the right middle cerebral artery, characterized by tissue swelling, blurring of the gray–white junction, and dusky discoloration. Note the compression of the right lateral ventricle and displacement of the right cingulate gyrus.

space-occupying lesion. Thus, there may be symptoms and signs of increasing intracranial pressure, and neuroimaging studies may show shifting of midline structures. When advanced, cerebral edema may lead to herniation of cerebral tissue and its complications: ipsilateral cranial nerve (CN) III palsy, compression of the contralateral cerebral peduncle, occlusion of the ipsilateral posterior cerebral artery, and fatal compression of the brain stem. Postmortem examination of the surface of the brain characteristically shows a large expansile supratentorial infarct, displacement of medial temporal lobe structures that is highlighted by prominently asymmetrical tentorial notches, and a softened brain stem with a flattened ventral surface. In some instances, contusion of CN III may be observed. Upon sectioning, the features of a recent infarct are apparent. In addition, midline structures are displaced and the brain stem, particularly the pons, is dusky and may contain slender Duret hemorrhages (Figs. 200-3 and 200-5).

Intraparenchymal Small Arteries and Arterioles

Lacunar Infarcts

The intraparenchymal arteries and arterioles that arise from the arteries at the base of the brain are particularly sensitive to a spectrum of pathologic changes. In older patients, these vessels characteristically show intimal thickening with stenosis as well as loss of muscle fibers from the media that are replaced by collagen. These changes become exaggerated in patients with chronic hypertension. Damaged endothelial cells cannot oppose the insudation of plasma proteins, and the result is a swollen, acellular, and homogeneously eosinophilic vessel wall. Subsequently, eosinophilic material, mostly fibrin, seeps deeper and deeper into the vessel wall and

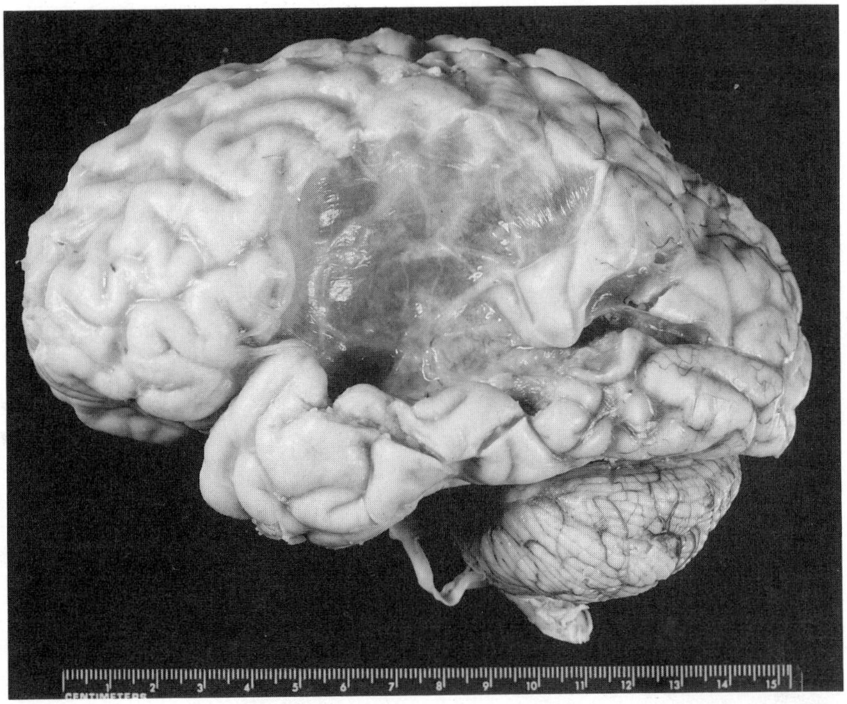

(*A*)

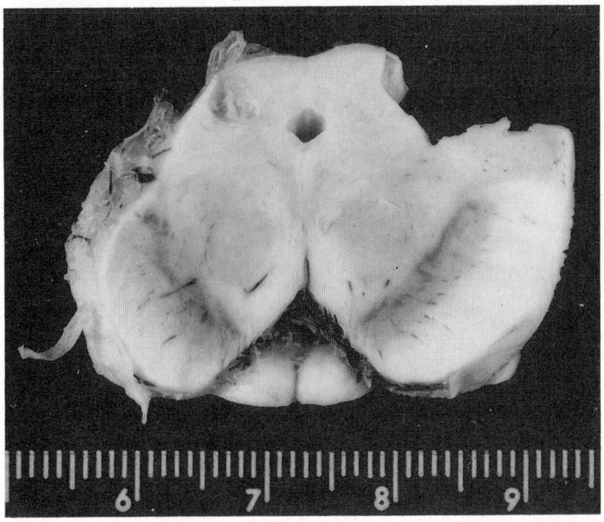

(*B*)

Figure 200-4 Cerebral infarct with tract degeneration. A 62-year-old man had neurological deficits of aphasia, right hemiparesis, and intractable right face and arm pain following an ictus 4 years prior to death. *A.* An external view of the brain shows intact leptomeninges that overlie a large cavitated infarct in the distribution of the left middle cerebral artery. *B.* An axial section of the midbrain highlights the asymmetrical cerebral peduncles. The small area of necrosis in the left mesencephalic tectum is secondary to a tracotomy for pain control.

may be accompanied by foam cells (fat-laden macrophages). The above-described changes in the vessel walls collectively are termed *lipohyalinosis* and commonly are associated with scattered perivascular monocytes and hemosiderin deposition.

The two major complications of lipohyalinosis are lacunar infarcts and microaneurysm formation that may lead to intracerebral hemorrhage. Lacunar infarcts are usually multiple, small (<2 cm) cavitated lesions that are observed, in decreasing order of frequency, in the lenticular nuclei, pons, thalami, internal capsules, and caudate nuclei (Fig. 200-6). Microscopically, these lesions display the features of focal cerebral necrosis: resorption of devitalized parenchyma leading to cavity formation, scattered macrophages within the cavity that sometimes contain hemosiderin pigment, and a thin astrogliotic rim with myelin pallor. Lipohyalinotic vessels typically are identified within the same microscopic field. While many of these lesions are thought to arise from ischemic injury secondary to lipohyalinosis and occlusion of arterioles, small hemorrhages from lipohyalinotic vessels may produce similar cavitated lesions. In addition, chronic hypertension not only foments lipohyalinosis, but it also accelerates atherosclerosis of large arteries. It is probable that a small subset of lacunar infarcts is due to thromboembolism of the parent or penetrating artery, and not a result of lipohyalinosis. Indeed, it seems most likely that all three potential causes, lipohyalinotic occlusion, microhemorrhages, and thromboembolism coexist to produce multiple lacunar infarcts.

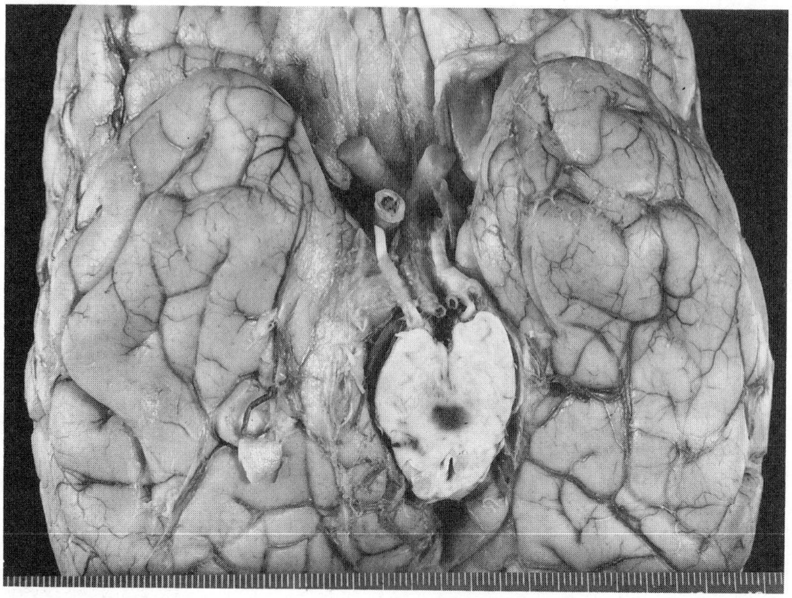

Figure 200-5 Tentorial herniation. External view of the base of the brain with the brain stem removed from a patient with markedly increased intracranial pressure 4 days after a right middle cerebral artery infarct. Note the prominent notching of the right medial temporal lobe, compression and displacement of the brain stem, and the Duret hemorrhage.

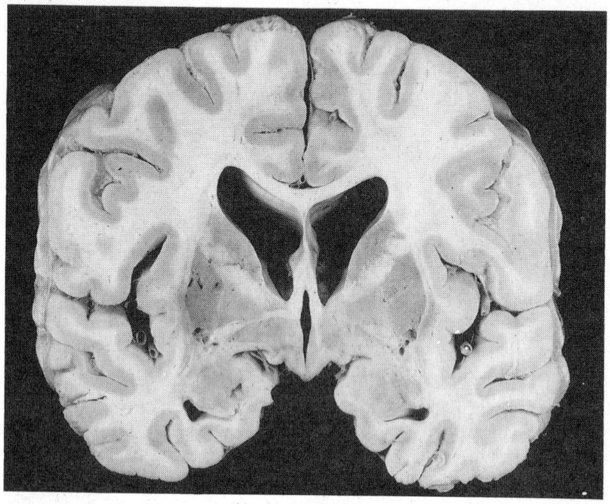

(*A*)

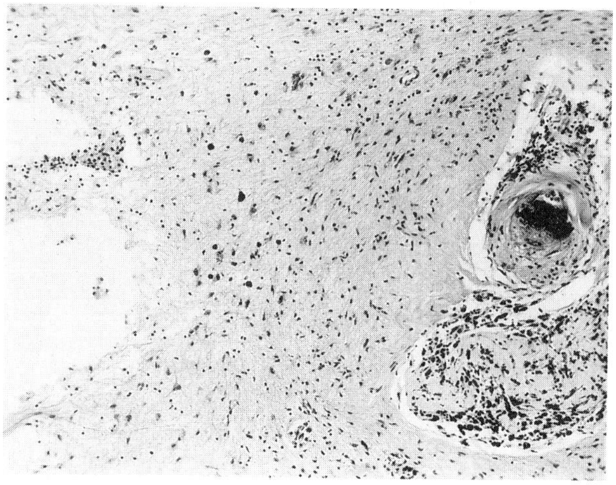

(*B*)

Figure 200-6 Lacunar infarcts. A 68-year-old man with longstanding diabetes and hypertension had a 5-year history of progressive neurological impairment. *A.* Coronal section of the brain demonstrating multiple lacunar infarcts that are most prevalent in the lenticular nuclei bilaterally. *B.* Photomicrograph of the edge of a lacunar infarct showing a cavity that contains a few macrophages and that is rimmed by astrogliosis and myelin pallor. Within the same field is a lipohyalinotic vessel with perivascular hemosiderin deposition (hematoxylin and eosin, Luxol fast blue, ×100).

Binswanger's Disease

Binswanger's disease, or subcortical arteriosclerotic encephalopathy, classically is an unusual form of subacute or chronic dementia seen in older patients with chronic hypertension. External examination of the brain from a patient with this disease typically shows advanced atherosclerosis in the circle of Willis and may reveal old, cavitated infarcts. On sectioning, the lateral ventricles are enlarged and the surrounding white matter is diffusely or focally degenerated, often with a pitted appearance. Multiple lacunar infarcts commonly coexist with these changes. Microscopically, the long penetrating vessels of the white matter, both small arteries and arterioles, show changes of medial hypertrophy and lipohyalinosis. The white matter lesions vary in severity from diffuse degeneration with astrogliosis to cavitated infarcts and probably reflect a varying severity of the insults from oligemia to ischemia.

Capillary Bed

Occlusion of cerebral capillaries, often with involvement of small arterioles and venules, leads to regional ischemic damage that is characterized by petechial hemorrhages, perivascular myelin pallor, and microinfarcts. Although they produce focal lesions, diseases that affect these small vessels tend to be widespread and to be associated with global neurological dysfunction. Thrombotic thrombocytopenic purpura preferentially involves the gray matter and shows engorgement of vessels with granular, hyaline material in addition to the above features. Rickettsial infections of the CNS produce a necrotizing vasculitis that also may yield this pattern of tissue damage, although the number of petechial hemorrhages are often relatively few when compared to the severity of neurological impairment. In contrast to thrombotic processes, minute emboli, *viz,* fat or air emboli, may pass through successive branches of the cerebral vasculature until they impede blood flow in the capillary bed; leading to damage of the distal endothelium. In cases of fat embolization, petechial hemorrhages are largely restricted to the white matter, while air emboli may produce lesions both in gray and white matter (Fig. 200-7).

Veins

Venous sinus thrombosis is observed most frequently as a complication of systemic dehydration, hypercoagulable states, or phlebitis, or as secondary to compression or infiltration by an adjacent tumor. Venous thrombosis leads to stagnation of blood flow in the territories being drained. Edema and diapedesis of erythrocytes are observed initially; however, venous thrombosis can lead to infarcts that are conspicuously hemorrhagic. Unlike arterial infarcts, hemorrhage from venous infarcts involves the leptomeninges, cortex, and white matter. The white matter hemorrhage is particularly prominent and, in cross section, appears triangular with the apex directed toward the ventricles. Thrombosis of the superior sagittal sinus, the most frequent form of venous thrombosis, characteristically produces symmetrical lesions in the cerebral hemispheres. Thrombosis of the vein of Galen leads to hemorrhagic infarction of periventricular white matter and the thalami.

Global Ischemia

Cerebral perfusion pressure is largely a function of the difference between mean arterial pressure and intracranial pressure. Therefore, disease processes that sufficiently decrease mean arterial pressure or increase intracranial pressure may compromise cerebral blood flow and lead to global ischemia.

Total Cerebral Necrosis

In its most extreme form, global ischemia culminates in total cerebral necrosis, or "respirator brain." The initial event is a dramatic and persistent increase in intracranial pressure from edema secondary to trauma, neoplasm, large infarct, inflammation, or hemorrhage. Although the patient's vital functions may be maintained artificially for some time, cerebral perfusion becomes blocked by the massively increased intracranial pressure, leading to necrosis of the entire brain.

Macroscopically, massive edema is manifested as a heavy softened brain with thinned subarachnoid space, flattened and broadened gyri, slitlike sulci, and compressed ventricles. The brain characteristically has a gray or dusky discoloration secondary to capillary dilatation and stagnation of blood. Herniation, often with sloughing of necrotic parenchyma, is observed commonly. Unlike the other lesions described in this chapter, the findings of total cerebral necrosis represent death of all tissue elements but without subsequent reperfusion. As a result, there is no inflammatory cell or macrophage infiltrate, no cavity formation, and no glial reaction. The microscopic features of total cerebral necrosis are tissue edema, autolysis, and possibly coagulative necrosis of neurons, depending on the length of survival.

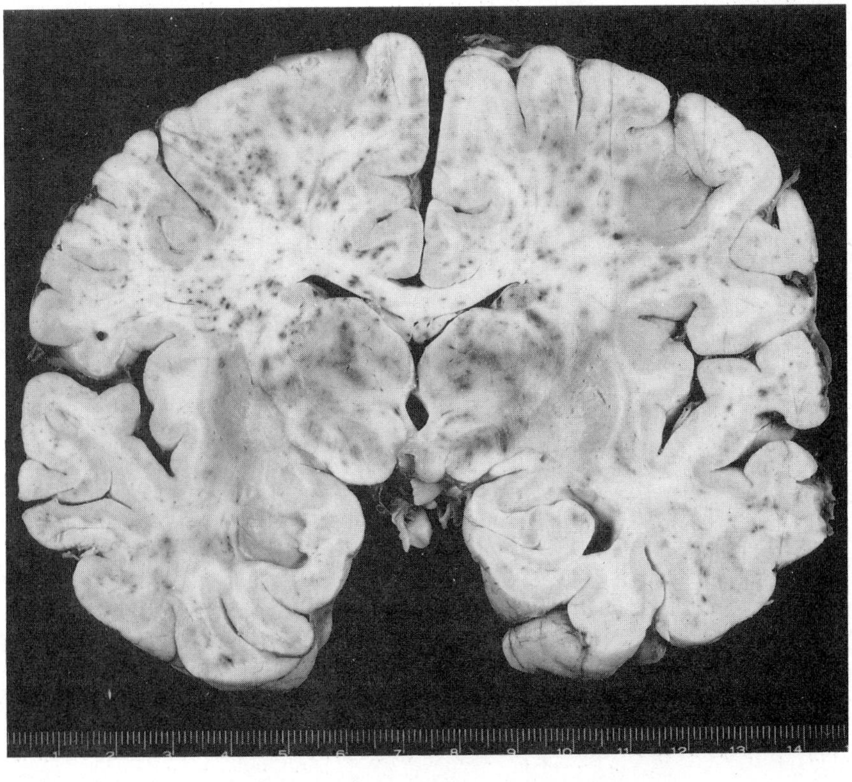

Figure 200-7 Fat embolism. A 62-year-old woman with severe osteoporosis died suddenly while undergoing repair of a fractured femur. Innumerable small hemorrhages were concentrated in the white matter of the cerebral hemispheres and brain stem.

Incomplete Global Ischemia

Global ischemia need not be so severe as to produce total cerebral necrosis. These instances are typified by sudden decrease in mean arterial pressure, *viz,* shock or cardiac arrest, from which the patient is resuscitated. The pattern of tissue damage reflects an exaggerated or selective vulnerability to ischemic injury. The most susceptible structures are the pyramidal neurons of the hippocampus and Purkinje cells of the cerebellum that may undergo incomplete infarction, or neuronal necrosis with astrogliosis. In more severe cases, complete infarcts of the hippocampus and cerebellar cortex as well as infarcts of the arterial border zones, laminar necrosis of the cerebral cortex, and bilateral necrosis of the thalamus and striatum may occur.

Arterial Border Zone Infarcts

Arterial border zone, or watershed, infarcts occur at the distal extreme of arterial territories, in regions of the brain and spinal cord where vascular territories overlap. When cerebral blood flow begins to ebb and the region of effective perfusion contracts, tissue in the border zone experiences the earliest and most profound ischemia that may progress to infarction. The areas of the brain that are most commonly affected in adults are those at the interface of the anterior and middle cerebral arteries. Thus, parasagittal infarcts of the cerebral hemispheres are observed, especially posterior to the interparietal sulcus (triple border zone); these are often bilateral. Although not occlusive in origin, these lesions follow the same pathologic progression as described above and are usually hemorrhagic. Less severe tissue damage with neuronal necrosis and astrogliosis but not cavity formation also may be seen with the same bilateral parasagittal distribution; this is termed *granular atrophy.*

Incompletely developed anastomoses between the cerebral cortical long penetrating arteries and the basal penetrating arteries produce a periventricular arterial border zone in premature infants that is inordinately sensitive to global ischemia. The resulting lesion, periventricular leukomalacia, typically is bilateral and is characterized by a spectrum of histopathologic changes that range from myelin pallor and astrogliosis to complete infarcts (Fig. 200-8).

Laminar Necrosis

Laminar necrosis is a consequence of abrupt loss of cerebral perfusion pressure leading to markedly reduced blood flow in the capillary plexus of the deep gray matter. Macroscopically, there is a grumous or cystic degeneration of the deeper layers of the cerebral cortical gray matter that faithfully follows the gyrations of the cortical ribbon. Unlike arterial infarcts, in which the necrotic tissue extends to the pial surface, laminar necrosis is surrounded by viable, albeit gliotic, brain parenchyma. The spared superficial cortical layers show neuronal necrosis and astrogliosis and the underlying white matter displays superficial astrogliosis (Fig. 200-9).

Selectively Vulnerable Neuron Groups

The Purkinje cells of the cerebellum and pyramidal cells of the hippocampus are inordinately prone to undergo necrosis with astrogliosis following ischemic injury. Purkinje cell necrosis is usually most severe in the region of overlap between the superior and inferior circulations. In the hippocampus, the pyramidal neurons in Sommer's sector (CA1) are most susceptible to necrosis, followed by those in CA3 and CA4 (end folium). The neurons of CA2 (dorsal resistant zone) are least likely to die following ischemia. Initially characterized by coagulative necrosis of neurons and tissue edema, ischemic damage to the hippocampus progresses to an astrogliotic scar. This pattern of injury is commonly referred to as *Ammon's horn sclerosis,* or *mesial temporal sclerosis* when the lesion extends into adjacent structures.

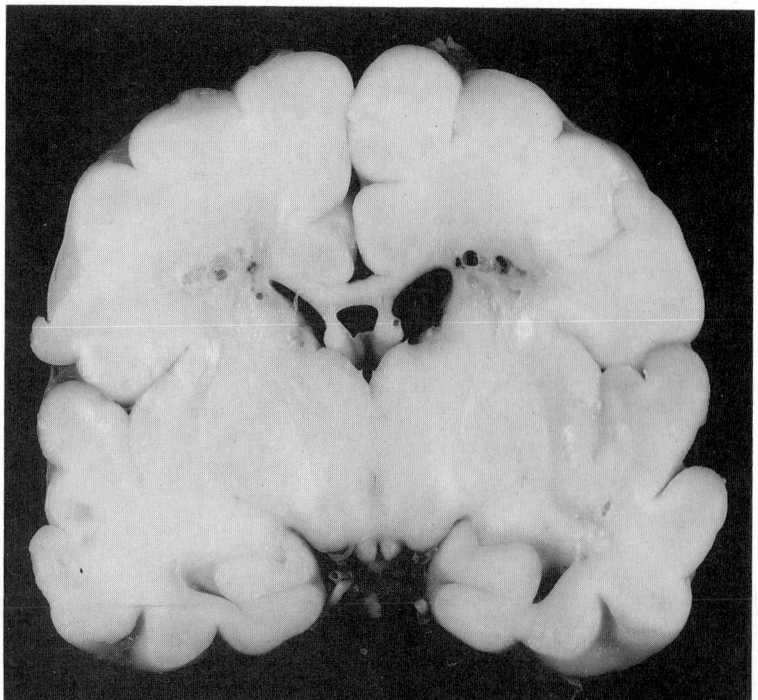

Figure 200-8 Periventricular leukomalacia. Coronal section of the cerebral hemispheres from a 28-week gestational-age infant who had a 1-month hospital course marked by multiple system failures. Small cavities were distributed bilaterally in the periventricular white matter, extending from the lenticular nuclei to the occipital lobes.

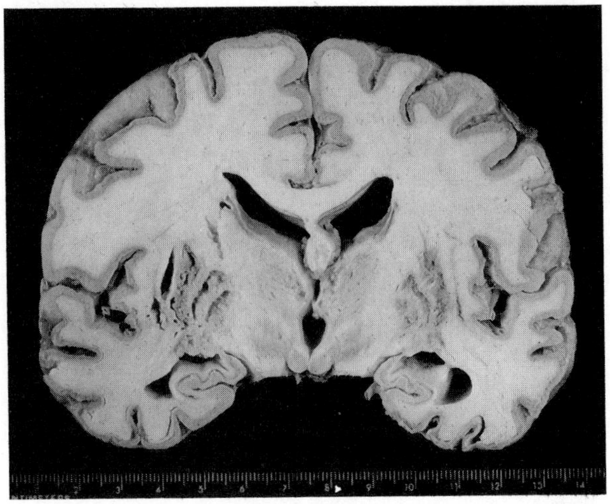

Figure 200-9 Laminar necrosis. A 73-year-old woman suffered cardiac arrest from which she was resuscitated; however, she remained comatose for 2 months before death. This coronal section of brain displays diffuse laminar necrosis of the cerebral cortices and hippocampi. Also present are cavitated infarcts in the basal ganglia.

References

1. Burger PC, Vogel FS. *Cerebrovascular Disease.* Bethesda: The American Association of Pathologists, 1978 [*Am J Pathol* 92(1):1–320].
2. Escourolle R, Poirier J. *Manual of Basic Neuropathology,* 2d ed. Philadelphia: Saunders, 1978.
3. Garcia JH. The evolution of brain infarcts: a review. *J Neuropathol Exp Neurol* 1992; 51:387–393.
4. Garcia JH, Anderson ML. Circulatory disorders and their effects on the brain. In Davis RL, Robertson DM (eds): *Textbook of Neuropathology,* 2d ed. Baltimore: Williams & Wilkins, 1991, pp 621–718.
5. Graham DI. Hypoxia and vascular disorders. In Adams JH, Duchen LW (eds): *Greenfield's Neuropathology.* New York: Oxford University Press, 1992, pp 153–268.
6. McCormick WF, Schochet SS Jr. *Atlas of Cerebrovascular Disease.* Philadelphia: Saunders, 1976.
7. Okazaki H. *Fundamentals of Neuropathology: Morphologic Basis of Neurologic Disorders,* 2d ed. New York: Igaku-Shoin, 1989.
8. Rorke LB. Anatomical features of the developing brain implicated in the pathogenesis of hypoxic-ischemic injury. *Brain Pathol* 1992; 2:211–221.
9. Toole JF, Patel AN. *Cerebrovascular Disorders: With Sections on Applied Vascular Anatomy and Physiology of the Brain and Spinal Cord.* New York: McGraw-Hill, 1967.

201

Clinical Syndromes of Brain Ischemia

David G. Sherman
J. Donald Easton

Stroke is a common cause of death and disability. Each year in the United States approximately 500,000 people suffer an initial stroke, and one-quarter of these individuals die as a consequence of their stroke and its attendant complications. Of those who survive beyond the first few weeks, the majority carry a persistent neurological deficit. A cost of over 20 billion dollars annually is incurred—in addition to incalculable human suffering. Unfortunately, the treatment of most strokes is woefully inadequate. Good supportive medical care and intensive rehabilitation have, however, improved the lot of many patients with stroke.[12]

Preventive measures such as control of hypertension, cerebral vascular surgery, and platelet antiaggregation therapy have an important role in reducing the likelihood of a stroke in the population at risk. Nevertheless, irreversible infarction occurs within minutes of a loss of blood flow to the brain, eliminating opportunities for prevention and setting into motion potentially devastating metabolic events.

Ischemic Stroke Syndromes

The clinical syndromes developing from focal brain ischemia are defined in terms of the arterial circulation involved and the time course of the resultant symptoms and signs. A patient's symptoms and signs (e.g., aphasia, amaurosis fugax, internuclear ophthalmoplegia) are the major testimony to the arterial circulation involved. This clinical assessment may be corroborated by diagnostic studies such as computed tomography (CT), magnetic resonance imaging (MRI), or cerebral angiography. However useful these and other diagnostic techniques may be, the stroke syndrome continues to be characterized by the nature and time course of the patient's clinical findings.

Within 10 s of a diminution in blood flow below about 15 ml/100 g per minute to an area of the brain, the affected neurons cease to function. This lack of metabolic reserve is the basis for the observation that clinical ischemic syndromes are almost invariably sudden in onset. If blood flow is re-established promptly, neuronal function recovers and neurological abnormalities resolve within a few minutes or hours. This brief disruption of function is termed a *transient ischemic attack* (TIA) if it is focal, or *syncope* if it is generalized. If perfusion is not restored, metabolic collapse occurs and ischemic infarction results in a clinical stroke. Thus the nature and time course of cerebral ischemic symptoms imply a particular underlying pathophysiology, which may in turn be linked to a presumed cause, prognosis, and therapeutic strategy.

Cerebral arterial occlusion or reduced flow may be the end result of a number of pathophysiologic processes culminating in focal brain ischemia (Fig. 201-1). Disease of the artery, whether

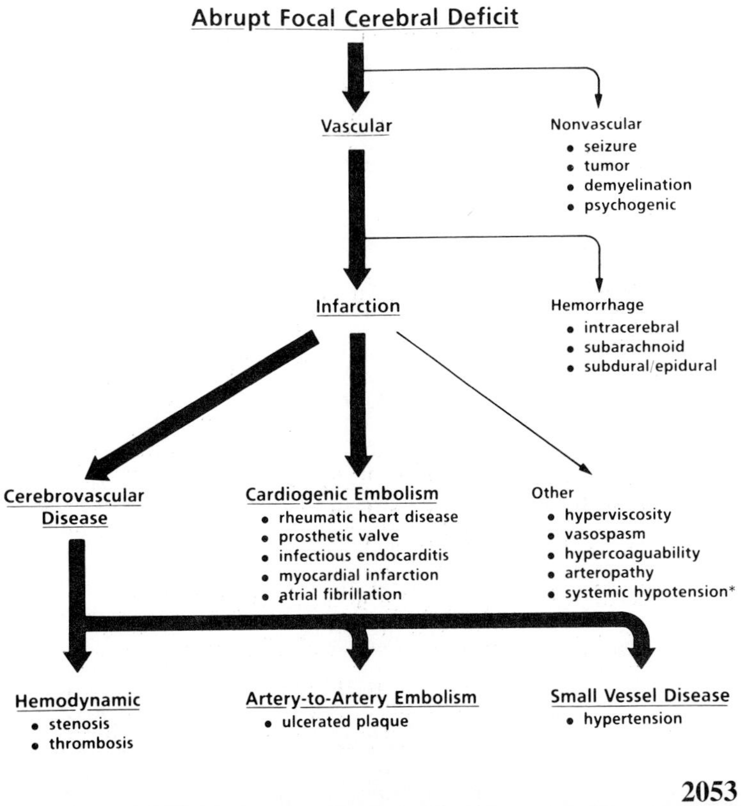

Figure 201-1 Pathophysiology of ischemic stroke.

atherosclerosis, arteritis, or trauma, may cause a flow-restricting stenosis or promote thrombus formation. A number of disorders of the cardiac rhythm, heart valves, and the myocardial muscle itself may also promote thrombus formation with the risk of systemic embolization, often to the cerebral vessels. Focal ischemic symptoms also occur associated with the cerebral arterial vasospasm of subarachnoid hemorrhage and possibly migraine. In addition, the production of vasoconstricting substances in an area of ischemic brain may accentuate and widen the ischemic injury produced by a thrombotic or embolic occlusion. Similarly, changes in the blood constituents, as seen in polycythemia and hyperviscosity states, may produce focal ischemia or cause deterioration of already ischemic brain by impairing flow in the microcirculation. It is testimony to the effectiveness of the brain's collateral circulation that many, if not most, patients with stenotic or occlusive arterial lesions do not suffer a brain infarction. Even when cerebral blood flow is further reduced by transient systemic hypotension, symptoms of global brain ischemia (presyncope or syncope), rather than focal ischemia, generally develop.[4]

Transient Ischemic Attack (TIA)

A transient ischemic attack is an episode of focal neurological dysfunction that results from ischemia and resolves completely within 24 h. Most TIAs last less than 10 to 15 min. One rarely has the opportunity to examine a patient during a TIA and therefore is dependent on the history for diagnosis. The onset of symptoms is sudden and focal in character. Monocular blindness, dysphasia, localized sensory loss, and hemiparesis are some of the symptoms that strongly suggest a focal ischemic episode, and the nature of the symptoms define the vascular distribution of the ischemia (Table 201-1).[16] Many other transient symptoms are far less specific and should not with confidence be attributed to focal brain ischemia (Table 201-2).[16] Still other symptoms are even less specific and are usually not symptoms of TIA (Table 201-3).[16]

TABLE 201-2 Uncertain TIA Symptoms

Vertigo alone	Dysphagia alone
Dysarthria alone	Diplopia alone

TIAs may occur as a consequence of any of the potential causes of focal ischemia, i.e., extracranial arterial disease, cardiac embolization, migrainous "vasospasm," etc. (Fig. 201-1). However, specific pathophysiologies are suggested by certain features of a TIA. Carotid system TIAs of short duration (i.e., less than 10 to 15 min) are more likely to occur from atheroembolic disease of the internal carotid artery, and those of an hour or more are more likely the result of a cardiac embolus. Transient ischemia producing prominent visual scintillations and the slow buildup and march of paresthesias over 5 to 30 min without major paralysis after the spell is typical of late-life migraine accompaniments. These transient migraine accompaniments are disturbing, but unlike TIAs they appear to be relatively harmless.[9] Sudden transient numbness of the face, arm, and leg on one side in the absence of weakness, homonymous hemianopsia, and aphasia is typically due to hypertensive arteriolar changes in small penetrating vessels, rather than to disease of the large vessels. It is sometimes the prelude to a lacunar infarct.[10]

The importance of TIAs lies in their role as harbingers of brain infarction. In some studies the incidence of TIA preceding cerebral infarction has been in the 10 to 20 percent range, while others have found an incidence as high as 80 percent.[2] Forty to 50 percent is quoted by most authors. It is quite likely that this variability is dependent on the type and location of the causative lesion (i.e., left atrial thrombus; internal carotid artery stenosis, ulceration, occlusion, plaque hemorrhage, dissection; carotid siphon disease; and small penetrating artery lipohyalinosis or arteriosclerosis). For carotid lesions amenable to carotid endarterectomy the incidence is probably 40 to 50 percent. Some patients experience multiple TIAs over an extended period of time and never suffer a brain infarction.

TABLE 201-1 TIA Symptoms

Carotid System	Vertebrobasilar System	Either System
Motor defect (paralysis, weakness, or clumsiness) of one extremity or of both extremities on the contralateral side	Motor defect (paralysis, weakness, or clumsiness) of any combination of extremities up to quadriplegia, sometimes changing from one side to another in different attacks	Dysarthria, if it occurs alone
Sensory defect (numbness, including loss of sensation, or paresthesia) involving one or both extremities on the contralateral side	Sensory defect (numbness, including loss of sensation, or paresthesia) in any combination of extremities including all four or involving both sides of the face or mouth; frequently bilateral; sometimes changes from side to side in different attacks	
Loss of vision in one eye or in part of one eye (amaurosis fugax)	Loss of vision, complete or partial in both homonymous fields (bilateral homonymous hemianopsia)	
Homonymous hemianopsia	Homonymous hemianopsia	Homonymous hemianopsia, if it occurs alone
Aphasia (language disturbance that may be only a minor defect or may be global)	Ataxia, imbalance, unsteadiness, or dysequilibrium not associated with vertigo	
	Either vertigo (with or without nausea and vomiting), diplopia, dysphagia, or dysarthria not considered as a TIA when any of these symptoms occurs alone; but in combination with one another or with any of the first four items above, the attacks should be considered a TIA	
Combinations of the above	Combinations of the above	

TABLE 201-3 Non-TIA Symptoms

Unconsciousness including syncope
Tonic and/or clonic activity
March of a sensory defect
Incontinence of bowel or bladder
Dizziness or wooziness alone
Loss of vision associated with alteration of consciousness
Focal symptoms associated with migraine
Scintillating scotomata
Confusion alone
Amnesia alone

However, most patients have fewer than four TIAs prior to their stroke. The period of greatest risk is the first hours and days following a first TIA, with about one-half of the strokes occurring within the first month. The risk is sustained, however, such that by 5 years approximately 35 percent of patients experiencing a TIA will have suffered a completed stroke.[7,15] Many clinicians view "crescendo TIAs" with particular alarm. This term describes a cluster of TIAs occurring at increasing frequency or duration over a few hours or days. Patients with crescendo TIAs are considered particularly unstable neurologically and at risk of imminent brain infarction.

Reversible Ischemic Neurological Deficit

Reversible ischemic neurological deficit (RIND) is the term used to describe a focal ischemic event lasting longer than 24 h but with complete resolution of the deficit within 3 weeks. These episodes are also referred to as *stroke with recovery* or *stroke with full recovery*. Greater diagnostic certainty exists with a RIND than a TIA because one can substantiate the focal neurological findings on physical examination.

From a management perspective a TIA and a RIND are viewed similarly, even though a RIND, like a completed stroke, is somewhat more likely to have a stuttering or gradual onset compared with the abrupt onset of a TIA. Some authors have found that cerebral angiograms are more often normal in RIND patients than in those with either TIA or completed stroke, suggesting that cardiogenic cerebral embolism, or some mechanism other than cervical artery atherosclerosis, is more likely to be causative in RINDs. It has also been suggested that compared with patients with TIA, those with a RIND are less liable to a subsequent stroke. Other authorities believe that TIA, RIND, and completed stroke are all on a continuum of worsening cerebral vascular disease and that the risk of subsequent stroke is substantial for all of them. Most experts manage all of these patients similarly, as threatening stroke patients, unless they have already suffered a major completed stroke.

The risk of having a stroke in the future is at least twice as high for patients with a completed stroke as for those with a TIA. The incidence of stroke is approximately 4 percent annually after a first TIA, although higher in the first year, and about 9 percent after a stroke.[15,17]

Progressing Stroke

The term *progressing stroke*, or *stroke in evolution*, describes the progression of focal ischemic symptoms over many minutes to several hours. The nature of the new neurological deficit suggests extension of the area of ischemia to encompass areas of brain immediately adjacent to the already involved area. Neurological worsening from ischemic edema should not be confused with progressing stroke. Hemispheric edema in the ischemic brain causes gradual worsening of the deficit from 48 h to 96 h after onset, whereas most progressing infarctions in the carotid territory have completed their evolution within 24 h, or occasionally 48 h.[13]

About 20 percent of patients with acute carotid system cerebral infarction experience clear progression within the first 48 h (Table 201-4).[13] Less than 5 percent show ischemic worsening after a stable period of 48 h or more. Progressing stroke appears to be more common in the vertebrobasilar territory where early progression occurs in about 40 percent of patients (Table 201-4).[14] In addition, there appears to be a longer period of risk for progression in vertebrobasilar strokes, with 15 to 20 percent of patients worsening between 48 to 96 h after onset.[14]

Worsening of an existing deficit may also arise from hypoxia or other metabolic disturbances and may be difficult to differentiate from a stroke in evolution. Consequently, in comparison to a TIA, RIND, or completed stroke, a progressing stroke conveys somewhat greater diagnostic uncertainty, and a neoplasm, or a subdural or intracerebral hematoma, is more often a real differential diagnostic consideration in progressing stroke than in the other ischemic syndromes.

A progressing stroke appears to forebode the gravest consequences of any of the ischemic syndromes. As many as one-half of patients with an evolving stroke in the vertebrobasilar distribution will die if untreated. The prognosis is better when the carotid distribution is involved.

Completed Stroke

A completed stroke is a stable, focal ischemic neurological deficit. Most embolic strokes have their maximal deficit appear suddenly and then stabilize or progressively improve over the subsequent hours, days, and months. Thrombotic infarctions may be just as sudden, but more commonly they evolve rapidly, over several minutes or a few hours, to a completed stroke. The most common presentation is for the patient to awaken from sleep with a complete focal neurological deficit that remains stable or progressively improves. If one sees a patient during the early hours following a cerebral infarction, it is important to observe the patient closely to determine whether one is dealing with a progressing stroke or a completed stroke. The earlier it is after the onset of an ischemic deficit, the less certainty there is that the stroke is complete. An apparent stable deficit observed at 4 to 6 h from onset may resolve by 24 h, proving to be a TIA, or it may suddenly worsen into a stroke in evolution.

TABLE 201-4 Temporal Profile of Cerebral Infarction (Clinical Course over 7 Days)

Course	Carotid, %	Vertebrobasilar, %
Stable (unchanged)	39	11
Improving	35	35
Progressing	19	43
Remitting-relapsing	3	11
Late worsening (>48 h)	4	0
Death	10.6	27

Source: Adapted from Jones and Millikan[13] and Jones, Millikan, and Sandok.[14]

Syndrome of Cardiogenic Embolic Occlusion

Possibly 20 to 30 percent of ischemic strokes originate from a cardiogenic embolus.[6–8,11] The determination that a stroke is embolic in origin generally results from the demonstration of an appropriate cardiac abnormality in a patient with a stroke featuring characteristics suggestive of an embolus.

Certain cardiac abnormalities are widely incriminated as sources of systemic and cerebral emboli (Table 201-5). Rheumatic mitral valvular disease with atrial fibrillation, prosthetic valves, infectious endocarditis, nonvalvular atrial fibrillation, acute myocardial infarction, and intracardiac tumor are universally recognized causes of emboli. The role of disorders such as patent foramen ovale, atrial septal aneurysm, and mitral valve prolapse is less clear. These latter abnormalities are relatively common, and although they are capable of producing systemic emboli, the frequency with which they do so remains unclear. The difficulty in identifying the role of the heart is magnified further when the cardiac abnormality may be episodic (e.g., atrial fibrillation) and perhaps not be recognized by either the patient or the physician.

Certain clinical features of a stroke suggest a possible cardiac embolic origin. Embolic strokes are usually sudden in onset with their maximal neurological deficit appearing immediately. A headache or seizure at the onset is more common with an embolic than a thrombotic stroke. Most cardiogenic emboli lodge in the stem or a branch of the middle cerebral artery with perhaps as few as one out of ten cardiac emboli coming to rest in a branch of the anterior cerebral or basilar artery. Emboli entering one of the vertebral arteries tend to lodge at the ''top of the basilar''[5] or in one or both posterior cerebral arteries. Thus, an infarction in the anterior cerebral artery distribution or in the brain stem is less likely due to a cardiogenic embolus than is an ischemic stroke in the middle cerebral artery distribution. Multifocal cerebral infarctions, especially in a patient with an associated systemic arterial occlusion, e.g., renal or limb, strongly suggest an embolic source. Additionally, certain radiologic and laboratory findings may corroborate the clinical suspicion of embolic infarction. CT or MRI may demonstrate an infarct in the middle or posterior cerebral artery distribution, it may reveal multiple infarcts, and it may demonstrate a hemorrhagic infarct. While hemorrhagic infarcts are infrequently demonstrated by CT or MRI, their presence strongly suggests a cardiac embolic source. A hemorrhagic infarct presumably develops when blood flow is re-established to an area of ischemia after the occluding embolus lyses. Cerebral angiography often shows an embolic occlusion of the stem or a branch of the middle cerebral artery within the first few hours or days, but it may show no occlusion thereafter. Also, there may be no cerebrovascular atherosclerosis.

TABLE 201-5 Most Common Causes of Cardiogenic Cerebral Embolism

Nonvalvular atrial fibrillation
Coronary heart disease
Myocardial infarction
Rheumatic heart disease
Mitral stenosis ± atrial fibrillation
Prosthetic valve
Other
Cardiomyopathy
Infectious endocarditis
Nonbacterial thrombotic endocarditis
Mitral valve prolapse
Congenital heart disease
Venous clots and intracardiac shunt
Mitral annulus calcification
Atrial myxoma
Fat emboli

Specific Vascular Syndromes

Stroke syndromes are defined not only by their temporal profile, e.g., TIA, progressing stroke, etc., but also by the vascular supply to the area of ischemic brain.[1] The amount of brain rendered ischemic by a particular vascular occlusion is very much dependent on the nature of collaterals to the affected region. An occlusion of the internal carotid artery may result in infarction of the entire cerebral hemisphere in one patient and cause no symptoms in another. In general, the more distally an occlusion occurs, the greater the likelihood an infarct will result. This must be partially explained by the diminishing opportunity for collateral circulation as one moves distal to the carotid bifurcation, the ophthalmic artery origin, and the circle of Willis. Thus, in order to be certain of the significance of a particular vascular lesion in a patient with an area of regional ischemia, one must visualize the relationships of several vessels to one another and to the area of ischemia.

Internal Carotid Artery Occlusion

An occlusion of the internal carotid artery (ICA) characteristically causes ischemia in the middle cerebral artery (MCA) territory. Areas of the brain supplied by the anterior cerebral artery (ACA), anterior choroidal artery (AchA), or posterior cerebral artery (PCA) are often involved in addition.

Symptoms of retinal and optic nerve ischemia are important clues to ICA disease. The ophthalmic artery is the first major branch of the ICA, and retinal ischemia may occur in response to diminished flow from an ICA stenosis or occlusion, or as a consequence of microemboli arising from an ulcerated ICA plaque. Episodic and transient monocular visual loss (amaurosis fugax) is the usual clinical correlate of ophthalmic artery ischemia. This transient loss of vision usually progresses from the periphery toward the center of vision. The visual loss often develops like a dark curtain descending from above or ascending from below, and it often abates in the reverse manner. The complete or partial blindness evolves over a few seconds and lasts only 1 to 5 min, rarely longer. Vision is usually back to normal within 5 to 15 min. While migraine, polycythemia, and other disorders may cause transient monocular blindness, most authorities believe that the majority of such episodes in patients over 40 years old is due to atherosclerosis at the origin of the internal carotid artery. These plaques may produce hemodynamic changes or emboli that cause the episodes of distal ischemia. Occasionally patients with an ICA occlusion may complain of transient, ipsilateral, monocular visual blurring following exposure to bright sunlight. This rare complaint presumably arises because of a limited retinal metabolic reserve on an ischemic basis.

Middle Cerebral Artery Occlusion

Ischemia to regions of the cerebral hemisphere supplied by one or more of the penetrating or cortical branches of the MCA is the basis for the most common stroke syndromes. The superior division of the MCA supplies the frontal and anterior parietal cortex (Fig. 201-2). Its several branches nourish the motor and sensory cortex about the central sulcus. Ischemia here produces a contralateral weakness of the face, hand, and arm. Sensory loss in a similar distribution may accompany the motor deficit. A nonfluent aphasia results when the frontal branches of the dominant cerebral hemisphere are involved. If only the more posterior parietal branches of the superior division are occluded, motor abnormalities may be limited primarily to limb apraxias, or a conduction aphasia if the dominant hemisphere is affected.

The inferior division of the MCA nourishes the posterior parietal and temporal cortex (Fig. 201-2). Occlusion of one of its branches may produce a Wernicke's aphasia in the dominant hemisphere, left-sided neglect in the nondominant hemisphere, and associated agnosias, apraxias, or visual disturbances including a contralateral homonymous hemianopsia.

Several small penetrating arteries arise from the proximal portion of the MCA and supply the internal capsule and parts of the basal ganglia (Fig. 201-3). Occlusion of these vessels, usually associated with hypertension, produces small infarcts called *lacunes*.[10] The most common stroke syndrome arising from these 1- to 1.5-mm lacunes is a *pure motor hemiplegia*.[10] Typically a hypertensive patient notes the stuttering onset of paralysis of the face, arm, and leg without accompanying sensory loss, aphasia, or hemianopsia. Striking recovery often occurs in the ensuing weeks. Other penetrating arteries arise from the circle of Willis, the stem of the anterior cerebral artery, the posterior cerebral artery, and the basilar artery. Occlusion of these vessels can also lead to lacunar infarction, producing a variety of other lacunar stroke syndromes.[10] A *pure sensory stroke* occurs with a lacunar infarct in the ventral posterior thalamus. Numbness and paresthesias affect one side of the body without motor, language, or visual abnormalities. A stroke syndrome consisting of slurred speech and clumsiness of one hand occurs with lacunar infarction and has been termed the *dysarthria–clumsy hand* syndrome. *Homolateral ataxia and crural paresis* is the designation for the occurrence of arm and leg ataxia with weakness of the foot and ankle. Both of these latter two syndromes have been attributed to lacunar infarctions of the brain stem or posterior limb of the internal capsule.

Anterior Choroidal Artery Occlusion

The anterior choroidal artery (AchA) arises from the ICA or proximal MCA and sweeps posteriorly to supply the medial temporal lobe, the internal capsule, and the geniculocalcarine tract (Fig. 201-3). Ischemia in the distribution of the AchA may produce contralateral hemiparesis, hemihypesthesia, or hemianopsia.

Anterior Cerebral Artery Occlusion

The anterior cerebral arteries (ACAs) supply the medial portions of the frontal and anterior parietal lobes (Fig. 201-4).[17] Collateral flow from the anterior communicating artery and the cortical branches of the MCA are variable from one person to the next and assume a pivotal role in determining the extent of infarction occurring after ACA occlusion. The characteristic pattern of an ACA infarct is paralysis of the opposite leg and foot with lesser weakness of the shoulder and arm. The face muscles are usually spared. Sensory loss over the leg and foot may accompany the weakness. Bilateral ischemia may produce paraplegia, urinary incontinence, and an apathetic, mute, "lobotomized" patient.

Heubner's artery arises from the proximal ACA and nourishes the anterior hypothalamus, a portion of the internal capsule, and the anterior portions of the caudate and putamen. Occlusion of Heubner's artery may produce a contralateral hemiparesis involving the face, arm, and leg. When the dominant hemisphere is affected, a transcortical motor aphasia may also result. This language disorder is characterized by nonfluent speech with retained comprehension and speech repetition.

Posterior Cerebral Artery Occlusion

The posterior cerebral arteries (PCAs) usually arise as the terminal branches of the basilar artery. However, about 25 percent of the time one or both PCAs are supplied by the ICA via the posterior communicating artery. Small penetrating arteries originate from the proximal PCA and supply the midbrain, subthalamus, and thalamus (Fig. 201-3). Cortical branches supply the parietal and occipital cortex and the inferior temporal regions (Fig. 201-4). A contralateral homonymous hemianopsia develops with unilateral cortical branch occlusion and the resultant ischemia of the ipsilateral calcarine cortex or optic radiation. Bilateral occipital infarction produces cortical blindness, usually accompanied by the patient's denial of visual impairment (Anton's syndrome).[18] Visual defects may take the form of illusions or unformed or simply formed imagery. More complex visual hallucinations usually arise from temporal lobe lesions. Dominant hemisphere parieto-occipital ischemia may produce reading impairment (alexia with or without agraphia) and defects of color naming. Transient or persistent memory loss has been attributed to bilateral ischemia of the inferomedial temporal lobes. Episodes of memory loss lasting several hours have been ascribed to this mechanism and designated *transient global amnesia*.[11]

Several neurological abnormalities may emerge from occlusion of the penetrating arteries originating from the proximal PCA. Infarction of the thalamus produces contralateral sensory impairment. This sensory loss may partially recover but be replaced after several weeks or months by pain and hyperpathia in the affected limbs. This *thalamic pain syndrome* of Dejerine and Roussy is often extremely difficult to treat.

Unilateral midbrain and subthalamic ischemia may produce a number of signs singly or in combination. These include an ipsilateral oculomotor paralysis and contralateral hemiparesis, ataxia, or hemiballismus. Bilateral infarction of the central reticular formation may produce stupor or coma.

Basilar Artery Occlusion

The basilar artery (BA) is formed by the two vertebral arteries (VA) at the pontomedullary junction. It ascends anterior to the base of the pons and bifurcates into the two PCAs. Deviations from this "normal" relationship of the basilar artery to the VAs and PCAs are common. Penetrating paramedian branches of the BA supply the medial pons, short circumferential branches nourish the anterolateral pons, and the superior and anterior inferior cerebellar arteries supply the posterolateral pons and much of the cerebellar hemispheres. These multiple branches supplying the many structures traversing the pons cause a variety of neurological signs with BA ischemia. If the rostral BA is occluded, there may be ischemia to the midbrain, subthalamus, thalamus, and portions of the temporal

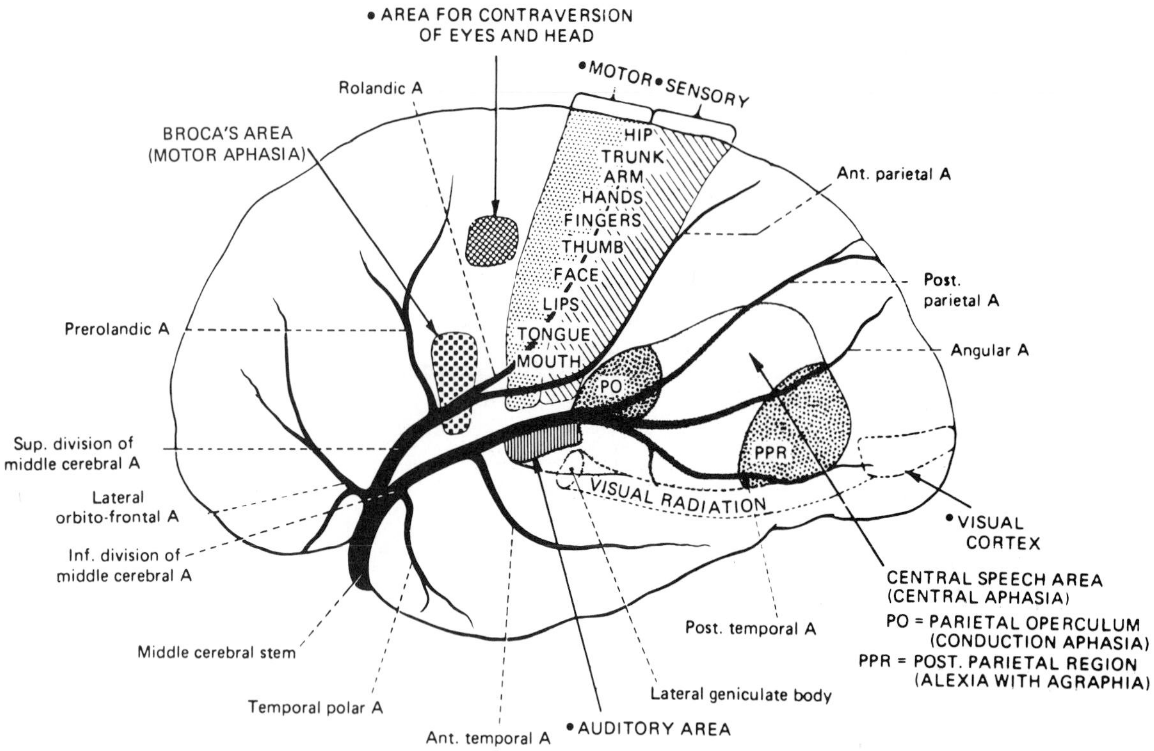

Signs and symptoms	Structures involved
Paralysis of the contralateral face, arm, and leg	Somatic motor area for face and arm and the fibers descending from the leg area to enter the corona radiata
Sensory impairment over the contralateral face, arm, and leg (pinprick, cotton touch, vibration, position, two-point discrimination, stereognosis, tactile localization, barognosis, cutaneographia)	Somatic sensory area for face and arm and thalamoparietal projections
Motor speech disorder	Broca's and adjacent motor area of the dominant hemisphere
"Central" aphasia, word deafness, anomia, jargon speech, alexia, agraphia, acalculia, finger agnosia, right-left confusion (the last four comprise the Gerstmann syndrome)	Central language area and parietooccipital cortex of the dominant hemisphere
Apractagnosia (amorphosynthesis), anosognosia, hemiasomatognosia, unilateral neglect, agnosia for the left half of external space, "dressing apraxia," "constructional apraxia," distortion of visual coordinates, inaccurate localization in the half field, impaired ability to judge distance, upside-down reading, visual illusions	Usually nondominant parietal lobe. Loss of topographic memory is usually due to a nondominant lesion, occasionally to a dominant one.
Homonymous hemianopia (often superior homonymous quadrantanopia)	Optic radiation deep to second temporal convolution
Paralysis of conjugate gaze to the opposite side	Frontal contraversive field or fibers projecting therefrom
Avoidance reaction of opposite limbs	Parietal lobe
Miscellaneous	
Ataxia of contralateral limb(s)	Parietal lobe
So-called Bruns ataxia or apraxia of gait	Frontal lobes (bilateral)
Loss or impairment of optokinetic nystagmus	Supramarginal or angular gyrus
Limb-kinetic apraxia	Premotor or parietal cortical damage
Mirror movements	Precise location of responsible lesions not known
Cheyne-Stokes respiration, contralateral hyperhidrosis, mydriasis (occasionally)	Precise location of responsible lesions not known
Pure motor hemiplegia	Upper portion of the posterior limb of the internal capsule and the adjacent corona radiata

Figure 201-2 Diagram of a cerebral hemisphere, lateral aspect, showing the branches and distribution of the middle cerebral artery and the principal regions of cerebral localization. Below the diagram is a list of the clinical manifestations of infarction in the territory of the middle cerebral artery and the corresponding regions of cerebral damage. (From Adams and Victor,[1] with permission.)

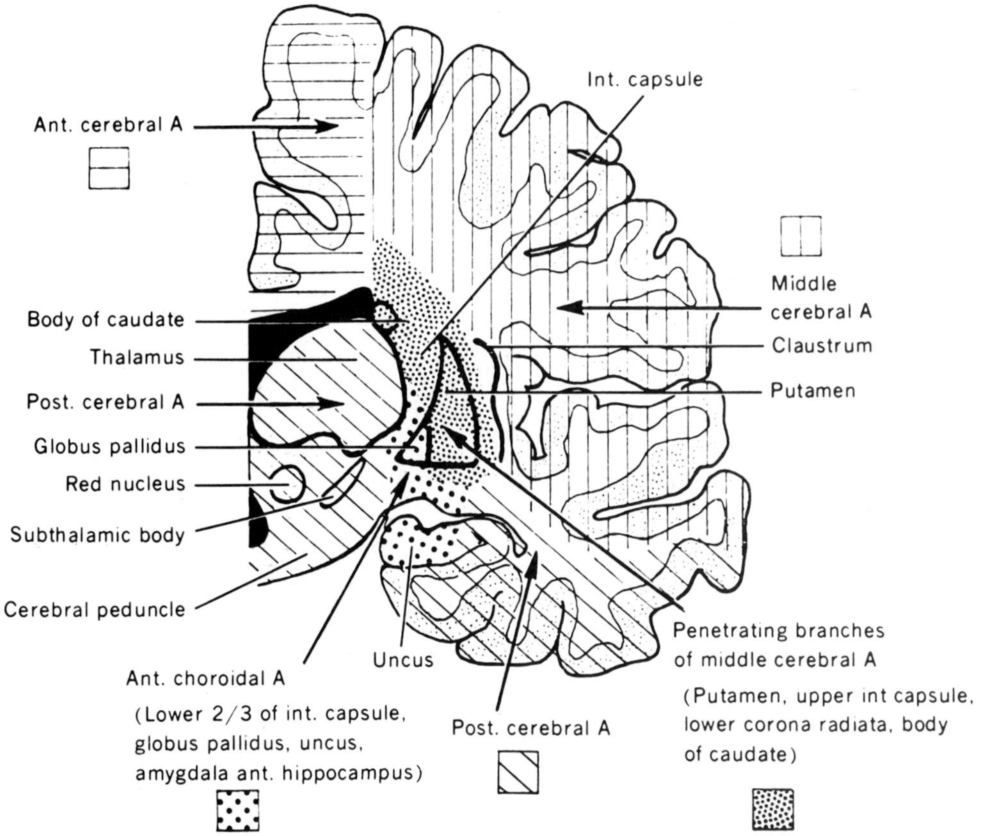

Figure 201-3 Diagram of a cerebral hemisphere, coronal section, showing the territories of the major cerebral vessels. (From Adams and Victor,[1] with permission.)

and occipital lobes. The resulting neurological abnormalities have been designated the *top of the basilar syndrome*.[5] This syndrome includes visual field defects, disorders of vertical gaze and convergence, slow deviation of the eyes, pupillary constriction, somnolence, and hallucinations in addition to bilateral weakness, ataxia, and sensory loss of the extremities.

Occlusion of the BA or one or more of its paramedian or short circumferential branches can lead to a wide variety of stroke syndromes. Some of the ocular abnormalities seen are nystagmus, internuclear ophthalmoplegia, gaze paresis, abducens palsy, ocular bobbing, and constricted pupils. Somnolence or coma occurs with reticular formation ischemia. Transient loss of consciousness in the absence of associated brain stem ischemic symptoms is rarely caused by vertebrobasilar ischemia. Weakness and hypesthesia of the face may be accompanied by similar impairment of the contralateral limbs, or all four limbs. Ischemia of the vestibular nuclei or pathways produces vertigo, nausea, vomiting, and nystagmus. Limb and gait ataxia occur following ischemia of the superior or middle cerebellar peduncles or cerebellar hemispheres. TIAs in the vertebrobasilar circulation are subject to greater diagnostic uncertainty than are those in the carotid circulation. This difference is easily appreciated in light of the varied symptoms of brain stem ischemia (Table 201-1). Dizziness, vertigo, light-headedness, loss of consciousness, and visual blurring represent some of the most common symptoms attributed incorrectly to vertebrobasilar ischemia (Tables 201-2 and 201-3). These symptoms occurring without other more definite symptoms of brain stem ischemia have such ubiquitous origins that they should not be attributed ipso facto to focal cerebrovascular disease.

The most characteristic syndromes resulting from basilar artery branch occlusions are the medial and lateral superior pontine syndromes, the medial and lateral midpontine syndromes, and the medial and lateral inferior pontine syndromes (Figs. 201-5 to 201-7). Each syndrome may be more or less complete. The usual artery involved in producing each of the syndromes is noted in the figure legends.

When all of the symptoms and signs of a posterior circulation ischemic episode can be accounted for by involvement of a single branch artery, the ischemic event can usually be attributed to occlusion of that specific artery. However, when the clinical features suggest multiple branch artery involvement, it is likely that the primary lesion is in the more proximal parent vessel, and one should be concerned about the possibility of a devastating basilar artery thrombosis (Fig. 201-8).[1,3]

Vertebral Artery Occlusion

The two vertebral arteries (VAs) ascend from the foramen magnum to nourish the rostral cervical spinal cord, the medulla, and the posterior inferior cerebellum before uniting to form the BA. There is considerable congenital variability in the diameter of the VAs. This fact, combined with the variability of collateral anastomoses

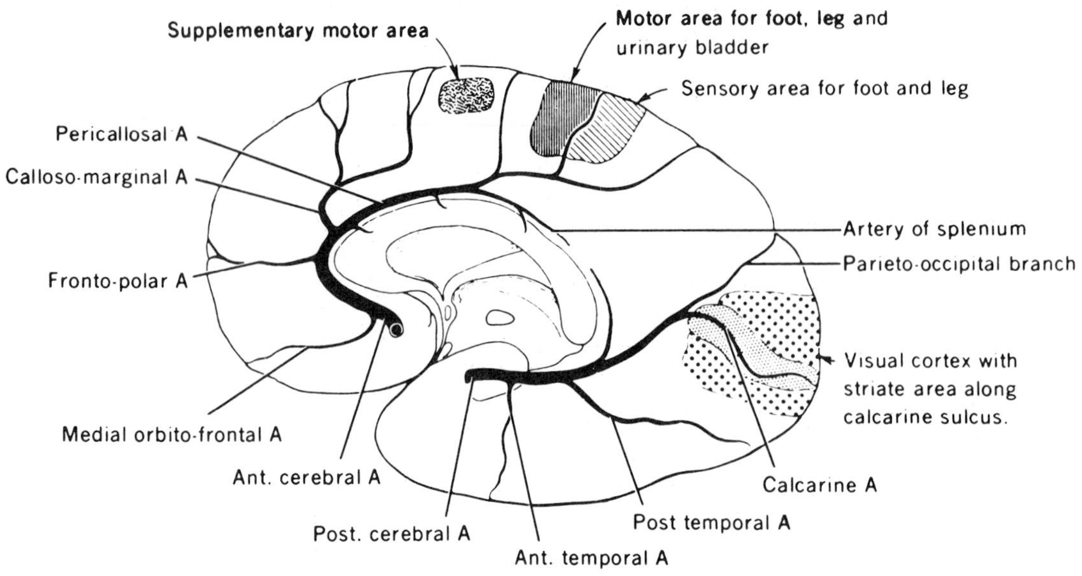

Signs and symptoms	Structures involved
Paralysis of opposite foot and leg	Motor leg area
A lesser degree of paresis of opposite arm	Involvement of arm area of cortex or fibers descending therefrom to corona radiata
Cortical sensory loss over toes, foot, and leg	Sensory area for foot and leg
Urinary incontinence	Posteromedial part of superior frontal gyrus
Contralateral grasp reflex, sucking reflex, gegenhalten (paratonic rigidity), "frontal tremor"	Medial surface of the posterior frontal lobe (?)
Abulia (akinetic mutism), slowness, delay, lack of spontaneity, whispering, motor inaction, reflex distraction to sights and sounds	Uncertain localization—probably inferomedial lesion near subcallosum
Impairment of gait and stance (gait "apraxia")	Inferomedial frontal-pallidal (?)
Mental impairment (perseveration and amnesia)	Localization unknown
Miscellaneous	
Dyspraxia of left limbs	Corpus callosum
Tactile aphasia in left limbs	Corpus callosum
Cerebral paraplegia	Motor leg area bilaterally (due to bilateral occlusion of anterior cerebral arteries)

Note: Hemianopia does not occur; transcortical aphasia occurs rarely.

Figure 201-4 Diagram of a cerebral hemisphere, medial aspect, showing the branches and distribution of the anterior cerebral artery and the principal regions of cerebral localization. Below the diagram is a list of the clinical manifestations of infarction in the territory of the anterior cerebral artery and the corresponding regions of cerebral damage. (From Adams and Victor,[1] with permission.)

from the external carotid and other neck arteries, the circle of Willis, and the BA, accounts for the diversity of neurological manifestations of VA disease. A VA occlusion may be asymptomatic, or it may cause a medullary infarction or ischemic symptoms throughout the BA or PCA distribution.

Infarction of the lateral medulla is usually caused by VA or posterior inferior cerebellar artery (PICA) occlusion, and it produces the Wallenberg syndrome, one of the most common ischemic syndromes of the vertebrobasilar circulation (Fig. 201-8). The syndrome may be more or less complete. Involvement of the spinothalamic tract and the descending tract and nucleus of the trigeminal nerve produces a loss of pain and temperature sensation in the ipsilateral face and contralateral body and limbs. Ischemia of the vestibular nuclei causes vertigo, nausea, vomiting, oscillopsia, and nystagmus. Ischemia of the cerebellum or its connections yields ataxia of the ipsilateral limbs. A Horner's syndrome arises from descending sympathetic tract involvement. Inclusion of the lower cranial nerve nuclei and nerves produces dysphagia, hoarseness, a diminished gag reflex, hiccups, and, rarely, loss of taste.

Infarction of the medial medulla is rare but produces paralysis of the contralateral arm and leg because of pyramidal tract involvement (Fig. 201-8). Loss of touch and proprioceptive sensation in a similar distribution arises from medial lemniscus ischemia. Ipsilateral tongue paralysis occurs when the hypoglossal nerve is injured.

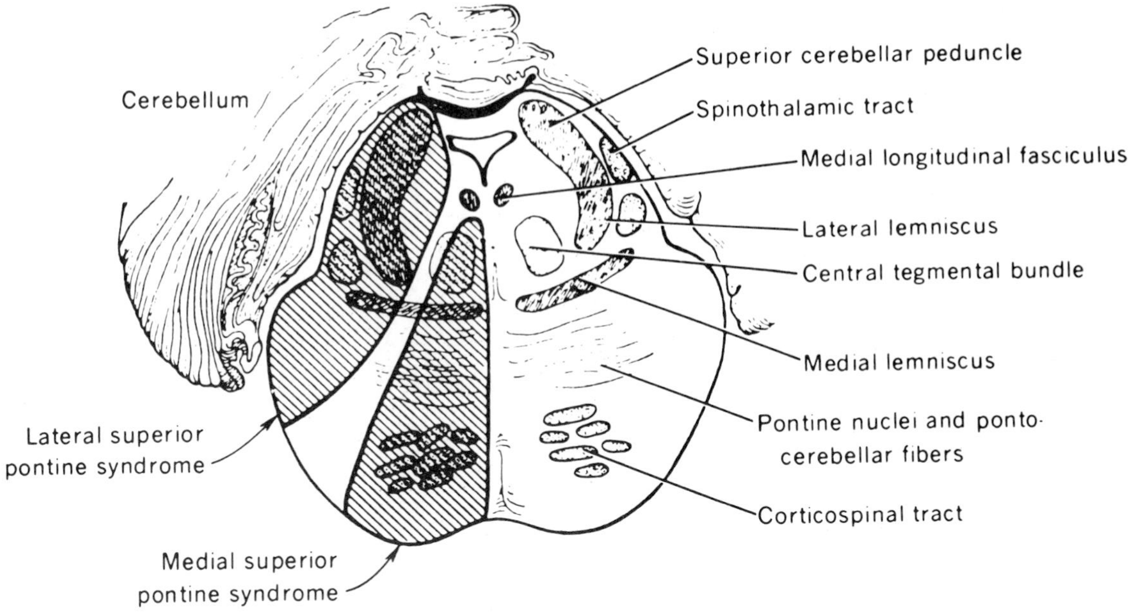

Signs and symptoms	Structures involved
1. Medial superior pontine syndrome (paramedian branches of upper basilar artery	
a. On side of lesion	
(1) Cerebellar ataxia	Superior and/or middle cerebellar peduncle
(2) Internuclear ophthalmoplegia	Medial longitudinal fasciculus
(3) Rhythmic myoclonus of palate, pharynx, vocal cords, respiratory apparatus, face, oculomotor apparatus, etc.	Central tegmental bundle
b. On side opposite lesion	
(1) Paralysis of face, arm, and leg	Corticobulbar and corticospinal tract
(2) Rarely touch, vibration, and position senses are affected	Medial lemniscus
2. Lateral superior pontine syndrome (syndrome of superior cerebellar artery)	
a. On side of lesion	
(1) Ataxia of limbs and gait, falling to side of lesion	Middle and superior cerebellar peduncles, superior surface of cerebellum, dentate nucleus
(2) Dizziness, nausea, vomiting	Vestibular nuclei } Territory of descending branch to middle cerebellar peduncle from superior cerebellar artery
(3) Horizontal nystagmus	Vestibular nuclei
(4) Paresis of conjugate gaze (ipsilateral)	Uncertain
(5) Loss of optokinetic nystagmus	Uncertain
(6) Skew deviation	Uncertain
(7) Miosis, ptosis, decreased sweating over face (Horner syndrome)	Descending sympathetic fibers
b. On side opposite lesion	
(1) Impaired pain and thermal sense on face, limbs, and trunk	Spinothalamic tract
(2) Impaired touch, vibration, and position sense, more in leg than arm (there is a tendency to incongruity of pain and touch deficits)	Medial lemniscus (lateral portion)

Figure 201-5 Diagram of a cross-section of the upper pons. Below the diagram is a list of the clinical manifestations of medial and lateral superior pontine infarction and their corresponding regions of damage. (From Adams and Victor,[1] with permission.)

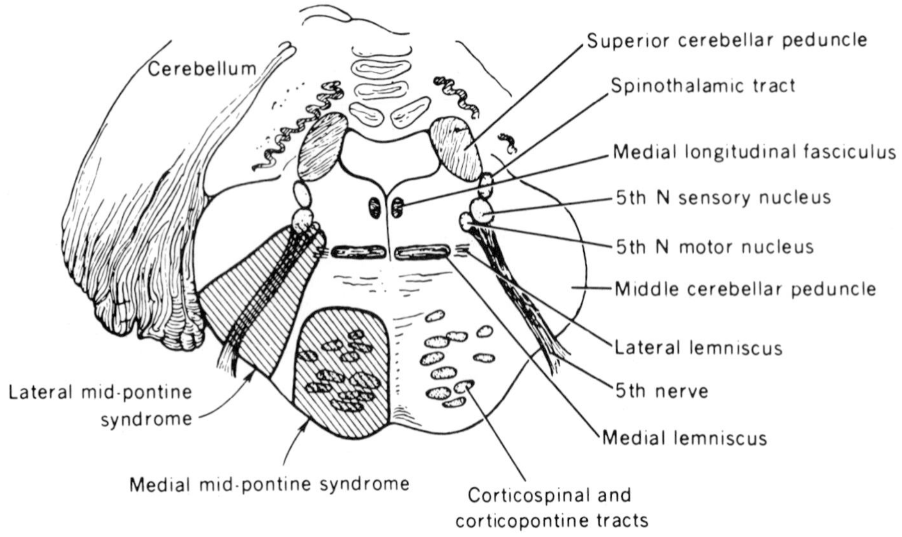

Signs and symptoms	Structures involved
1. Medial midpontine syndrome (paramedian branch of midbasilar artery)	
a. On side of lesion	
(1) Ataxia of limbs and gait (more prominent in bilateral involvement)	Middle cerebellar peduncle
b. On side opposite lesion	
(1) Paralysis of face, arm, and leg	Corticobulbar and corticospinal tract
(2) Deviation of eyes	
(3) Variably impaired touch and proprioception when lesion extends posteriorly. Usually the syndrome is purely motor.	Medial lemniscus
2. Lateral midpontine syndrome (short circumferential artery)	
a. On side of lesion	
(1) Ataxia of limbs	Middle cerebellar peduncle
(2) Paralysis of muscles of mastication	Motor fibers or nucleus of fifth nerve
(3) Impaired sensation over side of face	Sensory fibers or nucleus of fifth nerve

Figure 201-6 Diagram of a cross-section of the pons at the level of the fifth nerve. Below the diagram is a list of the clinical manifestations of medial and lateral midpontine infarction and their corresponding regions of damage. (From Adams and Victor,[1] with permission.)

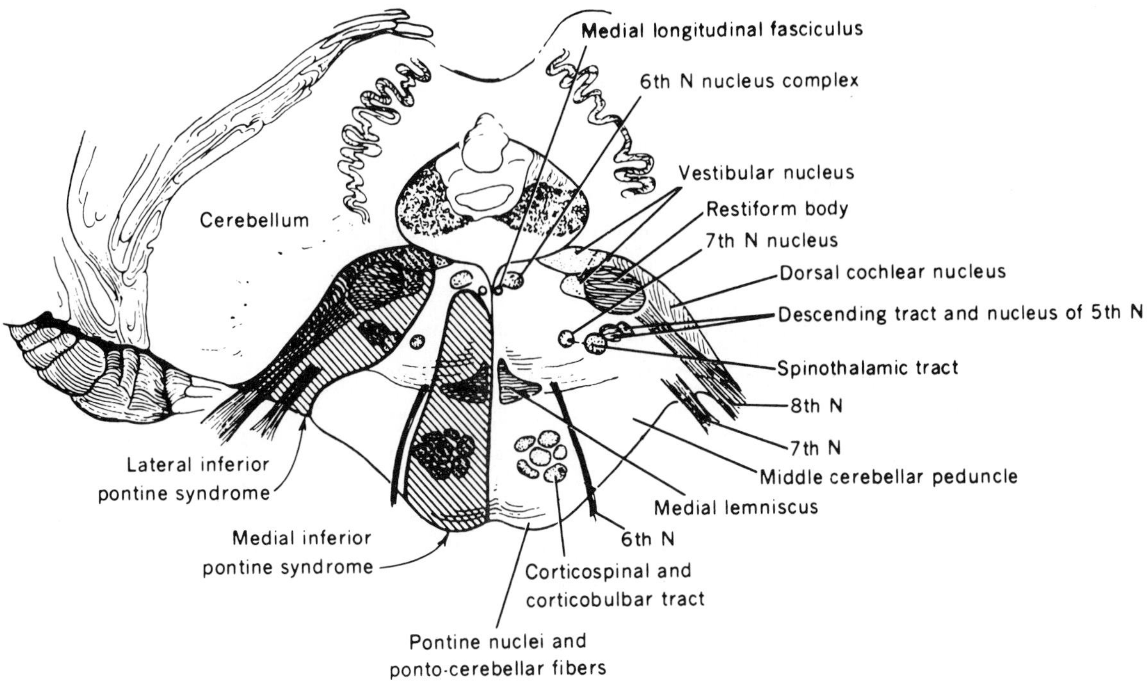

Signs and symptoms	Structures involved
1. Medial inferior pontine syndrome (occlusion of paramedian branch of basilar artery)	
a. On side of lesion	
(1) Paralysis of conjugate gaze to side of lesion (preservation of convergence)	Pontine "center" for lateral gaze (PPRF)
(2) Nystagmus	Vestibular nuclei and connections
(3) Ataxia of limbs and gait	Middle cerebellar peduncle (?)
(4) Diplopia on lateral gaze	Abducens nerve or nucleus
b. On side opposite lesion	
(1) Paralysis of face, arm, and leg	Corticobulbar and corticospinal tract in lower pons
(2) Impaired tactile and proprioceptive sense over half of the body	Medial lemniscus
2. Lateral inferior pontine syndrome (occlusion of anterior inferior cerebellar artery)	
a. On side of lesion	
(1) Horizontal and vertical nystagmus, vertigo, nausea, vomiting, oscillopsia	Vestibular nerve or nucleus
(2) Facial paralysis	Seventh nerve or nucleus
(3) Paralysis of conjugate gaze to side of lesion	Pontine "center" for lateral gaze (PPRF)
(4) Deafness, tinnitus	Auditory nerve or cochlear nucleus
(5) Ataxia	Middle cerebellar peduncle and cerebellar hemisphere
(6) Impaired sensation over face	Main sensory nucleus and descending tract of fifth nerve
b. On side opposite lesion	
(1) Impaired pain and thermal sense over half the body (may include face)	Spinothalamic tract
3. Total unilateral inferior pontine syndrome (occlusion of anterior inferior cerebellar artery); lateral and medial syndromes combined	

Figure 201-7 Diagram of a cross-section of the pons at the level of the sixth and seventh nerve nuclei. Below the diagram is a list of the clinical manifestations of medial and lateral inferior pontine infarction and their corresponding regions of damage. (From Adams and Victor,[1] with permission.)

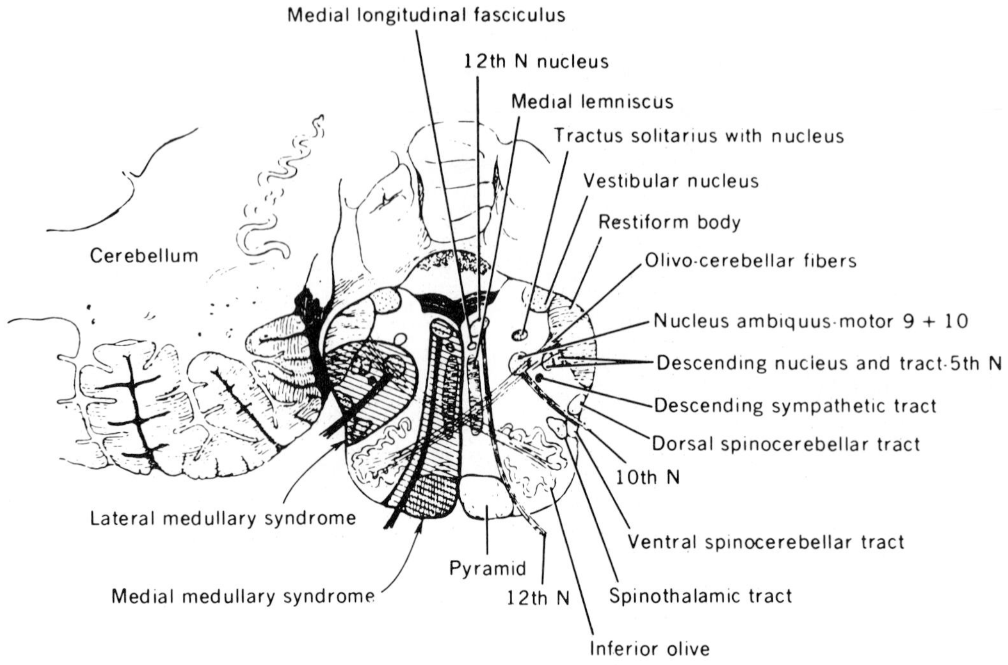

Signs and symptoms	Structures involved
1. Medial medullary syndrome (occlusion of vertebral artery or branch of vertebral or lower basilar artery)	
a. On side of lesion	
(1) Paralysis with atrophy of half the tongue	Issuing twelfth nerve
b. On side opposite lesion	
(1) Paralysis of arm and leg sparing face	Pyramidal tract
(2) Impaired tactile and proprioceptive sense over half the body	Medial lemniscus
2. Lateral medullary syndrome (occlusion of any of five vessels may be responsible—vertebral, posterior inferior cerebellar, or superior, middle, or inferior lateral medullary arteries)	
a. On side of lesion	
(1) Pain, numbness, impaired sensation over half the face	Descending tract and nucleus of fifth nerve
(2) Ataxia of limbs, falling to side of lesion	Uncertain—restiform body, cerebellar hemisphere, olivocerebellar fibers, spinocerebellar tract (?)
(3) Vertigo, nausea, vomiting	Vestibular nuclei and connections
(4) Nystagmus, diplopia, oscillopsia	Vestibular nuclei and connections
(5) Horner's syndrome (miosis, ptosis, decreased sweating)	Descending sympathetic tract
(6) Dysphagia, hoarseness, paralysis of vocal cord, diminished gag reflex	Issuing fibers ninth and tenth nerves
(7) Loss of taste (rare)	Nucleus and tractus solitarius
(8) Numbness of ipsilateral arm, trunk, or leg	Cuneate and gracile nuclei
(9) Hiccup	Uncertain
b. On side opposite lesion	
(1) Impaired pain and thermal sense over half the body, sometimes face	Spinothalamic tract
3. Total unilateral medullary syndrome (occlusion of vertebral artery); combination of medial and lateral syndromes	
4. Lateral pontomedullary syndrome (occlusion of vertebral artery); combination of medial and lateral syndromes	

Figure 201-8 Diagram of a cross-section of the medulla at the level of the twelfth nerve. Below the diagram is a list of the clinical manifestations of medial and lateral medullary infarction and their corresponding regions of damage. (From Adams and Victor,[1] with permission.)

Signs and symptoms	Structures involved
5. Basilar artery syndrome (the syndrome of the lone vertebral artery is equivalent); a combination of the various brainstem syndromes plus those arising in the posterior cerebral artery distribution. The clinical picture comprises bilateral long-tract signs (sensory and motor) with cerebellar and cranial nerve abnormalities.	
a. Paralysis or weakness of all extremities, plus all bulbar musculature	Corticobulbar and corticospinal tracts bilaterally
b. Diplopia, paralysis of conjugate lateral and/or vertical gaze, internuclear ophthalmoplegia, horizontal and/or vertical nystagmus	Ocular motor nerves, apparatus for conjugate gaze, medial longitudinal fasciculus, vestibular apparatus
c. Blindness, impaired vision, various visual field defects	Visual cortex
d. Bilateral cerebellar ataxia	Cerebellar peduncles and the cerebellar hemispheres
e. Coma	Tegmentum of midbrain, thalami
f. Sensation may be strikingly intact in the presence of almost total paralysis. Sensory loss may be syringomyelic or the reserve or involve all modalities.	Medial lemniscus, spinothalamic tracts or thalamic nuclei

Figure 201-8 (*Continued*)

References

1. Adams RD, Victor M. *Principles of Neurology*, 5th ed. New York: McGraw-Hill, 1993.
2. Barnett HJM. Progress towards stroke prevention: Robert Wartenberg lecture. *Neurology (NY)* 1980; 30:1212–1225.
3. Biemond A. Thrombosis of the basilar artery and the vascularization of the brain stem. *Brain* 1951; 74:300–317.
4. Byer JA, Easton JD. Therapy of ischemic cerebrovascular disease. *Ann Intern Med* 1980; 93:742–756.
5. Caplan LR. ''Top of the basilar'' syndrome. *Neurology (NY)* 1980; 30:72–79.
6. de Bono DP, Warlow CP. Potential sources of emboli in patients with presumed transient cerebral or retinal ischaemia. *Lancet* 1981; 1:343–346.
7. Easton JD, Hart RG, Sherman DG, Kaste M. Diagnosis and management of ischemic stroke: Part I. Threatened stroke and its management. *Cur Prob Cardiol* 1983; 8:1–76.
8. Easton JD, Sherman DG. Management of cerebral embolism of cardiac origin. *Stroke* 1980; 11:433–442.
9. Fisher CM. Late-life migraine accompaniments as a cause of unexplained transient ischemic attacks. *Can J Neurol Sci* 1980; 7:9–17.
10. Fisher CM. Lacunar strokes and infarcts: a review. *Neurology* (*NY*) 1982; 32:871–876.
11. Fisher CM, Adams RD. Transient global amnesia. *Acta Neurol Scand [Suppl]* 1964; 9:1–83.
12. Hart RG, Sherman DG, Miller VT, Easton JD. Diagnosis and management of ischemic stroke: Part II. Selected controversies. *Cur Prob Cardiol* 1983; 8:1–80.
13. Jones HR, Millikan CH. Temporal profile (clinical course) of acute carotid system cerebral infarction. *Stroke* 1976; 7:64–71.
14. Jones HR Jr, Millikan CH, Sandok BA. Temporal profile (clinical course) of acute vertebrobasilar system cerebral infarction. *Stroke* 1980; 11:173–177.
15. Millikan CH. Transient cerebral ischemia: definition and natural history. *Prog Cardiovasc Dis* 1980; 22:303–308.
16. National Institute of Neurological and Communicative Disorders and Stroke: a classification and outline of cerebrovascular diseases, III. *Stroke* 1990; 21:637–676.
17. Ostrowski AZ, Webster JE, Gurdjian ES. The proximal anterior cerebral artery: an anatomic study. *Arch Neurol* 1960; 3:661–664.
18. Symonds C, Mackenzie I. Bilateral loss of vision from cerebral infarction. *Brain* 1957; 80:415–455.
19. Wilterdink JL, Easton JD. Vascular event rates in patients with atherosclerotic cerebrovascular disease. *Arch Neurol* 1992; 49:857–863.

202 Noninvasive Diagnosis of Carotid Occlusive Disease

Robert M. Crowell
J. Philip Kistler
Christopher S. Ogilvy
Daryl R. Gress
Richard L. Robertson, Jr.

Occlusive disease of the cervical internal carotid artery (ICA) is an important cause of ischemic stroke. Controlled studies have demonstrated clearly that carotid endarterectomy is a safe and very effective measure to prevent stroke in patients with severe ICA stenosis. While conventional angiography is an effective study for identification of severe ICA stenosis, it carries a small but significant risk, even for experienced angiographers.

In this setting, noninvasive diagnosis, which avoids the risk of direct carotid injection, has great intuitive appeal. However, there has been a natural skepticism regarding the reliability of noninvasive techniques for detection of ICA stenosis and particularly for detection of intracranial pathology, such as carotid siphon or middle cerebral artery (MCA) stenosis or occlusion.

Recently there has been further refinement of carotid noninvasive studies (CNIS) for the detection of ICA and intracranial occlusive disease. In addition, transcranial Doppler (TCD) ultrasonography has been developed to detect with high reliability intracranial occlusive disease. Moreover, the maturation of magnetic resonance angiography (MRA) now provides reliable images of both extracranial and intracranial carotid atherosclerotic occlusive disease. By combining CNIS, TCD, and MRA, most cases of carotid occlusive disease, both symptomatic and asymptomatic, can now be adequately evaluated. Results from several centers confirm the reliability of this approach. Conventional angiography appears necessary for only a small minority of cases in which the results of CNIS/TCD/MRA are equivocal.

Atherosclerotic Lesions at the Origin of the Internal Carotid Artery

Pathology

The most common pathologic entities of the ICA that lead to stroke are atherosclerotic narrowing at its origin, atherosclerotic narrowing in the siphon, and dissection (usually beginning at the level of the first cervical vertebra). Less common causes include primary thrombosis at the origin, petrous carotid stenosis, compression of the distal internal carotid artery by tumor (usually meningioma), and fibromuscular dysplasia. Of all these entities, atherosclerotic narrowing at the origin of the internal carotid artery is by far the most common cause of stroke. The atherosclerotic plaque tends to form at the posterior aspect of the bifurcation and at the origin of the internal carotid artery. Plaque usually narrows the lumen in a concentric fashion, with the maximum narrowing usually located not more than 1 cm distal to the bifurcation and usually not extending for more than 1 to 2 mm. Rarely the maximal narrowing extends for up to 1 cm, and even more rarely the site of maximal narrowing from atherosclerotic lesions can be more distal in the internal carotid artery, up to the level of C1. Carotid siphon stenosis is an atherosclerotic lesion of the S-shaped portion of the intracranial internal carotid artery, either proximal or distal to the takeoff of the ophthalmic artery. When an atherosclerotic lesion narrows the origin of the internal carotid artery, a mural thrombus may form at or near the residual lumen.[20,46] Occasionally, blood from the lumen penetrates into the plaque. This penetration may be the mechanism by which an ulcer crater forms and becomes a nidus for the production of a mural thrombus.[46] Less often, hemorrhage into the plaque further narrows the lumen.

Pathophysiology

Often cervical carotid artery lesions are identified by the detection of a bruit, by the occurrence of a minor stroke, or by transient ocular or cerebral ischemic attacks in the territory of the carotid artery. Less often there may be a sudden disabling or fatal stroke. Bruits become audible when the residual lumen is narrowed to approximately 3 mm or less (about 50 percent stenosis). The higher the pitch of the bruit, the tighter the stenosis. A particularly high-pitched bruit that fades into diastole indicates a hemodynamically important stenosis of the internal carotid artery, with a residual lumen of less than 1.5 mm (75 percent stenosis or more). Retinal or cerebral ischemic symptoms are produced by either of two pathophysiologic mechanisms: transient decreases in already low blood flow or embolism.[18,34] Hemodynamic changes leading to transient retinal or cerebral ischemia or infarction occur less often than embolism. Symptoms caused by low flow require a hemodynamically important carotid stenosis (75 percent stenosis or more) in association with reduced collateral flow from either the external carotid–ophthalmic artery system or the anterior or posterior circle of Willis to the ipsilateral carotid territory. Under these conditions, repeated, short, stereotyped episodes of transient cerebral ischemia (true transient ischemic attacks)[18] or slowly evolving cerebral infarction[34] result.

Emboli

When emboli arise from an atherosclerotic plaque at the origin of the internal carotid artery, symptoms are usually caused by occlusion of the ophthalmic artery, the middle cerebral artery stem, the anterior cerebral artery, or one of their branches. The duration and nature of the symptoms depend on the location and size of the embolus, the duration of the arterial occlusion, and the amount of collateral flow to the cortical surface branches. Single episodes of transient symptoms may be referred to as *embolic transient ischemic attacks,* but if they persist longer than an hour, some element of infarction may have occurred. In the presence of a high-grade stenotic lesion (70 to 99 percent stenosis, with residual lumen diameter less than 2 mm), these symptoms suggest that the stenotic lesion was the source of the embolus.[13,18,19,20,30,34,46,47,53] Progression of the atherothrombotic lesion to high-grade stenosis that becomes hemodynamically important (stenosis of 75 percent or more) has been associated with a particularly high incidence of stroke, approaching 5 percent or more per year.[13,53] In the absence of stenosis at the origin of the internal carotid artery, the occurrence of an ischemic stroke or a single, prolonged transient ischemic attack suggests an embolus from another source, usually the heart.

Risk of Stroke

When a bruit is the only symptom or sign of an arteriosclerotic lesion at the bifurcation of the common carotid artery, concern arises as to whether the patient is at risk for stroke. To determine which patients with asymptomatic cervical bruits are the most likely to have severe strokes, it is important to determine the severity of the stenosis as well as its hemodynamic effects. Studies of cervical bruit that did not assess severity of stenosis and hemodynamic effect have not shown an increased rate of ipsilateral strokes, even among patients who underwent major cardiac surgery.[28,54,63] On the other hand, studies that have measured the severity and hemodynamic importance of the stenosis have shown that patients with a high-grade and hemodynamically important stenosis have an increased risk of stroke.[43] When collateral flow is available through the external carotid artery (ECA)-ophthalmic artery system or the circle of Willis, patients can maintain adequate flow in the ipsilateral carotid territory and avoid hemodynamically induced transient ischemic attacks or stroke. These patients may nonetheless face the threat of embolism, however, because reduced flow in the proximal internal carotid artery can result in the formation of a thrombus. Whether the thrombus does or does not occlude the artery is less important than the likelihood of embolism in such cases (probably higher than 3 percent per year).[13,34,43,53]

Carotid Endarterectomy

Carotid endarterectomy has now been shown to be effective in preventing subsequent ipsilateral strokes in patients with lesions at the origin of the internal carotid artery that are symptomatic and severely stenotic ($\geq$70 percent).[17,42,45] The treatment is effective only if surgical morbidity is sufficiently low.[32] Furthermore, endarterectomy is under study and may be considered in patients with hemodynamically significant asymptomatic atherosclerotic lesions at the origin of the internal carotid artery.[29,32]

Since safe, effective treatment is available, we must have accurate diagnostic methods to evaluate structural lesions and flow at the bifurcation of the common carotid artery (CCA), along the course of the internal carotid artery, and in its intracranial branches. While conventional cerebral angiography remains the gold standard for the diagnosis of cerebrovascular occlusive disease and assessment of collateral circulation, angiography has known risks and morbidity.[15] Furthermore, it cannot be practically repeated in serial fashion. The safety and reproducibility of carotid noninvasive tests are very attractive in this respect, especially for asymptomatic disease. An important problem has been skepticism regarding the reliability of noninvasive diagnosis, particularly for intracranial (''tandem'') lesions.

Noninvasive Testing

Recent advances in technology have persuaded us that a battery of three noninvasive testing modalities can in most cases accurately provide the required assessment of extracranial internal carotid artery occlusive disease and associated intracranial hemodynamic changes. As indicated above, these three noninvasive tests are (1) standard carotid noninvasive studies, (2) transcranial Doppler ultrasonographic assessment of intracranial arterial and ophthalmic artery flow, and (3) MRA of the cervical and intracranial artery system. This chapter will discuss these modalities, their relationships with each other, and the indications for their use. Finally, we will discuss indications for conventional angiography after combined assessment by these three noninvasive methodologies.

Carotid Noninvasive Studies

Carotid noninvasive tests are conveniently divided into those that directly assess flow and vascular morphology at the bifurcation of the common carotid artery (direct tests) and those that indirectly assess the hemodynamic effect of a stenotic lesion at the bifurcation of the common carotid artery or more distally in the internal carotid artery (indirect tests).

Direct Tests

Recently, direct tests have been narrowed to two principal modalities: *duplex ultrasound scanning* (B-mode ultrasound image combined with range-gated assessment of flow at the bifurcation of the common carotid artery) and *triplex ultrasound scanning* (duplex scanning combined with ''real-time'' two-dimensional flow images superimposed on the B-mode image). Continuous-wave Doppler spectral analysis of flow at the bifurcation of the common carotid artery (CW Doppler) is used less frequently.[33] Frequency-intensity fast Fourier spectral analysis of the bruit to calculate the residual lumen diameter of the stenotic lesion (quantitative phonoangiography)[33] is no longer used, although it provided an excellent assessment of the residual lumen diameter of bruit-producing stenotic lesions at the origin of the ICA. The equipment for this test was not manufactured in a way that would allow its generalized use.

Auscultation of the bruit is still the first step in noninvasive assessment. The quality of the carotid bifurcation bruit can provide reliable clues to the location and degree of narrowing of the stenotic lesion that produces it.[32,33] The bruit begins to be audible when the residual lumen diameter at the point of maximum stenosis is narrowed to 3 mm. The pitch of the bruit is a direct reflection of the degree of stenosis. Very high bruits that fade into diastole are indicative of a tightly stenotic lesion with a residual lumen diameter of 1.5 mm or less at the origin of the internal carotid artery. They may be loud, but as the residual lumen narrows to below 1 mm, the intensity of the bruit fades in both systole and diastole. This decrease in amplitude is directly related to a decrease in volume of flow as the lesion becomes progressively more hemodynamically significant. Palpation of the bifurcation of the common carotid artery offers no additional reliable information. It should be abandoned because of the theoretical hazards of dislodging a thrombus or changing the pulse rate.

Duplex Ultrasound Scanning

B-mode ultrasound 2-D images direct the range-gated pulse Doppler probe to the bifurcation of the common carotid artery, to the origins of the external and internal carotid arteries, and more distally along those vessels. The *range-gated pulse Doppler* samples a small volume of flowing blood inside the artery at a specific point. It is therefore able to analyze the frequency and intensity components of flow at the point of maximum stenosis (where the velocity of flow is maximal) and just distal to it, at the point of greatest turbulence, and yet further distally, where laminar flow is reconstituted. Laminar flow is detected when the range of frequencies throughout the cardiac cycle is similar. Turbulent flow is noted with many frequencies and/or velocities in systole and diastole (spectral broadening). The narrower the residual lumen diameter, the higher the peak frequency shift and the higher the velocity. In addition, with stenosis there is more turbulent flow. Spectral broadening and increases in both peak and end-diastolic frequencies are noted as the residual lumen diameter decreases.

B-mode images provide information about plaque morphology and the residual lumen diameter of the atherothrombotic lesion at the bifurcation of the common carotid artery. Calcium is echolucent. Soft atheromatous plaque is seen as shades of gray. An ulcer crater can also be seen as an irregular surface of the internal vessel wall. Dense fibrous tissue appears brighter and whiter, while a softer plaque with more fat appears less bright and more gray. For diagnosing the severity of the stenosis, the plaque morphology and spectral waveforms are both valuable. Attenuated spectral waveforms at the origin of the internal carotid artery suggest a lesion higher in the arterial system. Waveforms that have increased peak systolic and diastolic frequencies suggest a stenotic lesion at that site, which can be confirmed by the B-mode image.

The *carotid index* (the peak systolic frequency of the internal carotid artery divided by that of the common carotid artery) is used to quantify the degree of stenosis. This is possible because comparisons have been made between the carotid index obtained by the CW Doppler technique and the actual residual lumen diameter measured on the pathologic specimens removed intact.[12] For the normal internal carotid artery origin, the carotid index is less than 2.5, and there is minor spectral broadening but diastolic flow is present. For mildly stenotic lesions (up to 40 percent stenosis or a residual lumen diameter of 4 mm or greater), the carotid index ranges between 2.5 and 4.0. Moderately severe stenotic lesions, equivalent to 40 to 60 percent stenosis or a residual lumen diameter of 2 to 4 mm, have a carotid index of 4 to 6.9. Severely stenotic lesions, with residual lumen diameter of less than 2 mm, have a carotid index of 7 to 15 or more. Because flow velocities vary, a carotid index of 7 may not reflect a residual lumen diameter of 2 mm or less, but generally it does so. Further descriptions of duplex scanning are available elsewhere.[6,7,9,61,64]

Although duplex scanning can provide reasonably reliable estimates of the degree of narrowing at the origin of the internal carotid artery, its reliability is highly dependent on the technician. An uncooperative patient or unfavorable plaque morphology may prevent the range-gated pulse Doppler sampling area from being correctly placed, with the result that the point of maximal stenosis and highest velocity will not be detected. Furthermore, this technique cannot differentiate between complete occlusion and near occlusion with a thread of residual lumen.

Triplex Ultrasound Scanning

For triplex ultrasound scanning (color-flow Doppler), B-mode imaging is combined with a multigated pulse Doppler that insonates the entire vessel, thereby allowing flow measurements across the entire vascular structure.[35,51,59] The data are then subjected to spectral analysis by fast Fourier transformation, and the resulting frequency-intensity data are color-coded, making it possible to display two-dimensional color-flow images inside the B-mode image of the vessel (Fig. 202-1). The instrument simultaneously analyzes Doppler information from more than 300 small sample sites in the zone of insonation. The frequency-intensity information from the spectral analysis is subprocessed and displayed in the color-code format rather than the gray-scale format. This color depiction of the frequencies facilitates identification of focal areas of abnormal flow patterns with high peak frequency shifts. Turbulent flow is depicted as various shades of red (in the direction of blood flow in the insonated artery) and blue (in the opposite direction). The equipment also produces the conventional range-gated pulse Doppler spectral pattern, as in duplex scanning. It has the added advantage of showing the information in a color-flow spectral array over a large area of the vessel, thereby facilitating detection of flow in a vessel that is critically narrowed. Unfortunately, it still cannot differentiate a preocclusive lesion with a thread of flow from total occlusion.

Continuous-Wave Doppler Ultrasonography

Because of the advent of duplex and triplex scanning, CW Doppler ultrasonography is now used less frequently. It has the advantage of requiring only a small device, and it can be combined with the range-gated pulse Doppler technique in the same machine used to study intracranial arterial flow with transcranial Doppler ultrasonography. In addition, it has been used to correlate the peak frequency shifts and carotid index with the actual residual lumen diameter of the endarterectomy specimens removed en bloc by our neurosurgeons.[33] This information can be extrapolated to duplex and triplex Doppler flow frequency and velocity measurements, particularly when the carotid index is used.

Indirect Tests

Oculoplethysmography

Oculoplethysmography (OPG-Gee) is a technique that gives an indirect measure of the systolic pressure in the opthalmic artery, which reflects the pressure in the distal internal carotid artery.[21–23] Obstructive lesions in the internal carotid artery proximal to the ophthalmic artery that reduce the lumen diameter by 75 percent or more (to 1.5 mm or less) cause a reduction in pressure in the distal

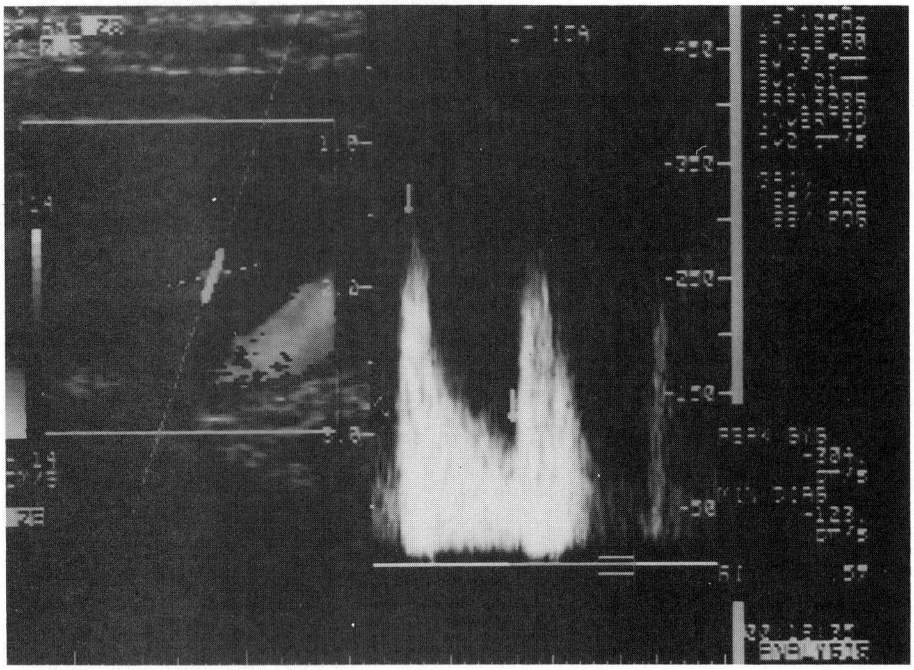

Figure 202-1 Doppler analysis of the internal carotid artery in a patient with severe stenosis. The panel on the left demonstrates the site of measurement and flow representation in a two-dimensional format of the flow through the carotid artery at an area of severe stenosis. On the right is shown the velocity of flow through one cardiac cycle. With the suggestion of this severe stenosis, the patient underwent carotid MRI/MRA analysis of the vasculature (Fig. 202-2).

internal carotid artery and therefore also in the ipsilateral ophthalmic artery. The OPG-Gee technique simultaneously measures the systolic pressure in both eyes and will therefore reveal a reduction in the eye ipsilateral to such a lesion. The test is accomplished by applying a vacuum (via an eye cup) significant enough to elevate the intraocular pressure above systolic pressure. The vacuum pressure is slowly reduced, and the peak systolic pressure reading is taken as the first pressure wave noted in the transducer from the eye cup.

Opthalmic artery pressure is considered reduced if there is a difference of 5 mmHg or more between the eye pressures. If bilateral hemodynamically significant lesions are present, then both ophthalmic artery pressures should lie below a value given by the formula OST = 39 + 0.436 × (brachial systolic blood pressure). A difference of 25 mmHg or more in brachial systolic pressure suggests innominate or subclavian disease.

The test is used to confirm the hemodynamic significance of a stenotic lesion. As such, it has been used to identify patients at greater risk of stroke.[13,43,53] It has the disadvantage of requiring direct scleral contact. The eye cups should be cleaned with alcohol and soap and water after each use to prevent the spread of viral diseases. Rarely, conjunctival hemorrhage occurs, and patients who are on anticoagulants should not have the test. Fortunately, transcranial Doppler assessment of ophthalmic artery flow also can provide reliable information as to the hemodynamic significance of a more proximal internal carotid artery stenotic lesion (see below).

Periorbital Doppler Ultrasonography

Periorbital Doppler ultrasonography is done by dynamically palpating the facial pulses while monitoring the direction of flow in the supraorbital and supratrochlear pulses by the CW Doppler technique. This test is highly technician-dependent and is reliable only in a few very experienced hands. False negatives occur frequently. It is therefore not widely used. Similarly, thermography has been largely abandoned.

Transcranial Doppler Assessment

Transcranial Doppler ultrasonography assesses intracranial arterial flow in the distal ICA, the middle, anterior, and posterior cerebral artery stems, and the ophthalmic artery. It can provide reliable estimates of the hemodynamic significance of extracranial or intracranial ICA occlusive disease and the availability of collateral flow through the intracranial circulation distal to the ICA stenotic lesion. In addition, it can detect the presence of significant occlusive lesions in the ipsilateral middle cerebral artery stem. TCD, therefore, has become a valuable technique in the noninvasive evaluation of patients with suspected carotid artery occlusive disease.

The test uses a 2-MHz range-gated pulse Doppler probe. Fast Fourier analysis of the incoming sampled Doppler shift signal derives a frequency-intensity flow spectrum at the point of insonation in the artery under study. Three-dimensional computer-assisted stereotactic head devices can be applied to allow for repeated insonation at the same point in the intracranial vessel. This method is usually reserved for patients undergoing repeated examination over time and is not necessary in the routine evaluation of extracranial carotid disease. For the latter purpose, flow is assessed in the opthalmic artery (transorbital approach), the distal ICA (transorbital and/or submandibular approach), the middle cerebral artery (MCA) stem, the anterior cerebral artery (ACA) stem, and the posterior cerebral artery (PCA) stem (transtemporal approach). Insonation of the vertebral and basilar arteries (foramen magnum approach) provides little information about the hemodynamic significance of carotid occlusive disease but can suggest occlusive lesions in those arteries that could account for symptoms mimicking carotid occlusive disease. The technique is briefly described below, and normal values are given. For more detailed information, the reader is referred to standard papers discussing normal and abnormal conditions.[1,2,5,10,11,24,27,36,37,40,44,48–50,52,56,57,60,62]

The *transorbital approach* is used to insonate the ophthalmic artery and the distal ICA. The intensity must be turned down to 25 percent of normal to prevent the possibility of retinal damage. The range-gated probe is set at 45 to 50 mm and placed superiorly on the covered globe. The probe depth is advanced to 60, insonating the ophthalmic artery. At 60 to 65 mm, the internal carotid artery siphon portion is insonated. The direction of flow in the ophthalmic artery and its mean and peak systolic velocities are recorded. Normal mean flow velocity is 21 ± 5 cm/s. Normal mean flow velocity for the carotid siphon is 41 ± 11 cm/s.

The *submandibular approach* is sometimes used to insonate the distal ICA. For this approach, the Doppler intensity is set at 100 percent. The distal ICA flow is usually met at a range-gated depth of 40 to 60 mm.

The *transtemporal approach* is attempted at the thinnest portion of the temporal bone cephalad to the zygomatic arch and immediately anterior and slightly superior to the tragus. The probe is then moved anteriorly toward the eye or superiorly to adjust for an anterior and a posterior window. Insonation depths are set at 40 mm for the bifurcation of the middle cerebral artery stem. The range gate is then advanced to 65 mm, which is generally where the internal carotid artery bifurcation is reached. The probe is then angled slightly anteriorly to locate the anterior cerebral artery stem (A1 segment). Most often the A1 segment of the anterior cerebral artery is insonated at a depth of 70 mm. The probe is then focused posteriorly to bring the posterior cerebral artery stem under insonation at 65 to 70 mm. Normal mean systolic velocities are 40 to 60 cm/s for the middle cerebral artery stem (M1), 45 to 55 cm/s for the anterior cerebral artery stem (A1), and 35 to 45 cm/s for the posterior cerebral artery stem (P1). The variation is 10 to 15 cm/s, and therefore it is most important to compare the right and left sides.

The *foramen magnum approach* allows for insonation of the vertebral and basilar arteries. The probe is placed suboccipitally just below the inion and is angled toward the nasion. It is then angled to the left and right and set at a range gate of 60 to 70 mm. Both vertebral arteries are insonated at that depth. The range gate is then advanced to 80 mm to obtain the vertebrobasilar junction. The basilar artery is insonated at 80 to 120 mm. Normal flow velocities for the vertebral artery are 35 to 45 cm/s and 30 to 45 cm/s for the basilar artery.

TCD signs of *hemodynamically significant ICA stenosis* in the proximal internal carotid artery or siphon include (1) flow reversal or reduction in the ophthalmic artery as compared to the contralateral side, (2) flow reduction in the ipsilateral middle cerebral artery (amplitude and pulsatility) compared to the contralateral side, (3) ipsilateral anterior cerebral artery flow reduction and/or reversal, and (4) increased flow velocity in the contralateral A1 cerebral artery, suggesting an increase in collateral flow across the anterior communicating artery. If the anterior communicating artery is atretic, then collateral flow across the anterior cerebral artery may not occur. In those special circumstances, (5) increase in velocity in the ipsilateral posterior cerebral artery may occur.

Middle cerebral artery stem stenosis may be associated with increased ipsilateral A1 anterior cerebral artery flow due to augmentation of flow through the anterior cerebral cortical surface branches to supply the middle cerebral artery cortical surface branches. Most important, middle cerebral stem stenosis is associated with an increased flow velocity distal to it, making the condition detectable by TCD in the face of ipsilateral ICA stenosis.

Uses of TCD

As noted, transcranial Doppler ultrasonography can now be used to diagnose hemodynamically significant occlusive disease in the ICA, ACA, and MCA. It can also be used to follow the progression of disease, particularly the progression of atherothrombotic disease or dissecting lesions. In addition, it can assess collateral flow during test occlusion of the internal carotid artery when therapeutic occlusion is required for the treatment of an intracranial aneurysm. Other potential uses include monitoring of middle cerebral artery flow during carotid surgery, monitoring the progress of thrombolytic therapy for middle cerebral artery embolic occlusive disease, or monitoring the spontaneous lysis of middle cerebral artery stem emboli. TCD is widely used for the detection and monitoring of cerebral vasospasm after subarachnoid hemorrhage. Also it is beneficial in adding another criterion for brain death. Lastly, CO_2 reactivity has been studied by TCD and may prove helpful in the analysis of complex cases of ICA occlusive disease.

Magnetic Resonance Angiography

Magnetic resonance angiography is a noninvasive imaging modality that makes use of the unique properties of moving protons in an applied magnetic field to provide a representation of blood flow. In the evaluation of carotid occlusive disease, MRA is emerging as an important tool for investigating both the cervical[3,4,26,31] and the intracranial[8,16,39,55] (Fig. 202-2) segments of the carotid system.

Two MRA bright-blood techniques, *time-of-flight* and *phase-contrast MRA,* are currently in widespread use. The most commonly employed technique, time-of-flight (TOF), uses repetitive radiofrequency pulses to suppress stationary tissues. The unsuppressed protons of inflowing blood are then used to create a vascular image. The second technique, phase-contrast (PC) MRA, is also widely available although less frequently used than TOF. Phase-contrast imaging is a subtraction technique in which moving protons acquire a phase shift proportional to their velocity during the application of a bipolar gradient. The net phase shift of stationary protons is zero. Phase-contrast sequences, therefore, provide excellent background tissue suppression and can also provide velocity and directional information. However, the technique is sensitive to only a limited velocity range, which must be specified prior to the initiation of a scan. (TOF sequences do not require selection of a velocity range.) The PC examination also requires longer scan time than TOF for the same spatial resolution. Both TOF and PC MRA may be performed as either individual-slice (2-D) or volume (3-D) acquisition.

Extracranial Carotid Imaging

The extracranial carotid system is most often evaluated by a combination of 2-D TOF gradient-echo MRA[3] with an axial T1-weighted spin-echo sequence. The use of this imaging protocol is based in part on the fact that the 2-D TOF technique is more sensitive for the detection of slow flow than the 3-D techniques. In addition, axially acquired 2-D TOF sequences are able to image long, relatively straight vascular segments without the progressive signal drop-off seen with volume (3-D) techniques, which results from repetitive excitation. The T1-weighted magnetic resonance images allow inspection of the vessel wall and corroborate the findings of the MRA.

The 2-D TOF sequence is acquired axially using contiguous 1.5 mm sections with a superiorly positioned saturation band to eliminate venous signal. The axial images are then analyzed using a maximum-intensity pixel projection algorithm which maps the

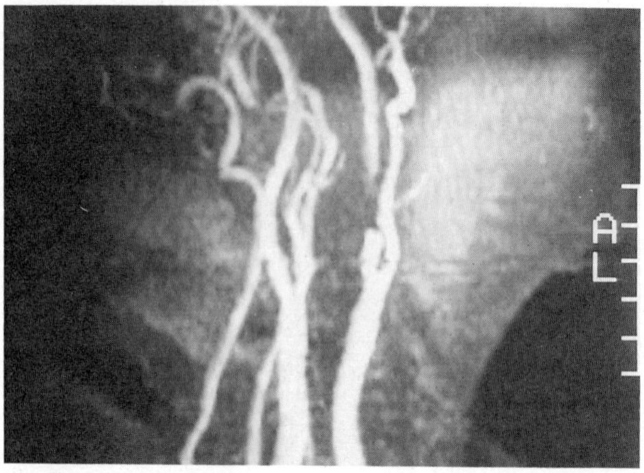

(*A*)

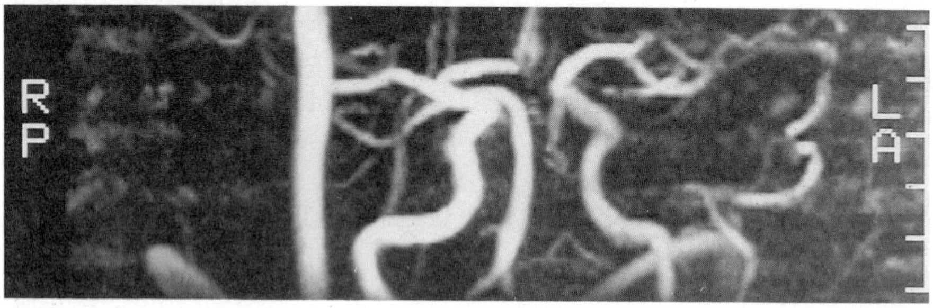

(*B*)

Figure 202-2 *A.* MRA of the neck in a patient with right stenosis suggested on carotid noninvasive testing. The MRA shows signal dropout above the bifurcation on the left side, and this corresponded with very high flow on noninvasive ultrasound testing. *B.* The intracranial MRA demonstrates an atretic A1 segment as well as an atretic posterior communicating artery on the left, suggestive of an isolated cerebral hemisphere. The patient required shunting at the time of endarterectomy crossclamping.

brightest pixels in each slice and projects the vessels in the sagittal and coronal planes. Individual vessels can be segmented from the initial (''raw'') data set to increase the detection of intraluminal signal, which may be lost in standard projection images. The axial and projection images are then reviewed in conjunction with the T1-weighted sequence to determine an approximate percent stenosis.

Intracranial Imaging

Intracranial imaging consists of 3-D TOF MRA in conjunction with sagittal T1- and axial T2-weighted spin-echo magnetic resonance imaging (MRI) sequences. The small vessel caliber and complex flow patterns of the circle of Willis pose special difficulties for MRA and to some extent limit its usefulness in this region; however, newer techniques that provide improved small vessel detection offer hope of better visualization of the intracranial circulation.[8,16] Evaluation of the circle of Willis is optimized by performing 3-D acquisition.[39] These sequences have better spatial resolution and suffer less signal loss in tortuous vessels than 2-D studies. The spin-echo sequences provide supportive information for the findings of MRA and also allow an assessment of the brain parenchyma.

The 3-D TOF sequence is obtained using a 6-cm axial volume with 1-mm individual partitions. A superior saturation band placed above the volume eliminates venous signal. Postprocessing of the data is similar to that performed with the cervical carotid arteries. Phase-contrast examination may be indicated to clarify equivocal findings on the TOF exam and to evaluate the direction of flow through the circle of Willis.[55]

Detecting Pathology

MRA studies can show characteristic patterns of flow signal that indicate the severity of a stenosis.[3,4,31,41] Although various classification systems have been used in the literature, the NASCET study threshold for a severe stenosis ($\geq$70 percent luminal narrowing) will be used in the following description of the MRA appearance of carotid stenosis.[45] Mild to moderate (10 to 69 percent) stenosis is indicated by vessel narrowing with a continuous flow column. Severe stenosis (70 to 95 percent) typically causes a focal signal loss (''skip sign'') in the flow column. A critical stenosis (95 to 99 percent) results in a ''slim sign'' with attenuation of the flow column above the zone of signal loss. At present, the reliability of MRA in distinguishing an extremely tight stenosis from an occluded vessel remains in doubt, with reported instances of occluded vessels misidentified as patent and extremely stenosed vessels misidentified as occluded.[38,41] An additional shortcoming of MRA is its inability to detect ulcerations. Huston and colleagues[31] reported that MRA detected only 1 of 24 common and internal carotid ulcers that were evident on contrast angiography.

Reliability of MRA

Multiple studies have confirmed the reliability of MRA in evaluating the carotid bifurcation, with reported sensitivities of 90 to 100 percent and specificities of 85 to 92 percent for the detection of a severe (>70 percent) internal carotid artery origin stenosis.[4,31,38,41] In most of the cases in which MRA was inaccurate in assessing the severity of stenosis as compared to conventional contrast angiography, the error resulted in overestimation of the degree and extent of the stenosis. This tendency for overestimation results largely from the disordered flow that occurs at and immediately distal to an area of stenosis, which results in loss of phase coherence and, in turn, loss of signal. Other factors that may add to the loss of signal include the specific sequence parameters employed, the configuration of the carotid plaque itself, and hemodynamic variables such as cardiac output and distal or contralateral ICA lesions.

Because of these potential pitfalls in MRA diagnosis, routine correlation with carotid ultrasonography should be obtained. In a small series of cases ($n = 41$), we found an excellent correlation among CNIS, MRA, and surgical pathology data regarding residual lumen diameter (Figs. 202-1 to 202-3).[14] Using a combined approach of MRA and duplex sonography, Mattle and colleagues[41] found in a small series of patients ($n = 20$) that MRA and sonographic examinations that agreed with each other also had a 100 percent rate of agreement with conventional contrast angiography. When MRA and sonographic data are not in agreement, conventional contrast angiography is indicated.

Using the techniques outlined above, the carotid system and intracranial vessels can be imaged reliably in a large percentage of patients. MRA is capable of providing accurate information regarding the carotid bifurcation as well as for assessing the existence of possible tandem lesions in the intracranial internal carotid artery and stenoses of the proximal anterior, middle, and posterior cerebral arteries.

Indications for CNIS, TCD, and MRA

The North American Symptomatic Carotid Endarterectomy Trial (NASCET)[45] and two other trials[17,42] demonstrated conclusively that carotid endarterectomy for high-grade (70 to 99 percent), symptomatic carotid stenosis is highly effective in preventing subsequent ipsilateral stroke. In NASCET, endarterectomy was safe (4 percent morbidity and 2.1 percent mortality). For endarterectomy performed with microsurgical techniques, 1 to 1.5 percent morbidity has been reported.[25,58]

It has been our practice to evaluate *symptomatic patients* with suspected occlusive disease at the carotid bifurcation with emergent carotid noninvasive studies and transcranial Doppler studies (Fig. 202-1). If the noninvasive studies are consistent with stenosis, we perform conventional MRI of the brain and MRA of the

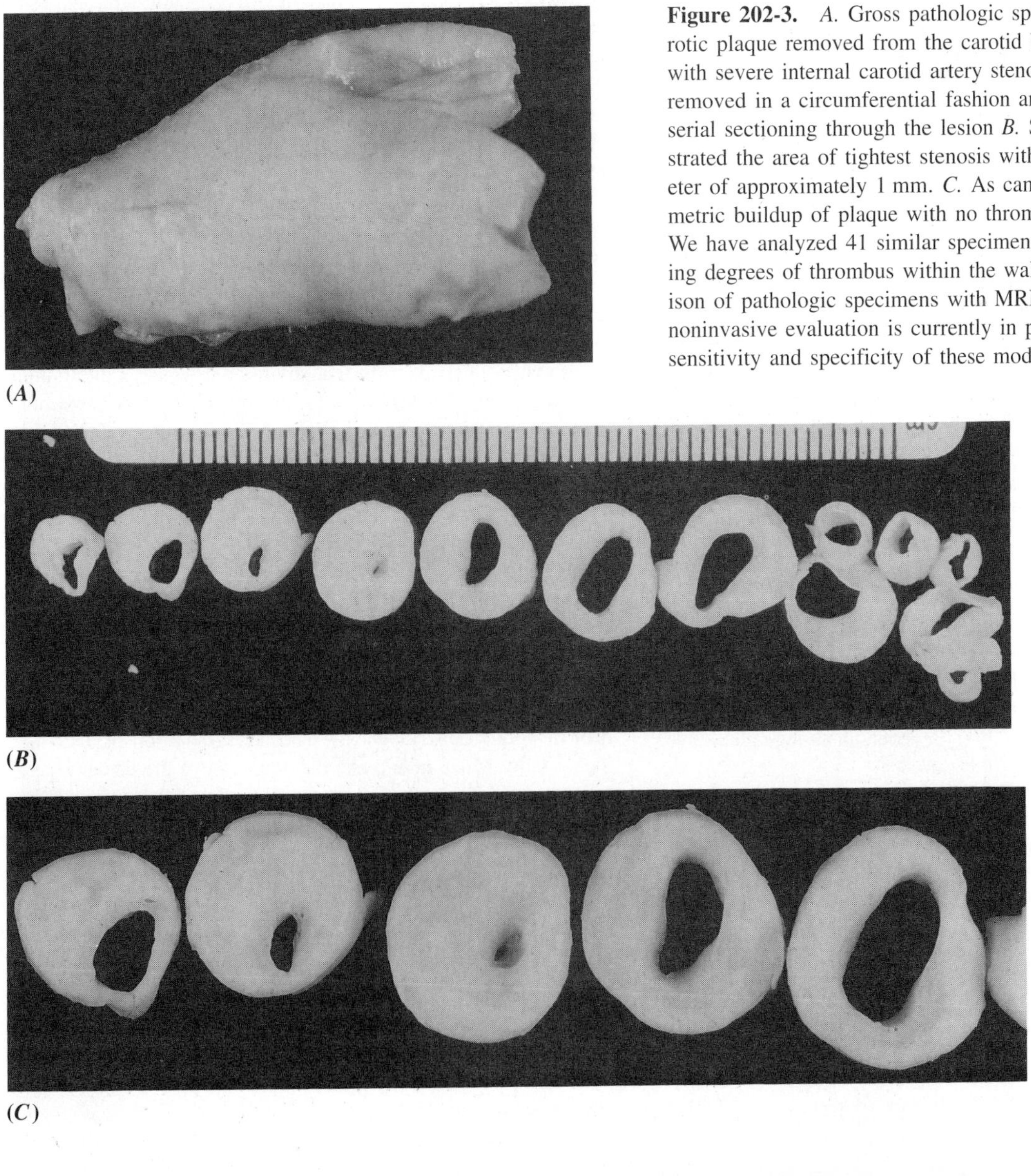

Figure 202-3. *A.* Gross pathologic specimen of the atherosclerotic plaque removed from the carotid bifurcation in a patient with severe internal carotid artery stenosis. The plaque was removed in a circumferential fashion and therefore allowed for serial sectioning through the lesion *B.* Serial sectioning demonstrated the area of tightest stenosis with a residual lumen diameter of approximately 1 mm. *C.* As can be seen, there is asymmetric buildup of plaque with no thrombus in this specimen. We have analyzed 41 similar specimens and have found varying degrees of thrombus within the wall of the vessel. Comparison of pathologic specimens with MRI studies and carotid noninvasive evaluation is currently in progress to evaluate the sensitivity and specificity of these modalities.

intracranial circulation and extracranial carotid circulation (Fig. 202-2). If the data from CNIS and MRA suggest a hemodynamically significant stenosis at the origin of the internal carotid artery, with a normal-appearing carotid siphon and middle cerebral artery stem, we then proceed to endarterectomy without angiography. However, if the noninvasive studies suggest that the ICA is occluded, or if there is any uncertainty with MRA, then cerebral angiography is performed to rule out a near-occlusion that could be corrected surgically. If the carotid siphon or the middle cerebral artery stem has a lesion visualized on MRA, then conventional angiography is strongly considered. Whenever the findings of the three noninvasive methods are equivocal, we proceed to angiography. If conventional angiography confirms a stenotic lesion at the ICA origin, endarterectomy is undertaken, provided the cardiac status is satisfactory.

For patients with an *asymptomatic bruit,* we begin with carotid noninvasive studies. If there is a suggestion of a lesion at the origin of the ICA that may be hemodynamically significant, we proceed to transcranial Doppler assessment of collateral flow across the circle of Willis and through the ophthalmic artery. Patients who are asymptomatic with very significant hemodynamic carotid stenosis generally have adequate collateral flow via the anterior circle of Willis, through the posterior communicating artery, or through the ophthalmic artery. If this is the case, the concern is that the carotid may progress to occlusion, with embolism at the time of complete occlusion. The natural history of these asymptomatic lesions is currently under study in ongoing randomized trials.[29] In the absence of extensive randomized data, however, we consider surgery in this situation. Accordingly, we proceed to MRA and careful cardiac evaluation. If there are no symptoms of coronary disease and the MRA confirms the stenotic lesion at the origin of the internal carotid artery with no stenosis of the distal ICA or middle cerebral artery, we generally proceed to surgery without conventional angiography.

When an asymptomatic stenotic carotid lesion is found not to be hemodynamically significant, we generally follow up every 6 to 8 months with conventional carotid noninvasive studies. If the lesion narrows to the point of severe stenosis as judged by our conventional carotid noninvasive study criteria, we proceed to transcranial Doppler to assess the presence or absence of collateral flow. If the transcranial Doppler study suggests that the internal carotid artery origin lesion is indeed hemodynamically significant, we then proceed to MRA; if the finding is confirmed, we recommend surgery.

When the MRA is in full agreement with the carotid noninvasive and transcranial Doppler studies, then angiography is not necessary before surgery. However, middle cerebral artery stem stenosis and siphon stenosis must always be carefully excluded. With either symptomatic or asymptomatic carotid stenosis, whenever the findings of MRA are equivocal, conventional angiography is always indicated.

Surgical Issues

Detecting Pathology at the Carotid Bifurcation

Of paramount importance is the reliable detection of hemodynamically significant stenosis (≥70 percent). CNIS consistently accomplishes this goal by detecting a high peak frequency (>14 kHz), diminished retinal artery pressure, and reversal of ophthalmic artery and A1 anterior cerebral artery flow. The precision of CNIS in the hands of an experienced technician/physician team is great enough to detect progression in serial studies. By detecting ''skip'' segments, MRA can offer confirmatory data, in itself demonstrative of significant stenosis. MRA is known to exaggerate stenosis, but CNIS can detect such an error. In our study of over 40 cases, we have not observed clinically important overestimation of the degree of stenosis by CNIS/MRA.[14] The experience of Mattle and colleagues is similar.[41]

It is important to identify a trickle of ICA flow for corrective surgery because total occlusion is usually not repairable. Therefore, these specific diagnoses are required with confidence. Today CNIS alone cannot distinguish between virtual and total occlusion, but 2-D TOF can sometimes demonstrate antegrade flow (often with a ''slim'' sign). When no flow can be detected with 2-D TOF, we suggest performing conventional angiography to both confirm the occlusion and to give an estimate of the extent of retrograde collateral filling of the intracranial ICA, to help guide the decision regarding surgery.

The diagnostic evaluation should also indicate the proximal and distal extent of the stenosis. Experience thus far suggests that MRA can give information that helps the surgeon obtain satisfactory exposure. In addition, the surgeon can adjust the exposure according to what is disclosed by exploration, including the findings of gentle palpation (e.g., proximal hard atheroma). Even in the case of far-cephalad plaque, the experienced surgeon can obtain good exposure by extending the incision, mobilizing the posterior belly of the digastricus, mobilizing the hypoglossal nerve, and even subluxing the jaw if needed.

Preoperative diagnosis of ulcerated plaque is desirable. In cases where CNIS and MRA detect significant stenosis, then overlooking an ulcer is unimportant since endarterectomy is already indicated. On the other hand, negative CNIS/MRA in the evaluation of transient ischemic attack or stroke may be followed by conventional angiography in search of a symptomatic ulcer.

Another aspect of pathoanatomy to be detected is intraluminal thrombus. Thus far, MRA cannot reliably identify such thrombi if they are small, but this diagnosis may be difficult even for conventional angiography.

Detecting Associated Pathology

Can this approach diagnose a ''tandem lesion'' with intracranial ICA or MCA stenosis? Until recently, this seemed the Achilles heel of noninvasive diagnosis. The recent addition of TCD and high-quality MRA now make the diagnosis of the tandem lesion reliable, even in the face of marked cervical ICA stenosis. When the studies are equivocal on this point, conventional angiography is still warranted. In addition, there are data supporting the performance of endarterectomy in the face of a tandem lesion.

The presence of other relevant pathology may challenge the system of CNIS/MRA. On one occasion we failed to identify a 360 degree ICA loop before surgery, and loop resection and patch grafting were required. While this eventuality caused the procedure to take more time than anticipated, surgical preparedness permitted satisfactory repair and good outcome. In the future, when a pattern of tortuous arteries is unclear on MRA, we will request conventional angiography.

Other Relevant Aspects of Anatomy and Physiology

The location of the bifurcation was formerly unclear from MRA, but we now routinely determine its level with respect to the cervical spine by reference to a midsagittal scout film and the raw MRA axial data. The transition from one dot (CCA) to two (ICA and ECA) indicates the bifurcation.

Identification of collateral circulation and its extent helps the surgeon by suggesting whether an in-lying shunt is likely to be needed during cross-clamping. CNIS can demonstrate reversal of flow in ophthalmic and A1 cerebral arteries. The base (''collapse'') 3-D MRA image shows the size of both A1 cerebral arteries well, and there may also be some image of posterior communicating artery flow, though this is less reliable. Moreover, the surgeon should be prepared to use a shunt if indicated by EEG criteria, regardless of the preoperative evaluation.

Indications for Conventional Angiography

When CNIS, TCD, and MRA do not clarify surgical issues, then conventional angiography is required to guide surgical decision-making. With increasing experience with noninvasive evaluation, and growing confidence in its reliability, we now resort to conventional angiography only in cases with (1) transient ischemic attack or stroke and negative CNIS/TCD/MRA, (2) CNIS, TCD, or MRA that are inadequate because of patient-related factors (marked obesity, severe claustrophobia), (3) no flow detected in the ICA on 2-D TOF evaluation, (4) discrepancy among the results of CNIS, TCD, and MRA, (5) complex or perplexing pathology (e.g., radiation-induced bilateral carotid stenosis), or (6) other inadequately understood pathophysiology.

Current Surgical Practice

We now rely on CNIS/TCD/MRA without conventional angiography in the evaluation of 90 percent of cases with symptomatic carotid stenosis and virtually all asymptomatic stenoses. Among 40 consecutive patients subjected to carotid endarterectomy without angiography, there have been no complications due to this approach, and the potential morbidity of 40 conventional angiograms has been avoided.[14] With the ongoing improvement of CNIS, TCD, and MRA, we expect to use this approach even more widely in the future. Such good results can be expected only for experienced CNIS/TCD technicians, neuroradiologists, and surgeons using late-model imaging instruments. In some hospital settings, conventional angiography may still provide the most reliable diagnostic information to guide carotid endarterectomy.

References

1. Aaslid R. *Transcranial Doppler Sonography.* New York: Springer-Verlag, 1986.
2. Adams R, McKie V, Nichols F, et al. The use of transcranial ultrasonography to predict stroke in sickle cell disease. *N Engl J Med* 1992; 326:605–610.
3. Anderson CM, Saloner D, Lee RE, et al. Assessment of carotid artery stenosis by MR angiography: comparison with x-ray angiography and color-coded Doppler ultrasound. *Am J Neuroradiol* 1992; 13:989–1003.
4. Anson JA, Heiserman JE, Drayer BP, Spetzler RF. Surgical decisions on the basis of magnetic resonance angiography of the carotid arteries. *Neurosurgery* 1993; 32:335–343.
5. Arnolds BJ, Von Reutern GM. Transcranial Doppler sonography. Examination technique and normal reference values. *Ultrasound Med Biol* 1986; 12:115–123.
6. Blackshear WM, Phillips DJ, Chikos PM, et al. Carotid artery velocity patterns in normal and stenotic vessels. *Stroke* 1980; 11:67–71.
7. Blackshear WM Jr, Phillips DJ, Thiele BL, et al. Detection of carotid occlusive disease by ultrasonic imaging and pulsed Doppler spectrum analysis. *Surgery* 1979; 86:698–706.
8. Blatter DD, Parker DL, Robison RO. Cerebral MR angiography with multiple overlapping thin slab acquisition. Part I. Quantitative analysis of vessel visibility. *Radiology* 1991; 179:805–811.
9. Bluth EI, Stavros AT, Marich KW, et al. Carotid duplex sonography: a multicenter recommendation for standardized imaging and Doppler criteria. *Radiographics* 1988; 8:487–506.
10. Brass LM, Duterte DL, Mohr JP. Anterior cerebral artery velocity changes in disease of the middle cerebral artery stem. *Stroke* 1989; 20:1737–1740.
11. Brass LM, Prohovnik I, Pavlakis SG, et al. Middle cerebral artery blood velocity and cerebral blood flow in sickle cell disease. *Stroke* 1991; 22:27–30.
12. Call GK, Abbott WM, Macdonald NR, et al. Correlation of continuous-wave Doppler spectral flow analysis with gross pathology in carotid stenosis. *Stroke* 1988; 19:584–588.
13. Chambers BR, Norris JW. Outcome in patients with asymptomatic neck bruits. *N Engl J Med* 1986; 315:860–865.
14. Crowell RM, Kistler JP, Ojemann RG, et al. Carotid endarterectomy without conventional angiography. Presented at the 60th Annual Meeting of the American Association of Neurological Surgeons, San Francisco, CA, April 11–16, 1992 (poster).
15. Dion JE, Gates PC, Fox AJ, et al. Clinical events following neuroangiography: a prospective study. *Stroke* 1987; 18:997–1004.
16. Edelman RR, Ahn SS, Chien D, et al. Improved time-of-flight MR angiography of the brain with magnetization transfer contrast. *Radiology* 1992; 184:395–399.
17. European Carotid Surgery Trialists' Collaborative Group. MRC European Carotid Surgery Trial: interim results for symptomatic patients with severe (70–99%) or with mild (0–29%) carotid stenosis. *Lancet* 1991; 337:1235–1243.
18. Fisher CM. Concerning recurrent transient cerebral ischemic attacks. *Can Med Assoc J* 1962; 86:1091–1099.
19. Fisher CM. Clinical syndromes in cerebral thrombosis, hypertensive hemorrhage, and ruptured saccular aneurysm. *Clin Neurosurg* 1975; 22:117–147.
20. Fisher M. Occlusion of the internal carotid artery. *Arch Neurol Psychiatry* 1951; 65:346–377.
21. Gee W. Ocular pneumoplethysmography. In Bernstein EF (ed): *Noninvasive Diagnostic Techniques in Vascular Disease,* 2d ed. St Louis: Mosby, 1982, pp 220–230.
22. Gee W. Ocular pneumoplethysmography (OPG-Gee). In Kempczinski RF, Yao JST (eds): *Practical Noninvasive Vascular Diagnosis.* Chicago: Year Book Medical Publishers, 1982, pp 167–180.
23. Gee W, Mehigan JT, Wylie EJ. Measurement of collateral cerebral hemispheric blood pressure by ocular pneumoplethysmography. *Am J Surg* 1975; 130:121–127.
24. Grolimund P, Seiler RW, Aaslid R, et al. Evaluation of cerebrovascular disease by combined extracranial and transcranial Doppler sonography. Experience in 1,039 patients. *Stroke* 1987; 18:1018–1024.
25. Halliday AL, Crowell RM, Ojemann RG, et al. One percent stroke morbidity and no mortality in 120 carotid endarterectomies. Presented at the 61st Annual Meeting of the American Association of Neurological Surgeons, Boston, MA, April 24–29, 1993 (poster).
26. Heiserman JE, Drayer BP, Fram EK, et al. Carotid artery stenosis: clinical efficacy of two-dimensional time-of-flight MR angiography. *Radiology* 1992; 182:761–768.

27. Hennerici M, Rautenberg W, Schwartz A. Transcranial Doppler ultrasound for the assessment of intracranial arterial flow velocity. Part 2. Evaluation of intracranial arterial disease. *Surg Neurol* 1987; 27:523–532.
28. Heyman A, Wilkinson WE, Heyden S, et al. Risk of stroke in asymptomatic persons with cervical arterial bruits: a population study in Evans County, Georgia. *N Engl J Med* 1980; 302:838–841.
29. Hobson RW II, Weiss DG, Fields WS, et al. Efficacy of carotid endarterectomy for asymptomatic carotid stenosis: the Veterans Affairs Cooperative Study Group. *N Engl J Med* 1993; 328:221–227.
30. Houser OW, Sundt TM Jr, Holman CB, et al. Atheromatous disease of the carotid artery. Correlation of angiographic, clinical, and surgical findings. *J Neurosurg* 1974; 41:321–331.
31. Huston J III, Lewis BD, Wiebers DO, et al. Carotid artery: prospective blinded comparison of two-dimensional time-of-flight MR angiography with conventional angiography and duplex US. *Radiology* 1993; 186:339–344.
32. Kistler JP, Buonanno FS, Gress DR. Carotid endarterectomy—specific therapy based on pathophysiology. *N Engl J Med* 1991; 325:505–507.
33. Kistler JP, Lees RS, Miller A, et al. Correlation of spectral phonoangiography and carotid angiography with gross pathology in carotid stenosis. *N Engl J Med* 1981; 305:417–419.
34. Kistler JP, Ropper AH, Heros RC. Therapy of ischemic cerebral vascular disease due to atherothrombosis. (Parts 1 and 2.) *N Engl J Med* 1984; 311:27–34, 100–105.
35. Kremkau FW. Principles of color flow imaging. *J Vasc Tech* 1991; 15:104–111.
36. Ley-Pozo J, Ringelstein EB. Noninvasive detection of occlusive disease of the carotid siphon and middle cerebral artery. *Ann Neurol* 1990; 28:640–647.
37. Lindegaard KF, Bakke SJ, Grolimund P, et al. Assessment of intracranial hemodynamics in carotid artery disease by transcranial Doppler ultrasound. *J Neurosurg* 1985; 63:890–898.
38. Litt AW, Eidelman EM, Pinto RS, et al. Diagnosis of carotid artery stenosis: comparison of 2DFT time-of-flight MR angiography with contrast angiography in 50 patients. *Am J Neuroradiol* 1991; 12:149–154.
39. Masaryk TJ, Modic MT, Ross JS, et al. Intracranial circulation: preliminary clinical results with three-dimensional (volume) MR angiography. *Radiology* 1989; 171:793–799.
40. Mattle H, Grolimund P, Huber P, et al. Transcranial Doppler sonographic findings in middle cerebral artery disease. *Arch Neurol* 1988; 45:289–295.
41. Mattle HP, Kent KC, Edelman RR, et al. Evaluation of the extracranial carotid arteries: correlation of magnetic resonance angiography, duplex ultrasonography, and conventional angiography. *J Vasc Surg* 1991; 13:838–844.
42. Mayberg MR, Wilson SE, Yatsu F, et al. Carotid endarterectomy and prevention of cerebral ischemia in symptomatic carotid stenosis: Veterans Affairs Cooperative Studies Program 309 Trialist Group. *JAMA* 1991; 266:3289–3294.
43. Meissner I, Wiebers DO, Whisnant JP, O'Fallon WM. The natural history of asymptomatic carotid artery occlusive lesions. *JAMA* 1987; 258:2704–2707.
44. Mohr JP. Sickle cell anemia, stroke, and transcranial Doppler studies. *N Engl J Med* 1992; 326:637–639.
45. North American Symptomatic Carotid Endarterectomy Trial Collaborators. Beneficial effect of carotid endarterectomy in symptomatic patients with high-grade carotid stenosis. *N Engl J Med* 1991; 325:445–453.
46. Ojemann RG, Crowell RM, Roberson GH, Fisher CM. Surgical treatment of extracranial carotid occlusive disease. *Clin Neurosurg* 1975; 22:214–263.
47. Pessin MS, Hinton RC, Davis KR, et al. Mechanisms of acute carotid stroke. *Ann Neurol* 1979; 6:245–252.
48. Petty GW. Transcranial Doppler ultrasonography. *Neurol Chron* 1991; 1:1.
49. Petty GW, Mohr JP, Pedley TA, et al. The role of transcranial Doppler in confirming brain death: sensitivity, specificity, and suggestions for performance and interpretation. *Neurology* 1990; 40:300–303.
50. Petty GW, Wiebers DO, Meissner I. Transcranial Doppler ultrasonography: clinical applications in cerebrovascular disease. *Mayo Clin Proc* 1990; 65:1350–1364.
51. Primozich JF. Color flow in carotid evaluation. *J Vasc Tech* 1991; 15:112–122.
52. Ringelstein EB, Sievers C, Ecker S, et al. Noninvasive assessment of CO_2-induced cerebral vasomotor response in normal individuals and patients with internal carotid artery occlusions. *Stroke* 1988; 19:963–969.
53. Roederer GO, Langloid YE, Jager KA, et al. The natural history of carotid arterial disease in asymptomatic patients with cervical bruits. *Stroke* 1984; 15:603–613.
54. Ropper AH, Wechsler LR, Wilson LS. Carotid bruit and the risk of stroke in elective surgery. *N Engl J Med* 1982; 307:1388–1390.
55. Ross MR, Pelc NJ, Enzmann DR. Qualitative phase contrast MRA in the normal and abnormal circle of Willis. *Am J Neuroradiol* 1993; 14:19–25.
56. Schneider PA, Rossman ME, Bernstein EF, et al. Effect of internal carotid artery occlusion on intracranial hemodynamics. Transcranial Doppler evaluation and clinical correlation. *Stroke* 1988; 19:589–593.
57. Schneider PA, Rossman ME, Torem S, et al. Transcranial Doppler in the management of extracranial cerebrovascular disease: implications in diagnosis and monitoring. *J Vasc Surg* 1988; 7:223–231.
58. Spetzler RF, Martin N, Hadley MN, et al. Microsurgical endarterectomy under barbiturate protection: a prospective study. *J Neurosurg* 1986; 65:63–73.
59. Steinke W, Kloetzsch C, Hennerici M. Carotid artery disease assessed by color Doppler flow imaging: correlation with standard Doppler sonography and angiography. *Am J Roentgenol* 1990; 154:1061–1068.
60. Tatemichi TK, Chamorro A, Petty GW, et al. Hemodynamic role of ophthalmic artery collateral in internal carotid artery occlusion. *Neurology* 1990; 40:461–464.
61. Taylor DC, Strandness DE Jr. Carotid artery duplex scanning. *J Clin Ultrasound* 1987; 15:635–644.
62. Wechsler LR, Ropper AH, Kistler JP. Transcranial Doppler in cerebrovascular disease. *Stroke* 1986; 17:905–912.
63. Wolf PA, Kannel WB, Sorlie P, McNamara P. Asymptomatic carotid bruit and risk of stroke. The Framingham study. *JAMA* 1981; 245:1442–1445.
64. Zwiebel WJ, Zagzebski JA, Crummy AB, Hirscher M. Correlation of peak Doppler frequency with lumen narrowing in carotid stenosis. *Stroke* 1982; 13:386–391.

203 Imaging of Ischemic Cerebrovascular Disease

Linda Gray
Neil C. Davey

Evaluation of cerebrovascular disease is directed toward examination of the heart, aortic arch, carotid and vertebral extracranial and intracranial vascular systems, brain, and orbits. Cardiac evaluation is beyond the scope of this chapter. Angiography remains the gold standard for evaluation of the aortic arch and extra- and intracranial vascular systems. However, noninvasive evaluation with magnetic resonance imaging (MRI) and magnetic resonance angiography (MRA), carotid Doppler ultrasound, and spiral computed tomography (CT), along with 3-D reconstruction and projection algorithms, are progressing rapidly; at present they constitute screening techniques at least, and they could eventually replace angiography in some cases. For evaluation of the brain, CT is used as a screening tool in the emergency setting to exclude acute changes such as subarachnoid hemorrhage. MRI is more often used to assess the extent of a stroke, to evaluate the posterior fossa, to evaluate flow in arteries and veins, and to image pathologic changes in multiple planes of section. MRI can be used in the setting of an acute stroke; although this application is a research tool at present, it may be used in determining stroke therapy in the future.

Techniques for Evaluation

Angiography

Angiography involves the injection of an iodinated contrast agent through a catheter and is performed as a cut-film technique or as digital subtraction angiography (DSA). The latter can also be performed with an intravenous injection (IV-DSA). Angiography techniques are discussed elsewhere in this text. Intraarterial DSA is considered the gold standard for the evaluation of carotid and cerebrovascular disease, although recent studies raise questions about this view. The risks associated with conventional angiography have been the major drawback to the procedure. They have been considered in several articles. For example, eight studies were evaluated retrospectively and the combined data from 8300 examinations of patients with cerebrovascular disease from 1968 to 1987 were analyzed. These data revealed a 4 percent risk of transient neurological complication, a 1 percent risk of a permanent stroke, and a 0.1 percent risk of death.[19,30] Two more recent studies, involving 1002 and 1095 patients, respectively, indicate lower risks for current conventional angiography, with approximately a 1.3 to 1.45 percent incidence of transient neurological deficit, a 0.1 percent risk of permanent stroke, and a very low death rate.[19,30] However, the risks associated with angiography make it undesirable as a screening technique. Therefore, carotid Doppler ultrasonography, MRA, and more recently spiral CT have been developed primarily as screening techniques for carotid vascular diseases.

Carotid Doppler Ultrasound

Carotid Doppler ultrasound is widely used as a screening technique for evaluating carotid vascular disease. The technique is well described in several articles.[10,11,48] Criteria for grading carotid stenosis by Doppler ultrasound are given in Table 203-1. Peak systolic velocities of 125 cm/s suggest a moderate degree of stenosis, and peak systolic velocities of 250 cm/s suggest high-grade stenosis. There are also other sonographic criteria for the evaluation of carotid stenosis.[10,11,48]

Magnetic Resonance Angiography

MRA is a noninvasive modality that uses various MRI techniques (TR, TE, flip-angle, and magnetic gradients) to produce angiographic images. Although a number of techniques are available, the two most commonly used are time-of-flight angiography (TOFA) and phase-contrast angiography (PCA).

Time-of-Flight Angiography

The principle behind TOF MR angiography is to increase the signal from moving protons (i.e., those flowing in blood) relative to stationary or static protons (i.e., those in stationary tissue). A brief discussion of the fundamentals of MR signal generation is necessary for a clearer understanding of TOF MRA.

Individual protons have a charge and a precession (spin) around an axis. When placed in a magnetic field, most protons will align themselves in the direction of the magnetic field, giving the tissue a net longitudinal magnetization vector. When energy in the form of a radio frequency (RF) pulse is applied to the tissue, the

TABLE 203-1 Doppler Ultrasound Criteria for Grading Stenosis

Percent Stenosis	ICA/CCA Ratio of Peak Systolic Velocities*	Peak Systolic Velocity, cm/s
41–50	<1.8	>125
60–79	>1.8	>130
80–99	>3.7	>250 or <25 (critical stenosis)

A peak velocity of ≥4.0 cm/s predicts 70 to 99 percent stenosis with 91 percent sensitivity and 88 percent overall accuracy.

Acute thrombus is hypoechoic; atherosclerosis is hyperechoic.

Ulcerations are predicted by color flow Doppler studies with 94 percent accuracy, 95.3 percent sensitivity, and 93.5 percent specificity.

*ICA, internal carotid artery; CCA, common carotid artery.

longitudinal magnetization vector is disturbed and displaced toward the transverse plane. The magnitude of the displacement depends on the duration and amplitude of the RF pulse: the longer the duration and the greater the amplitude, the larger the displacement of the longitudinal magnetization vector toward the transverse plane. The displacement is measured in degrees and is called the *flip angle.* When the RF pulse ceases, the transversely oriented vector returns to its equilibrium (longitudinal) position, aligned with the magnetic field. This process is called *relaxation.* During relaxation, the energy that has been transferred to the transverse magnetization vector by the RF pulse is liberated in the form of a signal (known as an echo). This signal, the amplitude of which depends on the size of the transverse magnetization vector, is used to generate an MR image. Full relaxation of the longitudinal magnetization takes a relatively long time (measured in seconds). Rapidly repeated RF pulses (at subsecond intervals) do not allow full relaxation between pulses. Each consecutive RF pulse thus displaces a smaller longitudinal magnetization vector, resulting in a smaller transverse magnetization vector, which in turn does not have sufficient time to achieve full relaxation before displacement by the next RF pulse. This process, known as *saturation,* results in a small transverse magnetization vector and hence a weak MR signal when the echo is measured. In TOF angiography, saturation pulses are applied to the tissue (slice or volume) of interest, resulting in a very weak signal from static protons. The flowing protons in blood, however, have not yet entered the slice or volume of interest while saturation is taking place. They are thus unsaturated and give a much stronger echo when the tissue signal is measured.

Presaturation slabs are used to distinguish arterial from venous flow. This technique is designed to saturate incoming venous flow (which is usually in the opposite direction to the arterial flow) before it enters the imaged slice or volume. This results in low or absent signal from protons in venous blood. The process can be reversed to saturate the incoming arterial flow, thus allowing imaging of only venous flow.[37,43,59]

Phase-Contrast Angiography

Spinning protons that are in motion during the application of a magnetic field gradient will experience an alteration in phase. The length of time that these protons are subjected to the gradient magnetic field determines the degree of phase alteration. When an RF pulse tips the longitudinal magnetization of a group of spins into the transverse plane, the spins begin to rotate (precess) around the longitudinal axis at the same rate (frequency) and in the same phase. The frequency of the precession is proportional to the magnetic field strength at any given position in the field. Thus, if a gradient magnetic field is applied, spins precess at different frequencies depending on their position in the field. The differing precession frequencies cause the spins to experience different magnetic field strengths and therefore to fall out of phase with one another.

When the gradient magnetic field is switched off, the spins experience the same magnetic field and precess at the same frequency but remain out of phase with each other. Precession in phase is restored if the initial gradient magnetic field is reversed and applied for the same length of time. It is important to note that spins will only return to their original phase (i.e., show no net phase shift) if they are static. Flowing spins will have moved during the application of the equal but opposite gradients and will not return to their original phase at the termination of the second gradient. This results in a net phase shift that is proportional to the speed of the flowing spins. To create an angiogram or an image of the flowing spins, the images resulting from the net phase shift are subtracted from the referenced image of the static spins.

Three phase-contrast techniques are commonly used: 2-D, 3-D, and ciné phase contrast. PCA gives both angiographic images and information on the direction and velocity of flow. Ciné-PCA images can be displayed in ciné form, providing a functional assessment of flow during the cardiac cycle.[21,29,59]

Although all the methods discussed can be applied to any vascular region, certain methods have proved more effective than others in specific vascular regions (Table 203-2).

There are limitations of both TOF and PC angiography that preclude either technique from, as yet, replacing conventional angiography as the definitive diagnostic tool. Slow flowing protons and protons within tortuous vessels are prone to saturation in TOFA because these protons remain within the saturated field for a relatively long period of time. Thus there is dropout of signal from flow in normal vessels which can mimic absent areas of flow or stenosis. Poor background suppression in TOFA may also degrade blood vessel visibility. The major disadvantages of PCA are the long image reconstruction times and the need to choose a velocity sensitivity for each study. Alterations in signal that can result from the ranges of velocity existing throughout vessels can cause inadequate evaluation of the true lumen.[21,29,59]

Spiral CT

CT angiography is an emerging technique that combines slip-ring CT technology with three-dimensional reconstruction algorithms. The technique is performed with the intravenous injection of approximately 100–150 ml of an iodinated contrast agent, after a 15–30 second delay, at the rate of 3 ml per second. Sixty slices can be obtained in sixty seconds and may be 1 to 5 mm in thickness. A distance of 6–30 centimeters can be obtained. Images are obtained on a 512 × 512 matrix with a field-of-view of 15–25 cm for improved anatomic resolution. Reconstructions are displayed in several different ways: (1) volume rendering, (2) surface rendering, (3) maximum intensity projection, or (4) curved planar reformation.

CTA has several advantages over MRA: (1) the total time of the examination is very short, approximately 1 minute, and 10 minutes are required for image reconstruction; (2) there is less susceptibility to motion artifact; and (3) images are less susceptible to eddy currents in the region of the carotid bulb; thus, more reliable depiction of carotid stenosis can be obtained. However, MRA has certain advantages over CTA: (1) no intravascular contrast material or ionizing radiation is necessary; (2) the examination can be repeated if there are technical difficulties; (3) cardiac output has little impact on the ability to detect flow, as it may have with CTA; and (4) the volume of tissue that can be evaluated by MRA is not limited, as it is with CTA. The volume limits of CTA will become less of an issue when slip-ring technology improves

TABLE 203-2 Optimal Uses of Magnetic Resonance Time-of-Flight (TOF) and Phase-Contrast (PC) Angiography Techniques

Method	Anatomic Region
2-D TOF	Carotid bifurcation or venous anatomy
3-D TOF	Circle of Willis
2-D PC	Localization of flow direction and velocity
	Extracranial and intracranial vascular structures
3-D PC	Intracranial vascular structures

so that four slices per second can be obtained; that will expand the length of tissue that can be examined.[56]

Disease Processes

Carotid Atherosclerosis

The incidence of stroke in the United States is approximately 400,000 to 500,000 per year, and stroke is the third leading cause of death in the United States, resulting in approximately 150,000 deaths per year. The large majority of cases of cerebral thromboembolic disease are caused by atherosclerosis. Recently, three trials have been performed: the North American Symptomatic Carotid Endarterectomy Trial (NASCET), the European Carotid Surgery Trial (ECST), and the VA Cooperative Symptomatic Carotid Stenosis Trial (VACS).[44] These studies demonstrated that, when carotid endarterectomy can be performed with reasonable rates of morbidity and mortality, patients with a high degree of carotid stenosis involving the internal carotid artery at the carotid bifurcation on the symptomatic side benefit from carotid endarterectomy more than patients treated strictly medically. Because of these recent studies, increased attention is given to evaluating carotid vascular disease and its potential impact on the brain. With the development of carotid Doppler ultrasonography, MR angiography, and spiral CT over the last 5 to 10 years, noninvasive evaluation of cerebrovascular disease has received greater attention.

Conventional Angiography

Atherosclerotic disease can cause transient ischemic attacks or strokes by means of either hemodynamic causes (stenosis) or embolism. Hemodynamic causes include atherosclerotic narrowing, subintimal plaque hemorrhage, and frank arterial occlusion. Embolic causes include plaque ulceration with or without superimposed thrombosis and emboli from cardiac or aortic arch disease.

Atherosclerotic stenosis can occur at the origins of the great vessels from the aortic arch (Fig. 203-1), or along the common carotid artery, especially at its bifurcation. The extent of such vascular disease can be assessed with conventional angiography or by noninvasive methods. Assessment of the degree of stenosis of the internal carotid artery (usually at its origin) can be made by the NASCET criteria; that is, the degree of stenosis is measured at the point of greatest stenosis and at the normal part of the artery beyond the carotid bulb. A 50 percent reduction reflects a 75 percent decrease in cross-sectional area; a 75 percent reduction, a 90 percent decrease in cross-sectional area. A "string sign" demonstrates a 90 to 99 percent decrease in diameter; delayed filming is often necessary to demonstrate antegrade filling of the internal carotid artery above a tight stenosis. While conventional angiography is the gold standard for carotid evaluation, interpreters can disagree significantly on the grade of stenosis present. Only complete occlusion produces high intra- and interobserver agreement.[12,33,41]

In addition to identifying carotid artery stenosis and assessing its severity, the radiologist and surgeon must also detect ulcera-

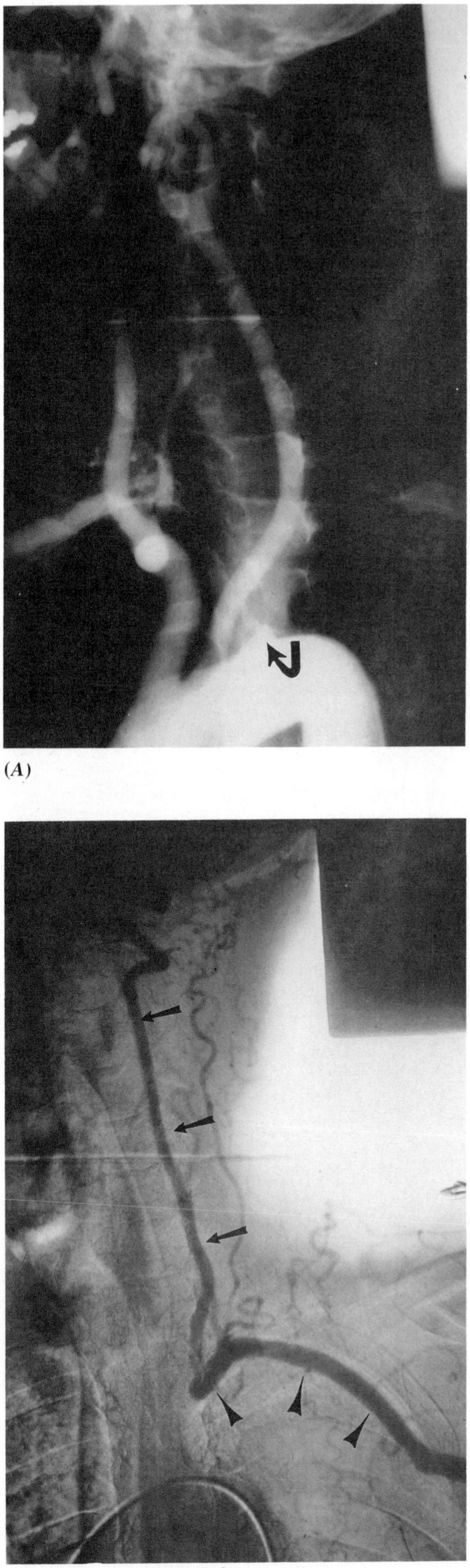

(*A*)

(*B*)

Figure 203-1 Subclavian steal in a patient with vertebrobasilar symptoms. Stenosis of the left innominate artery *(A, arrow)* results in retrograde flow in the left vertebral artery *(B, arrows),* which fills the left subclavian artery *(arrowheads).*

tions and tandem lesions. The extent of ulceration can be difficult to assess by either carotid angiography or any of the available noninvasive imaging methods. Ulcerations can give several appearances on imaging studies: (1) sharply undercut edges, (2) an irregular base to an excavated plaque, or (3) persistence of contrast material in an irregular base (Fig. 203-2). A depression between two plaques can mimic an ulceration, and a thrombus may hide an ulceration by covering it. A projecting thrombus can simulate an atherosclerotic plaque, or, if very large, can appear as an intraluminal filling defect (Fig. 203-2). Conventional angiography

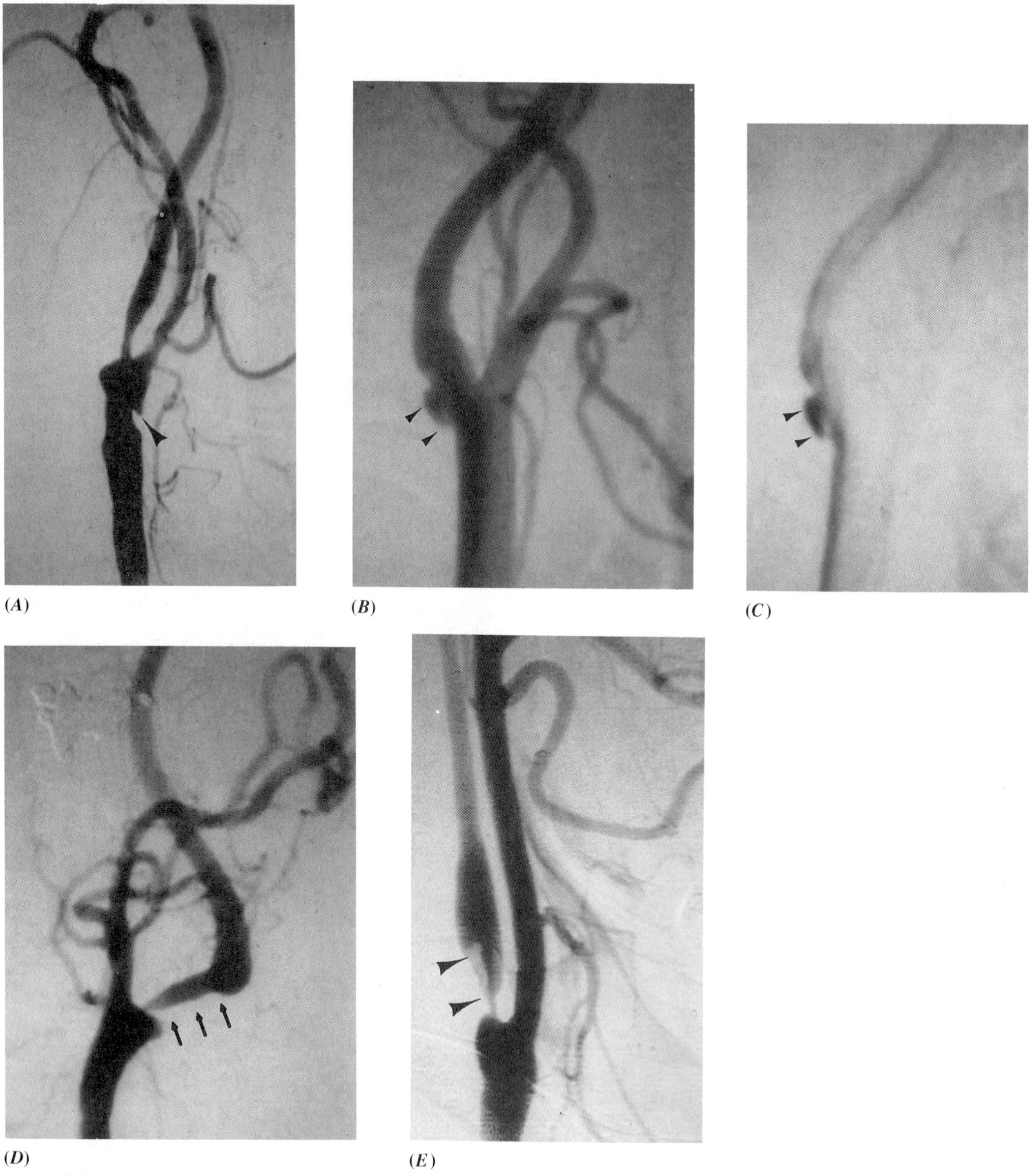

Figure 203-2 Conventional angiographic appearance of ulcers. *A.* Undercut edge of an ulceration confirmed at surgery *(arrowhead)*. *B, C.* Filling defect *(B)* in a plaque with persistence of contrast and undercut margins *(C)*; the ulceration *(arrowheads)* was confirmed at surgery. *D.* Marked smooth narrowing of the internal carotid artery. Thrombus superimposed on ulceration *(arrows)* was found at surgery. *E.* A filling defect in a contrast column representing intraluminal thrombus *(arrowheads)*.

easily misses ulcers. In one study, conventional angiography failed to identify 40 percent of ulcers later identified at surgery, and it was interpreted as showing ulcers in 34 percent of carotid arteries determined at surgery to be free of them.[23] In another study in which 155 carotid arteries were evaluated for ulceration, the results showed a sensitivity of only 73 percent, a specificity of only 62 percent, and an accuracy of only 67 percent.[24]

"'Tandem'' lesions may occur in the distal internal carotid artery, carotid siphon, or major branches of the circle of Willis and can increase the morbidity and mortality of carotid endarterectomy. It is therefore important to evaluate the distal internal carotid siphon and the proximal middle cerebral and anterior cerebral arteries before considering carotid endarterectomy.

Carotid Doppler Ultrasound

Carotid Doppler ultrasound is widely used as a screening technique for evaluating carotid vascular disease. Criteria for grading carotid stenosis by Doppler ultrasound are given in Table 203-1. Two studies have compared ultrasound to MR angiography and conventional angiography.[1,47] In the study by Anderson and colleagues, ultrasound over- and underestimated the degree of stenosis in a significant number of cases, as compared with conventional angiography.[1] These errors would have altered the medical and surgical management in 20 percent of patients (10 of 50). Mittl and colleagues evaluated 66 vessels using NASCET criteria and Moneta criteria for carotid Doppler evaluation of bifurcation stenosis.[47] Carotid duplex ultrasonography had a sensitivity of 81 percent and a specificity of 82.2 percent, giving a positive predictive value of 68 percent and a negative predictive value of 90.2 percent. Ultrasound overestimated the degree of stenosis in seven patients and led to the identification of one false-negative occlusion and two false-positive occlusions. In addition, it is difficult to differentiate ulceration from irregular plaque disease by ultrasound, and the technique is unable to identify tandem lesions.

Magnetic Resonance Angiography

MRA has been extensively evaluated over the last several years as a noninvasive way to evaluate both the extracranial carotid vascular system and the intracranial cerebral vascular system. Methods for evaluating the extracranial carotids include 2-D TOF, multiple overlapping thin slab acquisitions (MOTSA), and 3-D TOF. 2-D and 3-D phase-contrast studies can also be performed, but they are subject to more artifacts caused by dephasing. Black-blood techniques (i.e., spin echo techniques)[22,37] have also been used to determine the full extent of the lumen in an area of stenosis. While black blood techniques have had some success, they can falsely interpret calcifications as normal patent lumen. Overall, MRA depicts a normal lumen fairly well. Eddy currents in the posterior aspects of the bulb can occur and can mimic atherosclerotic disease (Fig. 203-3). An observer with some experience can easily identify these normal artifacts by looking at individual partition images. MRA will typically overestimate the length and degree of stenosis (Fig. 203-4). Moderate to severe stenoses are usually characterized by a flow gap between the proximal and distal portions of the internal carotid artery. Occlusion can be distinguished from moderate to severe stenosis by the fact that the internal carotid artery will be imaged distal to the flow gap in the latter case but not the former (Fig. 203-5). The length of the flow gap has been found to correlate with the degree of stenosis for stenoses of about 50 to 99 percent.[47,53,54] Ulcerations are poorly depicted by MRA, owing to dephasing in areas of disordered flow (Fig. 203-6). Tandem lesions are also not as well identified with MRA, because areas of in-plane flow in the carotid siphon and at the base of skull and areas of apparent flow gap at the base of the skull due to magnetic susceptibility artifacts make the technique insensitive in these regions.

Spiral CT

Spiral CT is a promising technique for the noninvasive evaluation of carotid vascular disease. High-resolution images are a must: images 1 to 2 mm thick with a pitch (table rate) of 1.5 will provide approximately 6 cm of coverage from C6 to C3. A short examination lasting 20 to 30 s, will make it possible to achieve filling of the carotid with less filling of the jugular veins. To detect tandem lesions, thicker slices and a higher pitch will provide greater longitudinal coverage.

Several studies have evaluated spiral CT as a technique for assessing carotid vascular disease.[18,57] Difficulties in distinguishing contrast in the vascular lumen from mural calcification can result in over- and underestimates of stenoses.[18,57] However, if bone and calcium are segmented out first, the result is an 89 percent correlation between CTA and conventional angiography, and a 100 percent correlation for severe stenoses (70 to 99 percent stenosis) and for occluded vessels. Evaluation of individual slices also aids in interpretation. The major limitation of spiral CT in the evaluation of the carotid arteries is the occurrence of partial voluming effects between mural calcification and contrast material in the lumen.

Intracranial Cerebral Vascular Disease

Abnormalities of the intracranial vessels can be evaluated with MRA and conventional angiography. The latter is the gold standard in this situation; it is the only technique by which very small vessels can be evaluated (Fig. 203-7). It has the disadvantage of being invasive and is also limited by the relatively small number of projections that can be obtained in a 2-D format. Stereo imaging can be performed to provide a 3-D perspective. MRA typically uses 2-D or 3-D TOF or 2-D or 3-D PC methods for evaluation of intracranial vessels. The proximal vessels—the internal carotid artery, the A1, A2, M1, and M2 segments, and the proximal vertebral arteries—can be evaluated adequately with a relatively high degree of sensitivity[34,63] (Fig. 203-8). As for the extracranial vessels, the length and extent of stenoses are overestimated. Phase-contrast techniques allow detection of the direction of flow in collateral vessels in the presence of proximal stenoses.

For patients with transient ischemic attacks (TIAs), evaluation of the extracranial and intracranial vasculature should be performed. In many cases this will demonstrate atherosclerotic disease (atheromatous plaque or stenosis), fibromuscular hyperplasia, arterial dissection, or arteritis.

CT and MRI are both used to screen the brain in patients having TIAs. CT scans are usually normal in patients with TIAs, but infarcts have been detected in up to 20 percent of these patients; these infarcts may occur in relatively silent areas of the brain. However, MRI is more sensitive than CT for the detection of ischemia and infarction.[5,6] Owing to the absence of bone artifact, MRI is superior for evaluating the brain stem and cerebellum.[5,6,8]

Lacunar-type infarcts range from 0.5 to 2.5 cm in diameter and are most common in the distribution of lenticulostriate and small

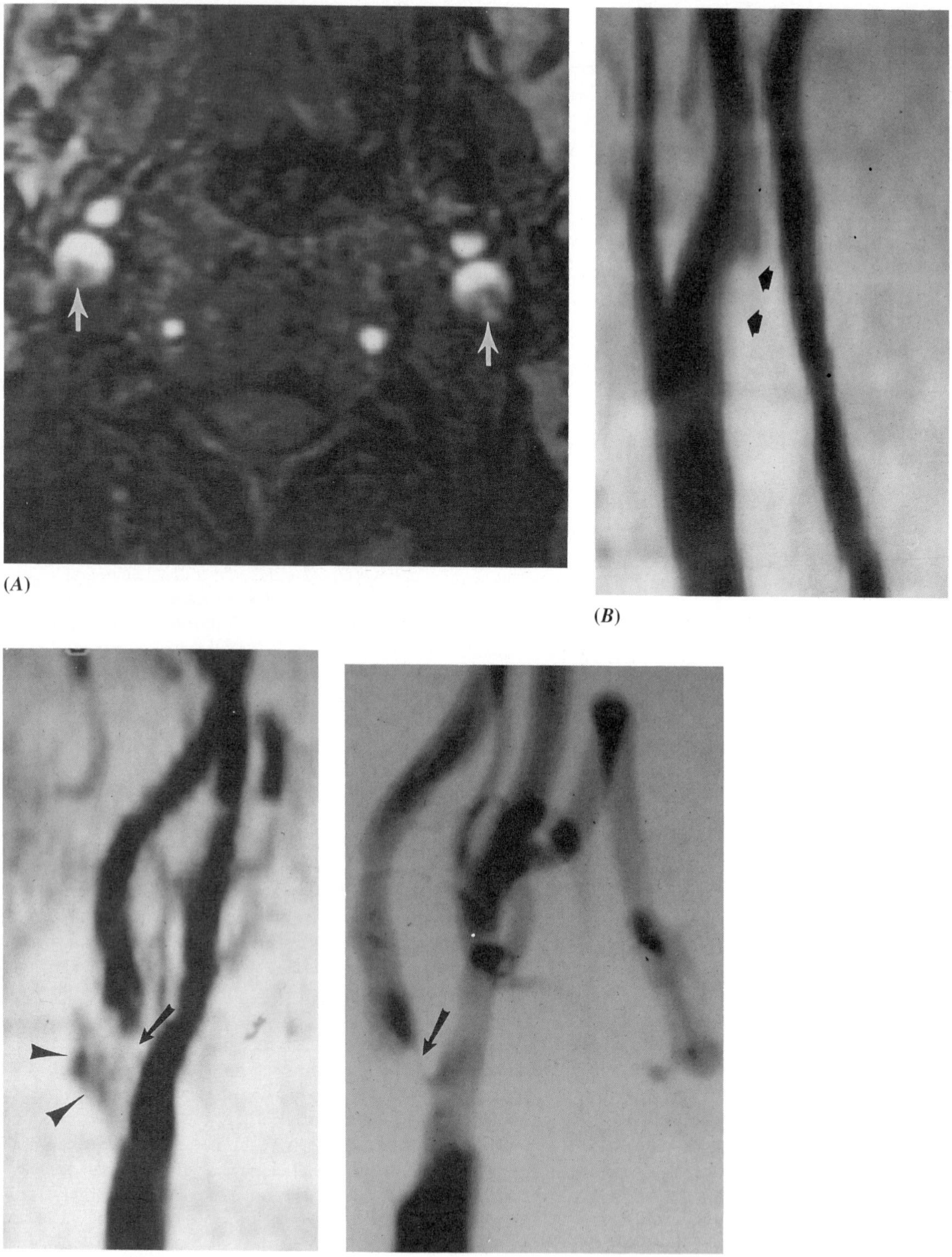

(*A*) (*B*) (*C*) (*D*)

Figure 203-3 Eddy currents mimicking atherosclerotic disease. *A*. An individual partition image (slice) from a MOTSA MRA demonstrates a low-signal abnormality *(arrows)* located posteriorly in each carotid bulb that simulates a filling defect and thus mimicks an atherosclerotic plaque. *B*. A maximum-intensity projection image from the same MOTSA MRA reveals the filling defect in the posterior bulb *(arrows)*, which is artifactual. MOTSA image *(C)* and conventional angiogram *(D)* of plaque disease *(arrowheads)* and 90 to 99 percent stenosis *(arrows)*. Atherosclerotic plaque *(arrowheads)* is visualized on the MRA.

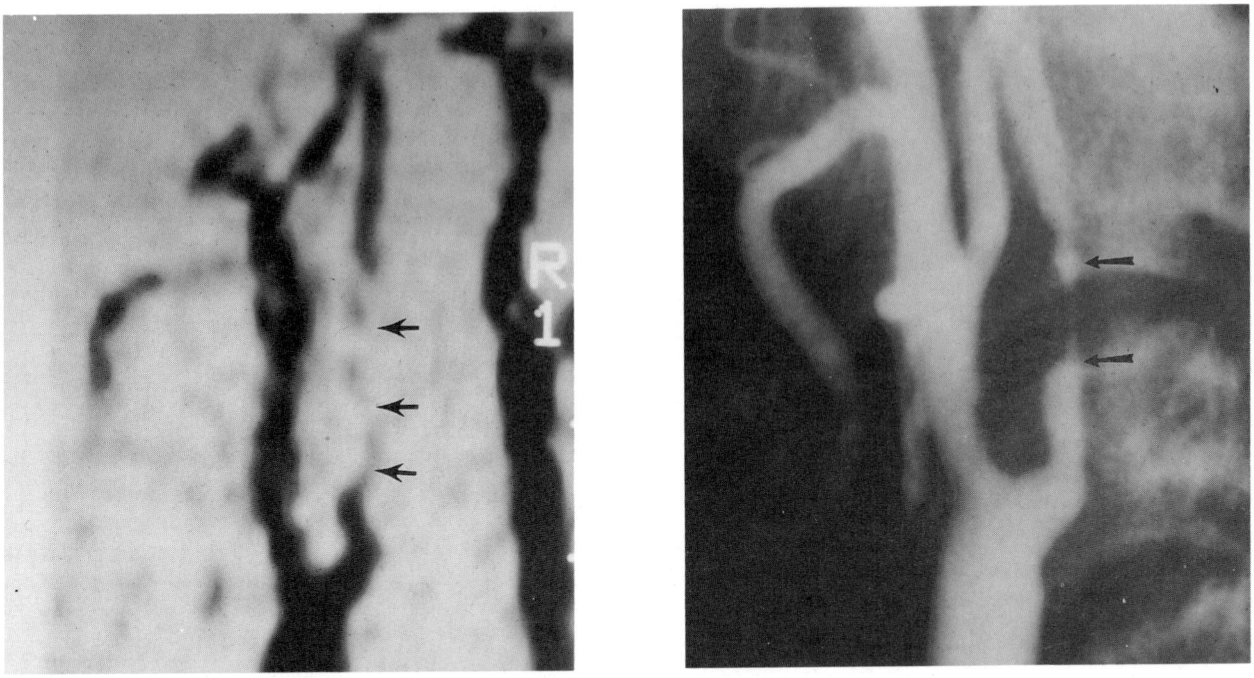

(*A*) (*B*)

Figure 203-4 A 2-D TOF MRA image *(A)* of severe stenosis of the internal carotid artery; a "flow gap" *(arrows)* is demonstrated which is longer and more severe than that depicted by the conventional angiogram *(B, arrows).*

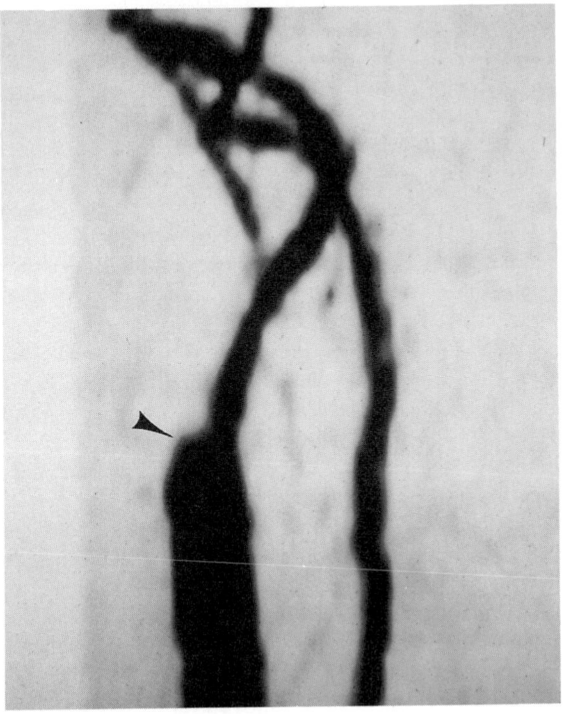

Figure 203-5 An occluded internal carotid artery *(arrowhead)*, showing the absence of any visualized distal internal carotid artery.

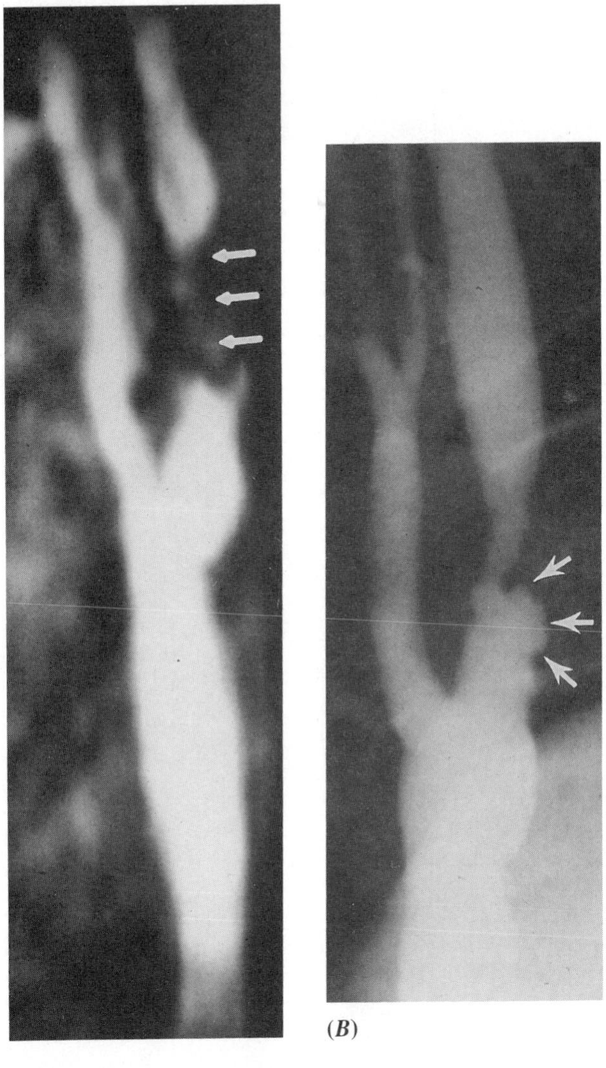

(*A*) (*B*)

Figure 203-6 3D TOF MRA image *(A)* and conventional angiogram *(B)* of an internal carotid artery with stenosis and ulceration. The ulceration is not seen on the MRA, but a flow gap due to the stenosis is present *(arrows)*. The conventional angiogram demonstrates an atherosclerotic plaque with an irregular base *(arrows)*, which was found at surgery to represent an ulcer.

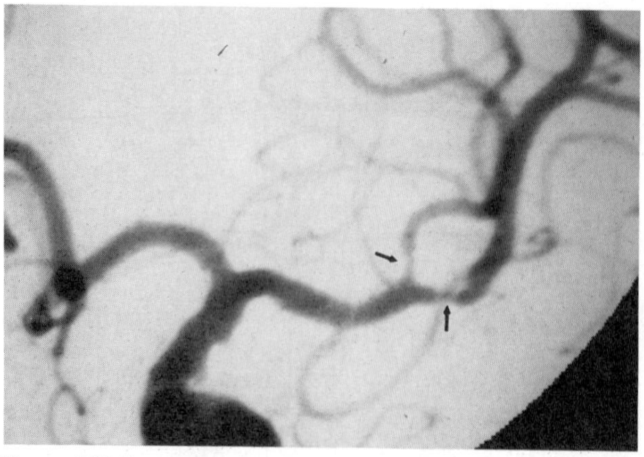

Figure 203-7 A case in which narrowing of branches due to atherosclerotic disease at the middle cerebral artery bifurcation *(arrows)* caused transient ischemic symptoms.

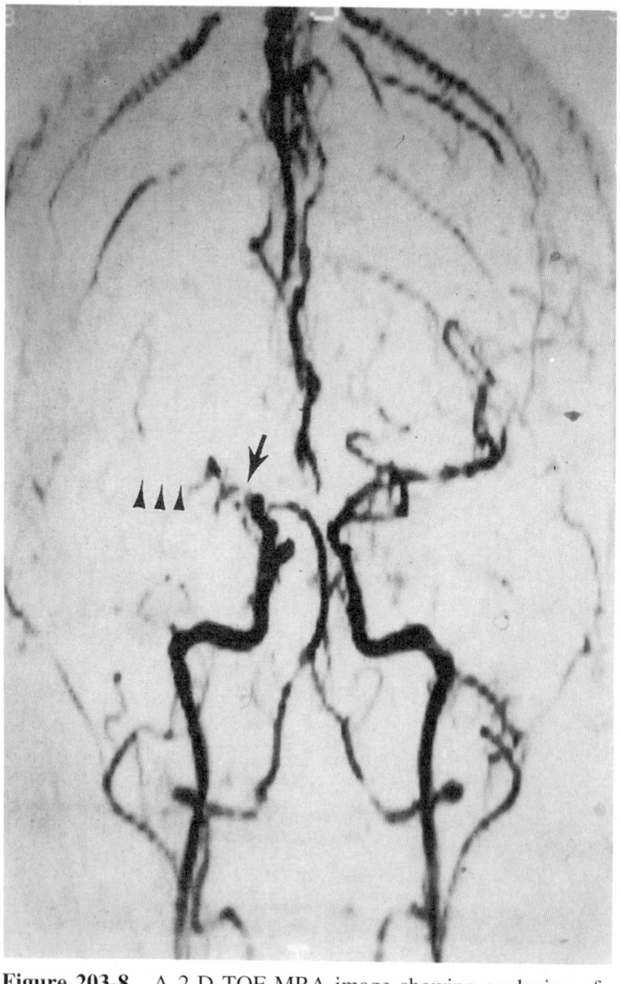

Figure 203-8 A 2-D TOF MRA image showing occlusion of the right M1 branch just distal to the internal carotid artery bifurcation *(arrow)*. No middle cerebral vessels can be clearly seen *(arrowheads)*.

penetrating vessels that supply the basal ganglia, thalamus, and brain stem. Lacunar infarcts result from the occlusion of a penetrating vessel by atheromatous plaque, fibrinoid necrosis, or embolic material. Small lacunar lesions are difficult to detect by CT; those 0.5 to 1 cm in diameter may be detected on CT within 24 to 48 h. They appear as round or ovoid areas of hypodensity.

The periventricular and deep white matter may also be involved, either focally or diffusely; the appearance is one of decreased density on CT in the periventricular and deep white matter regions. Although the changes can be secondary to vascular disease involving transmedullary arterioles, the appearance cannot be distinguished from that of gliosis or demyelination.

MRI is unable to distinguish ischemia, infarction, and edema; all cause increased T1 (low signal) and T2 (high signal) relaxation times. Lacunar infarcts are perceptible on T2-weighted images within 1 week (Fig. 203-9). Lesions older than one week can be seen on both T1-weighted and T2-weighted images. Lacunar infarcts and strokes cannot in general be detected with traditional spin echo MR imaging for 12 to 24 h. Diffusion-weighted imaging is a newer MR technique that allows detection of fluid shifts with the application of gradients. This technique can detect areas of ischemia and/or infarction within 30 min. With contrast administration, lacunar-type strokes may demonstrate enhancement beginning at 6 days and lasting 6 weeks. Enhancement of the meninges overlying the surface of the affected area may be noted first, followed by ring-like or parenchymal enhancement.[3,4]

Larger areas of ischemia or infarction are the result of thrombosis, embolism, or hypoperfusion. These cerebrovascular events can cause large cortical-based areas of thrombotic or hemorrhagic infarction, or watershed infarctions. MRI is the most sensitive technique for detecting infarction. Using animal models and *diffusion weighted* MR imaging, strokes can be detected within 30 min, and possibly sooner (Fig. 203-10).[7,15]

Diffusion imaging aside, MRI with contrast enhancement provides the earliest signs of infarction as described by Elster[25,26] and Moody. Intravascular enhancement of slow-flowing blood on T1-weighted images can be seen nearly immediately after the stroke and may precede T2-weighted changes by several hours. Meningeal enhancement occurs within the first 3 days and usually involves the overlying dura. It may be caused by arterial collaterals, by other vascular causes, or by local irritation from the adjacent infarction. Parenchymal enhancement is visible over the period from 6 days to 6 weeks and occasionally lasts longer; this type of enhancement is also evident on CT (Fig. 203-11).[25,26] The intensity of parenchymal enhancement depends largely on the extent of breakdown of the blood-brain barrier, with some contribution from increases in blood flow due to disordered autoregulation, collateral circulation, and the formation of granulation tissue in the area of infarction.[9] Chronic infarcts, periventricular white matter changes, and asymptomatic lacunar infarcts do not enhance. Symptomatic lacunar infarcts can enhance.

T2-weighted spin echo MRI can first detect strokes within 12 to 24 h. Although CT can also detect strokes in this period, the findings may be more subtle. Characteristic signal changes on MRI include prolonged T1 and T2 relaxation times distributed in a particular vascular territory. Acute and chronic infarcts give similar signal changes, but acute strokes are associated with effacement of sulci and gyri due to cytotoxic edema as well as with some degree of mass effect on adjacent structures. Chronic infarcts are associated with atrophy, including the cortex, and with dilation of the underlying ventricular system. Hemorrhagic infarcts may display characteristic signal changes depending on the age and location of

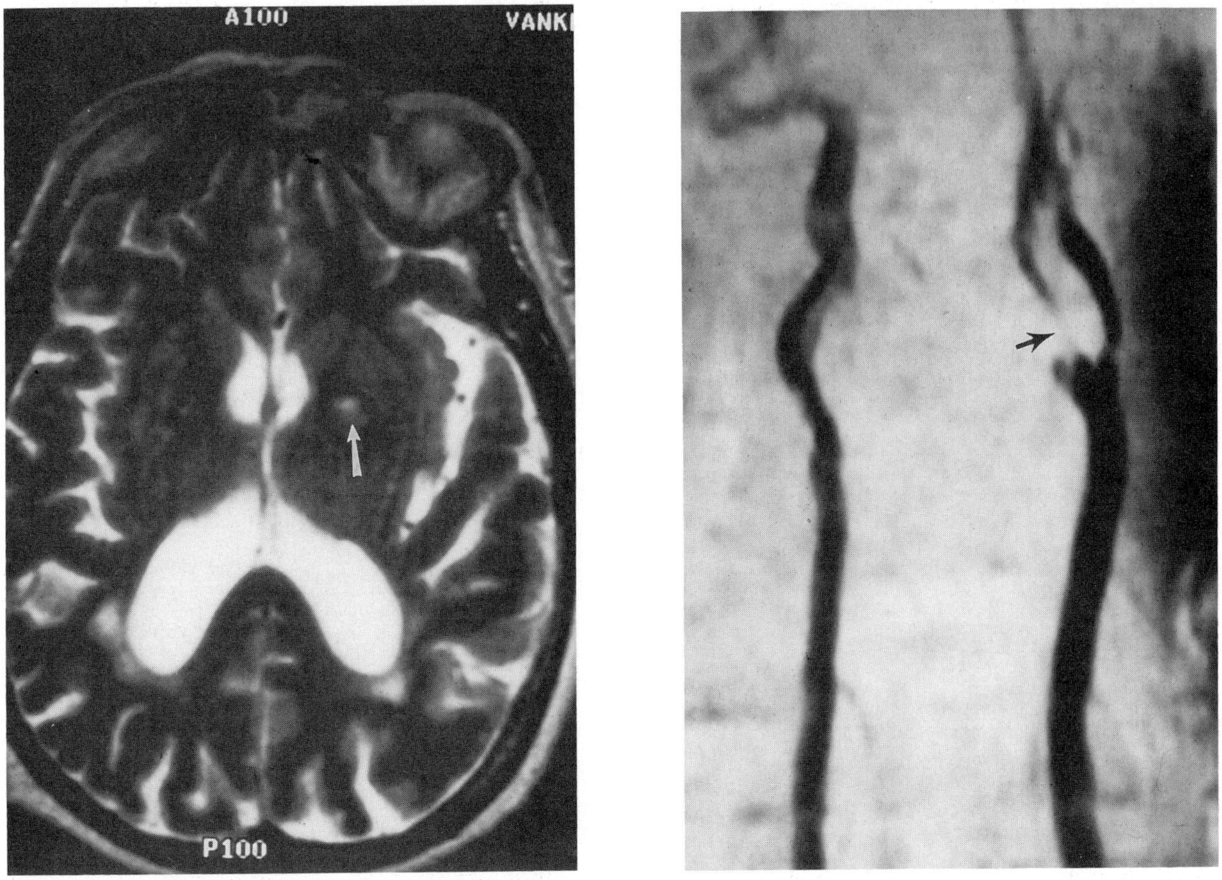

(*A*) (*B*)

Figure 203-9 *A.* A T2-weighted image of an acute lacunar infarct in the left putamen and globus pallidus *(arrow)*. *B.* A MOTSA MRA image revealing high-grade 70 to 95 percent stenosis of the left internal carotid artery *(arrow)*. A decision to operate was made on the basis of the MRA and carotid Doppler findings.

the infarct and the presence and nature of the degradation products of the blood.[16,17,20,28] MRI cannot distinguish transient ischemia from infarction, although it may be possible to make this distinction with spectroscopy in the future.

CT is often the first examination performed in the setting of an acute stroke because of its accessibility and its ability to readily exclude acute subarachnoid or parenchymal hemorrhage. The earliest changes of stroke may be seen within several hours, depending on the size and location of the stroke. These first changes consist of (1) loss of distinction between gray and white matter, (2) subtle effacement of sulci and gyri, and (3) a subtle mass effect on adjacent cisternal structures. In addition, (4) a ''dense middle cerebral artery'' may be present, and (5) hypodensity of the insular cortex may be an early sign in middle cerebral artery strokes. Within 24 h, the stroke becomes more hypodense, and the margins more distinct and sharply delineated (Fig. 203-12). Hypodensity and swelling are the result of cytotoxic edema, which becomes most marked between 5 and 7 days and then begins to decrease. It is during this acute period that marked shifts and herniations can occur.

Intravascular and meningeal enhancement is not readily apparent on CT, but parenchymal enhancement is seen, beginning at approximately 6 days and lasting to 6 weeks or sometimes longer. It generally resolves completely by 3 months. The mechanisms underlying CT contrast enhancement in stroke are the same as for MRI.

An embolus may be visible on a CT scan as a dense clot in a vessel or as a calcified nodule along the distribution of the middle or anterior cerebral artery. A hyperdense clot may only be visible for a few days, either because it undergoes lysis with distal migration of fragments or because breakdown of the hemoglobin in the clot reduces its density.[16,17,20,28] Embolic infarction differs from thrombotic infarction in that a multiplicity of lesions may be present in a variety of vascular territories, which may be unilateral or bilateral. In addition, embolic infarctions more often become hemorrhagic. This tendency to hemorrhage is thought to result from reperfusion at normal to increased pressures into tissue that has lost its autoregulatory capacity. The hemorrhage usually involves the gray matter initially but can later extend into the white matter. The hemorrhagic changes incite vasogenic edema, which contributes to the overall mass effect and shift (Fig. 203-13).

Watershed infarction is the result of hemodynamic changes in the circulatory system, which cause decreased blood pressure or cardiac output and lead to diminished cerebral blood flow. If diminished cerebral blood flow is superimposed on significant carotid or cerebrovascular stenosis, infarcts may occur in the watershed zones at the borders of specific vascular territories. Watershed infarcts generally occur at the borders between the territories of the middle and anterior cerebral arteries, the middle and posterior cerebral arteries, and the anterior and posterior cerebral arteries. The periventricular white matter region can also be involved (Fig. 203-14).

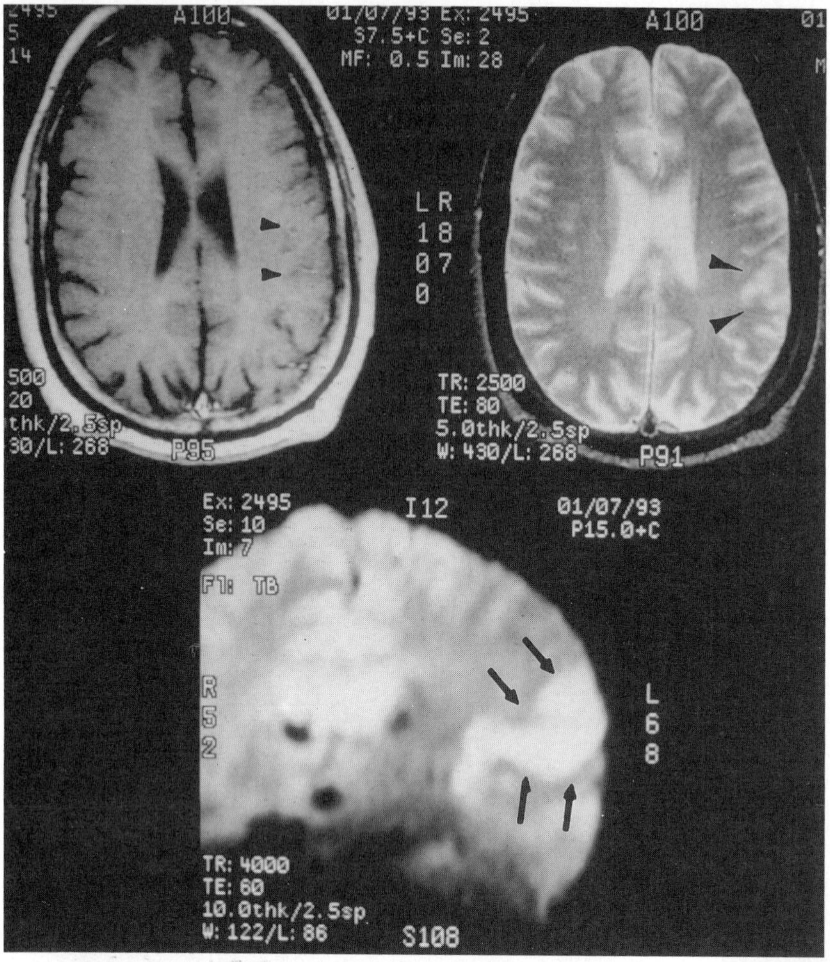

Figure 203-10 A stroke only 3 h old. *A.* A contrast-enhanced image showing the earliest changes of vascular enhancement and effacement of sulci and gyri *(arrowheads)*. *B.* Subtle T2 changes are present *(arrowheads)*. *C.* A diffusion image, which shows the area of ischemia *(arrows)* better than the other two MR techniques.

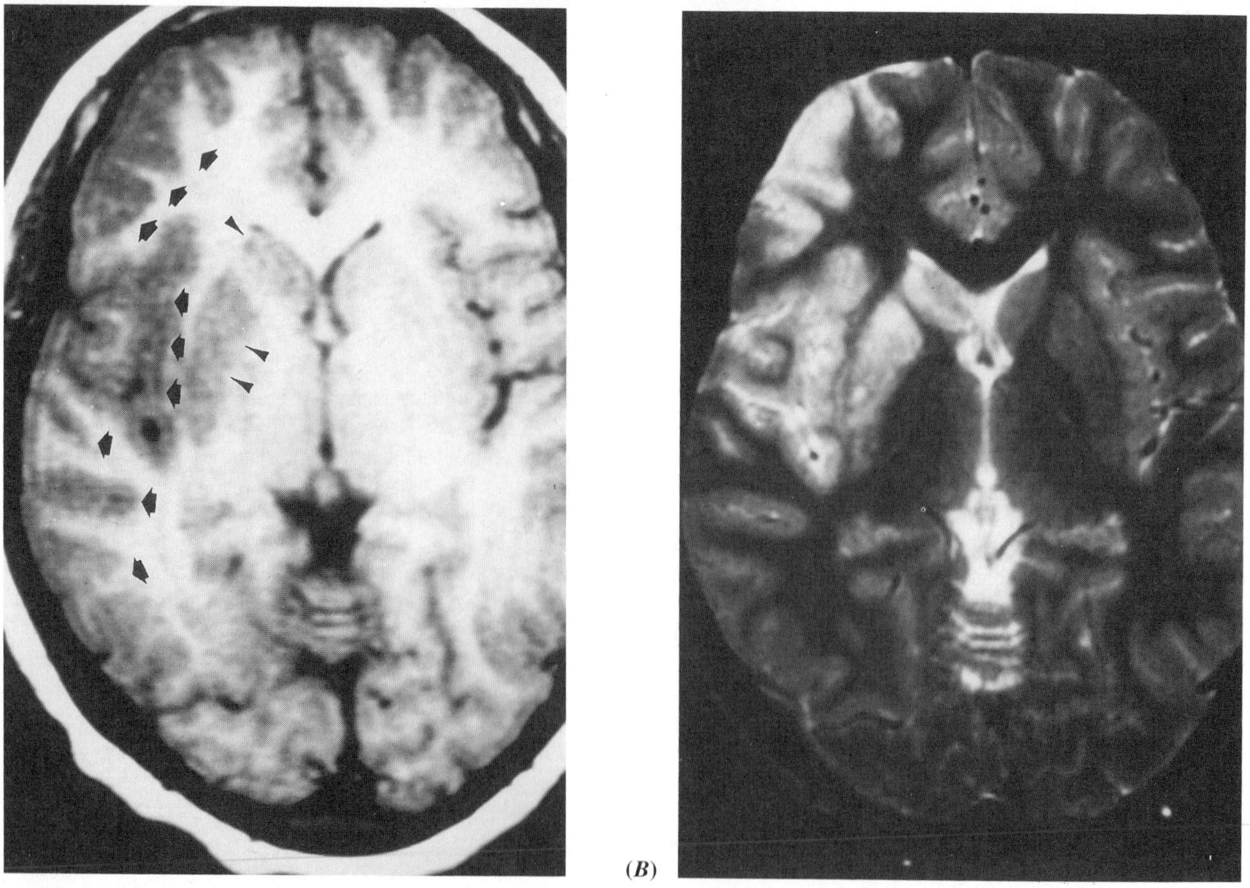

(*A*) (*B*)

Figure 203-11 MR enhancement pattern of stroke. T1-weighted *(A)* and T2-weighted *(B)* images at 24 h. The T1-weighted image shows a low-signal cortical abnormality in the right middle cerebral artery territory *(arrows)* and the right head of the caudate and putamen *(arrowheads)*. The T2-weighted image demonstrates a high signal in the same areas.

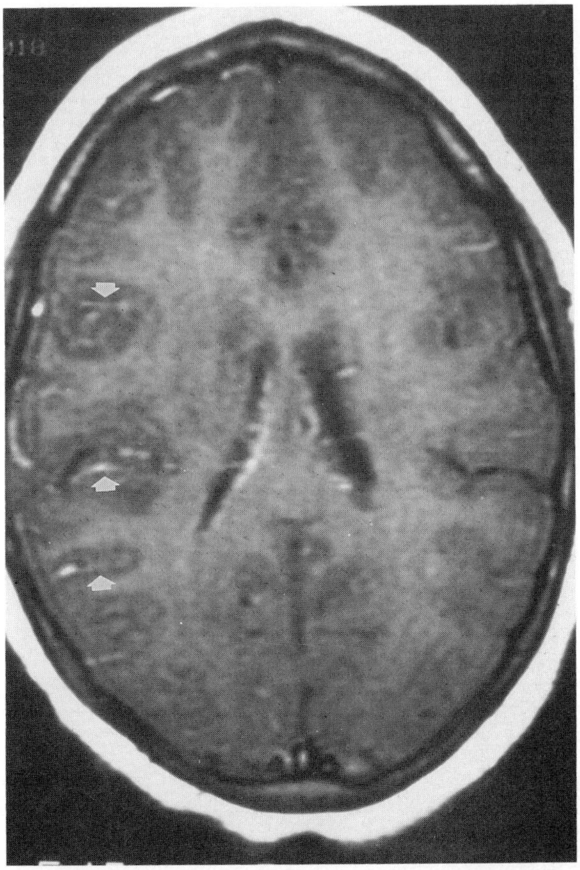

(*C*)

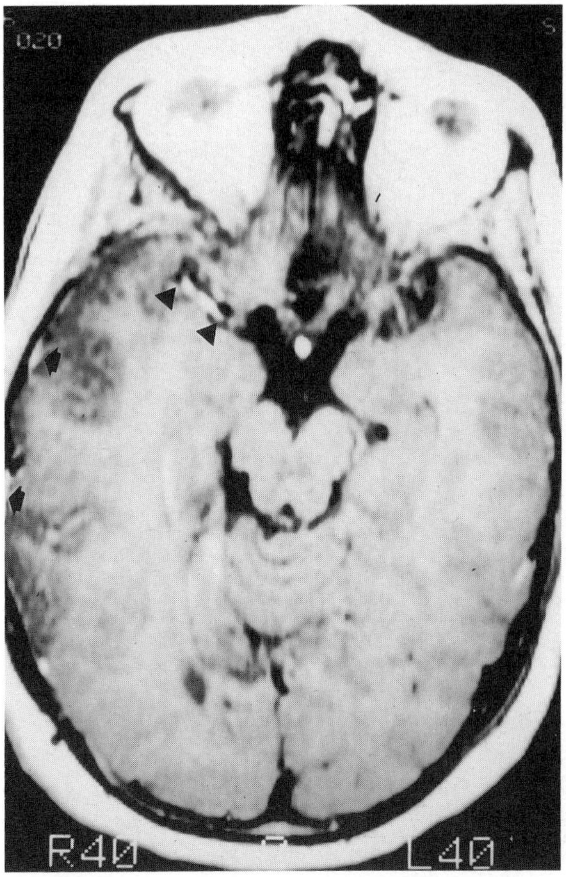

(*D*)

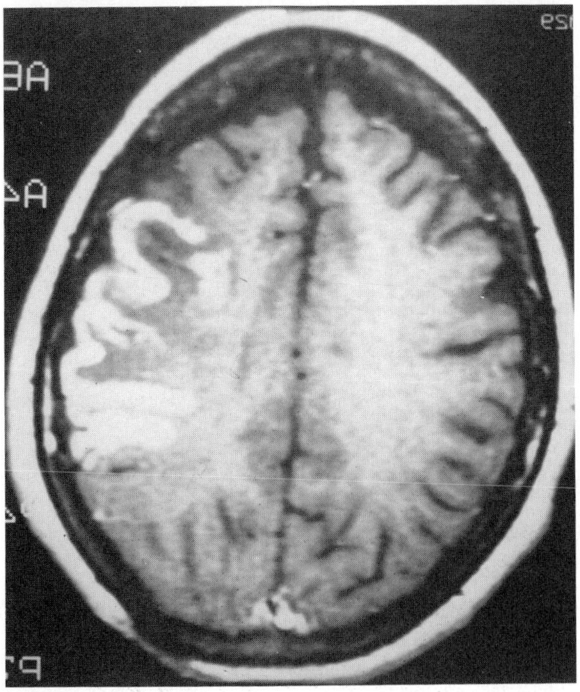

(*E*)

Figure 203-11 (*Continued*) *C.* A contrast-enhanced T1-weighted MR image showing enhancement of slow-flowing blood *(white arrows),* the earliest sign of a stroke. *D.* Leptomeningeal enhancement affecting the overlying dura *(arrows).* This sign appears within the first 3 days. Enhancement of the right middle cerebral artery is also present *(arrowheads). E.* The parenchymal enhancement of stroke at 2 weeks follows the gyri.

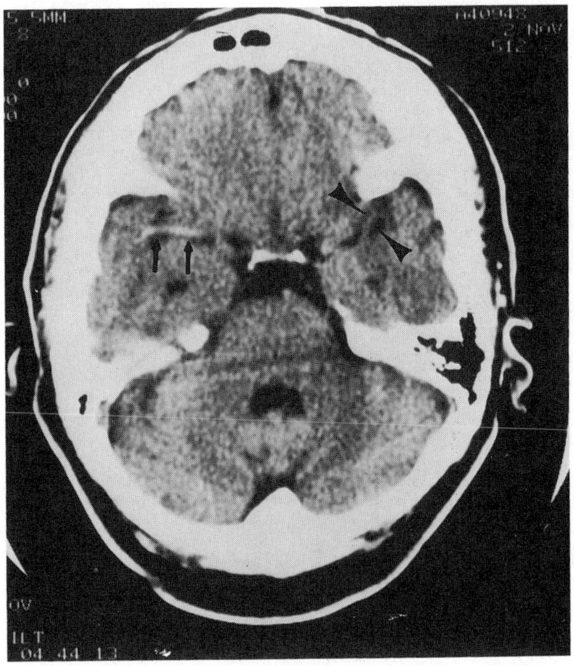

(*A*)

Figure 203-12 CT scans of an acute stroke in the right middle cerebral artery territory. *A.* The right middle cerebral artery shows increased attenuation secondary to thrombosis or slow flow *(arrows).* The normal left middle cerebral artery is shown for comparison *(arrowheads).*

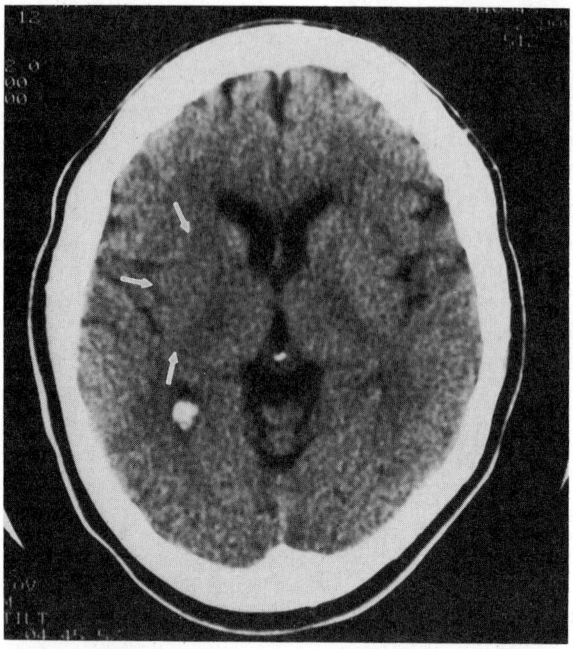

(*B*)

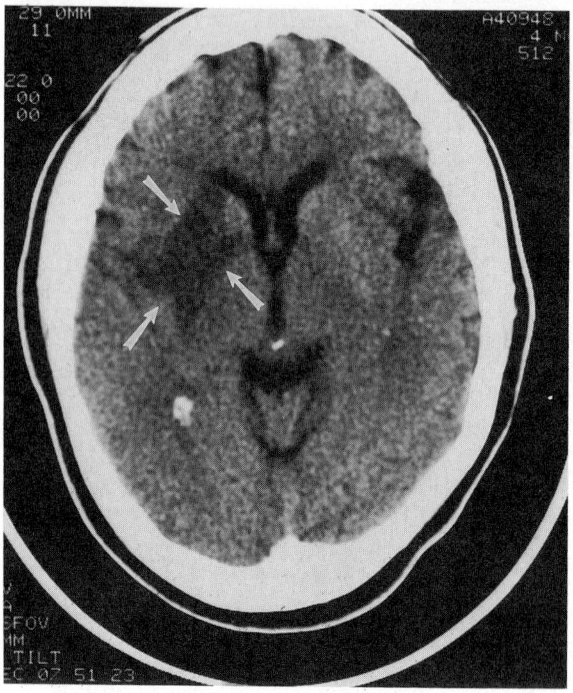

(*C*)

Figure 203-12 (*Continued*) *B.* A scan showing subtle hypodensity of the right putamen and insular cortex *(arrows)*. Notice the normal higher attenuation of the left putamen. *C.* Twenty-four h later, with evolution of the stroke, there is hypodensity of the putamen, the insular cortex, the anterior and posterior limbs of the internal capsule, and the anterior portion of the head of the caudate *(arrows)*.

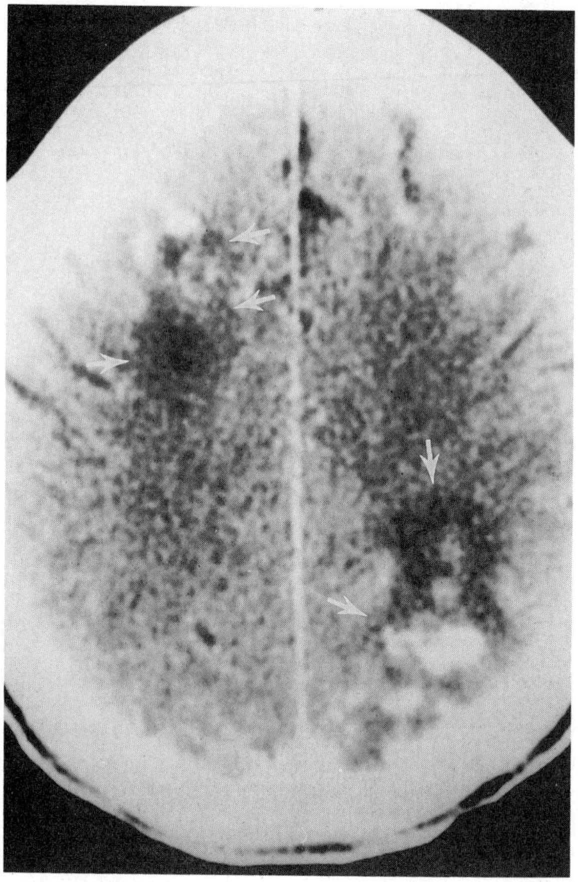

Figure 203-13 Bilateral hemispheric hemorrhagic infarcts secondary to emboli from a cardiac source *(arrowheads)*.

Fibromuscular Dysplasia

Fibromuscular dysplasia (FMD) is an uncommon, nonatheromatous angiopathy of unknown etiology. Small and medium-sized arteries are affected, and the disorder is characterized by abnormalities of smooth muscle and of fibrous and elastic tissue. The condition is usually diagnosed in the fourth or fifth decade of life, and it is more common among women, who account for about 85 percent of cases with cerebrovascular involvement.[13,14] Symptoms are usually those of TIAs, cerebral infarcts, or subarachnoid hemorrhage from intracranial aneurysms. Cervical bruits (which are evident in 70 to 100 percent of patients) are the most commonly identified physical abnormality.

FMD is a multifocal vascular disease, commonly affecting the renal and cephalic vessels. The pathology is characterized by hypoplasia or thinning of smooth muscle, destruction of elastic fibers, proliferation of fibrous tissue, and arterial wall disorganization.[31,32] Changes associated with atherosclerosis (necrosis, lipid accumulation, and calcification) are absent. Three histologic types can be identified. Disease of the media (medial FMD) accounts for most cases (90 to 95 percent) and is most common in women. The remaining cases represent intimal disease (about 5 percent) and adventitial disease (about 1 percent). These histologic abnormalities typically result in multifocal stenoses alternating with mural dilations, in focal or tubular stenoses, or, rarely, in asymmetrical diverticuli. Progressive disruption of the arterial wall may produce arterial dissection. Approximately one-third of patients have associated intracranial aneurysms,[35,46] which makes evaluation of the cerebrovascular system mandatory in patients with suspected FMD.

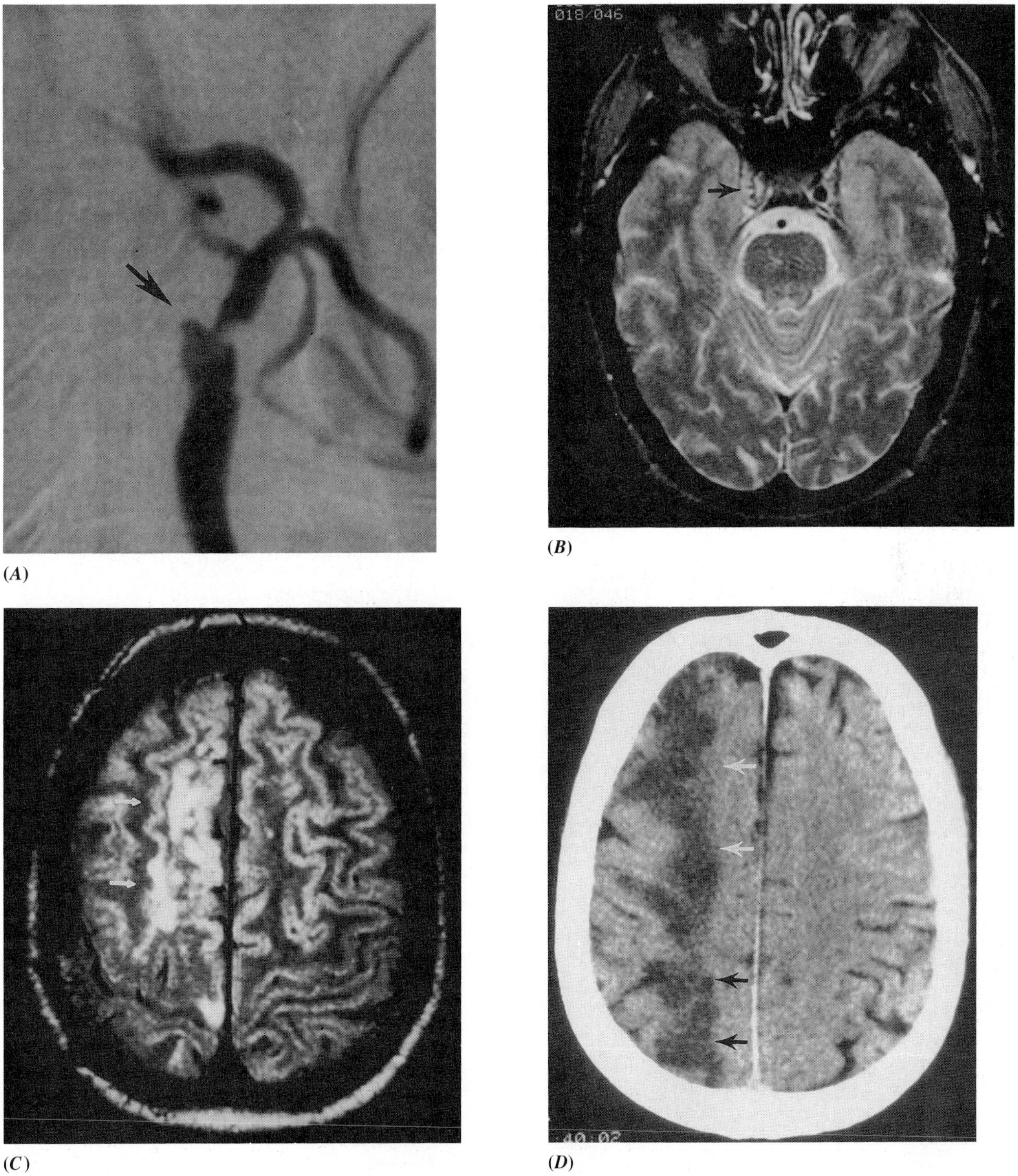

(*A*) (*B*) (*C*) (*D*)

Figure 203-14 A watershed infarct in the high right frontal region between the anterior and middle cerebral artery territories. It was caused by an occluded right internal carotid artery. *A.* A right common carotid angiogram demonstrating the occlusion *(arrow)*. *B.* A T2-weighted spin echo image shows the absence of a flow void in the right internal carotid artery *(arrow)*, which is consistent with the actual absence of flow. *C.* A T2-weighted spin echo image showing high-signal abnormalities in a distribution between the anterior and middle cerebral artery territories *(arrows)*, which are consistent with watershed infarcts. *D.* An axial CT scan showing watershed infarcts between the middle and anterior cerebral artery territories *(white arrows)* and between the middle and posterior cerebral artery territories *(black arrows)*.

Angiography of FMD

Lesions of the cerebrovascular system are typically located in the midportion of the internal carotid (75 percent) or vertebral (25 percent) arteries at the level of the first or second vertebra. Bilateral internal carotid artery involvement is seen in 65 percent of cases. Lesions rarely involve the petrous or intracranial internal carotid artery, and the common carotid bifurcation is usually spared. Classic cases show irregularly spaced areas of sharply localized concentric narrowing, which alternate with areas of dilation. This ''string of beads'' sign occurs in 80 to 90 percent of patients (Fig. 203-15). Smooth, concentric tubular stenosis is less common (6 to 12 percent or patients), and asymmetrical pseudoaneurysms/diverticula are the rarest angiographic manifestations. Despite the marked angiographic changes that are frequently seen, severe stenosis is uncommon, and complete occlusion is rare.

Although angiographic abnormalities consistent with FMD have been identified in the external carotid artery, in the anterior, middle, and posterior cerebral arteries, and in the basilar artery, these abnormalities have rarely been verified histologically. The arterial complications of FMD may be identified angiographically. Arterial dissection, pseudoaneurysms, or arteriovenous fistulae have been identified.

Although the angiographic findings in FMD are fairly characteristic, similar findings may be seen in arterial spasm, in standing arterial waves (which may be associated with distal arterial occlusion), or in Takayasu's arteritis. Smooth concentric stenosis, associated with tubular fibromuscular dysplasia, must be distinguished from arterial hypoplasia, vascular spasm, and, rarely, atherosclerosis or arterial dissection.

Moyamoya Disease

Initially identified in Japan, moyamoya disease (also known as idiopathic progressive arteriopathy of childhood) is a progressive occlusive cerebral vascular disorder of unknown etiology, which results in narrowing of the intracranial arteries at the base of the brain. The etiology of this disorder is unknown, and whether it is congenital or acquired is still debated. Moyamoya is most frequent in Japan, but cases have been reported from all over the world. The incidence in Japan is less than 1 per 100,000 persons per year, with a slight female dominance. Two age peaks have been identified, one at around 3 years of age and the other in the third decade. A familial tendency has been identified in some cases, and certain

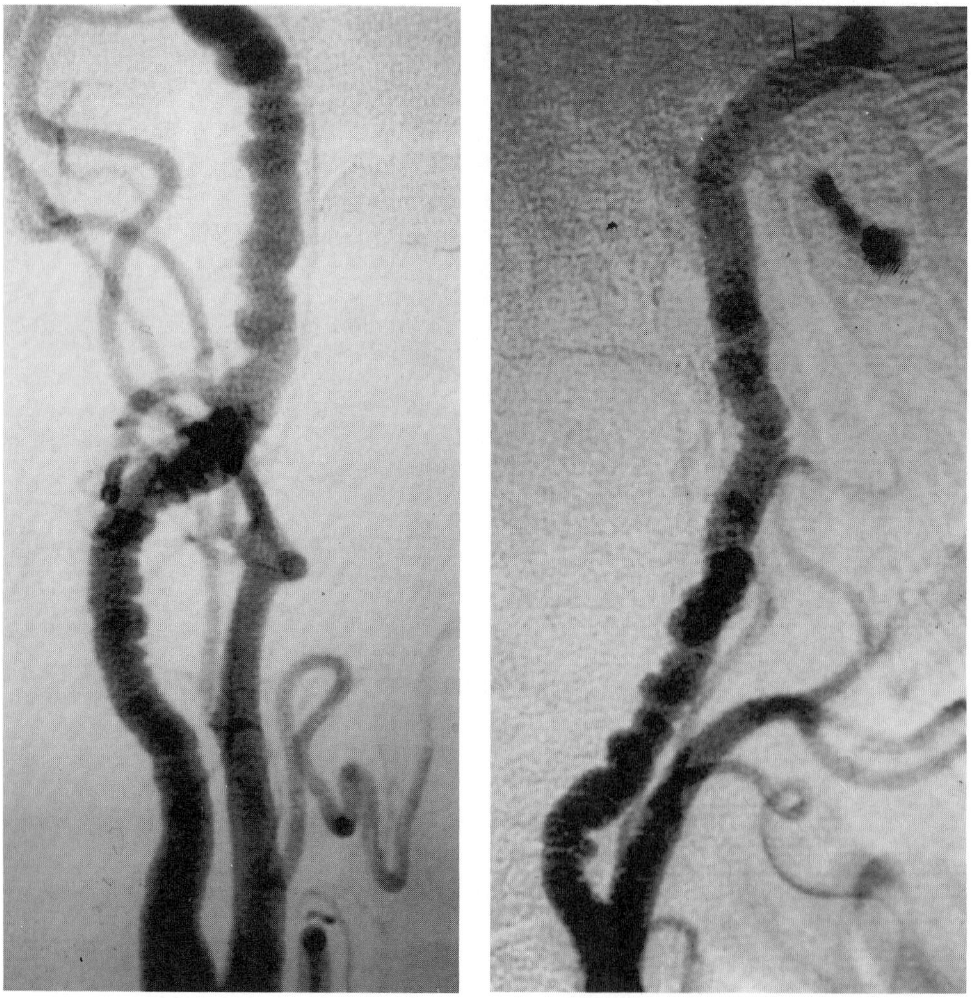

(A) *(B)*

Figure 203-15 Fibromuscular dysplasia. Anteroposterior *(A)* and lateral *(B)* views of a common carotid arteriogram demonstrating multiple alternating stenoses and dilations of the extracranial internal carotid artery.

human leukocyte antigen (HLA) antigens have been associated with the disease (HLA, antigen B40 in early-onset cases and HLA antigen B52 in later-onset cases).[38,58]

Clinical Manifestations

Various clinical manifestations have been reported, and the clinical course is thought to depend on the rapidity and extent of vascular occlusion versus the effectiveness of collateral circulation. Four groups of clinical conditions have been identified: TIA, infarction, hemorrhage, and epilepsy. TIAs and infarction are more common in the juvenile-onset group, whereas in adult cases, intracranial hemorrhage is a more prevalent clinical manifestation. Epilepsy has been observed in about 7 percent of all cases.

The nautral history of the condition is unclear. Whether the juvenile and adult types in fact represent the same disease entity is uncertain. If onset is before 4 years of age, prognosis is poor, whereas cases with TIAs of relatively late onset have a better prognosis.

Pathology

Four gross pathologic features are characteristic:

1. Narrowing or occlusion of the distal internal carotid arteries and proximal aspects of anterior and middle cerebral arteries
2. Multiple, extensive collateral vessels arising from the circle of Willis
3. Multiple leptomeningeal and transdural collateral vessels
4. Secondary changes in the brain parenchyma (infarction), commonly seen in the occipital and temporal lobes[42]

Histopathologic changes include intimal fibrous thickening (which may be associated with lipoid degeneration), widening of the internal elastic lamina, and thinning of the arterial media.

Imaging Findings

Although cerebral angiography is crucial in the diagnosis of moyamoya disease, CT and MRI provide useful information in the workup of patients, particularly in the identification of brain ischemia and infarction. CT and MRI demonstrate infarcts (multiple) in over 80 percent of patients. Most commonly affected is the anterior circulation, although the posterior cerebral artery territory may also be involved. MR images demonstrate collateral channels (most evident in the basal ganglia), while MR angiography shows large-vessel occlusions and major collateral flow patterns (Fig. 203-16). Intracranial hemorrhage is also identified by CT and MRI. Intraventricular bleeding (originating from the dilated perforating arteries in the ventricular wall, basal ganglia, and thalami) is the most commonly encountered type.

Catheter angiography demonstrates the following characteristic findings:

1. Symmetrical stenoses or occlusions of the terminal internal carotid arteries or the origins of the anterior and middle cerebral arteries

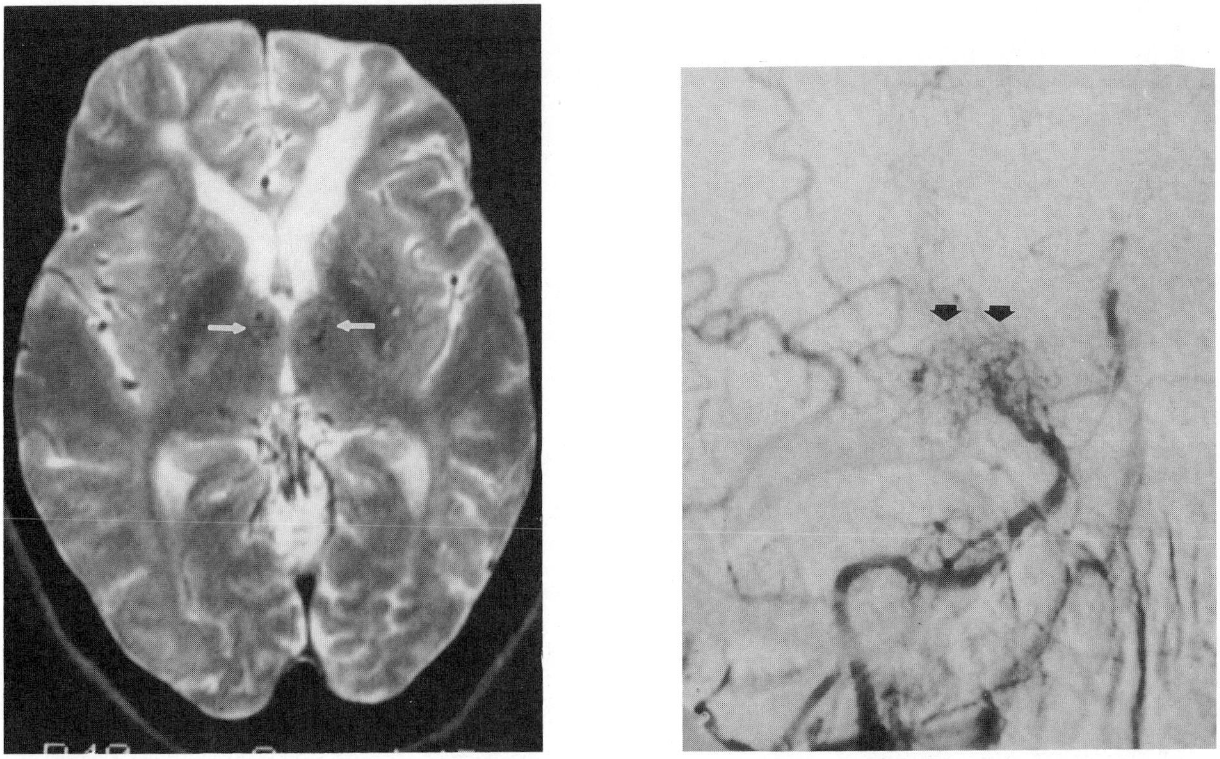

(A) ***(B)***

Figure 203-16 Moyamoya disease. *A.* T2-weighted MR image showing small, low-signal ''dots'' *(white arrows)* that represent dilated perforating arteries providing collateral circulation. *B.* Anteroposterior projection of a common carotid injection showing severe narrowing of the right internal carotid artery and occlusion of the anterior and middle cerebral arteries. A network of dilated collateral vessels at the internal carotid artery bifurcation create the characteristic ''puff of smoke'' vascular appearance *(arrows).*

2. Numerous enlarged lenticulostriate and thalamoperforating arteries (giving rise to the "puff of smoke" appearance after which the disease is named)
3. Numerous transdural, leptomeningeal, and pial collateral vessels (known as the rete mirabile)[61,62]

Although the moyamoya pattern of collateral blood flow is striking and easily recognized, it is important to remember that it is nonspecific and may be encountered in other occlusive vascular disorders (of slow onset), such as atherosclerosis or sickle cell disease.

Vasculitis

Inflammation and necrosis of blood vessel walls are the characteristics of this group of conditions, which are commonly divided according to whether the etiology is infectious or noninfectious. Infectious vasculitides include bacterial, fungal, and viral types, as well as vasculitides associated with tuberculosis and syphilis. Noninfectious vasculitides can be divided into conditions related to immune-complex disease (polyarteritis nodosa, systemic lupus erythematosus, and antiphospholipid antigen disease), cell-mediated disorders [Takayasu's arteritis (Fig. 203-17), temporal arteritis, Wegener's granulomatosis, neurosarcoidosis, and idiopathic arteritis], and miscellaneous vascular diseases, such as mucocutaneous lymph node syndrome (Kawasaki disease), thromboangiitis obliterans (Buerger's disease), and Behçet's disease.[52]

Imaging Findings

CT and MRI changes predominantly represent areas of ischemia and, occasionally, intraparenchymal hemorrhage. MRI is more sensitive than CT for identification of small ischemic foci. Although MRA images may show narrowing of the larger intracranial vessels, most cases will need cut-film conventional angiography for identification of the characteristic angiographic changes of vasculitis.

Angiographic changes are typically nonspecific, with multifocal segmental vascular stenoses (occasionally alternating with vascular dilations), which may be seen affecting all three major vascular territories. In severe cases the arteries may have a beaded appearance.[50] Vasculitis with an infectious cause may be associated with distal aneurysm formation. The angiographic changes of vasculitis are nonspecific and can be seen with meningitis or severe atherosclerotic diseases (Fig. 203-18).

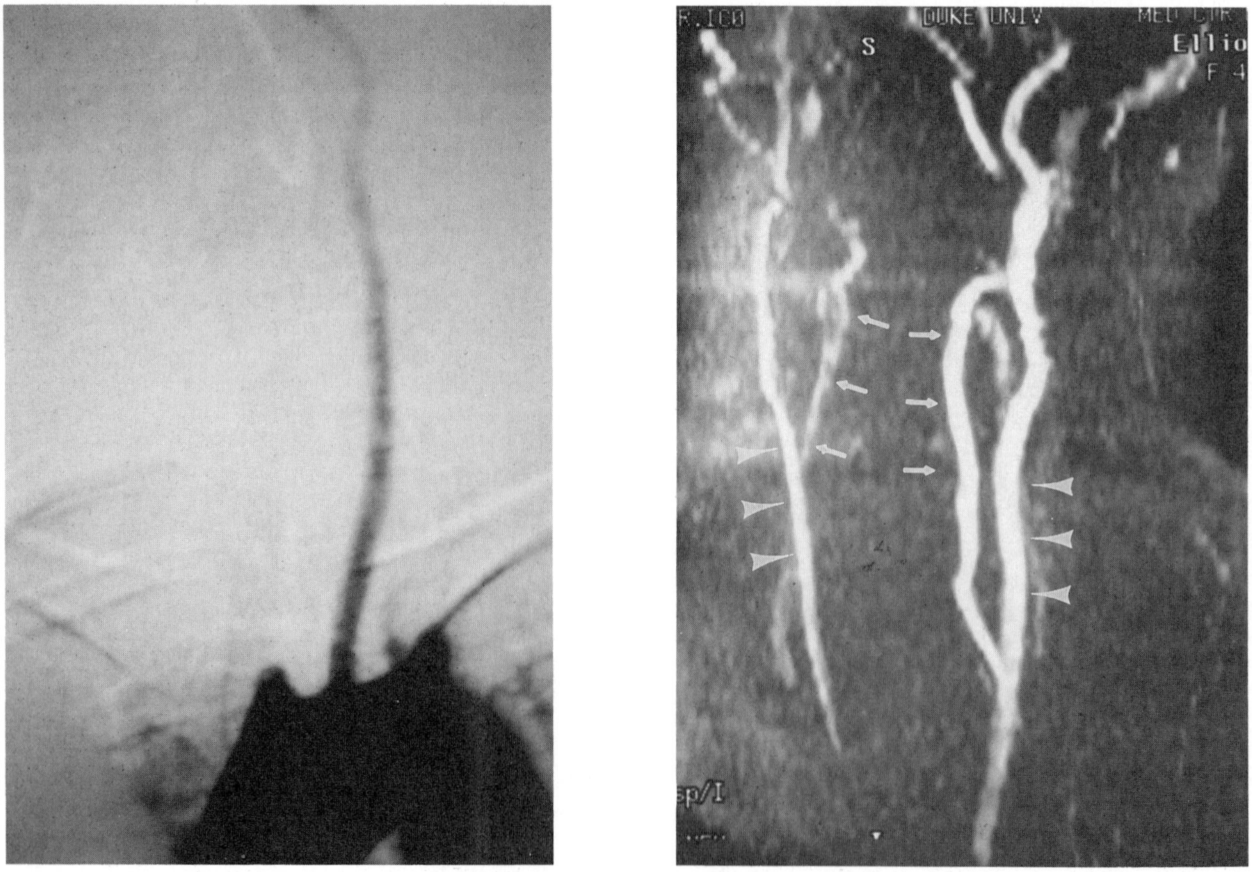

(*A*) (*B*)

Figure 203-17 *A.* A conventional aortic arch angiogram demonstrates cephalad flow only from the left common carotid artery; the right common carotid and both vertebral arteries appear to be absent. *B.* MRA demonstrates flow in both vertebral arteries *(arrows)* and both carotid arteries *(arrowheads)*, presumably via collaterals not perceptible by standard angiography.

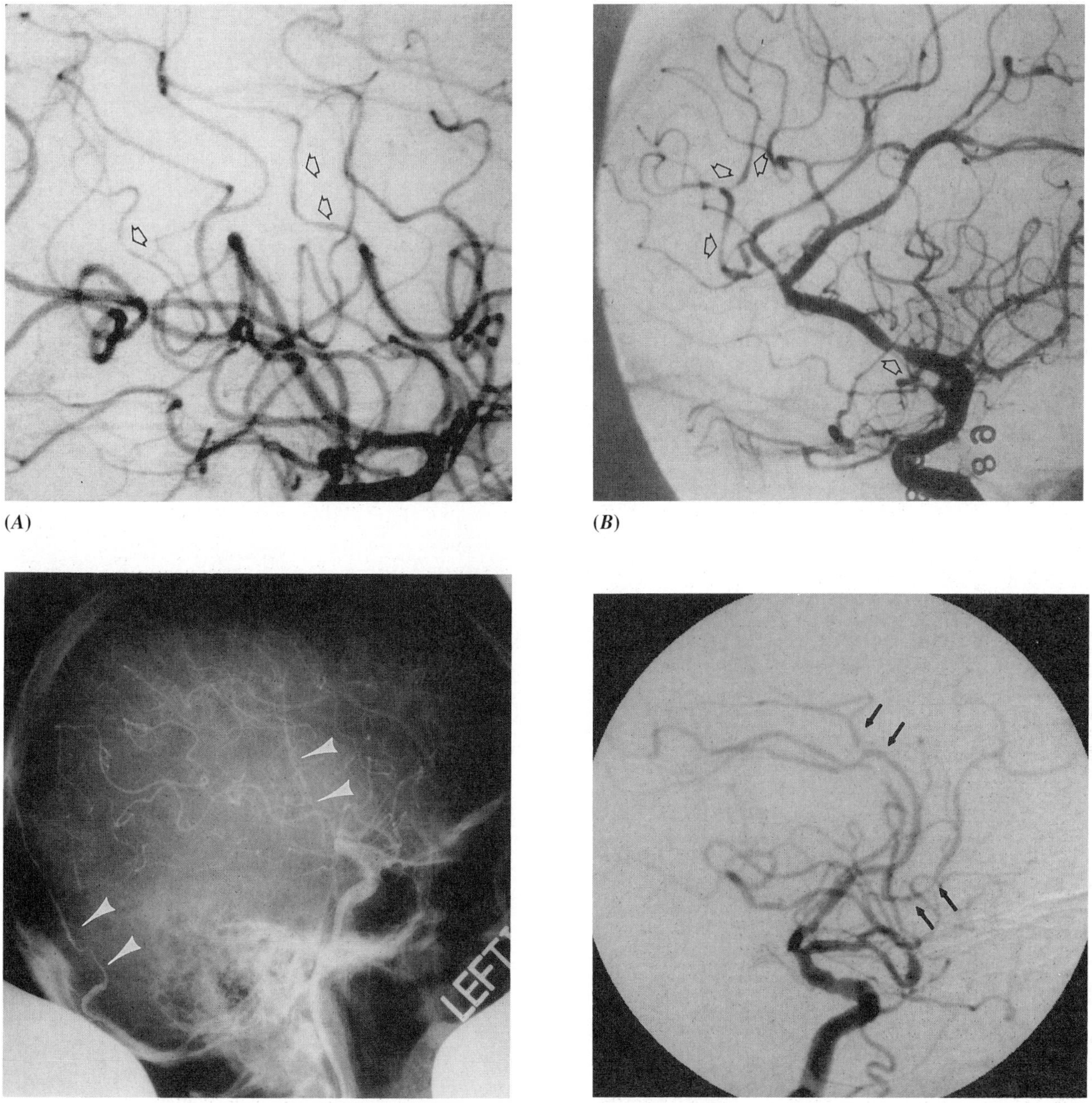

(*A*) (*B*) (*C*) (*D*)

Figure 203-18 Vasculitis. *A–D.* The luminal irregularities *(arrows* and *arrowheads)* of vasculitis can be subtle or marked.

Arterial Dissections

Carotid dissections can result from significant trauma to the neck (blunt or rotational cervical spine injury), from an underlying pathologic process of the extracranial vessels of the neck, such as FMD, or from what seems to be trivial trauma (vomiting, weight-lifting, or other strenuous activities). The dissection may begin at the origin of the common carotid artery, but more often it begins in the mid- to upper cervical region. The appearance on conventional angiography is that of a taper leading to a string-like zone. This abnormality may be focal or may extend over several centimeters; it can be seen in association with a pseudoaneurysm (Fig. 203-19).

Arterial dissections in the neck can also be diagnosed with MR (Fig. 203-20). MRA images will demonstrate absent or diminished flow in the affected vessel in association with tapering of the vessel. The intramural hemorrhage will form a rim or ellipse within the vessel wall and may appear concentric or eccentric in location. A curvilinear partition may be seen separating the intramural hemorrhage from the normal lumen. T1-weighted axial images may show blood products isodense or slightly hyperdense to muscle, depending on the age of the hemoglobin breakdown products. Acute hemorrhage (deoxyhemoglobin) gives a low signal on the MRA; subacute hemorrhage (methemoglobin) gives a bright signal.[27,40,51,55]

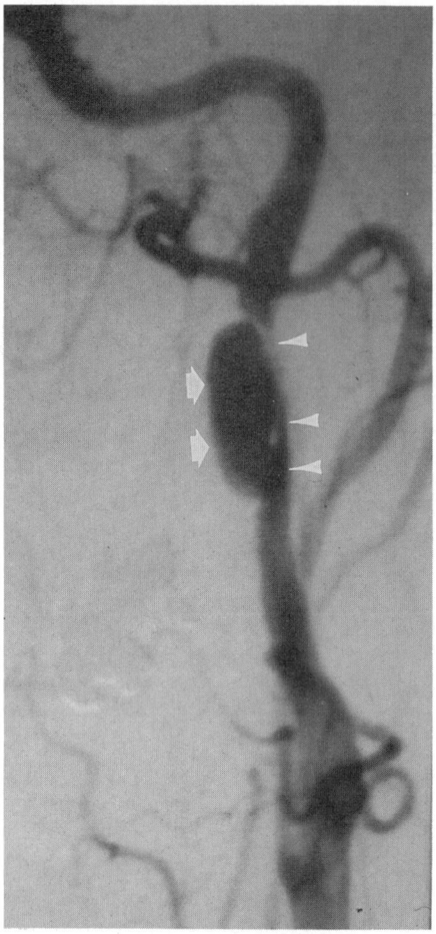

(*A*)

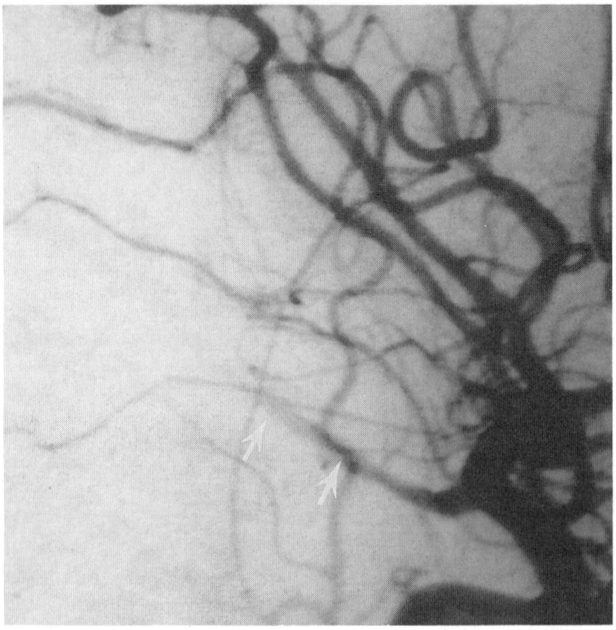

(*B*)

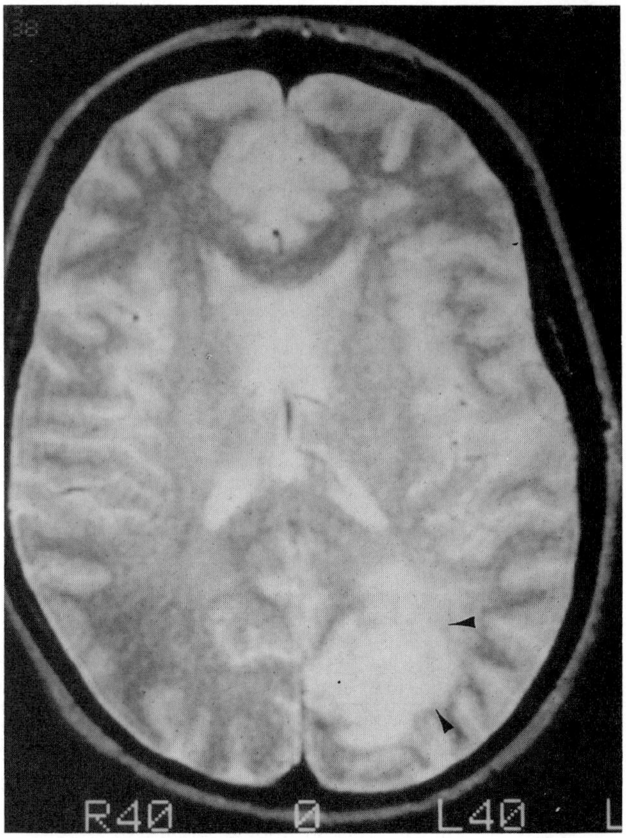

(*C*)

Figure 203-19 Dissection with resulting pseudoaneurysm. *A.* An oblique projection from a digital subtraction angiogram of the common and internal carotid artery demonstrates a large, rounded density *(arrows)*, which was found to be a pseudoaneurysm associated with an underlying dissection. The tapering of the proximal and distal ends of the dissection can be seen *(arrowheads)*. *B, C.* Additional studies demonstrate that an embolus from the dissection and pseudoaneurysm has led to *(B)* occlusion of the posterior cerebral artery *(arrows)* and *(C)* a resulting infarct in the posterior cerebral artery territory *(arrowheads)*.

Figure 203-20 (*Opposite*) Arterial dissections. *A.* 2-D TOF MR angiogram (axial partitioned image) showing luminal narrowing *(large arrow)* and intramural hemorrhage *(small arrow)* in a patient with left internal carotid artery dissection. *B.* Low-signal clot *(arrow)* impinging on the back wall of the internal carotid artery *(arrowhead)*. *C.* Dissection arising in the proximal portion of the left internal carotid artery *(large arrow)*. The 2-D TOF technique shows the carotid bifurcation well, but the intracranial internal carotid artery is poorly visualized owing to dissection *(small arrows)*. *D.* Angiography (MOTSA) showing the long segment narrowing *(arrows)* of the left internal carotid artery one year after arterial dissection. There is improvement in the flow to the intracranial internal carotid artery. *E.* In another case, a conventional angiogram of a carotid dissection shows marked tapering above the carotid bulb with occlusion.

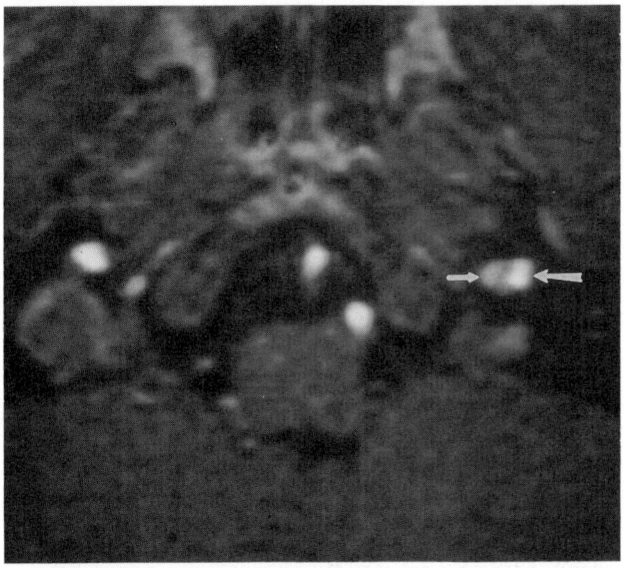

(*A*)

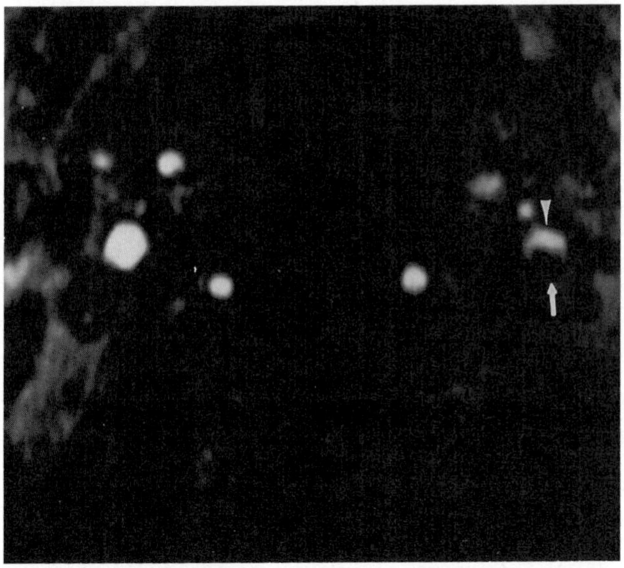

(*B*)

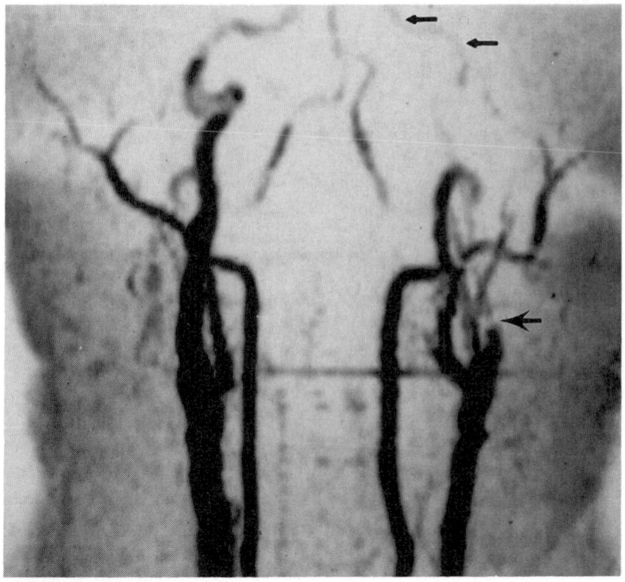

(*C*)

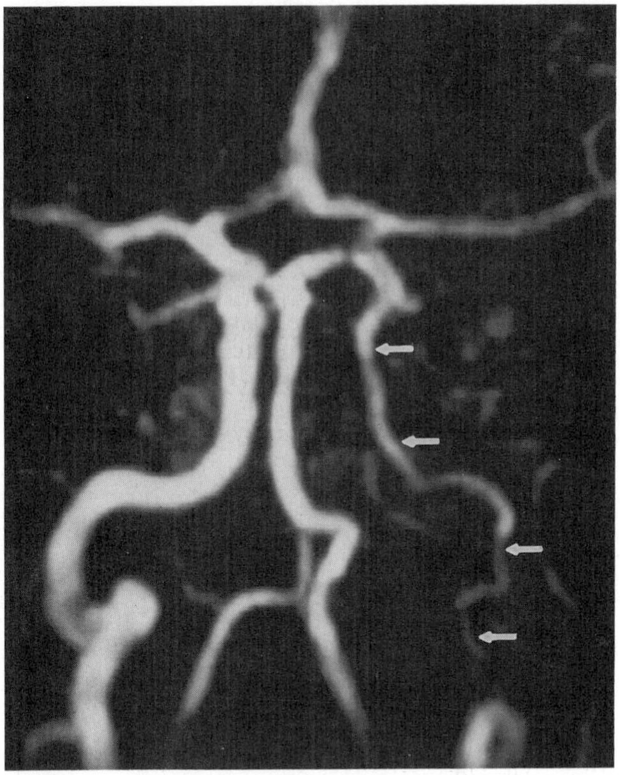

(*D*)

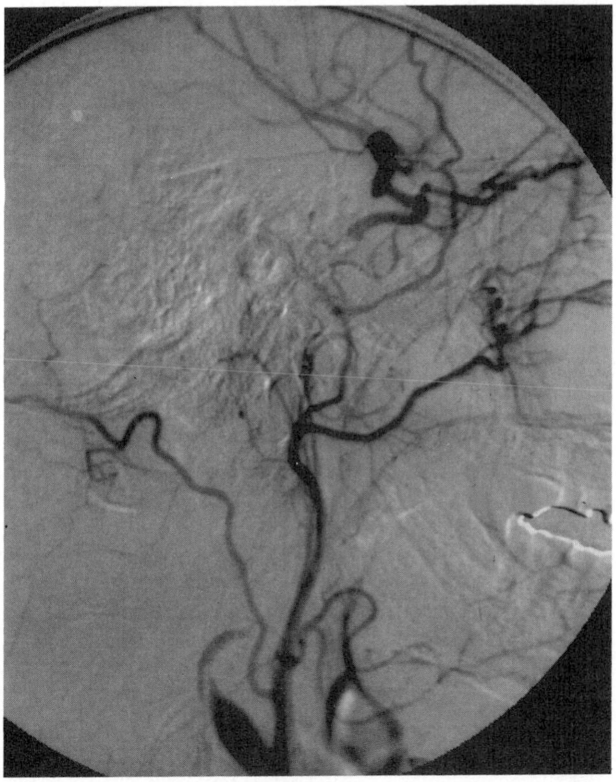

(*E*)

Hypertensive Encephalopathy

Hypertensive encephalopathy is caused by a marked increase in blood pressure, which results in characteristic findings on CT and MRI. Low attenuation in the periventricular white matter is seen on CT; both supra- and infratentorial white matter can be involved (Fig. 203-21). Associated with this finding is edema, which can cause a mass effect on the ventricular system and effacement of sulci, gyri, and basilar cisterns. On MRI the same findings are seen, but the edema is characterized by a low signal on T1-weighted images and a high signal on T2-weighted images. Once the hypertension resolves, incomplete reversal of the ''edema'' can be seen. The residual white matter changes most likely reflect gliosis and small infarcts from chronic hypertension.[39] Mechanisms for the changes seen on CT and MRI may involve disordered autoregulation of cerebral blood flow. Pathologically, focal and diffuse edema is present, as well as small infarcts with petechial hemorrhage and fibrinoid necrosis in small vessels.[60]

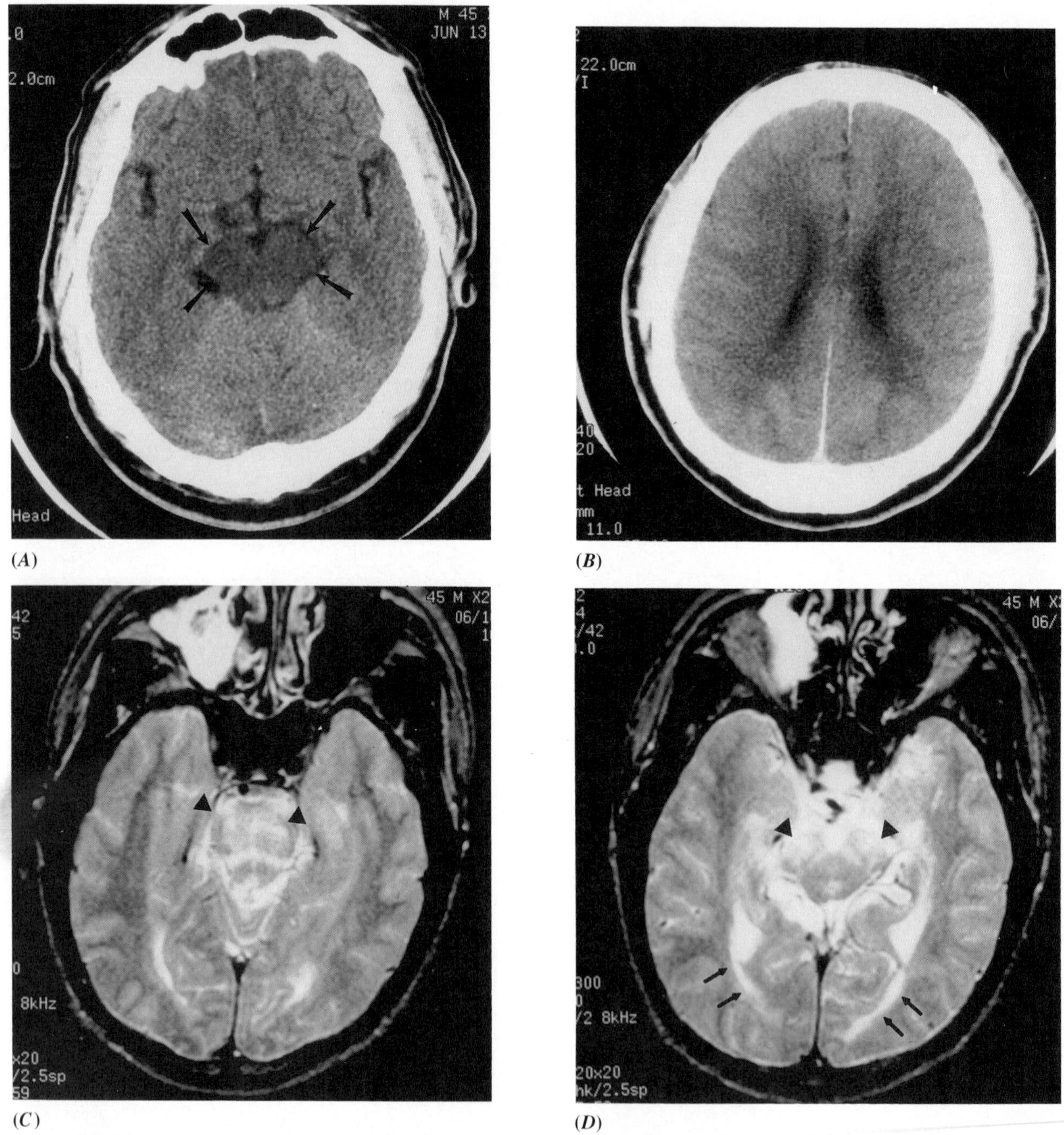

(*A*) (*B*) (*C*) (*D*)

Figure 203-21 CT and MRI appearance of hypertensive encephalopathy. *A, B.* Noncontrast CT scans of a 49-year-old man with a hypertensive crisis (arterial blood pressure, 240/130), showing periventricular and midbrain hypodensity *(black arrows)* caused by edema. *C, D.* T2-weighted MR images showing an increased T2 signal from the midbrain and pons *(arrowheads)* and adjacent to the occipital horns *(arrows)*, secondary to edema.

Venous Sinus Thrombosis and Infarction

An intracranial venous sinus may be compressed as a result of a fracture, a tumor, or some other extrinsic force, or it can be thrombosed, either partially or completely. Thrombosis may result from oral contraceptives, dehydration, infection, pregnancy, or other hypercoaguable states. Resulting symptoms include headache, nausea, vomiting, seizures, and symptoms resembling those caused by psuedotumor cerebri. In the past the prognosis was regarded as poor. Now, however, with improved detection by MR techniques, the incidence is probably higher and the morbidity and mortality lower. Treatment includes both treatment of the underlying disorder and systemic anticoagulation with heparin and warfarin. Direct lysis of the clot by invasive methods with an agent such as urokinase or streptokinase can be performed in extreme cases.[36,45,49]

Sagittal sinus thrombosis can be imaged by conventional angiography or CT but is now more typically evaluated with MRI and MRA. MRI and MRA are noninvasive, allow imaging of the brain parenchyma, and are more reliable than CT.[2] The MR signal abnormalities associated with venous sinus thrombosis go through a typically progression similar to that seen for the evolution of parenchymal hemorrhages. Acutely, the hemorrhage is in the deoxyhemoglobin state and is isointense to gray matter on T1-weighted images, replacing the normal flow void. On T2-weighted images the deoxyhemoglobin is hypodense and can be mistaken for a normal flow void. Subacutely, the thrombus becomes hyperintense (bright) on T1- and T2-weighted images, reflecting the progression of deoxyhemoglobin to methemoglobin (Figs. 203-22 and 203-23). The high signal could in some instances be misinterpreted as flow-related enhancement, as is seen in TOF angiography.

MRA techniques (2-D TOF or 2-D PC) are used to assist in detecting sinus thrombosis, and will allow diagnosis in most cases. The images are acquired in axial and coronal planes, perpendicular to the flow in the major sinuses. TOF images can lead to a false-negative diagnosis if bright clot (methemoglobin) projects onto the angiographic images, mimicking flow (Fig. 203-24). A false-positive diagnosis can also occur if (1) flow mimics clot by being too slow to produce a signal that projects onto the angiographic images or (2) an inferior saturation pulse results in absent flow in the anterior portion of the superior sagittal sinus, again mimicking clot. Phase-contrast techniques using a very low velocity (5 cm/s) are useful for diagnosing the presence and absence of flow. This MRA technique is not complicated by the presence of bright thrombus mimicking flow. Very slow flow, however—lower than the velocity encoded—could appear as a flow void and mimic clot.[49]

Venous sinus thromboses can be associated with venous infarctions (Fig. 203-24). These can be hemorrhagic, and they most often involve the subcortical white matter and traverse typical arterial vascular boundaries. In addition, sinus thrombosis can be associated with what appears to be meningeal enhancement when an MR contrast agent is administered. This appearance actually may reflect arterial engorgement or enhancement of flow in veins draining into the sinuses (Fig. 203-25).

In conclusion, the tools available for the evaluation and diagno-

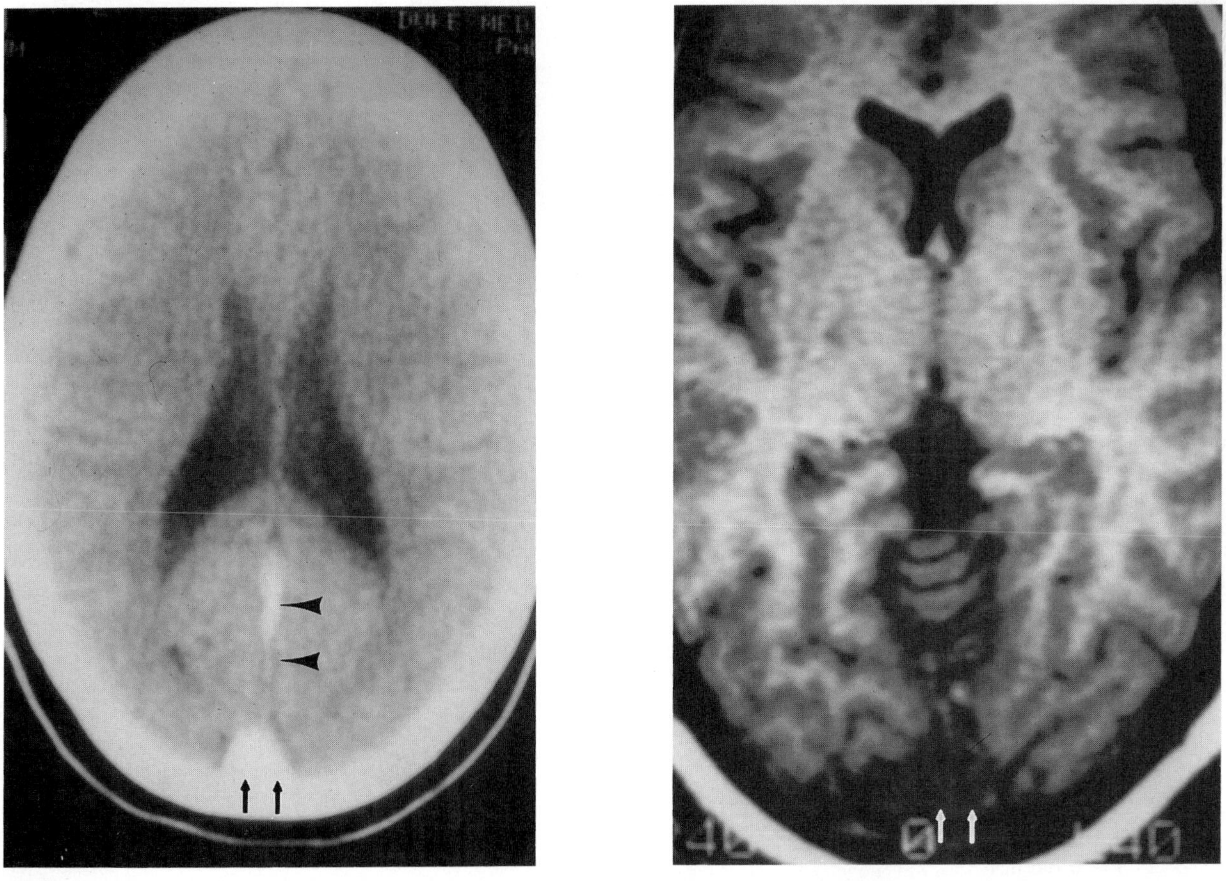

(*A*) (*B*)

Figure 203-22 Acute sinus thrombosis. *A*. A CT scan showing a hyperdense clot in the torcular *(arrows)* and straight sinus *(arrowheads)*. T1-weighted axial *(B)*

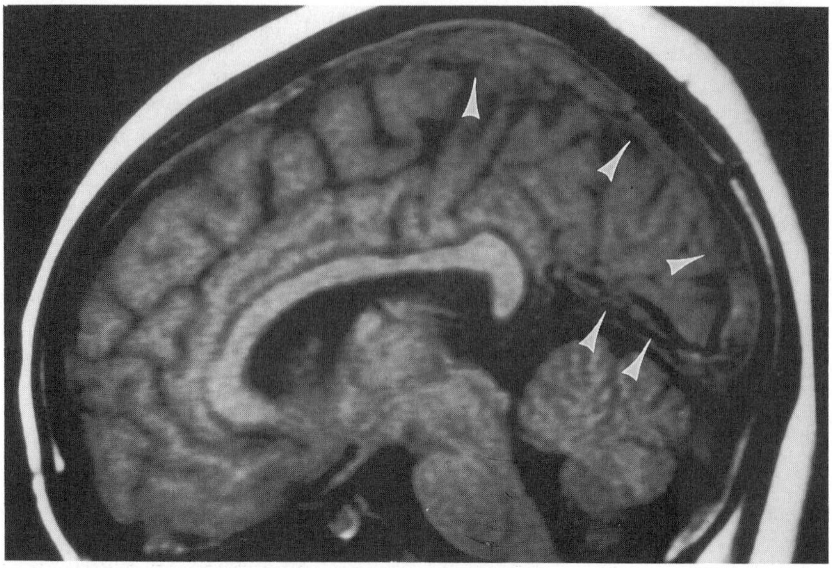

(*C*)

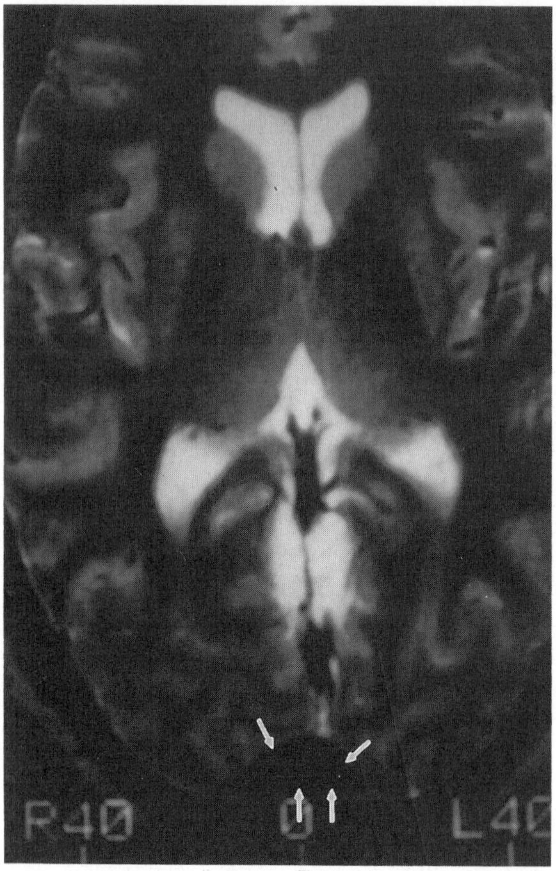

(*D*)

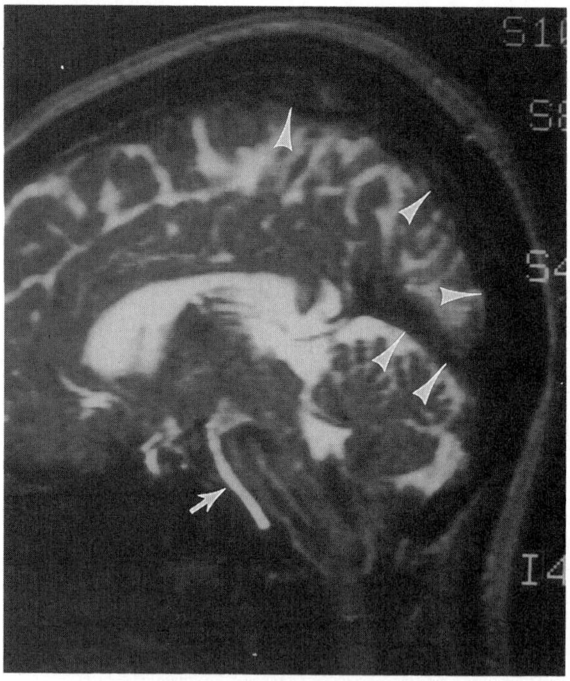

(*E*)

Figure 203-22 (*Continued*) and sagittal *(C)* spin echo MR images with iso- hypodense clot in the torcular *(arrows)* and superior sagittal and straight sinuses *(arrowheads)*. The clot is isodense or hypodense to gray matter because of deoxyhemoglobin. *D.* A T2-weighted spin echo MR image showing a low-signal (deoxyhemoglobin-containing) clot mimicking a normal flow void *(arrows)*. *E.* Gradient recalled echo (GRE) image showing flow in the basilar artery *(arrow)*. There is no flow in the straight or superior sagittal sinuses *(arrowheads)*.

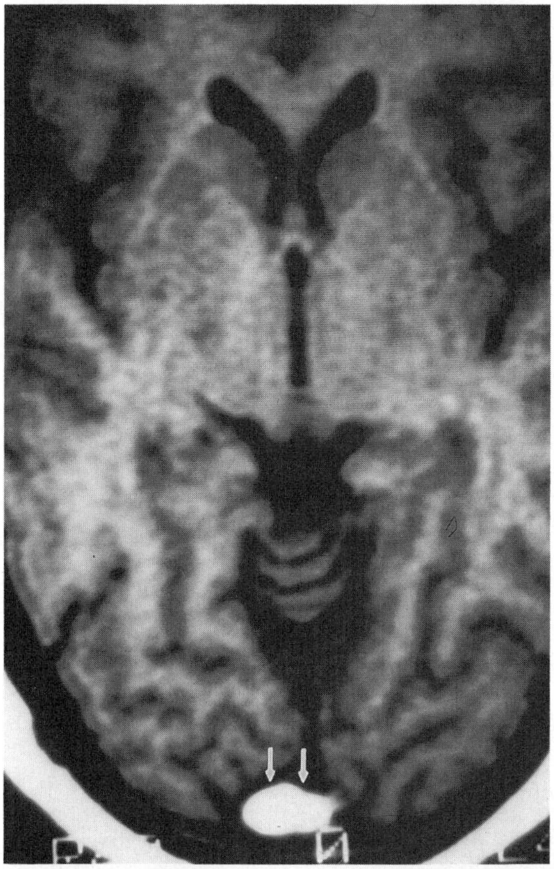

(*A*)

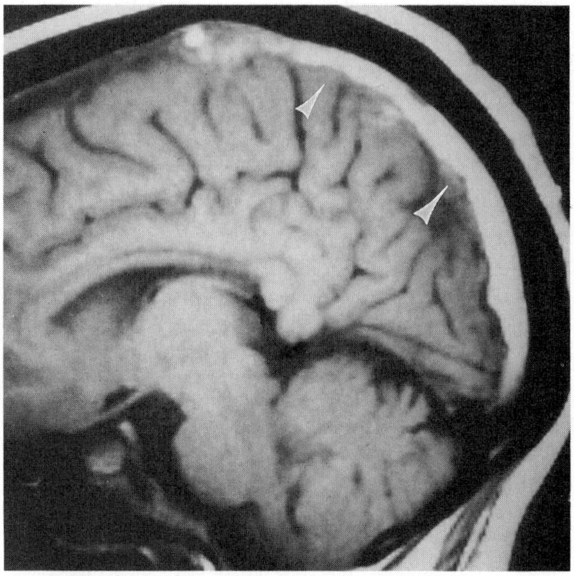

(*B*)

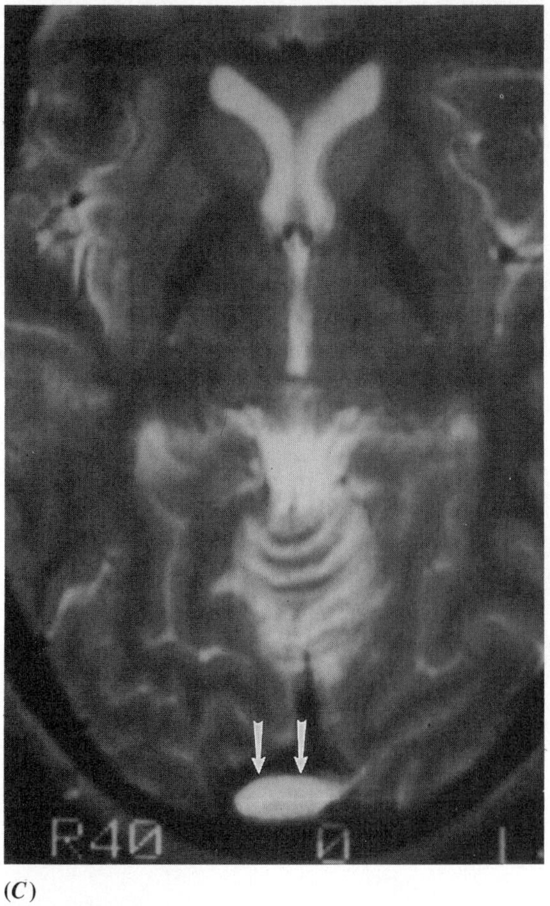

(*C*)

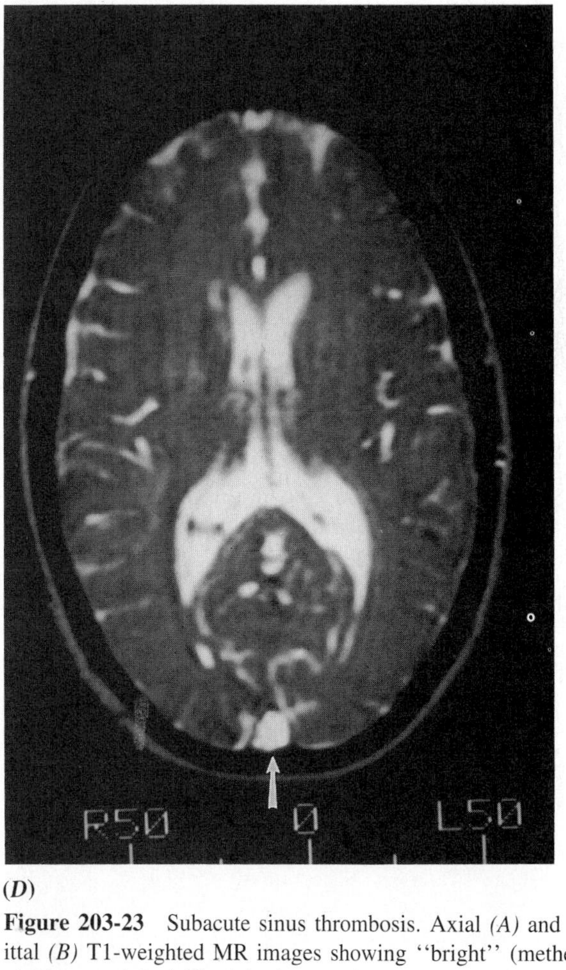

(*D*)

Figure 203-23 Subacute sinus thrombosis. Axial *(A)* and sagittal *(B)* T1-weighted MR images showing "bright" (methemoglobin-containing) blood in the torcular *(arrows)* and superior sagittal sinus *(arrowheads)*. *C.* A T2-weighted axial MR image showing bright clot in the torcular *(arrows)*. *D.* An axial GRE image showing a bright signal in the torcular *(arrow)*, which represents methemoglobin but could be mistaken for flow. T1-weighted images should be checked for bright clot to avoid making this misinterpretation.

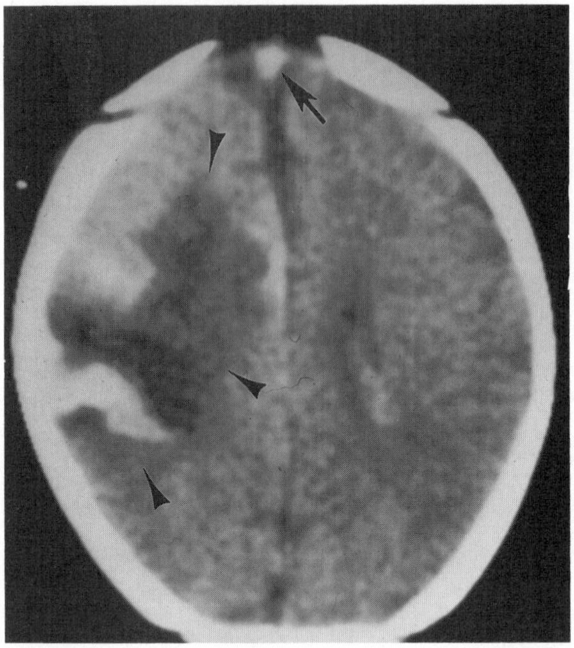

(*A*)

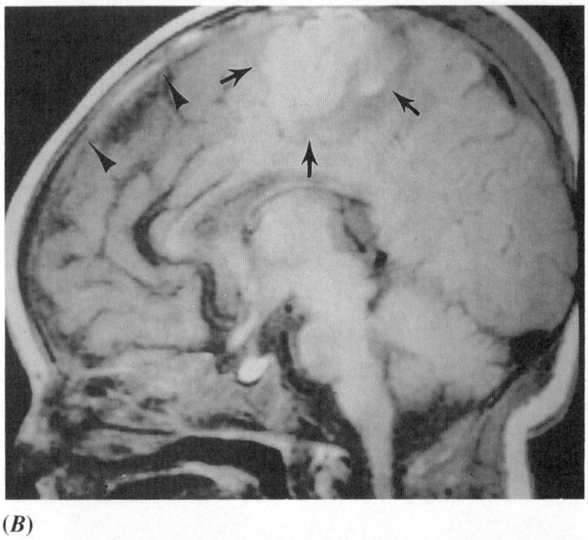

(*B*)

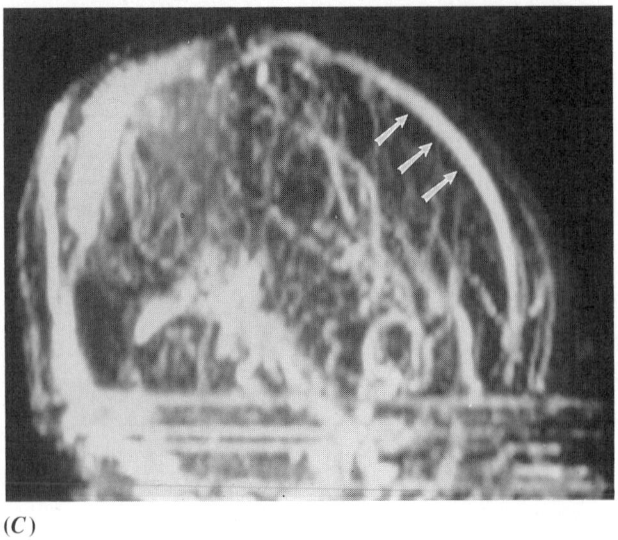

(*C*)

Figure 203-24 Images showing a superior sagittal sinus thrombosis that could give rise to a false-negative interpretation. *A.* An axial CT scan showing clot in the anterior sagittal sinus *(arrow)* in association with a hemorrhagic venous infarct *(arrowheads)*. *B.* A sagittal T1-weighted image showing bright clot in the anterior sagittal sinus *(arrowheads)* and the hemorrhagic venous infarct *(arrows)*. *C.* A sagittal 2-D TOF MRA showing a bright signal in the anterior sagittal sinus *(arrows)* that mimics flow but is actually due to methemoglobin-containing ''bright blood'' projecting onto the MRA image.

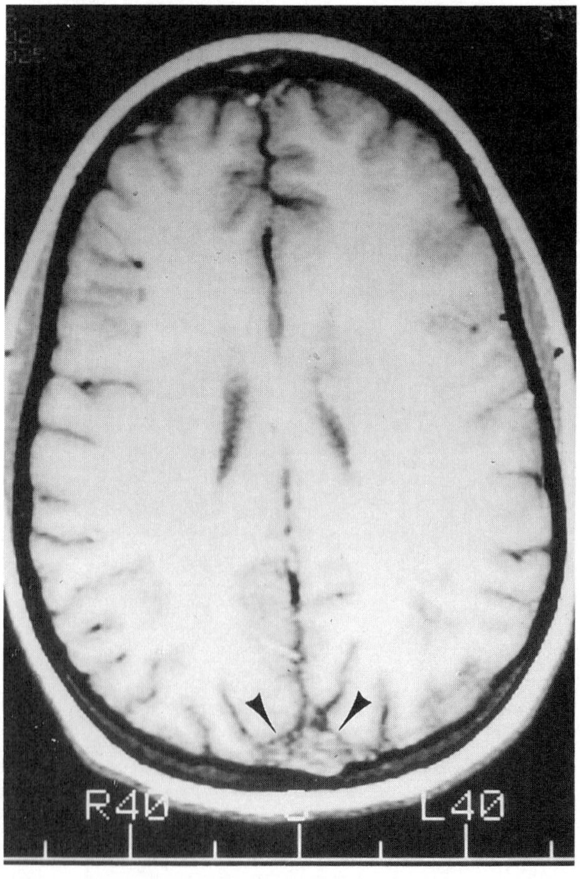

(*A*)

Figure 203-25 Superior sagittal sinus thrombosis. *A, B.* T1-weighted axial MR images without *(A)*

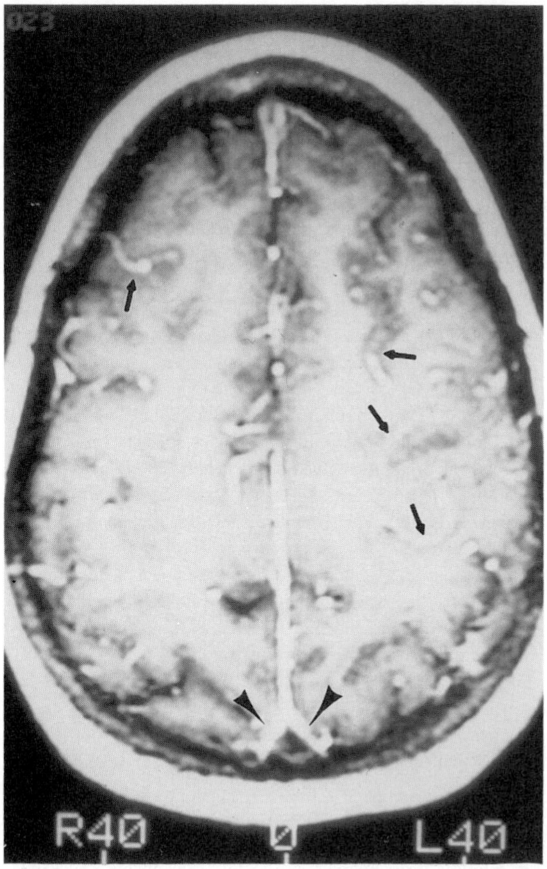

(*B*)

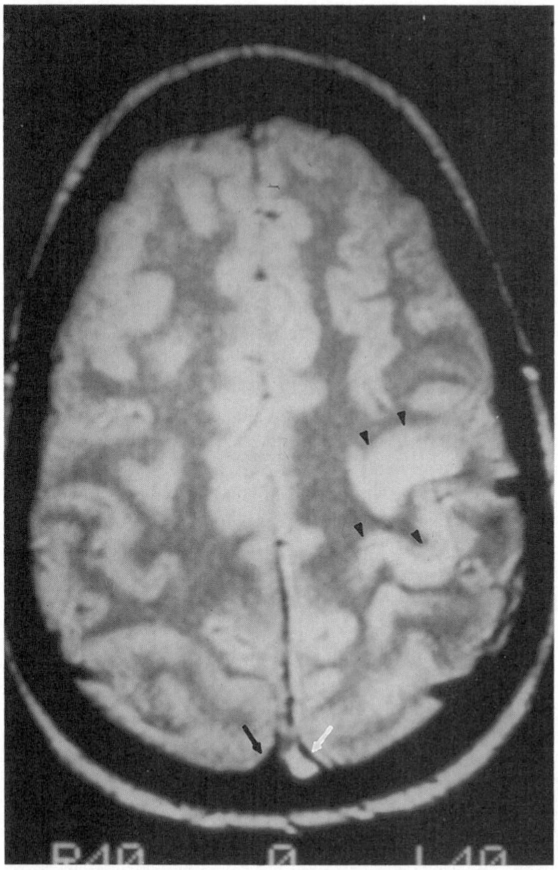

(*C*)

Figure 203-25 (*Continued*) and with (*B*) contrast. A deoxyhemoglobin-containing, hypodense or isodense clot is present *(arrowheads)*. *B.* The injection of a contrast agent leads to enhancement around the clot *(arrowheads)*. There is also bilateral leptomeningeal enhancement due to engorged arteries or veins *(arrows)*. *C.* A proton-density T2-weighted MR image shows bright *(white arrow)* and dark *(black arrow)* signals in the superior sagittal sinus, marking the presence of methemoglobin and deoxyhemoglobin, respectively. An increase in signal intensity and thickening of gyri *(arrowheads)* represent ischemia and/or edema due to congestion.

sis of cerebrovascular disease have vastly increased over the last 10 years. Although angiography remains the gold standard for vascular evaluation, noninvasive techniques are improving steadily and could supplant angiography in some instances. MRI remains the study of choice for evaluation of the brain parenchyma, particularly where the posterior fossa or brain stem is involved. New MR techniques such as diffusion and spectroscopy will add new power to this already important tool and may help change how we assess and treat stroke in the future.

References

1. Anderson CM, Saloner D, Lee RE, et al. Assessment of carotid artery stenosis by MR angiography: comparison with x-ray angiography and color-coded Doppler ultrasound. *Am J Neuroradiol* 1992; 13:989–1003.
2. Bauer WM, Einhäupl K, Heywang SH, et al. MR of venous sinus thrombosis: a case report. *Am J Neuroradiol* 1987; 8:713–715.
3. Braffman BH, Zimmerman RA, Trojanowski JQ, et al. Brain MR: pathologic correlation with gross and histopathology. 1. Lacunar infarction and Virchow-Robin spaces. *Am J Neuroradiol* 1988; 9:621–628.
4. Braffman BH, Zimmerman RA, Trojanowski JQ, et al. Brain MR: pathologic correlation with gross and histopathology. 2. Hyperintense white-matter foci in the elderly. *Am J Neuroradiol* 1988; 9:629–636.
5. Brant-Zawadzki M, Pereira B, Weinstein P, et al. MR imaging of acute experimental ischemia in cats. *Am J Neuroradiol* 1986; 7:7–11.
6. Brant-Zawadzki M, Solomon M, Newton TH, et al. Basic principles of magnetic resonance imaging in cerebral ischemia and initial clinical experience. *Neuroradiology* 1985; 27:517–520.
7. Bryan RN, Levy LM, Whitlow WD, et al. Diagnosis of acute cerebral infarction: comparison of CT and MR imaging. *Am J Neuroradiol* 1991; 12:611–620.
8. Bydder GM, Steiner RE, Thomas DJ, et al. Nuclear magnetic resonance imaging of the posterior fossa: 50 cases. *Clin Radiol* 1983; 34:173–188.
9. Cancilla PA, Frommes SP, Kahn LE, et al. Regeneration of cerebral microvessels: a morphologic and histochemical study after local freeze-injury. *Lab Invest* 1979; 40:74–82.
10. Carroll BA: Carotid sonography. *Radiology* 1991; 178:303–313.
11. Carroll BA: Carotid sonography. *Neuroimaging Clin North Am* 1992; 2:533–557.
12. Chikos PM, Fisher LD, Hirsch JH, et al. Observer variability in evaluating extracranial carotid artery stenosis. *Stroke* 1983; 14:885–892.
13. Collins GJ Jr, Rich NM, Clagett GP, et al. Fibromuscular dysplasia of the internal carotid arteries. Clinical experience and follow-up. *Ann Surgery* 1981; 194:89–96.

14. Corrin LS, Sandok BA, Houser OW. Cerebral ischemic events in patients with carotid artery fibromuscular dysplasia. *Arch Neurol* 1981; 38:616–618.
15. Dardzinski BJ, Sotak CH, Fisher M, et al. Apparent diffusion coefficient mapping of experimental focal cerebral ischemia using diffusion-weighted echo-planar imaging. *Magn Reson Med* 1993; 30:318–325.
16. De La Paz RL, New PFJ, Buonanno FS, et al. NMR imaging of intracranial hemorrhage. *J Comput Assist Tomogr* 1984; 8:599–607.
17. Di Chiro G, Brooks RA, Girton ME, et al. Sequential MR studies of intracerebral hematomas in monkeys. *Am J Neuroradiol* 1986; 7:193–199.
18. Dillon EH, van Leeuwen MS, Fernandez MA, et al. CT angiography: application to the evaluation of carotid artery stenosis. *Radiology* 1993; 189:211–219.
19. Dion JE, Gates PC, Fox AJ, et al. Clinical events following neuroangiography: a prospective study. *Stroke* 1987; 18:997–1004.
20. Dooms GC, Uske A, Brant-Zawadzki M, et al. Spin-echo MR imaging of intracranial hemorrhage. *Neuroradiology* 1986; 28:132–138.
21. Dumoulin CL. Phase contrast magnetic resonance angiography. *Neuroimaging Clin North Am* 1992; 2:657–676.
22. Edelman RR, Wentz KU, Mattle HP, et al. Intracerebral arteriovenous malformations: evaluation with selective MR angiography and venography. *Radiology* 1989; 173:831–837.
23. Edwards JK, Kricheff II, Riles T, et al. Angiographically undetected ulceration of the carotid bifurcation as a cause of embolic stroke. *Radiology* 1979; 132:369–373.
24. Eikelboom BC, Riles TR, Mintzer R, et al. Inaccuracy of angiography in the diagnosis of carotid ulceration. *Stroke* 1983; 14:882–885.
25. Elster AD. MR contrast enhancement in brainstem and deep cerebral infarction. *Am J Neuroradiol* 1991; 12:1127–1132.
26. Elster AD. Magnetic resonance contrast enhancement in cerebral infarction. *Neuroimaging Clin North Am* 1994; 4:89–100.
27. Goldberg HI, Grossman RI, Gomori JM, et al. Cervical internal carotid artery dissecting hemorrhage: diagnosis using MR. Radiology 1986; 158:157–161.
28. Gomori JM, Grossman RI, Goldberg HI, et al. Intracranial hematomas: imaging by high-field MR. *Radiology* 1985; 157–87–93.
29. Haacke EM, Smith AS, Lin W, et al. Velocity quantification in magnetic resonance imaging. *Top Magn Reson Imaging* 1991; 3:34–49.
30. Hankey GJ, Warlow CP, Sellar RJ. Cerebral angiographic risk in mild cerebrovascular disease. *Stroke* 1990; 21:209–222.
31. Harrison EG Jr, Hunt JC, Bernatz PE. Morphology of fibromuscular dysplasia of the renal artery in renovascular hypertension. *Am J Med* 1967; 43:97–112.
32. Harrison EG Jr, McCormack LJ. Pathologic classification of renal arterial disease in renovascular hypertension. *Mayo Clin Proc* 1971; 46:161–167.
33. Heiserman JE. The role of magnetic resonance angiography in the evaluation of cerebrovascular ischemic disease. *Neuroimaging Clin North Am* 1992; 2:753–767.
34. Heiserman JE, Drayer BP, Fram EK, et al. Carotid artery stenosis: clinical efficacy of two-dimensional time-of-flight MR angiography. *Radiology* 1992; 182:761–768.
35. Houser OW, Baker HL Jr, Sandok BA, Holley KE. Fibromuscular dysplasia of the cephalic arterial system. In Vinken PJ, Bruyn GW (eds): *Handbook of Clinical Neurology,* vol II. *Vascular Diseases of the Nervous System, Part I.* Amsterdam: North-Holland, 1972, pp 366–385.
36. Johnson BA, Fram EK. Cerebral venous occlusive disease. *Neuroimaging Clin North Am* 1992; 2:769–783.
37. Keller PJ. Time-of-flight magnetic resonance angiography. *Neuroimaging Clin North Am* 1992; 2:639–656.
38. Kitahara T, Ariga N, Yamaura A, et al. Familial occurrence of moyamoya disease: report of three Japanese families. *J Neurol Neurosurg Psychiatry* 1979; 42:208–214.
39. Kwong YL, Yu YL, Lam KS, et al. CT appearance in hypertensive encephalopathy. *Neuroradiology* 1987; 29:215.
40. Levy C, Laissy JP, Raveau V, et al. Carotid and vertebral artery dissections: three-dimensional time-of-flight MR angiography and MR imaging versus conventional angiography. *Radiology* 1994; 190:97–103.
41. Litt AW, Eidelman EM, Pinto RS, et al. Diagnosis of carotid artery stenosis: comparison of 2DFT time-of-flight MR angiography with contrast angiography in 50 patients. *Am J Neuroradiol* 1991; 12:149–154.
42. Maki Y, Makata Y. [Autopsy of hemangiomatous malformation of the internal carotid artery of the base of the brain.] *No To Shinkei* 1965; 17:764–766.
43. Masaryk TJ, Tkach J, Glicklich M. Flow, radiofrequency pulse sequences, and gradient magnetic fields: basic interactions and adaptations to angiographic imaging. *Top Magn Reson Imaging* 1991; 3:1–11.
44. Mayberg MR, Wilson SE, Yatsu F, et al. Carotid endarterectomy and prevention of cerebral ischemia in symptomatic carotid stenosis. Veterans Affairs Cooperative Studies Program 309 Trialist Group. *JAMA* 1991; 266:3289–3294.
45. Medlock MD, Olivero WC, Hanigan WC, et al. Children with cerebral venous thrombosis diagnosed with magnetic resonance imaging and magnetic resonance angiography. *Neurosurgery* 1992; 31:870–876.
46. Mettinger KL, Ericson K. Fibromuscular dysplasia and the brain: I. Observations on angiographic, clinical and genetic characteristics. *Stroke* 1982; 13:46–52.
47. Mittl RL Jr, Broderick M, Carpenter JP, et al. Blinded-reader comparison of magnetic resonance angiography and duplex-ultrasonography for carotid artery bifurcation stenosis. *Stroke* 1994; 25:4–10.
48. Moneta GL, Edwards JM, Chitwood RW, et al. Correlation of North American Symptomatic Carotid Endarterectomy Trial (NASCET) angiographic definition of 70 percent to 99 percent internal carotid artery stenosis with duplex scanning. *J Vasc Surg* 1993; 17:152–159.
49. Naidich TP, Righi AM. Neurovascular imaging. *Radiol Clin North Am* 1995; 33:115–166.
50. Osborn AG. *Introduction to Cerebral Angiography.* Hagerstown, MD: Harper & Row, 1980.
51. Pacini R, Simon J, Ketonen L, et al. Chemical-shift imaging of a spontaneous internal carotid artery dissection: case report. *Am J Neuroradiol* 1991; 12:360–362.
52. Petty GW, Mohr JP. Giant cell arteritis and isolated granulomatous angiitis of the central nervous system. In Barnett HJM, Stein BM, Mohn JP, et al. (eds): *Stroke, vol 2. Pathophysiology, Diagnosis, and Management.* New York: Churchill Livingstone, 1986, pp 789–803.
53. Polak JF. Noninvasive carotid evaluation: carpe diem. *Radiology* 1993; 186–329–331.
54. Polak JF, Bajakian RL, O'Leary DH, et al. Detection of internal carotid artery stenosis: comparison of MR angiography, color Doppler sonography, and arteriography. *Radiology* 1992; 182:35–40.
55. Provenzale JM. Dissection of the internal carotid and vertebral arteries: imaging features. Unpublished manuscript.
56. Rubin GD, Dake MD, Semba CP. Current status of three-dimensional spiral CT scanning for imaging the vasculature. *Radiol Clin North Am,* 1995; 33:51–70.
57. Schwartz RB, Jones KM, Chernoff DM, et al. Common carotid artery bifurcation: evaluation with spiral CT: work in progress. *Radiology* 1992; 185:513–519.
58. Sekiguchi S, Kobayashi K, Hattori M, et al. HLA antigen in spontaneous occlusion of the circle of Willis. In Gotoh F (ed): *Annual Report of the Ministry of Health and Welfare, Japan, Research Committee on Spontaneous Occlusion of the Circle of Willis.* Japan: Ministry of Health and Welfare, 1979, p 76.
59. Sheppard S. Basic concepts in magnetic resonance angiography. *Radiol Clin North Am* 1995; 33:91–112.
60. Skinhoj S, Strandgaard S. Patholgenesis of hypertensive encephalopathy. *Lancet* 1973; 1:461–462.
61. Suzuki J, Kodama N. Mineura K. [Etiological studies of cerebrovascular moyamoya disease.] *No To Shinkei* 1976; 28:459–470.
62. Suzuki J, Takaku A. Cerebrovascular ''moyamoya'' disease. Disease showing abnormal net-like vessels in base of brain. *Arch Neurol* 1969; 20:288–299.
63. Yamada I, Matsushima Y, Suzuki S. Moyamoya disease: diagnosis with three-dimensional time-of-flight MR angiography. *Radiology* 1992; 184:773–778.

204

Extracranial Carotid Artery Atherosclerosis; Carotid Endarterectomy

Robert M. Crowell
Christopher S. Ogilvy
Robert G. Ojemann

The diagnosis of extracranial carotid artery stenosis offers the possibility of medical or surgical treatment (or both) to prevent a stroke. Symptoms in patients with carotid atherosclerosis and the noninvasive techniques and the radiographic studies used in evaluating these patients are discussed in other chapters in this textbook.

In about 85 percent of patients undergoing carotid endarterectomy, we find that the combination of (1) carotid noninvasive studies, (2) magnetic resonance imaging (MRI) of the head, and (3) magnetic resonance angiography (MRA) of the head and neck satisfactorily defines carotid atherosclerosis and the cerebrovascular system.[1,18,19] In complex cases, digital subtraction angiography is needed to image the pathologic abnormalities and the vascular anatomy.

The indications for carotid endarterectomy have been controversial until recently. Several major controlled studies confirm a highly beneficial protection against stroke in symptomatic patients with severe ICA stenosis.[8,20,24] Studies are underway regarding asymptomatic stenosis.

Incidence

There is good evidence that transient ischemic attacks (TIAs) that include either transient monocular blindness (TMB) or transient hemisphere attack (THA) are related to carotid atherosclerosis. Data from the Harvard Stroke Registry indicate that significant stenosis (lumen <2 mm) or occlusion in the region of the common carotid artery (CCA) bifurcation or proximal internal carotid artery (ICA) is present in approximately 50 percent of the patients with TIAs in the territory of the carotid artery, while this is true in less than 10 percent of patients with stroke due to nonischemic cerebral disease.[27] Table 204-1 records the angiographic findings in 95 patients with TIAs. In addition to the 52 percent of patients with significant carotid stenosis or occlusion, six other patients (6 percent) had ulceration that may have been important in the symptomatology. When a patient has both THA and TMB, there is a very high probability of finding significant carotid atherosclerosis.

Pathogenesis

In patients with significant carotid atherosclerotic disease, TIAs may be caused by embolism arising from an atheromatous carotid lesion or from reduction in cerebral blood flow (CBF). It seems less likely that reduced CBF is caused by transient carotid occlusion, systemic reduction in blood pressure, or other factors.

When TMB is present, it has been suggested that embolism is the cause because of the observation of embolic material in retinal vessels. This pathologic mechanism can cause the wedge-shaped visual defects typical of central retinal artery branch occlusion, but this is an uncommon clinical finding. The common shade or curtain altitudinal symptoms suggest reduced circulation to the posterior ciliary arteries or circle of Zinn, an arterial network that could be occluded by emboli but is more likely to be susceptible to the effects of hypotension and diminished blood flow.[27]

The patient with a THA whose angiogram shows a normal carotid bifurcation or only minimal atherosclerosis and who has an intracranial branch occlusion is likely to have a cardiac embolic source. In the group of patients in the Harvard stroke study, 25 percent with THAs had intracranial branch occlusion on angiography.[27] The actual incidence is probably even higher because embolic occlusions are often transient. When significant carotid artery stenosis is present, THA is probably due to inadequate distal

TABLE 204-1 Angiographic Findings in 95 Patients with Transient Ischemic Attacks*

	Angiographic Findings				
Type of Attack	**Carotid Occlusion**	**Severe† Stenosis (<2 mm)**	**Moderate† Stenosis**	**Minimal† Stenosis**	**Normal Carotid**
Transient hemisphere attack (THA)	4	18	4	17	9
Transient monocular blindness (TMB)	5	14	1	5	8
Both THA and TMB	2	6	1	0	1
Total	11	38‡	6	22§	18

*Thirteen patients had intracranial branch occlusion, and nine of these did not have significant carotid disease.
†This refers to the proximal portion of the ICA.
‡Three patients also had an ulceration.
§Six patients had an ulceration.
Source: Adapted from Pessin et al.[27]

perfusion in most cases, but what part emboli play has not been established.[10]

There is also the possibility that lacunar disease may be the cause of TIA. This diagnosis has been considered because of the pure motor or sensory character of some THAs, features characteristic of the lacunar stroke, and the finding that TIAs may precede pathologically documented lacunar infarction.[27]

Indications for Treatment

In this section we consider the indications for treatment in patients with clinical syndromes due to carotid atherosclerosis and various combinations of angiographic abnormalities in the region of the carotid bifurcation. Previous publications have included an extensive review of the literature on this subject.[25,26] In the next section we consider general risk factors that relate to planning surgical treatment.

TIAs with Unilateral Carotid Stenosis and/or Ulceration

Carotid endarterectomy is usually indicated for the patient with TIAs and severe stenosis (>70 percent or lumen < 2 mm in diameter), and/or severe ulceration in the CCA bifurcation region or proximal ICA. These attacks are warnings of possible impending disaster. Removal of the pathologic lesion not only stops the attacks but reduces the chance of a future stroke. Controlled studies prove that for the patient with severe carotid stenosis and TIAs, carotid endarterectomy is associated with much less risk than the natural history of the disease or than medical therapy.[8,20,24] Moreover, the more severe the stenosis, the greater the benefit of surgery. Overall, surgery confers dramatic benefit for patients with TIAs and severe stenosis.

If the studies show severe ICA stenosis with reduced flow or a thrombus in the lumen, or if the clinical picture includes increasingly severe attacks in the preceding days, attention should be directed to performing the operation as soon as possible. If there is going to be a delay, the patient should be heparinized.

If ulceration is found with a nonobstructive plaque, a decision regarding surgical or medical therapy is made based on the severity of the lesion. In the past, carotid endarterectomy has been recommended for patients with TIAs who were found to have an area of ulceration, even though the lumen diameter was greater than 2 mm. When the ulceration is deep, surgery is the recommended treatment. There is some evidence that a shallow ulcer associated with nonobstructive atherosclerosis may have a low risk of future stroke. Such patients may be treated with antiplatelet therapy and be followed with noninvasive studies of the carotid circulation. Should there be evidence of the development of stenosis or should TIAs continue, then surgery is indicated.

TIAs with Bilateral Carotid Stenosis

In some patients who are studied because of symptoms due to stenosis in one carotid artery, significant narrowing of the carotid artery is found on the opposite side. Occasionally a patient may present with a history of TIAs related to both carotid arteries. Noninvasive studies can help the physician decide the hemodynamic significance of the lesions.

When only one side is symptomatic, it is generally treated first unless the asymptomatic side has a tighter stenosis with a more severe hemodynamic lesion as demonstrated by MRA and noninvasive tests. If both sides are symptomatic, the side with the more severe hemodynamic lesion is operated upon first. The second side is usually done within 7 to 14 days. When the second stenosis is very severe, heparin therapy may be indicated until the second operation is performed.

TIAs with Ipsilateral Carotid Stenosis and Contralateral Carotid Occlusion

Most patients with this combination of lesions present with TIAs related to the internal carotid stenosis. Occasionally patients will have had neurological symptoms related to the contralateral carotid occlusion.

The indications for surgery are the same as for TIAs associated with unilateral carotid stenosis. The patient with a contralateral occlusion is more likely to have an electroencephalographic (EEG) change and need a shunt at the time of the carotid occlusion for the endarterectomy than is the patient with an open contralateral ICA. However, our experience as well as that of others is that there is no increase in neurological complications in this group.[25,26]

TIAs with Tandem Stenosis

In a few patients with TIAs, angiography or MRA will show the stenosis at the carotid bifurcation or proximal ICA and a second stenosis in the intracavernous or intracranial portion of the ICA. The occurrence of this problem emphasizes the importance of complete angiography. Usually the stenosis in the neck is more severe than that found in the more distal lesion. If the stenosis in the neck is less than 2 mm, carotid endarterectomy is indicated for TIAs even if the distal lesion is also severe. Postoperatively, a decision is made between anticoagulation or antiplatelet therapy and follow-up noninvasive and MRA studies. In general, our plan has been to consider bypass surgery only in the rare case with symptoms persisting after carotid endarterectomy and a good program of medical treatment.

TIAs with Ipsilateral Internal Carotid Occlusion and the Problem of External Carotid Stenosis

TIAs can occur in the territory of a completely occluded ICA.[26] The cause of symptoms may be an embolus from the distal end of the occlusion, an embolus passing through the external carotid circulation from atheromatous stenosis of the external or distal CCA or from the stump proximal to the occlusion in the ICA, or a reduction of flow to the eye and/or cerebral hemisphere.

Studies should include angiography of the collateral circulation through the opposite carotid artery, in many cases the vertebrobasilar circulation, and lateral serial films of the head and neck over several seconds to determine the collateral flow and to see how far down the ICA the contrast agent flows. This is important in deciding about the cause of the symptoms and the probability of reopening the complete occlusion. If the angiogram shows retrograde flow below the carotid siphon, and especially if this is present to the base of the skull, there is a good chance of reopening the ICA with surgery.

If the occlusion of the ICA extends into the carotid siphon, a decision has to be made either to attempt to reopen the ICA, to use anticoagulation, or to perform a bypass graft. In general, patients with this angiographic finding will likely have had a carotid occlusion for some time, and we usually do not try to reopen the artery. Even if there is good collateral circulation, we have favored anticoagulation because of the risk of embolization.

If the angiogram shows a significant proximal stump in the occluded ICA in the neck and collateral flow from the external carotid via the ophthalmic artery to the ICA, this may be the source of embolus and should be treated with endarterectomy and "stumpectomy." If there is atherosclerosis with stenosis and/or ulceration at the origin of the ECA, this may also be the source of emboli and ischemia and should be treated with surgery. When the ICA is open, external carotid stenosis or occlusion does not cause significant clinical symptoms.

Posterior Circulation TIAs with Carotid Stenosis

When there is evidence of carotid artery disease either from physical examination or noninvasive studies in a patient with posterior circulation TIAs, angiography is indicated. This should include both the carotid and posterior circulations. Carotid endarterectomy is usually indicated if the angiogram shows (1) filling of the posterior cerebral artery via the stenotic ICA, (2) filling of the posterior circulation from the ICA because of vertebral artery occlusive disease, or (3) a persistent hypoglossal or trigeminal artery. We are not convinced that carotid endarterectomy will alter vertebrobasilar symptoms unless one of the conditions noted above is found on the angiogram. When severe carotid stenosis is present with no filling of the posterior circulation from that artery, the problem is viewed as an asymptomatic carotid stenosis. The optimal treatment for this lesion is then correlated with management of the vertebrobasilar occlusive disease.

Established Stroke and Carotid Stenosis

In a group of patients we treated who had suffered a stroke and were found to have carotid disease, more than half had had a prior history of TIAs due to carotid stenosis that had not brought the patient to medical attention.[26] Because these patients are at risk for further stroke, they should be studied. A CT scan is done to define the extent of the infarction and to look for other lesions. If there is any suspicion of carotid occlusive disease, noninvasive studies and MRA (or angiography) are indicated.

In general, the presence of severe stenosis or a deep ulcer is an indication for surgical treatment. If the angiogram shows a thrombus in the lumen or a carotid occlusion that may be reopened, then surgery is performed promptly. In those patients with a recent stroke who are continuing to show improvement, and if prompt surgery is not indicated from the angiogram, operation may be delayed to allow recovery from cerebral ischemia. How long one should delay has not been established. Some have advocated waiting several weeks to reduce the chance of postoperative brain hemorrhage. If the neurological deficit is mild, we operate within a few days. If the deficit is moderate to severe, the patient will usually have CT evidence of an infarct. In this circumstance, we wait 2 to 3 weeks to allow maximum recovery. Surgery can then be done safely as long as there is careful control of the blood pressure postoperatively.

If the patient has had a massive stroke with a severe fixed deficit, only a CT scan is done. These patients cannot be helped by carotid endarterectomy.

An occasional patient will have a slowly progressive neurological deficit due to chronic cerebral ischemia. A CT scan excludes an intracranial mass lesion. MRA or angiography usually shows multiple-vessel occlusion. A combination of endarterectomy and bypass procedures may need to be considered.

Acute Stroke with Carotid Stenosis or Occlusion

If the history and/or findings suggest carotid disease in a patient with increasing TIAs in preceding days, the sudden onset of a mild to moderate neurological deficit with or without prior TIAs, or a progressive or fluctuating neurological deficit, immediate MRA and noninvasive studies are indicated. In many cases, conventional angiography will be needed for clarification. If there is severe stenosis with delayed flow, a thrombus in the lumen distal to the stenosis, or carotid occlusion with reflux to the intrapetrous segment of the carotid artery, surgery should be done promptly to allow maximum blood flow to ischemic brain tissue, prevent extension of a thrombus, and remove a source of embolization. Information from several experienced centers suggests that results of surgery are superior,[14,16,22,25,26] but there are as yet no controlled data. A stenosis with a residual lumen diameter greater than 2 mm (not hemodynamically significant) or ulceration in a plaque at the carotid bifurcation suggests an embolus as the cause of the problem, and the patient should be considered for anticoagulation. If an acute neurological deficit occurs with loss of a previously documented carotid bruit, emergency endarterectomy should be undertaken without CT or angiography. With the careful control of postoperative blood pressure, the risk of postoperative intracerebral hemorrhage is very low.[26]

When there is the sudden onset of a severe neurological deficit that persists, it is likely that significant infarction has occurred. This is almost certainly the case if there is a decreased level of consciousness. In this situation, restoration of blood flow by emergency carotid endarterectomy has only rarely been beneficial.

Asymptomatic Carotid Stenosis

Reliable guidelines for the management of an asymptomatic carotid bruit have not been established. Consequently, controversies exist as to the value of antiplatelet or anticoagulant therapy and the indications for carotid endarterectomy. No data are available on the impact of antiplatelet or anticoagulant therapy on the eventual stroke rate in patients with asymptomatic bruit. A recent report suggests that carotid endarterectomy reduces the risk of stroke for patients with asymptomatic carotid stenosis of 60 percent or more, but only if the perioperative risk is 3 percent or less.[8a]

At the present time, we recommend MRA and noninvasive studies in those medically stable patients with an asymptomatic carotid bruit. If there is a very severe stenosis (residual lumen of 1.5 mm or less), we strongly consider endarterectomy. This recommendation is strengthened by definite evidence of progression, reduced oculoplethysmographic values, or reversal of flow in the ipsilateral A1 segment of the anterior cerebral artery—all ominous signs of impending occlusion and possible infarction. If the noninvasive tests do not demonstrate a hemodynamic lesion and the clinical assessment of the bruit is not worrisome, we recommend that the patient be followed on aspirin (650 mg bid) and that the noninvasive tests be repeated at 4- to 6-month intervals.

Preoperative Medical Evaluation

Many patients with carotid artery atherosclerosis have significant medical risk factors. These include symptomatic coronary artery disease, myocardial infarction within 6 months, severe peripheral arterial disease, rheumatic heart disease, congestive heart failure, severe hypertension (blood pressure > 180/110 mmHg), and chronic obstructive pulmonary disease. Other factors to consider are diabetes, hyperlipidemia, and obesity. Previous publications have documented that the operative risks are higher in certain groups of patients with significant medical risk factors.[7,26,31] In patients without significant risk factors, the combined operative morbidity and mortality is 1 to 2 percent. The major medical risk relates to cardiac disease, and when this is present, the operative risk is significantly higher.[11,30,31,35]

Whenever there is a concern about the patient's cardiac status, a cardiologist is called for consultation. Often a thallium-persantin exercise tolerance test will be performed; evidence of significant myocardial ischemia represents a relative contraindication to surgery. In some cases, coronary angiography may be recommended, and adverse findings may suggest monitoring with a pulmonary artery catheter or even deferral of endarterectomy. Occasionally, severe symptomatic coronary and carotid occlusive disease may warrant a combined coronary artery bypass and carotid endarterectomy.

Many patients will be on several drugs for treatment of the factors noted above. In general these drugs are continued. Patients receiving diuretic medication should have the serum potassium value checked prior to operation, and any deficiency should be treated. It is important that patients with severe hypertension be treated because the incidence of postoperative hypertension and morbidity is higher in this group. This is particularly true for those patients who have an associated cerebral infarction and are at risk to develop a cerebral hemorrhage.[7]

Other indications for intraoperative monitoring with a pulmonary artery catheter include left ventricular failure, a recent myocardial infarction, severe mitral valvular disease, and persistent angina after a coronary artery bypass. Patients with symptomatic heart block undergo placement of a temporary intravenous pacer.

Carotid Endarterectomy

Anesthetic Management

Preoperative medication is kept to a minimum because of the fragile cardiovascular state of many of these patients. We prefer general endotracheal anesthesia. This technique provides good airway control, maintenance of normal arterial blood gases, maximum patient comfort, optimal surgical exposure, and some protection against cerebral ischemia.

On a few occasions, we have performed carotid endarterectomy under regional block in patients with a strong medical contraindication to general endotracheal anesthesia (severe pulmonary or cardiac failure). This can be done successfully, especially in a cooperative patient, but the precision of surgery is reduced, especially when ischemia leads to movement in an agitated patient.

A radial intra-arterial cannula is inserted percutaneously for direct blood pressure recording and for blood gas measurement. The Pa_{CO_2} level is kept between 30 and 39 mmHg. If there is any indication of low blood volume or hypotension, central venous pressure (CVP) is monitored, and the patient is given fluid or colloid to raise the CVP to 8 to 10 cmH_2O. A vasopressor intravenous (IV) infusion is prepared, usually with 10 mg of phenylephrine hydrochloride (Neosynephrine, Winthrop Laboratories, New York, NY) in 250 ml of saline, and administered through a pediatric microdrip set as needed to maintain an adequate blood pressure.

Brain Protection and Monitoring

The best method of maintaining adequate cerebral circulation during the operation is to combine the benefits of general anesthesia with the maintenance of adequate blood volume and a normal or slightly elevated arterial pressure. At the time of carotid occlusion for carotid endarterectomy, the arterial pressure is elevated to an average systolic level of 170 mmHg if there is no cardiac contraindication.

The most effective method of monitoring the intracranial circulation during the time of vascular occlusion for the endarterectomy is continuous EEG recording with a full set of leads from both sides of the head.[3,25,26,32] A high degree of correlation has been found between CBF measurements during carotid occlusion and changes in the EEG.[32] If a significant EEG abnormality occurs, with severe slowing or loss of amplitude, a shunt should be placed promptly.

The question of whether a temporary shunt is indicated during carotid endarterectomy has been the subject of many articles. Some surgeons routinely use a shunt for cerebral protection.[13] Others never use a shunt, and some use a shunt selectively when monitoring indicates a need for it.[26,32] The use of a shunt carries with it a possible risk of embolization and of injury to the intima, although we have not seen this, and it does make the technical removal of the distal end of the plaque in the ICA a little more difficult. Everything should be done to reduce the morbidity of the operation to as low a level as possible. Every patient should be monitored. In only a small percentage of patients will a shunt be needed (about 10 percent in our series), but when it is indicated, it should be used. In some patients, the surgeon will know preoperatively that a shunt will be needed. These include patients in whom the vertebrobasilar circulation depends on the carotid artery or in whom there are multiple occlusions of major extracranial vessels.

Operative Technique

Since the original report of our operative approach[25] we have gradually revised and refined the technique.[15,26] The general layout of the operating room is shown in Fig. 204-1. The patient is placed in the supine position with a thyroid bag inflated under the shoulders. The head is extended slightly, placed on a firm head holder, and turned away from the side of the operation. The opposite calf (if nonischemic) is prepared and draped for possible saphenous vein harvesting. The entire operation is done using a headlight and magnifying loupes, with use of microsurgical instruments for improved precision of plaque removal and arteriotomy closure. We

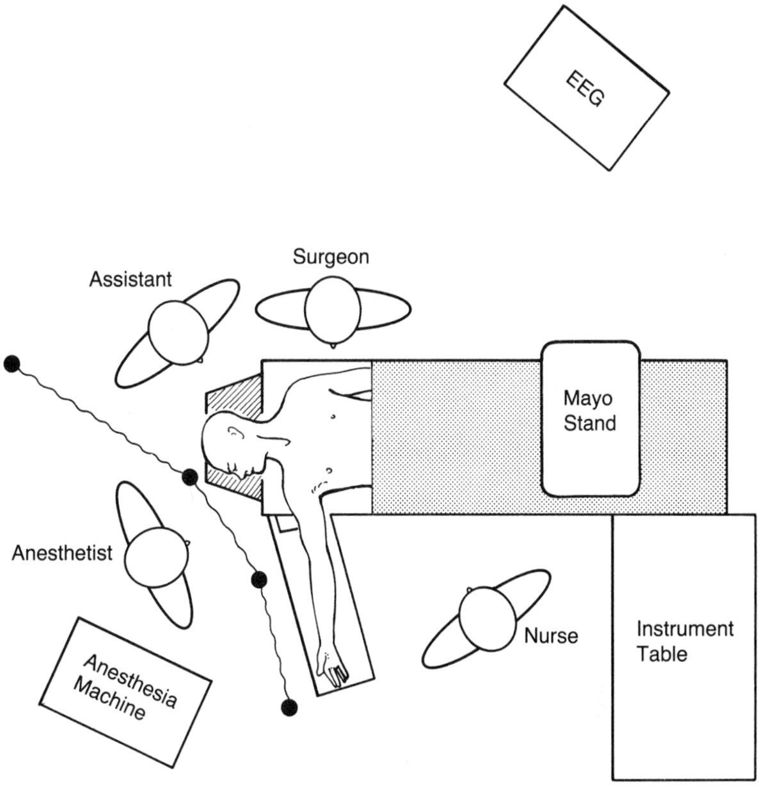

Figure 204-1 Operating room layout for a left carotid endarterectomy. We believe that it is helpful to have the scrub nurse stand across the table from the surgeon. (From Ojemann et al.,[26] with permission.)

prefer loupes and a headlight for greater mobility and an improved line of sight up the internal and external carotid arteries, especially with a high-lying bifurcation and plaque.

Some surgeons have recommended the use of the operating microscope for carotid endarterectomy,[9,29] and we have been impressed in 10 cases of the value of the approach for precise plaque removal and suturing. This may prove to be especially valuable for more proximal lesions in which the oblique upward line of sight is not important. Whether loupes or the microscope are employed, meticulous endarterectomy and closure are crucial.

The incision is made along the lower anterior border of the sternomastoid muscle and just below the level of the angle of the jaw and should be curved over the muscle posteriorly and superiorly toward the mastoid process (Fig. 204-2*A*). If necessary, this incision will allow maximum exposure to the base of the skull and helps avoid retraction on the lower branch of the facial nerve near the angle of the jaw.

After the initial incision and throughout the exposure, careful attention is paid to meticulous hemostasis. This is done to permit nonreversal of intraoperative heparinization and postoperative continuation of heparinization, in most cases. To avoid unwanted bleeding, bipolar cauterization of all bleeders, even to the most minute, is recommended.

After the skin incision is made, the platysma is incised. The external jugular vein is ligated, small transverse cervical nerves divided, and the great auricular nerve identified and spared at the upper end of the exposure. Deep dissection is continued along the anterior border of the sternomastoid muscle.[26] Self-retaining retractors are used to aid the exposure. The medial blades must be kept on the subcutaneous tissue and platysma. If they are placed too deeply against the paratracheal muscles, there may be tracheal and nerve injury.

The internal jugular vein is identified just medial and deep to the sternomastoid muscle. The dissection then extends along the medial border of the internal jugular vein; medial draining branches are ligated as necessary. The descendens hypoglossi nerve is often seen in the tissue just medial to the internal jugular vein and overlying the CCA. This nerve is reflected medially.

By opening the carotid sheath, the CCA is exposed medial to the internal jugular vein in the lower part of the incision. A vascular loop is placed around this vessel, which maintains its exposure and facilitates the further dissection. On rare occasions the vagus nerve lies anteriorly on the CCA, and one must be alert for this possibility.

The dissection is then extended superiorly along the medial border of the internal jugular vein. The descendens hypoglossi is kept medially and leads one to the hypoglossal nerve, which may swing low into the neck across the carotid bifurcation or lie high beneath the edge of the posterior belly of the digastric muscle. Sometimes it lies just beneath the common facial vein and may be adherent to this vessel. In some patients, nerve branches will come around the lateral side of the CCA to enter the descendens hypoglossi. Usually these branches are from the cervical plexus, but on rare occasions they seem to come from the vagus nerve. Vagal branches are preserved; they may be laryngeal. The descendens hypoglossi may be sacrificed for better exposure, without noticeable loss of function. This branch may be confirmed when bipolar stimulation causes contraction of the strap muscles (this is possible only when one or two twitches are evident on twitch monitoring). To give adequate exposure it may be necessary to remove a group of lymph nodes that are commonly present over the region of the carotid bifurcation.

When the carotid bifurcation is exposed, the region of the carotid sinus is blocked with lidocaine hydrochloride (Xylocaine,

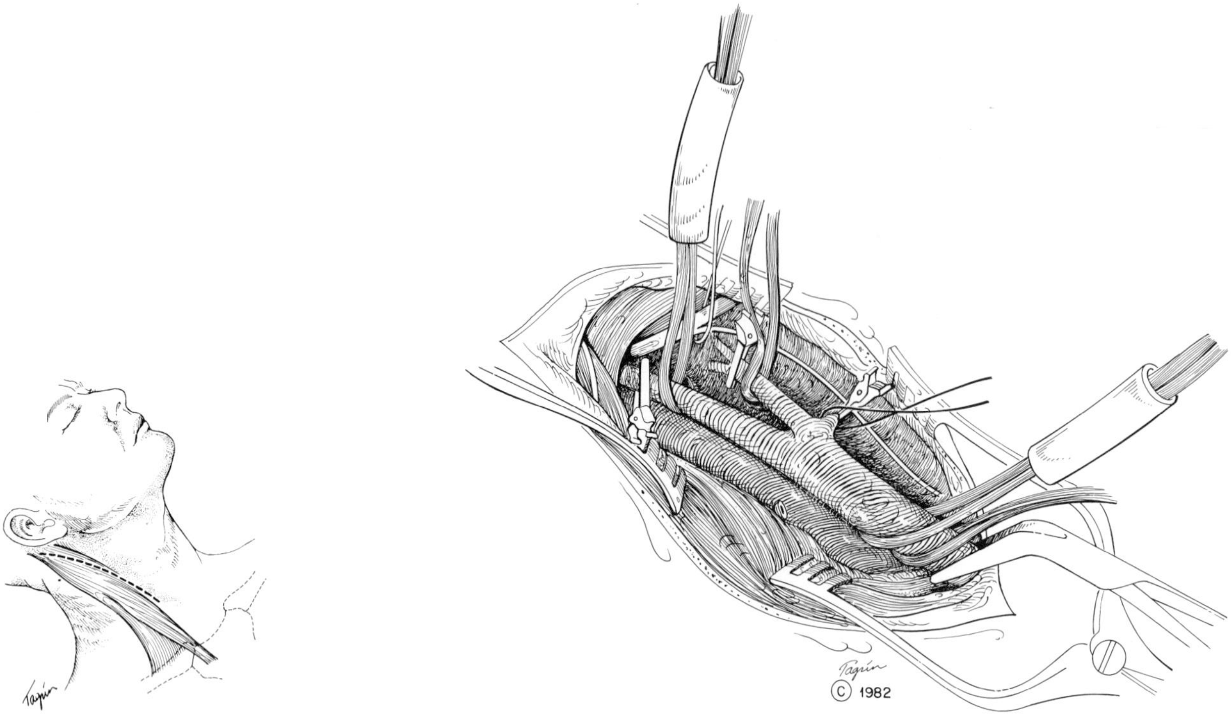

(*A*) (*B*)

Figure 204-2 Exposure for a carotid endarterectomy. *A.* The incision begins along the lower anterior border of the sternomastoid muscle and curves over the upper portion of the muscle toward the mastoid process. *B.* The region of the carotid bifurcation has been exposed. Appropriate loops and vascular occluding clamps have been placed. (From Ojemann et al.,[26] with permission.)

Astra Pharmaceutical Products, Inc., Worcester, MA) to avoid a carotid sinus reflex bradycardia and hypotension. Care is taken to leave the region of the distal common carotid artery, carotid bifurcation, and proximal ICA adherent to the posterior tissue. This avoids undue manipulation of the area, reducing the possibility of dislodging an embolus, lessening the chance of carotid sinus stimulation, and avoiding possible injury to the superior laryngeal nerve.

The superior thyroid artery is identified on the medial wall of the distal CCA or proximal ECA, and a miniloop is placed around it. The ECA is exposed to the level of the first major branching of this vessel, and a maxiloop is placed at this point. If the arteriogram shows an ascending pharyngeal artery coming off the region of the bifurcation, this will have to be exposed and controlled separately.

The distal ICA is carefully exposed, staying in the tissue plane between the hypoglossal nerve or descendens hypoglossi medially and the internal jugular vein laterally (Fig. 204-2*B*). If one follows these guidelines, the distal ICA can be nicely exposed. As the hypoglossal nerve swings medially, an arterial branch often comes across the inner side of the curve of the nerve and passes posteriorly. This fairly constant sternocleidomastoid artery, often accompanied by a vein, is ligated. The hypoglossal nerve can, if necessary, be reflected gently medially with a 4–0 suture through the transected descendens hypoglossi stump. If the carotid bifurcation is located high in the neck, dissection is carried along the medial border of the internal jugular vein and beneath the parotid gland. Up to 2 cm of distal ICA exposure can be obtained by dissection of the posterior belly of the digastric muscle, with firm retraction by a Cushing retractor attached to the drapes by elastics and an Allis clamp. (The drapes are clamped with towel clips to an IV pole which is stabilized by sand bags under its wheels.) Subluxation of the jaw by wiring of the teeth can give an additional 1 to 2 cm of distal exposure in selected cases. It may be necessary to retract the posterior belly of the digastric muscle. On occasion the occipital artery must be divided to free the hypoglossal nerve in order to expose the distal ICA. The exposure of the distal ICA is carried to a point at least 1 cm above the distal end of the plaque. In the majority of cases the atheromatous plaque extends several millimeters further up the posterior wall of the ICA than it does on the anterior wall. Great care is taken in exposing this vessel to avoid any undue pressure or manipulation of the artery. The vagus nerve may be closely adherent to the posterior wall of the artery; occasionally it will be lateral or superficial to the artery. It must be carefully dissected free before placing the loop around the vessel. Pump tourniquets are placed on the loops on the common and ICAs to use in case a shunt is needed.

With a marking pen, the proposed arteriotomy is marked on the common and ICAs. The line is smooth and stays lateral, away from the bifurcation. Marking in this way avoids zig-zag cuts if the arteriotomy is extended later on. A mark is made for a possible external carotid arteriotomy. Transverse hash marks are made at the expected distal end and distalmost possible end of the arteriotomy, and the external diameters are measured.

If the distal artery is very small (<4 mm in diameter), or if there is a tendency to kink (or if severe irregularity of the wall is disclosed after endarterectomy), we believe there is a higher likelihood of thrombosis, which warrants selective placement of a saphenous patch graft. Therefore, in case of a kinked or very small distal ICA, we next harvest the saphenous vein at the ankle. An incision is made longitudinally about 1 cm anterior and 1 cm proximal to the medial malleolus. After the saphenous vein is identified, the incision is carried proximally at least 10 cm. Hemostasis is obtained and Weitlaner retractors are placed. The vein is marked with a marking pen. Making every effort to avoid trauma to the vein, the surgeon opens the adventitia and dissects beneath the distal vein, placing a miniloop around it. By gently lifting the vein, attachments are put on stretch and divided sharply. Two or three large side branches are ligated with 4–0 silk and divided; small branches are coagulated with bipolar current. Finally the vessel is ligated distally and proximally, and excised. It is immediately irrigated gently (from distally) with heparinized saline. With a Potts scissors, the vein is opened along the longitudinal marking and placed in a bath of heparinized saline. The wound is closed with interrupted 3–0 coated Vicryl in the subcutaneous tissue and running 3–0 nylon in the skin. The patient is given an IV bolus of 5000 to 7000 units of heparin. The blood pressure is raised to at least 170 mmHg systolic, if there is no cardiac contraindication.

The common carotid artery is then occluded with an appropriate vascular clamp (usually an angled Fogarty hydro-grip), care being taken to avoid injury to the underlying vagus nerve. We prefer to use Sugita temporary aneurysm clips to occlude the other arteries, but on occasion a large ICA or ECA will require the use of a small bulldog clamp. Care must also be taken to avoid injury to the vagus nerve at this point because it lies in the tissue adjacent to the ICA. The clip on the ECA is placed at or just below the first major bifurcation.

A longitudinal incision is made along the previously placed mark in the distal CCA with a no. 15 knife blade (Fig. 204-3*A*). The incision is carried through the wall of the artery until the shiny yellow surface of the atheromatous plaque is seen. A Penfield no. 4 dissector is then used to develop the plane between the atheroma and the outer arterial wall (Fig. 204-3*B*). Often the atheroma is adherent to a relatively thin outer wall at the bifurcation. It is best to separate the plaque for a few millimeters and then extend the incision superiorly with a Potts scissors before attempting further dissection. The distal end of the incision extends up the ICA to approximately the distal end of the plaque. The proximal extent of the arteriotomy is usually 1 to 2 cm below the bifurcation. A thin layer of thickened intima will usually extend proximally in the common carotid artery and does not need to be of concern as long as one is proximal to the stenosis.

The atheromatous plaque is then separated carefully from the outer arterial wall in the CCA. A right-angled clamp is placed around the plaque, and the plaque is cut off and beveled with curved microscissors at the proximal end of the arteriotomy in the common carotid artery (Fig. 204-3*C*). The plaque is kept intact and is removed first from the origin of the superior thyroid artery and the proximal ECA. In some patients it is necessary to temporarily open the clamp on the ECA to remove the plaque, which may extend quite far distally. Additional bits of atheroma may be removed circumferentially with a Jacobson hemostat. The line of sight provided by loupes and a headlight is very helpful for this step. Once this removal has been accomplished, the atheroma is carefully dissected from the outer wall of the ICA, keeping gentle traction on the intact plaque. Often there is a very clean dissection plane. Great care is taken as the distal end of the plaque is reached (Fig. 204-3*D*). Usually the plaque will extend distally several millimeters further along the posterior wall of the artery. Care must be taken to remove this portion of the atheroma. Once the plaque has been separated, it usually comes away cleanly at the junction with normal intima and does not leave an intimal flap. The plaque may "feather" away from the wall, becoming ever thinner, then vanishing. Or it may extend along the posterior wall like a yellow tongue, with a clear-cut dissection margin. In both of these situations, there is no tendency to distal irregularity or intimal flap formation. Sometimes the plaque seems to extend further distally, without a clear-cut margin. In this case the surgeon should consider a circumferential bevelling incision of the thin plaque with the curved microscissors. When done properly, this results in a very smooth inner wall, without a significant shelf effect. Tiny distal irregularities, either longitudinal or transverse, may be excised flush with the microscissors (more cleanly than by avulsion). The distal artery is inspected under loupes or microscope, with jets of irrigation to reveal any possible tendency to intimal flap formation. Further revision of the endarterectomy margin can be made. Only occasionally do we use 6–0 double-armed tacking stitches to improve such a situation.

The area of the endarterectomy is irrigated with heparinized saline and inspected with the help of the headlight and magnification. There are almost always some loose fragments adherent to the wall, which are excised or removed by peeling them in a circumferential fashion with a Jacobson hemostat. The final inspection is made of the distal end of the endarterectomy in the ICA and ECA, visualizing the area directly using a headlight and fine suction.

The arteriotomy is then closed with a continuous 6–0 Prolene (Ethicon, Inc., Somerville, NJ) suture beginning at the distal end of the arteriotomy on the ICA and progressing down onto the CCA (Fig. 204-4*A*). The 6–0 suture permits very thin bites and interbite distance (0.3 to 0.4 mm) with virtually no arterial narrowing. To avoid fracture, the surgeon should never handle the brittle suture with instruments. Seven tight square throws are needed on the distal knot to prevent untying. The suture must be snugged down with each stitch to maintain a taut suture line. Each stitch must include, under direct vision, both the medial and intimal layers on both lateral and medial sides. As one reaches the bifurcation, the lumen becomes larger and the wall thicker, and a larger bite and interbite distance (0.6–0.8 mm) are appropriate. In the CCA, a 10 to 12 mm artery warrants even larger bites and intervals (1.0 to 1.2 mm).

Just before the final sutures are placed, backflow is allowed from both the ICA and the ECA so that air and any debris are flushed out of the area of the endarterectomy. If the backflow is poor, the arteriotomy is reopened and the problem corrected. In this situation there may be an intimal flap or narrowing at the distal end of the suture line. After the last suture is placed, backflow through the superior thyroid artery is permitted to exclude air from the lumen during the final tying of the suture. When the closure is completed, a rubber dam is placed over the suture line and held by a sponge with gentle pressure. Blood flow is allowed first into the ECA to wash out any further residual debris, and then into the ICA. Bleeding from the suture line is usually not a problem and is easily controlled by gentle pressure on the rubber dam. One should not be in any hurry to close small areas of leak from the suture line because most will clot with gentle pressure and patience. Surgicel (oxidized cellulose, Johnson and Johnson, New Brunswick, NJ) is placed on the suture line. If the hemorrhage persists, the surgeon may place an additional stitch at the point of leakage, with tiny bites to avoid narrowing; a small flap of periarterial tissue may be used.

Once flow has been re-established, the endarterectomy site is checked. The exposed arteries and the superficial temporal artery are palpated gently. If there is a thrill in the ICA, the clamps are

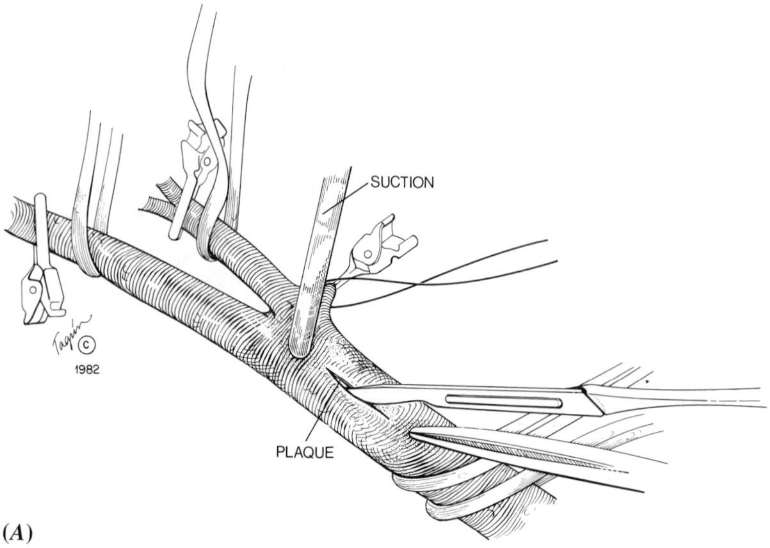

(*A*)

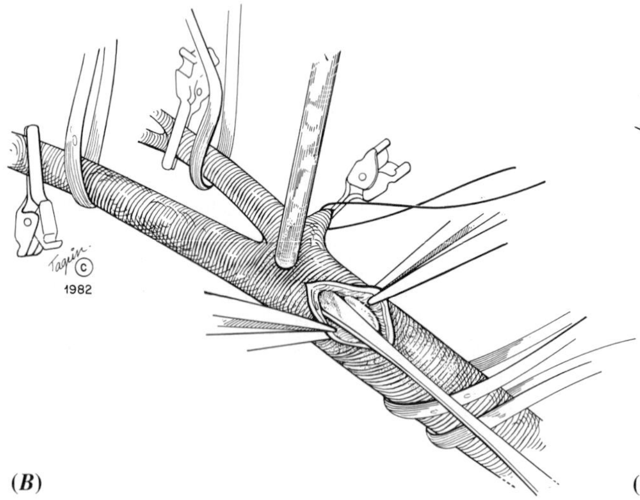

(*B*)

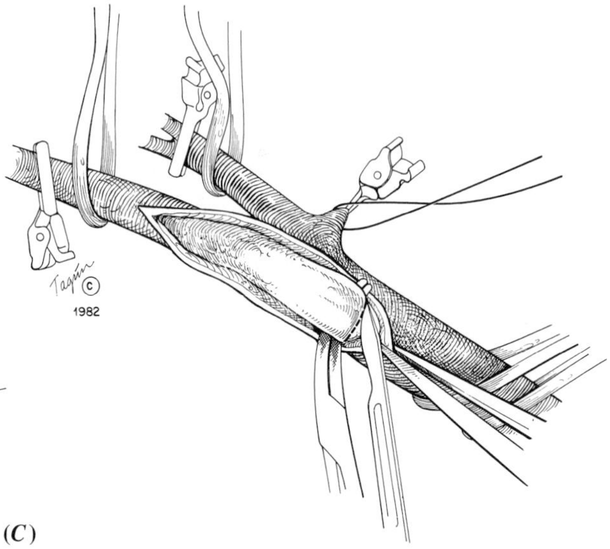

(*C*)

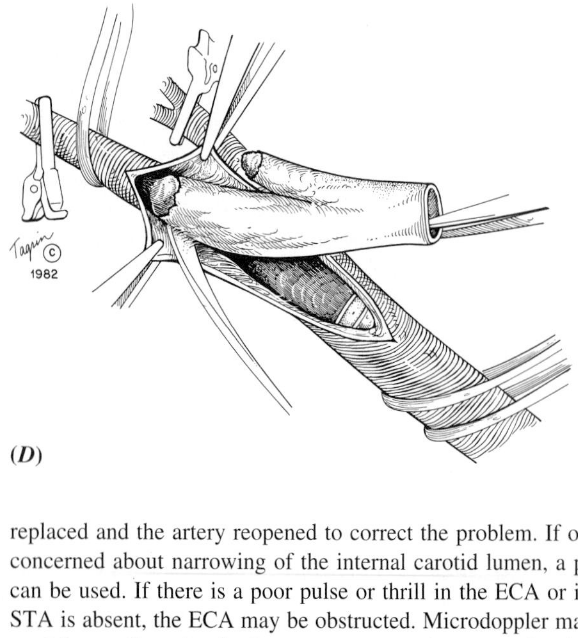

(*D*)

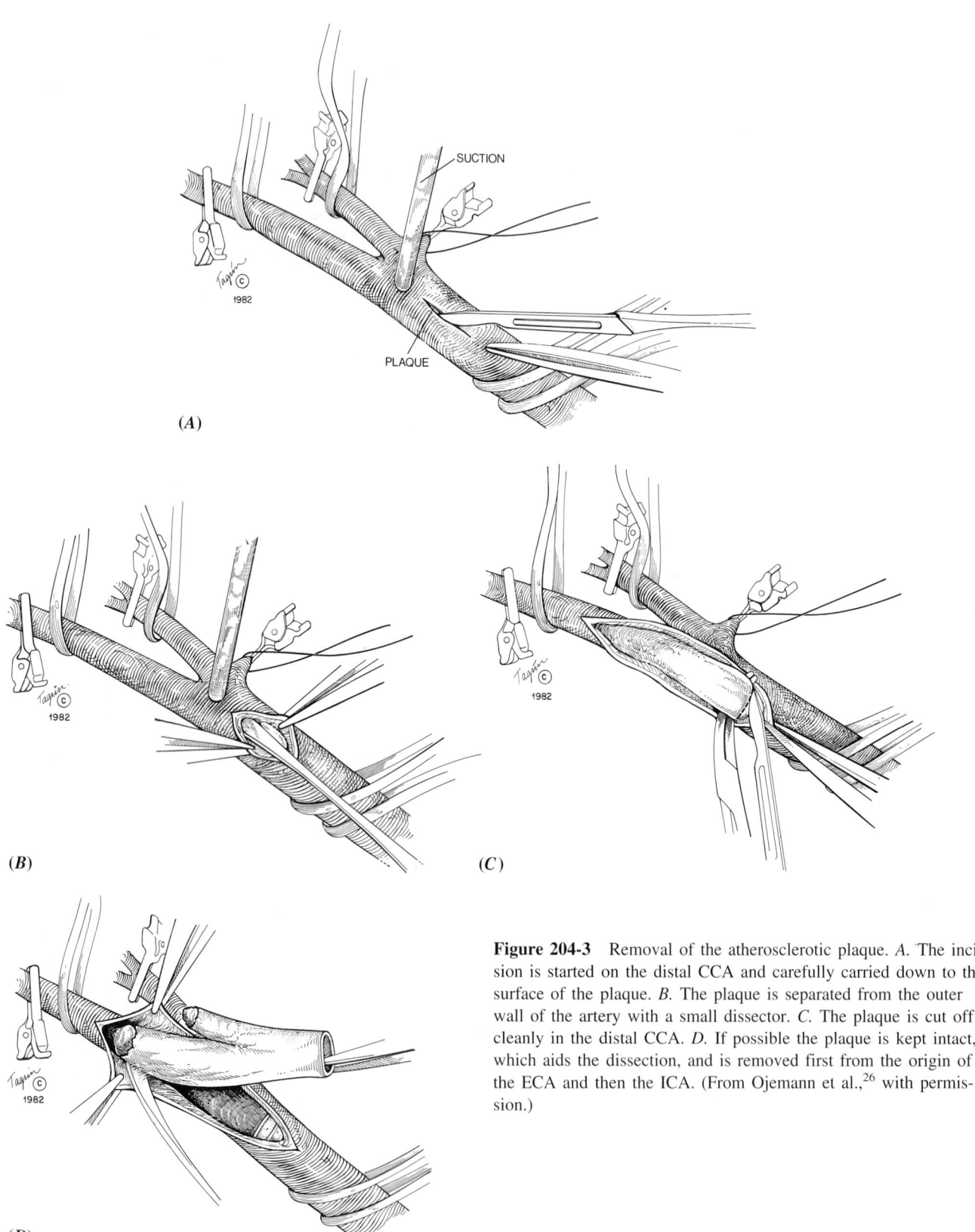

Figure 204-3 Removal of the atherosclerotic plaque. *A.* The incision is started on the distal CCA and carefully carried down to the surface of the plaque. *B.* The plaque is separated from the outer wall of the artery with a small dissector. *C.* The plaque is cut off cleanly in the distal CCA. *D.* If possible the plaque is kept intact, which aids the dissection, and is removed first from the origin of the ECA and then the ICA. (From Ojemann et al.,[26] with permission.)

replaced and the artery reopened to correct the problem. If one is concerned about narrowing of the internal carotid lumen, a patch can be used. If there is a poor pulse or thrill in the ECA or if the STA is absent, the ECA may be obstructed. Microdoppler may be used for confirmation in that a separate arteriotomy and endarterectomy may be needed.

We almost always do not reverse the heparin. Not reversing the heparin may protect against thrombus formation, particularly during the first hour after the closure.[32] Occasionally with extended cross-clamping of over 1 h, additional heparin may be needed. Rarely, bleeding at the time of closure demands (partial) reversal with protamine sulfate (Eli Lilly and Co., Indianapolis, IN). Re-

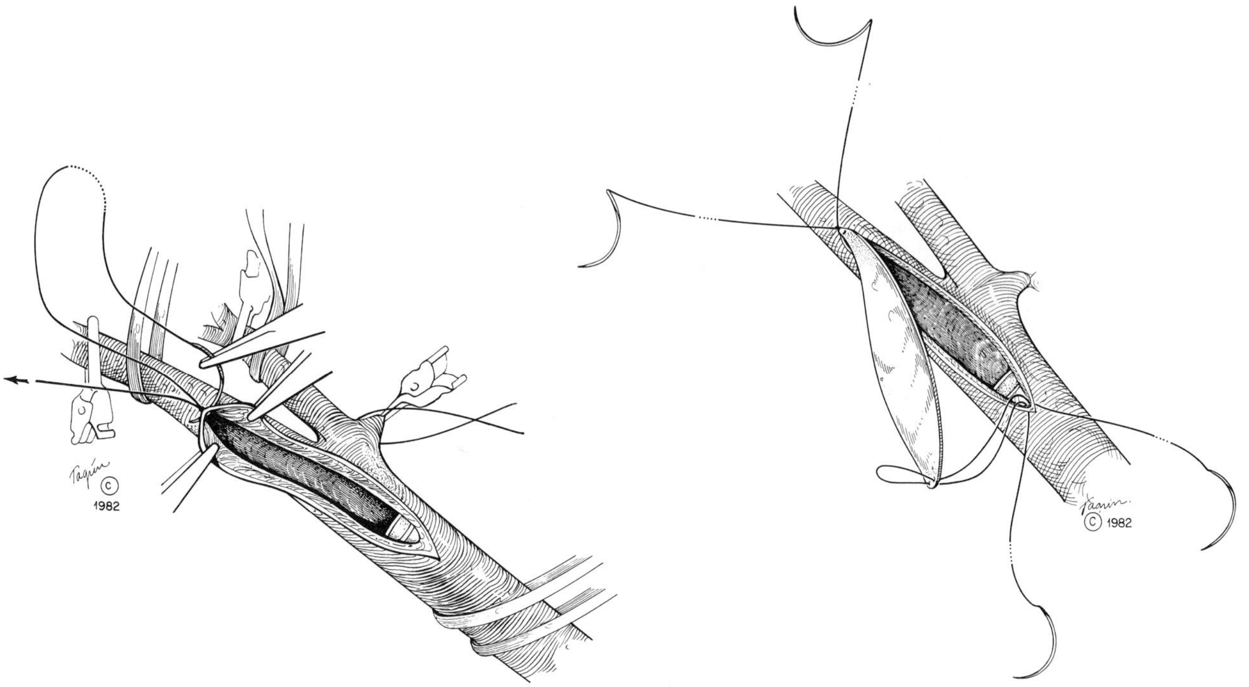

(*A*) (*B*)

Figure 204-4 Closure of the arteriotomy. *A.* Usually the incision in the artery can be closed with a running suture. This is placed with the aid of magnification. *B.* Technique for placing a patch if it is needed. (From Ojemann et al.,[26] with permission.)

cently we have gained some experience with activated clotting time (ACT) determinations during carotid endarterectomy. Because the test is done in the operating room by the anesthesiologist, with results within 5 min, data can be used to guide repetition of heparin administration or the use of protamine sulfate.

We generally place a no. 10 French Jackson-Pratt drain, attached to a grenade chamber put to 1½ psi wall suction. If the dressing is dry in the recovery room, heparin is restarted at 500 units/h for 48 hours. This program seems to reduce the risks of embolization and we have rarely experienced a wound hematoma.

Special Technical Problems

Insertion of a Patch Graft

With the routine use of magnification for the endarterectomy, we have found that in most cases the arterial incision can be closed with a continuous 6–0 Prolene running suture. When the ICA appears to be too small for satisfactory closure (≤4 mm in diameter) or it appears that closure will compromise the lumen (particularly with a tendency to kink or with a markedly irregular wall), we have no hesitation in using a patch graft.[26] In most patients with recurrent stenosis, a patch graft is used because of the scar formation in the wall of the artery. Some surgeons use a patch routinely.[32]

The patch is made from a collagen-impregnated knitted Dacron graft (Hemashield, Meadox Medicals, Inc, Oakland, NJ). This graft material is convenient, handles well, avoids needle hole leakage, and has not been associated with blow out.[11a] The patch is cut to fit the arteriotomy. The graft is usually about 4 mm in width near the distal end and tapers over 6 to 8 mm to a blunt distal end and gradually to a long 2-mm tail.

Double-armed sutures of 6–0 Prolene are used (Fig. 204-4*B*). One arm of the suture is placed through the distal end of the graft from the inner to the outer surface and the other arm is placed at the distal end of the arteriotomy from inside the lumen to the outer wall. Sutures are placed from the outside through the graft and then from the arterial wall lumen to the exterior, in order to accurately suture the intima and media. Four to five sutures are placed on one edge, then a similar number on the other to maintain smooth symmetry. Note that one edge will be done backhand. The graft should extend about 8- to 10-mm above the end of the remaining thickened intima to confer adequate expansion of the lumen at this critical spot. Note that in placing a patch graft, the bite size and interbite distance are larger (about 0.8 to 1.0 mm) than in primary closure. This is done to exclude the irregular wall edge from the lumen, and it can be done so because the patch offers extra material for adequate lumen maintenance. When suturing reaches the bifurcation, the tail of the graft is pulled taut and transected. The end of the patch is sewn to one side of the arteriotomy and tied. The other limb of suture is used for continuous closure of the CCA. If there is concern about a possible blow out (which we have not encountered), a 10-mm diameter Gore-tex sleeve (Gore and Co, Flagstaff, AZ) is placed around the entire graft and carotid artery.

Use of a Shunt

When the EEG demonstrates ischemic changes after cross-clamping (slowing, voltage loss), these can be reversed to prevent stroke by the use of a shunt. However, a shunt can cause intimal dissection or emboli, which can cause a stroke. Meticulous technique can prevent these problems.

We use the Argyle (St. Louis, MO) carotid shunt catheters.[26] The advantage of these sterile polyethylene catheters is that the surgeon has four sizes (nos. 8, 10, 12, and 14 French) immediately available that are the correct length (15 cm) and have smooth ends. Shunts are prepared by filling with heparinized saline and temporary cross-clamping with a hemostat. After arterial clamps and clips are placed, a rapid arteriotomy incision is made, including through the plaque, starting a few millimeters more proximally on the common carotid artery than usual and extending a few millimeters more distally on the ICA (Fig. 204-5). The shunt tube is first passed distally into the ICA; the surgeon visualizes the intima distal to the plaque so that a flap is not dissected by the tip of the catheter. A tape and tourniquet gently keep the arterial wall snug around the shunt. Rarely a Sundt-Kees clip graft can be used to provide a better view higher up. The shunt is checked to be certain there is satisfactory backflow of blood. The catheter is again temporarily occluded and is then passed proximally into the CCA, and the tourniquet is tightened. The plaque can then be dissected and removed as previously described. Great care is taken to ensure a smooth ending to the plaque removal, especially at the distal end. Sometimes the shunt will have to be removed temporarily to ensure a satisfactory margin. The arteriotomy is closed with two sutures that begin at either end. All but about 3 mm in the central portion of the arteriotomy is closed. The catheter is clamped and removed, and the closure of the arteriotomy is completed.

Complete ICA Occlusion

When the angiogram indicates a complete ICA occlusion, changes in the operative approach are indicated. Great care is taken to avoid hypotension. An incision is made on the ICA distal to the plaque after occluding the common and external carotid arteries. In the majority of patients a thrombus will be found, but in a few the lumen of the ICA will be open distal to the atheromatous plaque. If there is a long-standing occlusion, the artery may be a firm fibrous cord without backflow, and ligation with 0–0 silk is indicated.

If the thrombus can be removed and backflow established, the endarterectomy is completed as described. In some patients with complete occlusion of the ICA, the ECA may supply significant collateral flow to the brain. In some of these patients, flow can be maintained in the ECA by the application of a Satinsky clamp across the bifurcation at the origin of the ICA or by the use of a common to external carotid artery shunt.

Certain techniques may help in opening the completely occluded artery. If a thrombus is encountered in the ICA, an effort is made to withdraw it gradually with forceps using a hand-over-hand technique. Thrombi as long as 20 cm have been removed. If this technique fails, a smooth-ended suction catheter (a shunt tube attached to suction) is introduced into the internal carotid lumen until resistance is felt. Suction is then applied, and this may withdraw the thrombus. If this method fails, a no. 3 Fogerty catheter is passed gently as far as the base of the skull, inflated, and withdrawn. Care is required to avoid injuring the distal ICA with subsequent development of a carotid-cavernous fistula. Measurements on the angiogram from the internal carotid origin to the base of the skull may help in determining the safe length of catheter that may be inserted. An intraoperative angiogram is recommended to document restoration of flow without an intimal flap or distal thrombus. If good backflow with satisfactory angiography cannot be achieved, the ICA is doubly ligated with 0–0 silk sutures. When flow is re-established, anticoagulation should be continued in the postoperative period.

Postoperative Management

Systolic blood pressure is generally maintained in the range of 100 to 150 mmHg, with efforts to avoid both hypotension and hypertension. If hypotension develops, the electrocardiogram (ECG) is checked. Mild hypotension will usually respond to the administration of IV fluid or colloid. A phenylephrine drip is available if needed. If the hypotension does not immediately respond to volume replacement, a CVP catheter is inserted. If the CVP is maintained in the range of 5 to 10 cm with judicious utilization of fluid, this problem will generally resolve. On occasion, bradycardia may develop and the administration of atropine may be necessary. The blood pressure and pulse usually return to a normal level within a few hours.

Control of hypertension is also important. There is a significant incidence of postoperative hypertension.[4] Patients who develop postoperative systolic readings that are persistently above 170 mmHg require treatment with rapid-acting IV antihypertensive medication until long-acting medications become effective. We have encountered intracerebral hemorrhage with postoperative hypertension, as previously reported, but since the institution of careful postoperative blood pressure control, this complication has been rare.[4,25]

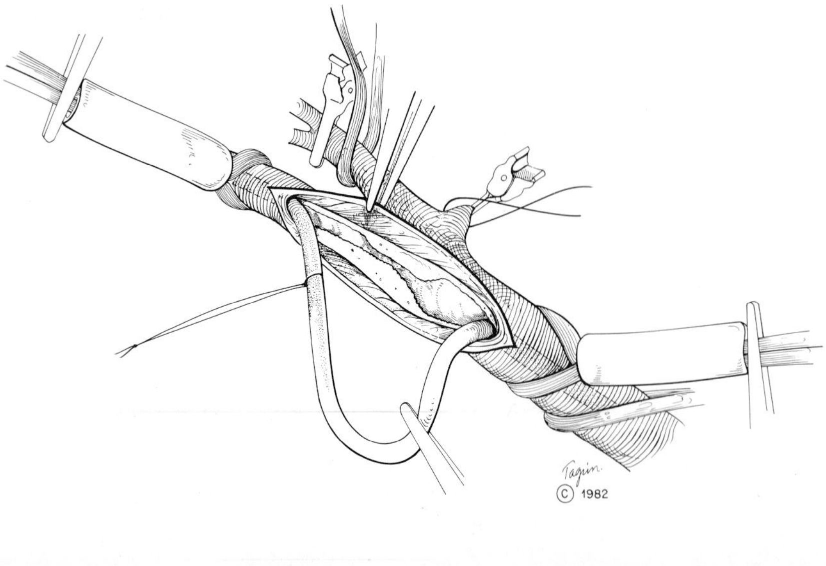

Figure 204-5 Placement of a shunt. The distal end of the catheter is placed first in the ICA. Then the proximal catheter is inserted into the common carotid artery. After the endarterectomy the shunt is placed internally until the closure is just about completed. (From Ojemann et al.,[26] with permission.)

In most cases, we use low-dose heparin for 48 h as described and then switch to aspirin. In patients with severe irregularity of the luminal wall after endarterectomy, we use therapeutic heparinization (partial thromboplastin time, 55 to 65 s) and then warfarin therapy for 3 months (prothrombin time, 15 to 17 s). In these cases, the dissection was difficult, the endarterectomy plane seemed roughened, the plaque was particularly long, or a complete occlusion was reopened. A special circumstance when anticoagulation should probably be continued is when the patient has a severely stenotic contralateral ICA stenosis.

Results

Our results for carotid endarterectomies done for carotid stenosis and/or ulceration in patients with TIAs have been reported.[25,26] The mortality rate was 1 percent, the incidence of major stroke 1 percent, and the incidence of minor stroke 1 percent. Virtually all other patients returned to their previous level of activity. In 120 elective endarterectomies over 3 years, we encountered no mortality, one disabling stroke, and three reversible strokes.[15] Several other reports of patients who have had elective carotid endarterectomies for TIAs have documented similar low morbidity and mortality rates when the operation is done by an experienced person in a center performing a significant number of operations.[2,3,6,7,13,28,31–33] For patients who have had a previous stroke there is a slight increase in risk.[25]

Reports of surgical treatment for asymptomatic carotid atherosclerosis include those of Thompson et al.,[34] who reported two strokes among 167 operations for asymptomatic bruit, and Moore et al.,[23] who reported no complications in 78 operations for asymptomatic carotid ulcerations. In our own series of 41 operations for asymptomatic carotid stenosis there was no morbidity or mortality.

Our results of operation for acute stroke in patients with carotid disease have been reported.[26] Among patients with crescendo TIAs, acute mild to moderate deficit, or fluctuating or progressive stroke, 29 enjoyed an excellent or good outcome. In this group there was one death; the patient had complete neurological recovery but then died of a cardiopulmonary complication. There were two occasions where the neurological deficit was worse after the operation, but there were also several spectacular recoveries in the immediate postoperative period after operation for both stenosis and occlusion. In another report of emergency carotid endarterectomy, 7 patients with crescendo TIAs all made a full recovery, and of 17 patients with stroke in evolution, none were worse, 4 were unchanged, 12 made a good recovery, and 1 died.[21] Encouraging results in selected cases have also been reported from other centers.[14,22,31]

Complications

Cerebral Ischemia and Infarction

The EEG electrodes are left on the patient until the patient awakens in the recovery room. If a neurological deficit is found as the patient awakens and a significant EEG change has occurred after leaving the operating room, the patient is returned immediately for exploration of the artery. If the deficit is present with no change in the EEG, a bedside ultrasound examination is performed immediately to look for occlusion and a CT scan is performed to look for hemorrhage. If these studies are normal, angiography is done. If studies show that the endarterectomy site is normal and that blood volume and blood pressure are maintained, a decision is made regarding anticoagulation. If the neurological deficit is mild and nonprogressive, usually no abnormality is found on angiography. In such patients it is assumed that an embolus was dislodged sometime during the dissection.

If the patient develops a substantial neurological deficit after an initial good recovery, it often indicates occlusion at the site of the operation. If the superficial temporal pulse is lost or the ultrasound shows occlusion, the patient should be taken immediately to the operating room to ascertain the status of the artery. If the deficit is mild and highly focal, a CT scan is done to look for hemorrhage, and if this study is normal, an angiogram is performed. The usual reason for postoperative carotid occlusion is a residual plaque or an intimal flap, but on rare occasions the problem may be associated with an ICA kink or an unrecognized hypercoagulable state.

Transient Ischemic Attacks

A small number of patients will have one or more transient ischemic episodes in the postoperative period. Usually it is a single attack, but if there is more than one it usually does not recur after 10 to 14 days and does not signify a serious problem in the operated artery. None of our patients who experienced this has gone on to have a stroke.

Noninvasive studies are done to ascertain whether there is a hemodynamic lesion. In our experience most patients will not have evidence of stenosis. They are treated with antiplatelet or anticoagulant therapy and usually do not have further problems. If TIAs persist or a significant abnormality is present on the noninvasive tests, angiography is indicated and may demonstrate a lesion that needs reoperation.

Intracerebral Hemorrhage

Early in our series a typical hypertensive hemorrhage occurred in the basal ganglia 4 days after surgery when the patient's blood pressure was 200/100 mmHg. Since that time careful and aggressive control of postoperative hypertension has reduced the incidence of this complication. However, occasionally even with a mild elevation in blood pressure, a hemorrhage may occur. In the single disabling postendarterectomy complication in the past 4 years, intracerebral hemorrhage occurred and upon evacuation, amyloid angiopathy was demonstrated. Intracerebral hemorrhage is also of concern when postoperative heparin or antiplatelet therapy is used and in patients who have had previous cerebral infarction.

Cranial Nerve Injury

If the incision is carried too near the angle of the jaw or retraction is too vigorous, the mandibular branch of the facial nerve can be stretched, causing weakness of the lower lip. This is an annoying problem; it causes a cosmetic change and may cause the patient to drool from the corner of the mouth. Spontaneous recovery almost always occurs. We have avoided this problem by curving the incision away from the angle of the jaw toward the mastoid process and being careful with placement of the self-retaining retractors.

Injury to the vagus or recurrent laryngeal nerve with vocal cord paresis has been reported to occur in about 1 percent of patients undergoing carotid endarterectomy.[25,36] Traction or pressure on the nerve is the usual cause. As noted in the discussion of operative technique, the vagus nerve can lie on the anterior surface of the common carotid artery and may be encountered early in the dissection. Another area where the vagus nerve is susceptible to injury is in dissection of the ICA, to which it may adhere. The majority of patients will show spontaneous recovery within a year.

Injury to the hypoglossal nerve is generally avoided by following the steps outlined in ''Operative Technique.'' When it does occur, it is usually due to excessive traction on the nerve. Nothing need be done. Usually there are no symptoms, and a majority of the patients will have a spontaneous recovery within a few months.

Other Complications

Cardiopulmonary complications have been reduced by following the guidelines described under ''Preoperative Medical Evaluation.'' Other neurological complications include seizures and headaches. When a headache occurs, it generally subsides in a day or so.

Recurrent Stenosis

Recurrent stenosis occurs in a small percentage of patients who have had a carotid endarterectomy.[5,12] There seem to be three groups of patients in which this problem arises:

1. Patients in whom surgical technique has contributed to the problem. This includes failure to remove the distal tongue of the plaque, narrowing of the lumen during the arteriotomy closure, and damage to the intima by vascular clamps.
2. Patients who have a tendency to excessive scar formation.
3. Patients who develop a combination of fibrosis, recurrent atherosclerosis, and, at times, an associated thrombus.

Symptomatic stenosis may recur within a few months of the operation. This usually relates to one of the problems in surgical technique or to the thickened fibrosis of the arterial wall, which is grossly and histologically distinct from the typical atherosclerotic plaque. Fortunately, this tendency to excessive scar formation is a rare happening. Recurrent stenosis that occurs after 2 years usually has significant atheroma formation as well as fibrosis.

Reoperation is often difficult because of the dense periarterial scar and the fibrosis of the vessel wall. Great care is required to avoid injury to the internal jugular vein and the vagus and hypoglossal nerves. The thickened intima is often densely adherent to the arterial wall, particularly in the region of the previous suture line. In most patients it is necessary to use a patch graft to repair the artery. In some instances where myofibrointimal hyperplasia is the problem, no dissection plane can be developed, and patch grafting alone is the best procedure.

References

1. Anson JA, Heiserman JE, Drayer BP, Spetzler RF. Surgical decisions on the basis of magnetic resonance angiography of the carotid arteries. *Neurosurgery* 1993; 32:335–343.
2. Bland JE, Lazar ML. Carotid endarterectomy without shunt. *Neurosurgery* 1981; 8:153–157.
3. Callow AD. An overview of the stroke problem in the carotid territory. *Am J Surg* 1980; 140:181–191.
4. Caplan LR, Skillman J, Ojemann R, Fields WS. Intracerebral hemorrhage following carotid endarterectomy: a hypertensive complication? *Stroke* 1978; 9:457–460.
5. Cossman D, Callow AD, Stein A, Matsumoto G. Early re-stenosis after carotid endarterectomy. *Arch Surg* 1978; 113:275–278.
6. Easton JD, Sherman DG. Stroke and mortality rate in carotid endarterectomy: 228 consecutive operations. *Stroke* 1977; 8:565–568.
7. Ennix CL Jr, Lawrie GM, Morris GC Jr, et al. Improved results of carotid endarterectomy in patients with symptomatic coronary disease: an analysis of 1546 consecutive carotid operations. *Stroke* 1979; 10:122–125.
8. European Carotid Surgery Trialists' Collaborative Group. MRC European Carotid Surgery Trial: interim results for symptomatic patients with severe (70–99%) or with mild (0–29%) carotid stenosis. *Lancet* 1991; 337:1235–1243.

8a. Executive Committee for the Asymptomatic Carotid Atherosclerosis Study. Endarterectomy for asymptomatic carotid artery stenosis. *JAMA* 1995; 273:1421–1428.

9. Findlay JM, Lougheed WM. Carotid microendarterectomy. *Neurosurgery* 1993; 32:792–798.
10. Fisher CM. Clinical syndromes in cerebral thrombosis, hypertensive hemorrhage and ruptured saccular aneurysm. *Clin Neurosurg* 1975; 22:117–147.
11. Fode NC, Sundt TM Jr, Robertson JT, et al. Multicenter retrospective review of results and complications of carotid endarterectomy in 1981. *Stroke* 1986; 17:370–376.

11a. Freischlag JA, Moore WS. Clinical experience with a collagen-impregnated knitted Dacron vascular graft. *Ann Vasc Surg* 1990; 4:449–454.

12. French BN, Rewcastle NB. Recurrent stenosis at site of carotid endarterectomy. *Stroke* 1977; 8:597–605.
13. Giannotta SL, Dicks RE III, Kindt GW. Carotid endarterectomy: technical improvements. *Neurosurgery* 1980; 7:309–312.
14. Goldstone J, Moore WS. A new look at emergency carotid artery operations for the treatment of cerebrovascular insufficiency. *Stroke* 1978; 9:599–602.
15. Halliday AL, Crowell RM, Ojemann RG, et al. One percent stroke morbidity and no mortality in 120 carotid endarterectomies. Presented at the 61st Annual Meeting of the American Association of Neurological Surgeons, Boston, April 24–29, 1993, poster 1090.
16. Heros RC, Ojemann RG. Emergency carotid endarterectomy. In Wood JH (ed): *Carotid Artery Surgery in Stroke*. Philadelphia: Hanley & Belfus, 1989, pp 171–178.
17. Hobson RW II, Weiss DG, Fields WS, et al. Efficacy of carotid endarterectomy for asymptomatic carotid stenosis: The Veterans Affairs Cooperative Study Group. *N Engl J Med* 1993; 328:221–227.
18. Masaryk TJ, Modic MT, Ross JS, et al. Intracranial circulation: preliminary clinical results with three-dimensional (volume) MR angiography. *Radiology* 1989; 171:793–799.
19. Mattle HP, Kent KC, Edelman RR, et al. Evaluation of the extracranial carotid arteries: correlation of magnetic resonance angiography, duplex ultrasonography, and conventional angiography. *J Vasc Surg* 1991; 13:838–845.
20. Mayberg MR, Wilson SE, Yatsu F, et al. For The Veterans Affairs Cooperative Studies Program 309 Trialist Group. Carotid endarterectomy and prevention of cerebral ischemia in symptomatic carotid stenosis. *JAMA* 1991; 266:3289–3294.
21. Mentzer RM Jr, Finkelmeier BA, Crosby IK, Wellons HA Jr. Emergency carotid endarterectomy for fluctuating neurologic deficits. *Surgery* 1981; 89:60–66.
22. Meyer FB, Sundt TM Jr, Piepgras DG, et al. Emergency carotid endarterectomy for patients with acute carotid occlusion and profound neurological deficits. *Ann Surg* 1986; 203:82–89.
23. Moore WS, Malone JM, Boren C, et al. Asymptomatic ulcerative lesions of the carotid artery: natural history and effect of surgical therapy compared. *Stroke* 1979; 10:96 (abstr).

24. North American Symptomatic Carotid Endarterectomy Trial Collaborators. Beneficial effect of carotid endarterectomy in symptomatic patients with high-grade carotid stenosis. *N Engl J Med* 1991; 325:445–453.
25. Ojemann RG, Crowell RM, Roberson GH, Fisher CM. Surgical treatment of extracranial carotid occlusive disease. *Clin Neurosurg* 1975; 22:214–263.
26. Ojemann RG, Heros RC, Crowell RM. *Surgical Management of Cerebrovascular Disease,* 2d ed. Baltimore: Williams & Wilkins, 1988.
27. Pessin MS, Duncan GW, Mohr JP, Poskanzer DC. Clinical and angiographic features of carotid transient ischemic attacks. *N Engl J Med* 1977; 296:358–362.
28. Robertson JT, Auer NJ. Extracranial occlusive disease of the carotid artery. In Youmans J (ed): *Neurological Surgery.* Philadelphia: Saunders, 1982, pp 1559–1583.
29. Spetzler RF, Martin N, Hadley MN, et al. Microsurgical endarterectomy under barbiturate protection: a prospective study. *J Neurosurg* 1986; 65:63–73.
30. Steed DL, Peitzman AB, Grundy BL, Webster MW. Causes of stroke in carotid endarterectomy. *Surgery* 1982; 92:634–641.
31. Sundt TM Jr, Sandok BA, Whisnant JP. Carotid endarterectomy: complications and preoperative assessment of risk. *Mayo Clin Proc* 1975; 50:301–306.
32. Sundt TM Jr, Sharbrough FW, Piepgras DG, et al. Correlation of cerebral blood flow and electroencephalographic changes during carotid endarterectomy: with results of surgery and hemodynamics of cerebral ischemia. *Mayo Clin Proc* 1981; 56:533–543.
33. Thompson JE, Garrett WV. Peripheral-arterial surgery. *N Engl J Med* 1980; 302:491–503.
34. Thompson JE, Patman RD, Talkington CM. Asymptomatic carotid bruit: long-term outcome of patients having endarterectomy compared with unoperated controls. *Ann Surg* 1978; 188:308–316.
35. Toronto Cerebrovascular Study Group. Risks of carotid endarterectomy. *Stroke* 1986; 17:848–852.
36. Wylie EJ, Ehrenfeld WK. *Extracranial Occlusive Cerebrovascular Disease: Diagnosis and Management.* Philadelphia: Saunders, 1970.

205

Vertebral Artery Atherosclerosis

James I. Ausman
Fernando G. Diaz
R.A. de los Reyes
Fady T. Charbel
Konstantin V. Slavin

Vertebrobasilar insufficiency (VBI) may result from atherosclerotic stenosis anywhere from the proximal subclavian artery to the distal basilar artery. This chapter will deal with those lesions of the vertebrobasilar system that are proximal to the origin of the posterior inferior cerebellar artery (PICA). We will thus focus on symptomatic structural lesions of the vertebrobasilar system, realizing that VBI may be secondary to or aggravated by extracerebrovascular causes, such as cardiac arrhythmias or hematologic causes, which should be adequately worked up and ruled out. It is similarly important that the clinical diagnosis of VBI be based upon at least two separate symptoms indicative of posterior circulation ischemia, and not just dizziness alone.[5]

Anatomy

The vertebral artery is the first and usually the largest branch of the subclavian artery and may be anatomically divided into four segments. The first segment extends from the vertebral origin to its entry into the intravertebral foramen of the sixth cervical vertebra. The second portion runs through the foramina of C6 through C1 to become the third segment as it passes over the superior surface of the posterior arch of C1, behind the articular process, and enters the atlanto-occipital membrane to become the fourth segment. This latter segment is intracranial and courses anteriorly and superiorly giving rise to its largest branch (PICA) and joins the opposite vertebral artery in the midline on the ventral aspect of the pontomedullary junction, forming the basilar artery. It is worthy of note that the vertebrobasilar system is the only major arterial system in the body in which two arteries converge to form a third, single artery.

Incidence

There are few data regarding the incidence of intracranial occlusive disease of the posterior circulation. Autopsy studies on "random" populations seem to indicate the incidence of extracranial vertebral artery disease to be in the neighborhood of 5 percent. Clinical and angiographic studies demonstrate posterior circulation disease in 25 to 50 percent of all patients with cerebral vascular disease.

This apparent discrepancy can be explained, as in the case of anterior (carotid) circulation disease, by the fact that (1) not all lesions are symptomatic, and (2) not all patients with symptoms have corresponding structural lesions (e.g., patients with cardiac sources of emboli). This picture is further complicated by the peculiar anatomy of the vertebrobasilar system (see above) and the fact that ischemia from structural lesions may be the result of either decreased flow or embolism from atherosclerotic stenosis.[6]

Perhaps the best clinical study on the incidence and natural history of VBI is that by Carlidge et al. in which the incidence of posterior circulation transient ischemic attacks (TIAs) was found to be half that of anterior circulation TIAs and approximately 35 percent of these patients developed a cerebral infarction within 5 years.[5] It should be recalled, however, that this study was based on a population that was not studied by angiography.

Diagnosis

The diagnosis of VBI should be entertained in any patient who complains of transient episodes of two or more symptoms that can be localized to the territory supplied by the posterior circulation. Thus brain stem symptoms such as diplopia, dysarthria, or dysphagia, cerebellar symptoms such as vertigo or ataxia, and occipital lobe symptoms such as bilateral amaurosis or hemianopsia with or without motor or sensory alterations involving any combination of the four extremities are consistent with this diagnosis.

The necessity to search for extracerebrovascular causes of VBI has already been discussed. Likewise, standard noninvasive neurological diagnostic studies, such as computed tomography or magnetic resonance imaging, should be performed. The definitive diagnostic test, however, remains the cerebral angiogram. Cerebral angiography should include bilateral carotid and vertebral runs with visualization of the origins of all the vessels as well as assessment of collateral intracranial circulation. After all the diagnostic information is obtained, consideration can be given to the risks and benefits of all the available modes of therapy.

Therapy

Given a patient with symptoms of VBI and structural disease in the posterior circulation, one must then decide on a course of therapy. The best available natural history study indicates a 35 percent incidence of cerebral infarction within 5 years.[5] Any treatment option must then be a significant improvement on this figure. There are to date no controlled randomized studies on an angiogrammed population with structural lesions in the posterior circulation to guide us in our choice of therapy, medical or surgical. It is evident then that this choice has to be made on an individual basis after obtaining a complete evaluation, including angiography, and weighing the potential risks and benefits of medical (anticoagulation, antiplatelet agents, etc.) versus surgical therapy. Clearly one must first decide what constitutes a significant structural lesion. Taking into account the above uncertainties, at present we believe that the following lesions of the vertebral system may result in VBI:

1. The subclavian steal syndrome (reversal of flow in a vertebral artery secondary to significant stenosis in the ipsilateral proximal subclavian artery).

2. Stenosis of one vertebral artery when the opposite vertebral artery is stenotic, occluded, or hypoplastic, or terminates in the PICA.
3. Single lesions in either vertebral artery causing stenosis and/or ulceration significant enough to cause decreased flow or embolism.

Beyond these general guidelines, the choice of therapy must be individualized. Certainly one would be more inclined to operate on a patient who has ongoing frequent episodes of vertebrobasilar insufficiency even while on anticoagulants, and who has angiographic demonstration of occlusion of one vertebral artery and severe stenosis of the distal portion of the remaining vertebral artery, than on a patient with infrequent episodes and a single lesion who has not been tried on antiplatelet therapy. We further believe that for surgery of the vertebrobasilar system to be considered, the patient should have ongoing episodes of VBI, because in our experience, patients who have had a single episode in the past and have been asymptomatic since have not significantly benefited from surgery, presumably because of the formation of adequate collateral circulation.

Surgical Therapy

Structural disease of the vertebral system may occur (1) in the subclavian artery proximal to the vertebral artery, causing the subclavian steal syndrome, (2) in the first portion of the vertebral artery, usually at the origin, (3) in the intraforaminal portion of the vertebral artery, and (4) in the third and fourth portions of the vertebral artery, and C1 to the origin of PICA or slightly beyond.

The Subclavian Steal Syndrome

The *subclavian steal syndrome* is the name commonly used to denote reversal of flow in a vertebral artery, usually secondary to stenosis in the ipsilateral subclavian artery proximal to the origin of the vertebral artery. This syndrome may not infrequently be angiographically demonstrated in otherwise asymptomatic patients. Symptomatic patients usually present with symptoms of neurological ischemia, most frequently in the posterior circulation, although a few patients may present with symptoms of brachial ischemia.[4] We refer here only to the symptomatic subclavian steal syndrome. Although a variety of operations have been designed to treat the subclavian steal syndrome (subclavian to subclavian artery bypass, axilloaxillary bypass, etc.), the principle for therapy of this condition should be that of restoration of antegrade flow to the cerebral circulation, or at least the prevention of retrograde flow therefrom. Because of a rich collateral supply, ischemic symptoms in the upper extremity are extremely rare during gradual occlusion of the subclavian artery by atherosclerosis.[4] Although vertebral artery ligation at its origin is relatively simple and quick, and may be the procedure of choice in the patient who is at high risk for surgery because of other medical problems, it does not restore antegrade flow in the vertebral artery. In our experience (Table 205-1) the procedure of choice for this syndrome is vertebral artery–common carotid artery end-to-side anastomosis. Anastomosis of the subclavian artery to the common carotid is also an attractive approach, but we have had no experience with this procedure.

Endovascular treatment of stenotic and occlusive vascular disorders is also very promising. In a series reported by Hebrang et al.,[8] the symptoms of VBI subsided in 72 percent of patients after percutaneous transluminal angioplasty (PTA) of a stenosed or occluded subclavian artery.

Surgical Technique

A vertical incision is made along the anterior border of the sternocleidomastoid muscle, extending from the sternoclavicular joint approximately 10 cm up the neck. The platysma is incised and the sternocleidomastoid is separated from the pretracheal fascia. The jugular vein is retracted laterally with the sternocleidomastoid muscle, and the carotid sheath is entered, exposing the common carotid artery. The sternocleidomastoid muscle is then displaced laterally, and the posterior cervical fascia is exposed. The transverse process of the sixth cervical vertebra is identified by palpating the carotid tubercle on its anterolateral aspect, and the vertebral artery is identified by dissecting the space between the anterior scalene muscle insertion and the insertion of the longus coli muscle onto the carotid tubercle. The inverted V that is left by the insertion of these two muscles marks the location of the entry of the vertebral artery into the foramen transversarium. The vertebral artery is usually covered by a spiral of veins, necessitating careful electrocoagulation and incision during the dissection from the carotid tubercle to the origin of the vertebral artery. Care must also be taken to identify, ligate, or coagulate the lymphatic channels draining into the subclavian vein, particularly the thoracic duct on the left side. On the right side special care must be taken to avoid injuring the recurrent laryngeal nerve, which is most frequently identified below the origin of the inferior thyroid vein. Once the vertebral artery has been completely dissected, the patient receives 5000 units of intravenous heparin. A ligature and silver clip are then placed at the origin of the vertebral artery, a temporary clip is placed on the vertebral artery at the level of the foramen transversarium, and the artery is then transected. If additional length of vertebral artery is needed in order to avoid a tense anastomosis, the anterior surface of the foramen transversarium may be removed with rongeurs. This is, however, usually not necessary. A fishmouth opening is then made at the origin of the vertebral artery. The site of anastomosis is then chosen on the common carotid

TABLE 205-1 Surgical Treatment of Subclavian Steal Syndrome

Operation	No. of Patients	Angiographic Patency	Postoperative Course	Permanent Complications
Vertebral–carotid transposition	5	5/5	Better	None
Vertebral artery ligation	1	—	?	Phrenic nerve injury; dysphagia

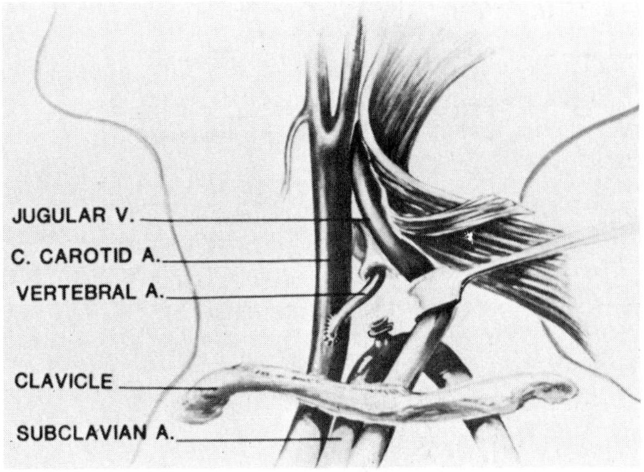

Figure 205-1 The anatomic relationships in vertebral–carotid transposition.

artery, and the appropriate segment of the common carotid is isolated between two clamps, below the bifurcation. A 4- or 5-mm stoma is then made with an aortic punch in the common carotid artery, and an end-to-side anastomosis is performed using no. 7–0 monofilament nylon and the operating microscope (Fig. 205-1). The clamps are then removed and the flow is restored. Clamp time is usually in the range of 20 to 30 min. The incision is then closed in layers in the usual manner (Figs. 205-2 and 205-3).

Results

Our experience with five such patients is summarized in Table 205-1. All symptoms were either significantly improved or resolved completely. A sixth patient, who was at high risk for surgery because of severe cardiovascular instability, underwent vertebral artery ligation because of crescendo TIAs of the posterior circulation. Although his TIAs ceased postoperatively, he was left with a persistent dysphagia, as well as an elevated left hemidiaphragm, presumably due to intraoperative phrenic nerve injury.

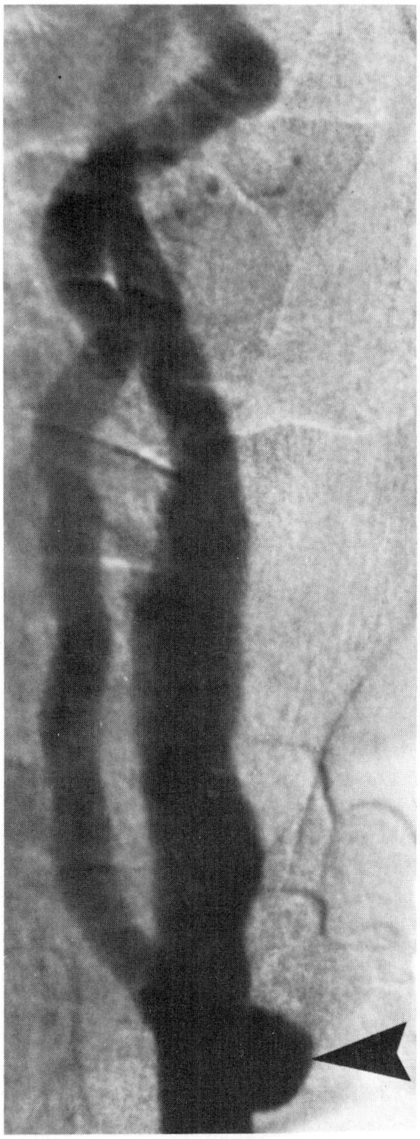

Figure 205-3 Postoperative left carotid angiogram (same patient as in Fig. 205-2) showing a patent vertebral–carotid transposition. The *arrowhead* points to the site of anastomosis.

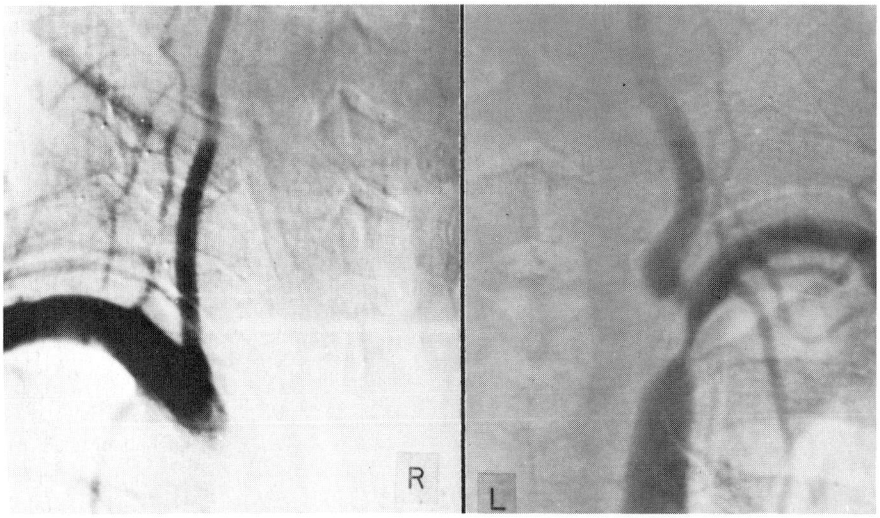

Figure 205-2 Preoperative bilateral subclavian–vertebral angiograms, demonstrating stenosis of the left subclavian artery proximal to the origin of the left vertebral artery. The patient had clinical as well as angiographic findings consistent with the subclavian steal syndrome.

TABLE 205-2 Surgical Treatment of Vertebral Origin Stenosis

Operation	No. of Patients	Angiographic Patency	Postoperative Course	Complications
Vertebral–carotid transposition	19	18/18	17 better 2 same	2 permanent Horner's syndrome
Vertebral–subclavian transposition	1	1/1	Better	None
Vertebral–thyrocervical transposition	1	0/1	Better	None
Vertebral origin endarterectomy	1	1/1	Better	None
Vertebral–carotid saphenous vein graft	1	1/1	Better	Transient upper brachial plexopathy

Vertebral Origin Stenosis

Vertebrobasilar insufficiency may result from atherosclerotic stenosis at the vertebral origin if the opposite vertebral artery is stenotic, occluded, or hypoplastic or terminates in the PICA. The presumed mechanism here would be hemodynamic compromise of the posterior circulation due to stenosis of the remaining vertebral artery. Whether the same can occur from a single lesion in one vertebral origin with an angiographically normal contralateral vertebral is open to speculation. Only slightly less controversial is the matter of embolization from an atherosclerotic vertebral artery plaque. Atherosclerotic emboli in the distal basilar system have been found at autopsy in patients with vertebral artery plaques,[6] and our own intraoperative experience has shown us that ulceration can occur in vertebral artery plaques, but there are no available data regarding the frequency of VBI secondary to atherosclerotic emboli.

Our experience with 23 cases of vertebral origin stenosis, associated in most cases with compromise of the opposite vertebral artery, is summarized in Table 205-2. Experience with several different types of vertebral origin surgery has shown us that, in our hands, vertebral–carotid transposition is the operation of choice for this condition, because it avoids the torsion and double anastomosis necessary for subclavian–vertebral artery vein grafts. Most patient's symptoms have improved or disappeared, and morbidity has been limited for the most part to the development of Horner's syndrome, which in all but two cases was transient. As advocated by Ogawa et al.,[11] vertebral–subclavian transposition achieved very impressive results; however, there may be some tension at the anastomosis site, which does not occur with vertebral–carotid transposition. We have, additionally, had experience with 13 patients who had ipsilateral vertebral and internal carotid artery stenosis (Table 205-3). In these cases we perform the vertebral–carotid transposition prior to proceeding with a standard carotid endarterectomy, as suggested by Bohmfalk et al.,[4] in order to restore antegrade flow in the vertebral artery prior to occluding the carotid artery.

Atherosclerotic stenosis in the second (intraforaminal) portion of the vertebral artery may result from intrinsic narrowing due to a plaque[7] or from extrinsic compression due to cervical spondylosis.[10] Symptomatic stenosis in this portion of the artery is, in our experience, much less frequent than that in the more proximal or distal portions. There have been case reports describing the resection of osteophytes[10] to relieve extrinsic compression or bypasses[7] for the treatment of intrinsic stenosis. Direct endarterectomy of intrinsic stenosis in this portion of the artery is another alternative. We have performed this twice in two patients with stenosis at C5, with patency of the endarterectomies (Table 205-4 and Figs. 205-4 and 205-5).

Becker et al.,[3] in 1989, mentioned that the overwhelming majority of vertebral artery atherosclerotic stenoses are morphologically suitable for PTA, but that is role in the treatment was still uncertain. In 1993, Higashida et al.[9] reported improvement in symptoms in 39 or 42 patients (92.9 percent) after transluminal angioplasty of hemodynamically significantly stenosed (>70 percent) vertebral and basilar arteries.

Discussion about the choice between endovascular and open surgical treatment still continues. However, there are not enough data to make a final decision. In our experience the dilatation of the stenosis by PTA is incomplete, and concern for restenosis is real.

Distal Vertebral Stenosis

Atherosclerotic stenosis in the third and fourth portions of the vertebral artery may be either bypassed (occipital artery–PICA anastomosis) or dealt with directly (C1–intracranial vertebral endarterectomy). Those procedures are designed primarily to treat disease proximal to the origin of PICA. The bypass procedure may be

TABLE 205-3 Surgical Treatment of Vertebral Origin Stenosis and Ipsilateral Internal Carotid Stenosis

Operation	No. of Patients	Angiographic Patency	Postoperative Course	Permanent Complications
Vertebral–carotid transposition; carotid endarterectomy	13	13/13	13 better	1 recurrent laryngeal nerve injury 1 permanent Horner's syndrome

TABLE 205-4 Surgical Treatment of Midvertebral Stenosis

Operation	No. of Patients	Angiographic Patency	Postoperative Course	Permanent Complications
Midvertebral endarterectomy	2	2/2	Better	None

performed to treat either stenotic or occlusive disease proximal to PICA, and it is discussed elsewhere.[2] Direct intracranial vertebral endarterectomy can be used only for stenotic disease, but it has the advantages of providing a larger channel for blood flow and removing the atheroma, with its (at least theoretical) potential for embolization.

Surgical Technique

The operation is done with the patient in the three-quarters prone position, with the involved side down to facilitate viewing the lumen of the artery after the arteriotomy is performed. A midline incision is made from the inion to the spinous process of C5 and carried down to expose the laminae of C2 and C1. Dissection is then carried out in the region of the foramen magnum, and extended laterally until the vertebral artery is palpated. The vertebral artery is then carefully dissected from the surrounding tissue and freed of its surrounding venous plexus. A suboccipital craniectomy is then performed on the involved side to expose the vertebral artery as it enters the posterior fossa. This allows exposure of the vertebral artery as it penetrates the dura next to the condyle. The dura is then opened from the point at which the vertebral artery penetrates it, thereby exposing the full length of the vertebral artery. The arachnoid is then opened. A vessel loop is placed around the vertebral artery for the purposes of retraction and, if necessary, temporary occlusion. Clips are placed at appropriate locations on either side of the plaque, and a longitudinal arteriotomy is performed. A no. 11 bladed knife is used for this, and the incision is extended with microscissors. The plaque is then dissected circumferentially using a Penfield dissector and microdissectors. The plaque may be cut flush using microscissors if necessary, and luminal tags are removed using a microbiopsy forceps. After adequate irrigation with heparin, the arteriotomy is closed with a running no. 7–0 Prolene suture (Ethicon Inc., Somerville, NJ), and the incision is closed in layers in the usual manner.

Results

This operation was first reported by Allen et al. in 1981,[1] and experience with it has been limited to date. We have attempted six such endarterectomies and were able to complete five (Table 205-5, Figs. 205-6 and 205-7). The sixth resulted in ligation of the vertebral artery as a result of technical factors in the dissection of the plaque. Of the five successful intracranial vertebral endarterectomies, one patient died on 11th day after cerebellar infarction and acute hydrocephalus had developed. In this case the patency of the endarterectomized artery was not known. Of the remaining four patients, two had patent arteries after the surgery. Interestingly

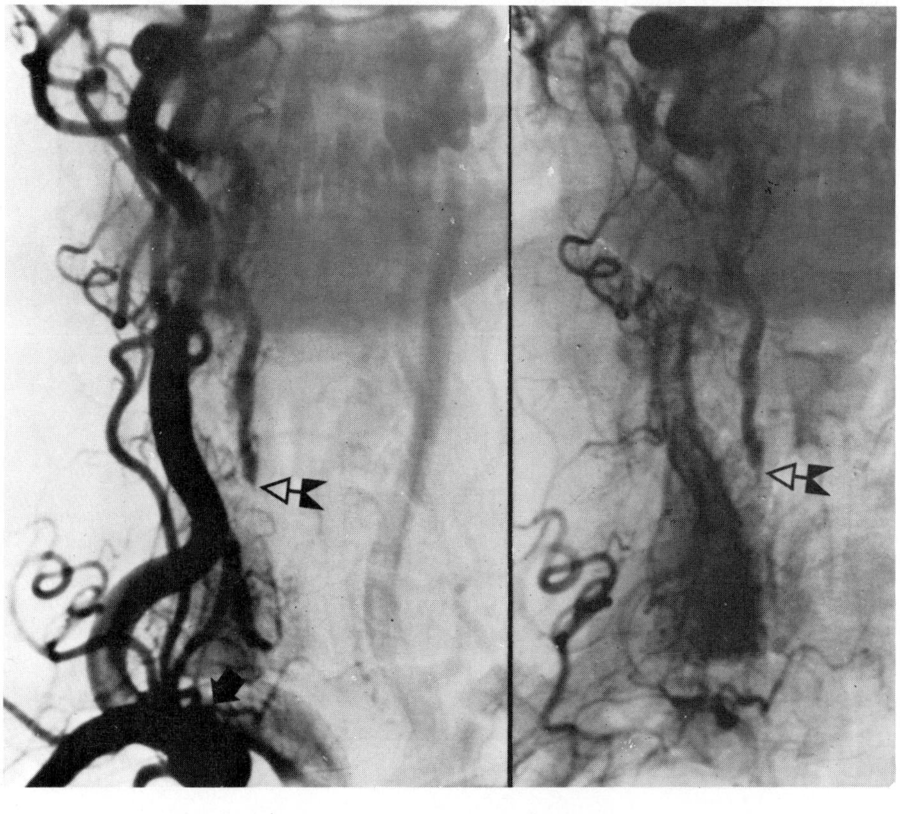

Figure 205-4 Right retrograde brachial cerebral angiograms demonstrating occlusion of the right vertebral artery at its origin (*solid arrow*) with reconstitution in the midcervical region (*open arrow*).

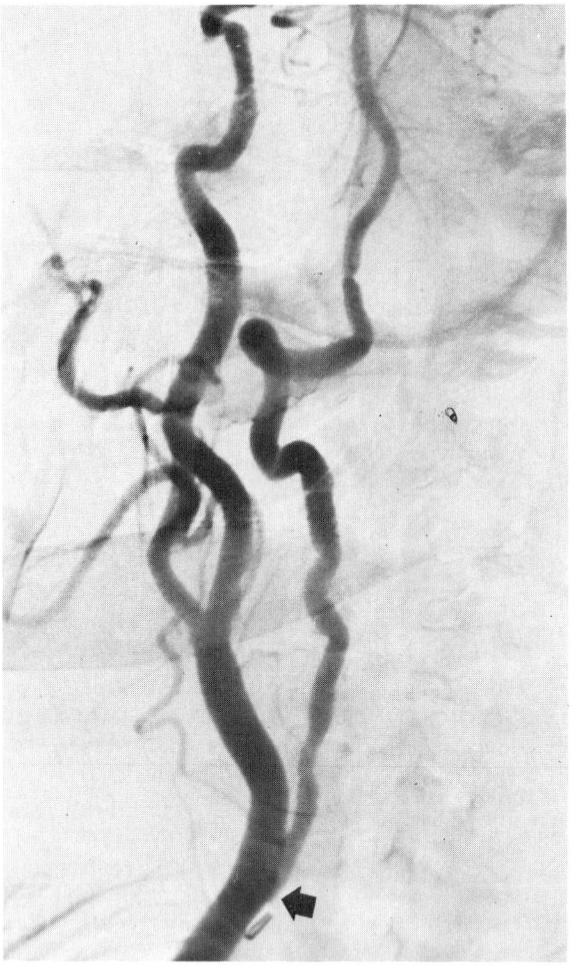

Figure 205-5 Postoperative right carotid angiogram (same patient as in Fig. 205-4) following endarterectomy of the right vertebral artery in the midcervical region and vertebral–carotid transposition. The *arrow* points to the site of anastomosis.

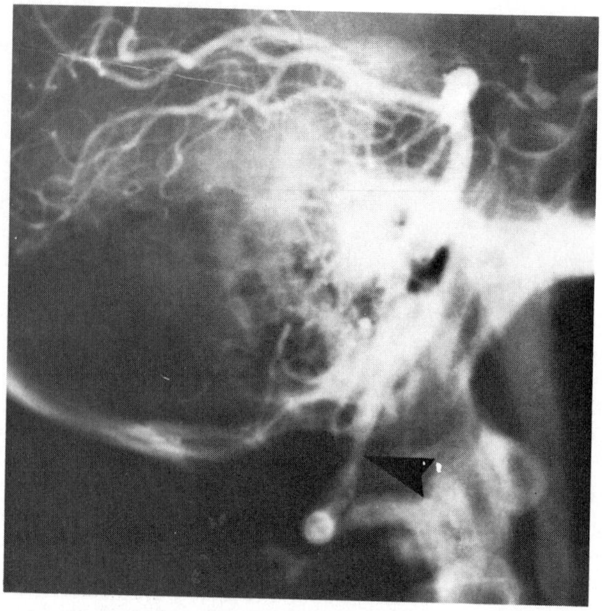

Figure 205-6 Preoperative right vertebral angiogram. The *arrowhead* points to the area of stenosis at the level of C1.

enough, three of these four patients were symptomatically improved, including the patient whose vertebral artery was not patent postoperatively, raising the possibility of embolization as a possible cause of the patient's intermittent ischemic symptoms. The fourth patient did improve after an occipital artery–PICA bypass was done. Our personal experience suggests that this is not a highly successful procedure and other methods of treatment should be pursued prior to consideration of this approach.

Conclusion

We have covered the surgical aspects of vertebral artery atherosclerosis. Although surgical procedures for the treatment of this disease have been performed since the late 1950s and early 1960s, it has only been with recent advances in neuroradiology and increased sophistication in diagnosis that adequate assessment of the entire vertebrobasilar system has been available on a routine basis. The indications for this type of surgery are, therefore, still in the stages of development. It is evident that full and complete diagnostic evaluation, including angiography, is essential before a rational management decision can be made for these patients. More data regarding the natural history of vertebral artery atherosclerosis in an angiogrammed population, as well as its course in populations treated medically and surgically, are needed. Pathologic and physiologic studies regarding the frequency of embolic versus hemodynamic causes of vertebrobasilar insufficiency are likewise necessary. In the meantime, however, one must make do with the available information when faced with a patient who meets the criteria for the diagnosis of vertebrobasilar insufficiency. Each case must be evaluated on an individual basis. Given a patient with vertebrobasilar insufficiency thought to be due to structural lesions

TABLE 205-5 Surgical Treatment of C1–Intracranial Vertebral Stenosis

Operation	No. of Patients	Angiographic Patency	Postoperative Course	Complications
Intracranial vertebral endarterectomy	5	2/4, 1 unknown	3 better 1 died 1 improved after occipital artery–PICA bypass	1 cerebellar infarction, hydrocephalus, death 1 CSF leak, meningitis
Intracranial vertebral artery ligation	1	—	1 worse	Wallenberg's syndrome

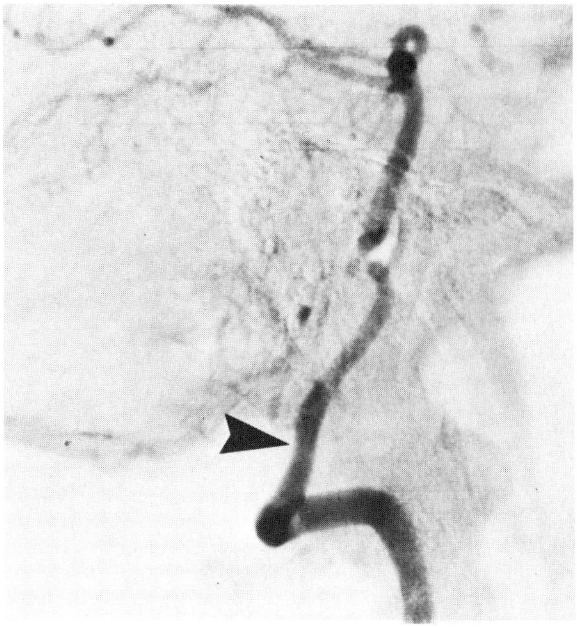

Figure 205-7 Postoperative right vertebral angiogram (same patient as in Fig. 205-6). The *arrowhead* points to the site of endarterectomy.

in the vertebral system, the surgical choices include vertebral to carotid transposition for the subclavian steal syndrome and for vertebral origin disease, decompression or bypass for disease in the intraforaminal portion of the artery, and bypass or direct endarterectomy for lesions in the distal vertebral artery. Further experience will reveal whether these operations are reasonable therapeutic alternatives in the management of vertebrobasilar insufficiency due to vertebral artery disease.

References

1. Allen GS, Cohen RJ, Prezoisi, TJ. Microsurgical endarterectomy of the intracranial vertebral artery for vertebrobasilar transient ischemic attacks. *Neurosurgery* 1981; 8:56–59.
2. Ausman JI, Diaz FG, Vacca DF, Sadasivan B. Superficial temporal and occipital artery bypass pedicles to superior, anterior inferior, and posterior inferior cerebellar arteries for vertebrobasilar insufficiency. *J Neurosurg* 1990; 72:554–558.
3. Becker GJ, Katzen BT, Dake MD. Noncoronary angioplasty. *Radiology* 1989; 170:921–940.
4. Bohmfalk GL, Story JL, Brown WE Jr, Marlin AE. Subclavian steal syndrome: Part I. Proximal vertebral to common carotid artery transposition in three patients, and historical review. *J Neurosurg* 1979; 51:628–640.
5. Cartlidge NEF, Whisnant JP, Elveback LR. Carotid and vertebral-basilar transient cerebral ischemic attacks: a community study, Rochester, Minnesota. *Mayo Clin Proc.* 1977; 52:117–120.
6. Castaigne P, Lhermitte F, Gautier JC, et al. Arterial occlusions in the vertebro-basilar system: a study of 44 patients with post-mortem data. Brain 1973; 96:133–154.
7. Corkill G, French BN, Michas C, et al. External carotid-vertebral artery anastomosis for vertebrobasilar insufficiency. *Surg Neurol* 1977; 7:109–115.
8. Hebrang A, Maskovic J, Tomac B. Percutaneous transluminal angioplasty of the subclavian arteries: long-term results in 52 patients. *Am J Roentgenol* 1991; 156:1091–1094.
9. Higashida RT, Tsai FY, Halbach VV, et al. Transluminal angioplasty for atherosclerotic disease of the vertebral and basilar arteries. *J Neurosurg* 1993; 78:192–198.
10. Nagashima C. Surgical treatment of vertebral artery insufficiency caused by cervical spondylosis. *J Neurosurg* 1970; 32:512–521.
11. Ogawa A, Yoshimoto T, Sakurai Y. Treatment of proximal vertebral artery stenosis. Vertebral to subclavian transposition. *Acta Neurochir (Wien)* 1991; 112:13–18.

206 Moyamoya Disease

David G. Piepgras
Keisuke Ueki

Starting in the late 1950s, individual case reports, particularly from Japan, accumulated concerning patients with progressive narrowing or occlusion of both internal carotid arteries associated with a fine network of neovascularity at the base of the brain. In 1968, Kudo first introduced the disease in the English literature as "spontaneous occlusion of the circle of Willis."[13] Later in the same year, Nishimoto and Takeuchi also described this disease with an extensive review of 96 cases.[19] Suzuki and Takaku first used the term "moyamoya disease" in the literature in their article of 1969, using the Japanese word "moyamoya" to describe the hazy, puff-of-smoke appearance of the neovascularization which develops and may be a prominent feature on cerebral angiography.[25] Since then, this entity has been widely known as "moyamoya disease."

Subsequent case reports, series analyses, and study of pathologic material have led to a clearer, but as yet incomplete, understanding of this rare condition. It now appears that the radiographic moyamoya appearance, which is due to numerous dilated collaterals of the basal perforating arteries and arterioles, is nonspecific and may be seen with chronic occlusive processes of the intracranial carotid circulation that arise from a variety of causes, including atherosclerosis, meningitis, sickle cell anemia, and radiation therapy.[23,24] Clearly, there is a distinct entity, moyamoya disease, that occurs most frequently in Japanese people but affects other populations as well, both children and adults and, seemingly, females more than males. The cause of moyamoya disease remains unknown, and theories of inflammatory and immunologic pathophysiologic mechanisms remain unproven. There is strong evidence for hereditary factors in the disease, with familial cases being reported especially among the Japanese but also from Europe and in identical twins. It has also been reported that children with Down's syndrome have a heightened risk for moyamoya disease.[5]

Radiologic Features

The diagnosis of moyamoya disease is made on the basis of angiographic findings, the features and progression of which have been well described by Suzuki and Takaku.[25] In its earliest stage there is stenosis of the supraclinoid portion of the internal carotid artery, frequently bilaterally. With progression, there develops some dilation of the main intracerebral arteries, and basal perforating vessels begin to enlarge to form the characteristic moyamoya. Carotid stenoses progress to occlusions, and there is extension of the occlusive process to the middle and anterior cerebral arteries with development of leptomeningeal collaterals and intensification of the moyamoya. This basal vascular network is contributed to by lenticulostriate, choroidal, thalamoperforating, premammillary, and thalamogeniculate arteries as well as by unnamed branches arising directly from the circle of Willis.

Later there may be extension of the occlusion into the posterior communicating and posterior cerebral arteries, with reduction of some of the moyamoya. Conversely, there is enlargement of extracranial transdural collaterals, including meningeal branches; superficial temporal, occipital, and internal maxillary arteries from the external carotid system; and ethmoidal, recurrent meningeal, and anterior falcine arteries from the ophthalmic circulation. Figures 206-1 and 206-2 show typical angiographic changes. In the late stages of the disease, there may be complete obliteration of the internal carotid artery intracranially, disappearance of the moyamoya, and complete dependence of the cerebral circulation on external carotid collaterals and the vertebrobasilar circulation. Serial angiography in moyamoya disease has shown progressive changes in most childhood cases, whereas the process is less predictable in adults and may arrest itself at any stage or, rarely, show some spontaneous improvement.[25]

Although not diagnostic, computed tomography may show characteristic changes, including multiple low-density areas in the brain and more general atrophy. With contrast enhancement, tortuous curvilinear vessels in the basal ganglia and cortical surface may be seen, corresponding to the moyamoya and leptomeningeal collaterals (Fig. 206-3). The proximal portions of the anterior and middle cerebral arteries are often poorly visualized.[26] Magnetic resonance imaging has proved to be superior to CT scanning in demonstrating the characteristic changes of moyamoya disease including the multiple collateral vessels in the basal ganglia, stenosis and occlusion of the major trunks, and parenchymal changes including both ischemic infarctions (predominantly in watershed regions) as well as evidence of previous hemorrhage.[4]

Pathology

The pathologic changes of the stenotic and occluded vessels of moyamoya disease are nonspecific, the most prominent features being intimal thickening and hyperplasia with irregularities and reduplication of the internal elastic lamina.[25] There is no evidence of inflammatory vasculitis per se. The moyamoya vessels appear to be markedly dilated intracerebral perforating arteries and arterioles. Aside from marked dilation, these vessels may be histologically normal; however, certain reports have noted pathologic changes, including marked thinning of the wall, mural fibrin deposits, fragmented elastic lamina, and microaneurysm formation.[23,24,27,30] These changes seem to predispose the perforating arteries to rupture, and according to Yamashita and colleagues,[30] they are the most likely cause of massive hemorrhage.

Hoshimaru and Kikuchi have found arterial segmental stenosis in extracranial vessels in 13 of the 66 moyamoya cases that they studied, which suggests that systemic factors may contribute to the pathogenesis of this condition.[6] Further, intriguing studies on patients undergoing surgery for moyamoya disease have found increased levels of basic fibroblast growth factor (FGF) in scalp arteries and dura and an altered response of cultured smooth muscle cells to platelet-derived growth factor.[1,6,7] The significance of

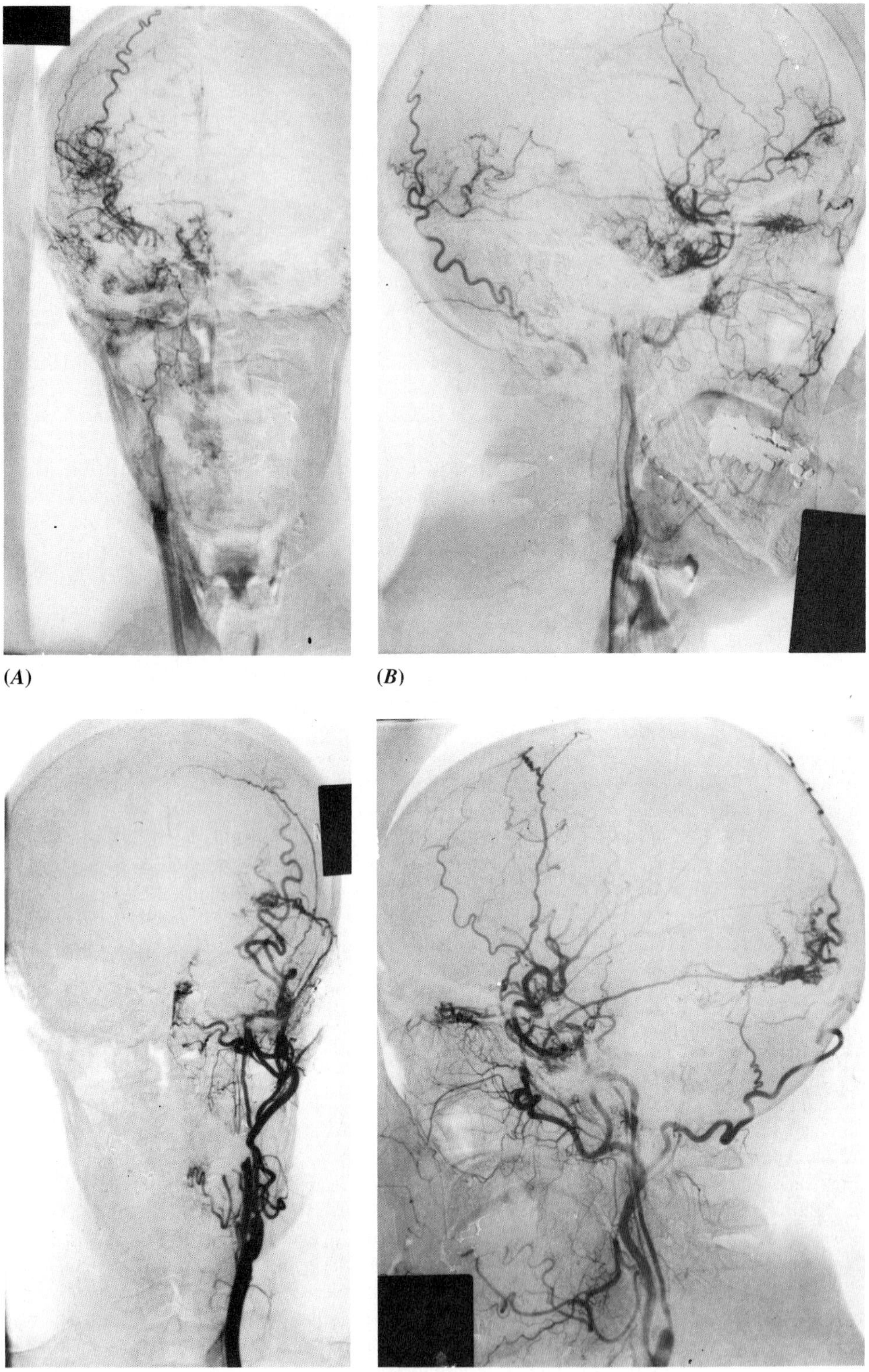

(*A*) (*B*)

(*C*) (*D*)

Figure 206-1 Bilateral carotid angiograms in a 52-year-old woman with moyamoya disease. The right carotid angiogram, anteroposterior (*A*) and lateral (*B*) views, shows occlusion of the entire right internal carotid artery and extensive external carotid and ophthalmic system collateralization. There is mild moyamoya development. The left carotid angiogram, anteroposterior (*C*) and lateral (*D*) views, shows left internal carotid occlusion at the level of the clinoid and similar extensive extracranial-to-intracranial collaterals.

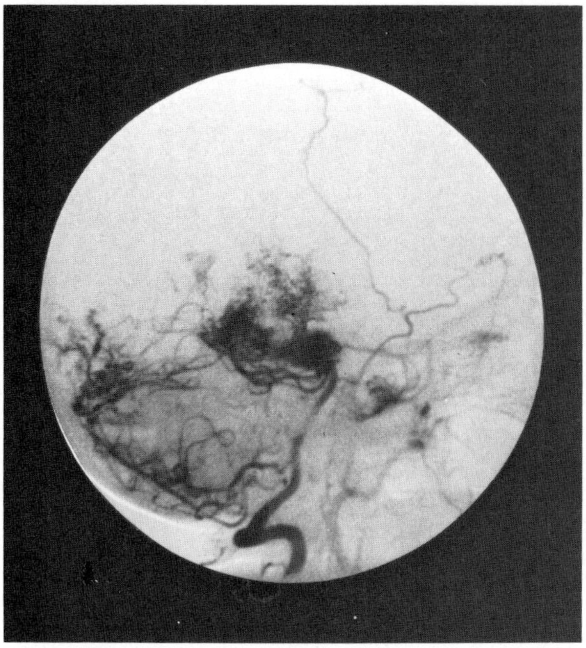

Figure 206-2 Vertebral angiogram, lateral view, of the patient shown in Fig. 206-1 showing normal vertebral and basilar arteries with extensive moyamoya development from the posterior choroidal and posterior perforating vessels.

these findings remains uncertain; however, a very important question is whether the increased levels of basic FGF are a secondary response to intracranial ischemia or a manifestation of a primary genetic change and the cause of pathologic changes in the intracranial arterial vasculature.[7]

Clinical Features

The age of onset of moyamoya disease shows a bimodal distribution, with one peak in the first decade of life and the other in the fourth decade.[23] In most cases, these patients present with either brain ischemia or hemorrhage. In children, the most typical symptoms are ischemic, consisting of recurrent, sometimes alternating episodes of focal cerebral deficit, especially hemiparesis but also speech and sensory disturbances. Seizures and involuntary movement disorders are also more common in children. It has been stated that the severity of moyamoya disease varies inversely with the age of onset; it is most severe in young children, in whom it may produce a progressive course of motor deficit and intellectual deterioration.[3] Although repeated ischemic attacks and stroke are the major cause of morbidity in children, mortality is most commonly related to intracranial hemorrhage. Such hemorrhage may be subarachnoid in location, but in most cases it occurs either within the brain in the basal ganglia or within the ventricular system.

In adult patients, intracranial hemorrhage is the most common presenting event, although ischemic symptoms may also occur. Hemorrhages may be caused by several different pathologic processes. Two sources of hemorrhage, moyamoya vessels and pseudoaneurysms, are peculiar to moyamoya disease. Bleeding may also occur from saccular aneurysms, which have a predilection for the vertebrobasilar circulation.

As already mentioned, the mechanism of hemorrhage may often be a breakdown of the greatly dilated perforating moyamoya vessels that form the extensive basal collateral network.[30] Pseudoaneurysms have also been described in cases of hemorrhage. They are identified angiographically as discrete vascular dilations, typically arising from the peripheral portions of the perforating and anterior and posterior choroidal arteries in a paraventricular loca-

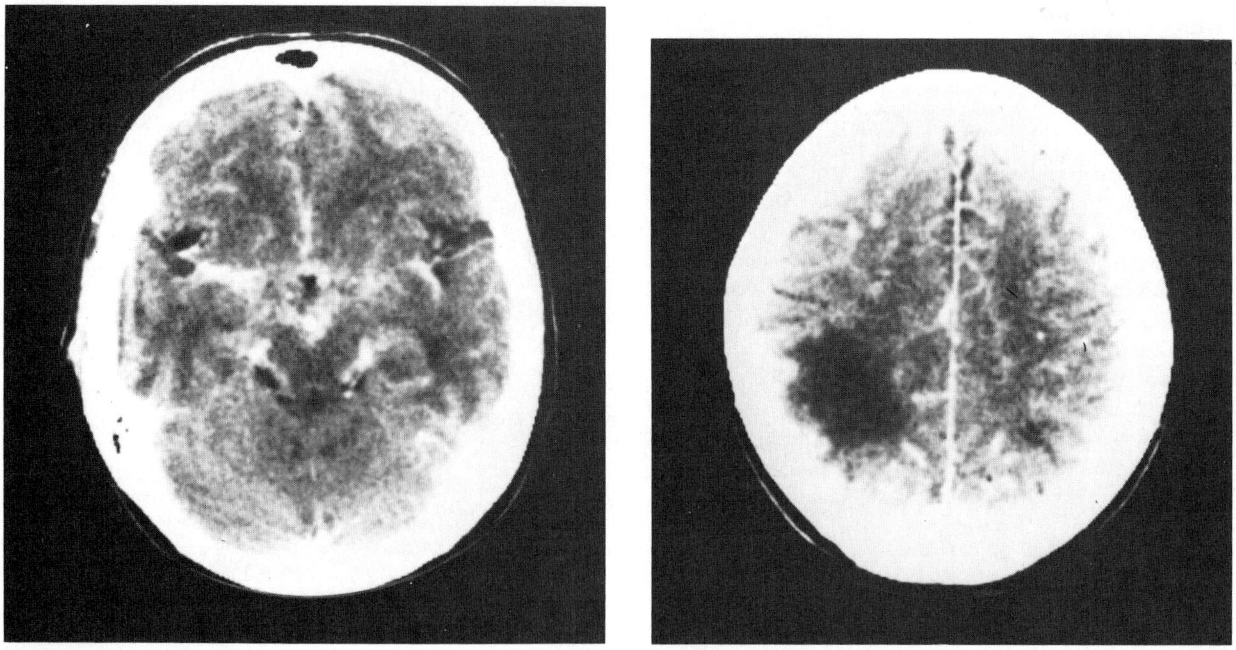

(A) *(B)*

Figure 206-3 A contrast enhanced CT scan of the same patient shown in Figs. 206-1 and 206-2 showing extensive basal collateral (moyamoya) vessels on the lower cut (*A*). On the higher cut (*B*), large right and smaller left parietal infarcts are present, and enlarged leptomeningeal collateral channels are visualized on the cortical surfaces.

tion.[11,18,24] It has been postulated that these pseudoaneurysms form along the abnormally dilated collaterals as a result of hemodynamic stress.[28,30] Commonly they will have disappeared by the time of follow-up angiography.

Saccular aneurysms also have been demonstrated in association with moyamoya disease. In a review of 903 cases, Nishimoto and colleagues found an incidence of aneurysm of 1 percent (4/391) in children and 6.2 percent (32/512) in adults.[20] Most of these aneurysms occur on major arterial trunks; however, they may also occur in smaller peripheral vessels. Nagamine and colleagues, like others, have found most of the major artery aneurysms to be located in the posterior circulation.[18] This increased frequency of vertebrobasilar aneurysms has also been attributed to hemodynamic factors of increased flow in the posterior circulation in these patients with compromised carotid circulation.

Physiologic Studies

In a study of 40 patients, including both adults and children, Ogawa and colleagues[22] reported a significant reduction in regional cerebral blood flow in patients with moyamoya disease compared to normal individuals. Cerebral blood flow measurements tended to be higher in the posterior head region, a tendency that increased with progression of the disease. These authors also documented an impairment in the autoregulatory response to hypotension and to hypercapnia, particularly in younger patients.[21] Positron emission tomography has been applied to the study of moyamoya disease but as yet has provided little additional insight into the pathophysiology.[23]

Therapy

Ischemia

Because of either limited experience or lack of success, there is little information regarding medical therapies for moyamoya disease, although Krayenbühl does allude to reported good results from vasodilator therapy.[12] It is clear, however, that at present no definitive treatment for moyamoya disease exists. Suzuki and Kodama have carried out perivascular sympathectomy and superior cervical ganglionectomy in the treatment of 48 patients, reporting ''encouraging'' results, with improvement in 61 percent of children and 47 percent of adults.[23,24] Other authorities have questioned the efficacy of such procedures, however.

Selected patients suffering from recurrent or progressive focal cerebral ischemic events in the distribution of an occluded or stenotic carotid artery have been successfully treated with superficial temporal-to-middle cerebral artery (STA-MCA) anastomosis.[8,29] Boone and Samson reported dramatic resolution of ischemic symptoms in one patient treated with a bypass. The improved venous drainage and the decrease in the moyamoya disclosed by follow-up angiograms were attributed to improved cerebral perfusion as well.[2] Karasawa and colleagues have reported on their extensive series of juvenile patients treated with a combination of STA-MCA anastomoses and/or encephalomyosynangiosis (EMS—a temporal muscle flap applied directly to the pial surface).[8] In a subsequent report by Karasawa and colleagues on 104 juvenile cases with a mean follow-up of 9.6 years, an excellent response with improved neurological condition was reported in 84 percent of the patients.[9] The ultimate neurological outcome was reported as good in 79 cases; 13 had moderate disability, 9 had severe disability, and 2 were in a persistent vegetative state. Psychometric testing was also carried out, with IQ reported as normal in 66 patients, borderline in 19, mildly decreased in 9, moderately decreased in 4, and severely or profoundly decreased in 7. These authors found that an onset of symptoms before age 6 and preoperative major stroke were associated with a poor outcome in spite of treatment.

Encephaloduroarteriosynangiosis (EDAS—direct application of a segment of the STA and adjacent strip of galea to the pial surface) was proposed as a treatment by Matsushima et al. in 1981.[15] Although this procedure was successful in producing effective indirect arterial anastomoses and improvement in symptoms,[14] the most recent review and series comparison by the authors[16] clearly demonstrated that STA-MCA anastomosis combined with EMS gives better results than the other procedures and led the authors to recommend this combined direct and indirect anastomotic procedure as the treatment of choice for symptomatic moyamoya disease in children. This viewpoint is also supported by the experience of Miyamoto et al. who found STA-MCA anastomosis with EMS to be the appropriate surgical treatment for refractory cases of moyamoya disease.[17]

In their most recent report, Karasawa et al.[10] described the limitations of the above procedures for ischemia in the anterior or posterior cerebral artery territories. They advocated omental transplantation as a more effective alternative in these specific situations.

Hemorrhage

Neurosurgical intervention may be indicated in the treatment of intracranial hemorrhage due to moyamoya disease. Indications for evacuation of intracerebral hematomas and ventricular drainage should follow the standard neurosurgical principles and guidelines used for patients without moyamoya disease. Operations directed at pseudoaneurysms are rarely indicated, however, inasmuch as these lesions usually obliterate themselves; follow-up angiography is advised in these cases.[11] Occasionally, patients with moyamoya disease will sustain subarachnoid hemorrhage due to a saccular aneurysm, and surgery directed at repair of these lesions, assuming the aneurysm is the likely source of hemorrhage, may be advisable. The surgeon must be aware, however, that the presence of moyamoya vessels may limit the exposure and increase the risks of ischemic complications in these patients.[18]

References

1. Aoyagi M, Fukai N, Sakamoto H, et al. Altered cellular responses to serum mitogens, including platelet-derived growth factor, in cultured smooth muscle cells derived from arteries of patients with moyamoya disease. *J Cell Physiol* 1991; 147:191–198.
2. Boone SC, Samson DS. Observation on moyamoya disease: a case treated with superficial temporal-middle cerebral artery anastomosis. *Surg Neurol* 1978; 9:189–193.
3. Carlson CB, Harvey FH, Loop J. Progressive alternating hemiplegia in early childhood with basal arterial stenosis and telangiectasia (moyamoya syndrome). *Neurology* 1973; 23:734–744.
4. Chang KH, Yi JG, Han MH, Kim IO. MR imaging findings of moyamoya disease. *J Korean Med Sci* 1990; 5:85–90.

5. Fukushima Y, Kondo Y, Kuroki Y, et al. Are Down syndrome patients predisposed to moyamoya disease? *Eur J Pediatr* 1986; 144:516–517.
6. Hoshimaru M, Kikuchi H. Involvement of the external carotid arteries in moyamoya disease: neuroradiological evaluation of 66 patients *Neurosurgery* 1992; 31:398–400.
7. Hoshimaru M, Takahashi JA, Kikuchi H, et al. Possible roles of basic fibroblast growth factor in the pathogenesis of moyamoya disease: an immunohistochemical study. *J Neurosurg* 1991; 75:267–270.
8. Karasawa J, Kikuchi H, Furuse S, et al. Treatment of moyamoya disease with STA-MCA anastomosis. *J Neurosurg* 1978; 49:679–688.
9. Karasawa J, Touho H, Ohnishi H, et al. Long-term follow-up study after extracranial-intracranial bypass surgery for anterior circulation ischemia in childhood moyamoya disease. *J Neurosurg* 1992; 77:84–89.
10. Karasawa J, Touho H, Ohnishi H, et al. Cerebral revascularization using omental transplantation for childhood moyamoya disease. *J Neurosurg* 1993; 79:192–196.
11. Kodama N, Suzuki J. Moyamoya disease associated with aneurysm. *J Neurosurg* 1978; 48:565–569.
12. Krayenbühl HA. The moyamoya syndrome and the neurosurgeon. *Surg Neurol* 1975; 4:353–360.
13. Kudo T. Spontaneous occlusion of the circle of Willis. A disease apparently confined to Japanese. *Neurology* 1968; 18:485–496.
14. Matsushima Y, Aoyagi M, Koumo Y, et al. Effects of encephalo-duro-arterio-synangiosis on childhood moyamoya patients—swift disappearance of ischemic attacks and maintenance of mental capacity. *Neurol Med Chir (Tokyo)* 1991; 31:708–714.
15. Matsushima Y, Fukai N, Tanaka K, et al. A new surgical treatment of moyamoya disease in children: a preliminary report *Surg Neurol* 1981; 15:313–320.
16. Matsushima T, Inoue T, Suzuki SO, et al. Surgical treatment of moyamoya disease in pediatric patients—comparison between the results of indirect and direct revascularization procedures. *Neurosurgery* 1992; 31:401–405.
17. Miyamoto S, Kikuchi H, Karasawa J, et al. Pitfalls in the surgical treatment of moyamoya disease. Operative techniques for refractory cases. *J Neurosurg* 1988; 68:537–543.
18. Nagamine Y, Takahashi S, Sonobe M. Multiple intracranial aneurysms associated with moyamoya disease: case report. *J Neurosurg* 1981; 54:673–676.
19. Nishimoto A, Takeuchi S. Abnormal cerebrovascular network related to the internal carotid arteries. *J Neurosurg* 1968; 29:255–260.
20. Nishimoto A, Ueta K, Onbe H. Cooperative study on moyamoya disease in Japan. *Abstracts of 10th Meeting on Surgery for Stroke*. Tokyo: Nyuuron-sha, 1981, pp 53–58.
21. Ogawa A, Nakamura N, Yoshimoto T, Suzuki J. Cerebral blood flow in moyamoya disease. Part 2: autoregulation and CO_2 response. *Acta Neurochir (Wien)* 1990; 105:107–111.
22. Ogawa A, Yoshimoto T, Suzuki J, Sakurai Y. Cerebral blood flow in moyamoya disease. Part 1: correlation with age and regional distribution. *Acta Neurochir (Wien)* 1990; 105:30–34.
23. Suzuki J. *Moyamoya Disease*. Berlin: Springer-Verlag, 1986.
24. Suzuki J, Kodama N. Moyamoya disease: a review. *Stroke* 1983; 14:104–109.
25. Suzuki J, Takaku A. Cerebrovascular ''moyamoya'' disease: disease showing abnormal net-like vessels in base of brain. *Arch Neurol* 1969; 20:288–299.
26. Takahashi M, Miyauchi T, Kowada M. Computed tomography of moyamoya disease: demonstration of occluded arteries and collateral vessels as important diagnostic signs. *Radiology* 1980; 134:671–676.
27. Takeuchi K, Hara M, Yokota H, et al. Factors influencing the development of moyamoya phenomenon. *Acta Neurochir (Wien)* 1981; 59:79–86.
28. Tanaka Y, Takeuchi K, Akai K. Intracranial ruptured aneurysm accompanying moyamoya phenomenon. *Acta Neurochir (Wien)* 1980; 52:35–43.
29. Ueki K, Meyer FB, Mellinger JF. Moyamoya disease: the disorder and surgical treatment. Subject review. *Mayo Clin Proc* 1994; 69:749–754.
30. Yamashita M, Oka K, Tanaka K. Histopathology of the brain vascular network in moyamoya disease. *Stroke* 1983; 14:50–58.

207 Medical Management of Ischemic Cerebral Vascular Disease

James N. Davis
Oded Gerber

Diagnosis of Acute Neurological Deficit

The first step in evaluating a patient with an acute neurological deficit is to come to a hypothesis about the pathophysiology underlying the deficit. Traditionally an attempt is made to classify patients with strokes into those with hemorrhages, thrombotic infarctions, or embolic infarctions. A few patients present with strokes from unusual causes. To arrive at the best understanding of pathophysiology, the clinician uses the history, sequential physical examinations, imaging studies, and laboratory tests.

In addition to the pathophysiologically based classification of stroke patients, a clinical classification based on the timing of the neurological deficit is also used. The terms *transient ischemic attack* (TIA), *reversible ischemic neurological deficit* (RIND), *stroke-in-evolution* (evolving stroke), and *completed stroke* refer to the tempo of the onset and resolution of the neurological deficit rather than to its underlying pathology. TIA was originally defined as complete resolution of symptoms within 24 h. With the advent of modern imaging techniques, it is now recognized that at least 50 percent of TIA patients have cerebral infarction. There is a reasonable relationship between the size of the infarct and the recovery rate, such that small infarcts (lacunes) commonly present as TIAs. Because TIAs are often associated with strokes, the more modern term *reversible ischemic neurological deficit* was defined. Patients with RINDs have a complete or nearly complete recovery, like TIA patients, but they may take longer than 24 h to recover.

Approximately 60 percent of patients report progression after the initial symptoms. In around 30 percent, this evolution occurs in the hospital and is classified as a stroke-in-evolution. It is important to recognize stroke-in-evolution, since, in many centers, it is treated with immediate anticoagulation (see below). Evolution of a stroke will usually occur at any time within 24 h after an anterior circulation event and 72 h after a stroke in the posterior circulation. Because of the potential for evolution, it is important that patients with stroke be observed closely, ideally in the hospital.

Stroke in the Young Adult

Patients under the age of 40 without a history of diabetes or a history of hypertension rarely suffer a stroke from atherosclerotic cerebrovascular disease. The most common cause of stroke in this population is cardiac emboli, but cocaine use, arterial dissections, fibromuscular dysplasia, and coagulation disorders must be carefully considered. Early arteriographic studies are often necessary in these patients to document the presence of emboli, and they can give important information about other causes of stroke as well. Echocardiography and special coagulation studies are frequently useful in the young adult with stroke. Arterial dissection and drug abuse, particularly cocaine and crack use, are more frequent causes of stroke than atherosclerosis in this age group.

Classification and Evaluation of Ischemic Cerebral Vascular Diseases

Infarction

Embolic Infarction

It has been increasingly recognized that many cerebral infarctions are embolic. Early classifications underestimated the frequency of embolic causes until it was recognized that thrombosis of the middle cerebral artery is a relatively infrequent event. A characteristic of embolic infarcts is the eventual lysis of the clot with reperfusion of the damaged distal vasculature. When lysis occurs, it can lead to bleeding into the substance of the infarct, producing a *hemorrhagic infarction.* Only 50 percent of hemorrhagic infarctions are detected on routine computed tomography (CT) scans, because they take time to develop and CT scans to look for hemorrhage are routinely performed early in the evaluation of stroke patients. The detection of a hemorrhagic infarction in a patient with a prior CT scan showing early infarction is termed a *hemorrhagic transformation.* The importance of identifying a hemorrhagic infarction lies in differentiating it from an intraparenchymal hemorrhage. The clinical significance of hemorrhagic transformation is not clear. In most cases, such a transformation is not associated with worsening or change in neurological symptoms.

It is important to identify the source of emboli. Evaluation of the large arteries supplying the brain can be done with reasonable efficiency using bimodal Doppler ultrasonography. However, noninvasive studies of the carotid can be negative when the source of emboli is in the carotid siphon above the neck. Thus, when an artery-to-artery embolus is considered likely, angiography may be necessary to determine the state of the artery and whether clot remains. Consideration should also be given to a careful evaluation of the cardiac chambers and aortic arch with transesophageal echocardiography (see below). In the event that a source of emboli is not found by these studies, one might evaluate the venous system as a source of paradoxical emboli through a patent foramen ovale.

Thrombotic Infarction

Thrombosis occurs in either *large arteries* or *small arteries.* Large-artery thrombosis is most common in the internal carotid in association with carotid stenosis. Thrombosis in the vertebral and basilar arteries is the cause of most posterior cerebral infarctions. Thrombosis of the anterior cerebral or middle cerebral arteries is less common. It should be noted that occlusion of the anterior cerebral artery is almost always thrombotic, while occlusion of the middle cerebral artery is usually embolic. Warning transient symptoms (TIAs or RINDs) are common in thrombotic occlusions and justify the search for narrowing of a large extracranial vessel in patients with these events.

There is increasing interest in thrombolysis of acute cerebral infarction, but in cases of moderate to severe stenosis, rethrombosis is likely after thrombolysis. The benefit of interventional correction of stenosis is being actively studied.

Small Artery Thrombotic Infarction

In contrast to the large-artery thrombotic and embolic events, small-artery thromboses often present with mild symptoms or TIAs. (However, such lesions can also be devastating depending on their location.) With the advent of magnetic resonance imaging (MRI), small-vessel infarcts have been identified in more than 50 percent of individuals over the age of 65 years. Only some of these individuals have hypertension, leaving a significant population of nonhypertensive patients with small-artery thrombosis. In recent years, there has been suggestive evidence that platelet clumps can produce small-artery infarcts. These small infarcts may not be seen on CT scans.

Laboratory Studies

Routine

When a patient presents with an acute neurological deficit, laboratory investigation should include a complete blood count, liver function tests, renal function tests, plasma glucose concentration, and coagulation parameters in order to determine if any other organs are involved in the process that has produced the neurological deficit. In young patients with infarcts, it is important to screen for coagulation abnormalities such as protein C or protein S deficiency, the presence of a lupus anticoagulant, or the presence of homocystinuria.

Cardiac Studies

In patients suspected of having embolic infarction, careful study of the cardiac chambers is warranted. This study is best accomplished with transesophageal echocardiography (TEE). TEE provides good images not only of the left side of the heart but also of the ascending aorta. The presence of a patent foramen ovale can be detected by the microinjection of small quantities of air into the venous circulation during the TEE examination. (A full discussion of noninvasive diagnostic tests is found elsewhere in this textbook.)

Intracranial and Extracranial Doppler Studies

Doppler ultrasonography studies of the extracranial carotid arteries are frequently requested. The examination has good, but not perfect, sensitivity and specificity. Furthermore, there is considerable variability between carotid ultrasound laboratories. If embolic infarction is suspected and no cardiac source is identified, carotid Doppler studies will often help in identifying sources of emboli in these arteries. The finding of significant (>70 percent) stenosis in a carotid study of a stroke patient is more difficult to evaluate. If the patient has suffered a severe, paralytic stroke in the distribution of the stenotic artery, surgery should be withheld for at least 3 months to allow the patient to recover from the stroke, because immediate surgery can produce an intraparenchymal hemorrhage in the area of a large infarction. In these patients, arteriography and ultrasound studies should be done later, when the surgery would be performed.

Transcranial Doppler studies have been widely employed in patients with stroke and can give information about the relative flow and patency of the middle cerebral arteries and, less often, the basilar and vertebral arteries. These studies suffer from a lack of standardization and thus cannot be reliably used to decide on specific treatments.

Radiologic Studies

A full discussion of imaging in cerebral vascular diseases is found elsewhere in this textbook. What follows is a brief discussion of the use of imaging in the medical management of patients presenting with ischemic cerebral vascular disease.

Computed Tomography

A CT scan is usually performed in the emergency room when a patient with an acute neurological deficit is seen. It has the advantage of being very sensitive to the presence of blood and, thus, is useful for distinguishing hemorrhage from infarct. CT scans are often done for convenience in the event of complications after a stroke. MRI scanning will almost always give more information, but for reasons of cost and convenience, CT is often used to evaluate progressing strokes and other complications. It is well established that small to medium-sized infarcts are not easily appreciated on CT scans in the first few hours after the infarction. Larger infarcts may cause sulcal effacement and loss of a readily discernible gray–white matter junction after a few hours. The identification of a large infarct is very important for planning therapy (see below).

Magnetic Resonance Imaging

Except in the acute period, MRI is the preferred imaging technique for studying cerebral infarcts and hemorrhages. Within a few hours after an infarction, T2-weighted MR scans will show hyperintensities at and around the area of infarction. MRI is sensitive enough to reveal small infarcts and is better than CT at visualizing the posterior fossa. MRI does require patient cooperation, which is often not possible in the acute setting.

Magnetic Resonance Angiography

Significant technical advances have made it possible to obtain reasonable images of the cerebral arteries by magnetic resonance angiography. This technique has the advantages of being noninvasive and giving a more detailed picture of the vasculature than can be obtained with duplex scanning. However, it often underestimates the diameter of blood vessels. This tendency results from the fact that magnetic resonance angiography measures blood flow, rather than blood per se, and therefore (depending on the protocol) may fail to image the slow-flowing blood near the periphery of an artery (laminar flow). The technique is thus useful as a screening test, because it will not miss vessel narrowing, but a finding of stenosis may need to be confirmed by angiography if therapy is contemplated.

Digital Subtraction Angiography

X-ray angiography remains the gold standard for defining vascular lesions such as emboli, vasculitis, and atherosclerotic narrowing. Digital subtraction techniques make it possible to use less contrast medium, thus presumably reducing the toxicity and risk of complications as compared to traditional ''cut film'' angiography.

Management of Acute Cerebral Infarction

Immediate Measures

Avoidance of Glucose Solutions

Over a decade ago, it was observed that primates who had been fasted before the production of an experimental cerebral infarction had smaller infarct sizes than animals who had been fed. These observations have been confirmed in a variety of species, and the phenomenon has been shown to be dependent on the plasma glucose concentration at the moment of vessel occlusion.[8,12] The mechanism appears to be related to the production of lactate in an infarcted area when the plasma glucose concentration is elevated. High lactate levels lead to tissue acidosis, which facilitates the development of free radicals, thus producing greater damage. Several epidemiologic studies have shown that the plasma glucose concentration at the time of infarction is an important predictor of infarct size and stroke severity, independent of other factors such as the presence or absence of diabetes or hypertension. Even though one large study was unable to confirm the association between glucose level and functional outcome after stroke,[6] it seems reasonable to avoid glucose solutions during the first 24 h after a patient presents with an anterior circulation cerebral infarction and for 72 h after a posterior circulation event. These are the periods during which evolution of the stroke may occur. It should be noted that it is the glucose concentration at the time of infarction that is critical in determining stroke severity, so the purpose of avoiding glucose is to prevent hyperglycemia at the time of any extension of the infarct. In brittle diabetic patients, it may be necessary to institute an insulin drip infusion to maintain the blood sugar level below 140 mg/dL during these critical times.

Caution with Respect to Oral Intake

In the past decade, silent aspiration in stroke patients has been increasingly recognized through fluoroscopic swallowing studies. Silent aspiration may not be detected by simple trials with liquids at the bedside. Aspiration should be suspected in patients with strokes that involve the pharyngeal, buccal, or facial musculature. Patients with facial palsy, dysarthia, or bulbar or pseudobulbar symptoms should be kept on nothing by mouth until evaluated by a speech therapist familiar with the diagnosis of silent aspiration or until a fluoroscopic swallowing study can be carried out. Special dysphagia diets with soft solid foods can help patients with potential silent aspiration through the first few days after a stroke until there is sufficient recovery of swallowing to allow a normal diet. Careful attention to the identification of silent aspirators can dramatically reduce the rate of aspiration pneumonia in stroke patients.

Neurological Monitoring

The treatment of the patient whose stroke evolves in the hospital remains somewhat controversial. There have been three prospective, randomized trials of heparin anticoagulation for stroke-in-evolution. Unfortunately, the studies are over 30 years old and were not done with the rigor of modern clinical trials. Each series showed a nonsignificant reduction of mortality in patients treated with anticoagulants compared to nonanticoagulated control patients. However, the numbers were small and the observers were not blinded to the treatment arm. Nonetheless, taken together, these studies do suggest a benefit from anticoagulation, and most centers use it for evolving stroke patients.

It thus becomes critical to know when a new stroke victim has progression of symptoms. Progression is best detected through frequent observation by experienced personnel. Stroke Acute Care Units (SACUs) with cardiac monitoring and sufficient nursing personnel to make frequent observations have been established at a number of medical centers. Prospective studies of patients randomized to such a unit compared to patients admitted to a regular ward have shown better outcomes with a shorter length of stay for patients in a SACU. The recent introduction of caremaps have further shortened length of stay and enhanced outcome. It appears that these improvements reflect earlier physical therapy, careful attention to avoiding glucose, care for potential aspirators, and prompt attention to evolving patients.

Fluid and Electrolyte Balance

Most stroke patients tend to lose fluid during the first few hours after an infarction. It is important to prevent hypovolemia by carefully monitoring the outputs. In most cases, intravenous replacement with 0.5 *N* saline is appropriate, as it avoids glucose solutions and helps maintain the patient on nothing by mouth. If the patient's cardiac and renal function can support larger volumes of fluid, it may be helpful to give in excess of 2 liters of fluid per day to prevent hypovolemia and its associated hyperviscosity.

Hyptertension

Stroke patients often are hypertensive during the first few days after an acute infarction. This condition occurs more often in hypertensive patients and may raise the question of intervention to lower the blood pressure. In general, administration of antihypertensive agents immediately after a stroke should be avoided at all costs. Many clinicians have observed progression of stroke symptoms associated with even a mild lowering of perfusion pressure during this critical time. Even hypertensive patients should have their medication withheld for a few days, since stroke is occasionally associated with correction of hypertension. Although the exact management remains controversial, most authorities would agree that intervention is unnecessary with diastolic pressures under 120 mmHg. A nitroglycerin patch can be conveniently applied to the patient whose blood pressure exceeds 120 mmHg, as the resulting vasodilation can be readily and rapidly reversed by removing the patch. For the rare refractory hypertensive patient, administration of other antihypertensives may be necessary.

Antiplatelet Agents

Aspirin remains the most widely prescribed antiplatelet agent used in the prevention of ischemic cerebral vascular disease. Although some physicians still prescribe two aspirin tablets twice a day (700 mg b.i.d.), as in the joint Canadian-American aspiring trial, one aspirin once a day (350 mg daily) has been shown to be as effective as the higher dose.[3,9] The latter dosage is associated with significantly fewer side effects than larger doses. Aspirin is used in patients with TIAs or RINDs and in those with atrial fibrillation. In TIA patients, aspirin reduces risk more effectively in men than in women, an effect that may have a biological basis or may be a statistical artifact resulting from the larger number of men in all trials. In patients with atrial fibrillation, aspirin alone has been proved to be effective in reducing stroke risk, but not as effective as warfarin.[1,7] Thus, anticoagulation is the recommended therapy for atrial fibrillation patients, but aspirin should be prescribed for those who cannot be put on anticoagulants. *Dipyramidole* has never proved useful in patients with cerebral vascular disease, in contrast to its efficacy in those with coronary disease.

Ticlopidine is a newer antiplatelet agent that is thought to work in a different way than aspirin. Several large trials of ticlopidine have shown it to be at least as effective as aspirin.[5] Ticlopidine administration clearly lowers stroke risk in women with TIAs or RINDs. In men, it is slightly more effective than aspirin. Unfortunately, ticlopidine is expensive and is associated with about a 20 percent rate of side effects. The principal side effects are rash and diarrhea, but rare neutropenia has been reported. Patients placed on ticlopidine require frequent blood tests during the first few months of therapy. If they can afford the medication and are free of side effects, it is probably a better choice than aspirin. Ticlopidine has not been tested in atrial fibrillation.

Anticoagulation

At present, anticoagulation with heparin or warfarin remains the primary mode of treatment for certain stroke syndromes and stroke complications (Table 207-1). Ideally, recommendations for anticoagulation should be based on careful, controlled studies.[10,11] However, reliable studies have not always been carried out, so one's confidence in the recommendation must be based on the quality of the studies that have been done. For example, anticoagulation of patients with valvular heart disease significantly reduces the risk of stroke and can be recommended with great confidence. Treatment for stroke-in-evolution probably reduces mortality in stroke patients, but only slight confidence should be placed in the studies that underlie this recommendation.

The syndrome of *crescendo TIAs* consists of a series of increasingly frequent transient attacks of neurological deficit in one vascular territory. Although rare and not vigorously studied, patients with crescendo TIAs are more likely to progress to a stroke and more likely to have embolic causes for their symptoms than patients with ordinary TIAs. Many of these patients suffer from a clot in a carotid artery, but a cardiac source for the emboli also occurs when symptoms relate to more than one vascular territory. Anticoagulation is indicated while a noninvasive evaluation with carotid duplex or MR angiography and, if those are negative, transesophageal echocardiography is being completed emergently. The presence of significant carotid stenosis may necessitate urgent carotid endarterectomy.

TABLE 207-1 Indications for Anticoagulation

Crescendo TIAs
Stroke-in-evolution
Cerebral emboli caused by
Atrial fibrillation
Valvular heart disease
Myocardial infarction
Paradoxical embolization

Definite cerebral emboli are an indication for anticoagulation in the presence of atrial fibrillation or valvular heart disease. Recent studies have indicated that the incidence of stroke can be reduced in these patients by the use of anticoagulation. Atrial fibrillation is occasionally diagnosed when the patient presents with a stroke and should be evaluated carefully. Anticoagulation of these stroke patients can prevent subsequent strokes.

About 3 percent of patients having *myocardial infarction* will also have a stroke. The cerebral infarction generally occurs 3 to 5 days after the myocardial infarction and is mainly seen in patients with myocardial infarcts involving the anterior wall. These types of myocardial infarcts develop subendocardial damage with accumulation of clot or can give rise to ventricular aneurysms with clot formation in areas of stagnant cardiac blood flow. The risk of a second stroke diminishes with time, so that anticoagulation is needed for only 3 to 4 months after a stroke in a patient with myocardial infarction.

Paradoxical embolism occurs when clots in the venous system gain entry to the arterial circulation by way of a right-to-left shunt, through either a patent foramen ovale, an atrial septal defect, or a ventricular septal defect. Paradoxical embolism is facilitated when there is a temporary increase in right atrial pressure associated with prior pulmonary embolism or with an event such as a cough. Estimates of a patent foramen ovale from autopsy studies range around 20 percent. A patent foramen ovale can be detected by the intravenous injection of a small bubble of air during echocardiography or transcranial or carotid ultrasonography. A diagnosis of paradoxical embolization should be treated as a medical emergency, and immediate anticoagulation considered. Anticoagulation should be continued until the venous thrombosis has resolved.

When Not to Anticoagulate

There are clear contraindications to anticoagulation. The most important is a large, lobar cerebral infarction. This recommendation stems from anecdotal reports of frank intraparenchymal hemorrhage after early anticoagulation in patients with such large infarcts. The presence of or a history of gastrointestinal, genitourinary, or respiratory bleeding are also contraindications for anticoagulation in stroke patients. Before anticoagulation is begun, the stool and urine should be checked for occult blood. Anticoagulation should be considered with caution in pregnant women with stroke, especially late in the pregnancy.

Treatment of Herniation after Cerebral Infarction

Transtentorial herniation is the most frequent neurological cause of death in the acute period after cerebral infarction or hemorrhage. The mechanism by which cytotoxic and, to a lesser extent, vasogenic edema occurs in infarction is not well understood. The edema begins to be clinically significant 8 to 12 h after the infarction and usually subsides in 24 h if no secondary ischemic damage occurs. Clinically, the patient may appear drowsy, and occasionally a contraleteral Babinski response will signal subfalcian herniation. Any change in the level of consciousness of a patient after stroke should be investigated radiologically with either CT or MRI. Either study will disclose the presence of herniation if it is the cause of the change in mental status. If herniation is present, aggressive treatment of the edema should be considered if the patient becomes stuporous or comatose.

Intravenous mannitol is the first-line therapy. Unfortunately, mannitol infusions will reduce edema for only a few hours before the osmolarity of cerebrospinal fluid and that of blood re-equilibrate. If symptoms of herniation continue after mannitol administration, steroids are usually administered, although the evidence that steroids help in this situation is not convincing.

Endotrachael intubation and hyperventilation are also used, on the rationale that lowering the P_{CO_2} will produce cerebral vasoconstriction and thus lower the intracranial pressure. This theory assumes that the cerebral vasculature will autoregulate normally. However, the response of infarcted brain to changes in P_{CO_2} is unpredictable. The area of infarction may not be autoregulated and may thus still serve as a source for edema, while vasoconstriction of adjacent areas may impair collateral circulation and produce an extension of the infarct.

Early Physical Therapy

An important intervention in the stroke patient is early physical therapy. Patients should be encouraged to be as active as possible during the acute period after a stroke, as long as blood pressure is not affected by the activity. When paralysis prevents mobilization, active movements should be encouraged as much as possible, and passive range of motion should be performed on affected extremities. Recent studies in animals and humans have shown that certain drugs can have a profound effect on the recovery of function after brain injury (Table 207-2).[2,4] While there has not been direct clinical testing of the drugs that are detrimental to recovery in animals, it is wise to avoid these agents wherever possible.

New Treatments

As this chapter is being written, there is considerable excitement about a series of new agents currently in clinical trials. One group of agents are antithrombolytics, which are discussed in another chapter. Several groups of agents have been designed to protect neurons from ischemic damage during a cerebral infarction. One group are antagonists of the neurotransmitter glutamate. While effective in animal studies, these glutamate antagonists have had side effects in preliminary clinical trials. Nonetheless, full trials of some of these agents are under way. Free-radical scavengers are another class of agents that are showing promise in trials against other forms of brain injury and are currently being tested in stroke patients. Trials of calcium channel blockers have yielded mixed results, and these agents have not been generally recommended in the treatment of cerebral infarction. Other ongoing clinical trials include agents that change the viscosity of blood, that have antiplatelet properties, or that block endothelial cell adhesion. Finally, a full-scale trial of warfarin therapy after stroke is being carried out.

To date, these studies have supported the concept that early therapy of stroke is very important. A number of agencies have started campaigns to make the public more aware of the early signs of stroke and of the importance of seeking diagnosis when they occur. There is a general feeling that several drugs will become available for stroke shortly and that they will accelerate the public's awareness of the need to go to emergency rooms with early stroke symptoms, much as patients with chest pain do today.

TABLE 207-2 Drugs Detrimental to Recovery in Animals

Phenytoin sodium
Clonidine hydrochloride
Haloperidol
Benzodiazepines

References

1. The Boston Area Anticoagulation Trial for Atrial Fibrillation Investigators. The effect of low-dose warfarin on the risk of stroke in patients with nonrheumatic atrial fibrillation. *N Engl J Med* 1990; 323:1505–1511.
2. Criostomo EA, Duncan PW, Propst MA, et al. Evidence that amphetamine with physical therapy promotes recovery of motor function in stroke patients. *Ann Neurol* 188; 23:94–97.
3. The Dutch TIA Trial Study Group. A comparison of two doses of aspirin (30 mg vs. 283 mg a day) in patients after a transient ischemic attack or minor ischemic stroke. *N Engl J Med* 1991; 325:1261–1266.
4. Goldstein LB, Matchar DB, Morgenlander JC, et al. The influence of drugs on the recovery of sensorimotor function after stroke. *J Neurol Rehabil* 1990; 4:137–144.
5. Hass WK, Easton JD, Adams HP Jr, et al. A randomized trial comparing ticlopidine hydrochloride with aspirin for the prevention of stroke in high-risk patients. Ticlopidine Aspirin Stroke Study Group. *N Engl J Med* 1989; 321:501–507.
6. Matchar DB, Divine GW, Heyman A, et al. The influence of hyperglycemia on outcome of cerebral infarction. *Am Intern Med* 1992; 117:449–456.
7. Petersen P, Boysen G, Godtfredsen J, et al. Placebo-controlled, randomised trial of warfarin and aspirin for prevention of thromboembolic complications in chronic atrial fibrillation. The Copenhagen AFASAK study. *Lancet* 1989; 1:175–179.
8. Pulsinelli WA, Levy DE, Sigsbee B, et al. Increased damage after ischemic stroke in patients with hyperglycemia with or without established diabetes mellitus. *Am J Med* 1983; 74:540–544.
9. The SALT Collaborative Group. Swedish Aspirin Low-Dose Trial (SALT) of 75 mg aspirin as secondary prophylaxis after cerebrovascular ischaemic events. *Lancet* 1991; 338:1345–1349.
10. Sherman DG, Dyken ML, Fisher M, et al. Antithrombotic therapy for cerebrovascular disorders. *Chest* 1989; 95 (2 suppl):140S–155S.
11. Stein B, Fuster V, Halperin JL, et al. Antithrombotic therapy in cardiac disease. An emerging approach based on pathogenesis and risk. *Circulation* 1989; 80:1501–1513.
12. Yip PK, He YY, Hsu CY, et al. Effect of plasma glucose on infarct size in focal cerebral ischemia–reperfusion. *Neurology* 1991; 41:899–905.

208 Thrombolytic Therapy for Occlusive Cerebrovascular Disease

Michael Chicoine
DeWitte Cross
Ralph G. Dacey, Jr.

Cerebrovascular disease is the third leading cause of death in the United States,[8] and a major cause of morbidity and disability in our society. Approximately 30 percent of all strokes are fatal, and another 20 to 30 percent cause permanent, severe disability.[4,58] In 1989, the National Institutes of Health reported 145,551 deaths secondary to cerebrovascular disease (nearly 7 percent of all deaths in the United States that year).[8] Until recently, treatment for acute stroke has been supportive and preventative in nature. Thrombolytic therapy offers an opportunity to intervene and change the natural course of cerebral infarction.[24] The application of thrombolytic therapy to stroke has progressed largely because of the recent advances of thrombolytic intervention in coronary artery disease.[11,33,57]

Thromboembolism

Eighty percent of all strokes are the result of either thrombosis or embolization (30 percent and 50 percent, respectively).[57] Thrombosis is a disease of large vessels, particularly the internal carotid arteries, the vertebral and basilar arteries, and to a lesser extent, the middle cerebral and posterior cerebral arteries. Atherosclerotic plaque formation leads to progressive stenosis, and creates a nidus for intraluminal thrombus formation and vessel occlusion.[19] An angiographic study of 80 patients within 6 h of the onset of stroke by Fieschi et al. demonstrated occlusion of cerebral or precerebral vessels in 76 percent.[22] del Zoppo et al. showed similar results in the rt-PA Acute Stroke Study Group, in which 81 percent of the patients demonstrated angiographic occlusions in the relevant carotid distribution 8 h after stroke.[3] The patients affected frequently have carotid artery bruits, angina, claudication, or other manifestations of large-vessel occlusive disease. The clinical course of neurological deficits in these patients is often gradual or stepwise, and is frequently preceded by transient ischemic attacks.

Embolic phenomena are generally more sudden in clinical presentation.[38] Artery to artery occlusive embolism often arises from the origins of the internal carotid or vertebral arteries. Emboli of cardiac origin occur in patients with conditions predisposing to thromboembolism, such as atrial fibrillation, valvular heart disease, recent myocardial infarction, endocarditis, or right-to-left intracardiac shunts.[19,38] It is often difficult to distinguish thrombosis from embolism, and even angiography or postmortem evaluation may not be able to make this distinction.[19]

The anterior circulation is most often affected by cerebral ischemia, especially in the distribution of the middle cerebral artery (MCA). The Harvard Cooperative Stroke Registry (a prospective registry of nearly 700 stroke victims) reported that 75 percent of emboli occurred in the MCA, 11 percent in the posterior cerebral artery (PCA), 5 percent in the basilar artery, and 3 percent in the anterior cerebral artery.[38]

Middle Cerebral Artery/Internal Carotid Artery Occlusion

The presenting symptoms of MCA or internal carotid artery (ICA) occlusion may include hemiparesis or hemiplegia, hemisensory changes, contralateral homonymous hemianopsia or other visual deficits, language disturbances such as dysphasia and aphasia or other higher cortical function abnormalities, ocular motor disturbances, hemineglect, and depressed level of consciousness. Disease affecting the MCA will generally impair the face and arm more than the leg. Less often, presenting symptoms are seizures, movement disorders, or merely headache.[49]

Posterior Cerebral Artery/Vertebrobasilar Artery Occlusion

Symptoms of occlusive disease in the posterior cerebral artery (PCA) distribution may include visual field deficits and other visual disturbances, dyslexia or alexia, hemiparesis secondary to cerebral peduncle involvement, sensory changes of thalamic injury, movement disorders, and memory difficulties. Vertebrobasilar artery (VBA) occlusive disease is varied in its clinical presentations, and may involve part or all of the elements of PCA occlusion, in addition to the numerous deficits related to the cranial nerves, the cerebellum, and the brain stem nuclei and tracts. Among the possible components of VBA occlusive disease are ocular motility disorders, nystagmus, ataxia, hemiplegia or quadriplegia, altered levels of consciousness, sympathetic impairment as manifest in Horner's syndrome, vocal cord paralysis, palate paralysis, hiccups, and respiratory failure (Ondine's curse). Other symptoms and signs that might be included are headaches, nausea, vomiting, depressed level of consciousness, and other evidence of increased intracranial pressure as occurs with large cerebellar infarcts leading to hydrocephalus.[49]

The Ischemic Penumbra

The rationale for thrombolytic therapy for occlusive cerebrovascular disease is based on the concept of the *ischemic penumbra,*[5] an ischemic region of brain in the periphery of an infarct that can be spared permanent insult if adequate perfusion is returned within a critical window of time. Extensive research in animal models and clinical observations indicate that the first 4 to 8 h are crucial if neurological function is to be preserved.[11,14,15,29] Fundamental to the implementation of thrombolytic therapy is the immediate recognition of acute occlusive cerebrovascular events and prompt initiation of thrombolytic treatment to restore perfusion.[19,24]

Thrombolytic Therapy

The physiologic and biochemical basis for thrombolytic intervention lies in the ability to affect the pathway of fibrinolysis. The conversion of fibrinogen to fibrin is activated by thrombin generated by the coagulation cascades. A thrombus is formed by the woven matrix of the fibrin–plasminogen complex (Fig. 208-1) in conjunction with platelet aggregation.[21] The endogenous process for removal of the thrombus involves enzymatic conversion of plasminogen to plasmin, which initiates fibrinolysis.[57] Thrombolytic agents, including fibrinolysin, thrombolysin, urokinase, streptokinase, and tissue plasminogen activator, serve as catalysts of this process of fibrinolysis.[13]

Thrombolytic therapy for occlusive cerebrovascular disease is passing from a phase of experimental application to use in routine clinical care.[17] Thrombolytic treatment for coronary artery disease, pulmonary emboli, and peripheral vascular thromboses has achieved considerable success and has therefore gained wide acceptance.[32] Many questions, however, remain unanswered with regard to thrombolytic therapy for occlusive cerebrovascular disease. Which patients should be selected for such therapy? Which agent and dose will achieve the greatest yield in terms of neurological recovery with the lowest rate of complications? Which is the most appropriate route of administration, intra-arterial or intravenous? Does recanalization of an occluded vessel correlate with improved neurological outcome?

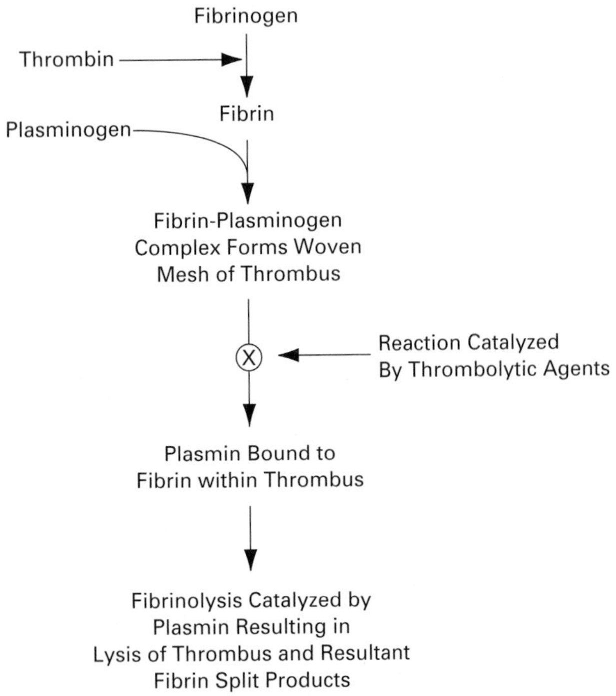

Figure 208-1 Schematic depiction of fibrinolysis. The circled x indicates the conversion of plasminogen to plasmin, which can be activated by any of the thrombolytic agents (tPA, uPA, scuPA, SK, and APSAC). Plasmin then activates lysis of the thrombus. (Adapted with modification from Craig and Stitzel.[13])

Patient Selection

The first step in thrombolytic treatment for occlusive cerebrovascular disease is patient selection. Optimal results are obtained with rapid recognition of the occlusive event, followed by prompt application of thrombolytic therapy. Evidence reveals that it is crucial for intervention to begin within the first 4 to 8 h from the onset of symptoms, and sooner if feasible. Prompt intervention serves to maximize neurological recovery as well as minimize reperfusion injuries. As Haley discusses in his review of thrombolytic therapy,[24] reperfusion injury is not fully understood, but may include exacerbation of vasogenic cerebral edema, introduction of injurious free radicals, enhancement of lipid peroxidation of cell membranes, and increased potential for intracerebral hemorrhage.[56]

The precise role of the cerebral angiogram in the patient selection process has not been defined.[3] If the thrombolytic agent is delivered intra-arterially, then angiographic confirmation will always be available. With intravenous administration of the thrombolytic agent, one must weigh the risks and benefits of angiography. When the diagnosis of an occlusive cerebrovascular event is uncertain, cerebral angiography should be considered in the algorithm. In the future, magnetic resonance imaging (MRI), magnetic resonance angiography (MRA), transcranial Doppler sonography, radionuclide cerebral blood flow measurements, or other diagnostic modalities may prove to yield information more rapidly than traditional angiography,[19,45] particularly as these alternative imaging studies continue to improve.

Additional factors to consider in patient selection include the exclusion of patients with lacunar infarcts, as they will not respond to thrombolytic treatment. Computed tomography (CT) scans should be obtained in all candidates to detect early evidence of infarction, hemorrhagic infarction, hemorrhage into mass lesions, subarachnoid hemorrhage, and other contraindications to thrombolytic therapy. Patients with bleeding disorders should be excluded as well, and screening with complete blood count, prothrombin time, and activated partial thromboplastin time is indicated. Rarely, an allergic response to the thrombolytic agent may contraindicate thrombolytic therapy.

Thrombolytic Agents

There is controversy regarding the optimal thrombolytic agent. Early trials in the late 1950s and early 1960s utilized thrombolysin and fibrinolysin.[19] These agents are nonselective for fibrinolysis, and some investigators have attributed to them a higher risk of creating a systemic lytic state and subsequent hemorrhages, both intracranial and extracranial. Fibrinolysin, for example, has been obtained from bovine sources,[27] and carries a significant, albeit nonserious, risk of antigenic response. These and other factors have led to the use of alternative thrombolytic agents with recent trials.[21]

Streptokinase

Streptokinase (SK) is a relatively inexpensive and readily available thrombolytic agent for which there is a considerable base of clinical experience in its experimental use for occlusive cerebrovascular disease, as well as extensive information on its use in coronary artery disease, pulmonary emboli, and occlusive peripheral vascular disease, both venous and arterial.[32,33,47] SK is an exogenous plasminogen activator produced by the *Streptococcus haemolyticus* bacterium, and has a half-life of 23 min. SK activates plasminogen conversion to plasmin[13,19] (Fig. 208-2), which promotes fibrinolysis and fibrinogenolysis, and inactivates other coagulation factors (V and VIII). The relative nonselectivity of SK, like that of urokinase, is a disadvantage that carries the additional risk of producing a systemic lytic state. Another disadvantage of SK relates to the variable presence of antistreptococcal antibodies, which inactivate SK in an unpredictable fashion. The patient's endogenous antibodies can lead to pyrexic or other antigenic reactions, or even to the creation of a completely refractory state, if SK is injected on multiple occasions.[19,33] Although thrombolytic trials in stroke have demonstrated the ability of SK to achieve recanalization with acceptable rates of intracerebral hemorrhage,[18,23,37,50] urokinase and the tissue plasminogen activators have become the agents of choice (Table 208-1).

Urokinase Plasminogen Activator

Urokinase plasminogen activator (uPA), an endogenous compound produced in renal cells, is found in low concentrations in serum and in high concentrations in urine, and serves in the natural mechanism of recanalization and clot resolution (Fig. 208-2). As an endogenous compound, uPA offers the advantage over SK of being less antigenic, although it is considerably more expensive. The half-life of the uPA ranges from 9 to 16 min. The proenzyme of uPA, single-chain urokinase (scuPA or proUK), can be produced in large quantities by recombinant techniques (rscuPA), and has a half-life of 7 min. Unlike SK and uPA, scuPA does not cause inactivation of coagulation factors V and VIII. Because of this fibrin selectivity, scuPA has less of a tendency to produce a systemic lytic state.[19,33,57] Thrombolytic trials in stroke with urokinase-type agents have been primarily with uPA[2,18,23,34,37,39,44,50,54,55] (Table 208-1), and therefore the role for scuPA remains to be determined.

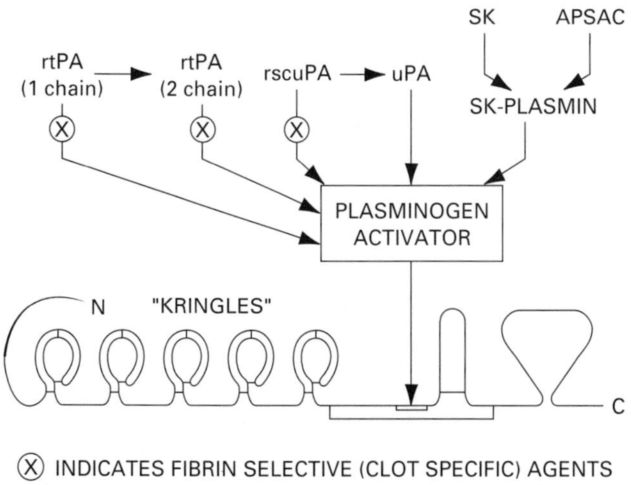

Figure 208-2 Schematic depiction of a plasminogen molecule including its fibrin-binding sites ("kringles"). Despite variations in the rate and specificity of the reaction, the different plasminogen activators all catalyze cleavage of the plasminogen molecule at the same site with resultant formation of plasmin. See text for explanation of acronyms. (Adapted with modification from Marder and Sherry.[32])

Tissue Plasminogen Activator

Tissue plasminogen activator (tPA) is an endogenous catalyst of the conversion of plasminogen to plasmin (Fig. 208-2), and is particularly active in the presence of fibrin.[19] This results in considerable selectivity in the cleavage of fibrin rather than fibrinogen (referred to by Papadopoulos et al. as *"clot-specific" thrombolysis*.[46] Endogenously tPA is produced predominantly by endothelial cells. Recombinant techniques now enable large-scale production of recombinant tissue plasminogen activator (rtPA). Two forms of tPA occur naturally, a single-chain form (alteplase) and a double-chain form (duteplase), the latter formed by plasmin-activated cleavage of the single-chain form. Duteplase has an apparent advantage of greater enzymatic effect upon fibrin. The half-life of these two agents ranges from 3 to 8 min.[19,33] The clot specificity of tPA makes it the preferred thrombolytic agent for intravenous administration, and many studies have demonstrated its utility intra-arterially as well (Table 208-1).

Newer Thrombolytic Agents

As Puri and Colman discuss in their review of thrombolytic therapies for myocardial infarction and stroke,[47] the second-generation plasminogen activators [e.g., staphylokinase and anisoylated plasminogen streptokinase (APSAC)] (Fig. 208-2) are largely unexplored in terms of the therapeutic advantages they may offer. The refinement of staphylokinase and APSAC, as well as of tPA mutants and tPA/uPA chimeras,[19] and the addition of other agents will further enhance the potential for therapeutic thrombolytic intervention.[33]

Clinical Trials

Early trials with thrombolytic agents in occlusive cerebrovascular disease some 30 years ago produced promising results, but their limited numbers of subjects made these studies difficult to interpret. Additionally, time intervals between the onset of symptoms and the initiation of thrombolytic therapy were as long as 3 to 6 days, much longer than the intervals now thought to be critical reperfusion times for the ischemic penumbra. Post-thrombolysis angiograms were often obtained after delays of many days, and it was difficult to determine whether a causal relationship existed between thrombolytic treatment and subsequent recanalization. Five patients reported by Clarke and Cliffton,[12] Atkin et al.,[7] and Meyer et al.[35] achieved recanalization after intra-arterial injections for carotid distribution occlusions. Additionally, Clarke and Cliffton[12] and Herndon et al.[27] together reviewed 20 patients, of whom 60 to 70 percent demonstrated clinical improvements after intravenous injection of the thrombolytic agents. Despite the limitations of these earlier studies, they did demonstrate that thrombolytic therapy could be utilized to achieve recanalization, but there was considerable concern regarding the hemorrhagic complications.

TABLE 208-1 Summary of Selected Thrombolytic Therapy Studies

Investigators (First Author, Reference, and Year)	Vascular Region Occluded	Thrombolytic Agent	No.	Interval to Treatment (Hours)	Result	Hemorrhage (%)
del Zoppo[19] (1991)	ICA/MCA/multiple	IV rtPA	94	<8	34% recanalized	31
Mori[40] (1991)	ICA/MCA/multiple	IV rtPA	19	<6	47% recanalized	52
	ICA/MCA/multiple	placebo	12		17% recanalized	42
Yamaguchi[53] (1991)	ICA/MCA/ACA	IV rtPA	52	<6	39% recanalized	29
von Kummer[52] (1991)	ICA/MCA	IV rtPA	22	<6	59% recanalized	36
Herderschnee[26] (1991)	BA	IV rtPA	2	<6	50% recanalized	50
von Kummer[52] (1991)	VBA	IV rtPA	5	<6	40% recanalized	0
Yamaguchi[53] (1991)	VBA	IV rtPA	5	<6	80% recanalized	0
Otomo[44] (1988)	ICA	IV rtPA	171	<120	59% clinical improvement	1
		IV uPA	184		55% clinical improvement	2
Abe[2] (1990)	ICA	IV rtPA	145	<72	66% clinical improvement	2
		IV uPA	77		45% clinical improvement	8
Brott[9] (1990)	ICA	IV rtPA	74	<1.5	39% clinical improvement	4
del Zoppo[18] (1988)	ICA/MCA/PCA	IA SK/uPA	20	<4	90% recanalized	20
del Zoppo[17] (1988)	MCA	IA rtPA	3	1	67% recanalized	67
Mori[39] (1988)	MCA	IA uPA	22	0.2–0.5	46% recanalized	18
Theron[50] (1989)	ICA/MCA	IA SK/uPA	12	<1	100% recanalized	25
Matsumoto[34] (1991)	ICA/MCA/PCA	IA uPA	40	.2–.5	60% recanalized	33
Hacke[23] (1988)	VBA	IA SK/uPA	43	<24	44% recanalized	9
Zeumer[54] (1989)	VBA	IA uPA	7	<48	100% recanalized	14
Mobius[37] (1991)	VBA	IA SK/uPA	10	<2	78% recanalized	0
Matsumoto[34] (1991)	BA	IA uPA	10	<7	40% recanalized	10
Zeumer[55] (1993)	BA	IA uPA/rtPA	28	<10	75% recanalized	7
Zeumer[55] (1993)	ICA	IA uPA/rtPA	31	<6	94% recanalized (59% partial)	19

ICA, internal carotid artery; MCA, middle cerebral artery; ACA, anterior cerebral artery; PCA, posterior cerebral artery; BA, basilar artery; VBA, vertebrobasilar artery(ies); SK, streptokinase; uPA, urokinase plasminogen activator; rtPA, recombinant tissue plasminogen activator; IV, intravenous; IA, intra-arterial.
Source: Adapted with modifications from del Zoppo et al.[19]

Intravenous Administration of Thrombolytic Agents

More recent studies of carotid distribution occlusion treated with intravenous rtPA within 6 h of the onset of symptoms have demonstrated recanalization (partial or complete) in 34 to 59 percent of patients.[3,19,40,52,53] Large multistudy series with combined totals of more than 1000 patients have examined the results of intravenous injections of rtPA or urokinase by correlating clinical outcomes without angiographic confirmations.[1,2,6,9,30,43,44] Excluding Koudstaal et al.,[30] who studied only two patients, neither of whom improved, clinical improvement was demonstrated in 39 to 70 percent. Many of these studies have the advantage of a control group to whom a placebo was administered. Control patients in these studies demonstrated clinical improvement rates of 41 to 47 percent. The trial by Brott et al.[9] was exceptional in that all the patients were treated with rtPA within 90 min of the onset of symptoms. Thirty-nine percent (29 of 74) of these patients demonstrated clinical improvement within 6 h, and smaller infarct volumes were documented on CT scans. Nonetheless, many of the other studies in this group had limitations, including significant numbers of patients with lacunar infarctions and delays between onset of symptoms and initiation of thrombolytic therapy as long as 5 to 10 days. Additionally, there was no angiographic demonstration of occlusion or recanalization in any of these studies, including the one by Brott et al.[9] Despite these limitations, such studies have demonstrated the relative safety of intravenous thrombolytic therapy on a large scale (0 to 7.8 percent incidence of intracranial hemorrhages compared to 0 to 1.1 percent in those studies with controls).

The experience with intravenous thrombolytic therapy for pure VBA occlusions is more limited, but some encouraging results have been seen. Of 12 patients reported in three series in which rtPA was administered within 6 h of the onset of symptoms, seven patients (58 percent) demonstrated recanalization.[26,52,53] In Yamaguchi's series alone, four of the five patients (80 percent) demonstrated angiographic evidence of recanalization.[53]

Intra-arterial Administration of Thrombolytic Agents

A number of studies have examined the role of intra-arterial administration of thrombolytic agents for cerebrovascular disease. Five patients reported in the early 1960s demonstrated good results from intra-arterial administration of fibrinolysin, plasmin, or thrombolysin for carotid distribution occlusions.[7,12,35] Recanalization was reported in all five patients and no intracranial hemorrhages were reported. Since these early reports, larger series of patients have been evaluated using urokinase, plasmin, streptokinase, and rtPA.[16,18,34,36,39,50] Recanalization rates ranged from 45 to 100 percent in these series. Intracranial hemorrhage rates ranged from 0 to 33 percent except in one study,[16] in which two of three (67 percent) patients with MCA occlusions treated with rtPA suffered intracranial hemorrhage, one being a hemorrhagic transformation of an infarct and the other being a frank intraparenchymal hematoma.

Intra-arterial injections for VBA occlusions have demonstrated encouraging results as well.[10,23,25,34,37,42,54] In these series, recanalization has been demonstrated in 40 to 100 percent of the patients in whom VBA administration of streptokinase, urokinase, or rtPA has been utilized. Intracranial hemorrhages occurred in 0 to 14 percent of the patients in these studies, except for that of Buteux et al.,[10] in which hemorrhage in the single patient discussed yielded a rate of hemorrhage of 100 percent.

In 1991, del Zoppo et al. presented an extensive review of the aforementioned studies (Table 208-1).[19] Of importance in their review is that in the sum total of patients in three of the larger series, 55 percent underwent recanalization, and a favorable outcome was associated in 64 percent of those patients demonstrating recanalization. Also of note, hemorrhagic transformations led to neurological deterioration in 0 to 17 percent of subjects in the intra-arterial urokinase and streptokinase studies reviewed, and in 4.1 to 11.1 percent of the intra-arterial rtPA studies. Hemorrhagic infarction was rarely associated with neurological deterioration, whereas parenchymal hemorrhage had a greater association with neurological decline. Parenchymal hemorrhage in the natural history of non-anticoagulated cerebral embolism is reported in up to 18 percent of patients[57] and therefore the hemorrhagic complications of thrombolytic therapy do not seem to vary greatly from those seen in untreated subjects with occlusive cerebrovascular events.

At this time, thrombolytic therapy to achieve recanalization and improve neurological outcome in occlusive cerebral arterial disease appears to be a promising modality. Continued research will be required before this therapy can be applied in routine clinical care. It is difficult to ascertain which thrombolytic agent is the most efficacious for thromboembolic cerebrovascular disease. Zeumer et al.,[55] for example, demonstrated no difference in the time to recanalization when comparing intra-arterial administration of urokinase and rtPA. Continued prospective randomized studies are needed to determine which thrombolytic agent is the most efficacious and safest treatment of occlusive cerebrovascular disease.

Additionally, further study needs to be undertaken to determine which route of administration is most appropriate. The intravenous route offers a simple method that permits prompt delivery of the thrombolytic agent. The intra-arterial mode of administration is a time-intensive process (120 min on average in the study by Zeumer et al.[55]) that further delays the interval between the onset of symptoms and the beginning of thrombolytic treatment. Intra-arterial administration, however, does enable direct angiographic visualization of the occluded vessels and confirmation of recanalization upon completion of the treatment (Fig. 208-3). If recanalization is not demonstrated, further thrombolytic agent may be administered. Intra-arterial injection also precisely places the thrombolytic agent at the source of the occlusion, thereby minimizing the effects on the systemic coagulation system. This can be performed by regional injections into the ICA for MCA occlusions, for example, or even more precisely by superselective catheterizations of a specific MCA branch (Fig. 208-4). No definitive study has shown greater efficacy or safety of one method over the other. It may be that one particular thrombolytic agent is best suited for the intra-arterial route, whereas another is more effective when introduced intravenously. These questions remain unanswered.

Another uncertainty is the true relationship between recanalization of the occluded vessel and improvement in neurological outcome. Many studies suggest a causal relationship between recanalization and improved outcome,[18,23,34,37,39,40,50,55] but this correlation is difficult to confirm. Spontaneous recanalization is well documented and, in fact, is thought by some authorities to be a common phenomenon.[19] In addition, reocclusion, thought to occur secondary to platelet aggregation, has been shown in up to 25 percent of patients undergoing thrombolytic therapy.[47] The occurrence of spontaneous recanalization, or reocclusion after recanalization, is difficult to assess, particularly in cases where there is no angiographic demonstration of recanalization, or when that documentation comes after significant delay from the completion of the thrombolytic treatment.

Many other factors make occlusive cerebrovascular disease difficult to study in a controlled fashion. Each patient's presentation is unique and there are multiple variables that might affect a patient's outcome. It is therefore difficult to even compare two patients with apparent identical presentations, because the variability of the vascular anatomy, the extent of collateral circulation, and the biochemical make-up and volume of the offending clot are important factors that will affect the patient's clinical course as well as the response to thrombolytic interventions. The rtPA Acute Stroke Study Group investigation demonstrated recanalization in 35 percent of patients with MCA occlusions, and only 8 percent of patients with ICA occlusions, thereby demonstrating that the anatomic location of the occlusion is an important factor in the treatment of stroke with thrombolytic agents.[3,20] To elucidate the effects that thrombolytic therapy may have upon occlusive cerebrovascular disease, continued investigation with large-scale controlled trials is needed. Morris et al.[41] reviewed 200 consecutive patients admitted with acute stroke and found that only 4.5 percent were eligible for the Multicentre Acute Stroke Trial of SK versus placebo (50 percent were ineligible because they presented after 6 h). This re-emphasizes the fact that thrombolytic therapy for acute stroke is most appropriately investigated by a multicenter study. Additionally, it demonstrates the need for education of the general public and the medical community to ensure that treatment for stroke is sought in the most expeditious fashion.

Venous Sinus Thrombosis

Another application of thrombolytic therapy for occlusive cerebrovascular disease is in the treatment of venous sinus thrombosis. Venous sinus thrombosis is an uncommon entity that may be found in association with infections, oral contraceptive use, pregnancy, trauma, dehydration, disseminated intravascular coagulation, polycythemia, and thrombocytosis. In cases of complete sagittal sinus thrombosis, mortality is reported to be as high as 80 percent, and patients may present with rapid neurological deterioration. Standard therapy has been supportive, directed at management of the intracranial hypertension that results from impaired venous drainage and poor CSF resorption. Anticoagulation, too, has often been utilized. Encouraging results, though limited in number, have been demonstrated with thrombolytic therapy for venous occlusive dis-

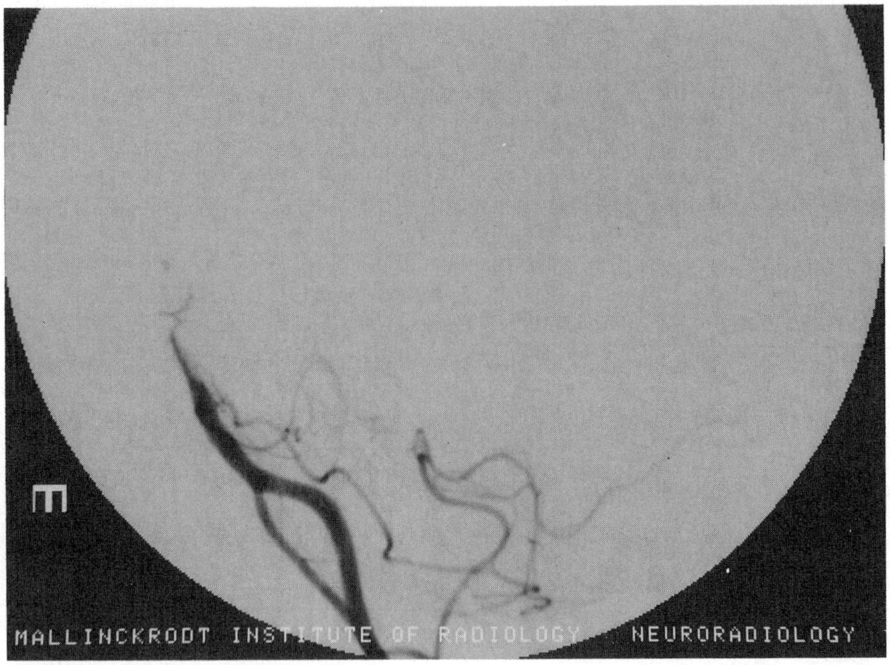

(*A*)

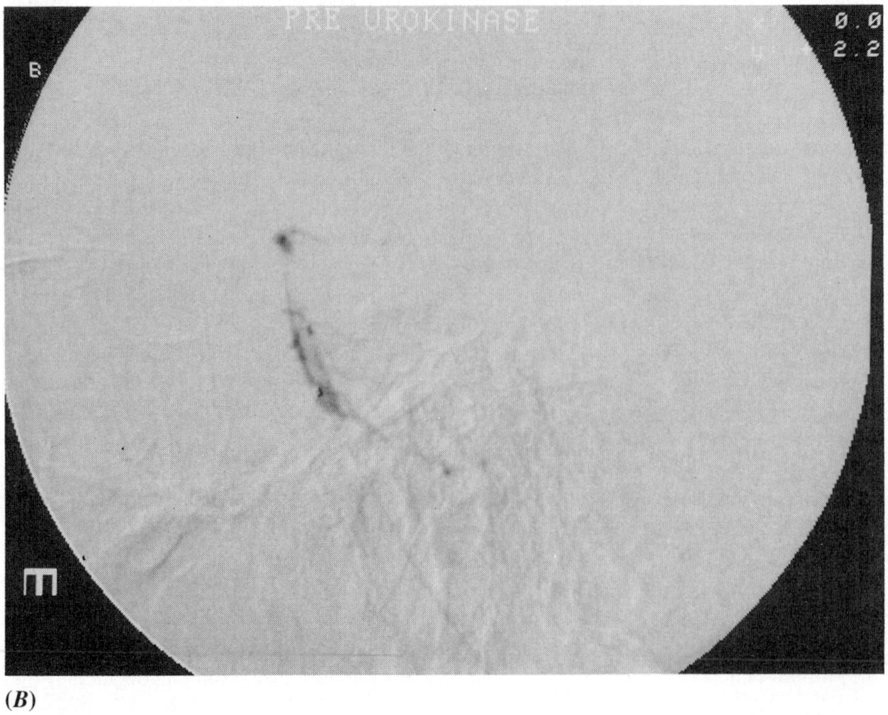

(*B*)

Figure 208-3 Intra-arterial fibrinolysis for basilar thrombosis. *A*. Lateral view of a vertebral artery angiogram before treatment demonstrating clot within the distal basilar artery and a basilar tip occlusion. *B*. Microcatheter in position proximal to the clot for infusion of the fibrinolytic agent.

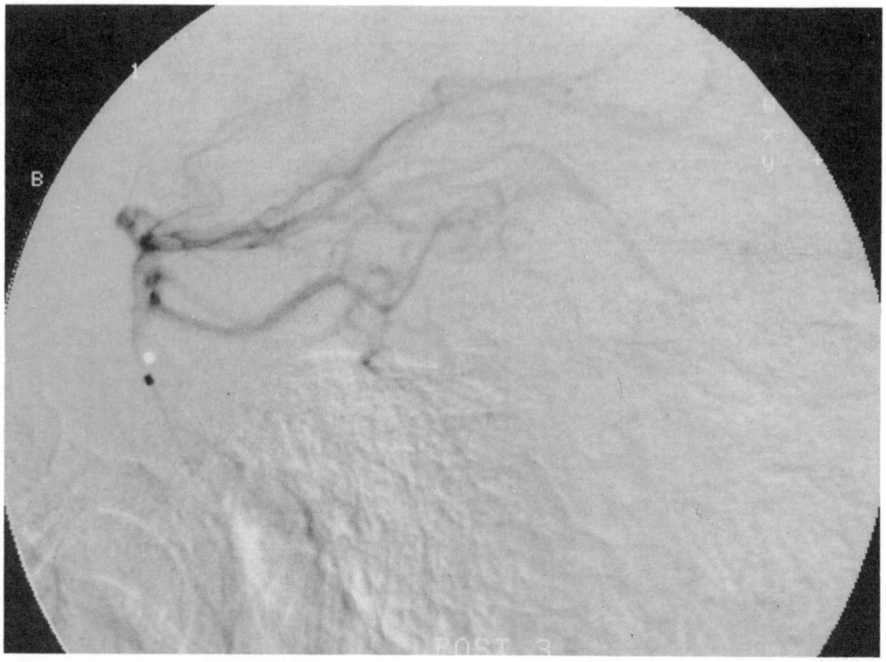

(*C*)

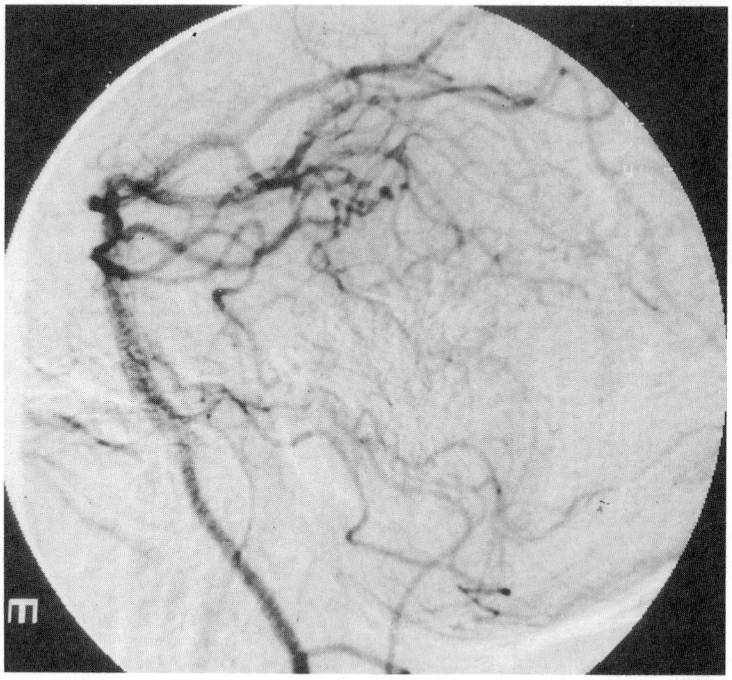

(*D*)

Figure 208-3 (*Continued*) *C.* Contrast injection through a microcatheter following delivery of 500,000 units of urokinase demonstrating recanalization of vessel. *D.* Lateral view of a vertebral artery angiogram after treatment.

ease (Fig. 208-5). Examples of thrombolytic therapy for venous sinus thrombosis include using intravenous urokinase in a 26-year-old postpartum woman,[31] infusing urokinase in the superior sagittal sinus via the anterior fontanelle of a neonate,[28] and infusing urokinase into the superior sagittal sinus of a 33-year-old man via a small midline frontal craniectomy.[48] In all three of these examples, the patients presented with profound neurological deterioration, and after thrombolytic therapy, made excellent neurological recoveries. Tsai et al.[51] present an additional five cases of superior sagittal or transverse sinus occlusion who had excellent outcomes after direct dural sinus administration of urokinase via a transfemoral approach. These results and others reported are primarily anecdotal, but offer encouragement for further investigations. Intraventricular hemorrhage and extensive subarachnoid hemorrhages have also been investigated as diseases potentially treatable with thrombolytic therapy. As with the thrombolytic treatment of occlusive cerebrovascular diseases, these modalities will require further investigation.

Summary

Thrombolytic therapy offers promise as a potential means to positively affect the natural course of acute occlusive cerebrovascular events. Laboratory and clinical investigations have demonstrated the ability to recanalize occluded vessels with a positive effect upon neurological outcome. Hemorrhagic complication is a risk, particularly hemorrhagic transformation of an infarction, but may not occur at a rate significantly higher than that seen in the natural history of cerebral infarctions. The specific agent, dose, and route of administration necessary for optimal results remain undeter-

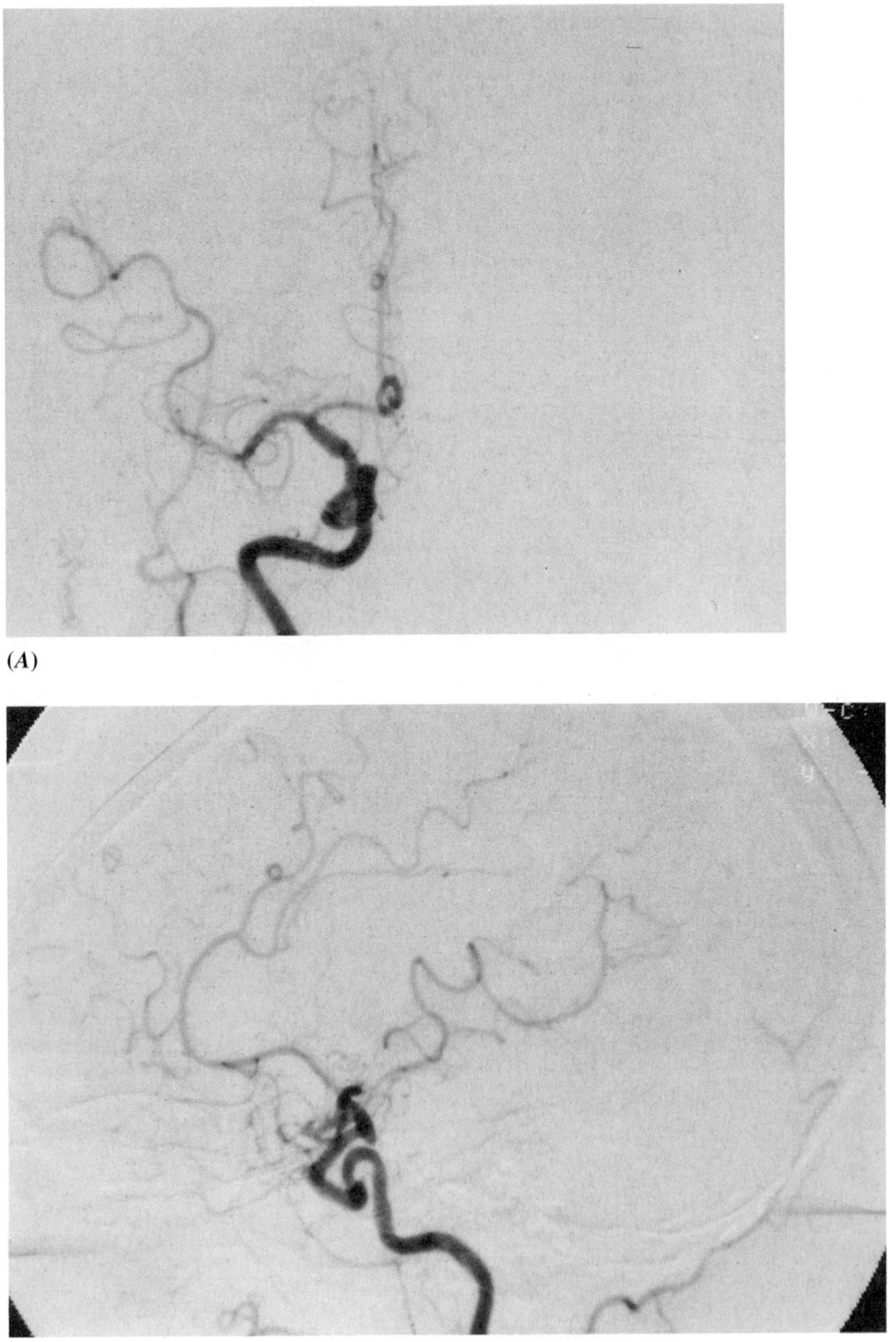

(*A*)

(*B*)

Figure 208-4 Intra-arterial fibrinolysis in a case of an acute MCA occlusion. A 67-year-old woman who was hospitalized for congestive heart failure developed sudden left-sided weakness and neglect, and an initial CT scan of the brain excluded hemorrhage. *A* & *B*. Anteroposterior (AP) and lateral views from the initial right common carotid angiography demonstrate an occlusion of most branches of the MCA. Only an anterior temporal branch and a posterior parietal branch fill.

mined. In addition, many other treatment options are also being evaluated for the treatment of acute stroke, including glutamate antagonists, free-radical scavengers, mannitol, and calcium channel blockers.[4,58] In addition, anticoagulant therapy has been used variably in the thrombolytic studies reviewed as well as in routine clinical management of stroke patients, and warrants further study. Determination of the most effective combinations of all of these modalities will come with continued investigation and will thus enable clinicians to optimize the neurological outcome of patients with occlusive cerebrovascular disease.

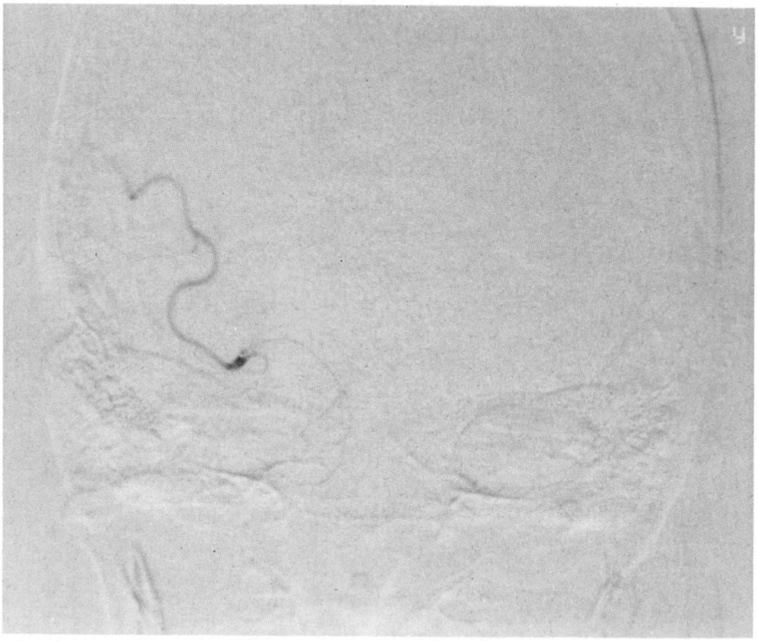

(*C*)

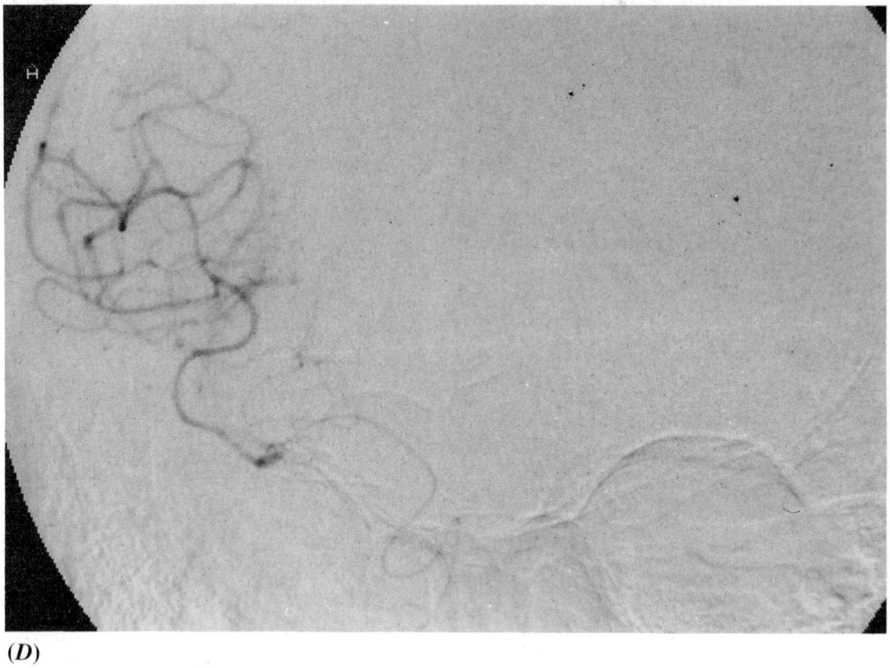

(*D*)

Figure 208-4 (*Continued*) *C.* A microcatheter was introduced. This AP view shows contrast injected through the microcatheter, which was placed in the MCA at the site of the occlusion. Contrast opacifies only the initially patent branches. *D.* Intra-arterial urokinase delivery was begun by intermittent 5000- to 10,000-unit boluses. After infusion of a portion of the total dose, contrast injected through the microcatheter demonstrates partial opacification of the branches missing on the initial examination.

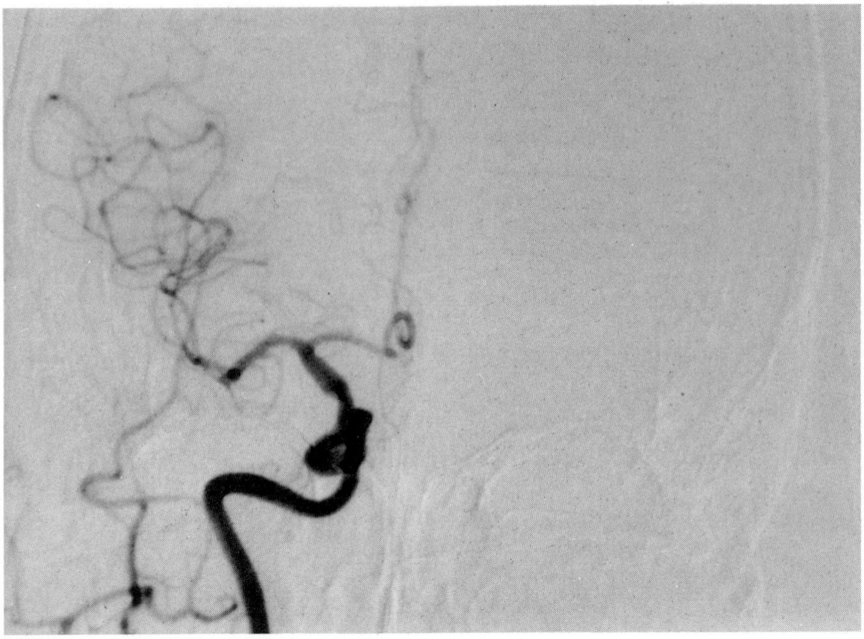

(*E*)

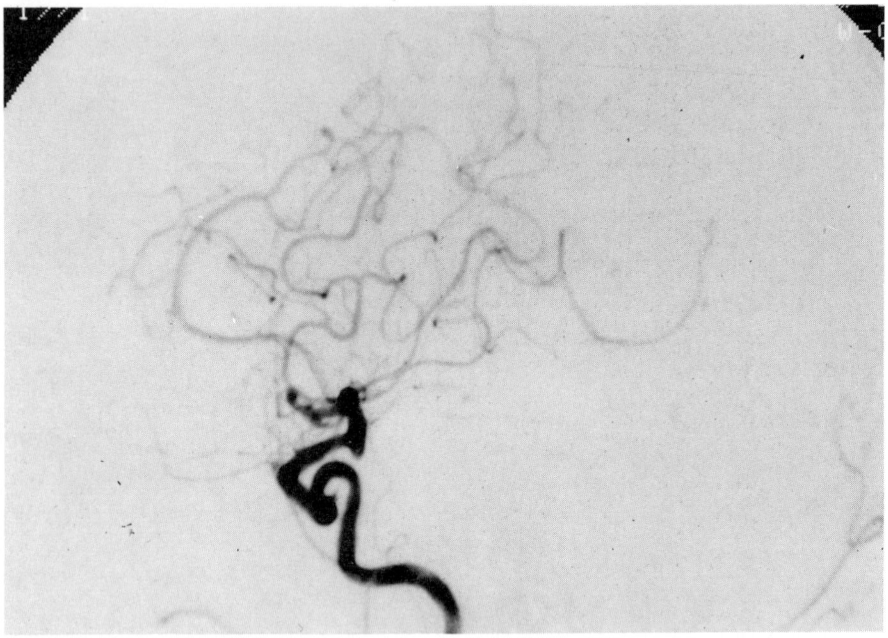

(*F*)

Figure 208-4 (*Continued*) *E* & *F*. The final AP and lateral views from the case following local intra-arterial delivery of a total of 2,000,000 units of urokinase. Total recanalization took 4 h to complete. There were no hemorrhagic complications. Subsequent CT scans confirmed a completed infarction in the right cerebral hemisphere, but the size of the infarct may have been reduced by the early restoration of flow.

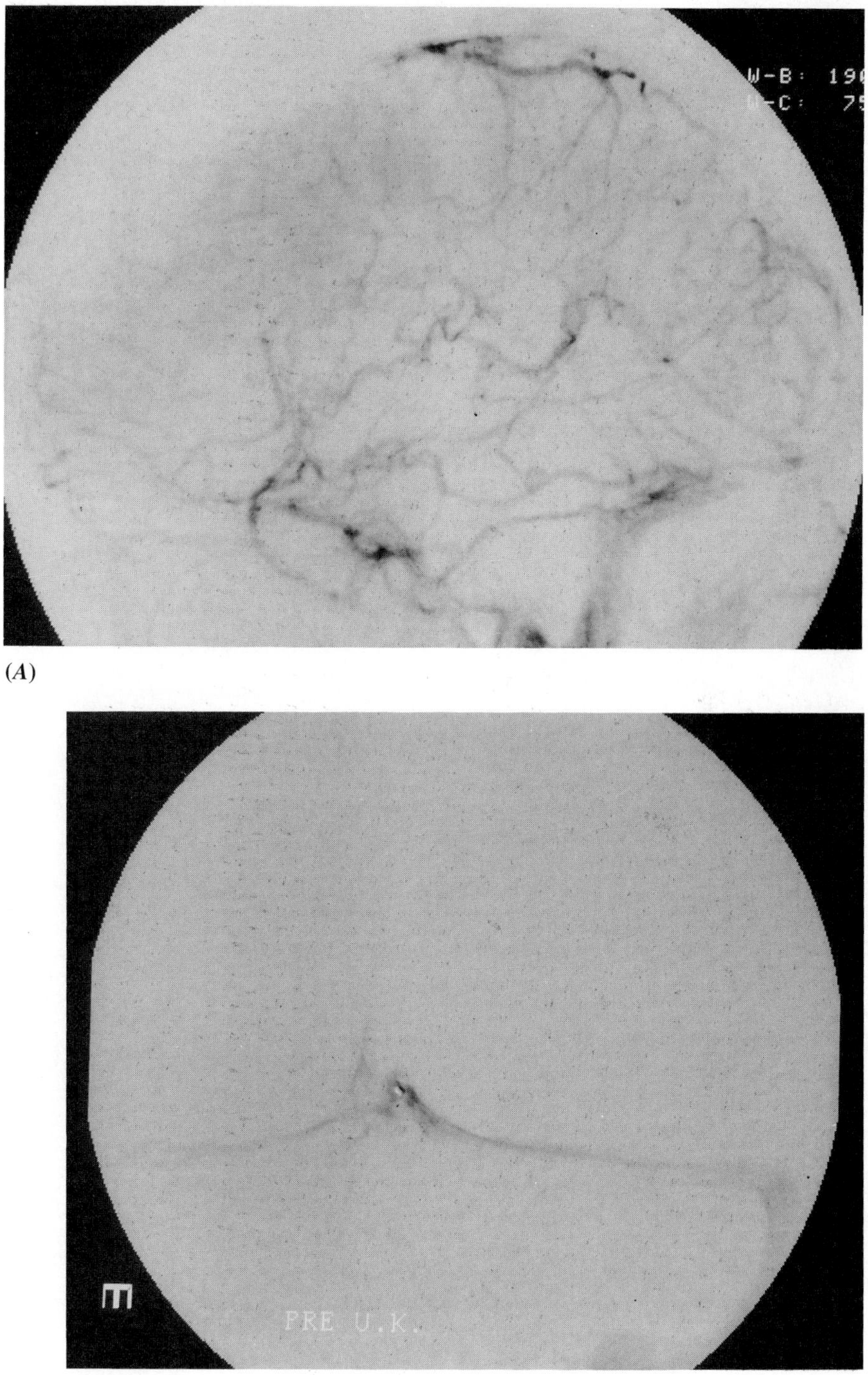

Figure 208-5 Local fibrinolysis for superior sagittal sinus thrombosis. *A*. Lateral view of venous phase of carotid angiogram before treatment demonstrating occlusion of the superior sagittal sinus. *B*. Anteroposterior (AP) view of the microcatheter positioned at the torcular for infusion of the fibrinolytic agent.

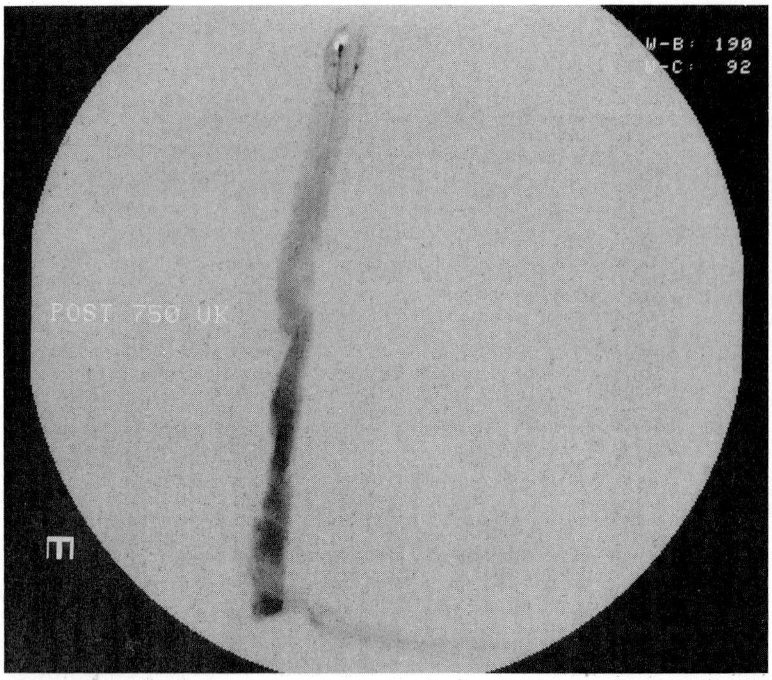

(*C*)

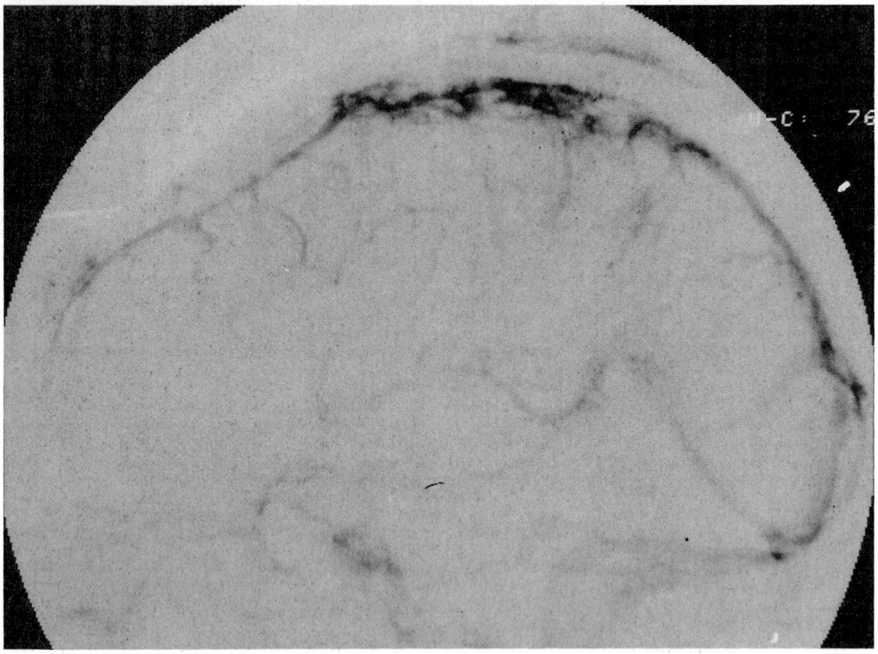

(*D*)

Figure 208-5 (*Continued*) *C.* AP view of the microcatheter in the superior sagittal sinus following progressive advancement and bolus local infusions of urokinase. Total Dose: 750,000 units. *D.* Lateral view of the venous phase of the carotid angiogram following treatment. The superior sagittal sinus is subtotally recanalized and irregular in appearance, but once again functions to drain cortical veins.

References

1. Abe T, Kazawa M, Naito I. Clinical effect of urokinase (60,000 units/day) on cerebral infarction—comparative study by means of multiple center double blind test. *Blood Vessels* 1975; 12:342–358.
2. Abe T, Terashi A, Tohgi H. Clinical efficacy of intravenous administration of SM-9527 (t-PA) in cerebral thrombosis. *Clin Eval* 1990; 18:39–69.
3. Acute Stroke Study Group. An open safety/efficacy trial of rt-PA in acute thromboembolic stroke: final report. *Stroke* 1991; 22:153 (abstr).
4. Adams HP Jr. Management of acute cerebral infarction. In Weinstein PR, Faden AI (eds): *Protection of the Brain from Ischemia.* Baltimore: Williams & Wilkins, 1990, pp 151–161.
5. Astrup J, Siesjo BK, Symon L. Thresholds in cerebral ischemia—the ischemic penumbra. *Stroke* 1981; 12:723–725.
6. Atarashi J, Otomo E, Araki G. Clinical utility of urokinase in the treatment of acute stage of cerebral thrombosis: multi-center double-blind study in comparison with placebo. *Clin Eval* 1985; 13:659–709.
7. Atkin N, Nitzberg S, Dorsey J. Lysis of intracerebral thromboembolism with fibrinolysin: report of a case. *Angiology* 1964; 15:436–439.
8. Boring CC, Squires TS, Tong T. Cancer statistics, 1993. *CA* 1993; 43:7–26.

9. Brott T, Haley C, Levy D. Safety and potential efficacy of tissue plasminogen activator (t-PA) for stroke. *Stroke* 1990; 21:181 (abstr).
10. Buteux G, Jubault V, Suisse A, et al. Local recombinant tissue plasminogen activator to clear cerebral artery thrombosis developing soon after surgery. *Lancet* 1988; 2:1143–1144.
11. Chehrazi BB, Seibert JA, Kissel P, et al. Evaluation of recombinant tissue plasminogen activator in embolic stroke. *Neurosurgery* 1989; 24:355–360.
12. Clarke RL, Cliffton EE. The treatment of cerebrovascular thromboses and embolism with fibrinolytic agents. *Am J Cardiol* 1960; 6:546–551.
13. Craig CR, Stitzel RE. *Modern Pharmacology,* 2d ed. Boston: Little, Brown, 1986.
14. Crowell RM, Jafar JJ. Surgical revascularization for acute occlusion: theoretical and practical considerations. In Weinstein PR, Faden AI (eds): *Protection of the Brain from Ischemia.* Baltimore: Williams & Wilkins, 1990, pp 285–297.
15. Crowell RM, Olsson Y, Klatzo I, et al. Temporary occlusion of the middle cerebral artery in the monkey: clinical and pathological observations. *Stroke* 1970; 1:439–448.
16. del Zoppo GJ. Thrombolytic therapy in cerebrovascular disease. *Stroke* 1988; 19:1174–1179.
17. del Zoppo GJ. Thrombolysis: new concepts in the treatment of stroke. In Hennerici M, Sitzer G, Weger HD (eds): *Carotid Artery Plaques.* Basel: S. Karger, 1988, pp 247–272.
18. del Zoppo GJ, Ferbert A, Otis S, et al. Local intra-arterial fibrinolytic therapy in acute carotid territory stroke. *Stroke* 1988; 19:307–313.
19. del Zoppo GJ, Pessin MS, Mori E, et al. Thrombolytic intervention in acute thrombotic and embolic stroke. *Semin Neurol* 1991; 11:368–384.
20. del Zoppo GJ, Poeck K, Pessin MS, et al. Recombinant tissue plasminogen activator in acute thrombotic and embolic stroke. *Ann Neurol* 1992; 32:78–86.
21. del Zoppo GJ, Zeumer H, Harker LA. Thrombolytic therapy in stroke: possibilities and hazards. *Stroke* 1986; 17:595–607.
22. Fieschi C, Argentino C, Lenzi GL, et al. Clinical and instrumental evaluation of patients with ischemic stroke within the first six hours. *J Neurol Sci* 1989; 91:311–321.
23. Hacke W, Zeumer H, Ferbert A, et al. Intra-arterial thrombolytic therapy improves outcome in patients with acute vertebrobasilar occlusive disease. *Stroke* 1988; 19:1216–1222.
24. Haley EC Jr. Thrombolytic therapy for acute ischemic stroke. *Clin Neuropharmacol* 1993; 16:179–194.
25. Henze T, Boeer A, Tebbe U, et al. Lysis of basilar artery occlusion with tissue plasminogen activator. *Lancet* 1987; 2:1391 (letter).
26. Herderschnee D, Limburg U, Hijdra A, et al. Recombinant tissue plasminogen activator in two patients with basilar artery occlusion. *J Neurol Neurosurg Psychiatry* 1991; 54:71–73.
27. Herndon RM, Meyer JS, Johnson JF, et al. Treatment of cerebrovascular thrombosis with fibrinolysin: preliminary report. *Am J Cardiol* 1960; 6:540–545.
28. Higashida RT, Helmer E, Halbach VV, et al. Direct thrombolytic therapy for superior sagittal sinus thrombosis. *Am J Neuroradiol* 1989; 10 (5 Suppl):S4–S6.
29. Kissel P, Chehrazi B, Seibert JA, et al. Digital angiographic quantification of blood flow dynamics in embolic stroke treated with tissue-type plasminogen activator. *J Neurosurg* 1987; 67:399–405.
30. Koudstaal PJ, Stibbe J, Vermeulen M. Fatal ischaemic brain oedema after early thrombolysis with tissue plasminogen activator in acute stroke. *Br Med J* 1988; 297:1571–1574.
31. Manthous CA, Chen H. Case report: treatment of superior sagittal sinus thrombosis with urokinase. *Conn Med* 1992; 56:529–530.
32. Marder VJ, Sherry S. Thrombolytic therapy: current status (1). *N Engl J Med* 1988; 318:1512–1520.
33. Marder VJ, Sherry S. Thrombolytic therapy: current status (2). *N Engl J Med* 1988; 318:1585–1595.
34. Matsumoto K, Satoh K: Topical intraarterial urokinase infusion for acute stroke. In Hacke W, del Zoppo GJ, Hirschberg M (eds): *Thrombolytic Therapy in Acute Ischemic Stroke.* Berlin: Springer-Verlag, 1991, pp 207–212.
35. Meyer JS, Herndon RM, Gotoh F, et al. Therapeutic thrombolysis. In Millikan CH, Siekert RG, Whisnant JP (eds): *Cerebral Vascular Diseases: Third Princeton Conference.* New York: Grune & Stratton, 1961, pp 160–177.
36. Miyakawa T, Sakuragawa N. Cerebral vessels and thrombosis. *Rinsho Ketsueki* 1984; 25:1018–1026 (Japanese).
37. Mobius E, Berg-Dammer D, Kuhne D, et al. Local thrombolytic therapy in acute basilar artery occlusion: experience with 18 patients. In Hacke W, del Zoppo GJ, Hirschberg M (eds): *Thrombolytic Therapy in Acute Ischemic Stroke.* Berlin: Springer-Verlag, 1991, pp 213–215.
38. Mohr JP, Caplan LR, Melski JW, et al. The Harvard Cooperative Stroke Registry: a prospective registry. *Neurology* 1978; 28:754–762.
39. Mori E, Tabuchi M, Yoshida T, et al. Intracarotid urokinase with thromboembolic occlusion of the middle cerebral artery. *Stroke* 1988; 19:802–812.
40. Mori E, Yoneda Y, Ohksawa S. Double-blind, placebo-controlled trial of recombinant tissue plasminogen activator (rt-PA) in acute carotid stroke. *Neurology* 1991; 41 (Suppl 1):347 (abstr).
41. Morris AD, Grosset DG, Squire IB, et al. The experiences of an acute stroke unit-implications for multicentre acute stroke trials. *J Neurol Neurosurg Psychiatry* 1993; 56:352–355.
42. Nenci GG, Gresele P, Taramelli M, et al. Thrombolytic therapy for thromboembolism of vertebrobasilar artery. *Angiology* 1983; 34:561–571.
43. Otomo E, Araki G, Itoh E. Clinical efficacy of urokinase in the treatment of cerebral thrombosis: multi-center double-blind study in comparison with placebo. *Clin Eval* 1985; 13:711–751.
44. Otomo E, Toghi H, Hirai S. Clinical efficacy of AK-124 (tissue plasminogen activator) in the treatment of cerebral thrombosis: study by means of multi-center double blind comparison with urokinase. *Yakuri To Chiryo* 1988; 16:3775–3821.
45. Overgaard K. Sperling B, Boysen G, et al. Thrombolytic therapy in acute ischemic stroke: a Danish pilot study. *Stroke* 1993; 24:1439–1446.
46. Papadopoulos SM, Chandler WF, Salamat MS, et al. Recombinant human tissue-type plasminogen activator therapy in acute thromboembolic stroke. *J Neurosurg* 1987; 67:394–398.
47. Puri RN, Colman RW. Reocclusion after thrombolytic therapy: strategies for inhibiting thrombin-induced platelet aggregation. *Blood Coagul Fibrinolysis* 1993; 4:465–478.
48. Scott JA, Pascuzzi RM, Hall PV, et al. Treatment of dural sinus thrombosis with local urokinase infusion: case report. *J Neurosurg* 1988; 68:284–287.
49. Sherman DG, Easton JD. Clinical syndromes of brain ischemia. In Wilkins RH, Rengachary SS (eds): *Neurosurgery.* New York: McGraw-Hill, 1985, pp 1199–1211.
50. Theron J, Courtheoux P, Casasco A. Local intraarterial fibrinolysis in the carotid territory. *Am J Neuroradiol* 1989; 10:753–765.
51. Tsai FY, Higashida RT, Matovich V, et al. Acute thrombosis of the intracranial dural sinus: direct thrombolytic treatment. *Am J Neuroradiol* 1992; 13:1137–1141.
52. von Kummer R. Intravenous tissue plasminogen activator in acute stroke. In Hacke W, del Zoppo GJ, Hirschberg M (eds): *Thrombolytic Therapy in Acute Ischemic Stroke.* Berlin: Springer-Verlag, 1991, pp 161–167.
53. Yamaguchi T. Intravenous rt-PA in acute embolic stroke. In Hacke W, del Zoppo GJ, Hirschberg M (eds): *Thrombolytic Therapy in Acute Ischemic Stroke.* Berlin: Springer-Verlag, 1991, pp 168–174.
54. Zeumer H, Freitag HJ, Grzyska U, et al. Local intraarterial fibrinolysis in acute vertebrobasilar occlusion: technical developments and recent results. *Neuroradiology* 1989; 31:336–340.
55. Zeumer H, Freitag HJ, Zanella F, et al. Local intra-arterial fibrinolytic therapy in patients with stroke: urokinase versus recombinant tissue plasminogen activator (r-TPA). *Neuroradiology* 1993; 35:159–162.
56. Zeumer H, Hundgen R, Ferbert A, et al. Local intraarterial fibrinolytic

therapy in inaccessible internal carotid occlusion. *Neuroradiology* 1984; 26:315–317.

57. Zivin JA. Thrombolytic therapy for stroke. In Weinstein PR, Faden AI (eds): *Protection of the Brain from Ischemia.* Baltimore: Williams & Wilkins, 1990, pp 231–236.
58. Zivin JA, Choi DW. Stroke therapy. *Sci Am* 1991; 265:56–63.

209
Surgery for Acute Brain Infarction with Mass Effect

Setti S. Rengachary

Many clinicians intuitively assume that brain infarcts are nonexpanding intracranial lesions. Indeed, this tenet forms the basis of differentiation of infarcts from expanding neoplastic lesions in brain imaging studies. Although this is true with old healed infarcts, some degree of brain swelling is present in the acute phase, the extent of the swelling depending on the size of the infarct. It ranges from virtually no discernible swelling such as in a small capsular infarct to a massive hemispheric swelling due to multilobar infarction from internal carotid or middle cerebral artery thrombosis (Fig. 209-1).[25] In the latter, there may be an increase in intracranial pressure and massive shift of structures across the midline, with intracranial pressure gradients and uncal or cingulate herniation. Because of the acute rise in intracranial pressure, the perfusion pressure is reduced, compounding brain ischemia. Distortion of the brain with obstruction of cerebrospinal fluid pathways further aggravates the problem.

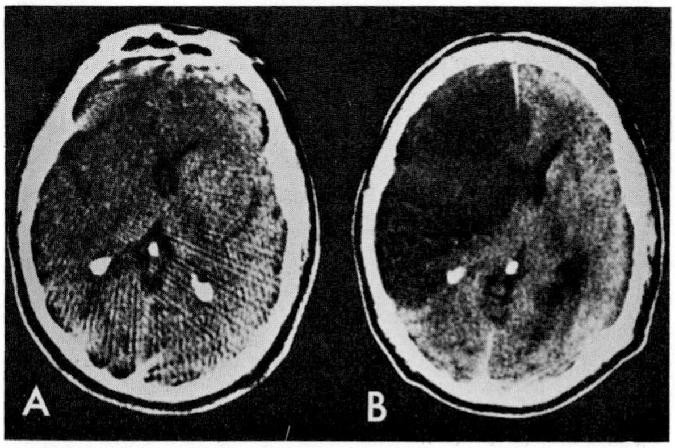

Figure 209-1 Axial CT scans of a patient with occlusion of the right internal carotid artery. *A*. This study, done on admission, is essentially normal. The ventricular system is in the midline. By retrospective analysis there is infarction of the right hemisphere, with cytotoxic edema, and no disruption of the blood-brain barrier (BBB). *B*. Four days later, with disruption of the BBB and superimposition of vasogenic edema, a large area of decreased density involving the frontotemporoparietal area has become evident. There is a massive shift of the midline structures. Note that the cortical mantle is involved but the thalamic area is spared (differentiation from neoplastic brain edema).

Experimental studies indicate that following acute focal ischemia with subsequent tissue necrosis there is at first accumulation of intracellular fluid (cytotoxic edema).[14] At this stage the blood–brain barrier (BBB) is not yet disrupted. This is indicated by a negative radionuclide brain scan, an essentially normal computed tomography (CT) scan with failure of enhancement (Fig. 209-1*A*), and a failure of extravasation of protein-bound dyes. Within a few hours to days, the BBB is disrupted and plasma-like fluid extravasates into the interstitial space (vasogenic edema) (Fig. 209-1*B*). Ischemic edema due to focal brain ischemia thus begins as a cytotoxic type, and the vasogenic component is superimposed on it subsequently.

Several clinical,[23,29] experimental,[12,18] and autopsy[1,21,26] studies have underscored the importance of brain swelling and herniation as a cause of death in the acute phase of ischemic stroke. Pressure gradients have been demonstrated in experimental models, the pressure being higher on the side of the infarct than on the opposite side, or the posterior cranial fossa.[22] In a study of 353 consecutive cases of supratentorial cerebral infarction, 45 (13 percent) showed severe brain swelling and marked herniation.[21] Brain swelling is maximal between the third and fifth days unless an extension of thrombus occurs later, with the delayed onset of signs of brain swelling and herniation.

Syndromes and Their Management

Supratentorial Compartment

Large cerebral hemispheric infarctions may present either as a syndrome simulating a brain neoplasm or a syndrome of uncal herniation. These two syndromes, of course, are not mutually exclusive.

Brain Infarction Simulating a Brain Tumor

Most neurosurgeons may be able to recount an occasional personal experience of operating on a patient with a cerebral infarct with a mistaken preoperative diagnosis of brain tumor. In such instances, the onset of symptoms may not be apoplectic and the clinical course may be stuttering. The patient may not be able to relate an accurate history either because of dysphasia or an impaired sensorium. The patient may live alone and be brought to the emergency room with no reliable history. Brain imaging studies may be equally confusing. A bizarre enhancing pattern and a mass effect in a CT scan (Fig. 209-2) may mimic a primary neoplasm such as a malignant glioma or lymphoma. Cerebral arteriography may show evidence of an avascular mass without definite occlusion of a major blood vessel.

If the diagnostic studies point to a tumor, it is inevitable that the patient will undergo an operative procedure, and the true diagnosis may not be established until after a biopsy. If a differential diagnosis of infarction is entertained based on diagnostic studies, then it would be prudent, if clinical circumstances permit, to wait 2 to 3 weeks, then reassess the patient and repeat the diagnostic studies.

Numerous helpful features have been suggested to differentiate an infarct from a tumor on a CT scan, but none is absolute.[20] They include the following:

1. Neoplastic white matter edema spares the cortex, whereas the low density due to infarction includes the cortex as well (Fig. 209-1).
2. The thalamic area is spared in infarction, especially those

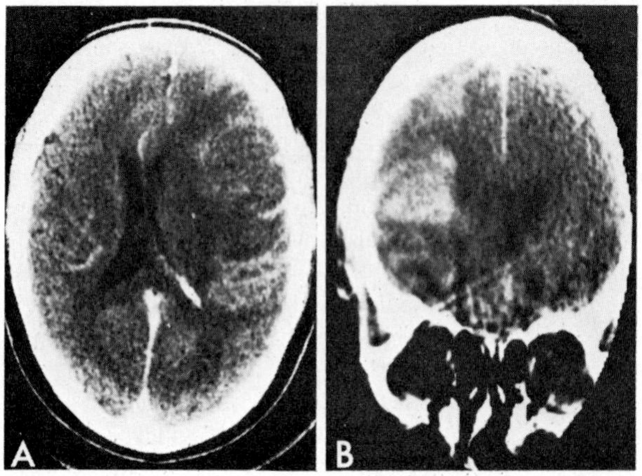

Figure 209-2 Axial (*A*) and coronal (*B*) views of a CT scan (after contrast enhancement), showing cerebral infarction with mass effect, marked ventricular displacement, and intense contrast enhancement. A diagnosis of neoplasm may be entertained, but the wedge shape of the lesion in the coronal view favors the diagnosis of infarction.

infarcts occurring in the middle cerebral or internal carotid artery distribution; such sparing is rare with peritumoral edema (Fig. 209-1).

3. Ring enhancement of the white matter is common in glioma and is rarely observed in recent infarcts.
4. Intense gray matter enhancement occurs in infarct but not in tumor.

Brain Infarction with Uncal Herniation

This generally follows massive multilobar infarction of the cerebral hemisphere from thrombotic or embolic occlusion of the internal carotid or the middle cerebral artery (Fig. 209-1). The etiologic factor may be atherosclerosis, trauma to the extracranial or intracranial vessels, thromboembolic disease secondary to the use of contraceptives, or arterial spasm following aneurysm rupture or clipping. The patient may be obtunded and densely hemiplegic at the outset. More commonly, the patient is admitted with an intermittent or mild fixed neurological deficit that, over a period of a few hours to days, progresses to a profound deficit with progressive depression in the sensorium. Transtentorial herniation and rostral brain stem compression are manifest clinically as an ipsilaterally dilated, nonreactive or poorly reactive pupil; contralateral decorticate or decerebrate posturing in the previously flaccid and paralyzed limbs; bradycardia; increase in pulse pressure; and altered respiratory pattern. If this condition is not treated, medullary failure usually culminates in death.

Aggressive medical therapy should be instituted in patients with massive cerebral infarction with early brain stem compression. Therapy is monitored with intracranial pressure measurements. The patient is intubated and hyperventilated, maintaining a Pa_{CO_2} of 30 mmHg. Mannitol is given in an initial bolus of 1 g/kg and is then repeated at 0.3 g/kg every 6 h. Furosemide used concurrently with mannitol may have a synergistic effect. Induced barbiturate coma has not conclusively been shown to be effective in reversing the changes following massive focal brain ischemia. If the patient does not show a significant response to therapy within several hours, consideration should be given to decompressive craniectomy.[6,13,16,24,30] One of the key factors determining the success of a decompressive procedure is judicious timing. It should not be attempted without the patient receiving full benefits of nonoperative therapy; yet, it should not be postponed so long that irreversible brain stem changes (such as Duret hemorrhages) occur.

The decompressive procedure of choice is ipsilateral hemicraniectomy (Fig. 209-3). The size of the hemicraniectomy may be tailored to the size of the infarct, but it is better to err on the generous side (subtemporal decompression through a small temporal craniectomy is ineffective). As the dura is opened, the pale infarcted avascular brain herniates outward into the wound. One notes conspicuous absence of pial circulation. A cortical biopsy may be done to confirm the diagnosis; there is usually no bleeding from the biopsy site. It is not necessary to resect the infarcted tissue unless necrotic material extrudes out under pressure. Resection of the necrotic brain is not advisable for two reasons: First, cranial decompression itself is adequate in allowing outward migration of the swollen brain and relieving the pressure on the rostral brain stem; second, in the acute phase of stroke, the margins of the infarct are poorly defined—if resection is attempted there is the risk of removing viable but nonfunctioning neural tissue (''idling neurons'') from the margins of the ''ischemic penumbra.'' The dura is not closed. A Silastic sheet may be laid on the brain to prevent cortical adhesions. The bone flap is preserved frozen in an antibiotic solution, to be replanted about 3 to 6 months later. The scalp is closed in watertight fashion. The recovery from the surgery is prompt. There is usually a striking and rapid improvement in the sensorium, although the focal motor deficit remains unchanged.

Hemicraniectomy seems to be more appropriate for patients with unilateral hemispheric swelling from stroke than for patients with head injury for several reasons:

1. In head injury, the brain herniating through the cranial defect tends to become incarcerated outside the skull, leading to impediment of venous drainage and contusion of the cortex at the margin of the defect, further aggravating brain edema; in stroke, the necrotic herniated brain has sluggish or nonexistent venous outflow.
2. In patients with hemispheric stroke, because the mass effect is strictly unilateral, hemicraniectomy corrects the brain displacement to relieve the pressure on rostral midbrain structures; head-injured patients tend to have diffuse brain swelling requiring bilateral decompressive procedures.
3. The brain stem is quite viable in patients with stroke unless irreversible changes such as Duret hemorrhages occur from the presence of uncal herniation that is not corrected. This is reflected in improvement in consciousness almost immediately after hemicraniectomy. Patients who have sustained trauma from severe acceleration–deceleration injuries tend to have associated brain stem injuries as well, and this adversely affects the prognosis.
4. In patients with head injury, if there is significant trauma to the posterior fossa contents in addition to the supratentorial structures, there is risk of upward herniation of the posterior fossa contents through the tentorial notch toward the zone of least pressure after hemicraniectomy. This phenomenon carries as bad a prognosis as does rostrocaudal tentorial herniation. Upward transtentorial herniation does not occur in stroke patients because the posterior fossa contents are normal.

One must consider four goals in the management of a patient with ischemic stroke: (1) preservation of life, (2) prevention of extension of thrombosis and ischemic infarction, (3) prevention of

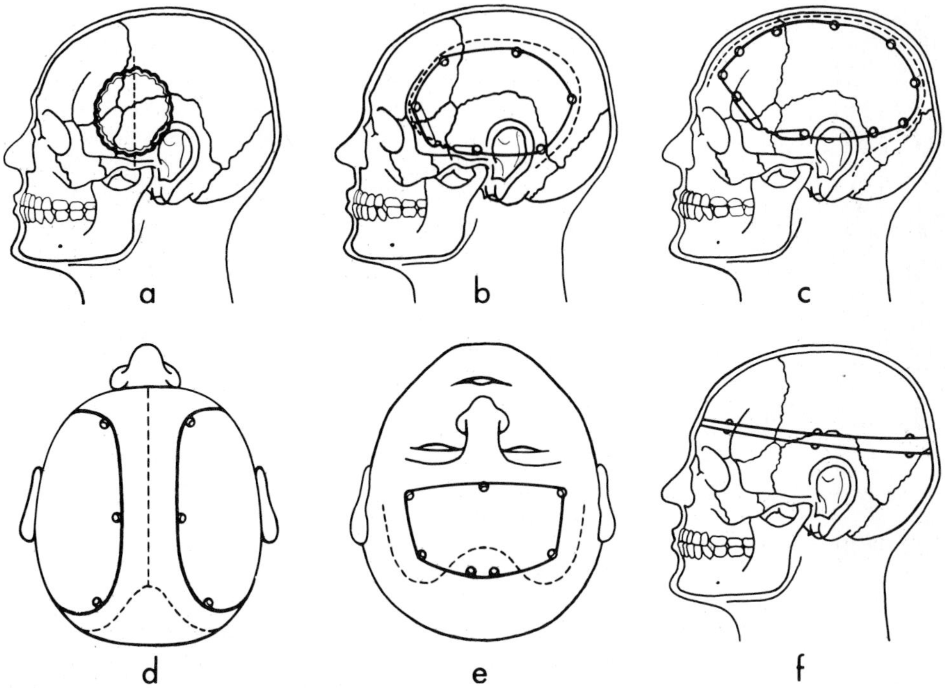

Figure 209-3 Cranial decompressive procedures for supratentorial masses: *a.* Subtemporal craniectomy: Popular in the Cushing era, this procedure is now of historic interest only. The size of the craniectomy is insufficient to alleviate increased intracranial pressure. Medium (*b*) and large (*c*) unilateral hemicraniectomy: This is ideally suited for patients with a large cerebral hemispheric infarct in whom medical therapy has failed. *d.* Bilateral hemicraniectomy: A bilateral decompressive procedure may be needed in situations where the brain swelling is diffuse and nonlateralizing, e.g., diffuse brain contusion, Reye's syndrome, lead encephalopathy, benign intracranial hypertension, etc. *e.* Bifrontal craniectomy: This procedure allows bifrontal decompression, but the temporal lobes are retained by the sphenoidal ridges and the anterior walls of the middle cranial fossa, preventing their forward migration. *f.* Circumferential craniectomy: This procedure carries the highest morbidity and mortality risk of all cranial decompressive procedures and should be avoided.

systemic complications, and (4) long-term rehabilitation. Hemicraniectomy helps to realize the first objective if the patient's life is threatened from an increase in intracranial pressure. One may philosophically argue whether preservation of life is worthwhile in the face of a severe neurological deficit. Every case must be reviewed individually to resolve this question, and no general statement is possible. The factors to be taken into consideration in deciding to operate are as follows:

1. The age of the patient—younger patients are more suitable candidates for surgery because of a reduced mortality risk, an increased likelihood of some neurological recovery, and a better potential for rehabilitation and vocational therapy.
2. Dominance of the hemisphere—stroke involving the nondominant hemisphere is more likely to have an acceptable neurological deficit because of the preservation of speech and other functions of communication.
3. Complicating illness—well-documented severe ischemic disease of the heart, uncontrolled diabetes mellitus, generalized arteriosclerosis, or dementing illness such as Alzheimer's disease will adversely influence prognosis.
4. The attitude of the immediate members of the family toward accepting attempts at preservation of life in the face of a severe neurological deficit.

Infratentorial Compartment: Cerebellar Infarction with Mass Effect

Since the initial description by Germain and Morvan in 1938[8] and with subsequent series of reports in the literature over the past four decades, cerebellar hemispheric infarction acting as an acute expansive process in the posterior cranial fossa with brain stem compression has come to be recognized as a clinically definable syndrome with a specific constellation of symptoms and signs.[10] The use of CT has permitted easier recognition and has enhanced the accuracy in the diagnosis of this syndrome (Fig. 209-4).

The disease generally affects older hypertensive men with diffuse atherosclerotic cardiovascular disease with clinical evidence of previous myocardial or cerebral infarcts.[28] Embolic occlusion of the vertebral or ipsilateral posterior inferior cerebellar artery from a thrombus in the heart is thought to be the etiologic factor in about one-half of the patients. The superior cerebellar artery is an uncommon site of occlusion. Other causative factors include penetrating or blunt trauma to the vertebral artery in the neck from chiropractic manipulation, football injuries, calisthenics, yoga exercises, bow hunting, stab or gunshot wounds of the neck, cervical dislocation, or anterior cervical discectomy. Spontaneous forced rotation of the head with occlusion of the vertebral artery has been

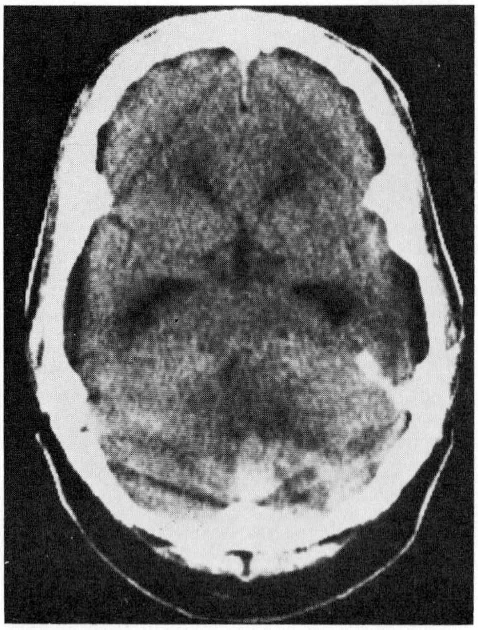

Figure 209-4 CT scan showing hemorrhagic cerebellar infarction with mass effect in the posterior cranial fossa. The fourth ventricle is compressed and there is early obstructive hydrocephalus. (Courtesy of Hilton I. Price, M.D.)

an occasional cause in infants. Rarer causes include basilar artery migraine, severe dehydration, congenital heart disease, sickle cell anemia, and (as a complication of) vertebral angiography. Cerebellar infarction in the pediatric age group is being recognized increasingly.[9]

The infarct is generally unilateral. The posteroinferior aspect of the cerebellar hemisphere in the territory of the posterior inferior cerebellar artery is the consistent site of softening.[19] Cerebellar infarctions sufficient to cause brain stem compression are always extensive, involving one-third to one-half of the hemisphere. In one-fourth of the cases, the infarction is hemorrhagic. A rich anastomotic network between the posterior inferior and the anterior inferior cerebellar arteries across the cerebellar hemispheric surface accounts for the rarity of cerebellar hemispheric infarction. The occurrence of infarction thus signifies poor development of this anastomotic network or spasm or atherosclerotic narrowing of the anastomotic vessels. The rapidity of embolic occlusion of the parent vessel may leave inadequate time for the collateral bed to expand sufficiently to carry the obligatory minimum volume of blood to sustain neural tissue. The cerebellar tonsil may undergo infarction as well and may herniate down to the level of C1. The ultimate cause of death is brain stem compression and medullary failure. Lateral medullary infarction may be associated with cerebellar infarction in about 15 percent of the cases.

The initial symptoms at onset may include dizziness or vertigo, nausea and vomiting, headache, ataxia of the limbs or trunk with inability to stand or walk, and dysarthria.[7] A history of transient ischemic attacks referable to the posterior circulation may be elicited in some patients. The subsequent clinical course is dependent on the size of the infarct. If the infarct is small, no further progression may occur, the symptoms resolve, and a mistaken diagnosis of labrynthitis may be made. In massive infarction with brain stem compression and obstruction of the fourth ventricle, the patient progressively becomes obtunded. Horizontal nystagmus when present denotes involvement of the vestibular connections of the cerebellum. Pontine compression is denoted by pinpoint and sluggish pupils, ipsilateral abducens or facial (lower motor neuron type) weakness, and forced conjugate deviation of the eyes to the opposite side that does not revert with cold caloric stimulation as a result of pressure on the ipsilateral para-abducens nucleus and ipsilateral horizontal-gaze paresis. Respirations may be ataxic or there may be central hyperventilation. Ocular bobbing, skew deviation of the eyes, decorticate or decerebrate posturing, bilateral Babinski signs, and Cheyne-Stokes respirations may occur preterminally.

Therapy should be initiated promptly. As with massive cerebral infarction, medical therapy consisting of hyperventilation and the administration of osmotic agents and steroids should be instituted. If there is no improvement, consideration should be given to surgical therapy.[2–5,15,17] The treatment options are external ventricular drainage or posterior fossa craniectomy and resection of infarcted cerebellar tissue.[11,27] The choice of therapy will depend on the clinical status of the patient; if the patient has significant hydrocephalus with minimal signs of brain stem compression, ventricular drainage may be the procedure of choice. If there is not a prompt clinical improvement, then posterior fossa surgery should be undertaken without much procrastination. In patients with significant brain stem compression from massive infarction, one should proceed directly with posterior craniectomy. A rapidly done craniectomy along with resection of avascular cerebellar tissue with the patient in the prone position is a relatively simple and definitive procedure. It quickly relieves the direct pressure on the brain stem, which is virtually the sole cause of death. Improvement is quick and dramatic, provided the brain stem has not undergone permanent changes from extrinsic pressure, or has itself undergone infarction from occlusive vascular disease.

References

1. Adams JH, Graham DI. Twelve cases of fatal cerebral infarction due to arterial occlusion in the absence of atheromatous stenosis or embolism. *J Neurol Neurosurg Psychiatry* 1957; 30:479–488.
2. Auer LM, Auer T, Sayama I. Indications for surgical treatment of cerebellar haemorrhage and infarction. *Acta Neurochir (Wien)* 1986; 79:74–79.
3. Bertalanffy H, De Vries J. Management of cerebellar infarction with associated occlusive hydrocephalus. *Clin Neurol Neurosurg* 1992; 94:19–23.
4. Chen HF, Lee TC, Wei CP. Treatment of cerebellar infarction by decompressive suboccipital craniectomy. *Stroke* 1992; 23:957–961.
5. Cioffi FA, Bernini FP, Punzo A, et al. Surgical management of acute cerebellar infarction. *Acta Neurochir (Wien)* 1985; 74:105–112.
6. Delashaw JB, Broaddus WC, Kassell NF, et al. Treatment of right hemispheric cerebral infarction by hemicraniectomy. *Stroke* 1990; 21:874–881.
7. Feely MP. Cerebellar infarction. *Neurosurgery* 1979; 4:7–11.
8. Germain A, Morvan A. Ramollissement cérébelleux pseudo tumoral. *Ann Med Interne (Paris)* 1938; 44:1695–1700.
9. Harbaugh RE, Saunders RL, Reeves AG. Pediatric cerebellar infarction: case report and review of the literature. *Neurosurgery* 1982; 10:593–596.
10. Heros RC. Cerebellar hemorrhage and infarction. *Contemp Neurosurg* 1980; 2 (25):1–6.
11. Horwitz NH, Ludolph C. Acute obstructive hydrocephalus caused by cerebellar infarction: treatment alternatives. *Surg Neurol* 1983; 20:13–19.
12. Iannotti F, Hoff JT, Schielke GP. Brain tissue pressure in focal cerebral ischemia. *J Neurosurg* 1985; 62:83–89.
13. Ivamoto HS, Numoto M, Donaghy RMP. Surgical decompression for cerebral and cerebellar infarcts. *Stroke* 1974; 5:365–369.

14. Katzman R, Clasen R, Klatzo I, et al. Brain edema in stroke: study group on brain edema in stroke. *Stroke* 1977; 8:512–540.
15. Klugkist H, McCarthy J. Surgical treatment of space-occupying cerebellar infarctions—4½ years post-operative follow-up. *Neurosurg Rev* 1991; 14:17–22.
16. Kondziolka D, Fazl M. Functional recovery after decompressive craniectomy for cerebral infarction. *Neurosurgery* 1988; 23:143–147.
17. Laun A, Busse O, Calatayud V, et al. Cerebellar infarcts in the area of the supply of the PICA and their surgical treatment. *Acta Neurochir (Wien)* 1984; 71:295–306.
18. Laurent JP, Molinari GF, Moseley JI. Clinicopathological validation of a primate stroke model. *Surg Neurol* 1975; 4:449–455.
19. Lehrich JR, Winkler GF, Ojemann RG. Cerebellar infarction with brain stem compression: diagnosis and surgical treatment. *Arch Neurol* 1970; 22:490–498.
20. Maseu JC. Infarct versus neoplasm on CT: four helpful signs. *Am J Neuroradiol* 1983; 4:522–524.
21. Ng LKY, Nimmannitya J. Massive cerebral infarction with severe brain swelling: a clinicopathological study. *Stroke* 1970; 1:158–163.
22. O'Brien MD, Waltz AG. Intracranial pressure gradients caused by experimental cerebral ischemia and edema. *Stroke* 1973; 4:694–698.
23. Plum F. Brain swelling and edema in cerebral vascular disease. *Res Publ Assoc Res Nerv Ment Dis* 1961; 41:318–348.
24. Rengachary SS, Batnitzky S, Morantz RA, et al. Hemicraniectomy for acute massive cerebral infarction. *Neurosurgery* 1981; 8:321–327.
25. Ropper AH, Shafran B. Brain edema after stroke. Clinical syndrome and intracranial pressure. *Arch Neurol* 1984; 41:26–29.
26. Shaw CM, Alvord EC Jr, Berry RG. Swelling of the brain following ischemic infarction with arterial occlusion. *Arch Neurol* 1959; 1:161–177.
27. Shenkin HA, Zavala M. Cerebellar strokes: mortality, surgical indications, and results of ventricular drainage. *Lancet* 1982; 2:429–432.
28. Sypert GW, Alvord EC. Cerebellar infarction: a clinico-pathological study. *Arch Neurol* 1975; 32:357–363.
29. Van Trotsenburg L, Vinken PJ. Fatal cerebral infarction simulating an acute expanding lesion. *J Neurol Neurosurg Psychiatry* 1966; 29:241–243.
30. Young PH, Smith KR Jr, Dunn RC. Surgical decompression after cerebral hemispheric stroke: indications and patient selection. *South Med J* 1982; 75:473–475.

210

Extracranial to Intracranial Bypass Grafting

Robert F. Spetzler
Mark N. Hadley

Cerebral revascularization is an important treatment option for the neurosurgeon in the treatment of selected patients with cerebral ischemia and patients with mass lesions (tumor, aneurysm) that compromise or involve the intracranial vasculature. The Cooperative Study of Extracranial/Intracranial Arterial Anastomosis (EC/IC Bypass Study) redefined the indications for cerebral revascularization procedures. The results of the study are clear: the routine use of an extracranial to intracranial (EC–IC) bypass without specific, documented indications is no longer valid. Although the EC–IC bypass study failed to identify a specific group of patients in whom revascularization (specifically a superficial temporal to middle cerebral artery bypass procedure) provided statistically significant benefit compared with medical therapy,[28] there nonetheless is a finite number of patients with cerebral ischemia for whom cerebral revascularization remains a valid therapeutic option.[9,17] These are patients who have persistent symptoms of cerebral ischemia with documented hypoperfusion, without infarction or other intracranial causative mass lesion, who are refractory to optimal medical management.

In addition, cerebral revascularization (either an EC–IC bypass or intracranial vascular interposition graft) is an important surgical adjunct in the treatment of patients with complex skull base tumors or intracavernous or giant or fusiform aneurysms that compromise hemispheral cerebral circulation or that require surgical occlusion of a major cerebral vessel as part of the treatment of the tumor or aneurysm. The prophylactic use of cerebral revascularization to prevent ischemia or stroke from such vascular occlusion has been well documented. Identification of the patients most likely to benefit from these procedures, and the therapeutic options available to the neurosurgeon in the treatment of these patients will be discussed.

Theoretical Considerations

Providing additional nutrient blood supply to the brain and/or brain stem in the treatment of ischemia has theoretical merit. A vascular conduit from the extracranial to the intracranial circulation (or an intracranial interposition graft) circumventing major cerebral arterial occlusion, whether acquired or performed as part of a surgical procedure, should be expected to provide significant additional nutrient blood supply and to ameliorate or prevent symptoms of ischemia secondary to hypoperfusion. Several individual series have documented improved neurological function following cerebral revascularization with long-term resolution of symptoms.[1,4,5,11,27] Cerebral blood flow (CBF) studies employing several measurement techniques have demonstrated an increase in regional CBF in previously ischemic regions following bypass surgery.[3,8,12]

This rationale and these observations appeared to be invalidated by the findings from the Cooperative Study of Extracranial/Intracranial Arterial Anastomosis.[28] Patients in that study who underwent bypass surgery had no better outcome than did patients randomized to medical treatment. At first glance, it appeared that cerebral revascularization was an excellent theoretical concept but was without specific indications and of no proven benefit.

Since the completion of the EC–IC bypass study, much has been learned about the pathophysiology of cerebrovascular ischemia. The results of the Cooperative Study have been analyzed in detail, and the indications for cerebral revascularization have been redefined.[2,9] Surgeons have learned that perioperative morbidity and mortality rates must be kept at an absolute minimum if the surgical treatment of cerebral ischemia is to have merit compared with medical therapy. They have developed surgical techniques to revascularize from more proximal (larger) vessels rather than distal branches. New treatment paradigms have been created to study patients more carefully and to optimize their individual care. Anterior and posterior EC–IC revascularization procedures as well as intracranial interposition grafting procedures are now being employed in a limited and rational manner, with excellent clinical results.

Cerebral revascularization procedures can divert additional nutrient blood flow to an ischemic region of the brain or brain stem and can circumvent vessel occlusion, ligation, or resection. High long-term patency rates have been achieved.[5,9,11,27,28] The Cooperative Study and multiple surgical series have demonstrated that the difficulty with these procedures lies not in completing the surgical exercise but in minimizing perioperative ischemic complications and in selecting the patient who is most likely to benefit from the operation. Patients with transient cerebral ischemia from thromboembolic sources or cardiovascular dysfunction are unlikely to realize long-term relief of their symptoms after EC–IC bypass. Revascularization procedures for patients without documented ischemic hypoperfusion, those who do not have definable angiographic causative vascular lesions, or those who have had cerebral infarction, are of little merit. Potential EC–IC bypass patients must be studied with care in a compulsive, comprehensive manner if the relatively rare patient with persistent transient ischemic symptoms from hypoperfusion is to be identified. Potential interposition graft patients must be evaluated with equal detail, for careful definition of intracranial anatomy and reasonable determination of procedure feasibility and long-term outcome.

Patient Selection

The majority of patients with cerebral ischemia have symptoms caused by thromboembolic events.[2,9] Still, patients with transient ischemic attacks (TIAs) or stroke from hemodynamic vascular insufficiency represent a significant minority. Often, multiple factors are operating simultaneously to produce symptoms in an individual patient. Great care must be taken to correctly diagnose patients with hemodynamic cerebrovascular insufficiency. Vague complaints such as a lightheadedness, dizziness, or headache must be accompanied by more concrete symptoms and signs of hemodynamic compromise which must correlate with a demonstrable abnormality on the radiologic studies. The evaluation of patients with cerebral ischemia involves a complex paradigm and includes angiography of the entire cerebral vascular tree, stable xenon computed tomography (CT)-CBF studies, and magnetic resonance (MR) imaging (Fig. 210-1).

Anterior Circulation Cerebral Ischemia

Patients with anterior circulation cerebral ischemia typically have symptoms due to thromboembolic events. Cardiac disease and atherosclerotic ulcerative disease involving the carotid artery bifurcations in the neck represent the most frequent sources of emboli. Patients with anterior circulation ischemic events must undergo angiographic study of their entire cerebral vascular tree. Detailed four-vessel head and neck angiography (including aortic arch views) is essential to document vascular occlusion or stenosis, the presence or absence of collateral blood supply (or a ''steal'' phenomenon), and the location and caliber of extracranial vascular channels.

All potential embolic sources must be identified and appropriately treated. Detailed medical evaluations should be performed, including a cardiologic assessment for cardiac arrhythmias or a potential cardiac embolic source. Attendant medical problems should be brought under optimal control. If patients with carotid artery disease (ulcer, stenosis, or occlusion) remain symptomatic despite aspirin therapy, then the appropriate carotid artery surgical procedure should be performed (endarterectomy, stumpectomy, external carotid endarterectomy) by an experienced neurovascular surgeon with a documented low perioperative complication rate.

If patients remain symptomatic despite aspirin or anticoagulation therapy after successful surgical treatment of their carotid artery bifurcation disease (stumpectomy or carotid endarterectomy), *and* if they have a documented causative vascular lesion (high-grade stenosis or occlusion of a major intracranial vessel), confirmed by angiography, then stable xenon CT-CBF studies should be utilized. These studies, without and with acetazolamide (Diamox; Lederle Laboratories, Wayne, NJ) activation,[25] document regions of hypoperfusion and limited autoregulatory reserve (Figs. 210-2 and 210-3). Acetazolamide, a carbonic anhydrase

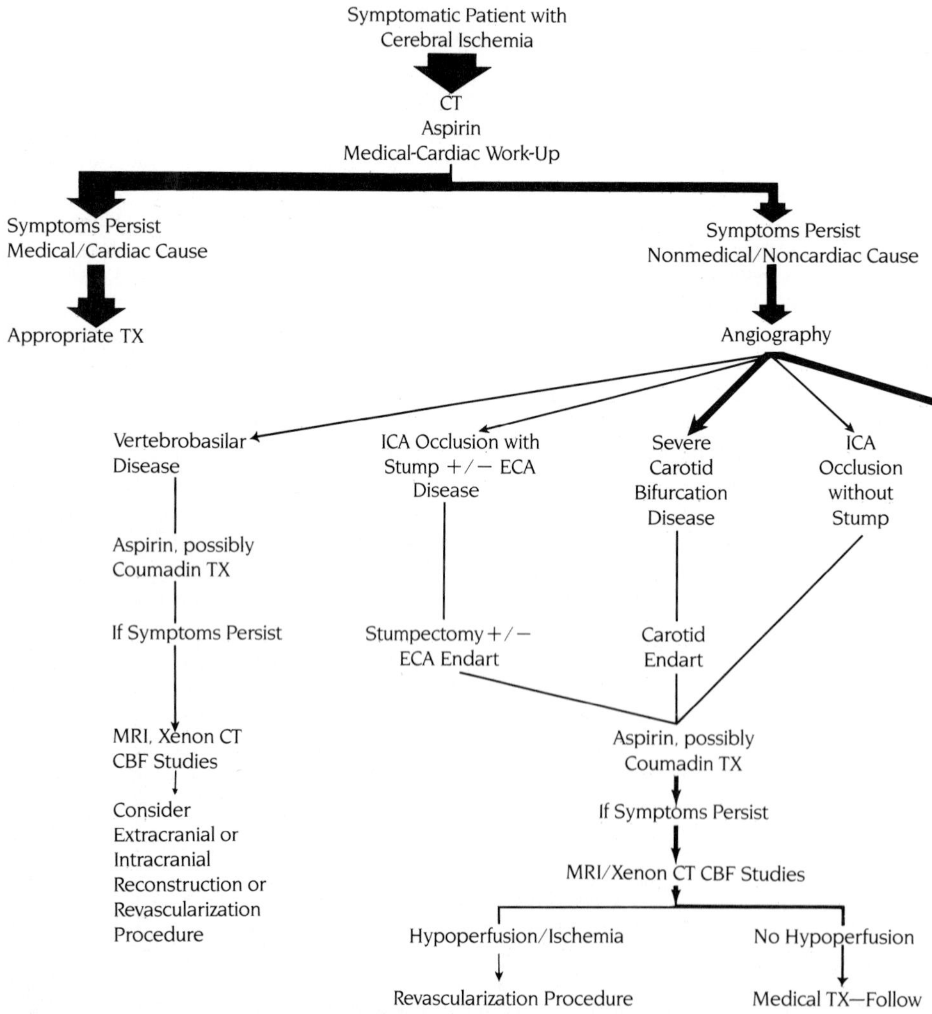

Figure 210-1 Graphic representation of an evaluation-treatment algorithm for patients with symptoms of cerebral ischemia. The size of the arrows indicates the relative numbers of patients. Endart, endarterectomy; TX, therapy. (From Hadley and Spetzler,[9] with permission.)

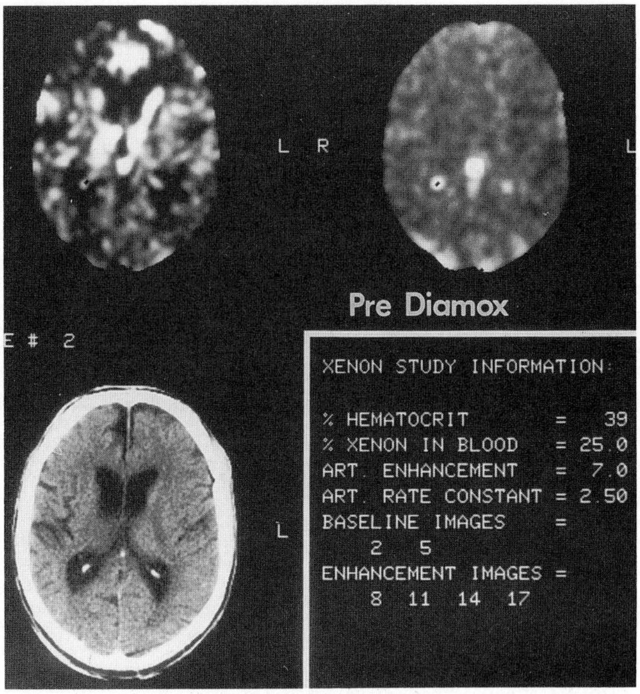

Figure 210-2 A xenon CT-CBF study prior to activation with acetazolamide in a patient with right MCA distribution ischemia.

inhibitor, causes an increase in CBF. In ischemic areas with limited autoregulatory reserve, relatively little (or no) increase in regional CBF will be visualized after acetazolamide activation, providing additional evidence that the region of cerebral tissue in question is indeed underperfused.[25]

MR imaging is utilized in the treatment algorithm to furnish critical information about infarction in the regions of the brain that appear ischemic on the xenon CT-CBF studies.[24] In addition, MR imaging provides precise views of the brain stem and posterior fossa structures (which traditionally are poorly visualized on CT studies) as well as documents ventricular size and the presence of mass lesions (e.g., cyst, tumor, hematoma, or arteriovenous malformation) that might mimic ischemic disease.[24]

The ischemic and hypoperfused region of cerebral tissue (determined by xenon CT-CBF) must not have evidence of cerebral infarction (determined by MR imaging) and must correlate with the patient's clinical picture if revascularization is to have the potential to reverse the cerebral ischemia.

Skull base or cavernous sinus tumors or giant or fusiform intracavernous–intracranial aneurysms often can be effectively managed with radical resection and/or vascular trapping. These procedures often include resecting or ligating the intracavernous or

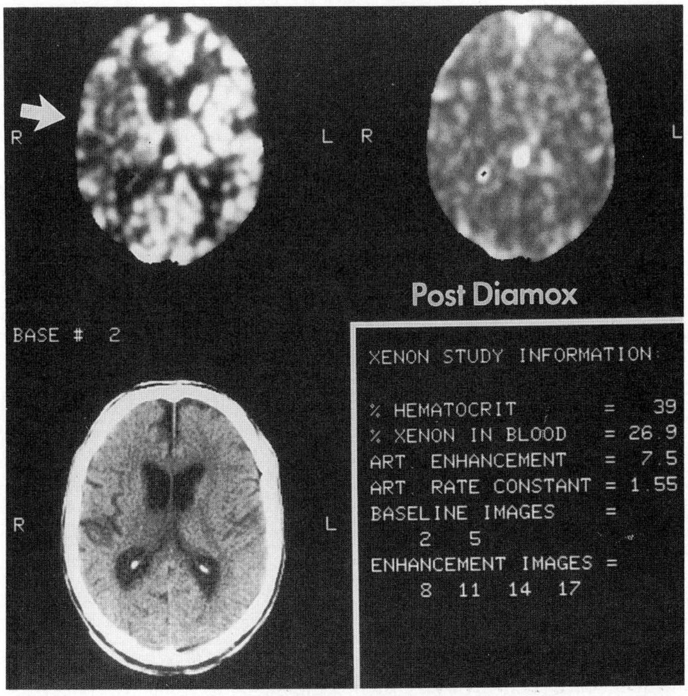

Figure 210-3 A xenon CT-CBF study after the administration of acetazolamide to the patient depicted in Fig. 210-2. Note the overall increase in CBF as measured by this technique (*upper left image*). The right MCA distribution does not reveal increased CBF with activation (*arrow*).

proximal intracranial portion of the internal carotid artery. A petrous carotid to intracranial carotid artery interposition graft revascularization procedure can be performed to maintain cerebral perfusion. Angiography, MR imaging, and occasionally MR angiography allow determination of vascular anatomy and definition of the size and extent of the pathologic lesion, and allow the surgeon to determine the feasibility of the procedure and predict long-term outcome.

If a prospective patient meets the criteria of each step of the evaluation–treatment paradigm as outlined and is an acceptable operative candidate from an anesthetic risk perspective, he or she may be considered for a cerebral revascularization procedure. The bypass to be performed on an individual patient is based on the unique pathologic and anatomic features of that individual as determined by the preoperative radiologic diagnostic studies and is directed at the ischemic region of greatest need. In general, a more proximal revascularization procedure is preferred over a more distal one.

Posterior Circulation Cerebral Ischemia

In contrast to patients with symptomatic anterior circulation ischemia, patients with posterior circulation ischemic symptoms have a lower incidence of atherosclerotic embolic disease and a higher incidence of ischemia due to hypoperfusion. Thromboembolic ulcerative disease is much less common in the vertebral and basilar arteries compared with that which occurs in the carotid arteries in the neck. True hypoperfusion, usually due to vertebral artery luminal compromise or occlusion *without* other major vascular collaterals to the posterior circulation (ie., patent posterior communicating arteries), is much more prevalent in the posterior vasculature compared with the anterior circulation (Figs. 210-4 and 210-5).

The evaluation–treatment paradigm for patients with posterior circulation ischemia is similar to that described for patients with anterior circulation disease (Fig. 210-1). If they remain symptomatic despite optimal medical therapy and if they have angiographic evidence of vertebrobasilar arterial disease, then MR imaging and xenon CT-CBF studies are obtained. If these studies support the diagnosis of vertebrobasilar insufficiency, are without evidence of infarction, and correlate with the patient's angiographic studies and clinical picture, then a posterior circulation reconstruction or revascularization procedure is considered.

Technical Aspects

The most heralded and most frequently performed EC–IC anastomosis has been the superficial temporal artery to middle cerebral artery (STA–MCA) bypass for anterior circulation disease. Several variations of this procedure have been performed, including STA to middle meningeal artery bypass, a "bonnet" bypass to the contralateral MCA, and the use of various interposition grafts (e.g., vein, artery, prosthetic grafts) in attempts to augment regional CBF.[2,5,11,13] We routinely attempt to direct STA–MCA anastomoses deep into the sylvian fissure to provide flow to the more proximal portions of the MCA rather than an anastomosis at a distal cortical branch. Occasionally double-limb bypasses will achieve similar high-flow results (Fig. 210-6).

Several reconstruction and revascularization options exist in the treatment of patients with posterior circulation ischemia. Every attempt is made to direct the surgical procedure at the offending

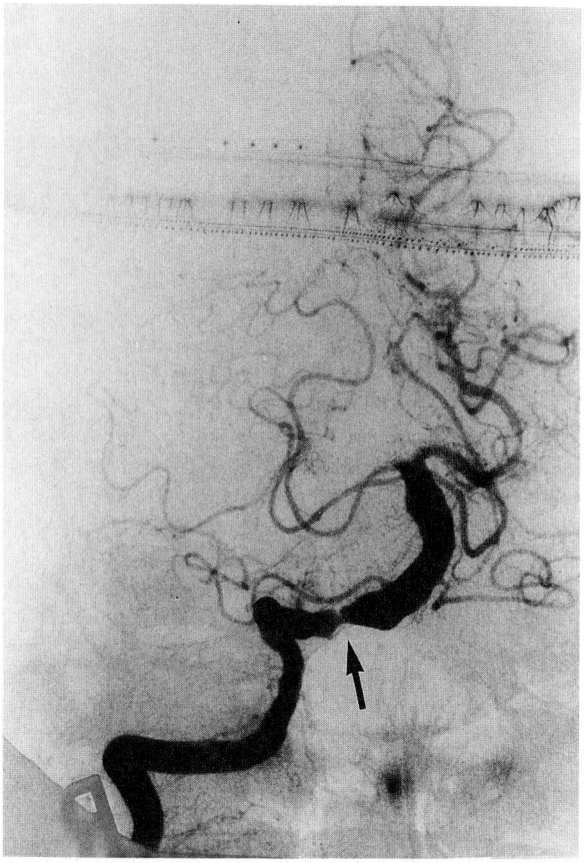

Figure 210-4 An angiogram of a patient with profound vertebrobasilar ischemia. The left VA was occluded above PICA. There was no other collateral supply to the basilar artery. The area of marked distal right VA stenosis could not be corrected surgically (*arrow*).

pathology, particularly in patients with first, second, or third portion vertebral artery (VA) disease. Procedures for these extracranial portions of the VA include proximal VA endarterectomy, VA to common carotid artery transposition, cervical osteophyte decompression of the VA, and third portion VA repair or endarterectomy.[19]

Intracranial VA compromise is rarely amenable to direct repair and usually requires (like basilar artery disease) an EC–IC bypass directed above the level of vascular compromise.[11] Revascularization options for intracranial vertebrobasilar insufficiency include STA to posterior cerebral artery (STA–PCA), STA to superior cerebellar artery (STA–SCA), STA to anterior inferior cerebellar artery (STA–AICA), and STA to posterior inferior cerebellar artery (STA–PICA) anastomoses.[9,11] Frequently, the occipital artery rather than the STA is used as the extracranial vascular conduit when attempting revascularization of the AICA or PICA vascular distributions.

Rarely, tumor masses may cause intracranial vascular compromise and resultant hemodynamic insufficiency (Figs. 210-7 to 210-9). More often, in an attempt to completely resect a skull base or cavernous sinus tumor, the surgeon must sacrifice the proximal intracranial portion of the internal carotid artery.

Occasionally, patients with giant or fusiform intracranial aneurysms require aneurysm trapping or excision. In rare circumstances, an aneurysmorrhaphy or end-to-end vessel reanastomosis is impossible. An EC–IC bypass to the distal vessel trunk can

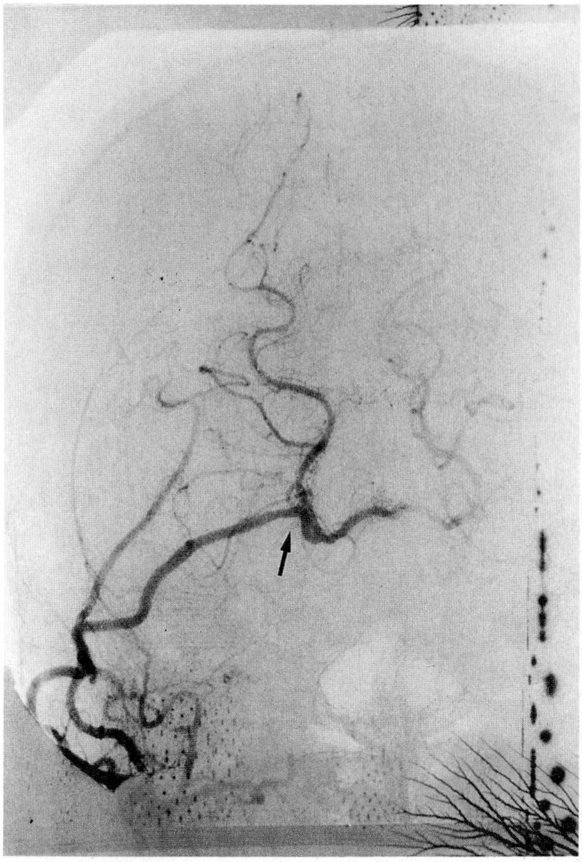

Figure 210-5 A postoperative selective external carotid artery injection in the same patient as shown in Fig. 210-4 reveals patency of the STA–PCA anastomosis (*arrow*) and filling of the posterior cerebral vessels. The patient's ischemic symptoms resolved.

prevent regional ischemia or stroke in the vascular distribution distal to the aneurysm trapping or excision site in these patients (Figs. 210-10 to 210-12).[10,17] A petrous carotid to intracranial carotid artery interposition graft will allow resection or trapping of a giant or fusiform intracavernous or proximal intracranial internal carotid artery aneurysm.[18]

Many aspects of the operative anesthetic management of patients undergoing cerebral revascularization procedures are the same irrespective of the specific anastomosis to be performed. All operations are performed under general anesthesia with maintenance of normotension, normocapnia, and adequate oxygenation ($P_{O_2} > 100$ mmHg). Intraoperative monitoring of the electroencephalogram (EEG) by compressed spectral analysis and of somatosensory and brain stem auditory evoked potentials are performed in all patients.[9,11,21,22] Aspirin (5 grains by mouth daily) is administered preoperatively and continued postoperatively.

Before vascular clamping of the recipient vessel, we administer barbiturates (thiopental, 1 to 3 mg/kg loading dose) to achieve EEG burst suppression. During the period of vessel occlusion, barbiturates are continued at a dose adequate to maintain burst suppression. If hypotension occurs before burst suppression, vasopressors (usually dopamine) are given to maintain normotension.[9,11,21,22]

A portable Doppler unit may be of value early in the procedure to map the course of the donor extracranial vessel when it is otherwise not apparent by inspection. The Shaw hemostatic scalpel

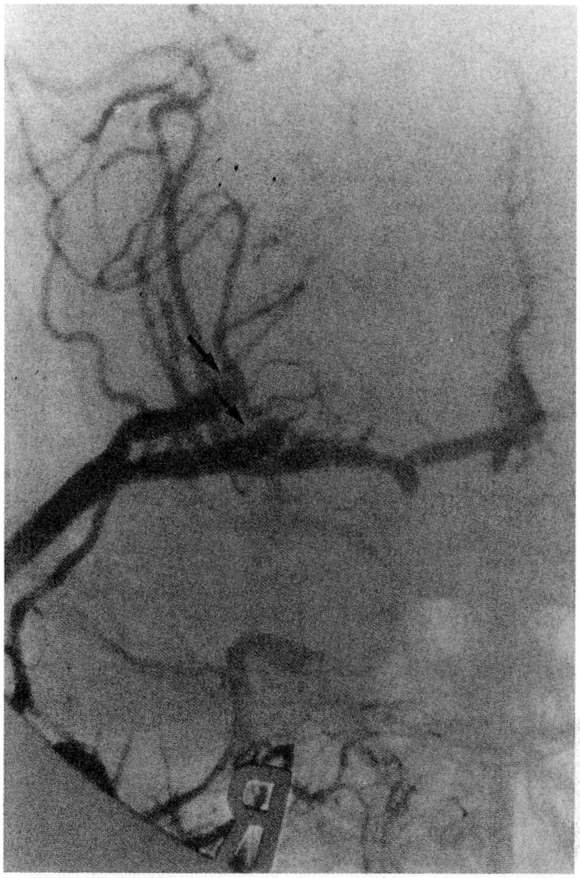

Figure 210-6 A double-limb (*arrows*) venous interposition graft to the deep middle cerebral artery. (From Awad and Spetzler,[2] with permission.)

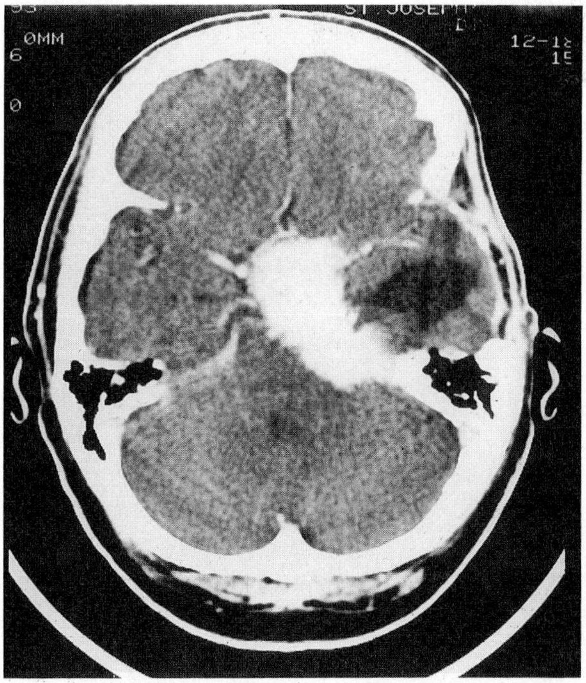

Figure 210-7 A large residual meningioma invading the cavernous sinus. The patient had been previously operated upon and irradiated, and was treated with iridium seeds within the tumor cavity.

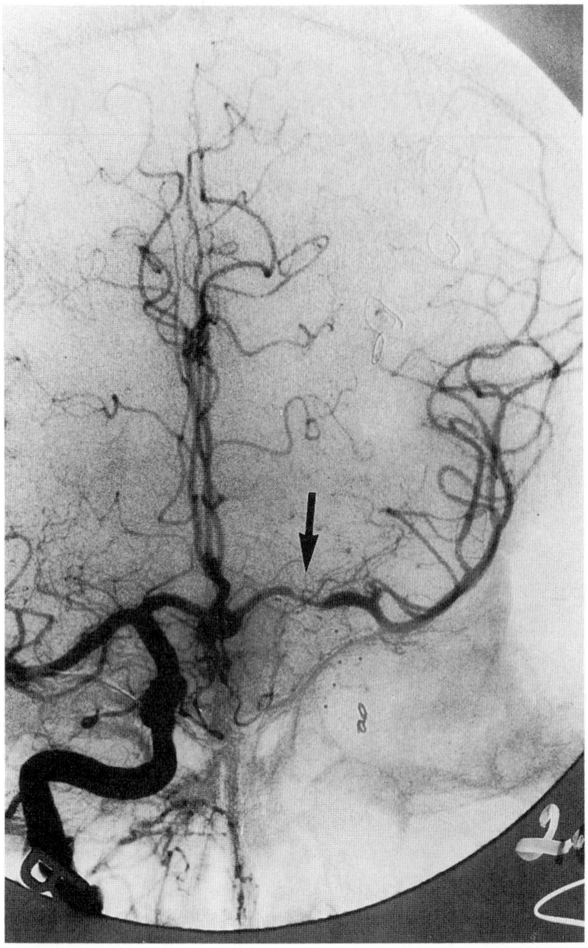

Figure 210-8 An angiogram of the same patient shown in Fig. 210-7 who presented with left hemispheric ischemic symptoms. Note the occlusion of the ICA with marked narrowing of the MCA (*arrow*).

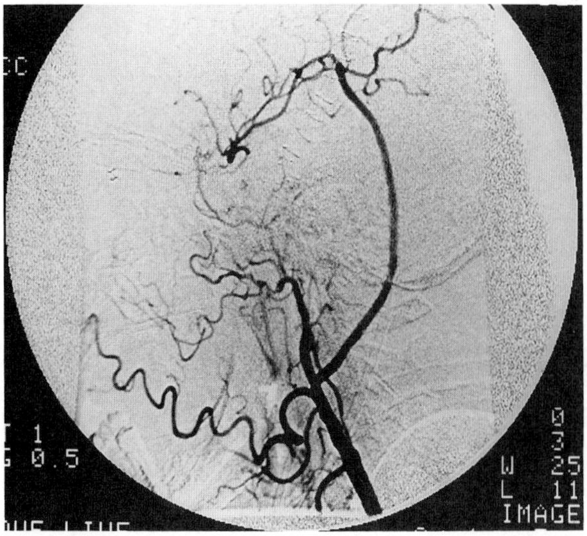

Figure 210-9 Same patient as depicted in Figs. 210-7 and 210-8. A postoperative digital subtraction angiogram reveals a saphenous interposition graft from the ICA stump in the neck to the MCA. The patient's ischemic symptoms resolved.

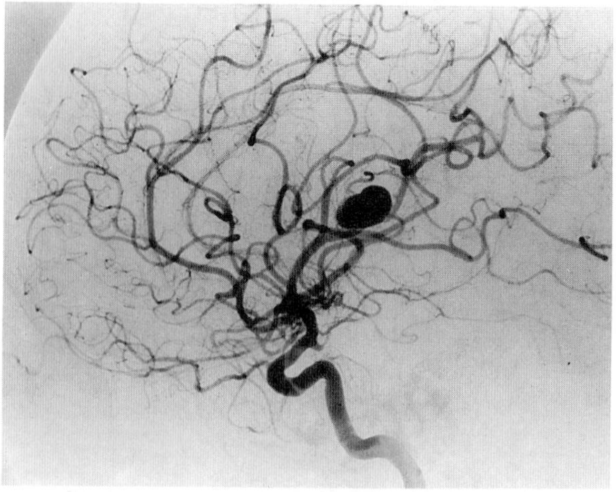

Figure 210-10 A mycotic aneurysm due to *Nocardia asteroides* in a patient with systemic lupus erythematosus. (From Hadley et al.,[10] with permission.)

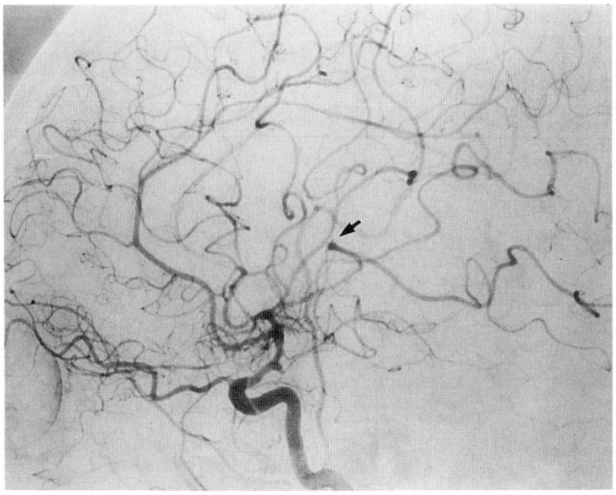

Figure 210-11 A postoperative angiogram of the same patient shown in Fig. 210-10 reveals absence of the aneurysm with loss of distal MCA branches. (From Hadley et al.,[10] with permission.)

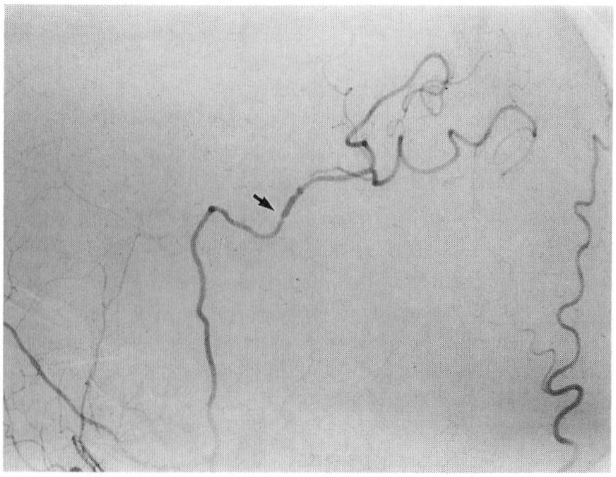

Figure 210-12 A selective external carotid artery injection of the patient depicted in Figs. 210-10 and 210-11 reveals an STA–MCA bypass filling the remaining MCA vasculature to the dominant parietal region. (From Hadley et al.,[10] with permission.)

(Oximetrix, Inc., Mountain View, CA) is utilized to make the skin incision and to perform the initial dissection. This instrument provides excellent hemostasis and allows a rapid, bloodless approach to both the donor and recipient vessels. When the intracranial anastomosis is performed, a small plastic dam is placed beneath the recipient artery and Microvac suction (Microvac, PMT Inc., Hopkins, MN) is placed beneath or near the dam to constantly clear cerebrospinal fluid from the operative field.[11,22] When using a vein interposition graft, great care must be taken to avoid damage to the vessel during harvest.[13,26] All side branches must be tied securely, and the orientation of the interposition graft once in place must be rechecked to avoid kinking or twisting and compromise of the lumen.[26]

All procedures are performed utilizing the operative microscope with a 250-mm lens, which provides excellent optics, lighting, and magnification. Following surgery, patients are monitored in the intensive care unit for the management of postoperative hypo- or hypertension. They usually undergo follow-up angiography within the first week after surgery. Follow-up stable xenon CT-CBF studies and/or MR imaging studies are performed selectively. The portable Doppler unit may be utilized at the bedside to assess blood flow through the extracranial donor vessel in the postoperative setting. Transcranial Doppler studies can be used to monitor flow through an internal carotid artery interposition graft.

Anterior Circulation

Superficial Temporal Artery to Middle Cerebral Artery Bypass

STA–MCA anastomoses are performed with the patient in the supine position with the head rotated to one side, exposing the temporoparietal region of the ischemic side. The parietal branch of the superficial temporal artery is most frequently used as the donor vessel. In our experience, the frontal branch is frequently already participating in the collateral supply to the region of ischemia. The donor vessel is dissected free from the scalp first, and then a small temporoparietal craniotomy is performed through the same scalp incision directly over the sylvian fissure. The EC–IC anastomosis is performed deep in the sylvian fissure.

Petrous Carotid Artery to Intradural Carotid Artery Bypass

An internal carotid artery interposition graft [petrous carotid artery, C5 segment, to intradural carotid artery, C3 segment (Fig. 210-13)] is accomplished with the patient in the supine position with the head rotated 30 degrees from the horizontal axis. A frontotemporal craniotomy is performed and the sylvian fissure

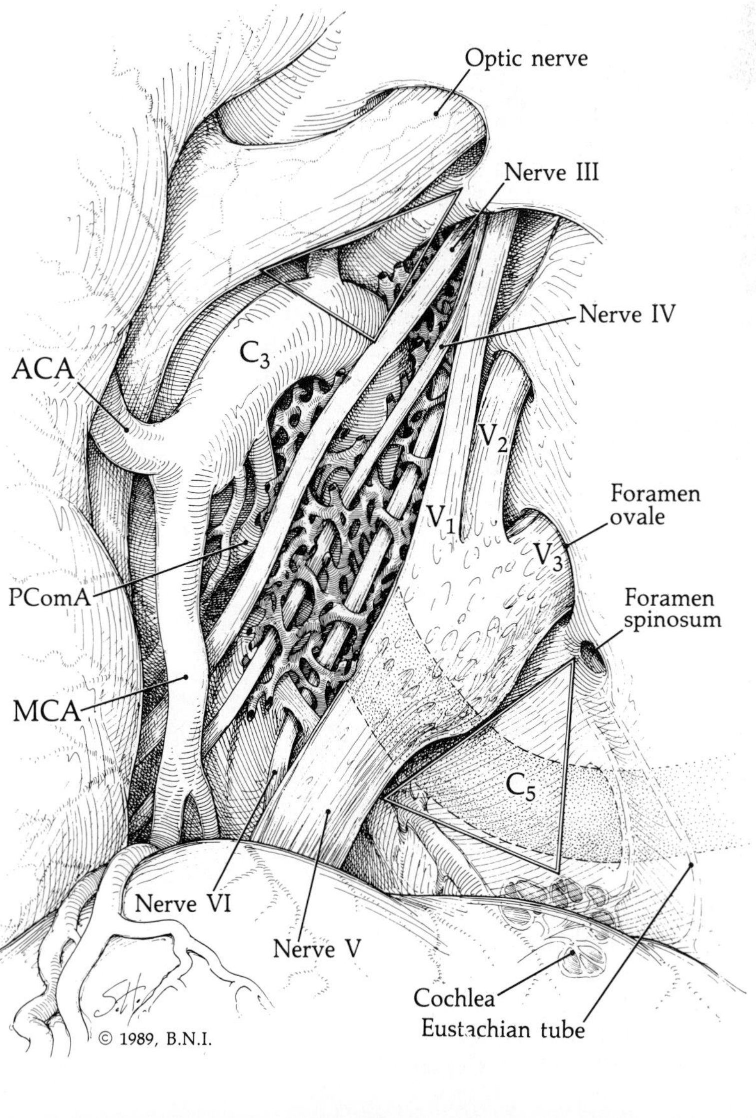

Figure 210-13 Artist's representation of the anatomy of the internal carotid artery (ICA) and the contents of the cavernous sinus as the ICA courses through the cavernous sinus. The C5 and C3 portions of the ICA are identified, and the avenues of exposure to the proximal and distal ICA are delineated by triangles. ACA, anterior cerebral artery; PComA, posterior communicating artery; MCA, middle cerebral artery; V_1, V_2, V_3 are the three branches of the trigeminal nerve; other cranial nerves are denoted by Roman numerals. (From Spetzler et al.,[18] with permission.)

opened. The sphenoid ridge, anterior clinoid process, and proximal optic canal are drilled away. The last aspect of the procedure is performed with a diamond-tipped burr. The dural fibrous ring at the intradural–extradural internal carotid artery junction is cut, allowing exposure of the C3 segment of the artery.[6,18] A clip can be placed across the internal carotid artery proximal to the origin of the ophthalmic artery with enough room to perform the saphenous vein interposition anastomosis between the ophthalmic artery and the posterior communicating artery.

The more proximal petrous (C5) portion of the internal carotid artery is exposed as described by Glasscock.[7,18] Care is taken to avoid stretching of the greater superficial petrosal nerve (which could cause ipsilateral facial palsy) and the eustachian tube (which could cause an ipsilateral decrease in hearing).[7,14,15,18] Ten to twelve millimeters of the internal carotid artery is exposed at this level. A saphenous interposition graft (harvested from the upper thigh for appropriate diameter) is sutured into position (after appropriate sizing and orientation of the graft). The proximal (C5) anastomosis is completed first, typically end-to-side, followed by the distal (C3) segment anastomosis, also end-to-side. The temporary vascular occlusion, anastomosis portions of the procedure are performed under barbiturate cerebral protection utilizing thiopental and anticoagulation with heparin.[18,20] The bypassed portion of the diseased internal carotid artery is left trapped (Fig. 210-14), or with cavernous sinus exenteration, can be resected.

Posterior Circulation

The patients who undergo a posterior circulation revascularization procedure are placed in the modified park bench or prone position, depending on the specific vascular anastomosis to be performed. The Midas Rex drill (Midas Rex, Ft. Worth, TX) is used to create the bony exposure and is particularly useful for a posterior fossa craniotomy. All bone flaps are replaced at the completion of surgery. Patients having a posterior circulation intracranial procedure have a modest incidence of postoperative aseptic meningitis and/or communicating hydrocephalus [6 of 35 (17 percent) of patients in our series] that must be treated appropriately.[11,27]

Surgical Results

The senior author has performed over 200 cerebral revascularization procedures (Tables 210-1 and 210-2). One hundred sixty-five procedures were directed at the treatment of anterior circulation disease, 45 of which involved vein interposition grafts. Ten procedures were performed after aneurysm excision or trapping and two were performed to ameliorate ischemic symptoms due to tumor stenosis or occlusion of the intracranial internal carotid artery. Thirty-five EC–IC bypasses have been performed in the treatment

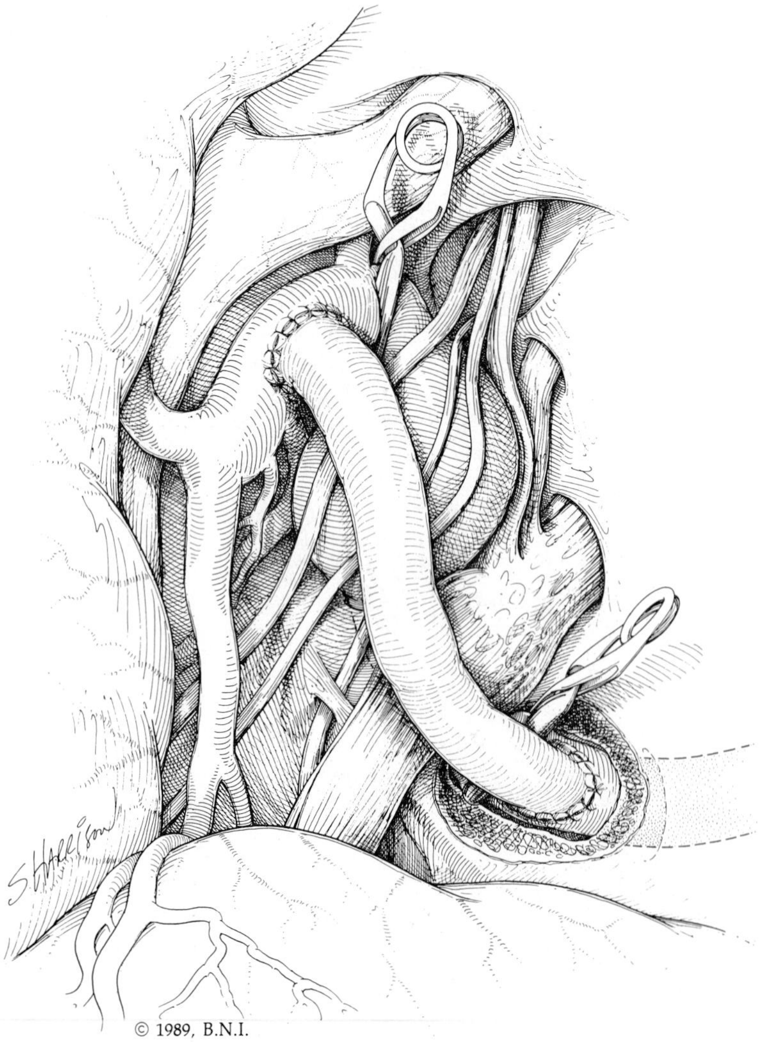

Figure 210-14 Artist's depiction of a completed C5–C3 saphenous vein graft interposition bypass. Aneurysm clips are placed across the ICA close to the ophthalmic artery (distally) and the proximal anastomotic site to eliminate any vascular dead space. (From Spetzler et al.,[18] with permission.)

TABLE 210-1 Revascularization Procedures Performed from 1978 to 1988

Procedures	Number
Anterior circulation	
STA–MCA bypass	120
Vein interposition	45
Posterior circulation	
Occipital–PICA	21
STA–SCA	9
STA–PCA	3
Vein interposition	2
Total	200

of vertebrobasilar insufficiency, two of which involved vein interposition grafts. The frequency with which these procedures have been performed has changed dramatically over time, particularly because the Cooperative Study results dictated a more rational, comprehensive approach to patients with cerebral ischemia. We have averaged less than four EC–IC bypass procedures per year in the treatment of cerebral ischemia since 1985, a marked reduction over the pre-bypass study years. More recently a more aggressive approach has been employed in the treatment of selected patients with skull base tumors or internal carotid artery aneurysms within the cavernous sinus.[18]

Follow-up was achieved in 180 of the 200 treated patients listed in Tables 210-1 and 210-2 (90 percent), with a median duration of 32 months. Eighteen patients died, most as a result of severe cardiopulmonary disease. The patency rate of the STA–MCA anastomoses was 95 percent, the patency rate of the posterior circulation anastomoses (excluding the vein interposition grafts) was 96 percent, and the patency rate of the vein interposition grafts (anterior and posterior) was 83 percent. Eighty-five percent of patients were relieved of their symptoms, 10 percent had a reduction in symptoms, and 5 percent had no improvement in their preoperative status. There was zero operative mortality and less than 5 percent morbidity for the series as a whole.

Although the number of patients is smaller and the follow-up is limited, the senior author's success rate with the petrous carotid to intracranial carotid artery interposition graft procedure has been good, with zero mortality and limited perioperative morbidity.[18]

TABLE 210-2 Variations on Autologous Venous Interposition Anastomoses

Procedure	Number
Anterior circulation	
SCA–MCA	25
CCA–MCA	4
SCA–ECA/STA–MCA	4
CCA–ICA	3
"Bonnet" (STA–contralateral MCA)	2
CCA–ECA/STA–MCA	1
ICA–MCA	1
ECA–MCA	1
SCA–CCA	1
ICA–ICA	3
Posterior circulation	
ECA–PCA	1
SCA–PCA	1
Total	47

CCA, common carotid artery; ICA, internal carotid artery; SCA, subclavian artery.

Discussion

EC–IC vascular anastomosis procedures remain a viable option in the treatment of a small group of selected patients with brain ischemia. The number of patients who are candidates for these procedures represents a small percentage of the total population of patients with symptomatic cerebrovascular ischemia. Prior to the EC–IC Bypass Study, a wide variety of patients with cerebral ischemia were treated with an EC–IC bypass (a maximum of 70 in 1 year by the senior author). The use of EC–IC revascularization is now restricted to a limited, select group of patients who meet the criteria of the evaluation–treatment cerebrovascular insufficiency paradigm as outlined. Utilizing this systematic approach to the evaluation and treatment of cerebral ischemia, we have averaged less than four EC–IC bypass procedures per year for cerebral ischemia since the results of the study were made available.

The revascularization procedures are technically straightforward and high patency rates have been documented (albeit lower with vein interposition grafts).[5,9,11,26–28] Several series have documented improvement in acute cerebral ischemic symptoms after bypass, a finding that suggests a possible reduction of stroke risk in treated patients.[1,4,5,9,11,26,27] For surgical treatment of cerebrovascular hypoperfusion to be considered efficacious compared with optimal medical therapy, two conditions must be realized. The first, as already discussed, is careful, judicious selection of patients. The second is to achieve morbidity and mortality rates of an absolute minimum for the revascularization procedures.

Several surgical adjuncts we routinely employ help to maintain morbidity and mortality rates at or near zero. Most important is the use of microneurosurgical techniques and the operative microscope. In addition, we believe the practices of intraoperative heparinization, barbiturate-induced suppression of cerebral electrical activity, and perioperative blood pressure control are important adjuncts for successful EC–IC bypass surgery.[9,11] Pre- and postoperative antithrombotic therapy (aspirin) helps to prevent thrombosis at the site of anastomosis. Several studies have documented the beneficial effects of heparin on platelet aggregation (inhibition) and fibrin formation (inhibition) during vascular surgery.[9,11,22] Avoidance of pharmacologic heparin reversal and the perioperative use of aspirin contribute to the protection from perioperative thromboembolic events.[22]

The rationale for the use of barbiturates is that they reduce the metabolic requirements of cerebral tissue and may be responsible for extending the tolerance of the brain for the reduction of substrate supply that occurs with ischemia.[11,16,21–23] Several investigators have reported that barbiturates, in particular thiopental and pentobarbital, have the capacity to modify or prevent cerebral injury due to focal ischemia.[11,16,21–23] Barbiturate therapy is most efficacious when the agent is administered before a period of temporary focal ischemia, which makes them a logical choice as a cerebroprotective agent during elective neurovascular surgery.[11,16,21,22] We use barbiturate protection to the point of EEG burst suppression in all major neurovascular procedures and have had no untoward reactions or complications.[9,11,21,22] Most importantly, in our experience barbiturate therapy has been effective in protecting the brain during surgery. No patient in this series had a postoperative neurological deficit from ischemia as a result of clamping the recipient vessel to perform the anastomosis. Our experience with the use of barbiturate cerebral protection during carotid endarterectomy and during complete circulatory arrest in the treatment of giant intracranial aneurysms has been similar.[21,22]

Strict blood pressure control during the operative and postoperative periods helps reduce the incidence of hypotensive ischemia (hypoperfusion) and hypertensive intracerebral hemorrhage.[11,22] In our experience, postoperative hypotension has been due to hypovolemia; close attention to the patient's intraoperative fluid balance and cardiac parameters will avoid this potential complication. Hypertension has been common in the immediate postoperative period and is effectively treated by a constant infusion of sodium nitroprusside. As noted, patients who undergo posterior fossa revascularization procedures (particularly occipital artery–PICA anastomoses) have an increased incidence of postoperative aseptic meningitis and/or communicating hydrocephalus.[11] Clinicians must be aware of these potential complications and treat them appropriately.

The decision to use a vein interposition graft is made when other anatomic collateral channels are unavailable, too small, or already involved in the collateral circulation process.[11,13,26] We commonly use the saphenous vein as the interposition graft because it affords a wide variety of potential anastomoses employing either long or short segments. The advantages of using a vein graft include its luminal diameter (much larger than that of the STA), the lack of atherosclerotic changes within the vein that are commonly found in the donor artery, the ability to provide immediate high flow rates to the recipient vascular bed, and the length of the vein (essentially unrestricted). It is the most suitable interposition graft substrate option when performing an internal carotid artery interposition bypass graft procedure. The disadvantages of using a vein as a donor vessel include the necessity of harvesting an additional vessel, the performance of two anastomoses, the luminal size discrepancy between the vein and the recipient vessel, and reduced long-term patency rates.[11,13,26] All of these factors must be considered in the treatment of an individual patient.

Summary

There remains a finite group of patients with recurrent transient cerebral ischemia without infarction who seem to benefit from extracranial to intracranial revascularization procedures. These are patients with persistent cerebral ischemia from hypoperfusion who are refractory to optimal medical management. The identification of these relatively infrequent patients can be facilitated by employing the evaluation–treatment paradigm we have outlined, which includes a comprehensive medical–cardiac workup and ''ischemia sensitive'' neuroradiologic diagnostic procedures (angiography, xenon CT-CBF studies, and MR imaging).

There exists another group of patients with intracavernous or intracranial mass lesions (tumor, aneurysm) who can benefit from resection of their offending pathology and reconstruction of their internal carotid artery with an interposition bypass graft. The selection of these patients has been described. For all those patients being considered for cerebral revascularization, conscientious perioperative patient management and meticulous microneurosurgical and anesthetic techniques can minimize perioperative morbidity and mortality and improve long-term survival.

References

1. Andrews BT, Weinstein PR, Chater NL. Emergency extracranial–intracranial arterial bypass for stroke in evolution. In Spetzler RF, Carter LP, Selman WR, et al. (eds): *Cerebral Revascularization for Stroke.* New York: Thieme-Stratton, 1985, pp 542–547.
2. Awad IA, Spetzler RF. Extracranial–intracranial bypass surgery: a critical analysis in light of the International Cooperative Study. *Neurosurgery* 1986; 19:655–664.
3. Carter LP, Hadley MN, Spetzler RF. Regional cortical blood flow during extracranial–intracranial bypass. In Spetzler RF, Carter LP, Selman WR, et al. (eds): *Cerebral Revascularization for Stroke.* New York: Thieme-Stratton, 1985, pp 136–142.
4. Day AL. EC–IC bypass for MCA obstruction. In Spetzler RF, Carter LP, Selman WR, et al. (eds): *Cerebral Revascularization for Stroke.* New York: Thieme-Stratton, 1985, pp 458–466.
5. Diaz FG, Umansky F, Mehta B, et al. Cerebral revascularization to a main limb of the middle cerebral artery in the sylvian fissure: an alternative approach to conventional anastomosis. *J Neurosurg* 1985; 63:21–29.
6. Dolenc VV. A combined epi- and subdural direct approach to carotid-ophthalmic artery aneurysms. *J Neurosurg* 1985; 62:667–672.
7. Glasscock ME III. Exposure of the intra-petrous portion of the carotid artery. In Hamberger CA, Wersall J (eds): *Disorders of the Skull Base Region: Proceedings of the Tenth Nobel Symposium, Stockholm, 1968.* Stockholm: Almqvist & Wiksell, 1969, pp 135–143.
8. Gratzl O, Schmiedek P, Spetzler R, et al. Clinical experience with extra-intracranial arterial anastomosis in 65 cases. *J Neurosurg* 1976; 44:313–324.
9. Hadley MN, Spetzler RF. Contemporary application of the extracranial–intracranial bypass for cerebral revascularization. *Contemp Neurosurg* 1988; 9(25):1–6.
10. Hadley MN, Spetzler RF, Martin NA, et al. Middle cerebral artery aneurysm due to *Nocardia asteroides:* case report of aneurysm excision and extracranial–intracranial bypass. *Neurosurgery* 1988; 22:923–928.
11. Hopkins LN, Martin NA, Hadley MN, et al. Vertebrobasilar insufficiency: Part 2. Microsurgical treatment of intracranial vertebrobasilar disease. *J Neurosurg* 1987; 66:662–674.
12. Laurent JP, Lawner PM, O'Connor M. Reversal of intracerebral steal by STA–MCA anastomosis. *J Neurosurg* 1982; 57:629–632.
13. Marano SR, Spetzler RF, Carter LP. Autogenous saphenous vein interposition grafts for high flow augmentation of cerebral blood flow. *BNI Q* 1985; 1(4):29–33.
14. Paullus WS, Pait TG, Rhoton AL Jr. Microsurgical exposure of the petrous portion of the carotid artery. *J Neurosurg* 1977; 47:713–726.
15. Sekhar LN, Schramm VL Jr, Jones NF. Subtemporal-preauricular infratemporal fossa approach to large lateral and posterior cranial base neoplasms. *J Neurosurg* 1987; 67:488–499.
16. Selman WR, Spetzler RF, Roski RA, et al. Barbiturate coma in focal cerebral ischemia: relationship of protection to timing of therapy. *J Neurosurg* 1982; 56:685–690.
17. Spetzler RF, Carter LP. Revascularization and aneurysm surgery: current status. *Neurosurgery* 1985; 16:111–116.
18. Spetzler RF, Fukushima T, Martin N, et al. Petrous carotid-to-intradural carotid saphenous vein graft for intracavernous giant aneurysm, tumor, and occlusive cerebrovascular disease. *J Neurosurg* 1990; 73:496–501.
19. Spetzler RF, Hadley MN, Martin NA, et al. Vertebrobasilar insufficiency: Part 1. Microsurgical treatment of extracranial vertebrobasilar disease. *J Neurosurg* 1987; 66:648–661.
20. Spetzler RF, Hadley MN, Raudzens PA. Barbiturate therapy for brain protection during temporary vascular occlusion. In Weinstein PR, Faden AI (eds): *Protection of the Brain from Ischemia.* Baltimore: Williams & Wilkins, 1990, pp 253–263.
21. Spetzler RF, Hadley MN, Rigamonti D, et al. Aneurysms of the basilar artery treated with circulatory arrest, hypothermia, and barbiturate cerebral protection. *J Neurosurg* 1988; 68:868–879.
22. Spetzler RF, Martin N, Hadley MN, et al. Microsurgical endarterectomy under barbiturate protection: a prospective study. *J Neurosurg* 1986; 65:63–73.
23. Spetzler RF, Selman WR, Roski RA, et al. Cerebral revascularization

during barbiturate coma in primates and humans. *Surg Neurol* 1982; 17:111–115.
24. Spetzler RF, Zabramski JM, Kaufman B. Clinical role of magnetic resonance imaging in the neurosurgical patient. *Neurosurgery* 1985; 16:511–524.
25. Sullivan HG, Kingsbury TB IV, Morgan ME, et al. The rCBF response to Diamox in normal subjects and cerebrovascular disease patients. *J Neurosurg* 1987; 67:525–534.
26. Sundt TM Jr, Piepgras DG, Marsh WR, et al. Saphenous vein bypass grafts for giant aneurysms and intracranial occlusive disease. *J Neurosurg* 1986; 65:439–450.
27. Sundt TM Jr, Whisnant JP, Fode NC, et al. Results, complications, and follow-up of 415 bypass operations for occlusive disease of the carotid system. *Mayo Clin Proc* 1985; 60:230–240.
28. The EC/IC Bypass Study Group. Failure of extracranial–intracranial arterial bypass to reduce the risk of ischemic stroke: results of an international randomized trial. *N Engl J Med* 1985; 313:1191–1200.

211 Fibromuscular Dysplasia

L. N. Hopkins
James L. Budny

Fibromuscular dysplasia (FMD) is a multifocal angiopathy of unknown etiology most commonly affecting aortic branch arteries with multiple constrictions and aneurysmal dilatations. The diagnosis is usually made by angiography. It is most commonly found in the renal arteries. Surgical correction with transluminal angioplastic techniques has been shown to reverse renovascular hypertension.

In the mid-1960s various reports demonstrated FMD in most of the branches of the abdominal aorta and in the cervical portion of the internal carotid artery (ICA). FMD has been described in the vertebral and, more recently, the intracranial vessels, although the most common cerebral vessel involved is the ICA at the level of the second cervical vertebra.[4] Cerebral FMD is most often diagnosed in middle-aged women and is associated with intracranial aneurysms in 20 to 50 percent of cases in reported series. The diagnosis is usually made by angiography in patients being evaluated for ischemic, hemorrhagic, or nonspecific neurological symptoms. Several articles provide an excellent review and comprehensive bibliography of cerebral FMD.[9,10,12]

Pathology

Histologic studies of FMD are somewhat limited in view of the fact that relatively few cases have been followed to autopsy, and surgical resection of the involved arteries is rarely indicated. The histologic pattern originally described by Harrison and McCormack in the renal arteries and later modified by Stanley et al. appears to be the same in all affected vessels.[14] There is a spectrum of lesions of mixed histologic pattern based on the location of lesions within the vessel wall. The most common type (medial hyperplasia) consists of areas of deficient smooth muscle or internal elastic membrane in which alternating ridges of fibroproliferative tissue or collagen disrupt the smooth muscle layer and protrude as webs into the vessel lumen. Microaneurysms are also seen in areas of deficient smooth muscle or internal elastic membrane.[14] This histologic pattern results in the angiographic "string of beads" pattern that is seen in 60 to 85 percent of the cases.[11] Other rare forms of FMD are seen, with dysplasia of intimal or adventitial layers predominating. Macroscopic aneurysms, outpouchings, and dissections probably represent complications of FMD and are not classified separately. Ultrastructural studies suggest that all forms of FMD are based on a uniform morphologic process of fibroblastic transformation of smooth muscle cells.[10,13]

Etiology

The etiology of FMD is unknown. Recent studies suggest a multifactorial origin in which minor congenital lesions of the smooth muscle and internal elastic membrane predispose the artery to an abnormal fibroproliferative response to mechanical and circulatory stimuli. Aneurysm formation and dissection probably result from defects in vessel walls caused by the disease. The characteristic location in the distal portion of the cervical ICA and associated findings of renal FMD in 15 percent and intracranial aneurysms in greater than 20 percent of patients along with occasional familial occurrence all suggest a congenital component. Hormonal, metabolic, and immunologic factors, in addition to vessel ischemia and repeated trauma, have all been implicated as etiologic factors.[9–11] FMD has been demonstrated to be progressive in some cases, which fits with the above hypothesis of mechanical and circulatory aggravation of congenital medial defects.[13] Mettinger's work with pedigrees of FMD patients shows a relatively high incidence of stroke, hypertension, and migraine and suggests that FMD is inherited as a dominant trait with reduced penetrance in males.[10]

Angiography

Angiographically, FMD is divided into three separate types (Fig. 211-1) based on Osborn and Anderson's classification.[11]

Type 1 The majority of FMD patients show an angiographic pattern of multiple, irregularly spaced, concentric constrictions alternating with normal or dilated intervening segments in the involved vessel described as the string of beads appearance (Figs. 211-1 and 211-2). Fibroplasia of the media is the histologic type

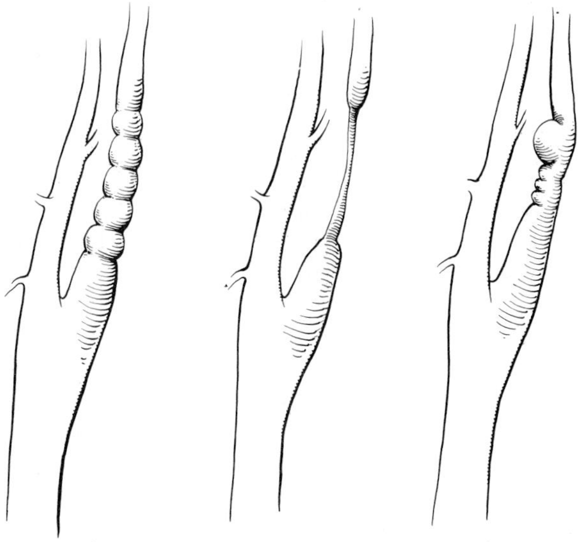

Figure 211-1 Angiographic appearance of carotid fibromuscular dysplasia. *Left.* Type 1, "string of beads." *Center.* Type 2, tubular stenosis. *Right.* Type 3, atypical fibromuscular dysplasia. (Modified from Osborn and Anderson.[11])

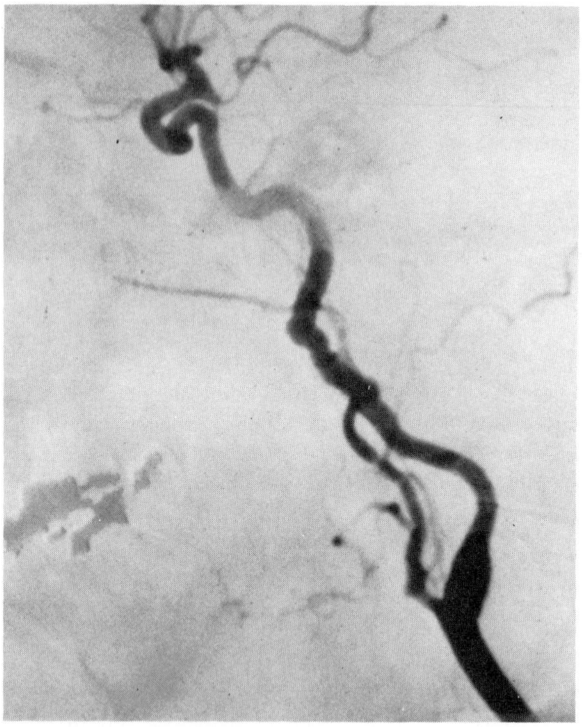

Figure 211-2 Angiogram of a 65-year-old woman who presented with a subarachnoid hemorrhage. The "string of beads," which was asymptomatic, is typical of cervical carotid FMD. Also note the small aneurysm of the carotid infundibulum intracranially. The opposite carotid angiogram showed a large aneurysm of the carotid artery, which was responsible for the subarachnoid hemorrhage.

usually associated with this angiographic finding. The angiographic differential diagnosis includes stationary arterial waves or circular spastic contractions in which the constrictions are more regular and evenly spaced without the intervening segmental dilatation usually seen in FMD. FMD lesions can also be confused with atherosclerosis and arteritis. Type 1 lesions are seen in 80 to 100 percent of reported cases in the literature.[10,11,13]

Type 2 Focal tubular stenosis (Fig. 211-1) is a much less common pattern that is seen in approximately 7 percent of reported cases. The smooth concentric tubular narrowing is less specific than the string of beads appearance and can be associated with any histologic type of FMD. The angiographic differential diagnosis includes Takayasu's or sclerosing arteritis, arterial hypoplasia, diminished vessel caliber secondary to decreased distal blood flow, and vascular spasm. The characteristic location of the FMD lesion in the distal ICA helps to distinguish it from other disease entities.

Type 3 "Atypical FMD" (Fig. 211-1) usually affects only one wall of the involved segment with a diverticulum-like smooth or corrugated outpouching of the vessel wall. Type 3 lesions are quite rare and are sometimes associated with typical type 1 lesions. Most type 3 lesions probably represent complications of type 1 FMD. There are numerous case reports of other atypical types of FMD, including several examples of fibrous webs at the common carotid bifurcation area and tubular stenosis of the common carotid artery.[11,13,17]

The great majority of cerebral FMD is located in the high cervical ICA, and is bilateral in 60 to 86 percent of reported cases. The vertebral arteries are affected in 10 to 33 percent of patients. Most patients with vertebral involvement also have carotid lesions. Intracranial disease is found in 7 to 20 percent of cases.[4,9,10,14] Angiographic studies reported in the literature rarely included pancerebral and renal studies. Thus, the above percentages may be somewhat low.

Clinical Aspects

Renal artery FMD is usually diagnosed before the age of 45 in patients undergoing a workup for hypertension, whereas cerebral FMD is usually found about one decade later. The incidence of FMD in autopsy and angiographic series ranges from 0.5 to 1.5 percent.[1,9,10,13] FMD is primarily a disease of Caucasians, although 30 of 1100 patients reviewed by Mettinger were black. There was a marked female preponderance of greater than 3:1 in Mettinger's review of 321 cases of cerebral FMD.[9]

Intracranial Aneurysms

The incidence of intracranial berry aneurysms in association with cerebral FMD varies from 20 to 50 percent in reported series. Subarachnoid or intracerebral hemorrhage occurs in 13 to 51 percent of cases.[1,3,9–11,13] Mettinger's review shows that the aneurysms are most commonly located ipsilateral to the cervical carotid lesion on the supraclinoid carotid or middle cerebral artery.[9] They are multiple in one-third of cases. Patients with FMD and intracranial aneurysm are noted to be hypertensive in less than one-half of the cases, which suggests that increased blood pressure alone is not the major etiologic factor. However, two-thirds of FMD patients with subarachnoid or intracerebral hemorrhage have a prior history of hypertension, implicating increased blood pressure as a cause of hemorrhage.[9] Aneurysms may occur with or without angiographic evidence of intracranial FMD. Usually the disease is limited to the cervical internal carotid artery (Fig. 211-2). Evidence that FMD is a widespread congenital mesenchymal disorder with multiple areas of defective media may help explain the development of intracranial aneurysms in FMD patients with otherwise normal intracranial vasculature.

Ischemic Symptoms

The relationship between cerebral FMD and ischemic symptoms is unclear. There is little doubt that FMD is responsible for symptoms of cerebral ischemia in selected cases. Patients presenting with symptoms and signs of cerebral ischemia are reported in 18 to 56 percent of cases. Often, there are no other associated lesions besides FMD to explain the symptoms; and in some cases, platelet and fibrin debris and even well-formed thrombi have been demonstrated on the fibrous webs, which suggest FMD as a source of emboli. Occasionally, the lesions are hemodynamically significant as well.[3,9,10,13,15] This may be especially significant in type 1 FMD. Each fibromuscular ring may represent a separate site of resistance to flow with the total resistance then being additive, and with blood flow beyond a diseased segment being decreased more than what might be expected from a relatively moderate stenosis.

FMD is also known to be associated with spontaneous dissection of the carotid artery with all of its ischemic complications.[9]

The angiographic diagnosis of FMD must be interpreted with caution. Up to one-half of these patients have associated atherosclerotic lesions located appropriate to the symptoms.[1,13] Corrin et al. have pointed out that patients with a known diagnosis of FMD followed up to 5 years rarely experience further cerebral ischemic events.[1] Their review suggests that in many cases cerebral FMD is an incidental finding that does not require aggressive treatment. It may well represent a benign condition, requiring no treatment in the majority of cases.

Additional Clinical Observations

Although most reports suggest a variable clinical presentation, Mettinger has defined a clinical syndrome associated with cerebral FMD where headache, ECG abnormalities, hypertension, mental distress, tinnitus, vertigo, arrhythmia, cerebral ischemic events, syncope, and subarachnoid hemorrhage are frequent components.[9] Headache is extremely common in both renal and cerebral FMD. It is quite commonly unilateral and occasionally presents as typical migraine. Atypical facial pain and pain in the cervical region are occasionally seen in patients with advanced disease. Horner's syndrome is occasionally seen and may relate to extension of the disease into the cervical sympathetic nerves. Involvement of the carotid sinus nerves may explain the occurrence of recurrent syncope in some patients. ECG abnormalities were seen in one-third of Mettinger's patients. They were usually confined to T-wave abnormalities and may be due to involvement of the coronary arteries. Carotid bruits are commonly seen in patients with FMD, although they are nonspecific and nondiagnostic. Hypertension is commonly seen in patients with cerebral FMD and is often associated with renal involvement. Noninvasive workup with Doppler imaging, etc., is unlikely to reveal the diagnosis because the dysplastic webs of tissue are thin and located high in the ICA. Good-quality digital subtraction angiography, however, can be diagnostic.[3,9–11,13,15]

Cerebral FMD is known to occasionally occur in children and to be progressive in one-third of cases where angiographic follow-up is available. The remainder of cases show no significant change, but there is no reported case of angiographic regression of the disease. Frens et al. revealed a 7 percent intracranial and a 10 percent vertebral artery incidence of FMD.[4] The true incidence is probably higher in view of the fact that many cases may have gone unrecognized.

When symptoms do occur in patients with FMD, extreme care must be taken to rule out other sources. Vague and confusing presentations should probably be treated conservatively with antiplatelet agents. Surgery most often should be reserved for patients with hard focal symptoms and those who have failed medical therapy.

Treatment

Various treatment modalities have been recommended—from medical therapy with anticoagulation and antiplatelet drugs to a multitude of surgical approaches. Early surgical procedures included endarterectomy of the affected segment or resection and interposition of vein grafts. These procedures were technically difficult and associated with relatively significant morbidity due to the usual location of cerebral FMD high in the cervical carotid artery near the base of the skull.[3,15] More recently, large numbers of patients have been treated effectively with transluminal dilatation procedures in which the fibromuscular rings are disrupted and normal flow restored (Fig. 211-3). The original technique involved operative exposure of the carotid bifurcation and internal carotid artery in the neck. A small arteriotomy was made near the bifurcation, and Bakes' gallbladder dilators were used to gradually dilate the arterial lumen from 2 mm up to 5 or 6 mm. The surgeon could feel the rings of tissue break loose as the dilators were passed up the vessel lumen.[3,15,17] Extreme caution had to be exercised to prevent embolization of fragments or disruption of the arterial wall with the dilators. Carotid cavernous fistulas and perforations were reported as complications.

Subsequent reports advocated the use of the Gruntzig percutaneous transluminal angioplasty technique for cervical carotid FMD.[6] Although preliminary reports were encouraging, potential embolic complications presented a formidable risk. The use of a Gruntzig balloon or Fogarty catheter to progressively dilate the involved segment could more safely be employed in an open technique where back bleeding could be allowed to occur and complications could be dealt with immediately and directly.[5]

Increasingly, percutaneous transluminal angioplasty (PTA) has emerged as the treatment of choice for FMD (Fig. 211-3).[2,7,8,16] PTA offers several advantages over open procedures. It can be performed under local anesthesia, allows greater access to distal as well as multiple sites, and permits angiographic control of the entire procedure. Results are encouraging, with clinical improvement, angiographic resolution of lesions, and good long-term results. PTA is not without complications, however, and cases have been reported of intimal dissection, pseudoaneurysm formation, and distal emboli. As endovascular techniques continue to develop, this procedure, in our opinion, will become the procedure of choice for FMD.

Most surgical interventional series show good resolution of symptoms (including unilateral headache and facial pain) with minimal recurrence of ischemic symptoms. However, the association between clinical symptoms and angiographic FMD must be interpreted carefully. There is considerable evidence to suggest that isolated cerebral FMD is a relatively benign disorder which rarely results in ischemic symptoms.[1] Interventional treatment should therefore be reserved for those patients with clear-cut clini-

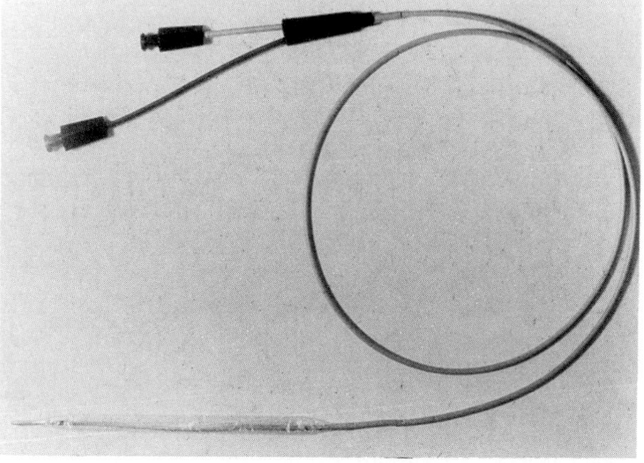

Figure 211-3 A 6-mm angioplasty catheter suitable for percutaneous transluminal angioplasty (Medi-tech, Watertown, MA).

cal symptoms referable to their angiographic disease in whom no other obvious cause can be found. Patients shown to have cervical carotid FMD should certainly be subjected to four-vessel cerebral angiography to rule out associated aneurysms, particularly in the face of hypertension. Renal arteriograms should also be performed in hypertensive patients.

References

1. Corrin LS, Sandok BA, Houser OW. Cerebral ischemic events in patients with carotid artery fibromuscular dysplasia. *Arch Neurol* 1981; 38:616–618.
2. Dubin AB, Baltaxe HA, Cobb CA III. Percutaneous transluminal carotid angioplasty in fibromuscular dysplasia. Case report. *J Neurosurg* 1983: 59:162–165.
3. Effeney DJ, Ehrenfeld WK, Stoney RJ, Wylie EJ. Fibromuscular dysplasia of the internal carotid artery. *World J Surg* 1979; 3:179–186.
4. Frens DB, Petajan JH, Anderson R, Deblanc HJ Jr. Fibromuscular dysplasia of the posterior cerebral artery: report of a case and review of the literature. *Stroke* 1974; 5:161–166.
5. Garrido E, Montoya J. Transluminal dilatation of internal carotid artery in fibromuscular dysplasia: a preliminary report. *Surg Neurol* 1981; 16:469–471.
6. Hasso AN, Bird CR, Zinke DE, Thompson JR. Fibromuscular dysplasia of the internal carotid artery: percutaneous transluminal angioplasty. *Am J Roentgenol* 1981; 136:955–960.
7. Jooma R, Bradshaw JR, Griffith HB. Intimal dissection following percutaneous transluminal carotid angioplasty for fibromuscular dysplasia. *Neuroradiology* 1985; 27:181–182.
8. Lord RSA, Graham AR, Benn IV. Radiologic control of operative carotid dilatation. Aneurysm formation following balloon dilatation. *J Cardiovasc Surg* 1986; 27:158–162.
9. Mettinger KL. Fibromuscular dysplasia and the brain: II. Current concept of the disease. *Stroke* 1982; 13:53–58.
10. Mettinger KL, Ericson K. Fibromuscular dysplasia and the brain: observations on angiographic, clinical and genetic characteristics. *Stroke* 1982; 13:46–52.
11. Osborn AG, Anderson RE. Angiographic spectrum of cervical and intracranial fibromuscular dysplasia. *Stroke* 1977; 8:617–626.
12. Sandok BA. Fibromuscular dysplasia of the internal carotid artery. *Neurol Clin* 1983; 1:17–26.
13. So EL, Toole JF, Dalal P, Moody DM. Cephalic fibromuscular dysplasia in 32 patients: clinical findings and radiologic features. *Arch Neurol* 1981; 38:619–622.
14. Stanley JC, Gewertz BL, Bove EL, et al. Arterial fibrodysplasia: histopathologic character and current etiologic concepts. *Arch Surg* 1975; 110:561–566.
15. Starr DS, Lawrie GM, Morris GC Jr. Fibromuscular disease of carotid arteries: long term results of graduated internal dilatation. *Stroke* 1981; 12:196–199.
16. Wilms GE, Smits J, Baert AL, De Wolf L. Percutaneous transluminal angioplasty in fibromuscular dysplasia of the internal carotid artery: one year clinical and morphological follow-up. *Cardiovasc Intervent Radiol* 1985; 8:20–23.
17. Wirth FP, Miller WA, Russell AP. Atypical fibromuscular hyperplasia: report of two cases. *J Neurosurg* 1981; 54:685–689.

212

Arterial Dissections

Allan H. Friedman

Although dissecting aneurysms of the head and neck were once thought to be extremely rare, they are now recognized with increasing frequency as a cause of stroke. Arterial dissection occurs when blood is forced between the tissue planes of a vessel wall, and although trauma or some disease states may predispose a vessel to dissection, a dissecting hemorrhage may also occur spontaneously in a seemingly normal artery. Arterial dissection always must be considered in the young patient who presents with cerebral ischemia, as well as in the trauma patient who has a focal neurological deficit and a normal initial CT scan.

Fortunately, the neurological deficit associated with a dissection frequently has a delayed onset. A patient with a dissecting aneurysm may present with a spontaneous severe headache, a transient ischemic attack, or a mild neurological dysfunction prior to developing a completed stroke. The diagnosis must therefore be made early so that appropriate therapeutic intervention can halt the evolution of the disease.

Internal Carotid Artery

Several reports have dispelled the misconception that idiopathic carotid dissections are rare. Dissection of the internal carotid artery may occur spontaneously in a seemingly healthy patient.[11] Alternatively, dissection may occur in blood vessels weakened by a primary arteriopathy such as cystic medial necrosis, fibromuscular dysplasia, Marfan's disease, Ehlers-Danlos syndrome type IV, or syphilitic arteritis. The coincidental occurrence of saccular intracranial aneurysms in patients harboring a spontaneous cervical artery dissection or in their family members suggests an underlying occult arteriopathy in this subset of patients. A rare cause of internal carotid dissection is the propagation of a dissection originating in the aortic arch.

Dissecting aneurysms of the internal carotid artery may result from trauma[16] such as after a direct blow to the neck. Similarly, the artery may be contused by a restraining shoulder harness during an automobile accident, or an intimal flap may be raised by an angiographer's catheter. Less violent activities such as coughing, chiropractic manipulation, and surgical manipulation have caused a carotid artery dissection as has hanging by the neck. A dissection more commonly results from the stretching of the internal carotid artery over the upper cervical vertebral bodies during abrupt hyperextension and lateral rotation of the neck.[20] Compression of the carotid artery between the angle of the mandible and the upper cervical vertebrae or against a long styloid process have also been proposed as mechanisms capable of initiating a carotid artery dissection. Longitudinal basilar skull fractures have also been implicated as a cause of arterial contusion and subsequent dissection, as has the rarer case of direct intraoral trauma to the carotid at the level of the tonsillar pillar.

The site of origin of the arterial dissection generally lies distal to the carotid bifurcation and proximal to the vertical petrous segment of the carotid artery.[3,5] Although it is generally believed that the hemorrhage initiating a dissection enters the media of the blood vessel through a tear in the intima, it is possible that some hemorrhages originate directly from the vasa vasorum. Once the media is broached, blood dissects upward within the media or between the media and adventitia of the vessel, narrowing the true lumen of the carotid artery and producing an abnormal dark blue or purple discoloration of the involved arterial segment. An aneurysm may result when the dissection tracks between the media and adventitia (Fig. 212-1). Dissections of traumatic origin and rarely "spontaneous" dissections of the internal carotid artery may occur bilaterally.[12]

In approximately 50 percent of patients, the dissection is heralded by a steady aching forehead or periorbital pain. Concomitant ipsilateral scalp tenderness is frequently noted. Some patients note upper neck pain which radiates to the mastoid process. A detailed analysis of the pain accompanying a spontaneous carotid artery dissection reveals that the pain is primarily ipsilateral to the dissection but may spread to any portion of the face, head, or neck.[2] Ipsilateral oculosympathetic paresis (ptosis, miosis) resulting from injury to the pericarotid sympathetic plexus is present in one-half of cases. Because the sympathetic fibers traveling along the external carotid artery are unaffected, anhydrosis is only found in a

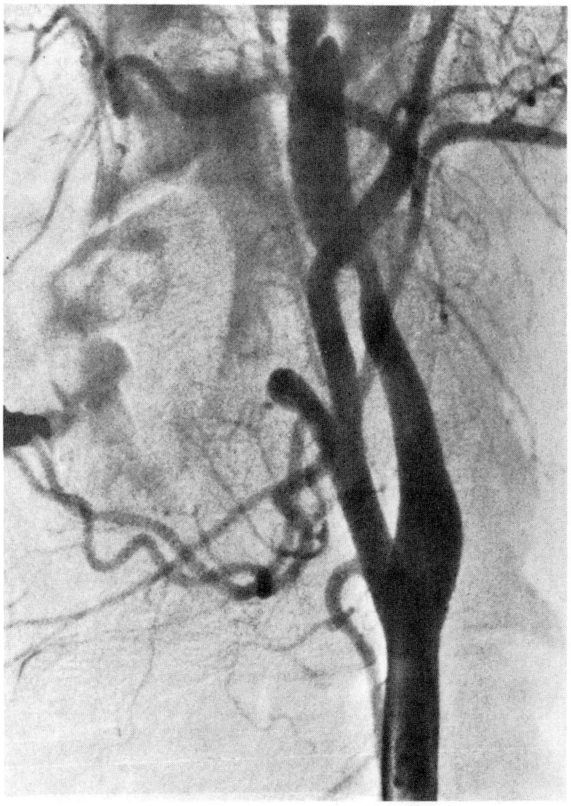

Figure 212-1 Carotid angiogram demonstrating a dissection of the internal carotid artery with a pseudoaneurysm.

small patch of skin over the eyebrow. A high cervical lesion may be associated with a bruit, and a lower cervical lesion may sometimes present as a pulsatile mass in the neck. Difficulty with taste or tongue movements can also result from injury to the adjacent chorda tympani or hypoglossal nerve.

Unfortunately, however, carotid dissection is not diagnosed in 90 percent of cases until the patient has suffered a neurological deficit in the form of a transient ischemic attack, a reversible ischemic neurological deficit, or a stroke.[20] Possible ocular manifestations include amaurosis fugax, scintillating scotomata, and retinal infarction. In the majority of patients, these neurological symptoms are delayed in onset, and only 10 percent of patients develop symptomatic cerebral ischemia coincident with the onset of dissection. In the case of dissecting aneurysms precipitated by trauma, the injury precedes the onset of neurological symptoms by an average of 10 h. A few reported cases describe latent periods of 1 to 2 years, although none of them documented an arterial dissection prior to the onset of symptoms.[12] Although carotid stenosis or complete occlusion of the arterial lumen is responsible for the development of a neurological deficit in some cases, embolization to the intracranial vessels has been documented angiographically in several cases. Evaluation of patients using a combination of MRI, Doppler sonography, and SPECT scanning confirms that infarcts can occur secondary to low blood flow or thromboembolic events.[19] Carotid artery dissection is a common cause of stroke in patients less than 30 years of age.

Although angiography is generally recognized as the "gold standard" for diagnosing an arterial dissection, newer techniques may suggest or even definitively demonstrate the dissection. Doppler sonography will frequently demonstrate a high grade stenosis of the internal carotid artery that begins at least 2 cm beyond the carotid bifurcation. If the vessel is completely or virtually occluded by the dissection, to and fro movements of the blood column will be detected in the proximal internal carotid artery. Transcranial Doppler sonography can detect arterial dissections that extend into the cranium. An intimal flap or false lumen can occasionally be demonstrated on B-mode imaging studies.

An enhanced CT scan may reveal an enhancing outer arterial wall and narrow lumen separated by an organizing subintimal clot of lower attenuation. Thin section dynamic CT scanning can be used to assess the size of the residual arterial lumen and to diagnose a partially thrombosed aneurysm.[14]

As the clot in the dissected arterial wall organizes, MRI demonstrates on T1- and T2-weighted images a hyperintense, intramural mass comprising the arterial lumen. MR angiography can demonstrate the compromised vessel lumen. Serial scans are useful in monitoring the resolution of the intramural hematoma.[6,13]

The angiographic picture of any arterial dissection depends on the relationship between the true carotid lumen and the dissection cavity (Fig. 212-2).[9] Occasionally the false channel caused by the dissecting blood will rupture back into the true lumen, and both channels will be patent to blood flow. On a carotid angiogram, the double lumen will appear as a double density of contrast material. More commonly, the true lumen is compressed by clotted blood lying within its arterial wall, and is therefore markedly thinned over the involved arterial segment. This segmental luminal constriction is known as the angiographic "string sign." In many cases, a small projection of the contrast column will extend into the wall of the artery at the proximal end of the dissection. Because the dissection normally involves only a portion of the arterial wall, the true lumen will not be concentrically narrowed, but rather will be asymmetrically compressed to one side. This asymmetrical focal constriction helps differentiate the luminal narrowing of carotid dissection from that of fibromuscular dysplasia, which concentrically narrows the vessel lumen (and more commonly involves multiple arteries). Carotid dissection must also be distinguished from atherosclerotic arterial disease. Atherosclerosis usually involves the carotid bifurcation and carotid siphon, whereas dissecting aneurysms generally begin 2 cm distal to the bifurcation. Both fibromuscular dysplasia and atherosclerosis are slowly progressive diseases, and thus sequential angiograms will show stable or slowly progressive lesions. With carotid dissection, however, sequential angiograms will generally show either rapid progression of the disease with arterial occlusion or, more commonly, restoration of normal arterial caliber 1 to 3 months later.[4]

The dissection may break into the plane between the media and adventitia, expanding the adventitia into an aneurysm. Aneurysms occur more commonly in association with dissections of traumatic origin. These aneurysms may not become radiographically apparent until several days following trauma.[17] If the dissection continues out through the adventitia, a pseudoaneurysm may result from flowing blood invaginating into a perivascular tamponading hematoma (Fig. 212-1). Pseudoaneurysms are usually the result of a penetrating injury. Evidence of fibromuscular dysplasia and distal embolization may also be demonstrated angiographically.

The natural history of carotid dissection is not fully known because the diagnosis may easily be missed in patients with neurologically asymptomatic lesions. In general, dissecting aneurysms

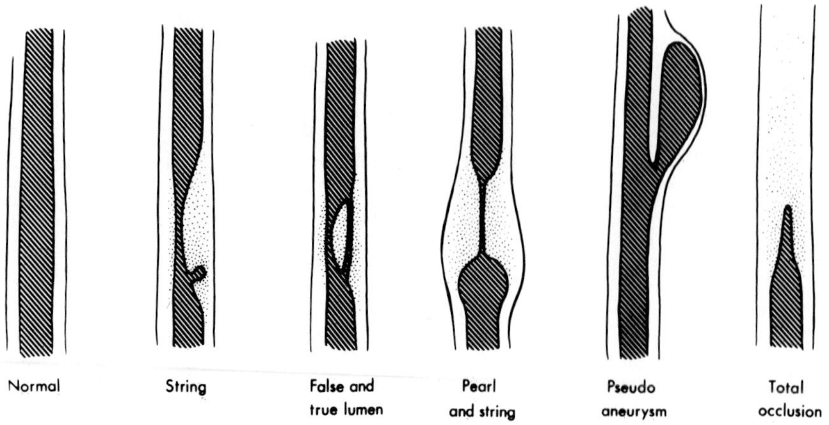

Figure 212-2 Types of dissections of cranial arteries. The patent lumen as it would appear on an arteriogram is represented by crosshatching. Hematoma within the vessel is represented by stippling. Note the small diverticulum accompanying the string sign. This diverticulum is commonly seen when the dissection involves the internal carotid artery.

that cause luminal stenosis without a concomitant pseudoaneurysm will frequently resolve in 1 to 3 months with restoration of the carotid lumen to normal. Distal embolization to branches of the middle cerebral artery has been demonstrated; however, it is prior to the resolution of the stenosis. Stenosed vessels will progress to complete occlusion in a small number of patients. This occurs most often in arterial dissections of traumatic origin. This group of patients tends to suffer more severe neurological deficits than do those patients whose carotid arteries remain patent.

If aneurysm formation occurs, the lesion may not resolve spontaneously. Serial angiography has demonstrated that most aneurysms have a propensity to enlarge or to remain stable.

The patient's ultimate neurological function is closely correlated to the degree of neurological dysfunction manifest by the patient at the time of diagnosis. A review of the literature demonstrates that 15 percent of patients are severely disabled or dead at the time of follow-up. This percentage is higher in patients who have suffered traumatic carotid artery dissection because of concomitant injuries.

A large number of patients may have spontaneous partial or complete resolution of their initial neurological deficits. As with all forms of cerebrovascular disease, there is no known effective therapy for a completed stroke. Treatment of carotid dissection is therefore aimed at preventing future cerebral or ocular ischemias. In order to prevent carotid occlusion or distal embolization, several authorities have advocated treating these patients with anticoagulant or antiplatelet agents. This type of therapy appears to be successful in thwarting future ischemic events. Although the number of cases reported is too small to establish firmly the benefits of any particular therapeutic modality, this method seems to be the treatment of choice for most lesions. It is unclear from reviewing the literature whether anticoagulants are superior to antiplatelet agents.

Most of these lesions are inaccessible to the surgeon because they extend to the base of the skull. However, a small number of localized dissections have been treated with endarterectomy and suturing of the distal intima to the media, or resection of the dissected arterial segment and interposition grafting. Carotid ligation with or without a superficial temporal to middle cerebral artery anastomosis should be considered for patients who have persistent emboli despite adequate anticoagulation. Distal aneurysms can be resected if they prove to be the source of recurrent emboli.[18]

Vertebral Artery

Like carotid artery dissection, the dissection of the vertebral artery may present with neck pain or a stroke. Because complete occlusion of a vertebral artery can often be tolerated without adverse effect, dissection of the vertebral artery may frequently pass detected.

Vertebral dissection most commonly results from cervical hyperextension and lateral cervical rotation, such as may occur with trauma or with chiropractic manipulation of the neck. Less commonly, vertebral dissection is due to less dramatic causes such as sports activities, archery practice, ceiling painting, sudden head turning, yoga exercises, or tonic-clonic seizures. Vertebral dissections may occur spontaneously or in association with fibromuscular dysplasia and other systemic diseases that affect the arterial wall.[1,10] Bilateral vertebral dissections have reportedly occurred in cases of traumatic or spontaneous origin.

The dissection is heralded by neck pain that radiates into the suboccipital region and is exacerbated by head turning. Neurological symptoms may include vertigo, ataxia, blurred vision, slurring of speech, memory loss, and drowsiness. In approximately one-third of cases, patients manifest elements of a lateral medullary syndrome with the physical examination revealing Horner's syndrome, facial and contralateral body numbness, dysarthria, ipsilateral palatal paresis, nystagmus, ataxia, and ipsilateral dysmetria. More widespread evidence of vertebrobasilar ischemia can occasionally be seen.

Although a neurological deficit may result solely from vessel occlusion, distal emboli have also been documented. Symptoms are delayed from minutes to days in 30 percent of patients. The syndrome evolves slowly or fluctuates initially in an additional 30 percent of patients.[1] An early diagnosis should be made so that prophylactic treatment can be instituted.

MRI demonstrates that the normal flow void of the vertebral artery is narrowed by material of increased intensity on both T1- and T2-weighted images. Gradient refocused images demonstrated the constricted column of flowing blood.[15] Angiographic studies have shown that although the dissection may occur anywhere along the cervical portion of the vertebral artery, the most common site of involvement is between the second cervical vertebra and the occiput.[7] The most common angiographic finding is irregular vessel narrowing at C1-C2, the seat of maximal head rotation. Pseudoaneurysm formation occurs at the site of dissection in 20 percent of patients. As with carotid dissection, the lesion generally heals spontaneously, although in some cases the vertebral artery may thrombose entirely.

In a small number of patients, anticoagulants have been shown to lower the morbidity associated with vertebral dissection. Successful resection of the affected segment has been reported. If symptoms result from inadequate collateral circulation, distal revascularization seems warranted.

Intracranial Arterial Dissection

The dissection of an intracranial artery is a rare event. Although virtually all named intracranial vessels have been reported to suffer a dissection, the process most frequently involves the middle cerebral or intracranial vertebral artery. The dissections are not confined to the larger trunk arteries at the base of the brain but extend peripherally into small peripheral arteries. Although many intracranial dissections have occurred in healthy patients with apparently normal intracranial arteries, the disease has also been associated with syphilitic arteritis, polyarteritis nodosa, fibromuscular dysplasia, and mucoid degeneration of the media. Other cases have been reported in connection with head trauma and surgical manipulation of the intracranial vessels. One investigator has noted an absence of reticular fibers adjacent to the internal elastic lamina in two patients with intracranial dissecting aneurysms. Although migraine headache has been identified as a possible risk factor in intracranial dissection, the number of reported cases is small. A curious theory that has been suggested is that a dissection represents the rupture of a small aneurysm into the media of a blood vessel.

The dissection causes severe headache in 95 percent of reported cases. Neurological deficits may be delayed up to 4 weeks from the onset of headache, and the resulting stroke frequently evolves over time. Middle-aged patients are most commonly affected, although intracranial arterial dissection may cause a juvenile stroke or infantile hemiplegia. Patients may present with a subarachnoid hemorrhage.[4] Eighty-five percent of intracranial dissecting aneurysms presenting with subarachnoid hemorrhage involve the vertebral or basilar artery. This fact reflects the propensity of the hemorrhage in dissections of the posterior circulation vessels to dissect between the media and the adventitia.

MR imaging demonstrates an abnormal high signal intensity within the wall of the dissected vessel and compromise of the vessel's lumen.[8] The angiographic findings are most often focal narrowing of the vessel lumen (string sign), preceded by a small aneurysmal dilatation of the vessel (pearl sign) (Fig. 212-3). This combination is frequently misdiagnosed as a congenital aneurysm with adjacent vasospasm. Occasionally the contrast medium will fill both the true and the false vessel lumens, thereby creating a double density on the angiogram film.[21]

Because of the paucity of cases, the optimum therapy for these lesions is unclear. Patients who present with a completed stroke are beyond primary therapy. They should be treated for brain swelling if it occurs, and then be rehabilitated. Patients presenting with subarachnoid hemorrhage have been treated most frequently by ligation of the involved vessel just proximal to the area of dissection or with wrapping of the dissected segment. Rare cases of a second hemorrhage from the dissection have been reported prior to therapy. The treatment of patients undergoing a stroke in evolution is speculative. Although it is possible that this group would benefit from revascularization of the ischemic area, the effect of this mode of therapy is unknown.

The patient's prognosis is influenced by the location of the dissection. For instance, dissection of the basilar artery has a mortality rate of 75 percent whereas dissection of the vertebral artery has a mortality rate of 8 percent.[8]

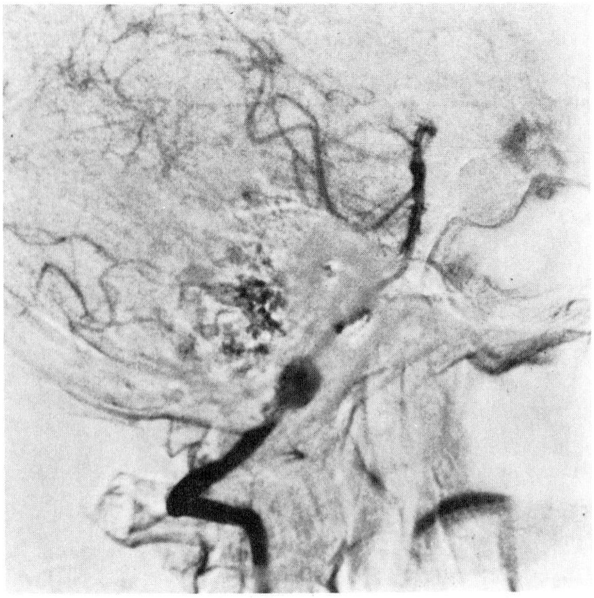

Figure 212-3 Lateral view of a vertebral angiogram demonstrating a dissection of the vertebral artery. Note the pearl and string sign. (Courtesy of Charles G. Drake, M.D.)

References

1. Caplan LR, Zarins CK, Hemmati M. Spontaneous dissection of the extracranial vertebral arteries. *Stroke* 1985; 16:1030–1038.
2. Fisher CM. The headache and pain of spontaneous carotid dissection. *Headache* 1982; 22:60–65.
3. Fisher CM, Ojemann RG, Roberson GH. Spontaneous dissection of cervico-cerebral arteries. *Can J Neurol Sci* 1978; 5:9–19.
4. Friedman AH, Drake CG. Subarachnoid hemorrhage from intracranial dissecting aneurysms. *J Neurosurg* 1984; 60:325–334.
5. Friedman WA, Day AL, Quisling RG, et al. Cervical carotid dissecting aneurysms. *Neurosurgery* 1980, 7:207–214.
6. Goldberg HI, Grossman RI, Gomori JM, et al. Cervical internal carotid artery dissecting hemorrhage: diagnosis using MR. *Radiology* 1986; 158:157–161.
7. Hinse P, Thie A, Lachenmayer L. Dissection of the extracranial vertebral artery: report of four cases and review of the literature. *J Neurol Neurosurg Psychiatry* 1991; 54:863–869.
8. Hosoda K, Fujita S, Kawaguchi T, et al. Spontaneous dissecting aneurysms of the basilar artery presenting with a subarachnoid hemorrhage. Report of two cases. *J Neurosurg* 1991; 75:628–633.
9. Houser OW, Mokri B, Sundt TM Jr, et al. Spontaneous cervical cephalic arterial dissection and its residuum: angiographic spectrum. *Am J Neuroradiol* 1984; 5:27–34.
10. Hugenholtz H, Pokrupa R, Montpetit VJA, et al. Spontaneous dissecting aneurysm of the extracranial vertebral artery. *Neurosurgery* 1982; 10:96–100.
11. Luken MG III, Ascherl GF Jr, Correll JW, Hilal SK. Spontaneous dissecting aneurysms of the extracranial internal carotid artery. *Clin Neurosurg* 1979; 26:353–375.
12. Mokri B, Piepgras DG, Houser OW. Traumatic dissections of the extracranial internal carotid artery. *J Neurosurg* 1988; 68:189–197.
13. Mullges W, Ringelstein EB, Leibold M. Non-invasive diagnosis of internal carotid artery dissections. *J Neurol Neurosurg Psychiatry* 1992; 55:98–104.
14. Petro GR, Witwer GA, Cacayorin ED, et al. Spontaneous dissection of the cervical internal carotid artery: correlation of arteriography, CT, and pathology. *Am J Roentgenol* 1987; 148:393–398.
15. Quint DJ, Spickler EM. Magnetic resonance demonstration of vertebral artery dissection. Report of two cases. *J Neurosurg* 1990; 72:964–967.
16. Stringer WL, Kelley DL Jr. Traumatic dissection of the extracranial internal carotid artery. *Neurosurgery* 1980; 6:123–130.
17. Sullivan HG, Vines FS, Becker DP. Sequelae of indirect internal carotid injury. *Radiology* 1973; 109:91–98.
18. Sundt TM Jr, Pearson BW, Piepgras DG, et al. Surgical management of aneurysms of the distal extracranial internal carotid artery. *J Neurosurg* 1986; 64:169–182.
19. Weiller C, Müllges W, Ringelstein EB, et al. Patterns of brain infarctions in internal carotid artery dissections. *Neurosurg Rev* 1991; 14:111–113.
20. Yamada S, Kindt GW, Youmans JR. Carotid artery occlusion due to nonpenetrating injury. *J Trauma* 1967; 7:333–342.
21. Yonas H, Agamanolis D, Takaoka Y, White RJ. Dissecting intracranial aneurysms. *Surg Neurol* 1977; 8:407–415.

213

Nonseptic Venous Occlusive Disease

Bermans J. Iskandar
John P. Kapp

Until recently, occlusions of the cerebral veins and dural sinuses, and especially thrombotic occlusions, had been underrecognized and thought to have a very poor prognosis. This was the result of the nonspecific and variable symptomatology associated with these disorders, the lack of adequate radiographic techniques, and the fact that most incidence reports were based on autopsy studies. Newer technology has effected the following important changes in the general understanding of the disease: (1) The widespread use of antibiotic therapy for infections of the face, cranial air sinuses, and meninges has significantly decreased the incidence of infection as a cause of cerebral venous thrombosis. Whereas dural sinus infection had previously been the most common cause of sinus thrombosis, it is now an infrequent occurrence, mainly in the cavernous sinus.[5] (2) The advent of digital subtraction angiography (DSA) and computed tomography (CT) has allowed the diagnosis of milder cases of venous sinus occlusion thereby providing earlier detection and a better overall prognosis. Recently, magnetic resonance imaging (MRI) and magnetic resonance angiography (MRA) have proven extremely sensitive in diagnosing this disorder, predicting that MR techniques may soon supplant the "invasive" angiogram as the definitive diagnostic method for cerebral venous occlusion. (3) Sophisticated laboratory analyses have revealed previously unknown, but potentially treatable causes of venous thrombosis, such as protein C deficiency. Finally, (4) recent literature strongly suggests that the use of anticoagulants in the treatment of cerebral venous thrombosis is effective and involves minimal risk, and that thrombolytic therapy shows promise. Conversely, surgery has always been, and still is, reserved for special circumstances.

Anatomic Considerations

One may speculate that the anatomic design of the cerebral venous system functions to keep the vascular channels from collapsing in the face of negative intracranial venous pressure. The veins bridging the brain to the venous sinuses usually enter the sinus in a direction opposite the flow of blood within the sinus. The Venturi effect, which would collapse the veins, is thereby minimized. The major sinuses are formed by splits in the dura of the cerebral convexity and the major intracranial partitions—the falx cerebri and tentorium cerebelli. They are thus triangular structures rigidly anchored at three points, and are accordingly noncollapsible. Anatomical features that are present in the cerebral venous system but not in the peripheral venous system include the lateral lacunae, which accept arachnoidal granulations and bridging veins, and the cords of Willis, or septations within the sinuses. These features must be accommodated in planning surgical operations on the sinuses (Fig. 213-1).

Etiology

Cerebral venous occlusion can be secondary to injury (e.g., laceration or contusion), compression (e.g., tumor or depressed skull fracture), infiltration (e.g., leukemia), blood disorders causing a hypercoagulable state (e.g., protein C deficiency), flow disturbances causing hyperviscosity and sludging (e.g., dehydration), and inflammation of the venous walls or meninges (e.g., vasculitis).[35] The most common etiologies are discussed below, and an exhaustive list is shown in Table 213-1.

Trauma

The superficial location of the major dural sinuses makes them susceptible to injury. Suspicion should arise when a fracture, especially a compound depressed fracture, overlies a sinus. If precautions are not taken, attempts at repair of such fractures may result

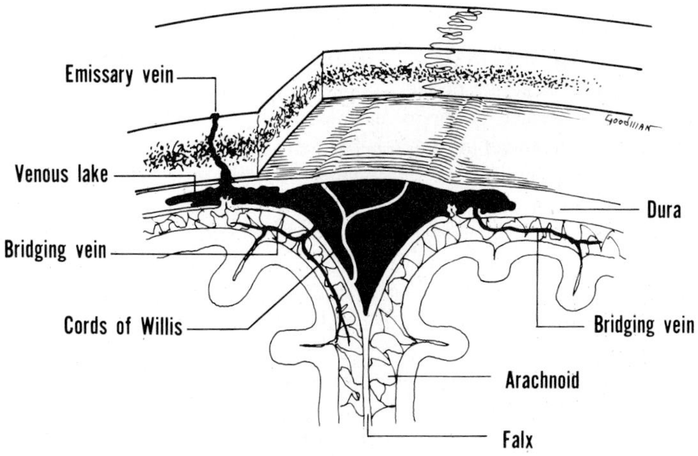

Figure 213-1 Drawing of a cross-section of a dural sinus showing triangulation, lateral lacunae, and cords of Willis. [From Kapp JP. Surgical management of dural sinus lacerations. In Schmidek HH, Sweet WH (eds): *Operative Neurosurgical Techniques: Indications, Methods, and Results.* New York: Grune & Stratton, 1982, pp 205–213, with permission.]

TABLE 213-1 Noninfective Diseases Associated with Thrombosis of Cerebral Veins and Dural Sinuses (with selected references)

Tumors	**Drugs and Toxins**
Meningiomas[104]	Danazol[55]
Metastases to the skull[104]	Methotrexate[35]
Metastases to the sinus[87]	L-Asparaginase[103]
Primary bone tumors[104]	Lead poisoning[122]
Leukemias[28,116]	Pentosan polysulfate[62]
Lymphomas[104]	Tranexamic acid[61]
Gynecological Disorders	Iopamidol (myelography)[50]
Pregnancy and puerperium[64,70,88,109]	Antifibrinolytic agents[2]
Use of oral contraceptive pills[8,38,40]	Others
Connective Tissue and Inflammatory Disorders	**Hematological Disorders**
Behçet's disease[127]	Protein C deficiency[128]
Systemic lupus erythematosus[123]	Protein S deficiency[77]
Sarcoidosis[20]	Antithrombin III deficiency[17]
Wegener's granulomatosis[85]	Paroxysmal nocturnal hemoglobinuria[121]
Periarteritis nodosa[72]	Sickle cell trait[41]
Ulcerative colitis[15]	Beta-Thalassemia[84]
Regional enteritis[112]	Polycythemias[93]
Trauma	Thrombocytosis[80]
Closed head injury[21,33,69,83]	Lupus anticoagulant[75]
Skull fracture[83]	Anticardiolipin antibodies[49]
Strangulation[106]	Plasminogen deficiency[107]
Iatrogenic	Heparin-induced thrombocytopenia[73]
Colloid cyst surgery[44]	Myeloproliferative disease[35]
Other intracranial surgery	Anemias[111]
Cannulation of neck veins[117]	Cryofibrinogenemia[32]
Cardiac catheterization[14]	**Other Etiologies**
Medications (see drugs)	Diabetes[7]
Spinal anesthesia[105]	Trichinosis[39]
Embolization of arteriovenous malformation[31]	Colon carcinoma[102]
Blood Flow Abnormalities	Nephrotic syndrome[74]
Dehydration[10,96,119]	Homocystinuria[24]
Congestive heart failure[119]	Cerebral arterial occlusion[10,64]
Congenital heart disease[76]	Hypertensive intracerebral hemorrhage[10]
	Dural arteriovenous fitula[12]
	Idiopathic

in hemorrhage or air embolism.[104] Dural sinus injuries may be immediate and obvious, or may become apparent when delayed thrombosis has occurred.[33,34,69] They occur in about 10 percent of combat wounds involving the brain, but their exact incidence in blunt trauma of the head is unknown. In a review[83] of 978 cases of head injury requiring surgery, Meier et al. found a 4 percent (38 patients) incidence of dural sinus injury. Thirty-one percent of those were associated with an open injury, and 69 percent with a closed head injury. Almost all patients had an associated skull fracture. There was damage to the anterior and central parts of the superior sagittal sinus (SSS) in 66 percent of cases, the transverse sinus in 18 percent, the posterior SSS in 8 percent, and multiple sinuses in 8 percent. Furthermore, among these 38 patients, the sinus injury was found to be the cause of all subdural hematomas, but only 27 percent of epidural hematomas. Mortality rates were as follows: posterior SSS—100 percent; multiple sinuses—67 percent; central SSS—50 percent; transverse sinus—29 percent; and anterior SSS—17 percent. However, it is important to realize that half of all deaths were intraoperative. The overall mortality was 41 percent in patients presenting with a midbrain syndrome versus 17 percent in patients without such a presentation.[83] In neonates, compression of the superior sagittal sinus by calvarial molding has been documented angiographically and has been proposed as a cause of intracerebral hemorrhage in infants.[91]

Tumors

Meningiomas and malignant tumors are the most common tumors to involve the dural sinuses. Unlike traumatic injuries, which often result in rapid occlusion of a dural sinus, tumors tend to cause a more gradual occlusion. This slow process allows enough time for collateral circulations to form, therefore minimizing the clinical manifestations due to the occlusion. This is especially true of slow-growing tumors, particularly meningiomas. Since it is often impossible to completely resect a tumor such as a parasagittal meningioma[65] unless part of the sinus is also resected, an important corollary follows: If the sinus is resected early (i.e., before the occurrence of significant occlusion), severe neurological problems may arise. However, if the surgery is delayed until such occlusion has time to develop slowly, and care is taken not to injure the collateral circulation intraoperatively, the deficits may be minimal. This obviously depends on the size of the tumor and its exact location (certain sinuses can be occluded, ligated, or resected with minimal clinical manifestations, whereas these same procedures on others may lead to severe disability or death).[104]

Two types of malignant tumors may invade the dural sinuses: (1) tumors extending locally from the scalp and skull (e.g., primary bone tumors, bone metastases, glomus tumors), and (2) metastatic lesions to a sinus wall.[87] The occlusion can result from either direct compression, infiltration, or a hypercoagulable state and/or thrombosis. Sinus thrombosis secondary to leukemic infiltration of the walls has been reported.[28,116] Finally, the involvement of arachnoidal granulations by an intraluminal tumor has been hypothesized to obstruct venous outflow, causing a syndrome comparable to benign intracranial hypertension.[18] This concept, however, is still controversial.[104]

Pregnancy/Oral Contraceptive Pills

Spontaneous thrombosis of cerebral veins and dural sinuses is seen during pregnancy and delivery and is most common during the first two postpartum weeks. The differential diagnoses include eclampsia, water intoxication, pituitary apoplexy, postlumbar puncture headaches, and postpartum headaches.[35,95] The new onset of seizures during pregnancy or puerperium should especially alert the physician to the possibility of cerebral venous thrombosis.[109] Spontaneous cerebral venous thrombosis has also been reported extensively in young women taking oral contraceptives (8 percent of patients with cerebral venous thrombosis in one study),[5] and a causal relationship has been suggested. The event commonly occurs within a few weeks of starting the medication. It is important to note that occasionally an event such as pregnancy will be merely a contributing cause of venous thrombosis, allowing a previously asymptomatic hematological defect such as protein C deficiency or the antiphospholipid syndrome[82] to express itself.

Retrograde Extension from Neck Veins

Thrombosis of a jugular vein may be associated with retrograde propagation of thrombus into the lateral sinus, torcular, and superior sagittal sinus. This complication has been reported to follow radical neck dissection,[42] transvenous pacemaker implantation,[43] internal jugular vein cannulation,[117] and even Greenfield filter placement.[58]

Collagen Vascular Diseases and Inflammatory Disorders

A variety of inflammatory diseases have been associated with cerebral venous thrombosis. Most commonly reported are Behçet's disease[127] and systemic lupus erythematosus,[123] in which the thrombotic occlusions are thought to be due to vasculitis. Since the intracranial abnormality may be the presenting feature,[35] these inflammatory disorders are often not recognized until other systemic manifestations arise late in the disease course. Therefore, at early stages, the thrombotic occlusions are frequently labeled "idiopathic."

Hematologic Disorders

Blood disorders causing a hypercoagulable state or high viscosity also frequently lead to cerebral venous thrombosis. The importance of diagnosing these diseases is that some of them are treatable, while others are familial, therefore allowing precautionary measures to be taken in affected family members. The most common blood disorders are the anemias,[111] thrombocytosis,[80] paroxysmal nocturnal hemoglobinuria,[121] protein C[128] and S deficiencies, antithrombin III deficiency,[17] lupus anticoagulant[75] and anticardiolipin[49] antibodies, the polycythemias[93] (including polycythemia due to high altitude[26]), leukemia, lymphoma, and sickle cell trait,[41] in addition to nonhematologic disorders causing blood flow abnormalities such as dehydration and congestive heart failure.[119] Since several of these disorders were recognized only recently, they had previously comprised a large proportion of the idiopathic category of cerebral venous thrombosis.

Iatrogenic Causes

Intraoperative dural sinus injury and postoperative sinus thrombosis, as well as different medication regimens (androgen, danazol,[55] or antifibrinolytic[2] therapy) can lead to venous thrombosis. Methotrexate is reported to cause sinus thrombosis, possibly secondary to arachnoiditis.[35] Colloid cyst excision through a transcallosal approach was also reported to cause SSS thrombosis. Hypothetical mechanisms have included aggressive electrocoagulation around the sinus, electrocoagulation of large draining veins, and excessive retraction on the SSS or falx. In these cases, preoperative MRI and MRA to map out the parasagittal veins is especially important.[44]

Idiopathic

About 25 percent of cerebral venous thrombosis cases show no obvious cause.[35] Before such a classification, these patients should have a complete hematologic, inflammatory, and rheumatologic work-up, as well as a minimal search for occult neoplasms.

An association with dural arteriovenous fistulae[12] was reported. However, it has been convincingly suggested that these fistulae are the result rather than the cause of the thrombosis, presumably representing a form of collateralization.[11,59]

Clinical Features

General Symptoms and Signs

Clinical manifestations of cerebral venous occlusion vary from no symptoms or signs, to coma and death. In a series of 110 patients with cerebral venous thrombosis, Ameri and Bousser[5] found the presentations to be acute (less than 48 h) in 28 percent, subacute (between 48 h and 30 days) in 42 percent, and chronic (over 30 days) in 30 percent of their patients. Acute onsets tended to follow infectious or obstetric causes, while more chronic manifestations occurred with inflammatory or idiopathic etiologies. In addition, focal symptoms and signs tended to present acutely, while nonfocal ones were usually chronic.[5] In a literature review of 306 articles, McLean[81] notes that almost all patients studied had presented with symptoms and signs of increased intracranial pressure, with or without focal deficits.

Regardless of the site of thrombosis, headaches occurred in the majority of patients (41 to 75 percent) in three reports.[5,67,81] Papilledema was the second most common manifestation and the most common sign (39 to 49 percent), followed by motor or sensory deficits (34 to 40 percent), seizures (29 to 45 percent), nonspecific mental status changes or coma (26 to 50 percent), aphasia (10 to 16 percent), cranial nerve palsies (2 to 12 percent), cerebellar signs, nystagmus, hearing loss, and other signs (2 to 3 percent each) (Table 213-2).[5,67,81]

TABLE 213-2 Symptoms and Signs of Cerebral Venous Thrombosis

	Frequency of Occurrence (%)
Headache	41–75
Papilledema	39–49
Motor or sensory deficit	34–40
Seizures	29–45
Mental status changes/coma	26–50
Aphasia	10–16
Cranial nerve deficits	2–12
Cerebellar signs	Rare
Nystagmus	Rare
Hearing loss	Rare
Cortical blindness	Rare
Hemifacial spasm	Rare
Visual "migraine"[90]	Rare

Source: Adapted from McLean[81] and Ameri and Bousser.[5]

Although 60 percent of children present with headaches as the most common manifestation, 80 percent of neonates present with seizures. When no asphyxia is present at birth, as in the majority of cases, the prognosis is excellent with no neurodevelopmental delay and low risk of persistent seizure activity beyond the neonatal period.[13,110]

Typical Presentations

The older literature erroneously suggested that the majority of cases of venous sinus occlusion presented with impaired consciousness, frequently followed by rapid deterioration into a comatose state and death.[10,64,70] Prior to CT, DSA, and MRI, such diagnoses were usually made very late, and often at autopsy. Currently, three main modes of presentation are recognized: (1) focal deficits with or without increased intracranial pressure (ICP); (2) increased ICP without focal signs; and (3) cavernous sinus thrombosis. The last consists of a very specific and easily recognizable set of symptoms and signs, which will be discussed briefly later in this chapter.[5]

The occurrence of focal signs or seizures (present in over 75 percent of published cases)[5,81] points to the occlusion of a cerebral vein with or without dural sinus involvement. These signs often resolve completely, however, indicating an ischemic rather than an infarctive etiology. Often, the thrombotic process involves several veins, and mimics the clinical presentation of subarachnoid hemorrhage. The ictal event may be immediately catastrophic, with headache, collapse, seizures, and coma with stiff neck and blood-tinged cerebrospinal fluid.

In contrast, the involvement of a dural sinus without extension into the cerebral veins (30 to 40 percent of cases) is more likely to cause increased intracranial pressure and no focal deficits. Without radiographic confirmation, this presentation is usually indistinguishable from the syndrome of benign intracranial hypertension (BIH). Hydrocephalus does not usually develop. Papilledema is usually present, and gradual loss of vision is an important consequence, although both are much less common than in BIH.[71,97,100] Cerebral venous thrombosis should therefore be suspected and ruled out in any patient thought to suffer from this syndrome. This becomes especially important in the presence of a hematologic or metabolic disorder which may predispose to thrombosis, or if the classic characteristics of BIH (e.g., female sex; 40 to 50 years of age; obesity; normal CSF composition) are not met.

Venous sinus injury is usually suspected in trauma patients, when (1) the wound or impact site overlies a dural venous sinus; (2) a fracture line crosses a venous sinus; or, (3) the path of a missile crosses a sinus. However, traumatic sinus thrombosis may occur in the absence of these signs, and the clinical examination alone is often unreliable in predicting such an occlusion.[21,69]

Symptoms due to Occlusion of Individual Dural Sinuses

Because it is common for venous thrombosis to simultaneously involve different sinuses, it is difficult to assign a particular set of symptoms and signs to the occlusion of a specific sinus. Certain general guidelines may apply, however. There is no clinical syndrome associated with occlusion of the *anterior portion of the superior sagittal sinus.* When the *midportion of the superior sagittal sinus* is occluded, an increase in muscle tone in the extremities innervated by the involved cortex is sometimes seen, which may range from spastic hemiparesis or quadriparesis to decerebrate rigidity. ICP may rise within minutes.[104] In lesions involving the *posterior aspect of the superior sagittal sinus,* visual field defects or cortical blindness are common, and coma is frequently seen. Occlusion of the *transverse sinus* produces no neurological deficit unless the contralateral sinus is hypoplastic or does not drain the torcular. In that case, the clinical syndrome may be identical to that produced by occlusion of the posterior portion of the sagittal sinus. *Cavernous sinus* thrombosis classically presents with ipsilateral, and occasionally bilateral chemosis, proptosis, and painful ophthalmoplegia.[5] Cranial nerve signs may be prominent. Occlusion of the *deep venous system* frequently results in diencephalic dysfunction and death. A few survivors have been reported, the majority of whom suffered from abulia, disorientation, vertical gaze dysfunction, and severe problems with memory and cognition. Some benign forms, however, produced only confusion.[5,54] Deep venous thrombosis is much more common in children than in adults. The thrombus has usually propagated from other dural sinuses, rarely occurring in isolation, and the patient has a poor prognosis.[124] *Cerebellar venous* thrombosis is also rare. Scattered reports in the literature mention the occurrence of papilledema, cerebellar ataxia, and cranial nerve palsies, all symptoms reminiscent of posterior fossa masses.[5] Occlusion of the *occipital sinus* exhibits no specific symptoms or signs.

Laboratory Studies

The most consistent hematological abnormality is moderate to extreme elevation of the erythrocyte sedimentation rate (50 percent of reported cases).[16,69] A lymphocytosis may be present, however, especially in the setting of a malignant or inflammatory etiology of the occlusion.[86] More specific coagulation abnormalities will be found depending on the causative disease process. These should be investigated in the cases with no obvious cause, or when clinically suspected (Table 213-3).[5] Lumbar puncture usually demonstrates an increased cerebrospinal fluid pressure, and occasionally bloody and xanthochromic cerebrospinal fluid. This will also help distinguish cerebral venous thrombosis from benign intracranial hypertension.[47,48,63]

TABLE 213-3 Suggested Laboratory Tests When the Etiology Is Questionable

1. Complete blood count
2. Erythrocyte sedimentation rate
3. Disseminated intravascular coagulation screen
4. Coagulation screen
Protein S assay
Protein C assay
Antithrombin III assay
5. Other hematological studies
Hemoglobin S titer
Serum protein electrophoresis
Urine protein electrophoresis
Lupus anticoagulant
Anticardiolipin antibodies
Hemolysis screen
6. Full rheumatological work-up, especially
Rheumatoid factor
Antinuclear antibodies
AntiDNA antibodies
Antimitochondrial antibodies
7. Infectious work-up, including HIV titer, VDRL, PPD
8. Cerebrospinal fluid studies
9. Urinalysis and urine sample for homocystinuria
10. Pregnancy test
11. Work-up for neoplasm

Source: Adapted from McLean.[81]

Other Associations

Cerebral venous thrombosis has been associated with other thromboembolic diseases. Among these is a striking association with pulmonary embolism in the absence of lower extremity deep vein thrombosis, suggesting that the pulmonary emboli may have originated from the intracranial thrombus.[25,29]

Radiographic Features

Computed Tomography (CT)

The importance of CT as an initial study in the diagnostic evaluation of cerebral venous thrombosis is threefold: (1) other intracranial anomalies need to be excluded, especially since the clinical manifestations of venous occlusive disease are nonspecific; (2) a combination of distinctive CT signs may highly suggest the disease, and thus would help with the diagnosis and choice of further studies,[5,16,35] and (3) since CT scans are readily available in most medical centers, and at the present time are much faster than MRI scans, they are preferred in an emergency situation. A normal CT scan is noted in 10 to 20 percent of cases[5] and does not exclude the diagnosis. Scans without and with contrast enhancement are necessary, and the findings depend on the timing of the scan in relation to the onset of symptoms.

The presence of the different CT signs may be based on one of three pathophysiological mechanisms: (1) the direct visualization of the thrombus (e.g., cord sign, dense vein sign, fresh clot, and filling defect); (2) a consequence of the thrombosis (e.g., infarcts, hemorrhages, small ventricles, and edema); and (3) the development of a collateral circulation (e.g., empty delta sign, tentorial and gyral enhancement, and dilated transcerebral medullary veins).[129] Patients with venous sinus thrombosis very commonly have *small ventricles* (13 to 50 percent).[5,129] This is an early and nonspecific sign. With time, however, the ventricles may become larger than normal. *Fresh clot* within the venous system may be visualized on a noncontrasted scan, while low-density *filling defects* are often seen on a contrast-enhanced scan. When the CT slice is perpendicular to the sagittal sinus, a high-density triangle (enhancing collaterals in the sinus wall)[98] with a low-density center (thrombus) creates the so-called *empty delta sign.*[5,16,35,124] Since its original description by Buonanno et al.,[19] this sign has been found at variable frequencies in different studies (2 to 35 percent, and even 70 percent in one study).[19,94,118] It usually appears about one week into the disease process, and disappears by two months,[79] which is the time it takes for the dural enhancement to resolve. By comparison, recanalization of the sinus may only take a few days. High splitting of the sagittal sinus (i.e., duplication of the posterior aspect of the sinus) may mimic the empty delta sign. This ''false delta sign'' may be recognized by reviewing several contiguous CT sections, and using different window settings. Similarly, the combination of a contrast-enhanced sinus and an adjacent process of low signal intensity (such as an epidural abscess) may look like an empty delta sign. *Venous infarcts*[23] are noted in about 20 percent of reported cases. Pathophysiologically, they reflect a rapid rise in venous pressure, and are more common in the brain than in other tissues in the body probably because of the brain's tendency to produce vasogenic edema. Only one-quarter of these are hemorrhagic. Most of these lesions, however, whether or not they are hemorrhagic on CT scan, disappear with time. This means that they more commonly represent ischemic rather than infarctive processes. The hemorrhage usually disappears within one month, and the enhancement and edema by two months.[23] The associated *parenchymal hemorrhages* are usually unilateral, and although nonspecific, they become suspicious for venous thrombosis when they occur in locations that are unusual for hypertensive or aneurysmal hemorrhages. *Gyral enhancement* following contrast infusion, also indicative of brain ischemia or infarction, is noted in about 30 percent of patients. When seen in combination with an empty delta sign, it is highly suggestive of sinus thrombosis. Intense *tentorial enhancement,* presumably representing tentorial collateral pathways, has been reported to occur with straight sinus thrombosis. The *cord sign* on unenhanced CT scans is a rare occurrence. It represents high-density clot in a cortical vein, and is considered pathognomonic of cerebral vein thrombosis.[94] Another rare and related sign on unenhanced scans is the *dense vein sign.* This represents thrombus in the deep venous and/or superior sagittal sinuses. A small percentage (4 percent in one study)[129] of patients presents with *dilated transcerebral medullary veins.* This is another phenomenon of enhanced collateral circulation, also pathognomonic of venous sinus thrombosis. Finally, *thalamo-ventricular hemorrhages* in term newborns have been reported to be caused by deep venous thrombosis.[51]

Angiography

Prior to the advent of MRI, four-vessel digital subtraction angiography (DSA) had been the method of choice[52] for diagnosing cerebral venous thrombosis. Currently, it is used mainly when MRI is either nondiagnostic, unavailable, or contraindicated. DSA allows excellent visualization of the major venous sinuses, including the deep venous system. In patients who have thrombosis of major venous channels, there is lack of filling of the thrombosed sinuses. In addition, the cerebral circulation time may be prolonged, and delayed filming may be required to adequately visualize the venous system. In the interpretation of intraluminal filling defects, it is important to remember that blood entering the sinus from a vessel that was not injected with the contrast agent may appear as an intraluminal defect in the contrast pool. Finally, the complete absence of a venous channel, particularly the transverse sinus, may be a normal anatomic variation. However, the visualization of stumps or of abnormal collateral pathways on the angiogram, and the presence of a normal jugular foramen and a lateral sinus groove on skull radiographs support the diagnosis of an occlusive process.

Magnetic Resonance Imaging (MRI)

MRI is the diagnostic modality of choice for cerebral venous thrombosis. Its advantages include the following: (1) noninvasiveness; (2) freedom from bone artifact; (3) good visualization of the cavernous sinus[27] and the deep venous system;[6] (4) capacity for multiplanar imaging; (5) sensitivity to the absence of flow; (6) ability to image the thrombus itself, as opposed to a filling defect (as in angiography); (7) possibility of assessing the approximate age of the clot; (8) ease with which frequent and noninvasive long-term follow-ups can be obtained; (9) ability, unlike with angiography, to simultaneously evaluate both neural and vascular structures (especially helpful in cases of dural sinus occlusion by tumor mass);[130] (10) ability to differentiate dural sinus hypoplasia from thrombosis (especially important with transverse sinus imaging); and finally, (11) availability of MRA for more problematic diagnoses.

Depending on the stage of evolution of the thrombus, MRI will show a variety of manifestations.[130] Early in the disease, absence of a flow void is the most prominent finding. A flow void indicates rapidly moving blood, and appears hypointense (dark) compared with brain on both T1- and T2-weighted images (WI). In contrast, the thrombus is usually isointense on T1WI (Fig. 213-2), and hypointense on T2WI. Collateral venous channels may be prominent at this point. In the intermediate or subacute stage (24 h to two weeks), the thrombus becomes hyperintense, first on T1WI (Fig. 213-3), then on T2WI. This reflects a change in the breakdown products of blood from deoxyhemoglobin to methemoglobin, which starts peripherally and spreads centrally. As recanalization starts (about two weeks into the disease process), the flow void reappears. Although gadolinium-DTPA (Fig. 213-4) may be useful in some circumstances, it is not used routinely. Its most prominent finding is enhancement of the sinus walls due to their vascularity.[56,98]

Conventional MRI (spin-echo imaging), however, admits some limitations. Since its signal reflects both blood clotting and blood flow velocity, the combination of these two indices may cause some ambiguity in interpretation.[89] For instance, on occasion, slow-flowing blood will have a hyperintense signal similar to methemoglobin. A relatively inexperienced observer may incorrectly interpret this as a thrombus. No perfect method exists to avoid this artifact in conventional MRI; however, one way to minimize it is to change the imaging plane (e.g., from axial to sagittal), thereby changing the direction of flow. The signal characteristics of slow-flowing blood will then change (usually becoming more hypointense), while the methemoglobin signal will stay hyperintense on

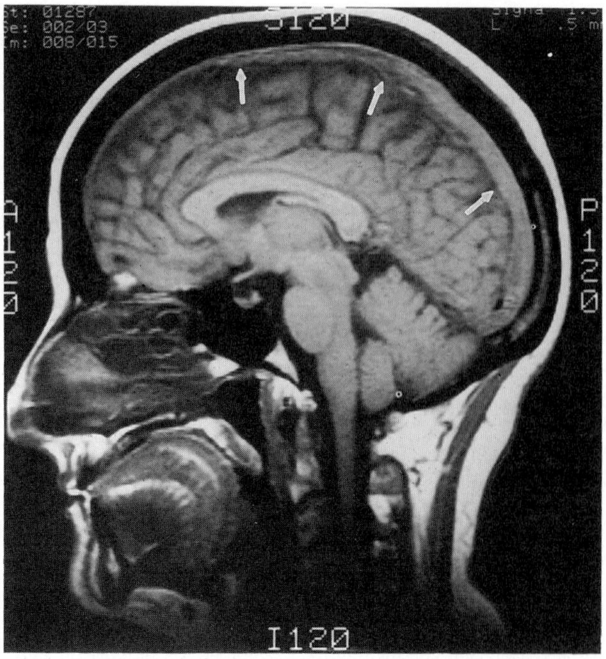

Figure 213-2 T1-weighted sagittal image. The normal flow void of the superior sagittal sinus (SSS) is replaced by abnormal signal, indicating thrombosis of the entire SSS (*arrows*). (Courtesy of E. Ralph Heinz, M.D., Duke University Medical Center.)

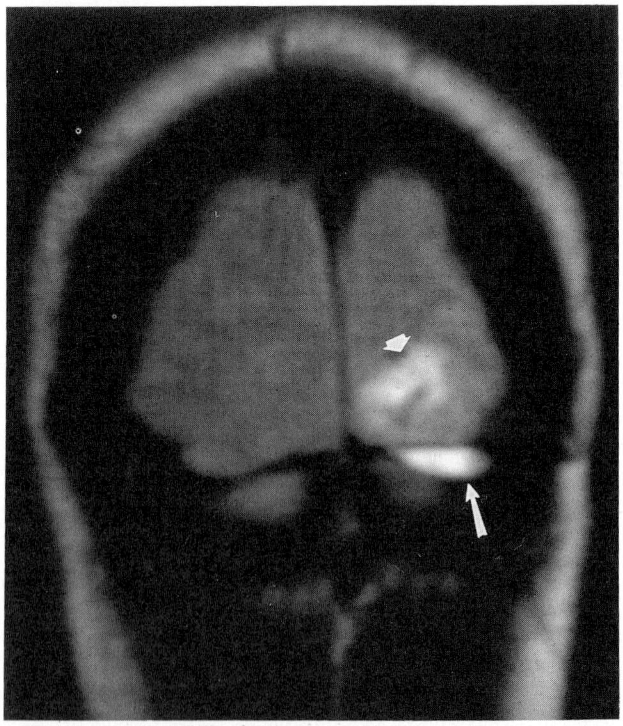

Figure 213-3 This is a T1-weighted coronal image from a patient with a 3-week history of headaches and a previous MRI showing sinus thrombosis. Following the acute onset of a motor deficit, a follow-up MRI scan (shown above) demonstrated a hemorrhagic venous infarction (*short arrow*) adjacent to a thrombosed left transverse sinus (*long arrow*). The venous infarction was absent on the MRI scan done prior to the development of the focal deficit. (Courtesy of E. Ralph Heinz, M.D., Duke University Medical Center.)

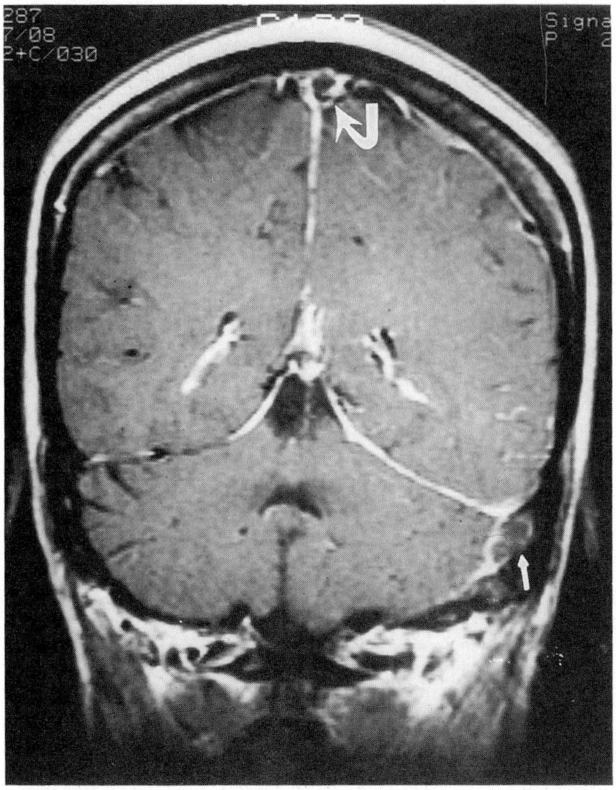

Figure 213-4 This is a gadolinium-enhanced T1-weighted coronal image showing nonenhancing thrombus in the left transverse (*straight arrow*) and superior sagittal (*curved arrow*) sinuses. Normal flow void is present in the right transverse sinus. (Courtesy of E. Ralph Heinz, M.D., Duke University Medical Center.)

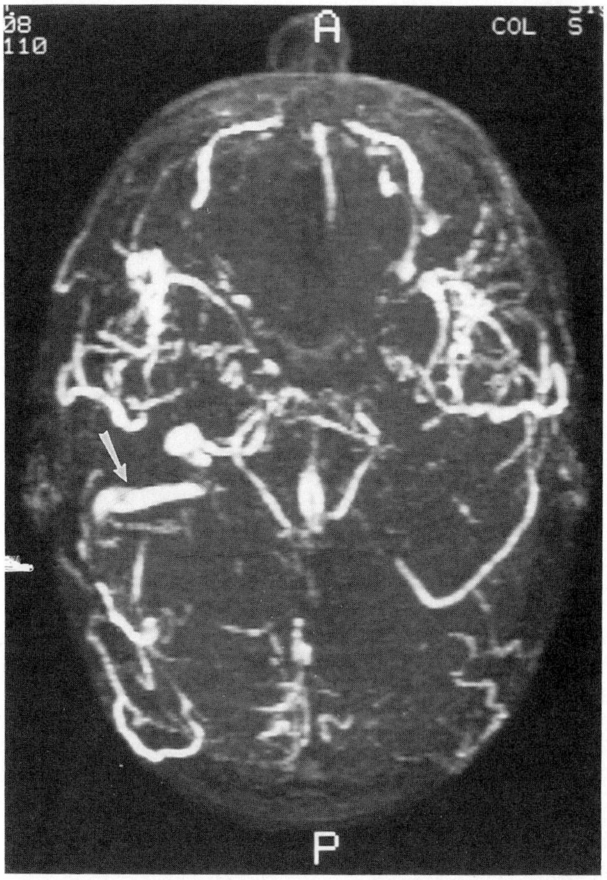

Figure 213-5 MR angiogram in which venous flow has been targeted. Normal signal is present in the right sigmoid sinus (*arrow*). There is absence of signal in the left sigmoid sinus and both transverse sinuses, indicating their occlusion. (Courtesy of E. Ralph Heinz, M.D., Duke University Medical Center.)

all imaging planes.[89] Another MRI caveat is that deoxyhemoglobin is usually hypointense on T2WI, similar to flow void; it is therefore essential to look at all sequences, particularly T1WI to make the correct diagnosis. Finally, the evolution of a thrombus does not always follow strict time intervals; for example, it may take several days, even up to two weeks, before the methemoglobin signal characteristics arise. These problems can be adequately resolved by the appropriate use of MRA.

Magnetic Resonance Angiography (MRA)

The basis of MRA is its ability to show flowing liquids to the exclusion of nonflowing structures. In MRA images, flowing blood displays a bright signal, whereas stationary tissues (e.g., brain) do not. This results in an appearance similar to a conventional angiogram (Fig. 213-5). MRA also has some practical advantages. Imaging time is not significantly prolonged when it is added to a routine MRI study, and there is often no need to reposition the patient.[78,89,101]

Two main MRA techniques are currently used in intracranial imaging: time-of-flight (TOF) and phase contrast (PC). Although both techniques are routinely used in venous cerebral disease, a few important differences stand out. (For a more detailed analysis, the reader is referred to the radiology literature.)[78] Although TOF is faster and less affected by patient motion than PC, it has two major drawbacks which generally make it less reliable than PC for evaluation of cerebral venous thrombosis.[89,101] (1) in TOF, a thrombus may occasionally mimic the appearance of flowing blood, and (2) unlike PC, TOF is not sensitive to slow flow; hence, slow-flowing blood in the sinuses may have a dark signal mimicking a thrombus. Both of these problems are avoided with PC.

Although MRA techniques allow the depiction of flow in a noninvasive manner, they have some limitations, including the inability to visualize very small vessels (e.g., in suspected vasculitis). However, the combination of conventional MRI and the currently available MRA investigations has been very reliable in confirming the presence or absence of cerebral venous thrombosis. Even though large scale controlled studies comparing DSA with MRI/MRA are unavailable—and probably difficult to accomplish—recent experience seems to show that the combination of MRI and MRA, when used in problematic cases, should obviate the need for an angiogram.[101]

Therapy

There are five main objectives in the treatment of cerebral venous occlusion: (1) to correct the basic pathologic process that caused the problem; (2) to prevent extension of the thrombus into patent veins; (3) to afford symptomatic control at least until the involved vessels have recanalized or collateral channels have developed (this is especially important in the setting of a seizure disorder and/or elevated ICP); and (4) when indicated, to chemically lyse or surgically remove the clot.

Anticoagulation

Anticoagulation prevents or delays the extension of the thrombus until collaterals form or until recanalization occurs. Once instituted, anticoagulation may have to be continued for 3 to 6 months, or longer and even lifelong in the occasional case with multiple recurrences. Anticoagulants take on even greater importance when it is realized that those same hypercoagulable states which cause cerebral venous thrombosis may also cause thromboembolic disease elsewhere in the body.[10,119]

With the tendency for venous infarcts to be hemorrhagic, the use of anticoagulants has been strongly debated. Despite occasional anecdotal reports to the contrary,[46] recent data based on several retrospective studies and one prospective study have suggested that the administration of heparin and coumadin in patients with cerebral venous thrombosis does not result in an increased risk of intracranial bleeding, even in the presence of a hemorrhagic infarct. Furthermore, anticoagulation has been shown to improve the outcome of the disease in a large majority of published cases, with minimal, if any, associated complications.[12,22,34,40,64,70,100,118] In fact, some patients who had been deteriorating prior to the institution of heparin therapy, showed dramatic improvement after starting the treatment.[16,35] In a retrospective review of 82 patients treated with dose-adjusted heparin, there were no complications or deaths associated with the use of heparin.[4] In a randomized, blinded, and placebo-controlled trial[34] in 20 patients with cerebral venous thrombosis, the clinical course of the group treated with dose-adjusted heparin showed a statistically significant improvement compared with the control group as early as 3 days into treatment. By 3 months, eight of the ten heparin-treated patients had recovered completely, while two had a partial recovery. In contrast, three patients in the control group died, one patient had a complete recovery, and six others suffered residual neurological deficits. Intracerebral hemorrhage occurring after institution of the heparin or placebo was seen only in the control group (three out of ten, two of whom had also bled before the start of the trial). The three patients in the heparin group who had bled prior to the institution of heparin did not rebleed afterward. These prospective data were corroborated in the same institution by a retrospective review of 43 patients who had both cerebral venous thrombosis and intracerebral hemorrhage. The mortality rate was 15 percent in the heparin-treated group, versus 69 percent in the untreated group. However, the study was criticized because the study size was small, the reliability of its severity scale was questioned,[114] and the authors did not take into account the different etiologies of the disease, which have different prognoses. Nonetheless, it is encouraging that only 3 of 56 heparin-treated patients had a hemorrhage, and that none of those were serious.[36]

The importance of knowing the cause of the thrombosis cannot be overemphasized, as we are constantly learning more about the different causal diseases. The following are some practical examples: (1) in paroxysmal nocturnal hemoglobinuria, heparin is contraindicated because of the coexistence of thrombocytopenia; (2) in protein C or S deficiencies, because warfarin can cause an initial worsening of the hypercoagulable state, full anticoagulation with heparin should take place before starting warfarin therapy; and (3) in antithrombin III deficiency, heparin is only effective if fresh frozen plasma is also administered.[35,36]

Treatment should obviously be tailored according to etiology, and on a case-by-case basis. However, until results of larger studies indicate otherwise, it is recommended that anticoagulation be used to manage cerebral venous thrombosis, although the use of long-term anticoagulation with warfarin is still debatable. The heparin dosage and schedule of administration may be crucial, and a schedule that minimizes peaks and troughs in the level of anticoagulation is preferable. In their prospective study, Einhaüpl et al.[34] used the following regimen, which they found both safe and effective: intravenous heparin 3000 IU bolus, followed by a continuous infusion of 25,000 to 65,000 IU/day, with an initial PTT that is at least doubled without exceeding 120 s. Clearer guidelines concerning dosage, timing, and length of treatment are expected from future studies.

Thrombolytic Therapy

The use of fibrinolytic agents for treatment of cerebral venous thrombosis is controversial, but shows promise. Multiple case reports convincingly demonstrate its efficacy and occasionally its necessity.[8,30,40] This is further substantiated by the successful, and relatively uncomplicated use of thrombolytic agents in myocardial infarction, peripheral arterial occlusion, and pulmonary embolism.[1] However, because of the unpredictable natural history of the disease and the lack of controlled studies, especially with regard to *fresh* occlusions, no conclusions or recommendations can be given at this time regarding this form of therapy.

Thrombolytic agents may be infused either systemically (intravenously),[3,46,99] or locally in or near the thrombus. Local thrombolysis has been performed through direct and indirect approaches to the sinus. Direct approaches have included puncture of the torcular through a craniotomy,[92] as well as puncture of the SSS through the anterior fontanel in infants[57] or a midline frontal craniectomy in adults.[108] These techniques have allowed the operators to gain access to other sinuses using an angiographic infusion catheter. The indirect methods have included transjugular[12,37] and transfemoral[120] approaches, also using an angiographic Tracker catheter (Target Therapeutics, Los Angeles) that is passed into the intracranial sinuses with the help of a steerable guidewire. It has been hypothesized that local infusions may minimize the systemic hemorrhagic complications of the thrombolytic agents, while achieving adequate recanalization of the sinus.[108] This has yet to be proven, however. In addition, the risks involved in directly invading a dural sinus have to be seriously contemplated before such a procedure is attempted.

In the late 1970s, Gettelfinger and Kokmen[46] and Rousseaux et al. each reported one death involving patients with extensive intracranial venous thrombosis who had received intravenous heparin and urokinase, although the cause of death could not be definitely attributed to these agents. Since that time, more encouraging studies have been done. Barnwell et al.[12] used a direct transjugular infusion of high-dose urokinase for 4 to 10 days in three patients with venous sinus thrombosis and an associated dural arteriovenous fistula. All three patients started to improve by 24 h, one ultimately showing partial radiographic resolution of the clot, and the other two showing significant clinical improvement accompanied by venographic evidence of sinus recanalization. All three patients were anticoagulated before, during, and for at least 6 weeks after the thrombolytic treatment. Scott et al.[108] reported the use of local urokinase infusion in a patient with a severe acute neurological deterioration from diffuse dural sinus thrombosis. The urokinase was administered through a frontal craniectomy and direct placement of an angiographic infusion catheter in the superior sagittal sinus, to be advanced later to the torcular. There was dramatic improvement in ICP and clinical status, and recanalization of the sinuses. Although the infusion was stopped 8 h later because of a hemorrhagic temporal lobe infarction, the patient continued to improve. A similar infusion through the anterior fontanelle was also successfully attempted in a newborn infant with diffuse dural sinus thrombosis by Higashida et al.[57] The decision for thrombolytic therapy was made because of the patient's active neurological deterioration and ongoing seizure activity despite supportive management. Again, the patient improved significantly—both clinically and radiographically. Similar successes with urokinase or streptokinase were reported by Eskridge and Wessbecher,[37] DiRocco et al.,[30] Tsai et al.,[120] and Persson and Lilja.[92]

Alexander et al.[3] induced sinus thrombosis in rabbits, and demonstrated total lysis of the clot in seven of eight animals treated with systemic tissue plasminogen activator (tPA), partial lysis in one, and no lysis in the control animals after saline infusions. tPA has high affinity for fibrin-bound plasminogen, low affinity for circulating plasminogen, and has proven very effective for treating myocardial ischemia.[3]

Surgical Therapy

Surgical thrombectomy of the superior sagittal and transverse sinuses is technically possible but has not yet received a place in the therapeutic armamentarium for cerebral venous thrombosis. This is because (1) the clot most frequently does not limit itself to the sinus; instead, it extends into tributary veins and lateral lacunae, and (2) recurrence of thrombosis is common after such a procedure.

Surgical Indications

The need for operative treatment of lesions involving the venous system of the brain, especially the dural sinuses, often arises in the management of head injuries and neoplasms. The involvement of a dural venous sinus by a localized malignant neoplasm involving scalp, skull, or dura would constitute a strong indication for resection of the involved sinus and, if necessary, its replacement with a graft. Indications for resection of dural sinuses involved by meningiomas are less definite. Conventional management dictates that if the sinus cannot be sacrificed, gradual occlusion will occur as the remaining tumor left attached to the sinus wall grows. The sinus can then be resected at a later date, at less risk of sudden neurological compromise. Resection of sinuses that have been totally occluded by meningiomas is not without risk, however, probably because of interference with collateral venous channels in the scalp, in the skull, or in the brain itself.[125] It appears likely that as surgeons become more comfortable with the techniques of dural sinus reconstruction, more aggressive attempts will be made to totally remove meningiomas involving the venous sinuses at the first operation.[53]

General Surgical Techniques

Before any surgical procedure on the dural sinuses is attempted, a detailed MRI/MRA scan should be obtained with the purpose of delineating the detailed anatomy of the sinuses, and localizing, as much as possible, the extent of the injury or thrombosis. The techniques for surgical reconstruction of dural venous sinuses are based on the established principles of peripheral vascular surgery (i.e., adequate exposure of all sides of the involved vascular structure, proximal and distal control of hemorrhage, and accurate approximation of the endothelial surfaces with fine suture material).[65]

However, certain accommodations must be made because of the unique anatomical features of the dural venous sinuses. Extensive mobilization of a dural sinus is hampered by rigid triangulation, by veins entering at frequent intervals along the course of the sinus, and by the lateral lacunae that may be opened when the dura is incised parallel to the lumen of the sinus. Therefore, intraluminal occlusion of a sinus by *inflation of a balloon* is usually used to control bleeding. Likewise, *shunts* (Fig. 213-6) for use in dural sinus reconstruction are held in place by *balloon cuffs* on each end rather than by tourniquets around the vessel. The passage of tubes and shunts may be obstructed within a sinus by the cords of Willis, unless a *rigid tube* is first inserted with sufficient force to break them. Finally, a shunt tube inserted into the lumen of a sinus may enter a lateral lacuna and fail to function.

Control of Bleeding

Control of hemorrhage is achieved by digital pressure in the case of small lacerations, or by inserting a balloon-tipped catheter (e.g., large Fogarty catheter) into the lumen of the sinus, and inflating the balloon. If occlusion of the involved sinus is not tolerated, a shunt, which can be fashioned from a pediatric anode endotracheal tube with a short pediatric tracheostomy tube cuff on each end, will provide control of the hemorrhage as well as diversion of the blood. The shunt must be prepared preoperatively, siliconized by the application of a thin layer of high vacuum silicone stopcock grease (Dow-Corning, Midland, MI) to both the lumen and the exterior surface, and gas sterilized prior to use.[66]

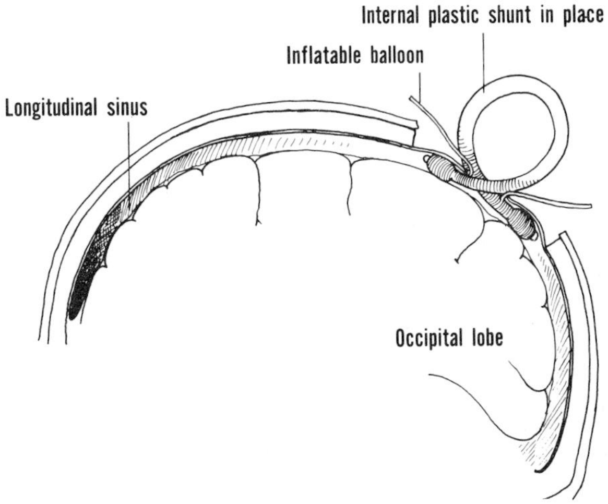

Figure 213-6 Shunt illustrating the balloon tips inflated within the sinus. [From Kapp JP. Surgical management of dural sinus lacerations. In Schmidek HH, Sweet WH (eds): *Operative Neurosurgical Techniques: Indications, Methods, and Results.* New York, Grune & Stratton, 1982, pp 205–213, with permission.]

Management of Sinus Wall Injuries

Small lacerations in the venous sinuses can often be closed with small interrupted sutures. Relaxing incisions in the dura on each side of the involved sinus may reduce tension on the closure. Some stenosis of the sinus at the suture line is acceptable. In our experience, venous sinus stenosis of up to 50 percent was well tolerated. It is also possible to tie the sutures over a small roll of pericranium or dura if the closure is particularly tight.

Ligation should be considered when (1) the lesion is in a noncritical area, (2) primary suture repair would result in stenosis of such magnitude that postoperative thrombosis would be expected, and (3) proximal venous flow is insignificant because of involvement of multiple bridging cortical veins. The areas that are considered *noncritical* are the portions of the superior sagittal sinus anterior to the entrance of the rolandic vein, the nondominant transverse or sigmoid sinus, the inferior sagittal and straight sinuses, and the minor sinuses on the floor of the skull. On the other hand, the *critical* sinuses include the superior sagittal sinus posterior to the rolandic vein, the torcular, and the dominant transverse sinus. When one or more walls of these (critical) sinuses are destroyed or invaded by tumor, the injured walls should be replaced by an autogenous vein graft.

Sinus Grafting Preparation

Autogenous veins have proven very effective in sinus grafting. In contrast, arterial grafts have been known to progressively fibrose and constrict, giving rise to a high incidence of late thrombosis.[113] There has been virtually no experience with the use of synthetic materials in the cerebral venous system. When the need to resect or graft a venous sinus is anticipated, the operation should be planned (1) to allow wide *exposure* of the injured sinus; (2) to provide means for rapid, massive *blood replacement* (for that purpose, a large intravenous tube is inserted into the proximal stump of the vein and threaded centrally); and (3) to provide tissue for use in sinus *reconstruction.* If the patient's condition is not urgent, a 20-cm segment of the proximal portion of the greater saphenous vein should be removed before the craniotomy is started. This procedure usually requires 20 to 30 min. If a delay of this magnitude is deemed unwise and the prone position is required for the cranial surgery, a segment of small saphenous vein below the knee can be removed by a second surgical team after the craniotomy has started. The segment is then flushed with heparinized saline, hydrostatically dilated to overcome spasm, and placed in the heparinized saline solution for later use.

In trauma cases, the injured area of the sinus should be left undisturbed until adequate exposure has been obtained. Prior to the introduction of the balloon catheter or shunt into the sinus, thrombi and foreign material must be removed from the lumen of the sinus. In the resection of tumors, the sinus wall involved with the tumor is usually removed after the bulk of the tumor has been excised.

Sinus Grafting Technique

Circulation through the operative area is controlled by the use of digital pressure, Fogarty catheters, or immediate insertion of the shunt. The lumen of the sinus is irrigated with heparinized saline, the anatomy of the lesion is defined, and if the shunt is not already in place, it is inserted at this time. If profuse hemorrhage from the sinus wound makes it impossible to define the lumen of the sinus, a small sinotomy is made that is just large enough to admit a no. 7 Fogarty catheter. The catheter is then introduced through the opening, and inflated within the sinus. Digital pressure is usually sufficient to control bleeding from the distal sinus and prevent air embolism. The previously prepared vein graft is opened. A 5-0 nonabsorbable synthetic vascular suture is used to approximate the end of the defect and the end of the graft. The graft must be properly oriented because of the possible presence of valves. One side of the graft is sutured into the defect with a continuous suture. The remainder of the graft is tailored to fit the defect, and the suture line is partially completed with a continuous suture to a point where the opening will allow easy removal of the shunt. Interrupted sutures are then placed at the shunt insertion site, but not tied (Fig. 213-7). The shunt is removed, a largebore sucker is passed in each direction within the sinus to remove clots, and the preplaced sutures are tied down to close the remaining defect and complete the suture line. Effort should be made to triangulate the

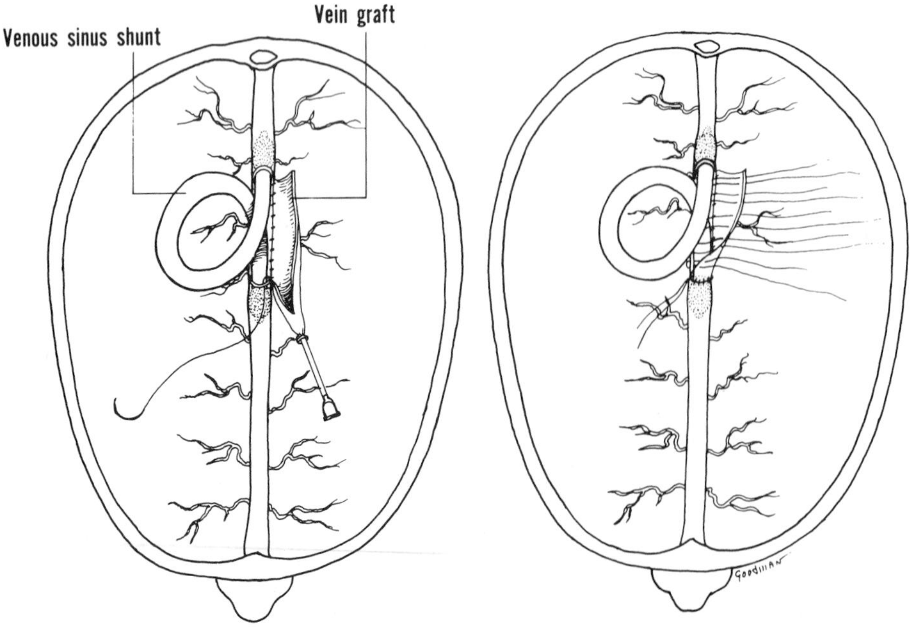

Figure 213-7 *Left.* The shunt has been placed, and the saphenous vein graft has been sutured into the defect on the right side with a continuous suture. *Right.* Interrupted sutures have been placed on the left side to be tied down when the shunt is removed. [From Kapp JP. Surgical management of dural sinus lacerations. In Schmidek HH, Sweet WH (eds): *Operative Neurosurgical Techniques: Indications, Methods, and Results.* New York, Grune & Stratton, 1982, pp 205–213, with permission.]

grafted segment of the sinus. This is accomplished by attaching it to dura or dural grafts at multiple points, with fine vascular sutures placed through the adventitia. Compression of the grafted sinus by tight scalp flaps or extradural fluid collections may lead to thrombosis. A soft suction drain should be placed in the epidural space and brought out through a stab wound in the scalp.

General Treatment

Theoretical or practical problems have arisen with virtually every approach to therapy, and most often an attempt to respond to one objective has created a problem in another area. For example, corticosteroids have been shown to interfere with reactive fibrinolysis.[45] The administration of corticosteroids to control increased intracranial pressure may interfere with clearance of intravascular thrombi, and thereby worsen an already abnormal coagulation state in some cases. Dehydration of the patient through fluid restriction or by the administration of diuretics or hyperosmolar agents (also as a treatment for increased ICP) may increase blood viscosity and sludging, resulting in the extension of the thrombus, and increasing an already high risk of thromboembolic complications elsewhere in the body. Treatment should indeed be tailored on a case-by-case basis, bearing in mind the patient's risk factors, the etiology of the disease, and the response to therapy. Based on the above discussions, the following are some general guidelines (also summarized in Table 213-4):

1. Medical management of increased ICP should be maximized (hyperosmolar agents, diuretics, and head elevation) and if necessary, a lumbo-peritoneal shunt inserted. Once collaterals have formed or sinus recanalization has occurred, the ICP will decline, although different reports disagree as to the speed of that decline (months versus years).[71,97,100]
2. Medical management of seizures should be continued for 6 to 12 months, or as deemed clinically appropriate.
3. The primary disorder responsible for the thrombosis should be corrected.
4. Full anticoagulation should be performed as outlined above, unless contraindicated.
5. Thrombolysis should be an experimental consideration under controlled circumstances.

Incidence, Risk Factors, and Outcome

As mentioned previously, the incidence of nonseptic cerebral venous thrombosis has been greatly underestimated; the true incidence is still unclear, however. Several risk factors seem to predispose to the development of this disorder: extremes of age (newborns and elderly), and especially men above age 60, probably reflecting a greater incidence of general thromboembolic disease in this group; women between ages 20 and 35, reflecting the occurrence of pregnancy and the use of oral contraceptive pills;[5] and the presence of other thrombotic sites or systemic diseases such as dehydration, debility, and congestive heart failure.[119]

Nonseptic thrombosis of a cerebral venous sinus has a variable mortality rate. In 1942, Stansfield reported a mortality of 56 percent in cases collected from the literature,[115] and in 1948, Kendall estimated that 30 percent of recorded cases were fatal.[68] The figures in other reports have ranged from 5 to 71 percent.[9,38,46,60,70,126] Recently, however, mortality rates have consistently been between 5 and 20 percent.[4,16,35,67] These numbers mainly reflect the earlier diagnoses afforded by the current imaging modalities, and anticoagulant use.[16] Multiple factors have been associated with a poorer prognosis: (1) the presence of focal symptoms, reflecting the involvement of cerebral veins; (2) the speed of evolution of the thrombus; (3) the presence of coma; and (4) extremes of age.[16]

Finally, while the mortality associated with the surgical management of lesions of the anterior portion of the sagittal sinus has not been influenced by changes in technique, the mortality associated with management of penetrating injuries of the posterior sagittal sinus has been reduced from 42 percent to zero, and the overall mortality in patients with dural sinus injury has been reduced from 27 to 6 percent by using the surgical techniques described in this chapter.[65]

TABLE 213-4 Treatment of Nonsurgical Cerebral Venous Thrombosis

1. Treat the etiology of the disorder
2. Treat the elevated intracranial pressure (medical management; intermittent lumbar punctures; consider lumbo-peritoneal shunt placement)
3. Treat the seizure disorder
4. Anticoagulate (unless specifically contraindicated)
5. Follow with frequent MRI scans

References

1. Abel H. Thrombolysis. The logical approach for the treatment of vascular occlusions. *Acta Cardiol* 1992; 47:287–295 (editorial).
2. Achiron A, Gornish M, Melamed E. Cerebral sinus thrombosis as a potential hazard of antifibrinolytic treatment in menorrhagia. *Stroke* 1990; 21:817–819.
3. Alexander LF, Yamamoto Y, Ayoubi S, et al. Efficacy of tissue plasminogen activator in the lysis of thrombosis of the cerebral venous sinus. *Neurosurgery* 1990; 26:559–564.
4. Ameri A. *Les Thromboses Veineuses Cérébrales* 110 cas. Paris: Thése, 1991, p 150.
5. Ameri A, Bousser MG. Cerebral venous thrombosis. *Neurol Clin* 1992; 10:87–111.
6. Ashforth RA, Melanson D, Ethier R. MR of deep cerebral venous thrombosis. *Can J Neurol Sci* 1989; 16:417–421.
7. Askenasy HM, Kosary IZ, Braham J. Thrombosis of the longitudinal sinus: diagnosis by carotid arteriography. *Neurology* 1962; 12:288–292.
8. Atkinson EA, Fairburn B, Heathfield KWG. Intracranial venous thrombosis as a complication of oral contraceptives. *Lancet* 1970; 1:914–918.
9. Averback P. Primary cerebral venous thrombosis in young adults: the diverse manifestations of an underrecognized disease. *Ann Neurol* 1978; 3:81–86.
10. Barnett HJM, Hyland HH. Non-infective intracranial venous thrombosis. *Brain* 1953; 76:36–49.
11. Barnwell SL, Halbach VV, Dowd CF, et al. A variant of arteriovenous fistulas within the wall of dural sinuses. Results of a combined surgical and endovascular therapy. *J Neurosurg* 1991; 74:199–204.
12. Barnwell SL, Higashida RT, Halbach VV, et al. Direct endovascular thrombolytic therapy for dural sinus thrombosis. *Neurosurgery* 1991; 28:135–142.
13. Barron TF, Gusnard DA, Zimmerman RA, Clancy RR. Cerebral venous thrombosis in neonates and children. *Pediat Neurol* 1992; 8:112–116.

14. Ben Achour D, Kchock M, Ben Miled K, Bouchami T. Rubrique iconographique: un cas de thrombose veineuse cérébrale et renale après un cathétérisme cardiaque. *Arch Fr Pediat* 1991; 48:641–642.
15. Borda IT, Southern RF, Brown WF. Cerebral venous thrombosis in ulcerative colitis. *Gastroenterology* 1973; 64:116–119.
16. Bousser MG, Chiras J, Bories J, Castaigne P. Cerebral venous thrombosis—a review of 38 cases. *Stroke* 1985; 16:199–213.
17. Brenner B, Fishman A, Goldsher D, et al. Cerebral thrombosis in a newborn with a congenital deficiency of antithrombin III. *Am J Hematol* 1988; 27:209–211.
18. Browder J, Kaplan HA, Howard EM. Hyperplasia of pacchionian granulations. *Arch Pathol Lab Clin Med* 1973; 95:315–316.
19. Buonanno FS, Moody DM, Ball MR, Laster DW. Computed cranial tomographic findings in cerebral sinovenous occlusion. *J Comput Assist Tomogr* 1978; 2:281–290.
20. Byrne JV, Lawton CA. Meningeal sarcoidosis causing intracranial hypertension secondary to dural sinus thrombosis. *Br J Radiol* 1983; 56:755–757.
21. Carrie AW, Jaffé FA. Thrombosis of superior sagittal sinus caused by trauma without penetrating injury. *J Neurosurg* 1954; 11:173–182.
22. Castaign P, Laplane D, Bousser MG. Superior sagittal sinus thrombosis. *Arch Neurol* 1977; 34:788–789.
23. Chiras J, Dubs M, Bories J. Venous infarctions. *Neuroradiology* 1985; 27:593–600.
24. Cochran FB, Packman S. Homocystinuria presenting as sagittal sinus thrombosis. *Eur Neurol* 1992; 32:1–3.
25. Crimmins TJ, Rockswold GL, Yock DH Jr. Progressive posttraumatic superior sagittal sinus thrombosis complicated by pulmonary embolism. Case report. *J Neurosurg* 1984; 60:179–182.
26. Cucinell SA, Pitts CM. Thrombosis at mountain altitudes. *Avia Space Environ Med* 1987; 58:1109–1111.
27. Daniels DL, Pech P, Mark L, et al. Magnetic resonance imaging of the cavernous sinus. *Am J Roentgenol* 1985; 144:1009–1014.
28. David RB, Hadfield MG, Vines FS, Maurer MD. Dural sinus occlusion in leukemia. *Pediatrics* 1975; 56:793–796.
29. Diaz JM, Schiffman JS, Urban ES, Maccario M. Superior sagittal sinus thrombosis and pulmonary embolism. A syndrome rediscovered. *Acta Neurol Scand* 1992; 86:390–396.
30. Di Rocco C, Iannelli A, Leone G, et al. Heparin-urokinase treatment in aseptic dural sinus thrombosis. *Arch Neurol* 1981; 38:431–435.
31. Duckwiler GR, Dion JE, Vinuela F, Reichman A. Delayed venous occlusion following embolotherapy of vascular malformations in the brain. *Am J Neuroradiol* 1992; 13:1571–1579.
32. Dunsker SB, Torres-Reyes E, Peden JC Jr. Pseudotumor cerebri associated with idiopathic cryofibrinogenemia: report of a case. *Arch Neurol* 1970; 23:120–127.
33. Ecker AD. Linear fracture of the skull across the venous sinuses. *NY State J Med* 1946; 46:1120–1121.
34. Einhäupl KM, Villringer A, Meister W, et al. Heparin treatment in sinus venous thrombosis. *Lancet* 1991; 338:597–600.
35. Enevoldson TP, Russell RW. Cerebral venous thrombosis. New causes for an old syndrome? *Q J Med* 1990; 77:1255–1275.
36. Enevoldson TP, Russell RW. Heparin treatment in sinus venous thrombosis. *Lancet* 1991; 338:1153–1154.
37. Eskridge JM, Wessbecher FW. Thrombolysis for superior sagittal thrombosis. *J Vas Interven Radiol* 1991; 2:89–94.
38. Estanol B, Rodriguez A, Conte G, et al. Intracranial venous thrombosis in young women. *Stroke* 1979; 10:680–684.
39. Evans RW, Patten BM. Trichinosis associated with superior sagittal sinus thrombosis. *Ann Neurol* 1982; 11:216–217.
40. Fairburn B. Intracranial venous sinus thrombosis complicating oral contraception: treatment by anticoagulant drugs. *Br Med J* 1973; 2:647.
41. Feldenzer JA, Bueche MJ, Venes JL, Gebarski SS. Superior sagittal sinus thrombosis with infarction in Sickle cell trait. *Stroke* 1987; 18:656–660.
42. Fielding IR, Grant JMF, Selby G. Lateral sinus thrombosis following radical neck dissection for malignant melanoma. *Aust NZ J Surg* 1973; 43:228–231.
43. Floyd WL, Mahaley MS. Cerebral dural venous sinus thrombosis following cardiac pacemaker implantation. *Arch Intern Med* 1969; 124:368–372.
44. Garrido E, Fahs GR. Cerebral venous and sagittal sinus thrombosis after transcallosal removal of a colloid cyst of the third ventricle: case report. *Neurosurgery* 1990; 26:540–542.
45. Gerrits WBJ, Prakke EM, Van der Meer J, et al. Corticosteroids and experimental intravascular coagulation. *Scand J Haematol* 1974; 13:5–10.
46. Gettelfinger DM, Kokmen E. Superior sagittal sinus thrombosis. *Arch Neurol* 1977; 34:2–6.
47. Gills JP. Pseudotumor cerebri from venous obstruction. *Ophthalmology* 1992; 99:1346 (letter).
48. Gills JP Jr, Kapp JP, Odom GL. Benign intracranial hypertension: pseudotumor cerebri from obstruction of dural sinuses. *Acta Ophthamol* 1967; 78:592–595.
49. Ginsburg KS, Liang MH, Newcomer L, et al. Anticardiolipin antibodies and the risk for ischemic stroke and venous thrombosis. *Ann Intern Med* 1992; 117:997–1002.
50. Glowinski J, Breuillard P, Delafolie A, Redondo A. Thrombosis of the superior longitudinal sinus after sacculoradiculography with iopamidol. *Rev Rhum Mal Osteoartic* 1986; 53:183.
51. Govaert P, Achten E, Vanhaesebrouck P, et al. Deep cerebral venous thrombosis in thalamo-ventricular hemorrhage of the term newborn. *Pediat Radiol* 1992; 22:123–127.
52. Grosman H, St. Louis EL, Gray RR. The role of CT and DSA in cranial sinovenous occlusion. *Can Assoc Radiol J* 1987; 38:183–189.
53. Hakuba A, Huh CW, Tsujikawa S, Nishimura S. Total removal of parasagittal meningioma of the posterior third of the sagittal sinus and its repair by autogenous vein graft: case report. *J Neurosurg* 1979; 51:379–382.
54. Haley EC Jr, Brashear HR, Barth JT, et al. Deep cerebral venous thrombosis. Clinical, neuroradiological, and neuropsychological correlates. *Arch Neurol* 1989; 46:337–340.
55. Hamed LM, Glaser JS, Schatz NJ, Perez TH. Pseudotumor cerebri induced by Danazol. *Am J Ophthalmol* 1989; 107:105–110.
56. Harris TM, Smith RR, Koch KJ. Gadolinium-DTPA enhanced MR imaging of septic dural sinus thrombosis. *J Comput Assist Tomogr* 1989; 13:682–684.
57. Higashida RT, Helmer E, Halbach VV, Hieshima GB. Direct thrombolytic therapy for superior sagittal sinus thrombosis. *AJNR Am J Neuroradiol* 1989; 10(Suppl 5):S4–6.
58. Hommel M, Vasdev A, Fouillet P, Perret J. Thromboses du sinus longitudinal supérieur complication d'une interruption de la veine cave inférieure par un filtre préventif de l'embolie pulmonaire. *Presse Med* 1984; 13:1156 (letter).
59. Houser OW, Baker HL Jr, Rhoton AL Jr, et al. Intracranial dural arteriovenous malformations. *Radiology* 1972; 105:55–64.
60. Huhn A. Die Differentialdiagnose der Hirnvenen- und Sinus-thrombose. *Acta Neurochir Suppl (Wien)* 1961; 7:355–361.
61. Humbert P, Gutknecht J, Mallet H., Dupond JL. Acide tranexamique et thrombose du sinus longitudinal supérieur. *Therapie* 1987; 42:65–66.
62. Jacquin V, Salama J, Le Roux G, Delaporte P. Thromboses veineuses cérébrales et des membres supérieurs associées à une thrombopénie, induites par le polysulfate de Pentosane. *Ann Med Interne (Paris)* 1988; 139:194–197.
63. Johnston I, Hawke S, Halmagyi M, Teo C. The pseudotumor syndrome. Disorders of cerebrospinal fluid circulation causing intracranial hypertension without ventriculomegaly. *Arch Neurol* 1991; 48:740–747.
64. Kalbag RM, Woolf AL. *Cerebral Venous Thrombosis.* London: Oxford University Press, 1967, pp 247–248.
65. Kapp JP, Gielchinsky I, Deardourff SL. Operative techniques for management of lesions involving the dural venous sinuses. *Surg Neurol* 1977; 7:339–342.
66. Kapp JP, Gielchinsky I, Petty C, McClure C. An internal shunt for use in the reconstruction of dural venous sinuses: technical note. *J Neurosurg* 1971; 35:351–354.

67. Karabudak R, Caner H, Oztekin N, et al. Thrombosis of intracranial venous sinuses. Aetiology, clinical findings and prognosis of 56 patients. *J Neurol Sci* 1990; 34:117–121.
68. Kendall D. Thrombosis of intracranial veins. *Brain* 1948; 71:386–402.
69. Kinal ME. Traumatic thrombosis of dural venous sinuses in closed head injuries. *J Neurosurg* 1967; 27:142–145.
70. Krayenbühl HA. Cerebral venous and sinus thrombosis. *Clin Neurosurg* 1966; 14:1–24.
71. Kristensen B, Malm J, Markgren P, Ekstedt J. CSF hydrodynamics in superior sagittal sinus thrombosis. *J Neurol Neurosurg Psychiatry* 1992; 55:287–293.
72. Kulawik H, Hoppe W. Thrombose der intrakraniellen Venen und Sinus bei Periarteriitis nodosa. *Schweiz Arch Neurol Neurochir Psychiatr* 1971; 109:237–244.
73. Kyritsis AP, Williams EC, Schutta HS. Cerebral venous thrombosis due to heparin-induced thrombocytopenia. *Stroke* 1990; 21:1503–1505.
74. Lau SO, Bock GH, Edson Jr, Michael AF. Sagittal sinus thrombosis in the nephrotic syndrome. *J Pediatr* 1980; 97:948–950.
75. Levine SR, Kieran S, Puzio K, et al. Cerebral venous thrombosis with lupus anticoagulants. Report of two cases. *Stroke* 1987; 18:801–804.
76. Lhermitte J, Lereboullet J, Kaplan B. Ramollissement hémorragipare d'origine nerveuse chez un enfant, atteint de malformations cardiaques. *Rev. Neurol (Paris)* 1936; 65:305–312.
77. Liedtke W. Inadequate antidiuretic hormone secretion after sagittal sinus thrombosis caused by protein S deficiency. *Stroke* 1991; 22:819 (letter).
78. Masaryk TJ, Ross JS. MR angiography. Clinical applications. In Atlas SW (ed): *Magnetic Resonance Imaging of the Brain and Spine.* New York: Raven Press, 1991, pp 1079–1097.
79. Matsumura A, Shinohara A, Komatsu Y, et al. Vanishing empty delta sign in cerebral venous thrombosis. *Am J Neuroradiol* 1988; 9(6):1239–1240.
80. McDonald TD, Tatemichi TK, Kranzler SJ, et al. Thrombosis of the superior sagittal sinus associated with essential thrombocytosis followed by MRI during anticoagulant therapy. *Neurology* 1989; 39:1554–1555.
81. McLean BN. Dural sinus thrombosis. *Br J Hosp Med* 1991; 45:226–231.
82. McLean BN, Whitehead PJ, Campbell MJ. Antiphospholipid syndrome in pregnancy. *Br J Hosp Med* 1992; 48:504–506.
83. Meier U, Gartner F, Knopf W, et al. The traumatic dural sinus injury—a clinical study. *Acta Neurochir (Wien)* 1992; 119:91–93.
84. Michaeli J, Mittelman M, Grisaru D, Rachmilewitz EA. Thromboembolic complications in beta thalassemia major. *Acta Haematol* 1992; 87:71–74.
85. Mickle JP, McLennan JE, Chi JG, Lidden CW. Cortical vein thrombosis in Wegener's granulomatosis: case report. *J Neurosurg* 1977; 46:248–251.
86. Milandre L, Gueriot C, Girard N, et al. Les thromboses veineuses cérébrales de l'adulte. Aspects diagnostiques et thérapeutiques à propos de 20 observations. *Med Interne (Paris)* 1989; 139:544–554.
87. Mones RJ. Increased intracranial pressure due to metastatic disease of venous sinuses: a report of six cases. *Neurology* 1965; 15:1000–1007.
88. Monteiro ML, Hoyt WF, Imes RK. Puerperal cerebral blindness. Transient bilateral occipital involvement from presumed cerebral venous thrombosis. *Arch Neurol* 1984; 41:1300–1301.
89. Nadel L, Braun IF, Kraft KA, et al. Intracranial vascular abnormalities. Value of MR phase imaging to distinguish thrombus from flowing blood. *Am J Roentgenol* 1991; 156:373–380.
90. Newman DS, Levine SR, Curtis VL, Welch KM. Migraine-like visual phenomena associated with cerebral venous thrombosis. *Headache* 1989; 29:82–85.
91. Newton TH, Goodling CA. Compression of superior sagittal sinus by neonatal calvarial molding. Radiology 1975; 115:635–639.
92. Persson L, Lilja A. Extensive dural sinus thrombosis treated by surgical removal and local streptokinase infusion. *Neurosurgery* 1990; 26:117–121.
93. Pouillot B, Pecker J, Guegan Y, et al. Hypertension intra-crânienne "bénigne" au cours d'une polyglobulie ayant entrainé une thrombose du sinus latéral. *Neurochirurgie* 1984; 30:131–134.
94. Rao KCVG, Knipp HC, Wagner EJ. Computed tomographic findings in cerebral sinus and venous thrombosis. *Radiology* 1981; 140:391–398.
95. Ravindran RS, Zandstra GC. Cerebral venous thrombosis versus postlumbar puncture headache. *Anesthesiology* 1989; 71:478–479.
96. Reddy CR, Rao MS. Cerebral infarction due to intracranial venous sinus thrombosis. *J Indian Med Assoc* 1968; 50:98–102.
97. Repka MX, Miller NR. Papilledema and dural sinus obstruction. *J Clin Neuroophthalmol* 1984; 4:247–250.
98. Roland J, Bernard C, Bracard S, et al. Microvascularization of the intracranial dura mater. *Surg Radiol Anat* 1987; 9:43–49.
99. Rousseaux P, Bernard MH, Scherpereel B, Guyot JF. Thrombose des sinus veineux intra-crâniens (à propos de 22 cas). *Neurochirurgie* 1978; 24:197–203.
100. Rousseaux P, Vieillart A, Scherpereel B, et al. Hypertension intrâcranienne bénigne (17 cas) et thromboses veineuses cérébrales (49 cas): étude comparative. *Neurochirurgie* 1985; 31:381–389.
101. Ruggieri PM, Masaryk TJ, Ross JS, Modic MT. Intracranial magnetic resonance imaging. *Invest Radiol* 1992; 27:S33–9.
102. Ryan J, Olmeadow M, Horne M, O'Donnell C. Cerebral venous thrombosis as the presenting feature of colonic adenocarcinoma. *Med J Aust* 1990; 153:234 (letter).
103. Schick RM, Jolesz F, Barnes PD, Macklis JD. MR diagnosis of dural venous thrombosis complicating L-asparaginase therapy. *Comput Med Imaging Graph* 1989; 13:319–327.
104. Schmidek HH, Auer LM, Kapp JP. The cerebral venous system. *Neurosurgery* 1985; 17:663–678.
105. Schou J, Scherb M. Postoperative sagittal sinus thrombosis after spinal anesthesia. *Anesth Analg* 1986; 65:541–542.
106. Schroeder BA, Czarnecki DJ, Wells RG, et al. Radiological case of the month. Poststrangulation cerebral sinovenous thrombosis. *Amer J Dis Child* 1988; 142:1235–1236.
107. Schutta HS, Williams EC, Baranski BG, Sutula TP. Cerebral venous thrombosis with plasminogen deficiency. *Stroke* 1991; 22:401–405.
108. Scott JA, Pascuzzi RM, Hall PV, Becker GJ. Treatment of dural sinus thrombosis with local urokinase infusion. Case report. *J Neurosurg* 1988; 68:284–287.
109. Shesser R, Kline P, Goodwin L. Seizures in pregnancy. *Am J Emerg Med* 1985; 3:551–555.
110. Shevell MI, Silver K, O'Gorman AM, et al. Neonatal dural sinus thrombosis. *Pediatr Neurol* 1989; 5:161–165.
111. Shiozawa Z, Ueda R, Mano T, et al. Superior sagittal sinus thrombosis associated with Evans' syndrome of haemolytic anaemia. *J Neurol* 1985; 232:280–282.
112. Sigsbee B, Rottenberg DA. Sagittal sinus thrombosis as a complication of regional enteritis. *Ann Neurol* 1978; 3:450–452.
113. Sindou M, Mazoyer JF, Fischer G, et al. Experimental bypass for sagittal sinus repair: preliminary report. *J Neurosurg* 1976; 44:325–330.
114. Stam J, Lensing AW, Vermeulen M, Tijssen JG. Heparin treatment for cerebral venous and sinus thrombosis. *Lancet* 1991; 338:1154 (letter).
115. Stansfield FR. Puerperal cerebral thrombophlebitis treated by heparin. *Br Med J* 1942; 1:436–438.
116. Steinherz PG, Miller LP, Ghavimi F, et al. Dural sinus thrombosis in children with acute lymphoblastic leukemia. *JAMA* 1981; 246:2837–2839.
117. Stephens PH, Lennox G, Hirsch N, Miller D. Superior sagittal sinus thrombosis after internal jugular vein cannulation. *Br J Anaesth* 1991; 67:476–479.
118. Thron A, Wessel K, Linden D, et al. Superior sagittal sinus thrombosis. Neuroradiological evaluation and clinical findings. *J Neurol* 1986; 233:283–288.

119. Towbin A. The syndrome of latent cerebral venous thrombosis: its frequency and relation to age and congestive heart failure. *Stroke* 1973; 4:419–430.
120. Tsai FY, Higashida RT, Matovich V, Alfieri K. Acute thrombosis of the intracranial dural sinus. Direct thrombolytic treatment. *Am J Neuroradiol* 1992; 13:1137–1141.
121. Van Vleyman B, Dehaene I, Van Hoof A, Pattyn G. Cerebral venous thrombosis in paroxysmal nocturnal haemoglobinuria. *Acta Neurol Belg* 1987; 87:80–87.
122. Viader F, Bakchine S, Gaudin H, et al. Encéphalopathie saturnine avec thrombose du sinus longitudinal supérieur. *Ann Med Interne (Paris)* 1985; 136:401–404
123. Vidailhet M, Piette JC, Wechsler B, et al. Cerebral venous thrombosis in systemic lupus erythematosus. *Stroke* 1990; 21:1226–1231.
124. Virapongse C, Cazenave C, Quisling R, et al. The empty delta sign. Frequency and significance in 76 cases of dural sinus thrombosis. *Radiology* 1987; 162:779–785.
125. Waga S, Handa H. Scalp veins as collateral pathway with parasagittal meningiomas occluding the superior sagittal sinus. *Neuroradiology* 1976; 11:199–204.
126. Weber G. Treatment of cerebral venous and sinus thrombosis. *Thromb Diath Haemorrh Suppl* 1966; 21:435–448.
127. Wechsler B, Vidailhet M, Piette JC, et al. Cerebral venous thrombosis in Behçet's disease. Clinical study and long-term follow-up of 25 cases. *Neurology* 1992; 42:614–618.
128. Wintzen AR, Broekmans AW, Bertina RM, et al. Cerebral hemorrhagic infarction in young patients with hereditary protein C deficiency. Evidence for ''spontaneous'' cerebral venous thrombosis. *Br Med J (Clin Res Ed)* 1985; 290:350–352.
129. Yee CW, Ping TK. Computerized tomography in dural sinus thrombosis. *Astralas Radiol* 1990; 34:24–31.
130. Zimmerman RA, Bilaniuk LT, Hackney DB, et al. Magnetic resonance imaging of dural venous sinus invasion, occlusion and thrombosis. *Acta Radiol* 1986; 369:110–112.

SECTION C

Aneurysms and Subarachnoid Hemorrhage

214

Intracranial Aneurysms and Subarachnoid Hemorrhage: An Overview

Bryce Weir
R. Loch Macdonald

The dawn of modern aneurysm surgery came in 1933 when Egas Moniz demonstrated an aneurysm by the technique of cerebral angiography, which he had discovered.[78] The first malleable hemostatic clips in neurosurgery had been introduced by Cushing in 1911, but they were not appropriate for aneurysms. Schwartz developed a spring clip with cross legs, which was modified by Mayfield by making a smaller, tweezer-like applicator for it.[72] This paved the way for the introduction of a host of different spring clips in a variety of strengths and configurations. Other brilliant technical progress included the demonstration by Lundberg in 1960 of the feasibility of intraventricular catheters to continuously record and control ventricular fluid pressure.[71] Two years later came the first report of an intracranial vascular procedure carried out with the aid of the operating microscope, which brought the twin blessings of magnification and illumination.[54] By 1971 the first computed tomographic (CT) head scanner was operational, having been developed by a group that included Godfrey Hounsfield.[14]

The first planned intracranial operation for a saccular aneurysm was conducted by Dott in 1933.[26] He stuffed a muscle fragment against an aneurysm that had ruptured intraoperatively and succeeded in stopping the bleeding and obtaining a good long-term result. Credit for the first definitive treatment of a preoperatively diagnosed intracranial aneurysm (by virtue of a third nerve palsy) goes to Dandy, who in 1937 clipped the neck of an aneurysm with a metal clip and shriveled the sac with electrocautery[21] (Fig. 214-1). Aided by technical advances and general progress in radiology, anesthesia, and intensive care, many neurosurgeons achieved progressively lower postoperative mortality rates after operations for intracranial aneurysms in the 1960s and 1970s. Preeminent among these workers are Yaşargil of Zürich[135] and Drake of London, Ontario,[28] who have established benchmarks of excellence in huge series of aneurysms in the anterior and posterior circulations, respectively. Their careful anatomic observations and technical advice will be of immense help to the generations of surgeons who follow them.

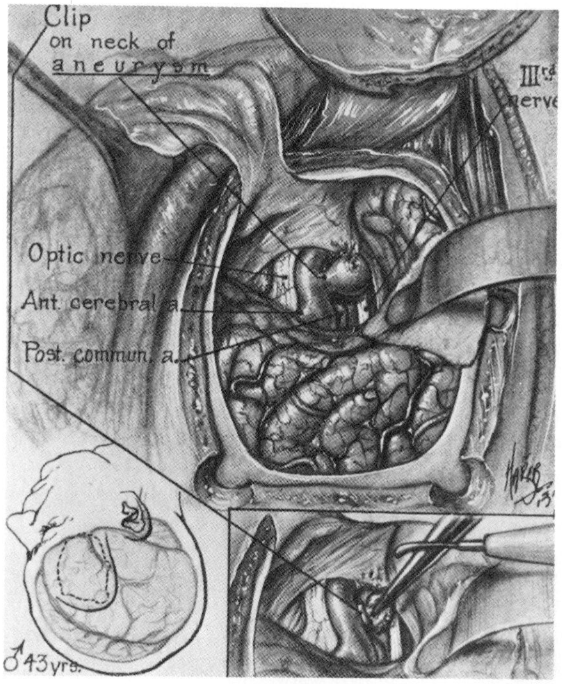

Figure 214-1 Operation of March 23, 1937: "The present effort is but a beginning or a suggestion that an aneurysm at the circle of Willis is not entirely hopeless . . . So far as I know this is the first attempt to cure an aneurysm at the circle of Willis by direct attack upon the aneurysm." (From Dandy.[21])

TABLE 214-1 Surgical Classification of Intracranial Arterial Aneurysms

- **I.** Morphology
  - **A.** Saccular
  - **B.** Fusiform
  - **C.** Dissecting
- **II.** Size
  - **A.** <3 mm
  - **B.** 3–6 mm
  - **C.** 7–10 mm
  - **D.** 11–25 mm
  - **E.** >25 mm (giant)
- **III.** Location
  - **A.** Anterior circulation arteries
    - **1.** Internal carotid
      - **a.** Carotid canal
      - **b.** Intracavernous
      - **c.** Paraclinoid (ophthalmic)
      - **d.** Posterior communicating region
      - **e.** Anterior choroidal region
      - **f.** Carotid bifurcation
    - **2.** Anterior cerebral
      - **a.** A_1 (main branch)
      - **b.** Anterior communicating region
      - **c.** A_2 (distal): callosomarginal region or distal pericallosal
    - **3.** Middle cerebral
      - **a.** M_1 (main branch) lenticulostriate or temporal branch regions
      - **b.** Bifurcation
      - **c.** Peripheral
  - **B.** Posterior circulation arteries
    - **1.** Vertebral
      - **a.** Main trunk
      - **b.** Posterior inferior cerebellar artery region
    - **2.** Basilar
      - **a.** Bifurcation
      - **b.** Superior cerebellar artery region
      - **c.** Anterior inferior cerebellar artery region
      - **d.** Basilar trunk
      - **e.** Vertebrobasilar junction region
    - **3.** Posterior cerebral
      - **a.** P_1 (first branches of basilar-distal to apex)
      - **b.** P_2 (distal posterior cerebral)

A step forward in understanding the course of this disease came with the introduction by Botterell, Lougheed, and others of a neurological grading system in 1956.[11] In May of the following year a central registry for aneurysm cases was begun at the University of Iowa, and a Cooperative Study was initiated. This has been a continual source of accurate data and an increasingly sophisticated guide to the efficacy of different therapeutic approaches.[56,57,81,96] The definitive study of the natural history of aneurysms was published by Pakarinen in 1967.[89] Lougheed later introduced the concept of management mortality rather than simple postoperative mortality in the assessment of surgical treatment.[69]

Classification, Characteristics, and Occurrence of Intracranial Aneurysms

A surgical classification of intracranial arterial aneurysms is proposed in Table 214-1. Such lesions can also be classified with respect to their presumed etiology. Some causative factors in intracranial arterial saccular and fusiform aneurysms are given in Table 214-2.

TABLE 214-2 Etiology of Intracranial Arterial Aneurysms

Saccular Aneurysms

- **A.** Hemodynamic
  - **1.** Uneven pulsatile pressure head distribution at apex of bifurcations, branchings, or outer aspect of curves, causing local degeneration of internal elastica
  - **2.** Increased flow from:
    - **a.** Distal arteriovenous malformation
    - **b.** Aplasia, hypoplasia, or ligation of contralateral vessel normally present
    - **c.** Persistent carotid-basilar anastomosis (trigeminal, otic, hypoglossal, proatlantal) and basilar-middle meningeal anastomosis
  - **3.** Increased blood pressure (and possibly associated vessel defect in)
    - **a.** Coarctation of aorta
    - **b.** Autosomal dominant polycystic kidney disease
    - **c.** Fibromuscular dysplasia, renal arteries
- **B.** Structural
  - **1.** Combined media and elastica defects
  - **2.** Preaneurysmal lesions: infundibula, thin areas, microaneurysms
- **C.** Genetic
  - **1.** Familial intracranial aneurysms—dominant inheritance
  - **2.** Genetic or possibly genetic syndromes associated with blood vessel abnormalities and reported with intracranial aneurysms: Ehlers-Danlos syndrome, Marfan's syndrome, pseudoxanthoma elasticum, Rendu-Osler-Weber syndrome, Klippel-Trenaunay-Weber syndrome, type III collagen deficiency
- **D.** Traumatic
  - **1.** Skull fracture
  - **2.** Penetrating foreign body
  - **3.** Surgical injury
- **E.** Infectious
  - **1.** Bacterial
  - **2.** Fungal
- **F.** Neoplastic
  - **1.** Metastatic: choriocarcinoma, atrial myxoma, undifferentiated carcinoma
  - **2.** Primary neoplasms
  - **3.** Aneurysms associated with neoplasm: pituitary adenomas
- **G.** Other disorders affecting blood vessels
  - **1.** Granulomatous (giant cell) angiitis
  - **2.** Systemic lupus erythematosus
  - **3.** Moyamoya disease
  - **4.** Sickle cell anemia
- **H.** Radiation-induced saccular aneurysm

Fusiform Aneurysms

- **A.** Atherosclerosis
  Most common cause of elongated, distended (dolichoectatic) cerebral vessels
  Posterior circulation most affected
- **B.** Structural
  - **1.** Long areas of loss of normal elastica and media
  - **2.** Diffuse arterial fibromuscular dysplasia
- **C.** Genetic
  Possibly genetic conditions associated with fusiform aneurysms include Marfan's syndrome, pseudoxanthoma elasticum
- **D.** Infectious
  Syphilis
- **E.** Other disorders of blood vessels
  Giant cell arteritis
- **F.** Hemodynamic
  Coarctation of aorta
- **G.** Radiation-induced fusiform aneurysm

The common saccular aneurysm is probably acquired by hemodynamically induced degeneration of the arterial wall. Bacterial aneurysms make up under 5 percent of all cases of intracranial aneurysms. The most common cause is a streptococcal infection in a patient with bacterial endocarditis. Mortality is relatively low in patients treated with appropriate high-dose antibiotics and surgery. The majority of these aneurysms are on the distal middle cerebral circulation.[123] Fungal aneurysms are considerably rarer, are usually associated with arteritis and thrombosis, and have so far been uniformly fatal.[115,123] Traumatic aneurysms are uncommon and can result from either blunt or penetrating head trauma. The majority of patients have associated skull fractures. Penetrating injuries result from a variety of missiles and surgical instruments. These aneurysms are usually located on the supratentorial circulation at sites other than branching points and are most commonly single. Their presence should be considered when there is a syndrome of delayed deterioration following head injury. The sac may have an irregular contour, a neck may be absent, and there may be delayed filling and emptying on angiography. The outlook is poor without direct surgical treatment.[123]

Embolization of tumor cells into the cerebral arteries may result in aneurysm formation. The most common neoplasm to metastasize to the brain and form an aneurysm is atrial myxoma, although it more commonly causes arterial occlusion with cerebral infarction. Choriocarcinoma and other metastatic neoplasms may rarely form aneurysms by tumor embolization. Gliomas may invade the walls of major cerebral arteries and form saccular aneurysms.[123] The possibility that some tumors stimulate the growth of aneurysms in nearby blood vessels has also been raised. However, it is not clear whether the incidence of such aneurysms exceeds what would normally be expected: brain tumors and aneurysms are both relatively common, so instances of both conditions in the same patient are inevitable. There is, nevertheless, considerable surgical relevance to the finding of an aneurysm in the intracavernous or supraclinoid portion of the carotid artery in 7.4 percent of 95 pituitary adenomas.[122] The increased incidence of aneurysms is seen particularly with growth hormone–secreting adenomas.[124] The association of aneurysms and pituitary tumors also includes aneurysms mimicking tumors, aneurysms occurring following intraoperative injury to the carotid artery, and aneurysms developing after irradiation of the sella. Distinguishing aneurysms and pituitary neoplasms is a diminishing problem in the era of magnetic resonance imaging (MRI).

Anatomic Sites of Aneurysms

The relative frequency of aneurysms at different anatomic sites is illustrated in Fig. 214-2 and Table 214-3. Use of routine three- or four-vessel angiography has increased detection of posterior circulation aneurysms from 5.4 percent to more than 8 percent, which is more in keeping with autopsy findings. Ninety-five percent of

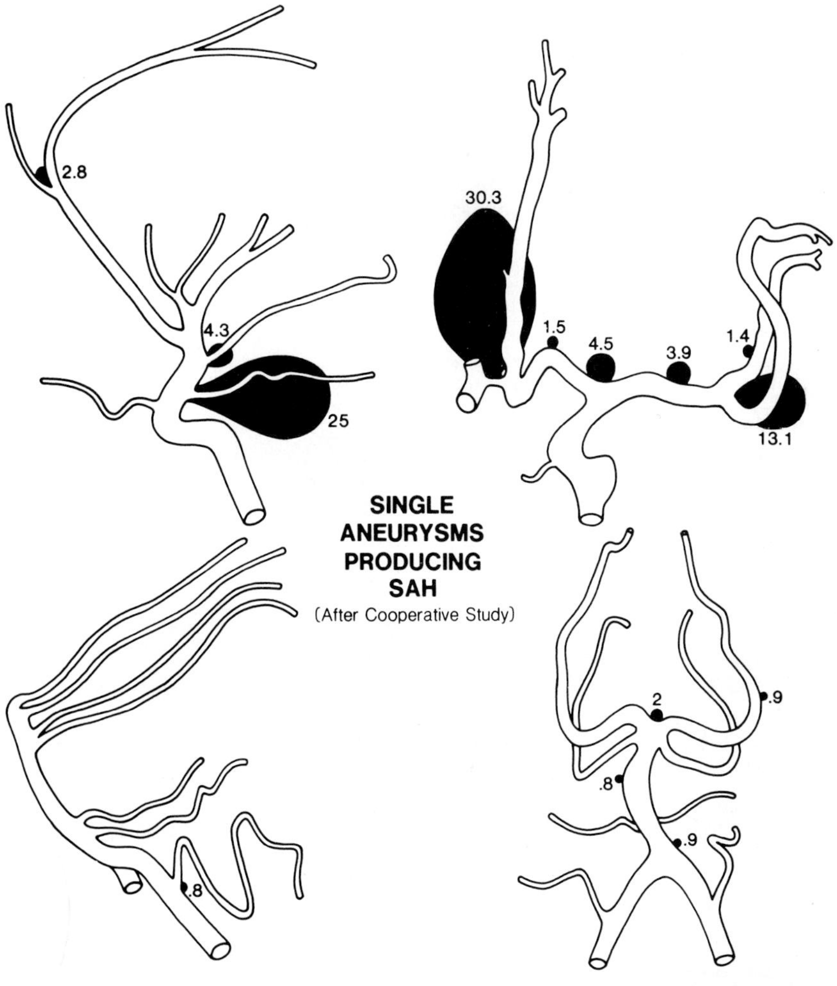

Figure 214-2 Schematic representation of the frequency (in percent) of single aneurysms producing subarachnoid hemorrhage, based on cooperative study data from Sahs et al.[96]

TABLE 214-3 Location of Intracranial Aneurysms by Artery (Numbers Are Percent of Total Aneurysms on Each Artery)

Author	Type of Study	Number of Cases	Middle Cerebral Artery	Anterior Cerebral Artery	Internal Carotid Artery	Vertebro-basilar System
Sahs et al.[96]	Cooperative	2630	20	34	41	4
Kassell et al.[56]	Cooperative	3521	22	39	30	8
Stehbens[101]	Clinical series	5267	20	31	38	5
Stehbens[101]	Autopsies	8000	33	30	24	12

aneurysms occur close to the circle of Willis in relation to the anterior and posterior communicating arteries and the bifurcations of the internal carotid, middle cerebral, and basilar arteries. Aneurysms usually arise from the distal carina of a bifurcation. They are usually on the convexity of a curve and point in the direction that the proximal axial bloodstream would have taken if the curve were not there.[93]

Size of Aneurysms

The frequency distribution of aneurysm size is illustrated in Fig. 214-3. Ruptured aneurysms tend to be larger than unruptured aneurysms, and symptomatic aneurysms are larger than asymptomatic aneurysms. The size at which aneurysms usually begin to rupture is about 3 mm in maximum diameter, and the size at which they begin to produce symptoms by means other than rupture is around 7 mm.[73] In a planned autopsy study, the mean size of ruptured aneurysms was 8.6 mm, almost twice the mean size of the nonruptured aneurysms, which was 4.7 mm.[18] In another pathologic series,[73] 16 percent of aneurysms 10 mm or less in size were ruptured, whereas 91 percent of aneurysms 11 mm or greater were ruptured. In 3521 patients with aneurysmal subarachnoid hemorrhage, the size distribution was as follows: under 12 mm, 78 percent; 12 to 24 mm, 20 percent; over 24 mm, 2 percent.[56]

Multiple Aneurysms

In Suzuki's personal series of 1080 cases, single aneurysms constituted 85 percent of the series, and multiple aneurysms 15 percent.[110] He reviewed seven other clinical series, totaling 10,795 cases, in which the incidence of multiple aneurysms was 14.1 percent overall, with a range of 7.7 to 29.8 percent. He similarly reviewed six autopsy series in which 1404 cases were studied to reveal multiple aneurysm cases in 23.5 percent (range 18.9 to 50 percent).[110] In two cooperative studies involving 6842 patients, 19 percent of patients had more than one aneurysm.[56,96] At autopsy, 22 percent of patients in the study of Sahs et al. had multiple aneurysms.[96] The lower rate of clinical detection probably reflects the fact that four-vessel angiography was not routinely carried out in 1969. In the multiple aneurysm cases of the conservatively managed patients in the cooperative study[96] and in Suzuki's personal series, patients having two aneurysms constituted 71 and 77 percent; three aneurysms, 23 and 15 percent; and four or more aneurysms, 7 and 6 percent of multiple aneurysm cases, respectively. Multiple aneurysms are relatively more common in females (74 percent) than males.[96] The same study showed that 47 percent of multiple aneurysms are on opposite sides, 21 percent are on the same side, 29 percent have one in the midline and one on the side, and 3 percent have both in the midline. When two internal carotid aneurysms coexist, the chance of their being "mirror" aneurysms

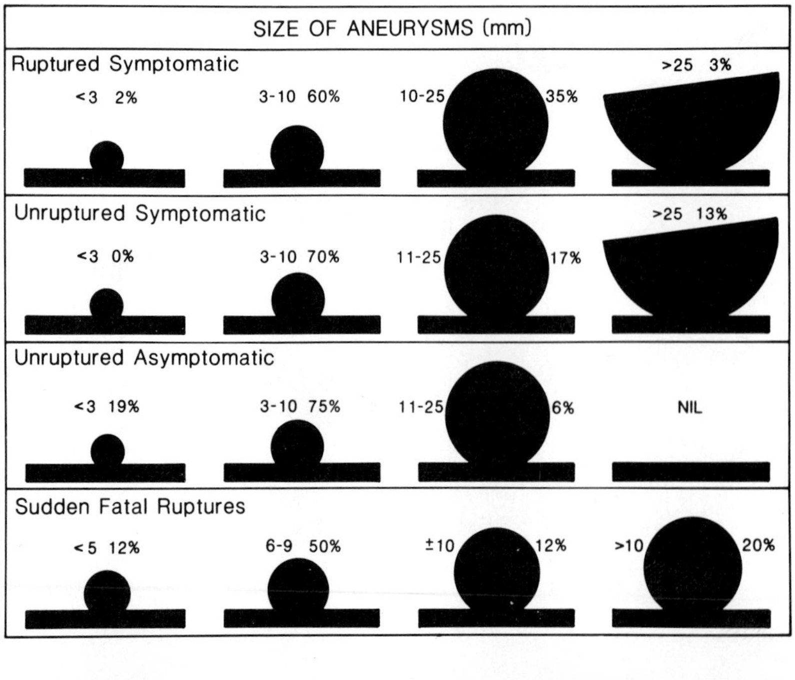

Figure 214-3 Size of aneurysms. The frequencies for ruptured aneurysms are those of 350 cases from the University of Alberta. The frequencies for unruptured aneurysms are from the cooperative study (Sahs et al.[96]) and those for sudden fatal ruptures are from Freytag.[39] Six percent of aneurysms could not be measured.

is three times greater than that of their both being on the same side. Similarly, with two middle cerebral aneurysms the chance is four times greater. When an aneurysm on the anterior circulation is found, the chance of a second aneurysm existing on the posterior circulation is between 3 and 5 percent. With internal carotid and middle cerebral aneurysms, there is a tendency toward either symmetric aneurysms or a second aneurysm on the same vessel.

How is it possible to tell which aneurysm has ruptured? No clinical method predicts with 100 percent accuracy which aneurysm has bled. Traditionally, the largest of the aneurysms has ruptured.[134] Other angiographic signs of rupture are a local mass or vasospasm, irregular aneurysm shape, or intra-aneurysmal clot. When two aneurysms are on the same vessel, unless the proximal aneurysm is thrombosed, the proximal aneurysm has ruptured.[19] Clinical signs are usually not helpful, although a third nerve palsy or unilateral retro-orbital pain, for example, would suggest that an aneurysm had ruptured at the origin of the posterior communicating artery. Localized collections of subarachnoid blood on a CT scan may point to the offending lesion. An algorithm for identifying the ruptured aneurysm, proposed by Nehls et al., was as follows: exclude extradural aneurysms, look for focal blood on the CT scan, check for focal mass or vasospasm on angiogram, observe size and shape (the larger aneurysm is more likely to bleed; if they are of similar size, look for irregularity of the sac or daughter loculus), use clinical signs, consider an EEG, repeat the angiogram later and look for changes in the aneurysms, and finally choose the aneurysm site with the highest probability of rupture.[79] Subtle local changes may appear on MRI.

Occurrence of Aneurysms

Age

Aneurysmal rupture is extremely uncommon in the first decade of life. The incidence gradually increases for each decade and peaks in the sixth decade. In Pakarinen's review of the literature, the prevalence in each decade was as follows: first, less than 1 percent; second, 2 percent; third, 6 percent; fourth, 15 percent; fifth, 26 percent; sixth, 28 percent; seventh, 16 percent; and eighth, 6 percent.[89] These data were from 15 series comprising 5679 cases. In another study, when correction was made for smaller numbers of elderly persons in a population, there was no decrease in age-specific incidence rates of aneurysmal subarachnoid hemorrhage in the elderly. Rates, by decade, were as follows: first and second, less than 1 percent; third, 9 percent; fourth, 16 percent; fifth, 22 percent; sixth, 32 percent; and seventh, 30 percent.[53]

Sex

Figure 214-4 shows the sex and age distribution of cases. There is no doubt that there is a clear female preponderance overall. The ratio of females to males was 1.6:1 in the cooperative study on timing of surgery.[56] Before age 40 males and females were equally affected. Above age 40, there was an increasingly strong predominance of females, with female/male ratios of 2.74:1 and 4.16:1 for 60- to 69-year-olds, and 70- to 87-year-olds, respectively. This late-life predominance of females may be partly, but probably not entirely, due to the increasing proportion of females in the population.

Geographic and Racial Factors

All races share a propensity to develop intracranial aneurysms, although the rates of aneurysm formation and subarachnoid hemorrhage in a given geographic area depend on the age distribution, the availability of medical care, and possibly on racial factors, smoking, alcohol intake, atherosclerosis, hypertension, and diet composition. The incidence of subarachnoid hemorrhage has been reported to be higher in Japan and Finland than in the United States.[3,52,123] Blacks in the Greater Cincinnati area had 2.1 times the risk of subarachnoid hemorrhage as whites (95 percent confidence interval, 1.3 to 3.6).[12]

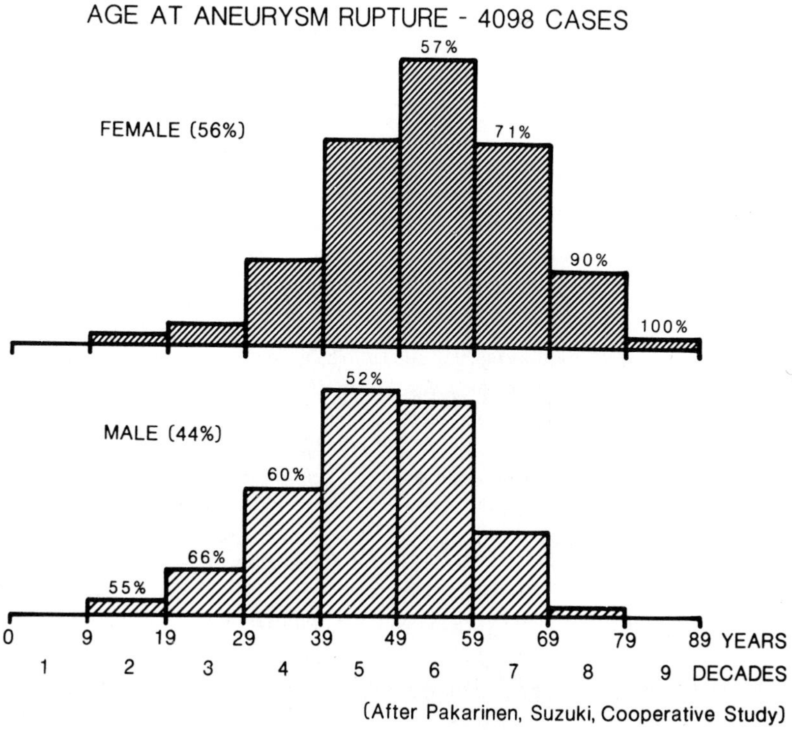

Figure 214-4 Age distributions of patients with ruptured aneurysms showing male predominance to the fifth decade and female predominance thereafter. Combined data of Sahs et al.[96] (cooperative study), Suzuki and Yoshimoto,[113] and Pakarinen.[89]

Incidence of Aneurysm Rupture

Aneurysmal subarachnoid hemorrhage accounts for 5 to 10 percent of strokes. The percentage of autopsied cases showing aneurysms will obviously be a function of the enthusiasm with which they are sought, as well as the age and sex mix of any particular institution's cases. Jellinger reviewed 12 series totaling 87,772 postmortem examinations, which revealed aneurysms in 1.6 percent of cases (range, 0.2 to 9 percent).[55] About 1 percent were ruptured and 0.6 percent were unruptured. Bannerman et al. reviewed eight autopsy series comprising 51,360 cases[4] in which the total prevalence of aneurysms was 1.43 percent, 0.34 percent being unruptured and 1.09 percent ruptured. The occurrence of aneurysms is higher in forensic pathologic series, since aneurysms are a relatively more important cause of unexpected sudden death. In four such series, Pakarinen found the incidence of aneurysms to be 2, 2.4, 4, and 4.7 percent.[89]

There are few studies of subarachnoid hemorrhage as the cause of death in whole populations. Brule (1958), in more than half a million deaths, found aneurysmal rupture to be the reported cause in 0.59 percent. Falconer (1950), in more than 50,000 deaths, found the corresponding figure to be 0.46 percent (both quoted by Pakarinen[89]).

The incidence of subarachnoid hemorrhage (new cases in a year) was reported to be between 6 and 10.9 per 100,000 population in the six series reported between 1950 and 1966 and reviewed by Pakarinen.[89] In those series, aneurysms constituted 77.2 percent of cases of subarachnoid hemorrhage. In five epidemiologic studies involving populations of 5184 to 1,460,000 studied between 1945 and 1984, the annual incidence of aneurysmal subarachnoid hemorrhage ranged from 9.3 to 28 per 100,000. Spontaneous subarachnoid hemorrhage occurred with an annual incidence of 6.5 to 26.4 per 100,000 in 13 studies reported between 1956 and 1984.[52]

In the pathologic study of McCormick and Acosta-Rua of 136 patients with aneurysms, 40 percent had ruptured aneurysms at autopsy.[73] In a similar pathologic study of Chason and Hindman of 137 autopsies in which aneurysms were found, 42 percent of the patients had ruptured aneurysms.[18]

Based on the above data, it is probably a reasonable first-order approximation to say that less than 2 percent of the entire population will have an aneurysm; an intracranial aneurysm will rupture in less than 1 percent of the population and will be the cause of death in 0.5 percent.

Familial Occurrence of Aneurysms

Because aneurysms are relatively common, about 5.6 percent of patients can be expected to have a first- to third-degree relative affected with an aneurysm by chance alone. There are, however, occasional families with aneurysms that appear to have been inherited by an autosomal dominant mechanism. The familial occurrence of intracranial aneurysms is usually defined by aneurysms occurring in two or more first- to third-degree relatives. In a retrospective review of 485 patients with aneurysmal subarachnoid hemorrhage, 16 of 237 (6.8 percent) who responded to a questionnaire reported having blood relatives with the same condition.[84] Lozano and Leblanc reviewed 243 aneurysms in 177 patients from 74 families.[70] There were 129 siblings, including eight identical twins. Fifty-six cases (28 pairs) were in parent and child. By comparison with sporadic aneurysm cases, familial aneurysms were found to rupture at a smaller size and when the patient was younger (peak decade, 40 to 49 years). The sex distribution and incidence of multiple aneurysms was the same as in reported series of sporadic aneurysms. Decision analysis was used to determine when family members should be screened for aneurysms.[9] The determinants for elective screening were age of patient and risk of harboring an aneurysm. Treatment would be determined based on estimated lifetime risk of rupture (related to patient age) and surgical risk. Surgical treatment was recommended for patients under 70 years of age with moderate or low surgical risk, and screening was recommended for family members aged 35 to 65 years (presumably when two other members have had hemorrhages). Magnetic resonance angiography may become a useful screening tool.

In an even smaller percentage of cases, there are familial aggregations with aneurysms due to the effects of known hereditary syndromes or suspected hereditary syndromes (see Table 214-2). The Ehlers-Danlos syndrome is characterized by fragmentation or absence of elastic tissue in small arteries and probably also by defects of type III collagen. There is hyperelasticity of the skin, subcutaneous nodules, and increased joint mobility, as well as easy bruisability. Angiography and surgery are extremely hazardous.

Patients with coarctation of the aorta also have a greatly increased chance of having intracranial aneurysms, which tend to rupture when the patients are in their twenties. There is a high incidence of multiplicity of aneurysms. Early diagnosis and treatment are imperative. It is uncertain whether there is a vascular intracranial anomaly associated with the aortic vascular lesion or whether the aneurysms result from the arterial hypertension secondary to the coarctation.

A similar problem exists in determining the relationship of autosomal dominant polycystic kidney disease to intracranial aneurysms. This relationship was studied in a selected group of 88 of a total population of 378 patients with polycystic kidney disease.[17] Cranial CT was performed in 60 patients, cerebral angiography in 21, and both procedures in 11. Aneurysms were found in four patients (4 percent; 95 percent confidence interval, 0.1 to 9 percent). Although the 95 percent confidence interval included the frequency of aneurysms in the general population, the results suggested an increased risk of aneurysms in patients with polycystic kidney disease. Previous studies found aneurysms in 0 to 40 percent of patients with polycystic kidney disease.

Aneurysms of Infancy and Childhood

A cooperative aneurysm study included one case of an aneurysm in a child under 4 years of age.[96] Pakarinen found no cases involving children among 511 patients.[89] Patel and Richardson found that among 3000 cases of aneurysms, only 58 patients were under 20 years of age and none were under 2 years of age.[91]

Despite their rarity, over 500 aneurysms are reported in the pediatric population, and they tend to differ from the usual adult aneurysm. Overall, patients under age 18 account for about 1 to 2 percent of cases of aneurysmal subarachnoid hemorrhage.[38] The male/female ratio is reversed: 60 percent of pediatric aneurysms occur in boys. Between 40 and 45 percent occur on arteries in the vertebrobasilar circulation, and perhaps 30 percent are giant. The sites do not differ greatly from those in adults, except that in the anterior circulation, the most common site is usually the internal carotid artery bifurcation. Traumatic and bacterial aneurysms are more common. Presentation is with subarachnoid hemorrhage in 72 percent, as a mass in 17 percent, and incidental in 4 percent. Multiple aneurysms appear to be less common.

Meyer and coworkers reviewed 24 aneurysms in 23 patients under the age of 18 years.[75] Seventy-four percent of the patients were boys; 42 percent of the aneurysms were on the posterior circulation, and 54 percent were giant. Subarachnoid hemorrhage occurred in 13 patients. A variety of treatments were required for these unusually difficult cases, including direct clipping (14 cases), trapping (4 cases), trapping plus bypass (4 cases), and excision (2 cases). Results were excellent in 87 percent, good in 8 percent, and poor in 4 percent.

Stehbens critically assessed the histology of published cases of aneurysms in infants.[102,103] He stated that inadequate pathologic examination or atypical histologic features in many of the cases gave little support to the theory of a congenital origin of these aneurysms. He thought that the existence of even a few authentic cases of saccular aneurysms at birth does not warrant the conclusion that all such aneurysms are due to a developmental defect.

Hemodynamics of Aneurysms

It is now generally considered that the impingement of an axial blood stream on a distal carina can generate forces that cause local destruction of the internal elastic membrane and initiate aneurysm formation. The resultant saclike outpouching increases the turbulence of flow in the area. This in turn may cause the wall to vibrate and accelerate the degenerative process.[35] Alternatively, aneurysms may enlarge by a passive yield of the sac to the prevailing blood pressure, with secondary reactive healing and thickening of the wall as the aneurysm increases in diameter.[104] Studies of tensile strength and elasticity of aneurysm walls and cerebral arteries of humans show that aneurysms are less elastic and much less able to withstand forceful stretch than normal arteries. Tension and stress in the aneurysm wall are greater than in the arterial wall because the aneurysm is stiffer and larger in diameter and its wall is thinner (law of Laplace). Large fluctuations in stress in the aneurysm wall result from the pulsating blood pressure, which produces structural fatigue in the wall and further degeneration of the elastica. In an animal model of aneurysms involving a tail artery, at all flow rates no flow occurred beyond 2.5 tube diameters downstream from the mouth of the aneurysm. This is probably why large aneurysms thrombose.[94]

In morphologic studies of the internal elastic lamina at the bifurcation of human cerebral arteries, the mean diameter of the fenestrations in the elastica was found to increase in the vicinity of the apex, and the proportion of the area of internal elastic lamina composed of fenestrations also increased significantly.[16] On the basis of a comparison of stress concentration factors, it was proposed that the presence of enlarged fenestrations weakens the lamina and contributes to the initiation of microaneurysms.

Pathologic observations relative to the hemodynamics of aneurysms have been made in 289 cases of fatal aneurysm rupture.[19] The actual site of aneurysmal rupture was most commonly the distal apex. Thin surface bubbles or multiloculations were present in 57 percent of ruptured aneurysms but in only 16 percent of unruptured aneurysms. Multiloculations were more common as aneurysms increased in size. In 88 percent of 90 cases with multiple aneurysms, the aneurysm with the greatest maximum external diameter had ruptured. The critical size beyond which aneurysms suddenly became unstable and likely to rupture was 4 mm. When combinations of middle cerebral and internal carotid aneurysms were present on the same side, the proximal aneurysm was the one that ruptured first in 70 percent of cases. Aneurysmal rupture is determined by an equation of enormous complexity, which includes factors such as the number of water hammer pulses delivered, the pressure configurations, the thickness, elasticity, and tensile strength of the wall, and the relative sizes and geometry of the aneurysm, its orifice, and the feeding artery.

Pathology and Pathogenesis of Aneurysms

Current concepts of the pathology of aneurysms are summarized in Table 214-4[20,41,48,55,73,96,101,102,111] and are illustrated in Figure 214-5. In 1930 it was suggested that elastica could herniate through areas of medial defects and then undergo degeneration secondary to the strain produced by overdistension.[37] However, a decade later Glynn[41] was unable to produce bulging of the unsupported elastic elements of arterial vessel walls even when these were subjected to a pressure of 600 mmHg. Since probably everyone has medial defects in the cerebral arteries and since probably fewer than 5 percent (more likely 2 percent) of all persons have aneurysms, some pathologic factor other than a medial defect must be at play. It is now widely accepted that damage to the internal elastic lamina by hemodynamic factors is the critical pathologic change. Stehbens reviewed the etiology of intracranial saccular aneurysms and concluded that there was no evidence for a congenital, developmental, or inherited weakness of the arterial wall.[103] He believed the most plausible explanation was that aneurysms are acquired lesions due to hemodynamic stress upon the relatively unsupported arterial bifurcations of the cerebral arteries. These arteries are predisposed to degenerate because of their thin walls and lack of abundant elastic tissue, including absence of external elastic lamina. Factors that alter blood flow, such as vessel occlusions, arteriovenous malformations, and hypertension and diseases that affect connective tissue may accelerate the degenerative process. It should not be forgotten, however, that in addition to absence of the elastica, all aneurysms show absence of media.

Crompton examined 149 cases at autopsy.[20] He found medial defects, intimal cushions, and even changes in the internal elastica in cerebral arterial forks at birth, although he did note that all these lesions increased in size and number with increasing age. Elastic degeneration appeared first in the intimal pads around the bifurcation, then in the elastica over medial defects. He found that large medial defects were unusual in the first decade but thereafter became progressively more common. Arterial hypertension and renal polycystic disease were associated with increased numbers of large medial defects. Atheromas were found in 52 percent of aneurysm cases—76 percent of such cases when there was evidence of hypertension and only 22 percent when there was not.

The consensus now is that atherosclerosis does not lead directly to the formation of aneurysms. When arteries feeding aneurysms were studied in 100 patients, in all but 12 atherosclerosis of the parent vessel was evident.[101] Intimal proliferations occurred at the mouths of all aneurysms and to some extent at the sites of early aneurysmal change. Elastic tissue alterations and loss in early aneurysmal changes were similar to, although greater than, the changes at forks without aneurysms. Apical regions were affected much more frequently than could be explained by chance alone. The absence of a distinct media in the sac wall was emphasized. The sac wall was still capable of organization and repair. Rather

TABLE 214-4 Pathology of Intracranial Arterial Saccular Aneurysms

A. Light microscopy: The aneurysmal sac lacks normal layers.
  1. Intima: Normal or shows subendothelial proliferations consisting of several layers of smooth muscle cells and connective tissue enveloped by internal elastic membrane usually situated at the mouth of the sac; there may be foam cells.
  2. Internal elastic lamina: Usually absent or reduced to fragments; may be hypertrophied and duplicated at margin of aneurysm.
  3. Muscularis layer of media: Ends abruptly at neck of aneurysm.
  4. Aneurysm wall: May vary greatly in thickness. Larger aneurysms with thick walls may have a laminated appearance, with fibrous tissue layers having hemosiderin deposits and cholesterol and foam cells interposed between them. Thin areas may consist of only endothelium and adventitial fibrous tissue, but usually some fibrohyaline tissue is interposed.
  5. Rupture site: Usually the thinnest area of the dome of the sac. Fibrin plug or layer is present at break in the wall. Thrombus is associated within the sac. In remote ruptures the fibrin is infiltrated by capillaries from the arachnoid. These can traverse the wall to regions of intimal proliferation. Microhemorrhages can occur in the wall from these capillaries.
  6. Lumen: May contain thrombus of varying degrees of organization; dense hyaline acellular tissue may occur in an organized thrombus.
  7. Adventitia: The loose fibrous tissue may be infiltrated by leukocytes, lymphocytes, and hemosiderin-laden phagocytes if there has been previous hemorrhage.
  8. Parent artery: Usually shows atherosclerotic changes, most marked in intimal pads at entrance to sac; foam cells, lipophages, and cholesterol clefts are seen.

B. Electron microscopy
  1. Scanning microscopy shows:
    a. Regressive changes in endothelium, such as ballooning, craters, and cytoplasmic bridges. At gaps between endothelial cell junctions, platelets and leukocytes adhere. Endothelium may be missing altogether.
    b. Adventitia may look normal.
  2. Transmission microscopy shows:
    a. Endothelial cells containing intracytoplasmic vacuoles, empty or full of lipid material.
    b. Beneath the endothelium there is often a grossly thickened basement membrane, which is multilaminar or reticulated.
    c. Fragments of elastica still present have lost their fibrillar structure.
    d. Scanty and sclerotic smooth muscle cells exist in the wall. Some contain hyaline patches, others autophagic vacuoles. Connective tissue contains some well-preserved fibroblasts. Extracellular lipid is common. Collagen fibers of variable length are arranged haphazardly. There is an abundant intercellular space containing lipofuscin granules.

than a medial defect being the earliest change, funnel-shaped dilatations, areas of thinning, and small evaginations were thought to be the essential preaneurysmal lesions, since they were associated with severe degenerative changes in the internal elastic lamina that had areas of thinning or evagination. Stehbens denied that small vessels arising from the apex of forks, vestiges of primitive capillary plexuses, or inflammatory processes are important in the pathogenesis of aneurysms.[101,103]

The role of abnormalities of type III collagen in the etiology of saccular aneurysms remains unclear. Ostergaard and Oxlund found a deficiency in type III collagen in middle cerebral arteries of 6 to 14 patients who died of aneurysmal subarachnoid hemorrhage.[88] This was accompanied by an increase in arterial extensibility but not an alteration in the mechanical strength of the arteries. Brachial arteries from the same cases were biomechanically normal even though they had less type III collagen. Other studies have not identified deficiencies of type III collagen produced by skin fibroblasts of patients with aneurysms.[65]

The pathologic sequelae of aneurysmal rupture are listed in Table 214-5. The most feared by neurosurgeons are rebleeding and focal ischemic infarction due to severe vasospasm. In the cooperative study of Sahs et al.[96] 13 percent of initial survivors who were not operated on rebled in the first week; 12 percent rebled in the second, 6 percent in the third, and 6 percent in the fourth. The mortality rate for the second bleeding episode was 43 percent. About 50 percent of patients rebleed in the first year, and 35 percent die. Six to 12 months after hemorrhage, the rate of rebleeding probably becomes 3 percent per year.[123]

Of 3521 patients admitted within 3 days of subarachnoid hemorrhage, a CT scan on admission showed subarachnoid hemorrhage in 85 percent, intracerebral hemorrhage in 17 percent, intraventricular hemorrhage in 17 percent, and hydrocephalus in 15 percent. Cerebral vasospasm was thought to cause death in 7.2 percent and disability in 6.3 percent, although 28 percent of patients developed cerebral ischemia at some time.[56]

Association of Aneurysms with Other Vascular Lesions

Because saccular aneurysms are probably acquired through hemodynamically induced stresses, any process altering blood flow may increase the propensity to form aneurysms. Obviously, blood flow may change in the absence of changes in systemic blood pressure, and vice versa. The interaction of pregnancy, the puerperium, and subarachnoid hemorrhage is discussed in another chapter.

Anatomic Variants

Figure 214-6 illustrates some of the structural anomalies that have been reported in association with intracranial aneurysms. It may be that such anomalies cause altered flow patterns, which generate aneurysms through hemodynamic mechanisms. An alternative explanation is that there are common embryonic processes that predispose patients to both the anatomic variants and the arterial wall defects that result in the aneurysms.

Of 232 patients with a primitive trigeminal artery, 14 percent had associated aneurysms; of these aneurysms, 13 percent were on the primitive trigeminal artery itself.[40] All the primitive carotico-basilar anastomoses have been reported in association with intracranial aneurysms, including the rare otic artery,[123] although like most predisposing factors for aneurysms, a propensity for these anastamoses to be associated with aneurysm is difficult to confirm statistically.

Figure 214-7 is based on an analysis of 143 ruptured and 39 unruptured aneurysms in 143 autopsy cases.[131] It is evident that hyperplasia of one anterior cerebral artery was associated with a relatively high incidence of aneurysms in the region of the anterior communicating artery. However, relative hyperplasia of one posterior communicating artery was not associated with a relative increase of aneurysms in that region. The meticulous operative findings of Yaşargil in aneurysms of the anterior communicating artery region substantiate the increased frequency of aneurysms when there is one hyperplastic or dominant A1 segment (84 percent of

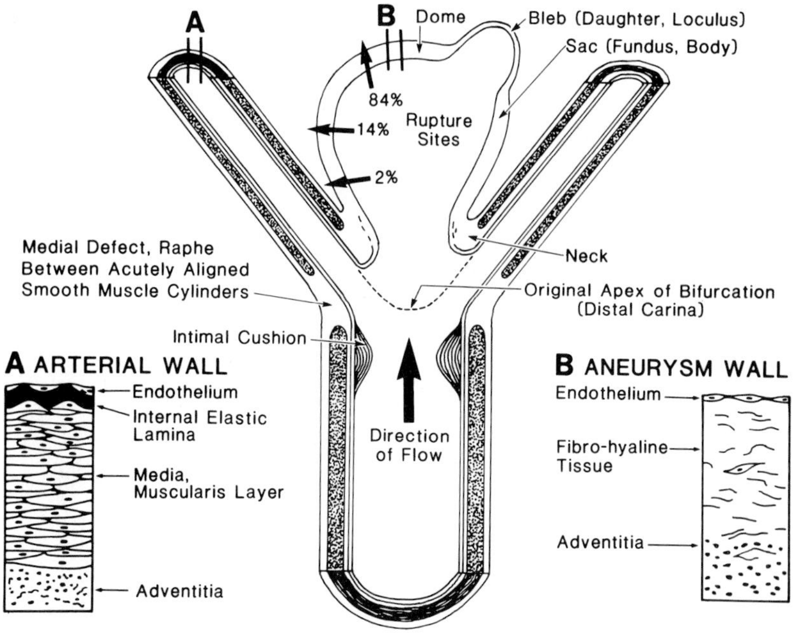

Figure 214-5 Diagram of aneurysmal pathology based on various authors. The data on frequency of rupture at different aneurysmal sites are from Crompton.[19]

375 cases).[135] The aneurysm in 97 percent of his 305 cases of unilateral hyperplasia was on the wall opposite the incoming dominant axial flow.

Arteriovenous Malformations

Of 3265 patients with intracranial aneurysms in the cooperative study, 1 percent also had intracranial arteriovenous malformations (AVMs)[96] (see Chap. 238). Conversely, between 6 and 12 percent of patients with intracranial AVMs have associated aneurysms; this is higher than the incidence of aneurysms in the general population, which is probably less than 5 percent. Aneurysms in patients with AVMs are multiple in 28 to 41 percent of cases. Aneurysms occur on arteries feeding the AVM in 37 to 77 percent of cases, in locations that statistically are significantly different from what a coincidental association of the lesions would suggest.[85] In 22 to 43 percent of cases, aneurysms are on arteries not hemodynamically related to the AVM. Three explanations have been advanced to explain the association of aneurysms and AVMs. The high incidence of aneurysms on arteries feeding the AVM, the presence of larger infundibula, the increased incidence of multiple aneurysms, and reports of regression of aneurysms on feeders following obliteration of the AVM all support the theory that these aneurysms are due to abnormally high blood flow. Some cases may be coincidental, and others may be due to a common developmental defect.[6,123]

In patients presenting with hemorrhage, it may be difficult to identify the responsible lesion, as most series find about equal rates of hemorrhage from each lesion. In general, the symptomatic lesion should be treated first, but aneurysms on feeding vessels may be at increased risk of rupture if they are not clipped before or when the AVM is obliterated.[6]

TABLE 214-5 Pathologic Sequelae of Aneurysmal Rupture

A. Immediate
- **1.** Hemorrhage
  - **a.** Subarachnoid
  - **b.** Intracerebral
  - **c.** Intraventricular
  - **d.** Subdural
  - **e.** Intra-aneurysmal
- **2.** Acute brain swelling
- **3.** Acute ventricular dilatation
- **4.** Brain shifts
  - **a.** Tentorial herniation
  - **b.** Foraminal impaction of cerebellar tonsils

B. Delayed
- **1.** Hemorrhage
  - **a.** Repeat aneurysmal rupture
  - **b.** Secondary midbrain hemorrhages
- **2.** Chronic hydrocephalus
- **3.** Arterial vasospasm
- **4.** Brain infarction
  - **a.** Direct pressure from space-occupying lesion
  - **b.** Vessel compression from brain shift
  - **c.** Severe diffuse vasospasm
  - **d.** Systemic hypotension, decreased cardiac output, decreased red cell mass and blood volume, hypoxia, acidosis, other fluid and electrolyte abnormalities

Infundibular Widenings of the Posterior Communicating Artery

Infundibula are pyramidal in shape, under 3 mm in maximum diameter, and located at arterial origins with small arteries coming from the apex. Miyasaka et al. studied 132 patients with AVMs, of whom 16.7 percent had associated aneurysms[76]; 10 patients had aneurysms and infundibula, and 20 had infundibula alone. Infundibula were more likely to occur in older patients and in patients with larger AVMs. Of the infundibula, 65 percent occurred at the junction of the internal carotid and posterior communicating arteries and 82 percent were located on arteries supplying the AVM or on the internal carotid artery ipsilateral to the AVM. In four patients the infundibulum decreased in size following successful

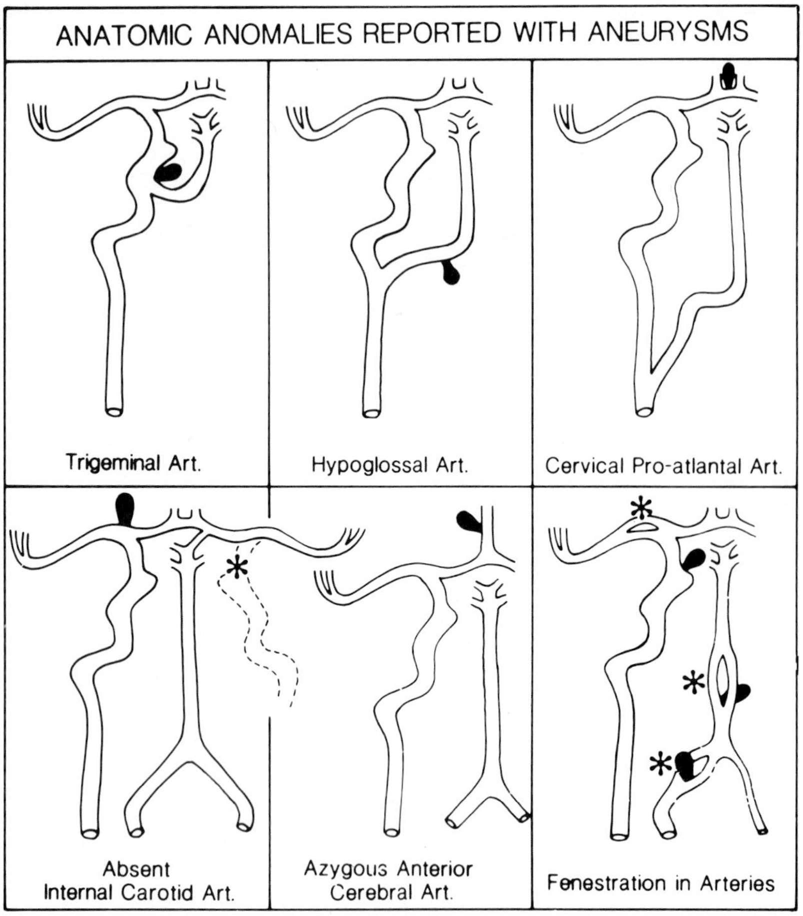

Figure 214-6 Synopsis of some of the anomalies that have been reported in association with intracranial aneurysms.

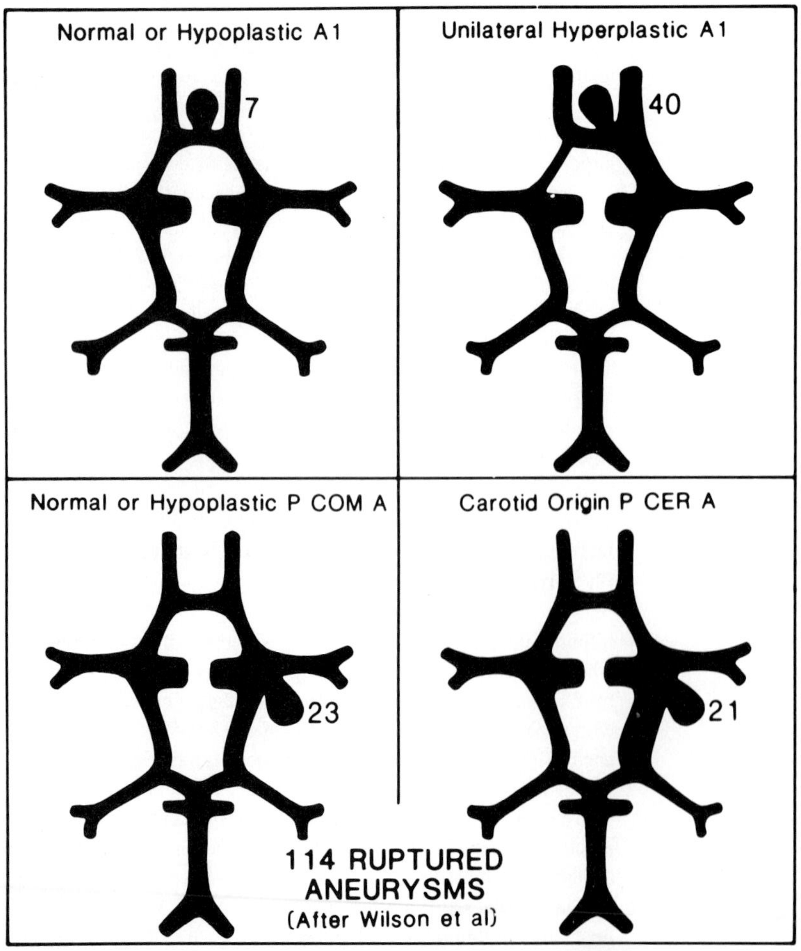

Figure 214-7 Pictorial depiction of data of Wilson et al.[131] showing the increased frequency of unilateral hyperplasia of the A1 segment of the anterior cerebral artery with anterior communicating aneurysms but no such association in the posterior circle.

treatment of the AVM. In the same study, 3 of 43 aneurysms decreased in size after removal of the AVM. It has been suggested that infundibula occur in about 7 percent of normal angiograms and that their frequency increases with age.[120] A case of infundibular enlargement over a period of 9 years with evolution into an aneurysm that was unruptured has been documented. There are eight similar cases reported in the literature, some of which developed subarachnoid hemorrhage.[123] Other authorities have assessed the gross and histologic findings in seven junctional dilatations discovered at autopsy.[32] No significant histologic abnormalities were found in any case, and it was concluded that a junctional dilatation was neither aneurysmal nor preaneurysmal. If an infundibulum does evolve into an aneurysm, it must be an unusual event. A rupture is even rarer.

Hypertension

The relationship between blood pressure and aneurysmal rupture was investigated in 212 cases seen between 1964 and 1976.[1] Blood pressures were determined by the patient's medical record before admission for aneurysmal rupture and/or by measurements of stable blood pressure taken as long as possible after the initial bleeding and while the patient was off medication. The series was compared with Department of Health and Human Services data for approximately 10,000 patients in each matched age group. Mean systolic and diastolic blood pressures were not elevated to a statistically significant extent in patients with aneurysms as compared with the general population, except for a minor elevation in systolic blood pressure in a few subsets of younger male and female patients. A hypertensive patient under 55 years of age of either sex was found to be twice as likely to have multiple aneurysms as a normotensive patient.

McCormick and Schmalstieg used both blood pressure records and myocardial hypertrophy found at autopsy to assess hypertension and reported no increase in hypertension in aneurysm patients, compared with controls.[74] In their 250 aneurysm patients, there was also no evident association of hypertension with multiplicity of aneurysms, age at which aneurysms presented clinically, or age at rupture.

A comparison was made of 319 cases of subarachnoid hemorrhage, with an equal number of controls and almost half a million discharges from the Veterans Administration hospitals of the United States.[58] Among the 173 patients in whom angiograms were performed, aneurysms were found in 74 percent of the 109 normotensive but only 58 percent of the 64 hypertensive patients. Conversely, hypertension existed in 49 percent of 55 patients without aneurysms but only 31 percent of 118 with aneurysms. The coexistence of aneurysms and hypertension was therefore uncommon. In 743 patients admitted with aneurysmal subarachnoid hemorrhage to one institution, the presence or absence of hypertension was assessed based on prior treatment with antihypertensive medication, elevated blood pressure while in the hospital, and signs of left ventricular hypertrophy on an electrocardiogram or at autopsy.[87] About 25 percent of aneurysm patients had high blood pressure according to these criteria. Hypertension was an important factor in explaining cases of multiple aneurysms. However, female gender was also a significant independent associated factor, and other unidentified causes were thought to be essential to aneurysm formation.

A case-control analysis was used to determine the relationship among subarachnoid hemorrhage, cigarette smoking, and hypertension.[10] Overall, 16 percent of controls had been treated for hypertension, compared with 38 percent of individuals with subarachnoid hemorrhage. People with hypertension were more than three times as likely to suffer subarachnoid hemorrhage.

In summary, four of five recent studies show that hypertension is not a major factor in the etiology of saccular aneurysms, although it may cause more aneurysms in susceptible individuals and may promote aneurysmal rupture. These findings should not be confused with the fact that immediately following the ictus of aneurysmal rupture, the occurrence of hypertension has been universally a very important negative prognostic factor (see Table 214-11). In these circumstances, however, it is probably partly a reflection of the Cushing response to intracranial hypertension.

Arterial Occlusions and Stenoses

Following cervical carotid artery ligation, 40 to 92 percent of aneurysms become smaller on follow-up angiography, 8 to 27 percent stay the same, 17 to 80 percent are not visualized, and 9 percent are larger.[123] Although thorough angiographic follow-up studies are not reported, the incidence of *de novo* aneurysm formation on arteries contralateral to the occluded carotid artery is estimated to be between 0 and 4 percent. A review of 14 cases found that 86 percent of the patients with new aneurysms presented with subarachnoid hemorrhage between 3 and 15 years after ligation.[30]

Fox reviewed 33 cases of aneurysms in association with carotid stenosis.[38] In most cases, the carotid stenosis was symptomatic and no treatment was directed toward the aneurysm. Endarterectomy did not seem to increase the risk of aneurysm rupture. Stenosis was ipsilateral to the aneurysm in 15 cases and contralateral in 18. The absence of an increased incidence of aneurysms contralateral to the side of the carotid stenosis suggested that hemodynamic mechanisms were not responsible for aneurysm formation in this situation. Common sites for aneurysms were the middle cerebral artery (24 percent of 38 aneurysms), the posterior communicating artery (32 percent), and the cavernous internal carotid artery (18 percent).

Fields and Weibel reported a 67-year-old patient who presented with an aneurysmal rupture and third nerve palsy.[36] A carotid endarterectomy was performed, and 10 months later the patient had a recurrent hemorrhage, which ultimately proved fatal.

In general, reported cases suggest there is little additional risk in performing carotid endarterectomy in patients with asymptomatic aneurysms, but this risk is considerably increased if the endarterectomy is being performed in the feeding vessel of a symptomatic or previously ruptured aneurysm. Initial treatment should be directed toward the symptomatic lesion. In cases of transient ischemic attacks with associated severe carotid stenosis and asymptomatic aneurysm, carotid endarterectomy can be performed, with due attention given to blood pressure perioperatively. The asymptomatic aneurysm should be dealt with based on the usual factors, including aneurysm size and location, and age of patient. However, symptomatic or ruptured aneurysms should be repaired before attention is given to an asymptomatic carotid stenosis, the management of which is still open to question pending results of randomized clinical trials.

A case of anterior communicating artery aneurysm associated with absence of a left cervical carotid artery was reviewed, and 15 previously published cases were analyzed.[121] Of these aneurysms, 63 percent were on the anterior communicating artery and 19 percent on the basilar bifurcation. In these cases two vessels would be subjected to increased flow to compensate for the unilateral carotid absence. The occurrence of an intracranial aneurysm in 9 of 36 patients with an absent internal carotid artery has been described.[99]

At least nine cases of pulseless disease (Takayasu's disease) associated with aneurysm rupture have been reported, all in Japanese people. Eight patients were female, and most aneurysms were ruptured posterior circulation lesions. There was a 20 percent mortality rate in patients undergoing aneurysm surgery.[123] Patients with carotid artery occlusion due to moyamoya disease also have a propensity to develop cerebral aneurysms, which occur in about 14 percent of adults with moyamoya disease. A review of 60 cases of bilateral moyamoya disease found aneurysms on collateral vessels in 33 percent, moyamoya vessels in 28 percent, the vertebrobasilar circulation in 25 percent, internal carotid artery in 12 percent, and middle cerebral artery in 2 percent. Aneurysms in moyamoya disease are about equally divided between true saccular aneurysms, which sometimes increase in size and never disappear, and pseudoaneurysms on the moyamoya vessels, which may disappear spontaneously.[123]

Experimental Aneurysms

Cerebral aneurysms have been induced in rats and monkeys by feeding them β-aminoproprionitrile, which causes a connective tissue abnormality due to defects in the cross-linkage between elastin and collagen. Both species were also rendered hypertensive by a variety of means. Flow was increased through one carotid system by ligation of the other common carotid.[47,59] The aneurysms induced in monkeys were histopathologically the same as aneurysms in humans.[59] Ligation of the carotid artery in rabbits induced exceptionally large defects in the media, especially at the distal end of the basilar artery.[48] Very rare reports of post-traumatic intracranial aneurysms in animals have also appeared in the literature. There is not yet a naturally occurring model of aneurysms in animals.

Predisposing Factors to Aneurysm Rupture

Activities at Time of Rupture

Among 2228 cases in the cooperative study, the onset of subarachnoid hemorrhage was associated with lifting or bending in 12 percent, emotional strain in 4 percent, defecation in 4 percent, coitus in 4 percent, trauma in 3 percent, coughing in 2 percent, urination in 2 percent, and parturition in 0.35 percent.[96] In about one-third of cases, rupture was said to have occurred during sleep or in unspecified circumstances. In the absence of data on the time age- and sex-matched individuals without aneurysms spend on these strenuous activities, it is not possible to prove that they precipitate aneurysmal rupture. Notwithstanding this, it is very likely that peaks of arterial hypertension, rapid oscillations in venous and CSF pressure, and possibly movement of brain structures in relation to one another can all precipitate aneurysmal rupture.

Smoking

A retrospective study of 208 patients with ruptured cerebral aneurysms found a highly significant excess of cigarette smokers compared with the expected incidence. It was suggested that continued smoking increases the risk of suffering a subarachnoid hemorrhage by a factor of 3.9 for men and 3.7 for women.[8] Smoking resulted in similar, significant increases in risk of subarachnoid hemorrhage in a case-control study.[10]

Alcohol Consumption

In 25 percent of 75 aneurysmal ruptures in a Finnish study, the bleeding was preceded within 24 h by a bout of alcohol consumption.[50] This intoxication preceding the ictus was two to four times as common in male patients and three to five times as common in female patients as alcohol intoxication in the general Finnish population of the same age and sex. This uncontrolled study suggests an association between acute alcohol intoxication and aneurysm rupture. A review of risk factors for subarachnoid hemorrhage concluded that further work was necessary to confirm an association of alcohol consumption with aneurysmal subarachnoid hemorrhage.[68]

Aneurysmal Rupture during Angiography

Clinical and experimental data indicate that significant but mild increases in blood pressure and blood flow rate occur during angiography, particularly during injection of large volumes of contrast material. These increases may be aggravated by a high flow rate of the contrast material, vasospasm, spasm at the tip of the catheter, increased blood pressure, and increased intracranial pressure.[123] Although angiography may precipitate aneurysm rupture, the hemorrhage is probably coincidental in some cases.

A review of 10 new cases of aneurysmal rupture during angiography and 20 other well-documented cases from the literature[61] indicated that internal carotid injections were not more dangerous than common carotid injections. Aneurysms were more likely to rupture during injection with cross-compression. Overall, these patients tended to be in poor condition, with 18 percent being grade 4 and 32 percent grade 5 at the time of angiography, which was performed in 53 percent within 12 h of admission to the hospital; 45 percent had common carotid injections and 42 percent had internal carotid injections. Of these patients, 84 percent died following the extravasation. The authors suggested that a mixture of blood and hyperosmolar contrast agent must be more toxic than blood alone. They found no correlation between the volume of contrast material and the number of injections given before the one associated with rupture. Unfortunately, detailed data on arterial blood pressure, injection pressures, and flow rates were not obtainable.

Diagnosis of Aneurysmal Rupture

Warning Symptoms and Signs

Symptoms and signs preceding aneurysmal rupture have been reported in 20 to 59 percent of patients. They are usually attributed to aneurysm expansion or minor subarachnoid hemorrhages.

In 2621 aneurysm cases from the cooperative study of Sahs et al.,[96] symptoms antedating the first subarachnoid hemorrhage occurred as follows: headache, 48 percent; dizziness, 10 percent; orbital pain, 7 percent; diplopia, 4 percent; and loss of vision, 4 percent. Signs antedating the first hemorrhage were motor or sensory disturbances, 6 percent; seizures, 4 percent; ptosis, 3 percent; bruits, 3 percent; and dysphasia, 2 percent. Of the total number of patients with unruptured symptomatic aneurysms, 68 percent had third cranial nerve involvement. It was suggested that only 10 to 15 percent of all aneurysm cases presented the opportunity for diagnosis before rupture.

In an analysis of 112 single aneurysm cases, the most frequent warning symptoms and signs prior to rupture were as follows: generalized headache, 25 percent; localized head pain, 18 percent; lethargy, 8 percent; impairment of extraocular movements, 7 percent; face and eye pain, 6 percent; and neck and back pain, 6 percent. Internal carotid–posterior communicating artery region aneurysms were associated with impairment of extraocular movements in 23 percent of cases and with visual field defects, eye pain, and face pain in 8 percent each. The average interval between the warning signs and major hemorrhage in these patients was 3 weeks. Patients with warning signs tended to be younger.[86]

Warning signs preceded aneurysm rupture in 74 (20 percent) of 364 patients admitted to 24 centers in Italy over 1 year.[5] These patients were compared with 78 patients who had similar symptoms but whose aneurysms were diagnosed at the time of their warning symptoms. Sudden, severe headache was the cardinal feature in both groups, although loss of consciousness occurred in 33 percent of diagnosed cases, compared with 12 percent of the undiagnosed cases. A group of 57 patients were seen by a physician and not diagnosed correctly. Major subarachnoid hemorrhage developed within 3 months in 78 percent of patients. The eventual outcome in patients with missed warning signs was much worse; they had a 24 percent mortality rate, compared with 4 percent among those diagnosed initially.

In another study, 34 of 87 consecutive patients with aneurysmal subarachnoid hemorrhage had a premonitory warning leak characterized by sudden, severe headache.[64] Half of the patients saw a physician but remained undiagnosed. CT findings were normal after a warning leak in 55 percent, but lumbar puncture always showed subarachnoid hemorrhage. In most of these cases, the sudden, severe headache should have been atypical enough to prompt a CT scan and, if necessary, a lumbar puncture. Although a variety of nonspecific symptoms are common in the general population and may precede subarachnoid hemorrhage, the significance of the classic warning headache would seem recognizable as serious, and the threshold for investigation in these cases should be minimal.

Clinical Presentation of Aneurysmal Rupture

About 89 percent of patients with aneurysms present with subarachnoid hemorrhage, and 7 percent with tumor symptoms with or without hemorrhage; in 4 percent the aneurysms are incidental findings.[38] Sarner and Rose studied 962 patients with ruptured aneurysms.[97] Symptoms and signs occurred with decreasing frequency as follows: meningism, 64 percent; coma, 52 percent; nausea and vomiting, 45 percent; generalized headache, 32 percent; classic occipital headaches, 21 percent; reflex changes, 19 percent; motor deficit, 17 percent; dysphasia, 13 percent; confusion, 12 percent; intraocular hemorrhage, 12 percent; anisocoria, 11 percent; papilledema, 9 percent; homonymous hemianopia, 9 percent; lateralized headache, 8 percent; third nerve palsy, 7 percent; and sensory disturbances, 5 percent. No localizing signs occurred in 39 percent.

The cardinal diagnostic feature remains a headache that is unusually severe for the patient and has a very sudden onset.

Symptoms and Signs Not due to Rupture

Distal Embolization from Partially Thrombosed Aneurysms

At least 30 cases of distal embolization from partially thrombosed aneurysms are known.[31,60,90,105,123] Transient ischemic attacks or stroke may be considered to be secondary to an aneurysm if no other lesion or predisposing risk factor is present, if the aneurysm is located proximal to the territory involved in the symptomatology, if there is thrombus in the sac, if the attacks cease when the aneurysm is excluded from the circulation, and if there is no evidence of subarachnoid hemorrhage or vasospasm. Reported patients ranged in age from 10 to 69 years (mean, 49 years). About 40 percent of the aneurysms were giant, and the most common locations were the internal carotid artery (23 percent) and middle cerebral artery (57 percent); only four reported cases involved posterior circulation aneurysms. In 92 percent symptoms ceased following definitive treatment of the aneurysm, in 25 percent symptoms continued or recurred when the aneurysm was not excluded from the circulation, and in 75 percent attacks stopped with no treatment or with administration of antiplatelet drugs.

Neurological Signs from Giant Aneurysms

Overall, about 5 percent of intracranial aneurysms are larger than 2.5 cm in maximum diameter and are called *giant*. Figure 214-3 illustrates the frequency with which such aneurysms are found in ruptured and unruptured groups as well as in symptomatic and asymptomatic groups. Of Drake's series of 174 giant aneurysms, 38 percent involved the anterior circulation and 62 percent involved the posterior circulation.[27] The high incidence of vertebrobasilar giant aneurysms probably was at least partly a reflection of his expertise in dealing with such aneurysms. Of his patients, 36 percent presented with subarachnoid hemorrhage.

The most commonly involved artery is the internal carotid artery, from which giant aneurysms arise in 59 percent of cases. Most giant aneurysms arise from sites similar to those of smaller saccular aneurysms. A review of 573 cases from six series in the literature reveals the following arterial distribution: intradural internal carotid–ophthalmic, 21 percent; middle cerebral, 16 percent; anterior cerebral, 12 percent; internal carotid bifurcation, 9 percent; basilar-superior cerebellar, 8 percent; basilar bifurcation, 7 percent; cavernous carotid, 6 percent; vertebral, 4 percent; other sites, 11 percent.[38,123] Over 60 percent are partially thrombosed, and females make up 60 percent of patients, although males predominate for every site except the internal carotid artery.

Symptoms and signs relate to the location of the giant aneurysm and include seizures, focal neurological deficits due to mass effect or embolization from the aneurysm, and pain. Subarachnoid hemorrhage occurs in between 14 and 76 percent of cases. In a cooperative study of 130 giant aneurysms, 45 percent of the patients presented with hemorrhage (subarachnoid, intracerebral, or intraventricular), 39 percent with focal deficit due to mass effect, 12 percent with sudden cranial nerve deficit, and a few percent each with ischemic episodes and seizures.[7] Giant cavernous aneurysms are extradural and are manifested differently, most commonly with cranial nerve deficits (58 percent) followed by subarachnoid hemorrhage (19 percent), and as an incidental finding (12 percent). They may produce carotid-cavernous fistulae and massive epistaxis.[123]

Cranial Nerve Signs from Nongiant Aneurysms

Patients with aneurysms that are not giant can present with symptoms and signs not due to subarachnoid hemorrhage. In the cooperative study there were 86 patients with unruptured, symptomatic posterior communicating–internal carotid artery aneurysms.[96] Of these patients, 87 percent had signs of third cranial nerve involvement. Only 2 and 1 percent had evidence of sixth and fourth cranial nerve palsies, respectively. The same study included 37 patients with ophthalmic–internal carotid artery aneurysms. Of these patients, 29 percent presented with loss of vision, and 19 percent had symptoms referable to the third cranial nerve, 13 percent to the fifth, 10 percent to the fourth, and 6 percent to the sixth. For unruptured symptomatic aneurysms of the internal carotid artery, the maximum frequency occurred with aneurysms 7 to 10 mm in size.

Of 570 patients who had aneurysms with or without subarachnoid hemorrhage, 58 had cranial nerve palsies; 48 were in the group of 534 with subarachnoid hemorrhage. The third nerve was affected most commonly (38 patients), followed by the sixth nerve (18 patients). In patients with unruptured aneurysms, these nerves were also the ones most commonly damaged.[63]

Differential Diagnosis of Sudden, Severe Headache

Subarachnoid hemorrhage should be searched for in a patient with headache that is of sudden onset and more severe than any prior headaches (Table 214-6). However, many other processes may mimic subarachnoid hemorrhage; in some cases, no cause of the headache is found. Vomiting and a headache that persists tend to differentiate subarachnoid hemorrhage from benign headache.[5]

TABLE 214-6 Causes of Sudden, Severe Headache

- Intracranial
  - Subarachnoid hemorrhage
    - Aneurysm
    - Arteriovenous malformation (cerebral, dural, spinal)
  - Pituitary apoplexy
  - Arterial dissection
  - Cerebral venous thrombosis
  - Other intracranial hemorrhages
  - Acute hydrocephalus
  - Other intracranial mass (neoplasm, abscess)
  - Meningitis, encephalitis
- Extracranial
  - Dental disease
  - Sinusitis
  - Ocular disease (glaucoma)
- Systemic
  - Hypertensive encephalopathy
  - Temporal arteritis
- Benign
  - Migraine (common, classic)
  - Cluster
  - Tension
  - Benign exertional headache
  - Benign coital headache

Clinical Grading of Subarachnoid Hemorrhage

The importance of assessing the neurological condition of patients after subarachnoid hemorrhage lies in the prediction of outcome. In the cooperative study on timing of aneurysm surgery involving 3521 patients, the most important factors predicting outcome were level of consciousness, which contributed to both death and disability, and presence of hemiparesis and/or aphasia, which was important in disability but had no effect on mortality.[29,56] Headache and stiff neck were not related to outcome as long as consciousness was normal. A grading scale was devised by the World Federation of Neurological Surgeons, incorporating the Glasgow coma score and presence or absence of motor deficit (Table 214-7).[29]

There are numerous other grading systems, including the Botterell and Hunt and Hess scales (see Table 214-7).[11,51] The latter includes assessment of headache and neck stiffness, and both scales rely on less consistent definitions of level of consciousness

TABLE 214-7 Grading Scales for Subarachnoid Hemorrhage

Grade	Description
	Botterell et al. Scale[11]
1	Conscious with of without signs of blood in the subarachnoid space
2	Drowsy without significant neurological deficit
3	Drowsy with neurological deficit and probably intracerebral clot
4	Major neurological deficit and deterioration due to large intracerebral clot, or older age with less severe neurological deficit but pre-existing cerebrovascular disease
5	Moribund or near-moribund with failing vital centers and extensor rigidity
	Hunt and Hess Scale[51]*
1	Asymptomatic or minimal headache and slight nuchal rigidity
2	Moderate to severe headache, nuchal rigidity, no neurological deficit other than cranial nerve palsy
3	Drowsiness, confusion, or mild focal deficit
4	Stupor, moderate to severe hemiparesis, possible early decerebrate rigidity and vegetative disturbances
5	Deep coma, decerebrate rigidity, moribund appearance
	World Federation of Neurological Surgeons Scale[29]
1	Glasgow coma score 15, no motor deficit
2	Glasgow coma score 13 to 14, no motor deficit
3	Glasgow coma score 13 to 14, with motor deficit
4	Glasgow coma score 7 to 12, with or without motor deficit
5	Glasgow coma score 3 to 6, with or without motor deficit

* Patients are moved into the next worst category if they have vasospasm on angiography or serious systemic disease, such as hypertension, diabetes, atherosclerosis, or chronic lung disease.

than does the Glasgow coma score. The interobserver variability in the Hunt and Hess scale is probably greater than in the Glasgow coma score.[66]

Natural History of Aneurysms

Table 214-8 summarizes some of the major contributions to our understanding of the prognosis when an aneurysm is present. The major observation is that the highest mortality rate occurs immediately following the hemorrhage and diminishes rapidly thereafter. A fact of paramount importance from the cooperative study was that for patients with single aneurysms, the mortality rate over the entire first week after subarachnoid hemorrhage was 27 percent.[96] Rebleeding is estimated to occur in 50 percent of cases of ruptured aneurysms within 6 months of the first hemorrhage, and thereafter at a rate of 3 percent per year.[123] The best available data suggest that asymptomatic aneurysms, either discovered incidentally or existing in patients with multiple aneurysms, bleed at a rate of 1 to 2 percent per year.[33,123] Fifty to 60 percent of patients die after rebleeding, and 20 to 25 percent are left disabled. Because the risk of surgery for unruptured aneurysms is low (mortality close to 0 percent, morbidity about 4 percent), it is recommended that asymptomatic aneurysms be clipped in most patients.[33]

Figure 214-8 is a graphic estimate of what might happen to the total population of patients with aneurysmal rupture in North America. The 1980–1981 census figures give a total population of about 251 million. The incidence of ruptured aneurysms in two careful studies in the United States and Europe was 10.5 and 10.3 per 100,000 population per year. About 15 percent of patients die before reaching a hospital. In the cooperative timing study, 27 percent of patients with subarachnoid hemorrhage were excluded because of admission more than 3 days after the ictus, and 7 percent had had more than one subarachnoid hemorrhage.[56] The number of cases initially misdiagnosed must have been greater than 7 percent, since some patients would not have had a second subarachnoid hemorrhage or would have died from the hemorrhage, again without a diagnosis. Drake reported that neurosurgeons were operating upon 1.6 per 100,000 per year in Japan and 3.6 per 100,000 per year in Ontario.[28] We are therefore not operating on the majority of aneurysm rupture cases and, for the most part, are probably simply treating the "survivors."

The natural history of a patient admitted to the hospital is still bleak. From the data presented in Table 214-9, it can be seen that for those patients admitted for neurosurgery very early, the postoperative mortality can be reduced by delaying operation, but this is a spurious gain because overall management mortality usually increases. The international cooperative study on timing of aneurysm surgery provides outcome data on 3521 patients admitted within 3 days of aneurysmal subarachnoid hemorrhage to 68 centers between 1980 and 1983. Of these, 75 percent were in good neurological condition on admission, and 83 percent underwent surgery. After 6 months, 26 percent of patients were dead and only

TABLE 214-8 Prognosis for Surgically Untreated Saccular Intracranial Aneurysms

A. Ruptured
1. *Unselected,* entire city, minimal surgical withdrawals, all sudden deaths autopsied. Helsinki 1954–1961, 363 cases. Mortality: 1 day 32%; 1 week 43%; 1 month 56%; 6 months 60%.[89]
2. *Selected* by virtue of surgical withdrawals, admissions to many hospitals. Cooperative study, 1958–1965, 830 single aneurysm cases. Mortality: 1 day 10%; 1 week 27%; 1 month 49%; 6 months 61%.[96]
3. *Unselected* since surgical withdrawals were randomized, admissions to two hospitals. London 1958–1967, 364 cases, anterior communicating aneurysms. Mortality: 6 months 41%; 5 years, 48%; 10 years, 51%.[133]
4. *Partly selected,* entire city, 27 surgical withdrawals at a mean time of 9 days postrupture. Rochester 1945–1974, 119 cases (estimated from an illustration). Mortality: 1 day 8%; 1 week 40%; 1 month 60%.[92]

B. Unruptured
1. *Asymptomatic* multiple aneurysms associated with other previously ruptured and clipped aneurysms. Helsinki, 1956–1970, 61 cases, follow-up 10 to 24 years. Mortality from rupture of different aneurysms at 10 years after original aneurysm rupture 6.6%. Mortality at last available follow-up 11.5%.[49]
2. *Asymptomatic* multiple aneurysms associated with other previously ruptured and clipped aneurysms. London, 38 cases. Mortality from rupture of different aneurysms at mean follow-up 8 years was 8%, about 1% per year.[132]
3. Combined *asymptomatic* (71%) and *symptomatic* (29%), no surgical withdrawals. Rochester, 1955–1975, 65 cases, follow-up mean 8 years. Mortality from aneurysm rupture 11%.[129]
4. *Asymptomatic,* no surgical withdrawals. Cooperative study, 1958–1965, 50 cases, follow-up not stated, said to be "less satisfactory" than for other groups. Mortality at 5 years 2%.[96]
5. *Asymptomatic,* estimates using prevalence averages and decremental life table analysis methods. 1982. Estimated mortality for a 20-year-old by age 75 years 16.6%. Estimated mortality for a 60-year-old by age 75 years 4.68%.[23]
6. *Symptomatic,* no surgical withdrawals. Cooperative study, 1958–1965, 32 cases. Mortality at mean follow-up 41 months 28%.[96]

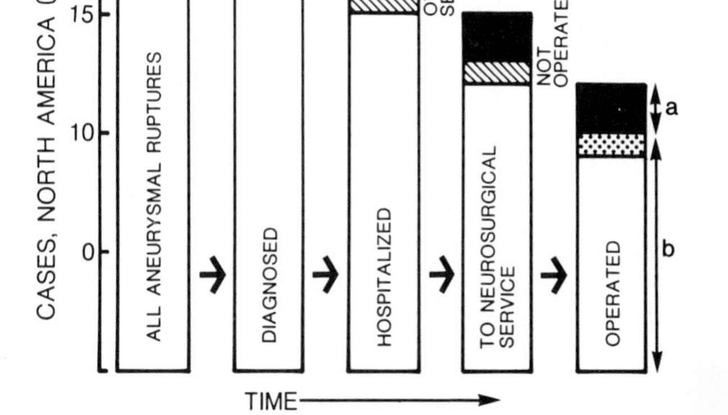

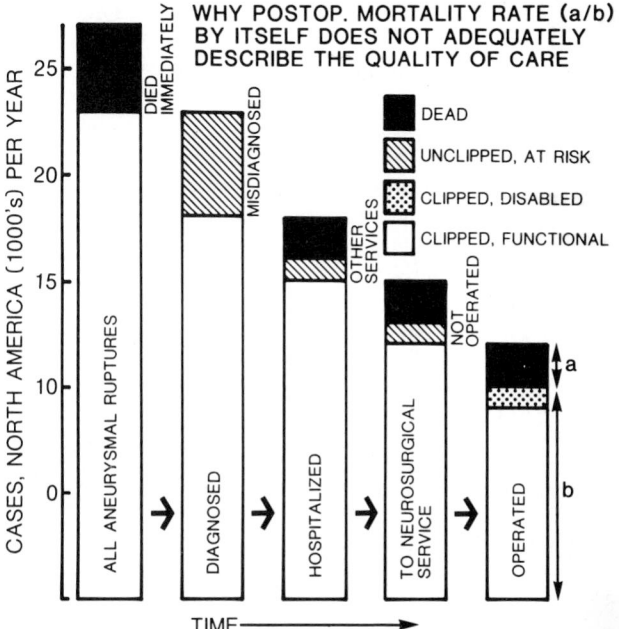

Figure 214-8 Schematic representation of patient flow follow-ing aneurysm rupture. The actual numbers can best be d scribed as an educated guess in the absence of any hard miologic data.

TABLE 214-9 Proportion of Early Operations and Occurrence of Intraventricular Hemorrhage as Determinants of Management Mortality. Admissions to Hospital Day 0–1 after Aneurysm Rupture

			Postoperative Mortality, %		Management Mortality, %	
Reference	**Types of Aneurysms**	**Number of Cases**	**≤7 days**	**>7 days**	**≤7 days**	**>7 days**
Weir and Aronyk[125]	All	224	30	7	53	64
Wheelock et al.[128]	With intracerebral hematoma	103	40	18	46	47
Mohr et al.[77]	With intraventricular hemorrhage	74	22	40	71	89
Kassell et al.[57]*	All	1463	17	11	21	24

*Patients admitted and operated upon within 3 days of subarachnoid hemorrhage.

58 percent were completely recovered. The main causes of morbidity and mortality were vasospasm and rebleeding.[56,57]

How can we reconcile these bleak figures with the reports of others who are obtaining very low postoperative mortality figures overall in very large series? The explanation in part lies in the delay in transfer to, and natural selection that occurs prior to arrival at, major tertiary referral centers. This can be seen in Table 214-10, in which the lower overall postoperative mortality rate in three large series was due to the delay in operation, compared with a smaller series in which the patients were more commonly admitted for neurosurgery immediately following their aneurysmal rupture.

It is of vital importance to a neurosurgeon to be able to advise patients and their relatives about the possible outcomes of different courses of action. In the past 2 decades, more sophisticated methods of analysis using multiple regression (or multivariant) techniques have permitted the simultaneous analysis of potentially important preoperative prognostic factors. Table 214-11 lists some of these studies. However, we are still a long way from predicting with 100 percent accuracy what is likely to happen to an individual patient.

Disney et al. used discriminant function analysis to determine the relative importance of prognostic indicators for outcome in 184 patients admitted in grades 3 to 5 within 96 hours of subarachnoid hemorrhage. Factors, in order of importance, were whether the patient was treated surgically, neurological grade on admission, age, initial systolic blood pressure, and aneurysm size. The discriminant function analysis correctly classified 80 percent of patients.[25] In the cooperative timing study, univariate analysis showed that a decreasing level of consciousness, increased age, aneurysm larger than 12 mm, and aneurysms on the anterior cerebral artery or posterior circulation were associated with worse outcome. Multivariate analysis found factors important for predicting death included level of consciousness, age, blood pressure on admission, subarachnoid blood distribution on CT, pre-existing medical illness, and aneurysm site. Good outcome was related to these factors in addition to vasospasm.[56,57]

The results that any given neurosurgeon can achieve in the treatment of aneurysmal rupture are as individual as fingerprints. Although most of us would wish otherwise, individual technical skill is probably of lesser importance than geographic, sociologic and organizational factors in our area of practice, which ultimately determine the nature of the patient group referred to us and the time at which this is done. In analyzing the reports of neurosurgical series, the reader should note whether it is stated when the patients were seen by the neurosurgeon in relation to the time of their aneurysmal rupture, what grade they were, whether there were any arbitrary exclusions of cases on the basis of age or neurological status, and whether all aneurysmal ruptures in that geographic area were likely to have been included.

Medical Complications of Aneurysmal Rupture

General

Table 214-12 lists experience from the cooperative study on the timing of aneurysm surgery.[56,57] The most frequently encountered medical complications are hypertension, cardiac arrhythmias and hypotension, pneumonia and atelectasis, syndrome of inappropriate secretion of antidiuretic hormone (SIADH), gastrointestinal hemorrhage, and anemia.

Infections can also be a major source of danger to a patient with

TABLE 214-10 Proportion of Early Operations as a Determinant of Total Postoperative Mortality Rate

Reference	Yaşargil[135]	Suzuki et al.[112]	Sundt[109]	Weir and Aronyk[126]
Number of cases	638	625	271	67
Postoperative mortality <7 days, %	15	16	18	10
Postoperative mortality 7–14 days, %	2	5	8*	0
Postoperative mortality >14 days, %	2	3	2†	0
Total postoperative mortality, %	4	5	6	7
Percent of cases operated <7 days	18	17	17‡	73

*7–9 days.
†≥10 days.
‡≤6 days.

TABLE 214-11 Relative Strength of Preoperative Factors as Predictors of Mortality after Aneurysmal Rupture (Multiple Regression Analyses)*

A. All Aneurysmal Ruptures	
1114 cases, 1970–1977, 14-day mortality[116]	
1. Neurological status	17.74
2. Diastolic blood pressure	11.66
3. Interval to treatment	9.44
4. Vasospasm	8.51
5. Medical condition	5.51
265 cases, 1972–1977, 5-year postoperative mortality, excluding preoperative deaths and postoperative deaths from unrelated causes[2]	
1. Botterell grade	0.65
2. Age	0.47
3. Blood pressure	0.31
4. Interval to operation	0.20
5. Aneurysm side	0.19
135 cases, 1968–1973, mortality 2 months after aneurysmal rupture[127]	
1. Neurological grade	0.36
2. Grade at operation	0.34
3. Preoperative vasospasm	0.28
4. Mass lesion	0.23
5. Blood pressure	0.20
6. Interval to surgery	0.10
7. Age	0.06
B. Aneurysmal Rupture Producing Intracerebral Hematoma	
132 cases, 1982, mortality during initial admission[128]	
1. Systolic blood pressure	0.37
2. Preoperative herniation	0.35
3. Grade at clipping	0.33
4. Grade at evacuation of clot	0.27
5. Diastolic blood pressure	0.16
6. Grade at initial CT scan	0.14
7. Size of hematoma	0.14
8. Vasospasm	0.13
C. Aneurysmal Rupture Producing Intraventricular Hemorrhage	
91 cases, 1982, mortality during initial admission[77]	
1. Size of ventricles	0.56
2. Systolic blood pressure	0.38
3. Age	0.37
4. Diastolic blood pressure	0.32
5. Grade on admission	0.31
6. Associated intracerebral clot	0.17
7. Location of aneurysm	0.15
8. Location of clot	0.11

*Numbers in each series are only relative within the series.

an aneurysm. Weir, in a study of 100 consecutive patients, found that 16 percent developed cystitis and 9 percent developed vaginitis.[123] Three percent showed evidence of gram-negative septicemia or fungal superinfection.

Pulmonary Complications

Among the most dramatic and dangerous acute complications of aneurysm rupture is pulmonary edema. Of 141 patients with fatal aneurysm rupture, 13 percent showed clinical evidence of this entity.[123] All patients had shown sudden onset of coma and virtually instantaneous onset of breathing difficulties. Respirations were irregular, and pink foam issued from the airways. Skin was cyanotic,

TABLE 214-12 Medical Complications of Aneurysm Rupture as Percent of 3521 Cases

Cardiovascular			
Hypertension	16.4	12.4	18.3
Arrhythmia	2.4	2.4	3.6
Hypotension	1.4	2.3	3.0
Cardiac failure	1.2	1.6	2.0
Angina	0.7	0.4	0.6
Myocardial infarct	0.6	0.4	0.7
Thrombophlebitis	0.6	1.7	1.4
Respiratory			
Pneumonia	2.9	5.7	7.0
Atelectasis	1.2	2.3	2.3
Adult respiratory distress syndrome	0.9	1.8	2.0
Asthma	0.8	1.0	1.2
Pulmonary edema	0.7	1.2	1.7
Pulmonary embolism	0.2	0.6	0.8
Endocrine			
Inappropriate ADH secretion	1.9	2.7	3.6
Metabolic			
Diabetes mellitus	1.6	1.8	2.2
Gastrointestinal			
Hemorrhage	1.3	3.2	3.7
Hepatic failure	0.4	1.6	1.9
Hepatitis	0.1	1.0	1.1
Renal			
Failure	0.9	1.2	1.4
Hematologic			
Anemia	1.9	5.5	4.9
Bleeding disorder	0.4	0.9	1.0

Source: Data from Kassell et al.[56]

moist, and cool. These patients tended to be young. The treatment of the pulmonary problem is intubation, artificial ventilation with positive end-expiratory pressure, and furosemide (Lasix; Hoechst-Roussel Pharmaceuticals Inc., Somerville, NJ).

Fluid and Electrolyte Disturbances

In a review of Suzuki's 1000 surgically treated aneurysms, hyponatremia (<130 meq Na/liter) occurred in 4 percent of cases, hypernatremia (>155 meq Na/liter) in 2.1 percent, both disorders in 1 percent, and polyuria in 0.7 percent.[114] These abnormalities occurred with aneurysms of the anterior communicating artery more commonly than with aneurysms at all other sites combined. The death rate associated with hypernatremia was 43 percent; with diabetes insipidus 25 percent; and with hyponatremia 15 percent, compared with the overall death rate of 6 percent. The abnormalities reached a peak (20 percent) between the third and seventh day after the last hemorrhage. Patients coming to autopsy showed hypothalamic hemorrhage.

Other authors have reported that hyponatremia is more common after subarachnoid hemorrhage, occurring in 25 to 34 percent of patients.[24,80,130] Hyponatremia after subarachnoid hemorrhage has usually been attributed to SIADH. Fluid restriction used to treat hyponatremia and SIADH is associated with an increased risk of neurological deterioration and cerebral infarction.[130] The classic features of SIADH are serum sodium < 135 meq/liter, serum osmolality < 280 mosmol/kg, urinary sodium > 25 meq/liter, and a urine osmolality greater than the plasma osmolality. The urinary sodium wasting must not be due to renal or adrenal disease, and there should be absent peripheral edema and dehydration and a poor response to hypertonic saline infusion.

It is now believed that hyponatremia after subarachnoid hemorrhage is not always due to SIADH. In contrast to mild volume expansion that occurs in SIADH, many patients with subarachnoid hemorrhage are volume-depleted and exhibit negative sodium balance.[24,80,130] Several studies have found significant decreases in red blood cell volume and total circulating blood volume in patients with subarachnoid hemorrhage.[80] Reasons for volume contraction include bed rest, supine diuresis, pooling in the peripheral vascular beds, negative nitrogen balance, decreased erythropoiesis, and iatrogenic blood loss. Identification of atrial natriuretic factors and data showing that these peptides are elevated in plasma after subarachnoid hemorrhage provide evidence that cerebral salt wasting occurs commonly after subarachnoid hemorrhage and may be the basis for natriuresis and volume depletion.[24] There is a complex and variable interaction of atrial natriuretic factors, antidiuretic hormone, renin, aldosterone, and catecholamines after subarachnoid hemorrhage, which will determine the sodium and water balance in any particular patient. In general, however, hyponatremia after subarachnoid hemorrhage should not be treated with volume restriction.

Diabetes insipidus is uncommon after aneurysmal rupture. When urinary output exceeds fluid intake or when absolute urine volume is in excess of 3 liters/day, diabetes insipidus should be suspected.[100] The urinary specific gravity is <1.005, urine osmolality is between 50 and 150 mosmol/kg, and serum sodium levels are usually normal or increased. Treatment consists of maintaining accurate fluid balance. Fluid intake should be almost solely dextrose and water solutions. Aqueous vasopressin is the preferred treatment in the early stages. Frequent, accurate monitoring of body weight and electrolyte levels is essential.

Cardiovascular Complications

In 15 series involving 256 patients with subarachnoid hemorrhage, electrocardiographic abnormalities occurred in at least 50 percent of patients and included T-wave abnormalities (47 percent), Q-T prolongation (37 percent), ST segment changes (30 percent), prominent U waves (25 percent), and rhythm disturbances (35 percent).[123] The basis of the changes is thought to be subendocardial ischemia, hemorrhages, and focal areas of myocardial necrosis due to increases in sympathetic tone and norepinephrine levels. The significance of the changes is uncertain, and one review concluded that use of sympathetic blockers had not altered outcome after subarachnoid hemorrhage.[123]

Serial electrocardiographic monitoring was carried out in 61 patients with subarachnoid hemorrhage.[13] All patients had at least one abnormal electrocardiogram, although cardiac disease did not directly contribute to morbidity or mortality. Sinus bradycardia, ST segment changes, ischemic T waves, and prominent U waves each occurred in up to 50 percent of patients. The effect of these changes on myocardial function has been infrequently studied. Davies and colleagues did electro- and echocardiography on 35 subarachnoid hemorrhage patients.[22] All patients with abnormal echocardiograms had abnormal electrocardiograms, although there was no relationship between severity of the electrocardiogram changes and myocardial dysfunction on echocardiogram. Myocardial dysfunction was most closely related to the neurological grade on the Botterell scale.

Neurological Complications of Aneurysmal Rupture

The neurological complications of aneurysmal rupture represent an infinite spectrum of brain dysfunction. In the cooperative timing study, focal ischemic neurological deficits occurred in 28 percent, hydrocephalus in 13 percent, recurrent subarachnoid hemorrhage and brain swelling in 11 percent each, intracerebral hematoma in 8 percent, and seizures in 4.5 percent. Overall causes of death and disability were almost all neurological (Table 214-13).[56,57]

Intracranial Pressure Elevations

Nornes and Magnaes recorded extradural pressure from nine patients during a subarachnoid hemorrhage.[83] In massive hemorrhage, there was an instantaneous rise in intracranial pressure with a leveling off at levels approaching the systemic blood pressure, which was associated with death. A second type was characterized by an instantaneous rise followed by a rapid fall to a level higher than the initial level, frequently followed by a lower secondary rise. Subsequently, it was noted that 77 percent of the hemorrhages started when the intracranial pressure was below 29 mmHg. Most hemorrhages arrested at or below the diastolic blood pressure. At the height of the hemorrhage, the forward flow in the carotid artery was arrested at the end of diastole but continued during systole; 1 or 2 min following the peak of the hemorrhage, diastolic blood pressure averaged 111 mmHg, and intracranial pressure averaged 128 mmHg.[82]

Intraventricular pressure in 52 cases of aneurysmal rupture was measured for a mean of 8 days each.[118] The ventricles were drained if pressure was greater than 25 mmHg for more than 30 min. Patients in clinical grades I and II had a mean intraventricular pressure of 10 mmHg; in grades II and III, 18 mmHg; and in grades III and IV, 29 mmHg. All patients who improved clinically had progressive reductions in their intraventricular pressure. Of 16 who deteriorated, 44 percent showed a progressive increase in intraventricular pressure. At angiography patients with no vasospasm had a mean intraventricular pressure of 16 mmHg, whereas those with severe vasospasm had a mean level of 27 mmHg. Eighteen patients with a mean intraventricular pressure greater than 25 mmHg had a 77 percent mortality rate; of 34 patients with a mean intraventricular pressure below 25 mmHg, only 26 percent died. B waves were recorded persistently at all intraventricular pressure

TABLE 214-13 Causes of Death and Disability in 3521 Patients Admitted within 3 Days of Aneurysmal Subarachnoid Hemorrhage and Assessed 6 Months after Hemorrhage*

Cause	Death	Disability	Total
Direct effect of primary hemorrhage	7.0	3.6	10.6
Vasospasm	7.2	6.3	13.5
Rebleeding	6.7	0.8	7.5
Hydrocephalus	0.3	1.4	1.7
Intracerebral hemorrhage	1.0	1.0	2.0
Complications of intracranial surgery	1.7	2.3	4.0
Other	2.0	1.2	3.2

*Disability includes moderate disability, severe disability, and vegetative state on the Glasgow outcome scale. Numbers are percent of 3521 patients developing death or disability due to the particular cause, from Kassell et al.[56]

levels. These are 1/s waves (range 0.5 to 2/s) with an amplitude of under 50 mmHg. A waves (plateau waves) were extremely rare or absent in patients with aneurysmal rupture. In five cases CSF was drained during the rebleeding episode.[119] The steady-state intraventricular pressure level after the repeat rupture was significantly increased in comparison with that of patients in whom CSF was not drained during the rupture. Four of five such patients died with large intracerebral hemorrhages. The usual profile for intracranial pressure changes based on their seven cases of observed ruptures without drainage was as follows: initial intracranial pressure, 18 mmHg, peaked at 2½ min to 95 mmHg; in another 3 min it fell to 40 mmHg, and in another 5 min to 22 mmHg. At peak, the intracranial pressure was 10 to 15 mmHg greater than diastolic blood pressure.

Many authors have noted clinical improvement coincident with ventricular drainage and reduction of elevated intracranial pressure. Continuous ventricular drainage to a level of 15 mmHg in 88 patients produced marked clinical improvement.[108] A reduction in intracranial pressure in cases of acute subarachnoid hemorrhage resulted in an increase in cerebral blood flow if the intracranial pressure had been initially elevated.[45]

Increased intracranial pressure after subarachnoid or intraventricular hemorrhage is usually due to an increase in CSF outflow resistance. In 17 patients with subarachnoid hemorrhage, intracranial pressure was elevated in all cases at some time.[62] Resistance to outflow of CSF was increased in all patients to 11.5 to 85 mmHg/ml per minute. Presumably, erythrocytes and fibrin debris from hemorrhage into the subarachnoid space acutely block the arachnoid villi, the main site of egress of the CSF. Late hydrocephalus is probably due to a fibrotic obliteration of CSF pathways at many points.

Hydrocephalus

Table 214-14 reviews some of the major series that have added to our understanding of hydrocephalus as it complicates aneurysmal rupture. Acute ventricular dilatation should be treated with external ventricular drainage as an emergency. The more insidious chronic hydrocephalus, if it is delaying full recovery or is associated with regression and neurological signs, should be treated with a ventriculoperitoneal shunt.

TABLE 214-14 Hydrocephalus Complicating Aneurysmal Rupture

1. All of 167 patients studied by computed tomographic (CT) scans were below 65 years of age and either never lost consciousness or regained it following subarachnoid hemorrhage; only 15 percent were grade 3, 4, or 5. Acute ventricular dilatation was associated with intraventricular clots in 35 percent of cases. Of 26 cases with early (<14 days after subarachnoid hemorrhage) ventricular dilatation, 35 percent showed progression, and surgery was carried out in 31 percent. Hydrocephalus developed in 10.5 percent of 210 cases in all types of subarachnoid hemorrhage after 2 weeks and was clinically significant in 7 percent. Indications for shunting were lack of improvement from a neurological plateau or deterioration with marked ventricular dilatation, periventricular lucencies, rounding of frontal horns, and obliteration of sulci.[117]
2. CT scans were used to study 91 patients with intraventricular hemorrhage. Of 54 having CT scan on same day as rupture, 85 percent had ventricular dilatation. The degree of dilatation was the most powerful preoperative indicator of mortality. Progressive chronic enlargement was more common in survivors than a spontaneous relapse to normal-size ventricles.[77]
3. Hydrocephalus was diagnosed at admission (within 3 days of ictus) in 15 percent of 3521 subarachnoid hemorrhage patients and was symptomatic in 13 percent. Using discriminate factor analysis to predict clinical hydrocephalus, the most important variables in order were the following: CT hydrocephalus, intraventricular hemorrhage, admission level of consciousness, pre-subarachnoid hemorrhage hypertension, increasing age, subarachnoid hemorrhage noted on CT scan, posterior circulation aneurysm, postoperative hypertension (canonical correlation = 0.399). Development of hydrocephalus was multifactorial. Patients treated with antifibrinolytic drugs and those with focal ischemic neurological deficit or hyponatremia were also at risk for hydrocephalus.[43]
4. Of 473 patients with aneurysmal subarachnoid hemorrhage, 19 percent had hydrocephalus on CT within 72 h of ictus. Hydrocephalus developed within 7 days in 11 more patients. Ventricular drainage was used in 31 percent of patients with acute hydrocephalus, resulting in improvement in consciousness in 78 percent. Rebleeding occurred significantly more often in 43 percent of patients with drainage, compared with only 15 percent of hydrocephalus patients without drainage and 20 percent of patients without hydrocephalus.[46]

Epilepsy

The problem of epilepsy after subarachnoid hemorrhage is reviewed in Table 214-15. It seems reasonable that most young patients with middle cerebral hematomas should be treated with anticonvulsants for at least 2 years following their aneurysmal rupture. Decisions about other patients should probably be individualized.

Psychiatric Complications of Aneurysmal Rupture

The most common psychiatric problems after aneurysmal rupture (Table 214-16) are intellectual impairment and depression. The psychiatric disability and the neurological deficits tend to go *pari passu*; however, the occasional patient can have a reactive depression out of proportion to the neurological dysfunction. Surgeons should be aware of this in order to obtain appropriate consultation.

The syndrome of disorientation and lethargy associated with damage to the small hypothalamic arteries leaving the posterior aspect of the anterior communicating artery has been described by Yaşargil.[135] His insistence on the careful preservation of these fine vessels will tend to reduce this complication.

Nonaneurysmal Subarachnoid Hemorrhage

Subarachnoid hemorrhage can be due to the rupture of any vascular structure that communicates in some fashion with the intracranial or intraspinal subarachnoid space. The ruptured vessel can be normal or pathologic. Numerous traumatic, infectious, neoplastic, toxic, inflammatory, and degenerative factors can induce the hemorrhage (Table 214-17). Trauma is the most common cause of

TABLE 214-15 Epilepsy Complicating Aneurysmal Rupture

1. Of 1009 cases, 1958–1962, with average follow-up of less than 5 years, 10.4 percent of patients developed epilepsy, according to clinic notes. A follow-up detailing examination and history of 61 cases showed a rate of 14.8 percent. Rate by decade: 3rd to 5th, 15.8 percent; 6th to 7th, 6.4 percent. Rate by location of aneurysm: middle cerebral artery, 25 percent; posterior communicating artery, 9 percent; anterior communicating artery, 2.5 percent. For cases with hematoma, 20 percent. The rate was not increased if a fit occurred at the time of aneurysm rupture. After aneurysm rupture, 72 percent of seizures began within 1 year, 94 percent within 2 years. No patients were on an adequate dosage of anticonvulsants at the time of first seizure.[95]
2. Of 152 patients operated upon 1945–1973 with a mean follow-up of 7 years, 22 percent developed epilepsy (28 percent rate for intracranial surgery, 5 percent for carotid ligation). Of those with a severe postoperative deficit, 50 percent developed epilepsy; of those with a mild or negligible deficit, 20 percent became epileptic. Of patients with middle cerebral aneurysm and moderate and severe neurological sequelae, 56 percent became epileptic. This was the highest-risk group.[15]
3. In 109 patients from neurological series, grade 1 to 3 only, with a follow-up time of 1½ to 5½ years, the only significant risk factor was younger age. Seizures developed 10 to 54 months postoperatively and occurred in 4.5 percent of patients. In four patients having seizures within less than 24 h, none developed late epilepsy. No patient was on anticonvulsants at the time of first seizure.[34]
4. Seizures occurred in 26 percent of 100 consecutive patients with ruptured aneurysm; 63 percent occurred near the onset of the first subarachnoid hemorrhage, and these early seizures were not related to aneurysm location or prognosis. Seizures with subarachnoid hemorrhage were usually brief, generalized, and associated with loss of consciousness and tonic posturing. No benefit was demonstrated for anticonvulsants during the acute phase after subarachnoid hemorrhage.[44]
5. In 100 consecutive survivors of surgery for ruptured aneurysm, three patients developed epilepsy. Prophylactic phenytoin did not decrease the risk of epilepsy. Five previous series involving 1772 patients who underwent intracranial operation recorded epilepsy after subarachnoid hemorrhage in 1 to 7 percent, similar to the rate in patients who had subarachnoid hemorrhage and were treated with carotid ligation (0 to 5 percent). Risk factors for epilepsy were intracerebral hematoma, resection of gyrus, medial temporal retraction, major postoperative deficit, middle cerebral artery aneurysm, and history of seizures.[98]

subarachnoid hemorrhage but, excluding this, the relative frequencies in one cooperative study were as follows: aneurysm 51 percent; AVM 6 percent; aneurysm and AVM 0.7 percent; and "other" causes 43 percent.[96] This latter group comprises hypertension and/or arteriosclerotic disease, 64 percent; brain tumors, 7 percent; endocarditis, 3 percent; anticoagulants, 3 percent; infections, 1 percent; and unknown, 22 percent. The latter category existed despite both angiographic and autopsy studies. The most important cause of fatal subarachnoid hemorrhage in cases not due to aneurysm or AVM is intracerebral hemorrhage associated with hypertension and arteriosclerotic disease in older persons. No particular tumor type in either primary or metastatic cases dominates the neoplasms with associated subarachnoid hemorrhage. Similarly, no specific infectious agents account for the majority of subarachnoid hemorrhages in this class.

TABLE 214-16 Psychiatric Illness after Aneurysmal Rupture

1. A study of 209 patients from 1958 to 1964, with a follow-up time of less than 3 years in 56 percent, revealed that 45 percent were normal, 24 percent had mild intellectual impairment, and 18 percent had moderate disability (could not do skilled work, had deteriorated personal relationships, showed severe depression); 10 percent showed severe disability (were unemployed, had markedly deteriorated family relationships, had personality damage, showed severe depression); 3 percent suffered from very severe disability (were demented, inaccessible, bedfast, grossly dysphasic).[107]
2. Of 203 patients with anterior cerebral artery aneurysms operated upon, 20 percent developed confusion, disorientation, dementia, and lethargy lasting days and rarely weeks; this was permanent in 4 percent of cases.[135]
3. Of 118 patients with apparently good neurological recovery, 40 were randomly subjected to neuropsychological tests an average of 3.5 years after aneurysmal subarachnoid hemorrhage. Slight to severe cognitive impairment persisted in 83 percent, as did social and personal disabilities. Casual assessment, however, might have classified the patients as having excellent or satisfactory recoveries.[67]
4. A group of 27 patients with repaired ruptured anterior communicating artery aneurysms were subjected to neuropsychological testing 12 to 84 months postoperatively. Preoperative clinical grades were 1 to 3. Three subgroups of patients were identified: those with persuasive cognitive deficits (six patients), those with residual frontal lobe damage (8 patients), and those with normal function (11 patients). Vasospasm was the most consistent predictor of long-term cognitive deficit.[106]

TABLE 214-17 Causes of Subarachnoid Hemorrhage Excluding Arteriovenous Malformations*

Angiopathy: atherosclerosis, hypertension, intra-arterial embolism, congophilic angiopathy (amyloid angiopathy), lupus angiitis, lupus erythematosus, giant cell arteritis, amyloidosis, focal vascular necrosis, polyarteritis nodosa, telangiectasia, Sturge-Weber syndrome

Venous thrombosis: pregnancy, oral contraceptives, trauma, infection, coagulopathy, marasmus, volume depletion

Blood diseases: leukemia, hemophilia, sickle cell anemia, pernicious anemia, aplastic anemia, agranulocytosis, thrombocytopenic purpura, polycythemia vera, Waldenström's macroglobulinemia, lymphoma, myeloma, hereditary spherocytosis, afibrinogenemia, hypofibrinogenemia (liver disease), consumption coagulopathy, disseminated intravascular coagulation, Hodgkin's disease, anticoagulants

Allergic diseases: anaphylactoid purpura, hemorrhagic nephritis, Shwartzman phenomenon, Henoch-Schönlein purpura

Infections: bacterial meningitis, tuberculous meningitis, syphilitic meningoencephalitis, fungal meningitis, leptospirosis, listeriosus, brucellosis, yellow fever, typhoid fever, dengue, malaria, anthrax, viral encephalitis (herpes simplex, influenza), cytomegalovirus inclusion disease, parasites (gnathostomiasis)

Intoxications: epinephrine, monoamine oxidase inhibitors, amphetamines, alcohol, ether, carbon monoxide, morphine, nicotine, lead, quinine, phosphorus, pentylenetetrazol, hydrocyanic acid, insulin, snake venom

Tumors: glioma, meningioma, hemangioblastoma, choroid plexus papilloma, chordoma, hemangioma, pituitary adenoma, sarcoma, osteochondroma, ependymoma, subependymoma, neurofibroma, bronchogenic carcinoma, choriocarcinoma, melanoma

Trauma: blows, electrical injury, electroconvulsive therapy, high altitude, caisson disease, radiation, strangulation, heat injury

Pediatric causes: germinal matrix hemorrhage

Miscellaneous: uremia, sunstroke, scurvy, Valsalva maneuver, vitamin K deficiency, hyperbilirubinemia, electrolyte imbalance, eclampsia

*From Weir[123]

Negative Workup for Aneurysm as a Cause of Subarachnoid Hemorrhage

With modern four-vessel angiography, subtraction, magnification, multiple projections, injection of external carotid arteries, and attention to lesions in the spinal canal as a possible source of subarachnoid hemorrhage, the proportion of patients who have a negative workup should be smaller than in previous decades. In five series reported between 1986 and 1989, a source of subarachnoid hemorrhage could not be identified in between 3.8 and 30 percent of patients.[42] This topic is discussed in detail in another chapter.

Workup of Patients Suspected of Having Recent Aneurysmal Rupture

Patients suspected of recent aneurysmal rupture should be admitted rapidly to a neurosurgical service experienced in their care. Intensive care measures should be instituted for those who are in very poor neurological condition with respiratory distress, and CT scanning should then be carried out immediately. Lumbar puncture is performed if the CT scan does not show unequivocal evidence of abnormal blood collections. Complete angiographic workup should be performed as soon as possible if the CT scan or lumbar puncture shows evidence of hemorrhage. There is no advantage in delaying the definitive investigation. At present, magnetic resonance angiography remains investigational, although it may be of more value to the workup of subarachnoid hemorrhage in the future.

References

1. Andrews RJ, Spiegel PK. Intracranial aneurysms: age, sex, blood pressure, and multiplicity in an unselected series of patients. *J Neurosurg* 1979; 51:27–32.
2. Artiola-Fortuny L, Prieto-Valiente L. Long-term prognosis in surgically treated intracranial aneurysms: Part 1. Mortality. *J Neurosurg* 1981; 54:26–34.
3. Bamford J, Sandercock P, Dennis M, et al. A prospective study of acute cerebrovascular disease in the community: the Oxfordshire Community Stroke Project—1981–86. 2. Incidence, case fatality rates and overall outcome at one year of cerebral infarction, primary intracerebral and subarachnoid haemorrhage. *J Neurol Neurosurg Psychiatry* 1990; 53:16–22.
4. Bannerman RM, Ingall GB, Graf CJ. The familial occurrence of intracranial aneurysms. *Neurology* 1970; 20:283–292.
5. Bassi P, Bandera R, Loiero M, et al. Warning signs in subarachnoid hemorrhage: a cooperative study. *Acta Neurol Scand* 1991; 84:277–281.
6. Batjer H, Suss RA, Samson D. Intracranial arteriovenous malformations associated with aneurysms. *Neurosurgery* 1986; 18:29–35.
7. Battaglia R, Pasqualin A, Da Pian R. Italian cooperative study on giant intracranial aneurysms: 1. Study design and clinical data. *Acta Neurochir Suppl (Wien)* 1988; 42:49–52.
8. Bell BA, Symon L. Smoking and subarachnoid haemorrhage. *Br Med J* 1979; 1:577–578.
9. ter Berg HWM, Dippel DWJ, Limburg M, et al. Familial intracranial aneurysms. A review. *Stroke* 1992; 23:1024–1030.
10. Bonita R. Cigarette smoking, hypertension and the risk of subarachnoid hemorrhage: a population-based case-control study. *Stroke* 1986; 17:831–835.
11. Botterell EH, Lougheed WM, Scott JW, Vandewater SL. Hypothermia, and interruption of carotid, or carotid and vertebral circulation, in the surgical management of intracranial aneurysms. *J Neurosurg* 1956; 13:1–42.
12. Broderick JP, Brott T, Tomsick T, et al. The risk of subarachnoid and intracerebral hemorrhage in blacks as compared with whites. *N Engl J Med* 1992; 326:733–736.
13. Brouwers PJAM, Wijdicks EFM, Hasan D, et al. Serial electrocardiographic recording in aneurysmal subarachnoid hemorrhage. *Stroke* 1989; 20:1162–1167.
14. Bull J. History of computed tomography. In Newton TH, Potts DG (eds): *Radiology of the Skull and Brain,* vol 5. *Technical Aspects of Computed Tomography.* St Louis: Mosby, 1981, pp 3835–3849.
15. Cabral RJ, King TT, Scott DF. Epilepsy after two different neurosurgical approaches to the treatment of ruptured intracranial aneurysm. *J Neurol Neurosurg Psychiatry* 1976; 39:1052–1056.
16. Campbell GJ, Roach MR. Fenestrations in the internal elastic lamina at bifurcations of human cerebral arteries. *Stroke* 1981; 12:489–496.
17. Chapman AB, Rubinstein D, Hughes R, et al. Intracranial aneurysms in autosomal dominant polycystic kidney disease. *N Engl J Med* 1992; 327:916–920.
18. Chason JL, Hindman WM. Berry aneurysms of the circle of Willis: results of a planned autopsy study. *Neurology* 1958; 8:41–44.
19. Crompton MR. Mechanism of growth and rupture in cerebral berry aneurysms. *Br Med J* 1966; 1:1138–1142.
20. Crompton MR. The pathogenesis of cerebral aneurysms. *Brain* 1966; 89:797–814.
21. Dandy WE. Intracranial aneurysm of the internal carotid artery: cured by operation. *Ann Surg* 1938; 107:654–659.
22. Davies KR, Gelb AW, Manninen PH, et al. Cardiac function in aneurysmal subarachnoid haemorrhage: a study of electrocardiographic and echocardiographic abnormalities. *Br J Anaesth* 1991; 67:58–63.
23. Dell S. Asymptomatic cerebral aneurysm: assessment of its risk of rupture. *Neurosurgery* 1982; 10:162–166.
24. Diringer MN, Wu KC, Verbalis JG, Hanley DF. Hypervolemic therapy prevents volume contraction but not hyponatremia following subarachnoid hemorrhage. *Ann Neurol* 1992; 31:543–550.
25. Disney L, Weir B, Grace M, Canadian Nimodipine Study Group. Factors influencing the outcome of aneurysm rupture in poor grade patients: a prospective series. *Neurosurgery* 1988; 23:1–9.
26. Dott NM. Intracranial aneurysms: cerebral arterio-radiography: surgical treatment. *Edinburgh Med J* 1933; 40:219–240.
27. Drake CG. Giant intracranial aneurysms: experience with surgical treatment in 174 patients. *Clin Neurosurg* 1979; 26:12–95.
28. Drake CG. Management of cerebral aneurysm. *Stroke* 1981; 12:273–283.
29. Drake CG, Hunt WE, Kassell N, et al. Report of World Federation of Neurological Surgeons Committee on a universal subarachnoid hemorrhage grading scale. *J Neurosurg* 1988; 68:985–986 (letter).
30. Dyste GN, Beck DW. De novo aneurysm formation following carotid ligation: case report and review of the literature. *Neurosurgery* 1989; 24:88–92.
31. Eller TW. MRI demonstration of clot in a small unruptured aneurysm causing stroke. Case report. *J Neurosurg* 1986; 65:411–412.
32. Epstein, F, Ransohoff J, Budzilovich GN. The clinical significance of junctional dilatation of the posterior communicating artery. *J Neurosurg* 1970; 33:529–531.
33. Eskesen V, Rosenorn J, Schmidt K. The influence of unruptured intracranial aneurysms on life expectancy in relation to their size at the time of detection and to age. *Br J Neurosurg* 1988; 2:379–384.
34. Fabinyi GCA, Artiola-Fortuny L. Epilepsy after craniotomy for intracranial aneurysm. *Lancet* 1980; 1:1299–1300.
35. Ferguson GG. Physical factors in the initiation, growth, and rupture of human intracranial saccular aneurysms. *J Neurosurg* 1972; 37:666–667.
36. Fields WS, Weibel J. Coincidental internal carotid stenosis and intracranial saccular aneurysm. *Trans Am Neurol Assoc* 1970; 95:237–238.

37. Forbus WD. On the origin of miliary aneurysms of the superficial cerebral arteries. *Bull Johns Hopkins Hosp* 1930; 47:239–284.
38. Fox JL. *Intracranial Aneurysms.* New York: Springer-Verlag, 1983.
39. Freytag E. Fatal rupture of intracranial aneurysms: survey of 250 medicolegal cases. *Arch Pathol* 1966; 81:418–424.
40. George AE, Lin JP, Morantz RA. Intracranial aneurysm on a persistent primitive trigeminal artery: case report. *J Neurosurg* 1971; 35:601–604.
41. Glynn LE. Medical defects in the circle of Willis and their relation to aneurysm formation. *J Pathol* 1940; 51:213–222.
42. Gomez PA, Lobato RD, Rivas JJ, et al. Subarachnoid haemorrhage of unknown aetiology. *Acta Neurochir (Wien)* 1989; 101:35–41.
43. Graff-Radford NR, Torner J, Adams HP Jr, Kassell NF. Factors associated with hydrocephalus after subarachnoid hemorrhage. A report of the Cooperative Aneurysm Study. *Arch Neurol* 1989; 46:744–752.
44. Hart RG, Byer JA, Slaughter JR, et al. Occurrence and implications of seizures in subarachnoid hemorrhage due to ruptured intracranial aneurysms. *Neurosurgery* 1981; 8:417–421.
45. Hartmann A, Alberti E, Lange D. Effects of CSF-drainage on CBF and CBV in subarachnoid hemorrhage and communicating hydrocephalus. *Acta Neurol Scand [Suppl]* 1977; 64:336–337.
46. Hasan D, Vermeulen M, Wijdicks EFM, et al. Management problems in acute hydrocephalus after subarachnoid hemorrhage. *Stroke* 1989; 20:747–753.
47. Hashimoto N, Handa H, Nagata I, Hazama F. Experimentally induced cerebral aneurysms in rats. V. Relation of hemodynamics in the circle of Willis to formation of aneurysms. *Surg Neurol* 1980; 13:41–45.
48. Hassler O. Experimental carotid ligation followed by aneurysmal formation and other morphological changes in the circle of Willis. *J Neurosurg* 1963; 20:1–7.
49. Heiskanen O. Risk of bleeding from unruptured aneurysms in cases with multiple intracranial aneurysms. *J Neurosurg* 1981; 55:524–526.
50. Hillbom M, Kaste M. Does alcohol intoxication precipitate aneurysmal subarachnoid haemorrhage? *J Neurol Neurosurg Psychiatry* 1981; 44:523–526.
51. Hunt WE, Hess RM. Surgical risk as related to time of intervention in the repair of intracranial aneurysms. *J Neurosurg* 1968; 28:14–20.
52. Inagawa T, Ishikawa S, Aoki H, et al. Aneurysmal subarachnoid hemorrhage in Izumo City and Shimane Prefecture of Japan. Incidence. *Stroke* 1988; 19:170–175.
53. Ingall TJ, Whisnant JP, Wiebers DO, O'Fallon WM. Has there been a decline in subarachnoid hemorrhage mortality? *Stroke* 1989; 20:718–724.
54. Jacobson JH II, Wallman LJ, Schumacher GA, et al. Microsurgery as an aid to middle cerebral endarterectomy. *J Neurosurg* 1962; 19:108–114.
55. Jellinger K. Pathology and aetiology of intracranial aneurysms. In Pia HW, Langmaid C, Zierski J (eds): *Cerebral Aneurysms. Advances in Diagnosis and Therapy.* New York: Springer, 1979, pp 5–19.
56. Kassell NF, Torner JC, Haley EC Jr, et al. The International Cooperative Study on the Timing of Aneurysm Surgery. Part 1: Overall management results. *J Neurosurg* 1990; 73:18–36.
57. Kassell NF, Torner JC, Jane JA, et al. The International Cooperative Study on the Timing of Aneurysm Surgery. Part 2: Surgical results *J Neurosurg* 1990; 73:37–47.
58. Keller AZ. Hypertension, age and residence in the survival with subarachnoid hemorrhage. *Am J Epidemiol* 1970; 91:139–147.
59. Kim C, Kikuchi H, Hashimoto N, Hazama F. Histopathological study of induced cerebral aneurysms in primates. *Surg Neurol* 1989; 32:45–50.
60. Kobayashi H, Hayashi M, Kawano H, et al. Magnetic resonance imaging of embolism from intracranial aneurysms. *Surg Neurol* 1989; 32:225–230.
61. Koenig GH, Marshall WH Jr, Poole GJ, Kramer RA. Rupture of intracranial aneurysms during cerebral angiography: report of ten cases and review of the literature. *Neurosurgery* 1979; 5:314–324.
62. Kosteljanetz M. CSF dynamics in patients with subarachnoid and/or intraventricular hemorrhage. *J Neurosurg* 1984; 60:940–946.
63. Laun A, Tonn JC. Cranial nerve lesions following subarachnoid hemorrhage and aneurysm of the circle of Willis. *Neurosurg Rev* 1988; 11:137–141.
64. Leblanc R. The minor leak preceding subarachnoid hemorrhage. *J Neurosurg* 1987; 66:35–39.
65. Leblanc R, Lozano AM, van der Rest M, Guttmann RD. Absence of collagen deficiency in familial cerebral aneurysms. *J Neurosurg* 1989; 70:837–840.
66. Lindsay KW, Teasdale GM, Knill-Jones RP. Observer variability in assessing the clinical features of subarachnoid hemorrhage. *J Neurosurg* 1983; 58:57–62.
67. Ljunggren B, Sonesson B, Saveland H, Brandt L. Cognitive impairment and adjustment in patients without neurologic deficits after aneurysmal SAH and early operation. *J Neurosurg* 1985; 62:673–679.
68. Longstreth WT Jr, Koepsell TD, Yerby MS, van Belle G. Risk factors for subarachnoid hemorrhage. *Stroke* 1985; 16:377–385.
69. Lougheed WM. Selection, timing, and technique of aneurysm surgery of the anterior circle of Willis. *Clin Neurosurg* 1968; 16:95–113.
70. Lozano AM, Leblanc R. Familial intracranial aneurysms. *J Neurosurg* 1987; 66:522–528.
71. Lundberg N. Continuous recording and control of ventricular fluid pressure in neurosurgical practice. *Acta Psychiatr Scand (Suppl)* 1960; 149:1–193.
72. Mayfield FH, Kees G Jr. A brief history of the development of the Mayfield clip: technical note. *J Neurosurg* 1971; 35:97–100.
73. McCormick WF, Acosta-Rua GJ. The size of intracranial saccular aneurysms: an autopsy study. *J Neurosurg* 1970; 33:422–427.
74. McCormick WF, Schmalstieg EJ. The relationship of arterial hypertension to intracranial aneurysms. *Arch Neurol* 1977; 34:285–287.
75. Meyer FB, Sundt TM Jr, Fode NC, et al. Cerebral aneurysms in childhood and adolescence. *J Neurosurg* 1989; 70:420–425.
76. Miyasaka K, Wolpert SM, Prager RJ. The association of cerebral aneurysms, infundibula, and intracranial arteriovenous malformations. *Stroke* 1982; 13:196–203.
77. Mohr G, Ferguson G, Khan M, et al. Intraventricular hemorrhage from ruptured aneurysm: retrospective analysis of 91 cases. *J Neurosurg* 1983; 58:482–487.
78. Moniz E. Anévrysme intra-cranien de la carotide interne droite rendu visible par l'artériographie cérébrale. *Rev Otoneuroophthalmol* 1933; 11:746–748.
79. Nehls DG, Flom RA, Carter LP, Spetzler RF. Multiple intracranial aneurysms: determining the site of rupture. *J Neurosurg* 1985; 63:342–348.
80. Nelson RJ. Blood volume measurement following subarachnoid hemorrhage. *Acta Neurochir (Wien) [Suppl]* 1990; 47:114–121.
81. Nibbelink DW, Torner JC, Henderson WG. Antifibrinolytic therapy in recent onset subarachnoid hemorrhage. In Sahs AL, Nibbelink DW, Torner JC (eds): *Aneurysmal Subarachnoid Hemorrhage: Report of the Cooperative Study.* Baltimore: Urban & Schwarzenberg, 1981, pp 297–306.
82. Nornes H. The role of intracranial pressure in the arrest of hemorrhage in patients with ruptured intracranial aneurysm. *J Neurosurg* 1973; 39:226–234.
83. Nornes H, Magnaes B. Intracranial pressure in patients with ruptured saccular aneurysm. *J Neurosurg* 1972; 36:537–547.
84. Norrgard O, Angquist KA, Fodstad H, et al. Intracranial aneurysms and heredity. *Neurosurgery* 1987; 20:236–239.
85. Okamoto S, Handa H, Hashimoto N. Location of intracranial aneurysms associated with cerebral arteriovenous malformation: statistical analysis. *Surg Neurol* 1984; 22:335–340.
86. Okawara S. Warning signs prior to rupture of an intracranial aneurysm. *J Neurosurg* 1973; 38:575–580.
87. Ostergaard JR, Hog E. Incidence of multiple intracranial aneurysms. Influence of arterial hypertension and gender. *J Neurosurg* 1985; 63:49–55.
88. Ostergaard JR, Oxlund H. Collagen type III deficiency in patients with rupture of intracranial saccular aneurysms. *J Neurosurg* 1987; 67:690–696.

89. Pakarinen S. Incidence, aetiology, and prognosis of primary subarachnoid haemorrhage: a study based on 589 cases diagnosed in a defined urban population during a defined period. *Acta Neurol Scand [Suppl]* 1967; 29:1–128.
90. Parenti G, Fiori L, Marconi F. Intracranial aneurysm and cerebral embolism. *Eur Neurol* 1992; 32:212–215.
91. Patel AN, Richardson AE. Ruptured intracranial aneurysms in the first two decades of life: a study of 68 patients. *J Neurosurg* 1971; 35:571–576.
92. Phillips LH II, Whisnant JP, O'Fallon WM, Sundt TM Jr. The unchanging pattern of subarachnoid hemorrhage in a community. *Neurology (NY)* 1980; 30:1034–1040.
93. Rhoton AL Jr. Anatomy of saccular aneurysms. *Surg Neurol* 1980; 14:59–66.
94. Roach MR. A model study of why some intracranial aneurysms thrombose but others rupture. *Stroke* 1978; 9:583–587.
95. Rose FC, Sarner M. Epilepsy after ruptured intracranial aneurysm. *Br Med J* 1965; 1:18–21.
96. Sahs AL, Perret GE, Locksley HB, Nishioka H (eds). *Intracranial Aneurysms and Subarachnoid Hemorrhage: A Cooperative Study.* Philadelphia: Lippincott, 1969.
97. Sarner M, Rose FC. Clinical presentation of ruptured intracranial aneurysm. *J Neurol Neurosurg Psychiatry* 1967; 30:67–70.
98. Sbeih I, Tamas LB, O'Laoire SA. Epilepsy after operation for aneurysms. *Neurosurgery* 1986; 19:784–788.
99. Servo A. Agenesis of the left internal carotid artery associated with an aneurysm on the right carotid syphon: case report. *J Neurosurg* 1977; 46:677–680.
100. Shucart WA, Jackson I. Management of diabetes insipidus in neurosurgical patients. *J Neurosurg* 1976; 44:65–71.
101. Stehbens WE. *Pathology of the Cerebral Blood Vessels.* St Louis: Mosby, 1972, pp 351–470.
102. Stehbens WE. Ultrastructure of aneurysms. *Arch Neurol* 1975; 32:798–807.
103. Stehbens WE: Etiology of intracranial berry aneurysms. *J Neurosurg* 1989; 70:823–831.
104. Steiger HJ. Pathophysiology of development and rupture of cerebral aneurysms. *Acta Neurochir Suppl (Wien)* 1990; 48:1–57.
105. Steinberger A, Ganti SR, McMurty JG III, Hilal SK. Transient neurological deficits secondary to saccular vertebrobasilar aneurysms. Report of two cases. *J Neurosurg* 1984; 60:410–413.
106. Stenhouse LM, Knight RG, Longmore BE, Bishara SN. Long-term cognitive deficits in patients after surgery on aneurysms of the anterior communicating artery. *J Neurol Neurosurg Psychiatry* 1991; 54:909–914.
107. Storey PB. Psychiatric sequelae of subarachnoid haemorrhage. *Br Med J* 1967; 3:261–266.
108. Sundbärg G, Pontén U. ICP and CSF absorption impairment after subarachnoid hemorrhage. In Beks JWF, Bosch DA, Brock M (eds): *Intracranial Pressure III.* Berlin: Springer, 1976, pp 139–146.
109. Sundt TM Jr. Cerebral vasospasm following subarachnoid hemorrhage: evolution, management, and relationship to timing of surgery. *Clin Neurosurg* 1977; 24:228–247.
110. Suzuki J. Multiple aneurysms: treatment. In Pia HW, Langmaid C, Zierski J (eds): *Cerebral Aneurysms: Advances in Diagnosis and Therapy.* Berlin: Springer, 1979, pp 352–363.
111. Suzuki J, Ohara H. Clinicopathological study of cerebral aneurysms: origin, rupture, repair, and growth. *J Neurosurg* 1978; 48:505–514.
112. Suzuki J, Onuma T, Yoshimoto T. Results of early operations on cerebral aneurysms. *Surg Neurol* 1979; 11:407–412.
113. Suzuki J, Yoshimoto T. Distribution of cerebral aneurysms. In Pia HW, Langmaid C, Zierski J (eds): *Cerebral Aneurysms: Advances in Diagnosis and Therapy.* Berlin: Springer, 1979, pp 127–133.
114. Takaku A, Shindo K, Tanaka S, et al. Fluid and electrolyte disturbances in patients with intracranial aneurysms. *Surg Neurol* 1979; 11:349–356.
115. Takeshita M, Izawa M, Kubo, et al. Aspergillotic aneurysm formation of cerebral artery following neurosurgical operation. *Surg Neurol* 1992; 38:146–151.
116. Torner JC, Kassell NF, Wallace RB, Adams HP Jr. Preoperative prognostic factors for rebleeding and survival in aneurysm patients receiving antifibrinolytic therapy: report of the Cooperative Aneurysm Study. *Neurosurgery* 1981; 9:506–513.
117. Vassilouthis J, Richardson AE. Ventricular dilatation and communicating hydrocephalus following spontaneous subarachnoid hemorrhage. *J Neurosurg* 1979; 51:341–351.
118. Voldby B, Enevoldsen EM. Intracranial pressure changes following aneurysm rupture: 1. Clinical and angiographic correlations. *J Neurosurg* 1982; 56:186–196.
119. Voldby B, Enevoldsen EM. Intracranial pressure changes following aneurysm rupture: 3. Recurrent hemorrhage. *J Neurosurg* 1982; 56:784–789.
120. Waga S, Morikawa A. Aneurysm developing on the infundibular widening of the posterior communicating artery. *Surg Neurol* 1979; 11:125–127.
121. Waga S, Okada M, Kojima T. Saccular aneurysm associated with absence of the left cervical carotid arteries. *Neurosurgery* 1978; 3:208–212.
122. Wakai S, Fukushima T, Furihata T, Sano K. Association of cerebral aneurysm with pituitary adenoma. *Surg Neurol* 1979; 12:503–507.
123. Weir B. *Aneurysms Affecting the Nervous System.* Baltimore: Williams & Wilkins, 1987.
124. Weir B. Pituitary tumors and aneurysms: case report and review of the literature. *Neurosurgery* 1992; 30:585–591.
125. Weir B, Aronyk K. Management mortality and the timing of surgery for supratentorial aneurysms. *J Neurosurg* 1981; 54:146–150.
126. Weir B, Aronyk K. Management and postoperative mortality related to time of clipping for supratentorial aneurysms: a personal series. *Acta Neurochir (Wien)* 1982; 63:135–139.
127. Weir B, Rothberg C, Grace M, Davis F. Relative prognostic significance of vasospasm after subarachnoid hemorrhage. *Can J Neurol Sci* 1975; 2:109–114.
128. Wheelock B, Weir B, Watts R, et al. Timing of surgery for intracerebral hematomas due to aneurysm rupture. *J Neurosurg* 1983; 58:476–481.
129. Wiebers DO, Whisnant JP, O'Fallon WM. The natural history of unruptured intracranial aneurysms. *N Engl J Med* 1981; 304:696–698.
130. Wijdicks EFM, Ropper AH, Hunnicutt EJ, et al. Atrial natriuretic factor and salt wasting after aneurysmal subarachnoid hemorrhage. *Stroke* 1991; 22:1519–1524.
131. Wilson G, Riggs HE, Rupp C. Pathological anatomy of ruptured cerebral aneurysms. *J Neurosurg* 1954; 11:128–142.
132. Winn HR, Almaani WS, Berga SL, et al. The long-term outcome in patients with multiple aneurysms. Incidence of late hemorrhage and implications for treatment of incidental aneurysms. *J Neurosurg* 1983; 59:642–651.
133. Winn HR, Richardson AE, Jane JA. The assessment of the natural history of single cerebral aneurysms that have ruptured. In Hopkins LN, Long DM (eds): *Clinical Management of Intracranial Aneurysms.* New York: Raven Press, 1982, pp 1–10.
134. Wood EH. Angiographic identification of the ruptured lesion in patients with multiple cerebral aneurysms. *J Neurosurg* 1964; 21:182–198.
135. Yaşargil MG. *Microneurosurgery,* vol 2. *Clinical Considerations, Surgery of the Intracranial Aneurysms, and Results.* Stuttgart: Thieme Verlag, 1984.

215 Microsurgical Anatomy of Saccular Aneurysms

Albert L. Rhoton, Jr.

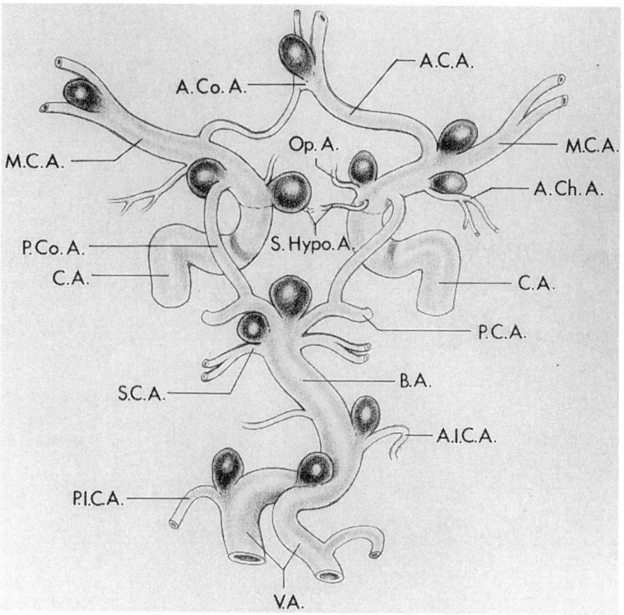

Figure 215-1 Most common sites of saccular intracranial aneurysms. Each aneurysm arises from the branching site of a large artery. Most are located on or near the circle of Willis. Over 90 percent are located at one of the following five sites: (1) the internal carotid artery (C.A.) at the level of the posterior communicating artery (P.Co.A.); (2) the junction of the anterior cerebral (A.C.A.) and anterior communicating (A.Co.A) arteries; (3) the proximal bifurcation of the middle cerebral artery (M.C.A.); (4) the junction of the basilar (B.A.) and posterior cerebral (P.C.A.) arteries; and (5) the bifurcation of the carotid artery into the anterior cerebral and middle cerebral arteries. Other aneurysm sites on the carotid artery are at the origins of the ophthalmic (Op.A.), superior hypophyseal (S.Hypo.A.), and anterior choroidal (A.Ch.A.) arteries. Other sites on the vertebral (V.A.) and basilar arteries include the sites of origin of the posterior inferior cerebellar (P.I.C.A.), the anterior inferior cerebellar (A.I.C.A.), and the superior cerebellar (S.C.A.) arteries and the junction of the vertebral and basilar arteries.

Basic Anatomic Principles

Three aspects of the anatomy of saccular aneurysms should be considered when planning the operative approach to these lesions.[9] These three aspects will be reviewed in relation to each of the common aneurysm sites.

First, these aneurysms arise at a branching site on the parent artery. This site may be formed either by the origin of a side branch from the parent artery, such as the origin of the posterior communicating artery from the internal carotid artery, or by subdivision of a main arterial trunk into two trunks, as occurs at the bifurcation of the middle cerebral artery. The operative approach should be planned so as to protect the flow through these branching sites, which seem to be a part of the basic substrate essential to the formation of a saccular aneurysm (Fig. 215-1).

Second, saccular aneurysms arise at a turn or curve in the artery. These curves, by producing local alterations in intravascular hemodynamics, exert unusual stresses on apical regions, which receive the greatest force of the pulse wave. The sites of the curves associated with the common intracranial aneurysms are reviewed in the discussion that follows.

Third, saccular aneurysms point in the direction that the blood would have gone if the curve at the aneurysm site were not present. The aneurysm dome or fundus points in the direction of the maximal hemodynamic thrust in the preaneurysmal segment of the parent artery. The operation to obliterate an aneurysm should be designed to allow the surgeon to control and reduce the hemodynamic thrust in the parent artery until after the aneurysm is obliterated. As a saccular aneurysm enlarges, it may encounter obstacles that change the direction of growth from that based solely on the direction of the maximal hemodynamic thrust.

Aneurysms are infrequently encountered on a straight, nonbranching segment of an intracranial artery. The aneurysms occurring on straight, nonbranching segments are more often found to have sacs that point longitudinally along the wall of the artery in the direction of blood flow and project only minimally above the adventitial surface. Aneurysms having these characteristics are of a dissecting type rather than of the congenital saccular type, and their development is heralded more frequently by the onset of ischemic neurological deficits than by the subarachnoid hemorrhage associated with congenital saccular aneurysms. It is rare to find an aneurysm on the concave side of an arterial curve or to find one that points in a direction opposite to that of the flow in the parent artery.

Internal Carotid Artery Aneurysms

These three facets of anatomy as they apply to aneurysm sites on the supraclinoid portion of the internal carotid artery are discussed first.[2,10] These aneurysms arise at five sites (Figs. 215-2 and 215-3): the upper surface of the internal carotid artery at the origin of the ophthalmic artery, the medial wall at the origin of the superior hypophyseal artery, the posterior wall near the origin of the posterior communicating artery, the posterior wall at the origin of the anterior choroidal artery, and the apex of the carotid artery bifurcation into the anterior and middle cerebral arteries.

An aneurysm at the carotid-ophthalmic artery junction arises from the superior wall of the carotid artery distal to the origin of the ophthalmic artery immediately above the roof of the cavernous

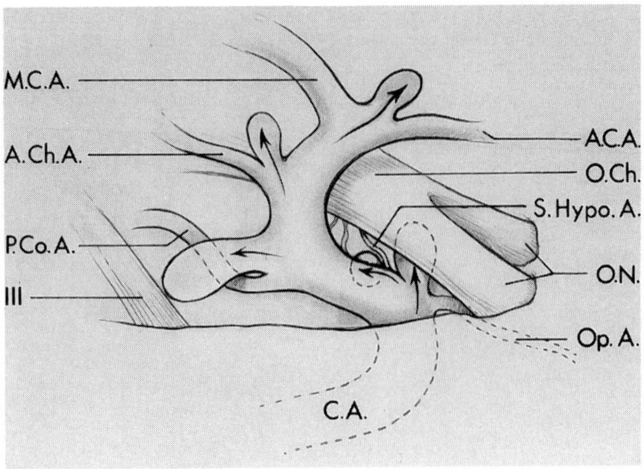

(*A*)

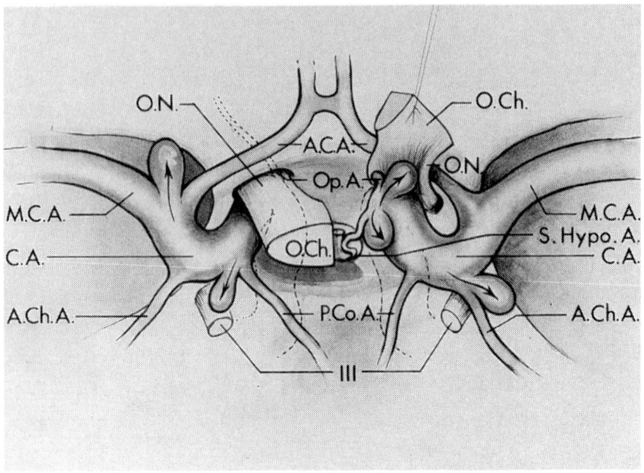

(*B*)

Figure 215-2 Lateral (*A*) and superior (*B*) views of common aneurysm sites on the supraclinoid portion of the internal carotid artery. *A*. Lateral view of the right internal carotid artery. *B*. Superior view of the internal carotid arteries, with the right optic nerve and right half of the optic chiasm reflected forward to expose the origin of the ophthalmic artery. The intracavernous portion of both carotid arteries and the course of the left ophthalmic artery are shown by dotted lines. The aneurysms arise on curves in the artery at the site of origin of its branches. The aneurysms point in the direction (*arrows*) of the maximal hemodynamic force immediately proximal to the aneurysm site and in the direction the blood would have gone if there were no curve at the aneurysm site. The aneurysm sites on the internal carotid artery (C.A.) are usually located immediately distal to the origins of its branches. Aneursyms arising at the origin of the ophthalmic artery (Op.A.) point upward into the optic nerve (O.N.). Aneurysms arising at the origin of the superior hypophyseal artery (S.Hypo.A.) point medially under the optic chiasm. Aneurysms arising near the origin of the posterior communicating artery (P.Co.A) point posteriorly toward the oculomotor nerve (III) and are usually located superolateral to the posterior communicating artery. Aneurysms arising near the origin of the anterior choroidal artery (A.Ch.A) point posterolaterally and are usually located immediately superior to the origin of the anterior choroidal artery. Aneurysms arising at the carotid bifurcation into the anterior (A.C.A.) and middle (M.C.A.) cerebral arteries point upward lateral to the optic chiasm (O.Ch.) toward the anterior perforated substance.

sinus where the superiorly directed intracavernous segment turns posteriorly. At this turn, the maximal hemodynamic thrust is directed toward the superior wall of the carotid artery just distal to the ophthalmic artery, and the aneurysm projects upward toward and eventually against the optic nerve (Figs. 215-2 and 215-3).

The segment of the carotid artery just distal to the origin of the ophthalmic artery has a medially convex curve as the artery passes backward in the area lateral to the pituitary stalk. The superior hypophyseal artery arises on this medially convex curve. The aneurysm arising at the carotid–superior hypophyseal junction arises from the medial wall of the carotid artery just distal to the origin of the superior hypophyseal artery and points medially into the area between the diaphragma sellae and the lower surface of the optic chiasm (Figs. 215-2 and 215-3). The next segment of the carotid artery after the origin of the superior hypophyseal artery turns upward toward the anterior perforated substance to form a curve which is posteriorly convex. The posterior communicating and anterior choroidal arteries arise from the posterior wall on this convex curve as the carotid artery passes upward toward its bifurcation (Figs. 215-2 and 215-3). An aneurysm at the carotid–posterior communicating artery junction usually arises from the posterior wall of the carotid artery near the apex of this turn immediately above the level of the origin of the posterior communicating artery. The aneurysm points posteriorly toward the oculomotor nerve. The posterior communicating artery is usually found on the inferomedial side of the aneurysm. The anterior choroidal artery is located superior or superolateral to the aneurysm arising at the level of the posterior communicating artery. The apex of the posteriorly convex curve may also be located at the level of origin of the anterior choroidal artery, which shifts the hemodynamic force distally from the level of origin of the posterior communicating artery to that of the anterior choroidal artery. An aneurysm arising at the level of the anterior choroidal artery is usually located superior or superolateral to the origin of the anterior choroidal artery (Figs. 215-2 and 215-3).

The aneurysm arising at the terminal bifurcation of the internal carotid artery most easily fits these principles (Figs. 215-2 and 215-3). It arises at the level of the T-shaped bifurcation formed by the origin of the anterior and middle cerebral arteries and points upward in the direction of the long axis of the prebifurcation segment of the internal carotid artery.

Middle Cerebral Artery Aneurysms

Aneurysms arising on the middle cerebral artery also conform to these three anatomic precepts (Fig. 215-4).[1] They arise at the level of the bifurcation or trifurcation of the artery. The angulation with which the bifurcating trunks arise from the main trunk forms the turn or curve. These aneurysms usually point laterally in the direction of the long axis of the prebifurcation segment of the main trunk.

Anterior Cerebral Artery Aneurysms

The most common aneurysm site on the anterior cerebral artery is at the level of the anterior communicating artery (Fig. 215-5).[6] The aneurysm usually arises at the point where the dominant proximal or precommunicating segment bifurcates at the level of the anterior communicating artery to give rise to both distal segments. These aneurysms usually point away from the dominant proximal segment toward the opposite side. They may also project in other

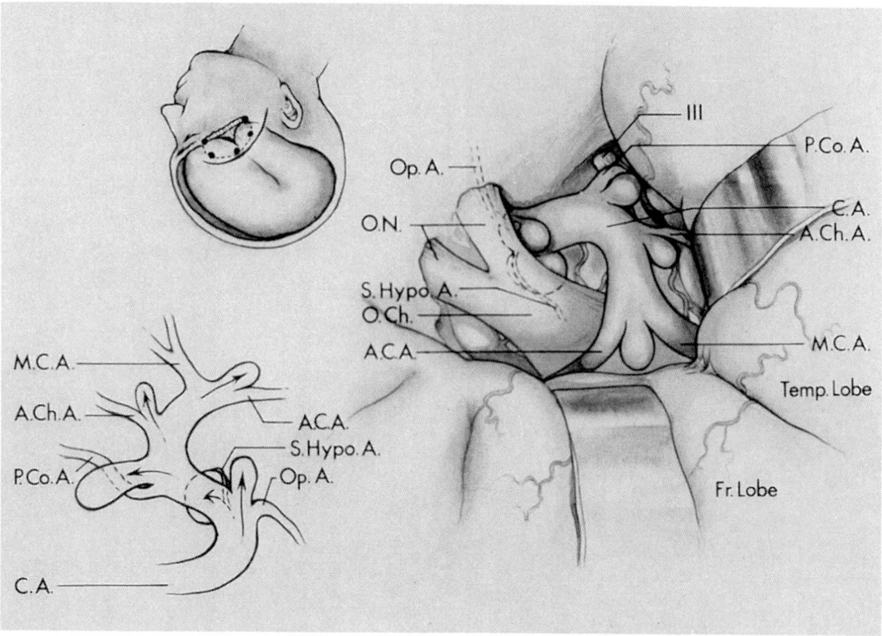

Figure 215-3 Operative view of common aneurysm sites on the supraclinoid portion of the internal carotid artery. *Upper left:* Head position, scalp incision (*solid line*), bone flap (*dotted line*), and craniectomy (*oblique lines*) used to approach internal carotid artery aneurysms. *Right:* Operative view provided by a right frontotemporal craniotomy with retractors on the frontal and temporal lobes. *Lower left:* Lateral view of the right internal carotid artery showing aneurysm sites. These aneurysms point in the direction (*arrows*) of the maximal hemodynamic force proximal to the aneurysm sites and in the direction the blood would have gone if there were no curve in the parent artery at the aneurysm site. The aneurysm sites on the internal carotid artery (C.A.) are usually located immediately distal to the origins of its branches. Aneurysms arising at the origin of the ophthalmic artery (Op.A.) point upward into the optic nerve (O.N.). Aneurysms arising at the origin of the superior hypophyseal artery (S.Hypo.A.) point medially under the optic chiasm (O. Ch.). Aneurysms arising near the origin of the posterior communicating artery (P.Co.A.) point posteriorly toward the oculomotor nerve (III) and are usually located superolateral to the posterior communicating artery. Aneurysms arising near the origin of the anterior choroidal artery (A.Ch.A.) point posterolaterally and are usually located immediately superior to the origin of the anterior choroidal artery. Aneurysms arising at the carotid bifurcation into the anterior (A.C.A.) and middle (M.C.A.) cerebral arteries point upward lateral to the optic chiasm toward the anterior perforated substance. Each of these aneurysms can be approached through a frontotemporal craniotomy.

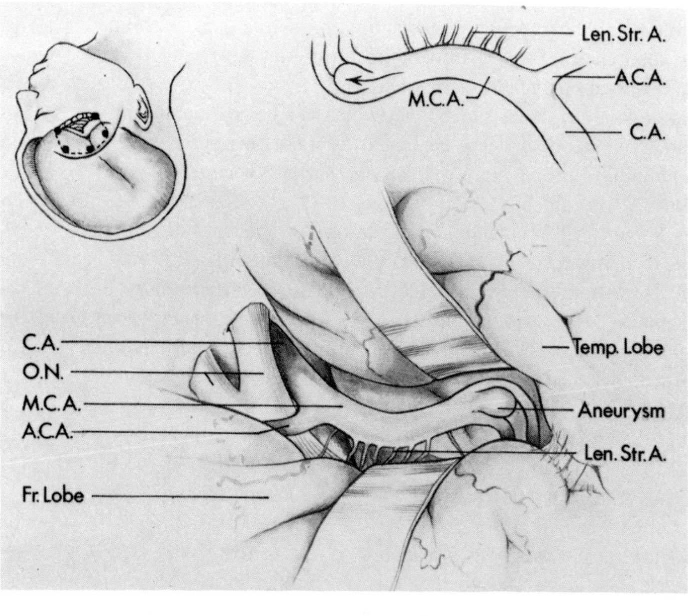

Figure 215-4 Middle cerebral artery aneurysm. *Upper right:* Anterior view of an aneurysm at the bifurcation of the right middle cerebral artery (M.C.A.). Aneurysms arising on the M.C.A. are usually located at the proximal bifurcation near the genu of the artery. The arrow shows the direction of hemodynamic force at the aneurysm site. *Upper left:* Head position, scalp incision (*solid line*), bone flap (*dotted line*), and craniectomy (*oblique lines*) for the approach to these aneurysms. *Lower center:* Operative view provided by a right frontotemporal craniotomy. The right sylvian fissure has been split to provide this view of the optic nerves (O.N.) and the carotid (C.A.) and anterior cerebral (A.C.A.) arteries. Retractors are on the temporal and frontal lobes. The lenticulostriate arteries (Len.Str.A.) arise proximal to the bifurcation of the M.C.A. and the aneurysm. (From Rhoton,[7] with permission.)

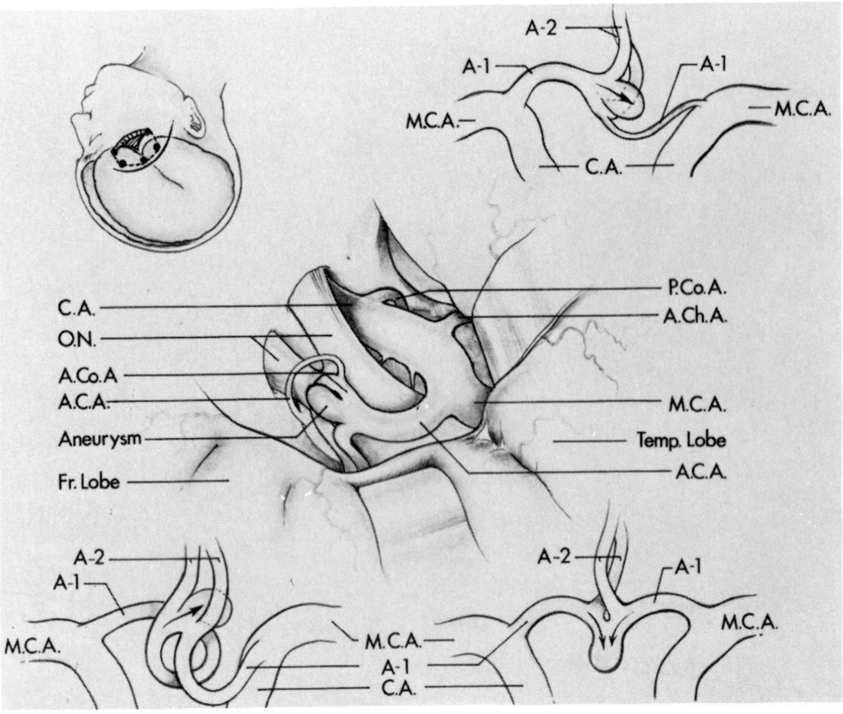

Figure 215-5 Anterior and operative views of anterior communicating artery aneurysms. *Upper right, lower right,* and *lower left:* Anterior views show three different aneurysm configurations created by the different hemodynamic forces (*arrows*) associated with the various sizes and shapes of proximal (A-1) and distal (A-2) segments of the anterior cerebral arteries. The most common configuration (*upper right*) is associated with a hypoplastic A-1 segment. Less common projections of these aneurysms are straight forward (*lower right*) or posterior (*lower left*). The direction in which the fundus points is determined by the course of the artery proximal to its junction with the anterior communicating artery. *Upper left and center:* Operative view of an anterior communicating artery aneurysm: scalp incision (*solid line*), bone flap (*dotted line*), and craniectomy (*oblique lines*). The aneurysm points downward and forward away from the dominant anterior cerebral artery. The anterior cerebral (A.C.A.) and anterior communicating (A.Co.A.) arteries are located above the optic nerve (O.N.) and optic chiasm. The carotid arteries (C.A.) also give rise to the middle cerebral (M.C.A.), posterior communicating (P.Co.A.), and anterior choroidal (A.Ch.A.) arteries. The retractors are on the frontal and temporal lobes. (From Rhoton,[7] with permission.)

directions. The direction in which the fundus points is determined by the course of the anterior cerebral arteries proximal to their junction with the anterior communicating artery. Tortuosity of the arteries may create a situation in which the hemodynamic thrust varies so that these aneurysms may project not only to the opposite side but also in the anterior, posterior, superior, or inferior direction.

The next most common aneurysm site on the anterior cerebral artery is at the level of origin of the callosomarginal artery from the pericallosal artery (Fig. 215-6). The curve is formed by the angulation of branching and the artery's passage around the rostrum of the corpus callosum. The aneurysm points distally into the interval between the junction of the pericallosal and callosomarginal arteries.

Vertebral and Basilar Artery Aneurysms

Aneurysms arising on the branches of the vertebral and basilar arteries also share the same three facets of anatomy: they arise at a branching site on a curve and point in the direction the blood would have followed if the curve were not present (Fig. 215-7). The basilar apex aneurysm arises at the branching of the posterior cerebral arteries from the basilar artery. The curve at the aneurysm site is related to the change from the vertical direction of the basilar artery to a lateral direction of the posterior cerebral arteries. These aneurysms project upward in the direction of the long axis of the basilar artery (Fig. 215-8*A*,*B*).

Aneurysms arising from the basilar artery at the level of origin of the superior cerebellar or anterior inferior cerebellar artery or from the vertebral artery at the level of origin of the posterior inferior cerebellar artery initially appear to conform poorly to the three facets of anatomy applicable to the other aneurysms because the basilar and vertebral arteries are often pictured as straight arteries, with the cerebellar arteries arising at right angles from them (Fig. 215-7).[9] Most of the arteries harboring aneurysms are tortuous, however, and the change in direction of flow associated with the curves creates hemodynamic stress on the wall of the basilar or vertebral arteries near the origins of the cerebellar arteries. These aneurysms point in the direction the blood would have gone had

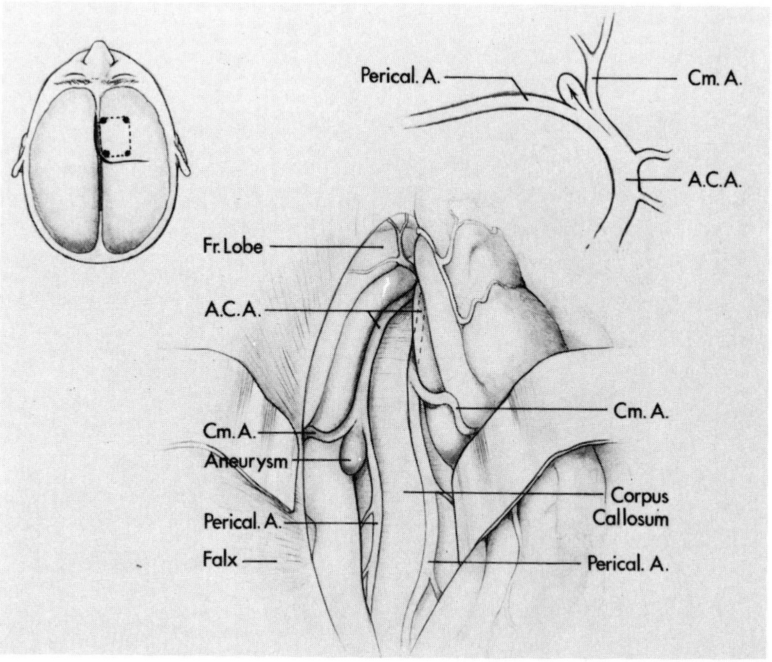

Figure 215-6 Lateral and operative views of the most common aneurysm site on the distal part of the anterior cerebral artery. *Upper right:* Medial surface of the right anterior cerebral artery. The aneurysm arises on the medial surface of the frontal lobe at the anterior margin of the corpus callosum. The hemodynamic thrust (*arrow*) and the aneurysm are directed distally in the interval between the pericallosal (Perical.A.) and callosomarginal (Cm.A.) arteries. *Upper left:* Scalp incision (*solid line*) and bone flap (*dotted line*). *Lower:* The right frontal lobe (Fr. Lobe) is retracted to expose the anterior cerebral arteries (A.C.A.), the falx, and the aneurysm arising above the corpus callosum at the origin of the callosomarginal and pericallosal arteries. (From Rhoton,[7] with permission.)

there not been a curve at the level of origin of the involved branch. For example, a basilar aneurysm at the level of the superior cerebellar artery often arises where there is a curvature and tilt of the upper basilar artery, so that the hemodynamic thrust created by flow along the basilar artery is just above the origin of the superior cerebellar artery rather than at the basilar apex (Fig. 215-8*C*).[3]

The aneurysm located at the origin of the anterior inferior cerebellar artery commonly arises from the convex side of the curve in the basilar artery and points in the direction of the long axis of the basilar segment immediately proximal to the aneurysm (Figs. 215-7 and 215-8*D*).[5]

The most common aneurysm site on the vertebral artery is at the level of origin of the posterior inferior cerebellar artery. The

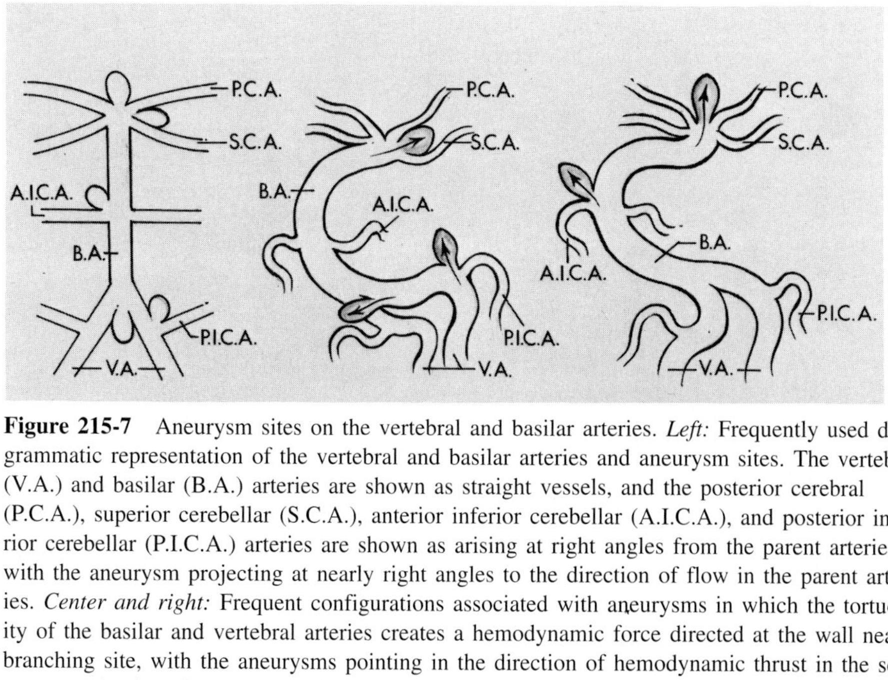

Figure 215-7 Aneurysm sites on the vertebral and basilar arteries. *Left:* Frequently used diagrammatic representation of the vertebral and basilar arteries and aneurysm sites. The vertebral (V.A.) and basilar (B.A.) arteries are shown as straight vessels, and the posterior cerebral (P.C.A.), superior cerebellar (S.C.A.), anterior inferior cerebellar (A.I.C.A.), and posterior inferior cerebellar (P.I.C.A.) arteries are shown as arising at right angles from the parent arteries, with the aneurysm projecting at nearly right angles to the direction of flow in the parent arteries. *Center and right:* Frequent configurations associated with aneurysms in which the tortuosity of the basilar and vertebral arteries creates a hemodynamic force directed at the wall near a branching site, with the aneurysms pointing in the direction of hemodynamic thrust in the segment proximal to the aneurysm site. The aneurysms of the vertebral artery arise at its junctions with the posterior inferior cerebellar and basilar arteries (*center*). The aneurysms of the basilar artery arise between the posterior cerebral and superior cerebellar arteries (*center*), at the basilar apex (*right*), and at the origin of the anterior inferior cerebellar artery (right). All point in the direction of the long axis of the preaneurysmal segment of the artery and in the direction of maximal hemodynamic thrust (*arrows*) at the aneurysm site. (From Rhoton,[7] with permission.)

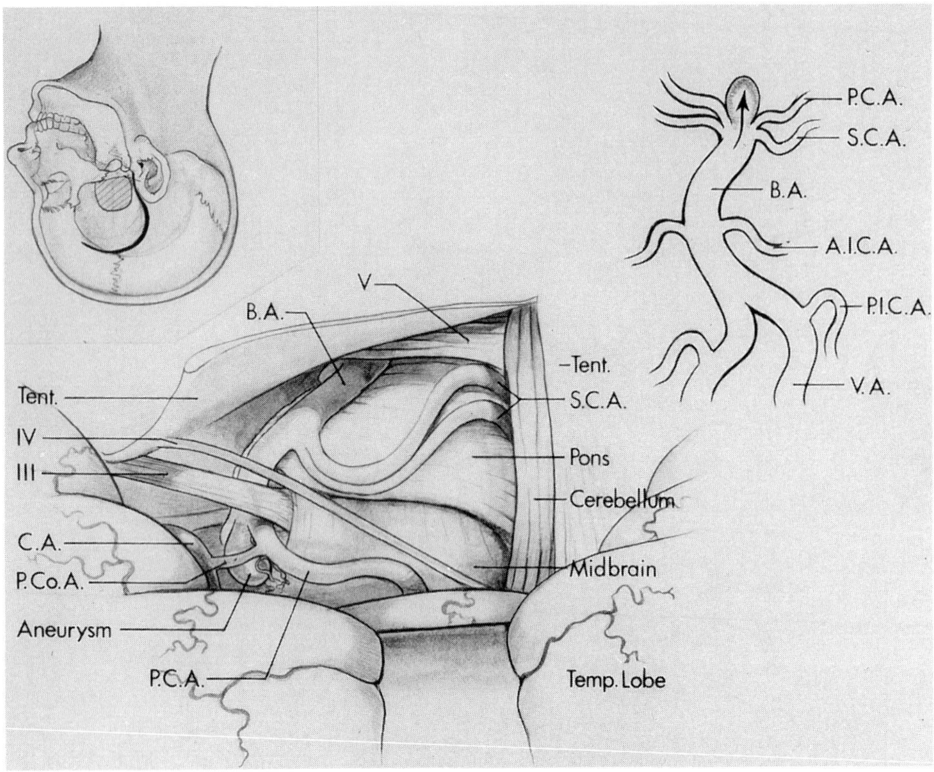

(*A*)

Figure 215-8 *A* to *E*. Common aneurysm sites in the posterior cranial fossa. Diagrams on the upper right show the basilar (B.A.), vertebral (V.A.), posterior cerebral (P.C.A.), superior cerebellar (S.C.A.), posterior inferior cerebellar (P.I.C.A.), and anterior inferior cerebellar (A.I.C.A.) arteries; the site of the aneurysm; and the direction of hemodynamic force (*arrow*) at the aneurysm site. Diagrams on the upper left show the scalp incision and bone flap or craniectomy used to expose the aneurysm.

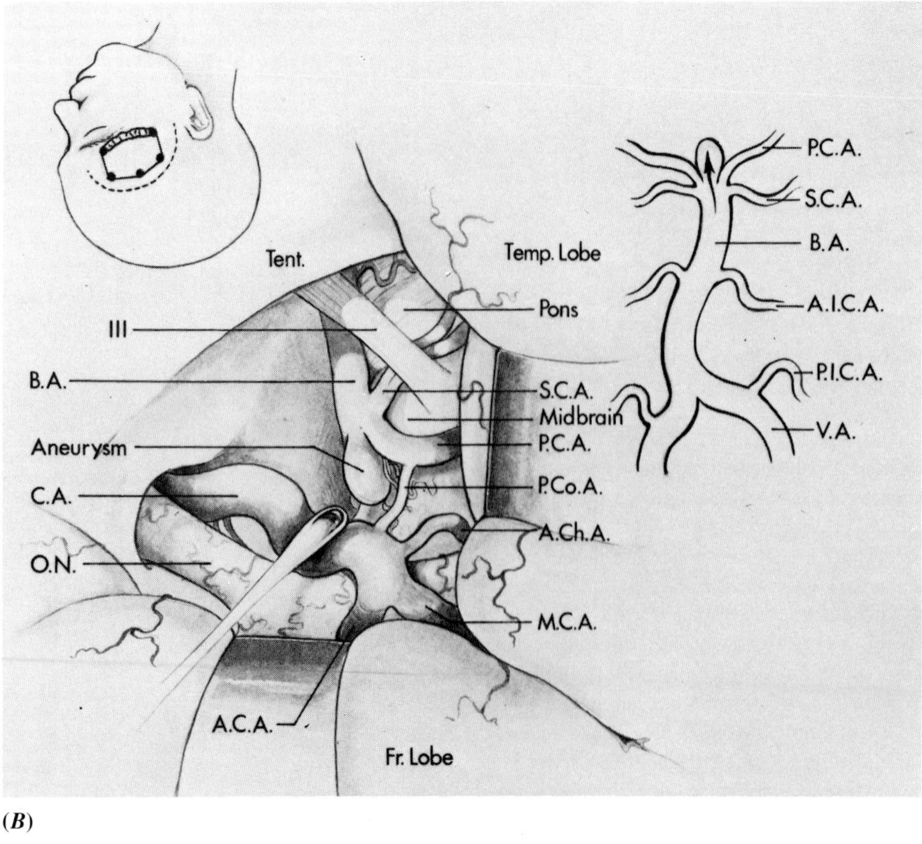

(*B*)

Figure 215-8 (*Continued*) *A*. A basilar apex aneurysm is shown arising at the origin of the posterior cerebral arteries as exposed by a right anterior subtemporal craniotomy. Note scalp incision and bone flap or craniectomy. The retractor is on the temporal lobe, and the tentorium cerebelli (Tent.) has been divided to expose the basilar, posterior cerebral, superior cerebellar, posterior communicating (P.Co.A.), and internal carotid (C.A.) arteries and the oculomotor (III), trochlear (IV), and trigeminal (V) nerves. *B*. A basilar apex aneurysm is exposed by a frontotemporal approach. The sylvian fissure has been split and the frontal and temporal lobes are retracted to expose the aneurysm. The middle cerebral (M.C.A.), anterior cerebral (A.C.A.), and anterior choroidal (A.Ch.A.) arteries and the optic nerves (O.N.) are also exposed. The carotid artery is retracted with a blunt dissector to expose the aneurysm.

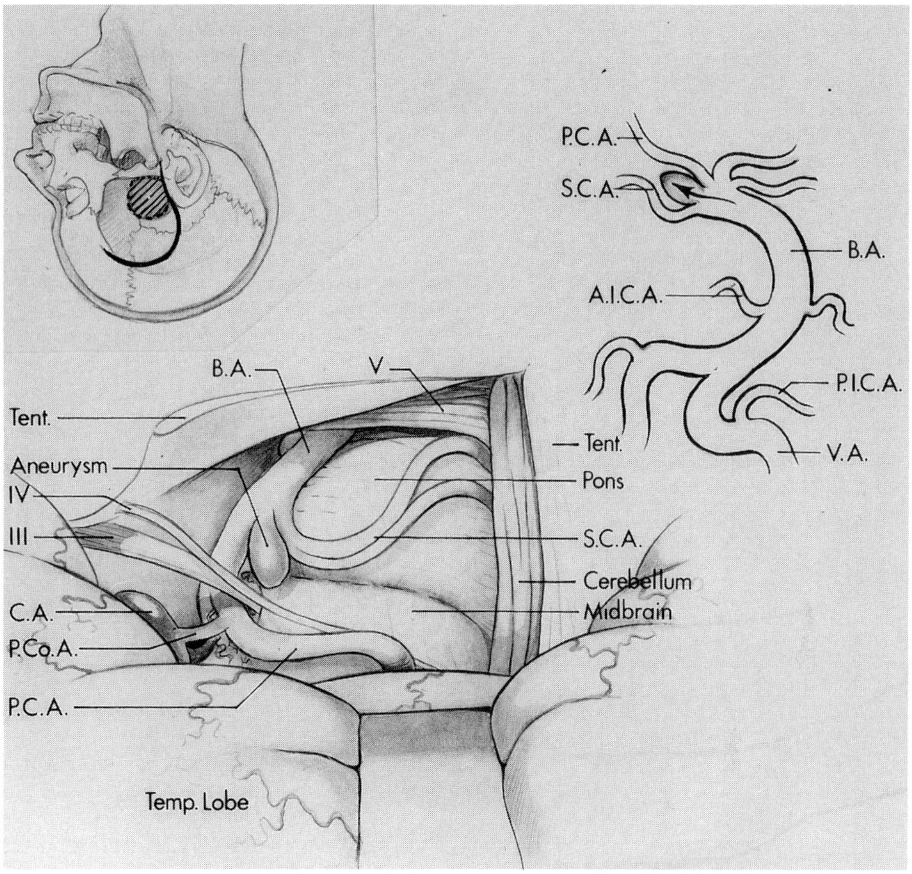

(*C*)

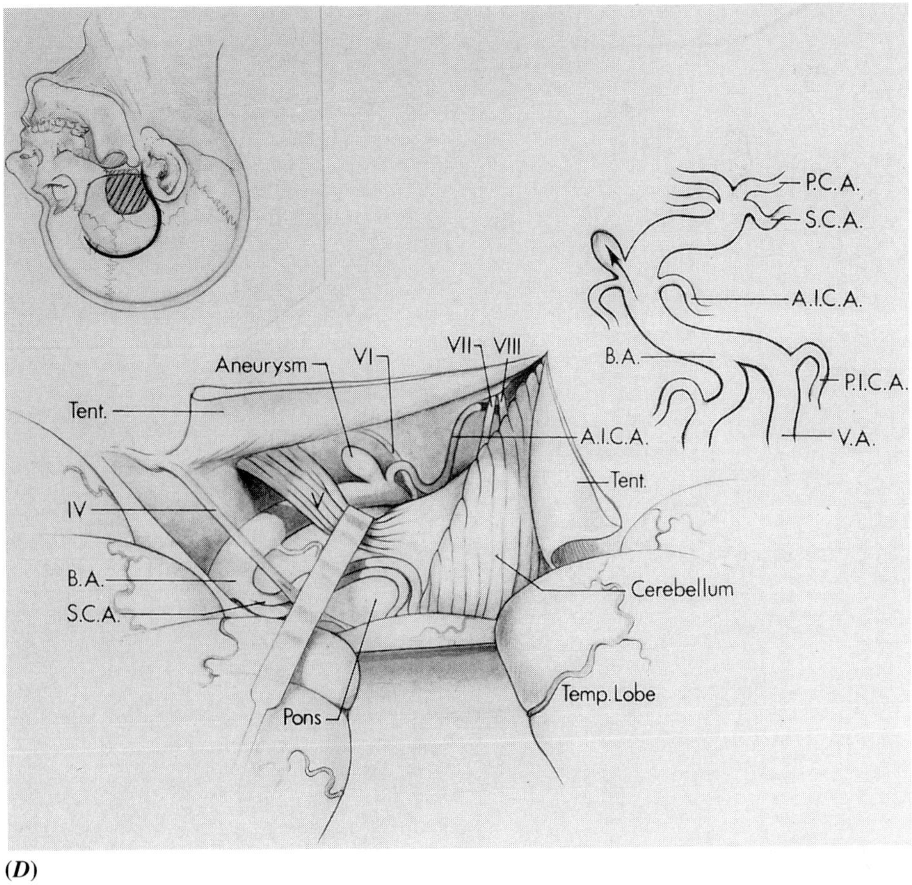

(*D*)

Figure 215-8 (*Continued*) *C.* Anterior subtemporal exposure of a basilar aneurysm arising between the origin of the superior cerebellar and posterior cerebral arteries. The basilar artery curvature creates a hemodynamic thrust (*arrow*) against the wall of the artery at the junction of the upper two branches of the basilar artery. The aneurysm projects laterally below or into the oculomotor nerve. *D.* Anterior subtemporal exposure of a basilar aneurysm arising at the origin of the anterior inferior cerebellar artery. The abducens nerve (VI) is below the anterior inferior cerebellar artery. The tentorium is split laterally above the trigeminal nerve to expose the facial (VII) and vestibulocochlear (VIII) nerves. The curvature of the basilar artery creates a hemodynamic thrust (*arrow*) against the wall of the artery at the junction of the basilar and anterior inferior cerebellar arteries.

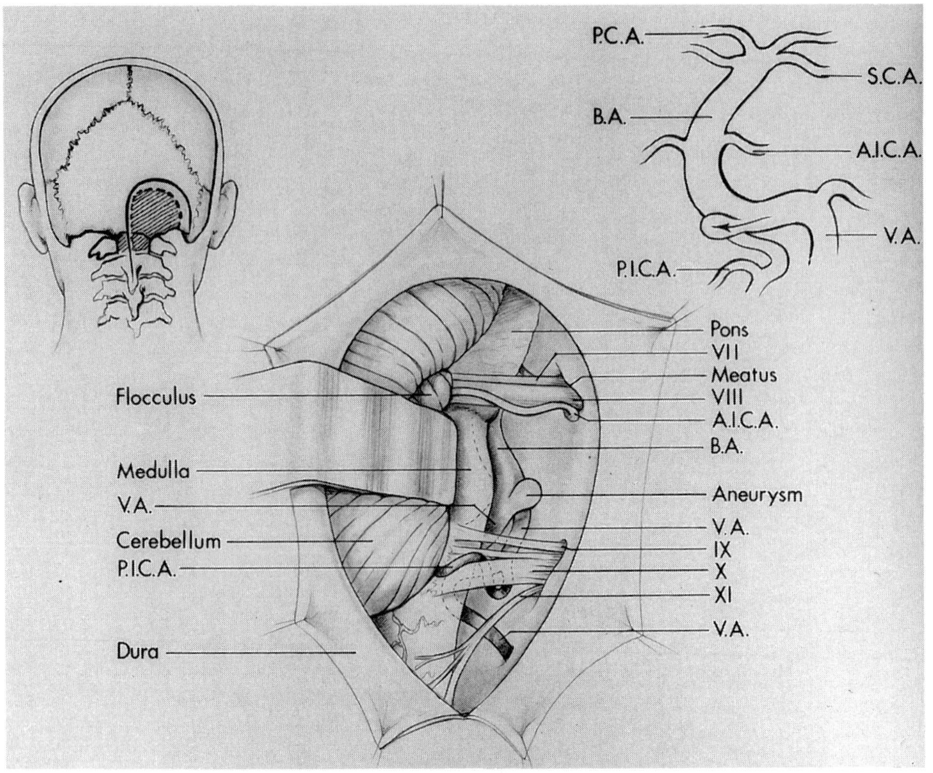

(*E*)

(*F*)

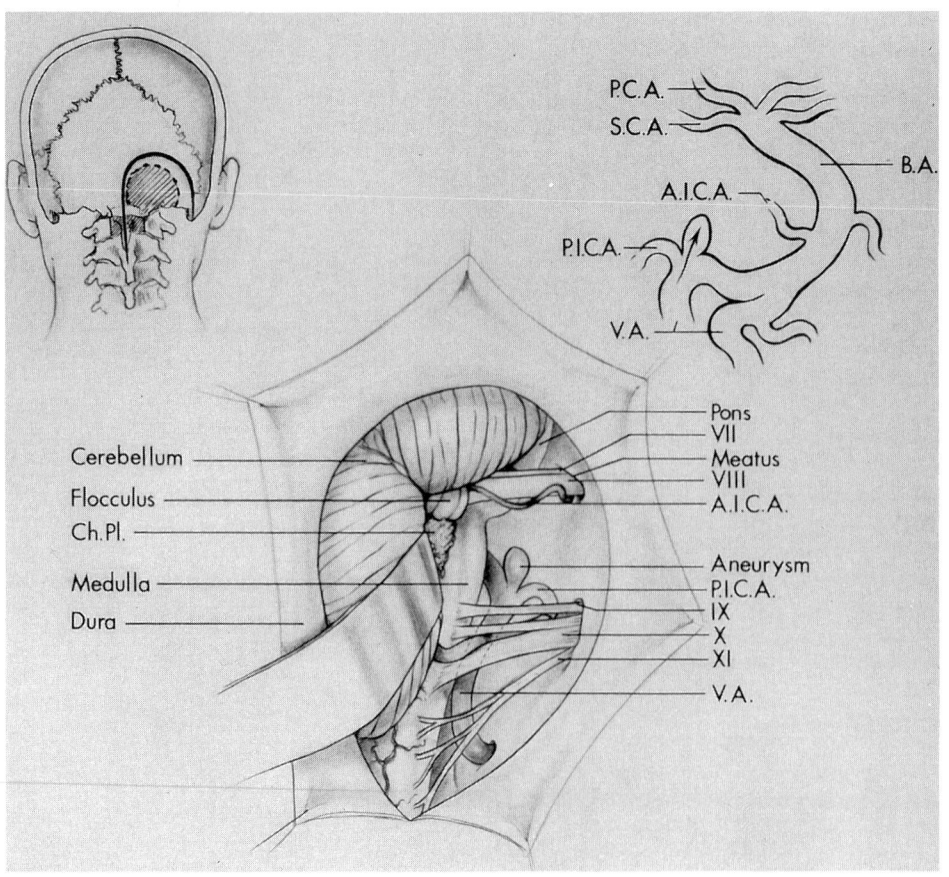

Figure 215-8 (*Continued*) *E.* Suboccipital exposure of an aneurysm arising at the junction of the vertebral and basilar arteries. The patient is in the sitting position. The right half of the cerebellum is retracted to expose the facial, vestibulocochlear, glossopharyngeal (IX), vagus (X), and spinal accessory (XI) nerves and the internal acoustic meatus. One of the vertebral arteries often joins the other in a configuration resembling the branching seen at other aneurysm sites. Angiographic views in multiple projections reveal the aneurysm pointing in the direction of flow in the preaneurysmal segment of the larger vertebral artery. *F.* Suboccipital exposure of an aneurysm arising at the origin of the right vertebral and posterior inferior cerebellar arteries. The angulation of the vertebral artery creates a hemodynamic thrust (*arrow*) in the direction in which the aneurysm points. The flocculus and choroid plexus (Ch.P1.) protrude into the cerebellopontine angle. (Part *B* from Rhoton,[7] with permission.)

vertebral artery is often depicted as being straight; however, if an aneurysm is present, the vertebral artery is often found to have a convex upward curve from the apex, where the posterior inferior cerebellar artery arises (Figs. 215-7 and 215-8*F*).[4] The aneurysm arises from the apex of this curve at the origin of the posterior inferior cerebellar artery and points upward.

Aneurysms arising infrequently at the junction of the two vertebral arteries with the basilar artery may initially seem difficult to fit into these precepts. When examined in multiple angiographic projections, however, they are often found to conform to these same anatomic principles applied in predicting the site and direction of projection of the more common saccular aneurysms. These aneurysms often arise on the convex side of a tortuous curve formed at the vertebrobasilar junction (Figs. 215-7 and 215-8*E*), and the junction of the two vertebral arteries with the basilar artery creates a configuration similar to the branching at other aneurysm sites. If this tortuous configuration is not present, it is likely that the aneurysm is associated with a fenestration in the lower part of the basilar artery.

Anatomic Principles Directing Surgery

The following basic anatomic principles are helpful in directing the surgical attack on intracranial aneurysms.

1. The parent artery should be exposed proximal to the aneurysm. This allows control of flow to the aneurysm if it ruptures during dissection. Exposure of the internal carotid artery above the cavernous sinus will give proximal control for aneurysms arising at the level of the posterior communicating or anterior choroidal artery. Exposure of the internal carotid artery at the level of the ophthalmic and superior hypophyseal arteries is commonly achieved by removing the anterior clinoid process, the adjacent part of the roof of the optic canal, and the posterior part of the orbital roof. The internal carotid artery should also be exposed initially to obtain proximal control of middle cerebral and anterior cerebral artery aneurysms. The exposure can be directed laterally from the internal carotid artery for middle cerebral aneurysms and medially over the optic nerves and chiasm for anterior communicating aneurysms. For basilar apex aneurysms, control of the basilar artery proximal to the aneurysm can be obtained by following the inferior surface of the posterior cerebral artery or the superior surface of the superior cerebellar artery to the basilar artery and then working up the side of the basilar artery to the neck of the aneurysm.
2. If possible, the side of the parent vessel opposite the side on which the aneurysm arises should be exposed before dissecting the neck of the aneurysm. The dissection can then be carried around the side of the parent vessel to the origin of the aneurysm.
3. The aneurysmal neck should be dissected before the fundus. The neck is the area that can tolerate the greatest manipulation, has the least tendency to rupture, and is to be clipped. Unfortunately, it is the portion of the aneurysm that is most likely to incorporate the origin of a vessel. Therefore, dissection of the neck and proximal part of the fundus should be done carefully with full visualization to prevent passage of a clip around the arterial branches, described previously, which arise near the neck of the aneurysm. The dissection should not be started at the dome because this is the area most likely to rupture before or during surgery.
4. All perforating arterial branches should be separated from the aneurysmal neck prior to passing the clip around the aneurysm. A detailed review of the important perforating arteries at each common aneurysm site has been presented elsewhere.[8] Prior to the use of magnification there was a tendency to keep dissection of aneurysms to a minimum because of the hazard of rupture. The use of magnification has permitted increased accuracy of dissection of the aneurysmal neck and more frequent preservation of the recurrent and other perforating arteries.[2,6,8,11] The risk of occlusion of perianeurysmal perforating arterioles that results from placement of a clip on an inadequately exposed aneurysm is greater than the hazard of rupture with microsurgical dissection.
5. If rupture occurs during microdissection, bleeding should be controlled by applying a small cotton pledget to the bleeding point and concomitantly reducing mean arterial pressure. If this technique does not stop the hemorrhage, a temporary clip can be applied to the proximal blood supply, but only for a brief time.
6. The bone flap should be placed as low as possible to minimize the need for retraction of the brain. Most aneurysms are located on or near the circle of Willis under the central portion of the brain. A low flap minimizes the amount of brain retraction needed to reach these areas.
7. A clip with a spring mechanism that allows it to be removed, repositioned, and reapplied should be used.
8. After the clip is applied, the area should be inspected to make certain the clip does not kink or obstruct a major vessel and that no perforating branches are included in it.
9. If an aneurysm has a broad-based neck that will not accept the clip easily, the neck may be reduced by bipolar coagulation. Nearby perforating arteries are protected with a cottonoid sponge during coagulation. The tips of the bipolar coagulation forceps are inserted between adjacent vessels and the neck of the aneurysm and are gently squeezed during coagulation. Short bursts of low current are used, and the tips of the forceps are relaxed and opened between applications of current to prevent them from adhering to the aneurysm and to evaluate the degree of shrinkage.

Operative Approaches

Ninety-five percent of aneurysms are found at one of five sites, all of which are located in close proximity to the circle of Willis (Fig. 215-1). These sites are (1) the internal carotid artery between the posterior communicating and the anterior choroidal arteries; (2) the anterior communicating artery area; (3) the proximal bifurcation of the middle cerebral artery; (4) the internal carotid bifurcation; and (5) the basilar bifurcation. The frontotemporal craniotomy with slight modifications is suitable for approaching all these aneurysms arising from the anterior circle of Willis and for some originating from the upper basilar artery (Figs. 215-2 to 215-5, 215-8, and 215-9).

A small frontotemporal flap centered at the pterion may be used for internal carotid artery aneurysms (Fig. 215-3). It may be enlarged posterosuperiorly for reaching aneurysms of the middle cerebral artery and of the internal carotid artery bifurcation (Fig. 215-4), forward for approaches to the anterior communicating area

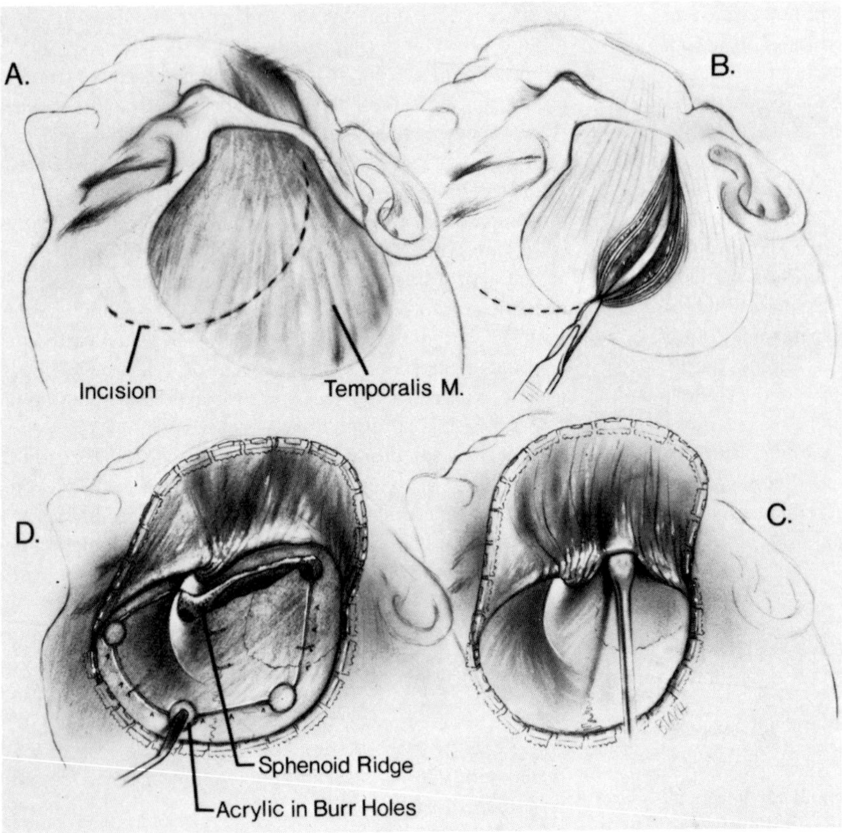

Figure 215-9 Frontotemporal craniotomy used to expose aneurysms on the anterior part of the circle of Willis. *A* to *C*. The scalp and temporalis muscle and fascia are elevated as a single layer. *D*. As the craniotomy flap is closed, soft acrylic is molded into the burr holes and allowed to harden under direct vision to minimize the cosmetic deformity associated with this bone removal. (From Rhoton,[7] with permission.)

(Fig. 215-5), and posteriorly to provide a pterion–anterior subtemporal approach for an aneurysm of the basilar apex (Fig. 215-8*B*).

The method of opening the scalp for the frontotemporal exposure varies depending on the site of the aneurysm (Figs. 215-9 and 215-10). If the aneurysm is located at the level or above the posterior communicating artery, the scalp, galea, pericranium, and temporalis muscle and fascia are reflected as a single layer. If the aneurysm is located at the level of the ophthalmic or superior hypophyseal artery, the scalp and galea are elevated in one layer and the temporalis muscle and fascia are elevated in a second layer. The two-layer scalp opening provides a lower exposure and better access to the anterior clinoid process and orbital roof than the single layer flap.

The scalp incision for this flap begins above the zygoma and extends across the temporal region and forward to the frontal region behind the hairline. The scalp, galea, pericranium, and temporalis muscle and fascia are reflected as a single layer if the aneurysm is located at or above the level of the posterior communicating artery (Fig. 215-9). A small bone flap having the center of its base at the pterion is elevated. The opening in the skull is extended inferiorly and medially by removing the lateral two-thirds of the sphenoid ridge. The time required to prepare this flap, in which all the soft tissue layers are reflected together, is less than that required to separate and reflect each layer individually. The incidence of weakness of the frontalis muscle is reduced because the layers superficial to the temporalis fascia are not disturbed. Decreased dissection around the temporalis muscle diminishes the incidence of contractions that limit opening of the mouth and reduces cosmetic deformities caused by scarring and atrophy of the temporalis muscle. Any burr holes or craniectomy site that would heal with a cosmetic deformity are closed with acrylic, mixed at the time the flap is replaced. The soft acrylic is molded into position and allowed to harden under direct vision to ensure that it fits the natural contour of the area (Fig. 215-9).

The frontotemporal scalp flap is modified so that the scalp and galea are elevated as one layer and the temporalis muscle and fascia are elevated as a second layer if the aneurysm is located at the origin of the superior hypophyseal or ophthalmic artery (Fig. 215-10). This allows the temporalis muscle to be reflected into the posterior-inferior part of the exposure and provides a lower exposure for removal of the anterior clinoid process, roof of the optic canal, and adjacent part of the roof of the orbit which are commonly needed to manage aneurysms that arise proximal to the posterior communicating artery.

After the bone flap is elevated, the dura mater is opened and the posterior-inferior frontal lobe is elevated with the use of a self-retaining brain retractor to expose the sphenoid ridge to the depth of the anterior clinoid process. The cistern over the optic nerve and carotid artery is opened, and a suction drain protected with a cottonoid pledget is inserted to remove cerebrospinal fluid to relax the brain and increase exposure. One is at the desired location if the aneurysm arises from the internal carotid artery (Figs. 215-2 and 215-3). For anterior communicating artery aneurysms, the dissection is directed superiorly to the bifurcation of the internal carotid artery and over the optic nerve and chiasm along the anterior cerebral artery to the neck of the aneurysm (Fig. 215-5). Middle cerebral artery aneurysms are exposed by splitting the sylvian fissure, beginning at the internal carotid artery (Fig. 215-4). Some basilar artery aneurysms may be exposed using this approach by working through the space between the optic nerve and the internal carotid artery if the interval between those two structures is sufficiently wide and the aneurysm projects superiorly or anteriorly (Fig.

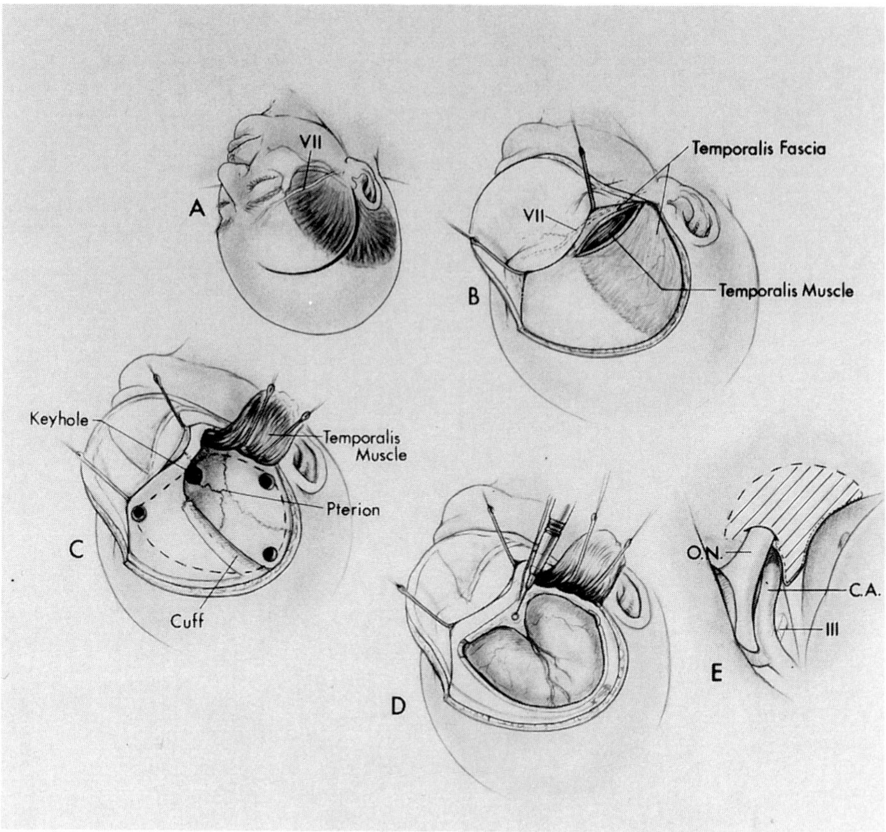

Figure 215-10 Modification of the frontotemporal craniotomy for exposing aneurysms arising at the origin of the ophthalmic and superior hypophyseal arteries. This two-layer scalp opening provides a lower exposure and easier access for removal of the anterior clinoid process and the adjacent part of the orbital roof as compared to when the scalp flap is turned as a single layer as shown in 215-9. Site of scalp incision (*solid line*) and bone flap (*interrupted line*). *A*. The branches of the facial nerve (VII) pass across the zygoma to reach the muscles of the forehead. *B*. The scalp, including the galea, is reflected downward by opening the plant between the pericranium and the galea. An incision is made in the temporalis fascia (but not the temporalis muscle), just above the fat pad containing the branches of the facial nerve to the forehead so that the fat pad and facial branches can be reflected downward with the scalp flap, thus reducing the possibility of damaging these branches of the facial nerve. *C*. The scalp flap and temporalis muscle have been reflected to expose the keyhole and pterion. A cuff of pericranium and temporalis fascia is preserved along the anterior part of the temporal line to facilitate closure of the temporalis muscle and fascia. *D*. The frontotemporal bone flap has been elevated and the lateral part of the sphenoid ridge is being removed. The temporalis muscle and fascia are reflected into the posterior-inferior margin of the exposure. *E*. The anterior clinoid process, roof of the optic canal, and adjacent part of the orbital roof and lesser wing of the sphenoid are commonly removed (*oblique lines*) to access the internal carotid artery proximal to ophthalmic and superior hypophyseal aneurysms.

215-11).[10] If this approach is used, care should be taken to preserve the vital perforating branches that arise on the internal carotid artery and cross this space to supply the optic nerve and tract and diencephalon.[2] Aneurysms arising on a high basilar bifurcation may also be exposed through the interval between the bifurcation of the internal carotid artery and the optic tract (Fig. 215-11). Care must be taken to protect the perforating arteries crossing this interval. The aneurysm is approached more commonly through the space between the internal carotid artery and the oculomotor nerve (Figs. 215-8*B* and 215-11). This exposure is facilitated by elevating the carotid artery with a dissector. After exposing the area between the carotid artery and the oculomotor nerve, a decision must be made about whether to expose the aneurysm by operating above or below the posterior communicating artery. If a basilar aneurysm arises from the posterior aspect of the upper basilar artery, it is best to elevate the temporal lobe and approach the area along the floor of the middle fossa (Fig. 215-8*A*).

Most basilar artery aneurysms are approached through a subtemporal craniotomy (Figs. 215-8*A* and 215-12). This approach under the temporal lobe gives better exposure of the perforating arteries that commonly arise from the posterior aspect of the basilar artery than does the frontotemporal approach along the sphenoid ridge. These perforating branches are especially important because they supply diencephalic areas controlling consciousness.

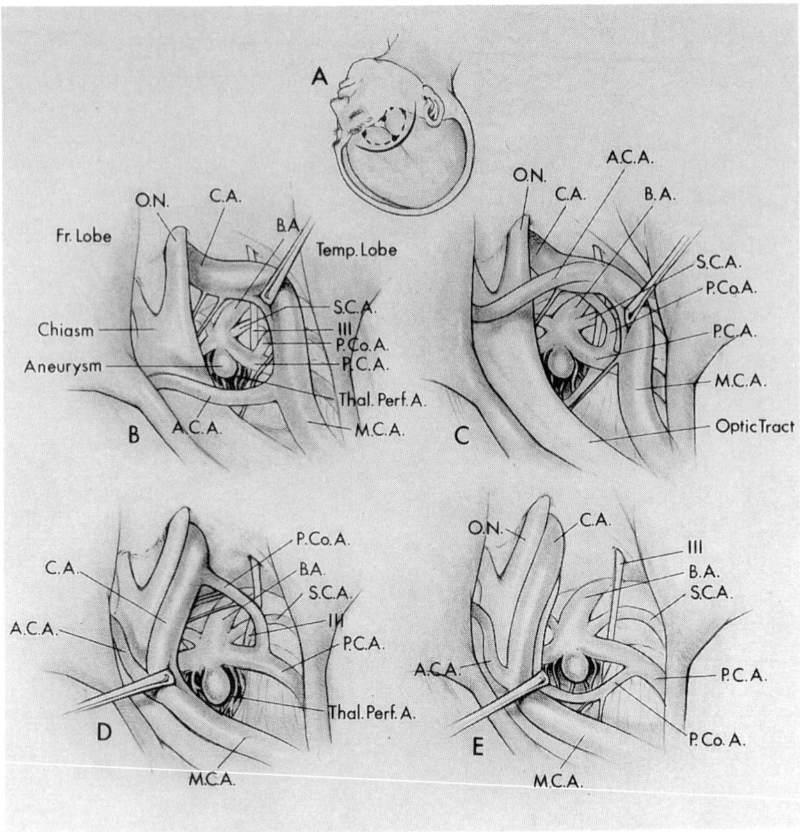

Figure 215-11 Four operative routes directed through a frontotemporal craniotomy to a basilar apex aneurysm. *A*. Site of the frontotemporal scalp incision (*solid line*) and bone flap (*interrupted line*). *B*. The basilar apex is exposed through the opticocarotid triangle which is located between the carotid artery (C.A.), optic nerve (O.N.), and anterior cerebral artery (A.C.A.). The frontal (Fr. Lobe) and temporal lobes (Temp. Lobe) have been separated along the sylvian fissure. This approach may be used if the carotid artery and the initial segment of the anterior cerebral artery are long, thus providing a wide opening through this triangular space. Other structures exposed include the middle cerebral (M.C.A.), posterior cerebral (P.C.A.), posterior communicating (P.Co.A.), thalamoperforating (Thal. Perf. A.), and superior cerebellar arteries (S.C.A.), oculomotor nerve (III), and optic chiasm (Chiasm). Perforating branches of the carotid and posterior communicating arteries may provide an obstacle and should be preserved in each of the four approaches. *C*. Approach through the interval between the carotid bifurcation and the optic tract. This approach may be used if the carotid artery is short, thus providing an opening between the bifurcation and the optic tract. The perforating branches arising in the region of the bifurcation of the carotid artery may limit access through this area. *D*. Approach directed behind the carotid artery and above the posterior communicating artery through the interval between the carotid artery and the oculomotor nerve. The perforating branches of the posterior communicating artery may need to be separated to reach the basilar apex. *E*. Approach directed below the posterior communicating artery through the interval between the carotid artery and the oculomotor nerve. The posterior communicating artery has been elevated with a small dissector.

The subtemporal approach, when combined with sectioning of the tentorium cerebelli posterior to the trochlear nerve, can be used to reach basilar aneurysms arising from the junction of the basilar artery and the superior cerebellar or anterior inferior cerebellar arteries (Fig. 215-8*C,D*).

Aneurysms arising at the vertebrobasilar junction are approached through a subtemporal exposure if the junction is high, through a combined supra- and infratentorial presigmoid exposure if the junction is deep in the mid part of the posterior fossa, or through a suboccipital craniectomy if the vertebrobasilar junction is low (Figs. 215-12 and 215-13). Vertebral aneurysms arising at the origin of the posterior inferior cerebellar artery are approached through a suboccipital craniectomy if they are located low in the posterior fossa and through a combined supra- and infratentorial presigmoid exposure if they are deep in the mid portion of the posterior fossa. If the suboccipital approach is selected, the arch of the C-1 vertebra is removed to provide adequate exposure of the segment of the vertebral artery proximal to the aneurysm. The side for the suboccipital approach should be selected only after carefully reviewing the angiogram since aneurysms of one vertebral artery may lie on the opposite side of the brain stem due to the extreme tortuosity of these arteries.

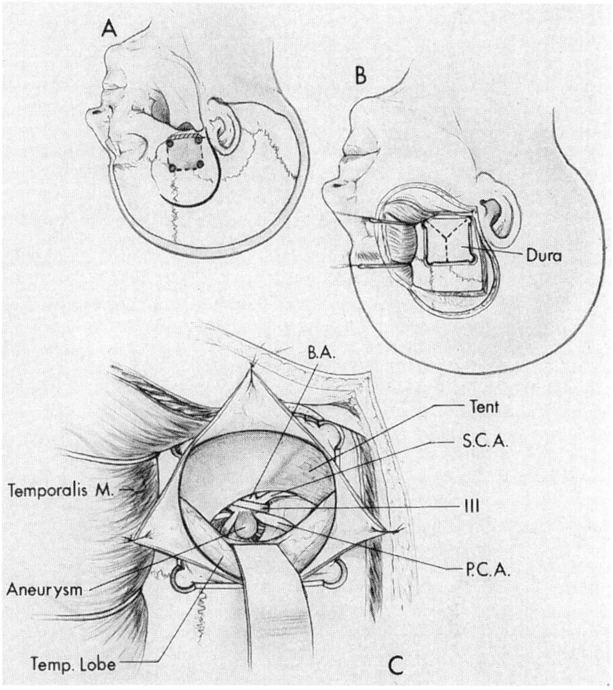

Figure 215-12 Anterior subtemporal exposure for aneurysms of the upper part of the basilar artery. *A*. The scalp incision (*solid line*) in the shape of a question mark and the bone flap (*dashed line*) are located above the zygoma. The upper edge of the zygoma (*oblique hatching*) is removed with a drill if it blocks access to a low exposure along the floor of the middle fossa. *B*. The bone flap has been elevated to expose the site of the dural opening (*interrupted line*). A small portion of the temporalis muscle is divided just anterior to the ear and the remaining fibers are reflected forward. A small craniectomy may be needed at the lower margin of the bone flap to bring the line of vision down to the floor of the middle cranial fossa. *C*. The temporal lobe (Temp. Lobe) has been elevated to expose the basilar (B.A.), posterior cerebral (P.C.A.), and superior cerebellar (S.C.A.) arteries, oculomotor nerve (III), and tentorium (Tent.). The temporalis muscle (Temporalis M.) is reflected forward.

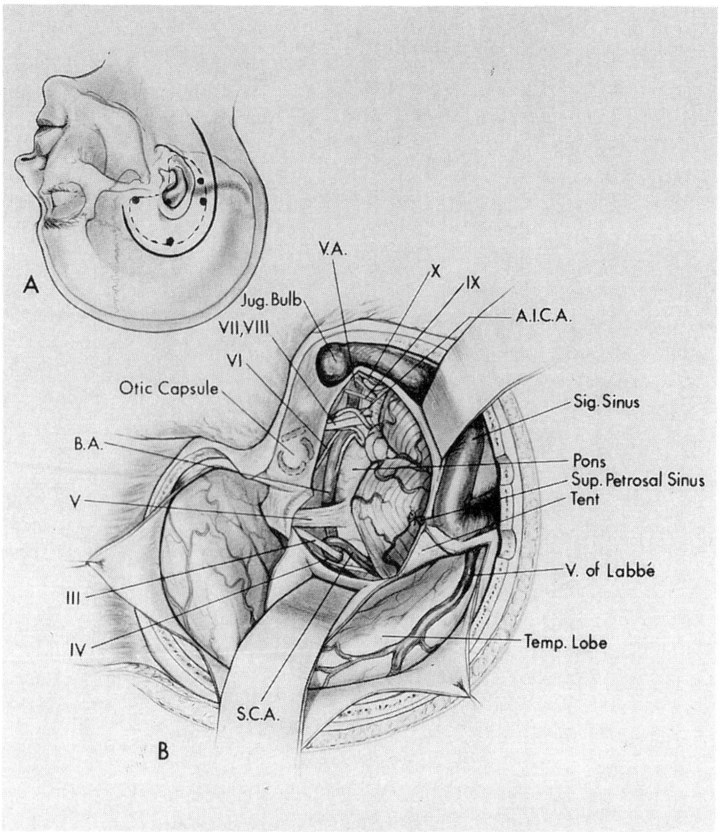

Figure 215-13 Combined supra- and infratentorial presigmoid approach to the basilar artery. *A*. Site of scalp incision (*solid line*) and bone removal (*interrupted lines*). *B*. The supra- and infratemporal areas have been exposed. A mastoidectomy has been performed with care being taken to preserve the otic capsule and bone over the semicircular canals. The dura is opened in front of the sigmoid sinus (Sig. Sinus). The dural incision is carried across the superior petrosal sinus (Sup. Pet. Sinus) and tentorial edge (Tent.) with care being taken to preserve the trochlear nerve (IV). This procedure accesses the upper part of the vertebral artery (V.A.) and the full length of the basilar artery (B.A.). This approach may be used for aneurysms arising from the basilar artery at the origin of the anterior inferior cerebellar artery (A.I.C.A.), or at the junction of the vertebral arteries with the basilar artery. This approach may also be selected for vertebral aneurysms arising at the origin of the posterior inferior cerebellar artery (P.I.C.A.), if the aneurysm is located high and deep in the posterior fossa. The jugular bulb (Jug. Bulb) may block access to the lower part of the intracranial part of the vertebral artery. A vertebral aneurysm located in the lower part of the posterior fossa would be approached through a suboccipital craniectomy. Care is taken to preserve the vein of Labbe (V. of Labbe) as the temporal lobe (Temp. Lobe) is elevated. Other structures in the exposure include the oculomotor (III), trigeminal (V), abducens (VI), facial (VII), vestibulocochlear (VIII), glossopharyngeal (IX), and vagus (X) nerves and the superior cerebellar artery (S.C.A.).

References

1. Gibo H, Carver CC, Rhoton AL Jr, et al. Microsurgical anatomy of the middle cerebral artery. *J Neurosurg* 1981; 54:151–169.
2. Gibo H, Lenkey C, Rhoton AL Jr. Microsurgical anatomy of the supraclinoid portion of the internal carotid artery. *J Neurosurg* 1981; 55:560–574.
3. Hardy DG, Peace DA, Rhoton AL Jr. Microsurgical anatomy of the superior cerebellar artery. *Neurosurgery* 1980; 6:10–28.
4. Lister JR, Rhoton AL Jr, Matsushima T, Peace DA. Microsurgical anatomy of the posterior inferior cerebellar artery. *Neurosurgery* 1982; 10:170–199.
5. Martin RG, Grant JL, Peace D, et al. Microsurgical relationships of the anterior inferior cerebellar artery and the facial-vestibulocochlear nerve complex. *Neurosurgery* 1980; 6:483–507.
6. Perlmutter D, Rhoton AL Jr. Microsurgical anatomy of the anterior cerebral–anterior communicating–recurrent artery complex. *J Neurosurg* 1976; 45:259–272.
7. Rhoton AL Jr. Anatomy of saccular aneurysms. *Surg Neurol* 1980; 14:59–66.
8. Rhoton AL Jr, Saeki N, Perlmutter D, Zeal A. Microsurgical anatomy of common aneurysm sites. *Clin Neurosurg* 1979; 26:248–306.
9. Saeki N, Rhoton AL Jr. Microsurgical anatomy of the upper basilar artery and the posterior circle of Willis. *J Neurosurg* 1977; 46:563–578.
10. Yaşargil MG, Fox JL. The microsurgical approach to intracranial aneurysms. *Surg Neurol* 1975; 3:7–14.
11. Zeal AA, Rhoton AL Jr. Microsurgical anatomy of the posterior cerebral artery. *J Neurosurg* 1978; 48:534–559.

216 Imaging of Intracranial Aneurysms

Eugene F. Binet
Edgardo J. C. Angtuaco

Aneurysms are the most common nontraumatic cause of subarachnoid hemorrhage in adults but they may also present as mass lesions or cause neurological symptoms and signs not secondary to hemorrhage.

In the past, plain skull radiography was the first radiologic procedure undertaken in a patient suspected of having an intracranial aneurysm. These roentgenograms were reviewed for displacement of the pineal body or choroid plexus secondary to an intracerebral or subdural hematoma. Very rarely, calcification was seen in the walls of a giant aneurysm. In a small percentage of patients, bony erosion of the clivus, pituitary fossa, or sphenoid wing indicated a giant aneurysm.

High-Resolution Computed Tomography

More recently, high-resolution computed tomography (CT) has become the procedure of choice for the detection of subarachnoid hemorrhage and the localization of intracranial aneurysms.[10,23,25] It may obviate lumbar puncture in a patient at risk for transtentorial herniation. The CT scan should be performed within the first 24 h of the ictus. Sections should be obtained both before and after intravenous injection of a contrast medium. Ultrathin sections encompassing the circle of Willis should be obtained following a second bolus injection to detect small aneurysms arising from the arteries at the base of the skull (Fig. 216-1).

Unenhanced CT Scans

On the unenhanced CT scan subarachnoid hemorrhage will be identified as areas of increased density in the subarachnoid spaces

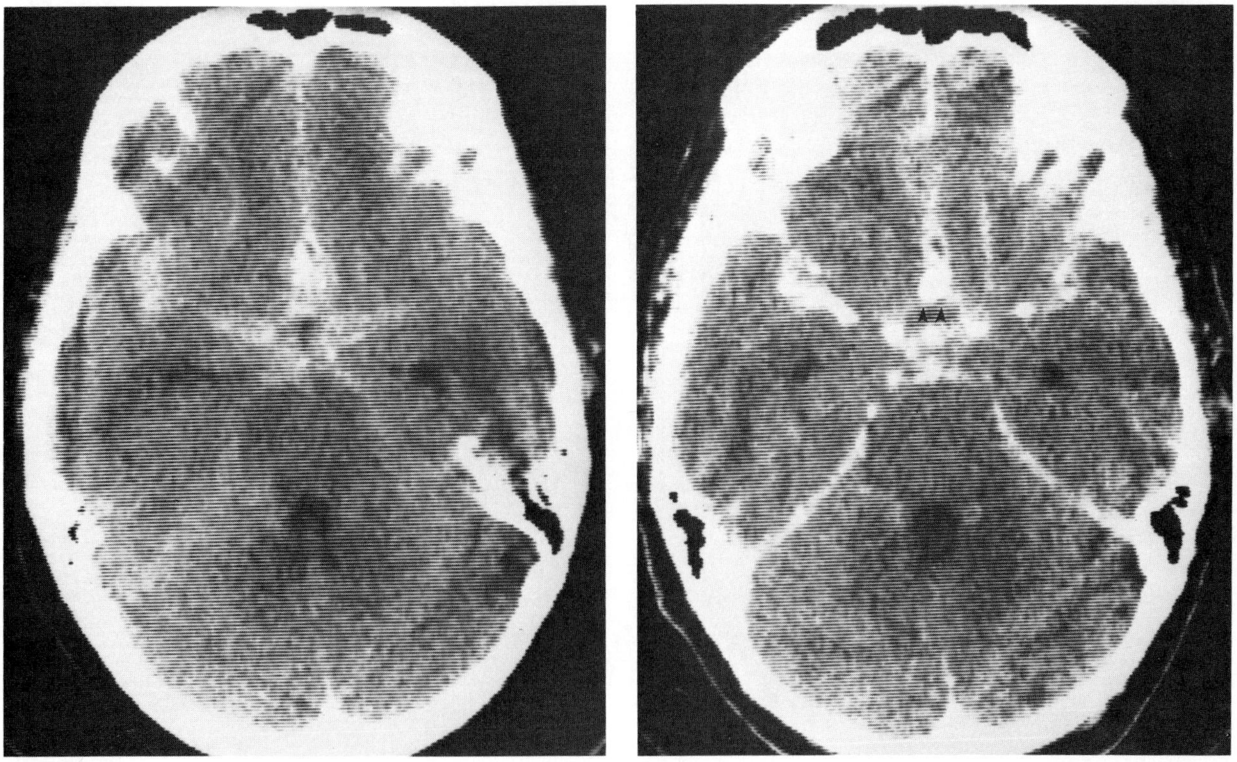

(*A*) (*B*)

Figure 216-1 *A*. Unenhanced 10 mm-thick CT scan at the level of the basilar cisterns shows subarachnoid hemorrhage in the interhemispheric fissure, the suprasellar cistern, and the interpeduncular cistern and along the tentorium. *B*. A 1.5 mm-thick enhanced high-resolution CT scan shows an anterior communicating artery aneurysm 5 mm in diameter (*arrowheads*).

along the base of the skull, within the sylvian fissures, within the sulci over the periphery of the brain, along the falx and tentorium, and even in the interhemispheric fissure (Figs. 216-1*A*, 216-11*A*, 216-14*A*). The development of a full-fledged appearance, with Hounsfield units ranging from 60 to 80 HU, may take several hours following the hemorrhage. The detection of subarachnoid hemorrhage on unenhanced CT scans depends on the cooperation of the patient, the time since the subarachnoid hemorrhage, and the use of a high-resolution CT scanner.[14]

In patients with severe anemia, subarachnoid, intracerebral, and intraventricular hemorrhages may be only slightly more dense than the surrounding brain tissue. Subarachnoid hemorrhage in the presence of a bleeding aneurysm will be detected in more than 90 percent of the patients in the first 24 h and in over 50 percent within the first week.[8] These percentages drop off dramatically following the seventh day. Significant subarachnoid hemorrhage seen 10 or more days after an episode of bleeding is suspicious for rebleeding. If the unenhanced CT scan does not demonstrate subarachnoid hemorrhage, a lumbar puncture should be done in the absence of an intracranial mass lesion.

In addition to subarachnoid hemorrhage, the unenhanced study should be evaluated for intraventricular or intracerebral hemorrhage (Figs. 216-2*A* and *B*, 216-3*A*). Extensive intraventricular hemorrhage may completely fill both lateral ventricles as well as the third and fourth ventricles. More commonly, however, the CT scan shows a thin layer of blood confined to the occipital horns. Intracerebral hemorrhage may be identified as a large area of increased density within the substance of the temporal or frontal lobes associated with edema and mass effect. Subdural hematomas occur in 1 to 8 percent of patients with subarachnoid hemorrhage due to bleeding aneurysms and these may be identified on CT scans as areas of increased density paralleling the inner table of the skull.[6]

The location of the subarachnoid blood may frequently suggest the site of the bleeding aneurysm. It is very common for anterior communicating artery aneurysms to bleed into the interhemispheric fissure. Hemorrhage into the septum pellucidum and adjacent frontal lobe alone is almost pathognomonic for an anterior communicating artery aneurysm (Fig. 216-2*B*). Unenhanced scans showing hemorrhage into the temporal lobe and sylvian fissure alone are frequently obtained with a ruptured middle cerebral artery aneurysm (Fig. 216-3*A*). Aneurysms at the internal carotid artery bifurcation may bleed into the basal ganglia, the frontal and medial temporal lobes, and the adjacent subarachnoid space. The location of the subarachnoid hemorrhage associated with bleeding posterior communicating artery aneurysms varies depending on the direction to which the aneurysm points. Hemorrhages into the sylvian fissure and temporal lobe are often present where the tip of the aneurysm points laterally. On the other hand, a tip pointing posteriorly may be associated with hemorrhage into the interpeduncular cistern. Hemorrhage into the brain stem as well as the interpeduncular cistern may be the presenting findings for distal basilar artery aneurysms, although hemorrhage into the third ventricle has also been recorded with these lesions. Posterior inferior cerebellar artery aneurysms often bleed into the medullary cistern, with blood also appearing in the fourth ventricle. In general, posterior fossa aneurysms do not frequently bleed into the supratentorial subarachnoid space or into the lateral ventricles. More blood is present in the fourth ventricle than the third ventricle with posterior fossa aneurysms.

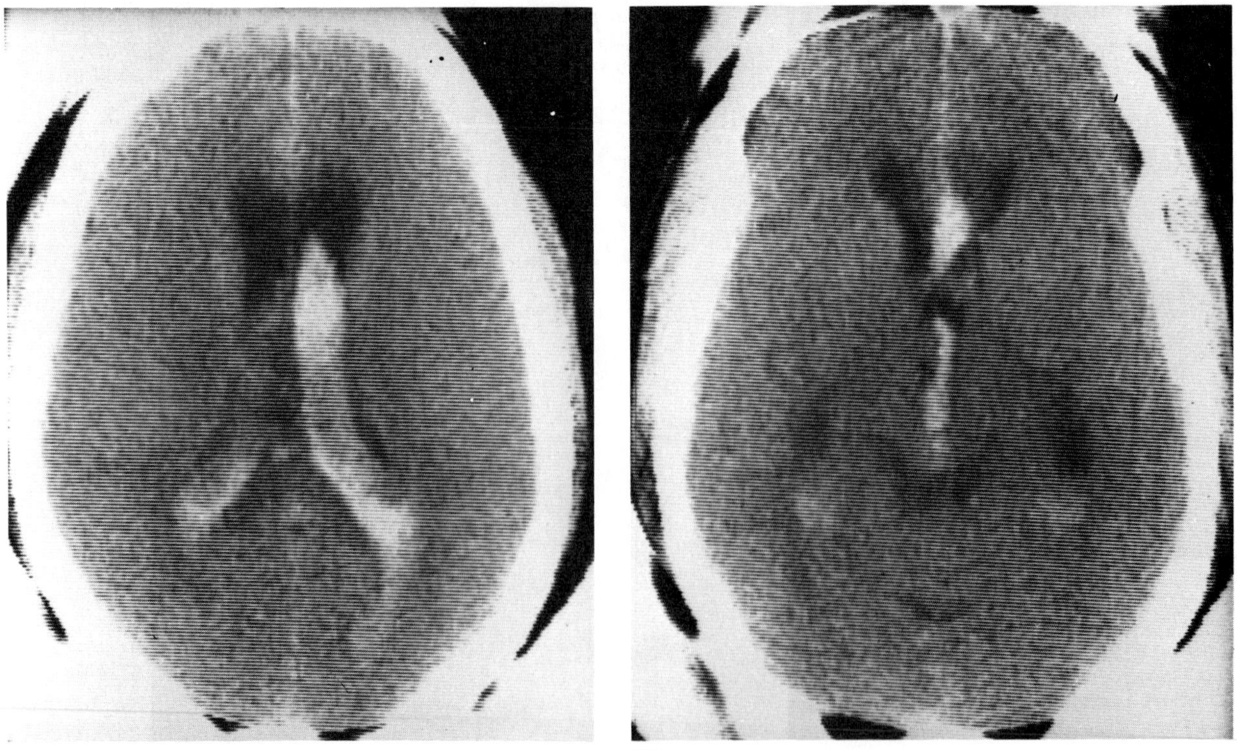

(*A*) (*B*)

Figure 216-2 *A*. Unenhanced CT scan shows massive hemorrhage within both lateral ventricles. *B*. Unenhanced CT scan shows hemorrhage into the septum pellucidum and the third ventricle.

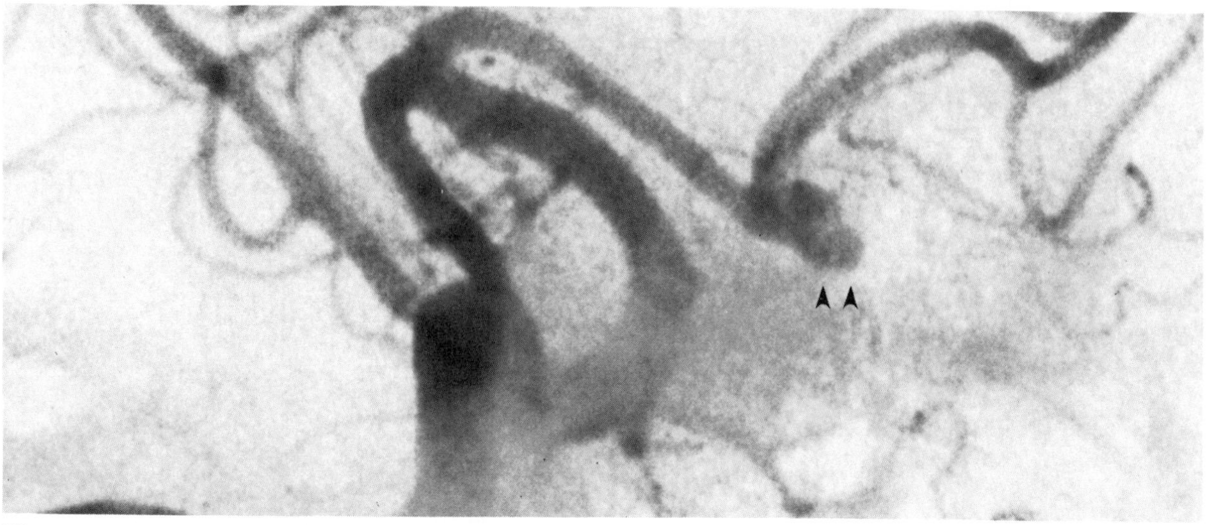

(*C*)

Figure 216-2 (*Continued*) *C*. Right common carotid angiogram, oblique projection, subtraction print, shows anterior communicating artery aneurysm (*arrowheads*).

Enhanced CT Scans

Following analysis of the unenhanced CT scans, intravenous contrast may be given and the routine sections repeated. Sequential high-resolution thin slices through the circle of Willis following a second IV bolus may also be performed. These maneuvers are especially helpful in very sick patients where immediate cerebral angiography or surgery is not contemplated or where the unenhanced CT has not localized the site of the aneurysm. The contraindications to enhanced CT scans include an absolute sensitivity to intravenous contrast material, renal shut down, or severe jeopardizing of the patient. The final decision as to whether a patient should have a postcontrast study lies with the referring physician after consultation with the supervising neuroradiologist. That decision should take into account the great amount of information that is provided on contrast enhanced high-resolution CT scans.

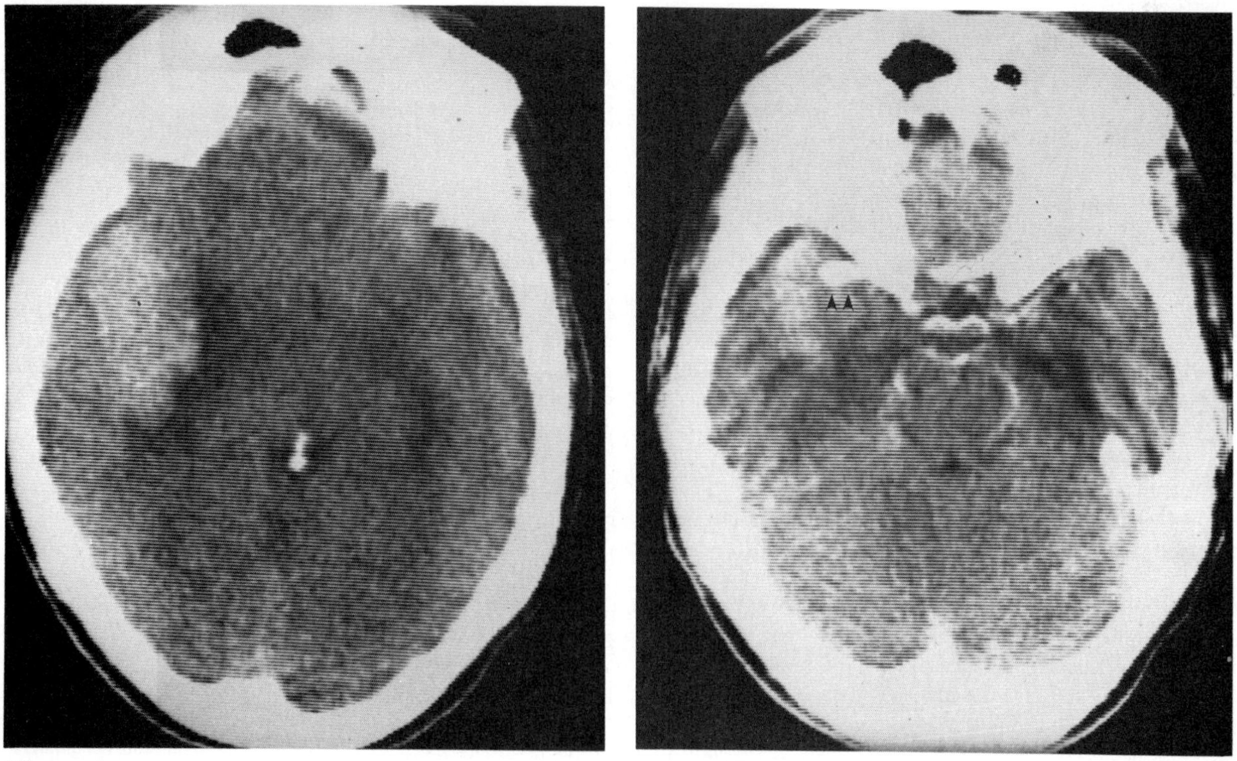

(*A*) (*B*)

Figure 216-3 *A*. Unenhanced CT scan shows intracerebral hematoma in the right temporal lobe. *B*. Thin-section high-resolution enhanced CT scan shows a right middle cerebral artery aneurysm projecting to the edge of the right temporal lobe hematoma (*arrowheads*).

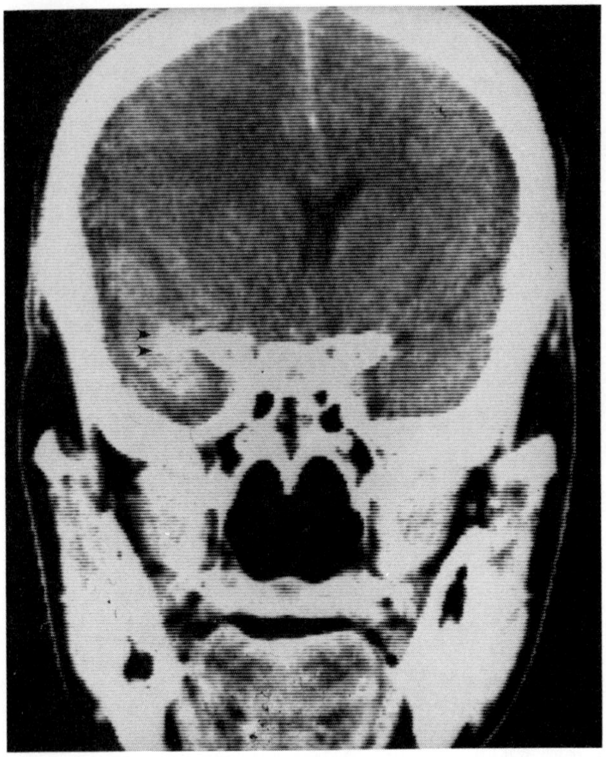

(*C*)

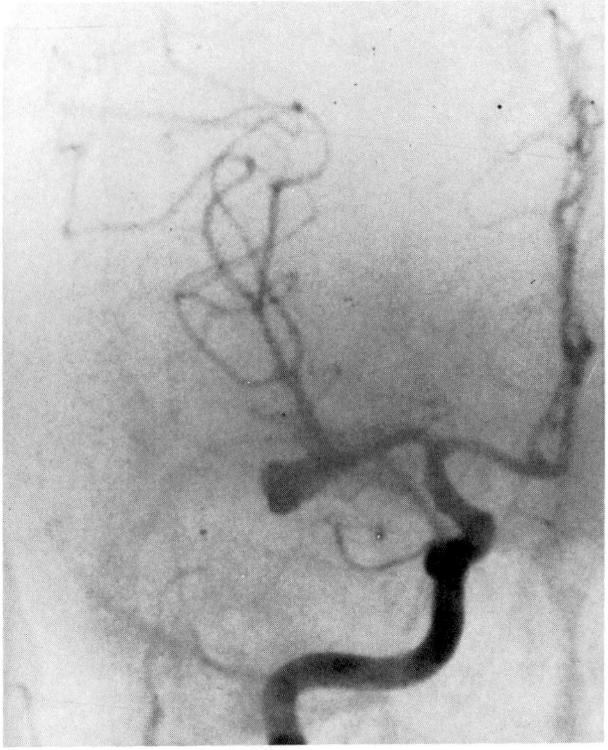

(*D*)

Figure 216-3 (*Continued*) *C*. Direct coronal, thin-section high-resolution enhanced CT scan shows the right middle cerebral artery aneurysm projecting into the right temporal lobe hematoma (*arrowheads*). *D*. Right common carotid angiogram, transorbital projection, subtraction print, shows the large right middle cerebral artery aneurysm. The large right temporal lobe hematoma causes medial displacement of the middle cerebral artery and contralateral displacement of the anterior cerebral artery.

Enhanced studies have several purposes. First and foremost, they identify the cause of subarachnoid hemorrhage in most patients (Figs. 216-1 and 216-3*A* to *C*). Although the localization of subarachnoid hemorrhage on unenhanced studies frequently points to the site of an aneurysm, enhanced CT scans confirm this location and may show the presence of a second aneurysm as well (Fig. 216-4*A* and *B*). The size, shape, and relationship of an aneurysm to its parent vessel can easily be determined with high-resolution techniques (Figs. 216-3*B* and *C*, 216-7). Aneurysms greater than 5 mm can be seen (Fig. 216-1*B*). The magnification mode is also helpful to delineate fine detail (Fig. 216-4*A* and *B*). The use of sagittal coronal reformatting or direct coronal scanning will provide additional information concerning the aneurysm's relationship to other vital structures at the base of the brain (Figs. 216-3*B* and *C*, 216-15*A* and *B*). The enhanced CT scan provides a road map for angiography when preoperative fine detail analysis of the aneurysm becomes necessary. In many patients, the localization of subarachnoid hemorrhage and its cause can therefore be made on a relatively noninvasive, low-morbidity study, and angiography can be deferred until the patient is more stable, the angiography team better prepared, and the angiographer better informed.

Enhanced studies will occasionally show that an aneurysm is not the cause of subarachnoid hemorrhage. An arteriovenous malformation may be identified on enhanced CT scans as a serpentine tangle of enlarged feeding arteries and draining veins. Cavernous hemangioma and venous angioma may present with subarachnoid hemorrhage; they also have distinctive CT appearances on enhanced studies. Even rarer lesions such as metastatic melanoma to the brain, which occasionally causes subarachnoid hemorrhage, can be detected on enhanced studies.

With present techniques, high-resolution CT scanning without and with contrast enhancement will detect the cause of nontraumatic subarachnoid hemorrhage in most patients. Utilizing this first radiological step, the neurosurgeon and neuroradiologist will be better prepared to evaluate the patient's status and plan the remainder of the patient's diagnostic workup. If immediate surgery is required to remove a subdural or intracerebral hematoma or to place an intraventricular catheter, the precise localization of the aneurysm on the enhanced CT scan will allow the surgeon to determine the approach to the problem without waiting for the corroborative angiogram (Fig. 216-3*B*, *C*).

Transfemoral Cerebral Angiography

The final step in the radiologic evaluation of patients with suspected subarachnoid hemorrhage due to a ruptured aneurysm is a complete transfemoral cerebral angiogram. This procedure can be performed immediately preceding surgery. A catheter study is indicated because it is the only method whereby complete evaluation of the vasculature to both cerebral hemispheres and the posterior fossa can be accomplished with one vessel puncture. In patients with aortofemoral grafts, axillary puncture with selective catheterization of the brachiocephalic vessels is easily accomplished. In older patients it may be necessary to evaluate the aortic arch and

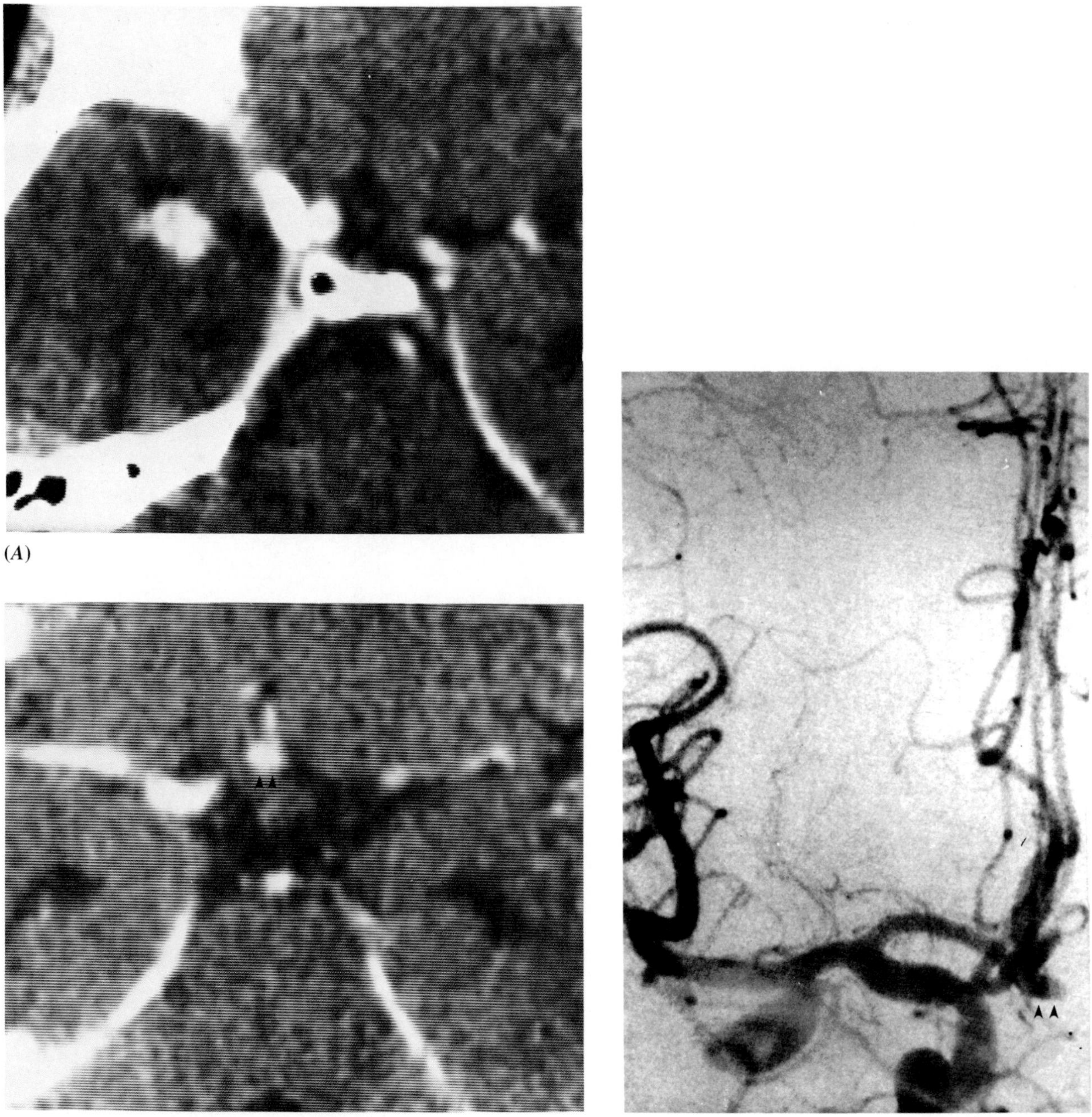

(*A*)

(*B*)

(*C*)

Figure 216-4 *A*. Enhanced high-resolution thin-section CT scan, magnification mode, shows a right middle cerebral artery aneurysm with irregular margins. A small clot is seen within the lumen of the aneurysm. *B*. Enhanced high-resolution CT scan, magnification mode, shows a second smaller anterior communicating artery aneurysm (*arrowheads*). *C*. Right common carotid angiogram shows the right middle cerebral artery aneurysm with clot within its lumen. Also note the small anterior communicating artery aneurysm (*arrowheads*).

carotid bifurcations in the neck to exclude the presence of significant vascular disease. Patients with an antecedent history of transient ischemic attacks or previous strokes should have an arch aortogram prior to selective catheterization of the neck vessels. It is not uncommon to find significant cervical lesions in older patients with a bleeding aneurysm (Fig. 216-5).

Selective injection of small amounts of contrast medium (6 to 10 ml) into the common carotid and vertebral arteries will usually suffice to demonstrate the circle of Willis in great detail. Selective injections into the internal carotid artery or high in the vertebral artery are usually unnecessary and are contraindicated, because they may cause intra-angiographic rupture of an aneurysm. Steps should be taken to correct any bleeding diathesis prior to angiography. Replacement blood transfusions should be considered for patients with sickle cell anemia.

The initial angiogram should be performed utilizing the standard anteroposterior and lateral projections. Biplanar magnification techniques should be used if available, and subtraction films

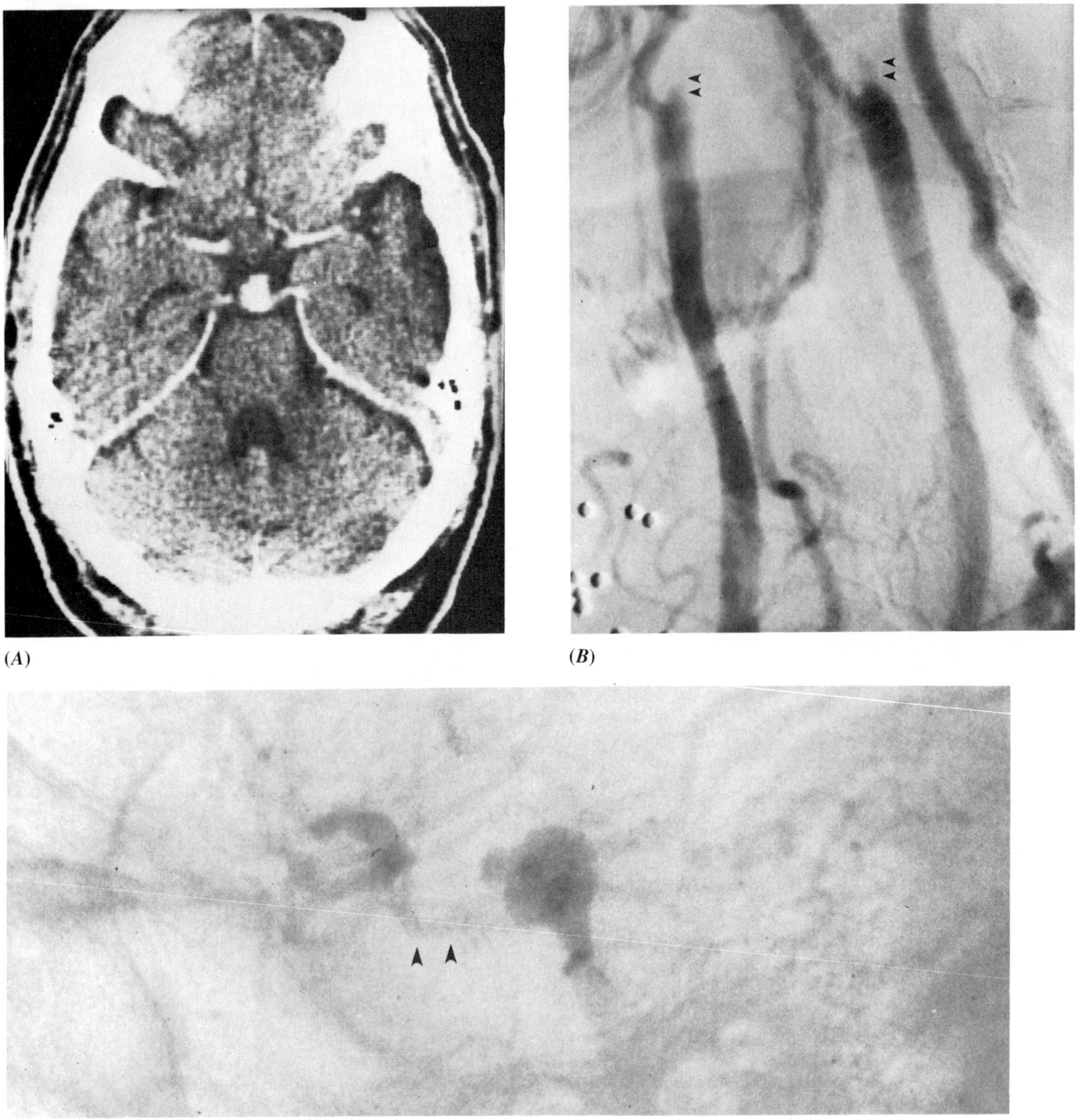

Figure 216-5 *A*. Enhanced thin-section CT scan shows a large basilar artery aneurysm. *B*. An arch aortogram, subtraction print, demonstrates complete occlusion of both internal carotid arteries at their origins (*arrowheads*). *C*. A vertebral angiogram, lateral projection, subtraction print, shows the basilar artery aneurysm. The supraclinoid portion of both the right and the left internal carotid arteries are filled via the posterior communicating arteries (*arrowheads*).

should always be obtained in all projections, not only to clarify details about observed aneurysms but also to exclude additional aneurysms obscured by overlying bone. The angiogram should be performed on the "side closer to the aneurysm" first. The side of the bleeding aneurysm can usually be discerned from the CT if the neurological findings are nonlocalizing. If the blood supply to the aneurysm is in the distribution of one carotid circulation, that vessel should be examined first. Then the contralateral common carotid artery and the larger or more accessible vertebral artery should be injected. If the aneurysm is in the posterior fossa, then the larger, more accessible vertebral artery should be cannulated first and this should be followed by selective injections into both common carotid arteries. There are several advantages to performing the angiogram first in the artery "closest to the aneurysm." If there is severe spasm of the cerebral vasculature on the first angiographic run, at least a "peek" at the aneurysm will have been obtained prior to terminating the study. In addition, if there is a technical malfunction of the equipment during or after the first angiographic run, again a peek will have been obtained. The same is true if the patient has an allergic reaction or a cardiorespiratory failure during the procedure. If all goes well, the films from the first run will be developed first and will be available for detailed scrutiny while the other vessels are being examined. The angiographer can then plan and carry out special views of the aneurysm while the additional routine runs are being processed. This plan of sequencing ensures a greater likelihood of a successful angiogram and reduces the length of time that the catheter is in the bloodstream, which is an important consideration in the prevention of complications.

Special views are often necessary to identify the neck of an aneurysm.[11] For suspected anterior communicating artery aneurysms, the patient's head should be turned away from the side of injection (Fig. 216-2*C*). Middle cerebral artery aneurysms are often best identified by placing the area of suspicion within the bony orbit (Fig. 216-3*D*). This is accomplished by utilizing the transorbital oblique view with the head in moderate extension. Basilar artery aneurysms are often best identified in the base view (Fig. 216-6*B*). The submentovertical view is also helpful in anterior communicating artery and middle cerebral artery aneurysms (Fig. 216-7*B*). The special view technique chart described by Lin and Kricheff should be used as a guide to the proper projection for any given aneurysm.[11]

If no aneurysm is identified on the routine studies, the other vertebral artery should be injected if it has not been already visualized adequately. If this is not helpful and the enhanced CT scan is not diagnostic, consideration should be given to obtaining additional special views of those areas demonstrating subarachnoid or intracerebral hemorrhage on the CT scan. For example, if the standard views do not demonstrate an aneurysm of the anterior communicating artery and the CT scan shows interhemispheric hemorrhage or hemorrhage into the septum pellucidum, either an oblique or base angiogram of the anterior communicating artery should be obtained, as most surely the aneurysm will be found in this location.

The standard angiographic runs should be carried out well into the venous phase of the cerebral circulation and analyzed for the presence of other lesions. If no aneurysm has been seen on the routine and special views, a careful analysis of the arterial, capillary, and venous phases of the angiogram may reveal a small, cryptic arteriovenous malformation that has not only bled but has defied detection by CT scanning. This important analysis is often overlooked in the flurry of activity to find the more dramatic saccular aneurysm.

Cross-compression techniques are seldom performed because they are not physiologic, do not accurately predict the change in flow patterns that will occur as a result of surgery, and are technically difficult to perform correctly.

The accuracy of the initial angiogram in detecting a bleeding aneurysm varies from investigator to investigator, depending on observer error, the use of magnification and subtraction techniques, and whether all four vessels are examined.[5] With modern techniques, one should expect to identify more than 75 percent of the aneurysms on the first study. Causes for nonvisualization of an aneurysm on the first study may be due to its being totally thrombosed or completely "blown out" at the time of the first hemorrhage. The cryptic arteriovenous malformation that has destroyed

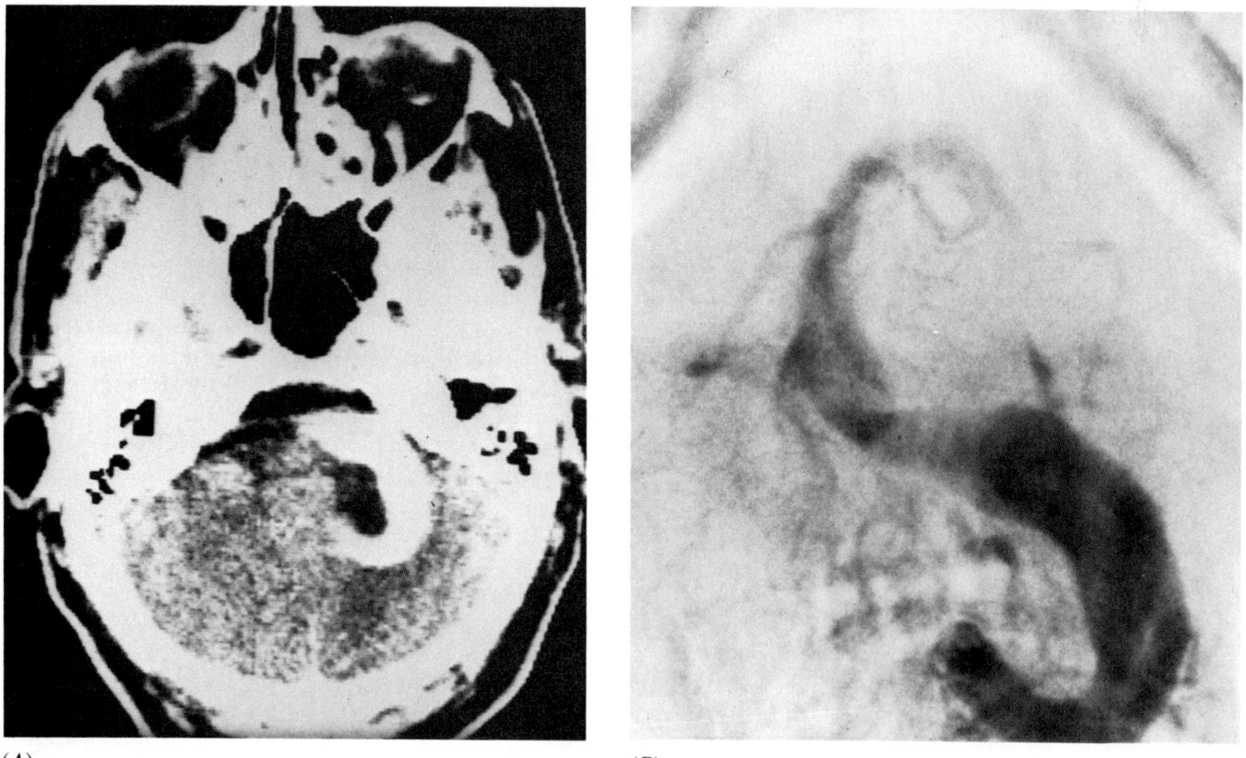

(*A*) (*B*)

Figure 216-6 *A*. Enhanced CT scan shows a large atherosclerotic aneurysm of the basilar artery. *B*. Left vertebral angiogram, submentovertical projection, subtraction print, shows the large atherosclerotic aneurysm of the basilar artery.

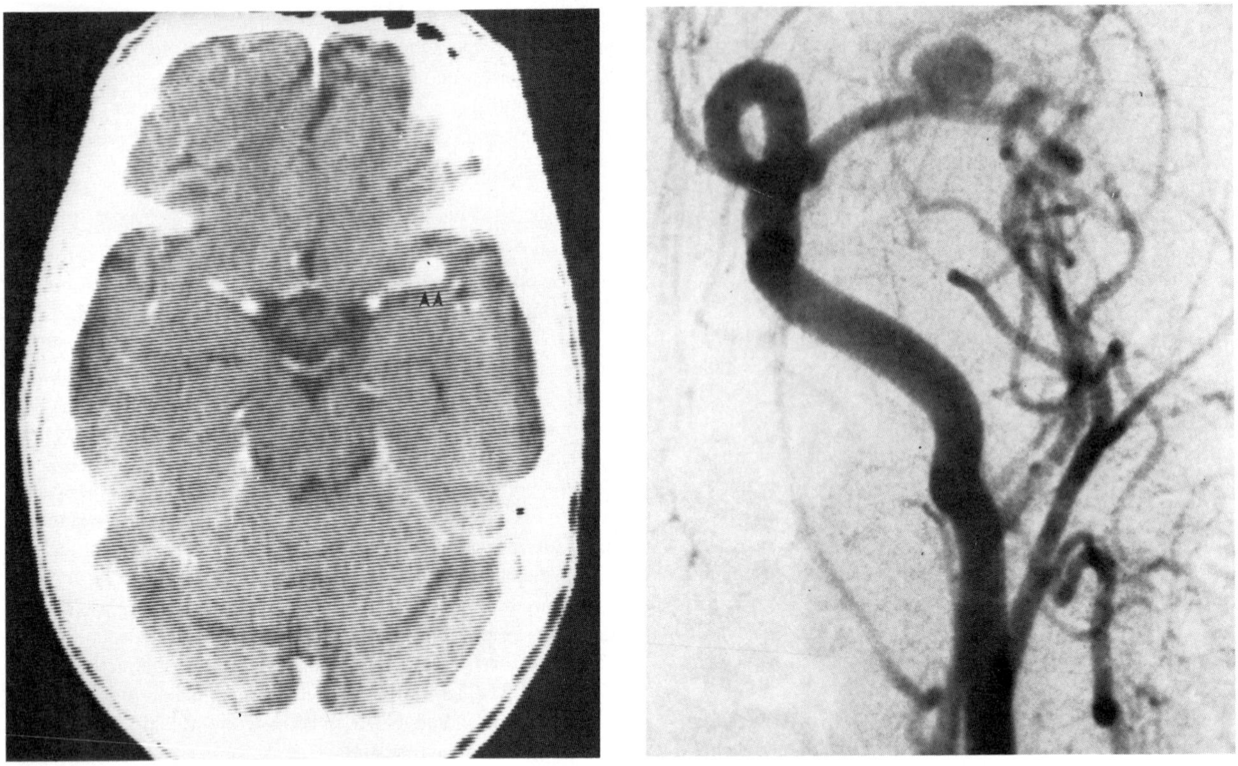

(*A*) (*B*)

Figure 216-7 *A*. Enhanced thin-section high-resolution CT scan shows a left middle cerebral artery trifurcation aneurysm (*arrowheads*). *B*. Left common carotid angiogram, submentovertical projection, subtraction print, shows an irregularly marginated aneurysm projecting anteriorly from the left middle cerebral artery.

itself at the time of first hemorrhage is also in this category. A second high-quality angiogram will usually discover 5 to 10 percent more aneurysms. Two high-quality cerebral angiograms should have been interpreted as normal before searching for a spinal arteriovenous malformation or spinal cord tumor. How soon a high-quality but completely negative angiogram should be repeated depends on several factors, not the least of which is the condition of the patient. It is said that the maximal spasm of the cerebral vasculature occurs between the fourth and fourteenth day after bleeding.[4] Certainly an angiogram should not be performed during this period of time unless absolutely necessary. The use of intra-arterial digital angiography as a screening procedure to rule out spasm before proceeding to a full-fledged second angiogram is helpful.

Magnetic Resonance Imaging and Magnetic Resonance Angiography

While CT scans remain the radiologic procedure of choice for detecting subarachnoid hemorrhage and transfemoral catheter cerebral angiography is still the gold standard for identifying cerebral aneurysms, magnetic resonance imaging (MRI) and magnetic resonance angiography (MRA) have become very useful in diagnosing and treating intracranial aneurysms. MRI scans do not consistently identify fresh subarachnoid hemorrhage due to the relatively high P_{O_2} in the CSF which prevents the formation of paramagnetic deoxyhemoglobin. Further, it is difficult to manage acutely sick patients within the environment of the MRI suite. Vascular spasm which often accompanies subarachnoid hemorrhage may significantly reduce the conspicuity of cerebral aneurysms or their parent vessels on MRA.[21] On the other hand, MRI and MRA are excellent screening procedures to detect and characterize unruptured intracranial aneurysms. They should be considered in patients who have an increased risk of aneurysm formation (e.g., those with polycystic kidney disease, fibromuscular dysplasia, or aortic coarctation).[19,20] Aneurysms as small as 3 mm have been identified in high-quality MRA studies.[19] The sensitivities of these studies have varied from 73 to 95 percent depending on the sequences performed and computer programs used.[19] Aneurysms smaller than 3 mm are of marginal clinical significance. MRI studies have also been helpful in quantifying the extent of the cerebral ischemia that accompanies arterial vasospasm due to subarachnoid hemorrhage.[12] MRI may also pinpoint which of many aneurysms has bled by identifying the presence of subacute hemorrhage adjacent to the offending lesion.[15] In the postoperative period, MRI studies clearly delineate postoperative complications such as small areas of ischemia or extra-axial fluid collections, as well as demonstrating the effectiveness of balloon occlusion techniques.[2,24] The usefulness of MRI in evaluating the status of "postclipped" aneurysm depends on the nonferrous nature of the aneurysm clip (susceptibility artifacts), and the availability of ultrashort echo times and very small voxels.[21]

Totally patent aneurysms are seen on MRI as saccular flow voids silhouetted against the white CSF of T2-weighted MRI images (Fig. 216-8*A*). They are most easily identified when located proximally in the circle of Willis. Peripherally located aneurysms

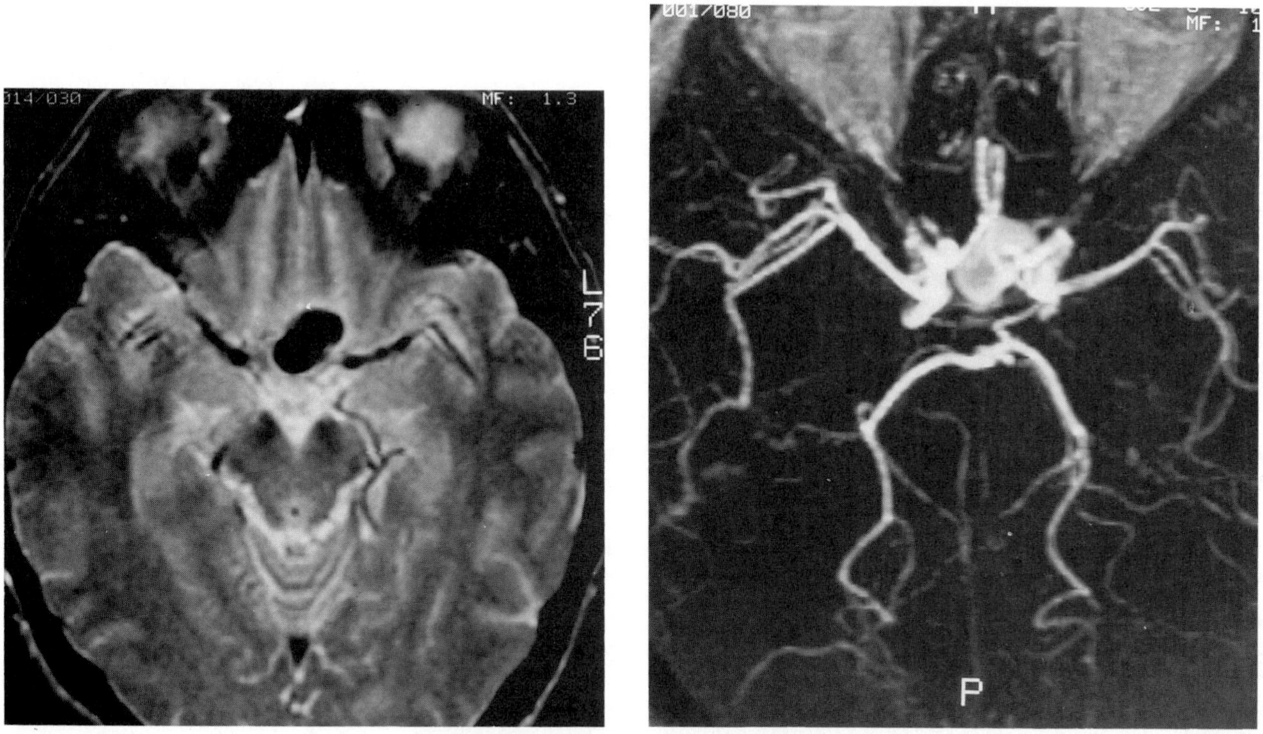

(*A*) (*B*)

Figure 216-8 *A*. An axial T2-weighted brain MR image shows a large internal carotid artery aneurysm projecting into the suprasellar cistern. *B*. An axial brain MRA shows a large, completely patent left internal carotid artery aneurysm projecting into the suprasellar cistern.

are more difficult to see because of the relative lack of surrounding high-intensity CSF. On spin echo images the black flow void is often less conspicuous due to the isointense surrounding CSF and brain signals. Giant aneurysms have varying appearances in MRI studies (Fig. 216-9). Many show the typical flow void of rapid flow while others demonstrate increased signal due to even echo rephasing or flow related entry phenomena.[7] Fresh laminated, eccentric thrombus will be seen as areas of increased signal.[1,13] Para-aneurysmal hemorrhage will demonstrate varying signal intensities depending on its age. Aneurysm calcification is seldom seen. Aneurysms have been falsely identified in instances where a normal blood vessel demonstrates a serpentine appearance as it passes in and out of the tomographic section. In addition, pulsatile flow within a vessel may be transmitted to the adjacent brain tissue, simulating an aneurysm.[7]

MRA is a technique whereby computer manipulated MRI slices can demonstrate the cerebral vasculature without interference from overlying brain and CSF signals. It is more sensitive to the presence of aneurysms than plain MRI and should be performed in cases where an aneurysm seen on MRI needs further clarification or when a negative MRI in a highly suspicious patient demands it. MRI and MRA should be seen as complementary procedures. Time-of-flight (TOF) or phase contrast (PC) are the two techniques for performing MRA. Both can be performed as two-dimensional or three-dimensional acquisitions. In TOF studies, fresh incoming unsaturated spins from flowing blood outside the imaging area generate a bright signal as these spins do not become saturated as they pass through the slice (Fig. 216-8*B*). In PC studies, the net phase shift induced by flowing blood generates the MR signal in contrast to the absent phase shift and consequent background suppression of the surrounding stationary soft tissue. For

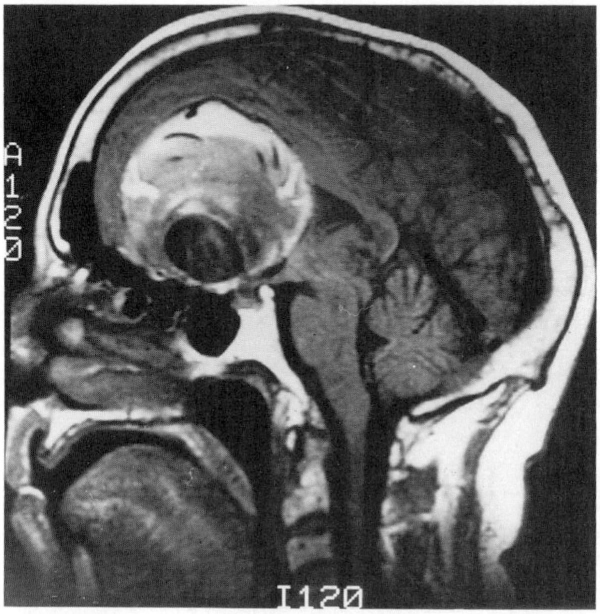

Figure 216-9 A sagittal brain MRI shows a giant internal carotid artery aneurysm. The large flow void at the center of the aneurysm represents its patent lumen. Enhancement due to slower flowing blood within the lumen is present. Surrounding the patent lumen are areas of differing intensity due to subacute and chronic hemorrhage in the wall of the giant aneurysm. Displaced cerebral blood vessels are identified as serpentine shadows at the very outer margin of the giant aneurysm.

studies of the arteries of the circle of Willis, the 3-D TOF studies are preferred due to the extremely thin individual slices (0.7 mm), shorter echo times, and higher spatial resolution. In larger aneurysms with slower or disturbed flow, 3-D PC studies are more sensitive in showing the lumen of the aneurysm. The individual slices or partitions are then subjected to a reconstruction algorithm, generally the maximum intensity projection (MIP) technique that allows the blood vessels to be displayed in multiple projections thereby providing better discrimination of the aneurysm (Fig. 216-10*A* to *C*). Occasionally, in giant aneurysms with very slow or turbulent flow, studies with intravenous contrast (gadolinium) help to demonstrate the lumen of the aneurysm. The question of which technique is applicable in a given case depends on the size and location of the aneurysm, its imaging characteristics, and the software programs available on various MRI devices. In the stable patient whose aneurysm has not yet ruptured, a combined MRI/MRA study is a noninvasive, cost-effective way to detect the presence of an aneurysm larger than 3 mm in diameter. It also serves as an excellent study to evaluate postoperative sequelae of aneurysm surgery or other forms of management.

Follow-Up Studies

Follow-up CT and MRI studies may determine the cause of neurological deficits that may occur during the waiting period before surgery. These include rehemorrhage, hydrocephalus, and vasospasm. A rebleed is identified as an area of increased density in the subarachnoid cisterns on CT. It may also extend into the ventricles or into the brain parenchyma. Hydrocephalus can be easily recognized by comparing the ventricular size with that shown by the initial scan. Frequently the hydrocephalus is accompanied by periventricular edema, occurring most prominently adjacent to the frontal horns. Hydrocephalus is caused by the blockage of the pacchionian granulations by erythrocytes, which prevent absorption of cerebrospinal fluid. The possibility of a rebleed or the development of hydrocephalus cannot be predicted either clinically or from the initial CT scan.

Vasospasm is related directly to the presence of blood in the subarachnoid space. It occurs when blood comes into direct contact with the adventitia of an artery. On the initial CT scan, the

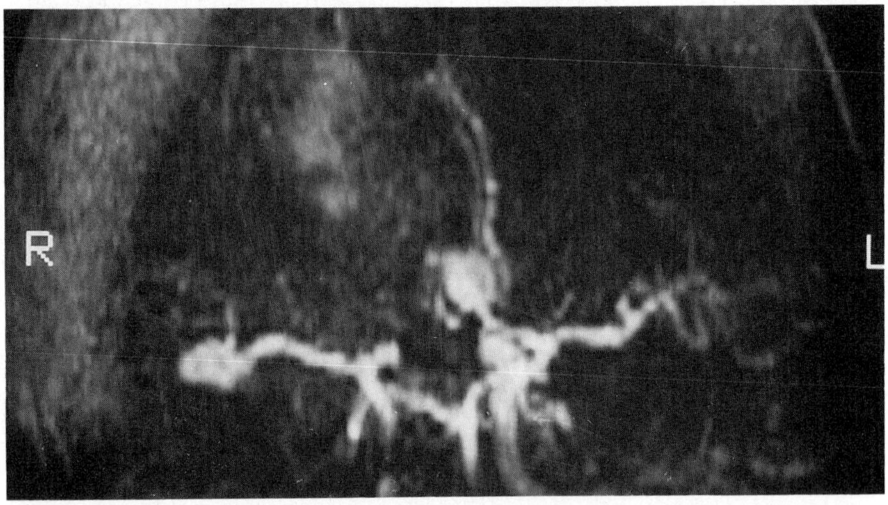

(*A*)

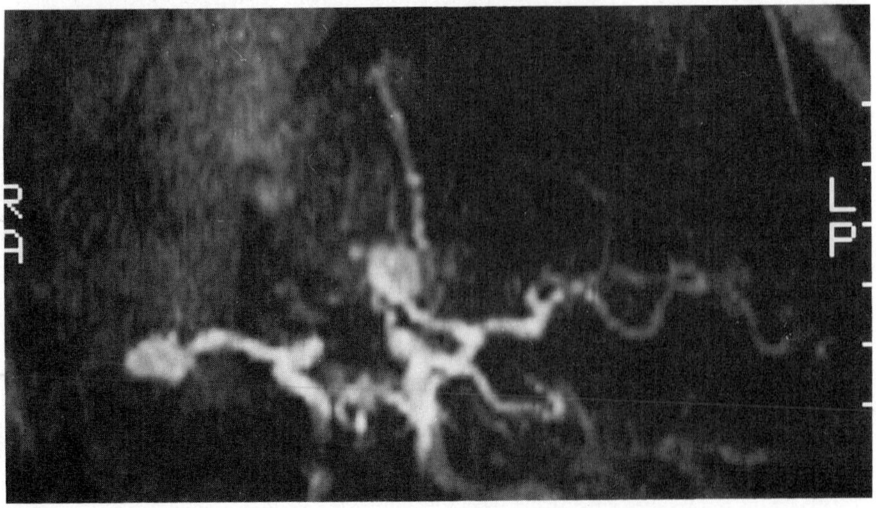

(*B*)

Figure 216-10 *A*. A coronal brain MRA shows a peripheral aneurysm located on the right middle cerebral artery and a large aneurysm at the level of the anterior communicating artery. A third aneurysm of the supraclinoid portion of the left internal carotid artery is suspected. A large frontal intracerebral hematoma due to the rupture of the anterior communicating artery aneurysm is identified as an irregularly margined area of increased density in the right frontal lobe. *B*. A coronal brain MRA with 15 degree rotation to the left shows the previously described right middle cerebral artery and anterior communicating artery aneurysms. The suspected aneurysm arising from the supraclinoid portion of the left internal carotid artery is now more clearly identified than in *A*. The right frontal lobe hemorrhage remains.

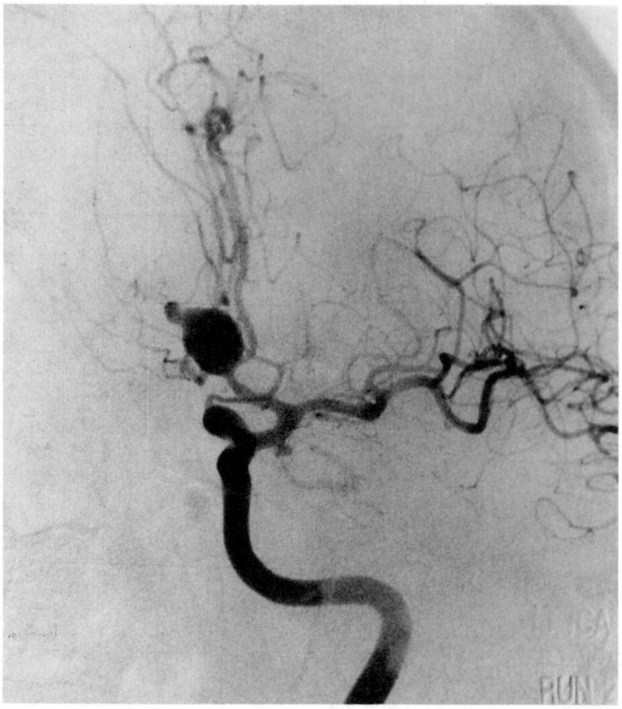

(*C*)

Figure 216-10 (*Continued*) *C.* A left internal carotid artery angiogram (subtraction print, 15 degree left posterior oblique projection) demonstrates good visualization of the large anterior communicating artery aneurysm which has hemorrhaged into the right frontal lobe. Note the excellent visualization of the supraclinoid carotid artery aneurysm projecting from the left internal carotid artery and the good correlation with *B*.

thickness of blood clot in the subarachnoid cisterns correlates highly with the severity of vasospasm seen at angiography (Fig. 216-11). The angiographic finding of severe vasospasm, judged as greater than 75 percent compromise of the vascular lumen with poor cephalad flow of contrast medium, directly correlates with the development of permanent neurological deficits. Transcranial Doppler ultrasonography is helpful in assessing the presence, location, and degree of cerebral vasospasm. Increasing mean flow velocities in excess of 120 cm/s may suggest the presence of vasospasm even before it becomes evident clinically. On CT scans, the effects of vasospasm are manifested as low-density changes within the brain parenchyma. These low-density appearances, however, do not represent permanent brain damage and may disappear with improvement in the neurological status. Delayed enhancement of the low-density areas on CT scans has been associated with permanent brain damage. In effect then, the severity of angiographic vasospasm is directly proportional to the thickness of the blood clot found on the initial scan following aneurysm rupture.[3] The development of cerebral infarcts following vasospasm directly correlates with the severity of angiographic vasospasm.

Postoperative CT has been useful in detecting residual lesions such as encephalomalacia or cerebral infarction (Fig. 216-12). In some instances faulty placement of the aneurysm clip may even be detected (Fig. 216-13). The development of postoperative hydrocephalus, whether due to the original bleeding insult or the operation itself, is best analyzed by serial CT scans. The ease of performance of postoperative CT has reduced the need for postoperative angiography.

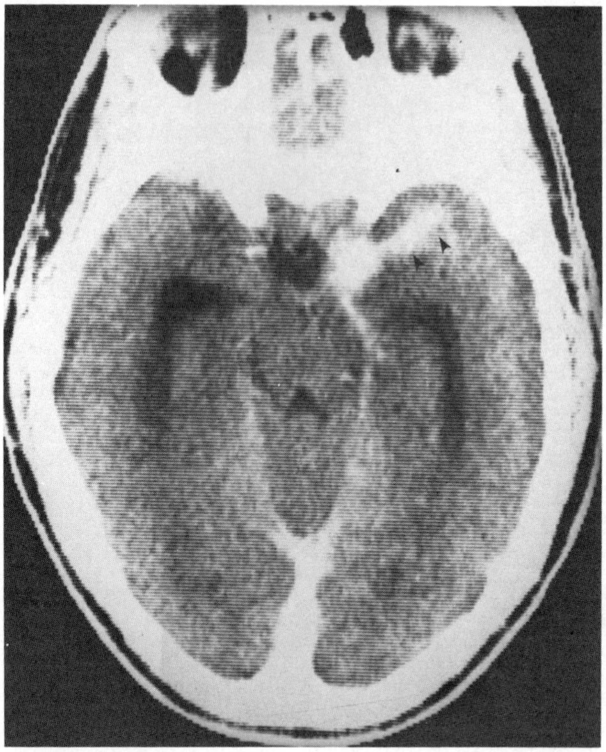

(*A*)

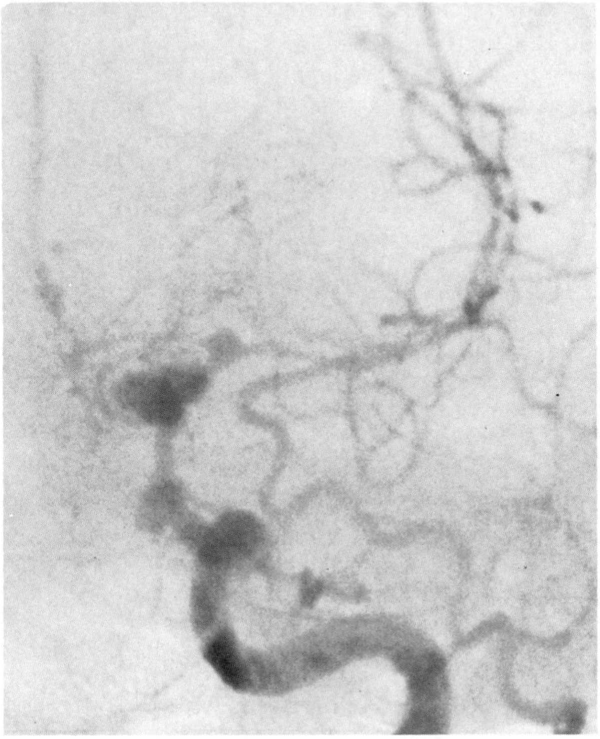

(*B*)

Figure 216-11 *A.* Enhanced thin-section high-resolution CT scan shows a left posterior communicating artery aneurysm with hemorrhage into the adjacent subarachnoid space (*arrowheads*). *B.* Left common carotid angiogram, subtraction print, demonstrates marked spasm of the supraclinoid portion of the left internal carotid artery and the horizontal rami of the left anterior and middle cerebral arteries. A large left posterior communicating artery aneurysm is seen.

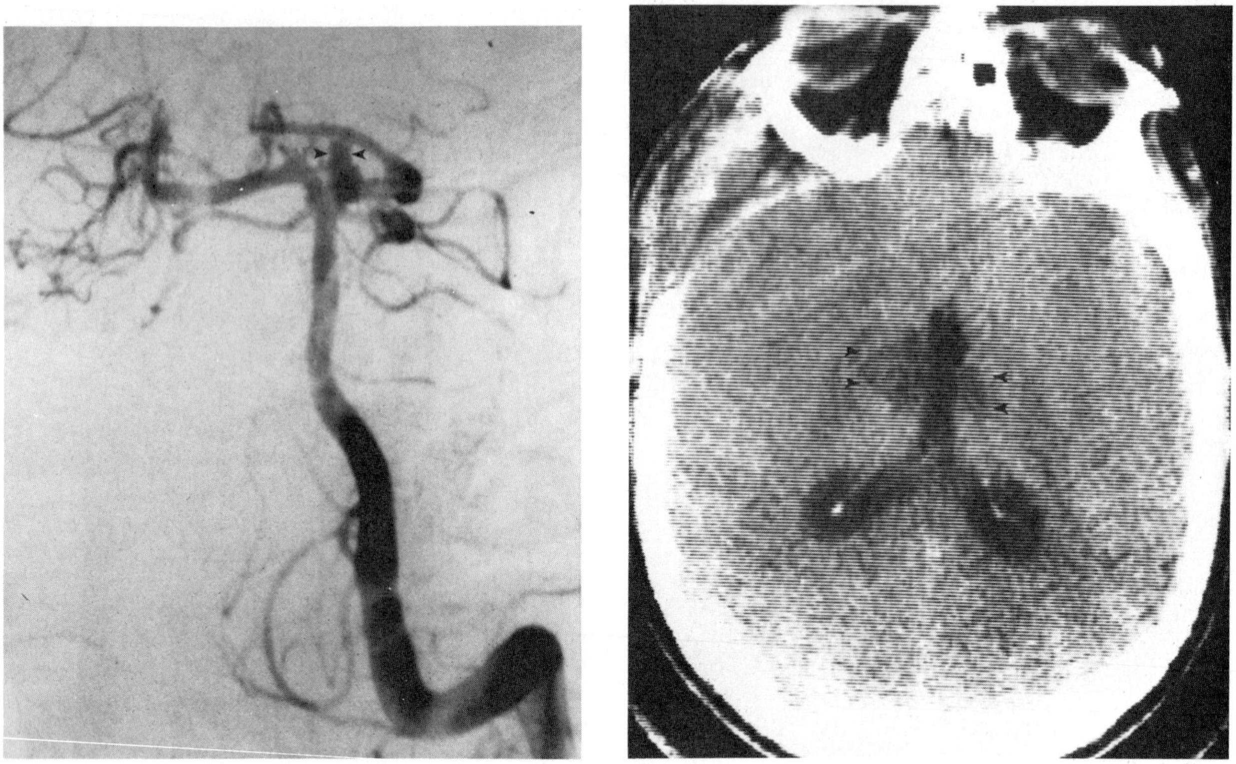

(*A*) (*B*)

Figure 216-12 *A*. Selective left vertebral angiogram, subtraction print, shows an irregularly marginated basilar artery aneurysm (*arrowheads*). *B*. Computed tomogram following successful aneurysm surgery shows areas of decreased density in the right and left thalami, representing thalamic infarctions (*arrowheads*).

Types of Intracranial Aneurysms

Congenital

The incidence of ''congenital'' aneurysms will vary from investigator to investigator depending on whether statistics were derived from a study of partial or complete angiograms, autopsy series, or autopsy series with selective injection of the arteries at the base of the skull with x-ray analysis and microdissection.[16] Estimates as low as 8 percent and as high as 20 percent have been recorded based on these differing analyses. It is not unreasonable to expect the incidence of congenital aneurysms to approach 15 percent. Etiologically, there is a definite relationship between atherosclerosis and aneurysm formation. Aneurysms are also seen in the presence of developmental anomalies such as polycystic kidneys, aortic coarctation, fibromuscular dysplasia, and lupus erythematosus. The precise statistic as to which is the most common location of an intracranial aneurysm also depends on the investigator being quoted. In the opinion of Taveras and Wood, middle cerebral artery aneurysms are most common, with posterior communicating artery aneurysms second in frequency and anterior communicating artery aneurysms third.[28] Up to 20 percent of aneurysms are multiple. Bilateral middle cerebral artery bifurcation and posterior communicating artery aneurysms are often symmetric.

Atherosclerotic

Atherosclerotic aneurysms also occur at the base of the brain and are most common on the basilar artery, where they may block the outlet of the third ventricle and produce hydrocephalus. They can occur on the internal carotid artery as well. The vessel involved with the atherosclerotic aneurysm is usually uniformly enlarged, somewhat irregular, tortuous, and elongated.[17] Atherosclerotic aneurysms seldom produce subarachnoid hemorrhage but more often present as masses, producing cranial nerve deficits and in some instances even mimicking extra-axial brain tumors.

Infectious

Infectious (mycotic) aneurysms represent approximately 6 percent of all intracranial aneurysms. They usually involve peripheral branches. They may produce an infected hematoma by bleeding into either the brain or the subdural space.[26]

Traumatic

Traumatic aneurysms are usually secondary to blunt trauma to the skull and result when a spicule of bone in a depressed skull fracture lacerates an adjacent cortical branch of the middle cerebral

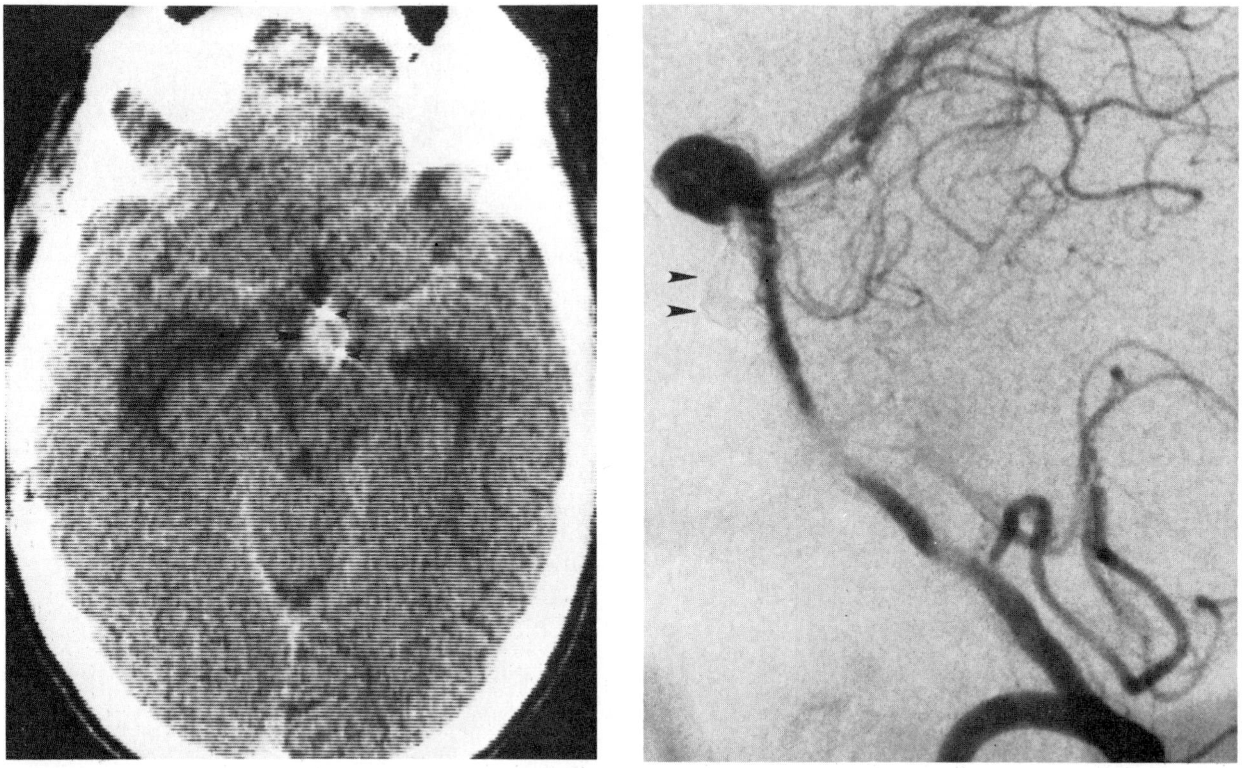

(*A*) (*B*)

Figure 216-13 *A*. Enhanced thin-section high-resolution CT scan performed following basilar artery aneurysm surgery shows persistent filling of a basilar artery aneurysm (*large arrowhead*). Two small metallic densities adjacent to the aneurysm are tips of the aneurysm clip (*small arrowheads*). *B*. Selective left vertebral angiogram, lateral view, subtraction print, shows persistence of the basilar artery aneurysm. The misplaced aneurysm clip is seen adjacent to the aneurysm (*arrowheads*).

artery. They may occur on the pericallosal artery where it lies adjacent to the rigid falx (Fig. 216-14).[27] Rarely, penetrating skull trauma may result in laceration of a cerebral vessel, producing a false aneurysm. Many of these lesions are associated with an adjacent intracerebral hematoma or cerebral edema.

Neoplastic

Neoplastic aneurysms have been reported in patients with metastatic atrial myxoma and choriocarcinoma. Infectious, traumatic, and neoplastic aneurysms are rare and may be suspected on the basis of clinical information. While they may rarely be centrally located, they usually lie peripherally in the distribution of the middle cerebral artery and can be easily identified on magnified subtracted cerebral angiograms. If the lesions are large, they may be seen on contrast-enhanced CT scans.[26]

Giant

Giant aneurysms by definition must be greater than 2.5 cm in greatest diameter. They represent 5 percent of all verified aneurysms. They most often present clinically as intracranial masses with focal neurologic signs. Lower cranial nerve deficits occur with posterior fossa giant aneurysms (Fig. 216-15). There are two

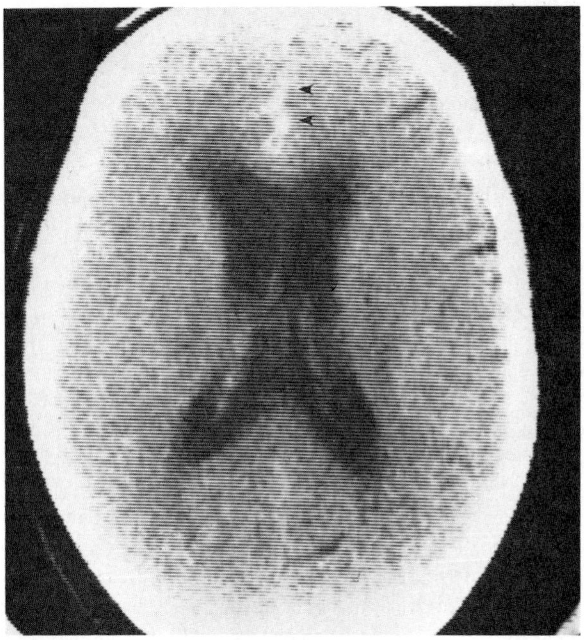

(*A*)

Figure 216-14 *A*. Unenhanced CT scan shows subarachnoid hemorrhage in the interhemispheric fissure (*arrowheads*).

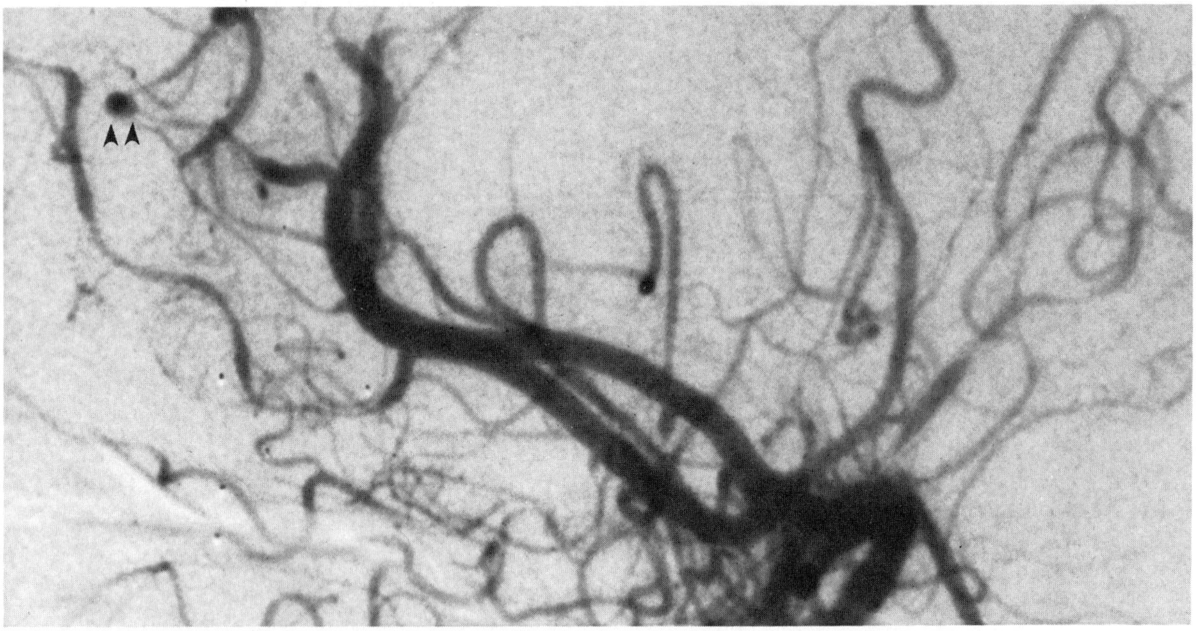

(*B*)

Figure 216-14 (*Continued*) *B*. Left carotid angiogram, lateral view, subtraction print, shows a small pericallosal artery aneurysm (*arrowheads*) with marked spasm of the adjacent pericallosal and callosomarginal arteries.

types of giant aneurysms, *globoid* and *serpentine*. The globoid are thought to be large examples of the more commonly seen small saccular aneurysms. They are congenital lesions with a defective internal elastic membrane and may contain either a central or an eccentric thrombus within their lumen with circumferential flow about the thrombus. By distinction, the serpentine aneurysm, also called *fusiform*, shows a snakelike vascular channel surrounded by a large thrombus. This variety should not be confused with diffuse arterial ectasia, in which a tortuous vessel with an enlarged lumen is present but without mass effect or thrombus (Fig. 216-6). The serpentine variety does not necessarily occur at arterial bifurcations and is not associated with atherosclerosis. It is commonly on the middle cerebral artery. An arteriovenous malformation should not be confused with the serpentine aneurysm as there are no early filling veins present. The etiology of serpentine giant aneurysms is not certain. They may be expansions of smaller saccular aneurysms or may arise by a different pathologic process and represent a congenitally different subgroup.

The characteristic plain radiographic findings in giant aneurysms include calcification and bony erosion. The calcification seen in approximately 18 percent of proven giant aneurysms may be either curvilinear, ringlike, or even shell-like but is usually thinner than that seen with intracranial tumors. In an additional 18 percent of cases the plain films will show bone erosion. This erosion may involve the petrous bone, the floor of the middle cranial fossa, the sella turcica, the anterior clinoid, or even the superior orbital fissure. Although bone erosion is not a specific finding for giant intracranial aneurysms, it should be carefully looked for and properly documented.

The CT findings of giant aneurysms will vary depending whether the lumen of the aneurysm is totally patent, partially thrombosed, or completely thrombosed. In the completely patent giant aneurysm the nonenhanced CT scan will show a round or oval mass of slightly increased density (as compared with the adjacent brain), with varying amounts of calcification at its circumference. Following intravenous contrast infusion, intense enhancement of the lumen occurs. While there is intense enhancement of the aneurysm wall as well as the lumen, it usually cannot be identified separately. This rim enhancement is due to the presence of increasing numbers of adventitial vessels in the rim of the giant aneurysm. In a completely thrombosed giant aneurysm, the unenhanced CT scan usually shows an area of increased density greater than the adjacent brain, with a somewhat mottled appearance again accompanied by varying amounts of calcification at its periphery. This area of significantly increased density represents the completely clotted lumen. Following the intravenous infusion of a contrast agent, the clotted lumen is not enhanced but the richly supplied vascular wall of the giant aneurysm is well luminated. In cases in which a partial thrombosis of a giant aneurysm has occurred, the CT appearance is more complex. The unenhanced CT study will usually show a round or oval lesion with mixed densities. There will be a central or eccentric area of significantly increased density, which is the thrombosed portion of the aneurysm surrounded or capped by a slightly less dense area (but denser than the adjacent brain), which represents the remaining patent lumen of the aneurysm. This in turn is surrounded by a peripheral zone of increased density containing variable amounts of calcification, which represents the aneurysm wall. Following intravenous contrast enhancement, the residual patent lumen enhances intensely, as does the vascular rim of the aneurysm. This has been referred to as the *target sign* and is quite specific for a partially thrombosed aneurysm on CT (Fig. 216-15).[18] As by definition giant aneurysms of the serpentine subcategory are partially thrombosed, their appearance fits into this last category.

The differential diagnosis of a giant aneurysm seen on computed tomography includes pituitary adenoma, craniopharyngioma, chordoma, germinoma, epidermoid tumor, chemodectoma, glioma, colloid cyst, choroid plexus papilloma, pinealoma, and metastasis. While angiography is usually required to make a definitive differential diagnosis, certain CT features of giant aneurysms

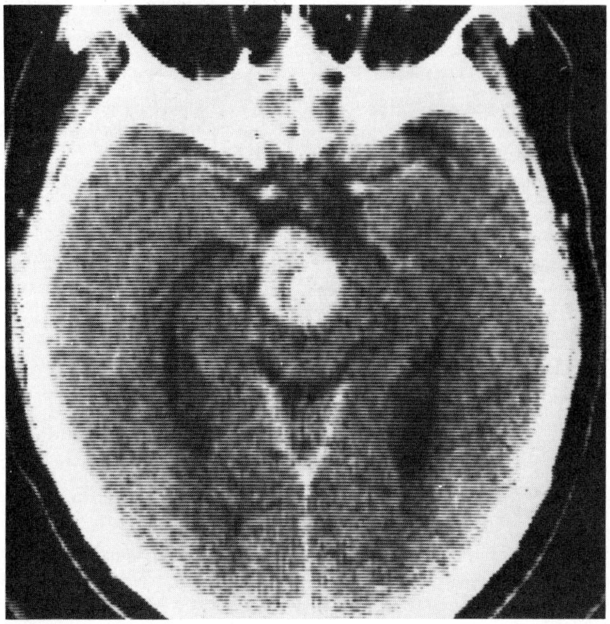

(*A*)

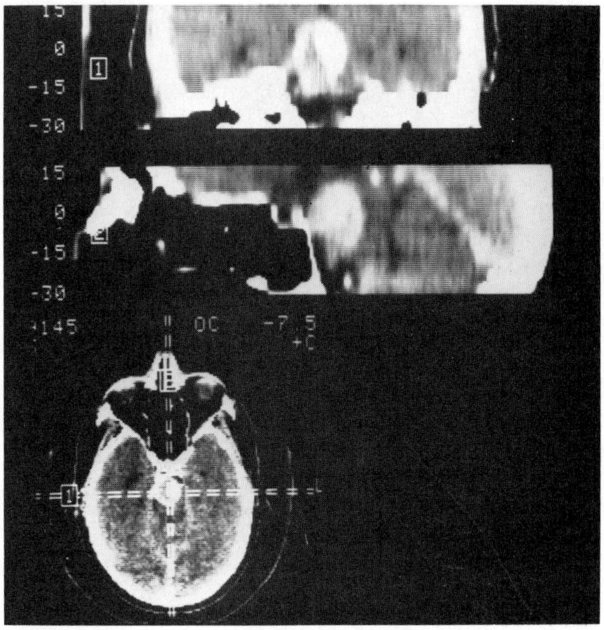

(*B*)

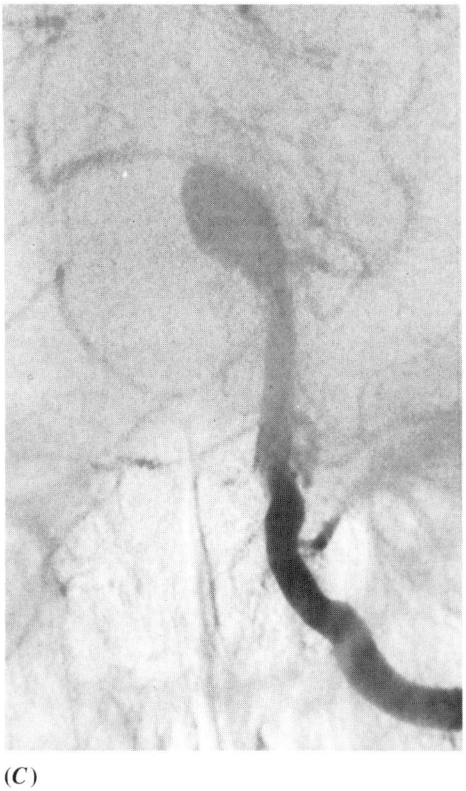

(*C*)

Figure 216-15 *A*. Enhanced high-resolution thin-section CT scan shows a giant basilar artery aneurysm. The area of marked enhancement is the residual lumen. The area of lesser density represents intraluminal thrombus. The markedly thickened wall of the aneurysm also enhances. *B*. Enhanced high-resolution thin-section CT scan with sagittal and coronal reformatting shows the partially thrombosed giant basilar artery aneurysm compressing the upper brain stem. *C*. Selective left vertebral angiogram, anteroposterior view, subtraction print, shows the giant basilar artery aneurysm. The mass of the aneurysm causes upward bowing of the right posterior cerebral artery and downward displacement of the right superior cerebellar artery. Only the residual lumen of the aneurysm is identified on the angiogram.

may allow a differentiation. Little or no surrounding edema is seen on the CT scan in patients with giant intracranial aneurysms. Giant aneurysms are found almost exclusively on the circle of Willis or occur only as far distally as the proximal middle cerebral artery bifurcation. Transit time analysis of patent giant aneurysms demonstrates washin and washout phases with timing similar to that of the larger adjacent cerebral vessels. This will allow distinction from vascular tumors which do not show this washin and washout phenomenon.[18]

Bleeding Aneurysms

The criteria for determining which of multiple aneurysms has bled were established in the neuroradiologic literature prior to CT scanning[29]; CT scanning has affected these criteria only minimally.[22] The most significant single criterion for concluding that a given aneurysm among several has bled is to see the aneurysm actually bleed during angiography (a rare event), or during the enhanced CT study (an even rarer event).[9] More often, the presence of a mass near or adjacent to an aneurysm indicts that aneurysm as the one having most recently bled. While classically this mass has been first detected at angiography, more recently CT scanning has disclosed the presence of even small hemorrhages adjacent to aneurysms, thereby affirming the bleeding lesion (Fig. 216-11). Much less localizing is the presence of spasm adjacent to a particular aneurysm. While it has been said that spasm localized to the vicinity of only one aneurysm strongly suggests that it is the bleeding site, in most instances the spasm may involve several vessels having aneurysms. It is usually wise not to attempt to determine which is the offending aneurysm in the presence of severe spasm but to wait for a more complete angiographic study of all intracranial vessels after the spasm has subsided. The more irregularly shaped, larger aneurysm is usually the offender (Fig. 216-4*A, B*). Bleeding aneurysms are often associated with a small hematoma within their lumen (Fig. 216-4*A, B*). Proximity to the circle of Willis is also a consideration. Regardless of the above criteria, if an anterior communicating artery aneurysm is present, it is often the offender.

References

1. Atlas SW. Intracranial vascular malformations and aneurysms: current imaging applications. *Radiol Clin North Am* 1988; 26:821–837.
2. Brothers MF, Fox AJ, Lee DH, et al. MR imaging after surgery for vertebrobasilar aneurysm. *Am J Neuroradiol* 1990; 11:149–161.
3. Davis JM, Davis KR, Crowell RM. Subarachnoid hemorrhage secondary to ruptured intracranial aneurysm: prognostic significance of cranial CT. *Am J Roentgenol* 1980; 134:711–715.
4. Davis KR, Kistler JP, Heros RC, Davis JM. A neuroradiologic approach to the patient with a diagnosis of subarachnoid hemorrhage. *Radiol Clin North Am* 1982; 20:87–94.
5. Forster DMC, Steiner L, Hakanson S, Bergvall U. The value of repeat pan-angiography in cases of unexplained subarachnoid hemorrhage. *J Neurosurg* 1978; 48:712–716.
6. Handel SF, Perpetuo FOL, Handel CH. Subdural hematomas due to ruptured cerebral aneurysms: angiographic diagnosis and potential pitfall for CT. *Am J Roentgenol* 1978; 130:507–509.
7. Hyman RA, Black KS. Aneurysms and vascular malformations. *Top Magn Reson Imaging* 1989; 2:49–62.
8. Inoue Y, Saiwai S, Miyamoto T, et al. Postcontrast computed tomography in subarachnoid hemorrhage from ruptured aneurysms. *J Comput Assist Tomogr* 1981; 5:341–344.
9. Jordan K, Lefkowitch J, Hays A, Sane P. Rupture of intracranial aneurysm during computerized tomography. *Arch Neurol* 1980; 37:465–466.
10. Liliequist B, Lindqvist M. Computer tomography in the evaluation of subarachnoid hemorrhage. *Acta Radiol [Diagn] (Stockh)* 1980; 21:327–331.
11. Lin JP, Kricheff II. Angiographic investigation of cerebral aneurysms. *Radiology* 1972; 105:69–76.
12. Matsumura K, Matsuda M, Handa J, et al. Magnetic resonance imaging with aneurysmal subarachnoid hemorrhage: comparison with computed tomography scan. *Surg Neurol* 1990; 34:71–78.
13. Matsumura K, Saito A, Nakasu Y, et al. Magnetic resonance imaging of large and giant intracranial aneurysms. *Neurol Med Chir (Tokyo)* 1990; 30:382–388.
14. Modesti LM, Binet EF. Value of computed tomography in the diagnosis and management of subarachnoid hemorrhage. *Neurosurgery* 1978; 3:151–156.
15. Mourier KL, Gelbert F, Assouline E, et al. MRI in multiple vascular lesions: identification of the ruptured malformation. *Acta Neurochir (Wien)* 1991; 112:83–87.
16. Newton TH, Potts DG. *Radiology of the Skull and Brain.* St Louis: Mosby, 1974.
17. Peterson NT, Duchesneau PM, Westbrook EL, Weinstein MA. Basilar artery ectasia demonstrated by computed tomography. *Radiology* 1977; 122:713–715.
18. Pinto RS, Cohen WA, Kricheff II, et al. Giant intracranial aneurysms: rapid sequential computed tomography. *Am J Neuroradiol* 1982; 3:495–499.
19. Ross JS, Masaryk TJ, Modic MT, et al. Intracranial aneurysms: evaluation by MR angiography. *Am J Roentgenol* 1990; 155:159–165.
20. Ruggieri PM, Masaryk TJ, Ross JS. Magnetic resonance angiography. Cerebrovascular applications. *Stroke* 1992; 23:774–780.
21. Ruggieri PM, Masaryk TJ, Ross JS, et al. Intracranial magnetic resonance angiography. *Cardiovasc Intervent Radiol* 1992; 15:71–81.
22. Schnapf DJ. Multiple aneurysms of the intracranial arteries: Computed tomography in detecting the site of bleeding. *JAOA* 1981; 81:208–211.
23. Scotti G, Ethier R, Melançon D, et al. Computed tomography in the evaluation of intracranial aneurysms and subarachnoid hemorrhage. *Radiology* 1977; 123:85–90.
24. Sevick RJ, Tsuruda JS, Schmalbrock P. Three-dimensional time-of-flight MR angiography in the evaluation of cerebral aneurysms. *J Comput Assist Tomogr* 1990; 14:874–881.
25. Silver AJ, Pederson ME Jr, Ganti SR, et al. CT of subarachnoid hemorrhage due to ruptured aneurysm. *Am J Neuroradiol* 1981; 2:13–22.
26. Simmons KC, Sage MR, Reilly PL. CT of intracerebral haemorrhage due to mycotic aneurysms—case report. *Neuroradiology* 1980; 19:215–217.
27. Smith KR Jr, Bardenheier JA III. Aneurysm of the pericallosal artery caused by closed cranial trauma: case report. *J Neurosurg* 1968; 29:551–554.
28. Taveras JM, Wood EH. *Diagnostic Neuroradiology*, 2d ed. Baltimore; Williams & Wilkins, 1976.
29. Wood EH. Angiographic identification of the ruptured lesion in patients with multiple cerebral aneurysms. *J Neurosurg* 1964; 21:182–198.

217

Intracranial Arterial Spasm

Marc R. Mayberg

Since its recognition over 40 years ago, cerebral vasospasm has remained an enigma to neurosurgeons. Laboratory and clinical research efforts have lent considerable insight into the etiology, pathophysiology, and potential therapeutic strategies for this disorder, yet the basic mechanisms of arterial narrowing after subarachnoid hemorrhage remain largely undiscovered and current treatments are mostly palliative. Even the term *cerebral vasospasm* may be imprecise, as controversy exists regarding the role of active vasoconstriction as a cause of decreased vessel caliber. Furthermore, the relationship between angiographic arterial narrowing and potentially reversible neurologic deterioration is poorly understood, further complicating the development of effective therapeutic modalities.

In its broadest sense, cerebral vasospasm can be defined as the insidious onset of delayed focal or diffuse narrowing of large capacitance arteries at the base of the brain following hemorrhage into the subarachnoid space. Aneurysmal subarachnoid hemorrhage (SAH) is the most common etiology for vasospasm, although it is seen after hemorrhage from arteriovenous malformations, tumors, or head trauma. The angiographic narrowing, which follows a relatively consistent temporal course, may be entirely asymptomatic or disguised by other complications related to the SAH. In about one-half of cases, however, vasospasm manifests by the occurrence of a delayed neurological ischemic deficit, which may resolve or progress to permanent cerebral infarction. Despite advances in diagnosis and treatment, cerebral vasospasm remains the greatest treatable cause of morbidity and mortality in patients who survive the ictus of SAH. In most contemporary series, up to 15 percent of such patients suffer stroke or death from vasospasm despite maximal therapy.[22,25,37,67–69,79,84]

The presumed mechanism of neurological deterioration in cerebral vasospasm is diminished regional or global cerebral blood flow (CBF) through narrowed segments of major capacitance arteries at the circle of Willis. Some authors have suggested that neurologic deficits in vasospasm are due to direct effects of blood on the brain, disorders of the cerebral microcirculation, or distal emboli. However, positron emission tomography (PET) has documented decreased CBF, increased blood volume, and increased oxygen extraction in the distribution of affected large arteries with vasospasm consistent with regional ischemia.[70] In addition, computed tomography (CT) or autopsy evidence of cerebral infarction after vasospasm is usually (but not invariably) consistent with ischemia in the distribution of major arteries.[14] The gradual onset and nonocclusive stenosis of cerebral arteries in vasospasm likely produces wide areas of marginal CBF analogous to the *penumbra* which occurs after vascular occlusion.[80] Neurons in this marginally perfused region may be nonfunctional at these CBF levels (10 to 20 ml/100 g per min), yet permanent damage may not occur for hours or days. This unique aspect of ischemia from cerebral vasospasm may explain several important features of the disorder, including its evanescent course and the effectiveness of therapeutic strategies such as hypervolemia and hemodilution and calcium-channel antagonists, as discussed below. With prompt recognition and institution of therapy, cerebral vasospasm is potentially the most treatable cause of cerebral ischemia.

Clinical and Angiographic Features

The angiographic correlate of cerebral vasospasm is narrowing of intracranial segments of major cerebral arteries at the base of the brain, usually in contrast to a prior angiogram documenting normal caliber of the involved vessels (Fig. 217-1). The arterial narrowing can be focal or diffuse, and is often associated with radiographic evidence of diminished flow in the distal territory of the affected artery. Angiographic vasospasm has a typical temporal course, with onset at 3 to 5 days after the hemorrhage, maximal narrowing at 5 to 14 days, and gradual resolution over 2 to 4 weeks (Fig. 217-2).[25,37,89]

Clinical features of vasospasm are less predictable, and depend on many variables including severity and location of the arterial narrowing, age and clinical condition of the patient, the presence of complicating factors (e.g., elevated intracranial pressure or hypotension), and the extent of collateral circulation to the ischemic brain.[6,31,36,84] For these and other indeterminate reasons, one-half of patients with angiographic vasospasm remain asymptomatic (see below). In symptomatic patients, clinical manifestations of vasospasm vary in their presentation, severity, and duration for similar reasons. The *delayed ischemic neurological deficit* associated with symptomatic vasospasm usually presents shortly after the onset of angiographic vasospasm with the acute or subacute development of focal or generalized symptoms and signs.[6,31,36] For lesions affecting the anterior circulation, these signs include hemiparesis, hemisensory deficits, visual disturbance, dysphasia, or change in level of consciousness. For vasospasm of the posterior circulation, manifestations may include dysarthria, diplopia, vertigo, ataxia, or altered sensorium. Frequently the onset of neurological signs is preceded by fever,[71] increased meningismus, and nonspecific light-headedness. Once manifest, symptoms and signs may progress in severity or fluctuate, and are often associated with changes in intravascular volume status or blood pressure. Progression to permanent cerebral infarction occurs in approximately 50 percent of symptomatic cases; recovery without deficit in the remaining individuals may occur despite the persistence of angiographic vasospasm.[25,37,84]

Incidence

Analysis of the incidence of cerebral vasospasm is complicated by the lack of consistent diagnostic criteria among reported studies. Nevertheless, the incidence of cerebral vasospasm following aneurysmal SAH has probably declined somewhat in recent years. The Cooperative Aneurysm Study in 1987 reported the incidence of angiographic vasospasm at over 50 percent, with symptomatic vasospasm in 32 percent of patients.[2] These values have remained

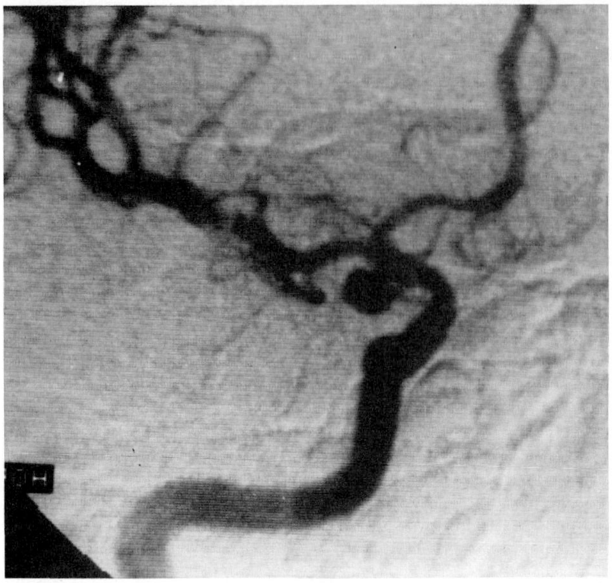

(*A*)

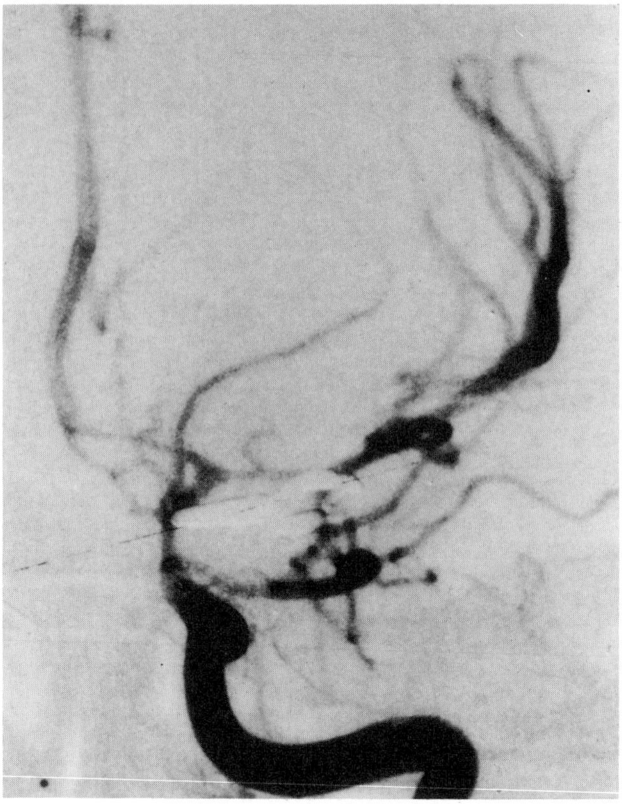

(*B*)

Figure 217-1 Angiographic appearance of cerebral vasospasm. Compared to the preoperative angiogram *(left)* there is marked narrowing of the supraclinoid internal carotid artery (ICA), anterior cerebral artery (ACA), and middle cerebral artery (MCA) at 6 days after SAH *(right)*. The posterior communicating artery aneurysm has been clipped in the interim.

consistent in numerous retrospective reviews.[4,5,23,62] Most patients in recent reports have been treated with regimens of volume expansion and hemodilution (see below). In recent major prospective trials for oral nimodipine,[3,68,69] angiographic (50 to 66 percent) and symptomatic (30 to 40 percent) vasospasm were

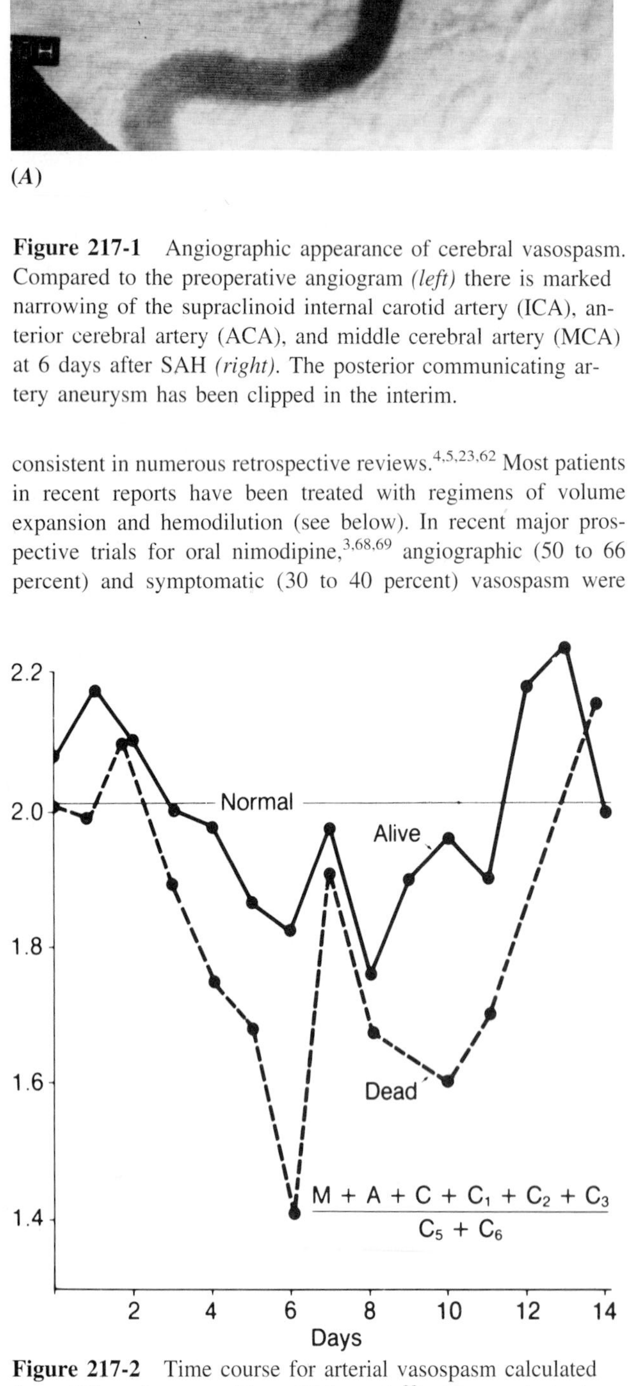

Figure 217-2 Time course for arterial vasospasm calculated from 429 angiograms. (From Weir et al.,[89] with permission.)

relatively consistent among both placebo and treatment groups. Recent uncontrolled retrospective studies utilizing intravenous calcium-channel antagonists have reported the incidence of symptomatic vasospasm lower than 10 percent.[4,21,23,56,77]

Vasospasm following head injury is less often recognized because of the declining use of angiography and the coexistence of significant neurological deficits which make diagnosis more difficult.[65] In a retrospective study, Wilkins and Odom[94] described angiographic vasospasm in 19 percent of 350 patients with moderate or severe head injury. The advent of the noninvasive technique of transcranial Doppler (TCD) sonography has renewed interest in vasospasm as a complication of head injury,[46] and may better define its incidence in this setting. Cerebral vasospasm following hemorrhage from arteriovenous malformations is considerably less frequent than that of aneurysmal subarachnoid hemorrhage, probably because of the absence of extensive subarachnoid blood collections in the former disorder.[36]

Predisposing Factors

Conditions associated with a higher incidence of cerebral vasospasm after SAH are listed in Table 217-1. The initial observations of Takemae et al.[86] regarding the relationship between the volume of subarachnoid blood on CT and the subsequent development of vasospasm have been subsequently confirmed in numerous reports. Fisher et al.[20] described a scaling system for the volume of subarachnoid hemorrhage which correlated highly with the risk of subsequent vasospasm. Clinical grade of the patient at the initial presentation also correlates with vasospasm risk,[60] probably because poor-grade patients tend to have more extensive subarachnoid bleeding.[33] The presence of intraventricular blood and coexis-

TABLE 217-1 Conditions Associated with Increased Risk of Cerebral Vasospasm

Increased volume of subarachnoid blood on CT
Worse clinical grade
Intraventricular blood and hydrocephalus
Fever/peripheral leukocytosis
Hyponatremia (hypovolemia)
Antifibrinolytic agents
Female with MCA aneurysm

tent hydrocephalus have been associated with an increased incidence of vasospasm.[9] Elevated peripheral white blood cell counts often predict an increased risk of vasospasm,[71,88] although this parameter usually manifests at the onset of symptoms (see below). Hyponatremia has been suggested as a predictor of vasospasm, probably due to the associated hypovolemia.[92] As discussed below, antifibrinolytic agents such as epsilon-aminocaproic acid increase the risk of vasospasm.[2,27] Several studies have not shown that increased risk of vasospasm is related to sex or aneurysm location; a single retrospective study suggested an increased risk for women with middle cerebral artery aneurysms.[95] Angiographic vasospasm may be more common in younger individuals, although it is less likely to be symptomatic in this age group.[64]

Diagnosis

Effective therapy for cerebral vasospasm depends on early recognition of clinical manifestations. Cognizance of predisposing risk factors for vasospasm (Table 217-1) is essential. In this regard, the CT scan within 48 h after SAH is a good predictor of vasospasm risk. The definitive diagnosis of vasospasm is made by angiography; however, the invasive nature of this procedure necessitates its use primarily to confirm a diagnosis which is based upon clinical and noninvasive measures. Comprehensive monitoring of patients after SAH, especially those at high risk for vasospasm, will increase the diagnostic accuracy.

Noninvasive Diagnosis

The recent advent of TCD has greatly facilitated the diagnosis of vasospasm. This modality uses range-gated pulsed Doppler insonation through thinner parts of the skull to determine blood velocity in large arteries at the cranial base.[1] With SAH, elevated cerebral arterial blood velocity correlates highly with angiographic vasospasm (Figure 217-3).[30,59,76] Normative values for major cerebral arteries have been established; the ratio of middle cerebral to cervical carotid artery velocity *(carotid index)* can help differentiate vasospasm from increased cerebral blood flow due to a hyperdynamic state.[58] A prominent increase in TCD velocity during the first week after SAH is highly characteristic of vasospasm and often precedes the onset of clinical symptoms by several hours. Similarly, restitution of normal TCD velocities usually signals the remission of vasospasm, and can aid in determining therapy duration. Additional noninvasive adjuncts to the diagnosis of vasospasm include methods to assess regional cerebral blood flow, including ^{133}Xe,[96] xenon-CT,[97] single photon emission tomography (SPECT)[43] and positron emission tomography (PET).[70]

Clinical Diagnosis

The diagnosis of cerebral vasospasm is largely based on careful sequential neurologic examinations by personnel familiar with its manifestations. A high index of suspicion can facilitate diagnosis, thereby accommodating estimated risk factors and the temporal course of the disease. Fever and a slight leukocytosis in peripheral blood frequently herald the onset of symptoms.[71,88] A sharp increase in TCD velocity (e.g., middle cerebral artery velocity > 120 cm/s) should alert physicians to impending symptoms.[76] At this stage, any change in neurological condition mandates a thorough evaluation to exclude other causes of deterioration, including hydrocephalus, seizures, cerebral edema, electrolyte abnormalities, drug reactions, respiratory insufficiency, or new intracranial hemorrhage (Table 217-2). Cerebral ischemia from other

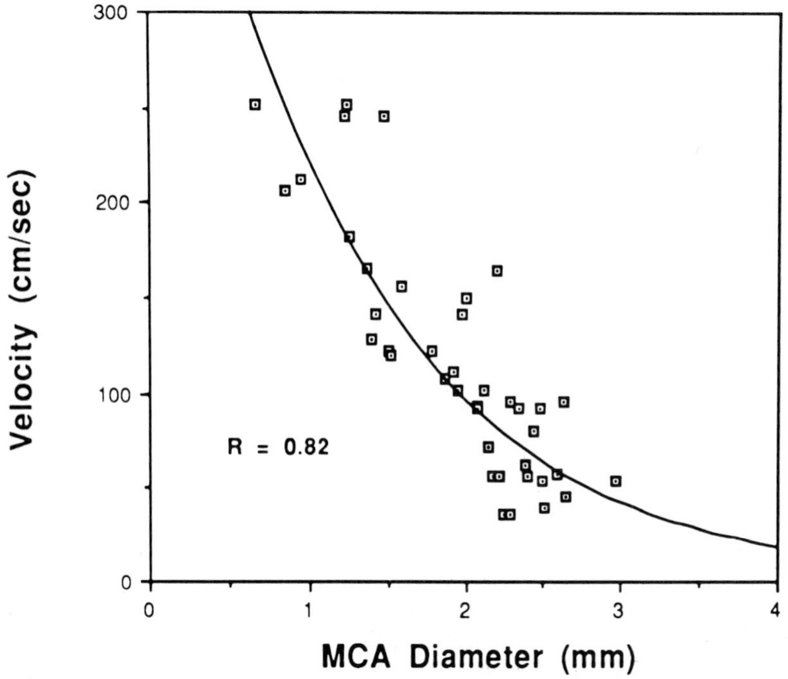

Figure 217-3 Correlation of middle cerebral artery dimeter and TCD velocity readings in 10 patients following SAH. (From Newell and Winn,[59] with permission.)

TABLE 217-2 Alternative Causes of Delayed Neurologic Deterioration after SAH

Rebleeding
Cerebral edema
Hydrocephalus
Seizures
Other causes of cerebral ischemia (emboli)
Metabolic disorders
Electrolyte imbalance
Hypoxia
Hepatic dysfunction
Drug withdrawal
Drug allergy

causes (e.g., emboli from the aneurysm) must also be considered. Appropriate tests include CT scanning, serum electrolyte and blood gas determinations, and monitoring of intracranial pressure. If alternative causes are excluded, delayed neurological deterioration in this setting is almost certainly due to ischemic consequences of vasospasm. Documentation of focal or global alterations in CBF by various noninvasive measures, as mentioned earlier, further substantiates the diagnosis.

Therapy

Several treatment strategies have emerged due to increased understanding of the pathophysiology of cerebral vasospasm. Nevertheless, no single therapy is a panacea for this disorder, and stroke or death related to vasospasm accounts for a significant proportion of poor outcome related to SAH in patients treated with maximal therapy. Therapy is often initiated prophylactically for some treatments (e.g., hypertension and hypervolemia, thrombolytic agents, and calcium antagonists), or at the onset of symptoms for other therapies (e.g., transluminal angioplasty). Prompt initiation of therapy often produces rapid improvement, again emphasizing the importance of prompt diagnosis of vasospasm.

Poiseuille's law describes theoretical flow through a blood vessel according to the formula:

$$Flow = \Delta p \pi r^4 / 8LN,$$

where Δp = pressure gradient, r = radius, L = length, and N = viscosity. From a simplistic standpoint, current therapies for vasospasm address flow through stenotic segments of cerebral arteries by either augmenting those variables comprising the numerator (i.e., increasing pressure gradient and radius), or by reducing components of the denominator (i.e., decreasing length and viscosity). Of these alternatives, changes in radius are clearly the most important variable in determining flow, yet they have proved to be the most resistant in the treatment of vasospasm.

Vasodilating Agents

Much of the early experimental work in vasospasm focused on developing agents to reduce the narrowing in cerebral arteries, which was presumed to be caused by focal vasoconstriction. In 1986, Wilkins[93] summarized three decades of research into prevention and treatment of intracranial arterial spasm; these methods included the use of vasodilators and antagonists to vasoconstrictors, as well as other pharmacologic means of inhibiting smooth muscle cell contraction. Despite occasional promising reports in experimental models, these agents were uniformly unsuccessful in reversing vasospasm in clinical trials. As discussed below, chronic exposure to perivascular blood renders cerebral vessels relatively insensitive to both vasoconstricting and vasodilating agents.[8,38] Calcium-channel antagonists, which were proposed as a therapy for vasospasm based on their ability to inhibit cerebral smooth muscle contraction, are probably effective because of mechanisms other than dilation of narrowed large vessel segments (see below). Thus, interest in vasodilating agents as a treatment for vasospasm waned in the past decade. Recent reports have renewed interest in this mode of therapy, however. In a prospective, randomized trial, intravenous nicardipine ameliorated angiographic vasospasm but failed to improve outcome at 3 months.[26] In uncontrolled trials, high dose intra-arterial papavarine (administered at the site of arterial narrowing) effectively reduced both angiographic and symptomic vasospasm in patients refractory to other therapies. Perhaps ongoing trials will determine the efficacy, durability, and safety of these new treatment modalities.

Hypertension/Hypervolemia/Hemodilution

The normal brain maintains CBF at relatively constant levels over a wide range of blood pressure *(autoregulation)* by intrinsic mechanisms controlling vascular tone in small arterioles. In ischemic brain, these arterioles are maximally dilated, so that CBF varies more directly with blood pressure (or cardiac output) in a passive manner. Additionally, augmentation of cardiac output by volume expansion with colloid or crystalloid typically lowers blood viscosity by hemodilution. In this manner "triple-H" therapy (hemodilution/hypervolemia/hypertension) potentially might improve CBF in vasospasm by affecting several variables of the Poiseuille equation.

Following the initial report of Kosnik and Hunt in 1976,[40] several reports described resolution of deficits from vasospasm following elevation of blood pressure and/or volume expansion.[5,35,42,55] In these cases, distinct changes in neurological deficits were occasionally observed with fluctuated depending on blood pressure. Outcome related to vasospasm in these uncontrolled series was considerably better than historical controls, leading to widespread application of triple-H therapy. Subsequent reports suggested further reduction in vasospasm when therapy was initiated prior to the onset of symptoms.[83]

Little is known regarding the specific mechanisms by which triple-H therapy affects cerebral vasospasm. Its efficacy has not been demonstrated in controlled trials, and studies of CBF after starting therapy have been equivocal. In addition, it is unclear which component of this therapy (hemodilution vs. hypervolemia vs. hypertension) is most important. Only a portion of patients with vasospasm respond to triple-H therapy, with stroke and death rates approaching 15 percent in the best series.[5,55]

Initiation of triple-H therapy is associated with significant risk, including cardiac failure, electrolyte abnormalities, cerebral edema, bleeding abnormalities, and rupture of an unsecured aneurysm.[42] Patients receiving this treatment should be monitored in an intensive care setting with Swan-Ganz catheter, arterial line, and frequent serum electrolyte determinations. Most protocols utilize measurements of left ventricular end diastolic pressure (LVEDP) and cardiac output to optimize hemodynamics according to the Starling curve.[42] Volume expansion is accomplished using either crystalloid or colloid to achieve LVEDP in the range of 12 to 16 mmHg, depending on the patient's age and cardiac status.

Hemodilution with reduction of hemocrit to less than 35 percent is usually coincident with volume loading. Blood pressure is most often maintained at physiologic levels; augmentation to supranormal values with dopamine or dobutamine may be reserved for neurologic deterioration refractory to hemodilution and hypervolemia. Therapy may be more effective if initiated prophylactically prior to the onset of symptoms (preferably after clipping of the aneurysm,[83] and should be continued beyond the period of risk for vasospasm or until vasospasm abates by clinical and TCD parameters.

Calcium-Channel Antagonists

Calcium-channel antagonists may affect pathologic processes in cerebral vasospasm by a number of mechanisms (Table 217-3). This class of drugs consists of dihydropyridines (nimodipine, nicardipine, nifedipine), diphenyl alkamines (verapamil), and benzothiazepines (diltiazam), which act to block receptor-mediated calcium channels (L-channels) on smooth muscle cells. Certain agents (diltiazam, nicardipine, and nimodipine) have affinity for cerebral arterial smooth muscle and effectively antagonize agonist-mediated vasoconstriction in vitro.[91] In this regard, calcium-channel antagonists might affect either spastic large cerebral arteries or augment collateral flow by dilatation of smaller pial or penetrating vessels. In addition, lipophilic calcium-channel antagonists readily cross the blood-brain barrier, bind to neurons, and inhibit calcium influx after stimulation of glutamate receptors during ischemia.[52] Finally, calcium-channel antagonists affect platelet aggregation and erythrocyte membrane deformability, thus potentially augmenting capillary flow in low-flow states.

Based on the multiple potential beneficial effects for calcium-channel antagonists in cerebral vasospasm, a number of prospective, randomized trials for nimodipine were initiated in the past decade.[3,56,67–69] The characteristics of these trials can be summarized as follows: (1) oral nimodipine consistently reduced poor outcome due to vasospasm in all grades of patients; (2) with the exception of one trial, the incidence of symptomatic vasospasm was not affected by nimodipine treatment; (3) vessel caliber by angiography was not affected by nimodipine therapy; and (4) complications and side effects of the drug were minimal. Combined with observations that nimodipine had no effect upon CBF in vasospasm,[56] these data suggest that the protective effect of nimodipine may have been due to limitation of calcium influx in marginally-ischemic neurons, rather than dilatation of large capacitance arteries.

Several uncontrolled trials[4,23,24,77] have reported even lower incidence of permanent deficit from vasospasm following the intranvenous administration of nimodipine, with rates ranging from 1 to 10 percent. In a prospective, randomized dose-escalation trial,[26] however, there was no significant difference in symptomatic vasospasm or outcome at 3 months for either 0.15 mg/kg per h or 0.3 mg/kg per h compared to controls. Of interest, angiographic vasospasm was significantly less in the nicardipine-treated group. Further studies to elevate the effectiveness of intravenous calcium-channel antagonists are ongoing.

A new class of calcium antagonists have been developed which act to sequester intracellular calcium and inhibit protein kinase C, both of which mediate contractile mechanisms in smooth muscle. One such agent, AT877, significantly reduced symptomatic and angiographic vasospasm and improved outcome at 3 months in a prospective randomized trial.[78]

TABLE 217-3 Potential Mechanisms by which Calcium-Channel Antagonists May Act in Vasospasm

Mechanism	Physiologic Consequence
Large vessel dilatation	↑rCBF, ↑collateral flow
Small vessel dilatation	↑rCBF, ↑collateral flow
Neuronal protection	↓Ischemic cell death
Erythrocyte deformability	↑Microcirculatory flow
Decreased platelet aggregation	↑Microcirculatory flow

Clot Removal and Agents Affecting Fibrinolysis

Antifibrinolytic agents (epsilon-aminocaproic acid, tranexemic acid) were widely employed in the 1970s and 1980s to reduce the risk of rebleeding in patients awaiting surgery. Presumably these agents stabilize the thrombus at the site of aneurysm rupture by inhibiting plasmin-mediated thrombolysis. However, they also probably inhibit the lysis of thrombus adjacent to arteries in the subarachnoid space, thus potentially exacerbating vasospasm. These concepts were substantiated by the results of the Cooperative Aneurysm Study in 1987.[2] In this trial, rebleeding rates among patients with delayed surgery were significantly less among those treated with antifibrinolytic agents (24 percent) as compared to nontreated patients (45 percent). However, this protective effect was negated by a significant increase in delayed ischemic neurological deficits for patients receiving antifibrinolytics (42 vs. 24 percent). The increasing practice of early surgery in patients with aneurysmal SAH has obviated somewhat the necessity for preventing rebleeding with antifibrinolytic agents; in those patients with delayed surgery the beneficial effect of antifibrinolytic agents must be weighed against the risk of exacerbating vasospasm.

Considerable clinical and experimental evidence has related the severity of cerebral vasospasm to the volume and duration of perivascular thrombus in the subarachnoid space, as described below. This concept led to aggressive clot removal at surgery, as first advocated by Suzuki et al.[85] However, subarachnoid clot is often tenaciously adherent to the brain and pial vessels, and many neurosurgeons are hesitant to perform additional dissection and retraction during surgery. Weir's group[19] postulated that intrathecal fibrinolytic agents [e.g., tissue plasminogen activator (tPA) and urokinase] might ameliorate vasospasm by hastening the lysis of subarachnoid clot. On the other hand, accelerated thrombolysis by these agents may also increase the risk of postoperative hemorrhage. Following encouraging results in a primate model of vasospasm,[18] this modality has recently been applied in selected clinical cases. Intracisternal recombinant tPA is currently under investigation in a prospective, randomized trial.[99]

Transluminal Angioplasty

Zubkov and colleagues[101] first reported successful resolution of symptomatic cerebral vasospasm by dilatation of the narrowed segment using an intravascular balloon. This report remained largely unnoticed until the late 1980s, when steerable balloon catheters enabled safe navigation into intracranial arteries. Since that time there have been numerous uncontrolled reports[7,16,32,57] describing profound improvement in neurological deficits for patients with vasospasm refractory to other modes of therapy. The effects of transluminal angioplasty can be summarized as follows:

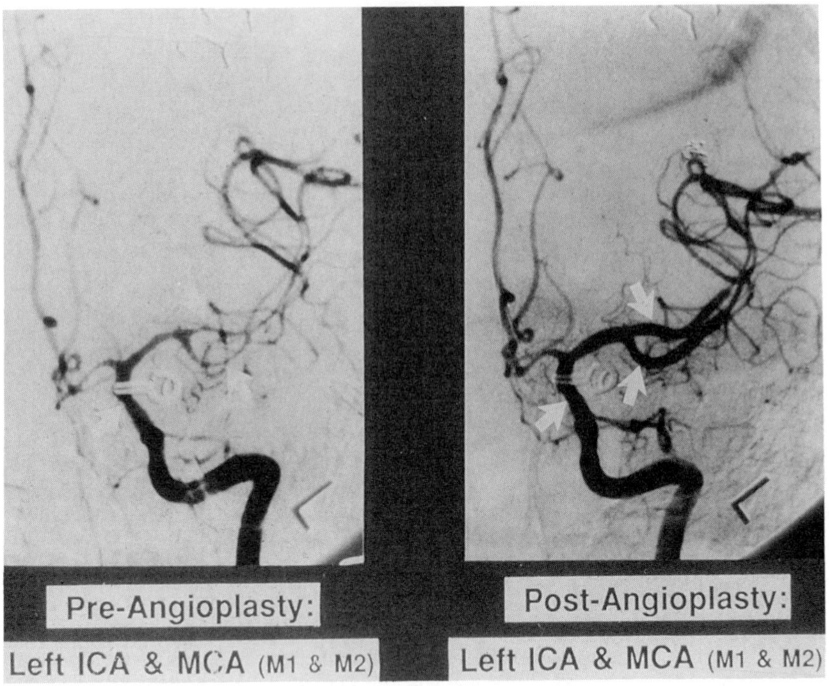

Figure 217-4 Cerebral angiograms before and after angioplasty. In the preangioplasty study *(left)* there is moderate to marked narrowing o the distal ICA, ACA, and MCA. Following angioplasty of the ICA and MCA, there is marked persistent dilatation of these vessels *(arrows)*. The ACA could not be dilated in this patient. Note the apparent increase in distal flow in the MCA distribution.

(1) significant improvement occurs in 60 to 80 percent of patients, often within minutes of the dilatation; (2) normal angiographic caliber (Fig. 217-4) is achieved in nearly all cases, which persists without recurrent vasospasm; (3) evidence of improved CBF by TCD or SPECT correlates with clinical improvement; and (4) complications (rupture of vessels or unsecured aneurysm) occur in approximately 5 percent of cases. Although controlled trials have not been done, the generally good outcome described in these reports is significant due to the ominous natural history of vasospasm in the subset of patients with symptomatic vasospasm refractory to conventional therapy. Several unresolved issues concerning transluminal angioplasty include its application in patients with asymptomatic vasospasm or those with unsecured aneurysms, its safety in widespread application, and its role in relation to intra-arterial papavarine infusion.

Timing of Surgery

Because mechanical stimulation causes transient constriction of cerebral arteries, it was assumed that surgery would exacerbate existing or developing vasospasm. In addition, inflammation and swelling of the brain were thought to coincide with vasospasm, thereby increasing surgical morbidity due to retraction injury. These concepts led to the practice of delaying surgery beyond the period of maximal therapy. Recently, there has been a trend toward early surgery, as discussed elsewhere in this text. Early surgery clearly reduces the risk of rebleeding, facilitates the removal of perivascular thrombus, and enables the institution of aggressive therapies for vasospasm such as triple-H therapy, thrombolytics, and angioplasty. The role of early surgery in exacerbating vasospasm remains unresolved due to conflicting reports from uncontrolled trials. Data from the Cooperative Aneurysm Study[25,37] suggested that surgical intervention in the risk period for cerebral vasospasm (4 to 14 days) was associated with higher morbidity and mortality rates. However, overall morbidity and mortality was not different for early (less than 3 days) or delayed (more than 14 days) surgery, presumably because of vasospasm in the early surgery group and rebleeding in the late surgery group.

For surgery prior to the onset of vasospasm (less than 3 days after SAH), the benefits of initiating early therapy probably outweigh the risks of worsening vasospasm. For patients considered for surgery during the period of peak vasospasm (days 4 through 10), the decision to operate may be based on a number of variables, including clinical status, assessment of risk factors for vasospasm, noninvasive indicators of vasospasm, and response to therapeutic intervention. In the setting of existing vasospasm, surgical management should include avoiding intraoperative hypotension or hypovolemia and maintaining aggressive therapy in the postoperative period. Surgery followed by immediate angioplasty has been proposed as an alternative strategy in this group of patients.[41]

Antioxidant and Anti-Inflammatory Agents

Experimental studies have implicated both free-radical-mediated lipid peroxidation and inflammatory responses in the pathogenesis of cerebral vasospasm (see below). Although improvement in vasospasm has been noted in animal models while using both anti-inflammatory agents (e.g., ibuprofen or methylprednisolone[10]) and antioxidants (21-aminosteroids[102] or deferoxamine[29])) clinical trials demonstrating efficacy are limited to date. In a prospective, nonrandomized study, Chyatte et al.[12] showed a reduction in cerebral vasospasm in patients treated with high-dose methylprednisolone. Current prospective, randomized trials are testing the efficacy of Tirilazad, a nonglucocorticoid 21-aminosteroid with antioxidant and iron-chelating properties.

Pathophysiology and Experimental Aspects of Vasospasm

An extensive literature regarding potential pathogenic mechanisms and experimental therapies for cerebral vasospasm has been reviewed elsewhere[48] and will be briefly summarized here. Despite considerable advances in this field, the precise mechanism by which SAH elicits delayed arterial narrowing remains uncertain. In fact, controversy persists as to (1) whether arterial narrowing is a consequence of active vasoconstriction or passive structural changes in vessel; (2) whether large vessel narrowing is integral to the pathologic process; or (3) the specific component of blood that elicits delayed arterial narrowing and the process by which this occurs.

Experimental Models

Much of the uncertainty regarding vasospasm relates to variability among several experimental models. Early work utilizing cerebral artery preparations in vitro did not account for important factors such as chronic exposure to putative spasmogens and the maintenance of intact endothelium. Animal models vary considerably in the time course of arterial narrowing after SAH. In nonprimates, this probably relates to the rapid clearance of subsarachnoid blood following intracisternal injection. This issue has been addressed by strategies such as multiple blood injection[87] or placement of barriers[49] to limit thrombus degradation. It is not clear whether short-term arterial narrowing observed in single-injection small animal models[61] corresponds to chronic vasospasm in humans. A primate model employing direct application of autologous thrombus to the middle cerebral artery probably best simulates human vasospasm.[45]

Blood Exposure to Cerebral Arteries

Several lines of evidence have suggested that the volume and duration of exposure for blood adjacent to cerebral arteries are critical to vasospasm development. Substances released from the perivascular thrombus have ready access to the vessel wall through a porous adventitia.[100] In humans, the volume of subarachnoid blood on CT scan is a strong predictor of vasospasm.[20] The critical period of blood exposure appears to be approximately 72 h; in animal models, the direct removal of thrombus prior to that time eliminates vasospasm.[28,98] Intracisternal administration of recombinant tPA during the same period effectively lysed subarachnoid thrombus and reduced cerebral vasospasm in a primate model.[17] Current application of this concept to human vasospasm includes the aggressive removal of thrombus at surgery and ongoing trials for tPA.

Potential Spasmogens in Blood

Approximately 20 agents which elicit vasoconstriction in cerebral arteries in vitro have been identified in whole blood,[90] including catecholamines, serotonin, prostaglandin derivatives, thrombin, and various kinins. However, the majority of these substances are not present in significant concentrations at the time of delayed arterial narrowing, and therefore are not likely participants in chronic vasospasm. One exception are the constituents of erythrocytes, most notably the reduced form of hemoglobin *(oxyhemoglobin)*. The temporal course of red cell lysis (3 to 5 days) in the subarachnoid space corresponds to the onset of clinical vasospasm, and bloody CSF at these time intervals is a potent vasoconstrictor for cerebral arteries. Extracts of lysed erythrocytes[63] and oxyhemoglobin[15] (but not its oxidized form methemoglobin) produce sustained contraction of cerebral arteries in vitro. Chronic in vitro exposure of cerebral arteries to washed erythrocytes,[50] or oxyhemoglobin[44,50] causes delayed arterial narrowing with angiographic and histologic features of vasospasm; exposure to leukocytes and platelet-rich plasma, erythrocyte membranes, methemoglobin, or bilirubin does not induce vasospasm in these models.

Although these data strongly implicate constituents of the erythrocyte cytosol (primarily oxyhemoglobin) in the pathogenesis of vasospasm, the specific mechanism producing delayed arterial narrowing remains uncertain. In addition to its direct vasoconstrictor effect, oxyhemoglobin generates activated oxygen species (i.e., superoxide anion radical, hydrogen peroxide, and singlet oxygen) through its autoxidation to methemoglobin.[54] In conjunction with free iron, these free radicals propagate the peroxidation of membrane lipids by the Haber-Weiss reaction. Lipid peroxidation may stimulate smooth muscle contraction or mediate structural changes in the vessel wall by cytoxic action.[72] Antioxidant agents reduced vasospasm in several experimental models[29,102]; clinical trials for their use in humans are forthcoming.

Structural Changes in Vessel Wall

Light and electron microscopic alterations in cerebral artery structure after SAH have been consistently described in human postmortem and intraoperative specimens, which correlated with angiographic vasospasm and cerebral infarction in the territory of the affected vessel.[13] Smith et al.[82] reported similar postmortem angiopathic changes in 24 of 28 patients autopsied after SAH from ruptured cerebral aneurysm. A number of animal models for SAH have shown that continuous exposure of large cerebral arteries to clotted blood over several days was associated with consistent ultrastructural changes in the vessel wall. Cerebral artery morphology was characterized by alterations in endothelial cell morphology, thickening and discontinuities of the elastica, smooth muscle vacuoles with occasional frank myonecrosis, proliferating "myointimal cells" migrating into the intima, and periadventitial inflammation with loss of perivascular axons (Fig. 217-5).[49,51,75,81]

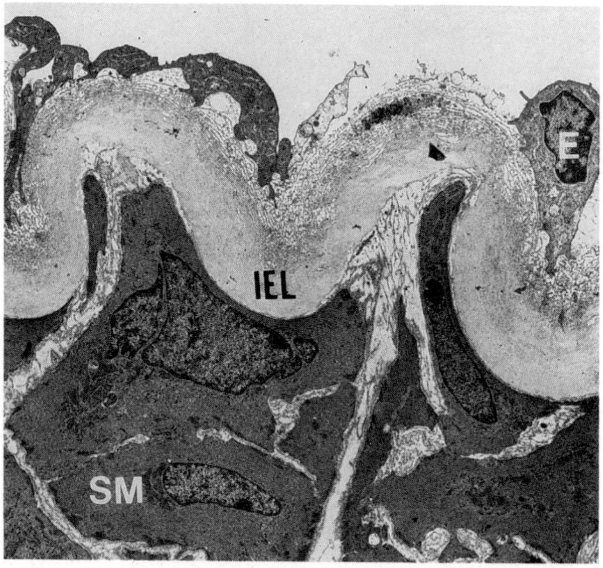

Figure 217-5 Transmission electron micrograph of pig MCA following exposure to perivascular blood for 7 days. There is marked convolution of the internal elastic lamina (IEL), vacuolization of the endothelium (E), and distortion of the smooth muscle (SM).

At 2 weeks to 6 months post-SAH, there was regression of the subintimal proliferation, increases in luminal diameter, and deposition of collagen in all three vessel layers.

Structural changes in cerebral arteries associated with vasospasm may determine in part the unique physiologic abnormalities seen in this disorder. Immunhistochemical studies showed loss of contractile protein[49] and increases in vessel wall collagen[49,82] associated with chronic arterial narrowing. Cerebral arteries exposed to subarachnoid blood for several days were less distensible than controls,[8] and were relatively insensitive to both vasocontricting and vasodilating agents.[8,38] This suggests that ''fibrosis'' of the vessel in its contracted state may represent one component of prolonged vasospasm. The effectiveness of angioplasty in reversing vasospasm may be based to this mechanism.

Endothelial Factors

Numerous changes have been demonstrated in cerebral endothelium after exposure to subarachnoid blood, including alterations in prostaglandin metabolism,[74] increased permeability,[73] and diminished secretion of endothelium dependent relaxation factor (EDRF).[34] *Endothelin* (ET) is a long-lasting, potent vasoconstrictor secreted by vascular endothelial cells. Both plasma and CSF endothelin concentrations were increased in patients after SAH,[47] and intracisternal injection of ET produced prolonged narrowing of cerebral arteries in vivo.[39,53] At present, however, the specific role of endothelial factors in the pathogenesis of vasospasm remains indeterminate.

Inflammation

As described above, inflammatory processes have been implicated in a number of putative mechanisms for cerebral vasospasm. Potental inflammatory mediators include eicosanoids (prostaglandins, leukotrienes), immune complexes (immunoglobin and complement), and cytokines (IL-1).[11,66] Inflammatory processes may also be linked to cytotoxic lipid peroxidation, as described above. Although effective in certain experimental models, anti-inflammatory agents have not been widely tested in clinical trials.

References

1. Aaslid R, Huber P, Nornes H. A transcranial Doppler method in the evaluation of cerebrovascular spasm. *Neuroradiology* 1986; 28:11–16.
2. Adams HP Jr, Kassell NF, Torner JC, Haley ECJ. Predicting cerebral ischemia after aneurysmal subarachnoid hemorrhage: influences of clinical condition, CT results, and antifibrinolytic therapy. A report of the Cooperative Aneurysm Study. *Neurology* 1987; 37:1586–1591.
3. Allen GS, Ahn HS, Preziosi TJ, et al. Cerebral arterial spasm—a controlled trial of nimodipine in patients with subarachnoid hemorrhage. *N Engl J Med* 1983; 308:619–624.
4. Auer LM. Acute operation and preventive nimodipine improve outcome in patients with ruptured cerebral aneurysms. *Neurosurgery* 1984; 15:57–66.
5. Awad IA, Carter LP, Spetzler RF, et al. Clinical vasospasm after subarachnoid hemorrhage: response to hypervolemic hemodilution and arterial hypertension. *Stroke* 1987; 18:365–372.
6. Barker FG II, Heros RC. Clinical aspects of vasospasm. *Neurosurg Clin North Am* 1990; 1:277–288.
7. Barnwell SL, Higashida RT, Halbach VV, et al. Transluminal angioplasty of intracerebral vessels for cerebral arterial spasm: reversal of neurological deficits after delayed treatment. *Neurosurgery* 1989; 25:424–429.
8. Bevan JA, Bevan RD, Frazee JG. Functional arterial changes in chronic cerebrovasospasm in monkeys: an in vitro assessment of the contribution to arterial narrowing. *Stroke* 1987; 18:472–481.
9. Black PM. Hydrocephalus and vasospasm after subarachnoid hemorrhage from ruptured intracranial aneurysms. *Neurosurgery* 1986; 18:12–16.
10. Chyatte D. Prevention of chronic cerebral vasospasm in dogs with ibuprofen and high-dose methylprednisolone. *Stroke* 1989; 20:1021–1026.
11. Chyatte D. Anti-inflammatory agents and cerebral vasospasm. *Neurosurg Clin North Am* 1990; 1:433–450.
12. Chyatte D, Fode NC, Nicholls DA, Sundt TM Jr. Preliminary report: effects of high dose methylprednisolone on delayed cerebral ischemia in patients at high risk for vasospasm after aneurysmal subarachnoid hemorrhage. *Neurosurgery* 1987; 21:157–160.
13. Conway LW, McDonald LW. Structural changes of the intradural arteries following subarachnoid hemorrhage. *J Neurosurg* 1972; 37:715–723.
14. Crompton MR. The pathogenesis of cerebral infarction following the rupture of cerebral berry aneurysms. *Brain* 1964; 87:491–510.
15. Dora E, Feher E, Farago M, et al. Mechanism of hemoglobin-induced spasm in the isolated middle cerebral artery of the cat. *Adv Exp Med Biol* 1989; 248:533–542.
16. Eskridge JM, Newell DW, Pendleton GA. Transluminal angioplasty for treatment of vasospasm. *Neurosurg Clin North Am* 1990; 1:387–399.
17. Findlay JM, Weir BKA, Kanamaru K, et al. The effect of timing of intrathecal fibrinolytic therapy on cerebral vasospasm in a primate model of subarachnoid hemorrhage. *Neurosurgery* 1990; 26:201–206.
18. Findlay JM, Weir BKA, Kassell NF, et al. Intracisternal recombinant tissue plasminogen activator after aneurysmal subarachnoid hemorrhage. *J Neurosurg* 1991; 75:181–188.
19. Findlay JM, Weir BKA, Steinke D, et al. Effect of intrathecal thrombolytic therapy on subarachnoid clot and chronic vasospasm in a primate model of SAH. *J Neurosurg* 1988; 69:723–735.
20. Fisher CM, Kistler JP, Davis JM. Relation of cerebral vasospasm to subarachnoid hemorrhage vizualized by computerized tomographic scanning. *Neurosurgery* 1980; 6:1–9.
21. Gaab MR, Haubitz I, Brawanski A, et al. Acute effects of nimodipine on the cerebral blood flow and intracranial pressure. *Neurochirurgia (Stuttg)* 1985; 28 (Suppl 1):93–99
22. Gilsbach JM, Harders AG. Morbidity and mortality after early aneurysm surgery—a prospective study with nimodipine prevention. *Acta Neurochir (Wien)* 1989; 96:1–7.
23. Gilsbach JM, Reulen HJ, Ljunggren B, et al. Early aneurysm surgery and preventive therapy with intravenously administered nimodipine: a multicenter, double-blind, dose-comparison study. *Neurosurgery* 1990; 26:458–464.
24. Grotenhuis JA, Bettag W. Prevention of symptomatic vasospasm after SAH by constant venous infusion of nimodipine. *Neurol Res* 1986; 8:243–249.
25. Haley EC Jr, Kassell NF, Torner JC, et al. The International Cooperative Study on the Timing of Aneurysm Surgery. The North American experience. *Stroke* 1992; 23:205–214.
26. Haley EC Jr, Kassell NF, Torner JC, et al. A randomized trial of nicardipine in subarachnoid hemorrhage: angiographic and transcranial Doppler ultrasound results. A report of the Cooperative Aneurysm Study. *J Neurosurg* 1993; 78:548–553.
27. Haley EC Jr, Torner JC, Kassell NF. Antifibrinolytic therapy and cerebral vasospasm. *Neurosurg Clin North Am* 1990; 1:349–356.
28. Handa Y, Weir BKA, Nosko M, et al. The effect of timing of clot removal on chronic vasospasm in a primate model. *J Neurosurg* 1987; 67:558–564.

29. Harada T, Mayberg MR. Inhibition of delayed arterial narrowing by the iron-chelating agent deferoxamine. *J Neurosurg* 1992; 77:763–767.
30. Harders AG, Gilsbach JM. Time course of blood velocity changes related to vasospasm in the circle of Willis measured by transcranial Doppler ultrasound. *J Neurosurg* 1987; 66:718–728.
31. Heros RC, Zervas NT, Varsos B. Cerebral vasospasm after subarachnoid hemorrhage: an update. *Ann Neurol* 1983; 14:599–608.
32. Higashida RT, Halbach VV, Cahan LD, et al. Transluminal angioplasty for treatment of intracranial arterial vasospasm. *J Neurosurg* 1989; 71:648–653.
33. Hijdra A, Braakman R, van Gijn J, et al. Aneurysmal subarachnoid hemorrhage. Complications and outcome in a hospital population. *Stroke* 1987; 18:1061–1067.
34. Hongo K, Kassell NF, Nakagomi T, et al. Subarachnoid hemorrhage inhibition of endothelium-derived relaxing factor in rabbit basilar artery. *J Neurosurg* 1988; 69:247–253.
35. Kassell NF, Peerless SJ, Durward QJ, et al. Treatment of ischemic deficits from vasospasm with intravascular volume expansion and induced arterial hypertension. *Neurosurgery* 1982; 11:337–343.
36. Kassell NF, Sasaki T, Colohan ART, Nazar G. Cerebral vasospasm following aneurysmal subarachnoid hemorrhage. *Stroke* 1985; 16:562–572.
37. Kassell NF, Torner JC, Jane JA, et al. The International Cooperative Study on the Timing of Aneurysm Surgery. Part 2: Surgical results. *J Neurosurg* 1990; 73:37–47.
38. Kim P, Sundt TM Jr, Vanhoutte PM. Alterations of mechanical properties in canine basilar arteries after subarachnoid hemorrhage. *J Neurosurg* 1989; 71:430–436.
39. Kobayashi H, Hayashi M, Kobayashi S, et al. Cerebral vasospasm and vasoconstriction caused by endothelin. *Neurosurgery* 1991; 28:673–679.
40. Kosnik EJ, Hunt WE. Postoperative hypertension in the management of patients with intracranial arterial aneurysms. *J Neurosurg* 1976; 45:148–154.
41. LeRoux PD, Newell DW, Eskridge J, et al. Severe symptomatic vasospasm: the role of immediate postoperative angioplasty. *J Neurosurg* 1994; 80:224–229.
42. Levy ML, Giannotta SL. Cardiac performance indices during hypervolemic therapy for cerebral vasospasm. *J Neurosurg* 1991; 75:27–31.
43. Lewis DH, Eskridge JM, Newell DW, et al. Brain SPECT and the effect of cerebral angioplasty in delayed ischemia due to vasospasm. *J Nucl Med* 1992; 33:1789–1796.
44. Macdonald RL, Weir BKA. A review of hemoglobin and the pathogenesis of cerebral vasospasm. *Stroke* 1991; 22:971–982.
45. Macdonald RL, Weir BKA, Runzer TD, et al. Etiology of cerebral vasospasm in primates. *J Neurosurg* 1991; 75:415–424.
46. Martin NA, Doberstein C, Zane C, et al. Posttraumatic cerebral arterial spasm: transcranial Doppler ultrasound, cerebral blood flow, and angiographic findings. *J Neurosurg* 1992; 77:575–583.
47. Masaoka H, Suzuki R, Hirata Y, Emori, T. Raised plasma endothelin in aneurysmal subarachnoid haemorrhage. *Lancet* 1989; 2:1402 (letter).
48. Mayberg MR (ed). *Cerebral Vasospasm* [*Neurosurg Clin North Am* 1(2)]. Philadelphia: Saunders, 1990.
49. Mayberg MR, Okada T, Bark DH. The significance of morphological changes in cerebral arteries after subarachnoid hemorrhage. *J Neurosurg* 1990; 72:626–633.
50. Mayberg MR, Okada T, Bark DH. The role of hemoglobin in arterial narrowing after subarachnoid hemorrhage. *J Neurosurg* 1990; 72:634–640.
51. Mayberg MR, Okada T, Bark DH. Morphologic changes in cerebral arteries after subarachnoid hemorrhage. *Neurosurg Clin North Am* 1990; 1:417–432.
52. Meyer FB. Calcium antagonists and vasospasm. *Neurosurg Clin North Am* 1990; 1:367–376.
53. Mima T, Yanagisawa M, Shigeno T, et al. Endothelin acts in feline and canine cerebral arteries from the adventitial side. *Stroke* 1989; 20:1553–1556.
54. Misra HP, Fridovich I. The generation of superoxide radical during the autoxidation of hemoglobin. *J Biol Chem* 1972; 247:6960–6962.
55. Muizelaar JP, Becker DP. Induced hypertension for the treatment of cerebral ischemia after subarachnoid hemorrhage. Direct effect on cerebral blood flow. *Surg Neurol* 1986; 25:317–325.
56. Neil-Dwyer G, Mee E, Dorrance D, et al. Early intervention with nimodipine in subarachnoid hemorrhage. *Eur Heart J* 1987; 8 (Suppl K):41–47.
57. Newell DW, Eskridge JM, Mayberg MR, et al. Angioplasty for the treatment of symptomatic vasospasm following subarachnoid hemorrhage. *J Neurosurg* 1989; 71:654–660.
58. Newell DW, Grady MS, Eskridge JM, Winn HR. Distribution of angiographic vasospasm after subarachnoid hemorrhage: implications for diagnosis by transcranial Doppler ultrasonography. *Neurosurgery* 1990; 27:574–577.
59. Newell DW, Winn HR. Transcranial Doppler in cerebral vasospasm. *Neurosurg Clin North Am* 1990; 1:319–328.
60. Nibbelink DW, Torner JC, Henderson WG. Intracranial aneurysms and subarachnoid hemorrhage: a cooperative study. Antifibrinolytic therapy in recent onset subarachnoid hemorrhage. *Stroke* 1975; 6:622–629.
61. Nihei H, Kassell NF, Doughtery DA, Sasaki T. Does vasospasm occur in small pial arteries and arterioles of rabbits? *Stroke* 1991; 22:1419–1425.
62. Öhman J, Heiskanen O. Effect of nimodipine on the outcome of patients after aneurysmal subarachnoid hemorrhage and surgery. *J Neurosurg* 1988; 69:683–686.
63. Osaka K. Prolonged vasospasm produced by the breakdown products of erythrocytes. *J Neurosurg* 1977; 47:403–411.
64. Østergaard JR, Voldby B. Intracranial arterial aneurysms in children and adolescents. *J Neurosurg* 1983; 58:832–837.
65. Pasqualin A, Vivenza C, Rosta L, et al. Cerebral vasospasm after head injury. *Neurosurgery* 1984; 15:855–858.
66. Peterson JW, Kwun BD, Hackett JD, Zervas NT. The role of inflammation in experimental cerebral vasospasm. *J Neurosurg* 1990; 72:767–774.
67. Petruk KC, West M, Mohr G, et al. Nimodipine treatment in poor-grade aneurysm patients: results of a multicenter double-blind placebo-controlled trial. *J Neurosurg* 1988; 68:505–517.
68. Philippon J, Grob R, Dagreou F, et al. Prevention of vasospasm in subarachnoid haemorrhage: a controlled study with nimodipine. *Acta Neurochir (Wien)* 1986; 82:110–114.
69. Pickard JD, Murray GD, Illingworth R, et al. Effect of oral nimodipine on cerebral infarction and outcome after subarachnoid haemorrhage: British Aneurysm Nimodpine Trial. *Br Med J* 1989; 298:636–642.
70. Powers WJ, Grubb RL Jr, Baker RP, et al. Regional cerebral blood flow and metabolism in reversible ischemia due to vasospasm: determination by positron emission tomography. *J Neurosurg* 1985; 62:539–546.
71. Rousseaux P, Scherpereel B, Bernard MH, et al. Fever and cerebral vasospasm in ruptured intracranial aneurysms. *Surg Neurol* 1980; 14:459–465.
72. Sano K, Asano T, Tamishima T, Sasaki T. Lipid peroxidation as a cause of cerebral vasospasm. *Neurol Res* 1980; 2:253–272.
73. Sasaki T, Kassell NF, Yamashita M, et al. Barrier disruption in the major cerebral arteries following experimental subarachnoid hemorrhage. *J Neurosurg* 1985; 63:433–440.
74. Sasaki T, Wakai S, Asano T, et al. Prevention of cerebral vasospasm after SAH with a thromboxane synthetase inhibitor, OKY-1581. *J Neurosurg* 1982; 57:74–82.
75. Seifert V, Stolke D, Reale E. Ultrastructural changes of the basilar artery following experimental subarachnoid haemorrhage. A morphological study on the pathogenesis of delayed cerebral vasospasm. *Acta Neurochir (Wien)* 1989; 100:164–171.
76. Seiler RW, Grolimund P, Aaslid R, et al. Cerebral vasospasm evaluated by transcranial ultrasound correlated with clinical grade and

CT-visualized subarachnoid hemorrhage. *J Neurosurg* 1986; 64:594–600.

77. Seiler RW, Grolimund P, Zurbruegg HR. Evaluation of the calcium-antagonist nimodipine for the prevention of vasospasm after aneurysmal subarachnoid haemorrhage. A prospective transcranial Doppler ultrasound study. *Acta Neurochir (Wien)* 1987; 85:7–16.
78. Shibuya M, Suzuki Y, Sugita K, et al. Effect of AT877 on cerebral vasospasm after aneurysmal subarachnoid hemorrhage. Results of a prospective placebo-controlled double-blind trial. *J Neurosurg* 1992; 76:571–577.
79. Shibuya M, Suzuki Y, Takayasu M, et al. The effects of an intracellular calcium antagonist HA 1077 on cerebral vasospasm in dogs. *Acta Neurochir (Wien)* 1988; 90:53–59.
80. Siesjö BK. Cerebral circulation and metabolism. *J Neurosurg* 1984; 60:883–908.
81. Smith RR, Clower BR, Cruse JM, et al. Constrictive structural elements in human cerebral arteries following aneurysmal subarachnoid haemorrhage. *Neurol Res* 1987; 9:188–192.
82. Smith RR, Clower BR, Grotendorst GM, et al. Arterial wall changes in early human vasospasm. *Neurosurgery* 1985; 16:171–176.
83. Solomon RA, Fink ME, Lennihan L. Early aneurysm surgery and prophylactic hypervolemic hypertensive therapy for the treatment of aneurysmal subarachnoid hemorrhage. *Neurosurgery* 1988; 23:699–704.
84. Sundt TM Jr, Kobayashi S, Fode NC, Whisnant JP. Results and complications of surgical management of 809 intracranial aneurysms in 722 cases. Related and unrelated to grade of patient, type of aneurysm, and timing of surgery. *J Neurosurg* 1982, 56:753–765.
85. Suzuki J, Onuma T, Yoshimoto T. Results of early operations on cerebral aneurysms. *Surg Neurol* 1979; 11:407–412.
86. Takemae T, Mizukami M, Kin H, et al. Computed tomography of ruptured intracranial aneurysms in acute stage: relationship between vasospasm and high density on CT scan. *Brain Nerve* 1978; 30:861–866.
87. Varsos VG, Liszczak TM, Han DH, et al. Delayed cerebral vasospasm is not reversible by aminophylline, nifedipine, or papaverine in a ''two-hemorrhage'' canine model. *J Neurosurg* 1983; 58:11–17.
88. Weir B, Disney L, Grace M, et al. Daily trends in white blood cell count and temperature after subarachnoid hemorrhage from aneurysm. *Neurosurgery* 1989; 25:161–165.
89. Weir B, Grace M, Hansen J, Rothberg C. Time course of vasospasm in man. *J Neurosurg* 1978; 48:173–179.
90. White RP. Responses of isolated cerebral arteries to vasoactive agents. *Neurosurg Clin North Am* 1990; 1:401–415.
91. White RP, Cunningham MP, Robertson JT. Effect of the calcium antagonist nimodipine on contractile responses of isolated canine basilar arteries induced by serotonin, prostaglandin $F_{2\alpha}$, thrombin, and whole blood. *Neurosurgery* 1982; 10:344–348.
92. Wijdicks EFM, Vermeulen M, Hijdra A, et al. Hyponatremia and cerebral infarction in patients with ruptured intracranial aneurysms: is fluid restriction harmful? *Ann Neurol* 1985; 17:137–140.
93. Wilkins RH. Attempts at prevention or treatment of intracranial arterial spasm: an update. *Neurosurgery* 1986; 18:808—825.
94. Wilkins RH, Odom GL. Intracranial arterial spasm associated with craniocerebral trauma. *J Neurosurg* 1970; 32:626–633.
95. Winn HR, Richardson AE, Jane JA. The long-term prognosis in untreated cerebral aneurysms. I. The incidence of late hemorrhage in cerebral aneurysm: a 10-year evaluation of 364 patients. *Ann Neurol* 1977; 1:358–370.
96. Yamakami I, Isobe K, Yamaura A, et al. Vasospasm and regional cerebral blood flow (rCBF) in patients with ruptured intracranial aneurysm: serial rCBF studies with the xenon-133 inhalation method. *Neurosurgery* 1983; 13:394–401.
97. Yonas H. Cerebral blood measurements in vasospasm. *Neurosurg Clin North Am* 1990; 1:307–318.
98. Zabramski JM, Spetzler RF, Bonstelle C. Chronic cerebral vasospasm: effect of volume and timing of hemorrhage in a canine model. *Neurosurgery* 1986; 18:1–6.
99. Zabramski JM, Spetzler RF, Lee KS, et al. Phase I trial of recombinant tissue plasminogen activator for the prevention of vasospasm in patients with aneurysmal subarachnoid hemorrhage. *J Neurosurg* 1991; 75:189—196.
100. Zervas NT, Liszczak TM, Mayberg MR, Black PM. Cerebrospinal fluid may nourish cerebral vessels through pathways in the adventitia that may be analogous to systemic vasa vasorum. *J Neurosurg* 1982; 56:475–481.
101. Zubkov YN, Nikiforov BM, Shustin VA. Balloon catheter technique for dilatation of constricted cerebral arteries after aneurysmal SAH. *Acta Neurochir (Wien)* 1984; 70:65–79.
102. Zuccarello M, Marsch JF, Schmitt G, et al. Effect of the 21-aminosteroid U-7400F on cerebral vasospasm following subarachnoid hemorrhage. *J Neurosurg* 1989; 71:98–104.

218

Timing of Aneurysm Surgery

Allan H. Friedman

The optimal time to obliterate a recently ruptured intracranial berry aneurysm has been debated in the neurosurgical literature. The persistence of the question despite numerous epidemiologic studies confirms the absence of a single answer which if applied to all patients will result in a marked improvement in outcome. When large populations of patients are studied, the timing of surgery has only a marginal effect on patient outcome. Still, it is the belief of many neurosurgeons that selective timing of aneurysm surgery can improve the overall results of management.

Many factors can theoretically affect the optimal timing of aneurysm surgery. Some of these are outlined in Table 218-1. The most obvious consideration is the propensity of the aneurysm to rehemorrhage. If rehemorrhage were the only consideration, all patients would be taken directly to the operating room upon admission to the hospital (Table 218-2).

A second important factor is the reduction of cerebral blood flow which coincides with the rupture of the aneurysm and is exacerbated by vasospasm.[17,19,29] This factor raises several theoretical questions. Can surgical manipulation of the cerebral vasculature or intracisternal blood exacerbate or mitigate the incidence or severity of vasospasm?[49] Is systemic hypotension which can occur in association with the induction of general anesthesia or premature rupture of the aneurysm, or focal hypotension induced by temporary occlusion of a parent blood vessel tolerated in the 2 weeks immediately following a subarachnoid hemorrhage? Because the propensity of the patient to develop vasospasm is proportional to the amount of cisternal blood seen in a post-hemorrhage brain CT scan, should surgery be postponed when no blood is visualized on the admission brain computed tomography (CT) scan? Can vasospasm be treated more safely with the aneurysm secured?

TABLE 218-1 Considerations in Timing of Aneurysm Surgery

Propensity for rehemorrhage
Influence of surgery on vasospasm
Likelihood of patient developing vasospasm
Effect of surgery on hemodynamically compromised brain
Patient's clinical grade
Amount of subarachnoid blood visualized on CT scan
Patient's age
Concurrent medical problems
"Tightness" of brain
Planned operative approach
Anatomy of aneurysm
Presence of intraparenchymal hemorrhage
Expertise of operating team
Timing of patient referral

TABLE 218-2 Theoretical Advantages of Early Surgery

Eliminates chance of rehemorrhage
Removes clots, possibly decreasing incidence of vasospasm
Allows hypertensive and endovascular treatment of vasospasm
Prevents complications of bed rest
Soft clot easier to dissect
Shortens hospital stay

The patient's age and preictal medical status could influence optimal timing of surgery. A perfectly performed operation is a hollow victory if the patient succumbs to medical complications. Does the clinical grade of the patient influence the most appropriate time for surgery? The rapid removal of mass-producing intracranial blood clots has been shown to improve results.[20]

Technical considerations include the "tightness" of the brain and the surgeon's anticipated need for brain retraction for optimal exposure of the neck of the aneurysm. A basilar bifurcation or posteriorly pointing anterior communicating artery aneurysm will require more brain manipulation than an internal carotid artery aneurysm. The dissection of important perforating vessels may be compromised because of poor exposure.[8] More brain manipulation is needed to adequately dissect and clip a large broad-based aneurysm than a small pliable aneurysm.

The condition of the operating team must be taken into account. Are experienced anesthesiologists and nurses available? Is the surgeon fatigued?

Finally, the actual timing of the patient's surgery is to some extent dictated by timely diagnosis of the subarachnoid hemorrhage (SAH). In the International Cooperative Study on the Timing of Aneurysm Surgery, 27 percent of patients were excluded because they were first admitted to the hospital more than 3 days after their subarachnoid hemorrhage. In several reported series, even though the surgeons advocated performing surgery within 3 days of the hemorrhage, less than one-half of the patients arrived within 3 days of their hemorrhage.[11,42]

Our present management of aneurysms and SAH has plenty of room for improvement. In a prospective epidemiologic survey of 3521 patients hospitalized within 3 days of an aneurysmal SAH, only 58 percent recovered to their premorbid state.[33] The cause of disability was vasospasm/ischemia in 13.5 percent, rehemorrhage in 7.5 percent, direct effect of the initial hemorrhage in 10.6 percent, and surgical complications in 4.0 percent. Timing of surgery could theoretically affect the incidence of vasospasm, rate of rehemorrhage, and incidence of surgical complications.

The Problem

After the development of cerebral angiography made possible the routine premortem diagnosis of berry aneurysms, it became clear that once an aneurysm ruptured it had a high propensity to rehemorrhage. In an attempt to stave off a second hemorrhage, pioneering neurosurgeons attempted surgery to obliterate the ruptured aneurysm as soon as the diagnosis was made. This strategy resulted in a high operative morbidity and mortality.[16,51] Some reviews even questioned whether surgical intervention changed the natural course of the disease.[16,41] It is not clear if these poor results

TABLE 218-3 Theoretical Advantages of Delayed Surgery

Improved hemodynamic status of brain
Brain slack
Proven excellent surgical results

were due to the patient's poor clinical condition, technical difficulties encountered at the time of surgery, or ischemic infarction from vasospasm.

In an attempt to improve surgical results, many neurosurgeons began to postpone surgery until 2 to 3 weeks after the hemorrhage (Table 218-3). Norlén and Olivecrona reported that "early surgery" (less than 22 days after the hemorrhage) resulted in eight deaths in 15 patients, whereas "late surgery" resulted in only two deaths in 63 patients (direct aneurysm neck ligation in 48).[47] They concluded that surgery in the first 3 weeks following aneurysm rupture was dangerous. The strategy of late surgery seemingly resulted in a sharp reduction in operative morbidity and mortality. For instance, Sundt and coworkers, who customarily delayed surgery for 7 to 10 days, reported a 4 percent overall operative mortality.[59,60]

Unfortunately, the improved operative results reported by surgeons delaying surgery did not translate into improvements in the results of overall patient care.[33,52] Ropper and Zervas reported on 112 consecutive Grades I to III patients treated by delayed surgery.[52] Despite good surgical results, only 46 percent of these patients had made a full recovery at a one year follow-up. In reviewing the Mayo Clinic experience of treating ruptured aneurysms with predominantly delayed surgery, Whisnant et al. noted that despite exemplary surgical results, there was only a modest improvement in the probability of surviving an aneurysmal SAH in the population served.[67]

Even though most surgeons adopted a policy of delaying surgery for at least 10 days, a few surgeons continued to investigate surgery within the first week following SAH. Pool advocated an early attack on the ruptured aneurysm, partially based on the erroneous assumption that vasospasm did not occur in the first week following an SAH.[50] He operated on 14 patients within 12 days of the SAH using hypothermia and temporary occlusion of the parent vessels which resulted in a 14 percent mortality rate and most surviving patients returning to gainful employment. In a 1968 paper, Hunt and Hess hypothesized that patients who entered the hospital in good condition following SAH would benefit from early surgery even though only 11 of their Grades I and II patients were actually operated on within 3 days of hemorrhage.[25] Fifteen of the 149 Grade I and II patients admitted to the hospital rebled while awaiting surgery. Of the 16 Grade III patients, only five deaths were due to subsequent hemorrhage; the predominant cause of death was cerebral infarction.[26] With increased experience, Norlén softened his opposition to surgery during the acute post-hemorrhage period on noncomatose patients.[46] He noted that 11 of 12 patients with a preoperative altered level of consciousness undergoing "early surgery" died, whereas only two of 12 patients who were allowed to regain consciousness before undergoing early surgery died.

In an influential paper, Suzuki et al. reviewed their results from treating 625 cases of aneurysmal SAH. In the 122 patients operated on in the first week following the hemorrhage, management mortality was noted to be highest at 15.6 percent but mortality was lower (9.6 percent) in the 53 patients operated on within 48 h of their SAH.[61] In a subsequent report from this same institution, 83 percent of Grades I and II patients, 62 percent of Grade III patients, and 50 percent of Grade IV patients operated on within 3 days of their SAH recovered to lead independent lives.[71] Corroborating these results, Sano and Saito reported no postoperative deaths in patients operated on within 72 h of suffering an aneurysmal SAH.[54] These papers rekindled interest in immediate surgery for patients who have suffered an aneurysmal SAH. Most surgeons presently advocate early surgery for young patients who are in good neurological condition, but the timing of surgery for older, neurologically impaired patients remains open to debate.[11,36]

Technical Considerations

Some of the problems encountered by the pioneering aneurysm surgeons have been eased by technologic advances. The operating microscope has facilitated the physician's ability to accurately dissect and clip the neck of a ruptured aneurysm while preserving the adjacent fine perforating arteries. Although great emphasis is placed on its magnification, the microscope more importantly provides stereoscopic vision and good lighting at the base of a deep, narrow operative field. Pioneering aneurysm surgeons occluded the neck of a ruptured aneurysm with silk sutures and malleable aneurysm clips. Spring-loaded, high-pressure aneurysm clips in various shapes allow surgeons to precisely reconstruct the parent blood vessels while excluding the aneurysm from the circulation and to reposition a poorly placed clip. Fenestrated aneurysm clips allow surgeons to circumvent blood vessels that are tightly adherent to the dome of the aneurysm. Today's surgeons are aided by the vast number of detailed anatomic studies that outline the variations in the vascular anatomy which can be encountered during aneurysm surgery.

In their early writings, Botterell and Drake prophesied that early surgery would pit the surgeon against a "tight," friable brain. While the brain is more likely to be tight when surgery is performed within 3 days of the SAH than when surgery is delayed for 10 days, controlled ventilation, CSF drainage, and the appropriate anesthetic agents and diuretics will allow the surgeon to approach most aneurysms without deleterious brain retraction. In the International Cooperative Study on the Timing of Aneurysm Surgery, the brain was reported to be tight in 50 percent of cases operated on within 72 h after the SAH but in only 20 percent of cases operated on more than 10 days postictal.[34] Still, surgeons in that study reported no increase in the rate of brain contusion, lacerations, or resections with early surgery. The incidence of intraoperative aneurysm rupture was not related to the timing of surgery. In their review of 244 patients, Chyatte et al. found no difference in the incidence of intraoperative aneurysm rupture or brain contusion after comparing groups of patients who had been operated on at different posthemorrhage times.[10] Neither Samson et al.[53] nor Öhman and Heiskanen[48] found intraoperative complications to be a function of surgical timing. Reporting on 160 patients operated on within 3 days of their SAH, Ljunggren et al. noted that the "red swollen" brain became treatable with the help of anesthetic techniques and the removal of CSF.[38,39] They noted that intraoperative complications resulted in poor results in 11 (7 percent) patients. Several other surgeons corroborated the observation that the "tight swollen" brain was largely a consequence of subarachnoid blood and that simple drainage of CSF will frequently facilitate "brain relaxation."[5,15,42] Auer noted two complications attributable to "brain tightness" in 65 patients operated on acutely; rupture of the aneurysm occurred prior to the completion of aneurysm dissection in five additional patients.[5] Milhorat and Krautheim found no greater propensity for the aneurysm to rupture during "early surgery" than during procedures delayed at least one week after the SAH.[42]

In summary, modern technology has aided the surgeon who stages an early attack on a ruptured aneurysm. The brain is clearly "tighter" during early surgery than during delayed surgery. In most cases, the brain will become tractable with appropriate anesthetic techniques and CSF drainage. Timing of surgery does not significantly affect the incidence of complications when surgery is performed on small or moderate sized aneurysms of the anterior circulation.

Rehemorrhage

If rehemorrhage were the primary complication incurred by patients who had suffered an aneurysmal SAH, early surgery would be expected to greatly improve management outcomes. Data accrued from the Cooperative Aneurysm Study demonstrated a peak rehemorrhage rate of 4.1 percent during the first 24 h after the initial hemorrhage.[31] The rate of rebleeding then drops to 1.5 percent per day for the next 48 h. The risk of rehemorrhage gradually diminishes so that the cumulative incidence of rehemorrhage at 2 weeks is 19 percent. Winn et al. have reported that the cumulative rebleeding rate of an untreated ruptured aneurysm is 50 to 60 percent at 6 months and then approximately 3 percent per year thereafter.[69] Antifibrinolytic agents reduce the rate of rehemorrhage at the expense of an increased propensity for ischemic infarction.[32] Overall, antifibrinolytic agents do not improve management mortality beyond that of the natural history. Öhman and Heiskanen reported a randomized study of 216 patients in which 3 percent of patients operated on within 3 days of their hemorrhage suffered a second SAH as compared with 11 percent of patients operated on more than 8 days after their initial SAH.[48] In an uncontrolled retrospective study, Chyatte et al. found that 16 percent of patients undergoing surgery more than 10 days after the initial aneurysmal hemorrhage rebled and that in-hospital rehemorrhage was associated with a 25 percent mortality.[10] In studying 251 noncomatose patients admitted to the hospital within 24 h of their SAH, Taneda found that 38 percent of patients rehemorrhaged in the 11 days following SAH.[62] He recorded an astonishingly high rebleeding rate of 20 percent within the first 24 h and then 8 percent in the second 24 h following the initial hemorrhage. In the International Cooperative Study on the Timing of Aneurysm Surgery, patients whose surgery was scheduled to take place within 72 h after the first hemorrhage suffered a rebleeding rate of 5.7 percent whereas the accrued rehemorrhage rate for patients operated on between days 11 and 14 was 13.9 percent.[34] Hillman et al. noted that even with a policy of early surgery, 9.6 percent of patients admitted within 24 h of an SAH experienced proven or suspected rehemorrhage during transportation or while preparations were being made for surgery.[21]

Cerebral Ischemia

Cerebral ischemia is the leading cause of morbidity and mortality once the patient with a ruptured intracranial aneurysm enters a tertiary care center.[33] On average, vasospasm has its onset on day 3 following an SAH, reaches its zenith between days 6 and 8, and begins its resolution on day 10.[66] Stornelli and French along with Allcock and Drake warned that early operation was likely to provoke postoperative vasospasm.[1,57] Sundt opined that surgical trauma exacerbated vasospasm.[58] Worsening vasospasm is not the only mechanism by which surgery can precipitate a stroke. The patient with compromised cerebral blood flow, dysautoregulation, and impaired reactivity to CO_2 may also develop a cerebral infarction secondary to the induction of general anesthesia or intraoperative manipulation such as brain retraction or temporary clipping of cerebral blood vessels.[17,22,63,64] This compromised hemodynamic state may also render the patient less tolerant of iatrogenic complications such as intraoperative hemorrhage or the inadvertent occlusion of a cerebral vessel. Pickard et al. demonstrated that patients with defective autoregulation and cerebral blood flow are at greater risk of developing postoperative cerebral ischemia.[49]

Some authors have theorized that potential spasmogens could be removed at the time of early surgery or that surgery on the aneurysm would make proven therapies for vasospasm such as systemic hypertension or balloon angioplasty safer.[30,45,61,62] In experimental models of vasospasm, removal of the blood clot within 48 h reduces vasospasm.[6,18] Taneda compared 91 patients who underwent surgery within 3 days of their SAH with 99 patients who underwent surgery during the same time interval but had aggressive removal of subarachnoid blood.[62] "Vasospasm" developed in 24 percent of patients undergoing early surgery with the aggressive removal of clot and in 58 percent of patients undergoing early surgery alone. Mizukami et al. attempted to remove all cisternal blood at the time of surgery performed within 4 days of SAH in 64 patients.[44] They found a correlation between residual cisternal blood and vasospasm. The failure of early surgery to reduce the incidence of vasospasm may be due to the difficulty in removing subarachnoid blood.[28] The use of fibrinolytic agents may provide a method of removing blood clot without injuring adjacent brain. Preliminary uncontrolled studies have demonstrated an impressive reduction in the incidence of vasospasm below the expected rate for patients with thick intracisternal clots as demonstrated on their CT scans. Success in using such agents should be another strong argument for early surgery.

Yasui et al.[70] and others have demonstrated that, beginning 4 days after the hemorrhage, cerebral blood flow reserves decrease and eventually cerebral blood flow itself decreases and does not return to normal until 3 weeks following the hemorrhage. Hori and Suzuki,[23] and Sano and Saito[54] noted that surgery undertaken soon after the onset of vasospasm worsened the postoperative condition.[23,54] If surgery was delayed until the patient's neurological deficits were clearing, no such postoperative worsening was noted. In the International Cooperative Study on the Timing of Aneurysm Surgery, the incidence of focal ischemic deficits was highest in patients undergoing surgery 4 to 10 days after their hemorrhage.[34] Solomon et al. reported that there was a trend toward a higher rate of ischemic deficits when surgery was performed later in the week following SAH in a series of 145 consecutive patients.[55] Unlike other series, the patient's grade only influenced the incidence of delayed ischemic deficit in those patients operated on within 24 h. Although 66 of 145 patients developed a delayed ischemic deficit despite postoperative blood volume expansion, with hypertensive therapy only 12 of these patients developed cerebral infarction and in only four was this the cause of a poor result. Most studies indicate that surgery undertaken between days 4 and 10 after an SAH carries an increased risk of exacerbating cerebral ischemia.

Not all authors report an effect of timing of surgery on the incidence of delayed ischemic deficits. In a randomized study of 216 patients, Öhman and Heiskanen reported that the incidence of vasospasm was unaffected by the timing of surgery.[48] Chyatte et al. noted a higher incidence of delayed ischemic complications in patients operated on 0 to 3 days after SAH than those operated on 4 to 7 days following an SAH.[10]

Even though it seems to be more hazardous to operate on patients between days 4 and 10 following an SAH, it is not clear that mechanical manipulation of blood vessels exacerbates vessel narrowing per se.[9,34,48] Using a primate model, Findlay et al. found that surgical manipulation and temporary clip placement on the sixth postoperative day did not exacerbate established angiographic vasospasm.[14] Other researchers using various animal models have shown that cerebral blood vessels exposed to extraluminal blood are actually hyporesponsive to vasoactive substances.[9,14,35] Macdonald et al. reviewed pre- and postoperative angiograms on 56 patients.[40] Thirty-four patients were operated on 4 to 12 days following their SAH. Postoperative blood vessel diameters were a function of preoperative diameters and not of the timing of surgery. These results question whether established vessel constriction per se is aggravated by surgery.

Ligation of the ruptured aneurysm does facilitate the treatment of vasospasm. Hypertensive therapy is of less risk when the risk of aneurysmal hemorrhage has been eliminated. Le Roux et al. reported a small series of patients who underwent clip ligation of an intracranial aneurysm while still evolving a neurological deficit from vasospasm.[37] Immediately after surgery, the patients were treated with hypervolemic therapy and balloon angioplasty for their spasm. This technique deserves further investigation.

In summary, it does not seem that surgery greatly influences the course of vasospasm. Eliminating the threat of aneurysmal hemorrhage facilitates the use of hypertensive therapy and possibly balloon angioplasty. Surgery undertaken during the evolution of vasospasm carried a higher risk of delayed ischemic neurological deficit. If thrombolytic agents fulfill their promise, it is possible that early surgery could decrease the incidence of vasospasm.

Management Results

Early reports focused the results of therapy on the complications of surgery for ruptured aneurysms. However, the only true measure is patient outcome; this measure is referred to as "management results." Alvord et al. definitively demonstrated that the outcome of the patient who has suffered an aneurysmal SAH is a function of the patient's neurological grade and the duration of time between the SAH and the patient's admission to the hospital.[2] The longer the patient survives, the better his chance of subsequent survival. Thus, a true assessment of management results requires that the patient come under observation soon after the aneurysm ruptures, and is assessed at a fixed period. There are only a small number of reviews in the literature that report management mortality as a function of timing of surgery.

Taneda reviewed the results of 251 patients, all of whom were admitted to the hospital within 24 h of their SAH.[62] The 61 patients treated with delayed surgery had a worse outcome than the 190 patients who were operated on within 3 days of their hemorrhage. Weir and Aronyk reported a retrospective review of 244 patients admitted into the hospital within 24 h of their SAH.[65] Timing of surgery made no difference in the outcome of patients admitted in Grades I, II, or V condition. Lower management mortality was achieved in Grades III and VI patients operated on within 96 h of their SAH. A subsequent report from that institution corroborated the finding that early surgery leads to a decline in management mortality.[13] Chyatte et al. reported on 244 patients admitted within 3 days of their SAH.[10] For these patients, there was a trend toward later operations for poor grade patients and technically difficult aneurysms. When the patients were segregated by grade, there was no significant effect of timing of surgery on management outcome. Artiola i Fortuny and Prieto-Valiente found that late surgery resulted in a slight decline of mortality.[3,4] This conclusion must be discounted because the authors did not include patients who had died prior to surgical therapy and because timing of admission was not specified. Solomon et al. operated on all patients upon arrival.[55] There was a trend toward worse results in patients operated on in the second half of the first week for Grades I and II patients, but there was no such trend in Grades III and IV patients. Similarly, Hugenholtz and Elgie in a nonrandomized study reported that management mortality and morbidity for Botterell Grades 1 and 2 patients were clearly lower in patients operated on within 48 h of hemorrhage only to rise again in patients operated on in the second half of the first week.[24] A similar trend was noted in Grade 3 patients. In a nonrandomized retrospective study of 106 good grade patients, Samson et al. noted no effect of the timing of surgery on good results, or mortality.[53] In a cooperative prospective observational epidemiological survey,[33,34] Kassell et al. reported no significant difference in management mortality in patients operated on early (0 to 3 days after hemorrhage) or late (11 to 14 days). Outcome was worse for patients operated on in the day 7 to 10 interval. Although these conclusions were significant for alert patients (Grades I and II), they did not hold for drowsy patients.

Miyaoka et al. retrospectively reviewed 1622 cases of aneurysmal SAH, 85 percent of whom were hospitalized by posthemorrhage day 3.[43] Outcome was not affected by the timing of surgery except for an increase in good results in Grade III patients undergoing early surgery. When 216 Grades I to III patients were randomized to surgery 0 to 3 days, 4 to 8 days, or more than 8 days following SAH by Öhman and Heiskanen, there was no effect of timing on surgery on mortality.[48] Significantly more patients remained dependent in the group of patients operated on between day 4 and 8 than those operated on early. There was a trend for patients who were operated on early (day 0 to 3) to be more likely to be independent.

Although many authors have reserved early surgery for good-grade patients, a few surgeons have reported the results of early surgery on poor-grade patients. Disney et al. reported that management mortality was lowest in Grades III, IV, and V patients operated on within 96 h as compared to those operated on at subsequent time intervals.[12] At 6 month follow-up, Auer reported that 86 percent of patients admitted at Grade III or IV and operated on within 48 h of their SAH were living independently.[5] Bailes et al. reported on 54 Grades IV and V patients.[7] Thirty-five patients who had blood flow on angiography, no massive infarction, and no basal ganglia or brain stem hemorrhage, and whose intracranial pressure could be lowered to below 30 cmH_2O by ventricular drainage underwent immediate clip ligation of the ruptured aneurysm. Thirty-five percent of patients (54 percent of those undergoing surgery) recovered to an independent life style. Winn et al. reported performing early surgery on 79 patients who were hospitalized in Grades III, IV, or V condition within 72 h of suffering a ruptured intracranial aneurysm.[68] The mortality at 6 month follow-up was 13 percent, 35 percent, and 41 percent in Grades III, IV, and V patients, respectively. Although these results are better than historical controls, the place for early surgery in Grades IV and V patients awaits a contemporary comparison.

Inagawa noted a significant adverse effect of age on the management of aneurysmal SAH.[27] Advocating early surgery (83 percent operated on before day 3), he found that 80 percent of Grades I to III patients less than 60 years of age enjoyed a good result but that a good result was only obtained in 51 percent of similar grade patients 70 to 79 years of age.

Most studies rate a patient who is either independent or grossly intact 6 months after their SAH as a good result. The question must be asked whether early surgery takes an exorbitant toll on the patient's cognition. Fifty-five patients with an ostensibly normal recovery following early surgery were compared with 38 patients with an ostensibly normal recovery following late surgery using sophisticated testing of emotional stability and cognition.[56] The alterations in cognitive and psychosocial disturbances did not differ substantially between the two groups of patients.

Conclusions

In summary, there is no compelling evidence that timing of surgery will greatly influence the outcome of aneurysm surgery in large patient populations. Thus far, early surgery has not been shown to significantly reduce the severity of vasospasm, although the use of fibrinolytic agents may change this verdict. Since vasospasm is less likely to occur in patients with little subarachnoid blood, it would seem reasonable to operate on good-grade patients without significant medical problems as quickly as an experienced operating team can be organized. If surgery is undertaken between the fourth and tenth posthemorrhage day, special care must be given to protect cerebral perfusion. In most other cases, timing of surgery should be dictated by the patient's medical condition, the presence of a large intracranial mass, and further data as they become available.

References

1. Allcock JM, Drake CG. Ruptured intracranial aneurysms—The role of arterial spasm. *J Neurosurg* 1965; 22:21–29.
2. Alvord EC Jr, Loeser JD, Bailey WL, et al. Subarachnoid hemorrhage due to ruptured aneurysms. A simple method of estimating prognosis. *Arch Neurol* 1972; 27:273–284.
3. Artiola i Fortuny L, Prieto-Valiente L. Long-term prognosis in surgically treated intracranial aneurysms: Part 1: Mortality. *J Neurosurg* 1981; 54:26–34.
4. Artiola i Fortuny L, Prieto-Valiente L. Long-term prognosis in surgically treated intracranial aneurysms: Part 2: Morbidity. *J Neurosurg* 1981; 54:35–43.
5. Auer LM. Acute operation and preventive nimodipine improve outcome in patients with ruptured cerebral aneurysms. *Neurosurgery* 1984; 15:57–66.
6. Aydin IH, Onder A. The effect of very early cisternal irrigation on basilar artery spasm after SAH in the rat model. *Acta Neurochir (Wien)* 1991; 113:69–73.
7. Bailes JE, Spetzler RF, Hadley MN, et al. Management morbidity and mortality of poor-grade aneurysm patients. *J Neurosurg* 1990; 72:559–566.
8. Batjer HH, Samson DS. Causes of morbidity and mortality from surgery of aneurysms of the distal basilar artery. *Neurosurgery* 1989; 25:904–916.
9. Bevan JA, Bevan RD, Frazee JG. Functional arterial changes in chronic cerebrovasospasm in monkeys: an in vitro assessment of the contribution to arterial narrowing. *Stroke* 1987; 18:472–481.
10. Chyatte D, Fode NC, Sundt TM Jr. Early versus late intracranial aneurysm surgery in subarachnoid hemorrhage. *J Neurosurg* 1988; 69:326–331.
11. Deruty R, Mottolese C, Pelissou-Guyotat I, et al. Management of the ruptured intracranial aneurysm—early surgery, late surgery or modulated surgery? Personal experience based upon 468 patients admitted in two periods (1972–1984 and 1985–1989). *Acta Neurochir (Wien)* 1991; 113:1–10.
12. Disney L, Weir B, Grace M. Factors influencing the outcome of aneurysm rupture in poor grade patients: a prospective series. *Neurosurgery* 1988; 23:1–9.
13. Disney L, Weir B, Petruk K. Effect on management mortality of a deliberate policy of early operation on supratentorial aneurysms. *Neurosurgery* 1987; 20:695–701.
14. Findlay JM, Macdonald RL, Weir BK, et al. Surgical manipulation of primate cerebral arteries in established vasospasm. *J Neurosurg* 1991; 75:425–432.
15. Gilsbach JM, Harders AG, Eggert HR, et al. Early aneurysm surgery: a 7 year clinical practice report. *Acta Neurochir (Wien)* 1988; 90:91–102.
16. Graf CJ. Results of direct attack on nonfistulous intracranial aneurysm with remarks on statistics. *J Neurosurg* 1955; 12:146–153.
17. Grubb RL Jr, Raichle ME, Eichling JO, et al. Effects of subarachnoid hemorrhage on cerebral blood volume, blood flow, and oxygen utilization in humans. *J Neurosurg* 1977; 46:446–453.
18. Handa Y, Weir BK, Nosko M, et al. The effect of timing of clot removal on chronic vasospasm in a primate model. *J Neurosurg* 1987; 67:558–564.
19. Heilbrun MP, Olesen J, Lassen NA. Regional cerebral blood flow studies in subarachnoid hemorrhage. *J Neurosurg* 1972; 37:36–44.
20. Heiskanen O, Poranen A, Kuurne T, et al. Acute surgery for intracerebral haematomas caused by rupture of an intracranial arterial aneurysm: a prospective randomized study. *Acta Neurochir (Wien)* 1988; 90:81–83.
21. Hillman J, von Essen C, Leszniewski W, et al. Significance of "ultra-early" rebleeding in subarachnoid hemorrhage. *J Neurosurg* 1988; 68:901–907.
22. Hino A, Mizukawa N, Tenjin H, et al. Postoperative hemodynamic and metabolic changes in patients with subarachnoid hemorrhage. *Stroke* 1989; 20:1504–1510.
23. Hori S, Suzuki J. Early and late results of intracranial direct surgery of anterior communicating artery aneurysms. *J Neurosurg* 1979; 50:433–440.
24. Hugenholtz H, Elgie RG. Considerations in early surgery on good-risk patients with ruptured intracranial aneurysms. *J Neurosurg* 1982; 56:180–185.
25. Hunt WE, Hess RM. Surgical risk as related to time of intervention in the repair of intracranial aneurysms. *J Neurosurg* 1968; 28:14–20.
26. Hunt WE, Kosnik EJ. Timing and perioperative care in intracranial aneurysm surgery. *Clin Neurosurg* 1974; 21:79–89.
27. Inagawa T. Management outcome in the elderly patient following subarachnoid hemorrhage. *J Neurosurg* 1993; 78:554–561.
28. Inagawa T, Yamamoto M, Kamiya K. Effect of clot removal on cerebral vasospasm. *J Neurosurg* 1990; 72:224–230.
29. Ishii R. Regional cerebral blood flow in patients with ruptured intracranial aneurysms. *J Neurosurg* 1979; 50:587–594.
30. Johnson RJ, Potter JM, Reid RG. Arterial spasm in subarachnoid haemorrhage: mechanical considerations. *J Neurol Neurosurg Psychiatry* 1958; 21:68 (abstr).
31. Kassell NF, Torner JC. Aneurysmal rebleeding: a preliminary report from the Cooperative Aneurysm Study. *Neurosurgery* 1983; 13:479–481.
32. Kassell NF, Torner JC, Adams HP Jr. Antifibrinolytic therapy in the acute period following aneurysmal subarachnoid hemorrhage: preliminary observations from the Cooperative Aneurysm Study. *J Neurosurg* 1984; 61:225–230.
33. Kassell NF, Torner JC, Haley EC Jr, et al. The International Cooperative Study on the Timing of Aneurysm Surgery. Part 1: Overall management results. *J Neurosurg* 1990; 73:18–36.
34. Kassell NF, Torner JC, Jane JA, et al. The International Cooperative Study on the Timing of Aneurysm Surgery. Part 2: Surgical results. *J Neurosurg* 1990; 73:37–47.

35. Kim P, Sundt TM Jr, Vanhoutte PM. Alterations of mechanical properties in canine basilar arteries after subarachnoid hemorrhage. *J Neurosurg* 1989; 71:430–436.
36. Krupp W, Heienbrok W, Muke R. Management results attained by predominantly late surgery for intracranial aneurysms. *Neurosurgery* 1994; 34:227–234.
37. Le Roux PD, Newell DW, Eskridge J, et al. Severe symptomatic vasospasm: the role of immediate postoperative angioplasty. *J Neurosurg* 1994; 80:224–229.
38. Ljunggren B, Säveland H, Brandt L. Causes of unfavorable outcome after early aneurysm operation. *Neurosurgery* 1983; 13:629–633.
39. Ljunggren B, Säveland H, Brandt L, et al. Early operation and overall outcome in aneurysmal subarachnoid hemorrhage. *J Neurosurg* 1985; 62:547–551.
40. Macdonald RL, Wallace MC, Coyne TJ. The effect of surgery on the severity of vasospasm. *J Neurosurg* 1994; 80:433–439.
41. McKissock W, Paine KWE. Subarachnoid haemorrhage. *Brain* 1959; 82:356–366.
42. Milhorat TH, Krautheim M. Results of early and delayed operations for ruptured intracranial aneurysms in two series of 100 consecutive patients. *Surg Neurol* 1986; 26:123–128.
43. Miyaoka M, Sato K, Ishii R. A clinical study of the relationship of timing to outcome of surgery for ruptured cerebral aneurysms. A retrospective analysis of 1622 cases. *J Neurosurg* 1993; 79:373–378.
44. Mizukami M, Kawase T, Usami T, et al. Prevention of vasospasm by early operation with removal of subarachnoid blood. *Neurosurgery* 1982; 10:301–307.
45. Newell DW, Eskridge J, Mayberg M, et al. Endovascular treatment of intracranial aneurysms and cerebral vasospasm. *Clin Neurosurg* 1992; 39:348–360.
46. Norlén G. Some aspects of the surgical treatment of intracranial aneurysms. *Clin Neurosurg* 1961; 9:214–222.
47. Norlén G, Olivecrona H. The treatment of aneurysms of the circle of Willis. *J Neurosurg* 1953; 10:404–415.
48. Öhman J, Heiskanen O. Timing of operation for ruptured supratentorial aneurysms: a prospective randomized study. *J Neurosurg* 1989; 70:55–60.
49. Pickard JD, Matheson M, Patterson J, et al. Prediction of late ischemic complications after cerebral aneurysm surgery by intraoperative measurement of cerebral blood flow. *J Neurosurg* 1980; 53:305–308.
50. Pool JL. Early treatment of ruptured intracranial aneurysms of the circle of Willis with special clip technique. *Bull NY Acad Med* 1959; 35:357–369.
51. Pool JL. Timing and techniques in the intracranial surgery of ruptured aneurysms of the anterior communicating artery. *J Neurosurg* 1962; 19:378–388.
52. Ropper AH, Zervas NT. Outcome 1 year after SAH from cerebral aneurysm. Management morbidity, mortality, and functional status in 112 consecutive good-risk patients. *J Neurosurg* 1984; 60:909–915.
53. Samson DS, Hodosh RM, Reid WR, et al. Risk of intracranial aneurysm surgery in the good grade patient: early versus late operation. *Neurosurgery* 1979; 5:422–426.
54. Sano K, Saito I. Timing and indication of surgery for ruptured intracranial aneurysm with regard to cerebral vasospasm. *Acta Neurochir (Wien)* 1978; 41:49–60.
55. Solomon RA, Onesti ST, Kelbanoff L. Relationship between the timing of aneurysm surgery and the development of delayed cerebral ischemia. *J Neurosurg* 1991; 75:56–61.
56. Sonesson B, Ljunggren B, Säveland H, et al. Cognition and adjustment after late and early operation for ruptured aneurysm. *Neurosurgery* 1987; 21:279–287.
57. Stornelli SA, French JD. Subarachnoid hemorrhage—factors in prognosis and management. *J Neurosurg* 1964; 21:769–780.
58. Sundt TM Jr. Cerebral vasospasm following subarachnoid hemorrhage: evolution, management, and relationship to timing of surgery. *Clin Neurosurg* 1977; 24:228–239.
59. Sundt TM Jr, Kobayashi S, Fode NC, et al. Results and complications of surgical management of 809 intracranial aneurysms in 722 cases. Related and unrelated to grade of patient, type of aneurysm, and timing of surgery. *J Neurosurg* 1982; 56:753–765.
60. Sundt TM Jr, Whisnant JP. Subarachnoid hemorrhage from intracranial aneurysms. Surgical management and natural history of disease. *N Engl J Med* 1978; 299:116–122.
61. Suzuki J, Onuma T, Yoshimoto T. Results of early operations on cerebral aneurysms. *Surg Neurol* 1979; 11:407–412.
62. Taneda M. The significance of early operation in the management of ruptured intracranial aneurysms—an analysis of 251 cases hospitalized within 24 hours after subarachnoid hemorrhage. *Acta Neurochir (Wien)* 1982; 63:201–208.
63. Tenjin H, Hirakawa K, Mizukawa N, et al. Dysautoregulation in patients with ruptured aneurysms: cerebral blood flow measurements obtained during surgery by a temperature-controlled thermoelectrical method. *Neurosurgery* 1988; 23:705–709.
64. Voldby B, Enevoldsen EM, Jensen FT. Cerebrovascular reactivity in patients with ruptured intracranial aneurysms. *J Neurosurg* 1985; 62:59–67.
65. Weir B, Aronyk K. Management mortality and the timing of surgery for supratentorial aneurysm. *J Neurosurg* 1981; 54:146–150.
66. Weir B, Grace M, Hansen J, et al. Time course of vasospasm in man. *J Neurosurg* 1978; 48:173–178.
67. Whisnant JP, Phillips LH II, Sundt TM Jr. Aneurysmal subarachnoid hemorrhage: timing of surgery and mortality. *Mayo Clin Proc* 1982; 57:471–475.
68. Winn HR, Newell DW, Mayberg MR, et al. Early surgical management of poor-grade patients with intracranial aneurysms (review). *Clin Neurosurg* 1990; 36:289–298.
69. Winn HR, Richardson AE, Jane JA. The long-term prognosis in untreated cerebral aneurysms. 1. The incidence of late hemorrhage in cerebral aneurysms: a 10-year evaluation in 364 patients. *Ann Neurol* 1977; 1:358–370.
70. Yasui N, Ito Z, Ohta H, et al. Surgical problems and pathophysiology in severe cases with ruptured aneurysm in the acute stage. *Acta Neurochir (Wien)* 1982; 63:163–174.
71. Yoshimoto T, Uchida K, Kaneko U, et al. An analysis of follow-up results of 1000 intracranial saccular aneurysms with definitive surgical treatment. *J Neurosurg* 1979; 50:152–157.

219 Pre- and Postoperative Management of a Patient with a Ruptured Aneurysm

Allan H. Friedman

A patient who has suffered a ruptured intracranial berry aneurysm can be injured by the initial hemorrhage or by the effects of subsequent aneurysmal hemorrhage, vasospasm, hydrocephalus, surgical complications, and medical complications. Like the patient who has suffered cerebral head trauma, the surgeon can do nothing to mitigate the permanent neuronal injury that occurred at the time of the initial hemorrhage. Care is aimed at avoiding subsequent compounding complications.

Diagnosis

The most prevalent remedial cause of morbidity and mortality following the rupture of an intracranial aneurysm is delayed diagnosis.[3] The hallmarks of a subarachnoid hemorrhage (SAH) are severe headache with or without nausea and vomiting, and alteration in consciousness. A seizure or vomiting may occasionally herald the rupture of an intracranial aneurysm. Nuchal rigidity frequently develops in the hours following the hemorrhage. In approximately one-third of patients, a devastating SAH will be preceded by a small leak of subarachnoid blood manifest as an unusually severe headache. The most significant intervention a physician can perform to avoid complications is to diagnose an intracranial aneurysm at the time of this warning leak.

Computed tomography (CT) demonstrates subarachnoid blood in 90 to 95 percent of patients scanned within 24 h of hemorrhage but becomes less effective with time, demonstrating subarachnoid blood in only 74 percent of patients scanned on the third posthemorrhage day and 50 percent of patients scanned on the seventh posthemorrhage day.[4,126,139] If the CT scan is negative, a lumbar puncture should be carried out.

The role of magnetic resonance imaging (MRI) scanning in the detection of acute subarachnoid blood is controversial. While some authors have reported that acute subarachnoid blood appears hyperintense on proton density weighted MR images, most observers find acute subarachnoid blood difficult to discern on an MRI scan.[8] A week after the hemorrhage when paramagnetic methhemoglobin evolves, the blood-stained subarachnoid space takes on a hyperdense appearance.

Grading

Patients suffering an SAH from a ruptured intracranial aneurysm are traditionally graded by the Hunt-Hess or Nishioka scale.[50,95] The patient's grade on admission is of prognostic value and for some surgeons it influences the course of therapy. Unfortunately, the symptoms used to determine the patient's grade such as degree of headache or degree of cognitive impairment are subjective and therefore result in interobserver variability.[73,74]

More recently, the World Federation of Neurological Surgeons proposed a scale based on the Glasgow Coma Scale that may result in a more reproducible grading of patients.[24] This scale is based on the observation that level of consciousness and focal neurological deficit are the most important predictors of outcome. Its efficacy awaits validation.[112]

Early Surgery

The best time to clip an aneurysm and eliminate the possibility of rehemorrhage remains controversial. Although the pendulum of opinion has swung toward immediate surgery, the question of whether all patients, regardless of age and clinical grade, are best served by immediate intervention is not proven.

In the rare patient with a large concomitant subdural or intraparenchymal hemorrhage, surgical evacuation of the hematoma may be life-saving.[13,144] In these cases, a CT scan combined with the continuous infusion of contrast material may demonstrate the ruptured aneurysm, obviating a preoperative cerebral angiogram.[93]

Prevention of Rehemorrhage

General Measures

The patient who survives the initial hemorrhage of an intracranial aneurysm is at significant risk of a second hemorrhage from the aneurysm.[60] If left untreated, at least 4 percent of patients will experience rehemorrhage within the first 24 h and 19 percent will have rehemorrhage within the 2 weeks following the initial rupture. The second hemorrhage has a 50 percent mortality.[44]

The mainstay of therapy to avoid a second hemorrhage is clip ligation of the aneurysm. While awaiting surgical repair of the aneurysm, therapy is aimed at avoiding elevations in systemic blood pressure, seizures, and straining. Rebleeding rates appear to be higher in patients with a systolic blood pressure above 160 mmHg.[94] Patients are traditionally kept at bedrest in a dark, quiet room with limited emotional stimulation. These maneuvers should not be so excessive as to cause the patient anxiety. Soft music, a comforting relative, or even access to cigarettes may be more effective than total isolation. In the immediate posthemorrhage period, hypertension can be treated without the risk of stroke from concomitant vasospasm. Hypertension from pain and anxiety is treated with narcotic analgesics such as codeine or intravenous morphine and sedatives such as midazolam or phenobarbital. Intravenous mexiletine or lidocaine can suppress the autonomic response provoked by painful procedures such as endotracheal suctioning. Short-acting hypotensive agents such as labetalol or sodium nitroprusside are reserved for labile hypertension or transient hypertension provoked by therapeutic maneuvers. Because ischemic areas of brain with altered autoregulation depend on arterial blood pressure for perfusion, hypotensive therapy should not be aggressively pursued, and only extreme elevations in blood pressure should be treated. Although treating hypertension seems to decrease the incidence of rehemorrhage, it does so at the expense of an increased rate of cerebral infarction.[94,147]

Antifibrolytic Agents

Antifibrinolytic agents have been used to retard rebleeding from ruptured intracranial aneurysms, using the reasoning that these agents would prevent dissolution of the clot tamponading the rent in the aneurysm.[140] The most commonly used agents, ϵ-aminocaproic acid and tranexamic acid, are small molecules structurally similar to lysine that block the binding of plasminogen onto fibrin.

Since their introduction, the efficacy of antifibrinolytic agents has been debated through numerous reports.[2,109,143] Some recent large studies have helped define their therapeutic benefits. In a nonrandomized survey of 872 patients, antifibrinolytic agents were found to significantly reduce the rate of acute rehemorrhage from 19.4 to 11.7 percent, but because of a concomitant increase in the rate of delayed ischemic cerebral infarction, the management mortality rate was unchanged by therapy.[61] In a randomized double-blind study of 285 patients with an aneurysmal SAH, patients receiving tranexamic acid had a lower rate of acute hemorrhage. Because of an increased rate of cerebral infarction in patients receiving the drug, there was no net difference in clinical outcome measured 3 months after the hemorrhage.[48] These findings have led most surgeons to abandon the use of these agents.

Can the beneficial effects of reduced acute hemorrhage be separated from the deleterious effects of increased cerebral infarction? The question of whether these agents increase the incidence of cerebral infarction by hampering the clearance of subarachnoid blood, by increasing the viscosity or coagulability of intravascular blood, or by simply dehydrating the patient remains unanswered. In a preliminary report of 42 patients treated with a combination of antifibrolytic agents and nicardipine only one patient (2 percent) developed a cerebral infarction attributable to vasospasm.[10]

If antifibrinolytic agents are delivered without a loading dose, therapeutic blood levels will not be reached for 24 to 36 h. This agrees with studies that demonstrate no reduction in the rehemorrhage rate during the first 2 to 3 days of drug administration. In order to rapidly achieve a therapeutic blood level, a 5 g bolus of ϵ-aminocaproic acid should be followed by 1 to 1½ g/h in a continuous infusion.

Antifibrinolytic agents are associated with a significantly increased incidence of diarrhea, hydrocephalus, and thrombophlebitis.

Nutrition

Although there are no nutritional studies specifically limited to patients with ruptured intracranial aneurysms, patients with CNS injuries have increased nutritional needs.[155] Nutritional support favorably influences the outcome of many serious diseases by decreasing rates of infection, decubitus ulcers, and gastric ulcers and by improving wound healing and pulmonary status. Obtunded or comatose patients should be fed enterally, through a tube passed nasally into the duodenum. Patients should be provided with at least 40 kcal/kg body weight per day.

Significant perioperative gastrointestinal hemorrhage occurs in approximately 2 percent of patients.[128] H2 antagonists or antacids are used to avoid gastrointestinal hemorrhage with resulting anemia or hypotension. Stool softeners are used to avoid straining on the passage of stool.

Hydrocephalus

Hydrocephalus occurs in approximately 20 percent of patients suffering an aneurysmal SAH and has an incidence that parallels the patient's neurological grade. Although acute hydrocephalus may be asymptomatic and resolve spontaneously, in selected cases, emergent drainage of CSF will greatly improve the patient's neurological status.[84] Hasan et al. found that 78 percent of patients with symptomatic hydrocephalus improved following ventricular drainage.[46] Ventricular drainage for acute hydrocephalus should be used with caution because it results in a higher incidence of rehemorrhage from the aneurysm.[84,101] Patients may develop a gradual worsening of their neurological condition from chronic hydrocephalus with or without an elevation in CSF pressure. CSF diversion improves neurological function in these patients after the aneurysm has been clipped.

Medical Complications

Hyponatremia

Hyponatremia with decreased serum osmolarity occurs in approximately 10 percent of patients after aneurysmal SAH. Although this had been thought to be due to inappropriate antidiuretic hormone (ADH) secretion, it is now clear that in most cases this is due to an elevation in serum atrial natriuretic factor.[23,145] Unlike patients with inappropriate ADH secretion, most patients are hypovolemic and their hyponatremia should be corrected with volume expansion.[146,148] Natriuresis can be reduced by the prophylactic use of fludrocortisone.[44] When serum sodium levels drop below 125 mEq/L, patients should be treated with intravenous hypertonic saline to avoid seizures and alteration in level of consciousness.

Deep Venous Thrombosis

Clinically apparent thrombophlebitis occurs in 1 to 2 percent of patients treated for a ruptured intracranial aneurysm. If ^{131}-I labelled fibrinogenic uptake or duplex ultrasonography are used to detect thrombus, the incidence of deep vein thrombosis (DVT) is considerably higher. Risk factors for developing DVT include advanced age, obesity, cardiac failure, lengthy surgery, lower extremity paralysis, previous history of thrombophlebitis, and various hypercoagulable states. Most surgeons employ prophylactic leg exercises and graduated compression stockings. Intermittent pneumatic compression of the calf has been demonstrated to lower the incidence of DVT in the neurosurgical population.[118,135] Low dose subcutaneous heparin, an effective prophylaxis of DVT, is seldom employed prior to or immediately after cerebral aneurysm surgery, but this form of therapy is appropriate for patients who are confined to bed for a prolonged period following surgery.[16,118,125]

The usual therapy of systemic anticoagulation is seldom employed to treat a DVT prior to or immediately following the clipping of an intracranial aneurysm. The available literature indicates that a patient may safely be anticoagulated one week following surgery for an uncomplicated aneurysm but the data supporting this tenet are not firm, and clearly this topic requires further investigation.[16] Anticoagulation should be further delayed in cases where there is a significant intraparenchymal hematoma, the surgical dissection was extensive, or the patient suffered a large (or multiple) cerebral infarction. In patients with DVT who are not suitable candidates for anticoagulation, a vena cava filter will decrease the incidence of pulmonary embolism to 2 to 3 percent.[35] Low molecular weight heparin and heparinoids, which seem to have a lower risk of bleeding complications, may prove to be an ideal alternative for DVT prophylaxis and treatment of postoperative patients.

Pulmonary Complications

Patients suffering an SAH an manifest respiratory arrest necessitating mechanical ventilation. Patients suffering apnea may return to normal following respiratory support.[49] Patients may aspirate abdominal contents at the time that the aneurysm ruptures or while in an obtunded state. Aspiration pneumonia should be treated with an aminoglycoside and a third generation cephalosporin. Therapy can be refined when sputum culture results become available.

Increased sympathetic activity is thought to be the mechanism by which patients with ruptured aneurysms acutely develop severe neurogenic pulmonary edema.[113] Because diuretic therapy with loss of intravascular volume makes the patient more susceptible to vasospasm, patients are initially managed best with positive airway pressure. Pulmonary edema may persist if intracranial pressure remains elevated.

Seizures

Early seizures appear in approximately 10 to 20 percent of patients with SAH.[43] In many cases, early seizures are the harbinger of aneurysmal hemorrhage.[43] Late seizures or epilepsy occur in approximately 8 percent of patients.[15,45,110] Epilepsy is most likely to manifest in patients who have a higher neurological grade, who experience rehemorrhage, who harbor a middle cerebral artery aneurysm, who have an intracerebral hematoma, or who suffer vasospasm.[97] A seizure occurring within 12 h of a hemorrhage does not increase the patient's risk for developing epilepsy.[45] As has been shown in patients suffering cranial trauma, prophylactic use of diphenylhydantoin is unlikely to affect the incidence of epilepsy following an SAH.[11,136] Some surgeons employ short-term anticonvulsants to avoid the hypertension and agitation associated with early seizures.

Cardiac Complications

EKG abnormalities including prolonged QT intervals, U-wave formation, elevated or depressed S-T segments, and T-wave flatting, commonly occur following SAH. These changes are believed to result from subendocardial ischemia and hemorrhage. Increased ventricular excitability with runs of ventricular arrhythmia can be life threatening.[26,27] This ventricular hyperexcitability is thought to result from the increased serum levels of catecholamines. Beta blocking agents will resolve most dysrhythmias associated with SAH.[79,90] Prophylactic propranolol or atenolol has been shown to reduce serum levels of creatinine kinase and improve outcome following SAH.[19,89,90]

Cerebral Ischemia; Vasospasm

Vasospasm is the leading cause of death and morbidity in patients admitted to a tertiary care center with a ruptured intracranial aneurysm.[59,62] Focal, thick collections of cisternal blood visualized on a CT scan are highly predictive of vasospasm.[5] Angiographic vasospasm can be detected in 70 to 90 percent of these patients and will have clinical consequences in 30 percent of them. The clinical picture of vasospasm varies from an insidious alteration in level of consciousness to an abrupt focal neurological deficit. This may be preceded by headache, fever, and leukocytosis. Clinical symptoms usually appear between the fifth and twelfth day following the hemorrhage. Although the presumptive diagnosis of vasospasm is made by the time course of the neurological deficit and the elimination of other sources for a deficit, an accurate diagnosis can only be established by angiography.

Transcranial Doppler Ultrasonography

Serial transcranial Doppler (TCD) ultrasound measurements, which can monitor blood velocity in the horizontally oriented blood vessels at the base of the brain, have been used to monitor patients at risk for developing vasospasm.[1] A wide variation in experience has been reported using TCD to predict vasospasm. While investigators at a few centers have reported an excellent correlation between angiographic vasospasm development and elevated blood flow velocities recorded by ultrasound, those at most centers note discrepancies.[51,71,72,115] A comparison of the diameter of the middle cerebral artery as measured on an angiogram and the blood flow velocity measured by TCD yields a correlation coefficient of approximately 0.5, which indicates a reasonable but not perfect correlation. Based on personal experiences, several investigators have decided that patients with a middle cerebral artery velocity of 150 cm/s or greater are considered to be at risk for developing a delayed neurological deficit. Using this criterion, TCD is reported by many groups to have a 80 to 100 percent sensitivity and a 60 to 70 percent specificity in diagnosing angiographic vasospasm.[36,37,119] Thus significant vasospasm may be missed by this method. Some of these false negatives reflect the inability of TCD to measure velocity in the vertically oriented or more distal vessels. It is estimated that 50 percent of patients with vasospasm will have significant involvement in these vertical arterial segments.[92] Grosset et al. found considerable overlap in middle cerebral artery flow velocities between asymptomatic patients and those with delayed ischemic deficit. In their patients, a rise in flow velocity of 50 cm/s in 24 h identified patients likely to develop delayed ischemia.[38] After reviewing the literature, it appears that TCD provides an early warning for vasospasm in some patients, but more recent reports expose the shortcomings of this technique.[68] In our hospital, TCD is performed every other day for

2 weeks, monitoring absolute values and changes in middle cerebral artery velocities as a possible early warning for vasospasm.

Free Radical Scavengers

Several investigators have theorized that free radicals play a role in the pathogenesis of vasospasm. The chemical degradation of hemoglobin follows the clinical time course of vasospasm. A free radical superoxide anion is released with the conversion of oxyhemoglobin to methemoglobin. In an iron-dependent process, free radicals induce peroxidation of polyunsaturated fatty acids in cellular membranes. The question of whether vasospasm is induced by free radical injury of the blood vessel or the release of eicosanoids is debated.

Asano et al. reported that the antioxidant 1,2-bis (nicotinamide) propane reduced vasospasm in an experimental dog model of SAH.[7] Suzuki and colleagues championed the use of mannitol, vitamin E, and dexamethasone as free radical scavengers for the treatment of cerebral ischemia (see Kudo et al.[67]). Travis and Hall demonstrated that a twofold increase in dietary antioxidant vitamin E reduced cerebral hypoperfusion in the cat model of SAH.[134] Vollmer et al. demonstrated that the iron chelator, deferoxamine, attenuated delayed arterial narrowing in the rabbit model of SAH.[141] High doses of methylprednisolone are known to inhibit CNS tissue lipid peroxidation. Chyatte et al.,[17,18] Lombardi et al.,[78] and others have demonstrated that high dose methylprednisolone reduces the risk of vasospasm following SAH. Ticlopidine, leukotriene antagonists, and thrombobane synthetase inhibitors have also been used to block or inactivate spasmogenic substances.[64,96,129] Nizofenane, a free radical scavenger, reduced neurological deficit following SAH in a small double-blind clinical trial.[114] The immunosuppressant cyclosporin A was effective in preventing vasospasm in the double SAH canine model.[104]

The 21-aminosteroid, U74006F, is a nonglucocorticoid, nonmineralocorticoid steroid compound that inhibits iron-dependent lipid peroxidation. In vivo, it can scavenge both lipid hydroperoxide and superoxide radicals. This agent may benefit the patient because of its antispasmodic properties or its ability to mitigate the effects of cerebral ischemia. Several investigators have demonstrated that U74006F inhibits clot-induced arterial constriction in the experimental rabbit and cat models of SAH.[42,142,158] In a series of experiments, researchers from the University of Alberta demonstrated the efficacy of U74006F in mitigating subarachnoid blood induced vasospasm in primates.[55,56,123] The European-Australian study reported a 44 percent decrease in mortality and 28 percent decrease in clinical vasospasm in 256 patients receiving 6 mg/kg per day of tirilazad as compared to 253 patients receiving only the vehicle.

Calcium-Channel Blockers

Calcium-channel blocking agents theoretically can avoid vasospasm-induced cerebral ischemic damage by blocking the entry of calcium into smooth muscle cells, a common pathway for smooth muscle contraction, and blocking the entry of calcium into ischemic neurons, a common pathway mediating cell death. Nimodipine, a calcium-channel blocker, also inhibits platelet aggregation. Small, randomized blinded trials of nimodipine have demonstrated a modest reduction in the incidence or severity of ischemic neurological deficits or an improvement in outcome.[6,52,83,98,106] A multicenter double-blind placebo-controlled trial of nimodipine in 154 poor grade aneurysm patients demonstrated a reduction in delayed ischemic deficits and an improvement in good outcome rate.[105] A second multi-institutional placebo-controlled study of 554 patients who had suffered an SAH reported that patients receiving oral nimodipine had a significant reduction in presumed cerebral infarction and poor clinical outcome.[107] On the contrary, a randomized controlled trial of high dose intravenous nicardipine in 906 patients suffering aneurysmal SAH revealed a reduction in symptomatic vasospasm in the nicardipine-treated group but no gross improvement in clinical outcome as measured by the Glasgow Outcome Scale 3 months following hemorrhage.[40,41] In summary, a 21-day course of calcium-channel blocking agents appears to reduce the incidence and severity of vasospasm but the magnitude of its effect on outcome is less certain.

Calcium-channel blocking agents can induce deleterious hypotension. Headache and acute colonic pseudo obstructions have been reported. The usual dose of nimodipine is 60 mg PO q 4 h but it must be decreased in patients with liver failure or hypotension secondary to the administration.

Clot Removal

Fisher et al. demonstrated that vasospasm was most likely to occur in patients harboring large blood clots in the CSF cisterns surrounding the large basal arteries;[33] a relationship confirmed by others.[21,39,86,102] Cisternal enhancement on CT scan has also been correlated with vasospasm.[130] This has led to the general belief that vasospasm is caused by some product of cisternal blood breakdown. Oxyhemoglobin is the agent most favored presently. While timely clot removal from animal models where the clot is focal has reduced vasospasm, this technique has not proven to have a significant impact when applied to diffuse subarachnoid clot encountered in the clinical situation.[14,103] Several surgeons advocated the slow removal of cisternal blood by cisternal or lumbar drains left in place at the time of surgery.[154] The effectiveness of this technique has not been proven in a controlled fashion. Peterson et al. proposed the use of fibrinolytics in the cat model of SAH.[103,124] Findlay et al. demonstrated that the incidence of vasospasm could be markedly reduced in baboons by lysing the subarachnoid clot within 48 h using intrathecal fibrinolytic therapy.[31] One-half mg of recombinant tissue plasminogen activator (rTPA) injected three times over 24 h lysed a 4.4 ml clot and virtually eliminated vasospasm in 12 animals at 7 days. Öhman and associates used escalating doses of rTPA (3 to 15 mg) in 30 patients administered in a single intracisternal injection at the end of the operation.[99] They found a significant reduction in the intracisternal hemorrhage visualized on postoperative CT scans and a significant reduction in postoperative vasospasm in patients receiving higher doses of rTPA. One patient suffered an intracerebral hemorrhage and another patient suffered an epidural hemorrhage. With experience in many centers, the intraoperative bolus dose of TPA has been replaced by lower dose injection of TPA in the postoperative period. This has the theoretical advantage of avoiding leakage into the epidural space. Using 1.5 mg of TPA injected in three postoperative doses into the cistern, Zabramski and associates found that only one of nine patients with thick intercisternal hemorrhage had severe vasospasm on a seventh day postoperative angiogram.[156] Using daily 2 mg intracisternal injection of TPA until clot lysis (as documented on daily CT scans), Mizoi et al. demonstrated that only 10 percent of 30 patients developed moderate vasospasm and one patient developed severe vasospasm.[85] No patient who received TPA developed a delayed ischemic neurological deficit. The clot persisted for almost a week after the initiation of the injections; however, no significant complications were reported. Findlay treated 10 patients with 7.5 to 15 mg rTPA in a single bolus at the time of surgery.[29] Repeat CT scans revealed resolution of the subarachnoid clot in all but three patients. Only one patient who also had residual clot developed symptomatic vasospasm. One patient developed a symptomatic epidural hematoma as a result of rTPA. Using a continuous subarachnoid irrigation of urokinase and ascorbic acid, Kodama et al. found symptomatic vasospasm in only three of 50 patients who had Fisher grade 3 clots on presentation.[65] In a retrospective comparison of rTPA, urokinase, and cisternal drainage, Usui et al. found that rTPA and urokinase reduced the severity of vasospasm and the incidence of infarctions.[137] TPA also reduced the incidence of symptomatic vasospasm. In addition to their effect on subarachnoid blood, rTPA and urokinase given into the ventricle appear to hasten the resolution of intraventricular hemorrhage resulting from a ruptured aneurysm.[30,132]

The initiation of hemorrhage into a fresh operative site is the major theoretical complication of rTPA therapy. Although hemorrhage has not been a problem in the small number of cases reported, it will have to be carefully monitored as larger experiences are reported. In the uncontrolled series published, fibrinolytic agents seem to significantly reduce the incidence of vasospasm. If these agents fulfill their potential, they will bolster the argument for early surgical intervention.

Hypertension, Hypervolemia, Hemodilution

The mainstay of medical therapy for treating vasospasm is hypertension, hypervolemia, and hemodilution. In 1951, Denny-Brown speculated that raised systemic arterial blood pressure would abate transient neurological deficits caused by cerebral vessel thrombosis.[22] The efficacy of this form of therapy for the treatment of ischemic cerebral vascular disease was documented in articles by Shanbrom and Levy,[116] and Farhat and Schneider.[28]

Kosnik and Hunt used hypertensive therapy to treat seven patients with symptomatic vasospasm, noting a mitigation of the neurological deficit in six.[66] These surgeons reasoned that blood flow to ischemic brain was no longer impeded by autoregulation but was a passive function of systemic blood pressure. Muizelaar and Becker confirmed this theory by demonstrating an increase in hemispheric cerebral blood flow concomitant with an improvement in neurological condition in four patients treated with arterial hypertension for symptomatic vasospasm.[88]

Hypervolemic Therapy

An increase in intravascular volume or cardiac output may reverse the ischemic symptoms of vasospasm independent of systemic arterial pressure. Vanderark and Pomerantz reported a patient who developed a neurological deficit whenever systolic pressure fell below 120 mmHg.[138] When the patient's heart rate rose to 80 and her cardiac output rose, the patient was able to tolerate a systolic pressure of 90 mmHg without developing a neurological deficit. Pritz et al. reported a reversal in neurological deficit secondary to vasospasm with intravascular volume expansion and increased cardiac output without concomitant hypertension.[108] Finn et al. corroborated this observation although the exact percentage of patients responding to intravascular volume expansion without a concomitant rise in blood pressure is not precisely reported.[32]

The observation that increased intravascular volume and cardiac output can augment cerebral blood flow has been corroborated by animal experiments. In their study of cerebral blood flow in normal cats, Davis and Sundt found that decreasing intravascular volume while maintaining a constant blood pressure led to a fall in cardiac output and CBF.[20] They reported that increasing intravascular volume increased cardiac output but CBF remained unchanged. Keller et al. noted that normotensive hypervolemia increased cardiac output and CBF in areas of primate brain rendered ischemic by middle cerebral artery occlusion.[63] The change in blood flow in areas that were nonischemic was not significant. Tranmer et al. increased cardiac output by hypervolemic hemodilution in eight primates that had undergone middle cerebral artery occlusion. Cardiac output was then lowered in these animals by exanguination which further decreased the animal's hemocrit.[133] In areas of the brain rendered ischemic by middle cerebral artery occlusion, CBF was a direct function of cardiac output but was not affected independently by reductions in hematocrit. It seems that increased cardiac output has little effect on cerebral blood flow in normal brain, but that it profoundly affects ischemic brain with altered autoregulation.

Hypovolemia in the Clinical Setting

Patients with clinical manifestations of vasospasm are frequently found to have a diminished intravascular volume.[66,67,148] Giannotta et al. noted that all 17 of their patients with symptomatic vasospasm had a central venous pressure (CVP) below 5 mmHg.[34] Maroon and Nelson found that plasma volume and red cell mass were diminished in patients who had suffered an SAH.[81] Solomon et al. demonstrated that patients with symptomatic vasospasm were more likely to have a low total blood volume and red cell mass than patients with asymptomatic angiographically documented vasospasm.[122] The deleterious effects of hypovolemia were underscored by Rosenwasser et al. who pharmacologically lowered the arterial blood pressure in patients with unclipped but ruptured aneurysms.[111] Sixty percent of patients whose arterial pressure was lowered without intravascular volume expansion developed symptomatic vasospasm, but symptomatic vasospasm developed in only 20 percent of patients treated simultaneously with vascular volume expansion and arterial hypotension. Wijdicks and associates demonstrated that fluid restriction instituted to correct hyponatremia in 26 patients suffering from an SAH was associated with cerebral infarction in 21 cases.[146] A regimen of 3 liters of intravenous fluid and discontinuation of hypertension treatment were shown to decrease the rate of delayed cerebral ischemic deficits.[47]

The prophylactic use of moderate blood volume expansion was advocated independently by Hunt, Schneider, and Giannotta. Fraioli et al. demonstrated that prophylactic hypervolemic hemodilutional therapy can elevate CBF for at least 2 weeks following an SAH.[117] Solomon et al. prophylactically maintained the CVP above 10 mmH_2O or the pulmonary artery wedge pressure above 12 mmHg for at least 7 days following surgery.[120] As a result, only one of 24 patients developed a transient delayed ischemic deficit.[121]

Hypervolemic therapy does more than just replace the inherent blood volume deficit that follows an SAH. Several authors have noted that this degree of hypervolemic therapy is important. Origitano et al. reported that 15 of 43 (35 percent) of patients in whom central venous pressure was maintained between 8 to 12

mmH_2O developed signs of delayed cerebral ischemia which resolved with more vigorous hypervolemic and hypertensive therapy.[100] Levy et al. also noted that 34 percent of patients suffering an SAH treated empirically with 500 to 1000 ml of intravenous 5% albumin on admission and 150 ml/h lactated Ringer's solution manifested neurological compromise presumedly due to vasospasm.[70] Sixty percent of these symptomatic patients improved when a Swan-Ganz catheter was placed and cardiac output was maximized by the administration of intravenous fluid. Eighty percent of the still recalcitrant patients had a reversal of their ischemic symptoms when cardiac output was further elevated with dobutamine. Solomon et al. reported delayed cerebral ischemia in 10 of 56 patients (18 percent) despite empirical treatment with volume expansion to a CVP of 10 to 12 mmH_2O or pulmonary artery wedge pressure to 12 to 16 mmH_2O.[120] The deficits resolved in six patients after blood volume and hypertension were maximized. These studies show that intravascular volume expansion beyond normovolemia is effective for treating delayed ischemic deficits.

Hemodilution

An alternate explanation for the successful treatment of ischemic neurological deficits with volume expansion is the improved rheology that occurs with hemodilution. Hematocrit is an important determinant of blood viscosity and its importance increases as blood flow velocity decreases.[149] In a series of dog experiments, Wood et al. found that intravascular volume expansion in the absence of hemodilution failed to increase cerebral blood flow or reduce the size of infarction in the area rendered ischemic by middle cerebral artery occlusion despite a significant increase in cardiac output.[152] In a complementary set of experiments, intravascular volume expansion with hemodilution increased cardiac output and significantly elevated blood flow to the ischemic brain. In these experiments, the increase in blood flow to nonischemic brain was insignificant.[150,151] To the contrary, Little et al. found no beneficial effects of hypervolemic hemodilution in protecting the cat brain rendered ischemic by middle cerebral artery occlusion.[76] As noted earlier, Tranmer found that CBF in ischemic brain was a function of cardiac output but not hematocrit.[133]

In patients with impaired cerebrovascular autoregulation secondary to closed head injury, Bouma and Muizelaar found that CBF was inversely correlated to blood viscosity.[12] Conversely, when Yamakami et al. transfused 500 ml of human albumin into each of 35 patients who had suffered an SAH, no increase in hemispheric CBF could be demonstrated despite a significant decrease in hematocrit.[153] The exact role of hemodilution below physiologic levels remains to be defined.

Although no controlled study has ever been instituted, the value of hypervolemic hypertensive therapy in reversing deficits associated with vasospasm has been documented by several groups. Kassell et al. noted that 43 of 58 patients with progressive neurological deterioration from angiographically confirmed vasospasm permanently improved with intravascular volume expansion and induced arterial hypertension.[58] Caution should be exercised in that three of 16 patients with an unsecured aneurysm sustained rehemorrhage with therapy. Awad et al. reported that 60 percent of patients with clinical manifestations of vasospasm improved at least one clinical grade using this type of therapy.[9] In summary, approximately two-thirds of patients with delayed ischemic neurological deficits from vasospasm will improve with hypervolemic hypertensive therapy.

Complications

Hypervolemic hypertensive therapy is not without risk. Insertion of the Swan-Ganz catheter can result in pneumothorax or hemothorax and the catheter itself can cause sepsis, cardiac arrhythmias, and pulmonary infarction.[58,87] Medlock et al. reported that 16 of 47 patients treated prophylactically with a Swan-Ganz catheter and hypervolemia developed pulmonary edema.[82] This group attributed one death to this therapy. Kassell et al.[58] reported that 10 of 58 patients developed pulmonary edema and Awad et al.[9] reported pulmonary edema in seven of 118 patients. These reports underscore the need for close hour-by-hour monitoring of patients being treated with maximal hypervolemic therapy.

Increased systemic arterial pressure can theoretically lead to rupture of an unclipped aneurysm, hemorrhage into an area of cerebral infarction, or the production of cerebral edema in infarcted areas of brain where the blood-brain barrier has been disrupted. Wood et al. reported that hemodilutional hypervolemia can result in increased intracranial pressure.[150] Shimoda and colleagues reported a 19 percent incidence of cerebral edema and 9 percent incidence of hemorrhage into an infarction which was attributed to hypervolemic therapy.[117] If the patient does not respond to hypervolemic therapy within 8 h, the surgeon must consider the possibility that the deficit is due to cerebral infarction and that further treatment can lead to cerebral edema or hemorrhagic infarction.

Suggested Therapy

Based on what has been published in the literature, patients at our hospital are maintained on 3 liters per day of intravenous fluids including approximately 500 ml of a colloid solution. If the patient has thick subarachnoid clots as demonstrated on a CT scan, or angiographic evidence of vasospasm without symptoms, the patient's central venous pressure is kept above 10 cmH_2O (or in a patient with cardiac or pulmonary disease, pulmonary artery wedge pressure is kept above 12 mmHg).

If the patient manifests a delayed ischemic deficit and brain CT shows no large areas of infarction, a Swan-Ganz catheter is placed and the pulmonary artery wedge pressure is raised to maximize cardiac output.[69] Cardiac output is further increased with dobutamine as necessary. The patient's hematocrit is maintained between 30 and 35. With this therapy most patients will maintain their systolic blood pressure above 180 mmHg so that additional dopamine or neosynephrine is rarely used. Angioplasty is employed if the patient's neurological deficit fails to resolve in 2 h or if the deficit relapses on maximal therapy.

Transluminal Angioplasty

Transluminal angioplasty, the mechanical distension of arteries, has been successfully applied to cerebral vessels manifesting vasospasm following SAH. Zubkov et al. introduced this technique for the treatment of vasospasm, successfully dilating all but one of 105 vessels in 33 patients.[157] Clinical results were not detailed in that report. Higashida et al. treated 33 vascular territories in 10 patients with vasospasm after SAH.[48] Six patients demonstrated clinical improvement. Treated vessels maintained their dilated state on follow-up angiography. Using this technique, Takahashi et al.[127] reported clinical improvement in 14 of 20 patients with refractory vasospasm and Newell et al.[92] found clinical improvement in 28 of

39 patients. Angioplasty has been limited to the more proximal arteries of the intracranial circulation although successful angioplasty of secondary vessels has been reported using smaller, softer balloons.[131] Clinical improvement reportedly occurred in approximately 70 percent of patients with vasospasm refractory to more conventional therapies.[91] Complications include vessel rupture, vessel thrombosis, hemorrhagic infarction, and hemorrhage from an unclipped aneurysm.[75] Although early results of transluminal angioplasty from a few experienced neuroradiologists and neurosurgeons are encouraging, the incidence of complications with more general use remains to be defined.

Intra-Arterial Papaverine

Intra-arterial papaverine has been used to successfully dilate cerebral blood vessels with acute vasospasm during angiography.[25] Kassell et al. used a 1-h intra-arterial infusion of papaverine to dilate 16 distal arteries in 12 patients who manifested clinical symptoms from vasospasm following an SAH.[57] A dramatic reversal of vasospasm was noted in eight patients. Two patients who had a recurrence of ischemic symptoms and arterial narrowing 5 days after the initial treatment responded to a second infusion of papaverine. Kaku et al. was able to dilate 34 of 37 vessels constricted from post-SAH vasospasm with intra-arterial infusions of 0.2% of papaverine.[54] Recurrent stenosis was not evident on follow-up angiography one to 7 days later. These observations have been corroborated by others.[7,80] The mechanisms of action and the duration of dilation obtained from intra-arterial papaverine remain uncertain.

Similarly, calcitonin gene-related peptide, a potent dilator of cerebral blood vessels, was demonstrated to transiently improve the neurological deficit in nine of 15 patients with vasospasm in a small, randomized placebo-controlled trial.[53] This improvement may have been secondary to increased cardiac output from infusion of this agent.

Conclusion

A patient who has suffered a ruptured aneurysm is at risk of secondary injury from rerupture of the aneurysm, cerebral ischemia, hydrocephalus, and several medical complications. Surgical clipping of the aneurysm will only treat the possibility of rehemorrhage, although if fibrinolytic agents fulfill their potential, it is also possible that each operation will reduce the incidence of delayed ischemia. Judicious medical management in terms of quickly diagnosing and treating secondary complications as they occur will improve patient outcome.

References

1. Aaslid R, Markwalder TM, Nornes H. Noninvasive transcranial doppler ultrasound recording of flow velocity in basal cerebral arteries. *J Neurosurg* 1982; 57:769–774.
2. Adams HP Jr. Antifibrinolytics in aneurysmal subarachnoid hemorrhage: do they have a role? Maybe. *Arch Neurol* 1987; 44:114–115.
3. Adams HP Jr, Jergenson DD, Kassell NF, et al. Pitfalls in the recognition of subarachnoid hemorrhage. *JAMA* 1980; 244:794–796.
4. Adams HP Jr, Kassell NF, Torner JC, et al. CT and clinical correlation in recent aneurysmal subarachnoid hemorrhage: a preliminary report of the Cooperative Aneurysm Study. *Neurology* 1983; 33:981–988.
5. Adams HP Jr, Kassell NF, Torner JC, et al. Predicting cerebral ischemia after aneurysmal subarachnoid hemorrhage: influences of clinical condition, CT results, and antifibrinolytic therapy. *Neurology* 1987; 37:1586–1591.
6. Allen GS, Ahn HS, Preziosi TJ, et al. Cerebral arterial spasm: a controlled trial of nimodipine in patients with subarachnoid hemorrhage. *N Engl J Med* 1983; 308:619–624.
7. Asano T, Sasaki T, Koide T, et al. Experimental evaluation of the beneficial effect of an antioxidant on cerebral vasospasm. *Neurol Res* 1984; 6:49–53.
8. Atlas SW. MR imaging is highly sensitive for acute subarachnoid hemorrhage. *Radiology* 1993; 186:319–323.
9. Awad IA, Carter LP, Spetzler RF, et al. Clinical vasospasm after subarachnoid hemorrhage: response to hypervolemic hemodilution and arterial hypertension. *Stroke* 1987; 18:365–372.
10. Beck DW, Adams HP, Flamm ES, et al. Combination of aminocaproic acid and nicardipine in treatment of aneurysmal subarachnoid hemorrhage. *Stroke* 1988; 19:63–67.
11. Bidzinski J, Marchel A, Sherif A. Risk of epilepsy after aneurysm operations. *Acta Neurochir (Wien)* 1992; 119:49–52.
12. Bouma GJ, Muizelaar JP. Relationship between cardiac output and cerebral blood flow in patients with intact and with impaired autoregulation. *J Neurosurg* 1990; 73:368–374.
13. Brandt L, Sonesson B, Ljunggren B, et al. Ruptured middle cerebral artery aneurysm with intracerebral hemorrhage in younger patients appearing moribund: emergency operation? *Neurosurgery* 1987; 20:925–929.
14. Brouwers PJ, Wijdicks EF, Van Gijn J, et al. Infarction after aneurysm rupture does not depend on distribution or clearance rate of blood. *Stroke* 1992; 23:374–379.
15. Cabral RJ, King TT, Scott DF. Epilepsy after two different neurosurgical approaches to the treatment of ruptured intracranial aneurysm. *J Neurol Neurosurg Psychiatry* 1976; 39:1052–1056.
16. Cerrato D, Ariano C, Fiacchino F. Deep vein thrombosis and low-dose heparin prophylaxis in neurosurgical patients. *J Neurosurg* 1978; 49:378–381.
17. Chyatte D. Prevention of chronic cerebral vasospasm in dogs with ibuprofen and high-dose methylprednisolone. *Stroke* 1989; 20:1021–1026.
18. Chyatte D, Fode NC, Nichols DA, et al. Preliminary report: effects of high dose methylprednisolone on delayed cerebral ischemia in patients at high risk for vasospasm after aneurysmal subarachnoid hemorrhage. *Neurosurgery* 1987; 21:157–160.
19. Cruickshank JM, Neil-Dwyer G, Degaute JP, et al. Reduction of stress/catecholamine-induced cardiac necrosis by beta-1 selective blockade. *Lancet* 1987; 2:585–589.
20. Davis DH, Sundt TM Jr. Relationship of cerebral blood flow to cardiac output, mean arterial pressure, blood volume, and alpha and beta blockade in cats. *J Neurosurg* 1980; 52:745–754.
21. Davis JM, Davis KR, Crowell RM. Subarachnoid hemorrhage secondary to ruptured intracranial aneurysm: prognostic significance of cranial CT. *Am J Roentgenol* 1980; 134:711–715.
22. Denny-Brown D. The treatment of recurrent cerebrovascular symptoms and the question of "vasospasm." *Med Clin North Am* 1951; 35:1457–1474.
23. Dóczi T, Bende J, Huszka E, et al. Syndrome of inappropriate secretion of antidiuretic hormone after subarachnoid hemorrhage. *Neurosurgery* 1981; 9:394–397.
24. Drake CG, Hunt WE, Sano K, et al. Report of World Federation of Neurological Surgeons Committee on a Universal Subarachnoid Hemorrhage Grading Scale. *J Neurosurg* 1988; 68:985–986.
25. Eckard DA, Purdy PD, Girson MS, et al. Intraarterial papaverine for relief of catheter-induced intracranial vasospasm. *Am J Roentgenol* 1992; 158:883–884.
26. Estañol Vidal B, Badui Dergal E, Cesarman E, et al. Cardiac arrhythmias associated with subarachnoid hemorrhage. Prospective study. *Neurosurgery* 1979; 5:675–680.

27. Estañol Vidal B, Marin OS. Cardiac arrhythmias and sudden death in subarachnoid hemorrhage. *Stroke* 1975; 6:382–386.
28. Farhat SM, Schneider RC. Observations on the effect of systemic blood pressure on intracranial circulation in patients with cerebrovascular insufficiency. *J Neurosurg* 1967; 27:441–445.
29. Findlay JM. Subarachnoid fibrinolytic treatment for the prevention of cerebral vasospasm (review). *Semin Neurol* 1991; 11:400–410.
30. Findlay JM, Grade MG, Weir BK. Treatment of intraventicular hemorrhage with tissue plasminogen activator. *Neurosurgery* 1993; 32:941–947.
31. Findlay JM, Weir BK, Kanamaru K, et al. The effect of timing of intrathecal fibrinolytic therapy on cerebral vasospasm in a primate model of subarachnoid hemorrhage. *Neurosurgery* 1990; 26:201–206.
32. Finn SS, Stephensen SA, Miller CA, et al. Observations on the perioperative management of aneurysmal subarachnoid hemorrhage. *J Neurosurg* 1986; 65:48–62.
33. Fisher CM, Kistler JP, Davis JM. Relationship of cerebral vasospasm to subarachnoid hemorrhage visualized by computerized tomographic scanning. *Neurosurgery* 1980; 6:1–9.
34. Giannotta SL, McGillicuddy JE, Kindt GW. Diagnosis and treatment of postoperative cerebral vasospasm. *Surg Neurol* 1977; 8:286–290.
35. Greenfield LJ, Michna BA. Twelve-year clinical experience with the Greenfield vena caval filter. *Surgery* 1988; 104:706–712.
36. Grolimund P, Seiler RW, Aaslid R, et al. Evaluation of cerebrovascular disease by combined extracranial and transcranial Doppler sonography: experience in 1039 patients. *Stroke* 1987; 18:1018–1024.
37. Grosset DG, Straiton J, McDonald I, et al. Angiographic and Doppler diagnosis of cerebral artery vasospasm following subarachnoid haemorrhage. *Br J Neurosurg* 1993; 7:291–298.
38. Grosset DG, Straiton J, McDonald I, et al. Use of transcranial Doppler sonography to predict development of a delayed ischemic deficit after subarachnoid hemorrhage. *J Neurosurg* 1993; 78:183–187.
39. Gurusinghe NT, Richardson AE. The value of computerized tomography in aneurysmal subarachnoid hemorrhage. The concept of the CT score. *J Neurosurg* 1984; 60:763–770.
40. Haley EC Jr, Kassell NF, Torner JC, et al. A randomized controlled trial of high-dose intravenous nicardipine in aneurysmal subarachnoid hemorrhage. A report of the Cooperative Aneurysm Study. *J Neurosurg* 1993; 78:537–547.
41. Haley EC Jr, Kassell NF, Torner JC, et al. A randomized trial of nicardipine in subarachnoid hemorrhage: angiographic and transcranial Doppler ultrasound results. A report of the Cooperative Aneurysm Study. *J Neurosurg* 1993; 78:548–553.
42. Hall ED, Travis MA. Effects of the nonglucocorticoid 21-aminosteroid U74006F on acute cerebral hypoperfusion following experimental subarachnoid hemorrhage. *Exp Neurol* 1988; 102:244–248.
43. Hart RG, Byer JA, Slaughter JR, et al. Occurrence and implications of seizures in subarachnoid hemorrhage due to ruptured intracranial aneurysms. *Neurosurgery* 1981; 8:417–421.
44. Hasan D, Lindsay KW, Wijdicks EF, et al. Effect of fludrocortisone acetate in patients with subarachnoid hemorrhage. *Stroke* 1989; 20:1156–1161.
45. Hasan D, Schonck RSM, Avezaat CJ, et al. Epileptic seizures after subarachnoid hemorrhage. *Ann Neurol* 1993; 33:286–291.
46. Hasan D, Vermeulen M, Wijdicks EF, et al. Management problems in acute hydrocephalus after subarachnoid hemorrhage. *Stroke* 1989; 20:747–753.
47. Hasan D, Vermeulen M, Wijdicks EF, et al. Effect of fluid intake and antihypertensive treatment on cerebral ischemia after subarachnoid hemorrhage. *Stroke* 1989; 20:1511–1515.
48. Higashida RT, Halbach VV, Cahan LD, et al. Transluminal angioplasty for treatment of intracranial arterial vasospasm. *J Neurosurg* 1989; 71:684–653.
49. Hijdra A, Vermeulen M, van Gijn J, et al. Respiratory arrest in subarachnoid hemorrhage. *Neurology* 1984; 34:1501–1503.
50. Hunt WE, Hess RM. Surgical risk as related to time of intervention in the repair of intracranial aneurysms. *J Neurosurg* 1968; 28:14–20.
51. Hutchison K, Weir B. Transcranial Doppler studies in aneurysm patients. *Can J Neurol Sci* 1989; 16:411–416.
52. Jan M, Buchheit F, Tremoulet M. Therapeutic trial of intravenous nimodipine in patients with established cerebral vasospasm after rupture of intracranial aneurysms. *Neurosurgery* 1988; 23:154–157.
53. Johnston FG, Bell BA, Robertson IJ, et al. Effect of calcitonin-gene-related peptide on postoperative neurological deficits after subarachnoid haemorrhage. *Lancet* 1990; 335:869–872.
54. Kaku Y, Yonekawa Y, Tsukahara T, et al. Superselective intra-arterial infusion of papaverine for the treatment of cerebral vasospasm after subarachnoid hemorrhage. *J Neurosurg* 1992; 77:842–847.
55. Kanamaru K, Weir BK, Findlay JM, et al. A dosage study of the effect of the 21-aminosteroid U74006F on chronic cerebral vasospasm in a primate model. *Neurosurgery* 1990; 27:29–38.
56. Kanamaru K, Weir BK, Simpson I, et al. Effect of 21-aminosteroid U-74006F on lipid peroxidation in subarachnoid clot. *J Neurosurg* 1991; 74:454–459.
57. Kassell NF, Helm G, Simmons N, et al. Treatment of cerebral vasospasm with intra-arterial papaverine. *J Neurosurg* 1992; 77:848–852.
58. Kassell NF, Peerless SJ, Durward QJ, et al. Treatment of ischemic deficits from vasospasm with intravascular volume expansion and induced arterial hypertension. *Neurosurgery* 1982; 11:337–343.
59. Kassell NF, Sasaki T, Colohan AR, et al. Cerebral vasospasm following aneurysmal subarachnoid hemorrhage. *Stroke* 1985; 16:562–572.
60. Kassell NF, Torner JC. Aneurysmal rebleeding: a preliminary report from the Cooperative Aneurysm Study. *Neurosurgery* 1983; 13:479–481.
61. Kassell NF, Torner JC, Adams HP Jr. Antifibrinolytic therapy in the acute period following aneurysmal subarachnoid hemorrhage. Preliminary observations from the Cooperative Aneurysm Study. *J Neurosurg* 1984; 61:225–230.
62. Kassell NF, Torner JC, Haley EC Jr, et al. The International Cooperative Study on the Timing of Aneurysm Surgery. Part I: Overall management results. *J Neurosurg* 1990; 73:18–36.
63. Keller TS, McGillicuddy JE, LaBond VA, et al. Volume expansion in focal cerebral ischemia: the effect of cardiac output on local cerebral blood flow. *Clin Neurosurg* 1982; 29:40–50.
64. Kobayashi H, Ide H, Handa Y, et al. Effect of leukotriene antagonist on experimental delayed cerebral vasospasm. *Neurosurg* 1992; 31:550–556.
65. Kodama N, Sasaki T, Yamanobe K, et al. Prevention of vasospasm: cisternal irrigation therapy with urokinase and ascorbic acid. In Wilkins RH (ed): *Cerebral Vasospasm.* New York: Raven Press, 1988, pp 415–418.
66. Kosnik EJ, Hunt WE. Postoperative hypertension in the management of patients with intracranial arterial aneurysms. *J Neurosurg* 1976; 45:148–154.
67. Kudo T, Suzuki S, Iwabuchi T. Importance of monitoring the circulating blood volume in patients with cerebral vasospasm after subarachnoid hemorrhage. *Neurosurgery* 1981; 9:514–520.
68. Laumer R, Steinmeier R, Gönner F, et al. Cerebral hemodynamics in subarachnoid hemorrhage evaluated by transcranial Doppler sonography. Part 1. Reliability of flow velocities in clinical management. *Neurosurgery* 1993; 33:1–9.
69. Levy ML, Giannotta SL. Cardiac performance indices during hypervolemic therapy for cerebral vasospasm. *J Neurosurg* 1991; 75:27–31.
70. Levy ML, Rabb CH, Zelman V, et al. Cardiac performance enhancement from dobutamine in patients refractory to hypervolemic therapy for cerebral vasospasm. *J Neurosurg* 1993; 79:494–499.
71. Lindegaard KF, Nornes H, Bakke SJ, et al. Cerebral vasospasm after subarachnoid haemorrhage investigated by means of transcranial Doppler ultrasound. *Acta Neurochir (Wien)* 1988; Suppl 42:81–84.
72. Lindegaard KF, Nornes H, Bakke SJ, et al. Cerebral vasospasm diagnosis by means of angiography and blood velocity measurements. *Acta Neurochir (Wien)* 1989; 100:12–24.
73. Lindsay KW, Teasdale GM, Knill-Jones RP. Observer variability in assessing the clinical features of subarachnoid hemorrhage. *J Neurosurg* 1983; 58:57–62.

74. Lindsay KW, Teasdale G, Knill-Jones RP, et al. Observer variability in grading patients with subarachnoid hemorrhage. *J Neurosurg* 1982; 56:628–633.
75. Linskey ME, Horton JA, Rao GR, et al. Fatal rupture of the intracranial carotid artery during transluminal angioplasty for vasospasm induced by subarachnoid hemorrhage. Case report. *J Neurosurg* 1991; 74:985–990.
76. Little JR, Slugg RM, Latchaw JP Jr, et al. Treatment of acute focal cerebral ischemia with concentrated albumin. *Neurosurgery* 1981; 9:552–558.
77. Livingston K, Guterman LR, Hopkins LN. Intraarterial papaverine as an adjunct to transluminal angioplasty for vasospasm induced by subarachnoid hemorrhage. *Am J Neuroradiol* 1993; 14:346–347.
78. Lombardi D, Gaetani P, Marzatico F, et al. Effect of high-dose methylprednisolone on anti-oxidant enzymes after experimental SAH. *J Neurol Sci* 1992; 111:13–19.
79. Marion DW, Segal R, Thompson ME. Subarachnoid hemorrhage and the heart. *Neurosurgery* 1986; 18:101–106.
80. Marks MP, Steinberg GK, Lane B. Intraarterial papaverine for the treatment of vasospasm. *Am J Neuroradiol* 1993; 14:822–826.
81. Maroon JC, Nelson PB. Hypovolemia in patients with subarachnoid hemorrhage: therapeutic implications. *Neurosurgery* 1979; 4:223–226.
82. Medlock MD, Dulebohn SC, Elwood PW. Prophylactic hypervolemia without calcium channel blockers in early aneurysm surgery. *Neurosurgery* 1992; 30:12–16.
83. Mee E, Dorrance D, Lowe D. Controlled study of nimodipine in aneurysm patients treated early after subarachnoid hemorrhage. *Neurosurgery* 1988; 22:484–491.
84. Milhorat TH. Acute hydrocephalus after aneurysmal subarachnoid hemorrhage. *Neurosurgery* 1987; 20:15–20.
85. Mizoi K, Yoshimoto T, Takahashi A, et al. Prospective study on the prevention of cerebral vasospasm by intrathecal fibrinolytic therapy with tissue-type plasminogen activator. *J Neurosurg* 1993; 78:430–437.
86. Mizukami M, Takemae T, Tazawa T, et al. Value of computed tomography in the prediction of cerebral vasospasm after aneurysm rupture. *Neurosurgery* 1980; 7:583–586.
87. Moser KM, Spragg RG. Use of the balloon-tipped pulmonary artery catheter in pulmonary disease. *Ann Intern Med* 1983; 98:53–58.
88. Muizelaar JP, Becker DP. Induced hypertension for the treatment of cerebral ischemia after subarachnoid hemorrhage. Direct effect on cerebral blood flow. *Surg Neurol* 1986; 25:317–325.
89. Neil-Dwyer G, Cruickshank J, Stratton C. Beta-blockers, plasma total creatine kinase and creatine kinase myocardial isoenzyme, and the prognosis of subarachnoid hemorrhage. *Surg Neurol* 1986; 25:163–168.
90. Neil-Dwyer G, Walter P, Cruickshank JM. Beta-blockade benefits patients following a subarachnoid haemorrhage. *Eur J Clin Pharmacol (Suppl)* 1985; 28:25–29.
91. Newell DW, Eskridge J, Mayberg M, et al. Endovascular treatment of intracranial aneurysms and cerebral vasospasm. *Clin Neurosurg* 1992; 39:348–360.
92. Newell DW, Grady MS, Eskridge JM, et al. Distribution of angiographic vasospasm after subarachnoid hemorrhage: implications for diagnosis by transcranial Doppler ultrasonography. *Neurosurgery* 1990; 27:574–577.
93. Newell DW, LeRoux PD, Dacey RG Jr. CT infusion scanning for the detection of cerebral aneurysms. *J Neurosurg* 1989; 71:175–179.
94. Nibbelink DW, Torner JC, Henderson WG. Randomized treatment study: drug induced hypotension. In Sahs AL, Nibbelink DW, Torner JC (eds): *Aneurysmal Subarachnoid Hemorrhage.* Baltimore: Urban & Schwarzenberg, 1981, pp 77–106.
95. Nishioka H. Report on the Cooperative Study of Intracranial Aneurysms and Subarachnoid Hemorrhage, Section VII. I: Evaluation of the conservative management of ruptured intracranial aneurysms. *J Neurosurg* 1966; 25:574–592.
96. Nishizawa S, Peterson JW, Shimoyama I, et al. Therapeutic effect of a new immunosuppressant, FK-506, on vasospasm after subarachnoid hemorrhage. *Neurosurgery* 1993; 32:986–992.
97. Notani M, Kawamura H, Amano K, et al. The incidence of postoperative epilepsy and prophylactic anticonvulsants in patients with intracranial aneurysms. *No Shinkei Geka* 1984; 12(Suppl 3):269–274.
98. Öhman J, Heiskanen O. Effect of nimodipine on the outcome of patients after aneurysmal subarachnoid hemorrhage and surgery. *J Neurosurg* 1988; 69:683–686.
99. Öhman J, Servo A, Heiskanen O. Effect of intrathecal fibrinolytic therapy on clot lysis and vasospasm in patients with aneurysmal subarachnoid hemorrhage. *J Neurosurg* 1991; 75:197–201.
100. Origitano TC, Wascher TM, Reichman OH, et al. Sustained increased cerebral blood flow with prophylactic hypertensive hypervolemic hemodilution ("triple-H" therapy) after subarachnoid hemorrhage. *Neurosurgery* 1990; 27:729–740.
101. Pare L, Delfino R, Leblanc R. The relationship of ventricular drainage to aneurysmal rebleeding. *J Neurosurg* 1992; 76:422–427.
102. Pasqualin A, Rosta L, Da Pian R, et al. Role of computed tomography in the management of vasospasm after subarachnoid hemorrhage. *Neurosurgery* 1984; 15:344–353.
103. Peterson EW, Choo SH, Lewis AJ, et al. Lysis of blood clot and experimental treatment of subarachnoid hemorrhage. In Wilkins RH (ed): *Cerebral Arterial Spasm,* Baltimore: Williams & Wilkins, 1980, pp 625–627.
104. Peterson JW, Nishizawa S, Hackett JD, et al. Cyclosporine A reduces cerebral vasospasm after subarachnoid hemorrhage in dogs. *Stroke* 1990; 21:133–137.
105. Petruk KC, West M, Mohr G, et al. Nimodipine treatment in poor-grade aneurysm patients. Results of a multicenter double-blind placebo-controlled trial. *J Neurosurg* 1988; 68:505–517.
106. Philippon J, Grob R, Dagreou F, et al. Prevention of vasospasm in subarachnoid haemorrhage. A controlled study with nimodipine. *Acta Neurochir (Wien)* 1986; 82:110–114.
107. Pickard JD, Murray GD, Illingworth R, et al. Effect of oral nimodipine on cerebral infarction and outcome after subarachnoid haemorrhage: British aneurysm nimodipine trial. *Br Med J* 1989; 298:636–642.
108. Pritz MB, Giannotta SL, Kindt GW, et al. Treatment of patients with neurological deficits associated with cerebral vasospasm by intravascular volume expansion. *Neurosurgery* 1978; 3:364–368.
109. Ramirez-Lassepas M. Antifibrinolytic therapy in subarachnoid hemorrhage caused by ruptured intracranial aneurysm. *Neurology* 1981; 31:316–322.
110. Rose FC, Sarner M. Epilepsy after ruptured intracranial aneurysm. *Br Med J* 1965; 1:18–21.
111. Rosenwasser RH, Delgado TE, Buchheit WA, et al. Control of hypertension and prophylaxis against vasospasm in cases of subarachnoid hemorrhage: a preliminary report. *Neurosurgery* 1983; 12:658–661.
112. Rowley G, Fielding K. Reliability and accuracy of the Glasgow Coma Scale with experienced and inexperienced users. *Lancet* 1991; 337:535–538.
113. Samuels MA. Cardiopulmonary aspects of acute neurologic diseases. In Ropper AH (ed): *Neurological and Neurosurgical Intensive Care,* 3d ed. New York: Raven Press, 1993, pp 103–119.
114. Sano K. Cerebral vasospasm and aneurysm surgery. *Clin Neurosurg* 1983; 30:13–58.
115. Sekhar LN, Wechsler LR, Yonas H, et al. Value of transcranial Doppler examination in the diagnosis of cerebral vasospasm after subarachnoid hemorrhage. *Neurosurgery* 1988; 22:813–821.
116. Shanbrom E, Levy L. The role of systemic blood pressure in cerebral circulation in carotid and basilar artery thromboses: clinical observations and therapeutic implications of vasopressor agents. *Am J Med* 1957; 23:197–204.
117. Shimoda M, Oda S, Tsugane R, et al. Intracranial complications of hypervolemic therapy in patients with a delayed ischemic deficit attributed to vasospasm. *J Neurosurg* 1993; 78:423–429.
118. Skillman JJ, Collins RE, Coe NP, et al. Prevention of deep vein thrombosis in neurosurgical patients: a controlled, randomized trial of external pneumatic compression boots. *Surgery* 1978; 83:354–358.

119. Sloan MA, Haley EC Jr, Kassell NF, et al. Sensitivity and specificity of transcranial Doppler ultrasonography in the diagnosis of vasospasm following subarachnoid hemorrhage. *Neurology* 1989; 39:1514–1518.
120. Solomon RA, Fink ME, Lennihan L. Early aneurysm surgery and prophylactic hypervolemic hypertensive therapy for the treatment of aneurysmal subarachnoid hemorrhage. *Neurosurgery* 1988; 23:699–704.
121. Solomon RA, Fink ME, Lennihan L. Prophylactic volume expansion therapy for the prevention of delayed cerebral ischemia after early aneurysm surgery. Results of a preliminary trial. *Arch Neurol* 1988; 45:325–332.
122. Solomon RA, Post KD, McMurtry JG III. Depression of circulating blood volume in patients after subarachnoid hemorrhage: implications for the management of symptomatic vasospasm. *Neurosurgery* 1984; 15:354–361.
123. Steinke DE, Weir BK, Findlay JM, et al. A trial of the 21-aminosteroid U74006F in a primate model of chronic cerebral vasospasm. *Neurosurgery* 1989; 24:179–186.
124. Stolke D, Seifert V. Single intracisternal bolus of recombinant tissue plasminogen activator in patients with aneurysmal subarachnoid hemorrhage: preliminary assessment of efficacy and safety in an open clinical study. *Neurosurgery* 1992; 30:877–881.
125. Swann KW, Black PM. Deep vein thrombosis and pulmonary emboli in neurosurgical patients: a review. *J Neurosurg* 1984; 61:1055–1062.
126. Swann KW, Black PM, Baker MF. Management of symptomatic deep venous thrombosis and pulmonary embolism on a neurosurgical service. *J Neurosurg* 1986; 64:563–567.
127. Takahashi A, Yoshimoto T, Mizoi K, et al. Transluminal balloon angioplasty for vasospasm after subarachnoid hemorrhage. In Sano K, Takakorn K, Kassell NF, et al. (eds): *Cerebral Vasospasm*. Tokyo: University of Tokyo Press, 1990, pp 429–432.
128. Tanaka S, Mori T, Ohara H, et al. Gastrointestinal bleeding in cases of ruptured cerebral aneurysms. *No Shinkei Geka* 1979; 7:977–981.
129. Tani E, Maeda Y, Fukumori T, et al. Effect of selective inhibitor of thromboxane A2 synthetase on cerebral vasospasm after early surgery. *J Neurosurg* 1984; 61:24–29.
130. Tazawa T, Mizukami M, Kawase T, et al. Relationship between contrast enhancement on computed tomography and cerebral vasospasm in patients with subarachnoid hemorrhage. *Neurosurgery* 1983; 12:643–648.
131. Terada T, Nakamura Y, Yoshida N, et al. Percutaneous transluminal angioplasty for the M2 portion vasospasm following SAH: development of the new microballoon and report of cases. *Surg Neurol* 1993; 39:13–17.
132. Todo T, Usui M, Takakura K. Treatment of severe intraventricular hemorrhage by intraventricular infusion of urokinase. *J Neurosurg* 1991; 74:81–86.
133. Tranmer BI, Keller TS, Kindt GW, et al. Loss of cerebral regulation during cardiac output variations in focal cerebral ischemia. *J Neurosurg* 1992; 77:253–259.
134. Travis MA, Hall ED. The effects of chronic two-fold dietary vitamin E supplementation on subarachnoid hemorrhage-induced brain hypoperfusion. *Brain Res* 1987; 418:366–370.
135. Turpie AG, Gallus A, Beattie WS, et al. Prevention of venous thrombosis in patients with intracranial disease by intermittent pneumatic compression of the calf. *Neurology* 1977; 27:435–438.
136. Ukkola V, Heikkinen ER. Epilepsy after operative treatment of ruptured cerebral aneurysms. *Acta Neurochir (Wien)* 1990; 106:115–118.
137. Usui M, Saito N, Hoya K, et al. Vasospasm prevention with postoperative intrathecal thrombolytic therapy: a retrospective comparison of urokinase, tissue plasminogen activator, and cisternal drainage alone. *Neurosurgery* 1993; 34:235–245.
138. Vanderark GD, Pomerantz M. Reversal of ischemic neurological signs by increasing the cardiac output. *Surg Neurol* 1973; 1:257–258.
139. van Gijn J, van Dongen KJ. The time course of aneurysmal haemorrhage on computed tomograms. *Neuroradiology* 1982; 23:153–156.
140. Vermeulen M, Lindsay KW, Murray GD, et al. Antifibrinolytic treatment in subarachnoid hemorrhage. *N Engl J Med* 1984; 311:432–437.
141. Vollmer DG, Hongo K, Ogawa H, et al. A study of the effectiveness of the iron-chelating agent deferoxamine as vasospasm prophylaxis in a rabbit model of subarachnoid hemorrhage. *Neurosurgery* 1991; 28:27–32.
142. Vollmer DG, Kassell NF, Hongo K, et al. Effect of the nonglucocorticoid 21-aminosteroid U74006F on experimental cerebral vasospasm. *Surg Neurol* 1989; 31:190–194.
143. Weir B. Antifibrinolytics in subarachnoid hemorrhage. Do they have a role? No. *Arch Neurol* 1987; 44:116–118.
144. Wheelock B, Weir B, Watts R, et al. Timing of surgery for intracerebral hematomas due to aneurysm rupture. *J Neurosurg* 1983; 58:476–481.
145. Wijdicks EF, Ropper AH, Hunnicutt EJ, et al. Atrial natriuretic factor and salt wasting after aneurysmal subarachnoid hemorrhage. *Stroke* 1991; 22:1519–1524.
146. Wijdicks EF, Vermeulen M, Hijdra A, et al. Hyponatremia and cerebral infarction in patients with ruptured intracranial aneurysms: is fluid restriction harmful? *Ann Neurol* 1985; 17:137–140.
147. Wijdicks EF, Vermeulen M, Murray GD, et al. The effects of treating hypertension following aneurysmal subarachnoid hemorrhage. *Clin Neurol Neurosurg* 1990; 92:111–117.
148. Wijdicks EF, Vermeulen M, ten Haaf JA, et al. Volume depletion and natriuresis in patients with a ruptured intracranial aneurysm. *Ann Neurol* 1985; 18:211–216.
149. Wood JH, Kee DB Jr. Hemorheology of the cerebral circulation in stroke. *Stroke* 1985; 16:765–772.
150. Wood JH, Simeone FA, Fink EA, et al. Hypervolemic hemodilution in experimental focal cerebral ischemia. Elevation of cardiac output, regional cortical blood flow, and ICP after intravascular volume expansion with low molecular weight dextran. *J Neurosurg* 1983; 59:500–509.
151. Wood JH, Simeone FA, Kron RE, et al. Rheological aspects of experimental hypervolemic hemodilution with low molecular weight dextran: relationships of cortical blood flow, cardiac output, and intracranial pressure to fresh blood viscosity and plasma volume. *Neurosurgery* 1982; 11:739–753.
152. Wood JH, Snyder LL, Simeone FA. Failure of intravascular volume expansion without hemodilution to elevate cortical blood flow in region of experimental focal ischemia. *J Neurosurg* 1982; 56:80–91.
153. Yamakami I, Isobe K, Yamamura A. Effects of intravascular volume expansion on cerebral blood flow in patients with ruptured cerebral aneurysms. *Neurosurgery* 1987; 21:303–309.
154. Yamamoto I, Hara M, Ogura K, et al. Early operation for ruptured intracranial aneurysms: comparative study with computed tomography. *Neurosurgery* 1983; 12:169–174.
155. Young B, Ott L, Norton J, et al. Metabolic and nutritional sequelae in the non-steroid treated head injury patient. *Neurosurgery* 1985; 17:784–791.
156. Zabramski JM, Spetzler RF, Lee KS, et al. Phase I trial of tissue plasminogen activator for the prevention of vasospasm in patients with aneurysmal subarachnoid hemorrhage. *J Neurosurg* 1991; 75:189–196.
157. Zubkov YN, Nikiforov BM, Shustin VA. Balloon catheter technique for dilatation of constricted cerebral arteries after aneurysmal SAH. *Acta Neurochir (Wien)* 1984; 70:65–79.
158. Zuccarello M, Marsch JT, Schmitt G, et al. Effect of the 21-aminosteroid U-74006F on cerebral vasospasm following subarachnoid hemorrhage. *J Neurosurg* 1989; 71:98–104.

220 Aneurysm Clips

Troy D. Payner
John M. Tew, Jr.
Hans Jacob Steiger

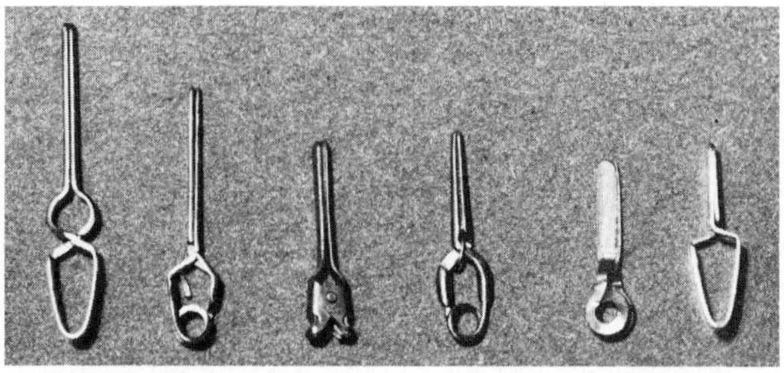

Figure 220-1 Various aneurysm spring clips. *Left to right:* Drake, McFadden, Heifetz, Yasargil, Scoville, and Mayfield designs.

In 1911, Cushing described the use of a malleable silver vascular clip. Malleable tantalum or gold clips were commonly used to obliterate most intracranial aneurysms until the first spring clips were developed by Schwartz and Mayfield in the 1950s. Despite early problems with these designs, such as slippage and a tendency to cut the aneurysm in the junction of the blades, the advantage of the easily removable clip was obvious—it did not commit the surgeon to a perfect clip application on the first attempt. The Mayfield clip was the first reappliable spring clip and was used for aneurysm surgery during the 1950s and 1960s. Subsequently, a new generation of spring clips—as many as 50 different brands—provided a more consistent occlusive force, corrosion resistance, and broad versatility in the blade configurations (Fig. 220-1). The advent of magnetic resonance imaging (MRI) in the 1980s resulted in another generation of change in available aneurysm clips based on MR compatibility. Since the early 1990s, only four major brands of aneurysm clips have withstood the dramatic changes in neurosurgery of the past 10 years: the McFadden Vari-Angle (Codman and Shurtleff, Inc., Randolph, MA), Sundt Slim-Line (Codman and Shurtleff, Inc.), Sugita (Mizuho, Tokyo, Japan), and Yasargil (Aesculap, San Francisco, CA) clips.

Several factors affect the neurosurgeon's choice of aneurysm clips. In addition to personal preference based on the variety of configurations, flexibility, closing force, and handling of the applier, the size and location of the aneurysm may also influence the selection of a clip. Cost may limit the number of different types of clips and appliers stocked in the operating room. Performance data such as mechanical properties, inertness, closing forces, metallic fatigue, corrosion resistance, and compatibility with MRI are also considered.[1,4,6,9–11]

In this chapter, we discuss the classification of clips, principles of clip selection, and objective data about performance (including MR capability). The four major aneurysm clips currently used in the United States are shown in the figures. Additionally, previously popular clips are included because many are still used in hospitals or remain in some patients who underwent surgical treatment for aneurysms.

Classification of Aneurysm Clips

Dujovny and Kossowsky pioneered the classification and mechanical study of aneurysm clips.[4,6,11] Clips are divided into three classes called alpha, pivot, and mobile fulcrum clips based on their mechanical principles.[5] The alpha class includes the four major clips presently available: the McFadden Vari-Angle, Sugita, Sundt Slim-Line, and Yasargil; this type is an integral crossed-leg design, which resembles the Greek letter alpha (α). The Mayfield clip was a prototype of this class. The Drake, McFadden, and Rhoton clips also have this configuration as well as the Sundt and Biemer clips used for temporary microvascular occlusion. The Mayfield, Drake, McFadden, McFadden Vari-Angle, Sundt, and Biemer clips consist of only one part, whereas the Yasargil, Rhoton, and Sugita clips have an additional small ringlet or strut that acts as an alignment guide.

In contrast, pivot clips consist of several parts. The blades rotate or rock around a central pivot, and a separate coil spring provides the closing force. The Heifetz clip is the prototype of the pivot class. Pivot (formerly V. Mueller & Co, Chicago, IL) and Kleinert-Kutz (formerly Edward Weck & Co., Inc., Research Triangle Park, NC) clips for temporary use were other popular members of this family. In the Scoville clip, an example of the mobile fulcrum clip, part of the integral spring coil acts as a fulcrum around which the blades rotate; the position of the fulcrum depends on the gap between the blades. Another example of this class is the Acland clip, which is designed for temporary microvascular occlusion.

Aside from the mechanical principle, spring clips are classified as permanent or temporary according to their closing force. Yasargil, Sugita, and Sundt clips offer reduced closing force for temporary vessel occlusion. The temporary Yasargil clip was originally designed as a pilot clip for preliminary clipping of an aneurysm, because the blades open wider than most other clips and permit easier application of the clip. Biemer, Acland, and Kleinert-Kutz clips are strictly designed for temporary occlusion and not for permanent implantation.

There are two additional Sundt clips that conform to the alpha class: (1) a reinforcing clip with an increased closing force enhances occlusion of the aneurysm neck (Fig. 220-2); and (2) the Sundt Slim-Line graft clips used to encircle an artery in which a hole has developed, either from trauma or a tear at the aneurysm neck (Fig. 220-3). These graft clips include a Teflon fabric that seals the bleeding site after clip application.

Despite the predominant use of spring clips, malleable clips are sometimes used, especially when dealing with broad-based or fusiform aneurysms that require aneurysmorrhaphy. The Weck Hemoclip (Edward Weck & Co, Inc.) and the Ethicon Ligaclip (Ethicon, Inc., Somerville, NJ), which are made of tantalum, are used primarily. The original silver clips have been abandoned because they induce an inflammatory tissue reaction and have poor functional properties.

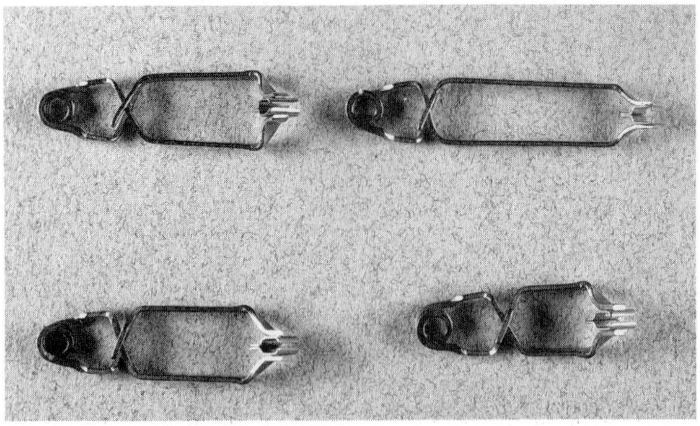

Figure 220-2 Sundt Slim-Line reinforcing clips are available in three blade lengths and three jaw angles—all with enhanced closing force. (Courtesy of Codman and Shurtleff, Inc., Randolph, MA.)

Principles of Aneurysm Obliteration

In the past only relatively small aneurysms not hidden behind vital structures could be eliminated directly by ligation or with simple clips. Large aneurysms were often dealt with indirectly by ligation of the parent vessel or by coating the aneurysm with muscle, gauze, or adhesives. Modern sophisticated clips permit direct ablation of almost all intracranial aneurysms, even large fusiform aneurysms hidden behind vital structures. Various clip configurations must be available in the operating room to permit selection of the proper method for clipping.

The size and geometric configuration of the aneurysm, parent artery, and surrounding structures determine the proper clipping technique. If the size of the aneurysmal neck is large compared with the diameter of the parent artery, the clip blade must be applied parallel to the parent artery to avoid constriction of the arterial wall or rupture of the aneurysm base. If the parent vessel, or vascular or neural structures obstruct direct access to the aneurysm, a fenestrated clip should be chosen.[5,7] Fenestrated clips were originally designed by Drake for clipping basilar-tip aneurysms hidden behind the posterior cerebral artery. Now, several manufacturers offer both straight and angled fenestrated clips for aneurysms found in a variety of locations (Fig. 220-4). If accessible, large broad-based aneurysms can also be dealt with effectively by aneurysmorrhaphy. After temporary occlusion of the proximal and distal parent artery, the aneurysmal sac is excised and the vessel is reconstructed with an appropriate aneurysm clip or a series of malleable clips or sutures. Temporary clips are useful not only to isolate an aneurysm during the ablation but also to test occlusion of the aneurysm. The blades of the temporary clips open wider than the blades of permanent aneurysm clips, and the blades slide more easily around a large aneurysm. Intraoperative systemic hypotension or temporary trapping with clip application may facilitate clipping of an aneurysm.

Difficulty may arise when operating in a deep surgical cavity. Because of the limited freedom of motion, it is often difficult to align the clip blades in the desired line of action. Careful selection of the optimal clip and applier combination is necessary. McFadden Vari-Angle clips are designed to rotate in a single plane in the jaws of the applier (Fig. 220-5). The clips can be loaded at any angle and even rotated while approaching the aneurysm neck; such variability also facilitates either clip removal or its repositioning after release even if the angle of the clip changes. The jaws can be sequentially locked into the two sides of the clip body and slid into locking position—not only straight over the top of the clip but also from any side. Pivot and Rhoton clips operate similarly.

Sundt Slim-Line (Fig. 220-6) and Sano (Fig. 220-7) clip appliers are available with angled or hinged shafts that increase the flexibility in applying a specifically shaped clip from a desired angle for optimal aneurysm occlusion. If the clip rotates or changes position after its release, it may be more difficult to recapture. Hinged appliers are available for Sundt, Sugita, Yasargil, and Heifetz clips. Yasargil clips are also available with pistol grip appliers that can be rotated along the axis of the shaft (Fig. 220-8). Despite such potential challenges, these clip appliers are smaller and allow the surgeon better visualization during clipping, especially in a deep surgical field.

Closing Force

Closing force is an important factor when choosing an aneurysm clip for a particular aneurysm. In practice, a clip may be too weak to occlude a large aneurysm. A trial-and-error method for clip selection is dangerous because manipulation of an aneurysm can

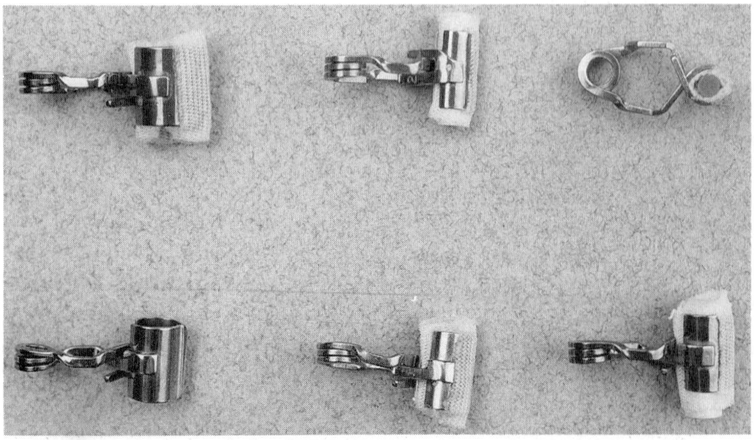

Figure 220-3 Sundt Slim-Line graft clips (available in diameters 2 to 5 mm) serve to encircle a partially torn artery. (Courtesy of Codman and Shurtleff, Inc., Randolph, MA.)

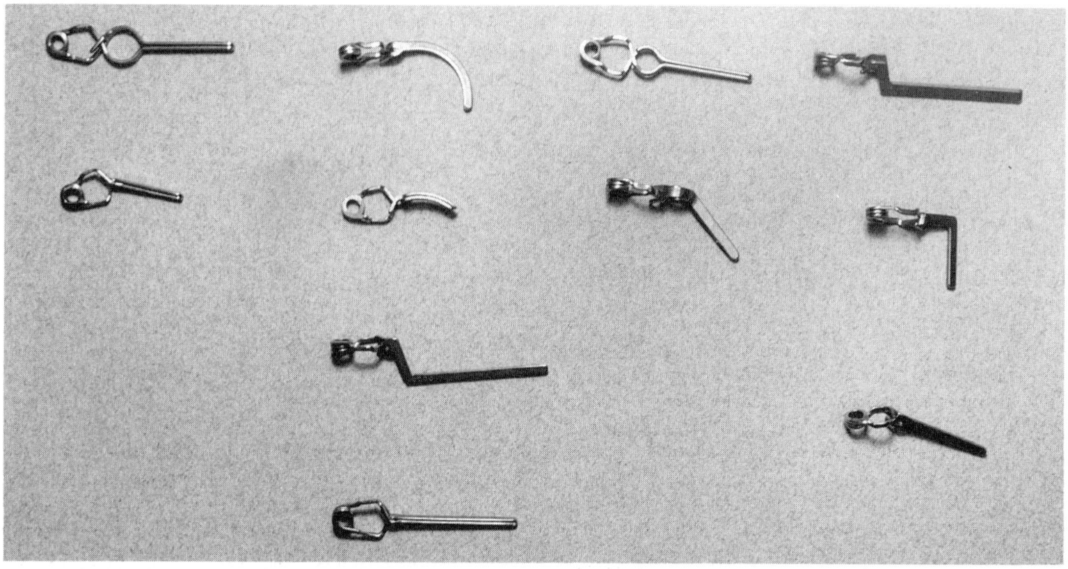

Figure 220-4 Representative clips from the Sundt Slim-Line series including fenestrated clips of various angles. (Courtesy of Codman and Shurtleff, Inc., Randolph, MA.)

lead to premature rupture. The neurosurgeon should know from performance data which clip will provide sufficient force for closing a given aneurysm but will not damage the vessel by applying excessive force.

The force necessary to occlude an aneurysm or artery is impossible to assess without a method for precise measurement. Additional factors such as blood pressure, clip blade width, diameter of the aneurysm, stiffness of the aneurysm wall, and geometrical configuration of the aneurysm must be considered. The orientation of the clip blades to the artery alter the transmitted force. Although the occlusive force to cross-clamp an artery can be established, the force of an artery against a clip placed parallel is more difficult to assess. Dujovny et al. have published tables of minimal occlusive forces for various vessel diameters, blood pressures, and clip blade widths. These data,[4] generated by a computer program, were verified by measurements in vivo. A study by the same group also indicates that small arteries do not tolerate excessive compression loads because endothelial disruption and clot formation may occur.

Although performance data for various clips need consideration, there is presently no industry standard to determine the opening and closing pressures of various clips. The opening force is the minimum force required to open a clip placed on an artery and the closing force is the amount of tension exerted by an aneurysm clip. Several factors affect these forces. As the gap between the blades increases, the closing force increases linearly according to the "spring law." The force exerted on a vessel increases exponentially with decreasing distance from the fulcrum of the clip, as determined by the "lever law." Although some distributors provide closing force measurements with package inserts, variations in the conditions of measurements make comparisons difficult.

Several independent studies have provided comparative data of clip performance. In a 1990 report, Atkinson et al. compared the

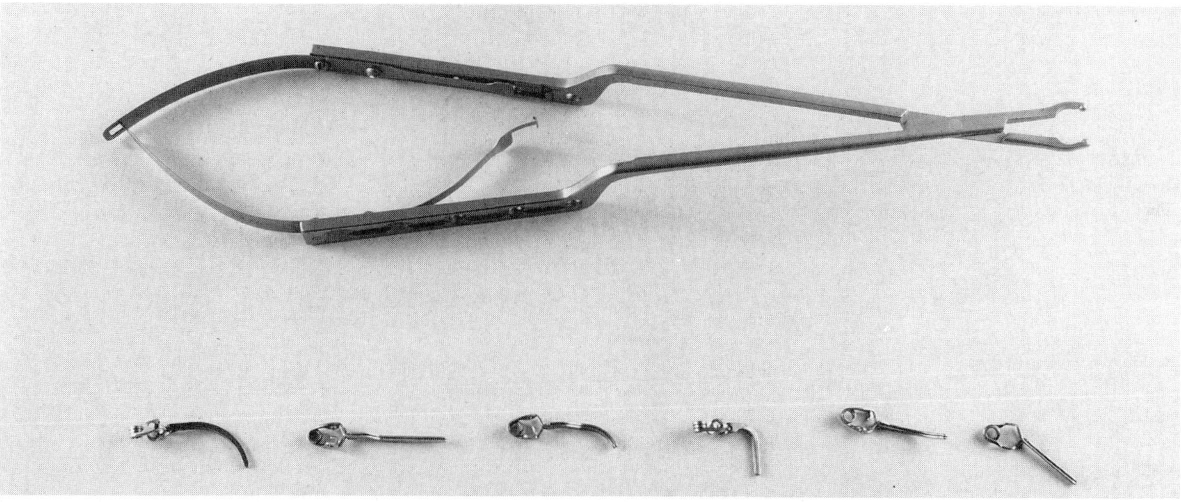

Figure 220-5 Representative clips from the McFadden Vari-Angle series including fenestrated clips of various angles. (Courtesy of Codman and Shurtleff, Inc., Randolph, MA.)

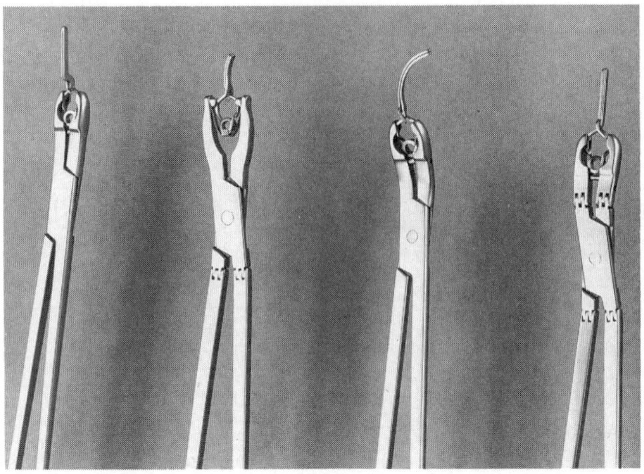

Figure 220-6 Sundt Slim-Line appliers, including angled and hinged shafts. (Courtesy of Codman and Shurtleff, Inc., Randolph, MA.)

opening and closing forces of five commonly used aneurysm clip brands.[1] The closing force of an 8 to 10 mm clip in decreasing order was Sundt, McFadden Vari-Angle, Yasargil, Heifetz, and Sugita clips. The closing forces for 20 to 21 mm clips were similar for Sugita, Yasargil, and Sundt clips; however, the measured forces differed significantly from those of smaller counterparts. The only definitively increased closing force was generated by a Sundt reinforcing clip, which increased the force by nearly 200 percent (Fig. 220-2). However, despite variations in closing forces, none of the clips studied failed to maintain occlusion of an artery when subjected to forces up to 300 mmHg.

Surgeon preference and experience remain the main factors in clip selection for routine aneurysms. Reinforcing clips or a second clip placed in parallel may be necessary for giant or atherosclerotic aneurysms, which are difficult to occlude.

Corrosion Resistance

Freedom from corrosion is the prime requirement for a metal suitable for biological implantation. Corrosion may lead to mechanical failure of the implanted device and cause unwanted inflammatory tissue reaction. Several authors reported slippage and fracture of older aneurysm clips due to corrosion.

Corrosion is an electrochemical reaction consisting of oxidation of an anodic metal (negative pole) and simultaneous reduction of a cathodic metal (positive pole). An alloy composed of different metallic elements may have a heterogeneous surface, which can form anodic and cathodic poles. Electrolysis may also be induced by scratches on the surface or by enclosure of the surface by foreign materials. Clips composed of several parts are more prone to corrosion than integral devices.[4,6,7]

Stainless steel and cobalt-based alloys form a passivated chromium oxide surface layer that inhibits corrosion. This layer depends on homogeneous availability of oxygen. Partial encasement of a clip with synthetic material interferes with oxygen contact.

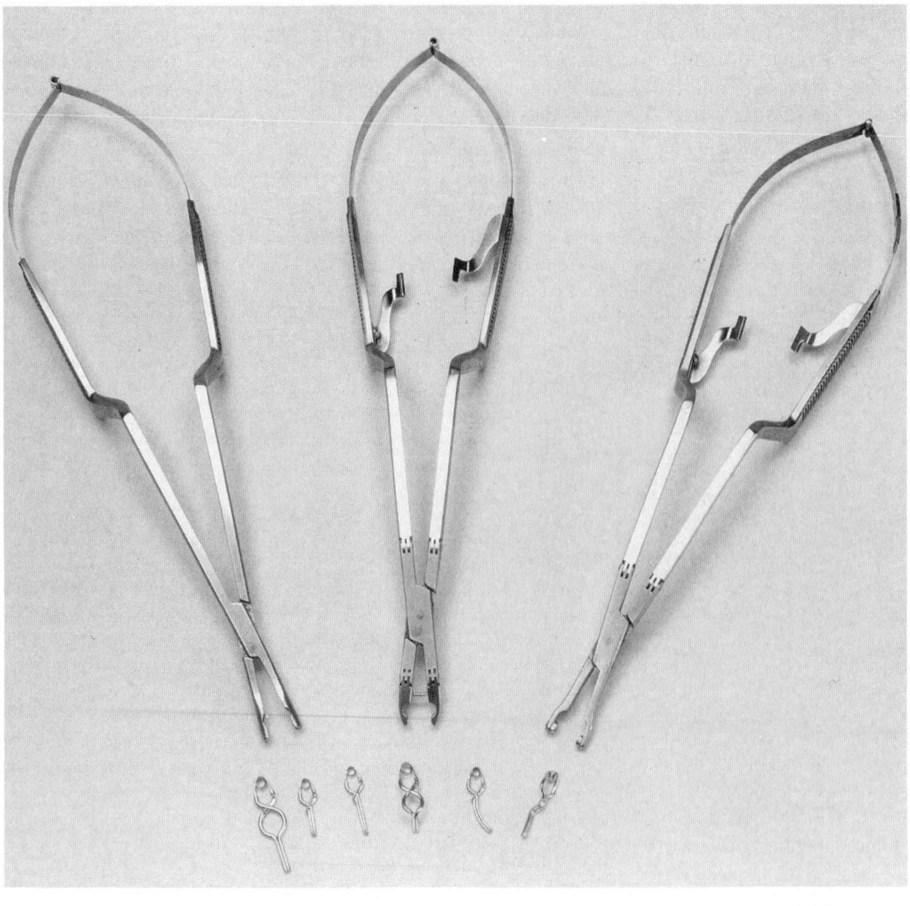

Figure 220-7 Sano clip appliers with hinged shafts for use with Sugita aneurysm clips. (Courtesy of Sims Surgical, Keene, NH.)

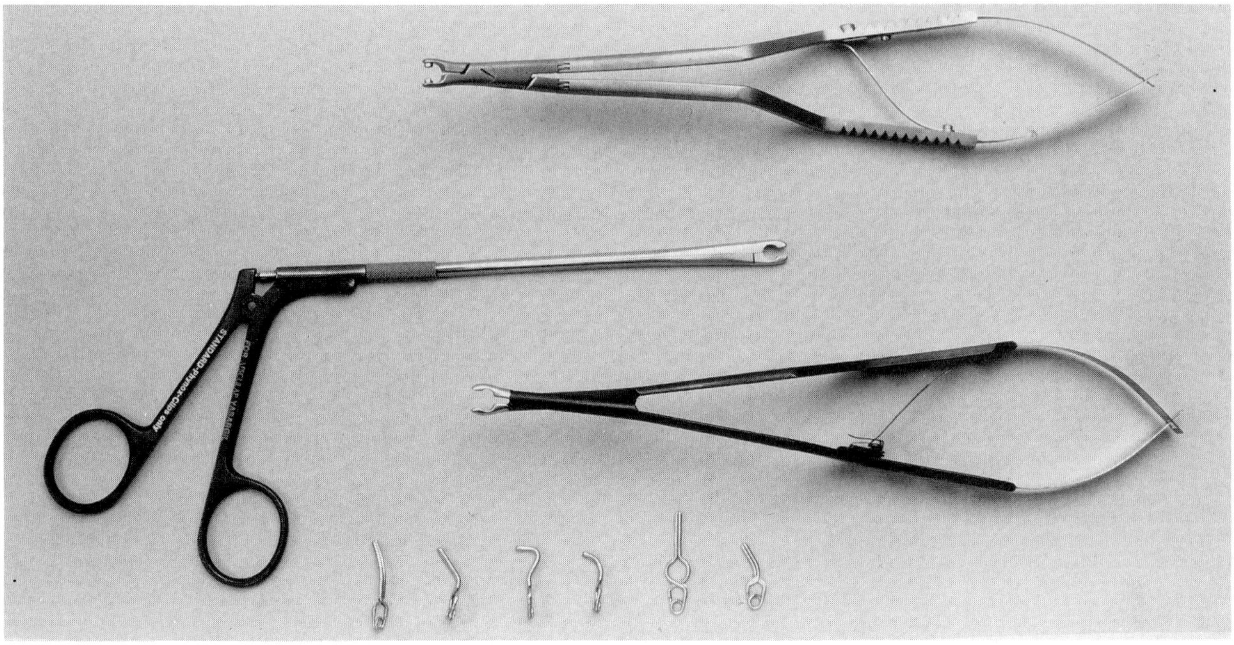

Figure 220-8 Various configurations of Yasargil clips and their appliers. (Courtesy of Aesculap, San Francisco, CA.)

Corrosion of aneurysm clips can be a result of partial oxygen deprivation.

The four major clips used today are composed of cobalt alloys that resist corrosion better than older stainless steel clips. Some researchers have reported a high risk of corrosion among Heifetz, Mayfield, and Pivot clips.[6,9] Although some aneurysm clips remain in stock in many hospitals, their use should be avoided.

Magnetic Resonance Compatibility

The routine availability of MRI requires a knowledge about clip compatibility. The two major concerns are heat absorption and rotation or movement of the clips. Davis et al. reported that heat effects do not appear to be clinically relevant.[3] Ferromagnetic objects are subject to two forces related to MRI: (1) displacement forces related to moving through a magnetic field gradient and (2) rotational forces generated within a uniform magnetic field.[12]

It is important to ascertain the clip type and its metal content before a patient undergoes MRI. Sundt, Sugita, McFadden Vari-Angle, and Yasargil clips available today are composed of nonferromagnetic cobalt alloys. Barrafato and Henkelman reported ferromagnetic properties in Drake, Heifetz, Mayfield, McFadden, Scoville, Sundt-Kees, Vari-Angle Micro, and Vari-Angle Spring clips.[2] Reports of serious complications caused by MRI in patients with ferromagnetic clips are rare; however, one fatality has been reported.[8] Additionally, some older clips are associated with a high degree of artifact that may render the images useless.[2] Therefore, the use of MRI in patients with these clips should be avoided. Clips composed of cobalt alloys are also associated with artifact but are small enough so as not to interfere with radiologic interpretation.[13] The Food and Drug Administration warns that a complete record of the clips used should be maintained for each patient. Additionally, patients with clips should undergo MRI only when the need is well established and the compatibility of the clip is ensured.

The use of aneurysm clips has become a standard treatment modality for cerebral aneurysms. Although technological advances have improved corrosion resistance, closing forces, variability in clip configuration, and MRI compatibility, the basic principles of clip application remain unchanged. It remains to be seen whether future technologies will establish effective treatments that lessen or eliminate the use of aneurysm clips.

References

1. Atkinson JL, Anderson RE, Piepgras DG. A comparative study in opening and closing pressures of cerebral aneurysm clips. *Neurosurgery* 1990; 26:80–85.
2. Barrafato D, Henkelman RM. Magnetic resonance imaging and surgical clips. *Can J Surg* 1984; 27:509–512.
3. Davis PL, Crooks L, Arakawa M, et al. Potential hazards in NMR imaging: heating effects of changing magnetic fields and RF fields on small metallic implants. *Am J Roentgenol* 1981; 137:857–860.
4. Dujovny M, Kossovsky N, Kossowsky R, et al. Intracranial clips: an examination of the devices used for aneurysm surgery. *Neurosurgery* 1984; 14:257–267.
5. Dujovny M, Kossovsky N, Laha RK, et al. Temporary microvascular clips. *Neurosurgery* 1979; 5:456–463.
6. Dujovny M, Kossowsky R, Kossovsky N, et al. Corrosion of aneurysm clips: evaluation and clinical implications. Part II: Individual performance. *Acta Neurochir (Wien)* 1984; 72:257–269.
7. Fujita S. Fenestrated clips for internal carotid artery aneurysms: technical note. *J Neurosurg* 1986; 65:122–123.
8. Klucznik RP, Carrier DA, Pyka R, Haid RW. Placement of a ferromagnetic intracerebral aneurysm clip in a magnetic field with a fatal outcome. *Radiology* 1993; 187:855–856.

9. Kossowsky R, Dujovny M, Kossovsky N. Metallurgical evaluation of the compatibility of surgical clips with their appliers. *Acta Neurochir (Wien)* 1981; 59:95–109.
10. Kossowsky R, Dujovny M, Kossovsky N, Keravel Y. Failure of a Heifetz aneurysm clip. *J Neurosurg* 1982; 57:233–239.
11. Kossowsky R, Dujovny M, Kossovsky N, et al. Corrosion of aneurysm clips: evaluation and clinical implications 1: metallurgical foundations of stress corrosion failure. *Acta Neurochir (Wien)* 1984; 72:31–43.
12. New PF, Rosen BR, Brady TJ, et al. Potential hazards and artifacts of ferromagnetic and nonferromagnetic surgical and dental materials and devices in nuclear magnetic resonance imaging. *Radiology* 1983; 147:139–148.
13. Romner B, Olsson M, Ljunggren B, et al. Magnetic resonance imaging and aneurysm clips: magnetic properties and image artifacts. *J Neurosurg* 1989; 70:426–431.

221

Intraoperative Aneurysm Rupture

H. Hunt Batjer
Duke S. Samson

Intraoperative bleeding from an intracranial aneurysm of a magnitude that interrupts the orderly progression of the operative procedure is an unwelcome event. Sequelae of the hemorrhage or of maneuvers directed at control of the bleeding can jeopardize the patient's chance for favorable recovery. Although voluminous literature exists dealing with perioperative management of subarachnoid hemorrhage patients as well as the technical aspects of aneurysm surgery, little information is available regarding the incidence of intraoperative rupture, techniques for management, and ultimate impact on patient morbidity and mortality.

The Cooperative Study dealing with 228 patients randomized to surgical treatment between June 1963 and February 1970 reported a surprisingly low 18 percent incidence of intraoperative aneurysm rupture, presumably without the benefits of microsurgical technique.[6] However, when intraoperative hemorrhage did occur, it resulted in significant postoperative complications in over 70 percent of such patients; the 14-day mortality was 38 percent and the overall 6-month mortality was 44 percent.

Pertuiset, in a thoughtful and well-documented study of his own material, examined the incidence of aneurysmal rupture in patients who underwent a conventional aneurysm operation and those who were operated on with microsurgical technique.[9] Among 159 patients with a supratentorial aneurysm operated upon without the microscope, hemorrhage occurred in 36 percent, with most hemorrhages (80 percent) occurring distally on the aneurysm fundus. In an additional 41 patients undergoing operation with induced hypotension and microscopic technique, intraoperative rupture was encountered in a surprising 61 percent, again with 90 percent of these occurrences being secondary to aneurysmal rupture distally along the fundus. Pertuiset did not, unfortunately, discuss the long-term outcome of the patients who suffered intraoperative aneurysmal rupture.

Pia, in a brief discussion of Pertuiset's report, commented that, in his experience, intraoperative rupture had lost much of its former risk as related to the production of subsequent neurological deficit.[10] Before the advent of microsurgery, over 50 percent of his patients suffering intraoperative aneurysmal rupture had a poor surgical result but, subsequent to the introduction of microtechnique, only 15 percent could be classified as having had a poor outcome. Kassell et al., in a study comparing management morbidity/mortality in patients undergoing early versus late microsurgical aneurysm surgery at the hands of one surgeon, reported intraoperative rupture in 26 percent of both patient populations but did not correlate its occurrence with any subsequent impact on management morbidity and mortality.[7]

Giannotta et al. reviewed an 8-year surgical experience in which 276 consecutive operations for 317 aneurysms were performed.[5] Forty-one cases of premature rupture were documented. Cases in which hemorrhage occurred during dissection or clipping were studied as regards techniques used to handle the complication. Although tamponade was found to be equally as effective as temporary clipping, the use of induced hypotension was found to be associated with a high risk of poor neurological outcome.

Occurrence of Intraoperative Aneurysm Rupture

We reviewed our experience over an 8-year period ending in 1986 and found that intraoperative rupture occurred in 19 percent of operated cases.[2] As will be discussed below, it is our impression that the increasing use of temporary clips has significantly decreased this frequency. This incidence is somewhat lower than that in other similar series.[6,7,9] We found this complication to occur in three distinct phases of the surgical procedure. These stages include the initial exposure (predissection), actual dissection of the aneurysm (dissection), and aneurysm clipping. The following discussion will focus on the causes of rupture during these periods and the surgical maneuvers that have proved most successful in both the prevention of hemorrhage and its safe correction.

Predissection

We have noted spontaneous subarachnoid hemorrhage occurring at the time of bony craniotomy, dural opening, or initial brain tissue retraction. This has fortunately been a relatively rare occurrence in our experience. Potential causes include increased turbulence due to transmitted vibrations from the power instruments, changes in transmural pressure brought about by the dural opening, initial brain tissue retraction, and blood pressure lability.

Each case complicated by hemorrhage at this time of the procedure was continued using either profound hypotension followed by temporary arterial clipping, or if proximal control was easily accessible through the carotid cistern or by occluding the internal carotid artery in the neck through the drapes, this was performed followed by temporary clipping once exposure was adequate. Occasionally it has been necessary to resect significant portions of the frontal or temporal lobe in order to obtain adequate exposure. Acquisition of proximal control following early rupture of a distal basilar aneurysm is extremely difficult and always requires brain resection. We have been impressed at how quickly the brain becomes very tight and tense even if the bleeding is generalized into the subarachnoid space. Despite these aggressive measures, the outcome in this group of patients has been disappointing. Less than half of these patients have had what we consider a good neurological outcome. In the series of Giannotta et al., four of five patients died whose aneurysm ruptured prior to dissection, highlighting the grave consequences of this occurrence.[5] One could argue that when rupture occurs at a time prior to dural opening it may be most appropriate to abort the surgical procedure and allow the rapid elevation of intracranial pressure to tamponade the bleeding as it does in spontaneous subarachnoid hemorrhage from which most patients survive. Once the dura has been violated or the brain retracted, however, there is very little evidence to support any approach other than a direct attack with early proximal control.

Obviously, these poor results mandate efforts to prevent the occurrence of predissection hemorrhage. Bleeding occurring at the time of preliminary craniotomy flap construction has been attributed by some to vibration from power instruments used for burr hole placement and bone cutting; this hypothesis has certainly never been proved and, in light of the high frequency of power instrument usage and the low incidence of aneurysm rupture at this time, it seems somewhat unlikely. On the other hand, this portion of the operative procedure could potentially produce significant amounts of pain if the patient were not under adequate anesthesia/analgesia. The resultant discomfort could potentially be reflected by alterations in systemic blood pressure and ventilatory pressure, both of which may conceivably lead to changes in transmural pressure. Theoretically, it is possible that early achievement and maintenance of an adequate depth of anesthesia coupled with infiltration of the planned scalp incision with a local anesthetic could be of benefit in the prevention of this catastrophe. Similarly, to maintain relatively stable transmural aneurysm pressure during the early stages of the operative procedure, one should defer until dural opening the maximal reduction of intracranial pressure produced by hypocarbia, spinal or ventricular drainage, and diuresis.

As the intradural portion of the procedure begins, the surgeon's conceptual focus shifts from emphasis on maintenance of normal transmural pressure to avoidance of shearing stresses on the aneurysm and its surrounding structures, which may be produced by preliminary brain retraction. One component of this effort is the well-planned use of appropriately situated craniotomies, which magnify the extent of subarachnoid exposure before the application of brain tissue retraction. Radical removal of the sphenoid ridge, extensive subtemporal craniectomy, and complete bony exposure of the sinodural angle are three examples of critical aspects of bone removal in three different aneurysm approaches. A second facet of the attempt to minimize brain tissue retraction involves the use of a variety of agents to reduce brain volume. We have had only minimal success with lumbar spinal drainage intraoperatively as these fragile catheters frequently become kinked during positioning for a pterional approach. In elderly patients, significant brain relaxation can be obtained by evacuating the cortical sulci but recent subarachnoid hemorrhage jeopardizes the efficacy of this maneuver. Placement of a catheter within the lateral ventricle, however, has been an extremely reliable and rapidly effective mechanism to achieve exceptional brain relaxation. A very effective landmark in our experience has been obtained by identifying a point 2.5 cm superior and posterior to the sphenoid ridge such that a perpendicular 2.5-cm line can be constructed to interface with the distal sylvian fissure. A directly perpendicular passage of a brain catheter from that point will consistently enter the lateral ventricle following a routine pterional craniotomy. In addition to ventricular drainage, the use of appropriate diuretics, generous hypocarbia, and, on occasion, the supplementation of maintenance anesthesia with large doses of barbiturates will in almost all cases produce significant decreases in brain distention. The technical advantages of dealing with a "slack brain" during the initial exposure and dissection of aneurysms, to say nothing of the avoidance of premature rupture at this moment, far outweigh any inconvenience produced by a few minutes' delay, as the surgeon allows these mechanisms sufficient time to become maximally effective.

Dissection

The majority of intraoperative aneurysm ruptures in our experience have occurred during the microsurgical dissection in the subarachnoid space prior to clip application. Most frequently, rupture has been produced by a variety of regrettable blunt dissection techniques involving dissectors, micronerve hooks, and forceps, and the inappropriate use of the arachnoid knife or scissors in divesting the aneurysm and adjacent vasculature of its arachnoid sheath and removing loculated hematoma from the subarachnoid space. Injuries to aneurysms acquired in this manner typically resulted in a large rent, often located in the proximal aneurysm sac and occasionally extending into the neck of the aneurysm itself. Bleeding from these large irregular tears was relatively profuse and unresponsive to gentle tamponade or mild hypotension. Typically, exposure of the aneurysm at the time of rupture in these circumstances was insufficient to permit definitive clipping without a high risk of further injury to adjacent arteries or cranial nerves, mandating the application of temporary clips for hemorrhage control.

This type of intraoperative bleeding was markedly different from that encountered in the small number of patients whose aneurysms were injured by sharp dissection techniques using an arachnoid knife or microscissor. Generally, bleeding encountered during this type of dissection has been modest, usually emanating from a punctuate bleeding site that can often be covered by a single small no. 5 or no. 7 sucker tip. These small lacerations tended to be focal and were not infrequently located distally on the fundus. This type of aneurysmal injury tended to occur late in the dissection as the final arachnoidal adhesions were being lysed and in no instance did the tear extend into the proximal neck or into the parent vessel.

The major technical problem secondary to aneurysmal rupture during dissection has been obscuration of important subarachnoid anatomy by the torrential hemorrhage encountered with a blunt tear, with the serious sequelae of severe neurological deficit secondary to premature and inappropriate permanent clip placement. When dealing with such large rents, we have found it unwise to attempt immediate definitive clip application without adequate aneurysm exposure. Instead, by using two suckers initially to clear the field, the surgeon should identify the site of rupture and then, by placing a single sucker immediately on the rent, prevent or minimize blood escaping into the subarachnoid space and obscuring the vascular anatomy. If, as is frequently the case, the anatomy is insufficiently defined to allow definitive clip placement, it is best to place temporary clips on afferent and efferent vessels, as far from the aneurysm as possible. Simultaneously, normotension is restored and a loading dose of a cerebral protective agent like etomidate (Amidate; Abbott Laboratories, North Chicago, IL) is administered.

When the bleeding has been controlled, it is important to resume meticulous sharp dissection of the aneurysm, parent vessel, and emerging arterial branches. When exposure is complete, careful inspection of the area of the aneurysm tear may demonstrate that one to several microsutures are necessary to close an extension of the rent beyond the neck of the aneurysm into the parent artery before applying a final clip. In our experience, little is gained and much is potentially lost by premature efforts to clip the aneurysm hastily to restore normal circulation; relatively extended periods of temporary arterial occlusion have been clinically demonstrated to be well tolerated,[1] and every attempt must be made to avoid compounding the previous injury to the aneurysm by inadvertent compromise of the adjacent vasculature.[8,12,13]

When sharp dissection has produced a small aneurysm tear, very frequently a single sucker tube can be used to cover the site of injury, clear the wound, and permit visualization of the remainder of the anatomy. Most commonly, bleeding of this nature responds to gentle tamponade with a small piece of cotton. This material can either soon be removed or simply retracted gently, allowing further dissection. Gentle and judicious use of the bipolar cautery often seals puncture wounds of this type, but even persistent hemorrhage is typically insufficient in volume to prevent continued dissection. Only when this maneuver has failed have we had to resort to temporary clipping in such instances.

In general, inadvertent aneurysmal rupture during dissection is much more amenable to corrective action than that occurring before aneurysm exposure. In our experience, hemorrhage at this point has been most frequently associated with blunt dissection techniques, and the occasional bleeding occurring as a result of sharp dissection has routinely been correctable by gentle tamponade. These observations have important implications for the selection of techniques for aneurysm exposure. First in importance is minimizing or eliminating blunt dissection in the area of the aneurysm itself. The surgeon should rely instead on extensive sharp arachnoidal opening over proximal and distal vessels as well as over the aneurysm itself before commencing aneurysm dissection. Delineation of the aneurysm neck is best done with microscissors or a sharp disposable arachnoid knife. We have found the simple straight knife blade preferable to the variety of curved and angled blades available. Simultaneously, gentle displacement of afferent or efferent arteries with the suction tube may accentuate the hidden subarachnoid space adjacent to the aneurysm, which must be entered and developed to expose the neck safely. Sharp dissection should also extend to the removal of adjacent subarachnoid clot which often is tenaciously adherent to underlying vessels and the aneurysm and should be cleanly removed piecemeal using scissors or an arachnoid knife. Once the aneurysm itself has been freed from its attachments to the surrounding brain tissue, clot, and adjacent vasculature, its complete mobilization for inspection before clipping is safer and more reliable than investigation of the hidden aspects of the aneurysm neck with blunt and blind palpation by microdissectors or nerve hooks. During the actual dissection of the aneurysm neck, an increase in magnification is of great benefit in permitting the surgeon to appreciate the delicate subarachnoid planes at the base of the aneurysm neck. When the aneurysm is extremely thin-walled and efferent vessels are densely adherent to the aneurysm fundus, we now resort to early planned temporary arterial occlusion. Using the previously described brain protective regimen[1] with normotension, normovolemia, and metabolic brain suppression, temporary clips can be applied either to the proximal vessel alone or to all afferent and efferent vasculature, permitting rapid and safe final dissection and clipping.

Clip Application

Following the completion of the microdissection, another relatively frequent stage of the procedure to be complicated by intraoperative bleeding was during clip application, a complication due to either inadequate exposure of the aneurysm before placement of the clip or poor technical clip application. The majority of these problems occurred because of incomplete dissection of the aneurysm before an attempt at definitive clipping. Typically, the surgeon was aware that the aneurysm was less than optimally exposed. Bleeding occurring at the time of clip application was markedly similar to that produced by blunt dissection techniques; that is, it tended to be from relatively large tears, proximally located, and associated with an excessive amount of bleeding as the clip blade punctured or sheared the aneurysm wall. Such hemorrhage occurred most commonly before complete closure of the aneurysm clip and often was exacerbated as the clip blades became approximated. As one would expect, closure of the clip at this time would increase the size of a puncture or shearing injury. Prompt removal of the clip at the time of hemorrhage and prior to clip closure has proved to be a key initial maneuver in managing this situation. On occasion, simply allowing the aneurysm to redistend has resulted in hemostasis as the lesion is tamponaded against adjacent structures.

On the other hand, aneurysms adherent to the skull base dura may rupture during clip closure owing to less sinister causes. Occasionally, proximal carotid or anteriorly projecting basilar apex or basilar trunk aneurysms may be avulsed from their dural adhesions as shearing stresses increase during clip closure. It is vital for the surgeon to be aware of this possibility as the resolution of this problem is quite different from the more dangerous circumstances of aneurysm puncture by the clip blade. If the surgeon is aware of the potential dural attachment, and the neck dissection and clip application are believed to be definitive, simple closure of the clip will abate the hemorrhage. This critical decision-making is absolutely dependent on the surgeon's knowledge that the clip placement is accurate.

When bleeding remains brisk, we have found it useful to employ two suction tips simultaneously to identify the bleeding site, and allow a rapid decision regarding the feasibility of definitive clipping at that time. In most cases, owing to the location of the laceration or the severity of bleeding, it has been most prudent to resort to temporary clipping to allow completion of the dissection and mobilization of the aneurysm so that the site of penetration could be identified and a more definitive and more proximal clip site identified.

Bleeding episodes due to technically inappropriate clip application were usually of less magnitude than those secondary to incomplete aneurysmal dissection; such bleeding occurred at the time of clip closure and markedly abated when the blades of the clip were approximated. We suspect that these hemorrhages have been manifestations of small tears in the distal aneurysmal sac produced by traction on the fundus associated with clip closure and persisted only because either the clip did not completely span the neck, the clip closing pressure was insufficient to occlude the neck, or differential thickness in the tissue comprising the neck prevented complete closure of the entire breadth. Regardless of etiology, bleeding at this point was usually quite minimal and thorough inspection of the length of the clip blades allowed definition of the mechanical problem at hand. In our experience with Yaşargil clips (Aesculap Instrument Corp., Burlingame CA), technical error has been by far the most common cause of hemorrhage during clip application. Although mechanical clip failure has occurred, this is a singularly rare event when using modern clips with documented closing force.

In the face of relatively modest hemorrhage occurring at the time of clip closure, it is most important to inspect the distal aspect of the clip blades to determine first whether they are indeed completely across the aneurysm neck and second whether they are in close apposition. When the surgeon determines that the aneurysm clip does not span the entire breadth of the neck and when the aneurysm is in a relatively uncomplicated site such as the middle cerebral bifurcation or the posterior carotid wall, a simple advancement of the clip several millimeters may remedy the situation. However, if the clip itself must actually be replaced by a second clip of a different length or shape or if the surgeon is dealing with a more complicated lesion such as a basilar bifurcation aneurysm, we have had success with a more conservative approach. In these situations we have found it most judicious to place a second longer clip parallel to the first to encompass the neck completely and then, with the surgeon's field of vision unobscured, to gently open and advance or replace the initial clip. In some distal basilar aneurysms when the anatomy was complicated by a very confining exposure or the presence of perforators from the P1 segments which were jeopardized by further manipulation of the initial clip or the addition of a second clip, we have seen angiographically proven instances of thrombosis of the lesion over the ensuing 48 h. Although this approach clearly places the patient at some risk in the short term, we do consider it a viable option when the risks of additional clip manipulation are deemed inappropriately high.

If careful inspection demonstrates that the initial blades seem to span the aneurysm neck completely but are not in close apposition or are obviously being distended by the systolic pulsations, placement of second "tandem" clip parallel to the first will usually adequately compress the residual patent neck. On occasion, two or more additional tandem clips may be necessary to compress large, complex, and calcified lesions. However, this maneuver may be ineffective when dealing with aneurysm necks that contain in a portion of their circumference, thick atherosclerotic plaque; complete apposition of thicker portions of such a neck may leave an adjacent thin-walled segment patent. If this residual neck lies toward the surgeon, it can readily be dealt with by a shorter clip; if the residual neck lies beyond the atheromatous plaque, a large fenestrated clip, as described by Drake, can be used to encircle the bulky neck and close the distal patent lumen.[3]

The operative results with rupture occurring at the time of clip application have mirrored those associated with rupture during the dissection phase of the procedure. If rupture was secondary to blunt trauma to the aneurysm associated with the premature clip application, it carried significant negative consequences. However, if the aneurysm had been completely dissected before bleeding that occurred because of technically poor clip application, almost routinely the patient's outcome was favorable. These findings simply reinforce the negative effect of a large tear occurring before the aneurysm neck has been exposed adequately to permit definitive clipping.

Sequelae of Intraoperative Aneurysm Rupture

Despite carefully thought out maneuvers which were largely effective in dealing with intraoperative bleeding, patients who suffered this complication had a significantly less favorable outcome than those who did not. Although the increasingly routine application of temporary clips in difficult aneurysm situations has favorably affected patient outcome, cumulative data from the past several years at our center suggest that management morbidity and mortality for patients suffering serious intraoperative rupture is in the range of 30 to 35 percent. Patients undergoing uneventful surgical procedures have been found to have morbidity and mortality rates of approximately 10 percent.

There are several potential reasons for the marked disparity between the ultimate outcome for these two groups of patients, the most striking of which is the surprisingly high incidence of postoperative complications in patients suffering intraoperative bleeding. We have noted a high incidence of symptomatic and often life-threatening vasospasm in these patients, presumably resulting from the addition of supplemental subarachnoid clot. The use of unplanned temporary arterial occlusion was required in greater than 50 percent of those patients with intraoperative rupture but in only 10 to 15 percent of the uncomplicated group as a whole. Over the past 5 years, our use of temporary clipping in both groups is increasing. In the uncomplicated surgical patients, these occlusions are elective maneuvers accomplished at normal levels of blood pressure and following the administration of agents to decrease cerebral metabolism, and episodes of temporary arterial interruption tend to be of shorter duration than in procedures complicated by intraoperative bleeding in which temporary clips were emergently applied.

Management of Intraoperative Aneurysm Rupture

From a technical viewpoint, each aneurysm surgeon develops a series of maneuvers to manage intraoperative rupture that reflects the surgeon's training, technical abilities, instinctive reactions, and surgical experience. Theoretically, each of these maneuvers is directed at elimination of hemorrhage, prevention of further damage to the aneurysm, preservation of associated vasculature and neural tissue, and facilitation of aneurysm obliteration. Unfortunately, these individual goals can be mutually exclusive. Certain maneuvers quite effective in the achievement of hemostasis may potentially injure the aneurysm or adjacent neural tissue. Large fragments of cottonoid, while certainly helpful in tamponading hemorrhage, markedly impair the surgeon's ability to obtain further exposure preparatory to final clip placement. Similarly, maneuvers developed to deal with relatively minor degrees of bleeding may be totally insufficient to provide hemostasis during torrential bleeding. Their unsuccessful trial may both prolong a period of uncontrolled hemorrhage and, by permitting subarachnoid spaces to become packed with fresh blood, complicate further exposure and increase the risk of vasospasm. Thus, the "appropriate" remedial measure to manage any intraoperative hemorrhage is determined not only by the surgeon's experience but also by the nature of the bleeding, the stage of dissection at which it occurs, and other anatomic and physiologic factors unique to the individual patient. A number of therapeutic gestures that have proved useful to us in dealing with intraoperative bleeding will be discussed briefly.

Suction Dissection of the Aneurysm

This technique, described by Poppen, relies on the aspiration of the entire aneurysm sac into a large sucker tube, where it is held as the exposed neck is then ligated with an aneurysm clip.[11] This technique has been advocated by various authors both before and after the advent of the microsurgical era. In our experience, the applicability of this technique is restricted either to those cases in which the aneurysm ruptures after nearly complete dissection of its circumference or to Pertuiset's type IV rupture, which he terms "bursting of the sac."[9] The dense arachnoidal adhesions that tether an aneurysm to the adjacent brain, cranial nerves, and vessels necessitate extensive sharp subarachnoid dissection of the aneurysm neck and fundus to permit accurate permanent clip placement. Attempts to accomplish this dissection by aspiration of the entire thin-walled sac into a large suction tube may result in shearing of the entire aneurysmal fundus and neck, thus eliminating any possibility of preserving the continuity of the parent vessel. An exception to this general feeling relates to middle cerebral aneurysms that project into a large temporal hematoma. Suction aspiration of the sac of an actively bleeding lesion of this type can permit early clipping of the distal fundus, allowing accurate microdissection to proceed.

Coagulation of the Aneurysmal Rent

This technique is uniquely modern, being developed and popularized by several of the initial exponents of microvascular surgery, including Drake, Pertuiset, and Yaşargil.[4,8,9,12,13] Its use requires the surgeon to clear the entire field of blood by the use of the two suckers and then, while holding one suction tip over the small aneurysmal rent, to apply the bipolar cautery across the rent repetitively, sealing and contracting the aneurysmal wall gently without producing additional injury. It is important to ask the surgical assistant to drip a small amount of irrigant into the exposure to prevent sticking of the forceps. We have had reasonable success in closing small lacerations produced by sharp dissection techniques. In using this technique, the surgeon is well advised to be gentle with the aneurysm, to use repetitive short bursts of low-intensity current, and to massage the intact aneurysmal wall between the jaws of the forceps and avoid the temptation to seal the laceration with a single protracted burst of cautery. Not infrequently, this technique is successful at diminishing the amount of bleeding and the residual bleeding can either be controlled by tamponade or be tolerated during the final stages of the dissection.

Clip Application to the Distal Sac

This innovative technique, initially described by Drake, involves isolation of the lacerated portion of the aneurysm by a permanent or temporary clip applied across the fundus well distal to the aneurysmal neck.[3] It is especially effective when dealing with a multiloculated giant aneurysm when bleeding occurs during the dissection or the mobilization of a distal lobe of the lesion. Often the bleeding site can be isolated by a large clip, permitting resumption of the dissection of the remainder of the aneurysm and final preparation of the neck for definitive clip placement. Our own experience suggests that this technique is best applied when the injured portion of the aneurysm has been well dissected from the surrounding arachnoid so that application of the distal clip does not inadvertently rupture an as yet undissected lobe of the aneurysm. Particularly in the circumstance of recent subarachnoid hemorrhage, this maneuver may be successful in eliminating even brisk hemorrhage and avoidance of temporary arterial occlusion which may be less well tolerated in this setting.

Severe Induced Hypotension

This technique has been recommended by many aneurysm surgeons but as microsurgical technology has expanded and further information has become available regarding the impact of dysautoregulation on ischemic tolerance, this technique is being used less. Surgeons accustomed to operating in the first and second weeks after subarachnoid hemorrhage have drifted well away from this practice even in excellent grade patients because of its deleterious impact on patients with angiographic narrowing. However, marked reduction in arterial pressure does frequently diminish bleeding and on occasion allow the neurosurgeon to regain control of a seemingly irretrievable situation. The adverse neurological and systemic effects of severe hypotension coupled with extreme blood loss suggest that this maneuver should be avoided whenever possible. In the series of Giannotta et al., the use of induced hypotension was associated with a high (>50 percent) incidence of poor outcome.[5] The same authors found that when hypotension was avoided, the patients had a much better result. The introduction of safe temporary clips by a variety of manufacturers as well as the increasing use of agents to decrease cerebral metabolism and therefore increase ischemic tolerance have provided a safer means for microsurgeons to both prevent and manage serious intraoperative hemorrhage.

Temporary Arterial Occlusion

There is little doubt that the planned elective use of temporary occlusion has advantages over its emergency institution in the face of sudden severe aneurysmal bleeding. Normotension, normovolemia, the administration of cerebral protective agents, and appropriate temporary clip placement all can be methodically utilized to minimize the risk of cerebral ischemia. Hypothermia to 32°C to 33°C when prophylactically instituted may provide even longer safe intervals of temporary arterial occlusion. However, the use of all these methods should be considered even when it is necessary to move rapidly to arterial occlusion to deal with an intraoperative rupture. This is especially important in the face of sudden hemorrhage because it is in this setting that the surgeon is least able to predict accurately whether a brief or a protracted period of local circulatory arrest will be required to deal with the problem. It has become our routine practice to employ intraoperative electroencephalographic monitoring, begun during the positioning of all aneurysm patients. We similarly make the attempt to optimize the rheologic properties of the intravascular volume by achieving a hematocrit in the range of 30 to 35 percent and administering a dose of mannitol during the late stages of the craniotomy. Etomidate has become our cerebral protectant of choice because of its favorable impact on the cerebral metabolic rate and its desirable properties of minimal cardiotoxicity and rapid reversibility such that patients awaken quickly in the intensive care unit and become neurologically examinable even after protracted usage.[1] In order to avoid the application of temporary clips without the benefit of brain protection, we routinely advise our anesthesiologists to administer a loading dose of 1.0 mg/kg etomidate as we enter the final stages of subarachnoid dissection in large and giant aneurysms and more recently have begun to generalize this technique as we approach more routine but ruptured lesions. With the patient normovolemic and normotensive and with the cerebral metabolic rate diminished by at least 50 percent with burst suppression doses, we have noted excellent tolerance of even protracted episodes of temporary arterial occlusion with and without recent subarachnoid hemorrhage. Intervals of up to 15 to 17 min have been routinely tolerated.

Dissection of an aneurysm and its associated vasculature after the placement of temporary clips should not be compromised by undue haste in completing the exposure, clipping the aneurysm, and reinstituting normal perfusion. Certainly the surgeon must proceed in the dissection without delay, but the main goal must remain the atraumatic complete exposure of critical vascular anatomy followed by judicious, accurate aneurysm obliteration. The surgeon must be aware of the passage of time, but cannot be distracted by repetitive announcements heralding every minute of temporary occlusion. With appropriate precautions and forethought, temporary arterial occlusion can be a very well-tolerated maneuver that enhances the surgeon's ability to deal with even the most difficult case of intraoperative aneurysmal rupture and in our recent experience has substantially diminished the frequency of this untoward occurrence.

Summary

Intraoperative aneurysm rupture remains an undesired, relatively infrequent, but unavoidable consequence of intracranial aneurysm surgery. For some patients suffering this complication the ultimate prognosis is negatively impacted. Therefore, the surgeon must diligently search for mechanisms both to decrease the overall incidence of this complication and to minimize its ultimate clinical significance. The use of careful microdissection techniques and the prior thoughtful development of a systematic contingency plan for dealing with this occurrence should serve to minimize its overall effect on management morbidity and mortality. A clear-headed and relaxed approach, allowing deliberate methodical remedial actions to this stressful intraoperative complication, together with the knowledge that inappropriate therapeutic gestures pose much more potential risk to the patient than the relatively small amount of blood entering the suction tubing, will consistently allow surgeons to maximally utilize their technical skills and creative thinking.

References

1. Batjer HH, Frankfurt AI, Purdy PD, et al. Use of etomidate, temporary arterial occlusion, and intraoperative angiography in surgical treatment of large and giant cerebral aneurysms. *J Neurosurg* 1988; 68:234–240.
2. Batjer H, Samson D. Intraoperative aneurysmal rupture: incidence, outcome, and suggestions for surgical management. *Neurosurgery* 1986; 18:701–707.
3. Drake CG. Giant intracranial aneurysms: experience with surgical treatments in 174 patients. *Clin Neurosurg* 1979; 26:12–95.
4. Drake CG. The treatment of aneurysms of the posterior circulation. *Clin Neurosurg* 1979; 26:96–144.
5. Giannotta SL, Oppenheimer JH, Levy ML, et al. Management of intraoperative rupture of aneurysm without hypotension. *Neurosurgery* 1991; 28:531–536.
6. Graf CJ, Nibbelink DW. Randomized treatment study: intracranial surgery. In Sahs AL, Nibbelink DW, Torner JC (eds): *Aneurysmal Subarachnoid Hemorrhage: Report of the Cooperative Study.* Baltimore: Urban & Schwarzenburg, 1981, pp 145–202.
7. Kassell NF, Boarini DJ, Adams HP Jr, et al. Overall management of rupture aneurysm: comparison of early and late operation. *Neurosurgery* 1981; 9:120–128.
8. Ojemann RG, Crowell RM. *Surgical Management of Cerebrovascular Disease.* Baltimore: Williams & Wilkins, 1983, pp 151–153.
9. Pertuiset B. Intraoperative aneurysmal rupture and reduction by coagulation of the sac. In Pia HW, Langmaid C, Zierski J (eds): *Cerebral Aneurysms: Advances in Diagnosis and Therapy.* Berlin: Springer-Verlag, 1979, pp 398–401.
10. Pia W. Discussion of Pertuiset B. Intraoperative aneurysmal rupture and reduction by coagulation of the sac. In Pia HW, Langmaid C, Zierski J (eds): *Cerebral Aneurysms: Advances in Diagnosis and Therapy.* Berlin: Springer-Verlag, 1979, pp 401.
11. Poppen JL. *An Atlas of Neurosurgical Techniques.* Philadelphia: Saunders, 1960, pp 160–161.
12. Yaşargil MG. *Microneurosurgery,* vol I. Stuttgart: Georg Thieme Verlag, 1984, pp 269–271.
13. Yaşargil MG, Smith RD. Management of aneurysms of anterior circulation by intracranial procedures. In Youmans JR (ed): *Neurological Surgery,* 2d ed. Philadelphia: Saunders 1982, pp 1663–1696.

222 Aneurysms within the Cavernous Sinus and Transitional Cavernous Aneurysms

Nayef Al-Rodhan
David G. Piepgras

Despite the advances in microneurosurgical and anesthetic techniques, as well as our increased understanding of the surgical anatomy of the cavernous sinus, the surgical approach to the cavernous sinus continues to be a major challenge. The earliest documented reference to the cavernous sinus was by Winslow in 1732,[56] who coined the term "cavernous" because he thought the structure resembled the corpus cavernosum.

In our series of intracranial aneurysms,[3] cavernous internal carotid artery (ICA) aneurysms represented 6 percent of all intracranial aneurysms, as well as 15 percent of all the ICA aneurysms treated in our institution during the same period. These percentages are similar to those in previous reports,[37,47] in which cavernous ICA aneurysms accounted for 3 percent of all intracranial aneurysms and 14 percent of ICA aneurysms.

Surgical Anatomy

There have been a number of excellent anatomic studies of the cavernous sinus (for review see Inoue et al.[31]). The cavernous sinuses are paired structures located on either side of the sella turcica. In the adult, each sinus measures 2.5 cm long by 2 cm high, extends from the petrous portion of the temporal bone posteriorly to the superior orbital fissure anteriorly, and is contained within dural folds. These dural folds attach to the anterior and posterior clinoid processes as well as to the sphenoid bone. A number of important neurovascular structures are found in the cavernous sinus itself—the ICA and its cavernous branches, the abducens nerve (VI), and the sympathetic fiber bundles that surround the carotid artery. In addition, the thickened lateral dural walls of the sinus contain the oculomotor nerve (III), the trochlear nerve (IV), and the ophthalmic and maxillary divisions of the trigeminal nerve (V_1 and V_2).

The intracavernous portion of the ICA begins at the foramen lacerum, where the vessel emerges from the carotid canal and enters the posterior-inferior aspect of the cavernous sinus. The ICA leaves the cavernous sinus by passing upward on the medial aspect of the anterior clinoid process until it pierces the dural roof of the cavernous sinus, entering the intracranial cavity and becoming the supraclinoid ICA. Within the cavernous sinus, the artery ascends toward the posterior clinoid process, then abruptly turns forward to run horizontally for about 2 cm. The length of the cavernous portion of the ICA ranges from 14.5 to 23.0 mm (average, 18.0 mm), and its diameter ranges from 4.0 to 7.0 mm (average, 5.4 mm).[31]

The cavernous segment of the ICA has several branches.[25,42] The longest and most proximal branch is the meningohypophyseal trunk, which is always present. This branch arises at the level of the dorsum sellae and divides into three branches: the tentorial artery of Bernasconi-Cassinari, the inferior hypophyseal artery, and the dorsal meningeal artery. The second cavernous branch of the ICA is the artery of the inferior cavernous sinus, which arises from the lateral wall of the horizontal segment, 8 mm distal to the meningohypophyseal trunk. The third branch is McConnell's capsular artery, which is present in about 30 percent of specimens. It arises 5 mm distal to the inferior cavernous branch and supplies the anterior and inferior pituitary capsule. Several additional branches are less consistently present. These include the persistent trigeminal artery (which joins the proximal cavernous ICA to the basilar artery between the superior and anterior inferior cerebellar arteries), the ophthalmic artery, and the dorsal meningeal artery.

Detailed anatomic studies have revealed that the cavernous sinus is not a trabeculated venous space but, rather, a plexus of veins.[43] It is connected by venous channels to a number of structures, including the face, eye, orbit, nasopharynx, mastoid, middle ear, brain stem, cerebellum, and cerebrum. While a number of neural structures are associated with the cavernous sinus, the abducens nerve (VI) and the sympathetic nerves are the only true intracavernous neural structures. The sixth nerve enters the cavernous sinus through Dorello's canal and ascends upward and laterally around the carotid. The sympathetic nerves (from the superior sympathetic ganglion) pass parallel to the carotid artery through the base of the skull to the parasellar region. At frequent intervals in the cavernous sinus, they send fibers to the wall of the carotid artery. The remaining sympathetic fibers first join the sixth nerve, then leave it and join the ophthalmic division of the trigeminal nerve before exiting through the superior orbital fissure and ultimately innervating the papillodilator and superior tarsal muscles.[44] The other neural structures that are contained in the dural fold forming the lateral wall of the cavernous sinus (nerves III, IV, V_1, and V_2) are also often implicated in cavernous sinus lesions.

Vascular lesions of the cavernous sinus are of two types: carotid-cavernous fistulae and nonfistulous arterial aneurysms. This chapter deals with the latter.

Clinical Features of Intracavernous Aneurysms

Cavernous aneurysms are found predominantly in middle-aged women. In our series (Al-Rodhan et al.[3] and Al-Rodhan et al., in preparation), the female-to-male ratio was 5:1 and the mean age was 53.4 years. These values are similar to those in other reports,[38,47] which have found a 6:1 female-to-male ratio. In our series, most of these aneurysms presented with compressive symptoms: headache (41 percent); retro-orbital pain (25 percent); and cranial nerve defects, including visual loss (22 percent) and field cuts (13 percent), third nerve palsy (36 percent), fourth nerve palsy (10 percent), facial numbness/pain (14 percent), and sixth nerve palsy (23 percent). Hypopituitarism was seen in 3 percent of patients and cerebrospinal fluid (CSF) leakage in 1 percent. Hemorrhagic symptoms included epistaxis (1 percent) and subarachnoid hemorrhage (11 percent; associated only with the transitional type of cavernous aneurysm, described below.) Cavernous aneurysms usually enlarge, resulting in ophthalmoplegia. Third nerve palsies secondary to cavernous sinus aneurysms, however, may not cause a dilated pupil because the sympathetic fibers responsible for dilating the pupil, which are located around the carotid, are also paralyzed. Pain and progression of symptoms tend to be episodic, with episodes lasting days or months, which suggests that compression may be caused by episodes of distension rather than by steady expansion. Retro-orbital pain, a very common presenting symptom, is caused by dural and trigeminal nerve compression. The trochlear and abducens nerves are also frequently affected, regardless of the location of the aneurysm in the sinus.[32,33] Occasionally, loss of taste may occur owing to compression of the greater superficial petrosal nerve and traction on the facial nerve at the petrous ridge.[55] Compressive symptoms frequently result in the ''cavernous sinus'' or ''parasellar'' syndrome, which consists of pain in the sensory fields of V_1 and V_2 and paresis of one or two extraocular muscles.

Medial projection of cavernous aneurysms results in bony erosion of the dorsum sellae, posterior clinoid process, anterior clinoid process, or sellar floor, with subsequent compression and dysfunction of the pituitary gland. Cavernous and other aneurysms cause 1 to 3 percent of all enlarged sellae. In our series, four cavernous aneurysms projected into the sella, causing hypopituitarism, and a fifth aneurysm eroded the planum sphenoidale and presented with a CSF leak.

The cavernous carotid artery is a frequent site of giant aneurysms (>25 mm) which enlarge insidiously. The cavernous carotid artery was the location of 14 percent of the giant aneurysms in Drake's series,[13] 59 percent of those in Morley and Barr's series,[39] 16 percent of those in the series of Linskey and colleagues,[36] and 75 percent of those in our series.

Classification of Clinoidal-Cavernous Region Aneurysms

Despite the many publications about aneurysms of the ICA in the region of the clinoid process, the nomenclature of these lesions has remained confused. Terms like *ophthalmic, carotid-ophthalmic, paraophthalmic, supraclinoid, subchiasmal, paraclinoid, ventral paraophthalmic, carotid cave,* and *cavernous* have been used to describe these aneurysms.[1,5,7,8,13–17,20,23,27,33,41,45] We recently proposed a classification system for these clinoid-cavernous region aneurysms,[2] which is described below and shown in Table 222-1 and Fig. 222-1.

Group I: Superior Hypophyseal (Subtype Ia) and Ventral Paraclinoid (Subtype Ib) Aneurysms

This group includes aneurysms with necks that arise intradurally from the ICA segment that is distal to the ophthalmic artery and proximal to the posterior communicating artery. The group is divided into two subtypes, Ia and Ib. Subtype Ia includes superior hypophyseal aneurysms,[7,8] that is, aneurysms that project superiorly while remaining entirely intradural. Subtype Ib includes what Fox[17] called *ventral paraclinoid aneurysms,* that is, aneurysms that project posteroinferiorly either intradurally, or extradurally into the cavernous sinus.

Group II: Ophthalmic Aneurysms

This group includes true ophthalmic aneurysms with necks that arise at the junction of the ophthalmic artery and the ICA. They tend to project anterosuperiorly and remain intradural.

Group III: Carotid Cave Aneurysms

This group includes what Kobayashi and coworkers[34] called *carotid cave aneurysms.* These are medial infraophthalmic and supracavernous aneurysms that arise from the ICA in the clinoid space (carotid cave), which is a pocket at the anterior clinoid process that measures about 5 mm. This space is totally extracavernous. These aneurysms are intradural where they arise from the carotid artery, and they either remain intradural as they project inferiorly or, occasionally, project into the cavernous sinus. They show many similarities in behavior to aneurysms of group Ib, owing to the ventral paraclinoid position of the intradural aneurysm neck in both types and to the fact that the aneurysm dome in both types sometimes extends into the cavernous sinus, which means that the cavernous sinus must sometimes be opened for the aneurysm to be clipped.

TABLE 222-1 Classification of ''Clinoidal-Region'' Aneurysms of the Internal Carotid Artery

	Group I: Supraophthalmic Infra-PComA		Group II: Ophthalmic (at Origin of Ophthalmic Artery)	Group III: Infraophthalmic Supracavernous (Carotid Cave)	Group IV: Transitional Cavernous	Group V: Cavernous
	Ia: Superior Hypophyseal	Ib: Ventral Paraclinoid				
Neck	Intradural	Intradural	Intradural	Intradural	Intracavernous	Intracavernous
Dome	Intradural (superior)	Intradural or intracavernous (inferior)	Intradural (superior)	Intradural or intracavernous (inferior)	Intradural (superior)	Intracavernous
Risk of SAH	↑	↑	↑	↑	↑	↓

Abbreviations: SAH, subarachnoid hemorrhage; PComA, posterior communicating artery.
Source: From Al-Rodhan et al.,[2] with permission.

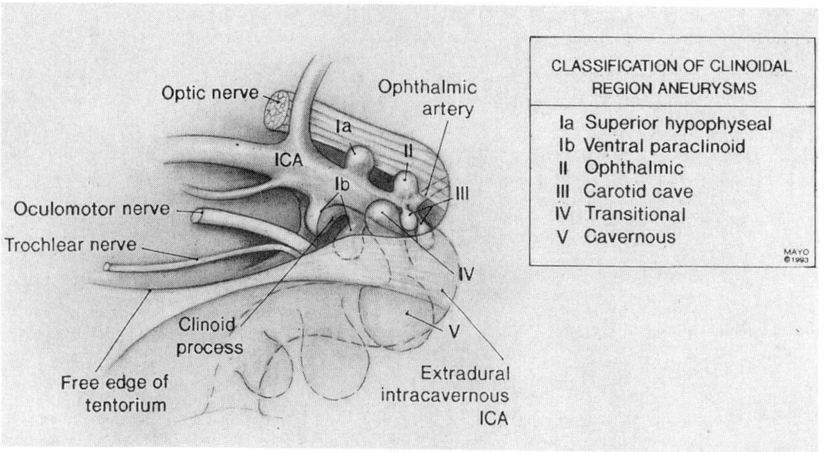

Figure 222-1 Our classification of clinoidal-region ICA aneurysms. (From Al-Rodhan et al.,[2] with permission.)

Group IV: Transitional Cavernous Aneurysms

This group includes what we have termed *"transitional" cavernous aneurysms*[2] (Fig. 222-2). These are by definition cavernous aneurysms in that their necks arise from the cavernous segment of the ICA, but their domes project superiorly into the intradural extracavernous subarachnoid space. These aneurysms deserve special attention because the projection of their domes into the intradural subarachnoid space means that they tend to present with subarachnoid hemorrhage (SAH). Clinically they are thus a different entity from purely cavernous aneurysms.

Group V: Cavernous Aneurysms

This group includes pure intracavernous aneurysms, in which the aneurysm neck and dome are both contained entirely in the cavernous sinus (Fig. 222-3). Since there is no direct communication with the intradural subarachnoid space, there is virtually no risk of SAH.

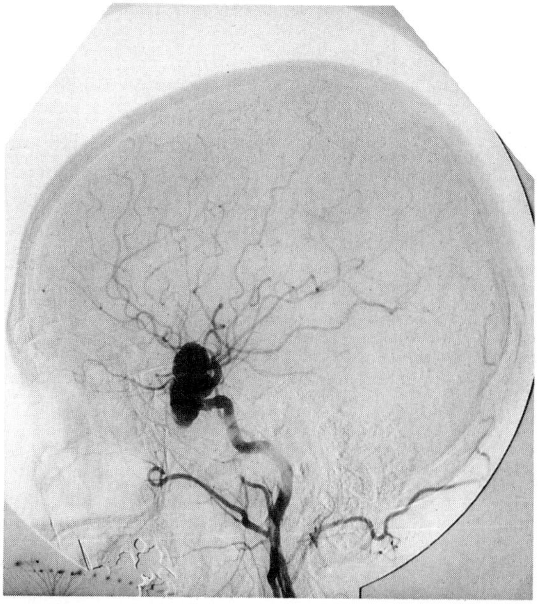

Figure 222-2 A lateral angiogram showing a transitional cavernous ICA aneurysm (clinoidal type IV) with the neck in the cavernous sinus and the dome projecting into the intradural subarachnoid space.

Transitional Cavernous Aneurysms and Subarachnoid Hemorrhage

True intracavernous aneurysms (group V), the neck as well as the dome of which are contained totally within the cavernous sinus, rarely bleed. Various series have reported an incidence of bleeding of 0 to 40 percent,[4,11,36,39] although in most of these series a clear distinction between true intracavernous aneurysms and paraclinoid noncavernous aneurysms was often not made. "Paraclinoid" aneurysms are a different group, with a higher bleeding rate and a different presentation and management.[27]

In our classification, groups I through IV are associated with SAH, whereas group V is not. In our series of cavernous sinus aneurysms (Al-Rodhan et al., in preparation), none of the nontransitional cavernous aneurysms presented with SAH. Our series of cavernous aneurysms included 23 "transitional" cavernous aneurysms, which represented 19 percent of the cavernous sinus aneurysms in the series as well as 7.8 percent of the ICA aneurysms and 1 percent of the intracranial aneurysms repaired at our institution during the same period. The patients with transitional cavernous aneurysms included 17 women and 6 men, ranging in age from 24 to 80 years, with a mean age of 50 years. Of the aneurysms, 6 were small (less than 15 mm), 6 were large (15 to 25 mm), and 11 were giant (more than 25 mm).

The clinical features of the 23 transitional aneurysms included compressive symptoms in nine patients (39 percent) and subarachnoid hemorrhage in 13 patients (57 percent); one patient (4 percent) was asymptomatic. The compressive symptoms included headache (30 percent), orbital pain (17 percent), visual loss (9 percent), visual field cut (9 percent), oculomotor palsy (9 percent), and abducens palsy (4 percent). Of the 13 patients with subarachnoid hemorrhage, seven were grade I, five were grade II, and one was grade III.

Surgical Options

The indications for treatment of cavernous aneurysms include subarachnoid hemorrhage, loss of vision, severe intractable facial

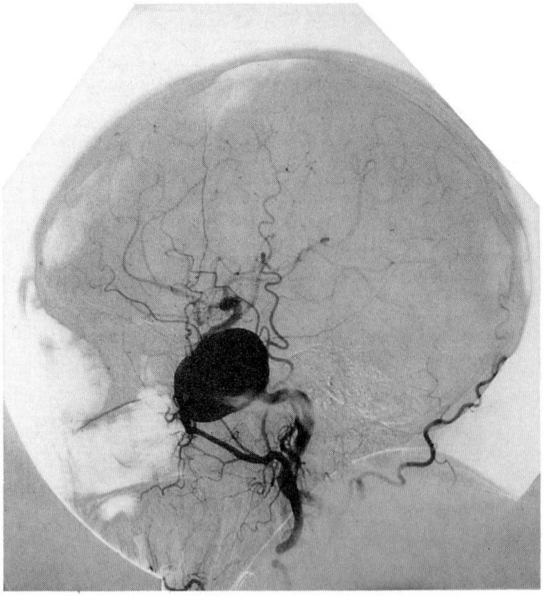

(*A*)

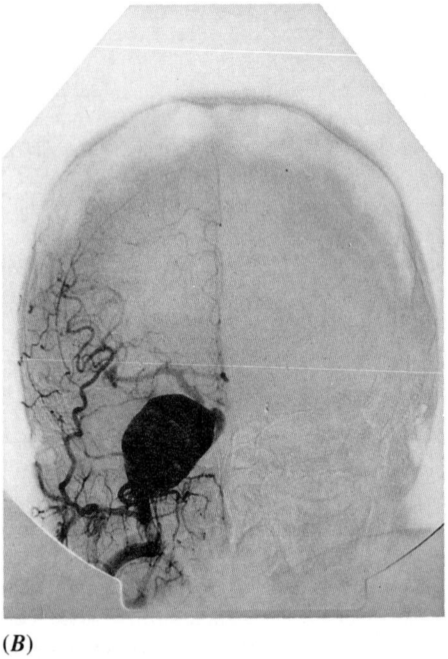

(*B*)

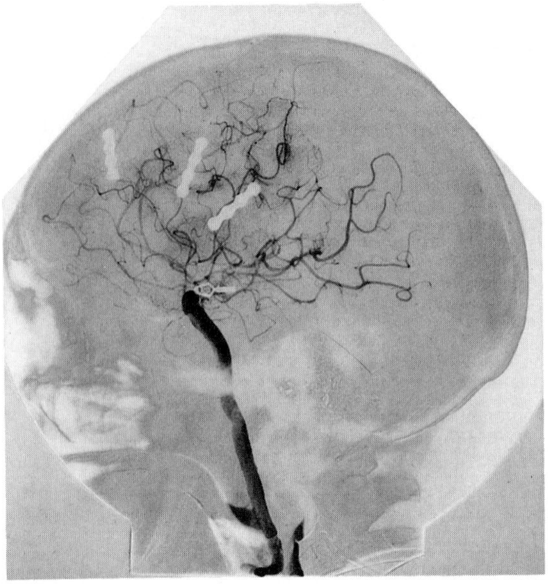

(*C*)

Figure 222-3 A cavernous aneurysm. Lateral (*A*) and anteroposterior (*B*) angiograms show a giant intracavernous ICA aneurysm (clinoidal type V) with the neck and the dome entirely within the cavernous sinus. A postoperative angiogram (*C*) shows an interposition saphenous vein graft.

pain, progressive ophthalmoplegia, and epistaxis. Most aneurysms that are asymptomatic or cause only minimal compressive symptoms can be followed with observation, especially in the elderly. There are a number of surgical options and, more recently, endovascular techniques for dealing with these lesions. The surgical options are listed in Table 222-2. Direct surgical methods (those involving intracavernous surgery) include direct clipping, direct obliteration with sacrifice of the ICA, exploration and reinforcement, or excision with repair of the ICA defect. Indirect methods—those in which the integrity of the cavernous sinus is not violated—include proximal ligation of the ICA, trapping, and proximal occlusion of the ICA with collateral augmentation by a superficial temporal artery–middle cerebral artery (STA-MCA) anastomosis or an interposition saphenous vein graft from the proximal carotid to the intracranial ICA or MCA segment. Although direct repair and preservation of the ICA is the preferred method, there are instances when it is not feasible or carries an excessive risk, and alternative indirect methods have to be used.

Our direct surgical approach to cavernous sinus aneurysms is similar to that advocated by Dolenc,[12] and has been described in detail elsewhere.[51] If the aneurysm has a definable neck and arises from the anterior genu segment, and especially if it is of the ''transitional'' variety, direct surgical clipping is recommended, regardless of the size of the aneurysm. If, however, the neck of the aneurysm is poorly defined or arises from a more proximal cavernous

TABLE 222-2 Surgical Methods for Treating Intracavernous Aneurysms

Direct	Indirect
1. Direct clipping	1. Proximal cervical ICA ligation
2. Direct obliteration with sacrifice of the ICA	2. Trapping
3. Exploration and reinforcement	3. STA-MCA bypass with proximal ICA ligation
4. Excision of the aneurysm and use of a saphenous vein patch graft	4. Interposition saphenous vein graft bypass with proximal ICA ligation

TABLE 222-3 Collateral Flow Assessment with Trial Carotid Balloon Occlusion

	Adequate	Inadequate
Clinical signs	None	Deficit
Angiography	Good	Poor
Electroencephalography	No change	Change
Cerebral blood flow	>35 ml/100 g/min	<20 ml/100 g/min
SPECT scan	Symmetric perfusion	Asymmetric perfusion

segment, or if the aneurysm is fusiform, then direct clipping may not be possible without significant cranial nerve morbidity and risk of sacrifice of the ICA. In these cases, we have favored indirect treatment methods.

Although proximal ICA occlusion either by balloon or by ligation in the neck seems attractive and simple,[19,24] it is not the preferred treatment option except in patients who, for reasons of age or medical risk, could not tolerate an intracranial procedure and who have a proven adequate collateral flow (Table 222-3). It is to be noted that some patients who tolerate ICA occlusion at first deteriorate up to several days later. These complications can take the form of an acute stroke due to hemodynamic insufficiency or infarction owing to thrombus propagation or embolism.[6,10,16,18,28,40,46] To minimize these risks, many surgeons now recommend using post-occlusion anticoagulation[10,26] in combination with increasing the circulatory blood volume and inducing hypertension.[10,16,40] Although occlusion of the ICA rather than the common carotid artery (CCA) is preferred because it gives the best reduction of aneurysmal pressure and a higher rate of aneurysm thrombosis,[35,40] it carries a higher risk of cerebral ischemia than CCA ligation, which preserves some ICA flow through the external carotid system.

If major hemorrhage or a mass effect are the presenting symptoms, trapping the aneurysm by balloon, either alone or in combination with ICA ligation, may be the best option. Distal ICA obstruction should optimally be carried out proximal to the ophthalmic artery, as this approach allows the emptying of the aneurysm to release the mass and also minimizes the risk of ischemia caused by propagated thrombus or embolism.

Before the ICA can be sacrificed, it is necessary to confirm the patient's hemispheric collateral flow. The best method is probably angiographic trial balloon occlusion of the ICA. We also supplement this technique with cerebral blood flow measurements using direct intracarotid injection of xenon as well as single photon emission computed tomography (SPECT) studies (Table 222-3).

If inadequate hemispheric collateral flow is suspected from the trial balloon occlusion studies, a bypass procedure is needed.[18,48,50–53] Although we have used STA-MCA bypass with proximal ICA occlusion with good success, our current preferred method of bypass is an interposition saphenous vein bypass graft from the proximal ICA with proximal ICA occlusion, because this bypass delivers a large volume of blood. We prefer to place these long saphenous vein grafts from the cervical segment of the ICA, rather than from the petrous segment as advocated by Fukushima and Spetzler.[49] Although short saphenous vein grafts have certain advantages, exposing the petrous segment of the ICA is technically more difficult and is associated with risk of injury to hearing and to facial nerve, eustachian tube, fifth nerve, and lacrimal gland function.[48,49] The harvesting and preparation of vein grafts and the technique of using them as arterial conduits have been described previously.[54]

In our series, 58 aneurysms were repaired directly. Of these, 49 were clipped, 3 wrapped, 3 directly obliterated with sacrifice of the ICA, and 2 excised with repair of the ICA. Sixty cases were managed indirectly: 18 had proximal ICA ligation, in 6 the aneurysm was simply trapped, 8 had an STA-MCA bypass with proximal ICA ligation, and 28 had an interposition saphenous vein bypass graft from the cervical ICA with proximal ICA ligation. Direct surgery gave an excellent outcome in 53 of the 58 cases (91 percent); major complications occurred in five patients, including one death. These complications included cardiopulmonary arrest (two patients), stroke (one), infection and vasospasm (one), and hemiparesis (one). Post-clipping angiograms showed that the parent vessel was patent in 93 percent of the patients. Retrospective analysis of the origin and projection of the necks of the 58 aneurysms that are operated on directly showed that 55 of them arose from the anterior genu.

Indirect surgery gave an excellent outcome in 54 of the 60 cases (90 percent); major complications occurred in six patients, including three deaths. In the proximal ligation group, all patients had an eventual excellent outcome except for one fatality from cerebral embolism. All eight cases managed with STA-MCA bypass with proximal ICA ligation as well as the six cases managed with trapping had an eventual excellent outcome. The saphenous vein bypass group had an excellent outcome in 23 of the 28 patients (82 percent). The complications in the remaining five patients included stroke (two patients), subdural hematoma with seizures and hypoxia (one), vasospasm (one) and contralateral intracerebral hemorrhage (one).

Overall, 11 of the 118 patients (9 percent) had complications, which were fatal in 4. The nonfatal complications in the other seven patients (6 percent) included stroke (three), cardiac arrest with anoxia (one), infection and vasospasm (one), subdural hematoma with seizures and hypoxia (one), and retraction hemiparesis (one). The causes of death in the four patients (3 percent) who died were embolic stroke (one), cardiopulmonary arrest (one), severe SAH and vasospasm (one), and contralateral multiple intracerebral hematomas (one). These results compare favorably with those of similar surgical series,[11,36] despite the facts that 75 percent of the aneurysms in our series were giant (>25 mm) and that, in contrast to other series, we excluded strictly noncavernous paraclinoid aneurysms from our analysis.

In summary, our recommendations are as follows: (1) Asymptomatic cavernous sinus ICA aneurysms should be managed with observation, especially in the elderly. (2) Distal or transitional cavernous aneurysms should be treated like intracranial aneurysms and repaired directly, owing to their high risk for SAH. (3) Anterior genu cavernous aneurysms with definable necks can usually be clipped successfully with preservation of the parent vessel and low morbidity. (4) Symptomatic proximal-segment cavernous aneurysms or distal aneurysms with indefinable necks should probably be treated with carotid occlusion or, in the absence of good collateral flow, indirectly with proximal carotid occlusion and bypass. (5) Proximal-segment cavernous aneurysms with .definable necks should probably be treated with platinum coils. (6) We currently prefer a long interposition saphenous vein graft bypass with acute ICA ligation over a short interposition saphenous vein graft or STA-MCA bypass with graded occlusion, although both of these options have merit and a role in the management of these aneurysms. (7) Proximal balloon occlusion of the ICA remains a good treatment option in selected patients with proven adequate collateral flow. If this option is chosen, postocclusion anticoagulant therapy should be instituted to minimize the risk of ischemia due to thrombus propagation and embolization. (8) In all cases, a careful preoperative evaluation, including full angiography to characterize the aneurysm and its neck as accurately as possible and trial balloon occlusion to assess the clinical sufficiency of the collateral circulation, is necessary.

Role of Endovascular Techniques

A number of endovascular techniques have been used in the management of these aneurysms.[9,16,21,22,29,30] However, the results of balloon occlusion for cavernous sinus aneurysms show that many of these lesions were ultimately managed by carotid occlusion.[9,16,30] In the recent series by Higashida and colleagues,[30] preservation of the parent artery was achieved in only 22 percent of cases, and total exclusion of the aneurysm from the circulation was accomplished in only 63 percent of cases. The rate of parent vessel patency with balloon techniques is lower than the rate achieved with direct surgical repair in our series, in which parent vessel patency was maintained in 93 percent of cases so handled.

Recent experience with detachable platinum coils,[21,22] however, has been promising for treatment of selected aneurysms, and this technique may prove especially suitable for intracavernous ICA aneurysms with small, well-defined necks.

The Future

We need to further refine the angiographic criteria for patient selection, especially in relation to the anatomy of the aneurysm neck. Further experience and familiarity with anatomy and surgical techniques will undoubtedly improve our ability to expose proximal segments of the ICA, making surgery in this area more efficacious, with less risk to the cranial nerves. Techniques for better cerebral protection during periods of temporary carotid occlusion are needed. These will undoubtedly involve not only pharmacologic but also temporary shunting techniques. Such techniques are likely to be useful not only for cavernous aneurysms but also for intracranial occlusive vascular disease and invasive tumors of the cavernous sinus.

In terms of endovascular techniques, the new platinum coils or a refined version thereof will be a useful adjunct in the treatment of selected cases of intracavernous ICA aneurysms, making possible thrombosis of the aneurysm sac with preservation of the parent ICA.

References

1. Almeida GM, Shibata MK, Bianco E. Carotid-ophthalmic aneurysms. *Surg Neurol* 1976; 5:41–45.
2. Al-Rodhan NRF, Piepgras DG, Sundt TM Jr. Transitional cavernous aneurysms of the internal carotid artery. *Neurosurgery* 1993; 33:993–998.
3. Al-Rodhan NRF, Piepgras DG, Sundt TM Jr, et al. The microsurgical management of cavernous sinus aneurysms. *J Neurosurg* 1991; 75:170 (abstr).
4. Barr HWK, Blackwood W, Meadows SP. Intracavernous carotid aneurysms: a clinical-pathological report. *Brain* 1971; 94:607–622.
5. Benedetti A, Curri D. Direct attack on carotid ophthalmic and large internal carotid aneurysms. *Surg Neurol* 1977; 8:49–54.
6. Brackett CE Jr. The complications of carotid artery ligation in the neck. *J Neurosurg* 1953; 10:91–106.
7. Day AL. Clinicoanatomic features of supraclinoid aneurysms. *Clin Neurosurg* 1990; 36:256–274.
8. Day AL. Aneurysms of the ophthalmic segment. A clinical and anatomical analysis. *J Neurosurg* 1990; 72:677–691.
9. Debrun G, Fox A, Drake C, et al. Giant unclippable aneurysms: treatment with detachable balloons. *Am J Neuroradiol* 1981; 2:167–173.
10. Diaz FG, Ausman JI, Pearce JE. Ischemic complications after combined internal carotid artery occlusion and extracranial-intracranial anastomosis. *Neurosurgery* 1982; 10:563–570.
11. Diaz FG, Ohaegbulam S, Dujovny M, et al. Surgical alternatives in the treatment of cavernous sinus aneurysms. *J Neurosurg* 1989; 71:846–853.
12. Dolenc VV. A combined epi- and subdural direct approach to carotid-ophthalmic artery aneurysms. *J Neurosurg* 1985; 62:667–672.
13. Drake CG. Giant intracranial aneurysms: experience with surgical treatment in 174 patients. *Clin Neurosurg* 1979; 26:12–95.
14. Drake CG, Vanderlinden RG, Amacher AL. Carotid-ophthalmic aneurysms. *J Neurosurg* 1968; 29:24–31.
15. Ferguson GG, Drake CG. Carotid-ophthalmic aneurysms: visual abnormalities in 32 patients and the results of treatment. *Surg Neurol* 1981; 16:1–8.
16. Fox AJ, Vinuela F, Pelz DM, et al. Use of detachable balloons for proximal artery occlusion in the treatment of unclippable cerebral aneurysms. *J Neurosurg* 1987; 66:40–46.
17. Fox JL. Microsurgical treatment of ventral (paraclinoid) internal carotid artery aneurysms. *Neurosurgery* 1988; 22:32–39.
18. Gelber BR, Sundt TM Jr. Treatment of intracranial and giant carotid aneurysms by combined internal carotid ligation and extra- to intracranial bypass. *J Neurosurg* 1980; 52:1–10.
19. Giannotta SL, McGillicuddy JE, Kindt GW. Gradual carotid artery occlusion in the treatment of inaccessible internal carotid artery aneurysms. *Neurosurgery* 1979; 5:417–421.
20. Gibo H, Lenkey C, Rhoton AL Jr. Microsurgical anatomy of the supraclinoid portion of the internal carotid artery. *J Neurosurg* 1981; 55:560–574.
21. Guglielmi G, Vinuela F, Dion J, Duckwiler G. Electrothrombosis of saccular aneurysms via endovascular approach. Part 2: Preliminary clinical experience. *J Neurosurg* 1991; 75:8–14.
22. Guglielmi G, Vinuela F, Sepetka I, Macellari V. Electrothrombosis of saccular aneurysms via endovascular approach. Part 1: Electrochemical basis, technique, and experimental results. *J Neurosurg* 1991; 75:1–7.
23. Guidetti B, La Torre E. Management of carotid-ophthalmic aneurysms. *J Neurosurg* 1975; 42:438–442.
24. Gurdjian ES, Lindner DW, Thomas LM. Experiences with ligation of the common carotid artery for treatment of aneurysms of the internal carotid artery. *J Neurosurg* 1975; 23:311–318.
25. Harris FS, Rhoton AL. Anatomy of the cavernous sinus, a microsurgical study. *J Neurosurg* 1976; 45:169–180.
26. Heros RC. Thromboembolic complications after combined internal carotid ligation and extra-to-intracranial bypass. *Surg Neurol* 1984; 21:75–79.
27. Heros RC, Nelson PB, Ojemann RG, et al. Large and giant paraclinoid aneurysms: surgical techniques, complications, and results. *Neurosurgery* 1983; 12:153–163.
28. Heyman A, Tindall GT, Finney WHM, Woodhall B. Measurement of retinal artery and intracarotid pressures following carotid artery occlusion with the Crutchfield clamp. *J Neurosurg* 1960; 17:297–305.
29. Hieshima GB, Higashida RT, Halbach VV, et al. Intravascular balloon embolization of a carotid-ophthalmic artery aneurysm with preservation of the parent vessel. *Am J Neuroradiol* 1986; 7:916–918.
30. Higashida RT, Halbach VV, Dowd C, et al. Endovascular detachable balloon embolization therapy of cavernous carotid artery aneurysms: results in 87 cases. *J Neurosurg* 1990; 72:857–863.
31. Inoue T, Rhoton AL Jr, Theele D, Barry ME. Surgical approaches to the cavernous sinus. A microsurgical study. *Neurosurgery* 1990; 26:903–932.
32. Jefferson G. On the saccular aneurysms of the internal carotid artery in the cavernous sinus. *Br J Surg* 1938; 26:267–302.
33. Jefferson G. The Bowman Lecture: concerning injuries, aneurysms, and tumours involving the cavernous sinus. *Trans Ophthalmol Soc UK* 1953; 73:117–152.
34. Kobayashi S, Kyoshima K, Gibo H, et al. Carotid cave aneurysms of the internal carotid artery. *J Neurosurg* 1989; 70:216–221.
35. Krayenbuhl H, Yasargil MG. Diagnosis and therapy of intracranial aneurysms. *Surg Annu* 1970; 2:327–343.
36. Linskey ME, Sekhar LN, Hirsch W Jr, et al. Aneurysms of the intracavernous carotid artery: clinical presentation, radiographic features, and pathogenesis. *Neurosurgery* 1990; 26:71–79.

37. Locksley HB. Natural history of subarachnoid hemorrhage, intracranial aneurysms, and arteriovenous malformations. Based on 6368 cases in the Cooperative Study. *J Neurosurg* 1966; 25:219–239.
38. Meadows SP. Intracavernous aneurysms of the internal carotid artery: their clinical features and natural history. *Arch Ophthalmol* 1959; 62:566–574.
39. Morley TP, Barr HWK. Giant intracranial aneurysms: diagnosis, course and management. *Clin Neurosurg* 1969; 16:73–94.
40. Nishioka H. Report on the Cooperative Study of Intracranial Aneurysms and Subarachnoid Hemorrhage, Section VIII, Part 1: Results of the treatment of intracranial aneurysms by occlusion of the carotid artery in the neck. *J Neurosurg* 1966; 25:660–704.
41. Nutik S. Carotid paraclinoid aneurysms with intradural origin and intracavernous location. *J Neurosurg* 1978; 48:526–533.
42. Parkinson D. Collateral circulation of cavernous carotid artery: anatomy. *Can J Surg* 1964; 7:251–268.
43. Parkinson D. A surgical approach to the cavernous portion of the carotid artery: anatomical studies and case report. *J Neurosurg* 1965; 23:474–483.
44. Parkinson D, Johnston J, Chaudhuri A. Sympathetic connections of the fifth and sixth cranial nerves. *Anat Rec* 1978; 191:221–226.
45. Pia HW. Classification of aneurysms of the intenal carotid system. *Acta Neurochir (Wien)* 1978; 40:5–31.
46. Roski RA, Spetzler RF, Nulsen FE. Late complications of carotid ligation in the treatment of intracranial aneurysms. *J Neurosurg* 1981; 54:583–587.
47. Sahs AL, Perret GE, Locksey HB, et al. (eds). *Intracranial Aneurysms and Subarachnoid Hemorrhage: A Cooperative Study*. Philadelphia: Lippincott, 1969.
48. Sekhar LN, Sen CN, Jho HD. Saphenous vein graft bypass of the cavernous internal carotid artery. *J Neurosurg* 1990; 72:35–41.
49. Spetzler RF, Fukushima T, Martin N, Zambramski JM. Petrous carotid-to-intradural carotid saphenous vein graft for intracavernous giant aneurysm, tumor, and occlusive cerebrovascular disease. *J Neurosurg* 1990; 73:496–501.
50. Spetzler RF, Roski Ra, Schuster H, et al. The role of EC-IC in the treatment of giant intracranial aneurysms. *Neurol Res* 1980; 2:345–359.
51. Sundt TM Jr. *Surgical Techniques for Saccular and Giant Intracranial Aneurysms*. Baltimore: Williams & Wilkins, 1990, pp 71–107.
52. Sundt TM Jr, Piepgras DG. Surgical approach to giant intracranial aneurysms: operative experience with 80 cases. *J Neurosurg* 1979; 51:731–742.
53. Sundt TM Jr, Piepgras DG, Marsh WR, Fode NC. Saphenous vein bypass grafts for giant aneurysms and intracranial occlusive disease. *J Neurosurg* 1986; 65:439–450.
54. Sundt TM III, Sundt TM Jr. Principles of preparation of vein bypass grafts to maximize patency. *J Neurosurg* 1987; 66:172–180.
55. White JC, Adams RD. Combined supra- and infraclinoid aneurysms of internal carotid artery: report of a case of unusual congenital dilatation of intracranial portion of carotid artery and injuries to visual, oculomotor, sensory, and taste fibers. *J Neurosurg* 1955; 12:450–459.
56. Winslow JB. *Exposition Anatomique de la Structure du Corps Humaine,* vol 2. London: Prevost, 1732, p 31.

223 Ophthalmic Segment Aneurysms

Arthur L. Day

Carotid-ophthalmic region aneurysms account for 5 to 10 percent of all intracranial saccular aneurysms.[5,27] First reported as a unique class of carotid aneurysm by Drake et al. in 1968, these lesions were originally defined as those aneurysms taking origin at the level of the ophthalmic artery.[8] Many aneurysms from this region, have no direct relationship to that named branch, however. As a result, these lesions are frequently described according to their shape (global), direction of projection (dorsal or ventral), or relationship to adjacent structures (proximal carotid, paraclinoid, supraclinoid, paraophthalmic, supraopthalmic, infraophthalmic, parachiasmal, subchiasmal, suprachiasmal).[1,8,16,18,24,26,28,30,36,41]

Recently, the anatomy of this region has been greatly clarified, thereby allowing the classification of ophthalmic region aneurysms according to more traditional nomenclature methods.[5,7,20,23,33] These lesions are no longer characterized solely by their relationship to the anterior clinoid process (supraclinoid vs. infraclinoid), but are now viewed according to their exact point of origin from the carotid artery, a factor which allows the treating surgeon to preoperatively define (1) the relationship of the aneurysm to the carotid artery and arterial branches and perforators; (2) the relationship of the aneurysm to the visual system; (3) the relationship of the aneurysm neck to the dural ring, clinoidal space, and cavernous sinus; and (4) the best approach and clip type for successful aneurysm obliteration.[5,6,23]

Pertinent Anatomy and Terminology

The ophthalmic segment (OphSeg) is the longest subarachnoid portion of the internal carotid artery (ICA), beginning below the level of the anterior clinoid process at the point where the ICA penetrates the dura to enter the subarachnoid space (the dural ring), and ending at the origin of the posterior communicating artery (PComArt) (Fig. 223-1).[14] There are two major arterial bends in this segment. The first occurs as the carotid artery ascends and then bends sharply posteriorly after penetrating the dural ring to enter the subarachnoid space. The second is a gentler medial-to-lateral curve as the ICA approaches its terminal bifurcation.

Two named branches arise from the OphSeg, both of which typically originate just above the dural ring. The first, larger, and better known is the ophthalmic artery (OphArt).[17,32] It usually arises from the dorsal or dorsomedial surface of the ICA just after the carotid enters the subarachnoid space. The OphArt typically originates immediately beneath the optic nerve, and subsequently travels through the optic canal to reach the orbit.

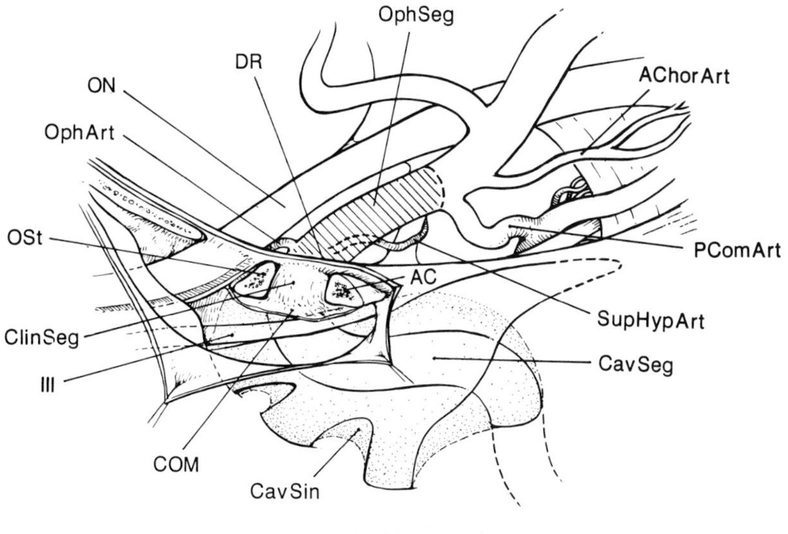

Figure 223-1 Ophthalmic segment anatomy, lateral view (schematic). All but the tip of the anterior clinoid process (AC) has been removed, but its dural/periosteal coverings have been preserved. The dura on the superior surface of the AC blends medially with the floor of the optic canal, chiasmal sulcus, and diaphragma sellae. The point where this medial dural continuance encircles the internal carotid artery (ICA) is known as the dural ring (DR), which marks the true point of emergence of the ICA into the subarachnoid space. The DR separates the ophthalmic segment (OphSeg) from the clinoidal segment (ClinSeg). The dura on the medial surface of the AC is adherent to the ClinSeg of the ICA. The dura covering the inferior surface of the AC reflects laterally to the oculomotor nerve (III), and this sheet is termed the carotid-oculomotor membrane (COM) or membranous ring. The COM is intimately attached to the venous channels of the cavernous sinus (CavSin), and separates the ClinSeg from the cavernous segment (CavSeg). The OphSeg begins just proximal to the ophthalmic artery (OphArt) origin and ends at the posterior communicating artery (PComArt) takeoff. In most instances, the OphArt and superior hypophyseal artery (SupHypArt) arise from the OphSeg, just above the dural ring. Note the posterior bend of ICA just beyond the OphArt. A second bend also occurs in this segment as the ICA emerges along the medial surface of the AC and then spirals laterally to approach the terminal carotid bifurcation. The origin of the OphArt is usually obscured by the AC, while the origins of the SupHypArt arise medially from the OphSeg, and are obscured at surgery by the ICA. (AChorArt, anterior choroidal artery; OSt, optic strut; ON, optic nerve).

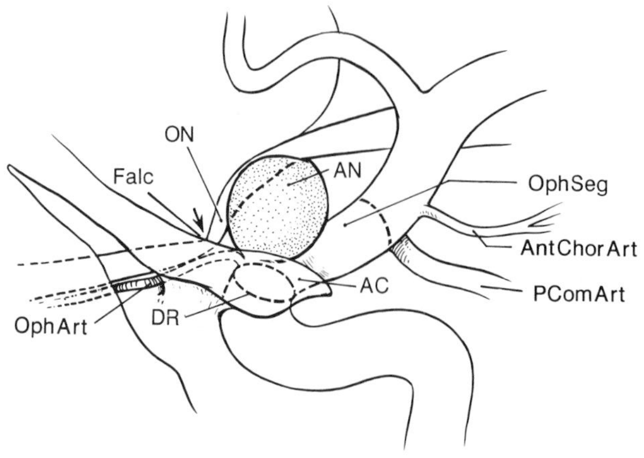

(*A*)

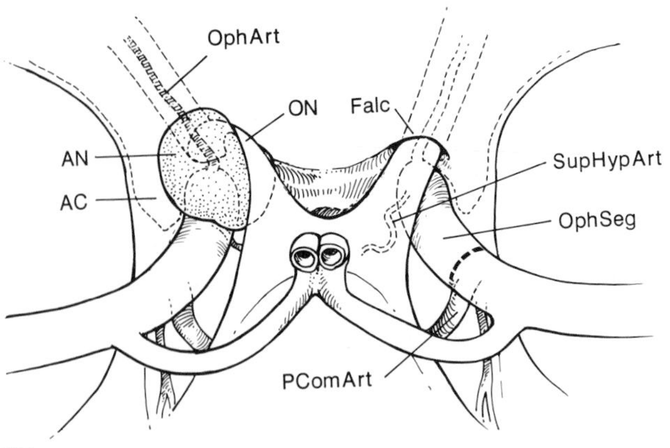

(*B*)

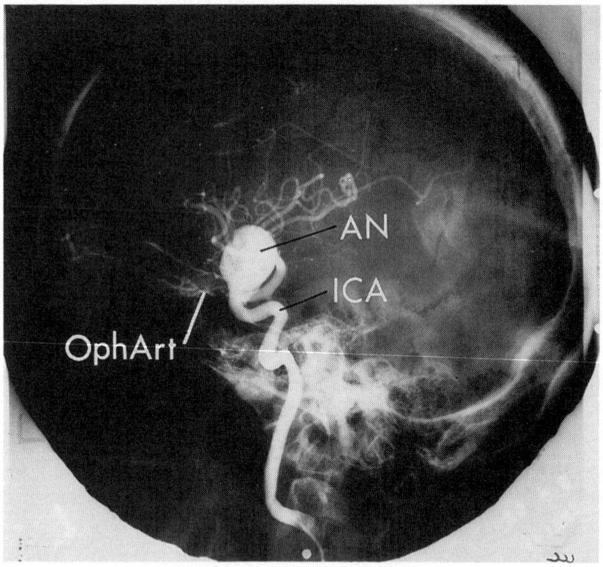

(*C*)

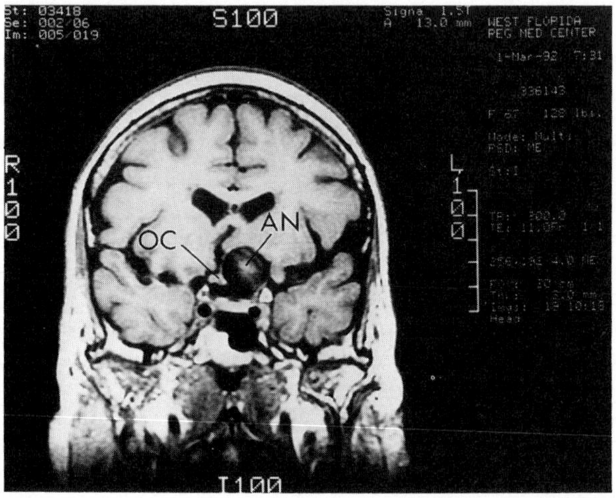

(*D*)

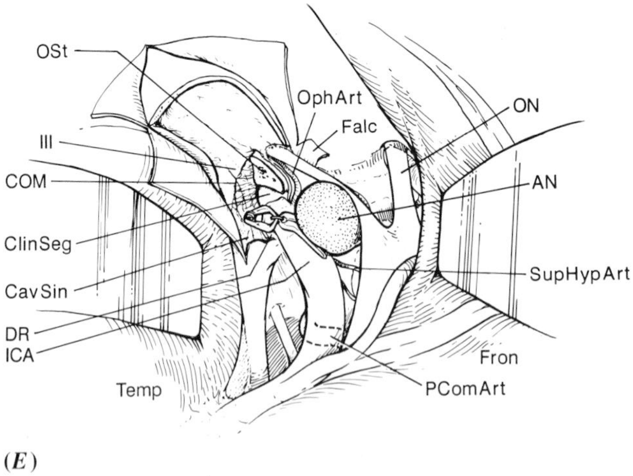

(*E*)

Figure 223-2 Large ophthalmic artery aneurysm: typical anatomy. *A*. Lateral view (schematic). Note the position of the optic nerve (ON), and the sharp angulation of its superior surface (*arrow*) against the edge of the falciform ligament (Falc). Note also that the anterior clinoid process (AC) limits the view of the proximal aneurysm neck and the origin of the ophthalmic artery (OphArt). (DR, dural ring; OphSeg, ophthalmic segment; AN, aneurysm; PComArt, posterior communicating artery; AChorArt, anterior choroidal artery). *B*. Dorsal view (schematic). Note the medial displacement of the lateral aspect of the optic nerve (ON). The optic nerve often creates a groove on the superomedial surface of the aneurysm (AN) and restricts its medial extension. (Falc, falciform fold; AC, anterior clinoid process; OphArt, ophthalmic artery; SupHypArt, superior hypophyseal artery; PComArt, posterior communicating artery; OphSeg, ophthalmic segment). *C*. Lateral view (arteriogram). Note that the aneurysm (AN) originates just beyond the ophthalmic artery (OphArt) take-off and projects dorsally, above the internal carotid artery (ICA). As the lesion expands, the superior restriction imposed by the overlying optic nerve tends to close the carotid siphon. *D*. Coronal view (MRI) of same case as *C*. Note that the aneurysm (AN) expands superomedially, but is restricted from contralateral extension by the optic nerve and optic chiasm (OC). *E*. Operative view, left side (schematic). The anterior clinoid (AC), roof and lateral wall of the optic canal, and adjacent orbital roof have been removed. Extensive removal of the optic strut (OSt) provides exposure of the clinoidal segment (ClinSeg) and permits temporary ICA clipping if necessary. The falciform fold (Falc) is sectioned before any manipulation of the aneurysm (AN) is undertaken. A side-angled clip has been placed parallel to the long axis of the ICA. (CavSin, cavernous sinus; III, oculomotor nerve; COM, carotid-oculomotor membrane; ON, optic nerve; OphArt, ophthalmic artery; SupHypArt, superior hypophyseal artery; PComArt, posterior communicating artery; Fron, frontal lobe; Temp, temporal lobe; DR, dural ring).

Several large perforating vessels also arise from the OphSeg, the largest of which is the superior hypophyseal artery (SupHypArt).[4,35] These perforators, which may be quite large, supply the dura around the cavernous sinus, the superior aspect of the pituitary gland and stalk, and the optic nerves and chiasm. They typically arise from the medial or inferomedial surface of this segment, usually along the second, lateral bend of the ICA prior to the PComArt origin. Their ventromedial origin, coupled with the gentle downward slope of the dural ring posteriorly, often places the SupHypArt origins on a horizontal plane below the level of both the anterior clinoid process and OphArt.

Ophthalmic segment aneurysms can be divided into two large categories, depending on association of the aneurysm neck with the named arterial branches within the segment.[5,6] Aneurysms arising in clear relation to the ophthalmic artery are termed OphArt aneurysms (Fig. 223-2). These lesions arise from the ICA just distal to the origin of the ophthalmic artery, and initially project dorsally or dorsomedially from the carotid surface toward the lateral half of the optic nerve.

Other aneurysms originating within this segment invariably incorporate the perforating branches to the hypophysis, and are herein called SupHypArt aneurysms (Figs. 223-3 and 223-4). Small SupHypArt aneurysms usually arise from the inferior or inferomedial surface of the ICA just opposite and slightly distal to the OphArt origin. These lesions may remain lateral to the sella, burrowing beneath and medial to the ICA under the anterior clinoid process.[5,25] Because the space beneath the carotid is limited, however, most larger lesions will eventually expand medially or superomedially above the diaphragma sella into the suprasellar space.

Clinical Features

From a recent series of over 700 patients with intracranial aneurysms seen at our institution, 80 cases (11 percent) were identified that harbored at least one OphSeg aneurysm.[5] The clinical features of these 80 lesions are summarized in Table 223-1. The series included 41 patients with OphArt aneurysms, and 39 with SupHypArt aneurysms. The average age of presentation was 54 years. There was a striking (86 percent) female to male predominance. Thirty-six of 80 patients (45 percent) had additional aneurysms elsewhere. Bilateral OphSeg lesions were identified in 10 to 20 percent of cases.

Size and Hemorrhage Risks

Table 223-2 lists the specific types of presentations, as related to aneurysm size and location. Approximately one-third of the patients presented with subarachnoid hemorrhage (SAH), one-third with visual symptoms, and one-third were discovered because of nonspecific symptoms such as headache, incidental CT findings, transient ischemic attacks, or hemorrhage from other lesions.

Sixty-two (78 percent) of the aneurysms were either large (1.0 to 2.4 cm) or giant (2.5 cm or greater), which is strikingly different

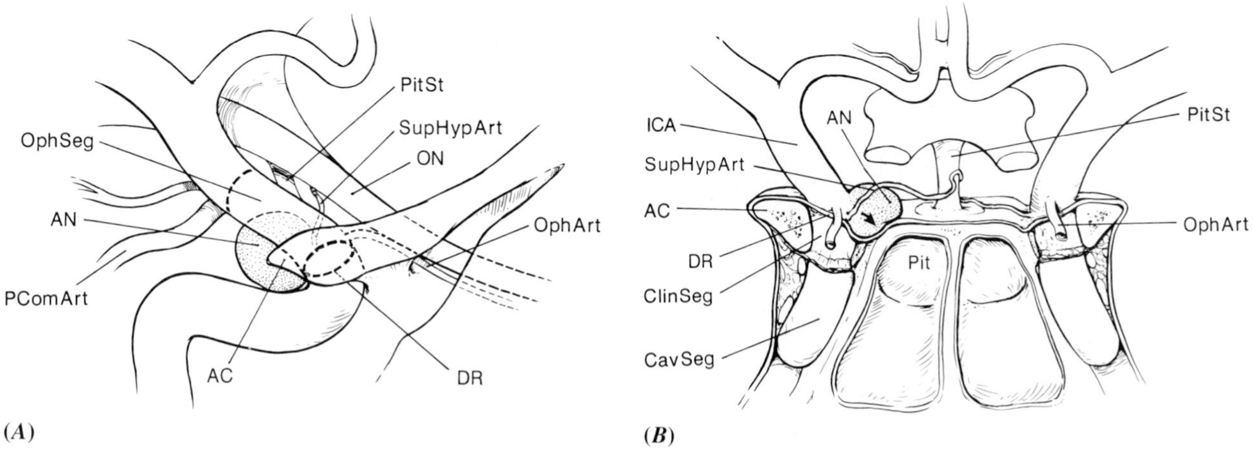

Figure 223-3 Small superior hypophyseal artery aneurysm: typical anatomy. *A*. Lateral view (schematic). The aneurysm (AN) arises ventromedially above the dural ring (DR), opposite the ophthalmic artery (OphArt) origin, and appears to project into the cavernous sinus. The AN lies partly below level of anterior clinoid process (AC), but is still within the subarachnoid space. (ON, optic nerve; PitSt, pituitary stalk; PComArt, posterior communicating artery; SupHypArt, superior hypophyseal artery; OphSeg, ophthalmic segment). *B*. AP view (schematic). The aneurysm (AN) projects ventromedially above the dural ring (DR) toward the lateral sellar wall. (SupHypArt, superior hypophyseal artery; OphArt, ophthalmic artery; Pit, pituitary gland; PitSt, pituitary stalk; ICA, internal carotid artery; ClinSeg, clinoidal segment; CavSeg, cavernous segment; AC, anterior clinoid process).

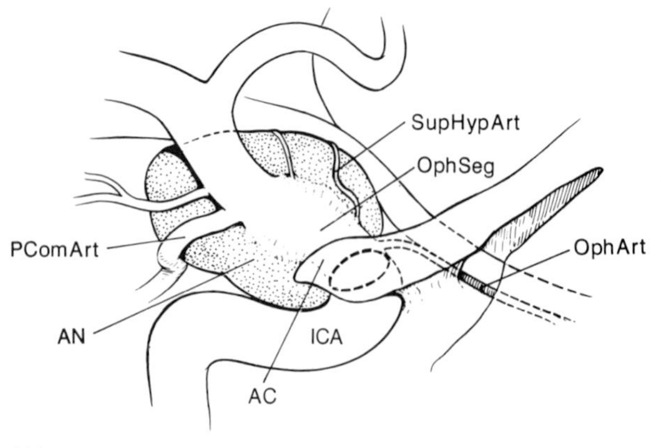

(*A*)

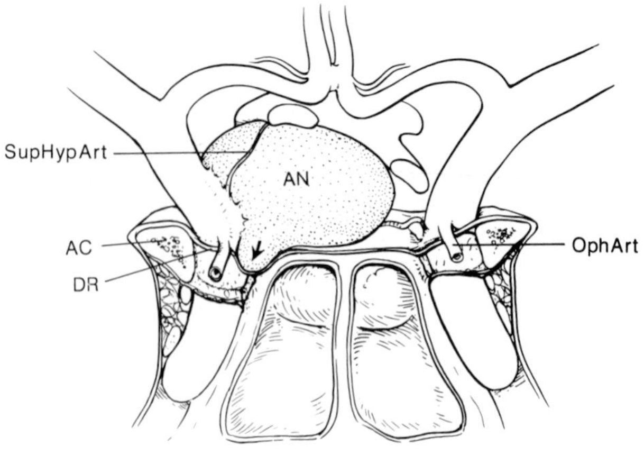

(*B*)

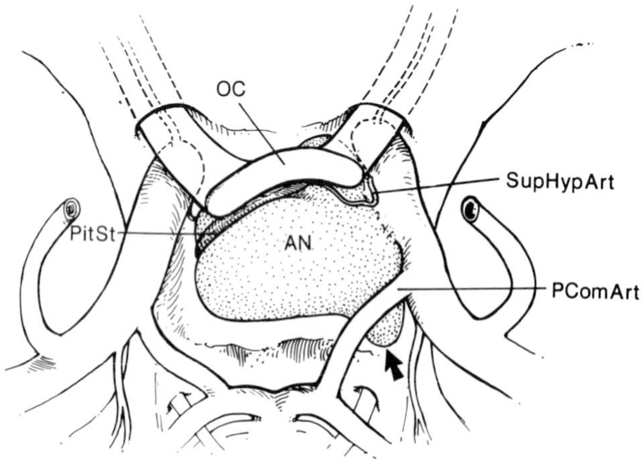

(*C*)

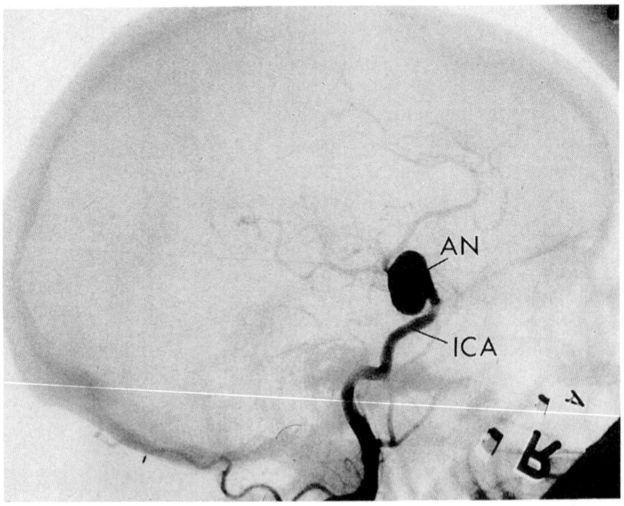

(*D*)

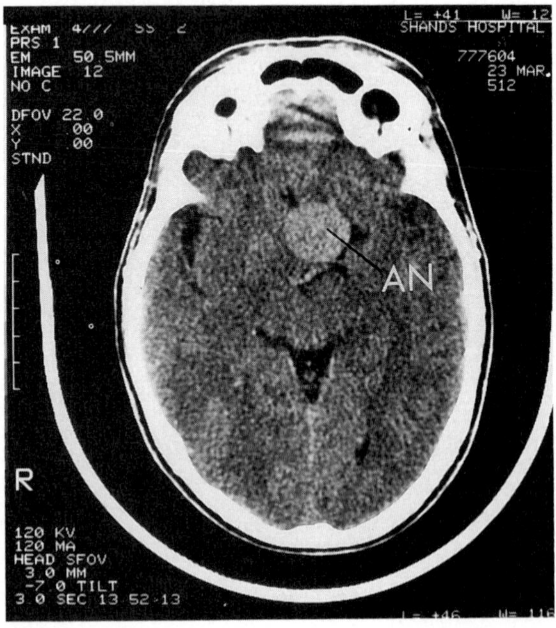

(*E*)

Figure 223-4 Large superior hypophyseal artery aneurysm. The lesion size now exceeds its ventral confines and expands into the suprasellar space below the optic chiasm. *A*. Lateral view (schematic). Note that the aneurysm (AN) projects both dorsal and ventral to the ophthalmic segment (OphSeg). The superior hypophyseal arteries (SupHypArt) drape over the aneurysm's superior surface, while the posterior communicating artery (PComArt) is displaced posteriorly and laterally. The anterior clinoid process (AC) limits the view of the ventral and medial aspects of the AN neck. Note also that the AN does not sharply angulate the optic nerve at the falciform fold. (OphArt, ophthalmic artery; ICA, internal carotid artery). *B*. AP view (schematic). Note the two bulges of the aneurysm (AN), one ventrally at the AN origin (*arrow*), and the other in the suprasellar space. (AC, anterior clinoid process; SupHypArt, superior hypophyseal artery; OphArt, ophthalmic artery; DR, dural ring). *C*. Dorsal view (schematic). Note the suprasellar extension of the aneurysm (AN) beneath the chiasm (OC), with the pituitary stalk (PitSt) displaced across the optic midline. *Arrow* marks the ventromedial AN origin. (PComArt, posterior communicating artery; SupHypArt, superior hypophyseal artery). *D*. Lateral view (arteriogram). The aneurysm (AN) balloons both above and below the projected course of the internal carotid artery (ICA), which appears to run through the aneurysm lumen. The part of the AN below the ICA represents the initial ventral origin, while the suprasellar extension lies superior. The carotid siphon appears to open as the lesion enlarges, due to the bulge beneath and medial to the ICA. Note that the region of the typical OphArt origin is independent of the AN. *E*. CT scan. Note the midline suprasellar aneurysm (AN) that somewhat resembles a pituitary tumor.

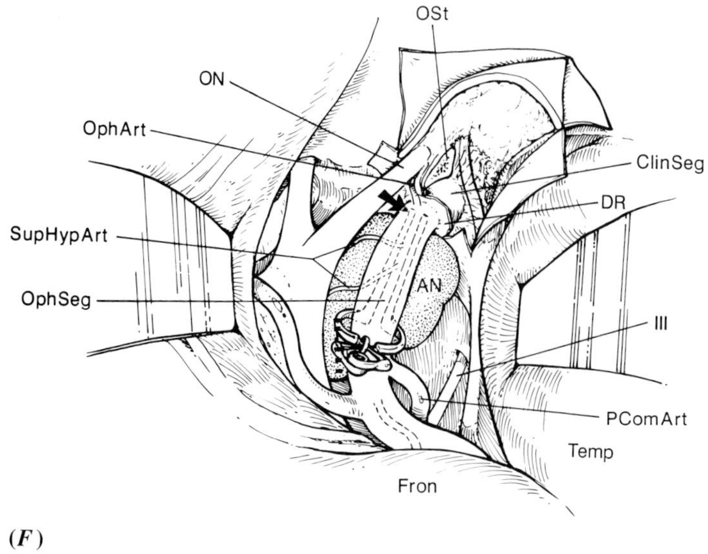

(F)

Figure 223-4 (*Continued*) *F*. Operative view, right side (schematic). The ophthalmic segment (OphSeg) and anterior clinoid process have been prepared as outlined in Fig. 223-2. Separation of the ventral aneurysm (AN) bulge from the dura adjacent to the dural ring (DR) is often aided by circumferential sectioning of the dura alongside the ring. A right-angled fenestrated clip is passed over the broadened carotid wall and carefully placed parallel to the internal carotid artery, with the fenestration reconstructing the parent vessel lumen. The butt of the clip must spare the posterior communicating artery (PComArt), while the tips of the clip are advanced to the ventromedial border (*arrow*) of the DR. If possible, the superior hypophyseal arteries (SupHypArt) should be spared, as they may provide critical blood supply to the optic nerve (ON) or chiasm. (OphArt, ophthalmic artery; ClinSeg, clinoidal segment; Fron, frontal lobe; Temp, temporal lobe; OSt, optic strut; III, third cranial nerve).

from subarachnoid aneurysms seen at other locations. The larger size and lower rupture rate of OphSeg aneurysms is probably related to the reinforcement that such lesions encounter. As an OphArt aneurysm expands upward, its fundus contacts and is subsequently capped by the overlying optic nerve, which allows it to reach giant proportions without bleeding. Similarly, SupHypArt aneurysms expanding medially or inferomedially encounter the dura of the lateral sellar wall and cavernous sinus (Figs. 223-3 and 223-4). Once this variant extends into the suprasellar space (usually after having reached a size greater than 1 cm), the dural investment becomes less protective, however, and hemorrhage risks rise.

Visual Loss

Table 223-3 lists the distribution of visual field deficits. They are usually predictive of aneurysm size and site of origin.[3,21,22,34] Aneurysms smaller than 1 cm rarely produce visual signs regardless of any association with bleeding. Six large aneurysms (four OphArt and two SupHyp suprasellar types) produced visual deficits, several of which presented with SAH and had hemorrhage directly into the optic nerve (OphArt types). The remaining patients exhibited visual deficits caused by giant aneurysms, two-thirds of which were OphArt types. No SupHypArt aneurysm that remained purely parasellar presented with visual symptoms, regardless of its size or association with SAH.

OphArt aneurysms typically trap the optic nerve immediately as it exits from the optic canal. Because this aneurysm type arises beneath the lateral aspect of the nerve, the nerve is deflected medially and is uplifted and angulated against the sharp falciform fold (Fig. 2*A*, *B*). The initial compressive forces on the lateral and superior surfaces of the optic nerve produce an early field defect in the inferior nasal quadrant—a clinical finding that is frequently overlooked by both the patient and examining physician. Further enlargement produces a nasal hemianopsia, later followed by a contralateral superior temporal quadrant defect as the anterior knee of Wilbrand is affected (junctional hemianopsia).

Because SupHypArt aneurysms arise farther along and ventromedial to the ICA, the optic nerve is usually not angulated against the falciform fold. Visual symptoms are therefore less common with this variant, even when giant proportions are reached. With enough suprasellar extension, however, inferior chiasmal compression occurs, which produces visual deficits more typical of pituitary tumors.[31,39]

Radiologic Features

Hemorrhage from OphSeg aneurysms typically appears in the subarachnoid space within the anterior chiasmatic cisterns, and occasionally in the orbitofrontal gyri.[38] Although many patients are

TABLE 223-1 General Characteristics (80 patients)

Age (mean)	54 years
Sex (F:M)	69:11 (86% F)
Presentation (type of symptoms)	
SAH only	23
Visual changes only	24
SAH + visual changes	5
Other	
Related to another aneurysm	8
Nonspecific symptoms*	20
Patients with multiple aneurysms	36/80 (45%)

*Transient ischemic attacks, headache, bruit, incidental finding, etc.
F, female; M, male; SAH, subarachnoid hemorrhage.

TABLE 223-2 Presentation vs. Size and Artery of Origin (80 patients)

	Location			Size		
Presentation	OA	SHA	Total	sm	lg	gt
SAH only	10	13	23	6	8	9
SAH + visual changes	4	1	5	—	3	2
Visual changes only	16	8	24	—	3	21
Other symptoms*	11	17	28	12	15	1
Total	41	39	80	18	29	33

*Other symptoms e.g., headache, transient ischemic attacks, bruit, incidental finding of another symptomatic aneurysm
OA, ophthalmic artery aneurysm; SHA, superior hypophyseal artery aneurysm; SAH, subarachnoid hemorrhage; sm, small (less than 10 mm); lg, large (10 to 24 mm); gt, giant (25 mm or greater)

TABLE 223-3 Visual Field Defects vs. Aneurysm Location (29 patients)

	OA	SHA
Unilateral		
Nasal	12*	0
Other	3	2
Bilateral		
Bitemporal	0	4
Homonymous	2	3
Unilateral blindness + contralateral loss	3	0
Total	20	9

* Includes 3 patients with SAH, two associated with hemorrhage into the optic nerve
† Includes 1 patient with SAH
SAH, subarachnoid hemorrhage; OA, ophthalmic artery aneurysm; SHA, superior hypophyseal artery aneurysm

quite ill from their SAH, they rarely develop an intraparenchymal clot large enough to be life-threatening. Small OphSeg aneurysms with SAH are not usually seen well on CT or MRI scanning. Aneurysms presenting with visual loss, however, are invariably defined by one of these modalities (Fig. 223-2*D*). The lesion is often larger on CT than the angiographically apparent lumen size, indicating a significant incidence of partial luminal thrombosis. Calcifications are common in giant lesions.

Arteriographically, OphArt aneurysms arise from the dorsal or dorsomedial surface of the proximal ophthalmic segment, just distal to the OphArt origin (Fig. 223-2*C*). With expansion, the lesion elevates the inferior and lateral aspects of the ipsilateral optic nerve, creating a notch or flattening on the superomedial aneurysm surface. This optic nerve position restricts expansion of the aneurysm across the midline until late in the clinical course, and often leads to inferior deflection of the ICA, with "closing" of the carotid siphon.

SupHypArt aneurysms that enlarge and extend into the suprasellar space may create a CT picture resembling that of a pituitary tumor (Fig. 223-4*E*). A flow-void seen on MRI will usually distinguish these two entities. As they extend beneath the chiasm, their medial expansion is not restricted by the optic nerve, and chiasmal-type visual deficits may be produced. Arteriographically, there is often some question on initial interpretation as to whether small SupHypArt aneurysms are actually within the subarachnoid space or are projecting into the cavernous sinus.[25,30] As this type enlarges, the ICA is often deflected laterally and superiorly, thereby "opening" the siphon (Fig. 223-4*D*). With further growth, the ventromedial parasellar space is exceeded, and the aneurysm begins to project medially into the suprasellar space. Most large and giant SupHypArt aneurysms have two "scalloped" basal surfaces, one in the parasellar region where the aneurysm originates, and the second more medially as the aneurysm extends over the diaphragma sellae beneath the chiasm.

Treatment

Direct Surgical Obliteration

The ideal treatment for symptomatic OphSeg aneurysms is clipping, with preservation of the ICA and its branches.[5,10,11,18,37] Because 40 to 50 percent of patients with one OphSeg lesion also have at least one other intracranial aneurysm, the surgeon often must decide which lesion bled. Small SupHypArt lesions that remain purely parasellar seem to have a very low hemorrhage rate compared to aneurysms at other locations. Small asymptomatic lesions are often best treated conservatively unless intervention is planned for other reasons. Larger aneurysms (greater than 1 cm—especially those with medial suprasellar extension), appear to bleed more frequently.

Bleeding is managed preoperatively in the same fashion as SAH from other aneurysm locations, using such measures as bedrest, calcium-channel blockers, hydration, ventricular drainage (when indicated), steroids, anticonvulsants, and perioperative prophylactic antibiotics. Surgery is performed on the earliest day possible following hemorrhage, provided the patient is not a poor medical risk or has not sustained significant and irreversible brain injury.

During surgery, the patient is placed in the supine position, with the head elevated above the heart to promote good venous drainage. The head is turned 45 degrees toward the opposite side, with the vertex lowered, to allow gravitational distraction of the frontal and temporal lobes from the skull base. The head and neck are draped in sterile fashion to permit visualization of the frontal and temporal regions from the midline to below the zygoma into the neck, and to allow access to the cervical carotid bifurcation for proximal control or bypass source as needed. An incision is marked over the cervical carotid bifurcation, but it need not be opened in all instances. Blood pressure, which is monitored with an indwelling radial artery catheter, is generally maintained at normal levels. If temporary ICA clipping is anticipated, intravenous barbiturates are administered until burst suppression is achieved on EEG, and are continued, together with induced hypertension, until patency in the carotid system is restored.

Bone Removal

A standard frontotemporal pterional craniotomy is used. The temporalis muscle is reflected inferiorly and posteriorly to facilitate visualization of the sphenoid ridge and orbital roof.[40] After a free bone flap is elevated, the sphenoid ridge is extensively removed, as is the posterior orbital roof and the lesser wing of the sphenoid bone covering the superior and medial surface of the superior orbital fissure.

While not always necessary for smaller lesions, removal of the anterior clinoid process is frequently required for safe and accurate clipping of large or giant lesions. With unruptured aneurysms, extradural clinoid removal can usually be done quite safely, without exposing the subarachnoid space to bone debris.[7] Generally, however, and especially following SAH, the clinoid tip is removed intradurally while the aneurysm is visualized simultaneously, thereby avoiding inadvertent rupture during extradural manipulation. As the base of the clinoid process and optic nerve are approached, a high-speed diamond drill is used to thin the bone, which is then fractured away with microcurettes. After the dura has been stripped away from the remaining clinoid tip, the process is grasped with a hemostat, gently rocked free of any remaining attachments, and removed. Bleeding is quite easily controlled with bone wax, Gelfoam (absorbable gelatin sponge; The Upjohn Company, Kalamazoo, MI), and Surgicel (oxidized regenerated cellulose; Johnson & Johnson Medical, Inc., Arlington, TX).

Intradural Technique

Proximal visualization of the carotid and ophthalmic arteries is mandatory for both OphArt and SupHypArt aneurysms. The sylvian fissure is split widely to allow an unobstructed view of the optic nerve, ICA, and aneurysm with minimal retraction. The falciform ligament should be sectioned before the aneurysm is approached, because dissection of the nerve against it may increase visual morbidity.

Although covered by thin reflections of periosteum and small venous channels, the clinoidal segment (ClinSeg) of the ICA can be freed from its loose attachments, thus providing proximal exposure for temporary ICA clipping if required.[23] This segment lies beneath the dural ring, but above the cavernous sinus, and is in clear view when the anterior clinoid process is widely resected. Although cervical carotid exposure is a reasonable alternative to proximal control within the clinoidal space, neither are substitutes for extensive clinoidal and optic strut removal.[2]

The proximal neck of OphArt aneurysms just distal to the OphArt can be separated with gentle retraction of the aneurysm base and spreading dissection using bayoneted microforceps (Fig. 223-2*E*). Although the distal neck is usually unencumbered by major branch attachments, any perforators to the optic nerves, chiasm, or hypophysis should be dissected free. A straight or side-angled clip, closed parallel to the course of the ICA and sparing the OphArt, satisfactorily secures most OphArt lesions. A clip placed perpendicular to the ICA is often ineffective in collapsing a larger lesion, and risks avulsion of the proximal aneurysm neck. Because of their superior or medial projection, small OphSeg aneurysms can often be clipped from a contralateral approach between or behind the optic nerves.[29] This capability may be important when deciding which side to treat first in a patient harboring bilateral lesions—one of which is an OphSeg type.

Small SupHypArt aneurysms may be initially hidden from the surgeon by the overlying ICA and anterior clinoid process.[5,25] In large and giant aneurysms, the ICA is displaced slightly laterally and superiorly toward the surgeon, and the entire carotid wall appears widened and incorporated into the aneurysm. By carefully following the dural surface, the part of the aneurysm wall that bulges beneath the clinoid process is separated from the parasellar dura, thus freeing the proximal neck. The PComArt or its thalamoperforating branches are often draped over the distal end of the aneurysm, and must be carefully identified, separated, and preserved. The hypophyseal stalk may be adherent to the posterior and medial aneurysm surface.

SupHypArt lesions are usually best obliterated with a fenestrated clip whose blades pass over and then run parallel to the ICA, spanning the distance between the PComArt and the dural ring (Fig. 223-4*F*). Although the OphSeg perforators (superior hypophyseal arteries) do not generally supply brain parenchyma, some reach the optic chiasm, and consequently every attempt should be made to spare them from the surgical clip.

The large type of both lesions (OphArt and SupHypArt aneurysms) tend to be associated with atherosclerosis in the carotid artery and/or adjacent aneurysm neck. Broad necks are commonplace, and are best secured by placing several clips parallel to the parent vessel (i.e., ICA). The lesion is then opened and its contents evacuated. The entire aneurysm wall does not need to be removed, but the visual apparatus must be thoroughly decompressed.

Some OphSeg lesions with marked calcification within their walls can be clipped by using barbiturate anesthesia and temporary ICA clipping, followed by removal of the laminated calcific walls through an incision into the aneurysm interior. Once the aneurysm is clipped and aspirated, an intraoperative arteriogram is frequently done to document good ICA patency, especially in giant lesions. Afterwards, all deep bone edges must be inspected, and any defects carefully sealed with muscle, bone wax, and acrylic to prevent CSF leakage. Once the dura is closed, a drain is left in the epidural space, and brought out posterior to the skin incision through a separate stab wound. Closure then proceeds in traditional fashion.

Indirect and Interventional Neuroradiologic Approaches

The term *unclippable* should not be applied to any OphSeg aneurysm until it has been surgically explored by an experienced surgeon, and until extensive removal of the sphenoid ridge, anterior clinoid process, and optic strut has been accomplished. Thereafter, or in cases where general medical risks are too high, the patient may become a candidate for one of several other types of procedures.[12,13,15,19] One option is to ligate the common carotid artery. The pressure reduction that follows this procedure is usually transient, and the reversed flow in the external carotid artery allows the ICA to remain patent and the aneurysm to continue to fill. Occlusion of the ICA is more reliable for achieving aneurysm thrombosis, but also is accompanied by a higher risk of stroke. These risks can be reduced by using trial balloon occlusion accompanied by clinical assessment and cerebral blood flow studies.[9] In patients with reduced collateral circulation and increased chances of hemodynamic stroke, a bypass procedure is indicated, although its use does not guarantee complete safety of the occlusion.

Detachable balloons are often effectively used to occlude the ICA, but their release within the aneurysm, without ICA occlusion, may be excessively hazardous. Newer coils can fill the aneurysm lumen and thrombose it, but their long-term effectiveness and safety, as well as their immediate impact on rebleeding rates and visual function (the aneurysm mass persists and may enlarge), remain to be clarified.

Results

Direct surgery and clipping leads to good neurologic outcome in most cases, including maintenance of at least stable visual function, regardless of the size of the aneurysm (Table 223-4).[5,10,11,18] Postoperative hemibody deficits are indicative of carotid compromise until proven otherwise, and occur more frequently in patients with calcified or partially thrombosed aneurysms with atherosclerosis within the ICA wall. Intraoperative digital subtraction arteriography allows documentation of ICA patency while the wound is still open and the clip can be adjusted.

Visual deterioration following surgery may be caused by intraoperative retraction of the optic nerve against the falciform fold, especially if the nerve is already distorted medially and superiorly by the underlying aneurysm. Dissection of the visual system away from the aneurysm may damage the blood supply to the optic nerve or chiasm, and should be kept to a minimum while obtaining enough exposure to ensure accurate clip placement. Inclusion of the superior hypophyseal arteries in the clip may also cause visual or hypophyseal morbidity.

The extensive removal of the anterior clinoid process, and exposure of the clinoidal segment, can lead to postoperative diplopia usually as a result of oculomotor nerve paresis. When the dural ring is opened, this nerve lies in a relatively superficial position within the wall of the clinoidal space, where it may be disturbed either by clinoid removal or by the proximally advancing clip blades.[20] Dissection of the clinoidal segment may also cause a

TABLE 223-4 Surgical Results (54 patients)

Overall Outcome*	
Excellent–good	47 (87%)
Poor	4 (7%)
Dead	3 (6%)
Visual Outcome†	
Improved	16 (73%)
Stable	6 (27%)
Worse	0 (0%)
Complications	
Death	3
Ischemic injury	6
Related to surgery (3)	
Vasospasm (3)	
Visual deficits	6
Decreased acuity (3)‡	
Transient diplopia (3)	
Infection	2
''Unclippable''	2

*Author's cases only (54 patients)
†Includes patients who presented with visual deficits only
‡Includes 3 patients without recognized preoperative visual deficits

mild ptosis and pupillary asymmetry from sympathetic nerve disturbance.

Aneurysms may arise from the clinoidal segment, and may be difficult to differentiate from OphSeg lesions.[23] These aneurysms account for some lesions formerly termed ophthalmic aneurysms that at surgery were ''unclippable'' or ruptured catastrophically. ClinSeg aneurysms frequently represent cases in which the OphArt or SupHypArt arises from the clinoidal segment. Proximal exposure is much more difficult to obtain in these lesions, because the dural ring does not define its neck. Clinoidal segment aneurysms often adhere to the undersurface of the anterior clinoid process and optic strut, and extradural clinoid removal may cause premature aneurysm rupture before proximal or distal vascular control has been established. If this type of aneurysm is anticipated, proximal ICA exposure in the cervical region is essential.

References

1. Almeida GM, Shibata MK, Bianco E. Carotid-ophthalmic aneurysms. *Surg Neurol* 1976; 5:41–45.
2. Batjer HH, Samson DS. Retrograde suction decompression of giant paraclinoid aneurysms; technical note. *J Neurosurg* 1990; 73:305–306.
3. Berson EL, Freeman MI, Gay AJ. Visual field defects in giant suprasellar aneurysms of internal carotid: report of three cases. *Arch Ophthalmol* 1966; 76:52–58.
4. Dawson BH. The blood vessels of the human optic chiasma and their relation to those of the hypophysis and hypothalamus. *Brain* 1958; 81:207–217.
5. Day AL. Aneurysms of the ophthalmic segment: a clinical and anatomic analysis. *J Neurosurg* 1990; 72:677–691.
6. Day AL. Clinicoanatomic features of supraclinoid aneurysms. *Clin Neurosurg* 1990; 36:256–274.
7. Dolenc VV. A combined epi- and subdural direct approach to carotid-ophthalmic artery aneurysms. *J Neurosurg* 1985; 62:667–672.
8. Drake CG, Vanderlinden RG, Amacher AL. Carotid-ophthalmic aneurysms. *J Neurosurg* 1968; 29:24–31.
9. Erba SM, Horton JA, Latchaw RE, et al. Balloon test occlusion of the internal carotid artery with stable xenon CT cerebral blood flow imaging. *Am J Neuroradiol* 1988; 9:533–538.
10. Ferguson GG, Drake CG. Carotid-ophthalmic aneurysms: the surgical management of those cases presenting with compression of the optic nerves and chiasm alone. *Clin Neurosurg* 1980; 27:263–308.
11. Ferguson GG, Drake CG. Carotid-ophthalmic aneurysms: visual abnormalities in 32 patients and the results of treatment. *Surg Neurol* 1981; 16:1–8.
12. Fox AJ, Vinuela F, Pelz DM, et al. Use of detachable balloons for proximal artery occlusion in the treatment of unclippable cerebral aneurysms. *J Neurosurg* 1987; 66:40–46.
13. Gelber BR, Sundt TM Jr. Treatment of intracavernous and giant carotid aneurysms by combined internal carotid ligation and extra- to intracranial bypass. *J Neurosurg* 1980; 52:1–10.
14. Gibo H, Lenkey C, Rhoton AL Jr. Microsurgical anatomy of the supraclinoid portion of the internal carotid artery. *J Neurosurg* 1981; 55:560–574.
15. Guglielmi G, Vinuela F, Duckwiler G, et al. Endovascular treatment of posterior circulation aneurysms by electrothrombosis using electrically detachable coils. *J Neurosurg* 1992; 77:515–524.
16. Guidetti B, La Torre E. Management of carotid-ophthalmic aneurysms. *J Neurosurg* 1975; 42:438–442.
17. Hayreh SS. The ophthalmic artery. In Newton TH, Potts DG (eds): *Radiology of the Skull and Brain. Angiography*, vol 2, book 2. St Louis: Mosby, 1974, pp 1333–1350.
18. Heros RC, Nelson PB, Ojemann RG, et al. Large and giant paraclinoid aneurysms: surgical techniques, complications, and results. *Neurosurgery* 1983; 12:153–163.
19. Hieshima GB, Higashida RT, Halbach VV, et al. Intravascular balloon embolization of a carotid-ophthalmic artery aneurysm with preservation of the parent vessel. *Am J Neuroradiol* 1986; 7:916–918.
20. Inoue T, Rhoton AL Jr, Theele D, et al. Surgical approaches to the cavernous sinus: a microsurgical study. *Neurosurgery* 1990; 26:903–932.
21. Jefferson G. Compression of the chiasma, optic nerves, and optic tracts by intracranial aneurysms. *Brain* 1937; 60:444–497.
22. Jefferson G. Further concerning compression of the optic pathways by intracranial aneurysms. *Clin Neurosurg* 1955; 1:55–103.
23. Knego RS, Day AL, Masson RL Jr. Aneurysms of the clinoidal segment. Presented at the 61st Annual Meeting of the American Association of Neurological Surgeons, Boston, MA, April 28, 1993.
24. Knosp E, Muller G, Perneczky A. The paraclinoid carotid artery: anatomical aspects of a microneurosurgical approach. *Neurosurgery* 1988; 22:896–901.
25. Kobayashi S, Kyoshima K, Gibo H, et al. Carotid cave aneurysms of the internal carotid artery. *J Neurosurg* 1989; 70:216–221.
26. Kothandaram P, Dawson BH, Kruyt RC. Carotid-ophthalmic aneurysms: a study of 19 patients. *J Neurosurg* 1971; 34:544–548.
27. Locksley HB. Natural history of subarachnoid hemorrhage, intracranial aneurysms and arteriovenous malformations. *J Neurosurg* 1966; 25:219–239.
28. Nakagawa F, Kobayashi S, Takemae T, Sugita K. Aneurysms protruding from the dorsal wall of the internal carotid artery. *J Neurosurg* 1986; 65:303–308.
29. Nakao S, Kikuchi H, Takahashi N. Successful clipping of carotid-ophthalmic aneurysms through a contralateral pterional approach. Report of two cases. *J Neurosurg* 1981; 54:532–536.
30. Nutik S. Carotid paraclinoid aneurysms with intradural origin and intracavernous location. *J Neurosurg* 1978; 48:526–533.
31. Raymond LA, Tew J. Large suprasellar aneurysms imitating pituitary tumour. *J Neurol Neurosurg Psychiatry* 1978; 41:83–87.
32. Renn WH, Rhoton AL Jr. Microsurgical anatomy of the sellar region. *J Neurosurg* 1975; 43:288–298.
33. Rhoton AL Jr. Anatomy of saccular aneurysms. *Surg Neurol* 1980; 14:59–66.
34. Riise R. Ocular symptoms in saccular aneurysms of the internal carotid artery. (A survey of 100 cases.) *Acta Ophthalmol* (Copenh) 1969; 47:1012–1020.

35. Rosner SS, Rhoton AL Jr, Ono M, Barry M. Microsurgical anatomy of the anterior perforating arteries. *J Neurosurg* 1984; 61:468–485.
36. Sengupta RP, Gryspeerdt GL, Hankinson J. Carotid-ophthalmic aneurysms. *J Neurol Neurosurg Psychiatry* 1976; 39:837–853.
37. Sundt TM Jr, Piepgras DG. Surgical approach to giant intracranial aneurysms: operative experience with 80 cases. *J Neurosurg* 1979; 51:731–742.
38. Vinuela F, Fox A, Chang JK, et al. Clinico-radiological spectrum of giant supraclinoid internal carotid artery aneurysms: observations in 93 cases. *Neuroradiology* 1984; 26:93–99.
39. White JC, Ballantine HT Jr. Intrasellar aneurysms simulating hypophyseal tumours. *J Neurosurg* 1961; 18:34–50.
40. Yasargil MG, Fox JL. The microsurgical approach to intracranial aneurysms. *Surg Neurol* 1975; 3:7–14.
41. Yasargil MG, Gasser JC, Hodosh RM, Rankin TV. Carotid-ophthalmic aneurysms: direct microsurgical approach. *Surg Neurol* 1977; 8:155–165.

224

Other Aneurysms of the Internal Carotid Artery

Eugene S. Flamm

This chapter will focus on the preoperative and operative management of patients with aneurysms located at the posterior communicating (PCA) and anterior choroidal (ACh) arteries and the internal carotid artery bifurcation (ICAB). Although there are many similarities in managing all patients with aneurysmal subarachnoid hemorrhage (SAH), specific details of these locations will be stressed. The aneurysms that will be discussed in this chapter constitute approximately one-third of all intracranial aneurysms and thus are among the most frequently encountered causes of SAH.

The diagnostic methods currently used to document the specific location of a cerebral aneurysm are discussed in another chapter. Computed tomography (CT) scanning, magnetic resonance imaging (MRI), and angiography are highly effective tools for arriving at a correct diagnosis of SAH, but they are only useful once the diagnosis has been suspected clinically. Although this is not usually a problem for the neurological specialist, it is important to realize that the first physician called to see a patient with the sudden onset of headache may not have the same high index of suspicion.

Preoperative Preparation

The preoperative care of patients with SAH is as important to their overall outcome as is the actual surgical procedure. Once the correct diagnosis is made, the major steps include determining the neurological status of the patient, localizing the site of the SAH, and embarking on a course that will prepare the patient for surgical obliteration of the aneurysm. Three major developments that must be looked for and dealt with should they occur during the pre- and postoperative period are rebleeding, vasospasm, and hydrocephalus.

Once diagnosed, the patient is placed at bed rest in the neurosurgical intensive care unit. Although this may not be the most quiet environment for these patients, it provides them with a team of skilled nursing personnel. Attention must be given to the patient's discomforts such as headache, bowel and bladder function, and the general apprehension associated with hospitalization.

The same principles are used for all aneurysm patients regardless of the location of the aneurysm. Thus, in patients who are awake and responsive after SAH or who improve to this level after ventricular drainage, we proceed to surgery within the first 48 h.[7] Surgery is delayed in those patients who are not conscious and are unable to follow some commands unless there is a history of more than one recent hemorrhage or the aneurysm appears to be particularly threatening. All patients are managed with a regimen that increases blood volume and maintains maximum perfusion through control of blood pressure, hemodilution, and the administration of a calcium-channel blocking agent.[8] The recent addition of transcranial Doppler (TCD) monitoring and balloon angioplasty has increased our ability to manage those patients who develop delayed ischemic deficits.[9,10] This has allowed us to be more aggressive about operating early in those patients who are at higher risk to develop cerebral vasospasm (CVS).

Control of Blood Pressure

If the patient is known to be hypertensive, the blood pressure is lowered from the known level by about 30 percent. In normotensive patients the aim is to reduce the systolic pressure by 30 percent. It is important not to use the blood pressure obtained on admission as an indication of the patient's usual pressure because it is often elevated by the SAH itself.

Anticonvulsants

All patients with SAH are placed on phenytoin as soon as they are diagnosed. This treatment is continued postoperatively for 1 month after discharge unless the patient has had a seizure in which case it is continued for at least 1 year.

With the use of diuretics and dehydrating agents such as mannitol, we have found that plasma levels of phenytoin may be well below therapeutic level at the completion of the operation. It is important to determine the plasma level at the end of surgery so that a therapeutic level of 10 to 20 μg/ml is maintained.

Steroids

In preparation for surgery, patients are started on methyl prednisolone. An intravenous dose of 250 mg every 6 h is given; this is continued at this level during the first 3 postoperative days and then tapered over the next 4 to 5 days. While on steroids, patients receive an antacid or a histamine blocker.

Fluids

Fluid management of patients is one of the main therapies for preventing and treating delayed ischemic events due to CVS. Although the current practice is to use a dihydropyridine calcium-channel blocker, randomized trials have not provided a clear indication that these substantially reduce strokes.[8] At the present time we do utilize nimodipine during the patient's hospitalization, but this is added to a vigorous regimen of hemodilution, hypervolemia, and maintenance of blood pressure at a moderately elevated level.[8]

Patients are maintained at fluid intake of about 3000 ml/day. In patients who are clinically stable, central venous pressure alone is measured and maintained from 6 to 8 cmH_2O. In cases in which fluid management is a problem because of underlying cardiac disease or in those patients with high potential for vasospasm, a Swan-Ganz catheter is used for 5 days.

TABLE 224-1 Distribution of Aneurysms

Location	Number	%
Ophthalmic	129	11.3
Posterior Communicating	266	23.3
Anterior Choroidal	55	4.8
Carotid Bifurcation	48	4.2
Anterior Communicating	209	18.3
Distal Anterior Cerebral	34	3.0
Middle Cerebral	236	20.7
Vertebrobasilar	165	14.4
Total	1142	100.0

Angiography

A variety of angiographic techniques are used today. Patients are often .transferred with a set of angiograms already performed. These are often digital studies which vary in quality and definition of the details needed for safe surgery. The surgeon must feel comfortable with these studies and be satisfied that he or she has the necessary information. Care must be taken to be certain that a complete, 4-vessel study has been performed; this can be completed postoperatively but is usually done at the time of the definitive angiogram. At the present time many magnetic resonance angiograms (MRA) are performed. We do not recommend that these be used in place of radiographic angiograms as the definitive study.

It is not our usual practice to carry out routine postoperative angiograms if the aneurysm has been punctured at the time of surgery and the patient is doing well. If the clinical course differs from what is expected, we do not hesitate to restudy the patient. This decision is often supported by increased flow velocity as noted on transcranial Doppler studies that are routinely performed. With the availability of balloon angioplasty to treat postoperative vasospasm, the use of follow-up angiography has greater importance since it is not just a method of documentation but one that can lead to further therapy.[10,11]

Case Material

This chapter is based on the author's experience with 1142 aneurysms (Table 224-1). In the past 5 years all patients were operated on soon after admission provided that they were alert or easily arousable. We continue to defer surgery in patients who are unconscious until it becomes apparent that they may improve and have a meaningful recovery. This approach is used for intracranial aneurysms in all locations. From this series, 23.3 percent of aneurysms were located at the origin of the posterior communicating artery, 4.8 percent at the origin of the anterior choroidal artery, and 4.2 percent at the carotid bifurcation. These 369 cases form the basis of this chapter and represent 33 percent of the entire series of 1142 aneurysms (Table 224-2). Aneurysms at other locations are discussed in other chapters.

Anesthesia

Preoperative Medication, Preparation, and Induction

Patients receive phenytoin, methyl prednisolone, and antibiotics 1 h prior to arriving in the operating room. The patient should arrive calm and without hypertension. This can be facilitated by premedication. The administration of morphine (5 to 10 mg) and scopolamine (0.4 mg) IM, 1 h prior to arrival in the operating room is helpful for patients with normal neurological status. Premedication should be avoided in patients with significant neurological dysfunction or changing neurological status.

Upon arrival in the operating room, single intravenous and arterial catheters are inserted. Electrocardiogram leads, precordial stethoscope, and pulse oxymeter are positioned. Capnography is also utilized. The patient is now ready for induction of anesthesia.

After preoxygenation, anesthesia is induced with fentanyl (1 to 2 μg/kg) in divided doses and thiopental (3 to 5 mg/kg) intravenously. After consciousness is lost, the patient is ventilated with oxygen. Vecuronium (0.1 mg/kg) is given for muscle relaxation. The combination of fentanyl and vecuronium commonly produces bradycardia and a mild reduction in blood pressure. Hypotension can be minimized by preinduction administration of 5% albumin or crystalloid with an osmotic pressure close to 300 osmol/kg. Additional fentanyl (up to 5 μg/kg total dose) is given in divided doses. Prior to laryngoscopy, additional thiopental (100 mg) is administered. This is followed by topical spraying of the trachea with 4% lidocaine. The laryngoscope is removed and any increase in blood pressure is treated with additional narcotic and thiopental. Laryngoscopy is repeated and the endotracheal tube inserted. This approach of a brief direct laryngoscopy for tracheal anesthesia followed by a more prolonged laryngoscopy for intubation allows excellent determination of the depth of anesthesia and prevents the very large increase in blood pressure that might otherwise occur if intubation is followed immediately upon laryngoscopy. Nitrous oxide (70% in oxygen) and isoflurane (0.2 to 4%) are typically added after intubation.

After intubation additional catheters are inserted: a central venous catheter, a large bore peripheral intravenous catheter, and a Foley catheter are inserted. In some cases a catheter is inserted into the lumbar subarachnoid space to allow intraoperative spinal fluid

TABLE 224-2 Internal Carotid Artery Aneurysms: Overall Outcome

Location	Number	Excellent and Good	Favorable (%)	Dead	Mortality (%)
PCA	266	228	86	17	6
ACh	55	48	87	2	4
ICAB	48	44	92	1	2
Total	369	320	86.7	20	5.4

drainage. It is important that an appropriate depth of anesthesia be maintained at all times to avoid hypertension during insertion of the head fixation pins. A local anesthetic is also used to minimize any painful stimulus during the application of the head holder. Any decreases in blood pressure should be treated with small amounts of phenylephrine or ephedrine rather than by reducing the depth of anesthesia.

Maintenance of Anesthesia and Hypotension

Anesthesia is maintained with a 70:30 mixture of nitrous oxide and oxygen to which isoflurane (0.2 to 1.0%) is added. With this regimen, blood pressure can be maintained at 100 to 110 mmHg systolic without difficulty. Additional blood pressure control can be obtained with trimethaphan, esmolol, or labetalol—alone or in combination.

An infusion of nitroprusside can be used if lower levels of blood pressure are desired. Although this was frequently used in the past, we do not routinely use it presently. The appropriate level of blood pressure during surgery and clipping is subject to debate. Most patients will tolerate an intraoperative blood pressure of 100 to 110 mmHg systolic. However, higher blood pressure in patients with CVS and moderate to severe hypertension may be more appropriate. Blood pressure should also be increased during periods of temporary vessel occlusion and after the final clipping of the aneurysm.

After aneurysm clipping, blood pressure should be maintained at the higher end of the patient's normal range to maximize cerebral perfusion. The amount of anesthesia should be reduced to facilitate a rapid, smooth emergence and a high degree of post-emergence awareness to allow a good neurological examination. During this period, blood pressure is best controlled by autonomic nervous system blocking drugs such as esmolol, rather than by anesthetic agents or narcotics.

Aids to Exposure

To maximize the exposure of the circle of Willis and reduce the amount of retraction required, several adjuncts are utilized. An infusion of 20% mannitol (0.5 to 1.0 g/kg) is begun at the time of the skin incision. This results in a slack brain even before the dura is opened.

The other important adjunct is spinal drainage. A catheter introduced through a Tuohy needle is inserted into the lumbar subarachnoid space after the induction of anesthesia. The drainage is not opened at this time. When the dura has been exposed and tented, the spinal drainage is begun. This delay prevents stripping away of the dura, which may cause epidural bleeding that is difficult to control. Furthermore, it is easier to open the leaves of the arachnoid in the sylvian fissure if there is some CSF present. In addition to the relaxation of the brain and reduction of the need for retraction, this method facilitates the microdissection because the surgeon can work in a drier field and does not constantly have to remove CSF while working on the aneurysm. A spinal catheter is used in all patients who have had a recent SAH. When operating on Grade 0 patients with carotid artery aneurysms we do not routinely employ spinal drainage in patients over 60 years of age or in patients who have large cisterns because adequate drainage can be achieved once the dura has been opened.

The final step to achieve a slack brain is to maintain a P_{CO_2} in the range of 25 to 30 mmHg before the dura is opened; thereafter P_{CO_2} is kept between 30 and 35 mmHg.

Equipment

Operating Microscope

Our preferred objective lens for the operating microscope is 300 mm because it allows ample room to work between the lens and the point of focus. A 20× ocular lens in an inclined *f*-160 eyepiece to achieve the maximum possible magnification with the 300-mm objective lens is preferred. Although the overall field is smaller, this poses no problem for aneurysm surgery and is offset by the advantage of the increased magnification. It is essential to be able to focus the microscope without using one's hands; this allows the surgeon to keep both hands in the field at all times and make minor adjustments of the focus as the dissection proceeds. This is particularly important when the arachnoid is being dissected from the neck of the aneurysm. The surgeon should be seated, and both the surgeon and the microscope should be free to move and change positions with minimal effort.

Instrumentation

Fairly rigid, moderately heavy bipolar forceps with different tip sizes and angulations are used. By using heavier stainless steel, rather than titanium, instruments, it is possible to use them for both dissection and coagulation. The lighter instruments do not have sufficient spring to be used in a spreading fashion to divide the arachnoid and do not provide enough proprioceptive feedback to the surgeon.

A variety of sharp arachnoid knives are an important part of the equipment needed. These can be used effectively in places that scissors cannot; small disposable blades such as the Beaver blades (Rudolph Beaver, Inc., Waltham, MA.) or the Karlin arachnoid knife (Codman & Shurtleff, Inc., Randolph, MA) can be used to good advantage for this purpose. Less traction is transmitted to the aneurysm if the arachnoid is divided sharply rather than tearing it with forceps.

It is necessary to have an adequate array of microsurgical instruments. In addition to the standard instruments, dissectors with various curved and straight tips, on both bayonet and straight handles, are helpful for retracting vessels and the aneurysm itself. A no. 7 vented Frazier-type suction tip is used on the left side with a vacuum of 100 mmHg. A larger tip is kept on the right side for the first assistant in the event the aneurysm ruptures.

Although aneurysm clips are discussed in another chapter, certain points should be stressed here. Several suitable clips should be selected and loaded by the surgeon before the dura is opened. My own preference is for larger clips that will fit the aneurysm. There is no advantage in stuffing a large aneurysm into a small clip. A complete range of sugita clips are always available, including the many varieties of fenestrated clips.

The use of a self-retaining system for brain retractors is essential for all microsurgery and particularly for surgery of aneurysms. Because the operative exposure is small, there is usually insufficient room for the hands of an assistant on a brain retractor. Furthermore the brain retraction must be gentle and precise; this can only be achieved with a mechanically secured retractor.

Surgical Technique

Preparation

The patient is positioned with the head secured in the Sugita head holder and frame. This procedure is necessary to reduce any movement of the head which will interfere with the microdissection that is carried out at 16× magnification. The head is turned to a full lateral position, and the vertex is dropped slightly toward the floor. This extension permits better direct visualization of the region of the optic nerve and carotid artery and reduces any obstruction to vision by the temporalis muscle or floor of the skull. The zygoma is almost parallel with the floor.

Initial Steps

A curvilinear incision begins at the upper border of the zygoma, 1 cm in front of the tragus. It is extended upward following the hairline in a gentle curve. It should be placed as low as possible, and yet remain behind the hairline (Fig. 224-1). The medial extent of the incision is the midpupillary line. It is not necessary to bring the medial portion of the incision onto the forehead. If a larger flap is required, the incision can be extended toward the midline. Because the incision is made in front of the ear, care should be exercised to avoid injuring the superficial temporal artery.

The scalp flap is reflected inferiorly in a single layer including the temporalis muscle. This eliminates any injury to branches of the facial nerve to the frontalis muscle; if the scalp is separated from the underlying muscle as would be necessary for an osteoplastic flap, such injury with a loss of frontalis movement usually ensues.

After the incision is made, scalp clips are applied. The temporalis fascia is incised with a scalpel so that a good closure can be achieved. The temporalis muscle is then incised with the cutting cautery and separated from the skull. The entire scalp flap is reflected in a single layer down to the level of the supraorbital ridge. The bony landmark for this step is the zygomatic process of the frontal bone; it is important to expose at least 2 cm of frontal bone along the supraorbital ridge in front of the zygomatic process. This is particularly important when the flap is on the left side. Failure to do this will limit the angle at which a right-handed surgeon can introduce instruments through this small craniotomy.

A single burr hole is placed in the temporal region. From this a free bone flap measuring 4 × 5 cm is created with the craniotome. An initial cut is made from the burr hole toward the sphenoid wing as far as is possible. The craniotome is then returned to the burr hole and the remainder of the flap created; it is usually necessary to crack the bone at the sphenoid wing by elevating the flap. It is essential that the bony opening be flush with the floor of the frontal fossa. The lateral aspect of the sphenoid wing is then rongeured away so that it will not obstruct the line of vision. It is not necessary to drill this away; 1.5 cm of the wing can easily be removed with rongeurs (Fig. 224-2). After dural tenting sutures have been placed, the spinal drain is opened.

It is difficult to describe all the nuances of the dissection techniques used in aneurysm surgery. Certain general maneuvers can be outlined for aneurysms of the carotid artery such as posterior communicating, anterior choroidal, and bifurcation locations. The first step is to identify the optic nerve. Once this has been seen, the exposure is maintained with a self-retaining retractor. The landmarks for identifying the optic nerve are the olfactory tract and the sphenoid wing. The nerve is found at the point of intersection of these two structures.

The operating microscope is now brought into use. Magnification is increased from a low setting initially to higher magnifications for dissection along the parent vessel and aneurysm. The first step of the microdissection is to divide various arachnoid connections. This frees the aneurysm from any undue traction and increases the room in which to operate within the subarachnoid space. The arachnoid between the frontal lobe and optic nerve is first divided. This plane is extended laterally into the medial portion of the sylvian fissure. As the arachnoid is divided, additional retraction increases the exposure of the carotid artery. The next step is to obtain control of the carotid artery; this is particularly important for carotid artery aneurysms. The best place to begin this portion of the dissection is between the optic nerve and the artery. Once this arachnoid is opened, the dissection can proceed along the carotid to the point of origin of the aneurysm.

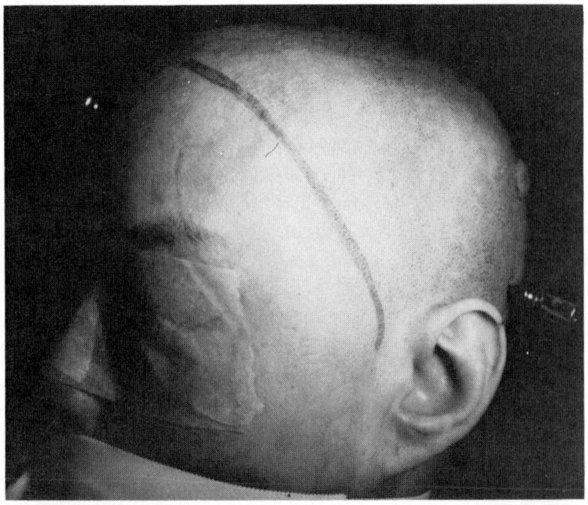

Figure 224-1 The scalp incision for the usual pterional approach. The incision is completely behind the hairline.

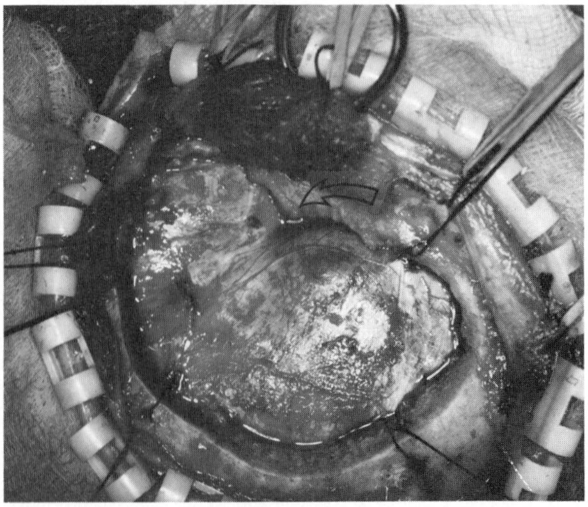

Figure 224-2 Dural exposure through a left pterional flap. The lateral aspect of the sphenoid wing (*arrow*) has been removed. The opening measures 4 × 5 cm.

TABLE 224-3 Large and Giant Cerebral Aneurysms*

Location	Number	Large and Giant	%
Ophthalmic	129	54	41.9
Posterior Communicating	266	18	6.8
Anterior Choroidal	55	8	14.5
Carotid Bifurcation	48	11	22.9
Anterior Communicating	209	20	9.6
Distal Anterior Cerebral	34	2	5.9
Middle Cerebral	236	37	15.7
Vertebrobasilar	165	34	20.6
Total	1142	184	16.1

*Diameter: 2.0–6.0 cm; Mean: 3.0 cm.

Proximal Control

With aneurysms of the carotid artery at the PCA and ACh, one can usually obtain proximal control of the intracranial carotid artery. In some situations the PCA aneurysm may be quite proximal or the aneurysm may be partially covered by the anterior clinoid process. In these situations, control of the carotid artery can only be obtained by exposing the carotid artery in the neck. While this is not often necessary, it should not be overlooked as a means of facilitating the clipping or increasing the safety of the procedure. With the widespread use of subtracted films, the relationship between the aneurysm and the anterior clinoid process and base of the skull may be overlooked.

Techniques for Large Aneurysms

In addition to these general methods that apply to the specific aneurysm sites discussed below, some special techniques for dealing with large aneurysms at these locations are necessary. Although large and giant aneurysms arising from the carotid artery are usually found at the origin of the ophthalmic artery, large and giant aneurysms may be found at the locations under discussion in this chapter (Table 224-3). Several problems that occur with aneurysms of 2-cm diameter or larger must be recognized before the clip application is attempted. The method and principles of the dissection are the same, but special attention must be given to the selection and application of the clip. Although Yasargil has advocated using bipolar coagulation of the aneurysm neck to reduce its size and permit safer clipping,[13] I do not often use this method. I prefer a larger clip when possible. The large variety of aneurysm clips now available makes it easier to find an appropriate clip for most aneurysms. Another alternative is to apply more than one clip, usually from different directions, to obliterate some of the larger aneurysms.

Another problem encountered with large aneurysms is that the wall of the neck is quite thick. This together with the large aneurysm sac may cause the clip to slip proximally and compromise the parent vessel.

An additional problem encountered with carotid aneurysms, especially large ones, is the tension within the aneurysm. This often prevents the clip from closing completely; there is also an increased chance of rupture if the clip does not completely obliterate the aneurysm when it is applied. Several techniques are available to reduce the tension within the aneurysm. Temporary occlusion of the internal carotid artery in the neck dramatically reduces the pressure in the supraclinoid carotid artery and within the aneurysm. The use of this method must be anticipated so that the carotid can be exposed in the neck before craniotomy. Although temporary clips can be applied directly to the supraclinoid carotid artery, this often reduces the working space necessary to clip the aneurysm and carries the risk of endothelial damage.

Another technique that has been helpful with large thick-walled aneurysms is suction decompression.[2] A 21-gauge scalp vein needle with the flanges removed is connected to the operating room suction. By puncturing the dome of the aneurysm where it is thick, blood can be suctioned through the aneurysm and the intraluminal tension reduced. Although this may not cause the thick-walled aneurysm to collapse, the aneurysm will become softer and more pliable. The clip can then be closed down easily and more safely. Blood loss has not been more than 150 ml when this technique is employed.

Another method is to suction through the carotid artery in the neck with the use of a flexible catheter inserted into the internal carotid artery. However, it is important to place a temporary clip distal to the aneurysm to avoid suctioning blood away from the brain.[1] Although this technique avoids putting a hole in the aneurysm, it is not always effective and does require the diversion of one of the members of the operating team from the intracranial field.

It is also important to remember that the length of the clip blade must exceed the diameter of the aneurysm neck because the collapsed neck will be longer than the distended diameter. This relationship is expressed in the formula $0.5\ \pi D = L$, where D is the diameter of the aneurysm neck and L is the length of the clip blade which indicates that the blades should be approximately 36 percent longer than the diameter of the neck.

Intraoperative Aneurysm Rupture

One of the most serious intraoperative complications of all aneurysm surgery is intraoperative rupture. This is particularly difficult to manage when it occurs during the initial exposure, prior to definition of the anatomy of the aneurysm. Aneurysms of the PCA may be particularly susceptible to this when they are adherent to the temporal lobe. In this situation, rupture of the aneurysm may occur when the temporal lobe is retracted to gain the initial exposure. The surgeon should be alert to this possibility in those patients with aneurysms of the PCA who do not have a third nerve palsy. This may indicate that the aneurysm is adherent to the temporal lobe rather than having the usual close relationship with the third nerve. This should also be suspected when the angiogram shows the aneurysm projecting lateral to the carotid artery. In these situations special attention to the placement of the temporal retractor is necessary. This should be delayed until good visualization of the aneurysm is available through the microscope. If still necessary, retraction of the temporal lobe should be done under direct visualization of the aneurysm to avoid tearing an adhesion that can safely be dissected and divided.

Even before the planes around the aneurysm are well established, the surgeon should develop a mental picture of the location of the neck. If rupture should occur before the dissection has been completed, it is helpful to have a good idea of where the neck is located so that a rapid and accurate dissection and application of the clip can be performed while bleeding is controlled by the suction. The first step in the case of a rupture is to maintain visualization of the operative field. This can often be accomplished with the accurate placement of a suction over the dome. Clip application should be attempted only after adequate dissection has been done. A temporary clip may be helpful if additional time is needed to complete the final delineation of the neck of the aneurysm as well as the branches of the carotid artery.

Posterior Communicating Artery Aneurysms

The most characteristic presentation of this aneurysm is the sudden appearance of a partial third nerve palsy at the time of the SAH. This almost always manifests itself with some pupillary abnormality. A recent report has described pupillary sparing with PCA aneurysms, but this is quite unusual.[12] In addition to anisocoria there may be ptosis and varying degrees of limitation of eye movements under the control of the third nerve. This is probably the only pathognomonic sign associated with SAH; with aneurysms in any other location it is usually not possible to be certain of the specific site.

Another common presentation of the PCA aneurysm is the development of a third nerve deficit in the absence of a SAH. The appearance of an enlarged pupil with or without involvement of other third nerve functions should be taken as diagnostic of a PCA aneurysm until proven otherwise. This usually requires angiography since neither CT scanning nor magnetic resonance angiography (MRA) is sufficient to rule out a small aneurysm in this location. Although this will undoubtedly result in some negative studies being performed, it can be fully justified because the greatest risk that such a patient can have is to sustain an SAH. If the diagnosis can be made before rupture of the aneurysm, the surgical management and overall prognosis are much improved.

About 10 percent of PCA aneurysms will not produce any third nerve deficit. When this occurs, special attention should be given to the angiogram since it often indicates that the aneurysm is projecting laterally onto the medial edge of the temporal lobe rather than in the more common downward position. This is of great importance in planning the surgical approach since care must be taken not to retract the temporal lobe prematurely and thereby rupture the aneurysm before the dissection has begun (Fig. 224-3).

The dissection for exposure of this aneurysm proceeds along the carotid artery.[4] The arachnoid between the optic nerve and the carotid artery is fully opened, as is the medial portion of the sylvian fissure. These steps are important to minimize brain retraction and the resultant forces applied to the aneurysm as well as to improve the visualization of the aneurysm and the pertinent branches of the carotid artery. The dissection should be carried out within the subarachnoid space. By elevating the arachnoid from the carotid artery, the region of the aneurysm can be easily identified. It is safer to enter this plane over the carotid artery than over the aneurysm itself.

The neck of the aneurysm is now freed of arachnoid both by sharp dissection and by the spreading of the dissecting forceps. The elevated arachnoid can be removed or coagulated to improve the exposure. Once a plane has been established on either side of the neck, attempts to identify the posterior communicating artery are made. Gentle lateral retraction of the carotid artery toward the aneurysm allows good visualization between the optic nerve and carotid artery. The communicating artery can usually be identified and spared. If necessary, this vessel can be included within the clip, provided it is truly a communicating artery and not a posterior cerebral artery arising directly from the carotid artery (Fig. 224-4). If the PCA aneurysm is somewhat distal on the carotid artery, an additional precaution is to identify the anterior choroidal artery. This vessel, unlike the posterior communicating artery, must always be preserved. Once the aneurysm has been clipped, it should be punctured not only to ensure that it is completely obliterated but also to achieve maximum decompression of the third nerve. Further dissection of the aneurysm from the third nerve is not necessary.

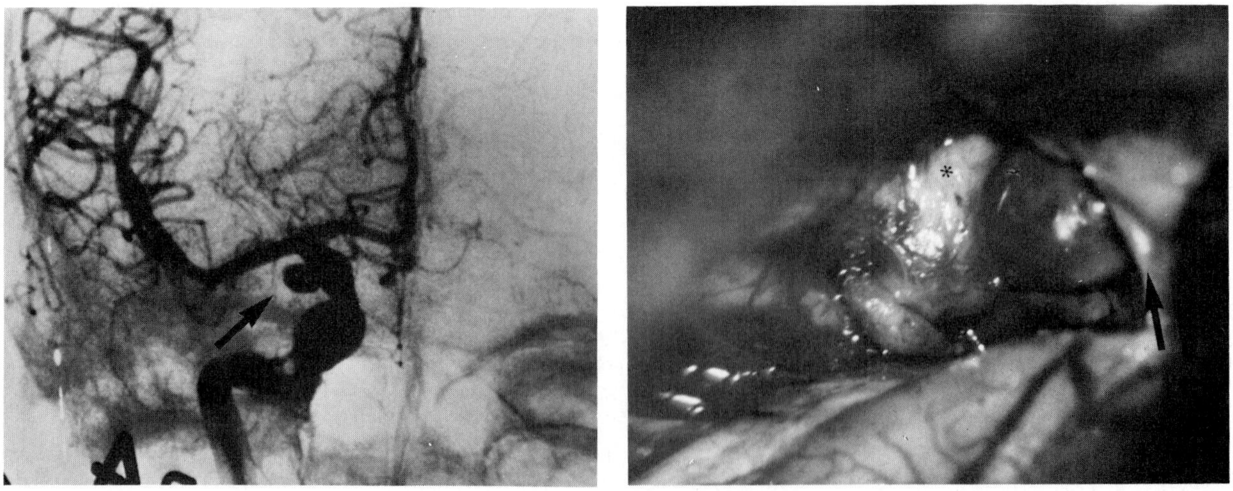

(*A*) (*B*)

Figure 224-3 *A*. A right carotid angiogram which shows a posterior communicating artery aneurysm (*arrow*) pointing laterally toward the temporal lobe. The patient did not have a third nerve palsy. *B*. The same aneurysm exposed at operation. *Right internal carotid artery; *arrow*, arachnoid of the sylvian fissure. The dome of the aneurysm is adherent to the medial aspect of the temporal lobe. (×12.)

Anterior Choroidal Artery Aneurysms

There is no specific clinical presentation of aneurysms that arise from the region of the anterior choroidal artery. They are relatively uncommon, composing less than 5 percent of the present series. Such aneurysms presented with SAH in 48 of 55 cases, temporal lobe seizures in 1, and a partial third nerve palsy in 1. They were found in association with another aneurysm in 16 cases, the most common association being with an adjacent PCA aneurysm. Seven cases were discovered by MRI performed for apparently unrelated symptoms.

Because of the important territory of the brain supplied by the anterior choroidal artery, every effort should be made preoperatively to identify the origin of this aneurysm and the artery itself.[5] At the time of the operation, great care must be taken to identify the anterior choroidal artery. Failure to do this will frequently cause the vessel to be included in the clip. In general, this is poorly tolerated and may result in an infarction in the internal capsule which produces a severe hemiparesis from which recovery is incomplete at best.

The dissection and clipping of aneurysms in this location are quite similar to the methods described for PCA aneurysms.[4] The major difference is the need to identify with certainty the anterior choroidal artery. An important aid to visualizing the anterior choroidal artery is to obtain adequate room to work at the distal end of the carotid artery. This is facilitated by widely opening the sylvian fissure. Although this is generally done as part of the initial approach to carotid aneurysms and certainly for aneurysms of the carotid bifurcation, an extra effort should be made in cases of anterior choroidal aneurysms because there is often a tendency to regard them as PCA aneurysms, which do not require the same amount of exposure. The anterior choroidal artery may course medial to the aneurysm; it becomes necessary to separate it from the aneurysm neck to prevent its inclusion in the clip. Often this can be done by working from the medial side of the carotid artery between the vessel and the optic nerve (Fig. 224-5).

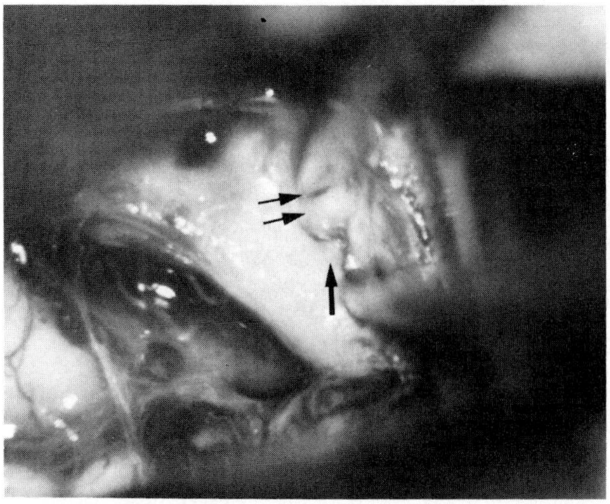

Figure 224-4 Dissection of the right posterior communicating artery from the aneurysm dome. The *arrow* indicates the origin of the right posterior communicating artery; the *double arrow* points to the wall of the aneurysm displaced by the forceps.

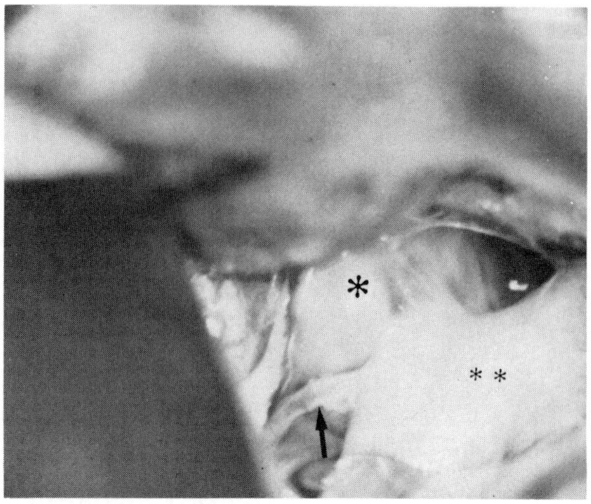

Figure 224-5 A left anterior choroidal artery aneurysm (*). The *arrow* indicates the anterior choroidal artery that has been separated from the neck of the aneurysm. **Left internal carotid artery.

Internal Carotid Bifurcation Aneurysms

Aneurysms at the distal end of the internal carotid artery are among the less frequent aneurysms of the anterior circulation. Nevertheless they can be a most challenging problem because of the size that they may attain, the increased likelihood of intraoperative rupture, and the involvement of several major vessels (i.e., the anterior and middle cerebral arteries, the anterior choroidal artery, and the internal carotid artery itself).

In most reported series and in my experience, aneurysms at the ICAB constitute about 5 percent of intracranial aneurysms (Table 224-1).[14,17] They may present as mass lesions or following SAH. There is no specific clinical presentation that increases the probability of finding an aneurysm in this location. The special considerations for this aneurysm revolve around the local anatomy, particularly the arrangement of the perforating arteries near the bifurcation of the carotid artery and the path of the anterior choroidal artery in relation to the aneurysm.[5,14]

It is imperative that the leaves of the sylvian fissure be opened so that good visualization of the artery and control of the related vessels can be obtained. This requires the use of two self-retaining retractors—one on the frontal lobe and one on the temporal lobe. Of particular importance is the exposure of the proximal anterior and middle cerebral arteries. To achieve this exposure, more retraction is needed than for other carotid artery aneurysms. These lesions often lie buried in the anterior perforated substance, a portion of the brain that should be carefully preserved.

The initial dissection is similar to that for other carotid aneurysms.[3] The carotid artery is exposed in its proximal supraclinoid segment, and dissection is carried up the sylvian fissure. It is important to divide the arachnoid bridging the lips of the sylvian fissure to gain adequate exposure. My own approach is not to proceed directly to the distal side of the bifurcation and the region of the aneurysm. When working up the carotid artery, one first encounters the anterior surfaces of the anterior and middle cerebral arteries. The dissection is then carried laterally along the middle cerebral artery and medially along the anterior cerebral artery to expose these segments before the aneurysm is confronted. By doing this, one can then return toward the aneurysm working along each of these vessels (Fig. 224-6). This allows one to identify and establish a cleavage plane between the dome of the aneurysm itself and the carotid bifurcation. The danger of proceeding directly to the bifurcation and dissecting the aneurysm is that one may enter the dome of the aneurysm while trying to establish the planes around the neck. By proceeding toward the aneurysm from the lateral and medial sides one can establish the cleavage plane and creep up on the neck of the aneurysm. It is important to keep in mind that the perforating arteries rarely arise in the immediate vicinity of the bifurcation.[5] While dissecting on these vessels, one should stay on the anterior and inferior surfaces of the vessels to avoid sacrificing any of the perforators. Once again, a path is established on either side of the neck. It is important that this be clearly visualized before attempts to pass a clip are made. Failure to do this may result in a tear of the aneurysm by one of the blades of the clip.

Even before these planes are well established, the surgeon should develop a mental picture of the location of the neck. Should rupture occur before the dissection has been completed, it is helpful to have a good idea of where the neck is so that a rapid and accurate dissection and application of the clip can be carried out while bleeding is controlled by the suction.

A point to remember is that the anterior choroidal artery passes behind the carotid artery as seen in this approach. This artery should be located before the clip is applied so that it is not included in the clip as it passes deep to the aneurysm. This is a small but important detail of this aneurysm's location.

Postoperative Management

The goals of postoperative care are to maintain adequate cerebral perfusion, reduce any postoperative cerebral swelling and increase in intracranial pressure, and prevent the occurrence of seizures. These aims can be accomplished by continuing the preoperative medical regimen of corticosteroids, anticonvulsants, and fluids.

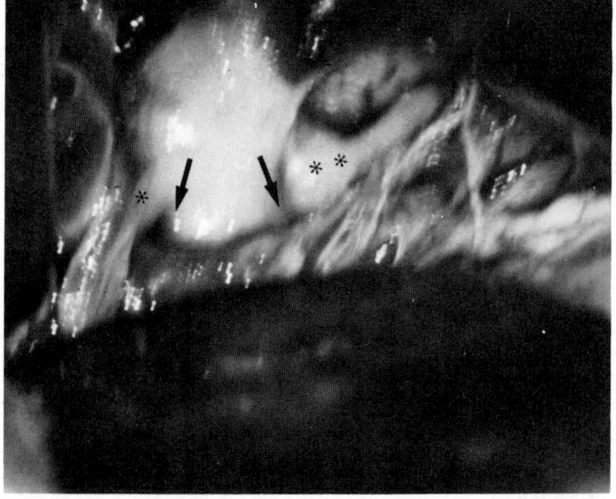

Figure 224-6 A left carotid bifurcation aneurysm. The *arrows* indicate both sides of the neck. *Middle cerebral artery; **anterior cerebral artery. Both vessels were separated before the neck was dissected.

Upon the patient's transfer to the recovery room, blood pressure is maintained at normal to slightly elevated levels. Central venous pressure is maintained at 6 to 8 cmH_2O by administering colloid and/or whole blood. Corticosteroids (in our practice, 250 mg of methyl prednisolone every 6 h) are maintained at this level for 3 days and then tapered over the next 5 days. Levels of anticonvulsants are determined initially after surgery and during the postoperative period.

Since most aneurysms have been opened intraoperatively, we do not routinely perform postoperative angiography. If there is any change in the patient's neurological condition, a rise in flow velocity with TCD measurements, or if the aneurysm was not opened at operation, angiography is performed. This is no longer only of academic interest. The availability of intra-arterial papaverine and balloon angioplasty has added important therapeutic modalities for the treatment of delayed ischemic complications.[10,11,16] In recent years we have become more willing to repeat angiography in the postoperative period since there is the option of changing the therapy.

Results

Table 224-2 summarizes the overall results. In general, the outcome follows closely the grade of the patient on admission. While this applies to those patients presenting with SAH, size of the aneurysm was related to poor outcome in those aneurysms 20 mm in diameter or larger (Table 224-3). Twelve of the 20 deaths occurred in patients with aneurysms of 20 mm or more. There were no deaths in Grade 0 patients who had not had a SAH. The remaining deaths and poor results were primarily related to the delayed ischemic events.

Future issues for patients with carotid artery aneurysms as well as patients with aneurysms at other sites are addressed in other chapters. It remains to be seen what the next few years will bring for the management of vasospasm beyond our current regimen of volume expansion. The role of intravascular procedures which address the lumen of the aneurysm but not the exclusion of the aneurysm from circulating blood still needs to be explored further.[6,15] In a separate review of 125 unruptured aneurysms at all locations operated on in the past 5 years at our institution, there have been no deaths. The direct clipping of aneurysms remains a safe, effective, and established method for dealing with these lesions. Newer technologies must improve on these results before they can be widely used or accepted. Just as beauty is in the eye of the beholder, an "unclippable aneurysm" can only be in the heart of a neurosurgeon.

References

1. Batjer HH, Samson DS. Retrograde suction decompression of giant paraclinoidal aneurysms. Technical note. *J Neurosurg* 1990; 73:305–306.
2. Flamm ES. Suction decompression of aneurysms: technical note. *J Neurosurg* 1981; 54:275–276.
3. Flamm ES. Cerebral aneurysms at the bifurcation of the internal carotid artery. In Rengachary SS, Wilkins RH (eds): *Neurosurgical Operative Atlas*. Park Ridge, IL: American Association of Neurological Surgeons, 1991, pp 87–96.

4. Flamm ES. Midcarotid artery (posterior communicating and anterior choroidal artery) aneurysms. In Apuzzo MLJ (ed): *Brain Surgery: Complication Avoidance and Management*. New York: Churchill Livingstone, 1993, pp 958–970.
5. Gibo H, Lenkey C, Rhoton AL Jr. Microsurgical anatomy of the supraclinoid portion of the internal carotid artery. *J Neurosurg* 1981; 55:560–574.
6. Guglielmi G, Vinuela F, Duckwiler G, et al. Endovascular treatment of posterior circulation aneurysms by electrothrombosis using electrically detachable coils. *J Neurosurg* 1992; 77:515–524.
7. Haley EC Jr, Kassell NF, Torner JC. The International Cooperative Study on the Timing of Aneurysm Surgery. The North American experience. *Stroke* 1992; 23:205–214.
8. Haley EC Jr, Kassell NF, Torner JC. A randomized controlled trial of high-dose intravenous nicardipine in aneurysmal subarachnoid hemorrhage. A report of the Cooperative Aneurysm Study. *J Neurosurg* 1993; 78:537–547.
9. Haley EC Jr, Kassell NF, Torner JC. A randomized trial of nicardipine in subarachnoid hemorrhage: angiographic and transcranial Doppler ultrasound results. A report of the Cooperative Aneurysm Study. *J Neurosurg* 1993; 78:548–553.
10. Hurst RW, Schnee C, Raps EC, et al. Role of transcranial doppler in neuroradiological treatment of intracranial vasospasm. *Stroke* 1993; 24:299–303.
11. Kassell NF, Helm G, Simmons N, et al. Treatment of cerebral vasospasm with intra-arterial papaverine. *J Neurosurg* 1992; 77:848–852.
12. Kissel JT, Burde RM, Klingele TG, Zeiger HE. Pupil-sparing oculomotor palsies with internal carotid-posterior communicating artery aneurysms. *Ann Neurol* 1983; 13:149–154.
13. Krayenbühl H, Yasargil MG, Flamm ES, Tew JM. Microsurgical treatment of intracranial saccular aneurysms. *J Neurosurg* 1972; 37:678–686.
14. Pia HW. Classification of aneurysms of the internal carotid system. *Acta Neurochir (Wien)* 1978; 40:5–31.
15. Setton A, Berenstein A. Interventional neuroradiology. *Curr Opin Neurol Neurosurg* 1992; 5:870–880.
16. Torner JC, Kassell NF, Haley EC Jr. The timing of surgery and vasospasm. *Neurosurg Clin North Am* 1990; 1:335–347.
17. Yasargil MG, Smith RD, Gasser C. Microsurgery of the aneurysms of the internal carotid artery and its branches. *Prog Neurol Surg* 1978; 9:58–121.

225 Middle Cerebral Artery Aneurysms

Roberto C. Heros

Clinical Aspects

Middle cerebral artery (MCA) aneurysms account for approximately 20 percent of all intracranial aneurysms.[13,15,17] The majority are located at the first major bifurcation of the MCA. A few arise more proximally on the main trunk, at the origin of an early frontotemporal or anterior temporal branch or in relation to the perforating lenticulostriate vessels. Another small proportion arise at a more distal bifurcation of one of the main divisions. A review of the literature and personal experience suggest that giant MCA aneurysms are more common than giant aneurysms in other locations, with the possible exception of the paraclinoid region of the internal carotid artery. This observation might relate to the fact that MCA aneurysms can reach massive proportions without producing symptoms from encroachment on vital structures.

When large enough, unruptured MCA aneurysms can produce clinical symptoms from mass effect.[7] Headaches associated with signs of increased intracranial pressure, including papilledema, occur rarely with the larger aneurysms. Temporal lobe epilepsy is another symptom that occurs rarely as a result of MCA aneurysms but only exceptionally as a result of aneurysms in other locations. Ischemic symptoms such as transient ischemic attacks and small strokes, although rarely due to aneurysms, occur more frequently with aneurysms of the MCA than with aneurysms in other locations. These symptoms are thought to result from intra-aneurysmal thrombosis with subsequent embolism. Only exceptionally has a major stroke occurred as a consequence of spontaneous thrombosis of the MCA or one of its major divisions as a result of aneurysmal expansion.

Rupture of an MCA aneurysm usually results in a syndrome indistinguishable from that associated with subarachnoid hemorrhage from rupture of an aneurysm in any other location. Certain clinical characteristics, however, favor the diagnosis of a ruptured MCA aneurysm. These characteristics were first described in detail by Höök and Norlén.[7] About 60 percent of patients with an MCA aneurysm lose consciousness at the onset of rupture—a higher proportion than with aneurysms at other locations. Diffuse headache is, of course, of no localizing significance, but about one-third of patients with a ruptured MCA aneurysm have primarily unilateral headache, which is much less commonly seen after rupture of aneurysms elsewhere. When such unilateral headache is present, it is almost always on the side of the aneurysm. About 80 percent of the patients in Höök and Norlén's series had focal neurological deficits when first seen. Such deficits were severe in half of the patients and usually consisted of hemiparesis, aphasia, visual field deficits, and central facial weakness. Only 34 percent of patients with ruptured aneurysms in other locations had such findings when first seen and only 7 percent had severe deficits.[7] When a patient with a ruptured aneurysm is first seen awake but with a severe hemiparesis, the most likely location of the aneurysm by far is the MCA. These aneurysms are also slightly more likely to result in seizures after rupture than aneurysms in other locations. In all likelihood, the propensity of MCA aneurysms to cause focal symptoms and signs is due to their tendency to bleed at least partially into the brain parenchyma as well as into the subarachnoid space. Thus, the incidence of intracerebral hematomas in patients with ruptured MCA aneurysms is between 30 and 50 percent, which is considerably higher than with aneurysms in other locations.[2,8] These intracerebral hematomas are frequently of great diagnostic value when identified by computed tomography (CT). A hematoma extending into both the frontal and the temporal opercula, bridging the sphenoid ridge, is virtually pathognomonic of a ruptured MCA aneurysm.

In terms of radiologic diagnosis, little can be said specifically for MCA aneurysms. An early CT scan is mandatory to establish the diagnosis of SAH, to localize and quantitate the amount of blood in the cisterns in order to predict the likelihood and location of vasospasm, and to determine whether an intracerebral hematoma is present. The timing of angiography is related to each surgeon's particular bias about the timing of surgery. My personal policy is to perform early angiography in all of these patients. This is particularly important for patients with a large intratemporal hematoma because their condition can deteriorate abruptly, and surgical evacuation of the clot may suddenly become mandatory. Under such circumstances, it is comforting to have in hand an angiogram delineating the anatomy of the lesion, which is usually dealt with when the clot is evacuated. Another reason for early angiography is that vasospasm is not likely to be present and thus the aneurysm and its surrounding anatomy can be demonstrated optimally. Angiography is, of course, essential in demonstrating the presence and location of the aneurysm and in providing a rough guide to the relation of the aneurysm to the major branches of the MCA. My experience indicates that it is not necessary to obtain multiple views to ascertain the presence or absence of a neck or the relationship of the MCA branches to the neck. Whether demonstrated or not, a neck is almost invariably present in all but the largest aneurysms. The anatomic details must be worked out at surgery by thorough exposure of the aneurysmal complex and cannot be predicted accurately even with the best angiographic technique. Magnetic resonance imaging (MRI) is of value in patients with giant aneurysms because it can show the true size of the lumen and anatomic relations optimally. In the acute stage, however, it should not be used instead of a CT scan because the presence and quantity of subarachnoid blood are better seen in the latter.

The question of early versus late surgery remains scientifically unsettled. However, it is clear that most experienced aneurysm surgeons throughout the world are currently operating early on most patients who are in good condition. With MCA aneurysms the rationale for early surgery is even stronger. As discussed earlier, these aneurysms are frequently associated with temporal lobe hematomas, which may require emergency drainage. It is possible, of course, to gently evacuate a portion of the clot, enough to effect adequate decompression, and to leave the clot around the aneurysm until the aneurysm is clipped at a later date. I prefer, however, always to clip the aneurysm at the time of evacuation of the clot. There is usually a large space to work through without brain retraction after the hematoma is evacuated and, in my opinion this facilitates dissection and clipping of the aneurysm. Also, I worry about rebleeding from the unclipped aneurysm once the clot has been evacuated. Additionally, in many of these patients the bleeding has been primarily into the brain parenchyma rather than into the subarachnoid space, and therefore vasospasm is not a significant problem. It is in this group of patients with large temporal lobe hematomas that we have seen our only successful outcomes after operation on grade 4 patients and even on one occasion on a moribund patient. These comments, of course, do not apply to patients with deep hematomas in the frontal lobe or basal ganglia, since evacuation of these clots does not necessarily facilitate exposure.

Even in the absence of a temporal lobe hematoma, patients with MCA aneurysms are ideal candidates for early surgery. These aneurysms are located peripherally, and therefore deep retraction is not necessary, since they can be exposed by opening the fissure peripherally or by suctioning some of the superior temporal gyrus without much retraction at all, as will be discussed below. In addition, the subarachnoid clots in these patients are frequently localized in the sylvian fissure, and removal of the clot can be accomplished more thoroughly through a unilateral exposure than with centrally located aneurysms. This more thorough clot removal may be a factor in decreasing the incidence of vasospasm. Even when vasospasm supervenes, it has been our clinical impression that its consequences are less devastating when the subarachnoid clot, and hence the resultant vasospasm, is limited to one major arterial territory.

The following section will describe the surgical approaches commonly used for MCA aneurysms. Problems and techniques specific to giant aneurysms will not be discussed since they are the subject of a separate chapter in this book.

Surgical Approaches

There are three basic approaches to MCA aneurysms. They involve (1) opening the sylvian fissure medially and following the MCA trunk distally or following the major divisions proximally either (2) by opening the fissure peripherally or (3) by subpial dissection after resection of a portion of the superior temporal gyrus. At times a surgeon can use a combination of these approaches or change from one approach to another when difficulties are encountered. It is important that the surgeon be familiar with each of these approaches because although he or she may use one preferentially, there are specific instances in which an alternative approach may be necessary.

Medial Trans-Sylvian Approach

When the aneurysm is approached by initially opening the sylvian fissure, the scalp incision and bone flap are the same as used for other aneurysms of the anterior circle of Willis. I use the basic pterional approach elaborated by Yaşargil and Smith[17] and described in detail elsewhere in this book. The importance of a thorough removal of the pterion and of the lateral wing of the sphenoid to achieve a low approach at the expense of bone removal rather than of brain retraction cannot be overemphasized. Just as important is the vigorous downward retraction of the muscle toward the temporal fossa, since nothing is gained by a thorough bone removal if overhanging muscle obstructs the view. I prefer to use a free bone flap and turn the flap of skin and muscle together by opening the fascia and the muscle along the same line of the skin incision posteriorly and then detaching the muscle from the bone by subperiosteal dissection and leaving it attached to the skin flap. I have found that cutting the anterior (frontal) attachments of the muscle fibers from within facilitates retraction of the muscle backward and downward toward the temporal fossa with barbless fishhooks or sutures attached to strong rubber bands. If this is done, it is important to resuture the muscle anteriorly during closure to avoid a cosmetically unpleasant depression over the pterional region. If the anterior incision of the muscle attachment is made only through the muscle fibers down to the plane of areolar and fatty tissue between the muscle and the temporalis fascia, the frontal branch of the facial nerve, which runs in this plane, will not be injured. Another step I have found useful in preventing injury to the frontalis nerve is to start the incision at the level of the zygoma just in front of the tragus, as opposed to 1 or 1.5 cm in front of the tragus as is frequently illustrated. By starting the incision just in front of the tragus, one spares not only the frontalis nerve, but also the superficial temporal artery, or at least its frontal branch, which may, on occasion, be used later for a bypass graft.

After the dura is opened and tented inferiorly to allow a flat subfrontal approach along the sphenoid ridge, cerebrospinal fluid (CSF) can be suctioned from the medial cisterns to facilitate exposure. I have not found it necessary to insert a lumbar CSF drain routinely, but this is a matter of preference. After adequate relaxation is obtained, the surgeon decides whether the exposure will proceed from medial to lateral or vice versa. In the former case, the carotid cistern is opened by sharp arachnoidal dissection, and then the medial aspect of the sylvian fissure is opened, preferably on the frontal side of the sylvian veins.[9] I have never hesitated to coagulate any vein that bridged the medial aspect of the fissure, regardless of its size. It must be pointed out that the exact location of the fissure medially is not always apparent and that the fissure does not always "open" in a clean arachnoidal plane, as is frequently illustrated. Occasionally, particularly in cases of recent hemorrhage, a small amount of brain must be suctioned in order to follow the carotid artery as it continues to curve laterally to become the MCA. The placement of the self-retaining retractors at this stage is critical. The frontal and temporal opercula must be gently retracted to put the medial aspect of the fissure under some stretch. This is best accomplished by gradually opening the tips of the retractors as the dissection proceeds. The vector of retraction is at 90 degrees, with the frontal lobe retracted superomedially and the temporal lobe posterolaterally. It is preferable to retract more on the temporal side, since excessive retraction of the frontal operculum can be harmful, particularly on the dominant side, where it can result in expressive aphasia.[11]

The MCA is followed along its anterior-inferior aspect, away from the perforating vessels. Usually one or two temporal or frontotemporal branches will be seen before the aneurysm is reached. When the aneurysm arises from the M_1 segment in relation to a perforating branch, it is necessary only to carefully separate the perforators from the neck enough to pass a clip. These aneurysms usually are not too large and point straight upward into the frontal lobe; it is not necessary to dissect the dome completely. In aneurysms of the bifurcation (or, rarely, trifurcation) of the MCA, however, complete dissection of the aneurysmal complex is usually preferable. This can be done with relative safety after a small portion of the MCA just proximal to the aneurysm has been prepared for temporary clipping in case of rupture. After preparing the neck as well as possible for clipping, the surgeon can advance the dissection distally, frequently in a subpial plane, leaving a small amount of adherent clot and brain with the dome. The relationship of the divisions to the dome is then worked out and, more frequently than not, at least one division must be separated carefully from the base of the aneurysm by sharp dissection to define the true neck. Particular care must be taken in sparing the important recurrent perforators that so frequently come from the origin of the major divisions.[3,9] Except in the case of small aneurysms, it is frequently necessary to replace the clip several times because of kinking of one division or ''slipping'' of the clip proximally onto the MCA. This frequently is an indication for further dissection to separate the divisions more proximally down to a narrower neck. With large aneurysms, I have found it helpful to use a small self-retaining retractor on the aneurysm itself. A small Rhoton-type dissector fits nicely into the arm of the Greenberg self-retaining retractor and can be used for this purpose, freeing both the surgeon's hands. With the aneurysm retracted in one direction, the surgeon can retract the vessel gently away from the aneurysm to stretch the arachnoid bands that must be sharply divided to separate the vessel from the aneurysm.[6]

One of the few recent technical refinements in aneurysm surgery has been the increased use of temporary clipping. Although introduced in 1960 by Pool and Housepian,[10] temporary clipping had not been widely used until recently.[1,14,16] Generally, we prefer to expose and prepare the neck as thoroughly as it appears safe and use a temporary clip as close to the aneurysm as possible only for the final dangerous aspect of the dissection and for clip application, which usually takes less than 5 minutes and for which we do not use any special protective measures. For many small straightforward aneurysms it is not necessary to use a temporary clip. In some giant aneurysms, temporary proximal clipping or complete temporary trapping will be necessary for considerably longer times, such as when aneurysmorrhaphy is required. In these instances some form of cerebral protection is indicated.[1,14,16] We usually use hypervolenia, mannitol, and temporary elevation of the blood pressure with or without barbiturates. Special low force clips are required for temporary clipping.

Lateral Trans-Sylvian Approach

In many instances it is preferable to open the sylvian fissure peripherally, find the distal divisions, and dissect proximally toward the aneurysm. This approach has the advantage of facilitating exposure of the distal anatomy of the aneurysmal complex, which is usually the difficult aspect of the case. The major disadvantage is that the surgeon reaches the aneurysm before achieving proximal control. To correct this situation, Yaşargil and Smith recommend starting the dissection medially on the fissure to expose the MCA and to achieve proximal control, and then moving laterally.[17] As mentioned previously, the exact location of the sylvian fissure may not always be obvious. A helpful maneuver is to pick a relatively large cortical vessel and follow it medially toward the fissure.[11,17]

Superior Temporal Gyrus Approach

When the fissure cannot be easily identified distally, as frequently happens with recent hemorrhage, it can be entered at a depth of 1.5 to 2 cm through a small incision, with subpial resection in the anterior portion of the superior temporal gyrus.[6] When this approach is planned, the patient is placed in the supine position with

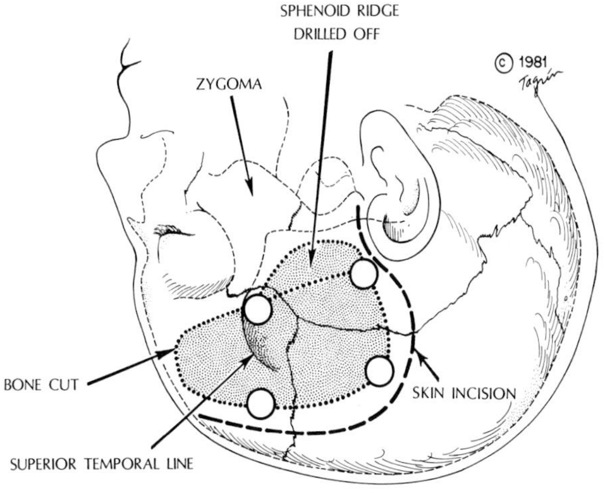

Figure 225-1 A diagram of the skin incision (*dashed line*) and bony opening (*stippled area*) for the superior temporal gyrus approach. (From Heros et al.,[6] with permission.)

the head turned about 60 degrees to the contralateral side, which is a slightly greater angle than for the usual pterional approach. A roll placed under the ipsilateral shoulder sometimes facilitates turning of the neck.

The incision is started at the level of the zygoma, just in front of the tragus, as discussed for the medial trans-sylvian approach. The only difference here is that the incision curves slightly backward above the ear before starting to swing forward to a point just about 1 cm in front of the hairline at about the level of the pupil (Fig. 225-1). As already discussed, this type of incision will preserve the frontalis branch of the facial nerve and the frontal branch of the superficial temporal artery. The muscle is turned down with the skin flap, as already discussed, and the anterior attachments of the muscles are cut so that the muscle can be retracted backward and downward into the temporal fossa. The bone flap is then cut in the same manner as for the standard pterional approach, but the cut is extended farther back into the temporal bone to expose more of the temporal lobe (Fig. 225-1). The pterion and the lateral aspect of the sphenoid ridge are totally removed. This step is important because it exposes the anterior aspect of the sylvian fissure, which allows dissection of the aneurysm and clip application from an anterolateral direction as well as from a posterior direction. If the pterion is not removed completely, the surgeon is forced to work only from behind, underneath the overhanging bone, which may be a significant handicap.

The dura is opened inferiorly in a crescentic fashion with a perpendicular posterior cut along the sylvian fissure, as illustrated in Fig. 225-2. When I use this approach, I do not open the medial cisterns, since brain relaxation is less critical with this approach than with the others because the exposure is obtained by suction of nonessential brain tissue. As soon as the dura is opened, the microscope is brought into the field, and a 1.5- to 2-cm incision is made in the superior temporal gyrus beginning just behind the front of the sylvian fissure and continuing posteriorly in a direction parallel to the fissure (Fig. 225-2). With suction and bipolar coagulation, the incision is extended medially into the vertical segment of the sylvian fissure over the insula. The sylvian veins are not disturbed. By microsurgical technique the branches of the MCA are followed proximally toward the aneurysm (Fig. 225-3). It is usually possible to follow one of the two major divisions toward the base of the aneurysm without disturbing the dome. This is done by following

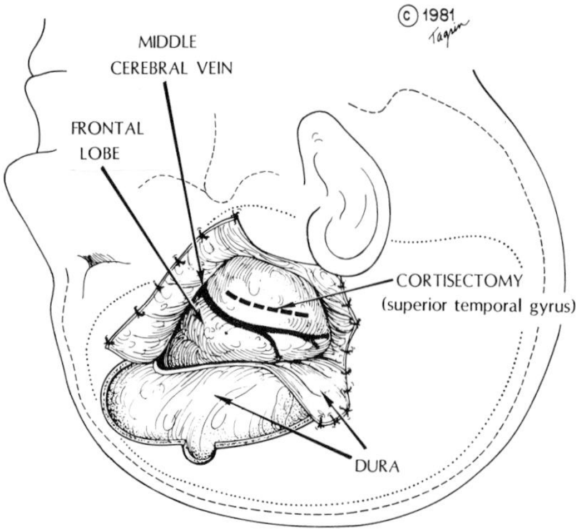

Figure 225-2 A diagram showing the dural opening and line of cortisectomy in the superior temporal gyrus (*dashed line*). (From Heros et al.,[6] with permission.)

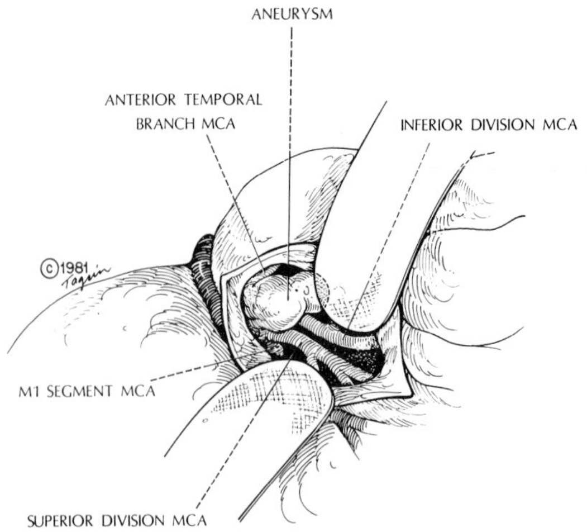

Figure 225-4 A diagram showing the exposure of the middle cerebral artery aneurysm through the superior temporal gyrus. (From Heros et al.,[6] with permission.)

the division on the side away from the aneurysm until the distal portion of the MCA can be seen. Only enough of the distal trunk of the MCA is exposed to allow the application of a temporary clip, should such become desirable. By this time the second division is usually in view and can also be followed to the aneurysm. Once the distal part of the trunk of the MCA and the origins of the main divisions have been identified, we usually proceed with a dissection of the entire aneurysmal complex, taking the precaution of leaving adherent brain and clot on the dome in the area of likely rupture (Fig. 225-4). In all but the simple, small aneurysms, we now use a temporary clip for these final stages of dissection and clipping.

Even though most of these aneurysms come from a true bifurcation, there is usually a third branch from the MCA just before the origin of the aneurysm or from one of the major divisions just after the origin of the aneurysm. Of course, every effort should be made to preserve each of these branches. In addition, it is very important to keep in mind the recurrent perforating vessels that can arise from the divisions, as discussed earlier. The approach through the superior temporal gyrus is particularly well suited to large aneurysms, since the surgeon has better circumferential access to the aneurysm and is able to retract it in any direction in order to expose the anatomy at the base and neck of the aneurysm.

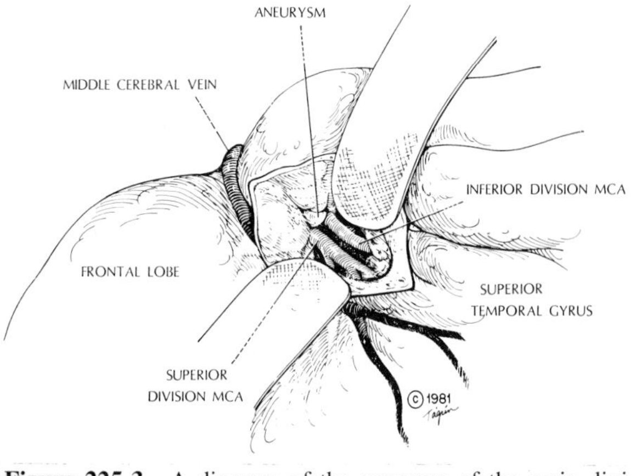

Figure 225-3 A diagram of the exposure of the main divisions of the middle cerebral artery through the superior temporal gyrus. (From Heros et al.,[6] with permission.)

The choice of approach to MCA aneurysms is determined by the individual surgeon's preference, by the position and configuration of the aneurysm, and by the ease of identification of the distal aspect of the sylvian fissure. Most MCA bifurcation aneurysms project laterally as a direct continuation of the MCA; less commonly they project caudally or rostrally.[6,12] In these cases, a distal to proximal approach, either by opening the sylvian fissure directly or through the superior temporal gyrus, allows the surgeon to expose the main trunk of the MCA without disturbing the dome of the aneurysm by following the branches proximally to the base of the aneurysm. In the rare cases in which the aneurysm projects mostly backward over the insula, the dome of the aneurysm is in the way when the aneurysm is approached from a distal direction. Therefore, we prefer to approach these aneurysms from a medial direction by splitting the sylvian fissure. It must be emphasized that this latter type of projection is unusual.

The superior temporal gyrus approach is not suited to aneurysms of the main trunk of the MCA proximal to the bifurcation or to those aneurysms that arise from the MCA at the point of origin of an early temporal branch. This approach is also not suitable for patients in whom the main trunk of the MCA is short and the aneurysm arises from an early bifurcation that occurs before the genu, that is, from the point at which the MCA starts to turn upward around the limen of the insula. In these instances, the aneurysm arises from the horizontal segment of the MCA beneath the insula, and nothing is gained by a temporal lobe resection because the surgeon must work from an anterior position to avoid damage to the insular region. The medial trans-sylvian approach is ideal for these cases.

One of the advantages of the superior temporal gyrus approach to MCA aneurysms is that significant retraction of the frontal operculum is avoided, and the exposure is achieved by suctioning nonessential brain tissue rather than by retraction. This advantage would seem to be particularly important in acute operations when the brain is swollen and hyperemic. There is also no doubt about the advantage of this approach in cases of a large anterior temporal

TABLE 225-1 Middle Cerebral Artery Aneurysms*

Preoperative Grade (Hunt)	Number of Cases	Surgical Result			
		Good	Fair	Poor	Dead
0, I, II	77	66	6	3	2
III	20	8	8	3	1
IV	6	1	3	1	1
V	5	0	2	0	3
Total	108	75	19	7	7

*Includes 27 patients with giant aneurysms.

hematoma, and even surgeons who routinely prefer to use the medial approach would ordinarily approach these aneurysms through the clot under such circumstances. Another relative advantage of working through the temporal lobe is that the sylvian veins are left undisturbed. Although we are not convinced that occlusion of these veins definitely leads to any difficulty, there is, of course, the theoretical possibility of venous congestion if the sylvian veins are injured, as occasionally occurs with the approach through the fissure. The transtemporal approach also avoids manipulation of the medial circle of Willis and of the proximal portion of the MCA with its important dorsal perforators. Whether such manipulation has any relationship to postoperative vasospasm is a question that remains unsettled.

The most important advantage of the distal to proximal approach, whether by opening the fissure directly or through the superior temporal gyrus, is that the distal, dorsal aspect of the aneurysmal complex is more thoroughly exposed. This is the most difficult portion of the aneurysmal anatomy to visualize, and it should be defined as well as possible before clipping is attempted, especially in the case of larger aneurysms. The distal approach combined with a thorough removal of the pterion allows, as discussed above, circumferential access to the aneurysm and placement of the clip from any direction. The main disadvantage is that the base of the aneurysm is encountered before proximal vessel control is assured. However, it is almost always possible to expose enough of the distal MCA to allow for the application of a temporary clip, should such become necessary, before exposing the dome of the aneurysm.

In conclusion, although early in my experience I used the superior temporal gyrus approach preferentially, I currently limit it to cases of large and giant aneurysms that are located relatively peripherally at the MCA bifurcation.

I also use this approach in cases of large temporal lobe hematomas or in other cases where, because of recent hemorrhage, there is difficulty identifying and opening the fissure distally. Most ordinary MCA bifurcation aneurysms are currently being exposed directly through the distal sylvian fissure. When the aneurysm is more proximal in the MCA trunk or at the bifurcation in cases of a short MCA trunk, I use the medial sylvian approach.

Results

Table 225-1 summarizes my surgical results with 108 consecutive MCA aneurysms operated on since 1980. Early in the series most patients were operated on late after SAH, usually on days 10 to 14; for the last 6 or 7 years, however, most patients in good neurologic condition (Hunt grades I, II, and III without neurological deficit) have been operated on early. In addition, patients in grades IV and V with a large intratemporal hematoma have usually been operated on emergently, sometimes without a preoperative arteriogram. The grade immediately before operation is compared with the result at the time of the last follow-up available, usually 6 months to a year after operation. A good result means a normal patient or a patient who had a minor neurological deficit that resolved completely within 3 months. A fair result indicates a patient who is ambulatory and independent but with a persistent mild to moderate neurological deficit. A poor result implies a patient incapacitated with a permanent moderate to severe neurological deficit. It should be emphasized that these are surgical resutls and not ''management'' results. The latter, of course, would be more meaningful but my personal records do not allow their compilation since data are missing for many patients with SAH who for one reason or another did not come to surgery.

Complications

With the exception of herniation from the mass effect of a temporal hematoma, no preoperative complication is peculiar to MCA aneurysms. The incidences of rebleeding, vasospasm, and hydrocephalus are probably not significantly different from those associated with aneurysms in other locations.[1] It has been our experience that the incidence of electrolyte disturbances and other evidence of hypothalamic dysfunction is a bit lower with MCA aneurysms than with aneurysms located more proximally in the circle of Willis, such as aneurysms of the anterior communicating complex.

Operative complications were seen mostly with large and giant aneurysms and include the gamut of technical problems typically encountered by other surgeons.[9,15–17] They include occlusion of the MCA trunk by an improperly placed clip in one patient and during aneurysmorrhaphy in another patient with a giant aneurysm, and occlusion of a major division in two other patients with giant aneurysms. Two other patients with preoperative hemiparesis from the mass effect of massive aneurysms did poorly.[5] The poor results and deaths in patients in grades 4 and 5 were from unsuccessful attempts at salvaging patients with herniation from a large temporal hematoma. Vasospasm accounted for several of the fair and poor results. Details of these complications have been discussed elsewhere.[4–6]

References

1. Charbel FT, Ausman JI, Diaz FG, et al. Temporary clipping in aneurysm surgery: technique and results. *Surg Neurol* 1991; 36:83–90.

2. Graf CJ, Nibbelink DW. Cooperative Study of Intracranial Aneurysms and Subarachnoid Hemorrhage: report on a randomized treatment study. III. Intracranial surgery. *Stroke* 1974; 5:559–601.
3. Grand W. Microsurgical anatomy of the proximal middle cerebral artery and the internal carotid artery bifurcation. *Neurosurgery* 1980; 7:215–218.
4. Heros RC. Middle cerebral artery aneurysms. In Wilkins RH, Rengachary SS (eds): *Neurosurgery.* New York: McGraw-Hill. 1985, pp 1376–1383.
5. Heros RC, Kolluri S. Giant intracranial aneurysms presenting with massive cerebral edema. *Neurosurgery* 1984; 15:572–577.
6. Heros RC, Ojemann RG, Crowell RM. Superior temporal gyrus approach to middle cerebral artery aneurysms: technique and results. *Neurosurgery* 1982; 10:308–313.
7. Höök O, Norlén G. Aneurysms of the middle cerebral artery. *Acta Chir Scand [Suppl]* 1958; 235:1–39.
8. Lougheed WM, Marshall BM. Management of aneurysms of the anterior circulation by intracranial procedures. In Youmans JR (ed): *Neurological Surgery: A Comprehensive Reference Guide to the Diagnosis and Management of Neurosurgical Problems,* 1st ed. Philadelphia: Saunders, 1973, pp 731–767.
9. Peerless SJ. The surgical approach to middle cerebral and posterior communicating aneurysms. *Clin Neurosurg* 1974; 21:151–165.
10. Pool JL, Housepian E. Temporary clip occlusion of major cerebral arteries during intracranial aneurysm surgery. *Surg Forum* 1960; 10:791–794.
11. Rand RW. Microneurosurgery in cerebral aneurysms. In Rand RW (ed): *Microneurosurgery*, 2d ed. St Louis: Mosby, 1978, pp 311–324.
12. Rhoton AL Jr, Saeki N, Perlmutter D, Zeal A. Microsurgical anatomy of common aneurysm sites. *Clin Neurosurg* 1979; 26:248–306.
13. Robinson RG. Ruptured aneurysms of the middle cerebral artery. *J Neurosurg* 1971; 35:25–33.
14. Samson DS, Batjer HH. Intracranial Aneurysm Surgery: Techniques. Mount Kisco, NY: Futura Publishing, 1990, pp 83–95.
15. Sundt TM Jr, Kobayashi S, Fode NC, Whisnant JP. Results and complications of surgical management of 809 intracranial aneurysms in 722 cases: related and unrelated to grade of patient, type of aneurysm, and timing of surgery. *J Neurosurg* 1982; 56:753–765.
16. Suzuki J, Kodama N, Fujiwara S, Ebina T. Surgical treatment of middle cerebral artery aneurysms: from the experience of 174 cases. In Suzuki J (ed): *Cerebral Aneurysms: Experience with 1000 Directly Operated Cases.* Tokyo: Tokyo Press, 1979, pp 278–283.
17. Yasargil MG, Smith RD. Middle cerebral artery aneurysms. In Youmans JR (ed): *Neurological Surgery: A Comprehensive Reference Guide to the Diagnosis and Management of Neurosurgical Problems*, 2d ed. Philadelphia: Saunders, 1982, pp 1663–1696.

226 Anterior Communicating Artery Aneurysms

Allan H. Friedman

The region of the anterior communicating artery is one of the most common sites for intracranial aneurysms to occur. These aneurysms are usually clinically silent until they rupture. The rare giant anterior communicating artery aneurysm can act as an intracranial mass, producing a loss of vision, endocrine deficiency, or altered mental status. Most frequently, anterior communicating aneurysms first come to clinical attention when they rupture and produce a subarachnoid hemorrhage. As with all aneurysms, a significant number of severe hemorrhages from anterior communicating artery aneurysms are preceded by a milder "warning leak" manifesting as a severe headache and sometimes a mild change in mental status.

Although the surgical treatment of anterior communicating artery aneurysms remains a formidable task, their treatment has benefited from advances in anesthetic techniques, microsurgical techniques, and instrumentation. A thorough knowledge of the anatomy of this region is the key to successful treatment of these lesions once they are diagnosed.

Anatomy

Although the textbook description of the anterior communicating artery complex is straightforward, the actual surgical anatomy is far more complicated. The simple textbook anatomy is complicated by perforating arteries, variations of vessel length and diameter, and vascular tortuosity brought on by atherosclerosis and hypertension.

The basic configuration is two anterior cerebral arteries, each arising from one of the internal carotid arteries and passing under the inferior frontal lobe. At the midline, each anterior cerebral artery turns upward to run in the interhemispheric fissure along the medial aspect of each hemisphere. The genu of the anterior cerebral arteries is joined by the anterior communicating artery.

A-1 Segment

The portion of the anterior cerebral artery that connects the internal carotid artery and the anterior communicating artery is termed the A-1 segment. The path which the A-1 segment takes is a function of the length of the intracranial internal carotid artery, the position of the anterior communicating artery, and the tortuosity of the A-1 vessel. The length of the intracranial segment of the internal carotid artery varies from 14 to 25 mm, and that of the A-1 segment varies from 7 to 18 mm.[15,50] The A-1 anterior communicating artery junction lies over the optic chiasm in 70 percent of cases and over the optic nerve in 30 percent of cases. The A-1 segment most commonly passes slightly anteriorly from its origin to its culmination at the anterior communicating artery. Its anterior angle is exaggerated when the parent internal carotid artery is long. If the intracranial internal carotid artery is short, the A-1 segment may pass horizontally over the optic nerve. Prior to crossing the optic chiasm, the A-1 segment passes through a thick arachnoid membrane marking the lateral wall of the lamina terminalis cistern.

Rarely the A-1 segment is replaced by a vessel which originates from the carotid artery at the level of the anterior clinoid and passes under the ipsilateral optic nerve.[44,49] This is probably not a misplaced A-1 segment, but a persistent embryologic vessel such as the ventral ophthalmic artery, since a hypoplastic A-1 segment usually persists. This anomaly is frequently associated with aneurysms.[14,44]

The diameter of the A-1 segment varies from 0.9 to 4 mm (average, 2.6 mm). The A-1 is less than 1.5 mm in diameter in only 10 percent of cases. Although a disparity between the diameter of the two A-1 segments is common, this disparity is greater than 1 mm in only 6 to 12 percent of the general population.[5,50,56] Some disparity between the A-1 segments has been noted in up to 90 percent of patients harboring an anterior communicating artery aneurysm.[31] In 50 percent of patients presenting with a ruptured anterior communicating artery aneurysm, the disparity is greater than 1 mm.[5,14,77] When such an inequality is present, the aneurysm originates from the junction of the larger A-1 and anterior communicating arteries in approximately 85 percent of cases. Fenestrations, duplications, and the complete absence of an A-1 segment have been reported.[46,71]

Two to 15 perforating vessels originate from the A-1 segment. When a small number of perforating vessels are present, one or more may be stem vessels which pass a short distance and then arborize into multiple perforating arteries. These stem vessels may be as large as the recurrent artery of Heubner which can cause confusion at the time of surgical dissection. Even thin A-1 segments give rise to important perforating arteries. Although the perforating arteries can arise from any part of the A-1, they are more prevalent along its proximal portion. The perforating arteries originating from A-1 pass to the dorsal optic chiasm, optic tract, hypothalamus, and medial portion of the anterior perforated substance. Perforating vessels originating at the bifurcation of the internal carotid artery irrigate the genu and contiguous posterior limb of the internal capsule, the adjacent globus pallidus, and the medial third of the anterior commissure. The more medial branches of the A-1 segment irrigate the paraolfactory nuclei, the medial inferior caudate, the anterior inferior putamen, the anterior limb of the internal capsule, and all hypothalamic nuclei anterior to the mamillary bodies.[10]

Special note must be made of the cholinergic nuclei located in the paraolfactory area and around the inferior third ventricle. The cholinergic innervation of the neocortex comes from the nucleus basalis and the cholinergic nucleus of the hippocampus originates in the diagonal band of Broca.[38] The latter is squarely in the vascular territory of the A-1 perforators. It has been postulated that destruction of these cholinergic fibers results in impaired memory and arousal.[20,52] Infarction of the nucleus accumbens is postulated to result in loss of volition.[52]

Anterior Communicating Artery

The anterior communicating artery is 2 to 3.4 mm in diameter (average 1.5 mm).[8,32,50] The diameter of this vessel is proportional to the disparity in the diameters of the two A-1 segments. Only 40 to 60 percent of anterior cerebral arteries are joined by a classic single anterior communicating artery.[72] This is not surprising considering that the anterior communicating artery forms from the coalescence of an embryologic multichannel plexus. Frequently there is residual branching, fenestration, or duplication of the vessel.[76] The artery varies from 0.8 to 4.6 mm in length.[32]

The anterior communicating artery is the origin of one to 13 perforating vessels.[8,10,32,50,57,74] Although these vessels may originate from any point around the circumference of the anterior communicating artery, 70 percent pass at an angle of 90 to 120 degrees posterior to the distal anterior cerebral arteries (A-2 segments) when measured in the sagittal plane.[74] Although most of these perforators are quite small, two larger vessels are frequently noted—the subcallosal and medial callosal arteries. Ninety percent of brains were found to have a subcallosal artery measuring 0.3 to 0.65 mm in diameter. This vessel appears to be a stem artery which arises from the caudal dorsal surface of the anterior communicating artery and gives rise to multiple perforating branches. Ten percent of brains have a medial callosal artery measuring 0.5 to 1.3 mm in diameter. The medial callosal artery is present in embryologic development and generally regresses along with the plexiform nature of the anterior communicating artery. This artery generally runs behind the plane of the A-2 vessels. It may give origin to hypothalamic and septal perforating arteries close to its origin, and if large, the terminal segment can irrigate parts of the medial frontal lobes bilaterally. This vessel can be difficult to identify on an angiogram.[46] The consequences of mistaking the vessel for an A-2 segment at the time of surgery have been documented.[14]

Perforating vessels originating from the anterior communicating artery provide blood supply to the lamina terminalis, anterior hypothalamus, septal nucleus, medial paraolfactory nuclei, subcallosal cingulum, and genu of the corpus callosum. It is important to note again the possibility of memory loss due to infarction of the septal and paraolfactory regions.[10]

A-2 Segment

The proximal A-2 segment varies from 1.7 to 3.7 mm in diameter (average, 2.6 mm). A single or azygous A-2 has been noted in approximately 2 percent of brains studied. This configuration is associated with a high incidence of aneurysms which reside proximally on that vessel.[18,28] The two proximal A-2 segments usually do not run perfectly parallel in the same coronal plane; instead, one runs posteriorly in the concavity of the other.[51] The recurrent artery of Heubner and a small number of perforating arteries originate from this segment. The smaller perforating vessels supply an area similar to that of the vessels originating from the anterior communicating artery.

The recurrent artery of Heubner originates from within 3 mm of the anterior cerebral-anterior communicating artery junction in 80 percent of brains examined. In 30 to 78 percent of brains examined, the origin is from the proximal part of the A-2 segment. In 7 to 55 percent of cases, the origin is from the lateral anterior cerebral artery diametrically opposite the junction with the anterior communicating artery, and in 14 to 40 percent of cases it originates from the superior surface of A-1.[42,50,77] The artery doubles back, passing anterior to the anterior cerebral artery in 60 percent of cases and superior to the A-1 segment in 40 percent of cases. Duplication of this artery is a frequent occurrence. The artery may have a common origin with, or give rise to, the frontopolar artery.[57] Branches of the artery enter the anterior portion of the anterior perforated substance over its entire mediolateral extent.

In 85 percent of brains, the recurrent artery of Heubner only perfuses structures anterior to the anterior commissure. This artery irrigates the anterior limb of the internal capsule, the anterior striatum and, to a varying degree, the nucleus accumbens and the precommissural septal gray mater. Critchley reported that occlusion of the recurrent artery of Heubner manifests as weakness of the upper extremity and face, alterations in emotions, and changes in personality.[7] Caplan et al. noted dysarthria and mild contralateral hemiparesis manifested more as neglect and lack of spontaneous movement than frank weakness.[3] Most patients were abulic with slowness to follow commands, a paucity of self-initiated speech and movement, and lack of persistence in performing tasks. This abulia may reflect infarction of the inferior striatum. A minority of patients demonstrated restlessness, agitation, or contralateral neglect.

Aneurysm Anatomy

Approximately 55 percent of anterior communicating artery aneurysms that receive clinical attention are 6 to 10 mm in diameter. Twenty percent are less than 6 mm in diameter and 25 percent are 11 to 25 mm in diameter. Giant aneurysms are rare.

Seventy to 80 percent of aneurysms originate at the junction of the anterior communicating and anterior cerebral arteries. In 85 to 97 percent of cases, the aneurysm arises from the side of the dominant A-1 vessel.[42,73,78] The remaining 20 to 30 percent of aneurysms originate from the midportion or along the entire length of the anterior communicating artery.

Ten to 15 percent of aneurysms project downward toward the optic chiasm while 20 to 25 percent project forward. The most common direction is upward between the A-2 segments. This accounts for 35 to 60 percent of cases. In eight to 15 percent of cases, the aneurysm points posteriorly.

By noting the direction to which the fundus projects, the surgeon will be alerted to particular problems which may occur at the time of surgery. Downward- or forward-pointing aneurysms may become tethered to the optic chiasm or tuberculum sellae. A bulbous downward- or forward-pointing fundus can obscure the surgeon's view of the contralateral A-1 segment. Retraction of the medial frontal lobe could precipitate a premature rupture of the aneurysm. A superior-pointing fundus can become adherent to the A-2, fronto-orbital, or frontopolar arteries. A large superior-pointing fundus will hinder the surgeon's view of the contralateral A-2 segment. Posterior-projecting aneurysms often adhere to the perforating vessels originating from the anterior communicating artery.

The surgeon must be aware of the multilobulated aneurysm. Particularly troublesome are aneurysms with a superior and posterior projection. The surgeon may clip the superior portion of the aneurysm between the two A-2 segments thereby obscuring the still patent posterior portion of the aneurysm.

Radiology

Computed tomography (CT) scanning will demonstrate hemorrhage in most but not all cases of ruptured anterior communicating artery aneurysm. The hemorrhage can permeate diffusely through the cisterns at the base of the brain or remain focal around the ruptured aneurysm in a characteristic pattern. Focal hemorrhage may be confined to the cistern of the lamina terminalis or may break into the interhemispheric cistern. Aneurysms which point laterally can hemorrhage into the gyrus rectus and base of the frontal lobe (Fig. 226-1). Aneurysms pointing toward the vertex can rupture into the septal nuclei, cavum septum pellucidum, hypothalamus, or putamen (Fig. 226-2). Such hemorrhages often extend into the ventricular system.[81]

Unruptured aneurysms can sometimes be seen on a CT scan of the brain. An enhancing anterior communicating artery aneurysm may stand out against the black background of the lamina terminalis cistern. A loop in an A-2 segment or an azygous A-2 segment can mimic this appearance and be mistaken for an anterior communicating artery aneurysm.[3] Giant aneurysms present on high-resolution brain CT scans as a pool of blood with a higher x-ray attenuation than the adjacent brain. Curvilinear calcifications and thrombosis within a large or giant aneurysm may also be visualized on the CT scan. Leaking vessels present in the thickened walls of a giant aneurysm frequently result in contrast enhancement around the circumference of the aneurysm.

Magnetic resonance imaging (MRI) is notoriously poor at demonstrating acute subarachnoid hemorrhage, although superficial hemosiderin may be seen long after the acute blood has disappeared. The lumen of the aneurysm may be demonstrated as a flow void; clotted blood within the aneurysm will have a varied appearance depending on the amount of methemoglobin and hemosiderin

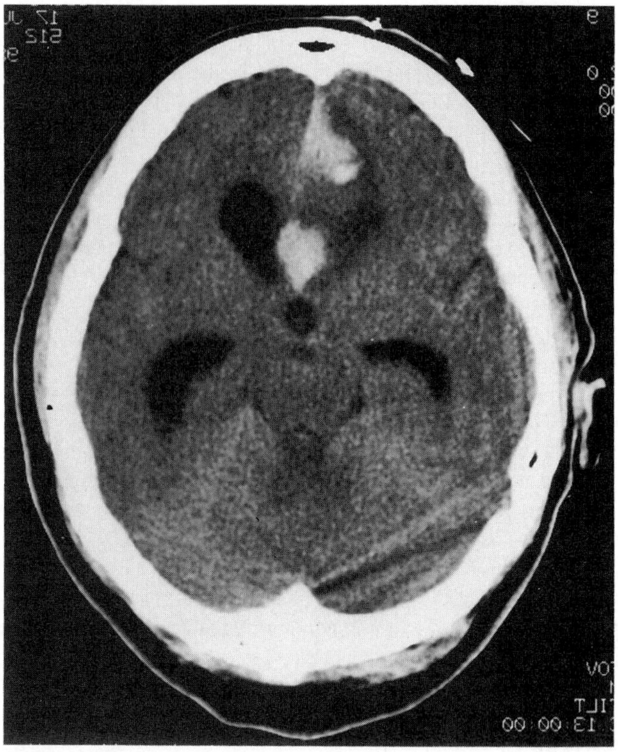

Figure 226-2 A CT scan following rupture of an anterior communicating artery aneurysm. A characteristic blood clot resides in the interhemispheric fissure and septal region.

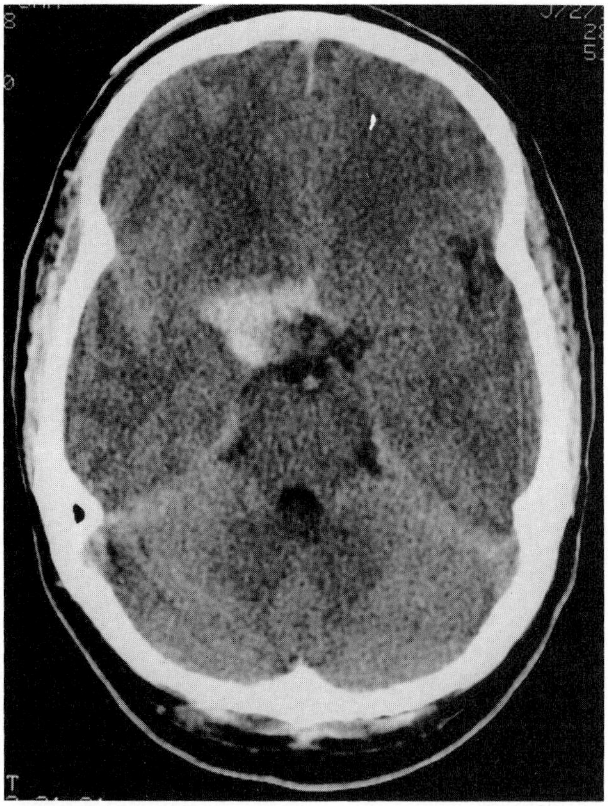

Figure 226-1 A CT scan of the brain following the rupture of an anterior communicating artery aneurysm. The aneurysm, which pointed to the right, caused hemorrhage into the gyrus rectus and basal forebrain.

present. MRI is an important adjuvant to angiography in delineating the anatomy of a partially thrombosed aneurysm.

Angiography will demonstrate all but completely thrombosed anterior communicating artery aneurysms. Basal and oblique views may be needed to delineate an aneurysm hidden among the tortuous loops of the anterior cerebral artery complex. Carotid angiography with compression of the contralateral carotid artery may be necessary to fill the anterior communicating artery. Using the angiogram, the surgeon should be able to discern the side of the dominant A-1 segment, the shape and axis of the aneurysm, and the relationship of the A-2 segments to themselves and to the aneurysm. Magnetic resonance angiography does not yet have the resolution to demonstrate the finer points of the anterior communicating artery complex.

Surgical Approaches

Bifrontal Craniotomy

The bifrontal approach to anterior communicating artery aneurysms was described by Tönnis in 1936.[70] His high craniotomy technique required resection of the genu of the corpus callosum to reach the anterior communicating artery complex. Pool subsequently reported a low bifrontal approach, with closure of the violated frontal sinuses with a vascularized pericranial flap.[53] French et al. advocated a right unilateral frontal craniotomy with a wedge resection of the mesial frontal lobe.[11]

More recently, Suzuki et al. reported their experience in treating 603 anterior communicating artery aneurysms through bifrontal craniotomy.[65] They employed a very low lying craniotomy and meticulously dissected the olfactory tracts from the undersurface of the frontal lobes, thereby preserving olfaction. Yasui et al. advocated a very basal opening of the interhemispheric fissure, affording early access to the A-1 segments.[79]

Using the operating microscope, an interhemispheric dissection can be performed through a small bony opening.[11,80] An interhemispheric approach through a 3-cm trephination was demonstrated to the author by Peerless in 1980. Fukushima et al. used a similar approach to treat 112 patients with anterior communicating artery aneurysms.[12]

Pterional Approach

Kempe and VanderArk described a lateral subfrontal approach with partial resection of the gyrus rectus.[24] Because earlier reports noted a very high incidence of ''premature'' aneurysm rupture, this approach was designed to isolate the neck of the aneurysm prior to encountering its fundus. Modifications such as Yaşargil's pterional and Chehrazi's[6] transylvian approach have been proposed. A variant of one of these approaches is employed by most surgeons to treat anterior communicating artery aneurysms.

Initial Approach

Some surgeons advocate approaching all aneurysms from the right side because of the absence of right brain language function and the unobstructed field afforded the surgeon's right hand.[59,78] Most surgeons approach the aneurysm from the side of the dominant A-1 segment. From the preoperative angiogram, the surgeon should have a mental three-dimensional vision of the anterior communicating artery complex, noting the direction in which the dome of the aneurysm is pointing, accessory lobulations, the side of the dominant A-1 segment, the anterior-posterior relationship of the A-2 vessels, the tilt of the anterior communicating artery, and the length of the internal carotid artery.

The patient's head is placed in three point fixation and rotated 60 degrees away from the side of the craniotomy for aneurysms which project inferiorly or anteriorly. For aneurysms projecting upward between the two A-2 segments, the working interval between the A-2 segments is increased by rotating the head only 30 to 45 degrees. The base of the frontotemporal bone flap is extended to a point above the mid orbit thereby giving the surgeon greater latitude in directing the aneurysm clip. The anterior, lateral, and inferior arachnoid of the sylvian fissure is opened, freeing the frontal lobe from the temporal lobe. This allows the surgeon to take a more lateral approach to the aneurysm and avoids lifting of the medial frontal lobe—a maneuver which can prematurely rupture an anterior- or inferior-pointing aneurysm. The A-1 segment is followed to the olfactory nerve where it is tethered by a thick arachnoid band which is the common wall of the olfactory, lamina terminalis, and carotid cisterns. A segment of the A-1 artery is freed to accommodate a temporary clip. Although some aneurysms can be visualized without cortical resection, it is usually safer to enter the cistern of the lamina terminalis through the gyrus rectus. The inferior pial surface of the gyrus rectus is opened and a subpial resection of the underlying tissue is performed. The fronto-orbital artery may be cauterized and divided. All vessels are cautiously inspected, because the recurrent artery of Heubner may run a tortuous course. The medial pia is carefully incised over the ipsilateral A-1 segment. The A-1 turns superiorly in the interhemispheric fissure, anastomoses with the anterior communicating artery, and proceeds as the A-2 segment. The ipsilateral recurrent artery of Heubner most often originates close to this junction. Unless the aneurysm is particularly bulbous or pointing downward, the anterior surface of the anterior communicating artery can be followed to the contralateral A-1 segment. If the aneurysm is adherent to the optic chiasm or tuberculum sellae, care must be taken not to avulse those adhesions by lifting up the aneurysm during this maneuver. Once both A-1 segments have been secured, the surgeon has the option of using temporary occlusion of these vessels to reduce the pressure within the aneurysm (Fig. 226-3).

Temporary Occlusion

Temporary occlusion of the blood flow to prevent intraoperative rupture of an aneurysm was first proposed by Jefferson in 1928.[53] Williamson and Brackett reported an excellent bloodless exposure of an anterior communicating artery aneurysm after temporarily occluding both A-1 segments.[75] Pool strongly advocated local control of circulation with temporary clips, citing experience in 40 cases of surgery for anterior communicating artery aneurysms.[53]

In the late 1970s, several well-known surgeons advocated using temporary clips to facilitate the final dissection and clipping of aneurysms. The exact duration in which temporary clips can safely be left in place is unknown. Charbel et al. left temporary clips in place for 6 to 32 minutes.[4] Seven patients had transient postoperative deficits while two patients suffered permanent deficits. In the two patients with permanent impairment, clips were left in place for more than 15 minutes. Using a combination of mannitol, vitamin E, and steroids for cerebral protection, Suzuki et al. reported safe circulatory arrest for up to 40 minutes.[65] Jabre and Symon used temporary occlusion in 22 cases: in 8 to control bleeding and in 14 to facilitate dissection.[21] Occlusion times ranged from 30 s to 23 min. Three of five patients with immediate postoperative deficits had subsequent resolution of their neurological deficits. Ljunggren et al. employed temporary occlusion for 5 to 15 min in

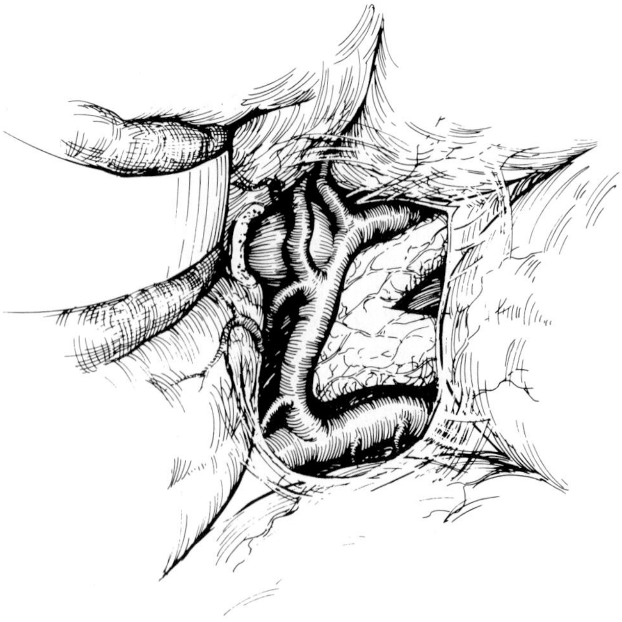

Figure 226-3 Surgical exposure of an anterior communicating artery aneurysm pointing posteriorly.

six patients, and noted no new deficits immediately following surgery.[29] The duration of focal circulatory arrest tolerated by an individual patient is probably a function of that patient's natural distal collateral supply. Unfortunately, methods used to monitor cerebral metabolism, such as evoked potentials and electroencephalography, and to monitor blood flow function poorly in the distribution of the anterior cerebral arteries. Recent laboratory studies indicate that intermittent clipping with intervening periods of reperfusion is better tolerated than continuous focal circulatory arrest.[16] Samson and Batjer[59] advocate temporary clipping of either A-1 segment and of the anterior communicating artery, but I have found placing a clip on the side of the aneurysm origin difficult.

Dissection and Clipping of the Aneurysm

The angiogram can show the relative position of the two A-2 vessels. The direction in which the aneurysm points and the direction the contralateral A-2 travels away from the anterior communicating artery will determine the best method of locating the contralateral A-2 segment (Fig. 226-4). A large contralateral frontopolar artery with a proximal origin should not be mistaken for the contralateral A-2 segment.

If the aneurysm points inferiorly toward the chiasm, the ipsilateral A-1 and bilateral A-2 segments are easily identified. The contralateral A-1 is often obscured by a bulbous sac. It can be identified, however, by following the contralateral A-2 to its junction with the anterior communicating artery and then gently depressing the aneurysm sac.

Anterior-projecting aneurysms are the easiest to manage. Once the position of the contralateral A-2 is determined from the angiogram, it can be identified within the interhemispheric fissure as anterior or posterior to the ipsilateral A-2 segment. Occasionally a large dome will obstruct the view of the most proximal portion of the A-2 segment. Gentle depression of the aneurysm will remove that obstacle. Before this maneuver is employed, however, enough of the aneurysm's dome must be dissected free so that depression of the dome will not pull on distal adhesions and rupture the aneurysm. Anterior- and inferior-projecting aneurysms can usually be obliterated by a straight clip placed parallel to the anterior communicating artery. The superior blade is placed anterior to the two A-2 segments. The tip of the clip should not extend beyond the dome of the aneurysm because it can occlude the contralateral frontopolar or perforating arteries.

Superior-projecting aneurysms tend to obscure the contralateral A-2 segment. If the contralateral A-2 segment sweeps more anteriorly than the ipsilateral A-2 segment, and if the distal anterior communicating artery is turned toward the surgeon, the aneurysm will appear to be framed by the two A-2 vessels. If the anterior communicating artery is not turned toward the surgeon, the anterior wall of the aneurysm must be dissected free and depressed posteriorly to reveal the origin of the contralateral A-2 vessel. Although vessels mildly adherent to the aneurysm will yield to very light blunt dissection, adhesions demonstrating **any** resistance should be dissected sharply. Manipulation of the adherent vessel will often demonstrate a fine tethering arachnoid band which when cut will release the adherent vessel. Injury to the aneurysm wall which occurs during sharp dissection produces small, focal, and more easily controlled rupture than the long, unpredicted tear that results from blunt dissection. When the contralateral A-2 segment courses posteriorly in an exaggerated fashion, it will be most easily identified by dissecting behind the aneurysm. The back wall of the aneurysm must be inspected for a "third" pericallosal artery or adherent perforating vessels. This can be accomplished by looking behind the ipsilateral A-2 or, in the case of very large aneurysms,

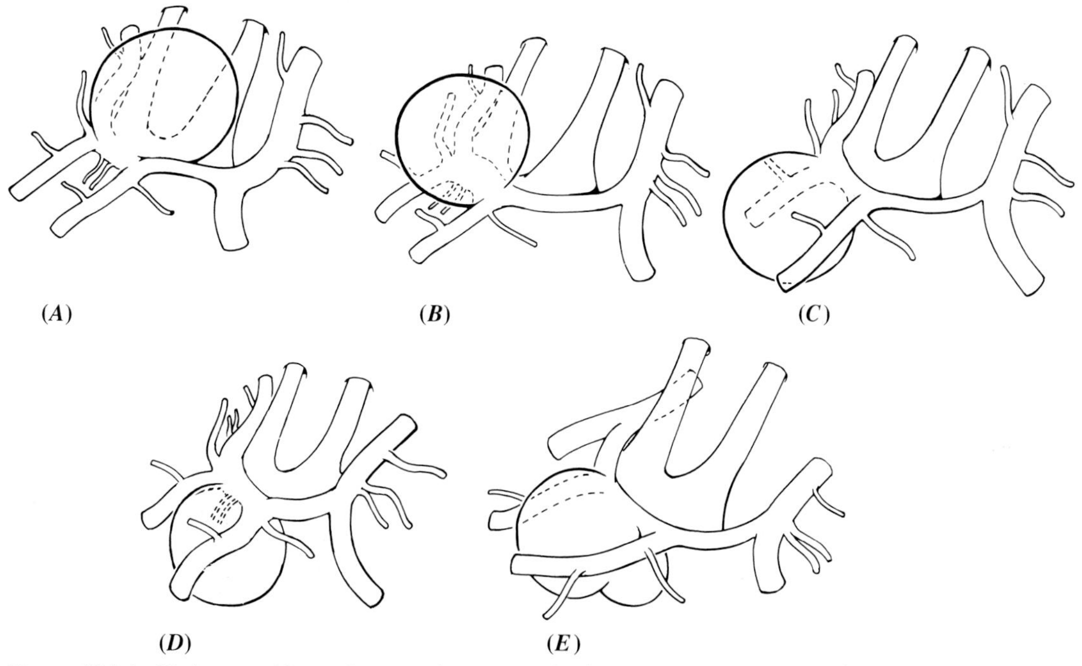

Figure 226-4 Various positions of an anterior communicating artery aneurysm. *A.* Inferior-pointing aneurysm which obscures the contralateral A-1 segment. *B.* Anterior-projecting aneurysm. *C.* Superior-projecting aneurysm which obscures the origin of the contralateral A-2 segment. *D.* Posterior-pointing aneurysms are often adherent to the perforating vessels. *E.* Multilobed aneurysm with two domes pointing in different directions.

by lifting the anterior communicating artery adjacent to the ipsilateral A-1 vessel. Fortunately, the perforating vessels originating from the anterior communicating artery travel perpendicular to the A-2 segments and are less likely to be firmly adherent to the aneurysm

The proximal A-2 segments may be firmly adherent to the dome of the aneurysm. Temporary clipping of the two A-1 vessels will reduce the turgor of the aneurysm and facilitate sharp dissection of the adhesions. Many superior-pointing aneurysms may be clipped perpendicular to the anterior communicating artery; each blade being placed between the aneurysm and one A-2 segment. If this technique is used, the surgeon must be certain that the aneurysm does not have a posterior projecting portion whose neck lies below the plane of the clip. The tips of the clip should not project beyond the aneurysm because a clip advanced too far may occlude perforating branches arising from the anterior communicating artery. If the aneurysm and A-2 segment are joined by a particularly recalcitrant adhesion at a fragile portion of the dome or if the neck of the aneurysm has incorporated the origin of an A-2 segment, the aneurysm may be obliterated using a fenestrated clip with the blades placed parallel to the anterior communicating artery.

The A-1 and A-2 segments are easily identified in aneurysms that project solely posterior to the plane of the anterior communicating complex. The problem lies in freeing the aneurysm from the perforating branches arising from the anterior communicating artery. This can be accomplished by working between the two A-1 segments and on both sides of the ipsilateral A-2 segment.

Overall Results

Natural History

Because most epidemiologic studies are based on those patients referred to specialized institutions, the exact natural history of the population of patients who suffer a ruptured anterior communicating artery aneurysm is imperfectly known. Ballantine reported that 14 of 16 patients followed for up to 8 years after the rupture of an anterior communicating aneurysm died from a recurrent subarachnoid hemorrhage.[54] Slosberg, treating patients with bedrest and induced hypotension, reported a 33 percent mortality from recurrent hemorrhage.[61] McKissock et al. observed 62 patients, who were treated without surgery, for 6 months to 10 years.[35] Fifty-two percent died and 40 percent returned to work. Logue followed 36 patients who had suffered a ruptured anterior communicating artery aneurysm.[30] Twenty (44.4 percent) of these patients died—15 from recurrent hemorrhage. Twenty of the 36 patients experienced a repeat hemorrhage. Richardson et al. noted that a patient's prognosis improved markedly as time elapsed from the most recent hemorrhage.[55] Forty-six percent of patients admitted within 24 h of their first hemorrhage died. Twenty-five percent of those admitted on the fourteenth post hemorrhage day died, but those patients who survived beyond 2 weeks experienced a marked decrease in mortality. Jane et al. noted that 50 percent of patients hospitalized with a ruptured anterior communicating aneurysm will rehemorrhage within the subsequent 6 months, and that after 6 months this patient population will rehemorrhage at a rate of 3.1 percent per year.[22] In an often quoted study, McKissock et al. compared surgical and nonsurgical therapy of ruptured anterior communicating artery aneurysms in patients admitted to their institution prior to 1960.[36] Although they found no difference in outcome between the two groups, clip ligation of the aneurysm was only performed in 15 percent of the surgically treated group.

Indirect Surgical Approaches

Several solutions were offered in the 1950s to circumvent the problems inherent in a direct attack on the aneurysm. Ley reported on eight patients treated by bilateral anterior cerebral occlusion, five of whom died and two of whom were severely disabled.[27] Pool also noted that trapping the aneurysm by ligating various elements of the anterior circle of Willis[30] resulted in a high rate of morbidity and mortality.[54]

Cognes' review of 37 patients treated with clipping of a single anterior cerebral artery demonstrated a lower than expected rate of recurrent hemorrhage.[70] Taylor et al. reviewed the long-term effects of unilateral A-1 ligation.[66] Although the methodology employed in this study was imperfect, the authors found that ligation of a single anterior cerebral artery significantly reduced the short- and long-term rate of rehemorrhage from a previously ruptured anterior communicating artery aneurysm.[66] The study found that approximately 25 percent of patients suffered a cerebral infarction, although the contribution of vasospasm is unclear. Höök and Norlén reported three deaths in 11 patients treated by trapping of the anterior communicating artery.[17] Surprisingly, six of the eight survivors returned to work.

Carotid ligation has been used in cases when the aneurysm only fills from a single A-1 on angiography or in conjunction with a contralateral A-1 ligation.[45,68] McKissock et al. noted that 11 percent of patients treated with carotid ligation suffered ischemic stroke and 22 percent died from recurrent hemorrhage.[36] Although this technique may give some protection against recurrent hemorrhage, insufficient data are present in the literature to evaluate its efficacy. For the most part, these Hunterian techniques have been replaced by direct microsurgical attack on the aneurysms.

Early experience with wrapping anterior communicating aneurysms with muscle was disappointing.[54] Studies looking at the long-term effect of aneurysm wrapping do not completely agree. In some studies, wrapping or coating seemed to reduce the chance of a subsequent hemorrhage; however, other long-term reviews showed only a partial or no protective effect.[23,40,69] Complications of wrapping have been reported.[33,47] The efficacy of wrapping technique is certainly influenced by the material used and the completeness of the wrap.

Early Surgical Series

The earliest series reported dismal results for the surgery of ruptured anterior communicating artery aneurysms.[27] In the 1960s, certain surgeons began to make progress. French et al. reported one operative death in 25 patients.[11] Seventeen patients (68 percent) returned to their original employment. French employed severe arterial hypotension and advocated rupturing the aneurysm, aspirating the dome into a suction aspirator, and clipping the exposed neck. Höök and Norlén reported two deaths among 43 operated patients.[17] Both patients were comatose prior to surgery. Twenty-nine (71 percent) patients returned to full employment. Pool reported excellent postoperative results in 68 percent of 56 patients who were grades I to III prior to surgery.[53,54] Forty-four percent of the patients were operated on more than 15 days after their hemorrhage.

Interhemispheric Approach

Suzuki et al. reported on 603 patients undergoing surgery for a single anterior communicating artery aneurysm.[65,82] Three hundred sixty-seven (61 percent) had an excellent outcome, 107 (18 percent) had a good outcome, and 30 (5 percent) died. Of 264 patients who were preoperative grades 0 to III (Hunt-Hess scale), 86 percent had a good to excellent outcome. Twenty-one percent of patients were operated on within 48 h of their hemorrhage and 61 percent were operated on within 1 week. Using a "micro" interhemispheric approach to treat 138 patients, Fukushima et al. reported that 119 (80 percent) patients were working and eight (6 percent) had died at follow-up.[12] Of 83 patients entering the hospital in grades I to III condition, 92 percent had an excellent or good result. Surgery was performed within 72 h of the hemorrhage in 40 percent of patients and within 1 week in 66 percent of patients.

Pterional Approach

Sengupta and McAllister reported on 160 patients harboring anterior communicating artery aneurysms, of which 115 were grade I or II.[60] Seventy-eight percent had a good postoperative outcome, and 14 percent had a fair outcome. Twenty-three patients developed postoperative ischemic complications. Yaşargil reported good results in 288 of 298 patients presenting in grade I or II condition; 38 of 73 patients presenting in grades III to V condition eventually had a good outcome.[78] In their series of 166 patients with anterior communicating artery aneurysm, Sundt et al. reported that 123 (74 percent) made an excellent recovery and 5 (3 percent) died.[64] Ljunggren et al. reported on 69 grades I to III patients who were operated on within 72 h of rupturing an anterior communicating artery aneurysm.[29] Seven patients had a permanent deficit that developed immediately following surgery, six patients developed a delayed ischemic deficit, four patients had a persistent deficit attributable to the initial hemorrhage, and two patients had hydrocephalus requiring CSF diversion.

Although results of surgery have improved dramatically, overall management results remain troublesome. Of 1374 patients who were hospitalized within 3 days of their hemorrhage and registered in the recent International Cooperative Study on the Timing of Aneurysm Surgery, 55 percent had a good result and 30 percent died.[23]

The incidence of recurrent hemorrhage following clip ligation of an aneurysm is seldom addressed. Todd et al. noted rehemorrhage in 4 of 120 patients followed for 10 years or until death.[69] Most of these patients were operated on prior to the routine use of the operating microscope. Yaşargil noted that 7 (2.9 percent) of 240 patients with anterior communicating aneurysms treated up to 1976 had symptomatic recurrent aneurysms.[78] None of the 214 patients who were treated between 1976 and 1982 and followed for up to seven years suffered a recurrent hemorrhage.

Intravascular Treatment

There are as yet only sporadic reports of anterior communicating aneurysms treated by intravascular techniques.[41] I am certain that in future editions, this section will become longer and more important.

Specific Neurological Deficits

Cognitive Defects

Early in their experience, Norlén and Olivecrona noted that some patients suffering a ruptured anterior communicating artery aneurysm manifest amnesia, confabulation, neglect, and abulia. Further investigations have reported a particular propensity for alterations in memory, personality, and mood following rupture of an anterior communicating aneurysm. Although early reports stressed amnesia and Korsakoff-like confabulation, most patients suffer only a mild to moderate memory impairment.[2,19,62–64] Gade found significant memory defects in 30 percent of patients treated for a ruptured anterior communicating artery aneurysm.[13] He found less severe deficits when the neck of the aneurysm was clipped than when the anterior communicating artery was ligated. Okawa et al. reviewed 85 patients operated on for a ruptured anterior communicating artery aneurysm, and found an amnestic syndrome in 66 percent of patients which persisted in 16 percent of patients followed for 2 to 3 years.[48] Sonesson et al. found that patients suffering a ruptured anterior communicating artery aneurysm were more likely to suffer decreased cognitive flexibility, decreased attention span, and decreased capacity to adopt to novel commands than patients who experienced a ruptured aneurysm elsewhere in the intracranial vasculature.[62] In a series of 27 patients, Stenhouse et al. found that vasospasm was the most consistent predictor of long-term cognitive defects.[63] The incidence of cognitive impairment could be correlated with the patient's age but was not affected by the timing of surgery. Recent reports note a higher percentage of patients returning to their premorbid level of employment following surgery.[26,67] Almost certainly a fixed percentage of patients will experience cognitive difficulties as a result of the initial hemorrhage and vasospasm and independent of surgical technique.

Several elements of the corticolimbic and corticostriatal circuits reside in the immediate vicinity or vascular distribution of the anterior communicating artery complex. These include the substantia innominata, diagonal band of Broca, ventral striation, cholinergic nuclei Ch3 and Ch4, columns of the fornix, medial forebrain bundle, and anterior hypothalamus.[3,20,52] Irle et al. attempted to localize the brain lesions responsible for cognitive deficits by correlating the results of psychological tests with lesions seen on CT in 30 patients.[20] They found that amnesia was most consistently found when the lesions involved the striatum and the basal forebrain structures. This finding agrees with primate studies demonstrating that the corticolimbic system including the basal forebrain structures and the corticostriatal systems participate in learning and memory. Personality and mood changes were most consistently demonstrated in patients with lesions of the striatum. Cognitive dysfunction rarely results from an unruptured giant anterior communicating artery aneurysm.[1]

Visual Loss

Although close to the anterior visual pathways, anterior communicating aneurysms only rarely compromise the patient's vision. Visual deficits resulting from mass effect can reflect compression of the optic nerves, chiasm, or tracts. A wide variety of visual field deficits have been described, but the most common patterns are bitemporal hemianopsia and monocular visual loss.[39] Following a subarachnoid hemorrhage, visual loss can result from periretinal or intravitreal hemorrhages. Vitreal hemorrhage generally clears spontaneously within one year. If bilateral hemorrhage results in functional blindness, a vitrectomy is indicated. Retinal ischemia secondary to vasospasm has also been proposed as a mechanism for vision loss.[58]

Endocrine Deficits

Because of their proximity to the hypothalamus and pituitary stalk, anterior communicating artery aneurysms can precipitate abnormalities in endocrine function. Diabetes insipidus, the most common endocrine abnormality, usually follows a severe subarachnoid and intraparenchymal hemorrhage.[37] Some minor endocrine dysfunction may be demonstrated in approximately 50 percent of patients who have suffered a ruptured anterior communicating artery aneurysm.[25,83] Panhypopituitarism has also been reported to occur following the rupture of an anterior communicating artery aneurysm.[43] Abnormalities in the endocrine system have rarely been reported as a manifestation of an unruptured aneurysm or immediately following surgery, presumedly from compromise of the hypothalamic vasculature.[34]

Conclusion

The treatment of anterior communicating artery aneurysms remains a formidable task.[9] The results of surgical therapy for these lesions have steadily improved. This belies the fact that a fixed percentage of patients will be irreversibly injured by their initial hemorrhage and a smaller number of patients will incur a neurological deficit from vasospasm. The medical community is challenged to improve early diagnosis of these lesions and neurosurgeons are challenged to improve surgical techniques and to prevent vasospasm.

References

1. Bokemeyer C, Frank B, Brandis A, et al. Giant aneurysm causing frontal lobe syndrome. *J Neurol* 1990; 237:47–50.
2. Bornstein RA, Weir BK, Petruk KC, et al. Neuropsychological function in patients after subarachnoid hemorrhage. *Neurosurgery* 1987; 21:651–654.
3. Caplan LR, Schmahmann JD, Kase CS, et al. Caudate infarcts. *Arch Neurol* 1990; 47:133–143.
4. Charbel FT, Ausman JI, Diaz FG, et al. Temporary clipping in aneurysm surgery: technique and results. *Surg Neurol* 1991; 36:83–90.
5. Charbel FT, Seyfried D, Mehta B, et al. Dominant A1: angiographic and clinical correlations with anterior communicating artery aneurysms. *Neurol Res* 1991; 13:253–256.
6. Chehrazi BB. A temporal transsylvian approach to anterior circulation aneurysms. *Neurosurgery* 1992; 30:957–961.
7. Critchley M. The anterior cerebral artery, and its syndromes. *Brain* 1930; 53:120–165.
8. Crowell RM, Morawetz RB. The anterior communicating artery has significant branches. *Stroke* 1977; 8:272–273.
9. Drake CG, Friedman AH, Peerless SJ. Failed aneurysm surgery: reoperation in 115 cases. *J Neurosurg* 1984; 61:848–856.
10. Dunker RO, Harris AB. Surgical anatomy of the proximal anterior cerebral artery. *J Neurosurg* 1976; 44:359–367.
11. French LA, Zarling ME, Schultz EA. Management of aneurysms of the anterior communicating artery. *J Neurosurg* 1962; 19:870–876.
12. Fukushima T, Miyazaki S, Takusagawa Y, et al. Unilateral interhemispheric keyhole approach for anterior cerebral artery aneurysms. *Acta Neurochir [Suppl] (Wien)* 1991; 53:42–47.
13. Gade A. Amnesia after operations on aneurysms of the anterior communicating artery. *Surg Neurol* 1982; 18:46–49.
14. Gibbons K, Hopkins LN, Heros RC. Occlusion of an "accessory" distal anterior cerebral artery during treatment of anterior communicating artery aneurysms: report of two cases. *J Neurosurg* 1991; 74:133–135.
15. Gibo H, Lenkey C, Rhoton AL Jr. Microsurgical anatomy of the supraclinoid portion of the internal carotid artery. *J Neurosurg* 1981; 55:560–574.
16. Goldman MS, Anderson RE, Meyer FB. Effects of intermittent reperfusion during temporary focal ischemia. *J Neurosurg* 1992; 77:911–916.
17. Höök O, Norlén G. Aneurysms of the anterior communicating artery. *Acta Neurol Scand* 1964; 40:219–240.
18. Huber P, Braun J, Hirschmann D, et al. Incidence of berry aneurysms of the unpaired pericallosal artery: angiographic study. *Neuroradiology* 1980; 19:143–147.
19. Hütter BO, Gilsbach JM. Cognitive deficits after rupture and early repair of anterior communicating artery aneurysm. *Acta Neurochir (Wien)* 1992; 116:6–13.
20. Irle E, Wowra B, Kunert HJ, et al. Memory disturbances following anterior communicating artery rupture. *Ann Neurol* 1992; 31:473–480.
21. Jabre A, Symon L. Temporary vascular occlusion during aneurysm surgery. *Surg Neurol* 1987; 27:47–63.
22. Jane JA, Winn HR, Richardson AE. The natural history of intracranial aneurysms: rebleeding rates during the acute and long term period and implication for surgical management. *Clin Neurosurg* 1977; 24:176–184.
23. Kassell NF, Torner JC, Jane JA, et al. The International Cooperative Study on the Timing of Aneurysm Surgery: Part 2: Surgical results. *J Neurosurg* 1990; 73:37–47.
24. Kempe LG, VanderArk GD. Anterior communicating artery aneurysms. Gyrus rectus approach. *Neurochirurgia (Stuttg)* 1971; 14:63–70.
25. Kuwayama A, Okada C, Takanohashi M, et al. Endocrine function in postoperative patients with anterior communicating aneurysm. *Neurol Med Chir (Tokyo)* 1977; 17:209–217.
26. Laiacona M, De Santis A, Barbarotto R, et al. Neuropsychological follow-up of patients operated for aneurysms of anterior communicating artery. *Cortex* 1989; 25:261–273.
27. Ley E Jr. Successful treatment of an aneurysm of the anterior communicating artery. *J Neurosurg* 1956; 13:294–298.
28. Lightfoote JB, Grusd RS, Nalls GA. Azygos anterior cerebral artery mimicking an anterior communicating artery aneurysm. *Am J Neuroradiol (Suppl)* 1989; 10:S74.
29. Ljunggren B, Säveland H, Brandt L. Causes of unfavorable outcome after early aneurysm operation. *Neurosurgery* 1983; 13:629–633.
30. Logue V. Surgery in spontaneous subarachnoid haemorrhage. Operative treatment of aneurysms of the anterior cerebral and anterior communicating artery. *Br Med J* 1956; 1:473–479.
31. Mackenzie JM. The anatomy of aneurysm-bearing circles of Willis. *Clin Neuropathol* 1991; 10:187–189.
32. Marinkovic S, Milisavljevic M, Marinkovic Z. Branches of the anterior communicating artery. Microsurgical anatomy. *Acta Neurochir (Wien)* 1990; 106:78–85.
33. McFadzean RM, Hadley DM, McIlwaine GG. Optochiasmal arachnoiditis following muslin wrapping of ruptured anterior communicating artery aneurysms. *J Neurosurg* 1991; 75:393–396.
34. McIver B, Connacher A, Whittle I, et al. Adipsic hypothalamic diabetes insipidus after clipping of anterior communicating artery aneurysm. *Br Med J* 1991; 303:1465–1467.
35. McKissock W, Paine KWE, Walsh LS. An analysis of the results of treatment of ruptured intracranial aneurysms. Report of 772 consecutive cases. *J Neurosurg* 1960; 17:762–776.

36. McKissock W, Richardson A, Walsh L. Anterior communicating aneurysms: a trial of conservative and surgical treatment. *Lancet* 1965; 1:873–876.
37. McMahon AJ. Diabetes insipidus developing after subarachnoid haemorrhage from an anterior communicating artery aneurysm. *Scott Med J* 1988; 33:208–209.
38. Mesulam MM, Mufson EJ, Levey AI, et al. Atlas of cholinergic neurons in the forebrain and upper brainstem of the macaque based on monoclonal choline acetyltransferase immunohistochemistry and acetylcholinesterase histochemistry. *Neuroscience* 1984; 12:669–686.
39. Miller NR. *Walsh and Hoyt's Clinical Neuro-ophthalmology,* 4th ed. Baltimore: Williams & Wilkins, 1991, pp 2044–2047; 2078–2082.
40. Minakawa T, Koike T, Fujii Y, et al. Long term results of ruptured aneurysms treated by coating. *Neurosurgery* 1987; 21:660–663.
41. Nakahara I, Taki W, Nishi S, et al. Treatment of giant anterior communicating artery aneurysm via an endovascular approach using detachable balloons and occlusive coils. *Am J Neuroradiol* 1990; 11:1195–1197.
42. Nathal E, Yasui N, Sampei T, et al. Intraoperative anatomical studies in patients with aneurysms of the anterior communicating artery complex. *J Neurosurg* 1992; 76:629–634.
43. Nukta EM, Taylor HC. Panhypopituitarism secondary to an aneurysm of the anterior communicating artery. *Can Med Assoc J* 1987; 137:413–415.
44. Nutik S, Dilenge D. Carotid-anterior cerebral artery anastomosis. Case report. *J Neurosurg* 1976; 44:378–382.
45. Odom GL, Tindall GT. Carotid ligation in the treatment of certain intracranial aneurysms. *Clin Neurosurg* 1968; 15:101–116.
46. Ogawa A, Suzuki M, Sakurai Y, et al. Vascular anomalies associated with aneurysms of the anterior communicating artery: microsurgical observations. *J Neurosurg* 1990; 72:706–709.
47. Ogilvy CS, Poletti CE. Clipping of an aneurysm 20 years after encasement with methyl methacrylate. Case report. *J Neurosurg* 1991; 75:305–307.
48. Okawa M, Maeda S, Nukui H, et al. Psychiatric symptoms in ruptured anterior communicating aneurysms: social prognosis. *Acta Psychiatr Scand* 1980; 61:306–312.
49. Onishi H, Yamashita J, Enkaku F, et al. Anomalous origin of the anterior cerebral artery and congenital skull dysplasia—case report. *Neurol Med Chir (Tokyo)* 1992; 32:296–299.
50. Perlmutter D, Rhoton AL Jr. Microsurgical anatomy of the anterior cerebral-anterior communicating-recurrent artery complex. *J Neurosurg* 1976; 45:259–272.
51. Perlmutter D, Rhoton AL Jr. Microsurgical anatomy of the distal anterior cerebral artery. *J Neurosurg* 1978; 49:204–228.
52. Phillips S, Sangalang V, Sterns G. Basal forebrain infarction. A clinicopathologic correlation. *Arch Neurol* 1987; 44:1134–1138.
53. Pool JL. Aneurysms of the anterior communicating artery. Bifrontal craniotomy and routine use of temporary clips. *J Neurosurg* 1961; 18:98–112.
54. Pool JL. Timing and techniques in the intracranial surgery of ruptured aneurysms of the anterior communicating artery. *J Neurosurg* 1962; 19:378–388.
55. Richardson AE, McKissock W, Walsh L. Anterior communicating aneurysms. In Fields WS, Sahs AL (eds): *Intracranial Aneurysms and Subarachnoid Hemorrhage.* Springfield, IL: Thomas, 1965, pp 467–485.
56. Riggs HE, Rupp C. Variation in form of circle of Willis. *Arch Neurol* 1963; 8:8–14.
57. Rosner SS, Rhoton AL Jr, Ono M, et al. Microsurgical anatomy of the anterior perforating arteries. *J Neurosurg* 1984; 61:468–485.
58. Ruben S, Afshar F. Visual failure following subarachnoid haemorrhage from rupture of an anterior communicating artery aneurysm. *J Neurol Neurosurg Psychiatry* 1991; 54:1017–1018 (letter).
59. Samson DS, Batjer HH. *Intracranial Aneurysm Surgery: Techniques.* Mount Kisco, NY: Futura Publishing, 1990, pp 97–120.
60. Sengupta RP, McAllister VL. *Subarachnoid Haemorrhage.* Berlin: Springer-Verlag, 1986, pp 249–250.
61. Slosberg PS. Medical treatment of intracranial aneurysms. An analysis of 15 cases. *Neurology* 1960; 10:1085–1089.
62. Sonesson B, Ljunggren B, Saveland H, et al. Cognition and adjustment after late and early operation for ruptured aneurysm. *Neurosurgery* 1987; 21:279–287.
63. Stenhouse LM, Knight RG, Longmore BE, et al. Long-term cognitive deficits in patients after surgery on aneurysms of the anterior communicating artery. *J Neurol Neurosurg Psychiatry* 1991; 54:909–914.
64. Sundt TM Jr, Kobayashi S, Fode NC, et al. Results and complications of surgical management of 809 intracranial aneurysms in 722 cases. Related and unrelated to grade of patient, type of aneurysm, and timing of surgery. *J Neurosurg* 1982; 56:753–765.
65. Suzuki J, Mizoi K, Yoshimoto T. Bifrontal interhemispheric approach to aneurysms of the anterior communicating artery. *J Neurosurg* 1986; 64:183–190.
66. Taylor W, Miller JD, Todd NV. Long-term outcome following anterior cerebral artery ligation for ruptured anterior communicating artery aneurysms. *J Neurosurg* 1991; 74:51–54.
67. Teissier du Cros J, Lhermitte F. Neuropsychological analysis of ruptured saccular aneurysms of the anterior communicating artery after radical therapy (32 cases). *Surg Neurol* 1984; 22:353–359.
68. Tindall GT, Kapp J, Odom GL, et al. A combined technique for treating certain aneurysms of the anterior communicating artery. *J Neurosurg* 1970; 33:41–47.
69. Todd NV, Tocher JL, Jones PA, et al. Outcome following aneurysm wrapping: a 10-year follow-up review of clipped and wrapped aneurysms. *J Neurosurg* 1989; 70:841–846.
70. Tönnis W. Erfolgreiche Behandlung eines Aneurysma der Art. commun. ant. cerebri. *Zentralbl Neurochir* 1936; 1:39–42.
71. Tracy PT. Unusual intercarotid anastomosis associated with anterior communicating artery aneurysm: case report. *J Neurosurg* 1987; 67:765–767.
72. Tulleken CA. A study of the anatomy of the anterior communicating artery with the aid of the operating microscope. *Clin Neurol Neurosurg* 1978; 80:169–173.
73. VanderArk GD, Kempe LC. Classification of anterior communicating aneurysms as a basis for surgical approach. *J Neurosurg* 1970; 32:300–303.
74. Vincentelli F, Lehman G, Caruso G, et al. Extracerebral course of the perforating branches of the anterior communicating artery: microsurgical anatomical study. *Surg Neurol* 1991; 35:98–104.
75. Williamson WP, Brackett CE Jr. Management of intracranial aneurysms of the anterior communicating artery. *Am Surg* 1956; 22:100–107.
76. Yamagami T, Kikuchi H, Higashi K, et al. Aneurysm arising at the triplicate anterior communicating artery—case report. *Neurol Med Chir (Tokyo)* 1992; 32:229–331.
77. Yaşargil MG. *Microneurosurgery,* vol I. New York: Thieme Stratton, 1984, pp 92–128.
78. Yaşargil MG. *Microneurosurgery,* vol II. New York: Thieme Stratton, 1984, pp 169–223.
79. Yasui N, Suzuki A, Sayama I, et al. A basal interhemispheric operative approach for anterior communicating artery aneurysms. *Neurol Med Chir (Tokyo)* 1987; 27:756–761.
80. Yeh H, Tew JM Jr. Anterior interhemispheric approach to aneurysms of the anterior communicating artery. *Surg Neurol* 1985; 23:98–100.
81. Yock DH Jr, Larson DA. Computed tomography of hemorrhage from anterior communicating artery aneurysms, with angiographic correlation. *Radiology* 1980; 134:399–407.
82. Yoshimoto T, Uchida K, Kaneko U, et al. An analysis of follow up results of 1000 intracranial saccular aneurysms with definitive surgical treatment. *J Neurosurg* 1979; 50:152–157.
83. Yoshimoto H, Uozumi T. Anterior pituitary function in cerebrovascular diseases, with special reference to ruptured cerebral aneurysm. *Neurol Med Chir (Tokyo)* 1985; 25:433–439.

227

Distal Anterior Cerebral Artery Aneurysms

Nelson M. Oyesiku
Daniel L. Barrow

Incidence, Anatomy, and Etiology

Distal anterior cerebral artery (DACA) aneurysms are rare (most series report fewer than 20 patients) and they comprise between 2.0 and 9.2 percent (mean 4.4 percent) of all intracranial aneurysms. As noted initially by Wilson and coworkers,[21] the earliest surgical report seems to be that of Sugar and Tinsley,[19] although this, in fact, was a vascular malformation involving the distal segment of the pericallosal artery and should not be included among reported DACA aneurysms. However, the aneurysm in Sugar's second case (reported by Hamby[6]) was an aneurysm of the pericallosal bifurcation.

A variety of diseases and anomalies are associated with DACA aneurysms, including other intracranial aneurysms.[8,24] The incidence of coexisting disorders is about 37.5 percent and involves most commonly, aneurysms of the middle cerebral[7,11,22] and internal carotid arteries, arteriovenous malformations,[8] azygos anterior cerebral arteries, bihemispheric anterior cerebral artery and a supreme anterior communicating artery,[22] polycystic kidney disease,[4] coarctation of the aorta,[8] hypertension,[7] craniosynostosis,[8] and agenesis of the corpus callosum.[21] In most series, the sex incidence is nearly equal.[1,3,7–9,11,18,20,22,24,25]

The DACA includes the anterior cerebral artery (ACA) and its branches distal to the anterior communicating artery. The anterior cerebral artery courses anteriorly and superiorly from the anterior communicating artery to the genu of the corpus callosum, where it bifurcates into the superior callosomarginal and the inferior pericallosal arteries. A few centimeters distal to the anterior communicating artery, the prefrontal and frontopolar arteries arise from the anterior cerebral artery. The two DACAs run parallel to each other a few millimeters apart on the medial surface of the olfactory area in the interhemispheric fissure. Beyond the origin of the callosomarginal artery, the anterior, middle, and posterior inferior frontal arteries arise as branches of the DACA. At about the midportion of the corpus callosum, the paracentral artery and, more distally, the precuneal and parieto-occipital arteries arise. About 25 percent of human brains have an anomalous pattern of the DACA, including an unpaired ACA, an artery feeding the opposite hemisphere, a triplicate vestigial vessel, and intercommunicating vessels between the DACAs beyond the anterior communicating artery.

Pertuiset and coworkers[13] classified the sites of origin (Fig. 227-1) of pericallosal aneurysms as follows:

1. Immediately distal to the anterior communicating artery
2. At the origin of the frontopolar artery
3. At the origin of the callosomarginal or anterior internal frontal artery (pericallosal bifurcation)
4. On the pericallosal artery distal to 3
5. On the callosomarginal artery distal to 3

Types 1 and 2 are infra- or subcallosal and Types 3 through 5 are supracallosal.

Like other intracranial aneurysms, DACA aneurysms can be categorized as saccular (berry, "congenital"), mycotic, atherosclerotic, or traumatic. The majority of DACA aneurysms are of the saccular type, presumably of congenital origin. The location of the aneurysm on the ACA is related to the etiology; for instance, proximally located aneurysms are most likely congenital in origin, whereas distal lesions may be mycotic or traumatic. Giant aneurysms of the DACA have been reported but are very rare.[15,18]

Approximately two-thirds[9] of DACA aneurysms are located near the genu of the corpus callosum at the bifurcation of the pericallosal and callosomarginal arteries, where the pericallosal artery frequently makes an abrupt bend posteriorly (Fig. 227-2); these are the so-called *malignant aneurysms* (Type 3 of Pertuiset). The proximal, distal, and frontobasal DACA aneurysms are less common (Fig. 227-1).[7] The etiology of most of these aneurysms is believed to be similar to that of berry aneurysms located on the circle of Willis, which occur at the bifurcations of vessels and are characterized pathologically by fragmentation and loss of the internal elastica and thinning of the media.[12] The description by Laitinen and Snellman[8] of the occurrence of a communication between the pericallosal arteries at the genu of the corpus callosum in conjunction with DACA aneurysms has been cited as evidence for a congenital etiology. These authors have termed this anomalous communicating vessel the *supreme anterior communicating artery.* Yaşargil and Carter noted similar arterial connections and

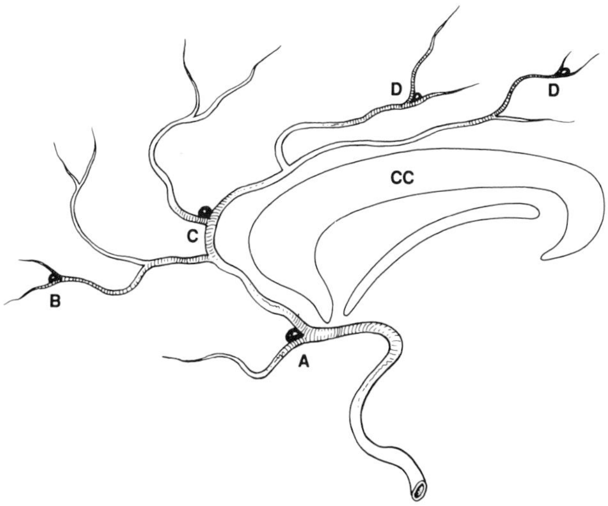

Figure 227-1 The different locations of DACA aneurysms. *A.* Proximal. *B.* Frontobasal (infracallosal). *C.* Genu/corpus callosum (infracallosal). *D.* Distal/supracallosal. CC, corpus callosum.

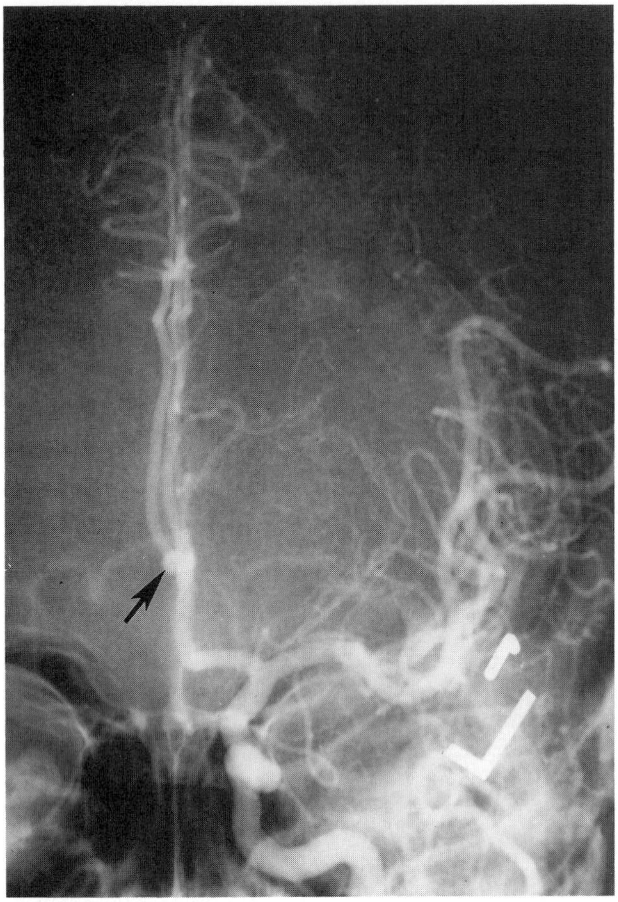

(*A*)

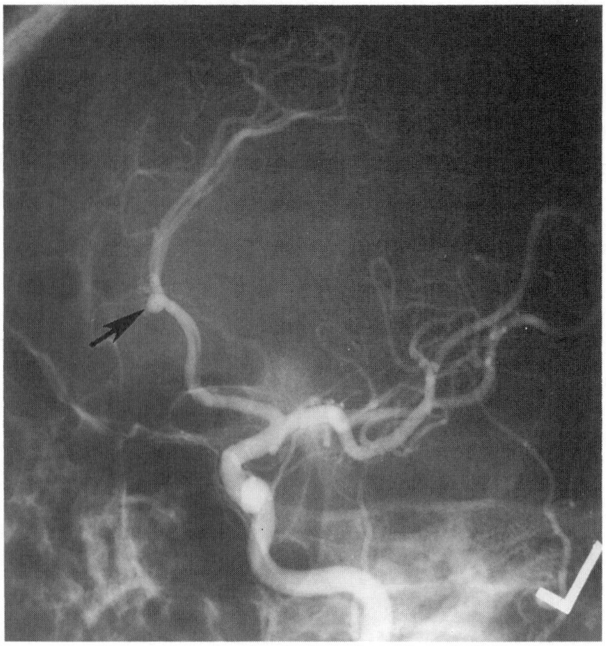

(*B*)

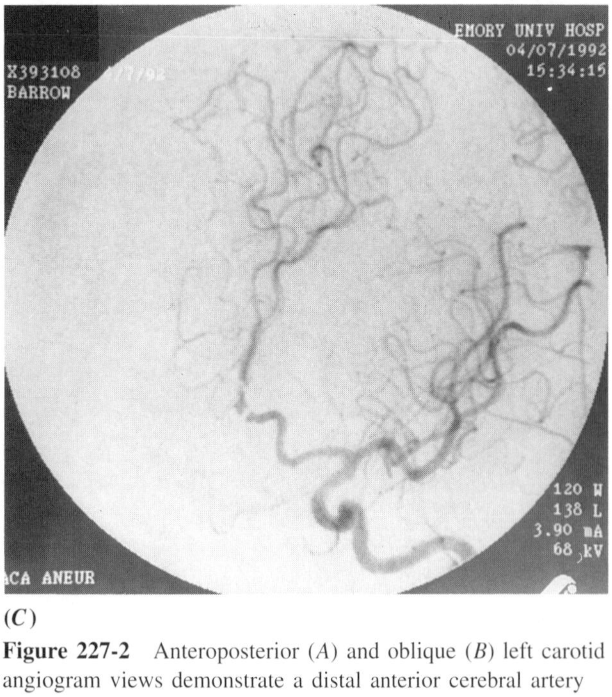

(*C*)

Figure 227-2 Anteroposterior (*A*) and oblique (*B*) left carotid angiogram views demonstrate a distal anterior cerebral artery aneurysm (*arrows*) arising at the bifurcation of an unpaired anterior cerebral artery. *C*. An intraoperative angiogram documents complete obliteration of the aneurysm with filling of normal surrounding arteries.

suggest that, although a developmental etiology is possible, it is just as likely that an anatomic variation may create a flow disturbance leading to aneurysm formation.[24] In support of this view, only five DACA Aneurysms have been reported in children under 5 years of age.

Most DACA aneurysms located beyond the genu of the corpus callosum are secondary to trauma, infection (mycotic), or tumor embolization, or are idiopathic.[12] A larger percentage of DACA aneurysms than aneurysms at other intracranial locations occur as a result of infection or trauma. Traumatic aneurysms, of which DACA aneurysms are second in incidence only to those of cortical branches of the middle cerebral artery, result from either direct or indirect trauma (Fig. 227-3). Direct trauma results in aneurysm formation when a penetrating object, surgical manipulation, or overlying skull fracture damages the wall of an artery in its pathway. Indirect vascular injury is usually associated with a significant closed head injury and is probably secondary to the deformity, shearing, and compression occurring with the traumatic acceleration and deceleration of the brain. The arterial injury producing DACA aneurysms may be secondary to compression of the vessel on the adjacent free edge of the falx during a transient shift of the brain beneath this rigid structure. If the injury to the arterial wall is incomplete, the damaged internal elastic lamina and media of the artery allow dilatation in a manner similar to a congenital (true) berry aneurysm. False aneurysms occur when all layers of the arterial wall are lacerated, with resultant hemorrhage. The hematoma is contained by surrounding brain and the periphery becomes organized over the next few days.[5]

Mycotic aneurysms result from infected emboli (usually from bacterial endocarditis) that infect the arterial wall by direct extension from the lumen.[16] DACA aneurysms of embolic infectious origin are usually located on the most distal branches. A DACA aneurysm located far from the genu of the corpus callosum should raise the suspicion of either a mycotic or traumatic origin.

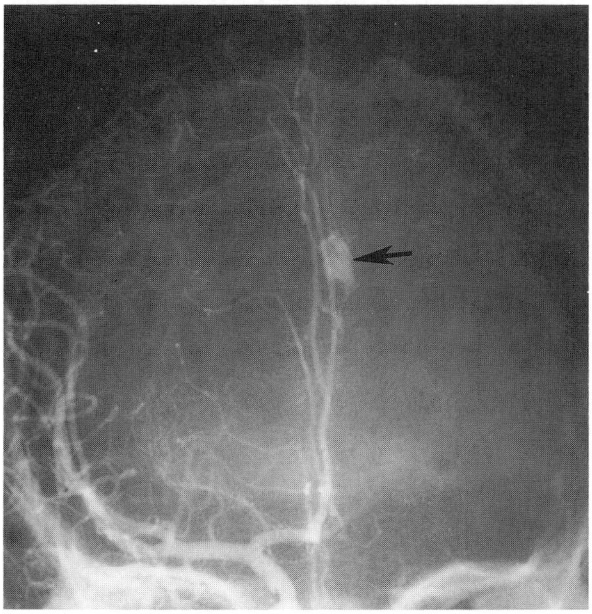

(*A*)

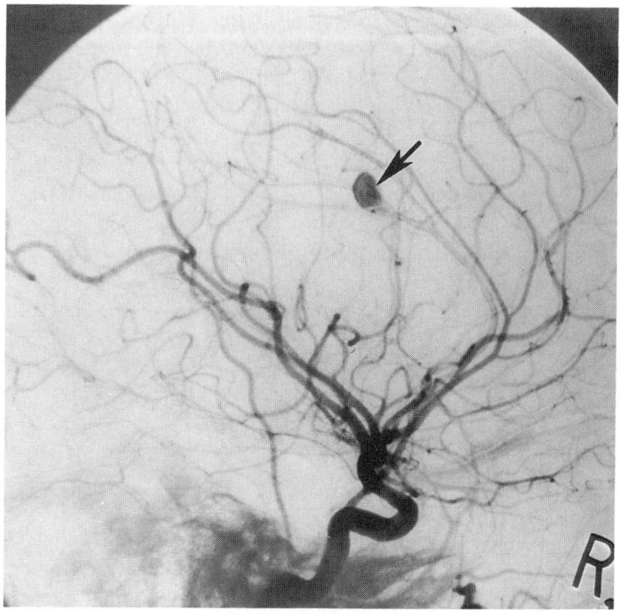

(*B*)

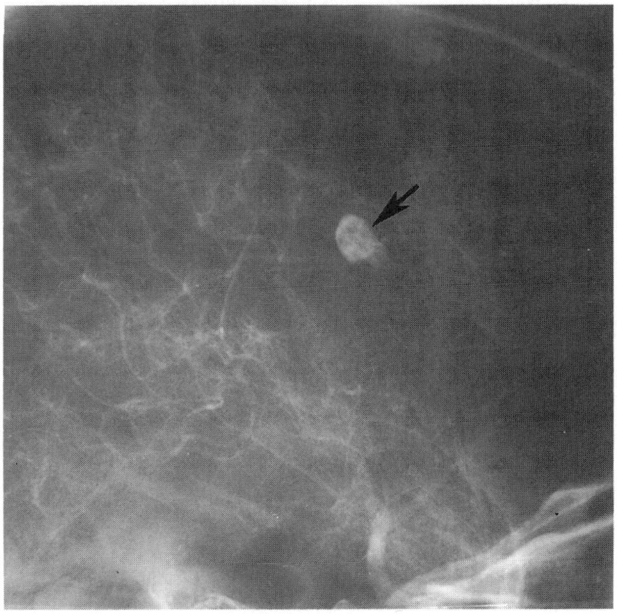

(*C*)

Figure 227-3 Anteroposterior (*A*) and lateral (*B*) right carotid angiogram views demonstrate an irregular aneurysm of the distal anterior cerebral artery in a patient who experienced a delayed hemorrhage following a closed head injury. *C.* A delayed lateral angiographic film demonstrates the delayed emptying which characterizes pseudoaneurysms.

Clinical Presentation

The most common presentation of DACA aneurysms is subarachnoid hemorrhage, with or without residual neurological deficit. However, intracerebral hemorrhage commonly occurs after rupture of DACA aneurysms,[7,8,18,20,21,24] presumably because the aneurysm is juxtaposed to the cerebral hemispheres, as well as because of the relative paucity of related subarachnoid cisterns. It is often difficult to clinically differentiate the subarachnoid hemorrhage caused by a DACA aneurysm from one resulting from other intracranial aneurysms, especially those of the anterior communicating artery. There is, however, a high incidence of pyramidal signs, especially a crural predominant hemiparesis[1] or contralateral lower extremity monoparesis.[8] This signature may be transient and should be looked for early. DACA aneurysms may also present with mental deterioration and urinary incontinence, simulating a frontal lobe tumor[14] or normal pressure hydrocephalus. The full syndrome produced by occlusion of the DACA with sparing of the recurrent artery of Huebner was first described by Critchley.[2] This consists of a variable neurological deficit, contralateral hemi- or monoplegia, superficial sensory impairments, transient aphasia, loss of memory or confusion, sphincteric dysfunction, catatonic posturing, forced grasping and hypokinesia, and visual agnosia if the occlusion extends posterior to the parieto-occipital fissure. Iatrogenic occlusion of a major branch of the distal anterior cerebral artery does not invariably result in a deficit, however. Snyckers and Drake reported four cases in which there was no deficit following occlusion of the pericallosal or callosomarginal artery.[18] Laitinen and Snellman reported mental confusion in one-half and papilledema in about one-third of their 14 patients, 13 of whom presented with a subarachnoid hemorrhage.[8] Other manifestations include intraventricular hemorrhage and compression of the optic nerves by an inferiorly directed frontopolar aneurysm, as well as the incidental finding of a DACA aneurysm during arteriography for unrelated symptoms.[1]

Management

Except for the surgical approach, the overall management of DACA aneurysms is the same as for other intracranial aneurysms. The results of an early cooperative study indicated that DACA aneurysms "appear to carry a worse prognosis for survival than aneurysms at any other site."[10] However, with the advent of microsurgical techniques, and improvements in neurosurgical anesthesia and postoperative care, the morbidity and mortality of these lesions has clearly improved.[7,9,11,17,23]

The etiology of the aneurysm will dictate the form of therapy in some instances. We believe that ruptured berry or traumatic aneurysms should be repaird surgically. Mycotic aneurysms occurring on the DACA should be treated with appropriate antibiotic therapy. If the aneurysm is not seen or appears smaller on a repeat angiogram performed 2 weeks after the start of therapy, antibiotics should be continued for a full course. If the aneurysm enlarges over this period, surgical intervention should be considered. Incidental DACA aneurysms should be managed in the same way as other incidental aneurysms.

Surgical Approaches

Aneurysms that arise immediately distal to the anterior communicating artery or at any point proximal to the middle of the genu of the corpus callosum are within the operating field of the anterior communicating artery and can be approached subfrontally or pterionally (Fig. 227-4). Laitinen and Snellman operated on 10 of their patients who had a DACA aneurysm through a subfrontal approach by locating the internal carotid artery and following the ACA to the pericallosal bifurcation.[8] These and other authors have pointed out the difficulty of this approach. All other series have used an interhemispheric approach as described by Yasargil and Carter[24] and Wilson et al.[21] We recommend this surgical approach for any DACA aneurysm distal to the midgenu of the corpus callosum. Preoperative treatment is identical to that for any other intracranial aneurysm.

The patient is placed in the supine position with the head slightly flexed in a brow-up manner. We do not use spinal drainage routinely. A coronal skin incision is made and reflected anteriorly. A rectangular bone flap is elevated on the right side of the midline. The dural flap is based on the superior sagittal sinus. Major bridging veins should be preserved, if feasible. Additional exposure may be provided by dividing the falx. A self-retaining brain retractor is used to maintain gentle lateral retraction on the right frontal lobe, exposing the interhemispheric fissure. The common occurrence of intracerebral hematomas with DACA aneurysms results in adhesions and may account for the increased frequency of intraoperative rupture reported by Snyckers and Drake.[18] This occurrence may be less common in recent series because of the popularity of early surgery. From this point on, the operating microscope is used and the ACA is located anterior to the aneurysm for proximal control in the event of a rupture. The aneurysm is then dissected from surrounding vessels and brain until its neck is well delineated. These aneurysms may be more difficult to dissect because of the limited space in the interhemispheric fissure, a broad base, sclerotic plaques at the neck, or the presence of multiple aneurysms.[8,18,24] The ACA and the pericallosal and callosomarginal arteries should be well visualized before clip application to avoid the potential significant morbidity associated with interruption of these vessels. If possible, a clip is applied across the base of the aneurysm to isolate it from the normal cerebral circulation. If the anatomy of the aneurysm precludes clip ligation, acrylic coating is indicated. If the aneurysm sac collapses after clipping, no further manipulation is necessary. Should it remain tense, a 27-gauge needle is used to aspirate the sac to ensure that it is adequately clipped. Postoperative angiography is not performed routinely.

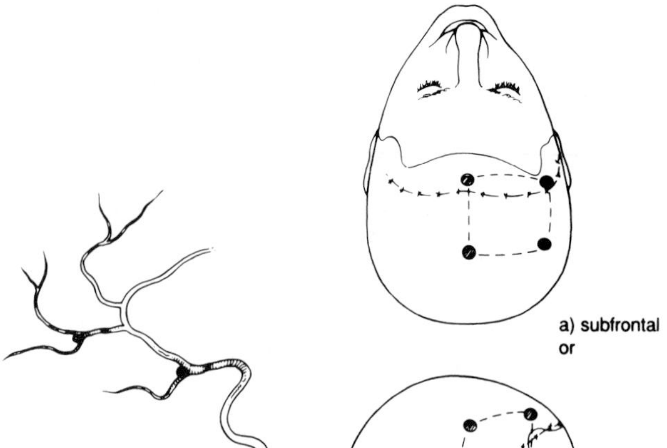

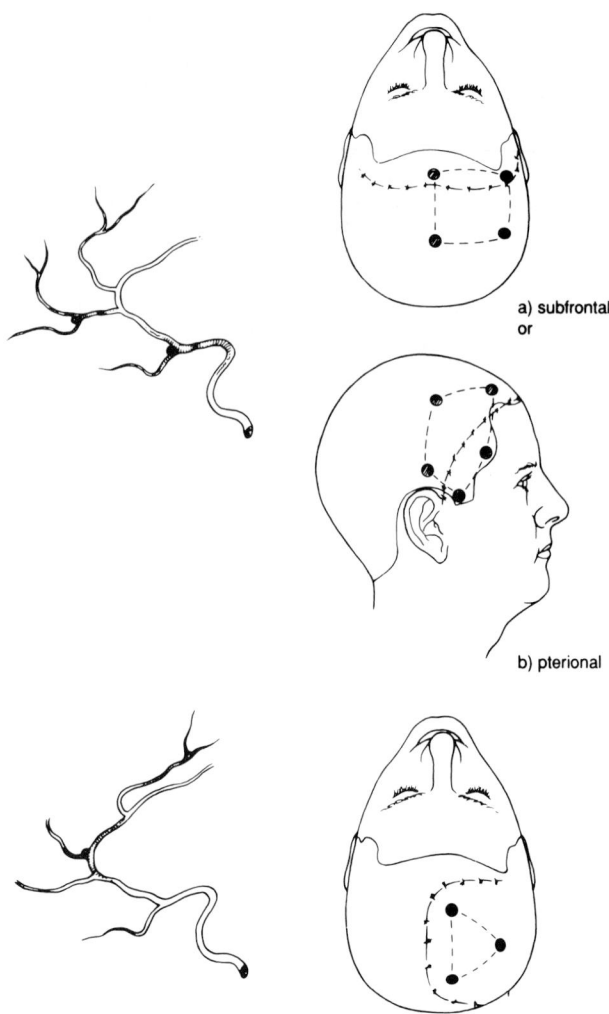

Figure 227-4 Operative approaches based on the location of DACA aneurysms.

The results of surgical treatment of DACA aneurysms have generally been good. In the literature, operative mortality ranges from 0 to 25 percent, with a morbidity of approximately 15 percent.[1,8,17,18,20,21,24] Fortunately, with technical advances in microsurgery and anesthesia, the mortality and morbidity are decreasing.[7,9,11,17,22]

References

1. Becker DH, Newton TH. Distal anterior cerebral artery aneurysm. *Neurosurgery* 1979; 4:495–503.
2. Critchley M. The anterior cerebral artery and its syndromes. *Brain* 1930; 53:120–165.
3. Dechaume JP, Aimard G, Michel D, et al. Les anévrysmes de l'artère péri-calleuse: a propos d'une série de 12 observations. *Neurochirugie* 1973; 19:135–150.
4. Fisher RG, Ciminello V. Pericallosal aneurysms. *J Neurosurg* 1966; 25:512–515.
5. Fleischer AS, Patton JM, Tindall GT. Cerebral aneurysms of traumatic origin. *Surg Neurol* 1975; 4:233–239.

6. Hamby WB. *Intracranial Aneurysms.* Springfield, IL: Thomas, 1952, p 329.
7. Hernesniemi J, Tapaninaho A, Vapalahti M, et al. Saccular aneurysms of the distal anterior cerebral artery and its branches. *Neurosurgery* 1992; 31:994–999.
8. Laitinen, L, Snellman A. Aneurysms of the pericallosal artery: a study of 14 cases verified angiographically and treated mainly by direct surgical attack. *J Neurosurg* 1960; 17:447–458.
9. Mann KS, Yue CP, Wong G. Aneurysms of the pericallosal-callosomarginal junction. *Surg Neurol* 1984; 21:261–266.
10. Nishioka H. Report on the Cooperative Study of Intracranial Aneurysms and Subarachnoid Hemorrhage. Section VII, Part 1. Evaluation of the conservative management of ruptured intracranial aneurysms. *J Neurosurg* 1966; 25:574–592.
11. Ohno K, Monma S, Suzuki R, et al. Saccular aneurysms of the distal anterior cerebral artery. *Neurosurgery* 1990; 27:907–913.
12. Olmsted WW, McGee TP. The pathogenesis of peripheral aneurysms of the central nervous system: a subject review from the AFIP. *Radiology* 1977; 123:661–666.
13. Pertuiset B, Lepoire J, Boudin G, Cabeza S. Les anévrysmes de l'artère péricalleuse. *Neurochirurgie* 1961; 7:321–338.
14. Petit-Dutaillis D, Cirilli M, Messimy R, Le Besherais Y. A propos de deux d'anévrisme de la péri-calleuse. *Neurochirurgie* 1959; 5:137–142.
15. Pozzati E, Nuzzo G, Gaist G. Giant aneurysm of the pericallosal artery: case report. *J Neurosurg* 1982; 57:566–569.
16. Roach MR, Drake CG. Ruptured cerebral aneurysms caused by microorganisms. *N Engl J Med* 1965; 273:240–244.
17. Sindou M, Pelissou-Guyotat I, Mertens P, et al. Pericallosal aneurysms. *Surg Neurol* 1988; 30:434–440.
18. Snyckers FD, Drake CG. Aneurysms of the distal anterior cerebral artery. A report on 24 verified cases. *South Afr Med J* 1973; 47:1787–1791.
19. Sugar O, Tinsley M. Aneurysms of terminal portion of anterior cerebral artery. *Arch Neurol Psychiatry* 1948; 60:81–85.
20. Thomas DGT, Paterson A. Results of treatment of pericallosal aneurysms. *J Neurol Neurosurg Psychiatry* 1975; 38:827.
21. Wilson CB, Christensen FK, Subrahmanian MV. Intracranial aneurysms at the pericallosal artery bifurcation. *Am Surg* 1965; 31:386–393.
22. Wisoff JH, Flamm ES. Aneurysms of the distal anterior cerebral artery and associated vascular anomalies. *Neurosurgery* 1987; 20:735–741.
23. Yasargil MG. *Microneurosurgery. II. Clinical Considerations, Surgery of the Intracranial Aneurysms and Results.* Stuttgart: George-Thieme Verlay, 1984, pp 224–231.
24. Yasargil MG, Carter LP. Saccular aneurysms of the distal anterior cerebral artery. *J Neurosurg* 1974; 40:218–223.
25. Yoshimoto T, Uchida K, Suzuki J. Surgical treatment of distal anterior cerebral artery aneurysms. *J Neurosurg* 1979; 50:40–44.

228 Carotid Ligation

Richard A. Roski
Robert F. Spetzler

Carotid artery ligation has been used for many years as an alternative method for treating intracranial aneurysms. Its place in the armamentarium of modern neurosurgery, however, constantly needs to be reassessed. As with many neurosurgical procedures, its role has been dramatically affected by the evolving changes in microneurosurgery. Improved techniques for intracranial aneurysm surgery have eliminated the necessity of carotid ligation for the treatment of most types of aneurysms. In contrast, the development of extracranial to intracranial (EC-IC) arterial bypass surgery has helped to augment the usefulness of carotid ligation in the treatment of difficult giant intracranial aneurysms. The present role of carotid ligation in the treatment of intracranial aneurysms will be reviewed, as well as the history, physiologic effects, and complications of the procedure.

History

The first reports of carotid ligation described its use in controlling severe hemorrhage from the neck.[36] This was most often encountered as a complication of a penetrating injury to the carotid artery, the rupture of an aneurysm of the extracranial portion of the internal carotid artery, or erosion into the carotid artery by a tumor of the head and neck region. One of the earliest such reports was by Paré in 1585, who reported the emergent use of carotid ligation to control life-threatening hemorrhage in a patient who had sustained a stab wound of the neck. In 1792 Lynn reported the use of common carotid ligation to control hemorrhage encountered during the removal of a tumor from the neck. Similar reports by Abernathy, Fleming, and Twitchell followed in the late 1700s and early 1800s. In 1805, Sir Astley Cooper performed the first "elective" ligation of the internal carotid artery in a patient with an extracranial internal carotid artery aneurysm. Although Cooper's first patient died, he subsequently reported a successful result in 1808. Carotid ligation continued to gain considerable popularity during the early 1800s. It was used not only for the treatment of hemorrhage but also for a variety of other problems, including trigeminal neuralgia, epilepsy, and psychosis. In 1868 Pilz published a series of over 600 common carotid artery ligations that had an operative mortality rate of 43 percent.[34] He stressed that the use of carotid ligation should be limited to controlling severe hemorrhage and to treating aneurysms of the carotid artery. Those two problems have subsequently remained its primary clinical indications.

The role of carotid ligation in treating intracranial aneurysms was questioned because of the high mortality that had been reported. In 1938 Jefferson stated that this poor reputation and high mortality resulted from its use in cases in which infection, secondary hemorrhage, and malignant disease of the neck were present. He suggested reevaluating its use for treating intracranial aneurysms. In 1940 Schorstein, following Jefferson's suggestion, reviewed 60 cases of intracranial aneurysm treated by carotid ligation.[39] That initial report included 27 cases from the literature as well as 33 previously unreported cases. The operative mortality and morbidity were each 13.3 percent. Schorstein's detailed analysis helped to highlight several important clinical factors regarding the use of carotid ligation. He noted that complications from internal carotid artery ligation were more common in patients with severe anemia from previous hemorrhage. He postulated that severe anemia, the mass effect of a giant aneurysm, or increased intracranial pressure produced poor cerebral perfusion. He observed better results in patients with infraclinoid as opposed to supraclinoid aneurysms and he noted a higher mortality rate in patients who had had a recent subarachnoid hemorrhage as compared with patients with a more remote hemorrhage. Although we are now better able to explain the operative risk factors in physiologic terms, very little has been added to the clinical observations of the complications of carotid ligation since Schorstein's excellent description. The relatively low operative morbidity and mortality rates helped to establish carotid ligation as a major method of treatment for intracranial aneurysms.

Physiologic Significance of Carotid Ligation

The rationale for using carotid ligation is based on the concept that ligating the carotid artery will produce a drop in blood pressure distal to the ligation and therefore help to potentiate thrombosis of the aneurysm. The effects of carotid ligation on the immediate and late changes in internal carotid artery pressure, the angiographic appearance of the aneurysm, and the blood flow changes in the carotid artery have all been studied extensively.

To document the change in the distal arterial pressure following carotid occlusion, Sweet et al. carried out pressure measurements in 26 patients who were undergoing cerebral arteriography.[46] When the internal carotid artery was occluded, the distal systolic pressure measured in the internal carotid artery dropped 49 percent, the pulse pressure dropped 69 percent, and the mean blood pressure dropped 43 percent. Extreme variability was seen. There were seven cases in which the systolic pressure drop was less than 30 percent and three cases in which the systolic pressure drop was greater than 70 percent. When the internal carotid artery pressure following common and external carotid artery ligation was measured, a minimal change in the distal internal carotid artery pressure was noted when the external carotid artery was opened. The minimal difference in distal internal carotid artery pressure observed in patients with a common carotid occlusion as contrasted with an internal carotid artery occlusion became an important point in later debates over whether to use common carotid or internal carotid artery ligation.

In subsequent work, Bakay and Sweet measured blood pressure in the intracranial vessels following carotid occlusion.[1] Mean pressures in the temporal branches of the middle cerebral artery averaged 86 percent of those measured in the common carotid artery. In five frontal branches and in three parietal branches, the pressures averaged 82 percent of the values measured in the common carotid artery. Bakay and Sweet demonstrated that carotid ligation could produce a reduction in the internal carotid artery pressure distal to the point of occlusion, as well as intracranially in blood vessels down to at least 0.4 mm in diameter. We have also reported that in patients with internal carotid artery occlusion secondary to atherosclerotic disease, the pressure measured in the middle cerebral artery showed a 42 percent reduction from normal.[37]

Bakay and Sweet assessed the prolonged effect of common carotid ligation by measuring internal carotid artery pressures in nine patients 6 days to 24 weeks following their initial ligation.[2] In the majority of patients, the repeat distal carotid pressure demonstrated a slight increase as contrasted with the immediate postocclusion pressure, except for two patients in whom there was a pronounced recovery of pressure almost to the preoperative level. Tindall et al. also recorded immediate and late pressure changes in the internal carotid artery following common carotid ligation.[47] The immediate pressure reductions ranged from 31 to 66 percent of the preocclusion values. The late pressure reductions, however, ranged from 25.5 to 30.8 percent. Retinal artery pressures, measured in the same group of patients, demonstrated an immediate drop in systolic and diastolic pressure of 40 and 33 percent, respectively, following ligation and 30 and 23 percent, respectively, on late follow-up examination. Others have found late pressure reductions in the internal carotid artery ranging from 16 to 44 percent.[16,52]

It is clearly established that ligation of either the common or internal carotid artery will produce a significant drop in the distal internal carotid artery pressure and that this drop in pressure is maintained well into the intracranial vasculature. With time, however, there appears to be an equilibration of the distal internal carotid artery pressure with a prolonged pressure reduction, which usually ranges from 20 to 30 percent of the mean systemic blood pressure.

The distal internal carotid artery pressure has also been correlated with the incidence of recurrent subarachnoid hemorrhage.[51] Among eight patients whose distal carotid pressure following ligation was greater than 100 mmHg, 80 percent had a recurrent hemorrhage. Of eight patients whose residual pressure ranged from 85 to 90 mmHg, two (25 percent) had a recurrent hemorrhage. Among 29 patients whose residual pressures ranged from 80 to 84 mmHg, two (7 percent) had a recurrent hemorrhage, and of 56 patients whose residual pressure was less than 70 mmHg, six (11 percent) had a recurrent hemorrhage.

Following common carotid ligation, blood flow in the internal carotid artery may be maintained in a forward direction or it may reverse, with flow coming down the internal carotid artery and proceeding up the external carotid artery.[49] With time, the reversed internal carotid artery flow will revert to a normal forward flow. The forward flow ranges from 24 to 50 percent of the preocclusion flow rate and it is usually stabilized by 9 h following ligation.[52]

Several authors have analyzed the angiographic change in intracranial aneurysms following carotid ligation. Table 228-1 summarizes 348 reported cases with follow-up arteriography.[10,13,25–27,32,41,47] Of the 348 patients, 30 percent were found on follow-up arteriography to have nonvisualization of their aneurysms and in 86 percent the aneurysms were found to be either nonvisualized or smaller than those seen preoperatively. Thirteen patients demonstrated nonocclusion of the carotid artery on follow-up arteriography. Interestingly, of these 13 patients only one was found on follow-up arteriography to have an aneurysm that was larger than that seen on the initial arteriogram. Despite the infrequent observation of an enlarging aneurysm in the series shown in Table 228-1, case reports have described late arteriographic enlargement of aneurysms following successful carotid ligation.[5]

Indications for Carotid Ligation

In the past, carotid ligation was considered an important alternative for the treatment of all types of intracranial aneurysms, excluding those of the posterior circulation. With present microsurgical techniques, however, most aneurysms of the internal carotid

TABLE 228-1 Arteriographic Changes Following Carotid Ligation

Authors	Year	Number Patients	Aneurysm Location	Artery Ligated	Change in Aneurysm on Follow-Up Arteriogram: Nonvisualized	Much Smaller	Smaller	Unchanged	Larger
Mount, Taveras	1956	10	ICA	ICA	8	—	0	2	0
		4	MCA	ICA	1	—	3	0	0
		8	ICA	Nonocc.	2	—	4	1	1
Harris, Udvarhelyi	1957	66	ICA-P. Com. A.	Various	7	8	51	0	0
Mount	1959	30	Various	Various	12	—	10	6	2
Morris	1963	13	ICA-P. Com. A.	ICA	0	10	2	1	0
		9	ICA-P. Com. A.	CCA	0	7	2	0	0
		5	ICA-P. Com. A.	Nonocc.	0	1	3	1	0
Gibbs	1965	24	ICA	Various	4	3	13	4	0
Stomach, Shenkin	1966	4	ICA	ICA	1	—	3	0	0
		7	ICA	CCA-ECA	4	—	2	1	0
		9	ICA	CCA	5	—	3	1	0
Tindall et al.	1966	58	ICA	CCA	17	—	26	14	1
Odom, Tindall	1968	67	ICA	CCA	25	—	27	14	1
		19	ACA	CCA	13	—	3	1	2
		5	ACA	CCA + ACA	3	—	0	2	0
		10	MCA	CCA	4	—	3	3	0
Total		348			106	29	155	51	7

ACA, anterior cerebral artery; ECA, external carotid artery; MCA, middle cerebral artery; P. Com. A., posterior communicating artery; ICA, internal carotid artery; Nonocc., vessel not occluded; CCA, common carotid artery.

artery distal to the cavernous sinus and those of the middle cerebral, anterior cerebral, and anterior communicating arteries can be treated by direct intracranial clipping. The direct approach offers both lower operative morbidity and mortality than does carotid ligation as well as definitive aneurysm neck occlusion and it avoids some of the long-term complications of carotid ligation that are discussed later in this chapter.

For aneurysms of the intracavernous segment of the internal carotid artery and for giant internal carotid artery aneurysms, which on intracranial exposure are found to be unclippable, carotid ligation remains a viable treatment.

One of the major problems encountered with carotid ligation is the selection of patients who will safely tolerate permanent occlusion. The Matas test was one of the earliest tests employed to select patients who could tolerate carotid occlusion. This technique involved manual compression of the carotid artery in the neck for a period of 10 to 15 min to determine if ischemic symptoms would develop. The test was helpful in predicting those patients who could not tolerate occlusion; however, it had very little predictive value in selecting patients who could tolerate occlusion. This is not surprising since many patients do not develop ischemic symptoms for 48 to 72 h following complete occlusion of the carotid artery.

The most comprehensive assessment to determine tolerance to carotid occlusion has been reported by Miller et al.[24] They established criteria for xenon cerebral blood flow (CBF) measurements, electroencephalography (EEG), and distal internal carotid artery pressure measurements that allowed them to select patients who could safely tolerate carotid occlusion. According to Miller et al., ligation is safe if: (1) CBF is greater than 40 ml/min per 100 g during carotid clamping; (2) CBF during carotid clamping ranges from 20 to 40 ml/min per 100 g, providing the reduction from the control flow is less than 25 percent, (3) CBF ranges from 20 to 40 ml/min per 100 g with up to a 35 percent reduction in flow from the control level, provided that the distal internal carotid artery pressure is greater than 60 mmHg in normotensive patients. Ligation is always considered unsafe if the CBF during clamping is less than 20 ml/min per 100 g. If adequate flow rates cannot be obtained during ligation of the internal carotid artery, then common carotid ligation with flow rate measurements performed can be used as an alternative. Using the criteria of Miller et al. approximately 20 percent of the patients will be unable to tolerate carotid occlusion. Using the above criteria and their surgical results, Miller et al. noted no correlation between tolerance of carotid ligation and preoperative arteriographic findings, including cerebral filling on cross-compression arteriography, jugular venous blood sampling, or EEG measurements, all of which have been used previously for determining the safety of carotid ligation. Unfortunately, patient selection does remain a very difficult problem despite all attempts to find a foolproof method.

Contraindications to the use of carotid ligation include

1. Severe hypovolemia
2. A poor rating on the Botterell or Hunt classification
3. Presence of a recent subarachnoid hemorrhage
4. Cerebral vasospasm noted on arteriogram
5. Presence of an intracerebral hematoma
6. Inability to tolerate carotid occlusion (positive Matas test)
7. Neurological deficit during temporary balloon occlusion of the internal carotid artery
8. Significant drop of CBF (measured by the xenon computed tomography technique) during temporary balloon occlusion even when there is no neurological deficit

The eight listed contraindications reflect situations in which collateral blood flow to the cerebral hemisphere may be severely impaired and therefore may increase the risk associated with carotid ligation. Cerebral vasospasm may already be limiting CBF, and a further decrease of CBF by occluding a carotid artery may cause marked cerebral ischemia or infarction. There is frequently a marked decrease in cerebral perfusion pressure noted in patients who have increased intracranial pressure from a recent hemorrhage or intracerebral hematoma, which may increase the patient's susceptibility to cerebral ischemic complications from carotid occlusion. A poor rating on the Botterell or Hunt classification often reflects a combination of the above situations. Severe hypovolemia is not as common in patients with intracranial aneurysms as in patients who have suffered severe neck hemorrhages. It can develop, however, when a patient has been maintained on severe fluid restriction for several days to reduce cerebral edema. Preoperatively, such patients need volume expansion to help prevent the potential ischemic problems of carotid ligation. It is apparent that the listed contraindications are similar in part to currently held contraindications for intracranial aneurysm surgery. Therefore, the choice of operative intervention, whether it be carotid ligation or intracranial surgery, should be based on the predicted acute and late morbidity and mortality of the operative procedure and not on the patient's immediate clinical condition.

Relative contraindications to carotid ligation include (1) the presence of a contralateral internal carotid artery aneurysm and (2) the presence of contralateral atherosclerotic carotid disease. Following ligation of a carotid artery, increased blood flow develops through the contralateral internal carotid artery. If a contralateral internal carotid artery aneurysm exists, increased flow through that artery may increase the likelihood of subsequent aneurysm rupture. Furthermore, the presence of severe contralateral atherosclerotic carotid artery stenosis may make carotid artery ligation a more dangerous procedure by diminishing the potential for increased flow on the contralateral side.

Selection of Artery

Over the years numerous types of carotid ligation have been performed to treat intracranial aneurysms. These include ligation of the common carotid artery, ligation of the internal carotid artery, ligation of the common carotid artery in conjunction with the external carotid artery, and ligation of the common carotid artery with subsequent ligation of the internal carotid artery. Since the pressure changes in the distal internal carotid artery are similar if either the internal carotid or the common carotid artery is ligated, many authors have recommended the preferential use of common carotid ligation. The incidence of complications from various types of carotid ligation vary considerably from series to series. When Brackett analyzed the complications of internal carotid versus common carotid ligation in patients with supraclinoid aneurysms, there was a considerably lower incidence of complications with internal carotid ligation.[4] When he compared the two types of ligation in patients with infraclinoid aneurysms, however, there was essentially no difference in the complication rate. Scott and Skwarok's review of 909 patients revealed that the operative mortality was 6 percent for internal carotid artery ligation as opposed to 11 percent for common carotid artery ligation.[40] The overall morbidity from internal carotid artery ligation, however, was 22 percent as compared to 11 percent for common carotid artery

TABLE 228-2 Morbidity and Mortality of Carotid Ligation

Authors	Date	Number Patients	Artery Ligated	Aneurysm Location	Morbidity, %		Mortality, %
					Temporary	Permanent	
Poppen, Fager	1960	101	ICA	ICA	6.9		3.9
German, Black	1965	35	Various	ICA	–0–		6.0
Somach, Shenkin	1966	20	CCA	ICA	5.0		5.0
Nishioka	1966	785	Various	Various	31.9		—
		814	Various	Various	—		23.9
Love, Dart	1967	20	Various	Various	5.0		5.0
Neill et al.	1968	146	CCA	ICA	—		13.0
Odom, Tindall	1968	220	CCA	Various	11.4	2.3	6.8
		143	CCA	ICA			16.7
Tindall et al.	1970	31	CCA + contralateral ACA	A. Com. A.	–0–		29.0
Kak et al.	1973	126	Various	ICA	27.0		4.7
Galbraith, Clark	1974	37	CCA	Various	5.4		2.7
Gurdjian et al.	1975	27	CCA	ICA	11.1		11.1
Miller et al.	1977	72	Various	ICA	21.0	5.0	–0–
		28	Nonocc.	ICA	32.0	11.0	–0–
Giannotta et al.	1979	21	Various	ICA	9.5		–0–
Roski et al.	1981	57	Various	Various	16.0		13.0
Jha et al.	1986	114	CCA	Various	42.9	46.4	–0–
Kapp et al.	1987	161	CCA	Various	26.1		15.5
Swearingen, Heros	1987	8	CCA	ICA	25.0	–0–	–0–

ICA, internal carotid artery; CCA, common carotid artery; ACA, anterior cerebral artery; A. Com. A., anterior communicating artery; Nonocc., vessel not occluded.

ligation. It is difficult to conclude from the literature whether internal carotid or common carotid ligation is the safer procedure. The data in Table 228-2 as well as the incidence of late rebleeding shown in Table 228-3 demonstrate the marked variability between the two procedures. We prefer to use internal carotid ligation in those patients with intracavernous internal carotid artery aneurysms or giant internal carotid artery aneurysms. This will often allow for an intracranial trapping procedure if the aneurysm is not completely obliterated following carotid ligation. In most cases we also prefer to perform carotid ligation in conjunction with a superficial temporal artery–middle cerebral artery bypass, as will be discussed in the last section.

Although many authors advocate gradual occlusion of the carotid artery with the use of either the Selverstone, Crutchfield, or Kindt clamp, Landolt and Millikan[22] as well as Nishioka[31] have reported no difference in morbidity from acute versus gradual occlusion of the carotid artery.

TABLE 228-3 Late Rebleeding Following Carotid Ligation

Authors	Date	Number Patients	Artery Ligated	Subarachnoid Hemorrhage
Hardy et al.	1958	54	CCA	3 Fatal (5.5%)
Poppen, Fager	1960	96	ICA	4 Fatal (4.2%)
Scott, Skwarok	1961	21	CCA	4 Fatal (19.0%)
German, Black	1965	18	CCA	2 Fatal (11.1%)
		15	ICA	3 Fatal (20.0%)
Somach, Shenkin	1966	19	Various	1 Fatal (5.3%)
Nishioka	1966	462	Various	16 Fatal (3.4%)
Love, Dart	1967	3	ICA	–0–
		13	CCA	2 Fatal (15.4%)
Neill et al.	1968	127	CCA	6 Fatal (4.7%)
Kak et al.	1973	84	Various	5 Fatal (5.9%)
Miller et al.	1977	72	Various	4 Fatal (5.5%)
Roski et al.	1981	39	Various	3 Fatal (7.5%)
Jha et al.	1986	46	CCA	11 Fatal (23.9%)

ICA, internal carotid artery; CCA, common carotid artery.

Procedure for Carotid Ligation

A patient who is considered appropriate for carotid ligation is one who has none of the aforementioned eight contraindications. We prefer to use a Selverstone clamp placed on the internal carotid artery. Giannotta et al. have stressed the importance of having the patient well hydrated prior to performing the carotid ligation and the use of volume expansion whenever ischemic symptoms occur.[9] If there is concern that a patient, because of age or previous cardiac symptoms, may not tolerate a rapid infusion of intravenous fluids, then a flow-directed catheter should be used to monitor cardiac output, and prophylactic preoperative administration of a digitalis glycoside may be necessary.

Surgery can be performed under local or light general anesthesia. The incision is made along the anterior border of the sternocleidomastoid muscle and dissection is taken down to the common carotid artery. The carotid bifurcation is identified and the carotid bulb is injected with 1% lidocaine. The hypoglossal nerve is identified and isolated from the field. The Selverstone clamp is placed around the internal carotid artery and the stem of the clamp is brought out through a separate stab wound in the skin. The clamp is partially closed to reduce the distal internal carotid artery pressure by 50 percent. This usually will require an 80 percent stenosis of the carotid artery. Postoperatively the clamp is further closed by increments over the next 3 days. If the patient develops focal cerebral ischemia, the clamp is immediately reopened and intravenous volume expansion with either low-molecular-weight dextran or Plasmanate (Cutter Laboratories, Inc., Berkeley, CA) is started. Vasopressors can be used along with volume expansion to increase cerebral perfusion should hypotension develop. When treating previously unruptured aneurysms, systemic heparinization can be used until the carotid artery is finally ligated.

Operative Complications

The operative morbidity and mortality for carotid ligation from previously reported series were reviewed by Scott and Skwarok in 1961.[40] The operative mortality in their review of 909 patients ranged from 0 to 18 percent. Table 228-2 summarizes the operative complications in the major series of carotid ligations reported since 1961.[6,8,9,11,18–20,23,24,30–32,35,38,41,45,48] Operative mortality still varies widely (from 0 to 29 percent). Significant variation in operative morbidity also exists.

Numerous factors have been shown to be significant in producing complications of carotid ligation. Some authors have suggested that older patients are at a higher risk; however, Schorstein, Brackett, and others believe that age is probably not a significant factor in the ability to tolerate carotid occlusion.[4,39] Higher morbidity and mortality rates have been reported when ligation is performed within 10 days of an acute subarachnoid hemorrhage whereas delaying ligation beyond 10 days seems to decrease the risks.

The two major causes of complications immediately following carotid ligation are aneurysmal rebleeding and cerebral ischemia. Kak and colleagues reviewed the incidence of early aneurysmal rebleeding after carotid ligation in the major series reported in the literature from 1953 to 1973.[19] Their review included a total of 1298 patients, 57 of whom had early rebleeding for an overall incidence of 4.4 percent. Several factors have been found to aggravate cerebral ischemia following carotid occlusion. These include systemic hypotension, anemia, and hypovolemia. Correction of anemia and the use of volume expansion have been shown to be beneficial in preventing the ischemic complications from carotid ligation and in treating such complications when they do occur. Although severe bradycardia has been noted following carotid ligation, there has been little documentation to implicate the carotid sinus reflex as a significant cause of early ischemic complications.[22] Another potential cause of ischemia is propagation of a thrombus up the occluded artery; however, Brackett suggests that there is very little evidence to implicate thrombus propagation as a major cause of ischemic complications.[4] Using xenon CBF measurements, Miller et al. have demonstrated that regional cerebral hypoperfusion can occur following carotid occlusion.[24] This may very well be the most significant factor in the development of early ischemic complications.

Late Complications

Late complications from carotid ligation following discharge from the hospital have included aneurysmal rebleeding and ischemic complications on the side of the carotid ligation.[36] Table 228-3 outlines the incidence of late aneurysmal rebleeding.[8,12,18,19,23,24,30,31,35,38,40,41] Wright and Sweet reviewed 112 patients who were followed for up to 16 years, 65 of them for more than 3 years.[51] During the time of follow-up, there were 19 subarachnoid hemorrhages from the treated aneurysms, 12 of those within a 4-year period, and 2 others from a contralateral aneurysm. German and Black followed 18 patients with common carotid artery ligation and 15 with internal carotid artery ligation.[8] Three patients in each group died from aneurysm-related causes, for an incidence of 17 percent in cases of common carotid artery ligation and 20 percent in cases of internal carotid artery ligation. There were also two fatal subarachnoid hemorrhages from other aneurysms in their series. In the report by Miller et al. of 72 patients with carotid ligation, there were 4 subarachnoid hemorrhages, 3 of which were related to a previously undiagnosed aneurysm.[24] Winn et al. compared the late follow-up results of patients with internal carotid–posterior communicating artery aneurysms that were treated either conservatively or with common carotid artery ligation.[50] Of the 41 conservatively treated patients, 8 had late rebleeding from their aneurysms, 3 of which were fatal. Of the 37 patients with common carotid ligation, 4 had fatal rebleeding and 1 had nonfatal rebleeding. There was also one late hemorrhage from a contralateral aneurysm that was treated with intracranial clipping. Winn et al. concluded that although the long-term morbidity was somewhat better in the patients with common carotid ligation, the prevention of aneurysmal rebleeding after 6 months was no different for the operated patients than for those patients who were treated conservatively. Jha et al. had a similar finding in their series of patients with common carotid ligation where the incidence of delayed subarachnoid hemorrhage was 2.4 percent per year.[18]

Several authors have reported the development of a delayed hemiparesis following carotid ligation. Black and German have recorded a 6 percent incidence of late ischemic problems following carotid ligation.[3] Roski and colleagues reported a late occurrence of transient ischemic attacks in 12.5 percent of their patients and a late occurrence of stroke in 7.5 percent.[38] Oldershaw and Voris reported hemiparesis developing in 2 of their 21 patients at 1 and 13 years following internal carotid artery ligation.[33] Love and Dart also reported two instances of delayed hemiparesis among the 40 patients in their series.[23]

Several other potential long-term effects of carotid ligation have been questioned.[50] Winn and associates have noted an increased incidence of hypertension following common carotid ligation.[50] Subarachnoid hemorrhage occurring from previously unrecognized contralateral aneurysms has also been reported.[8,50,51] Hassler[15] and Hashimoto and coworkers[14] have demonstrated in an experimental model that ligation of the carotid artery can lead to contralateral aneurysm formation.

Partial Carotid Ligation

The rationale behind the use of carotid ligation is to decrease the distal intraluminal pressure in an attempt to produce intra-aneurysmal thrombosis. These pressure changes occur following complete carotid occlusion. Other techniques have also been used to produce a similar change in the distal internal carotid artery. Early attempts were made to decrease the distal intraluminal pressure by inducing systemic hypotension. This proved to be difficult to control and did not provide significant protection against rebleeding. Two factors are known to affect a pressure and flow change across an area of stenosis. They are the cross-sectional diameter of the vessel and the length of the stenosis.[21] Very little alteration in the blood pressure across an area of stenosis is obtained until the stenosis reduces the cross-sectional diameter of the artery by at least 70 percent. The drop in pressure can be accomplished by increasing the degree of stenosis or by extending the stenosis over a longer area of the artery. Stenosis of the carotid artery that decreases the arterial diameter by 70 to 80 percent should produce a significant drop in the distal internal carotid artery pressure and potentially provide some protection from rebleeding.

Mullan et al. have reported using the Selverstone clamp to partially occlude the common carotid artery as a temporary means of preventing aneurysmal rebleeding in the period prior to craniotomy.[28,29] In Mullan's first series, all 16 patients were treated with partial ligation of the common carotid artery by using the Selverstone clamp, 24 g/day of epsilon-aminocaproic acid, and a hypotensive regimen of reserpine, chlorothiazide, and chlorpromazine.[28] None of the 16 patients suffered subsequent aneurysmal rebleeding prior to surgery; however, in one patient a contralateral intracavernous internal carotid artery aneurysm ruptured prior to operation and in one patient the treated aneurysm ruptured as the dura was being opened during her craniotomy. One additional patient developed a hemiplegia following the occlusion. It was unclear whether the partial occlusion or cerebral vasospasm caused the hemiplegia. Mullan et al. subsequently reported a series of 13 patients treated by subtotal carotid occlusion alone and 26 patients in whom partial occlusion was used in conjunction with other agents.[29] The average pressure reduction was 44 percent and the clamp was used for an average of 11 days. In five patients the clamp had to be reopened because of clinical deterioration. In two of those patients, symptoms progressed to hemiplegia despite the opening of the clamp. There were also two instances of embolization and three cases of infection. In patients in whom partial occlusion was used along with antifibrinolytic therapy and good control of blood pressure was obtained, there was no incident of rebleeding or death. Five of the six patients who did go on to rebleed from their aneurysm were patients who could not tolerate the hypotensive therapy. A definitive conclusion regarding the use of partial carotid ligation is currently unavailable. In selected cases of intracranial aneurysms, this therapy may prove to be beneficial.

EC-IC Bypass Surgery in Conjunction with Carotid Ligation

The advent of EC-IC arterial bypass surgery added a new dimension to the use of carotid ligation. The two major concerns regarding the use of carotid ligation are (1) the development of a hemiplegia hours to days following complete occlusion of the carotid artery and (2) the significant incidence of late ischemic complications. It has been proposed that providing collateral blood flow to the cerebral hemisphere with EC-IC bypass surgery may decrease the complications. Hopkins and Grand reported a series of 11 patients who were treated by a combination of both internal carotid artery ligation and superficial temporal to middle cerebral artery (STA-MCA) bypass.[17] Three patients developed a cerebral infarct following the EC-IC bypass but prior to ligation of the internal carotid artery. One of their patients died from a ruptured aneurysm. Gelber and Sundt reported excellent results in a series of 10 patients with the same combination of internal carotid ligation and STA-MCA bypass.[7]

Spetzler et al. described a series of 21 patients who had an STA-MCA bypass in conjunction with staged occlusion of the internal carotid artery.[43,44] No ischemic complications developed in the perioperative period or in a 6- to 41-month follow-up. They recommended that the STA-MCA bypass be performed at the same time as the placement of a Selverstone clamp on the internal carotid artery. The Selverstone clamp is partially closed at the time of operation, producing a 50 percent decrease in the distal internal carotid artery pressure. An arteriogram is performed on the third postoperative day to document bypass patency. The clamp is then

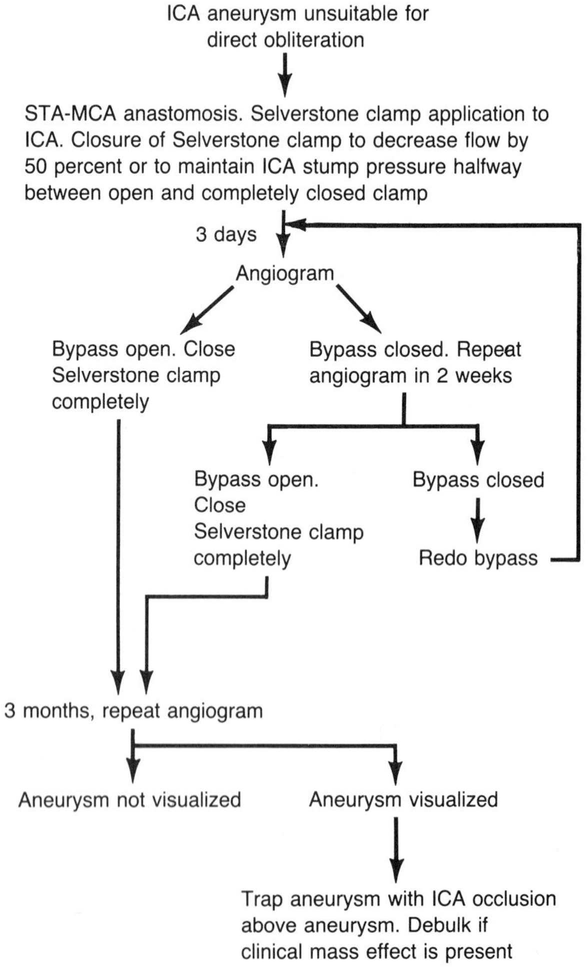

Figure 228-1 Summary of plan for treating internal carotid artery (ICA) aneurysms that are unsuitable for direct clipping. STA, superficial temporal artery; MCA, middle cerebral artery. (Modified from Spetzler et al.,[44] with permission.)

completely closed. The staged occlusion of the internal carotid artery allows time for maturation of the bypass to occur. The clamp is not closed unless a patent bypass has been well demonstrated arteriographically. Three days later the clamp is removed and triple ligation of the internal carotid artery is performed. A follow-up arteriogram is obtained 1 month later to ensure that the aneurysm does not visualize. If it does visualize, then an intracranial trapping procedure is performed. Figure 228-1 outlines our protocol for managing patients with an internal carotid artery aneurysm.

Occluding a portion of the ICA in conjunction with a short high-flow venous bypass is most appealing in dealing with giant unclippable cavernous sinus aneurysms. A petrous carotid-to-intradural carotid saphenous vein graft allows trapping of the cavernous portion of the ICA with elimination of the aneurysm while maintaining a high volume of flow through the remaining ICA.[42] This high-flow bypass has several distinct advantages over other methods. It establishes a high-flow venous graft entirely within the shell, thereby eliminating the stress of neck movement as seen with vein grafts that arise in the neck. The high-flow graft eliminates the risk of inadequate flow as may happen with an STA-MCA bypass. The short segment vein bypass decreases the risk of thrombosis of the graft. The clips that isolate the cavernous portion of the ICA are adjacent to the bypass, thus avoiding vascular dead space with its inherent risk of thrombosis formation.[42] Finally, the advantage of not having to manipulate the cranial nerves in the cavernous sinus as is necessary with the direct approach provides the best protection from further cranial nerve deficits.

References

1. Bakay L, Sweet WH. Cervical and intracranial intra-arterial pressures with and without vascular occlusion. *Surg Gynecol Obstet* 1952; 95:67–75.
2. Bakay L, Sweet WH. Intra-arterial pressures in the neck and brain: late changes after carotid closure, acute measurements after vertebral closure. *J Neurosurg* 1953; 10:353–359.
3. Black SPW, German WJ. The treatment of internal carotid artery aneurysms by proximal arterial ligation. *J Neurosurg* 1953; 10:590–601.
4. Brackett CE Jr. The complications of carotid artery ligation in the neck. *J Neurosurg* 1953; 10:91–106.
5. Cuatico W, Cook AW, Tyshchenko V, Khatib R. Massive enlargement of intracranial aneurysms following carotid ligation. *Arch Neurol* 1967; 17:609–613.
6. Galbraith JG, Clark RM. Role of carotid ligation in the management of intracranial carotid aneurysms. *Clin Neurosurg* 1974; 21:171–181.
7. Gelber BR, Sundt TM Jr. Treatment of intracavernous and giant carotid aneurysms by combined internal carotid ligation and extra- to intracranial bypass. *J Neurosurg* 1980; 52:1–10.
8. German WJ, Black SPW. Cervical ligation for internal carotid aneurysms: an extended follow-up. *J Neurosurg* 1965; 23:572–577.
9. Giannotta SL, McGillicuddy JE, Kindt GW. Gradual carotid artery occlusion in the treatment of inaccessible internal carotid artery aneurysms. *Neurosurgery* 1979; 5:417–421.
10. Gibbs JR. Effects of carotid ligation on the size of internal carotid aneurysms. *J Neurol Neurosurg Psychiatry* 1965; 28:383–394.
11. Gurdjian ES, Lindner DW, Thomas LM. Experiences with ligation of the common carotid artery for treatment of aneurysms of the internal carotid artery. *J Neurosurg* 1975; 23:311–318.
12. Hardy WG, Thomas LM, Webster JE, Gurdjian ES. Carotid ligation for intracranial aneurysm: a follow-up study of 54 patients. *J Neurosurg* 1958; 15:281–289.
13. Harris P, Udvarhelyi GB. Aneurysms arising at the internal carotid–posterior communicating artery junction. *J Neurosurg* 1957; 14:180–191.
14. Hashimoto N, Handa H, Hazama F. Experimentally induced cerebral aneurysms in rats. *Surg Neurol* 1978; 10:3–8.
15. Hassler O. Experimental carotid ligation followed by aneurysmal formation and other morphological changes in the circle of Willis. *J Neurosurg* 1963; 20:1–7.
16. Heyman A, Tindall GT, Finney WHM, Woodhall B. Measurement of retinal artery and intracarotid pressures following carotid artery occlusion with the Crutchfield clamp. *J Neurosurg* 1960; 17:297–305.
17. Hopkins LN, Grand W. Extracranial-intracranial arterial bypass in the treatment of aneurysms of the carotid and middle cerebral arteries. *Neurosurgery* 1979; 5:21–31.
18. Jha AN, Butler P, Lye RH, Fawcitt RA. Carotid ligation: what happens in the long term? *J Neurol Neurosurg Psychiatry* 1986; 49:893–898.
19. Kak VK, Taylor AR, Gordon DS. Proximal carotid ligation for internal carotid aneurysms: a long-term follow-up study. *J Neurosurg* 1973; 39:503–513.
20. Kapp J, Neill WR, Salter JE, Barnes TY. Systemic heparin in the early management of ruptured intracranial aneurysms: review of 104 consecutive cases and comparison with concurrent controls. *Neurosurgery* 1987; 20:564–570.
21. Kindt GW, Youmans JR. The effect of stricture length on critical arterial stenosis. *Surg Gynecol Obstet* 1969; 128:729–734.
22. Landolt AM, Millikan CH. Pathogenesis of cerebral infarction secondary to mechanical carotid artery occlusion. *Stroke* 1970; 1:52–62.
23. Love JG, Dart LH. Results of carotid ligation with particular reference to intracranial aneurysms. *J Neurosurg* 1967; 27:89–93.
24. Miller JD, Jawad K, Jennett B. Safety of carotid ligation and its role in the management of intracranial aneurysms. *J Neurol Neurosurg Psychiatry* 1977; 40:64–72.
25. Morris L. Arteriographic studies in aneurysm of the internal carotid artery treated by carotid occlusion. *Acta Radiol [Diagn] (Stockh)* 1963; 1:367–372.
26. Mount LA. Results of treatment of intracranial aneurysms using Selverstone clamp. *J Neurosurg* 1959; 16:611–618.
27. Mount LA, Taveras JM. The results of surgical treatment of intracranial aneurysms as demonstrated by progress arteriography. *J Neurosurg* 1956; 13:618–626.
28. Mullan S. Conservative management of the recently ruptured aneurysm. *Surg Neurol* 1975; 3:27–32.
29. Mullan S, Hanlon K, Brown F. Management of 136 consecutive supratentorial berry aneurysms. *J Neurosurg* 1978; 49:794–804.
30. Neill CL, Hodges LR, Neill WR. Cerebral aneurysms treated by common carotid ligation. *J Neurol Neurosurg Psychiatry* 1968; 31:87 (abstr).
31. Nishioka H. Results of the treatment of intracranial aneurysms by occlusion of the carotid artery in the neck. *J Neurosurg* 1966; 25:660–682.
32. Odom GL, Tindall GT. Carotid ligation in the treatment of certain intracranial aneurysms. *Clin Neurosurg* 1968; 15:101–116.
33. Oldershaw JB, Voris HC. Internal carotid artery ligation. A follow-up study. *Neurology* 1966; 16:937–938.
34. Pilz C. Zur Ligatur der Arteria carotis communis, nebst einer Statistik dieser Operation. *Arch Klin Chir* 1868; 9:257–445.
35. Poppen JL, Fager CA. Intracranial aneurysms: results of surgical treatment. *J Neurosurg* 1960; 17:283–296.
36. Roski RA, Spetzler RF. Carotid ligation in the treatment of cerebral aneurysms. In Hopkins LN, Long DM (eds): *Clinical Management of Intracranial Aneurysms.* New York: Raven Press, 1982, pp 11–19.
37. Roski RA, Spetzler RF. Middle cerebral artery perfusion pressure in occlusive cerebrovascular disease. Presented at the 51st Annual Meeting of the American Association of Neurological Surgeons, Honolulu, April 26, 1982.
38. Roski RA, Spetzler RF, Nulsen FE. Late complications of carotid ligation in the treatment of intracranial aneurysms. *J Neurosurg* 1981; 54:583–587.

39. Schorstein J. Carotid ligation in saccular intracranial aneurysms. *Br J Surg* 1940; 28:50–70.
40. Scott M, Skwarok E. The treatment of cerebral aneurysms by ligation of the common carotid artery. *Surg Gynecol Obstet* 1961; 113:54–61.
41. Somach FM, Shenkin HA. Angiographic end-results of carotid ligation in the treatment of carotid aneurysm. *J Neurosurg* 1966; 24:966–974.
42. Spetzler RF, Fukushima T, Martin N, Zabramski JM. Petrous carotid-to-intradural carotid saphenous vein graft for intracavernous giant aneurysm, tumor, and occlusive cerebrovascular disease. *J Neurosurg* 1990; 73:496–501.
43. Spetzler RF, Roski RA, Schuster H, Takaoka Y. The role of EC-IC in the treatment of giant intracranial aneurysms. *Neurol Res* 1980; 2:345–359.
44. Spetzler RF, Schuster H, Roski RA. Elective extracranial-intracranial arterial bypass in the treatment of inoperable giant aneurysms of the internal carotid artery. *J Neurosurg* 1980; 53:22–27.
45. Swearingen B, Heros RC. Common carotid occlusion for unclippable carotid aneurysms: an old but still effective operation. *Neurosurgery* 1987; 21:288–295.
46. Sweet WH, Sarnoff SJ, Bakay L. A clinical method for recording internal carotid pressure: significance of changes during carotid occlusion. *Surg Gynecol Obstet* 1950; 90:327–334.
47. Tindall GT, Goree JA, Lee JF, Odom GL. Effect of common carotid ligation on size of internal carotid aneurysms and distal intracarotid and retinal artery pressures. *J Neurosurg* 1966; 25:503–511.
48. Tindall GT, Kapp J, Odom GL, Robinson SC. A combined technique for treating certain aneurysms of the anterior communicating artery. *J Neurosurg* 1970; 33:41–47.
49. Tindall GT, Odom GL, Dillon ML, et al. Direction of blood flow in the internal and external carotid arteries following occlusion of the ipsilateral common carotid artery. *J Neurosurg* 1963; 20:985–994.
50. Winn HR, Richardson AE, Jane JA. Late morbidity and mortality of common carotid ligation for posterior communicating aneurysms. *J Neurosurg* 1977; 47:727–736.
51. Wright RL, Sweet WH. Carotid or vertebral occlusion in the treatment of intracranial aneurysms: value of early and late readings of carotid and retinal pressures. *Clin Neurosurg* 1962; 9:163–192.
52. Youmans JR, Kindt GW, Mitchell OC. Extended studies of direction of flow and pressure in the internal carotid artery following common carotid artery ligation. *J Neurosurg* 1967; 27:250–254.

229 Posterior Circulation Aneurysms

Sydney J. Peerless
Juha A. Hernesniemi
Charles G. Drake

Historical Review

Aneurysms arising from the posterior circulation are relatively uncommon, accounting for less than 15 percent of all intracranial aneurysms. As a result, few surgeons have had the opportunity to become familiar with their treatment, which requires manipulation in the confined space in front of the brain stem and cerebellum. Prior to 1950, a few tumor-like masses in the posterior fossa were explored and, when shelled out, were found to be thrombosed aneurysms.[3,15,21] The true nature of these lesions always came as a surprise to the pioneer surgeons of this era, and required hurried trapping and occlusion of the parent vessels with ligatures and crude clips to control the hemorrhage.[6,7] Schwartz is credited with the first direct attack on an aneurysm in the posterior fossa. Using simple silver clips, he trapped a large sac buried in the pons without the use of magnification and with a successful outcome for the patient.[17] In 1961, Drake first reported his own experience with four patients with aneurysms at the basilar bifurcation.[4] In reviewing the literature to that time, we find that 47 cases had been reported: 14 had been treated with vertebral artery ligation, and almost half of the remaining cases were unusual aneurysms arising peripherally off branches of the vertebral or basilar artery. Of the 10 aneurysms arising at the basilar bifurcation, only 4 were clipped; the remainder were packed with gauze.[11] In 1964, Jamieson published a gloomy report of the direct surgical treatment of 19 aneurysms of the vertebrobasilar system.[10] Postoperatively, only 4 of the patients were employable, 5 had significant neurological morbidity, and 10 died. In 1965, Drake expressed a note of optimism in the surgical treatment of aneurysms of the basilar trunk but emphasized the high morbidity and mortality of the direct surgical attack on aneurysms of the basilar bifurcation.[5] Of his first seven patients with terminal basilar artery aneurysms, four had died, one was severely disabled, and only two had returned to normal life. It was in this communication that Drake pointed out the absolute importance of identifying and protecting the perforating vessels arising from the proximal posterior cerebral arteries in dealing with aneurysms at the basilar bifurcation.

The advent of the operating microscope, fine instruments, and precise clips coupled with modern techniques of neuroradiology, neuroanesthesia, and patient care,[13] has remarkably improved the surgery of intracranial aneurysms. In the past 25 years, our experience has grown to more than 1750 surgically treated cases of vertebrobasilar aneurysms, and current results are comparable to the results of surgical treatment of aneurysms of the anterior circulation. Mortality and morbidity today are almost always limited to patients with giant aneurysms and those who are in a poor clinical state as a result of their initial subarachnoid hemorrhage.

Incidence

Aneurysms of the posterior circulation amount to approximately 15 percent of all intracranial aneurysms. With modern imaging techniques, aneurysms of 0.5 cm in diameter are commonly imaged with computed tomography (CT) scanning or magnetic resonance imaging (MRI). Bilateral injection of contrast substance into the vertebral arteries with anteroposterior (AP), Towne's, and lateral views, and occasionally basal views or angiotomography, are still necessary for precise determination of the surgical anatomy of these lesions.

The most common aneurysms of the posterior circulation are those arising at the basilar bifurcation (51 percent), with those arising from the basilar-superior cerebellar artery (SCA) junction and from the vertebral artery at the posterior inferior cerebellar artery (PICA) origin being the next most common. In our experience, those sacs arising off the posterior cerebral artery, at the vertebrobasilar junction, and off the midportion of the basilar artery in the region of the anterior inferior cerebellar artery (AICA) have been the least common aneurysms arising from this circulation (Fig. 229-1).

Clinical Features

Subarachnoid hemorrhage, caused by rupture of an aneurysm arising in the posterior circulation, can only occasionally be distinguished clinically from rupture of an anterior cerebral circulation aneurysm. Sudden onset of headache, neck pain, nausea, and vomiting are shared commonly by both groups. Abrupt loss of consciousness is perhaps somewhat more common following rupture of a posterior circulation aneurysm, and respiratory and, less often, cardiac arrest may be seen in rupture of an aneurysm nestled close to the medulla, such as the vertebral-PICA aneurysm.

There is a close proximity of some of the cranial nerves to the common sites of aneurysms in the posterior circulation. Aneurysms of the basilar bifurcation, or more commonly the basilar-SCA junction, are in close proximity to the oculomotor nerve as it exits from the interpeduncular fossa. The abducens nerve bears a close relationship to basilar-AICA aneurysms, and the hypoglossal nerve to vertebral-PICA aneurysms. Occasionally, sudden enlargement of the aneurysmal sac may compress and deform one of these nerves, producing a specific nerve palsy. More often, large or giant aneurysms of the terminal basilar artery or especially those arising at the origin of the superior cerebellar artery will deform and compress the peduncle as well as the third nerve, producing a Weber's syndrome. It is remarkable, though, how often even with a large

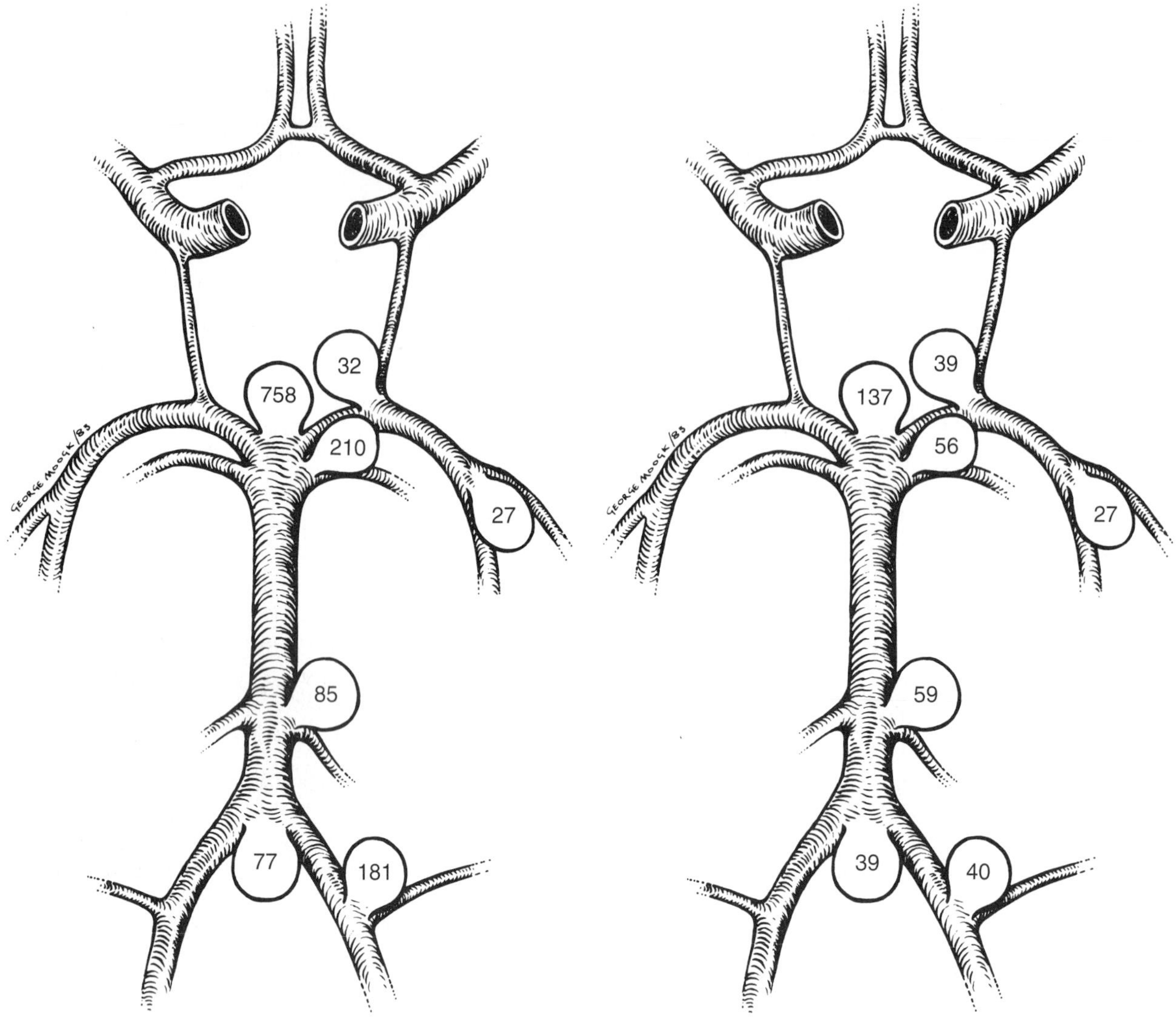

(*A*) (*B*)

Figure 229-1 *A.* Site of small and large aneurysms (<2.5 cm in diameter) arising from the posterior circulation. Numbers in circles indicate patients operated on in our series. *B.* Site of giant aneurysms (>2.5 cm in diameter) arising from the posterior circulation. Numbers in circles indicate patients operated on in our series.

sac and major deformities of the pons and medulla the patient is asymptomatic and has no signs of neurological dysfunction. We have seen deafness, facial palsy, hemifacial spasm, and glossopharyngeal neuralgia only rarely. Of course, with giant sacs and severe compression of the medulla and pyramids, one can see quadriparesis and severe respiratory dysfunction and even obstruction of CSF pathways.

In our experience, vasospasm is as common after subarachnoid hemorrhage from aneurysms of the posterior circulation as it is following rupture of anterior circulation aneurysms. The same relationship exists between the amount of blood spilled into the subarachnoid space and the development of spasm. Rupture of a posterior circulation aneurysm can produce spasm of vessels in the anterior circulation. Vasospasm involving vessels of the vertebrobasilar system results in ischemia in the brain stem, cerebellum, temporal lobe, and occipital pole.

Operative Approaches to Posterior Circulation Aneurysms

Anesthesia and Monitoring Techniques

Much of the success of modern aneurysm surgery is directly related to the development of precise scientific neuroanesthesia. We have been fortunate to work with dedicated neuroanesthetists who have been responsible for developing many of our current techniques.

The patient is brought to the operating room, lightly sedated and with an accurate assessment of fluid balance. A flexible needle is inserted into the radial or dorsalis pedis artery to provide a port for continuous monitoring of the systemic arterial pressure. In patients in whom cardiac function or fluid balance is in doubt, a

Swan-Ganz catheter is installed. The patient is gently induced with pentothal, paralyzed, and then intubated with an armored tube. The anesthetic techniques have varied over the years but basically they consist of assisted ventilation using nitrous oxide or a narcotic technique. In recent years, we have used isoflurane rather than halothane. Isoflurane has proved to be an excellent anesthetic, as well as a convenient way to induce hypotension. The anesthetic is kept reasonably light, with meticulous monitoring of blood gases to maintain the P_{CO_2} in the range of 35 to 45 mmHg and the P_{O_2} in excess of 100 mmHg.

After the patient is positioned, the anesthetist inserts a lumbar subarachnoid catheter through a Tuohy needle into the lumbar subarachnoid space and attaches it to an enclosed collection bag. Lumbar subarachnoid drainage is begun (only after the dura is opened) to aid intracranial relaxation. Adequate intracranial relaxation is essential for the success of surgical procedures at the base of the brain. To ensure a slack brain, we routinely administer 1 g/kg of 20% mannitol and double this dose if we contemplate temporary occlusion of a major intracranial vessel. If necessary, we will administer furosemide (1 mg/kg) intravenously shortly after induction, also to enhance the intracranial relaxation process. Because of this vigorous application of both an osmotic agent and a loop diuretic, meticulous monitoring of the fluid balance is essential and complete replacement of the fluid loss by the end of the procedure is mandatory.

Drug-induced hypotension (below 70 mmHg in half of the patients) for some period of the procedure is almost routine in our theater. The arterial line is connected to a transducer positioned at the level of the brain and connected to a monitor to provide readings of systolic, diastolic, and mean pressures. In the past, hypotension was induced by intravenous infusion of trimethaphan camsylate or sodium nitroprusside. Because of the great variability of the response to these drugs in some individuals and untoward toxic effects, we have, in recent years, abandoned these intravenous medications in favor of simply deepening the isoflurane anesthesia. This technique of isoflurane hypotension has proved to be safe, reliable, and, most importantly, precise. By increasing the concentration of the inspired isoflurane, the anesthetist can bring about an exact decrease in blood pressure and hold it precisely at the predetermined level. When higher pressures are required, the isoflurane concentration is simply reduced without the fear of overshoot or long delays before the pressure returns to normal. Normally, mean systemic arterial pressures of 50 to 60 mmHg are used during the initial dissection around the aneurysm. With manipulation of the sac, or application of the clip, the pressure is lowered to 40 to 45 mmHg. These low pressures have been well tolerated for 30 to 40 min and, even in the elderly, are unlikely to be responsible for neurological or cardiac dysfunction when used for as long as 60 to 90 min. Of course, to maximize collateral flow we do not use systemic hypotension if we contemplate temporary proximal clipping of the vertebral or basilar artery.

In more than 400 patients operated on since 1981, we have frequently come to rely on temporary occlusion of the parent (basilar or vertebral) artery as a means of softening the aneurysmal sac while we dissect and prepare the neck for clipping. In fact, only one-fifth of the patients were operated on under hypotension (below 70 mmHg) in the last 10 years. The new small, temporary clips designed by Suzuki and Sugita are best suited for this purpose, not only for their reliably soft closing pressures, but also for their relative ease of application and removal. The temporary clip must have a gentle closing pressure (less than 40 g) to prevent injury to the parent vessel, and it should not occlude any perforating vessels. Of course, before application of a temporary proximal clip, the patient should be normotensive and should receive an additional bolus of 1 g/kg 20% mannitol. Under these circumstances, temporary occlusion of the basilar artery for up to 10 min is well tolerated. In longer single occlusion times the mortality and morbidity seem to increase; admittedly, these cases have been technically more difficult. Occasionally, we have occluded the basilar artery intermittently for more than 1 h, with 6 or 7 occlusions of 10 min each interspersed with periods of reperfusion.

With the patient positioned, the anesthetist begins meticulous monitoring of fluid balance, electrocardiogram pattern, systemic arterial blood pressure, and blood gases. Occasionally we used brain retractor pressure monitoring but did not find it valuable. Electroencephalography, somatosensory evoked potential, and intraoperative cerebral blood flow (CBF) monitoring have been used in unique situations of giant aneurysms, or when we anticipate prolonged interruption of focal CBF.

Positioning

Most aneurysms of the basilar artery and its branches above the anterior inferior cerebellar arteries can be approached from the supratentorial compartment through the incisura. Normally, we use a subtemporal approach and, therefore, place the patient in the lateral decubitus or ''park bench'' position (Fig. 229-2). The patient is placed on the left side since we normally aim to retract the nondominant temporal lobe. The left axilla is supported on a sand bag, the chest is free, and the back is supported by a firm rest attached to the operating table. The head is attached to a pin headrest in a line so that the anteroposterior axis is precisely parallel to the floor and the sagittal plane angled 15 degrees toward the floor. Normally, we do not move the head again during the procedure, relative to the position of the body, but not infrequently we will tip the table head up or head down, or rotate it from side to side to enhance visualization of the upper basilar artery. The head clamp is positioned, and the operative area is clipped and prepared so as to permit extension of the normal tic craniectomy either forward or backward to fashion a frontotemporal or posterior temporal flap. As outlined below, most often a tic craniectomy has proved adequate to deal with most of the aneurysms of the upper basilar artery. In some circumstances, it will be necessary to convert the approach to the pterional trans-sylvian exposure, a combination of the subtemporal and trans-sylvian exposure, or the posterior temporal exposure. This flexibility must be planned for at the time of positioning.[14]

Prophylactic antibiotics are not used. Wound infection was seen in only 7 out of 1767 patients with more than 2000 intracranial procedures.

Subtemporal Approach to the Upper Basilar Artery

A small controversy exists regarding the optimum method of approaching aneurysms of the upper basilar artery. We have favored the subtemporal approach; others have suggested that the pterional approach is ideal. In reality, a true controversy does not exist. There are clear advantages and disadvantages to each method and to combinations of these methods, with certain configurations and positions of aneurysms clearly favoring one or another method.

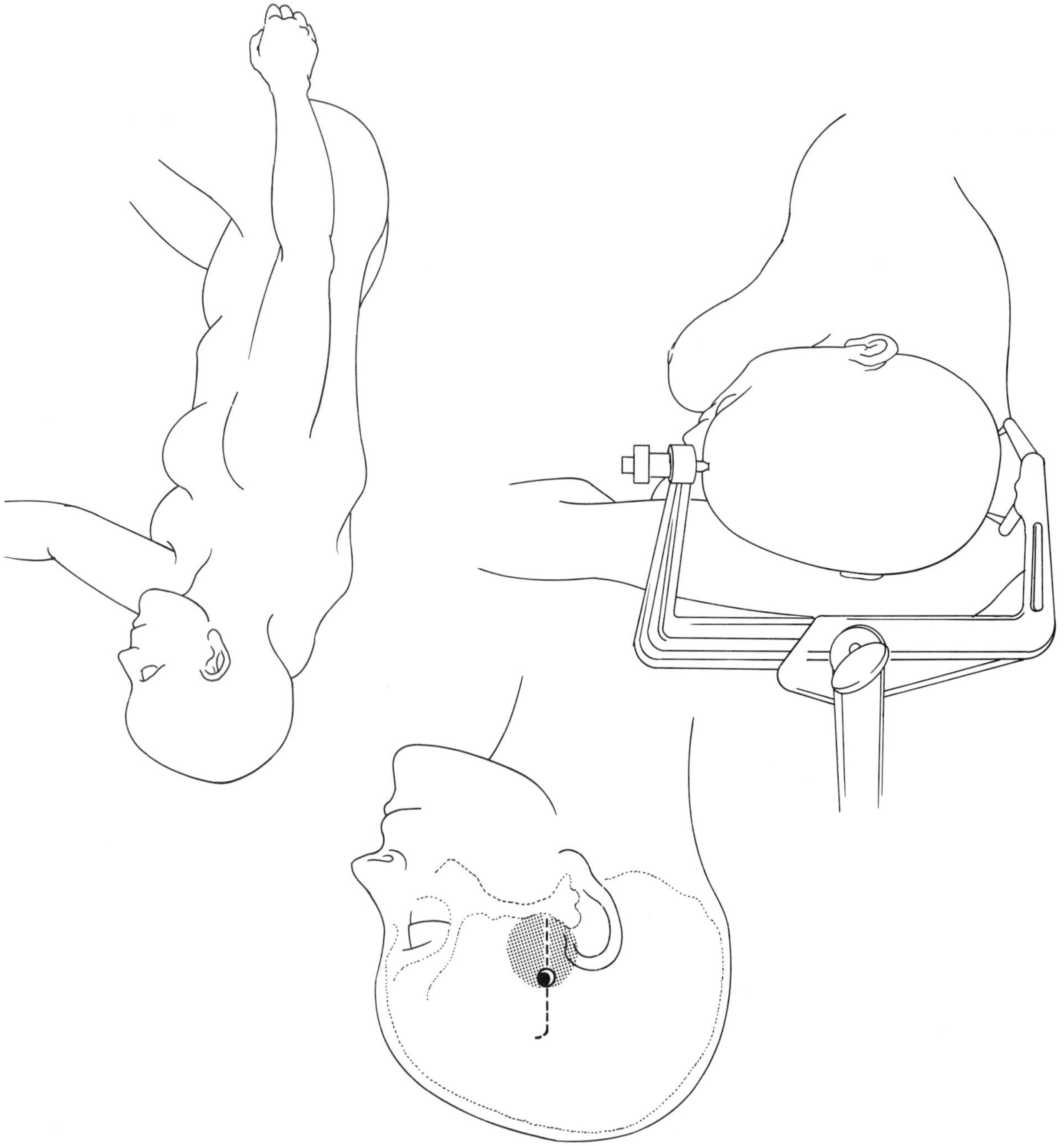

Figure 229-2 Lateral decubitus position for a subtemporal approach to the upper basilar artery. Note: The anteroposterior axis of the head is parallel to the floor. The dotted line and stippled area in the lower drawing show the scalp incision and craniectomy site, respectively.

Most important is the surgeon's familiarity with the method, the anatomy, the configuration of the aneurysm, the depths of the wound, and, in particular, certain fundamental hazards that must be recognized and guarded against with each of the methods.

In our early experience, we routinely turned sizable temporal bone flaps in the subtemporal approach to aneurysms of the upper basilar artery. However, in our more recent 1000 cases, this has proved unnecessary. With the routine use of the operating microscope, one needs a much smaller bony opening, large enough only to admit the light beam of the microscope, to manipulate the microinstruments, and to achieve sufficient retraction of the temporal lobe. The key to the exposure is to gain access to the base of the skull, at about the junction of the anterior and middle third of the temporal lobe where the temporal lobe has begun to turn upward to follow the convex floor of the middle cranial fossa. The surgeon gains nothing by exposing a large area of the lateral surface of the temporal lobe, either anteriorly or posteriorly, unless the exposure is to be converted to the frontotemporal approach or the posterior temporal approach. Certainly bone removal over the lateral surface of the temporal lobe is to no avail.

A linear incision extending vertically upward from the zygomatic process of the temporal bone, just in front of the main stem of the superficial temporal artery, for a distance of approximately 10 cm is sufficient. After the skin, subcutaneous tissue, and galea are divided, the temporalis fascia and muscle are incised using the monopolar cutting current, with the muscle fibers being cut at right angle to the vertical incision for about 5 mm on either side at the level of the zygomatic process. The scalp and soft tissue are then retracted, and a single burr hole is made in the squamous portion of the temporal bone. It is important to remove the temporal squama with rongeurs, or recently with a high-speed drill, down to the level of the zygomatic root so that the bony opening is as flush with the floor of the middle fossa as possible (Fig. 229-3*A*). The bony opening should be about 4 cm across at the base and 3 to 4 cm high. Recently, we have returned to a small bone flap the same size as the craniectomy with less posteoperative discomfort and deformity for better patient acceptance. The anterior branch of the superficial temporal artery will be divided, but the posterior branch is left intact because occasionally it may be necessary to use this scalp vessel to form a surgical collateral.

The triangular opening of the dura, based inferiorly, is fastened. The lumbar subarachnoid drain is normally opened at this point in the procedure, and drainage of cerebrospinal fluid is commenced. The undersurface of the temporal lobe is then gently inspected with a hand-held retractor to identify the position of any bridging veins anteriorly, and to identify and protect the vein of Labbé (Fig. 229-3*B*). We normally cover the vein of Labbé with several strips of Gelfoam (absorbable gelatin sponge; The Upjohn Company, Kalamazoo, MI) to protect it. This critical vein and those at the tip of the temporal lobe should be spared; tiny bridging veins on the undersurface of the temporal lobe, and particularly a commonly seen vein that runs between the uncus and the tentorial edge, may be coagulated and divided. The surface of the temporal lobe should then be covered with a compressed sheet of Gelfoam, and the temporal lobe gently retracted.

The key to this approach is to have sufficient intracranial relaxation. A slack brain is essential. The combination of mannitol and CSF drainage is usually sufficient to bring about relaxation, but if not, it is important to check the respiratory parameters, elevate the head, and wait until a little more CSF has been withdrawn, or give a second dose of mannitol. Although cerebral edema is the most likely cause for a persistently swollen and tight brain, corticosteroids have not been used because they have little effect on vasogenic edema and have many potential complications. Most maneuvers on the operating table will not adequately relieve this edema, and further retraction and manipulation run a high likelihood of aggravating it in the postoperative period. If retraction remains heavy, it is wise to abandon the procedure in favor of returning another day or to make the attempt through another approach. Occasionally, a swollen brain that cannot be adequately retracted will be encountered. Heavy retraction and damage to surface veins, combined with hypotension, will set the stage for disastrous brain swelling, infarction, or hemorrhage into the temporal lobe.

After a self-retaining retractor is inserted, the edge of the tentorium will come into view. Retractor pressure is deepened and increased slightly so that the uncus, seen through the layer of overlying arachnoid, is displaced away from the free edge of the tentorium by 2 or 3 mm. The free edge of the tentorium is now sutured back into the floor of the middle cranial fossa. By tensioning this suture, the free edge is rolled laterally, giving another 3 to 5 mm of exposure and obviating the need for division of the tentorium for most aneurysms of the upper basilar artery.

The operating microscope is now brought into position and, under 10 to 16 times magnification, the surgeon should focus on the layer of arachnoid covering the uncus and cerebral peduncle. The trochlear nerve will be seen shining through the outer layer of arachnoid as it runs around the peduncle to pass to the underside of the tentorium. The arachnoid should be picked up just superior to this nerve and sharply incised with a fine knife and the incision extended anteriorly, opening the double layer of arachnoid as it crosses to form the lateral boundary of the interpeduncular cistern. Following subarachnoid hemorrhage, the cistern is typically filled with clotted blood. This blood can be removed with suction and dissection, taking care to avoid the likely site of rupture of the aneurysm. We normally identify the superior cerebellar artery as it courses around the peduncle, and dissecting the old clot off its surface, we follow it down to the lateral aspect of the basilar artery. Then, after identifying the basilar artery, it is a simple matter to

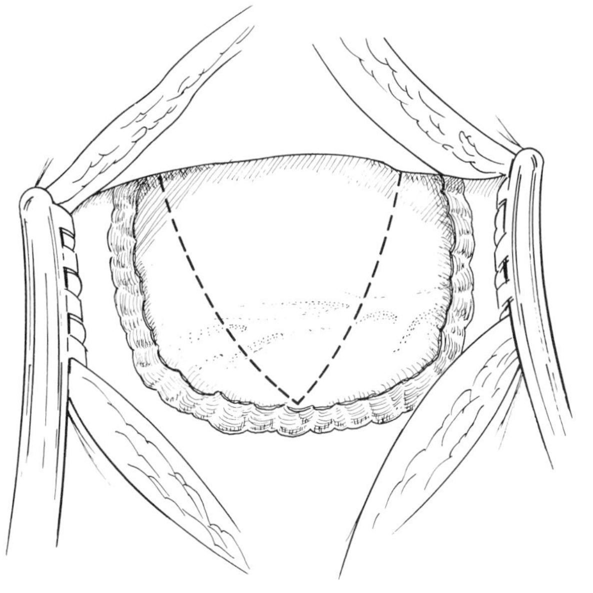

(*A*)

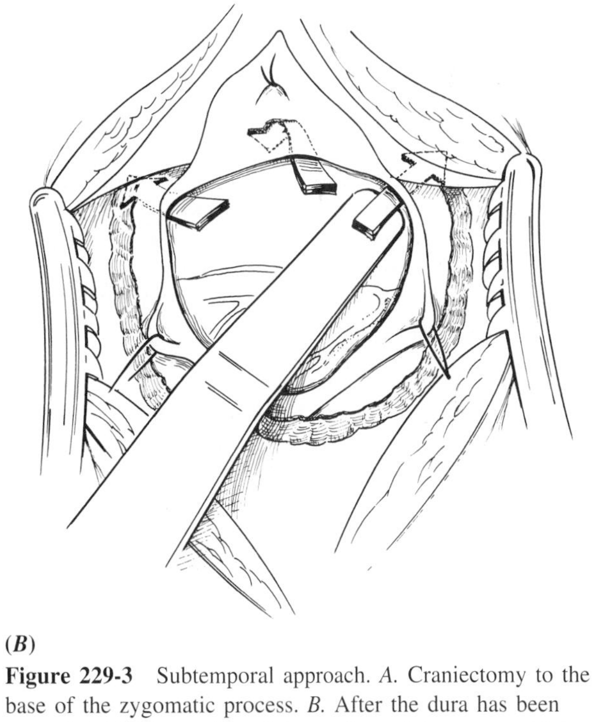

(*B*)

Figure 229-3 Subtemporal approach. *A*. Craniectomy to the base of the zygomatic process. *B*. After the dura has been opened, initial inspection of the surface of the temporal lobe for position of bridging veins.

move superiorly to expose the origins of the two posterior cerebral arteries on the near (right) side, on the left side, and on the anterior aspect of the neck of the aneurysm. By looking across the anterior aspect of the basilar artery, the origins of both proximal posterior cerebral (P1) arteries can be seen by gently compressing the neck and the ectatic basilar artery backward toward the pons. Similarly, with a small dissector, the terminal basilar artery can be gently lifted out of the interpeduncular fossa, bringing into view the posterior aspect of the neck and, more importantly, the fine perforating vessels that arise off the origins of each P1 segment (Fig. 229-4*A*).

The third cranial nerve frequently need not be manipulated at all during this exposure. It is left attached to the uncus by the double layer of arachnoid, and because the retractor has lifted the uncus, the third nerve is displaced out of the operative field. The site at which the posterior cerebral artery courses over the nerve is a useful reference point, as it is between this point and the origin of the P1 segment that all of the terminal perforating vessels will be found. It cannot be overemphasized that these perforating vessels must be identified and protected at all cost. They are frequently adherent to the posterior and lateral aspects of the aneurysm, and should be dissected free and clearly preserved during clip placement. Working from the lateral aspect in this approach, it is necessary to displace the terminal basilar artery for several millimeters out of the interpeduncular fossa so as to look behind the aneurysm and see the perforators off the opposite (left) P1, and ensure that they are also protected and free. Again from the lateral approach, we have found the aperture clip, designed originally by Drake, to be most useful. The clip blades are measured to be precisely long enough to obliterate the neck of the sac. We would normally place the right P1 segment into the aperture, often with one or two perforators (Fig. 229-4*B*). Occasionally, the third cranial nerve is included in the clip aperture to get an anatomic position of the blades across the neck of the aneurysm.

Several points need to be emphasized in dealing with basilar bifurcation aneurysms. First, the neck of such an aneurysm is almost always wider in the sagittal plane than in the anteroposterior dimension. This is another cogent reason for clipping from the subtemporal approach; one can compress the neck in its narrowest dimension without kinking or deforming the origins of the posterior cerebral arteries. It is critical always to review and identify the visible anatomy before applying the clip. It is easy to mistake the opposite superior cerebellar artery for the left P1, but by identifying the opposite oculomotor nerve, and recalling that this structure always runs between the superior cerebellar and posterior cerebral arteries, one should find that positive identification of the origin of the left P1 is not a problem. The precise length of the clip blade is essential. When too short, it will of course leave a portion of the neck open and the aneurysm still filling. A more troublesome error, however, is to place too long a clip blade, narrowing or occluding the origin of the opposite P1. We avoid this by actually measuring the width of the neck on its anterior and posterior surfaces with a slim dissector and choosing an appropriate clip or, if necessary, cutting and filing the blades of a clip to exactly the required dimension (Fig. 229-5).[14]

Typically, we place, remove, and replace the clip many times before we are satisfied. After the clip placement and careful inspection of the posterior and anterior surfaces to ensure that the major vessels and their perforators are free, the dome of the aneurysm is punctured and its contents aspirated. With the extra room afforded by the collapsed sac, the anatomy is carefully inspected again. If precision has not been achieved with the clip in position, it should be immediately removed and repositioned.

The length of the basilar artery varies considerably. The height of the bifurcation typically is just at or slightly above the level of the dorsum sellae. Occasionally, it may be much higher, reaching well above the mamillary bodies and indeed, at times, indenting the third ventricle. With a very high bifurcation aneurysm, the subtemporal approach may not be advantageous because more temporal lobe retraction is necessary, requiring dissection between the uncus and oculomotor nerve. With a very high bifurcation, it is occasionally prudent to choose the pterional trans-sylvian approach (Fig. 229-6). If, on the other hand, the bifurcation is low (i.e., a centimeter or more below the level of the dorsum sellae), the pterional trans-sylvian approach may be impossible because the bony barrier of the dorsum sellae will prevent exposure and visualization of the neck of the aneurysm.

With the low-lying bifurcation aneurysms, the dissection and

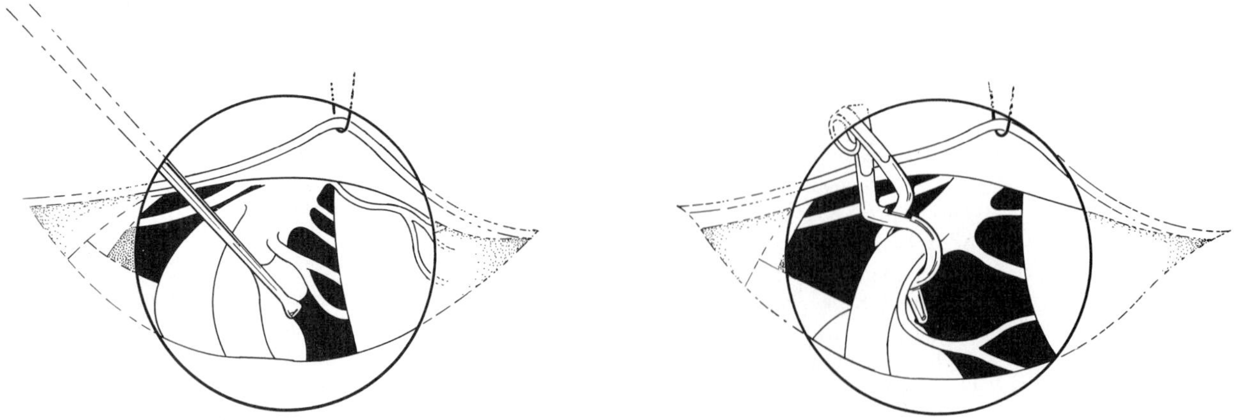

(*A*) (*B*)

Figure 229-4 Subtemporal approach. *A*. Exposure of a basilar bifurcation aneurysm. A dissector is displacing the aneurysm and terminal basilar artery away from the interpeduncular fossa. Note the perforating vessels arising from the P1 segment. The edge of the tentorium has been sutured back into the middle fossa. *B*. Placement of an aperture Sugita clip across the neck of the basilar bifurcation aneurysm. The P1 segment and one perforator are patent in the aperture.

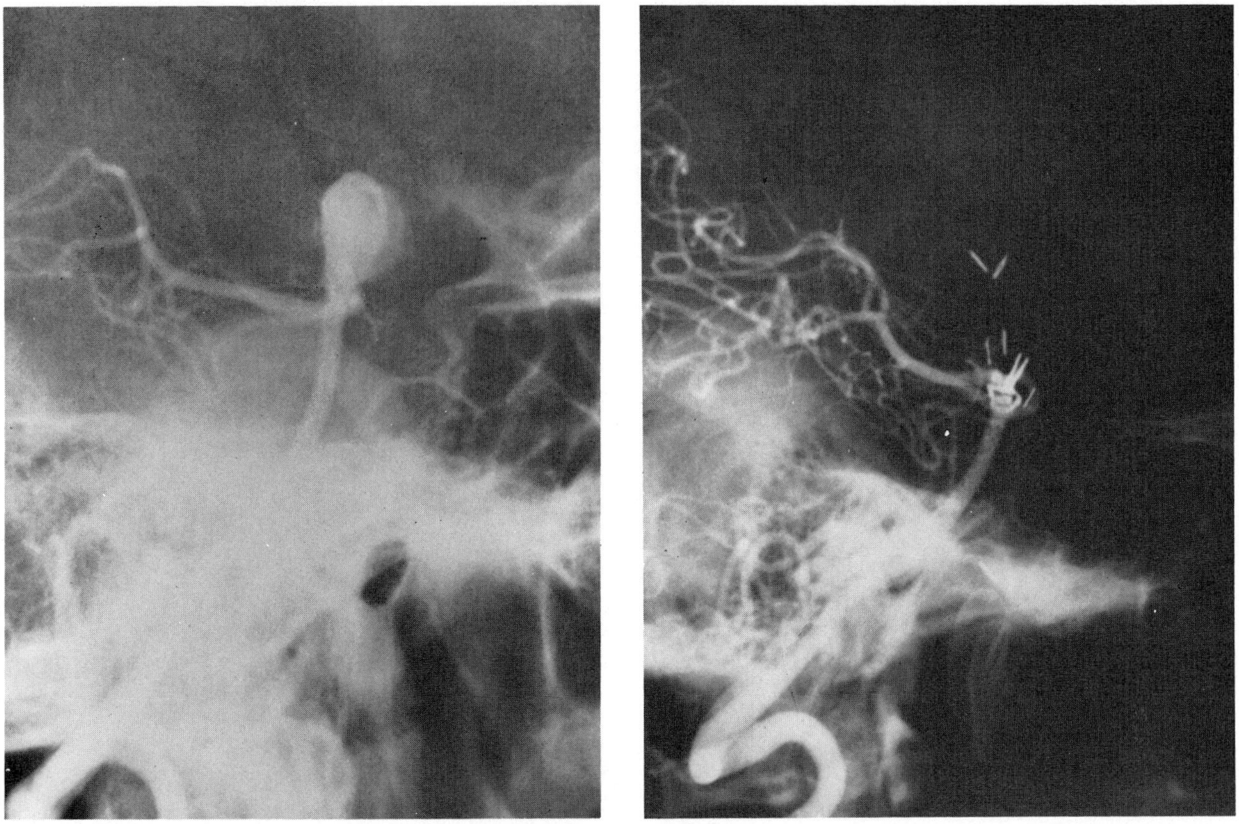

(*A*) (*B*)

Figure 229-5 *A.* Lateral vertebral angiogram showing a large basilar bifurcation aneurysm pointing upward. *B.* Postoperative angiogram after a subtemporal approach, showing the lateral orientation of the clip obliterating the neck of the aneurysm.

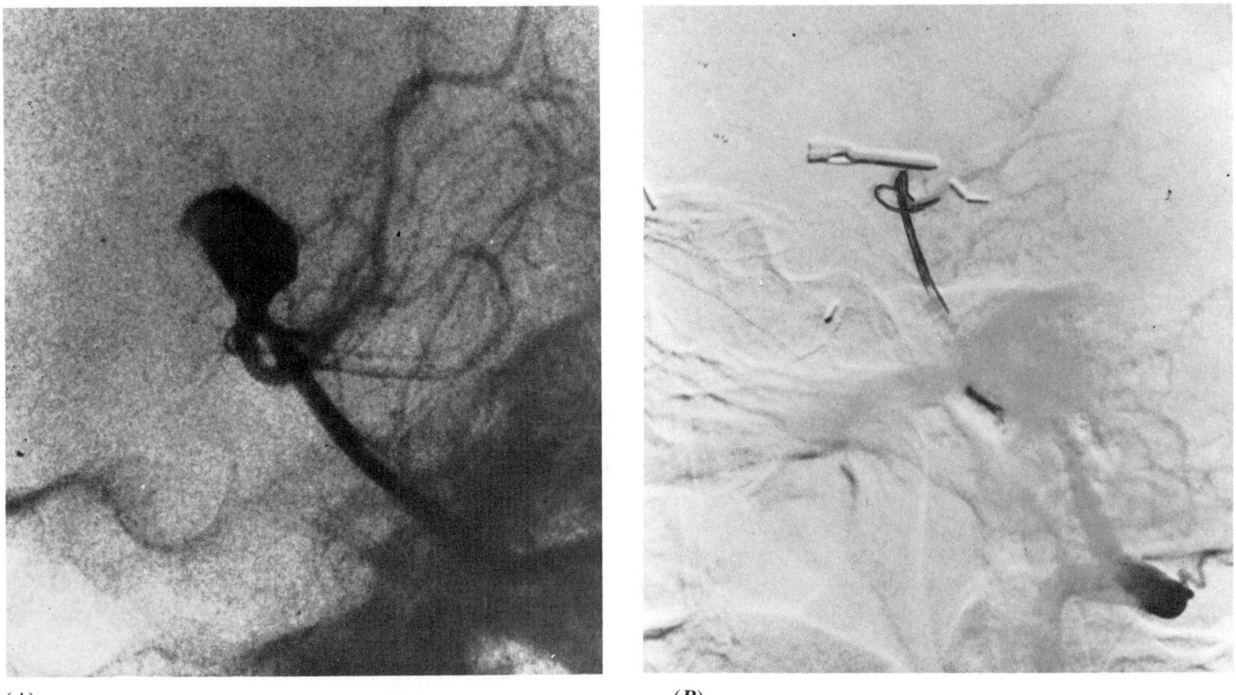

(*A*) (*B*)

Figure 229-6 *A.* Lateral vertebral angiogram showing an elongated basilar artery and the neck of a bifurcation aneurysm situated more than 1 cm above the dorsum sellae. *B.* This bifurcation aneurysm was clipped via the pterional trans-sylvian approach.

exposure are considerably more difficult, and indeed at times hazardous. The dome of the aneurysm and its original rupture site are often fused to the clivus or posterior aspect of the dorsum, making manipulation of the sac hazardous with an increased likelihood of intraoperative rupture. The space that contains these low-lying aneurysms is a narrow, truncated cone with the apex pointing downward. This forces the surgeon to gain visual access to the neck from the subtemporal approach, over the bulging belly of the pons in the depths of the wound. This approach is enhanced by retracting the temporal lobe somewhat more posteriorly to view the anterior aspect of the pons. Division of the tentorium is occasionally necessary to gain a better access to this region, and angled aperture clips are often essential to secure these low-placed aneurysms.

Another conceptual hazard in dealing with basilar bifurcation aneurysms is the appearance given by angiograms taken in the Towne's projection, which tend to show the P1 segments entirely separate from the neck of the aneurysm and coming straight laterally from the side of the basilar artery. In reality, and in particular when viewed from the surgical exposure of the subtemporal approach, the posterior cerebral arteries course forward, upward, and laterally before they turn out to cross above the oculomotor nerve and before swinging laterally around the peduncle under cover of the hippocampal gyrus. With the angiographic picture in mind, the surgeon will be surprised when faced with a large or bulbous bifurcation aneurysm to see from the lateral exposure what appear to be the P1 segments coming out of the side of the aneurysmal sac. As mentioned above, in the course of the development of the aneurysms, and particularly the larger ones, the terminal basilar artery becomes widened and ectatic. It is critical then for the surgeon to define the neck precisely, even though it may appear to be much wider than in the angiogram, and to spare the origins of both P1's and, of course, any adjacent perforators.

Superior Cerebellar Artery Aneurysms

Superior cerebellar artery aneurysms arise at the origin of the superior cerebellar artery off the basilar artery or seldom distally at the SCA itself. This aneurysm almost always projects laterally, forward, or backward with the fundus imbedded in the peduncle. As the sac and neck enlarge, the aneurysm will occupy the whole length of the basilar artery between the distal carina of the superior cerebellar artery and the proximal origin of the posterior cerebral artery. The fundus of the aneurysm almost always has an intimate association with the oculomotor nerve and will stretch this nerve over or below the dome of the sac. With large superior cerebellar artery aneurysms, deformity and dysfunction of the third nerve, as well as compression of the peduncle, produces the common Weber's syndrome.

Small and moderate-sized aneurysms of the basilar–superior cerebellar artery junction are usually quite straightforward to deal with. There are no perforators arising off the superior surface of the superior cerebellar artery, and the perforators arising off the inferior posterior surface of the posterior cerebral artery are usually displaced away from the sac and neck as the fundus enlarges. The subtemporal exposure gives an excellent exposure of this aneurysm. After defining the neck and being quite certain of the presence and position of the posterior cerebral perforators, the surgeon, following the natural line of the basilar artery as it turns to form the origin of the posterior cerebral artery, can usually work a clip across the neck of the aneurysm. The superior cerebellar artery tends to emerge from the inferior origin of the neck of the aneurysms rather than from the basilar artery, particularly as the sac enlarges, so that a clip must be applied with exquisite accuracy to preserve the orifice of this vessel (Fig. 229-7).

Small aneurysms of the left superior cerebellar artery will require a left subtemporal approach. There is a slight but additional hazard to the patient with retraction of the dominant temporal lobe, but, in our experience, this has not been significant. Very large aneurysms arising off the left side of the basilar artery at this site may be approached from the right side because the basilar artery is usually displaced toward the right as the aneurysm enlarges. The surgeon then performs the dissection over the front of the basilar artery, taking advantage of the shorter distances involved. The two major hazards of clipping these aneurysms are kinking or narrowing the basilar artery, and narrowing or occluding the origin of the superior cerebellar artery. These hazards may be avoided if, after the neck is secured with a clip, the sac is punctured and collapsed and careful inspection is made to ensure that both the basilar artery and the superior cerebellar artery are normally patent. The superior cerebellar artery normally has poor collateral circulation; narrowing or occlusion of this vessel with the tip of the clip blade will usually result in a devastating infarction of the midbrain and cerebellum.

Posterior Cerebral Artery Aneurysms

The four typical sites of origin of aneurysms from the posterior cerebral artery are (1) at the origin of the large perforating branches on P1; (2) at the junction of the posterior communicating artery and P1 segment; (3) at the origin of the anterior and posterior occipital-temporal arteries along the side of the brain stem; and (4) at the terminal branching of the vessel into its parietal and calcarine branches. The most common sites are at the origin of the large perforating branches on P1 and where the first major branching occurs along the side of the brain stem (P2).

The more proximal of these aneurysms can be dealt with conveniently via the subtemporal approach. These aneurysms are relatively easy to dissect, being somewhat distal to the main perforators going to the perforated substance and peduncle, but the surgeon must always take care to spare these vessels without exception. The more distal of these aneurysms are typically hidden under the hippocampal gyrus, requiring more retraction of this gyrus or occasionally resection of a small portion of the gyrus to gain exposure. Resection of a portion of the hippocampal gyrus is almost always necessary with those aneurysms lying in the origin of the choroidal fissure. With giant aneurysms arising off the posterior cerebral artery, we have found that it is usually safe to proximally occlude the posterior cerebral artery distal to the perforators that arise off the first and second segments and beyond the emergence of the major temporal branch of the posterior cerebral artery. The posterior cerebral artery normally has a rich collateral supply. In 47 cases where we have deliberately occluded the posterior cerebral artery, we have had only 5 incidences of a persistent visual field defect as the result of occipital infarction. Nevertheless, it is important to state that one must not occlude the posterior cerebral artery proximal to the origin of the posterior choroidal arteries or to trap any of the proximal perforators off the posterior cerebral artery because ischemia or infarction in the territory of these vessels will be devastating.

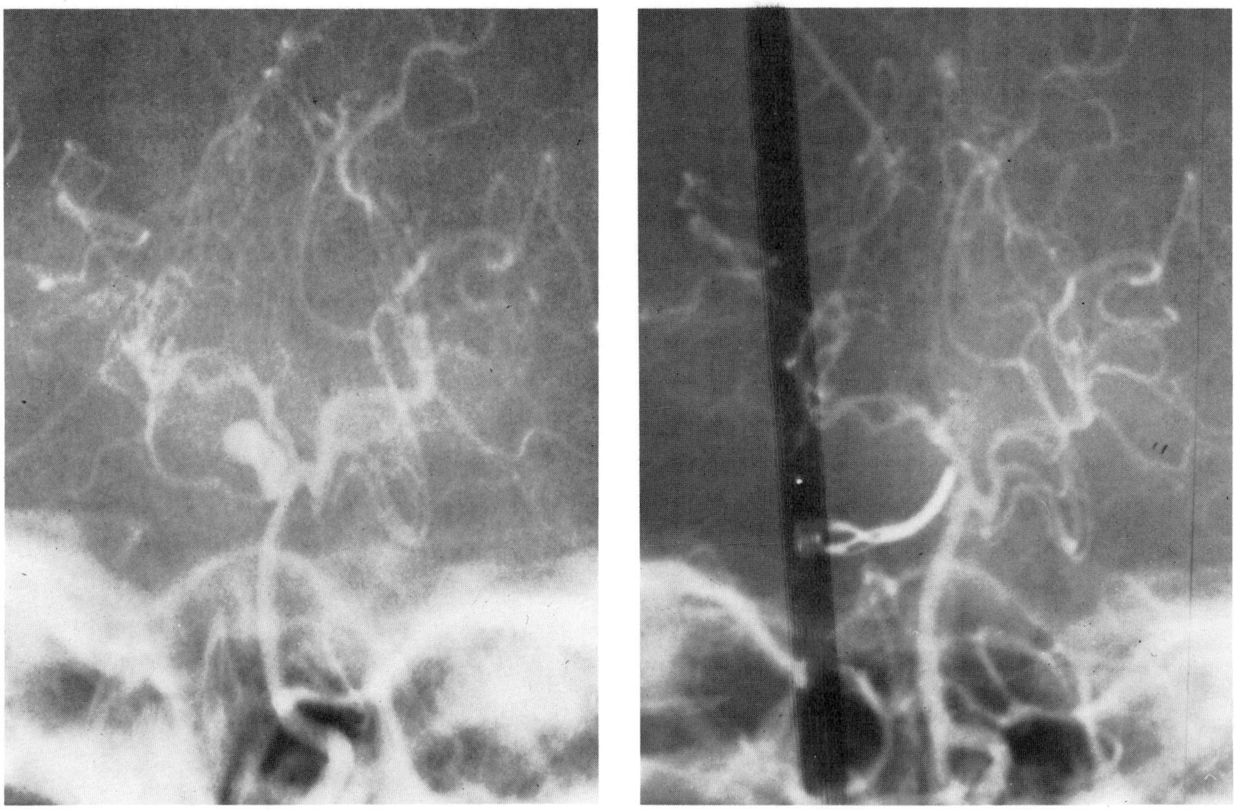

(*A*) (*B*)

Figure 229-7 *A*. Anteroposterior angiogram showing a partially thrombosed giant aneurysm arising from the right basilar-SCA junction. *B*. It was clipped with a curved Sugita clip.

Trans-Sylvian Pterional Approach to Aneurysms of the Terminal Basilar Artery

The pterional approach has many proponents and some distinct advantages (Fig. 229-8). The approach also has some hazards and disadvantages, which should be known and appreciated. As described by Yaşargil et al., this approach emphasizes a small frontotemporal craniotomy with removal of the lesser wing of the sphenoid at the pterion to give a greater exposure of the base of the brain by removing some of the base of the skull.[22,23] Although bone removal has been emphasized in this approach, the key to success is not only bone removal but a lengthy and careful splitting of the sylvian fissure. We think it would be more accurate to describe this as the trans-sylvian pterional approach to the basilar bifurcation, with the greater emphasis on opening the fissure. The fissure needs to be separated to the point where the carotid bifurcation and origin of the middle cerebral artery can easily be seen. Then with retraction of both the frontal and temporal lobes, and through the widely opened sylvian fissure, the dissection is carried deeply, usually on the lateral side of the carotid artery, following the posterior communicating artery backward to the posterior cerebral and thence to the bifurcation. Occasionally it will be necessary to clip and divide the posterior communicating artery (always between and sparing its vital perforators) to remove the curtain of vessels that will be between the operator and the operator's ultimate goal. With this exposure, the basilar artery and the bifurcation will appear obliquely oriented to the operator with the near (usually right side) P1 origin being clearly seen, with somewhat less visualization of the left P1. The neck of the aneurysm, in the case of the usual basilar bifurcation sac, will be nicely in view and easily dissected from this position. This immediate accessibility of the neck may prove a trap for the unwary. The hazard is that the P1 perforators are not immediately visible, arising as they do from the posterior aspect of the P1 segments, often wrapping around and behind the neck of the sac and often crossing the midline. A clip worked across the neck of the sac and closed, therefore, runs a considerable hazard of occluding one of these perforators without the vital vessel ever being seen.

In general, it is preferable to make this approach on the lateral side of the carotid artery. It has been suggested that the approach can also be made on the medial side of the carotid artery. We believe this is hazardous and rarely necessary. It requires retraction on the carotid artery, which can be troublesome, particularly if the vessel is atherosclerotic. Moreover, the space between the carotid artery and the optic nerve presents yet another shutter of vital structures between the surgeon and the ultimate goal, increasing the difficulty of visualization and instrument manipulation.[20]

Certain disadvantages of the trans-sylvian pterional approach need be emphasized. The basilar bifurcation is at least 1 cm deeper via the trans-sylvian approach as compared with the subtemporal

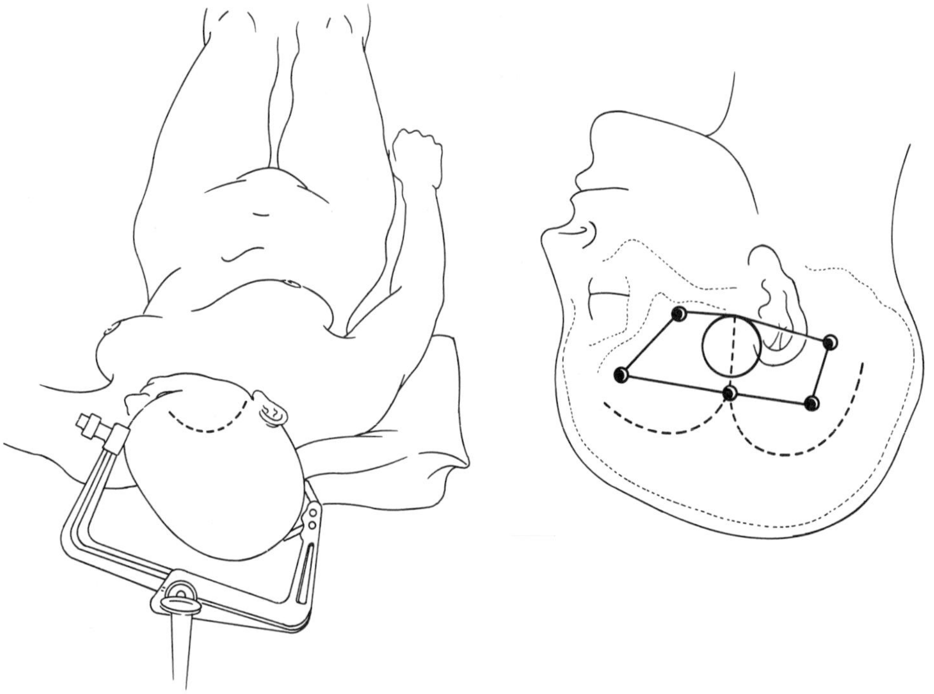

Figure 229-8 Position of a patient for a pterional trans-sylvian approach. The drawing on the right depicts the scalp incisions (*dotted lines*) and approximate craniotomy sites for the pterional, subtemporal, and posterior temporal approaches to the upper basilar artery.

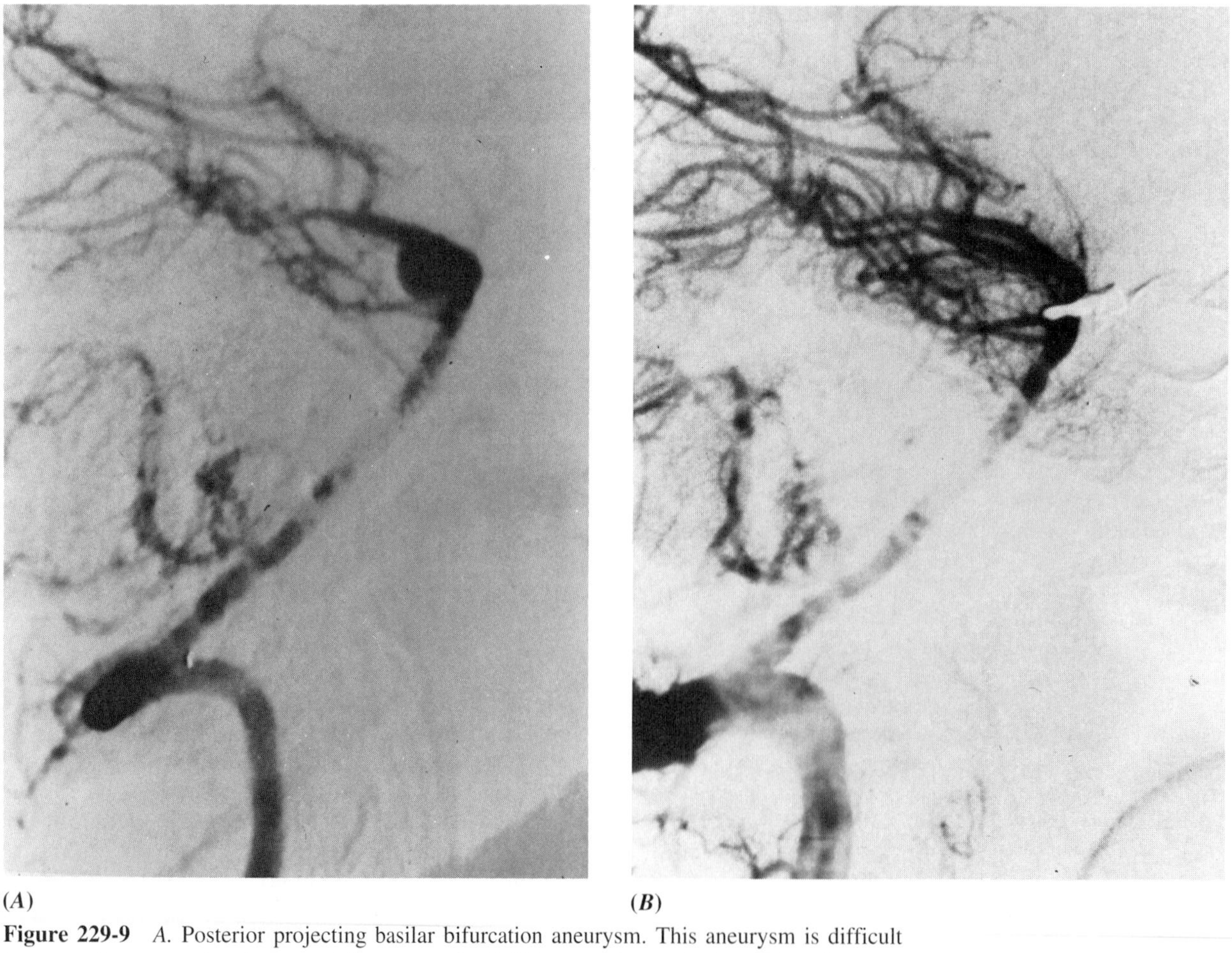

(*A*) (*B*)

Figure 229-9 *A*. Posterior projecting basilar bifurcation aneurysm. This aneurysm is difficult to secure from a pterional trans-sylvian approach. *B*. This posterior projecting bifurcation aneurysm was clipped from a lateral subtemporal approach.

approach. This greater distance, coupled with a curtain of vital structures (optic nerve, carotid artery, posterior communicating and anterior choroidal arteries and their perforators) in the path, will frequently make the exposure more technically demanding. The orientation of the basilar artery is oblique, and is addressed from the anterolateral aspect when using the trans-sylvian approach, increasing the possibility of anatomic confusion and always making it difficult to see the P1 perforators with certainly. Low-lying bifurcation aneurysms and those aneurysms arising off the basilar artery at the superior cerebellar origin may have their necks largely obscured by the dorsum sellae. Bilobed aneurysms of the bifurcation, or those that project entirely backward into the interpeduncular fossa, cannot be dealt with adequately by the trans-sylvian route (Figs. 229-9 and 229-10). Finally, a short, wide, or ectatic carotid artery may entirely block the operator's exposure of the terminal basilar artery.

On the other hand, the rare case of an aneurysm at the superior end of an elongated basilar artery with a high-lying bifurcation can most often be conveniently approached by splitting the sylvian fissure. Certainly, the most common bifurcation aneurysm, pointing directly upward at or above the dorsum sellae, can be dealt with quite satisfactorily if the surgeon has familiarity with the trans-sylvian approach. In the final analysis, experience with the approach and familiarity with the anatomy, with careful attention to the many small details, will be the major factors that determine the success of the surgeon's choice of approach to this remote site of aneurysms. Most (80 percent) of the frontotemporal approaches in our series were done in patients with associated aneurysms at the carotid bifurcation or on the middle cerebral artery or anterior communicating artery. The special *contraindications* for the trans-sylvian pterional approach remain (1) low basilar bifurcation, and (2) posterior projection of the aneurysm.

Aneurysms of the Basilar Trunk

Basilar-Anterior Inferior Cerebellar Artery Aneurysms

The anterior inferior cerebellar artery (AICA) aneurysms usually arise at the distal carina of the origin of the anterior inferior cerebellar artery from the basilar artery. Occasionally, however, these aneurysms will arise on the proximal side of this junction, or they will arise in the proximal or distal part of the AICA clearly separate from the basilar artery. These variations can usually be predicted on the preoperative angiogram. These aneurysms usually project laterally but may project anteriorly and be fused to the clivus, and occasionally may point backward and be buried in the pons or pontomedullary junction. Basilar-AICA aneurysms usually bear a close relationship to the abducens nerve.

These aneurysms may be approached subtemporally and transtentorially or, because of the variable site of origin of the AICA, suboccipitally, or occasionally by a combined subtemporal-suboccipital approach by dividing both the tentorium and the superior petrosal sinus. The choice of approach depends on the size, site of

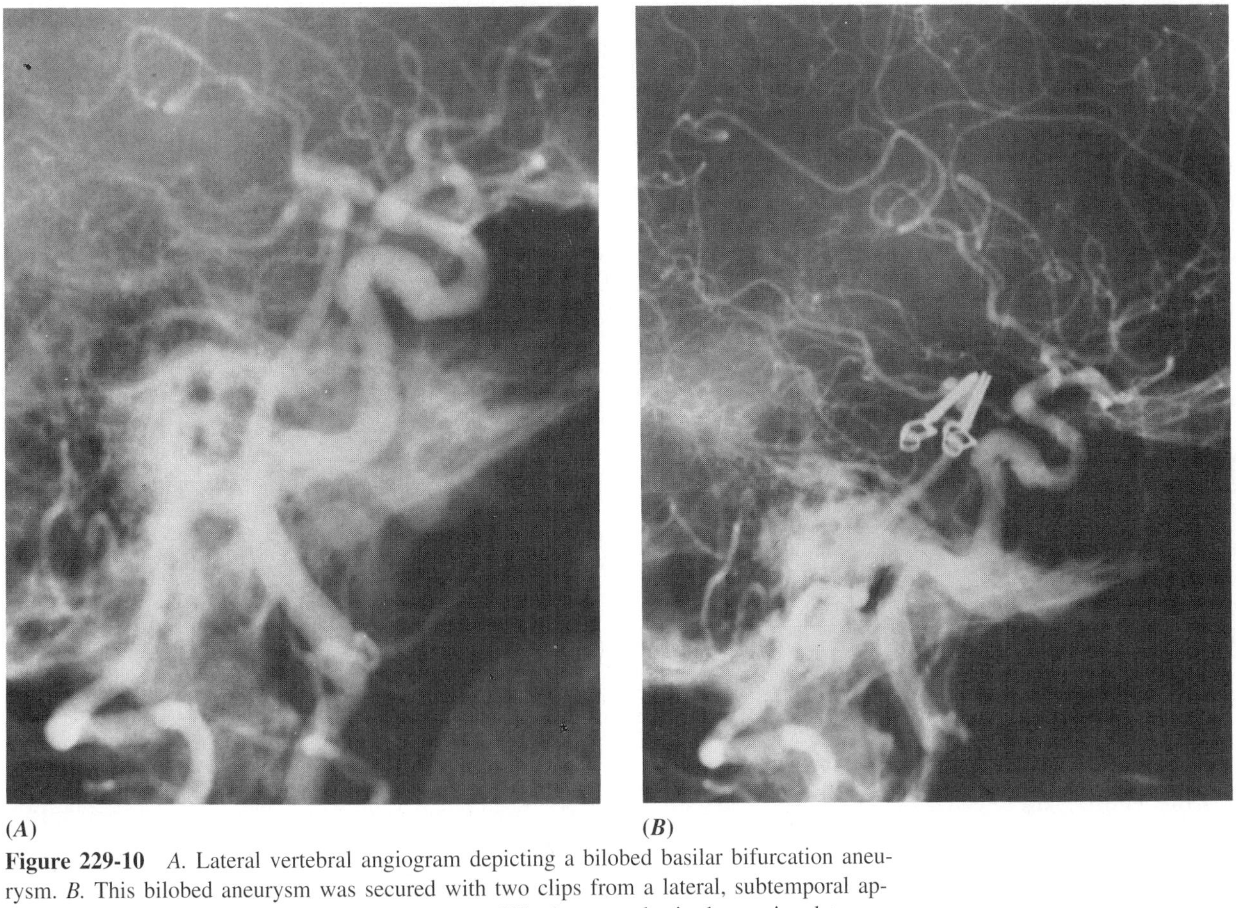

(A) *(B)*

Figure 229-10 *A.* Lateral vertebral angiogram depicting a bilobed basilar bifurcation aneurysm. *B.* This bilobed aneurysm was secured with two clips from a lateral, subtemporal approach. This aneurysm configuration is extremely difficult to attack via the pterional trans-sylvian approach.

origin, and configuration of the aneurysm. Basilar trunk aneurysms bulging forward and originating well along the trunk of the basilar artery are usually best approached subtemporally. Those originating more proximally on the basilar artery may be exposed more easily and directly through the suboccipital approach. Generally it is best to approach the aneurysm from an exposure closest to the neck and where the operator will have the best opportunity to visualize and spare with certainty the major branch vessels in the region. Whatever the approach, these aneurysms lie in a narrow and confined space at some distance from either a supra- or infratentorial exposure. It is always best, therefore, to plan the approach that will most readily bring the neck into view.

The subtemporal approach is centered to permit a direct line of sight down the posterior slope of the petrous bone and clivus. With this exposure, the vein of Labbé will be in the anterior third and must be protected. The tentorium is then divided sharply behind the attachment of the trochlear nerve, with the division carried almost to the junction of the petrosal and lateral sinuses. The anterior leaf of the tentorium is then sutured forward into the middle fossa, and the posterior leaflet coagulated to shrink it back out of view. After the tentorium is divided, the arachnoid that forms the roof of the posterior fossa cisterns will be exposed, and under it the trochlear and trigeminal nerves will be seen. The petrosal vein piercing this arachnoid layer should be coagulated and divided. After the arachnoid lateral to the trigeminal nerve has been opened, a narrow retractor blade can be used to gently displace the anterosuperior aspect of the cerebellum to expose the pons and the abducens, facial, and auditory nerves. With the anterior and superior aspects of the cerebellopontine angle now open, the basilar artery, partially obscured by the bulge of the pontine hemisphere, can be seen, and if this vessel is followed inferiorly, the aneurysm can be exposed. After removing clot and CSF, this narrow space will gradually open to expose the pertinent anatomy. It is usually necessary to separate the sixth nerve from the aneurysm, but because this structure is usually slack as it courses upward to gain the cavernous sinus, it can be easily displaced to clear the neck of the aneurysm. From the subtemporal transtentorial approach, the origin of the AICA will not usually be seen since it will be on the inferior aspect of the sac. We have found it useful to expose this vessel by gently grasping the neck of the aneurysm with bipolar forceps and tipping the sac away from the pons to expose the AICA, and then sharply dissecting this vessel free from the neck. Obviously the AICA must be spared with the clip placement. Because these aneurysms normally point anteriorly, the definition of the AICA, the basilar artery, and those perforatoring branches coming off the basilar artery to irrigate the pons is quite straightforward. With aneurysms that are buried into the pons, visualization of these vessels will be much more difficult. This exposure is always confining because at the critical moment of clip application the essential anatomy is usually obscured by the clip applier and the handle of the clip. Once the clip is applied, it is essential that the surgeon quickly inspect the position of the blades to ensure absolute accuracy of clip placement. To narrow or occlude the basilar artery, trap perforators, or obstruct the origin of the AICA will have catastrophic consequences for the patient.[14]

Midbasilar Trunk Aneurysms

A distinct group of nongiant aneurysms arise from the basilar artery trunk between the origins of the superior and anterior inferior cerebellar arteries, presumably at the site of origin of long or short pontine perforators. In 44 patients, no significant branch artery crotch of origin has been identified. In three of them, the aneurysm arose from the proximal carina of a short midbasilar fenestration.

Division of the inner one-third or half of the tentorium is nearly always required for their exposure. This is usually done through a generous posterior temporal bone flap on the side of their projection, so as to obtain a good line of sight behind the dorsum sellae and clivus in front of the pons. In one-third of patients, however, tentorial division could be done through a tic craniectomy or there was a high basilar artery origin. It is not usually necessary to divide the petrosal vein which will be near the lateral end of the tentorial cut. The aneurysm and adjacent structures can be exposed by working medial to the fifth nerve and usually on one or both sides of the slender fourth nerve. In those aneurysms arising from a fenestration and those with a forward projection, the dome, with the sealing clot, was often adherent to the clivus. Clip application should be perfect the first time so that if the dome is pulled away from its attachment, bleeding during clip reapplication is avoided.

Larger sacs, like those at AICA, often were adherent to the pontine pia, the integrity of which could not always be preserved during the dissection to free the neck. Basilar occlusion was used when it was not possible to clip the neck without kinking the perforators.

Vertebral-Basilar Junction Aneurysms

Because intracranial saccular aneurysms ordinarily arise at the carina of a bifurcation on which the higher velocity, axial arterial stream impinges, it would seem incongruous for aneurysms to arise in the region of the union of the vertebral arteries that forms the basilar artery. What has been realized is that in most cases these aneurysms so not arise at that carina projecting downward, but rather arise at the lower carina of a fenestration at the origin of the basilar artery, pointing upward. We believe it is likely that a complete, or incomplete, fenestration exists at the origin of all vertebral-basilar junction aneurysms.

Many "butterfly" aneurysms exist that have one saccule pointing backward and the other forward. In several of the small aneurysms, it seems that two separate aneurysms arose at the proximal fenestration. The larger ones were probably bilocular, but the locularity was not caused by pressure against the distal carina because the upper opening of the fenestration was usually open.

The vertebral-basilar union usually overlies the junction of the lower and middle one-third of the clivus. This region has been approached in most of this series either from above through the tentorium or below through the lateral posterior fossa.

The subtemporal transtentorial exposure is now seldom used unless another higher basilar aneurysm is to be obliterated too. The rewards of temporary clipping are such that it is imperative that both vertebral arteries are easily available, if need be, on either side of the medulla. Removal of the rim of the foramen magnum is usually necessary for identification of the origins of the vertebral arteries on both sides for bilateral temporary clipping. The temporary clip on the opposite vertebral can be left in place until neck clipping is completed, using brief periods of ipsilateral vertebral clipping when desired to slacken the aneurysm. Temporary trapping with another clip on the basilar artery above has been used in difficult cases.

The vertebral artery is followed upward and medially to where it disappears under the medulla. The remainder of the exposure under the medulla usually can be done just below the vagus nerve or between one or more medullary filaments of the eleventh cranial nerve. The importance of recognizing and preserving these filaments from the nucleus ambiguus cannot be overemphasized. Fortunately, they are not tense, and are attenuated enough to allow dissection in between with gentle manipulation.

Sometimes it is simple to expose the vertebral artery junction when the retroclival space is wide. But at other times, the medulla seems plastered over the arteries against the clivus. In these cases, the angle of attack narrows sharply and, to get better line of sight to the vertebrobasilar junction region, the "far lateral" subcerebellar exposure is helpful. This uses retraction that begins far out or at the anteroinferior aspect of the cerebellum near or at the sigmoid sinus, gradually displacing the cerebellum out of the lower lateral posterior fossa. In difficult exposures, spontaneous breathing is often used as the best guide to retractor pressure and medullary ischemia. Clipping can be awkward in the narrow exposure. The upper portion of the fenestration is usually quite evident. For backward-projecting sacs, even though the origin of the neck is at a fenestration, one or more perforators may arise here and must be searched for and preserved if present. In several cases where the origin of the neck at the fenestration was quite expanded, taking one limb of the fenestration with the blades made the clipping more complete.

The transmastoid transpetrosal approach provides wider exposure of these deep obscuring lesions while avoiding division of the lateral or sigmoid sinuses. The exposure is centered on the seventh and eighth nerves so that the basilar artery must be exposed above or below this nerve bundle. Even so, the whole of the basilar artery from near its apex to the vertebrobasilar junction can be seen as can both terminal vertebral arteries for temporary clip control.

Vertebral Artery Aneurysms

Aneurysms that arise from the vertebral artery usually arise just beyond the origin of the posterior inferior cerebellar artery (PICA). Some of these aneurysms arise from the vertebral artery more distal to the origin of the PICA, at the origin of unnamed branches, or at the origin of the anterior spinal artery. Two other groups of vertebral aneurysms are those with their origin from PICA usually within 1 cm or more from its origin, and those more distally located. As a rule, the anatomy of the PICA is extremely variable, and, as a result, we have seen vertebral-PICA aneurysms lying in or below the foramen magnum and as high as the middle of the clivus. Although these aneurysms are usually situated on the lateral aspect of the medulla, we have seen a left vertebral-PICA aneurysm lying largely in the right cerebellopontine angle. The aneurysms are typically nestled along the side of the medulla, with the twelfth cranial nerve intimately associated with the neck and, occasionally, even split by the sac as it enlarges. Frequently these aneurysms take origin from a significant portion of the proximal part of the PICA and, therefore, have a V-shaped neck, which presents a challenge to the surgeon in clip selection and placement so as to preserve the continuity of both the vertebral artery and the PICA.

Aneurysms arising off the vertebral artery are normally approached through the suboccipital exposure, with the patient in the lateral or "park bench" position, with the face turned slightly toward the floor. The "park bench" position has been used routinely for the lateral posterior fossa approach. It allows the surgeon to sit, while also providing a good angle for the dissection alongside, and then under the brain stem. It also reduces the risks of air embolism and allows a combined subtemporal-transtentorial or transmastoid-transpetrosal exposure, if necessary. A lateral, curvilinear paramedian incision is made, and after the muscle is reflected, with care to preserve the occipital nerves, a small craniectomy is made well lateral to expose the mastoid air cells. The rim of the foramen magnum is usually removed (Fig. 229-11). Because these aneurysms usually lie relatively close to the midline, extreme lateral or medial exposures are unnecessary; it is desirable only to have a moderate lateral exposure of the medulla to see the vertebral artery as it enters the subarachnoid space (after the cisterna magna is opened). With removal of CSF and gentle upward and medial retraction of the cerebellar tonsil, the ninth, tenth, and eleventh cranial nerves come into view. The caudal loop of the PICA is immediately apparent, and this need only be followed to its origin to expose the neck of the typical vertebral-PICA aneurysm. It is important to remove clot away from the proximal and distal vertebral artery, working across the neck of the aneurysm in order to gain appreciation of the configuration of the vertebral artery and the width of the neck. We have often found it necessary and useful to narrow the neck of this aneurysm with bipolar cautery, and to use aperture clips to enclose and protect the PICA and the twelfth nerve in the aperture to gain control of this aneurysm. It should be stressed again that dissection and exposure of aneurysms of the vertebral artery necessitate working between the filaments of the lower cranial nerves. This must be done gently and carefully to prevent their injury and the concomitant, disabling postoperative complications (Fig. 229-12).[14]

Transoral-Transclival Approaches to Basilar Trunk and Vertebrobasilar Aneurysms

These approaches are mentioned only to be condemned. Many years ago we attempted to expose aneurysms of the basilar trunk through the mouth and after removal of the clivus. This approach has many disadvantages. The exposure is always very confining. It

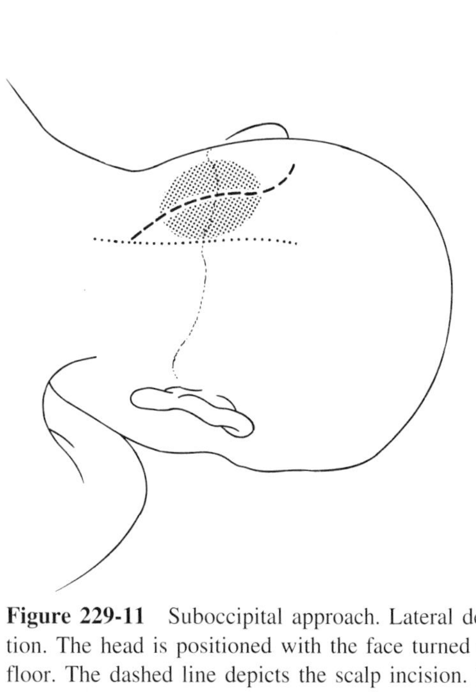

Figure 229-11 Suboccipital approach. Lateral decubitus position. The head is positioned with the face turned toward the floor. The dashed line depicts the scalp incision. The stippled area shows the bone removal.

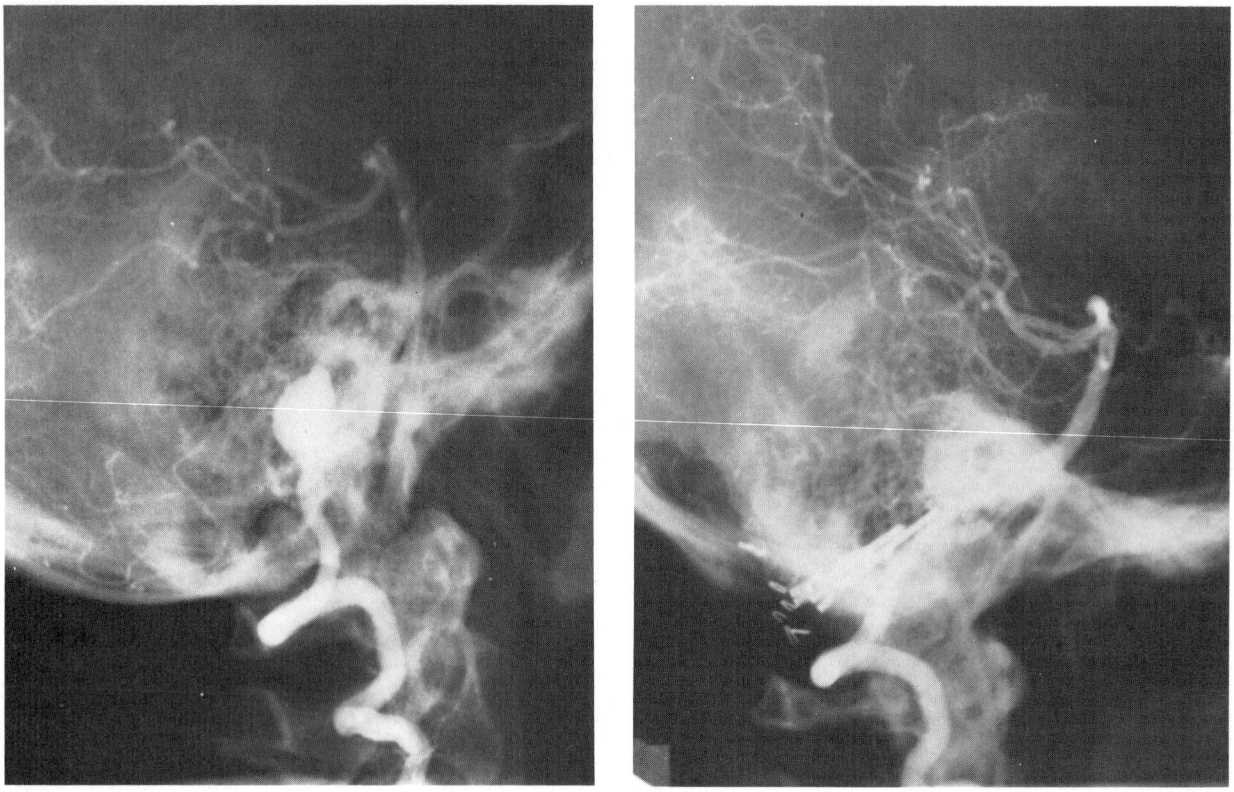

(*A*) (*B*)

Figure 229-12 *A.* Lateral vertebral angiogram showing a partially thrombosed giant vertebral-PICA aneurysm. *B.* This aneurysm was secured with tandem clips, maintaining the patency of the vertebral artery and the PICA.

almost always places the fundus of the aneurysm between the operator and the parent and branch vessels. Perhaps most importantly, there is real difficulty in obtaining a watertight closure, and the risk of CSF leakage and postoperative meningitis is very high. With refinements of the subtemporal and suboccipital approaches, we have not found it necessary to even consider the transoral-transclival exposure.

Results and Conclusions

A summary of our results over 34 years is given in Tables 229-1 to 229-5. These figures represent an experience that spans our original and, by comparison to today, crude efforts of direct attack on the aneurysms arising from the vertebrobasilar system. Until 1975, the operating microscope was not used routinely; microsurgical techniques were in their infancy, and clip technology was primitive. Moreover, neuroanesthesia and radiology have improved remarkably in the past decade. Nevertheless, our series is cumulative and historical, and the trials, tribulations, pitfalls, and complications of our original experience cannot be disregarded. They are, therefore, necessarily recorded in this summary (Tables 229-1 and 229-2).

In Table 229-3, small (up to 1.25 cm in diameter) and large (up to 2.5 cm in diameter) aneurysms are grouped and the results of surgical therapy indicated by the site of origin of the aneurysm. It

TABLE 229-1 Vertebrobasilar Aneurysms (All Sizes, All Grades): Summary of Results in Three Different Time Periods

Years	Total	Excellent	Good	Poor	Dead
1959–1970	87	53	9	11	14
		60.9%	10.3%	12.6%	16.1%
1971–1981	794	551	119	72	52
		69.4%	15.0%	9.1%	6.6%
1982–1992	886	608	142	86	50
		68.6%	16.0%	9.7%	5.6%
Total	1767	1212	270	169	116
		68.6%	15.3%	9.6%	6.6%

TABLE 229-2 Vertebrobasilar Aneurysms (Small or Large, Good Grade = Grades 1 or 2 or Unruptured): Summary of Results in Three Different Time Periods

Years	Total	Excellent	Good	Poor	Dead
1959–1970	58	45	2	5	6
		77.6%	3.4%	8.6%	10.3%
1971–1981	568	451	67	26	23
		79.5%	11.8%	4.6%	4.1%
1982–1992	609	490	67	35	17
		80.5%	11.0%	5.7%	2.8%
Total	1235	987	136	66	46
		79.9%	11.0%	5.3%	3.7%

TABLE 229-3 Vertebrobasilar Aneurysms (Small and Large): Results by Site, All Grades

Site	Number	Excellent	Good	Poor	Dead
Basilar bifurcation	758	554	109	63	32
Basilar–SCA junction	210	166	24	14	6
Midbasilar trunk	44	28	7	3	6
Basilar–AICA junction	41	30	6	3	2
Vertebrobasilar junction	77	53	12	7	5
Vertebral artery	181	150	17	6	8
Posterior cerebral					
P1	32	22	5	3	2
P2	27	20	3	1	3
Totals	1370	1023	183	100	64
		74.7%	13.4%	7.3%	4.7%

AICA, anterior inferior cerebellar artery; SCA, superior cerebellar artery.

is evident that the majority of the unsatisfactory results have occurred with aneurysms of the terminal basilar artery—a cogent reminder of the vital importance to normal brain function of the P1 perforating vessels. In these average-sized aneurysms in patients of all grades, we have experienced a surgical mortality of 4.7 percent; in the past 10 years and in more than 500 cases, the mortality has been less than 3 percent.

Table 229-4 summarizes our results with giant aneurysms (greater than 2.5 cm in diameter) arising from the various sites of the vertebrobasilar vessels. These lesions are clearly more hazardous due to their size, intraluminal thrombosis, sclerosis and calcification of the wall, incorporation of branch vessels, compression of the brain stem, and the confined space of the region. In patients harboring these large sacs, we have encountered a 13 percent mortality and 17 percent morbidity, although more than half of these poor results were present before surgery and were unaffected by the surgical effort.

TABLE 229-4 Giant Vertebrobasilar Aneurysms: Results by Site, All Grades

Site	Number	Excellent	Good	Poor	Dead
Basilar bifurcation	137	57	31	32	17
Basilar–SCA junction	56	20	16	9	11
Basilar trunk	59	27	12	8	12
Vertebrobasilar junction	39	17	7	7	8
Vertebral artery	40	21	10	7	2
Posterior cerebral					
P1	32	22	5	3	2
P2	27	20	3	1	3
Totals	397	189	87	69	52
		47.6%	21.9%	17.4%	13.1%

SCA, superior cerebellar artery.

TABLE 229-5 Vertebrobasilar Aneurysms (All Sizes, All Grades): Summary of Results

Size	Number	Excellent	Good	Poor	Dead
Small	939	736	113	56	34
Large	431	287	70	44	30
Giant	397	189	86	69	52
Total	1767	1212	270	169	116
		84%		16%	

Our total experience (until December 31, 1992) for all sizes of aneurysms and in all grades of patients is summarized in Table 229-5. We achieved excellent or good results in 84 percent of patients.

At the present time, if the surgical team has complete familiarity with the anatomy, technical experience, and excellence in neuroanesthesia, and pays particular attention to the many small details that encompass aneurysm surgery, it will find that most aneurysms of the vertebrobasilar system are amenable to surgical treatment.[1,2,8,9,12,16,18,19]

References

1. Batjer HH, Samson DS. Causes of morbidity and mortality from surgery of aneurysms of the distal basilar artery. *Neurosurgery* 1989; 25:904–916.
2. Canalis RF, Black K, Martin N, Becker D. Extended retrolabyrinthine transtentorial approach to petroclival lesions. *Laryngoscope* 1991; 101:6–13.
3. Dandy WE. *Intracranial Arterial Aneurysms.* Ithaca, NY: Comstock, 1944.
4. Drake CG. Bleeding aneurysms of the basilar artery: direct surgical management in four cases. *J Neurosurg* 1961; 18:230–238.
5. Drake CG. Surgical treatment of ruptured aneurysms of the basilar artery: experience with 14 cases. *J Neurosurg* 1965; 23:457–473.
6. Drake CG. Further experience with surgical treatment of aneurysms of the basilar artery. *J Neurosurg* 1968; 29:372–392.
7. Falconer MA. Surgical treatment of spontaneous intracranial hemorrhage. *Br Med J* 1958; 1:790–792.
8. Hernesniemi J, Vapalahti M, Niskanen M, Kari A. Management outcome for vertebrobasilar artery junction aneurysms by early surgery. *Neurosurgery* 1992; 31:857–862.
9. Ikeda K, Yamashita J, Hashimoto M, Futami K. Orbitozygomatic temporopolar approach for a high basilar tip aneurysm associated with a short intracranial internal carotid artery: a new surgical approach. *J Neurosurg* 1991; 28:105–110.
10. Jamieson KG. Aneurysms of the vertebrobasilar system: surgical intervention in 19 cases. *J Neurosurg* 1964; 21:781–797.
11. Logue V. Posterior fossa aneurysms. *Clin Neurosurg* 1964; 11:183–207.
12. Muizelaar JP. The use of electroencephalography and brain protection during operation for basilar aneurysms. *Neurosurgery* 1989; 25:899–903.
13. Peerless SJ. Pre- and postoperative management of cerebral aneurysms. *Clin Neurosurg* 1979; 26:209–231.
14. Peerless SJ, Drake CG. Surgical techniques of posterior cerebral aneurysms. In Schmidek HH, Sweet WH (eds): *Operative Neurosurgical Techniques.* New York: Grune & Stratton, 1982, pp 909–931.

15. Poppen JL. Vascular surgery of the posterior fossa. *Clin Neurosurg* 1959; 6:198–209.
16. Rice BJ, Peerless SJ, Drake CG. Surgical treatment of unruptured aneurysms of the posterior circulation. *J Neurosurg* 1990; 73:165–173.
17. Schwartz HG. Arterial aneurysm of the posterior fossa. *J Neurosurg* 1948; 5:312–316.
18. Solomon RA, Stein BM. Surgical approaches to aneurysms of the vertebral and basilar arteries. *Neurosurgery* 1988; 23:203–208.
19. Spetzler RF, Hadley MN, Rigamonti D, et al. Aneurysms of the basilar artery treated with circulatory arrest, hypothermia, and barbiturate cerebral protection. *J Neurosurg* 1988; 68:868–879.
20. Sugita K, Kobayashi S, Shintani A, Mutsuga N. Microneurosurgery for aneurysms of the basilar artery. *J Neurosurg* 1979; 51:615–620.
21. Tönnis W. Zur Behandlung Intrakraniellar Aneurysmen. *Arch Klin Chir* 1937; 189:474–479.
22. Yaşargil MG. *Microsurgery. II. Clinical Considerations, Surgery of the Intracranial Aneurysms and Results.* New York: Georg Thieme Verlag, 1984, pp 232–295.
23. Yaşargil MG, Antic J, Laciga R, et al. Microsurgical pterional approach to aneurysms of the basilar bifurcation. *Surg Neurol* 1976; 6:83–91.

230 The Far Lateral Inferior Suboccipital Approach

Roberto C. Heros

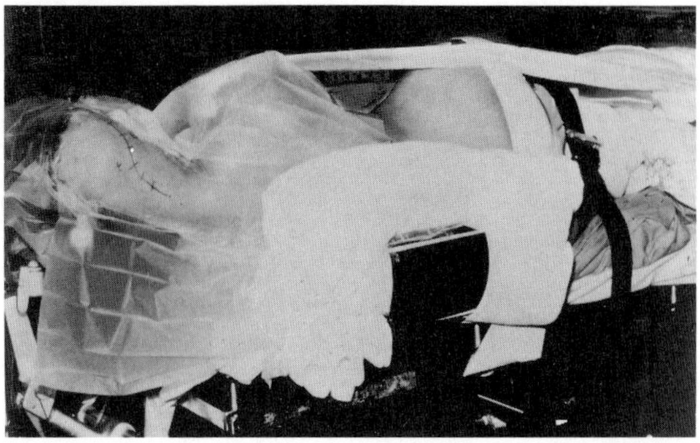

Figure 230-1 Position of the patient on the operating table. The head is in the straight lateral position; the ipsilateral shoulder is then pulled down and the head tilted toward the ipsilateral shoulder.

The standard lateral suboccipital approach is used routinely for lesions of the cerebellopontine angle, for microsurgical decompressive procedures for cranial neuropathies, and for vascular lesions of the vertebral artery. In approaching deeper aneurysms of the vertebral artery and the vertebrobasilar junction, some neurosurgeons prefer a more inferior approach along the lateral margin of the foramen magnum.[1,2,4,6,8,10] In 1986, I published a detailed description of the manner in which a surgeon can gain a satisfactory far lateral exposure when using this approach.[5] More radical lateral approaches that are sometimes necessary to deal with anteriorly placed tumors of the region of the foramen magnum have been described[3,9]; generally, however, these radical approaches are not necessary for aneurysms.

The subtemporal/presigmoid transtentorial approach is a satisfactory alternative for complex vertebrobasilar junction aneurysms.[7] Although I have used this approach occasionally, my experience is insufficient to make definite recommendations as to when to use it instead of the far lateral suboccipital approach.

Position and Incision

The patient is placed in the straight lateral position with a flat folded sheet as padding under the axilla (Fig. 230-1). The nose is straight ahead (at a 90-degree angle from the floor) and the head is tilted up in a 30-degree angle toward the ipsilateral shoulder. The lateral position is used to allow the cerebellum to fall away and minimize retraction. By tilting the head up, one brings the level of the head just slightly above the level of the heart which avoids venous engorgement and facilitates drainage of CSF by gravity. Because in this position the head is only slightly higher than the heart, air embolism is unlikely but possible and at least a Doppler monitor is recommended. Placement of a central venous line is optional but desirable.

The incision is illustrated in Fig. 230-2. It is started at about the level of the top of the ear about two finger breadths medial to the tip of the mastoid in the sagittal plane. The incision extends first straight downward toward the mastoid and then it curves sharply medial to the midline and then straight down toward the spinous process of C2. This incision cuts across some of the branches of the occipital nerve but so far this has not represented a problem in our experience. With this incision, the surgeon can expose as far laterally as the mastoid and also medially to the opposite side of the midline along the foramen magnum and the arch of C1. The muscle mass is opened with electrocautery along the line of the skin incision down to the occipital bone which is then exposed by subperiosteal dissection. Inferolaterally, sharp dissection is preferred in order to avoid injury to the vertebral artery. The posterior arch of C1 is exposed by subperiosteal dissection from just on the opposite side of the midline to the area of the sulcus arteriosus underlying the vertebral artery laterally. By opening the muscle mass along the line of the skin incision, one minimizes the muscle bulk laterally that would be in the way if one divided the muscles on the midline.

Craniectomy

The craniectomy extends from below the transverse sinus superiorly (there is no need for a high craniectomy) to the sigmoid sinus laterally and through the foramen magnum just to the opposite side of the midline inferiorly. The posterior arch of C1 can be removed either before or after the suboccipital craniectomy. It is removed from just beyond the midline on the opposite side to just underneath the vertebral artery laterally (Fig. 230-3). Laterally, the perivertebral venous plexus overlies the vertebral artery and venous bleeding from it is usually encountered before the artery can be exposed. This bleeding is easily controlled with bipolar coagulation and packing with Surgicel (oxidized regenerated cellulose; Johnson & Johnson Patient Care, New Brunswick, NJ) on both sides of the vertebral artery. I prefer to definitely identify the vertebral artery in order to be sure of its position, but this step may not be necessary if the surgeon is at least able to palpate the pulse from the artery and in this manner estimate its position. The removal of the arch of C1 allows a more inferior approach below the cerebellar tonsil which avoids the need for retraction of the cerebellar hemisphere located more lateral and superior.

Portions of this chapter, including the illustrations, have been reprinted with permission from Heros RC. Lateral suboccipital approach for vertebral and vertebrobasilar artery lesions. *J Neurosurg* 1986; 64:559–562.

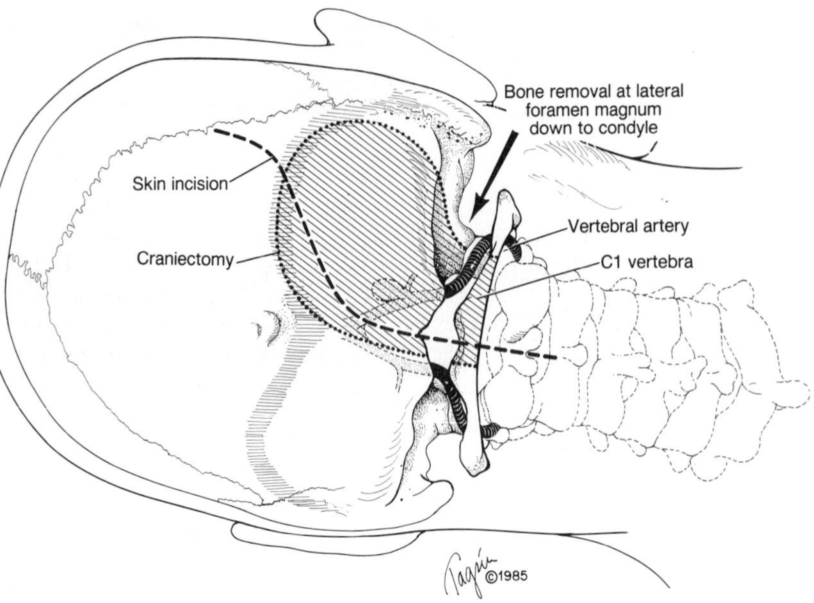

Figure 230-2 An artist's drawing showing the skin incision and craniectomy.

The most important aspect of this exposure is a very radical removal of bone in the area of the foramen magnum, going laterally as far as the condylar fossa just posterior to the occipital condyle and just above and behind where the vertebral artery enters the dura (Fig. 230-3). It is in this area that it is helpful to have the vertebral artery exposed so that the surgeon can feel confident of not injuring it. As one removes bone laterally, there is usually venous bleeding from the perivertebral plexus which again can be controlled with electrocoagulation and packing. Laterally, the bone edge becomes more vertical and it is impossible to reach under the bone with the footplate of a Kerrison rongeur. Therefore, a high-speed air drill can be used for the last 5 to 10 mm of exposure.

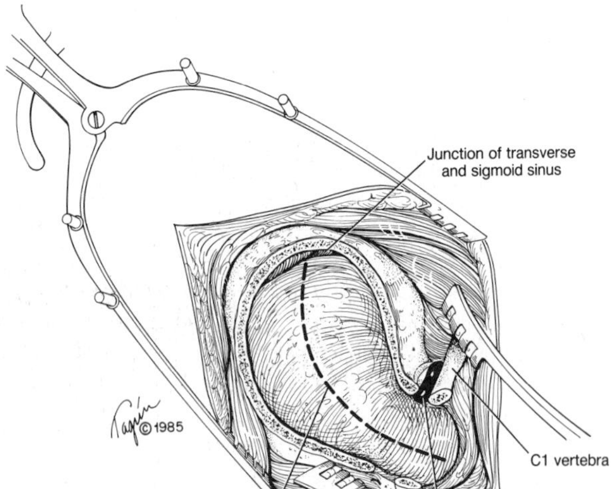

Figure 230-3 The dural incision starts superiorly at the junction of the sigmoid and transverse sinuses and comes down to the midline to just below the removed arch of C1.

Frequently, a small emissary branch of the vertebral artery is encountered perforating the bone behind the condyle in the condylar fossa. This is usually the limit of removal since to go beyond requires opening the capsule of the atlanto-occipital articulation; the latter, however, has not been a problem on several cases where I have removed part or most of the atlanto-occipital condyle to obtain a more lateral exposure to deal with tumors of this region. This extreme inferolateral removal of bone in the area of the foramen magnum is the key to being able to approach the front of the brain stem with minimal or no brain stem retraction. Each millimeter of the lateral rim of the foramen magnum removed gains for the surgeon several extra degrees in the lateral angle of exposure. In this respect, the lateral rim of the foramen magnum represents to the inferolateral suboccipital exposure what the pterion represents to the frontotemporal exposure.

Intradural Approach

The dura is opened in an oblique line starting superolaterally and coming down toward the midline in the area of the foramen magnum and then continuing straight down to about the level of C1 (Fig. 230-3). The lateral aspect of the dura is tented up tightly to the lateral muscle mass to maximize the lateral angle of exposure.

After the dura is opened, the procedure continues under the microscope. The first step is to open the arachnoid widely around the lower cranial nerves. It is helpful to cut the first dentate ligament to allow the medulla to fall away. The tonsil of the cerebellum is gently lifted upward and medially with a self-retaining retractor (Fig. 230-4). The vertebral artery is seen entering the dura immediately, sometimes even before retracting the cerebellar tonsil. In cases of proximal vertebral artery aneurysms, the aneurysm would be immediately obvious after lifting the tonsil. The posterior inferior cerebellar artery (PICA) is usually just proximal to the aneurysm. When applying a clip, one must be particularly careful to spare the PICA and also not to compromise the vertebral artery distally with the tip of the clip which is easy to do since the vertebral runs in a more superior course, usually tightly applied to the

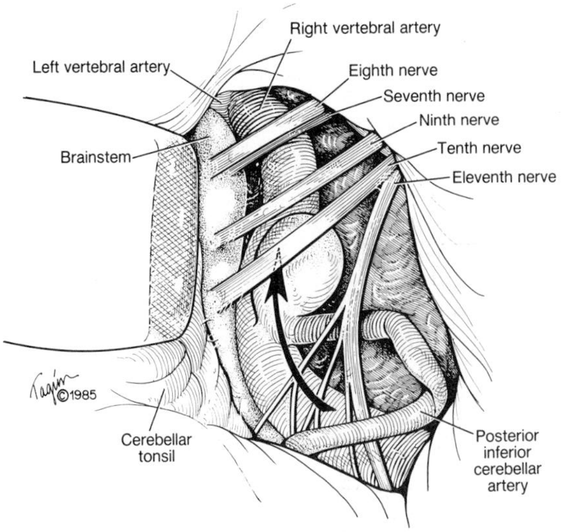

Figure 230-4 An *arrow* indicates the preferred direction of approach in the space between the eleventh cranial nerve inferiorly and the ninth and tenth cranial nerves superiorly.

back wall of the aneurysm. Dissection between the lower cranial nerves is necessary in order to gain access to the aneurysm. With this inferolateral approach, one can usually gain access to these aneurysms in the space between the eleventh cranial nerve inferiorly and the ninth and tenth cranial nerves superiorly. The more distal aneurysms are frequently intimately related to the twelfth cranial nerve which must be carefully preserved during clipping.

To reach aneurysms of the vertebrobasilar junction is more difficult and requires more retraction of the tonsil and the inferior aspect of the cerebellar hemisphere. Usually, if there is enough inferolateral bone removal, it is not necessary to directly retract the brain stem although the cerebellar retraction itself exerts some indirect retraction on the brain stem. I prefer to continue to follow the vertebral artery all the way to the vertebrobasilar junction, working from inferiorly between the eleventh cranial nerve below and the ninth and tenth nerves above (Fig. 230-4). However, if the basilar origin is high, one may need to change to a more superior angle of exposure between the ninth and tenth nerves inferiorly and seventh and eighth nerves superiorly. I try to avoid working in this space as much as possible because the seventh and eighth cranial nerves are quite intolerant of the slightest manipulation. The lower cranial nerves appear to be more tolerant although, of course, complete paralysis of these nerves is much more serious and life-threatening than paralysis of the seventh and eighth cranial nerves. When working with an aneurysm of the vertebrobasilar junction, I have frequently found it useful to direct the line of vision through the higher space (between the seventh and eighth nerves superiorly and ninth and tenth inferiorly) but to apply the clip through the inferior space (between the ninth and tenth nerves superiorly and the eleventh inferiorly). This has advantages of allowing an oblique line of vision to the clip applicator with better visualization of the blades as they are advanced. In addition, the lower space is wider and since the aneurysm is usually quite deep, the clip applier requires a wide space in order to open the blades of the clip and release it after placement. If one inserts the applier through the higher space, it is almost impossible to avoid some degree of distortion of the cranial nerves by the clip applier as its jaws are opened widely.

In cases of arteriovenous malformations located laterally in the cerebellum or in the cerebellar peduncles, one can follow the branches of the anterior inferior cerebellar artery and the PICA around the brain stem to the lesion. In addition, one can define well the critical anterior plane of these lesions by approaching them through this exposure.

Figure 230-5 shows postoperative computed tomograms of a patient operated on by this approach. The scans indicate the degree of bone removal in the suboccipital region (Fig. 230-5*A*) and at the level of the foramen magnum (Fig. 230-5*B*). One can appreciate from the arrow in Fig. 230-5*B* the lateral direction of approach that can be obtained with this exposure.

Indications

This far lateral inferior suboccipital approach is most useful for distal PICA aneurysms, aneurysms at the vertebrobasilar junction,

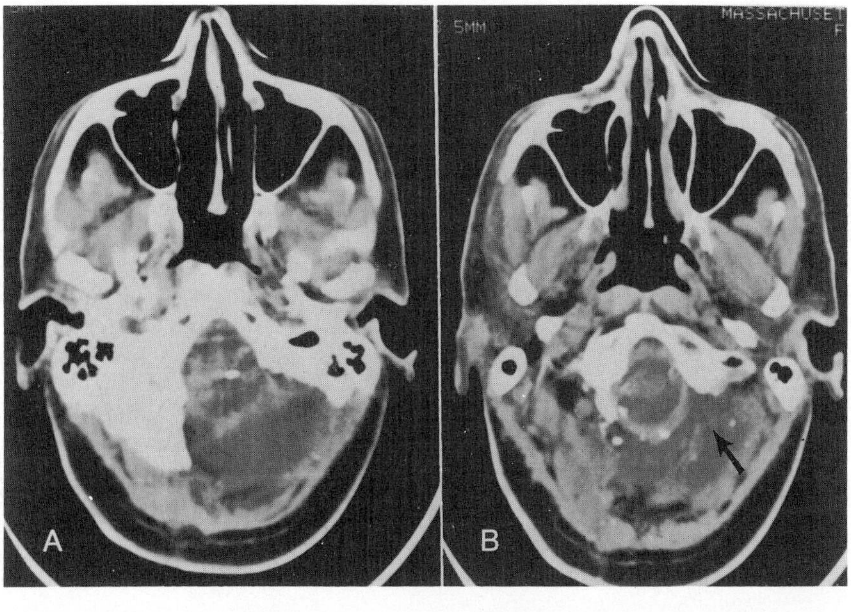

Figure 230-5 Postoperative computed tomography scans of a patient operated on by the inferolateral suboccipital approach. The amount of bone removal is shown at the suboccipital region *A* and at the level of the foramen magnum *B*. The *arrow* indicates the direction of the operative approach.

arteriovenous malformations of the lateral cerebellar hemisphere and the cerebellar peduncles, superficially located lesions in the lateral and anterolateral aspects of the medulla and the inferior pons, and anteriorly located tumors in the area of the foramen magnum. This approach can also be used for standard PICA aneurysms but for these aneurysms the extensive inferolateral bone removal all the way to the area of the condyle is not really necessary. Cerebellopontine angle tumors are more superior and laterally located and nothing is to be gained with the additional inferior bone removal described here.

References

1. Drake CG. The surgical treatment of vertebral-basilar aneurysms. *Clin Neurosurg* 1969; 16:114–169.
2. Fox JL. *Intracranial Aneurysms.* New York: Springer-Verlag, 1983, pp 1070–1102.
3. George B, Dematons C, Cophignon J. Lateral approach to the anterior portion of the foramen magnum: application to surgical removal of 14 benign tumors. Technical note. *Surg Neurol* 1988; 29:484–490.
4. Hammon WM, Kempe LG. The posterior fossa approach to aneurysms of the vertebral and basilar arteries. *J Neurosurg* 1972; 37:339–347.
5. Heros RC. Lateral suboccipital approach for vertebral and vertebrobasilar artery lesions. *J Neurosurg* 1986; 64:559–562.
6. Peerless SJ, Drake CG. Surgical techniques of posterior cerebral aneurysms. In Schmidek HH, Sweet WH (eds): *Operative Neurosurgical Techniques: Indications, Methods, and Results,* vol 2. New York: Grune & Stratton, 1982, pp 909–931.
7. Samii M, Ammirati M. The combined supra-infratentorial pre-sigmoid sinus avenue to the petro-clival region. Surgical technique and clinical applications. *Acta Neurochir (Wien)* 1988; 95:6–12.
8. Seeger W. *Microsurgery of the Brain: Anatomical and Technical Principles.* New York: Springer-Verlag, 1980, pp 506–507.
9. Sen CN, Sekhar LN. An extreme lateral approach to intradural lesions of the cervical spine and foramen magnum *Neurosurgery* 1990; 27:197–204.
10. Yaşargil MG. *Microneurosurgery.* Stuttgart: Georg Thieme Verlag, 1984, pp 234–244.

231

Giant Intracranial Aneurysms

H. Hunt Batjer
Thomas A. Kopitnik, Jr.
Phillip D. Purdy
Dana Matthews
Brandy Walker
Duke S. Samson
Daniel M. Meyer

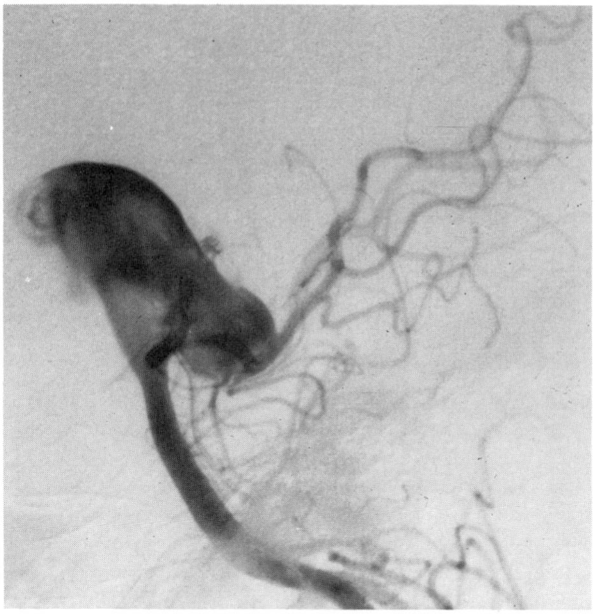

Figure 231-1 This case is an example of a broad-based, thrombotic giant basilar aneurysm whose efferent vessels were markedly displaced from the afferent basilar trunk.

By convention, those aneurysms which exceed 25 mm in maximal diameter are classified as "giant." There is adequate documentation that many aneurysms reach giant size as a dynamic evolution from smaller lesions. How this process occurs probably varies on a case-to-case basis. Clearly, many giant sacs in patients with no clear history of subarachnoid hemorrhage (SAH) are found by magnetic resonance imaging (MRI) or surgical exploration to be associated with considerable hemosiderin deposition in the subarachnoid space and in the surrounding pia or parenchyma. Perhaps, in these cases, intermittent breakdown of the wall with subsequent reinforcement by thrombotic, inflammatory, and, finally, dense connective tissue allows progressive enlargement. In patients with more generalized dysplastic cerebral (and systemic) vessels, it is likely that a true connective tissue disorder is the predisposing cause.

Giant aneurysms present formidable surgical challenges due to their varying etiology, the tendency for their necks to expand and incorporate efferent small and large vessels (Fig. 231-1), and a marked predisposition for intramural calcification and thrombosis. The majority of cases require temporary interruption of local or global cerebral circulation to allow vascular reconstruction. This requirement introduces iatrogenic cerebral ischemia into the host of potential difficulties that can befall the patient.

In this chapter, we will attempt to discuss management strategies in the context of many new diagnostic, surgical, and vascular developments. We believe the patient is best served by a multidisciplinary and carefully designed strategy involving the neurosurgeon, neurologist, neuroradiologist, endovascular therapist, and neuroanethesiologist. Morbidity from treatment can be minimized by developing clearly delineated goals for each patient. In many cases a perfect postoperative angiogram may be accomplished, but at the expense of a disabled patient. Experience teaches that appropriate goals must focus on alleviation of symptoms and successful competition with the natural history of this disease.

Etiology and Presentation

Perhaps some of the historical controversy regarding the natural history of giant aneurysms relates to their heterogeneous etiology and reliance on angiography as the sole diagnostic method in the pre-CT era. It is clear that a number of these lesions arise due to progressive expansion of previously small aneurysms. It is also likely that true arterial dissection may provide the initial violation of vessel-wall integrity, thereby leading to a complex giant aneurysm years later. Regardless of etiology, a large number of giant aneurysms harbor substantial degrees of intraluminal thrombosis and calcification, perhaps related to stasis within the sac, but perhaps also related to recurrent intramural hemorrhage, thrombosis, and enlargement. Reliance on angiographic methods may suggest that a thrombotic giant aneurysm is stable in size, when in fact it is substantially and progressively enlarging.[1,3,22]

In contrast to patients with small intracranial aneurysms, the giant aneurysm population may present with a variety of neurological symptoms. Stuttering neurological deficits, presumably due to ischemia, can result from either distal embolization from a giant sac or vessel stenosis or occlusion, simply due to mass effect as the lesion enlarges.[23] Epilepsy is an occasional complication, and may result from brain distortion or prior hemorrhage with hemosiderin deposition.[35] Some of our patients have presented with syndromes of generalized elevated intracranial pressure or focal mass effect in the presence of a giant sac. Clearly, cranial neuropathy is a frequent presentation with the specific nerve affected relating to the location of the aneurysm. Hydrocephalus, which may be acute in presentation, can also develop due to occlusion of the foramina of Monro, aqueduct, or fourth ventricular outlets. The most catastrophic clinical presentation obviously relates to acute SAH. Classical neurosurgical teaching is that as aneurysms enlarge to giant size the wall increases in thickness, thus protecting from hemorrhage. This is clearly not our experience, and it is commmonplace to see thick and calcific regions of a giant aneurysm adjacent to very attenuated tissue. All large series of giant aneurysms reflect that roughly one-third present with SAH.[12,35]

In our experience, the prognosis for patients with untreated giant aneurysms is quite poor. Intraluminal thrombosis, even if massive in degree, does not appear to protect against subsequent symptoms, and, in fact, may predispose to either progressive growth or embolization. This observation may have pertinence to the more recently advocated endovascular therapies.

Diagnostic Evaluation

The past decade has witnessed the tremendous potential of magnetic resonance technology to delineate a number of important features of giant aneurysms valuable in preoperative planning. Due to this development, some significant shifts have occurred in the practice habits at our center. Nevertheless, conventional diagnostic radiologic techniques remain invaluable in the overall evaluation of these patients.

The most common screening study yielding the diagnosis of giant intracranial aneurysm is the CT scan. Unenhanced studies can detect calcification in the walls of these lesions, as well as ischemic lesions from embolization or generalized edema in the region of the aneurysm. Obviously, the pressure of subarachnoid blood from a recent hemorrhage is clearly identifiable and quantifiable. The infusion of contrast provides more information which is invaluable in planning a surgical strategy. The homogeneous distribution of contrast enhancement, as seen in Fig. 231-2, allows visualization of the vessels adjacent to the mass and provides definitive evidence regarding the presence of intraluminal thrombosis.

Conventional selective cerebral angiography remains the gold standard of diagnostic methods for evaluating giant aneurysms, although substantial pitfalls remain. As seen in Fig. 231-3, conventional views from a vertebral arteriogram of a giant distal basilar artery aneurysm are ambiguous as to the origins and course of the efferent vasculature; oblique projections are extremely useful in picking up the origin of the posterior cerebral arteries (Fig. 231-4). These simple maneuvers can essentially resolve the issues surrounding the choice of operative approach. It is critical that the surgeon openly communicate with the radiologist regarding the specific items of information required in decision making for the individual case. This open communication ensures that each diagnostic angiogram will acquire the truly needed data and eliminates the possibility of the patient being subjected to multiple, unnecessary injections. The newer digital techniques with rapid sequencing are also extremely valuable for acquiring dynamic information. In addition, certain anatomic points can be established by this technique that would not be seen by conventional cut films.

As mentioned, the MR technology has provided major new insight into the diagnosis of giant aneurysms as well as their follow-up, if no specific therapy is recommended. Using standard MRI, the relationship of a vascular lesion to the skull base (Fig. 231-5) can be readily appreciated. More important, however, is the ability to precisely image the contents of a giant sac and its intimate relationship with other neurovascular structures. Figure 231-6 clearly shows a canalized channel through an otherwise thrombosed giant posterior circulation aneurysm. In addition, the

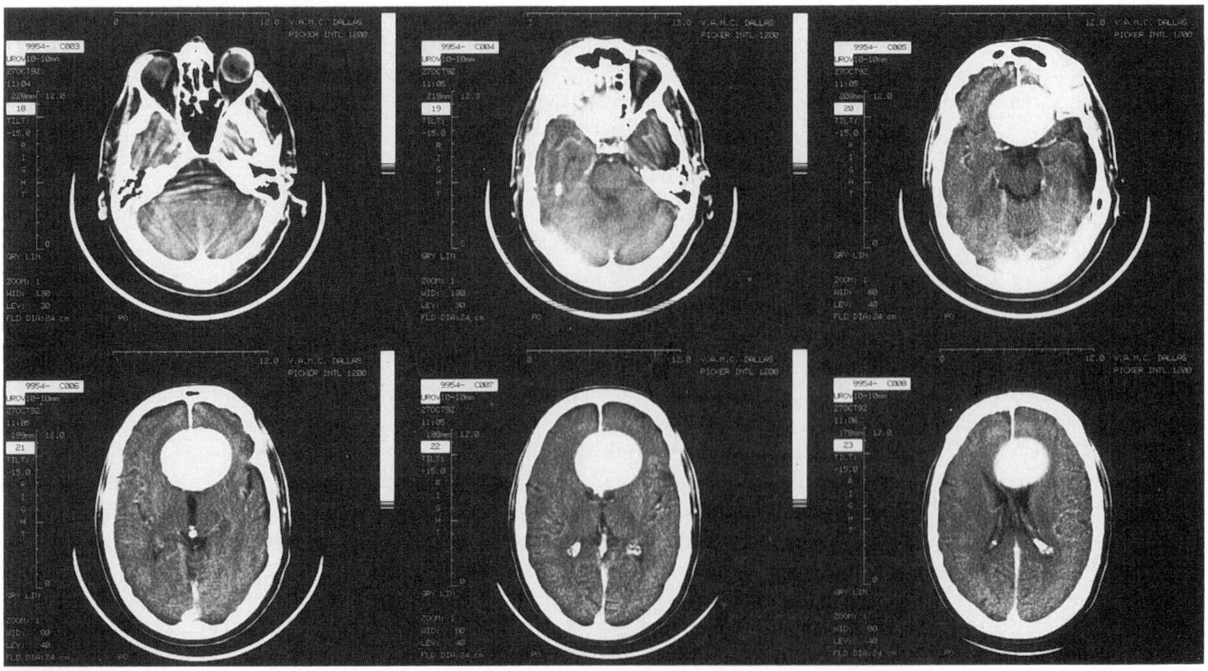

Figure 231-2 This enhanced CT scan clearly delineates the relationship of this giant aneurysm to the anterior communicating artery complex and strongly suggests that no intraluminal thrombosis is present.

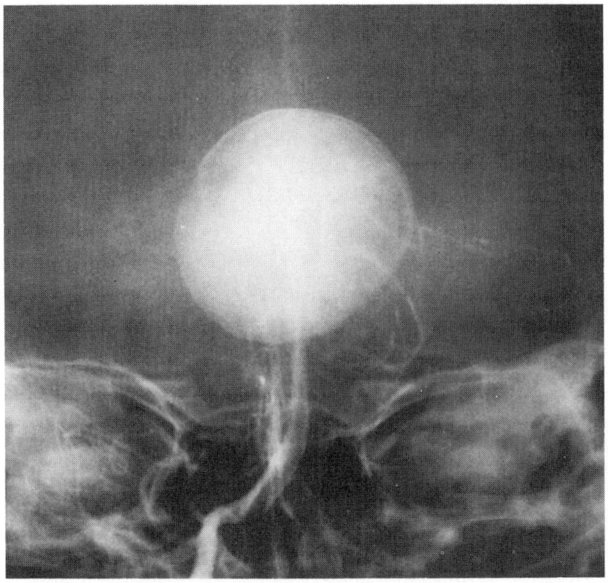

(*A*)

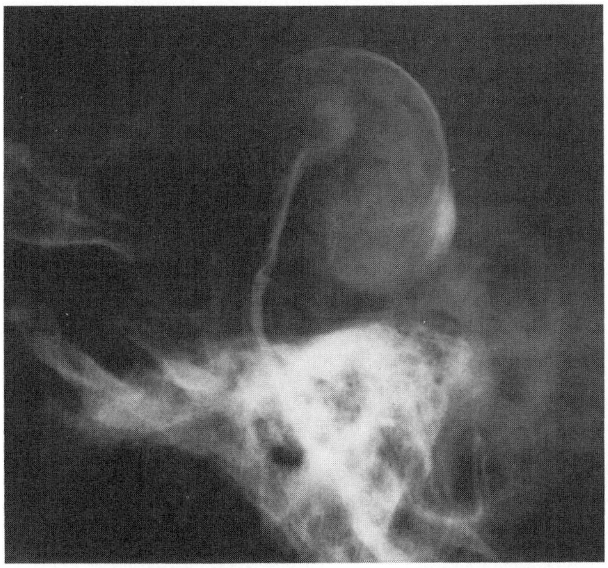

(*B*)

Figure 231-3 This case of giant distal basilar aneurysm illustrates the limitations of conventional angiography in the evaluation of giant aneurysms. Anteroposterior (*A*) and lateral (*B*) projections leave uncertainty as to the origin and course of efferent vessels.

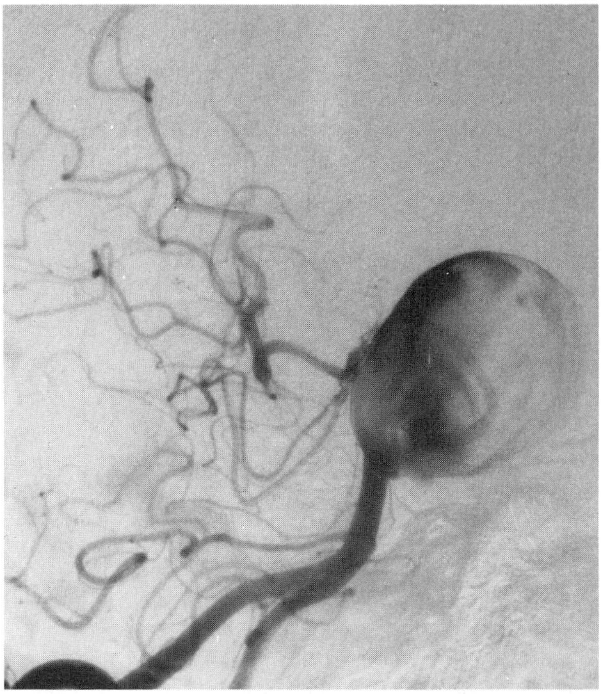

(*A*)

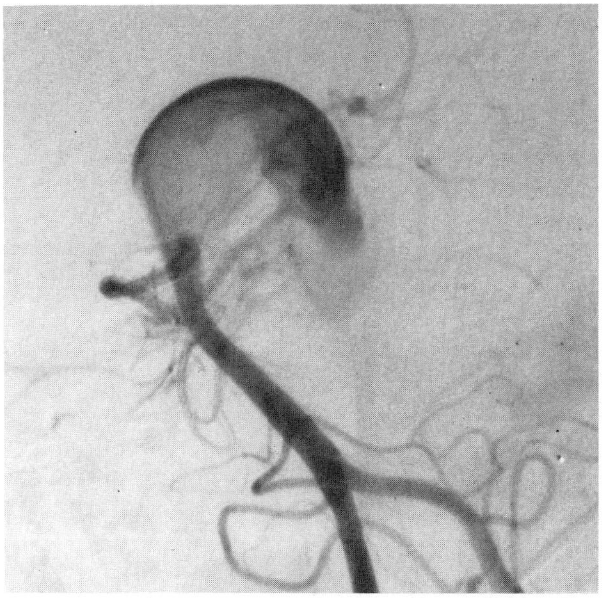

(*B*)

Figure 231-4 Oblique projections (*A* and *B*) are extremely helpful in giant distal basilar aneurysms, because the origins of the posterior cerebral arteries can be well seen.

distortion of the brain stem can be readily appreciated. It is occasionally possible, using thin-section sagittal and coronal reconstructions, to identify efferent vessels that are otherwise difficult to see on standard studies. We are still occasionally misled, however, by the suggestion of intraluminal thrombosis in certain high-flow giant sacs. In these cases the turbulence of the swirling blood within the sac gives rise to MR signals suggesting thrombosis. When this issue becomes important in determining the type of brain-protective strategy or operative procedure to be offered, we recommend supplementing the evaluation with a contrast-enhanced CT scan.

Our experience with MR angiography remains preliminary. Although these fascinating studies are clearly improving each year, it is our impression at this time that the frequent sluggish flow noted in giant aneurysms is disabling for this technology. We have had good success in identifying small aneurysms, but much more limited success in determining useful information on giant aneurysms. At this time we think that MR angiography is not a useful screening device for giant aneurysms, and clearly does not have the resolution to provide vital anatomic detail.

At the present time, most patients are referred to a neurosurgeon with either an enhanced CT or MRI demonstrating a giant aneurysm. From that point, it is critical that the neurosurgeon and neuroradiologist work closely together to ensure that subsequent investigations yield the vital anatomic detail to assist in therapeutic decision making.

Therapeutic Strategies

The availability of the plethora of treatment alternatives to be summarized in this section should suggest that universal solutions do not exist in the management of these challenging patients. Although historically most patients have been referred to neurosurgeons for "treatment," the availability of modern neuroimaging continues to identify more and more patients with minimal or trivial symptoms from what proves to be an intracranial vascular problem of great magnitude. Particularly in the elderly or frail patient, or those with an associated serious illness, it is occasionally appropriate to recommend no therapy at all. Induced hypotension has been reintroduced as a possible therapeutic alternative in this situation. Although the use of therapeutic hypotension has been abandoned in the acute SAH patient due to the risk of ischemic complications, this modality should perhaps be kept in mind in select cases. Two patients were reported in 1982 who were treated with diuretics and were noted to improve symptomatically.[32] The first patient noted resolution of her headaches and stabilization of a progressive visual deficit. The second patient presented with painful cranial neuropathy due to a giant aneurysm at the skull base; her symptoms reversed dramatically with medical management, allowing her to return to work as a nurse.

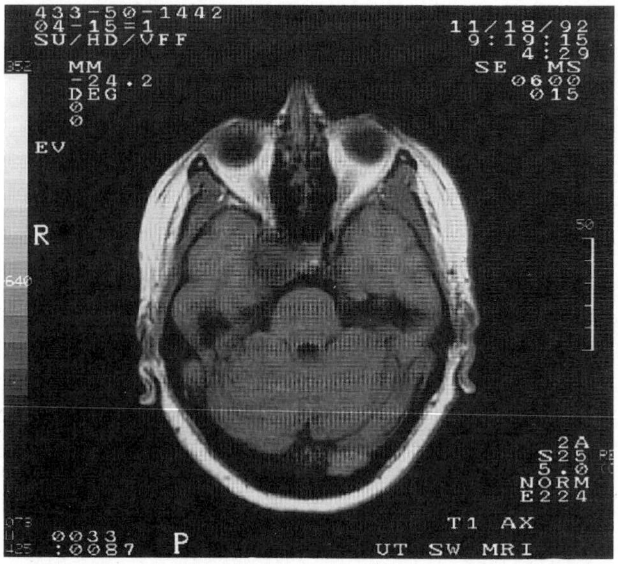

Figure 231-5 An MRI demonstrating a giant cavernous aneurysm.

Based on the observations of Hunter in 1784, the use of proximal arterial ligation has slowly gained momentum as an alternative method for treating intracranial aneurysms.[12] In 1885, Horsley applied this principle when a middle cranial fossa mass proved to be a giant aneurysm; internal carotid artery ligation stopped the bleeding and the patient made a good recovery.[13] Although this principle was widely used for treating SAH patients, hemispheral ischemia was quickly identified as a major limiting factor. Reversible occlusion clamps partially solved this problem, in that graded

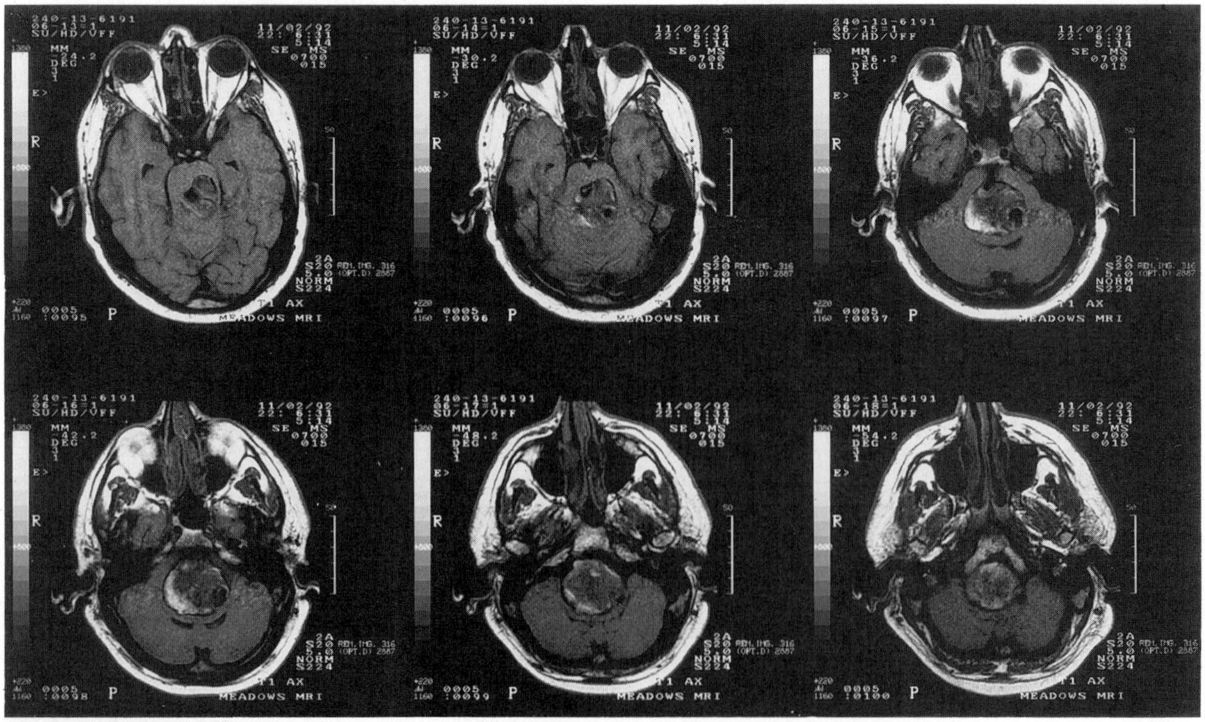

Figure 231-6 An MRI study demonstrating a patent channel through a giant vertebral confluens aneurysm. Also notable is the exquisite anatomic detail seen in the surrounding brain tissue.

occlusion was possible, allowing the patient's own collateral circulation to develop. Anticoagulation was subsequently added to this strategy to prevent embolic events.[12] In our unit we continue to employ graded carotid occlusion for patients failing endovascular trial occlusion, and have found that the use of transcranial Doppler ultrasonography allows much more precision during the final stages of arterial closure.[16] Drake is credited with applying the principle of proximal vessel occlusion to intracranial giant aneurysms on a large scale.[12] Considerable success was demonstrated in his institution in the management of otherwise inoperable lesions. The inevitable risk of ischemic sequelae in basilar artery occlusion led him to develop a tourniquet which allowed elective and awake basilar artery ligation during neurological surveillance.[12]

The use of endovascular methods (detailed below) has allowed even further application of the Hunterian principle, and at this point virtually all intracranial vessels have been occluded temporarily in awake patients. We use this technique frequently in the management of giant cavernous or basilar trunk lesions. The parent artery is occluded for 30 min, and the patient is carefully monitored neurologically. Dual-isotope regional cerebral blood flow (rCBF) studies are performed with single-photon emission CT, both during and after arterial occlusion. Patients who tolerate the occlusion neurologically as well as hemodynamically seem to be at little or no risk from definitive arterial sacrifice. However, those developing rCBF abnormalities in the absence of neurological events do appear to be at risk for the development of infarction, often several hours or even days after abrupt arterial sacrifice. These critical patients are now treated with either graded occlusion or prophylactic revascularization to minimize this ischemic risk. Our observation has been that trial basilar artery occlusion is plagued with false positives because the occlusive balloon itself blocks the orifice to numerous pontine perforating vessels, causing neurological symptoms in spite of adequate distal collateral blood flow.

One of the unfortunate aspects of proximal ligation, as well as other indirect methods of aneurysm treatment, lies in the inability of the surgeon to actually decompress the neurovascular tissues when mass effect may be solely responsible for the symptoms. The Hunterian principle can be expanded to allow decompression by the use of trapping procedures. In addition to allowing a definitive decompression to be performed, trapping also eliminates the occasionally noted risk of persistent aneurysm growth or recurrent hemorrhage due to persistent flow from collateral sources. The use of vascular trapping procedures seems to be most applicable in those lesions of the cavernous carotid artery with severe cranial neuropathy unresponsive to proximal occlusion, or in patients with complex distal vertebral artery lesions with severe brain stem distortion.

Definitive clipping of the aneurysm neck, with evacuation of its contents, allowing preservation of antegra e flow into all efferent vessels, remains the gold standard of therapy for all intracranial aneurysms. This goal is difficult to accomplish in the giant aneurysm, due to the frequent calcification noted in the aneurysm wall, intraluminal thrombosis, and wide expansion of the aneurysmal neck, occasionally with efferent vasculature emanating from the sac itself. In our experience, the achievement of precise neck clipping is often possible in giant aneurysms, but virtually always requires temporary arterial occlusion to facilitate the vascular reconstruction. The myriad of modern clips available, as well as the possibility of crushing the aneurysmal tissue with various instruments, allows the clipping of seemingly untreatable aneurysms, as long as either temporary proximal occlusion or temporary trapping is employed.

In some difficult lesions involving the skull base, direct clipping is either impossible or accompanied by undue risk to the cranial nerves, whose preservation is the actual goal of therapy. To circumvent this problem, direct interposition grafts with preservation of antegrade flow have been proposed and successfully accomplished.[33] This procedure, particularly involving the petrous and cavernous carotid segments, allows aneurysm evacuation as well as preservation of antegrade flow.

Over the past decade substantial developments have occurred in intravascular technology. Interventional neuroradiologists are now able to navigate safely and efficiently into virtually all intracranial vasculature. Serbinenko initially reported the use of the endovascular balloon.[29] This observation led to a series of innovative applications which have dramatically changed the way we approach patients with various forms of difficult cerebrovascular disease. This balloon technology was quickly applied for proximal ligation as well as definitive sac occlusion in the treatment of giant aneurysms.[7,9,10,14,15,18,20,28] In the past few years, numerous problems with the balloons themselves have become obvious. Numerous episodes of distal embolization, balloon deflation, and balloon rupture have been reported. Platinum microcoils have subsequently been developed, and can be elegantly placed within the sac of giant aneurysms.[19] These microcoils may prove to be substantially safer and offer more durable protection than the previously described balloons. It is clear that problems remain, however. It appears that the aneurysms which present the most difficult technical challenges to the surgeon and the highest risk to the patient offer the least possibility for definitive endovascular cure. The initial surgical procedure, when performed endovascularly, is safer than an open complex craniotomy for giant aneurysm, but most patients are left with less than complete aneurysm obliteration. It is not known if these patients are thus offered protection against subsequent aneurysm enlargement or rupture. In addition, the limitations concerning the lack of access for true decompression of the aneurysm sac are obvious. We have seen and reported a patient who was found to have a completely thrombosed giant distal basilar artery aneurysm, which despite its lack of patency, progressively enlarged and ultimately killed the patient.[3] It will be vital to achieve long-term follow-up in patients treated endovascularly.

Nevertheless, we remain convinced that major contributions to the management of the patient with a giant aneurysm will accompany these innovative procedures. Perhaps the most dramatic is the use of trial proximal occlusion with the awake patient, allowing neurological as well as hemodynamic surveillance. It is also clear that recurrent giant aneurysms (after previous therapy), present serious challenges to the neurosurgeon. It is very likely that microcoil therapy, if it proves to be durable, will offer a safer alternative. It is also obvious that patients with serious medical complications precluding a protracted general anesthetic can be offered some hope of symptom alleviation using endovascular methods.

Brain-Protective Strategies

The aforementioned physical characteristics of many, if not most, giant aneurysms renders them difficult and dangerous to clip while distended with normal arterial turgor. Pool's observations on the feasibility and tolerance of the intracranial vasculature to temporary arterial occlusion set the stage for successful direct treatment of intracranial giant aneurysms.[27] Due to their strong closing pressure, some early temporary clips and certainly the permanent aneurysm clips produced intimal injury when used on parent vasculature. These technical problems have now been circumvented by a new host of safe and effective clips.[21]

Numerous neurosurgeons have observed that virtually all intracranial vessels can be occluded for brief periods without fear of ischemic sequelae under modern neuroanesthetic conditions. Thus, when temporary occlusion is required to simply soften a sac slightly for clip closure or to finalize dissection, it is likely that no special precautions are needed to prevent ischemic injury. On the other hand, more complex aneurysms often require complete trapping of the afferent and efferent vessels with wide opening of the sac and evacuation of thrombus prior to clipping. In these circumstances the surgeon is confronted with the need for temporary occlusion of substantial duration and questions about the risk of infarction in the involved vascular territory. Unfortunately we have very few guidelines from which to base judgments about exactly how long each vascular territory may be safely rendered ischemic. Due to this uncertainty, a number of strategies have been developed and are now available to the clinician to prolong ischemic tolerance.

Barbiturates have been successfully employed in a number of animal models of cerebral ischemia, and have been shown to minimize permanent damage, but their associated cardiotoxicity in the clinical setting can jeopardize systemic blood pressure and collateral circulation.[17,24] Because of those concerns, particularly in elderly, fragile patients, we gained experience a number of years ago with another drug, etomidate (Amidate; Abbot Laboratories, North Chicago, IL), which was appealing due to its known cerebral metabolic depressant effects (similar to those of the barbiturates) without associated cardiotoxicity.[2] Abundant laboratory experience with etomidate has clearly demonstrated that it depresses cerebral metabolic rate incrementally until isoelectricity is reached. At that point the metabolic rate stabilizes at about 48 percent of control levels, as long as EEG silence is maintained.[25,26] Over time, our neuroanesthesiologists found that while EEG monitoring intraoperatively was critical to document burst suppression, most patients were appropriately suppressed with a dosage of 1 mg/kg initially, followed by 10 μg/kg per min, as necessary to maintain burst suppression.

Using additional techniques of normothermia, normoglycemia, and normotension, this local protocol was evaluated over a 2-year period, excluding patients in whom temporary occlusion was instituted emergently or in whom some vessel sacrifice was required. Several parameters were found to be associated with postoperative evidence of infarction. Patients older than 61 years of age and those in poor neurological condition clearly had a higher incidence of ischemic complications than did patients in better condition. The 95 percent confidence level for the tolerance of occlusion in patients in Hunt-Hess grades I and II was 19 min, while for those in grades III and IV, this safe period was decreased to 15 min. All patients whose arteries were occluded for longer than 31 min had both radiographic and neurological evidence of cerebral infarction. Patients with occlusion for less than 14 min routinely suffered no sequelae. A trend was noted in patients whose occlusion was longer than 14 min, suggesting a relationship between incomplete trapping and the development of ischemic consequence. It was also suggested that the distributions of the thalamoperforating and lenticulostriate vessels were uniquely sensitive to ischemia, and that increasing the number of episodes of temporary occlusion may predispose to permanent ischemic injury. It should be noted, however, that our standard practice does not involve repetitive and brief (1 or 2 min) episodes of temporary occlusion. Rather, our practice is to establish temporary occlusion and attempt to complete the dissection and reconstruction. When the ischemic interval is reaching the neighborhood of 15 min and the conclusion of the procedure is not in sight, if possible we will reestablish flow at that time for 1 to 10 min. Therefore, our data gave no particular insight into the commonly employed method of repetitive, brief ischemic intervals.

Although this study suffers from the inherent variability of the vascular territories involved and the heterogeneity of aneurysm patients in general, it is our belief that this experience suggests that the upper limits of safe ischemic tolerance, under the conditions utilized at our center, appears to be about 15 to 20 min. While most difficult vascular lesions can be successfully treated within this time frame, a number of thrombotic giant posterior circulation aneurysms do require more time to successfully complete the procedure.

It has been well known for years that hypothermia decreases cerebral metabolism profoundly, and seems to do so by a different mechanism than that of the pharmacologic agents. While neuronal activity is clearly depressed during incremental hypothermic challenges, cellular homeostatic mechanisms are also impaired. This difference in mechanism led us to hope that synergism between the pharmacologic agents and induced hypothermia might offer advantages for extended ischemic tolerance. Although profound hypothermia certainly has theoretical advantages, cardiopulmonary bypass is required when the temperature is depressed significantly below 30°C.

Procedures involving deep hypothermia (16°C) and complete circulatory arrest have been employed in the treatment of giant aneurysms for the past few decades.[6,30,31] Early attempts at this technique were abandoned, mainly due to hemorrhagic complications. Recently, improvements in the cannulation technique and the failure to surmount the technical and ischemic challenges with very difficult lesions have led to a resurgence of interest.[34] This procedure allows ischemic tolerance in the hypothermic state of up to approximately 50 min. An additional advantage is the attendant decompression of the aneurysm and adjacent vasculature when various fractions of the patient's blood volume are drained.

Our current practice involves use of purely pharmacologic metabolic suppression in routine and straightforward cases in which the surgeon anticipates temporary occlusion of less than 15 min. When ischemic intervals of between 15 and 20 min are anticipated, mild hypothermia (32 to 33°C) is added to that pharmacologic regimen. If occlusion times of greater than 20 min are anticipated, we now routinely employ deep hypothermia and circulatory arrest. One of the major pitfalls with this strategy, of course, is that in many circumstances it is quite difficult to accurately predict exactly the duration of temporary occlusion to be required for each case. We similarly believe that due to the inherent morbidity of circulatory arrest procedures, they should be used only for cases at the end of the spectrum of difficulty, in which experienced surgeons think that conventional techniques will not be successful.

Management of Specific Giant Aneurysms

The preceding discussions have focused on some of the strategic alternatives in the management of giant aneurysms; this section will attempt to focus on certain unique features of lesions at typical sites and to highlight some of our management biases. It should be obvious that many aspects of the treatment of these patients remain controversial, and that no universal solutions exist. We will attempt to highlight some of these controversies, and present some of the solutions that appear to be reasonably effective.

Giant Carotid Cavernous Aneurysms

This subgroup of giant aneurysms, which reside almost exclusively outside the subarachnoid space, is the focus of current neurosurgical controversy. As innovative efforts continue in the realm of skull-base surgery as well as interventional neuroradiology, we are somewhat handicapped by incomplete natural history data. The majority of patients with these aneurysms present to clinical attention with extraocular movement disorders due to cranial neuropathy. Occasionally headaches are a major portion of the clinical picture, and rarely the retro-orbital component of this pain is so severe as to warrant immediate intervention. A minority of patients present with distal embolic symptoms or spontaneous rupture, leading to carotid cavernous fistula. Only very rarely, in our experience and in the world's literature, is acute SAH a complication of this disorder. Therefore, the majority of patients evaluated in most neurosurgical centers present with non-life-threatening symptoms.

Direct and definite treatment of these aneurysms through either surgical or endovascular techniques is attractive, because carotid patency can be maintained. Dolenc[11] and a number of other investigators have developed anterior skull-base procedures capable of exposing the aneurysm anatomy within the cavernous sinus thereby allowing direct clipping in many cases. It should be kept in mind, however, that achievement of this goal is not without cost to the patient. As Dolenc noted, two deaths occurred in a series of seven patients, and the procedures ranged in length from 3 to 10 h.[11] As a flurry of subsequent literature extolling the virtues of this exposure and other modifications appeared, it was our impression that the incidence of severe postoperative cranial neuropathy may have been understated. In our own relatively modest experience with intracavernous open surgery, most patients suffered worsening of their extraocular dysfunction. The disability, occurring as a result of ophthalmoplegia, must be kept in mind as a patient with such a giant aneurysm is evaluated, either in an asymptomatic or minimally symptomatic state. A number of these lesions are clearly fusiform in nature and do not lend themselves well to direct clip reconstruction, regardless of the exposure achieved.

Endovascular technology has made a tremendous impact on our ability to manage these patients. As the detachable balloon technology developed, it was hoped that direct treatment of the aneurysm with preservation of carotid patency would be possible in a majority of cases. At least in our experience, detachable balloons have been a significant disappointment in this regard. We have had more than one complication related to distal embolism and have had one fatal SAH occurring 36 h following incomplete obliteration due to a ball-valve-type effect. A number of other lesions have been incompletely obliterated with balloons, resulting in a situation that may be hemodynamically unstable and has an unknown natural history. The detachable microcoils may improve this situation, although decompression of the sac is obviously not a component of this modality. It would appear possible that the use of some form of detachable sleeve to reconstruct the cavernous carotid artery might provide the ultimate solution for these lesions, but such a device has yet to be developed.

At the present time, however, we continue to use a historic form of therapy supplemented with modern technology. It is our belief that internal carotid artery occlusion offers the safest and most effective form of therapy for the most patients with symptomatic cavernous giant aneurysms. It is clear that in our experience, at least 80 to 85 percent of patients possess adequate collateral potential to tolerate abrupt carotid sacrifice, and despite the fact that the sacs are not deflated, symptoms of pain and cranial neuropathy tend to resolve surprisingly rapidly.

Our current protocol utilizes awake, trial internal carotid occlusion with a nondetachable balloon, accompanied by ongoing neurological monitoring during carotid occlusion, as well as dual-isotope single-photon emission computed tomography. For this procedure, the patient is taken to the angiography suite, where anticoagulation is induced and a nondetachable balloon is inflated in the internal carotid artery. The patient is examined for 30 to 45 min; toward the end of that challenge, a radioisotope is injected, permitting subsequent rCBF evaluation from that moment. At the completion of the trial the balloon is deflated and removed, and the patient is taken to the CBF laboratory. If that CBF determination discloses decreased flow in the involved hemisphere, a baseline study is obtained the following day for comparison. If the baseline study has reverted to normal, the patient is considered to be at hemodynamic risk from abrupt carotid sacrifice. Our current decision-making schema evolves from the results of the neurological as well as hemodynamic monitoring. In general, patients fall into three categories: (1) those remaining neurologically normal during occlusion with normal rCBF; (2) those remaining neurologically normal but with rCBF evidence of hemodynamic compromise; and (3) those developing a focal neurological deficit at the time of trial occlusion.

For those patients remaining neurologically well, with normal rCBF studies during occlusion (group 1), primary endovascular internal carotid occlusion is performed with detachable balloons reinforced by microcoils. For patients in group 2, who neurologically tolerate the procedure but develop flow abnormalities, an extracranial-intracranial bypass procedure is performed. Two days after the completion of that procedure, repeat cerebral angiography is performed to document patency of the graft and trial occlusion is repeated. If the flow through the graft is acceptable and clinical tolerance established, the patient is treated with abrupt carotid sacrifice. For the patients in group 3, who develop a focal deficit at the time of trial occlusion, a prophylactic bypass procedure is also performed with either a superficial temporal artery branch, if this vessel is large, or a short or long saphenous interposition graft. Forty-eight hours following this procedure the patient is again taken to the angiography suite for trial internal carotid artery occlusion. After documentation of graft patency, if the flow defect has been corrected by the bypass, abrupt carotid sacrifice is performed endovascularly. If the flow defect persists, graded occlusion with a Selverstone clamp is performed. It has proved quite helpful to monitor the use of the Selverstone clamp with transcranial Doppler studies to increase the precision of closure.[16]

This protocol has proven very effective in managing the majority of patients with this condition. We tend to use trapping only in those patients with visual symptoms due to optic nerve or chiasmal compression or persisting cranial neuropathy. If a trapping procedure is performed, the distal carotid clipping must occur proximal to the ophthalmic artery to preserve that source of collateral flow.

An important subgroup of patients harbor contralateral cavernous aneurysms. In this subgroup the potentially deleterious effect of ipsilateral carotid sacrifice must be kept in mind. It is likely that if anterior cerebral crossover flow is developed during carotid occlusion, the contralateral cavernous aneurysm may be at increased risk of subsequent distention and enlargement. Such a circumstance is illustrated in Fig. 231-7. Several treatment alternatives must be considered in these patients. One possible consideration for the asymptomatic or minimally symptomatic patient is to defer therapy at this time, until a detachable sleeve becomes available. For those mandating therapy, consideration must be given to the direct and selective occlusion of the aneurysm, by either surgical or interventional means, while preserving carotid patency. The patient illustrated in Fig. 231-7 has a relatively narrow base of the aneurysmal neck, and therefore is a good candidate for either surgical or endovascular aneurysm obliteration. In the unusual circumstance of a patient in whom direct therapy is unsuccessful or deemed impossible, who has a large ipsilateral posterior communicating artery, an alternative strategy may be considered. For these patients, occlusion of the anterior communicating artery and thus isolation of both carotid circulations may allow carotid occlusion to be performed on the symptomatic side without risk of increasing the hemodynamic stress on the contralateral lesion.

Giant Paraclinoidal Carotid Aneurysms

Giant aneurysms arising from the carotid immediately distal to the roof of the cavernous sinus are anatomically diverse and have been notoriously misunderstood. In our experience, these aneurysms arise from three aspects of the paraclinoidal carotid artery: the classic carotid ophthalmic origin, the superior hypophyseal artery origin, and the posterolateral carotid wall. Day has demonstrated the difference in origin between the carotid ophthalmic aneurysms and those associated with the superior hypophyseal artery.[8] In general, the carotid ophthalmic origin aneurysms arise from the anterior and superior aspect of the carotid artery as it emerges from the roof of the cavernous sinus. These lesions tend to project superiorly or superomedially, and the displacement of the optic nerve depends on the degree of medial growth of the sac. For those lesions extending predominantly superiorly, the optic nerve can be rotated and displaced medially. If the predominant projection is superomedial, however, the optic nerve may be slightly displaced laterally. Giant aneurysms originating from the superior hypophyseal origin project primarily medially, and often slightly posteromedially. These lesions, when giant sized, may displace the optic nerve medially and superiorly, and the carotid is typically elevated and displaced laterally. The unusual aneurysms associated with the posterolateral carotid wall pose somewhat more difficult surgical problems, in that they tend to be obscured more severely by the anterior clinoid process.

While strikingly different in angiographic, microsurgical, and technical characteristics, these aneurysms share the following common problems for the surgeon: (1) the acquisition of proximal arterial control; (2) appreciation of the exact site of emergence of the carotid from the roof of the cavernous sinus; (3) adequate deflation of the sac to allow clipping; and (4) delicate handling of the attenuated optic nerve to minimize the risk of iatrogenic visual loss. Each of these problems will be discussed in order, with specific reference to the individual projections of the three types of aneurysms.

For the overwhelming majority of paraclinoidal giant aneurysms, intracranial exposure of adequate proximal carotid artery to achieve definitive temporary clipping is difficult and achievable only after extensive bony resection. It has been our experience that the simplest and most efficient means of acquiring proximal control is to perform a cervical carotid exposure, isolating the internal carotid at its origin. Having access to a significant segment of the internal carotid, away from the intracranial exposure, also facilitates aneurysm deflation, as will be discussed below. This procedure similarly offers the surgeon the comfort of having proximal arterial control prior to initiating the craniotomy.

While these three specific aneurysm projections result in unique anatomic situations, all share the predictable location of the healthy proximal intracranial carotid artery. A common mistake in the technical approach to these giant aneurysms is to assume that the healthy proximal carotid is quite lateral to its actual location. This misconception results in excessive and unnecessary lateral bony resection of the anterior clinoid process. As one visualizes the anatomy, it is key to appreciate that the healthy carotid will be identified immediately beneath the lateral aspect of the optic canal. Once this important anatomic concept is appreciated, the technical problems associated with these aneurysms diminish substantially. A persistent controversy in the neurosurgical literature concerns the necessity for and the extent of bony resection in the treatment of paraclinoidal aneurysms. Our experience has been that many small carotid ophthalmic aneurysms can be clipped by incising the dural aspect of the optic canal laterally. For many, if not most, giant carotid ophthalmic artery aneurysms, this extension of the subarachnoid exposure is inadequate, and the proximal neck may only be defined by a focused resection of the bone of the lateral aspect of the optic canal and the optic strut. Once this bone has been resected and the dural ring incised, the ophthalmic artery origin may be visualized, which almost certainly represents healthy carotid tissue at the proximal neck. Surprisingly, most superior hypophyseal aneurysms, regardless of size, can be successfully clipped without bony removal. These aneurysms expand along the floor of the skull base within the subarachnoid space. Simple dural incision of the optic canal, with slight elevation of the optic nerve and depression of the aneurysm sac, allows identification of the ophthalmic artery, which defines the proximal neck. While classically the fenestrated clip has been recommended for this aneurysm, with adequate aneurysm deflation, traditional clipping beneath the carotid artery can usually be accomplished. The aneurysms arising at the posterolateral aspect of the carotid artery are, fortunately, unusual. The anatomic constraints imposed by the distal aspect of the anterior clinoid process obscure their exposure. We have found it necessary to radically resect the anterior clinoid under this circumstance, as well as to open the lateral aspect of the optic canal. It is only by such bony removal and the tedious elevation of the aneurysm from the roof of the cavernous sinus that an adequate appreciation of the proximal aspect of the neck can be achieved.

Although almost all giant aneurysms do require some degree of deflation prior to clipping, this necessity has proven virtually universal in the management of paraclinoidal giant aneurysms. Early in our experience we relied on either temporary cervical proximal occlusion or temporary trapping to adequately soften the neck. We were impressed and surprised by the residual turgor in the aneurysm sac despite trapping of the segment, and this distention was often enough to preclude precise neck clipping, allowing the clip to back down onto the parent artery. This persisting distention presumably arises from retrograde ophthalmic artery and cavernous branch artery flow. If the aneurysm is opened after trapping clips are applied, the surgeon loses the use of his nondominant hand to help manipulate the neck of the aneurysm to ensure safe clip passage. We stumbled upon a very helpful means of safely and reliably deflating the sac some years ago.[5] After dissection has been completed, a proximal occlusion clamp is placed on the cervical internal carotid, a temporary clip is applied to the intracranial carotid proximal to the posterior communicating artery, and, when

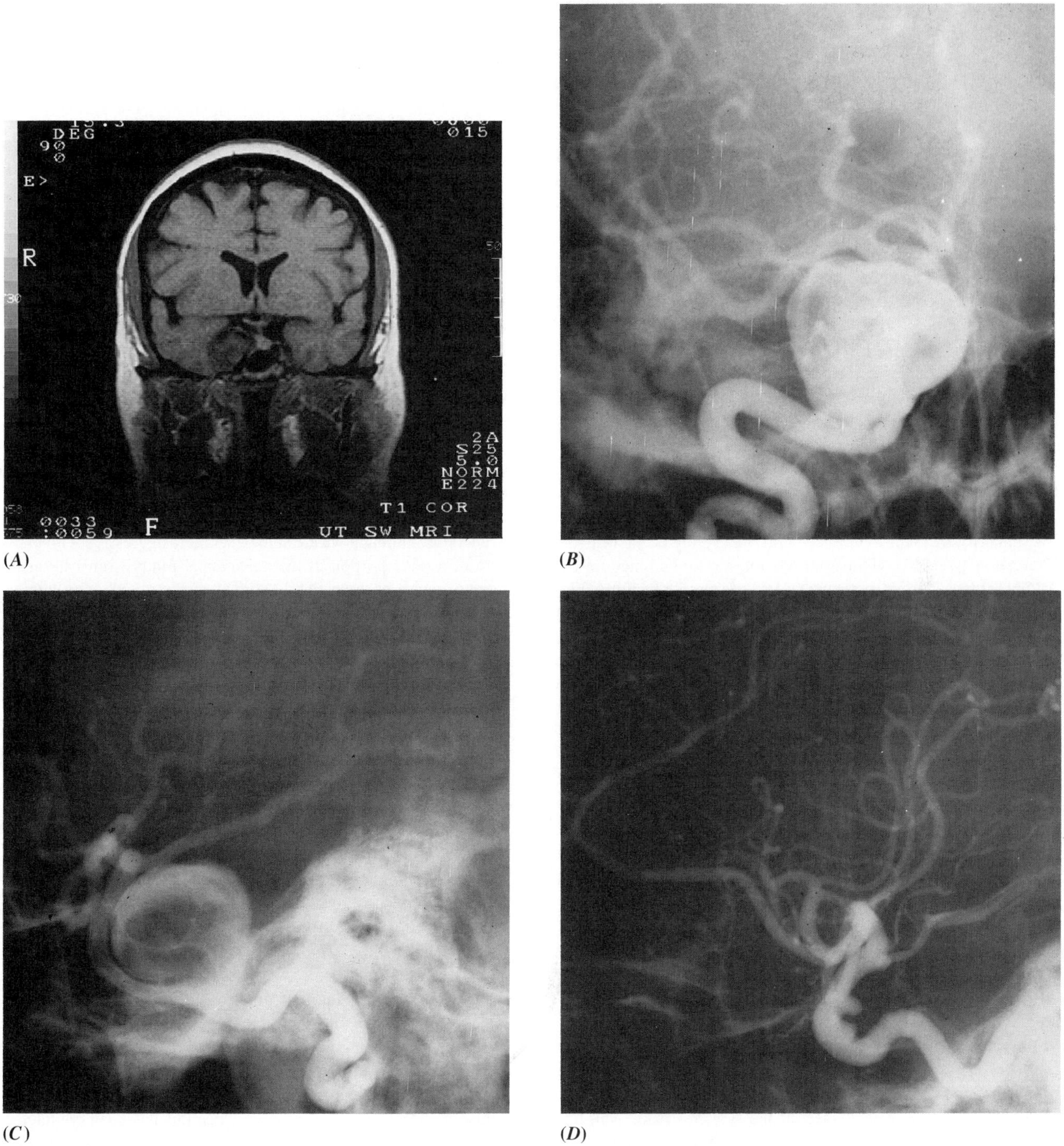

Figure 231-7 This case involves a 65-year-old woman with a near complete and painless right sixth nerve palsy. *A.* A coronal MRI demonstrates the presence of a right cavernous mass. *B.* An anteroposterior cerebral angiogram demonstrates the cavernous origin of a giant aneurysm. *C.* A lateral angiographic projection suggests a proximal cavernous neck with a relatively narrow base. *D.* A contralateral carotid angiogram discloses a small cavernous aneurysm and a small superior hypophyseal artery aneurysm that is probably at least partially within the subarachnoid space.

possible, a temporary clip is applied to the ophthalmic artery. Next, an 18-gauge Angiocath (IV catheter placement unit; Deseret Medical, Inc, Sandy, UT) is inserted into the cervical carotid distal to the clamp. Wall suction is then applied to that Angiocath through extension tubing. This simple technique facilitates dramatic aneurysm collapse and allows very rapid reconstruction of even difficult, thick-walled giant lesions. The advantages of this technique have been so pleasing that we have not sought other alternatives. We have also found that this technique greatly expedites the operative procedure and minimizes the degree of necessary resection.

The final problem previously alluded to concerns the manipulation of the optic nerve. It has become apparent that the key variable in allowing the safe mobilization of the optic nerve is the wide incision of the optic canal, and in many situations the extension of the optic canal by bony resection. This allows the optic nerve to be elevated gently, without producing undue angulation and stretching at the dural insertion.

While giving the appearance of extremely formidable challenges, these aneurysms can almost always be clipped definitively. It is vital in each case, however, to carefully individualize the primary concerns of proximal control, neck exposure, and aneurysm deflation. Although the means of achieving each of these goals may vary somewhat, depending on the individual characteristics of the aneurysm, they are vital for the safe and successful reconstruction of the paraclinoidal carotid artery.

Giant Middle Cerebral Artery Aneurysms

The majority of giant middle cerebral aneurysms occur near the bifurcation of the M1 segment in relationship to the limen insula. An important subgroup, however, involves a largely fusiform dilatation, often with significant thrombosis, incorporating much of the M1 segment. Thus, consideration of these lesions includes a continuum from the nonthrombotic saccular middle cerebral bifurcation giant aneurysm to the thrombotic yet saccular aneurysm of the middle cerebral bifurcation to the serpentine and fusiform lesion involving the proximal middle cerebral artery.

The most straightforward of this group of aneurysms is the nonthrombotic saccular aneurysm of the middle cerebral bifurcation. In our experience the overwhelming majority of the aneurysms project into the middle cranial fossa to a greater extent than the anterior cranial fossa. This anatomic feature makes the lateral trans-sylvian approach very appealing, because the dissection can be carried through the opercular-insular portion of the sylvian fissure down to an M2 segment, thus allowing identification of the aneurysm origin and the M1 segment totally within the subarachnoid space. A number of these lesions do require variable resection of the temporal lobe to facilitate their exposure, however, particularly in the setting of parenchymal hemorrhage from the aneurysm. In the setting of a large temporal lobe hematoma, we initiate the dissection in the anterior aspect of the temporal lobe to evacuate some hematoma and thus decompress the middle fossa somewhat prior to opening the lateral aspect of the sylvian fissure. This approach is also very worthwhile in the massive giant aneurysms in which exposure is greatly facilitated by simply uncapping the aneurysmal fundus by removing the rim of temporal lobe tissue. Regardless of whether the ultimate brain resection is performed from the cortical surface or in the subpial plane from within the sylvian fissure, we have found it extremely helpful to expose a very generous portion of the aneurysmal wall, and not just the neck, as is routine in smaller aneurysms. Once this exposure is accomplished, for the aneurysm with no or minimal intraluminal thrombosis, temporary clips are applied to the M1 and M2 segments, to effectively isolate the aneurysm. Early in our experience, we found that simple occlusion of the M1 segment gave relatively poor aneurysm decompression, and our ultimate occlusion times tended to be longer than when the lesion was isolated definitively. Following the application of temporary clipping, the aneurysm is opened. For the extremely thick-walled lesions, the use of the arachnoid knife to make a significant puncture wound through which the suction device can be introduced to quickly deflate the lesion is much more time efficient than using small spinal needles to accomplish this task. Once the aneurysm is definitively deflated, its reconstruction can be accomplished without undue delay, allowing preservation of efferent vasculature. While the specific aspects of the clipping itself depend on the nature of the lesion, the size of the giant aneurysm and the typical broad base often present the surgeon a difficult decision regarding whether to exclude *all* aneurysm tissue at the expense of stenosis of the efferent vessels, or to leave a small cuff of residual aneurysm and have widely patent outflow into the efferent branches. This is often a difficult decision, whose solution depends on a number of variables. For the elderly patient with an unruptured sac, there is little doubt that leaving a small amount of residual abnormal tissue is safer than producing an obvious stenosis in the efferent vasculature, which may be rendered more hemodynamically significant by unseen atheromatous change within these vessels.

The calcific and thrombotic middle cerebral giant aneurysms occurring at the bifurcation are more serious technical challenges to the neurosurgeon. The initial approach and exposure are not dissimilar from those for the previously mentioned patent saccular aneurysms, although we are somewhat more aggressive with exposure of a wide portion of the aneurysmal fundus. Intrinsic in the reconstruction of the patient's normal anatomy is the absolute necessity for evacuation of thrombus in the region of the neck. This requirement mandates the wide opening of the aneurysmal fundus. We have gone through a number of intermediate steps en route to our current preferred technique. We have found it dangerous and usually impossible to clip the aneurysm without definitive trapping. Without clearly visualizing the neck of the aneurysm (from within the sac), one cannot be certain that thrombus has not yet pushed into the lumen of the afferent and efferent vessels during clip closure. This type of aneurysm often has a calcific wall that is quite difficult to close while tethered to the distal sac, which is distended with thrombosis. We have found that the procedure is made much simpler and safer, and the intervals of temporary occlusion required are much shorter by applying definitive trapping temporary clips and excising the aneurysm throughout the circumference of the fundus. Once the temporary clips are applied, an incision is made circumferentially around the fundus at least 1 cm distal to the neck. It is critical to leave an adequate cuff for subsequent reconstruction, and the surgeon should always err on the side of leaving too much rather than too little. A number 11 knife blade has been found to be useful in initiating this incision, and the heavy bayoneted microscissors can then be used to quickly circumscribe the rest of the incision. Once this has been completed, attention should be directed to evacuating all material within the cuff. The distal sac should be ignored at this point, as the morbidity of the procedure will increase with prolonged occlusion times. Pancake curettes, as well as the ultrasonic aspirator, allow the cleavage of the thrombotic material from the aneurysmal wall. As the patent portion of the aneurysmal neck is entered, the intima should be treated with great care to avoid inadvertent injury which could lead to subsequent dissection and thrombosis of the middle cerebral complex. Once the material has been evacuated leaving a cuff, it is usually quite straightforward to clip the remaining cuff with conventional clips. If substantial calcification remains, it is occasionally necessary to crush the neck with a hemostat prior to application of the clips. Once clipping has been achieved and flow restored, the rest of the middle cranial fossa decompression can be performed, with excision of the aneurysm, thrombotic mass, and injured temporal lobe, if necessary. As mentioned, we advise the surgeon to err on the side of leaving a small residual neck rather than jeopardizing the middle cerebral outflow.

Our experience with the fusiform, thrombotic, and serpentine M1 aneurysm has been largely unsuccessful. It is likely that the initial pathophysiology of this aneurysm is that of repetitive dissection. We have tried numerous technical solutions including excision with distal bypass, temporary occlusion with opening and evacuation of the mass with clip reconstruction to preserve the lenticulostriates, and simple proximal ligation; we have been disappointed with the outcome of many of these attempts. It is likely that the majority of the morbidity occurs from loss of lenticulostriate vessels, whether or not the M1 trunk is preserved. We continue to search for solutions to this aneurysm but, to date, remain frustrated with our results. The use of circulatory arrest procedures with additional safe temporary occlusion time would not, on the surface, seem to offer much benefit because the reconstruction would still jeopardize perforator origins.

Giant Anterior Communicating Artery Aneurysms

Giant aneurysms involving the anterior communicating artery complex may be either completely patent or thrombosed to variable degrees. For the completely patent aneurysms, the principles of treatment would be similar to those for patent giant aneurysms of the middle cerebral bifurcation. Definitive isolation of the afferent and efferent vessels is an absolute prerequisite to adequate deflation. We have found that the unilateral pterional approach, with a slightly larger craniotomy than for smaller anterior communicating lesions, is sufficient in the overwhelming majority of cases. We believe strongly that temporary clips should be applied to both A1 and both A2 segments prior to aneurysm opening. Simple proximal occlusion of the A1 segments is occasionally helpful in softening the sac enough to identify and clip the A2 segments, but the aneurysm should not be opened after clipping of only the A1 vessels. In this setting as the contents of the aneurysm are evacuated through the suction, the collateral flow into the distal anterior cerebral circulation is also being removed. Therefore, we prefer aggressive gyrus rectus resection with clear isolation of the efferent vessels prior to the institution of temporary clipping. Once these four vessels are clipped, the completely patent aneurysm can be opened with an arachnoid knife and deflated, thereby allowing clip reconstruction of the anterior communicating complex. We remain convinced that the patient's future is much better with preservation of the anterior communicating artery and its associated perforating vessels than with simple trapping of the anterior communicating artery.

The giant anterior communicating aneurysm that is filled with thrombotic material requires more definitive dissection of the aneurysmal fundus, as was discussed for thrombotic middle cerebral aneurysms. We prefer to isolate all four vessels with temporary clips and completely excise the anterior communicating sac, leaving a cuff to be dealt with. The residual thrombotic material within the neck can be removed under direct visualization, allowing precise clip reconstruction. After perfusion is reestablished, the residual of the mass can be evacuated without undue haste.

Figure 231-2 illustrates the CT scan of a recently treated patient with a completely patent giant anterior communicating aneurysm that presented significant technical challenges. This patient is a 63-year-old man who had a several-year history of progressive personality changes with the precipitous onset of dense visual failure. Figure 231-8 illustrates the angiographic features of this patient's aneurysm. Both A1 segments were displaced superiorly and emptied into the giant sac. On none of the preoperative studies were the A2 segments visualized. The MRI, however, clearly identified the A2 segments as residing along the posterior aspect of the sac, being widely displaced from each other. Due to the size of this aneurysm and the severe compromise of the optic apparatus, we believed that it was going to be extremely difficult to identify the efferent vessels. We therefore elected to utilize the hypothermic circulatory arrest procedure for this relatively unique indication in the anterior circulation to capitalize on the decompressive aspect of the procedure so that all four vessels could be easily identified. The aneurysm was approached from the left side because the left frontal lobe appeared to have been most severely damaged by the growth of the aneurysm. At surgery we were extremely glad that provision had been made for the circulatory arrest procedure, as only the ipsilateral A1 and A2 segments could be seen prior to the use of circulatory arrest. As the blood volume was evacuated, the aneurysm was easily displaced to allow identification of the contralateral A1 and A2 segments. An interesting finding was noted intraoperatively that emphasizes another important aspect of giant aneurysm surgery. In addition to the predominantly anterior and superiorly projecting sac was a smaller, but very calcific posterior projecting fusiform enlargement of the anterior communicating artery. To actually perfectly exclude this tissue would have required an extremely aggressive mobilization and probably excision of that separate portion of the sac which was intimately associated with perforator origins. We therefore elected to leave a fusiform portion of the anterior communicating segment and exclude and evacuate the giant sac. As can be seen in Fig. 231-8*D* and *E*, this proved to be a relatively modest residual sac, apparent on postoperative angiography. It was encased in cotton to promote fibrosis. It is our belief that an aggressive attempt to exclude that final aneurysmal portion would have added substantially to the morbidity of the procedure.

Giant Vertebral Artery Aneurysms

Several regional anatomic features act in concert to render giant aneurysms of the vertebral artery conceptually and technically challenging. In addition to the invariable brain stem distortion by an aneurysm of giant size, the lower cranial nerves are always intimately related to the afferent and efferent vasculature or must be aggressively dissected to facilitate exposure. Both of these anatomic problems comprise major sources of perioperative morbidity to these patients. Unique features of the vertebral confluens, such that two major intracranial vessels merge into a single distal outflow channel, give the surgeon options of collateral flow not seen in most other intracranial situations. As has been discussed in other sites, giant aneurysms of this area are a continuum from the simple enlargement of a typical small aneurysm distal to the origin of the posterior inferior cerebellar artery (PICA) to the massive fusiform and serpentine thrombotic giants that encompass the vertebral confluens, and often much of the lower basilar trunk. Central to the surgeon's thought process during the planning for each case should be the preservation of the PICA, at least throughout its lateral medullary segment, as our experience has suggested that its loss is usually associated with medullary infarction. As subtle anatomic information can profoundly influence the type of surgical procedure to be offered, the preoperative evaluation of these patients must, at the very least, include selective bilateral vertebral arteriograms, usually with oblique and digital dynamic projections, evaluation of the patency and size of the posterior communicating ar-

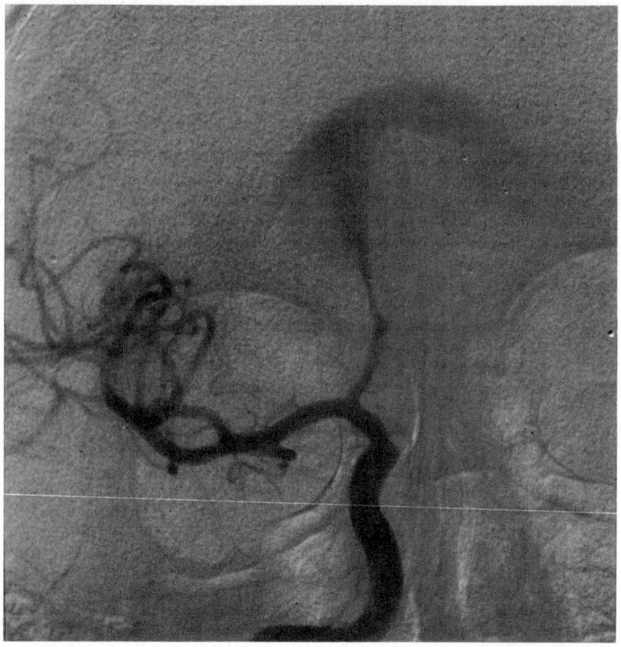

(*A*)

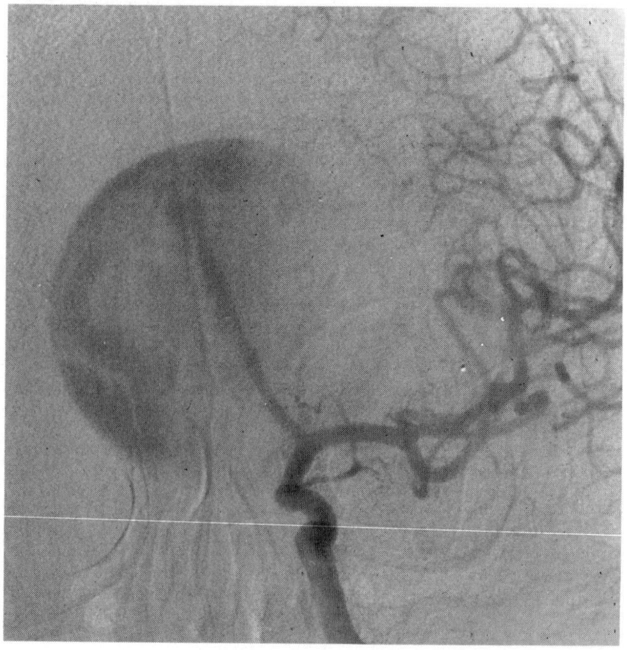

(*B*)

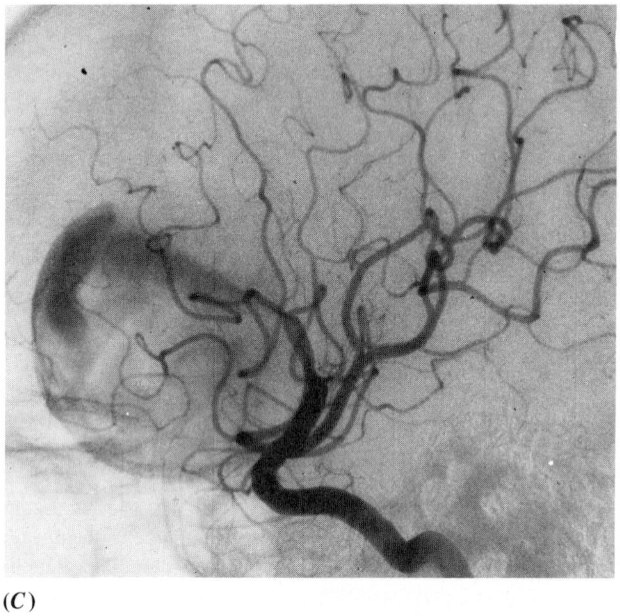

(*C*)

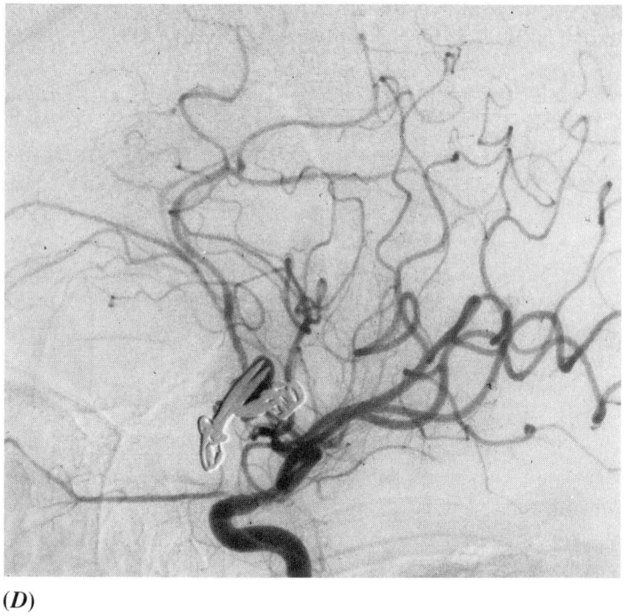

(*D*)

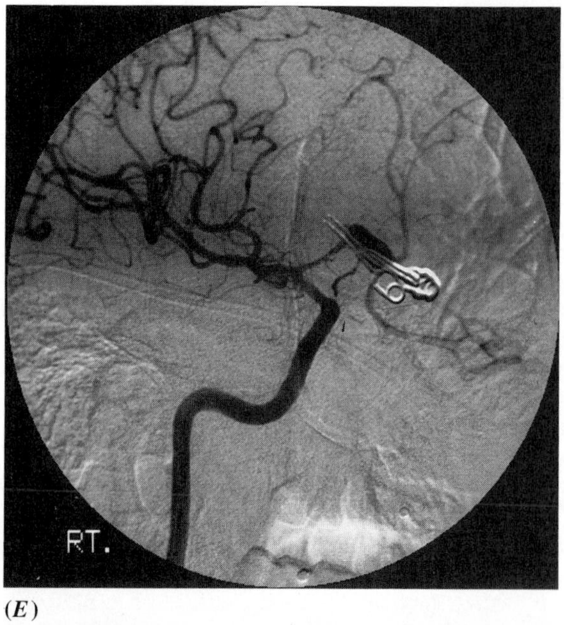

(*E*)

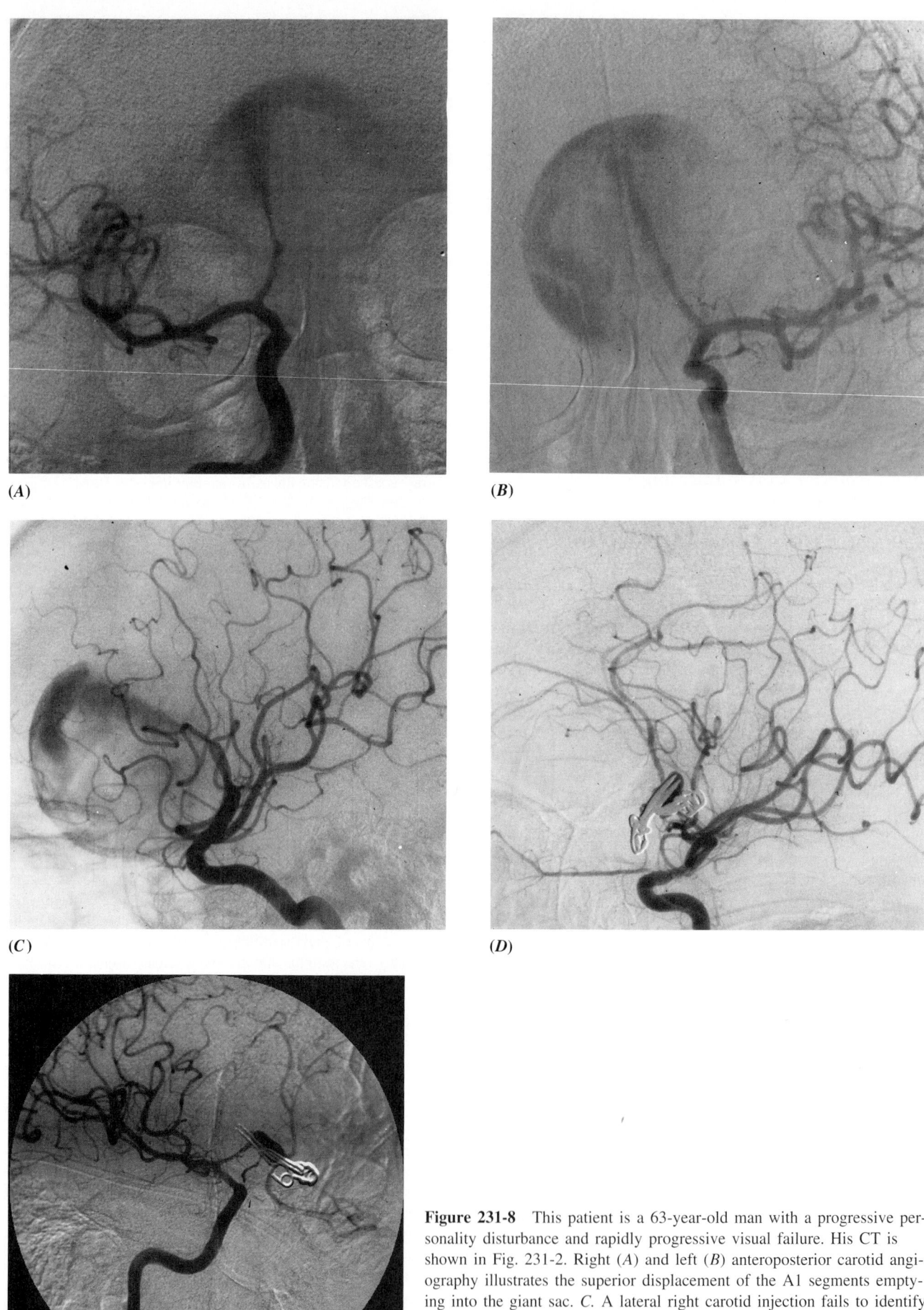

Figure 231-8 This patient is a 63-year-old man with a progressive personality disturbance and rapidly progressive visual failure. His CT is shown in Fig. 231-2. Right (*A*) and left (*B*) anteroposterior carotid angiography illustrates the superior displacement of the A1 segments emptying into the giant sac. *C*. A lateral right carotid injection fails to identify the A2 segment and demonstrates the extent of anterior-inferior projection of the aneurysm. *D*. A postoperative left carotid injection demonstrating a residual fusiform aneurysm and the patent A2 segment. *E*. A right transorbital oblique projection demonstrates the patency of the anterior communicating artery as well as the residual sac.

teries, and careful and focused MRI scrutiny of the posterior fossa, with sagittal and coronal reconstructions.

The demonstrated patency of a contralateral vertebral artery allows consideration of traditional Hunterian ligation as a potential therapeutic option. With this technique the ipsilateral PICA is usually supplied retrograde from the contralateral vertebral artery across the vertebral confluens. As in aneurysms of the cavernous carotid artery, the nondetachable balloon technology allows assessment of tolerance. Definitive occlusion can either be performed intravascularly or by an open surgical procedure. While proximal ligation procedures in the setting of a thrombotic giant aneurysm clearly do not allow for aneurysm decompression, we have seen surprising cases where simply elimination of the pulsation within a sac resulted in dramatic improvement in the patient's symptoms. There is also evidence that this form of therapy offers some hope that over the subsequent years some degree of thrombus resorption and thus decompression will occur spontaneously. In general, in our practice, proximal ligation has been used in those unusual aneurysms that appear to be fusiform enlargements of the vertebral artery immediately distal to he dural penetration and without a clearly demonstrated neck. We have also treated a few patients with giant thrombotic lesions who were too ill medically to withstand a major intracranial procedure.

For giant aneurysms that involve the vertebral artery distal to the origin of PICA, the presence of a patent contralateral vessel makes treatment surprisingly straightforward. The knowledge that the basilar artery will be irrigated during any period of temporary arterial occlusion permits an aggressive attempt at direct and definitive aneurysm clipping. A temporary clip can be applied proximal to the PICA, a second clip can be applied to the lateral medullary segment of PICA, and a final clip can be applied distally adjacent to the vertebral confluens. With such isolation, the aneurysm can then be aspirated dry, if nonthrombotic, and widely opened and evacuated, if filled with thrombus. The clipping can then be performed, allowing continuity of the distal vertebral artery. Another satisfactory solution to this problem would be to apply a clip distal to the PICA origin across the vertebral artery, and to definitively trap the aneurysm by a permanent clip at the confluens. The aneurysm can then be evacuated and the permanent clips left in place. If the PICA is incorporated into the mass itself, and definitive reconstruction is not possible to preserve this vessel, some form of bypass procedure should be entertained, using either an occipital-PICA anastomosis or a side-to-side, PICA-to-PICA anastomosis in the midline.

In our experience, the major difficulty with giant aneurysms in this region occurs with the thrombotic lesions that extend into the confluens area. These patients usually have a disabling mass effect and, thus, every attempt should be made to decompress the brain stem as part of the surgical strategy. When very protracted intervals of temporary occlusion are going to be necessary, involving both vertebrals and the lower basilar trunk, the hypothermic circulatory arrest procedure should at least be considered. We recently treated a patient (illustrated in Fig. 231-9), in whom the contralateral vertebral artery had been previously occluded endovascularly. Despite this therapeutic maneuver, the aneurysm continued to enlarge and progressively disable the patient. Using hypothermic circulatory arrest, the aneurysm was opened widely and all the thrombotic material evacuated. Nevertheless, the proximal vertebral appeared to enter the giant sac with the basilar trunk emerging 180 degrees from the afferent supply. Despite complete aneurysm decompression, it was not possible to reconstruct this patient's anatomy, and trapping had to be performed.

Despite persisting problems at the far end of the spectrum, most vertebral artery giant aneurysms have reasonable surgical or interventional alternatives that can provide reversal of neurological deficits and long-term protection. It is critical to leave no stone unturned in the preoperative evaluation of the patient's anatomy and the planning of a surgical strategy.

Giant Basilar Artery Aneurysms

Aneurysms of the distal basilar artery, even when modest in size, pose major challenges to the neurosurgeon. The neurological price of injury to the posterior thalamoperforating arteries arising from the posterior aspect of the basilar artery and the P1 segments is well known. Once an aneurysm of the distal basilar artery reaches giant size, the predictable expansion of the aneurysm neck, the intrinsic turgor of these lesions due to the direct continuity of the blood stream into the sac, and the progressive incorporation of the P1 origins into the base of the aneurysm itself within the confining space of the interpeduncular cistern create a formidable challenge. These aneurysms have had considerably higher risk to the patient in our hands than have the lesions of more typical size.[4]

A detailed discussion of the technical problems and solutions is beyond the scope of this chapter. A few pertinent points, are worthy of mention, however. The preoperative evaluation of the patient, including the size and projection of both P1 segments, the patency of both posterior communicating arteries, and the presence of any anomalies should be fully appreciated by complete preoperative angiography, including Allcock's maneuvers. MRI has proven invaluable with carefully planned sagittal and coronal views to alert the surgeon to the presence and location of intraluminal thrombosis. With this information, technical alternatives, including sacrifice of one or both P1 segments in rare circumstances, can be presumed safe.

The use of temporary arterial occlusion has proven invariably necessary for treating giant distal basilar aneurysms. For those lesions involving the origin of the superior cerebellar artery, proximal basilar occlusion is often adequate. For the more typical basilar bifurcation aneurysms, however, while allowing some increase in the surgeon's ability to manipulate and mobilize the aneurysm neck, this exposure is rarely adequate to definitively clear the thalamoperforating vessels from the posterior aspect of the neck. Clearly, in the management of the thrombotic giant distal basilar aneurysm in which aneurysm opening and evacuation prior to safe clipping is necessary, simple proximal basilar occlusion is inadequate. Therefore, in our experience we find the very frequent need for definitive trapping of the distal basilar complex during vascular reconstruction. While exposure of the basilar trunk and the ipsilateral P1 from either the pterional or the subtemporal view are quite acceptable, the contralateral P1 is often not safely clippable from a subtemporal view in the setting of a giant sac. It is our preference in the great majority of basilar apex giant aneurysms to expose the lesion from a trans-sylvian exposure using the half-and-half modification. By elevation of the uncus, the posterior reaches of the interpeduncular cistern can be seen from a nearly lateral exposure. This more anterior approach allows the routine and straightforward temporary clipping of the basilar trunk and both P1 segments. In addition, we believe there is somewhat improved access to a larger segment of the aneurysm fundus for opening and evacuation.

Two seemingly minor technical points should also be mentioned. Because of the thickness and turgor of the basilar trunk, particularly in older patients, it is often difficult to completely close this artery with a single temporary clip. We have had repeated frustration with persistent bleeding from a seemingly trapped basilar apex when it became clear that the proximal clip simply had not definitively closed the vessel. It has therefore be-

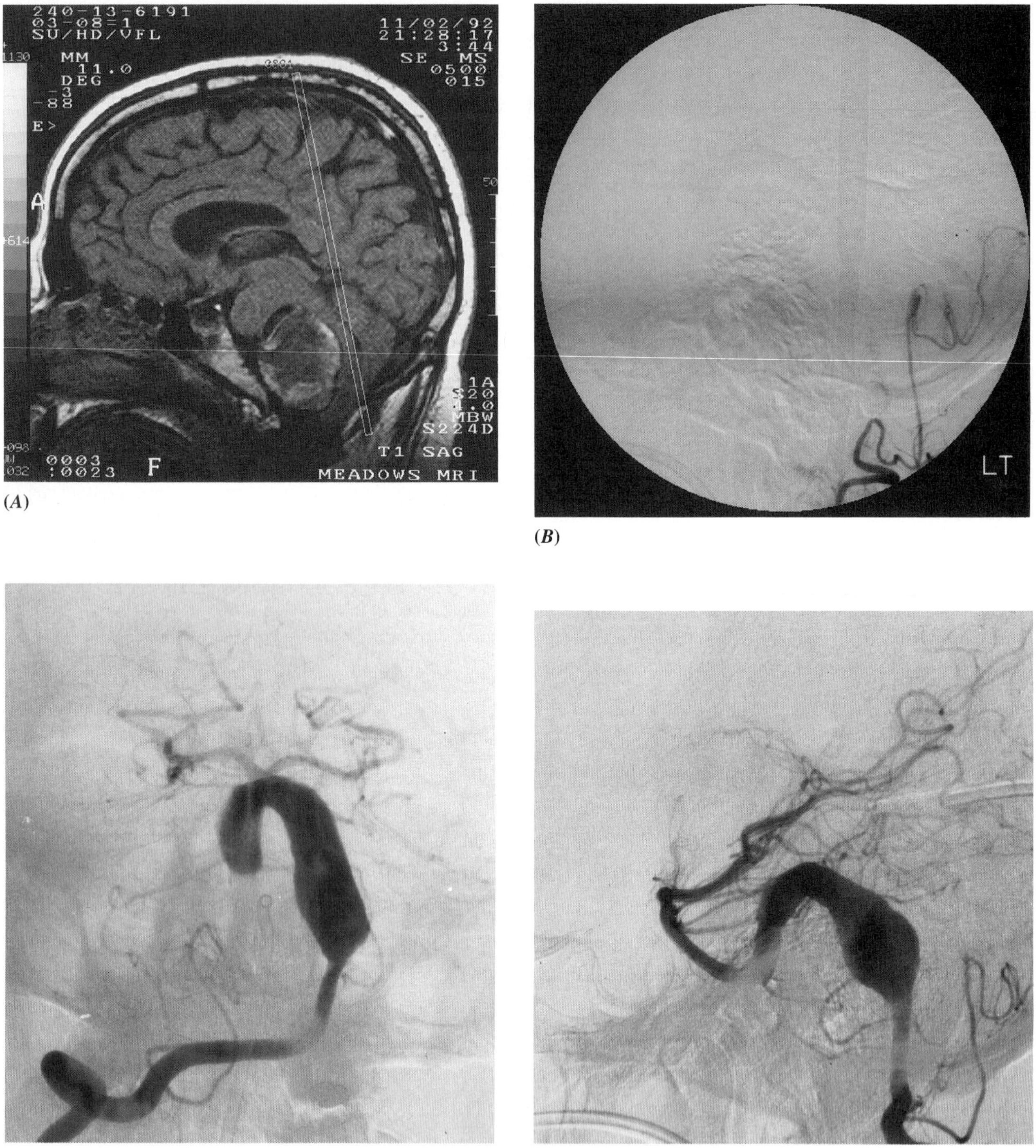

Figure 231-9 This patient presented with a disabling and progressive neurological deficit several years after left vertebral artery balloon occlusion. *A.* A sagittal MR image disclosing massive medullary and pontine displacement. *B.* A left vertebral artery injection revealing previous balloon occlusion distal to the PICA origin. Right anteroposterior (*C*) and lateral (*D*) vertebral angiograms showing a patent channel through a largely thrombosed giant aneurysm.

come our routine to apply two temporary clips to the basilar trunk in this setting. The second point concerns the application of the anatomic information derived preoperatively. When a posterior communicating vessel is known to be large, and temporary occlusion times are becoming prolonged, it is far safer to incorporate a particularly attenuated and tenacious P1 segment into the definitive clipping, relying on a healthy posterior communicating artery to supply the distal posterior cerebral artery territory as well as supply retrograde flow to the P1 segment and the associated perforating vessels.

Using the most modern technology, it is clear that standard surgical technique has not solved all the problems associated with these treacherous lesions. In that context, two additional strategies must be considered, particularly for the thrombotic giant masses. Classic Hunterian techniques with awake trial occlusion should be considered as a fallback option. It is our belief that the most appropriate application of the hypothermic circulatory arrest procedures is in the management of thrombotic giant basilar aneurysms. The features of prolonged tolerable ischemia time and easy decompression of patent portions of the mass are clearly advantages of this procedure. Despite its attractiveness, we and others continue to experience difficulties with the lesions that must be opened widely and evacuated of thrombotic contents prior to clip closure. Air embolism into the perforating vessels has resulted in basal ganglia damage despite what seemed to be perfect surgical procedures. It remains to be seen whether this technology, as it continues to evolve, will provide these unfortunate patients with a truly safe option.

The use of the detachable platinum microcoils is also quite feasible and appealing in the particularly difficult cases. The risk of subsequent aneurysm enlargement and growth and the inability to decompress the giant sac remain major obstacles. Nevertheless, this form of therapy deserves serious consideration in elderly or medically fragile patients.

Conclusion

The treatment of giant intracranial aneurysms remains difficult and associated with significant risk to the patient. We believe that the best available care at the present time involves a neurosurgeon experienced in cerebrovascular disease serving as the primary decision maker. He or she must receive input from an experienced interventional radiologist, both in the diagnostic workup of the patient and in the therapeutic decision-making process, as well as the actual definitive procedure when an endovascular strategy is planned. Input from the neuroanesthesiologist is also critical, so that the anesthetic is initiated anticipating the type of exposure required as well as the issues of the nature and duration of temporary arterial occlusion needed. Significant advances must be made both in the realm of ischemic brain protection as well as safety of the hypothermic circulatory arrest procedures. It is the neurosurgeon's challenge to keep all participants focused not on the creation of a perfect postoperative arteriogram, but on a functional and productive human being leaving the hospital and regaining his or her prior level of activity.

References

1. Artmann H, Vonofakos D, Muller H, et al. Neuroradiologic and neuropathologic findings with growing giant intracranial aneurysm: review of the literature. *Surg Neurol* 1984; 21:391–401.
2. Batjer HH, Frankfurt AI, Purdy PD, et al. Use of etomidate, temporary arterial occlusion, and intraoperative angiography in surgical treatment of large and giant cerebral aneurysm. *J Neurosurg* 1988; 68:234–240.
3. Batjer HH, Purdy PD. Enlarging thrombosed aneurysm of the distal basilar artery. *Neurosurgery* 1990; 26:695–700.
4. Batjer HH, Samson DS. Causes of morbidity and mortality from surgery of aneurysms of the distal basilar artery. *Neurosurgery* 1989; 25:904–916.
5. Batjer HH, Samson DS. Retrograde suction decompression of giant paraclinoidal aneurysms: technical note. *J Neurosurg* 1990; 73:305–306.
6. Baumgartner WA, Silverberg GD, Ream AK, et al. Reappraisal of cardiopulmonary bypass with deep hypothermia and circulatory arrest for complex neurosurgical operations. *Surgery* 1983; 94:242–249.
7. Berenstein A, Ransohoff J, Kupersmith M, et al. Transvascular treatment of giant aneurysms of the cavernous carotid and vertebral arteries: functional investigation and embolization. *Surg Neurol* 1984; 21:3–12.
8. Day AL. Aneurysms of the ophthalmic segment. A clinical and anatomical analysis. *J Neurosurg* 1990; 72:677–691.
9. Debrun G, Fox A, Drake C, et al. Giant unclippable aneurysms: treatment with detachable balloons. *Am J Neuroradiol* 1981; 2:167–173.
10. Debrun G, Lacour P, Caron JP, et al. Detachable balloon and calibrated-leak balloon techniques in the treatment of cerebral vascular lesions. *J Neurosurg* 1978; 49:635–649.
11. Dolenc V. Direct microsurgical repair of intracavernous vascular lesions. *J Neurosurg* 1983; 58:824–831.
12. Drake CG. Giant intracranial aneurysms: experience with surgical treatment in 174 patients. *Clin Neurosurg* 1979; 26:12–95.
13. Drake CG. Evolution of intracranial aneurysm surgery. *Can J Surg* 1984; 27:549–555.
14. Fox AJ, Vinuela F, Pelz DM, et al. Use of detachable balloons for proximal artery occlusion in the treatment of unclippable cerebral aneurysms. *J Neurosurg* 1987; 66:40–46.
15. Gianturco C, Anderson JH, Wallace S. Mechanical devices for arterial occlusion. *Am J Radiol* 1975; 124:428–435.
16. Giller CA, Stieg P, Batjer HH, et al. Transcranial Doppler ultrasound as a guide to graded therapeutic occlusion of the carotid artery. *Neurosurgery* 1990; 26:307–311.
17. Goldstein A Jr, Wells BA, Keats AS. Increased tolerance to cerebral anoxia by pentobarbital. *Arch Int Pharmacodyn Ther* 1966; 161:138–143.
18. Higashida RT, Halbach VV, Cahan LD, et al. Detachable balloon embolization therapy of posterior circulation intracranial aneurysms. *J Neurosurg* 1989; 71:512–519.
19. Higashida RT, Halbach VV, Dowd CF, et al. Interventional neurovascular treatment of a giant intracranial aneurysm using platinum microcoils. *Surg Neurol* 1991; 35:64–68.
20. Higashida RT, Halbach VV, Mehringer CM, et al. Giant cavernous aneurysm associated with trigeminal artery: treatment by detachable balloon. *Am J Neuroradiol* 1987; 8:757–758.
21. Jabre A, Symon L. Temporary vascular occlusion during aneurysm surgery. *Surg Neurol* 1987; 27:47–63.
22. Lyall A. Large aneurysm of the Circle of Willis with spontaneous cure by thrombosis. *Br Med J* 1936; 2:282.
23. Mehdorn HM, Chater NL, Townsend JJ, et al. Giant aneurysm and cerebral ischemia. *Surg Neurol* 1980; 13:49–57.
24. Michenfelder JD, Milde JH, Sundt TM Jr. Cerebral protection by barbiturate anesthesia: use after middle cerebral artery occlusion in Java monkeys. *Arch Neurol* 1976; 33:345–350.
25. Milde LN, Milde JH. Preservation of cerebral metabolites by etomidate during incomplete cerebral ischemia in dogs. *Anesthesiology* 1986; 65:272–277.
26. Milde LN, Milde JH, Michenfelder JD. Cerebral functional, metabolic, and hemodynamic effects of etomidate in dogs. *Anesthesiology* 1985; 63:371–377.
27. Pool JL. Aneurysms of the anterior communicating artery: bifrontal craniotomy and routine use of temporary clips. *J Neurosurg* 1961; 18:98–112.
28. Scialfa G, Vaghi A, Valsecchi F, et al. Neuroradiological treatment of carotid and vertebral fistulas and intracavernous aneurysms: technical problems and results. *Neuroradiology* 1982; 224:13–25.
29. Serbinenko FA. Balloon catheterization and occlusion of major cerebral vessels. *J Neurosurg* 1974; 41:125–145.
30. Silverberg GD. Giant aneurysms: surgical treatment. *Neurol Res* 1984; 6:57–63.
31. Silverberg GD, Reitz BA, Ream AK, et al. Operative treatment of a giant cerebral artery aneurysm with hypothermia and circulatory arrest: report of a case. *Neurosurgery* 1980; 6:301–305.

32. Slosberg PS. Symptomatic unruptured giant aneurysms: medical treatment. *Acta Neurochir (Wien)* 1982; 62:207–218.
33. Spetzler RF, Fukushima T, Martin N, et al. Petrous carotid-to-intradural carotid saphenous vein graft for intracavernous giant aneurysm, tumor, and occlusive cerebrovascular disease. *J Neurosurg* 1990; 73:496–501.
34. Spetzler RF, Hadley MN, Rigamonti D, et al. Aneurysms of the basilar artery treated with circulatory arrest, hypothermia, and barbiturate cerebral protection. *J Neurosurg* 1988; 68:868–879.
35. Whittle IR, Dorsch NW, Besser M. Giant intracranial aneurysms: diagnosis, management, and outcome. *Surg Neurol* 1984:218–230.

232 Surgery for Unruptured Intracranial Aneurysms

Duke S. Samson

Under the stewardship of neurologists and neurosurgeons, remarkable advances have been made in almost all phases of diagnosis, clinical treatment, and direct repair of ruptured and symptomatic intracranial aneurysms. The development of modern neuroanesthetic approaches coupled with the use of microsurgical techniques has significantly reduced the morbidity and mortality figures of patients undergoing surgical repair well below those levels that can be expected with conservative nonsurgical management of such symptomatic lesions.

The widespread and increasing use of sophisticated neurodiagnostic measures such as high resolution computed tomography (CT) scanning, magnetic resonance imaging (MRI), and angiography has subsequently brought to clinical attention a large and increasing group of patients with truly asymptomatic aneurysms—those without a prior history of subarachnoid hemorrhage or without symptoms or signs attributable to either direct mass effect or embolization from the aneurysm itself. As both the medical and general public have increased their awareness of the relatively bleak prognosis associated with aneurysm rupture (30-day mortality figure of greater than 50 percent), identification of such lesions focuses significant pressure on neurological surgeons to arbitrate the understandable conflict between a blanket recommendation of surgical resolution of all such lesions, and the adoption of an overly blasé approach of prophylactic management of each of these aneurysms.

Several issues deserve important consideration when assessing the relative merits of surgical management of asymptomatic unruptured aneurysms:

1. Natural History Much of the information available relating to the natural history of asymptomatic aneurysms is derived from the follow-up of subarachnoid hemorrhage patients with multiple aneurysms in whom only the ruptured lesion has been treated.[5,6,11,20] In evaluating a group of 61 patients with subarachnoid hemorrhage harboring multiple aneurysms in whom only the ruptured lesion was clipped, Heiskanen has found the long-term risks of rehemorrhage to be some 21 percent (mortality of 12 percent) over a follow-up period of more than 10 years.[5,6] After reviewing the available literature, Jane and colleagues have speculated that the natural history of an unruptured asymptomatic aneurysm parallels the natural history of a "healed" ruptured aneurysm, that is, a hemorrhage rate of some 3 to 4 percent per year,[7,23] figures not significantly different from Heiskanen's results or from the previously published statistical study of Bailey and Loeser.[1] In a second statistical study, Dell has projected a lifetime 16 percent risk of subarachnoid hemorrhage for a 20-year-old patient harboring an unruptured aneurysm.[3] All of these studies suggest a relatively low yearly incidence of hemorrhage in the range of 1 to 4 percent for incidental aneurysms, with a cumulative risk that is obviously of greatest significance in younger patients. All asymptomatic aneurysms do not share a common natural history, however. If the population at large has a prevalence of aneurysms of some 5 percent,[2,18] and an annual incidence of subarachnoid hemorrhage in the range of 10 to 14 per 100,000 persons per year of observation,[13] then it appears obvious that only some 15 to 20 percent of unruptured intracranial aneurysms are ultimately destined to hemorrhage; it is to that subset of lesions ideally that prophylactic clinical attention should be directed.[21,25]
2. Aneurysm Size The size of the aneurysm is one of the most important parameters in identifying the propensity of a given intact aneurysm to rupture.[21] Although lesions less than 5 mm in diameter certainly do bleed on occasion, and aneurysms 6 to 9 mm in diameter hemorrhage frequently, over a protracted period of observation, the greatest subset of asymptomatic unruptured aneurysms to ultimately become symptomatic by virtue of hemorrhage are aneurysms greater than 10 mm in diameter.[8,10,21]
3. Multiple Aneurysms An increased incidence of hemorrhage with asymptomatic unruptured aneurysms may occur, regardless of size, in patients who harbor multiple aneurysms, one of which has previously ruptured.[19] The reason for this observation is unclear, but it is reinforced by data from previous studies such as those of Heiskanen and Winn et al.[5,22] Thus, a solitary unruptured aneurysm which otherwise may be considered relatively innocuous because of its small size, may carry a more significant risk of hemorrhage when identified in the multiple aneurysm setting.
4. Patient Age The peak risk of aneurysmal rupture in patients lies between the ages of 40 and 60.[8,9] After age 65 the risk of subarachnoid hemorrhage seems to decline rather precipitously toward a level no greater than 1 percent annually as patients enter the ninth decade of life, suggesting that a more "benign" natural history should be attached to aneurysms discovered in later life.[9]

Just as all asymptomatic aneurysms are not equivalent in natural history, it would be fallacious to suggest that all surgery for such lesions, or that the surgery for each of these unequal lesions, carries a uniform risk of death or neurological morbidity. Large series collected over the past 15 years report a combined incidence of operative mortality and neurological morbidity associated with the surgery of asymptomatic unruptured aneurysms in the range of 5 to 8 percent.[4,12,15,16,24] Upon closer examination, however, such studies obviously include a prevalence of small aneurysms located almost exclusively on the branches of the internal carotid artery distribution in patients with mean ages of 50 to 60 years; when these series are further analyzed, morbidity and mortality rates seem to double with aneurysms greater than 2 cm in size.[24] In addition, notwithstanding the outstanding report by Rice et al.[15] of a combined management morbidity and mortality of less than 5 percent for unruptured aneurysms in the posterior circulation, the unique nature of Drake's personal experience[14,15] and the unlikely ability of other surgeons to approach this figure must be acknowledged. Thus, for the treatment of routine anterior circulation aneurysms less than 2 cm in size in patients in good health under age 65, a conservative figure anticipating 1 percent operative mortality and 7 percent operative morbidity would be reasonable for the competent microvascular-trained aneurysm surgeon. Aneurysms that are larger, located in more difficult anatomic areas, as well as lesions occurring in patients in more fragile clinical condition, must necessitate an upward revision of these optimistic estimates.

A surgeon with such general information must use these figures to draw a relative comparison between the estimated natural history of the specific aneurysm under consideration, and the anticipated management morbidity and mortality expectations appropriate to the situation, taking into account his own experience with aneurysms and recognizing always that the application of such broad statistical analysis to a single patient may be difficult. As an example, I personally believe that a competent aneurysm surgeon can justify an aggressive approach to unruptured aneurysms greater than 5 mm in diameter when the lesions are encountered in the anterior circulation, at the vertebral-PICA junction, or at the basilar bifurcation, if such lesions are identified in patients in good clinical condition with relatively long life expectancies (10 years or more). When treating patients over 65 years of age, I believe a more conservative approach is indicated with regard to aneurysms less than 1 cm in diameter, or larger lesions with calcified walls or whose fundi contain large portions of thrombus. The use of more extensive brain retraction/dissection and the necessity for protracted temporary arterial occlusion, both commonly necessary for the effective obliteration of such lesions, are not tolerated well in patients of advanced age.[17] In my opinion, the natural history of completely asymptomatic lesions in patients over 65 is sufficiently benign to warrant conservative management unless the patient strongly insists on surgical therapy.

References

1. Bailey WL, Loeser JD. Intracranial aneurysms. *JAMA* 1971; 216:1993–1996.
2. Chason JL, Hindman WM. Berry aneurysms of the circle of Willis; results of a planned autopsy study. *Neurology* 1958; 8:41–44.
3. Dell S. Asymptomatic cerebral aneurysm: assessment of its risk of rupture. *Neurosurgery* 1982; 10:162–166.
4. Freger P, DeSousa MM, Sevrain L, et al. Fait-il opérer les anévrysmes asymptomatiques? a prôpos de 114 añévrysmes asymptomatiques opérés. *Neurochirurgie* 1987; 33:462–468.
5. Heiskanen O. Risk of bleeding from unruptured aneurysms in cases with multiple intracranial aneurysms. *J Neurosurg* 1981; 55:524–526.
6. Heiskanen O, Marttila I. Risk of rupture of a second aneurysm in patients with multiple aneurysms. *J Neurosurg* 1970; 32:295–299.
7. Jane JA, Winn RH, Richardson AE. The natural history of intracranial aneurysms: rebleeding rates during the acute and long term period and implication for surgical management. *Clin Neurosurg* 1977; 24:176–184.
8. Locksley HB. Report on the Cooperative Study of Intracranial Aneurysms and Subarachnoid Hemorrhage. Section V, Part II. Natural history of subarachnoid hemorrhage, intracranial aneurysms and arteriovenous malformations. *J Neurosurg* 1966; 25:321–368.
9. Locksley HB, Sahs AL, Knowles L. Report on the Cooperative Study of Intracranial Aneurysms and Subarachnoid Hemorrhage. Section II. General survey of cases in the central registry and descriptions of the sample population. *J Neurosurg* 1966; 24:922–932.
10. McCormick WF, Acosta-Rua GJ. The size of intracranial saccular aneurysms: an autopsy study. *J Neurosurg* 1970; 33:422–430.
11. McKissock W, Richardson A, Walsh L, et al. Multiple intracranial aneurysms. *Lancet* 1964; 1:623–626.
12. Mount LA, Brisman R. Treatment of multiple intracranial aneurysms. *J Neurosurg* 1971; 35:728–730.
13. Pakarinen S. Incidence, aetiology and prognosis of primary subarachnoid haemorrhage: a study based on 589 cases diagnosed in a defined urban population during a defined period. *Acta Neurol Scand* 1967; (Suppl 29):1–28.
14. Peerless SJ, Drake CG. Posterior circulation aneurysms. In Wilkins RH, Rengachary SS (eds): *Neurosurgery*. New York: McGraw-Hill, 1985, pp 1422–1437.
15. Rice BJ, Peerless SJ, Drake CG. Surgical treatment of unruptured aneurysms of the posterior circulation. *J Neurosurg* 1990; 73:165–173.
16. Salazar JL. Surgical treatment of asymptomatic and incidental intracranial aneurysms. *J Neurosurg* 1980; 53:20–21.
17. Samson DS, Batjer HH, Bowman G, et al. A clinical study of the parameters and effects of temporary arterial occlusion in the management of intracranial aneurysms. *Neurosurgery* 1994; 34: 22–29.
18. Stehbens WE. Aneurysms and anatomical variation of cerebral arteries. *Arch Pathol* 1963; 75:45–64.
19. Wiebers DO, Torres VE. Screening for unruptured intracranial aneurysms in autosomal dominant polycystic kidney disease. *N Engl J Med* 1992; 327:953–955 (editorial).
20. Wiebers DO, Whisnant JP, O'Fallon WM. The natural history of unruptured intracranial aneurysms. *N Engl J Med* 1981; 304:696–698.
21. Wiebers DO, Whisnant JP, Sundt TM Jr, O'Fallon WM. The significance of unruptured intracranial saccular aneurysms. *J Neurosurg* 1987; 66:23–29.
22. Winn HR, Almaani WS, Berga SL, et al. The long-term outcome in patients with multiple aneurysms. Incidence of late hemorrhage and implications for treatment of incidental aneurysms. *J Neurosurg* 1983; 59:642–651.
23. Winn HR, Richardson AE, Jane JA. The long-term prognosis in untreated cerebral aneurysms: I. The incidence of late hemorrhage in cerebral aneurysm: a 10-year evaluation of 364 patients. *Ann Neurol* 1977; 1:358–370.
24. Wirth FP, Laws ER Jr, Piepgras D, et al. Surgical treatment of incidental intracranial aneurysms. *Neurosurgery* 1983; 12:507–511.
25. Yasargil MG. *Microneurosurgery*, vol 1. New York: Thieme Stratton, 1984.

233 Inflammatory Intracranial Aneurysms

John G. Frazee

Inflammatory intracranial aneurysms are divided into two forms: bacterial, which have traditionally been called mycotic aneurysms, and fungal, or true mycotic aneurysms. These lesions are uncommon but life-threatening and are often unsuspected until they produce a devastating hemorrhage. Historically, these lesions were fatal whether treated medically or surgically. As knowledge has increased, however, we have developed a better understanding of which patients are at risk to develop an aneurysm, of the period for which they are at risk, and of guidelines for treatment. In this chapter, information about both forms of aneurysm will be reviewed and the current controversies associated with treatment will be discussed.

Historical Perspective

It appears that Church in 1869 first traced a causal relationship between the formation of an intracranial aneurysm and vegetative endocarditis.[5] Osler first used the term *mycotic* in his ''Gulstonian Lectures on Malignant Endocarditis,'' given in 1885.[23] However, this term was used to refer to any process of infection and did not distinguish between bacterial and fungal infections.

Eppinger was the first to call the aneurysms associated with endocarditis *mycotic embolic.*[7] It has been only recently, most notably with Bohmfalk and colleagues[4] that the term *bacterial aneurysm* has been defined and substituted for mycotic aneurysm.

In 1923, Stengel and Wolferth reviewed 34 reported cases of bacterial aneurysm.[25] This was followed in 1954 by a report of 16 more by Shnider and Cotsonas.[24] The results were poor, with only 4 survivors from a group of 50. In the most recent comprehensive review, Bohmfalk and colleagues[4] found 85 reported cases from 1954 to 1978, with 4 of these cases being their own. The largest hospital experiences have been reported by Frazee and colleagues,[8] Monsuez and colleagues,[20] and Barrow and Prats.[2] In the last decade, at least 47 new bacterial aneurysm cases have been reported, bringing the documented experience to at least 142 patients.

Bacterial Aneurysms

Patient Population

The patients reported to have bacterial aneurysms ranged in age from 34 days[28] to 78 years.[4] The age distribution was uniform below the sixth decade and the average age of the patients was 30 years.[4]

When careful histories are obtained from those patients presenting with bacterial aneurysm, a majority of the patients are found to have either congenital heart disease or some other predisposing condition that might lead to bacterial endocarditis, including recent dental work, bronchitis, carious teeth, prolonged labor, and urological surgery. Less common causes include meningitis, immunosuppression, and cavernous sinusitis.[2]

Incidence

Bacterial intracranial aneurysms are thought to constitute between 2.5 and 6.2 percent of all intracranial aneurysms.[4] Those patients with bacterial endocarditis appear to have a risk of 4 to 15 percent of forming an intracranial aneurysm.[4] These figures are likely to underestimate the true incidence, however, because some aneurysms are asymptomatic and some patients present with multiple aneurysms.

Bacteriologic Studies

The diagnosis of a bacterial aneurysm is established either by the association of an intracranial aneurysm with positive blood cultures and other evidence of bacterial endocarditis or by pathologic study of autopsy or surgical specimens. Positive blood cultures commonly grow a *Streptococcus* or a *Staphylococcus* species. However, a variety of unusual organisms have been found including *Neisseria, Enterococcus,* and *Pseuodomonas.*[2] Other, extra-arterial infections responsible for bacterial aneurysms included meningitis and cavernous sinus thrombophlebitis.

Pathogenesis

In 1968, Nakata and colleagues published experimental results showing that after the introduction of bacteria into a dog aorta that had been isolated by temporary clamps above the renal arteries and at the aortic bifurcation, vascular wall destruction began in the vasa vasorum.[22] They concluded that stasis and sepsis in the vasa vasorum was a necessary initiating event for the formation of a bacterial aneurysm.

Molinari and coworkers pointed out that although the original site of infection might be the vasa vasorum, these are rarely present in cerebral arteries, particularly in distal branches where bacterial aneurysms are most likely to form.[18,19] Using experimental dog models with bacterial emboli introduced into the cerebral circulation, they were able to conclude that aneurysms consistently appeared at the site of the infected embolus and that the early changes in the vessel walls appeared in the adventitial layer and involved the media. They proposed that in the absence of the vasa vasorum, bacteria could escape through the occluded origins of thin-walled penetrating vessels to the Virchow-Robin spaces and then to the adventitia of a parent vessel. They explained that the aneurysmal enlargement was produced either by pulsation against the necrotic wall of the occluded vessel or by the same pulsation against the weakened wall of the recanalized vessel. This latter process might explain the late appearance of an aneurysm during antibiotic treatment for bacterial endocarditis.

Molinari and colleagues stressed the short time (1 to 3 days) between the lodging of an infected embolus in the cerebral vessel and an aneurysm formation in animals not treated with antibiotics or infected with virulent organisms.[18,19] However, they also noted that if dogs were partially treated with an appropriate antibiotic, aneurysm rupture no longer regularly occurred in the 1- to 3-day period, but aneurysms were present when the dogs were killed 7 or 8 days after embolization. These results would suggest that an aneurysm may develop in patients with bacterial endocarditis in as short as 1 week even if the patient is treated with appropriate antibiotics.

Clinical Presentation

The neurological symptoms and signs of patients who develop bacterial intracranial aneurysms are variable but are often secondary to either septic embolization, meningitis, or subarachnoid hemorrhage. The first two produce symptoms and signs before aneurysm formation and are infectious processes that may go on to aneurysm formation as noted by Molinari and colleagues.[18,19] The third is a direct result of aneurysm rupture and is frequently associated with disastrous results.

Most authors have expressed concern that there are no early warning signs to herald the aneurysm formation and that it is only subarachnoid hemorrhage which leads to the diagnosis. Thus, unless all patients with bacterial endocarditis undergo cerebral angiography, it is reasoned that the mortality rate cannot be reduced. Our experience suggests that most patients do present with symptoms or signs that herald the formation of a bacterial aneurysm.[8]

It has been reported that 28 to 39 percent of patients with bacterial endocarditis have some form of neurological involvement.[13] As this still constitutes a large population, it is important to select from this group of patients with neurological symptoms or signs those patients who are most likely to be at risk for aneurysm formation. In the review of 13 patients from our institution, each had premonitory symptoms or signs suggestive of intracranial disease. In six patients who survived, these events initiated angiography. One other patient who survived had early warning symptoms and signs but angiography was not done until she suddenly became hemiplegic. The six patients who died as a direct result of intracranial hemorrhage also had warning symptoms and signs. In two patients the symptoms occurred only a few hours before catastrophic events, and it is doubtful whether early diagnostic procedures would have changed their clinical course. However, the remaining four patients had symptoms and signs days before the catastrophic event, which if correctly interpreted would have led to early angiography and definitive treatment. These results suggest that patients who develop a sudden and severe headache, focal neurological deficits, or seizures should be selected for further study, including angiography. Comparing this set of symptoms and signs with those that have been reported for the population of patients with bacterial endocarditis as a whole, we could expect that 25 to 33 percent of patients with any of these three symptoms and signs would have an angiographically demonstrable intracranial bacterial aneurysm.

Serial Angiography

Several points should be noted from a review of the literature: (1) rupture of a bacterial intracranial aneurysm may occur at any time during a 6-week course of antibiotic therapy; (2) a new aneurysm may appear in subsequent angiograms even though previous angiograms have been negative; and (3) new aneurysms may appear after excision of a solitary aneurysm.

These facts emphasize the need for serial evaluation of patients throughout treatment for bacterial endocarditis. The experimental literature indicates that aneurysms may be present 7 days after a septic embolus to the brain in subjects treated with antibiotics and as early as 1 to 3 days following septic embolization in untreated subjects. The experience of our review suggests that there is a delay (averaging 10 days) from the onset of warning symptoms or signs to a catastrophic hemorrhage or to an angiographic demonstration of a cerebral aneurysm. If we assume that the early symptoms or signs are related to the lodging of the embolus in the cerebral vascular tree, then the time to formation of an aneurysm is similar to that noted in the experimental literature. Therefore, three-vessel cerebral angiography at the onset of symptoms or signs seems appropriate. It seems appropriate to repeat angiography every 7 to 10 days during a 6-week period of antibiotic therapy, even after surgical excision of one aneurysm, if aneurysms are to be detected before rupture. Some authors have suggested that this may be too aggressive an approach, citing reports that aneurysms disappear in some instances or decrease in others on follow-up angiography.[3] In fact, of 30 patients reported to have undergone more than one angiogram, the aneurysm resolved completely in 13 patients and decreased in size in another 5 patients (Table 233-1). However, 10 patients showed an enlargement of the original aneurysm or the appearance of a new aneurysm. These aneurysms, therefore, appear to be unpredictable in their course and the use of serial angiography seems justified in part by the high mortality from rupture of a bacterial aneurysm. However, with the advent of high resolution magnetic resonance imaging (MRI) and magnetic resonance angiography (MRA), a low risk alternative method for repeated evaluation is now available. This technique could be used frequently, with angiography reserved for unclear cases.

It is important to point out that a bacterial aneurysm is more likely to be located on the distal arterial tree, with most of these occurring in the distribution of the middle cerebral artery (Table 233-2). Those patients who demonstrate a proximal aneurysm may have developed that aneurysm from cavernous thrombophlebitis, in which case the aneurysm has an intracavernous location, or from infection of a previously present proximal berry aneurysm. It is also noteworthy that multiple aneurysms are not uncommon, having been reported in approximately 18 percent of cases.

Treatment—Surgical or Nonsurgical

The crux of the controversy surrounding the treatment of patients with bacterial intracranial aneurysms has been whether the risk of

TABLE 233-1 Results of Serial Angiography (30 Patients)

Aneurysm resolution	13
Decreased size of aneurysm	5
Aneurysm enlargement	6
New aneurysm	4
Aneurysm excised	2

TABLE 233-2 Documented Aneurysm Location (63 Patients)

Site	% of Total
Proximal artery	
Intracavernous segment, internal carotid artery	11
Intradural segment, internal carotid artery	21
Distal artery	
Anterior cerebral artery	16
Middle cerebral artery	43
Posterior cerebral artery	9

surgery is prohibitively high, particularly in light of the fact that many patients have aneurysms that either fail to rupture, become smaller, or disappear. In a review of 45 patients with intracranial bacterial aneurysms, Bingham emphasized that 11 of 21 patients followed with serial angiography had complete resolution of their aneurysms and an additional 6 patients had a decrease in aneurysm size.[3] This led him to suggest serial angiography for all patients with a documented aneurysm. He recommended an operation only if the aneurysm enlarged or did not change in size after 6 weeks of antibiotic therapy. He reported that 3 of 20 patients who received only antibiotic therapy died, and 6 of 25 patients who received combined antibiotic and surgical treatment died. He noted that the higher mortality rate associated with operation was not a true reflection of surgical mortality, however, for these patients were frequently moribund at the time of operation.

Bohmfalk and colleagues reviewed 85 patients, 45 of whom were included in the Bingham series.[4] They noted that an aneurysm resolved completely in 11 of 25 patients treated with antibiotics alone and followed with serial angiography. This group of patients, as with Bingham's series, was a selected population and excluded the majority of patients (60 of 85, 20 of 45, respectively) who were not followed by serial angiography. Therefore, it is important to emphasize that although intracranial bacterial aneurysms do resolve or decrease in size in some patients, the mortality with antibiotic therapy alone is still high. Bohmfalk and colleagues reported that 20 of 38 patients (53 percent) in this group died. This should be compared with surgical results. Combining the results of 78 patients with known outcome, we find that 34 patients underwent surgical therapy. Of these 16 were electively operated upon, with one death, not directly attributed to the surgery, and 13 underwent emergency surgery with 8 deaths, all of which were secondary to the moribund state of the patient. The emphasis should be on the low surgical mortality in elective cases.

Most authors[2,4,8] agree that indications for surgical treatment include

1. the presence of rupture
2. significant mass effect
3. enlargement with antibiotic treatment
4. an unresolved aneurysm after antibiotic treatment

However, consideration should be given to surgical treatment if the aneurysm is singular and easily approached.

Many authors recommend conservative, medical therapy if there are multiple aneurysms or the aneurysm is located in an area which is difficult to approach surgically.

Proximal and Multiple Aneurysms

The most recent comprehensive review has suggested that nonsurgical treatment for proximal and multiple aneurysms is the best approach, unless there is evidence of aneurysm enlargement.[4] A review of the outcome of 13 patients with proximal aneurysms, excluding those in the cavernous sinus, shows one surgical death in 3 patients and six deaths among 9 patients treated with antibiotics alone (Table 233-3). These groups are too small to allow us to draw conclusions as to the risks of therapy, but the trend seen in those patients treated with antibiotics alone suggests a high mortality for this therapy. It would again lead us toward the conclusion that the best alternative may be surgical intervention accompanied by antibiotic therapy. Cavernous sinus aneurysms should be considered differently. They carry less risk for death with hemorrhage although morbidity from cranial nerve compression may be frequent, severe, and prolonged. Conservative medical therapy is the best recommendation, although endovascular obliteration has been proposed.[16]

The concern for cerebral infarction as a complication of excision of a proximal bacterial aneurysm is reasonable, but there are other approaches that should be examined before relying on nonsurgical therapy alone. These would include clipping or trapping the aneurysm with the addition of a superficial temporal to middle cerebral artery bypass. Finally, there is the possibility of wrapping the aneurysm with muscle or muslin, but this would certainly be less than optimal therapy. The use of methyl methacrylate to coat bacterial aneurysms is undesirable because of its potential as a foreign body to harbor infectious organisms, and the difficulty of further surgical therapy should it be necessary.

Patients have presented with multiple aneurysms in 17 instances (Table 233-3), 6 of which were treated surgically and 11 nonsurgically. No patient died. It is generally agreed that multiple aneurysms should be treated medically unless there is evidence of rupture, or persistence or enlargement during or after treatment. If surgery is considered, all aneurysms easily approached at the time of surgery should be clipped. If they are bilateral, the largest aneurysm or the one presumed to have bled should be excised first. An appropriate recovery period should be allowed and angiography repeated to ensure that the remaining aneurysm(s) is still present before further surgery is planned.

Summary

In view of the serious consequences of a ruptured bacterial aneurysm, the high morbidity and mortality with nonsurgical therapy, the low elective surgical mortality rate, and the rapid appearance

TABLE 233-3 Treatment and Mortality for Proximal and Multiple Bacterial Aneurysms

Treatment	Total Cases	Died
Proximal aneurysms*		
Surgical	3	1
Nonsurgical	9	6
Multiple aneurysms		
Surgical	6	0
Nonsurgical	11	0†

*Treatment and outcome are unknown for one patient.
†Results of treatment for two patients are unknown.

of new aneurysms in some patients, aggressive management is indicated for those patients with bacterial endocarditis who develop sudden severe headache, focal neurological symptoms or signs, or seizures. Such patients should undergo cerebral angiography MRI, or MRA every 7 to 10 days. If an aneurysm is identified, it should be excised according to earlier suggested guidelines. Finally, patients with proximal or multiple aneurysms should also be considered for treatment (surgical or endovascular), if there is evidence of aneurysm rupture, or persistence or enlargement after antibiotic therapy.

Fungal Aneurysms

The first case of fungal aneurysm was reported in 1968[15] and since that time only a few more such cases have been reported.[1,2,6,9,10–12,14,17,21,26,27] The rarity of this disease is obvious, but the widespread use of cortical steroids and immunosuppressive drugs would suggest that fungal infections, including those of cerebral arteries, are increasing in number.

In each instance of fungal infection reported to date, the patient died from a severe, sudden, subarachnoid hemorrhage and in each case an autopsy report was available. The age of the patients varied significantly from 3 to 75 years of age.[2] The group is too small to draw any conclusions about sex distribution. The site of these aneurysms is much different from that of bacterial aneurysms. They involve the proximal major vessels such as the internal carotid artery or the basilar artery.

The most common infecting organism is *Aspergillus*, followed by *Candida* and *Phycomycetes*. The source of infection is by both direct extension and hematogenous spread. Autopsies have demonstrated a marked inflammatory disease of the cerebral vessels with invasion of the vascular wall by the fungus either from the intimal side or from the adventitial side. Vessels have shown infiltration by branching hyphae, with severe loss of the normal vascular layers.

Unlike the patients with bacterial aneurysms, these patients lack significant warning symptoms or signs that would suggest intracranial disease. The disease appears to progress rapidly and is quite lethal. To date there is no report of surgical intervention for this problem, yet it would seem that the approach recommended for proximal bacterial aneurysms might be appropriate in this situation if the diagnosis could be made early. In general, however, the outlook is very poor for fungal aneurysms of intracranial vessels.

References

1. Ahuja GK, Jain N, Vijayaraghavan M, Roy S. Cerebral mycotic aneurysm of fungal origin: case report. *J Neurosurg* 1978; 49:107–110.
2. Barrow DL, Prats AR. Infectious intracranial aneurysms: comparison of groups with and without endocarditis. *Neurosurgery* 1990; 27:562–573.
3. Bingham WF. Treatment of mycotic intracranial aneurysms. *J Neurosurg* 1977; 46:428–437.
4. Bohmfalk GL, Story JL, Wissenger JP, Brown WE Jr. Bacterial intracranial aneurysm. *J Neurosurg* 1978; 48:369–382.
5. Church WS. Aneurysm of the right cerebral artery in a boy of thirteen. *Trans Pathol Soc Lond* 1869; 20:109–110.
6. Davidson P, Robertson DM. A true mycotic (*Aspergillus*) aneurysm leading to fatal subarachnoid hemorrhage in a patient with hereditary hemorrhagic telangiectasia: case report. *J Neurosurg* 1971; 35:71–76.
7. Eppinger H. Pathogenesis (Histogenesis und Aetiologie) der Aneurysmen einschliesslich des Aneurysma equi verminosum. *Arch Klin Chir* 1887; 35:1–553.
8. Frazee JG, Cahan LD, Winter J. Bacterial intracranial aneurysms. *J Neurosurg* 1980; 53:633–641.
9. Hadley MN, Martin NA, Spetzler RF, Johnson PC. Multiple intracranial aneurysms due to Coccidioides immitis infection: case report. *J Neurosurg* 1987; 66:453–456.
10. Hadley MN, Spetzler RF, Martin NA, Johnson PC. Middle cerebral artery aneurysm due to Nocardia asteroides: case report of aneurysm excision and extracranial-intracranial bypass. *Neurosurgery* 1988; 22:923–928.
11. Horten BC, Abbott GF, Porro RS. Fungal aneurysms of intracranial vessels. *Arch Neurol* 1976; 33:577–579.
12. Iihara K, Makita Y, Nabeshima S, Fei T. Aspergillosis of the central nervous system causing subarachnoid hemorrhage from mycotic aneurysm of the basilar artery—case report. *Neurol Med Chir (Tokyo)* 1990; 30(8):618–623.
13. Jones RH Jr, Siekert RG, Geraci JE. Neurologic manifestations of bacterial endocarditis. *Ann Intern Med* 1969; 71:21–28.
14. Kikuchi K, Watanabe K, Sugawara A, Kowada M. Multiple fungal aneurysms: report of a rare case implicating steroid as predisposing factor. *Surg Neurol* 1985; 24:253–259.
15. Mahaley MS Jr, Spock A. An unusual case of intracranial aneurysm. In Smith JL (ed): *Neuro-ophthalmology*, vol 4. St Louis: Mosby, 1968, pp 158–166.
16. Micheli F, Schteinschnaider A, Plaghos LL, et al. Bacterial cavernous sinus aneurysm treated by detachable balloon technique. *Stroke* 1989; 20:1751–1754.
17. Mielke B, Weir B, Oldring D, von Westarp C. Fungal aneurysm: case report and review of the literature. *Neurosurgery* 1981; 9:578–582.
18. Molinari GF. Septic cerebral embolism. *Stroke* 1972; 3:117–122.
19. Molinari GF, Smith L, Goldstein MN, Satran R. Pathogenesis of cerebral mycotic aneurysms. *Neurology* 1972; 23:325–332.
20. Monsuez JJ, Vittecoq D, Rosenbaum A, et al. Prognosis of ruptured intracranial mycotic aneurysms: a review of 12 cases. *Eur Heart J* 1989; 10(9):821–825.
21. Morriss FH Jr, Spock A. Intracranial aneurysms secondary to mycotic orbital and sinus infection: report of a case implicating *Penicillium* as an opportunistic fungus. *Am J Dis Child* 1970; 119:357–362.
22. Nakata Y, Shionoya S, Kamiya K. Pathogenesis of mycotic aneurysm. *Angiology* 1968; 19:593–601.
23. Osler W. Gulstonian lectures on malignant endocarditis. *Lancet* 1885; 1:415–418, 459–464, 505–508.
24. Shnider BI, Cotsonas NJ Jr. Embolic mycotic aneurysms, complication of bacterial endocarditis. *Am J Med* 1954; 16:246–255.
25. Stengel A, Wolferth CC. Mycotic (bacterial) aneurysms of intravascular origin. *Arch Intern Med* 1923; 31:527–554.
26. Takeshita M, Izawa M, Kubo O, et al. Aspergillotic aneurysm formation of cerebral artery following neurosurgical operation. *Surg Neurol* 1992; 38(2):146–151.
27. Visudhiphan P, Bunyaratavej S, Khantanaphar S. Cerebral aspergillosis: report of three cases. *J Neurosurg* 1973; 38:472–476.
28. Whitfield PC, Bullock R. Infected intracranial aneurysm in an infant: case report. *Neurosurgery* 1991; 28(4):623–625.

234 Endovascular Treatment of Cervicocerebral Aneurysms

Jacques E. Dion
John M. Mathis
Fernando Viñuela

Intracranial arterial aneurysms were first imaged using angiography in 1933 by Egas Moniz.[54] Concurrently, the first direct surgical treatment of a saccular intracranial aneurysm was reported by Dott[15] who placed a muscle fragment against the aneurysm. The neck of an aneurysm was first surgically clipped by Dandy[10] in 1938. The initial reports of endovascular therapy of aneurysms appeared approximately 35 years later. In 1974, Serbinenko[68] reported his results pioneering the use of endovascular balloon occlusion techniques; he was later followed by Romodanov and Shcheglov,[64] Debrun,[11–13] Berenstein,[6] Higashida,[33,35] and Halbach et al.[26] Treatment was originally by balloon occlusion of the parent artery. In the last decade, however, an explosion in technologic developments and interest in these techniques has led to a variety of treatments which are aimed at the aneurysm sac with preservation of the parent artery. Intracranial arterial aneurysms have a reported incidence of 1.5 to 8 percent of the general population.[38,59,74] Therefore, as many as 5 million individuals in North America might harbor such an aneurysm and approximately 28,000 present with subarachnoid hemorrhage every year. There is an associated mortality which may be as high as 50 percent and a significant neurological morbidity of up to 25 percent.[8,41] Giant intracranial aneurysms commonly present with mass effect. Extracranial aneurysms located in the cervical region can be the cause of neurological or local morbidity. All aneurysms may be treated in one of two ways: (1) by indirect techniques, where the parent artery is occluded; or (2) by direct techniques, where the aneurysm is occluded and the parent artery preserved.

Basic Concepts of Endovascular Therapy

Aneurysms may be discovered incidentally at the time of a computed tomography (CT) or magnetic resonance imaging (MRI) scan performed for other reasons. In the symptomatic patient, noninvasive and/or invasive techniques may be used to demonstrate an aneurysm, or secondary findings such as hemorrhage. Ultimately, if treatment is considered, most or all patients will undergo cerebral angiography. Using modern angiographic equipment, nonionic contrast material, and skilled angiographers, these procedures are very safe[14] and greatly help in prognostication and therapeutic planning. State-of-the-art high-resolution digital angiography is considered by most endovascular therapists and surgeons to be equal to or superior to conventional angiography as it offers acceptable spatial resolution while improving contrast resolution and saving time. Because of the wide acceptance of intra-arterial digital subtraction angiography (DSA), it is rarely necessary to resort to conventional angiography. Using either method, the angiogram should carefully evaluate the following: (1) the exact location and size of the aneurysm, (2) its relation to adjacent vessels, (3) the presence or absence of an aneurysm neck, (4) the presence of intra-aneurysmal thrombus, and (5) the collateral circulation distal to the aneurysm in cases where occlusion of the parent artery might be considered. The presence of intraluminal thrombus may be more easily demonstrated on both CT and MRI. Calcification in the wall of the aneurysm or its neck is best shown on a CT scan; this finding is significant because the presence of calcification, especially in the neck of an aneurysm, may complicate surgery and may also prevent the aneurysm from regressing in size after appropriate treatment. The position of the aneurysm, its relationship to adjacent perforators, and potential distal collaterals should be carefully evaluated because they will affect the planning and risk of treatment.

Intracranial and extracranial aneurysms can be categorized as follows:

Aneurysm Type

Saccular: Outpouching from the arterial wall with a definable neck. Microscopically, an intima and adventitia are present.

Fusiform: Dilatation of the entire circumference of the arterial wall with no definable neck. Presence of intima and adventitia.

Pseudoaneurysm or false aneurysm (saccular or fusiform): Absence of all three layers—intima, media, and adventitia. These aneurysms are usually secondary to direct or indirect trauma or spontaneous dissection of a histologically abnormal vessel.

Dissecting: With or without direct or indirect trauma, it is possible for blood to track outside of the confines of the intima, sometimes through the media and even the adventitia. When this occurs extracranially, such as in the carotid or vertebral circulation, the patient can present with cerebral ischemic and embolic symptoms. If the dissection involves the intracranial circulation, especially the distal vertebral or basilar arteries, a subarachnoid hemorrhage may occur.

Aneurysm Size (Diameter)

Small:	up to 1.5 cm
Large:	1.5 to 2.5 cm
Giant:	larger than 2.5 cm

Additionally, in locations where there is an immediately adjacent vein, a ruptured aneurysm or pseudoaneurysm may be associated with *arteriovenous shunting*. Aneurysms in the cerebral circulation can be found *in association with a cerebral arteriovenous malformation* (AVM).[9,52] In up to 30 percent of patients harboring an AVM, aneurysms may be observed either on the circle of Willis, or on a feeder to the AVM. *Intra-nidal aneurysms* are also found and may result from dysplastic changes in elements of the AVM nidus.

Finally, *mycotic aneurysms* are usually fusiform in shape, occurring in the small intracranial arteries secondary to bacterial emboli which produce transmural necrosis.

Fusiform aneurysms are usually treated by parent artery occlusion with or without direct occlusion of the aneurysmal lumen. It is often impossible to treat saccular aneurysms with very wide necks while preserving the parent artery so that the treatment of choice may also involve indirect parent vessel occlusion. Saccular aneurysms with small or medium necks are usually treated by endosaccular obliteration with preservation of the parent artery.

The endovascular therapist may be called to deal with vasospasm which is found angiographically in up to 70 percent of patients following subarachnoid hemorrhage. This phenomenon usually occurs between days 3 and 12 after subarachnoid hemorrhage. Patients refractory to aggressive medical treatment consisting of hypertension, hypervolemia, and hemodilution (HHH) may require the intra-arterial infusion of a vasodilator agent (i.e., papaverine[39,40]), or the use of balloon angioplasty.[3,29,53,58]

Contemporary Materials Used in Endovascular Therapy of Aneurysms

Angiography Room

The modern interventional neuroangiography suite should be equipped with state-of-the-art DSA equipment capable of quality vascular road mapping. Skilled personnel to administer neuroleptic analgesia are required (nurse or anesthetist) because most interventional neuroradiologic procedures are performed under light sedation. The blood pressure, pulse rate, and oxygen saturation of patients undergoing neuroleptic analgesia should be constantly monitored in addition to clinical evaluation to detect any neurological change. In young children or uncooperative patients, one should not hesitate to use general anesthesia; thus, the facility should be spacious enough and appropriately equipped to satisfy the needs of a neuroanesthetist.

Catheter Systems

Embolization procedures almost universally utilize coaxial systems, and a variety of guiding catheters are available with the choice depending on the embolic agents and microcatheters employed. Catheters used as coaxial guides range from 4 French tapered diagnostic catheters to nontapered, dedicated guiding catheters which are thin-walled and vary in size from 5 to 10 French. The larger guides are used for the introduction of endovascular tools such as latex or silicone balloons or microangioplasty catheters. Nontapered guiding catheters have the advantage of allowing injection of contrast material from below for purposes of road mapping or control angiography without removal of the indwelling microcatheter system. Multiple microcatheters may be used to deliver embolic agents in the treatment of aneurysms; however, the most commonly used is the Tracker catheter (Target Therapeutics, Fremont, CA). It is a progressively flexible microcatheter which may be navigated into the cerebral vasculature over a microguidewire. Tracker systems used in the cerebral vasculature are the Tracker 18 and Tracker 10 representing a distal microcatheter outer diameter (O.D.) of 0.018 and 0.010 in., respectively. (It is beyond the scope of this chapter to discuss the details of the different Tracker microcatheters.) Flow-directed catheters (e.g., Magic catheter, Balt, Montmorency, France; Mini Torquer catheter, Ingenor-Nycomed, Paris, France) are flow-directed catheters with very flexible distal segments which are carried into the cerebral vasculature by blood flow without the use of a guidewire. The size of their lumen usually restricts compatibility with fluid agents. Finally, 1 and 2 French polyethylene microcatheters may be utilized without microguidewires for navigation of intracranial balloons.

Test occlusion of the cervical vessels[8,16,17,20,56,57,62] may be performed with 5 or 6 French Medi-tech test occlusion balloon catheters (Boston Scientific Corporation, Watertown, MA) or 5 French Swan-Ganz catheters. Test occlusion beyond tortuous cervical curves or in intracranial vessels is best performed by permanently attaching latex or silicone microballoons on 2 French microcatheters. Treatment of vasospasm with intracranial angioplasty is also performed with nondetachable microballoons mounted on 2 French microcatheters. Specially designed silicone microballoons generate only 1 atm of lateral wall pressure (compared with 6 to 8 atm of lateral wall pressure for latex balloons), which greatly decreases the risk of rupture during angioplasty of small intracranial vessels. The Stealth catheter (Target Therapeutics) (a dedicated microangioplasty catheter) may be used but it generates up to 8 atm of pressure and is more appropriate for angioplasty of atherosclerotic disease.

Embolic Agents

Parent Artery Occlusion

Parent artery occlusion is best accomplished using detachable latex or silicone balloons. Metallic coils are a less commonly used alternative. Latex balloons (Ingenor-Nycomed; Balt) come in a variety of sizes and shapes. They can be hand tied to the appropriate microcatheter using latex microligatures or can be fitted with a self-sealing valve (gold valve balloon, Ingenor-Nycomed). Balloons wih self-sealing valves are directly mounted onto a microcatheter without any external ligatures. Because the latex membrane is almost impermeable, these balloons can be filled with any strength contrast material. We prefer to use 50% dilution, which achieves adequate opacification but decreases the viscosity, allowing for more rapid inflation/deflation of the balloon. Silicone balloons (Interventional Therapeutics Corporation, San Francisco, CA) are also available in a variety of sizes and shapes and are equipped with an internal sealing miter valve.[30] Since silicone is a semipermeable membrane, these balloons need to be filled with an iso-osmotic contrast mixture to prevent osmotic passage of fluid across the balloon wall which will either increase or decrease the balloon size. A 2:1 mix of 300 mg % nonionic contrast and sterile water (not saline) approximates an iso-osmotic solution. With very few exceptions, balloons filled with contrast material eventually deflate over time. If permanent inflation of the balloon is required,[21] contrast material can be replaced by the permanent polymerizing material hydroxyethylmethacrylate (HEMA).[55] Some of the components of the HEMA mixture are incompatible with latex balloons and cause degradation of the membrane with subsequent rupture of the balloon. Therefore, HEMA is recommended for use only with silicone balloons. The advantage of balloons is that the occlusion is immediate and relatively large vessels can be occluded. Disadvantages include the possibility of distal embolization from unintentional detachment or a faulty valve mechanism with deflation. Additionally, relatively large introducer catheters are required for balloon introduction (up to 8 or 9 French).

Coils can be used for parent artery occlusion but they tend to be reserved for occlusion of smaller vessels. Coil occlusion is usually accomplished using platinum microcoils which are available in a variety of sizes, shapes, and lengths (Target Therapeutics; Cook, Inc, Bloomington, IN), with or without attached Dacron fibers for increased thrombogenicity. Platinum microcoils can be delivered through small, 2 French Tracker microcatheters. These coils are MRI compatible and produce little or no artifact. Larger, stainless steel coils are also available (Cook, Inc.) These are delivered through 4 or 5 French catheters for occlusion of larger vessels. They cause significant artifacts on MRI. The occlusion produced by coils is not immediate and there is also a risk of distal embolization during coil placement; usually multiple coils are required. The behavior of coils for parent vessel occlusion is less predictable than balloons, especially in larger vessels.

Endosaccular Occlusion

The lumen of a saccular aneurysm may be occluded using either detachable balloons or microcoils. Silicone or latex balloons may be navigated to an aneurysm on a microcatheter.[8,27,28,32] Balloons placed inside an aneurysm should be inflated with a permanent material such as HEMA in order to prevent subsequent balloon deflation which can lead to aneurysm recurrence. Silicone balloons are considered safer than latex balloons because they generate less lateral wall pressure and because they are compatible with HEMA.

Platinum microcoils may also be used to occlude aneurysms.[36,45] Although the standard platinum microcoils may be utilized, it should be noted that their behavior is difficult to predict and they cannot be withdrawn in the event that placement is suboptimal. They are also relatively stiff and the ideal goal of packing the lumen of an aneurysm cannot be achieved safely. This creates a high ratio of autologous clot to coil which often leads to recanalization of the clot and compaction of coils within the aneurysm lumen. The inherent stiffness of these coils as well as their unpredictable behavior increases the risk of aneurysm rupture or errant migration. In 1991, Guglielmi and associates[23,25] described a detachable platinum microcoil for use in the treatment of saccular aneurysms. This coil is much softer than the standard platinum microcoil and can be advanced into an aneurysm through either a Tracker 18 or Tracker 10 catheter. It is available in a variety of sizes and lengths. These coils should be individually tailored to the size of the aneurysm being treated. The coil is originally soldered to the end of a stainless guidewire pushing wire and is separated from this wire by passing a very small, direct current of 0.5 to 1 mA which causes electrolysis of the solder junction. Separation usually occurs within 2 to 10 min. Platinum microcoils which may be mechanically detached from the pusher are presently being investigated. Liquid polymers which may be introduced directly into the aneurysmal sac in order to achieve its occlusion[43,51] are also being investigated. The inherent disadvantage of this process is the difficulty in preventing the escape of the polymerizing material into the parent artery with resultant embolization.

Vasospasm

Papaverine is an opium alkaloid which causes vasodilatation of arteries through direct action on smooth muscle. We dilute 300 mg of papaverine (Eli Lilly Company, Indianapolis, IN) in 100 ml of nonheparinized saline. This is infused via microcatheter into an affected vascular territory superselectively over a period of 30 to 40 min. It is important to be aware that papaverine in certain concentrations and pH levels is incompatible with heparin or Hexabrix contrast material (ioxaglate meglumine and ioxaglate sodium solution; Mallinckrodt Medical, Inc., St. Louis, MO) and may form a white cloudy precipitate which could act as a distal embolus.[60] Therefore, the papaverine-saline mixture should not be heparinized, and care should be taken to flush the microcatheter with nonheparinized saline prior to infusion.

Indications for Treatment

Parent artery occlusion is sometimes utilized as a curative treatment for cervicocerebral aneurysms. Endovascular techniques have virtually replaced surgery for this purpose over the last 15 years.[2,11,18,28,31,37,49,50,55,69,72] Its advantages include the ability to test occlude a vessel with a balloon prior to permanent sacrifice. Compared to surgery, it is a much less invasive procedure with a shortened hospital stay. Aneurysms which would lend themselves to parent vessel occlusion include extracranial and intracranial pseudoaneurysms and fusiform aneurysms, extracranial saccular or dissecting aneurysms, and intracranial saccular aneurysms with large necks. Active interaction between the referring surgeon and the interventional neuroradiologist is needed to determine if a surgical procedure might be safer or more efficient, or have a higher probability of preserving the parent artery.

Endosaccular occlusion of intracranial aneurysms is usually recommended for patients who are nonoperable[22–25,27] (i.e., patients who have failed attempts at surgical clipping, have a medical condition resulting in an unacceptably high risk due to aneurysm location, or have a medical condition resulting in an unacceptable risk for general anesthesia). The endosaccular treatment of aneurysms is still in the investigational review stage and needs additional comparison to standard surgical treatment.

The goal of aneurysm eradication is to prevent future rupture and embolic phenomena from intrasaccular thrombus. When giant aneurysms thrombose, there is often a decrease in their size with an associated decrease in the symptoms associated with mass effect. The rate of rupture of partially occluded intracranial saccular aneurysms has not been adequately defined, however.[47,70]

Endovascular treatment of acutely ruptured aneurysms may be indicated as a temporizing measure to protect against repeat hemorrhage in patients who must undergo delayed surgical clipping (i.e., when acute medical problems or vasospasm prevent immediate surgery).

Finally, invasive endovascular techniques might be combined with surgery in order to facilitate clipping of technically difficult intracranial aneurysms.[4,66,69,72] Such a procedure (first reported by Scott et al.[66]) consists of positioning a double lumen, temporary balloon occlusion catheter in the cervical internal carotid artery during surgery. The aneurysm is exposed and a temporary occlusion clip placed distal to the aneurysm. The cervical internal carotid artery is then temporarily occluded with the balloon catheter while suction is applied to the internal lumen of the catheter, allowing decompression of the occluded ICA segment. The effect is usually quite dramatic, producing collapse and improved manipulation of the aneurysm and access to the neck for clipping. This technique has been most successful with large internal carotid, paraclinoid aneurysms or large, technically difficult aneurysms of the posterior fossa.

Technique, Results, and Complications

Intracranial Aneurysms, Parent Artery Occlusion

Carotid Circulation Aneurysms

The majority of aneurysms treated by parent artery occlusion in the carotid circulation are of the large or giant size variety and are located either in the cavernous sinus or in the paraclinoid area.[6,11] Rarely, aneurysms of the supraclinoid segment of the internal carotid artery which are not amenable to surgical or direct endosaccular treatment receive parent vessel occlusion as well. The aneurysms in this category usually have a broad neck or are fusiform.

As mentioned, the detachable balloon is generally considered the best embolic device for carotid artery occlusion. Prior to occlusion of the internal carotid artery, a test occlusion should be performed. For this purpose, a nondetachable balloon is positioned in the internal carotid artery. Ideally, the test occlusion should take place in the exact location where the permanent occlusion is desired. Therefore, the 5 French Meditech temporary occlusive balloon catheter and the 5 French Swan-Ganz catheter are somewhat at a disadvantage since they cannot be safely positioned above C1-C2. Prior to inflation of the test occlusion balloon, the patient should be fully heparinized with at least 5000 units of heparin. The interventionalist should verify that the patient's blood pressure at the time of the test occlusion does not exceed the baseline blood pressure recorded on the ward. This process is important since test occlusion with an artificially elevated blood pressure may invalidate a clinically normal response since the patient could still experience ipsilateral ischemia after carotid sacrifice with a lower blood pressure. The test occlusion is begun by carefully inflating the balloon to the point of minimal occlusion. This is verified by injection of contrast material either through the lumen of a double lumen balloon catheter or through the lumen of a guiding catheter below the occlusion balloon. When using a double lumen catheter with the end hole beyond the point of vessel occlusion, care should be taken not to flush the catheter with heparinized saline at a rapid rate because of the antegrade influx into the ophthalmic artery which may cause ocular symptoms that could be misinterpreted as a neurological change and a test failure. The test occlusion should last between 20 and 30 min, during which the patient is carefully examined for the development of neurological signs appropriate to the hemisphere being tested. In particular, ischemia to watershed areas may produce dysfunction of shoulder and hip muscles or mild cognitive abnormalities that could represent the only indication of subtle hypoperfusion. The addition of cerebral blood flow studies[8,17,56,57,62] and electroencephalography to detect subtle test occlusion failures is beyond the scope of this chapter. However, there exists much controversy over the actual ability of these additional tests to significantly improve the predictive ability of the clinical test occlusion. Some interventionalists actually induce hypotension during test occlusion as a way of measuring cerebral reserve.

After the temporary occlusion test, the temporary balloon system is replaced by a detachable balloon delivery system.[20] The permanent occlusion balloon is positioned as distal as possible in the vessel to be occluded, near the first collateral inlet, in hopes of decreasing the amount of dead space between the balloon and first collateral, thereby minimizing the possibility of clot propagation beyond the balloon. It is usually difficult to achieve this in the case of giant cavernous aneurysms because they usually have a wide neck into which the balloon will preferentially migrate during advancement. We usually attempt to navigate distal to the aneurysm; if this can be achieved simply, then the aneurysm is trapped with a balloon both distal and proximal to the aneurysm. A third security balloon is then detached in the cervical internal carotid artery, carefully avoiding the carotid bulb and the baroreceptor mechanism which could induce hypotension. In most cases, however, it is not possible to position the balloon distal to the aneurysm. The first balloon is therefore detached in the petrous internal carotid artery below but close to the aneurysm with a second security balloon positioned proximally. Reversed flow in the ICA does not create a problem because aneurysms with this anatomic configuration uniformly thrombose (Figs. 234-1 and 234-2). In the case of aneurysms situated distal to the ophthalmic artery and where parent artery occlusion is the treatment of choice, it is important to cover the ostia of possible collaterals proximal to the aneurysm. If this cannot be achieved, there is at least a 50 percent incidence of failure of the aneurysm to thrombose.

Rarely, a cavernous carotid aneurysm may rupture into the cavernous sinus and cause a carotid-cavernous fistula (Figs. 234-3 and 234-4). In these cases, great care should be taken to ensure that the fistula is occluded prior to carotid occlusion below the aneurysm, as this can lead to recruitment of blood flow to the aneurysm and fistula through collaterals or the ICA from above (posterior or anterior communicating arteries, ophthalmic artery, inferolateral

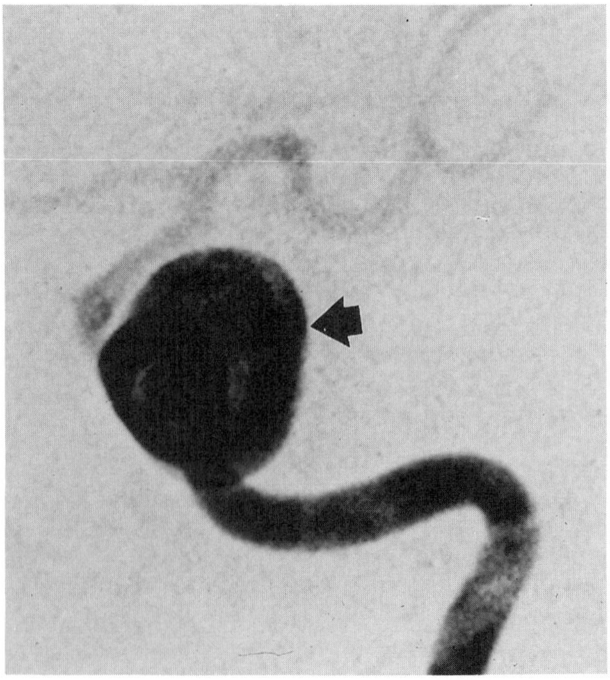

(*A*)

Figure 234-1 A 54-year-old woman with a giant aneurysm of the left cavernous internal carotid artery presenting with diplopia and retro-orbital headache. *A*. Oblique left internal carotid angiogram demonstrates a large cavernous segment internal carotid aneurysm (*arrow*).

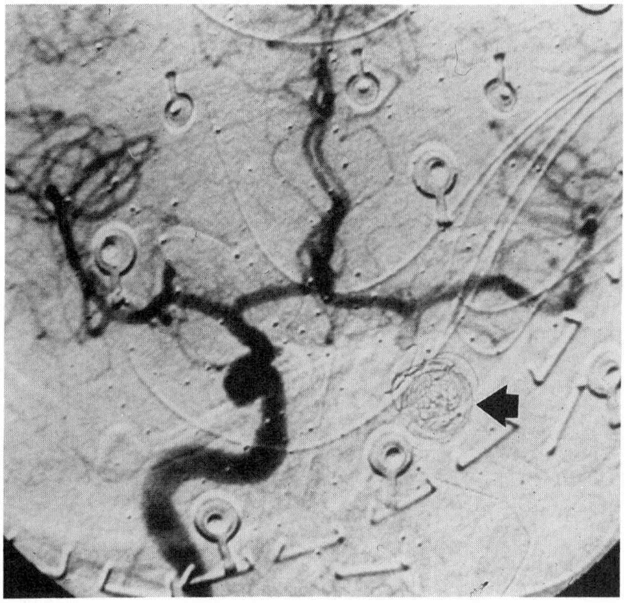

(*B*)

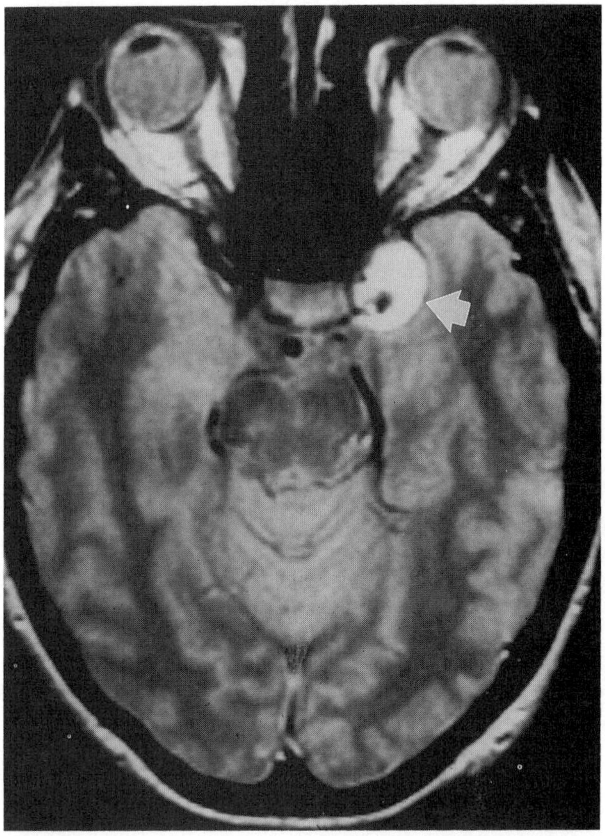

(*C*)

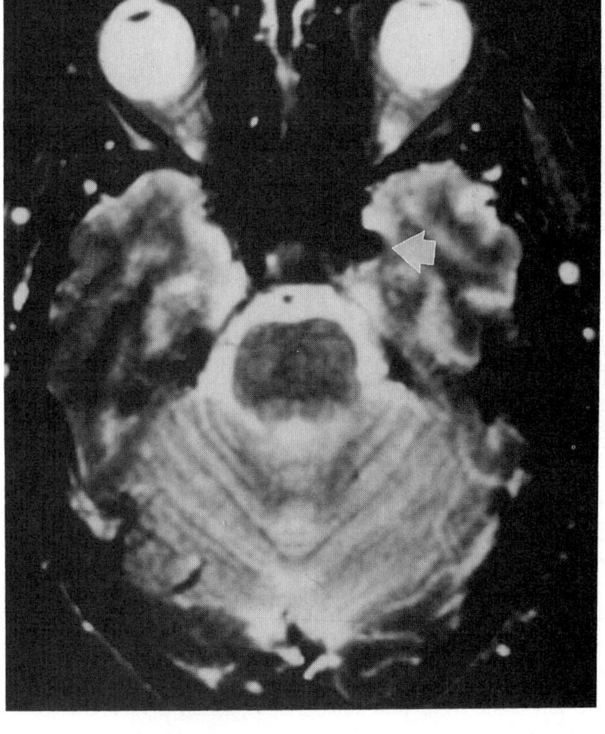

Figure 234-1 (*Continued*) *B*. Anteroposterior (AP) right internal carotid angiogram. For technical reasons, a detachable coil embolization (*arrow*) of the aneurysm was only partially completed. The left internal carotid artery was sacrificed with detachable balloons. The right internal carotid angiogram demonstrates good right to left cross flow and perfusion of the left hemisphere with exclusion of the aneurysm. *C*. T1-weighted axial MR image immediately after the left internal carotid occlusion demonstrates thrombosis of the aneurysm (*arrow*). *D*. Axial gradient echo MR image obtained 6 months after left carotid occlusion demonstrates marked reduction in the size of the aneurysm and no evidence of intra-aneurysmal flow (*arrow*). The alleviation of the mass effect resulted in clinical disappearance of the diplopia and the left retro-orbital headaches.

trunk or meningohypophyseal trunk). Occasionally, it is possible to occlude both the aneurysm and the fistula using a HEMA-filled balloon, thereby preserving the internal carotid artery. If this is not possible, multiple balloons may be needed to occlude the aneurysm, fistula, and internal carotid artery.

Sacrifice of the internal carotid artery, although not terribly elegant, is a very efficient way to treat inoperable aneurysms at the skull base. The failure rate is extremely low. In the case of giant aneurysms, occlusion of the ICA and thrombosis of the aneurysm is followed by eradication of symptoms related to pulsatile flow and mass effect.[18,32]

Unfortunately, clinically passing a test occlusion of the internal

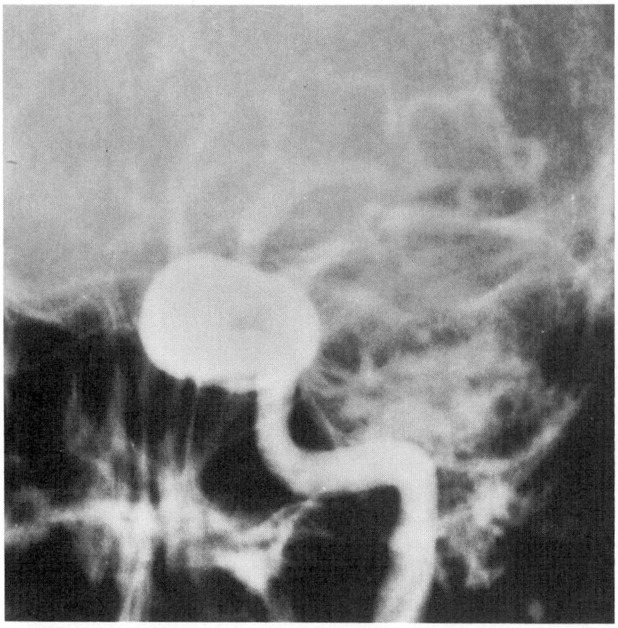

(*A*)

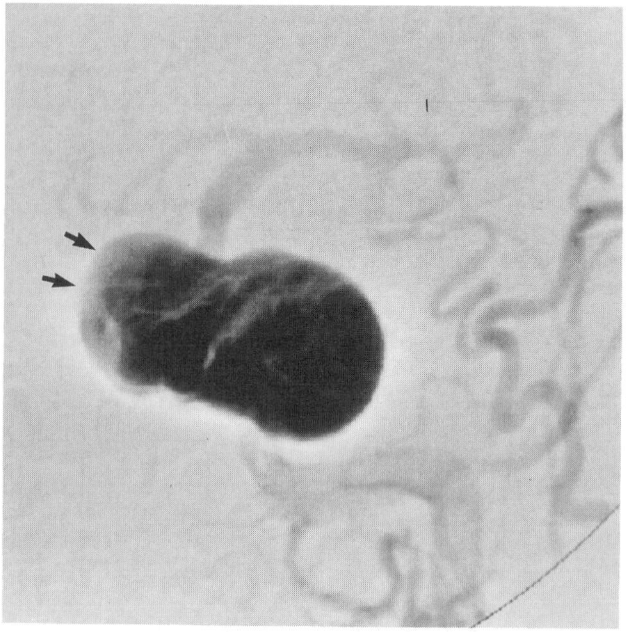

(*B*)

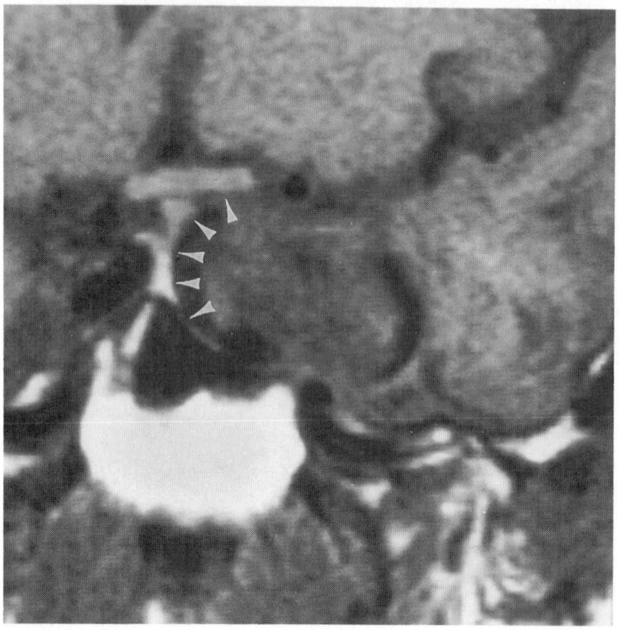

(*C*)

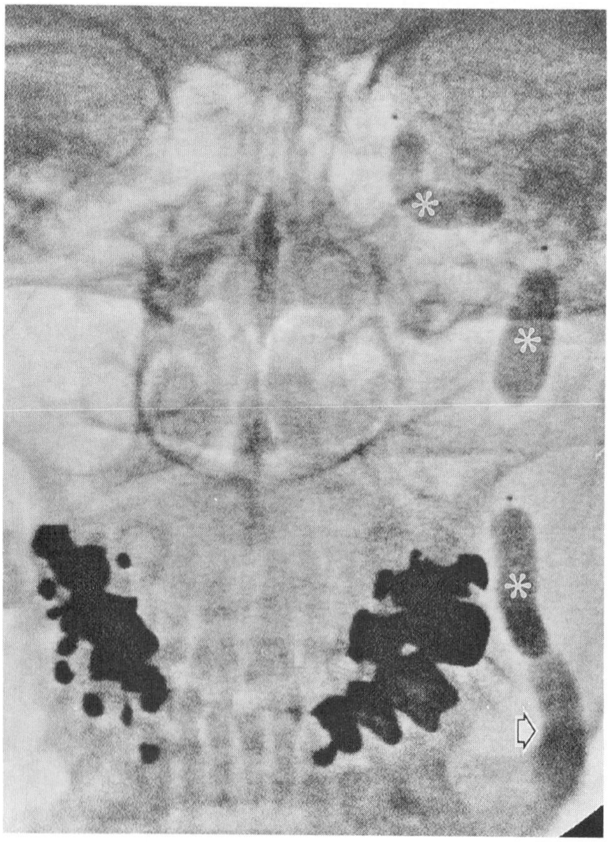

(*D*)

Figure 234-2 A 63-year-old woman with a left third nerve palsy and retro-orbital pain caused by rapid growth of a giant left internal carotid cavernous aneurysm. *A.* AP left internal carotid angiogram obtained 2 years prior to treatment demonstrates the intracavernous aneurysm. The patient was asymptomatic at this point and no treatment was deemed necessary. *B.* AP left common carotid angiogram obtained 2 years later demonstrates marked growth of the aneurysm. Note the intrasellar extension (*arrows*) which indicates communication with the subarachnoid space and increased morbidity from rupture. The patient now had severe left retro-orbital pain and a left third nerve palsy. *C.* Coronal T1-weighted MRI scan demonstrates the close relationship of the medial portion of the aneurysm (*arrowheads*) to the subarachnoid space, pituitary stalk, and optic chiasm. *D.* AP digital skull radiograph demonstrates three contrast-filled latex balloons (*asterisks*) occluding the left internal carotid artery. The most distal balloon is proximal to the aneurysm since it could not be navigated beyond it to perform a trapping procedure. There is static contrast material in the proximal internal carotid artery stump (*arrow*). The retro-orbital pain subsided within 24 h and the third nerve palsy gradually resolved over 3 months.

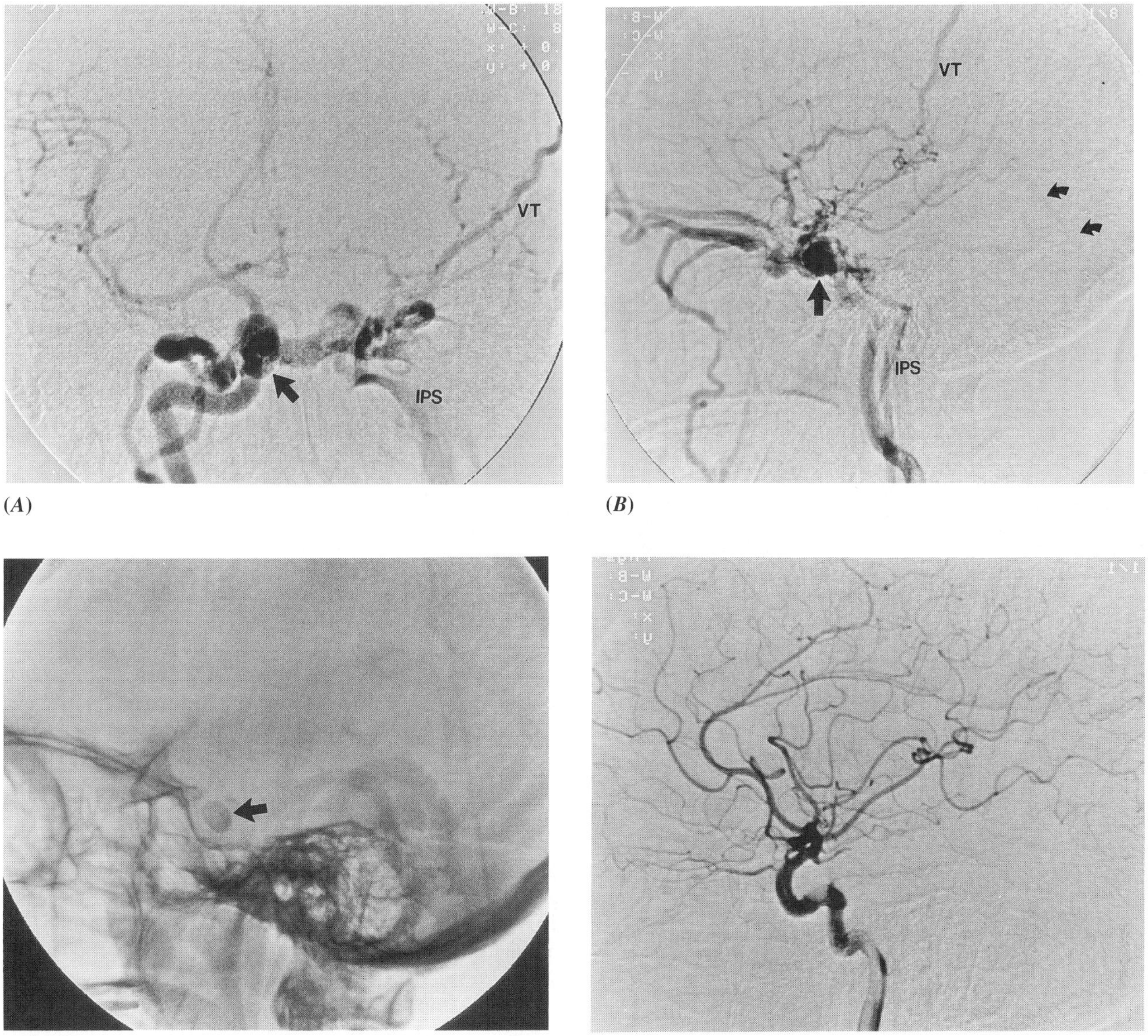

(*A*) (*B*) (*C*) (*D*)

Figure 234-3 A 61-year-old woman with spontaneous rupture of a right internal carotid cavernous aneurysm resulting in a carotid-cavernous fistula causing bilateral bruit, bilateral chemosis, and a right-sided decrease in visual acuity. AP *(A)* and lateral *(B)* right internal carotid angiograms demonstrate the cavernous carotid aneurysm (*arrow*), and carotid-cavernous fistula with anterior drainage to both superior ophthalmic veins and posterior drainage to the inferior petrosal sinuses (IPS). An important finding is the presence of pial venous drainage with recruitment of the left vein of Trolard (VT) and the deep venous system (*curved arrows*). Digital skull radiograph *(C)* and lateral right post-embolization internal carotid angiogram *(D)* demonstrate a HEMA-filled silicone balloon (*arrow*) which has been positioned in such a way as to occlude both the aneurysm and the fistula while preserving the internal carotid artery.

carotid artery does not preclude an ischemic event in the hemisphere distal to a subsequent permanent occlusion. After clinically passing temporary occlusion, the patient is subjected to permanent occlusion which has a reported early and late permanent neurological complication rate that ranges from 4 to 10 percent. Therefore, candidates for occlusive therapy should be carefully chosen; for example, certain large cavernous aneurysms which cause no or minimal symptoms and which do not exhibit rapid growth or extension into the subarachnoid space are often better left alone.[46,49]

Vertebrobasilar Circulation Aneurysms

Aneurysms in the vertebrobasilar circulation considered for treatment with parent artery occlusion are usually large, wide necked, saccular or fusiform aneurysms of either the distal vertebral or basilar arteries. Permanent balloon occlusion of one or both vertebral arteries may be performed following appropriate test occlusion.[2,28] Very rarely, permanent balloon occlusion of a short segment of the basilar artery may be attempted, but this is usually

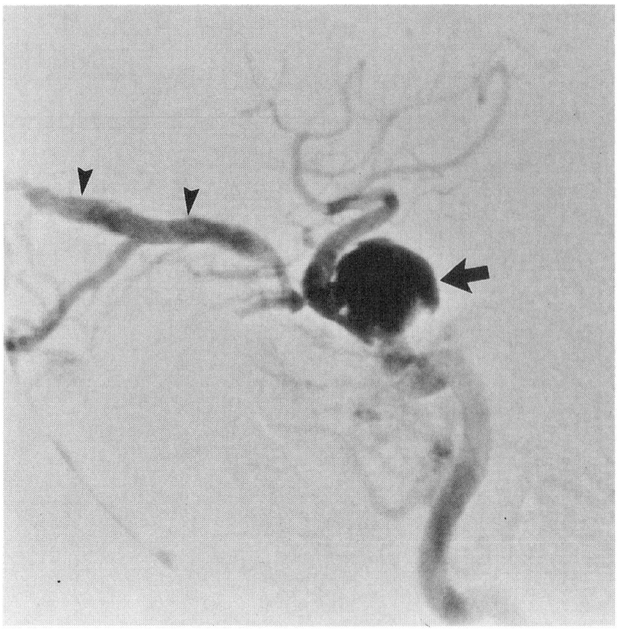

(*A*)

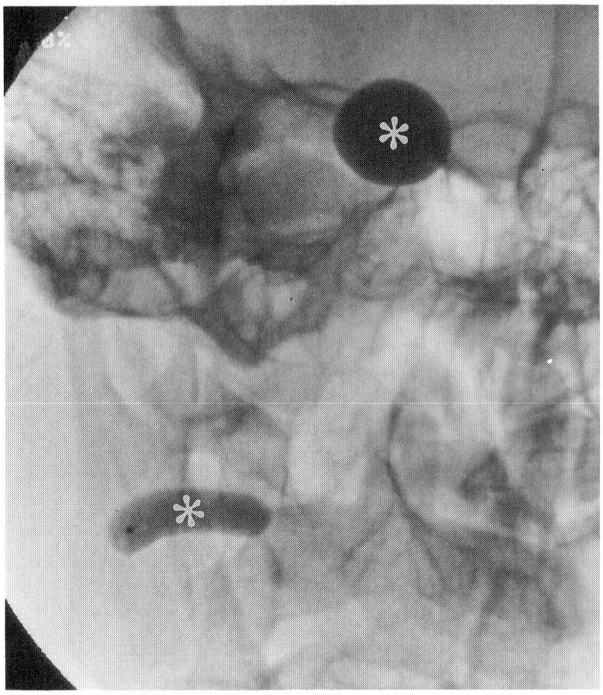

(*B*)

Figure 234-4 A 63-year-old woman with a ruptured large right cavernous carotid aneurysm, and resulting carotid-cavernous fistula causing right-sided chemosis and decreased visual acuity. *A*. Lateral right common carotid angiogram demonstrates the large aneurysm (*arrow*) and the carotid-cavernous fistula with anterior venous drainage to the superior ophthalmic venous system (*arrowheads*). *B*. AP digital radiograph showing detachment of two balloons (*asterisks*). One balloon occludes the carotid-cavernous fistula and upper carotid artery. The second balloon is placed at the level of C2-C3. There was resolution of the chemosis within 24 h and return to normal visual acuity within 1 week.

accompanied by high risks due to the presence of multiple perforators.

For aneurysms of the distal vertebral arteries, either a trapping procedure or occlusion of the vessel below the aneurysm may be performed. If the aneurysm is trapped with two balloons, thrombosis will ensue. There is a risk of perforator occlusion and ischemia if the occluded vertebral segment is known to carry perforating vessels [for example the vertebral artery situated between the posterior inferior cerebellar artery (PICA) and the basilar artery]. Occlusion of the vertebral artery below the aneurysm will result in either complete thrombosis or partial thrombosis due to the altered flow dynamics. For basilar aneurysms (fusiform or large saccular), occlusion of one or both vertebral arteries induces important changes in blood flow dynamics which may lead to partial or complete thrombosis of the aneurysm. This method can be very helpful for treatment of large inoperable aneurysms; in the case of fusiform aneurysms, partial thrombosis may be followed by reduction in mass and pulsation effects with preservation of basilar perforators. However, if the flow changes are sufficient to cause thrombosis of the basilar artery itself, this is usually a terminal event.

Occlusion of a single vertebral artery usually carries a very low morbidity unless the other vertebral artery is hypoplastic or absent and collateral supply from the circle of Willis is insufficient. Unfortunately, test occlusion in the vertebrobasilar system has less of an ability to predict future ischemia because it is only testing the ability of the vertebral-basilar system to withstand transient changes in perfusion dynamics following actual thrombosis of one of these vessels.

Serpentine Aneurysms

Serpentine aneurysms are usually giant, long, fusiform aneurysms found in the anterior circulation, most commonly in the middle cerebral artery M1 or M2 segments (Fig. 234-5). First, a test occlusion with a nondetachable balloon is performed just proximal to the aneurysm (if it is possible to do without occluding the perforating vessels). This will test the ability of the leptomeningeal collaterals to supply the territory distal to the aneurysm. If the patient fails the test occlusion, an extracranial to intracranial surgical bypass may be performed with a repeat test occlusion at a later date. If the patient tolerates the test occlusion, the nondetachable system is replaced by a detachable balloon system and the artery is sacrificed at the location of the test occlusion. It is also possible to use platinum microcoils for occlusion of the parent vessel just proximal to the aneurysm or, rarely, coils can be positioned both in the aneurysm and its parent artery. Because these aneurysms are often long, tortuous, and partially thrombosed, attempting to navigate distal to the aneurysm in order to perform a trapping procedure is usually contraindicated. Serpentine aneurysms are often found in younger individuals who have a good leptomeningeal capacity. Therefore, this type of treatment is usually successful with a low incidence of complications, especially in the anterior circulation. Even with incomplete aneurysm thrombosis, the change in flow dynamics can be sufficient to induce regression of the mass effect and to prevent distal embolic phenomena.

Mycotic Aneurysms

Mycotic aneurysms are caused by septic emboli that lodge at distal sites in the cerebral circulation, mainly in the middle cerebral or posterior cerebral arteries. The abnormality produced by

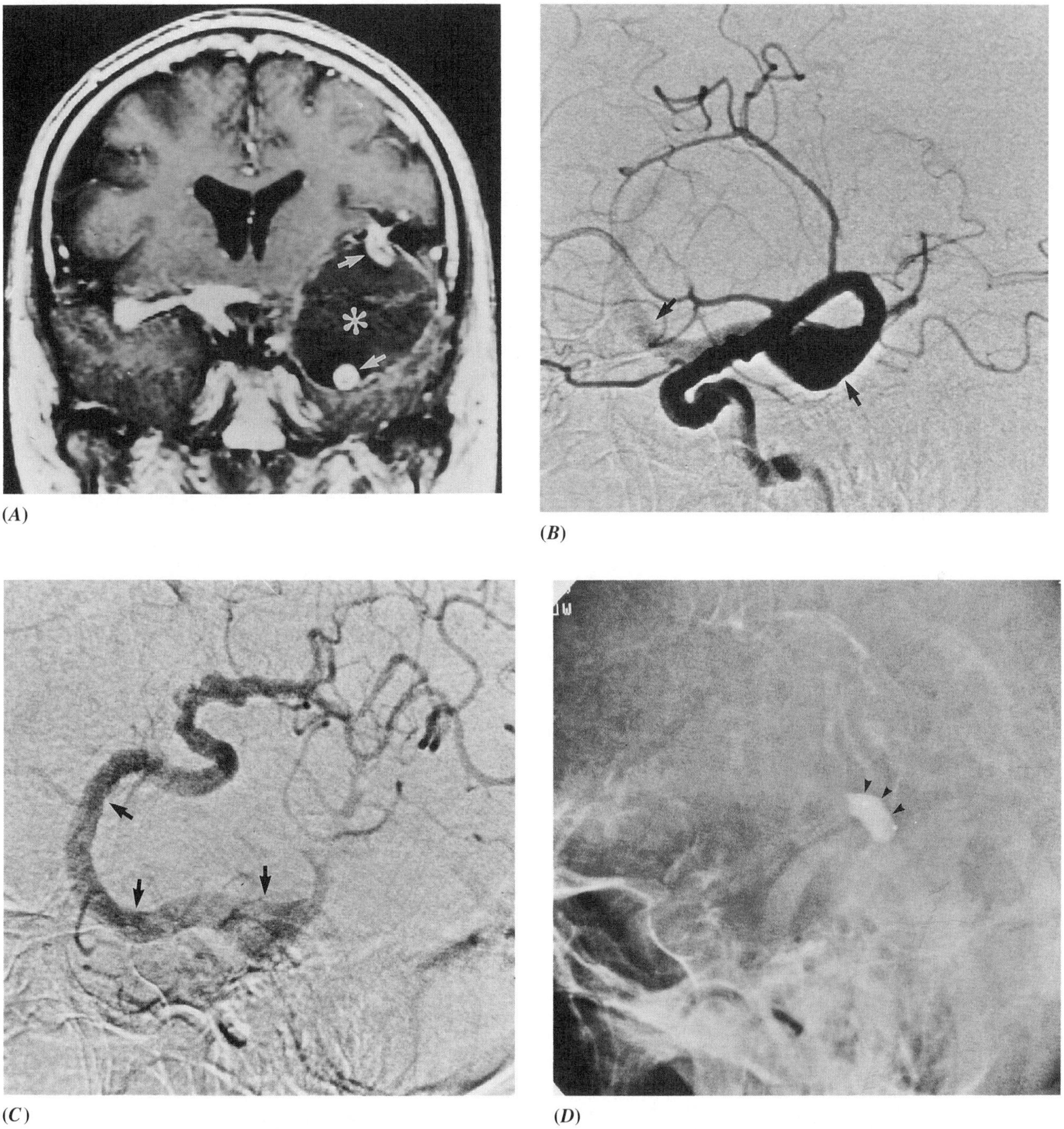

Figure 234-5 A 67-year-old man with a partially thrombosed fusiform, serpentine aneurysm of the left middle cerebral artery causing emboli responsible for dysphasia and right upper extremity weakness. *A*. Coronal T1-weighted, contrast-enhanced MRI scan demonstrates a largely thrombosed aneurysm (*asterisk*) with two enhancing vascular channels (*arrows*). Early *(B)* and late *(C)* phases of a left internal carotid angiogram demonstrate dolichoectasia of the aneurysmal parietal branch of the middle cerebral artery (*arrows*). The delayed phase demonstrates a large cortical area supplied by the distal portion of this artery. *D*. Lateral digital skull radiograph taken during test occlusion of the normal artery with a balloon (*arrowheads*) at the point of entrance into the aneurysm. Within 1 min of balloon inflation, the patient developed a dense right hemiplegia which was completely reversed by deflation of the balloon. In this case, leptomeningeal collaterals were insufficient to take over the territory distal to the aneurysm and no treatment could be offered to the patient, since an associated cardiac condition precluded surgery.

these emboli is usually transmural destruction of the vessel wall and the resulting appearance of aneurysmal outpouching. Aneurysms which persist despite medical therapy require intervention. Although neurosurgical methods have been successful at achieving resection and bypass of such aneurysms, it is also possible to effect a permanent cure using endovascular techniques.[42] A test occlusion of the small intracranial branch carrying the aneurysm may be performed by flow arrest using a Tracker catheter and the distal vascular territory assessed for adequate leptomeningeal collaterals. Alternatively, test occlusion might be performed with a small balloon (inflation may not be necessary for occlusion). If test occlusion is tolerated, the aneurysm and its parent artery can be occluded using small platinum coils or liquid acrylics such as N-butyl-cyanoacrylate (NBCA) glue.[42] Although at present no large series reporting the results of endovascular treatment of mycotic aneurysms exists, it would appear that embolization treatment is safe and efficient. Metastatic tumors such as choriocarcinoma[19] may also result in aneurysm formation which is possible to treat using endovascular techniques.

Intracranial Aneurysms, Endosaccular Occlusions with Balloons

As described earlier, endosaccular occlusion of aneurysms may be achieved using either silicone or latex balloons. It is generally agreed that latex balloons are incompatible with most HEMA preparations. Silicone balloons have the theoretical advantage of being softer and more adaptable to the aneurysm shape than latex balloons.[34] With either type, however, it is better to utilize a system whose internal sealing valve has been ''tucked'' inside the balloon so that it is less likely to protrude into the parent artery and be a source of future emboli.

When treating aneurysms with detachable balloons, the appropriate balloon is navigated into the aneurysm and then gently inflated to evaluate the fit of the balloon inside the aneurysm and its relation to the parent artery. The volume of contrast material required to inflate the balloon is then noted. If this volume is less than the dead space of the microcatheter, it will be impossible to replace the contrast material by HEMA. If this is the case, a small 1 French tubing (a vent tube) is placed into the balloon coaxially through the microcatheter in order to allow an exchange of contrast material for HEMA. In order for HEMA to polymerize properly, the ratio of contrast material to HEMA has to be at least 50 percent. The HEMA mixture can be mixed to polymerize anywhere between 20 and 60 min. Once the HEMA has polymerized (confirmed by a test quantity of HEMA immersed in a water bath at 37°C on the bench) the balloon is detached by gentle traction of the microcatheter. Some interventionalists prefer balloon introduction and HEMA exchange using a small 1 French polyethylene tubing which is permanently implanted in the body[61] bypassing the need for traction maneuvers which might displace the balloon. As with surgical clipping of aneurysms, the results and complications vary greatly depending on whether the aneurysm has previously ruptured and whether it is in the anterior or posterior circulation. In the series reported by Higashida et al.,[32] intrasaccular balloon embolization of aneurysms was associated with 18.2 percent mortality and 10.2 percent permanent neurological morbidity. Therefore, it is important that patients selected for this type of treatment by considered either nonsurgical candidates, or surgical candidates with a high estimated morbidity/mortality.

Long-term follow-up angiograms are needed in patients who have had intrasaccular balloon embolization of aneurysms because a large percentage of these patients will have aneurysmal recurrence caused by either the balloon shifting or aneurysmal regrowth from a weakened portion of the artery adjacent to the aneurysm neck.

Intracranial Aneurysms, Endosaccular Coil Occlusion

Electrolytically detachable microcoils have recently been developed by Guglielmi[23–25,37] (Figs. 234-6 and 234-7). They are constructed of soft platinum coils of varying lengths and diameters which are permanently soldered to a stainless steel coil pusher. These retrievable coils may be positioned inside the aneurysm and electrolytically detached if an acceptable fit and behavior of the coil is achieved. A small direct current produces the electrolysis of the solder joint. Using this technique, the soft microcoils allow a much denser packing of the aneurysm with less risk of perforation than is possible with fibered coils. At present, this technique remains investigational and is therefore only applicable in patients who are considered nonsurgical candidates. The best results have been achieved in patients harboring small aneurysms, in particular, with narrow necks. A permanent occlusion rate of over 80 percent has been observed in aneurysms with necks smaller than 4 mm. On the other hand, anatomic occlusion of the aneurysm has been achieved in only 20 percent of patients where the neck exceeded 4 mm in diameter. The presence of even a small residual aneurysm lumen at the end of an embolization procedure should be carefully followed. Repeat angiography over the course of several years

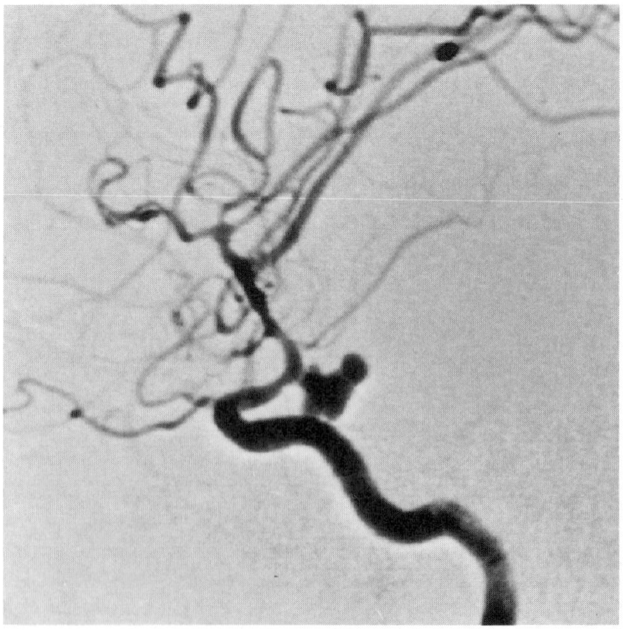

(*A*)

Figure 234-6 A 58-year-old woman with a ruptured left posterior communicating artery aneurysm, inoperable because of an acute myocardial infarct. *A*. Lateral left internal carotid angiogram demonstrates a multilobulated posterior communicating artery aneurysm. There is moderate supraclinoid internal carotid and left middle cerebral artery spasm which is asymptomatic at this point.

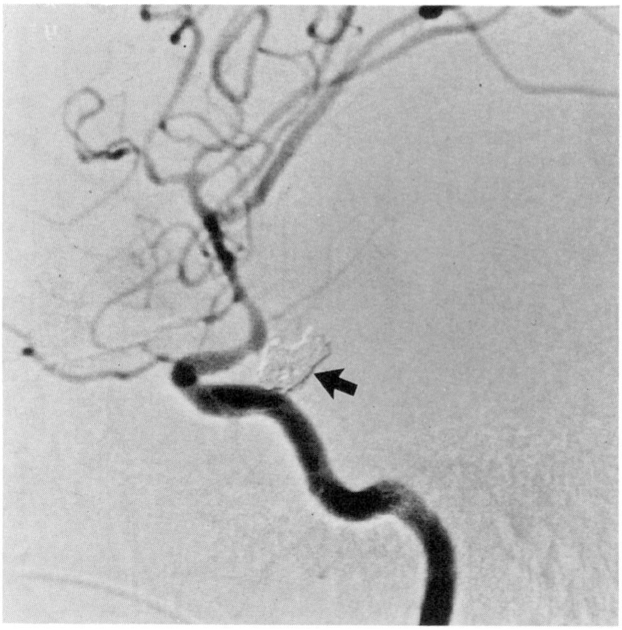

(*B*)

Figure 234-6 (*Continued*) *B*. Left internal carotid angiogram after embolization of the aneurysm with Guglielmi detachable coils shows almost complete obliteration of the aneurysm (*arrow*) with only a small residual neck.

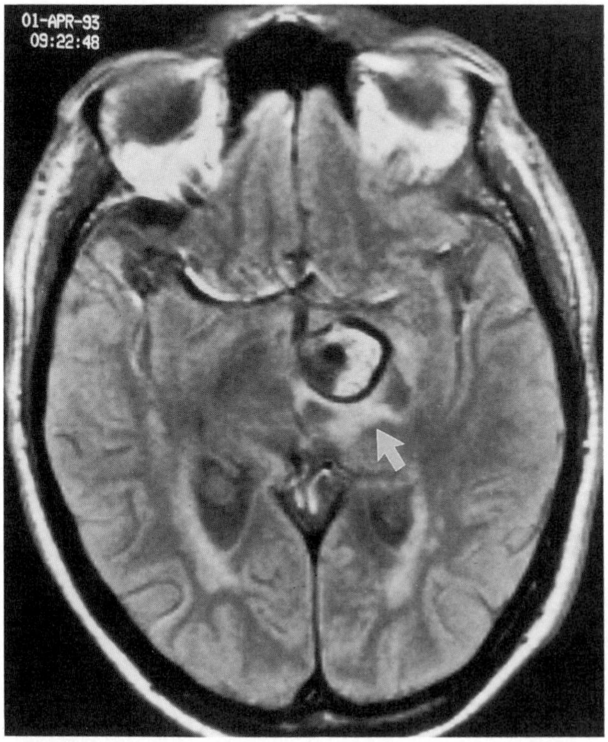

(*A*)

Figure 234-7 A 61-year-old man with a partially thrombosed giant basilar tip aneurysm and intractable headaches. *A*. Axial proton density MRI demonstrates a partially thrombosed aneurysm. There is surrounding hyperintensity of brain parenchyma from edema, probably secondary to the pulsation effect (*arrow*).

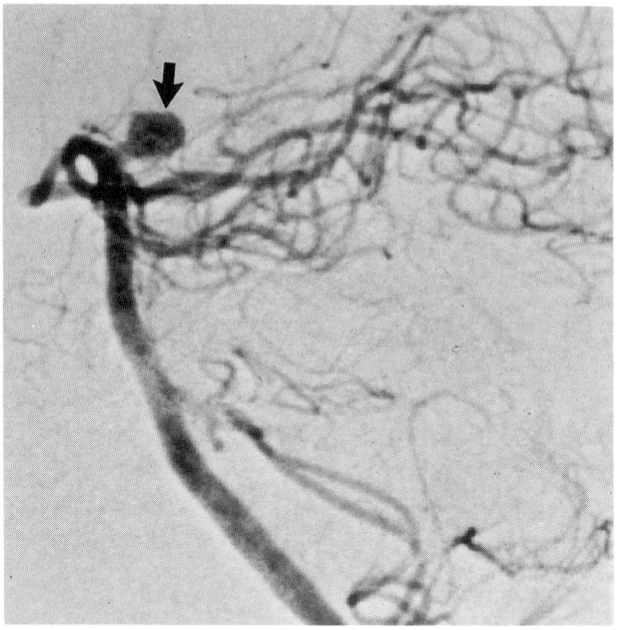

(*B*)

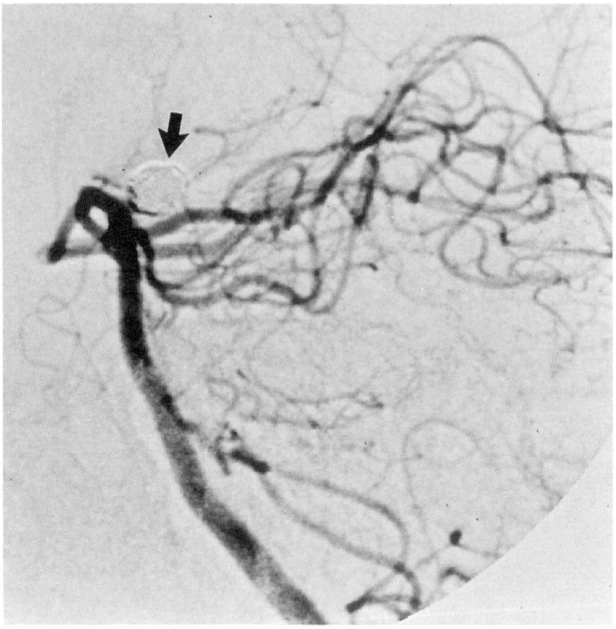

(*C*)

Figure 234-7 (*Continued*) *B*. Lateral left vertebral angiogram shows a small residual, posteriorly directed lumen of the aneurysm (*arrow*). *C*. Lateral left vertebral angiogram after embolization of the aneurysm with Guglielmi detachable coils reveals almost complete occlusion of aneurysm (*arrow*). The patient's intractable headache disappeared entirely within 24 h of the embolization.

may be necessary to demonstrate stability, further thrombosis, or aneurysm regrowth. Regrowth of an aneurysm cavity can occur from either compaction of platinum coils or true regrowth from a weak part of the artery at the neck. In a small proportion of aneurysms which appear occluded immediately postembolization, it is possible to observe recurrence of an aneurysmal cavity over time which points out the need for follow-up angiography.

In a recent series of 43 posterior circulation aneurysms (42 patients) by Guglielmi et al.,[24] overall morbidity and mortality rates related to treatment were 4.8 and 2.4 percent, respectively (2.6 and 0 percent considering only patients in Hunt-Hess grades I, II, and III). The complication rate associated with treatment of anterior circulation aneurysms is similar or slightly less. Longer follow-up will be essential in determining the long-term efficacy of this recently developed endovascular occlusion technique.

Anecdotal reports[36,45] have shown that it is possible to treat cerebral aneurysms using standard platinum microcoils. However, there are technical pitfalls associated with embolization of these coils (related to the lack of retrievability and relative stiffness which results in an increasing chance of perforation and decreasing possibility of tight packing). In particular, the inability to tightly pack the aneurysm is of concern since long-term follow-up in patients treated with standard platinum microcoils is showing a high percentage of aneurysmal recurrences (Jean-Pierre Pruvo, Lille, France, personal communication). Pruvo's findings showed a number of patients whose aneurysms were still anatomically excluded at 1-year follow-up but who showed recurrence on repeat 2-year studies; this finding should incide interventionalists to perform long-term follow-up studies in all aneurysm patients treated by any method of endosaccular occlusion.

Peri- or Intranidal Aneurysms Associated with Arteriovenous Malformations of the Brain

It has been shown[9,52] that the presence of intra- or perinidal aneurysms in brain AVMs are associated with an increased probability of cerebral hemorrhage. Therefore, selective occlusion of such aneurysms should prove beneficial in modifying the natural history of these patients. Endovascular therapy of these aneurysms can be performed alone, or, in association with radiosurgery (Fig. 234-8). Intranidal aneurysms are typically dysplastic with no distinct neck. Treatment must therefore consist of obliteration of both the aneurysm and the parent vessel. This can be accomplished using either liquid acrylic agents such as NBCA or platinum microcoils if a microcatheter can be navigated to the aneurysm.[73]

Dissecting Aneurysms (Extracranial or Skull Base)

Dissecting aneurysms of the anterior circulation rarely reach the subarachnoid space.[44] The dissection may be spontaneous or occur as a result of either minor or major trauma. The dissection can occur anywhere along the course of the cervical internal carotid artery and may extend to the skull base and exceptionally into the intracranial circulation. It is unusual for dissection to originate either at the skull base or in the subarachnoid course of the internal carotid artery. Patients with extra-arachnoid dissections of the anterior circulation usually present with ischemic or embolic events. Treatment is typically conservative in the form of anticoagulation; this treatment is often sufficient with the majority of patients who will demonstrate recanalization and improvement in the appearance of the internal carotid artery on follow-up angiography. However, some patients may present with ischemic or embolic episodes

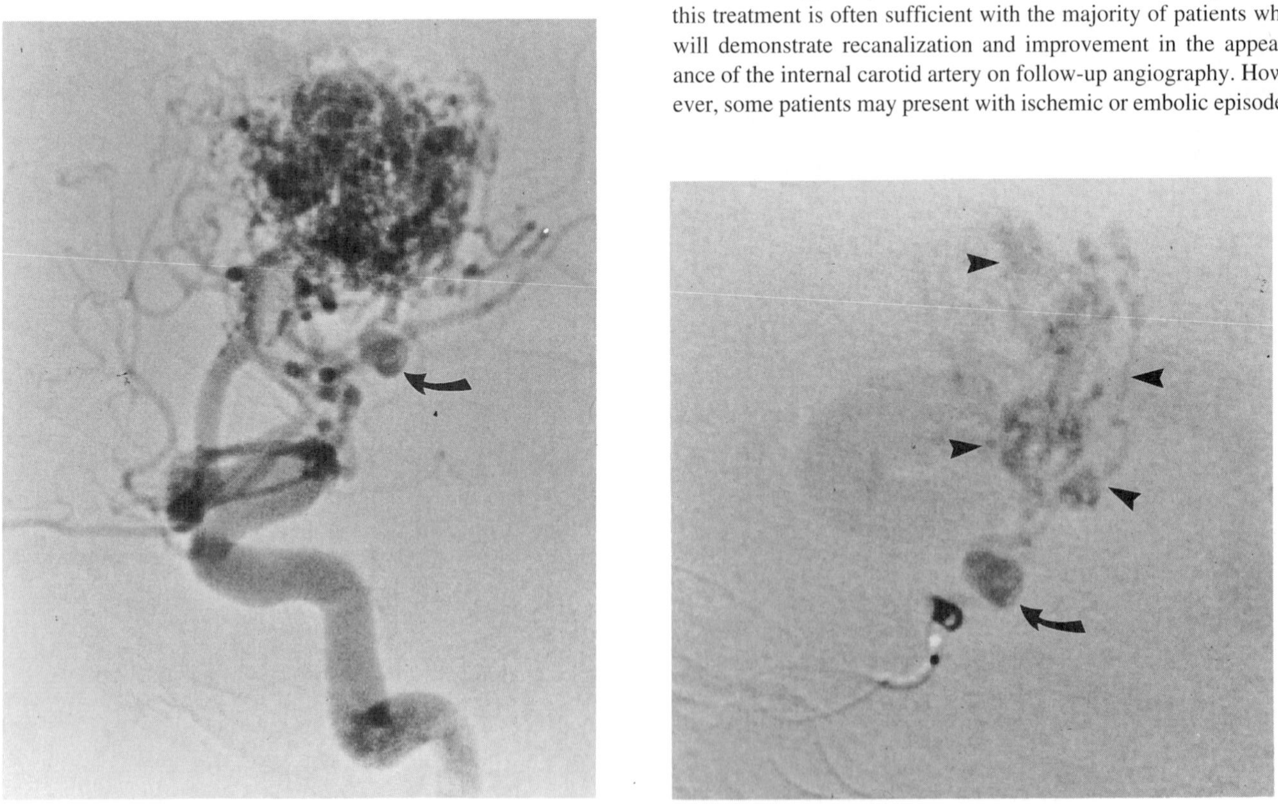

(*A*) (*B*)

Figure 234-8 A 46-year-old man with a right hemispheric deep-seated arteriovenous malformation and an associated lenticulostriate artery aneurysm. *A*. Lateral right internal carotid angiogram demonstrates both the AVM and the associated lenticulostriate artery aneurysm (*curved arrow*). *B*. Lateral superselective lenticulostriate angiogram demonstrates both the aneurysm (*curved arrow*) and the portion of AVM (*arrowheads*) fed by this vessel.

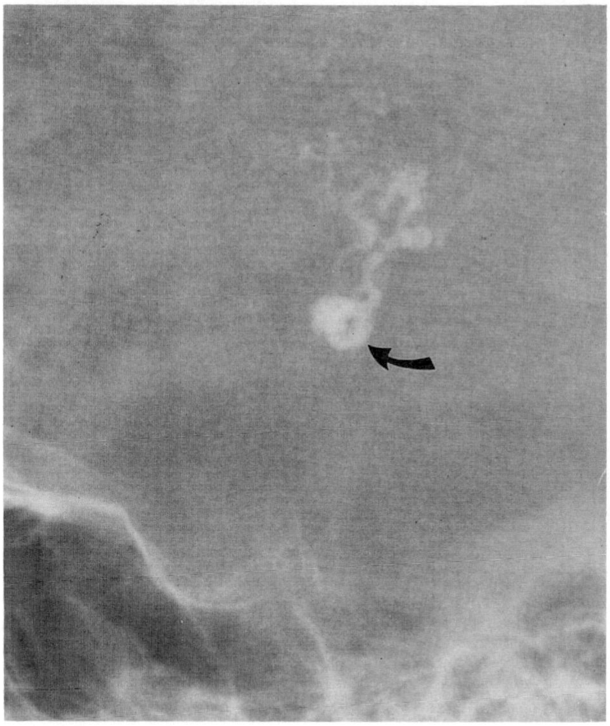

(*C*)

Figure 234-8 *(Continued) C*. Lateral skull radiograph after embolization with NBCA demonstrates the cast of glue in the aneurysm (*curved arrow*) and a portion of the AVM nidus. The remaining portion of the AVM was treated by stereotactic radiosurgery.

which are resistant to anticoagulation therapy. Rarely, it is necessary to occlude the internal carotid artery (Fig. 234-9). Despite successfully passing test occlusion, patients who have already suffered ischemic events may be at greater risk for delayed stroke due to decreased cerebral reserve.

Dissections in the vertebral-basilar circulation[75] should be divided into two categories: (1) extra-arachnoid, and (2) intra-arachnoid. Extra-arachnoid dissection of the vertebral arteries may also occur spontaneously or as a result of trauma. Patients usually present with ischemic or embolic events to the ipsilateral PICA or basilar territories. Treatment is usually medical[7] (anticoagulation) and only in rare cases is it necessary to occlude the vertebral artery with a balloon or coils. Dissections extending into the subarachnoid space have a very different natural history with a high proportion of these patients presenting with subarachnoid hemorrhage because the dissection commonly extends transmurally.[65] These patients are therefore not treated with anticoagulation. The preferred treatment is usually to occlude the ipsilateral vertebral artery in patients surviving the initial subarachnoid hemorrhage (Fig. 234-10).

Post-Traumatic Intracranial Aneurysms

It is rare that patients who suffer penetrating injuries (e.g., from gunshot or stab wounds or from surgery) will develop false aneurysms which need treatment by parent artery occlusion (Fig. 234-11). This treatment avoids placement of embolic material inside the false aneurysm which has no true wall. Both true and false

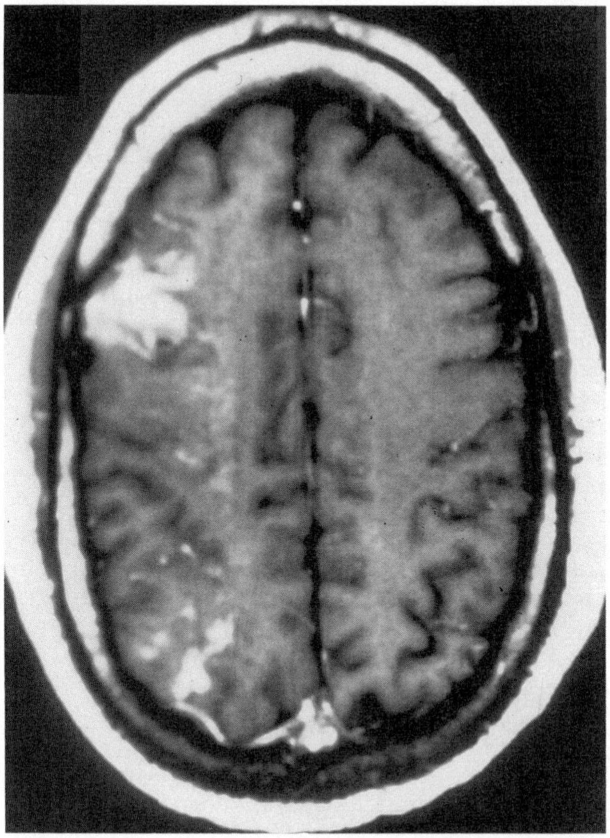

(*A*)

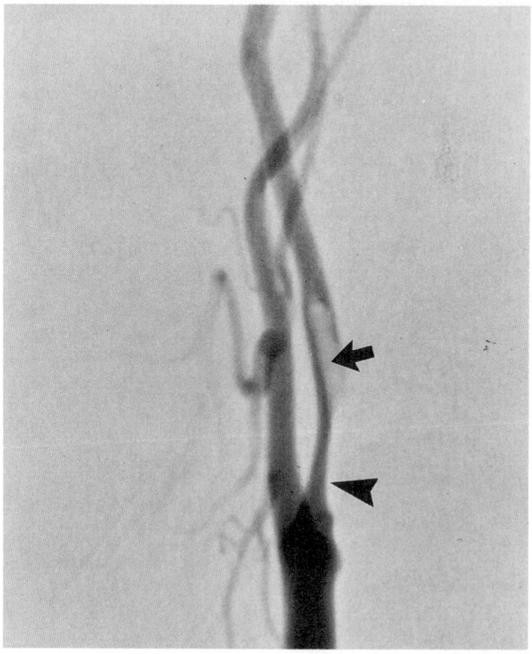

(*B*)

Figure 234-9 A 36-year-old man who sustained a right internal carotid artery dissection in a motor vehicle accident. An intraluminal, right internal carotid clot had caused multiple right hemispheric ischemic events despite systemic anticoagulation. *A*. Contrast-enhanced, axial T1-weighted MRI demonstrates multiple enhancing right hemispheric infarcts. *B*. Lateral right common carotid angiogram showing dissection of the origin of the right internal carotid artery (*arrowhead*) and the presence of an intraluminal thrombus (*arrow*).

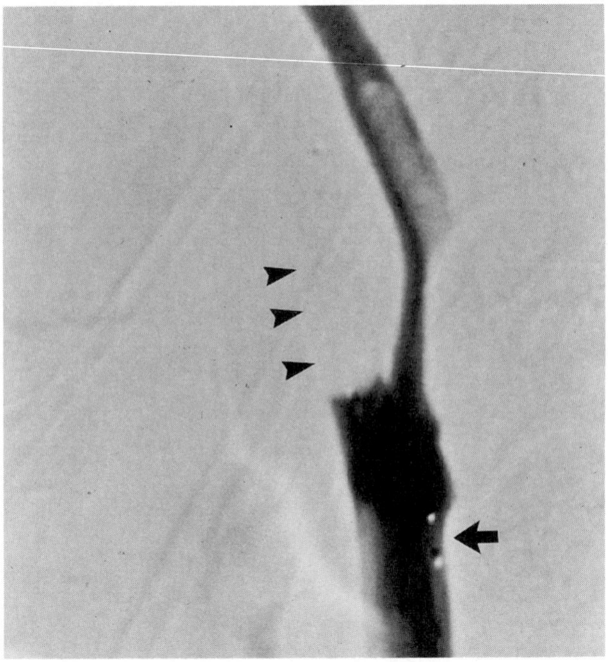

(*C*)

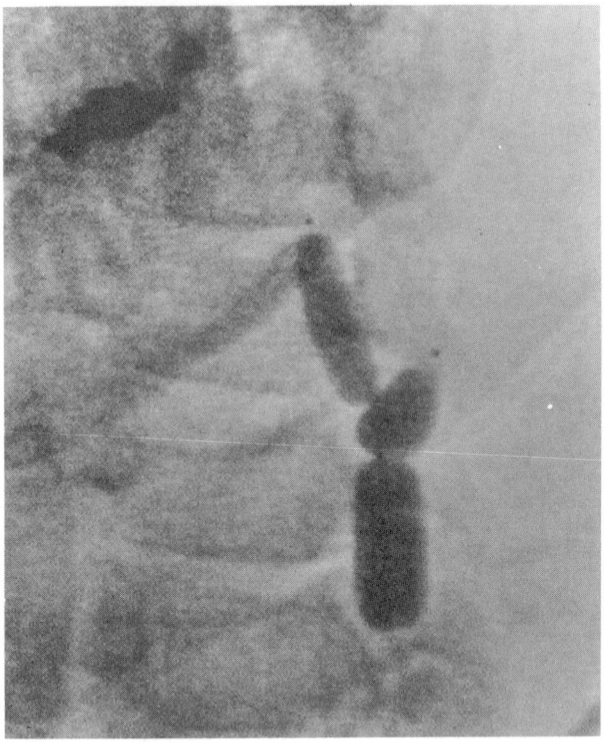

(*D*)

Figure 234-9 *(Continued) C.* Lateral right common carotid angiogram after placement of a balloon (*arrowheads*) in the origin of the right external carotid artery (which prevents reversal of blood flow into the internal carotid that might occur if only the common carotid were occluded). A second, simultaneously introduced, noninflated balloon (*arrow*) is positioned in the common carotid below and inflated immediately after the external carotid balloon. *D.* AP digital radiograph of the neck after detachment of the right external carotid and two distal, common carotid balloons, resulting in permanent occlusion of the right internal carotid artery. By using this maneuver, it was possible to avoid navigation beyond the friable thrombus.

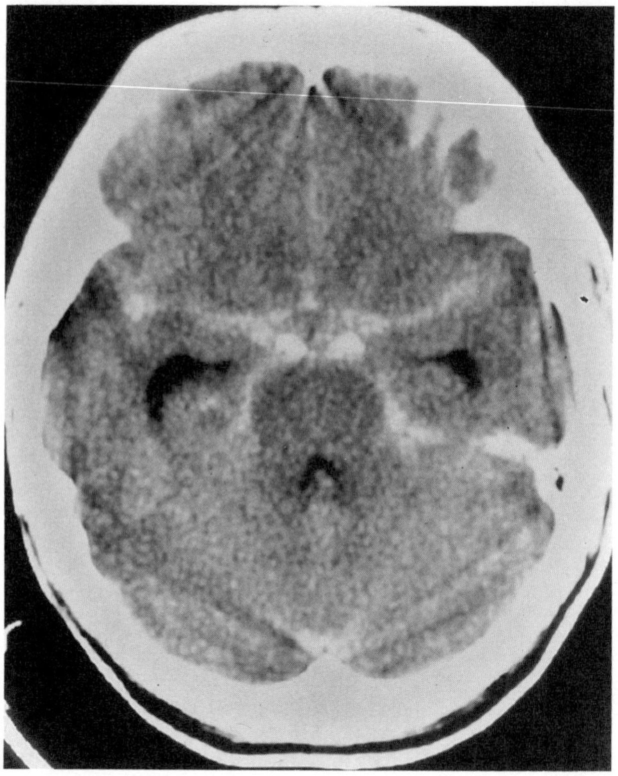

(*A*)

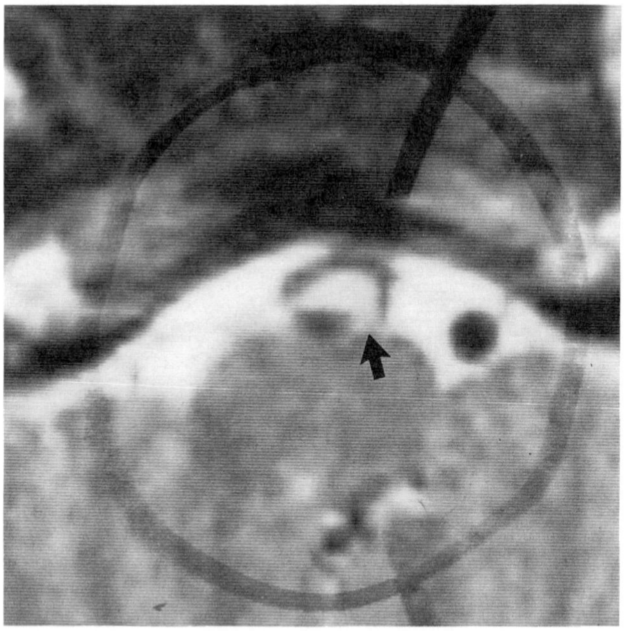

(*B*)

Figure 234-10 A 59-year-old man with subarachnoid hemorrhage caused by a dissecting right vertebral aneurysm. *A.* Unenhanced axial CT scan demonstrates subarachnoid and fourth ventricular blood. Early hydrocephalus is evidenced by dilatation of the temporal horns. *B.* Axial T2-weighted MRI scan at the level of the medulla demonstrates high intensity in the wall of the right vertebral artery consistent with dissection and a mural thrombus (*arrow*).

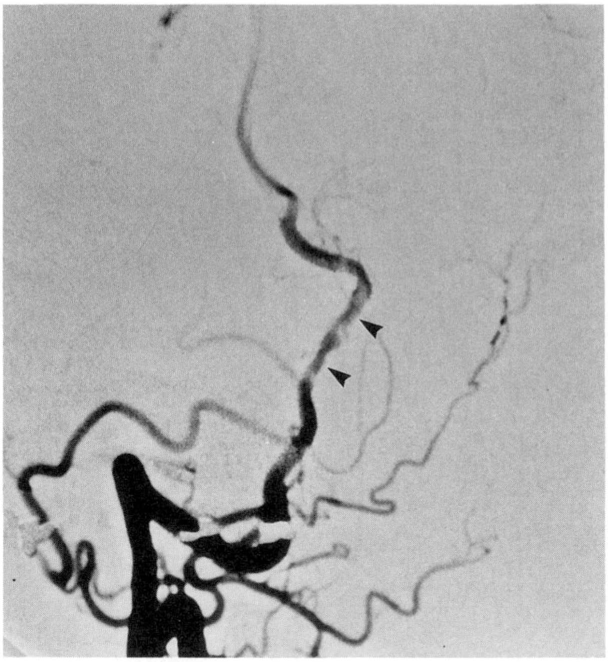

(*C*)

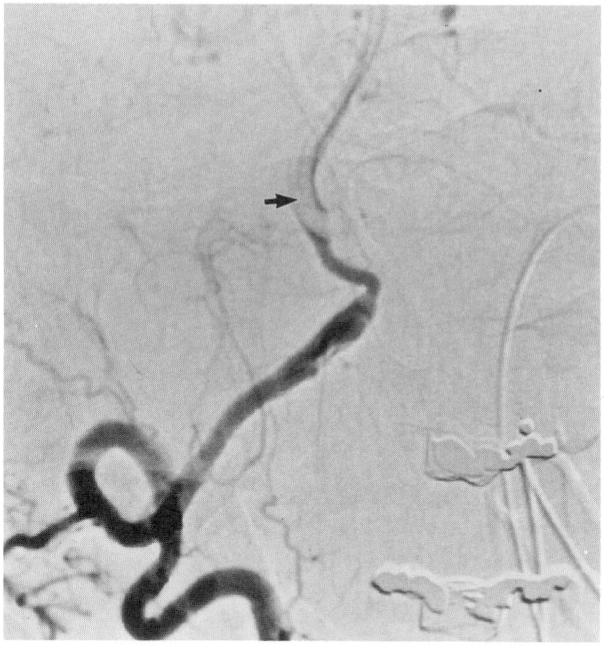

(*D*)

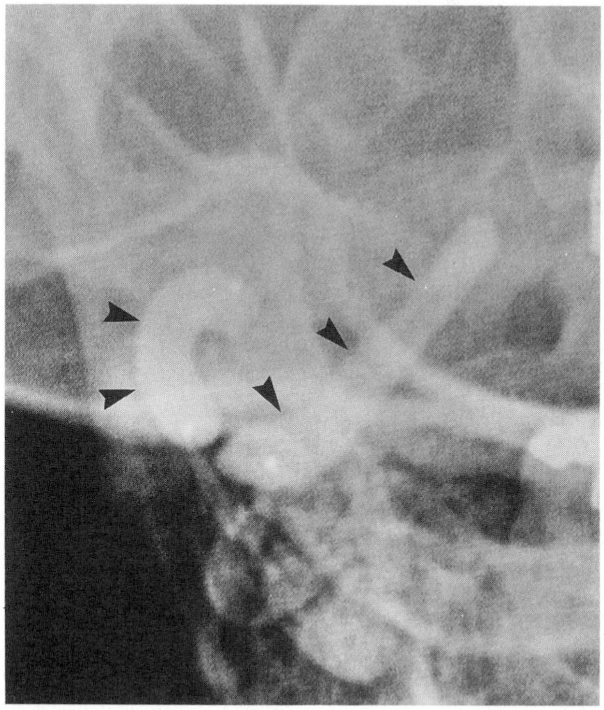

(*E*)

Figure 234-10 *(Continued) C.* Oblique transfacial right vertebral angiogram showing an irregular distal right vertebral artery (*arrowheads*) with some areas of narrowing compatible with dissection. *D.* Oblique right vertebral angiogram obtained 3 days later at the time of endovascular treatment shows irregular fusiform dilatation of the distal right vertebral artery. Notice inflow of unopacified blood (*arrow*) at the confluence of the normal left vertebral artery with the basilar trunk. *E.* Two detachable latex balloons (*arrowheads*) were positioned proximal to the aneurysm in order to achieve parent artery occlusion.

aneurysms may also develop after blunt trauma[63,67] (e.g., parts of the anterior cerebral artery may be damaged by the falx during a deceleration injury). Such aneurysms may be treated by either endosaccular occlusion or occlusion of the parent artery if they are not surgically correctable.

Extracranial Aneurysms

Penetrating trauma (e.g., gunshots, stabbing, needle punctures) as well as blunt trauma can result in the formation of aneurysms or pseudoaneurysms of the extracranial vessels. Penetrating injuries usually lead to the formation of pseudo or false aneurysms. In the external carotid circulation, occlusion of the parent artery as close as possible to the pseudoaneurysm is best accomplished with coils. Alternatively, NBCA may be utilized. Resorbable materials [i.e., Avitene (microfibrillar collagen hemostat, MedChem Products, Inc., Woburn, MA) or Gelfoam (absorbable gelatin sponge; The Upjohn Company, Kalamazoo, MI)] (Fig. 234-12) are occasionally utilized but may have a higher rate of recanalization.

Chronic, stable pseudoaneurysms of the internal carotid artery, if not associated with local or cerebral symptoms, may not need to

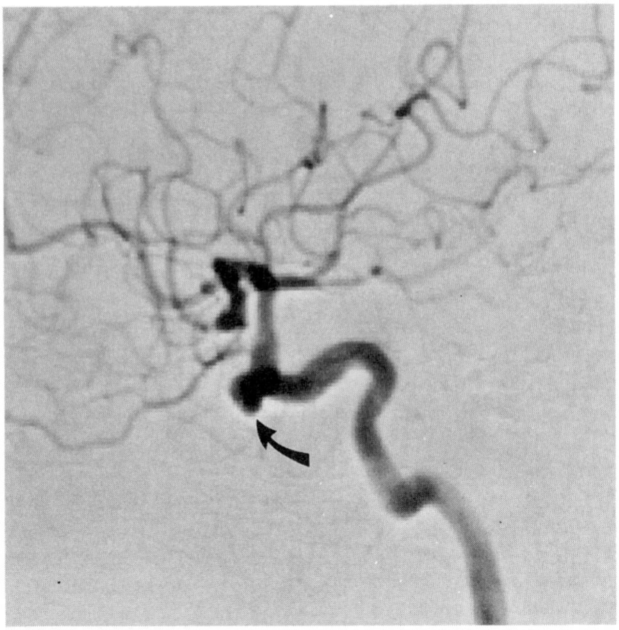

(*A*)

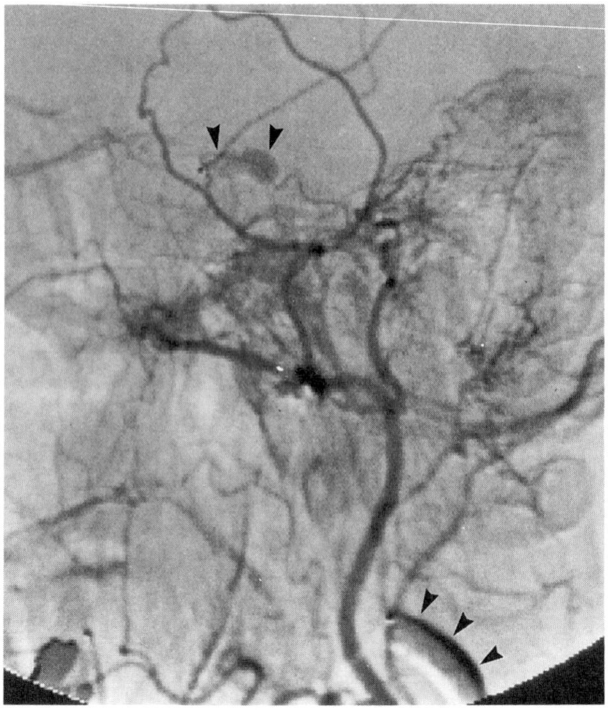

(*B*)

Figure 234-11 A 58-year-old woman with a right internal carotid artery (cavernous) pseudoaneurysm secondary to trans-sphenoidal pituitary surgery. *A*. Lateral right internal carotid angiogram demonstrates a pseudoaneurysm (*curved arrow*) in the anterior genu of the cavernous internal carotid artery. *B*. Lateral right common carotid arteriogram after test and permanent occlusion of the right internal carotid artery with two detachable balloons trapping the pseudoaneurysm (*arrowheads*).

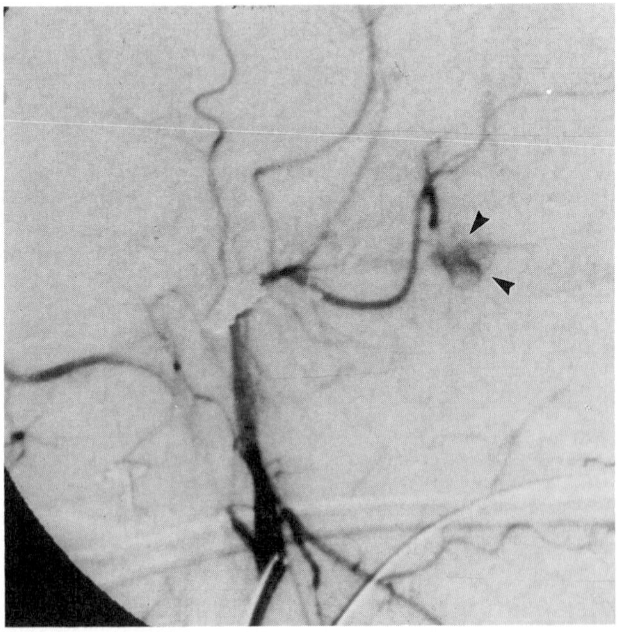

(*A*)

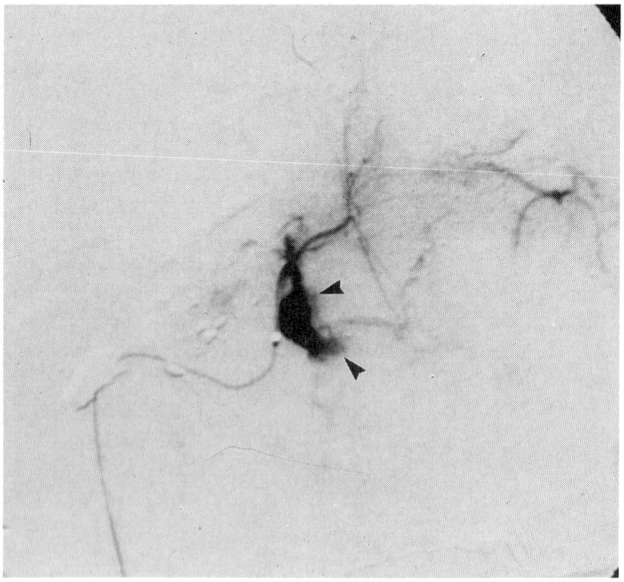

(*B*)

Figure 234-12 Epistaxis secondary to a pseudoaneurysm of the internal maxillary artery after a gunshot wound. *A*. Lateral external carotid angiogram demonstrates pseudoaneurysm formation with extravasation in the distal internal maxillary artery (*arrowheads*). *B*. Superselective lateral internal maxillary angiogram further demonstrates the pseudoaneurysm and extravasation (*arrowheads*).

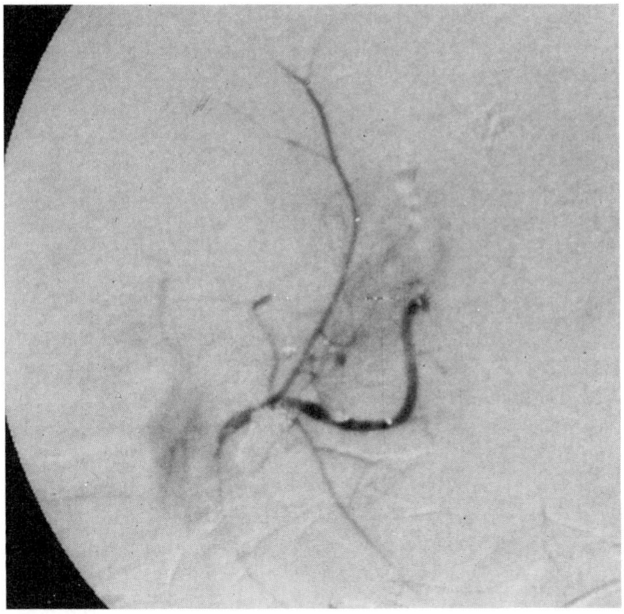

(C)

Figure 234-12 *(Continued) C.* Lateral internal maxillary angiogram obtained after embolization of three 2 × 4 mm Gelfoam pledgets shows obliteration of the pseudoaneurysm and absence of extravasation. The epistaxis stopped immediately.

be treated. In patients who present with an expanding neck hematoma or embolic phenomena to the ipsilateral hemisphere, the internal carotid artery may be sacrificed using balloons or coils if the patient demonstrates an adequate collateral reserve on test occlusion[71] (Fig. 234-13). Similarly, in the vertebral arterial system, pseudoaneurysms may not need to be treated endovascularly unless they produce symptoms. When indicated, the treatment should consist of occlusion of the vertebral artery. Penetrating injuries to the neck vessels may occasionally give rise to arteriovenous fistulae[53] which require closure. This can be achieved using coils, balloons, or NBCA (with or without preservation of the parent artery).

Endovascular Therapy of Vasospasm Secondary to Subarachnoid Hemorrhage

Following subarachnoid hemorrhage, spasm may be observed in the vessels of the circle of Willis or beyond in up to 70 percent of angiograms.[58] In approximately 30 percent of patients, such spasm may be symptomatic. Ischemia related to cerebral vasospasm significantly contributes to mortality and morbidity in patients who survive a subarachnoid hemorrhage. If spasm occurs prior to treatment of the aneurysm, the usual hypertensive, hypervolemic management, with resultant increase in cerebral blood flow and arterial pressure could lead to repeat hemorrhage. In patients who do not respond to aggressive medical treatment (hypervolemia, hypertension, and hemodilution), it may be necessary to employ endovascular techniques.

Microangioplasty has been described by numerous authors including Zubkov et al., Higashida et al., and Newell et al.[29,58,76] Generally speaking, the treatment consists of dilating vasospastic vessels with a small, low pressure balloon (Fig. 234-14). The small, 0.1 ml capacity, silicone balloon (Interventional Therapeutics) is probably the best suited for this form of treatment since it develops a maximum of 1 atm of lateral wall pressure. Alternatively, latex balloons (Ingenor-Nycomed, Balt) or dedicated microangioplasty catheters (Stealth, Target Therapeutics) may be utilized but they carry a higher risk of arterial rupture due to the high

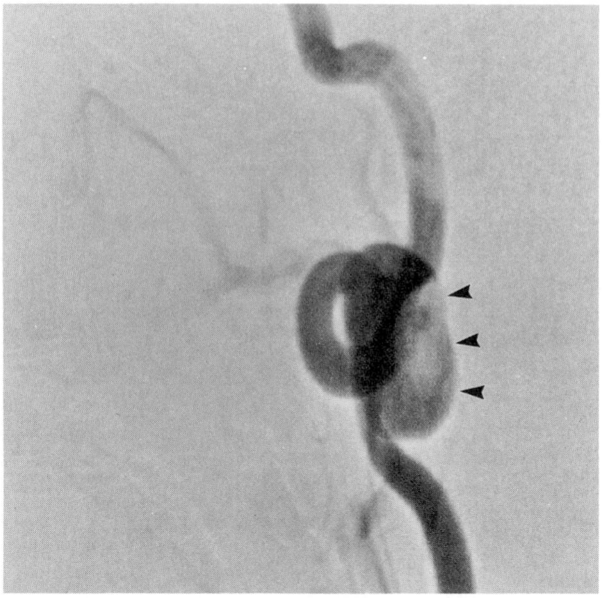

(A)

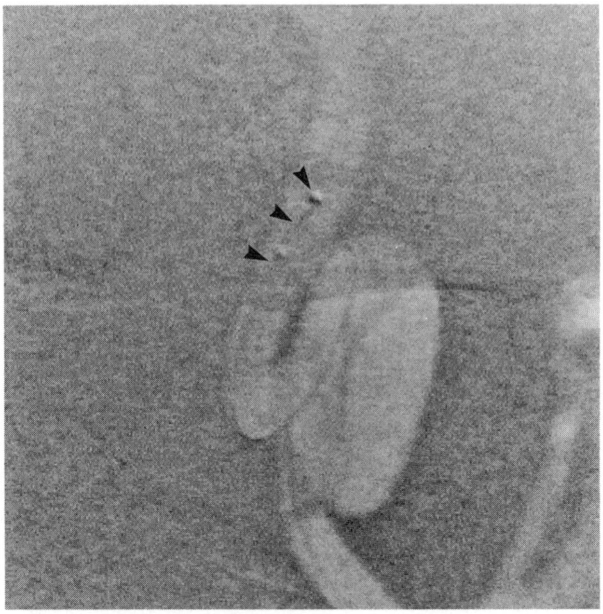

(B)

Figure 234-13 A 54-year-old man with a cervical left internal carotid artery aneurysm causing left hemispheric transient ischemic attacks and left amaurosis fugax. *A.* Lateral left common carotid angiogram demonstrates a wide-necked cervical internal carotid artery aneurysm at C1 *(arrowheads)*. *B.* Digital AP subtracted roadmap image shows that it was possible to navigate a microcatheter/latex detachable balloon combination *(arrowheads)* distal to the aneurysm to perform test and permanent balloon occlusion.

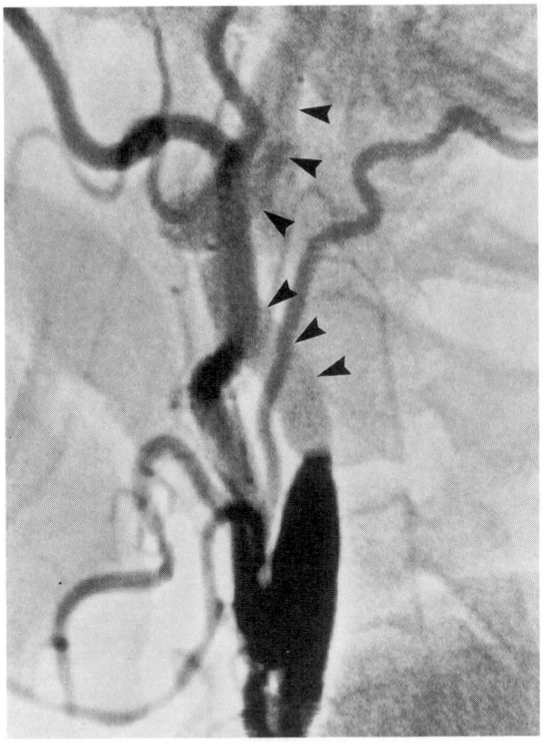

(*C*)
Figure 234-13 *(Continued) C.* Lateral left common carotid angiogram after detachment of two latex balloons (*arrowheads*).

lateral wall pressures (6 to 8 atm) capable with these systems. It is possible to decrease the amount of lateral pressure generated by latex balloons by creating a calibrated leak system, as described by Berenstein[5]; this has the added advantage of opacifying the vessel distal to the balloon and documenting improved flow. Microangioplasty for vasospasm may be problematic because of the difficulty of entering the anterior cerebral artery. Balloon catheters (with or without calibrated leaks) can, to some degree, be redirected by the use of a guidewire.[7] Mechanical dilation of a small blood vessel carries a risk of arterial rupture[48] which could be as high as 5 to 10 percent. Therefore, it is important not to dilate vessels whose native diameter is less than 2 to 2.5 mm. The presence of a recent infarct by CT or a fixed neurological deficit was initially considered a contraindication to angioplasty. However, there are anecdotal reports of such patients being treated without complications and an argument could be made that reperfusion will ultimately occur with time. Angioplasty for vasospasm has the best results when used early. Ideally, angioplasty should be pursued within 1 to 2 h after failure of medical therapy.

Recently, the infusion of papaverine hydrochloride, a potent vasodilator, has been described to be an effective alternative to mechanical dilation in the treatment of cerebral vasospasm.[39,40] Using this technique, 300 mg of papaverine hydrochloride (Eli Lilly, Indianapolis, IN), is diluted in 100 ml of nonheparinized saline. This total mixture is infused as close as possible to the area of vasospasm over approximately 30 to 40 min (Fig. 234-14). Because papaverine is unstable when mixed with heparin, Hexabrix,[60] and nonionic contrast materials at some concentrations and pH levels (Mathis JM, unpublished data), it is important to keep these materials separate during infusion, as this can result

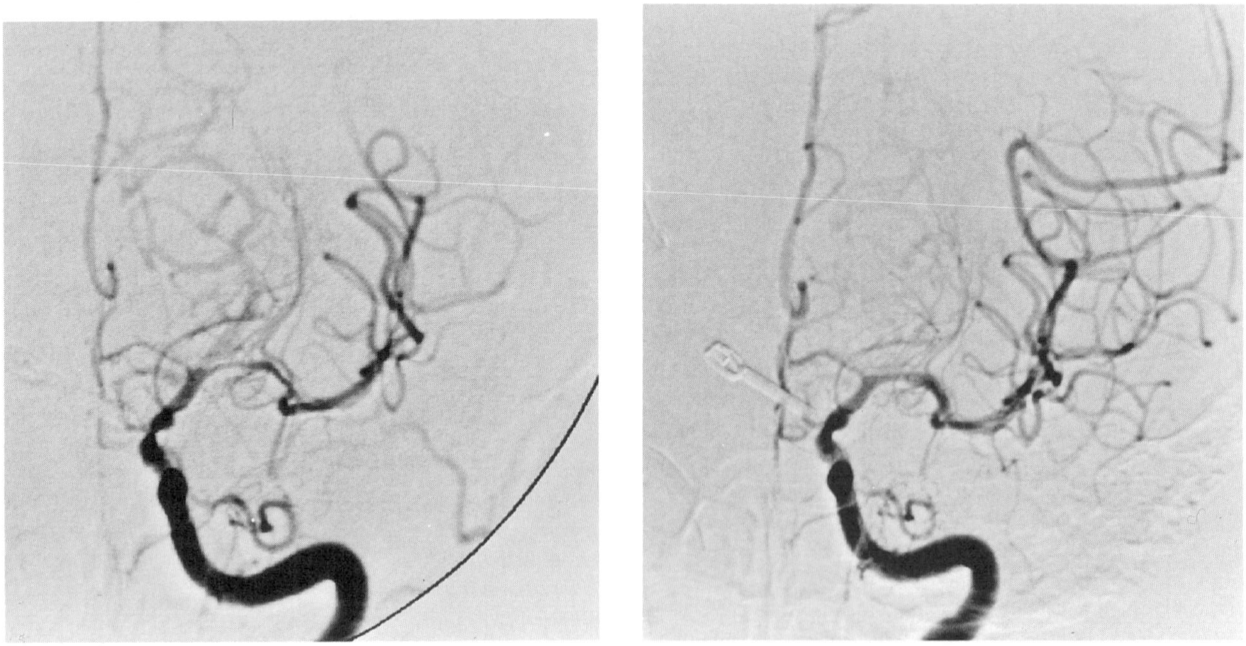

(*A*) (*B*)
Figure 234-14 A 50-year-old woman with recent SAH who presented with an altered level of consciousness and a right hemiplegia. *A.* AP angiogram of the left ICA reveals diffuse, severe vasospasm with markedly narrowed proximal ACA and MCA branches. Initial transcranial Doppler ultrasonography (TCD) revealed a peak velocity of 250 cm/s in the MCA. *B.* AP angiogram after papaverine infusion in the supraclinoid ICA shows diminished vasospasm. TCD flow velocity after papaverine was 180 cm/s.

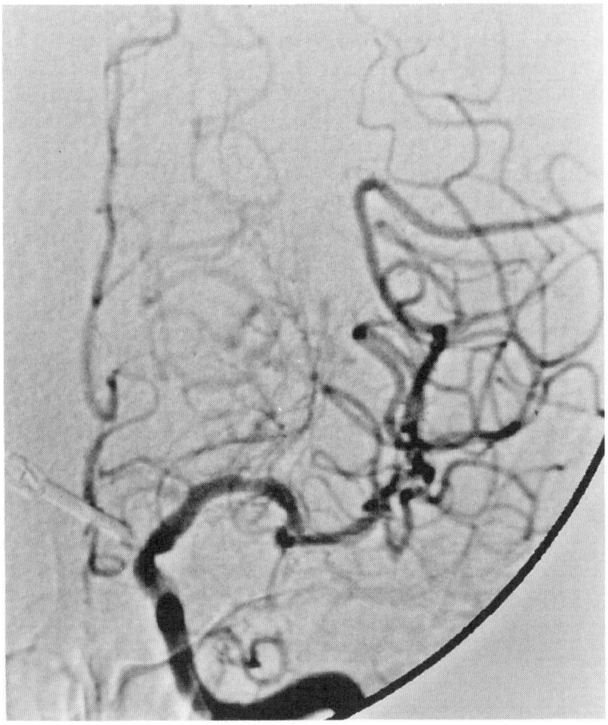

(*C*)

Figure 234-14 *(Continued) C.* AP angiogram following balloon angioplasty of the distal ICA and M1-MCA. Additional improvement in vessel caliber is noted. TCDs revealed additional improvement with a final MCA flow velocity of 130 cm/s.

in the formation of a precipitate which can act as an embolus. Up to three vascular territories may be infused in the same sitting; no adverse systemic effects have been demonstrated. If the infusion occurs below the ophthalmic artery, it is normal to observe an ipsilateral mydriasis which is caused by the papaverine. There have been anecdotal reports of medullary and brain stem dysfunction (Mathis JM, et al. unpublished data) within minutes of the beginning of papaverine infusions in the distal vertebral or basilar arteries. The exact mechanism of this process remains unclear but all patients have recovered over a period of minutes. The effects of papaverine are transient and it is possible for symptoms to reoccur 1 to 5 days after the initial infusion. If so, the infusion may be repeated or additional treatment may be employed in the form of angioplasty. However, the temporary increase in cerebral blood flow afforded by papaverine might be all that is needed to sustain viability until the spasm resolves on its own. A potential disadvantage of papaverine infusion is the discrepancy in blood flow between the anterior and middle cerebral arteries. Therefore, it may be necessary to selectively infuse the anterior cerebral artery when vasospasm significantly affects this territory. Papaverine infusion has the advantage of acting on the more distal, smaller vessels which cannot be reached by angioplasty. In can also be used in conjunction with angioplasty to partially dilate a vessel and permit easier passage of the angioplasty catheter.

Newell et al. reported sustained neurological improvement in 8 of 10 patients after angioplasty for the treatment of symptomatic vasospasm, as shown by the Glasgow Outcome Scale score at 1 month.[58] The percentage of clinical improvement occurring in the first 24 to 48 h is lower, between 40 and 50 percent. Best results should be expected in patients who are treated early and who have less severe deficits initially.

We have observed similar results with papaverine infusion; about 70 percent of patients have shown improvement at 1 week with approximately 30 to 50 percent showing improvement in the first 24 to 48 h. Similarly, the best results have been achieved in patients who were treated aggressively and who initially exhibited fewer neurological deficits.

The Future

The field of endovascular therapy for aneurysms of the CNS is still in its infancy. In the last 7 years there have been impressive developments in catheters and embolic devices which have improved both the safety and efficacy of endovascular treatment. One exciting area is the development of small endovascular stents which can be navigated through tortuous cervical and skull base vessels to bridge the ostia of aneurysms and exclude them from the circulation. This procedure should be particularly useful in the treatment of large or giant, wide neck aneurysms for which the present treatment is limited to occlusion of the parent artery. Undoubtedly, better coil devices or other agents will be developed which will facilitate endosaccular treatment of aneurysms.

References

1. Alom J, Matias-Guiu J, Padro L, et al. Spontaneous dissection of intracranial vertebral artery: clinical recovery with conservative treatment. *J Neurol Neurosurg Psychiatry* 1986; 49:599–600 (letter).
2. Aymard A, Govin YP, Hodes JE, et al. Endovascular occlusion of vertebral arteries in the treatment of unclippable vertebrobasilar aneurysms. *J Neurosurg* 1991; 74:393–398.
3. Barnwell SL, Higashida RT, Halbach VV, et al. Transluminal angioplasty of intracerebral vessels for cerebral arterial spasm: reversal of neurological deficits after delayed treatment. *Neurosurgery* 1989; 25:424–429.
4. Batjer HH, Frankfurt AI, Purdy PD, et al. Use of etomidate, temporary arterial occlusion, and intraoperative angiography in surgical treatment of large and giant cerebral aneurysms. *J Neurosurg* 1988; 68:234–240.
5. Berenstein A. Abstracts of the Annual Meeting of the American Society of Neuroradiology. 1990; 252.
6. Berenstein A, Ransohoff J, Kupersmith M, et al. Transvascular treatment of giant aneurysms of the cavernous carotid and vertebral arteries: functional investigation and embolization. *Surg Neurol* 1984; 21:3–12.
7. Brothers MF, Holgate R. Intracranial angioplasty for treatment of vasospasm after subarachnoid hemorrhage: technique and modifications to improve branch access. *Am J Neuroradiol* 1990; 11:239–247.
8. Camarata PJ, Latchaw RE, Rufenacht DA, et al. Intracranial aneurysms. *Invest Radiol* 1993; 4:373–382.
9. Cunha e Sa MJ, Stein BM, Solomon RA, et al. The treatment of associated intracranial aneurysms and arteriovenous malformations. *J Neurosurg* 1992; 77:853–859.
10. Dandy WE. Intracranial aneurysm of the internal carotid artery: cured by operation. *Ann Surg* 1938; 107:654–659.
11. Debrun G, Fox A, Drake C, et al. Giant unclippable aneurysms: treatment with detachable balloons. *Am J Neuroradiol* 1981; 2:167–173.
12. Debrun G, Lacour P, Caron JP, et al. Inflatable and released balloon technique: experimentation in dog—application in man. *Neuroradiology* 1975; 9:267–271.

13. Debrun G, Lacour P, Caron JP, et al. Detachable balloon and calibrated-leak balloon techniques in the treatment of cerebral vascular lesions. *J Neurosurg* 1978; 49:635–649.
14. Dion JE, Gates PC, Fox AJ, et al. Clinical events following neuroangiography: a prospective study. *Stroke* 1987; 18:997–1004.
15. Dott NM. Intracranial aneurysms: cerebral arterioradiography: surgical treatment. *Edinb Med J* 1933; 40:219–240.
16. Eckard DA, Purdy PD, Bonte FJ. Temporary balloon occlusion of the carotid artery combined with brain blood flow imaging as a test to predict tolerance prior to permanent carotid sacrifice. *Am J Neuroradiol* 1992; 13:1565–1569.
17. Erba SM, Horton JA, Latchaw RE, et al. Balloon test occlusion of the internal carotid artery with stable xenon/CT cerebral blood flow imaging. *Am J Neuroradiol* 1988; 9:533–538.
18. Fox AJ, Viñuela F, Pelz DM, et al. Use of detachable balloons for proximal artery occlusion in the treatment of unclippable cerebral aneurysms. *J Neurosurg* 1987; 66:40–46.
19. Fujiwara T, Mino S, Nagao S, et al. Metastatic choriocarcinoma with neoplastic aneurysms cured by aneurysm resection and chemotherapy: case report. *J Neurosurg* 1992; 76:148–151.
20. Gonzalez CF, Moret J. Balloon occlusion of the carotid artery prior to surgery for neck tumors. *Am J Neuroradiol* 1990; 11:649–652.
21. Goto K, Halbach VV, Hardin CW, et al. Permanent inflation of detachable balloons with a low-viscosity, hydrophilic polymerizing system. *Radiology* 1988; 169:787–790.
22. Guglielmi G. Embolization of intracranial aneurysms with detachable coils and electrothrombosis. In Viñuela F, Halbach VV, Dion JE (eds): *Interventional Neuroradiology: Endovascular Therapy of the Central Nervous System.* New York: Raven Press, 1992, pp 63–75.
23. Guglielmi G, Viñuela F, Dion J, et al. Electrothrombosis of saccular aneurysms via endovascular approach. Part 2: Preliminary clinical experience. *J Neurosurg* 1991; 75:8–14.
24. Guglielmi G, Viñuela F, Duckwiler G, et al. Endovascular treatment of posterior circulation aneurysms by electrothrombosis using electrically detachable coils. *J Neurosurg* 1992; 77:515–524.
25. Guglielmi G, Viñuela F, Sepetka I, et al. Electrothrombosis of saccular aneurysms via endovascular approach. Part I: Electrochemical basis, technique, and experimental results. *J Neurosurg* 1991; 75:1–7.
26. Halbach VV, Higashida RT, Hieshima GB. Treatment of intracranial aneurysms by balloon embolization therapy. *Semin Intervent Radiol* 1987; 4:261–268.
27. Higashida RT, Halbach VV, Barnwell SL, et al. Treatment of intracranial aneurysms with preservation of the parent vessel: results of percutaneous balloon embolization in 84 patients. *Am J Neuroradiol* 1990; 11:633–640.
28. Higashida RT, Halbach VV, Cahan LD, et al. Detachable balloon embolization therapy of posterior circulation intracranial aneurysms. *J Neurosurg* 1989; 71:512–519.
29. Higashida RT, Halbach VV, Cahan LD, et al. Transluminal angioplasty for treatment of intracranial arterial vasospasm. *J Neurosurg* 1989; 71:648–653.
30. Higashida RT, Halbach VV, Dormandy B, et al. Endovascular treatment of intracranial aneurysms with a new silicone microballoon device: technical considerations and indications for therapy. *Radiology* 1990; 174:687–691.
31. Higashida RT, Halbach VV, Dowd CF, et al. Endovascular detachable balloon embolization therapy of cavernous carotid artery aneurysms: results in 87 cases. *J Neurosurg* 1990; 72:857–863.
32. Higashida RT, Halbach VV, Dowd CF, et al. Intracranial aneurysms: interventional neurovascular treatment with detachable balloons—results in 215 cases. *Radiology* 1991; 178:663–670.
33. Higashida RT, Halbach VV, Hieshima GB. Treatment of complex intracranial aneurysms by interventional techniques. In Margulis AR, Gooding CA (eds): *Diagnostic Radiology.* Philadelphia: Lippincott, 1989, pp 357–360.
34. Higashida RT, Halbach VV, Hieshima GB. Endovascular therapy of intracranial aneurysms. In Viñuela F, Halbach VV, Dion JE (eds): *Interventional Neuroradiology: Endovascular Therapy of the Central Nervous System.* New York: Raven Press, 1992, pp 51–62.
35. Higashida RT, Hieshima GB, Halbach VV, et al. Intravascular detachable balloon embolization of intracranial aneurysms: indications and techniques. *Acta Radiol (Suppl)* 1986; 369:594–596.
36. Hilal SK, Khandji A, Solomon RW, et al. Obliteration of intracranial aneurysms with preshaped highly thrombogenic coils. *Radiology* 1989; 173(Suppl):250 (abstr).
37. Hodes JE, Aymard A, Gobin YP, et al. Endovascular occlusion of intracranial vessels for curative treatment of unclippable aneurysms: report of 16 cases. *J Neurosurg* 1991; 75:694–701.
38. Jellinger K. Pathology and aetiology of intracranial aneurysms. In Pia HW, Langmaid C, Zierski J (eds): *Cerebral Aneurysms: Advances in Diagnosis and Therapy.* New York: Springer, 1979, pp 5–19.
39. Kaku Y, Yonekawa Y, Tsukahara T, et al. Superselective intra-arterial infusion of papaverine for the treatment of cerebral vasospasm after subarachnoid hemorrhage. *J Neurosurg* 1992; 77:842–847.
40. Kassell NF, Helm G, Simmons N, et al. Treatment of cerebral vasospasm with intra-arterial papaverine. *J Neurosurg* 1992; 77:848–852.
41. Kassell NF, Torner JC. Epidemiology of intracranial aneurysms. *Int Anesthesiol Clin* 1982; 20:13–17.
42. Khayata MH, Aymard A, Casasco A, et al. Selective endovascular techniques in the treatment of cerebral mycotic aneurysms: report of three cases. *J Neurosurg* 1993; 78:661–665.
43. Kinugasa K, Mandai S, Terai Y, et al. Direct thrombosis of aneurysms with cellulose acetate polymer. Part II: Preliminary clinical experience. *J Neurosurg* 1992; 77:501–507.
44. Kitani R, Itouji T, Noda Y, et al. Dissecting aneurysms of the anterior circle of Willis arteries. *J Neurosurg* 1987; 67:296–300.
45. Knuckey NW, Haas R, Jenkins R, et al. Thrombosis of difficult intracranial aneurysms by the endovascular placement of platinum-Dacron microcoils. *J Neurosurg* 1992; 77:43–50.
46. Kupersmith MJ, Hurst R, Berenstein A, et al. The benign course of cavernous carotid artery aneurysms. *J Neurosurg* 1992; 77:690–693.
47. Lin T, Fox AJ, Drake CG. Regrowth of aneurysm sacs from residual neck following aneurysm clipping. *J Neurosurg* 1989; 70:556–560.
48. Linskey ME, Horton JA, Rao GR, et al. Fatal rupture of the intracranial carotid artery during transluminal angioplasty for vasospasm induced by subarachnoid hemorrhage: case report. *J Neurosurg* 1991; 74:985–990.
49. Linskey ME, Sekhar LN, Hirsch WL Jr, et al. Aneurysms of the intracavernous carotid artery: natural history and indications for treatment. *Neurosurgery* 1990; 6:933–938.
50. Linskey ME, Sekhar LN, Horton JA, et al. Aneurysms of the intracavernous carotid artery: a multidisciplinary approach to treatment. *J Neurosurg* 1991; 75:525–534.
51. Mandai S, Kinugasa K, Ohmoto T. Direct thrombosis of aneurysms with cellulose acetate polymer. Part 1: Results of thrombosis in experimental aneurysms. *J Neurosurg* 1992; 77:497–500.
52. Marks MP, Lane B, Steinberg GK, et al. Intranidal aneurysms in cerebral arteriovenous malformations: evaluation and endovascular treatment. *Radiology* 1992; 183:355–360.
53. Mehringer CM, Hieshima GB, Grinnell VS, et al. Therapeutic embolization for vascular trauma of the head and neck. *Am J Neuroradiol* 1983; 4:137–142.
54. Moniz E. Anévrysme intra-cranien de la carotide interne droite rendu visible par l'artériographie cérébrale. *Rev Otoneuroophtalmol* 1933; 11:746–748.
55. Monsein LH, Debrun GM, Chazaly JR. HEMA and latex balloons. Presented at the 29th Annual Meeting of the American Society of Neuroradiology, Los Angeles, CA, March 1990.
56. Monsein LH, Jeffrey PJ, van Heerden BB, et al. Assessing adequacy of collateral circulation during balloon test occlusion of the internal carotid artery with ^{99m}Tc-HMPAO SPECT. *Am J Neuroradiol* 1991; 12:1045–1051.
57. Moody EB, Dawson RC III, Sandler MP. ^{99m}Tc-HMPAO SPECT imaging in interventional neuroradiology: validation of balloon test occlusion. *Am J Neuroradiol* 1991; 12:1043–1044.
58. Newell DW, Eskridge JM, Mayberg MR, et al. Angioplasty for the treatment of symptomatic vasospasm following subarachnoid hemorrhage. *J Neurosurg* 1989; 71:654–660.

59. Pakarinen S. Incidence, aetiology and prognosis of primary subarachnoid haemorrhage: a study based on 589 cases diagnosed in a defined urban population during a defined period. *Acta Neurol Scand* 1967; 43(Suppl 29):1–28.
60. Pallan TM, Wulkan IA, Abadir AR, et al. Incompatibility of Isovue 370 and papaverine in peripheral arteriography. *Radiology* 1993; 187:257–259.
61. Partington CR, Graves VB, Rüfenacht DA, et al. Biocompatibility of 1-French polyethylene catheters used in interventional neuroradiology procedures: a study with rats and dogs. *Am J Neuroradiol* 1990; 11:881–885.
62. Peterman SB, Taylor A Jr, Hoffman JC Jr. Improved detection of cerebral hypoperfusion with internal carotid balloon test occlusion and ^{99m}Tc-HMPAO cerebral perfusion SPECT imaging. *Am J Neuroradiol* 1991; 12:1035–1041.
63. Piatt JH Jr, Clunie DA. Intracranial arterial aneurysm due to birth trauma. Case report. *J Neurosurg* 1992; 77:799–803.
64. Romodanov AP, Shcheglov VI. Intravascular occlusion of saccular aneurysms of the cerebral arteries by means of a detachable balloon catheter. *Adv Tech Stand Neurosurg* 1982; 9:25–49.
65. Sasaki O, Ogawa H, Koike T, et al. A clinicopathologic study of dissecting aneurysms of the intracranial vertebral artery. *J Neurosurg* 1991; 75:874–882.
66. Scott JA, Horner TG, Leipzig TJ. Retrograde suction decompression of an ophthalmic artery aneurysm using balloon occlusion: technical note. *J Neurosurg* 1991; 75:146–147.
67. Senegor M. Traumatic pericallosal aneurysm in a patient with no major trauma. Case report. *J Neurosurg* 1991; 75:475–477.
68. Serbinenko FA. Balloon catheterization and occlusion of major cerebral vessels. *J Neurosurg* 1974; 41:125–145.
69. Serbinenko FA, Filatov JM, Spallone A, et al. Management of giant intracranial ICA aneurysms with combined extracranial-intracranial anastomosis and endovascular occlusion. *J Neurosurg* 1990; 73:57–63.
70. Strother CM, Lund S, Graves V, et al. Late paraophthalmic aneurysm rupture following endovascular treatment. *J Neurosurg* 1989; 71:777–780.
71. Sundt TM Jr, Pearson BW, Piepgras DG, et al. Surgical management of aneurysms of the distal extracranial internal carotid artery. *J Neurosurg* 1986; 64:169–182.
72. Taki W, Nishi S, Yamashita K, et al. Selection and combination of various endovascular techniques in the treatment of giant aneurysms. *J Neurosurg* 1992; 77:37–42.
73. Terada T, Nakamura Y, Nakai K, et al. Embolization of arteriovenous malformations with peripheral aneurysms using ethylene vinyl alcohol copolymer. Report of three cases. *J Neurosurg* 1991; 75:655–660.
74. Weir B. *Aneurysms Affecting the Nervous System.* Baltimore: Williams & Wilkins, 1987, pp 1–60.
75. Yamaura A, Watanabe Y, Saeki N. Dissecting aneurysms of the intracranial vertebral artery. *J Neurosurg* 1990; 72:183–188.
76. Zubkov YN, Nikiforov BM, Shustin VA. Balloon catheter technique for dilatation of constricted cerebral arteries after aneurysmal SAH. *Acta Neurochir (Wien)* 1984; 70:65–79.

235 Subarachnoid Hemorrhage of Unknown Etiology

Allan H. Friedman

The diagnosis of spontaneous subarachnoid hemorrhage (SAH) alerts the physician to the possibility of a potentially life-threatening condition. Analogous to the situation which follows a closed head injury, the neurosurgeon can do little to ameliorate the direct consequences of the initial hemorrhage, but is most effective in avoiding or lessening the impact of further insults to the brain. Although some form of therapy can be offered to all patients, the neurosurgeon is especially concerned with maintaining the good condition of those patients who have survived their initial hemorrhage. Approximately 75 percent of patients who present with a spontaneous subarachnoid hemorrhage will be found to have an underlying intracranial aneurysm, and 5 percent will be found to have an intracranial arteriovenous malformation (AVM). Rarely, fibromuscular dysplasia or moyamoya disease will act as a source of an SAH. The accepted treatment of these lesions is discussed elsewhere. If the initial computed tomography (CT) or magnetic resonance imaging (MRI) of the brain and four-vessel angiography fail to reveal the source of the patient's hemorrhage, the physician must then decide what further diagnostic tests are indicated and what therapy should be instituted.

Differential Diagnosis

In patients who do not have an angiographically discernible cause for their subarachnoid hemorrhage, an extensive differential diagnosis must be considered. In any given patient, this long list can be winnowed by facts gathered from the patient's history and by the findings on the patient's brain CT scan.

Trauma is the most common cause of nonaneurysmal subarachnoid hemorrhage. Sometimes it it difficult to discern whether the patient's subarachnoid hemorrhage was the cause or result of the patient's injury. This is especially true when only a murky history accompanies the patient into the emergency room. Trauma must be considered as he cause of a subarachnoid hemorrhage when no other source can be identified.

A traumatic spinal tap in which successive tubes of cerebrospinal fluid have not been collected or in which the supernatant of the centrifuged fluid has not been examined can lead to the mistaken diagnosis of a spontaneous subarachnoid hemorrhage. The importance of a properly done spinal tap must be emphasized to referring physicians.

Subarachnoid hemorrhage is a well-recognized complication of several diverse medical conditions. It has been associated with deficiencies in each of the known coagulation factors and with therapeutic anticoagulation. Sickle cell anemia has been associated with subarachnoid hemorrhage, but in approximately 50 percent of these cases a concomitant aneurysm can also be found. Subarachnoid hemorrhage has been reported to occur in those congenital disorders in which there is either an increase in blood vessel fragility or an abnormality in the elastic tissue. Systemic collagen vascular diseases such as systemic lupus erythematosus or polyarteritis nodosa can also produce subarachnoid hemorrhage. These conditions sometimes give rise to aneurysmal dilatation of intracranial vessels. Rarely, an intracranial infection is associated with subarachnoid bleeding. Subarachnoid hemorrhage has been reported to occur with amphetamine abuse. Most commonly, the underlying medical condition has been diagnosed prior to the hemorrhage but the odd case report can be found in which a subarachnoid hemorrhage was the first manifestation of the disease.

Both intra- and extracerebral tumors can be a source of subarachnoid blood. Although these tumors are usually visible on an iodine-enhanced brain CT scan, they may be invisible on unenhanced brain CT scans or even on brain MR images. Similarly, hemorrhagic infarction, venous thrombosis, or hypertensive hemorrhage may manifest primarily as a subarachnoid hemorrhage originating from an undetectably small intraparenchymal source.

Certain intracranial vascular lesions which can be a source of intracranial hemorrhage are not visualized on intracranial angiography. Dural AVMs, an occasional source of subarachnoid blood, usually fill exclusively from the extracranial vasculature. The venous outflow of these lesions can frequently be seen on a contrasted brain CT scan. Cavernous angiomas usually come to clinical attention because of seizures or an intraparenchymal clot but can manifest as subarachnoid hemorrhage. Although these lesions are almost always invisible on intracerebral angiography, they have a distinct appearance on brain CT and MRI. Venous angiomas, which have a characteristic medusa head appearance on the venous phase of the angiogram, are only occasionally associated with hemorrhage. Some venous angiomas that have bled have been found at the time of pathologic examination to be associated with a small angiographically invisible AVM.[8] Mycotic aneurysms are known to disappear with time and thus may not be seen on a delayed angiogram. Finally, it must be noted that not all intracranial arteriovenous malformations are angiographically visible. Several examples of angiographically silent but histologically verified cerebral arteriovenous malformations have been reported.[13,23]

Rarely, subarachnoid hemorrhage may originate from within the spinal canal. Although ependymomas of the filum terminale are the most common spinal tumors to bleed, several other malignant and benign tumors have been reported to manifest as subarachnoid hemorrhage. Spinal AVMs and a rare spinal arterial aneurysm may present with a spinal subarachnoid hemorrhage. Classically, intraspinal hemorrhage manifests as spinal pain which may radiate into the chest, abdomen, or lower extremity. Physical examination reveals local spinal rigidity secondary to meningeal irritation and occasional evidence of local spinal cord compression or destruction. Hemorrhage within the spinal canal and especially that originating in the cervical canal may quickly spill into the cranium, causing headache, nausea, vomiting, and occasionally loss of consciousness. This last presentation is difficult to differentiate from subarachnoid hemorrhage of intracranial origin.

Even acknowledging these rare causes of subarachnoid hemorrhage, 7 to 27 percent of patients who have suffered a subarachnoid hemorrhage will demonstrate no source of that hemorrhage. It seems from reviewing the literature that improved neuroradiologic imaging techniques have reduced but not eliminated the number of patients in whom a source of hemorrhage cannot be found.

Clinical Presentation

As a group, patients who have suffered an SAH without a discernible etiology tend to present in better neurological condition than patients who show a well-defined source of their hemorrhage. In a recent cooperative study, approximately 49 percent of patients who had suffered a subarachnoid hemorrhage from an intracranial aneurysm were classified on admission as being in a Hunt-Hess clinical grade I or II. A review of the available literature reveals that 65 to 80 percent (average, 75 percent) of patients with a subarachnoid hemorrhage of undefined etiology were classified on admission as grade I or II by this same scale.

Also interesting is the high percentage of these patients who have no discernible subarachnoid blood as visible on a postictal brain CT scan. This finding varies from 30 to 62 percent in series reporting the results of CT scans on patients who have had a subarachnoid hemorrhage without discernible etiology. Because the CT scans in most series were performed at varying time intervals from the ictus, it is impossible to make a direct comparison between these results and the results of CT scanning following a ruptured aneurysm. However, the CT scan following a subarachnoid hemorrhage without discernible cause appears to be less likely to show blood than a CT scan done after a ruptured aneurysm, in which case 5 percent of scans performed on the first day and 16 percent of those performed on the third postictal day fail to demonstrate subarachnoid blood. In those cases of subarachnoid hemorrhage without a definable cause in which the postictal scan does demonstrate subarachnoid blood, several correlations have been drawn between the CT appearance and the patient's clinical course or diagnosis. First, the patient's clinical status correlates inversely with the amount of blood seen on the brain CT scan.[13] Second, patients with subarachnoid hemorrhage of undetermined etiology are less likely to have blood in the interhemispheric and sylvian fissures.[28] A third observation which has not gained universal acceptance is that blood confined to or found predominantly within the perimesencephalic cisterns indicates a subarachnoid hemorrhage without a discernible etiology (Fig. 235-1).

Etiology

The etiology of these hemorrhages remains open to speculation. In a single case, Hochberg and colleagues demonstrated a gap in the muscularis of a circumflex pontine vessel.[14] Alexander and colleagues theorized that such hemorrhages result from "leakage" of the thalamoperforating or lenticulostriate vessels,[1] but others have not found evidence to support this theory.[13] Another theory is that the hemorrhage is the manifestation of a small aneurysm or arteriovenous malformation which is either obliterated or thrombosed at the time of the hemorrhage. In support of this theory, rare cases have been reported in which an aneurysm spontaneously became thrombosed following a subarachnoid hemorrhage.[9] In addition,

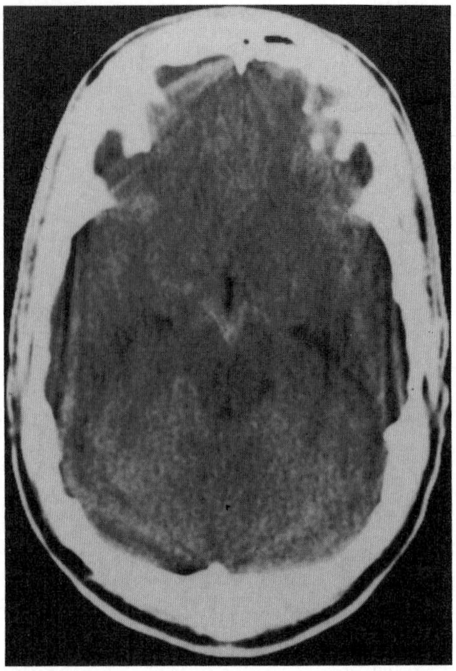

Figure 235-1 This 22-year-old patient's brain CT scan shows blood confined to the perimesencephalic cisterns. Although a basilar tip aneurysm was suspected, a detailed four-vessel cerebral angiogram failed to demonstrate the source of the hemorrhage.

several authors have demonstrated aneurysms seen on a second angiogram in a location clearly visualized on the first study.[29] However, autopsy studies of patients who had a subarachnoid hemorrhage without a defined source have only occasionally revealed an aneurysm not appreciated at the time of angiography. Most frequently, the autopsy does not reveal the source of the hemorrhage.[19] Thus, there are no conclusive data indicating that occult aneurysms are a major source of subarachnoid hemorrhage. The only identified risk factor for a subarachnoid hemorrhage of undetermined etiology is hypertension.

Further Diagnosis

When the initial brain CT scans and angiograms fail to demonstrate a source for the patient's subarachnoid hemorrhage, further diagnostic investigation should be tailored to each individual patient. The patient's history and physical examination should be reviewed, looking for evidence of an underlying medical condition that could be responsible for the hemorrhage or for a focal neurological deficit that might indicate an intraparenchymal brain lesion. The patient's CT and/or MRI study should be reviewed, looking for small areas of intraparenchymal blood or blood localized to a single cistern. The angiogram should be reviewed to be certain that all intracranial vessels have been clearly seen, that all "vessel loops" have been opened, and that no small aneurysms have been overlooked. When the patient suffers a subarachnoid hemorrhage, smaller aneurysms which would otherwise appear insignificant must be considered as a potential source of hemorrhage.

Although the spinal canal is a potential source of subarachnoid hemorrhage, most physicians only investigate the spine radiographically if the patient's history or physical examination raises the suspicion of a spinal subarachnoid hemorrhage. Additionally, the cervical spine should be investigated if the patient's CT scan shows a predominance of blood around the foramen magnum and if the intracranial angiograms are negative. Theoretically, the MRI could be helpful by imaging the upper cervical spine at the same time the brain is scanned.

The question of whether to repeat the angiography must be decided for each individual patient. The initial justification for second angiography comes from earlier studies, such as the cooperative survey conducted on cases of SAH. In one facet of this study, 13 of 72 patients with a subarachnoid hemorrhage and normal three-vessel angiography were found to have an intracranial aneurysm identified on the second study.[19] In another facet, the authors reviewed an autopsy series to verify the accuracy of cerebral angiography as performed at that time. In 23 of the 210 patients whose premortem angiograms failed to demonstrate the ruptured aneurysm, an aneurysm was identified at the time of autopsy.[23] More recent studies using refined neuroradiologic techniques indicate that repeat cerebral angiography has a lower yield. With improved radiographic technology, the cerebral vasculature can be more easily and completely surveyed. Despite these advances, two caveats persist. First, an occasional aneurysm does not fill with contrast material whether or not vasospasm is present.[11,27] Second, and probably more important, an aneurysm can be camouflaged by the surrounding vasculature; such aneurysms can often be seen in retrospect but missed when the study is first interpreted. Although these hidden aneurysms are reported to be found most often within the anterior communicating complex or middle cerebral artery trifurcation, occasionally an aneurysm of the distal internal carotid artery may be hidden.

Some authors have advocated abandoning the second angiographic study. For instance, Forster and colleagues reported that only 1 patient in 56 (1.8 percent) was found to have an aneurysm on a second study that was not seen on the first study.[11] Their patients were not studied using CT, however, and thus the denominator in this series may be inflated by patients with small intraparencymal hemorrhage- or tumor-related hemorrhages. In addition, 3 of their 94 patients who did not undergo a second angiogram had aneurysms that were only discovered in retrospect after the patient suffered a second hemorrhage.

A compilation of recent studies of patients who had suffered a subarachnoid hemorrhage and had had normal three- or four-vessel cerebral angiography reveals some trends. Table 235-1 is a comprehensive but not exhaustive list of studies published during the last 15 years and includes patients who had not had CT scanning of the brain. Among patients selected not to have a second angiogram, the rate of early rehemorrhage averages 4 percent. In patients selected to undergo a second angiogram, at least 3.6 percent will be found to have an aneurysm on repeat study.[4,11,17] This number does not include data from a report by Suzuki and colleagues that second angiography will reveal a previously undiscovered aneurysm in 22 percent of patients[29] or from the cooperative study in which 13 of 72 repeat studies revealed an unsuspected aneurysm.[19] Also excluded are the series reported by Ogasawara et al.[22] and Mehdorn et al.[18] Because the risk of a major complication following cerebral angiography is reported to be less than 0.3 percent and because the risk of death from a second hemorrhage is

TABLE 235-1 Incidence of Positive Repeat Angiogram or Rehemorrhage in Patients with Subarachnoid Hemorrhage and Negative Three- or Four-Vessel Angiography

First Author	Year of Publication	Positive Repeat Angiograms	Early Rehemorrhage (Within 6 Months)	Delayed Rehemorrhage	Number of Patients in Series	Reference
Forster	1978	1/56	†	†	56	11
Andrioli	1979	†	3.5%/year	3.5%/year	38	2
van Gijn	1980	0/11	0	†	28	30
Béguelin	1983	†	0	0.3%/year*	42	3
Ishii	1983	0/25	†	†	55	15
Eskesen	1984	†	2.2%	1.5%/year	44	10
Nishioka	1984	13/72	3.1–4.7%	0.2–0.86%/year	477	19
Alexander	1986	†	1%/year*	1%/year*	140	1
Juul	1986	2/17	3%	0	32	17
Spallone	1986	1/13	0.75%/year	0.75%/year	64	26
Biller	1987	1/11	†	†	11	4
Jain	1987	†, ‡	0	1.5%/year	43	16
Suzuki	1987	9/41§	0	0	41	29
Giombini	1988	0/7¶	7%	0.6%/year	58	13
Redfern	1988	†	0	1.3%/year	89	24
Cioffi	1989	3**	8	†	68	7
Gilbert	1990	0/24	0	0	24	12
Ogasawara	1990	8/25	0	1	25	22
Noterman	1991	0/7	3	†	59	20
Mehdorn	1992	71/143	7	1	143	18

*Approximated from graph.
**Three patients with aneurysm at postmortem examination.
†Insufficient information available.
‡One patient had a repeat subarachnoid hemorrhage 1 year later. Angiography revealed an AVM.
§One additional patient was found to have an aneurysm on an angiogram performed 9 months after the initial SAH.
¶One additional patient had a second SAH 4 years after first hemorrhage. Repeat panangiography demonstrated a small AVM.

relatively high, second angiography should not be universally abandoned, at least until more data have accumulated. At our institution, we repeat the angiogram in patients in whom vasospasm has compromised the original angiogram, in whom one portion of the cerebral vasculature is not optimally visualized, in whom there is a large amount of diffuse or a focal accumulation of subarachnoid blood as visualized by CT scans, or in whom a second subarachnoid hemorrhage has occurred. Although we have found aneurysms to be hidden in the region of the anterior communicating artery on second study, surprisingly we have also found two aneurysms on the internal carotid artery distal to the anterior choroidal artery.

Treatment

When no structural lesion is found, treatment is largely empirical. The possibility of a second hemorrhage and the fact that most patients suffer from severe headache and photophobia dictate that these patients be treated by the same methods used in the treatment of patients with an aneurysmal subarachnoid hemorrhage. Patients are kept at bed rest in a quiet environment with dim lighting for the 10 to 14 days which follow the subarachnoid hemorrhage. Patients should be kept well hydrated to ameliorate the effects of vasospasm.

Any change in neurological status during these 2 weeks must be investigated accordingly. Hydrocephalus may present as a subacute or chronic worsening in the patient's neurological status, as a chronic headache, or as the unexpected persistence of an altered mental status. The diagnosis of hydrocephalus may be confirmed by brain CT scanning. A persistent elevation in intracranial pressure is diagnosed by lumbar puncture. Persistent hydrocephalus should be treated with ventricular shunting. If the patient suffers a repeat hemorrhage, repeat radiographic examination for the source of hemorrhage is indicated. Vasospasm is generally treated by maximizing the patient's cardiac output with blood volume expansion. Although recently published data indicate that certain calcium channel blockers may be efficacious in prophylactically avoiding the complications of vasospasm, there is no indication that these agents will ameliorate established vasospasm. Whether these agents should be used in patients with extensive SAH of undetermined etiology has not yet been established.

Results

Patients who have suffered a subarachnoid hemorrhage of undetermined etiology have a markedly better prognosis than patients with a ruptured intracranial aneurysm.[25] Averaging the reported series, approximately 80 percent of patients with subarachnoid hemorrhage of undetermined etiology will have a good outcome and will return to full-time employment. Only 50 percent of patients with ruptured intracranial aneurysms fare as well. There is a positive correlation between the amount of subarachnoid blood seen on the postictal CT scan and the risk of complications such as persistent neurological deficit, vasospasm, hydrocephalus, and rehemorrhage in patients who have suffered a subarachnoid hemorrhage of undetermined etiology.[1,5] A prior history of hypertension, focal neurological deficit, and a Hunt-Hess grade greater than II prognosticate a late functional disability.[21]

Patients who are not found to have a structural lesion responsible for their initial hemorrhage rebleed at a rate of approximately 4 percent over the 3 months which follow the hemorrhage. This group then suffers rebleeding at a rate of 0.8 percent per year for at least the next 3 years.[1,17,19] This compares very favorably with the rate of rehemorrhage following the rupture of an aneurysm which are 50 percent for the first 6 months and then 3 percent per year.

Symptomatic vasospasm occurs in a small percentage of patients who have had a subarachnoid hemorrhage of undetermined etiology. The rate of symptomatic vasospasm is much lower than the 30 percent rate reported following a ruptured aneurysm.[7] The incidence of vasospasm appears to correlate with the amount of blood seen on the postictal brain CT scan and appears to be most devastating in those patients receiving antifibrinolytic agents.[17]

Persistent hydrocephalus requiring ventricular shunting occurs in approximately 3 percent of patients, although Juul and colleagues have reported a notably higher rate of 15 percent.[17] Epilepsy has occasionally been reported as a sequel to subarachnoid hemorrhage, and frequently patients report persistent headache, irritability, fatiguability, and memory loss following their hemorrhage.[1,6,21]

References

1. Alexander MSM, Dias PS, Uttley D. Spontaneous subarachnoid hemorrhage and negative cerebral panangiography: review of 140 cases. *J Neurosurg* 1986; 64:537–542.
2. Andrioli GC, Salar G, Rigobello L, et al. Subarachnoid haemorrhage of unknown etiology. *Acta Neurochir (Wien)* 1979; 48:217–221.
3. Béguelin C, Seiler R. Subarachnoid hemorrhage with normal cerebral panangiography. *Neurosurgery* 1983; 13:409–411.
4. Biller J, Toffol GJ, Kassell NF, et al. Spontaneous subarachnoid hemorrhage in young adults. *Neurosurgery* 1987; 21:664–667.
5. Boné G, Auer CM, Popsefthymiou G. Spontaneous subarachnoid hemorrhage of unknown origin—a prospective study. In Auer LM (ed): *Timing of Aneurysm Surgery.* New York: W. de Gruyter, 1985, pp 89–94.
6. Brismar J, Sundbärg G. Subarachnoid hemorrhage of unknown origin: prognosis and prognostic factors. *J Neurosurg* 1985; 63:349–354.
7. Cioffi F, Pasqualin A, Cavazzani P, et al. Subarachnoid haemorrhage of unknown origin: clinical and tomographical aspects. *Acta Neurochir (Wien)* 1989; 97:31–39.
8. Cohen HCM, Tucker WS, Humphreys RP, et al. Angiographically cryptic histologically verified cerebrovascular malformations. *Neurosurgery* 1982; 10:704–714.
9. Edner G, Forster DMC, Steiner L, et al. Spontaneous healing of intracranial aneurysms after subarachnoid hemorrhage: case report. *J Neurosurg* 1978; 48:450–454.
10. Eskesen J, Sorensen EB, Rosenorn J, et al. The prognosis in subarachnoid hemorrhage of undetermined etiology. *J Neurosurg* 1984; 61:1029–1031.
11. Forster DMC, Steiner L, Hakanson S. The value of repeat pan-angiography in cases of unexplained subarachnoid hemorrhage. *J Neurosurg* 1978; 48:712–716.
12. Gilbert JW, Lee C, Young B. Repeat cerebral pan-angiography in subarachnoid hemorrhage of unknown etiology. *Surg Neurol* 1990; 33:19–21.
13. Giombini S, Bruzzone MG, Pluchino F. Subarachnoid hemorrhage of unexplained cause. *Neurosurgery* 1988; 22:313–316.
14. Hochberg FH, Fisher CM, Roberson GH. Subarachnoid hemorrhage caused by rupture of a small superficial artery. *Neurology* 1974; 24:319–321.
15. Ishii R, Kuroki M, Tanaka R. Subarachnoid hemorrhage of unknown cause: clinical study. *Neurol Med Chir* 1983; 23:262–266.

16. Jain VK, Hedge T, Easwaran RK, et al. Benign subarachnoid haemorrhage (subarachnoid haemorrhage of unknown aetiology). *Acta Neurochir (Wien)* 1987; 86:89–92.
17. Juul R, Fredricksen TA, Ringkjøb R. Prognosis in subarachnoid hemorrhage of unknown etiology. *J Neurosurg* 1986; 64:359–362.
18. Mehdorn HM, Dietrich U, Kalff R, et al. Subarachnoid hemorrhage of unknown origin. Longterm prognosis. *Neurosurg Rev* 1992; 15:27–31.
19. Nishioka H, Torner JC, Graf CJ, et al. Cooperative study of intracranial aneurysms and subarachnoid hemorrhage: a long-term prognostic study. III. Subarachnoid hemorrhage of undetermined etiology. *Arch Neurol* 1984; 41:1147–1151.
20. Noterman J, Dewitte O, Baleriaux D, et al. Les hémorragies sous-arachnoidiennes (H.S.A.) d'étiologic inconnue: a propos de 59 cas. *Neurochirurgie* 1991; 37:383–387.
21. Oder W, Kollegger H, Zeiler K, et al. Subarachnoid hemorrhage of unknown etiology: early prognostic factors for long-term functional capacity. *J Neurosurg* 1991; 74:601–605.
22. Ogasawara K, Kayama T, Sakurai Y, et al. [Clinical analysis of etiology of spontaneous subarachnoid hemorrhage diagnosed by computed tomography.] *No To Shinkei* 1990; 42:399–404. [Japanese]
23. Perret G, Nishioka H. Cerebral angiography: diagnostic value and complications of carotid and vertebral angiography in subarachnoid hemorrhages. In Sahs AL (ed): *Intracranial Aneurysms and Subarachnoid Hemorrhage: A Cooperative Study*. Philadelphia: Lippincott, 1969, pp 109–124.
24. Redfern RM, Zygmunt S, Pickard JD, et al. The natural history of subarachnoid haemorrhage with negative angiography: a prospective study and 3 year follow up. *Br J Neurosurg* 1988; 2:33–41.
25. Shephard RH. Prognosis of spontaneous (non-traumatic) subarachnoid haemorrhage of unknown cause: a personal series 1958–1990. *Lancet* 1984; 1:777–779.
26. Spallone A, Farrante L, Palatinsky E. Subarachnoid haemorrhage of unknown origin. *Acta Neurochir (Wien)* 1986; 80:12–17.
27. Spetzler RF, Winestock D, Newton HT, et al. Disappearance and reappearance of cerebral aneurysm in serial arteriograms: case report. *J Neurosurg* 1974; 41:508–510.
28. Stober T, Emde H, Anstätt T, et al. Blood distribution in computer cranial tomograms after subarachnoid hemorrhage with and without an aneurysm on angiography. *Eur Neurol* 1985; 24:319–323.
29. Suzuki S, Kayama T, Sakurai Y, et al. Subarachnoid hemorrhage of unknown cause. *Neurosurgery* 1987; 21:310–313.
30. van Gijn J, van Dongen KJ. Computerized tomography in subarachnoid hemorrhage: difference in patients with and without aneurysm on angiography. *Neurology* 1980; 30:538–539.

236

Distal Extracranial Internal Carotid Artery Aneurysms

David G. Piepgras
Wouter I. Schievink

Aneurysms of the extracranial carotid artery have been recognized and reported in the medical literature for 300 years. Although their pathogenesis has changed through the centuries and the etiology as well as the spectrum and natural history of these lesions is now better understood than even a decade ago, they continue to be regarded as uncommon and potentially dangerous.

In a review of more than 20 years of surgical experience with 8500 aneurysms of the arterial system, McCollum and colleagues found only 37 cases of extracranial carotid artery aneurysms, over half of which were due to previous carotid endarterectomy (usually with patch angioplasty).[10] Our experience has shown that surgical treatment of extracranial internal carotid artery aneurysms comprises less than 1 percent of the surgical procedures performed on the extracranial carotid arteries. None of the 31 cases subsequently discussed in this review is related to previous carotid endarterectomy as we consider the latter to be a separate and unrelated category of lesions.

Etiology

Aneurysms of the extracranial carotid artery can best be classified under several main etiologic headings, including luetic aneurysms, mycotic aneurysms, aneurysms following endarterectomy, aneurysms due to atherosclerosis, aneurysms due to vasculitis or fibromuscular dysplasia, aneurysms associated with heritable connective tissue disorders, traumatic aneurysms, and aneurysms secondary to dissection.

Luetic aneurysms are seldom if ever encountered by neurovascular surgeons nowadays and will not be mentioned further in this discussion. Mycotic aneurysms of the extracranial carotid artery were one of the most common categories in the preantibiotic era, in part because of their association with paratonsillar abscess.[22,29] Today, mycotic aneurysms of the extracranial carotid artery constitute a very small percentage of the cases, these often related to previous neck operations, radiation therapy, and synthetic vascular grafts. When encountered, however, they usually demand urgent surgical and intensive antibiotic therapy owing to their risks for associated septicemia, mycotic embolization, and unpredictable expansion and hemorrhage.[4]

Postendarterectomy aneurysms are usually associated with faulty repair of the carotid artery and often involve a synthetic or venous patch graft.[2,10] The nature of these lesions at the carotid bifurcation region is usually self evident and the specific management of this subgroup is outside the scope of this discussion.

Although some atherosclerotic aneurysms may be saccular, atherosclerosis or vascular conditions such as cystic medial necrosis, pseudoxanthoma elasticum, Ehlers-Danlos syndrome, and Marfan syndrome, may predispose to the development of a fusiform expansion of the proximal carotid artery and bifurcation region. These aneurysms may be bilateral and associated with aneurysms of the arterial system elsewhere in the body. Most of the reports dealing with these lesions have appeared in the general surgical and peripheral vascular literature; they have been summarized in a review by Mokri and colleagues.[15]

Trauma to the neck or facial structures is also a relatively uncommon but important cause of focal extracranial carotid artery aneurysms. Cervical lacerating and penetrating injuries such as stab or gunshot wounds may produce direct carotid injury with acute hemorrhage and false aneurysm formation or delayed development of a true aneurysm. Iatrogenic carotid trauma may occur as a result of surgery such as tonsillectomy in the cervical levels or middle ear operations at the petrous level. Rarely, nonpenetrating trauma such as a blow to the neck, intraoral trauma, or mandibular fracture may result in vascular injury with true aneurysm formation which is typically delayed in its development and manifestations.

The last and nowadays seemingly the most recognized group of extracranial carotid (and especially internal carotid) artery aneurysms are those developing secondary to spontaneous or traumatic arterial dissections. For clarity, we have tried to clearly distinguish between the dissection process itself and the extraluminal outpouching (''dissecting aneurysm'' or ''aneurysm of dissection'') which may result.[12]

These aneurysms typically occur in the distal internal carotid artery near the skull base but may also develop in the mid or proximal internal carotid artery. They may have a saccular, elongated, or even fusiform appearance on angiography but rarely appear saccular on direct inspection of the artery inasmuch as the dissected vascular wall surrounds the pathologic lesion (Fig. 236-1).

The exact nature in which the aneurysms of dissection form is uncertain. Certainly it is part of the process of the intimal/medial disruption by the flowing blood with subadventitial expansion into an aneurysm, but whether this aneurysm forms at the site of the primary wall disruption, the distal site of termination of the dissection (typically near the skull base), or anywhere along the dissected segment has not been established. These aneurysms of dissection should not be designated as ''false'' or ''pseudo'' aneurysms inasmuch as their walls are formed by blood vessel elements.[12]

Mokri has found that aneurysms develop in more than one-third of the cases of spontaneous carotid dissection although nearly two-thirds of these will eventually resolve or diminish in size.[12] In a series of traumatic dissections involving 24 extracranial internal carotid arteries in 18 patients, Mokri and colleagues identified aneurysm formation in 14 of the arteries.[14] As in the spontaneous cases, the most common site of aneurysm formation was in the distal one-third of the internal carotid artery.

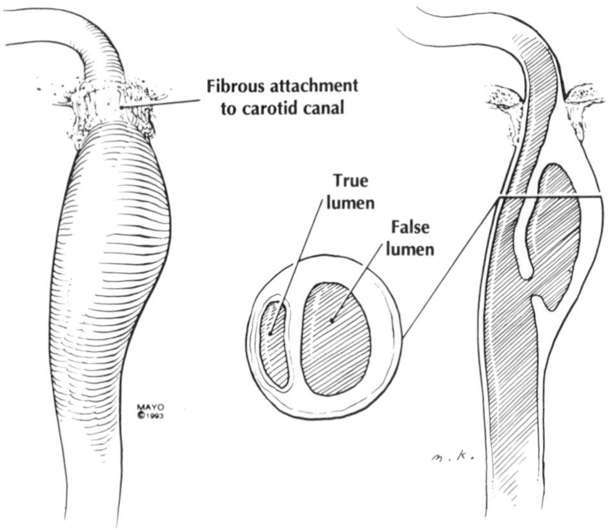

Figure 236-1 Illustration of a distal ICA dissection aneurysm near the skull base. Note that the aneurysm is, in fact, intramural and fusiform although on angiography it may give the misleading appearance of a saccular extramural aneurysm.

Clinical Features

The presenting symptoms in an ongoing series of extracranial internal carotid artery aneurysms treated on the neurovascular services at our institution since 1978 are presented in Table 236-1. Aneurysms of the extracranial internal carotid artery may present as a mass, with ischemic symptoms, or with hemorrhage, or they may remain asymptomatic. Rarely, headache or lower cranial nerve palsies may be the presenting complaint.

In his review of the reported cases of extracranial carotid aneurysm to 1925, Winslow emphasized the gravity of this condition and enumerated multiple instances of patients presenting with enlarging pulsatile pharyngeal or cervical masses, often obstructing swallowing or respiration.[29] Not surprisingly, there was often an erroneous diagnosis of paratonsillar abscess and in many instances incision of the mass was performed, resulting in fatal hemorrhage rather than release of expected pus. Spontaneous hemorrhage was also commonplace and was frequently the terminal event in patients treated conservatively. Among the patients not operated on, Winslow found a mortality of 71 percent, leading him to advocate internal carotid ligation proximal to the aneurysm as the treatment of choice. Today, hemorrhage is uncommon as a presenting symptom except for those aneurysms associated with acute penetrating trauma or infection. Undoubtedly, this change from the past experience results from earlier diagnosis and treatment as well as fewer mycotic lesions.

In modern experience with extracranial internal carotid artery aneurysm, most patients present with a cervical mass or ischemic symptoms.[2,10,15,18,30] The mass is typically pulsatile; it may or may not be painful or tender. It may project internally into the paratonsillar fossa and pharynx where it may cause dysphagia by its mere size or secondary to compression of nerves to the pharynx and tongue. Projecting laterally, the aneurysm may bulge into the cervical area below the sternocleidomastoid muscle or behind the angle of the mandible. A bruit may or may not be present over the mass.

In the past several decades, the widespread use of angiography has allowed the diagnosis of smaller extracranial carotid artery aneurysms. This advance, together with the recognition of the embolic etiology of focal cerebral and retinal ischemic events, has led to the recognition that these lesions may often present with ischemic symptoms. Of 21 patients reported by Zwolak and associates, half presented with focal neurological symptoms.[30] In series reported by Rhodes and colleagues[18] and by Busuttil and colleagues,[2] a transient ischemic attack or stroke was the presenting symptom in over two-thirds of the cases.

In our own experience with 31 cases of extracranial internal carotid artery aneurysm treated surgically since 1978, retinal or cerebral ischemia was the initial symptom in 15 (Table 236-1). These ischemic symptoms are unquestionably secondary to thrombus formation within the aneurysm and embolization of its fragments into the distal carotid circulation (Fig. 236-2). In one of our cases, an elderly patient presented after acute visual loss due to a calcific embolus to the retinal circulation, the fragment arising from old calcification in the wall of a giant cervical internal carotid artery aneurysm (Fig. 236-3). This source of a calcific embolus has been reported elsewhere as a unique presentation of an extracranial internal carotid artery aneurysm.[13]

Reports by Hodge and Lee,[8] Stringer and Kelly,[24] and Mokri and associates[12,14] have emphasized the importance of dissecting aneurysms as an embolic source. In Mokri's analysis, embolization seemed more frequent from aneurysms of traumatic dissection than from those of spontaneous dissection.[12] In this regard, it may be of importance that in follow-up of seven of the untreated traumatic dissection aneurysms, only one resolved completely; two decreased in size and four remained unchanged.[14] This contrasts with the follow-up of aneurysms secondary to spontaneous dissection of which one-third diminished in size and one-third resolved.[12]

It should be mentioned that cervical internal carotid artery aneurysms may present with ipsilateral headache and may be associated with oculosympathetic palsy. In three of our cases of

TABLE 236-1 Chief Presenting Complaint in 31 Cases of Surgically Treated Extracranial Internal Carotid Artery Aneurysm

Cause of Aneurysm	No. of Cases	Painful Cervical Mass	Cervical Mass with Dysphagia	Headache	Retinal or Cerebral Ischemia	Acute Injury	Asymptomatic
Atherosclerotic or degenerative	6	—	4	—	2	—	—
Fibromuscular disease	2	1	—	—	1	—	—
Infection	1	1	—	—	—	—	—
Traumatic dissection	11	—	—	1	8	—	2
Spontaneous dissection	9	—	—	2	3	—	4
Traumatic (GSW)	2	—	—	—	1	1	—

GSW, gunshot wound.

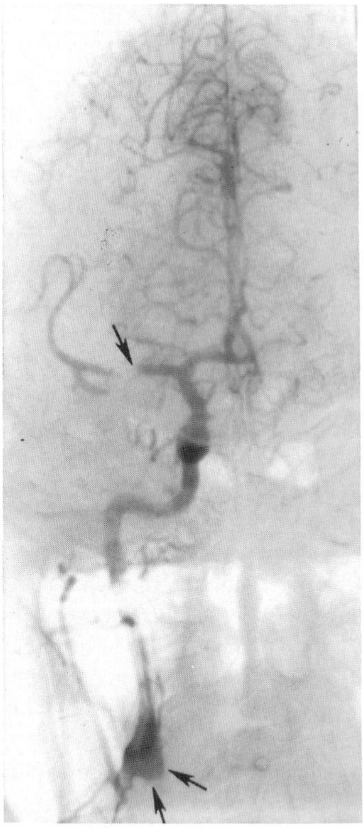

Figure 236-2 A right internal carotid artery angiogram (anteroposterior projection) demonstrating a traumatic aneurysm of the right cervical internal carotid artery (*double arrows*) and distal embolic occlusion at the middle cerebral artery bifurcation (*single arrow*). (From Sundt et al.,[25] with permission.)

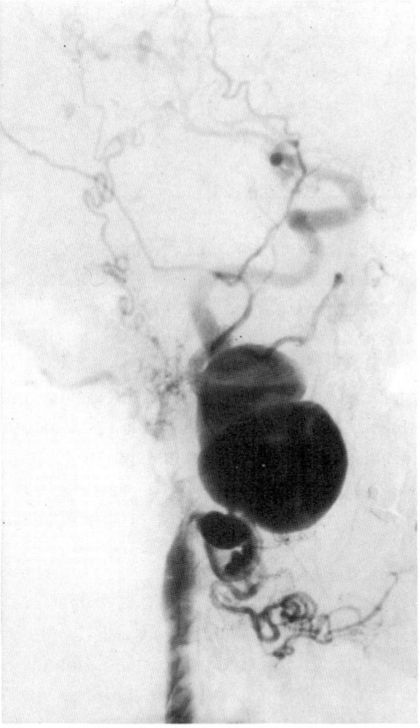

Figure 236-3 A right carotid angiogram, lateral view of the upper cervical area, showing a large atherosclerotic aneurysm of the right internal carotid artery. The wall of this aneurysm was partially calcified and was the source of a calcific retinal artery embolus. The surgical exposure and repair of this aneurysm are demonstrated in Figs. 236-8 and 236-9.

aneurysms secondary to dissection, headache was the primary complaint, although a cause and effect relationship is difficult to establish.

In addition, there are rare cases of internal carotid artery dissection which have presented with ipsilateral palsies of cranial nerves IX through XII (Collet-Sicard syndrome). Waespe and associates reported a case with bilateral internal carotid artery dissection and lower cranial nerve palsies on one side where there was also an internal carotid artery aneurysm at the skull base.[28] They attributed the nerve palsies to compression by the aneurysm mass, a conclusion supported by symptomatic improvement in their patient after internal carotid artery occlusion, but inconsistent with those cases of lower cranial nerve palsies occurring with dissection but without the presence of an aneurysm. Our experience has shown that lower cranial nerve palsies complicate spontaneous internal carotid artery dissection in approximately 5% of patients, the majority of whom do not have an associated aneurysm. Interruption of the nutrient arteries supplying these cranial nerves could also explain their involvement in internal carotid artery dissection.[16]

Imaging

As stated earlier, angiography has brought about improved detection and follow-up of extracranial as well as intracranial aneurysms and remains the gold standard for their demonstration as well as the depiction of associated or underlying vascular pathology. Only selective angiography can consistently show the subtleties of the aneurysm's relationship to the internal carotid artery, which may be redundant and ectatic. Furthermore, complete extracranial and intracranial cerebral angiography is indicated in these cases to detect evidence of other unsuspected vessel involvement (such as cases of bilateral carotid dissection or an associated intracranial aneurysm[19]) and of distal cerebral embolization, and to gain an understanding of the cerebral collateral circulation which becomes especially important if surgery is contemplated. As part of the preoperative angiographic evaluation, we have found trial balloon occlusion of the involved internal carotid artery to be helpful in certain instances to assess the patient's ability to tolerate temporary or even permanent occlusion of the internal carotid artery. This information has special significance in those cases where the aneurysm is very large or very high near or at the skull base so that intraoperative shunting may be difficult if not impossible.

The value of magnetic resonance imaging (MRI) and magnetic resonance angiography (MRA) in these lesions is only beginning to be appreciated. MRI plus MRA seems to be a sensitive test for imaging carotid dissection and is capable of elegantly demonstrating vascular anatomy and pathology including aneurysms both extracranially and intracranially.[3] At present, we believe that MRI and MRA may be useful in establishing the diagnosis and following these aneurysms but they do not supplant angiography for definition and surgical planning.

Computed tomography has been of limited usefulness in evaluating these lesions although a contrasted study may be helpful in determining the extent of an intra-aneurysmal thrombus when there is a discrepancy between the apparent size on angiography and what is appreciated on external examination.

Surgical Techniques

The surgical techniques which we have employed in the treatment of extracranial internal carotid artery aneurysms have evolved through knowledge and experience gained in our surgery for extracranial as well as intracranial vascular occlusive disease including over 3250 cases of carotid endarterectomy and over 750 cases of bypass procedures for treatment of both occlusive and aneurysmal disease. These techniques have been reported previously, including those specifically discussing the surgical management of aneurysms in the distal extracranial internal carotid artery.[20,25,26]

Intraoperative Monitoring

We consider intraoperative electroencephalography (EEG) and interval cerebral blood flow monitoring to be important adjuncts in the surgical procedure for these lesions. Together, these monitoring modalities give reliable information regarding the patient's ability to tolerate temporary occlusion of the involved internal carotid artery which may be prolonged in cases of complex, large, or distally located aneurysms. In cases where direct excision and repair is found to be difficult or involves higher risks, monitoring facilitates decisions regarding permanent carotid ligation and the need for a supplemental bypass.

Surgical Exposure of the Upper Cervical Carotid Artery

The operation is carried out under general anesthesia following the same anesthetic techniques that are employed for carotid endarterectomy. Patients are likewise positioned and the skin prepared in a similar fashion to that for carotid endarterectomy with the modifications that at least one entire leg is prepared for possible harvesting of a good-quality saphenous vein graft and the scalp is shaved in the temporal and retromastoid regions to facilitate superior extension of the incision if necessary.

The skin incision is outlined in Fig. 236-4. It proceeds along the anterior border of the sternocleidomastoid muscle to just below the ear lobe. In cases requiring high exposure of the internal carotid artery, the incision is carried forward and superiorly in the pretragal skin crease to the level of the zygoma. The superior cervical fascia is incised and the posterior border of the parotid gland exposed and elevated. The lower border of the external ear canal ("the pointer") serves as a guide in identifying the facial nerve trunk after its exit from the stylomastoid foramen between the mastoid process and the parotid gland. The branches of the facial nerve are dissected free as needed to allow mobilization of initially the superficial and then the deep portion of the parotid gland without undue stretching of the facial nerve.

Standard proximal dissection and exposure of the carotid artery and bifurcation as well as the vagus nerve is then accomplished. The hypoglossal nerve is readily identified in its familiar location below the belly of the digastric muscle and superficial to the external carotid artery. The descendens hypoglossi is divided below the hypoglossal nerve and the muscular branch of the occipital artery coagulated and divided to allow elevation of the hypoglossal

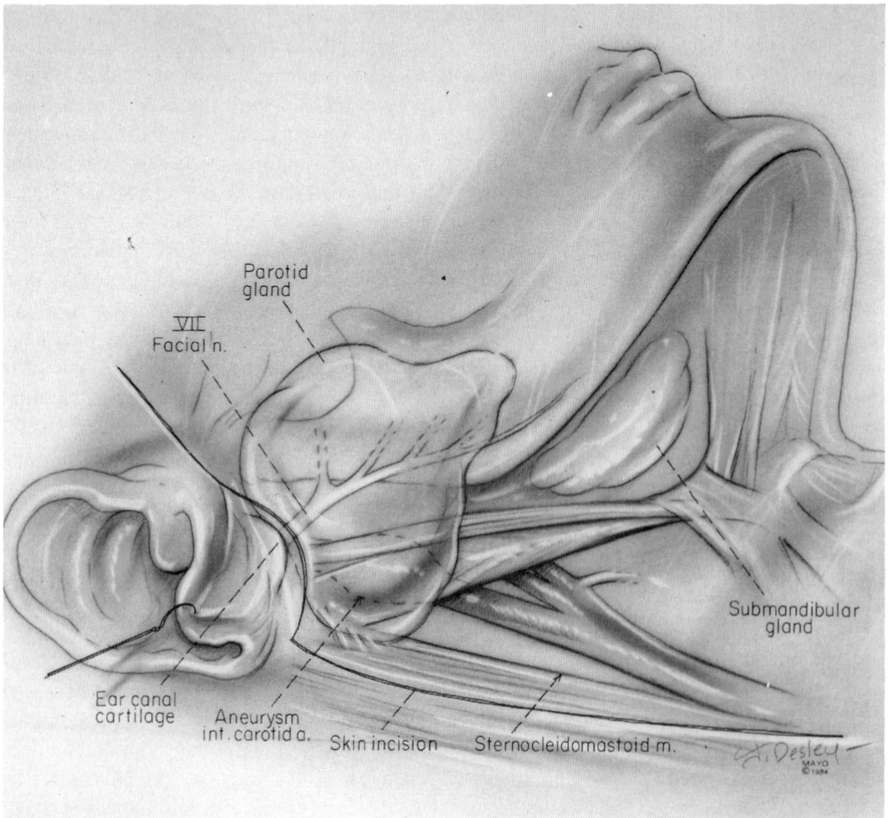

Figure 236-4 The skin incision for exposure of the distal internal carotid artery is illustrated, following the anterior border of the sternocleidomastoid muscle to the level of the mastoid process where it curves anteriorly into the pretragal skin crease. (From Sundt et al.,[25] with permission.)

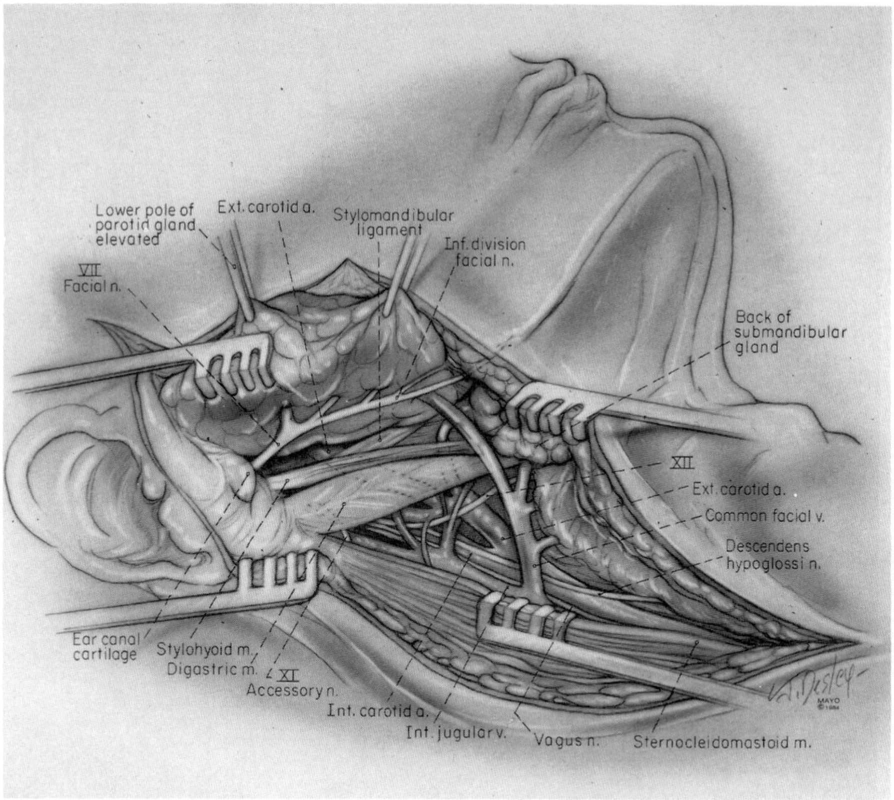

Figure 236-5 The cervical and temporoparotid fascia have been incised, the lower pole of the parotid gland elevated, and the facial nerve trunk dissected free between the "pointer" cartilage of the external ear and the parotid gland. The deep cervical veins to the jugular vein will be ligated and divided to expose the underlying carotid trunk, bifurcation, and internal carotid artery. The posterior belly of the digastric muscle, the stylohyoid muscle, and the stylomandibular ligament are exposed for transection. (From Sundt et al.,[25] with permission.)

nerve. For high exposure of the internal carotid artery, it is usually necessary to also ligate and divide the occipital artery as well as the digastric muscle near its insertion into the mastoid groove. Identification and division of the underlying stylomandibular and sphenomandibular ligaments is also essential in the exposure to allow forward displacement without dislocation or division of the mandible (Fig. 236-5). The styloid process may be excised if necessary to complete the exposure of the distal internal carotid artery to about 1 cm from its entrance into the carotid canal (Fig. 236-6). Higher exposure into the carotid canal itself can be obtained if necessary but requires a subtotal petrosectomy. It will be described later.[5,21]

Adequate distal exposure must provide not only access to the aneurysmal segment but also allow for carotid control and suture into uninvolved vessel wall. This usually requires exposure of at least an additional 1 to 2 cm of vessel above the aneurysm which for the distal-most lesions becomes difficult. Once accomplished, we proceed with baseline cerebral blood flow measurements and after heparinization of the patient, repeat the measurements with delayed occlusion of the internal carotid artery. Guided by information from preoperative temporary balloon occlusion studies, cerebral blood flow measurements, and associated changes in the EEG, if any, the surgeon can make knowledgeable decisions regarding the patient's tolerance of temporary internal carotid artery occlusion for even a prolonged period necessary for aneurysm excision and arterial reconstruction. If the EEG change is major and the reduction of cerebral blood flow profound with internal carotid artery clamping, a shunt will need to be used or, if not feasible because of the extent of the aneurysm, a preliminary bypass procedure will need to be accomplished before proceeding further. As previously stated, the patient's tolerance for prolonged temporary or even permanent ICA occlusion has been greatly facilitated by preoperative endovascular temporary balloon occlusion studies.

Aneurysm Resection and Interposition Saphenous Vein Grafting

In the majority of cases where the internal carotid artery is to be reconstructed following excision of the aneurysm, direct end-to-end anastomosis of the internal carotid artery segments is not possible and placement of an interposed saphenous vein segment is the most desirable reconstruction technique. Meticulous care must be given to harvesting a saphenous vein segment of adequate length and diameter. We have found it helpful to overlay the vein in situ with a papaverine-solution soaked cottonoid and, after its removal, to dilate the vein segment with cold heparinized saline solution at controlled distention pressure.[26,27]

The internal carotid artery is then clipped proximally and distally using weakened aneurysm clips or temporary vascular clips and the aneurysm is excised. If distal exposure of the internal carotid artery is not adequate for cross clipping, back bleeding from the internal carotid artery may be controlled with a Fogarty catheter passed through the vein segment and inflated in the carotid artery inside the carotid canal. The distal anastomosis is always performed first after spatulating both the vein and artery. Suturing is best accomplished under the operative microscope utilizing interrupted 7-0 or 8-0 nylon (Ethilon; Ethicon, Inc., Somerville, NJ) sutures and microvascular techniques. The proximal anastomosis may be accomplished in a similar fashion with 6-0 polypropylene (Prolene; Ethicon, Inc.) sutures (Fig. 236-7). The artery is thoroughly flushed before reestablishing flow through the graft. Following reconstruction of the internal carotid artery it is advisable to assess flow through the graft with an electromagnetic flow meter.

In some cases where the aneurysm is densely adherent to the adjacent tissues and especially to the cranial nerves, it is best to perform the necessary thrombectomy of the sac to allow placement

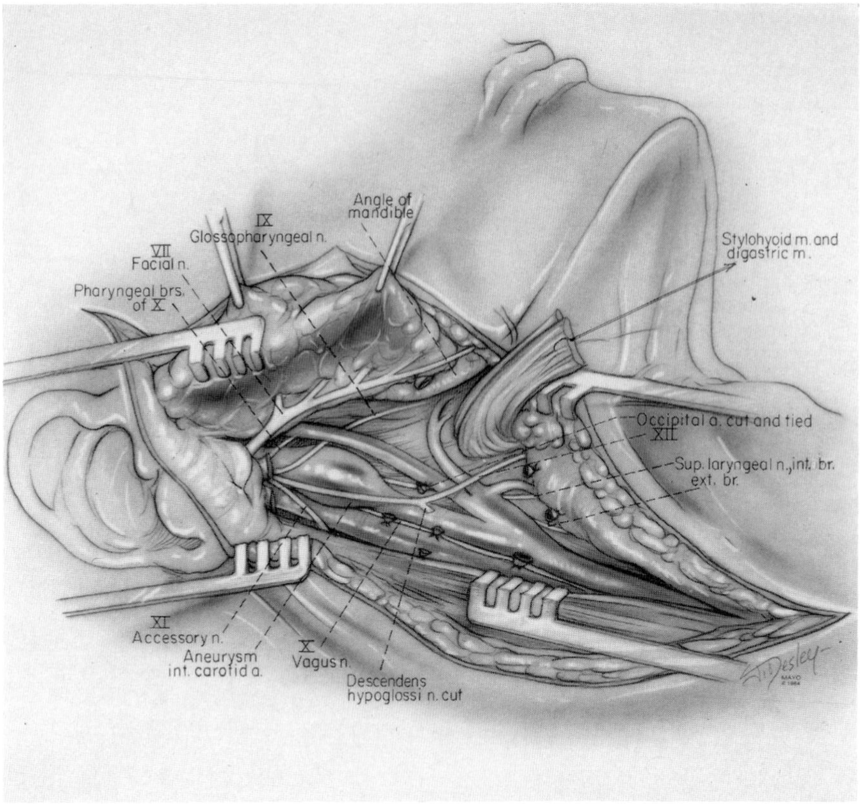

Figure 236-6 Division of the descendens hypoglossi nerve and ligation and division of the occipital artery allow elevation of the hypoglossal nerve. The stylohyoid and digastric muscles are divided and elevated to expose the underlying internal carotid artery and aneurysm. The styloid process has been resected and the stylomandibular ligament divided to facilitate anterior displacement of the mandible. (From Sundt et al.,[25] with permission.)

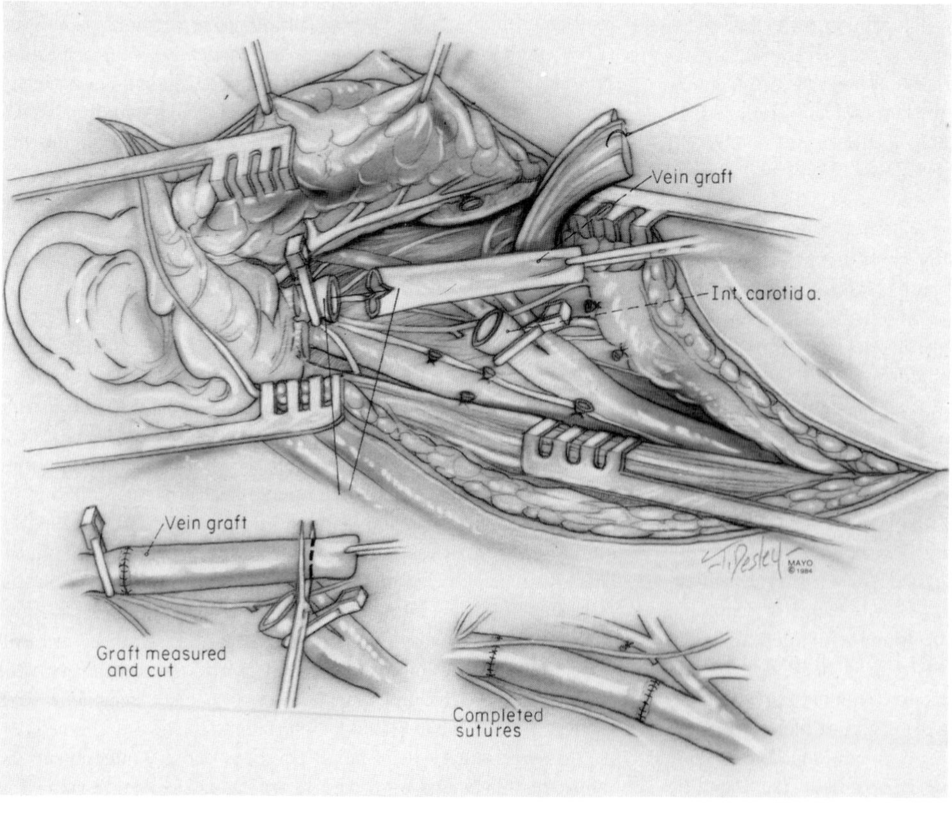

Figure 236-7 After systemic heparinization of the patient, the internal carotid artery has been temporarily occluded with low-pressure vascular clips and the aneurysm excised. The distal anastomosis is made first. "Fish-mouth" incisions are made in both the internal carotid and saphenous vein ends and suturing with 7-0 or 8-0 monofilament nylon sutures is performed under the operative microscope. The proximal anastomosis is usually made with 6-0 Prolene sutures utilizing a similar "fish-mouth" cut in both artery and vein as distally. (From Sundt et al.,[25] with permission.)

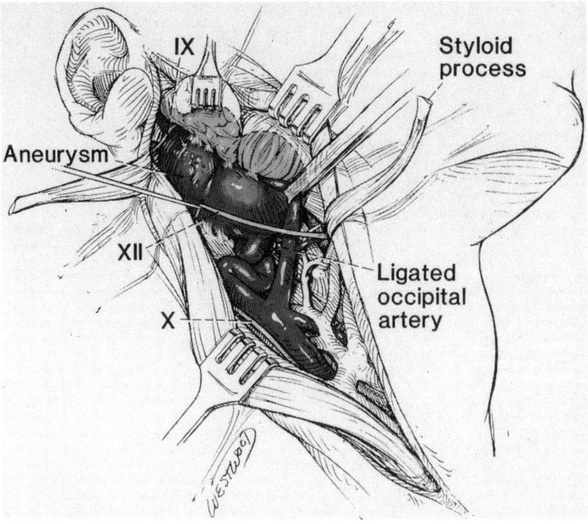

Figure 236-8 Exposure of the large atherosclerotic aneurysm demonstrated in the angiogram of Fig. 236-3. In this case the glossopharyngeal nerve (IX) was sacrificed to facilitate distal exposure of the aneurysm and internal carotid artery. (From Mokri et al.,[15] with permission.)

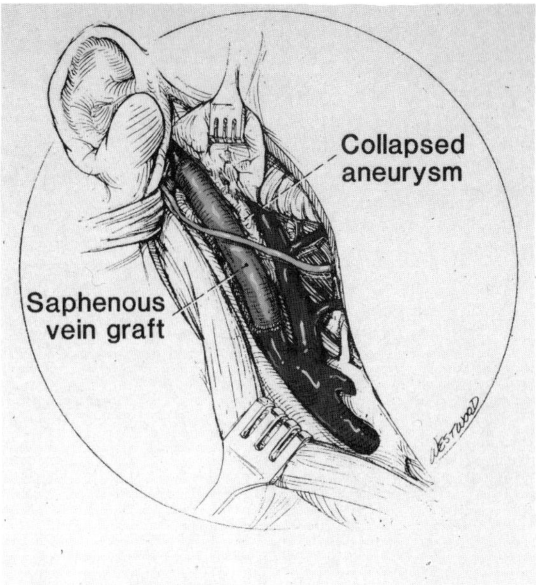

Figure 236-9 Because of the adherence of the aneurysm sac to the cervical structures, it was not excised but simply opened and the thrombus removed to allow placement of the saphenous vein graft. (From Mokri et al.,[15] with permission.)

of the interposition graft but to leave the walls of the aneurysm in place (Figs. 236-8 and 236-9). With very large and partially thrombosed aneurysmal sacs, it may be difficult to identify the internal carotid artery distal to the aneurysm until the sac has been opened and evacuated, a maneuver which carries the risk of major retrograde hemorrhage until the distal segment is controlled.

End-to-End Anastomosis

In certain patients, the pathologic process which results in aneurysm formation also is accompanied by elongation of the internal carotid artery so that the aneurysm may be simply resected and the proximal and distal ends of the internal carotid artery directly anastomosed. The two ends of the artery are opened with ''fishmouth'' cuts and are anastomosed under magnification with interrupted Prolene sutures. An alternative technique which could be employed if there is not ample internal carotid artery length but a large external carotid artery trunk is a direct end-to-end anastomosis between the external carotid artery proximally and the internal carotid artery distally after ligating the external carotid artery branches.[18] We have not used this repair for reconstruction of the ICA in our series of distal aneurysm cases.

Cervical-Cranial Internal Carotid Artery Reconstruction

In cases of very distal carotid aneurysms such as those typically associated with dissection and located immediately at the skull base or even within the proximal carotid canal (Fig. 236-10), excision of the aneurysm and reconstruction of the ICA requires exposure of the ICA in the petrous canal.[17] Basically two exposures are possible and selection of the appropriate technique must depend on the anatomy of the lesion to be treated, the preferences of the surgeons, and an understanding of the patient regarding the magnitude and side effects of the procedure.

For aneurysms immediately at or just below the skull base, the artery can be controlled and reconstructed as described by Fisch and colleagues[5] and Sekhar and colleagues.[21] This exposure is obtained through an extended incision behind the ear with division of the external auditory canal and mobilization of the mandible anteriorly. The participation of an otologic surgeon is usually advisable to then accomplish a partial petrosectomy to transpose the facial nerve out of its canal to the level of the geniculate ganglion. This may require sacrifice of the middle ear ossicles and at a minimum the exposure will deprive the patient of ipsilateral conductive hearing. The tympanic and mastoid portions of the petrous bone overlying the ICA can then be resected to provide exposure up to the proximal curve of the ICA as it enters the horizontal segment of the carotid canal. This exposure is illustrated in Fig. 236-11. The artery must be mobilized out of the proximal canal which also requires dissection of the fibrous ring which surrounds the artery immediately at its entrance into the canal. With proximal and distal control of the internal carotid artery thus achieved, the artery may be divided at healthy segments above and below the aneurysm and a vein graft interposed as previously described.

An alternative approach for more distal exposure of the ICA can be accomplished in its horizontal segment as first described by Glasscock.[7] Bypass into this segment was utilized initially by Fisch[5] and has subsequently been described and modified by others.[6,11,21] The cranial part of the procedure is entirely extradural and involves a small low temporal craniotomy that permits identification of the foramen spinosum and foramen ovale. After the middle meningeal artery and greater superficial petrosal nerve are divided, the floor of the middle fossa posterior to the foramen ovale and medial to the foramen spinosum is drilled off to expose the horizontal segment of the petrous portion of the internal carotid artery. A saphenous vein graft is anastomosed to this segment of the artery which is isolated over a length of approximately 1 to 2 cm between a permanent proximal clip and a temporary distal clip.

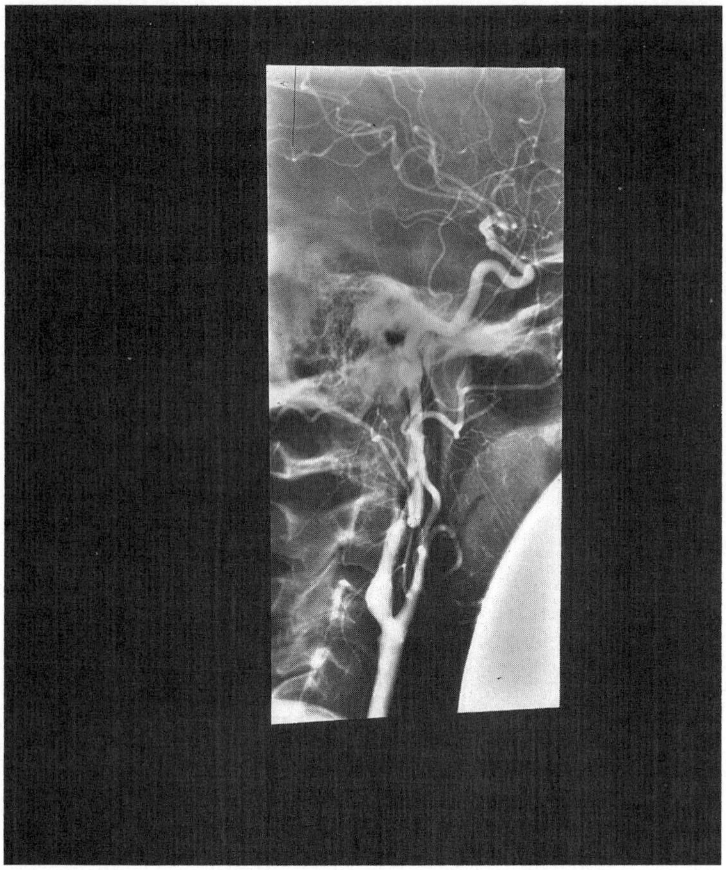

Figure 236-10 Lateral angiogram demonstrating a complex dissection of the ICA with an associated aneurysm at the entrance into the petrous carotid canal. This dissection and associated aneurysm were a source of recurring symptoms and were managed by an interposition sapheous vein graft from the cervical ICA to the horizontal petrous ICA in Glasscock's triangle.

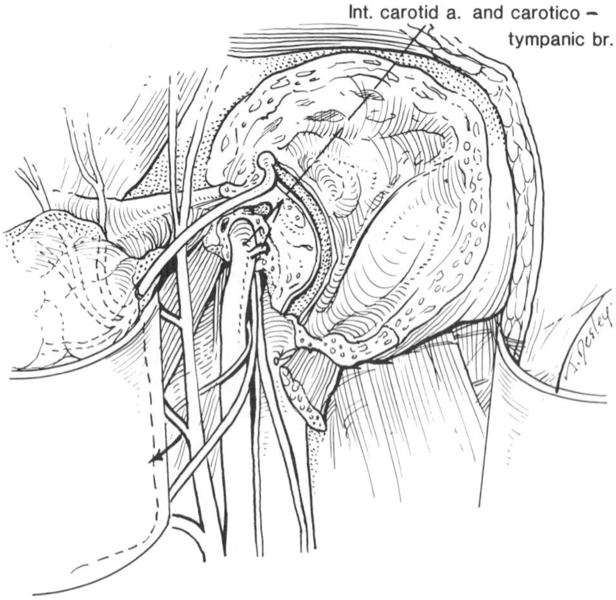

Figure 236-11 Illustration of the completed dissection after partial petrosectomy for exposure and control of the ICA at the skull base. The facial nerve has been mobilized from its canal and retracted forward with the parotid gland and mandible.

This anastomosis may be accomplished in an end-to-end or end-to-side fashion depending on the extent of the exposure. The graft is then tunneled subcutaneously, superficial to the zygomatic arch, into a previously fashioned cervical wound and is anastomosed end-to-end to the proximal internal carotid artery (Fig. 236-12). For high cervical or skull base ICA lesions there is a theoretical preference for this bypass procedure over the cervical-to-supraclinoid internal carotid artery bypass because the latter technique carries some increased risks related to an intradural exposure of the ICA as well as increased risk for distal thromboembolism should the anastomosis occlude. In our limited experience, however, the microsuture of the distal anastomosis may be easier for the intracranial than the intrapetrous ICA due to more space for vessel control and often a better vessel wall for anastomosis.

Internal Carotid Artery Occlusion and Bypass

Certain cases of extracranial internal carotid artery aneurysm, because of either their extent, an underlying infection, or the emergent nature of the situation, particularly in the face of an unstable patient, may require sacrifice of the internal carotid artery. If adequate collateral circulation can be guaranteed, either by existing collaterals or by the construction of a bypass, proximal occlusion of the internal carotid artery or trapping of the aneurysm may constitute the best therapeutic alternatives, as discussed by Hori and colleagues.[9] Widely available devices such as transvascular detachable balloons and coils have been used to control surgically inaccessible aneurysms or to prevent life-threatening hemorrhage, and their application to situations such as these should be kept in mind.[1]

Mycotic Aneurysms

In instances of mycotic aneurysm, carotid ligation, extensive debridement, and intensive preoperative and postoperative antibiotic therapy constitute the safest alternative, but only if adequate cerebral collateral blood flow can be assured. If not, reconstruction of the internal carotid artery with an interposed saphenous vein graft may be feasible but it is mandatory that the anastomoses be accomplished in an uncontaminated field and that the graft be placed in an extra-anatomic route with muscle layers protecting the graft from the areas of infection.[4] Spetzler and associates reported an innovative bypass with a long saphenous vein graft from the contralateral temporal artery to the ipsilateral middle cerebral artery; life-saving sacrifice of the ipsilateral infected carotid artery and associated aneurysm was then possible without cerebral ischemia.[23] We have used a variation of this technique in one case with an extra long vein graft from the contralateral external carotid artery to the intracranial middle cerebral artery on the involved side.

Complications and Results

The indications for surgery in the entire spectrum of extracranial internal carotid artery aneurysms have yet to be defined, but it seems clear that in most cases of symptomatic aneurysm, particularly when it is embolizing or enlarging, and always when it is infected, elimination of the aneurysm should be considered and the risk/benefit ratio assessed as carefully as possible. Surgery should also be considered for asymptomatic aneurysms caused by dissection to prevent future thromboembolic events, especially in young patients with aneurysms of traumatic dissection.

The major risks associated with surgical treatment of these aneurysms are cerebral ischemia, especially stroke, and cranial nerve injury causing permanent dysphagia and voice impairment. In the representative reports of modern surgical therapy of these lesions, the incidence of permanent ischemic neurological deficits ranges from 5 to 15 percent and that of major cranial nerve deficits is approximately 5 percent; the mortality rate ranges from 0 to 7 percent.[2,10,18,30]

Our complications from the surgical treatment of 31 cases of distal extracranial internal carotid artery aneurysm are summarized

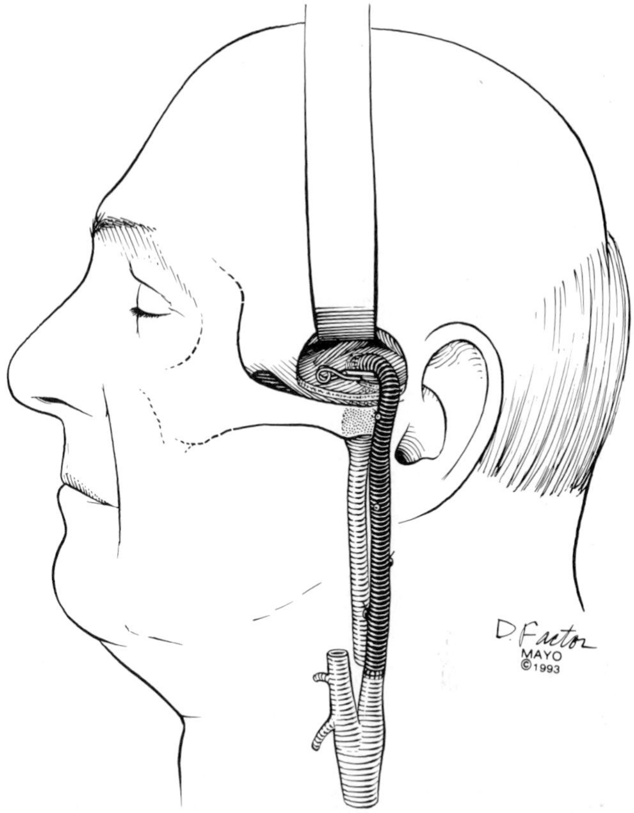

Figure 236-12 Illustration of the completed interposition vein graft from the cervical ICA to the petrous (horizontal segment) ICA.

in Table 236-2. We believe that our use of preoperative trial balloon occlusion studies and intraoperative monitoring with continuous EEG and serial cerebral blood flow assessment has been instrumental in reducing postoperative complications by identifying patients at risk for hemodynamic ischemia and allowing meticulous, unhurried vascular repair. One case of cerebral ischemia (3 percent) resulted because of embolization from the distal anastomosis site and was treated with anticoagulation, but only after endotracheal intubation to protect the airway in case of wound swelling. Follow-up evaluation including angiography after 3 months showed a satisfactory result in this case.

In seven patients treated with carotid ligation, there were no ischemic complications, protection against ischemia being assured

TABLE 236-2 Complications Related to Operative Procedure in 31 Cases of Extracranial Internal Carotid Aneurysm

Type of Procedure	No. of Cases	Ischemic Complications	Transient Dysphagia	Permanent Dysphagia
Resection of aneurysm, end-to-end ICA anastomosis	6	0	0	0
Resection of aneurysm, interposition vein graft	11	1	6	1
ICA ligation	7	0	1	0
Aneurysm clipping	1	0	1	0
STA-MCA bypass	3	0	0	0
ICA-ICA bypass	3	0	0	0

ICA, internal carotid artery; STA-MCA, superficial temporal artery-middle cerebral artery.

by the monitoring methods employed. Delayed ischemia due to a propagating thrombus and/or embolization is a potential threat in patients for whom heparin anticoagulation is administered for several days after occlusion; in selected cases, this is followed by a short course of oral anticoagulant therapy. In all patients with interposition saphenous vein grafts, long-term antiplatelet therapy with aspirin and dipyridamole is advised.

Avoidance of cranial nerve injury, especially to the ninth, tenth, and twelfth cranial nerves, may be difficult in certain of these aneurysms which are large or densely scarred to the adjacent structures. The glossopharyngeal nerve may be sacrificed without adverse effects, but injury to the vagus nerve and its pharyngeal branches may be particularly problematic. Permanent dysphagia occurred in one of our patients and necessitated a gastrostomy for nutrition. Particularly in the high carotid aneurysm where pathologic tissue and cranial nerves are in such close approximation, patients need to be well informed regarding this possible complication. Peripheral facial nerve palsies are almost invariably seen following a high cervical exposure, but these resolve over a 1- to 3-month period.

Hearing loss developed in both of our patients who underwent a cervical-to-petrous internal carotid artery bypass. Conductive hearing loss of varying degrees may occur due to injury to the tensor tympani muscle or eustachian tube, or due to hemotympanum but the occurrence of a complete hearing loss implies direct cochlear injury.

References

1. Braun IF, Battey PM, Fulenwider JT, et al. Transcatheter carotid occlusion: an alternative to the surgical treatment of cervical carotid aneurysms. *J Vasc Surg* 1986; 4:299–302.
2. Busuttil RW, Davidson RK, Foley KT, et al. Selective management of extracranial carotid arterial aneurysms. *Am J Surg* 1980; 140:85–91.
3. Dumoulin CL, Hart HR Jr. Magnetic resonance angiography. *Radiology* 1986; 161:717–720.
4. Ferguson LJ, Fell G, Buxton B, et al. Mycotic cervical carotid aneurysm. *Br J Surg* 1983; 70:245.
5. Fisch UP, Oldring DJ, Senning A. Surgical therapy of internal carotid artery lesions of the skull base and temporal bone. *Otolaryngol Head Neck Surg* 1980; 88:548–554.
6. Fitzpatrick BC, Spetzler RF, Ballard JL, et al. Cervical-to-petrous internal carotid artery bypass procedure. Technical note. *J Neurosurg* 1993; 79:138–141.
7. Glasscock ME III. Exposure of the intra-petrous portion of the carotid artery. In Hamberger C-A, Wërsäll J (eds): *Disorders of the Skull Base Region. Proceedings of the Tenth Nobel Symposium, Stockholm 1968.* New York: John Wiley & Sons, 1969, pp 135–143.
8. Hodge CJ Jr, Lee SH. Spontaneous dissecting cervical carotid artery aneurysm. *Neurosurgery* 1982; 10:93–95.
9. Hori T, Terao H, Eguchi T, et al. Huge intraoral aneurysm presenting with dysphagia and dyspnea successfully treated by STA-MCA anastomosis and ICA ligation: case report. *J Neurosurg* 1981; 55:625–628.
10. McCollum CH, Wheeler WG, Noon GP, et al. Aneurysms of the extracranial carotid artery: twenty-one years' experience. *Am J Surg* 1979; 137:196–200.
11. Miyazaki S, Fukushima T, Fujimaki T. Resection of high-cervical paraganglioma with cervical-to-petrous internal carotid artery saphenous vein bypass. Report of two cases. *J Neurosurg* 1990; 73:141–146.
12. Mokri B. Dissections of cervical and cephalic arteries. In Sundt TM Jr (ed): *Occlusive Cerebrovascular Disease: Diagnosis and Surgical Management.* Philadelphia: Saunders, 1987, pp 38–59.
13. Mokri B, Piepgras DG. Cervical internal carotid artery aneurysm with calcific embolism to the retina. *Neurology* 1981; 31:211–214.
14. Mokri B, Piepgras DG, Houser OW. Traumatic dissections of the extracranial internal carotid artery. *J Neurosurg* 1988; 68:189–197.
15. Mokri B, Piepgras DG, Sundt TM Jr, et al. Extracranial internal carotid artery aneurysms. *Mayo Clin Proc* 1982; 57:310–321.
16. Mokri B, Schievink WI, Olsen KD, et al. Spontaneous dissection of the cervical internal carotid artery. Presentation with lower cranial nerve palsies. *Arch Otolaryngol Head Neck Surg* 1992; 118:431–435.
17. Paullus WS, Pait TG, Rhoton AL Jr. Microsurgical exposure of the petrous portion of the carotid artery. *J Neurosurg* 1977; 47:713–726.
18. Rhodes EL, Stanley JC, Hoffman GL, et al. Aneurysms of extracranial carotid arteries. *Arch Surg* 1976; 111:339–343.
19. Schievink WI, Mokri B, Piepgras DG. Angiographic frequency of saccular intracranial aneurysms in spontaneous cervical artery dissection. *J Neurosurg* 1992; 76:62–66.
20. Schievink WI, Piepgras DG, McCaffrey TV, Mokri BM. Surgical treatment of extracranial internal carotid artery dissecting aneurysms *Neurosurgery* 1994; 35:809–816.
21. Sekhar LN, Schramm VL Jr, Jones NF, et al. Operative exposure and management of the petrous and upper cervical internal carotid artery. *Neurosurgery* 1986; 19:967–982.
22. Shipley AM, Winslow N, Walker WW. Aneurysm in the cervical portion of the internal carotid artery: an analytical study of the cases recorded in the literature between August 1, 1925, and July 31, 1936. *Ann Surg* 1937; 105:673–699.
23. Spetzler RF, Roski RA, Rhodes RS, et al. The "bonnet bypass": a case report. *J Neurosurg* 1980; 53:707–709.
24. Stringer WL, Kelly DL Jr. Traumatic dissection of the extracranial internal carotid artery. *Neurosurgery* 1980; 6:123–130.
25. Sundt TM Jr, Pearson BW, Piepgras DG, et al. Surgical management of aneurysms of the distal extracranial internal carotid artery. *J Neurosurg* 1986; 64:169–182.
26. Sundt TM Jr, Piepgras DG. Extracranial internal carotid aneurysms. In Sundt TM Jr (ed): *Occlusive Cerebrovascular Disease: Diagnosis and Surgical Management.* Philadelphia: Saunders, 1987, pp 303–314.
27. Sundt TM Jr, Piepgras DG, Marsh WR, et al. Saphenous vein bypass grafts for giant aneurysms and intracranial occlusive disease. *J Neurosurg* 1986; 65:439–450.
28. Waespe W, Niesper J, Imhof HG, et al. Lower cranial nerve palsies due to internal carotid dissection. *Stroke* 1988; 19:1561–1564.
29. Winslow N. Extracranial aneurysm of the internal carotid artery: history and analysis of the cases registered up to Aug. 1, 1925. *Arch Surg* 1926; 13:689–729.
30. Zwolak RM, Whitehouse WM Jr, Knake JE, et al. Atherosclerotic extracranial carotid artery aneurysms. *J Vasc Surg* 1984; 1:415–422.

237

Management of Intracranial Aneurysms and Arteriovenous Malformations during Pregnancy

Bryce Weir
R. Loch Macdonald

The catastrophe of intracranial bleeding poses an extraordinary challenge to the neurosurgeon at any time but the situation becomes even more poignant when the victim is a female with child or a just-delivered mother. This tragic event is fortunately rare and it is possible for busy obstetricians and neurosurgeons to pass their entire professional lives without encountering such a case. The difficulty which follows from this, however, is that the knowledge of any individual surgeon or center is necessarily limited and it is impossible to provide absolutely firm guidelines for the management of such cases from a study of past experience.

Incidence

In Fox's review of the world aneurysm literature up to 1979, there were 112 patients with 124 aneurysms who were either pregnant or in the immediate postpartum period.[9] The location of these aneurysms corresponded to the usual distribution in the nonpregnant female population. Only 7 percent of the patients were reported to have multiple aneurysms, which was attributed to the relative youthfulness of this subgroup of patients or the fact that inadequate investigation had frequently been performed. The mean month of aneurysm rupture was the seventh and the mode was the eighth. In 2 percent of patients, the aneurysm ruptured during labor and in 13 percent, in the postpartum period.

In four published papers on the frequency of subarachnoid hemorrhage (SAH) among pregnant women between the years 1945 and 1967, there were 46 intracranial hemorrhages in 245,914 pregnancies. This indicates a frequency of bleeding of 1 in 5345. This figure is probably fallaciously high and may have been influenced by the presence of well-known vascular surgeons or the chance occurrence of clusters of cases which resulted in their publication.

In a 1985 study of a well-defined population in Rochester, Minnesota, there were no instances of maternal intracranial hemorrhage in 26,098 live births.[36] In five large series of fatal SAH from aneurysms during pregnancy, the incidence ranged between 1/32,564 and 1/71,000 live births.[34] Aneurysm or arteriovenous malformation (AVM) accounted for 4.4 percent of all maternal deaths in Minnesota between 1950 and 1973. The incidence was 1 maternal death from SAH per 47,000 live births. Three deaths were associated with labor. Among 72 maternal deaths with intracranial bleeding, 51 percent were thought to be caused by a ruptured aneurysm or AVM and 35 percent were from eclampsia. Twenty-nine patients with SAH were autopsied; an aneurysm was found in 52 percent and an AVM in 34 percent. In 14 percent, the cause was not determined.[2] Between 1956 and 1965, one neurological institute in Scotland had 48 referred cases of stroke in women who were pregnant or in the puerperium; in 11 the stroke was due to hemorrhage.[6]

In the District of Columbia between 1950 and 1959, 6 percent of 131 maternal deaths were from a ruptured cerebral aneurysm.[10] In Chicago between 1956 and 1960, ruptured aneurysms accounted for 8 of 101 fatalities of patients who had nonobstetric causes of maternal death; at the same time, 19 patients died of toxemia of pregnancy.[17] In contrast, in only 2 of 149 maternal deaths reviewed by Heidrich and Niedner did the patient have symptoms of SAH.[12] Of 161 nonobstetric deaths in Michigan between 1960 and 1968, cerebral bleeding accounted for 22 maternal deaths (1 fatal SAH per 71,000 births).[32]

In the 52 cases of intracranial bleeding reviewed by Amias from the 1950s and 1960s in London, England, there were 21 aneurysm, 19 AVM, and 12 unknown etiology cases.[1] Forty of the hemorrhages occurred during pregnancy and 12 during the puerperium. Another British center reported 11 AVMs (history of 24 hemorrhages) and 14 aneurysms (history of 20 hemorrhages) shortly thereafter.[28] During similar time periods, Yaşargil operated on 7 aneurysm and 3 AVM patients who were pregnant.[38,39] Combining these figures suggests that the ratio of aneurysm to AVM as the cause of intracranial bleeding associated with pregnancy is 1.3 : 1.

The first cooperative study on intracranial aneurysms and SAH had 6368 cases.[29] Aneurysms comprised 51 percent and AVMs 8 percent of this series. The ratio of aneurysm to AVM was 6.4 : 1. The ratio of bleeding aneurysm to bleeding AVM was 8.4 : 1; the ratio of unruptured aneurysm to unruptured AVM was much lower at 2 : 1. The peak frequency of SAH for aneurysms occurred at 50 to 54 years of age, compared to the peak frequency of AVM SAH of 11 to 24 years. For the childbearing age (15 to 44 years), the ruptured aneurysms comprised 19 percent of all ruptured aneurysms. In comparison, the cases of ruptured AVM in the childbearing age were a much higher percentage of all ruptured AVMs, 60 percent. Aneurysms were more likely to present with SAH than AVMs. Intracranial aneurysms with SAH made up 46 percent of the total cases whereas AVMs with SAH made up only 6 percent of such total registered cases. Intracranial aneurysms without SAH were 5 percent of registered cases, and AVMs without SAH were 2 percent. The chance of a first SAH in females of childbearing age (15 to 44 years) being due to an aneurysm was 80 percent and being due to an AVM was 20 percent. The fact that in most series of SAH analyzed in pregnant females, the ratio of aneurysm to AVM is not 4 : 1 but closer to 1.3 : 1 suggests that the pregnant state is a greater stimulus to SAH from AVM than from aneurysm. Based on the first cooperative study, in females (pregnant and nonpregnant) 10 to 19 years of age having a first SAH, the chance of AVM is 2 : 1 compared to the chance of an aneurysm. For 20- to

29-year-old females, AVM and aneurysm have about an equal chance of being the cause of a first SAH, and for 30- to 34-year-old females, the ratio of aneurysm to AVM is 3.5 : 1.

Between 1974 and 1978 in the United States, there were 2067 pregnancies not associated with abortive outcomes in which the pregnant female died.[15] The causes of death were: embolism, 20 percent; hypertensive disease, 17 percent; obstetric hemorrhage, 13 percent; obstetric infection, 8 percent; and cerebral vascular accidents, 4 percent. In the last category, somewhat surprisingly 55 cases were postpartum; 19 were ante- or intrapartum, and 33 were unspecified.

Maternal mortality in the United States fell from 673/100,000 live births in 1932 to 7.8/100,000 live births in 1979.[11] Because many of the other causes of maternal mortality are steadily falling, it is likely that intracranial bleeding from aneurysm and AVM will become a relatively more significant cause of maternal mortality.

Natural History of Intracranial Aneurysms and Arteriovenous Malformations

Intracranial aneurysms commonly present with SAH. Tumor-like symptoms are uncommon. An unruptured incidental aneurysm has an unknown risk of rupture per year but is probably under 1 percent. The chance of rerupture of a previously ruptured but untreated aneurysm may be 2 to 3 percent per year after the first year. About 10 to 15 percent of patients with aneurysmal rupture die instantly. Without definitive therapy about 65 percent of patients are dead within 1 year. Rebleeding occurs during the first month in 10 to 20 percent of cases of ruptured aneurysm. The mortality rate increases sharply with each bleeding episode.[34]

Cerebral AVMs usually present with seizures or hemorrhage. Several studies found a 2 to 3 percent annual incidence of rupture, with a risk of death of about 1 percent per year. Follow-up data on 160 unoperated AVMs for a mean of 23.7 years found that major bleeding occurred in 4 percent per year, with mortality in 1 percent per year.[23] The mortality rate from the first hemorrhage is about 10 percent, 13 percent from a second, and roughly 20 percent from subsequent ones. Survivors from a hemorrhage have a 6 percent chance of rebleeding during the first year thereafter and a 2 to 3 percent annual risk after that.[37] At least these same risks are likely to apply in the pregnant as in the nonpregnant state.

Hemodynamics of Pregnancy and Pathophysiology of Hemorrhage

Blood volume increases in early pregnancy, peaks at 32 weeks, and remains level until term. The increase averages approximately 1600 ml or 50 percent above prepregnancy levels. It is greater in multigravidas and with multiple fetal pregnancies. The increase in plasma is 1300 ml and RBC mass, 400 ml. There is a dilution anemia. Vascular resistance decreases. Systolic blood pressure falls until midpregnancy (a decrease of 10 to 15 mmHg) and returns to normal around term; diastolic pressure falls more (a decrease of 20 to 25 mmHg). Cardiac output in the lateral recumbent position increases 30 to 50 percent over prepregnancy values to 4–4.5 to 6 liters/min; the greatest increase is in the first trimester and it peaks at about 20 to 24 weeks. The increase is mainly due to an increase in stroke volume. In late pregnancy, stroke volume declines but heart rate increases. During labor, cardiac output increases with each contraction, as does blood pressure. Cerebrospinal fluid pressure is also markedly elevated during uterine contraction, depending on the degree of analgesia and sedation, and whether the patient is pushing.[20] The rapid and sometimes large fluctuations in blood pressure and intracranial pressure make it difficult to know exactly what happens to transmural pressure across aneurysms or AVMs during pregnancy and labor and delivery, but it is perhaps surprising that intracranial catastrophes are not more common. Following delivery, cardiac output is increased, the heart slows, and an increased stroke volume is present. Blood volume decreases 10 percent in the first postpartum day and keeps declining over the subsequent few days. There is a relative hypercoagulable state, associated with a marked increase in fibrinogen and several other clotting factors. Several hormones increase substantially during pregnancy, including estrogen, progesterone, human chorionic gonadotropin, and relaxin, some of which are known to exert effects on connective tissue and the vasculature. The hematocrit falls from 37 to 48 percent to 32 to 42 percent in pregnancy.[11]

More than half of all types of arterial aneurysm rupture in females under 40 are related to pregnancy. The hemodynamic and endocrine changes appear to cause aneurysms to form and/or rupture. The most common types are cerebral, aortic, and splenic. All increase in frequency of presentation as pregnancy progresses.[2] Pregnancy increases the chance of aortic dissection in young people. In one literature review, up to 50 percent of such dissections in patients under 46 years of age occurred in the pregnant state. There are 100 or so reported cases. In 40 percent, the timing of occurrence was: first trimester, 2 percent; second trimester, 17 percent; third trimester, 49 percent; labor or first 24 h thereafter, 13 percent; and 2 days or more after delivery, 19 percent. Coronary artery aneurysms mainly present immediately postpartum. In one series of 25 cases, 17 were adult women and 7 were puerperal females. There have also been at least 90 reported cases of ruptured splenic artery aneurysm in pregnancy. Of these, 69 percent occurred in the third trimester, 13 percent during labor, and 16 percent during the puerperium. Twenty-four ruptured renal artery aneurysms have been reviewed; six occurred during pregnancy. Various other thoracic, abdominal, and pelvic arteries have been reported as the site of ruptured aneurysms during pregnancy.[11]

Because AVMs are relatively more common than aneurysms in pregnant rather than nonpregnant females of childbearing age, it seems as though the pregnant state per se has an adverse effect in causing these lesions to rupture. Changes in blood volume and pressure and in hormone levels have been suggested to contribute to this circumstance. The relationship of AVM rupture to pregnancy, however, has been difficult to confirm. In a retrospective analysis of 451 women with AVMs referred for proton beam therapy, the bleeding rate was 3.5 percent per year during pregnancy compared to 3.1 percent per year (not significantly different) in nonpregnant females. Pregnancy was not a risk for first hemorrhage from an AVM, although it did increase the risk of recurrent hemorrhage in patients who had already had one hemorrhage. The authors detailed the potential biases in this selected AVM population.[14]

Because aneurysms at any location present with increasing frequency as pregnancy advances, it seems likely that there is a real, increased tendency for such lesions to form and grow because the pregnant state results in a generalized and increasing laxity of blood vessel walls. This was vividly documented in the case of a

34-year-old woman who presented with headache, dizziness, and diplopia at 20 weeks of gestation. A superior cerebellar artery aneurysm was discovered, and subsequently clipped, leaving a small, residual aneurysm neck. This enlarged dramatically over the next 16 weeks when symptoms recurred; a giant aneurysm had formed from the previous aneurysm rest.[35]

The frequency of aneurysm rupture in relation to the time of pregnancy in several reviews of the literature is given in Table 237-1. Because the frequency of bleeding increases in late pregnancy and labor, changes in blood pressure and stroke volume are likely to be more important than changes in blood volume. Many authorities have suggested that aneurysm rupture during labor is rare, but they have generally considered the percentage of all of their cases who rupture during labor and compared this to percentages in preceding trimesters. If one considers that labor might last 12 or even 24 h and that the trimester can be roughly calculated as 90 days, it can be seen that even with a much smaller percentage occurring during actual labor, it is still the time of relatively greatest risk for the pregnant patient. From Table 237-1, the relative chance of hemorrhage per day within each series is calculated, assuming trimesters last 90 days, labor and delivery lasts 1 day, and the puerperium lasts 6 weeks.

At the time of hemorrhage, pregnant patients with an aneurysm are older on average than those with an AVM. The comparative figures are 30 years for 112 cases of aneurysm,[9] 29 years for 21 cases of aneurysm,[1] and 24 years for 19 cases of AVM.[1] In a review of 118 aneurysm ruptures and 36 AVM hemorrhages during pregnancy, the average ages were 29 and 27, respectively, the difference being statistically insignificant.[7]

Diagnosis

Any patient, regardless of the state of pregnancy, who has the very sudden onset of excruciating headache, faint feelings, or coma of unknown origin should have a CT scan performed. If the patient has not presented for several days after such an ictus, a magnetic resonance imaging (MRI) study may be more helpful than computed tomography (CT) because blood pigments are visualized for longer than on CT. Only after such a study has ruled out an intracranial mass lesion should lumbar puncture be performed if the diagnosis is still in doubt. The definitive examination remains angiography and pregnant patients should be considered for this on the same basis as any other suspect SAH case.

The differential diagnosis between eclampsia and SAH should not normally pose much difficulty. Eclampsia is an acute disorder, heralded by tonic-clonic convulsions, which is caused in some way by the hypertension induced or exacerbated by pregnancy. It is most commonly manifest in the last trimester. A hyperexcitable state commonly precedes the convulsion. The seizures may progress to status epilepticus. Generally in this catastrophic condition, diastolic blood pressure is elevated above 90 mmHg. A weight gain of more than 2 lb per week or 6 lb per month has occurred, and the patient may have physical signs of generalized edema. A gradually increasing proteinuria will have developed. Platelet numbers may fall and disseminated intravascular coagulation supervene. Headaches, epigastric and right upper quandrant pain, visual blurring, and decreased acuity may also be complained of. Table 237-2 lists the features differentiating eclampsia from SAH. The differential diagnosis includes idiopathic epilepsy, encephalitis, meningitis, cerebral tumor, acute porphyria, hysteria, intracranial venous thrombosis, arterial occlusions, and pituitary apoplexy.[8,27] Treatment of eclampsia includes sedation, antihypertensive medication, magnesium sulphate, and delivery of the fetus. There is growing use of antiepileptic drugs in this syndrome.

The definitive diagnosis of SAH from a ruptured aneurysm or AVM rests on the CT demonstration of subarachnoid blood and the subsequent angiographic demonstration of an aneurysm or AVM. If the CT is negative, lumbar puncture should be considered and a heavily blood-stained fluid would suggest the need for angiography even in the presence of a normal CT scan.[31]

TABLE 237-1 The Risk of Aneurysm Rupture in Relation to Time of Gestation Expressed as Percent of Total Cases Occurring During Each Time and as Number of Cases per Day within Each Time, Assuming Labor and Delivery Lasts 24 h

	Fox, 1983		Robinson et al., 1972		Walton, 1953		Copelan and Mabon, 1962	
	% of Cases	No. of Cases per Day	% of Cases	No. of Cases per Day	% of Cases	No. of Cases per Day	% of Cases	No. of Cases per Day
No. of cases	112		77		32		46	
Time of rupture								
1st trimester	8	0.1	8	0.07	}	}	}	}
2nd trimester	20	0.24	30	0.26	} 56	} 0.07	} 83	} 0.14
3rd trimester	55	0.75	60	0.51	}	}	}	}
Labor + delivery	2	2.24	2	2.0	13	4	4	2
Postpartum	15	0.37	—	—	31	0.2	13	0.13

	Pedowitz and Perell, 1957		Heiskanen and Nikki, 1963	
	% of Cases	No. of Cases per Day	% of Cases	No. of Cases per Day
No. of cases	79		37	
Time of rupture				
1st trimester	1	0.01	8	0.03
2nd trimester	15	0.13	22	0.09
3rd trimester	35	0.31	59	0.24
Labor + delivery	13	10	3	1
Postpartum	27	0.47	8	0.07

Source: Data from References 5, 9, 13, 24, 28, and 33.

However, 17 percent of fatal eclampsia cases have SAH at autopsy.[3] All but one of the more than 100 aneurysm patients reviewed by Fox presented with SAH during the pregnancy[9]; tumorlike symptoms are obviously very rare. The neurological grades at presentation were: I, 8 percent; II, 29 percent; III, 27 percent; IV, 24 percent; V, 11 percent.

Conservative Management of Aneurysms and AVMs in Pregnancy

In 1965, the neurosurgeon J. Lawrence Pool sent a questionnaire to several of his colleagues.[26] Of 11 patients with aneurysm rupture treated by ''bed rest,'' 8 (73 percent) died, all after initially recovering from the effects of their first SAH! This is very eloquent evidence in favor of an aggressive, early approach to aneurysmal clipping. Cannell reported nine conservatively treated patients with aneurysms and there was a 29 percent mortality, but the duration of follow-up was not stated.[3]

Robinson and colleagues reported 14 aneurysms in pregnancy.[28] There were no previous episodes of SAH. Eight patients were untreated and five had repeat SAH. Of the rebleeders, two rebled early, one in the same pregnancy, and two in the next pregnancy. There were three late rebleeds, one of which was during a pregnancy and two of which were in the nonpregnant state. The time of follow-up was not given, but a maximum of 16 years seems possible. Their cases with aneurysm rupture during pregnancy were six times as likely as their counterparts with AVM to have had a previously normal pregnancy. The impression of these workers was that aneurysms tended to rupture in older patients and were more likely in multiparous cases.[28] An extensive review of cases reported in the English literature found no significant difference in age and parity between women experiencing rupture of an aneurysm versus an AVM.[7] These authors also used logistic regression analysis to analyze the cases, finding that both maternal and fetal mortality were significantly lower if mothers had undergone aneurysm surgery as opposed to conservative management. The same authors reviewed case reports of 36 patients who had AVM rupture during pregnancy. Maternal mortality with surgery was 23 percent, compared to 32 percent with conservative treatment (not significantly different).[7]

In Amias' series of 10 conservatively managed ruptured AVMs, three rebled before delivery.[1] In the 11 AVM cases reviewed by Robinson and colleagues, six had a previous SAH (five while pregnant) and seven had a subsequent SAH after the one which brought them to medical attention.[28] Three of the subsequent SAH episodes were within 6 weeks and during the same pregnancy. Four patients rebled later when they were not pregnant. During the time from 1955 to 1979, no SAH from AVM was encountered in Rochester, Minnesota, in pregnant females but three occurred in nonpregnant 15- to 39-year-old females. These three had had five previous pregnancies with SAH and had been delivered vaginally.[36]

In Yaşargil's series of 414 operated AVMs, 45 percent were in females.[39] Of the female patients, 49 percent were under childbearing age and 24 percent had never been pregnant prior to surgery for their AVM. The remaining 26 percent had been pregnant prior to the surgery or were pregnant at the time of surgery. Of the latter group, 33 percent had symptoms from the AVM during a pregnancy. Of these patients who had been symptomatic during pregnancy, 75 percent had been symptomatic during their first pregnancy. Of this group of 12 cases, two had a further two or three pregnancies without further symptoms. There were two patients who had no symptoms in the first pregnancy and one who had no symptoms in the first two pregnancies who subsequently became symptomatic during pregnancy. In all of these cases harboring an AVM, there were 82 pregnancies without symptoms due to the AVM and 16 pregnancies with such symptoms. Of 82 asymptomatic pregnancies in AVM cases, 17 percent were first pregnancies; 34 percent, second; 26 percent, third; 15 percent, fourth; and 9 percent, fifth or greater. Considering the 16 pregnancies which were symptomatic in these patients with AVM, 38 percent of the patients had AVMs 4 to 6 cm in size; 50 percent, 2 to

TABLE 237-2 Differential Diagnosis of Eclampsia and Subarachnoid Hemorrhage

Feature	Eclampsia	Subarachnoid Hemorrhage
Clinical features	Insidious onset of moderate throbbing headache, excess weight gain, edema, epigastric distress, visual blurring, and decreased acuity. Generalized seizures are common and usually followed by coma; focal neurological deficits are rare; hypertension is usual and may be severe; diffuse hyperreflexia and clonus are characteristic.	Sudden, severe headache, nausea, and vomiting. Focal neurological signs in 20% including cranial nerve palsy. Seizures are uncommon; coma occurs in about 10%; meningeal signs are prominent; hypertension occurs in about 18%; no diffuse hyperreflexia and clonus.
Laboratory values	Proteinuria ubiquitous; may develop thrombocytopenia (25%) and elevated liver enzymes.	Proteinuria in about 15%; may develop hyponatremia and changes on electrocardiogram.
Lumbar puncture results	Usually clear with normal pressure; erythrocytes in 10%.	Erythrocytes present; pressure usually elevated.
Radiologic findings	CT scan usually normal, although intracerebral hemorrhage or petechial hemorrhages may be present. MRI shows small areas of increased signal intensity in white matter on T2-weighted images. Vasospasm is rarely seen on angiography.	SAH on CT scan and aneurysm or AVM on angiography. MRI may show SAH as well as source of hemorrhage. Vasospasm is common.

AVM, arteriovenous malformation; CT, computed tomography; MRI, magnetic resonance imaging; SAH, subarachnoid hemorrhage.

4 cm; and 13 percent, 1 to 2 cm. The most frequent sites were thalamic, 25 percent; frontal, 13 percent; and infratentorial, 13 percent. Only 3 (6 percent) of the patients who had been or were pregnant, were pregnant at the time of surgery.

Although there is obviously a risk, the chance of fatality is relatively much less by not operating on a ruptured AVM, compared to a ruptured aneurysm, during pregnancy.

Treatment

Surgical Treatment of Intracranial Aneurysm

Where the outcomes for the aneurysm cases in the literature prior to 1979 were given, they were: good, 48 percent; fair, 5 percent; poor, 9 percent, and fatal, 38 percent.[9] The outcome for 101 infants was known; 78 percent survived and 22 percent died. The outcomes for 42 patients having cesarean section were given. Forty-five percent had good outcome and 38 percent died; the remainder had intermediate results. For the 47 cases with known outcomes after vaginal delivery, 55 percent had a good outcome and 28 percent died. This difference could well reflect the fact that section was performed on more desperately ill patients. Very few patients had vaginal delivery done before their aneurysm surgery. Of five such cases, three had a good outcome, one had a fair outcome, and one died. Of 15 patients having vaginal delivery after aneurysm surgery, 73 percent had a good outcome and 27 percent a poor one. It seems clear that there were insufficient cases upon which to base really solid conclusions. Many of these cases were reported from the era before definitive microsurgical clipping of aneurysms.[9]

The large series of Amias does not reflect contemporary neurosurgical management of aneurysms. Of 21 cases presenting in pregnancy, only 4 (19 percent) had clipping of the lesion; 24 percent of cases had repeat hemorrhages following neurosurgical observation. Similarly, for the 19 patients with AVMs, only 37 percent had excision of the lesion and four cases (19 percent) had documented rebleeding after being treated initially.[1]

Seven of eight pregnant women with aneurysms in the series of Minielly and colleagues had their ruptured aneurysm operated on without postoperative mortality; one had a permanent serious deficit.[21] Seven living infants were delivered, six vaginally.

In Yaşargil's series of 1012 operated aneurysm cases, seven patients had one or more episodes of SAH during pregnancy.[38] The age range of the patients was 26 to 39 years and all the episodes occurred between 5 and 9 months of pregnancy. Two patients had a cesarean section followed by aneurysmal clipping. Five had clipping of the aneurysm carried out between 5 and 7 months and subsequent vaginal delivery at term. All of these patients were neurologically grade I or II at the time of their aneurysm surgery. There was no significant morbidity or mortality from the treatment for either the mothers or the fetuses.

As a general rule, patients who are pregnant and who have a ruptured aneurysm should be treated in the same fashion as if they are not pregnant. Those with a ruptured aneurysm should have the aneurysm clipped as rapidly as possible. During such clipping, general hypotension should be avoided if possible and reliance placed on temporary clips if that is deemed absolutely necessary. Consideration should be given in each case as to whether or not osmotic agents are vital. Once the aneurysm is successfully clipped, the pregnancy can be allowed to progress to term and the patient can be delivered vaginally if she is in good neurological condition. If labor begins or is likely to begin in the acute phase following aneurysmal clipping (when there is a higher risk of cerebral infarction, hemorrhage, or hydrocephalus), then serious consideration should be given to performing a cesarean section. In the unlikely event that a patient had a ruptured aneurysm and the preeclamptic state, one would be even more anxious to proceed to an expeditious delivery. If rupture of a known aneurysm occurs during labor, the simultaneous performance of a craniotomy and cesarean section should probably be undertaken. SAH from an aneurysm in the puerperium should be treated in the same way as if the female were not pregnant.

If the patient has an unruptured aneurysm diagnosed during pregnancy, consideration should be given to elective clipping if the aneurysm has shown signs of recent acute growth such as a painful third nerve palsy.[35] In that case, elective clipping should probably be carried out regardless of the state of pregnancy. If, however, the aneurysm is found incidentally and is small, is situated in a technically difficult site such as the basilar apex, or presents in a very young patient, one would probably not recommend surgery. The presence of an unruptured aneurysm which has become symptomatic would probably lead to a recommendation of cesarean section over vaginal delivery. It is impossible to make a strong recommendation for cesarean section versus vaginal delivery in a patient with an unruptured asymptomatic aneurysm. If, for instance, the patient has multiple aneurysms and a previously clipped ruptured aneurysm, discretion might dictate that a cesarean section would have less chance of rupturing the residual aneurysm(s). As with any other unruptured aneurysm, the patient would need to be well informed as to the risks and the aneurysm would have to be technically accessible and larger than 3 mm in size.

If an aneurysm has been well clipped and the patient is in good neurological grade, then there is certainly no contraindication to vaginal delivery. If there is doubt about the clipping or if the patient is in the acute postoperative period with a significantly damaged brain, then cesarean section should probably be done. If the decision has been made to proceed with vaginal delivery in the presence of an unsecured aneurysm, it might be wise to use epidural anesthesia to permit a shortening of the second stage of labor and a reduction in ''bearing down.''

Surgical Treatment of Intracranial Arteriovenous Malformation

Yaşargil operated on three patients with an AVM while they were pregnant and an additional 43 patients who had previously been pregnant.[39] The lesions of the pregnant patients included a 1- to 2-cm posterior fossa AVM which had ruptured to produce a state of somnolence and meningismus with cranial nerve VI and VII palsies. A second patient had had two episodes of SAH from a 2- to 4-cm supratentorial AVM which was not producing signs. The third patient had had two episodes of SAH from a 4- to 6-cm AVM which had ruptured to produce mild weakness. All three patients presented with SAH and did so at 3, 6, or 8 months of gestation. Following excision of the AVM, the postoperative courses were benign. The patients had normal vaginal deliveries of healthy children at 2, 3, and $6\frac{1}{2}$ months following their AVM excision.

In Yaşargil's total series, 62 percent of the AVMs occurred in patients less than 30 years of age. Seventy-nine percent of cases presented with bleeding. Of those that bled, 65 percent had intracerebral hematomas. In fewer than half were the hematomas greater than 4 cm in diameter. Thirty-three percent of all cases had a history of seizures; 12 percent of those who presented with bleeding had a history of epilepsy. Large intracerebral hematomas were operated upon in the acute phase in 2 percent of cases without a neurological deficit and 8 percent of cases with such a deficit. Alert patients with focal deficits were seen in 43 percent of AVM cases vs. only 15 percent of aneurysm cases. The AVM had at least one associated aneurysm in 11 percent of cases. The ruptured lesion was operated upon unless the proximity of both lesions allowed easy simultaneous surgical treatment.

Three ruptured AVMs in pregnancy were managed by Lee and colleagues.[18] Two of their patients had an emergency craniotomy with total excision of the AVM. One of these also had an emergency cesarean section because labor had commenced; the child survived. All of the women survived. One abortion was induced in early pregnancy and a spontaneous miscarriage occurred in the third case.

It is considered that the surgical resection of an AVM might be indicated if there are increasing signs of a space-occupying lesion (such as the progressive loss of consciousness), if the lesion is small, or if there has been multiple episodes of SAH. Surgery may be delayed with most AVMs pending a complete radiologic workup, resolution of associated intracerebral hematomas, and delivery of the child. Exceptions might exist when a significant mass effect from an associated clot worsened despite therapy or if the deterioration were of such a degree as to be life threatening. Such urgent clot evacuation is considered more likely to occur with cerebellar hematomas rather than those in other locations.

The symptoms and signs of herniation would need to be refractory to external ventricular drainage and medical measures. In AVMs as opposed to aneurysms, it is often reasonable to evacuate the intracerebral hematoma and leave the offending lesion alone. Excision of the AVM acutely is reasonable if the AVM is small (less than 2 cm), easily and completely defined, and does not impinge on the region of the basal ganglia, according to Yasargil.

Cesarean Section

Although cesarean section should not be undertaken lightly, it has become a more commonplace procedure over the past several decades and it seems to have become more readily utilized in the presence of an unclipped aneurysm or residual AVM, when severe SAH occurs after labor has begun, or if the patient has an acutely and severely injured brain after SAH or surgery.[4,16] Lennon and colleagues reported maternal and fetal survival in a case in which an emergency section was performed in a 23-year-old who presented at 40 weeks gestation following hemorrhage with active labor already begun.[19] Maternal mortality rates after cesarean section are very low in the hands of experienced operators in well-equipped institutions,[25] but cesarean section remains more hazardous than vaginal delivery. In some settings, however, large series of cesarean sections have been achieved with a zero maternal mortality rate. In the United States between 1977 and 1984, considering series of between 10,231 and 350,892 sections, the maternal mortality rates varied between 0 and 60/100,000 sections, while death attributable to the section alone varied between 0 and 59/100,000 sections. Section was associated with morbidity of the following types: endometritis, 6 to 18 percent; urinary tract infection, 1 to 8 percent; wound infection, 1 to 7 percent; transfusion complications, 0 to 6 percent; paralytic ileus, 0 to 1 percent; pulmonary embolus, 0.1 to 0.2 percent; and operative injury to the lower urinary tract, 0.2 to 0.3 percent. The performance of a section resulted in an average of 3 days longer in the hospital than vaginal delivery. Cesarean section by itself is no risk to the fetus. For instance, during the years 1973 to 1981, the section rate increased from 6 to 12 percent in Sweden.[22] At the same time, perinatal mortality declined from 12 to 7/1000 children. The incidence of section varied between 8 and 19 percent in different obstetric units. Despite this great difference, there was no significant difference in the rates of asphyxia or perinatal mortality. A section can therefore be undertaken with reasonable confidence that no great threat is being posed to the child. Evidence that it improves maternal and fetal survival in mothers with ruptured AVMs or aneurysms, however, could not be confirmed by Dias and Sekhar in their review of 154 patients.[7] Controlled, vaginal delivery with epidural anesthesia may approximate the risks of cesarean section.

Medical Aspects of Treatment

Anticonvulsant medication should be used with caution in a pregnant patient who has a convulsion associated with SAH. Such seizures occurring in close proximity to SAH are not prognostic of a long-term tendency toward convulsions. It is probably better not to treat them at that juncture but to await any subsequent seizures. However, patients with seizures and AVMs should receive anticonvulsants. Phenobarbital is probably the drug of choice. All antiepileptic drugs have been associated with an increased risk of fetal teratogenicity, neonatal coagulopathy, neonatal depression, and drug withdrawal syndromes. Moreover, drug pharmacokinetics are altered in pregnancy. There may be an increased tendency to folate deficiency in the mother who is on antiepileptic drugs. Few data are available as yet on the side effects of carbamazepine for the fetus and mother.[30]

Hypotension and hypothermia have been used during aneurysm clipping in many cases without apparent adverse effects on the fetus or mother. Notwithstanding this, it seems preferable to avoid their use if possible. Temporary clips accomplish the same role at operation and pose no risk to the fetus and probably less to the mother. The fetal heart rate should be monitored continuously for signs of distress, especially if hypotension or hypothermia are used. The utilization of osmotic diuretics would require a deliberate value judgment on the part of the surgeon. Mannitol predisposes to maternal hypovolemia and hypotension and may produce uterine hypoperfusion, fetal hypernatremia, and fetal hyperosmolarity.[7] The danger to the fetus of ordinary clinical dosages is probably small and has not been documented in clinical practice. Corticosteroids have been used in pregnancy, although their necessity following aneurysmal or AVM SAH is controversial. Nimodipine was teratogenic and embryotoxic in animals, although effects on human fetuses are unknown.[7]

In summary, there is more at stake when SAH occurs in pregnancy since two lives are in jeopardy. Youth and an increased blood volume are factors which are on the side of the neurosurgeon. The results should be at least as good as in the nonpregnant state. In the seriously ill mother, at or near term, with an unsecured lesion—either aneurysm or AVM—cesarean section has much to recommend it. A patient in good condition following aneurysmal clipping or excision of an AVM can be delivered normally in most circumstances. However, management decisions must be individualized and all generalizations are suspect.

References

1. Amias AG. Cerebral vascular disease in pregnancy: I. Haemorrhage. *J Obstet Gynaecol Br Commonw* 1970; 77:100–120.
2. Barno A, Freeman DW. Maternal deaths due to spontaneous subarachnoid hemorrhage. *Am J Obstet Gynecol* 1976; 125:384–392.
3. Cannell DE. Subarachnoid haemorrhage in pregnancy. *Proc R Soc Med* 1959; 52:950–952.
4. Conklin KA, Herr G, Fung D. Anaesthesia for caesarean section and cerebral aneurysm clipping. *Can Anaesth Soc J* 1984; 31:451–454.
5. Copelan EL, Mabon RF. Spontaneous intracranial bleeding in pregnancy. *Obstet Gynecol* 1962; 20:373–378.
6. Cross JN, Castro PO, Jennett WB. Cerebral strokes associated with pregnancy and the puerperium. *Br Med J [Clin Res]* 1968; 3:214–218.
7. Dias MS, Sekhar LN. Intracranial hemorrhage from aneurysms and arteriovenous malformations during pregnancy and the puerperium. *Neurosurgery* 1990; 27:855–866.
8. Estanol B, Rodriguez A, Conte G, et al. Intracranial venous thrombosis in young women. *Stroke* 1979; 10:680–684.
9. Fox JL. *Intracranial Aneurysms,* vol III. New York: Springer-Verlag, 1983, 1103–1463.
10. Fraser CK. Maternal mortality: District of Columbia, 1950–1959. *Med Ann D C* 1962; 31:456–469.
11. Gleicher N (ed). *Principles of Medical Therapy in Pregnancy.* New York: Plenum, 1985.
12. Heidrich R, Niedner K. Pregnancy and subarachnoid haemorrhage. *Eur Neurol* 1970; 3:38–49.
13. Heiskanen O, Nikki P. Rupture of intracranial arterial aneurysm during pregnancy. *Acta Neurol Scand* 1963; 39:202–208.
14. Horton JC, Chambers WA, Lyons SL, et al. Pregnancy and the risk of hemorrhage from cerebral arteriovenous malformations. *Neurosurgery* 1990; 27:867–872.
15. Kaunitz AM, Hughes JM, Grimes DA, et al. Causes of maternal mortality in the United States. *Obstet Gynecol* 1985; 65:605–612.
16. Kofke WA, Wuest HP, McGinnis LA. Cesarean section following ruptured cerebral aneurysm and neuroresuscitation. *Anesthesiology* 1984; 60:242–245.
17. Lane RE, Andelman SL. Maternal mortality in Chicago, 1956 through 1960: Part I. General analysis. *Am J Obstet Gynecol* 1963; 85:52–60.
18. Lee DF, Chen FT, Tsai MF, et al. Rupture of arteriovenous malformations during pregnancy: report of 3 cases. *J Formosan Med Assoc* 1983; 82:941–946.
19. Lennon RL, Sundt TM Jr, Gronert GA. Combined cesarean section and clipping of intracerebral aneurysm. *Anesthesiology* 1984; 60:240–242.
20. McCausland AM, Holmes F. Spinal fluid pressures during labor. Preliminary report. *West J Surg Obstet Gynecol* 1957; 65:220–233.
21. Minielly R, Yuzpe AA, Drake CG. Subarachnoid hemorrhage secondary to ruptured cerebral aneurysm in pregnancy. *Obstet Gynecol* 1979; 53:64–70.
22. Nielsen TF, Hökegard KH, Ericson A. Cesarean section and perinatal mortality in Sweden in 1981. *Acta Obstet Gynecol Scand* 1986; 65:865–867.
23. Ondra SL, Troupp H, George ED, et al. The natural history of symptomatic arteriovenous malformations of the brain: a 24-year follow-up assessment. *J Neurosurg* 1990; 73:387–391.
24. Pedowitz P, Perell A. Aneurysms complicated by pregnancy: Part II. Aneurysms of the cerebral vessels. *Am J Obstet Gynecol* 1957; 73:736–749.
25. Petitti DB. Maternal mortality and morbidity in cesarean section. *Clin Obstet Gynecol* 1985; 28:763–769.
26. Pool JL. Treatment of intracranial aneurysms during pregnancy. *JAMA* 1965; 192:209–214.
27. Pritchard JA, Macdonald PC (eds). *Williams Obstetrics,* 16th ed. New York: Appleton-Century-Crofts, 1980.
28. Robinson JL, Hall CJ, Sedzimir CB. Subarachnoid hemorrhage in pregnancy. *J Neurosurg* 1972; 36:27–33.
29. Sahs AL, Perret GE, Locksley HB, et al. (eds). *Intracranial Aneurysms and Subarachnoid Hemorrhage: A Cooperative Study.* Philadelphia: Lippincott, 1969, p 296.
30. Stempel LE, Rayburn WF. Anticonvulsant therapy during pregnancy. In Rayburn WF, Zuspan FP (eds): *Drug Therapy in Obstetrics and Gynecology,* 2d ed. Norwalk: Appleton-Century-Crofts, 1986, pp 53–72.
31. Tuttelman RM, Gleicher N. Central nervous system hemorrhage complicating pregnancy. *Obstet Gynecol* 1981; 58:651–656.
32. Visscher HC, Visscher RD. Indirect obstetric deaths in the state of Michigan 1960–1968. *Am J Obstet Gynecol* 1971; 109:1187–1196.
33. Walton JN. Subarachnoid haemorrhage in pregnancy. *Br Med J [Clin Res]* 1953; 1:869–871.
34. Weir B. *Aneurysms Affecting the Nervous System.* Baltimore: Williams & Wilkins, 1987.
35. Weir BKA, Drake CG. Rapid growth of residual aneurysmal neck during pregnancy. Case report. *J Neurosurg* 1991; 75:780–782.
36. Wiebers DO, Whisnant JP. The incidence of stroke among pregnant women in Rochester, Minn, 1955 through 1979. *JAMA* 1985; 254:3055–3057.
37. Wilkins RH. Natural history of intracranial vascular malformations: a review. *Neurosurgery* 1985; 16:421–430.
38. Yaşargil MG. *Microneurosurgery,* vol. II. *Clinical Considerations, Surgery of the Intracranial Aneurysms and Results.* Stuttgart: Georg Thieme Verlag, 1984.
39. Yasargil MG. *Microneurosurgery,* vol III B. *AVM of the Brain, Clinical Considerations, General and Special Operative Techniques, Surgical Results, Nonoperated Cases, Cavernous and Venous Angiomas, Neuroanesthesia.* Stuttgart: Georg Thieme Verlag, 1988.

238

Concomitant Intracranial Aneurysms and Arteriovenous Malformations

Wink S. Fisher III

Approximately 1 in 15 patients with an arteriovenous malformation (AVM) will harbor an intracranial aneurysm, and 1 in 100 aneurysm patients will have an AVM.[27] Balancing therapy between these lesions can be difficult, especially when the source of the hemorrhage is unclear. Treatment should be directed first toward the symptomatic lesion, and the surgical strategy should include both lesions whenever possible.[7,23,28,29]

Pathogenesis and Incidence

The causes of AVMs and aneurysms are not precisely known. AVMs are thought to be true congenital abnormalities that appear somewhere between the fourth and eighth weeks of embryonic formation.[9,29] At this stage, the primitive vascular network forms and differentiates into arteries, veins, and capillaries. The embryonic development of the primary pathologic abnormality of an AVM occurs during this time and is thought to be due to (1) the persistence of direct connections between the arterial and venous channels without development of the normal capillary network, (2) the development of an abnormal communication between the arterial and venous systems, or (3) agenesis of the capillary network (Table 238-1).[29] Aneurysms, on the other hand, are now thought to develop from degenerative processes rather than from congenital vessel wall defects. The congenital theory which is based on the idea that medial defects in the cerebral vasculature (medial defects of Forbus) allow for intimal outpouching with eventual aneurysm formation, has been refuted by Stehbens,[20–22] who proposes that defects occur in the vessel wall owing to degenerative changes as a component of the ''hypertensive complex,'' namely, elevated blood pressure. Supporting this argument are findings such as that (1) aneurysms occur most often in later life and have not been reported in the neonatal period and that (2) the medial defects of Forbus, which are natural locations in the vessel for the muscularis to anchor itself, become more common as the patient becomes older, implying that they are acquired. Also, (3) herniation of the mural wall near a defect of Forbus suggests that these medial raphes are actually drawn into the early aneurysm and are found fortuitously, rather than being the initiating site for aneurysm formation; (4) no statistically significant studies of congenital abnormalities confirm an association with aneurysm formation; the two most common disorders (coarctation of the aorta and polycystic kidney disease) frequently have the associated clinical finding of hypertension, which may be the etiologic link to aneurysm formation; and (5) the observation that aneurysms may not have associated atherosclerotic changes does not exclude degenerative causes for formation, since hypertension may play a considerable role.[20–22]

According to Boyd-Wilson,[4] Walsh and King, in 1942, reported the first case of an AVM associated with an aneurysm. Numerous small series of cases have been reported since that time. As cited by Weir,[27] Chason and Hindman carried out 2786 consecutive autopsies, and discovered that 5 percent of the individuals harbored intracranial aneurysms; if there were no developmental relationship between AVMs and aneurysms, no more than 5 percent of AVM cases should be associated with aneurysms. Perret and Nishioka[18] reported an 8 percent incidence of aneurysms in 490 cases, and Cronqvist and Troupp[6] found (in 150 patients with AVMs) a 9 percent incidence of aneurysms. Cunha e Sa et al.,[7] reporting on Stein's series of 400 AVM patients, found intracranial aneurysms in 10 percent; the proportion in other reports varies from 3 percent to as many as 18 percent of cases (Table 238-2).

Multiple aneurysms seem to be more common in patients with AVMs. Miyasaka and co-workers studied the angiograms of 132 consecutive patients with AVMs and found aneurysms in 17% of

TABLE 238-1 Pathogenetic Theories of AVM Formation

Author	Year	Theory of Formation
Dandy	1928	Retention of vascular connections between arteries and veins
Olivecrona & Landenheim	1957	Embryonic agenesis of the capillary system
Kaplan & Meier	1958	Perpetuation of a primitive communication between arteries and veins
Hamby	1958	Lack of vascular resistance (agenesis of capillary resistance)
Gold	1964	(1) direct anastomosis; (2) network of poorly differentiated vessels
Lagos	1977	(1) Direct anastomosis; (2) network of poorly differentiated vessels
Stein & Wolpert	1980	Arrest of normal development of arteries, capillaries, and veins
Parkinson & Bachers	1980	Local angioblastic error with the formation of a shunt
Warkany	1984	Arrest of normal development of arteries, capillaries, and veins
Garretson	1985	Persistence of direct connection between arteries and veins

This chart is a chronological listing of some of the different theories for AVM formation. Three general theoretical categories exist: persistence of direct connections between arterial and venous channels; development of abnormal communication between the arterial and venous systems; and agenesis of the capillary system.

TABLE 238-2 Chronological Listing of Reports of Concomitant AVMs and Aneurysms

Author	Year	Total number of Patients with AVMs	Total Number with Aneurysms (%)*	Aneurysms on Feeding Vessels†	Aneurysms on Unrelated Vessels‡	AVM/Aneurysm/?§
Paterson & McKissock[17]	1956	110	3 (2.7%)	—	—	0/1/2
Perret & Nishioka[18]	1966	490	37 (7.6%)	15/34 (37%)	18/34 (43%)	9/7/13
Cronqvist & Troupp[6]	1966	150	13 (8.6%)	9/13 (69%)	4/13 (30.8%)	—
Tsuchita & Miyazaki[25]	1976	—	—	—	—	28%/19%/53%
Suzuki & Onuma[23]	1979	140	9 (6.4%)	4/9 (44%)	2/9 (22%)	3/3/1
Higashi et al.[11]	1979	43	4 (9.3%)	4/4 (100%)	0/4 (0%)	—
Miyasaka et al.[14]	1982	132	22 (16.7%)	41/43 (95%)	2/43 (5%)	—
Tran-Dinh et al.[24]	1983	47	2 (4.3%)	1/2 (50%)	1/2 (50%)	0/1/0
Ostergaard (<age 10)[16]	1984	16	2 (12.5%)	—	—	1/1/0
Okamoto et al.[15]	1984	149	5 (3.4%)	2/5 (40%)	1/5 (20%)	2/1/1
Batjer et al.[3]	1986	157	22 (14%)	36/44 (82%)	8/44 (18%)	2/7/0
Yaşargil[29]	1987	414	45 (10.9%)	42/45 (93%)	3/45 (7%)	2/8/0
Brown et al.[5]	1990	91	16 (18%)	25/26 (96%)	1/26 (4%)	1/1/4
Cunha e Sa et al.[7]	1992	400	39 (9.75%)	63/64 (98%)	1/64 (2%)	33%/46%/21%
Total		2339	219 (9.4%)	242/289 (83.7%)	41/289 (14.2%)	

*These numbers represent the number of AVM patients that had aneurysms (incidence of aneurysms).
†These numbers represent the total number of aneurysms clearly on feeding vessels. Note that more aneurysms may be reported than the total number of patients in the preceding column; note also that the report of Miyasaka et al. includes infundibula and aneurysms.
‡These numbers represent all aneurysms clearly not related to the AVM and do not include those aneurysms proximal to the feeding vessels of the AVM (as well as aneurysms on feeding vessels).
§The number of AVMs that caused hemorrhage versus aneurysms or those cases where the cause of hemorrhage was not clear; some series only list percentages.

them.[14] Of these, 41 percent were found to have multiple aneurysms. In addition, the size of the AVM was related to the number of aneurysms found: 0 percent with small AVMs (less than 2 cm); 13 percent with lesions measuring 2 to 5 cm; and 37 percent with AVMs larger than 5 cm. Interestingly, an extremely high incidence of vertebrobasilar aneurysms was discovered in this series (33 percent of cases).[14] Brown et al., on the other hand, reported an increased frequency of aneurysm formation with AVMs of any size[5]; however, a higher frequency of atypical aneurysm locations was noted with larger AVMs. Batjer et al. reported that 50 percent of their patients with combined lesions had multiple aneurysms.[3]

Paterson and McKissock first introduced the hypothesis that increased blood flow is associated with the development of aneurysms.[17] In their three cases, they described a patient with multiple aneurysms and another with an aneurysm located peripherally on the posterior inferior cerebellar artery, which was feeding a cerebellar AVM. Alteration of cerebral flow to the AVM appears to directly affect aneurysms associated with AVMs.[2,11,17] Shenkin et al. reported a distinct reduction in the size of a large aneurysm located on a feeding vessel following removal of the AVM.[19] Koulouris and Rizzoli reported the angiographic disappearance of an aneurysm on a posterior cerebral artery feeding an occipital AVM three weeks after the latter was excised.[13] In addition, most studies have shown that aneurysms form more often on feeding vessels than on unrelated vessels (Table 238-2).

Three theories have been formulated to help define the association between AVMs and aneurysms: (1) a *congenital theory,* whereby a maldevelopment of the vascular system predisposes a patient to development of both lesions; (2) a *hemodynamic* or *degenerative theory,* whereby forces associated with blood flow to an AVM cause vessel wall weakening and formation of an aneurysm; and (3) a *coincidental theory,* according to which there is absolutely no pathophysiologic relationship between the two entities.[3,5,7,10] If AVMs are assumed to be congenital in origin, then the hemodynamic (degenerative) theory of association between AVMs and aneurysms seems most plausible, given the more recent theories of aneurysm formation.

Surgical Approach

Symptomatic Lesions

As is the case with all vascular lesions, symptomatic patients need to be differentiated from asymptomatic ones; patients with hemorrhagic or expanding lesions require more urgent decision making than those without. Most authorities agree that surgery of these combined lesions should be directed toward the symptomatic lesion first.[7,23,28,29] It is often difficult to discover the causative lesion; in addition, there does not appear to be any consensus on which of the two lesions (AVM or aneurysm) bleeds more frequently (Table 238-2). One of the largest series (that of Stein) had hemorrhage rates of 46 percent from aneurysms and of 33 percent from AVMs.[7]

Three hypothetical scenarios may arise with symptomatic lesions where the source of hemorrhage is either the AVM or the aneurysm, or is undetermined. (Although it is possible for both lesions to cause symptoms simultaneously, that would be quite unusual.) The surgical approach to patients who have experienced a hemorrhage from the AVM, particularly when associated with an intracerebral hematoma, is medical treatment until magnetic resonance imaging (MRI) indicates that the cerebral edema surrounding the hematoma has subsided (4 to 6 weeks). There is evidence that the risk of rehemorrhage from the AVM within this period is negligible. At the delayed AVM operation, all efforts are made to treat both lesions. Since most aneurysms are located on feeding vessels to the AVM (Table 238-2), the aneurysm(s) are clipped during the preliminary stages of vessel isolation for proximal control of the AVM. These vessels are, many times, quite fragile, are deeply located in sulci of fissures, and have extremely high flow, which necessitates careful dissection to avoid intraoperative rupture.

Drake (personal communication with Batjer[3]), Batjer et al.,[3] and Kassell[12] have all advised clipping aneurysms on feeding vessels even though primary therapy is directed toward the AVM. Postoperative hemorrhage from a feeding vessel aneurysm has been reported, despite other reports of aneurysm involution after resection or embolization of the AVM. Batjer et al. underscored this risk even in cases of unruptured AVMs associated with unruptured aneurysms.[3] Feeding vessel aneurysms that are exceedingly difficult to reach and anatomically remote may merit a staged approach; however, extraordinary efforts should be made to clip any aneurysm on a feeding vessel during surgery for a symptomatic AVM.

Symptomatic aneurysms [either enlarging lesions or ones causing subarachnoid hemorrhage (SAH)] require more urgent attention, since the natural history of these lesions includes early rehemorrhage. There are suggestions that aneurysms associated with AVMs may be more prone to hemorrhage than other solitary aneurysms and therefore may require even more urgent attention.[3] The justification for simultaneous removal of an AVM after aneurysmal hemorrhage and clipping may be lacking. Many factors play a role in the decision making in these cases: the patient's age, medical condition, and clinical grade; the amount of blood visible on scans at presentation; and the presence or absence of hydrocephalus, as well as size and location of the lesion. Difficult dissection coupled with fragile pial surfaces should dissuade the surgeon from an overly aggressive initial approach, especially when the source of hemorrhage is clearly the aneurysm. The sump effect of the AVM may assist in preventing vasospasm by enhancing cerebral blood flow in the area immediately surrounding the aneurysm. It also seems to follow that the flow characteristics in the asymptomatic AVM at the time of symptomatic aneurysm clipping will not be adversely altered by the aneurysm clipping itself, so that there is less chance of postoperative hemorrhage from the AVM. There are no statistics on AVM rupture in the immediate postoperative period after clipping of a symptomatic aneurysm.

The most difficult predicament for surgical decision making occurs when the source of hemorrhage cannot be identified. Most aneurysms are located on feeding vessels which, more often than not, are close to the AVM, making the source of hemorrhage difficult to identify (Table 238-1). CT scanning and occasionally MRI can assist in differentiating the source of hemorrhage: Parenchymal hemorrhages are usually associated with AVM hemorrhage, whereas SAH is usually associated with aneurysmal hemorrhage. The presence of multiple aneurysms further complicates the issue, since multiple aneurysms may be located in opposite hemispheres but in close proximity to each other (Fig. 238-1). Since the natural history of SAH due to aneurysms has a poor outcome, surgical efforts should be directed toward the aneurysm first, with treatment of the AVM delayed to a later date. There are no large series of cases with simultaneous excision of these lesions; in Stein's series, 13 of 27 patients had simultaneous excision of both lesions.[7] (Whether these cases presented as aneurysmal SAH or as AVM hemorrhage or were unruptured is not clear.)

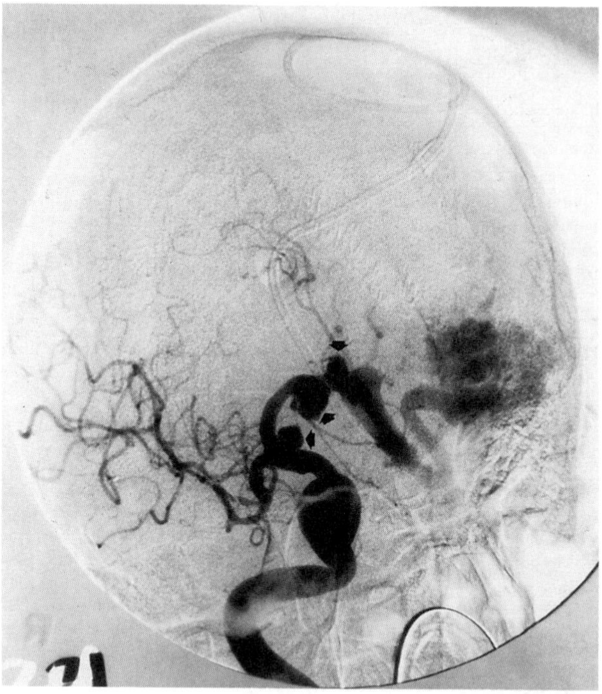

Figure 238-1 Right oblique internal carotid arteriogram of a left frontal AVM. The patient suffered a subarachnoid hemorrhage but had multiple ipsilateral and contralateral aneurysms on the circle of Willis. Determining the site of hemorrhage as well as the surgical approach in such cases is difficult.

Asymptomatic Lesions

Knowledge of the natural history of asymptomatic aneurysms and AVMs must be applied to patients who present with lesions that have never caused hemorrhagic symptoms. Once again, age, medical condition, and location of the lesion(s) all play critical roles in treatment strategy. In general, for patients older than age 65,[26] intervention for an asymptomatic aneurysm rarely makes sense; a similar stance is taken regarding treatment of unruptured AVMs in patients older than age 60.[1,8] In older patients (ages 60 to 65), clipping asymptomatic aneurysm(s) without resecting the AVM may be in the patient's best interest, because it will alter the natural history of the aneurysm without taking unnecessary risks with the AVM.

In younger patients, it makes sense to advise surgical resection of the AVM and clipping of the aneurysm in an attempt to improve on the natural history of both conditions. When anatomically feasible, the preferred treatment is a combined operation for both lesions, although when there are remote aneurysmal lesions, it may be best to occlude them first. Generally, we wait at least 6 weeks between operations in any staged procedure, unless radiologic investigations suggest otherwise.

Determining the surgical risk for treating the AVM or aneurysm alone or for treating both together is difficult (Table 238-3). Only a few surgical results have been reported, and no comparison between cases with hemorrhage and those without hemorrhage has been made. Clear-cut guidelines to therapy are not available; therefore, surgeons must rely on their own clinical experience to determine the appropriate therapy in these particularly difficult cases

TABLE 238-3 Chronological Listing of Surgical Results in Patients with AVMs and Aneurysms

Author	Year	AVM Mortality	AVM Morbidity	Aneurysm Mortality	Aneurysm Morbidity	Mortality for Both AVM and Aneurysm	Morbidity for Both AVM and Aneurysm
Paterson & McKissock[17]	1956	3/35	3/35	—	—	—	—
Perret & Nishioka[18]	1966	2/6	1/6	1/2	1/2	1/5	—
Cronqvist & Troupp[6]	1966	1/2	0/2	0/2	1/2	0/1	0/1
Suzuki & Onuma[23]	1979	—	—	0/1	0/1	0/8	2/8
Higashi et al.[11]	1979	—	—	0/1	0/1	1/1	—
Tran-Dinh et al.[24]	1983	—	—	0/1	0/1	—	—
Ostergaard (<age 10)[16]	1984	—	—	—	—	1/2	0/2
Okamoto et al.[15]	1984	0/2	0/2	—	—	—	—
Batjer et al.[3]	1986	2/3	—	1/8	—	1/8	—
Yaşargil[29]	1987	0/1	0/1	0/3	0/3	1/4	0/4
Cunha e Sa et al.[7]	1992	0/14	—	0/14	—	0/13	—
Total		8/63 (12.7%)	4/46 (8.7%)	2/32 (6.3%)	2/10 (20%)	5/42 (11.9%)	2/15 (13.3%)

Results are for resection of AVM and/or clipping of aneurysms. The small numbers of cases reported makes conclusions regarding mortality and morbidity difficult. Definitions: AVM mortality/morbidity: surgical mortality or morbidity for AVM resection alone, whether or not the aneurysm(s) were operated on later; aneurysm mortality/morbidity: surgical mortality or morbidity for aneurysm clipping alone, with or without later resection of the AVM; mortality/morbidity for both AVM and aneurysm: surgical mortality and morbidity for combined resection of both lesions.

References

1. Auger RG, Wiebers DO. Management of unruptured intracranial arteriovenous malformations: a decision analysis. *Neurosurgery* 1992; 30:561–569.
2. Azzam CJ. Growth of multiple peripheral high flow aneurysms of the posterior inferior cerebellar artery associated with a cerebellar arteriovenous malformation. *Neurosurgery* 1987; 21:934–939.
3. Batjer H, Suss RA, Samson D. Intracranial arteriovenous malformations associated with aneurysms. *Neurosurgery* 1986; 18:29–35.
4. Boyd-Wilson JS. The association of cerebral angiomas with intracranial aneurysms. *J Neurol Neurosurg Psychiatry* 1959; 22:218–223.
5. Brown RD, Wiebers DO, Forbes GS. Unruptured intracranial aneurysms and arteriovenous malformations: frequency of intracranial hemorrhage and relationship of lesions. *J Neurosurg* 1990; 73:859–863.
6. Cronqvist S, Troupp H. Intracranial arteriovenous malformation and arterial aneurysm in the same patient. *Acta Neurol Scand* 1966; 42:307–316.
7. Cunha e Sa MJ, Stein BM, Solomon RA, McCormick PC. The treatment of associated intracranial aneurysms and arteriovenous malformations. *J Neurosurg* 1992; 77:853–859.
8. Fisher WS III. Decision analysis: a tool of the future: an application to unruptured arteriovenous malformations. *Neurosurgery* 1989; 24:129–135.
9. Garretson HD. Intracranial arteriovenous malformations. In Wilkins RH, Rengachary SS (eds): *Neurosurgery*. New York: McGraw-Hill, 1985, pp 1448–1458.
10. Hayashi S, Arimoto T, Itakura T, et al. The association of intracranial aneurysms and arteriovenous malformations of the brain: case report. *J Neurosurg* 1981; 55:971–975.
11. Higashi K, Hatano M, Yamashita T, et al. Coexistence of posterior inferior cerebellar artery aneurysms and arteriovenous malformation fed by the same artery. *Surg Neurol* 1979; 12:405–408.
12. Kassell NF. Comment on Koulouris S, Rizzoli HV. Coexisting intracranial aneurysm and arteriovenous malformation: case report. *Neurosurgery* 1981; 8:222.
13. Koulouris S, Rizzoli HV. Coexisting intracranial aneurysm and arteriovenous malformation: case report. *Neurosurgery* 1981; 8:219–222.
14. Miyasaka K, Wolpert SM, Prager RJ. The association of cerebral aneurysms, infundibula, and intracranial arteriovenous malformations. *Stroke* 1982; 13:196–203.
15. Okamoto S, Handa H, Hashimoto N. Location of intracranial aneurysms associated with cerebral arteriovenous malformation: statistical analysis. *Surg Neurol* 1984; 22:335–340.
16. Ostergaard JR. Association of intracranial aneurysm and arteriovenous malformation in childhood. *Neurosurgery* 1984; 14:358–362.
17. Paterson JH, McKissock W. A clinical survey of intracranial angiomas with special reference to their mode of progression and surgical treatment: a report of 110 cases. *Brain* 1956; 79:233–266.
18. Perret G, Nishioka H. Report on the cooperative study of intracranial aneurysms and subarachnoid hemorrhage. Section VI. Arteriovenous malformations. An analysis of 545 cases of cranio-cerebral arteriovenous malformations and fistulae reported to the cooperative study. *J Neurosurg* 1966; 25:467–490.
19. Shenkin HA, Jenkins F, Kim K. Arteriovenous anomaly of the brain associated with cerebral aneurysm: case report. *J Neurosurg* 1971; 34:225–228.
20. Stehbens WE. Ultrastructure of aneurysms. *Arch Neurol* 1975; 32:798–807.
21. Stehbens WE. Etiology of intracranial berry aneurysms. *J Neurosurg* 1989; 70:823–831.
22. Stehbens WE. Pathology and pathogenesis of intracranial berry aneurysms. *Neurol Res* 1990; 12:29–34.
23. Suzuki J, Onuma T. Intracranial aneurysms associated with arteriovenous malformations. *J Neurosurg* 1979; 50:742–746.
24. Tran-Dinh H, Williams LM, Jayasinghe LS. Association of intracranial aneurysm and arteriovenous malformation. *Med J Aust* 1983; 1:521–523.
25. Tsuchita H, Miyazaki Y. A case associated with the combination of cerebral aneurysm and cerebral arteriovenous malformation originated from same artery in the same site. [Japanese] *No Shinkei Geka* 1976; 4:997–1003.
26. van Crevel H, Habbema JD, Braakman R. Decision analysis of the management of incidental intracranial saccular aneurysms. *Neurology* 1986; 36:1335–1339.
27. Weir B. *Aneurysms Affecting the Nervous System.* Baltimore: Williams & Wilkins, 1987, pp 379–384.
28. Yaşargil MG (ed): *Microneurosurgery,* vol I: *Microsurgical Anatomy of the Basal Cisterns and Vessels of the Brain. Diagnostic studies, General Operative Techniques and Pathological Considerations of the Intracranial Aneurysms.* New York: Georg Thieme Verlag, 1984, pp 309–312.
29. Yaşargil MG (ed): *Microneurosurgery,* vol IIIA: *AVM of the Brain. History, Embryology, Pathological Considerations, Hemodynamics, Diagnostic studies, Microsurgical Anatomy.* New York: Georg Thieme Verlag, 1987, pp 49–56, 182–189.

SECTION D

Vascular Malformations and Fistulas

239

Intracranial Arteriovenous Malformations

H. D. Garretson

Historical Review

Intracranial arteriovenous malformations were studied and classified as early as the mid-1800s (Luschka, 1854; Virchow, 1863), with the first surgical exposure of an arteriovenous malformation by Giordano occurring about three decades later in 1890.[45,52,73] Fedor Krause attempted to surgically eliminate an arteriovenous malformation by ligating its feeding arteries in 1908,[37] but Olivecrona appears to have been the first to actually completely excise a cerebral arteriovenous malformation (AVM) in 1932 and later a cerebellar AVM in 1938.[22] Except at a few major centers, however, an aggressive surgical approach to the larger examples of these lesions has awaited the major technological advances of neurological surgery, neuroradiology, and neuroanesthesia during the past several decades.

Embryologic Basis of Arteriovenous Malformations

Arteriovenous malformations of the brain are congenital lesions most likely developing during the late somite stages of the fourth week of embryonic life and almost certainly no later than the eighth week. The primary pathologic lesion consists of one or more persisting direct connections between the arterial inflow and venous outflow without an intervening capillary bed.

Early in the third week of embryonic life, cells (angioblasts) begin to differentiate from the mesoderm, forming small, syncytial islands.[54,64] These small clumps of syncytial cells develop tiny sprouts that extend to interconnect the cell groups, forming a syncytial plexus. Intercellular clefts appear within the syncytial masses.[49] These clefts fuse to form the primitive vascular lumen. The syncytial cells enveloping these clefts become the endothelium of the new vessels. Proliferative growth of this endothelium links the vascular lumina into a continuous irregular endothelial vascular meshwork over the surface of the developing brain. Further extension of this primitive network, present over the developing telencephalon of human embryos at 4 weeks of age, occurs through endothelial sprouting.

Sabin has described a fascinating alternative process for the development of the primitive vascular plexus.[54] She observed the appearance of intracellular vacuoles which coalesced to form the future vascular lumen, with the liquid of the vacuole becoming the primitive plasma. According to this schema, the first primitive vascular lumen is embryologically an intracellular structure, with the syncytial cells containing these interconnected vacuoles forming the primitive vascular endothelium.

The primordial vascular plexus first differentiates into afferent, efferent, and capillary components over the more rostral portion of the embryonic brain. The more superficial portion of the plexus forms larger vascular channels, eventually evolving into the arteries and veins, with the deeper portion resolving into the capillary component more closely attached to the brain surface. Beginning circulation to the brain appears around the end of the fourth week of embryonic life. Arteriovenous malformations arise from persistent direct connections between the future arterial and venous sides of the primitive vascular plexus, with failure to develop an interposed capillary network.

During the sixth and seventh weeks the third pair of aortic arches, together with the dorsal aorta, transform into the primitive internal carotid arteries, with the first and second arches undergoing early involution. The vertebral arteries arise from a longitudinal linkage of the dorsal rami of the intersegmental arteries of the neck during the fourth week. All the original proximal intersegmental artery stalks except the most caudal one atrophy, resulting in a longitudinal vessel taking origin along with the subclavian from the sixth cervical intersegmental artery. The vertebral artery establishes communication with the internal carotids through the basilar artery, which arises independently through the consolidation of two longitudinal vascular channels beneath the brain. This linkage is established by the sixth week of fetal life. Between the sixth and eighth week of fetal life, a compartmentalized brain, dural, and extracranial circulation has been established.[64] By the eighth week of fetal life the major venous sinus pattern of the adult has begun to emerge.

Pathologic Classification of Arteriovenous Malformations

The development of cerebral angiography catalyzed interest in the study of intracranial vascular anomalies, providing the first major new insights into the pathophysiology of these lesions. The first major classifications of intracranial vascular malformations, used extensively in the older European literature, consisted of four overall categories: (1) angioma cavernosum, (2) angioma racemosum, (3) angioreticuloma, and (4) angioglioma.[7,23] Angioma racemosum included the subheadings of *(a)* telangiectasis, *(b)* Sturge-Weber syndrome, *(c)* angioma racemosum arteriale, *(d)* angioma racemosum venosum, and *(e)* arteriovenous aneurysm. The term "arteriovenous aneurysm" corresponds to our current designation "arteriovenous malformation."

In 1966 McCormick proposed a more clinically oriented categorization into five pathologic types: (1) telangiectasia, (2) varix, (3) cavernous angioma, (4) arteriovenous malformation, and (5) venous angioma.[46] Telangiectasias are capillary angiomas, usually small and solitary and most frequently occurring in the pons and the roof of the fourth ventricle. They are only occasionally associated with hemorrhage. A varix is usually quite small and is occasionally invisible grossly, consisting of one or more dilated veins not associated with an arteriovenous shunt. These small lesions, found in either the parenchyma or the leptomeninges, may be associated with hemorrhage, occasionally massive. Cavernous angiomas are dilated sinusoidal vascular anomalies varying in size or diameter from 1 mm up to many centimeters and are associated with hemorrhage as well as seizures. They occur most often in the cerebrum but may occur in any part of the central nervous system. Brain parenchyma is absent between the sinusoidal vascular spaces. Calcium deposition and hyalinization of the vessel walls are common; spontaneous thrombosis of either part or all of the lesion may occur. The blood in a cavernous angioma is not arterialized. The term *venous angioma* defines a malformation consisting entirely of veins not associated with an arteriovenous shunt, though otherwise closely resembling an arteriovenous malformation in gross appearance,

The term *arteriovenous malformation,* the primary topic of this section, refers to a congenital maldevelopment of blood vessels, with preservation of one or more primitive direct communications between arterial and venous channels. The malformations are found throughout the central nervous system, occurring most commonly in the cerebral hemispheres, with from 70 to 93 percent found in the supratentorial structures in various reported series.[11,47,50,52] Arteriovenous malformations of the cerebral hemispheres most frequently involve the distribution of the middle cerebral arterial tree, followed in declining frequency by those of the anterior and then the posterior cerebral arteries. Hemispheral arteriovenous malformations can be further subclassified into those involving either one or a combination of the epicerebral, the transcerebral, and the subependymal circulations.

The epicerebral circulation consists of short perforating branches arising from the small pial arteries on the cortical surface and penetrating the cortex more or less at right angles to the brain surface (Fig. 239-1).[58] They form a distinct palisade of parallel short arteries of varying length, supplying the superficial, middle, and deep layers of the cortex. These slender cortical arteries show a grapnel-like pattern of branching, spreading outward and back upward toward the cortical surface as they terminate in a capillary bed. The longer transcerebral arteries (averaging 2 to 3 cm in length), traverse the cortex to feed an elongated capillary mesh or plexus paralleling the transcerebral arteries in the white matter. The transcerebral arteries terminate in the periventricular plexus.

Paralleling the arterial pattern, the venous drainage of the epicerebral circulation courses back outward to the veins on the pial surface.[59] The venous drainage of the transcerebral arterial circulation is predominantly inward toward the subependymal venous plexus of the lateral ventricles, though anastomotic connections with and associated flow to the epicerebral veins are also present.

Malformations involving only the transcerebral arteries are not visible on the cortical surface, although it is common to see arterialized venous channels on the pial surface of the cortex as a result of the anastomotic connections between the transcerebral and epicerebral venous draihages.

Pathology

The gross appearance of an arteriovenous malformation is that of a tangled mass of dilated tortuous vessels (Fig. 239-2). Small areas of hemosiderin staining and thickened, milky appearing pia-arachnoid are common in the immediate vicinity of the lesion in older patients. If the transcerebral circulation is involved in the malformation, the lesion presents a characteristic wedge-shaped appearance with the apex of the wedge at the ependymal surface of the lateral ventricle and the base of the wedge parallel to the overlying cerebral convexity (Figs. 239-3 and 239-4). There is a rare but surgically very favorable group of arteriovenous malformations limited entirely to the pial surface of the brain stem.[16]

Arteries emptying into the malformation become passively enlarged with time due to the high flow volume resulting from the abnormally low peripheral resistance of the A-V shunt.[14,25–27] The venous system draining the shunt similarly undergoes progressive enlargement with increasing tortuosity as a result of the high flow volume and sustained increased venous pressure produced by the A-V shunt. Atrophic changes of the cortex and subcortical white matter in the immediate vicinity of the malformation are also common findings in older patients. Secondary changes with time have been found in the arterial walls of the feeding arteries in the immediate vicinity of the malformation, with collagenous replacement of the normal smooth muscle component of the media.[26] Saccular aneurysms are an associated finding in between 10 and 15 percent of patients with arteriovenous malformations.[32,36,48] Between 60 and 95 percent of these aneurysms occur on arteries hemodynamically related to the arteriovenous malformation.

The external carotid artery may make a significant flow contribution to a cerebral arteriovenous malformation and occasionally may be the sole source of arterial inflow to the lesion.[12,19,53]

Incidence; Age and Sex Distribution

The cooperative study on intracranial aneurysms and arteriovenous malformations suggested that the frequency of intracranial arteriovenous malformations is about one-seventh that of saccular aneurysms.[50] This would indicate that about 0.14 percent of the U.S. population, or approximately 280,000 individuals, harbor one of

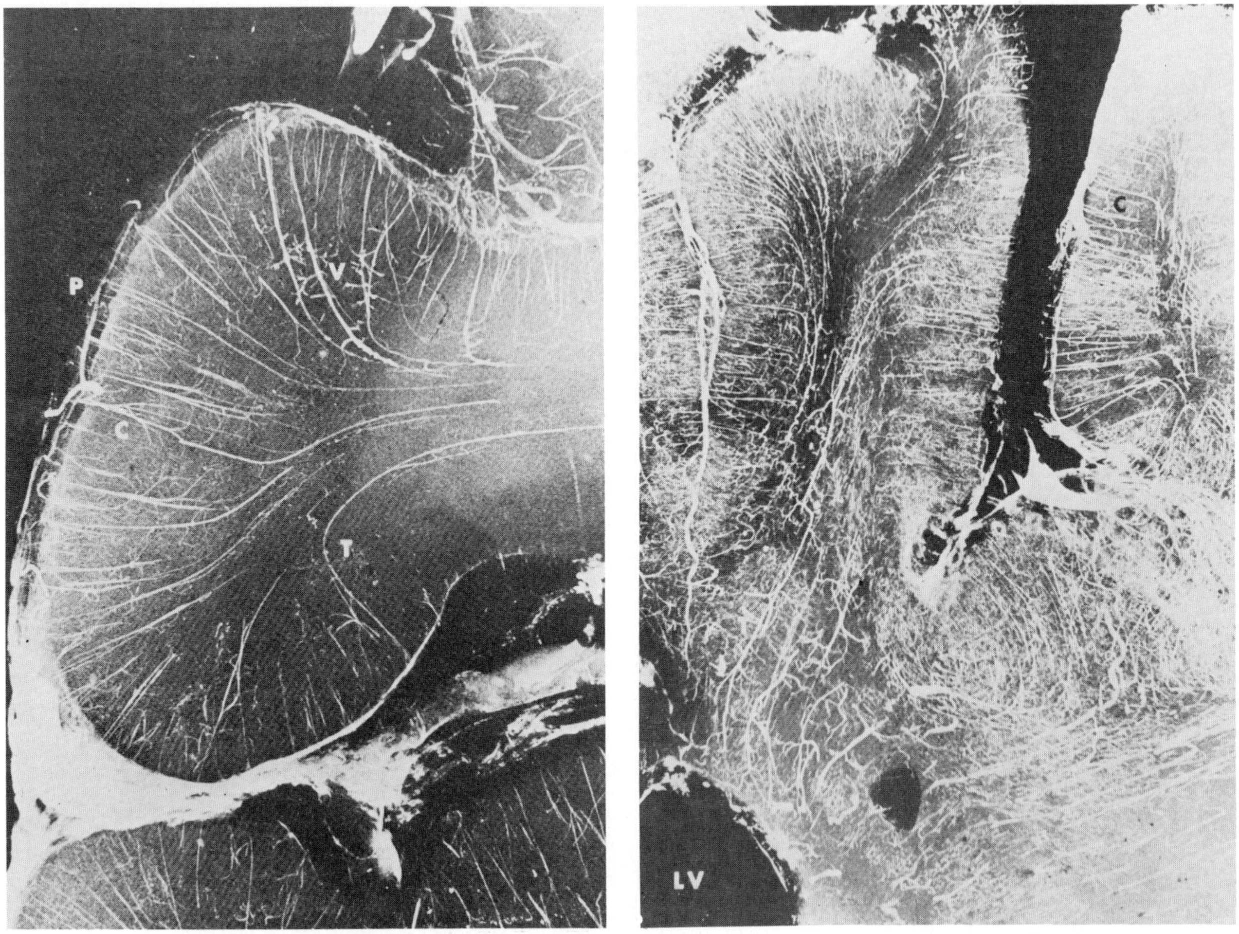

(*A*) (*B*)

Figure 239-1 *A*. Postmortem radiography of an intra-arterial micropaque barium injection (human cortex, ×11) showing short perforating epicerebral arteries (c) with ''grapnel-like'' endings, and sweeping curves of the transcerebral arteries (T). Several veins (V) are also filled. P, pial artery. *B*. Convergence of transcerebral arteries (T) on the periventricular vascular plexus (coronal section, ×5). LV, lateral ventricle. (From Saunders et al.,[58] with permission.)

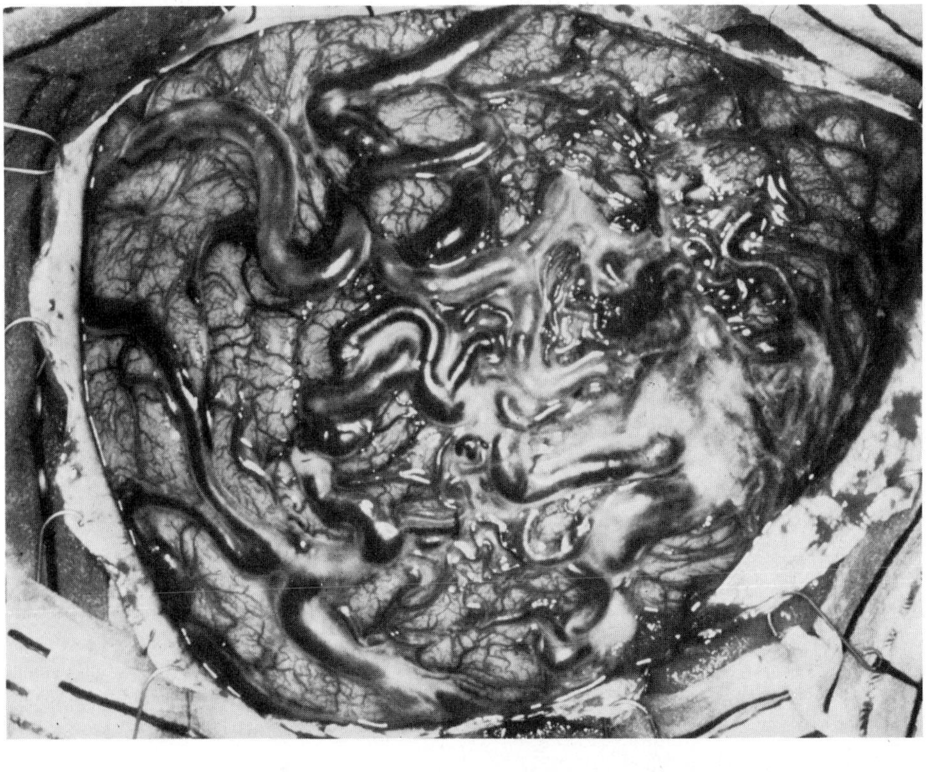

Figure 239-2 A parietal AVM involving both the epicerebral and transcerebral circulations with thickened pia-arachnoid and interstitial scarring from small, old focal hemorrhages.

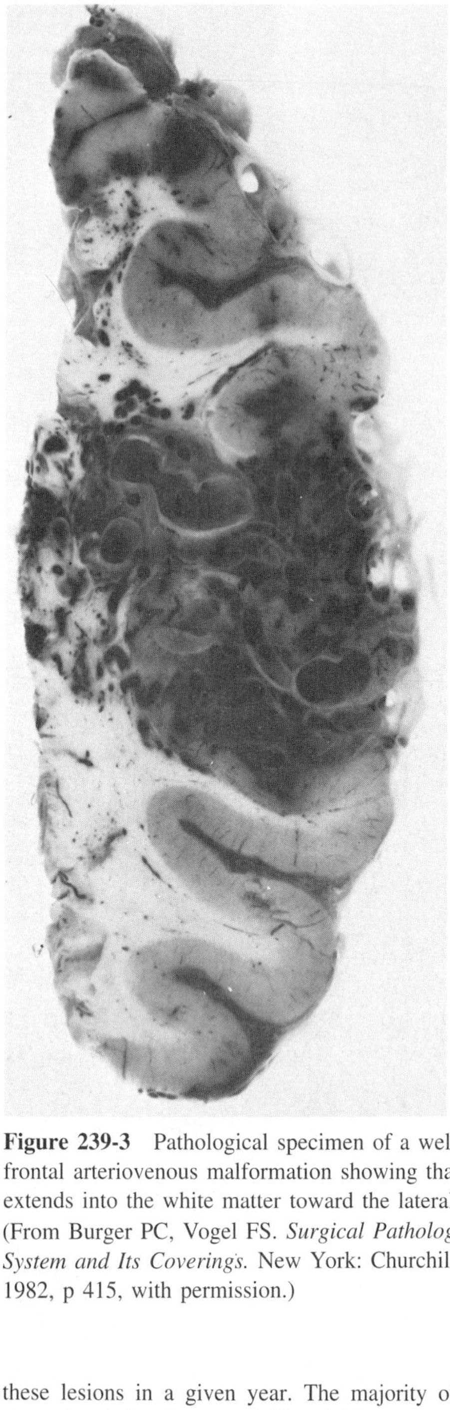

Figure 239-3 Pathological specimen of a well-defined right frontal arteriovenous malformation showing that it tapers as it extends into the white matter toward the lateral ventricle. (From Burger PC, Vogel FS. *Surgical Pathology of the Nervous System and Its Coverings*. New York: Churchill Livingstone, 1982, p 415, with permission.)

these lesions in a given year. The majority of lesions become symptomatic by the age of 40 and in most large series show no predilection for either sex. Although occasional reports of familial incidence are found in the literature, the larger series show no familial or genetic predisposition.[1,47,50]

Clinical Features

In adult life the first symptom of an arteriovenous malformation is usually either a hemorrhage or a seizure. These two types of presentation occur with about equal frequency. The average age of onset for epilepsy as the initial symptom is about age 25, with age 30 the corresponding figure for hemorrhage.[22,63] Patients with large arteriovenous malformations are more than twice as likely to

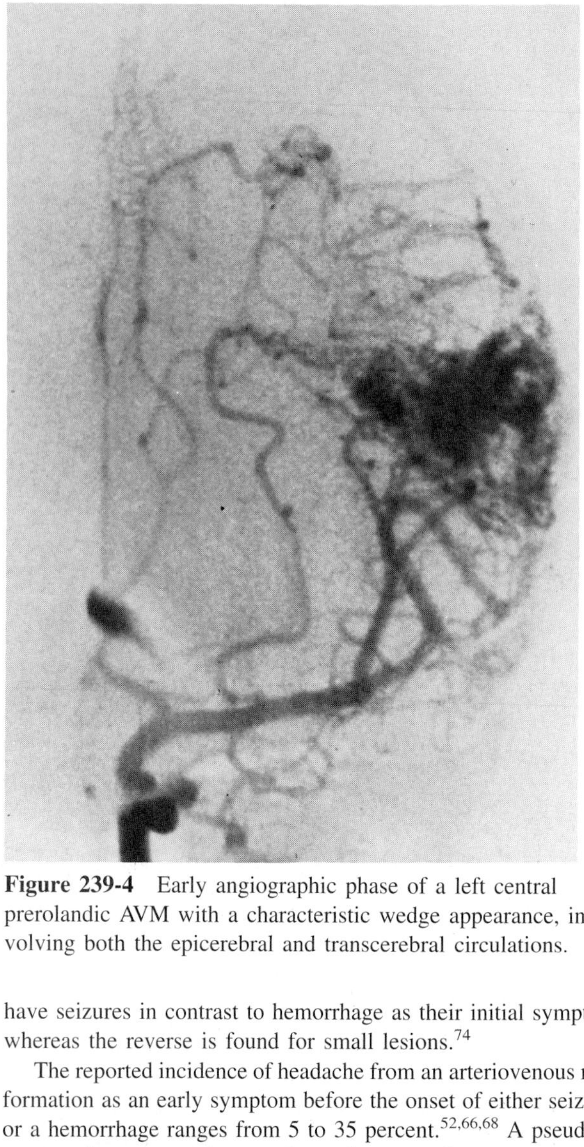

Figure 239-4 Early angiographic phase of a left central prerolandic AVM with a characteristic wedge appearance, involving both the epicerebral and transcerebral circulations.

have seizures in contrast to hemorrhage as their initial symptom, whereas the reverse is found for small lesions.[74]

The reported incidence of headache from an arteriovenous malformation as an early symptom before the onset of either seizures or a hemorrhage ranges from 5 to 35 percent.[52,66,68] A pseudotumor syndrome secondary to elevated venous sinus pressure from large A-V shunts, particularly if the shunts are near the torcular and transverse sinus, and hydrocephalus as a sequela to previously undiagnosed small subarachnoid hemorrhages are less common as a presenting feature.[71,75] Arteriovenous malformations may occasionally mimic a demyelinating disease or brain tumor, particularly when located in the brain stem or deep basal ganglia.[9] Intellectual deterioration tends to occur with large AVMs in the older age groups. This deterioration appears to be at least partially related to a cerebral steal phenomenon.[21,76]

In children, hemorrhage is seven times more likely than a seizure to be the initial presenting event.[31] An additional common presentation of an arteriovenous malformation in the neonatal period is high-output left ventricular cardiac failure. Detailed hemodynamic studies have shown that right heart failure may evolve as an additional complicating factor secondary to right side overload from the left to right shunt.[40]

The clinical course of an arteriovenous malformation, apart from hemorrhage, is usually one of slowly progressing symptomatology referable to the site of the lesion.[35] The mortality rate from hemorrhage in the cooperative study of 453 patients was 10 percent from the initial bleeding episode, 13 percent from a second episode, and 20 percent from a third episode.[50] The risk of recurrent hemorrhage after an initial bleeding episode is between 3.5

and 4.0 percent per year.[17,50,66] The risk of hemorrhage in a patient presenting with cerebral seizures but with no known previous hemorrhage has been variously reported as between 1 and 2.3 percent per year.[22,50] Forster et al. found, in a 15-year average follow-up of 35 patients presenting with epilepsy alone, a 17 percent mortality and 20 percent severe disability secondary to hemorrhage.[22] They further noted that if the patient had had one hemorrhage, there was a 25 percent risk of rebleeding over the next 4 years. If there had been two previous hemorrhages, the risk for further rebleeding was 25 percent within the year following the most recent hemorrhage. A review of 137 patients treated conservatively with a follow-up period ranging from a minimum of 10 years to a maximum of 25 years found that only 20 percent of the 137 were alive and well at the end of the study. Thirty-seven patients either had died or were severely incapacitated by the arteriovenous malformation.[69]

Vascular malformations presenting during pregnancy are more likely to rehemorrhage than those in the nonpregnant patient, with the frequency of rebleeding approaching that of saccular aneurysms.[70] The posthemorrhage mortality and morbidity figures, however, remain significantly lower than those for saccular aneurysms and comparable with those for the nonpregnant individual.[55] Surprisingly, the timing of rebleeding does not appear to peak or parallel the cardiovascular changes in pregnancy. The peak incidence of hemorrhage from AVMs occurs between the fifteenth and twentieth week of pregnancy as compared with the peak incidence of aneurysm rebleeding between the thirteenth and fourteenth week of gestation. Only 2 of 77 AVM hemorrhages during pregnancy in this series occurred during labor. Elective cesarian section at 38 weeks gestation was thought to carry the smallest combined risk to mother and child.

Occasional spontaneous disappearance of intracranial arteriovenous malformations has been reported, but this remains a very rare occurrence.[39,57]

Radiology

Cerebral angiography continues to be the definitive study for the assessment of intracranial vascular malformations (Fig. 239-5).

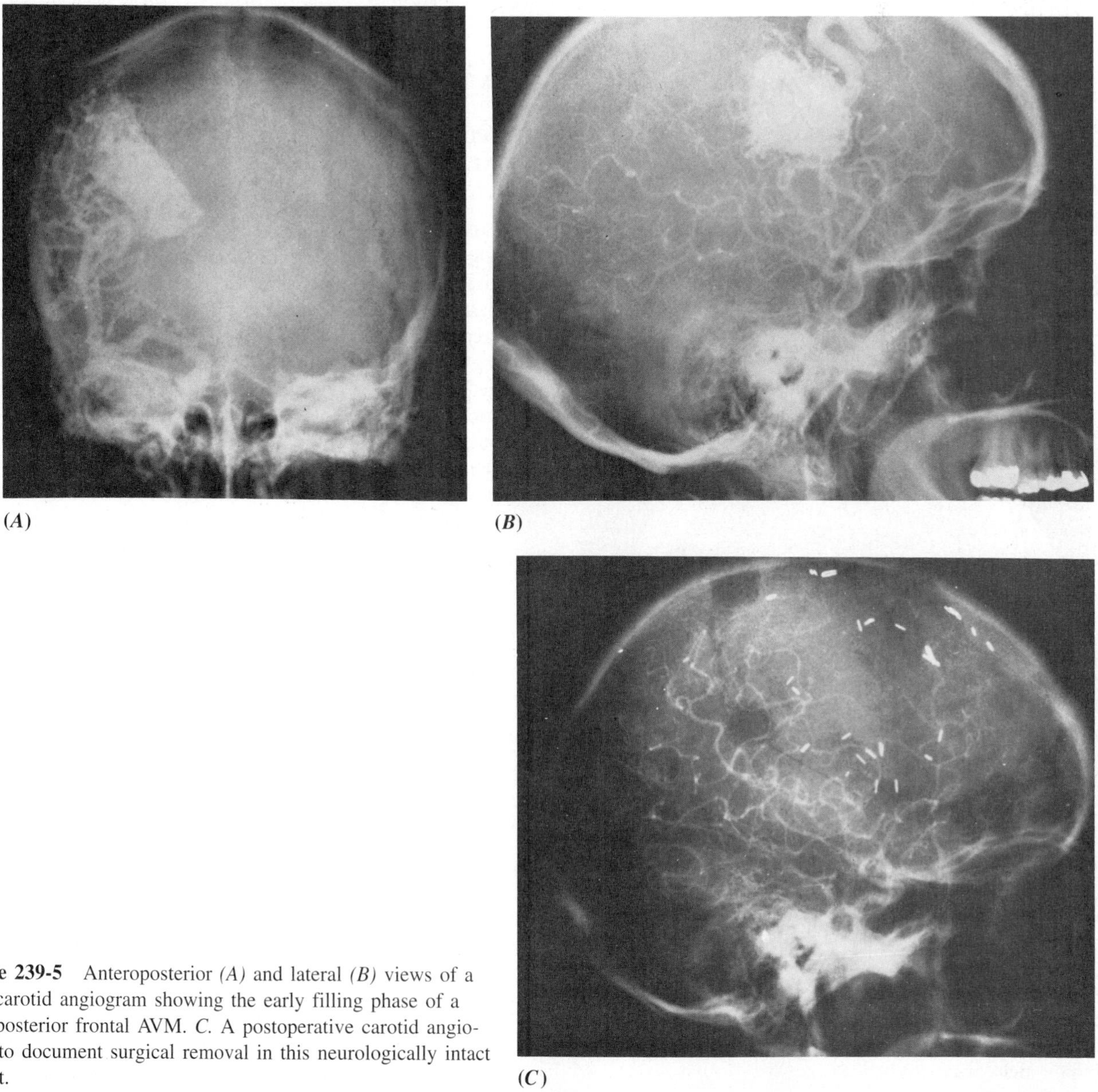

Figure 239-5 Anteroposterior *(A)* and lateral *(B)* views of a right carotid angiogram showing the early filling phase of a right posterior frontal AVM. *C.* A postoperative carotid angiogram to document surgical removal in this neurologically intact patient.

Careful bilateral carotid as well as vertebral angiography often demonstrates unexpected crossover or collateral filling of AVMs and is essential for adequate planning of therapy and assessment of risks to the patient. Computed tomography (CT) scanning or magnetic resonance imaging (MRI) have become common screening techniques for the diagnosis of vascular malformations (Fig. 239-6). Angiographically occult AVMs have been found using both imaging techniques. Intracerebral hemorrhage enhancing on CT scan, even when arteriography fails to demonstrate a vascular anomaly, should raise the suspicion of the presence of a small AVM.[8,41] Neither CT nor MRI reveals the anatomic detail necessary for surgical planning. They also do not reliably disclose the presence of associated vascular anomalies such as saccular aneurysms.

In a group of 43 patients with AVMs studied with unenhanced, enhanced, and 1-h postcontrast CT scans, the precontrast scan was abnormal in 81 percent of patients.[33] Two patients showed a venous angioma on the immediate postcontrast scan, which was not apparent on either the precontrast or the 1-h delayed scan. The 1-h delayed scan revealed one angiographically occult, thrombosed AVM not seen on the precontrast or immediate postcontrast scan. The 1-h delayed scan also showed additional pathologic changes in areas adjacent to the lesions shown on the precontrast and immediate postcontrast scans. Delayed high-contrast CT scanning was judged to show no advantage as the routine screening procedure and, if done as a sole procedure, might miss at least some venous angiomas.

The "flow void" seen on MRI of AVMs has become a useful, though not completely accurate, technique for assessing the degree of occlusion of AVMs after focused stereotactic radiation therapy.

Indications for Operation

The role of surgery in the clinical management of a given patient is based on a composite of the probable natural history of the patient's future clinical course, the risk of surgical management with particular reference to the patient's required occupational or daily activities, and finally, the patient's age.[4,65] Patients in the older age group who have seizures but who are otherwise neurologically intact and without a previous history of hemorrhage have comparatively a smaller cumulative risk of major morbidity and mortality with continued conservative management. An important factor in long-term planning for the younger patient is the problem that seizure foci secondary to AVMs tend to become progressively more resistant to medical management with time. Although most current surgical series show some reduction in seizure tendency after malformation excision, extirpation of the malformation more importantly may block the further development of medically intractable seizure activity.[15,51,77] In the younger patient, as is discussed in more detail below, the risk of mortality or major morbidity with surgery using current techniques is competitive with the 10-year prognosis for lesions that have not bled, and is better than the 5-year prognosis for malformations with a previous history of at least one hemorrhage. Malformations in areas of eloquent function are being found increasingly amenable to a surgical approach, with mortality or major morbidity risks of 10 percent or less.[27,28] Deep lesions involving the internal capsule, thalamus, midbrain, and lower brain stem are still usually found to be inoperable in terms of acceptable risks to neurological function.

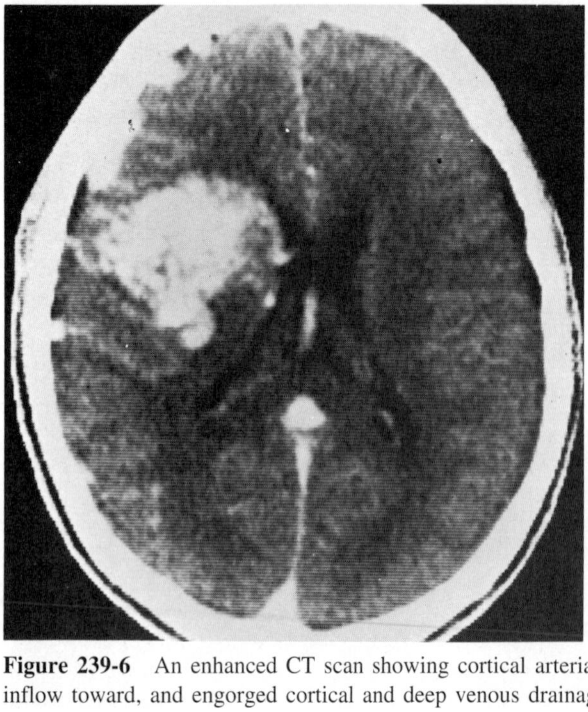

Figure 239-6 An enhanced CT scan showing cortical arterial inflow toward, and engorged cortical and deep venous drainage from, a right frontal AVM.

Role of Embolization in AVM Management

Embolization of larger AVMs has become an important therapeutic adjunct to their surgical management.[3,10,37,44,50,61] To date, the large majority of these lesions cannot be totally occluded by embolization techniques. Embolization does, however, permit a staged preoperative reduction in size of the arteriovenous shunt, producing significant circulatory readjustment and reducing the degree of hydraulic shock resulting from the final occlusion of the fistula at the time of surgical resection of the lesion.[18] Embolization, when practical, has largely replaced staged surgical occlusion of the feeding arteries to achieve this effect.[25,62]

Embolic agents are classified as either absorbable or nonabsorbable and as either solid or fluid. Solid embolic agents have been injected into the internal carotid or vertebral artery feeding the malformation, relying on the high-volume axial flow characteristics of the circulation to the AVM to carry the solid particles into its nidus. This technique is not satisfactory if the pellets, such as nonabsorbable barium-impregnated silicone spheres, have to leave the parent artery at a sharp angle to enter a branching vessel, such as would be required for a pellet entering the anterior cerebral artery from the internal carotid artery.

Gelfoam, cut into 1 × 2 mm strips, impregnated with tantalum powder and soaked in angiographic contrast material has been a common absorbable solid embolic agent. Although this material is relatively easy to handle, it has been more unpredictable in producing occlusion on the arterial side of the shunt and has no major advantages over silicone spheres.

Fluid embolic agents that have been employed have been nonabsorbable and of either the bucrylate or silicone types. Isobutyl-2-cyanoacrylate (ICBA) is a prototypic material of the bucrylate group. It is a rapidly polymerizing, low-viscosity tissue adhesive which is made radiopaque by adding tantalum powder. ICBA polymerizes rapidly on contact with ionic solutions such as blood or normal saline, while a 5% glucose solution will block polymerization. Considerable skill and experience are required in the use of this material. The speed of polymerization and rate of injection must be finely calculated to ensure that polymerization occurs on the arterial side of the malformation. Distal migration of this fluid into the major sinuses has occurred.[17] If the arterial inflow is not arrested by polymerization on the arterial side of the shunt, sudden swelling and rupture of the malformation with major hemorrhage may occur. Bucrylate produces a foreign body giant cell reaction with chronic inflammatory changes not only in the vessel wall but also to a lesser degree in the adjacent brain parenchyma.[72] The long-term effects of this material are not yet fully known. Occasional malformations have been completely occluded with bucrylate, although the success rate for total occlusion has not been high. There are several additional technical problems in using this material for occlusion of malformations in areas of eloquent function. Arterial branches to normally functioning eloquent cortex often depart from the parent artery distal to the first arterial branches going to the malformation. Total occlusion of the malformation would, of necessity, require sacrificing these normal branches, with potentially serious neurological sequelae. Additionally, the hardened, noncompressible prongs of bucrylate within an incompletely occluded malformation may significantly increase the difficulty of subsequent safe separation and surgical removal of the malformation from areas of critical function.

Silicone fluid mixtures have occasionally been used instead of bucrylate. The mixture consists of a silastic elastomer containing a filler necessary for vulcanization, and a medical-grade silicone fluid that acts as the diluent to the more viscous Silastic elastomer. These two silicones are mixed to the desired viscosity and then tantalum powder is added to permit radiographic visualization. A catalyst to produce vulcanization is required. The Silastic is injected just before vulcanization occurs. It has no adhesive properties, so that a complete filling or cast of the vascular lumen is required.

After embolization with attendant reduction in the sump effect of the AVM, some patients have been noted to show improvement in intellectual performance, suggesting the correction of some degree of symptomatic cerebral steal.[76] Wolpert et al. found, however, that embolization had no long-term effect on the progression of neurological symptoms or signs and no effect on seizure frequency.[76] Incomplete occlusion of the malformation by embolization has not reduced or modified the natural history of the lesion with respect to hemorrhage.[43]

In 1974, Serbinenko reported the use of detachable flow-directed balloons on the tips of catheters threaded into the proximal vessels to the malformation.[60] This technique has been a key factor in permitting selective catheterization of these vessels for the injection of embolic agents but has not been a satisfactory therapeutic occlusive maneuver in and of itself.[67]

Operative Management

Preoperatively, the patient is placed on an antiepileptic to minimize the risk of seizures during the early postoperative period of cerebral vasocongestion and cerebral swelling, even if the patient has no previous history of cerebral seizures. Serum antiepileptic levels are checked immediately before surgery to ensure that adequate antiepileptic levels are present. Dexamethasone is started 36 to 48 h preoperatively to help stabilize capillary membrane permeability during the early postoperative interval of hydraulic shock and local tissue reaction to surgical manipulation.[3,5,78,79]

If the malformation lies in or immediately adjacent to the expected location of the motor cortex or major speech centers, the surgical procedure may be carried out under local anesthesia with cortical mapping to ensure accurate localization of the areas of eloquent function and to permit the testing of these functions serially throughout the removal of the malformation.[10,28,30] In this latter situation, temporary clips are placed on the arterial feeders immediately proximal to the malformation, followed by function testing. The temporary clips are then replaced with permanent ones if no functional impairment has ensued.

Surgical resection should always be performed under magnification with appropriate microsurgical instrumentation. The dissection plane follows along the immediate margin of the malformation in the thin, gliotic nonfunctional zone between the malformation and the adjacent cortex and white matter. Particular care must be taken in occluding the small, thin-walled endothelial tubules composing the transcerebral venous drainage. These vessels are extremely fragile and, if torn, back-bleed profusely due to the increased venous pressure in the subependymal venous plexus from the A-V shunt. It is essential to avoid pursuing these vessels if unacceptable neurological deficit is to be avoided. Temporary placement of small fluffy cotton pledgets, accompanied by surgeon patience and by moving on to another area of the removal, will normally secure hemostasis of these individual venous bleeding points. Careful positioning of the head so that the major intracranial venous drainage is above heart level is a major factor in reducing venous congestion and attendant blood loss.

Selective identification and occlusion of the arterial inflow to the lesion with protection of the venous drainage as long as possible is important, although Malis advocates using one of the draining veins as a "handle" and a guide to resection when several major draining veins are present.[78] Major reduction in venous outflow before interruption of the arterial inflow must be avoided if malformation rupture with massive bleeding is to be avoided. High-contrast visual dye can be injected intra-arterially to aid in the identification of the feeding arteries to the malformation if the vascular tangle of the malformation makes selective identification of the arterial inflow otherwise difficult.[29] Significant fragility of the lesion persists down to the very end of the resection, making it essential that neither fatigue nor impatience results in a rush or hurry to complete the final stages of the removal.

A grid technique of localization of cortical function for a malformation lying in or adjacent to the central areas has been proposed by Kunc.[38] This technique presupposes a consistent pattern of cortical function with reference to standard anatomic landmarks. Experience with cortical mapping unfortunately has revealed significant deviation in location from the more common patterns of cortical function around the margins of arteriovenous malformations, especially with respect to speech localization. Modern techniques of anesthesiology have made a major contribution to increasing the safety of the surgical approach to, and manipulation of, these lesions. Moderate hypotension during critical periods of surgical resection is well tolerated, even under local anesthesia, and does not interfere with patient alertness and function testing.[30] The general anesthesia technique of jet ventilation can also essentially eliminate brain movement secondary to respiration.[24]

Preliminary experience with surgical lasers used on intracranial vascular lesions has appeared in the literature.[20] At present, the lasers seem to have limited application to the surgery of AVMs. This is particularly true of the CO_2 laser, which has relatively poor vessel coagulation ability because of its extremely shallow depth of penetration. The CO_2 laser tends to punch holes in the walls of larger vessels. The neodymium:YAG laser is more efficient in achieving hemostasis due to its greater depth of penetration. However, this latter laser type also is not effective in providing adequate hemostasis in dealing with the very thin-walled endothelial tubes of the engorged transcerebral circulation. The neodymium:YAG laser appears to provide adequate vascular occlusion when contractile elements are a significant component of the vessel walls being treated with the laser.

Gentle handling of the arteries proximal to the lesions is essential, particularly in the posterior fossa where proximal propagation of clot from the point of arterial occlusion can result in a disastrous outcome for an otherwise technically satisfactory surgical excision. After completion of the resection, the patient's blood pressure should be brought to normal levels and the operative field observed carefully to ensure that hemostasis is complete. Feeding arteries of 1 mm or larger must be securely clipped, if delayed postoperative hemorrhage is to be consistently avoided. Bipolar coagulation alone for these larger vessels is not adequate.

Postoperatively, the patient is nursed with the head of the bed elevated 30 to 40 degrees to maintain optimal venous outflow. It is helpful to maintain the systolic blood pressure between 90 to 110 mmHg, using a trimethaphan camsylate drip, to minimize the effects of hydraulic shock and attendant hyperperfusion around the margins of the resection during the first 24 h postoperatively. Crystalloids are restricted in order to produce a mild dehydration, with the goal of a serum osmolarity between 295 and 305. Blood volume is maintained with colloid administration. Dexamethasone is continued postoperatively for 8 to 10 days and is then rapidly tapered. Postoperative angiography is essential to confirm that complete removal of the malformation has been achieved (Fig. 239-5*C*).

Results

The type of patient screening before surgical referral as well as the aggressiveness of the consulting neurological and neurosurgical units are obvious factors in reported results. In larger series in which over 60 percent of all patients referred underwent surgical extirpation of the lesions, a mortality rate ranging from 7 to 14 percent is found.[2,16,27,34,65] The widespread use of the surgical microscope and the staged preoperative embolization of the lesions are major factors in the improving mortality and morbidity statistics. Surgical mortality rates now appear to compare favorably with the long-term mortality rates of these lesions managed conservatively in the younger patient. More information regarding the quality of postoperative survival, as compared to the quality of life with conservative management, is needed. In the few instances where this information is beginning to appear, preliminary indications are that the long-term quality of life is more favorable when surgical extirpation of the lesion has been carried out.

References

1. Aberfeld DC, Rao KR. Familial arteriovenous malformation of the brain. *Neurology (NY)* 1981; 31:184–186.
2. Albert P. Personal experience in the treatment of 178 cases of arteriovenous malformations of the brain. *Acta Neurochir (Wien)* 1982; 61:207–226.
3. Al-Rodhan, Sundt TM, Piepgras DG, et al. Occlusive hyperemia: a theory for the hemodynamic complications following resection of intracerebral arteriovenous malformations. *J Neurosurg* 1993; 78:167–175.
4. Aminoff MJ. Management of unruptured cerebral arteriovenous malformations. *Clin Neurosurg* 1986; 33:177–185.
5. Awad IA, Magdinec M, Schubert A. Intracranial hypertension after resection of cerebral arteriovenous malformations. Predisposing factors and management strategy. *Stroke* 1984; 25:611–620.
6. Berenstein A. Technique of catheterization and embolization of the lenticulostriate arteries. *J Neurosurg* 1981; 54:783–789.
7. Bergstrand H, Olivecrona H, Tönnis W. *Gefässmissbildungen und Gefässgeschwülste des Gehirns*. Leipzig: Georg Thieme Verlag, 1936, p 181.
8. Bitoh S, Hasegawa H, Fujiwara M, Sakurai M. Angiographically occult vascular malformations causing intracranial hemorrhage. *Surg Neurol* 1982; 17:35–42.
9. Britt RH, Connor WS, Enzmann DR. Occult arteriovenous malformation of the brainstem simulating multiple sclerosis. *Neurology (NY)* 1981; 31:901–904.
10. Burchiel KJ, Clarke H. Ojemann GA, et al. Use of stimulation mapping and corticography in the excision of arteriovenous malformations in sensorimotor and language-related neocortex. *Neurosurgery* 1989; 24:322–327.
11. Chou SN, Erickson DL, Ortiz-Suarez HJ. Surgical treatment of vascular lesions in the brain stem. *J Neurosurg* 1975; 42:23–31.
12. Dahl RE, Kline DG. Intraparenchymal arteriovenous malformations with predominant external carotid artery contribution. *J Neurosurg* 1974; 41:681–687.
13. Debrun G, Vinuela F, Fox A, Drake CG. Embolization of cerebral arteriovenous malformations with bucrylate: experience in 46 cases. *J Neurosurg* 1982; 56:615–627.
14. Delitala A, Delfini R, Vagnozzi R, Esposito S. Increase in size of cerebral angiomas: case report. *J Neurosurg* 1982; 57:556–558.
15. Dodick DW, Cascino GD, Meyer FB. Vascular malformations and intractable epilepsy; outcome after surgical treatment. *May Clin Proc* 1994; 69:741–745.
16. Drake CG. Surgical removal of arteriovenous malformations from the brain stem and cerebellopontine angle. *J Neurosurg* 1975; 43:661–670.
17. Drake CG. Cerebral arteriovenous malformations: considerations for and experience with surgical treatment in 166 cases. *Clin Neurosurg* 1979; 26:145–208.
18. Duckwiler G, Dion J, Vinuela F, et al. Intravascular microcatheter pressure monitoring: experimental results and early clinical evaluation. *Am J Neuroradiol* 1990; 11:169–175.
19. Faria MA Jr. External carotid component of AVMs. *J Neurosurg* 1982; 56:740 (letter).
20. Fasano VA. The treatment of vascular malformation of the brain with laser source. *Lasers Surg Med* 1981; 1:347–356.
21. Feindel W. The influence of cerebral steal: Demonstration of fluorescein angiography and focal cerebral blood flow measurement—pathophysiological aspects. In Pia HW, Gleave JRW, Grote E, Zierski J (eds): *Cerebral Angiomas: Advances in Diagnosis and Therapy*. Berlin: Springer-Verlag, 1975, pp 87–100.
22. Forster DMC, Steiner L, Håkanson S. Arteriovenous malformations of the brain. A long-term clinical study. *J Neurosurg* 1972; 37:562–570.
23. French LA, Chou SN. Conventional methods of treating intracranial arteriovenous malformations. *Prog Neurol Surg* 1969; 3:274–318.
24. Frost EAM. Anaesthetic management of cerebrovascular disease. *Br J Anaesth* 1981; 53:745–756.
25. Garretson HD. Surgical techniques in intracranial vascular malformation surgery. Presented at the Annual Meeting of the Society of University Neurosurgeons, Rochester, MN, May 1975.
26. Garretson HD. Postoperative pressure and flow changes in the feeding

arteries of cerebral arteriovenous malformations. *Neurosurgery* 1979; 4:544–545.
27. Garretson HD. Arteriovenous malformations. In Rosenberg RN, Grossman RG, Schochet S, Heinz ER, Willis WE (eds): *The Clinical Neurosciences.* New York: Churchill Livingstone, 1983, pp II:1089–II:1099.
28. Garretson HD, Geevarghese, G. Arteriovenous malformations of the dominant hemisphere. Presented at the Annual Meeting of the American Association of Neurological Surgeons, Miami, FL, April 6–10, 1975.
29. Garretson H, Perot P, Yamamoto YL, Feindel W. Intracarotid Coomassie blue dye as an aid in the surgery of intracranial vascular lesions. *J Neurosurg* 1967; 26:577–583.
30. Geevarghese KP, Garretson HD. ''Alert'' anesthesia for craniotomy. *Int Anesthesiol Clin* 1977; 15(3):231–251.
31. Gerosa MA, Cappellotto P, Licata C, et al. Cerebral arteriovenous malformations in children (56 cases). *Childs Brain* 1981; 8:356–371.
32. Hayashi S, Arimoto T, Itakura T, et al. The association of intracranial aneurysms and arteriovenous malformation of the brain: case report. *J Neurosurg* 1981; 55:971–975.
33. Hayman LA, Fox AJ, Evans RA. Effectiveness of contrast regimens in CT detection of vascular malformations of the brain. *Am J Neuroradial* 1981; 2:421–425.
34. Heros RC, Korosue K, Diebold PM. Surgical excision of cerebral arteriovenous malformations: late results. *Neurosurgery* 1990; 26:570–578.
35. Jane JA, Kassell NF, Torner JC, Winn HR. The natural history of aneurysms and arteriovenous malformations. *J Neurosurg* 1985; 62:321–323.
36. Koulouris S, Rizzoli HV. Coexisting intracranial aneurysm and arteriovenous malformation: case report. *Neurosurgery* 1981; 8:219–222.
37. Krause F. Krankenvorstellung aus der Hirnchirurgie. *Zentralbl Chir* 1908; 35(35):61–67.
38. Kunc Z. Surgery of arteriovenous malformations in the speech and motor-sensory regions. *J Neurosurg* 1974; 40:293–303.
39. Kuwahara S, Shima T, Ishikawa S, Uozumi T, Miyazaki M. A clinical study of intracranial AVMs with reference to their enlargement and regression—a follow-up study with angiography and CT scan. *Neurol Med Chir (Tokyo)* 1979; 19:149–161.
40. Lakier JB, Milner S, Cohen M, Levin SE. Intracranial arteriovenous fistulas in infancy—haemodynamic considerations: a review of 3 cases. *S Afr Med J* 1982; 61:242–245.
41. Leblanc R, Ethier R. The computerized tomographic appearance of angiographically occult arteriovenous malformations of the brain. *Can J Neurol Sci* 1981; 8:7–13.
42. Luessenhop AJ, Mujica PH. Embolization of segments of the circle of Willis and adjacent branches for management of certain inoperable cerebral arteriovenous malformations. *J Neurosurg* 1981; 54:573–582.
43. Luessenhop AJ, Presper JH. Surgical embolization of cerebral arteriovenous malformations through internal carotid and vertebral arteries. Long-term results. *J Neurosurg* 1975; 42:443–451.
44. Luessenhop AJ, Rosa L. Cerebral arteriovenous malformations. Indications for and results of surgery, and the role of intravascular techniques. *J Neurosurg* 1984; 60:14–22.
45. Luschka H. Cavernöse Blutgeschwulst des Gehirns. *Virchows Arch* 1854; 6:458–470.
46. McCormick WF. The pathology of vascular (''arteriovenous'') malformations. *J Neurosurg* 1966; 24:807–816.
47. Michelson WJ. Natural history and pathophysiology of arteriovenous malformations. *Clin Neurosurg* 1979; 26:307–313.
48. Miyasaka K, Wolpert SM, Prager RJ. The association of cerebral aneurysms, infundibula, and intracranial arteriovenous malformations. *Stroke* 1982; 13:196–203.
49. Moore KL. *The Developing Human: Clinically Oriented Embryology,* 3d ed. Philadelphia: Saunders, 1982.
50. Perret G, Nishioka H. Arteriovenous malformations. An analysis of 545 cases of cranio-cerebral arteriovenous malformations and fistulae reported to the cooperative study. *J Neurosurg* 1966; 25:467–490.
51. Piepgras DG, Sundt TM, Ragoowanse AT, Stevens L. Seizure outcome in patients with surgically treated cerebral arteriovenous malformations. *J Neurosurg* 1993; 78:5–11.
52. Pool JL, Potts DG. *Aneurysms and Arteriovenous Anomalies of the Brain: Diagnosis and Treatment.* New York: Harper & Row, 1965, pp 326–373.
53. Russell EJ, Berenstein A. Meningeal collateralization to normal cerebral vessels associated with intracerebral arteriovenous malformations: functional angiographic considerations. *Radiology* 1981; 139:617–622.
54. Sabin FR. Preliminary note on the differentiation of angioblasts and the method by which they produce blood-vessels, blood-plasma and red blood-cells as seen in the living chick. *Anat Rec* 1917; 13:199–204.
55. Sadasivan B, Malik GM, Lee C, Ausman JI. Vascular malformations and pregnancy. *Surg Neurol* 1990; 33:305–313.
56. Samson D, Ditmore QM, Beyer CW Jr. Intravascular use of isobutyl 2-cyanoacrylate. Part I: treatment of intracranial arteriovenous malformations. *Neurosurgery* 1981; 8:43–51.
57. Sartor K. Spontaneous closure of cerebral arteriovenous malformation demonstrated by angiography and computed tomography. *Neuroradiology* 1978; 15:95–98.
58. Saunders RL, Feindel WH, Carvalho VR. X-ray microscopy of the blood vessels of the human brain. *Med Biol Illus* 1965; 15:108–122.
59. Saunders RL, Feindel WH, Carvalho VR. X-ray microscopy of the blood vessels of the human brain, Part II. *Med Biol Illus* 1965; 15:234–246.
60. Serbinenko FA. Balloon catheterization and occlusion of major cerebral vessels. *J Neurosurg* 1974; 41:125–145.
61. Spetzler RF, Martin NA, Carter LP, et al. Surgical management of large AVM's by staged embolization and operative excision. *J Neurosurg* 1987; 67:17–28.
62. Spetzler RF, Wilson CB, Weinstein P, et al. Normal perfusion pressure breakthrough theory. *Clin Neurosurg* 1978; 25:651–672.
63. Stein BM, Wolpert SM. Arteriovenous malformations of the brain. I: current concepts and treatment. *Arch Neurol* 1980; 37:1–5.
64. Streeter GL. The developmental alterations in the vascular system of the brain. *Contrib Embryol* 1918; 8:5–38.
65. Sundt TM, Piepgras DG, Stevens LN. Surgery for supratentorial arteriovenous malformations. *Clin Neurosurg* 1991; 37:49–115.
66. Svien HJ, McRae JA. Arteriovenous anomalies of the brain: fate of patients not having definitive surgery. *J Neurosurg* 1965; 23:23–28.
67. Taki W, Handa H, Yonekawa Y, et al. Detachable balloon catheter systems for embolization of cerebrovascular lesions. *Neurol Med Chir (Tokyo)* 1981; 21:709–719.
68. Troost BT, Newton TH. Occipital lobe arteriovenous malformations: clinical and radiologic features in 26 cases with comments on differentiation from migraine. *Arch Ophthalmol* 1975; 93:250–256.
69. Troupp H, Marttila I, Halonen V. Arteriovenous malformations of the brain: prognosis without operation. *Acta Neurochir (Wien)* 1970; 22:125–128.
70. Tuttelman RM, Gleicher N. Central nervous system hemorrhage complicating pregnancy. *Obstet Gynecol* 1981; 58:651–656.
71. Vassilouthis J. Cerebral arteriovenous malformation with intracranial hypertension. *Surg Neurol* 1980; 11:402–404.
72. Vinters HV, Debrun G, Kaufmann JCE, Drake CG. Pathology of arteriovenous malformations embolized with isobutyl-2-cyanoacrylate (bucyrlate): report of two cases. *J Neurosurg* 1981; 55:819–825.
73. Virchow R. *Die Krankhaften Geschwülste* vol 3, Berlin: A. Hirschwald, 1863–1867, pp 345–463.
74. Waltimo O. The relationship of size, density and localization of intracranial arteriovenous malformations to the type of initial symptom. *J Neurol Sci* 1973; 19:13–19.
75. Weisberg L, Pierce JF, Jabbari B. Intracranial hypertension resulting from a cerebrovascular malformation. *South Med J* 1977; 70:624–626.
76. Wolpert SM, Barnett FJ, Prager RJ. Benefits of embolization without surgery for cerebral arteriovenous malformations. *Am J Radiol* 1982; 138:99–102.

77. Yeh H-S, Tew JM, Gartner M. Seizure control after surgery on cerebral arteriovenous malformations. *J Neurosurg* 1993; 78:12–18.
78. Young WL, Kader A, Prohovnik I, et al. Pressure autoregulation is intact after arteriovenous malformation resection. *Neurosurgery* 1993; 32:491–496.
79. Young WL, Pile-Spellman J, Prohovnik I, et al. Evidence for adaptive autoregulatory displacement in hypotensive cortical territories adjacent to arteriovenous malformations. Columbia University AVM Study Project. *Neurosurgery* 1994; 34:601–611.

240 Preoperative Evaluation of the Risk/Benefit Ratio for Arteriovenous Malformations of the Brain

Duke S. Samson
H. Hunt Batjer

In 1985 Robert Wilkins began a review of the natural history of intracranial vascular malformations with the succinct question, "Is this treatment likely to provide results that are better than the expected outcome of the disorder without such treatment?"[22] Although the intervening 5 years have not permitted an exact delineation of either the natural history of intracranial intradural malformations or a precise specification of the surgical efficacy and morbidity associated with their removal, a significant increase in the available clinical data base does currently permit a more precise estimation of both of these critically important parameters. A brief review of recent contributions to this field of vascular neurosurgery may benefit the difficult decision-making process that faces both neurosurgeons and their patients burdened with intracerebral arteriovenous malformations (AVMs).

Natural History

Historically, the major impediments to the identification of the natural history of AVMs have been problems in patient selection and long-term follow-up.[22] In many series reported prior to 1980, a substantial number of patients harboring AVMs underwent surgical treatment, leaving for follow-up a relatively small number of untreated lesions, the natural history of which may or may not be representative of the entire patient group.[14] Furthermore, many patients in the "natural history" group were not subjected to protracted, repetitive clinical evaluations; thus the reports may underestimate the true long-term morbidity and mortality of the lesions not surgically treated. Wilkins' comprehensive review of this issue began with a recognition of these drawbacks and attempted to minimize their effects by including 14 clinical series encompassing over 1500 patients.[22] From this broad and admittedly heterogeneous experience, Wilkins concluded that an unruptured AVM carries an annual risk of hemorrhage of some 2 to 3 percent, with an annual risk of death of about 1 percent. The rate of rebleeding following an initial hemorrhage was thought to be some 2 to 3 percent per year, after an initial 6 percent incidence of rebleeding during the first year after hemorrhage. Although this exhaustive review mentions that smaller AVMs have traditionally been thought to be more frequently associated with hemorrhage than large lesions and that a more malignant natural history (as regards hemorrhage) has been classically attributed to malformations that present with hemorrhage, in contrast to those presenting with seizures, no conclusive documentation of these suggestions could be identified.

In the years since Wilkins' publication, two important studies that may contribute to further delineation of the natural history of this disease have been concluded. Crawford et al. have reported a long-term study of 217 patients (from an AVM population of 343 patients) followed for a mean of over 10 years.[4] The comprehensive long-term risk of hemorrhage in this patient population was 42 percent (4 percent annually), and the major factors predictive of an increased incidence of hemorrhage were the patient's initial presentation with hemorrhage and the patient's age at presentation, with older patients being more likely to suffer hemorrhage or rehemorrhage. Patients diagnosed with an AVM on the basis of a seizure disorder were thought to be at significantly less risk of bleeding than those presenting with hemorrhage (33 percent vs. 51 percent), and temporal and occipital lobe lesions were believed to be at greater risk of ultimate hemorrhage than malformations in other locations. In contrast to prior studies, the size and depth of AVMs were thought to offer no predictive clues to the risk of bleeding.

Ondra et al. recently presented a long-term re-evaluation of the Helsinki series initially reported in 1970 and updated in 1977.[15] This group of 168 patients represents 64 percent of the total AVM patient population seen at Helsinki University between 1942 and 1975 and is relatively unique because of the completeness (98 percent) and the length (mean of 24 years) of clinical follow-up. These authors report an overall risk of AVM-related death of 23 percent, which translates to a 1 percent yearly mortality rate attributable directly to complications of AVM. This patient population had a "conservative" bleeding rate of 4 percent per year, and a combined annual morbidity and mortality of 2.7 percent related specifically to the AVM in question. Of special interest in this series was the lack of significant difference in either the annual risk of hemorrhage or the morbidity and mortality rate associated with hemorrhage when patients presenting with seizures were compared with those presenting with intracranial hemorrhage. Furthermore, the mean interval between presentation and subsequent hemorrhage (or rehemorrhage) was found to be almost 8 years, dramatically pointing out the importance of protracted re-evaluations of patients with this chronic disease problem. Insufficient data were available from this series to provide any significant information regarding long-term prognosis for asymptomatic patients harboring AVMs.

There are four critical components of the natural history of intracranial AVMs:

1. The risk of hemorrhage (or rehemorrhage) associated with the malformation.
2. The risk of death attributable to the malformation.
3. The risk of significant neurological morbidity directly related to the AVM.

4. The factors unique to the patient, the mode of presentation, and the individual AVM, which may influence the above three components.

Risk of Hemorrhage

Although it has traditionally been believed that the risk of hemorrhage is greatest in patients presenting with symptoms suggestive or diagnostic of prior bleeding, at least some recent information suggests that patients whose initial presenting symptom was hemorrhage or a seizure face a similar annual hemorrhage rate.[15] The data currently available suggest that subsequent to diagnosis, intraparenchymal AVMs carry an annual cumulative risk of subarachnoid or intraparenchymal hemorrhage of between 3 and 4 percent, or a risk per decade of 30 to 40 percent.[4,15,22] This risk may be slightly greater in the first year following an initial hemorrhage but would appear to remain relatively constant from that point for the remainder of the patient's life, with hemorrhages in many patients occurring years to decades following the initial diagnosis.[15] No information is currently available to identify precisely the hemorrhage risk faced by a patient whose presenting symptoms are other than intracerebral hemorrhage or seizures.

Risk of Death Attributable to the AVM

The overwhelming majority of deaths associated with intracranial AVMs are related to bleeding episodes.[8,10,16] Although some older series have reported significant differences in mortality rates for initial and sequential hemorrhages,[10,16] present data suggest that these differences are artifactual.[4,15] Currently the most reliable long-term studies place the risk of death associated with each hemorrhage at 10 to 15 percent, with the annual risk of death secondary to hemorrhage being roughly 1 percent and the decade risk being between 10 and 15 percent.[4,15] Recent information implies that episodes of bleeding may carry an increased risk of death for older patients,[4,10,15] but insufficient data are available to make this suggestion conclusive.

Risk of Permanent Neurological Morbidity Related to the AVM

Three potential sources of neurological morbidity in the AVM patient are readily apparent. First, and statistically of greatest importance, are the neurological sequelae of a nonfatal subarachnoid or intraparenchymal hemorrhage. The overall morbidity associated with each intraparenchymal hemorrhage has previously been estimated as twice the mortality rate (i.e., 20 to 30 percent per episode.[10,12]), and this figure is supported by recent longitudinal studies. Such data would suggest an annual neurological morbidity rate of 2 to 3 percent, without consideration of other potential causative etiologies.[15]

A second source of potential neurological morbidity is the poorly understood syndrome of progressive ischemic neurological deficit, most commonly seen in older patients harboring large high-flow malformations.[14,19,20] This debilitating neurological process, which may be manifested by a progressive focal neurological deficit or mental deterioration, is thought to be secondary to chronic hypoperfusion of normal brain parenchyma external to the margins of the AVM. As such, it represents a chronic state of cerebral ischemia produced by the "steal" effect of the AVM on the surrounding cerebral vascular network. The developmental incidence of this complication is unknown, and its potential for arrest and/or reversal by AVM removal, while suggested by several small clinical series, remains unproven.[7,23]

The final potential pathway for the occurrence of neurological morbidity in patients harboring an intracranial AVM is the development of an intractable seizure disorder. Once again, the incidence of this complication is unknown, although it must be extremely uncommon despite the large number of patients at risk. There is ample evidence available to suggest that younger patients, regardless of mode of presentation, are more likely to develop seizures than are elderly patients, and to imply that patients presenting with subarachnoid hemorrhage carry an approximately 1 percent annual risk of the development of epilepsy.[5] However, there are no data to provide even minimum indications as to the number of percentage of patients whose epilepsy ultimately proves refractory to medical therapy. Because the presence of intractable seizures has long been considered an indication for surgical treatment of AVMs, further studies to delineate the incidence of development of refractory epilepsy in the AVM population at risk are obviously important.

Factors That May Alter the Risk of Hemorrhage, Death, and Neurological Morbidity in AVM Patients

Age

Traditional neurosurgical wisdom has held that the majority of AVMs ultimately destined to become symptomatic have done so by the patient age of 50 years.[6,10,16] This supposition appears logical and consistent with current information but lacks conclusive proof. It is, however, apparent that patients who present with symptomatic AVMs in later life stand at substantially greater risk of subsequent or recurrent hemorrhage and that these hemorrhages may individually carry an increased risk of morbidity or mortality[4,10]; conversely, patients developing AVM-related symptoms at young ages obviously face a significant cumulative risk of hemorrhage and, as mentioned, a greater propensity to develop a symptomatic seizure disorder.[4,10,15] No current evidence supports the contention that AVMs presenting in childhood or adolescence carry an otherwise different natural history from lesions that come to clinical attention in the adult population.[8,22]

Site

It is well established that the anatomical location of many AVMs has some bearing on the mode of clinical presentation. For example, deep cerebral lesions and malformations of the posterior fossa most frequently present with hemorrhage, whereas "superficial" or cortical AVMs are more often associated with seizure disorders. However, no creditable data are available to lend prognostic importance to the location of such lesions for their subsequent risk of hemorrhage, death, or neurological morbidity.[4,10,15,22]

Size

Although small AVMs have traditionally been thought to carry an ominous prognosis as regards recurrent hemorrhage,[6,21] a careful review of the patient series to date fails to demonstrate any propensity for these malformations to produce initial or recurrent hemorrhage greater than that associated with all AVMs.[4,10,15,22]

Mode of Presentation

As mentioned, historically AVMs presenting with hemorrhage have been perceived to carry a greater risk of subsequent hemorrhage than those presenting with seizures,[10,16] a finding supported by the recent study of Crawford et al., which showed a 51 percent risk of recurring hemorrhage versus a 33 percent risk of initial bleeding in patients presenting with seizures.[4] The somewhat more complete data of Ondra et al. would refute this contention, suggesting a parallel and equal risk of initial and recurrent bleeding in these two patient populations.[15] The data are currently inadequate to forecast accurately the risk of hemorrhage, death, or ultimate neurological morbidity in the completely asymptomatic patient with an AVM of the brain.

Pregnancy

Insufficient data are available to suggest conclusively that pregnancy carries an increased risk of hemorrhage from an intracranial AVM.[4,22]

Surgical Therapy

The history of successful surgical management of AVMs begins with Olivecrona and Tönnis (as reported by Bergstrand et al.[3]) in 1936[3] and spans over a half century marked by tremendous diagnostic, technical, and therapeutic advances. Limitations of space preclude individual acknowledgments of the numerous neurosurgeons who have made significant contributions to the advancement of surgical therapy in this area, but an extensive review of these historic developments is given in the introduction of Yaşargil's own monumental work on intracranial AVMs.[24,25] His retrospective analysis of over 2000 reported operatives cases in over 100 individual surgical series yielded a collective operative mortality of some 11 percent. Even when cases done prior to the microsurgical era were included, serious operative morbidity was estimated to be in the range of 10 percent, with over 60 percent of all patients returning to full work capacity subsequent to surgery. Unfortunately, as the author points out, although such statistics may be useful in a general sense, they are, in themselves, insufficient to provide even minimal information about the current potential operative morbidity and mortality associated with a specific AVM being treated by an individual neurosurgeon.[24]

The present gold standard for such exact information is without question Professor Yaşargil's extensive two-volume work detailing his own personal experience with over 400 operative cases of intracranial AVMs. This tightly controlled, extremely descriptive, and completely documented personal series details the best currently achievable surgical results obtained with AVMs of diverse sizes located throughout the cerebrum, cerebellum, and brain stem, in a patient population of heterogeneous referral. To achieve an overall mortality rate of 2.4 percent and a morbidity rate of 2.9 percent in this extensive series of AVMs dominated by complex, deep, and large lesions represents an impressive and unparalleled tour de force, which other neurovascular surgeons must strive to equal.[25] Undoubtedly, the general mortality and morbidity rates associated with surgical therapy of these lesions are significantly greater than these landmark figures.

Lacking the depth and breadth of Yaşargil's surgical experience, other neurosurgeons have sought for some time to identify a shorthand method of classification of AVMs that would help quantify the difficulty of surgical resection of individual lesions and, by inference, their specific risk of operative morbidity and mortality. Beginning with Luessenhop and Gennarelli's initial grading system published in 1977,[13] four classifications of intracranial AVMs have been presented for evaluation by the neurosurgical community.[9,17,18] Each of these systems, by employing the sum of a specific set of variables, ultimately assigns a numerical designation to each individual AVM; these variables mainly are related to the angiographic and computed tomographic appearance and localization of the malformation and, when taken in sum, are purported to provide a relative indication of the risk of significant neurological morbidity and mortality associated with definitive surgical excision of the lesion in question. The specific parameters at issue do not in themselves represent potential technical problems, but rather have been found in the individual author's or authors' experience to be findings common to AVMs that have proved difficult to resect successfully. Each of these scales has been evaluated through application to the author's or authors' own surgical experience and has demonstrated validity within that limited context. These systems are presented in graphic form for comparison in Table 240-1 and are described briefly below.

The grading system of Luessenhop and Gennarelli is based solely on the number of angiographically identifiable "named" feeding vessels to the AVM in question.[13] In subsequent publications, the authors have indicated that this number correlates relatively well with the overall diameter of the malformation. In this system, grade 1 malformations are those less than 2 cm in diameter, grade 2 lesions are those 2 to 4 cm in diameter, grade 3 malformations are those 4 to 6 cm in diameter, and grade 4 lesions are those greater than 6 cm in diameter.

Garretson's grading system is perhaps the most complex of the

TABLE 240-1 AVM Grading Systems

Parameters	Luessenhop and Gennarelli[13]	Garretson[9]	Spetzler and Martin[18]	Shi and Chen[17]
AVM diameter	<2 cm 2–4 cm 4–6 cm >6 cm	—	<3 cm 3–6 cm >6 cm	<2.5 cm 2.5–5 cm 5–7.5 cm >7.5 cm
AVM location	—	—	Eloquent vs. noneloquent brain	Eloquence and depth
Arterial input	Number of angiographically named feeding arteries	1. Number of arterial systems 2. Number of branches of each system	—	Number and complexity of feeding arteries
Venous drainage	—	—	Presence/absence of deep drainage	Number and complexity of veins
Patient age	—	Decade of age	—	—

four and involves assigning a number to the malformation in each of three categories: (1) the number of principal circulations involved in feeding the AVM; (2) the number of branches in each circulation found to contribute to the malformation; and (3) the age of the patient by decade.[9] A sum of these three categories that is 10 or greater suggests that the risk of removing the malformation is greater than the risk of its natural history, in Garretson's experience.

The classification of Spetzler and Martin is based on three components: malformation size, location (as regards eloquence of brain tissue), and presence or absence of deep venous drainage.[18] When a numerical value is attached to each of these parameters, a sum is obtained that permits grading the malformation in terms of progressive operative difficulty from 1 to 6.

The fourth classification, authored by Shi and Chen, is based on four individual anatomical parameters of the AVM.[17] These include the size of the AVM, its location and depth, the complexity of its feeding arteries, and the complexity of its venous drainage. On this basis, malformations are graded from 1 to 4, again in ascending degree of technical difficulty.

In a somewhat different approach to identifying the factors predictive of postoperative morbidity and mortality following AVM surgery, Batjer et al. recently evaluated 70 patients undergoing resection of intraparenchymal AVMs over 6 years.[2] In this series, patients were studied extensively both pre- and postoperatively with routine imaging techniques in addition to regional cerebral blood flow analysis. The factors found to be statistically significant in predicting a relatively high incidence of postoperative morbidity and mortality were (1) AVM size of greater than 6 cm, (2) presence of preoperative angiographic and regional cerebral blood flow evidence of "steal," (3) involvement of perforating branches of either the middle cerebral or posterior cerebral arteries in supply of the AVM, (4) age of over 50 years, and (5) altered level of consciousness.

The efficacy of all of the above grading systems remains unproven; their ultimate utility will depend on both retrospective and prospective application of these individual systems to large series of AVMs operated upon by surgeons other than the systems' authors. Furthermore, the introduction of important new surgical adjuncts, such as preoperative AVM embolization and feeding artery occlusion,[1,11] may, when applied to a large series of AVMs, completely alter the parameters predictive of ultimate postoperative morbidity and mortality. In that light, pending further evidence to support the validity and utility of one or more of the above grading systems, or the development and widespread adoption of yet an additional system ultimately to be validated, the relatively unique nature and the variable complexity of AVMs seem best described narratively rather than numerically.

A judicious approach to the preoperative analysis of the risk and potential complications of surgical treatment of specific AVMs should begin with a review of Yaşargil's published results for similar size lesions in identical anatomical locations. These admittedly optimistic morbidity and mortality figures can then be modified, both by specific factors unique to the individual patient in question and by honest self-analysis by treating neurosurgeons of their own AVM operative experience and personal microvascular capabilities.

References

1. Andrews BT, Wilson CB. Staged treatment of arteriovenous malformations of the brain. *Neurosurgery* 1987; 21:314–323.
2. Batjer HH, Devous MD, Seibert GB, et al. Intracranial arteriovenous malformation: relationship between clinical factors and surgical complications. *Neurosurgery* 1989; 24:75–79.
3. Bergstrand H, Olivercrona H, Tönnis W. *Gefässmissbildungen und Gefässgeschwülste des Gehirns.* Leipzig: Georg Thieme Verlag, 1936.
4. Crawford PM, West CR, Chadwick DW, et al. Arteriovenous malformations of the brain: natural history in unoperated patients. *J Neurol Neurosurg Psychiatry* 1986; 49:1–10.
5. Crawford PM, West CR, Shaw MDM, et al. Cerebral arteriovenous malformations and epilepsy: factors in the development of epilepsy. *Epilepsia* 1986; 27:270–275.
6. Forster DMC, Steiner L, Häkanson S. Arteriovenous malformations of the brain: a long-term clinical study. *J Neurosurg* 1972; 37:562–570.
7. Fox AJ, Girvin JP, Viñuela F, et al. Rolandic arteriovenous malformations: improvement in limb function by IBC embolization. *Am J Neuroradiol* 1985; 6:575–582.
8. Fults D, Kelly DL Jr. Natural history of arteriovenous malformations of the brain: a clinical study. *Neurosurgery* 1984; 15:658–662.
9. Garretson HD. Intracranial arteriovenous malformations. In Wilkins RH, Rengachary SS (eds): *Neurosurgery.* New York: McGraw-Hill, 1985, pp 1448–1458.
10. Graf CJ, Perret GE, Torner JC. Bleeding from cerebral arteriovenous malformations as part of their natural history. *J Neurosurg* 1983; 58:331–337.
11. Hilal SK. Endovascular treatment of arteriovenous malformations of the central nervous system. In Wilson CB, Stein BM (eds): *Intracranial Arteriovenous Malformations.* Baltimore: Williams & Wilkins, 1984, pp 259–273.
12. Luessenhop AJ. Natural history of cerebral arteriovenous malformations. In Wilson CB, Stein BM (eds): *Intracranial Arteriovenous Malformations.* Baltimore: Williams & Wilkins, 1984, pp 12–23.
13. Luessenhop AJ, Gennarelli TA. Anatomical grading of supratentorial arteriovenous malformations for determining operability. *Neurosurgery* 1977; 1:30–35.
14. Michelsen WJ. Natural history and pathophysiology of arteriovenous malformations. *Clin Neurosurg* 1978; 26:307–313.
15. Ondra SL, Troupp H, George ED, et al. The natural history of symptomatic arteriovenous malformations of the brain: a 24 year follow-up assessment. *J Neurosurg* 1990; 73:387–391.
16. Perret G, Nishioka H. Report on the Cooperative Study of Intracranial Aneurysms and Subarachnoid Hemorrhage. Section VI. Arteriovenous malformations: an analysis of 545 cases of cranio-cerebral arteriovenous malformations and fistulae reported to the Cooperative Study. *J Neurosurg* 1966; 25:467–490.
17. Shi Y, Chen X. A proposed scheme for grading intracranial arteriovenous malformations. *J Neurosurg* 1986; 65:484–489.
18. Spetzler RF, Martin NA. A proposed grading system for arteriovenous malformations. *J Neurosurg* 1986; 65:476–483.
19. Spetzler RF, Selman WR. Pathophysiology of cerebral ischemia accompanying arteriovenous malformations. In Wilson CB, Stein BM (eds): *Intracranial Arteriovenous Malformations.* Baltimore: Williams & Wilkins, 1984, pp 24–31.
20. Stein BM, Wolpert SM. Arteriovenous malformations of the brain. II: Current concepts and treatment. *Arch Neurol* 1980; 37:69–75.
21. Waltimo O. The relationship of size, density and localization of intracranial arteriovenous malformations to the type of initial symptom. *J Neurol Sci* 1973; 19:13–19.
22. Wilkins RH. Natural history of intracranial vascular malformations: a review. *Neurosurgery* 1985; 16:421–430.
23. Wilson CB, U HS, Domingue J. Microsurgical treatment of intracranial vascular malformations. *J Neurosurg* 1979; 51:446–454.
24. Yaşargil MG. *Microneurosurgery,* vol III A. *AVM of the Brain, History, Embryology, Pathological Considerations, Hemodynamics, Diagnostic Studies, Microsurgical Anatomy.* New York: Georg Thieme Verlag, 1987, pp 10–20.
25. Yaşargil MG. *Microneurosurgery,* vol III B. *AVM of the Brain, Clinical Considerations, General and Specific Operative Techniques, Surgical Results, Nonoperated Cases, Cavernous and Venous Angiomas, Neuroanesthesia.* New York: Georg Thieme Verlag, 1988.

241 Surgical Resection of Medial Hemispheric Arteriovenous Malformations of the Brain

Robert A. Solomon
Bennett M. Stein

Anteriovenous malformations (AVMs) of the brain represent one of the most difficult challenges for the neurosurgeon. Patients with such lesions often come to medical attention because of devastating intracranial hemorrhage or a disabling seizure disorder. The natural history of these lesions is not fully known, yet the available evidence indicates that patients with AVMs that are left untreated frequently die prematurely or are left incapacitated.[7,8,17] This dismal prognosis has encouraged attempts at surgical obliteration.

An interesting and technically complex group of AVMs are located on the medial surfaces of the cerebral hemisphere.[15] These lesions are not visible on the convexities of the brain, and a series of specialized approaches is therefore required to achieve their resection.

Anatomic Considerations

Medial hemispheric AVMs are a diverse group of malformations that can involve all the different lobes of the brain. These lesions are unified by their location adjacent to the falx, the tentorium, and the structures that traverse the tentorial hiatus. In the temporal lobe this group of malformations involves the uncus, the amygdala, the hippocampal formation, and the parahippocampal and fusiform gyri. Moving more posteriorly and superiorly, the malformations often involve regions medial to the trigone of the lateral ventricle, incorporating the posterior parapeduncular region. Most posterior are the medial surfaces of the occipital lobes, including the precuneus and cuneus. Structures involved in the parietal and frontal lobes include the paracentral lobule, the cingulate gyrus, the medial frontal gyrus, and the septal region. Malformations on the medial side of the frontal and parietal lobes often involve the corpus callosum, even penetrating it to reach deep diencephalic structures such as the thalamus and corpus striatum.

The primary arterial supply to these lesions arises from the anterior cerebral artery for the superior and anterior lesions and from the posterior cerebral artery for the posterior and inferior lesions. Various contributions are also derived from the choroidal branches of the posterior cerebral artery, especially with lesions that are located near the splenium of the corpus callosum and extend into the posterior thalamus. The anterior choroidal artery is usually involved in lesions that arise far anteriorly on the medial and inferior surfaces of the temporal lobe. The venous drainage of these lesions is primarily into the deep galenic system, by either direct communication to the vein of Galen or indirect communication via the basal vein of Rosenthal. More superior and anterior lesions often have midline draining veins that ascend into the superior sagittal sinus. Larger malformations occasionally have multiple routes of venous drainage.

Patient Selection

The criteria for selecting surgical candidates from the group of patients that harbor medial hemispheric AVMs are not substantially different from the selection criteria that have been used for cerebral AVMs in general.[7,17] One difference is the greatly increased technical difficulty that attends surgical resection of the medial hemispheric AVM. Surgeons who are not experienced in the operative resection of lesions of this type would be ill advised to pursue this course.

In patients who present with intracranial hemorrhage from an AVM, the risk of recurrent hemorrhage and progressive neurologic demise would argue strongly in favor of surgical intervention in most cases. Patients who are elderly or have significant complicating medical illnesses might be candidates for conservative therapy. Very large malformations that encompass multiple lobes of the brain and extend deep into the diencephalon and internal capsule often must be considered surgically unresectable.

Patients who have a nonhemorrhagic presentation of a medial hemisphere AVM form a less clearly defined group in terms of the advisability of surgical intervention. The age of the patient, the size and complexity of the malformation, and the patient's desires must all be factored into a decision regarding operative intervention. Given the life expectancy of someone under the age of 50 and the likelihood that an untreated malformation will cause devastation within that patient's lifetime, surgical resection should be recommended even for patients who present with seizures or without symptoms.

There seems little doubt that individuals with malformations less than 3 cm in diameter, regardless of the mode of presentation, should be treated with operative resection. However, in older patients and with larger malformations, the indications for operation become more obscure.

Unless there are significant complicating factors, hemorrhage from a medial hemisphere AVM is a positive indication for surgery. Without a hemorrhagic presentation, the experience of the surgeon, the age of the patient, and the size of the AVM all must be factored into the decision of whether or not to operate.

Embolization Therapy

Preoperative intravascular embolization treatment has been a useful adjunct in the management of large supratentorial arteriovenous malformations.[17] The techniques and indications for embolization therapy have been well discussed in previous publications, and we will not review them here.

Malformations that are located primarily on the medial aspects of the cerebral hemispheres are generally not suitable for preoperative embolization therapy. These AVMs tend to be supplied by distal branches of the major arteries, such as the choroidal arteries, posterior cerebral arteries, and anterior cerebral arteries. These vessels generally have a small intraluminal diameter and arise from the parent vessel at a right angle. These factors make embolization hazardous, and therefore it is not usually indicated for malformations in this location.

In addition, when the malformations are small, the size of the arterial-to-venous shunt is relatively small and the possible flow-related complications of a one-stage resection are limited. Therefore, only malformations with very large shunts and multiple venous drainage routes require preoperative embolization. Even these malformations require advanced catheter techniques to position the embolic material into very distal branches of the cerebral circulation.

Radiation Treatment

Gamma radiation for the treatment of AVMs has recently been reported to be advantageous.[19,20] However, radiation of this type from external high-energy sources can be safely delivered only to small brain volumes. This point means that only malformations smaller than 3 cm in diameter are amenable to this form of therapy; larger malformations can at best be treated only partially or with a small probability of cure.[11,21] Moreover, radiation therapy requires at least 2 years to produce the desired vascular changes resulting in thrombosis of the malformation. During this latency period, the patient continues to be at risk for hemorrhage from the malformation, and partially treated lesions always carry a risk of rupture. In fact, recent reports indicate that the complication rate related to rupture of an AVM treated with high-energy radiotherapy may be higher than that from the natural history of the disease.[11,18,21] In addition, the long-term deleterious effects of high-energy radiation, which must pass through the normal brain before reaching the malformation, are as yet unknown. Radiation necrosis has been shown to be a complicating factor in patients treated by this approach.[18]

Because radiation therapy has been in use only for a relatively short time in the treatment of AVMs of the brain, the long-term benefits of this form of treatment have yet to be elucidated. Our own experience and that of others indicate that a group of patients have had complications related to the malformation many years after initial treatment with radiation therapy. These factors would argue against the use of radiation therapy as a first-line approach to AVMs of the brain under any circumstances. However, in a very small number of selected cases, in which the patient has not previously experienced a hemorrhage from the malformation, the malformation is less than 2 cm in size, and an experienced neurosurgeon has decided that the malformation is surgically inaccessible, radiation therapy may be indicated. Therefore, patients should be chosen very carefully for treatment by radiosurgery.

Surgical Approaches

Surgical resection of medial hemispheric AVMs should proceed according to the surgical principles that apply to AVMs in any location.[9–12,16] Adequate coaxial illumination, the operative microscope, and fine microinstruments are essential for the successful removal of these lesions. In addition, careful positioning of the patient and selection of the proper surgical approach are critical for operations on medial hemispheric AVMs. The specific elements of the approach to each location on the medial surfaces of the hemispheres will be discussed in detail.

Anterior Mesial Temporal Malformations

Malformations located on the anterior one-third of the mesial temporal lobe derive their blood supply primarily from the anterior choroidal artery and penetrating branches of the posterior communicating artery. The venous drainage for these lesions is into the basal vein of Rosenthal. At operation, the patient is positioned supine with the neck extended and the head turned 30 degrees away from the side of the craniotomy. Spinal drainage and mannitol administration are advantageous in producing adequate brain relaxation to assist with retraction. These malformations are best approached via a pterional craniotomy with microsurgical splitting of the anterior part of the sylvian fissure. This approach allows for visualization of the supraclinoid carotid artery and its branches that lead back to the malformation on the medial side of the temporal lobe.

The anterior choroidal artery serves as a useful guide back into the choroidal fissure and to the substance of the malformation. The main trunk of the choroidal artery must, of course, be preserved during any dissection, but the proximal penetrating branches that supply the malformation on the medial side of the temporal lobe can be sacrificed. Malformations in this location involve the uncus and the amygdala as well as portions of the anterior hippocampal formation. These regions are amenable to resection when involved by the AVM.

Posterior Mesial Temporal Malformations and Malformations on the Tentorial Surface of the Temporal Lobe

AVMs located in the posterior aspects of the temporal lobe in the parahippocampal gyrus and the fusiform gyrus generally are intimate with the superior aspect of the tentorium (Fig. 241-1). These lesions are supplied by the posterior temporal branch of the posterior cerebral artery, although the anterior choroidal artery often provides a significant supply when the malformation reaches to the temporal horn of the lateral ventricle. The venous drainage from these lesions is via the basal vein of Rosenthal and occasionally via bridging veins from the tentorium to the inferior surface of the temporal lobe.

The most appropriate surgical approach involves elevation of the temporal lobe and visualization of the malformation along its tentorial surface. The patient is positioned in the lateral position with the head flexed away from the side of the craniotomy. A low temporal craniotomy is fashioned to expose the entire length of the temporal lobe. Of course, care must be exercised in elevating the temporal lobe so that the critical vein of Labbé is not damaged. If it appears that this vein would be jeopardized by the necessary

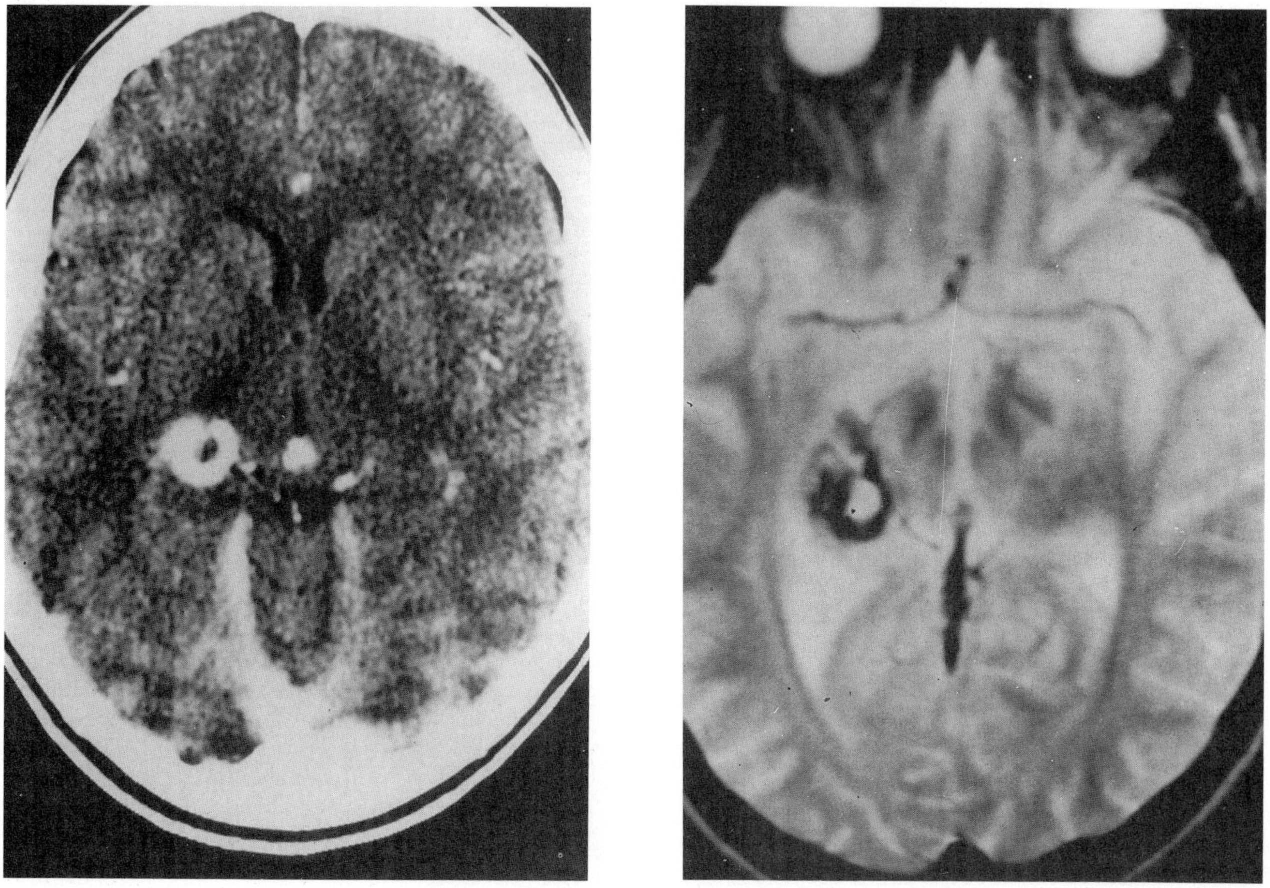

(A) (B)

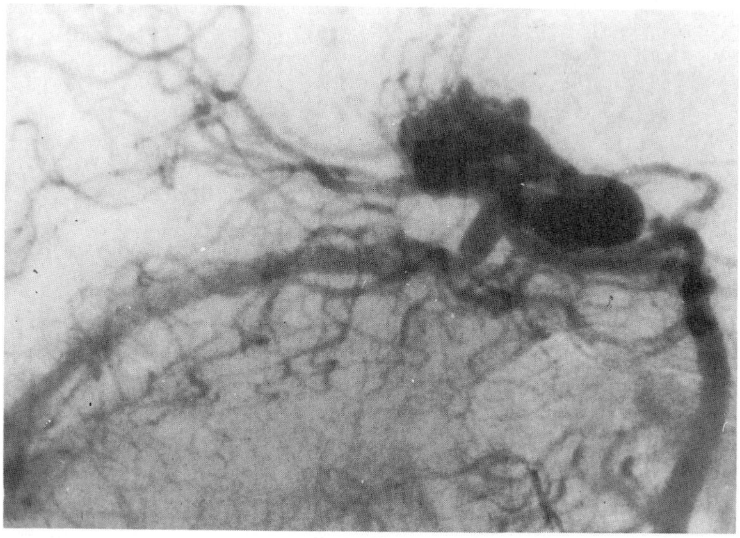

(C)

Figure 241-1 Representative radiologic studies of a patient with a posterior medial temporal AVM. *A.* Axial CT scan with contrast enhancement, demonstrating the location of the malformation on the tentorial surface of the temporal lobe. *B.* Axial MR image demonstrating the location of the malformation. *C.* Lateral vertebral angiogram demonstrating the arterial supply to the malformation from the posterior cerebral artery.

retraction, it is better to make an incision in the inferior temporal gyrus and approach the malformation through the substance of the temporal lobe. The latter approach has been used by Heros preferentially to treat malformations in this posterior inferior temporal region.[3] When the AVM is situated entirely below the atrium of the lateral ventricle, the subtemporal approach generally affords adequate visualization of the entire malformation and allows for appropriate resection. However, if the malformation extends medial to the atrium of the lateral ventricle, then the subtemporal approach generally is inadequate to reach its uppermost limit. This fact results from the sharp upward slope of the tentorium in the posterior temporal region.

Malformations Medial to the Trigone

AVMs adjacent to the trigone of the lateral ventricle (Fig. 241-2) have been approached by numerous routes by various surgeons over the years. Some degree of controversy, therefore, exists regarding surgical resection of these malformations.[4] Drake has

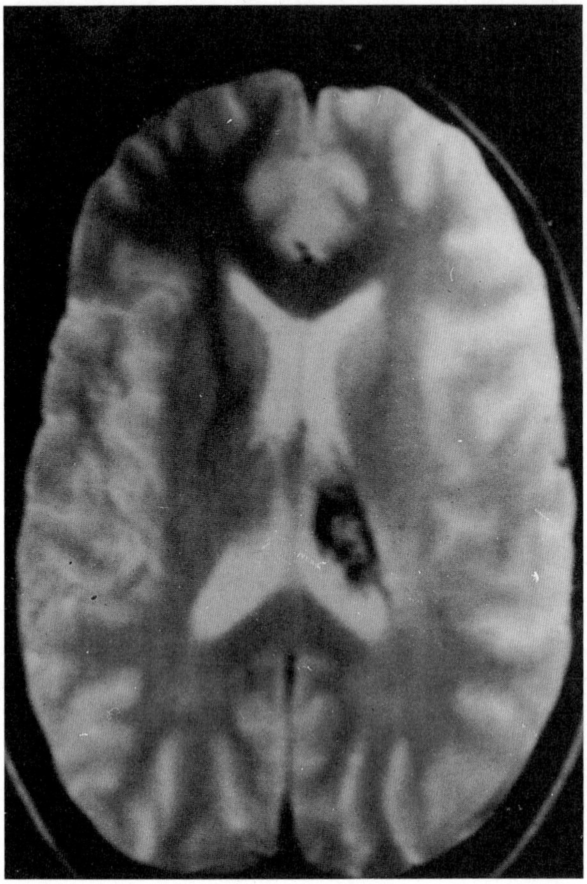
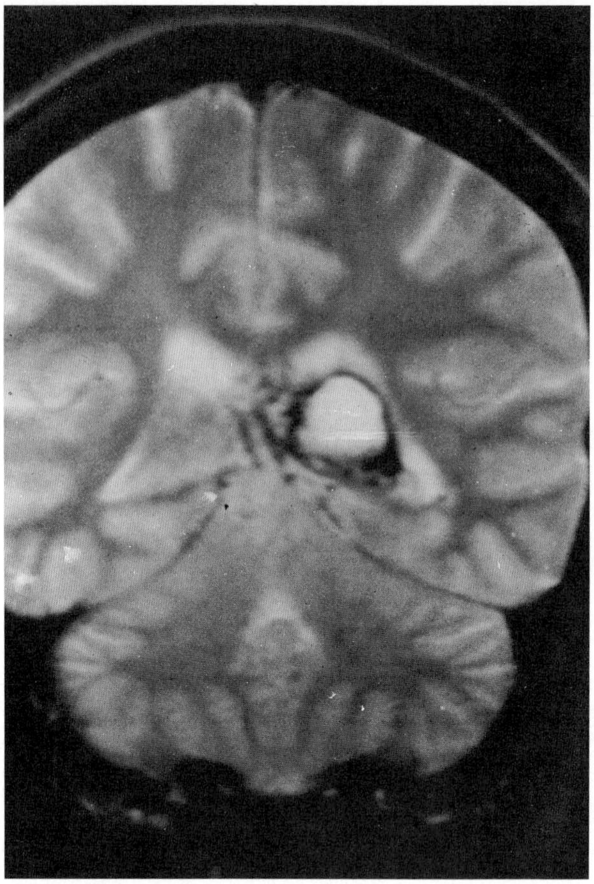

(*A*) (*B*)

Figure 241-2 Representative case of a medial hemispheric AVM located in the vicinity of the trigone of the lateral ventricle. *A*. Axial T1-weighted MRI indicating involvement of the posterior thalamus. *B*. Coronal T2-weighted MRI. Note the amount of neural tissue that would have to be violated in order to approach this lesion via a transcortical incision. The interhemispheric approach was used to advantage in this case.

approached malformations in the nondominant trigone via a transverse incision in the superior temporal gyrus,[2] and others have approached lesions in this location through the middle temporal gyrus.[22] Heros prefers a direct approach to the trigone through a small corticectomy in the parasagittal region, 7 to 8 cm above the occipital tip.[13] We have used an interhemispheric approach through a parietal craniotomy in a semisitting slouch position for malformations adjacent to the trigone of the lateral ventricle.[14]

The interhemispheric approach was originally designed for removal of tumors of the posterior third ventricle,[1] but it seems ideal for malformations located exclusively medial to the trigone of the ventricle. With retraction, one may reach the posterior cerebral artery as it courses around the lateral side of the brain stem and still have excellent visualization of the deep venous system. In contrast, approaches that traverse functional cortex to reach this region may increase the risk of postoperative neurological deficit; in addition, the surgeon first encounters the malformation at its body and must work around the margins to find the arterial supply that enters on the opposite side of the AVM. Because malformations near the trigone are supplied primarily by the posterior cerebral artery and its choroidal branches, an approach along the medial surface of the hemisphere affords control of the major feeding vessels before the malformation is dissected.

Larger malformations that extend inferior and lateral to the trigone region are often inaccessible by a pure interhemispheric route. When the malformations extend 2 to 3 cm lateral to the falx, a great deal of hemispheric retraction is necessary to reach them, and significant occipital damage can often be expected. Depending on the exact configuration of the malformation, the surgeon has two options. One is to approach the lesion via a transcortical approach and the other is to do a two-stage procedure.

We have found the two-stage procedure occasionally useful when malformations extend inferior and medial to the trigone.[13] The inferior aspect of the malformation can be removed by an infratemporal approach, whereas the medial component of the malformation must be approached via the interhemispheric route at a different operation. However, when the malformation is large and extends above the lateral portion of the trigone, an approach either through the middle temporal gyrus or through the superior parietal lobule is necessary.

The great majority of malformations located near the trigone of the lateral ventricle, including the small thalamic malformations and malformations involving the posterior aspect of the corpus callosum or cingulate gyrus, are best approached via a posterior interhemispheric exposure. Following the insertion of a spinal drainage catheter, the patient is placed in a semisitting slouched position. The head is straight and maximally flexed to bring the curved portion of the parietal bone parallel to the floor. A 4- by 4-in. bone flap is formed ipsilateral to the malformation, and the most medial burr holes are placed slightly to the opposite side of the superior sagittal sinus, with the posterior hole adjacent to lambda. A dural flap is created along the sinus, and medially draining veins are preserved whenever possible. However, in most instances, one or two of these veins must be sacrificed to gain adequate exposure of the interhemispheric region. Retractors are placed on the falx and on the parietal lobe to expose the medial side of the hemisphere. Visualization down to the splenium of the corpus callosum is easily achieved without disrupting any neural tissue. With division of the corpus callosum, the lateral ventricle can be entered, and deeper structures down to and including the posterior parts of the thalamus are accessible.

Medial Occipital Malformations

AVMs on the medial surface of the occipital lobe form a unique group of malformations (Fig. 241-3). These lesions have a propensity to cause migrainous headaches, and their location next to the visual cortex often accounts for the visual field defects that are seen in patients in whom they have hemorrhaged. Medial occipital AVMs are fed almost exclusively by branches of the posterior cerebral artery. The venous drainage of these malformations is primarily into the deep galenic system, although ascending veins to the

Figure 241-3 Medial occipital AVM. *A.* Contrast-enhanced axial CT scan demonstrating an AVM involving the medial surface of the occipital lobe. *B.* Confirmatory picture on the axial T2-weighted MRI. *C.* Anteroposterior vertebral angiogram demonstrating the arterial supply via the distal branches of the posterior cerebral artery.

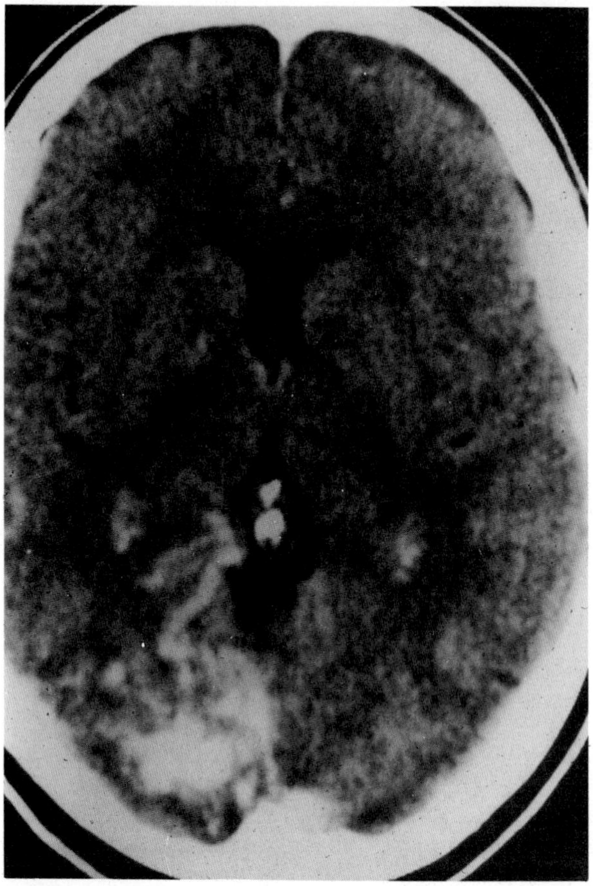

(*A*)

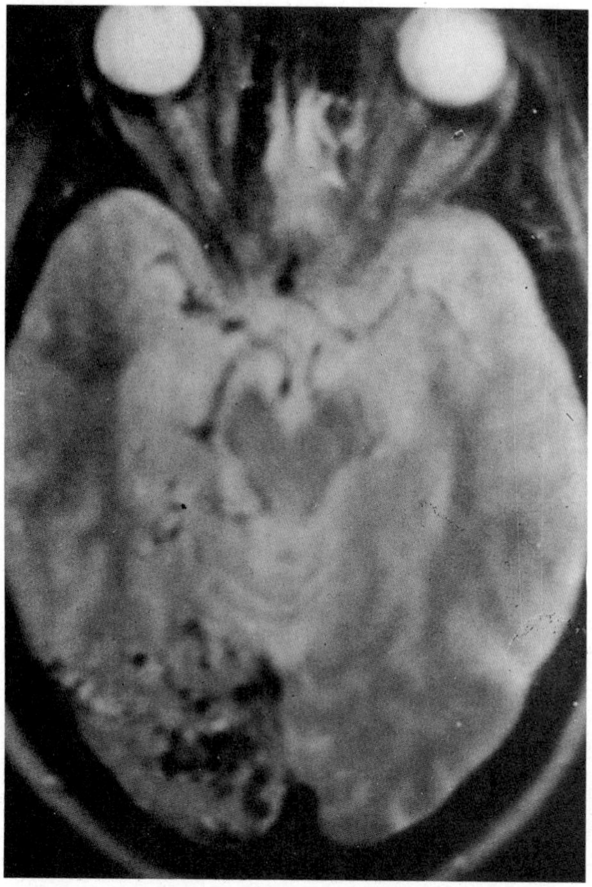

(*B*)

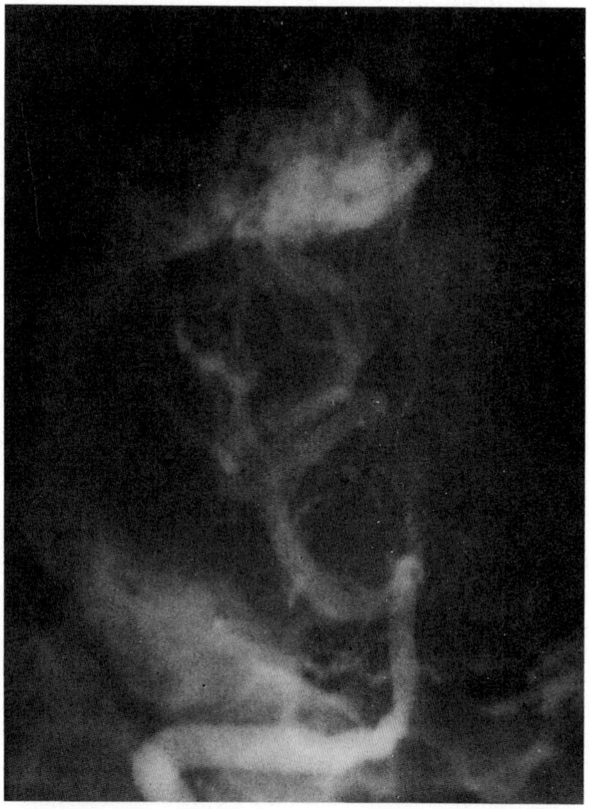

(*C*)

superior sagittal sinus may also contribute, especially when the malformations are more polar in location. The clinical features of, and the surgical approach to, medial occipital AVMs have been discussed in detail by Martin and Wilson.[6] Their experience as well as that of Kattah et al.[5] indicate that malformations in this location can be completely excised without additional damage to the visual fields. In some instances visual fields have improved following surgical resection of a medial occipital AVM. Headache, which has commonly been associated with AVMs of the brain, seems to be particularly prevalent in patients with occipital malformations. In seven of eight patients in Drake's series who presented with intractable headaches and cerebral AVMs, the malformation resided in the occipital lobe.[2] In Drake's series, as well as in the series of Martin and Wilson,[6] the presenting headaches either decreased significantly or disappeared in all patients who had excision of the malformation.

There are several surgical approaches to malformations in the medial occipital lobe. These lesions can be approached in a similar fashion as for lesions medial to the trigone of the lateral ventricle, with the patient in a semisitting slouch position. However, we now prefer to use a lateral position with the AVM side down. This position allows the hemisphere to retract by gravity and creates a more comfortable sitting position for the surgeon. The craniotomy is slightly more posterior than that used for the medial trigone lesions. The inferior border of the craniotomy must extend down to the tentorial surface at the superior aspect of the transverse sinus. The occipital pole is easily retracted laterally and/or superiorly, providing access along the falcotentorial junction all the way to the tentorial hiatus and the midbrain tegmentum. The posterior cerebral artery can be identified as it emerges from the tentorial hiatus to travel superior to the tentorium. At this point it can be followed distally into the malformation and used as a guide to the arterial side of the AVM.

Medial Parietal Malformations

Malformations located on the medial surface of the parietal lobe (Fig. 241-4) often involve the corpus callosum and cingulate gyrus.[23] The approach to this region is not dissimilar from that already discussed for malformations of the occipital lobe. The blood supply to AVMs in this location is primarily from terminal branches of the anterior cerebral artery, and occasionally from anastomotic branches of the middle cerebral artery over the convexity or from medial hemispheric branches of the posterior cerebral artery. Venous drainage is often divided between ascending veins that join with the superior sagittal sinus and veins that travel deeply into the vein of Galen. In some instances, with larger malformations that extend laterally toward the ventricle, venous drainage may also be directed into the subependymal veins.

Malformations in this location are approached in a lateral position with the AVM side down. A semisitting slouch position may also be used. A parietal craniotomy that exposes the midline is necessary for the interhemispheric approach to these lesions. Brain relaxation with mannitol and spinal drainage is essential for the degree of retraction of the parietal lobe that may be necessary to reach the lateral portions of the malformation.

Medial Frontal Malformations

The medial frontal malformations (Fig. 241-5) can extend into the anterior cingulate gyrus and the corpus callosum and often involve the latter structures exclusively. These malformations are supplied by large branches of the anterior cerebral arteries with occasional collateral branches from the middle cerebral artery or even transcallosal perforating vessels. Venous drainage is usually into the superior sagittal sinus and occasionally into the deep subependymal system which discharges into the internal cerebral veins. Resection of these lesions can often be quite difficult, especially when the malformation is located on the medial side of the rolandic fissure. Retraction on this region of the brain can produce contralateral hemiparesis, and profound motor deficits may ensue after interruption of the rolandic veins. Therefore, an approach to this region should be planned to avoid retraction on the motor strip and to avoid sacrificing the medial bridging veins in this region. Generally, this is accomplished by approaching the malformation tangentially from a very anterior craniotomy that permits retraction of the hemisphere anterior to the motor region. This approach is generally advantageous since the arterial supply approaches from the anterior side of the malformation and the venous drainage is generally posterior and superior. These patients can be operated on in the supine position through a craniotomy placed on the midline just anterior to the coronal suture. With neck extension, brain relaxation, and lateral retraction on the anterior frontal lobe, visualization back to the midportion of the corpus callosum can be achieved. Resection of these malformations must be carried out without damage to the anterior cerebral arteries, which usually supply important brain structures distal to the location of the malformation. At times this task can be made extremely difficult by extension of the malformation around and deep to the main trunk of the anterior cerebral artery, when the AVM penetrates the corpus callosum or approaches the frontal horn of the lateral ventricle.

Malformations in the septal region and the medial frontal lobe inferior to the rostrum of the corpus callosum are approached in a similar fashion. However, the craniotomy must be placed very low on the forehead to achieve an angle of vision beneath the genu of the corpus callosum. Special precautions must be taken in this area to preserve the main trunks of the anterior cerebral arteries and the numerous perforating vessels that return to the anterior perforated space and supply important anterior diencephalic structures.

Operative Results

In our series of 300 surgically treated AVMs of the brain, 55 lesions correspond to the categories discussed in this chapter. Seven malformations were located adjacent to the anterior mesial temporal lobe, 10 were in the region of the posterior temporal lobe on the tentorial surface, 12 were in the medial trigone and parapeduncular zone, 6 were on the medial occipital lobe, 9 were on the medial parietal lobe, and 11 were on the medial frontal lobe. Preoperative embolization treatment was performed on 12 patients because of the complexity and large size of their malformations. All patients then underwent operative resection and postoperative angiography. In four cases, a second operative procedure was carried out, either as part of a planned two-stage resection or to deal with residual malformation noted on the postoperative angiogram. All 55 patients eventually had total removal of the AVM.

Four patients in this group had a bad outcome, as judged by permanent neurological deficits postoperatively and loss of the ability to lead an independent life. The remaining 51 patients have been considered to have had a good outcome. However, 13 of these patients had residual neurological deficits that resulted from surgery or were worsened by surgery but that did not preclude an

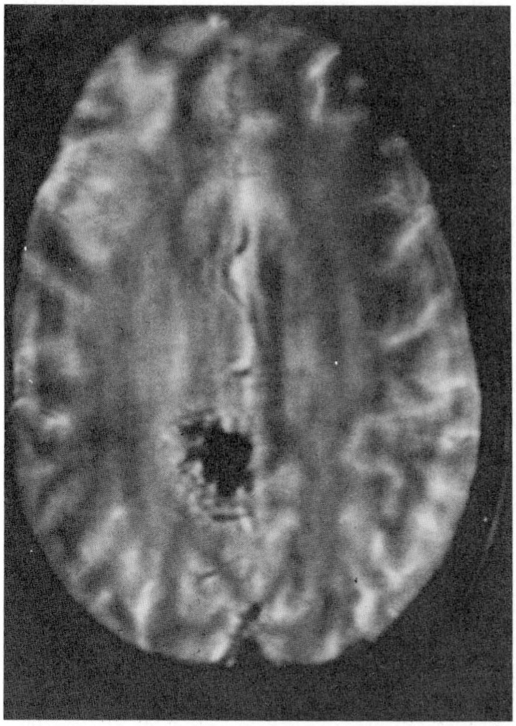

(*A*)

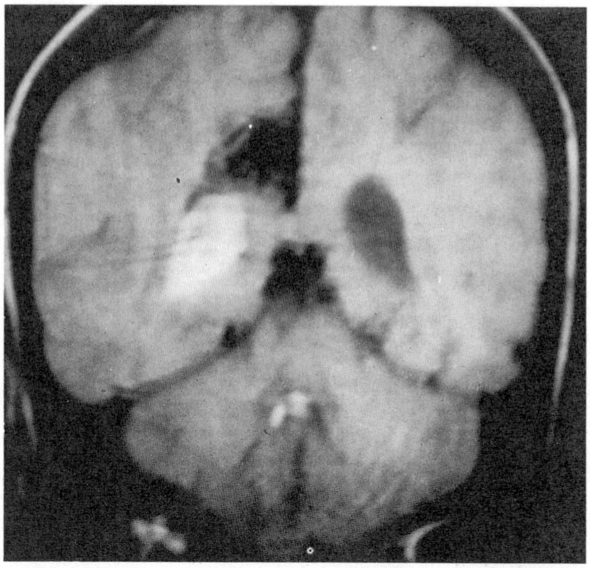

(*B*)

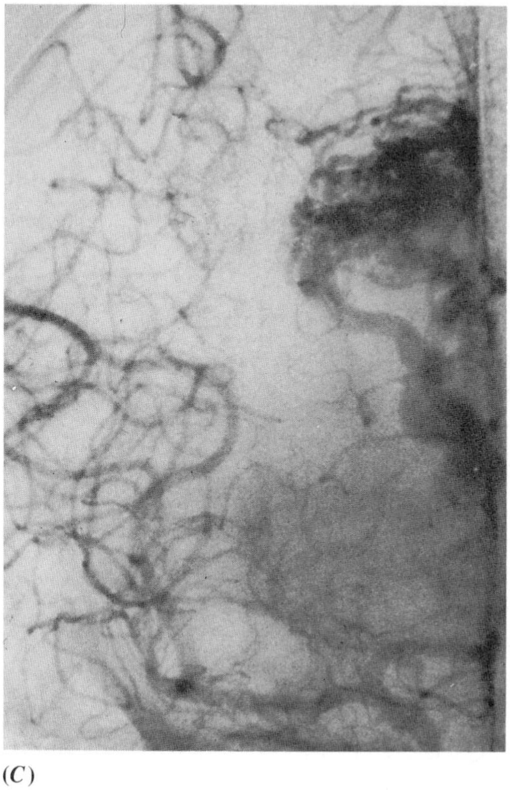

(*C*)

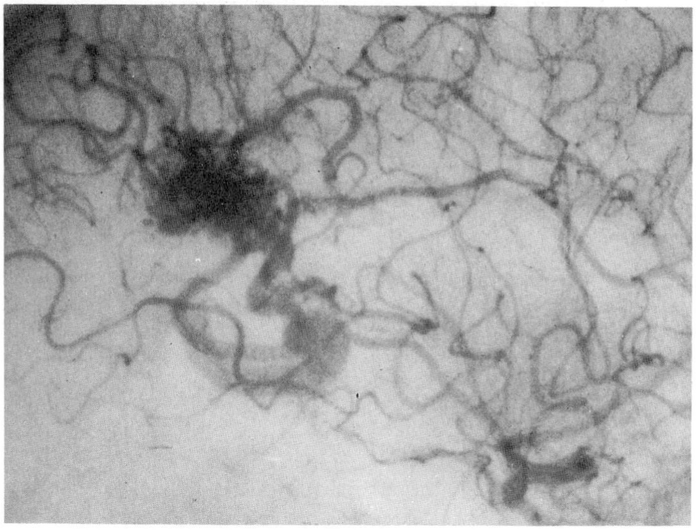

(*D*)

Figure 241-4 Medial parietal AVM. *A.* Axial T1-weighted MRI showing the signal void of a medial parietal AVM. Note the dilated, tortuous anterior cerebral artery on top of the corpus callosum approaching the malformation. *B.* Coronal T1-weighted MRI demonstrating the signal void of the malformation as well as the high signal area of the fresh hematoma. *C.* Anteroposterior carotid angiogram demonstrating the filling of the malformation via the anterior cerebral artery with venous drainage into the vein of Galen. *D.* Lateral carotid angiogram.

independent life. These complications have included homonymous hemianopsia, disturbance of recent memory, resolving hemiparesis, and a partial hemisensory loss. It would appear that since all of the patients in this series had a complete cure of their vascular malformation and less than 10 percent had an unsatisfactory neurological outcome, surgical resection of medial hemispheric AVMs of the brain is significantly better than the natural history of this disease.[8,17]

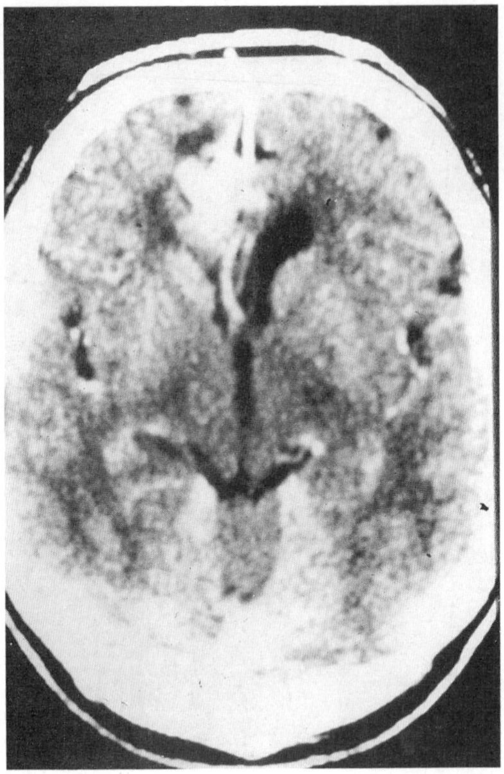

(*A*)

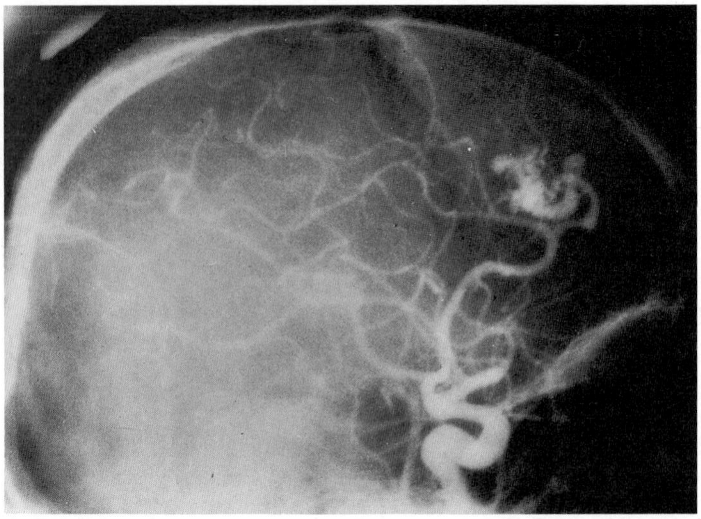

(*B*)

Figure 241-5 Medial frontal AVM. *A.* Contrast-enhanced CT scan demonstrating the nidus of the malformation on the medial side of the frontal lobe in the area of the cingulate gyrus. *B.* Lateral carotid angiogram demonstrating the supply to the malformation via the callosomarginal artery. (From Stein,[15] with permission.)

References

1. Dandy WE. Diagnosis, localization and removal of tumors of the third ventricle. *Bull Johns Hopkins Hosp* 1922; 3:188–189.
2. Drake CG. Cerebral arteriovenous malformations: considerations for and experience with surgical treatment in 166 cases. *Clin Neurosurg* 1979; 26:145–208.
3. Heros RC. Arteriovenous malformations of the medial temporal lobe: surgical approach and neuroradiological characterization. *J Neurosurg* 1982; 56:44–52.
4. Juhász J. Surgical treatment of arteriovenous angiomas localized in the corpus callosum, basal ganglia and near the brain stem. *Acta Neurochir (Wien)* 1978; 40:83–101.
5. Kattah JC, Luessenhop AJ, Kolsky M, et al. Removal of occipital arteriovenous malformations with sparing of visual fields. *Arch Neurol* 1981; 38:307–309.
6. Martin NA, Wilson CB. Medial occipital arteriovenous malformations: surgical treatment. *J Neurosurg* 1982; 56:798–802.
7. Mohr JP. Neurological manifestations and factors related to therapeutic decisions. In Wilson CB, Stein BM (eds): *Intracranial Arteriovenous Malformations.* Baltimore: Williams & Wilkins, 1984, pp 1–11.
8. Morello G, Borghi GP. Cerebral angiomas: a report of 154 personal cases and a comparison between the results of surgical excision and conservative management. *Acta Neurochir (Wien)* 1973; 28:135–155.
9. Riedel CJ, Solomon RA, Stein BM. Surgical management of deep arteriovenous malformations. *Neurosurgery: State Art Rev* 1988; 3:13–28.
10. Sisti MB, Kader A, Stein BM. Microsurgery for 67 intracranial arteriovenous malformations less than 3 cm in diameter. *J Neurosurg* 1994; 79:653–666.
11. Sisti MB, Solomon RA, Stein BM. Stereotactic craniotomy in the resection of small arteriovenous malformations. *J Neurosurg* 1991; 75:40–44.
12. Solomon RA, Stein BM. Management of arteriovenous malformations of the brain stem. *J Neurosurg* 1986; 64:857–864.
13. Solomon RA, Stein BM. Surgical management of arteriovenous malformations that follow the tentorial ring. *Neurosurgery* 1986; 18:708–715.
14. Solomon RA, Stein BM. Interhemispheric approach for the surgical removal of thalamocaudate arteriovenous malformations. *J Neurosurg* 1987; 66:345–351.
15. Stein BM. Arteriovenous malformations of the medial cerebral hemisphere and the limbic system. *J Neurosurg* 1984; 60:23–31.
16. Stein BM. General techniques for the surgical removal of arteriovenous malformations. In Wilson CB, Stein BM (eds): *Intracranial Arteriovenous Malformations.* Baltimore: Williams & Wilkins, 1984, pp 143–155.
17. Stein BM, Wolpert SM. Arteriovenous malformations of the brain: II. Current concepts and treatment. *Arch Neurol* 1980; 37:69–75.
18. Steinberg GK, Fabrikant JI, Marks MP, et al. Stereotactic heavy-charged-particle Bragg-peak radiation for intracranial arteriovenous malformations. *N Engl J Med* 1990; 323:96–101.
19. Steiner L. Treatment of arteriovenous malformations by radiosurgery. In Wilson CB, Stein BM (eds): *Intracranial Arteriovenous Malformations.* Baltimore: Williams & Wilkins, 1984, pp 295–313.
20. Steiner L, Lindquist C, Adler JR, et al. Clinical outcome of radiosurgery for arteriovenous malformations. *J Neurosurg* 1992; 77:1–8.
21. Wascher TM, Spetzler RF. Radiosurgery of arteriovenous malformations. *J Neurosurg* 1992; 76:1045–1057 (letter).
22. Wilson CB, Martin NA. Deep supratentorial arteriovenous malformations. In Wilson CB, Stein BM (eds): *Intracranial Arteriovenous Malformations.* Baltimore: Williams & Wilkins, 1984, pp 184–208.
23. Yasargil MG, Jain KK, Antic J, et al. Arteriovenous malformations of the splenium of the corpus callosum: microsurgical treatment. *Surg Neurol* 1976; 5:5–14.

242
Surgical Resection of Thalamocaudate Arteriovenous Malformations

Ghaus M. Malik
Patrick W. McCormick

Thalamocaudate arteriovenous malformations (AVMs) are commonly grouped under the heading of "deep-seated" malformations exclusive of those in the posterior fossa. These malformations are uncommon and represent 4 to 13 percent of all central nervous system AVMs. Drake reported five such AVMs in 166 cases (3 percent), of which four were thalamic and one involved the caudate nucleus.[1] Waga et al. reported nine periventricular AVMs in a series of 70 cases (13 percent),[7] and our experience has been with 25 AVMs (10 of the basal ganglia, 12 intra- and periventricular, and 3 thalamic) in a series of over 250 operated patients (10 percent).[2]

Because they are uncommon, the natural history of these lesions is only reasonably well understood. Most present at a young age with hemorrhage; and quite often, the hemorrhage is either predominantly or entirely intraventricular. If left untreated, 3 to 4 percent of AVMs bleed per year, and these deeper lesions may well have a higher incidence of rupture. The rate of rebleeding after an initial hemorrhage is thought to be 6 percent during the first year, with a subsequent return to 2 to 3 percent. The best natural history data available come from a population-based study conducted in Finland.[3] The annual rate of death and major neurological morbidity was 2.7 percent. This means that if an AVM is diagnosed now, then the chance of surviving 40 years without death or injury is 35 percent.

Given the apparent severity of this disease, which is identified most commonly in young patients, there has been a major impetus to treat and cure this condition. In addition to surgery, embolization alone, embolization with surgery, stereotactic gamma radiation, and proton beam therapy have all been proposed. We favor surgery because this approach (in an appropriate lesion) results in an immediate cure with a low morbidity and mortality. Surgery, if successful, is the only therapy that results in obliteration of the AVM with no further chance of bleeding in short- and long-term follow-up. Surgery is the time-honored "gold standard" mode of treatment, and long-term follow-up of patients treated with alternative means must be compared with surgical series. Recently, we have used superselective catheterization and embolization, if feasible, as an adjunct to surgery. This makes the technical aspects of surgery easier, but a favorable impact on overall management morbidity is yet to be shown.

On the other hand, surgery for these particular AVMs is complicated by the need for adequate deep exposure with minimal disruption of normal cortex, and by the fact that such deep lesions are surrounded by eloquent brain. Surgery is also complicated by anatomic restraints which dictate approaching most of these malformations from the side opposite their major vascular supply.

The following discussion will first outline general surgical principles pertaining to thalamic and periventricular AVMs, and will then consider the surgical approach to each anatomic location individually.

General Principles

The diagnosis of thalamic and periventricular AVMs is dependent on both traditional radiographic techniques and newer advanced imaging techniques. The initial evaluation is a contrast-enhanced computed tomographic (CT) scan of the head. This may show an enhancing area in the deep supratentorial structures, which is often obscured by recent hemorrhage. Four-vessel stereoangiography is the mainstay of radiologic evaluation. It is used to document the presence of the malformation, its supply, its drainage, and the anatomic relationship of vessels in the nidus. T1-weighted magnetic resonance imaging (MRI) is used to clearly demonstrate the anatomic location of the nidus in relation to important surgical landmarks. Using these studies to develop a good understanding of the malformation, including its anatomic location and its particular vascular geometry, is a fundamental step in designing a successful surgical approach to the problem.

It should be noted that in the event an AVM is highly suspect but fails to materialize on initial radiographic studies, we recommend repeat studies at a later date when the clot has resolved. The final preoperative evaluation for AVMs in these locations is neuro-ophthalmologic and neuropsychological baseline evaluations.

Patient selection is a difficult issue, but in light of the relative young age at presentation and the aforementioned poor natural history of the disease, the necessity of treatment is obvious, and the issue becomes the exact type of treatment. Surgery is the "gold standard" treatment, and competing therapies should be reserved for nonoperative candidates. Contraindications to surgery include: (1) devastating neurological sequelae from the initial hemorrhage; (2) a nidus located on or near the midline supplied by bilateral perforating arteries, the removal of which would probably involve bilateral damage to the fornices, ascending reticular tracts, or descending motor tracts (Fig. 242-1); or (3) a preexisting medical condition that limits the patient's survival to less than 5 years. The recommendation for surgery carries the implicit assumption that the operating surgeon believes that the total treatment morbidity and mortality will be better than the natural history.

Timing of the surgery depends on the subjective preferences of the surgeon. Obviously, life-threatening hemorrhages need immediate attention. It is our preference to treat other patients after a period of recovery from the initial hemorrhage. In patients who have intraventricular hemorrhage with associated hydrocephalus, it is advantageous to avoid shunting or performing ventricular drainage procedures if a transventricular approach is contemplated.

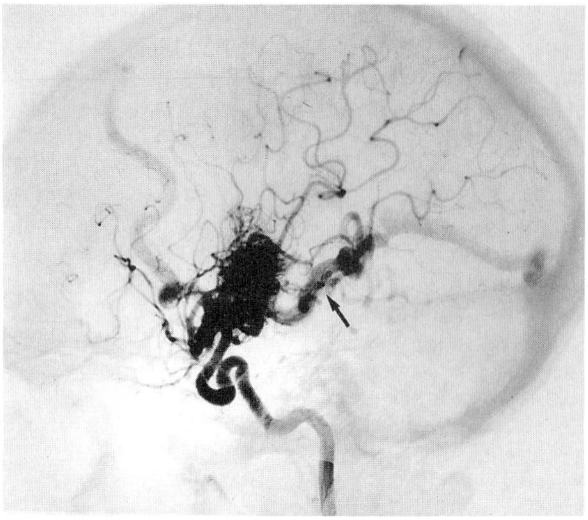

(*A*)

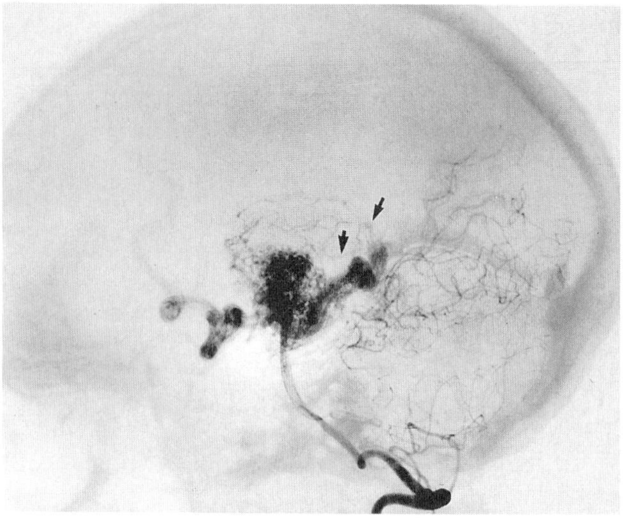

(*B*)

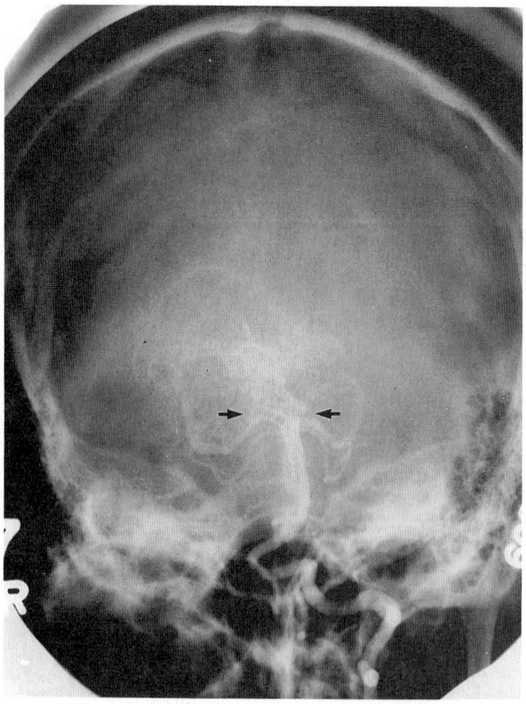

(*C*)

Figure 242-1 An AVM of the thalamus, judged to be inoperable, in a 37-year-old woman with a progressive hemiparesis and seizures. *A*. Selective injection of the internal carotid artery, lateral view, demonstrating the supply from the anterior choroidal artery and drainage through the basal vein of Rosenthal *(arrow)* to the straight sinus. *B*. Selective vertebral angiogram, lateral view, demonstrating the posterior extent of the AVM supplied by the posterior medial and lateral choroidal arteries *(arrows)*. *C*. Selective vertebral angiogram, anteroposterior view, demonstrating the supply from bilateral thalamoperforating arteries *(arrows)*.

Surgical Principles

The goal of the operation must be total removal of the AVM with minimal trauma to the surrounding structures. A detailed operative plan must be developed based on the radiographic studies and clinical assessment of the patient. The key to transforming this plan to a successful operation is anticipation of the expected anatomic landmarks and their orientation to the nidus, as well as anticipation of potential problems. Bleeding is a major concern with these lesions, and in our experience, AVM surgery (especially for supratentorial, superficial lesions) is made easier by preoperative superselective embolization. Unfortunately, deeper AVMs often have numerous deep perforating arteries from the circle of Willis that are not amenable to selective catheterization. In this circumstance, attempted embolization may add to rather than reduce morbidity.

The surgical approach falls into one of three categories: transcortical, transcortical-transventricular, or interhemispheric. Each has its own unique applications, depending on the anatomy of the malformation, which will be discussed in detail in the subsequent paragraphs. On occasion, stereotactic localization is necessary to guide the surgeon to the nidus. This requires that the nidus be visualized on CT, or that an advanced unit compatible with MRI equipment or digitalized angiographic data be used.

Once the approach is completed, a predetermined, systematic dissection of the AVM is carried out to initially remove arterial supply and ultimately venous drainage. The malformation does not contain functional brain, and is separated from the brain by a gliotic margin. The goal is to dissect within this margin.

Blood vessels are controlled using an irrigating bipolar forceps irrigated with normal saline. It has not been necessary in our experience to use aneurysm clips to control these vessels, and this is an advantage because it allows for follow-up magnetic and radiographic imaging without artifact. The most difficult vessels to control are the small arteries perforating the white matter to serve the malformation, usually on its deep surface. Magnified inspection shows these vessels to have extremely thin, delicate walls which are refractory to coagulation. Patience and persistence are required to ultimately coagulate them.

Angiographic demonstration of complete removal of a malformation is done either in the operating room prior to closure, in the angiogram suite immediately following surgery, or in approximately 5 to 7 days after the operation. The first two alternatives allow for further dissection in the event of persistent malformation. The advantages of that option are self-evident.

Postoperative care requires careful observation in an intensive care unit with well-trained personnel. The patient's blood pressure and coagulation profiles must be kept normal. There is often a surprising degree of recovery from neurological deficits associated with AVM surgery, and aggressive rehabilitation should be the rule.

Thalamic and Third Ventricular Malformations

Thalamic and third ventricular malformations generally present with headache and neurological deficits. Tomographic studies generally demonstrate intraventricular hemorrhage, a thalamic parenchymal hemorrhage, and often enlargement of the lateral ventricles. Angiographic studies can be expected to show a blood supply predominantly from the anterior and posterior choroidal arteries, the anterior and posterior cerebral arteries, and thalamic perforators from the circle of Willis. Venous drainage is uniformly deep through the internal cerebral veins to the vein of Galen and straight sinus. An example is shown in Fig 242-2. In this example, a 3.5- to 4.0-cm nidus in the posterior thalamus is fed by two large thalamic perforators and is drained by the deep venous system. The surgical approach is either interhemispheric or transcortical-transventricular.

For posteriorly located thalamic malformations, the interhemispheric approach is made using either a straight prone or three-quarter prone, operated-side-down position, as previously published. The advantage of the latter is that brain retraction is unnecessary because the occipital and posterior parietal lobes fall away from the falx with gravity. This is enhanced with spinal drainage. The semisitting position has been described for this exposure but, in our experience, it limits the comfort of the surgeon and carries a risk of venous air embolism. Regardless of the position, a horseshoe-shaped flap based posteriorly is made with the medial limb

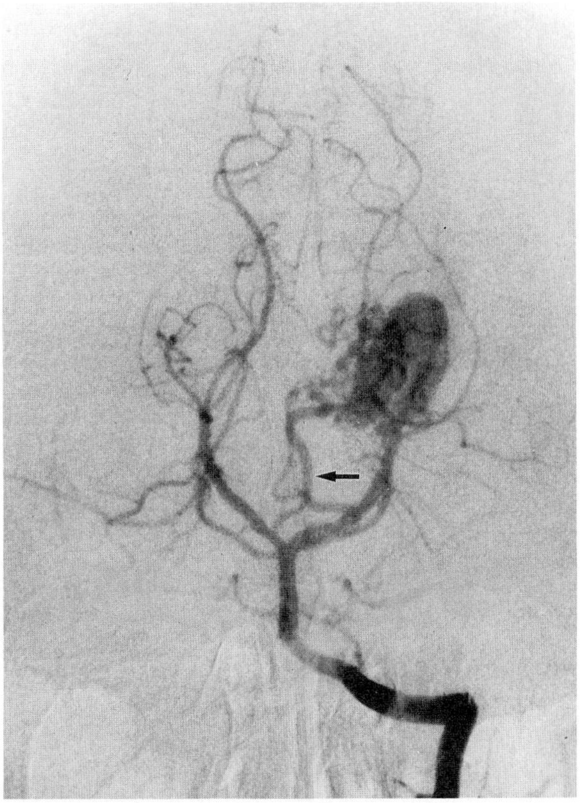

(*A*)

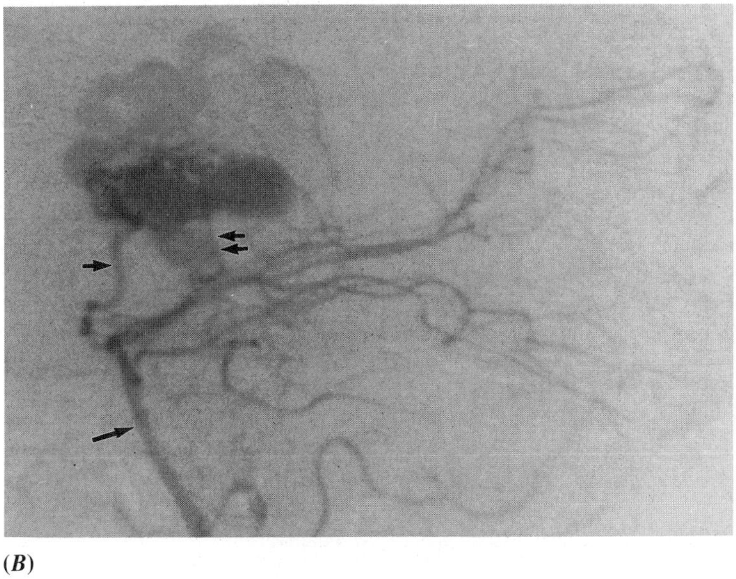

(*B*)

Figure 242-2 An AVM involving the pulvinar of the left thalamus in a 13-year-old boy presenting with hemorrhage. *A.* Selective left vertebral angiogram, anteroposterior view, demonstrating the AVM nidus and the supply from hypertrophied thalamoperforating branches *(arrow)*. *B.* Selective left vertebral angiogram, lateral view, showing the basilar artery *(long arrow)*, thalamoperforating artery *(short arrow)*, and posterior lateral choroidal artery *(double short arrow)*.

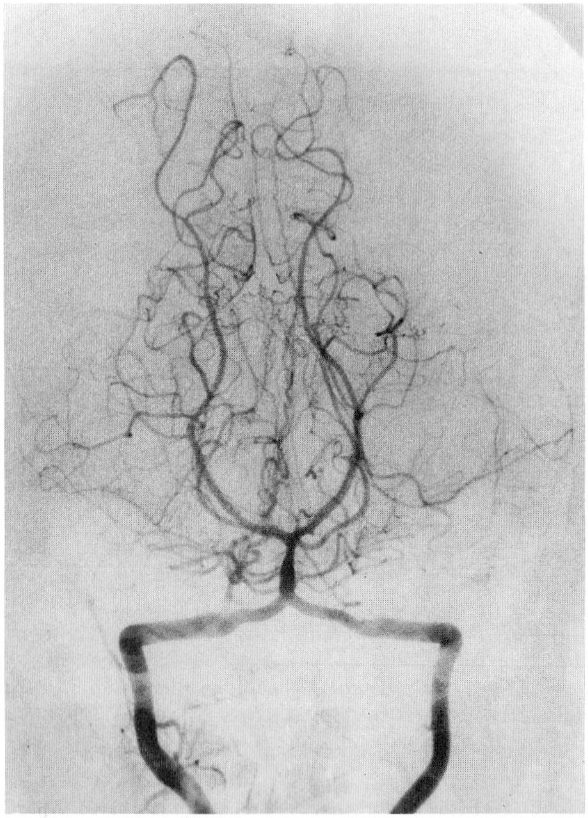

(C)

Figure 242-2 *(Continued)* *C.* Postoperative selective left vertebral angiogram, anteroposterior view, showing no residual AVM.

on the midline from the inion to 4 cm behind the coronal suture. The lateral limb is brought down in the line of the mastoid just behind the ear. We prefer to turn a free bone flap with the periosteum left on the bone in the event a dural patch is necessary. The bone flap is brought to the midline with burr holes placed just lateral to the sagittal sinus. These burr holes are closely spaced to allow easy dural dissection between them. The dural opening is based toward the sinus. Bridging veins represent a hazard of this approach, and it may be necessary to take one or two sizable veins draining the occipital and posterior parietal territories superficially to the superior sagittal sinus. The splenium is easily identified, and a 15- to 20-mm longitudinal leukotomy is made eccentric to the midline. With the aid of the microscope and long bayonetted instruments, the malformation can be dissected. The risks of this approach include memory deficits, a disconnection syndrome, visual field loss, hemiparesis, and hemianesthesia. The approach limits lateral exposure and necessitates approaching the malformation on the side opposite its arterial supply. The benefits include ease of orientation, minimal retraction, minimal cortical disruption, and excellent medial exposure.

The transcortical-transventricular approach to posterior thalamic AVMs is generally done in the prone position with a similar craniotomy flap except that the midline is not exposed nor are draining veins sacrificed. A corticotomy is made on the high medial parietal lobe, and dissection is carried out perpendicular to the cortical surface down to the occipital horn. Self-retaining retractors are placed, and the operative microscope is used to see the dorsal, posterolateral aspect of the thalamus. Often, tortuous, arterialized veins lead to the malformation. These veins may be more obvious after a portion of the choroid plexus is removed to adequately expose the thalamic surface.

Once the nidus is identified, dissection is carried out to isolate it from the surrounding brain and, again, one is forced to deal with the deep penetrating vessels. The ventricle is thoroughly rinsed with saline, and a ventricular catheter is left behind in the lateral ventricle to promote drainage. The risks of this approach include visual field deficits, hemiparesis, and hemianesthesia. The corticotomy is a potential epileptogenic focus, and here again the exposure is away from the deep penetrating arterial vessels. The benefits include better lateral exposure of the malformation than with the interhemispheric approach, and lower risk of venous infarction, which is occasionally associated with the sacrifice of bridging veins.

The exact location of the nidus from medial to lateral thalamus may influence a surgeon's choice between the two described approaches. Solomon and Stein have described a series of 20 malformations in the region of the trigone of the lateral ventricle operated on using an interhemispheric approach.[5] The most common postoperative problem was disturbance in recent memory (11 patients), which improved with time. Six patients had contralateral homonymous visual field deficits, and there were two cases of hemisensory deficit.

Anterior thalamic malformations involve similar surgical choices. An interhemispheric approach is accomplished by placing the patient supine with the head slightly flexed and not rotated. A standard question-mark frontal incision is made, and a bone flap extending to the midline is turned. Draining veins again present an obstacle to exposing the interhemispheric space. The corpus callosum is exposed, and the commisurotomy is larger here than the one described near the splenium. This approach gives better lateral exposure than is achieved in the posterior interhemispheric approach. The disadvantages of this approach are similar to the ones mentioned above for the interhemispheric approach, except that hemisensory and visual field deficits are not associated with the anterior exposure. A major risk is still injury to the fornix; moreover, because of its proximity, the contralateral fornix is also at risk.

The transcortical-transventricular approach is done using a standard frontal craniotomy with a 1.5- to 2.0-cm corticotomy in the middle frontal gyrus. Dissection is carried down to the frontal horn of the ventricle. Using the operative microscope, orientation is maintained by visualizing the structures of the foramen of Monro. The anterior, dorsal thalamus can be seen nicely, and manipulation of the operating table into the Trendelenburg position with slight rotation facilitates its exposure. Risks of this exposure include frontal lobe dysfunction with hemiparesis and, in the dominant hemisphere, dysphasia. In general, this approach is less direct than the interhemispheric approach, and the additional benefit of increased lateral exposure is often unnecessary.

There is no series of patients reported with AVMs in the anterior thalamic region resected by one approach. The anterior interhemispheric approach has been described for other lesions, most notably colloid cysts and craniopharyngiomas, with low morbidity. Dr. U's case reports include a case where a thalamic AVM was approached twice through a transcortical-transventricular exposure with good results.[6]

Malformations of the Basal Ganglia

Malformations of the basal ganglia are less common than thalamic AVMs. There are two basic types—those that present with predominantly intraventricular hemorrhage and those with intraparenchymal bleeding. Malformations on the ventricular surface that present with intraventricular hemorrhage generally involve the head of the caudate nucleus. Those with intraparenchymal hemorrhage tend to involve the putamen, globus pallidus, and internal capsule.

Malformations limited to the head of the caudate nucleus will be considered first. The vascular supply is from the lenticulostriate arteries, the recurrent artery of Heubner, and, occasionally, branches of the anterior choroidal artery. These may be approached either by a transcortical-transventricular exposure or by an interhemispheric-transventricular exposure. The former is identical to the one described for the anterior thalamic malformations. The latter is very similar to the one described for the anterior thalamic region; however, in this case, the lesion is more lateral and one must work across the ventricle from its medial to lateral surface to remove the AVM. This requires a larger opening in the corpus callosum, which is generally well tolerated; as long as the malformation is superficial, its dissection and removal should be straightforward. It is possible with either approach to design skin and bone flaps that allow a subfrontal exposure of the M1 segment of the ipsilateral middle cerebral artery. In this way, tortuous, hypertrophic feeding vessels can be identified and clipped before dissection of the nidus.

Waga et al. reported a series of four caudate AVMs, three of which were approached in a transcortical-transventricular fashion, two with excellent and one with good results.[7] The fourth AVM was approached via an interhemispheric-transventricular route, with excellent results. Drake has also described this approach for a caudate AVM with good results.[1] It has been stated that the interhemispheric-transventricular approach is ideal for lesions in the dominant caudate nucleus, but the risk of sacrificing draining veins and injuring the fornix seems prohibitive. In our experience, a corticotomy in the dominant middle frontal gyrus with careful white matter dissection carries a small morbidity. The transcortical-transventricular approach also allows better lateral exposure of the malformation without risk of injury to the fornix. Malformations of the basal ganglia that do not reach the ventricular surface often present with intraparenchymal hemorrhage. This event can be useful surgically, because evacuation of the hematoma leads the surgeon to the malformation.

The arterial supply to these AVMs includes perforating branches of the A1 and M1 segments of the anterior and middle cerebral arteries, respectively. The recurrent artery of Heubner, which generally arises at the junction of the A1 and A2 segments, also supplies these lesions.

The surgical approach to these malformations is guided by the principle of taking the shortest, safest route to the lesion. This includes the transcortical route through the superior or inferior surface of the frontal lobe, and the transinsular route through the sylvian fissure or through the temporal lobe. Our recent experience with these malformations has involved all of these approaches, a fact that demonstrates our belief that the operative plan must be tailored to the anatomy of the lesion.

In the case of lesions located near the middle cerebral artery, a transcortical approach through the inferior surface of the frontal lobe can be taken directly to the malformation. This approach has the additional advantage of allowing temporary or permanent occlusion of the perforators that feed the malformation. This approach is done through a standard frontotemporal craniotomy with dissection directed either subfrontally or along the sphenoid wing.

Malformations that are more laterally placed can be approached through the insular surface. This surface can be exposed either by widely splitting the sylvian fissure or by dissecting through the inferior temporal lobe. The necessary exposure would again allow for isolation and control of feeding vessels from the M1 segment of the middle cerebral artery. Direct exposure of the insular cortex may be complicated by focal neurological deficits due to frontal or temporal lobe retraction.

The more dorsal malformations are best approached via a convexity corticotomy with dissection through the deep white matter to the lesion. This approach may necessitate localization with stereotactic or ultrasonographic equipment, unless a large hematoma has already developed at the site. This approach is limited by lack of exposure of the deep surface of the malformation and the vessels feeding from below. However, if there are prominent identifiable feeding vessels, the surgical exposure can include dissection of the sylvian fissure and occlusion of large feeding vessels prior to excision of the AVM (Fig. 242-3).

We have previously reported on a series of six basal ganglia malformations treated with various surgical approaches.[2] Since then, four additional patients have been operated on, increasing the total to 10 patients. Of these 10 patients, 1 had hemiparesis, and, in another, the preexisting hemiparesis slightly worsened. A third patient with extension of the AVM into the anterior perforate substance has had a short-term memory deficit. Shi and Chen have described a series of 16 basal ganglia AVMs, most approached by widely splitting the sylvian fissure and dissecting transinsularly.[4] Eleven of their patients had an excellent outcome, four had increased deficits, and one died.

Malformations in the Region of the Trigone

These malformations are usually supplied by the anterior and posterior choroidal arteries, and occasionally by branches of the distal middle and posterior cerebral arteries. An example is seen in Fig. 242-4. Approaches to these malformations include the transcortical-transventricular, interhemispheric-transventricular, and direct transcortical.

The transcortical-transventricular exposure can be accomplished in the prone position and is then very similar to the approach described for the posterior thalamic exposure. Another transcortical-transventricular approach is via the posterior temporal horn ipsilateral to the lesion. This is done by positioning the patient with the head lateral. A flap is turned to expose the inferior and middle ipsilateral temporal gyri, and a corticotomy is made in either of these gyri. The temporal horn is entered and followed to the area of the trigone. This approach allows control of the choroidal vessels prior to dissection of the nidus. This temporal lobe approach has been described for the dominant hemisphere, but the risk of language deficits seems prohibitive, and there is almost always a homonymous quadrantanopsia with this approach. The transcortical-transventricular approach via the posterior medial parietal cortex is the safest exposure of this region. A more direct

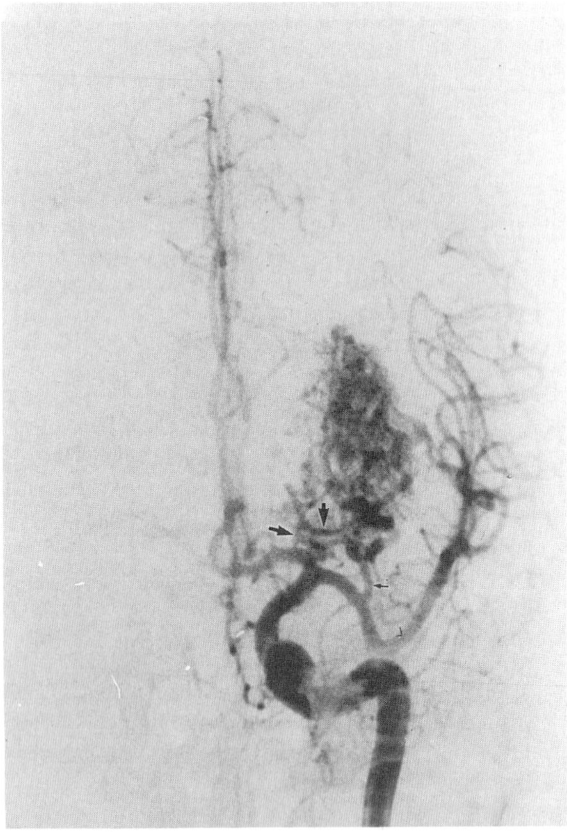

(*A*)

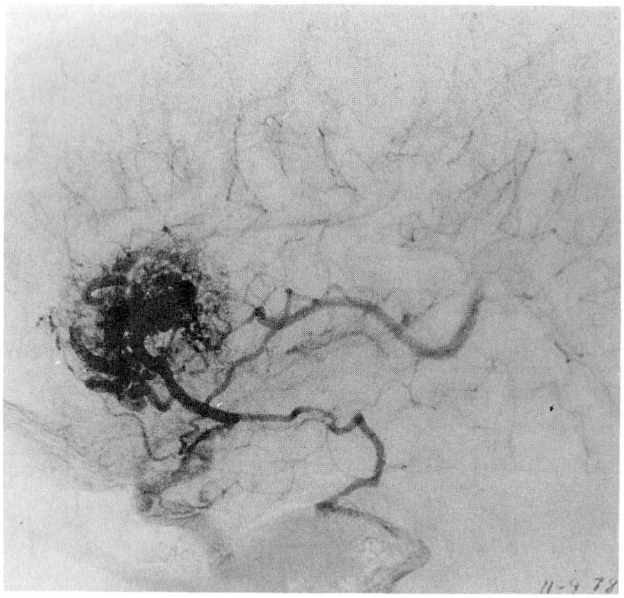

(*B*)

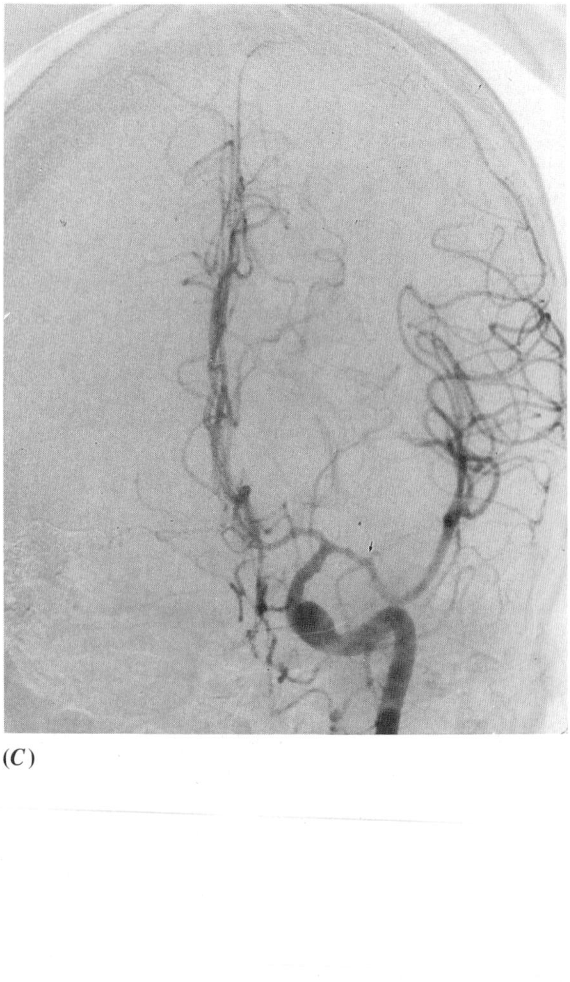

(*C*)

Figure 242-3 An AVM involving the head of the left caudate nucleus, the anterior limb of the internal capsule, and the putamen in a 21-year-old man who failed proton beam therapy. *A.* Left carotid angiogram, anteroposterior view, showing the medial striate supply *(large arrows)* and lateral striate supply *(small arrow)*. *B.* Left carotid angiogram, lateral view, demonstrating the nidus and the venous anatomy. *C.* Postoperative angiogram, anteroposterior view, showing no residual malformation. A *small arrow* points to the site of occlusion of the larger feeding vessels prior to the transcortical excision of the AVM. (From Malik et al.,[2] with permission.)

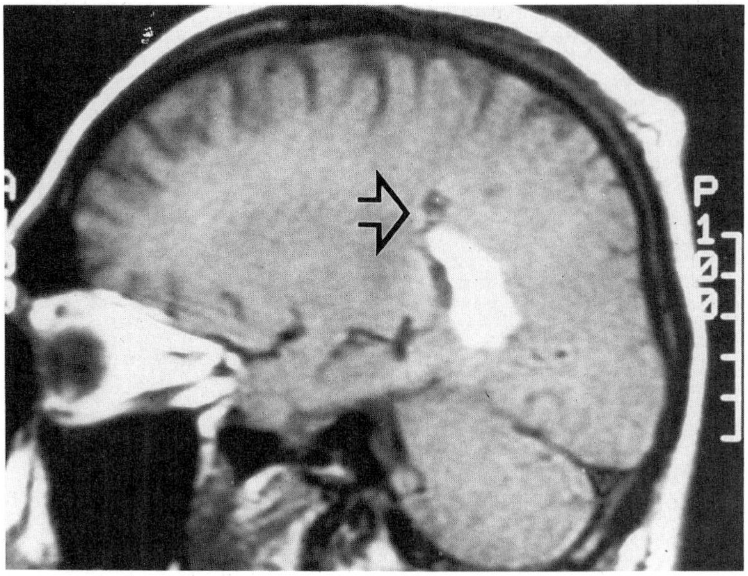

(*A*)

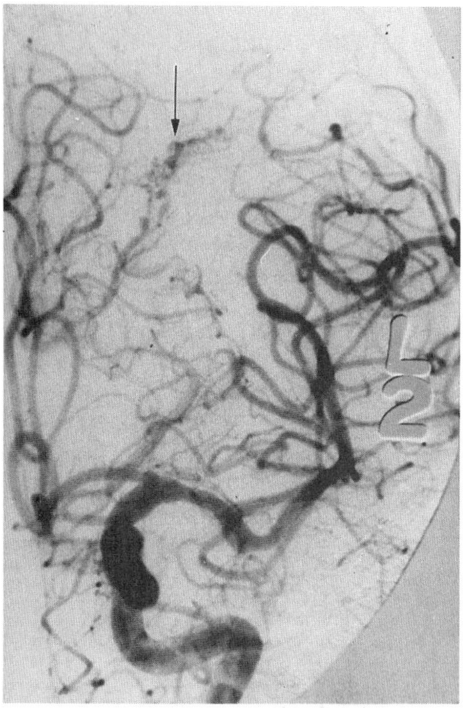

(*C*)

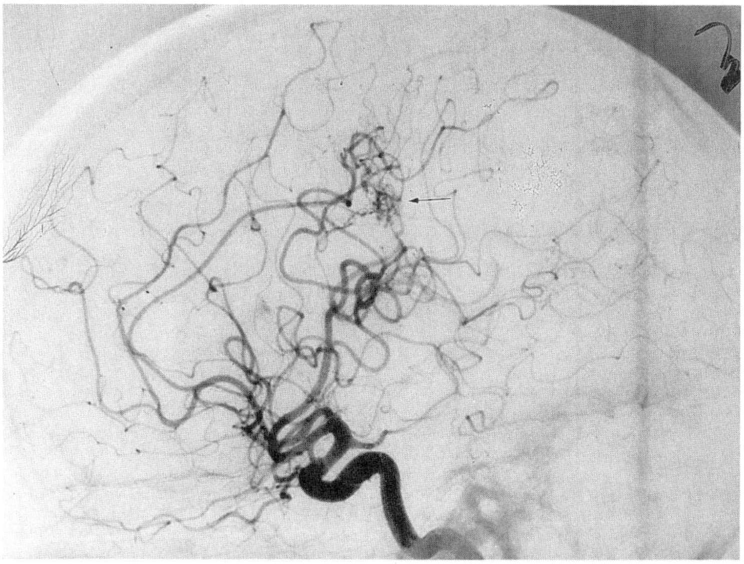

(*B*)

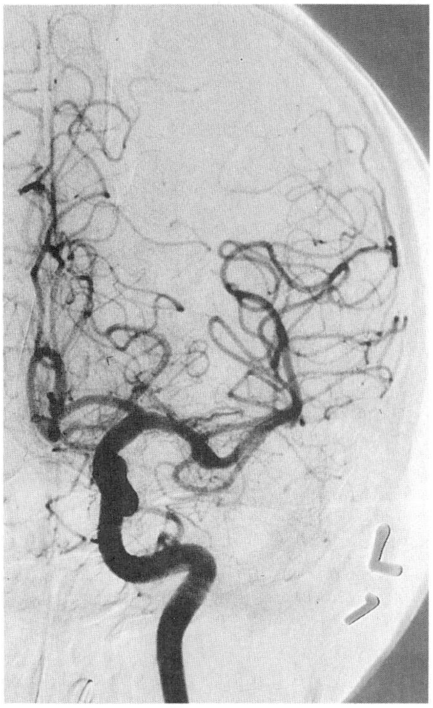

(*D*)

Figure 242-4 An AVM located in the roof of the trigone of the left lateral ventricle in a 34-year-old man. *A*. Parasagittal MRI detailing the nidus of the malformation *(arrow)* and associated hemorrhage *(white area)*. *B*. Selective left internal carotid angiogram, lateral view, demonstrating the nidus *(arrow)*. *C*. Selective left internal carotid angiogram, anteroposterior view, demonstrating the nidus of the malformation *(arrow)*. *D*. Postoperative angiogram, anteroposterior view, showing no residual malformation.

transcortical approach can be used for these malformations, especially those in the roof of the ventricle (as seen in Fig. 242-4). This, however, necessitates disruption of the white matter in the center of the centrum semiovale, including motor projections, and a resulting permanent hemiparesis is likely. This particular approach is best accomplished with the aid of stereotactic localization. U has described three cases of AVM in the trigone approached via the temporal lobe exposure, two with excellent and one with good results.[6] Our experience consists of 12 patients with intra- and periventricular AVMs that have been treated surgically. Resection was accomplished with no mortality or significant morbidity.

Finally, the interhemispheric approach has been described for malformations in this area, but theoretically this approach seems difficult because of the relative lack of exposure. Unless very unique indications are present, this approach cannot be recommended.

References

1. Drake CG. Cerebral arteriovenous malformations: considerations for and experience with surgical treatment in 166 cases. *Clin Neurosurg* 1979; 26:145–208.
2. Malik GM, Umansky F, Patel S, et al. Microsurgical removal of arteriovenous malformations of the basal ganglia. *Neurosurgery* 1988; 23:209–217.
3. Ondra SL, Troupp H, George ED, et al. The natural history of symptomatic arteriovenous malformations of the brain: a 24-year follow-up assessment. *J Neurosurg* 1990; 73:387–391.
4. Shi YQ, Chen XC. Surgical treatment of arteriovenous malformations of the striatothalamocapsular region. *J Neurosurg* 1987; 66:352–356.
5. Solomon RA, Stein BM. Interhemispheric approach for the surgical removal of thalamocaudate arteriovenous malformations. *J Neurosurg* 1987; 66:345–351.
6. U HS. Microsurgical excision of paraventricular arteriovenous malformations. *Neurosurgery* 1985; 16:293–303.
7. Waga S, Shimosaka S, Kojima T. Arteriovenous malformations of the lateral ventricle. *J Neurosurg* 1985; 63:185–192.

243 Arteriovenous Malformations of the Posterior Fossa

Sydney J. Peerless
Juha A. Hernesniemi
Charles G. Drake

Prior to the routine use of vertebral angiography, brain stem and cerebellar arteriovenous malformations (AVMs) were recognized unexpectedly during the removal of posterior fossa hematomas. Such an occurrence led to the first reported complete removal of an infratentorial AVM by Olivecrona in 1932.[3] As vertebral angiography became more widely used, the preoperative diagnosis of a posterior fossa AVM became possible, and further reports of complete removal came from the clinics of Logue and Moncton, Poppen, and others.[12,19,23] These surgeons were, however, disappointed that only very few of these lesions could be removed entirely without great risk, and other ineffectual techniques, such as vertebral artery or feeder ligation, were proposed as methods of treatment. In 1961, Verbiest's review of the literature identified 102 cases, to which he added 6 of his own.[23] His experiences, as well as those he reviewed, showed that small cerebellar AVMs could be removed safely, but that large posterior fossa AVMs, even if located outside the brain stem, could be extremely hazardous to remove. He and others thought that brain stem AVMs were unresectable by their very nature.

Since that report, the frequency of successful surgical removals of posterior fossa AVMs has kept pace with the development of microneurosurgical techniques, radiology (including interventional neuroradiology), neuroanesthesia, and intensive care. In the early 1970s, Green and Vaughan,[9] Chou et al.,[2] and Drake[5] reported that removal of AVMs in the more sensitive areas of the hindbrain could also be accomplished with excellent outcomes. Over the last 30 years, 116 patients harboring arteriovenous malformations in the posterior fossa have been treated at our institutions (Table 243-1). The successes and failures realized in the treatment of these patients are documented in this report and are the philosophical and practical basis for our current management plan for these relatively uncommon lesions.

TABLE 243-1 Posterior Fossa AVMs: Location and Size (Authors' Series)

Location	Totals	Size (Diameter, cm) <2.5	2.5–5	>5
Cerebellum	80	25	42	13
Cerebellopontine angle	16	12	4	0
Brain stem	19	15	4	0
Fourth ventricle	1	1	0	0
Totals	116	53	50	13

Pathology

McCormick et al. subdivided vascular malformations into four histologically distinct entities: arteriovenous malformations, cavernous hemangiomas, venous angiomas, and capillary telangiectasias.[15] This classification has withstood the test of time and is widely accepted. Capillary telangiectasias and venous angiomas rarely bleed, and we do not recommend operative therapy for either. In fact, these lesions may be variants of normal anatomy. There is no study on the natural history of cavernous hemangiomas. They are now frequently identified by magnetic resonance imaging (MRI). Some will hemorrhage repeatedly, and they may produce symptoms by enlargement and compression of surrounding structures. Many, even in the most eloquent parts of the brain and brain stem, can now be removed surgically. A fifth form of vascular malformation is the cryptic malformation, which is probably a small AVM or cavernous malformation that has obliterated itself by moderate to massive hemorrhage in the brain. The abnormal vessels cannot be identified on angiography but may be found at autopsy or in the surgical specimen. Certainly, in a few of our early cases treated before the advent of computed tomography (CT) and, more important, MRI studies, the lesions diagnosed at operation by removal of hematoma were cavernous malformations (see Table 243-6 and Fig. 243-6). The focus of this chapter, however, will be on AVMs because of their higher incidence and their significant associated morbidity and mortality.

Incidence

The incidence of all types of cerebral AVMs is estimated on the basis of small autopsy series to be about 3/100,000 population, or about one-seventh that of cerebral aneurysms. Nevertheless, cerebral AVMs are the most common vascular malformations seen in the clinic, with about 2500 new symptomatic cases presenting each year in the United States. Posterior fossa AVMs are uncommon lesions. Based on the following data, it can be roughly concluded that one-tenth of cerebral AVMs are located in the posterior fossa. Given that all of the reported surgical series comprise less than 100 patients, one must assume that most patients with posterior circulation AVMs are being managed conservatively. Of 453 cases of intracranial AVMs reported to the Cooperative Study of Intracranial Aneurysms and Subarachnoid Hemorrhage, only 32 (7 percent) were located infratentorially; however, vertebral angiography was only done in about 25 percent of cases with subarachnoid hemorrhage in this study.[18] Of more than 600 patients with AVMs

TABLE 243-2 Incidence of Posterior Fossa AVMs (Seven Reported Mainly Surgical Series)

		Posterior Fossa	
Series	Totals*	Number	Percent
Two Finnish series[10,17]	352†	15	4
Cooperative Study[18]	453‡	32	7
Yaşargil[24]	500	82§	16
Matsumura et al.[14]	84	14	17
Batjer and Samson[1]	171	32	19
Drake and Peerless	600+	116	19

*Total number of AVMs in each series.
†No admission biases, 49% with surgery.
‡41% with surgery.
§14 AVMs in this series were not operated on.

treated at our centers, 116 had their AVM in an infratentorial location. This group included 50 men and 66 women, whose ages ranged from 5 to 69 years (mean, 35 years). Thirteen patients were 16 years old or less. The relative frequency of these lesions in other centers is outlined in Table 243-2. As can be appreciated, the higher incidences in these series likely represent case selection owing to a referral bias, as is certainly true in our centers. More accurate epidemiologic data may be obtained from controlled populations. By combining two Finnish series without any admission biases, an incidence of posterior fossa AVMs of less than 5 percent in symptomatic patients was obtained; the incidence is 8 percent if one includes patients whose AVM was found incidentally on CT scans done for other indications.[10,17]

Location

The published series differ slightly, but AVMs localized to a cerebellar hemisphere or the vermis predominate (Table 243-3). Unfortunately, AVMs located in the brain stem are the next most common group. AVMs located in the cerebellopontine angle (CPA), flocculonodular lobe, and fourth ventricle are less common but pose their own unique technical challenges.

Clinical Features

In our experience, as in that of others,[1,13–15,18,24] hemorrhage, either subarachnoid, intraparenchymal, or intraventricular, is the most common presenting feature, occurring in 92 percent of patients (Table 243-4). The incidence of hemorrhage as a presenting feature of AVMs of the posterior fossa appears to be higher than that seen with AVMs above the tentorium—the reason being, of course, that posterior fossa AVMs do not cause seizures. Of the 421 supratentorial AVMs reported to the Cooperative Study, 281 (66.7 percent) presented with hemorrhage.[18] Similarly, in 264 (61 percent) of our 432 patients with supratentorial AVMs, the lesion manifested itself by hemorrhaging. However, it is difficult to draw conclusions regarding the relative likelihood of hemorrhage as a presentation because one can never be sure as to the actual value of the denominator, i.e., the population at risk for this occurrence.

The natural history of AVMs is uncertain because most series are small and selected and because the length of follow-up has been relatively short. Perhaps the longest and most complete follow-up came from Troupp and Ondra in Finland, where 160 cases were followed for an average of 24 years. The rebleeding rate in this series was 4 percent per year, with a mortality of 1 percent per year and a combined mortality and morbidity of 2.7 percent per year.[17] These rates were similar regardless of whether the patient presented with hemorrhage, seizures, or headache without hemorrhage. The natural history of posterior fossa AVMs is not specifically addressed in this latest follow-up. Earlier, Troupp stated that parietal, central, and posterior fossa AVMs rebleed far more frequently than those located in other regions.

Between 5 and 8 percent of all AVMs are accompanied by a co-existing aneurysm, and 1 percent of all aneurysm patients have a co-existing AVM. For posterior circulation aneurysms, this figure is higher (3.3 percent). In 3 percent of our series of 1767 patients with vertebrobasilar artery aneurysms there was an associated posterior circulation AVM, but only in one-third of the patients with AVMs had the vascular malformation been the source of the hemorrhage. Patients with both an AVM and an aneurysm have an elevated risk of hemorrhage. Of patients who have both an AVM and an aneurysm and who present with a subarachnoid hemorrhage (SAH), in two-thirds it is the aneurysm that has ruptured. Many times, the aneurysms will arise from vessels feeding the AVM; presumably in these cases it develops because the high flow through the feeding artery increases the hemodynamic stress on the vessel wall. Of the 23 patients in our series (20 percent) in whom one or more aneurysms were associated with the AVM, the aneurysm was the source of bleeding in 16. Emergent surgery was precipitated by intraparenchymal clots or acute hydrocephalus in 13 patients; 5 were treated by ventricular drainage and 8 by clot removal. In 80 percent of the patients with intraparenchymal hemorrhage and 58 percent of the patients with subarachnoid hemorrhage, the clinical findings localized the lesion to the posterior fossa.

Other forms of presentation included headache (not associated with hemorrhage) (31 patients), trigeminal neuralgia (4 patients), and hydrocephalus (3 patients). Progressive neurological deterioration, due most often to small recurrent hemorrhages, occurred in only two of our patients, both with lesions in the brain stem and

TABLE 243-3 Location of Posterior Fossa AVMs (Six Reported Series)

	Location			
AVM Series	Cerebellum	Cerebellopontine Angle	Brain Stem	Fourth Ventricle
Matsumura et al.[14]	10	2	2	—
Martin et al.[13]	16	—	2	—
Silber et al.[20]	22	—	7	—
Batjer and Samson[1]	26	2	4	—
Yaşargil[24]	46	10	10	2
Drake and Peerless	80	16	19	1

TABLE 243-4 Posterior Fossa AVMs: Clinical Presentation (Authors' Series)

Mode of Presentation	Number	Percent
Hemorrhage	107	92
Ruptured aneurysm	16	—
Unruptured aneurysm	7	—
Headache/incidental	7	6
Focal neurological deficit	2	2

initially diagnosed as having multiple sclerosis.[22] The incidental recognition of a posterior fossa AVM has become more common in recent years with the increasing use of modern imaging techniques.

Radiological Features

Computed tomography is an important initial mode of examination for patients presenting with a sudden ictus, particularly if the clinical examination points to a posterior fossa localization. In the case of a posterior fossa AVM that has bled, a noncontrast CT scan will show the location and amount of hemorrhage, as well as any associated mass effect or hydrocephalus. Calcification and evidence of prior hemorrhage may be seen and may serve as clues to the nature of the bleeding lesion. With the infusion of radiographic contrast agents, feeding arteries and draining veins may show as linear, vermiform, tubular, or serpentine high-density areas (Fig. 243-1). Occasionally, large venous varices will be seen (Fig. 243-2). When an intraparenchymal clot exists, careful inspection of its borders after contrast enhancement may reveal contiguous areas of enhancement that represent the vascular lesion. The nonenhanced CT scan will be abnormal in 60 to 75 percent of cases of posterior fossa AVM, the lesion usually appearing as an area of increased density. Contrast infusion will reveal nearly all AVMs and, in fact, might reveal cryptic AVMs not seen by angiography, especially in the brain stem.[16]

MRI using high field strengths provides exquisite detail of the anatomic relations of the AVM. This is particularly useful when the AVM lies in or near the brain stem or cerebellar peduncle, in order to determine operability or to plan the surgical approach. The MRI appearance of AVMs in the posterior fossa is similar to that seen with supratentorial lesions.[11] The nidus of the AVM is seen as an area of signal void and may have a honeycombed pattern.

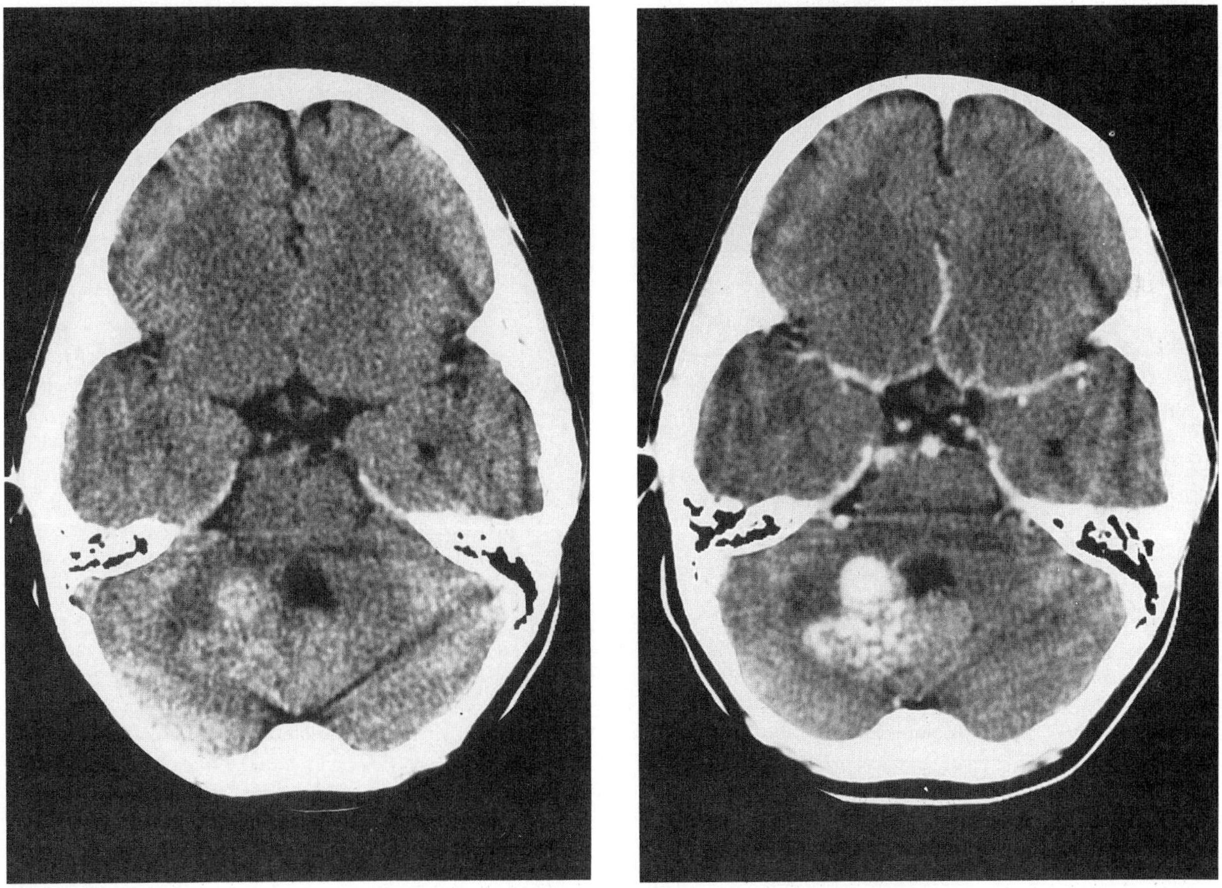

(*A*) (*B*)

Figure 243-1 *A*. Non-contrast-enhanced CT scan of a patient harboring a large right cerebellar AVM. A high-density lesion is seen in the right cerebellar hemisphere. An area of decreased density is seen anterolaterally and represents encephalomalacia secondary to a previous hemorrhage. *B*. Contrast-enhanced CT scan of the same patient. Numerous vermiform areas of increased density are seen, as well as a larger area of enhancement anteriorly, which represents an enlarged draining vein.

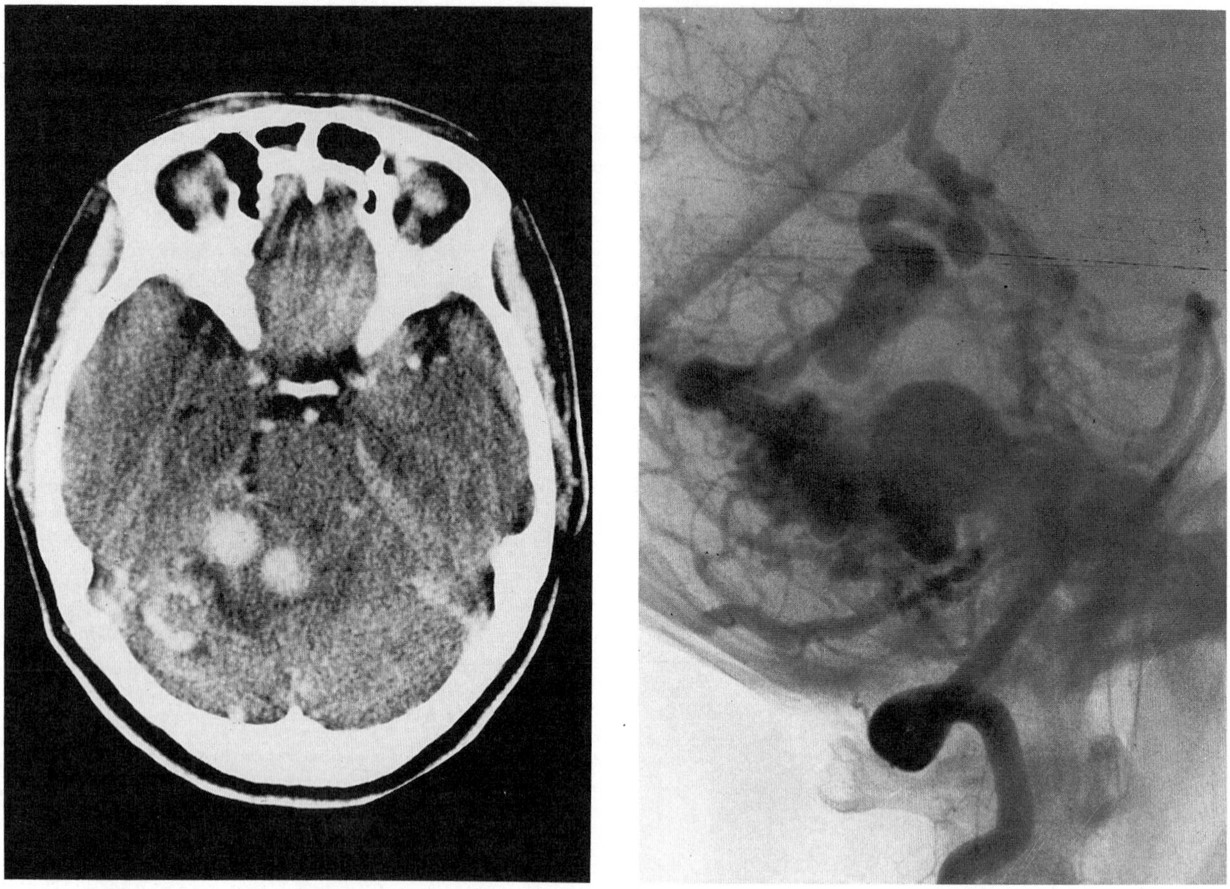

(*A*) (*B*)

Figure 243-2 Contrast-enhanced CT scan (*A*) and lateral vertebral angiogram (*B*). The large venous varices are well demonstrated on the contrast-enhanced CT.

Tubular signal void structures converging on the nidus represent the feeding arteries and draining veins (Fig. 243-3). Bony artifact is avoided with MRI, therefore allowing better identification of superficial supply to, or drainage from, the AVM. MRI is, however, an impractical imaging tool in critically ill patients harboring a cerebellar clot.

Angiography is essential in the diagnosis and subsequent management of all AVMs. All of the feeding arteries and draining veins must be visualized. This will necessitate selective injection of contrast material into both the external and internal carotid arteries as well as both vertebral arteries and, occasionally, superselective injection into the larger feeding arteries. Angiography is also vital in the detection of anatomic variants, associated aneurysms, and normal vessels of passage. The latter are arteries which feed the AVM but also continue on to irrigate areas of normal brain; these must be identified and protected at surgery.

Treatment

General Principles of Treatment

The natural history of untreated AVMs is modestly unfavorable. The decision of whether or not to treat these lesions and of what form of treatment to use is complex, and one must take into consideration the following factors: (1) the presentation and natural history of the lesion; (2) the known results of the available therapeutic alternatives; (3) the patient's age and general medical and neurological condition; (4) the presenting symptoms (hemorrhage, epilepsy, headache, or none); (5) the physical parameters of the AVM, including its location and size, the number and flow pattern of the feeding vessels, and the venous drainage; (6) whether there is a recent or remote hematoma; and (7) the site of the lesion—that is, the precise anatomic relationship of the malformation to the surrounding brain, cranial nerves, and pituitary gland.

For many patients, all that is necessary is symptomatic treatment for headache and firm reassurance that the risks involved in living with an AVM are small. This is particularly true in asymptomatic patients whose malformation has been detected during investigation of some other, unrelated complaint. It is also important to remember that the various therapies available for AVMs are primarily directed toward preventing hemorrhage. Furthermore, it is necessary to point out that incomplete treatment of AVMs (i.e., treatment after which some abnormal vessels remain) offers no significant protection to a patient against rebleeding.

Endovascular Techniques

In recent years, endovascular techniques have emerged as being not only diagnostic aids but also therapeutic tools in the management of AVMs. It was initially hoped that embolization of AVMs would obviate surgery; however, to date no embolic agent has

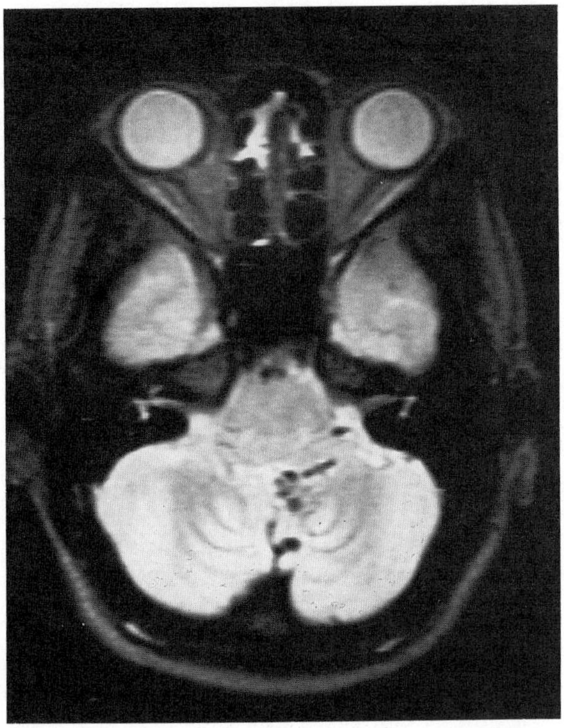

(*A*)

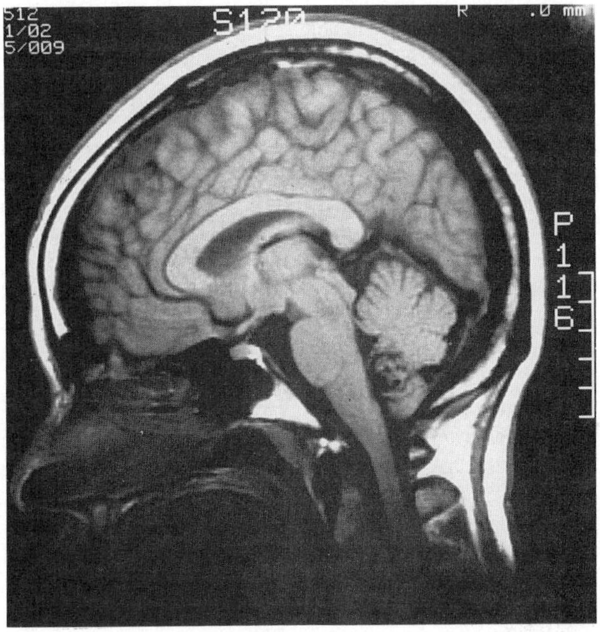

(*B*)

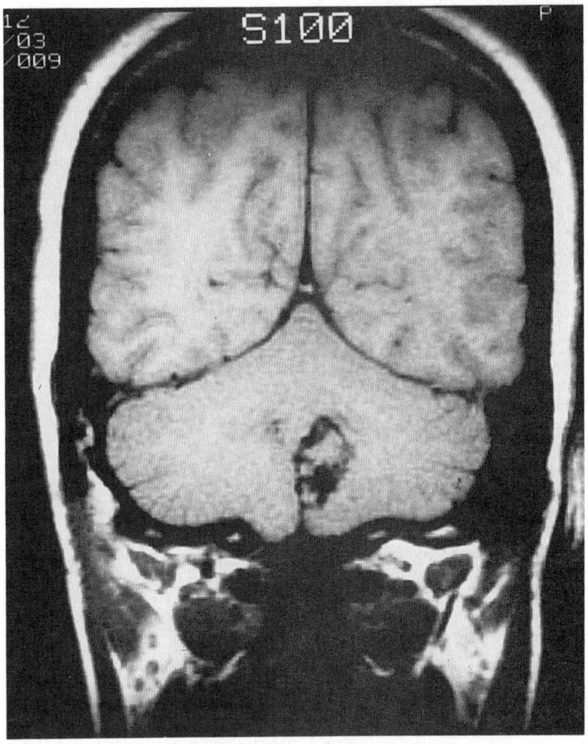

(*C*)

Figure 243-3 Axial (*A*) (TR = 2000 ms, TE = 70 ms), sagittal (*B*) (TR = 600 ms, TE = 20 ms), and coronal (*C*) (TR = 600 ms, TE = 20 ms) MR images of a patient with a vermian AVM. The T2-weighted axial image shows an enlarged inferior vermian vein draining the lesion. The nidus, best seen on the T1-weighted sagittal and coronal images, has a honeycombed appearance. These images clearly show the lack of brain stem involvement.

prevented the recanalization, reappearance, and rebleeding of these lesions. Partial obliteration of the AVM appears to afford no protection against hemorrhage. Therefore, we now use embolization only as a preoperative adjunct to surgical removal, to decrease intraoperative bleeding and reduce the ''sump'' effect of the AVM on the surrounding brain. However, embolization of AVMs is not without risk, which include premature venous occlusion with risk of AVM rupture, occlusion of arteries of passage, reflux of embolic material into normal arteries, and, rarely, the gluing of catheters into major cerebral arteries. Also, preoperative embolization with materials that form a hard mass may make dissection of the AVM more difficult, especially in the confined space of the posterior fossa.

Seven patients in our series underwent embolization as the primary mode of therapy. In five of these patients, the AVMs were cerebellar; in two they were in and around the brain stem. Four of the cerebellar AVMs and one of the two brain stem AVMs were embolized directly at craniotomy after cannulation of one of the feeding arteries.[8] The cannula was held in place either with a ligature or with a drop of *n*-butyl 2-cyanoacrylate. The lesions of the remaining two patients were embolized using a transfemoral technique. The embolic material used was Gelfoam (absorbable gelatin sponge; The Upjohn Company, Kalamazoo, MI) in the earlier two cases and isobutyl 2-cyanoacrylate (Bucrylate; Ethicon, Inc., Somerville, NJ) in the latter five. The degree of wipe-out achieved varied from 10 to 90 percent. There was no instance of complete obliteration. In one case, which initially had a near complete obliteration, a repeat study 2 months later revealed extensive recanalization. Five patients had good outcomes. In one patient, a rare anastomotic channel between the superior cerebellar and posterior cerebral arteries resulted in the aberrant embolization of Bucrylate into the posterior medial choroidal arteries, producing a thalamic infarction that has left the patient with a paralyzed and anesthetic left side. Another patient with a massive cerebellar and pontomesencephalic lesion was neurologically worsened by the embolization, with little recognizable decrease in the size of the lesion. This unfortunate young man has had at least two subsequent hemorrhages from his AVM and remains severely disabled (Fig. 243-4).

Radiosurgery

Irradiation causes endothelial cells and perivascular tissue to swell and degenerate, promoting thrombosis and proliferative fibroplastic repair. Progressive thickening and fibrosis of the abnormal vessel walls leads to occlusion of the shunt and, ultimately, to obliteration of the AVM. The success of these techniques depends on the ionizing radiation being delivered in a precise and focused manner to the malformation, using stereotactic principles and avoiding injury to surrounding brain. Over the past 20 years, Steiner has used these techniques to treat more than 1300 patients with small AVMs located in deep, eloquent areas of the brain. The malformation was totally obliterated in about 80 percent of these patients, and this percentage increased to 88 percent if the lesion was less than 1 cc in volume. Only 60 percent of malformations larger than 8 cc were completely obliterated, however. The process of AV shunt eradication takes up to 2 years. Recurrent hemorrhage in this period remains a risk; it occurs at least as often as if the lesion had been left untreated. It has been suggested that radiation treatment that does not result in complete occlusion of the AVM may nevertheless have some protective effect on the vessels, but, if this is so, the effect is small and probably does not appear for several years and, therefore, is of limited value. Of the patients treated with radiosurgery, 4 percent had permanent neurological injury due to radiation necrosis of surrounding brain.

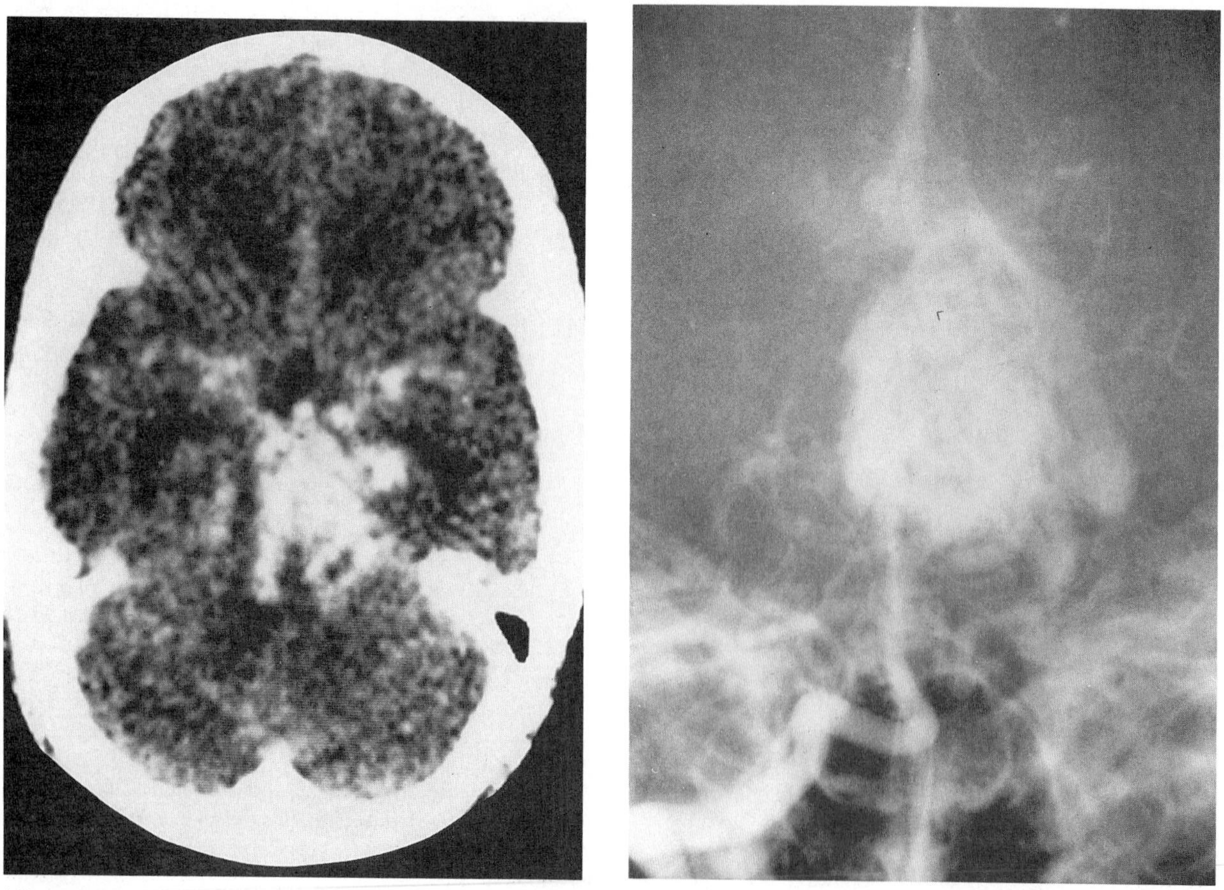

(*A*) (*B*)

Figure 243-4 Contrast-enhanced CT scan (*A*) of a large pontomesencephalic AVM, plus anteroposterior angiograms before embolization (*B*).

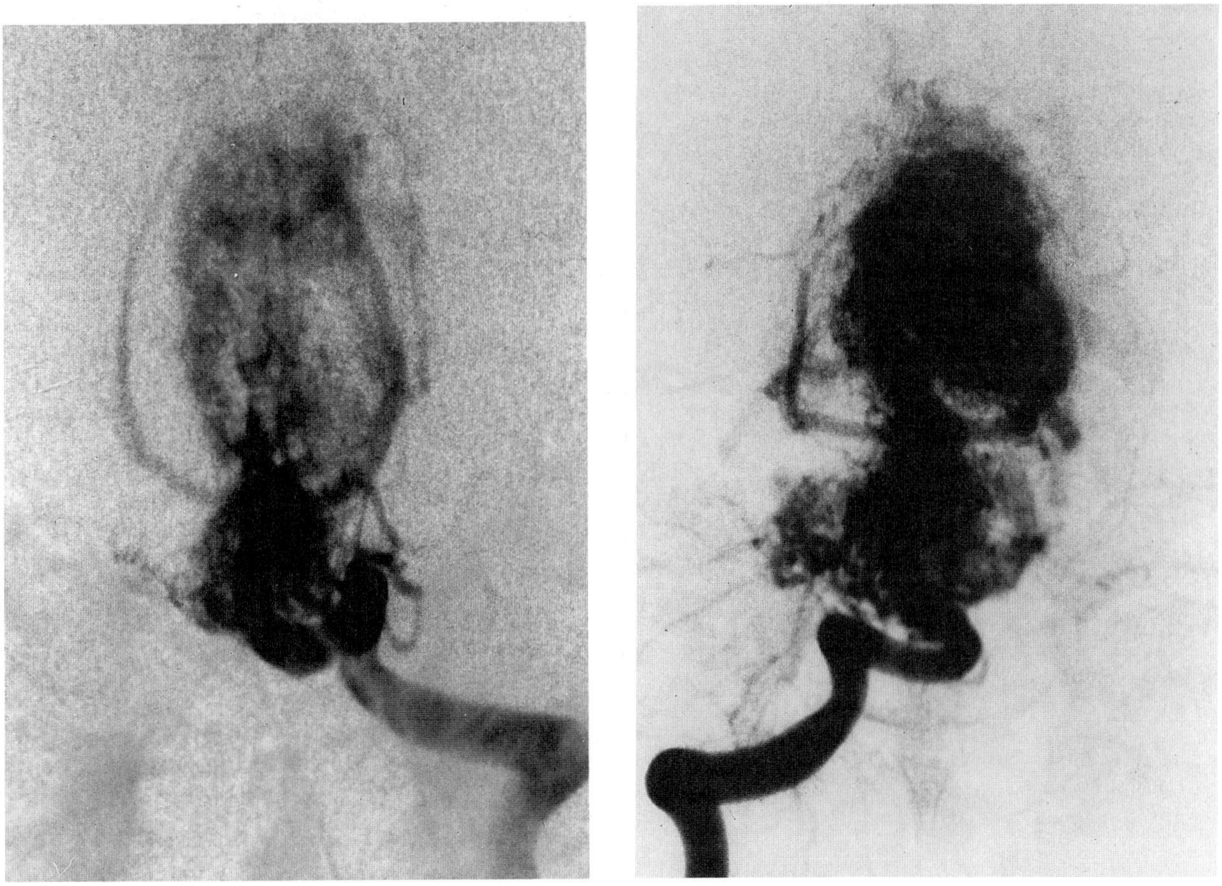

(*C*) (*D*)

Figure 243-4 (*Continued*) immediately after embolization (*C*), and at 1 year follow-up (*D*). Embolization with Bucrylate caused little reduction in the size of the AVM; however, the patient deteriorated neurologically after embolization and has subsequently suffered at least two further hemorrhages.

Microsurgery

Microsurgery is the ideal treatment for these lesions if it can be done safely, but the decision of whether or not to operate is based on three key variables—the size of the lesion, its anatomic site, and the surgeon's experience. The risk posed by surgical removal increases drastically with the size of the AVM. In our experience with good-grade patients, we have had no morbidity or mortality for small AVMs (<2.5 cm in diameter) and just over 15 percent morbidity and mortality for large AVMs (>5 cm in diameter). In addition, the site of the malformation is critical. A small, even tiny, malformation in the brain stem may be surgically inaccessible. Simple ligation of the feeding vessels of the malformation is completely ineffectual. The fistulous connection between arteries and veins in the nidus of the lesion will rapidly recruit surrounding vessels and make them as prominent as the ones that have been ligated.

Surgical Approaches

Anesthesia and Monitoring Techniques

Before the operation, the patient's fluid and electrolyte balance and coagulation parameters are assessed, and an attempt is made to achieve optimum physiologic homeostasis. Mild sedation only is used when the patient is taken to the operating room, to help relieve anxiety without leaving the patient sleepy postoperatively.

The patient is made somnolent with intravenous narcotics, and anesthesia is then gently induced with thiopental sodium and nondepolarizing muscle relaxants. The patient is intubated, and an inhalational anesthetic is given (usually isoflurane with or without nitrous oxide). If there are concerns regarding increased intracranial pressure, the inhalational agents are replaced by a combined barbiturate-narcotic technique. The patient is monitored with electrocardiography (ECG), intra-arterial and central venous catheters, a capnograph, and routinely with auditory and somatosensory evoked potentials. A P_{CO_2} of 30 to 40 mmHg and a P_{O_2} of over 100 mmHg is maintained. Frequently, but not routinely, 1 g/kg of mannitol is infused prior to dural opening to ensure a slack brain. It is important to accurately record fluid balance throughout the operation. A lumbar subarachnoid catheter is usually not necessary because posterior fossa approaches allow for early CSF drainage with opening of the cisterna magna.

The surgeon and anesthetist should be prepared to deliberately reduce the mean systemic arterial blood pressure (MAP) to 40 to 60 torr to facilitate the dissection and assist in the control of troublesome bleeding. To this end, isoflurane is both an excellent anesthetic and an ideal hypotensive agent. It can be readily and very accurately titrated.

At the end of the procedure, the anesthesia is gently reversed, and the patient is extubated while still unconscious to prevent coughing and gagging on the tube. The patient is transported to the recovery room and subsequently to the neurosurgical observation unit, where ECG, arterial blood pressure, and central venous pressure are recorded, and careful repeated neurological assessments are made. Use of postoperative hypotension to prevent postoperative hematomas has proved to be important. We attempt to maintain the MAP 20 percent below the patient's normal level by restricting fluid intake and using hypotensive medication for 3 to 7 days.

Positioning and General Operative Techniques

Both the park bench (lateral recumbent) and sitting or reclining positions are used in our unit. The relative merits of each have been debated extensively. There are two risks with the sitting position: air embolism and incomplete hemostasis. In any position, after removal of the AVM, hemostasis must be tested both on the venous side, by repeated Valsalva maneuvers, and on the arterial side, by raising MAP to more than 20 mmHg above normal pressure. The patient should be nursed sitting upright for at least 1 day following surgery to reduce intracranial arterial and venous pressure and brain swelling.

Only the operative area is shaved. Prophylactic antibiotics are not used. Adequate exposure of an AVM must give the surgeon access to the malformation, the feeding arteries, and the draining veins. This will usually be achieved by a posterior fossa craniectomy, or, more recently, by using a craniotomy with replacement of the bone flaps. Exposures through the tentorium or by a combined supratentorial-infratentorial approach can be used in some occasions. In addition to generous exposure, the chosen approach must assure minimal retraction of the delicate cerebellum, brain stem, and cranial nerves.

Initially, the AVM should be surveyed to determine the pattern of venous drainage and to define a plane of cleavage. If the latter is present, it will be marked by a yellow pseudocapsule of gliotic tissue formed as a reaction to the AVM as well as by previous hemorrhage from the AVM. The feeding arteries enter the AVM through this gliotic cleavage plane and should be coagulated and divided at this point. A long, coagulated stump of these feeding arteries should be left on the normal side of the dissection. Several pairs of nonsticking bipolar cauterizing forceps should be available so that they can be quickly interchanged when one becomes soiled. Hemostasis of tiny and fragile feeders remains the most difficult part of the procedure and is particularly taxing when these vessels are in close proximity to the ventricle. Bleeding from these vessels is difficult to control, as they have very little tissue for coagulation to act on. Unfortunately, the bleeding from these vessels usually occurs at the end of the procedure, when the surgeon may be exhausted. The microclips designed by Sundt and Sugita are useful for controlling bleeding from these troublesome vessels.

Occasionally there is no readily evident cleavage plane. In these cases, especially in critical areas in the brain stem, dissection must be precisely on the AVM, relying on the belief that no normal brain lies in between the coils. Bleeding from the AVM itself can usually be controlled with cautery or, if persistent, with gentle pressure from a retractor or surgical cottonoid. In addition, bipolar cautery may be used to shrink the coils of the AVM and to help define the plane of cleavage.

Larger arteries that feed the AVM usually also have branches that supply the normal cerebellum and/or brain stem. Inadvertent occlusion of these vessels may lead to devastating brain stem infarction. Before any such vessel is occluded, one should ensure that all branches to be divided terminate in the malformation. Obviously, nearby normal vessels should be carefully protected.

Unlike their supratentorial counterparts, posterior fossa AVMs do not always have deep periventricular draining veins; therefore, care must be taken to preserve at least one major surface draining vein. Loss of adequate venous drainage will cause the AVM to become tense and friable and even to burst, and may cause massive, uncontrollable swelling of the cerebellum. If a draining vein is impeding the progress of the resection, the surgeon can temporarily occlude it with the bayonet forceps, watching for swelling of the AVM or cerebellum. If this occurs, the vein cannot be safely divided at that time.

An immediate postoperative CT scan is always obtained, both to provide a baseline and to check for a postoperative clot which may have collected during closure. If a significant clot is identified, immediate evacuation is performed. Also, if there is any doubt whether the AVM has been resected completely, immediate postoperative angiography is performed under the same anesthetic. If residual AVM is seen, the patient is returned to the operating room and the removal completed. We equate residual AVM with untreated AVM, as hemorrhage continues to be a risk. This risk of hemorrhage from AVM remnants is particularly great in the immediate hours and days following the first operation. Because high-quality angiographic definition is necessary to rule out remaining AVM, we have abandoned intraoperative angiography in these cases.

Results and Special Considerations by Site

Cerebellar Hemispheric AVMs

Of the 39 AVMs in our series that were confined to a single cerebellar hemisphere, 33 were excised through a suboccipital craniectomy or craniotomy. One grade 5 patient was treated with a ventriculostomy without exposure of the posterior fossa. Of the remaining five cases, all large AVMs, three were exposed transtentorially after elevation of the temporal or occipital lobe. Two of these were excised; the third was directly embolized through the feeding superior cerebellar artery after an associated basilar-superior cerebellar artery aneurysm was clipped. The decision to use the transtentorial approach was made in two of these cases because of an associated upper basilar artery aneurysm and in one case because of the anteromedial location of the AVM. This approach allowed access to the basilar artery and to the feeding arteries that arose from the superior cerebellar artery. In the fourth patient, whom we treated early in our series, the AVM involved essentially the entire cerebellar hemisphere and was approached from both above and below the tentorium; several feeding arteries were ligated. Not surprisingly, this intervention caused essentially no change in the size of the AVM, with other feeders rapidly enlarging to supply the shunt. The last of these five cases was treated solely with transfemoral embolization with Bucrylate. An initially excellent, near complete wipe-out was achieved; however, extensive recanalization has subsequently occurred, with at least one documented subarachnoid hemorrhage.

Postoperative hemorrhage occurred in three patients 6, 10, and 53 h after completion of the operation. Only in one was residual AVM thought to have been the cause of the hemorrhage. One of the patients harbored a diffuse type of AVM with fine, corkscrew-like feeding vessels, which we have come to realize carries a high risk of associated morbidity.[6,7,10] These unusual and innumerable feeding vessels are extremely fragile, tear easily, and are difficult to secure with coagulation. We believe that postoperative hemorrhage from these vessels is more likely to be due to technically inadequate hemostasis than to theoretical physiologic dysfunction such as "breakthrough bleeding."[21] Two of these three patients had poor outcomes, remaining in a locked-in state. The third has made a good recovery.

Even with what amounted to resection of half of the cerebellum, the posteroperative development or worsening of cerebellar dysfunction has been mild and usually transient (Fig. 243-5). This can only be accounted for by the displacement of the roof nuclei by the AVM, which has its beginnings early in embryologic development.

Vermian-Paramedian AVMs

The AVMs were located in the vermis or adjacent medial portion of the hemisphere in 33 patients in our series. Of these lesions, 28 were approached through a wide suboccipital craniectomy or craniotomy that exposed the midline from C1 to the torcular. In 27 of these patients, the AVM was completely excised; in one patient, the feeding posterior inferior cerebellar artery (PICA) was cannulated and the AVM directly embolized with Gelfoam.

Postoperative hemorrhage occurred in six of the patients who underwent surgical excision; it was attributed to residual AVM in three of them. Four of these six cases had been operated on in a sitting position. Adequate hemostasis in this position may be very difficult to ensure. The arterial pressure may be as much as 20 mmHg lower than that measured in the extremity, and venous pressure will usually be negative. Postoperatively, increases in arterial or venous pressures for whatever reason may result in disruption of the triply coagulated vessels. Reoperation for clot removal was required in six patients: One of these patients died, two remain in poor condition, and three are well.

The subtemporal-transtentorial approach was deemed necessary for six patients. In three, the AVM lay in the anteromediosuperior vermis or the paramedian region, and the nidus and its feeding arteries could be best controlled from this vantage point. Three subtemporal exposures of the interpeduncular fossa were performed to make it possible to clip associated upper basilar aneurysms. In one case, the AVM was later excised through a suboccipital craniectomy. In the second case, the feeding superior cerebellar artery was cannulated and the AVM directly embolized with Bucrylate. Postoperatively, the patient was left with a Weber's syndrome thought to be due to backfilling of the superior cerebellar artery with glue. This woman made a good recovery over

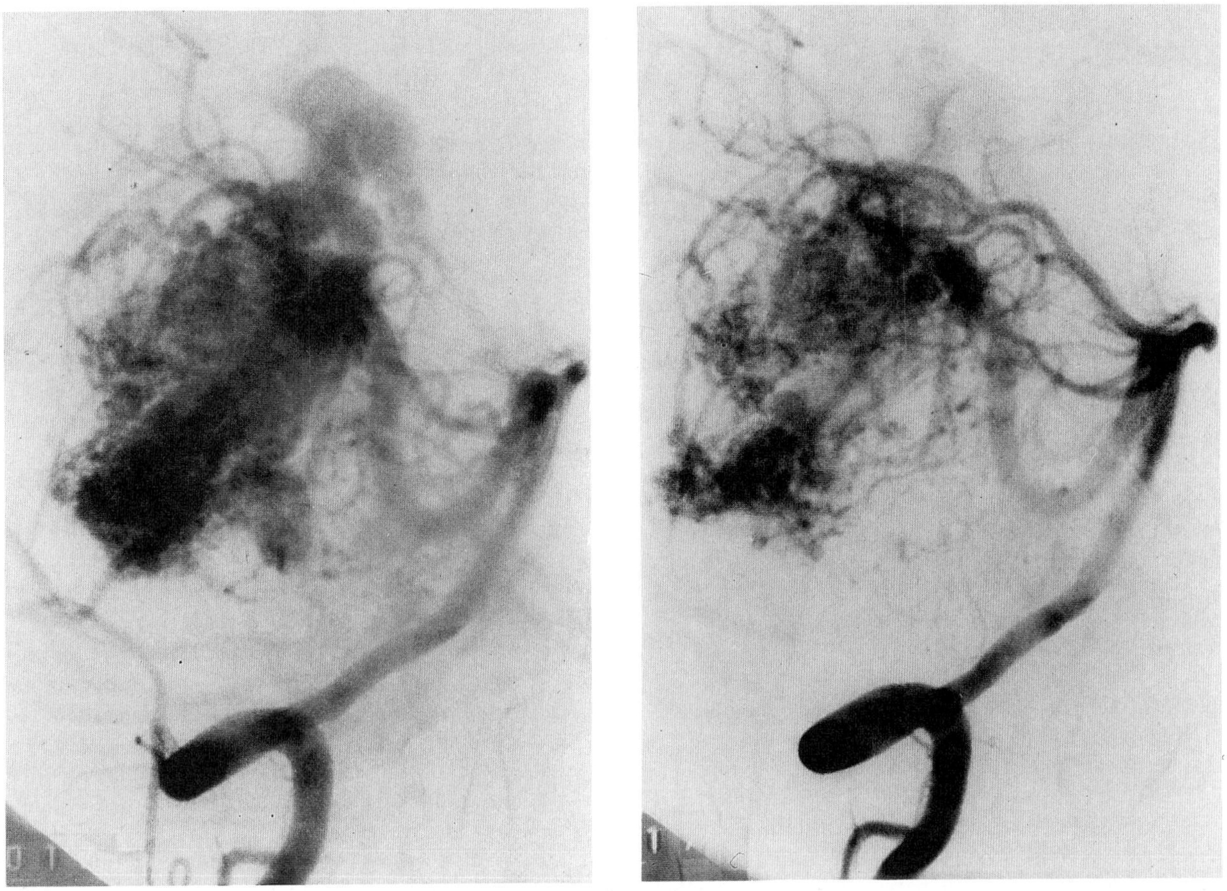

(*A*) (*B*)

Figure 243-5 Lateral vertebral angiograms before embolization (*A*), after the first embolization (*B*).

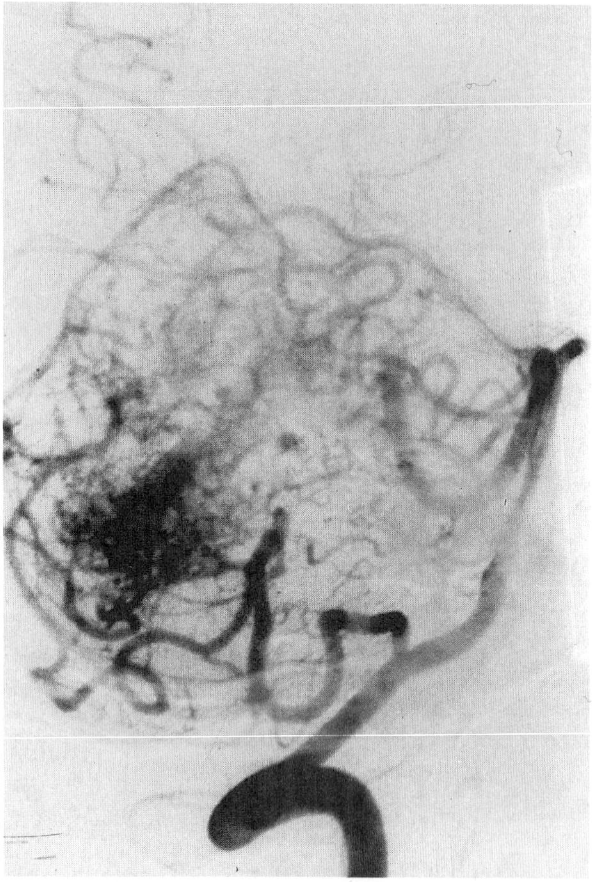

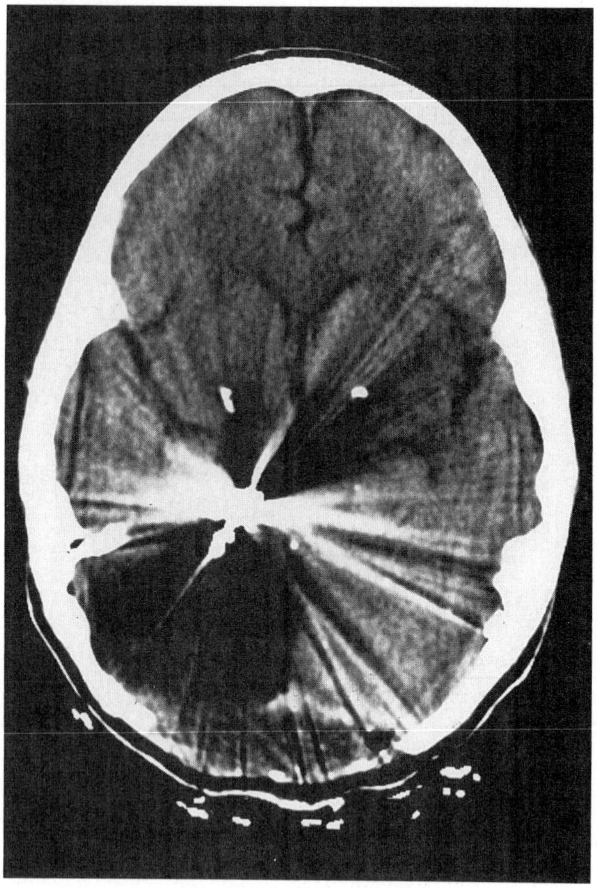

(*C*) (*D*)

Figure 243-5 (*Continued*) and after the second embolization (*C*) with Bucrylate. Note the large feeding right superior cerebellar artery and PICA. The AVM was subsequently resected completely. The surgeon thought that the preoperative embolization facilitated the removal. A postoperative CT scan (*D*) shows the extent of the cerebellar resection. The patient has been left with only very mild ipsilateral clumsiness. (The preoperative CT scan is shown in Fig. 243-1.)

several months. In one case, the subtemporal approach was used to explore the basilar bifurcation for a suspected aneurysm and to cannulate the superior cerebellar artery for direct Bucrylate embolization of the ruptured AVM. Postoperatively, 90 percent of the AVM was occluded; however, the patient developed a dense thalamic infarction from which he has made a poor recovery. Bucrylate could be seen filling the posterior medial choroidal arteries. An unusual and unrecognized anastomotic channel between the superior cerebellar artery and the posterior cerebral artery would seem to have been the cause of this tragedy.

Flocculonodular AVMs

With involvement of the flocculonodular lobe and the closely adjacent ninth, tenth, and eleventh cranial nerves, one must be concerned that resections in this area could lead to significant postoperative deficits in gait, eye movements, and lower cranial nerve function. In the eight patients in our series whom we treated for an AVM in this location—in all cases via a suboccipital craniectomy—the coils of the AVM could be separated readily from the lower cranial nerves, and postoperative dysfunction of gait or eye movements was mild and generally resolved with time. The AVMs in these patients were closely related to the foramen of Luschka, which was better visualized after splitting the inferior medullary velum on the involved side, permitting inspection of the floor of the fourth ventricle. A wide lateral bony exposure is necessary to gain proximal control of the vertebral artery and PICA and to permit precise identification and protection of both the cranial nerves and the arterial branches to the brain stem. The surgeon must make sure that each arterial branch is actually an AVM feeder before coagulating and dividing it. As a group, these patients have done well.

Fourth Ventricular AVMs

Only one patient in our series had an AVM that was confined to the fourth ventricle. Most of the feeding vessels arose from the tela choroidea and the choroid plexus. The lesion did not invade the floor of the ventricle, and the coils of the AVM could be gently dissected away and completely removed. The patient recovered with no neurological deficit.

Cerebellopontine Angle AVMs

Drake has described and characterized AVMs of the cerebellopontine angle, initially in 1975[5] and more recently in 1986.[7] Although these AVMs were initially considered unresectable, it was discovered that most of their bulk is actually located superficial to the pia of the pons and medulla and does not invade the brain stem, and that those AVMs that do invade the brain stem do so only minimally. We have often found that the coils of the AVM are intimately related to the trigeminal nerve, and, in fact, in several cases, they were embedded and passed between the fascicles of the nerve. In these cases, we divided the vessels on either side of the nerve, leaving short empty coils within the nerve in order to avoid extensive dissection and neural injury. However, it was generally been difficult to preserve hearing, because of dissection on the delicate eighth nerve.

These lesions may be approached either subtemporally through the tentorium, suboccipitally, or by a combination of approaches. The AVMs that lie higher up in the angle are best approached transtentorially. A transtentorial exposure is also used for associated upper basilar artery aneurysms.

Surgical morbidity and mortality in the 16 patients in our series who harbored this type of AVM was solely due to postoperative hemorrhage. Three such hemorrhages occurred, resulting in the deaths of two patients and a poor outcome for the third. In one case, the site of the hemorrhage was somewhat distant from the site of surgery and probably represented bleeding from a residual nidus of AVM. Technical difficulties in securing an arterial feeder passing through the foramen of Luschka were likely the cause of a postoperative hematoma in another. Since our experience with that case, we have routinely divided the inferior medullary velum to ensure adequate exposure of this area.

Brain Stem AVMs

We have treated 19 patients who harbored AVMs limited to the brain stem. These patients have proved to be the most difficult of all of our patients to treat and have had the least satisfactory outcomes. Four were simply explored, and the AVM was found not to be accessible to any surgical maneuver. One early patient in this group presented with a ruptured aneurysm of the anterior inferior cerebellar artery (AICA), which was successfully clipped, but unfortunately the patient died abruptly in the postoperative period from hemorrhage from a previously intact pontine AVM. Three patients presented with an intra-axial clot, and a cryptic AVM was found at operation. All were in a poor condition preoperatively, but two patients with pontomedullary clots have gone on to make good recoveries. One of these patients, who underwent clot evacuation and resection of a medullary cryptic AVM (Fig. 243-6), was quadriparetic and required ventilatory assistance preoperatively; the patient is presently walking and working and is able to swim. Feeder ligation was used in three patients in a desperate attempt to decrease the flow to essentially unresectable AVMs, although we have generally not found this intervention to be of any proven or lasting benefit. Three AVMs were located in the quadrigeminal cistern with involvement of the quadrigeminal plate. We were able to resect two of these AVMs with excellent outcomes, even with dissection through the midbrain tectum and into the posterior third ventricle. The third patient, whose associated incidental basilar bifurcation aneurysm was exposed subtemporally and easily clipped, died when bleeding occurred intraoperatively from a hidden, inaccessible part of the AVM.

Clearly, dissection in the brain stem is difficult and potentially very hazardous. In two patients, dissection was carried out within the pontomesencephalic region to disconcerting depths following bleeding coils of the AVM. Neither patient awoke from surgery, and both eventually succumbed. Postmortem examination revealed extensive hemorrhage through the pons and medulla.

Two patients with brain stem AVMs were treated with embolization. After clipping of an AICA aneurysm in one, an associated

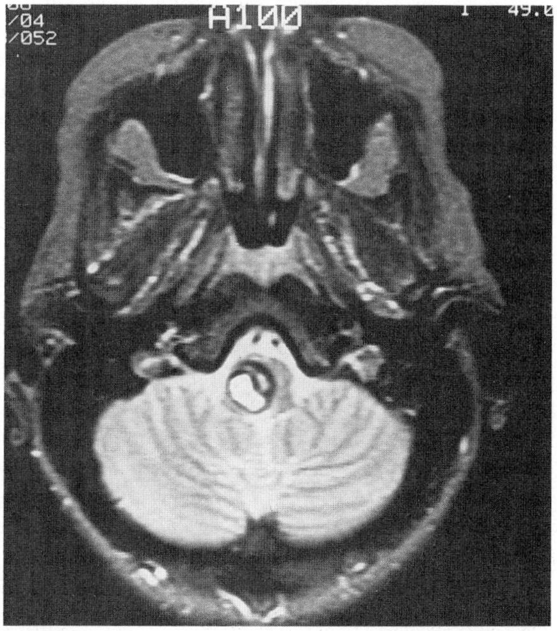

(*A*)

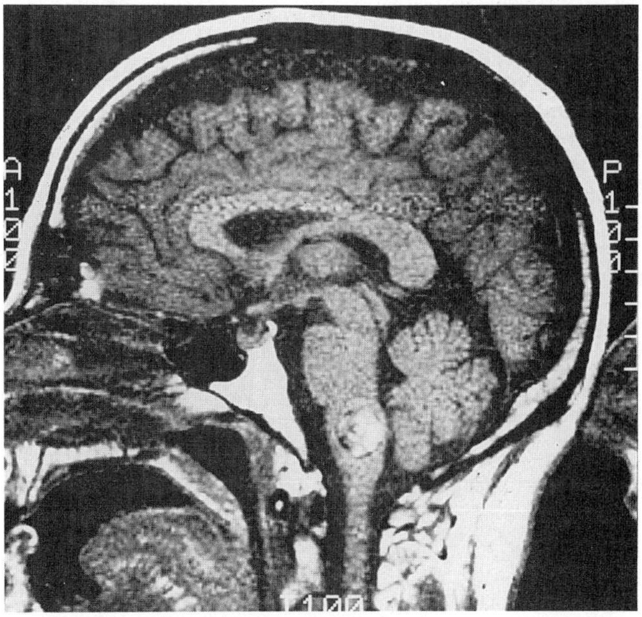

(*B*)

Figure 243-6 Axial (*A*) (TR = 2000 ms, TE = 70 ms) and sagittal (*B*) (TR = 500 ms, TE = 20 ms) MR images of a patient from whom a medullary clot and cryptic AVM were subsequently resected. These preoperative MR images beautifully demonstrate the location of the hematoma. The areas of lower signal intensity represent older hemorrhage (hemosiderin) and more recent hemorrhage (methemoglobin) corresponding to her stepwise neurological decline.

pontomedullary AVM was directly injected with Gelfoam after cannulation of the feeding PICA; 65 percent obliteration of the AVM was achieved and the patient did well. In another patient, a huge cerebellar hemisphere pontomesencephalic AVM was embolized with less than 10 percent of the malformation occluded. Unfortunately, this indirect procedure also caused worsening of the patient's neurological status, without protecting him from at least two further hemorrhages (Fig. 243-4).

Because of these difficulties experienced in attempted resections of AVMs within the brain stem, we now approach the management decisions of these lesions very cautiously. Without the presence of an associated hematoma to provide a surgical plane of cleavage, these AVMs (which now can be precisely placed in the brain stem by MRI) are generally not thought to be amenable to surgical resection. It would seem that patients presenting with medullary hematomas may represent a favorable subgroup in which clot evacuation and AVM removal may result in surprising recovery of function. Otherwise, we have been very cautious about recommending surgery for a brain stem AVM, but have several examples of complete angiographic obliteration of these AVMs following both conventional and focused cobalt therapy and believe the latter therapies may be ideally suited for these lesions.

TABLE 243-6 Posterior Fossa AVMs: Results by Treatment (Authors' Series)

Treatment	Totals	Results			
		Excellent	Good	Poor (Worse)*	Dead
Excision	97	54	25	11 (5)	7
Removal of clot and cryptic AVM	4	1	1	1 (0)	1
Feeding vessel ligation	3	1	1	1 (0)	0
Exploration only	4	2	0	1 (0)	1†
Ventriculostomy	1	0	0	0 (0)	1
Embolization only					
Direct	5	0	4	1 (1)	0
Transfemoral	2	0	1	1 (1)	0
Totals	116	58	32	16	10‡
		78%		22%	

* Worsened by treatment.
† Previously intact AVM ruptured postoperatively.
‡ Three deaths in poor-grade patients.

Results and Conclusions

Ours is a cumulative series, and the results reported here span three decades. The earlier cases were operated on before the advent of the operative microscope and modern neurosurgical techniques or contemporary neuroradiologic imaging. As improvements in surgical instrumentation, neuroanesthesia, and imaging have become available, the surgical results have improved. These improved results also certainly reflect the knowledge gained from our surgical experience.

The results of treatment in our series as a function of the site of the AVM are shown in Table 243-5. We define an excellent outcome as normal neurological function. Patients who are functioning at their premorbid level but may have minor residual deficits are classified as having a good outcome. A patient with residual neurological deficits that prevent return to premorbid function is defined as having a poor outcome; most of these patients remain dependent. As one might expect, the highest mortality and serious morbidity (47 percent) has occurred in patients with brain stem AVMs and, to a lesser degree, in patients harboring AVMs of the cerebellopontine angle (25 percent).

TABLE 243-5 Posterior Fossa AVMs: Results by Site, All Grades (Authors' Series)

Site	Totals	Results			
		Excellent	Good	Poor	Dead
Hemispheric	39	22	12	3	2
Vermian-paramedian	33	18	7	6	2
Cerebellopontine angle	16	6	6	2	2
Flocculonodular	8	5	3	0	0
Fourth ventricle	1	1	0	0	0
Midbrain	11	4	1	4	2
Pontomedullary	8	2	3	1	2
Totals	116	58	32	16	10
		78%		22%	

Table 243-6 summarizes outcome in relation to type of treatment for our series. We believe that only complete excision of the malformation is effective in changing the natural history of these lesions. The risks of surgical excision therefore need to be carefully weighed against the known natural history of AVMs and the patient's age. Crawford et al. followed 217 nonoperated patients, most with supratentorial AVMs, and found that 20 years after diagnosis, 27 percent were neurologically worse and a further 29 percent were dead.[4] Many authors have suggested that patients with infratentorial AVMs have a less favorable prognosis, but, because of the small numbers studied, this idea has not been adequately documented.[1,13–15,18,24]

The causes for the surgical morbidity and mortality in our series are listed in Table 243-7. Postoperative hemorrhage remains the primary cause of both poor outcome and death in patients who were of a good grade preoperatively. Similarly, Yaşargil had a 9 percent incidence of postoperative clots in his series of 68 patients operated on for posterior fossa AVMs.[24] Residual AVM was known to have resulted in postoperative hemorrhage in four of these patients and was the suspected cause in two others. In the remaining patients, this devastating complication was likely due to inadequate hemostasis and a marked afterload effect of high pressure on small, poorly secured feeding vessels. Although normal perfusion pressure breakthrough bleeding may have occurred, we

TABLE 243-7 Posterior Fossa AVMs: Surgical Morbidity and Mortality (Authors' Series)

Reason for Morbidity or Mortality	Outcome	
	Poor	Dead
Postoperative hemorrhage	5	5
Neurological worsening after embolization	2	0
Intraoperative hemorrhage	0	1
Postoperative rupture of previously intact AVM	0	1
Total	7	7

TABLE 243-8 Posterior Fossa AVMs: Results by Preoperative Neurological Grade (Authors' Series)

		Results			
Preoperative Grade	**Totals**	**Excellent**	**Good**	**Poor**	**Dead**
Good	96	56	27	6	7
		86%		14%	
Poor	20	2	5	10	3
		35%		65%	
Totals	116	58	32	16	10
		78%		22%	

do not favor this theory,[21] but rather look to technical failures as a cause of postoperative clots. It is of interest to note that we have not experienced a postoperative clot of significance in any patient who has successfully undergone preoperative embolization. Moreover, since the nonstick bipolar forceps and immediate postoperative angiography came into routine use 10 years ago, we have had no postoperative hematomas. When the results are grouped as to preoperative grade (Table 243-8), it can be seen that postoperative morbidity and mortality increases dramatically from 14 percent in good grade patients to 65 percent for patients in a poor preoperative grade.

AVMs of the posterior fossa pose unique problems. Hemorrhage from these AVMs within the confined space of the posterior fossa commonly results in death or significant and life-threatening neurological deficits. However, the decision to attack these lesions surgically is not to be taken lightly. AVMs over 5 cm in diameter represent a much greater technical challenge and a greater perioperative risk. Similarly, AVMs involving the pons, medulla, and midbrain may defy safe removal by any currently available surgical technique. We are also very cautious in recommending surgical removal of diffuse, small-vessel malformations, where effective permanent sealing of feeding or malformation vessels is more difficult and may be impossible with cautery or clips. A detailed appreciation of the anatomy and the relationships of the malformation and adjacent structures is imperative because operative injury to roof nuclei, peduncles, or cranial nerves is almost always associated with tragedy. Nevertheless, in our experience, it has been remarkable how little deficit is associated with removal of lone, large AVMs in the vermis, hemisphere, or flocculonodular lobe, reinforcing the notion that critical neural structures are displaced by the abnormal vessels.

For each patient, one should consider not only operative microsurgical extirpation of the malformation, but also the possibility of preoperative embolization for small lesions or focused gamma irradiation in relation to the AVM's location, history of previous hemorrhages, and the patient's age and current disability. The algorithm in Table 243-9—which depicts an annual hemorrhage rate of 4 percent per year, including a 1 percent mortality and 1.7 percent morbidity rate and a 1.3 percent rate of recovery without deficit after hemorrhage—allows the patient and the referring physician to grasp the risks of living with an AVM for a year or a decade. A more conservative estimate of risk of bleeding of 2 percent per year, with half of the patients returning to normal function and only 1 percent dead or disabled, strengthens the case for "leaving the AVM alone" and treating only the symptoms. Many more cases have been reviewed and rejected for any therapy than have been operated on.

TABLE 243-9 Natural History of AVMs*

Year x	Well		
	Well	Stroke	Dead
Year $x + 1$	98.0%	1.7%	1.0%
Year $x + 10$	73.0%	17.0%	10.0%

*Accruing 4 percent per year hemorrhage rate.

References

1. Batjer H, Samson D. Arteriovenous malformation of the posterior fossa: clinical presentation, diagnostic evaluation, and surgical treatment. *J Neurosurg* 1986; 64:849–856.
2. Chou SN, Erickson DL, Ortiz-Suarez HJ. Surgical treatment of vascular lesions in the brain stem. *J Neurosurg* 1975; 42:23–31.
3. Ciminello VJ, Sachs E Jr. Arteriovenous malformations of the posterior fossa. *J Neurosurg* 1962; 19:602–604.
4. Crawford PM, West CR, Chadwick DW, et al. Arteriovenous malformations of the brain: natural history in unoperated patients. *J Neurol Neurosurg Psychiatry* 1986; 49:1–10.
5. Drake CG. Surgical removal of arteriovenous malformations from the brain stem and cerebellopontine angle. *J Neurosurg* 1975; 43:661–670.
6. Drake CG. Cerebral arteriovenous malformations: considerations for and experience with surgical treatment in 166 cases. *Clin Neurosurg* 1979; 26:145–208.
7. Drake CG, Friedman AH, Peerless SJ. Posterior fossa arteriovenous malformations. *J Neurosurg* 1986; 64:1–10.
8. Girvin JP, Fox AJ, Vinuela F, et al. Intraoperative embolization of cerebral arteriovenous malformations in the awake patient. *Clin Neurosurg* 1984; 31:188–247.
9. Green JR, Vaughan RJ. Blood vessel tumors and hematomas of the posterior fossa in adolescence. *Angiology* 1972; 23:474–487.
10. Hernesniemi J, Keränen T. Microsurgical treatment of arteriovenous malformations of the brain in a defined population. *Surg Neurol* 1990; 33:384–390.
11. Leblanc R, Levesque M, Comair Y, et al. Magnetic resonance imaging of cerebral arteriovenous malformations. *Neurosurgery* 1987; 21:15–20.
12. Logue V, Moncton G. Posterior fossa angiomas. *Brain* 1954; 77:252–273.
13. Martin NA, Stein BM, Wilson CB. Arteriovenous malformations of the posterior fossa. In Wilson CB, Stein BM (eds): *Intracranial Arteriovenous Malformations.* Baltimore: Williams & Wilkins, 1984, pp 209–221.
14. Matsumura H, Makita Y, Someda K, et al. Arteriovenous malformations in the posterior fossa. *J Neurosurg* 1977; 47:50–56.
15. McCormick WF, Hardman JM, Boutler TR. Vascular malformations ("angiomas") of the brain, with special reference to those occurring in the posterior fossa. *J Neurosurg* 1968; 28:241–251.
16. McFerran DJ, Marks PV, Garvan NJ. Angiographically occult arteriovenous malformations of the brainstem. *Surg Neurol* 1987; 28:221–224.
17. Ondra SL, Troupp H, George ED, et al. The natural history of symptomatic arteriovenous malformations of the brain: a 24-year follow-up assessment. *J Neurosurg* 1990; 73:387–391.
18. Perret G, Nishioka H. Report on the Cooperative Study of Intracranial Aneurysms and Subarachnoid Hemorrhage. Section VI. Arteriovenous

malformations: an analysis of 545 cases of cranio-cerebral arteriovenous malformations and fistulae reported to the Cooperative Study. *J Neurosurg* 1966; 25:467–490.
19. Poppen JL. Vascular surgery of the posterior fossa. *Clin Neurosurg* 1959; 6:198--210.
20. Silber MH, Sandok BA, Earnest F IV. Vascular malformations of the posterior fossa: clinical and radiologic features. *Arch Neurol* 1987; 44:965–969.
21. Spetzler RF, Wilson CB, Weinstein P, et al. Normal perfusion pressure breakthrough theory. *Clin Neurosurg* 1978; 25:651–672.
22. Stahl SM, Johnson KP, Malamud N. The clinical and pathological spectrum of brain-stem vascular malformations: long-term course simulates multiple sclerosis. *Arch Neurol* 1980; 37:25–29.
23. Verbiest H. Arteriovenous aneurysms of the posterior fossa, analysis of six cases. *Acta Neurochir (Wien)* 1961; 9:171–195.
24. Yaşargil MG. *Microneurosurgery,* vol IIIB. New York: Thieme, 1988, pp 169–203, 358–366.

244

Vein of Galen Malformations

A. Loren Amacher

Aneurysmal malformations of the vein of Galen (VGAMs) are rare. Their absolute incidence is unknown, but they may be detectable in 10 to 12 per 100,000 living fetuses past the gestational age of 26 weeks.[3,11,16] Nevertheless, these lesions have important, frequently dramatic, clinical consequences. They tend to present in stereotyped patterns that depend on the age of the patient.[2] Most often the victim is very young, a neonate or infant, and the clinical features are those of actual or potential hemodynamic decompensation frequently coupled with ventriculomegaly. Terms such as ''spectacular'' or ''intimidating'' often are used to describe their radiologic and hemodynamic characteristics. Anyone who undertakes the obliteration of such a lesion, by whatever means, must approach the experience with some trepidation.

Anatomy and Embryology

During the past decade, a significant literature has accumulated relating to the arterial and venous anatomy of the galenic vicinity. The vein of Galen (VG) lies in the sagittal plane just within and then behind the transverse cerebral fissure, a choroidal and extraparenchymal space. It is formed by the confluence of several deep veins, including the internal cerebral, posterior thalamic, superior cerebellar, and basal veins (of Rosenthal). It lies a few millimeters above the pineal gland. After a short upward traverse of 10 to 20 mm, the VG penetrates the junction of the falx and tentorium, uniting with the inferior sagittal sinus to form the straight sinus. In its course, it sweeps around the posteroinferior aspect of the splenium of the corpus callosum.

Raybaud, Strother, and Hald[13] have collated and summarized relevant embryologic data with their own extensive survey of the vascular anatomy, normal and pathologic, of the quadrigeminal region. The vascular anomalies that give rise to VG fistulas and malformations arise during the 6th to 11th weeks of embryonic development, within the primitive vascular rete of choroidal origin, pial arteries, and overlying arachnoidal venous channels. The principal drainage channel of the region at this juncture is the median prosencephalic vein of Markowski. Early on, this vein does not communicate with the deep internal cerebral veins, apparently becoming confluent with them as its distal part regresses at about the 11th week. This rather arcane observation probably explains why sudden occlusion of a VG fistula usually does not cause catastrophic venous backpressure throughout the deep median cerebral drainage. It seems that ''primary'' VG malformations[2]—the VGAMs of Lasjaunias[6]—are not vein of Galen lesions in the strict sense, a distinction that may seem obscure but which has considerable power is explaining the venous drainage anomalies that so frequently accompany these lesions. Primitive venous outflow patterns from a VGAM may persist in the case of most VGAMs,[5,12,13] including persistence or reduplication of falcine sinuses and reduplication or absence of the straight sinus. The normal venous outflow from median telencephalic and diencephalic structures is often reversed into sphenopalatine and cavernous sinuses.

Appreciation of the embryologic anatomy and time of formation of VG fistulas has helped to clarify the vascular patterns seen, particularly in neonates.[13] The vascular matrix so frequently seen in very young patients, usually lying anteroinferior to the sac, probably represents perimesencephalic choroidal vessels that have persisted and are, in fact, an integral part of the fistula, on which their continued existence depends. Indeed, recognition of this fact has made understandable the success of transtorcular techniques in some of the neonatal cases that formerly were not treatable with any measure of success.

Other elements of vascular supply include the nearby arteries of posterior choroidal and posterior and anterior cerebral origin as well as occasional, persisting long branches of the middle cerebral and superior cerebellar arteries. An anterior choroidal supply is common only in neonates, as is contribution from lenticulostriate arteries. The thalamoperforating vessels may be drawn into supplying the fistula by a siphon effect. VGAMs do have a meningeal supply at times, and small feeders may run in the sac walls for some distance; both of these features are understandable from the embryogenesis of the lesion.

Classification

It is still worthwhile to think of VGAMs as being either primary or secondary, where these classes are defined as follows.

1. *Primary VGAM.* The arteries that feed directly into the sac of the aneurysm usually are huge, and through them most of the blood carried by the main-stem vessel may be diverted to the fistula. In cases that are symptomatic at birth, there may also be a myriad of small feeder vessels anteroinferiorly (see above). Occlusion of all arterial input to the fistula will obliterate the shunt and allow for collapse of the aneurysm. Excision of the sac is unnecessary. These lesions are the vein of Galen arteriovenous malformations (VGAMs) of Lasjaunias' nomenclature.[6]
2. *Secondary VGAM.* The dilated galenic system serves as the venous outflow for an adjacent (very occasionally remote) angioma. Usually, the angioma is situated in the medial posterior hemispheres, the superior cerebellum, the brain stem, or the deep ganglionic structures. Often, the inferior sagittal and straight sinuses are greatly dilated as well. With these lesions, the principles of angioma excision apply. The angioma must be obliterated; if the venous outflow from the lesion is occluded but the arterial component left intact, disaster will result. These lesions are referred to by Lasjaunias as vein of Galen aneurysmal dilatations (VGADs).[6]

Figures 244-1 through 244-4 show the radiological (VGADs) characteristics of VGAMs and VGADs by computed tomography (CT), angiography, magnetic resonance imaging (MRI), and magnetic resonance angiography (MRA). This chapter is concerned only with primary lesions.

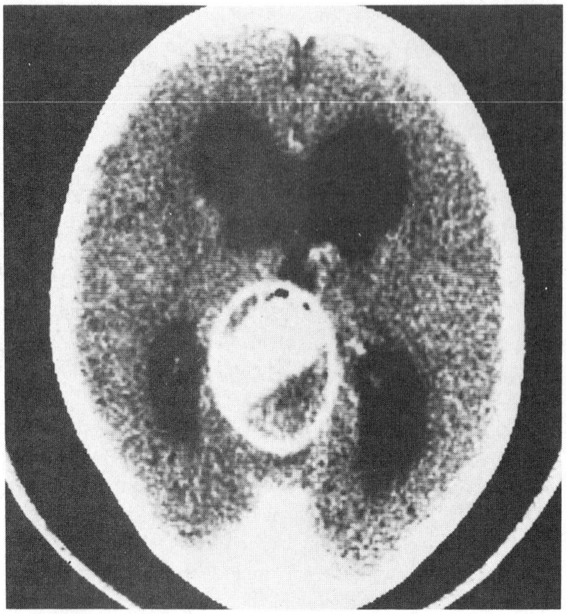

(*A*)

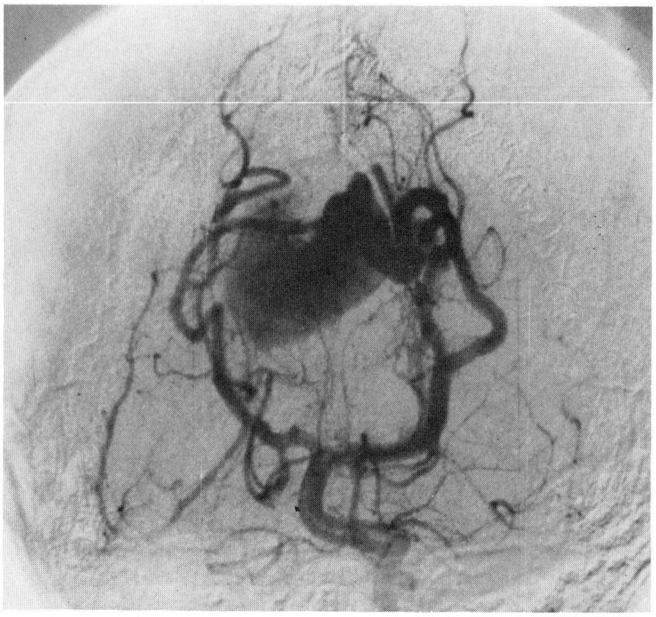

(*B*)

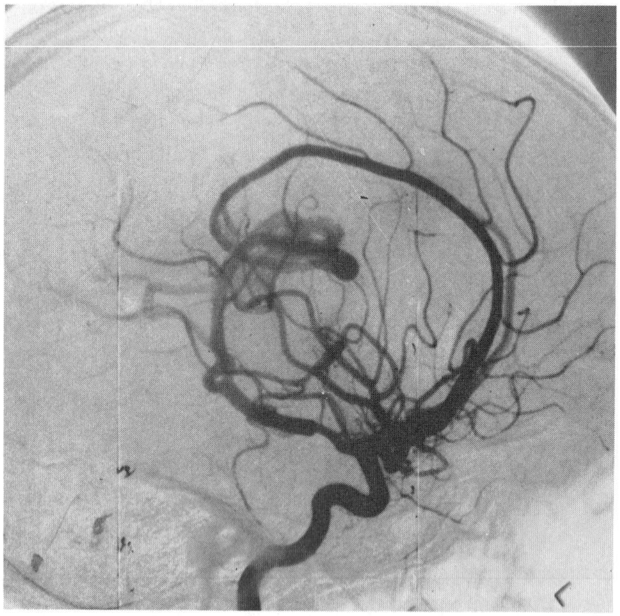

(*C*)

Figure 244-1 A partially thrombosed VGAM. *A*. CT appearance. *B*. Towne's projection from an angiogram. Note the very large left posterior cerebral artery with three fistulous connections to the vein of Galen. The right posterior cerebral artery also feeds directly into the vein. *C*. A lateral view from a carotid angiogram showing the sites of fistulous connection.

Clinical and Diagnostic Features

The clinical syndromes associated with primary vein of Galen aneurysmal malformations fall neatly into four groupings (Table 244-1), corresponding to the age of the patient at presentation.[2]

Neonatal Group

Almost universally, the children in this group present at or shortly after birth with overwhelming high-output, preload heart failure. As much as 80 to 90 percent of the infant's cardiac output may pass through the galenic fistula. Emergency investigation of such a child will show high jugular venous oxygen tension, and an angiogram or CT or MR images will reveal the aneurysm. Most commonly, there are numerous small feeders into the anterior and inferior aspects of the sac. There is usually a loud cranial bruit of virtually constant intensity. CT or MR scanning with or without contrast is diagnostic. Ultrasonic pulsed Doppler echoes are also very specific.[14] Continuous (rather than pulsatile) internal jugular blood flow is noted, along with an echo-free shadow in the region of the vein of Galen, in which the flow characteristics are similar to those of the internal jugular vein.

Operative attacks on these aneurysms in the face of intractable heart failure have been of little avail. The children die

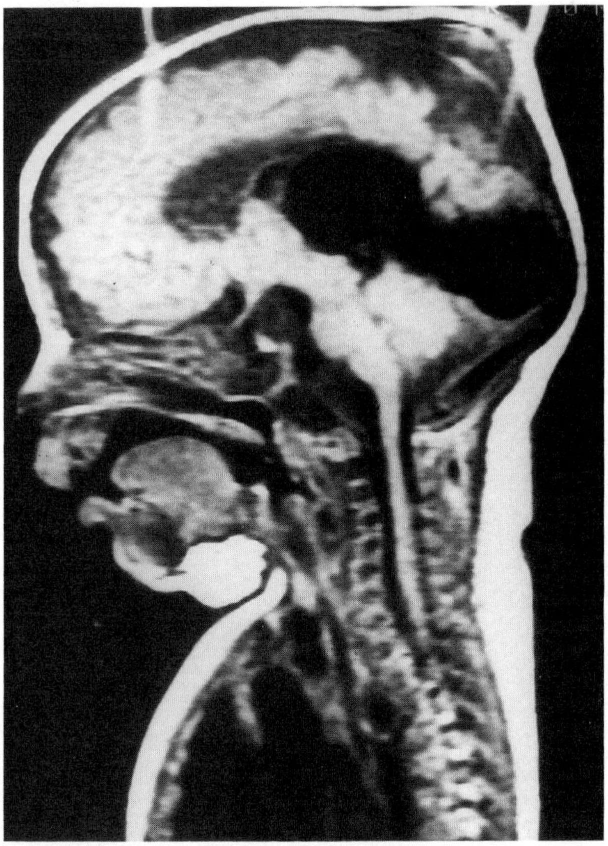

Figure 244-2 Sagittal MR image showing the typical appearance of a VGAM, symptomatic, in a 9-day-old infant, without MRI or MRA evidence of a major anteroinferior vascular network.

postoperatively of heart failure in spite of rigorous cardiac care, even including drastic reduction of circulating blood volume. Occlusion of the cervical carotid arteries has not helped. Myocardial infarction often occurs as a result of the low cardiac perfusion, which is aggravated by any intraoperative hypotension.[4]

Norman and Becker described the postmortem condition of the brain in seven neonates with this lesion.[10] Severe brain damage was seen in all, whether or not an operative procedure had been attempted. Neuropathologic findings included periventricular leukomalacia, deep parenchymal hemorrhages, numerous very small feeders to the sac, cortical gliosis and subcortical cavitation, and cortical infarction and calcification. As mechanisms of cerebral damage, they proposed arterial steal, ischemia secondary to heart failure, hemorrhagic infarction, compression atrophy, and operative trauma. They concluded that operative correction of the fistula in the neonate was futile, an opinion supported by the case reported by Sivakoff and Nouri.[14] This neonate survived operation for 10 months in a vegetative state, and an autopsy showed neuropathologic findings comparable with those mentioned above. Nevertheless, direct surgical attack on a neonatal VGAM has been carried out successfully on at least one occasion.[9]

Figure 244-5 demonstrates a neonatal VGAM scenario in which cerebral ischemia has been so severe as to produce a tiny, gliotic brain within a normal calvaria. Any therapy in such a situation is futile.

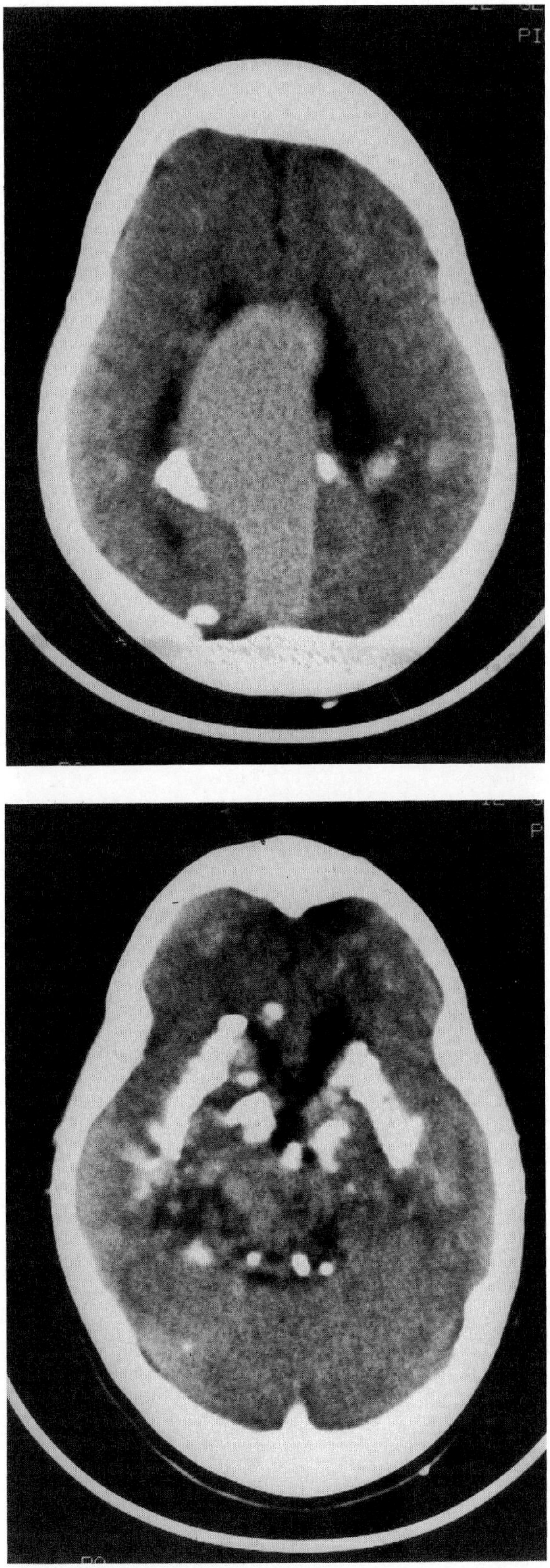

Figure 244-3 CT scans of a huge and uncontrolled high-flow VGAM (*upper scan*). Note the basal ganglia and thalamic calcifications, thought to be secondary to chronic ischemia (*lower scan*).

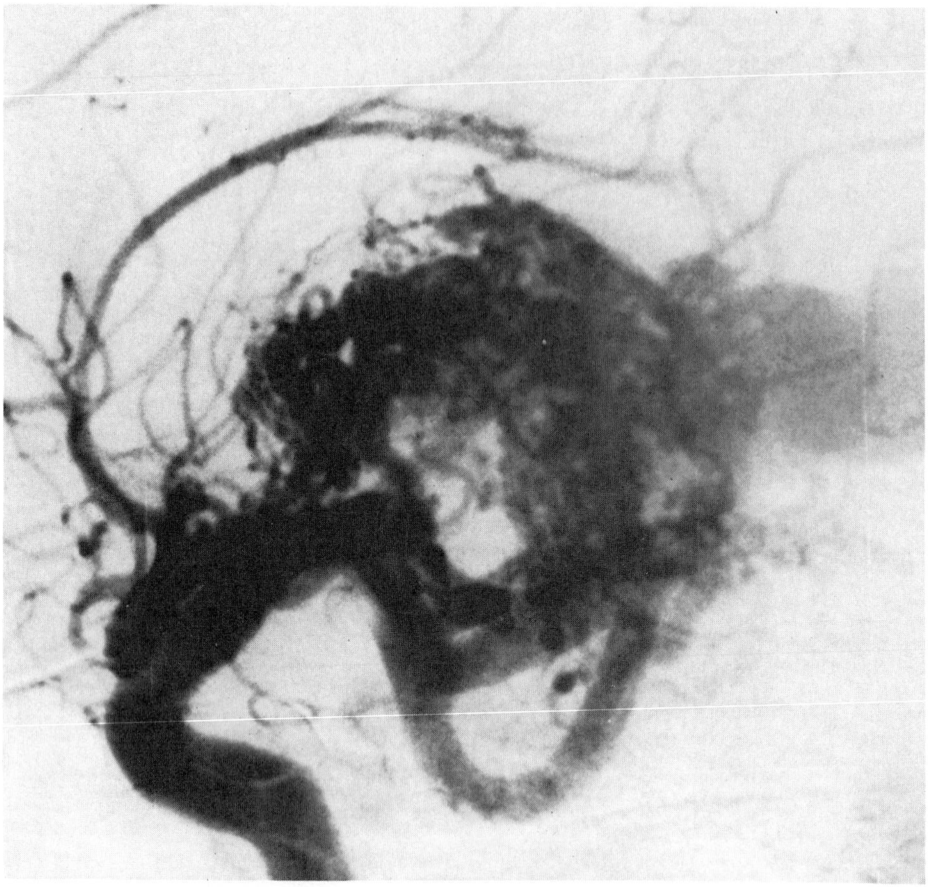

Figure 244-4 Lateral carotid angiogram, showing a VGAD draining a bilateral thalamic angioma.

Infantile Group

Two patterns are seen in this clinical grouping.

1. The child may have had mild cardiac decompensation neonatally, the condition settling down spontaneously or with treatment; later (usually at 1 to 12 months of age) the patient is found to have craniomegaly because of hydrocephalus. There is generally a loud bruit, which is audible over the entire head but is heard best posterolaterally. A CT scan will be diagnostic.
2. The patient has craniomegaly, and the cause of the hydrocephalus is discovered by CT scanning. The chest film frequently shows cardiomegaly. There is no history of cardiac decompensation.

TABLE 244-1. Clinical Groupings of Primary Vein of Galen Aneurysmal Malformations

Group	Presentation	Prognosis
Neonatal	Extreme high-output cardiac failure, usually lethal	Open procedure dangerous; transfusion embolization may save up to 50%
Infantile	Borderline cardiac status, early mild CHF, hydrocephalus	Careful preoperative assessment required; often need CSF shunt; may do well
Childhood	Hydrocephalus, +/− cardiomegaly, occasional SAH; pineal mass, occasional ring/bar calcification	Depends on degree of hydrocephalus
Mature	Headache, pineal mass, calcification, SAH, hydrocephalus	Good

Abbreviations: CHF, congestive heart failure; SAH, subarachnoid hemorrhage.

Very occasionally, the sac is discovered as a pineal-area ring calcification on a plain x-ray film of the skull. The aneurysm may not fill at angiography because of complete thrombosis[7] (unusual in a young child), or it may show the angiographic ''target'' sign if the periphery of the sac is thrombosed. In this situation, the calcified rim of the aneurysm is separated from the contrast ''bull's eye'' by clot—hence, the target appearance. Usually, the entire sac fills with contrast, often demonstrating the entering jets of contrast and the turbulent currents within.

The ventriculomegaly is usually pronounced, involving the lateral and third ventricles. The implications of this fact are discussed under Treatment, below.

Childhood Group

Most cases discovered past the age of 2 years have come to light during the investigation of craniomegaly. Some of these patients have presented with subarachnoid hemorrhage. There may be mild cardiomegaly as well. Cranial bruits are usually present. It must be pointed out, however, that flow bruits are commonly heard in normal infants and children with auscultation of the skull or ocular globes. These physiologic bruits are clearly identifiable as flow

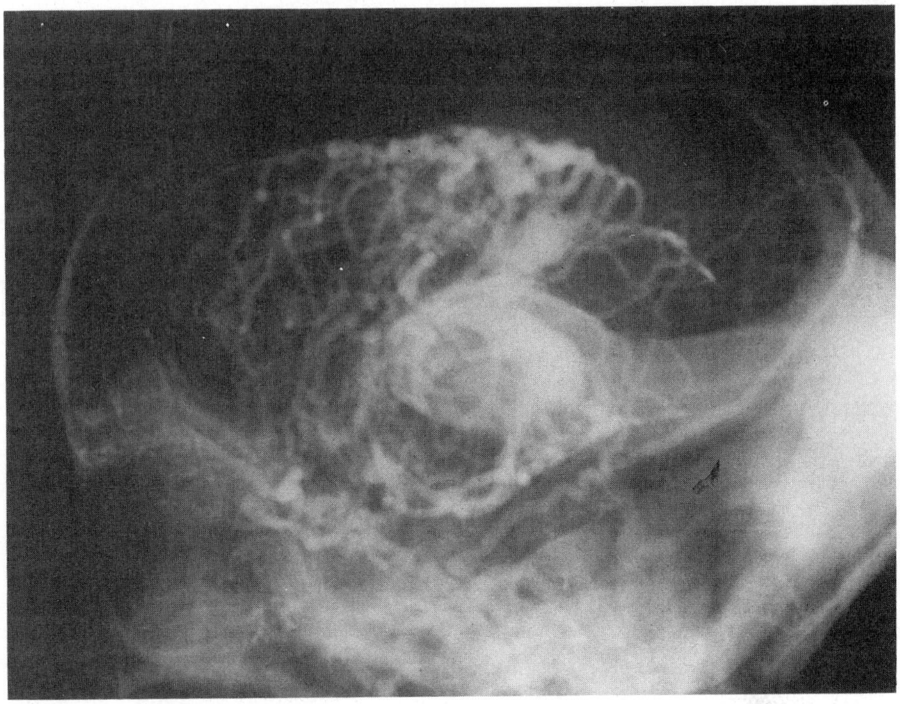

Figure 244-5 Lateral carotid angiogram, showing severe cerebral/calvarial size discrepancy and a high-flow VGAM.

phenomena by their maximum systolic intensity over the eyes and temples, as well as by their tendency to go away with minimal pressure over the cervical carotid arteries. In the child, the bruit associated with a vein of Galen aneurysm may be no more intense than a physiologic bruit, but it is heard best at the parietal apex or near the midline posteriorly. In the neonate and infant, the bruit usually is much louder, and it tends to run into diastole or may be virtually continuous.

Mature Group

In later childhood, adolescence, or young adulthood, these aneurysms present in a variety of ways: as subarachnoid hemorrhage, as a pineal area mass, as headaches usually associated with raised intracranial pressure, as a rim calcification near the pineal region, as syncopal attacks resembling those encountered occasionally with colloid cysts of the third ventricle, or as hydrocephalus. CT or MR scanning and angiography are diagnostic.

Treatment

In recent years, endovascular techniques of enviable precision and sophistication have been perfected.[6,12] Both transarterial and transvenous procedures are now frequently used to treat VGAMs. This development is mainly a great relief to the sensible surgeon, but there are reasons and opportunities still for direct, open surgical attack.[1] The remainder of this chapter will deal only with open operation.

The surgeon who takes on the obliteration of a vein of Galen aneurysm must do so with full awareness of the hazards involved. In general, the younger the child, the more risky the procedure. The problems to be considered and anticipated involve cardiac hemodynamics, hydrocephalus, operative blood loss, and aftercare.

Cardiac Hemodynamics

Even if no history of early cardiac decompensation is forthcoming, it is wise to have the infant or child assessed by a cardiologist. Of great importance is an accurate calculation of preoperative blood volume. Infants with a large fistula into the vein of Galen may have a greatly expanded blood volume in response to a very high cardiac output. Sudden occlusion of the fistula, with the resulting significant increase in peripheral vascular resistance, may precipitate disastrous intraoperative heart failure. The sudden increase in peripheral vascular resistance produces an afterload for which the myocardium cannot compensate. This, combined with the preload factor of a pathologically large blood volume, induces severe cardiac failure. Immediate reduction of blood volume, even coupled with inotropic stimulation of the myocardium, may not correct the problem. Precise and intensive cardiac monitoring is essential,[8] both intraoperatively and postoperatively. Swan-Ganz catheterization preoperatively is advisable when there is concern that central pressures may rise significantly during surgery.

Management of Hydrocephalus

The aneurysm sac produces hydrocephalus by compression of the midbrain and occlusion of the aqueduct, at least in part. It is reasonable to hope that release of the compression produced by the tense, distended aneurysm may allow reopening of the aqueduct, thereby curing the hydrocephalus. Several reported cases support this possibility, but in a significant number of patients, subsequent shunting will be necessary. This fact strongly suggests that the hydrocephalus is caused in a significant number of patients by hydrodynamic forces relating to venous hypertension.[17]

Although drainage of large ventricles at the time of craniotomy does facilitate a deep midline exposure, the collapse of a thin cerebral mantle is almost certain to lead to subdural fluid accumulation in the early postoperative period. For this reason, precraniotomy shunting of grossly distended ventricles is advisable. One should not wait until the ventricles have returned to normal, however, before getting on with the attack on the aneurysm. Doing so will simply make the exposure of the sac more difficult than need be.

Operative Blood Loss

Except in the young infant, operative blood loss should not be a problem. Children with VGAMs have an expanded blood volume to begin with, and some volume reduction may be beneficial for a heart on the verge of preload failure. The aneurysm sac is tough and resilient; it will not burst unless handled roughly. Intentional hypotension to a mean of 40 to 50 mmHg during dissection of the sac helps reduce sac tension and increases the surgeon's sense of security, but where myocardial ischemia is a risk, hypotension must be eschewed.

Aftercare

The need for careful cardiac monitoring has been stated. Seizures may occur, particularly if the cerebral mantle has sustained injury because it has sagged away from the skull. Persistent subdural effusions may require drainage, and unresolving hydrocephalus must be dealt with.

Surgical Technique

The consensus is that a posterior interhemispheric exposure of the aneurysm is best. The occipital approach along the falx is usually unencumbered, especially if the ventricles are drained of some volume. Magnified vision is essential. Transcallosal approaches are recommended for anteriorly placed fistulas.

The head should be positioned to facilitate exposure and provide a comfortable posture for the surgeon. In infants, the supine position with the head in neutral position or turned 45 degrees to either side is usually satisfactory. In older patients, the park-bench position has advantages, particularly for microscope placement. The semi-sitting position with the head flexed forward has the advantage of presenting the anatomy in a familiar manner but may allow collapse of the cerebral hemisphere if the ventricles are large. It is essential to use an exposure that is familiar to the surgeon, lest the three-dimensional anatomy of the region become confused. The subtentorial approach is disadvantageous because the major feeders into the sac will be unnecessarily remote from the point of first contact with the aneurysm, at least in the older infant and child.

Usual measures relating to pressure points and prevention of excessive hypothermia are taken. The bone flap should be generous, right to the midline, and placed over the posterior parietal and anterior occipital lobes. Bioccipital flaps will be favored by some surgeons but have not been necessary in my experience. Retraction of the occipital pole usually is not necessary.

With the operating microscope and self-retaining retractors, exposure down the falx is gentle and easy. Seldom is there extensive scarring in the vicinity of the sac, though arachnoid bands are encountered. These should be coagulated and divided; it is unlikely that they will contain feeder vessels of small caliber, except in neonates or very young infants.

Figure 244-6 shows the typical appearance of a sac and an entering artery. The feeders should be divided between clips far enough from the sac to allow the stumps to serve as handles for rotating the lesion. The arteries should be doubly secured proximally. By gently rolling the sac upward, feeders inferiorly are brought into view. This process is repeated until all communications on one side have been divided.

Depending on the size of the sac, the opposite-side feeders may be brought into view by rotating the aneurysm or by cutting a superiorly based flap in the falx to help in the visualization of those arteries. The latter maneuver is necessary only with a very large sac.

During this process, the anesthesiologist must keep a vigilant watch on the cardiac status, especially in young infants. Signs of incipient heart failure must be dealt with immediately and vigorously, by means including pharmacologic cardiac support, reduction of peripheral vascular resistance, and withdrawal of blood. In some situations, it may be safest to desist from further fistula reduction and to plan to resume the procedure in a few days when cardiac hemodynamics have stabilized. A two-stage procedure is preferable to a dead child. Alternatively, once the cardiac status appears to have stabilized, the surgeon may occlude the next visible feeder by a temporary clip; if cardiac stability persists, this feeder may be divided.

Upon completion of fistula closure, the sac will be soft, largely collapsed, and darker in color. Now, a needle may be introduced to collapse the sac further and to determine the oxygen tension of the blood in the sac. If all feeders have been divided, there is no need

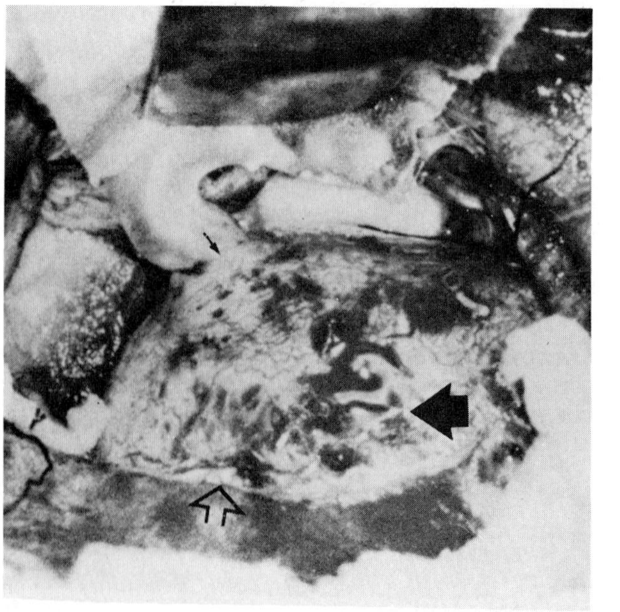

Figure 244-6 Operative photograph of a vein of Galen aneurysm. The small arrow indicates the site of an arterial fistula. The large dark arrow is on the aneurysm. The open arrow indicates the edge of the falx. The occipital lobe is behind the retractor at the top. (From Amacher and Shillito,[2] with permission.)

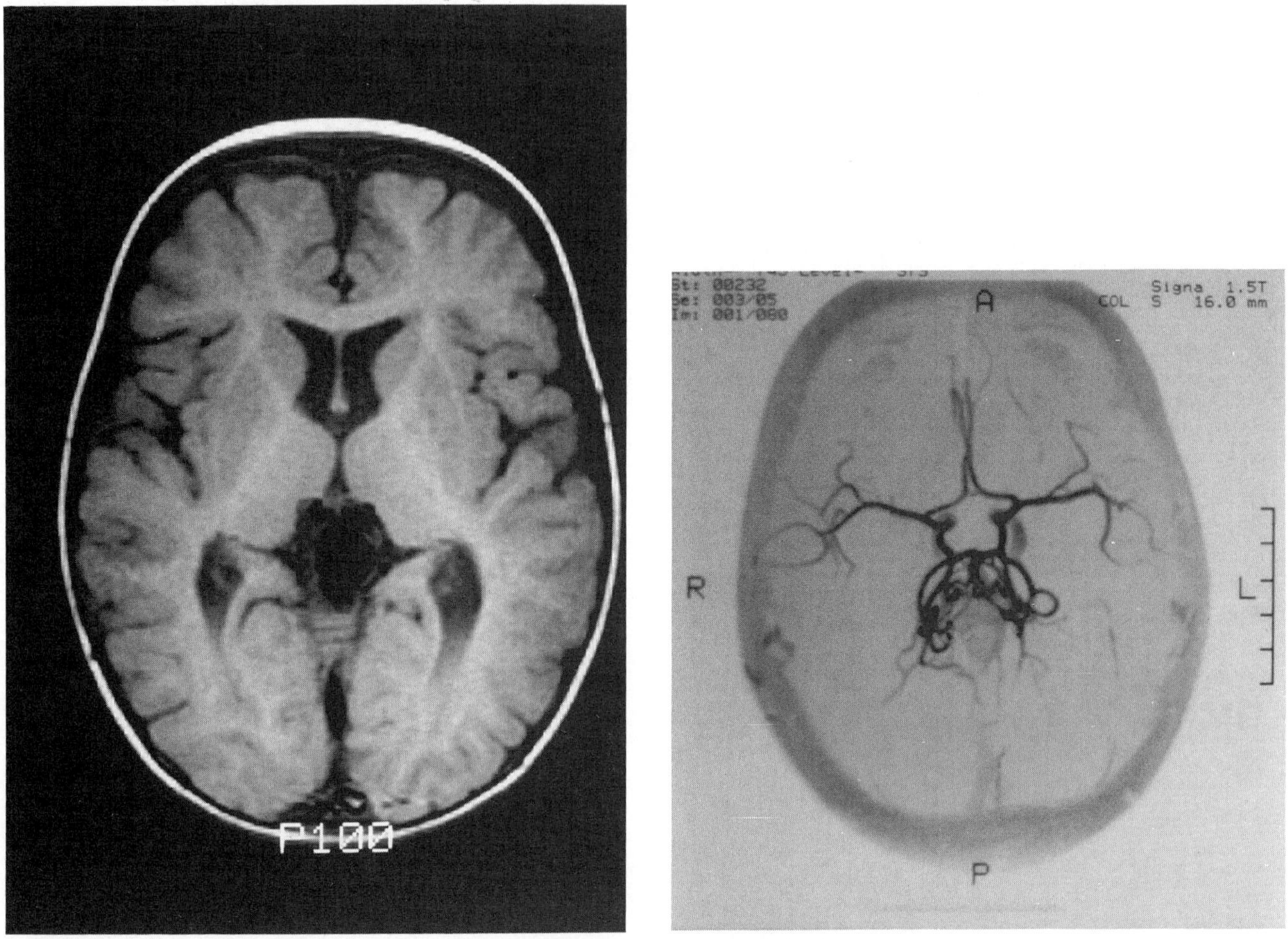

Figure 244-7 Axial MR image (*left*) and basal angiogram (*right*) of a VGAM that has remained stable clinically and radiologically for more than 3 years. The child remains normal.

to excise the aneurysm; however, if the sac wall is rigid with calcification or if the lesion is largely or totally thrombosed, partial or total excision for reduction of mass effect is reasonable.[15] There is no excuse for damaging the walls of the posterior hypothalamus and thalamus while attempting a total removal of one of these aneurysms.

If very large ventricles have been drained, they should be reexpanded with a physiologic solution at core temperature before the bone flap is secured. Even so, subdural effusions are likely to occur.

Postoperative angiography is necessary to confirm total closure of the fistula. Very small residual feeders may be watched for a time, as they are likely to disappear.[1]

In small children, the cardiac vigil must be maintained well into the recovery period. Of premier importance is the control of fluid and blood volumes. The surgeon must realize that these patients are at great risk intraoperatively and postoperatively. It is better to leave the fistula alone than to approach it with a cavalier attitude.

Prognosis

In recent years, the somber prognosis accompanying any form of treatment of this lesion[2] has been upgraded to one of cautious optimism. To a large extent, endovascular techniques deserve the credit for this welcome change. Even so, the treatment mortality for neonates probably will continue to exceed 50 percent, and a sober appraisal of outcomes for infants and children will acknowledge that many survivors are not, in fact, undamaged. In any event, the points of emphasis mentioned throughout this chapter must be observed if good outcomes are to be obtained.

1. For primary vein of Galen aneurysmal malformations, the fistula must be obliterated, though not necessarily in one session. Indeed, some evidence is accumulating that an occasional child may tolerate a VGAM of small size and stable flow characteristics without harm. Figure 244-7 shows the VGAM of a girl, now 4 years old, whose lesion remains unchanged since its discovery 3 years ago; the child continues to develop normally.
2. For secondary dilations of the galenic system that are caused by venous outflow from an adjacent angioma, the angioma must be the surgeon's target. The expanded galenic veins will collapse once the primary lesion is removed.
3. Strict attention to cardiac status and hemodynamics is critical during and after surgery. Intractable heart failure is the worst threat facing the child.
4. Proper control of hydrocephalus is necessary to optimize the patient's future.

References

1. Amacher AL. Vein of Galen malformations: an ongoing conundrum. *Crit Rev Neurosurg* 1993; 3:295–300.
2. Amacher AL, Shillito J Jr. The syndromes and surgical treatment of aneurysms of the great vein of Galen. *J Neurosurg* 1973; 39:89–98.
3. Comstock CH, Kirk JS. Arteriovenous malformations: locations and evolution in the fetal brain. *J Ultrasound Med* 1991; 10:361–365.
4. Hoffman HJ, Chuang S, Hendrick EB, Humphreys RP. Aneurysms of the vein of Galen. *J Neurosurg* 1982; 57:316–322.
5. Lasjaunias P, Garcia-Monaco R, Rodesch G, Terbrugge K. Deep venous drainage in great cerebral vein (vein of Galen) absence and malformations. *Neuroradiology* 1991; 33:234–238.
6. Lasjaunias P, Garcia-Monaco R, Rodesch G, et al. Vein of Galen malformation: endovascular management of 43 cases. *Child's Nerv Syst* 1991; 7:360–367.
7. Lazar ML. Vein of Galen aneurysm: successful excision of a completely thrombosed aneurysm in an infant. *Surg Neurol* 1974; 2:22–24.
8. Long DM, Seljeskog EL, Chou SN, French LA. Giant arteriovenous malformations of infancy and childhood. *J Neurosurg* 1974; 40:304–312.
9. Matjasko J, Robinson W, Eudaily D. Successful surgical and anesthetic management of vein of Galen aneurysm in a neonate in congestive heart failure. *Neurosurgery* 1988; 22:908–910.
10. Norman MG, Becker LE. Cerebral damage in neonates resulting from arteriovenous malformation of the vein of Galen. *J Neurol Neurosurg Psychiatry* 1974; 37:252–258.
11. Ordorica SA, Marks F, Frieden FJ, et al. Aneurysms of the vein of Galen: a new cause for Ballantyne syndrome. *Am J Obstet Gynecol* 1990; 162:1166–1167.
12. Quisling RG, Mickle JP. Venous pressure measurements in vein of Galen aneurysms. *Am J Neuroradiol* 1989; 10:411–417.
13. Raybaud CA, Strother CM, Hald JK. Aneurysms of the vein of Galen: embryonic considerations and anatomical features relating to the pathogenesis of the malformation. *Neuroradiology* 1989; 31:109–128.
14. Sivakoff M, Nouri S. Diagnosis of vein of Galen arteriovenous malformation by two-dimensional ultrasound and pulsed Doppler method. *Pediatrics* 1982; 69:84–86.
15. Smith DR, Donat JF. Giant arteriovenous malformation of the vein of Galen: total surgical removal. *Neurosurgery* 1981; 8:378–381.
16. Worswick L, Lamont RF, Thomas R, Gordon H. Prenatal ultrasonographic diagnosis of an aneurysm of the vein of Galen. *Br J Radiol* 1992; 65:609–610.
17. Zerah M, Garcia-Monaco R, Rodesch G, et al. Hydrodynamics in vein of Galen malformations. *Child's Nerv Syst* 1992; 8:111–117.

245 Vein of Galen Malformations: Transvenous Occlusive Therapy

J. Parker Mickle
Ronald G. Quisling

The central, high-flow arteriovenous malformations known as vein of Galen malformations have well-defined clinical presentations that are age-dependent.[1] The anatomic substrate for these clinical states exists early in development and involves the primitive circulation of the choroid plexus. Direct arterial connections into the vein of Galen result in a high-flow malformation of the type I variety. The number of arterial feeders in this situation may be limited, and this shunt lends itself to direct surgical extirpation. Type II malformations result when a complex arterial-to-venous malformation drains secondarily into the vein of Galen. These malformations involve the area around the midbrain, and some of them may lie within neural structures. This dangerous type of lesion is not easily approached surgically, and total removal is seldom accomplished.

The basic principle in arteriovenous malformation surgery has always been to interrupt the arterial feeders as close to the nidus as possible as the first step in eliminating the shunt. Certainly, acute venous outlet obstruction in these lesions carries a great potential for catastrophic hemorrhage. However, even in the more common brain angiomas, multiple venous outlets exist, and one can often use one or several of these outlets as handles for the stepwise removal of the angiomatous nidus.[7] By virtue of their deep central location adjacent to and within vital structures, vein of Galen malformations do not lend themselves to standard microneurosurgical techniques for their removal.

Because of this central location, the poor prognosis of untreated malformations, and the general poor results of standard surgical techniques, interventional endovascular manipulations have become attractive as an alternative way of approaching these lesions.[2] Again, the general principle has been to approach the lesions transarterially with various embolic materials, including glues, particulate embolization materials such as silk suture material, and balloons. The elegant efforts in this area are promising, and the techniques are usually used in conjunction with standard surgical procedures to eliminate some of these lesions.

The general concept of transvenous therapy for vein of Galen malformations arose because of the excellent results achieved in the treatment of high-flow carotid-cavernous fistulae by transvenous wire deposition.[11] Also, a case report presented at a neurosurgical meeting described the complete resolution of a vein of Galen malformation after the direct deposition of phosphor-bronze wire into the vein of Galen itself.[6] The important concepts for the transvenous approach to these high-flow fistulous states include the following[8–10].

1. Thrombogenic wires deposited in the vein of Galen aneurysm should accomplish a graded thrombosis or reduction in flow such that acute venous outlet obstruction does not occur.
2. In certain situations (the neonate in heart failure), the initial goal is to increase resistance in the high-flow, low-resistance system so that cardiac survival is encouraged.
3. Staged procedures and multiple embolizations may be required, depending on the clinical needs of the patient.
4. Other approaches (standard surgical approaches, transarterial embolization, stereotactic radiosurgery, etc.) may be required to totally eliminate some of these malformations.

These historical successes and the generally poor outcome for these unfortunate patients with standard surgical techniques led to our interest in the transvenous therapy for vein of Galen malformations. Our initial efforts are summarized below.

Indications, Contraindications, and Patient Selection

The prognosis of the patient with an untreated vein of Galen malformation is poor.[4] Generally, the neonate with high-output cardiac failure and the older child and young adult with subarachnoid hemorrhage from these lesions have very poor prognoses no matter which therapeutic modality is selected. The infant with a large head secondary to hydrocephalus or the asymptomatic patient with a bruit has a much better prognosis with standard surgical techniques. However, as evidenced by the high mortality even in this group, the surgeon should approach these lesions as a major technical challenge.

Over the past 8 years, we have had the opportunity to treat 24 patients with vein of Galen malformations. We have elected to treat all of them with the transvenous occlusive technique. Two patients whose high-flow fistulae were "asymptomatic" were at first followed expectantly. However, both of these patients became symptomatic and required therapy. As we and others have seen, some neonates with central high-flow fistulous states and heart failure have a major degree of structural damage to the brain. This damage usually can be seen on the initial computed tomographic scan as encephalomalacia and parenchymal calcification. The presence of such injury may be a relative contraindication to aggressive therapy of any form for this disease. However, there are patients who present even in the neonatal period with massive heart failure who have good neural development and have the potential for being competitive and educable.

Surgical Procedure

The advantages of the transtorcular approach to vein of Galen malformations are that it is technically simple and quick and is performed with commonly available materials (Fig. 245-1). We have elected to do all of these procedures initially in the operating room

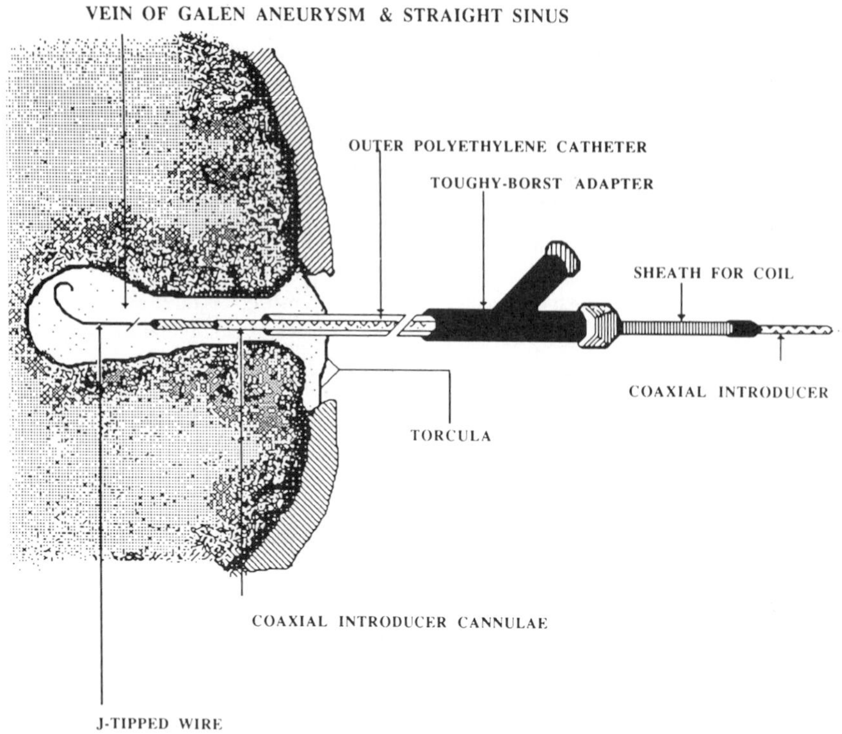

(*A*)

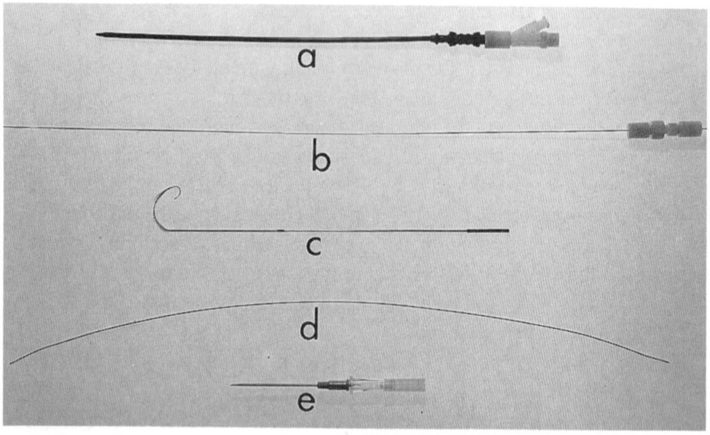

(*B*)

Figure 245-1 *A.* This semidiagram shows the surgical approach and equipment in situ for transvenous deposition of thrombogenic wires in a vein of Galen aneurysm. *B.* The basic pieces of equipment needed for the transtorcular approach to vein of Galen malformations are: *a,* a standard angiography catheter with a Toughy-Borst adapter; *b,* an optional introducer and tethering device for the initial wire deposition; *c,* a Gianturco sheath with a partially extruded coil (Cook, Inc., Bloomington, IN); *d,* a soft-ended guide wire; and *e,* a 16-gauge Angiocath.

through a small craniectomy over the capacious torcular. The aneurysm typically drains through a dilated straight sinus, but it may drain via alternate venous routes, because venous anomalies in this situation are common.[12]

The patient is positioned on the operating table or incubator with the head turned full laterally. If hydrocephalus exists before treatment, we recommend placing a ventriculoperitoneal shunt at this initial embolization.The lateral angiogram demonstrates the general location of the dilated torcular, but it is important to have an anteroposterior view of the torcular because its most dilated portion is often off the midline. It is also very important to have fluoroscopic capability during the operation. Furthermore, ultrasonography is useful in locating the torcular, the straight sinus, and the aneurysm after craniectomy.[3]

The craniectomy is easily accomplished with a small rongeur, and bleeding is minimal. The tense, red torcular is tapped with a standard 25-gauge needle, and a small amount of contrast material is injected under fluoroscopic observation. This assures identification of the torcular and its relationship to the straight sinus. A 16-gauge Angiocath (IV catheter placement unit; Deseret Medical, Inc., Sandy, UT) is then introduced through the 25-gauge needle puncture site, and the polyethylene sheath is advanced to the orifice of the straight sinus. Brisk bleeding through the Angiocath is encountered at this stage but is quickly controlled by the introduction of a standard soft-ended, straight guide wire, which under fluoroscopic control is advanced through the Angiocath into the vein of Galen aneurysm. The wire is fixed, and the Angiocath is removed under fluoroscopic control. Again, brisk bleeding occurs around the wire, but it is minimized with a tamponading finger fixing the wire in its length. A standard short angiography catheter is then advanced over the guide wire through the dural rent of the torcular and into the straight sinus and the aneurysm. All the while, the position of the guide wire is maintained stationary with fluoroscopic control. The guide wire is removed, and venography is performed through a Toughy-Borst connector via the indwelling catheter to confirm the position of the catheter tip in the middle of the aneurysm.

This catheter is easily advanced in and out of the aneurysm and straight sinus during the procedure as wire depositions dictate. Flow characteristics within the aneurysm are easily defined, and permanent records of them are made with small injections of a contrast agent during the embolization. Pressures within the aneurysm and straight sinus can be measured accurately, and the percent oxygen saturation of the blood can be measured at intervals. We now deposit a 90 to 145 cm demandreled Teflon-coated guide wire in the aneurysm. This tightly coiled mass acts as a retarding lattice, onto which coils, balloons, or bits of silk thread can be deposited (Fig. 245-2). Various sizes of standard Gianturco wire coils are deposited into the aneurysm through the indwelling catheter. We have developed a tethering introducer set which has allowed us to retrieve malpositioned coils during the embolization. At present, we use the tethering system only with the initial wire deposition, because malplacement subsequently is extremely rare with the use of the guide-wire basket described above.

Our therapeutic goal has been to reduce the intra-aneurysmal pressure to about one-half its initial value. In the neonate in severe heart failure, the pressure in the partially occluded aneurysm may actually increase owing to improved cardiac contractility after embolization. This usually is accomplished with multiple coil depositions (4 to 12) and has usually resulted in a substantial change in the flow characteristics as seen by fluoroscopic venography. The neurosurgeon and neuroradiologist work together very closely during the deposition of these wires to assure optimal localization. In the neonate, the clinical status will help dictate the end point of the embolization. Usually in this situation, the deposition of wires is accompanied by immediate improvement in the patient's blood pressure, arterial blood status, urinary output, and acidosis. In this situation, however, the improvement is short-lived, and repeat embolizations are required hours to days later.

At the termination of the procedure, the angiography catheter is removed and a tamponading finger is used to control the bleeding through the puncture site. A small piece of Gelfoam (absorbable gelatin sponge; The Upjohn Company, Kalamazoo, MI) may be used to encourage this control, but no dural sutures are required. The skin is closed in a standard fashion, and the patient recovers in the intensive care unit or the neonatal unit.

In the neonate, repeat embolization is required, and rarely does one embolization cure the malformation or assure survival. The repeat procedures can be done in the neuroradiology suite because access to the torcular, straight sinus, and aneurysm is easily accomplished through a transcutaneous approach.

This procedure is done under general anesthesia. The deposition of thrombogenic occluding wires in the vein of Galen malformation transvenously takes 30 min to 1 h, and so far no children have required transfusion as a result of the procedure.

Potential Hazards and Complications

The greatest potential hazard in this approach to vein of Galen malformations is acute thrombosis of the venous outlet with the potential for venous thrombosis and hemorrhage in and around the midbrain and thalamus. This potential risk is greatest in individuals with high pressure in the aneurysm and low flow as demonstrated by venography. We have seen this complication in one patient, in whom it resulted in a venous infarct in the right thalamus. This patient was treated aggressively with deep pentobarbital coma and survived. The small venous infarct was clearly demonstrable on CT scan, and no hemorrhage was seen.

Potentially, the thin venous sac and tenuous venous structures on the anterior and inferior portion of the aneurysm are at risk of being ruptured by misdirected wires at the time of deposition. This complication happened once early in our series.

If too small or too tightly coiled a wire is used, there is a chance of peripheral embolization. This complication has occurred in several of our patients without apparent effect. Usually the wires lodge at the junction of the lateral and sigmoid sinuses. There is a

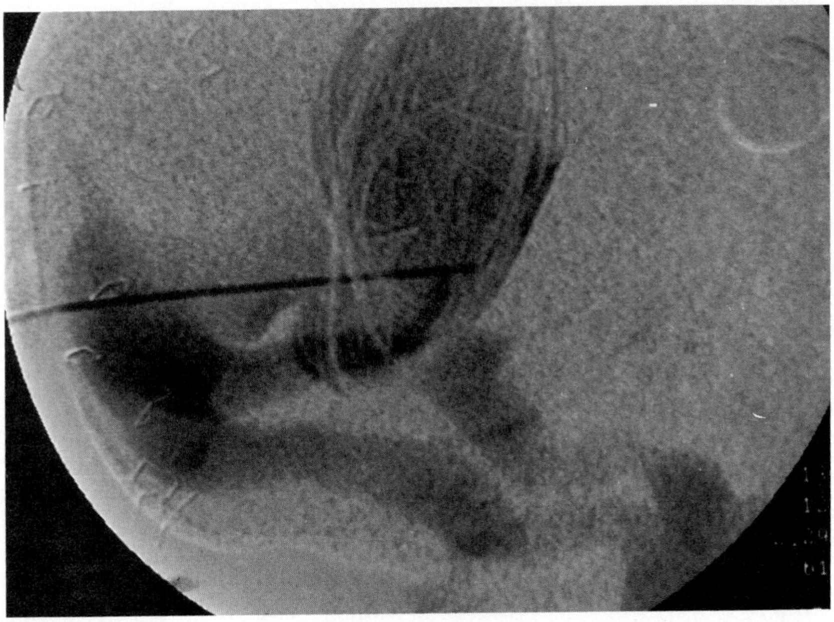

Figure 245-2 This lateral transtorcular venogram shows a wire basket in a vein of Galen aneurysm prior to the deposition of thrombogenic coils. This partially occluding lattice reduces the likelihood of inadvertent dislodgement of embolic coils or balloons.

potential for pulmonary embolization, but we have not observed it in our series of cases. We now reduce the possibility of this complication by introducing the wire lattice described above.

In patients with partially treated fistulae, the potential for injury to intravascular components such as platelets and red blood cells would appear to be real; however, no studies have been done to confirm or refute this idea. The long-term effects of indwelling stainless steel wires coated with Dacron (E.I du Pont de Nemours & Co., Wilmington, DE) in the deep midline structures of the brain are not known. Also, of major concern in this procedure is the potential of establishing as the major venous outlet of the deep structures of the brain the subependymal venous system and the potential risk of later hemorrhage from these structures.

Results

At this point in the evolution of the transtorcular approach to vein of Galen malformations, we are able to summarize our data for 24 patients.[8] We treated 10 of these patients with a single embolization and the remaining 14 with staged procedures. The number of wires inserted per patient ranged between 1 and 16, with a mean of 4.

Six patients, all neonates, died despite transtorcular embolotherapy: four of refractory heart failure and one of an acute subdural hematoma following attempted ventriculostomy for acute hydrocephalus. At postmortem examination, the vein of Galen straight sinus complex appeared to be completely thrombosed in all five of these patients. One patient died of massive hemorrhage caused by perforation of the aneurysm with a wire.

The 18 surviving patients have been followed for an average of 20 months, with a range of 7 to 72 months. Follow-up imaging studies have demonstrated a reduction of cerebral vessel size, a reduction in collateral venous drainage, and no progressive brain calcification. At this point, there have been four variations in treatment outcome in the survival group:

1. A single embolization with complete thrombosis of the malformation (Fig. 245-3).
2. Staged embolization resulting in complete thrombosis of the fistula and the vein of Galen aneurysm (Fig. 245-4).
3. Staged embolization resulting in thrombosis of the vein of Galen aneurysm but with some persistence of an arteriovenous shunt (Fig. 245-5).
4. Single embolization with a significant reduction in the size of the shunt and substantial reduction of periorbital venous distention (Fig. 245-6).

The clinical scenario with transtorcular embolization for the control of heart failure in the neonate is quite predictable. These patients respond temporarily to this therapy, but in our experience all of them require staged embolizations every 2 to 3 days to maintain the improvement in heart failure. One patient required multiple wire embolizations and, subsequently, multiple balloon embolizations in order to save him from recurrent heart failure. Unfortunately, this survivor succumbed to an acute subdural hematoma during an attempt to place a ventriculostomy for acute hydrocephalus. Another neonate (Fig. 245-7) required four embolizations over 3 months to save him from progressive and life-threatening cardiac failure. This neonatal survivor was completely normal at 14 months of age, with only a very small residual arteriovenous malformation present in the right thalamus.

Conclusions

The transtorcular approach to the control of vein of Galen arteriovenous fistulae is an evolving therapy. Many questions remain concerning its efficacy and indications, especially as related to patient selection and results. We are encouraged by our early successes in several cases and now realize that the initial primary therapeutic goal of total fistula elimination will not be feasible in all cases.

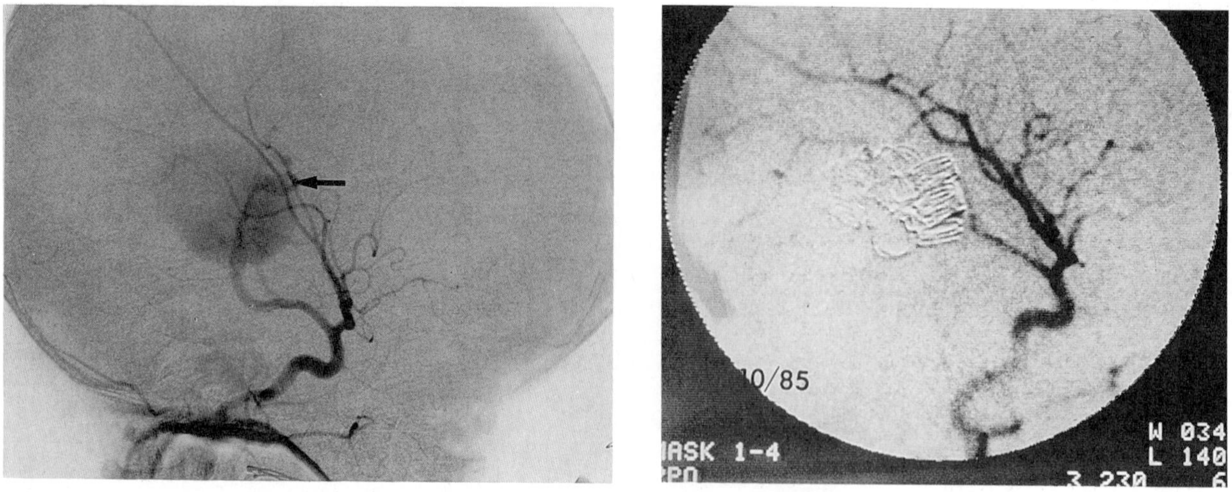

(*A*) (*B*)

Figure 245-3 *A.* A carotid angiogram showing a globoid vein of Galen aneurysm filling via multiple anterosuperior feeders *(arrow)*. *B.* A repeat angiogram taken 1 year after the deposition of 10 Gianturco coils, showing complete thrombosis of the malformation. This patient is presently 5 years old and normal.

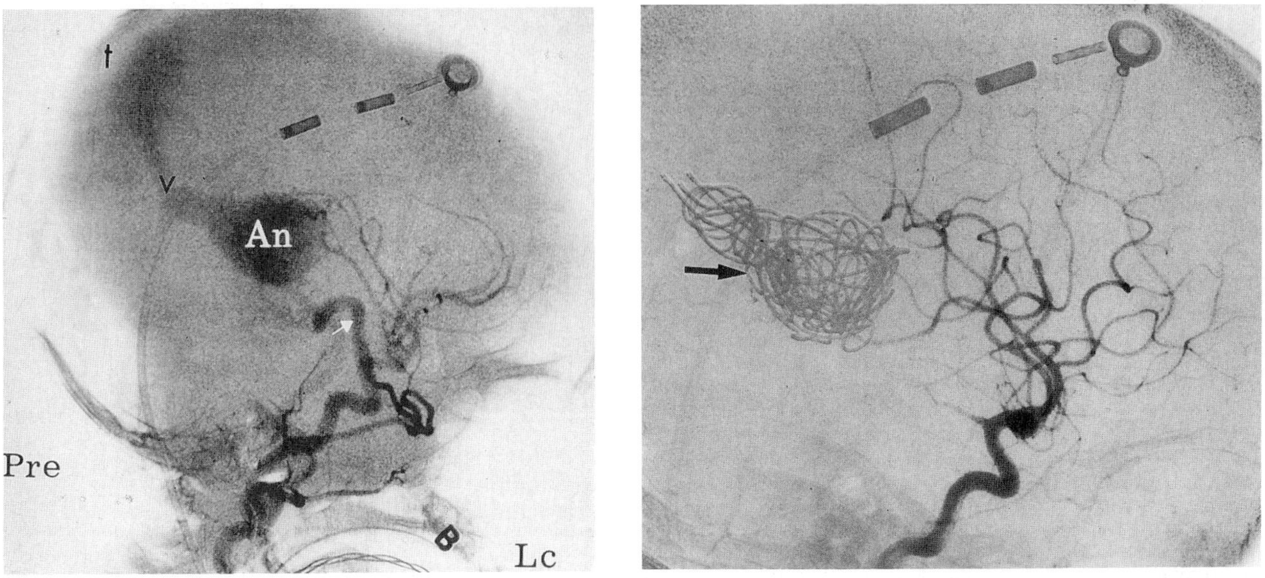

(*A*) (*B*)

Figure 245-4 *A*. The large aneurysm (An) in this 2-month-old drains via an abnormal venous structure (v) into a huge venous lake (t). *B*. Multiple wire depositions were required to rid the patient of the malformation *(arrow)*. This child is 5 years old and has a seizure disorder.

As noted above, there will be a variety of therapeutic outcomes, depending on the individual needs of each patient. Neonatal patients respond temporarily to this therapeutic modality and require repeated embolizations to effect survival and eventual cure. This situation is encouraging, and we continue to improve this therapeutic option in this group of patients.

As demonstrated by several cases in the literature concerning acute venous outlet obstruction in these lesions, this result can be devastating.[5] The goal in the transtorcular approach is to reduce flow in a stepwise, graded fashion and to avoid any acute thrombosis as an outcome. At this time we think that the patients at greatest risk for this outcome are those with vein of Galen aneurysms characterized as globoid with high intra-aneurysmal pressure and relatively low flow and with the potential for acute thrombosis after the deposition of wires.

For certain patients with high-flow vein of Galen malformations, the transtorcular approach offers a relatively safe way to substantially reduce the flow through the malformation. In certain

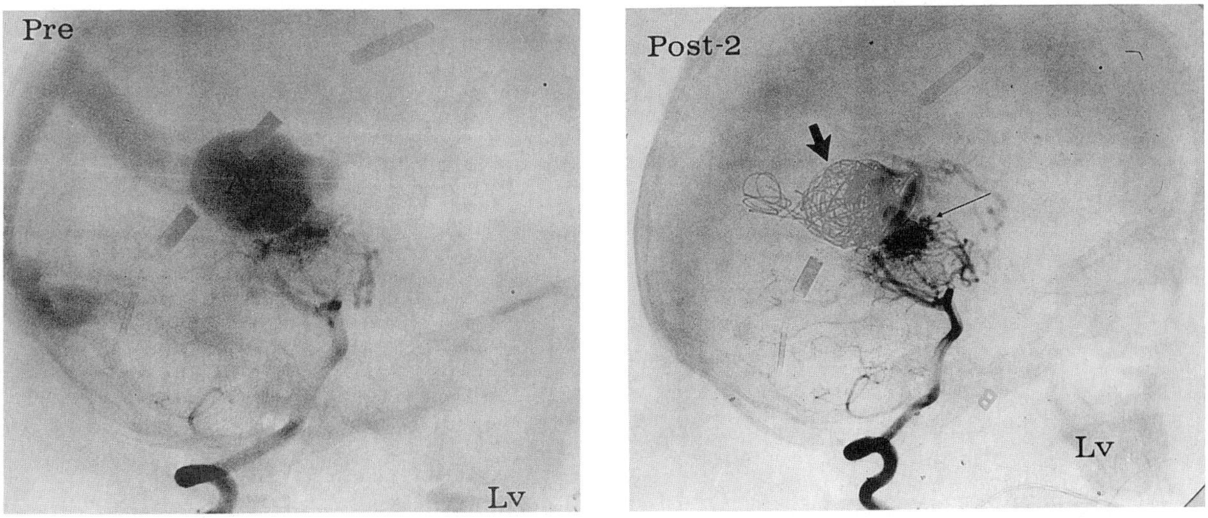

(*A*) (*B*)

Figure 245-5 *A*. This preoperative angiogram shows a large, complex angioma draining into a dilated vein of Galen. *B*. Multiple wire depositions transvenously *(large arrow)* resulted in thrombosis of the vein of Galen but persistence of a small fistula *(thin arrow)*. This child presented after three subarachnoid hemorrhages and is now 7 years old and doing well.

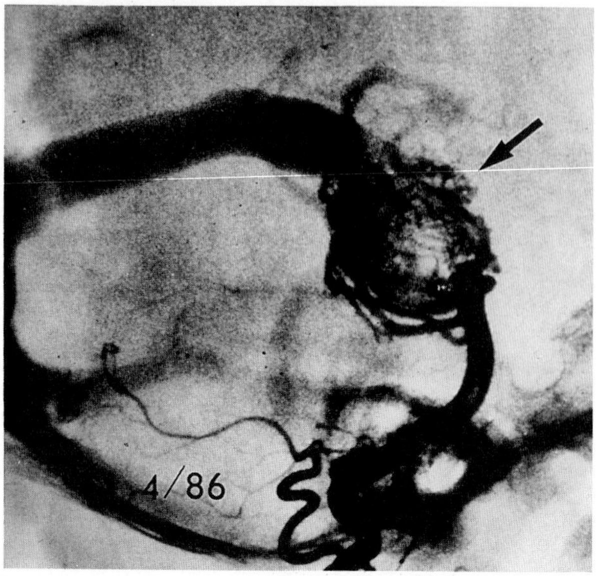

(*A*)

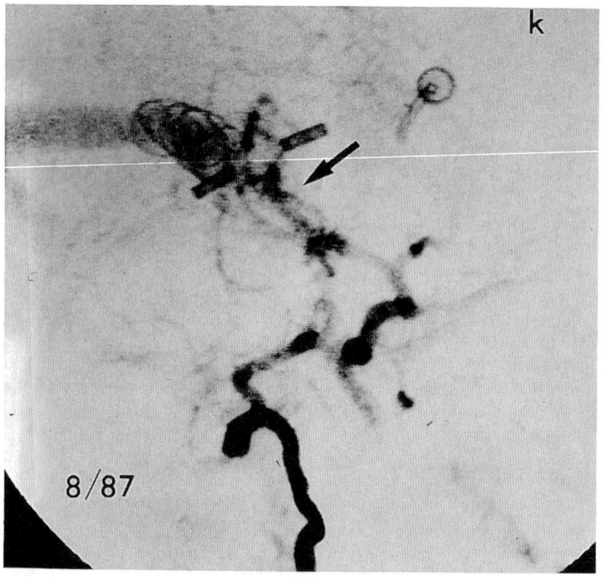

(*B*)

Figure 245-6 *A.* This lateral vertebral angiogram shows a complex angiomatous network *(arrow).* This patient had tremendous periorbital vein distention. *B.* After a single embolization and a ventriculoperitoneal shunt for hydrocephalus, the flow through the lesion is markedly reduced *(arrow).*

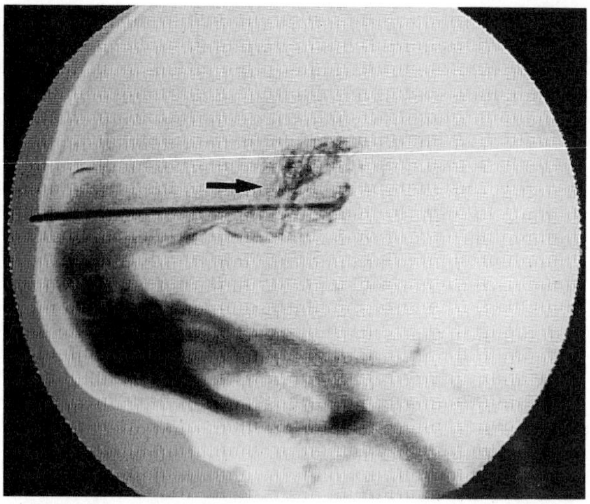

Figure 245-7 This venogram shows the typical flow pattern in a neonate with heart failure due to a vein of Galen aneurysm. Multiple wires *(arrow)* have been deposited to reduce the pressure and flow. After four embolizations, the patient is 14 months old and is doing well, with only a small arteriovenous malformation persistent in the right thalamus.

cases, graded thrombosis and cure are obtained. In other cases, there is marked improvement as judged by angiography; we have been extremely pleased with the clinical outcome in this group of patients. However, we think that in this group with a persistent fistula, other therapeutic modalities may be required for complete cure. Perhaps small residual arteriovenous niduses may require treatment with stereotactic radiation therapy to be eliminated completely.

We are encouraged by the outcome in our series of patients and think that the transtorcular approach to the treatment of vein of Galen malformations is an alternative for certain patients. This procedure is still an evolving therapeutic modality and requires refinement, principally in patient selection and in the degree of embolization required at any one sitting for optimal therapeutic outcome. The great advantages of this procedure remain its simplicity and the rapidity with which it can be accomplished. These patients are still critically ill after the transtorcular deposition of the thrombogenic wires and aggressive and expert intensive care are necessary to optimize survival.

References

1. Amacher AL, Shillito J Jr. The syndrome and surgical treatment of aneurysms of the great vein of Galen. *J Neurosurg* 1973; 39:89–98.
2. Berenstein A, Epstein F. Vein of Galen malformations: combined neurosurgical and neuroradiologic intervention. In Section of Pediatric Neurosurgery of the American Association of Neurological Surgeons: *Pediatric Neurosurgery: Surgery of the Developing Nervous System.* New York: Grune & Stratton, 1982, pp 637–647.
3. Ciricillo SF, Edwards MSB, Schmidt KG, et al. Interventional neuroradiological management of vein of Galen malformations in the neonate. *Neurosurgery* 1990; 27:22–28.
4. Hoffman HJ, Chuang S, Hendrick EB, et al. Aneurysms of the vein of Galen: experience at the Hospital for Sick Children, Toronto. *J Neurosurg* 1982; 57:316–322.
5. Johnson IH, Whittle IR, Besser M, et al. Vein of Galen malformation: diagnosis and management. *Neurosurgery* 1987; 20:747–758.
6. Laws ER Jr. Management of an aneurysm of the vein of Galen by insertion of phosphor-bronze wire. Paper presented at the Annual Meeting of the Neurosurgical Society of America, Marco Island, FL, 1982.
7. Malis LI. Arteriovenous malformations of the brain. In Youmans JR (ed): *Neurosurgical Surgery,* 2d ed. Philadelphia: Saunders, 1982, pp 1786–1806.
8. Mickle JP. The transtorcular embolization of vein of Galen aneurysms and update of the use of this technique in twenty-four patients. *Concepts Pediatr Neurosurg* 1991; 11:69–78.
9. Mickle JP, Quisling RG. The transtorcular embolization of vein of Galen aneurysms. *J Neurosurg* 1986; 64:731–735.
10. Mickle JP, Quisling R, Ryan R. Transtorcular approach to vein of Galen aneurysms. In Chapman PH (ed): *Concepts in Pediatric Neurosurgery,* vol 6. Basel: Karger, 1985, pp 230–238.
11. Mullan S. Treatment of carotid-cavernous fistulas by cavernous sinus occlusion. *J Neurosurg* 1979; 50:131–144.
12. Quisling RG, Mickle JP. Venous pressure measurements in vein of Galen aneurysms. *Am J Neuroradiol* 1989; 10:411–417.

246

Stereotactic Radiosurgery of Intracranial Arteriovenous Malformations

L. Dade Lunsford

Stereotactic radiosurgery is the closed-skull destruction of an intracranial target using ionizing beams of radiation, focused with the help of an intracranial guiding device. In 1951, Leksell defined the term and initiated investigation, first using an orthovoltage x-ray tube combined with his initial rectilinear stereotactic coordinate frame.[38] Working with Larsson, a physicist, Leksell subsequently reported the first clinical use of stereotactic guidance linked with a cyclotron-generated proton beam.[36] Similarly, in 1955, Lawrence, working with the Berkeley synchrocyclotron, began to use a proton beam to perform particle hypophysectomy in the treatment of metastatic breast carcinoma.[37] Beginning in 1957, alpha particles (accelerated helium ions) were used to treat more than 800 patients with a variety of neoplastic and metabolic conditions ranging from cancer to diabetes as well as secretory and nonsecretory pituitary tumors.[37]

In 1968, Leksell and Larsson arranged for the construction of the first in-hospital dedicated stereotactic radiosurgical unit, the gamma knife.[39] This unit contained 179 sealed sources of cobalt 60, which were collimated in such a way as to produce a discoid lesion at the intracranial target site. Its initial role was primarily for functional neurosurgical cases of intractable pain and medically unresponsive psychiatric conditions. In 1975, a redesigned second gamma unit entered routine clinical use at the Karolinska Hospital in Stockholm. Over the next 11 years, intracranial arteriovenous malformation (AVM) became the most common indication for this treatment at the Karolinska Institute.

Using the Boston-Harvard cyclotron, Kjellberg treated intracranial AVMs with a proton beam technique beginning in 1963,[29–31] and Fabrikant and coworkers in Berkeley expanded the application of the helium ion beam technique to the treatment of AVMs beginning in 1980.[14–17,47–51,61] In an attempt to make the radiosurgical technique available to a wider number of patients, recent investigators have explored the use of specially modified linear accelerators for single-treatment-session, photon irradiation of AVMs. By mid-1993, more than 5000 patients with intracranial AVMs had been treated with stereotactic radiosurgery using either a gamma knife,[1,2,4,40,43–45] a particle beam,[14–16,29–31] or a linear accelerator.[5–8,25,52,54,67,70] This chapter reviews the rationale, results, and risks of stereotactic radiosurgery for intracranial AVMs.

Rationale

It has been suggested that as many as 500,000 people in the United States and Canada have AVMs.[11,23,42] The growing use of precise new imaging tools [computed tomography (CT) and magnetic resonance imaging (MRI)] continues to increase the number of patients diagnosed. In fact, the availability of these sophisticated imaging tools provided one of the primary reasons for developing similarly sophisticated tools to obliterate AVMs with less morbidity than from microsurgical removal.

Various studies have attempted to define the natural history of cerebral AVMs.[3,9,11,23,24,32,53] Depending on the interval after diagnosis, the risk of hemorrhage from an AVM is 42 to 62 percent, with the average yearly probability of first hemorrhage between 2 and 4 percent.[9,53] The risk of death may be as high as 29 percent, and as many as 40.5 percent of patients who experience hemorrhage subsequently die as a result.[4,23] The likelihood of hemorrhage seems to be higher in the second through fourth decades of life[24] and has been linked to the size and location of the AVM. For example, the mortality rate may be as high as 67 percent after the first hemorrhage from a posterior fossa AVM.[23] In patients who already have experienced hemorrhage, the risk of rebleeding has been estimated to be 6 percent at 1 year, 13 percent in 5 years, and 47 percent in 20 years after the initial hemorrhage.[24] In addition to the risk of hemorrhage and death, Colombo et al. reported that epilepsy developed in at least 18 percent of the patients studied who were not treated surgically, and 27 percent had neurological handicaps by 20 years after diagnosis.[7]

The significant lifetime risks faced by patients with an untreated intracranial AVM must be balanced against the risks of intervention, whether by surgical removal, endovascular embolization, radiosurgery, or a combination of these methods. In general, microsurgical removal, when safe and feasible, is preferred, because it eliminates the risk of rebleeding (when postoperative angiography confirms a total excision). The patient takes the risks entirely "up front," provided that the lesion is removed. In contrast, adjuvant therapies (such as endovascular embolization) frequently are successful in improving symptoms such as intractable headaches and are a useful adjunct when either subsequent surgical removal or radiosurgical obliteration is planned. However, such techniques rarely succeed in totally obliterating the AVM.[10,22]

Patient Selection

Although the indications for stereotactic radiosurgery vary among institutions, in general, patients harboring an intracranial AVM are treated if they fulfill one or more of the following conditions:

1. The AVM is considered difficult to remove even with sophisticated microsurgical techniques, without an unacceptable risk of a new neurological deficit.
2. The patient is elderly or has another medical infirmity that would make surgical removal unacceptably dangerous.
3. Surgery alone or in combination with embolization already has been unsuccessful.

TABLE 246-1 Heavy Particle Stereotactic Radiosurgery for AVMs (U.S. Experience)

Investigators	Site	Source	Beam	Total No. of Patients Treated	Dates
Kjellberg et al.	Boston	165-MeV cyclotron	Proton*	1037	1963–1988
Fabrikant et al.	Berkeley	910-MeV synchrocyclotron	Helium*	375	1980–1991
Griffin et al.	Seattle	Synchrocyclotron	Neutron	20	Until 1991

*Bragg peak.

4. Despite the feasibility of open surgical removal, the patient is willing to undergo only the radiosurgical alternative.

Heavy particle stereotactic radiosurgery has been used primarily at two centers in the United States, the Boston cyclotron unit and the Berkeley cyclotron (Table 246-1). More recently, a neutron beam-generated radiosurgical technique was given an initial trial in Seattle.

Bragg Peak Proton Beam Therapy

Since 1963, Kjellberg and coworkers have treated more than 2550 patients using the Bragg peak proton beam generated by the 165-MeV cyclotron in Cambridge, MA.[29–31] This series includes 1037 patients with AVMs and 1105 patients with pituitary adenomas. Kjellberg has elucidated extensively his perception of the advantages of Bragg peak proton irradiation in comparison with photon irradiation. Kjellberg states that, in general, fractionated x-ray therapy, used in the treatment of AVMs since the late 1920s, has proved to be virtually ineffective. Although Kjellberg prefers to use the term "stereotactic Bragg peak proton beam therapy" as opposed to "radiosurgery," his use of a single-treatment-session technique combined with a stereotactic guiding device parallels the procedure described by Leksell in the 1950s. Kjellberg contends that, compared with photon irradiation, Bragg peak proton beam radiation has more compact isodose curves around the target, spares more brain surrounding the target, has no exit dose, and has a more "controllable uniform target dose."[29–31] The proton beam has been used to treat AVMs up to 123 mm (mean, 43.4 mm) in greatest dimension.

Kjellberg also believes that total obliteration of an AVM is not always a reliable indicator of outcome, because "total obliteration" after surgical excision has not always eliminated the risk of rebleeding, and because angiographically occult vascular abnormalities clearly can result in recurrent hemorrhage and disability. Instead, Kjellberg has based his assessment of the effectiveness of proton beam therapy on a "systematic periodic clinical follow-up" and an actuarial life table analysis. After proton beam therapy, the actuarial 20-year survival rate for AVM patients is 95 percent (RN Kjellberg, personal communication, 1988). Achievement of angiographic obliteration is related totally to the size of malformation treated (Table 246-2). In a series of 800 patients treated between 1965 and 1986, Kjellberg defined a 2-year obliteration rate of 15.3 percent in 360 patients studied. If the lesion was less than or equal to 30 mm in greatest diameter, the complete obliteration rate at 2 years was 42 percent; if 30 to 50 mm, the rate was 6 percent; and if greater than 50 mm in size, 1 percent. The risk of rebleeding after proton beam therapy is shown in Table 246-3. In a series of 800 patients, 5 percent had recurrent hemorrhage within 2 years of treatment, and 8.5 percent had recurrent hemorrhage 2 or more years after treatment.

Heavy Charged Particle (Helium Ion) Bragg Peak Stereotactic Radiosurgery

Since 1980, Fabrikant and coworkers have treated 375 patients (age range, 6 to 69 years) with an inoperable intracranial AVM.[14–17,50,51,61] A total of 262 adults and 44 children (age 18 years or younger) were treated using a multi-institution-approved protocol. As of 1990, more than 375 patients had been treated; the longest follow-ups were between 24 and 72 months (Table 246-4).

The helium ion beam technique results in a relatively homogeneous dose distribution,[47–49] and the 90 percent isodose is selected to treat the periphery of the lesion as defined by angiography and by MRI. The initial dose ranges varied from 45 to 35 GyE using the plateau phase of the Bragg peak. [Gray equivalent (GyE) is used because of the expected 1.3 to 1.5 greater radiobiological effect of accelerated heavy ions in comparison with photon irradiation.] Lesion volumes ranged from 120 to 54,000 mm^3. Thirty patients treated had an angiographically occult AVM. A specially designed irradiation stereotactic apparatus for humans was used for fixation.[47] This device is reported to have a 0.1 mm accuracy in three dimensions in positioning of the patient.

Fabrikant et al. have noted a relationship of the dose and volume to the complete obliteration rate (Table 246-4). By 3 years after treatment, obliteration had occurred in 90 to 95 percent of cases where the AVM volume was less than or equal to 4 cm^3. If

TABLE 246-2 Stereotactic Bragg Peak Proton Beam Therapy for AVM in 800 Patients

	Total No. of Patients Studied	Size of AVM	2-Year Complete Obliteration Rate (%)
	107/215	≤ 30 mm	42*
	150/341	> 30, ≤50 mm	6†
	103/244	> 50 mm	1‡
Total	360/800		15.3

*88% had > 50% reduction.
†37% had > 50% reduction.
‡16% had > 50% reduction.

TABLE 246-3 Hemorrhage after Stereotactic Bragg Peak Proton Beam Therapy for AVM

Size of AVM	No. of Patients	No. (%) of Hemorrhages within 2 Years	No. (%) of Hemorrhages after 2 Years
≤ 30 mm	215	13 (6)	11 (5)
> 30, ≤ 50 mm	341	15 (4.4)	33 (9.7)
> 50 mm	244	16 (6.5)	24 (9.8)
Total	800	44 (5)	68 (8.5)

TABLE 246-4 Stereotactic Heavy Charged Particle (Helium Ion) Bragg Peak Radiosurgery for AVM

Total No. of Patients Treated	Follow-up Duration	Size of AVM	Estimated Percentage of Complete Obliteration at 3 Years
375	24–72 months	< 2-cm diameter (volume ≤4 cm^3)	90–95
		< 3-cm diameter (volume > 4, ≤ 14 cm^3)	80–85
		Volume > 14 cm^3	70

the AVM volume was between 4 cm^3 and 14 cm^3, the total obliteration rate was 80 to 85 percent; and for volumes greater than 14 cm^3, a 70 percent total obliteration rate was achieved (JI Fabrikant, personal communication, 1991). Hemorrhage after helium ion beam treatment occurred in 6.5 percent of patients, 80 percent of whom were known to have bled prior to treatment. Of the patients who bled, 80 percent did so between 4 and 14 months after treatment; only 1 percent bled more than 24 months after treatment. Three percent of patients had hemorrhages from associated aneurysms during the first 12 months after treatment occurred.

More recently, Fabrikant significantly reduced the dose prescribed to the target, usually using a dose of 20 to 25 GyE, and, under special circumstances, 10 GyE. In addition to the institutions mentioned, the radiosurgical principle is reportedly being applied at cyclotron units in Moscow, Dubna, and Leningrad.

Neutron Beam Stereotactic Radiosurgery

Griffin and coworkers described an initial trial of neutron beam irradiation in the treatment of 20 patients. The neutron beam generated by the cyclotron at the University of Washington at Seattle was believed to have 2.4 to 2.8 times the radiobiological effect of photon irradiation. The accuracy of positioning the isocenter of the neutron beam was ±2 mm. The neutron beam was delivered from a gantry that could be rotated 360°. Various collimators were used to conform the beam size to the size of the malformation. Immobilization was accomplished with a fixation system compatible with CT, MRI, and angiography. A dose of 9 Gy was delivered in a single fraction, using multiple pathways (9 to 10 fixed beams). The treatment was performed in approximately 2 h on an outpatient basis. In these initial nine patients, no acute toxic effects were encountered in the treatment of AVMs ranging from 7 to 35 mm in greatest diameter. MRI done 5 to 6 months after treatment showed a reduction in AVM blood flow in three of five patients. Follow-up angiography was performed in nine patients, none of whom had complete AVM obliteration (Table 246-5).

TABLE 246-5 Results of Stereotactic Neutron Beam Irradiation

Total No. of Patients Treated	Total No. with Follow-up Angiography	Complete Obliteration
20	9	0*

*Three had 25–75% reduction; one had increase

Source: Stelzer K, Griffin B, Eskridge J, et al. Results of neutron radiosurgery for inoperable arteriovenous malformations of the brain. *Med Dosimetry* 1991; 16:137–141.

Stereotactic Radiosurgery Using the Gamma Knife

After the second gamma unit became available in Stockholm in 1975, Steiner greatly expanded the role of gamma knife radiosurgery in the treatment of AVMs (Table 246-6). Between 1971 and 1987, 900 patients were treated.[4,62–66] An additional 354 patients were treated at Buenos Aires, Argentina (Unit 3) and 615 at Sheffield, England[21,68] (Unit 4). From August 1987 to August 1988, 402 patients with an intracranial AVM were treated at the University of Pittsburgh site (Unit 5).

The current-generation Leksell gamma knife (Model U) consists of an 18,000-kg heavily shielded unit containing 201 gamma ray emitting sources of cobalt 60 (Fig. 246-1). The beams are directed at an intracranial target using a specially designed imaging-compatible stereotactic guiding device that is secured in the collimator helmet (Fig. 246-2). Four collimator helmets with 201 beam channels of 4-, 8-, 14-, and 18-mm diameter, respectively, are used to vary the size of the lesion as well as to conform the delivered dose to the outlines of the malformation as visualized by angiography. The Pittsburgh gamma unit is a self-contained site wherein frame application, imaging review, target selection, dose planning, and treatment are done (Fig. 246-3). Stereotactic imaging is performed off-site in the hospital radiology department.

Because the largest collimator available on the Stockholm Gamma 2 unit was 14 mm in diameter, Steiner generally treated malformations that were smaller than 20 to 30 mm at their widest points. The total obliteration rate at 1 year was 62.5 percent; at 2 years, 83.2 percent; and at 3 years, 93.9 percent (L Steiner, personal communication, 1988) (Table 246-7). Steiner found subtotal obliteration to be of no benefit, because patients hemorrhaged at a rate of approximately 2 to 3 percent per year during the latency period between treatment and total obliteration. Subtotal obliteration was defined to include even those patients in whom a tiny, early-filling vein was demonstrated on follow-up angiography. The selected target dose was 20 to 25 Gy at the periphery of the AVM using the 50 to 70 percent (occasionally the 90 percent) isodose at the margin. After angiographically demonstrated obliteration, no patients had recurrent hemorrhage; the rebleeding rate was 3 percent for the entire series. Twenty-five patients had angi-

TABLE 246-6 Stereotactic Gamma Knife Radiosurgery for AVM

Project Director	Location	Unit No.	Total No. of Patients Treated	Inclusive Dates
Steiner	Stockholm	2	900	1971–1987
Bunge	Buenos Aires	3	354	1984–1990
Forster	Sheffield	4	615	1985–1990
Lunsford	Pittsburgh	5	402	1987–1992
			2271	

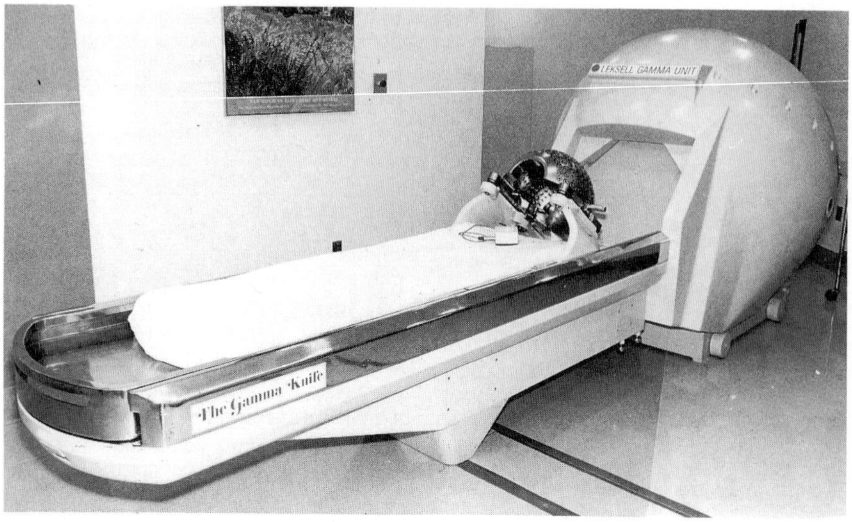

Figure 246-1 The Leksell 201 cobalt 60 source gamma unit for stereotactic radiosurgery. The sources are located in the 18,000-kg shielded central body. During treatment, the patient rests on the treatment couch with the head attached at the *X*, *Y*, and *Z* coordinates of the selected target. The 18-mm collimator helmet is shown.

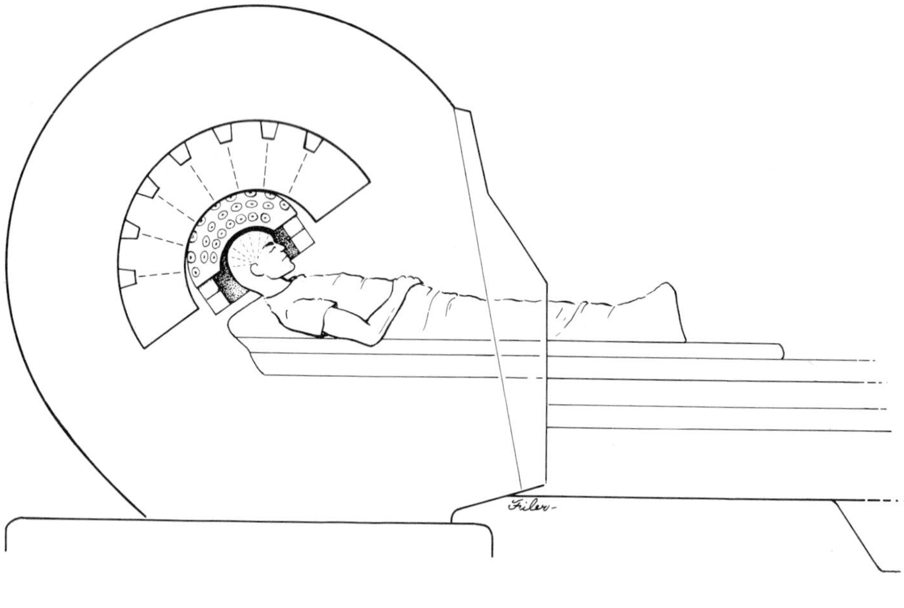

Figure 246-2 During treatment with the gamma unit, the 201 beams are focused through the apertures of the collimator helmet (diameter of 18, 14, 8, or 4 mm).

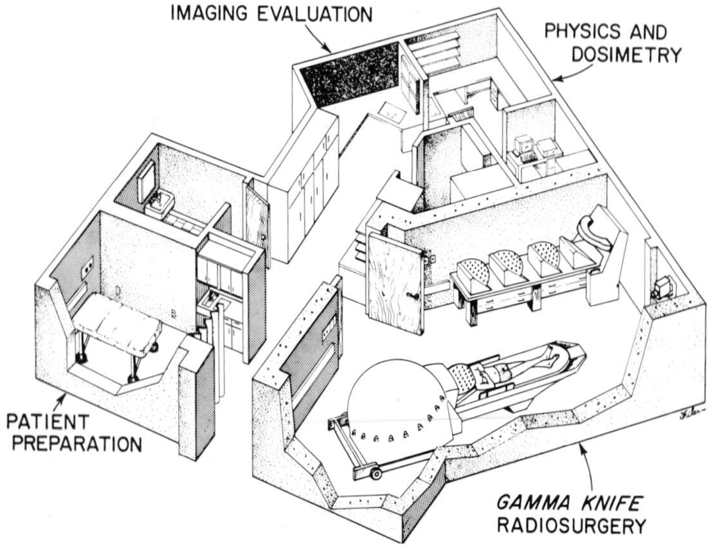

Figure 246-3 The University of Pittsburgh stereotactic radiosurgery suite. Stereotactic frame application, imaging review, dosimetry calculations, and radiosurgery are performed in the suite. Imaging is done off-site.

TABLE 246-7 Gamma Knife Stereotactic Radiosurgery for AVMs: Published 2-Year Obliteration Rates

Surgeon	Total No. of Patients Treated	Angiographically Confirmed 2-Year Obliteration Rate*	Study Interval
Bunge	354	40/47 (84%)	1984–1990
Forster	615	57/96 (59%)	1985–1990
Lunsford	348	80/112 (71%)	1987–1992
Steiner	600	258/310 (83.2%)	1971–1987

*Refers to entire series results regardless of AVM volume.

ography again 5 to 8 years after initially demonstrated obliteration; one patient had evidence of some recurrence in a calcarine branch of the posterior cerebral artery. Among the lesions that Steiner treated were seven angiographically occult angiomas, six dural AVMs, several carotid-cavernous fistulas, and a vein of Galen AVM.

Bunge treated 354 AVMs between October 1984 and August 1988 at the Buenos Aires (Unit 3) site (Table 246-7). Sixty-three patients were followed for more than 2 years. The patients were divided in three groups prospectively. Of the 47 patients in group 1 (optimal dose delivered to the nidus), an 84 percent total obliteration rate was observed after 2 years. Of the 14 patients in group 2 (partial coverage), subtotal angiographic obliteration was achieved in 8. Two patients were classified as group 3 (feeder therapy); in one, a vein of Galen AVM was obliterated successfully. Overall, Bunge noted a 1.27 percent rebleeding rate in the first year, including two deaths related to hemorrhage and another to delayed shunt malfunction.

In the 5-year interval between August 1987 and April 1992 we selected 348 patients (50 percent male, 50 percent female) for gamma knife stereotactic radiosurgery (Fig. 246-4). In every case the clinical symptoms, neuroimaging studies, and alternative treatment strategies were discussed at our multidisciplinary conference attended by neurological surgeons, radiation oncologists, interventional radiologists, and medical physicists. In this group of patients, 59 percent reported one or more prior hemorrhages, 47 percent had headaches, and 32 percent had seizures. Neurological deficits were found in 44 percent before radiosurgery, 13.5 percent had already undergone one or more attempts at removal, and in 16 percent intravascular embolization had been used in an attempt to reduce the AVM to a volume more suitable for radiosurgery.

Many patients had deep-seated AVMs, including 83 (24 percent) who were classified as inoperable (Spetzler-Martin grade 6). In all adult patients, frame application, angiography, and radiosurgery were performed under local anesthesia. We usually used general anesthesia in children age 13 or younger. Identification of the AVM nidus was performed using biplane-resolution magnification/subtraction angiography,[57] often supplemented by intraoperative MRI. Patients considered to be at relatively high risk for seizures (prior history or subcortical lobar location) were given anticonvulsants to obtain therapeutic levels. Selection of dose was based on prior published results, location of the AVM, and usage of the integrated logistic formula (which helps to relate selected dose, volume, and risk prediction).[18–20]

We requested serial MR imaging at 6-month intervals for the first 2 years after radiosurgery. Angiography was performed at either 2 years (if warranted because of regression of the AVM on MRI) or at 3 years. The angiograms of 112 evaluable patients were reviewed at our multidisciplinary conference for evidence of complete obliteration (complete disappearance of the pathologic shunting nidus and normalization of the intracranial vasculature), subtotal obliteration (residual early-draining vein), or no change. Radiosurgical obliteration was related to AVM volume: for AVMs 4 cm^3 or less in volume, 62 of 76 patients (82 percent) had complete obliteration.

Three additional factors were identified that influenced results. First, the interval that elapsed after radiosurgery was important—(in some patients, obliteration occurred only between 2 and 3 years). Second, we noted that clear definition of the AVM nidus facilitated dose planning and subsequent results. In two patients, a new AVM nidus not identified at the time of radiosurgery subsequently appeared. Third, the AVM dose selected probably also influences results, since the highest obliteration rate was observed in smaller AVMs that received marginal doses of 22–25 Gy. Dose selection continues to be made by balancing the twin goals of achieving obliteration and avoiding complications.[2,60,71]

The morbidity from radiosurgery was related to the risk of rebleeding during the latency interval between radiosurgery and obliteration and to the risk of developing a new neurological deficit caused by delayed radiation effects. Although no patient has had a hemorrhage after obliteration, 18 patients had an intracranial hemorrhage during the latency interval. We anticipated that during this interval 16 patients would hemorrhage. This estimate was made using a statistical model based on several assumptions: (1) a 4 percent annual risk of hemorrhage,[53] (2) an accrual rate of 70 patients per year, (3) a 1 percent yearly mortality due to hemorrhage,[53] and (4) an obliteration rate of 40 percent at 1 year and 80 percent at 2 years.[45] There was no statistical difference between the projected and observed rates of rebleeding ($p = .65$). Of our first 227 AVM patients, 4.4 percent developed new neurological deficits between 4 and 18 months after radiosurgery. Symptoms were location-dependent, with most occurring in patients whose AVM was located in an area of critical brain function.

Stereotactic Linear Accelerator Radiotherapy for AVM

Because of the scarcity, cost, and access limitations of dedicated radiosurgical units that are based on the cyclotron or gamma unit technology, since 1983 various investigators have modified existing linear accelerators to deliver a high dose radiation therapy in a single session. In 1983, Betti and Derechinsky described an initial experience,[5] as did Colombo et al. in 1985.[7] Heifetz et al. proposed an experimental model in 1984.[25] Throughout the world, various groups are now reporting different techniques to modify a conventionally available linear accelerator (Table 246-8).[6,8,46,54,55,67,70] Although each of these techniques has specific potential radiotherapeutic benefits, all cannot be described here. Initial data are available from several centers.

By 1988, Sturm had treated 180 patients with AVMs and brain tumors using a linear accelerator (reported at the Small Field Stereotactic Radiotherapy Workshop, Bethesda, MD, June 9, 1988). Using a 15-MeV linear accelerator with ±1 mm positioning accuracy, Sturm and colleagues delivered a single dose varying between 10 and 50 Gy (at the 80 percent isodose).[67] The field diameter of the AVM varied between 6 and 54 mm (mean size, 30 mm). Although single-dose treatment of less than 10 Gy met with no success, Sturm otherwise noted no clear relationship between outcome and the size of the malformation, finding success even in AVMs that were 40 mm in greatest diameter. Of the 41 patients treated for an AVM, 17 had postoperative angiography 1 to 1.5

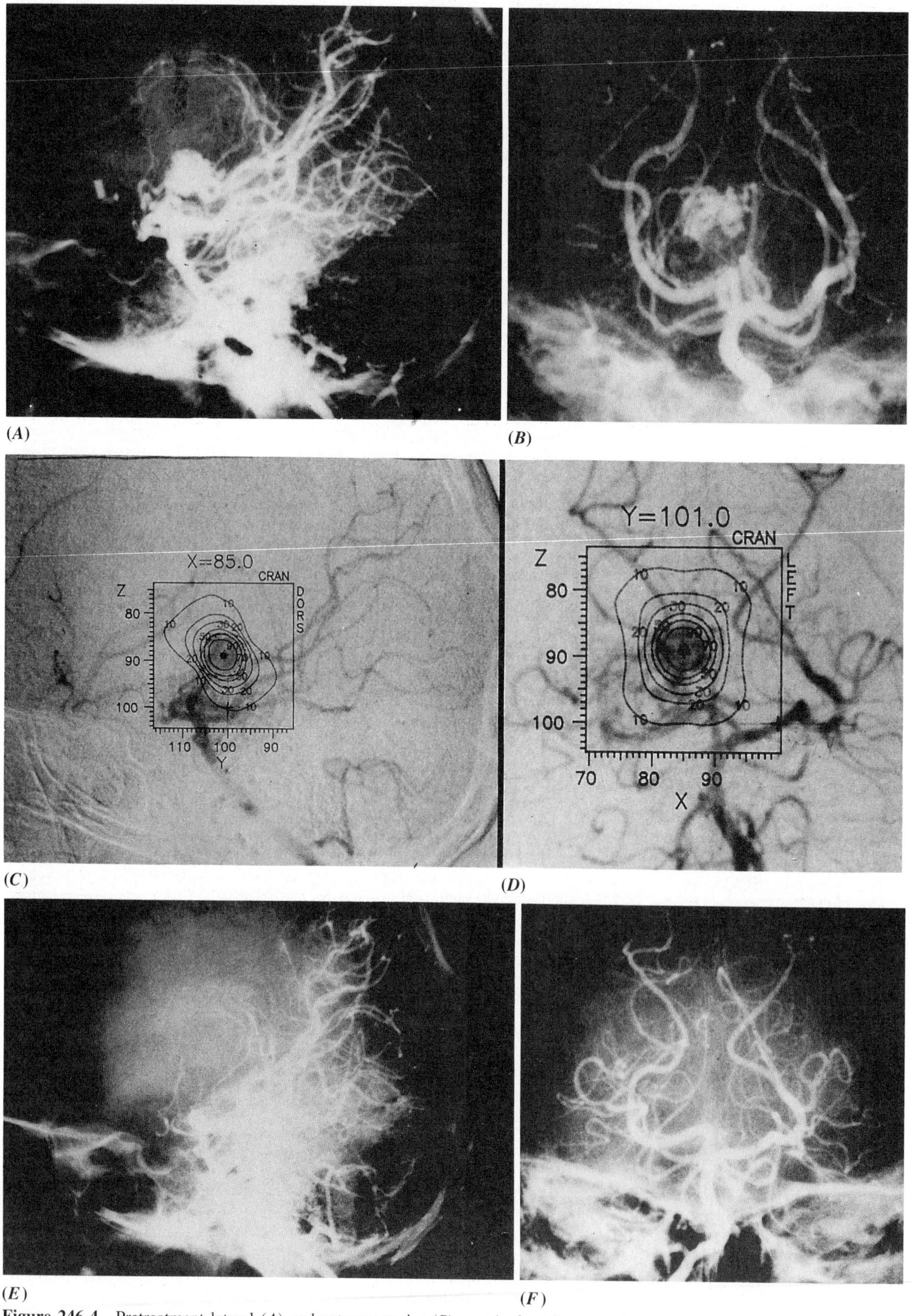

Figure 246-4 Pretreatment lateral (*A*) and anteroposterior (*B*) vertebral angiograms demonstrate a dorsal midbrain AVM. *C, D.* Multiplanar dose plan for treatment (using the 8-mm collimator helmet, 50 Gy was delivered to the AVM center and 25 Gy at the margin in a treatment session lasting 8.9 min). *E, F.* Total obliteration was confirmed at 4 months.

TABLE 246-8 Stereotactic Radiosurgery for AVMs: Linear Accelerator Technique

Project Director	Site	Technique	Total No. of Patients Treated	Date of Report
Betti	Buenes Aires	Multiple arcs	66	1989
Colombo	Vicenza	Multiple intersecting arcs	264	1992
Friedman	Gainesville	Intersecting arcs	119	1992
Merienne	Paris	Rotational	46	1991
Olivier	Montreal	Dynamic	28	1992
Sturm	Heidelberg	Multiple converging arcs	41	1991

years after treatment. In these 17 patients, total obliteration was found in 5, partial obliteration in 7, and no change in the remaining 5 (Table 246-9). Three patients hemorrhaged after treatment.

At Vicenza, Italy, Colombo et al. treated 146 patients with an AVM; the obliteration rate at 2 years was 80 percent (Table 246-9). A rebleeding rate of 3.5 percent was noted in the first 2 years after treatment. In Montreal, Olivier and Podgorsak (reported by Podgorsak et al.[55]) treated 28 AVM patients. Using a ''dynamic rotation'' technique, they delivered a heavy dose to a small volume without attempting to provide total coverage to the margins of the malformation. Multiple fractions were used in some patients. By 2 years, 11 of 27 patients (41 percent) had complete obliteration. Merienne and colleagues reported a 2-year obliteration rate of 34 percent in 36 patients who were treated with linear acceleration radiosurgery in Paris (Table 246-9).

Working at the Boston Joint Center for Radiation Therapy, Loeffler and colleagues treated 16 patients with an AVM using a specially designed collimator system for their linear accelerator, carrying on the efforts begun by Winston and Lutz.[46,70] A dose of 12 to 25 Gy was delivered to the margins of the AVM at the 80 to 85 percent isodose. At 1 year, 5 of 10 patients studied (50 percent) had total obliteration, and another had complete obliteration at 2 years. Additional experience has been reported by Friedman and colleagues (2-year obliteration rate of 84 percent) and Betti and colleagues (2-year obliteration rate of 68 percent).

To date, linear accelerator radiation therapy has been used at major tertiary medical centers that are committed to thorough quality assurance and careful analysis of results. Such results necessarily will be compared with the results established for the gamma unit and particle beam techniques. Concerns raised about the linear accelerator system include the homogeneous dose provided at isodose curves above 80 percent, the uncertain continuous accuracy of the stereotactic guiding system in relation to the linear accelerator isocenter, and the length of time required to perform the treatment (a feature that necessitates general anesthesia in some cases). There is no doubt, however, that the recent flurry of reports appearing to establish the role of the single-treatment-session stereotactic linear accelerator radiation therapy has greatly expanded the attention and assessment given the entire field of radiosurgery.

TABLE 246-9 Results of Linear Accelerator Radiosurgery for AVMs: Published 2-Year Complete Obliteration Rates

Project Director	Date of Report	Total No. of Patient Assessed	No. Obliterated at 2 Years	Percentage
Betti	1989	40	27	68
Colombo	1992	92	74	80
Friedman	1992	37	31	84
Merienne	1991	36	13	34
Olivier	1992	27	11	41
Sturm	1991	17	5	29

Complications of Radiosurgery

The risks of stereotactic radiosurgery for AVM are related to (1) hemorrhage (described previously), (2) transient radiation effects, and (3) permanent radiation-related effects. Table 246-10 demonstrates these risks with data recently supplied by the investigators listed. Because different investigators used different doses and techniques, this comparison must be interpreted cautiously. In addition, such complications must be balanced against the risk of conventional surgical removal.[11,27] Many of the patients treated with these techniques were deemed unsuitable for microsurgical removal.

In Kjellberg's series of 800 patients, 10 of the first 75 patients treated had complications. Kjellberg then significantly reduced the dose delivered to larger malformations in an attempt to keep the risk of cerebral radiation necrosis under 1 percent. In fact, of the last 725 patients treated, only 7(0.96 percent) sustained permanent radiation-related complications.

Using a helium ion beam technique, Marks and colleagues noted transient, asymptomatic white matter (vasogenic edema) MRI changes in approximately 10 percent of patients; this effect was not observed in any patient treated with a dose of less than 20 GyE.[50,51] During follow-up, all patients continued to do well, and the MRI changes resolved. An additional 4 percent of patients (who were asymptomatic) nonetheless required treatment with corticosteroids because of white matter changes (both reversible and irreversible, mild and severe). Patients treated with a dose of 25 GyE or less have not had this complication. Two to three percent of patients had occlusion of normal vessels (arterial and venous) associated with mild or severe permanent neurological deficits that were treated with corticosteroids. Again, Fabrikant states that this complication was not noted in patients treated with a dose of 25 GyE or less. Less than 1 percent of patients had permanent, symptomatic late-delayed radiation necrosis. Overall, total serious neurological complications accompanied by some permanent neurological deficit occurred in 3 to 4 percent of the patients within 2 years after treatment. Many of these complications and their appearance on serial imaging studies have been described recently.[50,51]

In a series of 600 patients treated with the gamma unit, Steiner noted a 3.3 percent rate of transient radiation-related complications.[62–64,66] In 3.1 percent of patients, a permanent radiation-related neurological deficit developed that was not present before gamma knife radiosurgery. Bunge observed that imaging or clinical changes compatible with a postirradiation effect developed in 8 (3.4 percent) of 236 gamma-knife-treated patients. Three patients

TABLE 246-10 Published Complication Rates for Stereotactic Radiosurgery for AVMs

Technique	Project Director	No. of Patients	Transient Radiation-Related (%)	Permanent Radiation-Related (%)	Rebleeding* (%)
Particle beam	Kjellberg	800	N/A	0.96	5
	Fabrikant	375	10	11	N/A
	Griffin	19	0	0	3
Gamma knife	Steiner	600	3.3	3.1	2.3
	Bunge	236	2.1	1.3	1.3
	Forster	339	N/A	4.4	3.2
	Lunsford	227	4.4	3.1	5.2
Linear accelerator	Betti	66	N/A	3	8
	Colombo	146	4.8	2.7	8.2
	Friedman	119	1.7	1.7	N/A
	Olivier	27	N/A	4	4
	Sturm	41	42	N/A	N/A

*Prior to obliteration or within 2 years.
N/A = not available.

(1.3 percent) had a contralateral hemiparesis; five (2.1 percent) had transient post-treatment CT evidence of edema but had no neurological deficits. In a recent series of 227 patients analyzed at the Pittsburgh gamma unit, we found a 4.4 percent incidence of transient radiation-related neurological deficits developing within 2 years; 3.1 percent of patients experienced new neurological deficits.[45]

After treatment by the linear accelerator technique, Sturm et al. found transient radiation-related complications in 17 (42 percent) of 41 patients; Colombo et al., in 4.8 percent of their patients. The rates of permanent radiation-related complications are not currently available for many linear accelerator centers.

Other delayed radiation-related complications, such as delayed carcinogenesis and the formation of cataracts, have not been adequately assessed. Steiner noted no increased rate of subsequent cancer diagnosis in his series of patients treated for AVMs with the gamma unit (L Steiner, personal communication, 1987). When either gamma unit or linear accelerator techniques are used, care is taken to avoid sending the beams through the lens of the eye.

The Advantages of Stereotactic Radiosurgery

Stereotactic radiosurgery has a number of advantages when compared with either nonsurgical therapy or direct surgical excision. Thus far, the complication rate appears to be acceptably low and is significantly less than the morbidity and mortality rates reported for the natural history of untreated AVMs. In contrast to open surgical removal, radiosurgery is not associated with such conventional surgical risks as blood loss, infections, or acute new neurological deficits. Instead, the risks are spread out over time and are related both to the probability of bleeding during the latency period before obliteration and to the likelihood of delayed radiation injury to the brain. Radiosurgery has significantly reduced the length of hospitalization required for the definitive treatment of an AVM.[43] For our patients, the average hospital stay was reduced from approximately 10.2 days (for surgical removal) to 1.5 days (for radiosurgery).[43] Our experience with an initial series of 62 patients also confirmed that hospitalization costs could be reduced between 40 and 75 percent when compared with craniotomy and AVM removal. We believe that an in-hospital stay is important for radiosurgery, because we perform angiography during the procedure for stereotactic localization of the AVM target, and because of the approximately 1 to 3 percent risk of perioperative seizures. Other centers have performed radiosurgery on an outpatient basis. Depending on the technique that is used, the length of actual surgical time required for radiosurgery is often considerably less than the time required for surgical removal. The primary advantage of radiosurgery, however, lies in the fact that definitive treatment is now possible for many intracranial AVM patients who previously were deemed inoperable and for whom the outlook in terms of hemorrhage and disability was indeed bleak.

Limitations

Many real concerns have limited the use of radiosurgical techniques for treating certain AVMs. The first concern is the size of the AVM, because the dose that can be used appears to be critical to achieve obliteration. Achieving a therapeutic result in large malformations would result in a potentially unacceptable (too high) dose to the brain. Kjellberg, however, maintains that total obliteration after radiosurgery is not an absolute goal (at least with the proton beam technique), because survival rates are superior to the natural history reported for untreated AVMs. Not all of the factors that result in delayed radiation-induced brain injury are understood.[2,34] Radiation injury is affected by the fractionation schedule, the dose, the volume treated, the patient's age,[1,33] the location and type (high flow versus low flow) of the AVM, the risk of early venous occlusion, and the danger to other surrounding cerebral vessels. It is clear that radiosurgery can result in AVM obliteration with preservation of the normal cerebral vessels. Because the radiosurgical technique does not instantaneously obliterate the AVM, the patient continues to be at risk of hemorrhage during the latency period. Extensive additional studies are necessary to further the understanding of these radiobiological issues as well as to assess the efficacy of all the available techniques over the long run. The benefits and hazards of the techniques relative to each other remain to be defined. If the results are to be evaluated in a scientific and orderly fashion, new studies must include detailed neurological, advanced imaging,[71] and multimodality electrophysiologic tests as well as long and persistent clinical follow-up.

The Future of Radiosurgery

All Arteriovenous Malformations?

At present, surgical removal, when possible and safe, remains the ideal neurosurgical approach for an AVM.[27,58,59] Using sophisticated localization and open microsurgical techniques, postoperative morbidity and mortality have been reduced significantly in the past 10 years. Results of such operations must be assessed objectively in relation to results for similar-sized AVMs treated by radiosurgical techniques, using the same parameters to judge the safety and efficacy of both modalities. Perhaps with increasing radiosurgical experience, more and more AVMs, especially those located in deep and critical areas of the brain, will prove to be best treated by radiosurgical techniques. Further analysis of seizure alleviation[26] and headache improvement after radiosurgery for AVM is warranted.

Angiographically Occult Angiomas?

The role of radiosurgery in the treatment of angiographically occult angiomas (AVMs and cavernous angiomas)—a group that is being recognized increasingly often—must be examined.[12,35] Angiography has been the benchmark technique in radiosurgery for defining AVM obliteration. However, because angiography cannot be used for occult or cryptic angiomas, obliteration of such lesions must be determined with CT or MRI.[13,56] There is currently debate about the risk of bleeding in the patient with an untreated occult angioma. Recent studies suggest that more than half of these lesions prove to be true AVMs on pathologic examination.[41] The recurrent hemorrhage rate may be as high as 2 percent per year (S. Peerless, personal communication, 1988), with an approximately 20 percent lifetime risk of hemorrhage (D. Rigamonti, personal communication, 1988). However, hemorrhages from occult vascular malformations usually are neither as severe nor as lethal as those occurring from angiographically demonstrated AVMs. Microsurgery has been advocated for even deep-seated cavernous-type malformations.[28,69]

In our gamma unit, we have treated 39 patients with angiographically occult cavernous-type malformations, all of which had bled for a second time after initial diagnosis. Using the gamma knife, Steiner treated 17 patients, with equivocal results. Fabrikant has treated 30 cryptic angiomas using helium ion beam radiosurgery. Treatment of occult angiomas needs to be scrutinized for an extended period in terms of both risk and efficacy. For the present, the long-term rebleeding rate and neurological outcome will be the only useful means for establishing a satisfactory clinical response. Combining the data from multiple radiosurgery sites will make it possible to gather this information more quickly.

New Energy Sources?

In addition to neutron beam techniques, radiophysicists have hypothesized that other heavy particle accelerated ions, such as neon or carbon ions, would have a more desirable beam configuration for radiosurgery than afforded by the ions currently available.[48] Extensive radiobiologic testing is necessary to confirm that the use of these beams actually will enhance the benefits to the patient without increased risk.

Widespread Availability?

The use of linear accelerators at multiple medical centers presages the rapid growth of radiosurgical techniques in the treatment of both AVMs and brain tumors. This innovative work must be monitored carefully to assess its efficacy and safety and to ensure that sufficient support is available from radiation oncologists, surgeons, and radiation physicists. A major commitment of time and a major financial investment are necessary to ensure the adequate functioning of such units. Because neither the total number of cases worldwide that are suitable for radiosurgical intervention nor the overall response rate is known, the scientific community must laboriously evaluate these newly devised systems. Quality assurance programs are of paramount importance.

Radiation Sensitizers?

There is a great need for agents that could enhance the dose-response effect, reduce the dose to the surrounding brain, and decrease the latency until obliteration occurs. The boron-neutron capture technique has been assessed periodically over several decades. One exciting area of future application that has not been explored fully, however, is the possibility of linking boron or some other radiation sensitizer to a monoclonal antibody directed at the AVM target endothelial cells during either particle or photon beam radiosurgery (B. Larsson, personal communication, 1986).

New Indications?

Beyond the treatment of AVMs, radiosurgical techniques will continue to be applied to intracranial tumors, both intra-axial and extra-axial, benign and malignant. The same principles that guided the treatment of 6000 AVM patients and the same follow-up detail and scrutiny must be applied to an increasing number of neoplastic conditions of the brain.

References

1. Atschuler EM, Lunsford LD, Coffey RJ, et al. Gamma knife radiosurgery for intracranial arteriovenous malformations in childhood and adolescence. *Pediatr Neurosci* 1989; 15:53–61.
2. Atschuler E, Lunsford LD, Kondziolka D, et al. Radiobiologic models for radiosurgery. *Neurosurg Clin North Am* 1992; 3:61–77.
3. Andersen EB, Petersen J, Mortensen EL, et al. Conservatively treated patients with cerebral arteriovenous malformation: mental and physical outcome. *J Neurol Neurosurg Psychiatry* 1988; 51:1208–1212.
4. Backlund EO. Stereotactic radiosurgery in intracranial tumors and vascular malformations. In Krayenbuhl H (ed): *Advances and Technical Standards in Neurosurgery,* vol 6. Vienna: Springer-Verlag, 1979, pp 3–37.
5. Betti O, Derechinsky V. Irradiation stéréotaxique multifasceaux. *Neurochirurgie* 1983; 29:295–298.
6. Betti OO, Munari C, Rosler R: Stereotactic radiosurgery with the linear accelerator: treatment of arteriovenous malformations. *Neurosurgery* 1989; 24:311–321.
7. Colombo F, Benedetti A, Pozza F, et al. External stereotactic irradiation by linear accelerator. *Neurosurgery* 1985; 16:154–160.
8. Colombo F, Benedetti A, Pozza F, et al. Linear accelerator radiosurgery of cerebral arteriovenous malformations. *Neurosurgery* 1989; 24:833–840.

9. Crawford PM, West CR, Chadwick DW, et al. Arteriovenous malformations of the brain: natural history in unoperated patients. *J Neurol Neurosurg Psychiatry* 1986; 49:1–10.
10. Dawson RC III, Tarr RW, Hecht ST, et al. Treatment of arteriovenous malformations of the brain with combined embolization and stereotactic radiosurgery: results after 1 and 2 years. *Am J Neuroradiol* 1990; 11:857–864.
11. Drake CG. Arteriovenous malformations of the brain: the options for management. *N Engl J Med* 1983; 309:308–310.
12. Ebeling JD, Tranmer BI, Davis KA, et al. Thrombosed arteriovenous malformations: A type of occult vascular malformation: magnetic resonance imaging and histopathological correlations. *Neurosurgery* 1988; 23:605–610.
13. Ehricke HH, Schad LR, Gademann G, et al. Use of MR angiography for stereotactic planning. *J Comput Assist Tomogr* 1992; 16:35–40.
14. Fabrikant JI, Frankel KA, Phillips MH, et al. Stereotactic heavy charged-particle Bragg peak radiosurgery for intracranial arteriovenous malformations. In Edwards MSB, Hoffman JH (eds): *Cerebral Vascular Diseases in Children and Adolescents.* Baltimore: Williams & Wilkins, 1989, pp 389–409.
15. Fabrikant JI, Lyman JT, Frankel KA. Heavy charged-particle Bragg peak radiosurgery for intracranial vascular disorders. *Radiat Res* 1985; 104(Suppl):S244–S258.
16. Fabrikant JI, Lyman JT, Hosobuchi Y. Stereotactic heavy-ion Bragg peak radiosurgery for intra-cranial vascular disorders: method for treatment of deep arteriovenous malformations. *Br J Radiol* 1984; 57:479–490.
17. Fabrikant JI, Lyman JT, Hosobuchi Y. Stereotactic heavy ion Bragg peak radiosurgery for intracranial vascular disorders. In Wilkins RH, Rengachary SS (eds): *Neurosurgery.* New York: McGraw-Hill, 1985, pp 1128–1132.
18. Flickinger JC. An integrated logistic formula for prediction of complications from radiosurgery. *Int J Radiat Oncol Biol Phys* 1989; 17:879–885.
19. Flickinger JC, Lunsford LD, Kondziolka D, et al. Radiosurgery and brain tolerance: an analysis of neurodiagnostic imaging changes after gamma knife radiosurgery for arteriovenous malformations. *Int J Radiat Oncol Biol Phys* 1992; 23:19–26.
20. Flickinger JC, Lunsford LD, Wu A, et al. Treatment planning for gamma knife radiosurgery with multiple isocenters. *Int J Radiat Oncol Biol Phys* 1990; 18:1495–1501.
21. Forster DE. The Sheffield ''gamma knife'' experience: results of arteriovenous malformations radiosurgery in 507 patients. In Lunsford LD (ed): *Stereotactic Radiosurgery Update.* New York: Elsevier, 1992, pp 113–115.
22. Fournier D, TerBrugge K, Rodesch G, et al. Revascularization of brain arteriovenous malformations after embolization with bucrylate. *Neuroradiology* 1990; 32:497–501.
23. Fults D, Kelly DL Jr. Natural history of arteriovenous malformations of the brain: a clinical study. *Neurosurgery* 1984; 15:658–662.
24. Graf CJ, Perret GE, Torner JC. Bleeding from cerebral arteriovenous malformations as part of their natural history. *J Neurosurg* 1983; 58:331–337.
25. Heifetz MD, Wexler M, Thompson R. Single-beam radiotherapy knife: a practical theoretical model. *J Neurosurg* 1984; 60:814–818.
26. Heikkinen ER, Konnov B, Melnikov L, et al. Relief of epilepsy by radiosurgery of cerebral arteriovenous malformations. *Stereotact Funct Neurosurg* 1989; 53:157–166.
27. Heros RC, Korosue K, Diebold PM. Surgical excision of cerebral arteriovenous malformations: late results. *Neurosurgery* 1990; 26:570–578.
28. Kashiwagi S, Van Loveren HR, Tew JM Jr, et al. Diagnosis and treatment of vascular brain-stem malformations. *J Neurosurg* 1990; 72:27–34.
29. Kjellberg RN, Abe M. Stereotactic Bragg peak proton beam therapy. In Lunsford LD (ed): *Modern Stereotactic Neurosurgery.* Boston: Martinus Nijhoff, 1988, pp 463–467.
30. Kjellberg RN, Davis KR, Lyons S, et al. Bragg peak proton beam therapy for arteriovenous malformation of the brain. *Clin Neurosurg* 1983; 31:248–290.
31. Kjellberg RN, Hanamura T, Davis KR, et al. Bragg-peak proton-beam therapy for arteriovenous malformations of the brain. *N Engl J Med* 1983; 309:269–274.
32. Kondziolka D, Dempsey PK, Lunsford LD. The case for conservative management of venous angiomas. *Can J Neurol Sci* 1991; 18:295–299.
33. Kondziolka D, Humphreys RP, Hoffman HJ, et al. Arteriovenous malformations of the brain in children: a forty year experience. *Can J Neurol Sci* 1992; 19:40–45.
34. Kondziolka D, Lunsford LD, Altschuler EM, et al. Biological effects of stereotactic radiosurgery in the normal primate brain stem. In Lunsford LD (ed): *Stereotactic Radiosurgery Update.* New York: Elsevier, 1992, pp 291–294.
35. Kondziolka D, Lunsford LD, Coffey RJ, et al. Stereotactic radiosurgery of angiographically occult vascular malformations: indications and preliminary experience. *Neurosurgery* 1990; 27:892–900.
36. Larsson B, Leksell L, Rexed B, et al. The high-energy proton beam as a neurosurgical tool. *Nature* 1958; 182:1222–1223.
37. Lawrence JH. Heavy particle irradiation of intracranial lesions: introduction. In Wilkins RH, Rengachary SS (eds): *Neurosurgery.* New York: McGraw-Hill, 1985, p 1113.
38. Leksell L. The stereotaxic method and radiosurgery of the brain. *Acta Chir Scand* 1951; 102:316–319.
39. Leksell L. Stereotactic radiosurgery. *J Neurol Neurosurg Psychiatry* 1983; 46:797–803.
40. Lindquist C, Steiner L. Stereotactic radiosurgical treatment of arteriovenous malformations. In Lunsford LD (ed): *Modern Stereotactic Neurosurgery.* Boston: Martinus Nijhoff, 1988, pp 491–505.
41. Lobato RD, Perez C, Rivas JJ, et al. Clinical, radiological, and pathological spectrum of angiographically occult intracranial vascular malformations: analysis of 21 cases and review of the literature. *J Neurosurg* 1988; 68:518–531.
42. Luessenhop AJ. Natural history of cerebral arteriovenous malformations. In Wilson CB, Stein BM (eds): *Intracranial Arteriovenous Malformations.* Baltimore: Williams & Wilkins, 1984, pp 12–23.
43. Lunsford LD, Flickinger JC, Lindner G, et al. Stereotactic radiosurgery of the brain using the first United States 201 cobalt-60 source gamma knife. *Neurosurgery* 1989; 24:151–159.
44. Lunsford LD, Kondziolka D, Bissonette DJ, et al. Stereotactic radiosurgery of brain vascular malformations. *Neurosurg Clin North Am* 1992; 3:79–98.
45. Lunsford LD, Kondziolka D, Flickinger JC, et al. Stereotactic radiosurgery for arteriovenous malformations of the brain. *J Neurosurg* 1991; 75:512–524.
46. Lutz W, Winston KR, Maleki PV. A system for stereotactic radiosurgery with a linear accelerator. *Int J Radiat Oncol Biol Phys* 1988; 14:373–381.
47. Lyman JT, Chong CY. ISAH: a versatile treatment positioner for external radiation therapy. *Cancer* 1974; 34:12–26.
48. Lyman JT, Howard J. Dosimetry and instrumentation for helium and heavy ions. *Int J Radiat Oncol Biol Phys* 1977; 3:81–85.
49. Lyman JT, Kanstein L, Yeater F, et al. A helium-ion bean for stereotactic radiosurgery of central nervous system disorders. *Med Phys* 1986; 13:695–699.
50. Marks MP, DeLaPaz RL, Fabrikant JI, et al. Intracranial vascular malformations: imaging of charged-particle radiosurgery. Part I. Results of therapy. *Radiology* 1988; 168:447–455.
51. Marks MP, DeLaPaz RL, Fabrikant JI, et al. Intracranial vascular malformations: imaging of charged-particle radiosurgery. Part II. Complications. *Radiology* 1988; 168:457–462.
52. McKenzie MR, Souhami L, Podgorsak EB, et al. Photon radiosurgery: a clinical review. *Can J Neurol Sci* 1992; 19:212–221.
53. Ondra SL, Troupp H, George ED, et al. The natural history of symptomatic arteriovenous malformations of the brain: a 24-year follow-up assessment. *J Neurosurg* 1990; 73:387–391.
54. Patil AA. Adaptation of linear accelerators to stereotactic systems. In

Lunsford LD (ed): *Modern Stereotactic Neurosurgery.* Boston: Martinus Nijhoff, 1988, pp 471–480.
55. Podgorsak EB, Olivier A, Pia M, et al. Dynamic stereotactic radiosurgery. *Int J Radiat Oncol Biol Phys* 1988; 14:115–126.
56. Rigamonti D, Dayer BP, Johnson PC, et al. The MRI appearance of cavernous malformations (angiomas). *J Neurosurg* 1987; 67:518–524.
57. Sadler LR, Jungreis CA, Lunsford LD, et al. Angiographic technique to precede gamma knife radiosurgery for intracranial arteriovenous malformations. *Am J Neuroradiol* 1990; 11:1157–1161.
58. Solomon RA, Stein BM. Management of arteriovenous malformations of the brain stem. *J Neurosurg* 1986; 64:857–864.
59. Spetzler RF, Martin NA. A proposed grading system for arteriovenous malformations. *J Neurosurg* 1986; 65:476–483.
60. Statham P, Macpherson P, Johnston R, et al. Cerebral radiation necrosis complicating stereotactic radiosurgery for arteriovenous malformations. *J Neurol Neurosurg Psychiatry* 1990; 53:476–479.
61. Steinberg GK, Fabrikant JI, Marks MP, et al. Stereotactic heavy-charged-particle Bragg-peak radiation for intracranial arteriovenous malformations. *N Engl J Med* 1990; 323:96–101.
62. Steiner L. Radiosurgery in cerebral arteriovenous malformations. In Fein JM, Flamm ES (eds): *Cerebrovascular Surgery.* New York: Springer-Verlag, 1984, pp 1161–1215.
63. Steiner L. Treatment of arteriovenous malformations by radiosurgery. In Wilson CB, Stein BM (ed): *Intracranial Arteriovenous Malformations.* Baltimore: Williams & Wilkins, 1984, pp 295–313.
64. Steiner L. Stereotactic radiosurgery with the cobalt 60 gamma unit in the surgical treatment of intracranial tumors and arteriovenous malformations. In Schmidek HH, Sweet WH (eds): *Operative Neurosurgical Techniques: Indications, Methods and Results,* 2d ed. Orlando: Grune & Stratton, 1988, pp 515–529.
65. Steiner L, Leksell L, Greitz T, et al. Stereotaxic radiosurgery for cerebral arteriovenous malformations. Report of a case. *Acta Chir Scand* 1972; 138:459–464.
66. Steiner L, Lindquist C, Adler JR, et al. Clinical outcome of radiosurgery for cerebral arteriovenous malformations. *J Neurosurg* 1992; 77:1–8.
67. Sturm VS, Kober BK, Höver KH, et al. Stereotactic percutaneous single dose irradiation of brain metastases with a linear accelerator. *Int J Radiat Oncol Biol Phys* 1987; 13:279–282.
68. Walton L, Bomford CK, Ramsden D. The Sheffield stereotactic radiosurgery unit: physical characteristics and principles of operation. *Br J Radiol* 1987; 60:897–906.
69. Weil S, Tew JM, Steiner L. Comparison of radiosurgery and microsurgery for treatment of cavernous malformations of the brain stem. *J Neurosurg* 1990; 72:336A (abstr).
70. Winston KR, Lutz W. Linear accelerator as a neurosurgical tool for stereotactic radiosurgery. *Neurosurgery* 1988; 22:454–464.
71. Yamamoto M, Jimbo M, Kobayashi M, et al. Long-term results of radiosurgery for arteriovenous malformation: neurodiagnostic imaging and histological studies of angiographically confirmed nidus obliteration. *Surg Neurol* 1992; 37:219–230.

247

Cavernous Malformations and Related Lesions

Daniele Rigamonti
Frank P.K. Hsu
Lee H. Monsein

Definition and History

The cavernous malformation (CM), also known as the cavernous angioma or cavernoma, is a vascular anomaly characterized by the presence of sinusoid-like capillary vessels. These capillaries are adjacent to one another, with little or no intervening brain parenchyma; the feeding arteries and draining veins are most often normal in size. The blood flow in the cavernous angioma is slow; therefore, standard angiography techniques usually fail to visualize this type of lesion. Stagnation of blood is also characteristic and is frequently the cause of thrombosis and calcification.

CMs can occur anywhere in the central nervous system. Their distribution seems to reflect the relative volume of the different structures. Multiple lesions are common: in a recent large series of 8131 magnetic resonance (MR) scans, the incidence of CMs was 0.4 percent; the incidence of multiple lesions in this group was 18.7 percent.[5] In patients with multiple cerebral CMs, similar lesions can be found in other organ systems.[49,50] Cerebral CMs are generally sporadic; at least 6 percent of cases are familial, however.[9]

On microscopic examination, the cerebral CM is a well-lobulated, circumscribed lesion; since it is either dark red or purple in color, often it is described as mulberry-like. An average diameter of 4.9 mm was reported in one large prospective autopsy series[22]; clinical descriptions usually give a greater diameter. The mean lesion size in a surgical series conducted by Giombini and Morello was 3.5 cm[8]; Yasargil reported a mean lesion size of 2.2 cm in a more recent surgical series.[52] There is a significant correlation between size and symptomatology.

CMs vary in consistency from soft to hard, depending on the relative proportions of blood-filled spaces, calcification, ossification, and areas of thrombosis. The surrounding brain parenchyma is typically gliotic and stained yellow by hemosiderin. This staining is the result of either frank hemorrhage or slow diffusion of pigment into the surrounding tissue following lysis of red blood cells. The presence of highly epileptogenic iron salts in the susceptible brain structures explains the high incidence of seizures in patients with CMs.[45]

Microscopically, the CM is characterized by enlarged capillaries, which are composed of a thin collagenous wall covered by a single layer of endothelium without smooth muscle fibers or elastic fibers. Typically, CMs do not have intermingled brain parenchyma; at the periphery, however, the dilated capillaries of many CMs may be separated by normal brain.[30] Hemosiderin-laden macrophages are invariably found secondary to previous hemorrhage or red blood cell lysis.[30] Varying degrees of thrombosis, fibrous scarring, calcification, and ossification are often present.[30]

Clinical Features

A comprehensive review of the literature shows that patients with symptomatic CMs have presented with seizures (39 percent), hemorrhage (32 percent), or a mass effect (29 percent).[43] A study of the members of six families with CMs, however, confirms that these malformations are asymptomatic in a significant percentage of cases (11 percent).[29] In this study, seizures were the most common symptom (55 percent), followed by progressive neurological deficit (15%), headache (15 percent), and hemorrhage (4 percent).[29] A more recent compilation of 664 patients assembled from the literature corroborates seizures as the predominant symptom (31 percent), followed by progressive neurological deficits (25 percent), hemorrhage (13 percent), and headache (6 percent); asymptomatic cases were more common than previously reported (21 percent).[9]

Two CM variants have been described: a cystic form and the so-called hemangioma calcificans. The cystic form tends to cause recurrent bleeding and is common in the posterior fossa, with a noticeable degree of surrounding edema.[1,44] In the absence of clear histologic confirmation, the hemangioma calcificans is presumed to be a calcified CM. Commonly located in the temporal lobe, it causes seizures and usually, because of its densely calcified structure, does not bleed.[23,37,38]

Imaging

The use of magnetic resonance imaging (MRI) means that CMs are now usually diagnosed at an earlier and much smaller stage than before, and rarely is calcification seen. Two old surgical studies reported the presence of calcification on conventional skull radiographs in 8 to 10 percent of the patients.[40,48] Similarly, earlier reports described angiographic abnormalities in 60 to 70 percent of cases[14,25,27,28]; this result also reflects a time before the advent of MRI, when patients typically had larger, symptomatic lesions. A capillary blush and early filling of the veins without enlargement of the arteries is very rarely seen.[13] Opacification of the cavernous spaces has been noted occasionally when using prolonged arterial injection.[19]

Computed Tomography

The computed tomographic x-ray (CT scan) can detect cavernous malformations and the distortions produced by a mass effect. On unenhanced CT scans, cavernous malformations appear as focal areas of increased attenuation[27,41,47]; only a few lesions appear hypodense.[40,47] An increase in density is characteristic of recent hemorrhage as well as of calcification, and increased attenuation can be observed on scans following an acute hemorrhage, which is frequently accompanied by a mass effect.[28] Areas of punctate calcification are visualized in 14 percent of cases.[40]

The intravenous (IV) administration of a contrast agent permits a faint enhancement.[27,40,41] The CT can outline abnormalities encroaching on the brain stem; however, an acute brain stem hemorrhage that produces subarachnoid or fourth ventricular hemorrhage is more likely to be due to a cryptic arteriovenous malformation (AVM) than to a CM.[53]

Magnetic Resonance Imaging

MRI yields extraordinary resolution and is particularly helpful in identifying CMs. On both T1- and T2-weighted images, the CM is represented as a well-defined, usually rounded lesion. The lesion is characterized by a rim of decreased signal intensity at the periphery and a heterogeneous central signal.[24,28] The hypodensity of the rim is produced by the presence of hemosiderin; the appearance of the central core is generated by blood and blood byproducts in various stages of evolution. Areas of increased signal outside the hemosiderin rim on T2-weighted images may represent edema.[28] Smaller CMs may appear only as petechial areas of decreased signal intensity (''black dots'').[28] Although enlarged vessels are not characteristic of CMs, a coexisting venous angioma has been identified now and then.[32,33]

It is important to recognize that these appearances are not limited to CMs and that a differential diagnosis is important to rule out the presence of a cryptic AVM or hemorrhagic neoplasm.[26,27] Hemorrhagic neoplasms, even when small, are accompanied by edema, which is usually absent from small CMs.[46] Magnetic resonance angiography (MRA) permits visualization of the CM by the time-of-flight technique but not by the phase contrast technique.[24]

Positron Emission Tomography

Positron emission tomography (PET) uses the uptake of radioisotopes to scan the brain. Both CT and MRI provide far more structural detail, but PET scanning can differentiate a CM from a tumor, since radioisotope uptake is markedly elevated in tumors but not in CMs.[24] One small series reported normal or decreased radioisotope uptake in CMs.[6]

Management

A prerequisite for the management of CMs is a knowledge of their natural history. Several prospective MRI series of patients harboring characteristic lesions have yielded a clearer understanding of the true risk of overt hemorrhage from a CM. A recent report estimates that the annual bleeding risk is 0.7 percent per patient.[36] Based on the assumption of uniform risk from birth to the age at which a hemorrhage is diagnosed, the risk is calculated to be 0.25 percent per lesion per year.[5] Although this information is useful, it is not necessarily accurate: The risk of hemorrhage may not be uniform and may depend on other factors, such as gender, age, and previous hemorrhage. It also is important to compare the lower risk of bleeding from a CM to the higher risk of bleeding from an AVM, which is calculated to be approximately 4.0 percent per year.[21] Furthermore, the consequences of a hemorrhage from a CM are rarely catastrophic, in contrast to the case with an AVM or aneurysm.

The course of a nonhemorrhagic lesion seems to correlate with the initial clinical presentation. In the absence of gross hemorrhage, one study reported a poor to fair outcome for 16 percent of patients.[36] Patients who present with seizures are very likely to become symptomatic again, and, frequently, seizure control becomes more difficult with time. The location of the lesion also may be significant; CMs in the infratentorial compartment may be associated with a more aggressive natural history (Fig. 247-1).[35]

Most lesions discovered incidentally require no therapy.[17] Occasionally, these lesions cannot be differentiated from tumors, and a biopsy is indicated. Surgical intervention can be attempted when a CM is identified as a seizure focus in patients with refractory seizures. In our opinion, surgery is not indicated as a measure to decrease the risk of bleeding in a patient who has never bled.

In children, surgical intervention is indicated to treat symptoms related to mass effect, hemorrhage, or seizures.[42] Surgery is favored more for children than for adults because of the higher risk of hemorrhage and greater epileptic potential in children.

The effect of pregnancy on CMs remains speculative. Although a statistically significant association between hemorrhage and pregnancy has yet to be established, pregnant women accounted for 86 percent of the hemorrhages (one-third in the first trimester) in one recent series.[36] There also are anecdotal cases of CMs expanding and becoming symptomatic during early pregnancy.[20,51] Based on our limited knowledge, it seems that an increased risk of lesion expansion and hemorrhage exists during pregnancy.

If the mother is stable, conservative management may be appropriate, and vaginal delivery is not contraindicated. Surgical resection before conception is preferred, provided the CM is located in a favorable location. Possible risks and management options should be discussed with women who plan to become pregnant, and surgical recommendations can be made at that time.

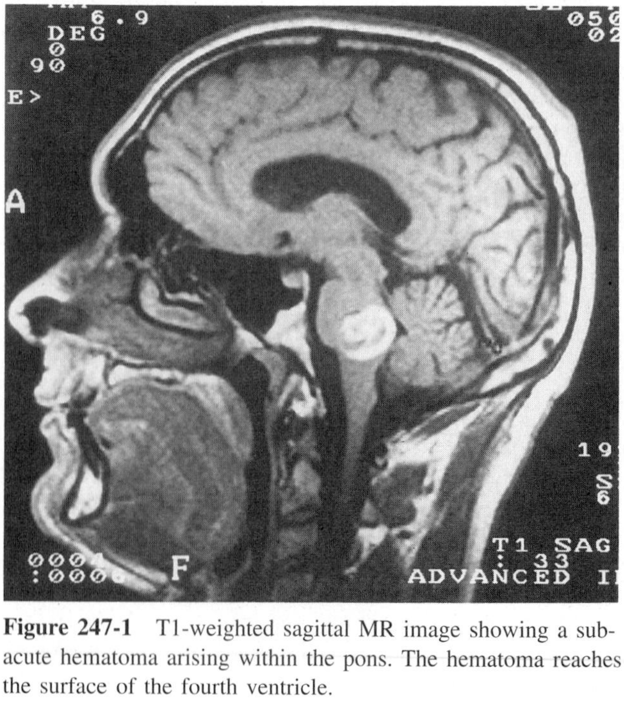

Figure 247-1 T1-weighted sagittal MR image showing a subacute hematoma arising within the pons. The hematoma reaches the surface of the fourth ventricle.

Surgical Intervention

A thorough medical history, family history, and physical examination, and detailed neuroimaging studies are crucial to the preoperative evaluation. MRI is particularly helpful in identifying the exact preoperative location of the lesion and detecting multiple lesions, which often are not detected by CT. For patients with a seizure disorder, electroencephalography (EEG) can confirm whether the epileptic focus is anatomically related to the CM, and can localize the seizure focus when multiple CMs are present.

Standard microsurgical techniques are employed for the resection of CMs. The surgical microscope and microsurgical instrumentation have revolutionized the surgical treatment of CMs, particularly the treatment of lesions located in the brain stem or deep in the cerebral hemispheres. Some authorities have recommended the use of the CO_2 laser, but it does not seem necessary for extirpation of these lesions. One useful addition to the surgical armamentarium is a stereotactic system, which can be used to precisely localize deep-seated lesions intraoperatively.

Usually, significant intraoperative bleeding does not accompany the resection of a CM. One area of notable exception is the extracerebral middle fossa CM. Significant bleeding in this area is probably due to intralesional pressures that are at once decidedly lower (38.2 ± 0.5 mmHg) than mean arterial blood pressures (99.6 ± 15.1 mmHg) and higher than central venous pressures (5.0 ± 1.0 mmHg).

In Giombini's first large, personal series accompanied by a review of the literature, 33 patients were known to have undergone radical resection of the lesion. All but three (10 percent) had improved or else continued with stable deficits after a follow-up averaging several years.[8] The two factors given as relating to surgical success were (1) the presence of a dissection plane and (2) a relatively scarce supply of blood to the CM.

A more recent publication reported 17 cases with an excellent outcome and 2 cases with a good outcome among 19 patients who had hemispheric lesions; on the other hand, the outcome in patients with lesions in the thalamus, pineal region, or spinal cord was consistently poor.[47] The higher surgical morbidity associated with deep-seated CMs has several distinct causes: damage to the internal capsule, injury to the lenticulostriate arteries, damage to the venous drainage, air embolism, and recurrent hemorrhage from a residual angioma.[3]

A fairly high incidence of surgical complications has chilled some of the initial enthusiasm.[3] The report on the largest series of brain stem CMs stresses the importance of combining clinical examination findings and MRI data to determine a safe surgical corridor for approaching the lesion (Fig. 247-2).[53] The authors recommend surgical resection for symptomatic brain stem CMs because the brain stem's ability to withstand expansion is poor.[53]

Deep CMs located in critical areas have been treated with radiosurgery. The results have not been favorable: the incidence of complications, presumably due to delayed radiation injury, is much higher than in a similar series of AVM patients.[12] We discourage radiosurgical treatment for CMs, as its efficacy is very difficult to evaluate. To start with, angiographic findings appear normal, even before radiosurgery, and any spontaneous reduction in the size of the CM following a hemorrhage would further complicate evaluation.

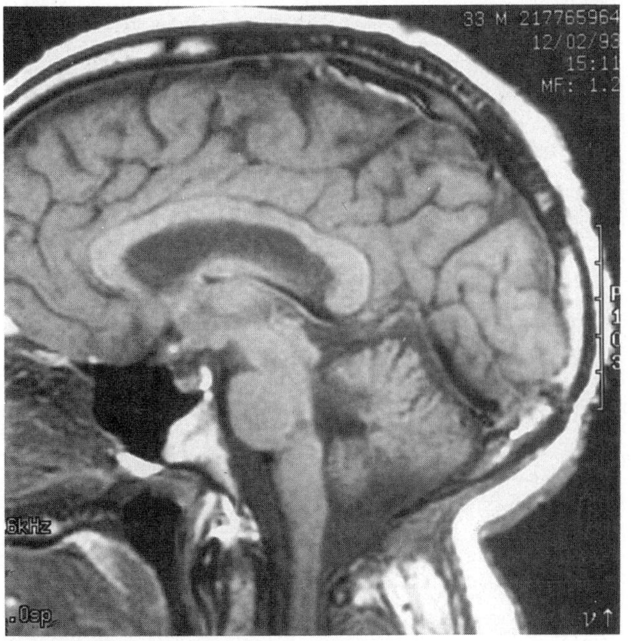

Figure 247-2 T1-weighted sagittal MR image demonstrating successful resection of the lesion shown in Figure 247-1. The pathologic diagnosis was cavernous malformation.

Middle Cranial Fossa Cavernous Malformations

Middle cranial fossa CMs are extraparenchymal and usually extradural. Histologically, these lesions are composed of dilated cavernous channels lacking mural smooth muscle.[11] They routinely surround the structures in the cavernous sinus, including the internal carotid artery and cranial nerves III through VI. These lesions are rare and primarily affect women.

The clinical presentation includes headaches and, more commonly, acute or subacute visual symptoms. Ocular findings include proptosis, visual loss, field cuts, and diplopia. Facial numbness and pituitary dysfunction are less common. Lesion growth often erodes the bone in the area of the cavernous sinus. Angiography outlines a vascular mass without an arteriovenous shunt. These lesions are a formidable surgical problem, as they tend to cause intraoperative, life-threatening hemorrhages. After biopsy, terminating attempts to further resect the lesion will drastically reduce mortality and morbidity, as will giving a course of radiotherapy prior to definitive surgical treatment.[32]

Retinal Cavernous Angioma

Retinal cavernous angiomas have been linked to one of four neurooculocutaneous syndromes (ophthalmic phakomatoses), characterized by disseminated hamartomas of the eye, skin, and brain.[7,40] On direct visualization of the retina, these lesions resemble clusters of grapes protruding from the inner retinal surface into the vitreous. The capillaries appear thin-walled and are similar to those of cerebral CMs. The arteries and veins surrounding the lesion are normal in appearance.

Fluorescein angiography is helpful, demonstrating a significant delay in the perfusion of dye through the lesion. This is why some workers recommend angiography with a very late venous phase to visualize these lesions.[18]

Calvarial Hemangioma

Calvarial hemangiomas occur more often in females than males and present as a painless, bony swelling usually in the parietal or frontal region. The scalp moves freely over the mass, and roentgenograms depict a well-defined lucent area with a trabeculated appearance. During angiography, the contrast agent pools within the lesion in the venous phase. Histologically, cavernous capillaries are separated by bony spicules.

Capillary Telangiectasias

The capillary telangiectasia (also called a capillary malformation) is a lesion characterized by the presence of capillary vessels with saccular and fusiform dilation interspersed among normal brain parenchyma. Capillary telangiectasias are punctate lesions composed of small dilated capillaries that are devoid of muscle and elastic fibers. On gross inspection, a capillary telangiectasia resembles a cluster of petechial hemorrhages. No abnormal arteries are present in the periphery of the lesion, but it may drain into an enlarged central vein.[4] The feature that most distinguishes these lesions from CMs is the presence of normal brain parenchyma between the dilated vessels. Typically, the parenchyma does not show evidence of gliosis or hemorrhage. Most of these malformations are clinically silent and are discovered at autopsy. They occur in the same locations as CMs and, like them, are frequently multiple. Observations of lesions transitional between capillary telangiectasia and cavernous malformation have been documented for years, which leads to the supposition that one lesion is the precursor of the other.[30] Radiologic studies were not able to detect capillary telangiectasias in the past; however, MRI can detect them as punctate areas of decreased signal intensity on T2-weighted images.[28] The hypodensity is due to the presence of small amounts of hemosiderin and, most likely, previous subclinical hemorrhages or diapedesis of red blood cells through the walls of the lesion. A true, massive hemorrhage is exceedingly rare, and only anecdotal cases have been reported. The importance of this lesion is that it represents a possible link between different types of vascular malformations.

Venous Angiomas

The venous angioma (venous malformation, medullary venous malformation) is characterized by an abnormal-looking but physiologically competent venous drainage. Venous angiomas are usually located in the deep white matter, drain an array of fine medullary veins that converge on them, and drain in turn into either the superficial or deep venous system[10]; most are located in the cerebral hemispheres or cerebellum.[39]

Macroscopically, a tuft of fine veins converge into an enlarged central venous trunk that appears much larger than the veins joining it. Microscopically, the vein appears normal in structure, except for occasional evidence of hyalinization and thickening. No abnormal arteries are associated with the venous malformation, and evidence of thrombosis, hemorrhage, or calcification is rare.[16] The intervening parenchyma appears normal.

The classic angiographic term for this lesion is *caput medusae,* coined because the numerous small veins appear in a radial arrangement around the enlarged central trunk; the arterial and capillary phases appear angiographically normal. By CT and MRI, the venous angioma typically appears as a linear or curvilinear structure with a nidus at the vessel origin resembling the spokes of a wheel.[33] Clinically, venous angiomas are usually asymptomatic and their discovery is incidental; however, venous malformations located in the posterior fossa tend to be more symptomatic (Fig. 247-3).

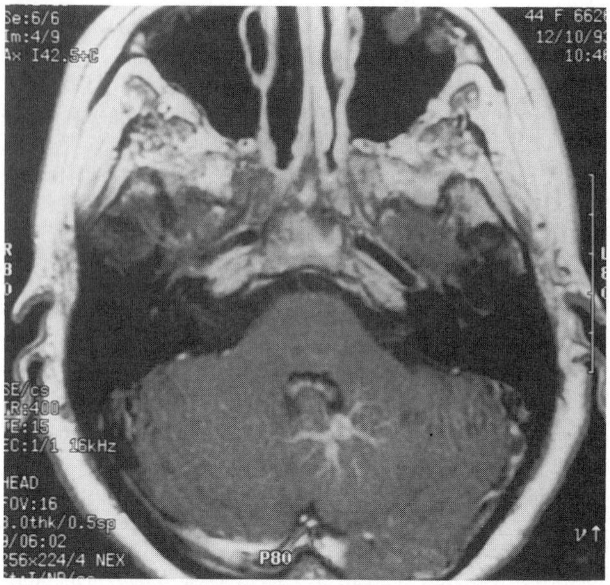

(*A*)

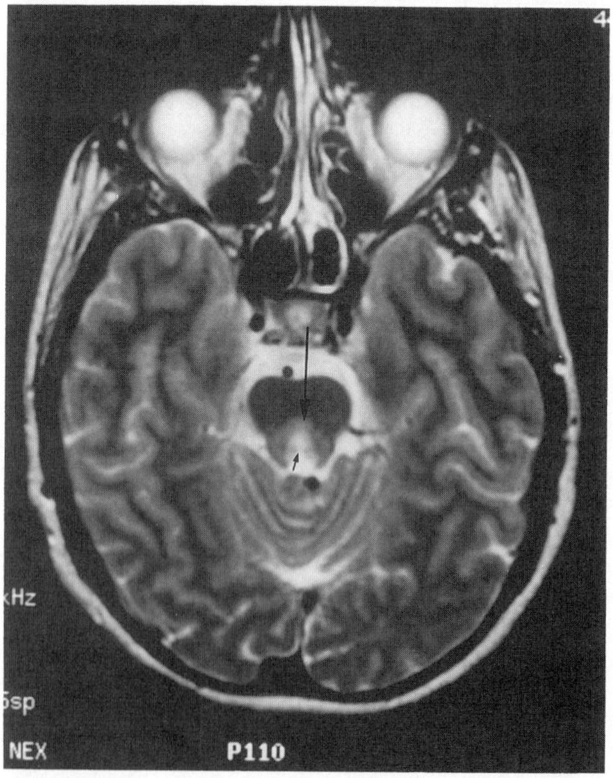

(*B*)

Figure 247-3 *A.* T1-weighted axial MR image, after administration of Gd-DTPA, demonstrating a venous angioma adjacent to the lateral recess of the fourth ventricle. *B.* T2-weighted axial MR image demonstrating increased signal in the midbrain tectum *(arrow).* The patient suffers from acute bilateral internuclear ophthalmoplegia.

Some authorities recommend more aggressive management of posterior fossa venous angiomas when they are associated with a hemorrhage.[2,15] This approach, however, carries a significant risk because the elimination of an abnormal-looking but functional draining vein, whether by surgical, endovascular, or radiosurgical techniques, can precipitate a venous infarction.[34] The natural history of this malformation seems to be quite benign, according to some initial follow-up studies. A most interesting and clinically relevant characteristic of this lesion is its relatively common association with a cavernous malformation.[32] This phenomenon is too common to be only coincidental. It raises several interesting questions regarding the possible genesis of cavernous malformations and the causative effect a venous angioma may have on the dilatation of the capillaries with which it is connected. Another important corollary to this previously underestimated association is that, if hemorrhage occurs, it most likely arises from the cavernous malformation rather than the venous angioma. Prior to the use of CT and MRI, a hematoma in the vicinity of a venous malformation was thought to be due to the venous malformation; any coexisting cavernous malformation could not be detected on the angiogram. Nowadays, it is standard to look for a cavernous angioma in the vicinity of a venous angioma. If a hemorrhage occurs, the clot and cavernous angioma are removed, while the venous malformation is best left alone.

References

1. Bellotti C, Medina M, Oliveri G, et al. Cystic cavernous angiomas of the posterior fossa. Report of three cases. *J Neurosurg* 1985; 63:797–799.
2. Berenstein A, Choi IS. Treatment of venous angiomas by direct alcohol injection. *Am J Neuroradiol* 1983; 4:1144 (abstr).
3. Bertalanffy H, Gilsbach JM, Eggert HR, et al. Microsurgery of deep-seated cavernous angiomas: report of 26 cases. *Acta Neurochir (Wien)* 1991; 108:91–99.
4. Blackwood W. Two cases of benign cerebral telangiectasis. *J Pathol Bacteriol* 1941; 52:209–212.
5. Curling OD Jr, Kelly DL Jr, Elster AD, et al. An analysis of the natural history of cavernous angiomas. *J Neurosurg* 1991; 75:702–708.
6. Ericson K, von Holst H, Mosskin M, et al. Positron emission tomography of cavernous haemangiomas of the brain. *Acta Radiologica Diagn (Stockh)* 1986; 27:379–383.
7. Gass JD. Cavernous hemangioma of the retina: a neuro-oculo-cutaneous syndrome. *Am J Ophthalmol* 1971; 71:799–814.
8. Giombini S, Morello G. Cavernous angiomas of the brain. Account of fourteen personal cases and review of the literature. *Acta Neurochir (Wien)* 1978; 40:61–82.
9. Hsu FPK, Rigamonti D, Huhn SL. Epidemiology of cavernous malformations. In Awad IA, Barrow DL (eds): *Cavernous Malformations.* Park Ridge, IL: American Association of Neurological Surgeons, 1993, pp 13–23.
10. Huang YP, Robbins A, Patel SC, et al. Cerebral venous malformations and a new classification of cerebral vascular malformations. In Kapp JP, Schmidek HH (eds): *The Cerebral Venous System and Its Disorders.* New York: Grune and Stratton, 1984, pp 373–474.
11. Johnson PC, Wascher TM, Golfinos J, et al. Definition and pathologic features. In Awad JA, Barrow DL (eds). *Cavernous Malformations.* Park Ridge, IL: American Association of Neurological Surgeons, 1993, pp 1–11.
12. Kondziolka D, Lunsford LD, Coffey RJ, et al. Stereotactic radiosurgery of angiographically occult vascular malformations: indications and preliminary experience. *Neurosurgery* 1990; 27:892–900.
13. Liliequist B. Angiography in intracerebral cavernous hemangioma. *Neuroradiology* 1975; 9:69–72.
14. Lobato RD, Perez C, Rivas JJ, et al. Clinical, radiological, and pathological spectrum of angiographically occult intracranial vascular malformations. Analysis of 21 cases and review of literature. *J Neurosurg* 1988; 68:518–531.
15. Malik GM, Morgan JK, Boulos RS, et al. Venous angiomas: an underestimated cause of intracranial hemorrhage. *Surg Neurol* 1988; 30:350–358.
16. McCormick WF, Hardman JM, Boulter TR. Vascular malformations (''angiomas'') of the brain, with special reference to those occurring in the posterior fossa. *J Neurosurg* 1968; 28:241–251.
17. Michelson WJ. Conservative management. In Awad IA, Barrow DL (eds): *Cavernous Malformations.* Park Ridge, IL: American Association of Neurological Surgeons, 1993, pp 81–85.
18. Numaguchi Y, Fukui M, Miyake E, et al. Angiographic manifestations of intracerebral cavernous hemangioma. *Neuroradiology* 1977; 14:113–116.
19. Numaguchi Y, Kishikawa T, Fukui M, et al. Prolonged injection angiography for diagnosing intracranial cavernous hemangiomas. *Radiology* 1979; 131:137–138.
20. Ondra SL, Doty JR, Mahla ME, et al. Surgical excision of a cavernous hemangioma of the rostral brain stem: case report. *Neurosurgery* 1988; 23:490–493.
21. Ondra SL, Troupp H, George ED, et al. The natural history of symptomatic arteriovenous malformations of the brain: a 24-year follow-up assessment. *J Neurosurg* 1990; 73:387–391.
22. Otten P, Pizzolato GP, Rilliet B, et al. A propos de 131 cas d'angiomes caverneux (cavernomes) du S.N.C., repérés par l'analyse rétrospective de 24,535 autopsies. *Neurochirurgie* 1989; 35:82–83.
23. Penfield W, Ward A. Calcifying epileptogenic lesions: hemangioma calcificans. Report of a case. *Arch Neurol Psychiatry* 1948; 60:20–36.
24. Perl J, Ross JS. Diagnostic imaging of cavernous malformations. In Awad IA, Barrow DL (eds): *Cavernous Malformations.* Park Ridge, IL: American Association of Neurological Surgeons, 1993, pp 37–48.
25. Rao VR, Pillai SM, Shenoy KT, et al. Hypervascular cavernous angioma at angiography. *Neuroradiology* 1979; 18:211–214.
26. Rapacki TF, Brantley MJ, Furlow TW Jr, et al. Heterogeneity of cerebral cavernous hemangiomas diagnosed by MR imaging. *J Comput Assist Tomogr* 1990; 14:18–25.
27. Requena I, Arias M, Lopez-Ibor L, et al. Cavernomas of the central nervous system: clinical and neuroimaging manifestations in 47 patients. *J Neurol Neurosurg Psychiatry* 1991; 54:590–594.
28. Rigamonti D, Drayer BP, Johnson PC, et al. The MRI appearance of cavernous malformations (angiomas). *J Neurosurg* 1987; 67:518–524.
29. Rigamonti D, Hadley MN, Drayer BP, et al. Cerebral cavernous malformations: incidence and familial occurrence. *N Engl J Med* 1988; 319:343–347.
30. Rigamonti D, Johnson PC, Spetzler RF, et al. Cavernous malformations and capillary telangiectasia: a spectrum within a single pathological entity. *Neurosurgery* 1991; 28:60–64.
31. Rigamonti D, Pappas CTE, Spetzler RF, et al. Extracerebral cavernous angiomas of the middle fossa. *Neurosurgery* 1990; 27:306–310.
32. Rigamonti D, Spetzler RF. The association of venous and cavernous malformations: report of four cases and discussion of the pathophysiological, diagnostic and therapeutic implications. *Acta Neurochir (Wien)* 1988; 92:100–105.
33. Rigamonti D, Spetzler RF, Drayer BP, et al. Appearance of venous malformations on magnetic resonance imaging. *J Neurosurg* 1988; 69:535–539.
34. Rigamonti D, Spetzler RF, Medina M, et al. Cerebral venous malformations. *J Neurosurg* 1990; 73:560–564.
35. Robinson JR, Awad IA. Clinical spectrum and natural course. In Awad IA, Barrow DL (eds): *Cavernous Malformations.* Park Ridge, IL: American Association of Neurological Surgeons, 1993, pp 25–36.
36. Robinson JR, Awad IA, Little JR. Natural history of the cavernous angioma. *J Neurosurg* 1991; 75:709–714.
37. Runnels JB, Gifford DB, Forsberg PL, et al. Dense calcification in a large cavernous angioma. Case Report. *J Neurosurg* 1969; 30:293–298.

38. Russell DS, Rubinstein LJ. *Pathology of Tumours of the Nervous System.* 5th ed. London: E. Arnold, 1989, pp 730–736.
39. Sarwar M, McCormick WF. Intracerebral venous angioma: case report and review. *Arch Neurol* 1978; 35:323–325.
40. Savoiardo M, Strada L, Passerini A. Cavernous hemangiomas of the orbit: value of CT, angiography, and phlebography. *Am J Neuroradiol* 1983; 4:741–744.
41. Savoiardo M, Strada L, Passerini A. Intracranial cavernous hemangiomas: neuroradiologic review of 36 operated cases. *Am J Neuroradiol* 1983; 4:945–950.
42. Scott RM, Barnes P, Kupsky W, et al. Cavernous angiomas of the central nervous system in children. *J Neurosurg* 1992; 76:38–46.
43. Simard JM, Garcia-Bengochea F, Ballinger WE Jr, et al. Cavernous angioma: a review of 126 collected and 12 new clinical cases. *Neurosurgery* 1986; 18:162–172.
44. Steiger HJ, Markwalder TM, Reulen HJ. Clinicopathological relations of cerebral cavernous angiomas: observations in eleven cases. *Neurosurgery* 1987; 21:879–884.
45. Sypert GW, Willmore LJ. A new model of post-traumatic epilepsy: iron cations. Presented at the 28th Meeting of the Congress of Neurological Surgeons, Washington, DC 1978. (abstr).
46. Sze G, Krol G, Olsen WL, et al. Hemorrhagic neoplasms: MR mimics of occult vascular malformations. *Am J Roentgenol* 1987; 149:1223–1230.
47. Vaquero J, Salazar J, Martinez R, et al. Cavernomas of the central nervous system: clinical syndromes, CT scan diagnosis, and prognosis after surgical treatment in 25 cases. *Acta Neurochir (Wien)* 1987; 85:29–33.
48. Voigt K, Yasargil MG. Cerebral cavernous haemangiomas or cavernomas. Incidence, pathology, localization, diagnosis, clinical features and treatment. Review of the literature and report of an unusual case. *Neurochirurgia (Stuttg)* 1976; 19:59–68.
49. Weskamp C, Cotlier I. Angioma del cerebro y de la retina con malformaciones capilares de la piel. *Arch Oftalmol (Buenos Aires)* 1940; 15:1–10.
50. Wood MW, White RJ, Kernohan JW. Cavernous haemangioma of the cerebrum. *Br J Surg* 1957; 38:245–246.
51. Yamasaki T, Handa H, Yamashita J, et al. Intracranial and orbital cavernous angiomas. A review of 30 cases. *J Neurosurg* 1986; 64:197–208.
52. Yaşargil MG. *Microneurosurgery.* Vol. IIIB: *AVM of the Brain, Clinical Considerations, General and Special Operative Techniques, Surgical Results, Nonoperated Cases, Cavernous and Venous Angiomas, Neuroanesthesia.* New York: Georg Thieme Verlag, 1988, pp 419–434.
53. Zimmerman RS, Spetzler RF, Lee KS, et al. Cavernous malformations of the brain stem. *J Neurosurg* 1991; 75:32–39.

248

Telangiectasias and Venous Angiomas

Setti S. Rengachary
Uma P. Kalyan-Raman

Vascular malformations of the nervous system can be divided into four major clinicopathologic categories (Fig. 248-1).

1. An *arteriovenous malformation* (AVM, racemose angioma, arteriovenous fistula, cirsoid aneurysm) consists of large feeding arteries, markedly dilated draining veins, and a vascular nidus consisting of tortuous dilated vessels but no capillary bed. Arterial blood directly shunts into the venous system, resulting in poor tissue perfusion and tissue ischemia.
2. A *cavernous hemangioma* (cavernoma, cavernous malformation) consists of a honeycomb of vascular spaces containing blood in very sluggish circulation. The blood is essentially stagnant and remains sequestrated in these vascular spaces. As a consequence, sedimentation, thrombosis, calcification, and ossification occur. The feeding artery and the draining vein are quite small and are not usually demonstrable on radiologic studies. There is no brain tissue in the malformation.
3. *Capillary telangiectasia* represents a collection of abnormally dilated, varicose capillaries with intervening brain parenchyma.
4. A *venous angioma* is a vascular malformation without an apparent arterial component. It consists of a myriad of small tapering veins arranged in a radial fashion in the deep white matter. These veins drain into a central vein, which in turn empties into a prominent cortical vein or dural sinus.

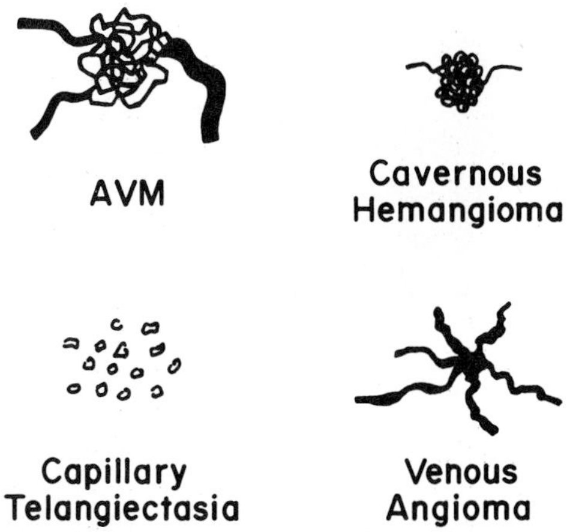

Figure 248-1 Types of vascular malformations that occur in the nervous system. AVM, arteriovenous malformation.

Only the latter two entities are discussed in this chapter.

Capillary Telangiectasias

Capillary telangiectasias are malformations composed of pathologically dilated capillaries. Most of these malformations are clinically silent, are not readily detectable on imaging studies, and are found incidentally at autopsy. They occur most commonly in the pons, near the midline. Other common locations are the cerebral cortex and the paraventricular white matter. On occasion they may be multiple[6] or may occur in association with other vascular malformations such as cavernous hemangiomas; indeed, in some instances transitional forms between telangiectasias, cavernous hemangiomas, and venous angiomas may occur.[26] In exceptional cases telangiectasias may calcify and may be diagnosed as hemangioma calcificans[34] in plain roentgenograms. In one unusual case, the medulla oblongata was extensively involved with this malformation, which resembled a sieve. The patient, who died of lymphosarcoma, had had a progressive unexplained neurological deficit for several years prior to death.[10] Massive hemorrhage from capillary telangiectasia into the brain parenchyma has been reported; the source of bleeding in such instances may be missed unless biopsy of the wall of the hematoma is undertaken.

Pathology

On gross inspection, the malformation appears as poorly defined punctate pink foci resembling an area of petechial hemorrhage. No dilated arteries or veins are seen leading to or from the malformation. Microscopically, the lesion consists of a group of variably dilated and varicose capillaries. In contrast to cavernous hemangiomas, there is intervening brain parenchyma (Fig. 248-2). This parenchyma generally appears normal, without evidence of gliosis, necrosis, or recent or remote hemorrhage.

Telangiectasias Presenting with Pontine Hematomas

The pons is the most common site of telangiectasias and related cryptic malformations in the posterior fossa. In certain instances, a patient with such a lesion may present with a primary pontine hematoma. It is imperative to differentiate this lesion from other causes of pontine hematoma such as hypertension, trauma, vasculopathy, coagulopathy, bleeding into a pre-existing tumor, and Duret hemorrhage, which follows tentorial herniation. Although most primary pontine hematomas are secondary to systemic hypertension, those occurring spontaneously in young, normotensive individuals should be assumed to be due to rupture of a cryptic malformation, even if such a malformation cannot be demonstrated by imaging studies or at operation.[27]

Based on a comprehensive postmortem study, McCormick and Nofzinger[21] found that, unlike large arteriovenous malformations, which are located predominantly in the supratentorial compartment, small cryptic malformations were distributed equally between supra- and infratentorial sites. In the infratentorial region, cryptic vascular malformations occur in the tegmentum of the

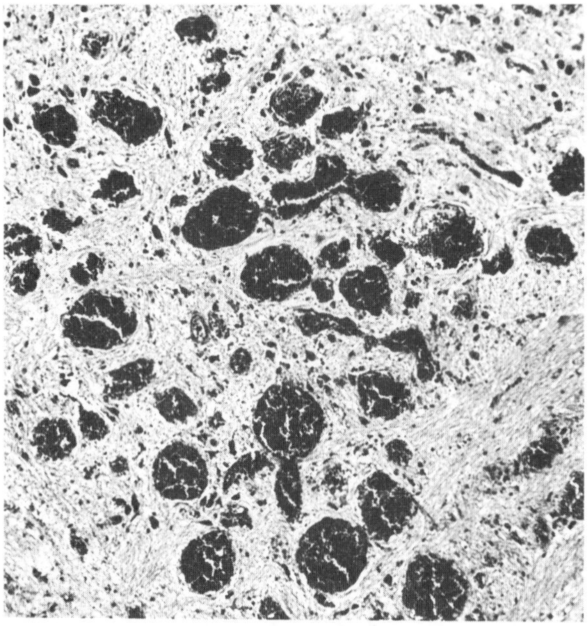

Figure 248-2 Capillary telangiectasia. The lesion consists of pathologically dilated capillaries with intervening brain parenchyma.

pons.[35] Less frequent sites include the cerebellum, midbrain,[9,14,29] and medulla.[15]

Major determinants of the clinical presentation of a pontine hematoma are its location and the extent of the clot within the pons (Fig. 248-3). The more common, large hematomas that result from systemic hypertension generally occupy the central pons and involve the reticular activating system, the basis pontis, the descending sympathetic pathways, and the pontine gaze center. They give rise to the syndrome that clinicians most commonly associate with pontine hematomas—namely, the abrupt onset of coma with quadriplegia, bilateral decerebrate posture, pinpoint pupils with a flicker of reaction to light, absence of horizontal eye movements (either spontaneous or reflexly induced), ocular bobbing, hyperthermia, and severe respiratory abnormalities. The outcome is almost invariably death. Patients in this category are seldom, if ever, considered for surgical therapy. The less common presentation shown by patients harboring telangiectasias of the pons is the partial pontine syndrome, which results from a hematoma restricted to the lateral half of the pons with sparing of the reticular activating system (Fig. 248-3). Thus, the cardinal features differentiating this from the preceding syndrome are preservation of consciousness and unilaterality of signs. The partial pontine syndrome may be divided into two subtypes[17]—a dorsolateral tegmental syndrome and a tegmentobasilar hemipontine syndrome. The principal difference between the two subtypes is the involvement of the basis pontis in the latter, with involvement of the corticospinal tract giving rise to contralateral hemiplegia. The main clinical manifestations of partial pontine syndrome are as follows: (1) ipsilateral conjugate gaze palsy, (2) ipsilateral internuclear ophthalmoplegia, (3) a combination of (1) and (2) resulting in a "one and half syndrome," (4) skew deviation of the eyes, (5) horizontal and vertical nystagmus, (6) ipsilateral facial sensory loss and contralateral hemisensory loss, (7) ipsilateral absence of the corneal reflex, (8) ipsilateral limb ataxia of the cerebellar type, and (9) ipsilateral abnormality in the brain stem auditory evoked responses.

The partial pontine syndromes run subacute or stuttering courses, although the onset of symptoms may be sudden and apoplectic. Small hematomas may resolve without surgical therapy. Surgical evacuation is considered under two conditions: (1) when the possibility of tumor cannot be ruled out on the basis of brain imaging, and (2) when progressive clinical deterioration occurs. The reported outcome after operative evacuation of partial pontine hematomas has been uniformly good.

Three surgical approaches have been used in the evacuation of pontine hematomas. The most commonly used is the posterior midline approach with splitting of the inferior vermis, exposure of the bulging discolored floor of the fourth ventricle, paramedian incision into the pons, and drainage of the hematoma.[13,23] In most instances, the liquefied clot extrudes under its own pressure. Pathologic demonstration of cryptic malformations has been limited to a few instances where the malformation extruded along with the clot.[28] This fact stresses the need to diligently examine the clot for evidence of vascular malformation. On other occasions, the malformation has been demonstrated in the wall of the hematoma cavity if a specific attempt had been made to biopsy the wall.

If the hematoma causes an asymmetric enlargement of the pons and the radiologic presentation is of a cerebellopontine angle mass,

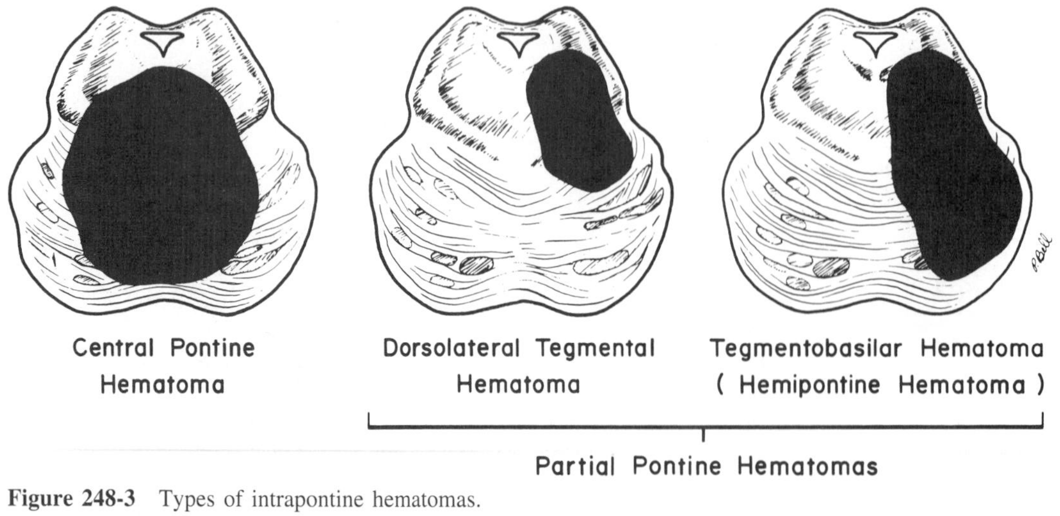

Figure 248-3 Types of intrapontine hematomas.

the surgical approach is naturally directed toward that anatomic site. The exposure is analogous to the one used for acoustic neuroma and other cerebellopontine angle masses. The incision is made at the maximal ventrolateral convexity of the pons near the root entry zone of the trigeminal nerve. It is important that the distended and discolored pons not be mistaken for tumor.

On at least two instances, pontine hematomas have been evacuated through stereotactic aspiration guided by computed tomography (CT), with excellent results in each instance.[4,8] Although a transcerebral transmesencephalic path was used, there were no reported serious complications except transient anisocoria. The possibility of injuring the vessels of the malformation and precipitating fresh bleeding is a risk, the likelihood of which remains unknown at present.

Hereditary Hemorrhagic Telangiectasia (Rendu-Osler-Weber Disease)

Hereditary hemorrhagic telangiectasia (HHT) is an autosomal dominant disorder characterized by the presence of vascular malformations of varying types in several tissues, including the brain, nasal mucosa, lungs, gastrointestinal tract, and liver.[24] The syndrome was first described by Rendu, a French internist; Sir William Osler stressed the familial nature of the disorder in 1901 when he was a Professor of Medicine at Johns Hopkins Hospital; Weber, an English dermatologist, recorded in detail the cutaneous manifestations of the syndrome. The clinical severity varies. It is estimated that 10 percent of affected individuals die from complications related to the disorder, but with diligent screening and prompt treatment, most complications may be prevented or treated effectively.

Genetics and Epidemiology

The incidence of HHT in the general population is currently estimated to be 1 to 2 per 100,000. This figure is generally considered to be an underestimate, because the disorder is rare and is unfamiliar to many health care professionals. The manifestations may be mild throughout life or may not appear until late in age, further contributing to underestimation. A realistic incidence is thought to be 10 to 20 affected individuals per 100,000 population. The disease occurs worldwide in all races but seems to be more common in persons of Western European origin; African-Americans and Asians are less frequently affected. Although uncommon, this disorder is thought to be the most common cause of vascular bleeding among genetically transmitted disorders. It is inherited as an autosomal dominant trait and exhibits all the characteristics of such an inheritance. On average, one-half of the children of an affected parent will exhibit the syndrome. Each affected individual will have a known affected parent, unless: (1) the affected individual is the product of an extramarital parentage; (2) the individual's disease results from spontaneous mutation of one allele of the gene; or (3) the disease is only weakly expressed in the transmitting parent.

Normal children of an affected individual will have only normal offspring. Vertical transmission of the condition through successive generations occurs because HHT is not lethal (except from its complications), and does not impair reproductive capacity. Males and females are affected equally. Each sex is equally likely to transmit the condition to male and female offspring, with documented male-to-male transmission.

Pathology

Three types of vascular malformations occur in HHT: telangiectasias, aneurysms, and arteriovenous malformations. In the brain, telangiectasia is the most common lesion. Roman and colleagues, in a study of 90 patients with HHT, noted cerebral telangiectasias in 40 percent, arteriovenous malformations in 19 percent, and aneurysms in 7 percent.

Telangiectasias consist of dilated capillaries with a single layer of endothelium attached to a continuous basement membrane. The mechanism of bleeding from these lesions in unknown. Tests of blood coagulation and platelet function are normal. Defects in endothelial cell junctions, deterioration of perivascular connective tissue, and endothelial cell degeneration are thought to be possible factors but are not proven. The strength of the supporting tissues around the telangiectasia may determine the propensity to bleed; thus, nasal telangiectasias bleed frequently whereas cutaneous lesions rarely do.

Detailed histologic studies comparing the structures of aneurysms and arteriovenous malformations in HHT with counterparts that are not genetically transmitted are not available. It is assumed that the lesions are histologically identical.

The Clinical Syndrome and Its Management

Five organ systems are the common sites of vascular malformations in HHT: the nasal mucosa, lungs, brain, gastrointestinal tract, and skin. This chapter will emphasize the central nervous system manifestations.

The central nervous system manifestations are summarized in Table 248-1. Neurological complications occur in 8 to 12 percent of patients with HHT. Neurological symptoms are caused in three ways.[25,31] The most common cause relates to complications of pulmonary arteriovenous malformations (PAVMs) and fistulae. Approximately 15 to 20 percent of patients with HHT have a PAVM. Because of the direct communication between the pulmonary artery and vein, the lung capillaries are bypassed. Thus, the oxygenating and filtering functions of the capillary bed are lost. Patients may be hypoxemic, with cyanosis, dyspnea, clubbing of fingers, and polycythemia, depending on the degree of shunting. Emboli that bypass the pulmonary filter and enter cerebral vessels may cause ischemic stroke. Septic emboli may cause single or multiple brain abscesses,[12] focal encephalitis, or mycotic aneurysms. An audible extracardiac bruit may be present over the chest.

TABLE 248-1 Central Nervous System Manifestations of Rendu-Osler-Weber Disease

1. Subarachnoid, intracerebral, or intraventricular hemorrhage due to rupture of arterial aneurysms, arteriovenous vascular malformations, telangiectasias, or other vascular dysplasias in the brain or spinal cord
2. Seizures
3. Sensory or motor deficits related to intracranial bleeding or to unruptured multiple vascular malformations
4. Ischemic strokes due to embolic events from pulmonary arteriovenous fistulae and right-to-left shunting
5. Ischemic cerebral events due to polycythemia and hypoxemia
6. Solitary or multiple brain abscesses due to septic emboli, also related to right-to-left shunting from pulmonary arteriovenous fistulae
7. Hepatic encephalopathy due to intrahepatic portosystemic shunts
8. Visual impairment due to intraocular hemorrhage from retinal telangiectasias

On chest radiographs, a PAVM is seen as a circumscribed, peripheral, noncalcified nodule connected to the hilum by vascular markings; fluoroscopy may demonstrate pulsations in the lesion. Determination of arterial blood gas values will give an estimate of the extent of right-to-left shunting. An air-contrast echocardiogram may show a "snow pattern" in the left heart, confirming the presence of the right-to-left shunt. This test is highly sensitive but not quantitative, unlike arterial blood gas values. Pulmonary angiography is the most definitive diagnostic test to confirm the presence, size, and morphology of a PAVM. High-resulution CT or magnetic resonance imaging (MRI) of the chest may be performed, but it will probably not yield any more information than provided by the tests listed earlier.[20] Selective embolization is the best available treatment modality for a PAVM. Recurrences may be treated by repeat embolization. Patients with a PAVM who are undergoing dental work should receive prophylactic antibiotics as recommended by the Committee on Endocarditis of the American Heart Association and the Council of Dental Therapeutics of the American Dental Association, to prevent septic embolic complications in the brain. The standard regimen consists of amoxicillin 3.0 g administered orally 1 h before the procedure, followed by 1.5 g 6 h after the initial dose.

The second way in which HHT may cause neurological complications is through the presence of telangiectasias, aneurysms, or arteriovenous malformations in the brain. There may be associated malformations in the scalp and skull. Rupture of an intracranial lesion may produce subarachnoid, intracerebral, or intraventricular hemorrhage. The presence of mutliple cerebral AVMs or of AVMs associated with arterial aneurysms should raise a high index of suspicion of HHT.[2] MRI and magnetic resonance angiography (MRA) are the best screening tests. Treatment options for these lesions include surgery, embolization, and focused beam radiation therapy or a combination thereof. Finally, HHT may cause hepatic encephalopathy as a result of portosystemic fistulae.

Telangiectasias in the Nasal Mucosa

Epistaxis is the most common and often the earliest manifestation of HHT. It occurs in 90 percent of affected individuals and appears before adolescence in 50 percent of patients. The duration and severity of bleeding varies. A third of the patients have severe recurrent bleeding requiring blood transfusion.

Treatment options include skin grafting (dermoplasty), laser coagulation, endovascular occlusive therapy, and hormonal therapy (estrogen, progesterone, and anabolic steroids). The relative merits of these treatment options await comparative clinical trials.

Gastrointestinal Tract

The spectrum of lesions encountered in the gastrointestinal tract includes mucosal and submucosal telangiectasias, arteriovenous malformations, aneurysms, varicosities of veins, and arteriovenous fistulas of the cardiac and mesenteric vessels. Painless upper or lower gastrointestinal bleeding is the rule but occurs late in the course of the disease, either in the fourth or fifth decade. Diagnosis is confirmed by endoscopy and celiac and mesenteric angiography.

Skin

Punctate telangiectasias measuring 1 to 3 mm across occur in the face, lips, tongue, nose, ears, hands, chest, and feet, generally appearing in the second or third decase of life. If they bleed or are cosmetically unacceptable, laser ablation is effective.

Clinical Diagnostic Criteria for HHT

The HHT foundation suggests that in order to make a diagnosis of HHT, two of the following three criteria must be met: (1) nosebleeds at least four times per month, (2) telangiectasias of the skin, and (3) a mother or father with a diagnosis of HHT

Optimal Timing for HHT Screening

If there are central nervous system or pulmonary manifestations among family members, the siblings should be screened before adolescence. Otherwise, screening may start after adolescence.

Venous Angiomas

A venous angioma may be defined as a vascular malformation without an obvious arterial component.[22] Generally it is clinically silent, often being diagnosed only incidentally on a contrast-enhanced CT scan, cerebral angiogram, or MR image. Subarachnoid hemorrhage or a seizure disorder may occur but is exceptional.[11,16] Most venous angiomas are located in the frontal or parietal lobe in the supratentorial space, or deep in the cerebellar white matter in the vicinity of the vein of Galen. Some workers consider that posterior fossa venous angiomas are not as benign as the supratentorial ones and are more likely to bleed.[5,30] Such bleeding may actually occur from coexisting adjacent cryptic malformations, rather than from the venous angiomas themselves.[1]

The cerebral angiographic appearance of a venous angioma has been described as resembling a caput medusae, a hydra, a spoked wheel, a spider, an umbrella, and a sunburst. The lesion consists of a myriad of small tapering veins arranged in a radial fashion in the deep white matter. These veins converge into a relatively large and centrally located draining vein, which in turn may empty into a larger cortical vein or a dural sinus (Fig. 248-4). Alternatively, the large collecting vein may drain into a subependymal vein in the wall of the lateral ventricle. Opacification of this anomalous venous network generally occurs in the venous phase of the arteriogram; the arterial and capillary phases usually appear normal even with magnification and subtraction techniques. Early filling of the venous angioma in the arterial or capillary phase is rare. The large transcerebral draining vein remains opacified through the late venous phase. The circulation time is in the normal range. No evidence of a mass effect is apparent unless the malformation has bled into the cerebral parenchyma.

A contrast-enhanced CT scan recapitulates the appearance seen on an angiogram.[19] The large draining vein is seen as a serpentine density, while the nidus of the malformation resembles the spokes of a wheel. A venous angioma may be visualized as a focal area of increased uptake in the venous phase of a dynamic radionuclide brain scan. The characteristic feature on MR imaging is a curvilinear streak of very low signal strength on T2-weighted images, corresponding to the transcerebral draining vein.[3,32,33,36]

On histologic examination, the vessels composing a venous angioma contain smooth muscle and elastic tissue, but to a much lesser extent than in arterial walls. Hyalinization and thickening of the vessel walls are common (Fig. 248-5). As with arteriovenous

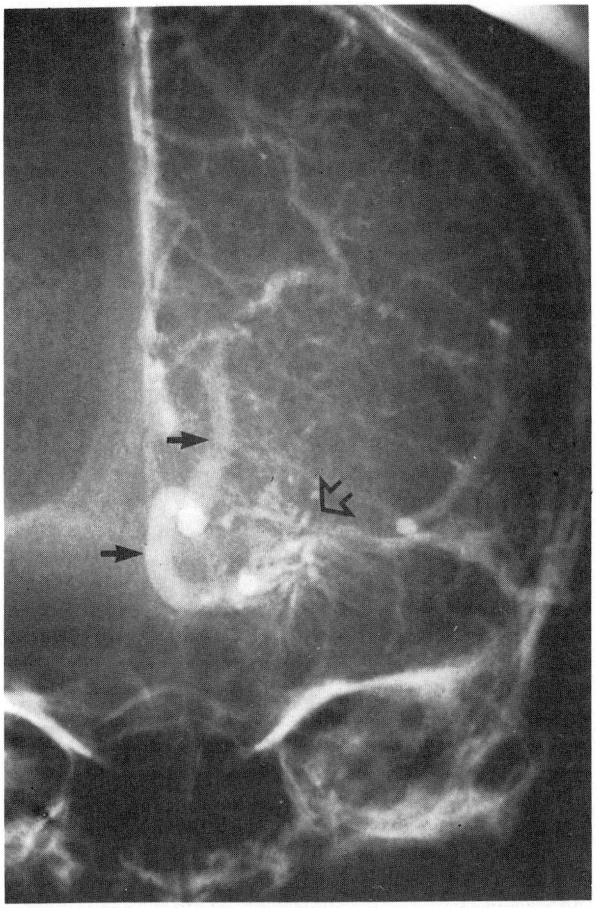

Figure 248-4 The typical angiographic appearance of a venous angioma. The angioma consists of a myriad of small tapering veins arranged in a radial fashion in the deep white matter *(open arrow)*. A prominent large cortical vein drains the malformation *(solid arrows)*. (Courtesy of K. Arjunan, M.D.)

malformations and telangiectasias, but unlike cavernous hemangiomas, neural parenchyma is found between the vascular elements of this malformation.

Some consider venous angiomas to represent anomalies of venous drainage. It is thought that in areas where angiomas occur there is a paucity of normal draining veins and that angiomas are no more than alternate venous drainage channels; indeed, if venous angiomas are removed, venous infarction in the affected territory may result.[30]

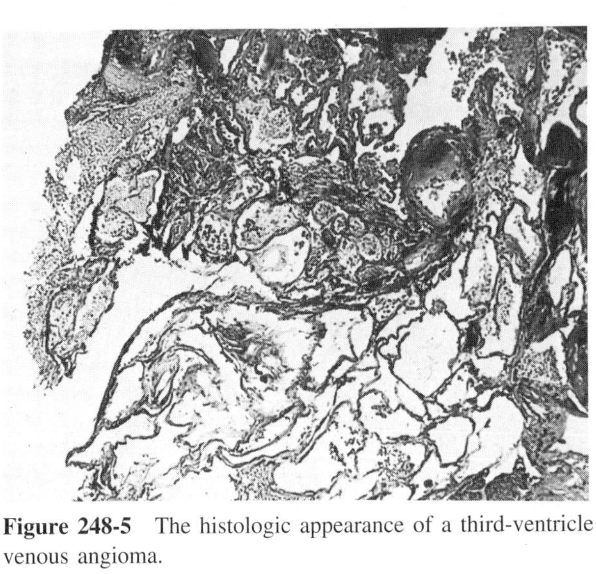

Figure 248-5 The histologic appearance of a third-ventricle venous angioma.

Since most venous angiomas are clinically silent and the risk of subarachnoid hemorrhage is quite small, a conservative approach is mandated if such a lesion is found incidentally on a cerebral angiogram.[5] The deep location of these lesions and the necessity of removing large segments of normal brain parenchyma along with the malformation further dictate a conservative approach unless bleeding is demonstrated from the malformation or an intractable seizure disorder is causally related to it.

Cryptic Vascular Malformations

The cryptic vascular malformations are a heterogeneous group of small angiomatous malformations (telangiectasia, venous angioma, cavernous hemangioma, arteriovenous malformation) that, although angiographically occult, can be detected by CT or MRI or at autopsy.[7,18] The failure of opacification during arteriography may be explained by small size or lack of arterial feeders, or by thrombosis in the malformation. A cryptic vascular malformation may induce seizures, mimic neoplastic lesions on CT scans, or produce spontaneous intracerebral hemorrhage. The following features characterize intraparenchymal hemorrhage from a cryptic vascular malformation: (1) occurrence in a relatively young individual; (2) absence of known predisposing factors, such as hypertension, trauma, or blood dyscrasia; (3) apoplectic onset with headaches; (4) delayed onset of loss of consciousness except with a hemorrhage occurring in the brain stem; (5) location of the bleeding usually in the periventricular white matter, ventricle, or the brain stem; and (6) absence of a demonstrable aneurysm, arteriovenous malformation, or other vascular lesion in the angiogram.

References

1. Abe M, Asfora WT, DeSalles AA, et al. Cerebellar venous angioma associated with angiographically occult brainstem vascular malformation. Report of two cases. *Surg Neurol* 1990; 33:400–403.
2. Aesch B, Lioret E, Toffol B, et al. Multiple cerebral angiomas and Rendu-Osler-Weber disease: case report. *Neurosurgery* 1991; 29:599–602.
3. Augustyn GT, Scott JA, Olson K, et al. Cerebral venous angiomas: MR imaging. *Radiology* 1985; 156:391–395.
4. Beatty RM, Zervas NT. Stereotactic aspiration of a brain stem hematoma. *Neurosurgery* 1983; 13:204–207.
5. Biller J, Toffol GJ, Shea JF, et al. Cerebellar venous angiomas. A continuing controversy. *Arch Neurol* 1985; 42:367–370.
6. Burke EC, Winkelman RK, Strickland MK. Disseminated hemangiomatosis. *Am J Dis Child* 1964; 108:418–424.
7. Cohen HCM, Tucker WS, Humphreys RP, et al. Angiographically cryptic histologically verified cerebrovascular malformations. *Neurosurgery* 1982; 10:704–714.
8. Dosch DA, Beute GN. Successful stereotaxic evacuation of an acute pontomedullary hematoma: case report. *J Neurosurg* 1985; 62:153–156.
9. Durward QJ, Barnett HJM. Presentation and management of mesencephalic hematomas. *J Neurosurg* 1982; 56:123–127.
10. Farrell DF, Forno LS. Symptomatic capillary telangiectasis of the brainstem without hemorrhage: report of an unusual case. *Neurology* 1970; 20:341–346.

11. Garner TB, Curling OD Jr, Kelly DL Jr, et al. The natural history of intracranial venous angiomas. *J Neurosurg* 1991; 75:715–722.
12. Gelfand MS, Stephens DS, Howell EI, et al. Brain abscess: association with pulmonary arteriovenous fistula and hereditary hemorrhagic telangiectasia: report of three cases. *Am J Med* 1988; 85:718–720.
13. Heffez DS, Zinreich SJ, Long DM. Surgical resection of intrinsic brain stem lesions: an overview. *Neurosurgery* 1990; 27:789–798.
14. Humphreys RP. Computerized tomographic definition of mesencephalic hematoma with evacuation through pedunculotomy: case report. *J Neurosurg* 1978; 49:749–752.
15. Kempe LG. Surgical removal of an intramedullary hematoma simulating Wallenburg's syndrome. *J Neurol Neurosurg Psychiatry* 1964; 27:78–80.
16. Kondziolka D, Dempsey PK, Lunsford LD. The case for conservative management of venous angiomas. *Can J Neurol Sci* 1991; 18:295–299.
17. Kushner MJ, Bressman SB. The clinical manifestations of pontine hemorrhage. *Neurology (NY)* 1985; 35:637–643.
18. Lobato RD, Perez C, Rivas JJ, et al. Clinical, radiological, and pathological spectrum of angiographically occult intracranial vascular malformations. Analysis of 21 cases and review of the literature. *J Neurosurg* 1988; 68:518–531.
19. Lotz PR, Quisling RG. CT of venous angiomas of the brain. *Am J Neuroradiol* 1983; 4:1124–1126.
20. Love BB, Biller J, Landas SK, et al. Diagnosis of pulmonary arteriovenous malformation by ultrafast chest computed tomography in Rendu-Osler-Weber syndrome with cerebral ischemia—a case report. *Angiology* 1992; 43:522–528.
21. McCormick WF, Nofzinger JD. Cryptic vascular malformations of the central nervous system. *J Neurosurg* 1966; 24:865–875.
22. Numaguchi Y, Kitamura K, Fukui M, et al. Intracranial venous angiomas. *Surg Neurol* 1982; 18:193–202.
23. Pau A, Viale S, Turtas S. Surgical removal of a pontine haematoma associated with a cryptic angioma. *Acta Neurochir (Wien)* 1979; 50:299–303.
24. Peery WH. Clinical spectrum of hereditary hemorrhagic telangiectasia (Osler-Weber-Rendu disease). *Am J Med* 1987; 82:989–997.
25. Press OW, Ramsey PG. Central nervous system infections associated with hereditary hemorrhagic telangiectasia. *Am J Med* 1984; 77:86–92.
26. Rigamonti D, Johnson PC, Spetzler RF, et al. Cavernous malformations and capillary telangiectasia: a spectrum within a single pathological entity. *Neurosurgery* 1991; 28:60–64.
27. Russell B, Rengachary SS, McGregor D. Primary pontine hematoma presenting as a cerebellopontine angle mass. *Neurosurgery* 1986; 19:129–133.
28. Scott BB, Seeger JF, Schneider PC. Successful evacuation of a pontine hematoma secondary to rupture of a pathologically diagnosed "cryptic" vascular malformation. *J Neurosurg* 1973; 39:104–108.
29. Scoville WB, Poppen JL. Intrapeduncular hemorrhage of the brain: successful operative approach with evacuation of clot and seven and one-fourth year observation period. *Arch Neurol Psychiatry* 1949; 61:618–694.
30. Senegor M, Dohrmann GJ, Wollmann RL. Venous angiomas of the posterior fossa should be considered as anomalous venous drainage. *Surg Neurol* 1983; 19:26–32.
31. Sobel D, Norman D. CNS manifestations of hereditary hemorrhagic telangiectasia. *Am J Neuroradiol* 1984; 5:569–573.
32. Truwit CL. Venous angioma of the brain: history, significance, and imaging findings. *Am J Roentgenol* 1992; 159:1299–1307.
33. Uchino A, Imada H, Ohno M. Magnetic resonance imaging of intracranial venous angiomas. *Clin Imaging* 1990; 14:309–314.
34. Vaquero J, Manrique M, Oya S, et al. Calcified telangiectatic hamartomas of the brain. *Surg Neurol* 1980; 13:453–457.
35. White RJ, Kernohan JW, Wood MW. A study of fifty intracranial vascular tumors found incidentally at autopsy. *J Neuropathol Exp Neurol* 1958; 17:392–398.
36. Wilms G, Marchal G, Van Hecke P, et al. Cerebral venous angiomas. MR imaging at 1.5 tesla. *Neuroradiology* 1990; 32:81–85.

249 Sinus Pericranii

Eben Alexander, Jr.
Marshall R. Ball

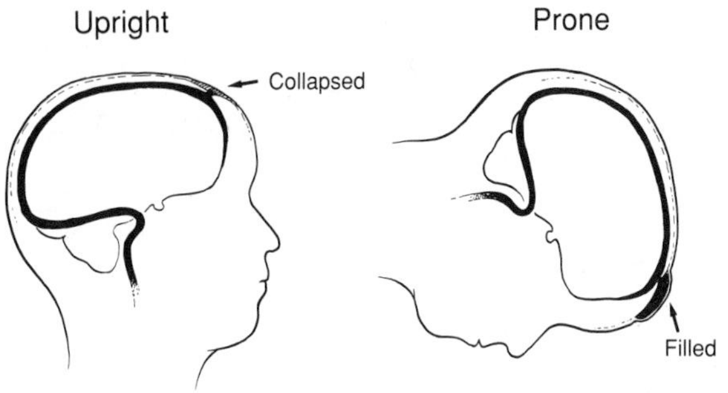

Figure 249-2 An artist's drawing demonstrating filling of the sinus pericranii with the head prone (or supine) at the level of the body; it collapses when the head is elevated.

The term "sinus pericranii" denotes a group of abnormal communications between the extracranial and intracranial venous systems, which usually involve the superior sagittal sinus (Fig. 249-1), and sometimes the transverse sinuses. They are uncommon.

In general, sinus pericranii is considered a congenital abnormality, although some cases have been attributed to trauma[2] or to unusual strain or stress. The entity was originally described by Stromeyer in 1950.[3]

Usually the patients are not symptomatic, and the problem is cosmetic. Most patients are seen as young infants, the others at a later age. Older patients sometimes complain of headache, dizziness, nausea, and vertigo, which may or may not be related to this abnormality.

A soft fluctuant mass usually is apparent on either the right or the left side in the frontal region. It may have a reddish or bluish hue, but many times it is not discolored. Anything that increases the intracranial pressure fills the lesion. If the patient sits up, the lesion disappears, and compressing the jugular veins bilaterally under those circumstances makes it reappear. The lesion is readily apparent when the patient is supine or prone, or when the head is held forward (Fig. 249-2).

A bony defect may be palpable beneath the lesion. More often, there are large venous openings in the skull adjacent to the midline, and it is through them that the veins enter the sagittal sinus (Fig. 249-3).

Sinus pericranii must be differentiated from encephalocele, meningocele, abscess, sebaceous cyst, and epidermoid cyst, as well as from arteriovenous fistula, which usually results from trauma or other arterial malformations draining into the scalp veins. Cavernous hemangiomas and angiomas are also usually easily differentiated from sinus pericranii.

Skull roentgenograms or computed tomographic scans usually demonstrate the large openings through the skull (Fig. 249-4). There may be complete absence of bone or small irregular crevices, sometimes even areas of fine honeycombing that are not clearly visible radiographically. The lesion is not seen by the usual angiographic technique, although digital subtraction studies and delayed films may show some filling. Direct injection of contrast medium through the wall of the structure will show a quick passage of medium into the superior longitudinal sinus (Fig. 249-5) or

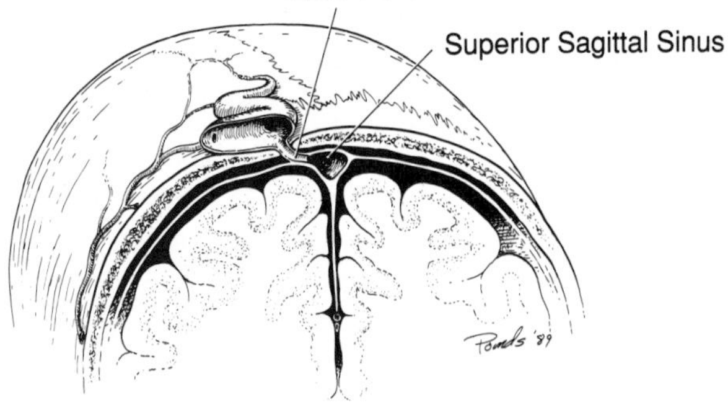

Figure 249-1 An artist's drawing of sinus pericranii, showing the communication with the sagittal sinus.

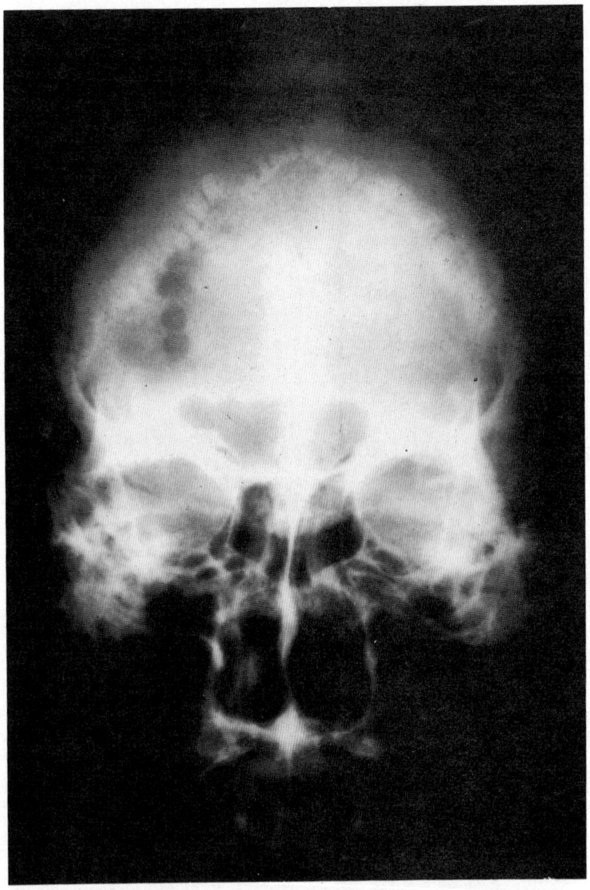

Figure 249-3 A posteroanterior radiographic projection demonstrates a series of vascular channels in the right frontal bone of this patient with sinus pericranii.

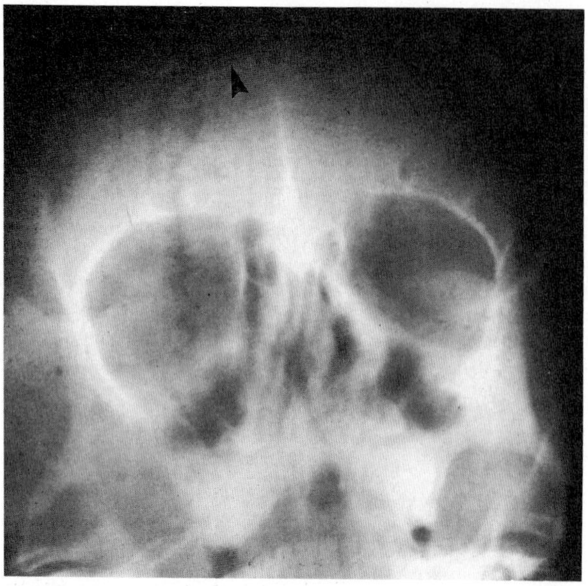

Figure 249-4 A Waters projection demonstrates an abnormal vascular groove and channel through the frontal bone (*arrowhead*) from the right inferiorly to the midline 3 cm above the nasion.

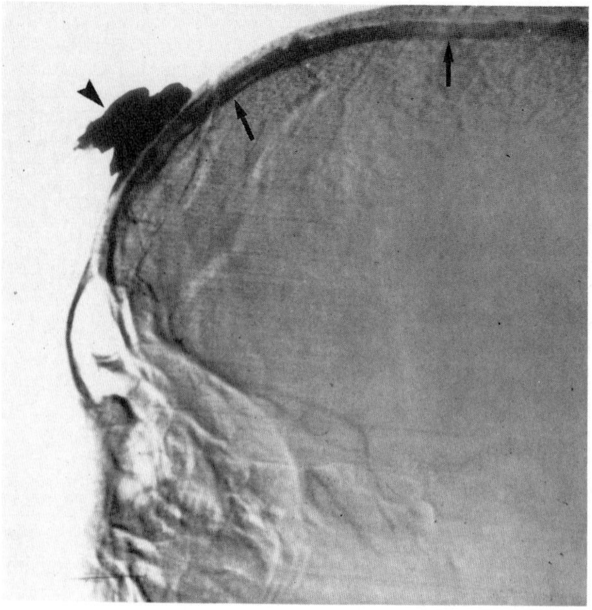

Figure 249-5 A lateral film made after the direct injection of a sinus pericranii in a 24-year-old man with a painless lump on the forehead that enlarged when he bent over. This subtraction venogram demonstrates a large venous structure (*arrowhead*) directly communicating with the longitudinal sinus (*arrows*).

the transverse sinus, as well as usually into the ordinary scalp veins (Fig. 249-6).

The sinus pericranii is found beneath or in the periosteum of the cranial vault and is connected with an intracranial sinus through anomalous emissary veins, which may be either congenital or acquired.[3] These lesions may gradually increase in size until they are cosmetically objectionable. There have been a few reports of spontaneous occlusion.

Bollar et al. have recently reported a case that resembled sinus pericranii except that the mass did not collapse when the patient sat up, and it was not compressible.[1] The excised specimen was called a benign mesenchymal neoplasm and may be categorized as a "pseudosinus pericranii."

The decision to operate on these lesions depends on the cosmetic appearance as well as the danger of hemorrhage from trauma; sometimes the cranial defect will need to be covered with a cranioplasty. Ohta et al. reported that Pott had treated a similar lesion in 1771 by trephining and packing the lesion with linen fibers.[3]

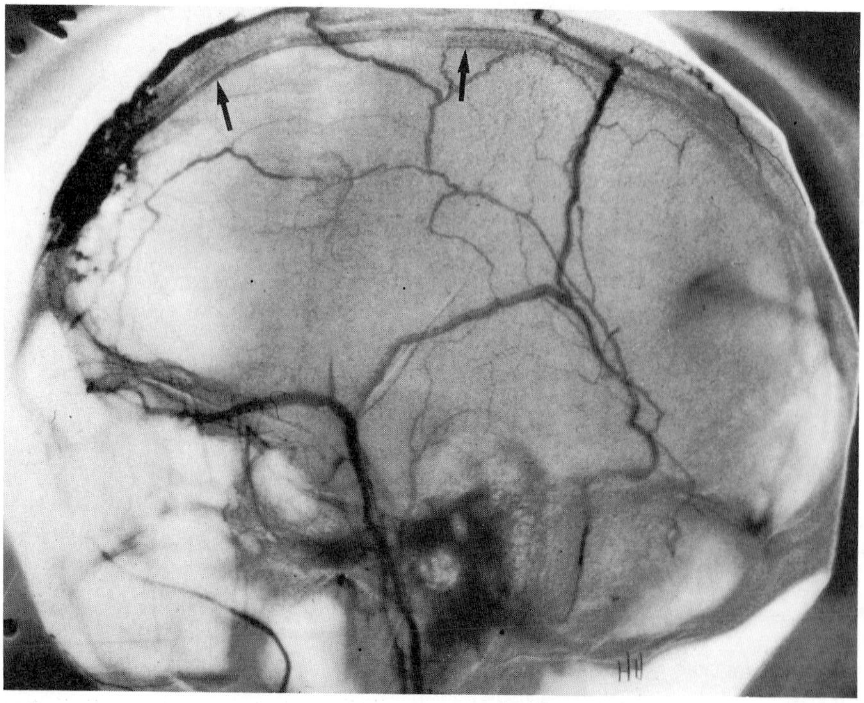

Figure 249-6 A lateral film made after the direct injection of a sinus pericranii. The abnormal vascularity of the soft tissue mass in the skin over the frontal bone communicates with the longitudinal sinus (*arrows*), and also freely with the veins of the scalp.

If the lesion is to be removed, the area adherent to the skull must be removed completely. This complete removal has resulted in one or two instances of extensive hemorrhage requiring about 3000 ml of blood replacement,[2] but such bleeding could be avoided by raising the patient's upper torso and head to the point that the veins collapse. Care must then be taken not to allow air to enter the venous sinuses, and great attention must be paid to obliterating all the communications with the superior longitudinal sinus, or, if the lesion is lateral, with the transverse sinus.

In one instance, a lesion recurred promptly after an operation performed by a surgeon who obliterated the communications with the sagittal sinus with bone wax. At the second removal (performed by the author), a craniectomy was done. There was very little blood loss, but operative findings included communications of the sinus pericranii not only through the openings in the skull to the longitudinal sinus, but also with some of the veins over the arachnoid of the frontal lobe. These were all obliterated, an acrylic cranioplasty was done, and there has been no recurrence of the lesion. Although the patient still had headaches, he returned to work and worked for several years until incapacitated by pulmonary problems. A follow-up examination 10 years later showed no recurrence of the lesion.

References

1. Bollar A, Allut AG, Prieto A, et al. Sinus pericranii: radiological and etiopathological considerations. Case report. *J Neurosurg* 1992; 77:469–472.
2. Mori K, Yoneda S, Handa H. Posttraumatic subepicranial varix. *Surg Neurol* 1976; 5:337–339.
3. Ohta T, Waga S, Handa H, et al. Sinus pericranii. *J Neurosurg* 1975; 42:704–712.

250 Intracranial Dural Arteriovenous Malformations

Issam A. Awad

A dural arteriovenous malformation (DAVM) is a region of arteriovenous shunting within the leaflets of dura mater (Fig. 250-1). The arterial supply to the lesion is recruited from dural arteries and from pachymeningeal branches of cerebral arteries.[17] Arterial branches within the dura mater, which may be seldom observed on normal angiographic studies, may be dilated and clearly visible when supplying a DAVM.[2,3,17,29] For example, an angiogram showing a prominent tentorial branch of the internal carotid artery (the artery of Bernasconi and Cassinari) or a visible meningeal branch of the posterior cerebral artery (the artery of Davidoff and Schechter) are strongly suggestive of a tentorial DAVM. Another defining feature of DAVMs is the visualization of venous structures during the arterial phase of the angiogram.

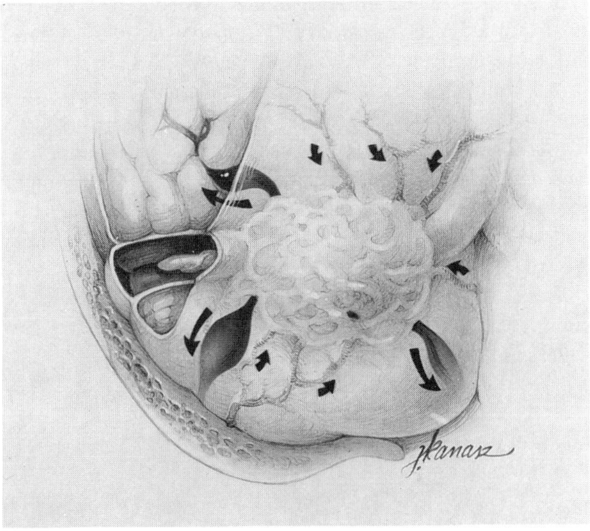

Figure 250-1 Artist's illustration of the gross pathoanatomy of a DAVM involving the region of the left transverse sinus (posterior view). Note the partial sinus occlusion, which is frequently encountered with such lesions and may play a role in their genesis. Note numerous pachymeningeal arteries converging on the region of dural pathology. There is arteriovenous shunting, which is contained solely within the leaflets of the dura mater. Drainage of the lesion is through the adjacent dural sinus and also via retrograde leptomeningeal venous drainage into the cortical venous circulation. Retrograde leptomeningeal venous drainage may be variceal or aneurysmal owing to chronic venous hypertension.

The nidus of arteriovenous shunting is contained solely within the leaflets of the dura mater, and this is an essential feature distinguishing DAVMs from other vascular malformations of the brain.[17] The nidus often is located close to a dural sinus, and the latter may appear narrowed or obstructed on angiography. The nidus of the DAVM is a region of dural pathology where all arterial feeders converge. Multiple injections of different arteries may be required to visualize the nidus and all contributing feeders.

A DAVM may drain through an adjacent dural sinus and/or other dural and leptomeningeal venous channels (Fig. 250-2). Retrograde leptomeningeal venous drainage is often tortuous and variceal, and may be frankly aneurysmal (Fig. 250-3). It is thought that arteriovenous shunting results in increased venous pressure within the dural leaflets, and that this pressure results in retrograde drainage through leptomeningeal veins which otherwise would drain blood from the leptomeningeal venous circulation into the dural leaflets.[2,10] In the setting of DAVMs, arterialized blood drains retrograde through these structures into the leptomeningeal circulation. These leptomeningeal veins become tortuous and variceal.

Diagnostic Studies

Catheter cerebral angiography is the best diagnostic study for defining DAVMs.[17,29] In cases of suspected DAVM, the study should include injection of both internal carotid arteries as well as separate injections of both external carotid arteries and both vertebral arteries. In cases of suspected clival or foramen magnum region DAVMs, arch injections may reveal additional ascending muscular or pharyngeal arterial feeders. Ultrarapid imaging started in the early arterial phase and continued well into the venous phase is necessary for visualizing all essential features of DAVMs. Digital subtraction and magnification techniques and the occasional use of superselective angiography have greatly enhanced the diagnostic potential of angiographic studies.

Other diagnostic tests may reveal indirect evidence of a DAVM (Figs. 250-2 and 250-3). Imaging with computed tomography (CT) or magnetic resonance (MR) is often performed as part of the initial investigation of presenting neurological symptoms.[2,16] These studies may reveal thickening of a region of dura mater or tortuosities of leptomeningeal venous drainage. More recently, magnetic resonance angiography (MRA) has been used to detect and follow DAVMs.[2] The radiologist should be alerted about the high index of clinical suspicion so as to focus on the region of interest and minimize false negative results with this modality. At present, these adjuvant diagnostic studies are incapable of totally excluding the presence of a DAVM, and they do not define relevant features of the lesion well enough for prognostic and therapeutic decisions. Only catheter cerebral angiography can provide the spatial diagnostic detail and dynamic flow information to identify arterial feeders and define in detail the pattern of flow and venous drainage in the DAVM. This information is essential for prognostication and therapeutic decisions. However, MR imaging and MRA may be used to screen patients with a low clinical suspicion of a DAVM and to follow specific features of DAVMs (i.e., development of or enlargement of leptomeningeal venous channels). Imaging studies

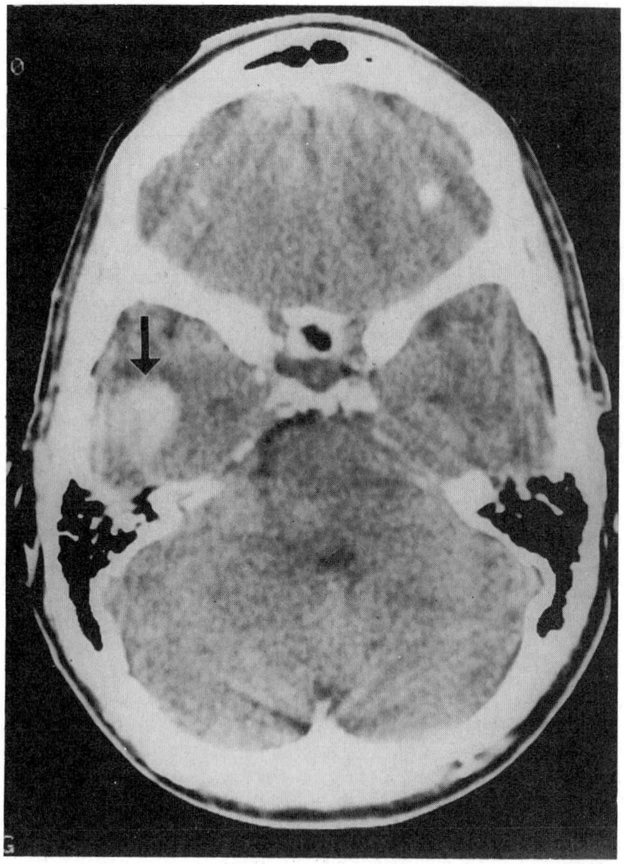

(*A*)

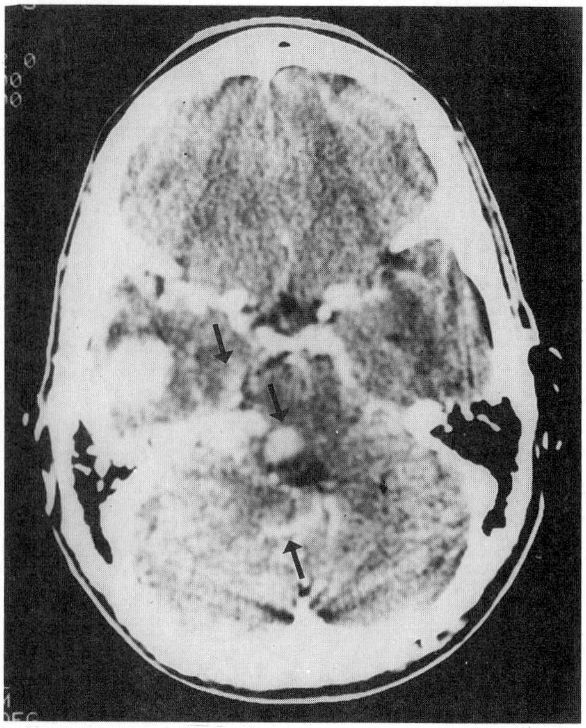

(*B*)

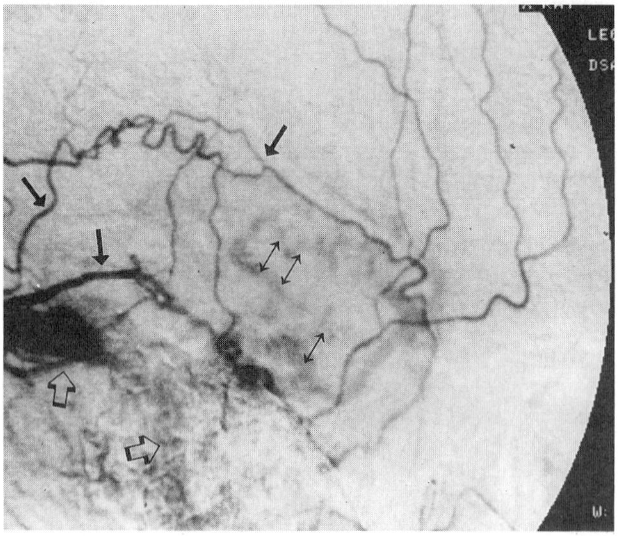

(*C*)

Figure 250-2 Right lateral tentorial-transverse sinus DAVM. This middle-aged woman was treated 10 years earlier with external carotid artery embolization for pulsatile tinnitus and a presumed DAVM. She had no further symptoms until she suddenly presented with a temporal lobe intracerebral hemorrhage. She had not been under medical follow-up despite her known residual DAVM. *A.* Unenhanced CT scan showing a focal temporal lobe hemorrhage (*arrow*). *B.* Enhanced CT scan showing numerous tortuous vascular structures in the temporal lobe, cerebellum, and perimesencephalic cistern (*arrows*), consistent with arterialized leptomeningeal venous drainage from the DAVM. *C.* External carotid arteriogram, lateral view, showing numerous scalp and meningeal feeders (*solid arrows*) converging onto a region of dural pathology near the transverse sinus. In the arterial phase of the angiogram there is premature visualization of the transverse and sigmoid sinuses (*open arrows*). In addition, there are numerous tortuous leptomeningeal venous structures (*double-headed arrows*).

should be evaluated with a high index of clinical suspicion in cases with vague clinical symptomatology so as to exclude subtle features possibly suggestive of DAVMs.

DAVMs are classified according to the adjacent dural sinus, the region of dura mater involved in arteriovenous shunting, or the pattern of venous drainage (dural sinus, galenic system, cortical pial, etc.).[3,16,19] A combination of the regional anatomic classification and the general pattern of venous drainage appears to be the most useful system clinically and has gained acceptance in the literature (Table 250-1).

Etiology

A few DAVMs present early in life and are thought to be congenital. These are usually associated with complex congenital anomalies, rare phakomatoses, or a vein of Galen malformation (actually a special form of DAVM).[17] In these cases, there is often gross malformation of dural sinuses with atresia of venous outflow from a region of dura mater involved in the DAVM.

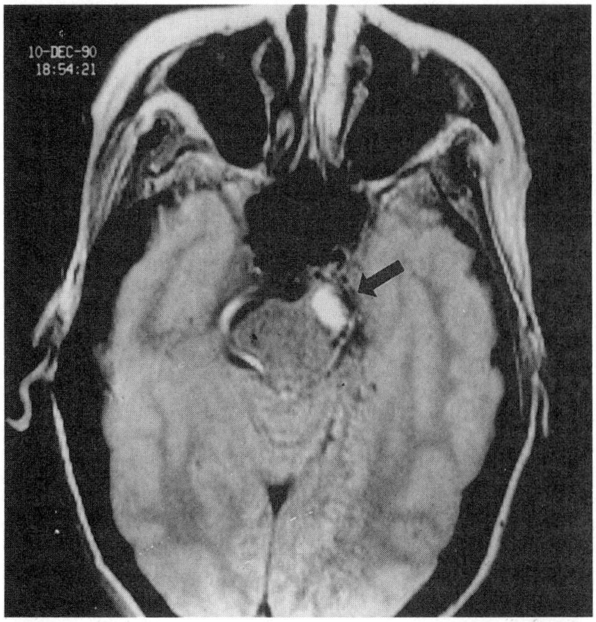

(*A*)

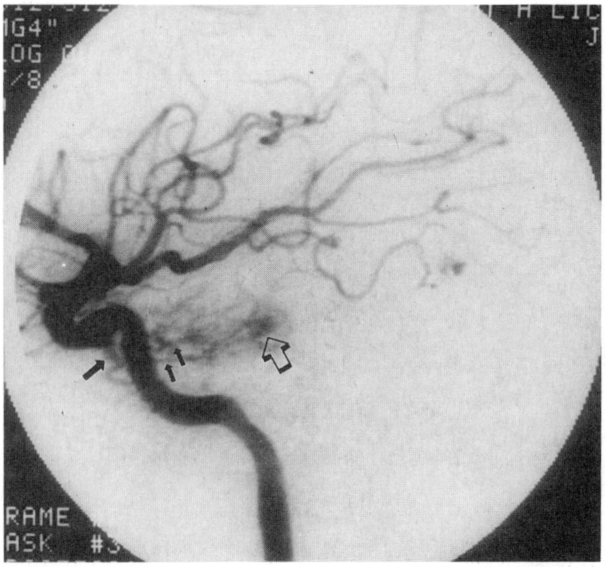

(*B*)

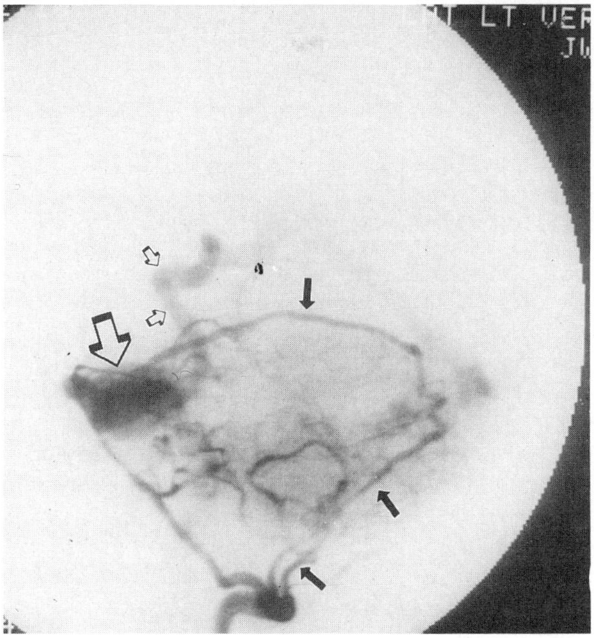

(*C*)

Figure 250-3 Tentorial incisura DAVM. This elderly woman presented with severe left facial pain and transient gaze and motor symptoms referable to the rostral brain stem. *A.* T1-weighted axial MR scan reveals hypertrophy of vascular structures in both perimesencephalic cisterns as well as signal characteristics of sluggish flow or thrombosis in a vascular structure near the left petrous apex (*arrow*). *B.* Internal carotid arteriogram, lateral view, reveals a venous blush in the region of the tentorial incisura, visible during the arterial phase of the angiogram (*open arrow*). There is hypertrophy of numerous arterial twigs from the petrous and cavernous segments of the internal carotid artery (*solid arrows*). *C.* Left vertebral arteriogram, lateral view, reveals hypertrophy of numerous muscular and pachymeningeal branches of the vertebral artery (*solid arrows*), converging onto the same region of dural pathology at the tentorial incisura. There is also premature visualization (during the arterial phase of the angiogram) of a giant venous varix in the same region (*large open arrow*), and leptomeningeal venous drainage into the galenic system (*small open arrows*).

Most DAVMs present later in life and are thought to be acquired.[6,14] Known or suspected etiologic factors include trauma and sinus thrombosis; other DAVMs are idiopathic.

Several lines of evidence suggest trauma as an etiologic factor in DAVMs.[1,2] Many cases clearly develop after a well-defined head injury, although it is rarely obvious whether the DAVMs developed de novo or were discovered incidentally after trauma. In other cases, new DAVMs have been reported to develop after cranial surgical intervention.[21,31] Most post-traumatic DAVMs (including most postsurgical DAVMs) do not develop at the site of dural injury and may be noticeably removed from the site of obvious trauma.

The role of dural sinus thrombosis in the development of DAVMs has been discussed by several authors.[2,3,6,14,25] Cases have been documented of angiographically proven dural sinus thrombosis in which DAVMs subsequently developed in relation to the obstructed sinus. Some investigators have shown ''early'' forms of DAVMs in the setting of dural vessel collateralization around a site of sinus obstruction.[6,14]

In normal dura mater there is microscopic communication between arteries and veins near venous sinuses.[15,28] Trauma, surgery, sinus thrombosis, or another factor might initiate the genesis of a DAVM within the dural leaflets next to a pathologic sinus.[2–4]

Pathophysiology and Natural History

An established DAVM may follow one of several unpredictable natural courses. Some lesions remain asymptomatic or maintain stable clinical symptomatology and angiographic features over

TABLE 250-1 Common Clinical and Angiographic Features of Intracranial DAVMs in Various Locations

Lesion Location	Clinical Presentation	Arterial Feeders	Venous Drainage
Lateral tentorium (transverse-sigmoid sinuses)	Pulsatile tinnitus; ear and neck ache; rarely hemorrhage*	ECA; VA; tentorial branches of ICA	Dural sinus†; rarely leptomeningeal to temporal lobe, cerebellum, or galenic system
Cavernous sinus (middle cranial fossa)	Pain, ophthalmoplegia (cavernous sinus syndrome); orbital or ocular symptoms; rarely hemorrhage*	Cavernous branches of ICA; internal maxillary branches of ECA	Anterior cavernous sinus to orbit; posterior or petrosal drainage; rarely leptomeningeal (usually to sylvian and basal veins)
Tentorial incisura	Hemorrhage,* focal neurological deficits,* facial pain	Tentorial branches of ICA, ECA, VA, meningeal branches of PCA and SCA	Leptomeningeal to galenic system
Anterior cranial fossa	Hemorrhage,* rarely orbital symptoms	Falcine branches of ethmoidal branches of ophthalmic artery (ICA), ECA	Leptomeningeal to frontal lobe; rarely to superior or inferior sagittal sinuses or to the orbit
Convexity dura, superior sagittal sinus, ocular	Headache, papilledema,‡ hemorrhage*	ECA (scalp and meningeal branches)	Dural sinus,† leptomeningeal to underlying cortex
Clival, petrosal	Pain; posterior cavernous sinus syndrome; rarely hemorrhage or focal neurological deficits*	ECA, VA, clival branches of ICA, ascending muscular branches from the arch	Jugular; petrosal; rarely leptomeningeal
Foramen magnum region	Focal neurological deficits (brain stem syndrome or myelopathy)*; hemorrhage*	ECA, VA, clival branches of ICA, ascending muscular branches from the arch	Leptomeningeal to medullary venous plexus

*Hemorrhage and focal neurological deficits only occur in lesions with leptomeningeal venous drainage.
†Dural sinus may be atretic or thrombosed.
‡Papilledema is more prevalent in high-flow lesions and in the setting of concomitant venous sinus outflow obstruction.
Abbreviations: ECA, external carotid artery; ICA, internal carotid artery; PCA, posterior cerebral artery; SCA, superior cerebellar artery; VA, vertebral artery.

many years.[1,8,14] Others undergo spontaneous regression, involution, and resolution with stabilization or improvement of neurological symptoms.[5,13,18,23] Features that may predispose to such spontaneous involution are not known. However, DAVMs in the region of the cavernous sinus are particularly prone to this phenomenon, with as many as 40 percent of reported cases having undergone spontaneous involution, usually after cerebral angiography.

In other cases, the lesion progressively recruits additional pachymeningeal arterial feeders.[2,3,7,17] These lesions seem to grow by recruitment of arterial feeders into the nidus, favored by the arteriovenous shunting (the sump effect) (see Fig. 250-5).[3] All arterial feeders appear to converge on the same region of dural pathology. The mechanisms behind this progressive recruitment of arterial feeders from numerous sources have not been elucidated. This phenomenon results in hypertrophy of dural arteries and the reappearance of involuted embryonic arteries that may not normally be visible in the adult dura mater.

There is also progression of pathology at the venous side of DAVMs (Figs. 250-1 through 250-3). Progressive arterialization of the pathologic dural leaflets results in hypertension in adjacent leptomeningeal venous channels. This may result in retrograde leptomeningeal venous drainage, as discussed previously, and under arterialized pressures these channels may become tortuous and, eventually, varicose or aneurysmal.

Clinical Features

Retrograde leptomeningeal venous drainage has been associated with serious neurological sequelae from DAVMs, including focal neurological deficits (foeal venous hypertension) and hemorrhage (rupture of arterialized leptomeningeal veins).[2,3,7,10,22] The natural course of DAVMs may result in other clinical phenomena as well.[3,16,30] Dilated venous structures may act as mass lesions, obstructing pathways of cerebrospinal fluid circulation in the ventricular system or basal cisterns. This obstruction may result in hydrocephalus. In other cases, dural venous hypertension may result in decreased absorption of cerebrospinal fluid and secondary intracranial hypertension and papilledema.[9] This latter complication appears to be more common in association with high-flow lesions draining into large dural venous sinuses, and in the setting of concomitant dural sinus outflow obstruction.[2,3]

Other clinical manifestations of DAVMs include pulsatile tinnitus or other subjective auditory symptoms, with or without pain, related to high flow through dural vascular channels at the base of the skull. Other painful complaints may be related to orbital congestion or stretching of dural leaflets by engorged vascular channels, or to compression of the trigeminal nerve by arterialized venous structures near the petrous apex.[16] A variety of neuro-ophthalmic manifestations of DAVMs include visual and gaze abnormalities caused by venous hypertension or by orbital or ocular venous hypertension with resulting orbital crowding, venous stasis retinopathy, frank optic disc edema, and/or glaucoma.[2]

DAVMs in various locations are associated with peculiar clinical presentations related to the region of dural pathology and the patterns of associated venous drainage (Table 250-1).[2,3,16,30] Regardless of lesion location or previous clinical presentation or other symptomatology, the most important factor determining the propensity for an aggressive clinical course seems to be the presence of leptomeningeal venous drainage.[3,16] DAVMs at the transverse or sigmoid sinuses or in the region of the cavernous sinus often drain into the associated venous sinus and may cause a variety of clinical manifestations due to flow or venous engorgement.

These do not bleed or cause focal neurological deficits unless there is associated retrograde leptomeningeal venous drainage. Lesions at the anterior cranial fossa or the tentorial incisura rarely drain into a patent dural venous sinus and are more frequently associated with leptomeningeal venous drainage, and they are more apt to cause serious clinical sequelae from venous hypertension and hemorrhage. Hemorrhage has not been reported in the absence of this feature, and in all published cases with carefully documented diagnostic studies, hemorrhage from DAVMs can be traced to the rupture of arterialized venous structures (Fig. 250-2). The prognosis of a first hemorrhage from DAVMs is ominous, and has been shown to be associated with greater than 30 percent mortality or serious disability. Hemorrhage from DAVMs in anticoagulated patients has uniformly been fatal.

Therapeutic Options

Table 250-2 summarizes the available therapeutic options for DAVMs and the general strategies of therapeutic decision making. Observation without invasive intervention is indicated for lesions with benign symptoms and for DAVMs without the aggressive features discussed above.[8,14] The decision to proceed with active therapeutic intervention depends on the patient's current clinical status and on the lesion's previous clinical manifestations, as well as its angiographic features. A natural history profile and an individualized risk-benefit ratio should be considered in each case. For example, a low-flow DAVM next to the transverse sinus in a middle-aged woman who presents with pulsatile tinnitus and without leptomeningeal venous drainage would not warrant invasive intervention unless the symptoms were absolutely disabling. In such a case, symptomatic and palliative measures short of complete lesion excision may be acceptable and may produce symptomatic relief with very low risk.

A similar conservative approach would be indicated in an elderly patient with a spontaneous carotid cavernous fistula (cavernous region DAVM) and facial pain or mild diplopia. In many such cases, the symptoms are more worrisome to the patient than truly disabling. With reassurance, the patient may tolerate the symptoms until they subside spontaneously, as they often do with this type of lesion.

Symptomatic treatment may include reassurance and counseling, biofeedback, and jugular massage (although the latter has never been shown to be effective in a controlled study and may be dangerous in elderly patients who have coexisting carotid disease or who may be vulnerable to vasovagal syncope). Patients with dull aching pain or bothersome pulsatile tinnitus may benefit from nonsteroidal anti-inflammatory agents, carbamazepine (for tic-like pain), or short courses of corticosteroids (particularly effective for retro-orbital discomfort). Patients with DAVMs and tic douloureux should not be treated by percutaneous methods involving puncture of the foramen ovale, since that may result in catastrophic hemorrhage.

Symptom palliation may also be accomplished by transarterial embolization of external carotid artery feeders to the DAVM, although such an intervention is not totally without risk and rarely succeeds in totally eliminating the DAVM. Arterial embolization may give a false sense of security that the lesion was "treated," while the DAVM may progress to acquire more aggressive features including leptomeningeal venous drainage (even in the absence of recurrent symptoms). DAVMs that are followed expectantly or treated palliatively should be monitored closely with serial diagnostic studies to watch for the development of leptomeningeal venous drainage, which may occur with no change in clinical symptoms. Noninvasive imaging methods, including MRI and MRA, may be used for interval studies, although these modalities may miss subtle development of leptomeningeal venous drainage, which may be clinically catastrophic. Depending on the clinical situation and the particular lesion, serial MR studies may be performed on a yearly basis, with formal angiography every few years, or sooner if symptoms change or there is a suggestion on MRI of new leptomeningeal venous drainage.

Transarterial embolization has been widely used in the treatment of DAVMs.[17,29] The introduction of newer flow-guided catheter technology and increased experience with particle and glue embolization have greatly improved the safety and efficacy of this method. However, transarterial embolization rarely succeeds in

TABLE 250-2 Treatment Approaches to Intracranial DAVMs.

Expectant or Symptomatic Treatment	Transarterial Embolization	Transvenous Obliteration	Open Surgery	Stereotactic Radiosurgery
Lesions with nondisabling symptomatology; incidentally discovered lesions	Accessible arterial feeders; may use chemical/sclerosing agents	Accessible venous drainage (via patent sinus or by direct puncture of venous varices)	Lesions with leptomeningeal venous drainage and/or recent aggressive neurological symptoms	Lesions near noneloquent brain; no recent hemorrhage
Lesions without leptomeningeal venous drainage	Rarely "curative"; may palliate disabling flow-related symptoms	Curative with occlusion of associated sinus	Typically curative; enhanced by preparatory embolization or open transvenous obliteration	Delayed effectiveness (does not protect against early rebleeding)
Close follow-up of lesions to exclude development of leptomeningeal venous drainage	Close follow-up of residual DAVM as in untreated lesions	Sudden obliteration may be associated with hemodynamic or thrombotic complications	Maximal resection and/or coagulation of pathologic dural leaflet; interruption of leptomeningeal arterialized veins	Close follow-up to verify effectiveness
Common approach to most transverse-sigmoid or cavernous sinus DAVMs	Useful as preparatory adjunct before transvenous, open, or radiosurgical treatment	Useful in cavernous sinus and transverse-sigmoid DAVMs	Useful for incisural, anterior fossa, and foramen magnum DAVMs	Useful for lateral tentorial, convexity, and middle fossa DAVMs

totally eliminating and curing a DAVM, except in rare instances of limited fistulae with a small number of accessible feeders. More commonly, DAVMs involve a multitude of feeders, which often arise as small twigs from major cerebral arteries that are not amenable to embolization. While transarterial embolization may obliterate the filling of the lesion after one injection, the DAVM often continues to draw feeders from other sources. Numerous instances are documented in the literature of DAVMs that were partially treated with transarterial embolization and later recurred and progressed to catastrophic hemorrhage.

Transarterial embolization may be effective in palliating disabling symptoms even when it does not totally cure the DAVM. Such lesions should continue to be followed as discussed above. Transarterial embolization also plays an important role in decreasing flow through DAVMs in preparation for surgical intervention, transvenous obliteration, or radiosurgery (see below). This adjunctive, preparatory use of transarterial embolization has greatly enhanced the safety and efficacy of other more definitive treatment measures. Embolization with sclerosing agents or hormones has been shown to cause progressive sclerosis resulting in the cure of certain DAVMs.[20,26] The safety and efficacy of these methods have not been scrutinized carefully in large controlled series.

Transvenous endovascular obliteration of DAVMs has recently been used with excellent results.[4,11,12,27] This modality aims at the thrombosis of the venous side of the lesion, often including the obliteration of the adjacent dural venous sinus. Occlusion of the venous side of DAVMs is usually well tolerated if the pathologic dural sinus is arterialized and does not serve as a site of drainage of cerebrovenous circulation. Instead, the pathologic dural segment is often associated with harmful retrograde leptomeningeal venous drainage, and these channels are secondarily obliterated with thrombosis of the venous side of DAVMs. This strategy has been used most successfully for the treatment of DAVMs with *accessible* venous drainage. Transvenous obliteration is particularly effective in the treatment of cavernous sinus DAVMs (access through the inferior petrosal sinus), although these lesions frequently do not require any therapeutic intervention because of their benign clinical symptomatology and tendency toward spontaneous regression. Transvenous obliteration has also been used in cases of transverse-sigmoid sinus DAVMs, and may be substantially safer than open surgical approaches to these lesions (Fig. 250-4). However, there may be no accessible transvenous route for many DAVMs, including tentorial incisura DAVMs and anterior cranial fossa DAVMs, which frequently behave aggressively. Transvenous obliteration may occasionally be performed after open surgical exposure, through puncture of the dural venous sinus or the arterialized venous varix and the injection of coils or glue. Rarely, transvenous occlusion may result in propagating venous thrombosis or altered hemodynamic patterns with paradoxical clinical deterioration or hemorrhage.[11,12,24]

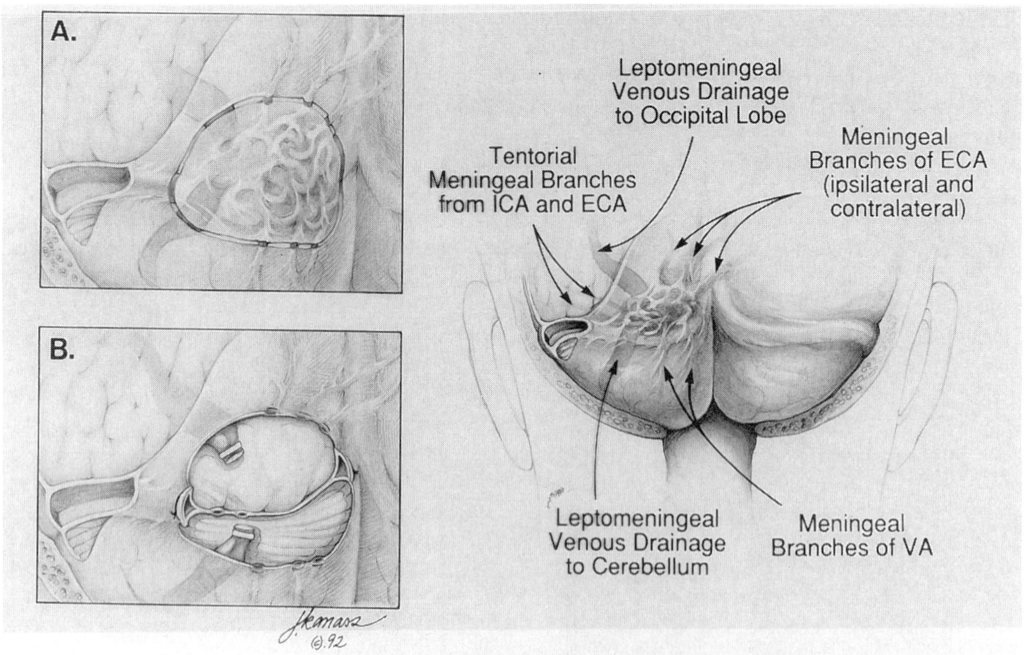

Figure 250-4 Surgical anatomy of a lateral tentorial-transverse sinus region DAVM (with leptomeningeal venous drainage) such as the ones illustrated in Fig. 250-1 and 250-2. *A.* Extent of durotomy of the tentorial leaflets to interrupt pachymeningeal arterial feeders and isolate and excise the pathologic region of dural arteriovenous shunting, including the involved segment of the transverse sinus. *B.* Extent of excision of the pathologic dural leaflets, with interruption of arterialized leptomeningeal venous connections to the adjacent occipital lobe and cerebellum. This same lesion can be treated by transvenous endovascular occlusion of the pathologic dural segment, which may result in thrombosis and obliteration of the whole DAVM. Transarterial embolization of external carotid artery feeders may greatly decrease blood loss during such an operation or may enhance the likelihood of obliterating the DAVM by transvenous occlusion. Transarterial embolization alone may palliate symptoms of pulsatile tinnitus and headache but is not likely to cure the DAVM.

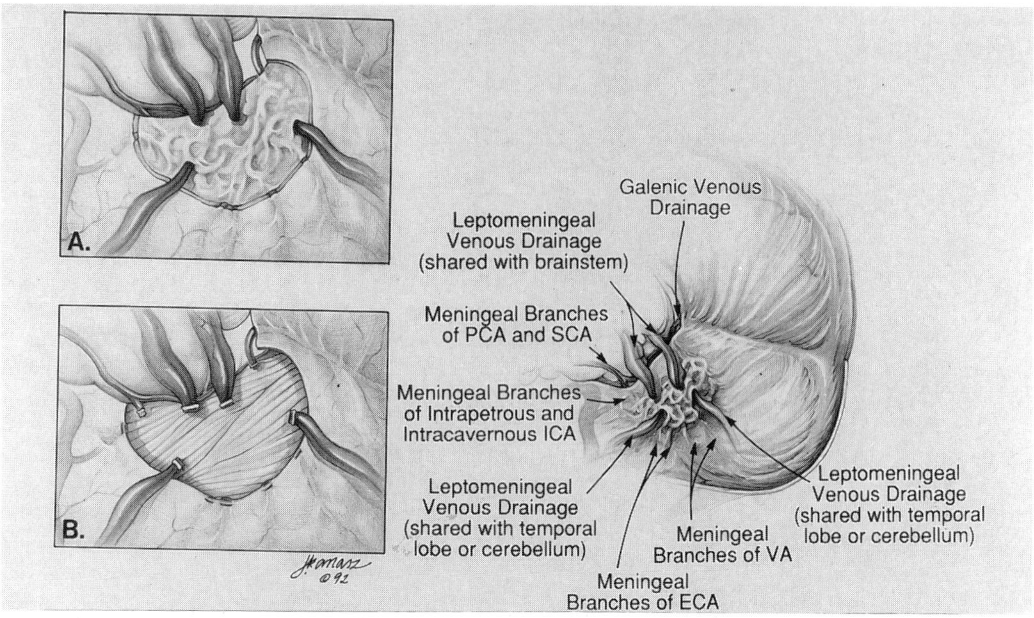

Figure 250-5 Surgical anatomy of a tentorial incisura DAVM (with leptomeningeal venous drainage) such as that illustrated in Fig. 250-3. *A*. Extent of durotomy of the tentorial leaflets to interrupt pachymeningeal arterial feeders and isolate and excise the pathologic region of dural arteriovenous shunting. *B*. Interruption of arterialized leptomeningeal venous drainage to the overlying temporal lobe, the perimesencephalic cistern, and the underlying cerebellum. Dural branches from the posterior cerebral artery and the superior cerebellar artery to the tentorial leaflets are frequently encountered and should be coagulated and divided. This type of lesion is often associated with aggressive neurological involvement, and is not usually amenable to endovascular therapy. Persistent giant arterialized venous varices (following tentorial excision) may be punctured under direct surgical exposure and injected with thrombogenic coils. Intraoperative angiography (internal and external carotid and vertebral artery injections) are extremely useful at confirming complete lesion obliteration.

Open surgical treatment with or without preparatory embolization remains the most versatile and effective therapeutic option for definitively treating DAVMs with aggressive features (Figs. 250-4 through 250-6). The surgical objectives include the isolation, coagulation, and resection of the pathologic dural leaflets (including in some instances the adjacent dural sinus), and disconnection of arterialized leptomeningeal venous drainage, which is typically the source of serious neurological sequelae.[2,3,10,25] Resection of the involved dural sinus can be accomplished without the risk of venous infarction if the resected segment is arterialized and collateral venous channels are well developed.[25] A careful and comprehensive angiographic analysis should be undertaken in each case. With careful planning, excellent surgical results may be achieved, despite the tediousness of the operation and the risk of morbidity from excessive blood loss and injury to brittle, engorged vessels in adjacent brain. Meticulous attention to hemostasis at every step is the key to an optimal technical outcome with these procedures.[2] Preparatory embolization can greatly reduce blood loss in such operations.

Stereotactic radiosurgery has recently been used to treat certain DAVMs, although reports are primarily anecdotal. Recent analysis of experience from a large stereotactic radiosurgery center (Steiner L: personal communication) suggests that this modality may lead to the obliteration of targeted pathologic dural leaflets within approximately 2 years after the procedure.[2] It appears that DAVMs respond like parenchymal arteriovenous malformations treated with radiosurgery. Optimal dosages have not yet been established, especially with regard to preventing radiation damage to adjacent neural structures. Lesions with aggressive clinical features remain prone to hemorrhage in the interval between radiosurgical treatment and obliteration. It is expected that increasing experience with this modality for the treatment of a variety of pathologic conditions will better define its safety and effectiveness. The author currently uses this modality for lateral tentorial DAVMs and for superior sagittal sinus DAVMs where there has not been recent hemorrhage and where other treatment options are judged to be more risky.

Lesions associated with intracranial hypertension and papilledema require special consideration.[2,3,9] Palliation or definitive cure of the DAVM frequently (but not always) results in reversal of papilledema and stabilization of visual symptoms. In other instances, the risks of definitively treating the DAVM may not be justified. Intracranial hypertension may be treated by lumboperitoneal shunting. Ventriculoperitoneal shunting may not be possible in view of small cerebral ventricles, and may be dangerous in the setting of arterialized cortical or subependymal veins. Optic nerve sheath decompression has also been used in cases of progressive papilledema and inoperable DAVMs.

Comprehensive Management Strategy

A DAVM may rarely be discovered on routine imaging studies or angiograms performed for other indications. Incidental lesions must be carefully assessed for features predisposing to aggressive

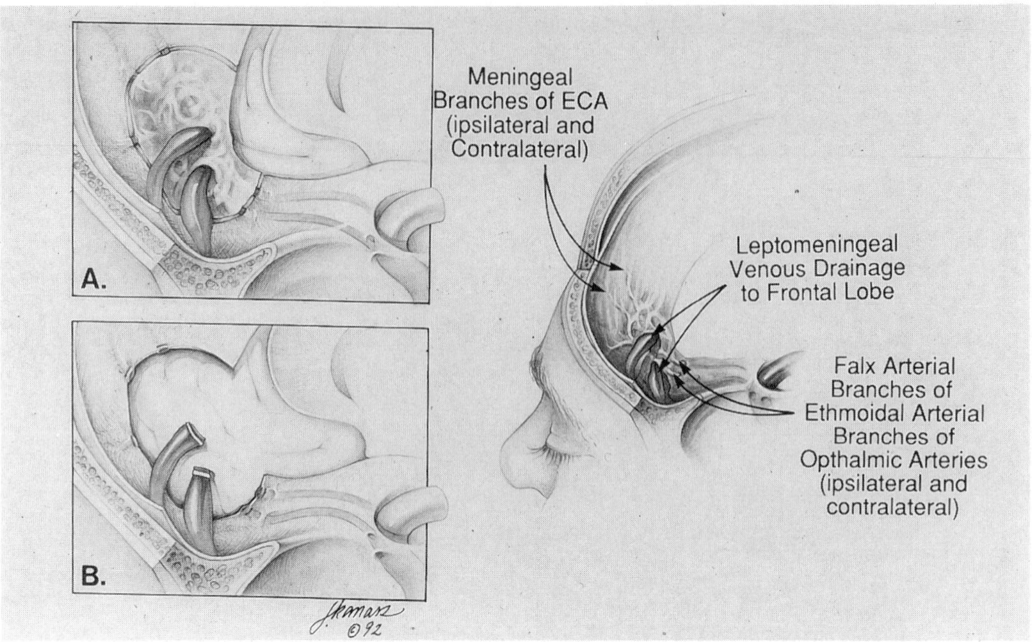

Figure 250-6 Surgical anatomy of an anterior cranial fossa-falx DAVM (with leptomeningeal venous drainage). *A.* Exposure via unilateral frontal craniotomy and outline of the pathologic dural leaflet and leptomeningeal venous connections. *B.* Following resection of the portion of the falx harboring the DAVM, all direct arterialized leptomeningeal venous connections are interrupted and divided. This type of lesion is particularly prone to leptomeningeal venous drainage and to aggressive neurological involvement (including hemorrhage). Preparatory embolization of external carotid artery feeders may reduce blood loss and enhance surgical safety.

clinical behavior. Complete angiographic evaluation is indicated in every case of suspected DAVM unless the patient is a poor candidate for therapeutic intervention or refuses invasive diagnostic studies. Lesions should be evaluated specifically for the presence of leptomeningeal venous drainage and for any variceal or aneurysmal changes in the venous circulation. In the absence of these features, the lesion should be followed expectantly. There is no evidence to justify prophylactic treatment of DAVMs that are not associated with leptomeningeal venous drainage. Expectant follow-up of these lesions should include serial MR imaging for any evidence of development of leptomeningeal venous dilations. Angiographic re-examination of the lesion every few years should be considered, especially for DAVMs at the anterior cranial fossa or the tentorial incisura, which very commonly result in leptomeningeal venous drainage.

Definitive prophylactic treatment should be strongly considered for asymptomatic and incidentally discovered DAVMs with leptomeningeal venous drainage. The patient should be given the option of open surgical intervention or such alternative radiosurgical or endovascular options as may be appropriate for the specific lesion type and location (Tables 250-1 and 250-2). If treatment does not succeed at totally eliminating leptomeningeal venous drainage, either further definitive therapy or very close follow-up of the lesion is indicated. It is our belief that anticoagulation is contraindicated in the setting of DAVMs with leptomeningeal venous drainage.

It appears easiest to justify definitive intervention for DAVMs that have already behaved aggressively. Nevertheless, the morbidity of a first hemorrhage with DAVMs is substantial, and many patients do not survive or do not recover to a condition suitable for therapeutic intervention. Furthermore, little is known about the risk either of subsequent hemorrhage or of the progression of neurological deficits in this clinical setting. However, there are numerous documented cases of progressive repeated hemorrhages or progression of focal neurological symptoms resulting in death or major disability unless the DAVM is obliterated. It is our recommendation that lesions that have hemorrhaged or that cause focal neurological symptoms due to parenchymal venous hypertension be considered for definitive treatment. Palliative therapy is not sufficient in this setting.

Lesions that present with pain or pulsatile tinnitus are evaluated and treated in the same way as incidental lesions. Nonspecific measures aimed at the symptoms are usually sufficient. Palliative treatment of the DAVM may be considered for the control of symptomatology. Rarely is definitive treatment indicated solely for pain or pulsatile tinnitus. We do not believe that the risk of definitive treatment is justified in such DAVMs if they do not exhibit leptomeningeal venous drainage.

Lesions associated with ophthalmoplegia are evaluated on a case-by-case basis. Frequently, painful ophthalmoplegia will resolve spontaneously, and many such lesions involute after angiography. In other cases, ophthalmoplegia may be progressive or associated with retinopathy and visual loss. In such situations, treatment of the associated DAVM is justified. Palliative treatment may be sufficient to stabilize visual symptoms. Again, a radical cure of the DAVM should not be pursued at any risk, and is generally not warranted unless the symptoms are truly debilitating or the DAVM is associated with leptomeningeal venous drainage.

The management of DAVMs associated with papilledema and increased intracranial pressure has been discussed previously.

Again, in the absence of leptomeningeal venous drainage, the risk of radical lesion treatment may not be justified, and may or may not result in subsequent control of intracranial hypertension. Lumboperitoneal shunting or optic nerve sheath decompression may effectively treat the secondary complications of papilledema while the DAVM is followed expectantly, treated palliatively, or subjected to radiosurgery.

In summary, clinical symptoms other than hemorrhage and focal neurological deficits rarely warrant radical treatment of a DAVM, unless the lesion is particularly accessible or is associated with features predisposing to subsequent aggressive clinical behavior. Patient reassurance, symptomatic treatment, or lesion palliation are frequently sufficient. In DAVMs with features predisposing to an aggressive clinical course, a more definitive treatment strategy should be adopted. It is obvious that the myriad of clinical manifestations of DAVMs and the wide spectrum of possible angiographic and pathophysiologic scenarios call for highly individualized management strategies. Diagnostic investigation should be thorough so as to identify DAVMs with features predisposing to aggressive clinical behavior. Treatment strategies should include a highly individualized choice of modalities from the available armamentarium of symptomatic treatment, lesion palliation, transarterial and/or transvenous endovascular therapy, open surgical intervention, and radiosurgery. For the foreseeable future, the treatment of DAVMs should preferably be entrusted to multidisciplinary teams with expertise in the recognition and management of these lesions, and with experience in a variety of treatment options and approaches.

References

1. Aminoff MJ, Kendall BE. Asymptomatic dural vascular anomalies. *Br J Radiol* 1973; 46:662–667.
2. Awad IA, Barrow DL (eds): *Dural Arteriovenous Malformations.* Park Ridge, IL: Am. Assoc. Neurol. Surg., 1993.
3. Awad IA, Little JR, Akarawi WP, et al. Intracranial dural arteriovenous malformations: factors predisposing to an aggressive neurologic course. *J Neurosurg* 1990; 72:839–850.
4. Barnwell SL, Halbach VV, Dowd CF, et al. A variant of arteriovenous fistulas within the wall of dural sinuses. *J Neurosurg* 1991; 74:199–204.
5. Bitoh S, Sakaki S. Spontaneous cure of dural arteriovenous malformation in the posterior fossa. *Surg Neurol* 1979; 12:111–114.
6. Chaudhary MY, Sachdev VP, Cho SH, et al. Dural arteriovenous malformation of the major venous sinuses: an acquired lesion. *Am J Neuroradiol* 1982; 3:13–19.
7. Enker SH. Progression of a dural arteriovenous malformation resulting in an intracerebral hematoma: a case report. *Angiology* 1979; 30:198–204.
8. Fermand M, Reizine D, Melki JP, et al. Long term follow-up of 43 pure dural arteriovenous fistulae (AVF) of the lateral sinus. *Neuroradiology* 1987; 29:348–353.
9. Gelwan MJ, Choi IS, Berenstein A, et al. Dural arteriovenous malformations and papilledema. *Neurosurgery* 1988; 22:1079–1084.
10. Grisoli F, Vincentelli F, Fuchs S, et al. Surgical treatment of tentorial arteriovenous malformations draining into the subarachnoid space: report of four cases. *J Neurosurg* 1984; 60:1059–1066.
11. Halbach VV, Higashida RT, Hieshima GB, et al. Transvenous embolization of dural fistulas involving the cavernous sinus. *Am J Neuroradiol* 1989; 10:377–383.
12. Halbach VV, Higashida RT, Hieshima GB, et al. Transvenous embolization of dural fistulas involving the transverse and sigmoid sinuses. *Am J Neuroradiol* 1989; 10:385–392.
13. Hansen JH, Sogaard I. Spontaneous regression of an extra- and intracranial arteriovenous malformation: case report. *J Neurosurg* 1976; 45:338–341.
14. Houser OW, Campbell JK, Campbell RJ, et al. Arteriovenous malformation affecting the transverse dural venous sinus: an acquired lesion. *Mayo Clin Proc* 1979; 54:651–661.
15. Kerber CW, Newton TH. The macro and microvasculature of the dura mater. *Neuroradiology* 1973; 6:175–179.
16. Lasjaunias P, Chiu M, ter Brugge K, et al. Neurological manifestations of intracranial dural arteriovenous malformations. *J Neurosurg* 1986; 64:724–730.
17. Lasjaunias P, Lopez-Ibor L, Abanou A, et al. Radiological anatomy of the vascularization of cranial dural arteriovenous malformations. *Anat Clin* 1984; 6:87–99.
18. Magidson MA, Weinberg PE. Spontaneous closure of a dural arteriovenous malformation. *Surg Neurol* 1976; 6:107–110.
19. Malik GM, Pearce JE, Ausman JI, et al. Dural arteriovenous malformations and intracranial hemorrhage. *Neurosurgery* 1984; 15:332–339.
20. Manaka S, Izawa M, Nawata H. Dural arteriovenous malformation treated by artificial embolization with liquid silicone. *Surg Neurol* 1977; 7:63–65.
21. Nabors MW, Azzam CJ, Albanna FJ, et al. Delayed postoperative dural arteriovenous malformations: report of two cases. *J Neurosurg* 1987; 66:768–772.
22. Nakada T, Kwee IL, Ellis WG, et al. Subacute diencephalic necrosis and dural arteriovenous malformation. *Neurosurgery* 1985; 17:653–656.
23. Olutola PS, Eliam M, Molot M, et al. Spontaneous regression of a dural arteriovenous malformation. *Neurosurgery* 1983; 12:687–690.
24. Sergott RC, Grossman RI, Savino PJ, et al. The syndrome of paradoxical worsening of dural-cavernous sinus arteriovenous malformations. *Ophthalmology* 1987; 94:205–212.
25. Sundt TM Jr, Piepgras DG. The surgical approach to arteriovenous malformations of the lateral and sigmoid dural sinuses. *J Neurosurg* 1983; 59:32–39.
26. Suzuki J, Komatsu S. New embolization method using estrogen for dural arteriovenous malformation and meningioma. *Surg Neurol* 1981; 16:438–442.
27. Takahashi A, Yoshimoto T, Kawakami K, et al. Transvenous copper wire insertion for dural arteriovenous malformations of cavernous sinus. *J Neurosurg* 1989; 70:751–754.
28. Vidyasagar C. Persistent embryonic veins in the arteriovenous malformations of the dura. *Acta Neurochir (Wien)* 1979; 48:199–216.
29. Vinuela FV, Debrun GM, Fox AJ, et al. Detachable calibrated-leak balloon for superselective angiography and embolization of dural arteriovenous malformations. *J Neurosurg* 1983; 58:817–823.
30. Vinuela F, Fox AJ, Pelz DM, et al. Unusual clinical manifestations of dural arteriovenous malformations. *J Neurosurg* 1986; 64:554–558.
31. Watanabe A, Takahara Y, Ibuchi Y, et al. Two cases of dural arteriovenous malformation occurring after intracranial surgery. *Neuroradiology* 1984; 26:375–380.

251 Carotid-Cavernous Fistulas and Intracavernous Aneurysms

Adam I. Lewis
Thomas A. Tomsick
John M. Tew, Jr.

Since this text was first published in 1985, the management of carotid-cavernous fistulas and intracavernous aneurysms has changed dramatically. Advances in interventional neuroradiology and skull base surgery have been chiefly responsible for the rapid evolution of treatment strategies. Coupled with a better understanding of cavernous sinus anatomy and pathophysiology, these advances make an update timely. Our expanded therapeutic armamentarium for carotid-cavernous fistulas and intracavernous aneurysms has led to a high rate of successful obliteration with minimal morbidity. This chapter first considers carotid-cavernous fistulas and then covers intracavernous aneurysms.

Carotid-Cavernous Fistulas

Historical Review

The earliest treatments for carotid-cavernous fistulas (CCFs) date back to 1809, when Travers successfully occluded a CCF by ligating the common carotid artery.[15] Although ligation often produced initially good results, collateralization from the external carotid artery (ECA) and cavernous segment of the internal carotid artery (ICA) and retrograde flow from the ophthalmic artery produced high recurrence rates. Ligation also led to arterial steal that resulted in cerebral ischemia and vision loss. In the 1930s, Brooks embolized CCFs with strips of muscle and Gardner trapped them by ligating both the cervical and intracranial portions of the ICA.[15] Variation of these early procedures continued into the 1960s with mixed success.

In 1971, the modern era of endovascular surgery began with Prolo and Hanberry, who successfully occluded CCFs with nondetachable balloons.[29] This technique required sacrifice of the ICA, but ischemic complications were less common because of compensated flow from the collateral sources. In 1973, Parkinson reported direct surgical repair of a CCF with preservation of the ICA.[27] Although successful at occluding the fistula, the operation was technically difficult, required cardiac standstill, and produced significant neurological morbidity. By 1974, Serbinenko had developed detachable balloons that occluded the fistula and preserved the ICA.[32] Later, Debrun and colleagues used latex detachable balloons to occlude direct CCFs and was able to achieve a carotid patency rate of 59 percent.[4]

Mullan recognized that symptoms were related to venous drainage. He obliterated CCFs by directly packing the cavernous sinus and was able to preserve the ICA in nearly every case.[25] In an attempt to avoid the morbidity and complexity of a skull base craniotomy, and drawing upon the early transvenous work of Debrun,[4] Halbach and co-workers obliterated CCFs with percutaneous transvenous obliteration techniques in the late 1980s.[11,14] By 1991, Guglielmi had introduced soft detachable platinum coils that were retrievable, and later used them to occlude CCFs (Figure 251-1).[8] Technical improvements in microcatheters, guide wires, and angiography (e.g., digital road-mapping, rapid-sequence imaging, magnification) have contributed greatly to recent advances in interventional neuroradiology and will continue to influence the treatment of CCFs.

No less significant was the work of Dolenc, who surgically repaired four carotid-cavernous fistulas and three cavernous sinus aneurysms without cardiac standstill.[6] His work renewed interest in surgical anatomy, techniques, and approaches to lesions of the cavernous sinus and the skull base. During the 1980s, numerous investigators advanced our understanding of cavernous sinus surgical anatomy and approaches. Today direct surgery for CCFs and intracavernous aneurysms is a safe and effective treatment alternative when endovascular techniques have failed.

Classification

Carotid-cavernous fistulas may be categorized according to pathogenesis, hemodynamic profile, or angiographic anatomy.[5] Barrow's classification for CCFs defines four types (A, B, C, and D) based on angiographic anatomy. It has become the most widely used classification scheme because each type has a characteristic vascular supply that determines the therapeutic approach and predicts outcome.[2]

Type A shunts are direct fistulas between the ICA and the cavernous sinus. These high-flow fistulas usually occur after trauma or rupture of a carotid-cavernous aneurysm (Fig. 251-2). Traumatic fistulas occur most often in young men, whereas ruptured aneurysms occur most frequently in elderly women. It is poorly understood how traumatic fistulas occur. A fracture of the skull base is often thought to be the cause, and occasionally a spicule of bone is seen adjacent to a tear in the carotid artery. Traumatic fistulas rarely resolve spontaneously and have a high cure rate with a single detachable balloon placed across the ostium of the fistula. Our series (1980 through 1992) included 100 type A fistulas; the patients were equally divided between males and females and ranged in age from 5 to 93 years (mean 42). Of the fistulas, 76 were traumatic, 22 resulted from a ruptured aneurysm, and 2 were iatrogenic. Eighty-six were closed with a detachable latex or silicone balloon, six resolved spontaneously after unsuccessful transarterial treatment attempts, five required direct surgery, two were closed with nondetachable balloons, and in the remaining case the patient died from related injuries. The permanent neurological complication rate was 4 percent: infarction occurred in one case, intracerebral hemorrhage in one case, aseptic cavernous sinus

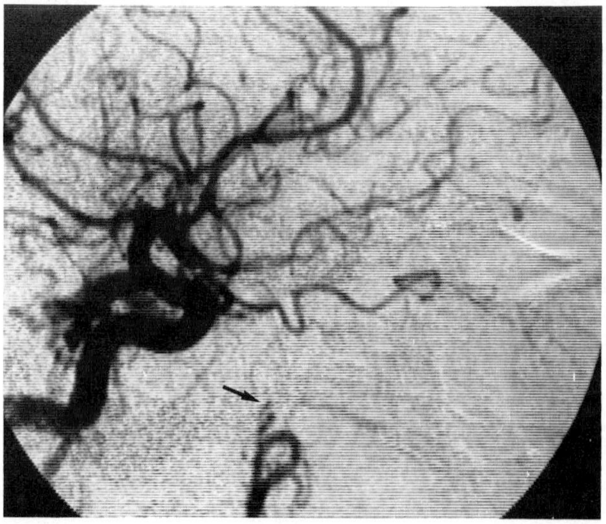

(*A*)

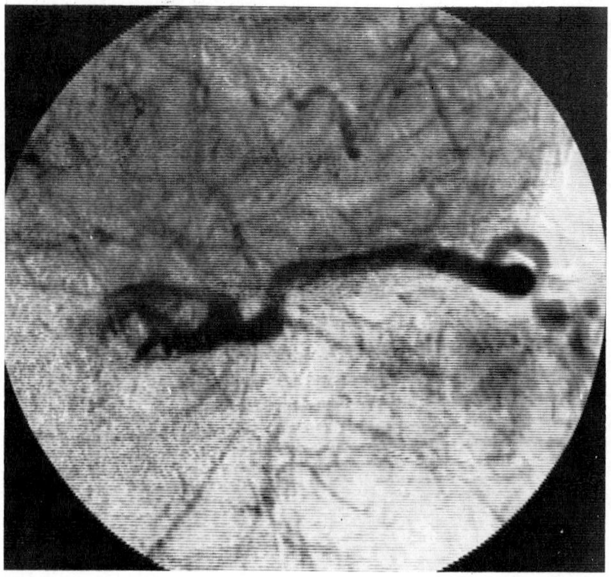

(*B*)

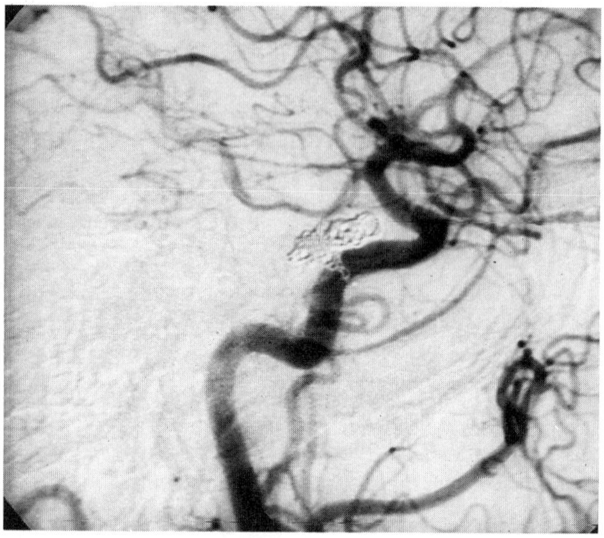

(*C*)

Figure 251-1 Digital subtraction angiograms show staged transarterial and transvenous embolization of a dural CCF. *A*. The fistula is fed by numerous branches of the ICA and ECA. Note the previously embolized branch of the internal maxillary artery (*arrow*). *B*. Late arteriogram of the common carotid artery with filling of the superior ophthalmic vein, which was catheterized in retrograde fashion. *C*. Complete obliteration of the fistula and preservation of the ICA after transvenous embolization with platinum microcoils.

thrombosis with unilateral vision loss in another case, and one death related to middle cerebral artery infarction from balloon movement and ICA occlusion. Overall, patency of the carotid artery was maintained in 74 percent of cases after the fistula was occluded with a detachable balloon.

Types B, C, and D are low-flow dural fistulas that arise spontaneously. They usually occur in middle-aged and elderly women, have an indolent natural history, and often resolve spontaneously. Type B shunts are fistulas between meningeal branches of the ICA and the cavernous sinus; type C shunts are fistulas between the meningeal branches of the ECA and the cavernous sinus; and type D shunts have connections between meningeal branches of both internal and external carotid arteries. To define the anatomy of dural CCFs, bilateral selective vessel angiography of both internal and external carotid arteries is required.

The origin of most dural carotid-cavernous fistulas is idiopathic. Atherosclerosis, hypertension, and mild trauma may predispose patients to rupturing of these meningeal vessels. A widely held theory is that sinus thrombosis leads to formation of dural fistulas, and, indeed, partial thrombosis of the cavernous sinus was found in 18 (90 percent) of 20 cases studied by Viñuela and associates.[34] Also, CCFs are linked to collagen vascular diseases such as Ehler-Danlos syndrome, Marfan's syndrome, fibromuscular dysplasia, and pseudoxanthoma elasticum.[9,16,18] Most investigators believe that dural CCFs are acquired lesions, but two cases of congenital CCFs have been reported.[20]

Clinical Features

The symptoms depend on the direction of venous drainage, and the severity depends on the rate of blood flow through the shunt. Type A, or high-flow, fistulas usually present with symptoms that are severe and rapidly progressive. A prominent orbital bruit is the most common initial symptom. In our series of 100 patients with type A fistulas, 80 had an orbital bruit, 72 demonstrated proptosis,

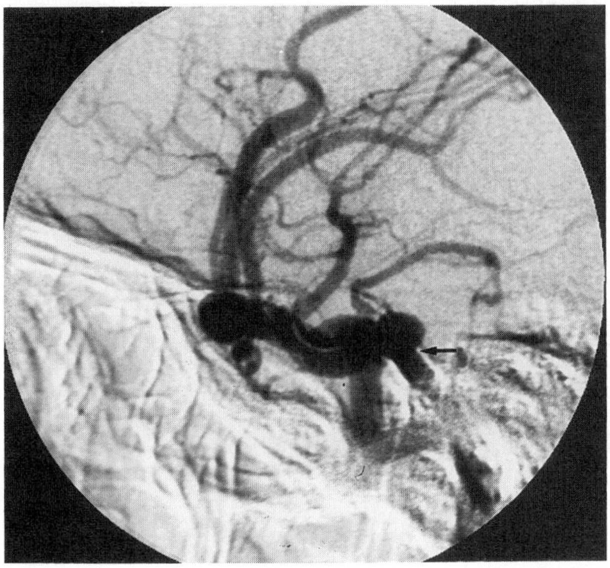

(*A*)

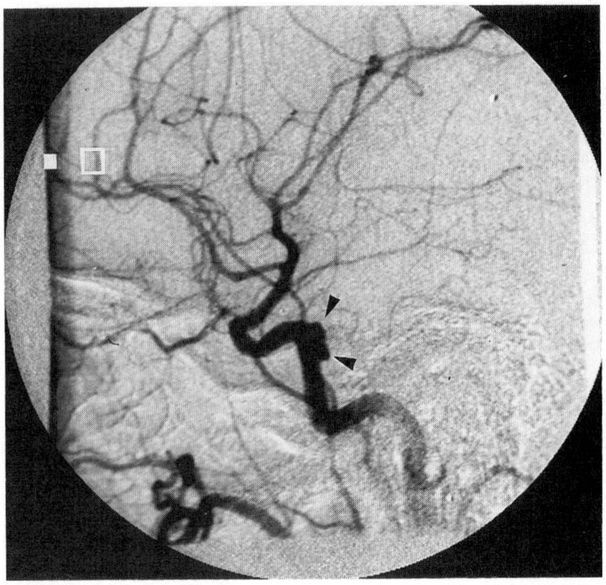

(*B*)

Figure 251-2 High-flow CCFs commonly arise from trauma or aneurysm rupture. *A*. Rupture of this spontaneous intracavernous aneurysm produced a CCF, which caused an intracerebral hemorrhage (*arrow*). *B*. After balloon embolization, the fistula was occluded and patency of the ICA was maintained (*arrowheads*).

55 had chemosis, and 49 presented with an isolated abducens palsy on the affected side. Patients complained of headaches or retro-orbital pain in 25 cases, of ophthalmoplegia in 24, and of visual loss in 17. Oculomotor and trigeminal nerve deficits occurred in 11 and 6 patients, respectively.

Eye signs (e.g., proptosis, chemosis, vascular congestion of the conjunctiva, diplopia, oculoparesis) are more prominent when the venous drainage is anteriorly through the ophthalmic veins. Proptosis is pulsatile, with distended veins pushing the globe downward and laterally. Chemosis results from the arterialization of the conjunctival and scleral veins. Extraocular muscle palsies may occur owing to cranial nerve ischemia or edema from venous distention. When the venous drainage is predominantly through the sphenoparietal sinus or superior and inferior petrosal sinuses, eye signs are minimal but cortical and brain stem dysfunction may be present. Fistulas that drain into cortical veins have a high risk for hemorrhage (Fig. 251-3). Most CCFs have a balanced anterior and posterior drainage pattern. When the anterior intracavernous sinus is patent, ocular symptoms and signs may be bilateral or contralateral to the fistula.

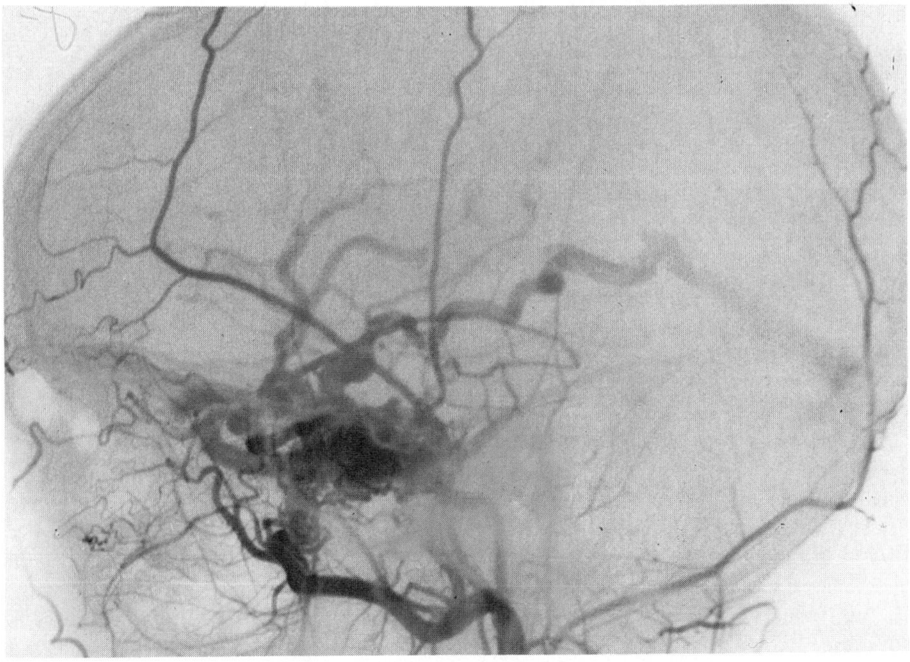

(*A*)

Figure 251-3 CCFs draining into cortical veins cause venous hypertension and are prone to hemorrhage. *A*. Angiogram shows a CCF with cortical venous drainage.

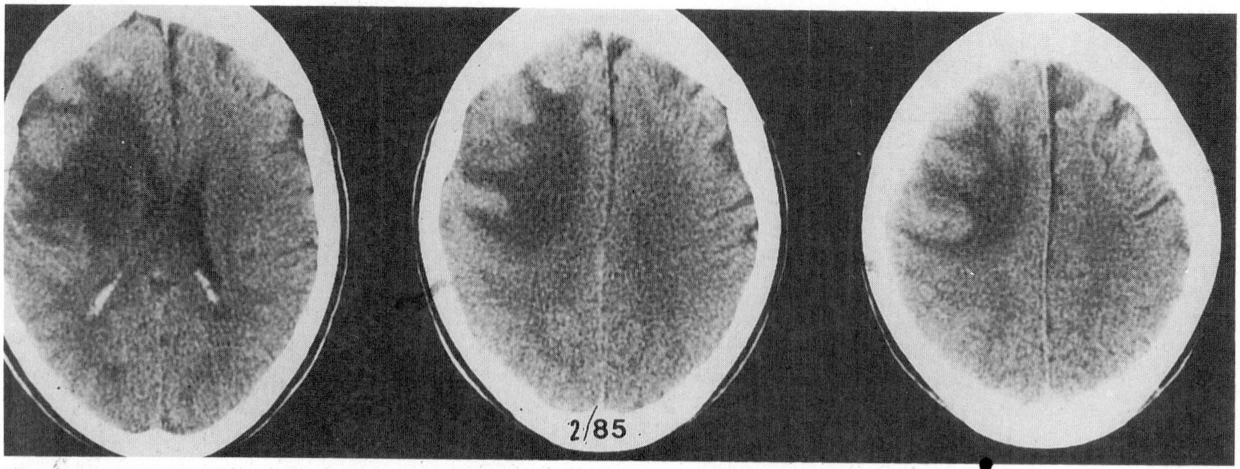

(*B*)

Figure 251-3 (*Continued*) *B*. Noncontrast CT scan of the same CCF shows significant right frontal lobe edema from venous hypertension and focal areas of hemorrhage caused by rupture of fragile cortical veins.

By comparison, dural CCFs are characterized by slow flow, low morbidity, and an indolent natural history. These shunts arise spontaneously, commonly present with mild retro-orbital headaches, and less frequently have cranial bruits. The conjunctival and scleral vessels are less dilated and the orbit is less proptotic and chemotic than with direct or type A fistulas. Symptoms may regress or change in character as the fistula undergoes thrombosis and other meningeal feeding vessels supplant the ones that have thrombosed. The rate of spontaneous resolution reported in the literature varies from 10 to 73 percent.[30] Although the cause of spontaneous occlusion is unknown, occasionally the fistula may thrombose during or after cerebral arteriography. Perhaps catheter-induced vasospasm or the thrombotic effects of the contrast material may cause the fistula to thrombose.

Radiologic Studies

Cerebral angiography is the best diagnostic study for CCFs. Selective catheterization of both internal and external carotid and vertebral arteries is essential to define the anatomy and develop the treatment plan. Rapid-frame sequencing is a useful angiographic tool for locating the shunt precisely. Slow ICA injection above carotid compression or vertebral injection with compression of the carotid artery on the ipsilateral side may achieve the same effect (Fig. 251-4). The characteristic angiographic features of direct CCFs are direct opacification of an enlarged cavernous sinus, early filling of ophthalmic veins, and diminished opacification of the distal arterial system. Angiography also determines the patency of the superior ophthalmic vein and the inferior petrosal sinus, information that is essential to planning a transvenous approach to the cavernous sinus.

Magnetic resonance (MR) imaging with MR angiography is useful for screening and routine post-treatment imaging. Computed tomography (CT) scans may be normal in small, low-flow fistulas. A flow void in the dilated superior ophthalmic vein, patency of the inferior petrosal sinus, and dilation of the intracavernous sinuses may be seen on MR images.

Transcranial Doppler ultrasound correlates well with angiography, detects flow changes in the orbit, and identifies collateral flow.[7] Color-coded images can differentiate zones of high and low flow. In the future, ultrasound may supplant MR imaging as a screening tool for CCFs because it is less expensive, provides accurate results, and shows blood flow in real time. In cases with classic history and physical findings of CCF, MR and CT studies can be bypassed in favor of angiography.

Indications for Treatment

Carotid-cavernous fistulas resulting from trauma or ruptured cavernous aneurysms rarely resolve because the shunts have a high rate of blood flow (Fig. 251-5). The goals of therapy are to preserve vision, eliminate the bruit, restore the orbit and its contents to

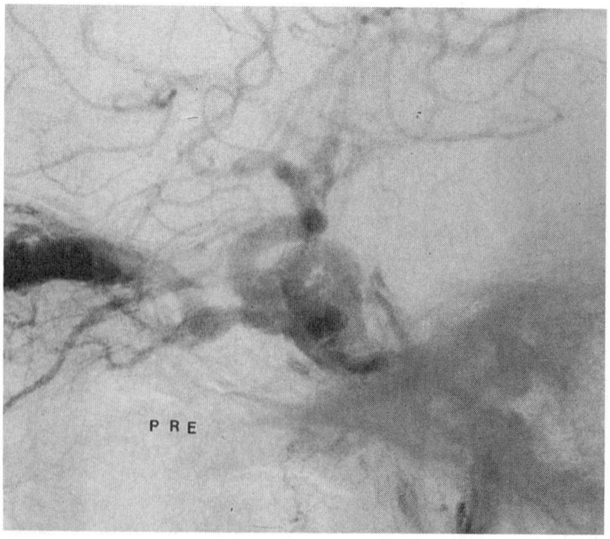

(*A*)

Figure 251-4 The size and location of the fistula must be identified precisely so that the balloon size can be matched to the size of the ostium. *A*. Angiogram of the ICA shows a traumatic CCF with poor filling of the cerebral vessels (arterial steal) and a prominent superior ophthalmic vein.

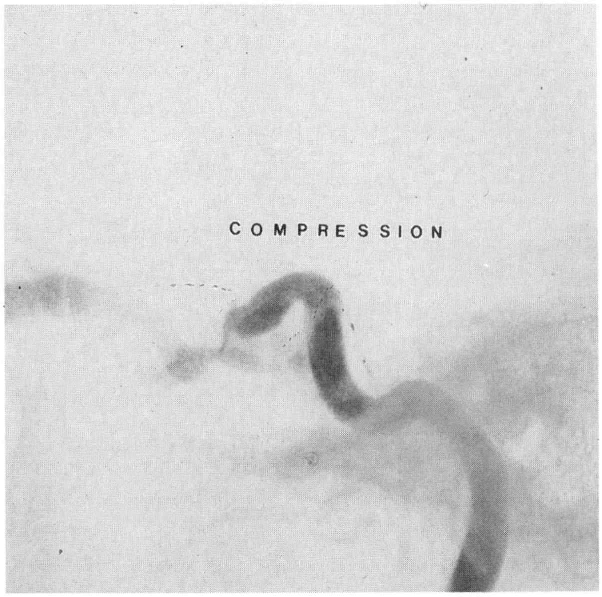

(B)

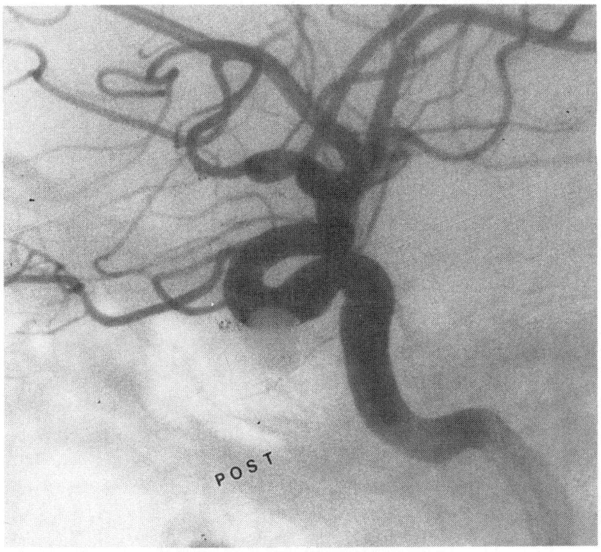

(C)

Figure 251-4 (*Continued*) *B*. Manual compression of the ipsilateral ICA is a useful technique for localizing the exact site of the fistula. *C*. The fistula is obliterated with two detachable balloons, and the ICA remains patent; normal flow to the distal cerebral vessels is restored.

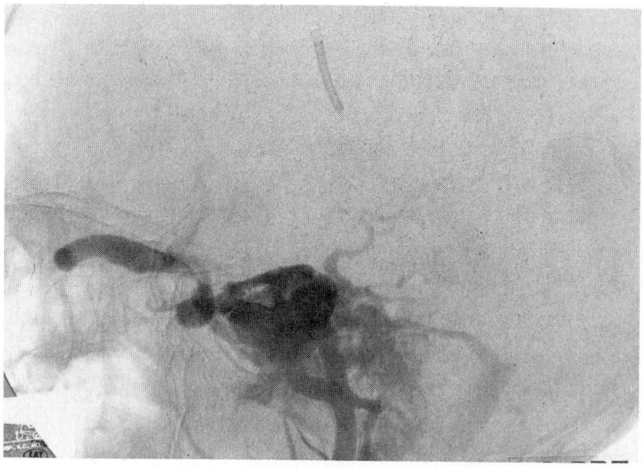

(A)

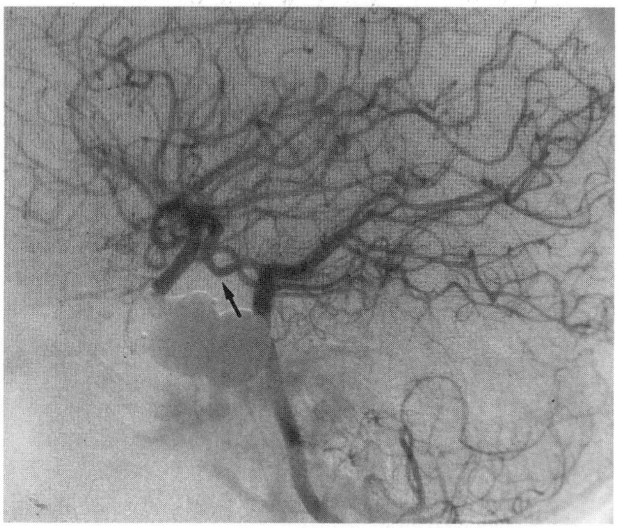

(B)

Figure 251-5 Detachable balloons are well suited to the treatment of high-flow, high-volume CCFs. *A*. This carotid angiogram shows a holocavernous carotid fistula with a dilated superior ophthalmic vein. *B*. The postocclusion angiogram shows obliteration of the fistula with collateral flow to the anterior circulation through the posterior communicating artery (*arrow*).

their normal architecture, and avoid cerebral ischemic complications. The surgical goal is to occlude the fistula and preserve the ICA. Urgent treatment is required when there is progressive visual loss, corneal exposure, cortical venous drainage, or epistaxis. If the patient is comatose and vision cannot be assessed, the fistula should be obliterated. Other less emergent but no less significant indications are medically intractable headaches, intolerable bruit, persistent extraocular muscle palsy, and cosmetically offensive chemosis.

By comparison, dural fistulas have an indolent natural history and a high rate of spontaneous cure. A trial of observation is warranted unless there is visual loss, increased ocular pressure, or corneal damage. Unlike traumatic, high-flow fistulas, with which vision loss occurs by vascular steal, direct injury to the optic nerve, or retinal detachment, vision loss from dural fistulas is caused by venous hypertension and ischemia from decreased perfusion. Chronically elevated intraocular pressure may produce optic atrophy, cataracts, glaucoma, and corneal neovascularity. Patients being observed should be monitored closely for visual acuity, pupillomotor activity, intraocular pressures, and visual fields; proptosis measurements, funduscopy, and gonioscopy should also be performed.

Treatment Options

Transarterial detachable balloon embolization is the treatment of choice for type A CCFs (Fig. 251-6). In our series, 86 percent of CCFs were occluded with detachable balloons, and in 74 percent of cases, patency of the ICA was maintained. In our early experience, the cervical carotid artery was punctured directly; however, this led to five cases of intimal dissection, fortunately without neurological injury. Presently, the standard endovascular approach is by percutaneous puncture of the femoral artery. Fistulas recurred from balloon movement in three cases and from premature deflation in one.

Type A CCFs may be treated transvenously when the ICA is narrowed or occluded. This situation is seen with traumatic dissections, atherosclerotic disease, a failed transarterial attempt, or fistula recurrence after trapping. The inferior petrosal sinus or superior ophthalmic vein must be patent for a transvenous approach to the cavernous sinus to be feasible. In our experience, a transvenous approach failed to occlude the fistula in three cases in which it was attempted because we were unable to navigate through the partitions of the cavernous sinus to the fistula site. Debrun and associates reported a similar experience.[4] Halbach et al., who treated 14 (8.5 percent) of 165 cases of type A CCFs from a transvenous approach, also had difficulty navigating through the partitions of the cavernous sinus.[11] In this series, 11 of the 14 fistulas approached transvenously were successfully occluded with a variety of embolic agents; one patient died after the occlusion of the fistula diverted flow into cortical veins and produced a pontine hemorrhage, and another patient suffered a subarachnoid hemorrhage after the inferior petrosal sinus was perforated during catheterization. A third patient's symptoms were palliated but the fistula remained patent. Since then, steerable guide wires and softer, smaller catheters that lessen the risk of vein perforation have been developed.

Embolic material deposited transvenously in the cavernous sinus may travel through the fistula into the ICA and lead to embolization of distal cerebral vessels. Temporarily inflating a balloon in the ICA at the ostium of the fistula prevents reflux into the ICA. The cavernous sinus may be converted into an aneurysm by blocking all venous drainage without occluding the fistula. Occluding posterior venous drainage may divert flow into the ophthalmic veins and cause vision loss or ocular symptoms. Currently, transarterial detachable balloons are the treatment of choice for type A or direct CCFs. In the future, the use of electrolytically detachable and retrievable platinum coils may overcome some of the limitations of detachable balloons.[8] These coils are soft enough to conform to the shape of the cavernous sinus and are less likely to damage or compress surrounding structures.

A direct surgical approach is indicated if the transarterial and transvenous approaches fail. For example, partial occlusion of a fistula with a single balloon may slow the flow and narrow the ostium so that another balloon will not flow into the fistula. Despite guide-wire-directed catheters, the ostium may be too narrow to allow a balloon to enter the cavernous sinus. To avoid a transvenous or surgical approach when the ICA is narrowed or occluded, percutaneous angioplasty[28] or high cervical-carotid puncture[13] are possible options.

Unless there is an emergent need for cure, dural CCFs should be managed conservatively. Manual compression of the cervical

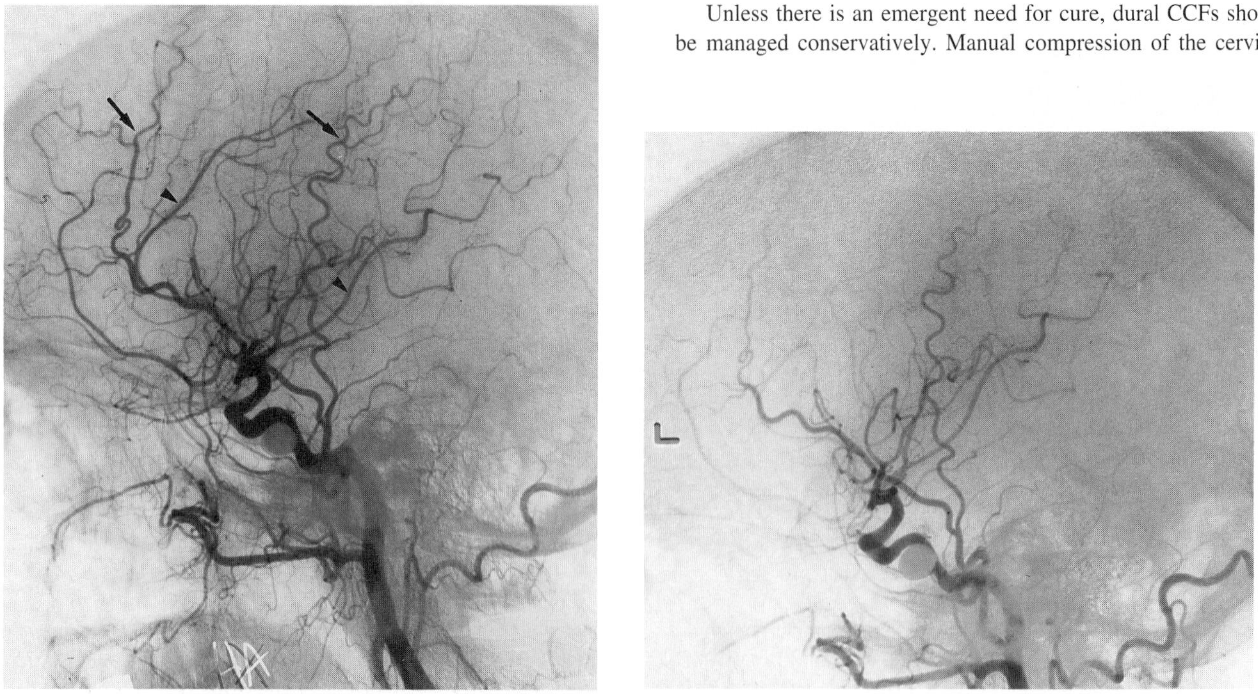

(*A*) (*B*)

Figure 251-6 Detachable balloons that protrude into the lumen of the parent artery may move or create thromboemboli. *A*. An ICA angiogram shows complete obliteration of a CCF. Although the ICA is patent, the balloon has caused a stenosis. Note that ECA branches (*arrows*) fill simultaneously with ICA branches (*arrowheads*), indicating diminished flow through the ICA. *B*. Angiogram repeated 2 days later shows movement of the balloon with near-complete ICA occlusion. Because of the risk for stroke, the ICA was occluded proximally with another detachable balloon.

carotid artery has been effective in 30 percent of cases and may be attempted initially if vision is not threatened and if there is no underlying atherosclerotic disease.[10] If symptoms persist or progress, more aggressive forms of therapy are required.

Symptomatic dural CCFs can be treated with a variety of endovascular approaches. Type C dural fistulas are derived entirely from the ECA and are most easily cured by transarterial embolization alone. Type B fistulas are very rare and are supplied entirely by dural branches of the ICA. Embolization of these branches carries a high risk for stroke; therefore, type B fistulas are best managed by transvenous approaches. Nevertheless, using superselective transarterial catheterization techniques, Halbach et al. successfully occluded four cavernous sinus dural fistulas that were fed primarily by branches of the ICA.[12] Type D fistulas have a mixed supply from both the internal and external carotid arteries. These shunts are initially treated with embolization of their external carotid component because partial occlusion in these slow-flow shunts may induce subsequent thrombosis of the remaining fistulous component. If that does not happen, then a transvenous or direct surgical approach is required.

Direct surgical packing of the cavernous sinus is a safe and effective option for treatment of types B and D dural CCFs.[25] Indications for packing of the cavernous sinus are the following: small-volume fistulas that will not accept a balloon; patients who will not tolerate carotid occlusion; fistulas with supply from the ICA; failed trapping or ligation methods; and failed endovascular transvenous attempts.[26] The goal of surgery is to completely thrombose the cavernous sinus.

Direct surgical packing of the cavernous sinus requires that the fistula be located precisely, in either the anteroinferior or posterosuperior compartment. The cavernous sinus is packed through the superior ophthalmic vein if the fistula is anterior, or through the superior petrosal sinus if it is posterior. If the superior petrosal sinus is not patent, Parkinson's triangle is opened. If the superior ophthalmic vein cannot be identified, then the cavernous sinus is opened through the anteroinferior triangle. A variety of thrombogenic materials are used to pack the cavernous sinus, including biodegradable Gelfoam (absorbable gelatin sponge; The Upjohn Company, Kalamazoo, MI) and Surgicel (oxidized regenerated cellulose; Johnson & Johnson Medical, Inc., Arlington, TX), platinum coils, copper wire, and strands of cotton.[26]

The pathophysiology of dural fistulas is primarily venous hypertension, and treatment is approached from the venous side. Despite the proven success of Mullan's surgical technique, percutaneous venous approaches have supplanted direct surgery. Advances in endovascular techniques now allow transvenous approaches to the cavernous sinus through the inferior petrosal sinus or the superior ophthalmic vein. Improved catheter and guide wire technologies have made navigation on the venous side much safer. Types B and D dural CCFs are now initially treated via the superior ophthalmic vein or inferior petrosal sinus. A percutaneous transvenous approach avoids the morbidity of a craniotomy and does not require the surgical expertise of skull base surgery. Nevertheless, direct surgery remains a complementary alternative for dural CCFs when percutaneous transvenous routes fail or are unavailable.

Radiosurgery may become a useful treatment alternative for dural CCFs, provided the symptoms are mild enough to allow a long latent period for occlusion. Radiosurgery has been shown to be safe and effective for dural CCFs.[1,36] However, further study of the long-term effects of irradiation on the cavernous sinus in a larger patient population is needed before radiotherapy can become a widely accepted treatment for dural CCFs.

Intracavernous Carotid Aneurysms

Historical Review

In 1928, Birley and Trotter first reported successful occlusion of a carotid-cavernous aneurysm after ligating the ICA and ECA. However, this form of treatment in other patients was associated with the same ischemic complications as occurred after carotid ligation for CCFs. Using nondetachable balloons, Weil et al. reported a significantly lower rate of ischemic complications (9.6 versus 24 percent) than with carotid ligation.[35] In 1981, Debrun et al. began trapping intracavernous aneurysms with detachable balloons[4] and, later, Higashida et al. were able to guide the balloon directly into the aneurysm and preserve the ICA in 19 (22 percent) of 87 cases.[17] To the same end, Dolenc surgically opened the cavernous sinus and directly clipped the aneurysm in three cases.[6] To preserve normal hemodynamics in cases where the carotid artery was sacrificed, Fukushima developed the petrous-to-supraclinoid carotid artery bypass in 1986.[33] Balloon test occlusion (BTO) was developed to provide a more rational approach to therapeutic decision making and the prevention of ischemic complications after ICA occlusion.

Classification

Intracavernous aneurysms are classified as congenital (saccular), atherosclerotic (fusiform), traumatic (pseudoaneurysm), or infectious (mycotic). Congenital aneurysms are caused by a defect in the vessel wall, arise at a bifurcation of the carotid artery, and occur in an older population, showing a strong association with hypertension. Fusiform aneurysms often contain a mural dissection that produces a circumferential dilation. The propensity for thrombus formation along the dissection may lead to transient ischemic attacks or stroke. Traumatic aneurysms arise from basal skull fractures or parasphenoidal procedures. Pseudoaneurysm formation and delayed massive epistaxis is well documented after ICA injury during transphenoidal pituitary surgery. Most mycotic aneurysms arise from direct extension of paranasal sinus infections. In a review of the literature, *Staphylococcus aureus* was the most commonly cultured organism; however, in nearly half of the cases no organism was identified.[19]

Intracavernous aneurysms account for approximately 5 percent of all intracranial aneurysms and occur mainly in women during the fifth and sixth decades. Most aneurysms arise from the C3 segment, or anterior genu (47 percent); followed by the C4, or horizontal, segment (34 percent); the C5, or posterior, portion (9 percent); and the ophthalmic segment (9 percent).[22] Morphologically, 90 percent of spontaneous aneurysms are saccular and 10 percent are fusiform. In comparison, traumatic aneurysms demonstrate delayed filling and emptying by angiography, have a sac with irregular contours, show an absence of a clear neck, and are not located at a vessel bifurcation. Nearly half (48 percent) are large (1 to 2.5 cm), 34 percent are small (<1 cm), and 16 percent are giant (>2.5 cm).[23] In our series of 72 patients with 77 cavernous aneurysms, 5 (7 percent) had bilateral intracavernous aneurysms, and 6 (8 percent) had multiple intradural aneurysms. In another series of 70 patients with 79 cavernous aneurysms, mirror-image cavernous aneurysms were present in 9 (13 percent) patients and intradural aneurysms in 7 (10 percent).[21]

Clinical Features

As the use of MR imaging increases, more asymptomatic intracavernous aneurysms are being discovered. When patients become symptomatic, the onset may be sudden, and symptoms may wax, wane, or progress slowly. In most cases, symptoms are related to a mass effect. For example, a cavernous aneurysm that enlarges medially may produce pituitary abnormalities; lateral displacement may cause a cavernous sinus syndrome; and anterior enlargement can manifest as a superior orbital fissure syndrome. Retro-orbital pain and headache caused by aneurysmal compression of the dura and trigeminal nerve was seen in 39 (54 percent) of 72 patients in our series. The abducens nerve was affected in 29 (40 percent), the optic nerve in 12 (17 percent), the oculomotor nerve in 10 (14 percent), and the trigeminal nerve in 8 (11 percent). Ophthalmoplegia occurred in 20 (28 percent) patients; in another large series it was seen in 59 (84 percent) of 70 patients.[21] Less frequently, patients may present with tinnitus, epistaxis, transient ischemic attacks, or subarachnoid hemorrhage. Vision loss occurs from compression of the optic nerve and is always preceded by signs of cavernous sinus dysfunction.[21] Transient ischemic attacks can occur when emboli dislodge from thrombus within the aneurysm; epistaxis occurs after the aneurysm has eroded into the sphenoid sinus and ruptures or after transnasal biopsy. In our series, 22 (31 percent) of 72 patients presented with aneurysmal rupture; in 17 cases the rupture was spontaneous and in 5 it was traumatic. In the literature, rates of spontaneous rupture with conversion to a direct CCF ranges from 3 to 9 percent.[17] The higher rate in our series probably reflects a referral bias. The rate of subarachnoid hemorrhage is 1.4 to 11 percent and varies according to the angiographic definition of an intracavernous aneurysm.[21] Some authors think that aneurysms that arise from the anterior genu or develop from trauma should not be counted as cavernous carotid artery aneurysms. Nevertheless, aneurysms arising from the anterior segment of the ICA are susceptible to subarachnoid hemorrhage and should be treated because angiography cannot predict if an aneurysm of the anterior genu is intra- or extracavernous in location; the exact origin requires surgical confirmation.

Radiologic Studies

Cerebral angiography demonstrates the origin of the aneurysm and the size of its neck, turbulent flow patterns, and collateral flow patterns of the circle of Willis. Magnetic resonance imaging and MR angiography complement the role of angiography by demonstrating the exact size of the aneurysm and its residual lumen, the occurrence of thrombosis, the relationship of the aneurysm to surrounding structures, and the resolution of mass effect and edema after treatment. In addition, MR imaging is a good screening tool for initial diagnosis. Computed tomography is useful to identify erosion of the anterior clinoid, inferior optic canal, and lateral wall of the sphenoid sinus, as well as to visualize calcium in the wall or neck of the aneurysm.

Indications for Treatment

Most intracavernous aneurysms have a benign natural history and may be observed if patients are asymptomatic[21] and if the aneurysm does not originate from the anterior genu of the ICA or extend into the subarachnoid space.[23] Treatment should be initiated emergently for subarachnoid hemorrhage, epistaxis, progressive visual loss, or worsening oculoparesis. Severe ipsilateral facial or retro-orbital pain, and radiographic evidence of aneurysm enlargement should be treated promptly. Stable cranial nerve palsies may be managed conservatively, because in 25 to 40 percent of patients they will improve spontaneously.[21,23]

Treatment Options

Aneurysms of the cavernous portion of the ICA are difficult to treat by direct surgery because of the surrounding cavernous sinus. The goal of treatment is to eliminate the aneurysm and reduce the mass effect. Historically, Hunterian ligation of the ICA or common carotid artery was the standard treatment for unclippable aneurysms. Unfortunately, this technique had a high morbidity and mortality rate from thromboembolic phenomena, vascular steal, hemorrhage, and persisting aneurysm.[17]

With improved endovascular techniques and cavernous sinus surgery, the treatment of intracavernous aneurysms has changed dramatically. Aneurysm occlusion by detachable balloons or thrombogenic platinum coils with preservation of the ICA is now the procedure of choice (Fig. 251-7). When the aneurysm neck is poorly defined, vascular bypass grafting of the aneurysmal segment followed by ICA occlusion maintains natural hemodynamics but involves an extensive surgical procedure. Another commonly employed approach involves trapping the aneurysm with detachable balloons. Among a patient population averaging over 60 years of age, ICA occlusion is well tolerated with minimal morbidity. Preoperative clinical balloon test occlusion (BTO) of the ICA is performed to assess cerebral blood flow and collateral circulation and to predict tolerance for occlusion.

In the management of cavernous carotid aneurysms or cavernous sinus lesions, the ICA may be sacrificed. We combine BTO with technetium-99m hexamethylpropyleneamineoxine (HMPAO) single-photon emission CT and nipride-induced hypotension to identify patients with poor collateral circulation who are at risk for stroke. HMPAO scanning is a radionucleotide cerebral blood flow study; the agent can be administered intravenously at the time of the BTO and scanning can be deferred until the catheter is removed. The HMPAO radionucleotide crosses the blood-brain barrier and is retained in cerebral tissue; its uptake is proportional to cerebral blood flow.[3] Our protocol begins with a 10-minute occlusion of the ICA followed by a 30 percent decrease in mean arterial pressure. We drop blood pressure with nipride to identify patients at risk for delayed stroke if they suffer a hypotensive episode during anesthesia induction, surgical blood loss, or other unforeseen situations. The HMPAO study is graded from 0 to 2 (none to minimal decrease in uptake) and 3 to 4 (moderate to severe decrease in uptake). This procedure is safe and the equipment is available in most radiology departments. Of other assessments of cerebral blood flow that can be done during BTO (quantitative stable xenon CT, transcranial Doppler sonography, EEG monitoring, and measurement of arterial back pressures), only xenon CT has contributed to patient management.

We placed our patients in three groups according to the results of the BTO and HMPAO scan. In 80 percent of cases (group 1), the BTO was negative and the HMPAO scan was graded 0 to 2. In 8 percent of cases (group 2), the BTO was negative and the HMPAO scan was graded 3 to 4. In 12 percent of cases (group 3), the BTO was positive and the HMPAO scan was graded 3 to 4. Our group percentages parallel the BTO results of Linskey et al. in that the risk for ipsilateral hemispheric ischemia after carotid occlusion was low in 75 percent, moderate in 15 percent, and high in

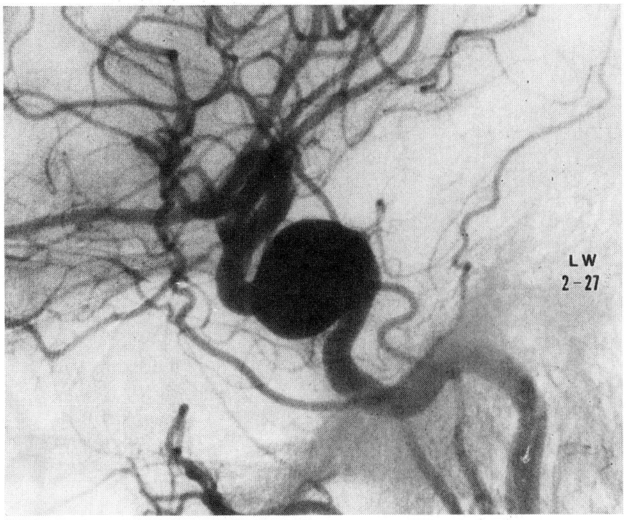

(*A*)

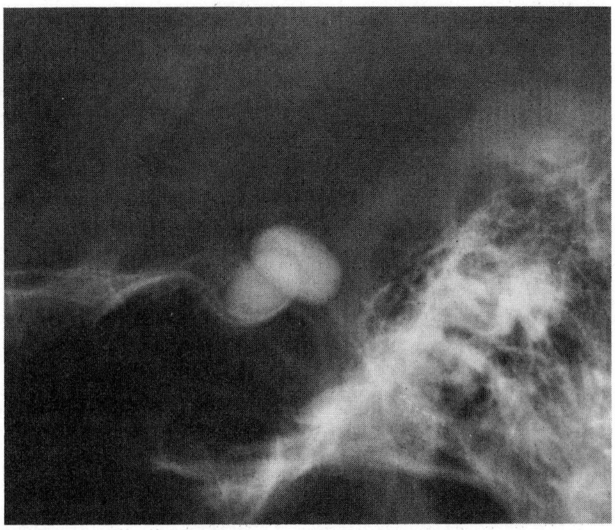

(*B*)

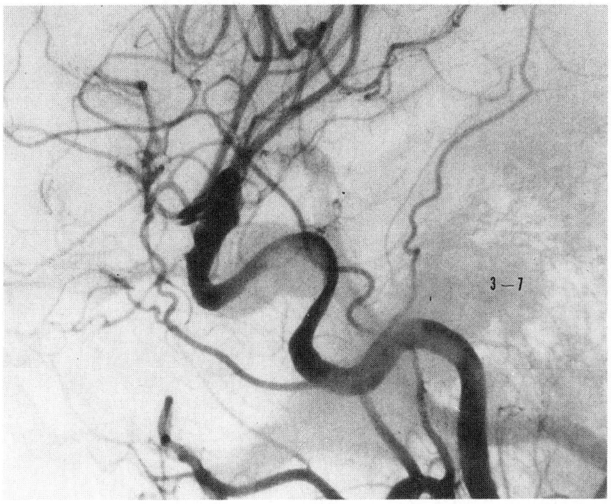

(*C*)

Figure 251-7 Occlusion of the aneurysm with preservation of the parent artery is the treatment goal for intracavernous aneurysms. *A*. Angiogram of a large intracavernous aneurysm. *B*. Plain film of two detachable balloons within the aneurysm taken on the first day after embolization to evaluate balloon placement and possible migration or deflation. *C*. Angiogram after balloon embolization shows complete obliteration of the aneurysm with preservation of flow in the ICA.

10 percent.[24] Of our last 50 patients who underwent ICA occlusion for ICA aneurysms, 6 percent of the group 1 patients suffered a stroke, possibly caused by factors such as hypotension or disruption of collateral flow. Maintenance of normal or hypertensive blood pressure and administration of low doses of heparin may help maintain collateral cross-flow. In the patients in groups 2 and 3, a bypass graft was created prior to carotid sacrifice. For patients who would not tolerate ICA occlusion, we performed extracranial-intracranial bypass grafts with good results. Alternative bypass procedures include saphenous vein bypass grafts from the superficial temporal artery to the middle cerebral artery and from the petrosal to the supraclinoid ICA. For direct surgical approaches to cavernous sinus lesions, some authors advocate a petrosal-to-supraclinoid ICA bypass graft because the saphenous vein is similar in size to the ICA, the bypass is performed through the same exposure, and the procedure takes only slightly longer than other bypass grafts.[31] Another advantage of the petrosal-to-supraclinoid ICA bypass graft is a relatively short bypass length, which reduces the risk for thrombosis and eliminates vascular dead space that might promote thrombus formation.[33]

Regardless of the BTO and HMPAO results, we attempt to preserve carotid patency, because the prevalence of long-term neurological sequelae after ICA occlusion with detachable balloons is not well known. In our series of 72 patients with cavernous carotid aneurysms, 3 suffered delayed transient ischemic attacks, 2 suffered subarachnoid hemorrhage from *de novo* aneurysm formation, and 1 suffered a major hemispheric infarction after carotid occlusion. If the neck of the aneurysm is well-defined and the risk for distal embolization is low, silicone detachable balloons or electrolytically detachable platinum coils are used to obliterate the aneurysm (Fig. 251-8). When the aneurysm neck is wide or poorly defined, the aneurysm is trapped between two balloons and the ICA is occluded. Trapping eliminates retrograde filling from the ophthalmic artery and reduces the amount of thrombus within the ICA. If the ICA is stenotic or tortuous and a catheter cannot be navigated through to the cavernous segment of the ICA, direct surgical exposure of the cavernous segment of the ICA is performed and the aneurysm is clipped or trapped. Traumatic aneurysms are best treated by placing detachable balloons in the parent artery above and below the false aneurysm. Occasionally, the balloon may not pass distal to the aneurysm, and carotid occlusion is then performed by placing the balloon proximal to and at the mouth of the aneurysm. Because traumatic aneurysms lack a true arterial wall, they are not amenable to clipping, and placing the

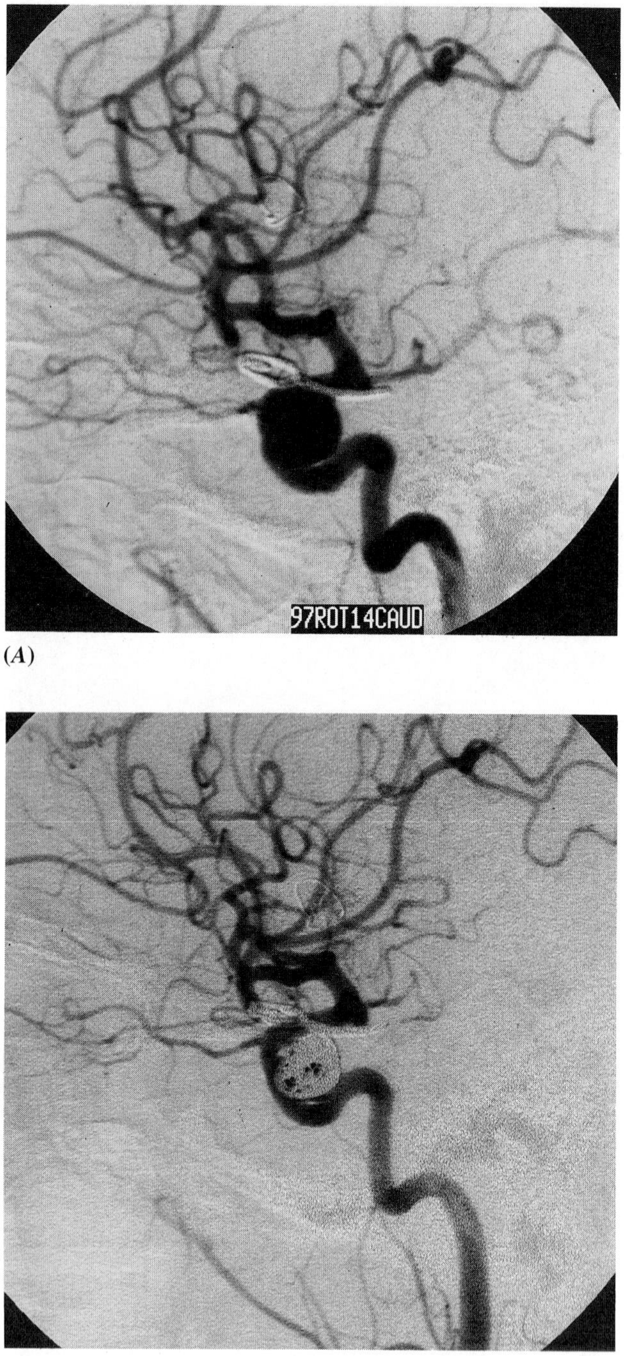

(*A*)

(*B*)

Figure 251-8 Guglielmi detachable platinum coils have proven useful for treating intracavernous aneurysms. *A*. Angiogram shows an intracavernous aneurysm with previous clipping of a posterior communicating aneurysm. *B*. After coil placement, minimal filling persists before thrombosis, and patency of the ICA is preserved.

balloon within the aneurysm may lead to rupture. Furthermore, the aneurysm neck is often wide and irregular, which makes it impossible to occlude the aneurysm while preserving the ICA.

In our series of 72 patients with 77 carotid cavernous aneurysms, 60 of the aneurysms were spontaneous, 13 were traumatic, and 4 represented complications of transphenoidal surgery. The patients ranged in age from 11 to 90 years of age. Patients with spontaneous aneurysms averaged 58 years of age and those with traumatic aneurysms averaged 28 years. Fifty-two (87 percent) of the 60 spontaneous aneurysms occurred in women, whereas 8 (61 percent) of the 13 traumatic aneurysms occurred in men. Five (7 percent) patients had bilateral cavernous carotid aneurysms, and 6 (8 percent) had associated intradural aneurysms. Twenty-two (31 percent) of all cavernous aneurysms were ruptured on presentation. Common presenting symptoms were retro-orbital headaches (in 38 patients), isolated abducens palsy (in 28), orbital bruit (in 21), and ophthalmoplegia (in 19). Of the unruptured aneurysms, 30 (65 percent) were treated with carotid occlusion, 15 (33 percent) were trapped, and 1 (2 percent) was occluded with balloons and the ICA preserved. Carotid patency was maintained in 18 (83 percent) of 22 patients with ruptured cavernous aneurysms using detachable balloons. Nine aneurysms were not treated. Transient complications occurring in 14 (19 percent) patients, including cranial nerve palsies in 5, transient ischemic attacks in 4, subarachnoid hemorrhage from *de novo* aneurysm formation in 2, and infarction in 3. One patient suffered a permanent left upper extremity weakness. Two patients died, one from thromboembolic infarction and another from delayed intracerebral hemorrhage. In most patients, serial postoperative CT or MR imaging demonstrated shrinkage of the thrombosed aneurysm and correlated positively with clinical improvement.

Antibiotic therapy for 6 weeks is the standard treatment for mycotic aneurysms. The aneurysm should be evaluated every 2 weeks by MR imaging during antibiotic therapy. If there is radiographic evidence of enlargement or progression of symptoms during antibiotic therapy, ICA trapping or ligation is indicated. Embolic materials should be avoided because they are foreign bodies that can potentiate an infection.

Complications

Each treatment approach has pitfalls. First, placement of platinum coils or balloons into the aneurysm may fail to relieve the mass effect and necessitate direct surgical clipping. Second, surgical clipping is contraindicated when the aneurysm neck is calcified or encrusted with atheromatous plaque. Third, patients require a repeat BTO after bypass grafting because a patent graft does not necessarily ensure adequate collateral flow. Fourth, when a patient has bilateral aneurysms of the cavernous segment of the ICA, treatment should be reserved for the symptomatic side. A contralateral berry aneurysm is a relative contraindication to sacrificing the ICA because a change in flow dynamics may precipitate aneurysm rupture.

Cerebral ischemia is the most common and feared treatment risk for cavernous-carotid aneurysms. Although uncommon, BTO may produce carotid dissection, stenosis, or occlusion. Despite systemic heparinization, thromboemboli from the balloon may cause a delayed stroke. The bypass graft is prone to pseudoaneurysm formation, thrombosis, or intimal dissection. Occlusion of the ICA may lead to propagation of a distal thrombus, *de novo* aneurysm formation, or accelerated atherosclerosis. Attempting to place embolic material into the aneurysm may dislodge thrombus within the aneurysm and produce distal cerebral infarction, which may also occur if the balloon is prematurely released or migrates out of the aneurysm. In addition, we have converted an intracavernous aneurysm into a CCF by overinflating a balloon within the aneurysm and causing its rupture. Incomplete clipping of the aneurysm may result in regrowth. Likewise, incompletely embolized aneurysms remain at risk for rupture.[17]

Conclusion

Over the past 10 years, management of CCFs and intracavernous aneurysms has improved significantly. Combining endovascular and skull base surgical techniques has fundamentally changed the treatment of these difficult lesions. The success of fistula or aneurysm obliteration is better than ever, and the morbidity and mortality rates continue to decline. Despite this success, current methods and materials will continue to evolve, changing our approach to these lesions. Currently, we are developing intraluminal vascular stents as a treatment alternative. Future studies will focus on the long-term radiographic occlusion rate and clinical outcome for patients with aneurysms embolized with Guglielmi detachable platinum coils. As experience with endovascular techniques increases and technology advances, prospective clinical trials comparing surgical and endovascular approaches to aneurysm treatment will help define the best treatment option for complex vascular lesions.

References

1. Barcia-Salorio JL, Soler F, Hernandez G, et al. Radiosurgical treatment of low flow carotid-cavernous fistulae. *Acta Neurochir Suppl (Wien)* 1991; 52:93–95.
2. Barrow DL, Spector RH, Braun IF, et al. Classification and treatment of spontaneous carotid-cavernous sinus fistulas. *J Neurosurg* 1985; 62:248–256.
3. Cordes M, Christe W, Henkes H, et al. Focal epilepsies. HM-PAO SPECT compared to CT, MR, and EEG. *J Comput Assist Tomogr* 1990; 14:402–409.
4. Debrun G, Lacour P, Viñuela F, et al. Treatment of 54 traumatic carotid-cavernous fistulas. *J Neurosurg* 1981; 55:678–692.
5. Debrun GM, Viñuela F, Fox AJ, et al. Indications for treatment and classification of 132 carotid-cavernous fistulas. *Neurosurgery* 1988; 22:285–289.
6. Dolenc V. Direct microsurgical repair of intracavernous vascular lesions. *J Neurosurg* 1983; 58:824–831.
7. Gomez CR, Gomez SM, Yoon KW, et al. Evaluation and follow-up of carotid-cavernous fistulas by transcranial doppler sonography: illustrative case. *Neurosurgery* 1989; 24:749–753.
8. Guglielmi G, Viñuela F, Briganti F, et al. Carotid-cavernous fistula caused by a ruptured intracavernous aneurysm: endovascular treatment by electrothrombosis with detachable coils. *Neurosurgery* 1992; 31:591–597.
9. Halbach VV, Higashida RT, Dowd CF, et al. Treatment of carotid-cavernous fistulas associated with Ehlers-Danlos syndrome. *Neurosurgery* 1990; 26:1021–1027.
10. Halbach VV, Higashida RT, Hieshima GB, et al. Dural fistulas involving the cavernous sinus: results of treatment in 30 patients. *Radiology* 1987; 163:437–442.
11. Halbach VV, Higashida RT, Hieshima GB, et al. Transvenous embolization of direct carotid cavernous fistulas. *Am J Neuroradiol* 1988; 9:741–747.
12. Halbach VV, Higashida RT, Hieshima GB, et al. Embolization of branches arising from the cavernous portion of the internal carotid artery. *Am J Neuroradiol* 1989; 10:143–150.
13. Halbach VV, Higashida RT, Hieshima GB, et al. Direct puncture of the proximally occluded internal carotid artery for treatment of carotid cavernous fistulas. *Am J Neuroradiol* 1989; 10:151–154.
14. Halbach VV, Higashida RT, Hieshima GB, et al. Transvenous embolization of dural fistulas involving the cavernous sinus. *Am J Neuroradiol* 1989; 10:377–383.
15. Hamby WB. *Carotid-Cavernous Fistula.* Springfield, IL: Charles C Thomas, 1966.
16. Hieshima GB, Cahan LD, Mehringer CM, et al. Spontaneous arteriovenous fistulas of cerebral vessels in association with fibromuscular dysplasia. *Neurosurgery* 1986; 18:454–458.
17. Higashida RT, Halbach VV, Dowd C, et al. Endovascular detachable balloon embolization therapy of cavernous carotid artery aneurysms: results in 87 cases. *J Neurosurg* 1990; 72:857–863.
18. Higashida RT, Halbach VV, Hieshima GB, et al. Cavernous carotid artery aneurysm associated with Marfan's syndrome: treatment by balloon embolization therapy. *Neurosurgery* 1988; 22:297–300.
19. Hurst RW, Choi IS, Persky M, et al. Mycotic aneurysms of the intracavernous carotid artery: a case report and review of the literature. *Surg Neurol* 1992; 37:142–146.
20. Konishi Y, Hieshima GB, Hara M, et al. Congenital fistula of the dural carotid-cavernous sinus: case report and review of the literature. *Neurosurgery* 1990; 27:120–126.
21. Kupersmith MJ, Hurst R, Berenstein A, et al. The benign course of cavernous carotid artery aneurysms. *J Neurosurg* 1992; 77:690–693.
22. Linskey ME, Sekhar LN, Hirch WL Jr., et al. Aneurysms of the intracavernous carotid artery: clinical presentation, radiographic features, and pathogenesis. *Neurosurgery* 1990; 26:71–79.
23. Linskey ME, Sekhar LN, Hirch WL Jr., et al. Aneurysms of the intracavernous carotid artery: natural history and indications for treatment. *Neurosurgery* 1990; 26:933–938.
24. Linskey ME, Sekhar LN, Horton JA, et al. Aneurysms of the intracavernous carotid artery: a multidisciplinary approach to treatment. *J Neurosurg* 1991; 75:525–534.
25. Mullan S. Treatment of carotid-cavernous fistulas by cavernous sinus occlusion. *J Neurosurg* 1979; 50:131–144.
26. Mullan S. Fistulas and vascular malformations of the dura and dural sinuses. In Apuzzo MLJ (ed): *Brain Surgery: Complication Avoidance and Management.* New York: Churchill Livingstone, 1993, pp 1117–1141.
27. Parkinson D. Carotid cavernous fistula: direct repair with preservation of the carotid artery: technical note. *J Neurosurg* 1973; 38:99–106.
28. Pilla TJ, Tantana S, Smith KR. Percutaneous transluminal angioplasty prior to carotid cavernous fistula embolization. *Am J Neuroradiol* 1988; 9:789–790.
29. Prolo DJ, Hanberry JW. Intraluminal occlusion of a carotid-cavernous sinus fistula with a balloon catheter: technical note. *J Neurosurg* 1971; 35:237–242.
30. Sasaki H, Nukui H, Kaneko M, et al. Long-term observations in cases with spontaneous carotid-cavernous fistulas. *Acta Neurochir (Wien)* 1988; 90:117–120.
31. Sekhar LN, Sen CN, Jho HD. Saphenous vein graft bypass of the cavernous internal carotid artery. *J Neurosurg* 1990; 72:35–41.
32. Serbinenko FA. Balloon catheterization and occlusion of major cerebral vessels. *J Neurosurg* 1974; 41:125–145.
33. Spetzler RF, Fukushima T, Martin N, et al. Petrous carotid-to-intradural carotid saphenous vein graft for intracavernous giant aneurysm, tumor, and occlusive cerebrovascular disease. *J Neurosurg* 1990; 73:496–501.
34. Viñuela F, Fox AJ, Debrun GM, et al. Spontaneous carotid-cavernous fistulas: clinical, radiological and therapeutic considerations. Experience with 20 cases. *J Neurosurg* 1984; 60:976–984.
35. Weil SM, van Loveren HR, Tomsick TA, et al. Management of inoperable cerebral aneurysms by navigational balloon technique. *Neurosurgery* 1987; 21:296–302.
36. Yasunaga T, Takada C, Uozumi H, et al. Radiotherapy of spontaneous carotid-cavernous sinus fistulas. *Int J Radiat Oncol Biol Phys* 1987; 13:1909–1913.

252 Spinal Vascular Malformations

Edward H. Oldfield

In the past few years, several advances have been made in the understanding of spinal arteriovenous malformations (AVMs). These findings indicate that prior conceptions of the site, the mechanism of cord injury, and the approach to treatment of the most common type of spinal AVM were based on incorrect assumptions. Accordingly, these recent findings have significantly altered the management of most patients with spinal AVMs and have led to new and more successful treatments.

Patients with spinal AVMs may present with acute spinal cord dysfunction as a result of hemorrhage, but subacute or chronic progression of myelopathy represents the more common clinical presentation. It is now apparent that the symptoms that affect patients with spinal AVMs depend on the mechanism of disruption of normal cord physiology. It is also clear that the clinical manifestations of the two major types of spinal AVMs—dural arteriovenous fistulas (AVFs) and intradural AVMs—differ, and that these differences often reflect different mechanisms of spinal cord injury caused by these two categories of spinal AVMs. Although the clinical course frequently indicates the pathophysiologic process involved (hemorrhage, venous congestion, vascular thrombosis, or ischemia) and suggests the type of AVM, it takes special diagnostic studies to determine that a spinal AVM is the cause of a given patient's myelopathy, as well as to determine the location and specific type of the AVM and its vascular anatomy and relationship to the blood supply of the spinal cord. These studies include myelography, magnetic resonance imaging (MRI), digital vascular imaging, and selective spinal arteriography. The decision to treat a patient with a spinal AVM and the choice of the specific treatment require consideration of (1) the natural history of progressive loss of neurological function with spinal AVMs, (2) the age and clinical condition of the patient, (3) the type of spinal AVM, (4) the vascular anatomy of the spinal cord and the AVM in the patient under consideration, and (5) the potential benefits and risks of treatment for that patient.

History and Classification

The first successful operation for a spinal AVM was performed in 1914 by Dr. Charles Elsberg.[17] His patient had a severe paraparesis and sensory loss to the level of the ninth thoracic dermatome. At surgery, Elsberg identified an abnormal "dilated spinal vein" that entered the dura adjacent to the dural penetration of the posterior root of the ninth thoracic intercostal nerve. He removed a 2-cm segment of the abnormal vessel as it entered the dura. Within 3 months after the surgical procedure, the patient regained normal neurological function.

The early classifications of spinal AVMs were based on the pathology of lesions examined at autopsy. In 1925, Sargent reviewed the previously reported patients and concluded that most spinal AVMs were venous angiomas.[41] Similarly, in 1943, Wyburn-Mason, after analyzing 110 patients with spinal AVMs, asserted that there were two main types of AVMs of the spinal cord, an arteriovenous type and a venous type.[51] The latter type, which he described as being formed of an abnormal mass of turgid, dilated, blue pial vessels embedded in the pia mater, he designated "angioma racemosum venosum" in keeping with Virchow's original classification of vascular abnormalities. He concluded that 75 of the 110 patients had the venous type of malformation. Thus, the early classifications, based on histologic analysis, indicated that most spinal AVMs were venous angiomas on the cord surface.

With the introduction of selective spinal arteriography in the 1960s, the vascular anatomy of spinal AVMs could be analyzed in vivo for the first time. A new classification of spinal AVMs developed that was based on the pattern of blood flow and vascular anatomy seen during arteriography. The result was a categorization of spinal AVMs into three types: the juvenile, glomus, and single coiled vessel types. In all three, the nidus of the malformation was thought to be within the spinal cord or pia. The juvenile type was considered to be analogous to cerebral AVMs. It was supplied by multiple feeding vessels and had rapid blood flow. This type of malformation was noted to usually affect children or young adults. The glomus type was a localized collection of fine blood vessels confined to a short segment of the spinal cord and was usually fed by a single feeding vessel. In the juvenile and glomus type AVMs, which comprised about 15 to 20 percent of all spinal AVMs, at least one of the feeding vessels was a medullary artery, which supplied the spinal cord in addition to providing blood to the AVM.

The "single coiled vessel" type—the most common type of spinal AVM, comprising 80 to 85 percent of all spinal AVMs—was described as consisting of a single, tightly coiled, continuous vessel on the cord surface. Flow through these lesions was slow; 16 to 20 s was often required for contrast to clear the lesion during arteriography. There was one feeding vessel, which usually supplied the AVM but not the spinal cord. Unlike the juvenile and glomus types, in which the nidus of the AVM was apparent at arteriography, in the single coiled vessel type the site of the transition from arterial to venous elements—the nidus of the AVF—was not identified; many small communicating vessels between the dorsolateral arterial plexus of the spinal cord and the long coiled vessel on the cord surface were considered to be the sites of vascular shunting. Later, with the introduction of microneurosurgery, the dilated, thin-walled pial vessels covering the cord surface seemed to be the glomus of the AVM, and surgical stripping of these engorged vessels from the dorsal surface of the spinal cord over multiple spinal segments became the treatment advocated.

In 1977, Kendall and Logue described nine patients in whom the nidus of the AVF was identified in the dura covering the proximal nerve root.[24] At operation, Logue excised the dural AVF. Most patients enjoyed considerable improvement postoperatively. It is now accepted that the lesions previously considered as venous angiomas on the cord surface and as the "single coiled vessel" type of AVM by the earlier classification are actually normal veins on the surface of the spinal cord that have been transformed by the reception of arterial blood from a dural AVF.

There are three biologically distinct types of vascular malformations of the spinal cord and its coverings: dural AVFs, in which

TABLE 252-1 Classification of Spinal Vascular Malformations

A. Dural arteriovenous fistulas
B. Intradural vascular malformations
   1. Juvenile arteriovenous malformations
   2. Glomus arteriovenous malformations
   3. Arteriovenous fistulas
C. Cavernous angiomas

the nidus of the AVF is embedded in the dural covering of the nerve root and the adjacent spinal dura; intradural vascular malformations of the spinal cord, in which the nidus either is within the tissue of the spinal cord or is embedded in the pia; and cavernous angiomas of the spinal cord.[37,40] The intradural vascular malformations are further subclassified into juvenile and glomus AVMs and direct AVFs (Table 252-1; Figs. 252-1 through 252-5). A knowledge of the vascular anatomy of the spinal cord is necessary for interpreting the diagnostic studies used to evaluate patients suspected of having a spinal AVM, for distinguishing the various subtypes of AVMs and the mechanisms by which they produce cord injury, and for implementing successful treatment.

Spinal Vascular Anatomy

Two arterial systems supply blood to the spinal cord: an anterior and a posterior arterial network (Fig. 252-1). The anterior arterial chain—the anterior spinal artery—extends along the entire anterior surface of the spinal cord in the anterior median fissure to supply the anterior two-thirds of the cord, including the corticospinal tracts. The posterior spinal arteries—two plexiform interconnecting channels that run along the posterior and posterolateral surfaces of the cord—perfuse the posterior one-third of the spinal cord.

In the developing fetus, two medullary arteries, one from each side, supply the spinal cord at each segmental level. Most of these regress during gestation, and only a limited number of medullary arteries, which provide blood to the anterior and posterior spinal arteries, remain. Unlike the medullary arteries, the embryonic ra-

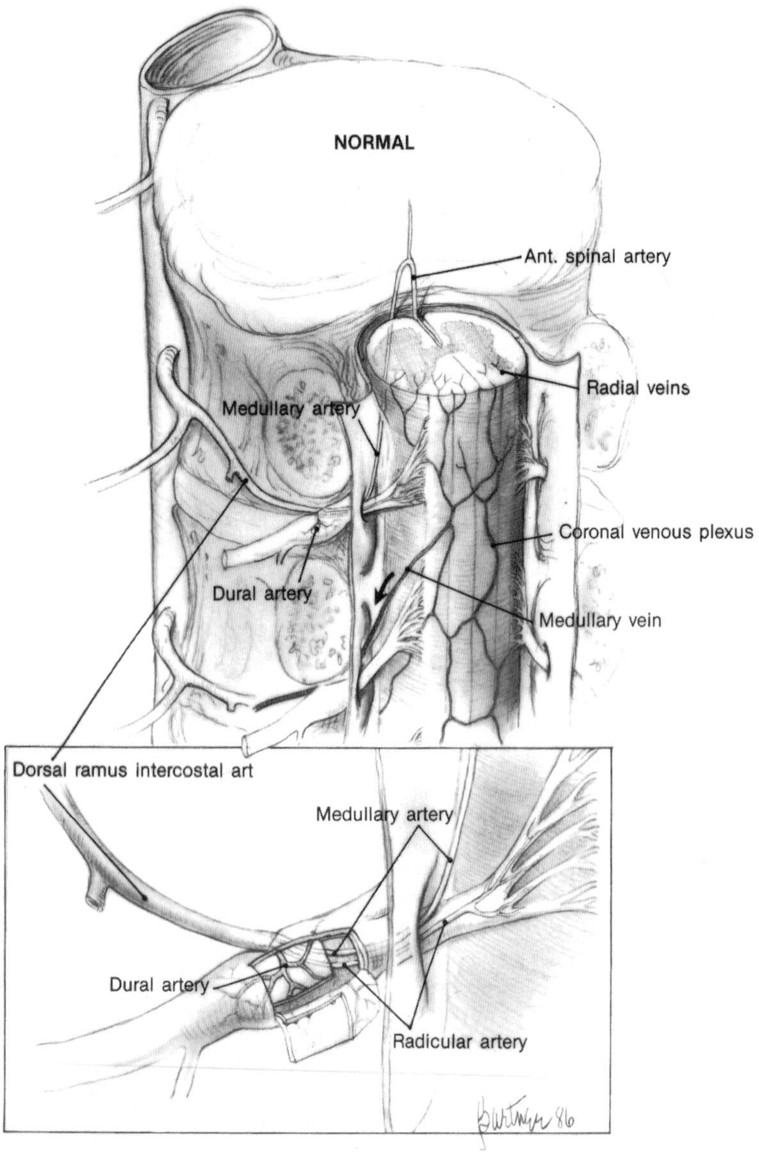

Figure 252-1 Normal arterial supply and venous drainage of the spinal cord. At each segmental level, the spinal ramus of each intercostal artery first enters the intervertebral foramen and penetrates the outer surface of the dura and then divides into dural arteries, which supply the root sleeve and spinal dura, and radicular arteries, which supply the anterior and posterior nerve roots. In addition, at some levels and sporadically, the spinal ramus of the intercostal artery also gives rise to a medullary artery, which enters the dura next to the nerve root ganglion, ascends, and joins an anterior or posterior spinal artery to supply the spinal cord. The cord is drained by radial veins, which carry blood to the coronal venous plexus or to longitudinal veins. These veins are drained by medullary veins which pierce the dura next to the dural penetration of the nerve roots. (From Oldfield and Doppman.[37])

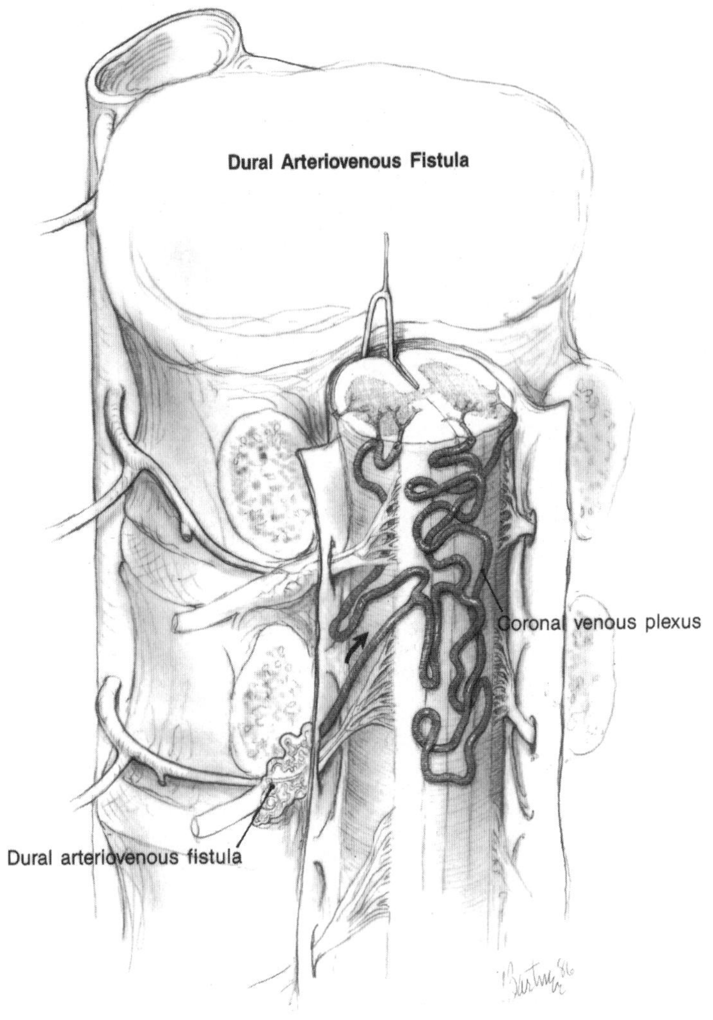

Figure 252-2 A dural AVF is supplied by a dural artery and is drained by a medullary vein, which carries blood retrograde to the normal direction of flow, to the coronal venous plexus, which becomes elongated, tortuous, and dilated by the reception of arterial blood. Increased venous pressure is transmitted to the spinal cord and causes myelopathy. (From Oldfield and Doppman.[37])

dicular and dural arteries persist at each level on both sides. Consequently, the adult has at each segmental level bilateral radicular arteries, which supply the anterior and posterior nerve roots, and dural arteries, which supply the proximal nerve root sleeve and the adjacent spinal dura. Medullary arteries, radicular arteries, and dural arteries are all derived from the intervertebral segment of the spinal ramus of the intercostal arteries or, in the cervical and lumbar regions, from their equivalents; these arteries arise from the aorta or from the vertebral, subclavian, or iliac arteries and enter the intervertebral foramen at each level. Particularly important is the artery of Adamkiewicz, a medullary artery that provides the anterior spinal artery with blood below the midportion of the spinal cord. This artery arises from an intercostal or lumbar artery between T8 and L4.

Therefore, at each segmental level, the spinal ramus of each intercostal artery first enters the intervertebral foramen and penetrates the outer leaflet of the dura and then divides into dural and radicular arteries. In addition, sporadically at some levels, the spinal ramus of an intercostal artery also gives rise to a medullary artery, which enters the dura next to the nerve root ganglion, ascends, and joins the anterior or posterior spinal artery to supply the spinal cord (Fig. 252-1).

The spinal cord is drained by radial veins, which carry blood centrifugally from the cord parenchyma to the surface, where they empty into the coronal venous plexus, a venous plexus in the pia on the cord surface. The venous blood passes from the intradural to the epidural veins via medullary veins. These traverse the subarachnoid space from the coronal venous plexus and the anterior median spinal vein to the dura, which they penetrate adjacent to the dural penetration of the nerve roots, to join the intervertebral veins of the epidural venous plexus (Fig. 252-1). The medullary veins, like the medullary arteries, are not present at every segmental level but have an inconstant occurrence along the long axis of the spine. Although functional valves at the level of the dura prevent retrograde flow of venous blood from the epidural to the intradural veins, there are no valves in the intrathecal or intraparenchymal veins.

Diagnostic Investigation

The goal in treating spinal vascular malformations is to permanently obliterate the nidus of the malformation without damaging cord tissue or compromising spinal cord blood supply. Because the different types of vascular malformations are managed differently, precise diagnosis of the malformation type is essential, and because successful treatment of the malformation preoperative requires knowledge of the anatomy of the blood supply to the malformation and to the spinal cord, a complete diagnostic investigation of the spinal cord is essential before deciding to undertake surgical or embolic treatment. The diagnostic approach is

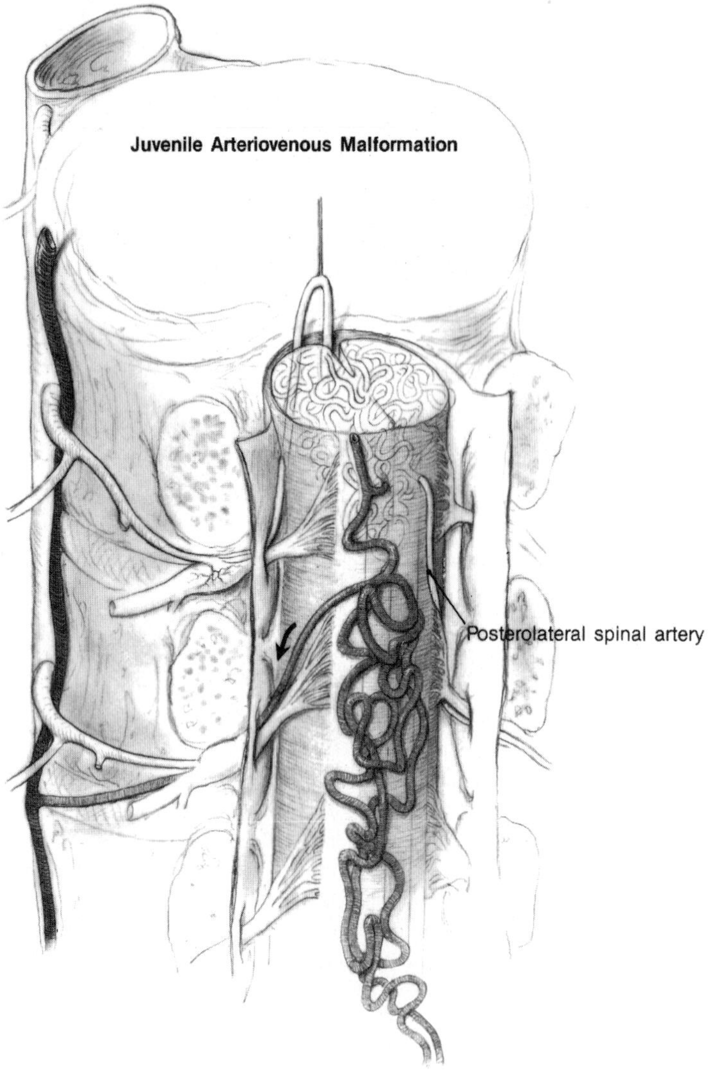

Figure 252-3 The juvenile type of intramedullary AVM is fed by medullary arteries via the anterior and posterior spinal arteries. The nidus of the AVM is large, often fills the spinal canal, and contains cord tissue interspersed among the vessels of the AVM. (From Oldfield and Doppman.[37])

performed in two stages. Screening studies with MRI or myelography detect or raise the suspicion of a vascular abnormality. Selective arteriography is then used to confirm the diagnosis, to precisely localize the lesion, and to define the vascular anatomy of the malformation and the blood supply of the spinal cord.

Until recently, myelography was the first special procedure performed in patients with progressive myelopathy. MRI has now replaced myelography as the first diagnostic procedure in these patients.

With spinal vascular malformations, abnormalities apparent on MRI may be produced by abnormal vessels in the subarachnoid space, by the nidus of an intramedullary AVM in the spinal cord, or by changes in the spinal cord resulting from venous congestion, myelomalacia, spinal cord infarction, or hemorrhage.[9,12,16,27,30,44] MRI may noninvasively yield the initial diagnosis of a vascular malformation and distinguish intramedullary AVMs from perimedullary and dural AVFs.

Because of the excess blood flow in the coronal venous plexus in patients with spinal AVFs and AVMs, T1- and T2-weighted MR images often show a serpentine pattern of low signal in the subarachnoid space.[12] This pattern is due to a signal flow void in the dilated, tortuous vessels of the arterialized coronal venous plexus or in an enlarged artery feeding an AVM of the spinal cord. Dilated, tortuous arterialized pial veins of the coronal venous plexus may focally indent the cord surface and produce a scalloped appearance on sagittal T1-weighted images. The abnormal signal produced by the enlarged coronal venous plexus is frequently more prominent in the posterior pia and subarachnoid space.

While MRI may provide enough evidence to suggest a spinal vascular malformation and the need for further spinal angiographic evaluation, *MR images may look normal or show only nonspecific changes in patients with dural or intradural perimedullary AVFs.* Since the dural AVF is the most common type of spinal vascular malformation, and because dural and intradural AVFs are also the most amenable to treatment, patients with an unexplained progressive myelopathy and normal MR images require additional diagnostic evaluation with myelography (Fig. 252-6).

In contrast to MRI, results of myelography are universally abnormal and demonstrate the presence of a lesion of excess vascularity in patients with all types of spinal vascular malformations except cavernous angiomas. Furthermore, there is no need to search for a spinal AVM or AVF with arteriography in a patient with a technically acceptable myelogram that does not reveal abnormal vessels.

After MRI or myelography has shown the presence of a vascular malformation, the diagnosis must be confirmed, the specific type of malformation must be established, and both the site of the nidus and the blood supply to the spinal cord and the malformation

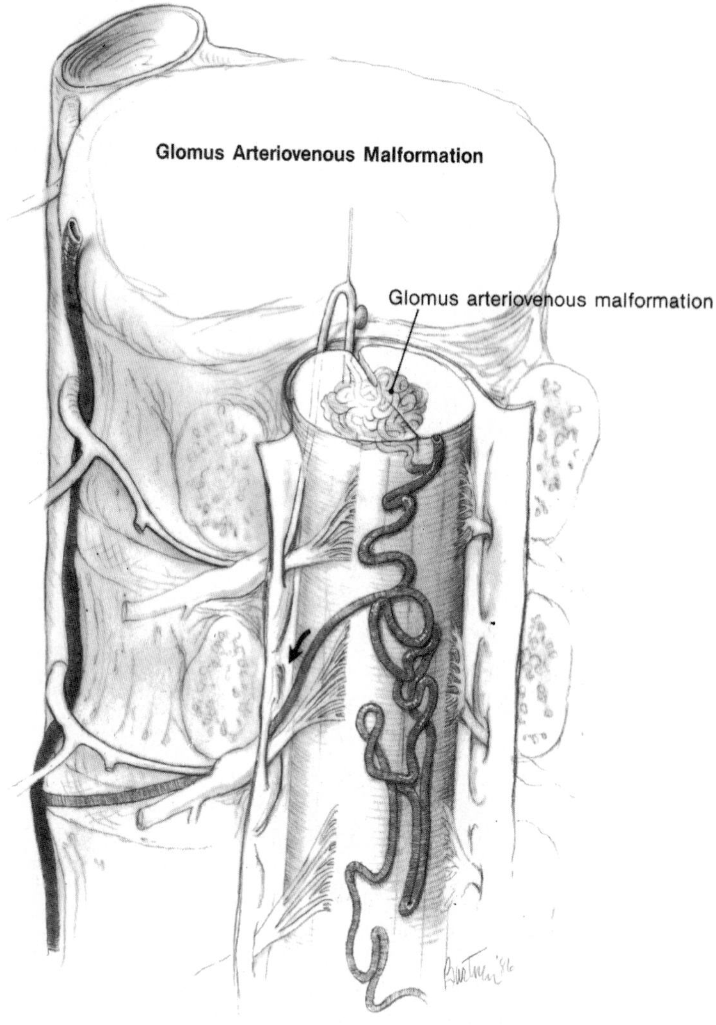

Figure 252-4 The nidus of the glomus type of intramedullary AVM consists of a tightly packed congerie of blood vessels confined to a short segment of the spinal cord. These AVMs, which are usually located in the anterior half of the cord, are supplied by medullary arteries. Intradural AVMs often have associated arterial or venous aneurysms. (From Oldfield and Doppman.[37])

must be defined. With modern instrumentation, selective spinal arteriography with intra-arterial digital vascular imaging (DVI), also known as digital subtraction arteriography, has high resolution and sensitivity. It confirms the presence of a spinal AVF or AVM, defines the segmental region of interest, and identifies the level of origin of feeding vessels. Furthermore, with the high-flow intradural types of AVMs, we have found high-resolution DVI with very rapid sequence imaging (6 to 10 per second) to be a valuable adjunct to conventional selective arteriography (''cut films''), because the early images permit the nidus of the AVM or AVF to be clearly demonstrated before opacification of the veins obscures it.[34] If performed before selective spinal arteriography, DVI often limits the region of interest to a short segment of the spinal axis and thus limits the extent of selective spinal arteriography required. However, it is always important that the normal arterial supply to the spinal cord in the region of the AVF or AVM be identified, so that inadvertent occlusion of a medullary artery, such as the artery of Adamkiewicz, does not occur when the malformation is occluded at operation or embolization. The normal cord vessels are often too small to be identified with DVI. Moreover, cut films make it much easier to orient the anatomy seen during operation with respect to the vascular anatomy revealed by preoperative arteriography, as is essential for successful surgery. Therefore, spinal arteriography with cut films should be performed in all patients with spinal AVFs and AVMs, even if the presence of the malformation has been established with other studies.

The preceding comments apply to all types of spinal vascular malformations except cavernous angiomas, which, unlike the spinal AVFs and AVMs, are not lesions of prominent hypervascularity. They usually are not apparent on myelography or spinal arteriography. These lesions have been recognized with increased frequency since (and because of) the introduction and widespread use of MRI, which consistently demonstrates the presence and site of a focal cord abnormality of increased, decreased, or mixed (high, low, and isointense) signal.[7]

Spinal Dural Arteriovenous Fistulas

Anatomic and clinical features distinguish the intradural types of spinal AVMs from the dural AVFs (Figs. 252-2 through 252-5, 252-7 through 252-9; Table 252-2).[37,40] Patients with intradural AVMs generally develop symptoms when they are less than 40 years old. They often have an acute onset of symptoms caused by hemorrhage. Males and females are affected about equally. In contrast, patients with dural AVMs are usually men older than 40 years of age, have a gradual onset and progressive worsening of symptoms, and experience exacerbations of symptoms or changes in posture or activity. Dural AVFs almost always affect the lower half of the spinal cord and produce symptoms only in the legs and the bladder and bowel.

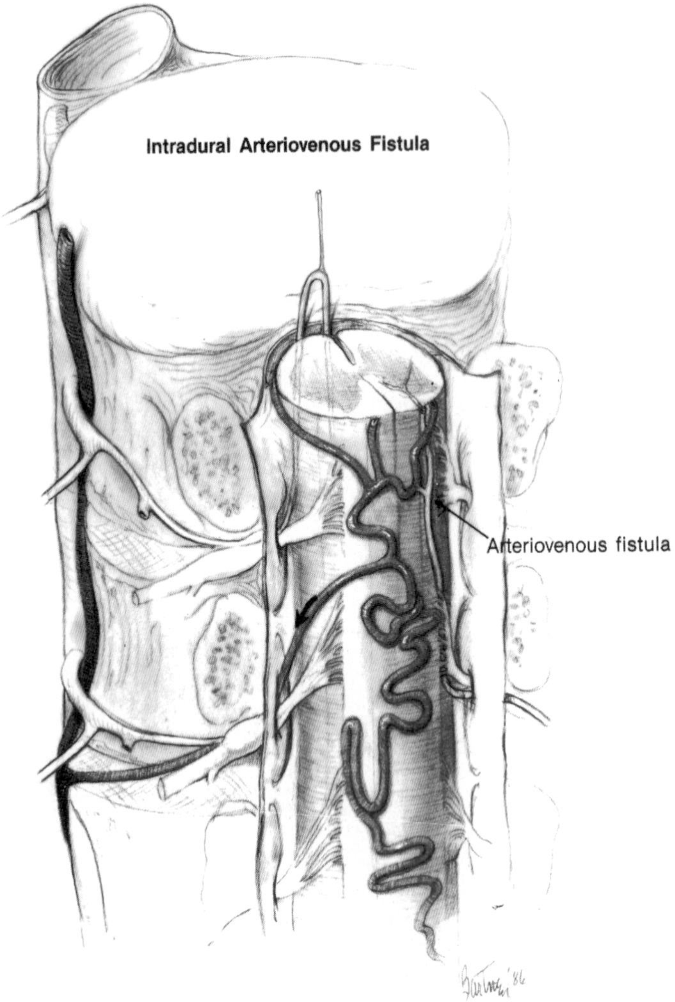

Figure 252-5 An intradural direct AVF in the pia. Medullary arteries provide the arterial supply. (From Oldfield and Doppman.[37])

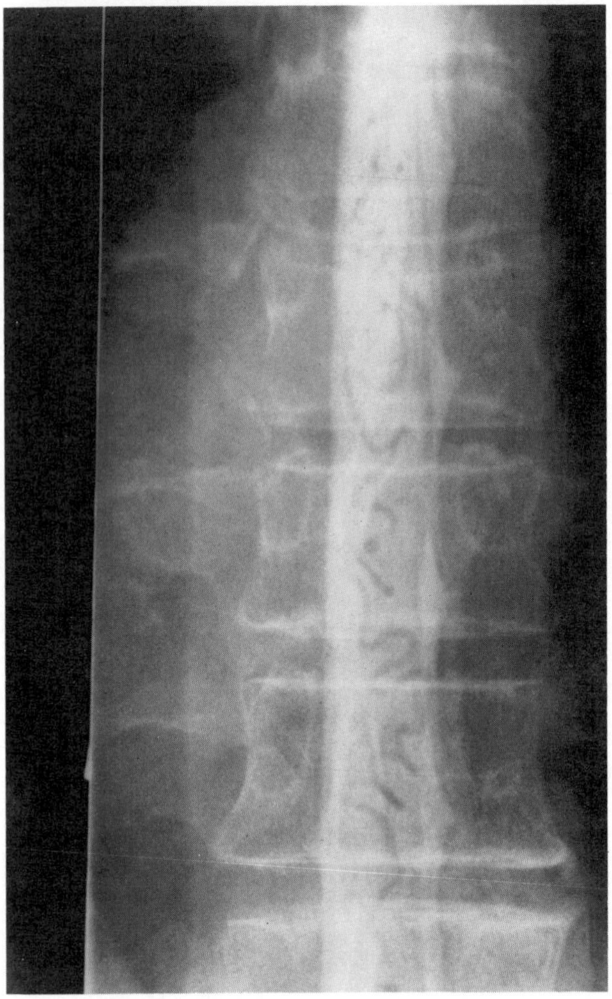

Figure 252-6 In patients with a spinal AVM or AVF, myelography always reveals abnormal vessels. The tortuous and dilated coronal venous plexus is evident on the dorsal surface of the spinal cord in this patient with a spinal dural AVF. Now that water-soluble contrast agents are available, supine myelography usually is not required. (From Muraszko and Oldfield.[31])

Pathophysiology, Epidemiology, and Clinical Presentation

Ninety percent of patients with dural AVFs are males and most are in the later half of life (Fig. 252-8). They generally have a gradual onset of neurological symptoms, including back pain, radiculopathy, and myelopathy, and these symptoms intensify in a progressive or stuttering manner. In many patients, the symptoms exacerbate with changes in posture or during physical activity. These AVFs commonly occur at lower thoracic and lumbar spinal levels (Fig. 252-9). Accordingly, patients are likely to present with symptoms that affect the legs and not the arms. Based on the extreme male predominance, the age of onset, and the distribution of dural AVFs along the lower half of the spine, these lesions are thought to be acquired.[37,40]

Figure 252-2 schematically shows the anatomic basis of spinal dural AVFs. The dural branch of the intervertebral artery (the spinal ramus of the intercostal artery) supplies the dural AVF. The medullary vein, the solitary venous outflow of dural AVFs, carries blood under high pressure in a retrograde manner to the coronal venous plexus. The latter becomes dilated, tortuous, and elongated as a result of excess blood flow under high pressure. Because there are no valves between the coronal venous plexus and the radial veins draining the spinal cord, the high pressure is transmitted directly to the spinal cord, and myelopathy results. Dural AVFs are low-flow shunts that impair cord physiology by inducing venous hypertension in the intrathecal venous system. Clinically, this produces gradually advancing loss of sensory and motor function (85 percent).[37,40,43] However, about 15 percent of patients present with acute or subacute symptoms. Rapid progression of myelopathy in these patients seems to indicate an advanced stage of venous congestion, which progresses to venous thrombosis and produces irreversible cord injury unless treatment to eliminate venous hypertension in the cord is carried out.[8]

In 1974, Aminoff and Logue reported the clinical features and the dismal natural history of patients with spinal vascular malformations.[2,3] Because this study began before the introduction of selective spinal arteriography and all patients were investigated and treated before the recognition of the dural AVF, the natural histories of the malformation subtypes were not compared. However, most patients now undergo treatment earlier, so the investigation by Aminoff and Logue is the most complete study of the untreated progression of patients with spinal vascular malformations. Because the great majority of such spinal malformations are

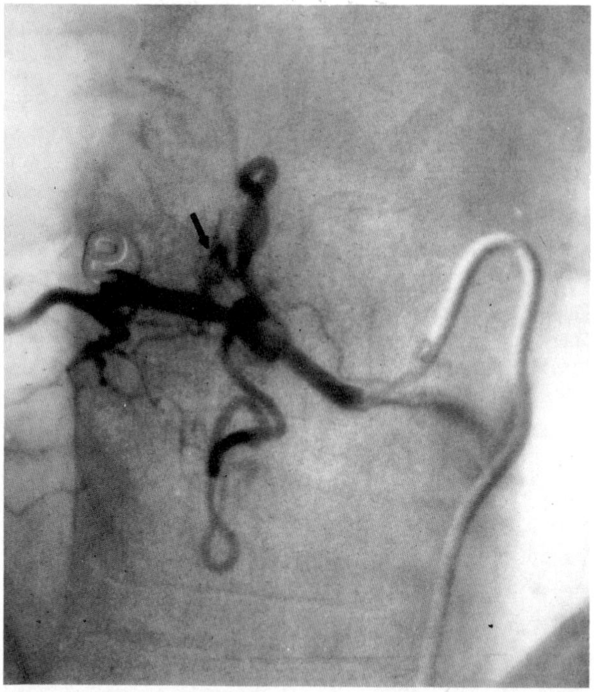

Figure 252-7 A selective spinal arteriogram of a spinal dural AVF (*arrow*) embedded in the root sleeve of the ninth thoracic nerve root and the adjacent spinal dura. The nidus of a spinal dural AVF typically lies in the intervertebral foramen and the lateral aspect of the spinal canal and drains into the dilated, tortuous intradural veins on the cord surface. (From Oldfield and Doppman.[37])

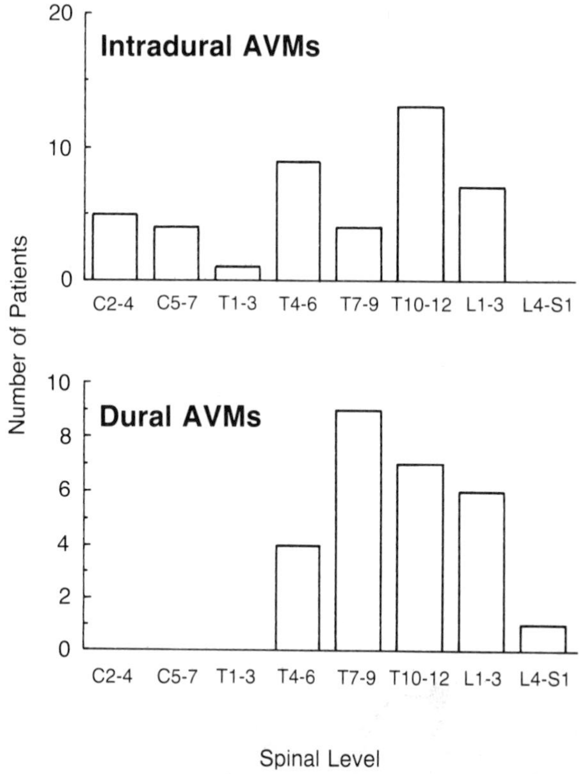

Figure 252-9 The site or the nidus in patients with dural AVFs is below the midthoracic level, whereas intradural AVMs are dispersed along the entire axis of the cord. (From Rosenblum et al.[40])

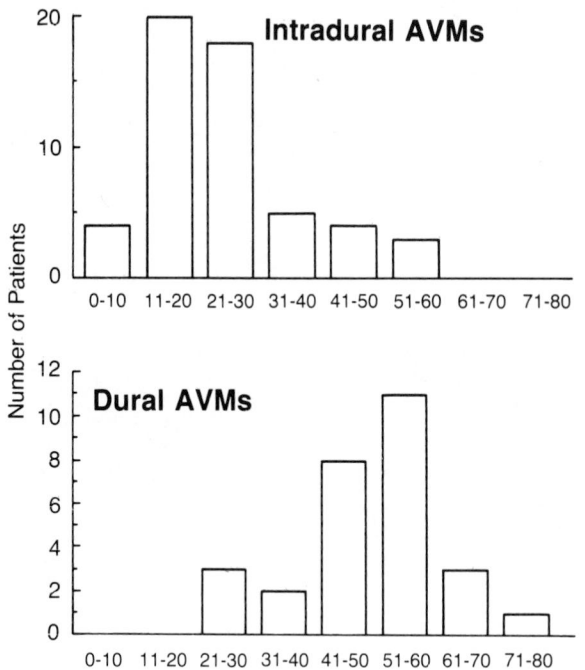

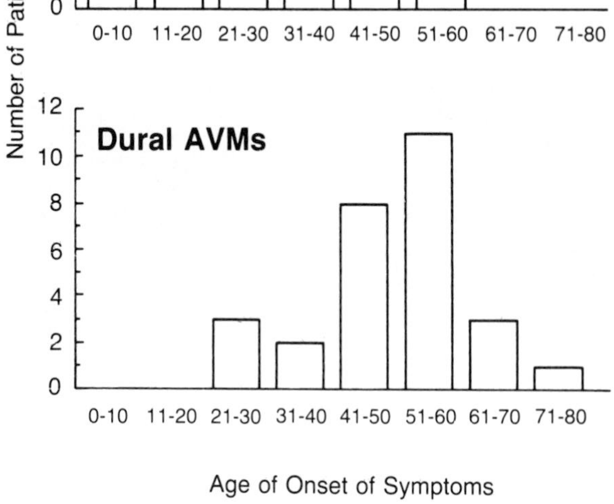

Figure 252-8 Intradural AVMs affect mainly children and young adults. Dural AVFs usually present in adults over 40 years old. (From Rosenblum et al.[40])

spinal dural AVFs, the study was strongly influenced by this type. The patients showed fluctuating symptoms against a background of steadily increasing disability. By 6 months after the onset of symptoms other than pain, 19 percent required crutches or were confined to a wheelchair or bed; within 3 years, 91 percent had restricted activity due to a disturbance of gait. The authors concluded that "once leg weakness or gait disturbance has developed, it is often progressive with great rapidity until the patient is severely disabled. Within three years of functional impairment of the legs, 50 percent of our patients were severely disabled."[2,3]

TABLE 252-2 Clinical Differences between Spinal Dural AVFs and Intradural AVMs

Clinical Parameter	**Dural AVF (n = 27)**	**Intradural AVM (n = 54)**
Gender	Predominantly male	Male or female
Mean age (years)	46	24
Onset of symptoms	Gradual (85%)	Acute (37%)
Subarachnoid hemorrhage	0	50%
First symptom	Paresis (44%)	Subarachnoid hemorrhage (32%)
Spinal bruit	0	6%
Exacerbation of symptoms by activity	70%	15%
Arms affected	0	11%

Source: Adapted from Oldfield and Doppman.[37]

Diagnostic Investigation

Patients with dural AVFs demonstrate a range of MRI findings (Figs. 252-10 and 252-11). In the thoracolumbar segments of a cord swollen from venous congestion, T1- and T2-weighted images reveal focal cord expansion, most commonly affecting the conus, with a central area of low or high signal intensity on T1 imaging and an increased signal intensity with T2 images (Fig. 252-10). Intravenous gadolinium-diethylenetriaminepentaacetic acid (DTPA) contrast often produces enhancement in this region on T1 images (Fig. 252-11), particularly if imaging is delayed until 40 to 45 min after the infusion of the contrast agent.[44] Immediately after injection of gadolinium, the vessels of the coronal venous plexus enhance (Fig. 252-10).[44] Elimination of the spinal dural AVF may or may not result in resolution of the abnormal appearance of the cord (Fig. 252-10). Whether the gadolinium enhancement indicates edema, venous congestion, or loss of integrity of the blood-brain barrier associated with irreversible ischemic injury has not been determined.

Selective spinal arteriography of dural AVFs shows that the nidus of the fistula is typically in the intervertebral foramen and the lateral aspect of the spinal canal, and that the fistula drains into the dilated, tortuous intradural veins on the cord surface (Fig. 252-7). Although most dural AVFs that cause myelopathy are located in the spinal dura, intracranial dural AVFs may also cause myelopathy. In fact, dural AVFs associated with myelopathy may be supplied by any artery that has the potential to provide arterial supply to the dura at a site where the venous drainage can reach the spinal veins. We have treated six patients with myelopathy resulting from spinal venous congestion in whom spinal arteriography was negative but internal and external carotid arteriography revealed dural AVFs of the tentorium with venous drainage caudally into the intrathecal spinal venous system.[46,50] Therefore, if spinal arteriography is negative but myelography indicates abnormal, tortuous spinal vessels, carotid arteriography should be performed.

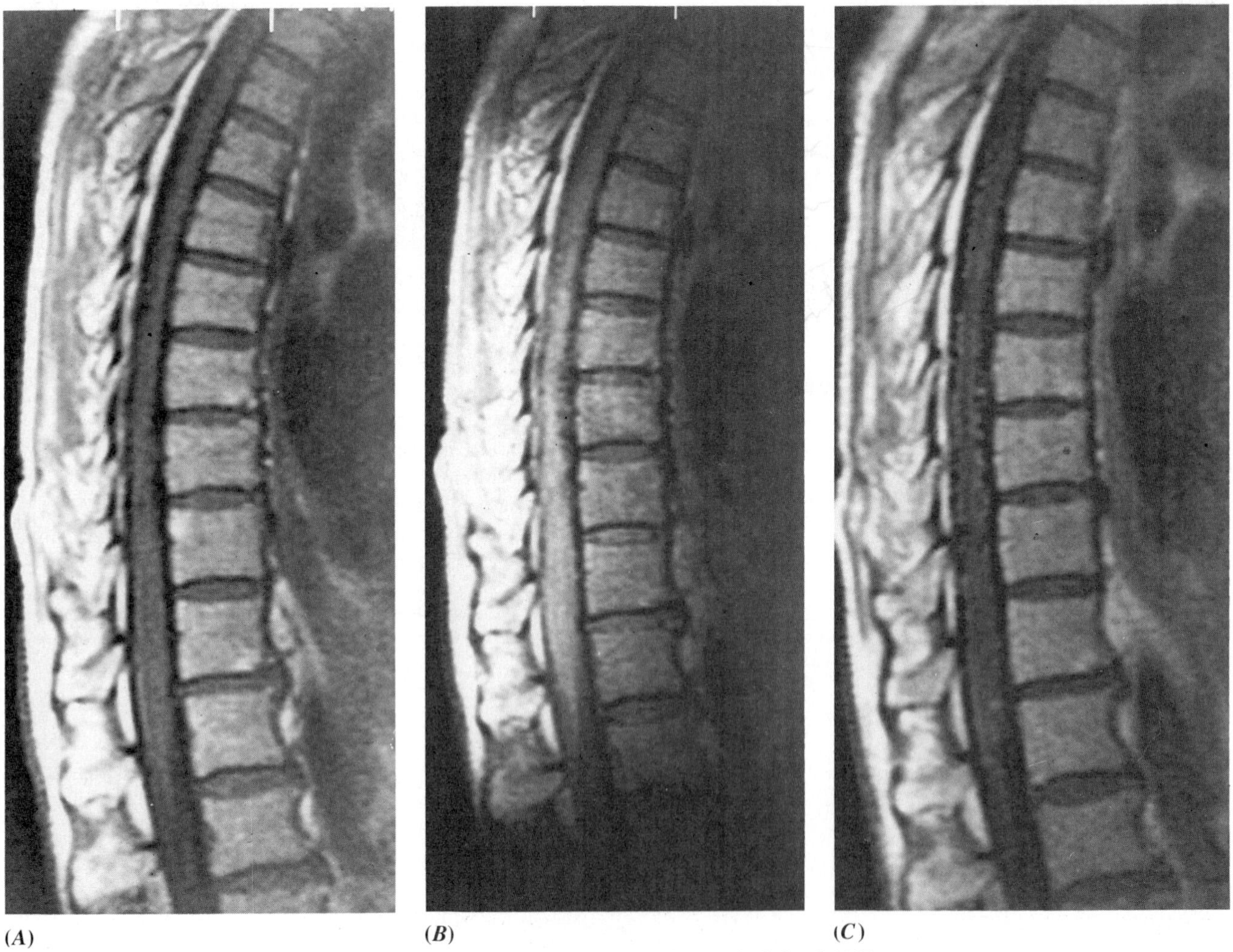

(*A*) (*B*) (*C*)

Figure 252-10 *A–E*. Sagittal spinal MRI scans of a 66-year-old man with a spinal dural AVF at T9-T10. *A*. T1-weighted (TE 400, TR 16) image taken before contrast injection reveals an area of focal cord expansion affecting the conus. *B*. T2-weighted proton density image (TR 2000, TE 20) of the thoracolumbar segments of a cord swollen from venous congestion shows an increased signal intensity. *C*. Immediately after injection of Gd-DTPA, a T1-weighted image (TR 400, TE 16) shows enhancement of the vessels of the coronal venous plexus (compare with the same MRI technique without enhancement in *A*).

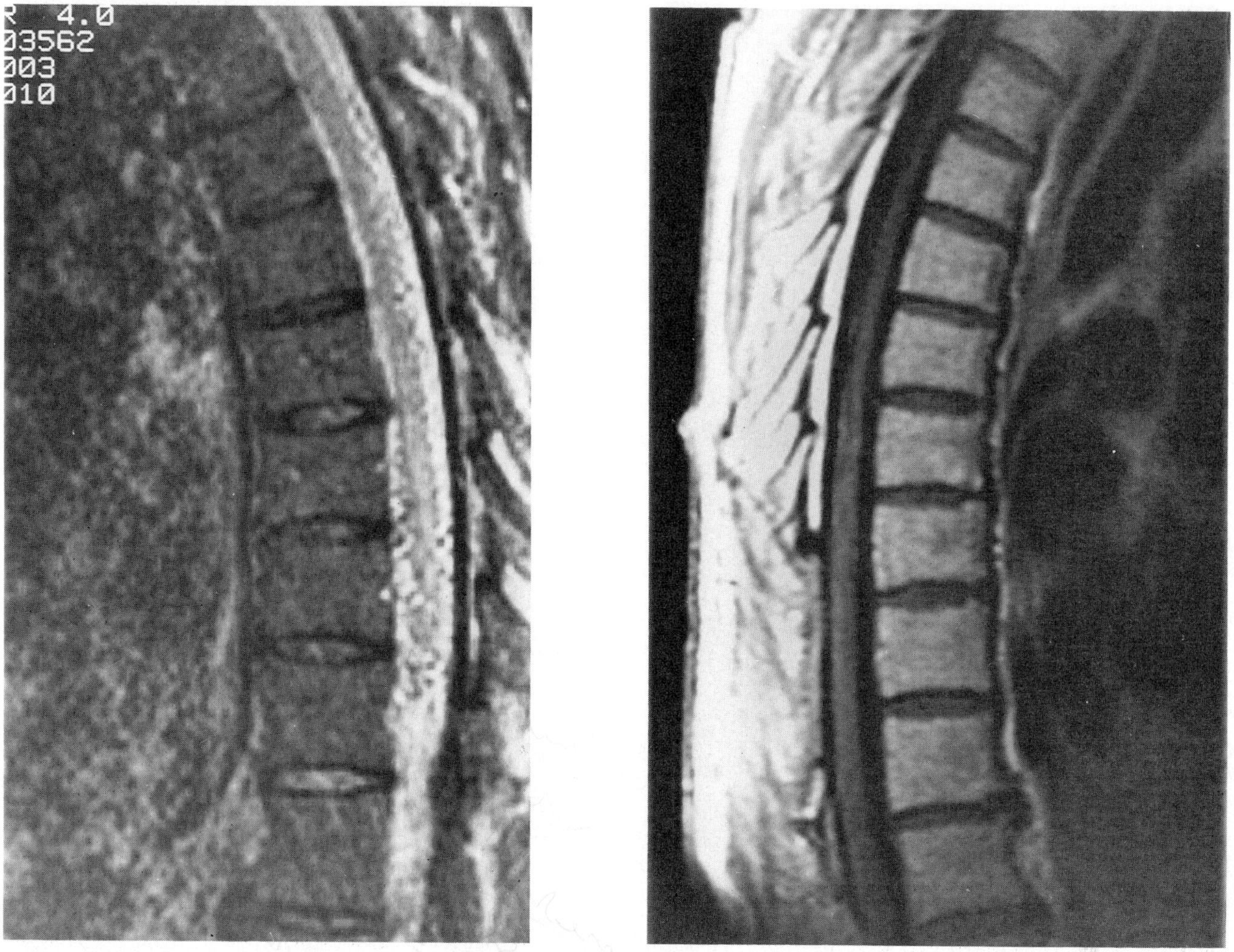

(*D*) (*E*)

Figure 252-10 (*Continued*) *D*. As in this image, T2-weighted techniques that show CSF brightly often prominently show the abnormal vessels on the surface of the cord and in the CSF. *E*. T1-weighted (TR 417, TE 16) image, taken after Gd-DTPA injection, of the site of a spinal dural AVF that had been excised 8 months earlier. As in this case, elimination of the fistula often results in resolution of the swollen appearance of the cord and disappearance of the abnormal enhancing vessels on the cord surface. (From Thompson BG, Oldfield EH. Spinal vascular malformations. In Carter LP, Spetzlar RF (eds): *Neurovascular Surgery*. New York: McGraw-Hill, 1995, pp 1167–1195.)

Treatment

The goal of treatment for patients with a dural AVF is to eliminate the venous congestion of the spinal cord. Before it was recognized that the nidus of the AVF with this type of malformation was in the dura, and not in the pia or the spinal cord, stripping the engorged coronal venous plexus from the spinal cord was used to treat this type of malformation. Since the engorged vessels on the posterior cord surface are the normal though transformed veins of the coronal venous plexus, stripping them from the cord surface removes a portion of the normal venous drainage of the cord and may cause further cord damage. For these reasons, and because the procedure requires an extensive laminectomy and a lengthy operation, this treatment is now discouraged.

By obliterating the dural AVF with an operation or embolization or by surgically interrupting the vessel that carries blood from the dural fistula to the coronal venous plexus, venous congestion can be eliminated and the normal venous drainage of the cord preserved. This procedure involves a simple two-level laminectomy, one level above and one level below the site of the intradural entry of the vein draining the AVF into the subarachnoid space. After the dura is opened, the site of intradural penetration of the vein draining the AVF is identified. This vessel is almost always adjacent to the site of dural penetration of the nerve root (Fig. 252-2). The intradural draining vessel is then divided, after bipolar coagulation, between the site of dural entry and the engorged coronal venous plexus. Thus, in most patients—that is, patients in whom the only venous drainage of the dural AVF is intradural—surgical excision of the dural fistula is unnecessary, as the fistula will undergo retrograde thrombosis and fibrosis after its only venous drainage is interrupted,[1a] as occurs in cranial dural AVFs with only intrathecal drainage.[46]

This approach is the only one that should be considered in patients in whom the intercostal artery provides a common origin for a medullary artery *and* the dural artery feeding the AVF,[13] because the origin of these vessels from the intervertebral artery is

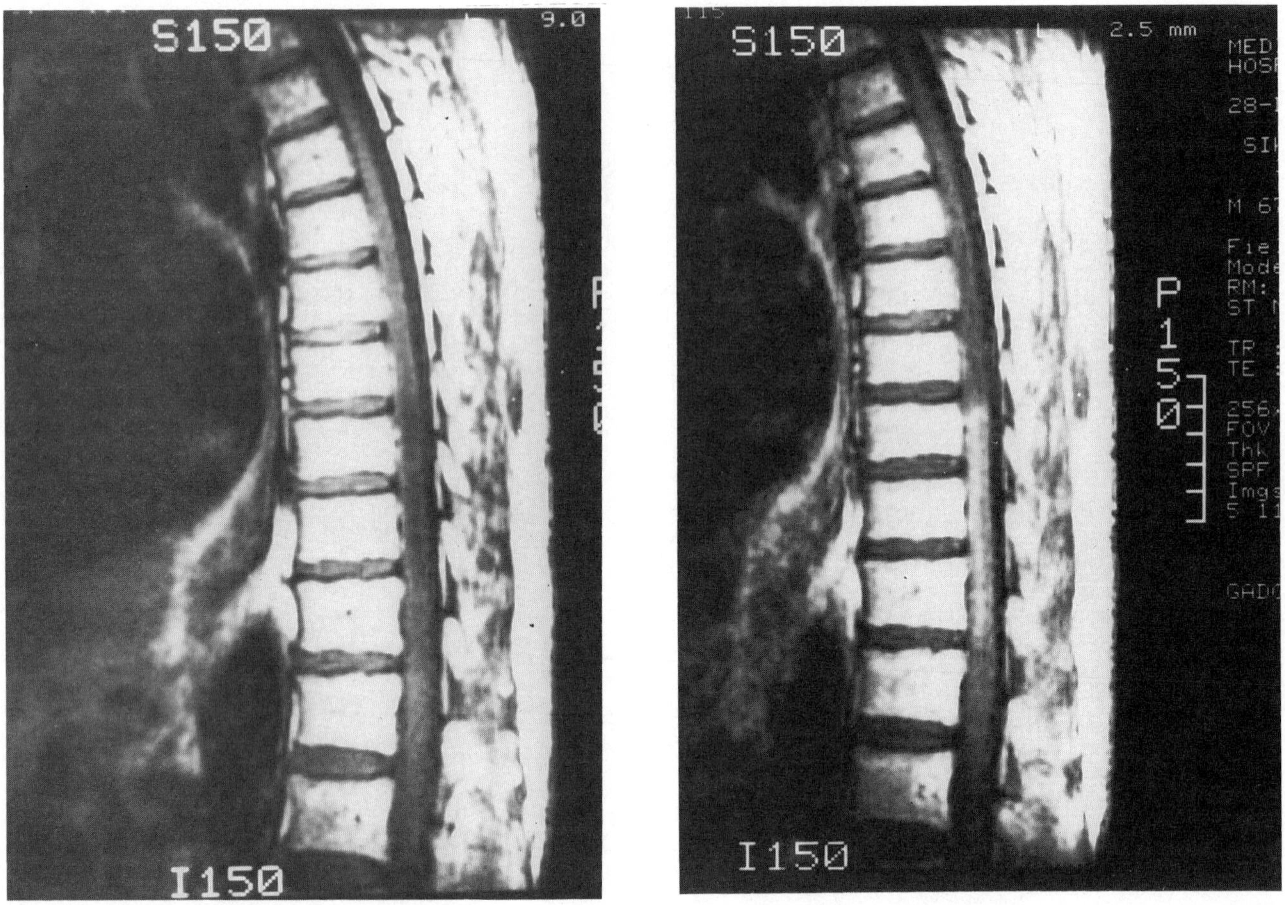

(*A*) (*B*)

Figure 252-11 T1-weighted images of a patient with severe paraparesis from a thoracic dural AVF. Note the nonspecific widening of the midthoracic portion of the cord and the low signal on the T1-weighted image before administration of gadolinium (*A*). The image after gadolinium enhancement (*B*) shows nonspecific enhancement in the region of the cord most severely affected. Note that the MRI findings in this patient do not lead to a clear diagnosis of a spinal AVM. MRI images may look normal in patients with spinal dural AVFs. (From Thompson BG, Oldfield EH. Spinal vascular malformations. In Carter LP, Spetzlar RF (eds): *Neurovascular Surgery.* New York: McGraw-Hill, 1995, pp 1167–1195.)

so close that it is not possible to separate them, either surgically or during embolization, without risking occlusion of the medullary artery. This simple procedure eliminates venous congestion of the cord without endangering the cord vascularity or the function of the nerve root at the involved level.[43] Dural AVFs appear only rarely to recanalize and find access to the venous system of the spinal cord at a later date after simple interruption of the draining vessel; this eventuality has occurred in only two of our patients, one at 6 months (a patient with intradural and extradural drainage of the dural AVF), and one at 17 years after treatment.[36]

The patients I have treated with simple interruption of the intradural draining vessel, and in whom the only venous drainage of the fistula was via a single intrathecal draining vein, have had retrograde thrombosis of the fistula and no further filling of it on spinal arteriography at least 1 year later.[1a] With patients who have both intradural and extradural venous drainage from the AVF, simple interruption of the intradural efferent vessel eliminates venous congestion of the cord but may not produce occlusion of the fistula, which still has patent pathways for venous drainage. These patients may require surgical excision of the fistula, if that can be done without sacrificing an important nerve root,[25] or embolic occlusion of the residual AVF during postoperative arteriography.

The dural AVF can also be occluded by transarterial embolization of the fistula during interventional arteriography.[11,14,29] However, embolic occlusion is often only temporarily effective, as the fistula frequently recanalizes and produces recurrent myelopathy.[20] Furthermore, embolization cannot be safely employed when the same segmental artery supplies both the AVF and the spinal cord, as was the case in 4 of our 27 patients with a spinal dural AVF.[13,37,40] In addition, patients occasionally become paraplegic after embolization,[29] possibly owing to retrograde thrombosis of the coronal venous plexus. Embolization can be used to interrupt the progression of venous congestion to thrombosis and irreversible cord injury in patients with the Foix-Alajouanine syndrome, permitting immediate reduction in venous congestion of the cord until surgery can be performed.[8]

Outcome

Dural AVFs are uniformly amenable to safe and successful treatment, which in most patients either produces improvement in function or halts clinical progression.[24,25,36,37,40,43] Most patients are able to ambulate independently following treatment, and micturition is improved in most.[40,43] The outcome after treatment is closely related to the preoperative neurological function; patients who are diagnosed early and treated before prominent neurological impairment occurs generally have a good outcome, whereas patients with little remaining function preoperatively fare less well (Fig. 252-12*A*).[37,40,43]

Spinal Intradural Vascular Malformations

In the intradural vascular malformations of the spinal cord (juvenile and glomus AVMs and direct intradural AVFs), the nidus of the fistula lies in the cord parenchyma or is embedded in the pia. In these lesions, one or more enlarged medullary arteries commonly supply both the malformation and the spinal cord (Figs. 252-3 through 252-5). These lesions are products of a defect in early vascular embryogenesis.

Juvenile and Glomus AVMs

Pathophysiology, Epidemiology, Clinical Presentation

Males and females are affected with equal frequency, and patients are generally less than 40 years old when symptoms begin (Fig. 252-8). Intradural AVMs are more likely to present in an apoplectic manner with pain and acute neurological dysfunction than are spinal dural AVFs (Table 252-2).[37,40] Unlike dural AVFs, these are AVMs of high flow. In 40 percent of patients, acute presentation is caused by subarachnoid or intramedullary hemorrhage, and 50 percent have subarachnoid hemorrhage before the diagnosis is established.[40] The acute disruption of cord function appears to result from the direct effects of the hemorrhage on or in the spinal cord. The increased risk of hemorrhage is partly attributable to the fact that a large proportion (44 percent) of intradural AVMs have associated arterial and venous aneurysms.[40] About half of the patients with intradural AVMs have a gradual onset and progression of symptoms and signs.[40] Whether this form of presentation results from arterial ischemia by a vascular steal phenomenon or from venous congestion remains unknown. Intradural AVMs more often occur in the cervical and upper thoracic segments of the spinal cord than do dural AVFs (Fig. 252-9) and are therefore more likely to produce symptoms affecting the upper extremities than are the dural lesions.

Diagnostic Investigation

Juvenile-type AVMs derive their blood supply from multiple medullary arteries via the anterior and posterior spinal arteries. The nidus is large and, as a rule, contains cord tissue interspersed among the AVM vessels (Fig. 252-3). These AVMs frequently also involve the vertebrae and paraspinous soft tissue. On examination, they may produce an audible spinal bruit at the level of maximum shunting. The nidus of the glomus type of intramedullary AVM is a tightly packed mass of blood vessels confined to a short segment of the spinal cord; it has a typical appearance on spinal MRI (Fig. 252-13). These lesions typically occur in the anterior half of the spinal cord and are supplied by the anterior spinal artery (Fig. 252-4).

Treatment, Outcome

The ideal therapy for intradural AVMs should be to completely and permanently obliterate the AVM while preserving the blood supply of the cord. This can be accomplished safely in some patients, but to preserve neurological function, many patients require treatment that only partially or temporarily occludes flow in the AVM.

Certain general principles apply to all operations for AVMs of the spinal cord.[6,26,52,53] To allow for lysis of clots and absorption of blood products, surgery is delayed if there has been recent subarachnoid hemorrhage. The operative microscope and appropriate microsurgical instruments and techniques are required for surgery of all spinal AVMs. Operative exposure of intramedullary spinal AVMs is performed with a complete laminectomy extending at least one segment above and one segment below the glomus of the malformation. A midline dural incision preserving the arachnoid allows for optimal exposure and avoids tearing the fragile, distended underlying blood vessels, which may adhere to the arachnoid, especially in patients with prior hemorrhage or surgery. Dural traction sutures are placed to include the arachnoid if the underlying engorged vessels of the AVM do not adhere to it. It is important to correlate the vascular anatomy as seen on the preoperative arteriogram with that seen intraoperatively to assure that all medullary arteries are preserved during dissection and to aid in the early identification and interruption of major feeding arteries where they enter the malformation. Intraoperative ultrasound, particularly with the new instruments that can distinguish the direction of blood flow in individual vessels, aids in the intramedullary localization of the AVM and in determining which vessels supply and which drain the high-flow malformations. Meticulous hemostasis is essential, as is liberal irrigation during bipolar coagulation. Larger feeding vessels may require ligatures or clips, but metallic clips impair postoperative imaging. They are rarely needed in the excision of spinal AVMs; most vessels can be managed with simple bipolar coagulation and interruption. As in intramedullary spinal surgery for all mass lesions, the malformation can be separated from the surrounding cord by dissecting in the gliotic plane between the malformation and the adjacent cord tissue. As the margins of the malformation are dissected, gentle bipolar coagulation is used to progressively shrink the AVM and render its periphery less friable. Pial traction sutures are used to maintain adequate separation of the spinal cord from the AVM to permit room for dissection. During the later stages of the dissection, the AVM is elevated to better expose the vessels that enter and leave it ventrally. At least one major draining vein is preserved until dissection around the periphery of the malformation has been completed and all arterial feeding vessels have been occluded. Postoperative spinal arteriography is used routinely to assess the success of complete excision of the AVM.

In juvenile AVMs or glomus AVMs that occupy the ventral half of the spinal cord, it may not be possible to remove the AVM without producing unacceptable neurological deficits. Under such circumstances, surgical excision should not be attempted. Plans to

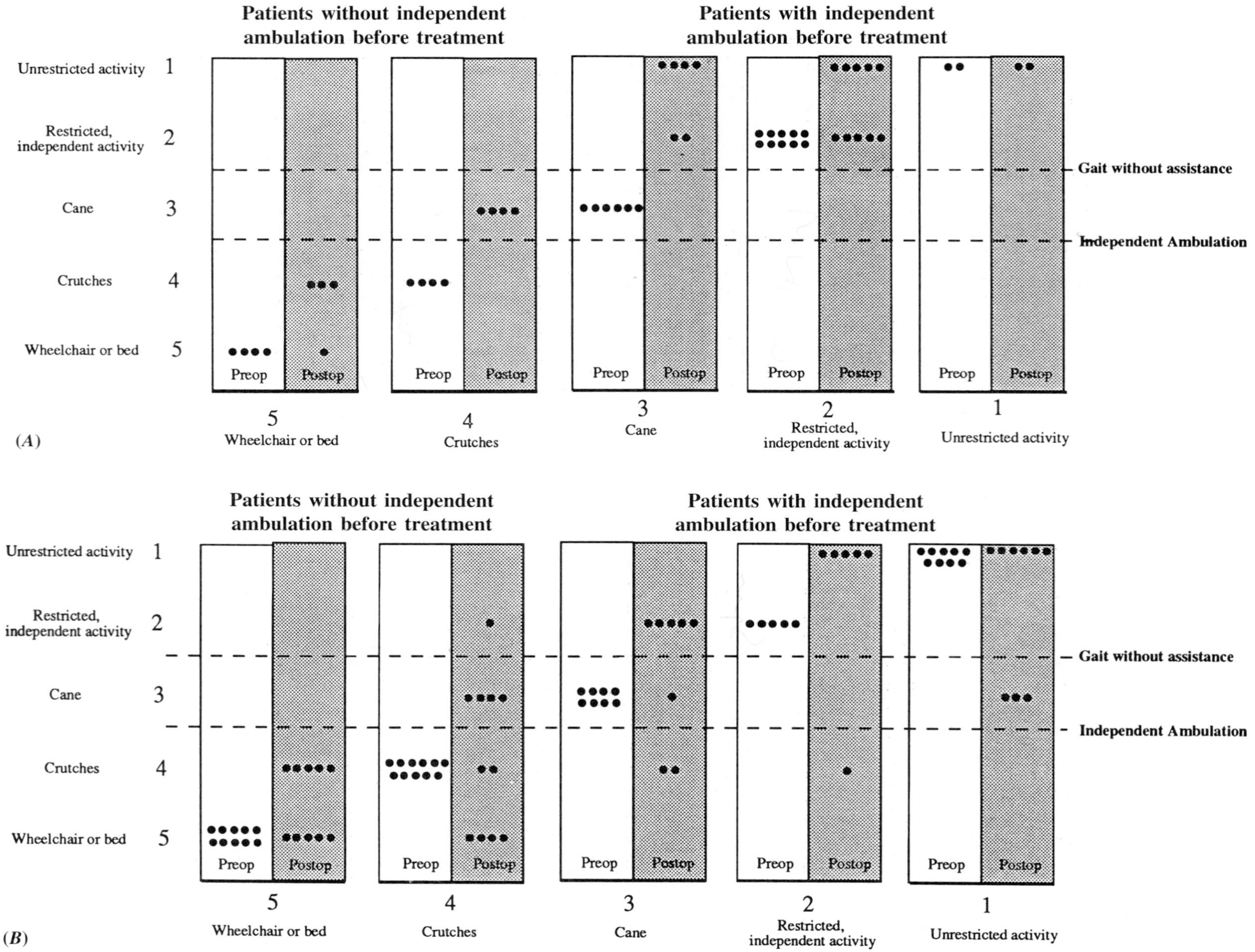

Figure 252-12 In patients with dural AVFs and intradural AVMs, the outcome after surgery is directly related to the preoperative neurological status. Early diagnosis and therapy offer the best outcome for patients in both groups. *A*. Relationship of preoperative functional state and postoperative outcome in patients with dural AVFs. *B*. Relationship of preoperative functional state and postoperative outcome in patients with intramedullary AVMs (n = 43). (From Muraszko and Oldfield.[31] Data from Rosenblum, Oldfield, and Doppman.[40])

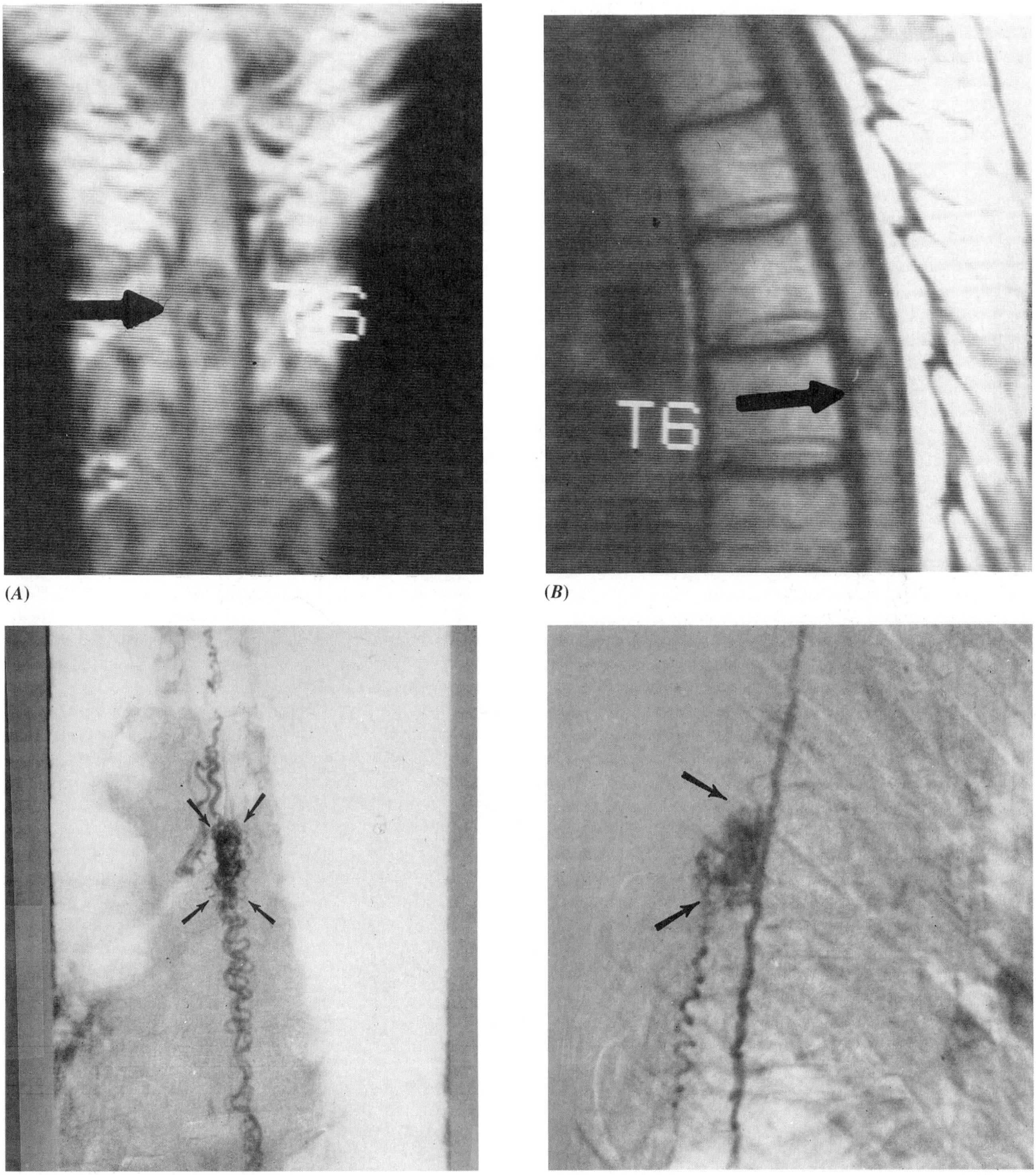

(*A*) (*B*) (*C*) (*D*)

Figure 252-13 MR images of an intramedullary AVM. Because of the rapid flow in the vessels of these lesions, they show areas of flow void on MRI. *A*. T2-weighted (1000/75) coronal scan reveals an intramedullary nidus (*arrow*) at the T6 vertebral level. *B*. T1-weighted (SE 600/25) sagittal scan shows the nidus (*arrow*) more clearly. On selective spinal arteriography, the anteroposterior (*C*) and lateral (*D*) views in the early venous phase confirm the intramedullary location of the nidus. (From Doppman et al.[12])

completely excise or obliterate the malformation may also have to be abandoned during the operation if it becomes apparent that carrying them out will pose an undue risk to cord function.

Surgery for intramedullary AVMs, which is usually performed for children or young adults, carries greater risks (particularly for lesions within the thoracic and lumbar segments), is more difficult, and generally is less rewarding than surgery for dural AVFs. Although the cervical lesions, which are typically partially intra- and extramedullary in a dorsal location, and which often are supplied mainly by posterior spinal arteries, are amenable to excision,[6,26,52,53] significant risks are associated with excision of lesions in the thoracic and lumbar segments of the cord supplied by the anterior spinal artery. Although there have been reports of successful surgery for these lesions, it is not clear to what extent patients with a good outcome have been disproportionately selected for publication.

Embolic occlusion of spinal AVMs is used alone or, because the incidence of recanalization after embolic occlusion is quite high,[20,47] before surgical excision. Deciding on embolization requires careful assessment of the anatomy of the blood supply, including the size of the vessels supplying the AVM, and the level of the lesion. For success, the nidus of the AVM must be occluded without obstructing the vessel supplying the AVM proximal to the nidus. The latter is often a medullary artery or the anterior spinal artery, occlusion of which may immediately interrupt the blood supply to the spinal cord, especially in lesions below the upper thoracic level. Cervical AVMs are safer to embolize because there are more collateral sources of blood for the spinal cord in that region. The progress of the embolization is assessed frequently during the procedure by high-resolution digital imaging. The selection of the catheter depends on how close the tip of the catheter must be to the nidus of the AVM to selectively occlude the AVM while preserving the blood supply of the spinal cord and, to a certain extent, on whether particulate or liquid embolic material will be used. For embolization with particulate material via an intercostal artery with the catheter tip in the proximal portion of the intercostal artery, the distal portion of the main trunk of the intercostal artery must be occluded with emboli, or with placement of a balloon-tipped catheter or an occlusive coil, before the particles will flow preferentially into the spinal ramus of the intercostal artery and to the AVM by a flow-directed phenomenon. For more distal catheterization, a wire-directable microcatheter, such as the Tracker catheter (Target Therapeutics, San Jose, CA), is used for selective arteriography and embolization.

Although several particulate materials have been used to occlude spinal AVMs, the most commonly used agent is polyvinyl alcohol (PVA) particles in the 150 to 250 μm diameter range. The size of the particles is chosen so that they will pass freely through the conducting vessel(s), medullary arteries, anterior or posterior spinal artery, and enlarged sulcal vessels to the AVM, without occluding the normal sulcal vessels. Since the diameter of the normal anterior spinal artery is 340 to 1100 μm, and the diameter of the normal sulcal arteries is 60 to 72 μm, PVA particles of 150 to 250 μm diameter should pass through the anterior spinal artery, not enter the normal sulcal arteries, and pass into the enlarged sulcal arteries supplying the AVM. When the vessel providing the most direct route to the AVM is particularly difficult to engage with a catheter, as is the case for feeding arteries from the cervical segment of the vertebral artery, the particles can be embolized in a flow-directed manner toward the nidus by means of temporary or permanent balloon occlusion of the artery just distal to the origin of the feeding vessel. Particulate embolization is terminated when the lesion is almost completely occluded (in-situ PVA particles continue to cause clot to form and propagate after completion of the procedure) or when there is retrograde reflux of the contrast medium proximal to the catheter tip, indicating that flow-directed targeting of the nidus will no longer occur. The liquid materials (isobutyl-2-cyanoacrylate), which are less embolic, require placement of the catheter tip at the edge of the nidus of the AVM and injection of a small amount of the polymer. Since, in our experience, the most common side effect of complete embolic occlusion of spinal AVMs is new neurological deficits that arise 24 to 48 h after embolization, and which may be related to propagation of venous thrombosis in the enlarged coronal venous plexus that is then sluggishly carrying only the venous drainage of the spinal cord, we routinely anticoagulate the patient with heparin for 48 to 60 h after the procedure. Repeat arteriography is performed 7 to 10 days later, with follow-up arteriography at intervals of 1 to 2 years or when neurological symptoms or signs recur, and additional embolization is performed as needed.

Despite the fact that embolization of spinal AVMs with PVA does not permanently eliminate flow through the AVM in most patients, it plays an important role in the current management of patients with intradural AVMs. Presurgical embolization makes the surgery easier, because it reduces blood supply to the AVM and transiently reduces the size of the AVM. Treatment of completely paraplegic patients may eliminate an intractable pain syndrome, reduce the risk of subsequent hemorrhage (which could cause quadriplegia or death), and ameliorate spasticity in some patients. Furthermore, the results of Biondi et al.[5] suggest that operative intervention is less effective for thoracic intramedullary AVMs[6,23,40,53] than is serial, yearly endovascular embolization with PVA. Their long-term follow-up (mean of 6 years) showed that, even though *none* of their patients had complete, permanent obliteration of the AVM (most patients had less than a 50 percent reduction in AVM size), nearly two-thirds of the patients were clinically better at the end of the study. We have several patients with thoracic or lumbar ventral intramedullary AVMs that receive their blood supply from the anterior spinal artery whose neurological status has been stabilized repeatedly by repetitive embolic occlusion of the AVM with PVA particles when recurrent symptoms arose. On the other hand, since further neurological disability may not be reversible, the approach of Biondi et al., who advocate routine yearly arteriography and embolization with polyvinyl alcohol (Ivalon), regardless of symptoms, appears to be safe and eliminates neurological progression in most patients.[5] As with surgery of intradural AVMs, the best results with embolization are obtained in patients who do not have major neurological deficits before treatments.[5,11,14,15,22,32,37,38,40,45,47] Selective catheterization and embolization is associated with risks of occluding the anterior spinal artery and causing paraplegia or quadriplegia; perforating an intradural vessel with the catheter and causing subarachnoid or intramedullary hemorrhage[47]; and having emboli pass (1) through the AVM into the venous system causing hemorrhage or venous infarction[11] or (2) into the distal vessels of the parent artery, such as the basilar artery when the vertebral artery is used to reach the AVM.

With the intradural AVMs, as with the dural AVFs, the better the neurological condition of the patient preoperatively, the better the outcome after treatment with surgery (Fig. 252-12*B*) or embolization.[5]

Direct Arteriovenous Fistulas

Direct AVFs are high-flow, extramedullary lesions that involve a direct shunt from an artery to a vein without an intervening nidus of abnormal vessels (Fig. 252-5). They are supplied by one or more arteries that also supply the cord and are frequently associated with large arterial or venous aneurysms, which may compress the cord or cause symptoms by vascular steal, hemorrhage, or venous congestion. The myelopathy is usually that of an anterior spinal artery syndrome or a Brown-Sequard syndrome.[10,19] Myelography demonstrates the dilated, serpentine vessels in the subarachnoid space and a focal filling defect or spinal block at the level of an aneurysm. As seen at arteriography, these lesions are on the cord surface or, rarely, may be free in the subarachnoid space. Anterior fistulae are perfused by the anterior spinal artery; lateral and posterior lesions may receive blood from the anterior and/or posterior spinal arteries.

High-resolution DVI with very rapid-sequence imaging (6 to 10 per second) often permits the nidus of these lesions to be clearly demonstrated. With this technique we have recently demonstrated that some of the intradural lesions that we would have considered to be AVMs on the basis of standard arteriography are actually the more easily and safely treated perimedullary AVFs.[34]

The goal of treatment is precise interruption of the abnormal communication between the artery and vein. Elimination of the extramedullary fistulous connection of perimedullary AVFs may be achieved by surgery[1,10,19,21,39] or embolization.[10,19,39] For purposes of treatment, these lesions can be categorized into three groups in relation to caliber, length, and the number of vessels supplying and draining the fistula: (1) small fistulas supplied by a long, thin anterior spinal artery, (2) larger fistulas fed by an enlarged anterior spinal artery, and (3) giant fistulas supplied by an enormously enlarged spinal artery.[19,39] Surgical intervention is typically reserved for posterior or posterolateral lesions or for circumstances in which embolization is inherently dangerous. The latter include lesions that are fed solely by a long anterior spinal artery of small caliber in which embolization may not be safe or effective and surgical intervention may entail lower risks.[1,21] Patients with larger fistulas and an enlarged anterior spinal artery can be treated by embolic occlusion with solid materials, by balloon occlusion, by surgery, or by a combination of embolic and surgical approaches. The giant fistulas are amenable to selective occlusion by detachable balloons, which permits a trial occlusion before disengagement.[19,38] In patients with an associated venous varix or aneurysm, treatment options include embolization, direct operative interruption, and temporary balloon occlusion as an adjunct to surgical extirpation. For these lesions, as in the other forms of AVMs, better results are obtained in patients who are diagnosed and treated early.[1,10,19,21,39]

Cavernous Angiomas

Cavernous angiomas are intramedullary lesions consisting of thin-walled vascular sinusoidal spaces without intervening nervous tissue. Affected patients are mostly middle-aged. Cavernous angiomas commonly cause progressive paraparesis and sensory loss with a stuttering, stepwise advancement of neurological deficits. They usually contain cysts of old blood and hemosiderin-laden macrophages, suggesting that the stepwise increases in cord dysfunction are related to repeated episodes of hemorrhage, as occurs in their cerebral counterparts.[7]

They can cause focal expansion of the cord, but are often not detected with myelography; results of arteriography are normal. Heretofore they have been diagnosed rarely, but they may be more common than previously thought. MRI is the most sensitive diagnostic test for these lesions.[7,18,42] The T1- and T2-weighted MRI appearances of intraspinal cavernous angiomas are similar to those of cavernous malformations in the brain. MR images typically demonstrate a well-delineated spherical or oblong intramedullary lesion of mixed signal intensity, predominantly low-signal with scattered areas of higher signal (Fig. 252-14). The findings with MRI depend on the age of the blood products. The low signal along the periphery of the angioma on T2-weighted imaging is due to hemosiderin deposition associated with chronic changes in the blood products. The punctate pattern of higher signal on T1 and T2 images suggests the presence of methemoglobin, and hence small hemorrhages that are subacute or chronic. On T2-weighted images, this mixed signal intensity produces the familiar "target" configuration (Fig. 252-14). Despite the foregoing description of the typical cavernous malformation of the spinal cord, exceptions occur, and the MRI appearance is nonspecific and depends on the timing of small foci of hemorrhage and the presence of blood in various stages of catabolism at distinct sites in the cavernous angioma. Enhancement with gadolinium is variable.

Most cavernous angiomas of the spinal cord are diagnosed after they cause myelopathy by a cycle of repeated small hemorrhages and gliosis. With cavernous angiomas, as with dural and intradural spinal AVFs and AVMs, the outcome after surgery depends greatly on the neurological function before surgery.[4,7,28,33] The usual considerations for surgery of intraparenchymal cord lesions must be considered: Lesions lying in the dorsal half of the cord, which are immediately accessible with a limited myelotomy over the most superficial aspect of the lesion (frequently indicated by bluish-gray discoloration of the pia), require less manipulation of the spinal cord for exposure and are associated with less risk of incurring additional neurological injury during surgery and a better prognosis for improvement after removal than are ventral lesions. At operation, these lesions are surrounded by a thin zone of gliosis that can be used to advantage for dissecting them from the surrounding cord. Since residual portions of cavernous angiomas that are left in situ during surgery tend to rehemorrhage and cause recurrent myelopathy, complete excision is mandatory and requires careful and complete inspection of the bed of the angioma in the spinal cord before closure.[4,7,33,48]

In contrast to lesions that cause significant or progressing neurological deficits, the question of whether asymptomatic spinal cord cavernous malformations should be excised is controversial, primarily because their natural history is unknown. Cavernous angiomas may remain asymptomatic and be detected incidentally during a spinal MRI screening evaluation in a patient with a symptom-producing cavernous angioma of the brain. One recent clinical-radiographic study of the natural history of *familial, mostly cerebral* cavernous malformations reported a 6.5 percent annual rate of symptomatic (re)hemorrhage,[49] but it is unclear whether these data can be extrapolated to treatment of *asymptomatic* cavernous malformations of the *spinal cord.* Therefore, recommendations for treatment must consider the patient's symptoms, evidence of progression, and the projected risks of surgery. Until more information is available, there is no compelling argument for treating asymptomatic cavernous angiomas.

Summary

Current techniques of diagnosis and treatment allow early detection, precise anatomic delineation, and successful treatment of

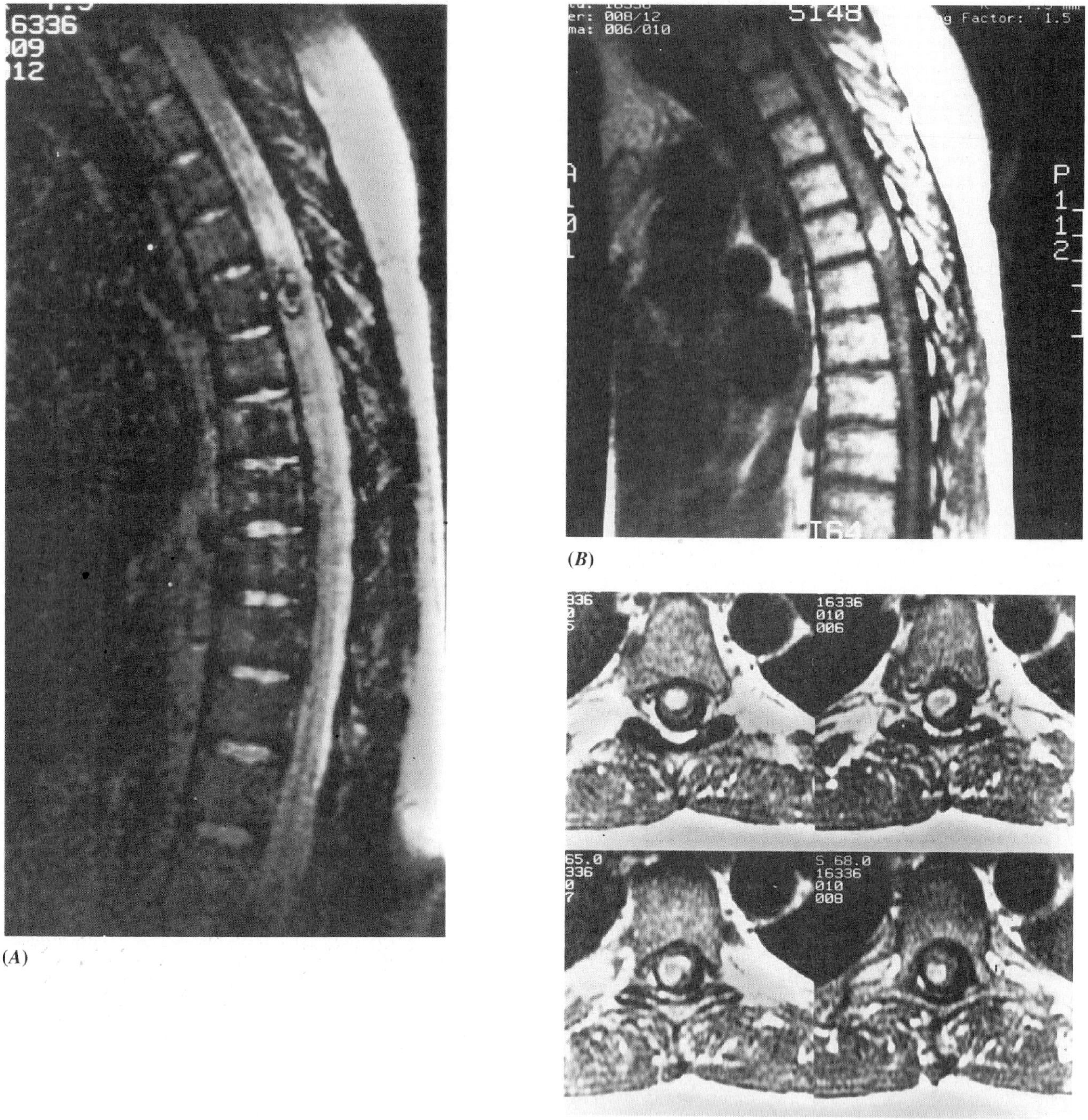

(*A*) (*B*) (*C*)

Figure 252-14 MR images of a cavernous angioma of the spinal cord. The increasing role of MRI in the diagnosis of spinal disorders has greatly enhanced the recognition of cavernous angiomas of the spinal cord. MRI is the most sensitive and specific diagnostic test for these lesions. T1- and T2-weighted MR images of the angioma, which show patterns similar to those of cavernous malformations in the brain, typically demonstrate a well-delineated spherical or oblong intramedullary lesion of mixed signal, usually with a low-signal area surrounding scattered areas of higher signal on T2-weighted images. The findings with MRI depend on the age of the blood products. These images show an angioma in the midthoracic portion of the spinal cord that was associated with chronic paraparesis that was progressing in a stuttering, subacute manner. *A*. T2-weighted (TR 2000, TE 40) sagittal image. *B*. T1-weighted (TR 500, TE 20) sagittal image. *C*. T1-weighted (TR 650, TE 25) axial images. The high signal on the T1-weighted images is consistent with methemoglobin accumulation in the subacute intramedullary hematoma, which was confirmed at surgery. (From Oldfield.[35])

most spinal vascular malformations. The prognosis for successful treatment of patients with spinal vascular malformations is a function of the type of malformation and the degree of preoperative neurological deficit. With spinal dural AVFs, the most common variety of spinal vascular malformation, myelopathy results from venous congestion, which can be eliminated by interrupting the vessel that drains the dural AVF as it enters the dura; this intervention also results in retrograde thrombosis and permanent occlusion of the AVF. Early treatment is usually successful. Even in patients with acute neurological deterioration, at least stabilization or partial reversal of neurological impairment can be expected.

Intradural spinal AVMs impair cord function by hemorrhage, ischemia, or venous congestion. The goal of treatment for intradural spinal AVMs is complete excision of the AVM or complete and permanent embolic obliteration of the nidus of the AVM. Because these lesions have a blood supply in common with the blood supply of the spinal cord (usually via the anterior spinal artery), treating them carries a significant risk of cord function impairment, particularly in the case of lesions in the ventral portion of the lower half of the spinal cord. Although embolic occlusion of intradural AVMs is usually not curative, it often temporarily improves or stabilizes neurological function and may reduce the risk of hemorrhage. Recent evidence suggests that most patients with ventral *thoracic or lumbar* intramedullary AVMs can be stabilized with serial yearly endovascular embolization with PVA. Certain malformations, particularly those in the posterior half of the spinal cord, the cervical glomus-type AVMs, and the posterior perimedullary AVFs, are best treated surgically after preoperative embolization. Symptom-producing cavernous angiomas should be excised.

The outcome after treatment of dural AVFs, intradural spinal AVMs and AVFs, and cavernous angiomas depends not only on the type and location of the lesion but also, closely, on the preoperative level of neurological function. Patients who are ambulatory before treatment are usually ambulatory after treatment. The best outcome requires early diagnosis and intervention before severe, irreversible cord injury has occurred.

References

1a. Afshar JK, Doppman JL, Oldfield EH. Surgical interruption of intradural draining vein as curative treatment of spinal dural arteriovenous fistulas. *J Neurosurg* 1995; 82:196–200.
1. Aminoff M, Gutin P, Norman D. Unusual type of spinal arteriovenous malformation. *Neurosurgery* 1988; 22:589–591.
2. Aminoff MJ, Logue V. Clinical features of spinal vascular malformations. *Brain* 1974; 97:197–210.
3. Aminoff MJ, Logue V. The prognosis of patients with spinal vascular malformations. *Brain* 1974; 97:211–218.
4. Anson J, Spetzler R. Surgical resection of intramedullary spinal cord cavernous malformations. *J Neurosurg* 1993; 78:446–451.
5. Biondi A, Merland J, Reizine D. Embolization with particles in thoracic intramedullary arteriovenous malformations: long-term angiographic and clinical results. *Radiology* 1990; 177:651–658.
6. Cogen P, Stein BM. Spinal cord arteriovenous malformations with significant intramedullary components. *J Neurosurg* 1983; 59:471–478.
7. Cosgrove GR, Bertrand G, Fontaine S, et al. Cavernous angiomas of the spinal cord. *J Neurosurg* 1988; 68:31–36.
8. Criscuolo GR, Oldfield EH, Doppman JL. Reversible acute and subacute myelopathy in patients with dural arteriovenous fistulas: Foix-Alajouanine syndrome reconsidered. *J Neurosurg* 1989; 70:354–359.
9. DiChiro G, Doppman J, Dwyer A, et al. Tumors and arteriovenous malformations of the spinal cord: assessment using MR. *Radiology* 1985; 156:689–697.
10. Djindjian M, Djindjian R, Rey A, et al. Intradural extramedullary spinal arteriovenous malformations fed by the anterior spinal artery. *Surg Neurol* 1977; 8:85–93.
11. Djindjian R. Embolization of angiomas of the spinal cord. *Surg Neurol* 1975; 4:411–420.
12. Doppman JL, DiChiro G, Dwyer AJ, et al. Magnetic resonance imaging of spinal arteriovenous malformations. *J Neurosurg* 1987; 66:830–834.
13. Doppman JL, DiChiro G, Oldfield EH. Origin of spinal arteriovenous malformation and normal cord vasculature from a common segmental artery: angiographic and therapeutic considerations. *Radiology* 1985; 154:687–689.
14. Doppman J, DiChiro G, Ommaya A. Obliteration of spinal-cord arteriovenous malformations by percutaneous embolisation. *Lancet* 1968; 1:477.
15. Doppman J, DiChiro G, Ommaya A. Percutaneous embolization of spinal cord arteriovenous malformations. *J Neurosurg* 1971; 34:48–55.
16. Dormont D, Gelbert F, Assouline E, et al. MR imaging of spinal arteriovenous malformations at 0.5 T: Study of 34 cases. *Am J Neuroradiol* 1988; 9:833–838.
17. Elsberg CA. *Diagnosis and Treatment of Surgical Diseases of the Spinal Cord and Its Membranes.* Philadelphia: Saunders, 1916, pp 201–204.
18. Fontaine S, Melanson D, Cosgrove R. Cavernous hemangiomas of the spinal cord: MR imaging. *Radiology* 1988; 166:839.
19. Gueguen B, Merland J, Riche M, Rey A. Vascular malformations of the spinal cord: intrathecal perimedullary arteriovenous fistulas fed by medullary arteries. *Neurology* 1987; 37:969–979.
20. Hall W, Oldfield E, Doppman J. Recanalization of spinal cord arteriovenous malformations following embolization. *J Neurosurg* 1989; 70:714–720.
21. Heros R, Debrun G, Ojemann R, et al. Direct spinal arteriovenous fistula: a new type of spinal AVM: case report. *J Neurosurg* 1986; 64:134–139.
22. Horton JA, Latchaw RE, Gold LHA, et al. Embolization of intramedullary arteriovenous malformations of the spinal cord. *Am J Neuroradiol* 1986; 7:113–118.
23. Hurth M, Houdart R, Djindjian R, et al. Arteriovenous malformations of the spinal cord: clinical, anatomical and therapeutic considerations—a series of 150 cases. *Prog Neurol Surg* 1978; 9:238–266.
24. Kendall BE, Logue V. Spinal epidural angiomatous malformations draining into intrathecal veins. *Neuroradiology* 1977; 13:181–189.
25. Logue V. Angiomas of the spinal cord: review of the pathogenesis, clinical features, and results of surgery. *J Neurol Neurosurg Psychiatry* 1979; 42:1–11.
26. Malis LI. Microsurgery for spinal cord arteriovenous malformations. *Clin Neurosurg* 1979; 26:543–555.
27. Masaryk T, Ross J, Modic M, et al. Radiculomeningeal vascular malformations of the spine: MR imaging. *Radiology* 1987; 164:845–849.
28. McCormick P, Michelsen W, Post K, et al. Cavernous malformations of the spinal cord. *Neurosurgery* 1988; 23:459–463.
29. Merland JJ, Riche MC, Chiras J. Intraspinal extramedullary arteriovenous fistulae draining into the medullary veins. *J Neuroradiol* 1980; 7:271–320.
30. Minami S, Sagoh T, Nishimura K, et al. Spinal arteriovenous malformations: MR imaging. *Radiology* 1988; 169:109–115.
31. Muraszko K, Oldfield E. Vascular malformations of the spinal cord and dura. *Neurosurg Clin North Am* 1990; 1:631–652.
32. Newton T, Adams J. Angiographic demonstration and nonsurgical embolization of spinal cord angioma. *Radiology* 1968; 91:873.
33. Ogilvy C, Louis D, Ojemann R. Intramedullary cavernous angiomas of the spinal cord: clinical presentation, pathological features, and surgical management. *Neurosurgery* 1992; 31:219–230.
34. Oldfield E. Editorial comment. *Neurosurgery* 1993; 33:1091.
35. Oldfield E. Spinal vascular malformations. In Rengachary SS, Wilkins

RH (eds):. *Neurosurgical Operative Atlas*, vol 4. Park Ridge, IL: American Association of Neurological Surgeons, 1995, pp 1–18.
36. Oldfield EH, DiChiro G, Quindlen EA, et al. Successful treatment of a group of spinal cord arteriovenous malformations by interruption of dural fistula. *J Neurosurg* 1983; 59:1019–1030.
37. Oldfield EH, Doppman JL. Spinal arteriovenous malformations. *Clin Neurosurg* 1988; 34:161–183.
38. Riche MC, Melki JP, Merland JJ. Embolization of spinal cord vascular malformations via the anterior spinal artery. *Am J Neuroradiol* 1983; 4:378–381.
39. Riche M, Scialfa G, Gueguen B, Merland J. Giant extramedullary arteriovenous fistulas supplied by the anterior spinal artery: treatment by detachable balloons. *Am J Neuroradiol* 1983; 4:391–394.
40. Rosenblum B, Oldfield EH, Doppman JL, et al. Spinal arteriovenous malformations: a comparison of dural arteriovenous fistulas and intradural AVMs in 81 patients. *J Neurosurg* 1987; 67:795–802.
41. Sargent P. Hemangioma of the pia mater causing compression paraplegia. *Brain* 1925; 48:259–267.
42. Simard J, Garcia-Bengochea F, Ballinger W, et al. Cavernous angioma: a review of 126 collected and 12 new clinical cases. *Neurosurgery* 1986; 18:162.
43. Symon L, Kuyama H, Kendall B. Dural arteriovenous malformations of the spine: clinical features and surgical results in 55 cases. *J Neurosurg* 1984; 60:238–247.
44. Terwey B, Becker H, Thron A, Vahldiek G. Gadolinium-DTPA enhanced MR imaging of spinal dural arteriovenous fistulas. *J Comput Assist Tomogr* 1989; 13:30–37.
45. Theron J, Cosgrove R, Melanson D, Ethier R. Spinal arteriovenous malformations: advances in therapeutic embolization. *Radiology* 1986; 158:163–169.
46. Thompson BG, Doppman JL, Oldfield EH. Treatment of cranial dural arteriovenous fistulae by interruption of leptomeningeal venous drainage. *J Neurosurg* 1994; 80:617–623.
47. Touho H, Karasawa J, Ohnishi H, et al. Superselective embolization of spinal arteriovenous malformations using the Tracker catheter. *Surg Neurol* 1992; 38:85–94.
48. Tyndel F, Bilboa J, Hudson A, Colapinto E. Hemangioma calcificans of the spinal cord. *Can J Neurol Sci* 1985; 12:321–322.
49. Wascher TM, Zabramski J, Johnson B, et al. Natural history of familial cavernous malformations. Presented at the 60th Annual Meeting of the American Association of Neurological Surgeons. San Francisco, CA, April 13, 1992. *J Neurosurg* 1992; 76:376A.
50. Wrobel CJ, Oldfield EH, DiChiro G, et al. Myelopathy due to intracranial dural arteriovenous fistulas draining intrathecally into spinal medullary veins: report of three cases. *J Neurosurg* 1988; 69:934–939.
51. Wyburn-Mason R. *The Vascular Abnormalities and Tumours of the Spinal Cord and Its Membranes.* London: Henry Kimpton, 1943.
52. Yasargil MG, DeLong WB, Guarnaschelli JJ. Complete microsurgical excision of cervical extramedullary and intramedullary vascular malformations. *Surg Neurol* 1975; 4:211–224.
53. Yasargil MG, Symon L, Teddy PJ. Arteriovenous malformations of the spinal cord. *Adv Tech Stand Neurosurg* 1984; 11:61–102.

SECTION E

Other Vascular Disorders

253 Spontaneous Intraspinal Hemorrhage

Hugh S. Wisoff

Spontaneous intraspinal hemorrhage is an uncommon event. It is most frequently heralded by the apoplectic onset of back pain. Hematoma formation in the epidural, subdural, and subarachnoid spaces causes compression of the underlying neural elements. Hemorrhage and hematomas also occur within the parenchyma of the cord unassociated with trauma, vascular lesions, or tumors. Bleeding in the three extramedullary compartments may be caused by lumbar puncture (including spinal anesthesia) and epidural anesthesia. Patients with an iatrogenic (anticoagulant-induced) or disease-related coagulopathy are at increased risk for both nontraumatic hemorrhage and hemorrhage associated with minor trauma and lumbar puncture.

The term *spontaneous* in the context of this chapter includes cases in which the onset is associated with activities of daily living: lifting, pulling, coughing, straining at stool or during micturition, dressing, shaving, turning over in bed, and trivial trauma.

The diagnosis and localization of an intraspinal hematoma previously required lumbar puncture to analyze the CSF and myelography to visualize the abnormalities produced by the mass. High-resolution computed tomography (CT) advanced the imaging of the intraspinal contents; diagnostic accuracy further improved with the development of water-soluble iodinated contrast agents that allowed CT of the spine to follow a myelogram. However, CT does not readily depict hematomas in the spine except in the acute phase, and the surrounding bone also interferes with CT imaging of the intraspinal contents.

Magnetic resonance imaging (MRI) revolutionized imaging and diagnosis of intraspinal pathology. MRI recognizes blood and the relative age of blood products, including hematoma formation. It identifies abnormal blood vessels, indicative of an arteriovenous malformation or associated with a neoplasm. (False-positive images consistent with abnormal intraspinal blood vessels have been reported. Myelography is recommended to confirm the MRI findings of abnormal vessels before spinal angiography is undertaken.) The ability of MRI to image multiple segments of the spine simultaneously in the sagittal projection is particularly valuable; the localization of the spinal level on clinical grounds may be difficult. Gadolinium-enhanced MRI usually reveals a neoplasm or cavernous angioma obscured by a hematoma. If available, MRI is currently the initial diagnostic study of choice.

Spinal Epidural Hemorrhage

The spinal epidural space is the most frequently reported site of spontaneous intraspinal hemorrhage. Such hemorrhage has been reported in more than 200 patients. This entity was first described by Blauby in 1808 according to Mayer.[47] Scholarly reviews of the subject were published in 1972 by Jellinger[35] and in 1976 by Bruyn and Bosma.[12] The true incidence is unknown; undoubtedly many cases are not reported. Bleeding without hematoma formation and compression of neural structures is not generally reported. In 1963, Gold[26] reported five cases from our institution seen during a 2-year period. We have not encountered more than one case every 2 to 3 years since his report.

Trauma as the cause of spinal epidural hematoma is also unusual. There are reports of epidural hematomas associated with vertebral fracture, significant injury without fracture (including birth injury), lumbar puncture (usually associated with a coagulopathy secondary to a blood dyscrasia, anticoagulants, alcoholism and liver disease, etc.), and spinal epidural anesthesia.

Among patients with spontaneous spinal epidural bleeding, arteriosclerosis and hypertension are reported frequently, particularly in the aged. Coagulopathy secondary to primary hematologic disorders is frequent; 25 to 30 percent of cases are associated with anticoagulants.[80] It has also been associated with pregnancy.[78] Rare causes of spontaneous spinal epidural bleeding include hemangioma of a vertebra, vascular anomalies of the epidural space,[19] Paget's disease of the spine,[41] ankylosing spondylitis,[32] familial cutaneous hemangiomas,[17] and streptokinase-heparin therapy for acute coronary artery thrombosis.[52]

Although simultaneous spontaneous extradural and intradural hematomas are theoretically possible—particularly in patients with a coagulopathy—they have never been reported.

Spontaneous spinal epidural hematoma is twice as common in males of all ages as in females. It is reported from early childhood to the eighth decade of life and is most frequent in the middle and older age groups. The lesion may occur at any spinal level. It is usually localized to two or three segments, although it may extend over eight to ten or more segments. In childhood, it is more common in the cervical and upper thoracic regions.

The hematomas are virtually always restricted to the posterior aspect of the epidural space, may be thicker on one side, and may extend into the lateral gutters. An anteriorly located hematoma was reported by Phillips et al.[56] in a 21-year-old man, extending from T2 to T6. Jackson's oft-quoted case report, frequently referred to as the first description of this entity, also described an anteriorly located hematoma: "The whole cervical portion of the spine, but particularly anteriorly and to the left side, was imbedded in an oblong clot of dark venous blood outside the membranes."[33] An anterior hematoma is more common following a vertebral body fracture; it is readily visualized on MRI.

The spinal epidural space is truly an intradural space between two leaves of the spinal dura mater. The cranial dura mater splits into two laminae at the foramen magnum: the internal lamina forms the dural sac; the external lamina lines the inner wall of the bony spinal canal. The external lamina is clearly defined in infants but rarely distinguishable in adults. The space external to the internal lamina of the spinal dura mater (between the two laminae) is the epidural space by traditional usage. The anterior portion of the dural tube is closely approximated to the bony canal and is fixed to the posterior longitudinal ligament by connective tissue strands. The posterior spinal epidural space is filled with fatty tissue that extends laterally to surround the nerve roots. The posterior epidural space is thinnest in the thoracic region; it may be as wide as 14 mm in the lumbosacral area and 3 to 6 mm in the cervical region. Small arteries and a complex venous network traverse the epidural fat. Large-caliber longitudinal veins run in the anterolateral epidural space, anastomose from side to side through an anterior and posterior transverse network, and contribute to the internal vertebral plexus, which anastomoses in turn with the external vertebral plexus. The epidural venous plexus anastomoses via the segmental veins with the inferior vena cava and azygos and hemiazygos veins.

The internal lamina of the spinal dura mater is supplied by two types of arterial networks originating from lateral spinal arteries: a longitudinal-oriented network on the posterior surface, which is more prominent in the cervical and lumbar regions, and small vascular clusters in the thoracic region.

The consensus of most authors is that spinal epidural hemorrhage is venous in origin. The lack of valves is a unique feature of the epidural venous plexus. This permits reversal of flow in the system and allows sudden increases in pressure during activities of normal daily living. This mechanism has been promulgated to explain spontaneous hemorrhage. Such an explanation is not satisfactory: one would expect this disorder to be much more common.

The intrathecal pressure is greater than the pressure in the epidural veins; venous bleeding should not compromise the cord under normal circumstances if the dura is intact. Elevated venous pressure, as caused by portal hypertension, is not associated with an unusually high incidence of epidural hemorrhage.

Beatty and Winston[7] suggested spontaneous rupture of a small epidural artery as the cause of epidural hemorrhage in the low cervical region. They hypothesized that erosion of a small artery was caused by the combination of disc disease, osteoarthritis, and nonrotary neck movement. Spontaneous rupture of a cryptic vascular malformation in the epidural fat or on the external surface of the dural tube is also possible. Failure to identify such a lesion is probably related to its destruction during the hemorrhage.

Premonitory symptoms are not associated with spontaneous epidural hemorrhage except in cases with an identifiable local lesion, such as a hemangioma of a vertebra, a vascular anomaly, or a vertebral or epidural neoplasm. The initial back pain is localized at the level of the lesion, and radicular pain may occur simultaneously with the episode of bleeding or develop minutes to hours later. Signs of neural compression appear rapidly in most cases. Chronic symptoms are most frequently associated with lesions involving the cauda equina.[9] A chronic epidural hematoma in the lumbar region may mimic the symptoms usually associated with lumbar stenosis[53] or herniated disc.[43,51] Brown-Séquard features were reported in several patients with posterior clots in the cervical canal.[18] Lack of pain is rare; pain was absent in Jackson's autopsy-proven case report of a 14-year-old girl.[33] On occasion, up to 2 weeks have elapsed between the onset of bleeding and the signs of myelopathy.

The differential diagnosis of spontaneous epidural hemorrhage includes all the disorders causing acute back pain with spinal cord and root dysfunction. Spinal epidural abscess most closely approaches bleeding in its onset and fulminant signs, but it is usually associated with symptoms of sepsis. Herniation of a thoracic intervertebral disc is uncommonly associated with the acute onset of paraplegia. Epidural and vertebral tumors most commonly have preceding back pain, though an apoplectic onset of pain and paraplegia is encountered with vertebral collapse and angulation. Dissecting aneurysm of the aorta, with rupture into the spinal canal, is associated with prominent cardiovascular signs. Spinal subdural hematoma is identical in onset and clinical symptomatology.

The CSF is usually clear and acellular; the protein content is generally increased. Bloody CSF is associated with coagulopathies and bleeding into more than the epidural space; it may result from myelomalacia of the cord and portends a poor prognosis.

The evaluation and treatment of patients with the acute onset of back pain and progressive neural dysfunction must proceed on an emergent basis. Recovery from spinal epidural hematoma is independent of age, although children seem to recover more readily than adults. Prognosis depends on the length of time between the first clinical symptoms and the onset of sensorimotor deficit; it worsens with the increasingly rapid development of cord dysfunction. The length of time between the onset of sensorimotor deficit and surgical decompression is critical. Recovery also varies directly with the severity of the neurological deficit at the time of decompression. In a review of 158 reported cases in 1981 (some of which were traumatic), it was concluded that 45 percent of patients (34 of 53) with complete sensorimotor deficit preoperatively made some motor recovery and 11 percent (6 of 53) made a complete recovery.[23] In an earlier study, it was concluded that useful motor recovery occurs in less than 50 percent of patients if paralysis is present for longer than 36 h.[48] The least favorable prognosis was in patients in whom the sensorimotor deficit developed rapidly and the clot extended over more than one segment in the thoracic region. The best outcome is in patients with lumbar hematomas.[45]

Plain x-ray films are usually normal. Myelography is no longer the diagnostic study of choice; it has been supplanted by MRI. Both lumbar and lateral C1-C2 punctures may be necessary to complete a myelogram and postmyelogram CT; the latter is particularly useful if a diagnostic lumbar puncture was performed earlier and a repeat attempt at lumbar puncture yields a "dry tap" or the injected contrast material is in other than the subarachnoid space. The use of a water-soluble contrast agent usually allows the study to be performed without turning the patient. The myelographic picture is most commonly that of a complete extradural-type block, infrequently an incomplete block except in the lumbar region, and rarely an enlongated defect with an irregular indented appearance. Anterior or posterior compression of the contrast column on frontal projections may suggest an intramedullary tumor;

the lateral projection shows the true nature of the extramedullary process and its anterior or posterior location within the spinal canal.

High-resolution CT has demonstrated epidural hematomas in the acute stage.[7] They appear as lesions of high attenuation and obliterate the adjacent epidural fat. Chronic lesions in the lumbar region are characterized by tapered convex margins, lesion greater than 2 cm in length, and a measurement of 60 to 70 HU.[43]

MRI usually shows the lesion extending over several segments; it has tapered convex margins, and CSF intervenes between the lesion and the spinal cord. The lesion's vertical extent is fully depicted. The axial images show the location of the lesion within the canal.[5,19,21,63] Smaller lesions in the lumbar region, mimicking a herniated disc, are also readily diagnosed.[51]

Figures 253-1 and 253-2 show the MRI of an epidural hematoma in the cervical region of a 73-year-old man. He had the spontaneous onset of neck pain 3 days previously and 48 h of progressive left-sided weakness. The prothrombin time was markedly elevated secondary to treatment with sodium warfarin (Coumadin) for heart disease and deep leg vein thrombosis. He made a good recovery after rapid correction of the coagulopathy followed by a laminectomy.

Treatment consists of prompt evacuation of the clot and decompression of the dural tube, usually by laminectomy. A rare anteriorly situated thoracic hematoma was localized by myelography and CT scanning by Phillips et al.[56] and treated successfully through a costotransversectomy. Isolated cases of recovery without operation have been reported.[5,69] These patients had mild symptoms, presented late in their course, and were beginning to recover spontaneously. Seepage of blood through a lumbar puncture needle track was the suggested mechanism if the lesion was in the lumbar canal. Temporary remission of symptoms in a few cases was attributed to dissection of blood in the epidural space, which created an internal decompression.[20] Solymosi and Wappenschmidt[72] reported the treatment of an anterior cervical hematoma, secondary to a vertebral fracture, by needle aspiration using an approach identical to that for discography. They proposed such treatment as an emergency measure until appropriate neurosurgical personnel and facilities became available. The urgent nature of the clinical problem usually requires evacuation of the hematoma even if a vascular malformation is suspected; angiography is then performed electively during the postoperative period.

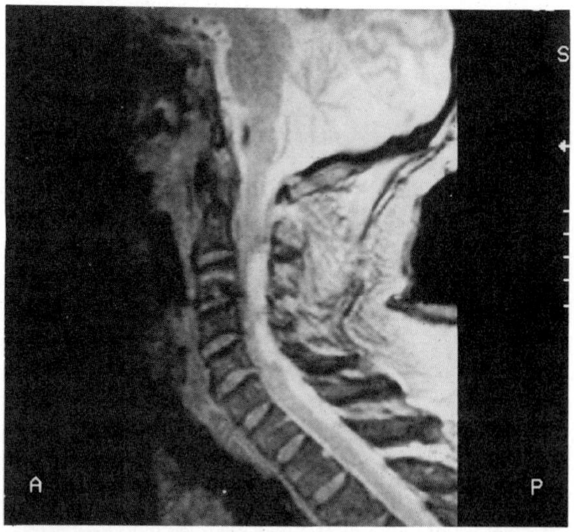

Figure 253-1 MRI, sagittal projection and gradient-echo image, of a cervical epidural hematoma. There is a hyperintense lesion in the posterior aspect of the spinal canal extending from C2 to C7. (The T1-weighted sagittal images showed an isointense lesion.)

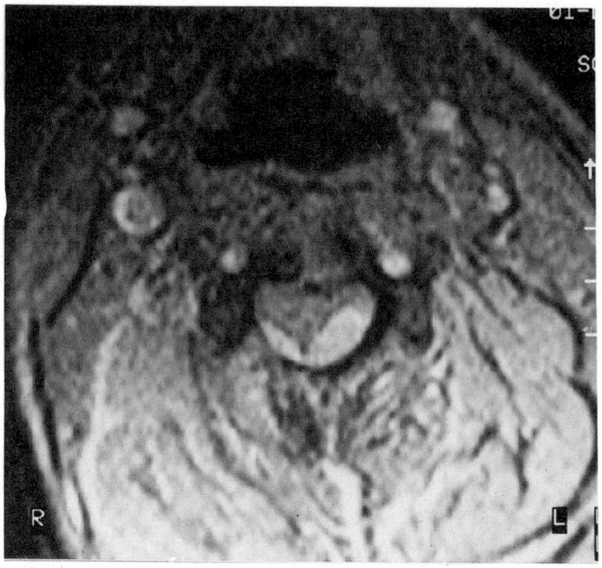

Figure 253-2 MRI axial projection through C5, gradient-echo image, of a cervical epidural hematoma. The posterior location of the hyperintense lesion is confirmed; it is thicker on the left. The spinal cord is displaced anteriorly and to the right. (See text for clinical description of case.)

Spinal Subdural Hemorrhage

Spontaneous spinal subdural hemorrhage is distinctly less common than bleeding in the spinal epidural space. Schiller et al.[68] are usually credited with reporting the first case in 1948. Their patient was a 16-month-old boy with hemophilia whose lesion was verified at laminectomy. Russell and Benoit,[65] in their 1983 review, stated that historical precedence should be given to Potts[59] in 1910 and Harris[29] in 1911 for the first description of the entity.

Potts' patient recovered after laminectomy and excision of a posteriorly situated thoracic subdural "cyst." The description of the lesion is compatible with a chronic lumbar hematoma. It is unclear to me whether the chronic lumbar hematoma in Harris's operated case was subdural or subarachnoid.

Most of the reported cases have been associated with trauma, including lumbar puncture in patients having hematologic disorders or receiving anticoagulants.[22] Spontaneous nontraumatic subdural hemorrhage and hematomas are also frequently associated with anticoagulants.[64] A coagulopathy was present in 38 percent of reported cases, and trauma coexisted with a coagulopathy in 84 percent.[37] Mattle et al.[45] estimated that about 60 cases of nontraumatic subdural hematoma have been reported. Unusual causes include tumor[71] and ventriculoperitoneal shunt[70]; in one case the hematoma developed 4 days after the patient had received epidural anesthesia for a delivery.[62]

Spontaneous hematomas appearing simultaneously in both intradural spaces, subdural and subarachnoid, are very rare. This combination was reported in two patients who were receiving anticoagulants.[8]

The spinal subdural space, in contradistinction to the cranial subdural space, does not normally contain bridging veins. Only extremely small veins are found on the surface of the spinal dura. It has been assumed that spontaneous bleeding in the subdural space originates from a radicular vessel. It has been postulated that a sudden rise in intravascular (venous) pressure might cause rupture of a vessel crossing the subdural space. Weinstein[76] suggested: "The occasionally observed bridging vessel from the pia of the spinal cord or the arachnoid of the caudal nerve roots to the dura is the responsible vascular channel."

A spontaneous spinal subdural hematoma is most commonly located in the lower thoracic or thoracolumbar region. Two cases of subdural hematoma in the cervical canal have been reported.[37,60]

Clinical presentation is either acute, indistinguishable from that of an epidural hematoma, or chronic, taking weeks to months for the development of paraplegia.[11] The acute presentation is usually associated with pain in a radicular distribution in addition to back pain.

A chronic spinal subdural hematoma develops membranes identical in appearance to those in the cranial cavity.[11,28,66] A fluctuating clinical course reminiscent of cranial subdural hematoma was reported in at least three cases; the lesions were one each in the cervical, low thoracic, and thoracolumbar regions.[3,37] A single case of a calcified subdural collection in the lower thoracic region was reported; the calcified portion was probably caused by an injury 35 years earlier.[61]

The CSF is usually clear and acellular; the protein content is generally increased. Bloody CSF is suggestive of primary subarachnoid hemorrhage and secondary rupture of the arachnoid. Lumbar puncture is frequently "dry" because of collapse of the subarachnoid space secondary to the frequent low thoracic or thoracolumbar location of the clot. Cisternal or lateral C1-C2 puncture may be necessary for myelography.

The CT of an acute thoracolumbar subdural hematoma typically shows a crescentic band of increased attenuation in the posterior portion of the canal. The longitudinal extent of the lesion can be appreciated on sagittal reformatted images.[74] A more chronic 10-day-old lumbar lesion was reported also to show increased attenuation in the posterior part of the canal. The MRI of the more chronic clot showed the lesion with greater clarity on gradient-echo axial images and T2-weighted sagittal images.[44] The MRI findings in several additional cases of spinal subdural hematomas have been reported.[13,34,36,46,70]

The MRI in the sagittal projection alone is not sufficiently typical to be differentiated from an epidural hematoma. A more diagnostic appearance is hyperintensity both anteriorly and posterolaterally in the axial images. The characteristic MRI image has been compared to an inverted Mercedes Benz® hood ornament.[36]

The myelographic appearance of a subdural hematoma may not be distinguishable from that of an epidural hematoma. The myelogram usually demonstrates a complete block, which is suggestive of an intradural extramedullary tumor, and less often a filling defect or displacement of the contrast medium to one side. Zilkha and Nicoletti,[79] in their discussion of a post-traumatic lumbar subdural hematoma, stated: "In rare cases of subdural lesions in which the contrast column is displaced to the opposite side, the ipsilateral axillary pouches of the nerve roots may remain in the normal position. In these instances the diagnosis of subdural lesion may be made."

The recommended treatment is laminectomy and drainage of the hematoma. Resolution of symptoms after spontaneous rupture into the subarachnoid space is possible.[46] (It seems obverse that the reverse, rupture of the arachnoid after subarachnoid hemorrhage which allows blood to enter the subdural space, is a proposed mechanism for the formation of a spinal subdural hematoma.) Two patients were relieved of symptoms after percutaneous drainage of lumbar collections.[44,73]

There are too few reported cases to discuss prognosis in a meaningful manner. It seems that good to excellent recovery follows drainage in 30 to 50 percent of cases if the preoperative deficit has not progressed to complete sensorimotor paralysis.

Spinal Subarachnoid Hemorrhage

Spontaneous spinal subarachnoid hemorrhage constitutes less than 1 percent of all cases of nontraumatic subarachnoid hemorrhage. The clinical manifestations were first described by Michon in 1928: "*Le coup de poignard rachidien*" (stab in the spine).[49] A clearly defined anatomical abnormality is usually demonstrable when bleeding is associated with an arteriovenous malformation, aneurysm[75] (including mycotic aneurysm), coarctation of the aorta with dilatation of collateral intraspinal vessels,[6] cavernous angioma,[1] or neoplasm (e.g., astrocytoma, ependymoma, glioblastoma multiforme, hemangioblastoma,[14] meningioma,[39] schwannoma,[15] and metastatic tumors of all types). The most common causes of spinal subarachnoid hemorrhage are intradural arteriovenous malformation and tumor. Hawkins and Heron[30] stated in 1988 that there had been reports of 56 cases of bleeding caused by tumor, 46 of which were located in the cauda equina; 33 of the tumors were ependymomas, and eight were schwannomas. The subject was also reviewed in 1989 by Kulali et al.[39] However, trauma, including lumbar puncture, particularly in patients receiving anticoagulants or having disorders of the coagulation mechanism, accounts for the bulk of cases with primary spinal subarachnoid hemorrhage and subarachnoid hematoma formation.

Rare causes of spontaneous spinal subarachnoid hemorrhage include Behçet's disease, endometriosis, systemic lupus erythematosus, the Sjögren syndrome, periarteritis nodosa, and generalized toxi-infective diseases (e.g., typhoid fever); hemophilia and anticoagulant use are somewhat more common.[31] No identifiable lesion or coagulopathy was determined in two patients reported by Plotkin et al., both of whom were treated by laminectomy for evacuation of subarachnoid hematomas.[58]

The onset of symptoms is apoplectic (*le coup de poignard rachidien*) with back pain referred to the site of bleeding. If the hemorrhage originates in the cervical region, the symptoms may mimic bleeding originating in the intracranial cavity because of the rapid spread of blood into the cranial subarachnoid space. Pain extends up and down the back with the spread of blood in the subarachnoid space, associated with signs of meningeal irritation. Pain and paresthesias in the lower limbs develop rapidly if the original site of the bleeding is in the low thoracic or thoracolumbar region. Bleeding into the parenchyma of the cord produces signs of an acute myelopathy.

The clinical differentiation of spinal subarachnoid hemorrhage from other apoplectic events involving the intraspinal contents is difficult. The development of a spinal subarachnoid hematoma sufficient in size to cause medullary compression is rare because dilution of the blood by CSF and defibrination by the normal pulsations of the fluid presumably prevent thrombus formation. When bleeding is massive and rapid or normal dilution is mechanically impeded, by tumor or arachnoidal adhesions, a frank hematoma may form more readily. Back pain followed by rapidly progressing paraparesis, a sensory level, meningismus, and a "dry" lumbar puncture characterize a subarachnoid hematoma.

In 1987, Gambacorta et al.[25] found reports of 32 cases of spinal subarachnoid hematomas. They added another case, which was a chronic lesion in the lumbar region; only three other cases were classified as chronic.

Myelography via the lumbar route is frequently impossible because of failure to obtain CSF. Introduction of the contrast medium via a cisternal or C1-C2 puncture is necessary under such circumstances. A small subarachnoid clot may appear as a nonspecific intradural extramedullary lesion. With increasing size, the clot envelops and displaces the cord with apparent widening of the cord shadow. The myelographic picture may mimic an intramedullary tumor. Capping of the contrast column on frontal and lateral views is the key radiographic feature that points to the extramedullary location of the clot. An intramedullary tumor with exophytic extension or hemorrhage may produce similar findings. Differentiation of a subarachnoid hematoma from a subdural or epidural hematoma is possible because the latter produces extra-arachnoidal myelographic defects. The epidural hematoma tends to displace the axillary pouches, whereas the subdural hematoma may not.[24] Absence of axillary pouches on the side of a high thoracic lesion was reported in one case.[4] Clots in the subarachnoid space, which cleared on repeat myelography, were reported in a pre-MRI case without a clear etiology for the hemorrhage.[73]

CT alone, done before myelography, failed to identify a subarachnoid hematoma in two cases.[38,39] No reports of the MRI appearance of a spinal subarachnoid hematoma, without an underlying arteriovenous malformation or tumor, were found in the literature through 1992.

If the etiology of a subarachnoid hematoma is not found at laminectomy, MRI with gadolinium enhancement is indicated (particularly if not done preoperatively). Postoperative myelography may also be necessary for further clarification of a suspected lesion (e.g., arteriovenous malformation; see above). Spinal angiography is necessary for the complete evaluation of a vascular lesion. However, the urgent nature of the clinical problem when associated with hematoma formation and compression myelopathy does not usually permit spinal angiography as an emergent preoperative undertaking.

Aneurysms of the spinal cord are rare and most commonly associated with arteriovenous malformations. Rupture invariably produces signs of myelopathy. Aneurysms in the high cervical region have been demonstrated during vertebral angiography. Vincent[75] reported successful clipping of an aneurysm, which had bled, arising from the anterior spinal artery at the C1-C2 level. He found five additional cases in a review of the literature: two aneurysms of the anterior spinal artery (T6 and T8, unruptured), one of a C4 radicular artery (unruptured), and ruptured aneurysms of a posterior spinal artery at C1-C2 and artery of Adamkiewicz at T6.

Recurrent episodes of spinal subarachnoid hemorrhage have been associated with arteriovenous malformations and tumors. The indications for repeat postoperative studies are discussed above. MRI of the spine is also indicated if a cranial source of subarachnoid hemorrhage is not identified.

Treatment is directed toward decompression of the spinal cord or cauda equina via laminectomy and evacuation of the hematoma. Plotkin et al.[58] reported full recovery following laminectomy in a 48-year-old man for evacuation of a thoracic hematoma, but an 81-year-old man remained totally paraplegic after evacuation of a thoracolumbar hematoma. Treatment of an underlying hematologic disorder or coagulopathy is indicated in patients who have bleeding without hematoma formation. Satisfactory to excellent postoperative recovery after drainage of thoracic and lumbar spinal subarachnoid hematomas has been reported.[4,25,38]

Spinal Intramedullary Hemorrhage

Spontaneous spinal intramedullary hemorrhage (hematomyelia) is very rare. The usual causes are (1) arteriovenous malformation,[40,54] (2) hemophilia and other disorders of coagulation,[10,16,57,67,77] (3) intramedullary tumor, (4) syringomyelia,[27,55,67] and (5) no demonstrable etiology.

Brandt[10] reported a 65-year-old woman in whom paraparesis developed 2 days after the appearance of interscapular pain and progressed to a complete T4 sensorimotor paraplegia over the ensuing 3 days. The myelogram showed a complete block at T2. The CSF was clear and colorless. The preoperative diagnosis was epidural hematoma. A coagulated intramedullary hematoma was removed via laminectomy and myelotomy. No vascular anomaly was identified intraoperatively. Postoperative angiography was not performed. The patient made no neurological recovery.

Schenk[67] reported the case of a 21-year-old man with known hemophilia whose low cervical intramedullary hemorrhage was operated on. At autopsy there were signs that the bleeding had taken place into a pre-existing syringomyelic cavity. Schenk stated that Tellegen in 1850 gave the first clinical description of spontaneous hematomyelia.

Gowers was the first to describe syringal hemorrhage. He first alluded to the subject in his 1886 textbook, *A Manual of Diseases of the Nervous System, Volume 1.* He stated that "The cavities in the cord into which blood may escape are sometimes of considerable vertical extent. I have known a fissure in the posterior column to be filled with blood through almost the whole length of the cord."[27] He amplified these observations in a later publication in 1904, as quoted by Perot et al.[55] They reported a 39-year-old man who developed a cervical hematomyelia, perhaps related to injury, and whose symptoms and myelogram 6 years earlier were compatible with syringomyelia. The patient improved after myelotomy and evacuation of the intramedullary clot.

Hemorrhage into a pre-existing syringomyelic cavity is possibly related to abnormal vascular channels in its walls. The finding of such abnormal vessels in autopsy studies led to the suggestion that syringomyelia is related to an intramedullary arteriovenous malformation.

The intramedullary hemorrhage in case 3 of Allen et al.[2] was identified on MRI; the patient's condition improved after the thoracic clot was evacuated. It was thought to be "related to radiation-treatment–induced vasculopathy." Improvement was also reported after evacuation of a cervical hematoma associated with factor XI deficiency[77] and a thoracolumbar hematoma in a patient with an iatrogenic coagulopathy.[57]

Hematomyelia associated with bleeding from a tumor is surprisingly infrequent. Tumors of the cauda equina, particularly ependymomas, are the most common to bleed; this causes only subarachnoid hemorrhage. The other tumors rarely associated with intraparenchymal hemorrhage include schwannoma, astrocytoma, hemangioblastoma, meningioma, and cavernous angioma. There may be no clinical significance to the finding of old hemorrhage in intramedullary tumors, particularly ependymomas, which occasionally can be identified on MRI.

Leech et al.[42] reported two cases studied at autopsy. No cause of a spontaneous hematomyelia was found in either case.

Lee and Kobrine[40] reported a case of neurogenic pulmonary edema associated with hematomyelia caused by a ruptured arteriovenous malformation. They suggested that the hemorrhage produced a stimulatory effect on the preganglionic sympathetic fibers in the cord, which caused a thoracolumbar sympathetic discharge leading to the pulmonary edema.

Milhorat et al.[50] reported their findings in an experimental model of hematomyelia in rats. They found that the injected blood was cleared by phagocytosis by microglial cells and drainage of blood products in a rostral direction through the central canal of the cord.

Very few reports describe either CT or MRI findings in cases of hematomyelia. MRI may help identify an arteriovenous malformation or tumor (with gadolinium enhancement) as the cause of the hemorrhage.

References

1. Acciarri N, Padovani R, Pozzati E, et al. Spinal cavernous angioma: a rare cause of subarachnoid hemorrhage. *Surg Neurol* 1992; 37:453–456.
2. Allen JC, Miller DC, Budzilovich GN, Epstein FJ. Brain and spinal cord hemorrhage in long-term survivors of malignant pediatric brain tumors: a possible late effect of therapy. *Neurology* 1991; 41:148–150.
3. Anagnostopoulos DI, Gortvai P. Spontaneous spinal subdural haematoma. *Br Med J* 1972; 1:30.
4. Arias MJ. Acute spinal cord compression by spontaneous subarachnoid haematoma. *Neurochirurgia (Stuttg)* 1986; 29:201–202.
5. Avrahami E, Tadmor R, Ram Z, et al. MR demonstration of spontaneous acute epidural hematoma of the thoracic spine. *Neuroradiology* 1989; 31:89–92.
6. Banna MM, Rose PG, Pearce GW. Coarctation of the aorta as a cause of spinal subarachnoid hemorrhage: case report. *J Neurosurg* 1973; 39:761–763.
7. Beatty RM, Winston KR. Spontaneous cervical epidural hematoma. A consideration of etiology. *J Neurosurg* 1984; 61:143–148.
8. Bernsen RA, Hoogenraad TU. A spinal haematoma occurring in the subarachnoid as well as in the subdural space in a patient treated with anticoagulants. *Clin Neurol Neurosurg* 1992; 94:35–37.
9. Boyd HR, Pear BL. Chronic spontaneous spinal epidural hematoma: report of two cases. *J Neurosurg* 1972; 36:239–242.
10. Brandt M. Spontaneous intramedullary haematoma as a complication of anticoagulant therapy. *Acta Neurochir (Wien)* 1980; 52:73–77.
11. Brandt RA. Chronic spinal subdural haematoma. *Surg Neurol* 1980; 13:121–123.
12. Bruyn GW, Bosma NJ. Spinal extradural haematoma. In Vinken PJ, Bruyn GW (eds): *Handbook of Clinical Neurology,* vol 26. *Injuries of the Spine & Spinal Cord.* Amsterdam: North-Holland, 1976, pp 1–30.
13. Calhoun JM, Boop F. Spontaneous spinal subdural hematoma: case report and review of the literature. *Neurosurgery* 1991; 29:133–134.
14. Cerejo A, Vaz R, Feyo PB, Cruz C. Spinal cord hemangioblastoma with subarachnoid hemorrhage. *Neurosurgery* 1990; 27:991–993.
15. Chalif DJ, Black K, Rosenstein D. Intradural spinal cord tumor presenting as a subarachnoid hemorrhage: magnetic resonance imaging diagnosis. *Neurosurgery* 1990; 26:631–634.
16. Constantini S, Ashkenazi E, Shoshan Y, et al. Thoracic hematomyelia secondary to coumadin anticoagulant therapy: a case report. *Eur Neurol* 1992; 32:109–111.
17. Cook RJ, Fearnside MR. Cervical cord extradural haematoma with familial cutaneous haemangiomas. *Br J Neurosurg* 1988; 2:265–268.
18. Crabbe DCG, Mendelow AD, Pharoh P, et al. Cervical spinal extradural hematoma causing a transient Brown-Séquard syndrome. *J Neurol Neurosurg Psychiatry* 1992; 55:239 (letter).
19. D'Angelo V, Bizzozero L, Talamonti G, et al. Value of magnetic resonance imaging in spontaneous extradural spinal hematoma due to vascular malformation: case report. *Surg Neurol* 1990; 34:343–344.
20. Davies KG, Weeks RD. Acute spontaneous spinal epidural haematoma with temporary resolution. *Br J Neurosurg* 1992; 6:63–66.
21. Di Lorenzo N, Rizzo A, Fortuna A. Spontaneous spinal epidural hematoma: pre-operative diagnosis by MRI. *Clin Neurol Neurosurg* 1990; 92:357–359.
22. Edelson RN. Spinal subdural hematoma. In Vinken PJ, Bruyn GW (eds): *Handbook of Clinical Neurology,* vol 26. *Injuries of the Spine & Spinal Cord.* Amsterdam: North-Holland, 1976, pp 31–38.
23. Foo D, Rossier AB. Preoperative neurological status in predicting surgical outcome of spinal epidural hematomas. *Surg Neurol* 1981; 15:389–401.
24. Frager D, Zimmerman RD, Wisoff HS, Leeds NE. Spinal subarachnoid hematoma. *Am J Neuroradiol* 1982; 3:77–79.
25. Gambacorta D, Reale F, De Falco D. Spontaneous chronic spinal subarachnoid hematoma. Report of a case and review of the literature. *Spine* 1987; 12:716–718.
26. Gold ME. Spontaneous spinal epidural hematoma. *Radiology* 1963; 80:823–828.
27. Gowers WR. *A Manual of Diseases of the Nervous System,* vol 1. *Diseases of the Spinal Cord and Nerves.* London: Churchill, 1886, p 283.
28. Guthikonda M, Schmidek HH, Wallman LJ, Snyder TM. Spinal subdural hematoma: case report and review of the literature. *Neurosurgery* 1979; 5:614–616.
29. Harris W. Two cases of spontaneous haematorrhachis, or intrameningeal spinal haemorrhage—one cured by laminectomy. *Proc R Soc Med* 1911; 5:115–122.
30. Hawkins CP, Heron JR. Subarachnoid haemorrhage from spinal tumour (in the absence of spinal symptoms or signs). *J Neurol Neurosurg Psychiatry* 1988; 51:305–307 (letter).
31. Henson RA, Croft PB. Spontaneous spinal subarachnoid haemorrhage. *Q J Med* 1956; 25:53–66.
32. Hissa E, Boumphrey F, Bay J. Spinal epidural hematoma and ankylosing spondylitis. *Clin Orthop* 1986; 208:225–227.
33. Jackson R. Case of spinal apoplexy. *Lancet* 1869; 2:5–6.
34. Jacquet G, Godard J, Orabi M, et al. Spinal subdural hematoma. *Zentralbl Neurochir* 1991; 52:131–135.
35. Jellinger K. Traumatic vascular disease of the spinal cord. In Vinken PJ, Bruyn GW (eds): *Handbook of Clinical Neurology,* vol 12. *Vascular Diseases of the Nervous System, Part II.* Amsterdam, North-Holland, 1972, pp 556–630.
36. Johnson PJ, Hahn F, McConnell J, et al. The importance of MRI findings for the diagnosis of nontraumatic lumbar subacute subdural haematomas. *Acta Neurochir (Wien)* 1991; 113:186–188.
37. Khosla VK, Kak VK, Mathuriya SN. Chronic spinal subdural hematomas. Report of two cases. *J Neurosurg* 1985; 63:636–639.
38. Koehler PJ, Kuiters RRF. Brown-Séquard syndrome caused by a spinal subarachnoid hematoma due to anticoagulant therapy. *Surg Neurol* 1986; 25:191–193.
39. Kulali A, von Wild K, Hobik HP. Subarachnoid haemorrhage with acute cauda symptom due to spinal tumour. *Neurochirurgia (Stuttg)* 1989; 32:87–90.
40. Lee DS, Kobrine A. Neurogenic pulmonary edema associated with ruptured spinal cord arteriovenous malformation. *Neurosurgery* 1983; 12:691–693.
41. Lee KS, McWhorter JM, Angelo JN. Spinal epidural hematoma associated with Paget's disease. *Surg Neurol* 1988; 30:131–134.
42. Leech RW, Pitha JV, Brumback RA. Spontaneous haematomyelia: a necropsy study. *J Neurol Neurosurg Psychiatry* 1991; 54:172–174.

43. Levitan LH, Wiens CW. Chronic lumbar extradural hematoma: CT findings. *Radiology* 1983; 148:707–708.
44. Levy JM. Spontaneous lumbar subdural hematoma. *Am J Neuroradiol* 1990; 11:780–781.
45. Mattle H, Sieb JP, Rohner M, Mumenthaler M. Nontraumatic spinal epidural and subdural hematomas. *Neurology* 1987; 37:1351–1356.
46. Mavroudakis N, Levivier M, Rodesch G. Central cord syndrome due to a spontaneously regressive spinal subdural hematoma. *Neurology* 1990; 40:1306–1308.
47. Mayer JA. Extradural spinal hemorrhage. *Can Med Assoc J* 1963; 89:1034–1037.
48. McQuarrie IG. Recovery from paraplegia caused by spontaneous spinal epidural hematoma. *Neurology (NY)* 1978; 28:224–228.
49. Michon P. Le coup de poignard rachidien. Symptome initial de certaines hémorragies sous-arachnoidiennes. Essai sur les hémorragies méningées spinales. *Presse Med* 1928; 36:964–966.
50. Milhorat TH, Adler DE, Heger IM, et al. Histopathology of experimental hematomyelia. *J Neurosurg* 1991; 75:911–915.
51. Mirkovic S, Melany M. A thoracolumbar epidural hematoma simulating a disc syndrome. *J Spinal Disord* 1992; 5:112–115.
52. Mustafa MH, Gallino R. Spontaneous spinal epidural hematoma causing cord compression after streptokinase and heparin therapy for acute coronary artery occlusion. *South Med J* 1988; 81:1202–1203.
53. Nehls DG, Shetter AG, Hodak JA, et al. Chronic spinal epidural hematoma presenting as lumbar stenosis: clinical, myelographic, and computed tomographic features. A case report. *Neurosurgery* 1984; 14:230–233.
54. Oyanagi K, Yamazaki K, Hinokuma K, et al. An autopsy case of intramedullary venous malformation of the spinal cord with spreading hematomyelia. *Clin Neuropathol* 1990; 9:148–151.
55. Perot P, Feindel W, Lloyd-Smith D. Hematomyelia as a complication of syringomyelia: Gowers' syringal hemorrhage: case report. *J Neurosurg* 1966; 25:447–451.
56. Phillips TW, Kling TF Jr, McGillicuddy JE. Spontaneous ventral spinal epidural hematoma with anterior cord syndrome: report of a case. *Neurosurgery* 1981; 9:440–443.
57. Pisani R, Carta F, Guiducci G, et al. Hematomyelia during anticoagulant therapy. *Surg Neurol* 1985; 24:578–580.
58. Plotkin R, Ronthal M, Froman C. Spontaneous spinal subarachnoid hemorrhage: report of 3 cases. *J Neurosurg* 1966; 25:443–446.
59. Potts CS. Intradural cyst of the spinal meninges removed by operation. Recovery of the patient. Remarks on the location of the spinal centers for testicular sensibility. *J Nerv Ment Dis* 1910; 37:621–625.
60. Reynolds AF Jr, Turner PT. Spinal subdural hematoma. *Rocky Mt Med J* 1978; 75:199–200.
61. Rieth KG, Quindlen EA. Calcified chronic spinal subdural hematoma demonstrated by computed tomography. *Spine* 1983; 8:812–816.
62. Roscoe MWA, Barrington TW. Acute spinal subdural hematoma. A case report and review of the literature. *Spine* 1984; 9:672–675.
63. Rothfus WE, Chedid MK, Deeb ZL, et al. MR imaging in the diagnosis of spontaneous spinal epidural hematomas. *J Comput Assist Tomogr* 1987; 11:851–854.
64. Russell N, Maroun FB, Jacob JC. Spinal subdural hematoma in association with anticoagulant therapy. *Can J Neurol Sci* 1981; 8:87–89.
65. Russell NA, Benoit BG. Spinal subdural hematoma: a review. *Surg Neurol* 1983; 20:133–137.
66. Sakata T, Kurihara A. Spontaneous spinal subdural hematoma. A case report. *Spine* 1984; 9:324–326.
67. Schenk VWD. Haemorrhages in spinal cord with syringomyelia in a patient with haemophilia. *Acta Neuropathol (Berlin)* 1963; 2:306–308.
68. Schiller F, Neligan G, Budtz-Olsen O. Surgery in haemophilia: a case of spinal subdural haematoma producing paraplegia. *Lancet* 1948; 2:842–845.
69. Sei A, Nakamura T, Hashimoto N, et al. Cervical spinal epidural hematoma with spontaneous remission. *J Spinal Disord* 1991; 4:234–237.
70. Silver JM, Wilkins RH. Spinal subdural hematoma formation following ventriculoperitoneal shunting for hydrocephalus. Case report. *Acta Neurochir (Wien)* 1991; 108:159–162.
71. Smith RA. Spinal subdural hematoma, neurilemmoma, and acute transverse myelopathy. *Surg Neurol* 1985; 23:367–370.
72. Solymosi L, Wappenschmidt J. A new neuroradiologic method for therapy of spinal epidural hematomas. *Neuroradiology* 1985; 27:67–69.
73. Swann KW, Ropper AH, New PFJ, et al. Spontaneous spinal subarachnoid hemorrhage and subdural hematoma. Report of two cases. *J Neurosurg* 1984; 61:975–980.
74. Tantana S, Pilla TJ, Luisiri A. Computed tomography of acute spinal subdural hematoma. *J Comput Assist Tomogr* 1986; 10:891–892.
75. Vincent FM. Anterior spinal artery aneurysm presenting as a subarachnoid hemorrhage. *Stroke* 1981; 12:230–232.
76. Weinstein PR. Comments. *Neurosurgery* 1979; 5:616.
77. Wisoff JH, Rovit RL, Ho V, et al. Spontaneous hematomyelia secondary to Factor XI deficiency. Case report. *J Neurosurg* 1985; 63:293–295.
78. Yonekawa Y, Mehdorn HM, Nishikawa M. Spontaneous spinal epidural hematoma during pregnancy. *Surg Neurol* 1975; 3:327–328.
79. Zilkha A, Nicoletti JM. Acute spinal subdural hematoma: case report. *J Neurosurg* 1974; 41:627–630.
80. Zuccarello M, Scanarini M, D'Avella D, et al. Spontaneous spinal extradural hematoma during anticoagulant therapy. *Surg Neurol* 1980; 14:411–413.

254 Spontaneous Intraparenchymal Brain Hemorrhage

Howard H. Kaufman

A spontaneous intracerebral hematoma (SICH) is a clot that arises without immediately preceding trauma. It may be *primary* (not due to other specific disease except indirectly as in the case of hypertension), or *secondary* (caused by a variety of congenital and acquired conditions). The evolution of the concepts of SICH can be gleaned from a number of sources.[54,63,142,143,193,208,215]

Interest in so-called *apoplexy* goes back to the dawn of written history. Apoplexy is a Greek word meaning "struck with violence as if by a thunderstorm" from which derives stroke, meaning a sudden loss of the senses with paralysis and the secondary fear it engenders.[193] Indeed, there are said to be 30 references to sanguinous apoplexy in the Hippocratic writings.[143] Gregor Nymman (1594–1638) published *De Apoplexia Tractus* (1658), the first monograph on apoplexy. Johann Wepfer (1620–1695) published *De Apoplexia* (1658), a discussion on postmortem examinations that includes the first recognition of cerebral hemorrhages. Giovanni Morgagni (1682–1771) published *De Sedibus* (1761) in which is found the first comprehensive clinical-pathologic correlations of SICH. Matthew Baillie (1761–1823) in his *Morbid Anatomy* suggested that diseased vessels cause hemorrhages. John Abercrombie categorized apoplexy into infarction, intracerebral hemorrhage, and subarachnoid hemorrhage. Duret (1874) believed that the lenticulostriate artery was responsible for cerebral hemorrhage. Charcot and Bouchard (1868) described miliary aneurysms in hypertension, although the significance of these structures was argued for many years.[54,208] Many cases of SICH in various anatomic locations were described in the late nineteenth and early twentieth centuries including hemorrhages in the cerebellum and pons.[114,142,215] Westphal (1925) suggested that hypertension caused SICH. Sir Charles Symonds (1931) emphasized that intracerebral hemorrhage should be distinguished from subarachnoid hemorrhage. Russell and Cole and Yates discussed the relationships of microaneurysms to hypertension and hemorrhage, including their common distribution.[114] Fisher expanded this discussion and also discovered that disruption of nearby vessels contributed to the enlargement of the hemorrhage.[114]

Macewen (1888) reported the first successful surgery for SICH (1883). By 1891 Chamboniere had reported 31 cases of SICH. Likewise, Lucas also had reported several cases. Cushing in 1903 successfully evacuated an SICH. In 1906 Ballance described the first successful evacuation of a cerebellar hemorrhage. Bagley in 1932 differentiated infiltrating deep hemorrhages from confluent superficial hemorrhages and suggested that the latter could be removed. Penfield in 1933 stated that solid clots could not be successfully aspirated.[142] A number of papers were published on surgical evacuation as well as aspiration. However, the reports of McKissock and colleagues around 1960 suggested that surgical evacuation produced worse outcomes than nonoperative treatment.[155,156,197] Neurosurgeons seemed to accept that little could be done to alter the natural history of SICH and consequently lost interest in this problem.

However, interest slowly increased, possibly because of the high incidence in such places as Japan, and new experimental and clinical studies were begun a little over a decade ago.[159,186] Much has been learned about the origin of SICH and its manifestations through human autopsies. The pathophysiology of SICH is being better understood through the use of animal studies. It has been often difficult to clinically differentiate infarctions from clots; however, clots can now be accurately diagnosed by computed tomography (CT) or magnetic resonance imaging (MRI), which also has permitted clinical/anatomic correlation of their clinical manifestations. Many changes in the population as well as changes in health care, ranging from improved treatment of hypertension to the increased use of cocaine and an aging population with a higher incidence of amyloid angiopathy, have changed the total incidence of SICH and relative incidence from different etiologies. The epidemiology of SICH cannot be fully understood, however, until all patients in large populations suffering strokes are studied by neuroimaging and/or autopsy. Since a large percent of victims of SICH die immediately or soon after their hemorrhage, prevention is the ultimate solution of the problem. Given the current situation, the question is how to optimize care. There is increased interest in treatment, both by controlling intracranial pressure and by evacuating the hematomas either with open surgery or by aspiration.

With growing interest, the literature dealing with SICH is increasing and now includes three monographs that were published in 1992,[9,78,117] several overview chapters[2,12,13,26,33,39,47,74,114,142,157,177,188,239,245] and review articles in journals,[30,31,53,175,176,233] and literally hundreds of more limited chapters and clinical and basic research articles published in the last few years. A comprehensive and critical review of the literature would require a monograph of several volumes.

Epidemiology

The epidemiology of SICH is problematic, although there have been many epidemiologic studies of stroke in general and SICH in particular.[62,99,114,233] Stroke is the third leading cause of death in the United States, accounting for 2 to 4 percent of all deaths. SICH is the cause of 8 to 13 percent of strokes and 15 to 20 percent of deaths due to strokes. There are about 37,000 incidences of SICH annually in the United States.[19] Hypertension is a contributing factor to at least 50 percent of SICH, with amyloid angiopathy beginning to assume more significance as the population ages. Risk factors include age, race, hypertension, prior cerebral infarction, coronary artery disease, diabetes mellitus, and a variety of diseases (discussed later).[2,19,62] The incidence of strokes, including SICH, declined in the 1970s, at least partly due to the more frequent detection and effective treatment of hypertension.[62,242]

Attempts to be more precise in detection are problematic for many reasons.[62] In order to properly understand the incidence of SICH, we would need national figures to eliminate population biases, and all cases would have to be diagnosed and all contributing factors would have to be identified. Current information does not meet these standards, however. Some hemorrhages are minimally symptomatic and not reported; small ones may be diagnosed as infarcts if neuroimaging is not done.[46,85,114,240] Large hematomas may be diagnosed but their cause not identified (e.g., hemorrhages into the basal ganglia from aneurysms). Patients may die suddenly from SICH but since they are not autopsied their deaths are attributed to other causes (it is thought that intracranial bleeding causes 10 to 15 percent of sudden deaths).[185] On the other hand, patients may die of conditions such as cardiac disease but be presumed to have suffered SICH. Regional statistics, where populations are atypical with regard to race, age, and socioeconomic factors, may not be representative of national statistics. Additionally, medical knowledge and practices are changing. For example, drug therapy for hypertension may be less aggressive, more hemorrhages may be detected because more stroke patients have CT scans, and less patients may be dying of other diseases and thus develop strokes.[62] Therefore, older statistics may not reflect current trends. Thus, when considering epidemiology, it is important to be aware of these problems and the limits of our current knowledge.

Some striking statistics have come from a recent study in Cincinnati where SICH was at least 1½ to 2 times as frequent as subarachnoid hemorrhage and equally as lethal.[19]

Etiologies

A unified theory for the etiology of SICH has been proposed based on acute increase in blood flow in areas of normal or ischemic arterioles or capillaries (or other vessels), or damage to penetrating blood vessels by chronic arterial hypertension.[28] This can be applied to most specific etiologies. Larger vessels may also be subject to weakening, or insignificant acute injuries may not seal in the face of impaired hemostatic mechanisms.

Table 254-1 outlines the etiologies of SICH. There are, however, some obvious overlaps: the bleeding diathesis in disseminated intravascular coagulation (DIC) contributes to delayed post-traumatic SICH, anticoagulants contribute to hemorrhages after cardiac surgery that are related to emboli, and trauma and infection lead to aneurysms. Etiologies listed after cerebral amyloid angiopathy in Table 254-1 are less common. Part of the "unknown" group may include many patients in whom bleeding was caused by acute rises of blood pressure due to a variety of causes.

As mentioned, chronic hypertension (i.e., known hypertension or left ventricular hypertrophy) is the most common cause of SICH,[114,240] and the incidence is related to the degree and duration of elevation of the blood pressure.[109] Racial (e.g., Japanese, African Americans) predisposition to hypertension and socioeconomic problems that have limited detection and treatment may explain the high incidence of SICH in certain racial groups.[2,18] The incidence of fatal intracranial hemorrhage is actually many times greater in Japan than in the United States, which probably explains the high level of interest, aggressive approach, and number of studies coming from that country. Although some series implicate hypertension in as many as 90 percent of patients with SICH, this may not be completely accurate and may be changing dramatically.[111] To put these issues in perspective, an approximation of frequency is indicated in Table 254-1. The future trends in the incidence of these problems are also projected based on assumptions that are fairly apparent (i.e., increased use of street drugs, aging of the population so that amyloid angiopathy will be more common, less use and better control of anticoagulants, and treatment of DIC to avoid delayed traumatic SICH).

TABLE 254-1 Etiologies of Spontaneous Intracerebral Hematoma

	Incidence	Trend
Hypertensive		
Chronic (Acute)	½	+
Not hypertensive		
Congenital vascular anomalies	¼	
Aneurysms		
Arteriovenous malformations		
Coagulopathy		−
Tumors		
Vasculopathy, vasculitis		
Cerebral amyloid angiopathy		+
Moyamoya		
Vasculitis		
Drug related		
Sympathomimetics		+
Anticoagulants		−
Fibrinolytics		+
Postoperative		
Intracranial		−
Carotid		−
Cardiac		
Stroke		
Arterial infarction		−
Venous occlusion		
Delayed post-traumatic		
Parenchymal		
Aneurysmal		
Postoperative		
Mycotic aneurysm		
Neonatal intraventricular*		
Other		
Unknown/none		
Secondary brain stem*		

*Not considered.

Source: From Kaufman HH. Spontaneous intracerebral hematomas. In Grossman RG (ed): *Principles of Neurosurgery*. New York: Raven Press, 1991, p 66, with permission.

SICH has traditionally been considered in a bipartite fashion. Because hematomas due to hypertension occur in typical locations (Table 254-2),[99,111,114] this group will be considered first by site. The remaining hematomas often originate in the subcortical white matter; each etiology will be considered separately. Although it is true that subcortical clots may have a variety of specific etiologies, a large proportion (45 percent) may still be related to hypertension. On the other hand, clots in locations typical for hypertensive hemorrhage may often be due to other causes. For example, clots in the cerebellum and pons may result from such problems as cryptic vascular malformations. Of course, hypertensive patients may have clots caused by other etiologies such as aneurysms.

Hypertensive Hemorrhage

Pathophysiology

The vasculopathy of chronic hypertension[114,122] affects the perforating arteries, 100 to 400 μm diameter, which arise directly from much larger trunks to enter the brain at right angles and which are end arteries. These vessels are subjected directly to changes in

TABLE 254-2 Relation of Hypertension to Location

	Hypertension 75 to 50% +	No Hypertension 25 to 50% −
Basal ganglia	65%	35%
Subcortical white matter	45%	55%
Thalamus	75%	25%
Cerebellum	62%	38%
Pons	90%	10%

Source: From Kaufman HH. Spontaneous intracerebral hematomas. In Grossman RG (ed): *Principles of Neurosurgery.* New York: Raven Press, 1991, p 67, with permission.

blood pressure, unlike cortical vessels which are protected by a series of bifurcations and have collaterals for run off.[65] These small arteries accumulate lipid and proteinaceous material in their walls (lipohyalinosis) that in turn can cause a scarring (hyalinosis) or, alternatively, focal necrosis and even Charcot-Bouchard or miliary "aneurysms." Target arteries include the lenticulostriate arteries, the thalamoperforating arteries, and the paramedian branches of the basilar artery as well as the superior and anterior inferior cerebellar arteries, in whose distributions SICH may develop. This process is more common in the proximal part of the artery (explaining why putaminal hemorrhages are more common than those in the caudate).[59] In addition, autoregulation of blood flow is altered in chronic hypertension, and the vessels are less able to compensate for increased blood pressure, predisposing to bleeding as well as impaired compensation after.[65,129,243]

Many other factors can contribute to bleeding. Damage to the parenchyma may compromise support to the vessels; the significance of this is not clear, however. Acute increases in blood pressure and flow may also be important, particularly where autoregulation may be compromised (as in trauma), or where pressure may be above the limits of autoregulation, as in toxemia. SICH generally occurs during the morning or early afternoon when a patient is active. Therefore, it has been postulated that the trigger for bleeding may be a diurnal rise or an acute increase in blood pressure from whatever cause.[53,177,216,245] Last, compromise of hemostatic mechanisms may play a role, as in delayed traumatic SICH, a bleeding diathesis, or anticoagulant usage.

It had been thought that the bleeding event is relatively acute.[80] However, angiograms have shown bleeding for several hours and, sometimes, even days from onset.[88,127] In one systematic study, it was shown that six of eight patients with serial CT scans had an increase of the volume of their clot of over 40 percent.[17] In another series, late deterioration was seen in a small proportion.[7] It seems that most bleeding takes place within 6 h, and clots larger than 5 cm in diameter are most likely to expand,[64] which fits with the theory of expansion due to tearing, which would be more likely to occur in a larger clot. Many authors believe that this secondary bleeding is a very important mechanism in clot development.[56,58,114,158,159] Small satellite hemorrhages, the marginal hemorrhages of Stemmer, may be due to similar disruption of more distant small vessels. The pathologic evidence of such bleeding is the fibrin-platelet masses found within and at the margin of the clots. Blood pressure (systemic and local), size and rigidity of the vessel involved, state of autoregulation, state of the hemostatic system, and physical condition of the surrounding parenchyma probably all play a role in determining the size of the hematoma. A small number of patients will develop new clots, usually in a different location.[212]

The ultimate clinical manifestations of the clot relate to the speed and volume of the hemorrhage as well as its location. The patterns of spread for each location have been described, as have the clinical manifestations related to location and extension.[29,101,114] A small hemorrhage may dissect along tissue planes (e.g., a lobar hemorrhage), splitting the tissue apart rather than destroying it, with limited compromise and/or with restitution of function when the blood is absorbed.[56] A very large hemorrhage may explode into the brain substance, destroying large amounts of tissue, raising intracranial pressure to the level of the blood pressure before the bleeding is tamponaded, and causing herniation of that part of the brain from its normal position under the falx, through the tentorial incisura, or through the foramen magnum, depending on the location of the bleeding. Even if there is not acute herniation, the brain is plastic and can further deform or "creep" due to pressure from the original mass. Local pressure and edema, disconnection, and more distant changes in metabolism and blood flow are also important.[29,245]

Blood may rupture into a ventricle (especially with caudate, thalamic, cerebellar, and pontine hemorrhages) and even cause hydrocephalus. On the other hand, the rupture may actually decompress the clot. Blood may also find its way into the subarachnoid space causing irritation and hydrocephalus as well. Distortion of the upper brain stem may also lead to hydrocephalus.

Death is due to distortion or compression of the brain stem, development of secondary brain stem hemorrhages, or direct extension of the clot into the brain stem.[33] With posterior fossa hemorrhage, there may be direct compression of the brain stem. Basal ganglia clots of more than 85 ml or more than 6 percent of the volume of the brain, or cerebellar clots more than 3 cm in diameter have a poor prognosis if left untreated.

If the patient lives, the clot will eventually be broken down and reabsorbed. A six-phase process based on evolution of the clot has been described. It includes invasion by macrophages, development of surrounding edema, and development of microvessels at the margin of the clot, followed by quieting of these processes and development of gliosis (Table 254-3).[127] In the case of a larger clot, this will take many months. A small number of patients will develop new clots, usually in a different location.[212]

Models have been used to study various aspects of SICH.[122] In vivo models mimic the natural dynamic milieu of human hematomas. But, animals are expensive, their hemostatic systems may be very different from those of humans, and their brains are too small to accept clots large enough to use to evaluate new surgical devices. However, animal studies have revealed many details about pathologic and physiologic changes after SICH. They have demonstrated that blood is irritating to the parenchyma, causing a progressive hemorrhagic necrosis with edema at the margin of the clot. This process is fixed by 6 h.[222] Animal studies have also demonstrated changes in local and distant blood flow and metabolism.[122] And, in animal studies, early evacuation of the clot has been shown to improve outcome.[222] In vitro models using human blood have been helpful in studying lytic drugs and aspiration devices, but they lack the dynamic setting of an animal model.

Supratentorial Hematomas

Statistics

Supratentorial hematomas constitute about 80 percent of SICHs.[2,26,27,29,33,47,57,114,142,162,177,197,245] Perhaps half of these hematomas are related to hypertension. Their highest incidence is in the fifth and sixth decades of life; males may predominate. Table 254-4 lists their distribution sites. They may be divided into

TABLE 254-3 Evolution of a Spontaneous Intracerebral Hematoma

		Stages in Development and Resolution						
				Subacute		Chronic		
Source	**Parameter**	**Hyperacute**	**Acute**	**Early**	**Late**	**Early**	**Late**	**Ancient**
Kirkpatrick and Hayman[127]	Histology	<6 h Evolution of clot	7 h–3 days Lysis of clot; entry of macrophages; brain edema	4–10 days Microvessels at margin		11 days–6 weeks Resorption of edema	7 weeks–6 months Processes quiet; lesion contracts; gliosis develops	>6 months Contracted glial scar; stained by hemosiderin
Chaney et al.[34]	Histology	0–24 h	1–7 days	1–2 weeks	2–4 weeks	>1 month		
Williams et al.[244]	Changes in hemoglobin		<1 week Intracellular deoxyhemoglobin	1–2 weeks Intracellular methemoglobin	2–4 weeks Extracellular methemoglobin	1–6 months Extracellular methemoglobin; hemosiderin	>6 months Hemosiderin	

gangliobasal and lobar. Gangliobasal hematomas may occur in the basal ganglia or thalamus. Those in the basal ganglia may be internal or deep (two-thirds) or external or superficial (one-third), depending on their relationship to the internal capsule. This classification may have considerable surgical significance. Lobar hematomas tend to be seen in younger patients. One-third are due to hypertension. Aneurysms and arteriovenous malformations (AVMs) are frequent causes, as are tumors and coagulopathies. There is no obvious etiology at the time of presentation in almost one-quarter of these hematomas.

Symptoms and Signs

Presentation is abrupt or acute with an altered level of consciousness and progression to death within hours to days in one-third to one-half of cases (although this is not a certain figure and reports vary considerably).[26,64] On the other hand, there may be only focal signs with preservation of consciousness with small hematomas.[53,114] There are subgroupings for each of the primary sites and degree of hematoma extension.[29,114,245] An excellent grading scheme based on level of consciousness has been developed (Table 254-5).[105,174] Initial symptoms may include headache, nausea, and vomiting. Seizures may be present, especially in lobar hematomas (50 percent or more) and may occur at onset or later; they may be an ongoing problem.[52,221] As mentioned, clinical manifestations relate to site of origin, direction and extent of further bleeding, secondary effects, and herniation, as well as to ventricular and subarachnoid extension with hydrocephalus and meningeal irritation.[2,26,29,113,114,178,245]

In putaminal hemorrhages, motor deficits predominate over sensory abnormalities. Depending on the extent of the hemorrhage, other symptoms may include frontal gaze paresis, homonymous hemianopsia, aphasia if the dominant hemisphere is involved, and hemineglect if the nondominant hemisphere is involved.[29,114] Caudate hematomas are less common and tend to be more benign. They do often extend into the lateral ventricle and cause hydrocephalus. However, some spread into the adjacent brain, which becomes problematic.[29,114,245]

Specific symptoms of thalamic hemorrhages include hemiparesis, sensory deficits, oculomotor and pupillary disturbances due to extension into the brain stem or hydrocephalus, a dysphasia characterized by fluctuation and paraphasia if the dominant hemisphere is involved, and neglect if the nondominant hemisphere is involved. Thalamic pain syndromes and hemisensory strokes may be seen. Specific syndromes have been described for small hemorrhages.[29,114,219,245] Ventricular extension (including that from paramedian and dorsal hematomas, size $>10\ cm^3$) warrants a poorer prognosis.[219]

Lobar hematomas commonly result from occult vascular malformations, microaneurysms (some not related to hypertension), cerebral amyloid angiopathy, or occult tumors (although many patients also have hypertension).[20,238] These causes might be anticipated based on previous hemorrhages, enhancement on CT, oval or round shape (malformations), or subarachnoid bleeding (amyloid angiopathy).[238] The clinical picture of lobar hematomas depends on their location and extent. The location of a headache may indicate the site.[13,200] Seizures are more common and coma is less common than with deep clots. The clinical pictures of all these lesions depend on site of origin, direction of spread, and size; prognosis is better than for deep clots.[29,114,245] An outcome grading scheme has been developed (Table 254-6).

TABLE 254-4 Distribution of Hypertensive Hemorrhages

Site	Percentage	Trends of Variation
Putamen	35–50	+
Subcortical white matter	30	−
Cerebellum	16	−
Thalamus	10–15	−
Pons	5–12	+

Source: Adapted from Kase et al.[114]

TABLE 254-5 Level of Consciousness

Grade	Criteria
1	Alertness or confusion
2	Somnolence
3	Stupor
4a	Semicoma without herniation*
4b	Semicoma with herniation*
5	Deep coma

*Herniation: unilateral or bilateral mydriasis (over 5 mm) and no reaction to light; unilateral or bilateral decorticate or decerebrate rigidity.

Source: From Kanaya and Kuroda,[103] with permission.

TABLE 254-6 Postoperative Evaluation of Patients

Grade	Activities of Daily Living
1	Well (full work)
2	Minimal disability (work, self-sufficient)
3	Partial disability (semi–self-sufficient)
4	Total disability (bedridden)
5	Vegetative
6	Dead

Diagnostic Studies

The general laboratory evaluation indicated for SICH may be extensive. Besides routine admission studies, there should be evaluation of the heart, peripheral vessels, and kidneys. The cause of hypertension might be investigated in patients with elevated blood pressure. It may be useful to screen for hematologic abnormalities, infectious processes, and vasculitides.

The most critical tests for the investigation of SICH are CT or MRI, both for initial diagnosis and for surgical planning.[88] The presence of primary intracranial lesions, including tumors and congenital vascular abnormalities, must be kept in mind.

Because of the high density of blood, hematomas just a few mm in diameter can be seen on CT. Indeed, recent studies have shown that many strokes formerly believed to be due to infarction are really due to hemorrhages.[126] In addition, details about the hemorrhage, including exact location, size, associated brain shifts, ventricular extension, and secondary hydrocephalus, aid in surgical planning and may provide the means for improving prognostication and understanding of the pathophysiology involved. A CT grading scheme has been developed for basal ganglionic hemorrhage (Table 254-7).[105] If the medial edge of the hematoma is less than 28 mm from the pineal, the posterior limb of the internal capsule is involved and the prognosis is worse.[103] A CT grading scheme has also been developed for thalamic hemorrhage (Table 254-8).[105] If the lateral edge of the hematoma is more than 32 mm from the pineal, the posterior limb of the internal capsule is involved and the prognosis is worse.[103] Contrast infusion may provide additional information about primary lesions and may be indicated in patients (1) less than 40 years of age, (2) without hypertension, (3) with neurological impairment increasing for more than 4 h, (4) with history of neoplasm, blood dyscrasia, vasculitis, or bacterial endocarditis, or (5) with blood in the subarachnoid space or an atypical location or appearance of the clot.[240]

The change in the CT appearance of the hematoma has been studied extensively.[26,33,37,47,88,114] Within hours, the clot becomes more dense and a ring of low density develops around it which may represent edema or fluid squeezed out as it retracts.[21,37,88] Initially hyperdense because of high protein content, acute clots are better seen with CT than with MRI. With time the clot becomes isodense with liquefaction and resorption. Small clots (<2 cm) are absorbed especially rapidly. Edema dissipates more slowly than clots resorb, but this is difficult to study in detail because the clot itself becomes more radiologically isodense.[45] Only a small proportion leave typical slit-like lesions, and in a number there may be no residual abnormalities.[61] More work remains to fully understand the time course of these changes and how they relate to the CT appearance.[37]

The high-field and midfield MRI appearance of SICH has been studied extensively in the last few years. We now know that there are many factors involving clotting and breakdown of the hematoma as well as the sequences used that relate to its appearance.[227] Because of the chemical and physical alterations within and around the clot, characteristic changes in its appearance in different sequences also permit its approximate dating. The appearance of the hematoma center, hematoma periphery, and adjacent and nearby brain have been looked at systematically. Acute clots have magnetic characteristics similar to brain on T1 and T2 sequences, so gradient echo sequences should be used.[227] They are better seen after a few days, however. MRI changes reflect lysis of erythrocytes, which occurs from the center outward, and chemical changes in the hemoglobin molecule (oxyhemoglobin, 0 to 12 h; deoxyhemoglobin, 1 to 7 days; methemoglobin, 5 days to months; and hemosiderin, 1 week to years). An area of "ring enhancement" develops around the margins of the clot, probably related to edema, which is maximal by 4 to 5 days and whose duration is between 3 and 64 days, and then inflammation occurs between 48 and 84 days. There is eventual resorption of the hematoma (weeks) and resolution of edema (months). One early schema based theoretically on changes in hemoglobin uses five time intervals (acute <1 week; early subacute 1 to 2 weeks; late subacute 2 to 4 weeks; early chronic 1 to 6 months; late chronic >6 months).[244] Another schema, derived from an extensive review of the literature and correlated with histologic changes,[127] uses five slightly different intervals (hyperacute 1 to 24 h; acute 1 to 7 days; subacute 1 to 2 weeks and 2 to 4 weeks; chronic >1 month).[34] Table 254-3 describes the time intervals and MRI appearances. It has been noted, however, that there may be considerable variability in the appearance of the clot, particularly early, because of differences in the many complex processes that contribute to the rapidly changing appearance[34,227] (Fig. 254-1). One great advantage of MRI is that

TABLE 254-7 CT Classification of Basal Ganglionic Hemorrhage

Class	Type	Criteria
I	External capsule	Localized at outside of internal capsule
II	Capsular (C)*	Extends to anterior limb of internal capsule
IIIa	Cp without V*	Extends to posterior limb of internal capsule
IIIb	Cp* with V	
IVa	Ca* + p without V	Extends to anterior and posterior limbs of internal capsule
IVb	Ca + p with V Th*	
V		Extends to thalamus or subthalamus

*V, massive ventricular hemorrhage; C, capsule; a, anterior; p, posterior; Th, thalamus.
Source: From Kanaya and Kuroda,[103] with permission.

TABLE 254-8 CT Classification of Thalamic Hemorrhage

Class	Criteria
Ia	Localized in thalamus without V*
Ib	Localized in thalamus with V
IIa	Extends to internal capsule without V
IIb	Extends to internal capsule with V
IIIa	Extends to hypothalamus or midbrain without V
IIIb	Extends to hypothalamus or midbrain with V

*V, massive ventricular hemorrhage.
Source: From Kanaya and Kuroda,[103] with permission.

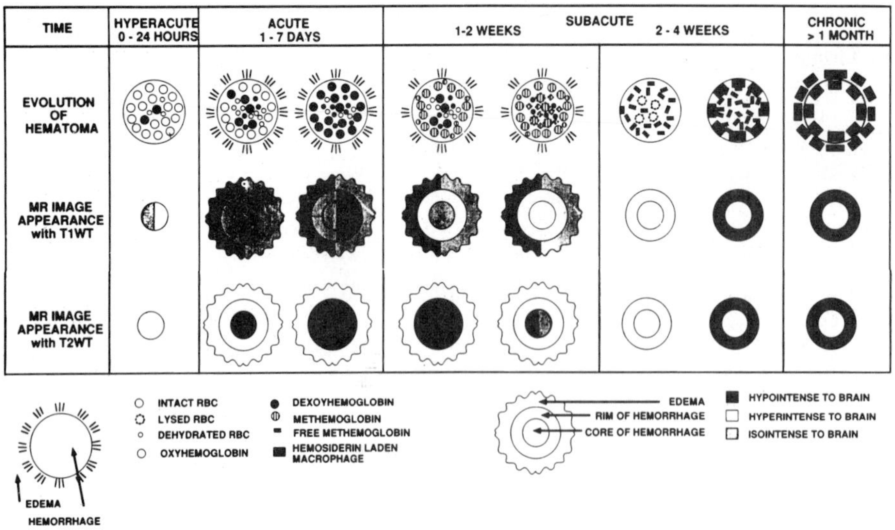

Figure 254-1 Magnetic resonance imaging of intracerebral hemorrhage. This schematic diagram shows the MR appearance of hematoma on T1- and T2-weighted images. Note: mixtures indicate that either intensity has been reported. (From Chaney et al.,[34] with permission.)

lesions such as AVMs or tumors are visualized better than on CT, particularly after enhancement with gadolinium.[88] Hemosiderin remains in the brain after the blood is absorbed and provides evidence of prior bleeding.[88] Also, the clots can be visualized in all planes.

Angiography may also be indicated if a primary lesion is suspected. It may be positive in 50 percent of younger patients.[88] Angiography provides evidence of mass effect and confirms the diagnosis of a primary lesion such as tumor, aneurysm, or AVM. Because edema as well as clot can contribute to mass effect, the volume of the clot may be overestimated by angiography. Conversely, where the brain is split, the angiographic changes may not fully reflect the size of the clot.

Natural History

Only one-third of patients present with an abrupt onset. The remaining patients deteriorate, and progression is usually maximum within hours. Decreased level of consciousness is seen in 60 percent, with coma in 40 percent.[114] Most who die do so within a few days.[2,26,33,114]

The patient's subsequent course may be one of deterioration, improvement, or even improvement with subsequent deterioration. Comatose patients with large clots can be expected to die.[85] Overall figures suggest more than 50 percent of hospitalized victims now survive,[2] which may be attributed both to more frequent identification of small clots and to improved treatment.[85] The level of consciousness, the size of the clot, the presence and degree of shift, and evidence of ventricular rupture are the most important prognostic indicators. Thalamic clots have the worst prognosis. Unfortunately, older patients fare worse. Any delay in treatment is harmful.[26,47]

Patients with marked focal neurological deficits and moderate-sized clots will survive with significant deficits. It is thought that most survivors are left with deficits, many of which may be incapacitating. Those with mild deficits and small clots will recover completely.

General Treatment

For severely affected patients, comprehensive management in an intensive care unit (ICU) seems warranted, especially to prevent the cardiac and pulmonary complications that often contribute to death.

Hypertension should be controlled. There is the possibility of increasing edema if the blood pressure is too high, and the risk of compromising cerebral blood flow if the blood pressure is too low in the face of increased intracranial pressure. The difficulty in patients with chronic hypertension, however, is that autoregulation may be altered with regard to the blood pressure required to sustain flow. It is not yet possible to individualize the blood pressure required to optimize cerebral blood flow given generally available technology.

Anticonvulsants should be used for lobar hemorrhages; indications for their use in deep clots is not clear.[53] Corticosteroids are contraindicated since they do not improve the patient but do cause increased complications.[192]

Intracranial Pressure Monitoring and Treatment

A French-Italian study demonstrated that patients with poor neurological status had a high ICP. However, some patients without high ICP did die, presumably from local damage. Patients with intermediate neurological status did or did not have increased ICP. Early surgery seemed to help reduce ICP and improve outcome, but delayed surgery did not. Patients in good clinical condition had low ICP.[97,98,183] Other authors have reported that ICP monitoring permitted optimal medical management of the patient,[26,48] as well as helped to successfully guide decision-making regarding whether surgery was necessary.[15,201] Ventricular drainage can be beneficial in treating the hydrocephalus seen in thalamic hemorrhage with ventricular extension.[101,114]

Stereotactic Aspiration with Fibrinolytic and Mechanical Assistance

There are two purposes for actually removing hematomas: (1) to preserve life, and (2) to maximize recovery of function. Both of these reasons may be threatened by the mass effect of the clot and progressive edema and tissue damage. The optimal approach for removal of an SICH would be a rapid simple method that combines a high success rate with low risk at minimal cost. One technique that may prove to have such characteristics is stereotactic aspiration.[119]

A number of features of clots make them suitable for stereotactic aspiration: (1) they can be easily detected by CT or MRI (vide supra); (2) they can be localized using stereotactic frames compatible with CT or MRI[3,23,69,199]; (3) their physical properties make them susceptible to aspiration with special devices and this can be facilitated by instillation of thrombolytic substances; and (4) their removal may be accomplished without high risk of rebleeding, or under circumstances where bleeding can be detected (including by intraoperative CT or ultrasonography) and treated. In addition, preliminary experimental and clinical trials show significant promise; future lines of research should further improve this approach.

Although the biophysical characteristics of clots and how these change over time have not been described in detail, early attempts at aspiration of fresh hematomas were recognized as being only partially successful because of difficulties in removing the more solid components of the clots.[22,41,92,130,156,209] On the other hand, a recent letter suggests that the use of a large (5 mm) cannula for aspiration with transventricular irrigation of deep clots may at times be successful.[1] More detailed information about the effectiveness of simple aspiration can be found in several reports from Japan, in which aspiration often yielded one-half to two-thirds of the clot volume.[89,94,152,153,166,169] To fully understand the meaning of this information would require more knowledge about the inner diameter of the catheters, the size of the ports, and the amount of vacuum applied as well as the age of the clot and its appearance on CT or MRI, and the hematocrit and clotting status of the patient. Simple aspiration does appear helpful for medium-sized (22 to 30 mm in diameter) pontine hematomas.[11,14,163,214]

To facilitate aspiration, a number of devices to physically morcellate hematoma material have been developed and used in both experimental and clinical investigations. The first such instrument was a 4-mm cannula in which there was an Archimedes screw. Suction was applied to bring the clot up into the cannula where it could be broken up by rotating the screw. The device was used successfully for subtotal removal.[5,6] It has been modified by other surgeons and used with some success,[86,87,107,181] but was never adopted widely. Another device involves high-pressure fluid irrigation to facilitate suction-aspiration of hematomas.[96,161] The authors who described the device suggested restricting its use to hematomas more than 24 h old, due to fears of rebleeding in operations done earlier. Other sophisticated mechanical approaches, namely breaking down the clot with ultrasonic aspirators, have been reported.[90,151]

We have experimented with a modified Nucleotome (Surgical Dynamics, San Leandro, CA), an instrument initially developed to carry out percutaneous aspiration of lumbar discs. The Nucleotome probe functions on the principle of a guillotine cutting instrument. Suction-aspiration and cutting occur concurrently.[179] From studies in an in vitro blood clot model, we found that with a vacuum of 150 mmHg, we could aspirate 75 percent of a 4-h old clot in 15 min.[120] A report about the use of this technique in humans was encouraging.[165] We expect to begin human studies of the devices in the near future.

Another approach has been to try to liquefy clots chemically to make them more amenable to aspiration. There is a great deal of activity in the development of thrombolytic drugs.[42,75,140,145] In experimental studies of subarachnoid, intracerebral, and intraventricular injections, urokinase appeared safe, and indeed promoted clot reabsorption.[49,50,55,160,164,182,211] Since 1980, several Japanese groups have had extensive experience using urokinase in spontaneous intracerebral hematomas in humans, including posterior fossa clots and intraventricular clots. They have indicated that it can be helpful, although it has been associated with rebleeding in 4 percent of cases.[51,89,94,95,152,166–170,232] In our experience in the laboratory, in vitro clot lysis is promoted to a modest extent by tissue plasminogen activator. This drug is safe when injected into the brain of rats and the CSF of rabbits. It also seems to promote clot absorption,[123] and has been used to dissolve intraventricular clots.[55]

An endoscope with irrigation, suction, and a laser for hemostasis was employed in a randomized series of 100 patients and was thought to be useful in removing subcortical as well as putaminal and thalamic hematomas.[4] Although in this report the endoscope was inserted using ultrasonography for guidance, a similar technique has been reported using stereotactic positioning of the endoscope.[247]

The aforementioned information suggests that eventually some form of stereotactic aspiration will be developed that will provide an optimum method for evacuating intracerebral hematomas. It is obvious that more needs to be known about the properties of clots, particularly regarding their susceptibility to morcellation and lysis at various intervals after formation, and the coagulation status of the patient. The capabilities of the various mechanical devices need to be studied in more detail, as do the fibrinolytic drugs now available and the new and improved drugs that certainly will be developed in the future.

Open Evacuation

Investigators in Japan, Europe, and South America have developed innovative techniques for the evacuation of clots in the basal ganglia, thalamus, and brain stem.[67,108,223]

Surgery is not indicated in the face of irreversible neurological damage suggested by greatly depressed level of consciousness, rapid clinical deterioration, or massive size of hematoma, and is generally not needed in the case of patients who are alert and have hematomas less than 2 cm in diameter. Some patients with clots between 2 and 3 cm may benefit from surgery.[33] Critical size may also be 85 ml.[26,217,218] One suggestion is that surgery is not needed if the clot occupies <4 percent of the intracranial space, should be based on the clinical status if 4 to 8 percent, should be done for 8 to 12 percent, and will not help if >12 percent. Not all agree on these guidelines, and there are certainly exceptions; for example, small clots in critical areas can be life threatening and large clots can be surprisingly well tolerated. Some authorities advocate immediate surgery (<6 h) to minimize ongoing bleeding, irritation of the brain, and edema. Others suggest waiting at least 6 h to minimize the possibility of rebleeding. If patients have not needed surgery by day 10, deterioration is infrequent.

Open surgery has been used for lobar hematomas with considerable success although hematomas due to amyloid angiopathy are more problematic.[238] Because of the risk of brain stem compression, temporal clots as small as 30 ml should be considered for evacuation.[147] Approaches should be made where the clot extends toward the surface or through ''silent'' areas of the brain. Surgery for deep clots has been facilitated by the development of transtemporal and trans-sylvian approaches.[67,108,223]

The general principles regarding skin, bone, and dura incisions should be followed.[33,39,74,177] Ultrasonography can be used to confirm localization of the clot. Modern technique includes the standard use of magnification and good illumination as well as gentle retraction to minimize difficult-to-control intraoperative bleeding. Most authors recommend that small amounts of adherent clot be left undisturbed, although some suggest that all clot should be removed,[239] which would allow examination of the entire cavity for evidence of an AVM or tumor. If there is any question of the etiology of the hematoma, surgery should include biopsy of the wall of the cavity. An interesting observation since CT has been available is that, with early surgery, the mass effect may actually increase after evacuation.

A number of developments from the 1970s make only recent series relevant when trying to understand the potential role of surgery. With modern neuroimaging, diagnosis is rapid and the anatomy clear. Medical care in an ICU setting can optimize cardiac and pulmonary function. ICP monitoring and control (although this has not been used frequently in SICH patients) is available. Clinical and CT grading scales as well as outcome scales (Tables 254-5 to 254-8) have been developed so that patients can be compared from series to series. Experimental design uses randomized clinical trials at best or closely matched controls in contemporary prospective trials. Even in current reports, however, information about these factors is not always available.

Some, although not all, of the recent literature is encouraging. For example, on the basis of matched controls (410 surgical patients vs. 204 medical controls), Kanaya et al. thought that surgery was helpful in all patients except those who were alert or only somnolent.[106] Using 165 medical controls for 187 surgical patients, Mizukami concluded that only grade III (i.e., moderately impaired) patients benefited from surgery.[157] Using internal controls ($N = 265$), Kanno et al. believed that moderate and severe cases who were operated on did slightly better; they did not come to a conclusion with regard to thalamic clots ($N = 135$).[110] Waga et al., comparing 44 patients who had surgery for putaminal hemorrhage with 130 who did not, decided that surgery was actually harmful.[237] Kaneko et al., comparing 100 patients with putaminal hemorrhage who had ultra-early operations with historical controls, believed that surgery was more beneficial than conservative management or delayed operations.[108] On the basis of a combined study in Japan using historical controls, Kanaya et al. believed that surgery for putaminal hemorrhage associated with stupor, semicoma, and coma ($N = 3216$) was definitely helpful. They also recommended operation for thalamic hemorrhages ($N = 639$).[104] Juvela et al. randomized 52 patients to surgery or conservative care. The only patients who did better with surgery had Glasgow Coma Scale scores between 7 and 10. However, although several survived, all were disabled.[100] In a small ($N = 21$) randomized study of putaminal hematomas (>3 cm) in hypertensive patients utilizing transinsular microsurgery, Batjer et al. concluded that evacuation was not helpful.[10] There were a higher proportion of survivors in those operated on, however, and the early termination of the study may have truly been premature. Fujitsu et al. concluded that the most important factor in determining the need for surgery was the time course in the first 6 h after bleeding. They believed that surgery was not beneficial for those with a fulminating course, but it could help those with a rapidly or slowly progressive course if done before irreversible damage, and was not needed if the patient was stable.[64]

Some authorities suggest delaying surgery 48 to 72 h until the clot is partially liquefied. The surgery is therefore technically easier, and the chance of rebleeding is reduced.[239] Also, there are some patients who either stabilize and then deteriorate, do not improve, or only improve slowly, and who may benefit from surgery even up to 4 weeks later to decompress nearby neurons.[39]

In the largest reported experience, Kanaya and Kuroda continued their work in the fifth all-Japan study in which 339 institutions participated. There were 7010 patients with putaminal hemorrhages studied, of whom 3375 were operated on and 3635 were not. Both aspiration and craniotomy were investigated. Using information from neurological examination, CT grading, clot volume, and deformity of cisterns, it was concluded that small hematomas did not require surgery, intermediate ones should be treated with serial aspiration with injection of urokinase, large ones causing "semicoma" or early herniation should have open surgery, and terminal patients should be treated expectantly. They also suggested that thalamic hemorrhages with hydrocephalus should be treated with ventricular drainage and possibly open surgery if they extended to the hypothalamus and midbrain and that lobar hematomas with semicoma benefited from surgery.[103] More formal and rigorous studies are needed to define precisely which patients should be managed aggressively and how to optimize treatment.

Intraventricular Hematoma

Intraventricular hemorrhage[2,24,26,39,43,66,137,176,177,245] may be an isolated (and often benign) problem and may be due to an AVM of the choroid plexus. However, almost 80 percent of intraventricular hematomas (IVHs) are related to intracerebral hematomas, and they are usually caused by hypertension, aneurysms, AVMs, and even pituitary apoplexy.[137] They are often accompanied by slightly enlarged ventricles. One-third of SICHs are accompanied by IVH, and these have a higher mortality rate. The primary hematoma and disease process are probably of more significance than the IVH. However, prognosis is also determined by the extent of the hemorrhage.[43] Headache, vomiting, confusion, decreased level of consciousness, and, in the case of secondary bleeding, hemiparesis, are common clinical findings.[33] The clots tend to disappear within 2 weeks. Recent CT studies suggest that IVH is more frequent than previously suspected, but it is often not significant clinically. When clots are symptomatic, intraventricular drainage (possibly bilateral) may be useful, but the blood often occludes catheters used for this purpose. Ultimately, a shunt may be required if permanent hydrocephalus develops. Intraventricular thrombolytic therapy has been shown experimentally to be useful and safe and has been used successfully in humans.[55,182] Direct surgery has not proved useful.[137]

Infratentorial

Cerebellum

Cerebellar hematomas constitute about 10 percent of SICH, a proportion coincident with the volume of brain in which they occur.[2,12,26,28,30,33,39,71,82,112,114,139,176,180,196,197,224–226,233,245] These occur more commonly in males. The highest frequency is in the sixth through eighth decades of life. Two-thirds of cerebellar hematomas are related to hypertension. These usually occur in the dentate nucleus which is irrigated by the superior cerebellar artery. There may be a left predominance. A small number originate in the vermis. Hematomas in the younger age group may be related to vascular malformations. Anticoagulants are another common predisposing factor.

Many of these hematomas are extensive and rupture into the fourth ventricle and also into the subarachnoid space. Secondary hydrocephalus may develop in up to 75 percent of patients. Death occurs in 60 to 80 percent of patients and is due to brain stem compression and tonsillar herniation.

Symptomatology is related to the rapidity of bleeding and the size and location of the hematoma as well as to compression of the brain stem, upward cerebellar herniation and tonsillar herniation, hematoma rupture into the fourth ventricle, and the development of hydrocephalus. The onset of symptoms is often abrupt, but may be subacute with progression over various times, or subacute with resolution. Symptoms and signs are protean and include headaches, alterations in level of consciousness, vomiting with or without nausea, dizziness, eye signs, including changes in pupils and gaze abnormalities, dysarthria, and motor signs, both cerebellar and pyramidal. The classic triad of signs includes appendicular ataxia, ipsilateral gaze palsy, and peripheral facial weakness. Two out of three of these findings are seen in 75 percent of patients.[180] A classic three-stage evolution has been described.[83]

The diagnosis can be difficult if the history is not known and the patient is stuporous. The differential diagnosis is again extensive and includes cerebellar infarction, brain stem hematoma or infarction, bleeding from an aneurysm or a tumor in the posterior fossa, as well as acute labyrinthitis. Clinical diagnosis is often difficult. In one series of 33 patients, 13 with cerebellar hemorrhages or infarctions were diagnosed correctly, 10 were not diagnosed initially, and 10 diagnosed as having cerebellar strokes actually had other problems.[202]

Diagnosis can now be readily made using CT, which can also be helpful in surgical planning.[139] The clot can be well visualized and other abnormalities including blood in the fourth ventricle, brain stem distortion, and hydrocephalus can also be seen. If the patient is not too sick and the test is possible, MRI can provide evidence of a vascular malformation and previous bleeding as well as to better define the anatomy. Angiography can demonstrate mass effect and might be employed if an AVM or other specified lesion is suspected, particularly in a young patient without a history of hypertension. (Even if this is negative, because of the high risk of rebleeding from a vascular malformation, surgery should also be considered.)[206]

Treatment includes control of blood pressure and respiratory support as needed. Surgery involves a posterior fossa craniectomy and evacuation of the clot. The indications for surgical therapy are probably better defined in this group of hematomas than in those in other locations. The key indicators are based on the level of consciousness,[63,79,234] clinical course, and size (2 to 3 cm) of the hematoma,[79,234,246] unless the patient is seen after doing well for a week. All clots 3 cm or larger and those between 2 and 3 cm (if the patient's level of consciousness is altered), should be considered for surgery, especially if there is deterioration, since some patients may decompensate rapidly.[177] Mortality is 72 percent if the patient is comatose.[226] Most patients without impaired consciousness will improve spontaneously. Indeed, CT scans have shown that clots tend to disappear in 2 to 6 weeks.

In the past, the use of ventricular drainage by itself was discouraged for two reasons: (1) it did not address the major problem, namely brain stem compression, and (2) because of the risk of upward cerebellar herniation. Indeed, it may delay definitive treatment and it has been suggested that it therefore be employed only in conjunction with clot evacuation.[234] But in cases with clots of borderline size, and possibly in conjunction with mannitol administration, this may be an alternate mode of treatment. A study concerning the implications for this therapy is underway.

Excellent surgical results with relatively low operative mortality have been described in patients with only moderately depressed levels of consciousness. Occasionally, patients with marked alterations in level of consciousness, particularly if they did not have too abrupt an onset and if operation was performed promptly, have improved with surgery. Patients in extremis are beyond help. Some patients with late deterioration or persistent deficits may also be helped by evacuation. Stereotactic aspiration has also been advocated.[103]

Although the guidelines for surgical treatment of cerebellar hematomas are probably better defined than for those in other locations, there may still be questions in those patients who are quite ill but not in extremis, or who are doing relatively well but are not improving rapidly.

Brain Stem

Brain stem hemorrhages tend to occur predominantly in the pons, although hemorrhages in the midbrain and medulla have been described.[2,12,29,33,39,103,112,114,136,177,215,224–226,233,235,245] Pontine hemorrhages constitute about 3 to 13 percent of SICH, far out of proportion to the volume of brain involved. Males and females are equally affected. The highest frequency is in the fourth and fifth decades of life. Ninety percent are related to hypertension and are believed to be due to vascular disease of penetrating branches of the basilar artery. Those hemorrhages seen in younger patients without hypertension may be related to cryptic vascular malformations, which are especially common in the pons but probably account for less than 10 percent of such hemorrhages.

In one series,[215] hematomas were present unilaterally in the basis pontis (at times with progression into the tegmentum) in 22 percent, in the basis bilaterally in 56 percent, and in the tegmentum in 22 percent (two-thirds bilaterally). Clots extended upward, even to the thalamus, but infrequently downward. The fourth ventricle was usually distorted. There was rupture into the fourth ventricle in at least 70 percent of cases. Extensive edema was often present, the cause of which was unknown. Local vascular disease was common, as was evidence of other cerebrovascular and cardiovascular disease.

Symptomatology is based on location, size, speed of development, and rupture into the fourth ventricle and subarachnoid space, as well as hydrocephalus secondary to ventricular occlusion or compression of the fourth ventricle and aqueduct. In the large postmortem series mentioned above, the onset was abrupt in one-half. In 30 percent, the initial symptom was severe headache, usually posterior. Symptoms and signs included alterations in level of consciousness, abnormalities of respiration, pulse, and blood pressure, hyperthermia, motor abnormalities that were often bilateral with posturing or paralysis, cranial nerve abnormalities, including pupillary and gaze changes with ocular bobbing, vertigo, vomiting, dysarthria, autonomic dysfunction, and ''seizures'' believed to arise from the basis pontis. The classic triad of miosis, hyperthermia, and bloody CSF was seldom seen. The diagnosis was suspected in only 25 percent of the cases. Seventy-five percent of patients died within 24 h.[115]

The common presentation of coma with neurological devastation involves an extensive differential diagnosis, including massive hemorrhages in other locations as well as posterior fossa infarcts and hypertensive encephalopathy. Definitive diagnosis can be made with CT scanning. The diagnosis may also be made with MRI. Angiography might be employed if a vascular malformation is suspected. Mortality is more than 80 percent in 48 h and more in the first week.

Treatment depends on the patient's condition. Most patients present with an acute onset of devastating symptoms and will die. One group has suggested that ophthalmologic findings as well as the size and location of the clot may be useful in predicting potential survivors.[229] In patients believed to be treatable, there should be immediate attention to respiratory support and control of blood pressure where needed. Ventricular drainage might be used if hydrocephalus is present, but the very presence of hydrocephalus may be a marker of a fatal hemorrhage. A major question concerns the role of direct surgery. On the one hand, hematomas have been followed by CT and have been seen to resorb, occasionally with a good result.[16] On the other hand, several cases, including a few with acute onset, have been thought to have been successfully operated on either through the fourth ventricle or subtemporally.[128,144] CT might suggest the best route.[235] Biopsy of the wall is thought to lead to deterioration.[233] Stereotactic aspiration has also proved helpful. Other series, however, have suggested that acute surgery does not improve outcome.[172,205] Patients with persistent symptoms from unresorbed clots might have direct or stereotactic aspiration, and patients with recurrent bleeding due to vascular malformations should be considered for open surgery. Collaborative studies will probably be needed to define those patients who are ill enough to require surgery but not yet beyond hope.

Finally, the usefulness of rehabilitation for many stroke victims appears well established and must be pursued when the patient is stable.

Nonhypertensive

Aneurysm, AVM

These anomalies are the second leading cause of SICH and there should be a high index of suspicion in young patients and those with superficial hematomas.[114,141,148,204] A history suggesting a sentinel hemorrhage, or in the case of AVMs, seizures, headaches, or focal findings may increase the index of suspicion.

It is thought that of those patients with aneurysms that bleed, 40 percent will have SICH, one-half of these >3 cm in diameter.[84] Aneurysms bleed into the brain when the aneurysm is typically imbedded in brain (i.e., internal carotid bifurcation, anterior cerebral artery, distal anterior cerebral artery), when it points into the brain (i.e., posterior cerebral artery), when surrounding structures are scarred from previous bleeding, or when the local brain is already damaged.[148,204,213] SICH is more common after the first hemorrhage.[204] Aneurysm should be suspected if the clot is frontal or temporal in location (Table 254-9), although even basal ganglia clots may originate from aneurysms.[114,148,204,213] Aneurysms >5 mm in diameter may be seen when enhanced CT scans are compared to unenhanced ones, especially with fine cuts which include the sites of typical aneurysms. Repeat CT may also be helpful to detect lesions not seen initially because of vasospasm and/or compression which could prevent filling. Angiography should be utilized aggressively and certainly for any patient who might be an operative candidate.[187] Repeat angiography may be necessary if no lesion is initially seen. Early surgery is indicated because of the risk of early rebleeding. The aneurysm should be clipped during the initial operation, preferably as the first step using subarachnoid dissection to initially obtain proximal control.[177,204] If the patient is moribund, there may not even be time for an angiogram, but the CT can provide some information about the aneurysm.[135] Patient outcomes are worse for aneurysm surgery in the presence of an intraparenchymal hematoma.[148,204]

Angiomatous malformations include AV fistulas, classic AVMs, telangectasias, cavernous angiomas, venous angiomas, and dural AVMs.[125,141,213] These lesions should be considered in younger patients without hypertension who have hemorrhages that are superficial, lobar, periventricular, or into the ventricle, clots that have a low density ring around them, or subarachnoid blood.[204,213] Hemorrhage is the presenting symptom in 30 to 55 percent, and 50 to 66 percent of patients with classic AVMs that bleed have SICH.[84,141,148,204,213] Ten to twenty percent of AVMs that bleed have aneurysms, which may or may not be associated with the AVM.[141,213] Bleeding from an AVM occurs most commonly from the draining veins or the nidus near the veins,[204] but can arise from the aneurysm. AVMs with central venous drainage, a periventricular or intraventricular location, and an intranidal aneurysm may be most likely to bleed.[146] Enhanced CT will often show the nidus and the draining veins. In some cases, however, the clot may compress the AVM and prevent its filling; repeat studies may be required. MRI is more sensitive for detecting AVMs. Some AVMs and cavernous angiomas may be occult (i.e., not seen on angiograms),[204] and studies may need to be repeated.

Eighty percent of AVMs can be resected.[213] It is best to delay surgery to allow neurological deficits to resolve. Also, it is easier to operate after the brain is less swollen, the AVM is better seen, and the clot has liquefied.[204,213] If immediate surgery is required, a flap should be turned that is large enough to permit resection of the AVM, and clipping of the feeding vessels.[204] However, if intraoperative bleeding is difficult to control, it is preferable to only remove the hematoma and to resect the AVM at a later time, since the early rebleeding rate is thought to be small.[204,213] The clot should also be sent for pathologic examination. On the other hand, if during surgery a cavernous angioma is seen, it should be resected if this seems easy.[115] The veins of venous angiomas may drain normal brain, and careful analysis of angiograms is required to determine if they can be safely resected.[204] Dural AVMs are only rarely the cause of SICH. They can be complex entities, and their treatment requires special considerations.[125]

Hematologic Disorders

Hemostasis is governed by complex interactions among blood vessels, platelets, and blood coagulation factors. Vessel disorders will be discussed elsewhere. Defects in hemostasis either exacerbate bleeding from other problems, such as trauma, or they lead to spontaneous bleeding if severe. Thus, spontaneous bleeding is most common if platelets are less than 10,000/ul or activity of a given clotting factor is less than 1 percent of normal. Abnormalities of the two entities can be classified as follows:

- Platelets
  - Thrombocytopenia
    - Peripheral destruction—immune (i.e., idiopathic thrombocytopenic purpura)
    - Decreased production (i.e., marrow injury or replacement)
  - Disorders of function
    - Inherited (i.e., von Willebrand's disease)
    - Acquired
- Coagulation Factors
  - Inherited deficiencies
    - Hemophilia—can be complicated by AIDS, inhibitors
  - Acquired disorders—involving deficiencies and inhibitors
    - Disseminated intravascular coagulation
    - Liver disease

It is important to have a consultation regarding treatment of the primary disease process, replacement of clotting factors and platelets, and decisions about surgery based not only on the acute but also on the ultimate prognosis of the patient. With the risk of transmitting various diseases, particularly AIDS, thresholds for prophylactic use of blood products and accepted replacement levels are changing.[2,188,195,198]

Tumors

Although intracranial tumors may bleed into a variety of sites,[2,26,111,134,138,171,177,188,191,203,210] they most commonly bleed

TABLE 254-9 Hemorrhage Patterns from Intracranial Aneurysms

Site	SAH (Cistern)	ICH	IVH (Ventricle)	SDH
ICA				
Oph Seg	Ant. suprasellar	Med. inf. frontal	Rare	Rare
PCom	Lat. suprasellar, ambient	Med. temporal	Temporal	Inf. lat. convexity
AChor				
Bifurc	Lat. suprasellar, prox. sylvian	Basal ganglia	Lat. vent	Rare
ACA				
ACOM	Interhemispheric, septal, ant. suprasellar	Inf. frontal (gyrus rectus), often opposite to lesion origin	Ant. III, frontal	Rare
Pericallosal	Interhemispheric	Med. frontal	Rare	Falcine
MCA				
Bifurc	Sylvian	Temporal	Temporal	Convexity
Prox	Lat. suprasellar, prox. sylvian	Temporal, basal ganglia	Temporal or frontal	Rare
Distal	Distal sylvian	Frontal or temporal	Rare	Convexity
V-B				
Bas apex	Interpeduncular, suprasellar	Rare (med. temporal)	Post. III, lateral	Rare
PICA	Cerebellopontine angle	Cerebellar hemisphere	IV	Rare

SAH, subarachnoid hemorrhage; ICH, intracerebral hemorrhage; IVH, intraventricular hemorrhage; SDH, subdural hemorrhage; ICA, internal carotid artery; PCom, posterior communicating artery; AChor, anterior choroidal artery; Bifurc, bifurcation; ACA, anterior cerebral artery; ACom, anterior communicating artery; MCA, middle cerebral artery; prox, proximal; V-B, vertebrobasilar arteries; bas apex, basilar artery apex; PICA, posterior inferior cerebellar artery; ant, anterior; post, posterior; med, medial; lat, lateral; inf, inferior; III, third ventricle; IV, fourth ventricle.
Source: From Masson and Day,[148] with permission.

into the brain, and even more specifically into the tumor.[134] Depending on the biases of the patient population, tumors may be the third or fourth most common specific cause of SICH. In one literature review, tumors caused 4.6 percent of all SICH, and 3.9 percent of patients with tumors had SICH.[203] Metastatic tumors (especially bronchogenic carcinoma, melanoma, choriocarcinoma, or renal tumors) most commonly, but also gliomas (especially more malignant ones), medulloblastomas,[228] and even benign tumors (meningiomas, pituitary tumors) have been associated with SICH. Factors leading to bleeding include hypervascularity, abnormal vessels, invasion of vessels, and tumor necrosis, as well as related disorders of hemostasis. Bleeding may occur after needle biopsy, shunting, decompression (even at a distance), and radiation therapy. The bleeding may be related to other factors such as anticoagulation or trauma. In many cases the patient was already known to have a tumor, or there was a prior history of progressive neurological dysfunction or headache. In one-third of cases, however, bleeding may have caused the onset of symptoms, which may have been abrupt or gradual.[171] On the other hand, many hemorrhages are small and asymptomatic.

CT abnormalities that may suggest a tumor include subcortical site, unusual appearance with abnormally appearing or enhancing tissue within or adjacent to the clot, and excessive edema or mass effect adjacent to the clot and extending even across the midline. Multiple lesions would also be suspicious. An angiogram may demonstrate abnormal vessels but is usually not required.

Surgery may be indicated depending on the clinical significance of the clot and the nature of the underlying disease. The surgeon should remove as much of the tumor as possible, not only to treat the underlying disease but also to minimize the risk of rebleeding. (If surgery is carried out for any clot, any suspicious tissue should be sent for histologic examination.) Patients often, but not invariably, do badly because tumors that bleed are often very malignant and because the prognosis for a large clot by itself is often poor.

Pituitary hemorrhages occasionally develop from a normal gland or nonadenomatous tumor, but generally arise from adenomas, both active and inactive endocrinologically. Indeed, <1 to >12 percent of pituitary adenomas give rise to pituitary apoplexy. Asymptomatic small hemorrhages are more common, and even large asymptomatic hemorrhages are seen. The bleeding may be spontaneous or may be precipitated by trauma, anticoagulant, estrogen, or bromocriptine usage, or radiotherapy. The etiology may not be clear. Clinical presentation includes sudden headache, nausea, stiff neck, decreased vision and field cuts, and impaired eye movements. CT and particularly MRI reveal the diagnosis; most hemorrhages extend above the sella. Steroid replacement and prompt surgery (generally transsphenoidal) are recommended. If some function is preserved, most deficits (except complete loss of vision) improve or clear even if the patient has been symptomatic for a few days.[76,154,191]

Vasculopathy, Vasculitis

Vasculopathy includes conditions that have proliferative changes or intramural deposits of adventitious materials.[131,132,207] Vasculitis includes conditions characterized by inflammation and necrosis of vessel walls.[36,207] A variety of classification schemes have been used.[36] There are a variety of types which may be of specific or nonspecific etiology, which involve the brain only or are generalized, which may involve vessels of different sizes, and which have different histologic appearances. They cause SICH by weakening vessel walls, by occluding vessels leading to infarction into which bleeding occurs, or by causing myocardial infarction, cardiac embolism, and a transforming infarction. The diagnosis is much more obvious when there is typical systemic involvement. The diagnosis is made by angiography and biopsy.

Cerebral amyloid angiopathy (CAA) may be the third leading cause of SICH. It predominates in the elderly population. Amyloid is deposited in the media and adventitia of small- and medium-sized superficial cortical and leptomeningeal arteries that become brittle and rupture and also lose the hemostatic function of their endothelia.[131] CAA is expected to be a more common cause of SICH as our population ages. Seen in 10 percent of those in their 70s, and in over 60 percent over 90, it leads to recurrent and multiple superficial hemorrhages from the weakened vessels. There are familial varieties. It is also associated with a variety of diseases from Alzheimer's disease to dementia pugilistica, and many patients have hypertension. The diagnosis must be made by biopsy or postmortem examination. The prognosis is usually poor, and surgery may be complicated by difficult hemostasis and rebleeding, although it can be done successfully.[2,26,33,73,111,114,131,132,142,150,207,236]

Fibromuscular dysplasia may lead to aneurysm formation. Secondary SICH may then occur.[116]

Moyamoya disease is a specific condition or a syndrome resulting from various diseases causing occlusion of proximal cerebral vessels. It is characterized by progressive stenosis of the anterior circle of Willis and compensatory transdural or posterior fossa anastomoses and collateral channels in the basal ganglia. Bleeding occurs from microaneurysms in the vessels in the basal ganglia or secondary proximal internal carotid and posterior fossa aneurysms. SICH is the most common cause of death.[2,131]

There are both multisystem (systemic lupus erythematosus, rheumatoid arthritis, giant cell arteritis) and isolated (granulomatous angiitis) vasculitides that can lead to cerebral vascular weakening and bleeding. The diagnosis can be suspected if the systemic disease is present; it can be confirmed by a picture of vascular stenoses and narrowings on angiography.[2,207]

Drugs

A number of sympathomimetic street drugs, including amphetamines and cocaine, as well as over-the-counter drugs, may cause SICH, generally after chronic abuse. This may be due to hypertension and/or vasculitis. At times, angiography will demonstrate vasculitis in the small- and medium-sized arteries. The arteritis will subside with cessation of drug use and the administration of cyclophosphamide and prednisone. However, blood pressure elevations per se may also precipitate rupture of preexisting aneurysms and AVMs. The clots tend to arise in the subcortical white matter.[2,33,72,111,114,195,233]

Anticoagulants can lead to SICH, especially if the clotting studies are especially prolonged (i.e., prothrombin time >1.5 times normal). The hemorrhage may evolve slowly and become very large. Related to age, hypertension, head injury (even minor), and infarction, it may be the cause of up to 10 percent of SICH; SICH may be seen in up to 2 percent of patients on anticoagulants. The parenchyma is the second most common site of intracranial bleeding (after the subdural space) that tends to occur in the lobar white matter or cerebellum. Treatment involves normalizing the hemostatic system with vitamin K in the case of oral anticoagulants and protamine sulfate for heparin. Patient outcome is often poor, with two-thirds usually dying.[2,33,60,72,111,114,194]

Thrombolytic drugs, particularly urokinase and tissue plasminogen activator, are now being used more extensively, particularly for treating coronary artery thrombosis. SICH has been identified as a complication of these drugs, but hemorrhagic transformation can occur after myocardial infarction without the drugs, and the increased risk is fairly small.[2,72] There is growing interest in using thrombolytic drugs to treat cerebral vascular occlusion, which will be discussed below. Treatment is problematic since reversing the effect of the drug might exacerbate the original thrombosis.

Alcohol, if used excessively, can predispose to SICH. This may be related to its causing hypertension or altering coagulation mechanisms.[70,72,241]

Postoperative

Bleeding after carotid endarterectomy, although it occurs in well under 1 percent of operations, may be devastating. Usually delayed a few days, it occurs especially after opening a severely stenotic artery (with hypoperfusion), particularly if the artery supplied an area of previous infarction. Postoperative hypertension with hyperperfusion exacerbates the risk, whereas optimal control of blood pressure minimizes it. Postoperative anticoagulants or antiplatelet agents increase the incidence.[2,177,190,220]

Postcraniotomy bleeding probably relates to a number of problems including inadequate hemostasis, low intracranial pressure which minimizes tamponade, local and generalized DIC, unrecognized platelet abnormalities (including inhibition by salicylates), breakdown of autoregulation, and postoperative hypertension.[68] In one series, such clots were seen in 0.5 percent of 4992 intracranial procedures; of these 24 patients, 8 died and 7 had a poor outcome.[102] Special problems arise in surgery for specific lesions.[68] Surgery for aneurysm may be complicated by bleeding after imperfect clip placement, and surgery for AVMs may be complicated by postoperative circulatory breakthrough. SICH occurs after extracranial to intracranial bypass surgery where there has been a prior infarct. Delayed traumatic ICH after craniotomy will be discussed below. The risk of hematoma formation after stereotactic surgery is 0 to 2.5 percent, but only one-quarter of patients require surgery.[68] Placement of monitoring devices through the brain may lead to direct injury to vessels, particularly in the face of DIC.[68,118,121] Diagnostic procedures, including lumbar puncture and angiography, and endovascular techniques such as embolization for tumor or AVM, occlusion of vessels or an aneurysm itself, and angioplasty for spasm may be complicated by hemorrhage.[68]

SICH after cardiac operations may be related to a number of factors unique to this kind of surgery. These include emboli, arterial hypertension, increased venous pressure, and anticoagulant use.[2]

Stroke

After an ischemic infarct, there may be transformation to a hemorrhagic infarct or even frank parenchymal hemorrhage, presumably due to reopening of the occluded vessel and leakage of blood from the vessels damaged from the ischemic insult.[28,33] Bleeding has been seen in more than one-half of autopsied patients.[86] Recent MRI studies have shown some hemorrhage in 69 percent; several CT and MRI studies have revealed small hematomas in about 15 percent and large hematomas in 10 percent of patients although they were often asymptomatic.[91] Risk is highest in patients with embolic strokes from carotid or cardiac disease, those who have large infarcts with significant mass effect and herniation, and those who have early hypodense changes or areas of contrast enhancement on CT.[91,149,230] Anticoagulants predispose to this problem, and their use in embolic disease of cardiac origin should be individualized.[77] This change is usually not seen in the first day, but often occurs within 4 days, although a certain number occur later. Angiography has revealed that many occlusions reopen within 24 h,[149] after which reperfusion leads to this bleeding. Later bleeding may relate to the development of collateral circulation.[230] The development of a parenchymous hemorrhage when accompanied by clinical deterioration has a poorer prognosis.[230] Specific treatment for this hemorrhage has not been discussed in detail. Since heparin can exacerbate the bleeding (but not change the incidence of hemorrhage), it may need to be stopped.[77,149,230]

Another issue involves the trials of thrombolytic therapy for occlusive stroke.[68,149,230,231] Although definitive studies are still ongoing, it appears this treatment is efficacious with acceptable risk.

Venous and sinus thrombosis, a complication of dehydration or congestive heart failure, hematologic problems, oral contraceptives, pregnancy, trauma, infection, or malignancies including leukemia, may also cause SICH. Venous thrombosis may involve the sagittal sinus, transverse sinus, cavernous sinus, or cortical veins. Clinical manifestations depend on the extent of the thrombosis and collaterals. There may be evidence of elevated intracranial pressure with or without obvious focal signs, depending on the sinus involved and the site of the hemorrhage. Seizures may be a prominent event. Sagittal sinus thrombosis can lead to SICH which is usually in the parasagittal white matter bilaterally. The CT and MRI appearance may be diagnostic for such occlusions because of bilateral clots. There may be a defect in filling of the sinus on contrasted CT or MRI scans. Angiography can be helpful. Venography is not necessary nor worth the risk. Treatment should be aimed at the underlying condition. The use of anticoagulants in the face of a hematoma is problematic. These hemorrhages have a significant mortality rate.[2,25,142,149,184,198]

Post-Traumatic

The so-called delayed traumatic intracerebral hematoma (DTICH) is discussed because it does occur spontaneously and differs from other etiologies only in that the primary initiating factor, the injury, occurs at a distinct point in time as opposed to being the result of ongoing or progressive disease.[38,118] There are actually three groups of such hematomas, depending on the vessel of origin: (1) clots from traumatic aneurysms on larger arteries, (2) classic DTICH from smaller arteries, and (3) clots from venous injuries (see above).

Traumatic aneurysms can be caused by penetrating injuries or closed head injuries (Table 254-10) and may be ''true,'' ''false,'' or mixed. At times rupture, often fatal, occurs within days after injury. They cause SICH in 10 percent of cases. The aneurysm may be detected by comparing an uncontrasted CT scan with a contrasted CT scan. Angiography should be performed if missiles or other objects have passed near major arteries. Early prophylactic clipping is suggested.

Classic DTICHs occur in 1.3 to 1.7 percent of patients with head injury judged significant enough to perform CT and 2.3 to 8.4 percent of those with Glasgow Coma Scale scores ≤8 and are generally seen 3 to 4 days after injury. A variety of mechanisms can play a role in their development (Table 254-11). As noted, decompressive surgery may contribute to their formation by releasing tamponade in areas of contusion. Treatment must be individualized. Prognosis depends on the size and location of the clot and the previous condition of the patient.

TABLE 254-10 Etiologies of Traumatic Aneurysms

I. Penetrating
Depressed fractures
Gunshot wounds
Knives, etc.
Iatrogenic
II. Closed head injury
Tethering
Supraclinoid carotid
Local injury
Anterior cerebral at falx
Middle cerebral at sphenoid ridge
Posterior cerebral at tentorium
Cortical vessels at adhesions or in linear fracture

Source: From Kaufman,[118] with permission.

Mycotic Aneurysm

SICH after infection may be due to disruption of a vessel wall, bleeding into an infarction, or (most commonly) rupture of an aneurysm arising from an infected vessel wall.[8,35,133,173,177] Aneurysms occur in perhaps 1.7 percent of patients with bacterial endocarditis, the most common cause, and they are multiple in 20 percent.[173] Neurological complications are seen in up to one-third of patients with bacterial endocarditis, one-half of which are vascular; and more than one-half of all victims die.[8] Mycotic aneurysms constitute 2.6 to 6 percent of all aneurysms, but their incidence is thought to be decreasing.[8]

Although called ''mycotic'' aneurysms, most aneurysms of infectious origin are secondary to bacterial infections, particularly subacute bacterial endocarditis. They are caused by infected emboli that lodge in distal intracranial arteries, particularly middle cerebral branches. Risk factors include subacute endocarditis, intravenous drug abuse, and immunosuppression. The type of infection is changing as the pattern changes in endocarditis.[8] Fungal

TABLE 254-11 Primary and Secondary Factors Leading to Delayed Traumatic Intracerebral Hematoma

Vessel damage
Neuropil damage
Vasospasm
Vasodilation
Vasoparalysis
Venous back pressure
Hypoxia, hypotension
Hypertension
Medical reduction of intracranial pressure
Surgical reduction of intracranial pressure
Disseminated intravascular coagulation
Effects of alcohol

Source: From Kaufman,[118] with permission.

aneurysms have also been reported.[189] They may also be the result of infections external to a vessel such as septic cavernous sinus thrombophlebitis[93] and meningitis.

Mycotic aneurysms present as SICH or subarachnoid hemorrhage, which have a high mortality,[35,173] or with just a headache. Bleeding may occur within 1 to 2 days or up to months after infection, but the average is about 17 days.[173] CT without and then with contrast enhancement or MRI may reveal the aneurysm as well as the hemorrhage. The workup should include complete cerebral angiography, which should be repeated until treatment is finished. Initial treatment should include antibiotics and correction of the cardiac lesion if indicated. Decisions about intracranial surgery should be based on the significance of the clot, details about the aneurysm, and the response to antibiotics. Based on their review of the literature, one group of authors suggest[173]:

1. If there is one distal middle cerebral artery aneurysm and the patient has bled, excise the aneurysm. The artery of origin will probably need to be sacrificed. An extracranial to intracranial bypass may be required as an adjunct.
2. If there is a proximal or unruptured aneurysm or an aneurysm on a critical branch, treat with antibiotics and obtain serial angiograms to see if the aneurysm is resolving, stable, or enlarging. Consider excising enlarging aneurysms and follow healing aneurysms until they disappear. The appropriate frequency for angiograms is not well established, but probably every 10 to 14 days is reasonable. A significant proportion of aneurysms will not disappear, but their walls will be stronger after they have had time to develop fibrosis.
3. Individualize if there are multiple aneurysms.

Endovascular occlusion has also been used successfully.[124]

Hemorrhage may occur with encephalitis, specifically *Herpes simplex* encephalitis and with brain abscess. SICH may also occur in a variety of circumstances in patients who are immunosuppressed, particularly by AIDS.[8]

Childhood

The most unique hemorrhage in childhood is the intraventricular and periventricular hemorrhage primarily seen in the premature.[40,81] Other predisposing conditions, such as vein of Galen malformations, leukemia, and idiopathic thrombocytopenic purpura, and inherited coagulation disorders may be seen especially in childhood.

Pregnancy

Intracranial hemorrhage, including SICH, is the leading nonobstetrical cause of maternal mortality in pregnancy. It may be related to normal changes in cardiovascular physiology, complications of pregnancy including hypertension in toxemia and eclampsia, coagulation disorders, and bleeding from preexisting lesions. Routine nonoperative and operative care are indicated, although it should be remembered that mannitol can dehydrate the fetus, hypotension can be detrimental, and anticonvulsants have teratogenic and depressant effects. Method of delivery does not influence bleeding and should be decided on obstetrical grounds.[32,44]

References

1. Acampora S, Profeta G, Troisi F. Stereotaxic evacuation of hematomas. *J Neurosurg* 1985; 62:460 (letter).
2. Adams HP Jr, Biller J. Hemorrhagic intracranial vascular disease. In Joynt RJ (ed): *Clinical Neurology*, vol 2. Philadelphia: Lippincott, 1988, pp 1–64.
3. Apuzzo MLJ, Sabshin JK. Computed tomographic guidance stereotaxis in the management of intracranial lesions. *Neurosurgery* 1983; 12:277–285.
4. Auer LM, Deinsberger W, Niederkorn K, et al. Endoscopic surgery versus medical treatment for spontaneous intracerebral hematoma: a randomized study. *J Neurosurg* 1989; 70:530–535.
5. Backlund E-O. Stereotaxic evacuation of hematomas. *J Neurosurg* 1985; 62:460–461 (letter).
6. Backlund E-O, von Holst H. Controlled subtotal evacuation of intracerebral haematomas by stereotactic technique. *Surg Neurol* 1978; 9:99–101.
7. Bae HG, Lee KS, Yun IG, et al. Rapid expansion of hypertensive intracerebral hemorrhage. *Neurosurgery* 1992; 31:35–41.
8. Baker R, Jones HR Jr. Intracranial hemorrhage in infectious diseases. *Neuroimaging Clin North Am* 1992; 2:213–220.
9. Batjer HH (ed). Spontaneous intracerebral hemorrhage. *Neurosurg Clin North Am* 1992; 3(3):497–713.
10. Batjer HH, Reisch JS, Allen BC, et al. Failure of surgery to improve outcome in hypertensive putaminal hemorrhage. A prospective randomized trial. *Arch Neurol* 1990; 47:1103–1106.
11. Beatty RM, Zervas NT. Stereotactic aspiration of a brain stem hematoma. *Neurosurgery* 1983; 13:204–207.
12. Borges LF. Management of nontraumatic brain hemorrhage. In Ropper AH, Kennedy SF (eds): *Neurological and Neurosurgical Intensive Care*, 2d ed. Rockville, MD: Aspen, 1988, pp 209–217.
13. Borges LF. Management of nontraumatic brain hemorrhage. In Ropper AH (ed): *Neurological and Neurosurgical Intensive Care*, 3d ed. New York: Raven Press, 1993, pp 279–289.
14. Bosch DA, Beute GN. Successful stereotaxic evacuation of an acute pontomedullary hematoma. *J Neurosurg* 1985; 62:153–156.
15. Brawanski A, Gaab MR, Fuhrmeister U, et al. Spontaneous intracranial hemorrhage, intracranial pressure and indications for operation: a clinical follow-up study. *Adv Neurosurg* 1983; 11:90–98.
16. Brismar J, Hindfelt B, Nilsson O. Benign brainstem hematoma. *Acta Neurol Scand* 1979; 60:178–182.
17. Broderick JP, Brott TG, Tomsick T, et al. Ultra-early evaluation of intracerebral hemorrhage. *J Neurosurg* 1990; 72:195–199.
18. Broderick JP, Brott T, Tomsick T, et al. The risk of subarachnoid and intracerebral hemorrhages in blacks as compared with whites. *N Engl J Med* 1992; 326:733–736.
19. Broderick JP, Brott T, Tomsick T, et al. Intracerebral hemorrhage more than twice as common as subarachnoid hemorrhage. *J Neurosurg* 1993; 78:188–191.
20. Broderick J, Brott T, Tomsick T, et al. Lobar hemorrhage in the elderly. The undiminishing importance of hypertension. *Stroke* 1993; 24:49–51.
21. Brott T, Broderick J, Barsan W, et al. Hyper-acute clot retraction in spontaneous intracerebral hemorrhage. *Stroke* 1992; 23:141 (abstr).
22. Browder EJ, Corradini EW. Surgical treatment of intracerebral hematomas. *Arch Neurol Psychiatry* 1951; 65:112–117.
23. Brown RA, Roberts T, Osborn AG. Simplified CT-guided stereotaxic biopsy. *Am J Neuroradiol* 1981; 2:181–184.
24. Bruce DA, Schut L, Zimmerman R, et al. Intraventricular hemorrhage: the clinical spectrum of the disease and implications for therapy based on the CT scan. Presented at the 44th Annual Meeting of the American Association of Neurological Surgeons, San Francisco, CA, April 6, 1976.
25. Busse O. ICH in sinus and cerebral vein thrombosis. In Pia HW, Langmaid C, Zierski J (eds): *Spontaneous Intracerebral*

Haematomas; Advances in Diagnosis and Therapy. New York: Springer-Verlag, 1980, pp 56–58.

26. Cahill DW, Ducker TB. Spontaneous intracerebral hemorrhage. *Clin Neurosurg* 1982; 29:722–779.
27. Caplan LR. Intracerebral hemorrhage. In Tyler HR, Dawson DM (eds): *Current Neurology*, vol 2. Boston: Houghton Mifflin, 1979, pp 185–205.
28. Caplan L. Intracerebral hemorrhage revisited. *Neurology* 1988; 38:624–627.
29. Caplan LR. Clinical features of spontaneous intracerebral hemorrhage. In Kaufman HH (ed): *Intracerebral Hematomas.* New York: Raven Press, 1992, pp 31–47.
30. Caplan LR. Intracerebral haemorrhage. *Lancet* 1992; 339:656–658.
31. Caplan LR, Mohr JP. Intracerebral hemorrhage: an update. *Geriatrics* 1978; 33:42–52.
32. Carmel PW, Swift DM. Spontaneous intracranial hemorrhage occurring during pregnancy. In Kaufman HH (ed): *Intracerebral Hematomas.* New York: Raven Press, 1992, pp 117–125.
33. Castel JP, Kissel P. Spontaneous intracerebral and infratentorial hemorrhage. In Youmans JR (ed): *Neurological Surgery: A Comprehensive Reference Guide to the Diagnosis and Management of Neurosurgical Problems.* 3d ed. Philadelphia: Saunders, 1990, pp 1890–1917.
34. Chaney RK, Taber KH, Orrison WW Jr, et al. Magnetic resonance imaging of intracerebral hemorrhage at different field strengths: a review of reported intraparenchymal signal intensities. *Neuroimaging Clin North Am* 1992; 2:25–51.
35. Clare CE, Barrow DL. Infectious intracranial aneurysms. *Neurosurgery Clin North Am* 1992; 3:551–566.
36. Cohen BA, Biller J. Hemorrhagic stroke due to cerebral vasculitis and the role of immunosuppressive therapy. *Neurosurgery Clin North Am* 1992; 3:611–624.
37. Cohen WA, Hayman LA. Computed tomography of intracranial hemorrhage. *Neuroimaging Clin North Am* 1992; 2:75–87.
38. Cooper PR. Delayed traumatic intracerebral hemorrhage. *Neurosurg Clin North Am* 1992; 3:657–665.
39. Crowell RM, Ojemann RG, Ogilvy CS. Spontaneous brain hemorrhage: surgical considerations. In Barnett HJM, Stein BM, Mohr JP, et al. (eds): *Stroke—Pathophysiology, Diagnosis, and Management,* 2d ed. New York: Churchill Livingstone, 1992, pp 1169–1187.
40. Dauser RC, McLone DG. Intracerebral hematomas in childhood. In Kaufman HH (ed): *Intracerebral Hematomas.* New York: Raven Press, 1992, pp 163–171.
41. Davidoff LM. Intracerebral hemorrhage associated with hypertension and arteriosclerosis. *J Neurosurg* 1958; 15:322–328.
42. Del Zoppo GJ. Thrombolytic therapy in cerebrovascular disease. *Stroke* 1988; 19:1174–1179.
43. de Weerd AW. The prognosis of intraventricular hemorrhage. *J Neurol* 1979; 222:46–51.
44. Dias MS, Sekhar LN. Intracranial hemorrhage from aneurysms and arteriovenous malformations during pregnancy and the puerperium. *Neurosurgery* 1990; 27:855–866.
45. Dolinskas CA, Bilaniuk LT, Zimmerman RA, et al. Computed tomography of intracerebral hematomas. I. Transmission CT observations on hematoma resolution. *Am J Roentgenol* 1977; 129:681–688.
46. Drury I, Whisnant JP, Garraway WM. Primary intracerebral hemorrhage: impact of CT on incidence. *Neurology* 1984; 34:653–657.
47. Ducker TB. Spontaneous intracerebral hemorrhage. In Wilkins RH, Rengachary SS (eds): *Neurosurgery.* New York: McGraw-Hill, 1985, pp 1510–1517.
48. Duff TA, Ayeni S, Levin AB, et al. Nonsurgical management of spontaneous intracerebral hematoma. *Neurosurgery* 1981; 9:387–393.
49. Dujovny M, Yokoh A, Cuevas P, et al. Experimental intracerebral hematoma: urokinase treatment. *Stroke* 1987; 18:280 (abstr).
50. Erickson RK, Dohrmann GJ, Wollmann RL. Experimental intracerebral hematoma: analysis of clot lysis and risk of rebleeding with urokinase therapy. Presented at the 55th Annual Meeting of the American Association of Neurological Surgeons, Dallas, TX, May 5, 1987.
51. Etou A, Mohadjer M, Braus D, et al. Stereotactic evacuation and fibrinolysis of cerebellar hematomas. *Stereotact Funct Neurosurg* 1990; 54–55:445–450.
52. Faught E, Peters D, Bartolucci A, et al. Seizures after primary intracerebral hemorrhage. *Neurology* 1989; 39:1089–1093.
53. Feldmann E. Intracerebral hemorrhage. *Stroke* 1991; 22:691 (abstr).
54. Fields WS, Lemak NA. *A History of Stroke. Its Recognition and Treatment.* New York: Oxford University Press, 1989.
55. Findlay JM, Weir BKA, Gordon P, et al. Safety and efficacy of intrathecal thrombolytic therapy in a primate model of cerebral vasospasm. *J Neurosurg* 1989; 24:491–498.
56. Fisher CM. The pathology and pathogenesis of intracerebral hemorrhage. In Fields WS (ed): *Pathogenesis and Treatment of Cerebrovascular Disease.* Springfield: Charles C Thomas, 1961, pp 295–317.
57. Fisher CM. Clinical syndromes in cerebral hemorrhage. In Fields WS (ed): *Pathogenesis and Treatment of Cerebrovascular Disease.* Springfield, IL: Charles C Thomas, 1961, pp 318–342.
58. Fisher CM. Pathological observations in hypertensive cerebral hemorrhage. *J Neuropathol Exp Neurol* 1971; 30:536–550.
59. Fisher CM. Capsular infarcts. The underlying vascular lesions. *Arch Neurol* 1979; 36:65–73.
60. Franke CL, de Jonge J, van Swieten JC, et al. Intracerebral hematomas during anticoagulant treatment. *Stroke* 1990; 21:726–730.
61. Franke CL, van Swieten JC, van Gijn J. Residual lesions on computed tomography after intracerebral hemorrhage. *Stroke* 1991; 22:1530–1533.
62. Frankowski RF. Epidemiology of stroke and intracerebral hemorrhage. In Kaufman HH (ed): *Intracerebral Hematomas.* New York: Raven Press, 1992, pp 1–11.
63. Freeman JW, Kennedy RM, Petty SS. Prognosis of nonoperated cerebellar hemorrhage. *Ann Neurol* 1978; 4:389–390.
64. Fujitsu K, Muramoto M, Ikeda Y, et al. Indications for surgical treatment of putaminal hemorrhage. Comparative study based on serial CT and time-cause analysis. *J Neurosurg* 1990; 73:518–525.
65. Garcia JH, Ho KL. Pathology of hypertensive arteriopathy. *Neurosurg Clin North Am* 1992; 3:497–507.
66. Gates PC, Barnett HJM, Vinters HV, et al. Primary intraventricular hemorrhage in adults. *Stroke* 1986; 17:872–877.
67. Gega A, Utsumi S, Terada H, et al. The posterior trans-sylvian approach for thalamic hemorrhage. *Neurol Med Chir (Tokyo)* 1979; 19:361–366.
68. Gibbons KJ, Guterman LR, Hopkins LN. Iatrogenic intracerebral hemorrhage. *Neurosurg Clin North Am* 1992; 3:667–683.
69. Gildenberg PL, Kaufman HH, Murthy KS. Calculation of stereotactic coordinates from the computed tomographic scan. *Neurosurgery* 1982; 10:580–586.
70. Gill JS, Shipley MJ, Tsementzis SA, et al. Alcohol consumption—a risk factor for hemorrhagic and non-hemorrhagic stroke. *Am J Med* 1991; 90:489–497.
71. Gilliard C, Mathurin P, Passagia JG, et al. L'hematome spontane du cervelet. *Neurochirurgie* 1990; 36:347–353.
72. Glick RP, Anson JA. Drug-induced intracranial hemorrhage. In Kaufman HH (ed): *Intracerebral Hematomas.* New York: Raven Press, 1992, pp 139–150.
73. Greene GM, Godersky JC, Biller J, et al. Surgical experience with cerebral amyloid angiopathy. *Stroke* 1990; 21:1545–1549.
74. Grubb RL Jr. Spontaneous cerebral hemorrhage. In Apuzzo MLJ (ed): *Brain Surgery. Complication Avoidance and Management.* New York: Churchill Livingstone, 1993, pp 1251–1269.
75. Haber E, Quertermous T, Matsueda GR, et al. Innovative approaches to plasminogen activator theory. *Science* 1989; 243:51–56.
76. Harsh GR, Wilson CB. Pituitary apoplexy in endocrine inactive pituitary adenomas. Presented at the 42nd Annual Meeting of the Congress of Neurological Surgeons, Washington, DC, November 3, 1992.

77. Hart RG, Easton JD. Hemorrhagic infarcts. *Stroke* 1986; 17:586–589.
78. Hayman LA, Taber KH (eds). Nontraumatic intracranial hemorrhage. *Neuroimaging Clin North Am* 1992; 2:1–250.
79. Heiman TD, Satya-Murti S. Benign cerebellar hemorrhages. *Ann Neurol* 1978; 3:366–368.
80. Herbstein DJ, Schaumberg HH. Hypertensive intracerebral hematoma. An investigation of the initial hemorrhage and rebleeding using chromium Cr-51-labeled erythrocytes. *Arch Neurol* 1974; 30:412–414.
81. Herman TE, Siegel MJ. Intracranial hemorrhage in the neonate. *Neuroimaging Clin North Am* 1992; 2:107–117.
82. Heros RC. Cerebellar hemorrhage and infarction. *Contemp Neurosurg* 1980; 2:1.
83. Heros RC. Cerebellar hemorrhage and infarction. *Stroke* 1982; 13:106–109.
84. Heros RC, Zervas NT. Subarachnoid hemorrhage. *Annu Rev Med* 1983; 34:367–375.
85. Hier DB, Davis KR, Richardson EP Jr, et al. Hypertensive putaminal hemorrhage. *Ann Neurol* 1977; 1:152–159.
86. Higgins AC, Nashold BS Jr. Stereotactic evacuation of large intracerebral hematomas. *Appl Neurophysiol* 1980; 43:96–103.
87. Higgins AC, Nashold BS. Stereotactic evacuation of intracerebral hematoma. In Lunsford LD (ed): *Modern Stereotactic Neurosurgery,* Boston: Martinus Nijhoff, 1988, pp 217–227.
88. Hogg JP, Gabriele OF. Radiology of nontraumatic hemorrhage of the brain. In Kaufman HH (ed): *Intracerebral Hematomas.* New York: Raven Press, 1992, pp 49–74.
89. Hondo H: CT-guided stereotactic evacuation of hypertensive intracerebral hematomas: a new operative approach. *Tokushima J Exp Med* 1983; 30:25–39.
90. Hondo H, Uno M, Sasaki K, et al. Computed tomography controlled aspiration surgery for hypertensive intracerebral hemorrhage: experience of more than 400 cases. *Stereotact Funct Neurosurg* 1990; 54–55:432–437.
91. Hornig CR, Bauer T, Simon C, et al. Hemorrhagic transformation in cardioembolic cerebral infarction. *Stroke* 1993; 24:465–468.
92. Howell DA. The surgical treatment of massive cerebral haemorrhage. A report of 33 cases. *Can Med Assoc J* 1957; 77:542–555.
93. Hurst RW, Choi IS, Persky M, et al. Mycotic aneurysms of the intracavernous carotid artery: a case report and review of the literature. *Surg Neurol* 1992; 37:142–146.
94. Itakura T, Komai N, Nadai E, et al. Stereotactic evacuation of hypertensive intracerebral hematoma using plasminogen activator. Presented at the 55th Annual Meeting of the American Association of Neurological Surgeons, Dallas, TX, May 6, 1987.
95. Itakura T, Komai N, Nakai E, et al. Stereotactic evacuation of hypertensive intracerebral hematoma using plasminogen activator. Surgical technique and long-term results. In Suzuki J (ed): *Advances in Surgery for Cerebral Stroke.* New York: Springer-Verlag, 1988, pp 443–448.
96. Ito H, Mukai H, Kitamura A, Yamashita J. Stereotactic AquaStream and Aspirator for hypertensive intracerebral hematoma. *Stereotact Funct Neurosurg* 1989; 53:77–84.
97. Janny P, Colnet G, Georget AM, et al. Intracranial pressure with intracerebral hemorrhages. *Surg Neurol* 1978; 10:371–375.
98. Janny P, Papo I, Chazal J, et al. Intracranial hypertension and prognosis in spontaneous intracerebral haematomas. A correlative study of 60 patients. *Acta Neurochir (Wien)* 1982; 61:181–186.
99. Jellinger K. Pathology and aetiology of ICH. In Pia HW, Langmaid C, Zierski J (eds): *Spontaneous Intracerebral Haematomas; Advances in Diagnosis and Therapy.* New York: Springer-Verlag, 1980, pp 13–29.
100. Juvela S, Heiskanen O, Poranen A, et al. The treatment of spontaneous intracerebral hemorrhage. A prospective randomized trial of surgical and conservative treatment. *J Neurosurg* 1989; 70:755–758.
101. Kagawa M. Thalamic hemorrhage. In Mizukami M, Kogure K, Kanaya H, et al. (eds): *Hypertensive Intracerebral Hemorrhage.* New York: Raven Press, 1983, pp 225–231.
102. Kalfas IH, Little JR. Postoperative hemorrhage: a survey of 4992 intracerebral procedures. *Neurosurgery* 1988; 23:343–347.
103. Kanaya H, Kuroda K. Development in neurosurgical approaches to hypertensive intracerebral hemorrhage in Japan. In Kaufman HH (ed): *Intracerebral Hematomas.* New York: Raven Press, 1992, pp 197–209.
104. Kanaya H, Saiki T, Ohuchi T, et al. Hypertensive intracerebral hemorrhage in Japan: update on surgical treatment. In Mizukami M, Kogure K, Kanaya H, et al. (eds): *Hypertensive Intracerebral Hemorrhage.* New York: Raven Press, 1983, pp 147–163.
105. Kanaya H, Yukawa H, Itoh Z, et al. A neurological grading for patients with hypertensive intracerebral hemorrhage and a classification for hematoma location of computed tomography. In *Proceedings of the 7th Conference of Surgical Treatment of Stroke,* Tokyo: Nyuronsha, 1978, pp 265–270.
106. Kanaya H, Yukawa H, Itoh Z, et al. Grading and the indications for treatment in ICH of the basal ganglia (Cooperative Study in Japan). In Pia HW, Langmaid C, Zierski J (eds): *Spontaneous Intracerebral Haematomas; Advances in Diagnosis and Therapy.* New York: Springer-Verlag, 1980, pp 268–274.
107. Kandel EI, Peresedov VV. Stereotaxic evacuation of spontaneous intracerebral hematomas. *J Neurosurg* 1985; 62:206–213.
108. Kaneko M, Koba T, Yokoyama T. Early surgical treatment for hypertensive intracerebral hemorrhage. *J Neurosurg* 1977; 46:579–583.
109. Kannel WB, Wolf PA, McGee DL, et al. Systolic blood pressure, arterial rigidity, and risk of stroke; the Framingham study. *JAMA* 1981; 245:1225–1229.
110. Kanno T, Sano H, Shinomiya Y, et al. Role of surgery in hypertensive intracerebral hematoma. A comparative study of 305 nonsurgical and 154 surgical cases. *J Neurosurg* 1984; 61:1091–1099.
111. Kase CS. Intracerebral hemorrhage: non-hypertensive causes. *Stroke* 1986; 17:590–595.
112. Kase CS, Caplan LR. Hemorrhage affecting the brain stem and cerebellum. In Barnett HJM, Mohr JP, Stein BM, et al. (eds): *Stroke.* New York: Churchill Livingstone, 1986, pp 621–641.
113. Kase CS, Mohr JP. Supratentorial intracerebral hemorrhage. In Barnett HJM, Mohr JP, Stein BM, et al. (eds): *Stroke.* New York: Churchill Livingstone, 1986, pp 525–547.
114. Kase CS, Mohr JP, Caplan LR. Intracerebral hemorrhage. In Barnett HJM, Mohr JP, Stein BM, et al. (eds): *Stroke—Pathophysiology, Diagnosis, and Management,* 2d ed. New York: Churchill Livingstone, 1992, pp 561–616.
115. Kashiwagi S, van Loveren HR, Tew JM Jr, et al. Diagnosis and treatment of vascular brain-stem malformations. *J Neurosurg* 1990; 72:27–34.
116. Kaufman HH. Fibromuscular hyperplasia of the carotid artery. In a case associated with an arteriovenous malformation. *Arch Neurol* 1970; 22:299–304.
117. Kaufman HH. *Intracerebral Hematomas.* New York: Raven Press, 1992.
118. Kaufman HH. Delayed posttraumatic intracerebral hematoma. In Kaufman HH (ed): *Intracerebral Hematomas.* New York: Raven Press, 1992, pp 173–179.
119. Kaufman HH. Stereotactic aspiration with fibrinolytic and mechanical assistance. In Kaufman HH (ed): *Intracerebral Hematomas.* New York: Raven Press, 1992, pp 181–185.
120. Kaufman HH, Herschberger JE, Maroon JC, et al. Mechanical aspiration of hematomas in an *in vitro* model. *Neurosurgery* 1989; 25:347–350.
121. Kaufman HH, Moake JL, Olson JD, et al. Delayed and recurrent intracranial hematomas related to disseminated intravascular clotting and fibrinolysis in head injury. *Neurosurgery* 1980; 7:445–449.
122. Kaufman HH, Schochet SS. Pathology, pathophysiology, and modeling. In Kaufman HH (ed): *Intracerebral Hematomas.* New York: Raven Press, 1992, pp 13–21.

123. Kaufman HH, Schochet S, Koss W, et al. Efficacy and safety of tissue plasminogen activator. *Neurosurgery* 1987; 20:403–407.
124. Khayata MH, Aymard A, Casasco A, et al. Selective endovascular techniques in the treatment of cerebral mycotic aneurysms. Report of three cases. *J Neurosurg* 1993; 78:661–665.
125. King WA, Martin NA. Intracerebral hemorrhage due to dural arteriovenous malformations and fistulae. *Neurosurg Clin North Am* 1992; 3:577–590.
126. Kinkel WR, Jacobs L. Computerized axial transverse tomography in cerebrovascular disease. *Neurology* 1976; 26:924–930.
127. Kirkpatrick JB, Hayman LA. Pathophysiology of intracranial hemorrhage. *Neuroimaging Clin North Am* 1992; 2:11–23.
128. Konovalov AN, Spallone A, Makhmudov UB, et al. Surgical management of hematomas of the brain stem. *J Neurosurg* 1990; 73:181–186.
129. Kotchen TA, Halbritter KA, Boegehold MA. Hypertension and the brain. In Kaufman HH (ed): *Intracerebral Hematomas.* New York: Raven Press, 1992, pp 23–29.
130. Lazorthes G. Surgery of cerebral hemorrhage. Report on the results of 52 surgically treated cases. *J Neurosurg* 1959; 16:355–364.
131. Leblanc R. Cerebral amyloid angiopathy and moyamoya disease. *Neurosurg Clin North Am* 1992; 3:625–636.
132. Leblanc R, Preul M, Robitaille Y, et al. Surgical considerations in cerebral amyloid angiopathy. *Neurosurgery* 1991; 29:712–718.
133. Lee KS, Liu SS, Spetzler RF, et al. Intracranial mycotic aneurysm in an infant: report of a case. *Neurosurgery* 1990; 26:129–133.
134. Leeds NE, Sawaya R, Van Tassel P, et al. Intracranial hemorrhage in the oncologic patient. *Neuroimaging Clin North Am* 1992; 2:119–136.
135. Le Roux PD, Lyndsey B, Dailey LA, et al. Emergent aneurysm clipping without cerebral angiography for the moribund patient. Presented at the 41st Annual Meeting of the Congress of Neurological Surgeons, Orlando, FL, October 26–31, 1991.
136. Link MJ, Bartleson JD, Forbes G, et al. Spontaneous midbrain hemorrhage: report of seven new cases. *Surg Neurol* 1993; 39:58–65.
137. Little JR, Blomquist GA Jr, Ethier R. Intraventricular hemorrhage in adults. *Surg Neurol* 1977; 8:143–149.
138. Little JR, Dial B, Belanger G, et al. Brain hemorrhage from intracranial tumor. *Stroke* 1979; 10:283–288.
139. Little JR, Tubman DE, Ethier R. Cerebellar hemorrhage in adults. Diagnosis by computerized tomography. *J Neurosurg* 1978; 48:575–579.
140. Loscalzo J, Braunwald E. Tissue plasminogen activator. *N Engl J Med* 1988; 319:925–931.
141. Lownie SP. Intracranial hemorrhage in aneurysms and vascular malformations. *Neuroimaging Clin North Am* 1992; 2:195–211.
142. Luyendijk W. Intracerebral haematoma. In Vinken PJ, Bruyn GW (eds): *Handbook of Clinical Neurology,* vol 11. New York: American Elsevier, 1972, pp 660–719.
143. Magladery JW. The natural course of cerebrovascular hemorrhage. *Clin Neurosurg* 1961; 9:106–113.
144. Mangiardi JR, Epstein FJ. Brainstem haematomas: review of the literature and presentation of five new cases. *J Neurol Neurosurg Psychiatry* 1988; 51:966–976.
145. Marder VJ, Sherry S. Thrombolytic therapy: current status. *N Engl J Med* 1988; 318:1512–1520; 1585–1595.
146. Marks MP, Lane B, Steinberg GK, et al. Hemorrhage in intracerebral arteriovenous malformations: angiographic determinants. *Radiology* 1990; 176:807–813.
147. Marshall LF, El-Hefnami M. Spontaneous intracranial hemorrhage. *Semin Neurol* 1984; 4:422–429.
148. Masson RL Jr, Day AL. Aneurysmal intracerebral hemorrhage. *Neurosurg Clin North Am* 1992; 3:539–550.
149. Mathews VP, Bryan RN. Intracranial hemorrhage in occlusive vascular diseases. *Neuroimaging Clin North Am* 1992; 2:221–233.
150. Matkovic Z, Davis S, Gonzales M, et al. Surgical risk of hemorrhage in cerebral amyloid angiopathy. *Stroke* 1991; 22:456–461.
151. Matsumoto K, Gyoten T, Yamashita S, et al. Clinical outcomes of burr hole and aspiration surgery for hypertensive intracerebral hemorrhage and a newly devised aspiration system. Presented at the 8th International Congress of Neurological Surgery, Toronto, July 7–13, 1985.
152. Matsumoto K, Hondo H. CT-guided stereotaxic evacuation of hypertensive intracerebral hematomas. *J Neurosurg* 1984; 61:440–448.
153. Matsumoto K, Hondo H, Tomida K. Aspiration surgery for hypertensive brain hemorrhage in the acute stage. In Suzuki J (ed): *Advances in Surgery for Cerebral Stroke.* New York: Springer-Verlag, 1988, pp 433–441.
154. McFadzean RM, Doyle D, Rampling R, et al. Pituitary apoplexy and its effect on vision. *Neurosurgery* 1991; 29:669–675.
155. McKissock W, Richardson A, Taylor J. Primary intracerebral haemorrhage. A controlled trial of surgical and conservative treatment in 180 unselected cases. *Lancet* 1961; 2:221–226.
156. McKissock W, Richardson A, Walsh L. Primary intracerebral haemorrhage. Results of surgical treatment in 244 consecutive cases. *Lancet* 1959; 2:683–686.
157. Mizukami M. Surgical treatment of hypertensive intracerebral hemorrhage. In Fein JM, Flamm ES (eds): *Cerebrovascular Surgery.* New York: Springer-Verlag, 1985, pp 1259–1282.
158. Mizukami M, Araki G, Mihara H, et al. Arteriographically visualized extravasation in hypertensive intracerebral hemorrhage. Report of seven cases. *Stroke* 1972; 3:527–537.
159. Mizukami M, Kanaya H, Kogure K, et al. (eds). *Hypertensive Intracerebral Hemorrhage.* New York: Raven Press, 1983.
160. Mohadjer M, Eggert R, May J, et al. CT-guided stereotactic fibrinolysis of spontaneous and hypertensive cerebellar hemorrhage: long-term results. *J Neurosurg* 1990; 73:217–222.
161. Mukai H, Yamashita J, Kitamura A, et al. Stereotactic AquaStream and Aspirator in the treatment of intracerebral hematoma: an experimental study. *Stereotact Funct Neurosurg* 1991; 57:221–227.
162. Mutlu N, Berry RG, Alpers BJ. Massive cerebral hemorrhage. Clinical and pathological correlations. *Arch Neurol* 1963; 8:644–661.
163. Nakai E, Komai N, Itakura T, Doi E. Stereotactic aspiration surgery for hypertensive pontine hemorrhage (Poster). American Association of Neurological Surgeons, Dallas, TX, May 3–7, 1987.
164. Narayan RK, Narayan TM, Katz DA, et al. Lysis of intracranial hematomas with urokinase in a rabbit model. *J Neurosurg* 1985; 62:580–586.
165. Nguyen JP, Decq P, Brugieres P, et al. A technique for stereotactic aspiration of deep intracerebral hematomas under computed tomographic control using a new device. *Neurosurgery* 1992; 31:330–335.
166. Niizuma H, Otsuki T, Johkura H, et al. CT guided stereotactic aspiration of intracerebral hematoma—result of a hematoma-lysis method using urokinase. *Appl Neurophysiol* 1985; 48:427–430.
167. Niizuma H, Shimizu Y, Yonemitsu T, et al. Results of stereotactic aspiration in 175 cases of putaminal hemorrhage. *Neurosurgery* 1989; 24:814–819.
168. Niizuma H, Suzuki J. Computed tomography-guided stereotactic aspiration of posterior fossa hematomas: a supine lateral retromastoid approach. *Neurosurgery* 1987; 21:422–427.
169. Niizuma H, Suzuki J. Stereotactic aspiration of putaminal hemorrhage using a double track aspiration technique. *Neurosurgery* 1988; 22:432–436.
170. Niizuma H, Yonemitsu T, Jokura H, et al. Stereotactic aspiration of thalamic hematoma. Overall results of 75 aspirated and 70 nonaspirated cases. *Stereotact Funct Neurosurg* 1990; 54–55:438–444.
171. Nutt SH, Patchell RA. Intracranial hemorrhage associated with primary and secondary tumors. *Neurosurg Clin North Am* 1992; 3:591–599.
172. Ochiai C, Sano K, Kobayashi S, et al. Clinical study of pontine hemorrhage with special reference to CT classification and surgical indication. *No To Shinkei* 1979; 31:803–811.
173. Ogilvy CS, Crowell RM. Infectious aneurysms and intracranial hemorrhage. In Kaufman HH (ed): *Intracerebral Hematomas.* New York: Raven Press, 1992, pp 85–93.

174. Ohta T, Waga S, Handa W, et al. New grading of level of disordered consciousness. *No Shinkei Geka* 1974; 2:623–627.
175. Ojemann RG. Spontaneous brain hemorrhage: what treatment should we recommend? *Stroke* 1983; 14:467.
176. Ojemann RG, Heros RC. Spontaneous brain hemorrhage. *Stroke* 1983; 14:468–475.
177. Ojemann RG, Heros RC, Crowell RM. *Surgical Management of Cerebrovascular Disease,* 2d ed. Baltimore: Williams & Wilkins, 1988, pp 435–449.
178. Ojemann RG, Mohr JP. Hypertensive brain hemorrhage. *Clin Neurosurg* 1976; 23:220–244.
179. Onik G, Helms CA, Ginsburg L, et al. Percutaneous lumbar diskectomy using a new 2 mm diameter aspiration probe. *Am J Neuroradiol* 1985; 6:290–293.
180. Ott KH, Kase CS, Ojemann RG, et al. Cerebellar hemorrhage: diagnosis and treatment; a review of 56 cases. *Arch Neurol* 1974; 31:160–167.
181. Pan DH-C, Lee L-S, Chen M-S, Manns AG. Modified screw-and-suction technique for stereotactic evacuation of deep intracerebral hematomas. *Surg Neurol* 1986; 25:540–544.
182. Pang D, Sclabassi RJ, Horton JA. Lysis of intraventricular blood clot with urokinase in a canine model: part 1, part 2, and part 3. *Neurosurgery* 1986; 19:540–572.
183. Papo I, Janny P, Caruselli G, et al. ICP time course in primary intracerebral hemorrhage. *Neurosurgery* 1979; 4:468 (abstr).
184. Persson L, Lilja A. Extensive dural sinus thrombosis treated by surgical removal and local streptokinase infusion. *Neurosurgery* 1990; 26:117–121.
185. Phillips LH II, Whisnant JP, O'Fallon WM, et al. The unchanging pattern of subarachnoid hemorrhage in a community. *Neurology* 1980; 30:1034–1040.
186. Pia HW, Langmaid C, Zierski J (eds). *Spontaneous Intracerebral Haematomas: Advances in Diagnosis and Therapy.* New York: Springer-Verlag, 1980.
187. Picard L, Roland J, Lepoire J, et al. The role of angiography in the neuroradiological diagnosis of intracerebral haematomas. In Pia HW, Langmaid C, Zierski J (eds): *Spontaneous Intracerebral Haematomas; Advances in Diagnosis and Therapy.* New York: Springer-Verlag, 1980, pp 171–177.
188. Piepgras DG, Redmond MJ. Surgical management of intracerebral hemorrhage. In Schmidek HH, Sweet WH (eds): *Operative Neurosurgical Techniques; Indications, Methods and Results,* 2d ed. New York: Grune & Stratton, 1988, pp 881–888.
189. Piotrowski WP, Pilz P, Chuang IH. Subarachnoid hemorrhage caused by a fungal aneurysm of the vertebral artery as a complication of intracranial aneurysm clipping. Case report. *J Neurosurg* 1990; 73:962–964.
190. Pomposelli FB, Lamparello PJ, Riles TS, et al. Intracranial hemorrhage after carotid endarterectomy. *J Vasc Surg* 1988; 7:248–255.
191. Post KD, Onesti ST, Wisniewski T. Intracerebral hemorrhage from pituitary lesions: pituitary apoplexy. In Kaufman HH (ed): *Intracerebral Hematomas.* New York: Raven Press, 1992, pp 107–115.
192. Poungvarin N, Bhoopat W, Viriyavejakul A, et al. Effects of dexamethasone in primary supratentorial intracerebral hemorrhage. *N Engl J Med* 1987; 316:1229–1233.
193. Quest DO. Stroke: a selective history. *Neurosurgery* 1990; 27:440–445.
194. Radberg JA, Olsson JE, Radberg CT. Prognostic parameters in spontaneous intracerebral hematomas with special reference to anticoagulant treatment. *Stroke* 1991; 22:571–576.
195. Renaudin JW, George RP. Coagulopathies causing intracranial hemorrhage. In Wilkins RH, Rengachary SS (eds): *Neurosurgery.* New York: McGraw-Hill, 1985, pp 1518–1520.
196. Richardson AE. Spontaneous cerebellar haemorrhage. In Vinken PJ, Bruyn GW (eds): *Handbook of Clinical Neurology,* vol 12. New York: American Elsevier, 1972, pp 54–67.
197. Richardson A. Spontaneous intracerebral and cerebellar haemorrhage. In Russell RWR (ed): *Cerebral Arterial Disease.* Edinburgh: Churchill Livingstone, 1976, pp 210–230.
198. Roach ES, Riela AR (eds). *Pediatric Cerebrovascular Disorders.* Mount Kisco, NY: Futura Publishing Company, 1988, pp 67–94; 143–160.
199. Roberts TS, Brown R. Technical and clinical aspects of CT-directed stereotaxis. *Appl Neurophysiol* 1980; 43:170–171.
200. Ropper AH, Davis KR. Lobar cerebral hemorrhages: acute clinical syndromes in 26 cases. *Ann Neurol* 1980; 8:141–147.
201. Ropper AH, King RB. Intracranial pressure monitoring in comatose patients with cerebral hemorrhage. *Arch Neurol* 1984; 41:725–728.
202. Rosenberg GA, Kaufman DM. Cerebellar hemorrhage: reliability of clinical evaluation. *Stroke* 1976; 7:332–336.
203. Salcman M. Intracranial hemorrhage caused by brain tumor. In Kaufman HH (ed): *Intracerebral Hematomas.* New York: Raven Press, 1992, pp 95–106.
204. Samson D, Batjer HH. Intracerebral hematomas secondary to ruptured aneurysms and intracranial vascular malformations. In Kaufman HH (ed): *Intracerebral Hematomas.* New York: Raven Press, 1992, pp 75–84.
205. Sano K, Ochiai C. Clinical aspects with reference to indications for treatment. In Pia HW, Langmaid C, Zierski J (eds): *Spontaneous Intracerebral Haematomas; Advances in Diagnosis and Therapy.* New York: Springer-Verlag, 1980, pp 366–371.
206. Sano K, Yoshida S. Cerebellar haematomas. Indications and prognosis. In Pia HW, Langmaid C, Zierski J (eds): *Spontaneous Intracerebral Haematomas; Advances in Diagnosis and Therapy.* New York: Springer-Verlag, 1980, pp 348–356.
207. Schochet SS Jr, Nelson J. Vasculitis and vasculopathies. In Kaufman HH (ed): *Intracerebral Hematomas.* New York: Raven Press, 1992, pp 127–137.
208. Schwartz P. Apoplectic lesions of the brain in adults. In Vinken PJ, Bruyn GW (eds): *Handbook of Clinical Neurology,* vol 11. New York: American Elsevier, 1972, pp 578–659.
209. Scott M. Neurosurgical treatment of spontaneous intracranial hemorrhage. Importance of differential diagnosis in "cerebral apoplexy" and evaluation of long-term postoperative results. *JAMA* 1960; 172:889–895.
210. Scott M. Spontaneous intracerebral hematoma caused by cerebral neoplasms. Report of eight verified cases. *J Neurosurg* 1975; 42:338–342.
211. Segal R, Dujovny M, Nelson D, Meyer J. Local urokinase treatment for spontaneous intracerebral hematoma. *Clin Res* 1982; 30:412A (abstr).
212. Seok K, Bae HG, Yun IG. Recurrent intracerebral hemorrhage due to hypertension. *Neurosurgery* 1990; 26:586–590.
213. Shah MV, Heros RC. Intracerebral hemorrhage due to cerebral arteriovenous malformations. *Neurosurg Clin North Am* 1992; 3:567–576.
214. Shitamichi M, Nakamura J, Sasaki T, et al. Computed tomography guided stereotactic aspiration of pontine hemorrhages. *Stereotact Funct Neurosurg* 1990; 54–55:453–456.
215. Silverstein A. Primary pontine hemorrhage. In Vinken PJ, Bruyn GW (eds): *Handbook of Clinical Neurology,* vol 12. New York: American Elsevier, 1972, pp 37–53.
216. Sloan MA, Price TR, Foulkes MA, et al. Circadian rhythmicity of stroke onset: intracerebral and subarachnoid hemorrhage. *Stroke* 1992; 23:1420–1426.
217. Steiner L, Lofgren J, Zwetnow NN. Characteristics and limits of tolerance in repeated subarachnoid hemorrhage in dogs. *Acta Neurol Scand* 1975; 52:241–267.
218. Steiner L, Lofgren J, Zwetnow NN. Lethal mechanism in repeated subarachnoid hemorrhage in dogs. *Acta Neurol Scand* 1975; 52:268–293.
219. Steinke W, Sacco RL, Mohr JP, et al. Thalamic stroke. Presentation and prognosis of infarcts and hemorrhages. *Arch Neurol* 1992; 49:703–710.
220. Sundt TM Jr, Piepgras DG, Ebersold MJ, et al. Postoperative evaluation and management of complications with illustrative cases. In Sundt TM Jr (ed): *Occlusive Cerebrovascular Disease: Diagnosis and Surgical Management.* Philadelphia: WB Saunders, 1987, pp 243–260.

221. Sung C-Y, Chu N-S. Epileptic seizures in intracerebral haemorrhage. *J Neurol Neurosurg Psychiatry* 1989; 52:1273–1276.
222. Suzuki J, Ebina T. Sequential changes in tissue surrounding ICH. In Pia HW, Langmaid C, Zierski J (eds): *Spontaneous Intracerebral Haematomas; Advances in Diagnosis and Therapy.* New York: Springer-Verlag, 1980, pp 121–128.
223. Suzuki J, Sato T. Surgery for the hypertensive intracerebral hematoma—trans-sylvian approach. *Neurol Med Chir (Tokyo)* 1976; 16:115–119.
224. Sypert GW. Cerebellar hemorrhage and infarction. *Compr Ther* 1977; 3(4):42–47.
225. Sypert GW. Posterior fossa hematomas. In Fein JM, Flamm ES (eds): *Cerebrovascular Surgery.* New York: Springer-Verlag, 1985, pp 1283–1297.
226. Sypert GW, Arpin-Sypert EJ. Spontaneous posterior fossa hematomas. In Kaufman HH (ed): *Intracerebral Hematomas.* New York: Raven Press, 1992, pp 187–196.
227. Taber KH, Ford JJ, Hayman LA. Magnetic resonance imaging appearance of hemorrhage. *Neuroimaging Clin North Am* 1992; 2:61–73.
228. Tachibana O, Oki H, Hayashi Y, et al. Repetitive intratumoral hemorrhage in medulloblastoma. A case report. *Surg Neurol* 1990; 33:378–383.
229. Tanaka Y, Nishiya M, Suematsu K, et al. Pontine hemorrhage. In Mizukami M, Kogure K, Kanaya H, et al. (eds): *Hypertensive Intracerebral Hemorrhage.* New York: Raven Press, 1983, pp 205–214.
230. Teal PA, Pessin MS. Hemorrhagic transformation: the spectrum of ischemia-related brain hemorrhage. *Neurosurg Clin North Am* 1992; 3:601–610.
231. Theron J, Courtheoux P, Casasco A, et al. Local intraarterial fibrinolysis in the carotid territory. *Am J Neuroradiol* 1989; 10:753–765.
232. Todo T, Usui M, Takakura K. Treatment of severe intraventricular hemorrhage by intraventricular infusion of urokinase. *J Neurosurg* 1991; 74:81–86.
233. Tsementzis SA. Surgical management of intracerebral hematomas. *Neurosurgery* 1985; 16:562–572.
234. Unwin DH, Batjer HH, Greenlee RG Jr. Management controversy: medical versus surgical therapy for spontaneous intracerebral hemorrhage. *Neurosurg Clin North Am* 1992; 3:533–537.
235. Vaquero J, Areitio E, Leunda G, et al. Hematomas of the pons. *Surg Neurol* 1980; 14:115–118.
236. Vinters HV, Duckwiler GR. Intracranial hemorrhage in the normotensive elderly patient. *Neuroimaging Clin North Am* 1992; 2:153–169.
237. Waga S, Miyazaki M, Okada M, et al. Hypertensive putaminal hemorrhage: analysis of 182 patients. *Surg Neurol* 1986; 26:159–166.
238. Wakai S, Kumakura N, Nagai M. Lobar intracerebral hemorrhage. A clinical, radiographic, and pathological study of 29 consecutive operated cases with negative angiography. *J Neurosurg* 1992; 76:231–238.
239. Weiner HL, Cooper PR. The management of spontaneous intracerebral hemorrhage. *Contemp Neurosurg* 1992; 14(21):1–8.
240. Weisberg LA. Computerized tomography in intracranial hemorrhage. *Arch Neurol* 1979; 36:422–426.
241. Weisberg LA. Alcoholic intracerebral hemorrhage. *Stroke* 1988; 19:1565–1569.
242. Whisnant JP. The decline of stroke. *Stroke* 1984; 15:160–168.
243. Williams JL, Furlan AJ. Cerebral vascular physiology in hypertensive disease. *Neurosurg Clin North Am* 1992; 3:509–520.
244. Williams KD, Drayer BP, Bird CR. Magnetic resonance imaging in the diagnosis of intracerebral hematoma. *BNI Q* 1989; 5:16–23.
245. Wityk RJ, Caplan LR. Hypertensive intracerebral hemorrhage: epidemiology and clinical pathology. *Neurosurg Clin North Am* 1992; 3:521–532.
246. Yoshida S, Sasaki M, Oka H, et al. Acute hypertensive cerebellar hemorrhage with signs of lower brainstem compression. *Surg Neurol* 1978; 10:79–83.
247. Zamorano L, Chavantes MC, Dujovny M, et al. Endoscopic laser stereotaxis: our indication for cystic or intraventricular lesion. Presented at the 57th Annual Meeting of the American Association Neurological Surgeons, Washington, DC, April 5, 1989.

255 Coagulopathies Causing Intracranial Hemorrhage

Justin W. Renaudin
Ralph P. George

Etiology

Hemostasis involves three basic elements: vessel wall, platelets, and coagulation factors. In this chapter, a coagulopathy will be defined as a disorder of blood coagulation involving plasma coagulation factors or platelets. The discussion will focus chiefly on the more common coagulopathies that result in intracranial hemorrhage (ICH). Rare disorders of coagulation, including disorders involving coagulation factor inhibitors and qualitative platelet abnormalities that do not often result in ICH, will be covered only briefly. Vasculopathy is the subject of the next chapter.

The process of blood coagulation is complex and interactive and—even after many decades of study—is incompletely understood. It has been described in detail in an earlier chapter. Briefly, a vessel is injured, and a reaction of platelets with the injured endothelial and subendothelial tissues results. The formation of plasma (intrinsic) thromboplastic activity follows. Prothrombin is converted to thrombin in the presence of thromboplastin and calcium. Finally, fibrinogen is converted to fibrin in the presence of thrombin.

Anticoagulation Therapy and Thrombolytic Therapy

The most commonly used anticoagulants are warfarin and heparin. Warfarin retards the synthesis of vitamin-K–dependent factors (factors II, VII, IX, and X). The effects of warfarin are not immediate, and the prothrombin time will lengthen to a therapeutic level over a couple of days. The maintenance dose is titrated against the desired level. Warfarin is taken orally and is used on a long-term, outpatient basis. Among the many drugs that enhance the effect of warfarin are alcohol, aspirin, and cimetidine.

Heparin is administered either intravenously or subcutaneously. It is used on a short-term, inpatient basis and can usually be neutralized promptly with protamine sulfate. It acts as an anticoagulant at several points along the coagulation sequence. There is individual variation in the response to most anticoagulants, and one needs to monitor treatment carefully. Patients receiving heparin are monitored by following the activated partial thromboplastin time (APTT). The effect of heparin is short-lived, a matter of 4 to 8 h, whereas it customarily requires 3 to 5 days before the effect of warfarin is eliminated.

Pharmacologic anticoagulants have prevented many deaths from thrombosis and embolism. Conversely, they have resulted in some very serious complications. ICH is far more common in patients treated with warfarin than with heparin.[6]

Evidence has accumulated over the past decade that thrombolytic therapy reduces the mortality rate in patients with evolving myocardial infarction , despite the increased risk of bleeding complications.[1] Streptokinase and tissue plasminogen activator (t-PA) have been the most commonly used thrombolytic agents. The reported risk of ICH is about 1 percent in patients receiving thrombolytic therapy. Thrombolytic therapy for occlusive cerebrovascular disease is discussed elsewhere in this text. ICH may occur in this setting, as well.

Blood Dyscrasias

Thrombocytopenia is a common hematologic abnormality. A reduction in the number of circulating platelets may be due either to decreased production of platelets by the bone marrow or to increased destruction or trapping of platelets.

Most platelets are produced from megakaryocytes in the bone marrow. The platelet life-span as estimated by isotope labeling is about 9 days. A large array of drugs, various chemical and physical agents, and several diseases can cause a reduction in the number of platelets. Generally, so long as the platelet count exceeds 60,000 per cubic millimeter, no untoward hematologic complications will ensue. Once the platelet count falls below 20,000 per cubic millimeter, the patient is distinctly at risk for hemorrhage.

Qualitative platelet disorders may be inherited or acquired. Von Willebrand's disease is an inherited hemostatic defect caused by lack of von Willebrand's factor (vWF), which is necessary for proper platelet function.[4] Aspirin will inhibit platelet aggregation to a significant degree and deserves mention because it is so commonly used. The inhibitory effect of aspirin lasts for the life-span of the platelet. Von Willebrand's disease and its variants, as well as aspirin use, will prolong bleeding time, but we have no personal experience of these conditions causing ICH.

Hemophilia is an inherited hemorrhagic disease caused by a deficiency of a clotting factor. Factor VIII deficiency (hemophilia A) accounts for 85 percent of hemophilia cases, and factor IX deficiency (hemophilia B) for about 14 percent of cases. The hemostatic level of the involved factor is about 30 percent, and abnormal bleeding usually ceases if the factor level is 30 percent or greater.

The liver is the main site of synthesis of the large majority of plasma coagulation factors. Therefore, a coagulopathy may be present in various types of severe liver disease; alcoholics with severe liver disease may be further burdened with thrombocytopenia and are particularly at risk for intracranial bleeding.

In leukemia, ICH accounts for about one-half of the serious bleeding episodes. ICH is more likely to develop in leukemia patients with very high leukocyte counts, and in granulocytic more than in lymphocytic leukemia. Leukostasis in the small cerebral vessels and disruption of the vessel wall is a serious risk in patients with white blood counts greater than 100,000 per cubic millimeter.

Thrombocytopenia, ranging from mild to severe, has been observed in 90 percent of leukemic patients with ICH. Other coagulation abnormalities also may be observed in patients with leukemia.

Clinical Presentation

As a general rule, hereditary coagulation factor deficiencies—hemophilias A and B—usually present at a younger age and almost exclusively affect males. A history of episodes of hemarthrosis is common.

Thrombocytopenic patients frequently manifest perechial hemorrhages. Acute immunologic thrombocytopenic purpura is more common in the younger population; medication-induced thrombocytopenia is usually seen in adults.

In some instances of ICH associated with a coagulopathy, the hemorrhage is caused by trauma, which may be mild or even unnoticed. The history may provide useful clues that a coagulopathy exists. The neurological symptoms and signs of ICH are similar in patients whether or not they have a coagulopathy. This fact merits emphasis, since patients suspected of ICH will be examined with computed tomography, and, if indicated, an operative procedure may follow promptly. A screening survey for patients who might have a coagulopathy and cannot give a history would include a complete blood count with a quantitative platelet count and measurement of prothrombin time, APTT, and bleeding time. Failure to recognize a coagulopathy before operation might lead to difficult, if not uncontrollable, bleeding during the operative procedure.

A review of the literature of published figures indicates that subdural hematoma is far more common than intracerebral hematoma in patients receiving anticoagulants. This has been the observation of Iizuka[3] and Silverstein[5] in large reviews. The most common presenting symptom is headache, and headache must be regarded seriously in any patient on anticoagulants. The presence of arterial hypertension, poorly controlled anticoagulation, and repeated episodes of trauma are important aspects of the history.

The incidence of ICH in patients with thrombocytopenia is between 1 and 4 percent. Bleeding may be intracerebral, subdural, or subarachnoid in location. Intracerebral bleeding is the most common.

Central nervous system bleeding is still a leading cause of morbidity and mortality among hemophiliacs. In an 11-year study from 1965 to 1976, there were 65 patients with ICH in a population of 2500 hemophiliacs.[2] Of this population, 2100 were factor-VIII–deficient and 400 were factor-IX–deficient. The most common presenting symptom was headache or vomiting. The site of ICH in the 65 patients was fairly evenly divided among the subdural, subarachnoid, and intracerebral spaces. Two-thirds of these patients were under 18 years of age; of this group, one-half were under 3. A symptom-free interval of greater than 24 h with a mean of 4 ± 2.2 days was noted in one-half of their patients with central nervous system trauma. Such an interval is common in patients with subdural hematoma, hemophiliac or not, but this longer latency period observed in some instances of intracerebral bleeding underlines the incidence of indolent bleeding in the hemophiliac population. Recurrent CNS bleeding will occur in 26 percent. The vast majority of patients with ICH had factor levels less than 2 percent.

Of patients with severe liver disease, alcoholics are at the highest risk. The coagulation abnormalities and thrombocytopenia are contributing factors to the known increased incidence of ICH in alcoholics.

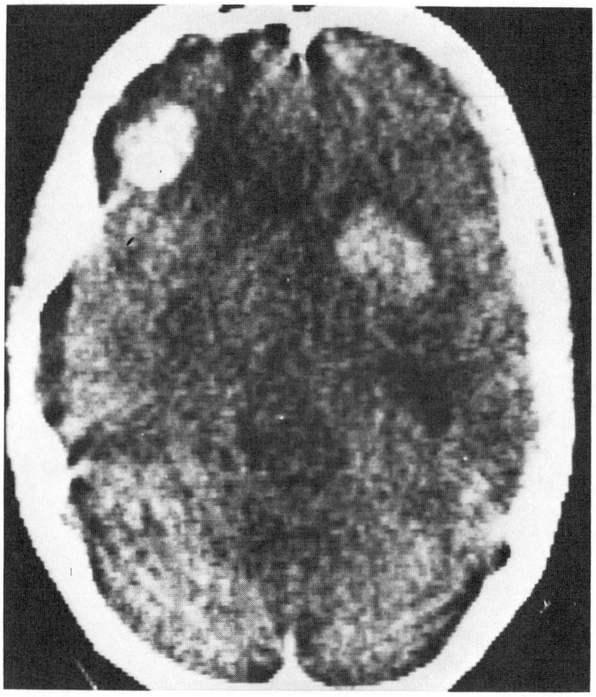

Figure 255-1 A CT scan without contrast enhancement, showing multiple hemorrhages in a patient with acute granulocytic leukemia. There were two more hematomas in other CT sections. The white blood cell count was 326,000 per cubic millimeter, and the platelet count was 29,000 per cubic millimeter.

ICH in leukemic patients is most often intracerebral; the subarachnoid space is the next most common site, and the subdural space is the least common. Almost half of patients with intracerebral bleeding will demonstrate multiple sites (Fig. 255-1).

Hematologic Therapy

Some of these disorders are complex. A close liaison with an expert in hematology is mandatory.

In patients receiving warfarin, the anticoagulant is stopped immediately, and vitamin K_1 is administered. If necessary, fresh frozen plasma may be given.

Thrombocytopenic patients may be treated with random donor platelet units. In theory, one unit of platelets should increase the platelet count of a 70-kg man by approximately 10,000 per cubic millimeter, although this increase is rarely obtained in practice. Patients in whom the thrombocytopenia is due to immunologic disturbances may benefit from corticosteroids. Some of these patients are candidates for splenectomy, and surgical consultation will be in order.

Assays for factors VIII and IX are available in most large hospital laboratories and are essential to the diagnosis and regulation of treatment in the hemophiliac. In classic hemophilia, the factor VIII level should be raised to 100 percent for operations and maintained at least 30 to 50 percent for 2 weeks after the ICH and operation. There are now available specific factors for factor VIII and IX replacement. These are purified by monoclonal antibody processing and significantly reduce the risk of transfusion transmitted disease.

Hematologic treatment of coagulation factor abnormalities in severe liver disease may be very frustrating. Vitamin K_1 should be administered, and fresh frozen plasma may be transfused. Coexisting thrombocytopenia is treated with platelet transfusion.

Thrombocytopenia in leukemic patients is managed with platelet transfusions.

Surgical Therapy

In treating patients with operable intracranial lesions, the neurosurgeon should establish a close working relationship with the hematologist. If the patient's condition will tolerate the procedure, and no contraindication exists, any nontrivial subdural or epidural hematoma should be evacuated. The timing of the operative procedure requires collaboration with the clinical laboratories and the blood bank. The clinical laboratories must ensure that clotting factors and platelet counts have reached at least acceptable levels. The blood bank must be prepared to meet estimated surgical requirements of whole blood, packed red blood cells, coagulation factors, and platelets.

The site, size, side, and shift measurements will influence the management of an intracerebral hematoma. Serial clinical examinations and CT scans are beneficial, and if an operation is indicated, coordination with the hematologist, clinical laboratories, and blood bank is essential.

Silverstein has recommended that anticonvulsants be administered to hemophiliacs with ICH, whether they are operated on or not.[5] Without anticonvulsants, the incidence of seizures in hemophiliacs with ICH is slightly over 50 percent. The margin of safety in these patients is low, and prophylactic anticonvulsant treatment is recommended. Hemophiliacs must be maintained for 2 weeks after operation with factor VIII or factor IX replacement so that their levels stay at 30 percent or higher.

Results

Many factors will influence the results. Among these are the severity of the underlying disease and the location of the intracranial hemorrhage. Intracranial hemorrhage associated with anticoagulant therapy has been found to be more often subdural than intracerebral, and the outcome has been good in about two-thirds of these patients.

The mortality from ICH in the hemophiliac population is 34 percent.[2] Among the patients reported by Eyster et al., of the group that died, one-fourth had inhibitors to the deficient factor. Of the hemophiliacs who survived, half showed motor impairment, mental retardation, or seizure disorders. The other half demonstrated no neurological deficit.[2]

The results of treatment are poor in patients with chronic severe liver disease or leukemia.

References

1. De Jaegere PP, Arnold AA, Balk AH, et al. Intracranial hemorrhage in association with thrombolytic therapy: incidence and clinical predictive factors. *J Am Coll Cardiol* 1992; 19:289–294.
2. Eyster ME, Gill FM, Blatt PM, et al. Central nervous system bleeding in hemophiliacs. *Blood* 1978; 51:1179–1188.
3. Iizuka J. Intracranial and intraspinal hematomas associated with anticoagulant therapy. *Neurochirurgia (Stuttg)* 1972; 15:15–25.
4. Miale JB. *Laboratory Medicine, Hematology,* 6th ed. St Louis: Mosby, 1982.
5. Silverstein A. Neurological complications in patients with hemorrhagic diathesis. In Vinken PJ, Bruyn GW (eds): *Handbook of Clinical Neurology,* vol 38. Amsterdam: North-Holland, 1979, pp 53–91.
6. Snyder M, Renaudin J. Intracranial hemorrhage associated with anticoagulation therapy. *Surg Neurol* 1977; 7:31–34.

256

Vasculopathies Affecting the Central Nervous System

Setti S. Rengachary
Abhay Sanan

A host of heterogeneous pathological processes affect blood vessels. Attempts to classify vascular disorders are hampered by poor understanding of the etiology and pathogenesis of many of them.[8] Current knowledge leads to the classification proposed in Table 256-1. Imperfect as this classification may be, it provides an overview of the spectrum of vascular disorders. The emphasis in this chapter is on the miscellany of vascular disorders that are not discussed elsewhere in the text and are of some relevance to the nervous system.

Temporal Arteritis

Temporal arteritis is a vasculopathy of unknown etiology affecting the elderly, past the age of 50.[11] It involves mainly the branches of the external carotid artery. When diagnosed early, the disease may be treated effectively with steroids, and blindness, a dreaded complication, may be averted.

Numerous synonyms have been used to describe this syndrome, but none is satisfactory. Thus, the terms "temporal arteritis" and "cranial arteritis" are topographically too restrictive, because in some individuals larger extracranial vessels, such as branches of the aorta, may be affected. "Giant cell arteritis" may be a misleading term, since giant cells are not always found, nor is their presence necessary to establish the histologic diagnosis if other criteria are met; even if found, they are not exclusive to this disease. Similar criticisms may be leveled against such terms as "arteritis of the aged," "granulomatous arteritis," and "polymyalgia arteritica."

The first ancient reference to temporal arteritis is in the *Tadkivat of Ali Ibn Isa* from the tenth century, in which headache and inflammation of the temporal muscle was related to blindness.[2] Certain paintings from around the fifteenth century depicting individuals with very prominent temporal arteries and other external features suggestive of temporal arteritis have not escaped the attention of present-day rheumatologists.[6] Notable among them are Jan Van Eyck's *The Virgin with the Canon* (1436) and Pieri di Cosimo's *Portrait of Francesco Gamberti* (1505) (Fig. 256-1). Redlich has proposed that Hitler may have suffered from the disease, but other authors find this diagnosis unconvincing and consider that he suffered from cluster headaches.[18]

Hutchinson was the first to describe this disease in 1890. His patient was an octogenarian who presented with inflamed, tender temporal arteries. Hutchinson believed that the disease was caused by a tight-fitting hat. Horton and colleagues reported seven cases in 1932. They emphasized the importance of headache and jaw

TABLE 256-1 A Classification of Vasculopathies

I. Degenerative arteriopathies
   A. Atherosclerosis
   B. Monckeberg's medial calcific sclerosis
   C. Arteriolosclerosis
      1. Proliferative
      2. Hyaline
II. Systemic necrotizing vasculitides
   A. Classic polyarteritis nodosa
   B. Allergic granulomatous angiitis (Churg-Strauss)
   C. Granulomatous angiitis of the nervous system
   D. "Overlap syndrome" (features of both polyarteritis nodosa and allergic granulomatosis)
III. Hypersensitivity vasculitides
   A. Drug-related vasculitides
   B. Henoch-Schönlein purpura
   C. Serum sickness and serum sickness-like reactions
   D. Vasculitis associated with malignancy (especially lymphoid neoplasms)
IV. Wegener's granulomatosis
V. Giant cell arteritides
   A. Temporal arteritis
   B. Takayasu's arteritis
VI. Intravascular lymphomatosis
VII. Specific disorders associated with vasculitis
   A. Arteritis associated with lupus erythematous
   B. Arteritis associated with rheumatoid arthritis
   C. Arteritis associated with acute rheumatic fever
   D. Arteritis associated with scleroderma
   E. Arteritis associated with sarcoidosis
VIII. Miscellaneous vasculopathies
   A. Amyloid angiopathy
   B. Thromboangiitis obliterans
   C. Vasculopathy induced by x-irradiation
   D. Neoplastic encirclement or invasion of vessels
   E. Moyamoya disease
IX. Infectious arteritides
   A. Bacterial
   B. Tuberculous
   C. Syphilitic (meningovascular and gummatous)
   D. Yeast, fungal, parasitic, viral, and rickettsial
      1. Actinomycosis
      2. Aspergillosis
      3. North American blastomycosis
      4. Candidiasis
      5. Cladosporiosis
      6. Coccidioidomycosis
      7. Cryptococcosis
      8. Histoplasmosis
      9. Nocardiosis
      10. Mucormycosis
      11. Cysticercosis
      12. Viral
      13. Rickettsial

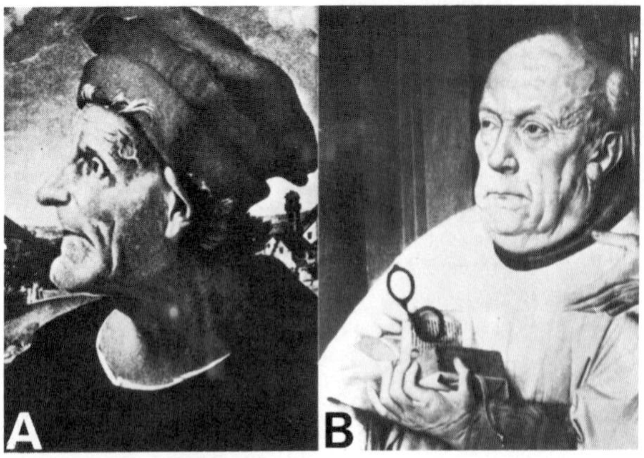

Figure 256-1 Paintings from around the fifteenth century depicting individuals with an appearance suggestive of temporal arteritis. *A. Portrait of Francesco Gamberti* by Pieri di Cosimo, 1505 (Rijkmuseum, Amsterdam). *B.* Canon Vander Paele in Jan Van Eyck's *The Virgin with the Canon,* 1436. (Groeningemuseum, Bruges, Belgium.)

claudication in this syndrome and presented the histologic findings for the first time. Numerous additional reports have appeared since then, especially from North America and Europe, emphasizing other facets of the disease, such as the occurrence of blindness, the association with polymyalgia rheumatica, and the involvement of larger systemic arteries.

Temporal arteritis appears to be more prevalent in northern climates and in persons of Scandinavian descent; it is quite uncommon in Asians, blacks, and American Indians. An incidence of 2.4 per 100,000 per year for the general population and 17.4 per 100,000 per year for those over the age of 50 and a prevalence rate of 233 per 100,000 in the latter age group have been recorded in Olmstead County, Minnesota. Of the affected individuals, 65 percent are women. The highest incidence occurs in individuals over 70 years of age.

Clinical Features

The onset may be abrupt, but quite frequently vague constitutional symptoms such as fatigue, malaise, weight loss, or low-grade fever have been present for weeks to months before a definitive diagnosis is made. "Occult malignancy," "fever of unknown origin," or "depression" is often the admitting diagnosis. Severe boring headaches localized to the temporal regions are seen as an initial symptom in 90 percent of affected individuals. Variations in the nature and location of the headache are sufficiently common to warrant a high index of suspicion of temporal arteritis in any elderly individual with the onset of a new headache. Scalp pain may be present, especially around the superficial temporal or occipital artery, which may worsen with combing the hair, wearing a hat, or laying the head on a pillow. The superficial temporal artery may be swollen, nodular, tender, and pulseless. Jaw claudication after chewing is thought to be pathognomonic of the disease. It results from involvement of the facial artery; less commonly, claudication in the tongue ("tongue angina"), pharyngeal muscles, calf, or arm may occur. Rarely, gangrene of the scalp, tongue, or an extremity may set in owing to vascular occlusion. Respiratory symptoms (cough, sore throat, hoarseness) are not uncommon, but their exact cause is not clear.

Visual symptoms are present in 25 to 50 percent of affected individuals, but permanent visual loss has been recorded in only 5 to 10 percent of patients. Patients generally have systemic symptoms for several weeks or months before visual symptoms set in. Although abrupt blindness frequently occurs, a history of amaurosis fugax, scintillating scotomata, ophthalmoplegia, or transient diplopia often precedes the onset of blindness. Visual loss is a reflection of ischemia of the retina or optic nerve secondary to involvement of the ophthalmic, the posterior ciliary, or, less commonly, the central retinal artery. Rarely, cortical blindness occurs from infarction of the calcarine cortex. Funduscopic examination will show evidence of ischemic optic neuropathy with a swollen, pale disc, small hemorrhages, and a few retinal cotton-wool patches. These features coupled with pallor of the opposite disc constitute the "pseudo Foster-Kennedy syndrome." In cases of central retinal artery occlusion, the retinal vessels appear obliterated, the disc is swollen, and the macula is cherry red. In retrobulbar ischemic neuropathy, the fundus may appear normal.

Involvement of the contralateral eye can occur within a few days or weeks. Blindness, once it occurs, usually is irreversible; thus, the primary goal in management is preventing blindness by prompt treatment with corticosteroids once the diagnosis is suspected or established. Extraocular muscle palsy or ptosis may occur owing to involvement of the vasa nervorum of the cranial nerves supplying these muscles.

Caselli and coworkers have reviewed the neurological manifestation of temporal arteritis in detail, and they report that 7 percent of their patients had cerebrovascular events and 14 percent had a neuropathic syndrome. Temporal arteritis seems to affect only the vessels that contain elastin. Because intracranial vessels lose elastin about 5 mm after penetrating the dura, the brain parenchymal vessels are not directly involved; thus, the central nervous system symptoms result from embolic disease of the extracranial carotid and vertebral arteries. A forme fruste variant is "occult" temporal arteritis. The patient presents with the sudden onset of blindness without any other associated symptoms, although a temporal artery biopsy is positive for arteritis.

One of the most underrecognized facts about temporal arteritis is that, despite its name, more than just the superficial temporal arteries are involved, and the aorta and its major branches are commonly affected. Involvement of the subclavian, axillary, and brachial arteries may produce claudication in the arm, bruits over the major arterial trunks, and decreased pulses. The common or internal carotid artery may be tender, swollen, and cordlike. Aortic dissection or rupture has been reported. Although the renal arteries may be involved, the renal parenchyma is rarely affected, thus differentiating this disease from polyarteritis nodosa. Occasional instances of myocardial infarction from coronary arteritis have been reported. The most severe involvement is found in the superficial temporal arteries, the vertebral arteries, and the ophthalmic and posterior ciliary arteries.

A localized eosinophilic vasculitis of the external carotid artery and its branches occurs rarely in children and young adults. This entity has been termed *juvenile temporal arteritis* and has a more benign course. It is distinguished from temporal arteritis by the absence of constitutional symptoms, the presence of a normal erythrocyte sedimentation rate, and a histopathology without granulomatous changes. The disease is self-limiting, and no treatment is needed. In particular, steroids are unnecessary and may be harmful.[22]

Polymyalgia Rheumatica

The symptom complex[5] of polymyalgia rheumatica occurs in about half of patients with temporal arteritis; it may begin before the symptoms related to arteritis develop, occur concurrently with them, or develop after they appear. The exact relationship between the two entities is unclear. Polymyalgia rheumatica consists of arthralgias and myalgias in the neck, shoulder, and hip girdle associated with an elevated sedimentation rate. The symptoms are worst on arising in the morning. The muscles are not tender to palpation. Muscle enzymes and the results of electrical and histologic studies of the muscles are normal. Inflammatory synovitis of the affected joints, which perhaps explains the clinical symptomatology, may be demonstrated with radionuclide scanning and with histologic examination. In about a third of the patients with polymyalgia rheumatica, temporal artery biopsy will show evidence of arteritis in the absence of specific clinical symptoms related to the arteries.

Pathology

Any one or a combination of the following features may be found (Fig. 256-2): (1) disruption of the internal elastic membrane; (2) the presence of Langhans giant cells in the region of the internal elastic membrane; (3) an inflammatory infiltrate consisting of lymphocytes (mostly T cells), eosinophils, plasma cells, and, less frequently, neutrophils through all layers of the vessel wall; and (4) intimal proliferation and thrombosis. The giant cells are not always present; their presence is unrelated to prognosis. The T-cell infiltrate has been characterized as being of the helper subset ($CD4^+$).

The exact etiology and pathogenesis of the disease are not understood, but various lines of evidence suggest a genetic predisposition with an overlying autoimmune process. The higher frequency of the disease in people of northern European descent and sporadic reports of familial aggregation suggest a genetic influence. Although no human leukocyte antigen (HLA) type consistently accompanies the disease, HLA-DR4 is associated with it more than would be expected by chance alone. A growing body of evidence implicates the immune system. Circulating immune complexes and levels of interleukin-6 (an immune mediator of inflammation) correlate with the clinical state of the disease. The lymphocytic infiltrate, and the immunoglobulin and complement deposition are most striking adjacent to the internal elastic lamina, and some have hypothesized that the disease is initiated by damage to elastin in the arterial wall, which results in an autoimmune response to elastin. The fact that the disease involves primarily extracranial branches of the carotid artery, which are rich in elastin, and spares intracranial vessels, which lack elastin, lends some support to this hypothesis. However, antielastin antibodies have not been identified, nor has clear phagocytosis of elastin been documented by electron microscopy, so the exact immunoactivating antigen remains a mystery.

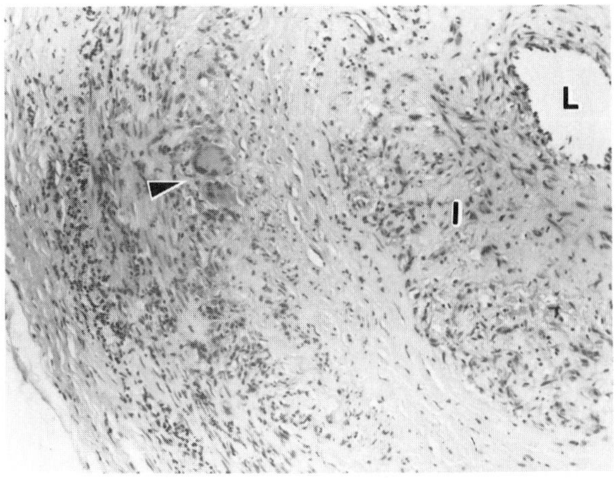

Figure 256-2 A cross-section of the superficial temporal artery showing features characteristic of temporal arteritis: narrowing of the lumen (L), fibrous thickening of the intima (I), giant cells *(arrowhead)* at the usual site of the internal elastic lamina, and diffuse mononuclear infiltration of the media and adventitia. (Courtesy of Venkata R. Challa, M.D.)

Laboratory Data

The erythrocyte sedimentation rate (by the Westergren method) is consistently elevated (usually greater than 50 mm/h), although occasional cases of biopsy-proven temporal arteritis with a normal sedimentation rate have been reported. Mild normochromic or hypochromic anemia with hemoglobin values in the range of 9 to 12 g/dl is common. The leukocyte count is usually normal, but mild elevation may occur. Serum protein electrophoresis reveals an increase in α-2 globulin and fibrinogen. Antinuclear antibodies and the rheumatoid factor are negative. Hepatocellular dysfunction, which is present in one-third of cases, may be reflected in an increase in serum glutamic oxaloacetic transaminase and alkaline phosphatase levels. A liver biopsy may show granulomatous hepatitis. Hypothyroidism seems to be the only autoimmune disease associated with giant cell arteritis, and patients with giant cell arteritis have three times the risk of developing hypothyroidism as age-matched controls.

Diagnosis

The American College of Rheumatology has published criteria for the diagnosis of temporal arteritis: (1) disease onset beginning at age 50 or older; (2) development of new headache; (3) temporal artery tenderness or decreased pulsation; (4) elevated sedimentation rate; and (5) temporal artery biopsy consistent with a granulomatous vasculitis. The presence of three or more of these criteria gives a better than 90 percent sensitivity and specificity for correct diagnosis.[10] Selective arteriography of the superficial temporal artery has been recommended in the past both for diagnosing the disease solely on the basis of angiographic abnormalities and for identifying pathologic segments of the affected artery to aid in the selection of a biopsy site (because in about 30 percent of patients "skip lesions" occur). Practical experience with arteriography, however, has been disappointing. No pattern of angiographic abnormality typical for giant cell arteritis has been found. The findings consist of nonspecific segmental narrowing of the vessel, a finding representative far more often of atherosclerosis than of giant cell arteritis in a geriatric population. Temporal arteriography is not a substitute for temporal artery biopsy.

Temporal artery biopsy is the most crucial and most specific diagnostic study. At least 3 to 5 cm of the artery should be removed to make sure that representative pathologic segments are included in the specimen. Before biopsy of the artery is undertaken, careful attention must be paid to the clinical data to make certain that the patient is not dependent on the superficial temporal artery as a major collateral channel for perfusing the brain owing to occlusion of the internal carotid artery in the neck, or that the patient may not require this artery for bypass grafting for the same reason. If the biopsy is negative and the clinical suspicion is high, biopsy of the contralateral temporal artery should be undertaken.

Treatment

Corticosteroid therapy should be instituted as soon as the diagnosis is suspected or established. If the clinical history and findings are suggestive of temporal arteritis, blood is drawn for a sedimentation rate and electrophoresis, the patient is started on 45 to 60 mg of prednisone daily in divided doses, and temporal artery biopsy is scheduled for the next elective day. One should not postpone the therapy with steroids until arterial biopsy is completed, because a few days of steroid therapy does not materially alter the histologic appearance of the lesion. Symptoms respond dramatically, and the sedimentation rate drops rapidly with prednisone. The effective starting dose should be continued until the clinical symptoms and laboratory data have normalized. This generally takes 3 weeks to a month. Thereafter, the prednisone dosage is tapered gradually to a maintenance level of 15 to 25 mg daily. Therapy should be monitored with clinical evaluations and sedimentation rate determinations. It is important to emphasize that the sedimentation rate is not always reliable in monitoring disease activity; indeed, clinical progression with normal sedimentation rates is a well-described phenomenon. In this regard, the interleukin-6 value may be more helpful, since it is much more sensitive in correlating with the disease state.[20] It remains to be seen whether this test will become practical enough to enter clinical practice. Occasional exacerbations may require a temporary increase in the dose of the steroid. Therapy may have to be continued for 6 months to 2 years. Alternate-day steroid therapy has been shown to be less effective than daily therapy. For patients who cannot tolerate high steroid doses because of side effects, oral methotrexate has been shown to reduce the steroid requirement. Once visual loss sets in, it is not generally reversed by steroid therapy, but high-dose intravenous pulse methyprednisolone should be tried if the visual loss has lasted less than 48 h, because recovery of sight has been documented in a few cases. In patients with polymyalgia rheumatica without vascular symptoms or signs, treatment with nonsteroidal anti-inflammatory drugs may be adequate. Long-term steroid therapy may be associated with certain well-known complications, for example, osteoporosis and compression fracture of a vertebra, the development of cushingoid features, gastrointestinal bleeding, aseptic necrosis of the femoral head, steroid myopathy, and an increased requirement for insulin in diabetics, to cite a few. The symptoms of this disease are effectively controlled with steroid therapy, and, once treated, patients can expect a normal life span.

Takayasu's Arteritis

Takayasu's arteritis (synonyms: pulseless disease, aortic arch arteritis, obliterative brachiocephalic arteritis, aortitis syndrome, Martorell's syndrome, Raeder-Harbits syndrome, reversed coarctation syndrome), a rarer form of giant cell arteritis, is named after the Japanese ophthalmologist who described in 1908 a wreath-like arteriovenous anastomosis around the optic disc induced by retinal ischemia (Fig. 256-3).[17] There are many similarities and differences between temporal arteritis and Takayasu's arteritis (Table 256-2).

Takayasu's disease has a strong predilection for young women (10 to 45 years), with a female-to-male ratio of 9:1. Although the disease has been reported from all parts of the world, most cases have been from Japan. It is also prevalent in India, Thailand, China, Korea, South America, and Israel. Among the Jews, the Sephardim are affected and the Ashkenazim are spared. The etiology of the disease is unknown, but the demonstration of high titers of antiaorta antibodies in a significant number of proven cases suggest an autoimmune process directed against the aorta and its major branches. Furthermore, a genetic susceptibility for the development and severity of the disease is suggested by recent HLA gene typing. Increased frequencies of HLA-Bw52 in Asians and of MB3 and DR4 in the North American population have been recorded. Very rarely, Takayasu's arteritis is seen in conjunction with systemic lupus erythematosus, but this occurrence is thought to be only coincidental.

Typically, the arch of the aorta and its major branches, the brachiocephalic, common carotid, and subclavian arteries, are afflicted (Fig. 256-4). In one-third of patients, there is evidence of involvement of the descending thoracic and abdominal aorta and their branches. Vertebral, mesenteric, renal celiac, pulmonary, iliac, and coronary arteries are less commonly involved. Interestingly, in Takayasu's arteritis the intracranial vessels do not show

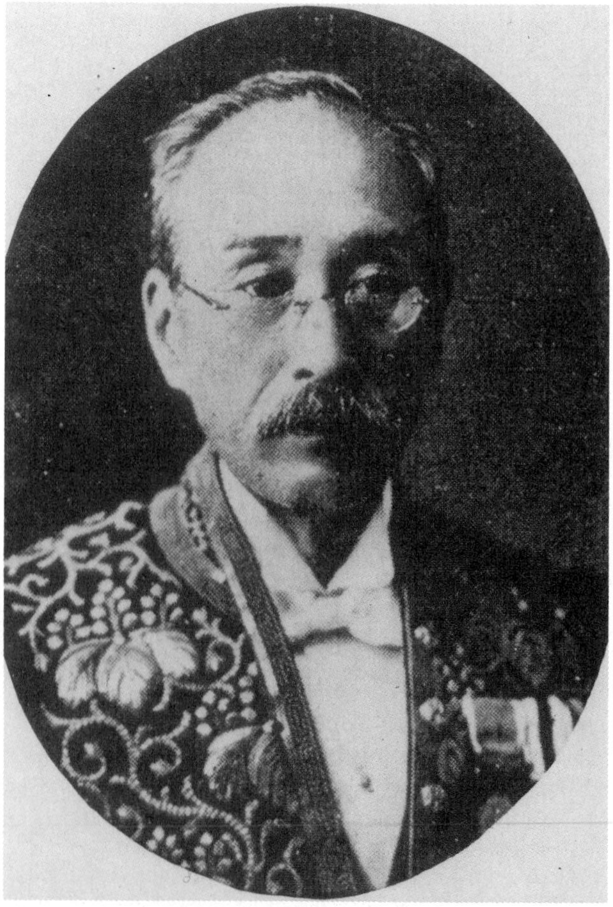

Figure 256-3 Dr. Mikito Takayasu (1860–1938).

TABLE 256-2 Comparison of Two of the Giant Cell Arteritides

	Temporal Arteritis	Takayasu's Arteritis
Epidemiology	Disease of the elderly (50–90 years); slightly higher prevalence in women; more prevalent in northern climates, especially in persons of Scandinavian descent; quite uncommon in Asians, blacks, and American Indians.	Disease of young women and children (10–45 years); male to female ratio is 1:9; although reported from all over the world, most cases are from Japan.
Arteries involved	Typically involves branches of the external carotid artery; involvement of the ophthalmic, posterior ciliary, or central retinal artery leads to blindness; the aorta or its branches may sometimes be involved.	Typically involves the arch of the aorta and its major branches; less commonly the abdominal aorta and its branches.
Pathology	Granulomatous panarteritis; disruption of the internal elastic membrane is an early feature; inflammatory infiltrate consists of lymphocytes, eosinophils, plasma cells, Langhans-type giant cells, and less frequently neutrophils, and involves all layers of the vessel wall.	Histologic changes are virtually the same as those of temporal arteritis except for the following subtle differences: infiltration by giant cells is less common in Takayasu's arteritis; in general, temporal arteritis begins in the media, whereas Takayasu's arteritis begins at the junction of the media and adventitia.
Etiology	Thought to be an autoimmune process directed against the elastic lamina of the arteries.	An autoimmune process directed against the aorta and its major branches; high titers of antiaorta antibodies support this hypothesis.
Clinical manifestations	Prodrome consisting of malaise, fatigue, loss of appetite, and anemia, followed by headaches. Half of patients have manifestations of polymyalgia rheumatica. Blindness is a dreaded complication.	Prodromal symptoms are present but may not be striking. Symptoms and signs related to decreased blood flow to the head and upper extremities: vertigo, syncope, convulsions, dementia, trophic changes in the skin and mucous membranes of the head, impaired or absent pulses in the upper extremities, bruit in the neck.
Laboratory data	Elevated sedimentation rate; mild anemia; increase in α-2 globluin, IL-6, and fibrinogen. Evidence of hepatocellular dysfunction. Temporal artery biopsy may show pathognomonic changes.	Elevated sedimentation rate; aortography may show stenosis or occlusion of the aortic arch or its major branches; results of arterial biopsy are pathognomonic.
Treatment	Dramatic response to steroid therapy. The disease is self-limited.	Moderate response to steroid therapy; the disease is usually relentlessly progressive; surgical excision of a stenotic segment and grafting may be necessary.

changes of vascular disease, despite major occlusions in the large arteries in the root of the neck, even among individuals who develop ischemic symptoms. Thus, the development of ischemic symptoms may not necessarily relate to the extent of angiographically demonstrated occlusion but, rather, to the presence or absence of collateral circulation between intracranial and extracranial vessels.

The histology of the affected vessel is one of granulomatous panarteritis. In the early stages, granulomatous inflammation with infiltration by lymphocytes, plasma cells, reticular cells, and multinucleate giant cells occurs at the junction of the media and adventitia. The inflammation then spreads through the thickness of the vessel wall. Lymphocytic infiltration and endothelial proliferation occur around the vasa vasorum. The elastic fibers and the smooth muscles in the media undergo necrosis and are replaced by collagen fibers. In the end stages, fibrosis of the media and adventitia and thickening of the intima lead to severe stenosis of the affected vessel. Diffuse calcification of affected areas is very common. Thrombotic occlusion of the lumen occurs terminally. Ectatic dilation and aneurysm formation from weakening of the vessel wall owing to scarring occur infrequently.

Early prodromal symptoms include asthenia, lassitude, weight loss, vague musculoskeletal pain, arthralgias, pain over the involved arteries, and low-grade fever. As the arteries become stenotic, symptoms and signs of ischemia of the head and upper extremities set in. These include dizziness, syncope, visual impairment, convulsions, dementia, and claudication in the upper limbs. All symptoms seem to worsen with activity. The upper limbs may feel cool and be pulseless. Bruits may be heard over the root of the neck. Trophic changes consisting of atrophic skin over the face and scalp, alopecia, loss of teeth, and ulcerations of the lips and the tip of the nose may occur in the late stages. Funduscopic examination may show preretinal hemorrhages and arteriovenous anastomoses around the optic disc. The patient may assume a stooped, head-low position in an attempt to improve the blood supply to the head. Despite the occlusion of major cervical vessels, stroke is not very frequent, because the slow progression allows for the development of a sufficient collateral blood supply. Hypertension occurs in about half of the patients and may result from narrowing of the thoracic or abdominal aorta, rigidity of the aortic wall, or renal artery involvement. To detect the hypertension, the blood pressure has to be recorded from the legs. Death usually occurs as a result of the cardiac involvement and, less commonly, from a cerebrovascular accident.

The erythrocyte sedimentation rate is elevated; a normochromic, normocytic anemia may be found, and α-2 globulin, fibrinogen, and γ-globulin values may be elevated. Carotid duplex imaging shows circumferential thickening of the common carotid artery with normal-appearing internal and external carotid arteries. Such thickening may reverse with steroid therapy.

Steroids are helpful in suppressing the early systemic symptoms and reducing the inflammation of the affected arteries. The pulse volume may improve, and the ischemic symptoms may subside. After fibrosis of the arterial wall and intraluminal thrombosis have occurred, the response to steroids is less dramatic. The roles of anticoagulants, platelet inhibitors, vasodilators, nonsteroidal

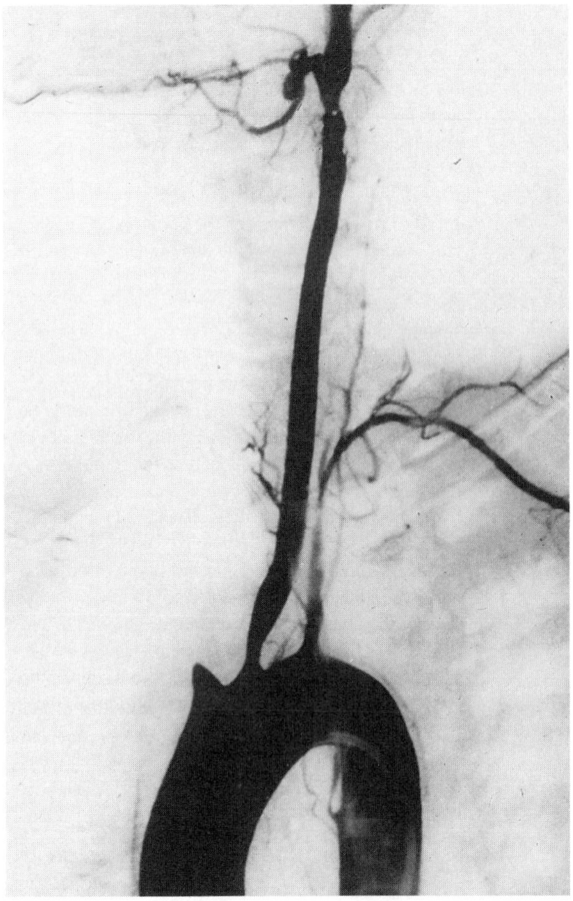

Figure 256-4 Arch aortogram showing a normal aortic arch but complete occlusion of the innominate artery. There is proximal stenosis of the left common carotid and subclavian arteries. (Courtesy of Richard E. Latchaw, M.D.)

anti-inflammatory agents, cytotoxic drugs, and balloon angioplasty in this disease remain to be elucidated.

After collagenization has occurred, surgical measures to resect or bypass a stenotic segment should be resorted to, particularly if symptoms of cerebral ischemia are present. It should be noted that cerebral ischemia is often secondary to stenosis of the thoracic aorta rather than the cervical vessels. Ideally, grafting should start from the ascending aorta and end in the major extracranial cerebral vessels. Surgical results are generally good in preventing stroke. Late complications of grafting include graft occlusion and graft stenosis or aneurysm formation at the suture line.[9]

Primary Cerebral Amyloid (Congophilic) Angiopathy

As its name implies, primary cerebral amyloid angiopathy is a clinicopathologic entity characterized by deposition of amyloid substance in the walls of cerebral and leptomeningeal vessels.[19] It is a part of a family of amyloid-depositing conditions, including Alzheimer's disease and the slow virus infections. The amyloid type (β-protein) found in primary cerebral amyloid angiopathy is also found in Alzheimer's disease, but the following distinguishing characteristics justify regarding the vessel condition as a distinct nosologic entity: (1) Patients with amyloid angiopathy do not necessarily have dementia; (2) senile plaques are not necessary for the diagnosis of amyloid angiopathy; and (3) most patients with the sporadic form of Alzheimer's disease do not have vascular deposition of amyloid. Nevertheless, most patients with Alzheimer's disease also have cerebral angiopathy, and approximately 50 percent of those with cerebral amyloid angiopathy have changes characteristic of Alzheimer's disease at autopsy.

Amyloid was originally thought to be a starchlike substance because of its characteristic reaction with iodine, but chemical analysis indicates that it is a protein. The nature of the protein varies in different disorders that involve amyloid deposition, thus accounting for different types of amyloid. In central nervous system amyloidosis, the viscera are spared; the reverse occurs in systemic amyloidosis with a few exceptions.

The cardinal clinical manifestation of amyloid angiopathy is dementia, although, as stated earlier, a subset of patients escape it. The clinical and radiologic features on occasion simulate the low-pressure hydrocephalus syndrome, but cerebrospinal fluid shunting fails to reverse the symptoms. Operative procedures on the brain in patients with cerebral amyloid angiopathy carry a higher than usual risk of postoperative hemorrhagic complications.[12] This is attributed to the inability of amyloid-laden vessels to contract normally. Another complication of neurosurgical interest is the occurrence of spontaneous intracerebral hematomas. It is estimated that cerebral amyloid angiopathy accounts for 5 to 10 percent of primary spontaneous cerebral hemorrhages, making it the third most common cause of this condition, after hypertension and aneurysmal rupture. The occurrence of nontraumatic intracerebral hemorrhage in a normotensive elderly person with dementia should arouse a suspicion of cerebral amyloid angiopathy. The extent of bleeding varies from small petechiae to massive intracerebral hematomas (Fig. 256-5). These hemorrhages are usually multiple in both time and location. In contrast to hypertensive hemorrhages, which occur predominantly in the basal ganglia, pons, or cerebellum, hematomas from amyloid angiopathy tend to be near the cortical surface in the parietal or occipital area. Weakening of the vessel wall owing to the deposition of amyloid is thought to permit rupture of cortical vessels. The presence of fibrinoid necrosis in the setting of cerebral amyloid angiopathy is a very significant and specific finding. In a large postmortem study by Vonsattel and colleagues, fibrinoid necrosis was only seen in patients who suffered cerebral hemorrhage. Moreover, the occurrence of fibrinoid necrosis and microaneurysms in hypertensive individuals worsens the problem.

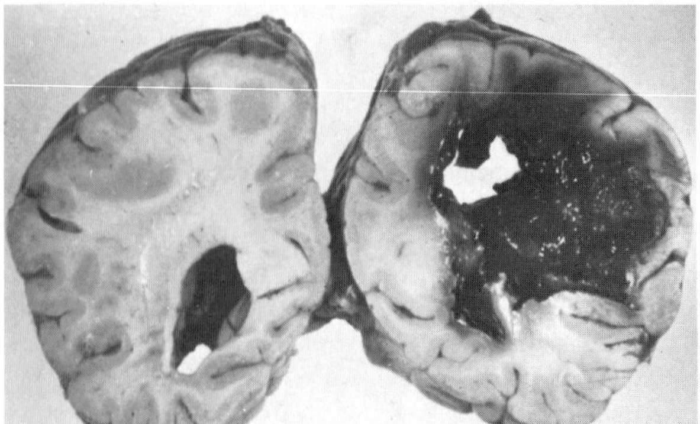

Figure 256-5 An intracerebral hematoma with rupture into the ventricular system in a patient with amyloid angiopathy.

TABLE 256-3 Comparison among the Cerebral Amyloid Angiopathies and Alzheimer's Disease

		Cerebral Amyloid Angiopathy		
	Alzheimer's Disease	**Sporadic**	**Dutch**	**Icelandic**
Amyloid type	β-Protein	β-Protein	β-Protein	Cystatin C (gamma trace)
Inheritance	Sporadic Rare autosomal dominant (familial) form	Sporadic	Autosomal dominant	Autosomal dominant
Mutation	The mutation is unknown in the sporadic form but is *not* within the β-protein gene The familial form has a point mutation of the β-protein precursor gene at codon 642 (valine for isoleucine substitution)	Unknown	Point mutation of β-protein precursor gene at codon 618 (glutamine for glutamic acid substitution at position 22 of protein)	Point mutation of cystatin C gene on chromosome 20 (glutamine for leucine substitution at position 68 of protein)
Age of onset	>60 years	>60 years	45–60 years	20–40 years
Clinical presentation	Dementia	Usually dementia	Usually hemorrhage	Usually hemorrhage
Amyloid in neuropil	Yes	Possible	Possible	No
Extracranial amyloid	No	No	No	Yes

Most cases of amyloid angiopathy reported from the United States are of the sporadic form. Familial forms of cerebral amyloid angiopathy have been described from throughout the world; however, two types have been well studied and genetically characterized—the Icelandic and the Dutch.[1,7,13] Both conditions are autosomal dominant with high penetrance. Clinically, they differ from the sporadic form by their propensity for causing massive, fatal hemorrhage at a young age. Alzheimer's disease and the sporadic, Icelandic, and Dutch forms of cerebral amyloid angiopathy are compared in Table 256-3. It should be noted that although the same amyloid type (β-protein) is deposited in Alzheimer's disease and in the sporadic and Dutch forms of cerebral amyloid angiopathy, the exact genetic and biochemical relationship among the three entities is still unclear. It is known that while the defect in the Dutch form is within the β-protein gene, the defect is outside this locus in Alzheimer's disease. To make matters more puzzling, the genetic defect in the familial, early-onset form of Alzheimer's disease is within the β-protein gene. The molecular biology of the sporadic form of cerebral amyloid angiopathy is still poorly characterized.

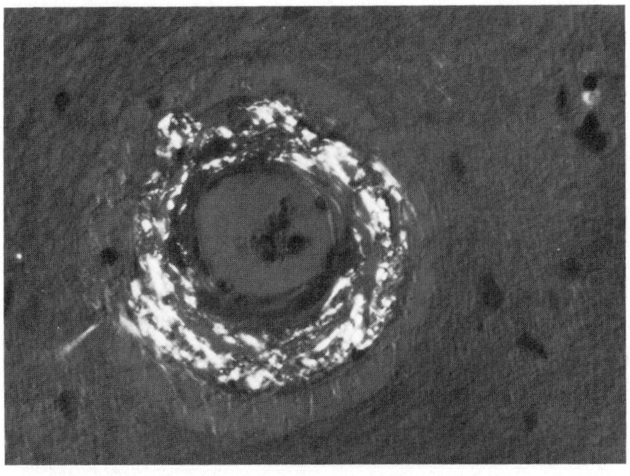

Figure 256-6 An amyloid-laden blood vessel in a section stained with Congo red and viewed with polarized light to show the birefringence of the amyloid.

In a report of 23 well-documented cases of amyloid angiopathy from the Mayo Clinic, Okazaki and colleagues emphasized the frequency of multiple ischemic cerebral lesions in their patients. The clinical picture was one of transient ischemic attacks, single or multiple strokes, or dementia. Dementia in amyloid angiopathy is thought to be due to the presence of senile plaques. Numerical correlations have been made between the senile plaques and dementia. Another explanation of the dementia is that amyloid accumulation may cause vascular occlusion and cortical infarction.

There are no specific diagnostic tests, other than brain biopsy, to establish the diagnosis of cerebral amyloidosis. The histologic diagnosis of amyloid angiopathy is made from certain specific tinctorial properties. With the hematoxylin and eosin stain, uniformly pink-staining hyaline amyloid material may be seen in the vessel wall. The outline of the vessel may be fuzzy and indistinct owing to the spread of the amyloid infiltrate into the adjacent neuropil. Sections stained with crystal violet will show evidence of metachromasia. With the Congo red stain, a deep purplish red

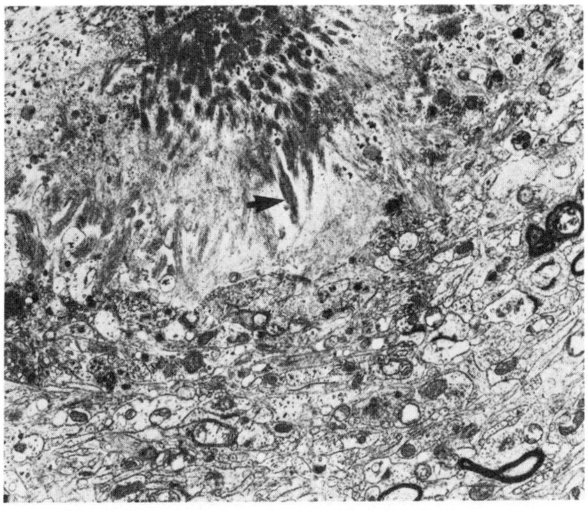

Figure 256-7 An electron microphotograph showing filamentous amyloid fibrils in the perivascular extracellular space *(arrow)*.

staining of the vessel may be noted; when the same section is viewed under polarized light, a greenish yellow birefringence will be apparent (Fig. 256-6). The birefringence is a result of the β-pleated sheet structure assumed by the amyloid fibrillar component. With electron microscopy, characteristic filamentous amyloid fibrils measuring 90 to 95 Å in diameter may be noted in the vessel wall and the adjacent perivascular extracellular space (Fig. 256-7).

Vasculopathy Associated with Drug Abuse

Numerous intracranial complications are known to occur among drug abusers. These are attributable to "behavioral toxicity," pharmacologic toxicity, or infectious complications. Behavioral toxicity refers to the irrational acts committed by the drug abuser under the influence of the drugs which may lead to physical injuries such as a high-speed automobile accident, drowning, or a fall from a height. Infectious complications resulting from the injection of drugs under unsterile conditions may lead to bacterial endocarditis, septic emboli, infectious intracranial vasculitis, mycotic aneurysm, subarachnoid hemorrhage, and brain abscess. A summary of the possible complications associated with drug abuse is listed in Table 256-4.[4]

A noninfectious necrotizing vasculopathy that has histologic features similar to those of polyarteritis nodosa and involves multiple organ systems, including the brain, has been reported among drug abusers. Since most abusers use multiple drugs, it is hard to incriminate a single agent in the induction of vasculopathy, but amphetamine or methamphetamine seems to be the most likely causal agent.[24] Despite cocaine's ability to produce stroke, it is rarely associated with a vasculitis. The clinical picture may be one of acute intracerebral hemorrhage or ischemic cerebrovascular stroke. A computed tomogram may confirm the presence of a hematoma in the brain parenchyma or ventricular system, and a cerebral arteriogram may show beading from segmental luminal irregularities, indistinctness of vessel outlines, microaneurysm formation, or arterial spasm or thrombosis. Histologic examination of the involved arteries may show fibrinoid necrosis with cellular infiltration.

TABLE 256-4 Possible Complications of Drug Abuse of Neurosurgical Importance

Complication	Commonly Associated Drugs
Vasculitis	Amphetamines, heroin
Hypertension	Amphetamines, cocaine
Hypotension	Opioids, barbiturates
Vasopasm	Cocaine, LSD, phencyclidine
Coronary artery disease	Cocaine, ethanol, tobacco
Cardiac arrhythmia	Cocaine, ethanol, tobacco
Atheroma	Tobacco
Mycotic aneurysm	Any injected drug
Foreign body embolus	Any injected drug
AIDS	Any injected drug
Hepatitis	Any injected drug

Source: Adapted from Brust.[4]

Drug-induced vasculopathy responds to steroid therapy with reversal of the abnormal features seen on arteriography. An intracerebral hematoma may need to be removed surgically.

Transverse myelopathy may occur with abuse of narcotics (morphine or heroin). The abuse involved may range from a single exposure to many years of addiction. Symptoms referable to the spinal cord generally appear on resumption of narcotic use following a period of enforced abstinence in a prison or hospital. This sequence of antigenic sensitization and challenge suggests a hypersensitivity reaction to the narcotic or adulterant. In a typical sequence, an addict goes to sleep or becomes comatose after self-administration of the drug. It is thought that during this interval he may become severely hypotensive from the effect of the drug, although this is not well documented. He awakens to find that he is unable to move his legs or void. Neurological examination indicates a transverse myelopathy involving the midthoracic cord with flaccid weakness of muscles, an atonic bladder, and absent muscle stretch reflexes. Over a period of days to weeks the weakness may improve, or it may remain unchanged, progressing to spastic paraplegia. The cerebrospinal fluid may show mild pleocytosis and an increase in protein content. A myelogram may be normal or may show widening of the spinal cord. In the instances where the latter is mistaken for a tumor, biopsy has yielded only necrotic tissue. In autopsy specimens, necrosis is frequently restricted to the gray matter, although segmental infarction in the distribution of a spinal artery may occur. On rare occasions, vasculitis involving the small arteries and arterioles with fibrinoid necrosis and proliferating thickening of the vessel wall is present. Doubly refractile foreign particles seen in histologic sections may represent adulterants present in black-market drugs. The involvement of the midthoracic segment of the spinal cord is attributed to the marginal blood supply of this "watershed," region which presumably is reduced to ischemic levels by severe hypotension after intravenous opiate administration. Associated vasculopathy may further compound the ischemia.

Intravascular Lymphomatosis

Intravascular lymphomatosis is a rare malignancy that affects the smaller vessels of virtually every organ system. The proliferation of neoplastic cells within the lumina of blood vessels results in reduction of blood flow, which causes end-organ ischemia. The malignant cells remain confined to the lumina; extravascular invasion or distant metastasis is unusual. The disease is relentlessly progressive and usually fatal. Previously called neoplastic angioendotheliomatosis, it has been renamed *intravascular lymphomatosis* because the cell of origin has been characterized as lymphocytic instead of endothelial.[16]

Since the original description of the Viennese authors Pfleger and Tappiner in 1959, who documented the cutaneous manifestations of the disease, numerous case reports have appeared in the literature, allowing this disease to be recognized as a distinct clinicopathologic entity. Strouth and his associates were the first to emphasize the nervous system manifestations of the disease. Although vascular involvement is generalized, with virtually no tissue being spared, the clinical manifestations broadly fall into two equally frequent classes, one in which cutaneous involvement dominates and the other in which central nervous system involvement dominates. Extraneural involvement is occasionally severe enough to cause cardiomyopathy, hepatosplenomegaly, dyspnea, or addisonism.

Although most patients have been in their fifth through eighth decades at the time of the onset of symptoms, no age group is exempt; the sexes are affected about equally. As with other lymphomas, the disease preferentially affects immunosupressed patients (e.g., transplant recipients and patients with acquired immunodeficiency syndrome). The most frequent and dominant symptom of central nervous system involvement is confusion and rapidly progressing dementia. Although certain specific intellectual faculties appear to be involved in the initial phases, relentless progression of the multi-infarct syndrome leads to global dementia. Lethargy and stupor may set in in the later stages, ultimately culminating in coma. Superimposed on this background of intellectual impairment are numerous focal neurological symptoms and signs, such as transient ischemic attacks with brief episodes of paralysis, numbness, or blindness. A strokelike syndrome with the sudden onset of hemiparesis may occur. Dysphasia and abulia have been reported. Seizures are not uncommon. Infarction of the spinal cord may result in the sudden onset of a flaccid paraplegia. Thus, the rapid clinical progression of an array of generalized or multifocal neurological symptoms and signs with negative laboratory data and virtually nondiagnostic radiologic tests frustrates the clinician, who feels helpless until a tissue diagnosis is established by brain biopsy. Indeed, in many instances, the diagnosis is made only after death.

Laboratory studies show only certain nonspecific findings, which are not helpful in arriving at the diagnosis. They include an elevated erythrocyte sedimentation rate, increased lactate dehydrogenase level, mild anemia, and increased cerebrospinal fluid protein level. Though there may be a mild lymphocytosis in the cerebrospinal fluid, the cytology has consistently been negative. Curiously, the peripheral blood smear and marrow examination are unrevealing. If computed tomography shows any abnormality at all, it consists of low-density areas in the brain parenchyma consistent with infarction; in rare instances, the infarction is massive or hemorrhagic and may produce a mass effect. The magnetic resonance imaging appearance is more helpful, because the lesions enhance with gadolinium administration; this can help direct a brain biopsy. Cerebral arteriograms do not show any changes; in an isolated instance, a picture of arteritis has been seen.

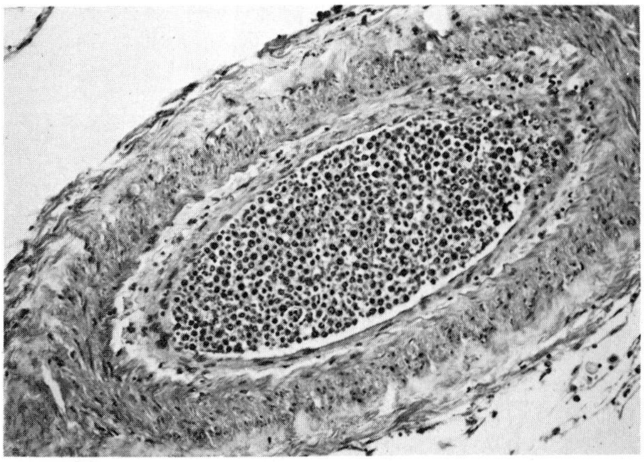

Figure 256-8 A section of a leptomeningeal artery in a patient with proven intravascular lymphomatosis. The vessel is occluded by malignant cells. The endothelial cells appear normal, indicating secondary accumulation of tumor cells at this site. (Courtesy of Bernd W. Scheithauer, M.D.)

Pathologic examination of affected brain tissue is the only way to reliably diagnose the disease.[21] There is a massive proliferation of pleomorphic, mononuclear neoplastic cells within the lumina of leptomeningeal or cerebral vessels (Fig. 256-8). All vessels appear abnormal, but the neoplastic cells show a predilection for capillaries and venules. The nuclei are large and vesicular, with prominent nucleoli. Mitotic figures are commonly seen. Fibrin deposition occurs between tumor cells. The endothelial lining of the blood vessel is histologically normal. An inflammatory reaction consisting of plasma cells and lymphocytes occurs around the adventitia of the vessels. There is an unexplained respect for the vessel wall, and transmural invasion of neoplastic cells is a rare occurrence. This failure to invade extravascularly distinguishes the tumor from angiosarcoma. Affected vessels are greatly distended by the noncohesive tumor cells, which can lead to occlusion or thrombosis. Areas of infarction may appear around the blood vessels, and this is the basis for the clinical symptomatology.

There has been a great deal of controversy regarding the histogenesis of the neoplastic cells. Based on positive immunoperoxidase staining for factor VIII-related antigen and the ultrastructural presence of Weibel-Palade bodies, both of which are endothelial cell markers, the cells were erroneously labeled as being of endothelial origin. Further studies failed to confirm these findings. Bhawan and coworkers were the first to describe the neoplastic cells as a large-cell lymphoma.[3] Immunoperoxidase staining has been positive for the leukocyte common antigen, and Southern blot analysis has confirmed the true lymphoid origin of the malignant cells. Detailed immunophenotyping has demonstrated that the overwhelming majority are B-cell lymphomas, although there have been a few tumors of T-cell lineage.

The prognosis is dismal and survival is generally measured in months. Frequently the definitive diagnosis is made late in the course of the disease, if at all. Early administration of steroids and polychemotherapy designed for large-cell non-Hodgkin's lymphoma is the most rational therapy.

Granulomatous Angiitis

Granulomatous angiitis is an uncommon noninfectious necrotizing vasculopathy of unknown etiology affecting predominantly or exclusively the central nervous system.[14,23] The disease is more appropriately termed *primary angiitis of the central nervous system,* because less than 50 percent of the cases show granulomatous change in histologic section, most having a necrotizing or lymphocytic infiltrate. Extracerebral vessels are rarely affected. Although frequently fatal and not diagnosed until after death, there are recent reports of cases diagnosed on the basis of surgical biopsy that have been successfully treated.

The disease presents as a diffuse or multifocal encephalopathy or transverse myelopathy. It generally affects middle-aged or elderly adults, with no predilection for sex or race. The onset is characterized by confusion, loss of memory, disorientation, and intellectual impairment. Progressive impairment of consciousness occurs as the disease progresses. Focal cerebral manifestations and seizures may be present during the course of the disease. Any region of the central nervous system can be affected, and the presentation can mimic tumor or encephalitis. Past or current herpes zoster and Hodgkin's lymphoma are the most noteworthy associations, occurring in nearly all afflicted patients. Other associated conditions include non-Hodgkin's lymphoma, sarcoidosis, amyloidosis, and infection with human immunodeficiency virus (HIV). A casual relationship with these entities has been postulated but not proved. Patients with granulomatous angiitis who harbor a lymphoma show improvement in the vasculopathy if the lymphoma is brought to remission, even if no specific therapy is directed toward the angiopathy. In patients with herpes zoster ophthalmicus, the virus is thought to spread along the first division of the trigeminal nerve to the internal carotid siphon and its proximal branches, inducing focal granulomatous angiitis. Contralateral hemiplegia may result. Spread through the subarachnoid space is thought to result in diffuse angiitis.[15] A causal relationship to the zoster virus is suspected but not proved.

Small arteries, arterioles, and venules less than 200 μm in diameter are generally affected. Leptomeningeal vessels are especially involved. Histologic changes include fibrinoid necrosis of the vessel wall, and a variable inflammatory infiltration consisting of polymorphonuclear leukocytes, lymphocytes, epithelioid-appearing histiocytes, and multinucleated foreign body or Langhans-type giant cells (Fig. 256-9). It should be emphasized that the absence of a granulomatous infiltrate does not exclude the diagnosis. The segmental vasculitis may be associated with parenchymal ischemic or hemorrhagic infarcts.

Laboratory tests, including the erythrocyte sedimentation rate, are usually normal. The disease lacks a characteristic clinical presentation, so cerebral angiography and brain biopsy are required for diagnosis. Angiography reveals nonspecific signs of vasculitis. Computed tomographic scans show multiple areas of poorly defined, nonenhancing, low-density lesions. Magnetic resonance imaging is more sensitive, and the lesions readily enhance with gadolinium. Because of the segmental nature of the disease, biopsy is specific but not very sensitive; therefore, an isolated negative biopsy does not exclude the diagnosis. Since the leptomeningeal vessles are primarily affected, a deep stereotactic biopsy is unlikely to reveal diagnostic tissue.

Treatment with steroids and immunosupression has proved beneficial in some cases. Nevertheless, the overwhelming majority of cases are fatal, with death occurring within weeks to months after diagnosis.

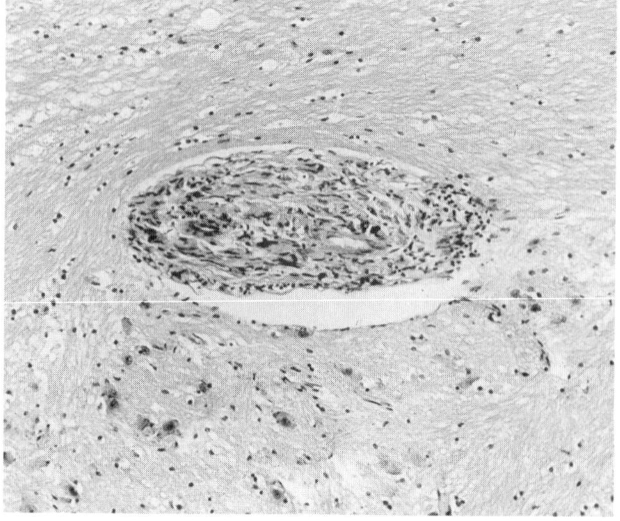

Figure 256-9 A section of a vessel from a patient with primary angiitis. The vessel wall has undergone fibrinoid necrosis and there is a mixed cellular infiltrate. (Courtesy of Joo H. Sung, M.D.)

References

1. Abrahamson M, Jonsdottir S, Olafsson I, et al. Hereditary cystatin C amyloid angiopathy: identification of the disease-causing mutation and specific diagnosis by polymerase chain reaction based analysis. *Hum Genet* 1992; 89:377–380.
2. Bengtsson BA. Epidemiology of giant cell arteritis. *Baillieres Clin Rheumatol* 1991; 5:379–385.
3. Bhawan J, Wolff SM, Ucci AA, et al. Malignant lymphoma and malignant angioendotheliomatosis: one disease. *Cancer* 1985; 55:570–576.
4. Brust JCM. Clinical, radiological, and pathological aspects of cerebrovascular disease associated with drug abuse. *Stroke* 1993; 24(12 Suppl): I129–I135.
5. Chuang TY, Hunder GG, Ilstrup DM, et al. Polymyalgia rheumatica: a 10 year epidemiologic and clinical study. *Ann Intern Med* 1982; 97: ′18. 672–680.
6. Dequeker JV. Polymyalgia rheumatica with temporal arteritis, as painted by Jan Van Eyck in 1436. *Can Med Assoc J* 1981; 124:1597–1598.
7. Duchen LW. Current status review: cerebral amyloid. *Int J Exp Pathol* 1992; 73:535–550.
8. Fauci AS, Haynes BF, Katz P. The spectrum of vasculitis: clinical, pathologic, immunologic, and therapeutic considerations. *Ann Intern Med* 1978; 89 (Part 1):660–676.
9. Giordano JM, Leavitt RY, Hoffman G, et al. Experience with surgical treatment of Takayasu's disease. *Surgery* 1991; 109:252–258.
10. Hunder GG, Bloch DA, Michel BA, et al. The American College of Rheumatology 1990 criteria for the classification of giant cell arteritis. *Arthritis Rheum* 1990; 33:1122–1128.
11. Huston KA, Hunder GG: Giant cell (cranial) arteritis: a clinical review. *Am Heart J* 1980; 100:99–107.
12. Leblanc R, Preul M, Robitaille Y, et al. Surgical considerations in cerebral amyloid angiopathy. *Neurosurgery* 1991; 29:712–718.
13. Levy E, Carman MD, Fernandez-Madrid IJ, et al. Mutation of the Alzheimer's disease amyloid gene in hereditary cerebral hemorrhage, Dutch type. *Science* 1990; 248:1124–1126.
14. Lie JT. Primary (granulomatous) angiitis of the central nervous system: a clinicopathologic analysis of 15 new cases and a review of the literature. *Hum Pathol* 1992; 23:164–171.
15. MacKenzie RA, Forbes GS, Karnes WE. Angiographic findings in herpes zoster arteritis. *Ann Neurol* 1981; 10:458–464.
16. Molina A, Lombard C, Donlon T, et al. Immunohistochemical and cytogenetic studies indicate that malignant angioendotheliomatosis is a primary intravascular (angiotropic) lymphoma. *Cancer* 1990; 66:474–479.
17. Moriwaki R, Numano F. Takayasu arteritis: follow-up studies for 20 years. *Heart Vessels [Suppl]* 1992; 7:138S–145S.
18. Redlich FC. A new medical diagnosis of Adolf Hitler. Giant cell arteritis—temporal arteritis. *Arch Intern Med* 1993; 153:693–697.
19. Rengachary SS, Racela LS, Watanabe I, et al. Neurosurgical and immunological implications of primary cerebral amyloid (congophilic) angiopathy. *Neurosurgery* 1980; 7:1–9.
20. Roche NE, Fulbright JW, Wagner AD, et al. Correlation of interleukin-6 production and disease activity in polymyalgia rheumatica and giant cell arteritis. *Arthritis Rheum* 1993; 36:1286–1294.
21. Smadja D, Mas JL, Fallet-Bianco C, et al. Intravascular lymphomatosis (neoplastic angioendotheliosis) of the central nervous system: case report and literature review. *J Neurooncol* 1991; 11:171–180.
22. Tomlinson FH, Lie JT, Nienhuis BJ, et al. Juvenile temporal arteritis revisited. *Mayo Clin Proc* 1994; 69:445–447.
23. Vollmer TL, Guarnaccia J, Harrington W, et al. Idiopathic granulomatous angiitis of the central nervous system: diagnostic challenges. *Arch Neurol* 1993; 50:925–930.
24. Yu YJ, Cooper DR, Wellenstein DE, Block B. Cerebral angiitis and intracerebral hemorrhage associated with methamphetamine abuse. *J Neurosurg* 1983; 58:109–111.

Part VIII

Cranial and Spinal Trauma

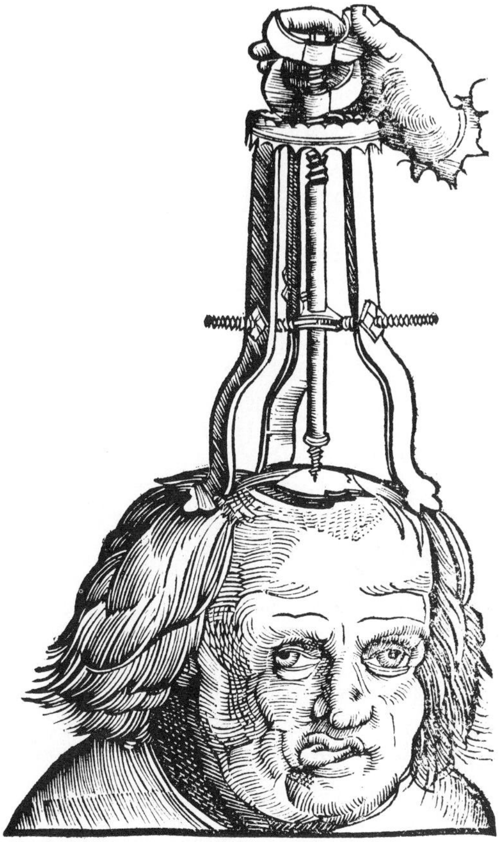

von Gersdorff H. *Feldtbuch der Wundartzney.* Strassbourg: J. Schott, 1517. An illustration showing the method of elevating depressed skull fractures. Right third and twelfth nerve palsies and left facial weakness are present.

SECTION A

General Information

257 THINK FIRST: The National Head and Spinal Cord Injury Prevention Program

E. Fletcher Eyster
Diana B. Kelker
Randall W. Porter

If disease were killing our children in the proportions that accidents are, people would be outraged and demand that this killer be stopped.—Former U.S. Surgeon General C. Everett Koop

When meditating over a disease, I never think of finding a remedy for it, but instead, a means of preventing it.—Louis Pasteur

Traumatic injuries are a major public health problem, imposing a greater burden on modern society than other diseases, but are the most preventable of major public health problems. In children, and in adults under age 45, injuries remain the leading cause of death, each year claiming more than 142,000 American lives[16] and causing more than 62 million Americans to seek medical attention.[17] The total health care bill for injuries in 1988 was approximately $170 billion.[22] (1988 was the most recent year for which statistics were available at the time this chapter was written.) Prevention and control efforts must be expanded to reflect the magnitude of this health problem.

Head and spinal cord injuries, in particular, are the leading causes of morbidity and mortality among America's youth. Such catastrophes result in enormous human and economic costs. Every year approximately 2 million Americans suffer a traumatic brain injury[10]; one injury occurs every 15 s. Of those brain-injury victims, 75,000 to 100,000 die within hours of injury; 500,000 require hospitalization; and 70,000 to 90,000 develop irreversible loss of function. Additionally, 10,000 to 12,000 spinal cord injuries occur each year,[2,9,12,14] of which more than half occur to individuals less than 24 years old.

Lifetime costs for spinal cord and head injuries can exceed $600,000 and $4 million, respectively.[22] These figures do not include loss of potential work income; more important, they place no monetary value on the pain and suffering that patients and families endure. The total national bill for traumatic brain injury is approximately $25 billion per year for rehabilitation, support services, and lost income for injured patients.[10,11]

Motor vehicle crashes are the primary cause of spinal cord injuries, accounting for about 50 percent of cases.[3] Most of these are alcohol-related. Falls are the second leading cause,[28] followed by diving injuries. More than 25 percent of spinal cord injuries and 12 percent of brain injuries[10,11] result from violent assaults. These figures vary considerably among geographic areas and populations.[22] Sports and recreation injuries are also important causes of morbidity and mortality, accounting for 10 percent of brain injuries and 7 percent of spinal cord injuries.[13] Approximately 1000 diving-related incidents occur each year,[15] which account for 10 percent of all spinal cord injuries and 60 to 65 percent of all recreationally incurred spinal injuries.[5,27,28] Furthermore, it is reported that 95 percent of these incidents result in quadriplegia.[27]

Prevention of injuries to the head and spinal cord appears to be the most effective means of improving survival rates. Unlike many other major health problems, a variety of effective preventive measures are available; unfortunately, they are not applied.[23]

Despite significant research on central nervous system regeneration and improved treatment of spinal cord damage with methylprednisolone, the medical and scientific communities have been unsuccessful in significantly reversing the effects of injury to the brain and spinal cord. Society cannot afford the loss of young lives, the high cost of medical treatment of head and spinal cord injuries, and the cost of supporting those permanently disabled by these injuries. Efforts to prevent this tragedy can be justified either by moral and ethical, or by economic, considerations. As neurosurgeons treating these individuals, we become frustrated at how little we can do to improve neurological deficit. Therefore, it is logical that we should take an active role in trying to prevent these injuries.[6]

The THINK FIRST® prevention program is an attempt on the part of the American Association of Neurological Surgeons and the Congress of Neurological Surgeons to fulfill this role.[6] For consistency with strategic objectives for health promotion and disease prevention in the United States, the messages of THINK FIRST® have been synchronized with the 1992 national document "Healthy People 2000." Two objectives of "Healthy People 2000" are to reduce nonfatal head injuries so that hospitalizations are required for no more than 106 persons per 100,000 and to reduce nonfatal spinal cord injuries so that hospitalizations are limited to no more than 5 persons per 100,000. The current rates are 124 and 5.9 per 100,000, respectively.[22]

Formerly called The National Head and Spinal Cord Injury Prevention Program, THINK FIRST® combines the experiences of model educational programs run in Florida by Dr. E. Fletcher Eyster and in Missouri by Dr. Clark Watts. These two programs were carefully designed and implemented over a multi-year period and have shown the potential for reductions in brain and spinal cord injuries. THINK FIRST® was founded on the principle that educating those at risk for injury as to the consequences of risky behavior can foster life-style changes that may decrease the likelihood of spinal cord and/or head injuries.

Injuries can be prevented effectively by three methods. The most effective is the provision of automatic protective devices in product and environmental design, such as installation of airbags, antilock brakes, and restraint systems in cars. The second method is the mandating of behavioral change by force of law or administrative rule (e.g., laws requiring safety belt and helmet use). In one of the major public health successes of recent decades, all 50 states now require safety restraints for young children riding in automobiles. This has contributed to a 36 percent decline in motor vehicle fatalities in persons aged 1 to 14 between 1980 and 1984.[21] The effectiveness of safety belts in preventing injury and death in motor vehicle crashes is well documented. Safety belts reduce motor vehicle fatalities by an estimated 40 to 50 percent and serious injury by 45 to 55 percent.[20] In addition, one study found that safety belt use reduced hospital bills by 67 percent.[4] Conversely, the rescission of laws mandating use of helmets by motorcyclists was a major setback; it resulted in a 40 percent increase in the numbers of fatally injured motorcyclists.[19,30]

The third, and most difficult, way to prevent injuries is to persuade individuals at risk to alter their behavior. The Centers for Disease Control stated that from 1984 to 1988, "universal use of helmets by all bicyclists could have prevented as many as 2,500 deaths and 757,000 head injuries."[26] Fewer than 10 percent of all cyclists, and fewer than 2 percent of those under 15 years old, wear helmets.[8] Riders wearing helmets reduce their risk of brain injury by 85 percent.[29] Other reports show that bicyclists who die with serious head injuries often do not sustain other life-threatening or potentially disabling injuries in fatal crashes.[2] It is apparent that attitudes of children and parents must change so that helmet use becomes just as acceptable in bicycling as in other sports, such as football and ice hockey.[22]

The national THINK FIRST® Program has four components: (1) a basic education program, (2) reinforcement activities, (3) general public education efforts, and (4) public policy initiatives.

The primary component of THINK FIRST® is an educational curriculum directed at the teenage population. The program defines vulnerability and the consequences of risk-taking behavior. Teenagers, who are at the greatest risk for brain and spinal cord injuries, are unaware of the potential consequences of these injuries, and often view themselves as invincible. Teenagers are easily influenced by their peers to engage in risky behavior; they wear safety belts less often than adults.[2] The THINK FIRST® Program is based on the health belief model of Rosenstock,[25] which proposes that teenagers must be made aware of risk and its consequences. Second, they must believe that there are actions they can take to avoid these risks. Third, they must realize that the barriers to such actions do not outweigh their benefits. In the context of THINK FIRST®, the major barrier to success is peer pressure.[6]

The THINK FIRST® education program is delivered primarily through the public school system to students in large assemblies or in a classroom format. The presentation has four parts. The first is an 18-minute award-winning film, *Harm's Way*. Through interviews with young people who have survived head and spinal cord injury, the film depicts the youthful risk-taking behaviors that led to their injuries, and the consequences of their injuries. The second part is a presentation of the definition and epidemiology of head and spinal cord injuries by a health professional. Types and causes of injuries are discussed, including those involving motor vehicles, drinking, diving, all-terrain vehicles, action sports, and violent crimes. Third, after that presentation, a young person who has sustained a spinal cord or brain injury discusses his or her injury—its cause and its physical, emotional, and social consequences—and answers questions from the student audience. Paramedics or emergency medical technicians are often on hand to discuss secondary injuries to the spinal cord that can occur after accidents because of inappropriate handling of victims. An optional fourth feature is a wheelchair obstacle course where students can experience some of the problems confronted in everyday life by persons confined to wheelchairs.

The second major component of the THINK FIRST® Program involves reinforcement activities. These are an invaluable feature, since no matter how effective a one-hour presentation may be, it is unlikely to change adolescents' behavior. A continued prevention message helps to reinforce the education program within the school. Areas of risk, such as swimming pools, ponds, creeks, and beaches, are marked with appropriate preventive signs placed by local civic groups. Other reinforcement activities include essay and poster contests, repeated exposure to the program, skills training for bystander response to accidents, school and community bulletin boards, school health fairs, bicycle rodeos, alcohol-free graduation events, and the creation of safety clubs.

The third and fourth components of the THINK FIRST® Program concentrate on general public awareness initiatives and support of state and federal public policy efforts. Injury prevention programs such as THINK FIRST® face numerous challenges. They must increase awareness among key decision-makers and the general public, who often are unaware of the magnitude of the injury problem in comparison with other public health problems. THINK FIRST® enhances its education efforts on safety with the general public through public service announcements, television talk shows, newspaper feature articles, position papers, and other media events. Additionally, the glorification of risk-taking behaviors by the media and society must be combatted.[18]

Public policy initiatives help to ensure that injury prevention issues are addressed at both community and state levels. The THINK FIRST® national office and local programs keep abreast of, and speak to, policy issues that can lead to laws enhancing the prevention effort. One of the most pressing goals of the National THINK FIRST® Program is the establishment of central nervous system injury registries in all states. Such registries can provide better data from which meaningful prevention, therapeutic, and rehabilitation programs can be developed. There are legislative efforts under way to increase funding for the prevention, treatment, and rehabilitation of brain and spinal cord injuries. Additionally, a major provision in pending bills is to establish a national traumatic brain injury registry.[11] The THINK FIRST® office provides technical assistance and referrals for state agencies undertaking the establishment of such registries. Also, the national office provides information on issues such as safety belt and motorcycle helmet laws.

THINK FIRST® encourages government research and programs geared to reduce injuries to the brain and spinal cord. More than one-fourth (28 percent) of direct costs for treatment of these injuries are borne by federal, state, and local governments. In marked contrast to societal burdens, total federal research expenditures for injury were estimated at $160 million, compared with National Cancer Institute expenditures of $1,400 million and National Heart, Lung, and Blood Institute expenditures of $930 million.[2]

It was recognized quickly that because of the magnitude of the problem, it would be difficult for neurosurgeons alone to make a substantial impact on the lack of public awareness of the devastation caused by brain and spinal cord injuries. Therefore, in addition to the implementation of the THINK FIRST® Prevention Program within neurosurgery, the THINK FIRST® Foundation was created in October 1990 to enlist other interested persons in a tax-free foundation dedicated to prevention. The foundation has facilitated involvement of both lay people and professionals outside neurosurgery in efforts to influence public policy, to collaborate with other prevention organizations, and to ensure that funding levels are maintained. The building and maintaining of strong links with other agencies and organizations is essential.[18] THINK FIRST® programs across the country are actively collaborating with SAFEKIDS, the National Head Injury Association, the National Spinal Cord Injury Association, the National Safety Council, Mothers Against Drunk Driving (MADD), the National Highway Traffic Safety Administration, the Consumer Product Safety Commission, and the Centers for Disease Control. Additionally, in 1992, the Medical Student Section of the American Medical Association passed a resolution vowing to increase medical students' involvement in spinal cord and head injury prevention.

The THINK FIRST® board of directors is strongly committed to measuring and evaluating the program's success in positively influencing teenagers' behavior, the incidence of injury, and public and legislative attitudes. Demonstration of efficacy, though not an easy task, is essential for any prevention program. Efficacy is measured in three ways. First, the message is transferred and the knowledge gain is measured. Second, the effect of knowledge on behavior is measured; participants are tested to determine if they use the newly gained knowledge to actually change their behaviors. Finally, the incidence of the disease or injury is monitored to show the result—hopefully, a decrease in injuries.

Socially oriented programs have many intangible variables making studies more difficult to standardize and study in a controllable fashion.[6] Several local programs have conducted studies to critically evaluate the impact of their programs on the behavior and knowledge of young people. The Missouri Heads Up Program, a THINK FIRST® local program under the direction of Dr. Clark Watts, conducted several studies that showed a positive influence on behavior as well as increased awareness. Another study by that group indicated that several years after exposure, the risk-taking attitudes of 445 students were favorably modified, compared with a control group of 379 students who had not been exposed to the program.[7]

In 1989 a THINK FIRST® Program led by Dr. Edward Neuwelt of Portland, Oregon, examined that program's impact on the knowledge, attitudes, and behavior of high school students. After the program, students were more likely to believe that there were actions they could take to keep from getting injured.[1] In a 1984 Florida study, a decrease in the incidence of spinal cord injuries was reported for counties using the Florida THINK FIRST® model compared to counties not using an intervention program.[27]

In 1993 the THINK FIRST® Program began its first national efficacy study to evaluate knowledge and behavior changes in the high school population. The questionnaire was created with the assistance of the injury prevention and research statistician staff at the Rehabilitation Institute of Chicago; clinical psychologists; and injury control specialists from the Florida Department of Health and Rehabilitative Services. In the 1993-1994 school year local programs began to use this national tool to measure program impact. Incidence of injury, however, cannot be adequately evaluated until more states have mandatory head and spinal cord injury registries.

Since the program's creation in 1986, much has been accomplished and many milestones have been achieved. In 1990 J.S. Richards, of the University of Alabama, wrote that THINK FIRST® was the major force and role model for head and spinal cord injury prevention in the United States.[24] In 1993 there were seven funded model training centers conducting train-the-trainer sessions. Training for new coordinators is provided free of charge. To date, 251 groups have been trained; 165 groups are actively presenting the program in 47 states, plus the District of Columbia, Canada, and Santiago, Chile. Since 1986, more than 3.4 million students have received the THINK FIRST® message.

Other accomplishments include the production of the award-winning film *Harm's Way.* This film has been purchased by more than 1500 groups since 1986. A shorter version, *Reflections,* has been produced. The film has won numerous awards and is continually updated.

Now there are several other age groups being targeted. During recent years, THINK FIRST® has increasingly received requests from elementary and middle school teachers. To determine if the program would be appropriate for the younger age levels, Avolio et al., in Oregon, demonstrated that, in fact, THINK FIRST® is an effective program for middle school audiences.[1] To better reach this age group, plans are underway to develop an elementary-school version of the curriculum.

THINK FIRST® is also active in Canada. With the help of US THINK FIRST®, THINK FIRST® Canada was founded in 1991 and has successfully launched its own fundraising efforts and program expansion.

The United States national office of the THINK FIRST® Program and Foundation is located near Chicago, in Park Ridge, Illinois. The staff are responsible for raising funds to implement the program and also serve as a technical resource for local program coordinators, assisting with curriculum development, program material development, coordinator training, program expansion, and national coalition building. The quarterly newsletter, *Prevention Pages,* is distributed to over 8000 persons. Further, the staff contribute articles for neurological newsletters, books, and injury prevention journals. Persons interested in more information about THINK FIRST® should call the national office at (708) 692–2740, or write to THINK FIRST®, 22 South Washington Street, Park Ridge, Illinois 60068.

References

1. Avolio AE, Ramsey FL, Neuwelt EA. Evaluation of a program to prevent head and spinal cord injuries: a comparison between middle school and high school. *Neurosurgery* 1992; 31:557–562.

2. Baker SP, O'Neill B, Karpf RS. *Injury Fact Book,* 2d ed. New York: Oxford University Press, 1992, p 289.
3. Carter RE Jr. Traumatic spinal cord injuries due to automobile accidents. *South Med J* 1977; 70:709–710.
4. Chorba TL, Reinfurt D, Hulka BS. Efficacy of mandatory seat-belt use legislation. *JAMA* 1988; 260:3593–3597.
5. Elder J. Human factors in drowning and near-drowning injuries. In Brill D, Micik S, Yuwiler J (eds): *Childhood Drownings: Current Issues and Strategies for Prevention.* Orange, CA: California Drowning Prevention Network, 1987, pp 27–28.
6. Eyster EF, Watts C. An update of the National Head and Spinal Cord Injury Prevention Program of the American Association of Neurological Surgeons and the Congress of Neurological Surgeons: Think First. *Clin Neurosurg* 1992; 38:252–260.
7. Frank RG, Bouman DE, Cain K, et al. A preliminary study of a traumatic injury prevention program. *Psychol Health* 1992; 6:129–140.
8. Goldsmith MF. Campaigns focus on helmets as safety experts warn bicycle riders to use—and preserve heads. *JAMA* 1992; 268:308–311.
9. Griffin MR, Opitz JL, Kurland LT, et al. Traumatic spinal cord injury in Olmstead County, Minnesota, 1935–1981. *Am J Epidemiol* 1985; 121:884–895.
10. Interagency Head Injury Task Force Reports. National Institute of Neurological Disorders and Stroke; National Institutes of Health, Bethesda, MD, 1989.
11. Jones L. Bill aims to curb brain injury. *Am Med News* 1992; 35 (October 19):3,9.
12. Kalsbeek WD, McLaurin RL, Harris BS III, et al. The National Head and Spinal Cord Injury Survey: major findings. *J Neurosurg* 1980; 53 (suppl):S19–S31.
13. Kraus JF, Conroy C. Mortality and morbidity from injuries in sports and recreation. *Annu Rev Public Health* 1984; 5:163–192.
14. Kraus JF, Franti CE, Riggins RS, et al. Incidence of traumatic spinal cord lesions. *J Chronic Dis* 1975; 28:471–492.
15. Maiman D, Kunelius D, Weiss H, et al. Diving-associated spinal cord injuries during drought conditions: Wisconsin, 1988. *MMWR* 1988; 37:453–464.
16. National Center for Health Statistics. *Advance Report of Final Mortality Statistics, 1985.* Washington, DC: US Government Printing Office, 1987.
17. National Center for Health Statistics. *Current Estimates from the National Health Interview Survey, United States, 1985.* Washington, DC: US Government Printing Office, 1986.
18. National Committee for Injury Prevention and Control. Injury prevention: meeting the challenge. *Am J Prev Med* 1989; 5(Suppl 3):1–303, pp. 106–108.
19. National Highway Traffic Safety Administration. *A Report to the Congress on the Effect of Motorcycle Helmet Use Law Repeal: A Case for Helmet Use.* Washington, DC: US Dept. of Transportation, 1980.
20. National Highway Traffic Safety Administration. Final Rule, FMVSS208: Occupant Crash Protection, 49 CFR, Part 571. Washington, DC: US Dept. of Transportation, 1984.
21. National Highway Traffic Safety Administration. *Fatal Accident Reporting System, 1987.* Washington, DC: US Dept. of Transportation, 1988.
22. Public Health Service. *Healthy People 2000.* National health promotion and disease prevention objectives—full report with commentary. Washington, DC: U.S. Department of Health and Human Services, Public Health Service, 1991; No. PHS 91-50212.
23. Rice DP. Cost of Injury in the United States: Report to Congress, 1989. San Francisco, CA: Institute for Health and Aging, University of California; and Injury Prevention Center, The Johns Hopkins University, 1989.
24. Richards JS. *Resources: A National Directory of Spinal Cord Injury Prevention Programs.* Birmingham, AL: University of Alabama at Birmingham, 1990.
25. Rosenstock IM. Historical origin of the health belief model. In Becker MH (ed): *The Health Belief Model and Personal Health Behavior.* Thorofare, NJ: CB Slack, 1974.
26. Sacks JJ, Holmgreen P, Smith SM, et al. Bicycle-associated head injuries and deaths in the United States from 1984 through 1988: how many are preventable? *JAMA* 1991; 266:3016–3018.
27. Shaw LR, McMahon BT, Bruce JH. The Florida approach to spinal cord injury prevention. *Rehabil Lit* 1984; 45:85–89.
28. Stover SL, Fine PR (eds). *Spinal Cord Injury: The Facts and Figures.* Birmingham, AL: University of Alabama at Birmingham, 1986.
29. Thompson RS, Rivara FP, Thompson DC. A case-control study of the effectiveness of bicycle safety helmets. *N Engl J Med* 1989; 320:1361–1367.
30. Watson GS, Zador PL, Wilks A. The repeal of helmet use laws and increased motorcyclist mortality in the United States 1975-1978. *Am J Public Health* 1980; 70:529–585.

258

Electrical Injuries of the Nervous System

Ralph G. Dacey, Jr.
Dennis G. Vollmer

Injuries caused by contact with electrical power sources or transmission lines and injuries caused by lightning are relatively unusual. When these injuries do occur, however, the neurosurgeon is often asked to see the patient because they commonly affect the nervous system. Their pathophysiology is complex and incompletely understood, and they often leave the patient with major disabilities.[1]

Electrical injuries account for approximately 5 percent of burn unit admissions in the United States, and electrocution is the fifth leading cause of fatal occupational injury. Most victims of electrical accidents are young males (mean age, approximately 30 years) working as construction workers, electricians, or truck drivers. Injury usually occurs when the worker or the equipment he is using comes in contact with energized transmission lines. The extended booms of transport and construction vehicles, sailboat masts, and ladders are frequent conduits of electrical power to the injured worker. Children account for approximately one-third of all victims of electrical injuries. Toddlers are frequently injured when their mouth comes in contact with electrical appliances, causing perioral burns.[18] Adolescents climbing trees or poles near high-tension electrical lines are also susceptible.

Lightning accounts for approximately 300 to 400 deaths per year in the United States, more than all other weather-related fatalities combined.[6,7] Inhabitants of rural areas are several times more susceptible to lightning injury than people living in cities. Farmers and other outdoor workers, golfers, hikers, and swimmers are especially susceptible. Approximately 30 to 40 percent of people struck by lightning die. Lightning strikes to the head are often fatal.

Electrical Aspects of High-Voltage Current and Lightning Injuries

In commercial distribution systems, electricity is the flow of electrons from atom to atom. The rate of flow of electrons, amperage, is determined by the voltage or driving force for electron movement and the resistance to flow in the conducting substance. Most commercial electric power sources generate a cyclic reversal of the direction of electron flow with a frequency of 50 to 60 cycles/s. Compared with direct current, alternating current is more useful in commercial power distribution systems because its voltage can be raised or lowered more easily by transformers. Electric power is most efficiently distributed at high voltages. Large regional power transmission lines carry voltages of about 750,000 V. Area distribution substations reduce voltage to about 12,500 to 138,000 V for industrial use. Local distribution systems use voltages in the range of 2000 to 34,500 V before further local voltage reduction to 110 to 220 V. For special applications, such as in rail transport systems, direct current is used.

Lightning is direct current, and voltage in a lightning strike may exceed 100 million volts. Temperatures in the core of a lightning strike may exceed 30,000°C. Air that is rapidly heated to such high temperatures expands, producing sound (thunder) and a concussive pressure pulse wave. However, the elevated temperature and current flow are of short duration—usually less than 100 μs. In various weather conditions, the lower sections of cumulonimbus clouds may become negatively charged relative to upper cloud layers and the earth, when many negatively charged large ice crystals and water droplets accumulate there. When the potential difference between the earth and negatively charged areas exceeds approximately 30,000 V, the resistance of the atmosphere to the conduction of electric current is overcome and a "leader stroke" originates in the cloud and travels toward the ground. This initial stroke is met by a "pilot stroke" coming from the ground, and positive current flows from the earth to the cloud.

Lightning injury may occur by three mechanisms. In a *direct strike,* current may flow from an elevated skin surface, such as the head or outstretched arm, through the trunk and legs to earth. However, indirect injury may also occur. *Splash injury* occurs when a nearby vertical object, such as a tree, has a relatively high resistance to current flow and the current arcs to a standing human, seeking a path of less resistance to the ground. Lightning may also cause a *ground strike* near a standing person. As current diffuses through the earth, a stride potential may be formed and current may pass through the lower extremities. Because of these indirect mechanisms of lightning-induced injury, persons should seek protection from severe electrical storms in grounded buildings and closed vehicles. A person caught in the open should not seek protection under isolated tall trees or areas of ground elevation but should lie on one side with the extremities drawn into the body in a recessed area of local terrain. Flash injury may occur from telephone lines and plumbing fixtures within homes and other structures. For this reason these devices should be avoided by persons who are indoors during thunderstorms.

Electrical injuries are frequently considered as either high (greater than 1000 V) or low (less than 1000 V) tension injuries. Thermal injury caused by the conduction of electrical energy through tissue is determined by Joule's equivalent (I^2RT), where I is the current passing through the tissue in amperes, R is the resistance of the tissue in ohms, and T is the time of contact in seconds. Resistance of skin and other tissue to transmission of electrical energy is quite variable and depends on a number of factors. For example, the average resistance of normal skin is 5000 ohms/cm^2. If the hands are wet, skin resistance may decrease to 1000 ohms/cm^2, whereas the formation of heavy callus may increase resistance to 1,000,000 ohms/cm^2.[15] However, tissue resistance and duration of contact rarely can be determined after an electrical injury. For this reason, voltage remains the most important electrical parameter in determining the severity of electrical injury.

Pathogenesis and Neuropathology of Electrical Injuries

In high-tension injury, tissue resistance is such that the body acts as a volume conductor. Heat generation is proportional to current density (amperage per cross-sectional area). Destructive injuries of the extremity are therefore much more frequent than those of the thorax and abdomen because of differences in cross-sectional area.[2] Bone has extremely high resistance to the passage of electric current, whereas peripheral nerves, spinal cord, and blood vessels have little resistance and therefore may be susceptible to relatively less thermal injury. In most electrical injuries the patient is interposed within a circuit. Current entering the body typically produces charring, whereas the exiting current may destroy tissue in an explosive pattern. As charring at the entrance point progresses, skin resistance drops and current flow increases. Often there is little evidence of tissue damage between entrance and exit points. When an upper extremity contacts the power source, current may arc to. the forearm and axilla, producing locally severe thermal injury.

Alternating current produces more severe injury than does direct current because of two characteristics. Tetanic contraction of extremity musculature may ''fix'' the hand or arm to alternating current sources, thereby lengthening the duration of contact. Alternating current is also much more likely to produce ventricular fibrillation than is direct current; as a result, arm-to-arm current flow with alternating current may be lethal at relatively low voltages.

In low-voltage electric shock, the central nervous system is almost always spared. In higher-tension injuries, a relatively common pattern of injury occurs, in which contact with the head may produce severe burns of the scalp and bone, after which current exits through the hand or foot. Because resistance to current flow through bone is high, severe local scalp and bone tissue destruction or devitalization may occur—sometimes without permanent injury to the underlying brain. However, thermal injury may occur with the formation of cavities and fissures in the cerebral hemispheres, especially immediately subjacent to the cranial vault.

Most information about the neuropathology of electrical injury comes from the postmortem examination of criminals subjected to judicial electrocution or laboratory animals after experimental electric shock. Extravasation of blood ranging from local petechial hemorrhage to diffuse subarachnoid hemorrhage is frequently observed on neuropathologic examination of the nervous system after electrical injury. Necrosis occurs in the white matter with relative preservation of gray matter, especially in the spinal cord. The brains of criminals examined after judicial electrocution show evidence of myelin sheath injury, chromatolysis of cell bodies, and petechial and subarachnoid hemorrhage. Examination of the spinal cords of patients with the delayed onset of a neurological deficit after electrical injury shows evidence of demyelination, neuronal cell death, and vasculopathy with intimal thickening and obliteration of intraparenchymal vessels.

Most of the neuropathologic changes reported in electrical injury are consistent with nonspecific effects of thermal heating of tissue: the formation of parenchymal vacuoles and fissures, neuronal death and chromatolysis, demyelination, and damage to the cerebral microcirculation. The occurrence of nervous system dysfunction distant from directly affected brain (such as brain stem deficits with an arm-to-arm current path) and delayed-onset neurological deficits suggest, however, that injury may also occur at the molecular level. Ionizing radiation is known to produce long-lasting changes in nucleic acid and membrane enzyme system macromolecular structure, and it is likely that electrical injury causes similar changes.[11] Such macromolecular structural changes may make cells less resistant to perturbation in their microenvironment and accelerate cell death. Cerebral endothelial cells may be particularly susceptible to such injury, causing delayed intimal proliferation and thrombosis in vessels supplying the brain and spinal cord, eventually resulting in ischemia.[11] In experimental electrical injury, current density in the lower cervical spinal cord was highest among regions sampled along a forepaw-to-forepaw injury in cats.[16] Despite these concepts, the pathophysiology of delayed neurological deficit after electrical injury remains incompletely understood.

In the extremities, high current densities may lead to extensive (explosive) injuries with damage to surrounding peripheral nerves. Arcing of electric current (usually occurring at an upper extremity entrance wound) is associated with extremely high temperatures and may cause thermal injuries to peripheral nerves in the upper extremities. Thus, the function of peripheral nerves may be impaired by at least three mechanisms in electrical injury. A neurapraxic injury may occur, probably related to the direct effects of electric current on the maintenance of ionic gradients in axons. Thermal injury may cause permanent disruption of axons and myelin sheaths in addition to causing complete neurotmesis. Lastly, peripheral nerves may be compressed as part of compartment syndromes associated with massive thermal injuries to the extremities.

Electromechanical factors may also cause injury. Lightning strikes are associated with a cylindrical pressure pulse wave, which may produce contusion of the brain or spinal cord underlying the strike area. Also, large charge differences occur between the victim and the surrounding environment, resulting in electrorepulsive or electroattractive forces violently propelling the victim to the ground or against fixed objects. Such propulsion and the effects of involuntary muscle contraction may lead to secondary injury of the brain or spinal cord and resulting parenchymal damage or development of intracranial hematomas.

The physics and pathophysiology of high-voltage electrical and lightning injuries differ to some extent. The energy level in lightning injuries is much higher and the time of exposure much shorter than in commercial high-voltage electrical injuries. Burns resulting from lightning injuries tend to be superficial and of minor severity, whereas those caused by high-voltage injuries may be associated with major destructive injuries of tissue planes deep within the limb. For this reason, fasciotomy and amputation are often necessary to treat high-voltage injuries, whereas they are rarely needed in lightning injuries. Finally, myoglobinuric renal failure occasionally occurs after high voltage injuries, but it is rare after lightning injuries.[5]

Clinical Presentation

Acute Course and Early Deficits

Approximately 30 percent of persons who are struck by lightning die of their injuries, and approximately 70 percent of lightning strike survivors have significant morbidity.[4,6] Patients having sustained electrical or lightning injuries may have variable external manifestations of their injury, depending on skin resistance, voltage, and duration of contact. Arcing wounds in the upper extremity may affect the forearm, anterior elbow, and axilla and cause extensive tissue destruction. Exit points, especially in the lower extremity, may be subjected to explosive forces with extensive tissue destruction. Victims of lightning injury may have dendriform figures over the skin of the trunk and extremities, indicating surface conduction or flashover of current.

Neurological symptoms at the time of lightning or other electrical injury can range from immediate death due to a head strike with brain injury, to minor sensory disturbances. Patients may report witnessing a loud crack or flash or may have no recollection of the lightning strike. However, retrograde amnesia in victims of lightning injury is unusual. Patients often report that immediately after the lightning strike they regained awareness of their environment but were unable to move or feel their body, even despite witnessing that their clothes were aflame. Temporary deafness frequently occurs and victims often report that they saw their rescuer's lips moving but heard no speech. Consciousness may be clouded and may spontaneously deteriorate, only to improve hours to several days later.

Victims of electrical injury may or may not lose consciousness during contact with the current; nevertheless, later they may have symptoms of bulbar or even cerebral dysfunction, indicating that the current path may not necessarily need to traverse the brain for neurological deficit to occur.

Paralysis is common after lightning strike or electrical injury. Hemiplegia, paraplegia, or quadriplegia may be observed. Recovery after paralysis of immediate onset usually occurs within 24 h and almost always occurs within a few days. Visual changes may be present immediately after injury. Late vision loss from delayed cataract formation has been documented. Weakness in some patients appears to be a combination of central and peripheral nervous system impairment as indicated by prolonged nerve conduction velocities during the immediate postinjury period.

Spinal cord injury can present with either immediate or delayed onset. Para- or quadriplegia that begins at the time of current contact often resolves within hours or days. Transient paralysis is particularly typical for patients struck by lightning and is usually associated with an initial brief loss of consciousness. Permanent spinal cord impairment is more likely in patients whose paralysis is delayed in onset.

Neurological Deficits of Delayed Onset

A variety of neurological syndromes with delayed onset may affect patients after electrical or lightning injury. Hemiplegia and aphasia occurring up to 9 months after injury have been reported.[8] Movement disorders with delayed onset, including tremor, parkinsonian syndromes, and cerebellar ataxia have also been reported as individual cases and are unusual.[16] Homonymous hemianopsia has also been reported.[13]

The most common form of delayed-onset neurological syndrome affects the spinal cord and may resemble progressive spinal muscular atrophy, amyotrophic lateral sclerosis, or transverse myelitis.[11,16,17] After initially sustaining an apparently mild injury, often with only minor sensory disturbances, permanent neurological deficits occur with a latency of days to months and progress slowly. Relatively localized progressive atrophy often affects the contact limb. Quadri- or paraplegia may have an abrupt or gradual onset. When spinal cord involvement occurs with a delayed onset after electrical injury, the prognosis for return of function is generally poor, although unusual cases of recovery have been reported.[3] Cases resembling amyotrophic lateral sclerosis have been described, especially in patients with current paths traversing the arm, hand, shoulder, or neck.[12]

Management

The extrication or rescue of a victim of an electrical accident can be hazardous to the rescuer. Many modern electrical systems are equipped with circuit breakers to interrupt the current flow that caused the injury. The electric current should be interrupted before the victim is separated from the source. Rescuers have been injured by using such "nonconducting" implements as wooden poles and ropes to extricate victims of electrical injury.

Lightning injury (direct current) and high-voltage injury produce cardiac asystole, whereas low-voltage alternating current injuries more often produce ventricular fibrillation. Cardiopulmonary resuscitation is often successful in such patients.

During the initial evaluation of the victim of electrical or lightning injury, the differential diagnosis of mechanical injury to the nervous system should be considered. As noted above, victims of such injuries are frequently propelled and may therefore sustain penetrating or blunt head injury or fracture-dislocation of the spine. In patients unable to protect their airway because of coma, endotracheal intubation should be performed. The initial neurological findings should be documented carefully and compared with the development of later deficits because a combination of immediate and delayed central and peripheral nervous system impairment otherwise may produce a confusing picture.

High-tension injuries frequently produce significant thermal injuries of the scalp and calvarium. Despite significant extracranial injury, the underlying brain may not be severely affected because the resistance of the bony skull is extremely high. Damage to the scalp and cranium may be more extensive than is apparent on initial examination. If full-thickness scalp tissue loss occurs, some bone destruction is likely. The outer table of the devitalized skull can be removed with a high-speed drill. The residual bone must be kept moist to limit the extent of bone necrosis. In some patients, additional procedures may be necessary to remove more necrotic bone. The general approach to management of electrical burns of the skull is conservative. Even if the full thickness of calvarium is lost, the dura will slowly generate granulation tissue, which can be covered initially by split-thickness skin grafts. Later reconstruction with split rib or split-thickness calvarial grafts and scalp flaps can be considered.

Many patients who are initially comatose will slowly regain consciousness. This usually begins during the first day after injury. Supportive care should be provided. Cerebral contusions from electrical and lightning injuries have been reported,[14] and a computed tomography (CT) scan of the head should be performed to identify these lesions and exclude the possibility of associated intracranial mass lesions as a result of unsuspected mechanical trauma at the time of the electrical injury. The usefulness of intracranial pressure monitoring has not been determined in these patients, but it may be indicated in patients with diffuse swelling or mass lesions.

Quadriplegia and paraplegia of immediate onset usually resolve in a similar fashion during the hours and days after injury. For these patients the possibility of fracture-subluxation of the spine due to mechanical injury should be considered in the differential evaluation.

Because of the high currents, the peripheral nerves and vessels that travel with them are often disproportionately injured. In the upper extremity, injuries of the median and ulnar nerve are most common, whereas radial nerve injuries are rather rare.[9] Decompression of the carpal tunnel and Guyon's canal has been advocated,[10] although the therapeutic efficacy of this procedure in these patients is yet unproved.

Patients presenting with a delayed occurrence of spinal cord injury or motor neuron disease after electrical injury should undergo an evaluation including CT-myelography and/or magnetic resonance imaging, and electrodiagnostic studies when indicated, to exclude a possible unrelated, treatable cause of deficit. Symptomatic and supportive treatment should then be provided as appropriate.

References

1. Apfelberg DB, Masters FW, Robinson DW. Pathophysiology and treatment of lightning injuries. *J Trauma* 1974; 14:453–460.
2. Bingham H. Electrical burns. *Clin Plast Surg* 1986; 13:75–85.
3. Christensen JA, Sherman RT, Balis GA, et al. Delayed neurologic injury secondary to high-voltage current, with recovery. *J Trauma* 1980; 20:166–168.
4. Cooper MA. Lightning injuries: prognostic signs for death. *Ann Emerg Med* 1980; 9:134–138.
5. Cooper MA. Electrical and lightning injuries. *Emerg Med Clin North Am* 1984; 2:489-501.
6. Cooper MA. Lightning injuries. In Auerbach PS, Geehr EC (eds): *Management of Wilderness and Environmental Emergencies,* 2d ed. St Louis: Mosby, 1989, pp 173–193.
7. Craig SR. When lightning strikes: pathophysiology and treatment of lightning injuries. *Postgrad Med* 1986; 79:109–112, 121–124.
8. Critchley M. Electrical injuries. *Trans Med Soc Lond* 1936; 59:19–31.
9. Dendooven AM, Lissens M, Bruyninckx F, et al. Electrical injuries to peripheral nerves. *Acta Belg Med Phys* 1990; 13:161–165.
10. Engrav LH, Gottlieb JR, Walkinshaw MD, et al. Outcome and treatment of electrical injury with immediate median and ulnar nerve palsy at the wrist; a retrospective review and a survey of members of the American Burn Association. *Ann Plast Surg* 1990; 25:166–168.
11. Farrell DF, Starr A. Delayed neurological sequelae of electrical injuries. *Neurology* 1968; 18:601–606.
12. Gallagher JP, Sanders M. Trauma and amyotrophic lateral sclerosis: a report of 78 patients. *Acta Neurol Scand* 1987; 75:145–150.
13. Gans M, Glaser JS. Homonymous hemianopia following electrical injury. *J Clin Neuro Ophthalmol* 1986; 6:218–221.
14. Iob I, Salar G, Ori C, et al. Accidental high voltage electrocution: a rare neurosurgical problem. *Acta Neurochir (Wien)* 1986; 83:151–153.
15. Nichter LS, Bryant CA, Kenney JG, et al. Injuries due to commercial electric current. *J Burn Care Rehabil* 1984; 5:124–137.
16. Panse F. Electrical trauma. In Vinken PJ, Bruyn GW (eds): *Handbook of Clinical Neurology,* vol 23. *Injuries of the Brain and Skull, Part I.* New York: Elsevier, 1975, pp 683–729.
17. Petty PG, Parkin G. Electrical injury to the central nervous system. *Neurosurgery* 1986; 19:282–284.
18. Robinson M, Seward PN. Electrical and lightning injuries in children. *Pediatr Emerg Care* 1986; 2:186–190.

SECTION B

Cranial Trauma

259

Mechanisms of Primary Head Injury

Thomas A. Gennarelli
David F. Meaney

The complex pathophysiologic phenomena encountered in patients with head injuries can be viewed ultimately as the response of the brain and its coverings to an external mechanical insult. Therefore, an understanding of the causative mechanical factors that result in the multitude of head injuries observed clinically is necessary for establishing both effective prevention strategies and therapeutic treatments to mitigate the short- and long-term consequences of head injury. In this chapter we will review the primary mechanical forces that act on the head, the manner in which these forces can damage the intracranial contents and, finally, the contribution of these forces in producing commonly observed head injuries. It is intended as an introductory description of the mechanisms for primary head injuries, and can serve as a prelude to more detailed engineering and mathematical investigations of head injury.[3,10,13,15]

Clinical Classification of Head Injuries

From a clinical standpoint, primary head injuries can be classified into three categories: skull fractures, focal injuries, and diffuse brain injuries (Table 259-1). *Skull fractures* may occur with or without concomitant damage to the brain, but a skull fracture is usually not a direct cause of neurological disability. *Focal brain injuries,* in comparison, are found in approximately one-half of all patients with severe head injuries and are responsible for nearly two-thirds of deaths associated with head injury.[1,5,7] They are defined as macroscopically visible damage to the parenchyma that is generally limited to a well-defined area; examples of focal head injuries include cortical contusions and subdural, epidural, and intracerebral hematomas. *Diffuse brain injuries* differ fundamentally from focal injuries and are associated with widespread brain dysfunction, often without macroscopic structural damage. Observed in approximately 40 percent of patients with severe head injuries, diffuse brain injuries account for one-third of deaths due to head injury and are the most prevalent cause of persisting neurological disability in survivors.[5] Diffuse brain damage may not necessarily be structural in nature, as in the case of concussion, and may involve complex alterations in neural excitability or in neurotransmitter receptor dysfunction. However, in more severe cases of diffuse brain injury such as prolonged coma without mass lesions, the damage involves some degree of structural derangement. Because of the widespread damage to axons in cases of prolonged coma without mass lesion, this clinical condition has been termed *diffuse axonal injury.*[2,9]

Mechanisms of Injury

Head injuries contained within these three clinical classification categories can be produced from very specific forms of mechanical input. Characteristics of the mechanical input, such as the direction, magnitude, application rate, duration, and point of action of the force contribute to the type and severity of the head injury(s) caused by the input. Table 259-2 classifies the mechanical loading experienced by the head, the effect of these inputs on the intracranial contents, and the possible resultant damage to the skull and brain.

The complex mechanical loading experienced by the head can be either classified as static or dynamic in nature (Fig. 259-1). *Static loading* (an uncommon occurrence), refers to loading which is applied to the head slowly, typically occurring in periods greater

TABLE 259-1 Primary Head Injuries

Skull Fractures	Focal Brain Injuries	Diffuse Brain Injuries
Vault	*Contusion*	*Concussion*
Linear	Coup	Mild
Depressed	Contrecoup	Classic
	Intermediate	
Basilar		*Diffuse Axonal Injury*
	Hemorrhage/Hematoma	*Other*
	Epidural	
	Subdural	
	Intracerebral	
	Petechial	

TABLE 259-2 Mechanistic Types of Head Injuries

Contact Injuries*	Head Motion Injuries†
Skull Deformation Injuries	*Skull-Brain Relative Motion*
Local Skull Bending	Subdural hematoma
Skull fracture (linear, depressed)	Contrecoup contusion
Epidural hematoma	Intermediate coup contusion
Coup contusion	
	Brain Deformation
Skull Volume Changes	Concussion syndromes
Vault, basilar fracture	Diffuse axonal injury
Contrecoup contusion	Intracerebral hemorrhage
	Tissue tear hemorrhage
Shock Wave Propagation	
Intracerebral hemorrhage	

*Blow to head required; head motion not necessary.
†Head motion required; direct blow to head not necessary.

than 200 ms. Events such as avalanches, earthquakes, and slowly moving vehicles that trap the head against rigid structures produce these events. Characterized by a squeezing or slow crushing of the skull, static loading usually results in numerous, comminuted fractures of the vault or base of the skull, often occurring while consciousness is preserved. Interestingly, severe neurological deficits do not appear until the level of static loading is sufficient to cause substantial distortion or deformation of the brain. At this point, serious or fatal compressive brain damage occurs.

Dynamic loading is the more common type of mechanical loading to the head and is characterized by an input applied rapidly to the head, typically in durations of less than 50 ms. As described later, the precise duration of the loading input is a critical factor in determining the type of head injury produced. Dynamic loading can be of two types: impulsive or impact. *Impulsive loading* occurs when the head is set into motion or when the moving head is arrested without its being struck or impacted. These conditions are not infrequent since a blow to the thorax or face can often set the head into violent motion without direct impact to the skull. In these circumstances, there is no impact to the cranium and thus no contact forces occur. The resulting head injuries are caused solely by the inertial forces produced by the way in which the head moves. Although there is no doubt that facial impact can cause sufficient inertial forces in the brain to result in any of the inertial injuries, recent evidence has raised the question as to whether this is true for situations not involving impact to the face. Although theoretically possible, it is uncertain that, in ''real-world'' accident circumstances, sufficiently high levels of inertial forces occur to produce the most serious inertial injuries if impact to the head or face does not occur. Thus, when the head is stopped or set into motion by indirect impact to the chest, it is unclear whether situations occur in which the head moves in the appropriate manner to generate the high intensity strains necessary to cause the full spectrum of inertial injuries. On the other hand, lesser degrees of diffuse brain injury and cerebral concussion can occur by impulsive loading.

Impact loading is the more frequent type of dynamic loading and usually results in a combination of contact forces and inertial forces. The response of the head to impact conditions depends on the object that strikes the head. For example, inertial effects can be minimal in certain impact conditions, especially if the head is prevented from moving when it is struck. The result is that most of the impact energy is delivered to the head as contact force and results in a complex set of effects collectively known as contact phenomena. The contact phenomena are a group of mechanical events that occur both near and distant from the point of impact. The magnitude and importance of these phenomena vary with the size of the impacting device and with the magnitude of the force delivered to the contact point. The latter is determined by the mass, surface area, velocity, and hardness of the impacting object. These factors determine the manner in which energy is transferred to the head. For objects larger than 2 sq in, localized skull deformation occurs with in-bending of the skull immediately beneath the point of impact and out-bending of the skull peripheral to the impact site. If the degree of local skull deformation exceeds the tolerance of the

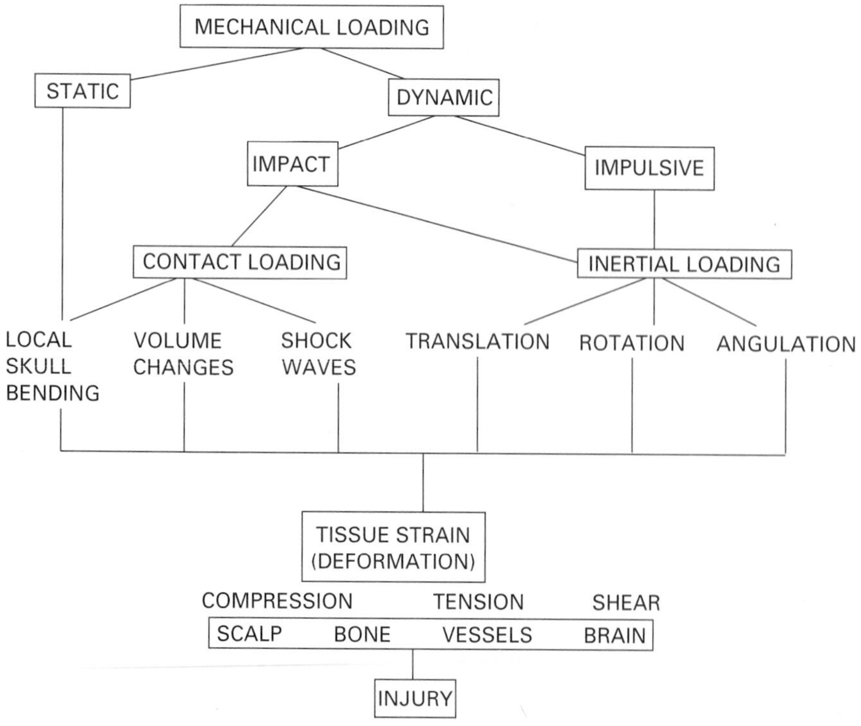

Figure 259-1 Classification of the types of mechanical loading to the head.

skull, fracture occurs. Penetration, perforation, or localized depressed fracture of the skull is more likely if the object has a surface area less than 2 sq in. Additionally, shock waves that travel at the speed of sound propagate throughout the skull from the point of impact, as well as directly through the brain substance. The shock waves cause local changes in tissue pressure. If these changes result in sufficient brain distortion, localized intraparenchymal brain damage, usually in the form of small hemorrhages, results.

Although these definitions highlight the etiologic differences between impact and impulsive loading, the fundamental means of damaging the skull and brain are the same: by distorting or straining the bony or soft tissues beyond their functional or structural tolerance. Strain, considered the proximal cause of tissue damage, can be either compressive, tensile, or shear in nature (Fig. 259-2). In general, strain can be considered as the amount of deformation that the tissue undergoes as a result of an applied mechanical force. Compressive strain is the amount of contraction observed when a material is compressed. For instance, if a stout cylindrical rod is placed upright on a tabletop and a stack of books is placed on the top circular face of the cylinder, the rod would shorten with respect to its original, unloaded length. If the rod was originally 10 cm in length and became 8 cm when the books were placed on top, the material is said to have a 20 percent compressive strain. Tensile strain, on the other hand, is the amount of elongation that occurs when a material is stretched. If a column of rubber 10 cm in length becomes 11 cm long when stretched by hanging a 100-g weight from it, it undergoes a 10 percent tensile strain (stretched length − original length ÷ by original length). Finally, shear strain can be considered the amount of distortion that occurs in response to forces applied along the surface of a material. A common illustration of shear strain is the distortional change that occurs in a deck of playing cards when a hand is placed on the top of the deck and moved lengthwise. None of the cards is compressed or stretched as a result of this motion, but the side profile of the deck changes to a ''slanted'' rectangle. The degree to which the deformed side profile varies from a normal rectangle indicates the state of shear strain.

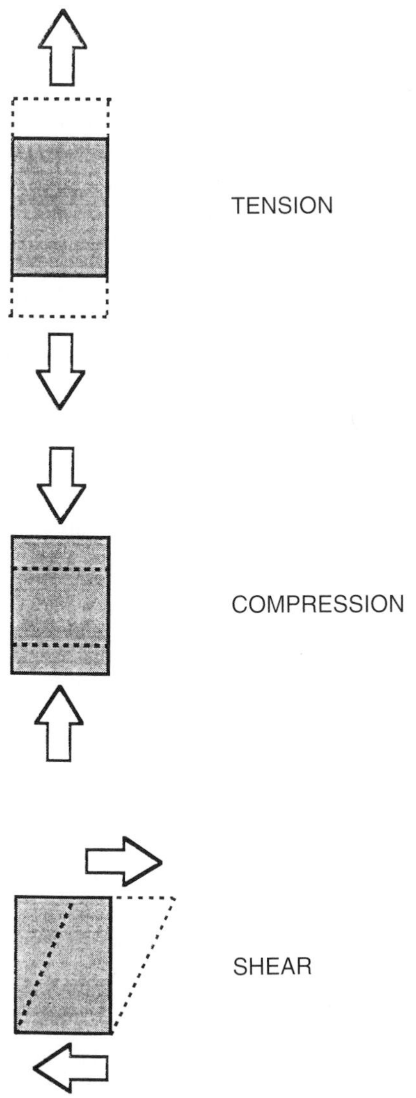

Figure 259-2 Types of strain that may cause damage to the skull and brain. Forces are applied to an object at rest (*shaded block*), causing the object to deform (*broken lines*).

The amount of tolerable strain depends on not only the magnitude of the applied force, but also on the mechanical properties and time-dependent behavior of the material. A steel rod is capable of sustaining substantial compressive loads because of its inherent strength, but it typically fails at relatively low strain levels. In contrast, rubber has an exceptionally high failure limit that is usually two to three times its original length, but it cannot sustain the stresses experienced by steel. Furthermore, the time-dependent, or viscoelastic, behavior of materials is a necessary consideration when determining the tolerable strain that applies to the more common dynamic loading situations. A viscoelastic material is one whose tolerance to strain changes with the rate at which the material is loaded. Perhaps the most recognizable viscoelastic material is Silly Putty (Binney & Smith, Inc., Easton, PA), a compound that can be easily kneaded into various shapes using one's hands. If pulled slowly from its ends, Silly Putty can deform substantially before breaking. If, however, this material is pulled very quickly, the material breaks at a much smaller length. Biological tissues typically display such viscoelastic behavior, and can therefore withstand strain better if they are deformed slowly rather than quickly (i.e., they become more brittle and will break at lower strain levels under rapidly applied loads). Thus, the type of injury that occurs as a result of a given loading condition is determined collectively by the nature, location, and time course of the induced strains and by the ability of the tissue to withstand those particular strains.

The three principal tissues involved in head injury (bone, vascular tissue, and brain tissue) vary considerably in their tolerances to compression, tension, and shear. Bone, for example, is considerably stronger than vascular or brain tissue and more force is therefore required to induce injurious levels of strain. The amount of strain that bone can tolerate is actually less than that needed to injure brain tissue (i.e., bone breaks at 1 to 2 percent strain, whereas brain and vascular tissue may not tear unless 10 to 20 percent strain is applied). However, it takes considerable force to cause 1 to 2 percent strain in bone. Bone shares with vascular and brain tissue the common property of being better able to withstand compressive strain than shear strain, with a tensile strain tolerance somewhere in between, although much closer to the shear tolerance. There is proportionately less difference between the three strain tolerances for bone, whereas there is a considerable difference in the ability of brain tissue to withstand compression and shear.

Since brain is virtually incompressible in vivo and since it has a very low tolerance to tensile and shear strain, the latter two types of strain are the usual causes of brain damage. The same is true for vascular tissue. Whether vascular or brain tissue damage occurs depends on the exact properties of these two tissues. As will be discussed later, vascular tissue tends to fail under more rapidly applied loads than does brain tissue, and, depending on the type of input to the head, conditions exist that can cause relatively pure injury to the vascular elements and to the neural elements within the head.

Mechanistic Causes of Head Injuries

Most head injuries are due to one of the two basic mechanisms: contact or inertial loading. Contact injuries require that the head strikes an object or is struck, regardless of whether the blow causes the head to move afterward. Inertial injuries are often called head motion or acceleration injuries because they result from violent head motion, regardless of whether the head moves because of a direct blow or not (Table 259-2).

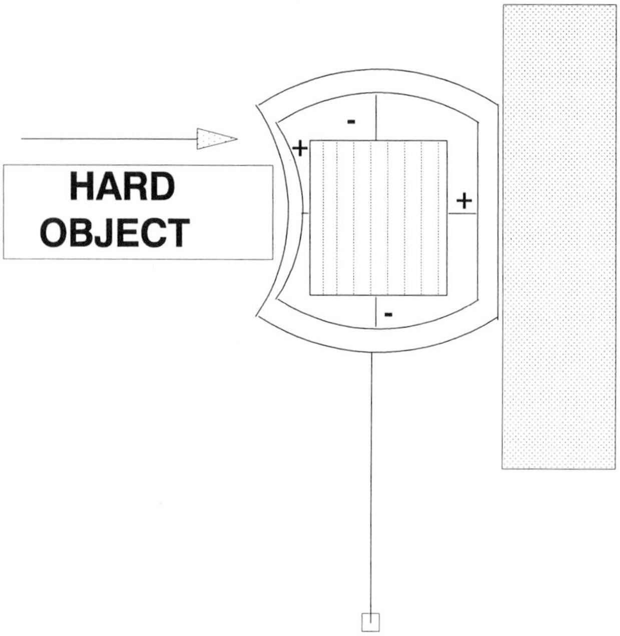

Figure 259-3 Impact loading with no head motion. Impact to the idealized, immobile head causes both local and remote skull deformation. Local skull inbending creates an area of high pressure immediately beneath the impact site, while simultaneous outbending outside the impact location causes negative pressures at the top and bottom of the idealized skull.

Contact Injuries

Contact injuries, in general, are caused by forces that occur during impact. These injuries result solely from contact phenomena and have nothing to do with head motion or head acceleration. Since most impacts also set the head into motion to some degree, trauma rarely occurs clinically in pure form; more frequently, contact injuries have superimposed acceleration injuries as well. Many times, however, the injuries received by a patient are predominantly contact related. Contact injuries can therefore be considered trauma that would occur if the head were prevented from moving (Fig. 259-3).

Contact forces are of two types: (1) effects that occur locally at or near the site of impact, and (2) effects that occur remote from the area of impact. In both instances, contact forces cause focal injuries that are either surrounding or remote from the impact site. Contact forces do not cause diffuse brain injury.

Local Contact Effects

Examples of injuries due to the local contact effects include most linear and depressed skull fractures, some basilar skull fractures, epidural hematomas, and coup contusions. The event producing linear skull fractures is the local skull bending occurring at the site of impact which exceeds the strain limit for the bony tissue. Since it has been explained that the strain tolerance for a material is related to the inherent mechanical properties of the material, it is not surprising to find that the occurrence of skull fracture depends in part on the material properties of the skull and the thickness of the skull in the impact region. Additional contributing factors include the magnitude and direction of impact, and the size of the impacted area.[12] Mechanistically, the local inbending caused by the impact creates compressive strains on the outer skull surface and tensile strains on the inner surface. Bone, naturally resistant to compressive forces and strains, is weaker to the tensile forces on the inner skull surface and thus the initial fracture begins at the inner table. Once initiated, the fracture follows a path of least resistance that is dictated by the geometric and strength characteristics of the surrounding skull. During the continuing fracture process, energy from the impacting object is being transferred to the skull via the fracture. The linear fracture is complete when the energy in the impact process is dissipated completely.

Depressed skull fractures occur when the striking or struck object is small enough to cause a concentration of strain and stress immediately beneath the impacting object. These concentrated strains produce a highly localized fracture pattern that does not emanate from the contact site. Unlike a linear skull fracture, energy is not absorbed by a fracture propagating away from the loading point but instead is dissipated by the localized failure of bone. For highly concentrated contact forces, these depressed skull fractures penetrate completely through the skull.

Impact to the skull base or nearby regions can occur and cause *basilar skull fractures* from local contact effects. Direct impacts to the occiput or mastoid are common methods for this type of skull fracture. Energy transferred to the basilar skull via impact to the facial bones is a way to produce similar fractures by indirect impact and local contact effects.

Vascular damage caused by local contact effects (i.e., epidural hematoma and coup contusions), is intimately linked to the causative phenomena for the preceding skull fracture types. The epidural hematoma can be considered a complicated form of the skull bending that could result in skull fracture. In the limiting case, dural vessels are torn as the fracture propagates and travels past a vessel. The mechanical failure of these vessels can occur without fracture, however, if skull deformation and bending are sufficient to cause vascular tears.

Coup contusions occur beneath the site of impact under certain conditions. They are due to either direct injury to the brain and its surface vessels that lie beneath the area of skull deformation or to the high negative pressures that develop when an area of inbent skull rapidly snaps back into place. The first mechanism causes highly focused compressive strains, whereas the second subjects the brain to very high tensile strains. In either case these strains are sufficient to cause tissue failure of the pia and cortical vessels and of the brain tissue itself. The localized contusion that results is therefore due to a combination of vascular and brain disruption. Brain laceration is an extension of the same phenomenon but may also occur if skull inbending is sufficient to actually perforate the pia.

Remote Contact Effects

Contact phenomena that are as equally important are remote injuries caused by two mechanisms: (1) local and global skull distortion, and (2) stress waves. These contribute to vault fractures that occur away from the impact site, to basilar skull fractures, and to contrecoup and intermediate coup contusions. Remote *vault fracture* can develop if the impact occurs over a thick portion of the skull or if the striking object is relatively broad. Since the thick skull can withstand the impact force, little inbending occurs. However, as the local bending travels away from the impact site as a means of dissipating energy, thinner sections of skull remote from the loading point may experience larger local bending due to their inherently weaker characteristics. If the strain tolerance for skull is exceeded, skull fracture at this distant site occurs. Once initiated, this fracture will usually propagate along the lines of least resistance that may or may not point toward the impact site. Typically, regions such as the basilar skull area have thin skull sections which offer this path of least resistance. As a result, various types of basilar skull fractures may occur from remote contact loading.

Occasionally, head contact is severe enough that global changes in skull shape occur in addition to local skull bending effects (Fig. 259-3). These global changes are particularly apparent if the skull structure is compliant, such as in infants and developing children. This type of large skull deformation results in increases or decreases in intracranial volume. These changes are usually transient and, due to the elastic nature of the skull and its contents, the skull returns to its normal shape immediately after the force is removed. Two phenomena that may appear at these large deformations (i.e., localized pressure changes and intracranial volume fluctuations), can cause a variety of injuries. The rapid changes in skull shape can be sufficient to produce levels of negative pressure at points where the skull has pulled away from the brain (Fig. 259-3, *top* and *bottom*); the resulting tensile loading of the brain surface at these locations can then cause *contrecoup contusions.* This localized pressure mechanism has also been impugned as a cause of small petechiae surrounding the ventricles, presumably as they expand in response to brief negative intracranial pressures. A sudden fluctuation or decrease in intracranial volume caused by the global skull deformations can prompt herniation of the intracranial contents through various foramina, primarily the foramen magnum. The action of herniation may place an excessive amount of strain on structures within the lower brain stem, and therefore cause tissue injury remote from the impact site. These intracranial volume fluctuations may explain part of the distinct neurological and pathological observations found in infants or children with developing skulls that maintain a fair degree of flexibility. However, the frequency with which trauma contributes to global skull deformation in the adult is still debated, and these injuries are probably much more commonly due to inertial effects.

The second mechanism for remote damage due to contact loading is stress waves originating at the point of impact. Radiating in a three-dimensional manner from the loading point at an exceedingly rapid speed, stress waves that spread through the skull cause local skull distortions that, if excessive, produce basilar and remote vault fractures. Stress waves also spread through the brain and, like waves in water, may reflect from the opposite side of the head and reverberate within the brain. The manner in which these waves reverberate within the brain depends on, among other factors, the ability of the brain tissue to absorb or dissipate these disturbances and the severity of impact. If the stress waves in the brain are amplified by this reverberation or local skull bending, high-intensity, localized pressure differences occur. These localized pressures result in strain on tissue that may be sufficient to exceed the brain's tolerance. Damage to vascular elements or to brain tissue at sites of strain concentration result. In theory, the areas of strain concentration due to reverberating shock waves lie deep within the brain and not at its surface. Therefore, shock waves have been used to explain the formation of intermediate coup contusions (a name sometimes used to describe hemorrhages occurring on nonconvexity surfaces), scattered deep petechial hemorrhages, and traumatic intracerebral hematomas. However, this mechanism remains a matter of debate, since it is argued that because these waves travel so rapidly through the brain, their effects are quickly dissipated and therefore they are not an important mechanism of injury.

Head Motion (Inertial) Injuries

Inertial loading of the head, whether from impact or from impulsive loading, causes such rapid movement of the head that resultant injuries are due only to the manner in which the head moves. These are commonly called acceleration-deceleration injuries because acceleration is an important physical measure of the loading. Other factors may be equally important (e.g., head velocity), and although this category should perhaps be called "head motion injuries," the term "acceleration injuries" remains with us. From the mechanical point of view, acceleration and deceleration are the same physical phenomenon and differ only in direction. Thus, the effects of accelerating the head in the sagittal plane from posterior to anterior are exactly the same as the effects of decelerating the head from anterior to posterior (Fig. 259-4).

Similar to contact injuries, head motion results in strains within the brain tissue that can cause either functional or structural damage by one of two mechanisms. First, differential movement of the skull and brain can be produced by head acceleration or motion. This relative movement occurs because the brain is free to move to some degree within the skull and because, as a result of inertia, the brain lags behind the skull for a brief moment after acceleration begins. When combined, these factors allow the skull and dura to move relative to the brain surface which thereby causes a localized strain at the brain surface. Particularly susceptible to this localized strain are the parasagittal bridging veins between the brain surface and dura, which may tear if the strain exceeds the vascular tolerance (Fig. 259-5, *top* and *bottom*). Furthermore, the movement of the brain away from the skull creates regions of low pressure (tensile strain) that, if sufficiently intense, cause contrecoup contusions (Fig. 259-5, *right*). The second way that head motion is injurious is that it can produce strain within the brain parenchyma, and therefore can cause widespread disturbances to brain function or structures that are manifest as classic cerebral concussion, diffuse axonal injury and associated tissue tear hemorrhages (deep petechial hemorrhages), and most intermediate coup contusions. In each type of injury, the acceleration or movement of the head causes

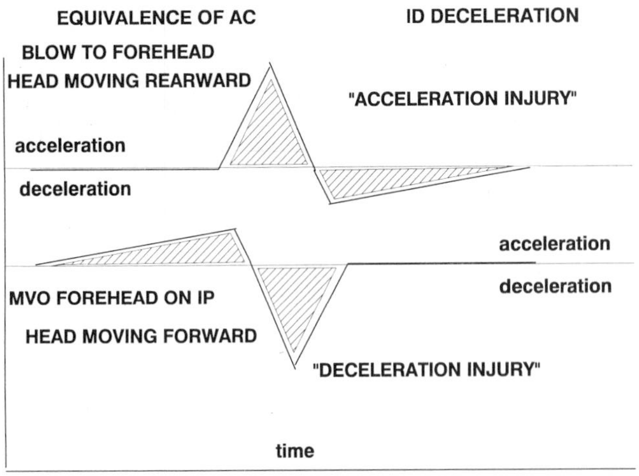

Figure 259-4 Equivalence of acceleration and deceleration. Two different situations that appear to be quite different are actually very similar. If the head is moving rearward as a result of a blow to the forehead (''acceleration injury''), the head experiences an acceleration shown in the top graph. In comparison, if a motor vehicle occupant (MVO) strikes his/her moving forehead on an automotive interior part (IP) or structure (''deceleration injury''), the head experiences an acceleration shown in the lower graph. Both situations cause the brain to deform within the skull and are capable of causing similar brain injuries due to the induced head motions. Differences arise when the impacting surface is hard and thus causes additional contact effect injuries (i.e., coup contusion, skull fracture, epidural hematoma), which is usually the case for the ''acceleration injury'' condition (see text).

either a functional or structural failure of neural and/or vascular structures, where the severity and extent of disruption are intimately linked to the magnitude, rate, duration, direction, and type of inertial loading.

Types of Head Acceleration

Three types of acceleration can occur: translational, rotational, and angular (Fig. 259-6). *Translational acceleration* occurs when the center of gravity of the brain (which is approximately in the pineal region) moves in a straight line. Purely translational acceleration is uncommon, since, because of the head-neck connections, this type of movement is not physiologic. Translational movements can occur for short periods of time during head motions, or the head can become arrested before other motions occur. An exception may be vertex impact, during which superior-inferior motion can occur. The brain motions that take place during translational acceleration are primarily due to the relative brain-skull motions previously described and not to strain produced deep within the brain. It has been shown that concussive injuries do not occur if the head is not accelerated or if it undergoes a purely translational acceleration.[4,14] For concussion or diffuse axonal injury to develop, the brain must undergo angular acceleration. Therefore, translational acceleration does not cause diffuse brain injuries but it can produce various focal injuries, including contrecoup contusion and intracerebral and subdural hematomas. It is not surprising, therefore, that situations exist in which substantial brain damage has occurred without primary loss of consciousness.

Rotational acceleration occurs when there is rotation about the center of gravity of the brain without the center of gravity itself moving. Since the center of gravity of the brain is in the pineal area, pure rotational acceleration is a virtual impossibility in clinical situations. For the brain to pivot around an axis that goes through the pineal area, the entire body would have to swing around the head. The only exception is in the horizontal plane, where pure rotation may occur about a vertical axis running through the pineal area. Rotational acceleration is a very important and highly injurious mechanism because it produces not only the high surface strains seen in translational motions but also is the only mechanism capable of producing high levels of strain deep within the brain itself. However, because of the infrequency of pure rotational motions in clinical situations, the effects of rotational acceleration are usually seen only in association with angular acceleration.

Angular acceleration occurs when components of translational and rotational acceleration are combined. In this situation the center of gravity moves in an angular manner. Because of the head-neck anatomy, angular acceleration is the most common head motion encountered clinically, the center of rotation most often being

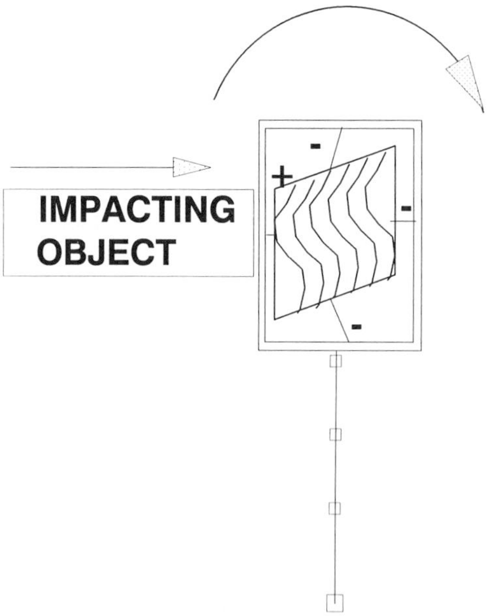

Figure 259-5 Impact loading with head motion. In contrast to Fig. 259-3, allowing head motion after impact causes the brain to deform as a result of including rotational acceleration. Impact to the idealized skull pictured above causes the brain to move slightly toward the impact site, creating areas of high pressure beneath the contact site and negative pressures opposite the impact location. In addition, the head rotational acceleration caused by allowing the head to angulate about a point in the lower to midcervical spine creates shear strains within the brain tissue. Injuries caused by these rotational acceleration effects include tearing of parasagittal bridging veins, cerebral concussion, and diffuse axonal injury.

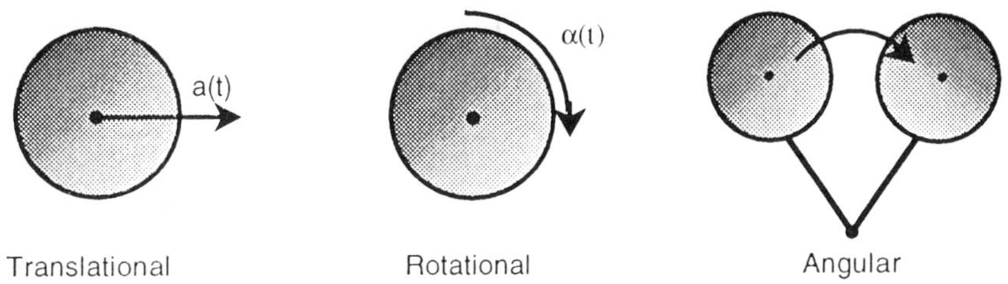

Figure 259-6 Types of acceleration experienced by the head. Translational acceleration occurs when the center of mass of the head is moved or slowed in a straight line, whereas rotational acceleration occurs when the head is rotated about its center of mass. With the exception of horizontal plane movements, pure rotational acceleration of the head is uncommon. Rather, the most common form of acceleration is angular acceleration, where the head's center of mass angulates about a point in the lower or midcervical spine. Angular acceleration contains components of both translational and rotational acceleration.

in the lower cervical region. The exact location of the center of angulation determines the proportion of translation and rotation that the brain undergoes. As the center of angulation moves higher up the cervical spine, there is a proportionately greater rotational component, and when the center of angulation moves lower, there is proportionately more translational acceleration. As might be expected, angular acceleration is the most injurious brain injury mechanism because it occurs most frequently and because it combines the injurious mechanisms of both translational and rotational movements (especially the latter). Except for skull fracture and epidural hematoma, virtually *every known type of head injury can be produced by angular acceleration.*[1,5]

Determinants of Acceleration Injury

The amount of acceleration damage depends not only on the type of acceleration to the head but also on several other factors. Because of the viscoelastic nature of biological tissue, the response of the tissue is determined by a combination of the acceleration magnitude and the rate at which acceleration occurs. The acceleration magnitude can be viewed as proportional to the amount of strain delivered to the brain, and the acceleration rate as proportional to the strain rate. If the acceleration magnitude is constant, the rate of acceleration varies inversely with the duration for which the acceleration is applied. Conversely, if the acceleration duration is constant, the acceleration rate varies directly with the acceleration magnitude.

Three zones of clinical interest are encountered as the acceleration duration increases at a constant amount of acceleration (Fig. 259-7). First, at very high strain rates (i.e., short acceleration durations), the properties of the brain are such that many of the inertial effects are damped, and, as a result, the brain actually experiences very little strain. Therefore, extremely high accelerations are required to produce injury. The second zone begins as the acceleration duration is slightly longer. Less damping occurs, and it therefore requires less acceleration to produce injurious strains within the head. However, the strain that occurs during these conditions is confined to the surface, since the acceleration is present for such a brief time that the strains cannot penetrate deeply. The types of injury that can be produced in these circumstances are those at the brain surface and those principally to vascular tissue (i.e., subdural hematoma). As the duration of acceleration increases further, the third zone begins; fewer of the inertial effects are damped and the resulting strains are able to propagate deeper into the brain. Accelerations of longer duration are more injurious to the brain and cause concussion and axonal injury that manifests as prolonged traumatic coma.

The strain rate also increases if the acceleration magnitude is increased while the acceleration duration remains constant. In the first zone described, the strain rate is already so high that increasing it further adds little to the pattern of injury. In the second zone, vascular tissues at the brain surface are already jeopardized; therefore, increasing the strain rate further can exceed the vascular tissue tolerance and cause damage to previously uninjured areas or can increase the number of disrupted vessels. In the third zone, in which the strain rate produces damage to brain tissue but is insufficient to produce damage to vessels, increasing the acceleration magnitude can increase the strain rate sufficiently to cause vascular injury. The result can be the combination of diffuse axonal damage with tissue tear hemorrhages or subdural hematoma.

Therefore, acceleration damage to the brain can be of several types depending on the amount and type of acceleration, its duration, and the rate at which acceleration is applied to the head. The last two variables are interrelated because for a constant level of acceleration, as one variable increases, the other must decrease.

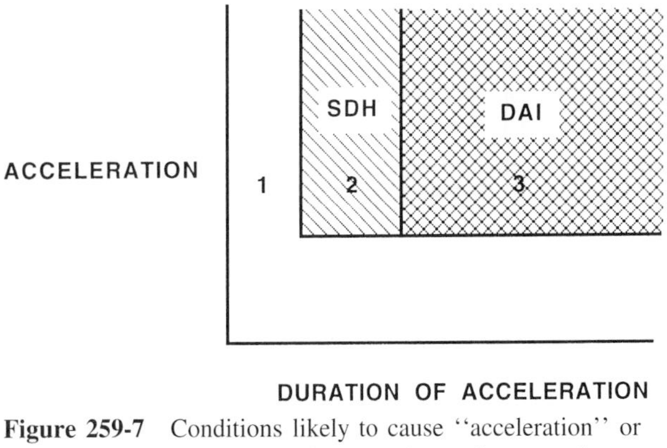

Figure 259-7 Conditions likely to cause "acceleration" or head motion brain injuries. If the head experiences a short-duration rotational acceleration, strains appear primarily along the brain periphery and the most likely injury is tearing of parasagittal bridging veins, creating a subdural hematoma (SDH). If the duration of rotational acceleration is increased as the magnitude remains constant, strains propagate deeper within the brain and cause widespread axonal damage (diffuse axonal injury; DAI).

Since the integral of the acceleration time curve represents velocity, head velocity increases with acceleration duration and decreases with acceleration rate. Thus, the brain's tolerance to head movement could equally be viewed in terms of two variables: head acceleration and head velocity. Structural damage to superficial vascular tissue, especially to bridging veins and pial vessels, occurs in high-acceleration, high-strain rate conditions (short acceleration duration, low velocity), whereas brain tissue damage (primarily axonal) occurs in circumstances in which high-acceleration levels are present with lower strain rates, longer pulse durations, and thus higher velocities.

Injuries and Their Mechanisms

This section uses the preceding concepts to explain the mechanisms responsible for frequently observed primary head injuries. The clinical classification system for head injuries described in the beginning of this chapter is used to separate individual classes of injury. It is clear that many of these injuries may occur in combination, and isolated occurrences of these injuries, particularly severe head injuries, are rare. Moreover, these injuries usually occur in accident situations where the head experiences a primary mechanical loading in which a particular mechanism (e.g., local or remote contact phenomena, inertial effects) is predominant. As a result, it is not uncommon to find particular head injuries occurring primarily in motor vehicle accidents, in cases of falls or assaults, or in pedestrian accidents.[5]

Skull Fracture

Linear Fracture

Linear fractures occur solely because of the contact effects due to impact. Head motion, acceleration, and inertial effects play no role in the genesis of fracture. A linear fracture is caused by a hard impacting object, with most of the energy from this object used to deform the skull locally. Little energy is used to move or accelerate the skull. To prevent the more localized depressed skull fracture, the impacting object must be larger than approximately 2 sq in. However, if the impacting object or surface is considerably larger, then contact is distributed across a broad area of the scalp and the local bending effects necessary for fracture to occur are not present. Acceleration injuries may occur in parallel with fracture, since most impact situations involve some form of inertial loading superimposed on the contact loading.

Depressed Fracture

Depressed fractures are caused by small, hard impactors that create concentrations of stresses and strains immediately beneath the impact point. Energy management of the impact occurs through fracture of the skull immediately beneath the impactor. If the impacting force is substantial, all bone under the impactor is damaged and skull perforation occurs. Due to the focused loading, little or no propagation of the fracture exists.

Basilar Fracture

Due chiefly to either direct impact or the propagations of stress waves through the skull as a result of the remote impact, basilar fractures may also occur as a consequence of impact to facial bones. The thin basilar skull is particularly susceptible to remote contact effects, since the structure of this region is considerably weaker and not as effective in managing local skull deformations initiated by remote impact. Common impact points for producing basilar skull fracture include the skull base (occiput, mastoid, supraorbital area), facial or mandibular bones, and remote skull impact points.

Focal Brain Injury

Epidural Hematoma

Epidural hematoma can be considered a more complex case of linear skull fracture. During the fracture initiation or propagation period, vessel(s) in the underlying dural membrane are torn and bleeding ensues in the epidural space. Epidural bleeding is also possible without skull fracture, since the local skull bending caused by impact may be sufficient to tear dural vessels without exceeding the failure limit of the bone. No head motion or inertial effects are causal to the occurrence of an epidural hematoma.

Coup Contusions

Immediately under the impact point, coup contusions arise principally from the local skull bending or fracture caused by impact from a relatively small, hard object. These phenomena in turn subject the underlying cortical and pial vascular network to strains that, if excessive, cause bleeding at or near the brain surface. Damage is likely to occur when the skull is "rebounding" from the impact and the vessels are experiencing tensile strain. For cases of skull fracture, the localized strains from the skull contacting the cortical surface provide a means for the vascular damage noted in the pia and cortex.

Contrecoup Contusions

Two phenomena have been attributed to the pathogenesis of contrecoup contusions: cavitation effects and inertial loading. Of the two, the more likely mechanism of the contrecoup damage is translational or angular head motion. On impact, the brain moves toward the impact site and creates an area of negative pressure directly opposite the point loading. This negative pressure may in turn cause damage by exceeding the tensile strength of water, which is the primary fluid component of the brain. This phenomenon, termed cavitation, has little experimental support and does not explain contusions located outside the region considered opposite the impact. Instead, it appears that regions of vascular disruption and cortical damage in contrecoup regions are due primarily to acceleration (inertial) effects and can result from either translational or angular head motions. Each head motion (particularly angular movement), is capable of producing tensile strains in regions throughout the brain. If the tensile strains that result are greater than the vascular tolerance in a given region, contusion occurs. However, due to this inertial or head motion mechanism, impact is not necessary for contrecoup contusions to occur. The term "contrecoup" can therefore be considered misleading, since the critical mechanism is most often acceleration and not impact, which is the necessary ingredient for coup contusions. In situations in which the head undergoes impulsive loading, contrecoup contusions occur solely because of the strains generated in the cortical brain region as a result of the head acceleration. Concentrations of strain may occur in specific regions of the brain due to geometric effects, and are responsible in part for the high incidence of frontal and temporal lobe contusions observed clinically. Although global skull deformation caused by impact may create tensile strains and contusion damage in regions remote from impact, the predominant mechanism for contrecoup contusions is head acceleration.

Due to their macroscopic and easily identifiable nature, contusions have been used periodically to characterize the biomechanical input to the head. However, several points deserve mention when using contusions as a tool to reconstruct the direction of the impact force or to classify the inertial loading as either acceleration or deceleration. First, the line of action of an impact force cannot be ascertained simply by connecting a line between the coup and contrecoup damage. The discussions in the preceding paragraphs highlight the significance and predominance of inertial head motions in producing the pattern of contrecoup damage, as compared to the role of local contact effects in dictating the extent and severity of coup contusions. Thus these two injuries, although differing only slightly in name, arise from fundamentally different mechanisms. Because of the complexity of head motions that occur in any accident situation and because of the anatomic irregularities of the inner surface of the skull, contrecoup contusions are often not exactly opposite the point of impact. In fact, the most frequently occurring contusions of the temporal and frontal poles are contrecoup in almost every instance, regardless of impact site. In consideration of these differences, it is more appropriate to consider a contrecoup contusion as one that is simply not immediately below the impact site; it should not be considered as appearing immediately opposite the point of impact. Second, in a similar manner, coup and contrecoup contusions should not be viewed as arising from acceleration and deceleration of the head, respectively. Rather, the relative proportion of coup vs. contrecoup contusions depends solely on the response of the head impact (i.e., on how much of the impact energy is converted into head motion and how much energy is attenuated in local skull bending). Due to its pathogenesis, the acceleration of the head caused by a concentrated blow to the head has led to the proposal that acceleration causes coup contusions. However, a hard, small impact object (e.g., a hammer) typical in the "acceleration" cases tends to produce focal skull deformation with underlying coup contusion, and a large portion of the energy is dissipated at the impact site. Local skull deformation produces a noticeable coup contusion, and the lack of substantial head motion produces slight or very limited contrecoup contusion. On the other hand, a softer or larger impact object occurs commonly in cases of "deceleration injury" (e.g., head striking pavement or padded motor vehicle interiors), that cause less local injury beneath the point of impact since a proportional increase in energy is used in setting the head into motion or stopping it from moving. In this case, a large contrecoup lesion occurs, with the coup contusion being smaller or nonexistent. Thus, most "acceleration" injuries have a greater proportion of contact phenomena and less head acceleration than do "deceleration" injuries, in which the proportion is usually reversed.

Intermediate Coup Contusions

This name has been given to vascular disruptions of brain surfaces that are not adjacent to the skull. Although the mechanism of these lesions has not been studied extensively, it is likely that they are due to strain concentrations resulting from impact-generated stress waves or from inertially generated brain movements. In the latter case, the brain is thought to strike or be pulled away from adjacent structures that are relatively immobile, resulting in focal compressive or tensile strains, respectively. Thus, intermediate contusion of the cingulate gyrus can be due to interactions with the falx, and, similarly, those of the inferomedial temporal lobe can result from involvement with the tentorium or petrous ridge.

Intracerebral Hematoma

Large traumatic intracerebral hematomas are uncommon and are most often associated with extensive cortical contusions. They can therefore be considered contusions in which larger, deeper vessels have been disrupted. Smaller, single hematomas that are not associated with contusion probably occur because of stress wave concentration resulting from impact or because of acceleration-induced tissue strains deep within the brain. These hematomas are poorly studied but may represent a forme fruste of the tissue tear hemorrhages that accompany diffuse axonal injury.

Tissue Tear Hemorrhages

Tissue tear hemorrhages are multiple areas of intracerebral damage to blood vessels and axons occurring in association with diffuse axonal injury. As such, these hemorrhages are considered to be due to inertial or head motion effects, and therefore are not related to contact phenomena. They are distinct from the intracerebral hematomas just described, and are actually a part of the pathologic picture of the severe form of diffuse axonal injury that results in immediate prolonged coma. Tissue tear hemorrhages are typically numerous, small (usually varying from petechial to 1 cm in diameter), and located parasagittally in the central (not polar) portion of the brain.

They are caused by high levels of shear and tensile strains as a result of head acceleration and are not related to stress wave concentration due to contact forces. Tissue tear hemorrhages appear to be small areas where the brain's tolerance to shear and tension forces has been exceeded, allowing the tissue to separate sufficiently to tear both axons and small vessels. Their locations are characteristically in the superomedial frontoparietal white matter (where they are called gliding contusions), corpus callosum, centrum semiovale, periventricular white and gray matter, internal capsule, and basal ganglia. In the brain stem, they occur in the dorsal area of the midbrain and upper pons. Several factors contribute to these multiple foci of damage, including the presence of intracranial partitioning membranes, the geometric irregularities of the skull, and the plane of motion experienced by the head. Tissue tear hemorrhages represent areas of maximum acceleration-induced brain damage.

Subdural Hematoma

Three varieties of acute subdural hematoma are found clinically. The first two are associated with contusion and laceration and are sometimes called complicated subdural hematomas. These result from the contact or acceleration effects that cause the primary lesion. The third type of subdural hematoma is the most common form of vascular disruption; it involves tearing of the parasagittal bridging veins located along the superior margin of the brain. It results entirely from inertial, and not from contact, forces. Because of their superficial location, the parasagittal bridging veins are susceptible to damage during short duration angular acceleration of the head.[8] Common situations of this acceleration condition include falls, when the head strikes a broad, hard surface, and in cases of assaults where a majority of the impact energy is used to set the head in motion. Under these loading conditions, the strain within the brain is concentrated along the outer margins where the parasagittal bridging veins reside. If the vascular tolerance is surpassed, subdural bleeding occurs. Due to its similar mechanism, subdural hematoma may coexist with underlying hemispheric or bihemispheric brain damage, usually diffuse axonal injury. This explains the frequency of cases in which the subdural hematoma is small but the brain damage underlying it is more than expected because of the brain compression from the hematoma.

Diffuse Brain Injury

Cerebral Concussion

All gradations of concussion (transient reversible neurological dysfunction due to trauma) are produced entirely by inertial forces. Brain motion causes these injuries, not contact phenomena. It is probable, however, that concussion is observed in concert with injuries arising from the contact phenomena caused by a likely impact. Unlike subdural hematoma, concussion does not occur with purely translational motion of the head (i.e., angular or rotational acceleration of the head must be present to produce the clinical entity known as concussion).[6] Angular or rotational head motions cause the deeper structures within the brain to deform and thus cause the classic widespread disruption of brain function that occurs in concussion. In this type of injury, most of the strain is insufficient to cause structural damage. Instead, the damage to the structures may be either partially or completely reversible depending on the severity of the inertial loading. The precise location of the functional derangement in concussion continues to be debated. It remains unsettled as to whether the effects of angular acceleration are principally to the brain stem, to the cerebral hemispheres, or to both regions.

Diffuse Axonal Injury

Axonal damage appears to be an important pathologic substrate of prolonged traumatic coma that is not due to mass lesions and, like cerebral concussion, is caused only by angular or rotational acceleration and not by contact phenomena.[9] Considered a more severe form of cerebral concussion, diffuse axonal injury nearly universally coincides with other forms of contact or inertial injuries. Furthermore, recent evidence has suggested that the magnitude of rotational acceleration needed to produce diffuse axonal injury requires the head to strike an object or surface, a requirement that raises the likelihood of superimposed contact injuries. The amount and location of axonal damage as a consequence of rotational acceleration probably determines the severity (depth and duration) of injury as well as the quality of recovery. Critical factors in estimating the amount and extent of axonal damage are the magnitude, duration, and onset rate of the angular acceleration, as well as the direction of head motion. In particular, diffuse axonal injury is produced by longer acceleration loading compared to the relatively brief loading duration that produces acute subdural hematoma. Thus, diffuse axonal injury is most likely when the head is impulsively loaded or when impact is due to a relatively soft, broad object (e.g., motor vehicle interiors). The former is not common, clinically, because of the levels of rotational acceleration needed for it; instead, the latter is the most frequent circumstance producing diffuse axonal injury.[2] In fact, although the mechanisms causing subdural hematoma and diffuse axonal injury are closely related, there is a marked difference in the type of accident that produces each condition. Almost all cases of diffuse axonal injury, especially its severe form, arise from vehicular injury (e.g., impact to padded dashboards, resilient windshields, deformable hoods, energy-absorbing steering columns) in which acceleration is long. Conversely, most subdural hematomas occur because of falls or assaults in which the impact duration is short and the angular acceleration is abrupt.

The direction that the head moves plays an important role in the amount and distribution of axonal damage in a given situation. For equivalent levels of angular acceleration, the brain is most vulnerable to axonal damage if it is moved laterally (Fig. 259-8). The brain tolerates sagittal movement best, and horizontal plane head motions are somewhere between lateral and sagittal movements. However, sagittal motions are the most effective in producing vascular injuries to the superior margin of the brain, since the motion of the brain in this plane and location is not severely restricted by intracranial membranes. To this end, the full-blown picture of widely scattered damage to the cerebral hemispheres and brain stem, along with tissue tear hemorrhages, occurs most likely because of spatial changes in the strain pattern induced by the falx and tentorium during lateral motions. Furthermore, the gyral geometry of the cerebrum and brain stem plays an important role in the response of the brain to rotational motions.[11] In response to a lateral head motion (clockwise in Fig. 259-8), small centers of rotation occur in the superior frontal and temporal lobes. Although the induced clockwise motion is the same for all centers of rotation, at the periphery of the rotations brain tissue is moving in opposite directions. The cross-hatched regions in Fig. 259-8 indicate the regions where the brain experiences intense levels of strain and, as a consequence, the areas most prone to axonal damage.

Summary of the Mechanisms of Primary Head Injuries

The complex clinical injury patterns observed in patients with head injuries can be attributed primarily to two phenomena: contact forces and inertial forces. These two phenomena cause damage to the brain and skull by causing a local deformation, or strain, of the bony or soft tissue that can result in either a functional or structural derangement. As the name implies, contact phenomena appear when the head strikes or is struck by an object. These contact phenomena include local deformations of the skull that result in local or remote compressive, shear, and tensile strains in the underlying skull and brain. Shock waves emanate from the point of impact and travel rapidly through the skull and brain, creating additional tissue strains. These strains within the brain tissue can add to the strains already caused by local deformation to produce a spectrum of injuries such as skull fracture, contusion, and some of the intra- or extra-axial hematomas.

In comparison, inertial forces are generated by head motions that occur during the traumatic event. The most common form of inertial loading appears with contact phenomena (i.e., the head is struck by or strikes a rigid object). Most commonly, these motions are described by acceleration or deceleration of the head as it is set into motion or is stopped from moving. Head accelerations or decelerations of appropriate magnitude, rate of onset, and direction together contribute to the type and severity of the inertial injuries. Although common in clinical situations, impact over the brain is not necessary provided that sufficient head motion occurs to cause injurious levels of strains within the head. Concussive injuries, diffuse injury without hematoma (diffuse axonal injury), and most

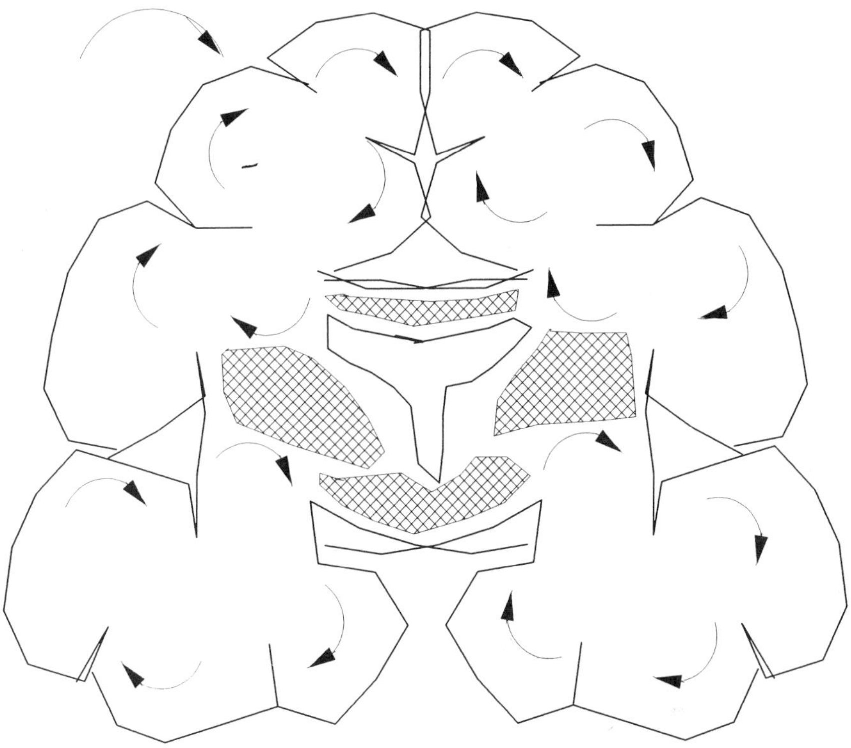

Figure 259-8 Brain motion caused by a lateral plane angular acceleration. A lateral head motion (*clockwise*) causes the frontal and temporal lobe regions of the brain to "swirl" within the vault. The *cross-hatched regions* indicate where the brain experiences intense levels of strain and, as a consequence, the areas most prone to axonal damage. If the duration of acceleration is sufficient, areas such as the corpus callosum and deep white matter are susceptible to axonal damage.

acute subdural hematomas and contrecoup contusions are produced solely as a result of acceleration of the head. In "real-world" situations, it is probable that some form of head contact is necessary to achieve the levels of rotational acceleration and velocity considered responsible for acute subdural hematoma and severe forms of diffuse axonal injury.

Using the guidelines presented in this chapter, it is possible to separate and explain the numerous head injuries observed clinically based on two fundamental mechanisms of injury: contact and inertial forces. Although instances of pure contact or inertially induced injuries can be found, the overwhelming majority of patients with head injuries exhibit a select constellation of lesions described in this chapter. This admixture of injuries, of course, suggests that contact and inertial mechanisms are often present simultaneously. In most trauma situations, however, a predominant mechanism is present and the major clinical injury can often be categorized into one of the two principal types.

References

1. Adams JH, Gennarelli TA, Graham DI. Brain damage in non-missile head injury: observations in man and subhuman primates. In Smith W, Cavanagh JB (eds): *Recent Advances in Neuropathology*. Edinburgh: Churchill Livingstone, 1982, pp 165–190.
2. Adams JH, Graham DI, Murray LS, Scott G. Diffuse axonal injury due to nonmissile head injury in humans: an analysis of 45 cases. *Ann Neurol* 1982; 12:557–563.
3. Backaitis SH (ed). *Biomechanics of Impact Injury and Injury Tolerances of the Head-Neck Complex.* Warrendale, PA: Society of Automotive Engineers, 1993.
4. Denny-Brown D, Russell WR. Experimental cerebral concussion. *Brain* 1941; 64:93–164.
5. Gennarelli TA. Head injury in man and experimental animals: clinical aspects. *Acta Neurochir (Wien) [Suppl]* 1983; 32:1–13.
6. Gennarelli TA. Mechanisms and pathophysiology of cerebral concussion. *J Head Trauma Rehab* 1986; 1:23–29.
7. Gennarelli TA, Spielman GM, Langfitt TW, et al. Influence of the type of intracranial lesion on outcome from severe head injury: a multicenter study. *J Neurosurg* 1982; 56:26–32.
8. Gennarelli TA, Thibault LE. Biomechanics of acute subdural hematoma. *J Trauma* 1982; 22:680–686.
9. Gennarelli TA, Thibault LE, Adams JH, et al. Diffuse axonal injury and traumatic coma in the primate. *Ann Neurol* 1982; 12:564–574.
10. Goldsmith W, Ommaya AK. Head and neck injury criteria and tolerance levels. In Aldman B, Chapon A (eds): *The Biomechanics of Impact Trauma.* Amsterdam: Elsevier, 1984, pp 149–187.
11. Grcevic N. Topography and pathogenic mechanisms of lesions in "inner cerebral trauma." *Rad Jazu (Med)* 1982; 402/18:265–331.
12. Gurdjian ES, Lang WA, Patrick LM, Thomas LM (eds). *Wayne State University Symposium on Impact Injury and Crash Proection: Impact Injury and Crash Protection:* Springfield, IL: Charles C Thomas, 1970.
13. Liu YK. Biomechanics and biophysics of CNS trauma. In Odom GL (ed): *Central Nervous System Trauma Research Status Report-1979.* Bethesda: National Institute of Neurological and Communicative Disorders and Stroke, NIH, 1979, pp 36–52.
14. Ommaya AK, Gennarelli TA. Cerebral concussion and traumatic unconsciousness: correlation of experimental and clinical observations on blunt head injuries. *Brain* 1974; 97:633–654.
15. Thibault LE, Gennarelli TA. Biomechanics and craniocerebral trauma. In Becker DP, Povlishock JT (eds): *Central Nervous System Trauma Research Status Report-1985.* Bethesda: National Institute of Neurological and Communicative Disorders and Stroke, NIH, 1985, pp 379–389.

260

Pathophysiology of Traumatic Brain Injury

A. John Popp
Paul J. Feustel
Harold K. Kimelberg

The initial event in craniocerebral trauma involves direct impact injury to the brain that produces parenchymal contusion and shearing injury of axons in the white matter of the cerebral hemispheres and brain stem. These primary injuries trigger a sequence of secondary alterations in brain metabolism and ion homeostasis, intracranial hemodynamics, and brain water compartmentation that develop during the hours following traumatic brain injury (TBI). These evolving pathophysiological processes can produce changes in the intracranial pressure-volume relationship with resulting intracranial hypertension and brain herniation. Satisfactory outcome for the patient often requires recognition and successful treatment of these secondary derangements.

The problems cited above may be complicated further both by traumatic injury to other organs and by the complex systemic response to TBI. In this chapter we present an overview of the cerebral and systemic pathophysiologic changes following TBI and the dynamic interaction among cerebral metabolism, altered intracranial hemodynamics, brain edema, and increased intracranial pressure (ICP). Other chapters in this textbook on cerebral edema, increased ICP, cerebral blood flow (CBF), and normal cerebral energy metabolism serve as a background for this chapter.

Cellular Metabolism and Ion Homeostasis

Normal cellular function requires the continual generation of energy in the form of adenosine triphosphate (ATP). Cellular respiration is usually limited by the adenosine diphosphate (ADP) supply, with oxygen and glucose being available in excess. Thus, ATP levels are normally high (3 m*M*), whereas ADP levels are relatively low (<1 m*M*). Phosphocreatine (PCr) serves as a buffer for ATP because it is readily hydrolyzed into inorganic phosphate (P_i) and creatine (Cr), converting ADP to ATP in the process. Thus, a reliable indicator of energy availability is the PCr/P_i ratio, which will decrease prior to ATP depletion. In animal studies involving direct impact injury alone, energy levels have been found not to be significantly affected.[59] However, major effects have been reported when the initial injury is followed by a secondary insult, such as ischemia or hypoxia.[1,25,40,43] For example, a study of fluid percussion head injury in rats[25] revealed significant decreases in the PCr/P_i ratio only when hypoxia was imposed after trauma (Fig. 260-1).

Autopsy results provide considerable clinical evidence of secondary ischemia or hypoxia accompanying TBI.[21] In head injury, ischemia and hypoxia are secondary events, but it is difficult to determine clinically the extent to which they have actually occurred. Ischemia after TBI may result from several causes, including generalized increased ICP, local brain distortion secondary to space-occupying lesions, or excessive vasoconstriction of blood vessels. One important cause of this latter effect is likely depolarization-induced release of neurotransmitters as a result of high levels of extracellular [K^+]. Loss of K^+ from cells to the extracellular space is known to occur after head injury. Hypoxia can be caused

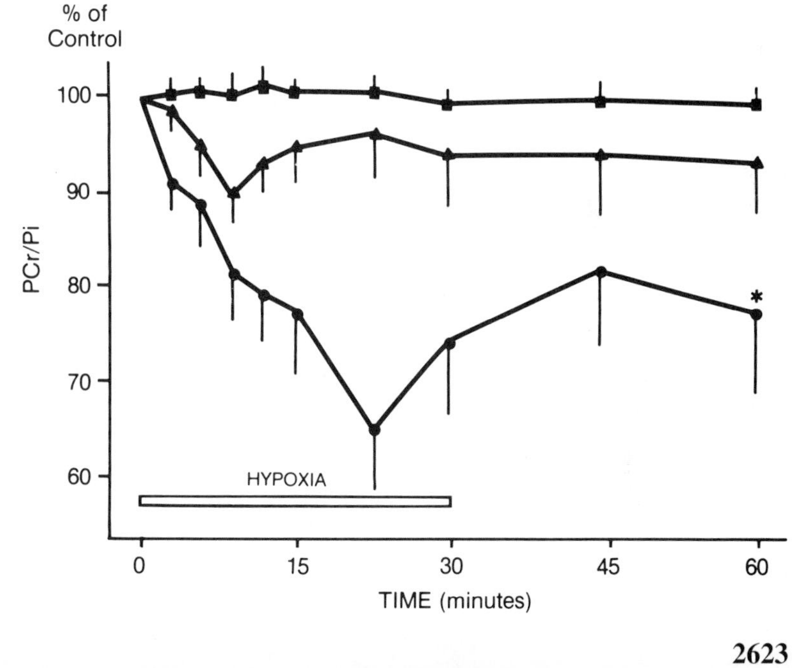

Figure 260-1 The time course of the change in the PCr/P_i ratio, as measured by ^{31}P magnetic resonance spectroscopy, in rats subjected to a fluid percussion injury at the outset (0 time). Rats with hypoxia alone are represented by the squares (■), rats with impact injury alone by the triangles (▲), and rats with impact injury plus hypoxia (Pa_{O_2} of 40 mmHg for 0 to 30 min) by the circles (●). The PCr/P_i ratio in the rats with combined insults was significantly lower at 60 min than that in rats that had suffered impact injury alone (*, $p < .05$). After the induction of hypoxia was completed, only at the 60-min point was there a significant difference in the PCr/P_i ratio between the rats with hypoxia alone and those with either trauma plus hypoxia or impact injury alone. The lowest value in the PCr/P_i ratio during hypoxia in the injury plus hypoxia group was also significantly different from the value recorded in the rats with impact alone. (Adapted from Ishige et al.[25])

by several mechanisms, including respiratory dysfunction, inadequate ventilation, or problems of oxygen delivery. Although the multifactorial effects of head injury cannot all be explained by ischemia or hypoxia, these are important components of secondary brain injury and must be considered in any discussion of TBI. The following is an overview of the general metabolic effects of ischemia and hypoxia and their applicability to human head injury.[54,55]

ATP Production

The energy in ATP is chemical energy in the form of hydrolyzable high-energy phosphate bonds. ATP is produced in two major ways. The less efficient method is anaerobic glycolysis, whereby glucose is metabolized to pyruvate and subsequently to lactate (Fig. 260-2). In the presence of oxygen, the metabolic path is extended from pyruvate via a series of decarboxylations (loss of CO_2) and oxidations (loss of reducing equivalents in the form of H) that constitute the reactions of the Krebs, or tricarboxylic acid, cycle. Glycolysis occurs in the cell cytoplasm, whereas the Krebs cycle occurs within the mitochondria; thus pyruvate must enter the mitochondria to be metabolized oxidatively. Reducing equivalents, released from glucose by the reactions of glycolysis or the Krebs cycle, are initially transferred to nicotinamide (NAD^+) or flavin nucleotides. In the presence of oxygen the energy in these reducing equivalents is converted to ATP within the membrane-embedded respiratory chain of the mitochondria by a process known as oxidative phosphorylation.

Cytochrome oxidase, which is the last step of the mitochondrial respiratory chain, has a very high affinity for O_2, and O_2 levels must be reduced dramatically before O_2 concentration becomes the limiting step in this process. This occurs when the rate of O_2 utilization is greater than the supply of O_2. A decrease in the ATP level will result from head injury because of the decreased supply of O_2 secondary to either hypoxia or ischemia. O_2 utilization continues because of the continued supply of substrate in hypoxia or the availability of substrate from substrate stores in ischemia, such as the glycogen stores found principally in astrocytes.

Ion Gradients

One important effect of an inadequate energy supply in the CNS is on transmembrane ion gradients. The major ion transport pathways seen in most cell plasma membranes, including those of the CNS, are depicted in Figure 260-3.[54] The (Na^+,K^+) pump (see Fig. 260-3 *#1*) directly utilizes ATP to pump $2K^+$ into the cell and $3Na^+$ out, per ATP hydrolyzed. Thus the pump is electrogenic, that is, there is a net transmembrane transfer of charge; in this case excess positive charge is pumped out of the cell. This positive charge needs to be accompanied passively by outward movement of an anion for electroneutrality, such as Cl^- or HCO_3^-. This net

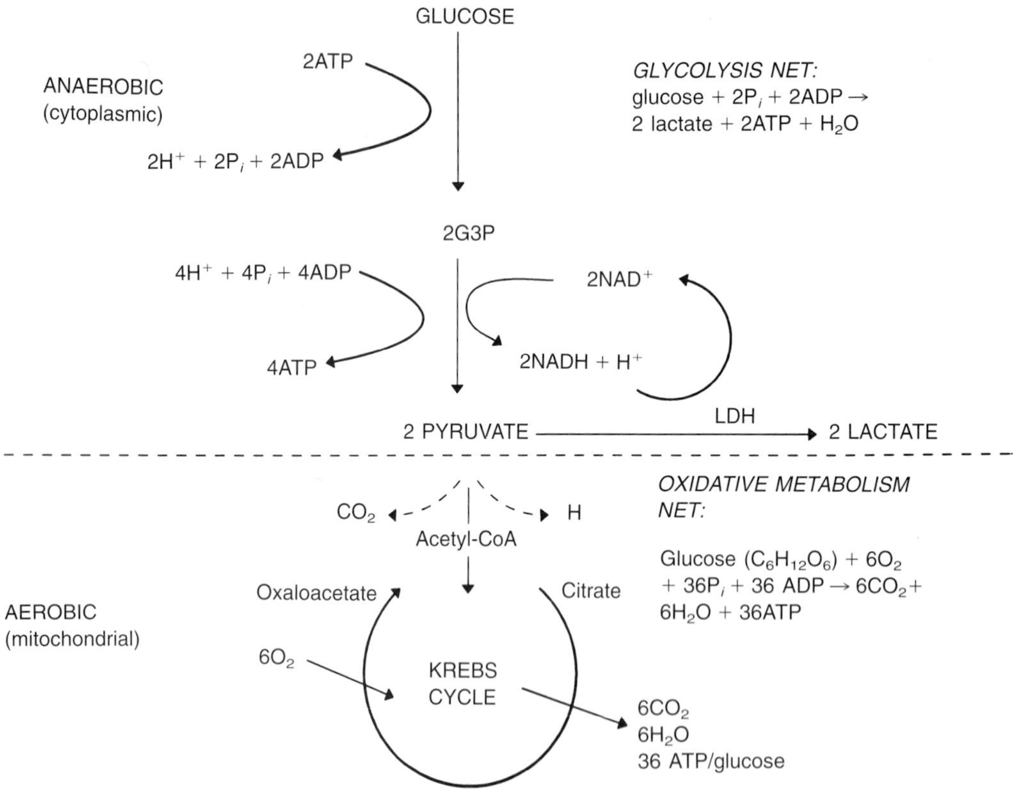

Figure 260-2 Outline of anaerobic and aerobic metabolism of glucose. In the absence of oxygen, glucose oxidation proceeds to lactate production *(top)*. Anaerobic glycolysis is not limited by the total NAD^+ pool because the reduced $NADH + H^+$ generated by oxidation of the intermediates of glycolysis is reoxidized to NAD^+ by the reduction of pyruvate to lactate. Glycolysis produces a net 2 moles of ATP per mole of glucose. In the presence of O_2 (bottom), pyruvate is further oxidized through the reactions of the Krebs cycle, generating a net 36 moles of ATP per mole of glucose by the reactions of oxidative phosphorylation. Each mole of glucose is completely oxidized to CO_2 and H_2O, with the intermediates of the Krebs cycle serving a catalytic role. G3P = glyceraldehyde-3-phosphate; LDH = lactate dehydrogenase.

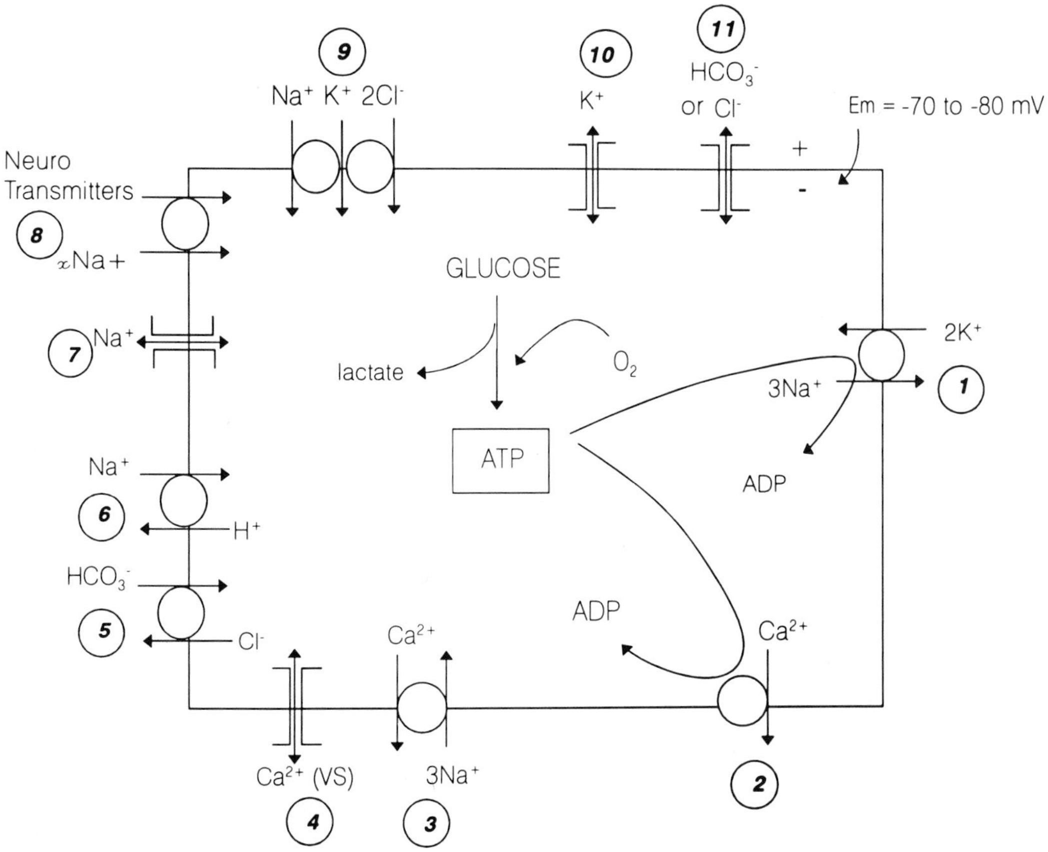

Figure 260-3 Plasma cell membrane ion transporting systems that are likely to be affected by diminished ATP levels. The ion transporting systems can be classified as *active* (requiring energy: 1, 2, 3, 6, 8, and 9) or *passive* (responding passively to ion gradients plus electrical gradients: 4, 5, 7, 10, and 11). Active transport is further divided into two subcategories: *primary* (ATP-dependent pumps utilizing ATP directly: #s 1 and 2) and *secondary* (those utilizing any driving force that depends on the ATP-dependent pumps—usually, the inward NA^+ gradient (#s 3, 6, 8, and 9). Inhibition of the primary Na^+,K^+-ATPase pump (1) leads to failure to pump out Na^+ and take up K^+. Because the membrane potential (E_m) is usually a few millivolts more positive than E_K, the K^+ equilibrium potential (E_K is -90 mV, whereas E_m is approximately -80 to -70 mV), there is always a small net outward efflux of K^+, which is normally balanced through uptake by the pump. Na^+ has a very large inward driving force ($E_{Na} = +50$ mV), but its influx is limited because the Na^+ channels (7) are either closed in the resting state or are present at very low density. Thus failure of the (Na^+,K^+) pump will lead to a loss of K^+ and a gain of Na^+. Secondary active systems utilize the inward driving force of Na^+ by coupling the transport of the substrate to inward Na^+ movement, as seen in Na^+-dependent neurotransmitter uptake (8) or outward H^+ (6) or Ca^{2+} exchange for Na^+ (3). Thus the gain of Na^+ and loss of K^+ that occurs as a result of the inhibition of the (Na^+,K^+) pump has widespread effects. The transport systems depicted include the ATP-driven Ca^{2+} pump (2); voltage-sensitive Ca^{2+} channels (4); HCO_3^-/Cl^- exchange transporter (5, of which there are several different types, some dependent on Na^+, not shown); coupled Na + K + 2Cl uptake (9); K^+ channels (10); and anion channels (11).

loss of Na^+ plus Cl^- or HCO_3^- will also be accompanied by an osmotically obligated movement of water. The Ca^{2+} pump (see Fig. 260-3 *#2*) pumps out one or two Ca^{2+} per ATP hydrolyzed. The Ca^{2+} pump operates against a large concentration gradient with $[Ca^{2+}]_i$ being around 10^{-7}M and $[Ca^{2+}]_o$ being 10^{-3}M.

The pumps just described are *primary* active transport systems, because they derive energy directly from the hydrolysis of ATP. The uptake and extrusion of many other ions and substrates into and out of the cell depend upon the Na^+ gradient generated by the (Na^+,K^+) pump, processes collectively referred to as *secondary* active transport. For example, glutamate accumulation into both neurons and astroglial cells occurs by cotransport with two or three Na^+ ions per glutamate. With failure of the (Na^+,K^+) pump after injury, these secondary Na^+-dependent processes will be progressively inhibited as the Na^+ gradient dissipates.

The passive ion permeability of most cells is predominantly that of K^+, as there are a greater number of open K^+ channels than there are channels for either Na^+ or anions in the membrane—at least under resting conditions. Channels are large proteins inserted through membranes that have water-filled pores formed by several protein subunits. These channels may be open or closed. Selectivity for specific ions is thought to depend on the topography and surface charge of the inside surface of the pore. Ions move passively through these channels under the influence of their transmembrane concentration gradients and the membrane potential. The Nernst equation gives the equilibrium potential for such movement, which is the electrical potential at which the concentration gradient tending to move an ion in one direction is exactly offset by the electrical potential difference driving it in the opposite direction. Under these conditions, there can still be rapid equal and opposite transmembrane ion movements but no net movement. Normally, the membrane potential is close to but slightly more positive than the K^+ equilibrium potential, which is around −90 mV, negative inside the cell. Thus when $[K^+]_i$ decreases or $[K^+]_o$ increases, the membrane potential becomes less negative, a change referred to as *depolarization.* This depolarization, in turn, causes the opening of numerous channels, known as *voltage-activated channels.* For example, as the membrane potential depolarizes from −70 to −10 mV, voltage-sensitive Ca^{2+} channels open, allowing Ca^{2+} to enter the cell (see Fig. 260-3 *#4*). In nerve terminals, this entry of Ca^{2+} is essential for exocytoxic release of transmitters. In its role as a prominent second messenger Ca^{2+} also has numerous cellular effects. However, with excessive influx, increased $[Ca^{2+}]_i$ can lead to cell death due to stimulation of Ca^{2+}-dependent enzymes, such as phospholipases (particularly phospholipase A_2) and proteases.[55,65] Excessive $[Ca^{2+}]_i$ is thought to be a principal cause of neuronal cell death in a number of pathologic states, including stroke and TBI. Other important voltage-activated channels include specific types of Na^+ and K^+ channels that are, for example, responsible for the action potential.

Failure of the (Na^+,K^+) pump results in the accumulation of intracellular Na^+. This occurs either as a result of the exchange of intracellular K^+ for extracellular Na^+ or by influx of Na^+ accompanied by Cl^- or another anion when both Na^+ and anion permeabilities are relatively high. Uptake of Na^+ plus anions leads to cellular swelling, and influx of Na^+ by either route leads to a reduction of the inward Na^+ gradient on which secondary active transport systems depend. Secondary active transport systems not only cotransport Na^+ plus other substances, such as transmitters, inward; they can also remove other ions from inside the cell by exchange transport with Na^+. The Na^+/H^+ exchanger (see Fig. 260-3 *#6*) transports H^+ out of the cell and helps maintain the pH inside the cell at close to 7.0. The Na^+/Ca^{2+} exchanger (see Fig. 260-3 *#3*) moves three Na^+ in for every one Ca^{2+} moved out. Together with the Ca^{2+} pump (see Fig. 260-3 *#2*), the Na^+/Ca^{2+} exchanger helps keep intracellular Ca^{2+} low. Thus, the results of a cellular increase in Na^+ are wide-ranging and include (1) intracellular accumulation of Ca^{2+}, (2) intracellular acidification, and (3) a reduced capacity to take up neurotransmitters. Acidosis (see below) also inhibits glycolysis via inhibition of phosphofructokinase, leading to a further decrease in energy supply. Thus a vicious circle is established; energy depletion leads to failure of ion pumps, which results in additional energy depletion. These effects are not unique to neurons but occur in all cells of the central nervous system. Changes in energy metabolism may be more or less significant in different cells owing to differing energy demands and/or ion fluxes. For example, the choroid plexus epithelia are particularly sensitive to a decline in ATP because of their high energy-requiring, ion-pumping properties. In ischemia or TBI, ion influx secondary to excessive excitation of *N*-methyl-D-aspartate (NMDA) receptors by glutamate causes an influx of Ca^{2+} and Na^+, and the cells will use their dwindling ATP supplies to pump out these ions.

For brevity, we have discussed only the multitude of effects that ATP depletion has on plasma membrane ion transport. In addition, $[Ca^{2+}]_i$ is controlled by ATP-dependent pumps, which pump Ca^{2+} into intracellular stores, principally the endoplasmic reticulum and mitochondria.

Acidosis

Acidosis is also thought to be an important consequence of ischemia and hypoxia following head injury. During ischemia, glycogen stores in astrocytes are converted to lactate plus protons, producing acidification.[24,54] Hypoxia may be even more deleterious than ischemia, because the continued supply of blood-borne glucose leads to continual glycolysis and lactate formation with acidosis. As noted earlier, acidosis further decreases ATP supply by inhibiting phosphofructokinase. Acidosis generally alters protein function through conformational changes induced by altered ionization of surface amino acid side groups. The displacement of Ca^{2+} from intracellular binding sites[55] may be an example of this process. This displacement, coupled with the inability of mitochondria deprived of oxygen to take up Ca^{2+}, leads to large increases in intracellular Ca^{2+} levels; this activates Ca^{2+}-dependent proteases and phospholipases, causing proteolysis and breakdown of membrane phospholipids, respectively. Phospholipases are also directly activated by G proteins through stimulation of specific receptors by transmitters, but such hydrolysis is far more limited and usually functions as a normal intracellular signaling system. Activation of phospholipases leads to liberation of free fatty acids, such as arachidonic acid, produced by the action of the highly Ca^{2+}-sensitive phospholipase A_2. Free fatty acids disrupt the lipid portion of cell membranes by exerting a detergent-like effect, breaking apart the hydrophobic packing between the lipids needed to maintain the integrity of the lipid bilayer. This process breaks down the normal selective permeability properties of the cell membrane and alters the activity of ion pumps and channels because of their dependence on their membrane lipid environment.

Free Radicals

With the re-establishment of blood supply, reperfusion injury may occur because the supply of reducing equivalents exceeds the supply of oxygen. This leads to the production of free radicals. The appearance of measurable free radicals and the protective effects of antioxidants, such as the 21 aminosteroids, have led to free radicals being considered an important component of secondary damage during ischemia and trauma.[55] There are a number of oxygen-based free radicals, such as the superoxide anion ($O_2^{\bullet -}$), that are produced by incomplete reduction of oxygen by cytochrome oxidase ($a + a_3$), as well as from other sources. Hydrogen peroxide (H_2O_2) can also be formed. The very short-lived hydroxyl free radical ($^{\bullet}OH$) is formed from H_2O_2 by a reaction catalyzed by free iron. Free iron can be liberated from the heme groups of hemoglobin or released from ferritin and transferrin after hemorrhage. Free radicals are damaging because of their ability to form an oxidative cascade involving the fatty acid side chains of membrane phospholipids, leading to peroxidatic breakdown of these fatty acids and the generation of more free radicals. These reactions can ultimately result in complete membrane breakdown.

Free radicals also can directly affect proteins. For example, the enzyme glutamine synthetase, which is predominantly localized in astrocytes, is known to be susceptible to attack by free radicals.

This enzyme is important in the conversion of neuroactive glutamate plus potentially toxic ammonia to glutamine in astrocytes. Thus, inhibition of this enzyme leads to greater levels of intracellular or extracellular glutamate and ammonia in the brain. The excitotoxic effect of glutamate has serious consequences, as discussed below. The toxicity of ammonia in the brain is not established clearly, but serum ammonia does increase following trauma.

Release of Transmitters

The large increases in extracellular $[K^+]$ (50 to 80 m*M*) that can accompany ischemia and trauma[26] will result in membrane depolarization. This depolarization opens voltage-gated Ca^{2+} channels, resulting in release of neurotransmitters. Uptake of released transmitters is also compromised because secondary active transport systems depend on an inwardly directed $[Na^+]$ gradient for their energy (as discussed above and depicted in Fig. 260-3 *#8*). Catecholamines are principally removed by reuptake into nerve terminals, whereas glutamate is thought to be taken up mainly by astrocytes and then converted to glutamine.

Massive release of the neurotransmitter glutamate has been shown to occur in a fluid percussion model of brain injury in the rat.[14,26] Neuronal toxicity resulting from excessive release of glutamate is thought to be primarily due to activation of NMDA receptors, leading to increased influx of Ca^{2+} into neurons that have a high density of those receptors.[6] The Ca^{2+} can then kill the cells by the mechanisms outlined above. The significance of these processes has been supported by the fact that NMDA antagonists are protective in experimental ischemia.

Adenosine is another neurotransmitter or neuromodulator that increases in the extracellular space under ischemic conditions. Adenosine is thought to be released primarily as ATP which is often colocalized with other transmitters. This ATP is then broken down by ectoenzymes to adenosine. Adenosine has several important effects, particularly in increasing CBF. Adenosine may also be viewed as being neuroprotective because of its inhibition of glutamate release by activation of presynaptic adenosine receptors.

Mechanosensitive Ion Transport

The sudden blow(s) causing TBI results in short-lived acceleration-deceleration forces acting on the brain. Aptly termed *commotio cerebri,* this type of injury produces shear forces within the brain as well as bruising or laceration secondary to the brain's impact on the internal surfaces of the skull. Such shear forces are thought to be one cause of the diffuse axonal injury seen clinically in TBI. However, even in experimental TBI delays have been found between the initial impact and the onset of diffuse axonal injury. There is a major question as to how the purely mechanical initial forces can result in delayed effects, such as ischemia and hypoxia. One possibility is a recently discovered class of ion channels termed *mechanosensitive,* or "stretch-activated," channels. These channels are activated by pressure or shear forces applied to the membrane and were first described in patch-clamp, electrophysiologic experiments. Mechanosensitive channels have been observed at high densities in cultured astrocytes.[4] The most common seem to be nonspecific cation channels that allow the passage of Ca^{2+}, Na^+, and K^+.[22] The entry of Ca^{2+} into arteriolar smooth muscle by such channels may be one basis of the myogenic mechanism of autoregulation described in the following discussion. Under pathologic conditions, the entry of excessive Ca^{2+} through such channels could result in vasoconstriction, leading to cerebral ischemia and further compromising the injured brain.

CBF Regulation

Following the initial disruptions occurring in primary TBI, alterations in the relationship between cerebral energy metabolism and CBF may cause additional brain injury. The direct relationship of CBF to metabolic demand is a fundamental aspect of normal cerebral circulatory control. This relationship is supported by studies demonstrating increased regional CBF in areas where neural and metabolic activity is increased. About 50 percent of the cerebral metabolic rate of oxygen ($CMRO_2$) is believed to be attributable to neural activity, because barbiturate-induced depression of neural activity can result in a 50 percent reduction in $CMRO_2$ and in associated CBF. The remaining 50 percent of $CMRO_2$ and CBF is presumably that required for resting cellular metabolism. The mechanism linking CBF to neural activity and metabolism is currently thought to involve increases in extracellular concentrations of the vasodilator adenosine, perhaps acting together with extracellular $[K^+]$, $[H^+]$, or prostaglandins.[23,47]

Unlike the linear dependence of CBF on $CMRO_2$, CBF is normally independent of cerebral perfusion pressure (CPP) in the range of approximately 50 to 150 mmHg. When CPP is rapidly increased or decreased but remains within these limits, CBF likewise will be transiently increased or decreased, but adjustment in vascular tone occurs within seconds and returns CBF toward resting levels. This vascular response, termed *autoregulation,* results in a relatively constant steady state of CBF (Fig. 260-4). The mechanism for autoregulation may be the same as that for the metabolism-CBF coupling (metabolic hypothesis) cited earlier, or there may be an intrinsic arterial vascular response to transluminal pressure gradients (myogenic hypothesis).

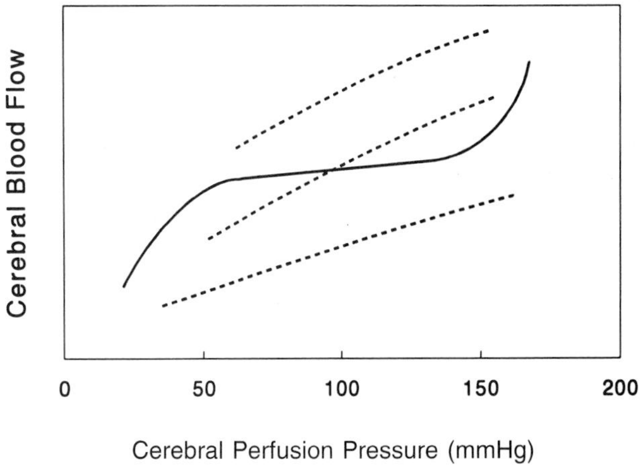

Figure 260-4 Normally, steady-state blood flow is relatively independent of CPP in the range of approximately 50 to 150 mmHg *(solid line).* Disordered autoregulation *(dashed lines)* may occur following traumatic brain injury, causing the CBF to become passively dependent on CPP. Disturbed autoregulation may accompany high, normal, or low levels of CBF at normal perfusion pressure, as shown by the upper, center, and lower dashed lines, respectively.

CBF Response to Changes in $CMRO_2$ and CPP

Although TBI is a complex injury with varying severity and distribution of lesions, disruptions in both the independence of CBF in relation to CPP (see Fig. 260-4, dashed lines) and the dependence of CBF on $CMRO_2$ (Fig. 260-5) are frequently found. Such alterations in CBF regulation may be diffuse or local and vary according to the severity of the TBI and the time elapsed since the injury. As a result of disrupted CBF regulation, normally innocuous episodes of hypoventilation, hypoxia, or decreased CPP can have devastating effects on O_2 delivery to the brain. Indeed, much of neurosurgical care is directed at avoiding these episodes to minimize additional brain injury.

Following TBI, autoregulation is absent, diminished, or delayed in about 50 percent of patients sustaining severe head injury.[2] Defective autoregulation may occur in association with any CBF level (see Fig. 260-4). In the absence of an autoregulatory response, moderate or transient hypotension can cause ischemia. This may explain the greatly increased susceptibility of the post-TBI brain to early hypotension.[40]

Following TBI, metabolism-CBF coupling has been found to be abnormal in more than 50 percent of patients with severe head injury.[38,45] The occurrence of disrupted metabolism-CBF coupling is not necessarily associated with disrupted autoregulation.[16] Measurements of CBF and $CMRO_2$ in injured humans generally have been obtained relatively late after injury (>6 h), and most have been obtained from severely injured individuals. The lowest Glasgow coma scores in these patients have been found to be associated with the lowest $CMRO_2$.[45] Despite a low $CMRO_2$, CBF is often within a normal range. This state is termed *relative hyperemia* because although the CBF is within a normal range, it is high in relation to the depressed $CMRO_2$. Higher-than-normal CBF in relation to a normal $CMRO_2$ is termed *absolute hyperemia*. Relative or absolute hyperemia has been found in up to two-thirds of post-TBI patients at some time during their hospital stay. Low CBF more than 24 h after injury is relatively rare and is associated with a poor prognosis.[46]

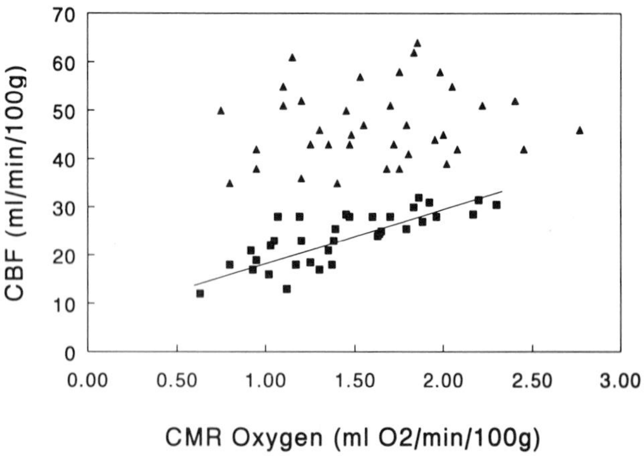

Figure 260-5 CBF plotted against $CMRO_2$. Data are from the results of a study of 75 adults with severe head injuries reported by Obrist et al.[45] The "reduced flow" group (■ indicates with regression) shows CBF values that are decreased in proportion to $CMRO_2$. Because arteriovenous oxygen content differences in these patients were within the normal range, the decrease in blood flow was considered to reflect the dependence of CBF on $CMRO_2$. The hyperemic group (▲) exhibits high CBF when considered in relation to their $CMRO_2$. There was no significant relationship between $CMRO_2$ and CBF in this group. (Adapted from Obrist et al.[45])

The mechanism that uncouples CBF from metabolism is unknown. Although commonly accepted mediators of coupling, such as extracellular adenosine, $[H^+]$, and $[K^+]$, have been elevated either in humans or experimental animals immediately following TBI,[13,26,42] these acute changes probably subside before absolute or relative hyperemia develops. In human CSF, a potential vasodilator, lactate, is elevated for days after injury,[13] but the lactate level does not correlate well with global CBF measurements.[2]

Hyperemia most often has been assessed by CBF measurements utilizing the clearance of diffusible indicators from brain tissue. Continuous jugular venous bulb oxygen saturation (S_{jvO_2}) measurements have been used to estimate the $CMRO_2$/CBF ratio.[10,53] High S_{jvO_2} is a consequence of relative or absolute hyperemia and implies more than adequate CBF relative to $CMRO_2$. According to the Fick principle as applied to the cerebrovascular bed:

$$\frac{CMRO_2}{CBF} = (C_aO_2 - C_vO_2)$$

where $CMRO_2$ is expressed in (milliliters of O_2) × $(\text{minutes})^{-1}$ × $(100\text{ g of tissue})^{-1}$, CBF is expressed in (liters of blood) × $(\text{minutes})^{-1}$ × $(100\text{ g tissue})^{-1}$, and C_aO_2 and C_vO_2 represent the arterial and jugular venous O_2 contents, respectively, expressed in (milliliters of O_2) × $(\text{liter})^{-1}$.

With normal hemoglobin concentration, the O_2 content difference is between 50 and 75 ml O_2 $(\text{liter})^{-1}$, and metabolism-CBF coupling and autoregulation keep this difference relatively constant. A high $(C_aO_2 - C_vO_2)$ level indicates insufficient blood flow for a given metabolic rate.

Most of the human data related to metabolism-CBF coupling have been acquired hours to days after injury, when hyperemia is a common finding. However, recent research[3,33] has shown that, when measured within 6 h after TBI, CBF may be low regionally, either approaching or entering the ischemic range. This is an important finding for two reasons. First, although ischemia has long been suspected as a mechanism of injury on the basis of ischemic-hypoxic changes found at autopsy,[21] few measurements of CBF in patients have actually demonstrated ischemia. Second, the finding that late hyperemia follows early ischemia suggests that the brain of patients sustaining TBI may be subject to reperfusion injury with the production of oxygen free radicals and lipid peroxidation. In this setting, relative hyperemia may be similar to the "luxury perfusion" that follows stroke, and drugs designed for intervention in ischemic situations may become important in arresting or preventing the secondary injury of TBI.

Following TBI, brain distortion or elevated ICP will result in ischemia and hypoxia secondary to decreases in CPP. Tissue hypoxia may be attenuated by either increasing O_2 supply or decreasing O_2 demand. Metabolic demand can be reduced by barbiturate-induced coma, which in animal models of ischemia, increases the local availability of O_2 in borderline ischemic cortex, provided CPP is maintained.[17] However, clinical trials using barbiturates generally have been disappointing.[60] Nevertheless, limiting O_2 demand by appropriate drug therapy seems prudent. One element of this treatment is the prevention of seizures, because seizures can increase metabolic activity to such an extent that ATP is depleted,[66] a situation that does not occur in the normal brain until the Pa_{O_2} decreases to less than 20 mmHg.

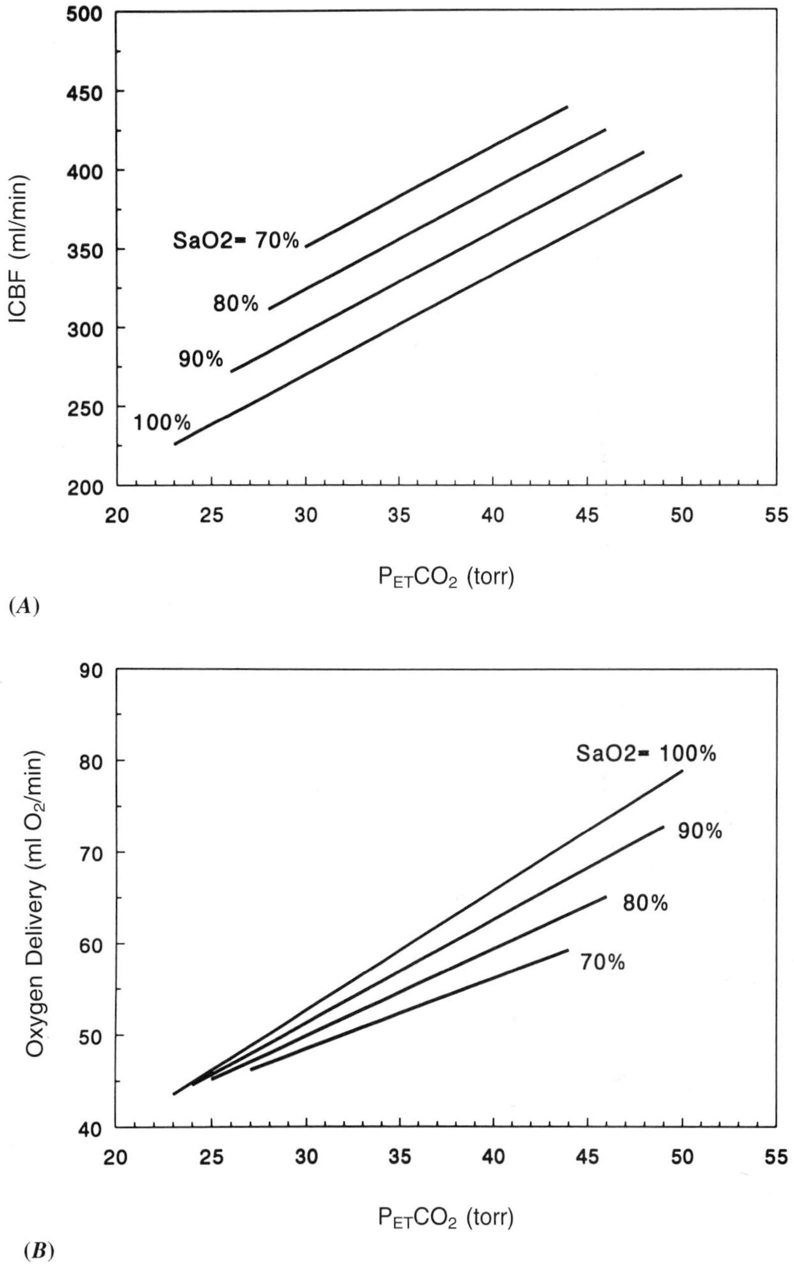

Figure 260-6 Unilateral internal carotid artery blood flow (ICBF) *(A)* and oxygen delivery to brain *(B)* as a function of end-tidal P_{CO_2} (PET_{CO_2}) at different levels of arterial oxygen saturation in normal humans. ICBF was measured by duplex ultrasound, and lines were drawn by multiple linear regression. (Data from Fortune et al.[19])

CBF Response to Changes in Blood Gases

The normal cerebral circulation responds to arterial carbon dioxide pressure (P_{CO_2}) and oxygen pressure (P_{O_2}) changes. Within the physiologic range of Pa_{CO_2} (20 to 60 mmHg), CBF normally increases 2 to 4 percent for each unit of increase in Pa_{CO_2} and 2 percent for each percent of arterial oxygen desaturation of arterial blood (Fig. 260-6*A*).[19] Regulation of cerebral vasculature by CO_2 occurs via a mechanism that is different from autoregulation or CBF-metabolism coupling. CO_2 diffuses across the blood-brain barrier and alters CBF by changing extravascular [H^+] concentration.[23] Experiments altering CSF [HCO_3^-] demonstrate that pial artery diameter depends upon [H^+] rather than P_{CO_2}. Hypocapnic vasoconstriction stops at about 20 mmHg, when O_2 delivery becomes insufficient to meet tissue requirements and the vasodilators lactic acid and adenosine prevent further vasoconstriction.

Following TBI, the CO_2 reactivity of CBF generally has been found to be preserved, even when CBF-metabolism coupling and autoregulation are disrupted.[37,45] The resilience of hypocapnic arterial vasoconstriction is also demonstrated by the usually rapid reduction in ICP that accompanies hyperventilation. The rapidity of this effect suggests that ICP is reduced by cerebral blood volume reduction. The CBF remaining unaffected by hyperventilation indicates complete vasomotor paralysis and is associated with a poor prognosis.[44]

In normal brain, the vasoconstriction that occurs with hyperventilation is short-lived, gradually diminishing over a period of 16 h (Fig. 260-7).[39] Normalization of pial artery diameter coincides with decreased CSF [HCO_3^-] and a return of the CSF [H^+] toward normal. If injured brain acts like normal brain in its adaptation to CO_2, hyperventilation is initially effective in reducing cerebral blood volume and ICP but progressively loses its effectiveness over 16 h of continuous hyperventilation.

Following TBI, local CBF can be affected by neighboring areas of altered CBF regulation because of the unusual distribution of cerebral vascular resistance. Unlike most other peripheral

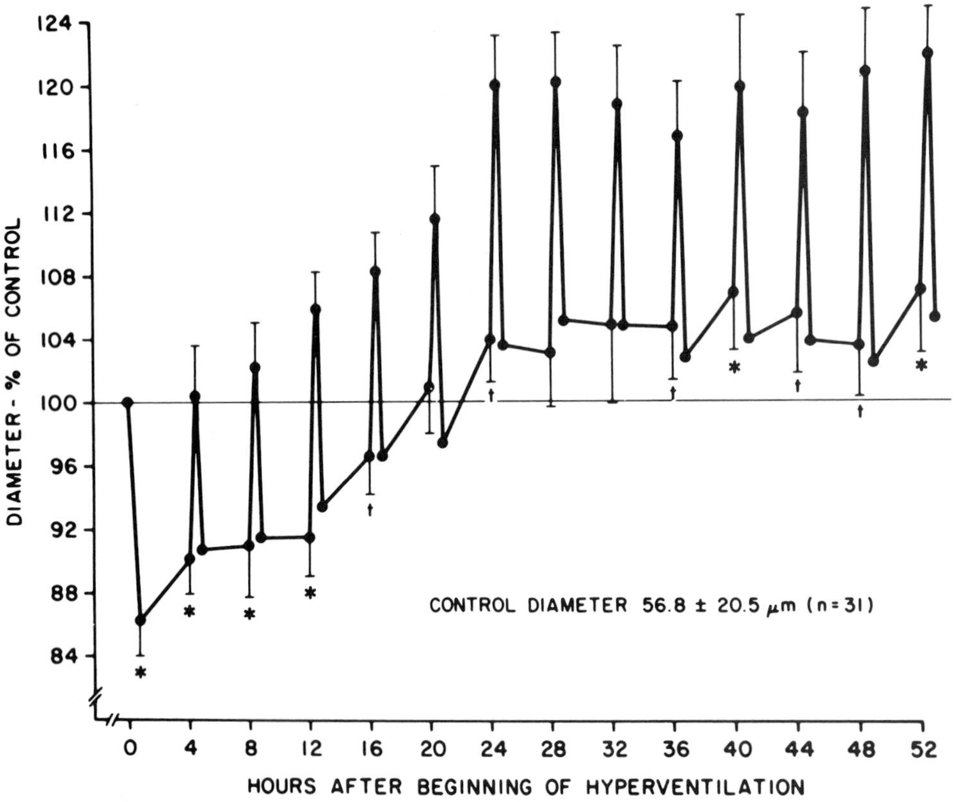

Figure 260-7 Pial artery diameters in rabbits as measured at 4-h intervals after the onset of sustained hyperventilation. The lower values are those associated with a Pa_{CO_2} of 25 mmHg. The upward spikes show the diameter with acute normocapnia (Pa_{CO_2} = 38 mmHg). Hyperventilation was effective for 12 to 16 h in reducing vessel diameter and, presumably, cerebral blood flow and cerebral blood volume. Acute normocapnic episodes cause vasodilation, as shown by the upward spikes. (From Muizelaar et al.,[39] with permission.)

circulations, the cerebral circulation has an appreciable percentage (>50 percent) of vascular resistance in arteries having diameters of greater than 30 μm.[15] This arrangement allows for the possibility of a significant "steal" effect (Fig. 260-8). Because the high resistance of large arteries causes the pressure in medium-sized arteries to be below arterial pressure, if one of several distal daughter arteries becomes dilated, the pressure in a medium-sized vessel can drop appreciably, even when arterial pressure is maintained. Flow in a second daughter vessel decreases because of the decrease in perfusion pressure—the steal effect. Unless proximal large arteries can dilate or the second daughter vessel is capable of further vasodilation, the flow through the second daughter vessel remains decreased. During the CBF dysregulation that occurs in the injured brain, ischemia may result by this steal mechanism.

The proximal distribution of resistance elements also facilitates the postulated "inverse steal" mechanism. The inverse steal hypothesis maintains that vasoconstriction of healthy areas (as with hypocapnia) increases perfusion pressure in medium-sized arteries, thereby increasing flow to areas with vessels incapable of vasoconstriction. This mechanism has been proposed as a benefit of hyperventilation following TBI. However, it has also been suggested that inverse steal leads to hyperperfusion of dilated vessels, resulting in vasogenic edema.[11]

An unanswered question of clinical importance is whether the loss of CBF-metabolism coupling means that unopposed hypocapnic vasoconstriction may result in hypoxia or ischemia or both. To protect against the possibility of hypocapnia-induced ischemia, it has been suggested that S_{jvO_2} should not be allowed to fall below 50 percent during hyperventilation.[53]

Normally, hypoxia causes vasodilation in direct proportion to hemoglobin desaturation, and the increased blood flow maintains oxygen delivery to the brain (see Fig. 260-6*B*). After TBI in animals, the CBF response to hypoxia is severely attenuated and short-lived.[18,29] This impaired oxygen delivery may be the mechanism for increased susceptibility of the traumatized brain to postinjury hypoxia.[25]

Much remains unknown about the complex interaction among the described CBF regulatory mechanisms following TBI. Furthermore, potential vasoregulators, which seem to have little effect under normal conditions, may play a role following TBI. For example, under normal conditions stimulation of sympathetic efferents to brain vessels causes constriction of larger vessels; however, more distal vessels vasodilate, presumably via the CBF-metabolism coupling system, and CBF remains unchanged.[23] However, after TBI metabolic regulation may be disrupted, and little is known about the importance of neural innervation in this setting. Similarly, blood-borne humoral agents (e.g., catecholamines) normally have little influence on CBF or metabolism because they do not cross the blood-brain barrier. However, following TBI and in the absence of an intact blood-brain barrier, humoral agents have access to vascular smooth muscle and brain parenchyma, potentially altering CBF and neural activity. This has been demonstrated in animal models in which intracarotid norepinephrine increases $CMRO_2$ and CBF after blood-brain barrier disruption.[31] Thus,

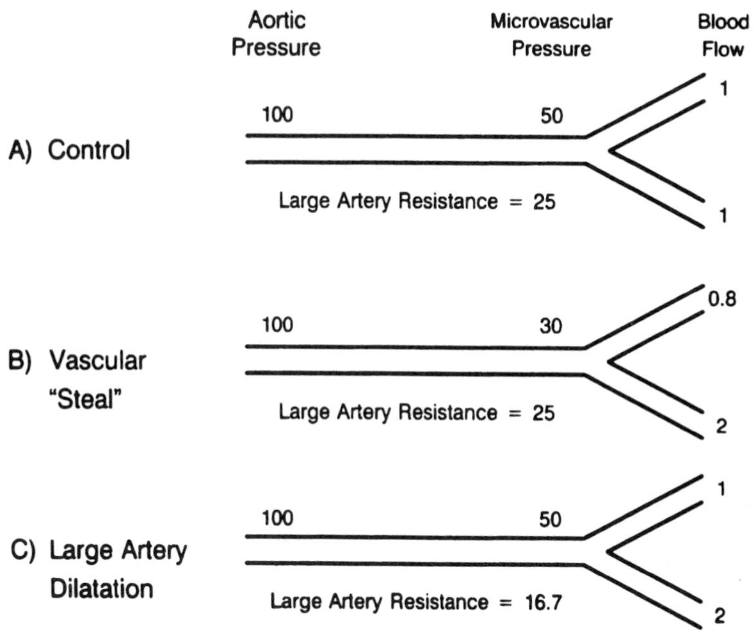

Figure 260-8 Diagram illustrating the vascular "steal" effect. Panel A shows normal conditions, with a microvascular pressure of 50 mmHg. In Panel B the lower daughter vessel has dilated, and pressure at the bifurcation has decreased to 30 mmHg. As a result, the perfusion pressure in the upper daughter vessel has decreased and, in the absence of vascular dilation, flow has also decreased to 0.8. The upper daughter vessel can restore flow by dilating or, as shown in Panel C, flow may be restored by dilation of the large artery. (From Faraci and Heistad,[15] with permission.)

TBI-induced disruption of CBF-metabolism coupling and autoregulation creates numerous possibilities for propagation of tissue damage, edema, and cell death into areas unaffected by the primary insult.

Brain Edema and ICP

Uncontrolled intracranial hypertension is a frequent cause of mortality in severely head-injured patients, and brain edema is an important component of this problem. Brain edema can be classified into two major categories, according to its characteristics and mechanisms of formation (Fig. 260-9):

1. Vasogenic edema, in which the blood-brain barrier is opened, producing a net gain of water, initially in the extravascular-extracellular compartment; it can be caused by hypertension.
2. Cellular (or cytotoxic) edema, in which cellular swelling occurs without opening of the blood-brain barrier; it is primarily metabolic in origin.

The term "brain swelling" can then be used to refer to increases in brain volume caused by increased intracranial blood volume as well as brain edema.

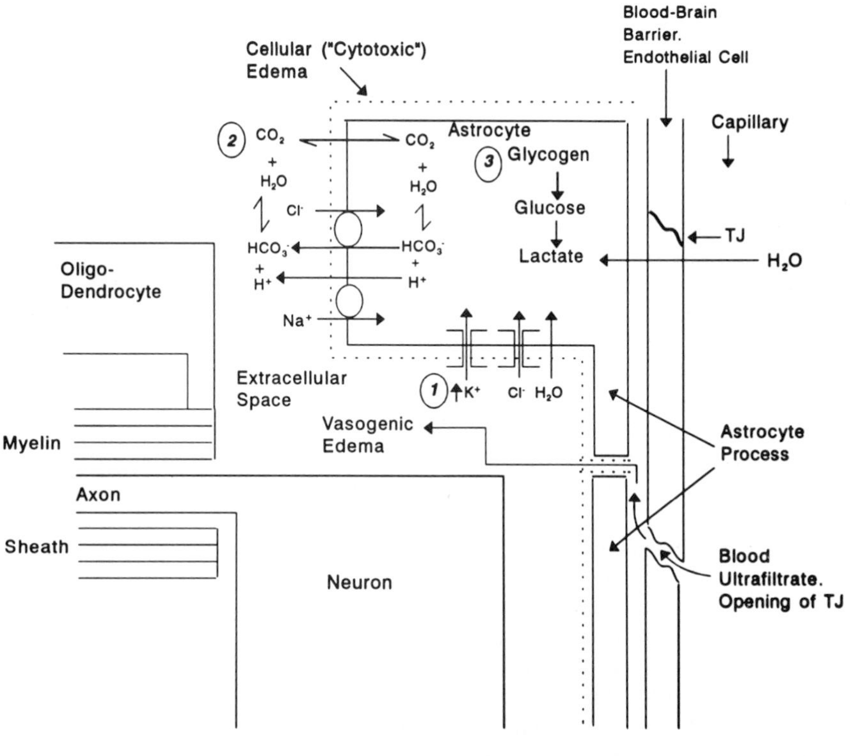

Figure 260-9 Cellular versus vasogenic edema. Cellular edema is thought to be principally attributable to cellular swelling (predominantly involving astrocytes and neuronal cell bodies and dendrites), whereas vasogenic edema is the result of the "opening" of the tight junctions (TJ) between the endothelial cells (the principal feature of the blood-brain barrier) with movement of a blood ultrafiltrate into the brain, driven by blood pressure. Cellular or vasogenic edema can coexist (see text). In its purest form, cellular edema need not result in a net gain of brain water because the cells swell only at the expense of the extracellular space. Three postulated causes of this cellular swelling are depicted in the diagram and numbered as follows: *1*, influx of K^+ and Cl^- driven by increased extracellular $[K^+]$; *2*, intracellular hydration of CO_2, producing H^+ and HCO_3^-, and their exchange for extracellular Na^+ and Cl^- respectively; *3*, generation of osmoles within the cell (e.g., by metabolism of macromolecular glycogen in astrocytes to a number of moles of lactate).

Vasogenic Edema

In vasogenic edema, solutes and water enter the brain as a result of the breakdown of the blood-brain barrier. The blood-brain barrier exists primarily as a result of the tight junctions between the endothelial cells lining blood vessels, the low pinocytotic activity of the brain endothelial cells themselves, and the absence of fenestrations, which are seen in capillaries in the choroid plexus, area postrema, and a few other regions in the central nervous system. These tight junctions exclude even small ions, and only lipid-soluble substances can freely diffuse across the cell membranes. Thus, transport systems are needed for moving polar substrates, such as glucose and the products of metabolism, into and out of the brain. These transport systems are located principally in the cell membranes of the endothelial cells and include the D-glucose carrier and a number of different amino acid carriers. When the blood-brain barrier remains intact, ions are restricted from entering the brain, and this contributes to the osmotic forces that retard movement of water into the brain.

In vasogenic edema the blood-brain barrier is breached. The extravasated fluid is a blood ultrafiltrate, essentially blood plasma with varying amounts of protein. Blood cells are usually retained, except when there is injury sufficient to lead to hemorrhage. Most fluid in edema accumulates in white matter, which can expand more easily than gray matter to accept an increased volume, in part because of the greater ease of separation of the parallel-oriented white matter tracts. Clinically, this is demonstrated by hypodensity of the white matter on computed tomography (CT).

Cellular (Cytotoxic) Edema

The origin of cellular swelling is less clear. Originally, cellular edema was termed *cytotoxic edema* because it could be produced by cell toxins, such as triethyl tin. More recently, cellular swelling has been found to occur in a number of non–toxin-induced pathologic states. For example, astrocytic swelling has been described as a prominent and early feature associated with cerebral contusion in head-injured patients, compared with its lower incidence in control patients operated on for epilepsy or glial tumors. Bullock et al.[5] noted the following: "Massive astrocytic swelling ("cytotoxic" oedema) was seen three hours to three days after injury, maximal in perivascular foot processes and compressing some of the underlying capillaries. The tight junctions were not disrupted. Neuronal damage was most marked 3 to 11 days after injury."

In its most limited form, cellular swelling could consist simply of a shift of osmoles from extracellular to intracellular compartments, followed by osmotically obligated water. The extracellular space would then be proportionately decreased in volume as the intracellular space expands. Microscopically, cellular edema consists principally of swelling of the astrocytic soma and processes as well as swelling of the neuronal dendrites. In addition, a reduction of the extracellular space is observed, as measured by increased electrical impedance and increased concentrations of extracellular membrane-impermeable molecules. Swelling of the neuronal cell soma and axon or of oligodendroglia generally is not seen.

One mechanism of cellular swelling involves the uptake of KCl when extracellular $[K^+]$ increases following TBI, as depicted for astrocytes (see Fig. 260-9 *#1*). Another proposed mechanism is the transport of HCO_3^- and H^+ out of the cell in exchange for Cl^- and Na^+, respectively, on the appropriate exchangers (see Fig. 260-9 *#2*). The HCO_3^- and H^+ can turn over many times by cycling as follows: membrane-permeable CO_2 diffuses into the cell, where it is hydrated to HCO_3^- and H^+; it is then exchanged for extracellular Na^+ and Cl^- and is dehydrated back to CO_2 in the extracellular space.[27] Cell swelling in astrocytes can also result from ischemia because of the breakdown of macromolecular glycogen, primarily localized in astrocytes, to a number of moles of lactate (see Fig. 260-9 *#3*). Fatty acids and free radicals can also cause swelling secondary to breakdown of the selective permeability of the cell membranes, resulting in the influx of Na^+ and Cl^-. Cellular swelling or shrinkage can also occur when systemic hypo- and hypernatremia are encountered after TBI (see below). Cellular swelling can produce numerous deleterious secondary effects in the cell, including (1) membrane depolarization secondary to loss of intracellular K^+, which in turn leads to influx of Ca^{2+} through voltage-gated channels; (2) activation of mechanosensitive channels, leading to an influx of Ca^{2+}; and (3) release and decreased uptake of excitatory amino acids, as seen in astrocytes.[27]

Treatment of vasogenic edema is directed toward reducing the swelling. One common clinical approach is the intravenous infusion of mannitol, in an attempt to increase the osmolality of blood and thereby withdraw water from the brain. However, this occurs only in areas of the brain retaining an intact blood-brain barrier. Also, a delayed rebound phenomenon often occurs as a result of delayed entry of mannitol into the brain. Therapies designed to limit the secondary effects that could be encountered in either vasogenic or cellular edema include administration of glutamate receptor antagonists, Ca^{2+} transport blockers, and free radical scavengers or antioxidants. Mannitol also functions as a free radical scavenger. Other therapeutic strategies have been designed to inhibit astrocyte swelling. In an experimental closed-head injury model, a significant decrease in mortality and an improvement in the rate of neurological recovery were associated with the administration of drugs that were nondiuretic derivatives of ethacrynic acid. These drugs inhibited astrocytic swelling in this same model, probably by blocking anion channels or anion exchange transport systems.[27,40] Information now appearing on the deleterious consequences of cell swelling would seem to make inhibition of such swelling an important therapeutic strategy.

Intracranial Pressure

ICP is often elevated after serious head injury. A distinction should be made, however, between the effects of elevated ICP associated with damaged brain and the effects of it in normal brain. Intracranial hypertension by itself may not be harmful, as exemplified by patients with pseudotumor cerebri, who can have ICPs of greater than 40 mmHg yet have little clinical neurological dysfunction. However, an ICP of the same magnitude in a patient with contused brain, altered cerebrovascular regulation, incipient hypoxic or ischemic injury, and/or cerebral edema can cause decreased CPP, a cycle of further CBF dysregulation, increasing edema, and death.

The intracranial compartment in adults is of fixed volume and contains three incompressible constituents: blood, CSF, and brain parenchyma. Any process that increases the volume of one of these will increase ICP if compensatory mechanisms fail. The extent to which increases in brain, CSF, or blood volume increase ICP is measured as intracranial compliance or Δvolume/ΔICP.

Intracranial compliance can provide important information about displaceable volume available for volume buffering. Volume buffering capacity is measured by injecting (or withdrawing) a known volume of saline or CSF and observing the resultant pressure change. The pressure-volume relationship is such that compliance decreases as ICP rises and displaceable volume is depleted.

This relationship means that compliance varies with pressure, even in normal brain. To evaluate pathologic changes in the volume buffering capacity of the intracranial compartment independent of the starting pressure, Marmarou et al.[35] defined the pressure volume index (PVI) as follows:

$$PVI = \Delta V/\log(P_{final}/P_{initial})$$

where ΔV is the change in volume in milliliters, and P_{final} and $P_{initial}$ are the ICP values after and before the change in volume. The PVI is thus the volume necessary to raise pressure by a factor of 10. A low PVI (<13 ml) indicates a "tight" brain, in which small changes in volume result in large increases in ICP (Fig. 260-10). Unlike compliance measurements, the PVI is relatively independent of the ICP at which it is measured. According to this formulation, a reduction in intracranial compliance is attributable to two interrelated but separate processes. First, compliance decreases as ICP rises, as it would in normal brain when volume is added. Second, the intrinsic ability to buffer volume changes at any given ICP can be abnormal, and this loss of compliance is reflected by a decreasing PVI. Such a loss of volume buffering ability may occur, for example, if brain volume starts out as a greater than normal proportion of the intracranial compartment. Following TBI, PVI is reduced; furthermore, a low PVI correlates well with a patient's tendency toward an unstable and rising ICP as well as a poor outcome.[36]

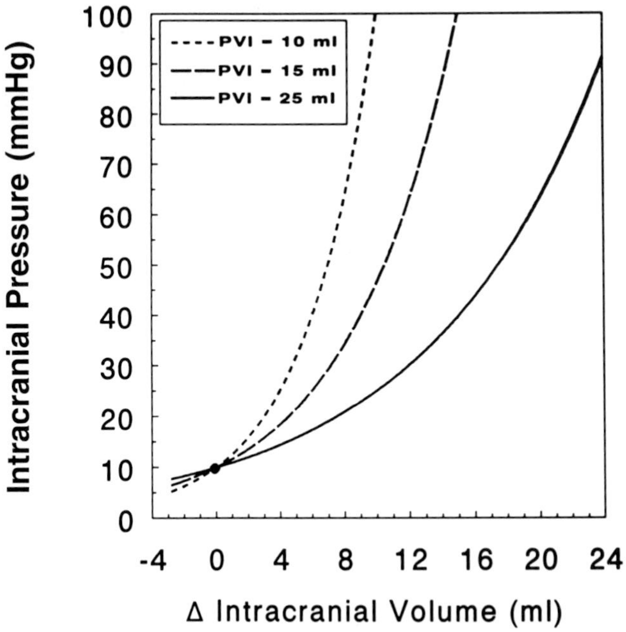

Figure 260-10 The ICP that results from a change in intracranial volume depends upon both the initial ICP and the available volume buffering (quantitated by the PVI; see text). The three curves show the effect of adding volume when ICP starts at 10 mmHg and intracranial volume buffering is normal (PVI = 25 ml), moderately decreased (PVI = 15 ml), or severely decreased (PVI = 10 ml). Compliance (the inverse slope of the curve) may decrease by (1) moving along a curve with increasing volume or (2) shifting from the normal curve to one with a lower PVI. After traumatic brain injury, the brain often has a near-normal ICP but a depressed PVI. Such individuals are at risk for labile or dangerously elevated ICP when intracranial volume changes minimally.

Following TBI several compensatory mechanisms can operate to keep ICP low. Initially after brain injury, increases in ICP are dampened by a reduction in the volume of intracranial CSF (approximately 10 percent of intracranial volume). This occurs as a result of increased CSF resorption and displacement of CSF from the intracranial compartment to the spinal compartment with distention of the spinal dura. The rate of CSF resorption is determined by the driving pressure (ICP minus venous pressure) divided by the resistance of CSF resorption pathways. Increases in ICP increase driving pressure and CSF resorption. Further compensation is afforded when increasing pressure compresses veins, thereby decreasing intracranial blood volume. During the initial compensation there is little change in ICP.

As compensatory mechanisms that modulate initial increases in ICP are depleted, intracranial compliance decreases. During this phase, the ICP may be normal or slightly increased, but small increases in intracranial volume produced by vasodilation, CSF obstruction, or increased edema produce comparatively greater increases in ICP. In this early phase of decompensation, elevations in ICP can be reversed by hyperventilation, which decreases Pa_{CO_2} and produces vasoconstriction in responsive vessels, resulting in a decreased intracranial arterial blood volume.[34] The rapid effectiveness of mannitol during this period may depend upon autoregulatory and CBF-metabolism coupling mechanisms. "Viscosity autoregulation" refers to a phenomenon related to pressure autoregulation in which a decrease in blood viscosity, such as that induced by mannitol, results in a transient increase in CBF followed by compensatory metabolic vasoconstriction that returns blood flow toward normal. The rapid effect of mannitol administration on reduction of ICP may be attributed to this vasoconstriction with an accompanying decrease of cerebral blood volume.[2]

As ICP continues to increase, compliance decreases further, and small changes in volume result in larger increases in pressure. Evidence of this phenomenon may be found in the episodic increases of ICP—termed *plateau waves*—that last for fractions of an hour and are thought to occur with small increases in intracranial blood volume. The final stage in the decompensation of protective mechanisms often occurs concurrently with vasomotor paralysis of the cerebral vasculature. In this phase little or no volume buffering is available, hyperventilation becomes ineffective, and the elevation in ICP is sustained.

Increased ICP due to edema to actually somewhat more complex because of the compartmentation of brain intracellular fluid, brain extracellular fluid, and CSF. Extracellular edema fluid may eventually move from extracellular space to drain via CSF channels. Brain tissue consists of a complex mosaic of cells and extracellular space that resist fluid flow; thus, small intracerebral pressure gradients may develop. Intracellular edema fluid must first be removed from cells by osmotic forces before it can be removed from the intracranial compartment.

Vascular engorgement and increased cerebral blood volume can also elevate ICP following TBI. However, absolute or relative hyperemia as described above is not necessarily associated with raised cerebral blood volume.[2] It is also possible for cerebral blood volume to be high but for CBF to be low. Cerebral blood volume is not commonly measured, but estimates of blood volume changes derived from measurements of PVI and the effect of hyperventilation on ICP suggest that, in some patients, two-thirds of the raised ICP can be attributed to blood volume changes.[34]

The physician managing a patient with progressive loss of intracranial compliance should repeatedly attempt to identify the causes of reduced compliance, many of which are medically or surgically treatable. A rapidly developing space-occupying lesion, such as a hematoma, is more poorly tolerated than a slowly evolving mass lesion, because compensatory mechanisms, such as CSF resorption, have less time to develop fully in the former case. Obstruction of the CSF pathways, such as can occur with hemorrhage, accelerates the increase in ICP by increasing resistance to CSF resorption or CSF flow into the spinal dural sac. Patients whose cardiovascular status is unstable have an increased risk in terms of their response to ICP elevations when their arterial blood pressure is low. Well-oxygenated blood, an adequate cardiac output, and maintenance of CPP at a level greater than 40 mmHg help ensure that the patient does not succumb to injury because of regionally insufficient cerebral perfusion.

Systemic Manifestations of Head Injury

Injury to the brain may cause abnormalities in systemic homeostasis and organ function. Systemic responses to head injury may occur immediately, or they may evolve over hours or days. Immediately after head injury occurs, cardiorespiratory function is often precarious. Ventilatory dysfunction, including apnea or hypoventilation, may occur. Cardiovascular function is also often impaired, and bradycardia, systemic hypotension or hypertension, reduced cardiac output, or cardiac arrhythmias may be identified.[50,58] These immediate responses are thought to result from the direct effect of TBI on the brain stem centers for cardiorespiratory function. Thus, the potential for hypoxemia and ischemia produced by cardiorespiratory compromise begins immediately after TBI and may lead to worsening of the brain injury. This exemplifies only one of the ways in which post-TBI systemic dysfunction may influence the clinical outcome. Other systemic abnormalities that may affect outcome and are covered in this discussion are water, electrolyte, and hormonal dysfunction; the post-TBI hypermetabolic state; and cardiopulmonary malfunction. A related topic, coagulopathy induced by head injury, is discussed in another chapter.

Abnormalities of Water and Electrolyte Homeostasis

Lesions in the hypothalamus, pituitary stalk, and pituitary gland occur in patients sustaining fatal head injury. Such injuries can result from several different mechanisms. Hypothalamic and pituitary stalk lesions are usually secondary to shearing stresses to the brain following impact. Pituitary gland injury may be secondary to infarction following damage to the hypothalamic-hypophyseal portal system. None of these injuries is necessarily associated with fractures involving the sella turcica.[9]

Abnormalities of water balance, evidenced by either excessive water retention or loss, are the most common manifestations of hypothalamic-hypophyseal dysfunction occurring after head injury. Diabetes insipidus follows direct injury of the supraoptic-paraventricular hypothalamic nuclei or injury to the pituitary stalk with damage of the axons carrying antiduretic hormone to the neurohypophysis.

Polyuria is usually the first manifestation of diabetes insipidus, although other signs may include polydipsia, low urine specific gravity, and elevated plasma osmolality. Most patients sustaining a head injury who are found to have polyuria may be assumed to have an antidiuretic hormone deficiency if simultaneous testing of urine osmolality reveals a level less than 300 mosmol/kg and serum osmolality tests reveal a level greater than 300 mosmol/kg. Post-traumatic diabetes insipidus may be permanent, but more frequently, only transient polyuria occurs. In awake patients with an intact thirst mechanism, oral intake often maintains fluid balance. In comatose patients, diagnosis before the onset of severe dehydration with resultant hypernatremia may be difficult. Early treatment includes fluid replacement and administration of vasopressin, but care must be taken to avoid excessive water replacement when vasopressin is used, as inhibition of urinary water loss may lead to water intoxication with worsening of pre-existing cerebral edema. Systemic volume depletion secondary to diabetes insipidus can be associated with a reduction of mean arterial pressure and a possible decrease in CPP. Hence, systemic water balance must be monitored carefully. Patients with chronic, incomplete loss of antidiuretic hormone may be treated with chlorpropamide, a sulfonylurea that seems to potentiate the effect of antidiuretic hormone on the kidney tubules.

Hypernatremia may also occur in the absence of diabetes insipidus when the comatose patient is unable to drink sufficiently to replace free water loss. This condition is accentuated by increased water loss associated with the administration of osmotic diuretics or by increased insensible loss associated with fever.

The opposite condition, hyponatremia, occurs in patients with the syndrome of inappropriate antidiuretic hormone (SIADH) secretion. Patients with SIADH characteristically present with the following features: hyponatremia ($[Na^+] < 135$ meq/liter), low serum osmolality (<280 mosmol/kg), a urinary $[Na^+]$ level exceeding 20 meq/liter, increased urinary osmolality (>100 mosmol/kg), and the absence of other causes of hyponatremia, such as adrenal, thyroid, or renal insufficiency.[28] The effects of profound hyponatremia ($[Na^+] < 120$ meq/liter) include nausea, vomiting, confusion, seizures, lethargy, and coma. Presumably, these effects are produced by water intoxication, accompanied by CNS cellular swelling and increased ICP. Systemic hypo-osmolality may be magnified by the use of loop and osmotic diuretics followed by rehydration with saline-poor fluid. Fluid restriction is the treatment of choice for asymptomatic or mildly symptomatic patients with serum $[Na^+]$ levels of greater than 120 meq/liter. In symptomatic patients or in those with a serum $[Na^+]$ level of less than 120 meq/liter, fluid restriction should be augmented by infusion of 3% or 5% NaCl in calculated amounts. (For example, the administration of 3% saline at a rate of 0.1 ml/kg per minute for 2 h will raise plasma $[Na^+]$ by 10 meq/liter.) During infusion, plasma $[Na^+]$ levels should be monitored to ensure that they do not increase by more than 25 mmol/liter, or rise above 130 mmol/liter, in a 24-h period. More rapid correction is dangerous because of the risk of causing central pontine myelinolysis.

The cerebral salt-wasting syndrome (CSWS) was described before SIADH by investigators who observed continued urinary sodium loss despite serum hyponatremia, but the subsequent description of SIADH appears to have distracted attention from CSWS. Recent evidence identifying patients with all of the criteria for SIADH but with decreased plasma and blood volume has again focused attention on CSWS. Atrial natriuretic polypeptide (ANP), found in the mammalian hypothalamus and lamina terminalis, produces prompt natriuresis and is thought to be the hormone responsible for CSWS. Recent studies of neurosurgical patients with hyponatremia have, in fact, identified reduced plasma and total blood volumes more frequently than the expanded blood volumes expected in SIADH.[30,41] In such patients, water restriction (the traditional mode of treatment for SIADH) would be hazardous; rather, correction of the sodium deficit should be managed by calculated saline replacement. Determining which patients with hyponatremia have SIADH and which have CSWS is often difficult because some patients have features of both disorders. Furthermore, in patients with CSWS, hypovolemia enhances ''appropriate'' secretion of antidiuretic hormone; likewise, antidiuretic hormone may increase ANP secretion. Because of the complexity of these interactions, diagnosis and treatment of patients with post-TBI hyponatremia should focus on assessing and correcting the patient's blood volume and electrolyte status, rather than assigning the patient to a particular nosological group. The hyponatremic and hypernatremic states described above may lead to volumetric changes of brain cells, especially astrocytes, activating either regulatory volume decrease or increase and associated membrane transport processes.

Other Hormonal Abnormalities

Symptomatic deficiency of anterior pituitary hormones after head injury is far less common that abnormalities of water balance and usually is not identified until long after the injury occurs. Generally, anterior pituitary dysfunction is thought to occur after trauma because injury to the hypothalamic-hypophyseal portal system produces pituitary ischemia. In some instances, however, hypothalamic injury may be causative because of a deficiency of releasing factors. Deficiencies of all of the adenohypophyseal hormones have been reported. Diabetes insipidus may also be associated with anterior pituitary dysfunction but may be masked by thyroid-stimulating hormone and adrenocorticotropic hormone (ACTH) insufficiency. The subsequent use of glucocorticoid therapy in these patients produces polyuria and polydipsia.

Hypersecretion of adenohypophyseal hormones, including ACTH, prolactin, and growth hormone, occurs as part of the physiologic response to TBI. Following injury, corticotropin-releasing factor is liberated from the median eminence, causing release of ACTH, which in turn stimulates cortisol secretion from the adrenal gland. Normally, an increased level of serum cortisol inhibits production of ACTH by negative feedback, thereby reducing cortisol production. However, after head injury, although the negative feedback loop often remains intact, dexamethasone suppression tests have demonstrated that it is set at a higher level, accounting for the lack of inhibition of ACTH by higher levels of circulating cortisol.[56] Steroid-induced negative nitrogen balance often results.

Metabolic Responses to TBI

In addition to serum cortisol, levels of other humoral mediators, including catecholamines, enkephalins, and cytokines, have been found to be increased after TBI. These increases are the most likely causes of the systemic metabolic derangements found in head-injured patients, which include hypermetabolism, depressed cellular immunity, hyperglycemia, hypercatabolism, increased counter regulatory hormones, and specific organ dysfunction involving such target organs as the lungs, heart, liver, and gut. Despite the potential utility of some of these metabolic responses, the impact of these changes is often deleterious.

TBI is associated with increased sympathetic neuronal activity and adrenal medullary stimulation, resulting in increased levels of circulating epinephrine and norepinephrine. This response occurs within seconds of injury, and its magnitude is related directly to the severity of the brain injury.[51] This hyperadrenergic state is presumed to be responsible for the hypermetabolic response observed after head injury and characterized by elevated oxygen consumption, hypertension, tachycardia, increased cardiac output, and increased resting energy expenditure with the development of a negative nitrogen balance and hyperglycemia.[7]

Judicious nutritional replacement after head injury may be important in determining the outcome for some patients.[49] Increased energy supply is required to support an energy expenditure that, in some injured patients, is greater than 50 percent above normal. A principal source of energy is derived from skeletal muscle catabolism, resulting in a negative nitrogen balance and increased urinary nitrogen loss. This occurs independent of steroid use.[8,63]

In addition to the catecholamine effect, enkephalins and cytokines may mediate some of the systemic metabolic responses after TBI. Both enkephalins and cytokines have been found to be increased in the cerebral ventricular fluid and serum after TBI.[64] Cytokines—particularly interleukin-1, interleukin-6, and tumor necrosis factor—have also been proposed as mediators of some of the features of the hypermetabolism-hypercatabolism that occurs after TBI.[65]

Hyperglycemia occurs commonly after head injury and correlates negatively with severity and outcome.[62] Serum glucose levels increase within minutes in experimental TBI, and they closely parallel circulating catecholamine levels. Catecholamines stimulate glucagon secretion, and both stimulate glycogen breakdown into glucose in the liver. Catecholamines also decrease the amount of insulin released from the pancreas and inhibit glucose uptake in muscle. Cytokines may also play a role in this response because of stimulation of glucagon secretion. Hyperglycemia after TBI may be deleterious because if there is diminished oxidative metabolism, this increased glucose will be metabolized to lactate. In experimental ischemia, hyperglycemia is known to worsen brain injury.[20]

Cardiopulmonary Malfunction

Increased levels of circulating catecholamines may also have a deleterious effect on certain target organs, especially the heart and lungs. Myocardial injury, in the form of cytolysis and subendocardial hemorrhage, occurs after head injury in humans, and similar abnormalities have been described in experimental animals following the infusion of norepinephrine. These findings may explain the arrhythmias, electrocardiographic changes, and decreased cardiac output observed in some patients after head injury. Cholinergic dysfunction mediated by the vagus nerve has also been implicated as one cause of the bradyarrhythmia and hypotension that may occur after TBI. In the presence of intracranial hypertension, these derangements of cardiac function may produce a lower mean systemic arterial pressure and CPP, thereby worsening the severity of the cerebral injury.

Lung dysfunction may also occur as a systemic manifestation of isolated head injury. The following discussion focuses on ''neurogenic'' pulmonary dysfunction and not on lung dysfunction occurring concomitantly with head injury as a result of aspiration, lung contusion, or hemothorax or pneumothorax. ''Neurogenic'' pulmonary dysfunction may occur within minutes after head injury. This fulminant condition is characterized by alveolar and tracheobronchial flooding by a blood-tinged, protein-rich fluid. This type of lung dysfunction, termed *neurogenic pulmonary edema,* is relatively uncommon and is generally associated with life-threatening head injuries or other catastrophic intracranial processes.

The syndrome is associated with decreased lung compliance, and chest radiographs usually demonstrate diffuse infiltration of the lung parenchyma ("white lung"). The rapid development of hypoxemia is the most serious manifestation of this disorder. Timely endotracheal intubation and mechanical ventilation delivering an increased fraction of inspired oxygen (FiO_2) under conditions of positive and expiratory pressure (PEEP) can succeed in preventing a dangerously low Pa_{O_2}, which could impair further the delivery of oxygen to the injured brain.

More often, if pulmonary dysfunction occurs after head injury, it is delayed by 24 to 48 h.[61] It is unknown whether this represents a less serious form of the fulminant variety just described or whether it is an entirely different entity. The principal manifestation of delayed pulmonary dysfunction is a gas exchange abnormality in the absence of overt pulmonary edema, as identified by either chest radiography or auscultation. Lung compliance is usually normal. Evaluation of ventilation-perfusion compartments of the lung by using multiple inert gases has demonstrated ventilation-perfusion mismatch with increased dead space and increased intrapulmonary shunt.[48,52] Continued perfusion of areas of the lung with little or no ventilation results in hypoxemia that may be difficult to correct using PEEP and increased Fi_{O_2}. Because lung compliance is normal, PEEP-related injury to the alveoli (barotrauma) is much more likely to occur in patients with delayed-onset pulmonary dysfunction than in patients with fulminant pulmonary edema.

The etiology of pulmonary dysfunction after isolated head injury is a source of controversy.[12,57] One theory, based on the post-injury hyperdynamic state, maintains that hypertension with increased peripheral vascular resistance produces an increased left ventricular afterload, resulting in increased left atrial pressure and pulmonary capillary pressure with resultant lung edema secondary to unbalanced Starling forces. Animal experiments and studies in humans, however, have shown that pulmonary capillary wedge pressure is not necessarily elevated when post–head-injury pulmonary edema occurs. In humans, this observation does not fully negate the peripheral hemodynamic theory, because significant cardiovascular hemodynamic changes occurring immediately after head trauma may produce capillary injury and capillary leakage, but the patient's hemodynamic status may subsequently return to normal by the start of monitoring.

Another purported cause of post–head-injury pulmonary dysfunction is the direct effect of circulating catecholamines or sympathetic stimulation on lung microvasculature, resulting in increased vascular permeability.[32] A third theory postulates that the lung vasculature may be injured by substances released from platelet, fibrin, and/or neutrophil microaggregates occurring in post–head-injury disseminated intravascular coagulation. This cause, if valid, is unlikely to account for the fulminant variety of pulmonary dysfunction because a longer period of time would be necessary to produce lung injury by this mechanism.

References

1. Andersen BJ, Unterberg AW, Clarke GD, Marmarou A. Effect of posttraumatic hypoventilation on cerebral energy metabolism. *J Neurosurg* 1988; 68:601–607.
2. Bouma GJ, Muizelaar JP. Cerebral blood flow, cerebral blood volume and cerebrovascular reactivity after severe head injury. *J Neurotrauma* 1992; 9(Suppl 1):S333–S348.
3. Bouma GJ, Muizelaar JP, Stringer WA, et al. Ultra-early evaluation of regional cerebral blood flow in severely head-injured patients using xenon-enhanced computerized tomography. *J Neurosurg* 1992; 77:360–368.
4. Bowman CL, Ding JP, Sachs F, Sokabe M. Mechanotransducing ion channels in astrocytes. *Brain Res* 1992; 584:272–286.
5. Bullock R, Maxwell WL, Graham DI, et al. Glial swelling following human cerebral contusion: an ultrastructural study. *J Neurol Neurosurg Psychiatry* 1991; 54:427–434.
6. Choi DW. Glutamate neurotoxicity and diseases of the nervous system. *Neuron* 1988; 1:623–634.
7. Clifton GL, Robertson CS, Grossman RG. Management of the cardiovascular and metabolic responses to severe head injury. *J Neurotrauma* 1992; 9(Suppl 1):139–160.
8. Clifton GL, Robertson CS, Grossman RG, et al. The metabolic response to severe head injury. *J Neurosurg* 1984; 60:687–696.
9. Crompton MR. Hypothalamic lesions following closed head injury. *Brain* 1971; 94:165–172.
10. Cruz J, Miner ME, Allen SJ, et al. Continuous monitoring of cerebral oxygenation in acute brain injury: assessment of cerebral hemodynamic reserve. *Neurosurgery* 1991; 29:743–749.
11. Darby JM, Yonas H, Marion DW, et al. Local "inverse steal" induced by hyperventilation in head injury. *Neurosurgery* 1988; 23:84–88.
12. Demling R, Riessen R. Pulmonary dysfunction after cerebral injury. *Crit Care Med* 1990; 18:768–774.
13. DeSalles AAF, Muizelaar JP, Young HF. Hyperglycemia, cerebrospinal fluid lactic acidosis and cerebral blood flow in severely head-injured patients. *Neurosurgery* 1987; 21:45–50.
14. Faden AI, Demediuk P, Panter SS, Vink R. Role of excitatory amino acids and NMDA receptors in traumatic brain injury. *Science* 1989; 244:798–800.
15. Faraci FM, Heistad DD. Regulation of large cerebral arteries and cerebral microvascular pressure. *Circ Res* 1990; 66:8–17.
16. Feustel PJ, Fortune JB, Weigle CGM. Continuously measured internal jugular venous oxygen saturation responses to increased arterial blood pressure in head-injured patients. *J Cereb Blood Flow Metab* 1991; 11:S832 (abstr).
17. Feustel PJ, Ingvar MC, Severinghaus JW. Cerebral oxygen availability and blood flow during middle cerebral artery occlusion. Effects of pentobarbital. *Stroke* 1981; 12:858–863.
18. Feustel PJ, Nelson LR. Cortical blood regulation during hypoxemia in experimental head injury. *J Surg Res* 1987; 43:86–93.
19. Fortune JB, Bock D, Kupinski AM, et al. Human cerebrovascular response to oxygen and carbon dioxide as determined by internal carotid artery duplex scanning. *J Trauma* 1992; 32:618–628.
20. Ginsberg MD, Welsh FA, Budd WW. Deleterious effect of glucose pretreatment on recovery from diffuse cerebral ischemia in the cat. I. Local cerebral blood flow and glucose utilization. *Stroke* 1980; 11:347–354.
21. Graham DI, Ford I, Adam JH, et al. Ischemic brain damage is still common in fatal non-missile head injury. *J Neurol Neurosurg Psychiatry* 1989; 52:346–350.
22. Hamill OP, Lane JW, McBride DW Jr. Amiloride: a molecular probe for mechanosensitive channels. *Trends Pharmacol Sci* 1992; 13:373–376.
23. Heistad DD, Kontos HA. Cerebral circulation. In Shepherd JT, Abboud FM (eds): *Handbook of Physiology: Section 2: The Cardiovascular System.* Bethesda, Md: American Physiological Society, 1983, pp 137–182.
24. Hochachka PW, Mommsen TP. Protons and anaerobiosis. *Science* 1983; 219:1391–1397.
25. Ishige N, Pitts LH, Pogliani L, et al. Effect of hypoxia on traumatic brain injury in rats. Pt 2: Changes in high energy phosphate metabolism. *Neurosurgery* 1987; 20:854–858.
26. Katayama Y, Becker DP, Tamura T, et al. Massive increases in extracellular potassium and the indiscriminate release of glutamate following concussive brain injury. *J Neurosurg* 1990; 73:889–900.

27. Kimelberg HK. Astrocytic edema in CNS trauma. *J Neurotrauma* 1992; 9(Suppl 1):S71–S81.
28. Kovacs L, Robertson G. Syndrome of inappropriate antidiuresis. *Endocrinol Metab Clin North Am* 1992; 21:859–875.
29. Lewelt W, Jenkins LW, Miller JD. Effects of experimental fluid-percussion injury of the brain on cerebrovascular reactivity of hypoxia and to hypercapnia. *J Neurosurg* 1982; 56:332–338.
30. Lolin Y, Jackowski A. Hyponatraemia in neurosurgical patients: diagnosis using derived parameters of sodium and water homeostasis. *Br J Neurosurg* 1992; 6:457–466.
31. MacKenzie ET, McCulloch J, O'Keane M, et al. Cerebral circulation and norepinephrine: relevance of the blood-brain barrier. *Am J Physiol* 1976; 231:483–488.
32. Malik AB. Mechanisms of neurogenic pulmonary edema. *Circ Res* 1985; 57:1–18.
33. Marion DW, Darby J, Yonas H. Acute regional cerebral blood flow changes caused by severe head injuries. *J Neurosurg* 1991; 74:407–414.
34. Marmarou A, Maset AL, Ward JD, et al. Contribution of CSF and vascular factors to elevation of ICP in severely head-injured patients. *J Neurosurg* 1987; 66:883–890.
35. Marmarou A, Shulman K, Rosende RM. A nonlinear analysis of the cerebrospinal fluid system and intracranial pressure dynamics. *J Neurosurg* 1978; 48:332–344.
36. Maset AL, Marmarou A, Ward JD, et al. Pressure-volume index in head injury. *J Neurosurg* 1987; 67:832–840.
37. Messeter K, Nordstrom CH, Sundbarg E, et al. Cerebral hemodynamics in patients with acute severe head trauma. *J Neurosurg* 1986; 64:231–237.
38. Muizelaar JP, Marmarou A, DeSalles AA, et al. Cerebral blood flow and metabolism in severely head-injured children. Part 1: Relationship with GCS score, outcome, ICP, and PVI. *J Neurosurg* 1989; 71:63–71.
39. Muizelaar JP, van der Poel HG, Li ZC, et al. Pial arteriolar vessel diameter and CO_2 reactivity during prolonged hyperventilation in the rabbit. *J Neurosurg* 1988; 69:923–927.
40. Nelson LR, Auen EL, Bourke RS, et al. Comparison of animal head injury models developed for treatment modality evaluation. In Grossman RG, Gildenberg PL (eds): *Head Injury: Basic and Clinical Aspects.* New York: Raven Press, 1982, pp 117–127.
41. Nelson PB, Seif SM, Maroon JC, Robinson AG. Hyponatremia in intracranial disease: perhaps not the syndrome of inappropriate secretion of antidiuretic hormone (SIADH). *J Neurosurg* 1981; 55:938–941.
42. Nilsson B, Hillered L, Ponten U, Ungerstedt U. Changes in cortical extracellular levels of energy-related metabolites and amino acids following concussive brain injury in rats. *J Cereb Blood Flow Metab* 1990; 10:631–637.
43. Nilsson B, Ponten U. Experimental head injury in the rat. Part 2: regional brain energy metabolism in concussive trauma. *J Neurosurg* 1977; 47:252–261.
44. Nordstrom CH, Messeter K, Sundbarg G, et al. Cerebral blood flow, vasoreactivity, and oxygen consumption during barbiturate therapy in severe traumatic brain lesions. *J Neurosurg* 1988; 68:424–431.
45. Obrist WD, Langfitt TW, Jaggi JL, et al. Cerebral blood flow and metabolism in comatose patients with acute head injury. Relationship to intracranial hypertension. *J Neurosurg* 1984; 61:241–253.
46. Overgaard J, Mosdal C, Tweed WA. Cerebral circulation after head injury. Part 3: Does reduced regional cerebral blood flow determine recovery of brain function after blunt head injury? *J Neurosurg* 1981; 55:63–74.
47. Phillis JW. Adenosine in the control of the cerebral circulation. *Cerebrovasc Brain Metab Rev* 1989; 1:26–54.
48. Popp AJ, Shah DM, Berman RA, et al. Delayed pulmonary dysfunction in head-injured patients. *J Neurosurg* 1982; 57:784–790.
49. Robertson CS, Clifton GL, Grossman RG. Oxygen utilization and cardiovascular function in head-injured patients. *Neurosurgery* 1984; 15:307–314.
50. Rosner MJ. Systemic response to experimental brain injury. In Becker DP, Povlishock JT (eds): *Central Nervous System Trauma Status Report.* Bethesda, MD: National Institute of Neurological and Communicative Disorders and Stroke, 1985, pp 405–415.
51. Rosner MJ, Newsome HH, Becker DP. Mechanical brain injury: the sympathoadrenal response. *J Neurosurg* 1984; 61:76–86.
52. Schumacker PT, Rhodes GR, Newell JC, et al. Ventilation-perfusion imbalance after head trauma. *Am Rev Respir Dis* 1979; 119:33–43.
53. Sheinberg M, Kanten MJ, Robertson CS, et al. Continuous monitoring of jugular venous oxygen saturation in head-injured patients. *J Neurosurg* 1992; 76:212–217.
54. Siesjö BK. Pathophysiology and treatment of focal cerebral ischemia. Part I. Pathophysiology. *J Neurosurg* 1992; 77:169–184.
55. Siesjö BK. Pathophysiology and treatment of focal cerebral ischemia. Part II. Mechanisms of damage and treatment. *J Neurosurg* 1992; 77:337–354.
56. Steinbok P, Thompson G. Serum cortisol abnormalities after craniocerebral trauma. *Neurosurgery* 1979; 5:559–565.
57. Theodore J, Robin ED. Speculations on neurogenic pulmonary edema (NPE). *Am Rev Respir Dis* 1976; 113:405–411.
58. Torbati D, Jacks AF, Carey ME, et al. Cerebral cardiovascular and respiratory variables after an experimental brain missile wound. *J Neurotrauma* 1992; 9(Suppl 1):S143–S155.
59. Unterberg AW, Andersen BJ, Clarke GD, Marmarou A. Cerebral energy metabolism following fluid-percussion brain injury in cats. *J Neurosurg* 1988; 68:594–600.
60. Ward JD, Becker DP, Miller JD, et al. Failure of prophylactic barbiturate coma in the treatment of severe head injury. *J Neurosurg* 1985; 62:383–388.
61. Yen JK, Rhodes GR, Bourke RS, et al. Delayed impairment of arterial blood oxygenation in patients with severe head injury: preliminary report. *Surg Neurol* 1978; 9:323–327.
62. Young B, Ott L, Dempsey R, et al. Relationship between admission hyperglycemia and neurologic outcome of severely brain-injured patients. *Ann Surg* 1989; 210:466–473.
63. Young B, Ott L, Norton J, et al. Metabolic and nutritional sequelae in the non-steroid treated head injury patient. *Neurosurgery* 1985; 17:784–791.
64. Young B, Ott L, Yingling B, McClain C. Nutrition and brain injury. *J Neurotrauma* 1992; 9(Suppl 1): S375–S383.
65. Young W. Role of calcium in central nervous system injuries. *J Neurotrauma* 1992; 9(Suppl 1):S9–S25.
66. Younkin DP, Delivoria-Papadopoulos M, Maris J, et al. Cerebral metabolic effects of neonatal seizures measured with in vivo ^{31}P NMR spectroscopy. *Ann Neurol* 1986; 20:513–519.

261 Pathology of Closed Head Injury

William F. McCormick

Closed head injury has reached epidemic proportions in Western societies owing both to the tremendous carnage engendered by our poorly controlled vehicular traffic and to the rising violence of citizens against each other in times of social unrest. The variety and severity of the types of closed head injury encountered will differ considerably from one study population to the next. Physicians and paramedical personnel who deal primarily with vehicular-generated CNS trauma will see a spectrum of lesions that will be different from those seen by physicians who usually deal with patients who have sustained accelerative-type head injuries from blows to the head. Furthermore, medical examiners and coroners will see a spectrum of lesions considerably different in both type and severity from those usually encountered by hospital-based physicians. Several types of direct brain stem lesions are rarely seen in hospital populations but are relatively common in a medical examiner's population, owing to their almost universally rapid lethality. Other types of lesions, such as some of the cranial nerve disorders resulting from closed head trauma, have been little discussed or studied by pathologists. Many are infrequently lethal, and detailed evaluation of these injuries using usual autopsy procedures is difficult.

Two other major changes in our understanding of closed head injury have occurred in recent years: the appreciation that the brain of an infant or young child responds very differently from that of an older child or an adult,[2,3,32,41,58,61,66,71,76,87,97,105] and the concept of "diffuse impact injury."[1–6,9,16,17,34,37,66,73,83,85,91,92,101,104,105] These two areas of rapidly expanding knowledge will be discussed in some detail in this chapter.

Two difficulties that commonly discourage the study of the pathology of head trauma are the fact that a lethal injury normally will bring the decedent to the attention of the coroner or medical examiner rather than to the hospital-based (academic) pathologist or neuropathologist,[1,3,17,66] and the all too frequent reluctance on the part of hospital pathologists to become involved in cases with a high probability of litigation.

It is critical that as much information as possible be available to the pathologist regarding the probable physical mechanisms responsible for the production of the head wound—whether the head injury resulted from the decedent being in a vehicular crash, or being hit with a hard object (pipe, brick), or being involved in a fall, etc. The often exceedingly complex patterns of vehicular trauma, with their multiple accelerative- and decelerative-type injuries, have been stressed previously. The pattern and extent of soft tissue injuries to the face and head and neck should be known by the pathologist before completing the evaluation of the injuries of the skull and brain and their pattern. The extent, distribution, and type of skull fractures, if present, should be known in detail (not just that a skull fracture was or was not present). The naive belief that the type of head injury can be determined with any degree of precision by the examination of a formalin-fixed brain should be vigorously corrected.

It should be kept in mind that the pathologist, like the clinician, is subject to a number of constraints when examining a cadaver. These constraints make it difficult at times to carry out as thorough an examination as both the clinician and the pathologist might desire. While this is less often true in cases that involve trauma victims than in cases that involve other types of patients (owing to the legal nature of the problem), there are still imperatives not to blatantly disfigure the body or to extensively delay the completion of the autopsy. Perhaps an even more serious problem is the pressure brought by police and attorneys to render a final report in an unrealistically short time. In order to do the most accurate evaluation possible, the autopsy findings must be documented thoroughly with photographs, x-ray films, and diagrams, when applicable. An examination that involves sectioning the fresh, unfixed brain and taking only a few, or no, blocks for histologic (microscopic) examination, as is common practice in many forensic settings, should be strongly discouraged.

The pathologist of record should personally carefully examine the soft tissues and bone, and the skull as well as the brain. It is highly desirable to remove (or closely supervise the removal of) the brain and spinal cord. The pathologist should see that the dura is stripped from the base of the skull so that careful evaluation of otherwise hidden skull fractures can be made. The paranasal sinuses and the petrous portion of the temporal bones should be opened and examined for bleeding into these structures. It is particularly important that careful examination, with as little manipulation as possible, be made of the cranio-cervical junction and the upper cervical spine and cord. This area is not well examined in the great majority of autopsies. An attempt should be made to carefully estimate the volume of blood in membrane hematomas (epidural or subdural); all clots should be weighed and the weight recorded. Careful evaluation of midline shifts and hernias should be made in the fresh state, but the fresh brain should not (as previously noted) be dissected further. The brain weight should be recorded in the fresh state (without the dura attached to the brain). The weight of the brain changes with fixation, and the amount of change is quite variable and unpredictable. All handling of fresh material should be done with great care. There are very few lesions that can be seen in the fresh, unfixed brain that are not seen more clearly with better delineation in a properly fixed specimen.

The necessity of using "special stains" in the detailed evaluation of brain trauma cases should be understood by all. These necessarily increase the interval between death and the completion of the report, just as they appreciably increase the cost in both time and consumable supplies. An accurate assessment of diffuse impact injury is not possible with only the routine hematoxylin- and eosin-stained sections.

The variety of lesions, both focal and diffuse, that can be found in patients sustaining closed head injury is far greater than was appreciated for many years. Moreover, the correct interpretation of the causative factors and the sequence of events in the pathogenesis of these various lesions is changing. The organization of this chapter will be somewhat different from the classic presentations of the neuropathology of trauma, and an attempt will be made to group most brain lesions under one of three major headings: focal, diffuse, and secondary.

Soft Tissue Injuries of the Head and Neck

Careful evaluation and recording of all soft tissue injuries of the head and neck are important in the evaluation of patients with head trauma. Some of these injuries, such as periorbital ecchymoses and postauricular ecchymoses (Battle's sign), are well-known indicators of orbitofrontal and petrous basilar skull fractures, respectively. Both periorbital ecchymoses and Battle's sign can develop very rapidly, but both, especially the postauricular ecchymoses, may be delayed for several days. All wounds (abrasions, lacerations, and contusions) should be described as to size, freshness, and location, using carefully defined anatomical landmarks. The hair of the head will often largely or partially obscure scalp lesions; the hair should be carefully shaved away from such lesions, allowing their clear delineation. The patterns of soft tissue injuries often suggest the type as well as the location and direction of various forces applied to the head.[33,66]

A significant number of patients who have sustained closed head injury will have facial fractures. These are generally neither easily nor well examined at autopsy. Their primary significance, insofar as closed head trauma is concerned, is that they may be associated with severe or fatal hemorrhage, either external (exsanguination) or internal, the latter having the potential to drown the patient. Nasogastric tubes can enter the cranial cavity through such compound facial and basilar skull fractures. Peripheral cranial nerve injuries can result from soft tissue injuries to the head and face. These injuries are usually clinically obvious, and the pathologic lesion is that of a traumatic nerve contusion or avulsion. Retinal hemorrhages are often present in cases of closed head injury, particularly in "shaken" children; retinal hemorrhage may be one of the few physical findings in such battered children. Small, apparently innocuous wounds in the soft tissues can be the entrance wounds of penetrating objects. Such wounds have often been sutured or taped closed without it being realized that a retained foreign body or severe intracranial injury might exist.

While a contusion, laceration, or incision of the soft tissues of the face or head is a mark of trauma and is thus helpful in localizing the site of impact, the extent of these lesions is often not a good indication of the seriousness of the intracranial (particularly brain) lesions.

Skull Fractures

A skull fracture is a laceration of bony tissue. It indicates significant trauma to the head (skull), but in and of itself it is not lethal. The likelihood of a fracture being produced varies with the site and area of impact, but is largely dependent on the force applied. In my material, slightly over 80 percent of patients with fatal closed head injuries have an associated skull fracture.

A simple working classification of skull fractures is to group them as "open," "closed," "linear," or "depressed," and then to specify the extent, the location, and the degree of bone fragmentation and bone fragment displacement. The proximity of a fracture to the underlying envelopes and the brain itself is important to note, as it explains some of the causes of membrane hematomas, fracture contusions, and cranial nerve and vascular lacerations.

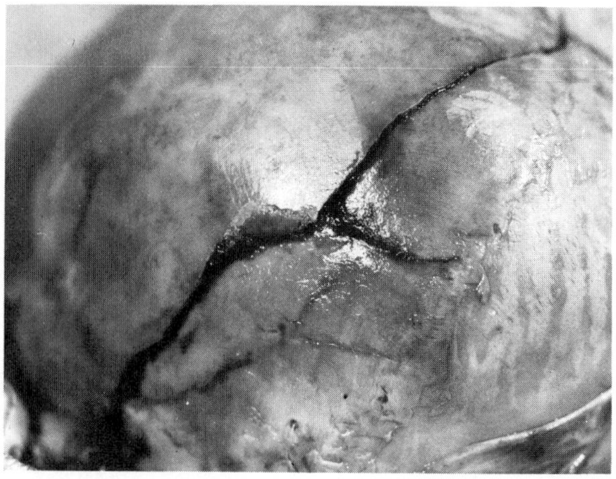

Figure 261-1 Typical linear ("bursting") skull fracture caused by outbending of the bone at a distance from the impact site.

Linear (bursting) fractures are the type most commonly seen in severe head injury and are caused by outbending of the bone at a distance from the impact site as a result of general deformation of the skull (Fig. 261-1). These fractures typically run toward the area of impact but may not reach it. *Depressed (bending) fractures* are due to more localized forces, and may be stellate, comminuted, and so forth. (Figs. 261-2 and 261-3). *Diastatic fractures* are linear fractures along suture lines resulting in separation of the cranial sutures (Fig. 261-4). Because of the structure of the calvaria, consisting of a soft diploe separating relatively rigid outer and inner tables, depressed (bending) fractures that result from short-duration forces of limited strength can leave the outer table intact while markedly fracturing the inner table.

It is sometimes possible to demonstrate a precise impact point in even an extensive depressed comminuted fracture if the skull is reconstructed. The lines of fracture usually radiate out from the apex of the cone of deformation and may be surrounded by a circular ring or concentric rings (Fig. 261-5). When a fracture is evaluated along with the overlying soft tissue injuries, the impact

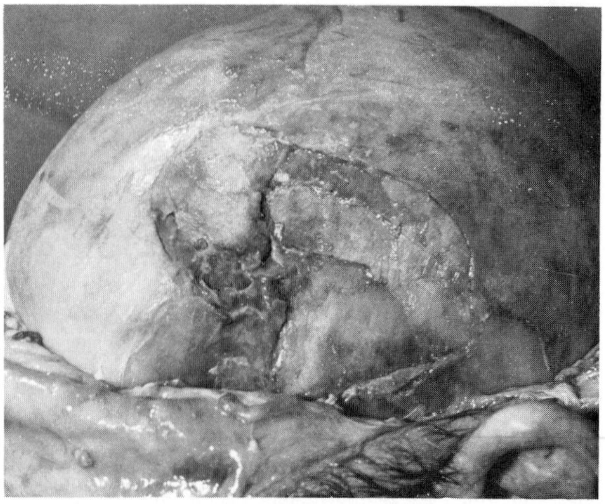

Figure 261-2 Depressed (bending) skull fractures from a localized blow to the side of the head.

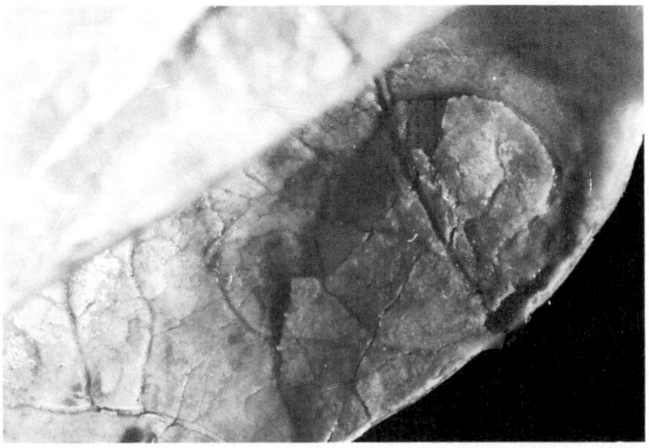

Figure 261-3 The inner surface of the skull from the patient with the depressed skull fracture seen in Fig. 261-2, illustrating the displacement of fragments of the inner table without complete separation.

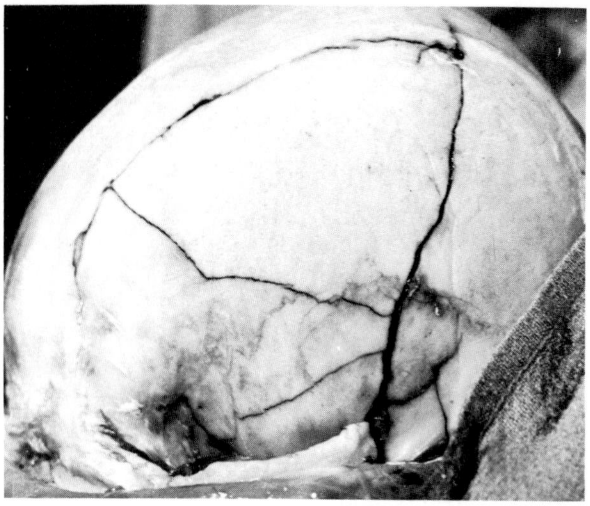

Figure 261-5 Linear (''bursting'') fractures with concentric rings encircling the area of impact.

site can sometimes be very accurately localized. However, the general pattern of a skull fracture is not always highly predictive of impact site. Impacts to the chin or occiput, for example, can produce hinge fractures of the base of the skull identical in appearance to those produced by lateral crushing-type injuries (Fig. 261-6).[38] While anatomic features, such as bony buttresses and much thinner ''plates,'' influence fracture patterns, the strength (magnitude) of the forces is most important. Gurdjian et al. have noted that the same amount of force (energy) can produce different fractures in different people, and that once sufficient energy has been absorbed to produce one linear fracture, very little additional energy can produce massive skull destruction (Fig. 261-7).[36] The force needed to produce a fracture varies with such factors as the area of skull involved, its thickness, and the integrity of the overlying soft tissues, but may be as little as 5 ft · lb.[36] It must be kept in mind that severe and fatal brain injuries can occur in the absence of external evidence of trauma.

Crushing skull injuries often result in direct cranial injuries

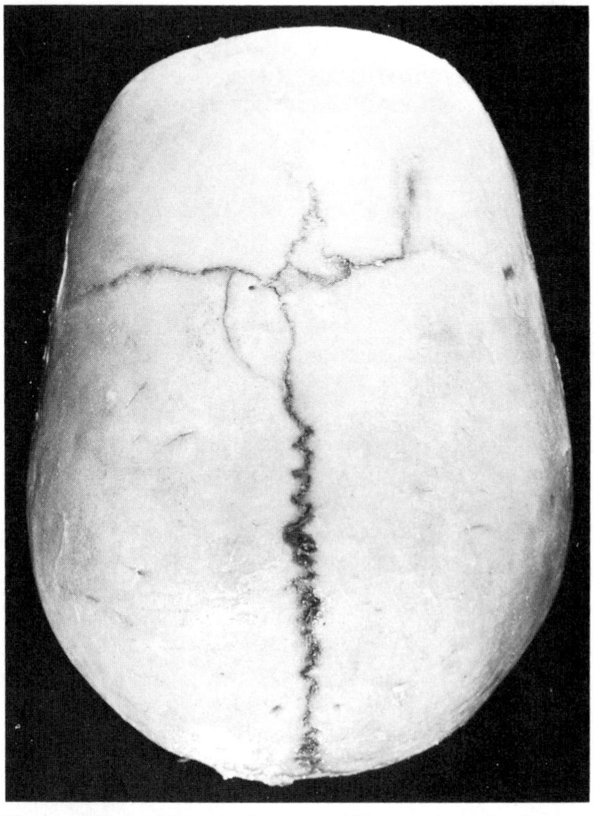

Figure 261-4 Diastatic fracture with extension of a linear fracture into the coronal suture and hemorrhage into the slightly separated suture. Focal diastatic fracturing of a metopic suture is also seen.

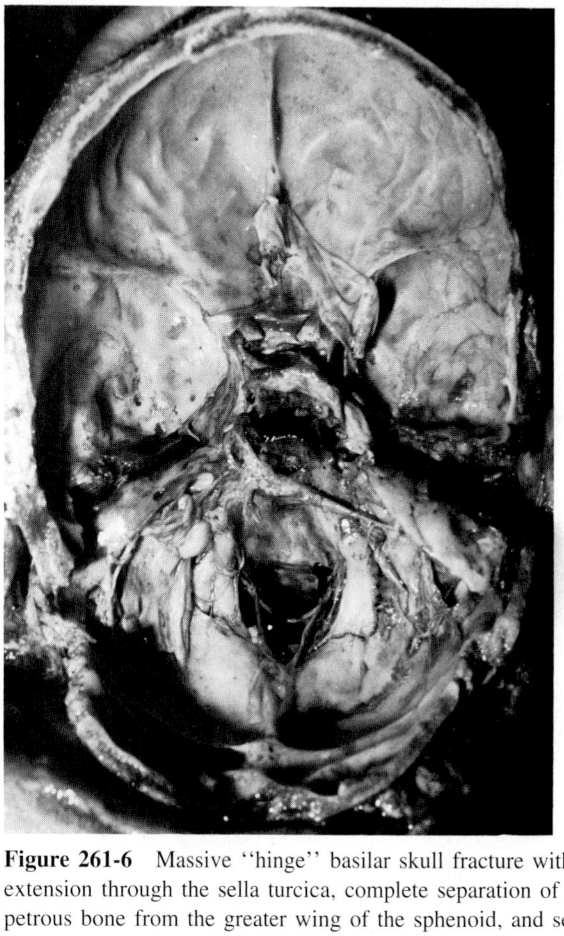

Figure 261-6 Massive ''hinge'' basilar skull fracture with extension through the sella turcica, complete separation of the petrous bone from the greater wing of the sphenoid, and separation of the temporal squama at the petrosquamous fissure. This pattern of skull fractures can be produced by either lateral crushing injuries or impact to the chin or occiput.

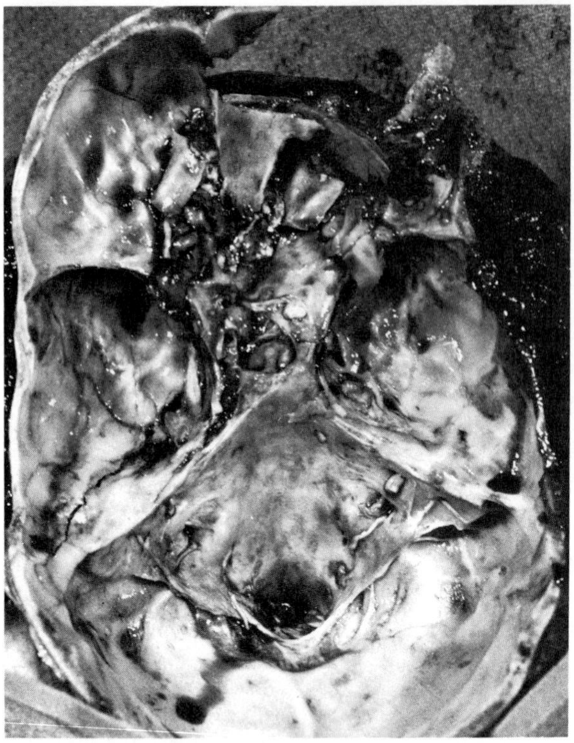

Figure 261-7 Massive skull fractures involving the vertex and base. Once there has been sufficient energy to produce one linear fracture, very little additional force is required to produce such massive bone shattering.

caused by extension of fractures across basilar foramina. Russell and Schiller demonstrated experimentally that bilateral crush produces bilateral, or occasionally unrelated, separation of the petrous bone from the greater wing of the sphenoid and from the temporal squama along the petrosquamous fissure.[84] The carotid canal is typically opened. The tegmen tympani is fractured in about half the cases, and the tympanic membranes may be torn. Fractures often extend across the dorsum sellae (Fig. 261-6). A transverse "hinge" fracture running in the direction of compression results. Such crushing injuries are seen in patients whose heads have been overrun by vehicles. While this pattern is typical of lateral compression, impacts to the chin or skull base can result in identical fractures, as seen in Fig. 261-6.[38]

Fractures extending through the cribriform plate into the paranasal sinuses, or through the petrous portion of the temporal bones breaking through the mastoid air cells or eustachian tube, can give rise to cerebrospinal fluid (CSF) leaks. Such CSF leaks are encountered only if the dura is lacerated. They are of primary importance as a route for intracranial spread of bacteria.

If the dura and underlying brain are lacerated, it is possible for leptomeninges and/or brain to become trapped in the line of a calvarial fracture at the brief moment when the inner skull table opens, thereby giving rise to a "growing" fracture. This uncommon event occurs almost exclusively in children; the great majority are less than 3 years of age. These fractures are usually parietal in location and are almost always associated with significant underlying brain damage.[51,63,86]

Depressed skull fractures may lacerate the dura and underlying brain. The resulting problems are essentially those of the direct brain wound; the question of whether all depressed fractures should be elevated is beyond the scope of this chapter.

Brain Injuries

Traumatic lesions in the brain will be discussed under three headings: focal, diffuse, and secondary. Focal lesions are those that manifest themselves structurally in a limited area and are the direct result of trauma to the tissues. Diffuse injuries are those that are manifested over all or a very large portion of the brain and are the result of very widespread shearing or rotational-type forces. Secondary lesions are those that result from dynamic changes in the brain initiated by either focal or diffuse brain injury, usually ischemic in nature. A few patients will have all three types of brain lesions; many will have two; and a few will have exclusively or overwhelmingly the first or second type.

Focal lesions of the brain include membrane hematomas (epidural and subdural hematomas and subarachnoid hemorrhages), parenchymal contusions and lacerations, intraparenchymal hematomas (including "burst" or "pulped" temporal or frontal lobes), direct cranial nerve lacerations and contusions, direct lacerations and contusions of the brain stem, and direct lacerations of major intracranial vessels (dural sinuses, arteries, veins). Diffuse impact injuries are those with alterations that are predominantly microscopic but include focal necrosis (hemorrhagic or ischemic) and tears of the corpus callosum and hemorrhagic necrosis of the dorsolateral quadrants of the rostral pons. Associated with those two macroscopic features of diffuse impact injury are reactive axons ("Stritch" lesions) and microglial clusters ("stars"). The most common secondary lesions resulting from trauma are due to vascular disruptive events secondary to brain hernias and to hypoxic/ischemic complications of closed head injury resulting from severe hypotension with perfusion failure.

Focal Intracranial Lesions

Intracranial Hemorrhages

Four major categories of traumatic intracranial hemorrhage must be considered. The accumulation of blood between the calvaria and the dura results in epidural (or extradural) hematomas. Bleeding between the dura and the arachnoid gives rise to subdural hematomas, whereas bleeding into the subarachnoid space itself gives rise to the typical subarachnoid hemorrhage. Of these, the subarachnoid hemorrhage is by far the most common in patients who sustain closed head trauma, but it is rarely in and of itself lethal, nor is it often as focal as epidural and subdural hemorrhages tend to be. These three types of hemorrhages are considered "membrane" hemorrhages. The fourth type of traumatic intracranial hemorrhage is the intraparenchymal hematoma, including what has been called "burst" or "pulped" lobes.[2,5]

Epidural (Extradural) Hematomas

The great majority of epidural hematomas are traumatic in origin and represent collections of blood between the calvaria and the dura, which has been stripped from the overlying bone both by the direct trauma and by the hydrostatic force of the blood (Fig. 261-8). Although usually encountered as acute lesions, both delayed-onset (as judged by clinical features and tomographic examination) and chronic epidural hemorrhages do occur and are being recognized and described increasingly often.[10,40,42,49,66,78,82] Especially

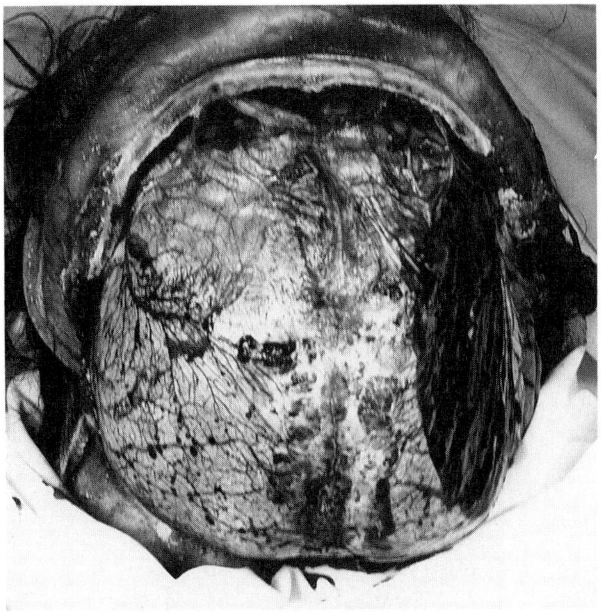

Figure 261-8 Vertex view of the dura after removal of the skull cap. There is an extensive concave deformity of the right frontoparietal region of the brain caused by an acute epidural (extradural) hematoma.

in adults, epidural hematomas are typically located in the temporal or frontal regions and are associated with an overlying skull fracture (Fig. 261-9). The association of a skull fracture with an epidural hematoma occurs in 65 to 90 percent of patients.[8,20,23,29,33,37,58,66,78,82] These hemorrhages most often arise from lacerations of branches of the meningeal arteries inflicted by fractured bone edges. The ultimate size of these hematomas depends on several variables, including how tightly the dura adheres to the inner table of the skull, how deeply the meningeal arteries are incorporated into the inner table of the skull, and how large the lacerated meningeal artery is. Associated traumatic lesions of the brain, once considered relatively uncommon, are quite frequent in my material,[66] as well as in several other reported series (Fig. 261-10).[82] These coexisting lesions include subdural hematomas, cortical contusions, and cortical lacerations. Traumatic lesions in the brain have been associated with epidural hemorrhage in about one-third of my cases.[66]

The blood in the typical epidural hematoma is clotted (Fig. 261-11), in contrast to blood in subdural hematomas, which is often a mixture of liquid and clotted blood. True encapsulation of epidural hematomas can occur in the more chronic forms, as in chronic subdural hematomas. Larger epidural hematomas, particularly those occurring in the temporal region, tend to be distinctly lens-shaped, as illustrated in Figs. 261-8 through 261-10; those that occur in the posterior fossa tend to be more flattened in configuration. Epidural hematomas due to the laceration of dural sinuses or of the veins of the diploe tend to be relatively thin and much less lens-shaped.

Two ''special'' types of epidural hematomas should be briefly mentioned, those that are located in the posterior fossa and those that are bilateral. Posterior fossa epidural hematomas seem to be more common in infants and children than in adults[8,23] and are more often than not associated with skull fractures. Bilateral hematomas—which are typically bifrontal—also are more commonly encountered in children.[29] Many if not most of these bilateral hematomas are of venous origin,[29,52] and they do not as often have the typical lens-shaped configuration.

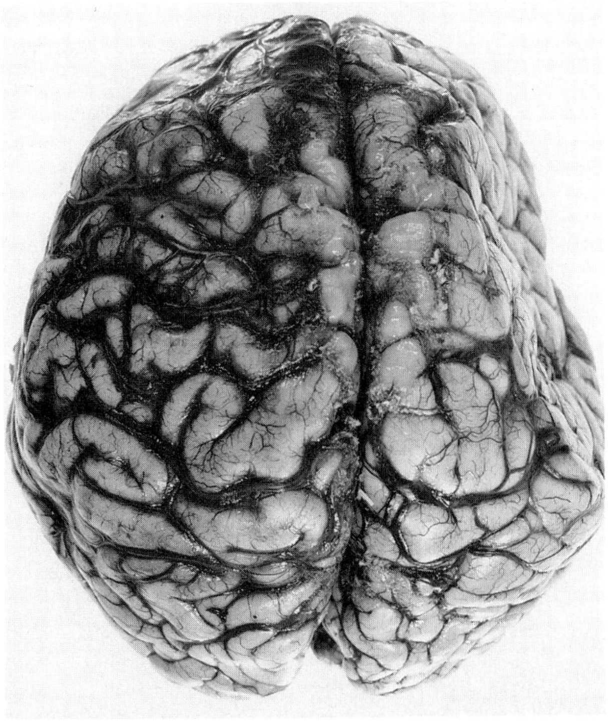

Figure 261-9 Dorsal view of the cerebral hemispheres showing a prominent deformity of the right frontoparietal area due to the epidural hematoma seen in Fig. 261-8. There are no contusions or lacerations of the brain subjacent to this lens-shaped blood clot.

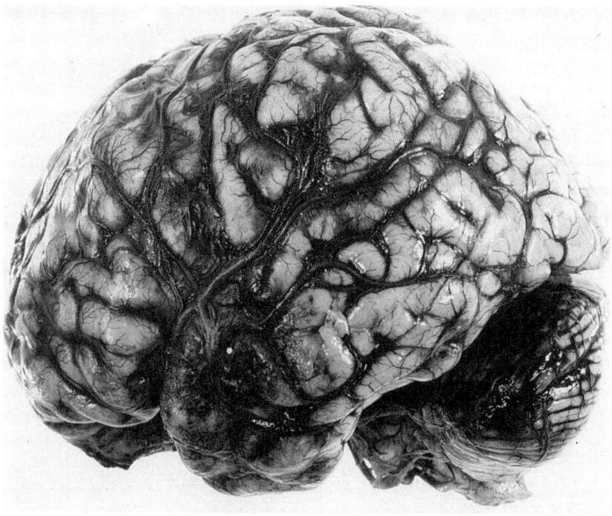

Figure 261-10 Left lateral view of the brain seen in Fig. 261-9. Note contusions and focal superficial lacerations of the left temporal lobe. Traumatic brain injuries are commonly found in patients with an epidural hematoma.

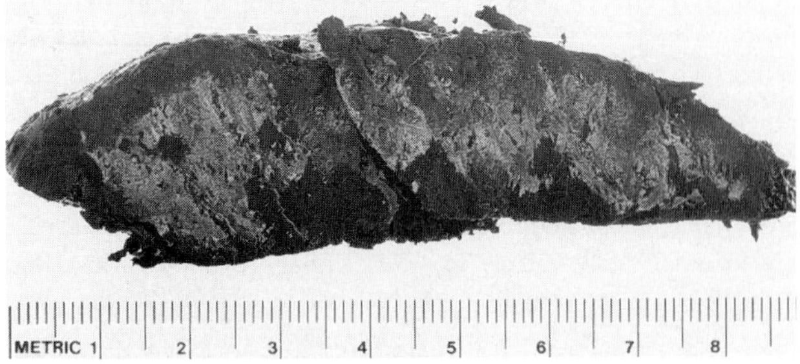

Figure 261-11 Cross-section of the planoconvex blood clot from the epidural hemorrhage in the case illustrated in Figs. 261-8 to 261-10. The blood in epidural hemorrhages is often extensively clotted.

An epidural hematoma will organize if its volume is insufficient to produce brain herniation. Such hematomas may so completely organize as to appear as fibrous plaques along the external surfaces of the dura.[40,46,66]

Subdural Hematomas

Hemorrhage occurring into the dura-arachnoid interface produces subdural hematomas (Fig. 261-12). These lesions are far more common than epidural hemorrhages and are less often clearly the result of head trauma.[47,100] Moreover, acute subdural hematomas are much more likely to be associated with other, often very significant, focal brain lesions (contusions, lacerations).[1,23,37,47,58,66,79,90,96,100] This high association with serious brain wounds is at least partially responsible for the frequently quoted mortality rate of up to 60 to 70 percent in series of patients with acute subdural hematomas.[66,90]

Subdural hematomas can be subdivided into acute, subacute, and chronic forms, but this division is quite arbitrary and may have little or no special pathologic significance.[2,79] Some authors have used very discrete time intervals for these three types, designating subdural hematomas that produce symptoms within 3 days of the initiating trauma as acute, those whose symptoms begin between 3 days and 3 weeks after trauma as subacute, and those with the onset of symptoms after 3 weeks as chronic.[79] For practical purposes, acute subdural hematomas are so often associated with skull fractures[90,100] and very significant underlying focal traumatic brain lesions that they should be considered separately from the chronic subdural hematomas, which are much less often associated with clear evidence of significant closed head trauma. (Subdural hematomas may arise from a variety of nontraumatic causes—ruptured saccular aneurysms with lacerations of the arachnoid, blood dyscrasias, etc.[66,80])

One question that pathologists are often asked is the age of a subdural hematoma. Estimates are based on the degree of lysis of the erythrocytes, the degree of formation and organization of encapsulating neomembranes, and the amount of resolution or extension of the hematoma (Figs. 261-13 and 261-14).[37,66] The use of computed tomography (CT) has considerably expanded our knowledge of the evolution of these membrane hematomas. Table 261-1 summarizes the sequence of events in the histologic aging of subdural hematomas. It is tempting to be overly precise in dating these lesions; the times given in Table 261-1 are as accurate as I can make them, but results this precise require adequate material

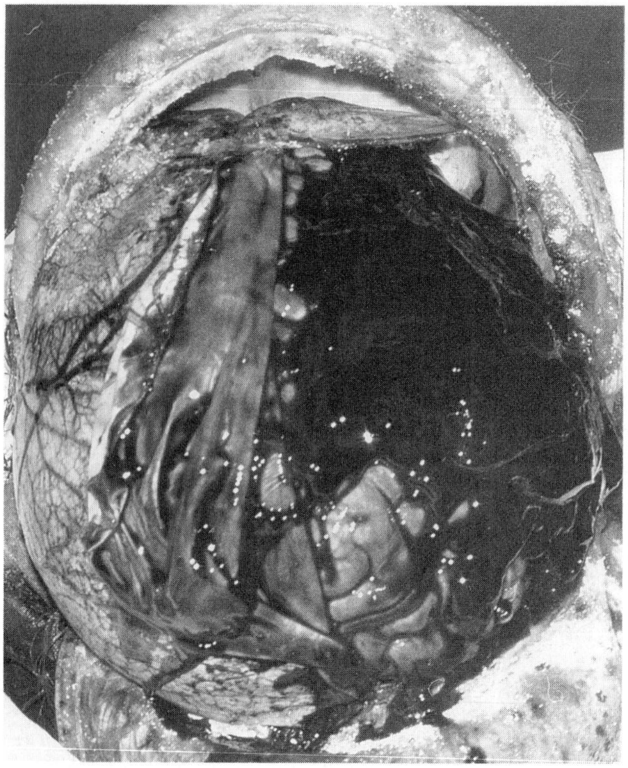

Figure 261-12 An acute right cerebral subdural hematoma. Both liquid and clotted blood are typically present. Brain contusions are very common in patients with acute subdural hematomas.

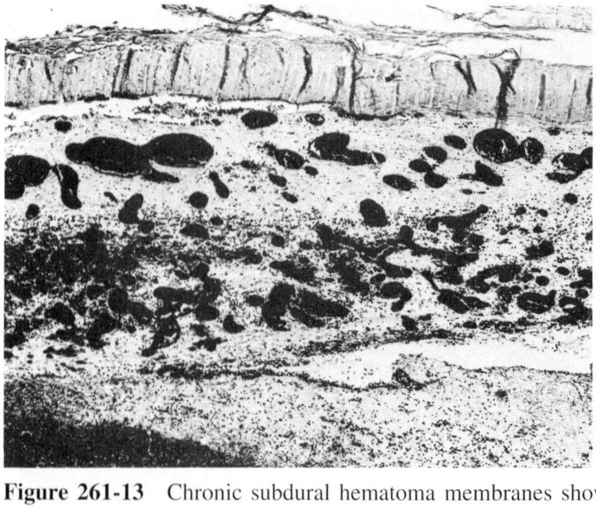

Figure 261-13 Chronic subdural hematoma membranes showing markedly vascular granulation tissue and hemorrhage. At this stage, the hematoma membranes are considerably thicker than the overlying dura. This hematoma was 7 weeks old by history. (Trichrome; × 14.)

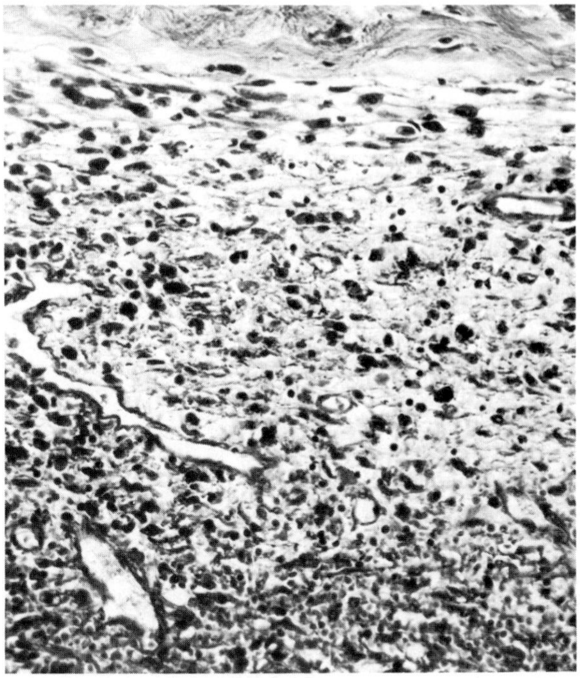

Figure 261-14 Photomicrograph of a subdural membrane showing numerous capillaries, erythrocytes (both intact and lysed), and hemosiderin-laden macrophages entrapped in the vascular granulation tissue. (H&E; × 76.)

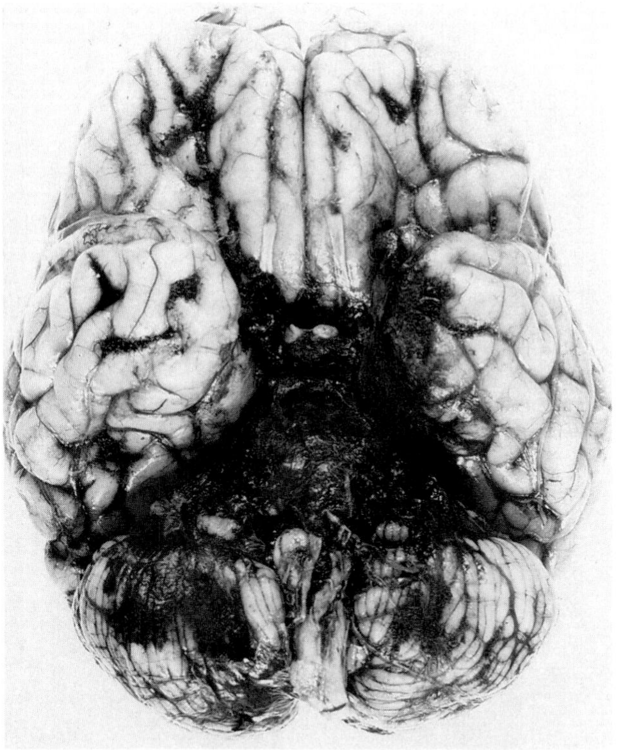

Figure 261-15 A massive basilar subarachnoid hemorrhage secondary to closed head trauma. Such traumatic hemorrhages may closely mimic those found in patients who have had ruptured saccular aneurysms. Such extensive basilar subarachnoid hemorrhages are usually due to demonstrable laceration of an artery, often a vertebral artery.

for examination and cannot be achieved in many clinical-pathologic situations.

Subarachnoid Hemorrhage

Bleeding into the subarachnoid space is the most common "lesion" resulting from closed head trauma.[66] It is often trivial, although it may be truly massive (Fig. 261-15) and life-threatening.[72] It can be found in the absence of cortical contusions or lacerations, but significant subarachnoid hemorrhage is almost always associated with cortical contusions.[95] Truly massive basilar subarachnoid hematomas usually result from the laceration of relatively large arteries, often the vertebrals.[2,72,95] Depending on the size and type of the vessels lacerated (veins, venules, arteries, arterioles), the accumulation of blood in the subarachnoid space may become so extensive as to produce mass lesions. More often, subarachnoid hemorrhage may impede the normal circulation of the

TABLE 261-1 Microscopic Features of Subdural Hematomas

Time after Injury	Clot	Dural Side	Arachnoid Side
0–36 h	Erythrocytes intact	Fibrin	Fibrin
36–60 h	Erythrocytes intact	A few fibroblasts at the dural junction	Fibrin
4–5 days	Erythrocytes lysing, with a few pigment-laden macrophages	Fibroblastic layer 2 to 5 cells thick	Fibrin
1–2 weeks	Erythrocytes lysing; angiofibroblastic invasion of clot	Fibroblastic layer 10 to 15 cells thick	May be a single layer of flat, epithelioid-like cells
2–3 weeks	Clot breaks up; vascular sinusoids ("giant capillaries") apparent	Fibroblastic layer now up to one-half the thickness of the dura	Fibroblastic membrane and rare capillaries
3–4 weeks	Vascular sinusoids well developed		
4–6 weeks	Liquefied clot	Fibroblastic membrane equal to the dura in thickness; pigment-laden macrophages	Well-formed membrane; relatively avascular
½–3 months	There is compaction and fibrosis of the membranes of both the dural and the arachnoid sides. There are large capillaries early, and there are often secondary hemorrhages.		
3–12 months	The neomembranes become fused, consist of more mature fibrous tissue, and contain numerous pigment-laden macrophages. Beyond 3 months, it is not possible to give a very accurate estimate of the age of the hematoma.		
Beyond 1 year	The neomembrane forms a distinct, fibrous connective-tissue layer, which closely resembles the adjacent dura mater. Occasionally calcification and/or ossification can appear after approximately 3 years.		

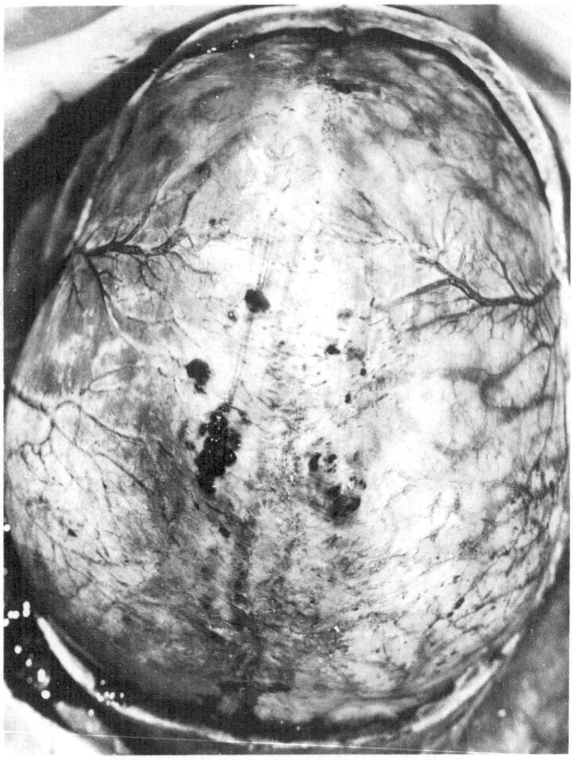

Figure 261-16 The pacchionian (arachnoid) granulations are distended by packed erythrocytes in a patient with a traumatic subarachnoid hemorrhage.

cerebrospinal fluid, blocking the exit of the CSF from the ventricular system or impeding its absorption by packing the pacchionian granulations over the vertex of the brain (Fig. 261-16). Such a blockage of cerebrospinal fluid passage or absorption can give rise to increased intracranial pressure with resulting brain herniation and secondary brain lesions. This is an example of how focal traumatic brain lesions, often themselves rather trivial, can result in serious secondary brain lesions.

Contusions and Lacerations

Contusions are bruises of the neural parenchyma and are always traumatic. Most often involving the crown of a gyrus (Fig. 261-17), they tend to be wedge-shaped, with the apex extending into the neural parenchyma.[1–3,37,58,60,66] They represent extravasation of erythrocytes around small lacerated vessels in the neural parenchyma (Fig. 261-18). In a simple contusion, the pial-glial membrane is intact. If this membrane is disrupted, a *laceration* is produced. While contusions occur in the absence of lacerations, lacerations are almost always associated with contusions.

Contusions have commonly been classified into one of six types, depending on their spatial relationship to trauma or a specific anatomic structure.[2,66] These are *coup, contrecoup, intermediate coup, gliding, herniation,* and *fracture* contusions. Coup contusions are those that occur beneath the immediate area of impact. Contrecoup contusions are those that are thought to be confined to areas remote from and most often directly opposite the impact site on the other side of the brain. The distinction between coup and contrecoup contusions appears less sharp now than in the past. The principal reasons for this lack of clear differentiation have been well summarized by Adams et al., who note that frontal and temporal contusions are the predominant ones regardless of the site of head impact.[2,3]

Although the classification of contrecoup contusions still has some utility in a consideration of the distribution of lesions caused by closed head injury, too great an emphasis on the distribution of contrecoup contusions should not be made. The concept of the intermediate coup contusion has arisen primarily from the publications of Lindenberg and Freytag, who described them as occurring within the neural parenchyma between the impact site and the opposite side of the brain.[58,60,61] These lesions often occur along areas of intermediate tissue density. At least some of the contusions classically called intermediate coup are quite clearly due to secondary vascular phenomena, largely tearing of thalamostriate and thalamoperforating arteries. I think that true intermediate coup contusions do occur in the sylvian fissure, where the temporal and frontal cortices may be forcibly ''slapped'' against each other during the transmission of force from one side to the other (Fig. 261-19). Gliding contusions have been described as those that occur at

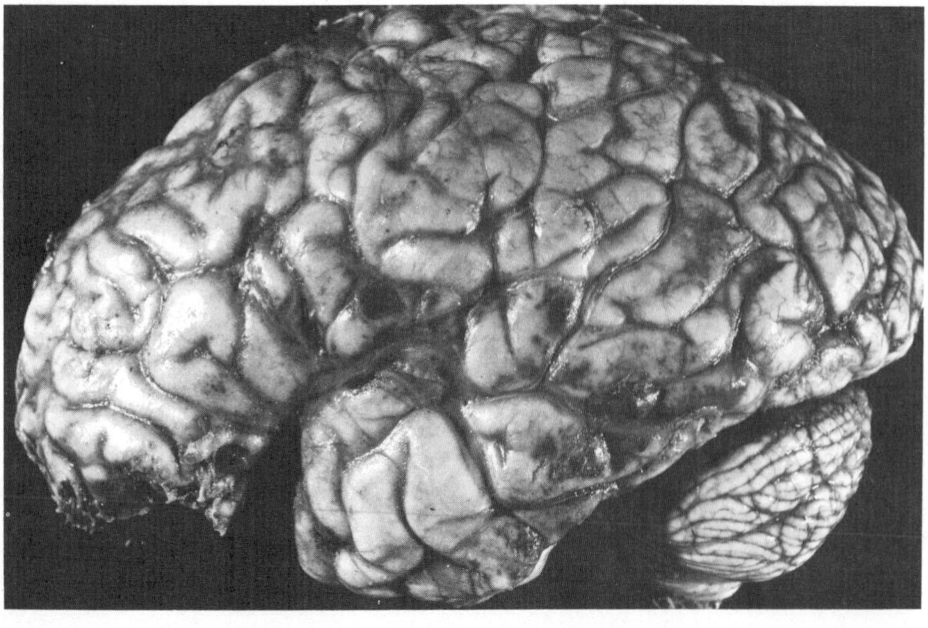

Figure 261-17 Lateral surface of the left cerebral hemisphere, showing numerous fresh cortical contusions involving maximally the crowns of the inferior frontal and temporal gyri.

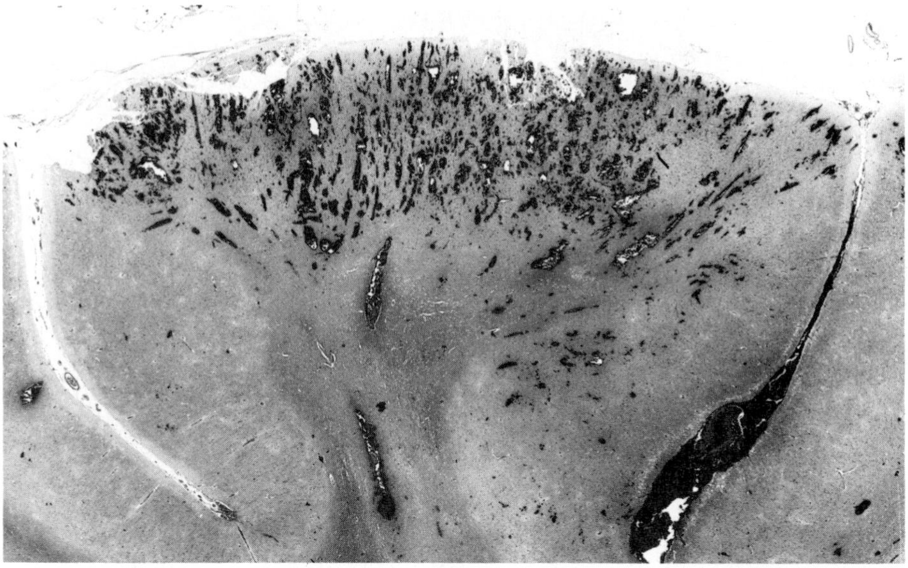

Figure 261-18 Photomacrograph of an acute cortical contusion with minute foci of pial laceration and pallor of staining (early ischemic necrosis) of the adjacent cortex. Note the location of this typical traumatic lesion at the crown of the gyrus and its approximately wedge shape. (H&E; × 6.)

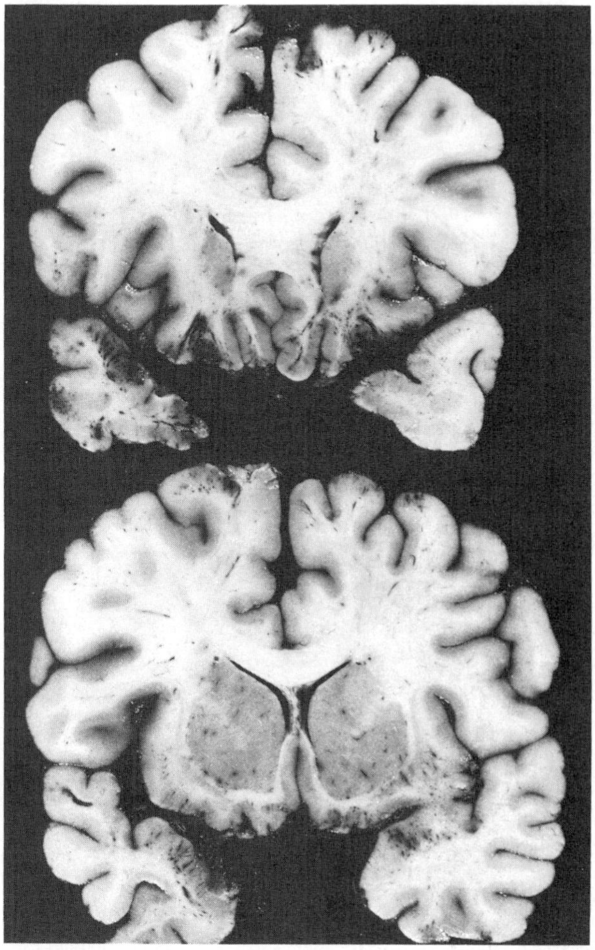

Figure 261-19 Acute contusions in the temporal and frontal gyri in the sylvian fissure. These are sometimes called intermediate coup contusions.

the vertex of the brain and are produced by a rostral-to-caudal movement of the brain during decelerative injuries. Unlike typical contusions, they tend to involve the deeper layers of the cortex more than the surface of the gyrus, with extension into the convolutional white matter (Fig. 261-20).[2,3,66] Herniation contusions are produced by the sudden forcing of a portion of the brain against a rigid opening, most often the incisura of the tentorium. These contusions are thus seen along the medial portion of the temporal lobes (unci and hippocampi) in the great majority of cases (Fig. 261-21). They occur at the moment of brain impact and do not represent the type of herniation necrosis that is seen so often after relatively long-standing transtentorial herniation. Fracture contusions are coup contusions that lie immediately under the fracture line. The term *fracture contusions* is usually restricted to contusions located immediately under a bursting fracture and does not include the contusions and lacerations that occur under a depressed skull fracture. Typical coup, contrecoup, and gliding contusions have been produced in the experimental monkey model discussed by Adams et al.[2,3]

Contusions are the classic and primary hallmark of brain trauma. However, they may be totally absent in patients who have sustained severe and even lethal closed head injury.[1,2,66]

The characteristic gross appearance of a contusion (of all types except the so-called gliding contusion) is an area of hemorrhage beneath the pia, extending into and usually through the cortex into the convolutional white matter. Contusions tend to be roughly wedge-shaped and are most often located over the crowns of gyri rather than involving the banks or depths of gyri within sulci. When the patient has survived for a significant period of time, there is breakdown of erythrocytes and of the directly traumatized neural parenchyma, with phagocytosis of the debris. This ultimately results in an area of tissue shrinkage, so that the old contusion is depressed below the adjacent surface (Fig. 261-22). The overlying leptomeninges are often discolored by hemosiderin pigment and may be adherent to the underlying shrunken brain. The ability of the pathologist to accurately guess the age of a contusion is quite limited. Acute inflammation is very transient. Lysis of erythrocytes is evident within 48 to 72 h, and infiltrated macrophages increase in abundance from 24 h to several weeks. Reactive gliosis can be seen as early as 48 h around a contusion, and it increases with the passage of time. After several months, it is no

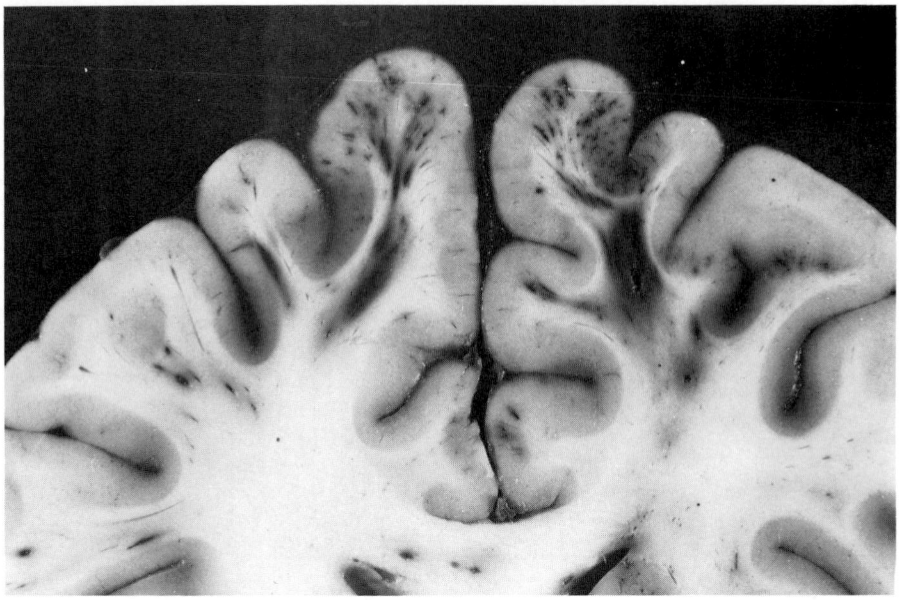

Figure 261-20 A gliding contusion involving the superior frontal convolutions. The hemorrhage has not extended to the pial surface of the cortex and is most prominent in the convolutional white matter.

longer possible to estimate the age of a contusion. The white matter surrounding a contusion is swollen and microscopically pallid and fenestrated.[66] Reactive axons can be seen in the convolutional white matter surrounding a contusion in a remarkably short time (Fig. 261-23), having been clearly demonstrated in some of our cases within 2 or 3 h of the time of injury,[9,58,66] and they are usually obvious by 12 h.[2] Homogenizing necrosis of neurons, manifested by cell shrinkage with hypereosinophilia of the cytoplasm and pyknosis of nuclei, can be seen within 2–3 h of the injury, and becomes truly conspicuous in 18 to 24 h. Capillary endothelial swelling begins early and increases with the passage of time. It is usually quite prominent in contusions 48 to 72 h old or older. It is not uncommon to find small foci of mineral within the neural parenchyma and encrusting neuronal and glial cell bodies and processes in old contusions. This phenomenon is rarely seen in contusions of less than a month's age.[66]

Finally, it is important to understand that patients who die immediately after massive head trauma may have minimal bleeding into the neural parenchyma. Such cases are rarely seen in hospital practices, but they are relatively common in medical-legal services that deal with large numbers of massively traumatized vehicular-injured patients. The longer the post-trauma survival period, the more obvious most lesions become.

Brain *lacerations* are physical disruptions of brain integrity at the macroscopic level. They are often but not invariably associated with obvious contusions and can occur in virtually any part of the

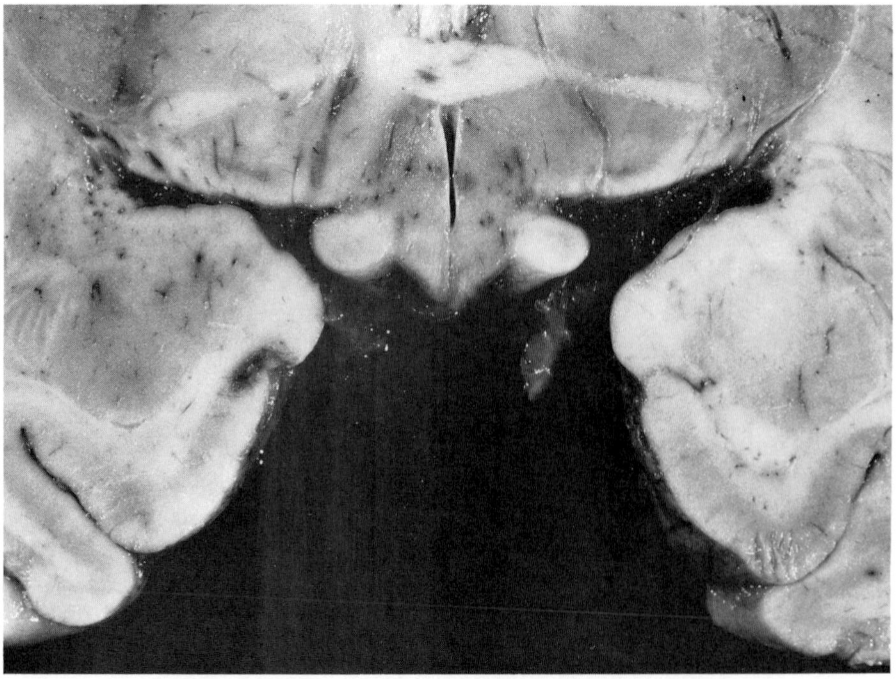

Figure 261-21 Typical herniation hemorrhagic contusion of the left uncus at the point of impaction at the tentorium cerebelli. A much smaller and less hemorrhagic groove is present on the right.

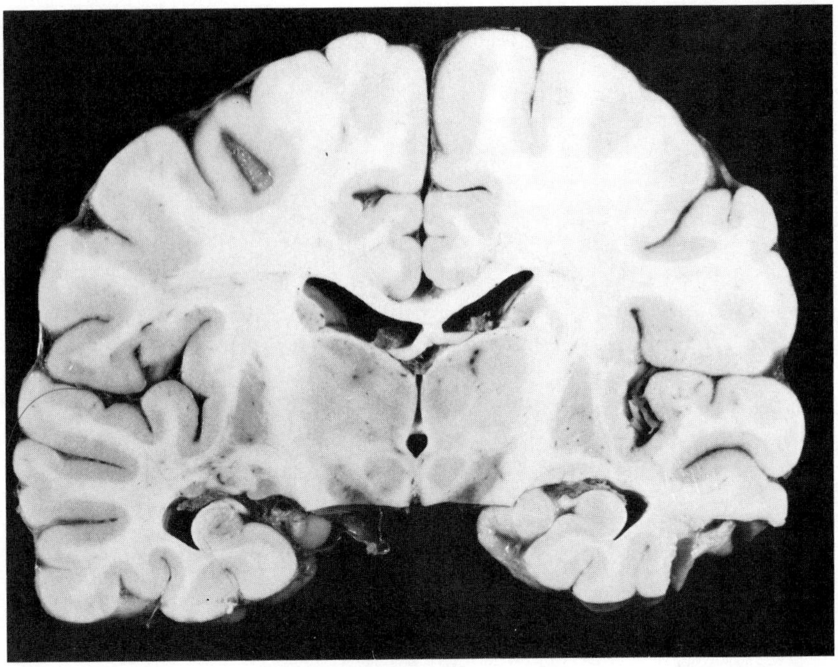

Figure 261-22 Remote contusion in the right middle temporal convolution showing the roughly cone-shaped area of necrosis and tissue loss typical of an old, resorbed contusion.

brain, including the brain stem. (The so-called pontomedullary tear or rent, an example of such a brain laceration, will be discussed below in the section, Direct Brain Stem Trauma.)

Intraparenchymal Hemorrhages

Hemorrhages within the parenchyma of the brain that form discrete hematomas, as distinct from contusions with diffusion of blood into the neural parenchyma, occur most often in the cerebral hemispheres, with most lying in the frontal and temporal lobes (Figs. 261-24 and 261-25). Intraparenchymal brain hemorrhages are often multiple, with patients harboring two or more hematomas of various sizes. The overall prevalence of intraparenchymal brain hemorrhages in closed head trauma patients reported in the literature ranges from less than 0.5 percent to approximately 15 percent.[2,66,81] In 110 cases of fatal closed head trauma examined on my clinical autopsy service, 24 had massive intraparenchymal hematomas, which were multiple in 10 cases and solitary in 14. The high prevalence of massive hematomas (22 percent) in this material reflects its origin from a hospital autopsy series. Clinically derived series of intraparenchymal hemorrhages have, as would be expected, a much lower prevalence, as would a series from a purely medicolegal autopsy service.

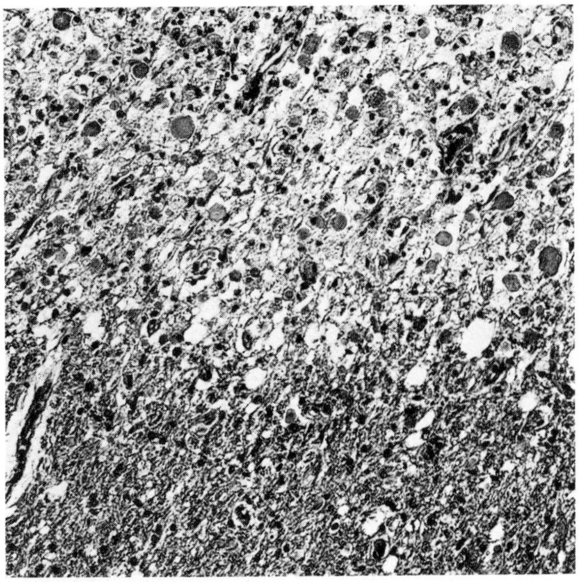

Figure 261-23 Photomicrograph through a small subacute contusion illustrating the numerous reactive axonal balls secondary to axonal transection. This contusion is approximately 120 h old. (Bodian; × 160.)

The great majority of massive traumatic intraparenchymal brain hemorrhages are accompanied by cortical contusions and lacerations. The great majority of them are also ''lobar'' in distribution; they are not commonly ganglionic unless arising in obvious extension from severely contused and lacerated cortex.[2,37,58,66,70,81,102] A significant number of patients with intraparenchymal hematomas will also have membrane hemorrhages, most commonly acute subdural hematomas and subarachnoid hemorrhage. Epidural hemorrhages may be present in these patients, but are relatively uncommon.

Adams et al. have discussed the entity they call ''burst lobes'' and have made a distinction between them and traumatic intraparenchymal hematomas (Fig. 261-26).[1,2,5] This distinction is based on whether or not the intraparenchymal hematoma is in direct continuity with overlying lacerated, contused brain, which in turn is in continuity with an acute subdural hematoma. ''Burst lobes'' should be distinguished, in my opinion, from true intraparenchymal hematomas, in that they represent progressive bleeding into contused and lacerated cortex and subcortical white matter.

The rapidity with which intraparenchymal hematomas accumulate after head trauma has been of considerable interest to a number of investigators. With the advent of CT, it has been possible to observe serially the progress of hematoma development and resolution.[102] It is now clear that many hematomas are not present in

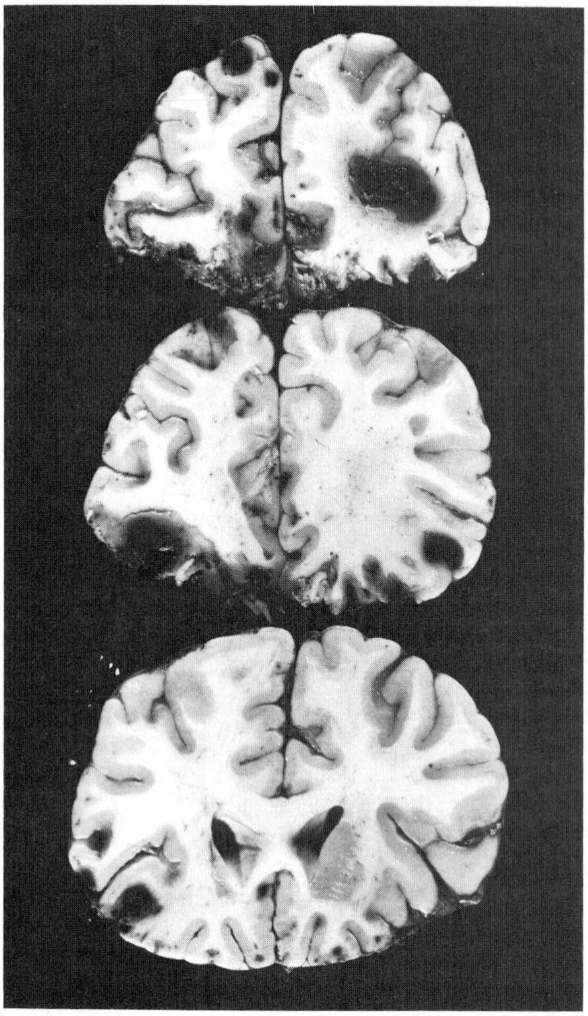

Figure 261-24 Coronal sections of the cerebral hemispheres through the frontal lobes revealing multiple fresh cortical contusions, concentrated in the orbital frontal gyri, and a portion of a right frontal hematoma.

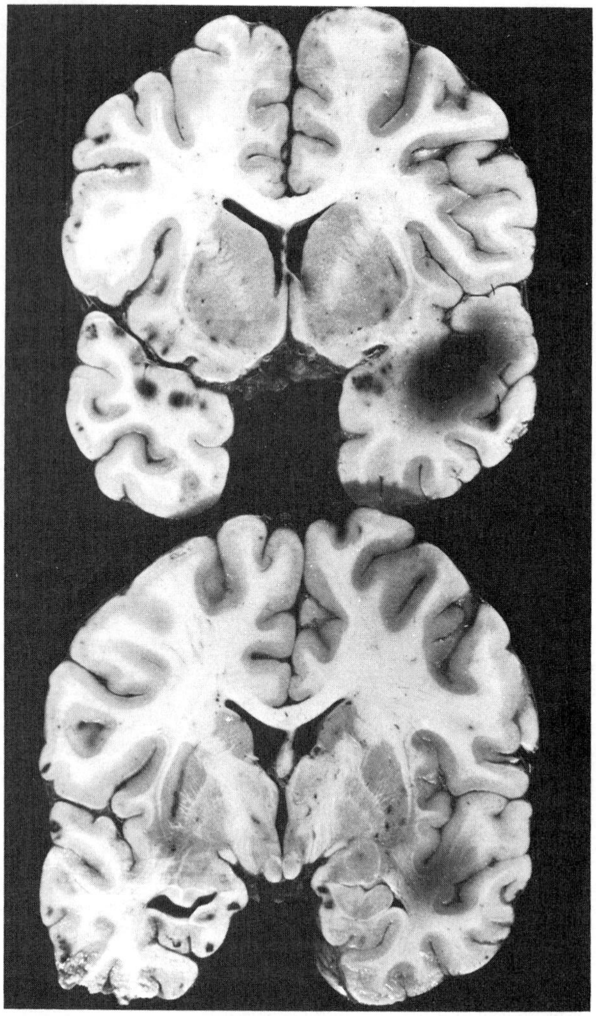

Figure 261-25 Same brain as in Fig. 261-24, demonstrating a second independent right temporal hematoma. Small ''intermediate coup'' contusions are evident in the temporal lobes in the mouth of the sylvian fissure on the right. Herniation contusions are evident in the herniated unci in the bottom section.

the first few hours after head trauma but develop subsequently.[2,12,19,27,50,56,57,70,81,102,103] This observation is also substantiated by the fact that victims who are dead on the scene or die within an hour or two have massive intraparenchymal hematomas far less often than patients who survive for a significant period of time.

Delayed post-traumatic hematomas (Bollinger's ''Spät-apoplexie'') have been of interest for a number of years. These hematomas typically become symptomatic a week or more after the traumatic event.[19,27] Although these hematomas once were considered rare, CT has demonstrated that the development of even massive intraparenchymal hematomas weeks after head trauma occurs more often than had been appreciated.

A distinction should be made between Bollinger's Spät-apoplexie and the far more common ''delayed'' traumatic intracerebral hematomas. The classic Bollinger's apoplexy occurs weeks or even months after trauma, and the patient is often relatively neurologically intact. The far more common delayed intracerebral hematomas typically occur within 72 h of injury, and the patient is rarely if ever asymptomatic between the time of injury and the discovery of the intracerebral hematoma. Such hematomas are typically associated with the obviously more serious head wounds. Among the factors that influence the delayed development of an intracerebral hemorrhage are hypotension due to shock,[57] preexisting areas, often extensive, of cerebral contusion,[19,70] decompression of the brain following evacuation of a subdural or extradural hematoma with release of the tamponade effect,[103] and the development of disseminated intravascular coagulation.[19,88,89] The usual delayed intracerebral hemorrhage (occurring 1 to 4 days after trauma) does not usually produce a perplexing medicolegal situation—whereas the true Spät-apoplexie often does.

Most traumatic intraparenchymal hemorrhages have a lobar distribution, but massive hemorrhage can occur in the region of the basal ganglia.[7,64] The common forensic quandary in such cases is whether the ganglionic hemorrhage was ''spontaneous,'' possibly giving rise to the accident that brought the patient to the attention of physicians, or whether it was caused by the trauma. I have encountered several cases with both closed head trauma and ganglionic brain hemorrhages where the forensic implications were truly significant. MacPherson and colleagues[64] found 41 cases of ganglionic hematomas in a series of 2,000 head-injured patients studied by CT. They concluded that there was a close relationship between these deep ganglionic hemorrhages and diffuse white

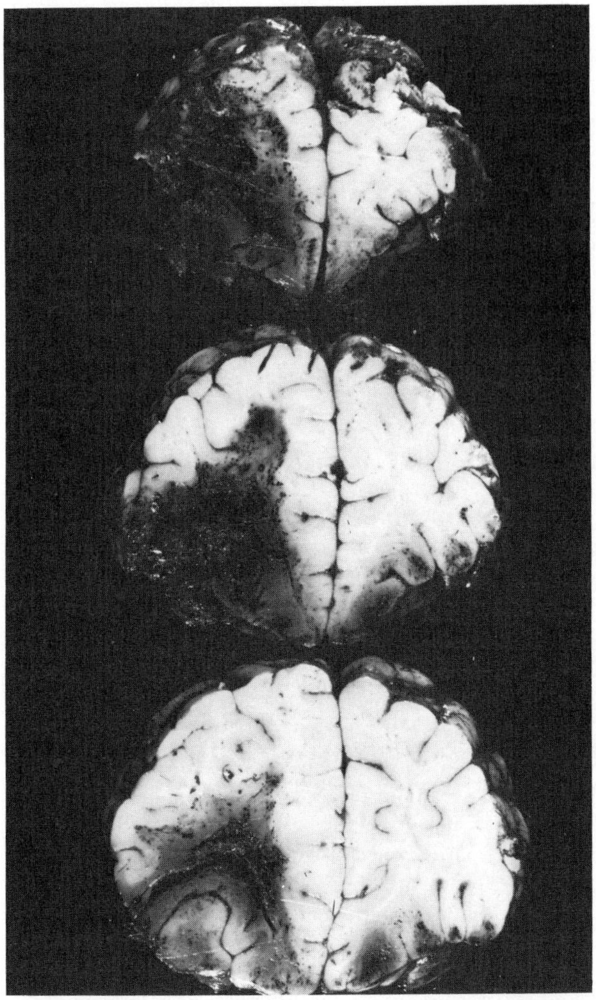

Figure 261-26 Massive hemorrhage, hemorrhagic necrosis, and pulping of the right frontal lobe (left side of photograph) in a patient with a "pulped" or "burst" frontal lobe. Acute contusions are prominent in the orbitofrontal gyri on the opposite side.

matter injury and proposed that the hemorrhages were the result of shearing of blood vessels in the white matter in most cases. Many of these "central" hemorrhages were only 1 to 2 cm in size. Agyeman and Huber[7] observed 20 patients with CT evidence of "primary basal ganglia and/or periventricular hemorrhage without notable cortical contusions." These 20 patients sustained decelerative-type injuries in which significant shear forces would be expected. Noteworthy was the observation that all 20 patients had traumatic subarachnoid hemorrhage and that several (number not stated) had CT-demonstrable cortical contusions; autopsy revealed even more of these lesions. These basal ganglionic hemorrhages, either unilateral or bilateral, were described as "extensive" in 12 patients. The authors believed that the ganglionic hemorrhages resulted from tearing ("rupture") of the lenticulostriate arteries caused by shear from rotational and translational movements of the freely mobile head. Judging by their report, these lesions were very similar in appearance to those described by Lindenberg[58] as "intermediary coup contusions."

The association of disseminated intravascular coagulation (DIC) with closed head trauma is becoming increasingly evident.[66,67,88,89,99] This DIC is apparently triggered by tissue thromboplastins derived from neural parenchymal destruction and is probably responsible for the development of hematomas from small contusional hemorrhages.

Another type of coagulopathy often encountered in patients with closed head injury is that associated with alcohol intake.[17,28,66] It has been demonstrated that alcohol ingestion has a direct effect on blood clotting,[26] and statistical evidence suggests that it plays a major role in the development of intraparenchymal hematomas in some trauma victims. Of the 24 decedents with massive intraparenchymal hematomas in my hospital-autopsy–derived material referred to previously, 16 were alcoholics and had alcohol in their blood at the time of hospitalization.

Both intraparenchymal hematomas and typical contusions of the coup-contrecoup type are much less often seen in infancy and early childhood than in adulthood. The most typical alterations found at autopsy in infants dying of closed head injuries are fresh membrane hemorrhages, slitlike intraparenchymal hemorrhages (most frequent in the frontal white matter, dissecting along the radiations of the medullary veins),[1-3,37,61,66,101] and diffuse, often severe brain hyperemia and swelling.[1,2,13,32,41,58,61,66,71,87] Less frequently encountered lesions in the brains of such infants are focal areas of decreased density (ischemia) in arterial border zones, particularly between the distributions of the posterior and middle cerebral arteries; tears of the corpus callosum, usually with minimal associated hemorrhage; and small areas of subependymal hemorrhage with or without intraventricular extension.[66] Acute subdural hematomas are common and should alert the physician to the probability of trauma even in the absence of other external stigmata. They are a common finding in battered children and may be caused by shaking.[2,32,76,101]

The typical slitlike frontal white matter hemorrhagic lesions have been described by Lindenberg and Freytag as "contusional tears."[61] They noted that these tears are largely confined to the white matter with little or no extension into either the overlying cortex or the ventricular system. The amount of blood associated with these small tears is often small, and with the passage of time, only a smooth-walled cleft remains (Fig. 261-27).

In summary, traumatic intracerebral hematomas are relatively common, being reported in 1 to 3 percent of patients in clinical series and up to 25 percent of victims of fatal closed head injuries in autopsy series. They are often associated with acute subdural hematomas, this association being seen in over 50 percent of cases in some series. They are associated with decelerative-type head injuries in the great majority of cases, are often multiple, and are typically "lobar," with frontal and temporal locations predominating. They are only uncommonly confined to the basal ganglia/internal capsule areas. Massive traumatic intraparenchymal hematomas are associated with a coexisting skull fracture in 60 to 90 percent of patients. Contusions, either coup or contrecoup, are conspicuous in the brains of the great majority of patients with traumatic hematomas. Their absence, particularly in a patient with a ganglionic hemorrhage, should strongly suggest that the cause of the hematoma is not trauma. The gross and microscopic changes seen in traumatic intraparenchymal hematomas seem similar in all respects to hematomas of the same size due to causes other than trauma.

Direct Brain Stem Trauma

Contusions and lacerations of the brain stem usually occur in association with traumatic lesions elsewhere in the brain (i.e., as a part of more diffuse injury).[1-7,17,37,66,77,83] However, they can occur as essentially solitary lesions as a result of head trauma.[2,17,30,31,37,45,62,66,77]

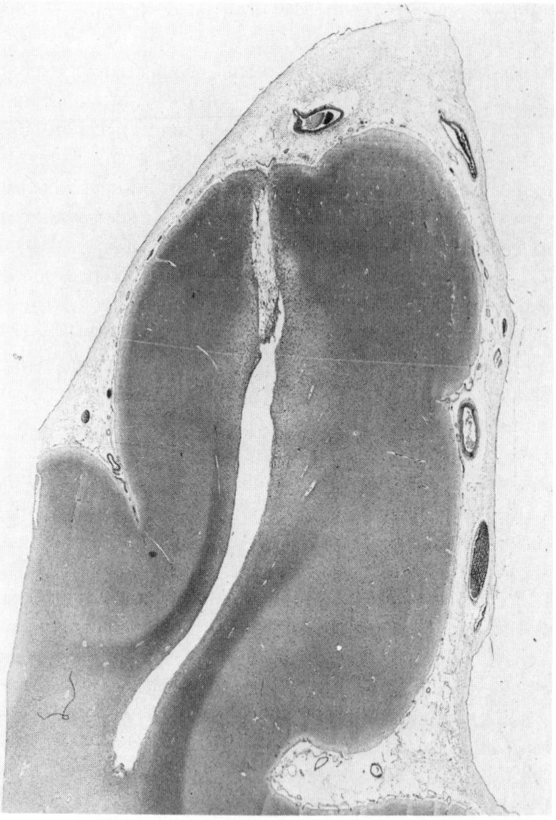

Figure 261-27 Photomacrograph of a frontal lobe gyrus revealing an old, slitlike cavity resulting from a closed head injury in an infant who survived for 3 months. A minimal amount of blood remains in this linear cavity. Unlike many of these lesions, this one extended through the cortex. (Trichrome; × 6.)

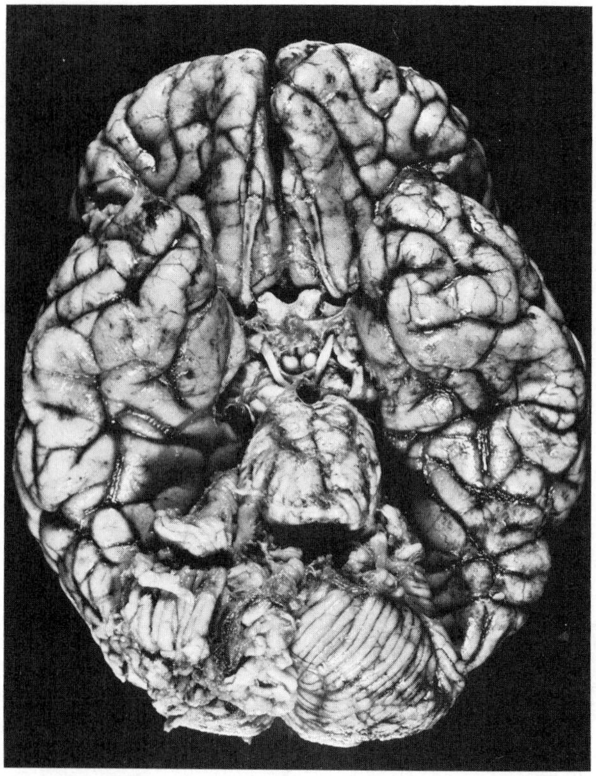

Figure 261-28 Ventral surface of the brain in a patient who sustained a brow impact with hyperextension of the body over the fixed brow. There is deep laceration at the junction of the pons with the rostral medulla.

One of the primary reasons that the existence of isolated direct brain stem trauma has been questioned is the origin of the cases available for study. Primarily on the basis of the experimental work of Ommaya and Gennarelli, Rosenblum et al.[83] have summarized the reasons for this debate over the existence of primary ("isolated") brain stem lesions in the absence of cerebral hemispheric lesions. Extensive direct brain stem trauma is so typically fatal that its victims do not live long enough to be admitted to a hospital and thus are not examined by hospital-based or academic pathologists.[66] It is only when significant material from medical examiners is available for examination that many cases of extensive direct traumatic brain lesions will be found.

Although direct isolated brain stem trauma is far more common in forensic pathology cases, a significant number of patients with this type of trauma have survived long enough to reach a hospital.[30,31] Indeed, Pilz and colleagues have described a patient who survived for 26 days after head trauma and who was found to have a large pontomedullary rent.[77] This lesion, the pontomedullary tear or rent, is now so well known that most pathologists associated with an active trauma service will have encountered it (Figs. 261-28 through 261-30). Among the larger reported series are those of Lindenberg and Freytag[62] with 21 cases, Britt et al.[11] with 24 cases, and Hardman[37] with 12 cases, as well as my own hospital-derived material with 12 cases.[66] I have now collected 38 such cases, 26 from my current forensic material. The great majority of these patients—over 97 percent in the series mentioned above—have had a skull or upper spinal fracture. These pontomedullary

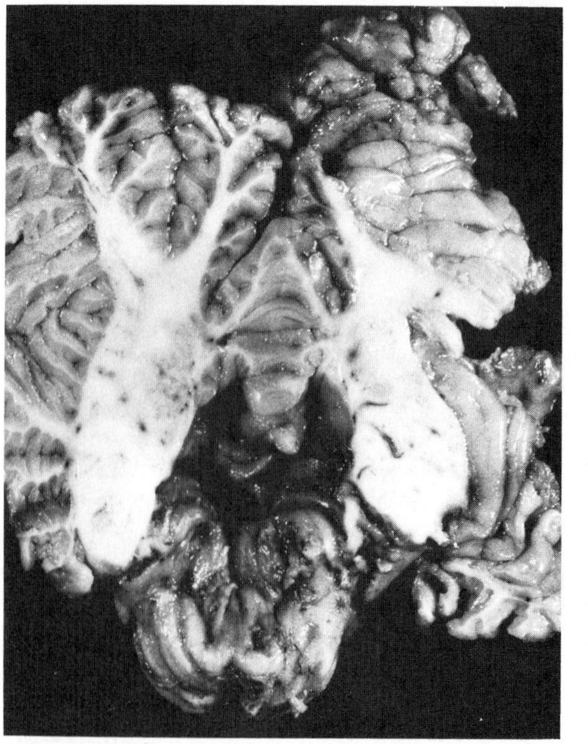

Figure 261-29 Same case as shown in Fig. 261-28; a section of the pons and cerebellum at the level of the pontomedullary separation. A relatively small amount of hemorrhage is typically seen in this area of laceration.

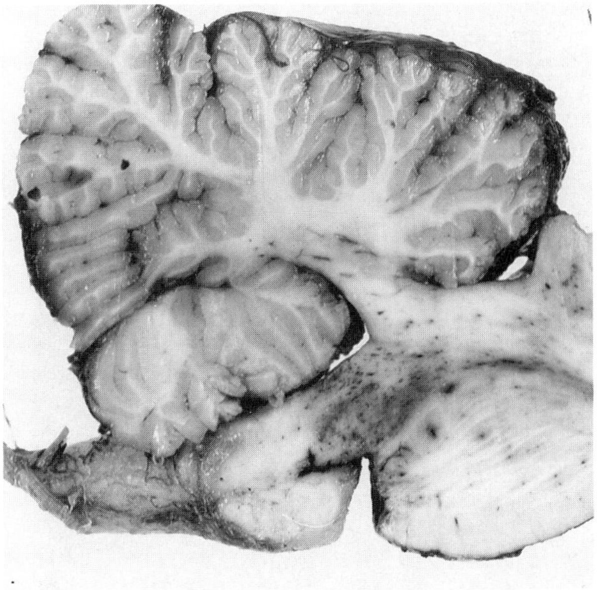

Figure 261-30 A sagittal section of the brain stem and cerebellum of a patient with a pontomedullary rent. Notice the fresh hemorrhage about this laceration.

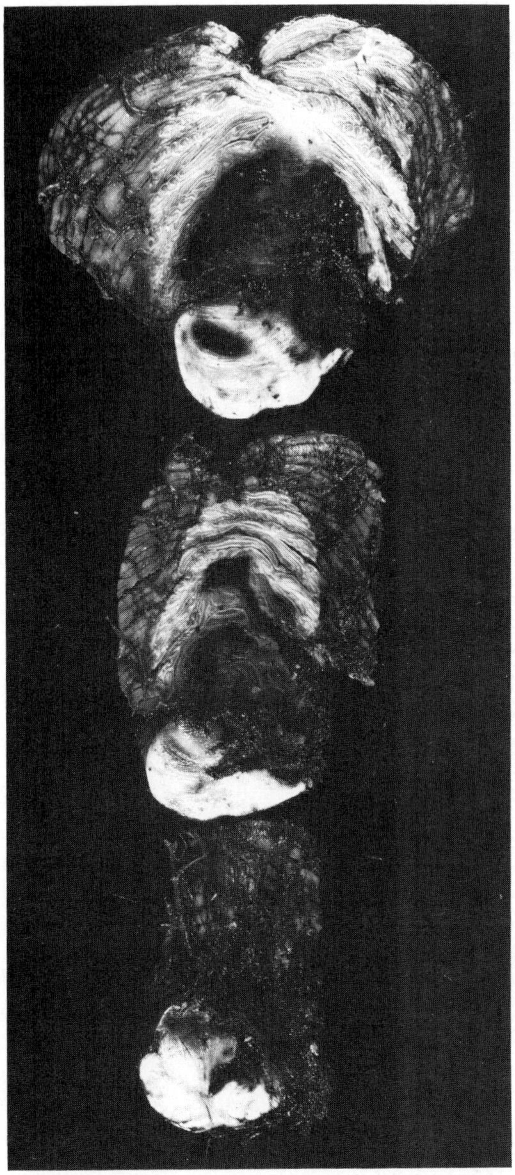

Figure 261-31 Coronal sections of the brain stem and cerebellum through the mesencephalon *(bottom section)* and rostral pons *(middle and upper sections)* showing extensive laceration and hemorrhage in and about the rostral brain stem.

junction tears are most often due to marked hyperextension of the head on the neck, most often with trauma directed to the brow while the legs and torso bend forward over the temporarily immobile head.[37,62,66,77] It is of great interest to note that Adams and his colleagues have been able to produce pontomedullary rents in monkeys subjected to severe angular acceleration of very short duration.[3]

Another distinct form of direct brain stem trauma, although one that is considerably less often observed and described, is focal or massive laceration at the mesencephalic-pontine junction (Figs. 261-31 and 261-32). In my own hospital material, such lacerations have been found in 4 patients in the same study population that contained 12 decedents with pontomedullary rents. There have been 3 additional cases with mesencephalic lacerations in my exclusively forensic material, as well as 26 additional cases of pontomedullary rents. Britt et al. had 8 patients with such mesencephalic-pontine junction lacerations as compared with their 24 with pontomedullary rents.[11]

A third distinct type of direct focal injury to the brain stem, typically associated with fractures of the clivus, is direct contusion, occasionally with focal superficial lacerations, of the striate portion of the pons (Fig. 261-33). I have encountered four such cases in my forensic (nonhospital) material. One of these cases was associated with transtentorial herniation. None of the decedents had evidence of diffuse impact injury, such as necrosis and/or hemorrhage in the corpus callosum or the upper outer quadrant of the rostral pons, or diffuse axonal swelling. These cases were also distinctly different from the "diffuse vascular injury" described by Adams[2] and others.

A fourth distinct type of primary traumatic brain stem lesion is the traumatic laceration or even complete separation (transection) of the medulla from the upper cervical spinal cord. Britt et al. reported that 1 of 41 patients with primary brain stem injury had this type of lesion.[11] In my hospital practice I had only one patient with complete spinal-medullary separation—a young man who sustained trauma to the left side of his neck in a motorcycle accident[66]—but I had no less than nine in my forensic practice. This type of lesion is thus quite common in dead-at-the-scene trauma victims and has been produced in experimental animal models.[98] Indeed, it appears to be one of the more common types of lethal lesions and is due to separation of the atlas from the skull.[98]

Rosenblum and his colleagues have described hemorrhagic and nonhemorrhagic necrotic lesions of various sizes in the mesencephalon in 88 percent of a series of 26 brains from patients dying from head trauma.[83] All patients had survived for "several days or more." These lesions were not considered to be secondary to transtentorial herniation and were thought to have occurred at the moment of impact, thus being primary lesions. Typically confined to the tegmentum or the lateral or superior margins of the mesencephalon and rostral pons, they showed a "spectrum of ages" that agreed with the time lapse between trauma and death, rather than all being fresh as in secondary brain stem hemorrhage (Figs. 261-34 and 261-35). They were found in patients without elevated

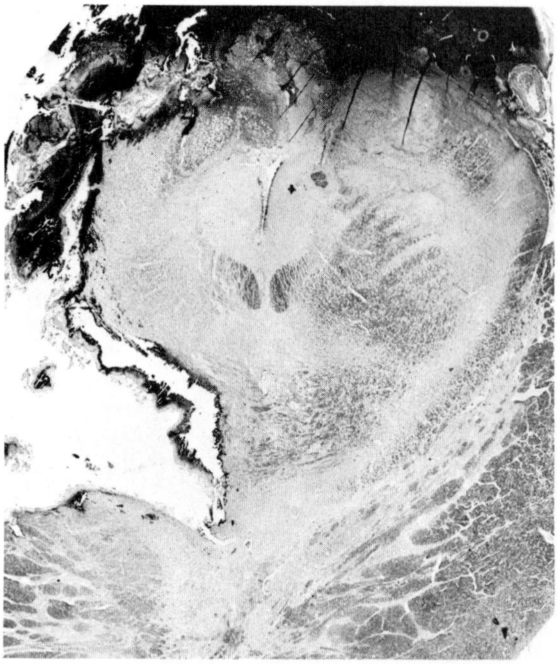

Figure 261-32 Photomacrograph of a typical mesencephalic and rostral pontine laceration in a patient with mesencephalic-pontine separation. This patient lived approximately 1.5 h after the injury, with ventilatory and circulatory assistance. (Trichrome; × 7.)

intracranial pressure and in patients without gross evidence of brain herniation. These authors summarized their findings and interpretations as follows:

> We can say that brain stem lesions, particularly of the midbrain, are extremely common in fatal closed head injury, that they are readily found at autopsy, that they can be detected with MEPs during life, and that their presence or absence provides a prognostic indicator at least as accurate [as] or better than other clinical findings. We agree that midbrain lesions rarely occur in "isolation" (that is, in the absence of hemispheric lesions). The almost universal occurrence of hemispheric damage when brain stem damage is present is consonant with the concept of a centripetal spread of forces in closed head injury with resultant "primary" midbrain damage. However, the primary midbrain lesions are common rather than rare, and this fact should not be obscured by the argument concerning the presence or absence of "isolated" brain stem lesions.[83]

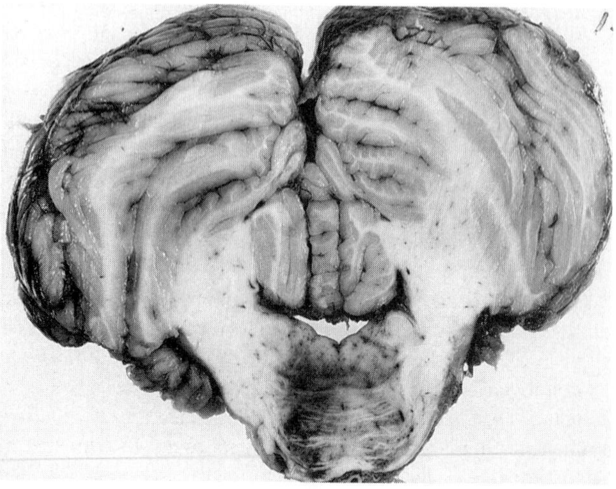

Figure 261-33 An isolated contusion with focal laceration of the pons in a patient with a transclival fracture. This patient did not have morphologic evidence of a diffuse impact injury.

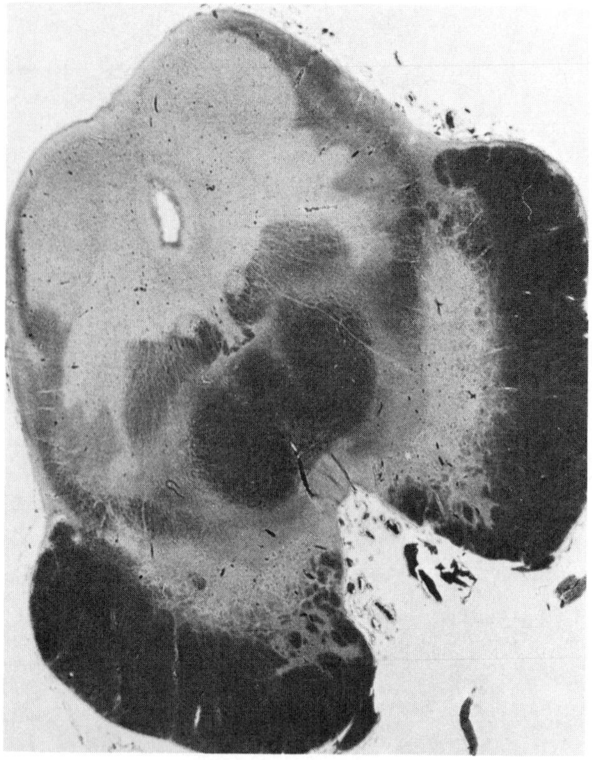

Figure 261-34 Photomacrograph of the mesencephalon of a patient with an extensive acute infarct in the tectum and periaqueductal gray matter. The patient survived 8 h. (Luxol fast blue—PASH; × 3.)

I have also found such minute lesions in a number of my 110 hospital cases, but with less frequency and more typically in patients with increased intracranial pressure and cerebral contusions. They are not typical secondary brain stem hemorrhages. At present I consider them to be not primary brain stem traumatic lesions but rather a combination of diffuse impact and secondary ischemic injury or, in some patients, a form of secondary vascular lesion (Fig. 261-34), a view apparently held by Adams[2] (see below). Regardless, their documentation by the Rosenblum group is an important contribution to our expanding knowledge of the lesions found in head trauma.

In the past, Adams and his colleagues maintained that traumatic brain stem injuries do not occur in the absence of diffuse brain injury. They stated, "In a personal series of 600 brains from patients dying as a result of head injury, we have never identified a primary traumatic lesion in the brain stem in isolation: when one was present, there was always evidence of DAI (diffuse axonal injury)."[3] Interestingly, in the same paper they recorded one patient with a pontomedullary separation (among "several hundred" fatal head injuries) and stated, "There is little doubt that these lesions occurred at the time of injury, and it would appear that this is one—and possibly the only—type of primary damage to the

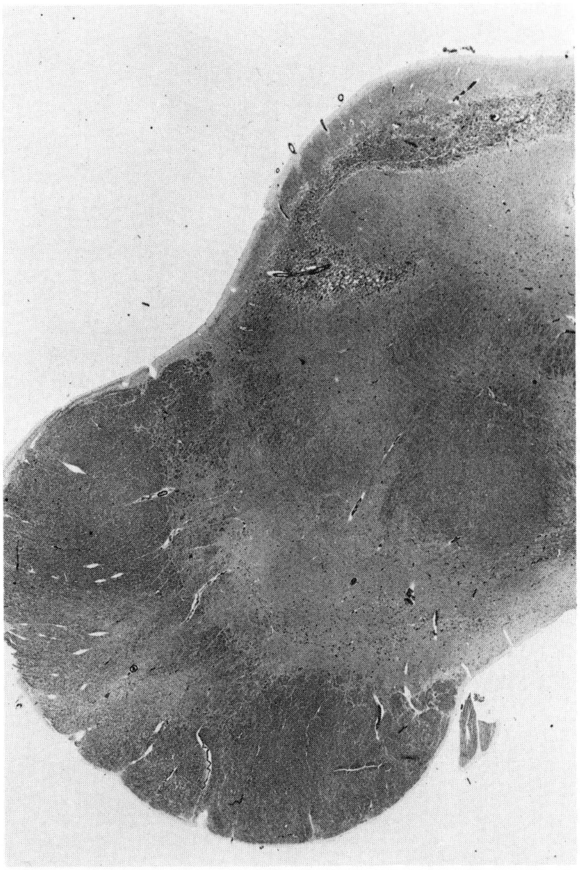

Figure 261-35 Mesencephalic tectal necrosis with features of both diffuse impact and secondary vascular injury. There were typical diffuse impact injuries in the pons and corpus callosum. (Luxol fast blue—PASH; × 7.)

brain stem that may occur in isolation.'' As now amply documented, this statement is not correct. Table 261-2 summarizes the types of brain stem trauma.

TABLE 261-2 Traumatic Brain Stem Lesions

- **I.** Primary brain stem injury
  - **A.** Direct focal injury
    - **1.** Fracture lacerations and contusions
    - **2.** Pontomedullary separations
    - **3.** Medullocervical separations
    - **4.** Mesencephalic-pontine separations
  - **B.** Diffuse impact injury (Strich lesions), including gross hemorrhagic necrosis of the dorsolateral pons
- **II.** Secondary brain stem injury due to herniations (including rare lateral medullary infarcts due to entrapment of the posterior inferior cerebellar artery)

Direct Cranial Nerve Injuries

Contusions, lacerations, and/or avulsions of cranial nerves can occur either as isolated lesions or, more commonly, as part of more severe and diffuse skull and brain damage. We have encountered patients with nerve avulsions involving one or more of almost all the cranial nerves.[66] Undoubtedly the most common traumatic cranial nerve lesion is contusion, sometimes to the point of destruction, of the olfactory bulbs and tracts, occurring in patients with orbitofrontal damage and often associated with orbital plate fractures. Optic nerve and chiasm lacerations have been reported in patients both with and without basilar skull fractures, usually as a result of severe frontal head trauma. Traumatic lesions of the optic chiasm are often associated with hypothalamic injury.

Heinze has described laceration and partial avulsion of the third cranial nerves.[39] I have seen the same type of injury in one patient with a mesencephalic-pontine laceration. Far more commonly encountered in trauma victims is hemorrhage and necrosis of the third nerves secondary to transtentorial herniation.

Lacerations and avulsions of the fourth, fifth, sixth, seventh, and eighth cranial nerves have been described (Figs. 261-36 to 261-38).[39,66,84,93] With all these injuries, basilar skull fractures are the rule. The separation of the occipitosphenoid synchondrosis has been observed to result in direct abducens nerve injury.[93] Petrous fractures, especially those that run perpendicular to the long axis of the petrous portion of the temporal bone (transverse fractures), are quite apt to involve portions of the seventh and eighth cranial nerves. Such fractures are most often caused by frontal or occipital impacts and are considerably rarer than (about one-fifth as common as) the longitudinal petrous fractures that result from lateral head impacts.

Traumatic cranial nerve injuries are undoubtedly more common than the pathology literature would suggest. Very few pathologists make examinations detailed enough to reveal them.

Direct Arterial Trauma

Another form of focal direct traumatic intracranial lesion is one in which arteries, veins, and/or dural sinuses are lacerated, avulsed, or thrombosed.[68] Traumatic carotid-cavernous fistulae have been described extensively during the past 150 years and have been estimated to occur in as many as 1 to 2 percent of patients who sustain severe head injuries.[48,66] Typically associated with a basilar skull fracture that traverses the cavernous sinus, they are most often the result of a frontotemporal impact, with the fracture extending through the sphenoid bone.

Traumatic aneurysms of the intracranial arteries are also well known, although distinctly uncommon.[14,43,44,66,69,74,75] These have been divided into both ''true'' and ''false'' types. ''True'' traumatic aneurysms occur when the artery wall is lacerated but not completely penetrated. ''False'' aneurysms result when there has been mural rupture and organization of the surrounding hematoma, with the interior of the hematoma communicating with the penetrated artery. The false aneurysms are the more common. Traumatic aneurysms were described as occurring in five anatomic locations by Jackson and colleagues: scalp, adjacent cranial vault, arteries traversing the cranium, intracranial arteries, and meningeal arteries.[43] Only the latter two will concern us. Most traumatic aneurysms have been found to occur on superficial branches of the middle cerebral arteries; the next most common site is the peripheral branches of the anterior cerebral arteries. Traumatic aneurysms have been found on other arteries, including the internal carotid, anterior choroidal, posterior cerebral, vertebral, superior cerebellar, and posterior inferior cerebellar. When traumatic aneurysms occur in their usual location on a peripheral branch of either the middle or anterior cerebral artery in an area of known trauma, they are not too likely to be confused with the far more common nontraumatic saccular (''medial defect,'' ''congenital'') aneurysm. The distinction can be difficult to make, however, when a

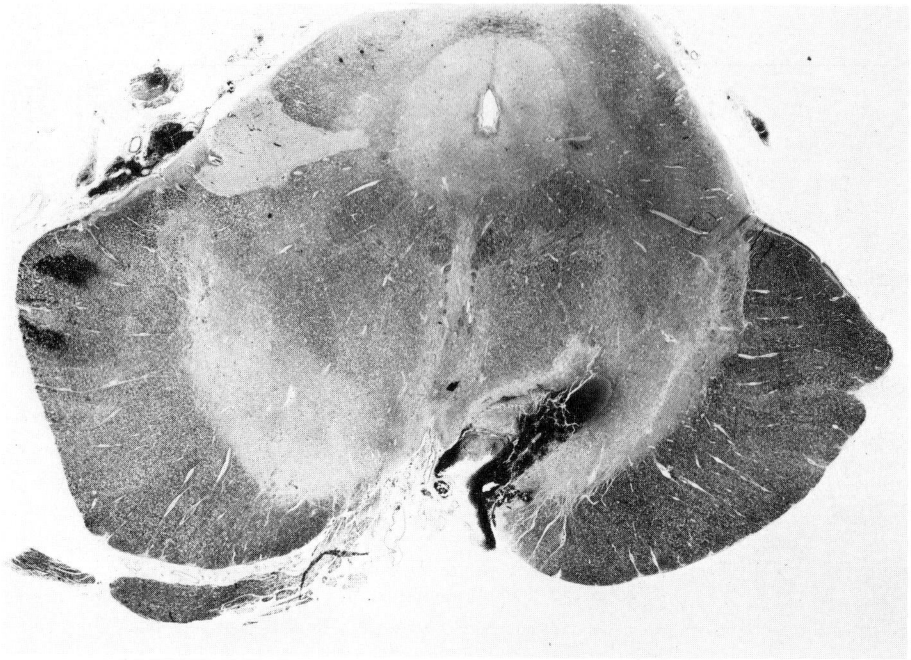

Figure 261-36 Complete avulsion of the third cranial nerve with a hematoma in the parenchyma along the nerve root. Note the wedge-shaped area of acute infarction in the left dorsolateral quadrant of the mesencephalon and the focal hemorrhages into the dorsal aspect of the left cerebral peduncle, together with myelin pallor in much of the left peduncle. The patient survived 2 days.

major artery at the base of the brain contains the aneurysm in a patient with severe head trauma. At times, the cause of the aneurysm can be determined only through detailed microscopic examination and a critical review of all clinical and anatomic evidence. The features that have proved most useful in differentiating traumatic from nontraumatic saccular aneurysms are (1) location of the aneurysm at a peripheral branch of an intracranial artery and usually not at a bifurcation point, (2) the absence of a demonstrable neck to the aneurysm, (3) an irregular contour of the aneurysm sac, and (4) a delay in angiographic filling and emptying of the aneurysm sac.[74] Many arteries (perhaps the great majority) with a traumatic aneurysm will also have multiple discrete wall injuries adjacent to but separate from the tear that produced the aneurysm.[75] Finally, it should be noted that because of the relatively high frequency of both saccular aneurysms and trauma in our population, patients with both nontraumatic saccular aneurysms and significant closed head trauma will be seen. While this problem has been addressed in several publications[65] and will not be discussed extensively in this chapter, it has been found that closed head trauma is unlikely to cause rupture of a pre-existing saccular aneurysm.

Thrombosis of major intracranial and extracranial cervical vessels secondary to trauma is well known. The initiating trauma may be quite trivial. The event leading to the production of the occluding thrombus is thought to be an intimal tear resulting from stretching of the vessel over a bony prominence. The most common sites of thrombotic occlusion in the internal carotid artery are a few

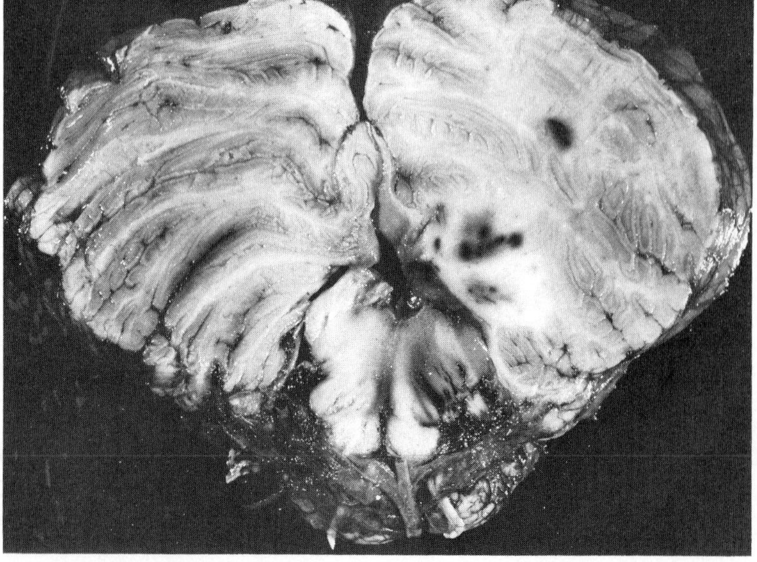

Figure 261-37 Section of the medulla and cerebellum showing hemorrhages extending into the medulla at the point of avulsion of cranial nerve roots.

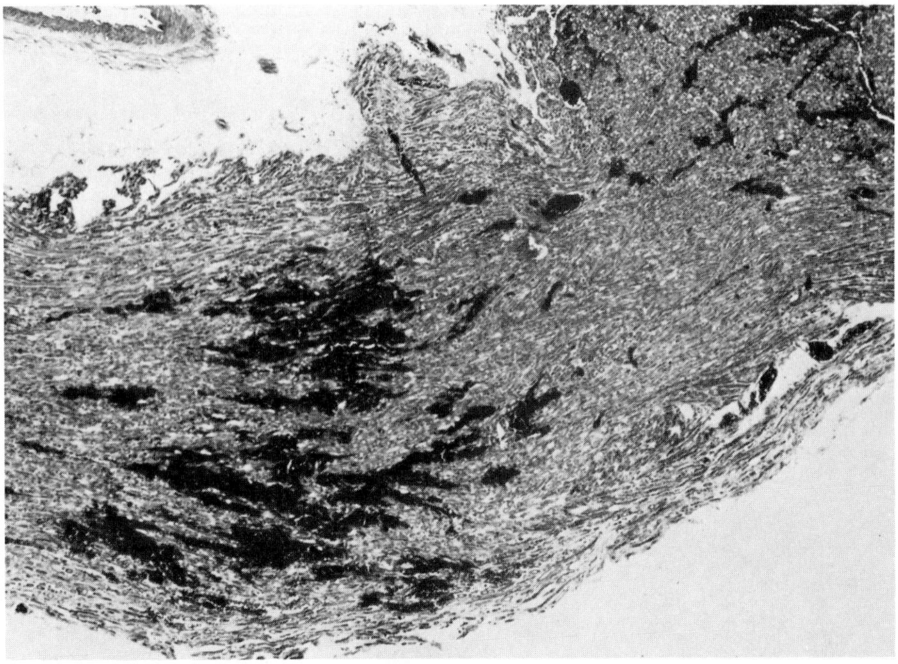

Figure 261-38 Photomicrograph of hemorrhage into an acutely traumatized cranial nerve root. (Trichrome; × 60.)

centimeters above the carotid bifurcation and in the carotid canal at the base of the skull. Traumatic rupture of the vertebral artery with high lateral neck injuries is being reported with increasing frequency.[2] Traumatic thrombosis of the vertebral arteries also occurs, most commonly at the C5-6 interspace, at the atlantoaxial joint, or at the atlanto-occipital joint. A rare form of intracranial artery occlusion secondary to head trauma is entrapment of the basilar artery in a transclival fracture, the basilar artery being trapped in the fracture when it opens and then closes at the instant of impact. The result is occlusion of the artery.[35,48] Traumatic thrombosis of the dural sinuses occurs less often than thrombosis of either the carotid or the vertebral artery in the neck.[94]

Direct laceration of cerebral arteries and veins is common in many forms of closed head injury. Lacerations of smaller branches or tributaries are almost invariably seen in patients with acute subdural hematomas with their associated cortical lacerations and contusions and are obviously the origin of the subdural and subarachnoid hemorrhages seen in these patients.

Pituitary and Hypothalamic Lesions

Traumatic lesions of the pituitary and hypothalamus are common consequences of closed head injury. Clinically, syndromes of diabetes insipidus or hypopituitarism, ranging from severe panhypopituitarism[53] to selective deficiency of a single pituitary hormone, may be observed. Over two-thirds of patients dying with closed head injury will be found to have structural abnormalities in the hypothalamus and pituitary if these areas are examined carefully.[25,66] In the combined series of Daniel and Treip,[24] Ceballos,[15] Kornblum and Fisher,[55] and McCormick,[66] involving a total of 434 trauma victims, pituitary lesions were found, consisting most often of hemorrhages into the posterior lobe (Fig. 261-39) or infarction in the anterior lobe (Fig. 261-40), with a smaller number of cases of anterior lobe hemorrhage or stalk hemorrhages and lacerations. Posterior lobe hemorrhage was recorded in 160 cases (37 percent), and anterior lobe infarction in 74 (17 percent). In a hospital series of 110 cases of closed head injury from my service, a pituitary lesion of some type (severe capsular hemorrhage, hemorrhage within the stalk, posterior lobe hemorrhage, or anterior lobe infarction) was found in 94, or 85 percent.

Lesions of the hypothalamus are also common, having been found in slightly over 42 percent of 106 patients with closed head injury studied by Crompton.[21,22] In the group of 106 patients, the pituitary was examined in only 53, of whom 14 (28 percent) had lesions. In 110 of my hospital cases, 22 had grossly evident lesions in the hypothalamus (Fig. 261-41), but an additional 6 patients had microscopic damage consisting of severe neuronal ischemia, focal minute perivascular hemorrhages, and tissue rarefaction (Fig. 261-42). Adams et al. state:

> There is no doubt that the pituitary stalk can occasionally be torn at the time of head injury, this invariably leading to massive infarction of the anterior lobe of the pituitary gland, but our own study suggests that most of the damage sustained by the hypothalamus and the pituitary stalk is secondary to raised intracranial pressure, a shift and distortion of the brain. We examined the pituitary glands routinely and have found infarcts of varying size in the anterior lobe in about 40 percent of fatal head injuries.[3]

Their contention that the pituitary and hypothalamic lesions are most often caused by elevated intracranial pressure rather than directly by trauma is difficult to refute in many cases; clearly some cases are caused in that way. We have seen some patients who had no significant increase in intracranial pressure and who at the time of autopsy manifested little or no evidence of secondary ischemic brain lesions but who had had some pituitary hemorrhages and necrosis. It is my impression that direct damage to this system is more common than the paper of Adams and colleagues would suggest, but I concur with the belief that a significant number (if not most) are totally or partially caused by increased intracranial pressure and secondary ischemic events. Thus, hypothalamic and

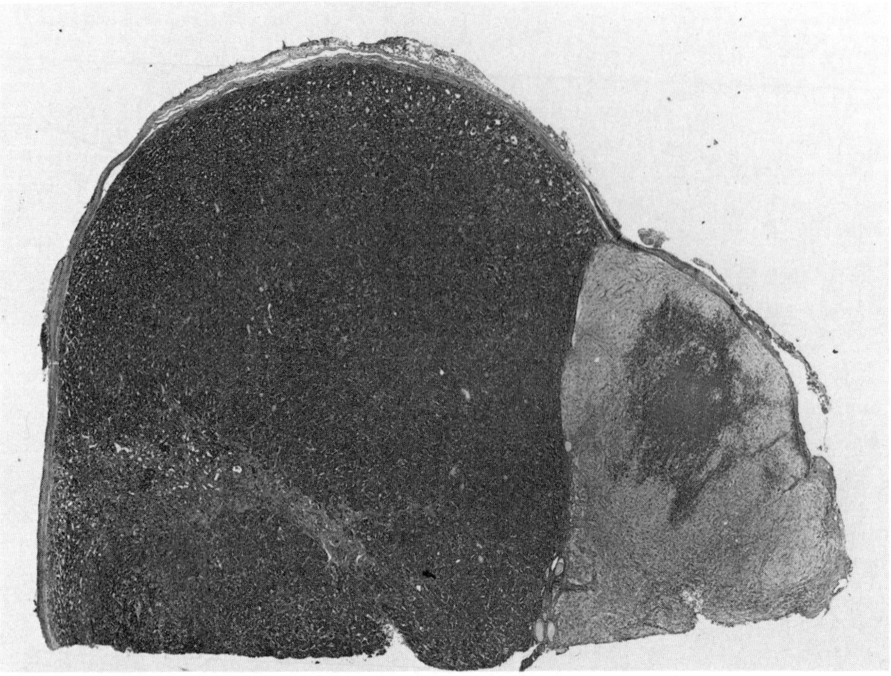

Figure 261-39 The pituitary gland with an acute focal posterior lobe hemorrhage in a case of acute closed head trauma. (H&E; × 10.)

pituitary lesions are very common in patients with severe closed head injury but rarely, if ever, occur in isolation; they are part of a spectrum of multifocal brain damage. Of 106 patients studied by Crompton, 82 percent had skull fractures. In my hospital series of 110 patients, 86 percent had skull fractures.

Diffuse Impact Injury (Diffuse Axonal Injury)

The most rapid expansion in both interest and knowledge has perhaps concerned the study of widespread damage to the brain caused by trauma and not presenting as localized injuries or as a consequence of herniation and perfusion failure. This type of injury, referred to by Adams and colleagues[1–6] as "diffuse axonal injury," was first clearly delineated by Strich.[91,92]

The brains of patients dying with diffuse impact injury (DII) may show minimal gross alterations at the time of their examination. Microscopically, characteristic lesions consisting of reactive axonal swellings secondary to distraction ("shearing") of nerve fibers (Fig. 261-23), scattered microglial clusters ("stars"), and debris-laden macrophages are found. Many brains with DII have hemorrhagic and/or necrotic lesions in the corpus callosum (Figs. 261-43 to 261-46) and in the dorsolateral quadrant of the rostral pons (Figs. 261-47 to 261-49).

Adams and colleagues compared many of the major findings in 45 patients with diffuse impact injury with those from 132 patients with other types of head injury.[3] They found that rotational accelerations were more constantly a factor in the production of DII than of focal brain lesions. None of their patients with diffuse impact injury had a lucid interval, whereas nearly half of their patients with focal brain lesions did. Fractures of the skull were

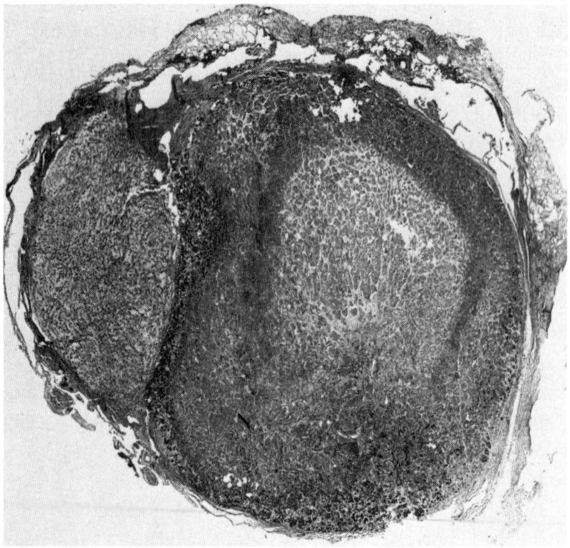

Figure 261-40 Extensive acute infarction of the anterior pituitary in a patient who died of acute head trauma. (Trichrome; × 9.)

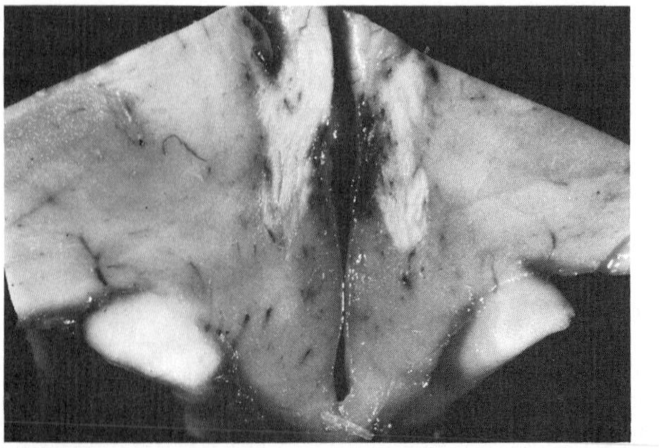

Figure 261-41 Cross section of the brain at the level of the optic tracts, mamillothalamic tracts, and hypothalamus, revealing hemorrhagic necrosis of the anterior hypothalamus.

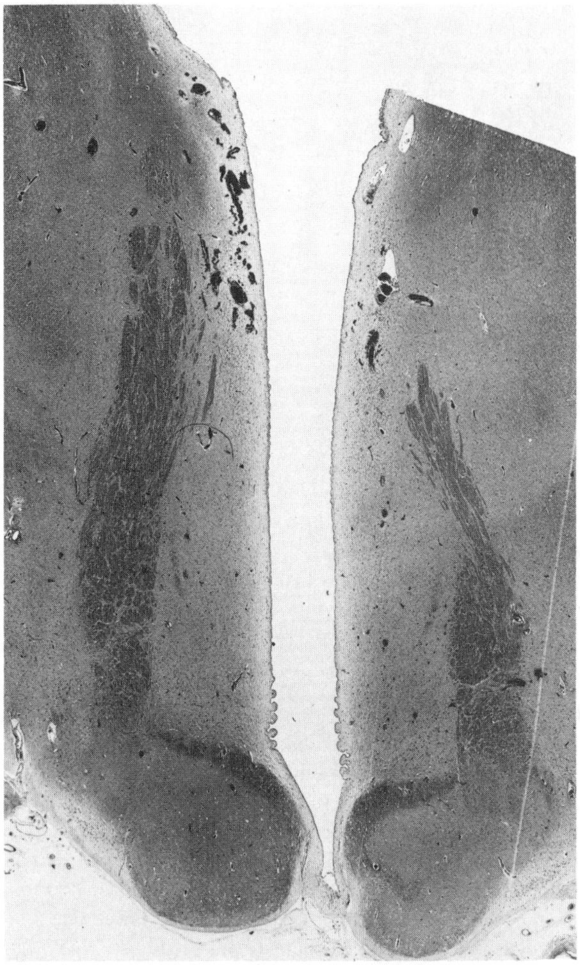

Figure 261-42 Section of the hypothalamus at the level of the mamillary bodies in a patient who died of closed head trauma. Note the small, fresh petechial hemorrhages in the subependymal region. Gross damage to the hypothalamus was not noted in this patient. (H&E; × 6.)

considerably less often encountered in the DII patients than in those with focal injury patterns (29 versus 86 percent). They found no difference in either the amount or the prevalence of hypoxic brain damage between the two groups, nor did there appear to be a significant difference in the presence of brain swelling—in spite of the fact that there was elevation of intracranial pressure in 86 percent of the patients with focal brain lesions and in only 56 percent of the patients with diffuse impact injury. There was a striking difference in the ''mean total contusion index'' between DII patients and the focal injury cases, with an index of 8.3 for the diffuse impact injury patients and 17.8 for the trauma patients with other types of head injury.

Of the three ''classic'' lesions seen in diffuse impact injury, focal necrosis and/or hemorrhage in the corpus callosum was the first to be clearly delineated, although it was not then recognized as part of the pattern now known as DII (Figs. 261-43 to 261-46).[1-6,9,37,54,58,59,66,73,85,104] The 1955 publication of Lindenberg and colleagues was perhaps the paper most instrumental in introducing the concept of significant callosal lesions in closed head injuries to the American audience.[59] Fifteen percent of the patients reported in that publication were noted to have gross callosal lesions. The prevalence of gross callosal damage in my own closed head trauma material is approximately 30 percent. Microscopic lesions in the corpus callosum are far more common, having been reported in 100 percent of the cases examined by Strich.[91]

Originally described by Lindenberg and colleagues as hemorrhage (Fig. 261-44), hemorrhagic necrosis (Figs. 261-43 and 261-46), and anemic necrosis (Fig. 261-45), these gross callosal lesions range in size from minute, barely visible ones to ones that involve nearly all the corpus callosum.[104] These callosal lesions are considered to be caused by lateral stretching of the corpus callosum owing to dorsoventral flattening of the head at the moment of impact. No constant relationship between gross callosal tears and skull fractures has been noted. Focal contusion- and laceration-type injuries in adjacent structures (fornix, cingulate gyri, septum pellucidum, caudate nuclei, and dorsal thalamus) are common (Fig. 261-46).

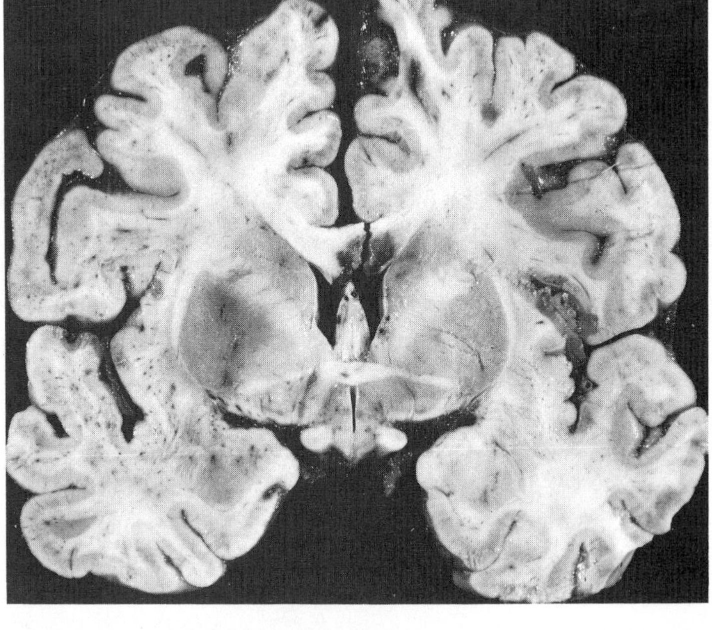

Figure 261-43 Hemorrhagic necrosis in the body of the corpus callosum seen in a section taken at the level of the anterior commissure. There is also conspicuous hemorrhagic necrosis secondary to a herniation contusion in the left uncus. This type of callosal lesion is a typical component of diffuse impact injury but can be found in some patients without other evidence of diffuse impact injury.

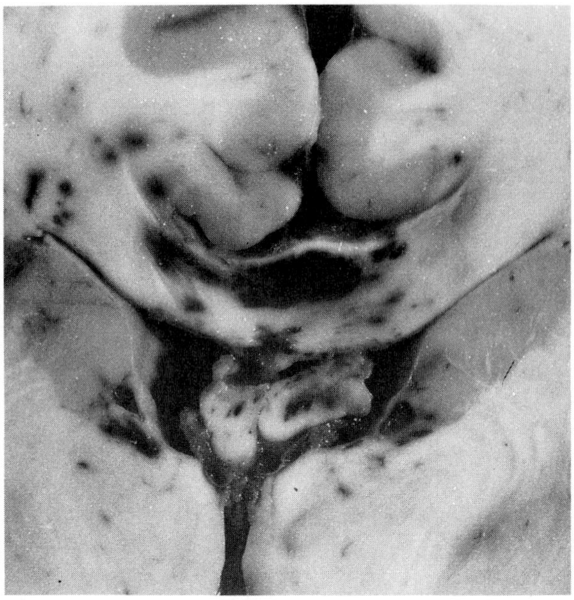

Figure 261-44 A small hematoma within the fibers of the body of the corpus callosum in a patient without other signs of diffuse impact injury. This patient sustained a fall with impaction at the vertex of the head.

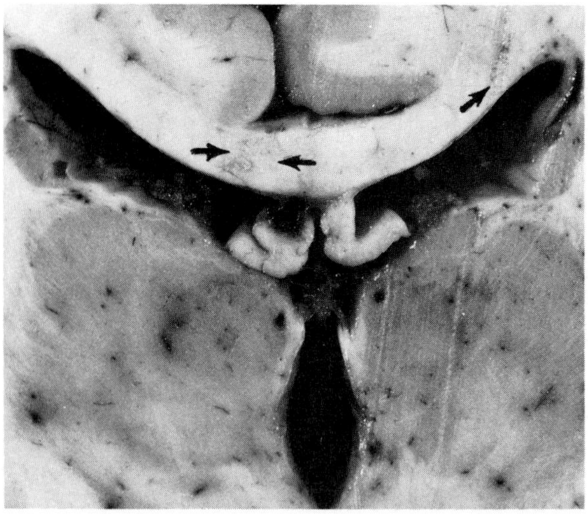

Figure 261-45 Area of ischemic (anemic) necrosis to the left of the midline in the body of the corpus callosum and along the right border *(arrows)*. This patient died approximately 72 h after sustaining a closed head injury.

The second classic gross finding in patients with diffuse impact injury is hemorrhagic necrosis in the dorsolateral quadrant of the rostral pons in and next to the brachium conjunctivum (Figs. 261-47 to 261-49). This lesion was once considered to result from direct impaction of the pons against the incisura of the tentorium,[46] but Adams and colleagues[1–6] now vigorously maintain that it is an indirect lesion associated with diffuse impact injury, a conclusion that I and others share.[9,66] These brain stem lesions vary considerably in size and conspicuousness. In patients who survive only briefly, they are almost always hemorrhagic, sometimes appearing as discrete hematomas. With the passage of time, the hemorrhagic malacia resorbs, leaving only hemosiderin-stained, shrunken malacic areas (Fig. 261-49).

The third lesion characteristic of the triad making up diffuse impact injury is the reactive axonal swelling from tearing of the axon. Reactive axonal ''retraction'' balls are most easily seen with silver impregnation techniques and increase in prominence with prolonged survival time. Retraction balls can be found very shortly after disruption of the axon (Fig. 261-50), having been demonstrated to occur in less than 3 h.[9,58,66] Degeneration of the corticospinal and corticobulbar tracts may become so advanced that these tracts appear very pallid when stained with Luxol fast blue or silver preparations (Figs. 261-36 and 261-49).

Experimental observations coupled with observations on human material have led Adams and colleagues to delineate a sequence of events giving rise to diffuse impact injury.

> At the moment of injury, stresses induced by movements of the head are sufficient to injure numerous axons throughout the brain, and it is clear from the experimental studies that

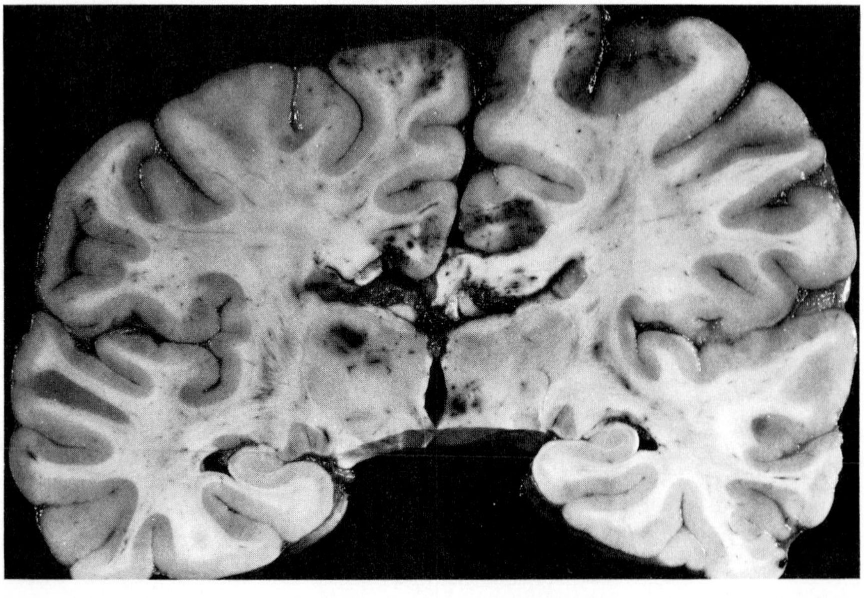

Figure 261-46 Hemorrhage and necrosis with transection of the body of the corpus callosum. There are associated hemorrhagic lesions in the cingulate and superior frontal gyri and small hemorrhages in the left thalamus and right hypothalamus. The impact was to the frontal vertex.

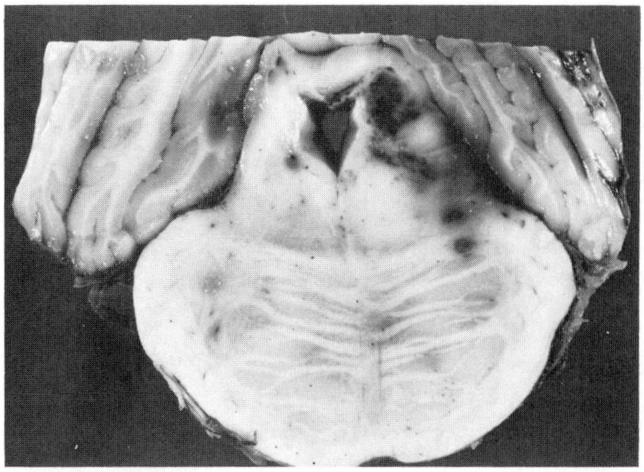

Figure 261-47 Typical gross appearance of the areas of hemorrhage and hemorrhagic necrosis in the dorsolateral aspect of the rostral pons seen in patients with diffuse impact injuries.

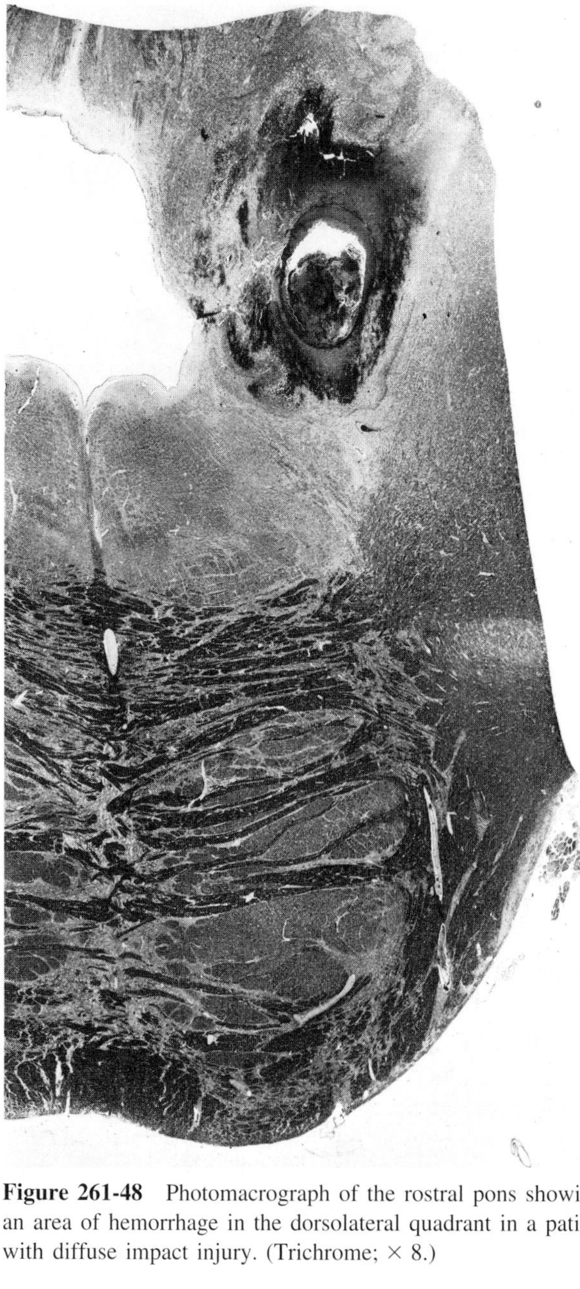

Figure 261-48 Photomacrograph of the rostral pons showing an area of hemorrhage in the dorsolateral quadrant in a patient with diffuse impact injury. (Trichrome; × 8.)

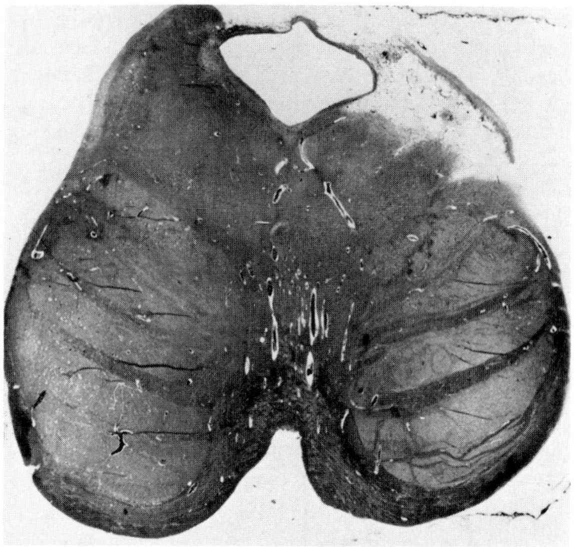

Figure 261-49 A Bodian-stained section of the rostral pons showing a remote cavitary dorsolateral quadrant lesion in a patient with diffuse impact injury and prolonged (120-day) survival. There is marked pallor of staining of the corticospinal and corticobulbar tracts bilaterally. Microscopically, large numbers of reactive axonal swellings were still present in these long tracts. (×5.)

contact phenomena are not essential in the pathogenesis of these injuries. Rather the head must undergo appropriate acceleration in particular directions to cause DAI. If the injury is of sufficient magnitude, many axons are physically disrupted, and small vessels—presumably capillaries—may also be torn. Thus, tissue tears appear in the corpus callosum and rostral brain stem and are characterized by the presence of small hemorrhages and axonal retraction balls. Invariably other axons must be injured and appear abnormal, but may not be completely disrupted; this may be represented by tuberosities on axons, where axonal damage is minimal, by the

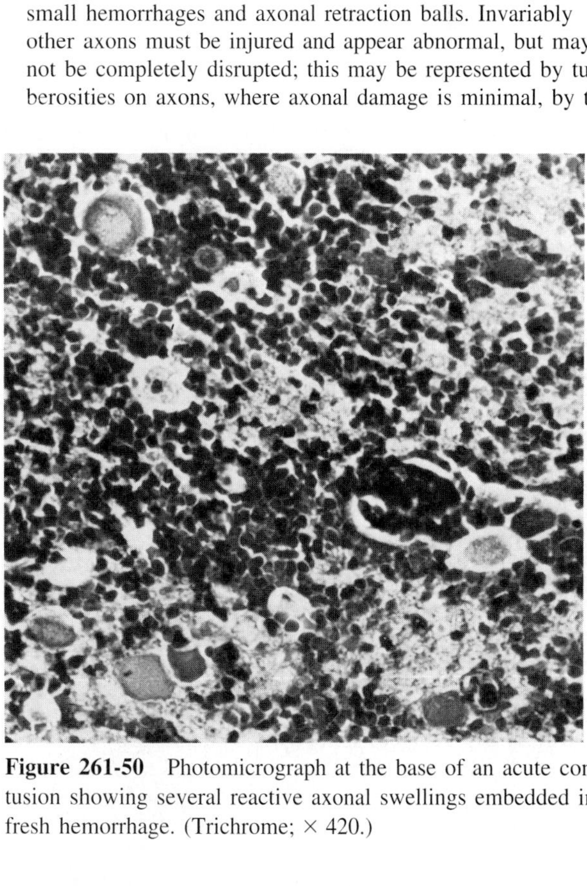

Figure 261-50 Photomicrograph at the base of an acute contusion showing several reactive axonal swellings embedded in fresh hemorrhage. (Trichrome; × 420.)

Fink-Heimer technique. Later, microglia migrate into the areas of axonal damage (microglial stars); and still later degeneration of the myelin associated with the destroyed axons leads to the production of lipid stainable by the Sudan dyes and the Marchi technique. Total brain mass is subsequently reduced and an atrophic appearance of the brain ensues.[3]

Secondary Post-Traumatic Brain Lesions

The brains of victims of fatal closed head trauma typically contain a variety of vascular/ischemic lesions that result from increased intracranial pressure, herniation-induced vascular occlusions, or systemic hypotension.[1-6,34,58,66,68] Morphologically, these alterations differ in no important respect from ischemic/anoxic lesions in nontraumatized brains. They occur in arterial border zones and terminal perfusion beds, in the hippocampi (especially Sommer's sector) (Fig. 261-51), and in the Purkinje layer of the cerebellum. An example is the herniation-induced necrosis in the distribution of the calcarine branch of the posterior cerebral artery (Fig. 261-52). When the cerebral cortex is involved, maximal damage is evident along the banks and in the depths of the sulci rather than over the crowns of the gyri. Areas of brain necrosis may be wedge-shaped, with the base of the wedge at the cortical surface and the apex deep in the parenchyma. Both cortex and convolutional white matter are involved, with some extension into the central white matter in the larger and necrotic lesions. Both grossly and microscopically, these wedge-shaped areas of necrosis resemble typical infarcts.

Adams and colleagues, in examining the brains from a series of patients whose intracranial pressure had been carefully monitored before death, observed that pressure necrosis in the hippocampal area ("parahippocampal gyri") occurred in the brains of all patients whose intracranial pressure had exceeded 40 mmHg and in most whose intracranial pressure had been between 20 and 40 mmHg; this change was absent in patients whose intracranial pressure had remained below 20 mmHg.[3] Adams and colleagues also noted, as have many others, that a clear majority of patients with increased intracranial pressure also had hemorrhages and hemorrhagic softenings (secondary or Duret hemorrhages) in the mesencephalon and pons (Fig. 261-53).

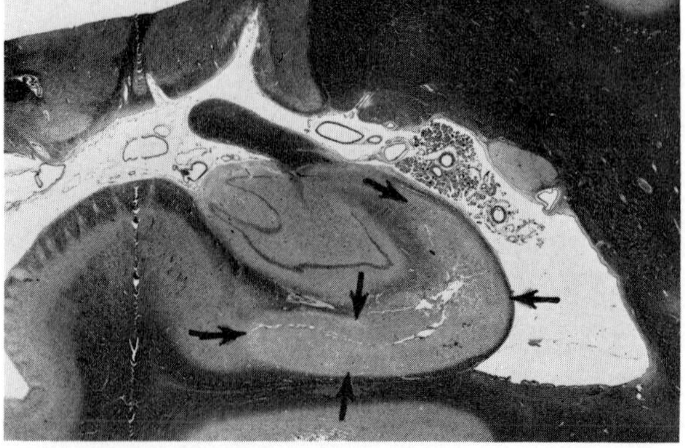

Figure 261-51 Acute sector necrosis as a secondary ischemic/anoxic lesion in a patient with closed head trauma. The swollen, pale necrotic sector is outlined by arrows. (Luxol fast blue—PASH; × 4.)

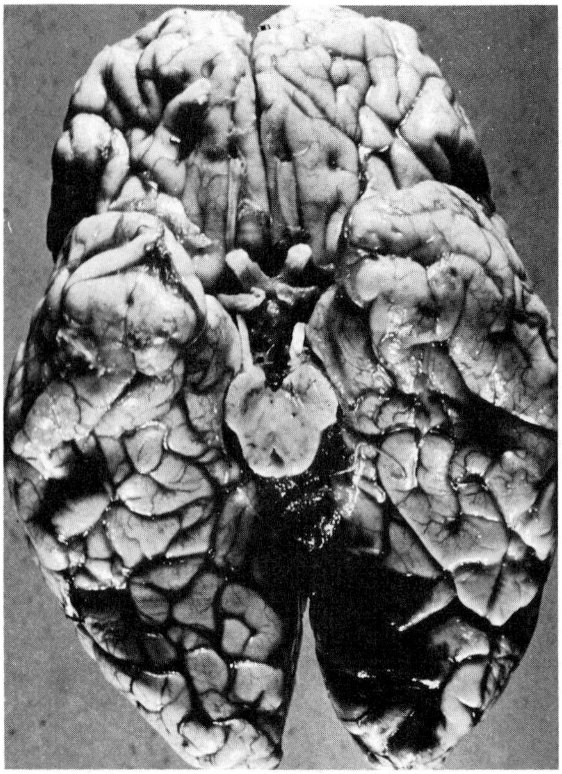

Figure 261-52 Calcarine artery distribution infarction secondary to lateral transtentorial herniation is a common secondary vascular lesion in head trauma patients.

Focal ischemic lesions occurring in arterial border zones are commonly encountered in patients who had episodes of systemic hypotension that were clinically apparent and in patients who developed ventilatory compromise owing to aspiration airway occlusion. Discrete, wedge-shaped border zone malacic foci are sometimes unilateral but more often bilateral and are most commonly located between the anterior and middle cerebral artery perfusion beds. Areas of anoxic tissue necrosis that appear quite similar are found at the terminal perfusion beds of the middle cerebral artery in a significant number of patients.

In addition to the very focal anoxic/ischemic lesions, diffuse hypoxic changes ranging from widespread homogenizing necrosis of neurons to widespread pseudolaminar necrosis of the cortex are seen in some patients (Figs. 261-54 and 261-55). In their 1978 study of ischemic brain damage in patients with closed head trauma, Graham and colleagues found anoxic/hypoxic lesions in 70 of 151 patients.[34] These were described as severe in 29, moderate in 35, and mild in 6 patients. In addition, 68 of these 151 victims of fatal closed head injury had focal ischemic lesions. Only 13 (8.6 percent) of them had neither anoxic nor ischemic brain damage. The location of the hypoxic damage in this series was the hippocampus in 80 percent, the basal ganglia in 79 percent, and the cerebellum in 44 percent. In a published report of 56 autopsied cases of closed head trauma from my service, it was noted that among the 25 that died less than 48 h after injury, 17 had diffuse homogenizing necrosis of neurons throughout the brain, 6 had a progressive mass effect, 1 (an infant) had a diffusely and massively swollen and congested brain, and 1 had a massive direct pontine laceration secondary to a transclival fracture.[17] In contrast, examination of the brains of 31 patients who survived for more than 48 h after their injury revealed similar diffuse homogenizing

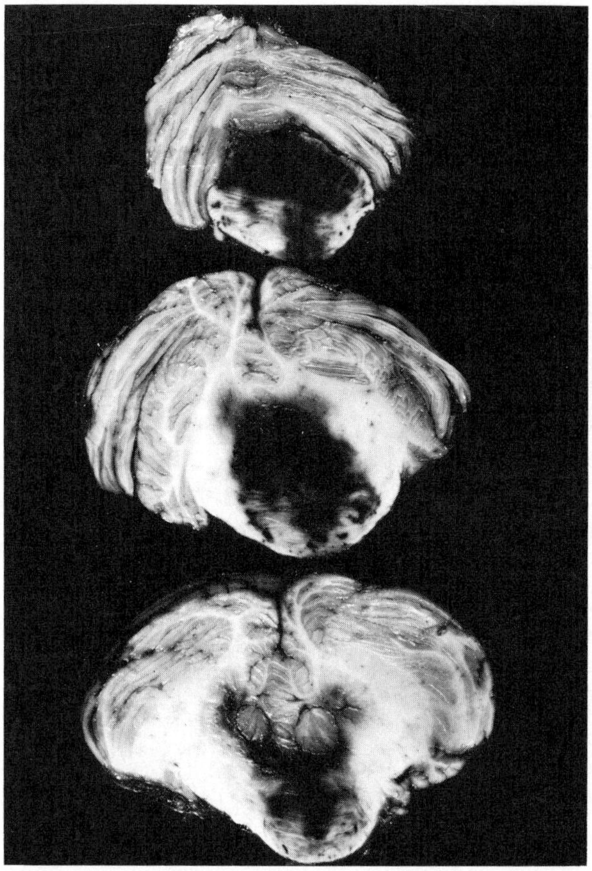

Figure 261-53 Typical extensive secondary (Duret) brain stem hemorrhages associated with transtentorial herniation. These are not direct (primary) brain stem lesions in trauma patients.

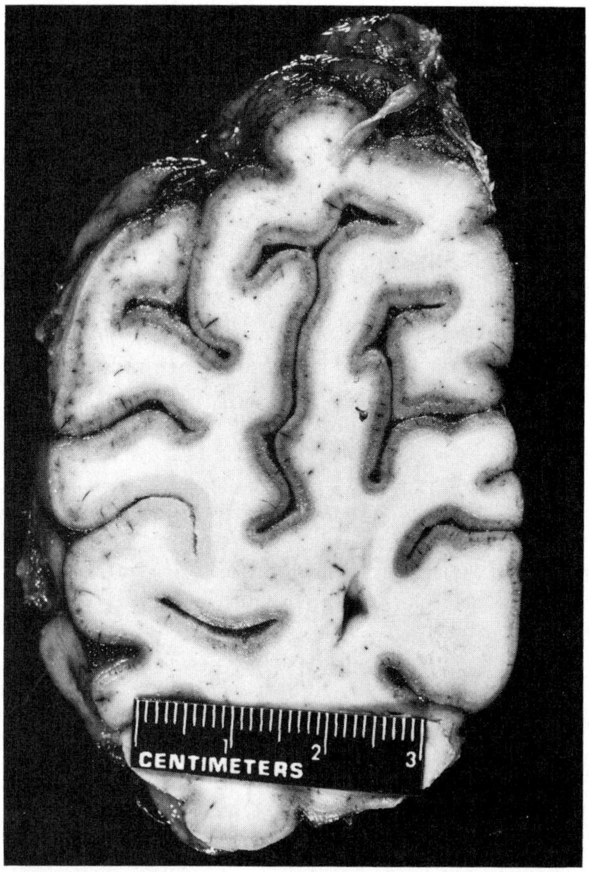

Figure 261-54 Diffuse "anoxic decortication" in a head trauma patient who survived 5 days after an episode of severe circulatory collapse.

necrosis of neurons in only 6, all of whom were deeply comatose from the time of injury and who undoubtedly would have died in the immediate post-trauma period if not for complete ventilatory support and pressor agents. The remaining 25 patients had only focal lesions, meningitis, severe suppurative bronchopneumonia with sepsis, or massive gastrointestinal bleeding with exsanguination. Among these 25 patients who survived more than 48 h, 7 died as the result of a progressive mass effect and had secondary brain stem hemorrhages from their hernias. All of the patients with diffuse homogenizing necrosis of neurons had a measured elevation of intracranial pressure.

The presence of many types of secondary vascular lesions in the brain stem in patients dying of closed head trauma is so familiar as to make a detailed discussion in this chapter unnecessary. Most often taking the form of hemorrhage with surrounding hemorrhagic necrosis, these lesions are generally considered to be due to displacement of the brain stem with an occluding/shearing effect on the paramedian and short circumflex arteries at the time of transtentorial brain herniation (Fig. 261-53). This development is most commonly seen in patients with significantly elevated intracranial pressure. Although the lesions are usually overtly hemorrhagic, severe localized pale infarctions of the brain stem can occur in patients with transtentorial herniation.

Generally, small ischemic lesions are found in the mesencephalon in many patients with fatal closed head injury. Rosenblum and colleagues think they occur at the moment of impact[83]; I consider them to be a secondary ischemic event or part of a diffuse impact injury.

Focal discrete infarctions of the brain in specific arterial territories constitute a relatively common and well-known complication of increased intracranial pressure and brain herniations in trauma patients. The best known of these lesions is undoubtedly the hemorrhagic infarction occurring in the distribution of the posterior cerebral artery following lateral transtentorial herniation (Fig. 261-52). Infarcts in the perfusion beds of the anterior choroidal, posterior inferior cerebellar, and posterior choroidal arteries are also

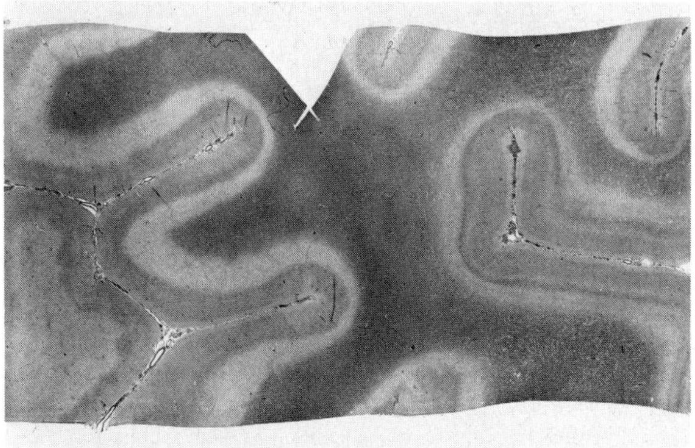

Figure 261-55 Photomacrograph of a cerebral section showing early cortical necrosis and severe convolutional white matter pallor. (Luxol fast blue—PASH; × 3.)

encountered. Table 261-3 summarizes the major types of secondary post-traumatic brain damage encountered.

A complication of fatal closed head injury found in many autopsies is fresh subendocardial hemorrhage along the intraventricular septum of the left ventricle (Fig. 261-56).[17,66] These hemorrhages range in extent from a few millimeters to 5 to 6 cm and in thickness from only a few erythrocytes to 3 mm. The hemorrhages are known to be associated with conduction defects in the electrocardiograms of patients when the appropriate studies are carried out during life. Such subendocardial hemorrhages were noted in 16 of the 56 patients dying of closed head injury in a previous report from this laboratory.[17] In 110 autopsies on hospitalized patients dying with closed head injury, such hemorrhages were observed in 38. Among nearly 200 head-injured patients who were ''dead at the scene'' or died within 30 min of injury, only about 5 percent had grossly recognizable subendocardial hemorrhage. The etiology and pathogenesis of these hemorrhages are not clear. The hemorrhages are not confined to victims of head trauma, being frequently encountered in patients with any mass in the brain (neoplasm, hematoma) that causes herniation, and in patients with massive subarachnoid hemorrhage from a ruptured saccular aneurysm. It seems probable that these hemorrhages are due to subendocardial ischemia secondary to the marked vasoconstrictive effect of norepinephrine, which is known to circulate in greatly increased amounts in patients with closed head trauma.[18]

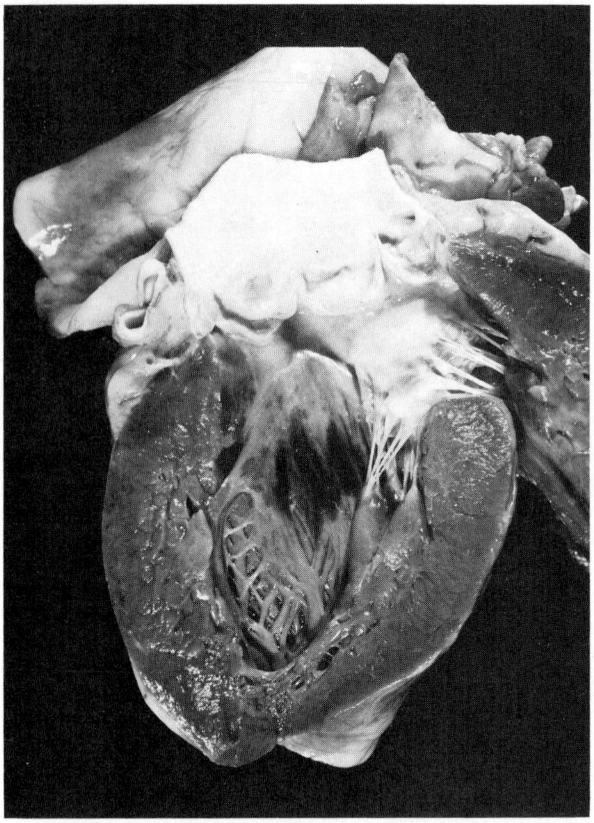

Figure 261-56 Acute subendocardial hemorrhage in the left ventricle of the heart along the interventricular septum. These lesions are found in about two-thirds of patients dying with acute closed head injuries.

Interpretation of Closed Head Injury: Problems and Pitfalls

A number of major practical problems confront the physician who attempts to interpret traumatic brain lesions. These problems include the attempt to be overly precise in guessing the age of a given lesion; unfounded dogmatism in rendering an opinion without regard to historical data on how the injury occurred; and the attempt to classify every lesion without proper consideration of the clinical features, including intracranial pressure measurements, hypotensive episodes before death, aspiration episodes, etc. It is necessary for the pathologist to be forceful in withstanding pressure to render a detailed opinion before the completion of all studies. It is the unfortunate situation in many forensic services that brains from trauma victims are examined and cut in the fresh state and a final opinion rendered without microscopic (or even detailed gross) examination. This is a major error, and one that has held back our knowledge of the pathology and pathophysiology of head trauma. It is also important to remember that different and totally unrelated disorders may be present in the brain of a patient dying with head trauma; trauma in no way precludes natural disease.

TABLE 261-3 Secondary Post-Traumatic Brain Damage

1. *Medial temporal (parahippocampal) necrosis*—caused by vascular compression in the brain as it is displaced against the tentorial edge during transtentorial herniation in a patient with elevated intracranial pressure (ICP)
2. *Focal infarction due to specific artery compression*—caused by transforaminal arterial compressions, the best known and most common being the calcarine infarcts due to posterior cerebral artery compression during lateral transtentorial herniation
3. *Border zone infarcts and focal hypoxic damage*—caused by circulatory failure secondary to systemic hypotension (''pump failure'') or direct traumatic arterial thrombosis or laceration
4. *Diffuse ischemic necrosis of neurons* in patients who die rapidly (within approximately 48 h) with increased ICP
5. *Secondary brain stem (Duret) hemorrhages*—caused by transtentorial herniation in patients with elevated ICP

References

1. Adams JH. The neuropathology of head injuries. In Vinken PJ, Bruyn GW (eds): *Handbook of Clinical Neurology,* vol 23. Amsterdam: North-Holland, 1975, pp 35–65.
2. Adams JH. Head injury. In Adams JH, Duchen LW (eds): *Greenfield's Neuropathology,* 5th ed. New York: Oxford University Press, 1992, pp 106–152.
3. Adams JH, Gennarelli TA, Graham DI. Brain damage in nonmissile head injury: observations in man and subhuman primates. In Smith WT, Cavanagh JB (eds): *Recent Advances in Neuropathology,* No. 2. Edinburgh: Churchill Livingstone, 1982, pp 165–190.
4. Adams JH, Graham DI, Murray LS, Scott G. Diffuse axonal injury due to nonmissile head injury in humans: an analysis of 45 cases. *Ann Neurol* 1981; 12:557–563.
5. Adams JH, Graham DI, Scott G, et al. Brain damage in fatal nonmissile head injury. *J Clin Pathol* 1980; 33:1132–1145.
6. Adams JH, Mitchell DE, Graham DI, Doyle D. Diffuse brain damage of immediate impact type: its relationship to ''primary brain-stem damage'' in head injury. *Brain* 1977; 100:489–502.
7. Agyeman JF, Huber P. Computer tomographical analysis of central cerebral haemorrhage resulting from closed head injury. *Eur Neurol* 1982; 21:298–304.

8. Ammirati M, Tomita T. Posterior fossa epidural hematoma during childhood. *Neurosurgery* 1984; 14:541–544.
9. Blumbergs PC, Jones NR, North JB. Diffuse axonal injury in head trauma. *J Neurol Neurosurg Psychiatry* 1989; 52:838–841.
10. Borovich B, Braun J, Guilburd JN, et al. Delayed onset of traumatic extradural hematoma. *J Neurosurg* 1985; 63:30–34.
11. Britt RH, Herrick MK, Mason RT, Dorfman LJ. Traumatic lesions of the pontomedullary junction. *Neurosurgery* 1980; 6:623–631.
12. Brown FD, Mullan S, Duda EE. Delayed traumatic intracerebral hematomas: report of three cases. *J Neurosurg* 1978; 48:1019–1022.
13. Bruce DA, Alavi A, Bilaniuk L, et al. Diffuse cerebral swelling following head injuries in children: the syndrome of "malignant brain edema." *J Neurosurg* 1981; 54:170–178.
14. Buckingham MJ, Crone KR, Ball WS, et al. Traumatic intracranial aneurysms in childhood: two cases and a review of the literature. *Neurosurgery* 1988; 22:398–408.
15. Ceballos R. Pituitary changes in head trauma (analysis of 102 consecutive cases of head injury). *Ala J Med Sci* 1966; 3:185–198.
16. Cervós-Navarro J, Lafuente JV. Traumatic brain injuries: structural changes. *J Neurol Sci* 1991; 103(Suppl S3–S14).
17. Clifton GL, McCormick WF, Grossman RG. Neuropathology of early and late deaths after head injury. *Neurosurgery* 1981; 8:309–314.
18. Clifton GL, Ziegler MG, Grossman RG. Circulating catecholamines and sympathetic activity after head injury. *Neurosurgery* 1981; 8:10–13.
19. Cooper PR. Delayed traumatic intracerebral hemorrhage. *Neurosurg Clin North Am* 1992; 3:659–665.
20. Cordobés F, Lobato RD, Rivas JJ, et al. Observations on 82 patients with extradural hematoma: comparison of results before and after the advent of computerized tomography. *J Neurosurg* 1981; 54:179–186.
21. Crompton MR. Hypothalamic lesions following closed head injury. *Brain* 1971; 94:165–172.
22. Crompton MR. Hypothalamic and pituitary lesions. In Vinken PJ, Bruyn GW (eds): *Handbook of Clinical Neurology,* vol 23. Amsterdam: North-Holland, 1975, pp 465–469.
23. Crooks DA. Pathogenesis and biomechanics of traumatic intracranial haemorrhages. *Virchows Arch [A] Pathol Anat Histopathol* 1991; 418:479–483.
24. Daniel PM, Treip CS. Lesions of the pituitary gland associated with head injuries. In Harris GW, Donovan BT (eds): *The Pituitary Gland,* vol 2. London: Butterworth, 1966, pp 519–534.
25. Edwards OM, Clark JDA. Post-traumatic hypopituitarism. Six cases and a review of the literature. *Medicine (Baltimore)* 1986; 65:281–290.
26. Eichner ER. The hematologic disorders of alcoholism. *Am J Med* 1973; 54:621–630.
27. Elsner H, Rigamonti D, Corradino G, et al. Delayed traumatic intracerebral hematomas: "Spät-apoplexie": report of two cases. *J Neurosurg* 1990; 72:813–815.
28. Flamm ES, Demopoulos HB, Seligman ML, et al. Ethanol potentiation of central nervous system trauma. *J Neurosurg* 1977; 46:328–335.
29. Frank E, Berger TS, Tew JM Jr. Bilateral epidural hematomas. *Surg Neurol* 1982; 17:218–222.
30. Galyon DD, Winfield JA. An unusual syndrome of pediatric brainstem trauma. *Pediatr Neurosci* 1988; 14:272–276.
31. George B, Thurel C, Pierron D, Ragueneau JL. Frequency of primary brain stem lesions after head injuries: a CT scan analysis from 186 cases of severe head trauma. *Acta Neurochir (Wien)* 1981; 59:35–43.
32. Gjerris F. Head injuries in children—special features. *Acta Neurochir (Wien) [Suppl]* 1986; 36:155–158.
33. Gordon A, Maloney AFJ. Blunt head injury. In Mason JK (ed): *The Pathology of Violent Injury.* London: Edward Arnold, 1978, pp 197–217.
34. Graham DI, Adams JH, Doyle D. Ischaemic brain damage in fatal non-missile head injuries. *J Neurol Sci* 1978; 39:213–234.
35. Guha A, Fazl M, Cooper PW. Isolated basilar artery occlusion associated with a clivus fracture. *Can J Neurol Sci* 1989; 16:81–83.
36. Gurdjian ES, Webster JE, Lissner HR. The mechanism of skull fracture. *J Neurosurg* 1950; 7:106–114.
37. Hardman JM. The pathology of traumatic brain injuries. *Adv Neurol* 1979; 22:15–50.
38. Harvey FH, Jones AM. "Typical" basal skull fracture of both petrous bones: an unreliable indicator of head impact site. *J Forensic Sci* 1980; 25:280–286.
39. Heinze J. Cranial nerve avulsion and other neural injuries in road accidents. *Med J Aust* 1969; 2:1246–1249.
40. Hirsh LF. Chronic epidural hematomas. *Neurosurgery* 1980; 6:508–512.
41. Humphreys RP, Hendrick EB, Hoffman HJ. The head-injured child who "talks and dies." A report of 4 cases. *Child's Nerv Syst* 1990; 6:139–142.
42. Iwakuma T, Brunngraber CV. Chronic extradural hematomas: a study of 21 cases. *J Neurosurg* 1973; 38:488–493.
43. Jackson FE, Gleave JRW, Janon E. The traumatic cranial and intracranial aneurysms. In Vinken PJ, Bruyn GW (eds): *Handbook of Clinical Neurology,* vol 24. Amsterdam: North-Holland, 1976, pp 381–398.
44. Jakobsson KE, Carlsson C, Elfverson J, von Essen C. Traumatic aneurysms of cerebral arteries. A study of five cases. *Acta Neurochir (Wien)* 1984; 71:91–98.
45. Jani NN, Laureno R, Mark AS, Brewer CC. Deafness after bilateral midbrain contusion: a correlation of magnetic resonance imaging with auditory brain stem evoked responses. *Neurosurgery* 1991; 29:106–109.
46. Jellinger K, Seitelberger F. Protracted post-traumatic encephalopathy: pathology, pathogenesis and clinical implications. *J Neurol Sci* 1970; 10:51–94.
47. Jones NR, Blumbergs PC, North JB. Acute subdural haematomas: aetiology, pathology and outcome. *Aust N Z J Surg* 1986; 56:907–913.
48. Joslyn JN, Mirvis SE, Markowitz B. Complex fractures of the clivus: diagnosis with CT and clinical outcome in 11 patients. *Radiology* 1988; 166:817–821.
49. Kars Z, Benli K, Sağlam S, Gürcay Ö: Chronic extradural haematoma: a late complication of head injury. *Neurochirurgia (Stuttg)* 1985; 28:145–146.
50. Kaufman HH, Moake JL, Olson JD, et al. Delayed and recurrent intracranial hematomas related to disseminated intravascular clotting and fibrinolysis in head injury. *Neurosurgery* 1980; 7:446–449.
51. Kingsley D, Till K, Hoare R. Growing fractures of the skull. *J Neurol Neurosurg Psychiatry* 1978; 41:312–318.
52. Kissel P, Boggan JE, Wagner FC Jr. CT evolution of an acute venous epidural hematoma. *J Emerg Med* 1989; 7:365–368.
53. Klingbeil GEG, Cline P. Anterior hypopituitarism: a consequence of head injury. *Arch Phys Med Rehabil* 1985; 66:44–46.
54. Komatsu S, Sato T, Kagawa S, et al. Traumatic lesions of the corpus callosum. *Neurosurgery* 1979; 5:32–35.
55. Kornblum RN, Fisher RS. Pituitary lesions in craniocerebral injuries. *Arch Pathol Lab Med* 1969; 88:242–248.
56. Koulouris S, Rizzoli HV. Delayed traumatic intracerebral hematoma after compound depressed skull fracture: case report. *Neurosurgery* 1981; 8:223–225.
57. Lee ST, Lui TN. Delayed intracranial haemorrhage in patients with multiple trauma and shock-related hypotension. *Acta Neurochir (Wien)* 1991; 113:121–124.
58. Lindenberg R. Trauma of meninges and brain. In Minckler J (ed): *Pathology of the Nervous System,* vol 2. New York: McGraw-Hill, 1971, pp 1705–1765.
59. Lindenberg R, Fisher RS, Durlacher SH, et al. Lesions of the corpus callosum following blunt mechanical trauma to the head. *Am J Pathol* 1955; 31:297–317.
60. Lindenberg R, Freytag E. The mechanism of cerebral contusions: a pathologic-anatomic study. *Arch Pathol Lab Med* 1960; 69:440–469.
61. Lindenberg R, Freytag E. Morphology of brain lesions from blunt trauma in early infancy. *Arch Pathol Lab Med* 1969; 87:298–305.

62. Lindenberg R, Freytag E. Brainstem lesions characteristic of traumatic hyperextension of the head. *Arch Pathol Lab Med* 1970; 90:509–515.
63. Lye RH, Occleshaw JV, Dutton J. Growing fracture of the skull and the role of computerized tomography: case report. *J Neurosurg* 1981; 55:470–472.
64. MacPherson P, Teasdale E, Dhaker S, et al. The significance of traumatic haematoma in the region of the basal ganglia. *J Neurol Neurosurg Psychiatry* 1986; 49:29–34.
65. McCormick WF. The relationship of closed-head trauma to rupture of saccular intracranial aneurysms. *Am J Forensic Med Pathol* 1980; 1:223–226.
66. McCormick WF. Trauma. In Schochet SS Jr (ed): *Clinical Neurosciences,* vol 3. New York: Churchill Livingstone, 1983, pp 241–283.
67. Miner ME, Kaufman HH, Graham SH, et al. Disseminated intravascular coagulation fibrinolytic syndrome following head injury in children: frequency and prognostic implications. *J Pediatr* 1982; 100:687–691.
68. Mirvis SE, Wolf AL, Numaguchi Y, et al. Posttraumatic cerebral infarction diagnosed by CT: prevalence, origin, and outcome. *Am J Roentgenol* 1990; 154:1293–1298.
69. Morard M, de Tribolet N. Traumatic aneurysm of the posterior inferior cerebellar artery: case report. *Neurosurgery* 1991; 29:438–441.
70. Ninchoji T, Uemura K, Shimoyama I, et al. Traumatic intracerebral haematomas of delayed onset. *Acta Neurochir (Wien)* 1984; 71:69–90.
71. Ordia IJ, Strand R, Gilles F, Welch K. Computed tomography of contusional clefts in the white matter in infants: report of two cases. *J Neurosurg* 1981; 54:696–698.
72. Otsuka S, Nakatsu S, Sato S, et al. Study on cases of traumatic subarachnoid hemorrhage. *Nippon Geka Hokan* 1988; 57:84–91.
73. Parker JR, Parker JC Jr, Overman JC. Intracranial diffuse axonal injury at autopsy. *Ann Clin Lab Sci* 1990; 20:220–224.
74. Parkinson D, West M. Traumatic intracranial aneurysms. *J Neurosurg* 1980; 52:11–20.
75. Paul GA, Shaw CM, Wray LM. True traumatic aneurysm of the vertebral artery: case report. *J Neurosurg* 1980; 53:101–105.
76. Pietrzak M, Jagoda A, Brown L. Evaluation of minor head trauma in children younger than two years. *Am J Emerg Med* 1991; 9:153–156.
77. Pilz P, Strohecker J, Grobovschek M. Survival after traumatic pontomedullary tear. *J Neurol Neurosurg Psychiatry* 1982; 45:422–427.
78. Poon WS, Rehman SU, Poon CYF, Li AKC. Traumatic extradural hematoma of delayed onset is not a rarity. *Neurosurgery* 1992; 30:681–686.
79. Ramamurthi B. Acute subdural haematoma. In Vinken PJ, Bruyn GW (eds): *Handbook of Clinical Neurology,* vol 24. Amsterdam: North-Holland, 1976, pp 275–296.
80. Rengachary SS, Szymanski DC. Sudural hematomas of arterial origin. *Neurosurgery* 1981; 8:166–171.
81. Rivano C, Borzone M, Carta F, Michelozzi G. Traumatic intracerebral hematomas: 72 cases surgically treated. *J Neurosurg Sci* 1980; 24:77–84.
82. Rivas JJ, Lobato RD, Sarabia R, et al. Extradural hematoma: analysis of factors influencing the courses of 161 patients. *Neurosurgery* 1988; 23:44–51.
83. Rosenblum WI, Greenberg RP, Seelig JM, Becker DP. Midbrain lesions: frequent and significant prognostic feature in closed head injury. *Neurosurgery* 1981; 9:613–620.
84. Russell WR, Schiller F. Crushing injury to the skull: clinical and experimental observations. *J Neurol Neurosurg Psychiatry* 1949; 12:52–60.
85. Sasiadek M, Marciniak R, Bem Z. CT appearance of shearing injuries of the brain. *Bildgebung* 1991; 58:148–149.
86. Sekhar LN, Scarff TB. Pseudogrowth in skull fractures of childhood. *Neurosurgery* 1980; 6:285–289.
87. Snoek JW, Minderhoud JM, Wilmink JT. Delayed deterioration following mild head injury in children. *Brain* 1984; 107:15–36.
88. Stein SC, Spettell C, Young G, Ross SE. Delayed and progressive brain injury in closed-head trauma: radiological demonstration. *Neurosurgery* 1993; 32:25–31.
89. Stein SC, Young GS, Talucci RC, et al. Delayed brain injury after head trauma: significance of coagulopathy. *Neurosurgery* 1992; 30:160–165.
90. Stone JL, Rifai MHS, Sugar O, et al. Subdural hematomas. I. Acute subdural hematoma: progress in definition, clinical pathology, and therapy. *Surg Neurol* 1983; 19:216–231.
91. Strich SJ. Diffuse degeneration of the cerebral white matter in severe dementia following head injury. *J Neurol Neurosurg Psychiatry* 1956; 19:163–185.
92. Strich SJ. Shearing of nerve fibres as a cause of brain damage due to head injury. *Lancet* 1961; 2:443–448.
93. Summers CG, Wirtschafter JD. Bilateral trigeminal and abducens neuropathies following low-velocity, crushing head injury: case report. *J Neurosurg* 1979; 50:508–511.
94. Taha JM, Crone KR, Berger TS, et al. Sigmoid sinus thrombosis after closed head injury in children. *Neurosurgery* 1993; 32:541–546.
95. Takahara T, Terai C, Okada Y, et al. Fatal traumatic subarachnoid hemorrhage due to rupture of the vertebral artery. *Intensive Care Med* 1993; 19:172–173.
96. Tandon PN, Prakash B, Banerji AK. Temporal lobe lesions in head injury. *Acta Neurochir (Wien)* 1978; 41:205–221.
97. Teasdale GM, Murray G, Anderson E, et al. Risks of acute traumatic intracranial haematoma in children and adults: implications for managing head injuries. *Br Med J* 1990; 300:363–367.
98. Unterharnscheidt F. Neuropathology of rhesus monkeys undergoing $-G_x$ impact acceleration. In Ewing CL, Thomas DJ, Sances A Jr, et al. (eds): *Impact Injury of the Head and Spine.* Springfield, IL: Charles C Thomas, 1983, pp 94–176.
99. Van der Sande JJ, Emeiss JJ, Lindeman J. Intravascular coagulation: a common phenomenon in minor experimental head injury. *J Neurosurg* 1981; 54:21–25.
100. Vicario S, Danzl D, Thomas DM. Emergency presentation of subdural hematoma: a review of 85 cases diagnosed by computerized tomography. *Ann Emerg Med* 1982; 11:475–477.
101. Vowles GH, Scholtz CL, Cameron JM. Diffuse axonal injury in early infancy. *J Clin Pathol* 1987; 40:185–189.
102. Yamaki T, Hirakawa K, Ueguchi T, et al. Chronological evaluation of acute traumatic intracerebral haematoma. *Acta Neurochir (Wien)* 1990; 103:112–115.
103. Young HA, Gleave JRW, Schmidek HH, et al. Delayed traumatic intracerebral hematoma: report of 15 cases operatively treated. *Neurosurgery* 1984; 14:22–25.
104. Žarković K, Jadro-Šantel D, Grčević N. Distribution of traumatic lesions of corpus callosum in ''inner cerebral trauma.'' *Neurologia Croat* 1991; 40:129–155.
105. Zimmerman RA, Bilaniuk LT, Bruce D, et al. Computed tomography of pediatric head trauma: acute general cerebral swelling. *Radiology* 1978; 126:403–408.

262

Neurological Evaluation of a Patient with Head Trauma: Coma Scales

Dennis A. Turner

Rationale for Coma Scales

The initial evaluation of the patient with a head injury includes serial neurological assessment for the detection of signs of head trauma and nervous system involvement and signs of deterioration. However, this initial evaluation may be brief, particularly if the patient is unstable, and may require multiple additional neurological assessments by both physicians and allied health personnel. A number of coma scales have been developed and refined to permit a rapid assessment of the patient's status and to increase the reliability of examinations performed by various personnel.[1,2,14,16–18,20–22] Although such scales are primarily an abbreviation of the full neurological examination, they may permit quantification of the patient's status, both to obtain a serial index and to predict outcome.[1,2,6,7,9,10,19] Thus, the rationale for developing and using coma scales is the need for sequential follow-up (particularly by allied health personnel) to assess potential worsening, the need for a standardized baseline measure for comparison with later measures to determine prognosis, and the need for planning a rational medical approach (such as intracranial pressure recording) to prevent secondary worsening. Thus, a coma scale (or the fuller neurological examination) may assist in the triage of difficult patients, in the allocation of scarce resources toward patients with a better prognosis, and as an early guide as to the aggressiveness of medical care. There is clearly a trade-off between sequential neurological examinations, which may be more reliable but less reproducible between examiners, and the simpler coma scale, which may decrease interobserver variability and provide a global view of neurological status but may not be sufficiently comprehensive.

The development of a coma scale is facilitated by the simpler neurological examination which can be performed on a stuporous patient. Using the neurological examination as a guide, Plum and Posner have detailed extensively the types of brain injury leading to impaired consciousness and alertness, the differentiation between various levels of stupor and coma, and the types of deterioration that may occur.[15] Critical neurological parameters include state of consciousness, pupil and eye movements, response to sensory input, best motor response, and nature of respiratory effort. Clear levels of nervous system function can be ascribed to each of these parameters, from no response to a fully appropriate response. The quantification of some or all of these parameters into an easily codable system is a coma scale. The first widely available (and now almost universally recognized) coma scale was the *Glasgow Coma Scale (GCS),* which was developed as a practical evaluation for repeated assessment of neurologically impaired patients.[20] This scale, shown in Table 262-1, is split into three main parts: eye opening, best motor response, and best verbal response. However, the GCS demonstrates a number of severe limitations, particularly the assessment of best verbal response in a patient who is either intubated or severely aphasic and the highly nonlinear and unequal summing. Two GCS scores may be similar yet reflect vastly different neurological examinations, because of the various ways components are added. Thus, although the GCS remains widely used and is often a key indicator of outcome (because of the critical use of this index), its limitations have led to the proposal of a variety of additional coma scales.[1,2,7,16–19,22] These newer scales include more of the critical components of the neurological examination than the GCS, for example, alertness and arousal indices. Thus, several new scales have been compared with the classical GCS and assessed in terms of outcome measures.[1,2,9,10,17–19,21]

General Examination in Head Trauma

It is widely recognized that systemic instability, such as decreased perfusion and hypoxia, may lead to a blunted neurological examination. Thus, the first aspect of triage of head injury is systemic stabilization, often including a rapid overall neurological assessment to note critical aspects, such as alertness, pupil size and reactivity, extraocular movements, motor and sensory responses, and respiration. Serial examination is critical during initial resuscitation and evaluation because the patient may show a decline rather than an expected improvement as the status is stabilized, suggesting a rapid neurological worsening that may require immediate attention. During and after the systemic stabilization of the airway

TABLE 262-1 Glasgow Coma Scale

Eye opening	
Spontaneous	E4
To speech	3
To pain only	2
No eye opening	1
Best motor response	
Obeys commands appropriately	M6
Localizes to stimulation	5
Withdraws from stimulation	4
Abnormal flexion response	3
Abnormal extension response	2
No motor response	1
Best verbal response	
Oriented and appropriate	V5
Confused conversation	4
Inappropriate words	3
Incomprehensible sounds	2
No verbal response	1

Total score = sum of eye opening + best motor response + best verbal response (minimum score = 3).

and circulatory system and the initial triage into major injury categories, a more detailed general examination may be performed. This general examination should include the external aspects of the body, including the head, neck, and back, searching in particular for neurological injuries.

Overt signs of head injury should be noted, including scalp contusions, lacerations, palpable fractures, changes in facial skeletal orientation, and drainage from the ear and nose, which may be related to basilar skull fractures. The several signs of occult basilar fractures may include Battle's sign (ecchymosis behind the ear), representing a likely petrous fracture; raccoon's eyes, suggesting an anterior basilar fracture; CSF rhinorrhea or otorrhea; and hemotympanum. This general examination should extend to the extremities, neck, and back and should include the thorax, abdomen, and perineal region. Clues may also be taken from the vital signs, such as unexplained hypotension or hypertension—particularly with bradycardia—which may indicate that the nervous system is the origin of the systemic instability. Acute quadriplegia (above the T1 level) is usually accompanied by an immediate sympathetic blockade and increased parasympathetic tone, resulting in bradycardia and hypotension from decreased vasoconstriction and blood pooling in the extremities. On the other hand, hypertension and bradycardia may suggest the attempt of the brain stem to maintain brain stem perfusion, in spite of severely increased intracranial pressure or direct injury. Tandem injuries, such as abnormalities of both the brain stem and spinal cord levels, may also be detected by unusual discrepancies among facial and upper and lower extremity responses. For example, a grimace on the face in response to a pinprick of the lower extremities but not accompanied directly by lower extremity movement may be suspicious for paralysis at a spinal level.

The reason behind the trauma and the presence of other contributing factors must also be considered. For example, a motor vehicle accident may follow a stroke or cardiac arrhythmia, yet the bulk of the neurological abnormalities may be due to the spontaneous event rather than the subsequent trauma. Thus, a severe hemiparesis from the time of the trauma may indicate a spontaneous intracerebral hemorrhage, since many of the trauma-related abnormalities may actually require some time after the injury to be fully noticeable or to mature. However, the initial postresuscitation neurological evaluation may still be clouded by the systemic instability, so that the examination at 24 h after the injury may be more accurate and predictive of long-term outcome than immediate scores. This delay allows both the systemic instability (e.g., hypotension, hypoxia) to be treated adequately and also leads to the maturation of the head injury to a more stable point.[8,9] However, early GCS scores and lowest postresuscitation GCS scores may also correlate with outcome.[8]

Neurological Assessment in Head Trauma

Circumstances surrounding trauma usually preclude a detailed neurological examination, especially the need to triage multiple injuries and the lack of patient cooperation. This leads to an abbreviated evaluation but one that can be repeated frequently to observe for improvement or deterioration. The initial neurological examination frequently leads to a conclusion of either focal or nonfocal changes. Together with the general examination for signs of trauma and the presence or absence of focal abnormalities, further assessment may focus on traumatic or spontaneous etiological factors. A frequent confounding issue with acute trauma is intoxication, due to ethanol or other neuroactive substances, which effectively worsens the clinical picture but clearly confuses initial examinations and may unduly influence early attempts at prognosis. However, these intoxicating influences may wane by 24 h, again indicating that this later evaluation may more accurately assess overall status. Because mental status can be assessed only occasionally in the population with more severe head trauma, the mental status may not be obtainable. The abbreviated neurological examination feasible in these instances is detailed below, including the elements of state of consciousness and awareness, the cranial nerve examination (particularly pupillary function), motor response and spontaneous movements, sensory responses that can be detected, the presence of normal and abnormal reflexes, and the status and rhythm of respiration.

State of Consciousness

Consciousness includes two separate elements: alertness, or arousal level, and the content of consciousness, or awareness.[15,17] These two elements are usually defined operationally, that is, by the actions that demonstrate them. Alertness may be identified by spontaneous eye opening, the patient's response to voice commands, and purposefulness of spontaneous activity and reactions to stimuli. However, as seen easily in infants, alertness may be separable from awareness and the ability to respond meaningfully to the environment; this separation is also seen in patients with aphasia and a decreased ability to understand and follow commands (in spite of being alert). The intensity of the stimulus required to bring the patient to alertness, similar to that needed to arouse a person from sleep, may represent the level of consciousness. Thus, a fully alert person responds quickly to voice, whereas a patient with depressed consciousness requires a stronger stimulus, such as pain, to become alert. The range of stimuli required to bring the patient to alertness may thus vary from voice alone to deep pain, with grades of lesser consciousness often being labeled as *clouding, delirium, stupor,* and *coma,* the latter requiring more severe stimuli to obtain a response. On the other hand, awareness rapidly becomes difficult to measure as alertness wanes, and full awareness of the environment and self (as assessed by the mental status) may not be detectable if consciousness is clouded significantly.

As defined by Plum and Posner, consciousness may not be affected by an insult to a single cerebral hemisphere but becomes progressively clouded as both hemispheres become involved, and particularly so if the brain stem undergoes pathological pressure or injury.[15] It is common in significant brain stem injuries, such as that following an irreversible transtentorial herniation syndrome, for spontaneous eye opening to occur after some recovery time, although no content of consciousness or awareness can be demonstrated. The eye opening may include day and night cycling, which is termed *coma vigil.* However, awareness may be preserved but the injury to the pons may be sufficiently severe as to block any effective motor output, except voluntary eye movements; this unfortunate condition is termed *locked-in state,* since the patient may be alert but almost completely unable to communicate. An EEG may differentiate this condition by the presence of a normal and reactive alpha rhythm, observed to be suppressed with eye opening. On the other hand, *alpha coma* indicates a persistent severe injury with preserved alpha frequency EEG, but neither awareness nor modulation of the frequency content occurs with eye opening. The role of aphasia and changes in mental status must be constantly considered in assessing arousal and awareness because difficulty in communication may be mistaken for either confusion or decreased responsiveness.

Pupils and Cranial Nerve Examination

Some aspects of cranial nerve function may be evaluated in a stuporous or comatose patient; this evaluation serves particularly to assay functioning levels of the brain stem using segmental reflexes. In this manner, the cranial nerve examination parallels assessment of other aspects of alertness, the motor and sensory examination, and respiratory capabilities. The aspects of the optic and oculomotor systems that can be tested include the pupillary light reflex, which requires the afferent link of the optic nerves and tracts to be intact as well as the parasympathetic oculomotor outflow for the efferent link. Extraocular movements may be tested by rotating the head in various directions (only if the cervical spine is not injured). The globes will be fixed at a particular point in space, regardless of head rotation, and the eyes kept passively at a certain gaze if the "doll's eye" response (oculocephalic reflex) is preserved. The extraocular muscles also receive a strong input from the vestibular system, so that caloric testing of labyrinth function also tests the efferent eye yoking responses, assuming that the vestibular system is intact. For the direct light reflex to be present, the mesencephalon must be functionally preserved, while the oculocephalic and caloric responses require the medulla and pons also to be functioning. The light reflex in particular is an excellent index of midbrain function, assuming that the afferent arc is intact. The pupillary fibers in the third nerve may also be compressed in the transtentorial herniation syndrome, leading to dilation due to the external location of these fibers on the surface of the nerve.

The trigeminal and facial nerves may be tested with corneal responses to a light cotton wisp or response to more severe facial stimuli, to assess for facial grimace and eye closure. Although hearing cannot be tested directly in a comatose patient (except by evoked potentials using audiometric inputs), vestibular function can be assessed through caloric testing (injecting cold water into one external ear canal if the tympanic membrane is intact) and through observing for abnormal extensor posturing reflex movements in the extremities. Because the increased extensor tone stems primarily from the lateral vestibular nucleus, such reflex posturing implies a functioning vestibulospinal system. Assessment of gag, swallowing, and vocal cord function will partially evaluate the glossopharyngeal and vagus nerves; this can be observed in manipulating the endotracheal tube in a comatose patient. The presence of a gag reflex implies that the medulla can integrate the reflex arc.

Motor Responses

The motor output of the extremities is tightly linked to the level of alertness and the functioning circuits within the brain stem. Normally a hierarchy of motor control exists, with cortical input being superimposed onto various levels of subcortical input, particularly enhancement of flexor tone by the red nucleus and the pontine reticular formation and driving of extensor (antigravity) tone by the vestibular nucleus. The output of these nuclei, together with corticospinal inputs, are superimposed on basic spinal reflexes, particularly myotatic reflexes and antagonist muscle inhibition. If this hierarchy is functionally decreased at any stage, then the less precise subcortical inputs may exert more final control over motor output, with the lowest level being the presence of spinal reflexes only, such as occurs following recovery from a spinal cord injury. This hierarchy of motor control, which can be observed clinically in many patients with head trauma, is divided into the following levels: purposeful movement, semipurposeful movement, flexor posturing, extensor posturing, and either flaccidity or expression of spinal reflexes (such as a mass reflex). Purposeful movement is rated as the relative force in relation to gravity and the examiner's resistance, with +3 representing motions against gravity only. On this scale, +1 represents a detectable motion, +2 a motion not sufficient to overpower gravity, +4 nearly normal strength, and +5 normal strength. Semipurposeful movement implies that movement may be purposeful in one direction (for instance, toward the head and neck) but not purposeful or directed to equally noxious stimuli in other directions (such as the lower extremities). Such semipurposeful movement often represents increased flexor tone, particularly in the upper extremities.

Flexor posturing may occur either spontaneously (without an overt external stimulus) or as a reflex response to noxious somatic input. Flexor posturing usually includes flexion at the elbow and extension at the knees, similar to that shown by a patient who has experienced a hemiplegic deficit from a deep hypertensive hemorrhage. This increased flexor tone likely results from decreased cortical control over the red nucleus and the reticular formation of the pons, with subsequent driving of motoneurons. Extensor posturing demonstrates often severe, full extension of both the upper and lower extremities and is dependent upon abnormal (unsuppressed) input from the vestibular nuclei to the spinal cord. Both types of posturing are reflex in nature with responses occurring both spontaneously and after painful stimuli. Because the lack of supratentorial control indicates a functional lesion at either the mesencephalic or pontine level for these types of reflex posturing, the motor output demonstrated upon examination shows a significant correlation with poor outcome measurements. As additional supratentorial motor control recovers with time after the initial injury, the increased flexor or extensor tone and reflex posturing may subside, leading to decreased tone overall before volitional control is established.

Sensory Responses

Sensory input may be considered a critical mechanism to demonstrate alertness, and the severity of the stimulus required to arouse a patient measures the depth of the coma or stupor. As in arousing a normal person from sleep, initially the examiner tries voice input at different levels of intensity, then attempts light shaking, and progresses to more severe pain if the milder stimuli fail to result in arousal. Deep or severe noxious stimuli commonly include nail bed pressure or nipple pinching, since skin bruising may result from direct skin pinching.

Reflexes

A variety of reflexes may be elicited in the abbreviated examination of the comatose patient. Special sensory and proprioceptive reflexes have been described above, including the pupillary light reflex, the oculocephalic reflex, and the vestibular caloric response. Myotatic (muscle stretch reflexes, evoked by tendon tap) are also tested, as are superficial reflexes, including the cremasteric and Babinski responses. As indicated above, the flexor and extensor posturing responses can also be evoked as a reflex, with pain input as the afferent arc. With various aspects of brain stem injury, pathological reflexes may be demonstrated, such as the posturing responses and the presence of a Babinski reflex. However, the cranial nerve reflexes and abnormal motor output may be the most critical in the comatose assessment because these are a direct assay, in a sense, of brain stem functioning. Thus, spinal reflexes may persist even after brain death and are of little prognostic importance.

Respiration

Plum and Posner have described levels of respiration, particularly the pattern of respiration and resulting systemic blood gas changes.[15] Diffuse, bilateral cortical dysfunction, sufficient to result in drowsiness, often may lead to the waxing and waning respiratory pattern termed *Cheyne-Stokes breathing,* which demonstrates intermixed shallow and deep respirations in a cyclical fashion. This type of respiration may result in overall hypoventilation and possibly hypercarbia, leading to increased intracranial pressure secondary to vascular stasis and blood pooling. As the level of injury becomes lower in the brain stem, spontaneous hyperventilation may occur at a pontine level of injury, with uniform, deep respirations, often resulting in hypocarbia from the hyperventilation. More caudal injury to the pons and particularly the medulla may result in ataxic or irregular respirations, which may be interpreted as agonal if not controlled. Clearly the next level is complete lack of respiration, although partial pressure of carbon dioxide (P_{CO_2}) is critical in determining the extent of the respiratory drive in effect. For example, a P_{CO_2} of at least 60 mmHg is the minimum necessary to determine if respiratory efforts occur, and higher levels may stimulate respiratory drive even further. Thus, damage to the medulla from the injury may result in a blunted response to hypercarbia, and patients occasionally may show ataxic respirations following removal from controlled ventilation, even with a negative apnea test for respiratory effort.

Summary

These various examination techniques may be blended into an overall assessment of brain stem function as assessed by arousal and content of consciousness; segmental reflexes (such as the pupillary examination; evaluation of long tracts coursing through the brain stem, such as motor output and sensory responsiveness; and respiration. As discussed below, salient features of the neurological examination are included in various coma scales, which more or less accurately reflect the overall examination.

Herniation Syndromes

Increased intracranial pressure is not harmful or dangerous unless associated with a mass lesion or shift of the brain; such distortion may result in a secondary ventricular outlet obstruction or CSF subarachnoid block, such as at the tentorial notch. The presence of a mass may compromise the brain and significantly decrease the buffering capacity to even minimal stimuli, such as a cough or Valsalva maneuver. This loss of buffering may lead to an irreversible, vicious circle in which CSF accumulation results in further mass, until the brain is severely compromised at various anatomical points of fixation. These anatomical tethering points include the falx cerebri, the tentorial notch between the middle and posterior fossa, and the foramen magnum. The frontal lobes may squeeze under the falx, resulting in a *subfalcine* herniation. More serious herniation of the brain occurs with side-to-side shift at the tentorial notch, usually secondary to a temporal mass effect pushing against the mesencephalon and displacing the midbrain to the opposite tentorial edge. If the tentorial notch is tight, then the ipsilateral third nerve is pushed on and the contralateral mesencephalon becomes tight against the notch, resulting in an ipsilateral hemiparesis. A central mass from both hemispheres may displace the entire mesencephalon inferiorly through the tentorial notch, resulting in a *central* herniation syndrome. This syndrome consists primarily of decreased consciousness and small pupils and may rapidly progress to a pontine level. The most inferior syndrome is coning of the cerebellum and tonsils through the foramen magnum, which may result in sudden loss of respiration and death from irreversible medullary compression. All of these herniation syndromes may progress rapidly to an irreversible state within a few minutes with a critical mass, and decompression after this time may not result in any functional improvement because of the irreversible brain stem changes.[15]

Use and Validity of Coma Scales

The abbreviated neurological examination of the comatose patient may be difficult to correlate directly with long-term outcome after head trauma. Therefore, codified scales of outcome have been developed, primarily for outcome prediction and for following patients during an acute hospitalization, particularly by allied health personnel. The oldest and most prominent of these scales is the GCS (Table 262-1), developed by Teasdale and Jennett as a practical scale.[20] Eye opening was included as a measure of arousal and alertness, and the best motor response as a measure of brain stem injury. However, the numbers assigned to verbal output are difficult to decipher for most severe head injury patients, in that endotracheal intubation prevents scoring on this subsection. Additionally, a patient may be very alert but aphasic, again giving rise to difficulties in scoring the verbal response section. Also, there are several different paths to arrive at the same GCS score, depending on eye opening and motor output; this implies that comparing various patients with different characteristics but similar GCS scores may be difficult. In response to these criticisms, multiple additional scales have been proposed, such as the Reaction Level Scale (Table 262-2), the Edinburgh Coma Scale, the Innsbruck Coma Scale, and the Coma Recovery Scale; validation of these scales has been studied primarily in relation to the GCS.[1,2,10,14,16–19,21,22]

Each of these alternative scales consolidates a few critical features from the neurological examination into a simplified index,

TABLE 262-2 Reaction Level Scale (RLS85)

1. Alert, no delay in response
2. Drowsy or confused; responsive to light stimulation
3. Very drowsy or confused; responsive to strong stimulation
4. Unconscious; localizes but does not ward off pain
5. Unconscious; withdrawing movements on pain stimulation
6. Unconscious; stereotyped flexion movements on pain stimulation
7. Unconscious; stereotyped extension movements on pain stimulation
8. Unconscious; no response to pain stimulation

particularly alertness, pupillary examination, and motor output. The usefulness of an index should be related to its correlation with outcome predictions, to increase the accuracy of early outcome predictions following an injury, when the level of aggressiveness of care can be altered according to the prognosis. However, the GCS does not include critical information about pupillary reactivity, other signs of damage to cerebral hemispheres, additional brain stem injury, and respiratory capability. Likewise, the Reaction Level Scale is highly abbreviated, although it does include an improved resolution of alertness. Additional features of the injury and examination that may improve the outcome predictions include etiological factors of the injury (such as a mass or surgical lesion), vital signs, and better descriptions of extremity strength and functioning. Of all these features, however, the best indicator of functioning brain stem levels continues to be the best motor response, although predictive accuracy may be increased with the addition of further brain stem indicators, such as pupillary reactivity and extraocular movement parameters.[2,3,9,17,21]

The GCS continues to be a valuable adjunct to all clinical investigations of severe head injury, particularly as a baseline for comparison of patients and later outcome studies.[1,8–11,13,18,21] Although validity of the scale has been questioned extensively,[17] newer scales require further validation, both in comparison to the GCS and with respect to outcome.[1,17–19,21,22] However, newer study designs have recommended using the GCS motor score in combination with age for randomization schemes, rather than the entire, ''lumped'' scale, which may be less representative.[3] These coma scales are useful primarily for study design and assisting with later outcome predictions; they are considerably less useful for measuring significant changes in the patient's clinical status over hours or days after the injury, except by allied health personnel as a rapid evaluation of the patient's status. Thus, unlike cardiac or respiratory function, the neurological examination cannot be codified easily or replaced with continuous on-line measures (such as intracranial pressure measurements[5,12]) because of the inherent complexity of the nervous system and the variety of responses of the brain to severe injury.

Brain Death Examination

Many severely head-injured patients already may have initiated a severe herniation syndrome as a consequence of the initial injury and early mass effect before medical intervention. Alternatively, patients may develop an irreversible picture of untreatable intracranial pressure but without a focal mass lesion, which also may lead to the vicious circle of herniation and secondary brain dysfunction. Once irreversible transtentorial herniation has occurred, then decompression of the mass lesion may do little to alter the brain stem injury, and the patient may persist indefinitely in a permanent vegetative state. The intracranial swelling and initial damage may lead to cessation of all evaluable brain function, which is termed *brain death.* A number of criteria for the determination of brain death have been published, but the outcome from this lack of evident brain function is extremely poor.[4] The declaration of brain death generally includes definition of a lesion (such as evidence of severe trauma on a computed tomography [CT] scan), lack of any known drug overdose, relative normothermia, and no identifiable brain function on clinical examination, confirmed by an apnea test with a P_{CO_2} of at least 60 mmHg at the end of the apnea test (usually performed with a 100% O_2 cannula in the endotracheal tube for oxygenation). The lack of identifiable brain function requires unreactive pupils, no oculocephalic responses, no responses to caloric testing, and no motor output or response to pain, in addition to the requirement for no spontaneous respirations. A number of confirmatory tests have also been suggested, including an angiographic or radionuclide study showing no cerebral blood flow and an electrically silent EEG. A critical criterion in many of the brain death guidelines is an additional clinical examination at 6, 12, or 24 h after the first one, to confirm that the condition is indeed permanent and will not suddenly reverse.

There are two primary reasons for declaring brain death. The first is for the possibility of organ donation. In this situation, the patient may be declared brain dead and the cadaver maintained so that individual organs remain viable until they are harvested. The declaration of brain death indicates the nonviability of the organism (as a functioning and living person) in contrast to the viability of individual organs, perfused by a functioning cardiovascular system. Brain death must be declared before organs are harvested.[4] The second reason for declaring brain death is for the removal of a patient from life support mechanisms when the outlook appears bleak and continuing medical care futile. The declaration of brain death implies that the prognosis is so poor that no functional survival can be expected, making further aggressive medical treatment futile and unwarranted. Once this state is reached and the patient declared to be a cadaver, life support systems may be removed if the cadaver is not appropriate for organ donation because of lack of consent or poor organ viability. If there is any question about the nature of the coma (i.e., no structural lesion identified on the CT scan) and possible reversibility (such as with a drug overdose), further observation time is warranted until the neurological status becomes clearer.

Adjunct Diagnostic Modalities

Electroencephalography

The EEG occasionally may be useful for diagnosing seizures in a comatose patient, particularly when the question of status epilepticus arises. Additionally, in some instances of coma vigil or persistent vegetative state, there are characteristic EEG patterns, such as alpha coma (an unmodifiable alpha frequency EEG pattern), which may confirm the lack of content of consciousness. The EEG may also be helpful in the declaration of brain death, although strict requirements for determining electrocerebral silence may be required because of electrical noise in intensive care units.

X-Ray Films and Ventriculography

Plain x-ray films may be useful for diagnosis of linear skull fractures, which are often missed on CT scans because of an odd plane of occurrence and lack of displacement of the fragments. Also, tangential x-ray films may assist in the diagnosis of depressed skull fractures, usually supplemented by bone windows on the CT scan. Ventriculography has almost been completely supplanted by CT scans and is primarily performed to evaluate CSF loculation within the ventricular system or the subarachnoid space, such as intraventricular cysts or septations and arachnoid cysts. The positive contrast medium injected for the ventriculogram may not fully enter trapped CSF spaces or may be delayed in emptying from such spaces, suggesting either a trapped or loculated CSF cavity that, if symptomatic, may benefit from surgical drainage.

Angiographic and Radionuclide Blood Flow Studies

Although severe head trauma is routinely accompanied by subarachnoid hemorrhage, this hemorrhage is likely due to pial oozing and rarely to a major vessel injury or rupture. Thus, the subarachnoid hemorrhage on CT scans following injury is usually of slight severity and is much less dense than that observed in a patient with subarachnoid hemorrhage from a berry aneurysm. However, occasionally an angiogram may be helpful to evaluate a potential internal carotid lesion, such as a carotid dissection or carotid-cavernous fistula. Additionally, an angiogram may help in deciding whether blood is flowing to the intracranial vessels to confirm brain death. Radionuclide blood flow studies may also confirm the presence or absence of supratentorial intracranial blood flow, although they are much less sensitive to posterior fossa blood flow.

CT and MRI Scanning

Although CT scans have become a standard and critical diagnostic tool in the evaluation of head-injured patients, magnetic resonance imaging (MRI) is not very useful. Most patients undergoing CT scans require emergent study, which usually cannot be arranged easily with MRI. Additionally, the life support equipment required for head-injured patients precludes the sheltered, nonmagnetic MRI environment. The newest generation of CT scans can image and process an entire set of brain CT scans within a few minutes, so the diagnostic results are available more rapidly than with an MRI imaging study. Additionally, the CT scan shows bone and fractures, which are common in the head-injured population, much more clearly than does MRI scanning, in addition to being much less expensive. Overall, the CT scan remains an important and easily obtainable imaging modality for initial and follow-up evaluations of the head-injured patient.

Outcome Scales and Relationship to Coma Scales

Two outcome scales are used commonly to assess head-injured patients at a time after the injury when the brain function is stable and most improvement has occurred. These include the Glasgow Outcome Scale (GOS, Table 262-3) and the Disability Rating Scale (DRS).[3,6] The GOS splits patients into five categories, ranging from death (1) to good recovery (5), whereas the DRS is more sensitive to milder head injuries. Both have been commonly used to assess patients at 3 or 6 months after injury, although 1 year may be a somewhat more stable end point. These two outcome scales have been highly validated and correlated with the initial GCS score and entry examination in multiple large population groups. Additional measures of cognitive function have been used, including tests of attention, memory, language, mental processing, and motor behavior, although no universal test has been applied to head injury patients, and many patients cannot undergo even simple neuropsychological testing because of the severity of their deficit. However, these tests are recommended, if possible in the context of clinical studies of head injury, as being uniform assessment measures across the highly variable patient population.[2,3,7,9,19]

A critical question arises soon after injury occurs: Which severely injured patients are likely either to die or to remain permanently in a chronic vegetative state? Considerable acute hospital resources, rehabilitation, and chronic care may be required for the maintenance of such a patient, for whom there is little hope of regaining any functioning as an individual. If such individuals could be clearly identified, resources could be applied to patients likely to have a better outcome. Unfortunately, apart from a patient declared to be brain dead, it is difficult to predict patient outcome by using current assessment techniques except in a general sense; it is also difficult to relay to families sufficiently detailed information to help them make informed choices about acuity of care. Although prognosis becomes clearer by 2 to 3 weeks after the injury, the patient already may have reached a chronic vegetative state but be past the initial instability of the injury. Thus, many decisions about aggressiveness of treatment are postponed until the chronic care stage, when changes in care level may have little effect on eventual outcome. Thus, development of more comprehensive early predictors of later poor outcome would be very helpful in the early, critical management of the severe head-injured patient, whereas currently the medical management is often influenced by the difficulty in clearly predicting outcome.

TABLE 262-3 Glasgow Outcome Scale

5. Good recovery
4. Moderate disability (disabled but independent)
3. Severe disability (conscious but disabled)
2. Persistent vegetative state
1. Death

References

1. Benzer A, Mitterschiffthaler G, Marosi M, et al. Prediction of nonsurvival after trauma: Innsbruck Coma Scale. *Lancet* 1991; 338:977–978.
2. Choi SC, Muizelaar JP, Barnes TY, et al. Prediction tree for severely head-injured patients. *J Neurosurg* 1991; 75:251–255.
3. Clifton GL, Hayes RL, Levin HS, et al. Outcome measures for clinical trials involving traumatically brain-injured patients: report of a conference. *Neurosurgery* 1992; 31:975–978.
4. Guidelines for the determination of death. *JAMA* 1981; 246:2184–2186.
5. Hickey JV. *The Clinical Practice of Neurological and Neurosurgical Nursing*, 2d ed. Philadelphia: Lippincott, 1986.
6. Jennett B, Bond M. Assessment of outcome after severe brain damage. *Lancet* 1975; 1:480–484.
7. Langfitt TW. Measuring the outcome from head injuries. *J Neurosurg* 1978; 48:673–678.
8. Levin HS, Aldrich EF, Saydjari C, et al. Severe head injury in children: experience of the Traumatic Coma Data Bank. *Neurosurgery* 1992; 31:435–444.
9. Levin HS, Gary HE Jr, Eisenberg HM, et al. Neurobehavioral outcome one year after severe head injury: experience of the Traumatic Coma Data Bank. *J Neurosurg* 1990; 73:699–709.
10. Lieh-Lai MW, Theodorou AA, Sarniak AP, et al. Limitations of the Glasgow Coma Scale in predicting outcome in children with traumatic brain injury. *J Pediatr* 1992; 120:195–199.
11. Luerssen TG, Klauber MR, Marshall LF. Outcome from head injury related to patient's age, a longitudinal prospective study of adult and pediatric head injury. *J Neurosurg* 1988; 68:409–416.
12. Lyons MK, Meyer FB. Cerebrospinal fluid physiology and the management of increased intracranial pressure. *Mayo Clin Proc* 1990; 65:684–707.
13. Marshall LF, Becker DP, Bowers SA, et al. The National Traumatic Coma Data Bank: Part 1: Design, purpose, goals, and results. *J Neurosurg* 1983; 59:276–284.

14. Murray GD. Assessing the clinical impact of a predictive system in severe head injury. *Med Inf (Lond)* 1990; 15:269–273.
15. Plum F, Posner JB. *The Diagnosis of Stupor and Coma,* 3d ed. Philadelphia: FA Davis, 1980.
16. Rowley G, Fielding K. Reliability and accuracy of the Glasgow Coma Scale with experienced and inexperienced users. *Lancet* 1991; 337:535–538.
17. Segatore M, Way C. The Glasgow Coma Scale: time for change. *Heart Lung* 1992; 21:548–557.
18. Starmark J-E, Stalhammar D, Holmgren E, et al. A comparison of the Glasgow Coma Scale and the Reaction Level Scale (RLS85). *J Neurosurg* 1988; 69:699–706.
19. Sugiura K, Fukuya R, Kunimoto K, et al. Significance of different levels of the Edinburgh 2 Coma Scale calculated from the outcome of neurosurgical patients. *Neurosurgery* 1992; 31:1023–1029.
20. Teasdale G, Jennett B. Assessment of coma and impaired consciousness: a practical scale. *Lancet* 1974; 2:81–84.
21. Tesseris J, Pantazidis N, Routsi C, et al. A comparative study of the Reaction Level Scale (RLS85) with Glasgow Coma Scale (GCS) and Edinburgh-2 Coma Scale (modified) (E2CS(M)). *Acta Neurochir (Wien)* 1991; 110:65–76.
22. Yates DW. ABC of major trauma: scoring systems for trauma. *BMJ* 1990; 301:1090–1094.

263 Radiologic Evaluation of Head Trauma

Chi Shing Zee
Hervey D. Segall
Sylvie Destian
Jamshid Ahmadi

Since its clinical introduction in the 1970s, computed tomography (CT) has become the primary diagnostic imaging procedure in the evaluation of head trauma patients. With the advent of CT, the roles of skull roentgenography (Fig. 263-1), cerebral angiography (Fig. 263-2), pneumoencephalography, and radionuclide brain scanning have diminished markedly. The advantages of CT over these imaging modalities (for example, in resolution, safety, and speed) have made CT an integral part of trauma patient evaluation.

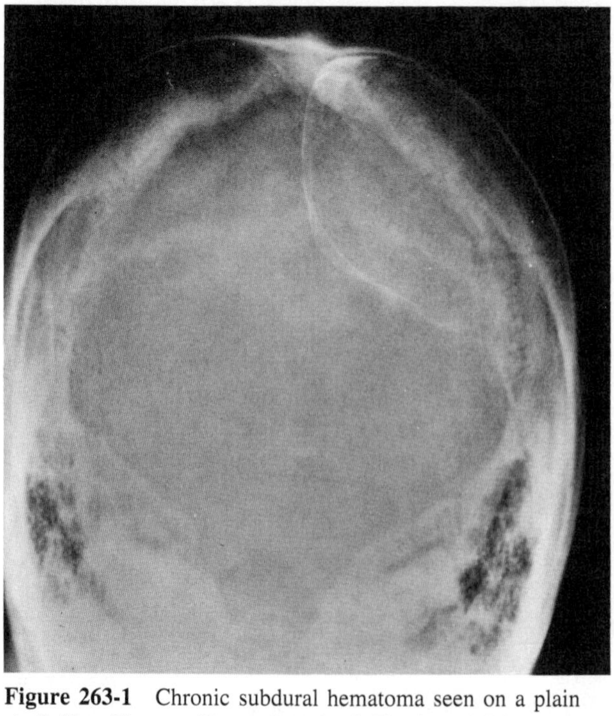

Figure 263-1 Chronic subdural hematoma seen on a plain skull film. The curvilinear rim of calcification visible on the patient's left side is consistent with the calcified membrane of a chronic subdural hematoma.

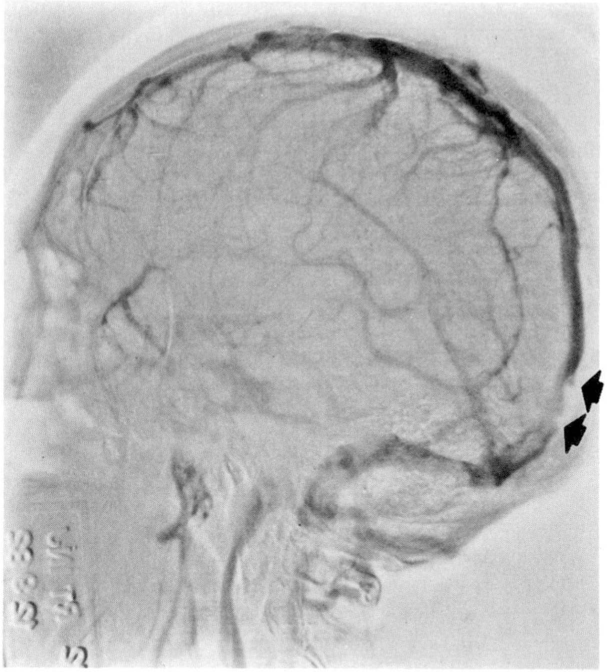

Figure 263-2 A depressed skull fracture compressing the superior sagittal sinus. This cerebral angiogram (venous phase) shows an irregularity of the superior sagittal sinus (*arrows*) just above the torcular.

The advantages and pitfalls of CT scanning for evaluating patients with head trauma are summarized in Table 263-1.

Since its introduction in the early 1980s, magnetic resonance imaging (MRI) has assumed a major role in the evaluation of CNS disorders. MRI was found to be better than CT at detecting traumatic lesions in head injury (Fig. 263-3).[7,12] Despite the success of MRI, however, CT has remained the primary imaging method in acute head trauma because of its sensitivity to acute intracranial hemorrhage and its speed. Monitoring the vital signs of acutely injured patients in the MR unit requires a completely different life support system, which is costly and not readily available in most facilities. Table 263-2 summarizes the advantages and pitfalls of MRI for evaluating patients with head trauma.

Technique

Standard transaxial CT is performed with slices angled conventionally relative to the orbitomeatal line. Our discussion will relate almost exclusively to the axial plane. Since motion is an important problem in scanning patients with head trauma, it is advisable to use the fastest scanning available. Newer instruments can complete a slice within a few seconds. The elimination of motion artifacts will outweigh any slight image degradation that may result from fast scanning. Motion can also be minimized by immobilizing the patient's head with tapes secured to the head holder. The use of sponge padding around the head holder is important in ensuring patient cooperation. Severely head-injured patients who have a depressed level of consciousness are usually intubated before CT scanning, so that total immobilization can be achieved by using muscle relaxants. This technique completely eliminates motion artifacts and also lessens the risk of hypoxia during the study.

TABLE 263-1 Advantages and Pitfalls of Computed Tomography in Head Trauma Evaluation

Advantages	Pitfalls
A noninvasive and rapid procedure.	Traumatic intracranial aneurysms are likely to be missed.
Helps define the nature of an acute mass lesion (hematoma, contusion, edema, etc.).	Other vascular lesions (such as carotid-cavernous fistula or arteriovenous fistula of the scalp) may be missed if contrast enhancement and proper window settings are not used.
Provides accurate anatomic localization of blood clots or other space-occupying lesions.	Unable to show findings related to neck vessel injuries initially.
Anatomic displacements and hydrocephalus resulting from trauma can be identified.	Depressed skull fractures may be confused with epidural hematomas if expanded windows are not used.
Delineates bony fractures as well as changes in the sinuses and soft tissues.	Depressed skull fractures at the vertex may be missed by axial CT scanning.
In assessing depressed skull fractures it is better than skull roentgenograms except for vertex fractures.	A lesion or lesions can be missed unless one has obtained a complete series of slices ranging from the foramen magnum to the vertex.
More sensitive than skull roentgenograms at detecting small amounts of intracranial air.	Motion may degrade the images.
Much better than skull films in anatomic localization of multiple metallic foreign bodies.	Artifacts can simulate pathologic lesions; they may obscure and prevent the identification of some abnormalities.

A complete examination is critical in evaluating head trauma. Contiguous CT slices should be obtained, including all areas from the foramen magnum to the vertex. This approach will permit accurate intracranial localization of traumatic lesions or foreign bodies as well as complete delineation of multiple lesions.

CT may be performed with or without the intravenous administration of a water-soluble contrast material. The decision to use contrast enhancement is dictated by a number of factors, but mainly by the clinical setting. Most acute traumatic intracranial lesions can be assessed without it, although in certain circumstances it may be most helpful. MRI makes it possible to readily detect vascular lesions without using a contrast agent and has significantly decreased the importance of contrast-enhanced CT for patients with head trauma.

The protocol we find most practical for MR imaging of patients with head trauma is as follows: (1) sagittal T1-weighted images (short TR/short TE spin echo); (2) axial multi-echo (long TR/short TE/long TE spin echo); (3) coronal T1-weighted (short TR/short TE spin echo). A unit with high field strength (1.5 T) should be used to evaluate patients with head trauma for two reasons: because it permits the quickest scanning and because it is best for evaluating blood and its temporal evolution. The capacity of MRI for multiplanar imaging is a distinct advantage over CT. This feature makes it easy to differentiate extra-axial from intra-axial

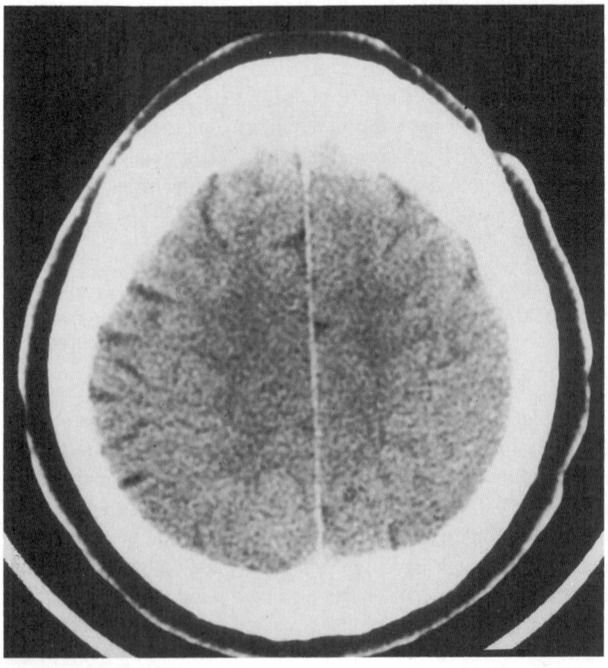

(*A*)

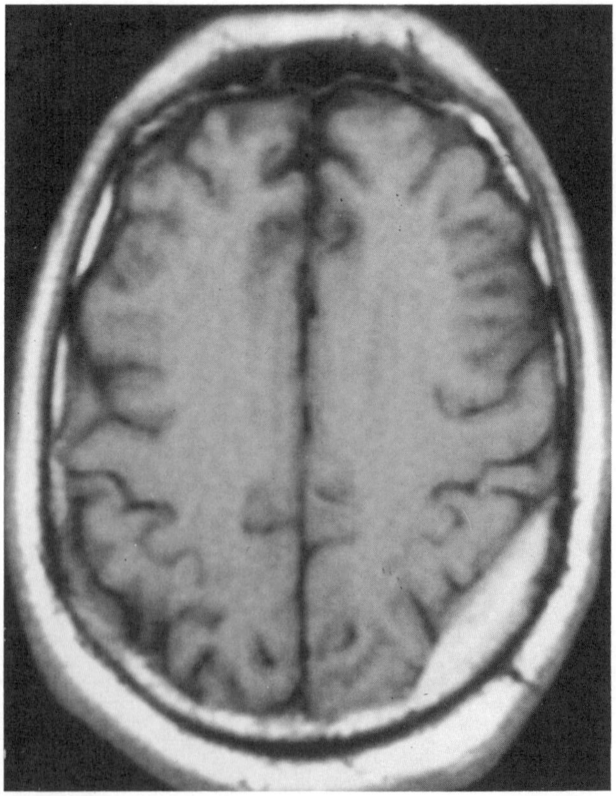

(*B*)

Figure 263-3 A subdural hematoma seen on MRI but not CT. *A.* An axial CT shows slight effacement of cortical sulci in the left parietal region but no definite lesion. *B.* An axial MR image (obtained in an axial plane slightly different from that for the CT) shows a high signal intensity subdural hematoma in the left parietal region.

TABLE 263-2 Advantages and Pitfalls of MRI as Compared to CT for Head Trauma Evaluation

Advantages	Pitfalls
Better at detecting subacute injuries, including shearing injuries, hemorrhagic and nonhemorrhagic contusions, and subdural hematomas	Longer imaging time
Better for localizing and assessing the extent of contusions and hematomas, owing to the capacity for multiplanar imaging	Less sensitive at detecting acute hemorrhage
In the case of small, subacute subdural hematomas, better at differentiating the hematoma from the calvaria	Special patient monitoring equipment required
Better at visualizing brain stem injuries	Bony fractures not well seen
Can visualize traumatic intracranial aneurysms without the use of contrast material; also easily reveals other vascular lesions, such as carotid-cavernous fistulae and arteriovenous fistulae of the scalp	Subarachnoid hemorrhage not well seen
	Small amounts of intracranial air may be missed

hematomas by MRI.[7] When vascular injuries are suspected, an MR angiogram may be obtained in conjunction with conventional MR images.

Injuries to the Skull

In general, we have found that CT is better than skull roentgenography for assessing depressed skull fractures.[2] Most such fractures are located low enough in the calvaria that axial CT studies can depict their extent and severity. The depth of the depression is usually easy to assess because axial CT images are tangential to most of the areas where depressed fractures tend to occur. Standard skull films frequently do not include a projection tangential to the depressed fracture, and the special effort needed to obtain such a view may not have been made.

However, axial CT does have some limitations in the evaluation of depressed skull fractures. Axial slices may fail to demonstrate vertex fractures. Fortunately, in these cases the depressed vertex fragment can usually be appreciated on skull roentgenograms. A scout view might also show such a fracture, or one could resort to coronal cuts. Overlying metallic foreign bodies may cast artifacts that interfere with the evaluation of important features underlying the calvarial depression.

Fractures of the skull base can be seen on CT evaluation, as can indirect evidence of trauma to the skull base. An air-fluid level may be demonstrated in the sphenoid sinus, indicating the presence of blood or cerebrospinal fluid. Persistence of the air-fluid level or clinical evidence of a cerebrospinal fluid (CSF) leak would suggest that the air-fluid level is of CSF origin. Although most CSF leaks resolve spontaneously, occasionally we have found the use of intrathecal nonionic contrast material to be helpful in evaluating chronic post-traumatic CSF leaks before they are treated surgically.[11]

The manipulation of window width is critical in studying skull trauma with CT. The term *window width* refers to the range of attenuation values between the ends of the gray scale. Any value above the selected window width appears pictorially in peak white; anything below appears in peak black. Thus, a narrow window will have a smaller range of absorption values between peak white and peak black, whereas a wide window will include a larger range of attenuation values.

The *window level* is the attenuation value that represents the center of the window. Like the window width, the window level may be adjusted by controls on the CT console. Some skull fractures will escape detection unless a wide window is used. We have also encountered cases in which a depressed skull fracture mimicked an epidural hematoma on scans displayed at standard window widths. Once the window was expanded, the depressed fragments were easily seen. Depiction of foreign bodies may also be improved by changing the window width.

CT may be superior not only to plain skull x-ray films but also to complex motion tomography, because it can delineate not only bony fractures but also changes in the sinuses and soft tissues. With an expanded window width, fractures of the lamina papyracea (Fig. 263-4), blowout fractures of the orbit, and fractures of the petrous bone can be clearly demonstrated (Fig. 263-5).

CT is also better than MRI for evaluating skull fractures. On MRI, the bony cortex appears as an area of low signal intensity on

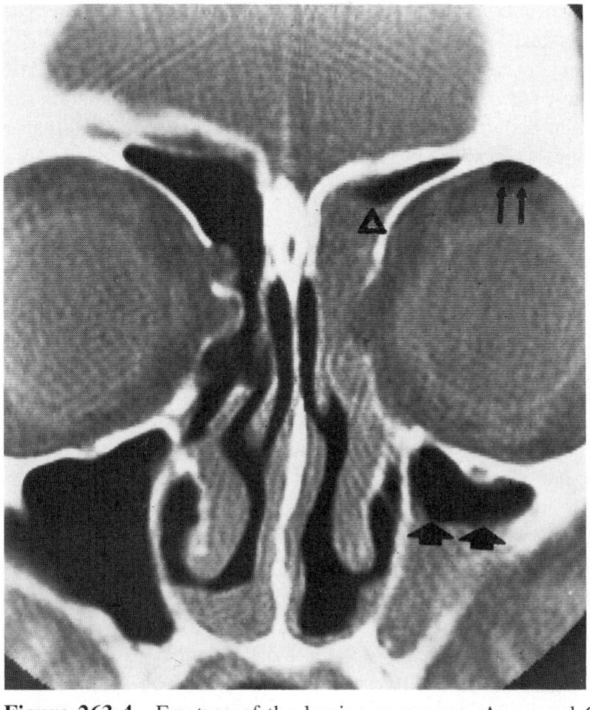

Figure 263-4 Fracture of the lamina papyracea. A coronal CT slice demonstrates an air-fluid level in the left ethmoid sinus (*arrowhead*), orbital emphysema (*small arrows*), and an air-fluid level in the left maxillary sinus (*large arrows*) secondary to a fracture of the lamina papyracea. An air-fluid level is also seen in the inferior nasal cavity below the inferior turbinate and above the hard palate on the right.

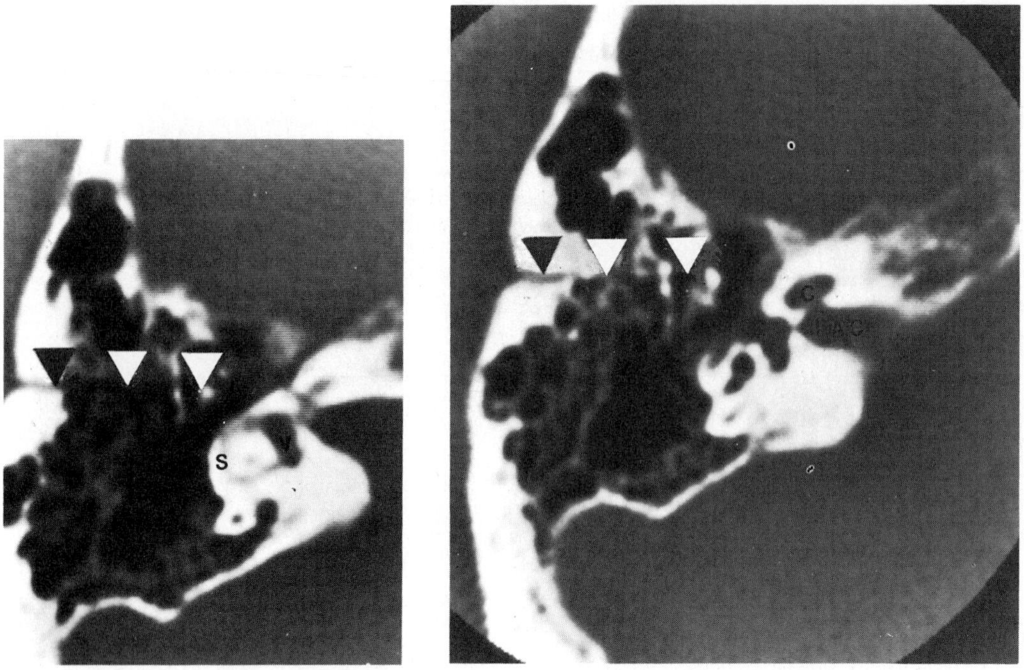

(*A*) (*B*)

Figure 263-5 Fracture of the petrous portion of the temporal bone shown by CT. *A,B.* Axial high-resolution scans show a longitudinal fracture of the petrous bone, extending into the middle ear cavity (*arrowheads*). The cochlea (C), vestibule (V), lateral semicircular canal (S), and internal auditory canal (IAC) are well seen.

both T1- and T2-weighted images. Detection of skull fractures depends entirely on the detection of a disruption in the bone marrow signal, which can vary in intensity as well as thickness throughout the calvaria. Skull fractures are easy to miss on MR studies. However, MRI may be better than CT for evaluating depressed skull fractures in the vertex region owing to its multiplanar imaging capability.

Intracranial Mass Lesions

Before the development of CT, angiography was frequently used to evaluate whether a surgically treatable intracranial mass was present. Although angiography can define the size and approximate location of a mass lesion, it cannot be relied on to differentiate hematomas from other space-occupying lesions, which may or may not require surgical evacuation. The ability of CT to distinguish different attenuation values aids in defining the nature of most mass lesions. For example, it is easy to distinguish edema from acute hematoma by CT. Thus, important management decisions can be made much more readily and with more confidence.

The major advantage of CT scanning is that it makes it possible to identify collections of blood in a manner previously not possible. New and Aronow have shown that whole blood with a hematocrit of 45 has an average attenuation value of 56 HU, which is greater than that of normal brain tissue.[9] Furthermore, these authors made the interesting observation that the high attenuation value of blood is due largely to the protein fraction of hemoglobin; the iron fraction contributes only about 7 to 8 percent of the attenuation value, and the contribution of the calcium in serum and red blood cells is negligible. In addition, it has been established that there is a linear relationship between hematocrit and radioattenuation.

Accurate anatomic localization of blood clots in the brain is now routine. Extracerebral blood collections can usually be identified as being subarachnoid, subdural, or epidural. Intraventricular blood can be readily appreciated as such (Fig. 263-6). Extra-axial blood collections will be discussed in detail in another chapter.

Acute traumatic hematomas appear in the brain as areas of increased attenuation. These areas tend to be fluffy, irregular, and poorly marginated compared with those from "spontaneous" hemorrhage. Also, intracranial hematomas in head trauma patients are often multiple and scattered in different areas of brain, whereas spontaneous hemorrhages are generally solitary.[11]

When an intracranial hematoma is monitored by serial scanning, the attenuation is frequently seen to rise by 14 to 28 HU over a very short period, which is consistent with clot formation.[9] Thereafter, the attenuation decreases progressively and at a variable rate. The area of increased attenuation in a hematoma usually persists from 1 to 3 weeks, and the subsequent decrease in attenuation starts at the periphery and moves inward. Eventually, the hematoma may pass through an isodense phase (having the same CT density as adjacent cerebral tissue), and finish by becoming an area of hypodensity. Usually, the latter state is reached after about 4 weeks.

Intravenous contrast enhancement may show a ringlike area of enhancement around the hematoma, which appears from 6 days to 6 weeks after the bleeding and disappears by approximately 2 to 6 months.[18] This ring of enhancement, a response of the brain to hemorrhage, represents contrast leakage secondary to breakdown of the blood-brain barrier and should not be confused with neoplasm or abscess (Fig. 263-7).

The complex biochemistry underlying hematoma evolution is

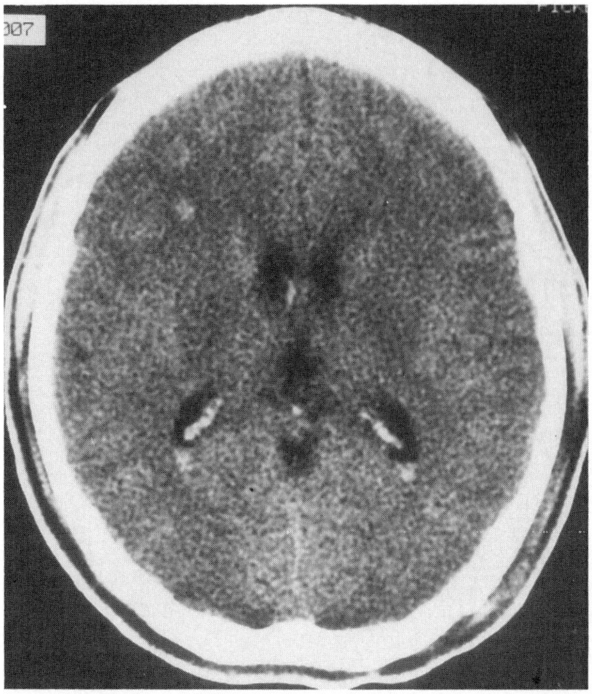

Figure 263-6 An acute intracerebral hemorrhage that was seen on CT. This axial CT scan shows high-density blood in the occipital horns of both lateral ventricles. Note the small hemorrhage in the right frontal white matter.

reflected in sequential MRI changes. In a simplified way, the evolution of a hematoma may be explained as follows. Hyperacute hemorrhage (the first few hours after the incident) involves proteinaceous fluid and appears as areas of hypointensity on T1-weighted images and of hyperintensity on T2-weighted images. In an acute intracranial hematoma, the deoxyhemoglobin in the blood creates areas that are hypointense or isointense to gray matter on T1-weighted images and of low signal intensity on T2-weighted images (Fig. 263-8). After oxidation to intracellular methemoglobin, the hematoma shows hyperintensity on T1-weighted images and hypointensity on T2-weighted images. When methemoglobin is released after lysis of the red blood cell membrane, extracellular methemoglobin exhibits hyperintensity on both T1-weighted and T2-weighted images (Fig. 263-9). As with CT, these changes start at the periphery and work inward. As the hematoma breaks down and macrophages begin removing blood products, a marked hypointense rim, consisting of hemosiderin phagocytized by macrophages, appears at the periphery of the hematoma.[6] This phenomenon can develop at anywhere from 13 days to 2 years after the hemorrhage.[8] In the clinical setting, the above-mentioned changes are frequently observed simultaneously, and various combinations of signal intensity patterns may be observed.

Usually there is little difficulty in distinguishing a peripherally situated intracerebral hematoma from an extracerebral hematoma. An intracerebral hematoma tends to have its widest point at some distance from the inner table of the skull, whereas an extracerebral hematoma will have its greatest dimension and its edges in close contact with the inner table of the skull. MRI, because of its multiplanar imaging capability, is better than CT for distinguishing intracerebral from extracerebral hematomas.

In patients with severe head injury who present with coma or focal neurological deficit, CT findings are sometimes normal. Superficial contusions of the cortex are frequently obscured on CT by volume averaging with the calvaria. Shear injuries of the white matter, unless hemorrhagic, are usually not identified. MRI is better than CT for detecting and characterizing subacute injuries, including shearing injuries. Contusions and subdural hematomas are better shown by MRI, as are old hemorrhages.[17]

Shear injuries commonly occur at junctions between gray and white matter but are also seen in the white matter of the centrum semiovale, corpus callosum, internal capsule, basal ganglia, brain stem, and cerebellum. In a clinicopathologic study of white matter shear injuries, Zimmerman and colleagues found that CT often shows generalized cerebral swelling, subarachnoid hemorrhage, eccentric hemorrhage at the corpus callosum, and hemorrhage adjacent to the third ventricle and in the white matter.[16] Focal, low-density lesions are hard to identify on CT. CT often fails to show more rostral shear injuries in the internal capsule and brain stem. MRI is far superior to CT at demonstrating shear injuries. Increased water in the form of vasogenic edema makes shear injuries

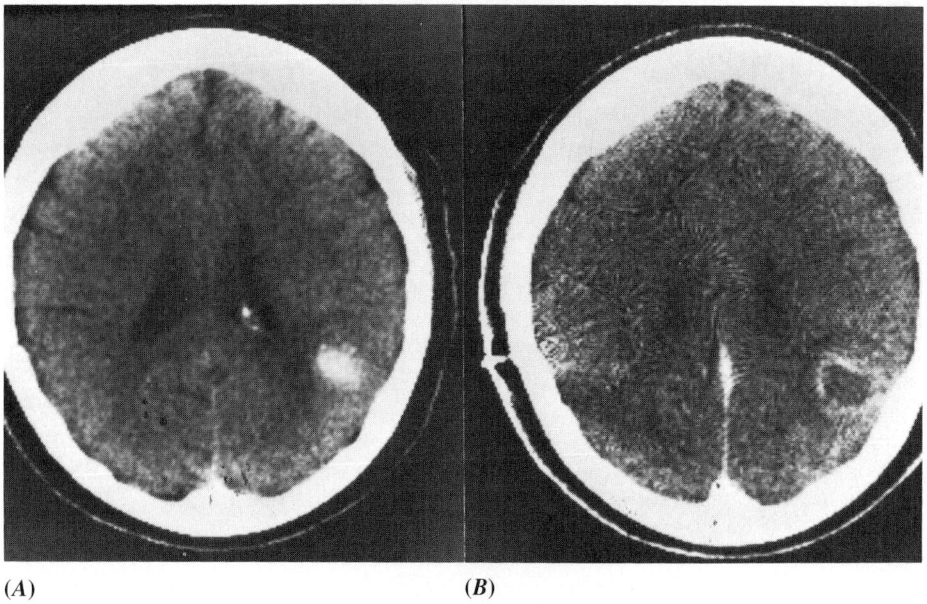

Figure 263-7 Ring enhancement in a resolving intracerebral hematoma. *A*. A post-traumatic intracerebral hematoma is seen in the left parietal region as a high density area on this CT slice. *B*. A follow-up CT slice (at a slightly higher level) obtained 2 weeks later shows a ringlike area of enhancement after contrast infusion in the same location as the hematoma (an unenhanced CT scan showed no abnormal densities).

(*A*) (*B*)

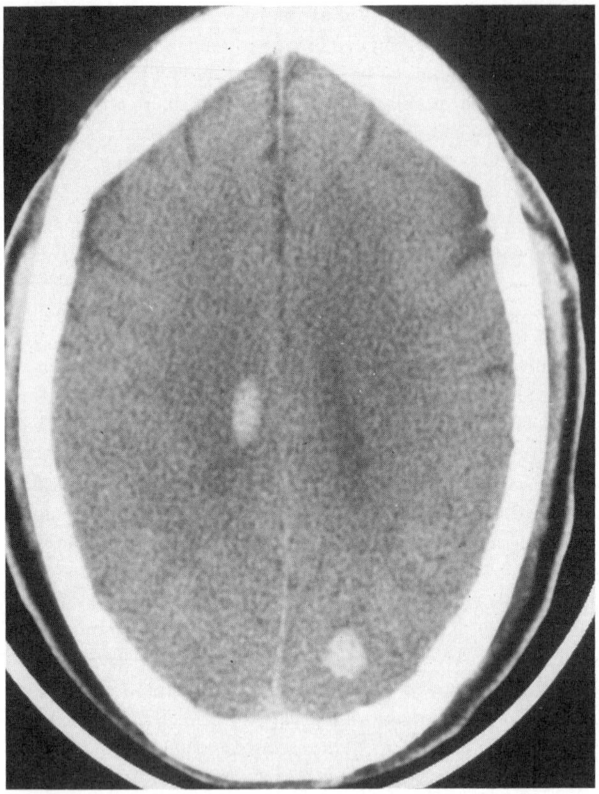

(*A*)

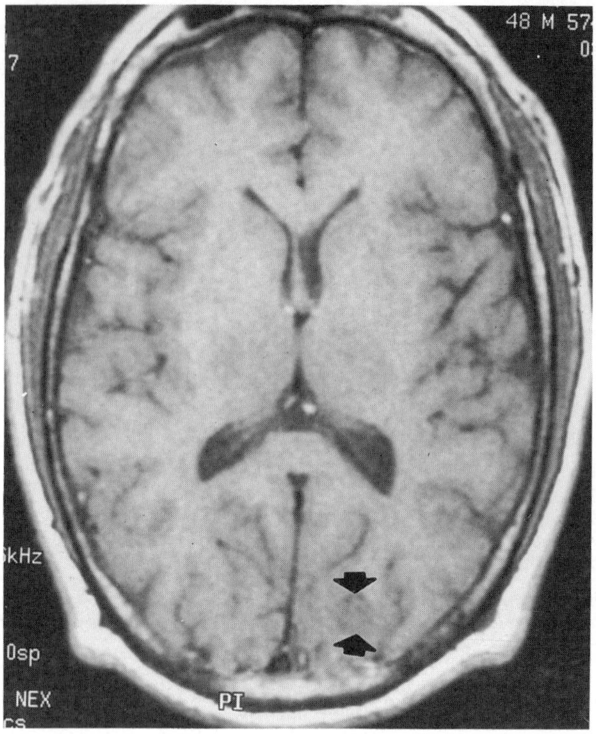

(*B*)

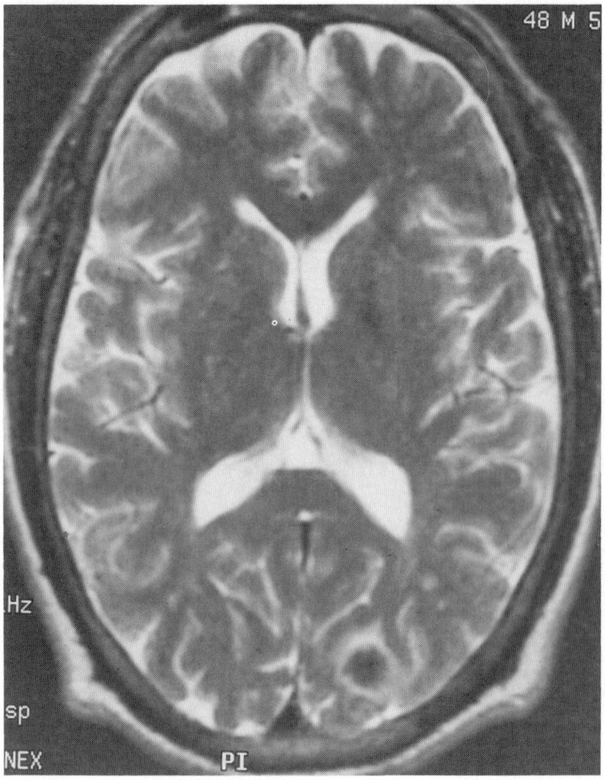

(*C*)

Figure 263-8 Intracerebral hemorrhage. *A.* An axial CT scan shows two small areas of hemorrhage. *B.* On this T1-weighted MR image, the left parietal hemorrhage (*arrows*) is isointense. (The right frontal hemorrhage is not seen because the image is in a different plane than the CT scan.) *C.* On this T2-weighted MR image the hemorrhage shows a low signal intensity consistent with deoxyhemoglobin in the acute stage of hematoma evolution.

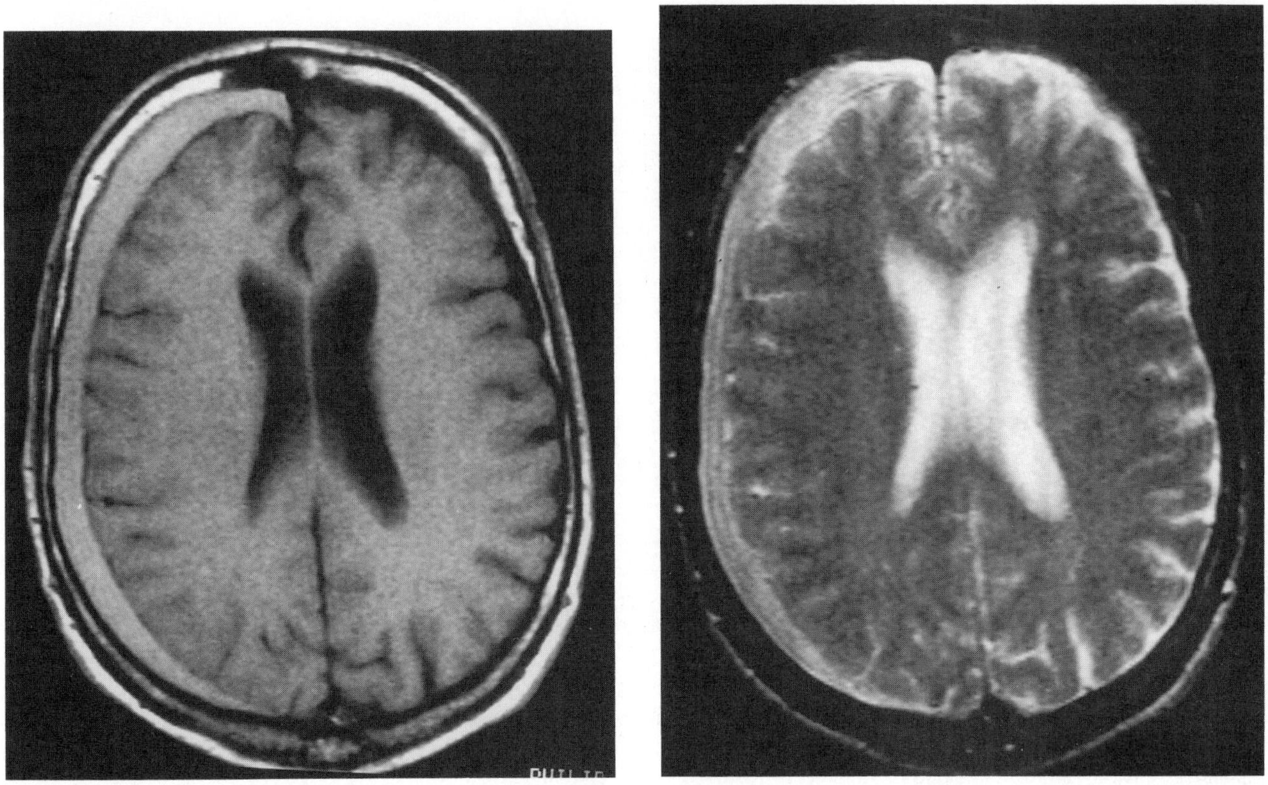

(*A*) (*B*)

Figure 263-9 Subacute subdural hematoma. *A.* This T1-weighted axial MR image shows a subdural hematoma of slight hyperintensity on the right side. *B.* On a T2-weighted axial MR image, the subdural hematoma is slightly hyperintense. This signal intensity pattern is consistent with a mixture of intracellular and extracellular methemoglobin and deoxyhemoglobin.

readily visible on T2-weighted images (Fig. 263-10). Areas of focal hemorrhage are also readily detected.

Cerebral contusion is a pathologic term that implies loss of integrity of cerebral tissue, usually without interruption of the physical continuity of the cerebral cortex or pia. Contusions are usually found where the dura is not perforated or lacerated. Minor hemorrhages that accompany contusions result from torn or ruptured arterioles, capillaries, or veins. The CT appearance of cerebral contusion may overlap that of intracerebral hematoma or cerebral edema, depending on the relative contribution of hemorrhage. Therefore, a contusion may have a "salt and pepper" appearance consisting of high-attenuation areas intermixed with low-attenuation zones.[3] As is the case with larger hemorrhages, high-density areas diminish with time, and the low-attenuation areas that remain persist for a protracted period.

Cerebral contusions are most common in the frontal and temporal regions but can occur anywhere. They may also occur in the side of the brain opposite from the direct blow, owing to the so-called contrecoup mechanism. Since cerebral contusion involves disruption of vessels, infusion of iodinated contrast may cause the area to enhance (Fig. 263-11.)[14]

Vasogenic cerebral edema occurs when fluid accumulates in the extracellular space as a result of loss of vascular integrity and extravasation of plasma proteins. On CT studies, cerebral edema appears as an area of homogeneously decreased attenuation (15 to 25 HU), which may be accompanied by a mass effect. Ventricular compression or obliteration can result. Also, the normal interface between gray and white matter may disappear. Cerebral edema is usually most intense at 12 to 24 h after the trauma. Edema may be mild and focal or multifocal and diffuse. It is to be borne in mind that low-attenuation areas on CT may also be caused by contusion or by cerebral infarction secondary to a vascular injury caused by the trauma. On MRI, cerebral edema shows as a loss of the distinction between gray and white matter; diffuse hypointensity is seen on T1-weighted images and hyperintensity on T2-weighted images.

The superior sensitivity of MRI for detecting subacute and chronic cerebral contusion is well documented.[8] T2-weighted images are more sensitive than T1-weighted images in detecting cerebral contusion. The increased water content in areas of cerebral edema and associated hemorrhage makes contusions easy to detect on T2-weighted images. The MR appearance of cerebral contusion varies, depending on the amount of hemorrhage in the area of contusion (Fig. 263-12). Hemorrhagic contusion is very dynamic, its appearance changing as the hematoma evolves. Nonhemorrhagic contusions change less. During the acute phase, the increased water content of the area of contusion results in hypointensity on T1-weighted images and hyperintensity on T2-weighted images. Cerebral edema increases over the first few days and then slowly decreases over the subsequent few weeks.

Acute generalized cerebral swelling manifests itself shortly after trauma.[15] This condition is most common in childhood and has certain CT characteristics and pathologic features. CT scans show compression or obliteration of the lateral ventricles, the third

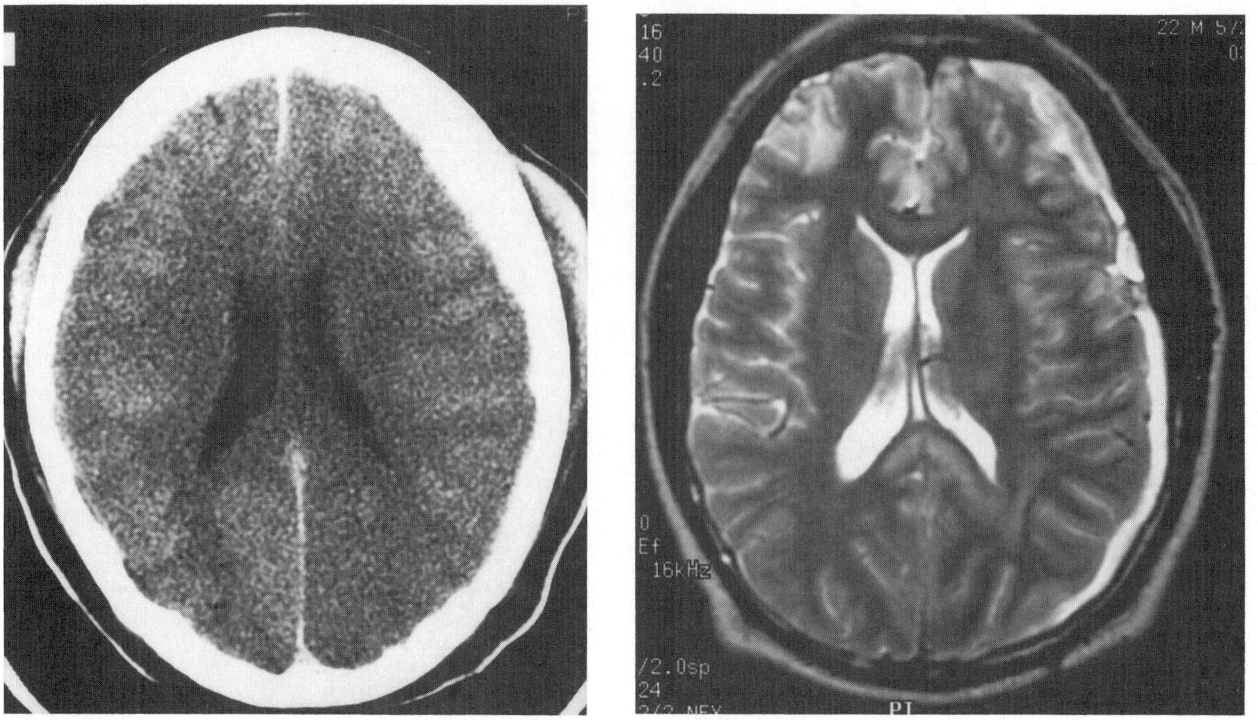

(*A*) (*B*)

Figure 263-10 A shearing injury of the splenium of the corpus callosum in a comatose, quadriparetic patient who only responded to deep, painful stimuli. *A.* An axial CT scan shows a small subdural hematoma on the left side. Obviously, the patient's clinical condition cannot be explained by this lesion. *B.* An axial T2-weighted MR image shows high signal intensity in the splenium of the corpus callosum and the left parietal white matter, consistent with shearing injury. The left subdural hematoma is much better seen than on the CT scan.

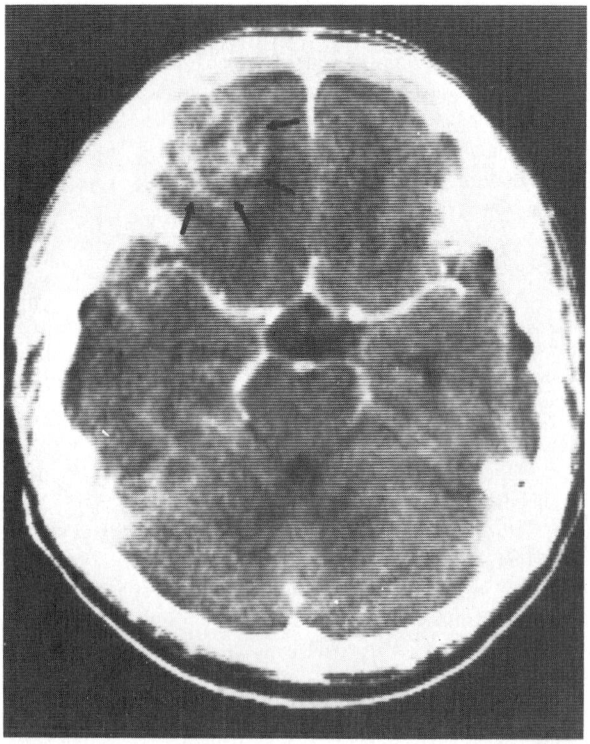

Figure 263-11 An enhancing cerebral contusion. A CT scan following contrast infusion shows a patchy, irregular focus of enhancement within an area of cerebral contusion (*arrows*). An unenhanced CT scan showed no abnormal density.

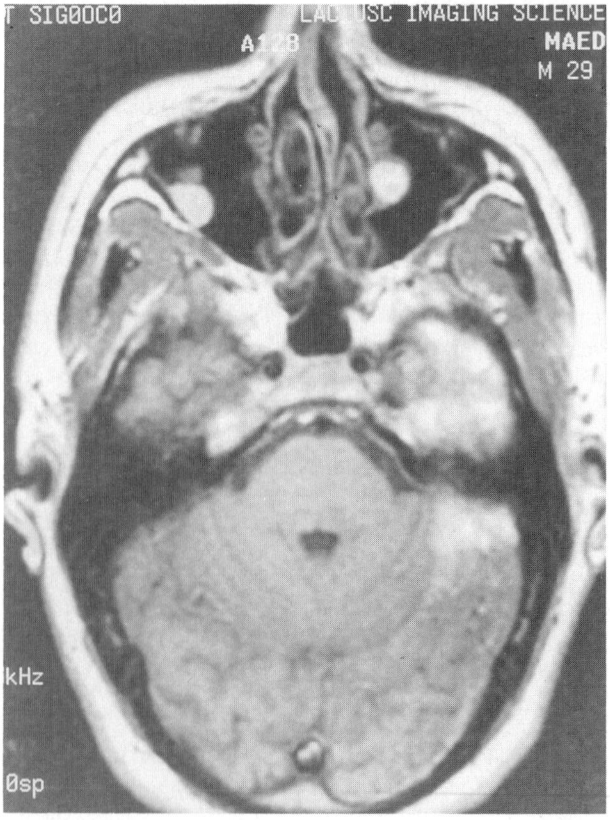

Figure 263-12 Hemorrhagic contusion. On this T1-weighted axial MR image, the lesion appears as an area of high signal intensity in the left temporal lobe.

ventricle, and the perimesencephalic and quadrigeminal cisterns. There is also an increase in the average density of the white matter (by about 3 HU) (Fig. 263-13).[15] The slightly increased density seen on CT in this condition appears to be due to hyperemia and correlates with increased regional blood flow as determined by xenon 133 radionuclide measurements. On MRI, cerebral edema manifests the changes described above. Clinically, almost all patients with acute generalized cerebral swelling are semicomatose or comatose. Many eventually recover with minimal residual dysfunction. However, intellectual loss, spastic quadriparesis, or death may occur.

Brain Stem Injury

Brain stem injuries (BSIs) may be divided into primary and secondary lesions. Primary BSI can result from direct or indirect mechanisms. The dorsolateral aspect of the brain stem may be directly contused by the free edge of the tentorium during severe injuries involving shear and strain caused by rotational acceleration of the head. Indirect primary BSI is caused by stretching and tearing of the small penetrating arteries supplying the brain stem, which most likely results from rotationally induced shear and strain that cause petechial hemorrhage in the brain stem.

Secondary BSI can arise from anoxia, hypotension, ischemia, or transtentorial herniation. Necrosis or ischemia develop as a result of mechanical compression of the brain stem. Direct hemorrhage can result from the disruption of the small perforating vessels in the interpeduncular cistern.

MRI is significantly more sensitive than CT for demonstrating, localizing, and characterizing brain stem lesions and associated cerebral lesions in patients with head trauma.[4,5]

Cerebral Herniation

Intracranial shifts of cerebral structures and cerebral herniation may also be identified using CT scanning.[13] The earliest sign of transtentorial herniation is encroachment of the uncus on the lateral aspect of the suprasellar cistern. This is followed by widening of the ipsilateral crural and ambient cisterns. With more advanced herniation, the cisternal spaces at the tentorial level are obliterated. There may be hydrocephalus of the portions of the ventricular system not directly exposed to the mass effect, which is believed to be caused by obstruction at the aqueduct or at the level of the third ventricle. Thus, dilation of the temporal horn, atrium, and occipital horn may occur on the side contralateral to the herniation when the alterations are sufficiently severe. Infarction in the distribution of the posterior cerebral artery can also result from vascular kinking and compression due to tentorial herniation and may produce CT or MR changes.

Pneumocephalus

Because of its low attenuation, air is readily visualized by CT. Air may be recognized on MRI as an area of low signal with adjacent paramagnetic artifact. Pneumocephalus usually results from fractures involving the paranasal sinuses or mastoid air cells, but fractures elsewhere that involve the entire thickness of the cranial vault

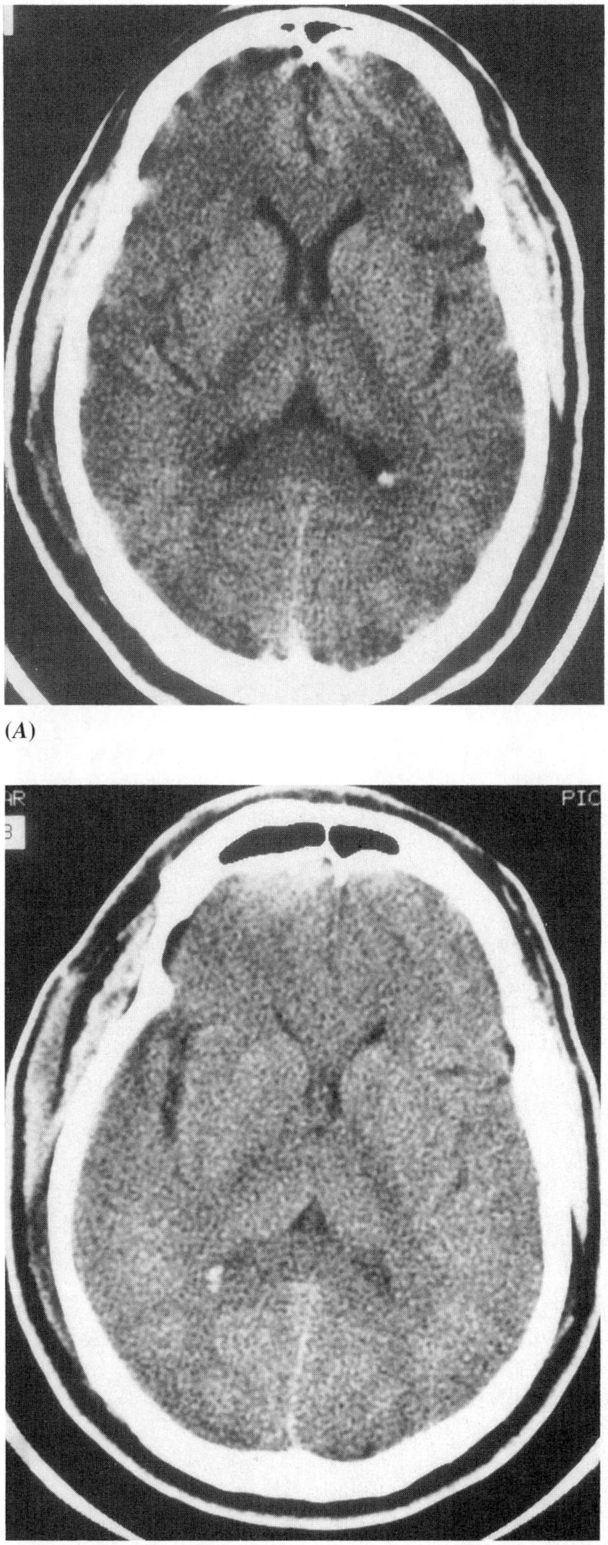

(*A*)

(*B*)

Figure 263-13 Diffuse cerebral edema. *A.* An axial CT scan taken immediately after the head trauma shows slight soft tissue swelling involving the scalp. No intracranial abnormality is visible. *B.* An axial CT scan obtained 24 hours later shows compression of both lateral ventricles and increased white matter density.

(scalp, skull, and meninges) may also permit air to enter the intracranial space. Air may be seen in the extradural, subdural, or subarachnoid space or within the brain parenchyma or ventricular system. Air is absorbed with time; therefore, if the pneumocephalus persists, a continuing cerebrospinal fluid leak should be suspected. CT may also dramatically demonstrate small but significant collections of air outside of the intracranial compartment. Rarely, the collection of air may expand because of a check valve mechanism producing tension pneumocephalus (Fig. 263-14).

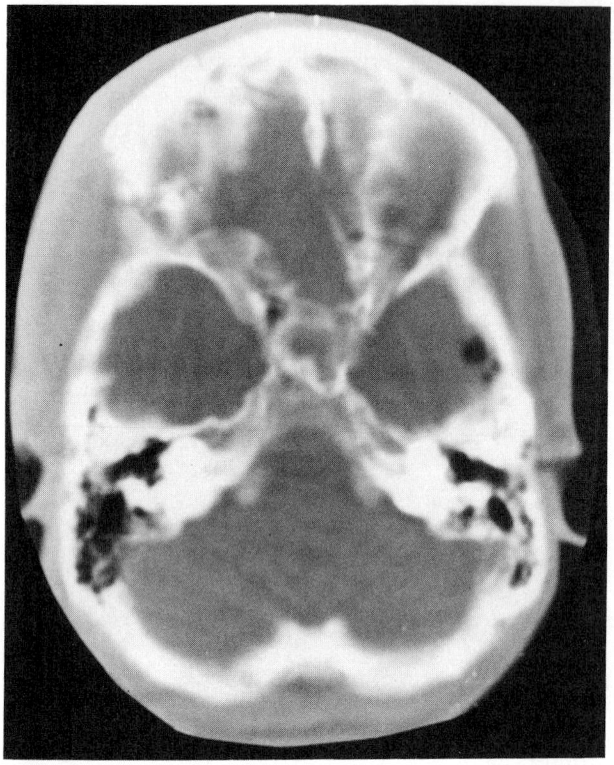

(*A*)

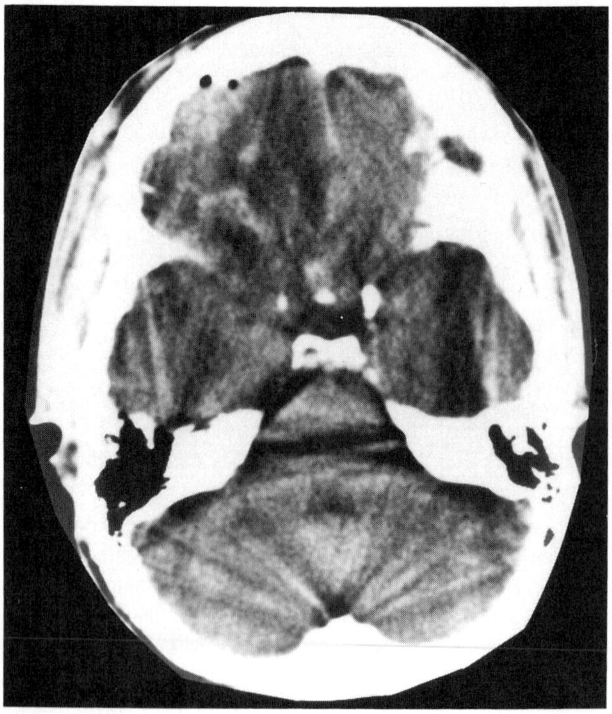

(*B*)

Hydrocephalus

CT and MRI are very sensitive tools for monitoring the size of the ventricular system. Subarachnoid or intraventricular hemorrhage caused by head trauma or penetrating injuries may, if severe enough, result in a communicating or noncommunicating hydrocephalus. A communicating hydrocephalus may begin as soon as the first week after trauma and may be revealed by serial CT or MRI. Thus, serial CT or MRI can give important information regarding the management of hydrocephalus as a sequela of head trauma. MRI is more sensitive than CT for determining the presence or absence of transependymal edema.

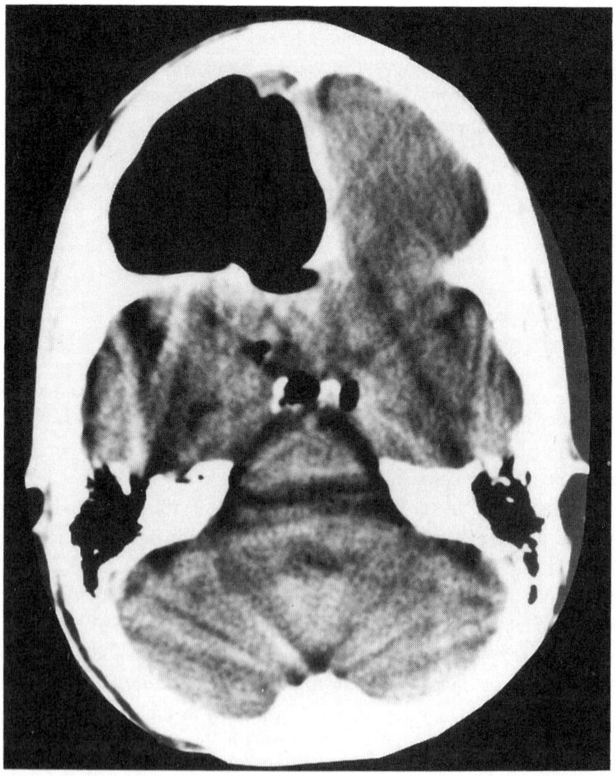

(*C*)

Figure 263-14 Tension pneumocephalus. *A*. An axial CT scan (bone window) shows fracturing of both orbital roofs. A small amount of air is visible in the left temporal fossa, and there is soft tissue swelling in the right scalp. *B*. An axial CT scan located slightly cephalad to the previous one shows a small epidural hematoma with a small amount of air in the right frontal region. *C*. An axial CT scan taken 3 days later shows a large air collection occupying most of the right frontal fossa, consistent with a tension pneumocephalus.

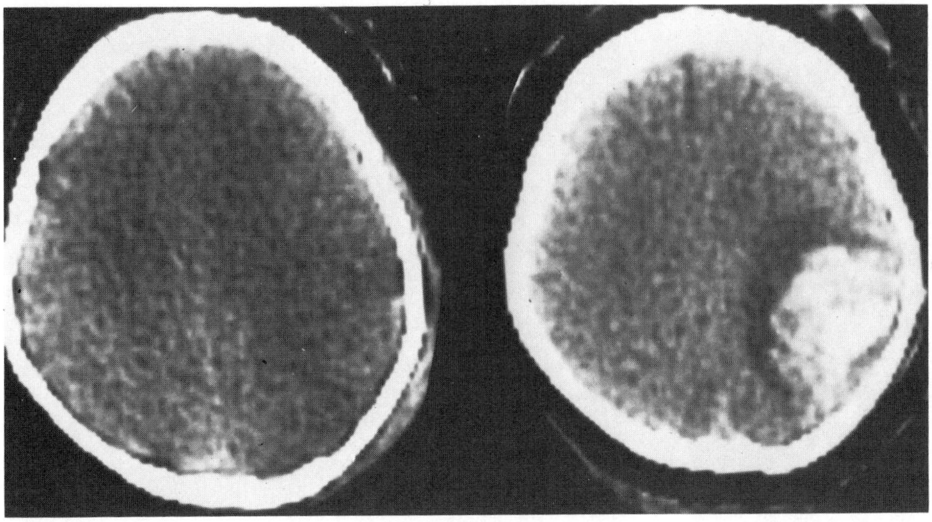

(*A*) (*B*)

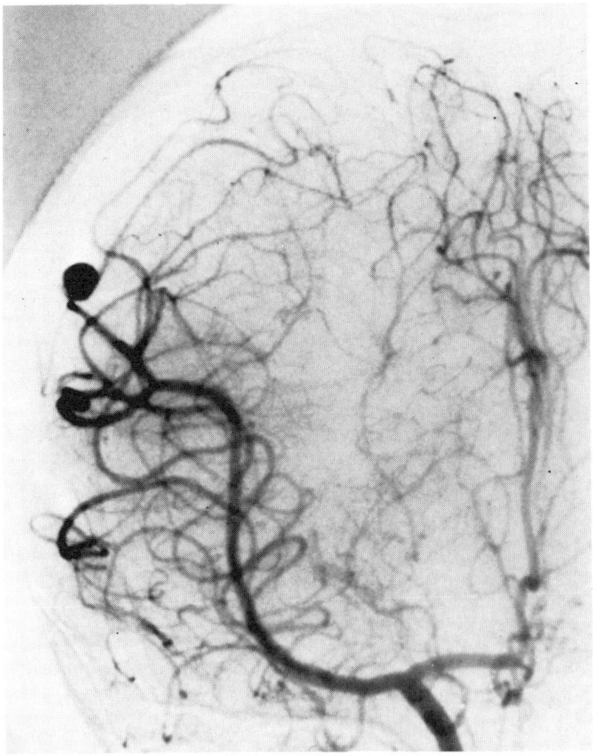

(*C*)

Figure 263-15 Intracerebral hematoma secondary to a traumatic cortical aneurysm. *A.* The initial CT scan following head trauma showed an area of low attenuation in the right parietal region, consistent with cerebral contusion. *B.* A follow-up CT scan taken 2 weeks later, before discharge, shows an intracerebral hematoma. Note that the hematoma appears to involve the cortical surface and comes into contact with the calvaria. A low density area surrounds the higher density hematoma. *C.* A cerebral angiogram demonstrates a peripheral aneurysm involving a cortical branch of the right middle cerebral artery. This traumatic aneurysm was successfully treated surgically.

Vascular Lesions

CT clearly has a number of advantages over cerebral angiography in the neuroradiologic evaluation of head trauma. However, CT can fail to show certain vascular complications of trauma. It is important to be aware that traumatic intracranial aneurysms can be easily missed if CT is the sole study and angiography is not performed. Before the CT era, nine traumatic cortical aneurysms were diagnosed at our institution in the 5 years from 1965 through 1969.[10] After the advent of CT, during the years 1977 through 1982, only three such aneurysms were found. No factors have been found to explain this statistic aside from the marked decrease in the use of cerebral angiography for head trauma.

Rumbaugh et al. described nine cases of traumatic aneurysm, all but one of which were associated with a subdural, epidural, or intracerebral hematoma, and four of which were associated with skull fracture.[10] The interval between the traumatic episode and the diagnosis of the aneurysm varied from a few hours to 3 weeks.

Figure 263-15*A* depicts the CT scan of a patient who presented with an area of cerebral contusion following head injury. Two weeks later, a routine follow-up evaluation (Fig. 263-15*B*) showed a hematoma at the area of the contusion. Because the hemorrhage extended to the surface of the brain, angiography was performed, revealing a cortical aneurysm (Fig. 263-15*C*). Follow-up CT evaluations are strongly recommended within 3 weeks of injury in patients found to have a skull fracture, intra- or extra-axial hematoma, or contusion. If there is any reason to suspect a traumatic vascular lesion, a cerebral angiogram should be performed. Needless to say, CT or MRI should be performed on any patient whose condition deteriorates suddenly after head trauma; however, if those modalities do not provide diagnostic information, angiography should be strongly considered.

Another vascular complication of head trauma is venous sinus occlusion. Although CT may demonstrate dural sinus filling defects, MRI and MR angiography are more sensitive and definitive. MRI shows high signal intensity filling the entire superior sagittal sinus, in place of the signal void seen in the normal sagittal sinus.

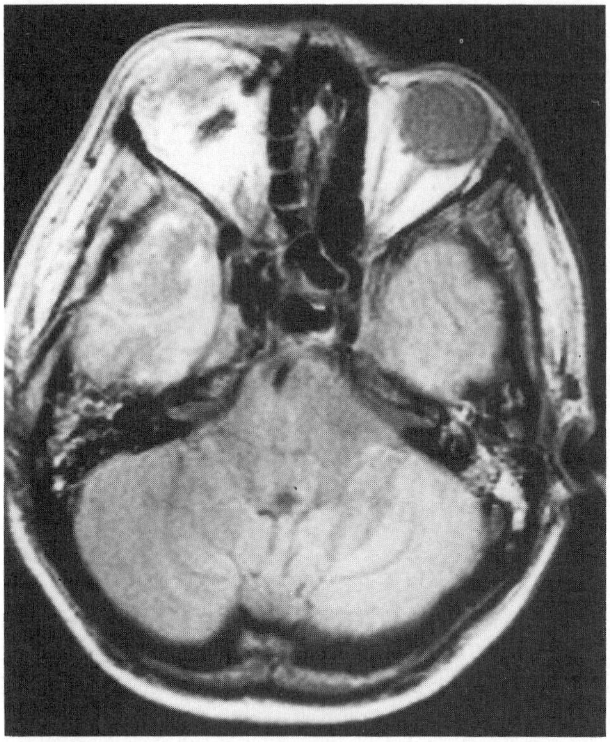

(*A*)

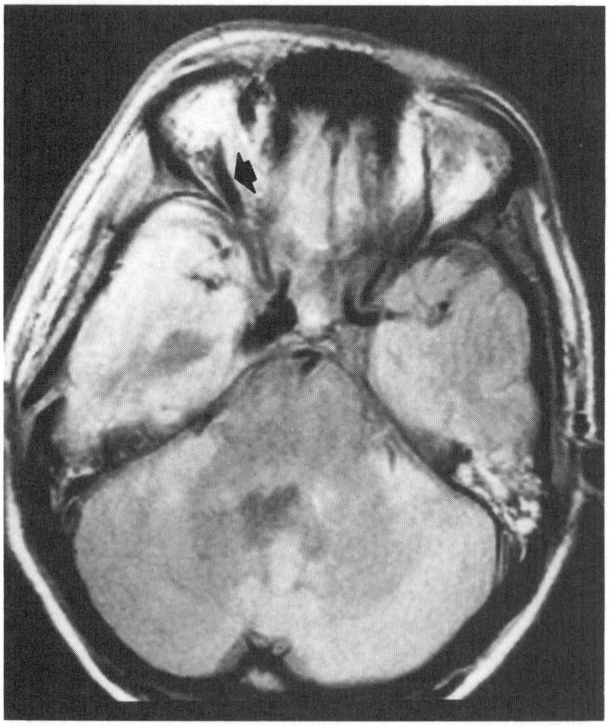

(*B*)

Figure 263-16 Carotid-cavernous fistula. *A.* An axial proton density weighted image shows an irregular area of signal void in the right cavernous sinus, which is much larger than the signal void seen in the left carotid artery. A segment of the dilated superior ophthalmic vein is visible. *B.* An adjacent axial proton density weighted image again shows a large signal void in the right cavernous sinus as well as the dilated right superior ophthalmic vein (*arrow*). *C.* An MR angiogram shows the right carotid-cavernous fistula as well as a large superior ophthalmic vein (*arrow*).

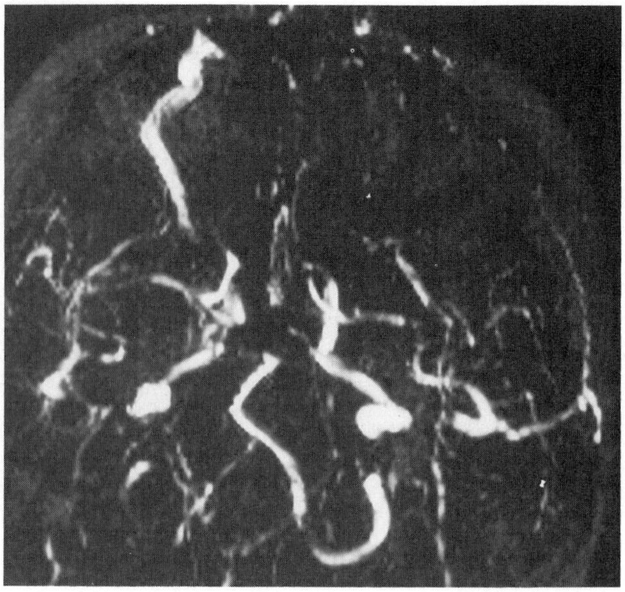

(*C*)

MR angiography is much less invasive than venography. Superior sagittal sinus occlusion may present with bilateral hemispheric hemorrhagic infarctions on CT or MRI.

Other vascular lesions, such as a carotid-cavernous fistula or an arteriovenous fistula of the scalp, might be suspected or even diagnosed with CT if adequate contrast-enhanced studies are obtained and properly scrutinized.[1] MRI can detect these anomalies without the use of any intravenous contrast material, as the mobile protons in the fast-flowing blood create a low signal intensity on T1-weighted, T2-weighted, and proton-density-weighted sequences. An MR angiogram can be obtained to better evaluate these vascular lesions (Fig. 263-16). Nevertheless, to appreciate important anatomic vascular details and to provide the information necessary for surgical treatment, a definitive angiographic study is required.

Some patients exhibit a profound localized neurological deficit after trauma that is out of proportion to the abnormalities seen on the initial CT evaluation. These features may also be observed in patients who have sustained a direct or indirect neck injury. These cases call for a high index of suspicion for an underlying vascular injury, and the clinician must bear in mind the pitfalls of CT in evaluating patients with vascular injuries. Blunt trauma to, or sudden distortion of, the neck may cause a thrombus or embolus to form in the internal carotid or vertebral artery, which could result in brain infarction; also, a hematoma in the soft tissues may lead to stenosis or occlusion of the carotid artery by external compression. Brain infarction caused by one of these mechanisms may not yet be apparent on an early CT scan.

Before the advent of MRI, contrast-enhanced CT was used to supplement the information obtained in evaluating vascular lesions associated with head trauma. It is exceedingly important to remember that intracranial hemorrhage found in a head trauma victim may actually have been caused by a primary underlying aneurysm or arteriovenous malformation, or even by a neoplasm, and that intracranial bleeding of this lesion may have precipitated the event leading to the head injury. Contrast enhancement, used judiciously, may lead one to suspect an underlying vascular disease as a cause of the traumatic event. Also, a number of other nontraumatic conditions might be revealed by CT. Incidental findings such as venous angiomas have been picked up in otherwise routine evaluations of head trauma patients, again with judicious use of contrast enhancement. With the availability of MRI, vascular lesions such as arteriovenous malformations, cavernous angiomas, venous angiomas, and neoplastic lesions can be detected without using contrast material. Intracranial aneurysms, when large enough, may also be seen on MRI as a round area of signal void. Failure to appreciate the possibility of incidental intracranial lesions may have tragic consequences. A case in point relates to a man who had a precontrast and postcontrast CT study for symptoms attributed to head trauma. The CT studies were interpreted as normal, and no further studies or neuroradiologic examinations were performed, despite the presence of headache and a stiff neck. The patient later died of a ruptured anterior communicating artery aneurysm. A review of the CT studies showed a rounded area of enhancement in the region of the anterior communicating artery. Presumably, had angiography been performed, the correct diagnosis would have been made and the proper treatment rendered.

The Value of Serial CT or MRI Scans

Serial CT or MRI scans can be useful in patients with small subdural or epidural hematomas treated conservatively. CT or MRI can clearly demonstrate the resolution or enlargement of these lesions.

Occasionally, an intracerebral hematoma may not appear until days or weeks after the trauma. Serial CT or MRI is very useful in detecting delayed intracerebral hemorrhage.

Finally, CT and MRI are also very helpful in ascertaining whether or not hydrocephalus is developing after head trauma. Other post-traumatic conditions involving the brain, such as atrophy, porencephaly, or leptomeningeal cyst formation, can also be detected by late imaging with CT or MRI.

References

1. Ahmadi J, Teal JS, Segall HD, et al. Computed tomography of carotid-cavernous fistula. *Am J Neuroradiol* 1983; 4:131–136.
2. Cowan BF, Segall HD, Zee CS, et al. Neuroradiological assessment of depressed skull fractures: axial CT vs skull roentgenography. Presented at the Annual Autumn Meeting of the Western Neuroradiological Society, Coronado, CA, Oct. 9, 1980.
3. French BN, Dublin AB. The value of computerized tomography (CT) in the management of 1000 consecutive head injuries. *Surg Neurol* 1977; 7:171–183.
4. Gentry LR, Godersky JC, Thompson B. MR imaging of head trauma: review of the distribution and radiopathologic features of traumatic lesions. *Am J Neuroradiol* 1988; 9:101–110.
5. Gentry LR, Godersky JC, Thompson B. Traumatic brain stem injury: MR imaging. *Radiology* 1989; 171:177–187.
6. Gomori JM, Grossman RI, Goldberg HI, et al. Intracranial hematomas: imaging by high-field MR. *Radiology* 1985; 157:87–93.
7. Han JS, Kaufman B, Alfidi RJ, et al. Head trauma evaluated by magnetic resonance and computed tomography: a comparison. *Radiology* 1984; 150:71–77.
8. Hesselink JR, Dowd CF, Healy ME, et al. MR imaging of brain contusions: a comparative study with CT. *Am J Neuroradiol* 1988; 9:269–278.
9. New PFJ, Aronow S. Attenuation measurements of whole blood and blood fractions in computed tomography. *Radiology* 1976; 121:635–640.
10. Rumbaugh CL, Bergeron RT, Talalla A, Kurze T. Traumatic aneurysms of the cortical cerebral arteries. *Radiology* 1970; 96:49–54.
11. Segall HD, McComb JG, Tsai FY, Miller JH. Neuroradiology in head trauma. In Gwinn JL, Stanley P (eds): *Diagnostic Imaging in Pediatric Trauma.* Berlin: Springer International, 1980, Chap 3.
12. Snow RB, Zimmerman RD, Gandy SE, et al. Comparison of magnetic resonance imaging and computed tomography in the evaluation of head injury. *Neurosurgery* 1986; 18:45–52.
13. Stovring J. Descending tentorial herniation: findings on computed tomography. *Neuroradiology* 1977; 14:101–105.
14. Tsai FY, Huprich JE, Gardner FC, et al. Diagnostic and prognostic implications of computed tomography of head trauma. *J Comput Assist Tomogr* 1978; 2:323–331.
15. Zimmerman RA, Bilaniuk LT, Bruce D, et al. Computed tomography of pediatric head trauma: acute general cerebral swelling. *Radiology* 1978; 126:403–408.
16. Zimmerman RA, Bilaniuk LT, Gennarelli T, et al. Computed tomography of shearing injuries of the cerebral white matter. *Radiology* 1978; 127:393–396.
17. Zimmerman RA, Bilaniuk L, Hackney DB, et al. Head injury: early results of comparing CT and high-field MR. *Am J Neuroradiol* 1986; 7:757–764.
18. Zimmerman RD, Leeds NE, Naidich TP. Ring blush associated with intracerebral hematoma. *Radiology* 1977; 122:707–711.

264 Resuscitation of the Multiply Injured Patient

R. Lawrence Reed II

Blunt vehicular trauma accounts for a large proportion of the injured patient population in current society. Of all injuries, roughly half result from vehicular accidents involving multiple injuries. Of these, a significant proportion have simultaneous spinal cord injuries. The leading single cause of death in multiply injured patients is head injury. Thus, the evaluation and resuscitation of multiply injured patients will confront the practicing neurosurgeon on a constant and probably escalating basis.

Over the past 15 years the initial evaluation and resuscitation of the multiply injured patient have been refined into established protocols by the Advanced Trauma Life Support Course of the American College of Surgeons' Committee on Trauma.[2] These protocols break down the process into several phases: the primary survey, resuscitation and treatment, secondary survey, and stabilization and transport.

Primary Survey and Resuscitation

In the primary survey immediately life-threatening conditions are quickly assessed and treated. Anoxia and cardiac arrest result in the cessation of oxidative phosphorylation within 15 to 20 s,[1] making the brain and other tissues depend upon anaerobic metabolism and the depletion of adenosine triphosphate (ATP) stores. In the trauma setting, it is often difficult to know when a loss of airway of anoxia actually occurred. Thus, the best response is immediately to provide an airway if an adequate one does not exist.

Airway Establishment

An immediate airway is required in acute airway obstruction, apnea, hypoxia, and rapidly expanding neck hematomas. Determination of the immediate need for an airway is based purely upon clinical grounds. Cervical spine films can be obtained before intubation *only* when there is no immediate need for an airway. Fortunately, the incidence of an unstable cervical spine in trauma is surprisingly low. A review of the San Diego Regional Trauma System trauma registry found cervical spine injuries in 58 (0.83%) of 6963 trauma patients admitted over 2½ years.[56] Yet the serious consequences of spinal cord injury require the assumption that the cervical spine is unstable until proven otherwise. If an x-ray film to rule out cervical instability can be obtained, then orotracheal intubation can be performed with greater security. However, if time does not permit the performance of a lateral cervical spine x-ray study, then orotracheal intubation is best avoided.

Aprahamian et al. created a model of severe cervical spine injury in a human cadaver and found that all maneuvers to establish an airway produced some positional changes in the vertebral elements, especially if no cervical collar was in place.[3] A normal-sized soft cervical collar or a rigid Philadelphia collar offered no protection, but a larger-than-normal soft collar minimized displacement. Nasopharyngeal tube and "blind" nasotracheal tube insertion appeared to be the safest maneuvers. Furthermore, in-line traction may offer no protection. Bivins et al. documented significant osseous distraction in recently deceased trauma patients with known cervical injuries when traction (6.8 kg by head halter) was employed during intubation attempts.[8] The similarity of these models to the clinical situation is speculative, given the severity of the neck instabilities studied and the absence of muscle spasm in the fresh cadaver. These studies probably represent the extremes that can be encountered with intubation attempts. Still, simple maneuvers, such as removal of foreign material from the mouth, chin lift, jaw thrust, and the insertion of oropharyngeal and nasopharyngeal airways, require caution for the cervical spine.

Esophageal obturator airways and the esophageal gastric tube airway were developed as tools for prehospital personnel to establish a more secure airway with minimal training. Unfortunately, the experience with these devices has not been entirely successful. Yet, recent design modification of these devices shows promise.

If the patient is not spontaneously ventilating, orotracheal intubation may be attempted. However, manual stabilization of the cervical spine is necessary during this procedure. Specifically, traction should be avoided because severe distraction and subsequent spinal cord damage may result if the spine is unstable. With proper precautions and manual stabilization, orotracheal intubation may be performed safely in the apneic patient. Orotracheal intubation with manual stabilization is often considered the gold standard for the provision of an airway,[2] but may be less safe than originally presumed.[3,8]

Blind nasotracheal intubation may be safer than orotracheal intubation with manual stabilization, but it is less likely to be successful.[68] However, effective nasotracheal intubation requires a patient who is spontaneously ventilating, and this may not always be the case. Additionally, nasotracheal intubation cannot be performed effectively if there is evidence of significant midface fractures and should be performed cautiously or avoided altogether if there are suspected fractures of the skull base, because the tube may be misdirected into the cranium. Thus, nasotracheal intubation without a prior cervical spine radiograph may not be an appropriate maneuver when an immediate airway is needed.[73] Direct access to the trachea by percutaneous transtracheal ventilation has been introduced and extensively studied. Although the technique is simple in concept, recent studies have indicated the potential for catheter misplacement or inadequate ventilation, especially in cases of airway obstruction and low flow rates; it is now contraindicated in cases of suspected airway obstruction. Other promising techniques involve tactile intubation and lighted stylet-guided intubation, although extensive experience with these techniques is lacking.

Surgical cricothyroidotomy was little used for over half a century, following a scathing condemnation by Chevalier Jackson in

1921,[41] in which he cautioned against the ultimate development of laryngeal stenosis. In 1976 Brantigan and Grow questioned Jackson's condemnation of cricothyroidotomy by reviewing their experience with 655 cricothyroidotomy patients.[11] The overall complication rate was 6.1%, and no cases of chronic subglottic stenosis occurred. Cricothyroidotomy has since been used with increasing popularity, perhaps partly because of its defined role as the ultimate back-up for airway provision in the Advanced Trauma Life Support (ATLS) Course.[2] It is still considered unwise to use it in children because of the higher risk of subglottic stenosis.[2] Furthermore, the technique seems to have a higher complication rate (39%) in the emergency setting and may be difficult for some to perform.[73] Part of this problem could be overcome by adequately training physicians and nurses in the technique. It is clearly unwise to use tracheostomy if an immediate airway is required.[2,73] However, recent percutaneous tracheostomy devices show some promise in simplifying the technique for direct tracheal access.

Ventilation

After an airway is established, breathing or ventilation must be assured by auscultation of both lung fields. Should either side be inadequately ventilated, assessment should be made for a mainstem bronchial intubation, other forms or airway obstruction, or potential life-threatening conditions, such as tension pneumothorax or massive hemothorax. If encountered, these should be corrected quickly, first by using a needle to provide an air vent through an intercostal space. Usually a thoracostomy tube should then be inserted because of the frequency with which pneumothoraces following multiple blunt trauma are actually hemopneumothoraces. In some selected cases of simple pneumothorax, however, it may be appropriate to drain the air with only a small multiperforated catheter.

Circulation: Assessment and Management

Once adequate ventilation is assured, attention is next turned to the circulation. The vital signs provide a quick and effective method to evaluate the adequacy of the circulation. The initial response to hemorrhage is a tachycardia that attempts to maintain cardiac output despite a reduced stroke volume. Subsequently, the pulse pressure narrows. This reflects the differential vasoconstriction that occurs in various tissue beds during hemorrhage in an effort to preserve vital organ flow. Once these compensatory mechanisms of tachycardia and vasoconstriction fail to provide a minimally effective circulation to vital organs, hypotension results as a function of decompensated shock.

The relative amount of blood lost and the fluid requirements for effective resuscitation can be estimated from the patient's vital signs and physical findings (Table 264-1). Initially, two large-bore intravenous lines are inserted, using antecubital or saphenous vein cutdowns if necessary. Isotonic crystalloid solutions (such as lactated Ringer's solution) are infused initially. Crystalloid solutions are preferred for the initial treatment of hemorrhage for two primary reasons. First, such solutions provide an inexpensive and effective means of expanding the circulating blood volume. Second, crystalloid fluid replacement is necessary for the effective management of shock because of the interstitial fluid deficit that usually accompanies cellular hypoperfusion.[83] Typically, crystalloids are infused using the "3:1 rule," in which three times the estimated volume of blood loss is administered as crystalloid solutions. This is because crystalloid solutions will distribute throughout the interstitium to replenish the interstitial loss, and the interstitial volume is roughly three times greater than blood volume in the body's fluid composition.

Should a class III or IV hemorrhage be present (see Table 264-1), blood transfusion is added to the crystalloid infusion. The signs of a class III or IV hemorrhage indicate inadequate organ function, primarily as a result of reduced circulatory oxygen delivery. Therefore, blood is given to increase oxygen-carrying capacity. Type-specific or O-negative blood are acceptable alternatives if the patient has not been adequately cross-matched and shows signs of a class III or more severe hemorrhage. All infused fluids should be warmed because massive infusions of refrigerated fluids or fluids stored at room temperature can produce a profound hypothermia, with resultant coagulopathies and dysrhythmias. Crystalloid solutions can be warmed in a microwave oven, but rapid infusion of blood products usually requires a rapid warming infuser, as microwaves usually denature protein structures.

Over the past 3 decades controversy has raged about the choice of crystalloid or colloid solutions. Colloid solutions seem to resuscitate to identical physiological end points with a smaller volume of infusate, and thus may appear to be more effective than crystalloids. Yet colloid solutions are typically 40 to 80 times more expensive than crystalloids. Because clinical comparison studies have failed to show any significant difference in outcomes—certainly none that would justify such a huge difference in costs—crystalloid solutions are usually adequate.

TABLE 264-1 Estimated Fluid and Blood Requirements Based on Initial Presentation

	Class of Hemorrhage			
Physiologic Indicator	**I**	**II**	**III**	**IV**
Blood loss (ml)	<750	750–1,500	1,500–2,000	>2,000
Blood loss (% blood volume)	<15%	15–30%	30–40%	>40%
Pulse rate	<100	>100	>120	≥140
Blood pressure	Normal	Normal	↓	↓
Pulse pressure	Normal or ↑	↓	↓	↓
Capillary refill test	Normal	+	+	+
Respiratory rate (breaths/min)	14–20	20–30	30–40	>35
Urine output (ml/h)	≥30	20–30	5–15	Negligible
Mental status	Slightly anxious	Mildly anxious	Anxious, confused	Confused, lethargic
Fluid replacement (3:1 rule)	Crystalloid	Crystalloid	Crystalloid and blood	Crystalloid and blood

Source: Adapted from the Advanced Trauma Life Support Course for Physicians.[2]

Yet, there remain some residual questions about the potential advantages of using colloid solutions in certain patients. It may be advantageous to administer colloid solutions preferentially to patients with associated head injuries to minimize cerebral edema. Although clinical evidence is insufficient to defend this approach, some experimental work supports the concept, especially with the use of agents such as hydroxyethyl starch.[91] In comparison to new agents, traditional albumin-containing colloid solutions exert relatively weak colloid effects. In the pulmonary circulation especially, albumin can diffuse through the normal pulmonary capillary endothelium, producing an interstitial albumin concentration that is roughly 60 to 70 percent of normal plasma concentration.[17] In contrast, newer, larger synthetic colloids, such as hydroxyethyl starch, seem to be less permeable across normal and injured endothelium.[34,69,102,103] Clinicians occasionally express concern that the use of colloid agents in the presence of capillary damage will promote leakage of the colloid agent into the interstitium and a resultant pull of fluid into the interstitium. Although such interstitial leakage certainly can occur, the interstitial concentration will never exceed circulating plasma concentrations; such a condition would imply active transport of the colloid agent into the interstitium, which has not been described.[54] Furthermore, it seems that larger synthetic colloids leak into the interstitium less ably than does albumin under conditions of capillary damage. These synthetic agents are also usually cheaper than albumin-containing solutions. Thus, they may offer advantages to patients with intracranial injury, although no clinical experience has been published. Additionally, experimental work indicates that the return of electrocortical activity following hemorrhage may improve when the subject is resuscitated with hydroxyethyl starch.[16]

Concerns have been expressed about the potential anticoagulant effects of synthetic colloids. This effect is seen with dextran-containing solutions, in which platelet aggregation seems to be inhibited. Hydroxyethyl starch appears to have a smaller anticoagulant effect than dextran.[87] Anecdotal reports exist of severe coagulopathies that followed the administration of large volumes of hydroxyethyl starch.[13,52] It is difficult to know whether concern about these reports is justified. Extensive analysis of the potential anticoagulant properties of hydroxyethyl starch indicates that most, if not all, of the effects seen are purely dilutional.[57,96] Such effects can be seen with any resuscitative fluids (other than clottable blood component solutions, such as fresh-frozen plasma or platelet concentrates) when they are rapidly infused in massive volumes. In fact, one comparison trial of cardiopulmonary bypass priming solutions found that albumin had a more adverse effect upon platelet aggregation than did hydroxyethyl starch.[81] Prospective clinical trials failed to show any significant clinical bleeding problems when large volumes of hydroxyethyl starch were infused.[14,19,33,39,48,97]

Another alternative for fluid resuscitation of shock is the use of hypertonic (7.5%) saline. This solution seems to restore vital signs effectively following a period of hemorrhagic shock, but it must be combined with an agent such as dextran to provide an effect that is more than transient.[85] This solution may also benefit the head-injured patient in that its hypertonicity may help minimize the cerebral edema that appears to result from more hypo-oncotic isotonic resuscitation.[16,74] Hypertonic saline has been shown to effectively lower intracranial pressure. However, it possesses vasodilator properties that may reduce mean arterial pressure, thus resulting in a lower cerebral perfusion pressure. This effect of hypertonic saline has been shown to correlate with inferior electrocortical recovery after hemorrhage, in comparison with hydroxyethyl starch.[16] Interestingly, hypertonic saline appears to exacerbate active bleeding through vasodilation if administered soon after hemorrhage starts, although this effect may not persist.[49–51] It also possesses significant intrinsic anticoagulant effects when excessive amounts are administered, probably through the effects of ionic potential on enzymatic action.[38,75] Thus, its use in head-injured patients should be studied further before it is recommended.

Secondary Survey

After the primary survey is completed and the initial resuscitation is underway, attention is turned to a secondary survey involving a more detailed examination of individual body regions. Throughout this evaluation, however, one should be warily vigilant to ensure that the patient's cardiorespiratory status remains stable: the airway must be maintained, ventilation and oxygenation ensured, and circulatory status monitored. Sudden deteriorations before a thorough evaluation can be completed are not unusual.

The secondary survey should be completed quickly and efficiently to determine promptly the evaluation and treatment priorities for the multiple injuries that could coexist. A consistent head-to-toe assessment that can be performed repeatedly is usually best because it reduces the likelihood that anything will be overlooked.

Head and Neck

The head is evaluated for external signs of trauma: contusions, ecchymoses, lacerations, or soft tissue swellings. Scalp lacerations and even cranial gunshot wounds can be hidden by overlying hair, and occipital locations of wounds are often overlooked because of their dependent location in the supine individual. Specific attention should be given to determining the presence of an ecchymosis over the mastoid region (Battle's sign), indicative of a basilar skull fracture. The presence of blood or CSF in the nares and external auditory canals should be sought. Palpation is performed carefully to detect any bony step-off abnormalities or crepitance. In assessing the facial bony structure, it is useful to determine symmetry by simultaneously palpating both sides of the facial skeleton. The presence of a maxillary (LeFort) fracture can be detected by grasping the upper incisors and pulling anteriorly to determine if there is any instability in the attached facial bones. With a LeFort I fracture, an instability will be noted that has a joint between the nose and the upper incisors. A LeFort II fracture will show instability through the bridge of the nose, and a LeFort III fracture is demonstrated by complete craniofacial dysjunction. Combinations of these fractures are common. If the patient is conscious, a standard cranial nerve examination should be performed.

The neck is inspected and carefully palpated for obvious abnormalities. The presence of hematomas should be noted and the presence of subcutaneous air should be felt for by carefully compressing the overlying skin; this finding could be a sign of esophageal or tracheal injury. As mentioned, care should be taken to ensure that the cervical spine is not manipulated until skeletal stability has been confirmed. Auscultation for bruits should be performed, although detection is often difficult in a noisy emergency center; this fact should be noted so that reassessment can be performed later in quieter surroundings.

Penetrating neck injuries present a controversial management issue. These injuries can appear relatively innocuous superficially, yet major structures such as the esophagus or carotid artery may be injured. Undetected, such injuries could lead to major morbidity, whereas their prompt repair can often protect against such complications. Because of this possibility, it is not uncommon for routine surgical exploration to be performed to evaluate deeper structures. Unfortunately, many such explorations yield negative results, thus prompting a search for less invasive diagnostic maneuvers. Techniques such as esophagoscopy, esophagography, arteriography, laryngoscopy, and bronchoscopy are all useful adjuncts for detecting the presence of injuries of major structures of the neck. Usually, these maneuvers are employed in some combination because no one study effectively evaluates all the neck structures that could be injured. However, it is not clear whether such a complex and expensive evaluation is an improvement over routine neck exploration. Indeed, a neck exploration may be less expensive (and perhaps less stressful for the patient), especially in the case of discharge from the hospital recovery room after a negative exploration.[89] Nevertheless, the decision to perform a routine neck exploration for a penetrating injury does not eliminate the need for further studies. Patients with zone I (from the suprasternal notch to the lateral clavicular head) or zone III (superior to the angle of the mandible) injuries usually should undergo arteriography, because arterial injuries in these regions are best handled by planning the operative approach to assure vascular control. Vascular injuries in zone II (from the lateral clavicular head to the angle of the mandible) usually can be adequately controlled and managed operatively without obtaining a preliminary arteriogram.

Chest

The chest should be inspected for wounds and for the symmetrical expansion of both hemithoraces with each ventilatory effort. Auscultation for breath sounds should be assessed rapidly over both sides of the chest cavity. Palpation for subcutaneous emphysema, bony step-offs, tracheal deviation, and symmetrical lung expansion is performed next, and any tender regions noted. Sternal tenderness, for example, can sometimes be a clue to the presence of a myocardial contusion from a compressive blow to the anterior chest, whereas tenderness of the lower left rib cage can suggest a ruptured spleen. Percussion for hyper-resonant areas or regions of dullness may help in the evaluation of pneumo- or hemothoraces.

The physical evaluation of the chest is useful in determining the presence of potentially life-threatening conditions following injury. These include tension pneumothorax, massive hemothorax, cardiac tamponade, open pneumothorax, and flail chest.

Tension pneumothorax occurs when the lung ruptures in such a way that air leaks out of it and into the pleural space during one phase of ventilation but cannot escape in the subsequent ventilatory phase. Thus, intrapleural pressure progressively rises, compressing the ipsilateral lung, shifting the mediastinal contents, and compromising expansion of the contralateral lung. Venous return ultimately is compromised, producing hypotension and shock. This condition can be recognized by noting an asymmetrical chest wall expansion, absence of breath sounds on the affected side, and often (although not always) tracheal deviation away from the side of accumulating intrapleural air. The condition is emergently relieved by rapidly inserting a large-bore needle into the second interspace in the midclavicular line on the affected side. This vents the pleural space and converts the condition into a simple pneumothorax that subsequently can be treated with a thoracostomy tube. The tube can be attached to an underwater seal or protected suction to re-establish negative intrapleural pressure.

An open pneumothorax, also known as a "sucking chest wound," can produce a progressive hypoxemia from progressive pulmonary collapse. This is best managed by sealing the wound opening with a taped airtight dressing and inserting a thoracostomy tube through a separate opening to evacuate the accumulated air.

A massive hemothorax can be detected in a patient who shows signs of hemorrhagic shock and has percussive dullness and absent breath sounds on one side. A chest radiograph can confirm the presence of a unilateral effusion. In the supine patient, this is often seen as a diffuse unilateral increase in radiographic density, compared with the opposite side, as opposed to the more familiar fluid meniscus or air-fluid level. Blood volume resuscitation should already be underway, based upon the patient's physiological response to hemorrhage. A thoracostomy tube that releases blood in excess of 1500 ml or a flow that is in excess of 200 ml/h for 4 h or longer confirms the diagnosis of massive hemothorax. Such findings should prompt an immediate operative thoracotomy to find and control the source of hemorrhage. With such massive bleeding, there is little likelihood that spontaneous cessation of hemorrhage is likely. Thus, emergent thoracotomy is indicated. In general, however, only about 15 percent of patients with thoracic injuries require thoracotomy.

Cardiac tamponade should be suspected in patients with penetrating trauma in whom there is a wound near the precordium. Blunt trauma occasionally produces a tamponade, although it occurs infrequently. Beck's triad, used in identifying the presence of pericardial tamponade, is defined as a low arterial pressure, an elevated central venous pressure, and muffled heart sounds.[7] Additionally, an accentuation of the normal pulsus paradoxus to a more than 15 mmHg decrease in systolic pressure during inspiration can make the astute clinician suspect cardiac tamponade. Unfortunately, the multiply injured patient frequently has confounding problems that can confuse the interpretation of these diagnostic signs. A central venous catheter can sometimes help differentiate hypovolemic shock from shock produced by tamponade, especially when trends in response to fluid challenges are evaluated.[101] If the diagnosis of cardiac tamponade is suspected, immediate pericardiocentesis should be performed, for diagnostic and therapeutic reasons. A long plastic catheter is threaded through or over a long pericardiocentesis needle inserted at a 45-degree angle through the skin just lateral to the xiphoid process, while it is aimed toward the lateral aspect of the left clavicle. Although aspiration of as little as 30 ml of blood may provide evidence of improvement, one must try to remove as much as possible. Repeated aspirations are often necessary to maintain an adequate blood pressure; thus, placement of a plastic catheter is preferred over repeated needle sticks because of the propensity to injure the heart with the latter. It is also important to ensure that the blood obtained is actually pericardial blood and not intracardiac blood. Because of defibrination, pericardial blood does not usually clot, unless flow into the pericardium is rapid. Most patients with pericardial tamponade from injury develop recurrent problems; therefore, pericardiocentesis is best thought of as a temporizing maneuver performed while an emergent operative decompression is being arranged.

Myocardial contusion should be suspected in a patient with injuries to the anterior chest wall.[43] In the past, a history of a collapsed steering column was associated with a likelihood of a significant chest injury. This may be observed less frequently with modern automotive designs that include an energy-absorbing steering column. The primary complications resulting from myocardial contusion are mechanical heart failure and arrhythmias. The former is often a fatal event at the scene of the accident and is infrequently observed. However, the latter is occasionally observed in the hospital. Until recently there has been a great tendency to admit such patients to electrocardiographically monitored beds and to obtain serial myocardial enzyme levels over several days in an attempt to document the presence or absence of a myocardial contusion. However, the overall value of this practice has been questioned in a number of studies.[6,12,15,24,60,63,67,99] Unlike in the patient with acute myocardial infarction, monitoring myocardial enzyme levels in a multiply injured patient seems to offer little help in diagnosing myocardial contusion.[94] The potential for arrhythmias usually can be safely excluded by observing no abnormalities on the patient's monitored electrocardiogram in the emergency room for at least 4 h.[24] Essentially all complications of myocardial contusion become apparent within 24 h of injury.[4,6,24,63]

Abdomen

In both blunt and penetrating forms of trauma, it is essential that the patient's physiological status be considered in determining the most effective route of management for abdominal injuries. Simply put, unstable victims of penetrating abdominal injuries require immediate laparotomy to control intra-abdominal hemorrhage. Diagnostic maneuvers in such situations merely delay effective management. Rarely, coexistent injuries in other body areas may need concomitant attention, but few should take precedence. Similarly, unstable victims of blunt abdominal trauma also require immediate efforts to stop hemorrhage, but in these patients it is necessary to determine from which body area the blood is being lost. The initial assessment rarely can identify the abdomen as the only site of bleeding.

Hemodynamically stable victims of blunt and penetrating trauma should undergo a different approach, because immediate exsanguination is less threatening. Rather, these patients require some form of evaluation or observation for potential later complications of abdominal injury, such as delayed hemorrhage or infection. Some controversy exists about their proper management. Significant cost savings may be realized in these stable patients by defining a standard, organized approach.

Evaluation of penetrating abdominal trauma is often a straightforward process. It is sometimes helpful to define the course of the penetration to identify the structures and organs at risk. This is usually done carefully with a sterile gloved finger or a sterile cotton-tipped applicator. In the case of gunshot wounds, the trajectory can sometimes be ascertained from the entrance and exit wounds, although deviation from a straight path occasionally occurs. For patients in whom there is no exit wound, there is often a temptation to determine the location of the projectile with a plain abdominal x-ray film, but that is usually unnecessary.

In contrast to the evaluation of penetrating abdominal trauma, whether to use an operative or nonoperative approach is controversial. The etiology of the penetrating injury is important in deciding whether a laparotomy should be performed. Gunshot wounds of the abdomen have a very high (roughly 85 percent) propensity to penetrate the peritoneal cavity and usually cause visceral damage requiring surgical correction.[64] On the other hand, approximately one-third of stab wounds to the abdomen fail to penetrate the peritoneum; of those that penetrate, only half do enough damage to require repair.[90] Thus, a patient with a gunshot wound to the abdomen should undergo emergent laparotomy, whereas some controversy exists over the proper management of abdominal stab wounds because only one-third of patients with this type of injury benefit from an operative approach. Therapeutic options range from mandatory exploration for all abdominal stab wounds to a "selective conservatism," in which patients are observed closely for signs of hemorrhage or peritoneal irritation.[59,65,104] Some authorities have argued for a systematic diagnostic approach involving local wound exploration and diagnostic peritoneal lavage.[28,37,70] No one approach has yet been shown to have any clear advantage, prompting at least one group to deem an expectant nonoperative course to be the most cost-effective one.[84]

The evaluation and management of a patient with blunt abdominal trauma is much more complex than those for penetrating abdominal injuries. In the early 1900s, before the onset of an aggressive diagnostic approach to abdominal trauma, the consequences of internal hemorrhage were a frustrating capitulation for the surgeon. All too often, patients rapidly deteriorated and died despite minimal external signs of injury. The recognition that loss of circulating blood volume could produce the clinically recognized pattern of progressive shock alerted clinicians that ongoing fluid losses had to be responsible for an otherwise mysterious condition.[9,71]

This realization prompted a more aggressive diagnostic approach for internal hemorrhage, especially in the case of blunt abdominal trauma. Initially, paracentesis had been advocated as a potential method.[80] Other suggestions for diagnostic approaches included a four-quadrant aspiration of the abdominal cavity and culdocentesis.[100] Yet, when scientifically analyzed, the reliability of such aspiration methods seemed to offer no significant improvement over the physical examination.[29] In 1965 Root et al. introduced the method of diagnostic peritoneal lavage (DPL), which had a 100% accuracy rate in their first 28 patients.[79] Subsequently, Fischer et al. reviewed their experience with the technique in 2,586 patients over a 14-year period and found it to have a 1.2% false-negative rate and a 0.2% false-positive rate.[22] Peritoneal lavage is thus quite sensitive for injuries following blunt trauma. Yet false-negative results occasionally occur, such as those associated with diaphragmatic tears that can allow for drainage of abdominal blood into the chest.[92] Fortunately, these conditions are rare.

DPL has since become a standard method for evaluating occult blunt abdominal trauma and has also been advocated for stab wounds of the abdomen. Its benefits seem greatest in the patient in whom the physical examination cannot be relied upon because of obtundation or in whom physical examination findings are equivocal.[72]

As computed tomography (CT) developed, it was evaluated as a diagnostic tool for abdominal injuries. Initial reports from the San Francisco General Hospital indicated high levels of sensitivity and specificity for CT evaluation of blunt abdominal trauma.[20,21] The role of this technique in the evaluation of abdominal trauma has been the subject of some controversy. CT clearly provides better information about the existence of retroperitoneal injuries than does DPL. Most authors agree that unstable patients with abdominal trauma do not benefit from CT because of the inherent delay a trip to the scanner incurs in most institutions.[93] Rather, as previously mentioned, unstable patients with penetrating abdominal injuries should undergo immediate laparotomy (assuming resuscitation is already underway). Similarly, unstable patients with blunt injuries require a rapid assessment of the potential bleeding areas. DPL, especially with the closed technique, is generally considered to be a quick and sensitive method to determine if intra-abdominal hemorrhage exists. Its expediency often makes DPL the preferred method of evaluating the abdomen as a potential source of hemorrhage in the hemodynamically unstable blunt trauma victim.

If CT has a role in the evaluation of abdominal trauma, it should be relegated to the assessment of hemodynamically stable patients, often those who are already obtaining a CT scan for evaluation of their head injury. In such circumstances, it may be possible for CT to delineate the nature and extent of an injury of the liver, spleen, or pancreas. CT has been used frequently in a similar manner in the injured child, in whom its imaging of splenic injuries allows for nonoperative management and resultant splenic salvage to prevent overwhelming postsplenectomy sepsis.[44,46,95] There are often minor liver injuries that have stopped bleeding by the time of laparotomy, for which a nonoperative approach could save the patient significant discomfort and expense. The occurrence of such nontherapeutic laparotomies provoked by a positive DPL result keeps active the search for a more satisfying approach.

Unfortunately, in comparison studies, CT seems relatively more likely to miss significant injuries than does DPL.[18,58,62] Yet there are also studies that find that CT detects a greater number of significant injuries of the abdomen than does DPL.[30,66] This inconsistency among studies can be explained in part by the relatively greater variability in interpreting CT scans, compared with DPL, depending on the interpreter's experience and the quality of the scan.[93] Such special CT expertise is not available in many institutions. Furthermore, the CT scan does not reliably eliminate the presence of a hollow viscus injury.[76] Thus, even though the patient is hemodynamically stable, the opportunity to prevent significant peritoneal infection at an early stage may be lost. This is most important in the injured adult, who appears more likely to sustain hollow viscus injuries from blunt trauma than is the injured child.[23] Thus, one could question the value of CT in injured adults who are hemodynamically stable.

Ultrasonography is being evaluated as a potential diagnostic method for injured patients. The advantages of its improved technology include portability of the unit, which can now be based in the emergency center itself. Additionally, the images are of better quality than ever, making interpretation less difficult. Finally, the controls on the newer devices are simple enough to be learned quickly by any interested clinician. Nevertheless, the overall benefit of ultrasonography in the setting of abdominal trauma is currently undetermined; evaluations thus far have indicated that it does not meet the diagnostic sensitivity of DPL.[32]

Radionuclide scanning and arteriography are other potential diagnostic modalities. Yet they offer no particular advantage in the acute setting over the physical examination combined with DPL and/or CT. Their usefulness lies mostly in the evaluation of posttraumatic complications of liver injuries, such as biliary duct leakage and hemobilia.[35,53]

Extremities

Because of their number and exposure, extremities are more frequently injured from major trauma than are other body parts.[5] Initial evaluation of extremity trauma is focused on hemorrhage and perfusion. Open bleeding wounds can frequently be a cause of hypovolemic shock and should be controlled with direct pressure until definitive operative control can be performed. Tourniquet application is generally discouraged and direct pressure preferred because of the more global ischemia produced by tourniquets. Definitive control is best achieved in an operating room environment, in which adequate lighting and exposure can minimize iatrogenic damage.

Even without open wounds, extremity trauma can usually produce a significant degree of hypovolemia. It is usually estimated that tibial fractures can produce a blood loss equivalent to 1 U of blood and that femur fractures can be accompanied by the loss of more than 2 U of blood into the thigh. Although there are different degrees of injury of different parts of the pelvis, it is common for closed pelvic fractures to produce hypovolemic shock if the patient is unresuscitated with blood volumes in the range of 6 U.

Extremity fractures sometimes produce ischemia through damage to major vascular structures. Injuries notorious for their propensity to produce ischemia are vascular injuries and fractures about the knee or elbow (i.e., knee dislocations, "floating" knees, supracondylar fractures of the elbow), extremity crush injuries and compartment syndromes, and dislocations of the hip. Evidence of vascular disruption often can be ascertained through the physical findings of pulselessness, pallor, coolness, and loss of sensation and motor strength. An overlying hematoma, bruit, or thrill can also indicate major vascular damage. In some cases, however, the determination of a vascular injury is less clear; although the extremity may appear viable, an intimal flap or vessel contusion may cause later problems. Generally, a high suspicion for vascular injury has prompted arteriography at an early stage when a fracture or penetrating injury is in the proximity of a major vessel.[40,47] Recently, the value of this approach has been questioned because of its relatively low yield.[25,27,36,45,86,98] One study determined that it cost $66,420 to detect one clinically occult vascular injury requiring surgery.[26] Because of this, the use of noninvasive Doppler ultrasound to screen patients for evidence of occult vascular injury has been evaluated. A recent prospective study determined the arterial pressure index (API) by calculating the Doppler arterial pressure distal to the injury relative to the Doppler arterial pressure in an uninvolved arm. Sensitivity and specificity (confirmed by arteriography) were 95 and 97 percent, respectively, when API was compared with clinical outcome, thus making this index a useful tool in evaluating "proximity" injuries.[55]

Interstitial tissue pressures sometimes rise above capillary perfusion pressure (generally estimated at roughly 25 mmHg) as a result of damaged vessels and permeability changes, especially when contained by tough nonyielding fascial compartments. In such situations, progressive ischemia and tissue necrosis of nerve and muscle will occur, with the ultimate result being a viable, although functionless, extremity. The fascial compartments of the leg and forearm are notorious for their potential to produce compartment syndromes, although such syndromes have been seen in compartments of the thigh, upper arm, and digits as well. Early identification of a risk for a compartment syndrome and prompt recognition of its presence are key in the effective management of the condition. Time is critical; it appears that permanent residual effects can be seen with a compartment syndrome of 6 or more hours' duration. Clinical evidence of a compartment syndrome is apparent when there is pain, especially with passive muscle stretching, diminished sensation in the involved peripheral nerve's distribution, tense swelling of the involved region, and muscle weakness. Occasionally, these signs are difficult to elicit, particularly in the obtunded patient. In such cases, the insertion of a handheld inexpensive solid-state transducer allows for rapid and either repeatable or continuous compartmental pressure monitoring. Normal compartment pressures are less than 10 mmHg. The absolute threshold above which compartmental pressure readings should prompt an emergent fasciotomy is somewhat controversial, although any pressure high enough to be above capillary perfusion pressure should be a concern. Thus, pressures above 30 to 45 mmHg usually indicate the need for a fasciotomy.

Fractured extremities are usually splinted or placed in traction for immobilization until definitive stabilization or fixation occurs. In the past, definitive fracture fixation was often delayed for days or weeks to enable stabilization of other, more vital functions. However, there is a growing body of evidence to indicate that definitive immobilization should occur as soon as possible following injury. One of the first observations was that there appeared to be a reduction in the incidence of pulmonary dysfunction from 22 to 4 percent when long bone fractures were fixed soon (within 24 h) after an injury occurred.[78] Subsequent studies confirmed this initial impression.[31,61,77,88]

Seibel et al.[82] conducted an exhaustive analysis of 56 patients with multiple blunt trauma to evaluate the effects of immediate versus delayed internal fixation of femoral or acetabular fractures. Ten days of femur traction doubled the duration of pulmonary failure and a clinical septic state, whereas 30 days of traction multiplied the duration by a factor of 3 to 5. Johnson et al.[42] reported on 132 consecutive patients with long bone fractures, in whom they compared the effects of fixation done within 24 h to that of fixation done more than 24 h following the injury. For all patients, a delay in fixation was associated with a fivefold increase in the incidence of the adult respiratory distress syndrome (ARDS). Interestingly, in patients who were more severely injured, as demonstrated by an injury severity score (ISS) over 40, there was a marked improvement in outcome if their fractures were fixed immediately, with a 17 percent incidence of ARDS versus 75 percent following delayed fixation. This finding was corroborated in a prospective randomized clinical study in which patients with an ISS above 18 had a reduced risk of ARDS and pneumonia as well as a reduced length of stay in the intensive care unit and the hospital.[10]

It seems that the major contribution provided by early fracture fixation is that of earlier patient mobilization, ventilator weaning, and ambulation. Prolonged bed rest, mechanical ventilation, and immobilization set the stage for retained secretions, atelectasis, and bacterial colonization of the respiratory tract, with resultant pneumonia and sepsis. The potential also exists for other complications to develop, such as venous thromboembolism, decubitus ulceration, and bacterial overgrowth of the gut as a result of gastrointestinal atony and stasis. Early mobilization provides the opportunity to counteract many of these adverse consequences.

References

1. Aitkenhead A. Cerebral protection. *Br J Hosp Med* 1986; 35:290–298.
2. American College of Surgeons Committee on Trauma. *Advanced Trauma Life Support Course for Physicians, 1988 Instructor Manual.* Chicago: American College of Surgeons, 1989.
3. Aprahamian C, Thompson BM, Finger WA, et al. Experimental cervical spine injury model: evaluation of airway management and splinting techniques. *Ann Emerg Med* 1984; 13:584–587.
4. Attenhofer C, Vuilliomenet A, Richter M, et al. Contusio cordis: Pathologische Befunde und Klinischer Verlaut. Schweiz Med Wochenschr 1992; 12:1593–1599.
5. Baker CC, Oppenheimer L, Stephens B, et al. Epidemiology of trauma deaths. *Am J Surg* 1980; 140:144–150.
6. Baxter BT, Moore EE, Moore FA, et al. A plea for sensible management of myocardial contusion. *Am J Surg* 1989; 158:557–562.
7. Beck CS. Wounds of the heart: the technic of suture. *Arch Surg* 1926; 13:205–227.
8. Bivins HG, Ford S, Bezmalinovic Z, et al. The effect of axial traction during orotracheal intubation of the trauma victim with an unstable cervical spine. *Ann Emerg Med* 1988; 17:25–29.
9. Blalock A. Experimental shock: the cause of the low blood pressure produced by muscle injury. *Arch Surg* 1930; 20:959–996.
10. Bone LB, Johnson KD, Weigelt J, Scheinberg R. Early versus delayed stabilization of femoral fractures: a prospective randomized study. *J Bone Joint Surg [Am]* 1989; 71-A:336–340.
11. Brantigan CO Sr, Grow JB Sr. Cricothyroidotomy: elective use in respiratory problems requiring tracheotomy. *J Thorac Cardiovasc Surg* 1976; 71:72–81.
12. Cachecho R, Grindlinger GA, Lee VW. The clinical significance of myocardial contusion. *J Trauma* 1992; 33:68–73.
13. Chang JC, Gross HM, Jang NS. Disseminated intravascular coagulation due to intravenous administration of hetastarch. *Am J Med Sci* 1990; 300:301–303.
14. Diehl JT, Lester JL III, Cosgrove DM. Clinical comparison of hetastarch and albumin in postoperative cardiac patients. *Ann Thorac Surg* 1982; 34:674–679.
15. Dubrow TJ, Mihalka J, Eisenhauer DM, et al. Myocardial contusion in the stable patient: what level of care is appropriate? *Surgery* 1989; 106:267–274.
16. Ducey JP, Lamiell JM, Gueller GE. Cerebral electrophysiologic effects of resuscitation with hypertonic saline-dextran after hemorrhage. *Crit Care Med* 1990; 18:744–749.
17. Erdmann AJ III, Vaughn TR Jr, Brigham KL, et al. Effect of increased vascular pressure on lung fluid balance in unanesthetized sheep. *Circ Res* 1975; 37:271–284.
18. Fabian TC, Mangiante EC, White TJ, et al. A prospective study of 91 patients undergoing both computed tomography and peritoneal lavage following blunt abdominal trauma. *J Trauma* 1986; 26:602–608.
19. Falk JL, Rackow EC, Astiz ME, Weil MH. Effects of hetastarch and albumin on coagulation in patients with septic shock. *J Clin Pharmacol* 1988; 28:412–415.
20. Federle MP. Computed tomography of blunt abdominal trauma. *Radiol Clin North Am* 1983; 21:461–475.
21. Federle MP, Goldberg HI, Kaiser JA, et al. Evaluation of abdominal trauma by computed tomography. *Radiology* 1981; 138:637–644.
22. Fischer RP, Beverlin BC, Engrav LH, et al. Diagnostic peritoneal lavage: fourteen years and 2,586 patients later. *Am J Surg* 1978; 136:701–704.
23. Fischer RP, Miller-Crotchett P, Reed RL II. Gastrointestinal disruption: the hazard of nonoperative management in adults with blunt abdominal injury. *J Trauma* 1988; 28:1445–1449.
24. Foil MB, Mackersie RC, Furst SR, et al. The asymptomatic patient with suspected myocardial contusion. *Am J Surg* 1990; 160:638–642.
25. Francis H III, Thal ER, Weigelt JA, Redman HC. Vascular proximity: is it a valid indication for arteriography in asymptomatic patients? *J Trauma* 1991; 31:512–514.
26. Frykberg ER, Crump JM, Vines FS, et al. A reassessment of the role of arteriography in penetrating proximity extremity trauma: a prospective study. *J Trauma* 1989; 29:1041–1052.
27. Frykberg ER, Dennis JW, Bishop K, et al. The reliability of physical examination in the evaluation of penetrating extremity trauma for vascular injury: results at one year. *J Trauma* 1991; 31:502–511.
28. Galbraith TA, Oreskovich MR, Heimbach DM, et al. The role of peritoneal lavage in the management of stab wounds to the abdomen. *Am J Surg* 1980; 140:60–64.
29. Giacobine JW, Siler VE. Evaluation of diagnostic abdominal paracentesis with experimental and clinical studies. *Surg Gynecol Obstet* 1960; 110:676–686.
30. Goldstein AS, Sclafani SJ, Kupferstein NH, et al. The diagnostic superiority of computerized tomography. *J Trauma* 1985; 25:938–946.
31. Goris RJA, Gimbrere JSF, van Niekerk JLM, et al. Early osteosynthesis and prophylactic mechanical ventilation in the multitrauma patient. *J Trauma* 1982; 22:895–903.
32. Grüessner R, Mentges B, Düber C, et al. Sonography versus peritoneal lavage in blunt abdominal trauma. *J Trauma* 1989; 29:242–244.

33. Harke H, Thoenies R, Margraf I, Momsen W. The influence of different plasma substitutes on blood clotting and platelet function during and after operations. *Anaesthesist* 1976; 25:366–373.
34. Harms BA, Rosenfeld DJ, Pahl AC, et al. Pulmonary transvascular fluid filtration response to hypoproteinemia and Hespan infusion. *J Surg Res* 1990; 48:408–414.
35. Heimbach DM, Ferguson GS, Harley JD. Treatment of traumatic hemobilia with angiographic embolization. *J Trauma* 1978; 18:221–224.
36. Henderson V, Nambisan R, Smith ME, et al. Anigographic yield in penetrating extremity trauma. *West J Med* 1991; 155:253–255.
37. Henneman PL, Marx JA, Moore EE, et al. Diagnostic peritoneal lavage: accuracy in predicting necessary laparotomy following blunt and penetrating trauma. *J Trauma* 1990; 30:1345–1355.
38. Hess JR, Dubick MA, Summary JJ, et al. The effects of 7.5% NaCl/6% dextran 70 on coagulation and platelet aggregation in humans. *J Trauma* 1992; 32:40–44.
39. Hicks GL Jr, Jensen LA, Norsen LH, et al. Platelet inhibitors and hydroxyethyl starch: safe and cost-effective interventions in coronary artery surgery. *Ann Thorac Surg* 1985; 39:422–425.
40. Itani KM, Burch JM, Spjut-Patrinely V, et al. Emergency center arteriography. *J Trauma* 1992; 32:302–307.
41. Jackson C. High tracheotomy and other errors the chief causes of chronic laryngeal stenosis. *Surg Gynecol Obstet* 1921; 32:392–398.
42. Johnson KD, Cadambi A, Seibert GB. Incidence of adult respiratory distress syndrome in patients with multiple musculoskeletal injuries: effect of early operative stabilization of fractures. *J Trauma* 1985; 25:375–384.
43. Kahn D. Myocardial contusion due to steering wheel injury. *JAMA* 1967; 200:255–257.
44. Kakkasseril JS, Steward D, Cox JA, Gelfand M. Changing treatment of pediatric splenic trauma. *Arch Surg* 1982; 117:758–759.
45. Kaufman JA, Parker JE, Gillespie DL, et al. Arteriography for proximity of injury in penetrating extremity trauma. *J Vasc Interv Radiol* 1992; 3:719–723.
46. King DR, Lobe TE, Haase GM, et al. Selective management of the injured spleen. *Surgery* 1981; 90:677–682.
47. King TA, Perse JA, Marmen C, Darvin HI. Utility of arteriography in penetrating extremity injuries. *Am J Surg* 1991; 162:163–165.
48. Kirklin JK, Lell WA, Kouchoukos NT. Hydroxyethyl starch versus albumin for colloid infusion following cardiopulmonary bypass in patients undergoing myocardial revascularization. *Ann Thorac Surg* 1984; 37:40–46.
49. Krausz MM, Bar-Ziv M, Rabinovici R, Gross D. ''Scoop and run'' or stabilize hemorrhagic shock with normal saline or small-volume hypertonic saline? *J Trauma* 1992; 33:6–10.
50. Krausz MM, Kablan M, Rabinovici R, et al. Effect of injured vessel size on bleeding following hypertonic saline infusion in ''uncontrolled'' hemorrhagic shock in anesthetized rats. *Circ Shock* 1991; 35:9–13.
51. Krausz MM, Landau EH, Klin B, Gross D. Hypertonic saline treatment of uncontrolled hemorrhagic shock at different periods from bleeding. *Arch Surg* 1992; 127:93–96.
52. Lockwood DN, Bullen C, Machin SJ. A severe coagulopathy following volume replacement with hydroxyethyl starch in a Jehovah's Witness. *Anaesthesia* 1988; 43:391–393.
53. Lockwood TE, Schorn L, Coln D. Nonoperative management of hemobilia. *Ann Surg* 1977; 185:335–340.
54. Lyden PD, Alving LI, Zivin JA, Rothrock JF. Hemodilution with low-molecular-weight hydroxyethyl starch after experimental focal cerebral ischemia in rabbits. *Stroke* 1988; 19:223–227.
55. Lynch K, Johansen K. Can Doppler pressure measurement replace ''exclusion'' arteriography in the diagnosis of occult extremity arterial trauma? *Ann Surg* 1991; 214:737–741.
56. Mackersie RC, Shackford SR, Garfin SR, et al. Major skeletal injuries in the obtunded blunt trauma patient: a case for routine radiologic survey. *J Trauma* 1988; 28:1450–1454.
57. Martin E, Armbruster I, Fischer E, et al. The influence of different plasma substitutes on blood clotting in isovolaemic haemodilution. *Anaesthesist* 1976; 25:181–184.
58. Marx JA, Moore EE, Jorden RC, et al. Limitations of computed tomography in the evaluation of acute abdominal trauma: a prospective comparison with diagnostic peritoneal lavage. *J Trauma* 1985; 25:933–937.
59. McAlvanah MJ, Shaftan GW. Selective conservatism in penetrating abdominal wounds: a continuing reappraisal. *J Trauma* 1978; 18:206–212.
60. McLean RF, Devitt JH, Dubbin J, McLellan BA. Incidence of abnormal RNA studies and dysrhythmias in patients with blunt chest trauma. *J Trauma* 1991; 31:968–970.
61. Meek RN, Vivoda E, Crichton A, Pirani S. Comparison of mortality of patients with multiple injuries according to method of fracture treatment. *J Bone Joint Surg [Br]* 1981; 63-B:456 (abstr).
62. Meyer DM, Thal ER, Weigelt JA, Redman HC. Evaluation of computed tomography and diagnostic peritoneal lavage in blunt abdominal trauma. *J Trauma* 1989; 29:1168–1172.
63. Miller FB, Shumate CR, Richardson JD. Myocardial contusion. When can the diagnosis be eliminated? *Arch Surg* 1989; 124:805–808.
64. Moore EE, Moore JB, van Duzer-Moore S, Thompson JS. Mandatory laparotomy for gunshot wounds penetrating the abdomen. *Am J Surg* 1980; 140:847–851.
65. Nance FC, Wennar MH, Johnson LW, et al. Surgical judgment in the management of penetrating wounds of the abdomen: experience with 2212 patients. *Ann Surg* 1974; 179:639–646.
66. Nelson EW, Holliman CJ, Juell BE, et al. Computerized tomography in the evaluation of blunt abdominal trauma. *Am J Surg* 1983; 146:751–754.
67. Norton MJ, Stanford GG, Weigelt JA. Early detection of myocardial contusion and its complications in patients with blunt trauma. *Am J Surg* 1990; 160:577–582.
68. O'Brien DJ, Danzyl DF, Hooker EA, et al. Prehospital blind nasotracheal intubation by paramedics. *Ann Emerg Med* 1989; 18:612–617.
69. Oppenheimer L, Landolfo KP. Treatment of permeability edema with macromolecular solutions. *J Trauma* 1991; 31:1036 (abstr).
70. Oreskovich MR, Carrico CJ. Stab wounds of the anterior abdomen: analysis of a management plan using local wound exploration and quantitative peritoneal lavage. *Ann Surg* 1983; 198:411–419.
71. Parsons E, Phemister DB. Haemorrhage and ''shock'' in traumatized limbs: an experimental study. *Surg Gynecol Obstet* 1930; 51:196–207.
72. Parvin S, Smith DE, Asher WM, Virgilio RW. Effectiveness of peritoneal lavage in blunt abdominal trauma. *Ann Surg* 1975; 181:255–261.
73. Phillips TF. Airway management. In Moore EE, Mattox KL, Feliciano DV (ed): *Trauma*, 2d ed. Norwalk, CT: Appleton & Lange, 1991, pp 127–145.
74. Prough DS, Whitley JM, Taylor CL, et al. Regional cerebral blood flow following resuscitation from hemorrhagic shock with hypertonic saline; influence of a subdural mass. *Anesthesiology* 1991; 75:319–327.
75. Reed RL II, Johnston TD, Chen Y, Fischer RP. Hypertonic saline alters plasma clotting times and platelet aggregation. *J Trauma* 1991; 31:8–14.
76. Rehm CG, Sherman R, Hinz TW. The role of CT scan in evaluation for laparotomy in patients with stab wounds of the abdomen. *J Trauma* 1989; 29:446–450.
77. Riska EB, Myllynen P. Fat embolism in patients with multiple injuries. *J Trauma* 1982; 22:891–894.
78. Riska EB, von Bonsdorff H, Hakkinen S, et al. Prevention of fat embolism by early internal fixation of fractures in patients with multiple injuries. *Injury* 1976; 8:110–116.
79. Root HD, Hauser CW, McKinley CR, et al. Diagnostic peritoneal lavage. *Surgery* 1965; 57:633–637.
80. Salomon H. Die diagnostische Punktion des Bauches. *Klin Wochenschr* 1906; 43:45–46.

81. Saunders CR, Carlisle L, Bick RL. Hydroxyethyl starch versus albumin in cardiopulmonary bypass prime solutions. *Ann Thorac Surg* 1983; 36:532–539.
82. Seibel R, LaDuca J, Hassett JM, et al. Blunt multiple trauma (ISS 36), femur traction, and the pulmonary failure-septic state. *Ann Surg* 1985; 202:283–295.
83. Shires GT, Carrico CJ, Canizaro PC. Response of the extracellular fluid. *Major Probl Clin Surg* 1973; 13:15–41.
84. Sirinek KR, Page CP, Root HD, Levine BA. Is exploratory celiotomy necessary for all patients with truncal stab wounds? *Arch Surg* 1990; 125:844–848.
85. Smith GJ, Kramer GC, Perron P, et al. A comparison of several hypertonic solutions for resuscitation of bled sheep. *J Surg Res* 1985; 39:517–528.
86. Smyth SH, Pond GD, Johnson PL, et al. Proximity injuries: correlation with results of extremity arteriography. *J Vasc Interv Radiol* 1991; 2:451–456.
87. Strauss RG, Stump DC, Henriksen RA, Saunders R. Effects of hydroxyethyl starch on fibrinogen, fibrin clot formation, and fibrinolysis. *Transfusion* 1985; 25:230–234.
88. Talucci RC, Manning J, Lampard S, et al. Early intramedullary nailing of femoral shaft fractures: a cause of fat embolism syndrome. *Am J Surg* 1983; 146:107–111.
89. Thal ER, Meyer DM. Penetrating neck trauma. *Curr Probl Surg* 1992; 29:1–56.
90. Thompson JS, Moore EE, van Duzer-Moore S, et al. The evolution of abdominal stab wound management. *J Trauma* 1980; 20:478–484.
91. Tranmer BI, Iacobacci RI, Kindt GW. Effects of crystalloid and colloid infusions on intracranial pressure and computerized electroencephalographic data in dogs with vasogenic brain edema. *Neurosurgery* 1989; 25:173–178.
92. Tribble JB, Julian S, Myers RT. Rupture of the liver and right hemidiaphragm presenting as right hemothorax. *J Trauma* 1989; 29:116–118.
93. Trunkey D, Federle MP. Computed tomography in perspective. *J Trauma* 1986; 26:660–661.
94. Unkle DW, Smejkal R, O'Malley KF. Myocardial contusion without creatine kinase—MB elevation. *Heart Lung* 1989; 18:539–541.
95. Upadhyaya P, Simpson JS. Splenic trauma in children. *Surg Gynecol Obstet* 1968; 126:781–790.
96. Vinazzer H, Bergmann H. The influence of hydroxyethyl starch on postoperative alterations of blood coagulation. *Anaesthesist* 1975; 24:517–520.
97. von Bormann B, Sticher J, Ratthey K, et al. Volumensubstitution wahrend akuter normovolamischer Haemodilution (ANH). Humanalbumin 5% vs. Hydroxyathylstarke 6%. *Infusionstherapie* 1990; 17:142–146.
98. Weaver FA, Yellin AE, Bauer M, et al. Is arterial proximity a valid indication for arteriography in penetrating extremity trauma? A prospective analysis. *Arch Surg* 1990; 125:1256–1260.
99. Wisner DH, Reed WH, Riddick RS. Suspected myocardial contusion. Triage and indications for monitoring. *Ann Surg* 1990; 212:82–86.
100. Wright LT, Prigot A, Hill LM Jr. Traumatic rupture of the liver without penetrating wounds: a study of thirty-two cases. *Arch Surg* 1947; 54:613–632.
101. Yao ST, Carey JS, Shoemaker WC, et al. Hemodynamics and therapy of acute hemopericardium from stab wounds of the heart. *J Trauma* 1967; 7:783–792.
102. Zikria BA, King TC, Stanford J, Freeman HP. A biophysical approach to capillary permeability. *Surgery* 1989; 105:625–631.
103. Zikria BA, Subbarao C, Oz MC, et al. Macromolecules reduce abnormal microvascular permeability in rat limb ischemia-reperfusion injury. *Crit Care Med* 1989; 17:1306–1309.
104. Zubowski R, Nallathambi M, Ivatury R, Stahl W. Selective conservatism in abdominal stab wounds: the efficacy of serial physical examination. *J Trauma* 1988; 28:1665–1668.

265 Intensive Management of Traumatic Brain Injury

Michael J. Caron
Daniel F. Kelly
Ehud Shalmon
Donald P. Becker

Intensive management of traumatic brain injury (TBI) is directed toward prevention of further damage to an already compromised brain and maintenance of an optimum biological environment to promote neuronal recovery. Intensive management of TBI includes all therapeutic maneuvers performed for nonoperative brain resuscitation. The primary focus of intensive management is directed toward patients suffering severe brain injury, defined as patients who demonstrate a Glasgow Coma Scale (GCS) score of 8 or less following initial resuscitation. An additional goal of intensive management is vigilant care to prevent patients suffering moderate injuries from deteriorating into unresponsive coma.[20,40] Therefore, the focus of this chapter is on the early, aggressive, nonoperative management of TBI and its complications.

It is crucial for all medical personnel involved in the care of TBI patients to understand the concept of vulnerability if they are to provide vigilant care and optimize recovery. It is universally agreed that a population of neurons is irreversibly damaged at initial impact. Neuronal demise continues unchecked until brain resuscitation is initiated. It is also accepted that the primary injury initiates a cascade of metabolic derangements affecting the cerebral vascular system, glial supporting cells, and neurons, which leaves the brain vulnerable to secondary injury. The concept of vulnerability to secondary injury has been demonstrated in animals by the administration of a moderate brain injury, followed by a transient episode of global ischemia. When either the brain injury or transient ischemia is administered alone, complete behavioral, electrophysiologic, and histologic recovery occurs. In dramatic contrast, the combination of tandem insults results in widespread neuronal demise, significant mortality, and obvious behavioral and electrophysiologic changes.[36,37] It is clear from these and other experimental studies that the traumatized brain is metabolically deranged and particularly vulnerable to hypoxia and ischemia. This metabolic derangement has been documented to persist up to 10 days following a mild fluid percussion injury in experimental animals with no light microscopic evidence of histologic damage.[34,38]

These findings are not unique to the laboratory setting.[6] The study of large populations of TBI patients in the United States and the United Kingdom has demonstrated that secondary injury in humans is responsible for increased morbidity and mortality.[11,17,48,49,60] Transport time to definitive neurosurgical care,[19,41] admission systemic oxygenation value,[66] admission systemic blood pressure,[47] timing of operative decompression of an intracranial hematoma,[75] length of time spent with an intracranial pressure (ICP) greater than 20 mmHg,[47] presence of traumatic arterial vasospasm,[13–15,51] episodes of jugular oxygen desaturation,[69,70,76] and, more recently, level of cerebral perfusion pressure[14,21,54,71,72,80] have all been demonstrated to play a role in outcome. Systemic insults other than hypoxia and hypotension are also factors in outcome. Untoward systemic events, such as cardiopulmonary arrest, hypovolemia, disseminated intravascular coagulopathy,[78] electrolyte imbalance, renal failure, adult respiratory distress syndrome, pneumonia, and systemic sepsis, are sources of secondary brain insults.[18,30,66,73]

Appropriate triage of head-injured victims from the scene of an accident to medical center facilities is essential to begin proper aggressive management and to prevent secondary insults. Vigilant medical care, providing an environment in which partially injured cells receive adequate oxygen and appropriate nutrition, can result in improved patient recovery. This places a great responsibility on the neurosurgeon managing these critically ill patients.

Initial Effects of Head Injury

The initial intracranial and systemic effects of closed head trauma have been carefully evaluated by Ommaya and Gennarelli.[31,64,65] The biomechanics, pathophysiology, and pathology of closed head injury are elaborated in other chapters in this textbook. A review of aspects pertinent to brain resuscitation emphasizes the need for prompt evaluation and management. Various biological changes are seen in graded severity of injury. Alterations of cardiovascular function occur before other physiologic changes; an initial bradycardia and hypotension are seen, followed by mild elevation of mean arterial pressure. Respiratory irregularity and periods of apnea then can actually precede loss of responsiveness to external stimuli. More severe trauma is necessary to alter consciousness than to change cardiorespiratory patterns, and experimental unconsciousness is related to brain stem trauma with subsequent loss of corneal and pupillary response. Arterial hypertension occurs at the higher injury levels, instead of the hypotension seen at lower levels of trauma.

With increasing levels of injury, loss of consciousness persists longer, and definite focal neurological alterations are seen from involvement of upper brain stem and cortical structures; these are often associated with cortical contusions and ischemic injury of the hippocampus. At the most severe levels of injury, intracranial hematomas, particularly subdural hematomas, occur and result in the worst outcome.

The histologic findings seen in animals subjected to increasing severity of injury are paralleled in humans. In patients who expire following TBI, 30 to 40 percent of examined brains reveal evidence of diffuse axonal injury and ischemic injury.[60] These findings at autopsy further underscore the need for aggressive management and monitoring to avoid secondary insults. Clinical studies of cerebral blood flow and metabolism following severe injury suggest that the most vulnerable period for cerebral ischemia is the first 24 h.[8–10,46] Both bedside xenon radioisotope studies and stable xenon computed tomography (CT) have revealed that the lowest blood flow values occur in the first 24 h. Monitoring of jugular venous oxygen saturation confirms these findings; the highest number of episodes of desaturation to ischemic levels occurs in the first 8 to 12 h following injury.[15,69,70,76] Transcranial Doppler examinations of blood flow velocity have emphasized the potential adverse effects of post-traumatic arterial vasospasm. Initial CT findings for all patients admitted to the United States Traumatic Coma Data Bank (TCDB) were examined for the presence or absence of traumatic subarachnoid hemorrhage. Upon detailed isolation of all other known outcome variables, the presence of traumatic subarachnoid hemorrhage independently was associated with increased mortality.[27] In one study, the combination of severe arterial spasm measured by transcranial Doppler ultrasonography, and a hemispheric cerebral blood flow (CBF) value below 30 ml/100 g brain/min, uniformly resulted in death, a vegetative state, or a severe disability.[51]

Changes in brain energy metabolism also occur, reflected by CSF acidosis and changes in CBF, as well as the development of cerebral edema and increased ICP. Dysfunction of neuroendocrine pathways may occur, and there are major systemic metabolic alterations in response to the physical trauma. Delayed effects of sustained hypoxia, dysregulation of CBF, intracranial hypertension, fat embolism, seizures, and disseminated intravascular coagulation may all occur within the initial 24 h, or may occur later.[58]

Initial Management of Acute Closed Head Injury

At the Accident Site and during Transit to the Hospital

Neurosurgeons and all emergency care physicians must realize that brain resuscitation must begin immediately after trauma and not just on arrival in the emergency room (ER) or intensive care unit (ICU). Systematic, rapid resuscitation must begin at the site of injury and be maintained during each phase of the patient's transport to a definitive neurological care unit. The concern for achieving optimal levels of support for head-injured patients is well founded, as there is a significantly adverse outcome for patients who sustain hypoxia, arterial hypotension, or other systemic compromises that add to the initial morbidity of cranial trauma.[5,66]

Two studies of the impact of prehospital emergency medical services on outcome reveal the magnitude of improvement provided by early, skilled resuscitation in the field. One study compared outcomes in two relatively rural areas; both areas had advanced neurosurgical care at the receiving hospital, but one did not provide emergency medical services in the field. Mortality was 11 percent without and 7.2 percent with trained prehospital caregivers. More dramatic was the fact that in patients who initially had a GCS motor score of 5 (localizing pain), a group expected to do well, mortality rose from 4.8 to 12.5 percent in the absence of organized prehospital care.[20] In a second study, head injury mortality decreased 24 percent in the 2 years following establishment of advanced prehospital emergency medical services. The reduced mortality was credited to early reversal of apnea and hypotension.[41]

The first echelon of care is to anticipate and prevent further cerebral damage due to pathologic systemic physiology, a common occurrence in patients with severe head injury. On admission of such patients to the ER, Miller et al. have observed a 35 percent incidence of hypoxia ($Pa_{O_2} \leq 65$ mmHg), a 15 percent incidence of arterial hypotension (systolic blood pressure <95 mmHg), and a 12 percent incidence of anemia (hematocrit less than 30).[60] Analysis of data from the TCDB initial patient contact through resuscitation indicates that hypotension with or without systemic trauma is the most deadly systemic insult. In this group of patients with severe TBI, the presence of one episode of hypotension increased mortality from 27 to 50 percent. Hypoxia alone was not as devastating as hypotension, although it did increase mortality, particularly when associated with systemic trauma.[47] Because up to 20 percent of trauma victims die as a result of inadequate treatment at the scene or during transport, early recognition of these phenomena and their treatment are crucial to improve outcome.[59]

Triage and resuscitation of respiration and blood pressure should proceed simultaneously with the initial diagnostic evaluation. A definitive outline for this has been prepared by the American College of Surgeons (Advanced Trauma Life Support [ATLS]). The "ABC" system, where A = airway, B = breathing, and C = circulation, is aimed at rapidly assessing and initiating the life supports urgently needed, followed by more detailed diagnostic examination and adjustment of treatment.

Transport of an unconscious patient should never begin until a patent, functioning airway and adequate ventilation are assured. Transport to a definitive neurological care facility following the resuscitation and assessment phase is urgent, but the distance to be traveled is of secondary concern unless shock with uncontrolled hypotension is present and requires stopping at an outlying medical facility to prevent death. Prolonged delays at intermediate hospitals are to be avoided in the face of severe neurological injury that requires immediate and optimal treatment.

Two guiding questions for decision making in airway management are (1) Is protection of the airway necessary? (2) Is assistance in ventilation necessary? It is absolutely necessary that a patent airway be maintained to provide adequate tidal volume and oxygenation. Hypoxia and hypercarbia must be avoided because both lead to increased ICP through vasodilation of the cerebrovascular system. Likewise, excessive hyperventilation by hand with an AMBU (air-mask-bag unit) is to be avoided. Although hyperventilation reduces ICP, the mechanism is through a reduction in CO_2, resulting in reflex cerebral vasoconstriction. Excessive hyperventilation can therefore result in cerebral ischemia. Recent studies support the recommendation that controlled ventilation to maintain a partial pressure of carbon dioxide (P_{CO_2}) in the range of 30 to 35 mmHg should be a target in both the emergency room and the intensive care environment.[61] Patients with a GCS score of less than 8 (unresponsive to commands and not verbalizing) should receive endotracheal intubation and mechanical ventilatory assistance as soon as possible to achieve proper oxygenation and mild hypocapnia. Apnea or respiratory arrest followed by irregularity of rate and depth of ventilation is a part of the concussive response, with more severe injuries resulting in prolonged apnea.[65] In some instances, this prolonged apnea may itself be the reason for death at the scene. Apnea of longer than 8 to 10 min in humans treated by intubation and successful respiratory resuscitation can, on occasion, result in a functional recovery.[44]

Airway management begins with clearing the upper airway of vomitus, blood, or foreign bodies such as false or loose teeth and using the jaw lift or thrust to align the airway anatomically. In less severely injured patients, the placement of an oral airway or nasal trumpet often opens the upper airway enough to provide oxygen by mask. This procedure assumes the patient is arousable, is making normal respiratory excursions, and appears to have preserved swallowing, cough, and gag reflexes. Immediate oxygenation of inspired air in all patients is necessary because atelectasis, aspiration, or pulmonary contusion may be undetected by the external examination and, despite normal respiratory excursion, can decrease the transfer of oxygen to the blood because of intrapulmonary shunting. Nasal oxygen alone can often raise the Pa_{O_2} despite a slow voluntary respiratory rate, and it should always be given as a minimum. If a patent airway cannot be obtained with simple oral or nasopharyngeal tubing, the use of an endotracheal tube is indicated. Endotracheal intubation requires special skill and, because of the risk of misplacement into the esophagus, should be performed only by those qualified to do so. The use of esophageal obturator airways is no longer recommended.[82] These techniques should be applied cautiously in unconscious patients or those suspected of cervical spine trauma (injury to or above the clavicles) to preclude potential spinal cord damage. A rapid-sequence induction and oral endotracheal intubation with minimal axial traction, no rotation, and maintenance of a neutral chin position does not seem to increase the risk of cervical spinal cord injury.[68,79]

A surgical alternative to endotracheal intubation is cricothyroidotomy. A linear incision placed transversely across the cricothyroid membrane will allow rapid placement of a small (no. 4 French) tracheostomy tube into the upper airway. It may be used effectively for patients in whom trauma to the face prevents laryngeal intubation, but it should be reserved for patients over 12 years of age and used only by those skilled in the technique.

Severely injured patients who are not making adequate respiratory efforts after establishment of airway protection require assisted ventilation to provide required levels of systemic oxygenation. Individual trauma systems must establish guidelines for the use of sedation and paralysis of combative patients who are initially minimally responsive and become combative once they are intubated and well oxygenated. If sedation and paralysis are used in the field, ultra–short-acting or reversible agents are preferred. This allows a more accurate initial neurological assessment on arrival in the emergency room.

Most intensive care specialists believe that the best method of mechanical ventilation is volume ventilation under positive pressure. Positive-pressure ventilation helps prevent the progressive pulmonary failure often seen in severe injuries and results in early resolution of atelectasis. It also counteracts the potential development of pulmonary edema that can develop as a result of excess catecholamine release that follows the brain injury. Early intubation and respiratory support also prevent aspiration of gastric contents in a patient who may have a depressed pharyngeal and laryngeal ''gag'' response, as well as the respiratory insufficiency that can occur in the event of seizure activity or soft tissue swelling of the neck, which could occlude the upper airway. Following intubation, the use of temporary paralysis by administering pancuronium will help in obtaining an artifact-free CT scan and aid in controlling respiration in the combative or restless patient.

Circulation is the next priority, once an adequate airway and breathing (ventilation) are established. Blood pressure can be supported by the placement of multiple (two or more) peripheral intravenous routes and the infusion of a 0.9% saline solution to achieve a minimum systolic pressure of 100 mmHg. The use of military antishock trousers (MAST) for elevation of systemic arterial pressure in the prehospital setting remains controversial. Proposed mechanisms for improvement in the hemodynamic status and hemostasis of the trauma patient include increased vascular resistance, autotransfusion of blood from the lower extremities, tamponade of bleeding vessels, and fracture stabilization. Insufficient evidence to support these physiologic mechanisms in trauma patients and a failure to demonstrate improved survival in a large series of patients prospectively randomized to MAST versus no MAST challenge the utility of these garments.[3,52,74] In a prospective study of 12 patients with severe head injury, MAST did not cause any abnormal increase in ICP with moderate inflation pressures to 45 mmHg in each compartment.[29] MAST should not be used in patients with thoracic injury, overt cardiac failure, or pulmonary edema. Release of MAST should be done only when the blood pressure is stabilized and there exists ample access for fluid support, should it be required.

Maintenance of a ''normal'' blood pressure is essential to evaluate fully the neurological status. Raising the blood pressure to a normal range may convert ''coma'' to purposeful responsiveness, totally altering the diagnostic and therapeutic approach. Patients with brain injury almost always have some impairment of cerebral autoregulation. Thus, if the blood pressure falls (even to levels of only 85 or 90 mmHg systolic), CBF may fall *pari passu* to levels that will not adequately support nerve cell function. Therefore, blood pressure must be maintained above 100 mmHg systolic to maintain adequate cerebral perfusion pressure.[2,71]

Prolonged hypotension from brain damage is a preterminal event associated with medullary failure and other signs of brain stem death. The hypotension seen following experimental and human head injury is transient (<3 min) and usually resolves before the first clinical evaluation. The most common cause of shock in trauma is the hypovolemia of hemorrhage. Restoring normal volume is crucial to protecting the brain and overcoming the dysregulation of CBF and cerebral vasospasm, which may lead to ischemic infarction of the brain.

Lactic acidosis commonly occurs with hypotension, apnea, and hypercapnia, resulting in a mixed (metabolic and respiratory) systemic acidosis. This can be treated with intravenous sodium bicarbonate (1 meq per kilogram of body weight, and repeated every 15 min as needed). However, a proper airway with adequate ventilation and blood pressure maintenance usually quickly corrects the acidosis.

Management in the Emergency Room

The role of the ER in the management of moderate and severe brain injury is to continue the brain resuscitation initiated in the field, treat any life-threatening systemic injuries, and promptly initiate imaging studies for diagnosis of cerebral and spinal injuries. ER management begins with the patient's arrival and ends with transfer to the operating room, ICU, or hospital ward. Emergency room management, therefore, includes transportation for diagnostic procedures. The goal of emergency room management is to prevent secondary insults due to either systemic abnormalities or the primary CNS injury.

Following arrival in the ER, the patient should be rapidly assessed by a brief neurological examination during stabilization of the airway, ventilation, oxygenation, and blood pressure. A lateral x-ray film of the cervical spine should be obtained in all unconscious patients and those with moderately severe trauma at or above the level of the clavicle. Documentation of the neurological examination provides the baseline for observing change in CNS status and should be continued on a regular and frequent basis.

The immediate evaluation of head injuries requires a systematic approach that defines the problems requiring urgent diagnostic or therapeutic action. Such an approach includes neurological evaluation of the level of consciousness as determined by the Glasgow Coma Scale (eye opening, motor response, and verbal response);

pupillary examination for size and reactivity, to assess potential or impending herniation and the status of the upper brain stem; eye movements (either oculocephalic or oculovestibular), to evaluate the midbrain region in the area of the reticular activating system; and motor power using the international five-level scale—normal = 5, moderate weakness = 4, severe weakness (no antigravity function) = 3, trace movement = 2, and flaccid = 1. External evaluation of the head may reveal signs of a basal skull fracture, such as mastoid ecchymosis (Battle's sign), hemotympanum, periorbital ecchymosis (raccoon eyes), and otorrhea or rhinorrhea.

This examination can be performed in less than 2 min and allows placement of patients into management protocols according to severity of injury during early resuscitation. For classification purposes and triage decisions, mild (GCS score, 13 to 15), moderate (GCS score, 9 to 12), and severe (GCS score, 3 to 8) injuries have been used as a simple scheme. Intensive management as described in this chapter should be provided for all patients with severe and moderate TBI. These patients have had a serious brain injury, reflected by the alteration of consciousness. All patients with severe TBI should have immediate endotracheal intubation and controlled respiration using a slow rate (12 breaths per minute) and adequate tidal volume (15 ml per kilogram of body weight), usually 750 to 1000 ml in adults. This should provide adequate oxygenation and mild hypocapnia. A CT scan to detect a possible intracranial mass lesion is indicated immediately for patients with severe TBI and as soon as possible for patients with moderate TBI (the delay should be no longer than 4 h). It should be performed at once in the patient with moderate TBI patient if his or her condition deteriorates to severe with unresponsiveness to verbal command. The ability to obey commands is a key indicator of the function of the nervous system and a major neurological boundary between moderate and severe intracranial disorders. If CT is unavailable, angiography or air ventriculography should be done to determine the presence of intracranial mass lesions causing a shift of the midline structures in excess of 5 mm. This is an indication for decompressive craniotomy because such lesions may exist without localizing clinical signs of focal neurological deficit or tentorial herniation, and these patients may suddenly and unexpectedly deteriorate rapidly to an unrecoverable level. Should signs of herniation or mass lesion appear before CT scanning is done, mannitol in a large-bolus intravenous dose should be used (1 g/kg) followed by a single-view CT scan at the level of the foramina of Monro across the supratentorial space. If a mass lesion is detected, immediate decompressive craniotomy should be performed without further delay for additional CT scanning. Surgery should never be delayed beyond 15 min, and an additional bolus dose of mannitol (0.5 to 1.0 g/kg) may be required en route to the operating room.

If transtentorial herniation is not developing, a complete CT scan of the cranial structures should be done, starting at the level of the orbits, to visualize possible facial fractures, basal fractures, and pneumocephalus. A noncontrast scan is usually sufficient unless there is a suspicion of a nontraumatic cause of brain damage, such as subarachnoid hemorrhage from an aneurysm or arteriovenous malformation, in which case a contrast scan is performed as well.

In all patients with moderate and severe TBI not requiring an immediate craniotomy, the transfer from the CT scanner to the intensive care unit is to be rapid and with close attention to monitoring adequate ventilation and circulatory support.

The measurement of arterial blood gases is useful in adjusting ventilatory therapy to normalize oxygenation and acid-base balance. In acutely head-injured patients, the early blood pH usually reflects a respiratory alkalosis secondary to hyperventilation, although shock and hypotension or respiratory arrest may cause a metabolic or respiratory acidosis, which if prolonged may increase the risk of death.[22] The studies of McLaurin and King indicated that patients with severe head injuries have a normal or mildly acidotic systemic pH initially, followed by respiratory alkalosis and bicarbonate loss within 24 h.[55] Overall, a primary initial mixed acidosis is replaced by respiratory alkalosis if hypoxia is treated and fluid balance maintained. Despite spontaneous hyperventilation, hypoxia may exist in 30 percent of severely injured patients as a result of ventilation-perfusion inequalities of the lungs resulting from aspiration, atelectasis, pulmonary contusion, or excessive catecholamine sympathetic discharge with vasoconstriction and intrapulmonary shunting.[60] The peripheral vasoconstrictive response may increase peripheral resistance beyond the capacity of left ventricular function, causing left-sided heart failure and subsequent pulmonary edema.[32]

Patients with an undamaged brain may tolerate a Pa_{O_2} level as low as 70 mmHg, but those with cerebral trauma are very sensitive to even moderate hypoxemia (90 mmHg). Gordon and Ponten proposed two reasons for this:

1. Respiratory alkalosis shifts the oxygen-hemoglobin dissociation curve to the left, decreasing effective oxygen transfer to the tissues.
2. Dysregulation of CBF and focal vasospasm can create severe relative ischemia and uneven perfusion in the brain.[32]

Both may lead to infarction. Aggressive and timely respiratory support is simple enough therapy to prevent such a severe complication.

Systemic arterial pressure must be measured and recorded at short intervals and kept in a normal range to maintain the cerebral perfusion pressure. MAST trousers, if already applied, may be continued or applied in the operating room as indicated. Intravenous fluid infusion continues with balanced crystalloid solution. Hypotonic fluids are to be avoided because they lead to decreased serum osmolality and sodium levels, which can precipitate brain edema. Although extensive edema does not usually occur within the first 24 h, it may be aggravated by the administration of an excess of hypotonic fluid.

A central venous line or pulmonary artery catheter can help the physician determine the intravascular volume status and the adjustments needed to maintain balance and avoidance of fluid overload or dehydration. Hypotension or shock from head injury alone is rare and is usually due to hypovolemia. With the exception of severe hemorrhage from scalp or facial trauma, the source of blood loss will be in the chest, abdomen, extremities, or pelvis.[35] Physical examination and x-ray films of the chest, abdomen, and pelvis may determine the site of hemorrhage, and in all patients who are unconscious or have reduced responsiveness to pain, a diagnostic peritoneal lavage (DPL) should be done. This simple technique has a low incidence of false-positive or false-negative results. Among 225 patients with severe head injuries, Miller et al. found 49 percent with one or more additional systemic injuries, the most common injury being limb fracture (30 percent) or chest trauma (29 percent).[59] Abdominal injuries occurred in 17 percent as diagnosed by DPL, and spinal injuries in 6 percent.[57]

Additional studies in the ER include x-ray films of the skull, chest, and all long bones that may be fractured. Arterial blood gases are determined as frequently as the clinical situation dictates, to direct treatment of acid-base imbalance or hypoxia. The central venous line is to be used for evaluation of the intravascular fluid volume state. It should not be considered a main site for infusion, however, as this is best accomplished through short, large-bore peripheral intravenous catheters inserted percutaneously or by cutdown. An exception to this is a triple-lumen central catheter inserted by subclavian vein puncture, which allows both volume infusion and central venous pressure monitoring. A central venous pressure maintained at 5 to 10 mmH_2O is recommended, and patients should not be kept in a hypovolemic dehydrated state.[16]

Venous blood is drawn for laboratory studies, including complete blood count, electrolyte determinations, blood typing and matching, alcohol assay, and coagulation studies. A Foley catheter is placed for urinary bladder drainage, for evaluation of adequate urine output, and to accommodate increased urinary volume should mannitol be required. Urine is sampled for urinalysis and drug screening. Nasogastric intubation is done to decompress the stomach, prevent aspiration, and detect any gastrointestinal hemorrhage. Based on the hematocrit, central venous pressure, arterial blood pressure, and urinary output, infusion of blood products or crystalloid is used to maintain a systolic arterial blood pressure of at least 100 mmHg.

Management in the Intensive Care Unit

All patients with severe brain trauma and those who are postoperative from removal of an intracranial hematoma should be treated in an ICU with a systematic protocol that includes management of respiratory and cardiovascular parameters, ICP monitoring and control, and cerebral metabolic support.[16,18,46,71,83,84]

Hypoxia and hypercapnia must be avoided; controlled ventilation in severe head injury has been shown to improve outcome.[83] The early need for an artificial airway to ensure oxygenation was recognized in 1950 by Echols et al., who recommended tracheostomy.[25] If endotracheal intubation is required beyond 72 h, tracheostomy may be considered, although intubation with a large cuffed tube has been successful for 10 to 12 days without complications.

Controlled ventilation at a slow rate assists in the re-expansion of collapsed alveoli, preventing intrapulmonary shunting due to atelectasis, and allows time for adequate venous return despite positive intrathoracic pressure. The minute volume is adjusted to bring the Pa_{CO_2} level to 30 to 35 mmHg, and the Pa_{O_2} value is maintained above 80 mmHg by adjusting oxygen flow. Medication such as chlorpromazine or morphine may be used to sedate the patient, reduce the effects of noxious stimuli, and "phase" the patient into this respiratory pattern. Pancuronium is a useful neuromuscular blocker, but it should not be used solely to synchronize the patient to the respirator, because it interferes with neurological testing and does not relieve pain from noxious stimuli that may increase ICP, especially laryngeal stimulation. Percutaneous catheterization of the radial or dorsalis pedis artery allows for continuous monitoring of blood pressure and easy access for arterial blood gas monitoring. Pulmonary toilet and chest physiotherapy should be used, with bronchoscopy if needed for removal of mucous plugs. During all pulmonary therapy, careful attention to ICP and systolic arterial pressure is required, because head-injured patients usually have an elevated baseline ICP, and this may be elevated further during pulmonary therapy, compromising cerebral perfusion pressure and causing further brain damage. Increases in arterial blood pressure may result in ICP increases to dangerous levels in patients who have impairment or loss of autoregulation.

Treatment with controlled ventilation is justified for several reasons. It may prevent sudden, unexpected hypoxic events and reduce elevated ICP by maintaining a low Pa_{CO_2} with a normal Pa_{O_2}, resulting in a decrease in cerebrovascular volume while effectively providing adequate oxygen delivery to the brain. When begun early, controlled ventilation tends to deter the development of pulmonary edema and atelectasis by expanding collapsed alveoli. Additionally, it relieves the patient of energy-dissipating and exhausting respiratory work during this critical period. The spontaneous, vigorous hyperventilation that is not due to hypoxia may be controlled to the patient's benefit by decreasing muscle fatigue and overwork. Sedation and pharmacologic neuromuscular paralysis are added as necessary to control severe rigors, posturing, agitation, or elevated intracranial pressure.[18]

Positive end-expiratory pressure (PEEP) is required for advanced pulmonary insufficiency and pulmonary shunting when the Pa_{O_2} level cannot be brought to normal by increasing inspired oxygen concentration (Fi_{O_2}). Despite the fact that it can decrease cardiac output and increase ICP, PEEP can be used without adverse effect up to a pressure of 10 cmH_2O.[28] Positioning of the patient in a 15- to 30-degree head-up position is useful if the ICP is above 15 mmHg.

Recent studies recommend using less hyperventilation, despite its effectiveness in reducing cerebral blood volume and ICP. This change is based on evidence that maintaining Pa_{CO_2} in the range of 25 to 30 mmHg can result in significant cerebral vasoconstriction leading to ischemia. Such levels of hypocapnia, which previously had been considered moderate, have been associated with a worse outcome than milder degrees of hypocapnia. Additionally, in the vast majority of patients, significant hyperventilation is not essential for control of ICP.[46,61,71,72,81] Furthermore, in recent studies of severely head-injured patients, the lowest CBF values consistently occurred within the first 6 to 12 h after injury and then progressively increased over the ensuring hours and days.[1,8,46,63] Thus, hyperventilation may have its most deleterious effect during the first 24 h after injury, when relative or absolute cerebral ischemia may already exist. A Pa_{CO_2} 30 to 35 mmHg is recommended until ICP returns to normal.

Systemic arterial pressure (SAP) should be controlled when hypertensive levels reach over 180 mmHg systolic. Lewelt et al. have shown that abnormalities of cerebral autoregulation correlate with the severity of injury,[45] and Langfitt et al. have demonstrated increased cerebrovascular volume secondary to loss of autoregulation as a prime cause of intracranial hypertension.[43] Furthermore, increases in SAP may contribute to the disruption of the blood-brain barrier with extravasation of protein into the extracellular space and the development of cerebral edema.[33] Percutaneous arterial catheterization affords instantaneous monitoring, and control of SAP over 180 mmHg usually can be accomplished with sedatives in small doses. In patients requiring pharmacologic lowering of blood pressure, the choice of agents depends upon the cause of the hypertension and any pre-existing cardiac, pulmonary, or renal disease. The need for minute-to-minute control and the expected duration of blood pressure management assist in selecting intravenous or enteral administration. Andrews reviewed the agents currently used under these varying conditions.[2] Nifedipine, esmolol, and labetalol all provide rapid onset of action and relatively short duration for titrated control in the ICU. Nitroprusside is not recommended when the ICP is elevated, because of its cerebral vasodilating effect and potential for causing a further increase in ICP.

Before the initiation of any centrally or peripherally acting agent to lower blood pressure, an accurate assessment of overall volume status is mandatory. In a patient who is intravascularly volume-depleted and in whom reflex tachycardia and mild hypertension may be protecting cerebral perfusion, administration of a peripheral vasodilator may result in profound hypotension. For this reason, Swan-Ganz catheterization may be useful in more complicated cases with the potential for pulmonary or cardiac compromise. The information gained will allow for better titration of fluid balance during the acute phase of injury than if only a CVP line is used. An adequate hemoglobin level is necessary for oxygen transport, and patients with hematocrit levels below 30 percent (hemoglobin < 10 g) should be transfused with blood components as needed. A low hematocrit reduces the oxygen-carrying capacity of the blood, can retard wound healing, and can increase CBF, with possible increases in ICP.

Proper fluid balance and maintenance of adequate intravascular volume will help prevent hypotension, intravascular clotting, and electrolyte abnormalities. In multiply traumatized patients, loss of intravascular volume may reduce cerebral perfusion pressure. Davis and Sundt experimentally demonstrated that in hypovolemic hypotension, it is cardiac output, not SAP, that determines CBF.[23] Severe dehydration may predispose an individual to particularly severe electrolyte abnormalities if inappropriate antidiuretic hormone secretion or diabetes insipidus follows head injury. If sedatives are used in patients with a contracted intravascular volume, sudden episodes of hypotension may occur as a result of their cardiac depressive effects. Cerebral edema should be managed by means other than generalized severe dehydration.

Intravenous fluid should be infused at the usual maintenance volume. This usually can be started with a 5% dextrose and 0.45% normal saline solution at a rate of 125 ml/h for adults, totaling 3000 ml/day. Central venous pressure is maintained at 6 to 8 cmH_2O, and urinary output is kept between 0.5 and 1.0 ml/kg per hour (approximately 30 to 60 ml/h).

Electrolyte imbalance, particularly hyponatremia, is a serious but preventable complication. Abnormalities of serum sodium (<125 or >150 meq/liter) and serum osmolarity (<260 or >320 mosmol/liter) should be avoided. Overhydration, *per se,* will not cause brain edema if the serum sodium value is normal (135 to 145 meq/liter); however, when combined with hyponatremia (<130 meq/liter), it can cause edema at brain injury sites. A frequent source of a low serum sodium concentration is the syndrome of inappropriate antidiuretic hormone (SIADH), secretion, possibly related to hypothalamic trauma. This may occur at any time up to 14 days following injury and produces a rapid drop in serum sodium values. Urinary and serum sodium and osmolarity values should be checked to make an early diagnosis (normovolemia with hyponatremia, and serum hypo-osmolarity with hyperosmolar urine and increased urine sodium concentration). A low serum sodium value may persist despite sodium loading, and the primary approach to treatment is to eliminate the excess water by fluid restriction. If hyponatremia is severe, serum osmolarity may be raised quickly by using a 3% NaCl infusion (500 ml given over 4 to 5 h) with frequent electrolyte checks. The administration of urea at a dose of 40 g in 150 cc of normal saline over 2 h with dosing every 8 h until serum sodium rises is an alternative to 3% NaCl infusion. This agent provides Na and also inhibits renal Na excretion.[39,67] In addition, steroids that increase sodium retention can be given along with furosemide, which accelerates water excretion. The differentiation of SIADH from the hyponatremia of salt depletion is possible, because none of the signs of hypovolemia (lowered blood pressure, increased blood urea nitrogen) associated with salt depletion exist. A condition frequently confused with SIADH is isotonic fluid loss with hypotonic fluid replacement, during which the preservation of volume takes precedence over tonicity. This condition is iatrogenic and is preventable by careful monitoring of serum and urine electrolyte levels, nasogastric output, and other fluid intake and output.

Diabetes insipidus is an infrequent but serious result of head injury and may be associated with a poorer prognosis. Treatment requires early diagnosis and administration of vasopressin. It may be difficult to regulate the large volumes of intravenous fluid required to keep up with urine output. In these patients, vasopressin must be used cautiously because it can cause arterial hypertension with subsequent increases in ICP and excessive fluid retention. A synthetic vasopressive substance, desmopressin (DDAVP), has fewer side effects than vasopressin and may be used as an alternative.[85]

Seizure prophylaxis is a high priority in all moderately or severely head-injured patients. Early seizures can be prevented with a 13 mg/kg (approximately 1000 mg in average-size individuals) loading dose of diphenylhydantoin. This is administered intravenously as a 500-mg intravenously bolus (50 mg/min) along with ECG monitoring and followed at 6-h intervals with two doses of 250 mg each. By 24 h, effective plasma levels are usually reached. Maintenance doses of 100 mg given intravenously at 6- to 8-h intervals are continued after loading. In children the loading dose is 10 mg/kg, followed by a maintenance dose of 5 mg/kg. Breakthrough seizures are treated with additional doses of phenytoin if serum levels are determined to be subtherapeutic, or with phenobarbital added to the antiepileptic therapy in doses adequate to achieve therapeutic serum levels (20 to 30 mg/100 ml). Certain individuals appear to hypermetabolize these agents, and interval measurement of serum levels is a method of ensuring adequate prophylaxis. Many neurosurgeons believe that the medications should be continued after the acute phase for at least 1 year in the case of severe head injury; the EEG is useful in determining the need for their extended use. In patients with a normal initial CT scan who regain consciousness within 12 to 48 h and have no clinically detected seizure activity, weaning from antiepileptics can begin within weeks of discharge.

Pulmonary therapy is aimed at preventing infection and edema while maintaining mild hypocapnia. Continued or recurrent hypoxia may be a warning of impending acute respiratory distress syndrome and requires prompt preventive measures. In this case, dyspnea, tachypnea, and a decreasing Pa_{O_2} value despite an adequate oxygen supply and assisted ventilation are associated with a normal Pa_{CO_2} value and a chest film showing patchy and fluffy interstitial pulmonary edema that may progress to a total loss of air space. Pulmonary artery catheterization with a Swan-Ganz catheter reveals a progressively increasing pulmonary vascular pressure despite a relatively normal ''wedge'' pressure that reflects left atrial function.

The clinical syndrome of acute respiratory distress is probably the result of several factors, such as central neurogenic pulmonary edema, shock with aggressive fluid resuscitation, hypoxia, and possibly fat embolism. The intravenous fluids used in resuscitation have been implicated as a cause; however, there does not seem to be a clear advantage to using colloids over crystalloids.

A Pa_{O_2} value of less than 70 mmHg should be managed with an increased Fi_{O_2} and positive-pressure volume ventilation with PEEP up to 15 cmH_2O for as long as the ICP tolerates it. In patients with a pulmonary wedge pressure (PWP) over 15, diuretics and digitalis may be helpful. It is difficult to differentiate neurogenic pulmonary edema from acute respiratory distress syndrome on clinical grounds, although brain-injured patients with a neurogenic type of pulmonary insufficiency readily respond to therapy.

Fat embolism can be an overlooked cause of acute respiratory distress, and although described as occurring in three forms—pure pulmonary, pure cerebral, and systemic with renal and hepatic involvement—it usually is recognized clinically because of its pulmonary effects. The diagnosis can be made on the basis of clinical criteria.[42] The syndrome is primarily pulmonary with associated cerebral symptomatology, and the pathologic changes include pulmonary edema, hemorrhagic parenchymal necrosis, and fat globules in the alveoli.[24] Petechiae may appear on the chest and in the conjunctivae. Fat embolism is reported to occur in 1 percent of major trauma victims, with the brain being the second most commonly affected organ.[59]

The most likely causes of fat embolism include fat that is embolized into the venous circulation from traumatized tissue and spontaneous intravascular lipid droplet formation caused by alterations in the blood resulting from the primary traumatic insult. Fat droplets may be formed from existing intravascular free lipids, and this has been shown to occur in nontraumatic conditions.[7]

Regardless of the etiology of fat embolism, the pulmonary circulation seems to serve as a filter for circulating fat globules, and this is the primary cause of the pulmonary dysfunction. Early recognition of hypoxia in patients with multiple trauma and long bone fractures allows aggressive early treatment, which may prevent serious complications.

Oxygen therapy with positive pressure, if necessary, combined with adequate intravenous volume replacement, including blood as required, prevents hypotensive shock and reduces catecholamine release, which contributes to increased lipid metabolism and release. Corticosteroids may reduce the pulmonary effects if given in high doses (at least 16 mg/day of dexamethasone).[4] Therapy designed to improve the microcirculation and reduce plasma lipid levels is controversial. Heparin, intravenous alcohol, and low-molecular-weight dextran have all been used, with mixed and often contradictory results.[42] In general, the best treatment after early recognition appears to be pressurized oxygen therapy to restore alveolar function to normal.

ICP Monitoring and Management

There is evidence that the monitoring of ICP and the management of elevated ICP in comatose brain-injured patients may significantly improve the outcome of severe head injuries. Intracranial hypertension is a major cause of death in severely head injured patients, and early recognition of an abnormally high intracranial pressure with immediate intervention to return it to normal should be part of any intensive neurological care program.

Institutions vary in management protocols for raised ICP. A guiding physiologic concept is that of cerebral compartmentalization. Directed therapy to reduce CSF volume, cerebral blood volume, brain interstitial fluid, intracellular brain water, and intracranial mass lesions as needed in an individual patient represents an ideal theoretical treatment course. In practice, current intensive care monitoring cannot define the precise contribution of each compartment to the overall level of raised ICP. Therefore, a balanced stepwise progression of therapy that does not immediately exhaust all options is preferred.[18]

Immediate evacuation of hematomas larger than 25 cc in volume and not located in eloquent brain is a priority.[75] Early placement of a subarachnoid or intraventricular monitoring device is recommended; techniques are discussed in other chapters. We prefer a ventricular catheter; fiberoptic intraparenchymal catheters are being used in patients with very small ventricles, as determined on CT scan, that would be difficult to catheterize. With rapid surgical decompression accomplished and ICP monitoring established, intensive management to control ICP and prevent cerebral ischemia is instituted.

Generally, ICP values above 20 mmHg in the resting patient are considered abnormally high, and those above 40 mmHg represent very serious and dangerous levels of intracranial hypertension. Controlled ventilation to maintain a level of 30 to 35 mmHg P_{CO_2} is capable of reducing ICP. Additional sedation with morphine sulfate (2 mg/h intravenously) may be used to reduce agitation and help synchronize respirations with the ventilator. If ICP remains elevated despite normothermia and repositioning of the head at a 20- to 30-degree head-up posture with avoidance of compression of the jugular venous system, then ventricular drainage is indicated. Continuous ventricular drainage is to be avoided because during drainage ICP readings are not accurate, and excessive drainage can collapse the ventricles against the catheter, leading to catheter failure. Ventricular drainage can be set to allow drainage of fluid when ICP elevates above 15 or 20 mmHg. This is done by setting the drainage catheter at 15 cm above the level of the foramen of Monro. Setting the drainage catheter at this level prevents ventricular collapse. ICP readings sustained above 20 mmHg for 1 to 2 min and not associated with patient movement or suctioning warrant opening of the ventricular drain for 5 to 10 min. This procedure can be repeated several times per hour if necessary. If this still fails to control ICP, osmotic diuretics (mannitol) in conjunction with loop diuretics (furosemide) may then be employed. Most authorities prefer to give mannitol as an intravenous bolus in a dose of 0.25 to 1.0 g/kg of a 20% solution. Furosemide (0.5 mg/kg given intravenously) may assist the bolus in its effectiveness in lowering ICP. Use of furosemide should be restricted to patients with a known positive fluid balance and high central venous or pulmonary capillary wedge pressures. Patients with concomitant brain and abdominal injuries may displace (third-space) a significant portion of their intravascular volume into the viscera and peritoneal cavity. Therefore, daily input and output, and body weight measurements are as critical to examine as the various intravascular pressures when diuretics are considered. Following the use of diuretics, serum electrolyte and osmolarity values should be checked, because serum values in excess of 320 mosmol/liter preclude further use of osmotic therapy in order to prevent renal damage.

Precipitous increases in ICP unresponsive to therapy should be investigated with a CT scan to detect emergent intracranial hematomas or acute hydrocephalus. In addition, repeat CT scanning 4 to 8 h after admission is recommended for patients harboring cerebral contusions not operated on and for those who demonstrate an abnormal initial coagulation profile.[53,77,78] New hematoma formation or contusion expansion requiring operative decompression may occur before ICP rises indicate their presence.[12]

If all ventilation, drainage, osmotic, and surgical therapies have been exhausted and ICP remains high, the use of high-dose barbiturate therapy may be indicated in a patient with severe head injury and a GCS score of less than 7 who has no medical contraindication such as liver or renal disease.[50,56] Although a trial of early barbiturate therapy in a mixed group of severely injured patients failed to show an improvement in outcome over conventional therapy, several observations suggest a role for barbiturates in a subset of patients.[18,26,62] Barbiturate therapy consistently lowers ICP; it is the complications of this therapy that cause poor outcomes. Hypotension and sepsis are the predominant secondary insults that lead to failure. Therefore, it is recommended that arterial and Swan-Ganz monitoring be instituted and that normal or slightly increased intravascular volume and normal temperature be achieved before barbiturates are administered. During therapy, vigilant maintenance must be enforced to avoid any hypotension. Barbiturate therapy should be reserved for young patients with no evidence of traumatic cardiac or pulmonary impairment. Additionally, a patient with an initial Glasgow motor score demonstrating flexion withdrawal or better and a CT scan that does not reveal severe bilateral hemispheric or brain stem injury has a greater chance of a good recovery if barbiturates lower ICP to nonischemic levels. Therefore, it is a select group—patients who do not have poor initial demographic, neurological, and CT findings but who develop uncontrolled ICP—that may benefit from barbiturate therapy. In this group, its is suggested that barbiturates be given as soon as ICP cannot be managed by other modalities and before physical signs of brain stem impairment develop. Continuous monitoring of ICP is required to regulate dosage, which can begin with 50 to 100 mg of intravenous pentobarbital, the EEG being observed continuously. Treatment should continue at least until a burst suppression pattern is obtained on the EEG or the mean arterial blood pressure (MABP) falls below 80 mmHg. At blood pressures less than this, cerebral perfusion pressure (CPP = MABP − ICP) may be reduced below a level of 60 to 70 mmHg, which can cause cerebral ischemia. If the blood pressure tolerates such dosage and burst suppression is obtained, a serum pentobarbital level of 2 to 4 mg/100 ml is maintained by using a 1- to 2-mg/kg intravenous bolus dose each hour. During active barbiturate therapy, the neurological examination remains less reliable; however, barbiturates in general cause small pupils, and if large, irregular pupils persist, they usually are associated with increased ICP, the development of an intracranial mass lesion with potential herniation, or advanced brain stem dysfunction.

Maintenance of adequate intravenous fluid balance and oxygenation with a pressure-volume ventilator is critical to prevent the pulmonary problems occasionally associated with barbiturate coma. The intermittent use of mannitol in addition to pentobarbital may be required and is permissible, provided that the serum osmolarity is less than 320 mosmol and the systolic blood pressure is maintained above 100 mmHg. Treatment is continued for 24 to 48 h after the ICP is controlled to less than 20 mmHg, and the patient is gradually weaned. Reduction of the barbiturate dose by 50% each day is recommended. If the ICP rises again, therapy may be reinstated for an additional 24-h interval prior to weaning. Patients who cannot tolerate weaning or are unresponsive to barbiturate therapy have a poor prognosis.

Cerebral Perfusion Pressure Management

An increasing number of reports suggest that cerebral perfusion pressure (CPP) management for patients suffering severe TBI is of greater importance than focusing solely upon tight control of ICP. The rationale for CPP management is to ensure adequate cerebral perfusion without the need for frequent measurement of CBF or cerebral metabolic rates. Monitoring can rely on well-established methods of measuring mean arterial pressure and ICP.

Previous studies of head-injured patients indicated that a CPP of as low as 40 to 50 mmHg was adequate for maintaining relatively normal CBF; more recent work showed that 60 mmHg was the critical CPP.[15,62,80] However, several of the latest investigations indicate that a CPP of at least 60 to 70 mmHg, if sustained, after severe head injury significantly improves long-term outcome. No further improvement in outcome or cerebral hemodynamics was seen if perfusion pressure was pushed beyond 70 mmHg.[14,15,21] Some proponents of this form of therapy think that CPP should be pushed until cerebral autoregulation is captured and improvement in ICP or jugular oxygen saturation is observed. This can occasionally require pushing CPP to as high as 100 mmHg.[71] It is recommended, based on recent evidence, that volume status be scrutinized carefully to ensure adequate cardiac filling pressures and to maintain CPP above 60 mmHg at all times, with a target CPP of about 70 mmHg or higher considered optimal. Many researchers continue to investigate the optimal management of CPP and CBF.

The strictest advocates of CPP management advocate nursing all head-injured patients in the flat position.[71] Others have demonstrated an improvement in ICP control with the head elevated to 45 degrees. Recent evidence using multimodality monitoring suggests that the maximum benefit to ICP occurs by a head elevation of 30 degrees. It seems reasonable to recommend positioning the head from flat to a maximum of 30 degrees, with careful attention given to the effect on ICP.

Nutritional Support and Rehabilitation

Nutritional considerations are important, and an extensive review supports the idea that patients with early nutritional supplementation have an improved outcome, compared with patients who are starved. It is not yet clear whether parenteral or enteral nutrition provides a greater benefit.[84] Feeding via nasogastric tube should not be started before the fourth or fifth day after injury. Total parenteral nutrition (TPN) may be started earlier and can be effective in reducing negative nitrogen balance and generalized inanition. Head-injured patients normally have an elevated metabolic rate, which increases progressively for 1 week to levels as high as 160 to 180 percent of normal. Major trauma and isolated severe head injury usually result in a marked depression of the patient's immune competence. However, properly administered TPN can bring immune responsiveness back toward normal within 2 weeks. There is preliminary evidence that TPN may reduce mortality; if this proves to be true, it is probably the result of a reduced infection rate. Adults should usually receive between 2200 and 2750 kcal/day. The blood sugar level should not be permitted to rise over 180 to 200 mg/100 ml. Higher levels may contribute to increased cerebral lactic acidosis, which can further injure the already-damaged brain.

Rehabilitation programs should begin during the first week of admission, even while the patient is in intensive care. Nonfractured extremities should be put through a full range of motion repeatedly during each day. Patients who are posturing can have this done during the muscle paralysis and relaxation used for ventilatory control. Many rehabilitation specialists recommend the early institution of controlled visual, auditory, and tactile stimuli, claiming this may hasten and improve recovery. Documentation that this is indeed true remains to be developed, but it certainly cannot be considered detrimental. Careful and gentle, yet direct and honest, family counseling must also begin early to prepare the family for an appropriate response to the ordeal ahead.

References

1. Aggarwal S. Time course of cerebral blood flow and metabolic changes following severe head injury. Presented at the 61st Annual

Meeting of the American Association of Neurological Surgeons, Boston, Mass, April 1993 (poster).
2. Andrews BT. The control of blood pressure in the neurosurgical intensive care unit. *Contemp Neurosurg* 1993; 15:1–5.
3. Aprahamian C, Gessert G, Bandyk DF, et al. MAST-associated compartment syndrome (MACS): A review. *J Trauma,* 1989; 29:549–555.
4. Ashbaugh DG, Petty TL. The use of corticosteroids in the treatment of respiratory failure associated with massive fat embolism. *Surg Gynecol Obstet* 1966; 123; 493–500.
5. Becker DP, Miller JD, Ward JD, et al. The outcome from severe head injury with early diagnosis and intensive management. *J Neurosurg* 1977; 47:491–502.
6. Becker DP, Miller JD, Young HF, et al. Diagnosis and treatment of head injury in adults. In Youmans JR (ed): *Neurological Surgery.* Philadelphia: Saunders, 1982, pp 1938–2083.
7. Bergentz SE. Studies on the genesis of posttraumatic fat embolism. *Acta Chir Scand (Suppl)* 1961; 282:5–72.
8. Bouma GJ, Muizelaar JP, Bandoh K, et al. Blood pressure and intracranial pressure-volume dynamics in severe head injury: Relationship with cerebral blood flow. *J Neurosurg* 1992; 77:15–19.
9. Bouma GJ, Muizelaar JP, Choi SC, et al. Cerebral circulation and metabolism after severe traumatic brain injury: the elusive role of ischemia. *J Neurosurg* 1991; 75:685–693.
10. Bouma GJ, Muizelaar JP, Stringer WA, et al. Ultra early evaluation of regional cerebral blood flow in severely head-injured patients using xenon-enhanced computed tomography. *J Neurosurg* 1992; 77:360–368.
11. Bowers SA, Marshall LF. Outcome in 200 consecutive cases of severe head injury treated in San Diego County: a prospective analysis. *Neurosurgery* 1980; 6:237–242.
12. Bullock R, Hannemann CO, Murray L, et al. Recurrent hematomas following craniotomy for traumatic intracranial mass. *J Neurosurg* 1990; 72:9–14.
13. Chan KH, Dearden NM, Miller JD, et al. Transcranial Doppler waveform differences in hyperemic and nonhyperemic patients after severe head injury. *Surg Neurol* 1992; 38:433–436.
14. Chan KH, Dearden NM, Miller JD, et al. Multimodality monitoring as a guide to treatment of intracranial hypertension after severe brain injury. *Neurosurgery* 1993; 32:547–553.
15. Chan KH, Miller JD, Dearden NM, et al. The effect of changes in cerebral perfusion pressure upon middle cerebral artery blood flow velocity and jugular bulb venous oxygen saturation after severe brain injury. *J Neurosurg* 1992; 77:55–61.
16. Chesnut RM. Medical complications of the head-injured patient. In Cooper PR (ed): *Head Injury,* 3d ed. Baltimore: Williams & Wilkins, 1993, pp 459–501.
17. Chesnut RM, Marshall LF, Klauber MR, et al. The role of secondary brain injury in determining outcome from severe head injury. *J Trauma* 1993; 34:216–222.
18. Chesnut RM, Marshall LF, Marshall SB. Medical management of intracranial pressure. In Cooper PR (ed): *Head injury,* 3d ed. Baltimore: Williams & Wilkins, 1993, pp 225–246.
19. Colohan AR, Alves WM, Gross CR, et al. Head injury mortality in two centers with different emergency medical services and intensive care. *J Neurosurg,* 1989; 71:202–207.
20. Colohan AR, Oyesiku NM. Moderate head injury: an overview. *J Neurotrauma* 1992; 9(Suppl 1):S259–S264.
21. Contant CF, Robertson CS, Gopinath SP, et al. Determination of clinically important thresholds in continuously monitored patients with head injury. *J Neurotrauma* 1993; 10(Suppl 1):S57, O4 (abstr).
22. Cook AW, Browder EJ, Lyons HA. Alterations in acid-base equilibrium in craniocerebral trauma: A determinant in survival. *J Neurosurg* 1961; 18:366–370.
23. Davis DH, Sundt TM Jr. Relationship of cerebral blood flow to cardiac output, mean arterial pressure, blood volume, and alpha and beta blockade in cats. *J Neurosurg* 1980; 52:745–754.
24. Dines DE, Burgher LW, Okazaki H. The clinical and pathologic correlation of fat embolism syndrome. *Mayo Clin Proc* 1975; 50:407–411.
25. Echols DH, Llewellyn R, Kirgis HD, et al. Tracheostomy in the management of severe head injuries. *Surgery* 1950; 28:801–811.
26. Eisenberg HM, Frankowski RF, Contant CF, et al. High-dose barbiturate control of elevated intracranial pressure in patients with severe head injury. *J Neurosurg* 1988; 69:15–23.
27. Eisenberg HM, Gary HE Jr, Aldrich EF, et al. Initial CT findings in 753 patients with severe head injury. A report from the NIH Traumatic Coma Data Bank. *J Neurosurg* 1990; 73:688–698.
28. Frost EAM. Effects of positive end-expiratory pressure on intracranial pressure and compliance in brain-injured patients. *J Neurosurg* 1977; 47:195–200.
29. Gardner SR, Maull KI, Swensson EE, Ward JD. The effects of the pneumatic antishock garment on intracranial pressure in man: A prospective study of 12 patients with severe head injury. *J Trauma* 1984; 24:896–900.
30. Gennarelli TA, Champion HR, Sacco WJ, et al. Mortality of patients with head injury and extracranial injury treated in trauma centers. *J Trauma* 1989; 29:1193–1202.
31. Gennarelli TA, Segawa H, Wald U, et al. Physiological response to angular acceleration of the head. In Grossman RG, Gildenberg PL (eds): *Head Injury: Basic and Clinical Aspects.* New York: Raven Press, 1982, pp 129–140.
32. Gordon E, Ponten U. The non-operative treatment of severe head injuries. In Vinken PJ, Bruyn GW (eds): *Handbook of Clinical Neurology,* vol 24. Amsterdam: North-Holland Publishing Company, 1975, pp 599–626.
33. Häggendal E, Johansson B. On the pathophysiology of the increased cerebrovascular permeability in acute arterial hypertension in cats. *Acta Neurol Scand* 1972; 48:265–270.
34. Hovda DA, Yoshino A, Kawamata T, et al. Diffuse prolonged depression of cerebral oxidative metabolism following concussive brain injury in the rat: a cytochrome oxidase histochemistry study. *Brain Res* 1991; 567:1–10.
35. Illingworth G, Jennett WB. The shocked head injury. *Lancet* 1965; 2:511–514.
36. Jenkins LW, Marmarou A, Lewelt W, Becker DP. Increased vulnerability of the traumatized brain to early ischemia. In: Baethmann A, Go KG, Unterberg A (eds): *Mechanisms Of Secondary Brain Damage.* New York: Plenum, 1986, pp 273–282.
37. Jenkins LW, Moszynski K, Lyeth BG, et al. Increased vulnerability of the mildly traumatized rat brain to cerebral ischemia: the use of controlled secondary ischemia as a research tool to identify common or different mechanisms contributing to mechanical and ischemic brain injury. *Brain Res* 1989; 477:211–224.
38. Katayama Y, Becker DP, Tamura T, Hovda DA. Massive increases in extracellular potassium and the indiscriminate release of glutamate following concussive brain injury. *J Neurosurg* 1990; 73:889–900.
39. Kelly DF, Laws ER Jr, Fossett DT. Fluid and sodium abnormalities after trans-sphenoidal surgery for pituitary adenomas with emphasis on delayed hyponatremia: a review of 99 patients. Presented at the 43rd Annual Meeting of the Congress of Neurological Surgeons, Vancouver, October 6, 1993.
40. Klauber MR, Marshall LF, Luerssen TG, et al. Determinants of head injury mortality: importance of the low risk patient. *Neurosurgery* 1989; 23:31–36.
41. Klauber MR, Marshall LF, Toole BM. Cause of decline in head-injury mortality rate in San Diego County, California. *J Neurosurg* 1985; 62:528–531.
42. Kramer J, Klawans HL. Fat embolism. In Vinken PJ, Bruyn GW (eds): *Handbook of Clinical Neurology,* vol 24. Amsterdam: North-Holland Publishing Company, 1975, pp 563–574.
43. Langfitt TW, Weinstein JD, Kassell NF. Vascular factors in head injury: Contribution to brain-swelling and intracranial hypertension. In Caveness WF, Walker AE (eds): *Head Injury: Conference Proceedings.* Philadelphia: Lippincott, 1966, pp 172–194.
44. Levine JE, Becker D. Reversal of incipient brain death from head-injury apnea at the scene of accidents. *N Engl J Med* 1979; 301:109.
45. Lewelt W, Jenkins LW, Miller JD. Autoregulation of cerebral blood

flow after experimental fluid percussion injury of the brain. *J Neurosurg* 1980; 53:500–511.
46. Marion D, Obrist WD, Penrod LE, et al. Treatment of cerebral ischemia improves outcome following severe traumatic brain injury. Presented at the 61st Annual Meeting of the American Association of Neurological Surgeons, Boston, MA, April 26, 1993.
47. Marmarou A, Anderson RL, Ward JD, et al. Impact of ICP instability and hypotension on outcome in patients with severe head trauma. *J Neurosurg* 1991; 75(Suppl):S59–S66.
48. Marshall LF, Gautille T, Klauber MR, et al. The outcome of severe closed head injury. *J Neurosurg* 1991; 75(Suppl):S28–S36.
49. Marshall LF, Marshall SB, Klauber MR, et al. The diagnosis of head injury requires a classification based on computed axial tomography. *J Neurotrauma,* 1992; 9 Suppl 1:S287–S292.
50. Marshall LF, Smith RW, Shapiro HM. The outcome with aggressive treatment in severe head injuries. Part I: The significance of intracranial pressure monitoring: Part II. Acute and chronic barbiturate administration in the management of head injury. *J Neurosurg* 1979; 50:20–25, 26–30.
51. Martin NA, Doberstein C, Zane C, et al. Posttraumatic cerebral arterial spasm: transcranial Doppler ultrasound, cerebral blood flow, and angiographic findings. *N Neurosurg* 1992; 77:575–583.
52. Mattox KL, Bickell W, Pepe PE, et al. Prospective MAST study in 911 patients. *J Trauma* 1989; 29:1104–1111.
53. McBride DQ, Patel AB, Caron M. Early repeat CT scan: importance in detecting surgical lesions after closed head injury. *J Neurotrauma* 1993; 10(Suppl):S227, P203 (abstr).
54. McGraw CP. A cerebral perfusion pressure greater than 80 mmHg is more beneficial. In Hoff JT, Betz AL (eds): *Intracranial Pressure VII.* Berlin: Springer-Verlag, 1989, pp 839–841.
55. McLaurin RL, King LR. Recognition and treatment of metabolic disorders after head injuries. *Clin Neurosurg* 1972; 19:281–300.
56. Miller JD: Barbiturates and raised intracranial pressure. *Ann Neurol* 1979; 6:189–193.
57. Miller JD. Physiology of trauma. *Clin Neurosurg* 1982; 29:103–130.
58. Miller JD. Head injury and brain ischaemia: implications for therapy. *Br J Anaesth* 1985; 57:120–129.
59. Miller JD, Butterworth JF, Gudeman SK, et al. Further experience in the management of severe head injury. *J Neurosurg* 1981; 54:289–299.
60. Miller JD, Sweet RC, Narayan R, Becker DP. Early insults to the injured brain. *JAMA* 1978; 240:439–442.
61. Muizelaar JP, Marmarou A, Ward JD, et al. Adverse effects of prolonged hyperventilation in patients with severe head injury: a randomized clinical trial. *J Neurosurg* 1991; 75:731–739.
62. Nordstrom CH, Messeter K, Sundbarg G, et al. Cerebral blood flow, vasoreactivity, and oxygen consumption during barbiturate therapy in severe traumatic brain lesions. *J Neurosurg* 1988; 68:424–431.
63. Obrist WD, Marion DW, Aggarwal S. Time course of cerebral blood flow and metabolic changes following severe head injury. Presented at the 61st Annual Meeting of the American Association of Neurological Surgeons, Boston, Mass, April 1993 (poster).
64. Ommaya AK, Gennarelli TA. Cerebral concussion and traumatic unconsciousness: correlation of experimental and clinical observations on blunt head injuries. *Brain* 1974; 97:633–654.
65. Ommaya AK, Gennarelli TA. Experimental head injury. In Vinken DJ, Bruyn GW (eds): *Handbook of Clinical Neurology,* vol 23. Amsterdam: North-Holland Publishing Company, 1975, pp 67–90.
66. Piek J, Chesnut RM, Marshall LF, et al. Extracranial complications of severe head injury. *J Neurosurg* 1992; 77:901–907.
67. Reeder RF, Harbaugh RE. Administration of intravenous urea and normal saline for the treatment of hyponatremia in neurosurgical patients. *J Neurosurg* 1989; 70:201–206.
68. Rhee KJ, Green W, Holcroft JW, et al. Oral intubation in the multiply injured patient: the risk of exacerbating spinal cord damage. *Ann Emerg Med* 1990; 19:511–514.
69. Robertson CS, Contant CF, Gokaslan ZL, et al. Cerebral blood flow, arteriovenous oxygen difference, and outcome in head injured patients. *J Neurol Neurosurg Psychiatry* 1992; 55:594–603.
70. Robertson CS, Contant CF, Narayan RK, Grossman RG. Cerebral blood flow, AVDO2, and neurologic outcome in head-injured patients. *J Neurotrauma* (Suppl 1) 1992; 9:S349–S358.
71. Rosner MJ. Pathophysiology and management of increased intracranial pressure. In Andrews BT (ed): *Neurosurgical Intensive Care.* New York: McGraw-Hill, 1993, pp 57–112.
72. Rosner MJ, Daughton S. Cerebral perfusion pressure management in head injury. *J Trauma* 1990; 30:933–941.
73. Ruff RM, Marshall LF, Crouch J, et al. Predictors of outcome following severe head trauma: follow-up data from the Traumatic Coma Data Bank. *Brain Injury* 1993; 7:101–111.
74. Schneider PA, Mitchell JM, Allison EJ Jr. The use of military antishock trousers in trauma—a reevaluation. *J Emerg Med* 1989; 7:497–500.
75. Seelig JM, Becker DP, Miller JD, et al. Traumatic acute subdural hematoma. Major mortality reduction in comatose patients treated within four hours. *N Engl J Med* 1981; 304:1511–1512.
76. Sheinberg M, Kanter MJ, Robertson CS, et al. Continuous monitoring of jugular venous oxygen saturation in head-injured patients. *J Neurosurg* 1992; 76:212–217.
77. Stein SC, Spettell C, Young G, et al. Delayed and progressive brain injury in closed-head trauma: radiological demonstration. *Neurosurgery* 1993; 32:25–31.
78. Stein SC, Young GS, Talucci RC, et al. Delayed brain injury after head trauma: significance of coagulopathy *Neurosurgery* 1992; 30:160–165.
79. Talucci RC, Shaikh KA, Schwab CW. Rapid sequence induction with oral endotracheal intubation in the multiply injured patient. *Am Surg* 1988; 54:185–187.
80. Tsutsumi H, Ide K, Mizutani T, et al. The relationship between intracranial pressure, cerebral perfusion pressure and outcome in head-injured patients: The critical level of cerebral perfusion pressure. In Miller JD, Teasdale GM, Rowan JO, et al. (eds): *Intracranial Pressure VI.* Berlin: Springer-Verlag, 1986, pp 661–666.
81. van Helden A, Schneider GH, Unterberg A, et al. Monitoring of jugular venous oxygen saturation as a guide to therapy of severe head injury. *J Neurotrauma* 1993; 10(Suppl):S103, O74 (abstr).
82. Weigelt JA. Resuscitation and initial management. *Crit Care Clin* 1993; 9:657–671.
83. White RJ. Programmed management of severe head injuries revisited. *J Trauma* 1975; 15:779–784.
84. Young B, Ott L, Phillips R, McCllain C. Metabolic management of the patient with head injury. *Neurosurg Clin North Am* 1991; 2:301–320.
85. Ziai F, Walter R, Rosenthal LM. Treatment of central diabetes insipidus in adults and children with desmopressin: a synthetic analogue of vasopressin. *Arch Intern Med* 1978; 138:1382–1385.

266 Pediatric Head Injury

Derek A. Bruce

Trauma is the most frequent cause of death in children. In the United States each year, 300,000 to 400,000 children are hospitalized for treatment of head trauma (230 per 100,000 per year), and many more, (12,000 per 100,000 per year) are seen for medical care. There are 6,000 to 7,000 deaths from trauma each year in children under 14 years of age.[2,5–7,45,48] The most common cause of head trauma in children is a fall; the most common cause of severe head injury is motor vehicle–related trauma. Although certain predisposing factors have been identified—inner city living, single-parent families, behaviorally or emotionally disturbed parents or children—the epidemic of injuries in children covers all levels of our society. For white male teenagers, suicide is the second leading cause of death, and for black and Hispanic male teenagers, homicide. Most of these fatalities are the result of gunshots. The overwhelming costs in loss of life, loss of independent function, and dollars spent must be controlled. Prevention is the only effective strategy. In Sweden,[8] as a result of coordinated efforts in the society, the rate of childhood accidental trauma has been reduced manyfold. We must improve the situation for the children in the United States. We have made a start by introducing car seat laws, seat belt laws, a push for children to wear bicycle helmets, the Look First program, and the Safe Kids campaign. Much more remains to be done, and all physicians caring for children should encourage the production of a safer environment for our children and teenagers.

From birth through adolescence the brain and the intracranial compartment undergo a multiplicity of physiologic and anatomic changes that influence the type of head injury and the child's response to it. The water content of the brain is 90 percent at birth and 75 percent by adolescence. The newborn's brain has almost no myelination, yet by 4 years of age most of the major tracts are already myelinated. The ratio of brain to CSF is smaller in the newborn and approaches the adult ratio by 4 to 5 years. The sutures are open and mobile, and the fontanel present through the first year of life. The normal intracranial pressure (ICP) with an open fontanel is only 3 to 5 mmHg. The cerebral blood flow (CBF) is initially less than that of the adult, with a lower cerebral metabolic rate for oxygen ($CMRO_2$); then from early childhood (3 to 4 years of age), the CBF increases to 50 percent or more than the adult with a higher $CMRO_2$. Finally in the midteens, the CBF and $CMRO_2$ reach the adult levels. In the first year the head is large and heavy compared with the body, and the neck muscles are weak. Because all these differences modify the effects of trauma on the head and brain, the physician caring for the head-injured child must be aware of them.

As the child ages and develops independent gait and functioning, the mechanism of trauma to which the child is exposed changes. Thus falls from the parents' arms, from the changing table, out of the stroller—usually low-impact injuries—are the common causes of head injury in the first year of life. As the child learns to walk, falls from greater heights occur. With the onset of independent exploratory skills, automobile-pedestrian accidents become increasingly frequent. The incidence of bicycle accidents, sports injuries, motor vehicle accidents with the child as driver, and suicide and homicide increases in the older child.

General Physiological Differences of Children

For the first months of life the heart muscle has little ability to alter the force of contraction; therefore, cardiac output can be increased only by increasing the rate of contraction. Thus the underperfused infant may maintain blood pressure as a result of increased heart rate, then suddenly develop frank irreversible shock without displaying the gradual drop in pressure one would expect in an older child.

Glomerular filtration rate is limited in the infant, and it is easy to overload the small child if fluid resuscitation is not regulated in a controlled fashion. Heat loss can be rapid in children because of the large surface area/weight ratio, and cooling should be avoided during resuscitation. Spinal cord injuries in children under 8 years of age have a predilection for the upper cervical region of the spinal cord and often occur without radiographic abnormalities (SCIWORA).[37] During resuscitation and intubation, this risk of spinal trauma must be kept in mind. The child's airway is different in size and anatomy, and appropriate endotracheal tube sizes must be available. It is neither necessary nor beneficial to hyperextend the child's neck for endotracheal intubation, and because of the risk of SCIWORA, it should not be done. Multiple trauma is common in children, and the most frequent site of occult blood loss is the abdomen because of the relatively large abdominal organs, the absence of a lot of subcutaneous fat, and the lower position of the liver and spleen in the abdomen such that the lower ribs do not protect them as well as in adults and older children.

A clear understanding of the pathophysiology is necessary to delivering the best possible care to the child and family. The traumatic event affects the whole family, and supportive services should be mobilized as soon as possible after the injury to help the family cope with it. A thorough history ascertains whether preventive strategies are required to limit the risks of further injury in the household; the family is helped to cope with the immediate life-threatening problems, and the stage is set for rehabilitation of the child and family. This highlights the three phases, each equally important, of trauma care in childhood: prevention, acute treatment, and rehabilitation.

Birth Injuries

Traumatic injuries to the skull and brain in utero are rare and rarely become the province of the neurosurgeon. The first common exposure to trauma is during delivery.[1,35,42] Birth injuries fall into two categories: injuries produced by the normal forces of labor and those produced by obstetrical intervention, usually complications of forceps applications. All newborns delivered vaginally and with vertex presentation have some scalp swelling, caput succedaneum. The most common of the former type of injuries is the "ping-pong" fracture. This typically occurs in the region of the parietal boss, is not associated with visible scalp trauma, and rarely, if ever, has any associated intracranial injury. The lesion is probably produced by steady pressure of the ischeal tuberosity against the skull with in-bending of the elastic skull. The lesion is diagnosed on clinical examination; plain x-ray films usually show the degree of deformation, although tangential views may be required. Computed tomography (CT) is not necessary unless there is reason to suspect some intracranial lesion. The suspicious findings include a full fontanel, early seizures, unexplained drop in hematocrit, or general failure to progress satisfactorily. Small lesions often resolve on their own if given a few days. Larger lesions, greater than 3 cm in diameter, usually require corrective surgery in the first 7 to 10 days. Most lesions that are going to resolve on their own show improvement during this time, although they rarely complete resolution. The reason for proceeding to surgery early is that the longer the fracture remains depressed, the harder it becomes to elevate through a small incision, and a simple procedure may become a craniotomy. The surgery is done through a small incision positioned close to the edge of the fracture and over the closest suture line. The scalp is infiltrated with 0.5% lidocaine with 1:200,000 epinephrine. The incision is only 3 to 5 cm long. The suture can be freed from the underlying dura along the nearest suture line, and this point used to insert the periosteal elevator between the dura and the inner surface of the cranial bone. The distal portion of the elevator must be passed beyond the deepest part of the depression to get adequate leverage to pop the fracture out. The only other precaution is to lever the periosteal elevator over one's finger and not deform the brain by levering directly against the deformable skull. Occasionally the fracture does not reduce, and a craniotomy is required.

Other traumatic lesions that occur with delivery are subarachnoid hemorrhage; intratentorial hemorrhage due to tearing of the tentorial artery as a result of deformation of the skull; and epidural, subdural, and intracerebral hemorrhage. In the full-term neonate, intraventricular hemorrhage occurs from the choroid plexus—not the germinal plate as in the premature infant; hemorrhage rarely enters the cerebral parenchyma or produces brain injury but is accompanied by a high incidence of hydrocephalus over the next 1 to 2 months.

The incidence of intracranial hemorrhage is higher in children with neonatal clotting disorders, and early seizures in this group of patients should be an indication for a CT scan. Most of these pathological events require no neurosurgical intervention, but the continuation of seizures, progressive neurological deterioration, or occasionally continuing blood loss may be indications for surgery to decompress the hematoma.

With continuing improvement in obstetrical care, the incidence of forceps-related injuries is low and the contribution of neonatal cranial trauma to neonatal mortality is small (2 to 3 percent).[20,39] The worst injuries result from the application of high forceps with improper positioning such that the cranium is severely deformed, resulting in dural tears that at worst include the dural sinuses with resultant hemorrhage from the ear and often death. These lesions are associated with bruising and contusion of the skull and with subgaleal hematomas.

In most cases surgical intervention is not necessary and conservative treatment is recommended. The major indications for obtaining a CT scan in the newborn suspected of harboring an intracranial clot are seizures not related to metabolic disturbances (e.g., hypoglycemia, hypocalcemia) and lethargy or progressive neurological deterioration. If surgery is required, the clotting studies should be normal if possible, blood should be available, and anesthesia should be given by someone trained and experienced in the care of the newborn surgical patient. The brain at this age is mostly water; therefore, massive herniation of cerebral tissue can occur when the dura is opened. The bleeding is not uncommonly from close to the major venous sinuses, and major hemorrhage resulting in cardiac arrest can occur in seconds. One must be prepared for these dramatic occurrences.

No effort is made to remove contused brain, because there is a chance of it recovering, and often bleeding within the cerebrum is difficult to control because of the fluid nature of the brain tissue. The pial membrane, including the cortical blood supply, is easily stripped by the sucker, resulting in further risk of brain damage from ischemia, and care must be exercised to avoid this. The rarity of the need for intracranial surgery in this age group of children suggests that such surgery should, whenever possible, be done in specialized pediatric neurosurgical units. The frequency of such birth trauma is low, representing only 1 to 3 percent of admissions for trauma to a busy pediatric neurosurgical unit. The prognosis for children who do require surgery is poor, with a 10 percent mortality and 30 percent poor outcome.[10]

Injuries in the First 2 Years

The most common cause of head injury in the first 2 years of life is a fall. These falls are usually from a low height, frequently onto a soft surface, and are rarely associated with disturbance of consciousness or intracranial damage. Recent studies have made it abundantly clear that minor falls and even many major falls of 10 feet or more do not produce intracranial damage, although skull fractures are very common.[14,16,27,28,34,36,49] Among children admitted to the Children's Hospital of Philadelphia and seen by the pediatric neurosurgical service between 1978 and 1983, 50 percent of those younger than 1 year of age had a skull fracture. These fractures are often extensive and may cross suture lines. If the fall was witnessed and disturbed consciousness and retinal hemorrhages are absent, there is no reason to suspect that these injuries are other than accidental. The delayed appearance of a subgaleal hematoma some days after minor trauma often is what prompts obtaining a skull x-ray film on which a skull fracture is noted. If there is no good history of trauma, child abuse may be suspected. If there are no other fractures (e.g., long bone or rib), no alteration of consciousness, and a normal funduscopic examination, child abuse is rarely the cause of these fractures.

Epidural hematomas are seen after accidental trauma in the child younger than 2 years of age; a fall down a flight of steps or in or out of a walker, and a child being fallen on by an adult (e.g., a slip on the ice) are often reported. The only two situations in which acute subdural hematomas are found in this age group are high-speed impacts, such as in an automobile accident, or child abuse, whether a direct blow or a shaking-impact injury. When a history of minor or unobserved trauma is given as an explanation for severe brain injury or for a child with a subdural hematoma or retinal hemorrhages, the story is almost always untrue and nonaccidental trauma (i.e., injury done to the child by a caretaker) is the etiology. Minor injuries do not produce severe brain injuries in infants.

Early post-traumatic seizures either at the time of impact or in the first hour occur in 1 to 30 percent of children.[23,24,26,41] The greatest frequency is in the more severely injured children; for all those sustaining head trauma of sufficient severity to come to medical attention, the average frequency is 2 to 3 percent. These seizures do not require medication unless they are ongoing or occur after the first hour. Post-traumatic status epilepticus can occur in children; this requires therapy. The prognosis is good, not ominous as that for adults.[19] Probably the most common constellation of significant symptoms and signs in the infant or young child is pallor, somnolence, and vomiting—the "pediatric concussion syndrome."[30,40,44,46] This scenario is reported in 10 percent of pediatric head trauma admissions[44] but probably occurs in a minor form in a much higher number. The onset may be delayed from hours to a day after injury and mimics an intracranial mass. The vomiting may be severe enough to require intravenous fluids. A soft fontanel is the norm, and an intracranial mass is rare. If the fontanel is full, the plain x-ray films show split sutures, vomiting is prolonged, or a low hematocrit is found, then a CT scan is indicated. This is a transient syndrome, and the parents can be assured that it will pass without residual neurological problems.

Child Abuse

It is appalling to realize that most severe head injuries [Glasgow Coma Scale (GCS) score <8] in children in the United States during their first year of life are the result of child abuse. The incidence of abuse in infants and toddlers hospitalized for trauma is 10 to 30 percent and accounts for 80 percent of the deaths.[10,16] Recent data show that homicide is the most frequent cause of death in children between 1 month and 1 year of life[48]: 17 percent versus 8 percent for children 10 to 14 years of age and 1 percent for adults. The most common history given for a child admitted following an abusive injury is either no trauma or a presumed but unwitnessed fall. Other common histories include seizures or respiratory arrest. The usual scenario for such an injury is that of a child crying inconsolably and a frustrated caretaker. The caretaker picks up and shakes the child to stop its crying. This usually aggravates the crying, and, still angry, the caretaker discards the child forcibly into a crib, onto a sofa, or at worst strikes the child's head against an object such as a wall. This impact, even against a soft surface, produces the deceleration forces that are adequate to produce subdural hematomas and brain damage.[17] Disturbance of consciousness occurs immediately, the caretaker panics, and the child is placed in a crib or on the floor in the hope of recovery. As the brain swells and ICP increases, the child's condition worsens; ventilation is suppressed with increasing Pa_{CO_2} and decreasing Pa_{O_2} until seizures or ventilatory arrest occurs. At this point medical care is sought, often too late, and the history of only the seizure, respiratory arrest, or minor fall is given.

It is important to understand the mechanism of shaking and impact injuries for clinical identification and care of the child and family, for public health training, and for legal proceedings should prosecution occur. An understanding attitude toward the caretaker believed to have caused the injury is necessary to finding the real cause of the injury. Such an event is usually a single episode that results from frustration and sudden loss of control rather than a pattern of systematic abuse, although the latter certainly occurs. When there is suspicion of child abuse, a skeletal survey should be obtained once the child is stable. Although the finding of other long bone or rib fractures helps confirm chronic abuse, the absence of these does not rule out nonaccidental trauma. Such injuries must be reported to a child abuse investigation team.

The pathophysiology of infant child abuse is rarely purely a shaking injury but almost always is associated with some form of impact, either a direct blow[22] or that described above. Pure shaking may result in death due to cervicomedullary injury, apnea, and cerebral ischemia.[21] The subdural hematomas are rarely large enough to require surgical evacuation, but this seems to depend on the mechanism of injury in that direct blows to the side of the infant's head or face are associated with unilateral hematomas that may require surgical decompression.

The final cause of severe head injury in the infant is an accident while the infant is a passenger in an automobile, either in a care seat or unrestrained. Unrestrained infants are thrown around the cab like a missile and frequently are found under the seat or dashboard, often apneic. The cause of fatal injury is usually cervicomedullary damage followed by apnea and cerebral ischemia.

Injuries in Older Children

After 1 year of age, most minor head injuries are the result of short falls, and most severe head injuries are the result of automobile-pedestrian accidents or falls from windows (the latter particularly in large urban areas). As the child gets older, major head injuries more frequently result from bicycle or automobile accidents. Thus, from infancy to 10 years of age, the major causes of severe head trauma are not impact, but acceleration-deceleration forces. Between 10 and 15 years, the frequency of trauma from impact increases (e.g., falls from bicycles or sports injuries). Unless a mass accumulates, with increased ICP, and cerebral herniation occurs, the damage done by impact injuries is most frequently local. In contrast, that produced by acceleration-deceleration trauma is almost always diffuse.

Clinical Features

In children and adolescents, a careful history that elucidates the type of injury, height of fall, condition of floor (carpeted or not), initial stage of consciousness (crying or not), occurrence of seizures, and occurrence of apnea must be obtained. A serial history is vital: Did the child's general condition improve, stabilize, or worsen? Did vomiting ensue? Did late seizures occur? Whenever the history is thought to explain the neurological picture poorly, child abuse must be suspected.

For the child younger than 2 years of age, the Glasgow Coma Scale can be applied but with some limitations. The portion on speech is most easily completed by giving the child a score of 5 if there is any vocalization at all, and 0 if no crying is elicited. Similarly, stereotypic eye opening occasionally occurs in the severely head-injured child younger than 12 months of age. This is not the normal spontaneous eye opening seen in older children, and too much reliance on this may lead the examiner to under-rate the severity of the child's injury. The motor portion of the GCS is applicable after the first few months of life, except for the response to command. However, in children, by and large, the GCS score gives a good indication of the initial depth of coma.

In the first few months of life, the neurological examination includes palpation of the fontanels and sutures, examination of the baby for postural changes in tone or clonus, and examination for the presence of primitive reflexes (e.g., the Moro reflex). Spontaneous bicycling movements of the lower extremities are seen in association with major head injuries in this age group and must not be misinterpreted as normal spontaneous motor movements. Vital signs usually reveal a normal blood pressure with tachycardia. Bradycardia is highly suggestive of intracranial hypertension in this age group. A necessary part of the child's examination is visualizing the fundi to seek evidence of retinal hemorrhage and papilledema. Acute deterioration of consciousness is common in the child after moderate or severe head injury and may be due to seizures, acute brain swelling, or, less frequently, to an expanding intracranial clot. Pallor, vomiting, and tachycardia are all extremely common after concussive injury in the child.

Hypotension is rarely due to the head injury and must be assumed to be due to blood loss elsewhere, such as the abdomen or long bone fractures. Occasionally, hypotension or shock in the small child is due to head injury. This may occur in a child under 1 year of age who has a large linear skull fracture and an epidural hematoma. The intracranial blood can leak through the fracture, producing an ever-enlarging subgaleal or subperiosteal hemorrhage, which, in association with the intracranial blood, may be sufficient to produce anemia and hypotension. The second situation is a head injury in a child with hydrocephalus. In infants and toddlers with functioning shunts, a large amount of intracranial blood may accumulate without much evidence of elevated ICP. The ventricular CSF is displaced down the shunt as the clot accumulates, preventing the usual symptoms and signs of slowly increasing ICP. These children usually present to the emergency room drowsy and irritable with a blood evaluation suggesting acute blood-loss anemia. Finally, hypotension can result from spinal cord injury.

Radiologic Evaluation

Skull x-ray films are particularly valuable as a screening procedure in children younger than 1 year of age with a history of a short fall. Rather dramatic-appearing fractures are frequently seen, often crossing suture lines and sinuses. In the absence of x-ray evidence of split sutures and in the presence of a normal neurological examination and soft fontanel, CT scanning is unnecessary. These children rarely develop a delayed chronic subdural or epidural hematoma and rarely have evidence of underlying brain injury. The only late complications are subgaleal hematomas and growing skull fractures or leptomeningeal cysts. These latter complications occur only when there is laceration of the dura and contusion of the underlying cerebral cortex.[25] They are uncommon and usually follow an accident in which the level of consciousness was significantly altered. Rather than obtaining routine follow-up x-ray films of the skull, we recommend that these children with extensive linear fractures be re-examined 2 to 3 months after injury. If the area of the fracture site is not enlarged or swollen, then it is unlikely that repeat skull films are necessary. A persistent fracture line with local swelling suggests a leptomeningeal cyst, and a CT scan is recommended to identify the relationship of the brain to the fracture and the subgaleal swelling. Routine skull films in older children are rarely helpful unless a specific lesion is being sought (e.g., pneumocephalus or a depressed fracture). The importance of a skull fracture on x-ray films in this age group continues to be the subject of debate.[15,43]

Lateral x-ray films of the cervical spine are obtained in all comatose head-injured children, usually before endotracheal intubation. However, because inadequate ventilation is life-threatening, the intubation, if required, *should not be delayed until a spine film can be obtained.* Children most likely to have combined cervicocranial trauma are those who have been unrestrained passengers in an automobile, those involved in a motor vehicle accident, or those who have fallen from higher than thirty feet. If one spinal fracture is found, x-ray films of the whole spine are required, because 10 to 30 percent of the time multiple levels of injury are found.

As in adults, the CT scan is the definitive initial study. All children who are unconscious, show clinical evidence of a deteriorating level of consciousness, have a focal neurological deficit, or have a depressed skull fracture require immediate CT scanning. In a child with minor trauma, a persisting or increasing headache over hours or days and persistent vomiting are indications for a CT scan.

Several CT patterns are unique to the child. The shaken baby typically has a CT scan showing an acute subarachnoid hemorrhage and a posterior interhemispheric triangular subdural hematoma (Fig. 266-1). These hemorrhages are rarely large enough to require surgical evacuation. Areas of low density may be seen on the initial CT scan, and in children, these are usually major vessel infarctions. Radioisotope perfusion scans usually demonstrate patency of the vessels, suggesting that the infarction was due to distortion and temporary vascular occlusion at the time of injury,

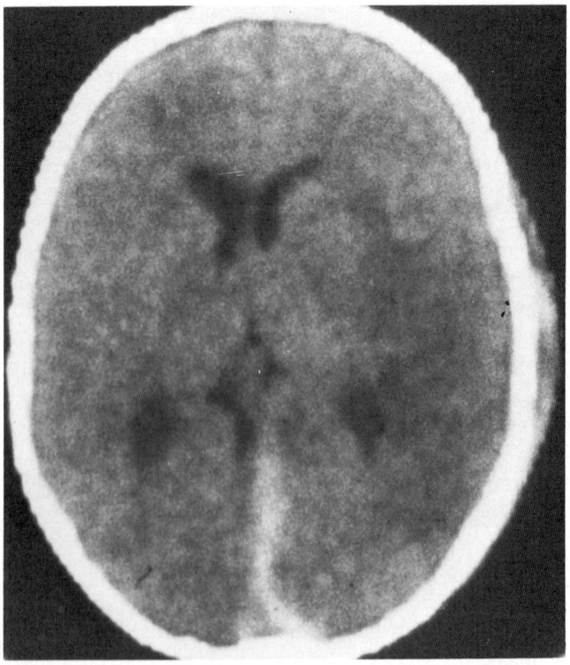

Figure 266-1 A posterior interhemispheric subdural hematoma and decreased density of the right hemisphere secondary to infarction.

transient vascular spasm, or some combination thereof. Cerebral transtentorial herniation can be responsible for infarction in the distribution of the posterior cerebral artery, and it is possible that retroalar herniation of the frontal lobes may result in middle cerebral or anterior cerebral territory infarction.

Diffuse axonal injury is seen on the CT scan in a small percentage of children. This is diagnosed by the finding of small hemorrhages in the head of the caudate nucleus, in the corpus callosum, in the region of the superior cerebellar peduncle, or around the aqueduct. Despite evidence of primary midbrain periaqueductal hemorrhage, children can make a significantly good recovery (Fig. 266-2). However, this finding should not be considered an indication for withholding therapy. Children with evidence of diffuse axonal injury frequently go on to develop severe brain swelling after 24 h, and ICP monitoring is indicated. Within hours of head injury, 20 to 40 percent of children who are comatose show a primary CT pattern that has been described as diffuse cerebral swelling.[12] It has been shown to be associated with increased CBF and current information suggests that early swelling is associated with vasodilation and is not due to cerebral edema. In children the swelling is bilateral, rarely associated with any other lesion except primary subarachnoid hemorrhage, and usually unassociated with skull fracture. Two types of early diffuse swelling occur and need to be separated. Diffuse swelling with a low-density brain suggests ischemic injury, and the outcome is likely to be poor—death or severe disability.[50] Most studies showing normal or increased density of the brain are correlated with a good recovery or minimal disability.[4,12,32]

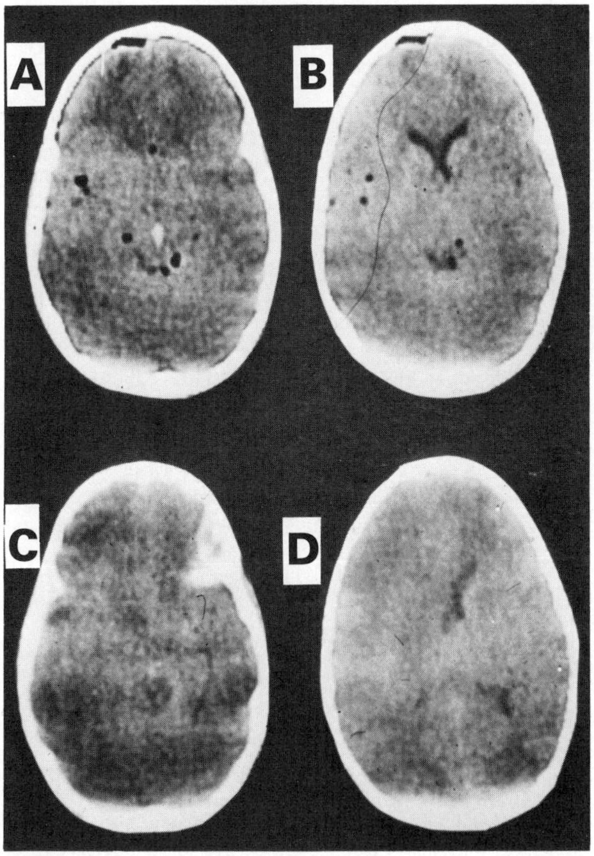

Figure 266-2 CT scans of a 4-year-old child presenting with bilateral fixed and dilated pupils and bilateral decerebrate posturing. *A, B.* Scans obtained on the first day show subarachnoid air from a petrous fracture and focal periaqueductal hemorrhage. *C, D.* Repeat CT scans at 24 h showing severe brain swelling. This was associated with increased intracranial pressure. This child is now walking independently but requires special schooling.

Delayed CT scans, 7 to 10 days after injury, frequently show mild ventricular dilatation and often collections of extracerebral CSF in the frontal areas. These CSF collections do not represent subdural hygromas and do not require surgical drainage.

Management

The initial management of the comatose child is not significantly different from that of the adult.[11,38] The initial resuscitation fulfills the usual ABCs of management: open and clear the airway, ensure adequate ventilation, and stabilize the circulation. *In children it is not necessary to hyperextend the neck to intubate.* Gentle pressure on the cricoid cartilage prevents air from entering the stomach during bagging of the patient before endotracheal intubation and also prevents regurgitation of the stomach contents into the lungs. The timing of passing a nasogastric (NG) tube depends on the level of consciousness of the patient and the type of injury. With severe facial trauma, an NG tube should not be passed until x-ray films of the skull demonstrate that the cranial base is intact. An oral gastric tube may be used in this situation, if necessary. In children with a markedly diminished or absent gag response, it is safer to pass the NG tube after an endotracheal tube is in place. In children with a good gag reflex, it is probably safer to pass the NG tube and evacuate the stomach before muscle paralysis and intubation. Intubation of the trachea should be performed as it would be in the operating room, with hyperventilation using 100% O_2, intravenous injection of pancuronium bromide followed by thiopental sodium, and then endotracheal intubation. After intubation, moderate hyperventilation to a Pa_{CO_2} level around 25 mmHg is performed.

Circulatory support with intravenous fluids should never involve the use of 5% glucose in water, and rarely one-quarter strength saline, because inappropriate antidiuretic hormone secretion is common in children with severe head trauma. The preferred intravenous solution is one-half normal saline or Ringer's lactate, run at one-half to two-thirds the normal maintenance volume. If both shock and coma are present, we suggest the insertion of an ICP monitor during resuscitation, because the large swings in ICP that will occur when large volumes of fluid are infused cannot otherwise be monitored. To establish a good circulation at the expense of an ICP that is equal to blood pressure makes little sense.

In the emergency room, the standard lines required for children with a GCS score of 8 or less are intravenous lines (usually 2) of as large a bore as possible, an arterial line, an endotracheal tube, and (if there is no evidence of perineal trauma) a Foley catheter. In those with a GCS score of 5 or less, an ICP monitor is also inserted. There is no evidence of benefit from steroids. Mannitol is not used unless the history or the clinical examination suggests an expanding mass lesion (e.g., an epidural hematoma) manifest by a rapid decrease in level of consciousness or a severe or worsening headache.

The management of epidural hematomas is the same as for adults, except that in the child a craniotomy, rather than a craniectomy, should always be performed. Furthermore, the location of the typical epidural hematoma in a child is higher in the parietal region than it is in adults, and the typical low temporal burr hole may miss such a lesion. Acute subdural hematomas usually do not require surgery in childhood. Cerebral contusion, in my opinion, should rarely be operated upon in childhood, and most intracerebral hematomas are small, again not requiring surgical evacuation.

The most common indication for surgical intervention in the child with a severe head injury is a depressed skull fracture. Over the last few years, our practice has been to do a craniotomy, elevate the depressed fracture, and then replace the fracture fragments, wiring them together into the cranium. This has been done even in the face of open compound fractures. It is a valuable way of avoiding a second operation, and with adequate antibiotic coverage we have had no problems with infection.

In the child younger than 1 year old who presents with a bulging fontanel and retinal hemorrhages (i.e., child abuse), the indications for fontanel tap are apnea, decerebrate posturing, or fixed dilated pupils. In these children, rapid intubation and hyperventilation are followed by bilateral fontanel taps with a 20-gauge, short-bevel spinal needle. Often, 10 to 15 ml of bloody CSF that does not clot is obtained from either side. This is usually adequate to reestablish spontaneous ventilation and return of responsive pupils, and it may reduce the decerebrate posturing. CT then usually shows blood in the interhemispheric fissure and brain swelling, but rarely a significant surgical mass lesion. In our experience it is very rare for these lesions to progress to chronic subdural hematomas, and usually no further subdural taps or surgical intervention is necessary. Children with acute subdural hematomas and subarachnoid hemorrhage frequently develop severe brain swelling, and monitoring of ICP along with excellent intensive care management is required to ensure that these children survive with the least possible damage.

The intensive care management of elevated ICP aims at keeping the ICP below 20 mmHg or if changes in pupil function are present, at levels below 15 mmHg.[13] The initial therapy is elevation of the head to 30 degrees with the head kept in the midline,[18] moderate hyperventilation to a Pa_{CO_2} level of 25 mmHg, and muscle paralysis. Muscle paralysis can be used only if the ventilator is equipped with an alarm system. If this is inadequate to control ICP, further therapy will depend upon the CT findings. In children with diffuse swelling, we prefer to avoid the use of mannitol in the first 24 h if possible. Thus, following hyperventilation to Pa_{CO_2} values as low as 18 to 20 mmHg, furosemide in doses of 1 mg/kg or ethacrynic acid is given. If this is still inadequate to maintain an ICP below 20 mmHg, then doses of pentobarbital are used to produce blood levels of 20 to 30 mg/liter. The dose is designed to control the ICP rather than to establish a specific serum level. If despite barbiturate therapy the ICP continues to be a problem, then mannitol is given.

In children in whom a midline shift is seen in conjunction with an elevated ICP, mannitol will be used after hyperventilation. If this is ineffective, then once again, barbiturates are used in an effort to lower ICP (Table 266-1). It is not uncommon to see a child's ICP become elevated again around the third to fifth days. This is believed to be a reflection of some anoxia or ischemia occurring at the time of trauma, and the CT scan may show continued brain swelling. If after 6 to 10 days the ICP is still elevated, a repeat CT scan will often show enlargement of the CSF spaces, and now ventricular drainage or lumbar punctures may be more than adequate to control the ICP. Specific therapy against oxygen free radicals and/or excitotoxic neurotransmitters (e.g., glutamate and aspartate) are being evaluated and are likely to be the next step in therapy.

TABLE 266-1 Selection of Therapy for Brain Swelling versus Brain Edema

Diffuse Swelling	Brain Edema
Head up	Head up
↓CO_2	Steroids?
Furosemide	Mannitol
Barbiturates	Furosemide
Mannitol	↓CO_2
	Barbiturates

Complications

Early complications after head injury include transient cortical blindness, seizures, pediatric concussion syndrome, cranial nerve palsy (most frequently VI), diabetes insipidus (rare), inappropriate antidiuretic hormone secretion syndrome, post-traumatic migraine, and carotid occlusion. Late complications include post-traumatic aneurysms, pituitary dysfunction, seizures (5 percent), CSF leakage and meningitis, hydrocephalus, and finally a whole series of neurocognitive, social, and behavioral deficits.

Outcome

If only mortality and gross neurological morbidity are considered, the outcome after head trauma in children is good. Mortality is 10 to 20 percent for all children with a GCS score less than 8. In many series the mortality rates for children with a score of 5 or above and no shock is 0 to 10 percent. Below 5, the mortality is 50 to 70 percent. At all GCS scores, shock worsens the outcome. The incidence of the vegetative state is 1 to 3 percent. Through the spectrum of head injury, the return to independent function should be 90 percent. Children under 3 years have a worse outcome; this may be related to the high incidence of child abuse in this group.[3,9,13,29,47]

Recent studies[31] demonstrate a high incidence of frontal lobe contusions in children who recover from moderate or severe head injury. These injuries are associated with disturbances of cognition and behavior that clearly interfere with the child's scholastic and social development. Rehabilitation of the head-injured child should include psychological and educational support as well as physical and occupational therapy. Finally, resources must be found to help the whole family cope with the altered child.

References

1. Abroms IF, McLennan JE, Mandell F. Acute neonatal subdural hematoma following breech delivery. *Am J Dis Child* 1977; 131:192–194.
2. Accident Facts. Chicago: National Safety Council, 1982.
3. Alberico AM, Ward JD, Choi SC, et al. Outcome after severe head injury: relationship to mass lesions, diffuse injury, and ICP course in pediatric and adult patients. *J Neurosurg* 1987; 67:648–656.
4. Aldrich EF, Eisenberg HM, Saydjari C, et al. Diffuse brain swelling in severely head-injured children. A report from the NIH Traumatic Coma Data Bank. *J Neurosurg* 1992; 76:450–454.
5. Anderson DW, McLaurin RL. The National Head and Spinal Cord Injury Survey. *J Neurosurg* 1980; 53(Suppl):S1–S43.

6. Annegers JF. The epidemiology of head trauma in children. In Shapiro K (ed): *Pediatric Head Trauma.* Mount Kisco, NY: Futura Publishing Co, 1983, p 1.
7. Annual Summary for the United States 1979. *Monthly Vital Statistics Report,* vol 28, Nos 13, 28. Washington, DC: Government Printing Office, Nov 13, 1980.
8. Bergman AB, Rivara FP. Sweden's experience in reducing childhood injuries. *Pediatrics* 1991; 88:69–74.
9. Brink JD, Imbus C, Woo-Sam J. Physical recovery after severe closed head trauma in children and adolescents. *J Pediatr* 1980; 97:721–727.
10. Bruce DA. Central nervous system injuries. In Welch KS, Randolph JG, Ravitch MM, et al (eds): *Pediatric Surgery.* Chicago: Year Book, 1986, pp 209–215.
11. Bruce DA. Scope of the problem: early assessment and management. In Griffith ER (ed): *Rehabilitation of the Adult and Child with Traumatic Brain Injury.* Philadelphia: FA Davis, 1990, pp 521–538.
12. Bruce DA, Alavi A, Bilaniuk L, et al. Diffuse cerebral swelling following head injuries in children: the syndrome of "malignant brain edema." *J Neurosurg* 1981; 54:170–178.
13. Bruce DA, Raphaely RC, Goldberg AI, et al. Pathophysiology, treatment and outcome following severe head injury in children. *Childs Brain* 1979; 5:174–191.
14. Chadwick DL, Chin S, Salerno C, et al. Deaths from falls in children: how far is fatal? *J Trauma* 1991; 31:1353–1355.
15. Chan KH, Mann KS, Yue CP, et al. The significance of skull fracture in acute traumatic intracranial hematomas in adolescents—a prospective study. *J Neurosurg* 1990; 72:189–194.
16. Duhaime AC, Alario AJ, Lewander WJ, et al. Head injury in very young children: mechanisms, injury types, and ophthalmologic findings in 100 hospitalized patients younger than 2 years of age. *Pediatrics* 1992; 90:179–185.
17. Duhaime AC, Gennarelli TA, Thibault LE, et al. The shaken baby syndrome: a clinical, pathological, and biomechanical study. *J Neurosurg* 1987; 66:409–415.
18. Feldman Z, Kanter MJ, Robertson CS, et al. Effects of head elevation on intracranial pressure, cerebral perfusion pressure, and cerebral blood flow in head injured patients. *J Neurosurg* 1992; 76:207–211.
19. Grand W. The significance of post-traumatic status epilepticus in childhood. *J Neurol Neurosurg Psychiatry* 1974; 37:178–180.
20. Gresham EL. Birth trauma. *Pediatr Clin North Am* 1975; 22:317–328.
21. Hadley MN, Sonntag VK, Rekate HL, et al. The infant whiplash-shake injury syndrome: a clinical and pathological study. *Neurosurgery* 1989; 24:536–540.
22. Hahn YS, Raimondi AS, McLone DG, et al. Traumatic mechanisms of head injury in child abuse. *Childs Brain* 1983; 10:229–241.
23. Hauser WA. Post traumatic epilepsy in children. In Shapiro K (ed): *Pediatric Head Trauma.* Mount Kisco, NY: Futura, 1983, pp 271–287.
24. Hendrick EB, Harris L. Post-traumatic epilepsy in children. *J Trauma* 1968; 8:547–556.
25. Ito H, Miwa T, Onodra Y. Growing skull fracture of childhood: with reference to the importance of the brain injury and its pathogenetic consideration. *Childs Brain* 1977; 3:116–126.
26. Jennett B. Trauma as a cause of epilepsy in childhood. *Dev Med Child Neurol* 1973; 15:56–62.
27. Joffe M, Ludwig S. Stairway injuries in children. *Pediatrics* 1988; 82:457–461.
28. Luerssen TG, Huang JC, McLone DG, et al. Retinal hemorrhages, seizures and intracranial hemorrhages: relationships and outcome in children suffering traumatic brain injury. *Concepts Pediatr Neurosurg* 1991; 11:87–94.
29. Luerssen TG, Klauber MR, Marshall LF. Outcome from head injury related to patient's age: a longitudinal prospective study of adult and pediatric head injury. *J Neurosurg* 1988; 68:409–416.
30. Mealy J Jr. *Pediatric Head Injuries.* Springfield, IL: Charles C Thomas, 1968, pp 53–87.
31. Mendelsohn D, Levin HS, Bruce D, et al. Late MRI after head injury in children: relationship to clinical features and outcome. *Childs Nerv Syst* 1992; 8:445–452.
32. Muizelaar JP, Marmarou A, DeSalles AAF, et al. Cerebral blood flow and metabolism in severely head-injured children. Part 1: Relationship with GCS score, outcome, ICP, and PVI. *J Neurosurg* 1989; 71:63–71.
33. Muizelaar JP, Ward JD, Marmarou A, et al. Cerebral blood flow and metabolism in severely head-injured children. Part 2: Autoregulation. *J Neurosurg* 1989; 71:72–76.
34. Musemeche CA, Barthel M, Cosentino C, et al. Pediatric falls from heights. *J Trauma* 1991; 31:1347–1349.
35. Natelson SE, Sayers MP. The fate of children sustaining severe head trauma during birth. *Pediatrics* 1973; 51:169–174.
36. Nimityongskul P, Anderson LD. The likelihood of injuries when children fall out of bed. *J Pediatr Orthop* 1987; 2:184–186.
37. Pang D, Wilberger JE Jr. Spinal cord injury without radiographic abnormalities in children. *J Neurosurg* 1982; 57:114–129.
38. Raphaely RC, Swedlow DB, Downes JJ, Bruce DA. Management of severe pediatric head trauma. *Pediatr Clin North Am* 1980; 27:715–727.
39. Salonen IS, Uusitalo R. Birth injuries: incidence and predisposing factors. *Z Kinderchir* 1990; 45:133–135.
40. Schnitker MT. A syndrome of cerebral concussion in children. *J Pediatr* 1949; 35:557–560.
41. Snoek JW, Minderhoud JM, Wilmink JT. Delayed deterioration following mild head injury in children. *Brain* 1984; 107:15–36.
42. Takagi T, Nagai R, Wakabayashi S, et al. Extradural hemorrhage in the newborn as a result of birth trauma. *Childs Brain* 1978; 4:306–318.
43. Teasdale GM, Murray G, Anderson E, et al. Risk of acute traumatic intracranial haematoma in children and adults: implications for managing head injuries. *BMJ* 1990; 300:363–367.
44. Todorow S, Feller AM. Benign secondary disturbance of consciousness (posttraumatic stupor) in children after cerebral trauma. *Z Kinderchir* 1982; 36:83–87.
45. *Vital Statistics of the United States.* Washington DC: Government Printing Office, 1981.
46. Vitzthum HE, Willenberg E, Lampe J, Minda R. Delayed encephalopathy. *Zentralbl Neurochir* 1986; 47:131–133.
47. Walker ML, Meyer TA, Storrs BB, Hylton PD. Pediatric head injury: factors which influence outcome. *Concepts Pediatr Neurosurg* 1985; 6:84–97.
48. Waller AE, Baker SP, Szocka A. Childhood injury deaths: national analysis and geographic variations. *Am J Public Health* 1989; 79:310–315.
49. Williams RA. Injuries in infants and small children resulting from witnessed and corroborated free falls. *J Trauma* 1991; 31:1350–1352.
50. Yoshino E, Yamaki T, Higuchi T, et al. Acute brain edema in fatal head injury: analysis by dynamic CT scanning. *J Neurosurg* 1985; 63:830–839.

267

Outcome Prediction in Severe Head Injury

Lawrence F. Marshall
Sharon B. Marshall

Outcome prediction after severe head injury continues to be an area of intense interest. In part, this reflects the natural curiosity of the neurosurgeon, but, as increasing attention is paid to resource allocation in all societies, our ability or inability to predict outcome accurately becomes very important to the targeting of scarce resources. Relatively accurate predictions of likely outcome allow specific populations who are failing our present therapeutic regimens to be identified so that new and experimental therapies can be targeted to them. Furthermore, as we increasingly recognize the heterogenous nature of the process called head injury, the likelihood that therapies will be selective for various patterns of brain injury becomes more apparent.

It has generally been accepted that the patient's neurological status (a marker of the severity of injury) and age are the two most important factors in outcome prediction. There is increasing evidence that to these two classic variables should be added the pattern of structural brain injury as visualized by computed tomography (CT), and the depth and duration of ischemia and/or ischemic hypoxia. Data from the Traumatic Coma Data Bank, using a recently introduced classification of head injury based on CT scanning (described later in this chapter)[12] have been useful in more clearly defining different patterns of brain injury and their relationship to outcome. Moreover, there is some evidence that recognition of these patterns has led to a reduction in mortality in at least some of these subgroups, because the lethality of a specific pattern of injury is more easily recognized and treatment initiated sooner.[9] Thus, in the mid-1990s, outcome prediction depends increasingly on a multivariate approach incorporating information not only about the patient's neurological status and age, but also from the results of serial CT scanning and from the influence of the secondary insults of ischemia and ischemic hypoxia.

Neurological Assessment

Glasgow Coma Scale

Many methods of neurological assessment are available, but none has been as extensively tested as the Glasgow coma scale (GCS) as a means of rapidly assessing the patient and making an early and accurate prediction of outcome.[17] The Glasgow coma scale, which is described in another chapter, has received widespread acceptance throughout the world. This scale, which assesses eye opening, verbal response, and motor response, is simple and, despite the absence of any specific assessment of brain stem function, yields an early and quite accurate prediction of outcome. The accuracy of the GCS, however, is center-specific rather than internationally specific. One pitfall in the neurological examination is the time when the examination is done. In a considerable number of patients suffering traumatic brain injury, an initial examination done in the field will indicate that the patient's clinical status is worse than it really is because of significant improvement during and after resuscitation. It is therefore extremely important to record the time at which the neurological examination is done relative to the time of injury for the prediction to be as accurate as possible. A patient with a motor score of 1 on the GCS after resuscitation has a much poorer outlook than a patient who has a motor score of 1 immediately or shortly after injury. The relationship of post-resuscitation GCS and outcome is shown in Table 267-1.[11]

As the GCS score rises, there is a precipitous decline in mortality. In approximately 15 percent of patients, the GCS is above 8 at first but then declines, usually because of an expanding mass lesion. The availability of rapid CT scanning and neurosurgical services has substantially reduced the mortality in this population over the last 15 years.

TABLE 267-1 Outcome at Last Contact Correlated with Postresuscitation Glasgow Coma Scale Score*

Outcome at Last Contact	Postresuscitation Glasgow Coma Scale Score																			
	Unknown		3		3.3†		4		5		6		7		8		≥9		Total Cases	
	No.	%	No.	%	No.	%	No.	%	No.	%	No.	%	No.	%	No.	%	No.	%	No.	%
Good	746	0	4	4.1	16	25.4	7	6.3	10	12.2	33	29.2	69	46.6	34	54.8	25	40.3	198	26.5
Moderate disability	0	0	3	3.1	12	19.0	9	8.1	14	17.1	24	21.3	33	22.3	14	22.6	13	21.0	122	16.4
Severe disability	0	0	10	10.3	11	17.5	21	18.9	19	23.2	26	23.0	17	11.5	4	6.5	8	13.0	116	15.6
Vegetative	0	0	4	4.1	5	7.9	12	10.8	6	7.3	6	5.3	3	2.0	3	4.8	0	0	39	5.2
Dead	8	100	76	78.4	19	30.2	62	55.9	33	40.2	24	21.2	26	17.6	7	11.3	16	25.8	271	36.3
Totals	8	100	97	100	63	100	111	100	82	100	113	100	148	100	62	100	62	100	746	100

*Outcome classified by the Glasgow Outcome Scale. Significance of difference (Kruskal–Wallis): $p < 0.001$.
†Patients who are untestable owing to paralytic agents.

Abnormalities of Brain Stem Function and Pupillary Dysfunction

The addition of tests of brain stem function to the GCS scale adds surprisingly little to initial accurate prediction. This reflects the fact that severe injuries which result in significant primary brain stem injury usually are associated with decerebrate or flexor responses, which by themselves indicate a very poor outcome. In the absence of such abnormal motor movements, however, the assessment of brain stem function becomes much more important in making an early prediction of outcome.

Traditionally, pupillary abnormalities have been reported as if they were static events. It is important to recognize that rapid recovery of pupillary responsiveness after injury, either spontaneous or because of systemic and brain resuscitation, has important implications when such patients are compared to those in whom the pupils remain abnormal after resuscitative efforts.[2,11] In patients whose pupils are bilaterally unreactive at first, the mortality is approximately 15 percent if pupillary function recovers immediately after resuscitation; if the pupils do not become reactive, mortality or vegetative survival occurs in 82 percent. The emphasis, therefore, is on the persistence of the loss of pupillary reactivity rather than on transient, early observations of pupillary abnormality.

The Influence of Age on Outcome

The influence of age on outcome after severe head injury has been extensively reviewed by Vollmer and colleagues.[20] Infants and very young children have a high mortality, most likely because many of their head injuries represent nonaccidental trauma due to abuse, which is associated with prolonged episodes of hypoxia. After this early peak, mortality from head injury remains relatively constant until age 35 and then begins to rise quite dramatically (Table 267-2). Mendelow (personal communication) has identified no favorable outcomes from severe head injury in patients over 65 who had abnormal motor movements at the time of admission or after resuscitation. In fact, the presence of abnormal motor movements in patients over 45 usually carries a dire prognosis.

TABLE 267-2 Comparison of Observed and Predicted Percentages of Patients Vegetative or Dead by Age Groups*

Age Group	No. of Cases	Observed	Predicted	95% Confidence Interval
15–25 yr	263	32.7%	31.2%	25.6%–36.8%
> 25–35 yr	119	30.3%	32.9%	24.4%–41.4%
> 35–45 yr	66	42.4%	45.6%	33.6%–57.6%
> 45–55 yr	39	59.0%	59.5%	44.1%–74.9%
> 55 yr	57	80.7%	78.7%	68.0%–89.4%

*Cases with missing data were excluded.

Vital Signs

As we have developed a better understanding of the influence of shock and hypoxia in patients with severe injury, it has become apparent that shock has a dramatic and very important effect on outcome. While the GCS in part incorporates the influence of shock and/or shock and hypoxia, the rather detailed studies of Chesnut and colleagues and Marmarou and colleagues indicate that one must separately take into account the presence or absence of shock.[3,10] These recent observations have been in part responsible for the intense interest in resuscitating the cerebral perfusion pressure (CPP), defined as the mean arterial pressure minus the intracranial pressure (ICP), to greater than 60 mmHg and maintaining it at substantially higher levels if at all possible. The adverse consequences of shock are shown in Table 267-3. Note that a combination of shock and hypoxia both still present at the time of initial hospital assessment carries a mortality more than two times greater than if neither of these secondary complications is present.

Abnormalities in respiratory function are often seen with severe head injury and complicate management, but their presence is not terribly useful in predicting outcome. Also of interest is the observation that bradycardia (defined as a heart rate of 50 or less) at the time of admission is associated with a nearly fourfold increase in the likelihood of death or severe disability.

Pathophysiology of the Lesion and CT Scanning

Until the introduction of CT in the general management of head-injured patients, the outcome for patients with mass lesions was much poorer than for those with diffuse injuries of the brain, but this gap has progressively narrowed as CT has been used both earlier and more often in the same patient. Because a number of investigators observed that the status of the cisterns and the degree of shift seen on CT were helpful in outcome prediction,[16,18,19] the Traumatic Coma Data Bank developed a new classification of head injury based on CT results. This classification is shown in Table 267-4, and its relation to outcome in patients is shown in Table 267-5. It is apparent that increasing intracranial volume, due either to brain swelling and/or edema or to an intracranial mass lesion (or, obviously, to a combination of these factors), directly

TABLE 267-3 Influence of Shock and Hypoxia Prior to Hospitalization on Outcome of Severe Head Injury

Secondary Insults	No. of Patients	% Total Patients	Outcome (%) Good or Moderate	Severe or Vegetative	Dead
Total cases	717	100.0	43.0	20.2	36.8
Neither hypoxia nor hypotension	308	43.0	53.9	19.2	26.9
Hypoxia	161	22.4	50.3	21.7	28.0
Hypotension	82	11.4	32.9	17.1	50.0
Both hypoxia and hypotension	166	23.2	20.5	22.3	57.2

TABLE 267-4 Diagnostic Categories of Types of Abnormalities Visualized on CT

Category	Definition
Diffuse injury I (no visible abnormality)	No intracranial abnormality visible on CT scan
Diffuse injury II	Cisterns are present with midline shift of 0–5 mm and/ or: • Lesion densities are present • No high- or mixed-density lesion of volume >25 ml is present • Bone fragments and foreign bodies may be present
Diffuse injury III (swelling)	Cisterns are compressed or absent with midline shift 0–5 mm; no high- or mixed-density lesion of volume >25 ml is present
Diffuse injury IV (shift)	Midline shift >5 mm, no high- or mixed-density lesion of volume >25 ml is present
Evacuated mass lesion	Any lesion surgically removed
Non-evacuated mass lesion	High- or mixed-density lesion of volume >25 ml, not surgically removed

and significantly influences outcome. For example, patients who have diffuse injury but no mass lesion have a remarkably good prognosis for survival. The importance of rapid removal of mass lesions was demonstrated by Seelig and colleagues in patients with acute subdural hematomas[15]; as emergency medical services systems have improved in all advanced societies, mortality for such lesions has progressively declined.

Now entering its third decade of use, CT has had an almost immeasurable influence on neurotraumatology. Patients who once would have died of mass lesions are now diagnosed before even becoming unconscious, and their lesions are rapidly removed. As we develop better ways to image the functional capacity of the brain and further refine the classifications shown here, it is likely that outcome prediction will get better.

Intracranial Pressure Measurements

ICP monitoring has yielded useful information regarding the pathophysiology of brain injury. It is also apparent that an inability to control ICP gives very reliable predictive information. Patients in whom the ICP exceeds 30 mmHg at the time of admission have an extremely high death rate. Furthermore, patients whose ICP exceeds 30 mmHg after the evacuation of a hematoma or during intensive management of diffuse brain injury, have a markedly worse prognosis than patients whose ICP is lower. The concept of the intensity of therapy, which has been called the therapy intensity level by Marmarou and colleagues, has been useful in comparing patients.[10] Thus, an ICP of 25 in a patient who requires no therapy has a remarkably different implication than it would in a patient in whom extensive treatment is failing.

Multimodality Evoked Potentials

The use of multimodality evoked potentials, including brain stem auditory evoked responses and somatosensory evoked potentials, has been the subject of intense scrutiny. However, in spite of more than 20 years of effort, the recording of these responses has not had a measurable impact on our ability either to identify patients in whom aggressive therapy will be of no avail or to refine outcome predictions beyond more than very gross categorization. Much of the initial work by Greenberg and colleagues, which demonstrated that significant abnormalities in somatosensory evoked potentials are almost always associated with a poor outcome and that approximately 20 percent of patients with head injuries who reach the hospital alive have irreversible brain stem injuries and are likely to die or do very poorly, has been confirmed.[5,6,13] It is clear that one can correlate evoked response data with the results of postmortem examinations and show that brain stem injuries are more common as a primary cause of deterioration than was previously thought; that deterioration in neurological function resulting in medical complications can to some extent be detected by multimodality evoked potentials; and that a combination of evoked response measurements is more useful than the measurement of one modality alone.[14] Nevertheless, we have not made significant progress in using these responses in outcome prediction. While abnormal brain stem auditory evoked responses reliably indicate the likelihood of a poor outcome, the presence of intact brain stem auditory evoked responses is much less useful in prediction because these responses tend to be quite robust.

More recently, Becker and colleagues have reported on their experience using multimodality evoked potentials in a highly sophisticated intensive care unit.[1] They were able to demonstrate that recording these evoked potentials and the electroencephalogram using computer compression techniques yields useful information for patient management. This is in keeping with the observations of Karnaze and colleagues, who demonstrated that a combination

TABLE 267-5 Outcome at Discharge in Relation to Intracranial Diagnosis*

Outcome at Discharge	Diffuse Injury I		Diffuse Injury II		Diffuse Injury III		Diffuse Injury IV		Evacuated Mass		Non-evacuated Mass		Brain-Stem Injury		Unknown		Totals	
	No.	%	No.	%	No.	%	No.	%	No.	%	No.	%	No.	%	No.	%	No.	%
Good	14	27.0	15	8.5	5	3.3	1	3.1	14	5.1	1	2.8	0	0	0	0	50	70
Moderate	18	34.6	46	26.0	20	13.1	1	3.1	49	17.7	3	8.3	0	0	1	5.9	138	18.5
Severe	10	19.2	72	40.7	41	26.8	6	18.8	72	26.1	7	19.4	1	33.3	0	0	209	28.0
Vegetative	5	9.6	20	11.3	35	22.9	6	18.8	34	12.3	6	16.7	0	0	0	0	106	14.0
Dead	5	9.6	24	13.5	52	34.0	18	56.2	107	38.8	19	52.8	2	66.7	16	94.1	243	32.5
Totals	52	100	177	100	153	100	32	100	276	100	36	100	3	100	17	100	746	100

*Outcome classified by the Glasgow Outcome Scale.

of multimodality evoked potentials with recording of the compressed spectral array can yield useful information.[7] The recent ability of Becker's group to digitally display electrical information about the brain may represent a significant advance, because it converts a somewhat user-unfriendly wave form to a display that is likely to be much more useful to the intensive care unit nurse.

Outcome after Penetrating Craniocerebral Injury

The rapid proliferation of firearm injuries of the brain in the United States has, unfortunately, provided an opportunity to study the outcome of these injuries, particularly in urban neurosurgical centers. In a recent report from Levy and colleagues, only 24 of 190 consecutive patients survived.[8] The important predictors of a poor outcome in these patients were not dissimilar to those for nonpenetrating injury, and included Glasgow coma scale scores at admission and after resuscitation, the status of the pupils, and the presence or absence of subarachnoid hemorrhage. A number of investigators have now shown that the latter variable is important in nonpenetrating injuries as well. The dismal outcome of penetrating missile wounds reflects both the tremendous destructive force of these injuries and the rapid development of secondary insults in these patients.

Profile of Outcome

There is an obvious need to predict outcome as early as possible. In an attempt to determine at which point the outcome is relatively fixed in patients with severe nonpenetrating injury, Choi and colleagues carried out a series of analyses, which demonstrated that the 6-month outcome point is the most stable end-point for clinical trials and for making overall statements with regard to prognosis.[4] The continued striking improvement over time in patients during the first 6 months and the number of patients in a vegetative state who improve after discharge also indicate that decisions regarding the withdrawal of supportive care in patients under 40 should be postponed until at least 6 months after injury. This recent study clearly demonstrates that the outcome for a significant number of patients who are considered to be vegetative, severely disabled, or moderately disabled at discharge will improve over the subsequent several months.

Outcome Prediction in the 21st Century

The addition of a new CT classification and a better understanding of the influence of shock and hypoxia on the outcome of severe head injury have materially improved our ability to predict outcome. Although electrophysiological monitoring has been quite disappointing to date, it appears that there may now be better mechanisms to analyze and display such information. If we can use these data more meaningfully, they might well improve our ability to predict outcome in marginal patients who are unlikely to die but for whom it is impossible to tell whether the outcome will be poor or not. It is apparent that we cannot remain dependent on the clinical examination. In a population of young patients, the clinical examination is unlikely to yield a highly accurate outcome prediction until many weeks after the injury, and by that time resource expenditure has usually been enormous.

An information base that includes the results of the clinical examination, detailed detection of secondary insults both before and during hospitalization, serial electrophysiological assessments, subsequent CT scans, and, where indicated, ICP and CPP measurements, is likely to result in significantly better outcome prediction for patients whose prognosis is not obvious from the clinical examination alone. It is important to recognize that prediction requires a very high degree of specificity and sensitivity. It is unsatisfactory to identify all patients who will do poorly but to include in the group some patients who ultimately do well. The clinical examination has not been adequate to allow such sensitivity.

As we learn more both about the pathophysiology of brain injury at the cellular level and about the microenvironments in which we care for such patients, it is likely that we will be able to detect events that adversely affect outcome and have not been identified before. That should allow us both to make sharper outcome predictions and to reverse or modify these adverse events so that outcomes are improved—which, after all, remains the major objective of the treating clinical neuroscientist.

References

1. Becker DP. New trends in head injury intensive care management. Presented to the Scandinavian Neurosurgical Society, Uppsala, Sweden, June, 1993.
2. Chesnut RM, Gautille T, Blunt BA, et al. The localizing value of asymmetry in pupillary size in severe head injury: relation to lesion type and location. *Neurosurgery* 1994; 34:840–846.
3. Chesnut RM, Marshall LF, Klauber MR, et al. The role of secondary brain injury in determining outcome from severe head injury. *J Trauma* 1993; 34:216–222.
4. Choi SC, Barnes TY, Bullock R, et al. Temporal profile of outcomes in severe head injury. *J Neurosurg* 1994; 81:169–173.
5. Greenberg RP, Becker DP, Miller JD, Mayer DJ. Evaluation of brain function in severe human head trauma with multimodality evoked potentials. Part 2: Localization of brain dysfunction and correlation with posttraumatic neurological conditions. *J Neurosurg* 1977; 47:163–177.
6. Greenberg RP, Newlon PG, Hyatt MS, et al. Prognostic implications of early multimodality evoked potentials in severely head injured patients: a prospective study. *J Neurosurg* 1981; 55:227–236.
7. Karnaze DS, Marshall LF, McCarthy CS, et al. Localizing and prognostic value of auditory evoked responses in coma after closed head injury. *Neurology* 1982; 32:299–302.
8. Levy ML, Masri LS, Lavine S, Apuzzo MLJ. Outcome prediction after penetrating craniocerebral injury in a civilian population: aggressive surgical management in patients with admission Glasgow coma scale scores of 3, 4, or 5. *Neurosurgery* 1994; 35:77–84.
9. Luerssen TG, Hults K, Klauber M, et al. Improved outcome as a result of recognition of absent or compressed cisterns on initial CT scans. In Hoff JT, Betz AL (eds): *Intracranial Pressure VII.* Berlin: Springer-Verlag, 1989, pp 598–602.
10. Marmarou A, Anderson RL, Ward JD, et al. Impact of ICP instability and hypotension on outcome in patients with severe head trauma. *J Neurosurg* 1991; 75(Suppl):S59–S66.
11. Marshall LF, Gautille T, Klauber MR, et al. The outcome of severe closed head injury. *J Neurosurg* 1991; 75(Suppl):S28–S36.
12. Marshall LF, Marshall SB, Klauber MR, et al. A new classification of head injury based on computerized tomography. *J Neurosurg* 1991; 75(Suppl):S14–S20.
13. Newlon PG, Greenberg RP, Hyatt MS, et al. The dynamics of neuronal dysfunction and recovery following severe head injury assessed with

serial multimodality evoked potentials. *J Neurosurg* 1982; 57:168–177.

14. Rosenblum WI, Greenberg RP, Seelig JM, Becker DP. Midbrain lesions: frequent and significant prognostic feature in closed head injury. *Neurosurgery* 1981; 9:613–620.
15. Seelig JM, Becker DP, Miller JD, et al. Traumatic acute subdural hematoma: major mortality reduction in comatose patients treated within four hours. *N Engl J Med* 1981; 304:1511–1518.
16. Teasdale E, Teasdale G, Cardoso E, et al. CT scan correlations in severe diffuse head injury. Presented at the International Conference on Recent Advances in Neurotraumatology, Edinburgh, UK, 1982.
17. Teasdale G, Jennett B. Assessment of coma and impaired consciousness: a practical scale. *Lancet* 1974; 2:81–84.
18. Toutant SM, Klauber MR, Marshall LF, et al. Absent or compressed basal cisterns on first CT scan: ominous predictors of outcome in severe head injury. *J Neurosurg* 1984; 61:691–694.
19. van Dongen KJ, Braakman R, Gelpke GJ. The prognostic value of computerized tomography in comatose head-injured patients. *J Neurosurg* 1983; 59:951–957.
20. Vollmer DG, Torner JC, Jane JA, et al. Age and outcome following traumatic coma: why do older patients fare worse? *J Neurosurg* 1991; 75(Suppl):S37–S49.

268

Minor Head Injury Management and Outcome

Eric M. Gabriel
Dennis A. Turner

Closed head injury represents a common aspect of trauma, often requiring neurosurgical evaluation in the emergency room. Subsequent treatment of affected individuals varies according to the severity of injury. The severity of head injury often is assessed by the Glasgow Coma Scale (GCS), a point value system ranging from 3 to 15.[11] To further elucidate the severity and associated outcome differences in head injury, the GCS score may be divided arbitrarily into three categories: severe, less than 8; moderate, 9 to 12; and mild, 13 to 15. Although much literature exists on the outcome of severely injured patients, the assessment of morbidity from minor head injuries has been relatively recent.[8] This lack of attention is partly due to the belief that patients with minor head injury do not sustain permanent or irreversible brain injury. The notion that minor closed head injury is benign is often reinforced by normal imaging studies, such as computed tomography (CT) scans.

Minor, or mild, head injury (these terms are often used interchangeably) defines a subset of closed head injuries with casualties ranging from simple scalp lacerations or contusions without brain involvement to those incurring a loss of consciousness. Rimel et al. defined minor head injury as cranial trauma resulting in a loss of consciousness for 20 min or less, an admission GCS score of 13 to 15, and the need for 48 h or less of hospitalization.[8] Williams et al. proposed a variant of the mild head injury classification by adding a separate category of severity between that of mild and moderate closed head injury: complicated mild head injury.[12] This group would consist of mild head injury with radiographic evidence of a focal brain lesion or depressed skull fracture, or both.

Minor head injury can be subclassified further by the presence and duration of unconsciousness and/or post-traumatic amnesia. The latter terms are generally associated with concussion; however, neither is mandatory for the diagnosis. *Concussion,* as defined by the Congress of Neurological Surgeons, is a "clinical syndrome characterized by immediate and transient impairment of neural function such as alteration of consciousness, disturbance of vision, equilibrium, etc., due to mechanical forces."[1] Concussions can be associated with alterations ranging from a mildly affected sensorium to a loss of consciousness for more than 1 min. More severe concussion producing loss of consciousness constitutes the majority of mild head injuries, whereas less severe concussion may not prompt the injured person to seek medical attention.

Of all brain-injured hospitalized patients, those with mild head injury predominate, constituting 50 to 80 percent of the group; one epidemiological study reported a hospitalization rate of 131 per 100,000 population per year.[6] The incidence is higher in males, with peak occurrence at ages 11 to 20 except in complicated mild head injury, in which the patients tend to be older.[6,8,12] Minor head injuries are most often related to motor vehicle accidents (40 to 50 percent of cases), with falls, sports, and assaults being the remaining causes; alcohol use is a major contributing factor.[8]

Pathophysiology

Before improved diagnostic neuroimaging, minor head injury was believed to be reversible or transient without persistent sequelae, over the time span of 3 to 6 weeks. This was partly due to the lack of detectable objective neurological deficits and unremarkable imaging studies. Because the mild nature of the injury precluded postmortem evaluations, pathological diagnosis was performed only in the rare cases in which mortality was attributable to comorbid disease. Many of the post-traumatic subjective complaints were often thought to be psychosocial rather than attributable to the brain injury. A growing body of evidence pathologically and physiologically documents neuronal dysfunction after minor head injury, although usually on a scale below the resolution of current imaging studies.

The study of biomechanics indicates that a force applied to the skull results in acceleration of the brain in either a translational or a rotational direction. Ommaya and Gennarelli provided evidence that translational or linear acceleration produces essentially focal effects, such as coup-contrecoup contusions of the brain, whereas rotational or angular acceleration results in concussions.[7] Morphological studies have identified central chromatolysis of neurons, most commonly in the brain stem, but also in the upper cervical spinal cord and cerebral cortex, as the typical pathological lesion.[10] Degenerating axons in the brain stem were also found after experimentally induced concussions.[5] Neurophysiological studies also lend credence to a clear structural etiology of concussion. Although most delayed EEG studies failed to demonstrate abnormal activity after minor head injury, some experimental data using brain stem auditory evoked responses (BAER) suggest prolonged brain stem conduction time and impaired choice reaction time.

With the increased detectability of axonal pathology using magnetic resonance imaging (MRI), parenchymal lesions not visualized on CT scans may be apparent. The increased detection of the pathological effects of minor head injury, especially in the frontal and temporal regions, probably will not influence the outcome of these patients but certainly clarifies the biological mechanisms underlying mild head trauma and the requirement for recovery time following such an injury.

Management

Much controversy has surrounded the initial evaluation and treatment of minor head injury. Rational decisions about neuroimaging and admission criteria for this group of patients are compounded by the ever-increasing cost-consciousness of the current practice climate. Clearly, a certain morbidity exists despite the relatively benign nature of mild head trauma. In a study performed by Dacey et al., 3 percent of 610 minor head injury patients eventually required a neurosurgical procedure.[3] The goals of initial evaluations are to ensure a good outcome by early diagnostic intervention in the few patients susceptible to serious complications and to inform and educate patients about expected sequelae and recovery time.

A number of algorithms reported in the literature use skull radiography, CT, MRI, or a combination thereof to assist with treatment plans. Although a fractured skull increases a patient's risk of having intracranial sequelae, most radiologists believe that skull radiography is not necessary and is often redundant, as a CT scan often is obtained in this situation. Some advocate routine CT scanning for all patients seen in the emergency room for minor head trauma, because this method detects the minority of patients with an acute lesion not necessarily requiring surgery, whereas a negative CT study with a normal neurological examination provides sufficient data to allow discharge.[9] A negative study permitting discharge would be more cost-effective than admitting a patient overnight for observation. MRI may provide a tool for delineating lesions undetectable by other modalities; however, the cost and logistics of obtaining a scan on a patient in the emergency room would likely negate any additional useful information in the acute setting. Nevertheless, MRI scanning may define a subset of the population at increased risk for long-term sequelae.

A more commonly accepted method of management for these patients entails selected neuroimaging and clinical acumen. The history of the trauma, use of alcohol or drugs, and the initial plus follow-up serial neurological examinations should be important factors in the decision to obtain a CT scan. The combined clinical and radiological data will influence the caretaker's further management (i.e., extended observation versus discharge). A multidisciplinary study has developed a management strategy for head-injured patients by dividing them into different risk group categories (Table 268-1). According to this scheme, a patient with a simple scalp laceration, no loss of consciousness, and normal neurological examination would not require a CT scan and could be discharged home with a head injury instruction sheet under the supervision of an adult. Loss of consciousness that has resolved upon presentation may represent a particular dilemma in deciding whether to admit the patient for observation. If the CT scan is normal and the patient has adequate monitoring supervision near a hospital, it is probably safe to discharge that patient.[9] However, a patient with a GCS score of 15 who is disoriented in place or time should be observed until the sensorium clears. A focal neurological deficit or a GCS score less than 15 should warrant a head CT scan and admission to observe for possible deterioration.

Another clinical aspect of minor head injury is the management of patients with repeated trauma. Rimel et al. reported that 31 percent of their patients had suffered prior head injury.[8] Because minor head injury may involve structural brain damage at a microscopic level, repeated injuries may lead to serious cumulative effects with poorer outcomes. Athletes who have suffered a cerebral concussion are four times more likely to suffer a second concussion.[2] The second impact syndrome, a variant of pediatric malignant brain edema syndrome, is a condition limited to adults who sustain fatal brain swelling after they incur a minor head injury while still suffering from symptoms of a previous head injury.[2] It is thought to be due to a defect in cerebrovascular autoregulation after the first head injury, which predisposes the patient to massive hyperemia and congestion after a second injury. This raises the question of when an athlete who has sustained a concussion should be permitted to return to the contest. Ultimately this is a clinical judgment made by the team physician. Table 268-2 offers some guidelines based on an expected recovery time of 3 to 4 weeks.

TABLE 268-1 Management Strategy for Radiographic Imaging in Patients with Head Trauma*

Low-Risk Group	Moderate-Risk Group	High-Risk Group
	Possible Findings	
Asymptomatic Headache Dizziness Scalp hematoma Scalp laceration Scalp contusion and laceration Absence of moderate-risk or high-risk criteria	History of change of consciousness at the time of injury or subsequently History of progressive headache Alcohol or drug intoxication Unreliable or inadequate history of injury Age <2 years (unless injury very trivial) Post-traumatic seizure Vomiting Post-traumatic amnesia Multiple trauma Serious facial injury Signs of basilar fracture Possible skull penetration or depressed fracture Suspected physical child abuse	Depressed level of consciousness not clearly due to alcohol, drugs, or other cause (e.g., metabolic and seizure disorders) Focal neurological signs Decreasing level of consciousness Penetrating skull injury or palpable depressed fracture
	Recommendations	
Observation alone: discharge patients with head injury information sheet (listing subdural hematoma precautions) and a second person to observe them	Extended close observation (watch for signs of high-risk group) Consider CT examination and neurosurgical consultation Skull series may (rarely) be helpful if positive, but does not exclude intracranial injury if normal	Patient is a candidate for neurosurgical consultation or emergency CT examination, or both

*Physician assessment of the severity of injury may warrant reassignment to a higher-risk group. Any single criterion from a higher-risk group warrants assignment of the patient to the highest-risk group applicable.

Source: From Masters SJ, McClean PM, Argarese JS, et al. Skull x-ray examinations after head trauma. *N Engl J Med* 1987; 316:84–91, with permission.

Outcome

Most patients with minor head injury leave the hospital without any serious neurological deficits and return to their normal activities of daily living. However, there is considerable evidence that

TABLE 268-2 Guidelines for Return to Play After Concussion

Grade	Loss of Consciousness	Duration of Post-Traumatic Amnesia	First Concussion	Second Concussion	Third Concussion
1 (mild)	None	<30 min	May return to play if asymptomatic* for 1 week	If asymptomatic for 1 week, then return to play in 2 more weeks	Terminate season; may return to play next season if asymptomatic
2 (moderate)	<5 min	30 min to <24 h	May return to play if asymptomatic for 1 week	May return to play after minimum of 1 month if asymptomatic for 1 week; consider terminating season	Terminate season; may return to play next season if asymptomatic
3 (severe)	≥5 min	≥24 h	Minimum of 1 month, may return to play if asymptomatic for 1 week	Terminate season; may return to play next season if asymptomatic	

*No headache, dizziness, or impaired orientation, concentration, or memory during rest or exertion.
Source: Adapted from Cantu RC,[2] with permission.

these injuries yield significant morbidity in the more subtle aspects of head and neck function. Common sequelae of mild head injury are listed in Table 268-3. A collection of symptoms referred to as the *postconcussion syndrome* encompasses complaints held by many who have sustained mild head trauma. These symptoms most often include headaches, fatigue, memory problems, difficulty concentrating, irritability, and light or noise sensitivity. Once considered secondary to psychogenic factors (anxiety, secondary gain), the symptomatology is now believed to be probably the result of cellular or macroscopic lesions identified on neuroimaging studies, BAER studies, and histopathological findings. This collection of symptoms may hinder the ability of many patients to conform to societal demands. In the study by Rimel et al., 34 percent of previously employed patients were not working 3 months after the injury.[8] The degree of unemployment correlated with either lower socioeconomic class or a lack of buffers to minimize stressors at the job site. This finding is consistent with the observation that premorbid chronic social adversity is more commonly associated with the postconcussion syndrome. Although young men are at greatest risk of minor head injury, older women are at greatest risk of chronic sequelae.[4]

The duration of the postconcussion syndrome is debatable, with some patients reporting symptoms after 1 year. The data in the literature suggest that although a significant impairment may persist for several weeks after the injury, the trend is toward gradual improvement, which suggests a recovery process. Because of the occasionally slow recovery of patients with the postconcussion syndrome and the cost incurred by society for unemployment disability, susceptible patients must be identified and optimally treated. One of the key features of treatment is patient education. Frequently, patients are discharged home after being informed that nothing is wrong. Perhaps if patients were informed of the common postconcussive complaints, they would experience less anxiety about these symptoms when they occur. The knowledge that symptoms of headache, memory disturbances, and concentration difficulties are common after minor head injury may reduce pressure on patients to justify their condition to family and peers, and decrease patients' performance anxiety when they do not meet premorbid standards. Neuropsychological testing may help justify patient complaints and document improvement over time, particularly for those whose symptoms persist over 3 to 4 weeks. Individ-

TABLE 268-3 Sequelae of Mild Head Injury

- Headaches
  - Muscle contraction type
  - Migraine
  - Cluster
  - Occipital neuralgia
  - Supraorbital and infraorbital neuralgia
  - Secondary to neck injury
  - Secondary to temporomandibular joint syndrome
  - Due to scalp laceration or local trauma
  - Mixed
- Cranial nerve symptoms and signs
  - Dizziness
  - Vertigo
  - Tinnitus
  - Hearing loss
  - Blurred vision
  - Diplopia
  - Convergence insufficiency
  - Light and noise sensitivity
  - Diminished taste and smell
- Psychological and somatic complaints
  - Irritability
  - Anxiety
  - Depression
  - Personality change
  - Fatigue
  - Sleep disturbance
  - Decreased libido
  - Decreased appetite
- Cognitive impairment
  - Memory dysfunction
  - Impaired concentration and attention
  - Slowing of reaction time
  - Slowing of information processing speed
- Rare sequelae
  - Subdural and epidural hematomas
  - Seizures
  - Transient global amnesia
  - Tremor
  - Dystonia

Source: From Evans RW. Post-concussion syndrome. In Evans RW, Baskin DS, Yatsu FM (eds): *Prognosis of Neurological Disorders.* New York: Oxford University Press, 1992, with permission.

ualized treatments (i.e., analgesics, antidepressants, muscle relaxants, biofeedback), may be beneficial for specific complaints. However, most patients recover fairly quickly, and these adjunct treatments only occasionally are needed.

Summary

Although minor head injury represents a lesser degree of severity than some other injuries, the frequently observed sequelae should be viewed with seriousness. The high incidence of these injuries in conjunction with distinct immediate and long-term sequelae warrants considerable attention. Also, the cost to society of these minor injuries can be substantial. As interest in minor head injury has increased over the past decade, much has been learned about the pathophysiology of the injury. However, further research is necessary to develop correlates between structural (and usually microscopic) lesions and clinically subjective complaints. The evaluation of these patients must also be clarified. As the United States health care system evolves, a more cost-conscious approach to this group of patients is warranted, but care must not be compromised, because the morbidity can be devastating. Finally, the role of the neurosurgeon can be crucial in reducing long-term morbidity related to trauma anxiety. Because they are often involved in initial patient care, neurosurgeons can positively affect the layperson's perception of the injury and its expected outcome.

References

1. *Ad Hoc* Committee to Study Head Injury Nomenclature. Report. *Clin Neurosurg* 1966; 12:386–387.
2. Cantu RC. Cerebral concussion in sport: management and prevention. *Sports Med* 1992; 14:64–74.
3. Dacey RG Jr, Alves WM, Rimel RW, et al. Neurosurgical complications after apparently minor head injury: assessment of risk in a series of 610 patients. *J Neurosurg* 1986; 65:203–210.
4. Fenton G, McClelland R, Montgomery A, et al. The postconcussional syndrome: social antecedents and psychological sequelae. *Br J Psychiatry* 1993; 162:493–497.
5. Jane JA, Steward O, Gennarelli T. Axonal degeneration induced by experimental noninvasive minor head injury. *J Neurosurg* 1985; 62:96–100.
6. Kraus JF, Nourjah P. The epidemiology of mild, uncomplicated brain injury. *J Trauma* 1988; 28:1637–1643.
7. Ommaya AK, Gennarelli TA. Cerebral concussion and traumatic unconsciousness: correlation of experimental and clinical observation of blunt head injuries. *Brain* 1974; 97:633–654.
8. Rimel RW, Giordani B, Barth JT, et al. Disability caused by minor head injury. *Neurosurgery* 1981; 9:221–228.
9. Shackford SR, Wald SL, Ross SE, et al. The clinical utility of computed tomographic scanning and neurologic examination in the management of patients with minor head injuries. *J Trauma* 1992; 33:385–394.
10. Shetter AG, Demakas JJ. The pathophysiology of concussion: a review. *Adv Neurol* 1979; 22:5–14.
11. Teasdale G, Jennett B. Assessment of coma and impaired consciousness: a practical scale. *Lancet* 1974; 2:81–84.
12. Williams DH, Levin HS, Eisenberg HM. Mild head injury classification. *Neurosurgery* 1990; 27:422–428.

269 Scalp Injuries

L. Scott Levin
William J. Barwick

The scalp is a specialized structure of skin, muscle, and fascia that is unique. In addition to providing coverage for the cranium, it contains some 100,000 hairs, which provide insulation in addition to having esthetic value.

The superficial location of the scalp puts it first in line for injuries from a variety of physical and chemical agents. Injuries to the scalp vary from minor lacerations to total loss, either by scalping (avulsion) or by burning.

The ability to treat severe scalp injuries has been enhanced by developments in musculocutaneous flaps and microsurgery. Injuries that would have been fatal 100 years ago can now be handled with relative ease. This chapter will present a general overview of the anatomy of the scalp and the treatment of scalp injuries and defects.

Anatomy

General Considerations

A sound working knowledge of scalp anatomy is necessary for treating scalp injuries effectively. The scalp extends from the supraorbital ridges to the inferior nuchal line. Laterally it extends to the auriculocephalic angle. In most individuals, the scalp is completely covered with hair except for the anterior portion, which is the forehead.

In cross section, the scalp contains five distinct layers (Fig. 269-1). The skin of the scalp is the thickest in the body, making it a good, if infrequently used, donor site for split-thickness skin grafts. Immediately subjacent to this is a layer of dense fibrofatty tissue into which the roots of the hairs extend. In the deep portion of this layer are the main blood vessels that supply the scalp. Just beneath it is the galea aponeurotica, which forms a continuous layer of tough fascia connecting the anterior, posterior, and lateral parts of the epicranius muscle. The epicranius muscle has two main divisions: the occipitofrontalis and temporoparietalis. Both the occipital and frontal portions of the occipitofrontalis consist of a pair of broad, quadrilateral muscles that are continuous with the galea. These muscles act to move the scalp forward and backward. The frontal portion also elevates the eyebrows and wrinkles the skin of the forehead. The epicranius muscle is innervated by branches of the seventh cranial nerve.

The first three layers of the scalp adhere firmly to one another and may be considered a single unit. Beneath the galea is a layer of loose areolar tissue. This tissue can be easily separated and is the plane in which scalp flaps are raised and scalp avulsions occur. The final layer is the pericranium (the periosteal layer of the outer table of the skull), which adheres firmly to the skull, particularly at the cranial sutures.

Vascular Anatomy

The creation of dependable scalp flaps as well as the repair of avulsion injuries to the scalp require a thorough knowledge of its blood supply. Blood reaches the scalp through terminal branches of the internal and external carotid arteries. Five major arteries enter the scalp on each side, anastomosing freely with each other and with those on the opposite side (Fig. 269-2). The anterior portion of the scalp is supplied by the supraorbital and supratrochlear (frontal) arteries, which are branches of the ophthalmic artery. These vessels pass around the supraorbital ridge into the frontalis muscle and supply the skin of the forehead.

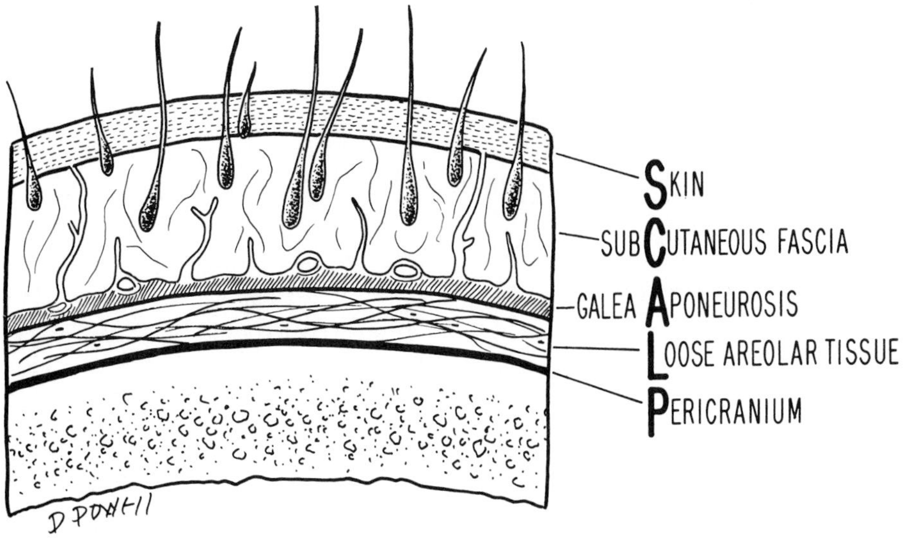

Figure 269-1 The scalp in cross section. The five layers can be remembered by using the mnemonic SCALP. The outer three layers function as a single unit.

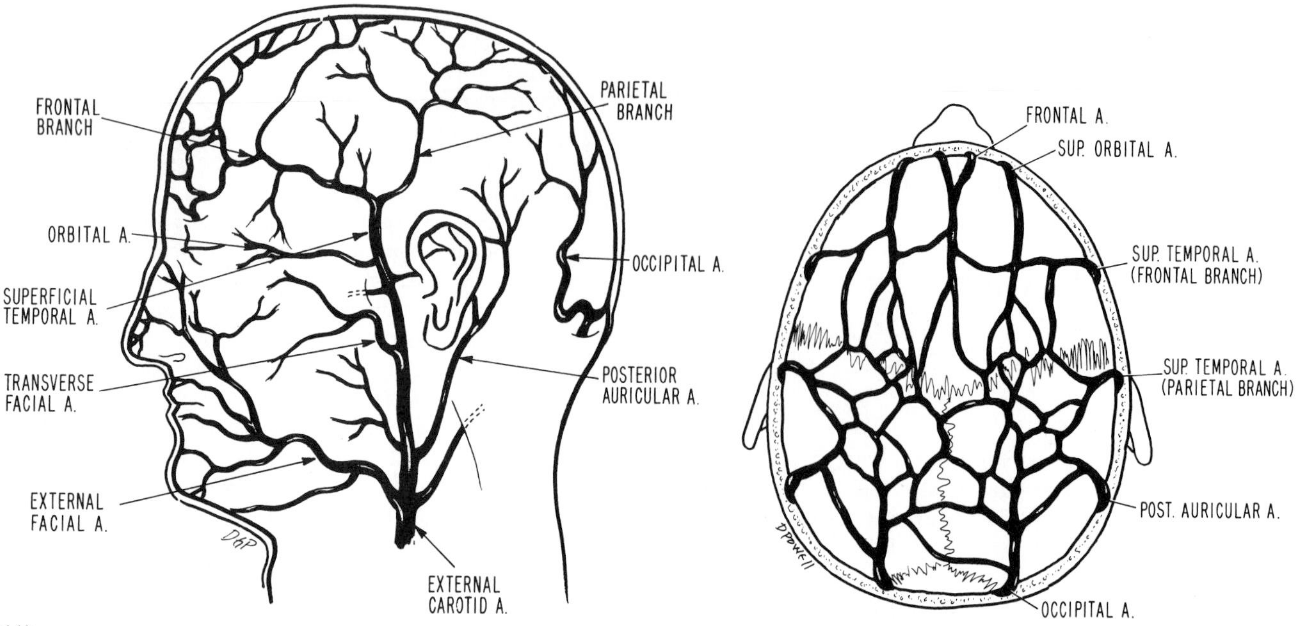

(*A*) (*B*)

Figure 269-2 The arteries supplying the scalp. *A.* Lateral view. All the vessels are branches of the internal and external carotid arteries. *B.* Vertex view, showing the five pairs of arteries supplying the scalp. There is an extensive interconnecting network of vessels across the top of the head.

The major vessel entering the scalp laterally is the superficial temporal artery, one of the two terminal branches of the external carotid. The superficial temporal is the largest artery supplying the scalp and is the most useful for anastomosis in scalp replantation. This artery passes over the zygoma anterior to the tragus. At approximately the level of the superior pole of the ear, the artery divides into an anterior (frontal) branch and a posterior (parietal) branch. The frontal branch joins with branches of the supraorbital artery, and the parietal branch anastomoses freely with the posterior auricular and occipital arteries.

The posterior portion of the scalp is supplied by two branches of the external carotid artery: the posterior auricular artery and the occipital artery. The posterior auricular artery is a small branch of the external carotid which passes cephalad and posteriorly behind the ear over the mastoid process. The occipital artery is larger and enters the scalp posteriorly on each side at approximately the superior nuchal line.

After entering the scalp, the arteries form an extensive interconnecting network of vessels across the most cephalic portion of the scalp (Fig. 269-2*B*). The vessels are located in the deep portion of the fibrofatty layer of the scalp just above the galea. It is convenient therefore to think of the scalp as having an axial pattern. Because of this fact, large scalp flaps can be developed without a prior delay procedure (Fig. 269-3). In designing scalp flaps, however, one should attempt to base the flaps laterally and to include the major vessels where possible (Figs. 269-4 and 269-5). The use of a Doppler device may be helpful.

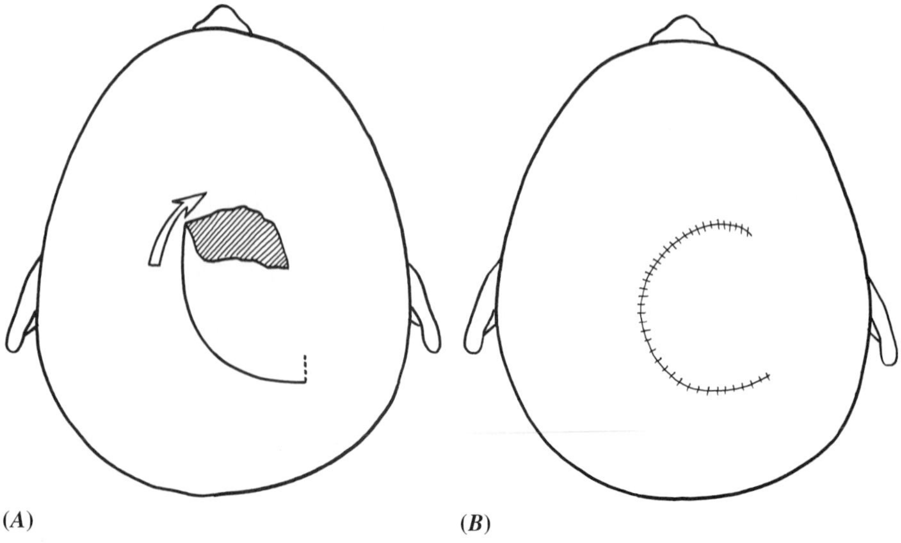

(*A*) (*B*)

Figure 269-3 A simple rotation flap. *A.* Many defects in the scalp that are too large for primary approximation can be closed by a simple rotation flap. The *dotted line* indicates a back cut, which may sometimes be necessary. *B.* If the rotation flap is large enough, the defect can be closed without using a skin graft.

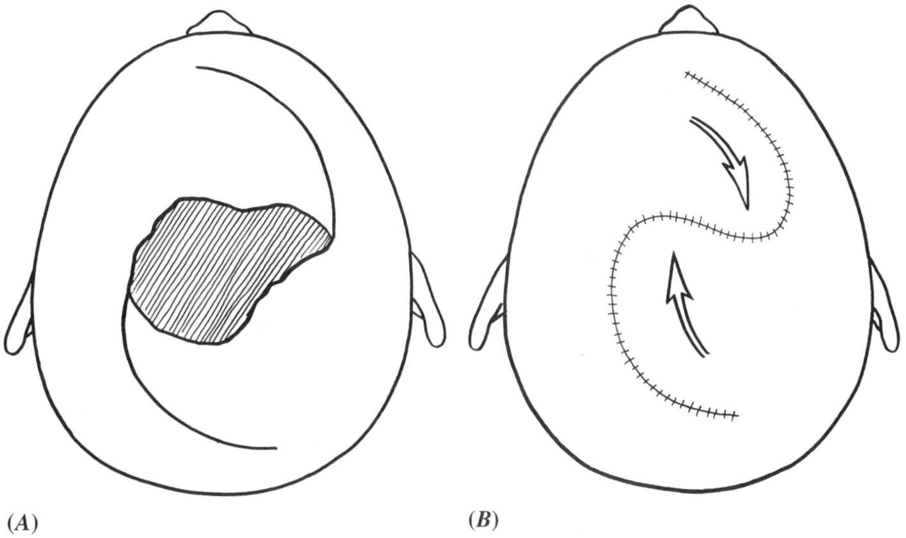

Figure 269-4 Larger defects (*A*) can be closed using multiple rotation flaps (*B*). The base of each flap should include major arteries if possible.

Nerve Supply

Sensation over the scalp is supplied by branches of the fifth cranial nerve anteriorly and by branches of dorsal rami of cervical nerves posteriorly. Anteriorly, the major cutaneous nerves are the supraorbital and supratrochlear nerves, which are branches of the ophthalmic division of the fifth cranial nerve. These accompany the arteries of the same name and supply the scalp as far posteriorly as a line drawn across the top of the head from one ear to the other. Posterior to this line, the scalp is supplied by the greater and lesser occipital nerves and a portion of the greater auricular nerve, all branches of the dorsal rami of C2 through C4. The parietal area on both sides is supplied by the zygomaticotemporal nerve (a branch of the maxillary division of the fifth cranial nerve) and the auriculotemporal nerve (a branch of the mandibular division of the fifth cranial nerve).

Lymphatics

The lymphatic drainage of the scalp, in general, parallels the neurovascular supply. The lower portion of the forehead drains through the face into the submandibular nodes. The upper frontal and parietal areas drain into the superficial parotid group of nodes,

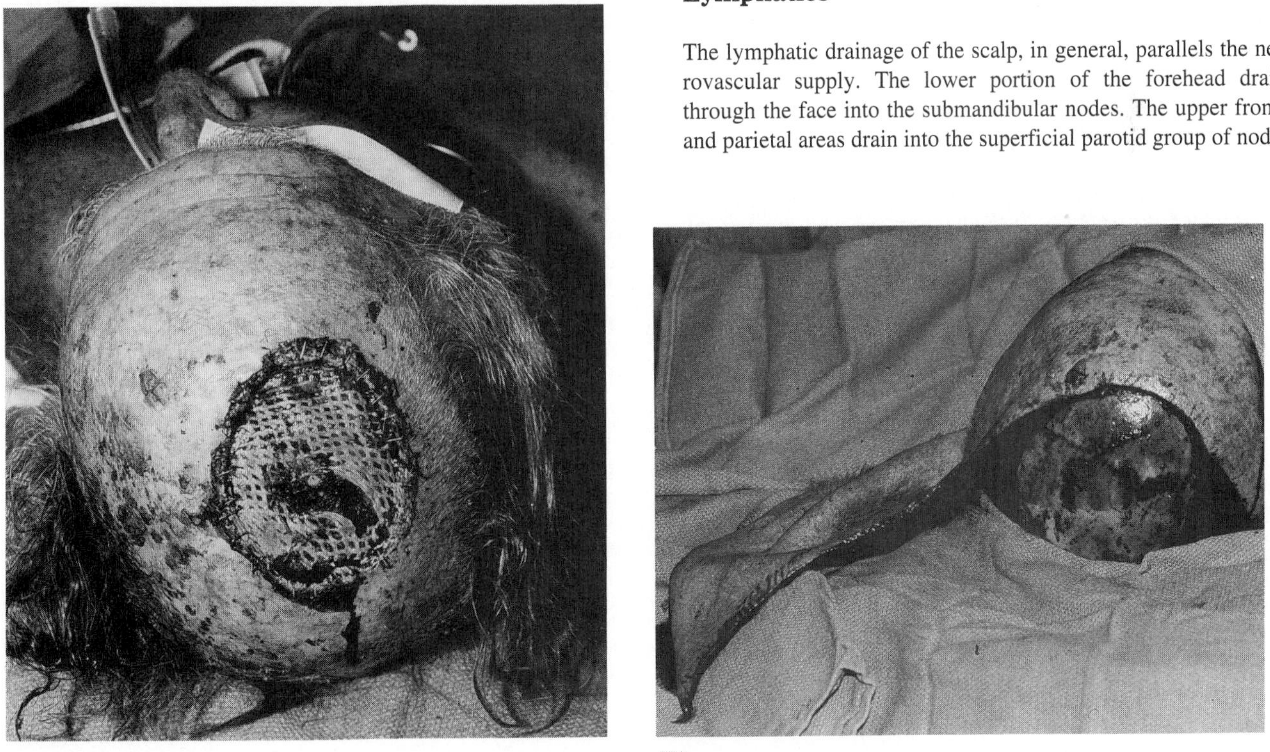

Figure 269-5 *A*. A recently excised squamous cell carcinoma in a 73-year-old man. The patient had positive deep margins on resection. He was not a candidate for a microvascular transplant, so a scalping/rotation flap was created. *B*. The secondary tumor resection included the pericranium; the large posterior rotation flap was based on the superficial temporal artery and branches of the occipital artery.

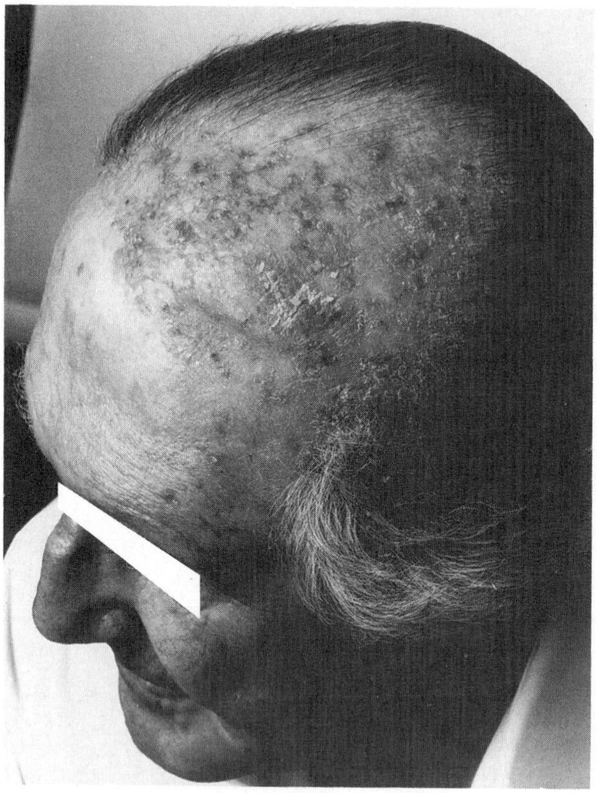

(C)

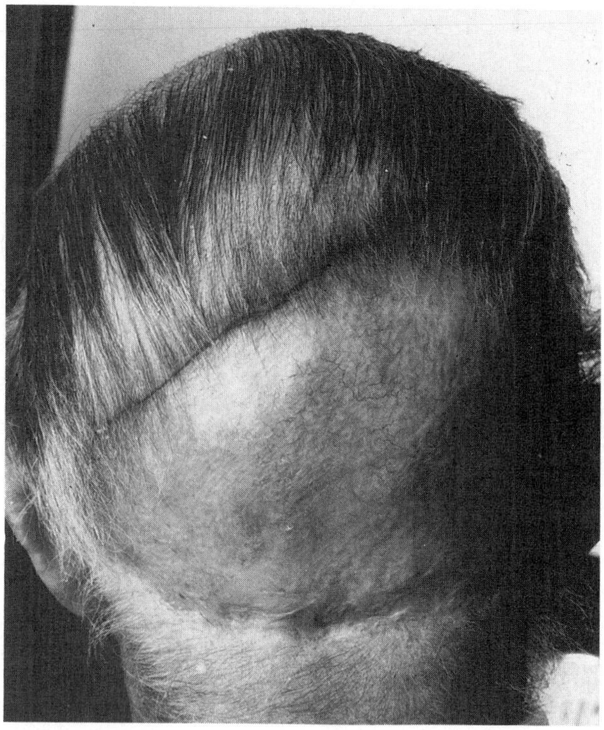

(D)

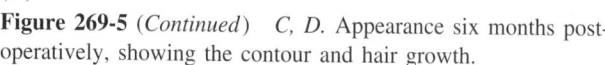

Figure 269-5 *(Continued)* *C, D.* Appearance six months postoperatively, showing the contour and hair growth.

which is located superficial to the parotid gland, just in front of the tragus. Both the submandibular and superficial parotid nodes drain to the deep cervical nodes. The coronal and occipital portions of the scalp drain to the retroauricular nodes and thence to the superficial cervical nodes. Thus it can be seen that the anterior portion of the scalp drains to the deep cervical nodes and the posterior portion to the superficial cervical nodes. The watershed generally follows a line connecting the superior poles of the two ears.

Examination and Primary Care of Scalp Injuries

The basic principles of trauma care are rarely more important than in the examination and treatment of scalp injuries. Injuries severe enough to damage the scalp may also damage the underlying skull. Injuries to the scalp are usually obvious and spectacular, but it should be kept firmly in mind that they may not be the most lethal injuries present. A complete examination of the whole patient is mandatory since life-threatening, but perhaps less obvious, injuries of the chest or abdomen take precedence over scalp lacerations. As with any trauma to the head and neck, attention should be given to the possibility of cervical spine injuries. If there is any question of injury to this area, a cross-table lateral x-ray film of the cervical spine should be obtained before the patient is moved.

All examinations of scalp wounds should be performed using sterile technique. Many times an underlying skull fracture can be palpated in the depths of a scalp laceration.

Because of the rich blood supply to the scalp, there may be copious bleeding. In the absence of an underlying skull fracture, the best method for controlling scalp bleeding is pressure directly over the wound. The pressure should be firm and continuous, and one should resist the temptation to keep dabbing at the wound. Because of the tendency for scalp wounds to gape, many irregular lacerations give the initial impression that tissue has been lost. However, after cleaning and sorting out the "jigsaw puzzle," one frequently finds that most of the tissue is present. Most scalp injuries can be dealt with immediately, but it is possible to delay closure of scalp wounds for up to 24 h if necessary if the patient is in poor condition or if other, more life-threatening injuries are present.[4] In such cases, a sterile saline-soaked gauze can be applied to the wound and a head dressing applied. Dressings for wounds of the scalp usually involve an external compression dressing that is applied as follows. The ears are padded with cotton, both in the external auditory meatus and the posterior auricular areas. Following this, 4 × 8 inch gauze pads can be placed on top of the ear. Next a Kling (conforming gauze bandage; Johnson & Johnson Medical Inc, Arlington, TX) or Kerlix (Kendall Healthcare Products Company, Mansfield, MA) wrap is wrapped around the chin to the vertex of the scalp and then transposed anteriorly to posteriorly above the eyebrows to the posterior nuchal area. Following this, a second layer of gauze is applied, taking care to avoid compression in the supraorbital areas. The posterior nuchal area is used as the anchor to keep the dressing from slipping. Following this, an elastic dressing retainer (Nylon and Spandex dressing retainer; American Hospital Supply, McGaw Park, IL) can be applied to keep the dressing in place. This is the standard dressing that should be applied to major scalp lacerations as well as to skin grafts applied to the scalp.

Lacerations

Lacerations of the scalp can take many forms. They may be small and linear, which can make them difficult to detect beneath matted, blood-soaked hair, or they may be large and stellate, giving the often erroneous impression that tissue is missing. Because of the tension in the galea, wounds that include this layer tend to gape considerably. However, the tendency of the galea to retract offers a form of protection. Since the main blood vessels are located in the subcutaneous fascia, they do not contract. If the galea is lacerated, however, the contraction of this layer will cause retraction of the vessels also. Thus, superficial lacerations with the galea intact may bleed more profusely than deep lacerations with the galea cut.

The best technique for stopping bleeding in scalp lacerations is circumferential pressure of the surrounding scalp against the skull. One should always make sure that no underlying skull fracture is present. In very large and gaping wounds, another useful technique is to place clamps on the galea and draw it back over the dermis, thereby compressing the vessels.

Most simple lacerations can be closed under local anesthesia. Scalp lacerations should be closed in two layers. The first layer approximates the galea and should be closed with an absorbable suture such as one of polyglycolic acid. The galea is the strongest layer of the scalp and should always be repaired if possible. It is unnecessary to place other stitches in the subcutaneous fascia. The skin is then closed with monofilament nylon suture or skin staples. Interrupted or running sutures may be used, and one should take fairly healthy bites of tissue on each side of the wound. Varying the depth of the stitch from one side of the wound to the other can help make the skin edges come together evenly.

In the case of extensive and stellate lacerations, or in very young children, it is necessary to use general anesthesia in the operating room. Because of the rich blood supply of the scalp, extensive debridement is both unnecessary and unwise, but all obviously devitalized tissue should be removed. Following closure, a compression dressing is helpful, particularly if there has been undermining of the subgaleal space, since subgaleal hematomas may take weeks to resorb. Drains beneath the galea are rarely necessary. Sutures should remain in place for 7 to 10 days.

Reconstructive Ladder

The reconstructive ladder given in Table 269-1 (Table 262-1) is a concept used by plastic surgeons to select the techniques to use in closing a given wound. An algorithm can be followed that facilitates treatment of wounds of the scalp from the simplest to the most complex.

Simple lacerations that are sharp without tissue loss and gross contamination can be approximated by *primary closure*. Wounds with tissue loss as deep as the pericranium can be debrided and the wound edges sutured in place, with the resulting smaller wound "marsupialized." If the resulting wound defect is not large, it can be left to granulate and heal by *secondary intention*.

If there is extensive tissue loss but the pericranium is intact, the wound can be debrided. Subsequently, a split-thickness skin graft can be applied to re-epithelialize the scalp surface. The skin graft can be harvested from a variety of sites and should be maintained by a moist bolster dressing containing Bunnell's solution or saline cottonoid sponges. In 48 to 72 h, the bolster can be removed and the skin graft treated in routine fashion. The skin graft will provide epithelialization of the scalp surface. Following this, if the patient so desires, tissue expanders can be used under the normal adjacent scalp to expand normal scalp skin. The surgeon can readvance flaps once they are created by tissue expansion, eliminating the skin-grafted area to improve the scalp covering as well as the cosmetic effect.

If there is extensive soft tissue loss and periosteal stripping, local flaps can be used to transpose normal scalp areas to the areas that are devoid of pericranium. If transposition flaps result in defects adjacent to flap donor areas, these can be skin-grafted. The main objective in such cases is to provide well-vascularized cover for the denuded pericranium (Figs. 269-3 and 269-4).

If local flaps are not sufficient for coverage, pedicle flaps of tissue such as the latissimus dorsi muscle or trapezius muscle can be used, but these are usually reserved for smaller defects in the occipital and nuchal areas.

In cases of massive or anterior defects, free tissue transplantation should be considered. Microsurgical techniques have made this a common practice, and the treatment goal is to replace "like with like." In instances of gross infection or contamination, or instances involving cranial osteomyelitis, muscle flaps are usually selected owing to their ability to bring an improved blood supply and combat infection. In addition, they can be used to fill a cranial defect after traumatic injury or tumor extirpation. The muscle flap is usually covered with a split-thickness skin graft. If the scalp defect was caused by tumor resection with skin ablation or pericranial stripping, a variety of skin flaps, such as the scapular flap, lateral arm flap, or radial forearm flap, can be used for coverage. The revascularization of these flaps is made possible by the rich arcade of vessels. Recipient vessels include the superficial temporal artery and vein and the facial artery and vein. If the scalp has been completely stripped by avulsion and there is no possibility of replantation, the omentum can be used to completely resurface the scalp. It is usually covered by split-thickness skin grafts. After reconstruction of the scalp with omentum, the patient will need to use a wig to camouflage the cosmetic defect.

Microsurgical techniques are commonly used after tumor extirpation and should be considered in instances of squamous cell carcinoma, melanoma, and other cutaneous malignancies.

TABLE 269-1 Reconstructive Ladder

1. Primary closure
2. Delayed primary closure
3. Secondary intention healing
4. Split-thickness skin graft
5. Local transposition flaps
6. Island pedicle flaps (trapezius, latissimus dorsi, temporalis)
7. Free autogenous tissue transplantation (skin, muscle, omentum)

Avulsions

Avulsions of the scalp usually occur in the loose areolar tissue between the galea and pericranium. Most scalp avulsions occur when a portion of hair is pulled at a tangential angle (Fig. 269-6). Perpendicular pulling may result in avulsion of hair only.

The treatment of scalp avulsions depends largely on the amount of scalp avulsed. If the defect is small, it can be repaired using either single or multiple rotation flaps (Figs. 269-3 and 269-4). Many times the wounds can be closed without leaving a donor defect that requires grafting. When constructing either single or multiple flaps in the scalp, additional length can be obtained by carefully incising the galea with parallel cuts on the underside of the flap perpendicular to the axis of pull of the flap, and allowing the flap to expand like an accordion. Extreme care should be taken when performing this maneuver, since the blood vessels are located just above the galea.

If the defect is too large for multiple rotation flaps and the avulsed segment too badly damaged for replantation, a skin graft should be applied if the pericranium is intact. It will provide wound coverage and prevent desiccation and infection of the tissues and will allow more definitive reconstruction at a later date. Split-thickness skin grafts take readily on pericranium, due to its excellent blood supply. Skin grafts may be harvested from any suitable donor site, such as the anterior thigh. However, with scalp avulsions that are too large for closure with local scalp tissue, every attempt should be made to replant the avulsed scalp using microvascular surgical techniques. If an avulsed segment cannot be replanted, it may still yield a split-thickness skin graft, which is taken with a dermatome.

Replantation of an Avulsed Scalp

Total avulsion of the scalp has declined in frequency since the closure of the western frontier, but the injury still occurs as a result of industrial or other types of accidents. Before the age of micro-

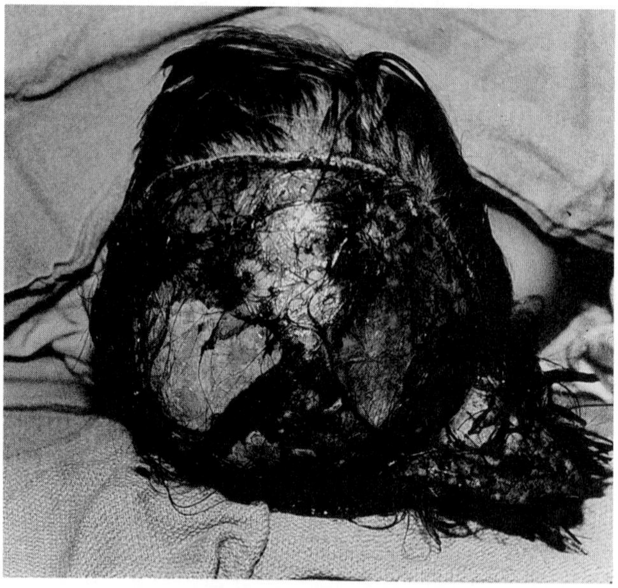

(*A*)

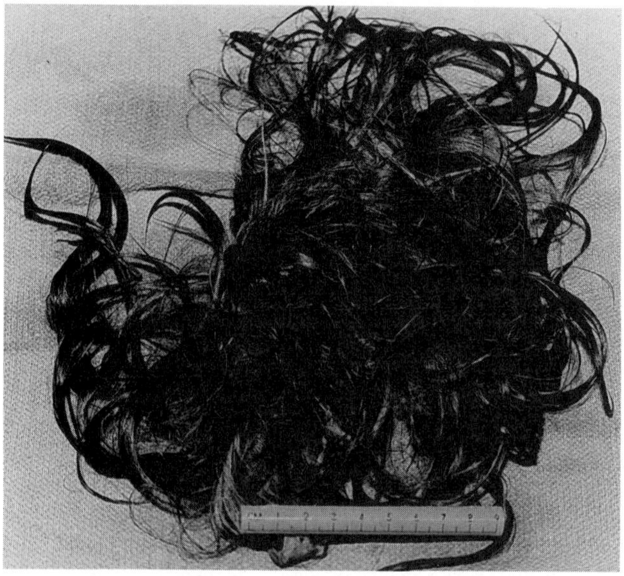

(*B*)

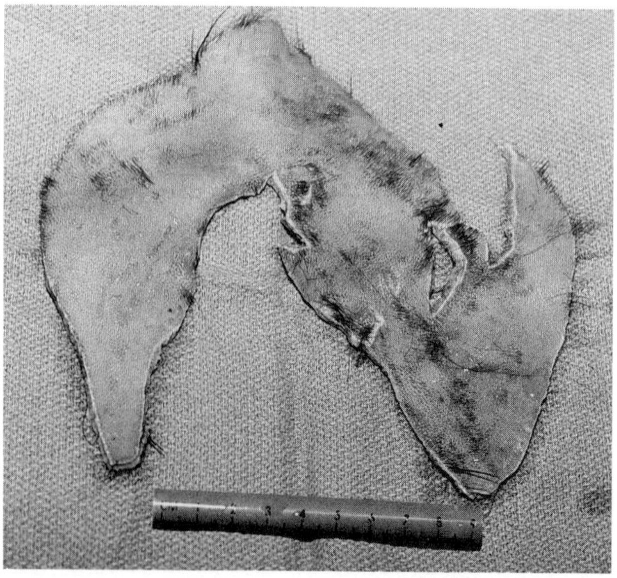

(*C*)

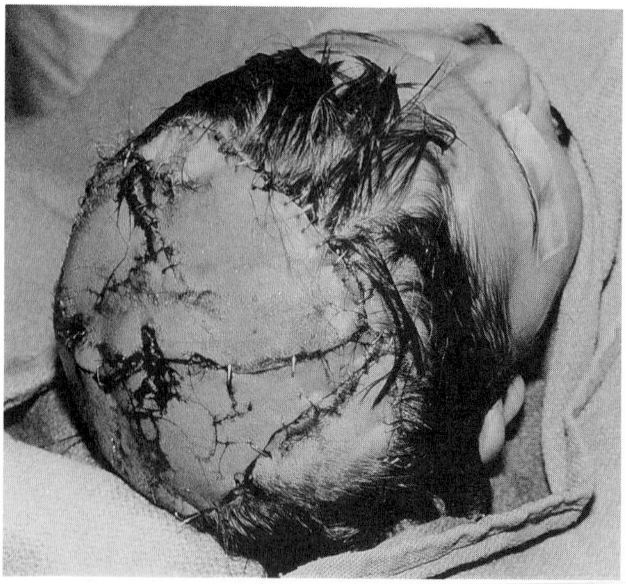

(*D*)

Figure 269-6 Avulsion of the scalp. *A.* Preoperative view showing exposed cranium and the extent of the injury. *B.* Hair-bearing scalp. *C.* Geographic pattern of the avulsed scalp. *D.* Scalp immediately after replantation, with all portions appearing viable.

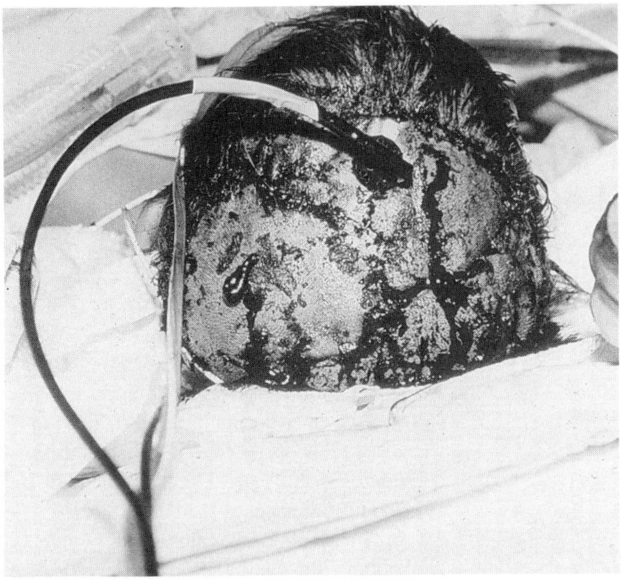

(*E*)

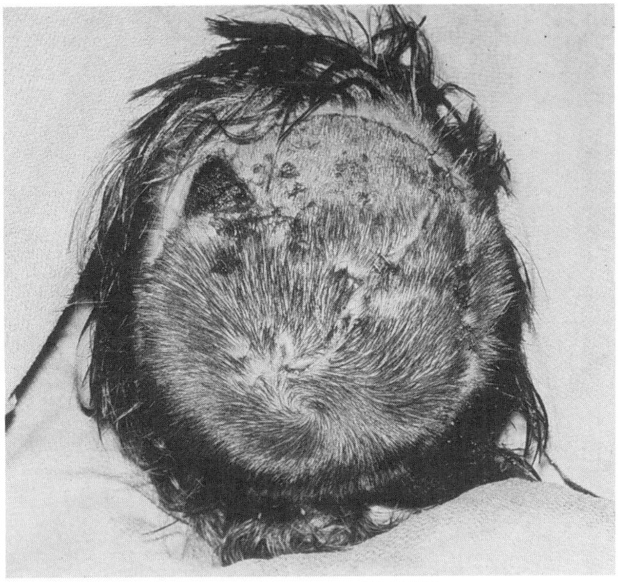

(*F*)

Figure 269-6 (*Continued*) *E.* Laser Doppler monitoring of the replant. Medicinal leeches are used to augment venous outflow. *F.* Early postoperative view.

vascular surgery, many scalp avulsions were treated by simply replacing the scalp as a free graft. The success rate of this treatment was dismally low; perhaps only one case has been reported where it succeeded without the use of vascular anastomoses.[6] The first report of the successful replantation of a scalp using microvascular anastomoses appeared in 1976.[8] Since then, there have been many reported cases of successful microvascular replantation of the scalp.[1] The extent of initial scalp loss has varied from 20 to 100 percent, with only three cases of successful replantation where more than 90 percent of the scalp had been avulsed.

Despite the difficulties inherent in performing it, scalp replantation should now be considered the procedure of choice for significant scalp avulsions, since the alternatives are much less satisfactory, both physiologically and aesthetically. The principles and technique of scalp replantation can be best illustrated by a representative case.

Figure 269-6 shows a previously unreported case of avulsion of the scalp in a 6-year-old child. The child was attacked by a dog with avulsion of the scalp. The scalp was packed with ice and transported with the patient to our unit, where she arrived approximately 3 hours after the injury. While the patient was being resuscitated in the emergency department, the avulsed scalp was immediately transferred to the operating room. The scalp was first shaved and cleansed on an iced table. An anterior branch of the superficial temporal artery on the left side was dissected out until normal vessel was found (diameter, 0.5 mm).

By the completion of this preparation, the patient had arrived in the operating room and was anesthetized. The proximal superficial temporal vessels were then dissected out on both sides and the scalp tacked in place with several stay sutures. Although in many cases of digital replantation it is advisable to repair the veins first, in most scalp avulsions it is advisable to repair the artery first, which helps in identifying the veins. Following the repair, the scalp immediately became pink. A demonstration that a single good artery can support the whole scalp was given by the fact that after successful completion of the arterial anastomosis, oxygenated blood and venous blood were seen coming from the opposite superficial temporal artery and vein. In this case, a cutaneous vein was repaired. Anticoagulants, including heparin, were used postoperatively. Medicinal leeches were used to augment venous outflow, which may be helpful in avulsion injuries.

A question that arises in scalp avulsions is whether one should attempt to repair the nerves. It is probably better not to do this, because the dissection necessary to isolate the nerves may put the already completed anastomoses at risk.

In cases of extensive scalp avulsion in which the pericranium has also been avulsed and in which a scalp replantation is impossible, one must resort to other measures. Obviously a skin graft will not take on bare bone. Several techniques have stood the test of time for promoting the formation of granulation tissue that will accept a skin graft. One is to make multiple drill holes through the outer table of the skull into the diploic space (Fig. 269-7*A*). This tactic will result in the development of granulation tissue, but the process may take several weeks or months. Another technique is to remove the outer table of the skull using an osteotome (Fig. 269-7*B*). In this case a skin graft may be applied immediately; however, hematomas are more common after immediate application of the graft, and it is usually advisable to wait several days until granulation tissue has formed.

Because of the length of time required for granulation tissue to develop and also because of the long-term instability of a split-thickness skin graft on the skull, the preferred technique now is placement of a distant flap of skin and subcutaneous tissue, with or without muscle. Recent developments in musculocutaneous flaps and in microvascular surgery have made it unnecessary to do multiple-staged pedicle flap techniques.

Some scalp defects can be reached easily by musculocutaneous flaps such as a latissimus dorsi flap or a trapezius flap. However, the safe arc of rotation of most musculocutaneous flaps does not reach beyond approximately the level of the upper pole of the ear. Defects in the central superior or anterior portion of the scalp are probably best handled by a microvascular free tissue transfer (Fig. 269-8). A number of donor sites are available that will provide durable functional skin cover for this area without excessive bulk.

The patient shown in Fig. 269-9 sustained deep thermal burns to the superior portion of the scalp. A portion of the wound was of

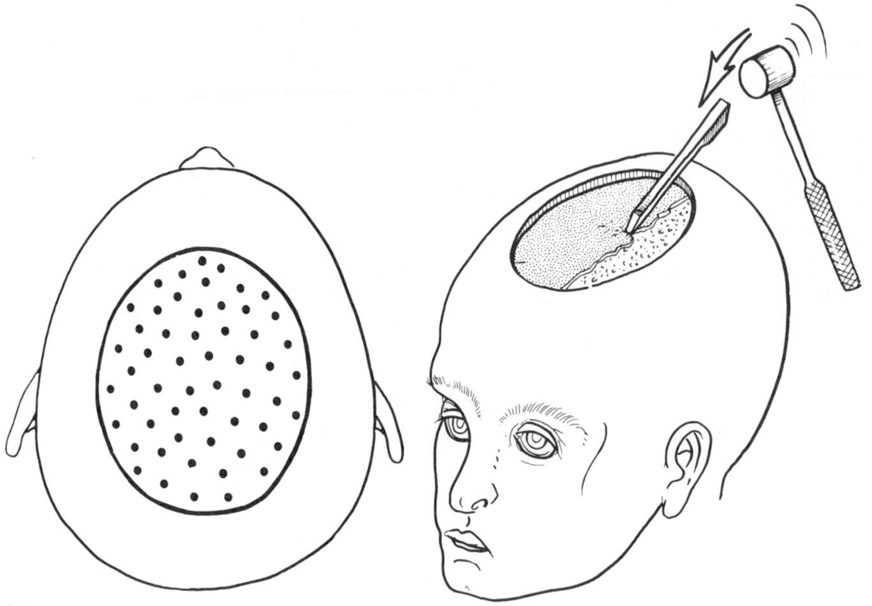

(*A*) (*B*)

Figure 269-7 Methods of promoting granulation tissue on bare skull. *A.* The method of using multiple drill holes into the diploic space. The holes should be approximately 1 to 2 mm in diameter and should be no more than 1 cm apart. *B.* The method of removing the outer table of the skull. The immediate or delayed application of a skin graft may be done.

partial thickness and healed in the usual fashion; however, the central portion of the wound was of full thickness, including pericranium. An attempt was made to stimulate the development of granulation tissue by removing the outer table of the skull; over a 4-week period, this resulted in only spotty development of granulations. The area was then resurfaced using a free scapular flap based on the circumflex scapular vessels, which were anastomosed to the superficial temporal vessels (Fig. 269-9*B*). Other potential free flaps for this situation are the groin flap and the dorsalis pedis flap. The groin flap is hampered by having a short pedicle which frequently requires a vein graft, and the dorsalis pedis flap is difficult to dissect and has considerable donor site morbidity. In addition, any free flap requires special techniques which are not available in most hospitals.

Injuries by Physical and Chemical Agents

Thermal Burns

Because of its exposed and prominent position, the scalp is frequently injured by physical and chemical agents. Thermal injury to the scalp may occur alone or, perhaps more frequently, in conjunction with burns elsewhere. For this reason, the initial resuscitation involves close attention to fluid and electrolyte balance as well as wound care. The reader is referred to standard works on the treatment of burns. The scalp represents only about 4 percent of the total body surface in adults (slightly more in children), and, for this

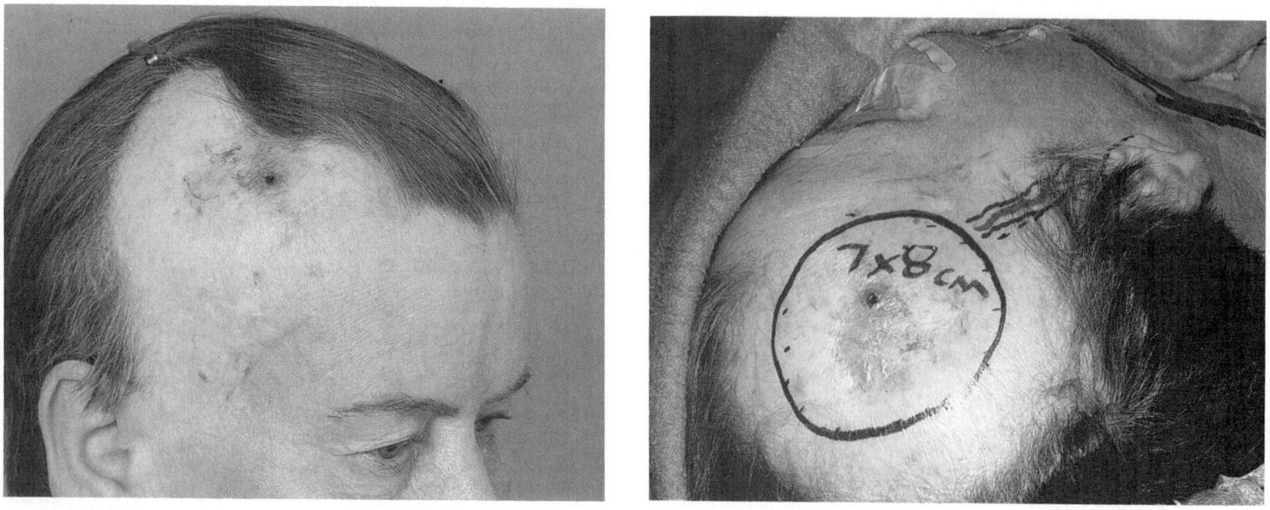

(*A*) (*B*)

Figure 269-8 *A.* A melanoma of the scalp previously excised with incomplete margins. *B.* Proposed area of resection and of dissection of the superficial temporal artery and vein for anastomosis.

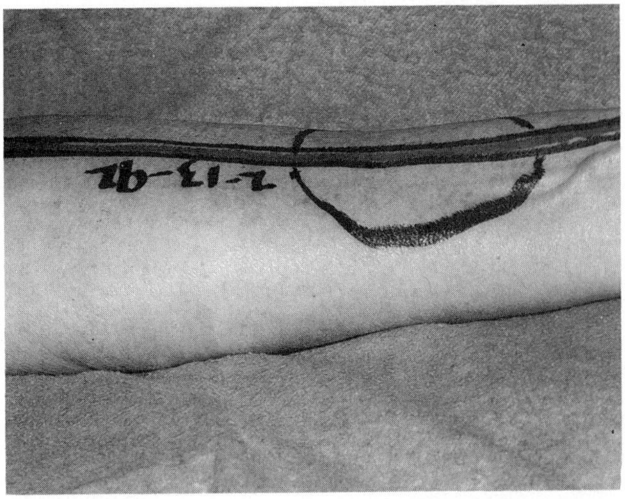

(*C*)

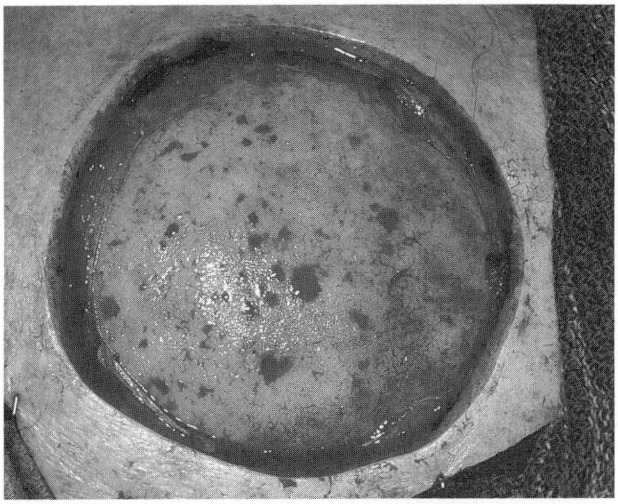

(*D*)

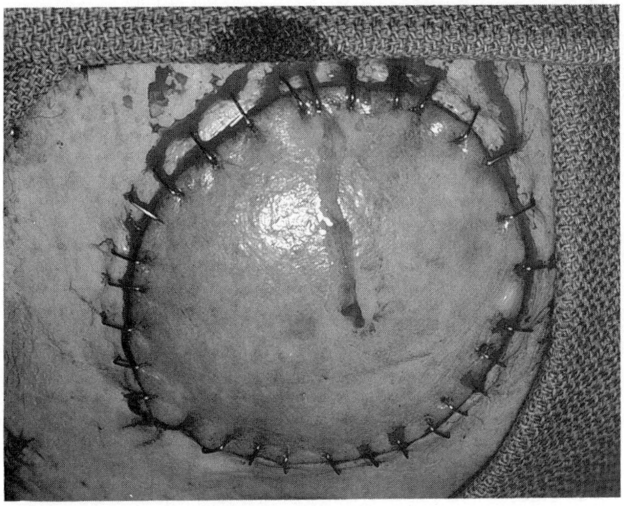

(*E*)

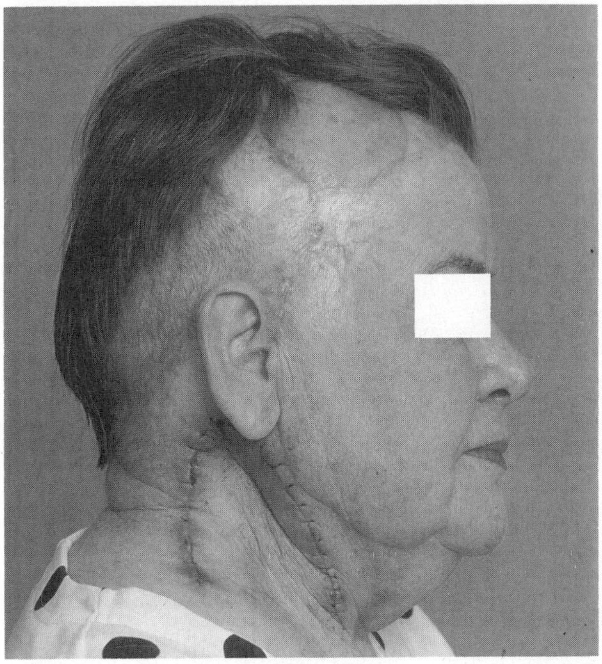

(*F*)

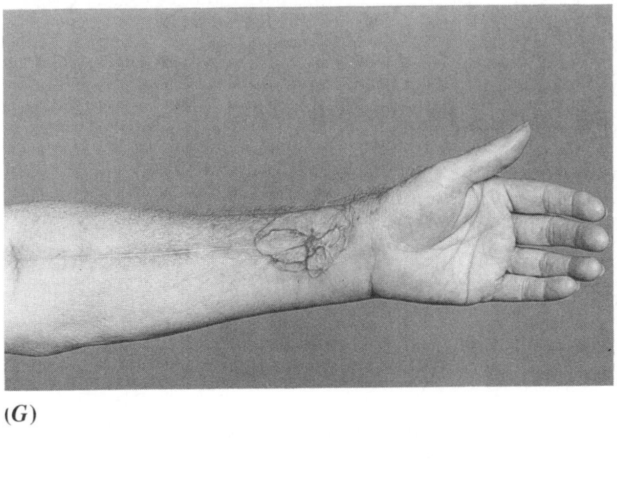

(*G*)

Figure 269-8 (*Continued*) *C.* Donor site (radial forearm flap) demonstrating the long vascular pedicle. *D.* The tumor resection included the pericranium. *E.* Free flap in place showing excellent contour and esthetic result. *F.* The patient subsequently had a radical neck dissection for positive lymph nodes. *G.* Donor site at six months with a well-healed split-thickness skin graft over the distal flexor tendons.

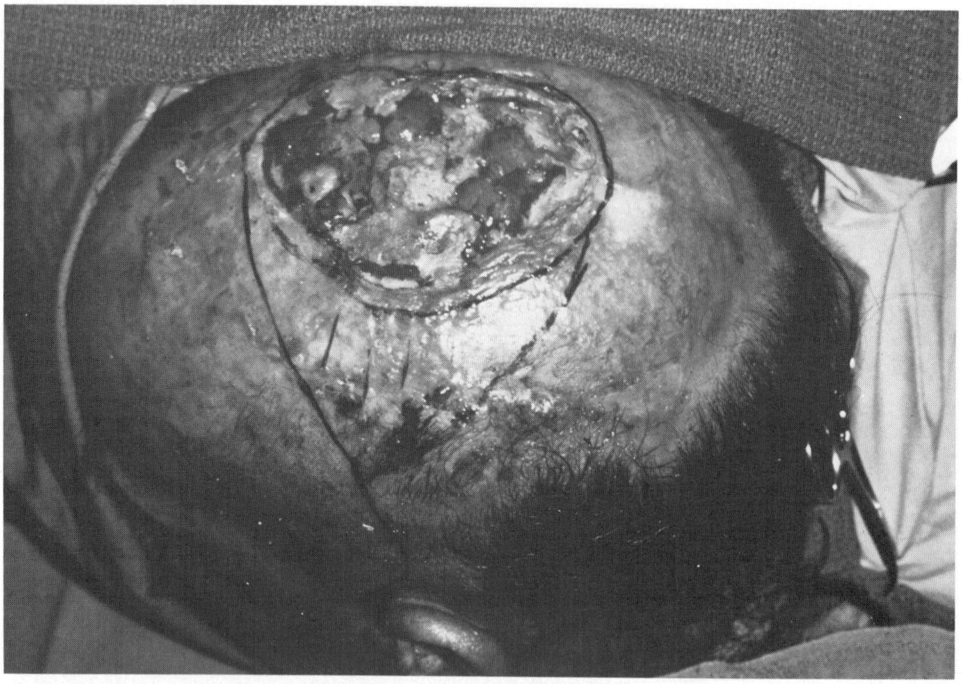

(*A*)

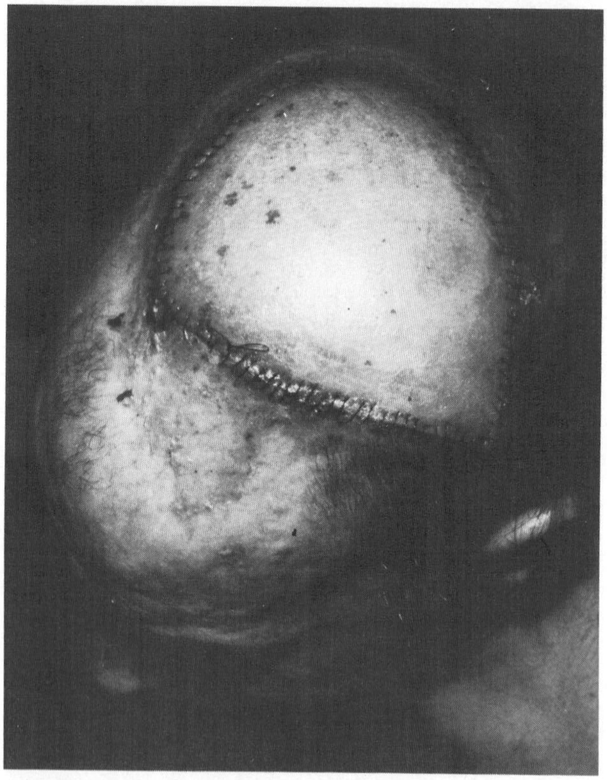

(*B*)

Figure 269-9 Thermal burns of the scalp. *A*. The central superior portion of the burn included the pericranium. After removing the outer table of the skull, only spotty granulation tissue developed over a 3-week period. *B*. The defect was repaired using a vascularized scapular cutaneous flap. The flap was anastomosed to the superficial temporal vessels.

reason, isolated burns of the scalp do not necessitate a great deal of attention to systemic effects.

The scalp has thick skin with a remarkable capacity to regenerate epithelium. This capability is due to the presence of many hair follicles and other epithelial adnexal structures. For these reasons, burns that would be full thickness in other parts of the body will eventually re-epithelialize in the scalp.

The treatment of scalp burns should, therefore, be conservative. Burn wounds may be covered with topical antibiotic agents such as silver sulfadiazine or povidone-iodine, but these dressings are frequently messy and difficult to keep in place. Another alternative is exposure. The wounds are cleansed initially, with removal of any devitalized debris. They are allowed to dry and are protected until re-epithelialization takes place.

Full-thickness scalp burns that include the pericranium, such as the one sustained by the patient shown in Fig. 269-9, are unusual. In these situations, although some areas may re-epithelialize, it is frequently necessary to resort to one of the techniques described earlier for repair.

Electrical Burns

Electrical burns of the scalp occur when a person's head comes into contact with high tension wires, and usually involve several thousand volts of electricity. Most authorities consider the damage to be the result of heat generated by the resistance of the tissues to the passage of the electric current. The amount of heat generated for a given current depends on the resistance of the specific tissue (Joule's law). Skin and bone, both abundant in the head, have a higher resistance than other tissues. The resistance of the skin is further influenced by its thickness and moistness, and the amount of vessels and nerves present. The injury may be further compounded by the phenomenon of "arcing," in which a spark is generated between the wire and the contact point. It should be kept in mind that damage will also be produced elsewhere in the body, at the exit point, although usually it is less severe owing to dissipation of the current. Damage to respiratory centers and the heart must also be anticipated, and respiration and cardiovascular functions supported if necessary.

The treatment of electrical burns of the scalp is based on the principle of removing devitalized tissue and replacing it as necessary to provide durable skin coverage and underlying bony support. The characteristic cross-sectional shape of the devitalized area has been well described.[9] The lesion is usually crescent- or saucer-shaped, with the burn deepest at the center and becoming more superficial toward the periphery. High-tension electrical burns of the scalp are always of full thickness, extending to and including bone.

The traditional treatment has been to debride the dead scalp and cranium and then await sequestration of bone. If the diploe is affected, a full-thickness section of the skull will be removed. Occasionally, only the outer table will require removal, with subsequent granulation of the underlying diploe. This sequence of debridement, sequestration, sequestrectomy, and repair can take many weeks or months, with the constant danger of infection of the underlying dura.

More recently, several authors have advocated a more radical approach, which may give better results.[7,10] They suggest thorough debridement of devitalized scalp and pericranium followed by immediate flap coverage of the underlying bone, regardless of its apparent nonviability. The rationale is that the bone will still function as a perfectly shaped ''in-situ'' bone graft even if it is dead. Coverage can be provided by local scalp flaps or by distant flaps. Follow-up by x-ray studies and bone biopsy have shown regeneration of normal bony architecture, thus obviating the need for future cranioplasty.

Chemical Burns

Injuries of the scalp by chemical agents may occur intentionally, as in an assault, but much more frequently are accidental, particularly in children. Lye burns are more common than acid burns. Several characteristics of chemical burns make them different from other types of burns. Damage to tissues in chemical burns is due to the action of free hydroxide or hydrogen ions in the tissues. Once these compounds come in contact with the skin, damage will continue until the agent is removed or neutralized by combining with ions in the tissues. It has been shown that irreversible cellular changes will take place if the pH is below 2.5 or above 11.5.[5] The ability of tissues to withstand this wide range of pH is due to the buffers present in them.

In general, the effects of different chemicals on the skin are determined by (1) the duration of contact and by (2) the concentration, (3) the penetrating ability, (4) the quantity, and (5) the manner of action of the compound.[2] In addition, especially in the case of lye burns, there is a latency period before the damage begins to be apparent. On the basis of these factors, the rationale for treatment is readily apparent. The only factor that can be influenced by the action of a physician is the duration of contact. One should therefore institute immediate, copious, and continuous irrigation of chemical burns with sterile water. Following this, an attempt can be made to neutralize the offending agent. For lye burns, dilute acetic acid can be used, and, for acid burns, a dilute sodium bicarbonate solution. It is important to remember that one should not attempt to neutralize the agent before thoroughly irrigating with water, since the neutralization reaction may cause further damage from the heat produced.

The depth of damage is sometimes difficult to determine in chemical burns, and for this reason debridement should be conservative. When the damaged area is well demarcated, however, it can be excised and a skin graft applied.

Radiation Injuries

Radiation burns usually occur as a result of accidental over-exposure due to lack of filtration or to intentional or unintentional overlapping of fields. The result may be both an acute and chronic radiodermatitis. Acute radiodermatitis is characterized by initial erythema and edema of the skin, with blanching in the areas of greatest exposure. This may last up to 48 h and then subside rapidly. During this period the lesions are exquisitely painful. This phase may be followed by a period of several days in which symptoms and signs disappear, but after approximately 1 week, a secondary erythema begins to develop, which may be complicated by extravasation of blood into the erythematous areas. This may progress to blisters with necrosis and ulceration of the underlying skin.[3] These ulcers are very reluctant to heal owing to radiation-induced endarteritis in the adjacent skin. The usual treatment for acute radiation ulcerations of the skin is excision and grafting, but this measure should be delayed until final demarcation has taken place.

References

1. Alpert BS, Buncke HJ, Mathes SJ. Surgical treatment of the totally avulsed scalp. *Clin Plast Surg* 1982; 9:145–159.
2. Bromberg BE, Song IC, Walden RH. Hydrotherapy of chemical burns. *Plast Reconstr Surg* 1965; 35:85–95.
3. Cairns RJ, Champion RH, Wilkinson DS. Cutaneous reactions to physical agents. In Rook A, Wilkinson DS, Ebling FJG (eds): *Textbook of Dermatology,* 1st ed. Philadelphia: FA Davis, 1968, pp 323–361.
4. Dingman RO, Argenta LC. The surgical repair of traumatic defects of the scalp. *Clin Plast Surg* 1982; 9:131–144.
5. Friedenwald JS, Hughes WF Jr, Herrmann H. Acid-base tolerance of the cornea. *Arch Ophthalmol* 1944; 31:279–283.
6. Lu MM. Successful replacement of avulsed scalp: case report. *Reconstr Surg* 1969; 43:231–234.
7. Luce EA, Hoopes JE. Electrical burn of the scalp and skull: case report. *Plast Reconstr Surg* 1974; 54:359–363.
8. Miller GDH, Anstee EJ, Snell JA. Successful replantation of an avulsed scalp by microvascular anastomoses. *Plast Reconstr Surg* 1976; 58:133–136.
9. Stuckey JG Jr. The surgical management of massive electrical burns of the scalp. *Plast Reconstr Surg* 1963; 32:538–543.
10. Worthen EF. Regeneration of the skull following a deep electrical burn. *Plast Reconstr Surg* 1971; 48:1–4.

270 Cephalhematoma and Subgaleal Hematoma

Derek A. Bruce

Understanding and diagnosing the various scalp masses that are associated with head trauma in children requires an understanding of the anatomy of the scalp. The scalp consists of five layers of tissue. For ease of remembering they can be represented by the mnemonic SCALP. The layers are skin, connective tissue, aponeurosis (galea), loose connective tissue, and pericranium (Fig. 270-1). The first three layers are held tightly together, and collections of blood therefore form between the deeper layers of tissue: subgaleal hematomas between the galea and the pericranium in the loose connective tissue layer, and cephalhematomas (subperiosteal hematomas) between the periosteal layer and the cranial bone. Swelling of the superficial layers of the scalp can occur; it is most common in the form of caput succedaneum in newborn babies after vaginal delivery.

Caput Succedaneum

Caput succedaneum is a localized swelling of the skin of the scalp, typically located in the midline posterior parietal area over the part of the cranium that leads the way down the birth canal during delivery. The swelling is intimately within the superficial layers of the scalp and usually consists of tissue fluid—edema—rather than being a true hematoma. Depending on the presentation of the head, the swelling may be over the anterior scalp or (with a face presentation) in the face. With prolonged labor or difficult delivery, the swelling may be associated with hemorrhage into the superficial scalp and frank bruising of the skin. These lesions are not associated with skull injury and require no therapy.

Cephalhematoma

Cephalhematoma[1] is the result of bleeding between the periosteum and the skull and is found almost exclusively in the newborn. This fact suggests that the mechanism of the injury is not impact but, presumably, shearing stress between the periosteum and the bone during passage through the birth canal, resulting in separation of the pericranium from the bone and bleeding from the bone into the subperiosteal space. Another but less likely explanation is distortion of the skull resulting in separation of the periosteum. Any attempt to free the pericranium from the underlying cranium in the newborn or small infant results in bleeding from the external surface of the skull and from the deep surface of the pericranium. It is this bleeding that forms the cephalo- or subperiosteal hematoma.

The presentation is of a localized, initially hard mass, usually over one or both parietal bones (the site varies with the presentation of the head at delivery). The scalp can be moved over the mass, which itself is fixed. Because the blood has collected under the pericranium, and the pericranium is attached at the sutures (Fig. 270-2), the mass is limited to one cranial bone and does not cross the suture lines. Bilateral cephalhematomas can occur, but they do not cross the sagittal suture. The limitation of the hematoma by the sutures makes the diagnosis straightforward in most cases. Occasionally, an early localized caput succedaneum or subgaleal hematoma can be very circumscribed and may be confused with a cephalhematoma. The differentiating factor is that the former two kinds of mass can be moved with the scalp, whereas a cephalhematoma is fixed, and the scalp can be moved over it. Shortly after delivery there may be both a caput and a cephalhematoma, and the diagnosis of the latter becomes clear only after the caput has resolved.

The skull bone is usually intact, with no fracture, and it is rare that there is any intracranial injury, since the cause of the hematoma relates to the normal mechanisms of delivery. The skin overlying the lesions is normal unless the hematoma results from forceps application, in which case contusion of the skin and a subgaleal hematoma may coexist with the cephalhematoma. Under these circumstances—forceps delivery with skin contusion—the risk of an associated depressed skull fracture is much higher, and skull films should be taken. If the baby shows depressed consciousness or has seizures or a full fontanel, a computed tomography (CT) scan is required to ascertain whether an intracranial hematoma or contusion is present.

With typical cephalhematomas, plain films will show only the soft tissue swelling deep to the scalp and therefore are not necessary. The initial therapy is to leave the lesion alone. It should not be tapped because of the risk of introducing infection with the possible occurrence of osteomyelitis. Typically, the lesion becomes soft and fluctuant over several weeks as the hematoma is

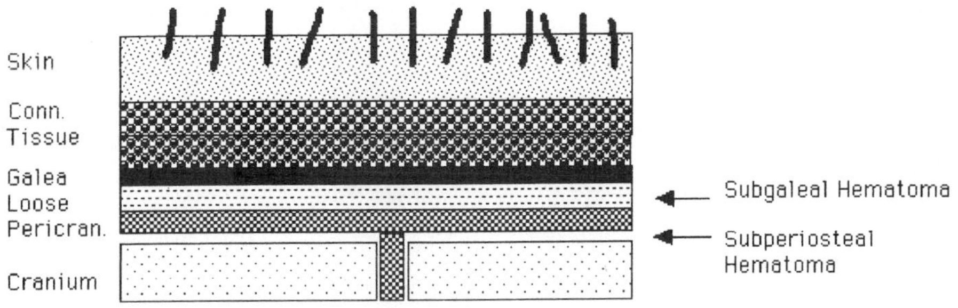

Figure 270-1 The five layers of the scalp and the sites of subgaleal and subperiosteal hematomas.

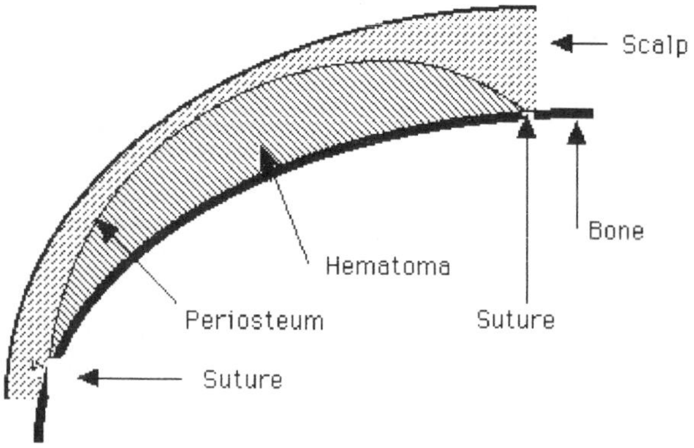

Figure 270-2 The structure of a cephalhematoma.

gradually reabsorbed. The only complication is that a small percentage (3–5 percent) of these lesions do not reabsorb but ossify and leave a prominent, hard mass on the skull that may be cosmetically unsatisfactory. If the lesion has not resolved by 6 weeks, plain skull films will show whether it is calcifying (Fig. 270-3). If a significant lump is present and calcifying, it should be removed surgically. Occasionally, a cephalhematoma becomes fluctuant but is not fully reabsorbed, and can mimic a depressed skull fracture. CT scanning may be required to ascertain that the skull is normal.

If surgery is necessary, the cephalhematoma can be separated from the underlying skull, and there is no need to remove normal skull bone. A curvilinear incision (as invisibly located as possible) is made around the lesion. It is not necessary to shave or clip the hair. The periosteum bounding the lesion is opened, and the mass external to the skull removed. Often there is a central cavity filled with organizing or liquid hematoma. Once this is identified, the level of the external skull table can be identified and the remainder of the mass removed with either a drill bit or an osteotome. The underlying skull must be preserved, the external table smoothed with the drill, and any oozing from the bone controlled with bone wax to prevent reaccumulation of the hematoma. The scalp is closed in two layers using 4-0 Vicryl (polyglactin 910; Ethicon, Inc, Somerville, NJ) in the galea and 4-0 chromic catgut in the scalp. The sutures do not need to be removed, and the hair is washed on the second postoperative day.

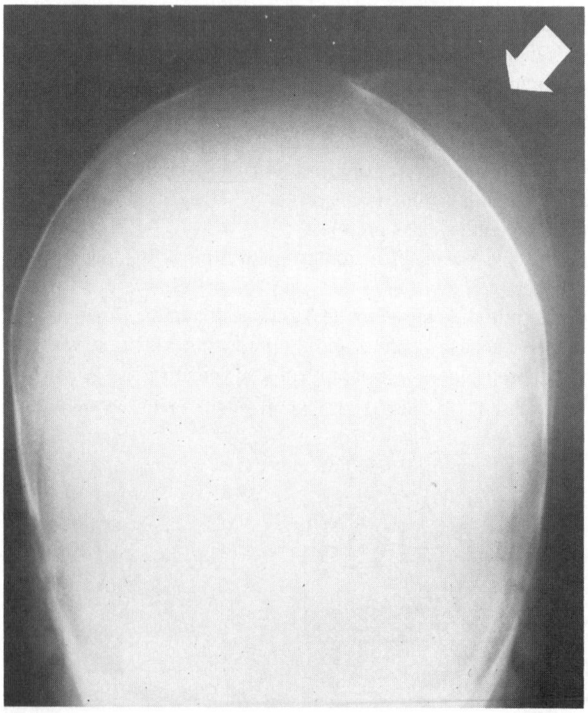

Figure 270-3 X-ray film of the skull showing a calcified cephalhematoma *(arrow)* in an 8-week-old boy.

Subgaleal Hematoma

Subgaleal hematomas are very common after head injury in children. They result from bleeding into the loose connective tissue layer between the galea aponeurotica and the pericranium. They may be caused by a variety of traumatic events, including fairly minor trauma and hair pulling episodes. Initially, because the clot is firm and localized, the lump may not be noticed by the parents. As the hematoma liquefies, the loose connective tissue is separated and a soft fluctuant swelling occurs that can spread extensively around the scalp. Since the boggy mass is often not noticed until several days after the trauma, no clear-cut history of trauma may be obtained. These lesions can spread across half the head or even all around the scalp. Because the parents often do not notice them until some days after the trauma, the parents may be accused of neglect or abuse because they did not bring the child for medical care sooner. It must be realized that this delayed presentation results from the pathophysiology of the lesion, not parental abuse or neglect. In children over 1 year of age, there is rarely a skull fracture, and in most cases radiologic studies are not necessary. In children under 1 year of age, the cause of the injury is usually a fall—for example, from the parent's arms or off a changing table—and linear skull fractures are common. These fractures can be extensive and can cross suture lines, but if there is no disturbance of consciousness, and if the fontanel and fundi are normal, they are most likely the result of accidental injury and not child abuse. The most common error in diagnosis is to assume—because of the skull fracture and the delayed appearance of a watery swelling—that the fluid under the scalp is cerebrospinal fluid. It is for this reason that it is useful to take plain skull films at the time of first presentation for any child under 1 year old with a history of a fall—because, if a fracture is seen, the physician will be able to warn the parents to expect a subgaleal hematoma and will not mistake the later watery mass for a cerebrospinal fluid leak.

In children under 1 year old, blood loss into the trapped space can occasionally be severe enough to produce anemia, and transfusion is sometimes necessary. These collections should not be tapped because of the high risk of infection. The treatment is to reassure the parents that the mass will resolve and, if the collection is large, to obtain serial hemoglobin and hematocrit determinations. If the child is seen at the time of minor trauma, it is advisable to tell the parents that a soft, fluctuant mass may appear over the subsequent few days. That will allay parental concern and prevent the doctor's being forced into unnecessary treatment.

Reference

1. Kendall N, Woloshin H. Cephalohematoma: associated with fracture of the skull. *J Pediatr* 1952; 41:125–132.

271 Skull Fractures

Fred H. Geisler

Skull fractures result from large energy forces applied to the head during injury. The extent and type of skull fracture is determined by the kinetic energy of the striking object, the direction of the impact force, the geometry of the striking object, and the anatomic site of the impact. Forces greater than 1000 lb in 1 ms are necessary to produce a fracture. Forces that are smaller or take longer to develop cause acceleration of the head rather than a skull fracture.[10,11] There is only a poor correlation between skull fracture and brain injury. Despite the large forces necessary to produce it, a patient with a skull fracture may have no signs of brain injury, and conversely, a patient with massive brain injury may have no skull fracture. The thickness and pliability of the skull vary among individuals and with age, as does the thickness of the dura and its adhesion to the skull. These variations result in differences in the injuries that follow trauma. For example, neonates have greenstick, depressed fractures because of the flexibility of the bone; epidural hematomas without skull fracture occur in children and young adults because of the relative ease with which the dura strips from the calvaria. Early definitive diagnosis and management of skull fractures decrease morbidity and mortality as well as achieving maximal functional and aesthetic rehabilitation.

Skull Fracture Classification System

Skull fractures[2–4,6,7,9,12,14,21–23] are classified in three ways: by pattern (linear, diastatic, comminuted, depressed); by anatomic location (convexity, base); and by type (open, closed). Either type of fracture can occur in either anatomic location and in any of the patterns.

The pattern of a skull fracture is affected by three factors. The first is the amount (or energy level) of the impact force. A linear fracture results when the skull fails to undergo elastic deformation during impact. A comminuted fracture results when the impact force is large enough to break the bone under the point of impact into multiple pieces. With even larger impact energies, the comminuted pieces can be driven inward and can penetrate the dura and cortical surface of the brain to create a depressed fracture.

The second factor is the ratio of the impact force to the impact area. If a high impact energy is dispersed over a large area, as when an individual wearing a motorcycle helmet strikes the head, there is often no skull fracture even in the presence of severe brain injury. However, an impact of considerably lower energy but concentrated in a small area, as when an individual is assaulted with a hammer or hit with the corner of a brick, can produce multiple linear skull fractures radiating from the site of impact.

The third factor is the location and physical properties of the skull at the contact point. Local indentation of the contact point occurs first with the impact. This deformation produces a compressive strain on the outer cortical table and a tensile strain on the inner cortical table. The cortical bone fails under tensile load and the fracture usually originates in the inner table near the contact site and propagates in a complex manner determined by the local dynamic forces, three-dimensional bone geometry, and physical properties of the skull. The injury also causes both skull distortion and shock waves, which can produce fractures distant from the impact site.[8]

The location of a skull fracture is divided into two areas for discussion: the skull convexity (where fractures are generally termed "skull fractures") or the base of the skull (where fractures are generally termed "basilar fractures"), but any one of the patterns can occur in either or both areas. For example, trauma to the head can produce a comminuted basilar fracture, a depressed convexity fracture, and/or a linear convexity/basilar fracture.

A skull fracture can be further classified as open or closed by the presence or absence, respectively, of an overlying scalp laceration, which provides a direct route for communication and contamination between the fractured bone and the environment. In addition, a fracture extending into the skull base with violation of the paranasal sinuses, mastoid air cells, or middle ear structures is, by definition, an open fracture.

Linear Skull Fractures

Description

A *linear skull fracture* is a single fracture line in the skull, which passes through the entire thickness of the skull.

Diagnosis

Although it is generally accepted that clinical indications for radiologic examination include loss of consciousness, retrograde amnesia, discharge from the nose or ear, eardrum discoloration, Babinski reflex, or cranial nerve abnormalities, there is controversy (based on a cost/benefit analysis) regarding the use of radiographs to diagnose linear skull fractures. Scalp trauma (abrasion, laceration, contusion, or avulsion) often marks the site of the impact and raises the suspicion of an underlying skull fracture. The presence of a linear skull fracture serves as a definitive indication that the head has received an impact of considerable energy, but the patient's eventual neurological outcome or disability depends on the brain injury, not the linear fracture. Therefore, knowledge of the absence or presence of a linear skull fracture will affect the clinical management and eventual outcome of only a small percentage of patients. For those few patients, however, it may make a crucial difference. For example, the presence of a linear fracture crossing the path of the middle meningeal artery in a mild head injury indicates that the patient is at risk for late neurological deterioration from an epidural hematoma. Furthermore, skull films can reveal depressed fractures, puncture wounds, and intracranial foreign objects that might otherwise elude prompt diagnosis. On the other hand, if a computed tomography (CT) scan is obtained, then skull radiographs add little information that would affect management or ultimate neurological outcome. Therefore, each medical facility needs to establish guidelines for obtaining skull radiographs and CT scans of the head based on experience with its own patient population.[3] A *diastatic fracture* is a separation of a cranial suture line. Diastatic fractures are common in infants under 3 years old and rare in older age groups except as part of a more extensive skull fracture.

Management

Linear skull fractures require no stabilization or exploration if the scalp is closed. An open linear fracture is inspected and vigorously debrided of foreign material; damaged soft tissue at the edges of the laceration is also debrided and then the scalp laceration is closed. When a scalp laceration is contiguous with the linear skull fracture, very seldom is surgical exploration with bone removal necessary. An exception, where bone removal would be indicated, is a machete injury to the skull producing a linear skull fracture with underlying dural laceration and brain damage. The presence of a skull fracture does serve as a marker that significant head trauma has occurred and that a careful assessment of the brain, facial structures, and cervical spine is required.

Comminuted Fractures

Description

A fracture is called *comminuted* when more than one linear fracture is present. These linear fractures often radiate from the impact point. Some of the fractures may involve suture lines (diastatic fractures) or stop at the suture lines. There may also be free bone fragments at the central impact point.

Diagnosis

The diagnosis is made on the basis of skull radiographs and CT scans of the head with bone windows.

Management

If the skin is closed and no depression of the bone fragments greater than the thickness of the skull is demonstrated on the CT scan, then the management is the same as for linear skull fractures, with no surgical exploration for the fracture itself. In many of these cases, surgery is performed for an underlying intracranial lesion such as an epidural hematoma (Fig. 271-1). After the intracranial abnormality has been corrected, the bone fragments are replaced as a cranioplasty, as in depressed skull fractures.

If the skin is open and free bone fragments are present, debridement of the contaminated fragments is performed along with vigorous debridement of the soft tissue before scalp closure (and, if necessary, dural closure) (Fig. 271-2). Massive comminuted skull fractures are usually associated with a fatal brain injury (Fig. 271-3).

Depressed Skull Fractures

Description

In a *depressed skull fracture,*[3–5,7,22] the outer table of one or more of the fracture edges lies below the normal anatomic level of the inner table as determined by the surrounding intact skull. The greatest bone depression can occur at the interface of the fracture with the intact skull or near the center of several fracture fragments that are displaced inward. A depressed fracture results when the impact energy is applied over a relatively small contact area. Typical situations include assaults with a hammer, club, or pipe; sports injuries caused by a hockey stick, golf club, or golf ball; or motor vehicle accidents in which the victim's head strikes either the interior of the car or an object outside the car upon being thrown from the vehicle.

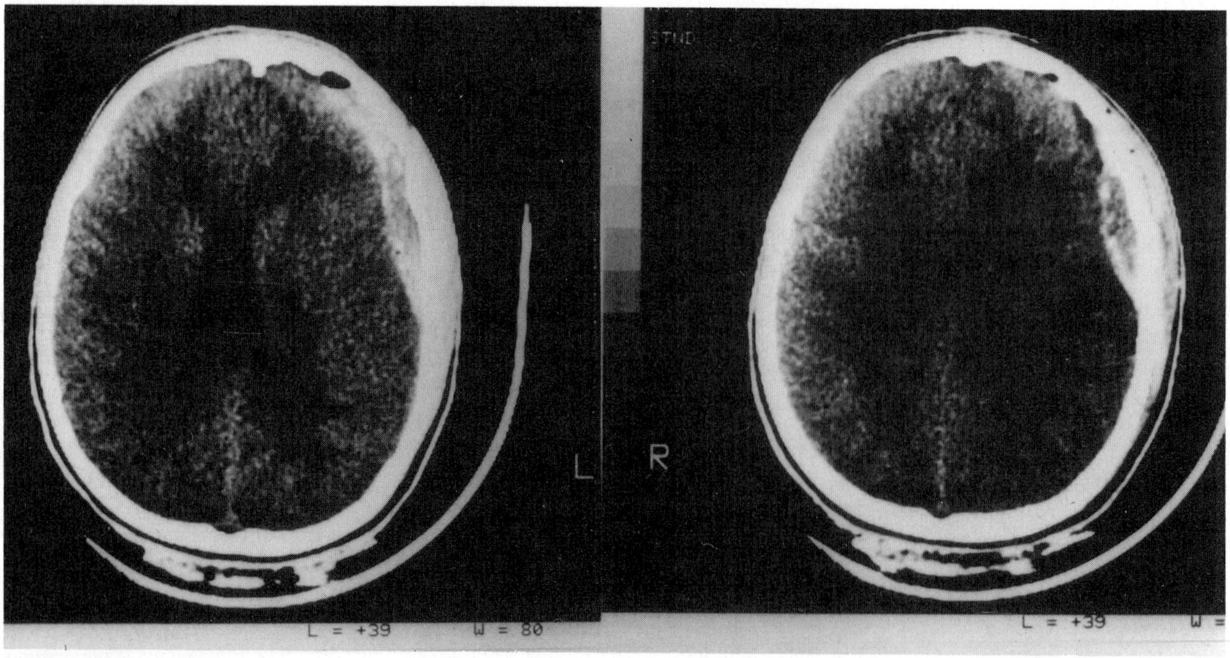

(*A*)

Figure 271-1 A comminuted open skull fracture with an underlying epidural hematoma. *A.* CT scan of the head through the center of the fractured region. Note the small amount of air at the anterior edge of the epidural hematoma.

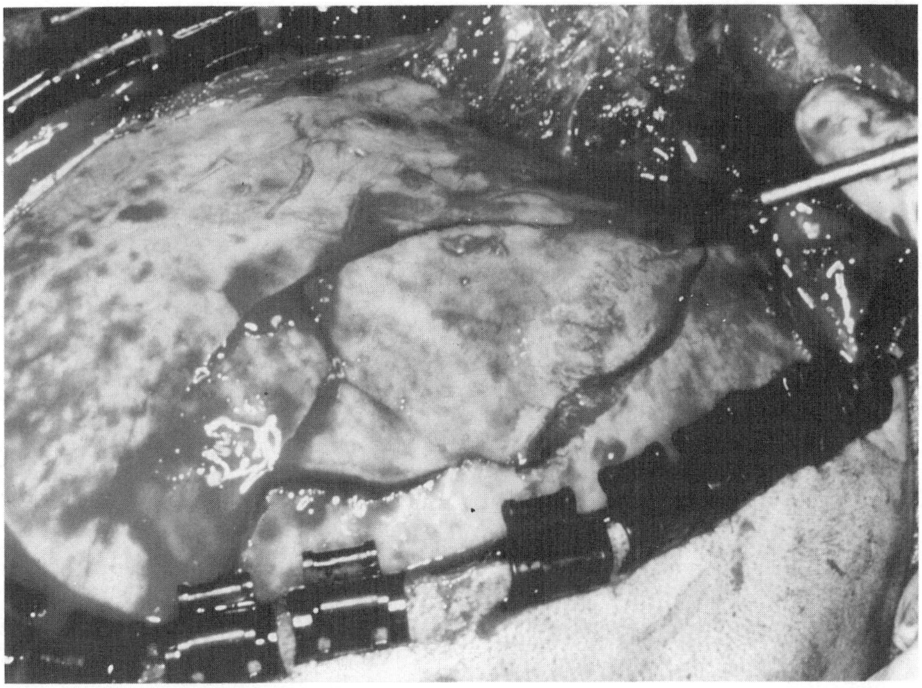

(*B*)

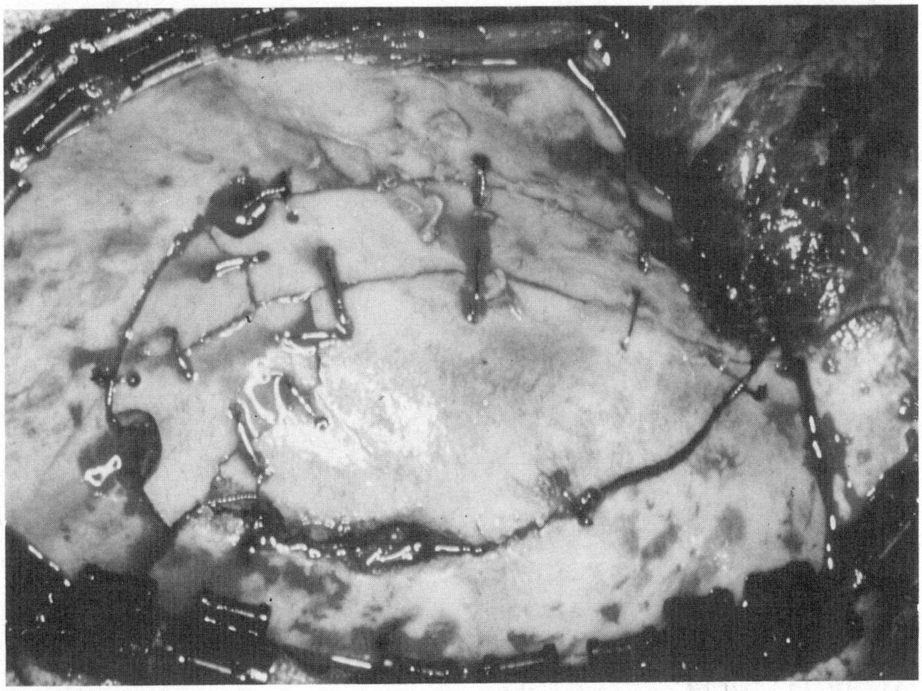

(*C*)

Figure 271-1 (*Continued*) *B.* Intraoperative view of the skull fracture before removal of the fragments. The bone fragments were removed, then the epidural hematoma was evacuated. *C.* The skull fragments were next wired together, and then they were replaced in the defect as a cranioplasty.

Diagnosis

Many patients with depressed skull fractures experience initial loss of consciousness and subsequent neurological recovery to an extent determined by the brain injury. However, one-quarter of the patients experience neither loss of consciousness nor neurological deficit and another quarter experience only brief loss of consciousness. Although the diagnosis of a depressed skull fracture is often made on routine skull radiographs by noting either an area of double density (suspicious for overlying bone fragments) or the presence of multiple or circular fractures, the full extent and depth of the fracture fragment is rarely appreciated on these studies unless tangential views are made.

Physical examination of patients with depressed skull fractures is difficult because of scalp mobility during injury and swelling at the time of examination. A scalp laceration accompanies the depressed fracture in 85 percent of the cases. Scalp mobility can result in considerable nonalignment of the scalp laceration and the depressed skull fracture during the examination. Thus, normal skull under a scalp laceration does not exclude a depressed fracture a centimeter or two under one edge of the laceration. Furthermore, traumatic scalp swelling minimizes the palpable and visual

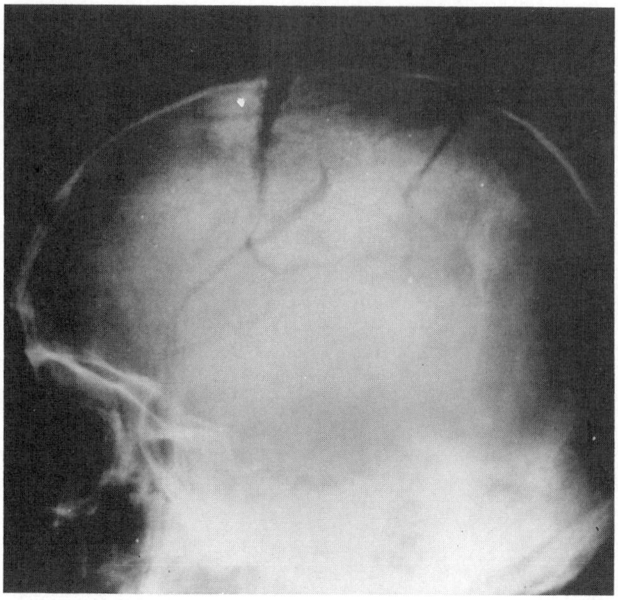

(*A*)

Figure 271-2 A comminuted fracture including a diastatic fracture of both coronal sutures and additional fractures of the frontal and parietal bones bilaterally. In this case the skin was open and CSF was coming from the wound. *A.* Lateral skull radiograph demonstrating the comminuted fracture. *B.* CT scan with bone windows near the top of the head showing the comminuted fracture.

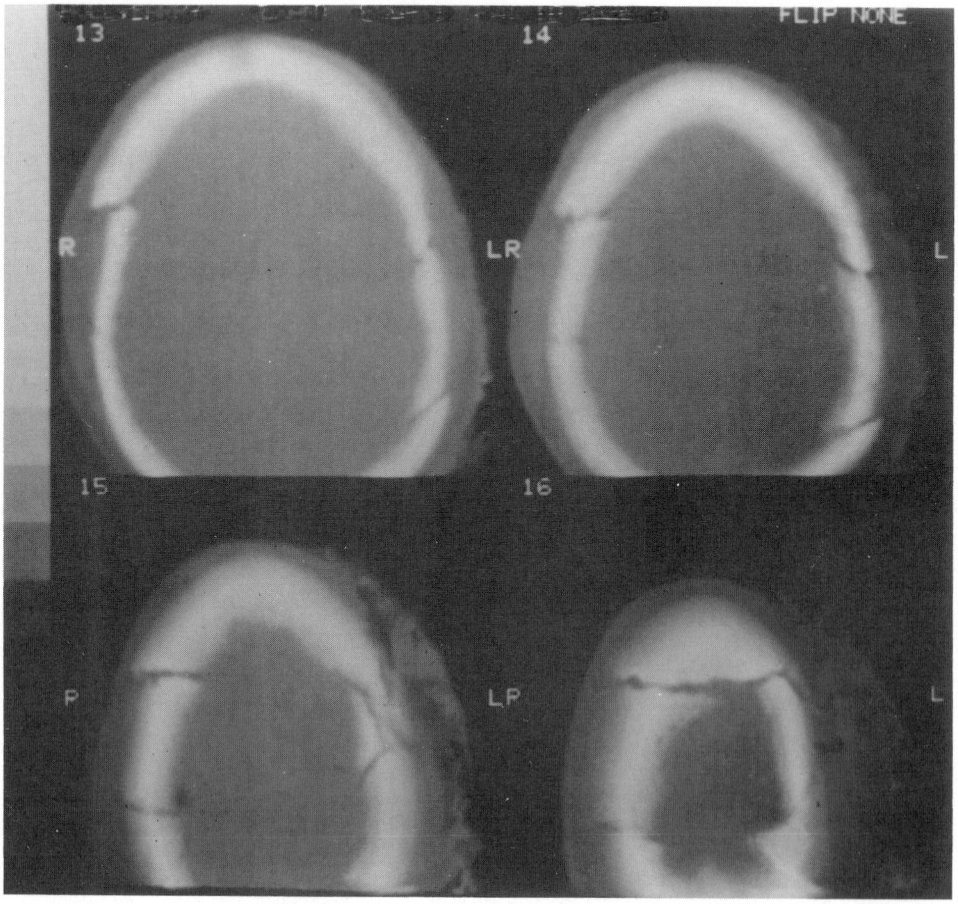

(*B*)

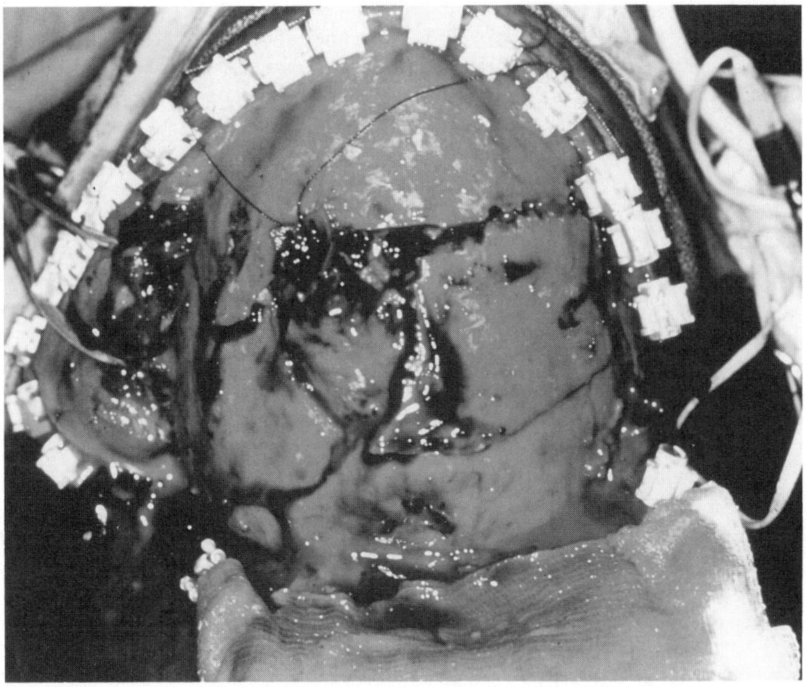

Figure 271-2 *(Continued)* *C.* Intraoperative view of the fracture after the scalp was opened by extending the scalp laceration. **(*C*)**

appearance of the step-off at the bony edges, preventing accurate clinical assessment of the extent of skull deformity for the first few days.

A CT head scan is the diagnostic method of choice. When the image display windows are adjusted to optimize bony detail, they display the position, extent, and number of fractures as well as the presence and depth of depression. With the imaging windows set to optimize the visualization of intracranial contents, the same CT scan also allows an assessment of the underlying brain for contusion or hematoma caused by indentation of superficial bone fragments, indriven small bone pieces, or foreign bodies within the brain substance, as well as of other traumatic intracranial lesions. Occasionally, coronal CT images through fractures near the vertex of the head or extending into the skull base are used to supplement the standard CT images, since the depth of a depression is more accurately measured on CT images perpendicular to the depression. Differences between the amount of dural laceration and cortical damage appearing on similar CT scan images occur because the position of the brain, bone fragments, and remaining intact skull at the time of the scan may differ from the actual maximum depth of the fragments at the time of impact. The brain, for example, may undergo linear or rotational movement and the skull can temporarily deform during the impact. Immediately after the injury, the depressed bone fragments tend to partially rebound or spring back as the deformed skull attempts to resume its anatomic shape. Also, only crude estimates of the sharpness of the bone edges can be made from the CT pictures, since these images have a resolution of 1 mm.

Management

When a depressed skull fracture is on the convexity and extends to include facial fractures, the intracranial injury is typically repaired first, with removal of an intracerebral hematoma and repair of a dural laceration if present. The facial fractures are then treated, during the same operation or subsequently.

Although elevation of bone fragments occasionally improves a focal neurological deficit originating in the cortex directly under a depressed bone fracture (presumably by increasing local cortical blood flow), this procedure usually produces no neurological change, implying that the impact itself produced the cortical damage. The brain dysfunction generally undergoes a neurological recovery phase of several weeks to months, similar to that after a stroke or a head injury without a depressed fracture. The incidence of epilepsy[3,4,9] after a depressed skull fracture (7 to 9.5 percent) is apparently determined by the cortical damage at the time of impact since it is not altered by elevation of the fragments. Thus, the treatment of depressed skull fractures is based not on initiating

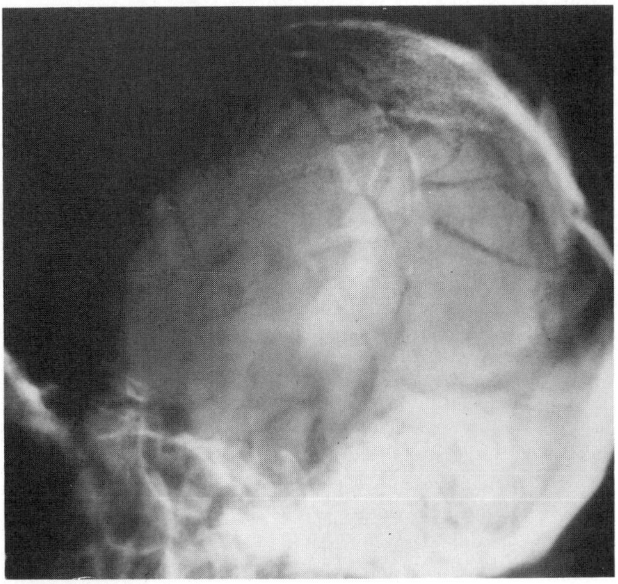

Figure 271-3 A massive comminuted skull fracture with a fatal brain injury.

neurological recovery or preventing epilepsy but, rather, on correcting a cosmetic deformity as well as preventing infection in open fractures.[4] The treatment of an individual depressed skull fracture depends on the presence or absence of (1) cosmetic deformity (and on its extent); (2) scalp laceration; (3) dural laceration; (4) contusion or laceration of the underlying brain; (5) extension of the fracture over a venous or paranasal sinus; and (6) coexistence of other traumatic intracranial lesions including epidural, subdural, and intracerebral hematomas and cerebral contusions, midline shift, and ventricle compression.

The indication for surgery in closed depressed fractures is usually cosmetic. The procedure is performed on an elective basis within the first few days after the trauma when the patient is cleared for elective anesthesia. The location of the depression, the thickness of the scalp, and the patient's body image perspective are critical to the decision to perform surgery. The forehead is the area where patients are most sensitive to cosmetic deformity. Depressions of 3 mm or more result in deformities for which most patients request correction. When the orbital rim is involved or the forehead scalp is thin, repair of smaller depressions is often requested. Exploration is more urgent in a patient with a large closed depressed fracture where the radiologic appearance suggests dural laceration, brain penetration, simultaneous frontal sinus fracture, a mass effect, or an underlying epidural, subdural or intracerebral hematoma. The hematoma is evacuated, the dura is repaired, and the bone fragments are replaced and wired in anatomic position.

An open depressed fracture represents a neurosurgical emergency because of the risk of bacterial infection of the cranial cavity. The initial operation is performed within 24 h and usually within the first 12 h after the accident. The major objectives of the surgery are to (1) remove contaminated bone fragments and foreign material (hair, cloth, dirt, etc.) from within the scalp wound, between the bone fragments, and within the cortex; (2) debride devitalized scalp, dura, and brain; and (3) provide a watertight closure of the dura. Removing devitalized tissues and contaminated material is essential to reduce the incidence of infection. Often, foreign material or hair wedged between bone fragments is not seen through the overlying scalp incision. Thus, simple wound irrigation and closure may be inadequate for the debridement of the foreign material. Dural closure is essential to prevent cerebrospinal fluid leaks from the wound and herniation of the brain into the fracture area. The closed dura also acts as a bacterial barrier, preventing the intracranial spread of infection from a scalp wound. Cosmetic correction is performed during the initial surgery only if considered safe; otherwise, a cranial defect is left and the cosmetic repair is performed later. The major reasons to postpone the cosmetic repair are when additional anesthesia is precluded by major head injury or multiple trauma, when the wound is grossly contaminated and the bone fragments cannot be adequately cleaned, or when there is a delay of more than 24 h for the initial surgery. This management plan decreases both the final neurological deficit and the incidence of epilepsy by reducing the potential for these complications from intracranial infection and intracerebral hematoma.

The patient is positioned (Fig. 271-4) with the center of the skull depression in a horizontal plane, which means that fractures in different locations have to be positioned quite differently: for depressions on the forehead the patient is placed in the supine position, whereas for depressions in the occipital area the patient is positioned prone. The head is held in place by either the Mayfield three-point head holder or the Mayfield horseshoe. When using the three-point head holder, one must be certain that no fracture lines are located where the pins will be placed. If a pin is positioned on a loose fragment or into a fracture line, it will not only be mechanically unstable but may even increase the fracture or cause displacement of fragments as it is applied. The surgical draping should allow for extension of the wound should additional exposure be required during the surgical exploration. When facial fractures and depressed skull fractures are both undergoing initial surgical correction, the patient's position and draping are coordinated between the two surgical regions. This can involve draping in layers to gradually expose different areas as the surgery progresses, or it may involve repositioning the patient and redraping. Generally, the intracranial portion of the combined surgery is performed first to establish a watertight dural closure and remove life-threatening intracranial lesions, and then the facial and nasal sinus fractures are repaired.

In an elective elevation of a closed depressed fracture for cosmetic improvement, the surgeon uses one of several standard scalp incisions behind the hairline. The exact size and placement are determined by (1) the need to expose the intact skull for at least 2 cm circumferentially around the depressed fragment, including the larger inner table splinters; and (2) the need to provide pericranium or temporal fascia for a dural graft should it prove necessary to repair the dura. The ''S'' incision is useful for depressions that are 1 to 6 cm in diameter and located behind the hairline, because

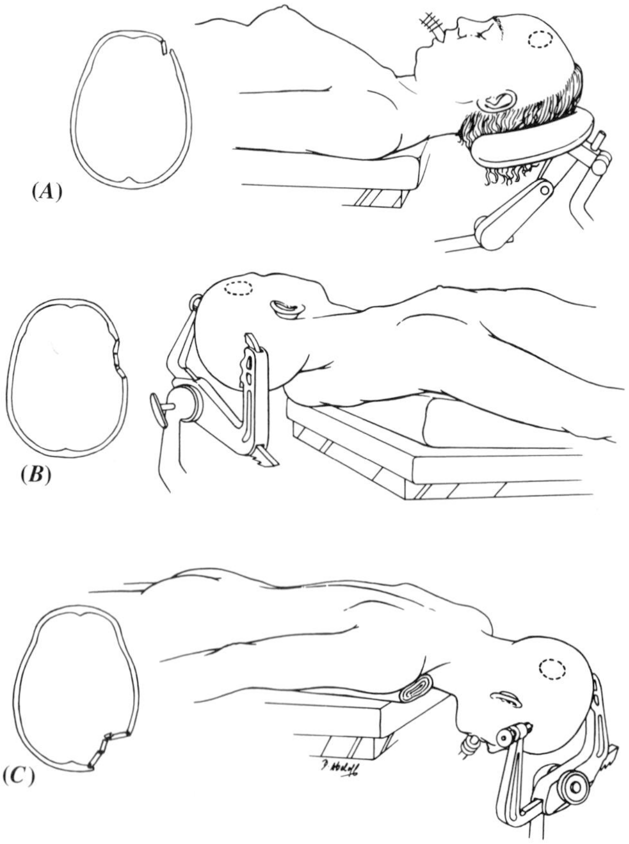

Figure 271-4 Line drawings of CT images of three depressed skull fractures and the different surgical positions used for each. Note that the center of the depressed region is at or near the horizontal plane. The skin incision and the location of the midline are marked before draping. *A.* An anterior frontal depressed skull fracture. *B.* A posterior frontal depressed skull fracture. *C.* A posterior parietal/occipital depressed skull fracture. (From Geisler,[5] with permission.)

it is easy to extend should more exposure be required. A flap incision must be large enough initially because it cannot be enlarged without adding a ''T'', with its potential healing problems, to the incision. In cases where an underlying intracranial lesion requires surgical attention, a large frontotemporoparietal scalp flap allows exposure of both the intracranial lesion and the depressed skull fracture.[4,9]

The scalp laceration associated with a compound depressed skull fracture is usually stellate and may contain areas of contused or devitalized tissue. These areas require debridement to normal scalp to allow prompt healing and prevent breakdown of the scalp covering the depressed fracture site. If scalp breakdown occurs, it usually cannot be treated with local care measures and often involves removal of the underlying cranial bone flap, skin debridement rotation of one or more scalp flaps, and delayed cranioplasty. The skin flap is planned with consideration of the strategy for scalp closure after debridement. The ''S'' incision allows local debridement by increasing the width of its center; it is then closed by sliding the two sides together. Either the flap incision has to be very large to allow for debridement and suturing in its center (for example, a bicoronal skin flap for a forehead laceration with the debridement, and repair of the forehead scalp), or the debrided area must be one of the edges so that the two sides of the incision can be slid together. When intact, the pericranium is opened carefully and saved for later harvesting as a dural graft or for closure over the fracture site as an additional barrier to protect the bone cranioplasty and the brain from scalp infection. However, if the pericranium is shredded and/or contaminated, it is debrided.

Once the depressed skull fracture is exposed with a margin of 2 cm circumferentially, a decision as to how to remove the bone fragments is made based on (1) how firmly the bone chips are wedged together and to the surrounding skull and (2) how much angulation or twisting will be necessary to remove the individual fragments. The surgeon must consider the likelihood that the visible fragments are only the top portions of far larger fragments that have razor-sharp edges already in, or directly on top of, the cortex. Fractures have a larger area on the inner table, and some fragments can extend a considerable distance under an intact outer table.

Occasionally, the fragments are loose and are easily removed from the wound in a straight linear fashion outward from the brain. These fragments are not wedged in place and do not tamponade vessels since they exert no compressive force. More often, the bone fragments are wedged firmly in place as a result of the mechanical configuration of the diploic bone of the skull: the outer table locks either into the diploic space or under the inner table; the inner table can lock under itself. The diploic layer is soft and compressible in comparison to the cortical tables. During the impact, the diploic layer adjacent to the fracture edges undergoes compression and remodeling, filling the spaces between the locked tables and firmly fixing them in place (Figs. 271-5*B*, *C*, *D*, 271-6*B*, and 271-7*D*). In most cases, to establish the normal skull/dura relationship, a burr hole is made adjacent to the depressed area in the outer table away from the areas shown by CT to have radial fracture splinters in the inner table and also away from the venous sinuses. The burr hole is then extended into a small slot craniectomy with a 2- or 3-mm Kerrison punch. To accomplish this, the dura is first stripped from the skull for a few millimeters in the direction of the planned slot craniectomy using a small, smooth dissector. Then the overlying bone is removed with the Kerrison punch, taking care not to inadvertently place the lower jaw of the Kerrison punch into the subdural space and debride dura. The skull/dural interface is carefully followed to the edge of the fracture of the outer table. Occasionally, the skull/dura relationship is seen first between fracture fragments and the strip craniectomy can be started there. The outer table limit of the fracture is then followed circumferentially in both directions with a Kerrison punch. As this circumferential, thin, ring-shaped craniectomy cut is being completed, pieces of the fractured bone will become separated from the other pieces and the intact skull, allowing atraumatic removal. When the circumferential cut has been completed with the Kerrison punch and all the bone fragments in the center of the depressed fracture have been removed, the skull edges are all inspected for remaining inner table splinters and dural lacerations. Remaining splinters of bone under the skull edge are debrided with a Kerrison punch, reaching under the edge. Care is taken to keep the bone in as large fragments as possible and to carefully note the interrelationship of the fragments if the cranial defect is to be repaired during the initial procedure. Repair is not necessary if the operative goal is to leave a craniectomy and perform a delayed secondary cosmetic repair. In these cases, the depressed fragments can be reduced in size for atraumatic removal with a rongeur or a Kerrison punch.

After the bone fragments have been completely removed, the dura is inspected. If the dura is intact, it is not opened unless the CT scan indicated an intracerebral or subdural lesion requiring further operative therapy. Shredded dura is debrided. Small dural lacerations are enlarged to allow inspection of the cortex. Superficial hematomas on the cortex and debris are removed with gentle irrigation and suction. Brain that has been pulped by the indriven fragments is removed with gentle suction until normal brain is exposed and the fragments and debris are removed. Gentle irrigation with normal saline via a 10-ml syringe with a #18 angiocatheter with the tip positioned in the depth of a cortical laceration can often deliver deep bone chips and debris, minimizing the amount of cortical resection. Bipolar coagulation is used for hemostasis. The dura is then closed watertight using 4-0 silk or braided nylon suture, with a dural graft of pericranium or temporal fascia if necessary. After the dura is closed, the wound is irrigated with copious quantities of an antibiotic irrigation solution for mechanical debridement of the skull and scalp before scalp closure. Figures 271-7 and 271-8 are diagrams of the surgery for depressed fractures.

In most cases, the large bone fragments are replaced as a cranioplasty at the end of the operation (Figs. 271-1 and 271-8). These fragments are first washed in 10% povidone-iodine or antibiotic solution to remove all visible hair, dirt, foreign debris, and devitalized tissue and then are rinsed thoroughly in normal saline. They are then reassembled into the shape of the skull before the fracture to resemble a craniotomy flap. They are attached with stainless steel wire (3-0, #24, or #26 monofilament surgical suture) with the twists on the inside of the bone and flush with the inner table. Dural tacking sutures of 4-0 silk or braided nylon are used to hold the dura to the skull edges. In larger repairs, a central dural tacking suture is also used. This is inserted by first making a single pass through the dura directly below two holes in the assembled cranioplasty. The two ends of this central dural stitch are then passed through these two holes and tied to fix the center of the dura to the cranioplasty after it has been secured in final position.The reconstructed craniotomy flap is then wired into place at several circumferential points and the scalp is closed with absorbable sutures in the galea layer and skin staples or nylon sutures in the cutaneous layer. A subgaleal drain is used for 24 h in patients whose fracture lines or contused scalp continue to bleed at closure. Postoperative radiographs of the skull and a CT scan of the head with both soft-tissue and bone imaging display windows are

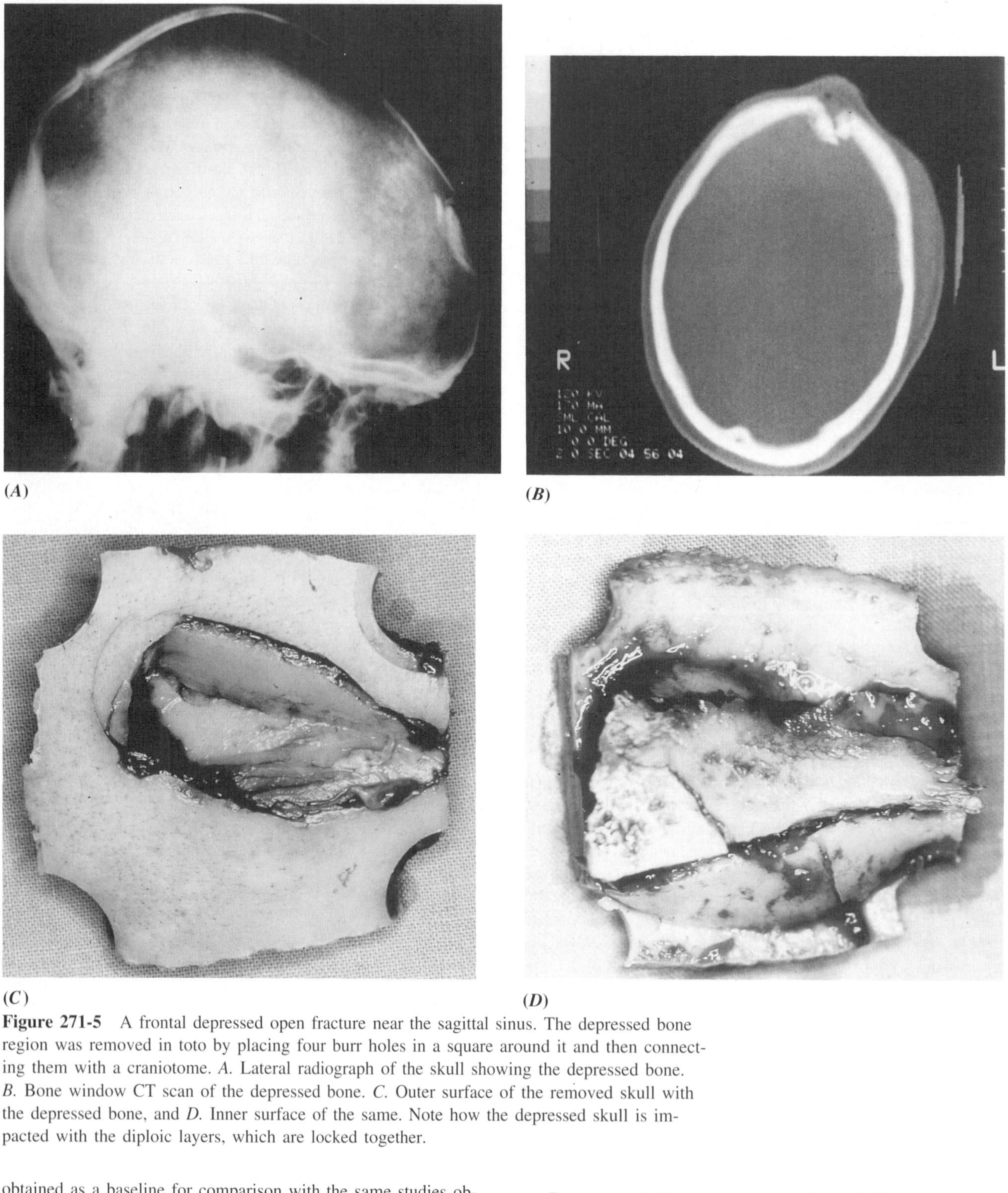

Figure 271-5 A frontal depressed open fracture near the sagittal sinus. The depressed bone region was removed in toto by placing four burr holes in a square around it and then connecting them with a craniotome. *A*. Lateral radiograph of the skull showing the depressed bone. *B*. Bone window CT scan of the depressed bone. *C*. Outer surface of the removed skull with the depressed bone, and *D*. Inner surface of the same. Note how the depressed skull is impacted with the diploic layers, which are locked together.

obtained as a baseline for comparison with the same studies obtained several months or years later for assessing the incorporation/absorption of bone and the cranial shape. Infection rates of 2.5 to 10.6 percent have been reported for operative treatment of open depressed fractures.[3]

If the skull defect left after removal of the bone fragments is small or was grossly contaminated, if a debrided scalp laceration must be closed under tension over the skull defect, or if the surgical repair was delayed until more than 24 h after the injury, then the bone fragments are not replaced at the time of surgery, and a delayed cranioplasty is planned (Fig. 271-6).

Depressed Fractures over Dural Sinuses

Depressed skull fractures located over a venous sinus require special handling.[13] The surgical elevation of fractures over a venous sinus may involve massive blood loss if a depressed fragment has been plugging a sinus tear. Unless such a fracture is grossly contaminated with foreign material, creates a major cosmetic deformity, or causes intracranial hypertension as a result of sinus occlusion, it should be managed with scalp debridement and massive irrigation, and then followed for at least a year by serial CT for signs of brain abscess. If the fracture requires debridement and

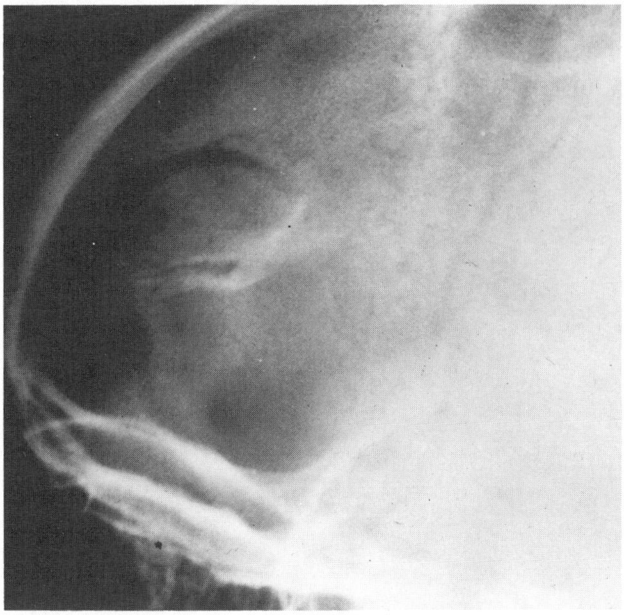

(*A*)

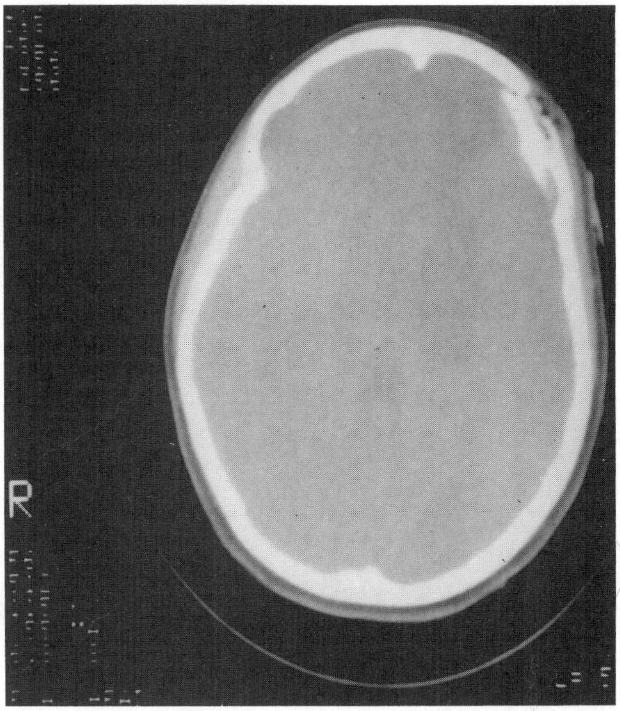

(*B*)

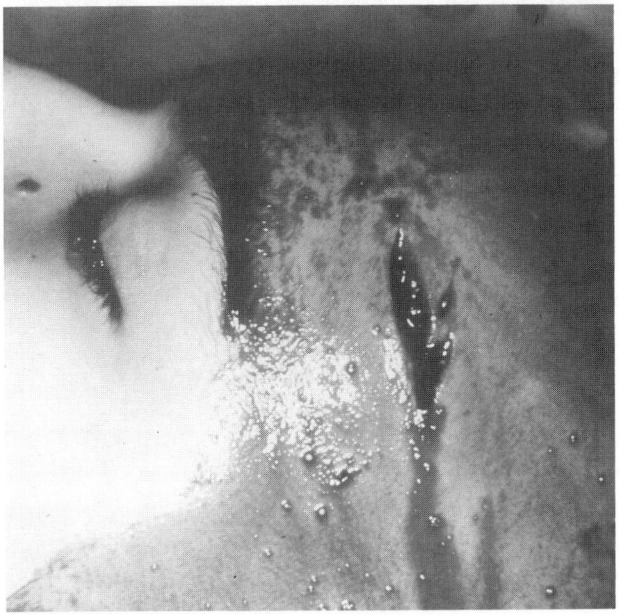

(*C*)

Figure 271-6 An open depressed frontal fracture from a golf club injury. This was operated on through a coronal incision scalp flap. *A*. Lateral skull radiograph showing the fracture. *B*. CT scan showing the locking of the fracture fragment below the level of the surrounding skull. *C*. Preoperative view of the scalp wound.

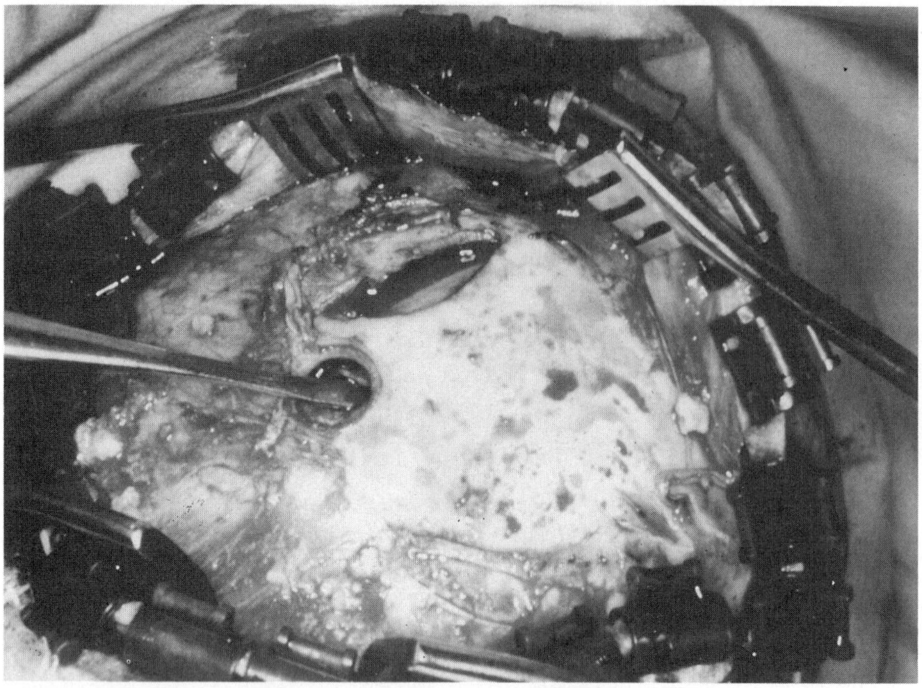

(*D*)

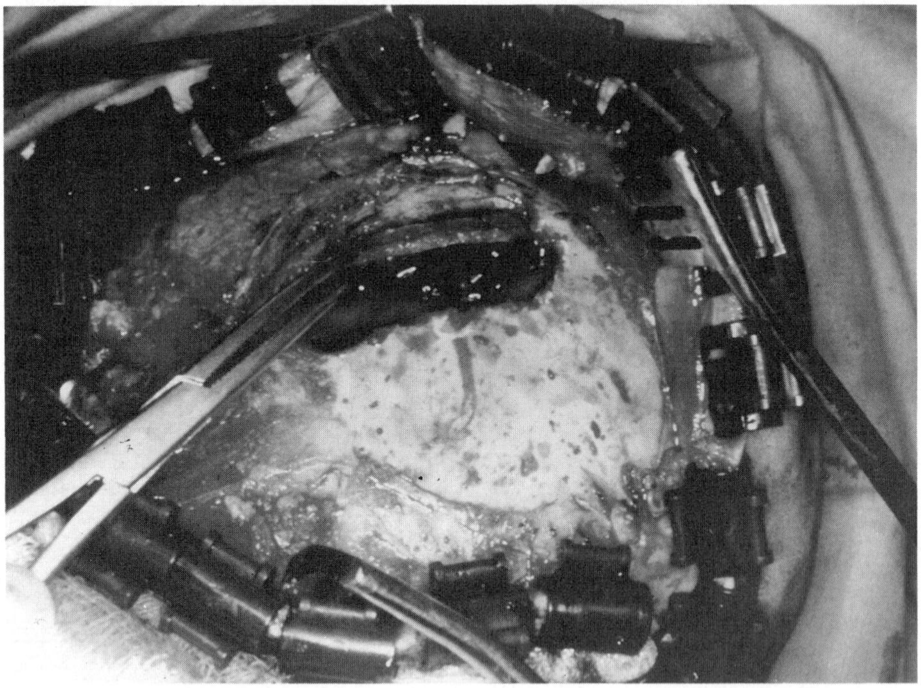

(*E*)

Figure 271-6 (*Continued*) *D.* View of the fracture after elevation of the scalp flap. An adjacent burr hole has been drilled and a Penfield dissector is defining the normal skull-dura relationship and stripping the dura from the inner surface of the skull in the direction of the depressed fracture. *E.* The bone from the burr hole to the depressed area has been removed with a Kerrison punch, and a slot circumferential craniectomy has been performed to free the large depressed fragment. The bone is being gently slid out of the skull as the locking portion of the fracture has been removed by the slot craniectomy.

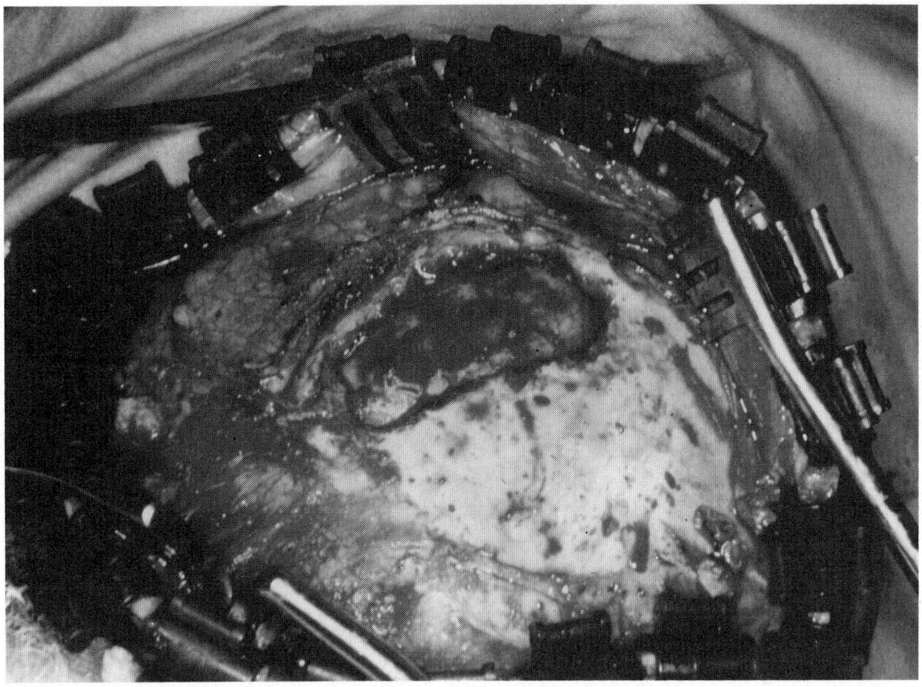

(*F*)

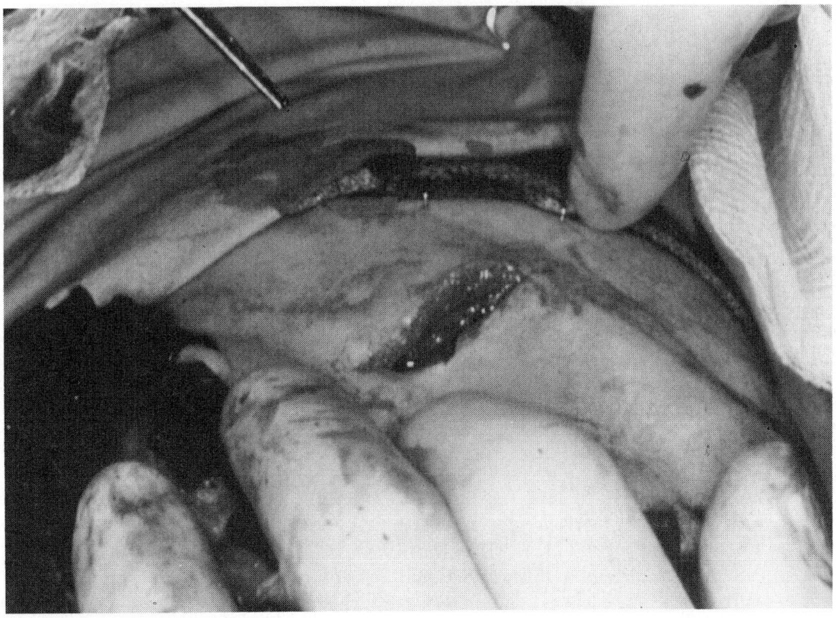

(*G*)

Figure 271-6 (*Continued*) *F.* Intact dura after removal of the depressed bone and before dural tacking sutures were placed circumferentially. *G.* Closure of the scalp laceration after debridement by sliding the scalp. This lacerated region was closed before the coronal scalp incision. The cranioplasty was delayed for 9 months because of the initial contamination of the wound with dirt.

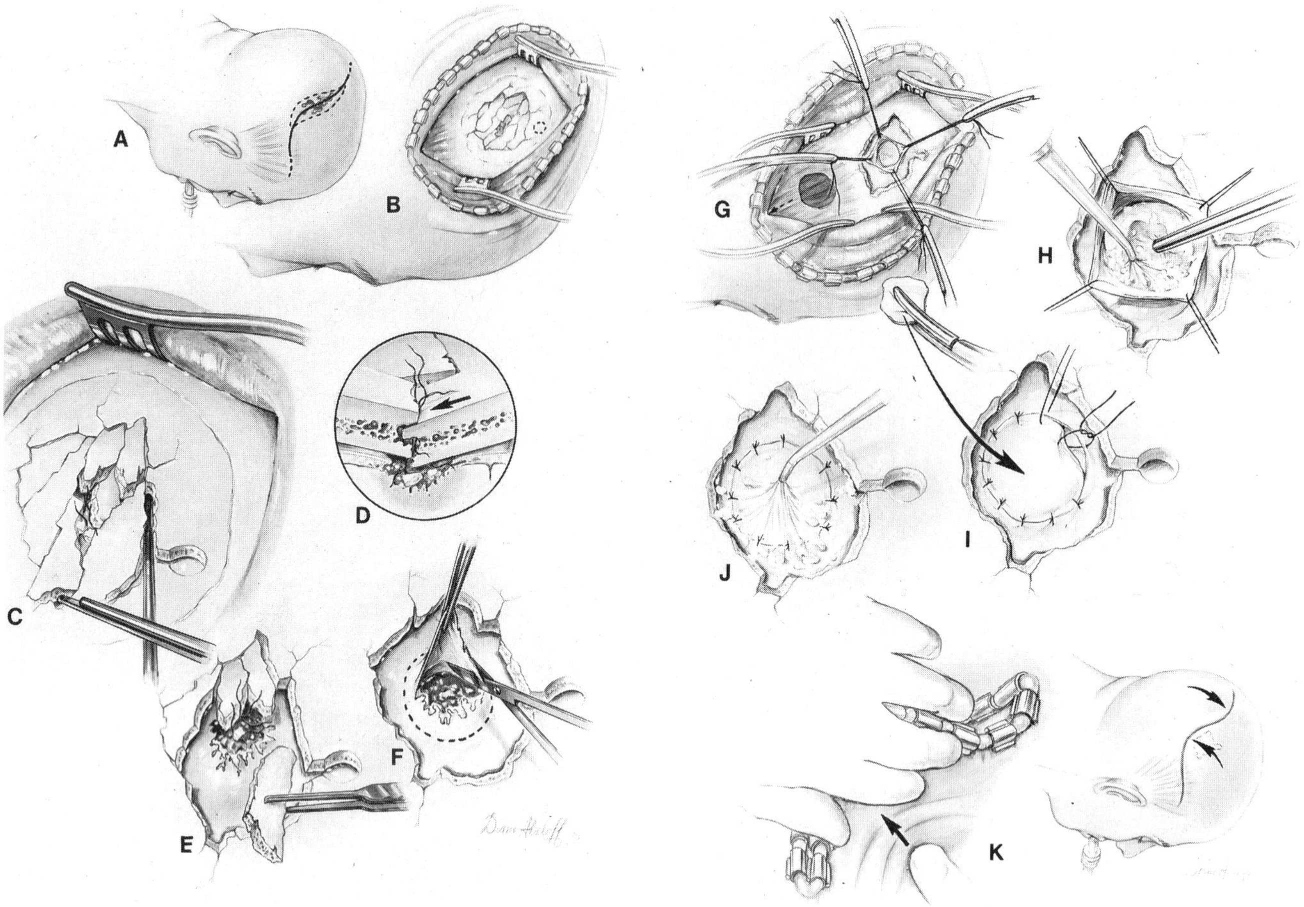

Figure 271-7 The steps in the treatment of an open depressed skull fracture with dural penetration and brain laceration. *A.* The scalp debridement lines. *B.* Initial burr hole placed slightly beyond the edge of the depressed skull fracture to expose normal dura. *C.* Enlargement of the burr hole into a slot craniectomy by proceeding circumferentially in both directions around the edge of the depressed skull fracture. *D.* The bone fragments are locked together, hair is wedged between the bone fragments, and a sharp edge of the fracture has lacerated the underlying dura and cortical surface. *E.* Removal of fracture fragments with a gentle, outward, nontwisting motion. *F.* Debridement of the dura. *G.* Harvesting temporalis fascia for a dural graft. *H.* Gentle debridement of pulped and contaminated cerebral cortex with normal saline irrigation and suction. *I.* Watertight closure of the dura. *J.* Irrigation of the wound after dural closure. *K.* Sliding together of the debrided skin edges to close the scalp wound. (From Geisler,[5] with permission.)

elevation, then four burr holes (two proximal and two distal, one on each side of the sinus) are made, with the fracture area in the center of the rectangle, and then connected with a cranial saw (Fig. 271-5). The entire craniotomy flap containing the depressed fracture is then elevated. Massive bleeding can occur during this elevation until proximal and distal control of the sinus is achieved. The laceration in the dural sinus can usually be repaired with direct suturing. A patch graft of rotated dura, pericranium, or vein is used to repair an avulsed section.

Depressed Fractures in Neonates and Children

The immature skull is more flexible and therefore harder to fracture than the adult skull.[16] When a fracture occurs in a child, it is usually a linear or diastatic fracture involving the coronal or lambdoid suture. Depressed fractures in the neonatal period are typically greenstick fractures located in the frontal or parietal areas. They have been termed ''ping-pong'' fractures because they show indented bone without a fracture in the cortical layers.[22] These fractures sometimes elevate spontaneously, and they have also been elevated with external suction and by surgery.[20] The surgical elevation of depressions greater than 5 mm involves introducing a smooth elevator through an adjacent burr hole and reducing the depressed area to a normal configuration by upward levering. The dura near the depression can be torn, allowing the elevator to contact the underlying cortical surface. It is wise to convert this procedure to a standard depressed fracture elevation if difficulty is encountered in this relatively blind elevation.

Basilar Skull Fractures

Description

Fractures of the skull base have been reported to occur in 3.5 to 24.0 percent of head-injured patients. This wide variation results both from differences in study patient populations and from the difficulty of obtaining radiographic verification of the fractures.

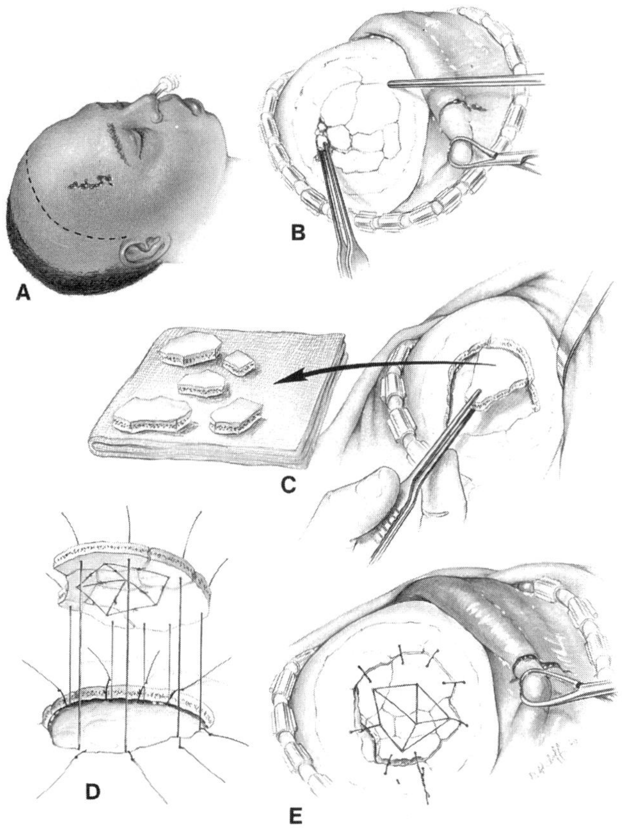

Figure 271-8 Treatment of an open depressed skull fracture with intact dura in which the large bone fragments were reassembled and used as a bone cranioplasty. *A.* A bicoronal scalp incision is used for the frontal open depressed fracture. *B.* Debridement of multiple pieces of fractured bone including smaller loose ones. *C.* Removal of large bone fragments with gentle force in an outward direction without angulation. *D.* Reassembly of the bone fragments with wire in anatomic position to form a bone cranioplasty. *E.* Cranioplasty wired to the skull. (From Geisler,[5] with permission.)

Basal skull fracture with CSF rhinorrhea is common after head injury and has an estimated incidence of 150,000 cases per year in the United States.[7] Although these fractures often are part of a convexity fracture that has extended into the skull base, they can occur alone.

Linear fractures in the skull base carry a risk of intracranial infection, whereas in fractures of the convexity the risk of an infection is extremely low unless the scalp, bone, and dura are all violated. On the convexity, an intact scalp suffices as a barrier against infection even when the dura is punctured by bone fragments. However, the dura covering the base of the skull, which is easily torn in association with a basal skull fracture, places the subarachnoid space in direct contact with the paranasal sinuses, middle ear structures, or mastoid air cells, providing a pathway for infection. A persistent fistula, allowing a continuous CSF leak, may develop with a basal skull fracture. This tract constitutes a persistent pathway for bacteria to the subarachnoid space and continually exposes the patient to the risk of meningitis or brain abscess if left untreated. An infectious complication (early or delayed by months or years) can occur after a basal fracture when the leaking of CSF is not apparent clinically and intracranial air is not visualized.

Diagnosis

Basal skull fractures are suspected when clinical signs related to the site of the fracture are present: bilateral periorbital ecchymosis, anosmia, or CSF rhinorrhea in anterior skull base fractures; and hemotympanum, blood in the external auditory canal, seventh or eighth nerve palsies, ecchymosis over the mastoids, or CSF otorrhea in temporal bone fractures.

Basal fractures often traverse foramina and thereby damage cranial nerves[18,24] and blood vessels by either direct contusion or stretching.[1] Temporal bone fractures are associated with injuries to the facial and vestibulocochlear nerves, which are damaged in half the cases in which the fracture is transverse to the long axis of the petrous pyramid. Hematotympanum is seen in most of these cases. The transverse pattern of fracture occurs in one-quarter or less of temporal bone fractures. In the more common longitudinal pattern (75 to 90 percent of all cases), the fracture is parallel to the long axis of the petrous bone. These fractures often do not injure the seventh or eighth nerves because the fracture line runs anterior to them, but they can disrupt the ossicular chain. Up to half of the patients with transverse and a quarter of the patients with longitudinal petrous bone fractures have associated facial nerve injury. The nerve is commonly injured in the internal auditory meatus or the horizontal portion of the fallopian canal on the medial wall of the tympanum in transverse fractures. In longitudinal fractures, injury occurs at the geniculate ganglion or just distal to it in the tympanic section of the facial canal. Since most patients spontaneously recover from the facial paralysis, most physicians treat with watchful expectancy. The technique and timing for decompressing and/or grafting the damaged facial nerve remain controversial.

The olfactory nerve is commonly injured in association with fractures of the anterior fossa floor. Optic nerve injury can follow fractures in the anterior fossa that involve the optic canal. Because the results of surgical decompression of the optic nerve in the optic canal are similar to spontaneous recovery rates, the only indication for decompression is documented deterioration of initially good vision following head trauma. The abducens nerve can be damaged in clivus fractures, either directly or because skull deformation at the time of impact stretches where it passes below the petroclinoid ligament.[18]

Basal fractures can cause traumatic carotid-cavernous fistulae, traumatic aneurysms of the carotid artery in its petrous or cavernous portion, or occlusion of the internal carotid artery. Carotid-cavernous fistula causes chemosis, headache, and bruit and can progress to pulsatile exophthalmos, ophthalmoplegia, and visual loss. Traumatic aneurysms of the carotid artery usually do not cause symptoms initially and are found incidentally. Later, clinical signs of cranial nerve palsy, pain, epistaxis, or effects of embolization can develop. When the internal carotid artery is damaged in the petrous pyramid in association with a basal fracture, 85 percent of the patients are left with a major neurological deficit related to the cerebral ischemia.[1]

Frequently, a CSF leak is first detected several days to weeks after the trauma. Usually this delay is due to the fact that the CSF leak was initially hidden in bloody nasal discharge from facial fractures; less frequently, it is due to the delayed development of hydrocephalus with rupture of the arachnoid at the fracture site. A "double-ring" sign of the bloody nasal discharge is used as a bedside test to indicate that CSF is mixed with the blood. When a few drops of bloody discharge containing CSF are placed on a paper towel, a larger clear ring surrounds a central blood-tinged clot. This double-ring sign can also be noted on the patient's pillow on morning rounds.

A clear watery nasal discharge is suggestive of CSF rhinorrhea. Recently, a beta 2-transferrin has been demonstrated to be a specific marker for CSF. In the situation of a bloody or nonbloody nasal discharge or an intermittent leak, the test for the beta 2-transferrin is more sensitive than either chemical analysis of the discharge fluid for glucose, protein or electrolytes, or a radioactive cisternography test.[17,19] An intermittent CSF leak originating in the paranasal sinuses can often be made apparent by having the patient sit on the edge of the bed with the head close to the knees for 2 min and watching for clear fluid to drip from the tip of the nose.

Management

The management of a basal skull fracture is usually determined by the presence or absence of a CSF leak. A patient with a basal skull fracture but no initially noted leak is managed by observation for 2 to 3 days. During this time, repeated checks for rhinorrhea or otorrhea are made to verify the absence of a CSF leak. Otorrhea is more likely than rhinorrhea to resolve spontaneously. Because antibiotics are not effective in preventing meningitis and may select for resistant organisms when an infection occurs, making treatment more difficult, prophylactic antibiotics are not used in patients with basal skull fractures with or without a CSF leak. Details of CSF fistula management are presented in another chapter.

CSF otorrhea usually occurs with a fracture of the petrous bone and perforation of the tympanic membrane, although it can occasionally occur with a laceration of the external canal via fractured mastoid air cells. If the tympanic membrane remains intact, CSF that has gained access to the middle ear can flow through the eustachian tube and present as rhinorrhea. In these cases, the CT scan typically images both a fracture in the temporal bone and fluid in the mastoid air cells and middle ear structures.

A patient with CSF otorrhea often presents with hearing loss or blood in the external ear canal. Irrigation and probing of the ear in cases of suspected otorrhea are not indicated initially because they increase the risk of intracranial infection. Such a patient is managed by placing a sterile gauze pad over the ear; the pad is changed every nursing shift and saved as an indicator of the amount of drainage from the ear. Most cases of otorrhea stop spontaneously within the first few days. A detailed auditory and vestibular examination is performed 6 to 8 weeks after trauma to diagnose abnormalities and determine treatment.

Fractures in the Posterior Wall of the Frontal Sinus

Fractures in the frontal area often extend to include the frontal sinus and floor of the anterior fossa.[15] The symptoms of a frontal sinus fracture include localized bruising, hematoma, or laceration; these fractures often extend into the orbit causing both palpebral and subconjunctival hematomas. When the posterior wall of the frontal sinus is fractured, injury to the cribriform plate with CSF leakage is a frequent occurrence. The surgical treatment involves removing the posterior wall of the frontal sinus, repairing the dural tear, removing all mucous membrane in the frontal sinus, and plugging the nasofrontal duct with muscle or layers of bone chips. Complete removal of the sinus mucosa requires light burring with a drill of all remaining sinus walls. The removal of the posterior wall of the frontal sinus "cranializes" it. Without complete removal of the frontal sinus mucosa and permanent obliteration of the nasofrontal duct, a mucocele (from an obstructed remnant of frontal sinus mucosa) can occur and infection (early or delayed) in the ethmoid sinus can spread to the anterior epidural space.

References

1. Aarabi B, McQueen JD. Traumatic internal carotid occlusion at the base of the skull. *Surg Neurol* 1978; 10:233–236.
2. Bakay L, Glasauer FE. *Head Injury.* Boston: Little, Brown, 1980.
3. Cooper PR. Skull fracture and traumatic cerebrospinal fluid fistulas. In Cooper PR (ed): *Head Injury,* 3d ed. Baltimore: Williams & Wilkins, 1993, pp 115–136.
4. Gade GF, Becker DP, Miller JD, et al. Pathology and pathophysiology of head injury. In Youmans JR (ed): *Neurological Surgery,* 3d ed. Philadelphia: Saunders, 1990, pp 1965–2016.
5. Geisler FH. Depressed skull fractures in adults. In Rengachary SS, Wilkins RH (eds): *Neurosurgical Operative Atlas,* vol 1. Baltimore: Williams & Wilkins, 1991, pp 25–35.
6. Geisler FH, Greenberg J. Management of the acute head-injury patient. In Salcman M (ed): *Neurologic Emergencies: Recognition and Management,* 2d ed. New York: Raven Press, 1990, pp 135–166.
7. Geisler FH, Salcman M. The head injury patient. In Siegel JH (ed): *Trauma: Emergency Surgery and Critical Care.* New York: Churchill Livingstone, 1987, pp 919–946.
8. Gennarelli TA. Mechanisms of cerebral concussion, contusion, and other effects of head injury. In Youmans JR (ed): *Neurological Surgery,* 3d ed. Philadelphia: Saunders, 1990, pp 1953–1964.
9. Gudeman SK, Young HF, Miller JD, et al. Indications for operative treatment and operative technique in closed head injury. In Becker DP, Gudeman SK (eds): *Textbook of Head Injury.* Philadelphia: Saunders, 1989, pp 138–181.
10. Gurdjian ES, Lissner HR. Deformations of the skull in head injury studied by the "stresscoat" technique: quantitative determinations. *Surg Gynecol Obstet* 1946; 83:219–233.
11. Gurdjian ES, Webster JE. *Head Injuries: Mechanisms, Diagnosis, and Management.* Boston: Little, Brown, 1958, pp 76, 211.
12. Jennett B, Teasdale G. *Management of Head Injuries.* (Contemporary Neurology Series, Vol 20.) Philadelphia: Davis, 1981.
13. Kapp JP, Gielchinsky I, Deardourff SL. Operative techniques for management of lesions involving the dural venous sinuses. *Surg Neurol* 1977; 7:339–342.
14. Lipper MH, Kishore PRS. Radiological investigation of acute head trauma. In Becker DP, Gudeman SK (eds): *Textbook of Head Injury.* Philadelphia: Saunders, 1989, pp 102–137.
15. Manson PN. Maxillofacial injuries. In Siegel JH (ed): *Trauma: Emergency Surgery and Critical Care.* New York: Churchill Livingstone, 1987, pp 983–1047.
16. Mealey J Jr. Skull fractures. In McLaurin RL, Venes JL, Schut L, et al. (eds): *Pediatric Neurosurgery: Surgery of the Developing Nervous System,* 2d ed. Philadelphia: Saunders, 1989, pp 263–270.
17. Meurman OH, Irjala K, Suonpaa J, et al. A new method for the identification of cerebrospinal fluid leakage. *Acta Otolaryngol (Stockh)* 1979; 87:366–369.
18. Rovit RL, Murali R. Injuries of the cranial nerves. In Cooper PR (ed): *Head Injury,* 3d ed. Baltimore: Williams & Wilkins, 1993, pp 183–202.
19. Ryall RG, Peacock MK, Simpson DA. Usefulness of beta 2-transferrin assay in the detection of cerebrospinal fluid leaks following head injury. *J Neurosurg* 1992; 77:737–739.

20. Saunders BS, Lazoritz S, McArtor RD, et al. Depressed skull fracture in the neonate. Report of three cases. *J Neurosurg* 1979; 50:512–514.
21. Tyson GW. *Head Injury Management for Providers of Emergency Care.* Baltimore: Williams & Wilkins, 1987.
22. Vollmer DG, Dacey RG, Jane JA. Craniocerebral trauma. In Joynt RJ (ed): *Clinical Neurology,* vol 3. Philadelphia: Lippincott, 1991, pp 1–79.
23. Wilberger J, Chen DA. Management of head injury. The skull and meninges. *Neurosurg Clin North Am* 1991; 2(2):341–350.
24. Williams GH, Giordano AM. Temporal bone trauma. In Becker DP, Gudeman SK (eds): *Textbook of Head Injury.* Philadelphia: Saunders, 1989, pp 367–377.

272

Growing Skull Fractures of Childhood

Tadanori Tomita

Simple skull fractures in childhood ordinarily heal without sequelae. However, in rare cases, the fracture lines widen with time and appear to be growing. This condition is called "growing fracture." A growing fracture is a rare complication of skull fracture and occurs mainly in infancy and early childhood. It is characterized by progressive diastatic enlargement of the fracture line. This late complication of skull fracture is also known as "leptomeningeal cyst" because of its frequent association with a cystic mass filled with cerebrospinal fluid (CSF). Although skull fractures are common in pediatric practice, the incidence of the growing fracture is reportedly only 0.05 to 1 percent among skull fractures in childhood.[4,18]

Pathogenesis

The "growth" of the fracture line is due to resorption of adjacent bone as a result of continuous pulsatile wedge pressure from tissue herniating through the fracture line. A dural laceration along the fracture line is always noted at the surgical repair, and it is an essential factor for development of the growing fracture. A growing fracture was produced in puppies at a craniotomy site by linearly cutting the dura.[6,19] At the site of a growing fracture, the dural gap is also enlarged, and grows larger than the fracture line.[8,14,25] The lack of resistance at both the dura and the skull defect results in a local amplification of intracranial pressure pulse waves, causing herniation of the cerebral tissue or subarachnoid space through the fracture line. The brain extrusion may be present shortly after diastatic linear fracture in neonates and young infants.[24] This fact accounts for the focal dilation of the lateral ventricle near the growing fracture that is seen on neuroimaging studies. This focal porencephalic dilation may be reversible and may normalize after the repair of a growing fracture.[20] Cranial defects never increase if the underlying dura is intact. Moreover, a craniotomy performed without watertight closure of the dura, for any reason, does not cause a growing fracture. Therefore, for a growing fracture to develop, a dural laceration must coincide with the fracture line.

Growing skull fractures usually occur during the first 3 years of life (particularly during infancy), and almost never after 8 years of life. During this early stage of life, brain volume increases very rapidly, which is a necessary factor for the development of a growing fracture. Other evidence indicates that growing fractures, after reaching a maximum extent, stop growing and remain stable through adulthood.[17,18] The rapidly developing brain of an infant contributes an outward driving force that can cause the brain to herniate through the dural and skull defect. Therefore, the development of the growing skull fracture is multifactorial: The pulsatile force of the brain during its period of maximum growth produces cerebral or subarachnoid herniation through the dural laceration at the fracture line, which causes the fracture in the thin skull to enlarge.

One risk factor for the development of a growing fracture is the severity of the head trauma. A linear fracture associated with a hemorrhagic contusion of the subjacent brain suggests a trauma significant enough to cause dural laceration. The brain at the growing fracture site frequently shows cerebromeningeal cicatrix formation. In some cases, loculated subarachnoid CSF cyst(s) may be noted with underlying gliotic, atrophic brain. Although some workers consider that the loculated subarachnoid space becomes cystic (a leptomeningeal cyst) and causes the growing fracture,[20,23] others have never found a leptomeningeal cyst at operation.[11,22] These leptomeningeal cysts may not be in communication with the subarachnoid space.[19] Cystic changes at the growing fracture site may be considered to result from cystic encephalomalacia. Post-traumatic aneurysms and subdural hematomas have also been reported to accompany growing fractures.[2,13] Although most patients show damage to the underlying brain,[12] this finding is not a prerequisite for development of a growing fracture. An unusual leptomeningeal cyst in the posterior fossa without evidence of cerebellar damage has been reported.[15] Others have reported an expanding cranial defect with herniation of uninjured brain through dural lacerations created in humans and animals.[19,25]

A depressed fracture usually does not become a growing fracture,[1] but a linear fracture extending from the depressed fracture can become one.[14] A fracture with a diastasis of more than 4 mm may be considered at risk of developing a growing fracture.[8,23,24] However, a post-traumatic diastasis of a cranial suture is an unusual site for a growing fracture.[9]

A growing fracture can occur in the skull base even in older individuals. If a linear fracture is accompanied by a dural laceration in the thin areas of the skull base, such as the orbital roof, ethmoid plate, and frontal sinus, a growing fracture and meningoencephalocele can develop.[3,7,16]

Clinical Features

A growing fracture commonly presents as a progressive, often pulsatile, scalp mass that appears several months to years after head trauma sustained during infancy or early childhood. The initial trauma often was significant enough to have caused the clinician to obtain skull radiographs or neuroimaging studies, but in other cases it was clinically insignificant.

Neurological disorders related to growing fractures include seizure disorder, hemiparesis, and psychomotor retardation. Seizures may be resistant to medical management. However, not infrequently, an asymptomatic palpable mass is the sole sign. These palpable scalp masses usually occur in the parietal region. A growing fracture in the skull base may present with ocular proptosis or CSF rhinorrhea or otorrhea.

Radiologic Studies

Skull radiographs show a wide diastasis of the fracture line. If initial skull films are available, the subsequent growth of the fracture line can be confirmed (Fig. 272-1). If the original trauma caused multiple fractures, a combination of a healing fracture with a growing fracture may be found (Fig. 272-2). A fracture line can cross coronal or lambdoid sutures, but it is usually limited to the parietal bone.[11,23]

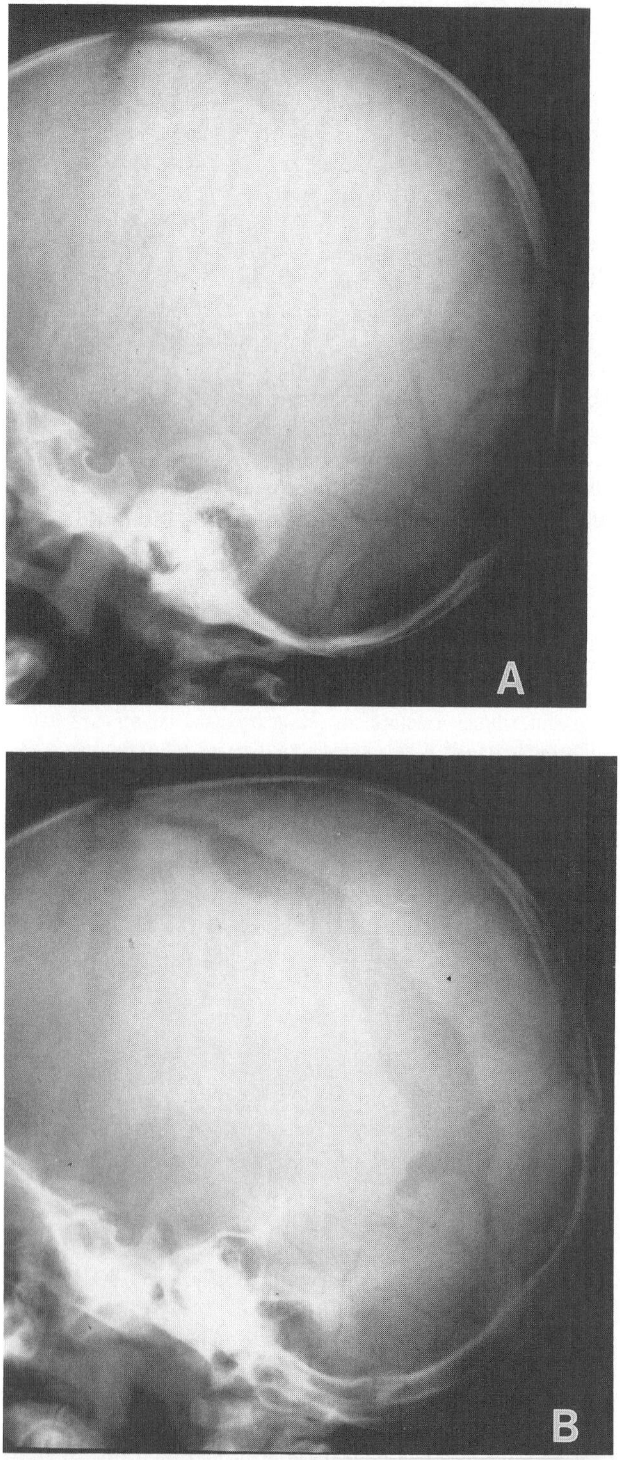

Figure 272-1 Lateral skull radiographs taken at the time of initial injury (*A*) and 10 months later (*B*), showing a growing fracture of the parietal bone.

Computed tomography (CT) provides more information on the contents of the growing fracture, and on intracranial pathologic changes. Furthermore, if CT scans are available from the time of the initial trauma, progressive soft tissue changes can be well appreciated. It is not unusual for hemorrhagic contusion or subarachnoid or extraparenchymal hemorrhage to be visible at the time of trauma. At the time of diagnosis of the growing fracture, CT scans will show the diastasis of the fracture line and often a hypodense lesion near the fracture site (Fig. 272-3). The intracranial hypodensity may represent encephalomalacia, arachnoidal loculation, or cortical atrophy. The ipsilateral lateral ventricle tends to show

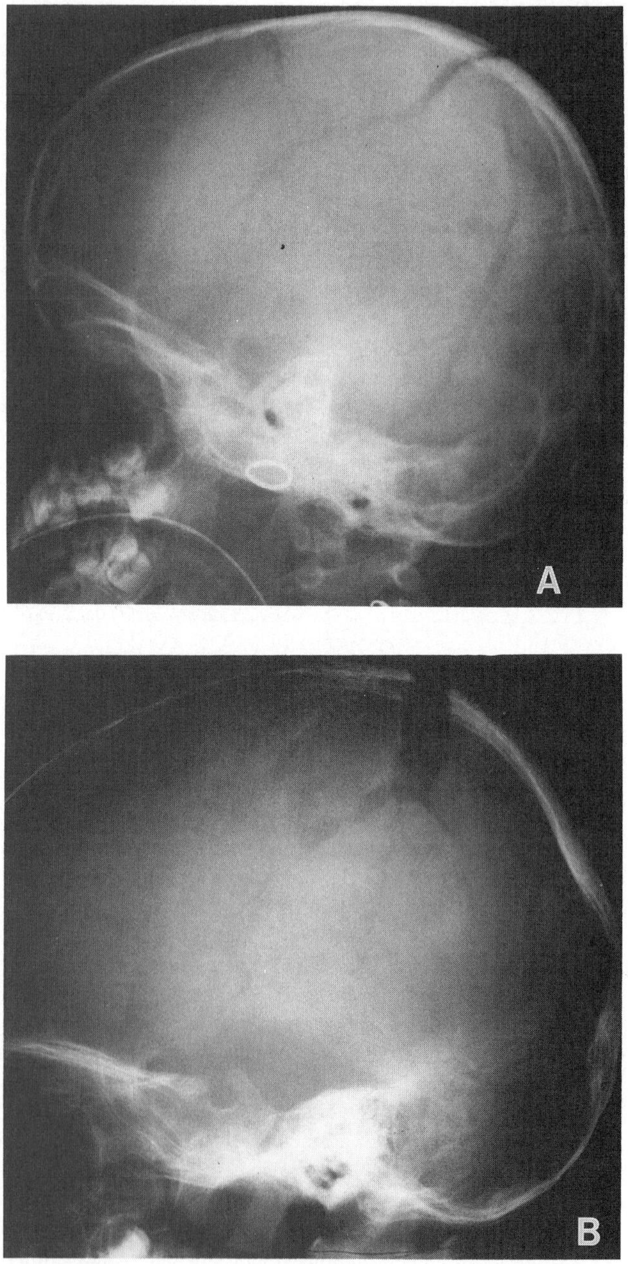

Figure 272-2 *A*. Lateral skull radiograph taken at the time of initial injury showing multiple fractures. *B*. Follow-up skull radiograph showing a growing fracture in one area and a healing fracture in another.

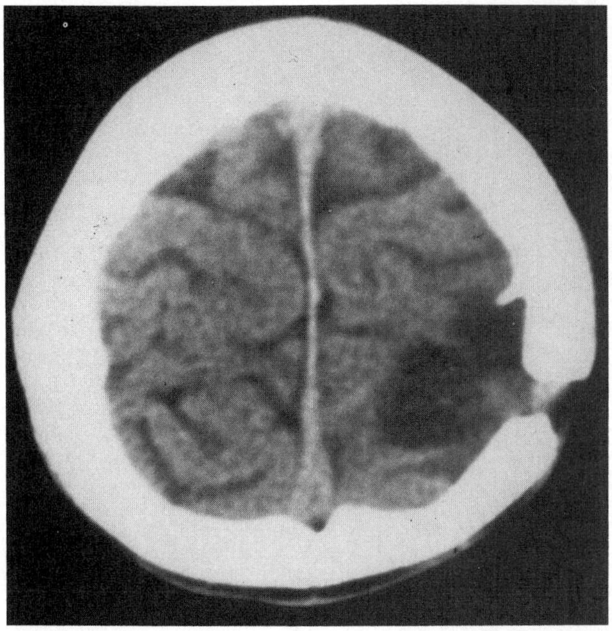

Figure 272-3 Axial CT scan showing a growing fracture with subjacent encephalomalacia.

focal porencephalic dilation. This phenomenon may be related to lack of dural resistance. Magnetic resonance imaging (MRI) provides further information on pathologic processes associated with a growing fracture (Fig. 272-4).

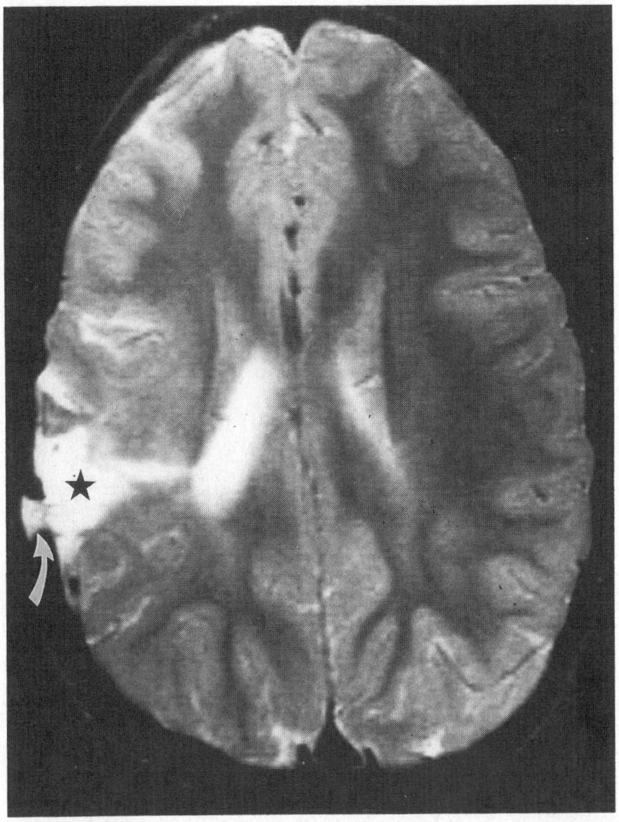

Figure 272-4 T2-weighted MR image showing a growing fracture (*arrow*) and encephalomalacia (*asterisk*). Note the brain tissue herniating through the fracture and the porencephalic dilation of the ipsilateral ventricle.

Management

Most authors recommend early surgical correction of growing skull fractures. Experimental data from rabbits showed progressive cystic degeneration in brain herniated through dural and cranial defects[5]; thus, early recognition and treatment of growing fractures should prevent further neurological deterioration. Attempts to control growing fractures by repetitive lumbar punctures or punctures of the leptomeningeal cyst have failed.[24] However, Ramamurthi and Kalyanaraman reported four patients whose growing fractures underwent spontaneous stabilization without surgical correction.[18] Others also have reported late discovery in adulthood of growing fractures that had become stable.[17] Transient progression and subsequent spontaneous healing of neonatal diastatic fractures has also been reported.[21] Nevertheless, owing to the risks of neurological deterioration and the development of a seizure disorder, surgical correction of growing fractures is recommended. In particular, intractable seizures often respond to surgical treatment. The goals of surgery are to repair the dural and cranial defect, to debride cerebromeningeal cicatrix, and to remove leptomeningeal cysts.

Surgical Technique

The scalp incision should be large enough to expose the entire length of the growing fracture. A scalp flap is turned subgaleally, exposing the pericranium covering the cranial defect, and the edge of the cranial defect is then dissected by incising the pericranium along the edge of the defect in the bone (Fig. 272-5*A*).

The pericranium is directly adherent to the underlying cerebral tissue, forming a cerebromeningeal cicatrix. Because the dural defect is wider than the cranial defect, no attempt should be made to identify and expose the dura by cutting back the edges of the growing fracture. Instead, to identify the dura, several burr holes are made at a distance from the cranial defect, and through them the dura is separated from the inner skull table toward the defect. The pericranium is separated from the outer skull table, and a wide craniotomy is made around the skull defect.

Once the intact dura and dural defects are identified (Fig. 272-5*B*), the cerebral tissue adhering to the reactive periosteal tissue is exposed by removing the cerebromeningeal cicatrix tissue. In this region, abnormal tissue, such as cystic changes or xanthochromic discoloration caused by previous hemorrhage, are often noted. These tissues should be removed until normal white matter is exposed.

After appropriate debridement and removal of abnormal tissues, the dural defect is closed by using a pericranial graft (Fig. 272-5*C*). Watertight closure of the dura is important to avoid recurrence of the growing fracture or postoperative CSF leakage. The cranial defect is repaired with the autologous split skull grafts that were obtained at the time of craniotomy. If the skull defect is too large for this method or if the skull is too thin to be separated into inner and outer tables, one may consider using an autologous rib graft. These autologous bone grafts are well incorporated. Foreign materials are best avoided for cranioplasty in growing skulls.

The growing fracture may extend toward a dural venous sinus, such as the superior sagittal or lateral sinus. Even though the

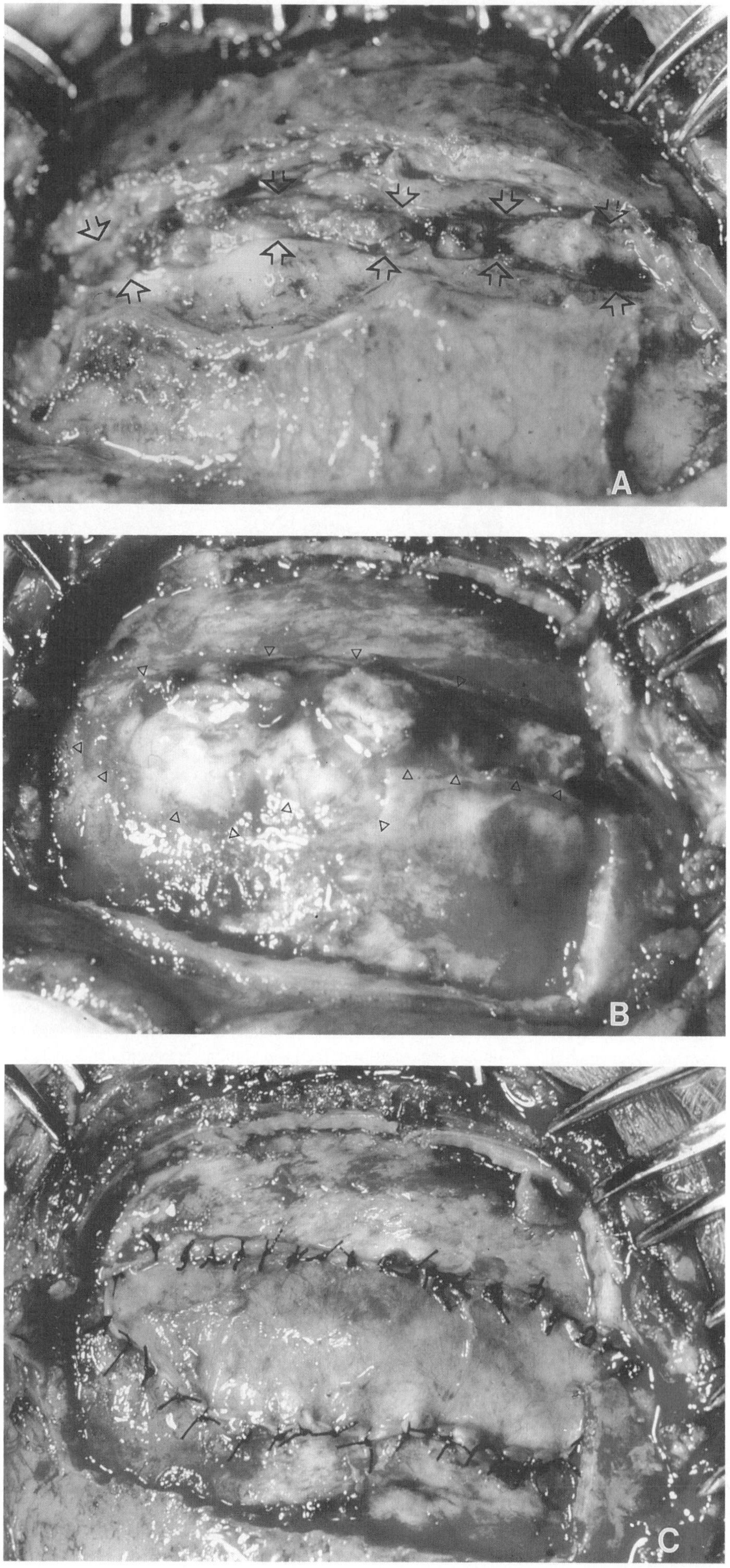

Figure 272-5 Operative photographs of the repair of a growing fracture. *A*. A diastatic fracture line is exposed after the separation of pericranium from the fracture edge (*arrows*). *B*. After a craniotomy around the growing fracture, a wide dural defect is identified (*triangles*). Note that the dural defect is larger than the cranial defect. *C*. The dural defect is repaired with a pericranial graft after debridement of the cerebromeningeal cicatrix.

venous sinus was not harmed in the initial trauma, it may pose problems for the repair of the growing fracture. When the fracture line extends perpendicularly to the sinus, the end closest to the sinus does not need dural repair. However, if the growing fracture is parallel to and near the sinus, dural repair may be difficult owing to the narrowness of the dural edge next to the sinus. In these cases, one may repair the dural defect with a pericranial graft, which is sutured either directly to the skull edge above the sinus or to the dura across the sinus.

A CSF diversion shunt has been recommended for postoperative CSF leakage.[10,14] It is justified if there is coexisting hydrocephalus or if CSF leakage occurs despite adequate repair of the growing fracture. Although some workers recommend a CSF diversion shunt as a primary therapy for growing fractures, direct repair of the fracture is the definitive treatment.

References

1. Arseni C, Ciurea AV. Clinicotherapeutic aspects in the growing skull fracture. A review of the literature. *Childs Brain* 1981; 8:161–172.
2. Buckingham MJ, Crone KR, Ball WS, et al. Traumatic intracranial aneurysms in childhood: two cases and a review of the literature. *Neurosurgery* 1988; 22:398–408.
3. Cook PG, Norman PF. Intradiplopic leptomeningeal cyst of the frontal bone occurring as a complication of head injury in an adult. *Clin Radiol* 1988; 39:214–215.
4. DesChamps GT Jr, Blumenthal BI. Radiologic seminar CCXLIX: growing skull fractures of childhood. *J Miss State Med Assoc* 1988; 29:16–17.
5. Falconer MA, Russell DS. Experimental traumatic cerebral cysts in the rabbit. *J Neurosurg* 1944; 1:182–189.
6. Goldstein FP, Rosenthal SAE, Garancis JC, et al. Varieties of growing skull fractures in childhood. *J Neurosurg* 1970; 33:25–28.
7. Greenwald MJ, Lissner GS, Tomita T, Naidich TP. Isolated roof fracture with traumatic encephalocele. *J Pediatr Ophthalmol Strabismus* 1987; 24:141–144.
8. Gruber FH. Post-traumatic leptomeningeal cysts. *Am J Roentgenol* 1969; 105:305–307.
9. Hansen KN, Pedersen H, Petersen MB. Growing skull fracture—rupture of coronal suture caused by vacuum extraction. *Neuroradiology* 1987; 29:502.
10. Kashiwagi S, Abiko S, Aoki H. Growing skull fracture in childhood. A recurrent case treated by shunt operation. *Surg Neurol* 1986; 26:63–66.
11. Kingsley D, Till K, Hoare R. Growing fractures of the skull. *J Neurol Neurosurg Psychiatry* 1978; 41:312–318.
12. Lende RA, Erickson TC. Growing skull fractures of childhood. *J Neurosurg* 1961; 18:479–489.
13. Locatelli D, Messina AL, Bonfanti N, et al. Growing fractures: an unusual complication of head injuries in pediatric patients. *Neurochirurgia (Stuttg)* 1989; 32:101–104.
14. Lye RH, Occleshaw JV, Dutton J. Growing fracture of the skull an the role of computerized tomography. Case report. *J Neurosurg* 1981; 55:470–472.
15. Nemoto S, Hoffman HJ. Leptomeningeal cyst of the posterior fossa. Case report. *J Neurosurg* 1986; 65:704–705.
16. Probst C. Growing bone defects of the skull-cap and the base of the skull. *Neurochirurgia (Stuttg)* 1975; 18:58–68.
17. Rahimizadeh A. Growing fracture of the skull in the elderly. *Neurosurgery* 1986; 19:675–676.
18. Ramamurthi B, Kalyanaraman S. Rationale for surgery in growing fractures of the skull. *J Neurosurg* 1970; 32:427–430.
19. Rosenthal SAE, Grieshop J, Freeman LM, Goldstein FP. Experimental observations on enlarging skull fractures. *J Neurosurg* 1970; 32:431–434.
20. Scarfo GB, Mariottini A, Tomaccini D, Palma L. Growing skull fractures: progressive evolution of brain damage and effectiveness of surgical treatment. *Childs Nerv Syst* 1989; 5:163–167.
21. Sekher LN, Scarff TB. Pseudogrowth in skull fractures of childhood. *Neurosurgery* 1980; 6:285–289.
22. Stein BM, Tenner MS. Enlargement of skull fracture in childhood due to cerebral herniation. *Arch Neurol* 1972; 26:137–143.
23. Taveras JM, Ransohoff J. Leptomeningeal cysts of the brain following trauma with erosion of the skull: a study of seven cases treated by surgery. *J Neurosurg* 1953; 10:233–241.
24. Thompson JB, Mason TH, Haines GL, Cassidy RJ. Surgical management of diastic linear skull fractures in infants. *J Neurosurg* 1973; 39:493–497.
25. Winston K, Beatty RM, Fischer EG. Consequences of dural defects acquired in infancy. *J Neurosurg* 1983; 59:839–846.

273

Facial Fractures

Gregory L. Ruff
Ronald Riefkohl
Gregory S. Georgiade
Nicholas G. Georgiade

Fractures of the facial skeleton consequent to violent accidents may cause tragic facial deformities in addition to significant disruption of vital physiologic processes. It is imperative that the physician treating these facial fractures understand the anatomy, pathology, and surgery of the head and neck and have had extensive training in the management of trauma victims.

Etiology and Incidence

The most common causes of facial fractures are high-speed motor vehicle accidents, assaults, and sporting injuries.[2,6,14] Usually motor vehicle accidents account for 40 to 50 percent of all fractures, and assaults account for another one-third. In 70 to 80 percent of the patients with midfacial fractures, the cause of injury is a high-speed motor vehicle accident.[2] The mandible is the bone most commonly fractured[6] (discounting nasal fractures). Next in frequency is the zygomaticomaxillary complex, then the nasoethmoid complex, and, finally, the maxilla.

Emergency Room Management

The first consideration is the assurance of a patent airway. The oropharynx should be cleared of tooth fragments, blood clots, dentures, and other foreign bodies. Anterior mandibular fractures may be associated with airway obstruction caused by the tongue falling into the pharynx because of lost anterior fixation.[6] Treatment is forward traction of the tongue with either a heavy stitch or a towel clamp.

Emergency tracheal intubation is necessary in some patients. It is futile to attempt orotracheal intubation in the presence of bleeding intraoral lacerations, and nasotracheal intubation may be difficult in the presence of midface fractures. A tracheostomy is often the safest and quickest means of establishing an airway, but it should be executed under optimum conditions. Tracheostomy may increase the risk of infection of facial fractures and should be reserved for cases where prolonged intubation is anticipated, as with severe brain injury or airway compromise due to a hematoma.

After an airway is secured, hemorrhage from wounds of the face, scalp, and mouth is stopped, if possible by simple pressure, although larger vessels may be temporarily suture-ligated until definitive operative exploration of the wound is made. A considerable volume of blood may be swallowed and thus be unaccounted for in estimating the patient's blood loss.

After the patient's condition is stabilized, a careful neurological examination is performed, and then the chest, abdomen, and extremities are evaluated. Finally, the facial injuries and the head and neck are examined.

In the emergency room, preliminary facial roentgenograms are obtained to confirm the clinical impression of facial fracture. In addition, views of the skull, cervical spine, and chest are essential if there is a history of significant trauma or an unreliable examination. *If a computed tomography (CT) scan to evaluate the brain is required—especially if the neck is immobilized—then plain films are obviated by scanning the entire head from the vertex through the mandible.*[5] Coronal and 3-D reformation are usually good enough to permit diagnosis of condylar fractures and to distinguish orbital fat from hematoma, as in the case of orbital herniation into the antrum.

Many patients with facial fractures, especially those caused by great violence, have other associated injuries that may be life-threatening. The incidence of associated injuries depends on the nature of the causative factors, with a higher incidence of associated injuries occurring in victims of high-speed accidents.[14,19] Major injuries that are often associated with facial fractures include pneumothorax, hemothorax, adult respiratory distress syndrome, basilar skull fracture, intra-abdominal injuries, cervical spine fractures, genitourinary injuries, and extremity fractures.[6]

Specialty consultations should be obtained while the patient is in the emergency room so that other injuries are managed immediately. Life-threatening injuries have treatment precedence over facial fractures, although temporary measures are occasionally required to facilitate later definitive fracture treatment.

Early repair is warranted given the fact that facial fractures often involve colonized mucosa and are thus compound fractures by definition. However, the patient must be stabilized and the facial injuries fully assessed. Treatment should be deferred if there is marked soft tissue edema, particularly in the case of the orbital contents, which are often compressed when the orbital walls are restored. On the other hand, the possibility of infection increases proportionally with the time interval between the injury and the time of treatment.[6] If definitive treatment of jaw fractures must be deferred, it may be necessary to implement temporary fixation by application of dental arch bars. Leakage of cerebrospinal fluid is not a contraindication to early surgery, since accurate reduction is the primary precept of treatment. The source of the leak must be addressed by the neurosurgeon to ensure adequate closure of the defect; in some cases a vascularized flap, such as a frontal pericranium or frontalis muscle flap, should be used, which may warrant involving the plastic surgeon.

After the clinical and radiologic evaluation, photographs are taken and soft tissue wounds are managed appropriately. The question of tetanus prophylaxis should be resolved, and prophylactic antibiotics should be administered if there are open fractures or if there is severe contamination of the wound.

General Principles of Treatment

The method selected for managing the injury should be the simplest and most direct. Basic operative principles include exposure of the fractures through existing lacerations or esthetically placed incisions, wound irrigation and debridement, gentle handling of tissues, perfect hemostasis, aspiration of blood and other debris from sinus cavities, obliteration of dead space by accurate layered wound closure, and accurate operative reduction and internal fixation of fractures. An adequate airway is critical postoperatively, as the surgical trauma will compound the edema from the initial injury.

Patients who have a tracheostomy are unable to communicate except by writing; thus they should be provided with pen and paper. Early ambulation prevents thrombophlebitis and pulmonary embolism and improves patient morale. Soft tissue wounds are kept clean by daily care.

If intermaxillary fixation is necessary, initial postoperative feedings are administered through a nasogastric tube, and after several days feedings may be in the form of a blenderized oral diet. Oral hygiene is maintained with a dilute peroxide mixture or commercial mouthwash. Wire cutters or strong scissors are taped to the bed or hung around the neck for immediate use in case the intermaxillary fixation must be released temporarily. The gums and buccal mucosa may become irritated from wires or arch bars; if irritation develops, wax is applied to the arch bars and wires.

The most significant recent advance in fracture repair is the use of rigid fixation. Screws and plates made of titanium or Vitallium undergo little oxidation-reduction reaction with the tissues and may firmly incorporate into the bone. The use of rigid fixation has profoundly reduced the rate of wound infection and has led to similar improvements in the degree of relapse, the union of bone grafts, and the endorsement by patients of early mobilization of the jaws.

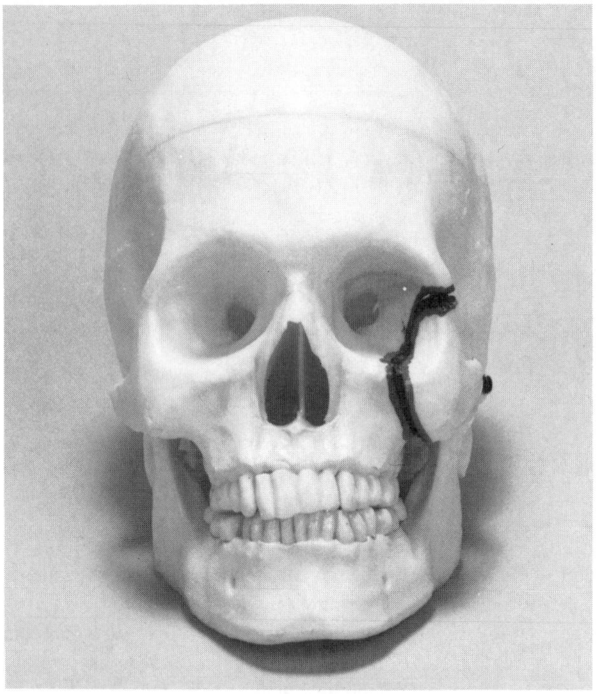

Figure 273-1 Zygomatic bone fracture. The most common site for fracture is actually through the infraorbital foramen of the adjacent maxilla.

Specific Fractures

Zygomatic Fractures

The prominence and architecture of the zygoma render it highly susceptible to fracture. A zygomatic fracture is the most common facial fracture in many series, but isolated fractures of the zygoma are not common.[2,6,18,22]

The zygomatic bone is a strong buttress between the maxilla and the cranium. Its articulations with the maxilla and frontal bone are broad and strong, but the articulations with the sphenoid and temporal bones are thin and weak. The zygomatic bone forms a portion of the lateral wall and floor of the orbit, and in occasional individuals forms the lateral superior wall of the maxillary sinus.[6] Zygomatic fractures should therefore be broadly lumped into fractures of the arch alone and zygomaticomaxillary or "tripod" fractures (Fig. 273-1). There are numerous classification schemes for zygomaticomaxillary fractures,[15] but a simple system based on the displacement and stability of the zygoma is the most applicable to treatment planning.[17]

Clinical findings depend on when the patient is first seen. If the patient is seen immediately after injury when there is minimal edema, there may be flattening of the malar eminence, bony irregularities, abnormal motion, crepitation, and anesthesia of the cheek. If the patient is seen later, periorbital edema and ecchymosis and subconjunctival hemorrhage may be the only obvious findings. With posterior and downward displacement of the zygoma, the lateral canthus, the lower eyelid, and the globe are also displaced inferiorly. The fracture through the orbital floor will tear the maxillary sinus mucosa and may result in epistaxis. There may be trismus because of impingement of the mandibular coronoid process against the posteriorly displaced zygoma, or because of medial displacement of the zygomatic arch with impingement of the fragments on the temporalis muscle and coronoid process. Anesthesia in the distribution of the infraorbital nerve is probably the most common finding and is only rarely absent. Diplopia may also be present.

The Water's view roentgenogram best demonstrates the fracture and the degree of zygomatic displacement, but the submentovertex view is necessary to visualize a fracture of the zygomatic arch. Commonly seen is opacification of the maxillary sinus; in nondisplaced fractures, this may be the only radiographic finding.

After the patient has been stabilized satisfactorily and an ophthalmologist has evaluated the eye, treatment may be instituted. Nondisplaced and minimally displaced fractures do not require treatment; however, many fractures are actually displaced more than is evident from clinical and radiographic examination. Displaced arch fractures may be treated by simple elevation, but, because there is a high incidence of redisplacement owing to the pull of the masseter, displaced tripod fractures should be reduced and rigidly fixed. Old, impacted fractures may require considerable force for reduction because of organization and fibrous union. If treated within 4 weeks, however, the bones may still be repositioned.

If there is unstable posterior displacement of the zygoma, since one review indicated that malunion was found in one-third of the patients treated with transosseous wires alone,[18] plating of the zygomatic frontal fracture is recommended. Unstable fractures of the zygomatic arch are difficult to manage. The fragments may be skewered by a small K pin or held in place by Penrose drain packing, or they may be exposed and wired directly through a coronal incision.

If the orbital floor is extensively comminuted, it must be reconstructed by autogenous tissue or by an artificial implant. Packing placed in the maxillary sinus must be removed in 7 to 10 days and, therefore, does not provide permanent stabilization of the orbital floor.[6] Packing also increases the likelihood of infection with an implant, and the implant should therefore be sufficiently rigid to prevent reherniation of orbital fat with postoperative edema.

The most common complication of zygomatic fractures is persistent infraorbital nerve anesthesia. In most cases, this gradually resolves over a 6- to 12-month period, but if there is no recovery, or if annoying dysethesia and anesthesia are present, then the infraorbital nerve may be explored. Other common complications include malunion with facial deformity, diplopia, and enophthalmos. Ocular complications include blindness, extraocular muscle dysfunction, and permanent diplopia. Nonunion and infection are rare. Chronic maxillary sinusitis may occur, particularly if sinus packing was a component of treatment. Fibro-osseous ankylosis involving the coronoid process is also rare.

Orbital Fractures

Patients who have suffered trauma in the vicinity of the orbit that was severe enough to cause a fracture should have a complete ophthalmologic evaluation prior to manipulation of the fractured bones.

Orbital fractures may be divided into fractures of the walls alone such as a blow-out fracture and those involving the rim as well.[3,6] A pure blow-out fracture involves the adjacent maxillary and/or ethmoid sinus. The basis of this classification is the contention that a blow-out fracture is a distinct injury having a specific pathophysiology and clinical presentation. The blow-out fracture supposedly is caused by an impact to the globe, which in turn transmits the force by hydraulic pressure to the orbital floor, causing a fracture.[6] This mechanism may be incorrect, since the inferior orbital rim may bend without fracturing, yet buckling and fracturing of the orbital floor results.[6]

The most common clinical finding in a blow-out fracture is diplopia. It may be present on admission but absent the following day or several days later. Diplopia, a result of deviation of the visual axis, may be caused by entrapment of soft tissues, such as the inferior rectus or inferior oblique muscle, in the fracture line.[6] However, since the orbital fat surrounding the globe and extraocular muscles has an intricate fibrous system that apparently has an important role in movements of the globe and gliding of the extraocular muscles,[16] incarceration of orbital fat rather than muscle may be the cause of diplopia. Diplopia may also be caused by downward displacement of the globe, although the binocular fusion mechanism easily compensates for globe displacement.[16] Injury to the motor nerves to the inferior oblique or inferior rectus muscle may also result in diplopia. Additional possible causes are injury to other cranial nerves or extraocular muscles, or disruption of muscle attachments. Edema and hemorrhage within the muscles may also play a role.

Enophthalmos, a common finding with blow-out fractures, may be difficult to recognize clinically and is seldom noticed by the patient. It is significant when there is a discrepancy of more than 2 mm in the distance from the cornea to the lateral orbital rim as compared with the normal side, and is disfiguring when this discrepancy is greater than 5 mm.[6] The precise cause of enophthalmos is unclear but is probably related to enlargement of the orbital cavity and escape of orbital fat through the fracture. Progressive late enophthalmos is probably due to orbital fat necrosis, resolution of edema and hematoma, and a low-grade inflammatory process. Enophthalmos results in a pseudoptosis of the upper eyelid, a deepening of the superior tarsal fold, and a shortening of the horizontal dimension of the palpebral fissure.

Other possible clinical findings with a blow-out fracture are subconjunctival hemorrhage, bleeding from the lacrimal canaliculus, periorbital ecchymosis, and anesthesia of the infraorbital nerve. With impure blow-out fractures, there may be a palpable bone irregularity, abnormal motion, soft tissue crepitation, and bone tenderness.

Radiographic opacification of the maxillary sinus without other signs of injury is not reliable evidence of a blow-out fracture.

The presence of diplopia is important to management decisions. However, in many patients, diplopia that is present immediately after the injury will resolve spontaneously without treatment.[8,21] Thus, diplopia alone is not necessarily an indication for surgery. Patients with diplopia alone should be treated by observation. If diplopia is still present after 2 weeks, then orbital exploration is indicated. A limitation of forced rotation of the eyeball (positive forced duction test), particularly if associated with significant enophthalmos or radiologic evidence of a large defect in the orbital floor, is a definite indication for operation.

Treatment principles for blow-out fractures include release of entrapped structures, replacement of escaped orbital fat into the orbital cavity, and restoration of the orbital cavity to its former size and shape.[6]

The orbital floor is usually exposed through a short incision through the lower eyelid, but many surgeons prefer a transconjunctival approach despite the reduced exposure.[6] Perhaps a transconjunctival incision is preferable for individuals with a tendency for hypertrophic scars or keloids. After exposing the inferior orbital rim, the periosteum is incised and elevated, and the entire fracture and adjacent undamaged bone are exposed. Large angulated fragments are repositioned, and, if the orbital floor defect is sizable, the floor must be reconstituted with either autogenous bone or an artificial implant. Release of entrapped structures should improve rotation of the globe as demonstrated by the forced duction test.

In many instances there is an associated blow-out fracture of the medial orbital wall, and perhaps this is the cause of late enophthalmos. Medial wall fractures are suspected if there is radiographic evidence of air in the orbit, clouding of the ethmoid sinus, or displacement of the medial orbital wall. Fractures through the lateral orbital wall and roof of the orbit are rare and usually are associated with more severe injuries.[6] Fractures involving extensive bone disruption are treated by placing an implant over the defect to prevent exophthalmos caused by herniation of intracranial contents—a so-called blow-in fracture.

The clinical findings for orbital fractures associated with high maxillary, naso-orbital, or zygomatic fractures are similar to those of the blow-out fracture, except that the forced duction test is usually negative.[6] Treatment is similar to that for blow-out fractures.

Orbital floor fractures may be complicated by late structural deformities resulting from malunion or nonunion. Artificial implants may become infected and extrude, may cause extraocular muscle dysfunction, or, rarely, may compress the optic nerve.[6] Bone graft implants may resorb, resulting in enophthalmos. There may be permanent damage to the extraocular muscles and, consequently, muscle imbalance that requires subsequent corrective surgery. Enophthalmos and its sequelae are unfortunately common after orbital fractures. Ocular complications have been reported in 15 to 30 percent of orbital fractures, with loss of vision the most severe problem.[14,19] If the patient arrives in the emergency room with loss of vision, then routine or computed tomography should be done immediately to determine if optic nerve or orbital exploration is indicated.[5] Blepharoptosis due to injury to the levator muscle or its innervation is uncommon. Vertical shortening of the lower eyelid occurs with severely displaced inferior orbital rim fractures and results in disfiguring scleral show, ectropion, or entropion.

The superior orbital fissure syndrome is associated with severe orbital, naso-orbital, or zygomatic fractures. There is interference with the function of cranial nerves III, IV, V_1, and VI because of direct bony impingement or because of bleeding into the orbital muscle cone space between the intermuscular membrane and Tenon's capsule which results in compression of the nerves against the margins of the superior orbital fissure. The syndrome consists of ophthalmoplegia, blepharoptosis, and anesthesia of the cornea and skin in the distribution of the supratrochlear and supraorbital nerves. If there is a parasympathetic block, there will be a fixed, dilated pupil. Because of paralysis of the motor nerves, the eye does not move and is proptotic. The maxillary division of the trigeminal nerve may also be involved if the fracture extends through the foramen rotundum. The syndrome may be complete, but in most instances it is partial. There is also an orbital apex syndrome, which consists of the superior orbital fissure syndrome plus blindness due to optic nerve injury. The generally accepted algorithm for intervention when there is bony contact with the optic nerve is similar to that for spinal trauma; high dose corticosteroids are used for acute blindness or a stable loss of visual acuity, while operative intervention is reserved for documented decrease in visual acuity that is refractory to steroids.[1]

Naso-Orbital Fractures

With a naso-orbital fracture, the nasal bones are forced back into the interorbital space, which is formed by the ethmoid sinuses, the superior and middle turbinates, and the perpendicular plate of the ethmoid bone.[4] The thin and fragile medial orbital walls may comminute extensively, and fragments of the roof of the interorbital space may enter the anterior cranial fossa, either at the cribriform plate or at the roof of the ethmoid sinuses. Laceration of the dura or olfactory nerve sheath, perforation of the brain, or necrosis of brain tissue may occur in serious injuries.[4] The levator palpebrae muscle, the medial canthal ligament, the lacrimal sac, or the lacrimal canaliculus may also be injured.

Clinical findings may include flattening and shortening of the nose, edema and distortion of the medial canthal region, ecchymosis and edema of the eyelids, subconjunctival hemorrhage, epistaxis, traumatic telecanthus, crepitation, and possibly CSF rhinorrhea. Plain roentgenograms are deceiving since abnormalities may be missed. Computed tomography is necessary to precisely define the full extent of the fracture.[4]

Treatment of naso-orbital injuries should be delayed until a thorough evaluation is completed and extensive edema has subsided. CSF rhinorrhea is not a contraindication to surgery, and in many instances will cease after reduction of the fracture.[4]

Although it is possible to expose these fractures through a transverse nasal incision plus bilateral medial canthal incisions, the facial scarring and interior exposure associated with this approach favor a coronal incision. Preoperative anticipation of the need for a frontalis or pericranial flap based on the supratrochlear or supraorbital vessels is important to avoid injury to them as they emerge from the orbit.[4] The medial canthal ligaments must be identified and reattached with transnasal wires, although occasionally primary bone grafts may be necessary to properly secure the canthi.[4] The medial canthi usually remain attached to the frontal process of the maxilla and should not be detached, because it is difficult to esthetically secure them and avoid lacrimal injury. Rather, the medial orbital rim must be reduced anatomically.[12] Also, a primary bone graft may be incorporated to restore the nasal dorsum.

Complications of naso-orbital fractures include structural deformities if treatment is delayed, medial canthal displacement, nasal saddle deformity, ocular complications, lacrimal system injuries (such as canalicular interruption, mucocele, and inflammatory conditions involving the lacrimal sac), blepharoptosis subsequent to loss of function of the levator muscle, and CSF rhinorrhea with recurrent meningitis.[4]

Supraorbital and Frontal Sinus Fractures

The paired frontal sinuses within the frontal bone are formed by the frontal bone and supraorbital rims. The posterior wall of the sinus is thin, yet it rarely is fractured.[20] These fractures may occur independently, but ordinarily they are associated with naso-orbital fractures or other serious facial fractures.

The clinical diagnosis is based on the findings of edema, tenderness, ecchymosis, deformity, crepitation, and abnormal motion. There may be anesthesia of the forehead because of injury to the supratrochlear and supraorbital nerves, or the trochlea of the superior oblique muscle may be injured, resulting in diplopia. There may also be CSF rhinorrhea.

Roentgenograms often fail to delineate the posterior wall of the sinus, but intracranial aerocele is pathognomonic for a posterior wall fracture and dural tear.[20]

Treatment nearly always consists of operative reduction and internal fixation, but it is advisable to observe the patient's neurological signs for 48 to 72 h prior to the operation.[6] A coronal incision is preferred for fracture exposure and to provide access for an intracranial procedure, if necessary. Intervention is dictated by the area injured: Anterior wall defects merit repair for esthetic reasons; posteriorly, the dural integrity must be assured; and severe comminution of the nasofrontal duct necessitates obliteration of the sinus mucosa. Stenting of the duct is associated with subsequent stenosis and mucocele formation. To expose the dura, the posterior wall is often resected with rongeurs, and the sinus is then "cranialized" by completely removing the mucosa and all the remaining wall. As with obliteration of the sinus for ductal injury, it is essential to burr the entire bony lining of the sinus to remove rests of mucosa. In one study, mucoceles formed in 72 percent of cats in which the lining was simply stripped.[7] Although free fat grafting to obliterate the sinus may reduce the incidence of mucocele to 4 percent (as opposed to 10 percent with spontaneous osteogenesis),[10] the most important intervention is closing the nasofrontal duct,[23] preferably with a local vascularized flap. The duct is poorly imaged if only nasofrontal reduction is used for repair; its patency is confirmed by postoperative demonstration of aeration.

Nasal Fractures

Nasal fractures usually occur at the junction of the thick and thin sections of the nasal bone and are rare in the upper, thick section except when associated with naso-orbital, Le Fort II, or Le Fort III fractures.[6]

Nasal fractures are classified into unilateral fractures with or without displacement, bilateral fractures with fracture of the septum, and open book fractures with severe comminution.[6,11] There may be concomitant injury to the nasolacrimal system, the perpendicular plate of the ethmoid bone, the ethmoid sinus, the cribriform plate, or the orbital plate of the frontal bone. The margins of the piriform aperture may also be involved. Nasal fractures rarely occur without injury to the cartilaginous septum; however, septal injuries are easy to miss, particularly in children.

Clinical findings may include edema and tenderness, deformity, periorbital ecchymosis and edema, subconjunctival hemorrhage, nasal obstruction and epistaxis, mobility, and crepitation. Intranasal evaluation is facilitated by the application of a vasoconstrictor agent to the mucosa. Standard facial roentgenograms may not reveal the nasal fracture; soft tissue technique or xeroradiograms are preferable.

Nasal fractures are treated by closed reduction, either immediately after injury, if edema is not marked, or a week to 10 days later, when edema has subsided. An Asche forceps is used to elevate and manipulate the fragments into position. Telescoping of the septum may require open reduction; for unstable septal fractures, intranasal silicone splints are necessary until fixation occurs. The nasal cavities are packed with medicated gauze, and an external plaster splint is placed on the nose for 7 days. Rarely, a nasal fracture requires open reduction, but probably this should be undertaken as an elective procedure later.

Complications of nasal fractures include hematoma of the septum and its possible sequelae, infection, synechiae between the septum and turbinates, nasal obstruction, malunion and deformity, and nonunion.

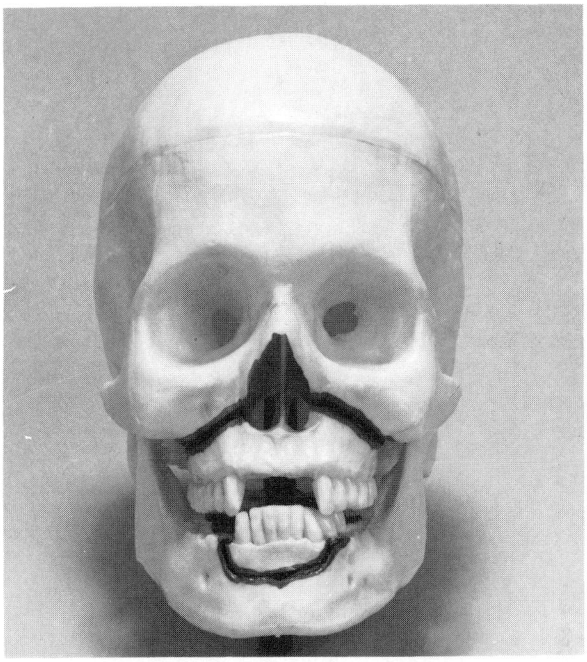

Figure 273-2 Le Fort I (transverse) maxillary fracture. The model also depicts an alveolar fracture of the mandible.

Maxillary Fractures

Owing to its mass and architectural arrangement, the maxilla is capable of resisting considerable violence. Most maxillary fractures are caused by direct impact, although some result from forces transmitted through the mandible. Muscular contraction has a minimal effect on displacement of maxillary fragments, but in the Le Fort II and III fractures, mastication may have a small role.[6]

Le Fort's experimental work with cadavers evolved into the classification of maxillary fractures into the following groups: (1) alveolar fractures; (2) transverse fractures (Le Fort I), in which the fracture line crosses the pterygoid plates and maxilla just above the apices of the teeth (Fig. 273-2); (3) pyramidal fractures (Le Fort II), in which the transverse fracture line extends obliquely upward across the inferior orbital rim and orbital floor to the medial orbital wall and then across the nasofrontal suture (Fig. 273-3); (4) craniofacial disjunction fractures (Le Fort III), in which the fracture involves the zygomatic arches, the zygomaticofrontal suture line, the nasofrontal suture line, the pterygoid plates, and the orbital floors, thus separating the entire maxilla from its cranial attachment (Fig. 273-4); and, finally, (5) vertical fractures, which occur just off the midline and are associated with other fractures of the maxilla.

Le Fort II fractures are the most common and Le Fort III are the least common type of maxillary fracture.[6] The most common cause of maxillary fractures is the automotive "guest passenger" injury, in which the individual is thrown forward during a collision and strikes the middle third of the face.[6] The consequent fracture depends on the direction and level of the impact. In many patients, multiple maxillary fractures occur together; this is especially common with the more serious injuries. Also, most patients with a fractured maxilla have another facial bone fracture.

Clinical findings may include epistaxis, periorbital ecchymosis, subconjunctival hemorrhage, facial edema, malocclusion often associated with an anterior open bite, submucosal hemorrhage or mucosal lacerations, a "dish-face" or "donkey-face" appearance, palpable bony irregularities, abnormal mobility unless the segments are impacted, crepitation, and CSF rhinorrhea. With Le Fort II and III fractures, the cribriform plate may be injured, and thus the nasal cavities should not be packed. With high Le Fort fractures there may be damage to the ethmoid bones, the nasal septum, and the lacrimal area, resulting in traumatic telecanthus. The nasolacrimal apparatus and cribriform plate are also frequently injured.

Radiographic evidence of maxillary fractures may be minimal; in many instances changes are absent entirely. There may be clouding of the maxillary or ethmoid sinuses, and in the Le Fort II and III types the fractures of the orbits and nasal bridge may be visible. The best radiographic view is the Water's view, but computed tomography will further define the fracture.

Proper reduction and fixation of jaw fractures depends on restoring and maintaining occlusion for a period of time. The maxillary and mandibular first molars are the guides for determining the correct establishment of normal occlusion,[6] but the abraded surfaces on occlusal and incisal areas of the teeth serve as useful landmarks. Fracture realignment will not be possible unless accurate occlusion is first restored.

Arch bars are ligated to all teeth, but traction should not be applied to the incisor region because the conical shape of these teeth and their roots may result in loosening. If traction in the anterior region is necessary, a circumferential mandibular wire and a maxillary suspension wire to the anterior nasal spine or piriform aperture will provide the required stability.

The timing of treatment depends on the extent of injury, but if definitive treatment is deferred, it may be appropriate to apply an arch bar for temporary stabilization, particularly if there are alveolar or vertical fractures. Isolated alveolar fractures are managed by applying an arch bar or by simply ligating teeth on the fracture fragment to adjacent teeth.[6] Six weeks of intermaxillary fixation may be necessary if good occlusion is not achieved with simple arch bar application.

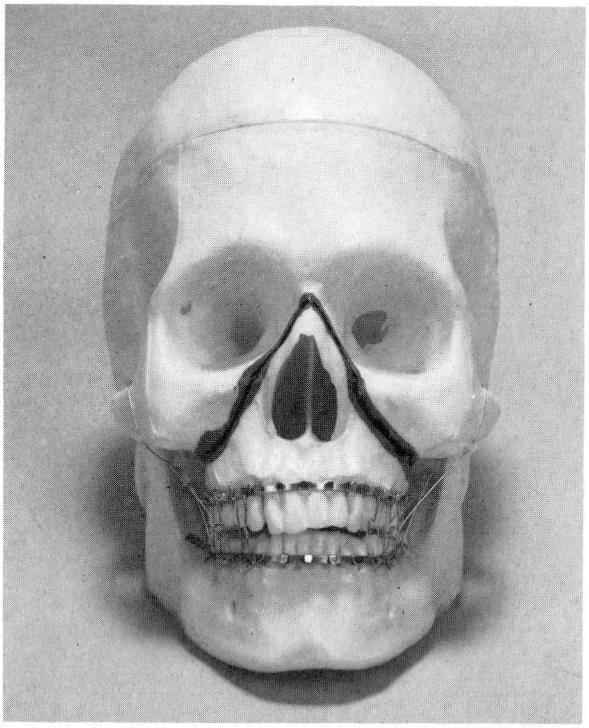

Figure 273-3 Le Fort II (pyramidal) maxillary fracture Arch bars have been ligated to the teeth and to one another. Note the two suspension wires looped around the zygomatic arches and secured to the mandibular arch bar.

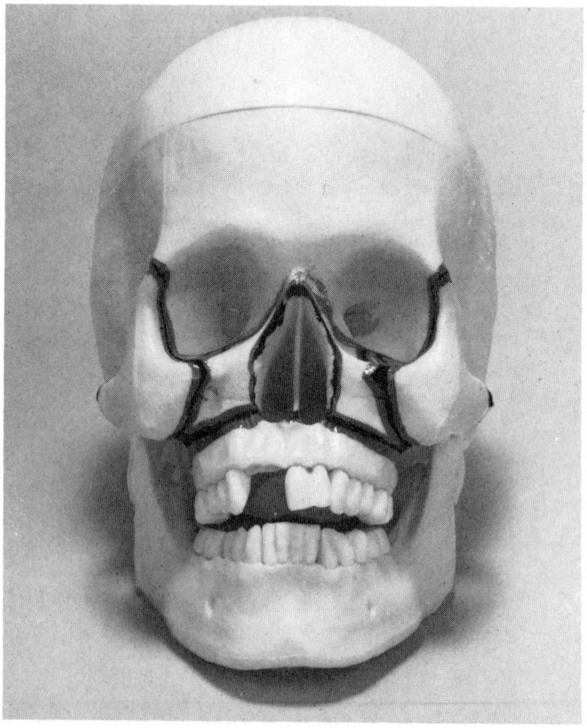

Figure 273-4 The model demonstrates a combination of Le Fort I, II, and III fractures. The Le Fort III lines extend across the zygomaticofrontal suture, then across the lateral orbital wall to the pterygomaxillary suture, which is disrupted.

Intermaxillary fixation with suspension of the arch bars to the intact skeleton superior to the fracture is one option for simple injuries. However, comminuted bone may be impacted by this technique, with consequent telescoping of the midface and loss of incisor show, so rigid fixation is indicated where comminution is present. Rigid fixation is also indicated for simple fractures in patients who would be unable to remove their intermaxillary wires in the event of emesis, such as in substance abusers, epileptics, and those of limited intellect.

Le Fort I fractures, provided there are sufficient teeth, are treated by application of arch bars and intermaxillary fixation.[6] Maxillary suspension to solid bone above the line of fracture is also necessary. Secure fixation may be obtained by permanent wires to either the piriform aperture or inferior orbital rims, or by temporary external suspension wires secured to the zygomatic arches or zygomatic processes of the frontal bone. Temporary suspension wires should be ligated to the mandibular arch bar. Open reduction is accomplished by degloving the maxilla through the upper gingival sulcus as with Le Fort II fractures.

Conservative treatment of Le Fort II and III fractures is similar to that for Le Fort I fractures, but in these more complex fractures it is best to internally ligate the fracture fragments at the infraorbital rims, the nasofrontal region, and the zygomaticofrontal region. As with the Le Fort I fracture, suspension to solid bone above combined with intermaxillary fixation is necessary. When opened, Le Fort III fractures may be best visualized by a coronal approach, although plating the lateral orbital rim through incisions below the eyebrow may suffice for minimally displaced injuries.

Fractures of edentulous maxillae are associated with extensive fractures of the middle third of the face.[6] The absence of teeth results in osteoporosis and hence fragile bone, but if little displacement occurs, treatment is unnecessary since the maxillary-mandibular relationship may be adjusted 4 to 6 weeks later by fabrication of new dentures. When there is significant displacement, however, the fracture fragments should be operatively reduced and immobilized; prefabricated dentures are secured and suspended above to solid bone as with other maxillary fractures.

When the anterior maxillary wall is crushed into multiple small fragments, resulting in deformity, packing of the maxillary sinus through a Caldwell approach has been supplanted by rigid fixation including bone grafts, preferably split cranium grafts.

Complications of maxillary fractures are rare. Profuse hemorrhage may be treated by direct ligature or packing. Uncontrolled bleeding from the internal maxillary artery is managed angiographically; removal of the posterior wall of the maxilla through a Caldwell approach and direct ligation of the vessel serves as the last alternative. Nasal airway obstruction is common with maxillary fractures, especially once intermaxillary fixation is implemented. Infection is rare and usually involves the maxillary sinus. Nonunion and malunion are rare unless there is considerable destruction of bone. Extraocular muscle imbalance is also a possibility if the fractures transgress the orbits.

Mandibular Fractures

Although the mandible is a strong bone, it has inherent areas of weakness in the region of the mental foramina, the condylar necks, and at the angles where the bodies join the rami. With resorption of alveolar bone consequent to loss of teeth, the mandible thins and is more prone to fracture.[6]

The most common site for mandibular fractures is the angle,

accounting for 30 percent of fractures. Next in frequency is the body (27 percent) followed by the condyle (20 percent). The least common location for fracture is the coronoid process.[13] About 60 percent of patients with a mandibular fracture have other mandibular fractures; of these 80 percent have two or more fractures, 50 percent have three or more fractures, 4 percent have four fractures, and 3 percent have more than four fractures. In 95 percent of the patients with multiple mandibular fractures, the fractures occur in separate areas of the mandible.[13]

Mandibular fractures may be classified on the basis of fracture direction and displacement.[6] Another useful classification is based on the presence or absence of serviceable teeth in the fracture segments, since this circumstance is so critical for treatment.[6]

Clinical findings with mandibular fractures may include pain with motion, tenderness, soft tissue edema, subcutaneous or submucosal hematoma, deformity, malocclusion, abnormal mobility, and crepitation. Deviation of the chin when the mouth is opened suggests a fracture of the condyle. The mandible deviates toward the side of the fracture (owing to loss of translation anteriorly because the lateral pterygoid muscle inserts on the condylar neck), and there will also be premature occlusion on the same side plus an open bite on the opposite side. There may also be tenderness of the temporomandibular joint. If there are bilateral condylar fractures, there is a bilateral open bite with occlusion only on the posterior teeth. The patient also complains of pain on attempting to open the mouth, but the mandible does not deviate.

Posteroanterior and lateral roentgenograms of the mandible may reveal a fracture, but pantomography x-ray films are more informative. Fractures involving the condyle may require computed tomography for precise delineation, and occlusal dental views are necessary to visualize small alveolar fractures.

The factors that influence displacement of fracture segments include the site of the fracture, the direction and angulation of the fracture, the presence or absence of teeth adjacent to the fracture, the direction of pull of muscles attached to the fragments, and the direction and intensity of the impact.[6] The muscles attaching to the mandibular fragments are mainly responsible for displacement. The strong posterior group of muscles pulls the jaw up, forward, and medially, and the weak anterior group depresses the jaw. A fracture may be favorable or unfavorable depending on both its orientation and its bevel (Fig. 273-5). Muscle action on the two fragments either distracts or impacts the fragments.

Treatment of mandibular fractures is based on the type of fracture, its location, and whether it is favorable or unfavorable. When teeth are in the mandibular fracture line, they should be extracted if there is extreme mobility, fracture of the root of the tooth, or preexisting apical disease.

A fracture between the teeth is treated with intermaxillary fixation provided the fracture is favorable. However, if the fracture is unfavorable, operative reduction and internal fixation are necessary. With proper open reduction and internal fixation, the teeth usually assume good alignment and interdigitation, but occasionally good interdigitation is not achieved with initial reduction and several days of rubber band traction are necessary to bring about normal occlusion. After normal occlusion is achieved, the rubber bands are removed and stainless steel wires are applied.

Muscular forces become much more significant for fractures in which one segment has no teeth which can be secured to an arch bar. Rigid fixation may be necessary, particularly for comminuted fractures in the region of the angle. These latter techniques have the disadvantage of greater periosteal dissection and also risk damage to teeth from drilling holes through the bone.

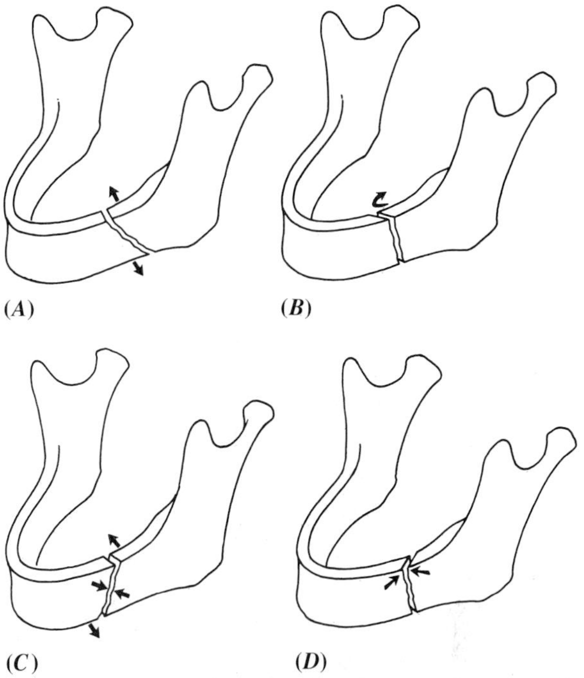

Figure 273-5 The effects of mandibular fracture orientation on fragment displacement. *A*. The posterior fragment will be displaced cephalad and the anterior fragment caudad by muscle contraction. *B*. The bevel of a vertical fracture may permit medial displacement of the posterior fragment because of muscle contraction. *C, D*. In these fractures, muscle contraction impacts the fracture fragments.

Fractures of edentulous mandibles usually occur in areas of the bone where atrophy is most marked. Because of the redundant soft tissue overlying the mandible, these fractures are rarely compound. In general, these fractures require an intraoral appliance even if there is minimal or absent displacement.[6] Again, rigid fixation is warranted for patients in whom intermaxillary fixation is contraindicated (e.g., the patient's dentures).

Direct circumferential wiring of the fragments may suffice if the fracture is sufficiently oblique, but transosseous wiring is more reliable. The fracture may be exposed through either intraoral or extraoral incisions. Wire ligatures may require removal later if there is mucosal irritation caused by a denture.

Fractures of the mandibular condyle usually occur by indirect trauma, as the condyle is protected by the overlying zygomatic arch. The fracture may occur either above or below the insertion of the lateral pterygoid muscle on the condylar neck. A fracture above the insertion is intra-articular. However, if the fracture is below the insertion, then the lateral pterygoid muscle will distract the proximal fragment anteriorly and medially. The proximal fragment may be minimally displaced or, rarely, completely dislocated out of the joint capsule. Usually the proximal fragment gradually returns to its normal position, but there may be some absorption and remodeling after fracture healing. Ordinarily, intermaxillary fixation alone is adequate treatment.[6] Direct reduction is necessary if dental occlusion cannot be reproduced, if there is an alteration in the vertical dimension of the face, or if the fragment is dislocated.[13] If the proximal fragment is displaced more than 90 degrees, particularly in children and edentulous patients, open reduction and internal fixation is indicated through either a preauricular or a Risdon incision.[6]

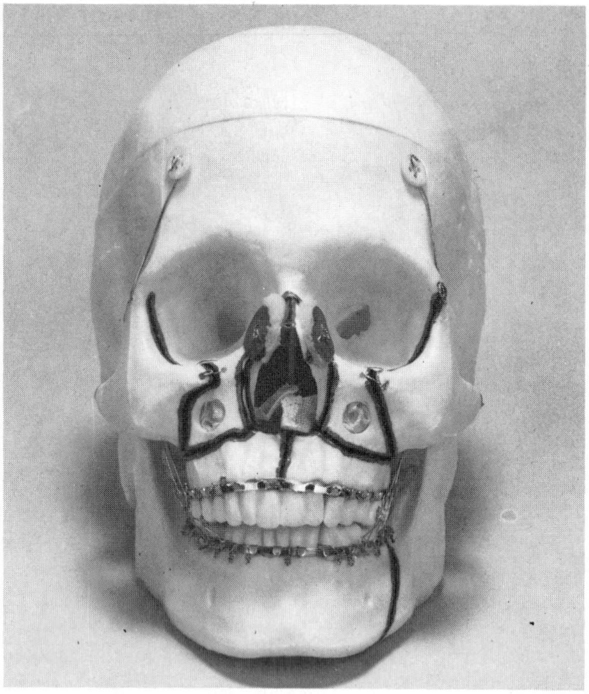

Figure 273-6 This model illustrates the repair of multiple facial fractures. The mandibular fracture is favorably oriented, and thus internal ligation is unnecessary. Arch bars have been applied to the teeth, and the inferior orbital rims and zygomaticofrontal sutures are internally ligated. Transnasal wires are secured over padded lead plates to support the naso-orbital fracture. Two suspension wires pass from the mandibular arch bar and behind the body of the zygoma to holes just above the zygomaticofrontal sutures. "Pull-out" wires are looped around the suspension wires, then passed subcutaneously upward to pierce the skin high on the forehead. These pull-out wires are tied over plastic buttons, and when the intermaxillary fixation is released, these wires are used to retrieve the two maxillary suspension wires.

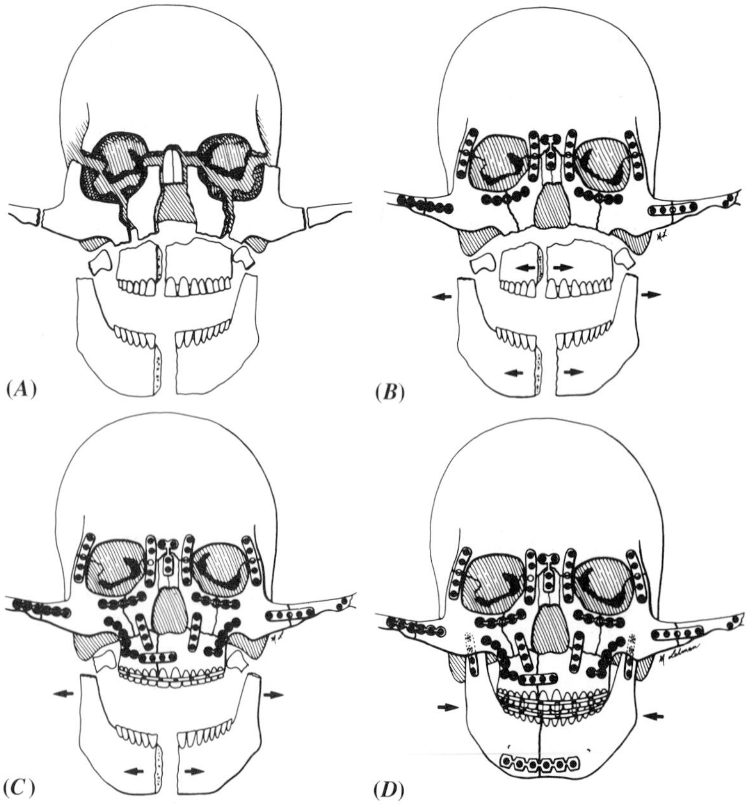

(*A*) (*B*) (*C*) (*D*)

Figure 273-7 *A* through *D* show sequential repair of a panfacial injury. The zygomatic arches first establish the anterior projection and facial width. Palatal fixation then is required to accurately align the mandible. Perhaps the most difficult aspect of such a reconstruction is reproducing facial height and, hence, the former degree of incisor show. (From Gruss et al.,[9] with permission.)

Mandibular fractures (especially with fractured, abscessed, or carious teeth) may be complicated by infection, which is minimized by wound debridement, accurate fixation, and the intravenous administration of antibiotics. Avascular necrosis, osteitis, and osteomyelitis are rare. However, nonunion, malunion, delayed union, anesthesia in the distribution of the inferior alveolar nerve, facial deformity, and malocclusion may occur. Ankylosis of the temporomandibular joint may result from condylar injury, and for this reason early motion is used, provided the closed occlusion can be maintained with light elastics on the arch bars.

Multiple Complex Fractures

Multiple facial fractures are usually a result of high-speed vehicular accidents. Serious life-threatening associated injuries are common, and the treatment of facial fractures has a low priority in the overall management of the patient.

Initial radiographic evaluation is usually not possible because of the nature of the associated injuries, but after the patient is stabilized and other injuries have been managed, a proper and thorough evaluation may be undertaken. The best time for fracture treatment is within the first 6 h, before massive edema develops, but this may not be practical when there are other injuries.

The most important principle of treatment of multiple facial fractures is direct operative reduction and rigid internal fixation (Figs 273-6 and 273-7). Unstable mandibular fractures are first operatively reduced and internally fixed, and arch bars are applied to the teeth. Next, the orbits are explored, and, finally, the central face is addressed—much as one assembles a jigsaw puzzle by first putting together the outside and then filling in the center.

Exceptions to this scheme are made in the most severe injuries, in which the palate is fractured and must be restored to properly reduce the mandible (Fig. 273-7) and when fractured condyles prevent the mandible from registering midfacial position.[9]

References

1. Anderson RL, Panje WR, Gross CE. Optic nerve blindness following blunt forehead trauma. *Ophthalmology* 1982; 89:445–455.
2. Barclay TL. Four hundred malar-zygomatic fractures. In Wallace AB (ed): *Transactions of the International Society of Plastic Surgery, Second Congress.* Edinburgh: Churchill Livingstone, 1960, pp 259–265.
3. Converse JM, Smith B, Wood-Smith D. Orbital and nasoorbital fractures. In Converse JM (ed): *Reconstructive Plastic Surgery.* Philadelphia: Saunders, 1977, pp 748–793.
4. Cruse CW, Blevins PK, Luce EA. Naso-ethmoid-orbital fractures. *J Trauma* 1980; 20:551–556.
5. Daffner RH, Gehweiler JA Jr, Osborne DR, et al. Computed tomography in the evaluation of severe facial trauma. *Comput Radiol* 1983; 7:91–102.
6. Dingman RO, Converse JM. The clinical management of facial injuries and fractures of the facial bones. In Converse JM (ed): *Reconstructive Plastic Surgery,* 2d ed. Philadelphia: Saunders, 1977, pp 599–747.
7. Donald PJ. The tenacity of the frontal sinus mucosa. *Otolaryngol Head Neck Surg* 1979; 87:557–566.
8. Emery JM, von Noorden GK, Schlernitzauer DA. Orbital floor fractures: long term follow-up of cases with and without surgical repair. *Trans Am Acad Ophthalmol Otolaryngol* 1971; 75:802–812.
9. Gruss JS, Bubak PJ, Egbert MA. Craniofacial fractures: an algorithm to optimize results. *Clin Plast Surg* 1992; 19(1):195–206.
10. Hardy JM, Montgomery WW. Osteoplastic frontal sinusotomy: an analysis of 250 operations. *Ann Otol Rhinol Laryngol* 1976; 85:523–532.
11. Harrison DH. Nasal injuries: their pathogenesis and treatment. *Br J Plast Surg* 1979; 32:57–64.
12. Jackson IT. Classification and treatment of orbitozygomatic and orbitoethmoid fractures: the place of bone grafting and plate fixation. *Clin Plastic Surg* 1989; 16:77–91.
13. James RB, Fredrickson C, Kent NJ. Prospective study of mandibular fractures. *J Oral Surg* 1981; 39:275–281.
14. Jurkiewicz MJ, Nickell WB. Fractures of the skeleton of the face. *J Trauma* 1971; 11:947–958.
15. Knight JS, North JF. The classification of malar fractures: an analysis of displacement as a guide to treatment. *Br J Plast Surg* 1961; 13:325–339.
16. Koornneef L. Current concepts on the management of orbital blow-out fractures. *Ann Plast Surg* 1982; 9:185–200.
17. Larsen OD, Thomsen M. Zygomatic fractures: I. A simplified classification for practical use. *Scand J Plast Reconstr Surg* 1978; 12:55–58.
18. Larsen OD, Thomsen M. Zygomatic fractures: II. A follow-up study of 137 patients. *Scand J Plast Reconstr Surg* 1978; 12:59–63.
19. McCoy FJ, Chandler RA, Magnan CG Jr, et al. An analysis of facial fractures and their complications. *Plast Reconstr Surg* 1962; 29:381–391.
20. Newman MH, Travis LW. Frontal sinus fractures. *Laryngoscope* 1973; 83:1281–1292.
21. Putterman AM, Stevens T, Urist MJ. Nonsurgical management of blow-out fractures of the orbital floor. *Am J Ophthalmol* 1974; 77:232–239.
22. Tempest MN. The surgical management of displaced fractures of the malar bone and zygomatic arch: a review of 275 consecutive cases. In Wallace AB (ed): *Transactions of the International Society of Plastic Surgery, Second Congress.* Edinburgh: Churchill Livingstone, 1960, p 259.
23. Walsh TE. Experimental surgery of the frontal sinus. The role of the ostium and nasofrontal duct in postoperative healing. *Laryngoscope* 1943; 53:75.

274

Cerebrospinal Fluid Fistula and Pneumocephalus

Ayub Khan Ommaya

Management of cerebrospinal fluid (CSF) leakage from the nose or ear demands a clear understanding of the etiology and pathogenesis of such dural fistulae. Most such leaks occur through the base of the skull, a fact undoubtedly related to the particular anatomy of the area and the inexorable force of gravity. The fundamental cause of CSF leakage is a meningeal fistula caused by a number of factors that will be discussed below. It should also be emphasized, however, that a second critical factor is impaired tissue repair, which may be due to lack of proper closure, inadequate support of weak healing tissues, and poor healing of tissues owing to infection, metabolic disorders, or other chronic diseases. Leakage is facilitated when the intracranial pressure (ICP) is elevated from any cause.

Although traumatic leakage of CSF is overwhelmingly more common, the first published case of CSF rhinorrhea was of a nontraumatic "high-pressure" type due to hydrocephalus.[46] This report by Miller in 1826 was followed by that of King in 1834,[34] and of Thomson in 1899 on so-called spontaneous rhinorrhea.[63] Neurosurgical treatment of such dural fistulas began much later with the work of Grant[26] and Dandy.[14] Three cases of traumatic leakage treated surgically were reported in 1927 by Cushing.[13] The first series of cases treated by a transcranial extradural repair using fascia lata was published by Cairns in 1937.[8] The transnasal approach to this problem was limited to cauterization until 1948, when Dohlman described a transnasal (transethmoidal) approach that could seal off leaks through the cribriform plate with a septal and middle turbinate flap.[18] The intradural repair technique that is currently the most widely used method was first used by Taylor, as reported by Eden in 1941.[21]

Classification

We previously published an etiologic classification developed some years ago that has been generally accepted (Fig. 274-1).[50,53,60] The categories shown are for didactic purposes and are certainly not mutually exclusive as far as the mechanism of leakage is concerned. Certain cases of delayed-onset traumatic CSF rhinorrhea have symptoms and signs identical to those of nontraumatic cases, and the actual precipitating cause of the leak may be identical. Voena has described such cases in which a congenital anomaly was found.[66] Analogously, the onset of nontraumatic CSF rhinorrhea in certain cases of pituitary tumor not subjected to surgery but treated with x-irradiation suggests atrophy of tissues as a common etiologic factor with delayed-onset traumatic leaks. However, the mode of onset, complications, and role of raised ICP in the traumatic and nontraumatic groups are significantly different. Nontraumatic leaks are much less common, are insidious in onset, and may persist for years. In most traumatic cases (>50 percent), rhinorrhea stops within 1 week and in most within 6 months. The flow of CSF is greater in the nontraumatic type, the side affected is not constant, aeroceles rarely develop intracranially, and anosmia, found in 78 percent of traumatic cases, is rare. Headache is common in nontraumatic cases. Traumatic CSF leaks bear no relationship to age or sex, whereas the nontraumatic variety affects adults mainly over 30 and females twice as often as males. Meningitis, the main danger in traumatic cases, is much less common in the nontraumatic variety. These and other contrasts between the two major subdivisions of dural fistula are given in Table 274-1.

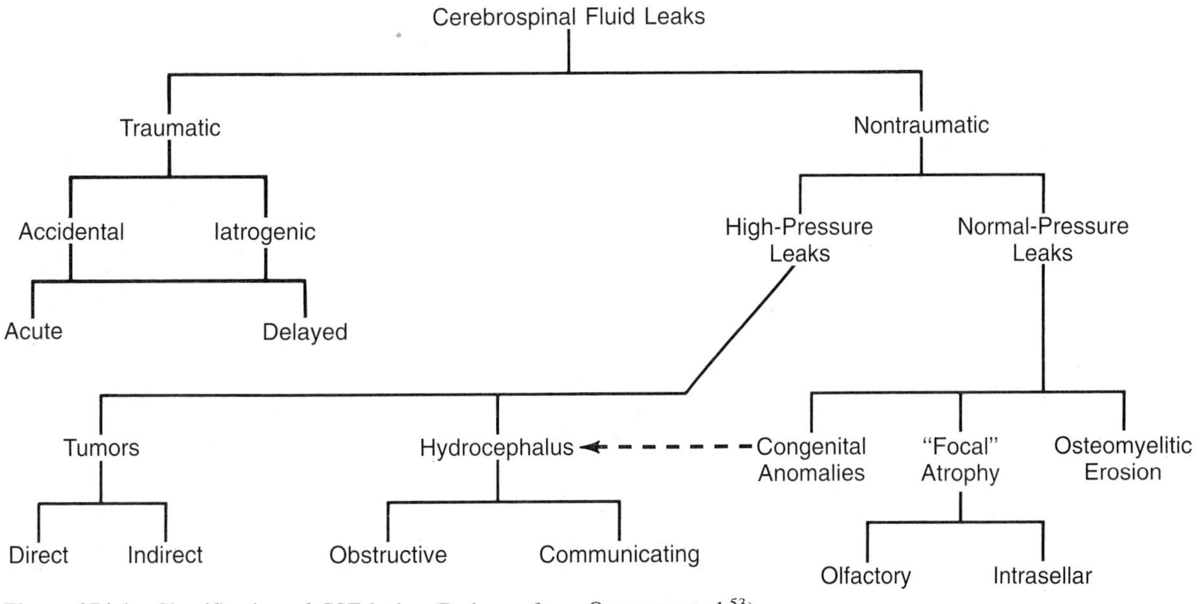

Figure 274-1 Classification of CSF leaks. (Redrawn from Ommaya et al.[53])

TABLE 274-1 Features of Traumatic and Nontraumatic CSF Leakage

Traumatic	Nontraumatic
Incidence	
Approximately 2% of unselected head injuries; relatively common condition	Rare condition; relatively few cases cited in literature
Age and Sex	
Irrespective of age, sex	Usually in mature adults (over 28); average age 43; females predominate (2:1)
Onset	
Usually within 48 h of trauma; occasionally after a few weeks; rarely after months; longest interval reported is 4½ years; onset is always abrupt	Insidious, often mistaken for allergic rhinitis; later becomes profuse flow; in a few cases, after bout of headache, sneezing
Duration of Leakage	
Over 70 percent cease within 1 week, 20–30% may continue for months; it is very unusual for flow to persist for years; nearly all stop within 6 months; recurrent leakage is very rare	Untreated leak may persist for years; in about one-third of cases spontaneous arrest occurs; flow is characteristically intermittent; recurrent leak after long stoppage is common
Amount of Leakage	
From few drops to few ounces daily; profuse leakage extremely unusual	Usually profuse flow; varies from few ounces to over 30 oz daily
Laterality	
Usually unilateral, and this often indicates side of fistula, but side of fracture is better index	Variable; bears no relation to side of fistula
Aerocele and Intracranial Air	
Found in about 20% of cases	Unusual
Anosmia	
Present in 78% of cases	Sense of smell usually preserved
Headache	
Relatively uncommon; in about 10% of cases, usually when marked aerocele or profuse flow is present; this headache is not relieved by flow	Fairly common; characteristically, cessation of flow associated with headache, then relieved by onset of flow, particularly seen in the high-pressure category
Risk of Infection	
High, from 25% to 50% of untreated cases	Lower when factor of longer duration is taken into consideration; appears to be especially true of those cases due to intracranial tumors, that is, high-pressure leaks

Source: Adapted from Ommaya et al.[53]

There is a certain degree of semantic confusion in the literature concerning the nasal leakage of CSF when trauma is not the cause. The term *spontaneous CSF rhinorrhea* has been used more or less consistently to describe such cases since the monograph by St. Clair Thomson in 1899.[63] Further subdivision of this category into *primary spontaneous* (or *idiopathic*) *rhinorrhea* when no precipitating cause could be found and *secondary spontaneous rhinorrhea* when a cause, usually a tumor, was discovered clearly reveal the nosological inadequacy of such a term as *spontaneous* CSF rhinorrhea, which indicates neither the pathogenesis nor the natural history of the disease. The word *spontaneous* means "arising from natural impulse, without external stimulant, or having a self-contained cause or origin, or arising from or entirely determined by the internal operative or directive forces of the organism" (*Shorter Oxford English Dictionary,* 1962). Careful study of the natural history of patients suffering from nontraumatic CSF leaks reveals no actual case that can fit such a definition—that is, in being truly "spontaneous"—hence our preference for the more general term *nontraumatic CSF rhinorrhea.* This category may then be subdivided etiologically as shown in Fig. 274-1.

A very important subdivision of the nontraumatic group is into *high-pressure* and *normal-pressure* categories. In the high-pressure category the leakage of cerebrospinal fluid is usually acting as a safety valve, closure of which may worsen the patient's condition if the causative lesion is not treated.

Diagnosis

Identification of CSF as the leaking fluid usually must precede demonstration of the cause as well as localization of the fistula itself. Biochemical tests on the collected fluid must show values for sugar of more than 30 mg/dl to be conclusive. It should be noted, however, that although a test with a Dextrostix reagent strip (Ames Division, Miles Laboratories, Inc., Elkhart, IN) has a 45 to 75 percent chance of positive results with normal nasal secretions, a negative test is often very useful, particularly in traumatic cases with serosanguinous leaks.[24] Positive identification of CSF necessitates introduction of suitable tracers into the CSF cavities and their recovery in the nasal discharge and is combined with the methods of fistula localization considered below.[43]

Over half of the cases with nontraumatic rhinorrhea are high-pressure leaks due to tumors, and the diagnostic approach to such patients should therefore be the same as that for patients with epilepsy of late onset, i.e., to vigorously pursue the possibility of a space-occupying lesion with the added proviso that the fistula must also be located.

The precise localization of the leakage is often a difficult and challenging problem. Possible leaking sites may be numerous and may occur in the anterior, middle, and posterior fossae. Most frequently the CSF reaches the nasal cavity through the frontal sinus, the lamina cribrosa, the sphenoidal roof, or the petrous bone via the middle ear and the eustachian tube. Lateralization of the leak according to nostril side is not reliable.

Table 274-2 summarizes the techniques available for localizing and lateralizing CSF fistulas. These include the use of dyes, fluorescent substances, radioactive tracers, and radiographic techniques.[3] Dyes (methylene blue, phenolsulfonphthalein, indigo carmine) have been introduced before or during surgery within the subarachnoidal spaces or intranasally for visual localization of the fistula. Fluorescein has also been used. However, most of these dyes, and particularly methylene blue, can cause significant morbidity.[70] In 1956, the use of radioactive sodium (^{24}Na) injected into the cisterna magna and detected by cotton pledgets distributed against the walls and roof of the nose and nasopharynx and the openings of the eustachian tubes was reported by Crow and colleagues.[12] Similar isotope-counting techniques have been reported employing radioiodinated serum albumin (RISA). Isotope cisternography was introduced by our group at the National Institutes of Health and has been used successfully to visualize the fistula in

TABLE 274-2 Diagnostic Procedures for CSF Fistula Localization

Modality	Agent	Comment
A. Dyes	1. PSP 2. Indigo carmine	Dyes are not recommended unless radioisotopes are not available
B. Photoluminescence	Fluorescein	As for A
C. Radiography with x-ray films and computed tomography	1. Conventional films of skull base 2. Tomography (pluridirectional) 3. Pneumoencephalography 4. Subdural pneumography (with tomography) 5. Positive contrast radiography	All are useful procedures. Provisos are: 1. Must show paranasal sinuses 2. Is particularly of value in traumatic leaks and in high-pressure nontraumatic leaks 3. Useful mainly for anterior leaks communicating with ventricles 4. Applicable only to frontal traumatic leaks 5. Especially of value in posterior and middle fossa leaks using metrizamide CT cisternography
D. Radioisotopic assessment	1. ^{99m}Tc-labeled albumin 2. Chelated ^{169}Yb-labeled diphosphothiamine	Fistula track only seen if leak is profuse and track large; accumulation of nuclide in sinus also helps localization; anteroposterior views are essential
E. Surgical methods	Retrograde air insufflation via nasopharynx while surgeon looks for bubbles intracranially	Carries risk of introducing infection and is therefore not recommended

many cases of traumatic and nontraumatic CSF rhinorrhea.[15,17,53] In 1972, a review of the use of isotopes in the assessment of CSF pathways was published by Holman and Davis.[28]

Plain roentgenograms may demonstrate air-fluid levels in the sphenoid sinus and may also reveal an enlarged sella turcica, and tomography may demonstrate suspicious bone defects. Pneumoencephalography has also been used to show a dilated intrasellar subarachnoid pocket, which, by acting as a tense, pulsating cyst, may be responsible for a rupture in the sellar floor.[7,22] The use of a pneumoencephalogram to decide between such a cyst and a pituitary adenoma has now been completely replaced by computed tomography (CT). Subdural pneumography may be useful in traumatic cases with leaks through the anterior cranial fossa. Various attempts have been made to localize a CSF fistula by Pantopaque or metrizamide injected into the subarachnoid space,[58] into the ventricular system, into a pneumocephalic cavity, or intranasally.[61] After the injection of such media, the passage of the opaque material is observed with fluoroscopy and radiography. The use of less irritating water-soluble positive contrast media such as metrizamide combined with CT scanning and suitable image reconstruction can often be extremely useful in pinpointing leak locations. However, despite the foregoing, it should be noted that the dictum of Dandy that visualization of the fistula may on occasion be impossible is still true today.

Traumatic CSF Leaks

Diagnosis of Traumatic Leaks

CSF leaks after trauma produce a risk of meningitis, which on occasion is fulminant in onset. Lewin has reported one patient with a fracture involving the frontal sinus, who died within 36 h after CSF rhinorrhea following head injury.[37] Pyogenic meningitis developed and the patient died in spite of antibiotics started within a few hours of the injury. Wehrle and coworkers reported a 21 percent incidence of meningitis after traumatic CSF leaks.[68] Lewin noted that in two-thirds of the patients in his extensive series, leaks started within 48 h of the trauma, while in most of the remainder delayed leaks occurred up to 3 months after head injury. In a few cases the onset was delayed by many months or even years, the longest delay being 9 years in this series. The longest published delayed onset of CSF rhinorrhea was 14 years.[38] Spontaneous closure of such fistulae occurs by adhesions or herniations of brain into bony crevices or by granulation tissue resulting from local meningitis. The quality of closure is thus often inadequate, and the risk of meningitis may remain in some cases of spontaneous closure. It is imperative, therefore, to search for evidence of CSF leakage in all patients with head injury, particularly those with fractures of the skull base. Specific fracture patterns that should be looked for are a fracture that passes through the frontal or ethmoidal sinuses or the common middle fossa fracture that passes parallel to the long axis of the petrous bone. The latter type of fracture almost always involves the middle ear, and if the tympanic membrane is torn, CSF otorrhea is evident. If the tympanic membrane is not torn, fluid will be visible through it in the middle ear. Transverse temporal bone fractures pass at right angles to the petrous pyramid and thus damage the membranous labyrinth but rarely tear the tympanic membrane. Meningitis is usually of delayed onset in such cases. Many cases of meningitis may be due to an undiagnosed transverse temporal fracture, the healing of endochondral bone being notoriously poor. An episode of otitis media at any time following such a fracture is capable of causing meningitis because of the communication between the middle ear and the subarachnoid space.[32]

In acute traumatic leaks, the CSF invariably is bloody initially and then becomes clear. Delayed leaks may present with a fairly sudden copious gush or as an attack of meningitis without an obvious leak. The rate and constancy of the leakage are probably key factors in determining the onset of meningitis. Copious, continuous leakage is probably less likely to be associated with meningitis than is a scanty, "stop and go" type of leak.

The overall incidence of CSF leaks with meningitis in head-injured patients varies between 0.25 to 0.5 percent. In Lewin's series of 100 unselected patients with head injury, 7 percent had basal skull fractures, of which one-third, or 2 percent of the total, had CSF leaks.[37] One-quarter of these patients (i.e., 0.5 percent of the total) developed meningitis. MacGee and associates reported a lower incidence of 0.25 percent in their series.[39]

In addition to the clinical search for evidence of a CSF leak or meningitis, the skull films should also be carefully examined for the presence of fluid levels in the sinuses[53] and for the presence of intracranial air. In Lewin's series, air was present intracranially in one-third of the patients with CSF leakage.[37] Marc and Schecter have described a pneumoencephalographic technique by which positioning the patient with a leak can create an air-fluid level in the sphenoid sinus if that is the site of the fistula.[41] A similar maneuver can also be used prior to CT scanning. Other clinical evidence may also alert one to the possibility of a fractured sinus and thus the risk of CSF leakage and meningitis. Thus, CSF escaping via the ethmoidal sinuses may collect in the periorbital tissues to cause local edema. In 50 percent of patients with fractures involving the sphenoid sinus, nearby structures are damaged and form the presenting neurological deficit, e.g., visual defects due to chiasmatic injury and evidence of trauma to the hypothalamus or internal carotid artery. However, one-third of patients with fractures involving the paranasal sinuses but with no obvious leak will be found to have no dural tear on intracranial exploration of the sinus fracture.

Although gamma scintigraphic display of the CSF fistula is eminently desirable, there is still a place for the simpler method of Crow and colleagues, particularly when plain x-ray films show a fracture passing through the cribriform plate and a gamma camera is not available.[12,31] A quantitative variant of this technique using chelated ^{111}In-labeled diethylenetriaminepentaacetic acid (DTPA) has also been published.[49] Results of a detailed analysis of the use of isotope cisternography in CSF rhinorrhea by Oberson[49] are summarized in Table 274-3. There were a total of 71 patients referred with a clinical suspicion of CSF rhinorrhea. The necessity for persistance and care in the use of this method is illustrated by the fact that of 29 definite leaks displayed, the majority (i.e., 7 of 11 large and 10 of 18 small fistulas) were seen only on the 24-h scan. A basal cisternal pouch was not thought to be diagnostic unless it was retained on the 24-h scan. Lateralization of the leak, a key need of the surgeon, was possible in only one-third of cases, an experience in keeping with our own.[16] Measurable isotope contamination of the nasopharynx was variable and did not correspond to the side of the fistula in 10 percent of cases. The 34 patients who had negative radioisotope signs in spite of a clinical suspicion of CSF rhinorrhea or otorrhea had no subsequent evidence of a leak in their clinical course, and none developed meningitis. All patients with a positive scan had radioactive handkerchiefs. Washing of the nostrils with physiologic water demonstrated contamination of the mucosa in eight cases of CSF fistula without evidence of rhinorrhea. In cases where the handkerchiefs were equivocal, radioactivity in the saliva was compared with the activity of the rinsing water. The test is considered positive only if the radioactivity of the handkerchief is greater than that of the saliva. The saliva is always somewhat radioactive because the resorption of radioiodine varies from one solution to another depending on the stability of the preparation. Alazraki and associates have recommended the use of 10 percent dextrose in water as a vehicle for the radioisotope in order to provide a hyperbaric medium, which apparently results in fewer scan failures, higher count efficiency, and decreased radiation exposure.[2] The most commonly used radioisotope is ^{99m}Tc-DTPA. PET scanning with ^{68}Ga ethylenediaminetetraacetic acid (EDTA) has been used to demonstrate a leak in one case.[5]

TABLE 274-3 Radioisotope Signs and Incidence in CSF Rhinorrhea

Sign	No. of Cases	Time of Positive Scan (No. of Cases): On First Day	On Second Day
No visible fistula	34	0	0
Large fistula	11	4	11
Small fistula	18	6	16
Basal cisternal pouch	22	13	20
Rhinopharyngeal contamination	19	6	17
Radioactive handkerchiefs	29	15	29
Rinsings from nostrils	8	–	8

Source: Summarized from Oberson.[49]

In difficult cases where the side and site of the fistula are not obvious, and particularly in cases of CSF otorrhea where it is not clear whether the leak is via the middle fossa or posterior fossa, positive contrast myeloencephalography and ventriculography are recommended.[19] Special care must be taken to use small amounts of the contrast medium and careful x-ray techniques. The risk of meningeal inflammation must always be kept in mind. (This caveat is true for all methods used to display the fistulous tract using chemical substances.)

Manelfe and colleagues have shown that one disadvantage of CT metrizamide cisternography is that leaks are not detected unless there is active drainage during the procedure.[40] A comparison of contrast-enhanced CT cisternography and isotope cisternography for the detection of CSF leaks in children showed the latter to be more sensitive.[69] Further details on the technical aspects of isotope cisternography may be found in one of our recent publications.[54]

Iatrogenic Traumatic Fistulae

CSF leakage through the nose after pituitary surgery and through the ear after surgery in the cerebellopontine angle were much more common in the past. With the introduction of the surgical microscope and the enormous facilitation of technique, this complication has been markedly reduced. In recent series, CSF leakage has been reported in only 5 to 10 percent of patients having an operation for acoustic neuroma[30,71] and in 3 to 6 percent of patients undergoing microneurosurgical pituitary surgery.[10,65] The routine use of fat grafts and fascial and muscle stamps to close any fistula created at the time of surgery has significantly reduced the incidence of this complication in contemporary practice.

Treatment of Traumatic Leaks

The surgical approach to traumatic leaks ranges from the vigorous one of Cairns[8,9] and Lewin,[37] who recommended exploration and repair of all leaks as soon as the patient is fit for surgery, to the more moderate approach of waiting to see if spontaneous arrest will occur. Apart from the special case of fractures involving the frontal sinus, which have a high risk of meningitis, the data are inadequate to justify immediate repair of dural fistulae caused by trauma. Five areas of controversy that do require further discussion are as follows.

1. Duration of Conservative Management before Surgery Most leaks stop spontaneously, and a significant number do not develop complications. Moreover, no surgical repair guarantees closure of all possible leaks. It is reasonable, therefore, to wait for the general condition of the patient to stabilize after the head injury. During the first week to 2 weeks, indications for surgery are:

(1) no decrease in the rate of CSF flow over 6 to 8 days, (2) an initial decrease of flow followed by continuation of flow for more than 10 to 12 days, (3) the presence of intracranial air on x-ray examination, (4) meningitis (surgery to follow medical control and recovery from meningitis), or (5) a special circumstance, e.g., a very extensive skull fracture involving the sinuses, especially frontal, or, in the course of surgery for a compound skull fracture, discovery of a dural tear.

2. *Antibiotics* Nose and throat cultures should be taken immediately, and all patients should be placed on antibiotics immediately thereafter. The antibiotics should be changed according to the culture results as they are discovered. Postoperative antibiotics are required only for 3 to 5 days. Broad-spectrum antibiotics are not recommended, and all cultures must be repeated at 48-h intervals in the first week.

3. *Timing of Sinus Repair* It is not necessary that sinus repair should precede the fistula repair. Cairns showed that sinusitis rarely follows sinus injury, whereas meningitis is a real risk.[8,9] The only exception to this advice is in the case of mastoid sinus injuries. Repair of the mastoid sinuses should precede closure of a related CSF fistula.

4. *CSF Drainage* This should not be used because of the high risk of reversing the flow gradient and inducing infection.

5. *Timing of Reduction of Facial Fractures in Association with CSF Rhinorrhea* Collins has reviewed 19 patients of this type and recommends early reduction (within 48 h) of the facial fractures to avoid poor primary healing of the fracture as well as the risk of meningitis. This author also emphasizes the increased difficulty of reducing partly healed fractures and the supportive advantage of a reconstituted bony support structure at the time of surgical closure of the CSF fistula.

Conservative management while waiting for the decision about operation should consist of total bed rest, 15 to 20 degree elevation of the head to decrease ventricular pressure, cultures of the nose and throat, and penicillin, 1 to 2 million units per day. In children, ampicillin is of value because of the risk of *Haemophilus influenzae* infection. Traumatic otorrhea stops spontaneously more frequently than traumatic rhinorrhea and, if persistent, is suggestive of raised intracranial pressure.

Nontraumatic CSF Leaks

Diagnosis of Nontraumatic Leaks

The clinical presentation of nontraumatic leaks is clearly different, as indicated earlier and as summarized in Table 274-1. Patients may present either with a leak as part of a neurological picture of a space-occupying lesion (i.e., a high-pressure leak), as a simple "leaky nose" often mistaken for a "rhinitis," or as recurrent meningitis without an obvious leak. The flow of CSF is usually more copious than with a traumatic leak and is often heavier on arising in the morning. This type of CSF leakage seldom stops spontaneously, and thus the first aim in diagnosis is to determine whether a high-pressure or normal-pressure type of mechanism is causative. Our experience with 19 cases of nontraumatic leaks in these two major subcategories is summarized in Tables 274-4 and 274-5.

TABLE 274-4 Summary of Case Material, Normal-Pressure Leaks

Case No.	Age	Lesion*	Surgery for: Lesion	Surgery for: Rhinorrhea	Result: Lesion	Result: Rhinorrhea	Follow-up Results
1	54	Hole in cribriform plate with arachnoid hernia	Yes	Yes (same operation)	Recurred	Recurred	Leak persists minimally 10 yr after surgery with no attacks of meningitis.
2	58	Arachnoid hernia into enlarged "empty sella"	Yes	Yes (same operation)	Cured	Cured	No further leak 6 yr after surgery; patient well.
3	32	Hole in cribriform plate with meningeal hernia	Yes	Yes (same operation)	Cured	Cured	No further leak 25 yr after surgery; patient well.
4	4	Nasal encephalocele	Yes	Yes (same operation)	Cured	Cured	No further leak 16 yr after surgery; patient well.
5	24	Hole in cribriform plate with brain and meningeal hernia	Yes	Yes (same operation)	Cured	Cured	No further leak 16 yr after surgery; patient well.
6	52	Hole in anterior cranial fossa with meningeal hernia	Yes	Yes (5 operations)	Recurred	Recurred	Leak persisted until death 11 yr after first operation; autopsy confirmed congenital hole; no evidence of tumor.
7	50	Hole in front of sella turcica	Yes	Yes (same operation)	Cured	Cured	No further leak 6 yr after surgery; patient well.
8	48	Hole in floor of sella with arachnoid hernia into sella	Yes	Yes (same operation)	Cured	Cured	No further leak 6 yr after surgery; patient well.
9	43	Hole in posterior aspect of sella floor in patient diagnosed as having "pituitary tumor" but having an empty sella with 3 yr of scanty CSF leak	No	Yes	Unchanged	Cured	No further leak at 1 yr after surgery.

*Analysis of 50 cases of normal-pressure nontraumatic leaks suggests that the fistula is equally likely to be located in the cribriform zone or in the floor of the sella and through the sphenoid sinus.

TABLE 274-5 Summary of Case Material, High-Pressure Leaks

Case No.	Lesion*	Surgery for Lesion	Surgery for Rhinorrhea	Result Lesion	Result Rhinorrhea	Follow-up Results
10	Pituitary adenoma; leak via sella floor	Yes (1)†	Yes (2)	Cured	Recurred	Leak persists 6 yr after surgery; on replacement therapy and penicillin.
11	Acoustic neurinoma; leak via eustachian tube?	Yes (1)	No	Cured	Cured	No leak for 6 yr.
12	Acoustic neurinoma; leak via eustachian tube?	Yes (2)	No	Cured	Cured	No leak for 9 yr.
13	Nasopharyngeal carcinoma	Yes (1)	No	Persisted	Stopped	Died after 1 yr; no autopsy.
14	Pituitary adenoma	Yes (1) +DXr‡	No	Persists	Stopped	No leak 5 yr later.
15	Pituitary tumor	No DXr only	No	?Cured	Persists	Minimal leak persists; patient refuses surgery; 6 yr.
16	Pituitary adenocarcinoma; leak via sellar floor	Yes (2) +DXr	Yes	?Cured	Cured	Massive tumor regressed after irradiation; no tumor recurrence for 3 yr; leak arrested.
17	Third ventricle tumor; leak in cribriform plate	No	Yes (shunt)	Persists	Cured	No leak for 11 yr.
18	Cerebellar glioma; leak via cribriform plate	Yes (3)	Yes (1)	?Cured	Cured	No leak or tumor recurrence for 6 yr.
19	Cerebellar glioma; leak via cribriform plate	Yes (3)	Yes (2)	?Cured	Persisted	Died from pulmonary embolism after second leak surgery.

* Analysis of 50 cases of high-pressure leaks suggests the following distribution for sites of fistulae: cribriform zone, 75%; sellar floor, 21%; via the eustachian tube, 4%. This distribution did *not* correspond to the sites of tumors, most of which were pituitary lesions.

† Numbers in parentheses refer to number of operations.

‡ DXr, Deep x-ray therapy.

Each of the etiologic factors in the two categories will now be reviewed in turn. Leakage caused by tumors is subdivided in our classification into *direct* and *indirect* types. This indicates the two ways in which the fistula may be created by the tumor—that is, either directly by tumor eroding the meninges and bone (cases 10 to 16 in Table 274-5) or indirectly via high intracranial pressure causing erosion of anatomically fragile areas of the skull base (cases 17, 18, and 19 in Table 274-5). It is significant that in all three of these indirect rhinorrheas the fistula was in the cribriform plate, an indication of the fragility of this area. Previous reports on tumor-induced CSF rhinorrhea[25,56,62] have emphasized that pituitary tumors are the most common lesions, and in our series of 10 patients with high-pressure leaks there were four such cases (cases 10, 14, 15, and 16 in Table 274-5). It should be stressed that CSF rhinorrhea is an extremely rare complication of such tumors.

Congenital anomalies and hydrocephalus are much less common than tumors in causing CSF rhinorrhea. The earliest report, by Miller, was of a case in which the hydrocephalus was the communicating type.[46] Occasionally hydrocephalus is associated with a congenital anomaly as the cause of a *high-pressure* CSF leak, and such an association has been reported with Crouzon's disease and Albers-Schoenberg disease (osteopetrosis). In most cases, however, congenital anomalies are etiologically more important for *normal-pressure* leaks. Here, nasal encephalocele is the usual lesion discovered (case 4 in Table 274-5), and such patients are the usual examples of normal pressure leaks occurring in childhood.

Congenital anomalies may also play a role in the next category of our classification, namely ''focal atrophy.'' We first proposed this speculative idea in 1968, suggesting that the normal contents of the cribriform plate or sella turcica areas are reduced in bulk. This atrophy may be due to ischemia, and the empty space thus created is filled with an arachnoidal pouch. This pouch, which is simply an extension of the normal CSF space—for example, the intrasellar cistern—enables the normal CSF pressure pulse to exert a focal and continually erosive effect analogous to the creation of cranial vault excavations by the arachnoidal granulations. This concept of focal atrophy was developed to explain the mechanism of CSF rhinorrhea in three of our patients with sellar leaks (cases 2, 8, and 9 in Table 274-4). It may also be invoked to explain normal-pressure CSF leaks from any site in adults. In this it agrees quite well with the hypothesis advanced by O'Connell.[51] He described in two patients a combination of an excavated lamina cribrosa plus a shrunken olfactory bulb, which made possible the development of a pulsating pocket of CSF over the fistula. In our series, case 1 in Table 274-4 appeared to have a similar lesion. A recent report by Front and Penning described three cases of recurrent meningitis without obvious rhinorrhea in whom a pouch of arachnoid bulged through the floor of the anterior cranial fossa into the nasal cavity.[23]

Leclercq and colleagues reviewed the ''empty sella'' syndrome and presented arguments indicating that a more suitable name for this example of focal atrophy would be *intrasellar arachnoidocele.*[36] They argued that the sella is filled with a fluid pouch of arachnoid overlying a normal though shrunken pituitary gland. The syndrome is relatively benign, as noted earlier by others.[6,20,27,33,45] These authors would reserve the term *empty sella* for the sella ''emptied'' by surgery.

Drolet and colleagues reported one additional case of empty sella with a CSF leak that illustrates important points in the diagnosis and treatment of such lesions.[20] Because of the posterolateral position of the fistula, it required three operations to stop the leak. The third, successful operation, which approached the fistula via the transnasal trans-sphenoidal route, was the only one that could truly disclose the site of the fistula. Our most recent case in this category is given as case 9 in Table 274-4.

The anatomy of the sphenoid bone in relation to CSF leaks has been carefully studied by AC Hooper.[29] In 138 adult sphenoids, 27 defects were found that could become potential sites for fistulae associated with CSF rhinorrhea. Fourteen holes were located at the site of the superior opening of the transient lateral craniopharyngeal canal. The remaining 13 were along the pathway of the internal carotid artery. Hooper concluded that the gross and microscopic appearances of these defects were consistent with their production by a process of focal atrophy, as suggested by us in 1968.

Minor degrees of congenital meningeal and meningocerebral hernia can also act as actual or potential pathways in the anterior skull base and present in adult life with CSF rhinorrhea, for example, cases 3, 5, and 6 in Table 274-4. Most case reports of "primary spontaneous" rhinorrhea are explicable by this etiology. The genesis of such a leak, aside from the role of focal atrophy, is probably related to the fact that CSF pressure attains its maximum in adulthood, and is then almost three times that of infants, as well as to factors such as sneezing, coughing, or other normal causes of fluctuations in CSF pressure.[51]

The final etiologic category is that of osteomyelitic erosion. This is a very rare cause,[47] and we have not had a single patient with this condition.

Nontraumatic Otorrhea

CSF fistulas of the temporal bone without preceding trauma are rare. They usually present as otorrhea, but, just like traumatic fistulas, they may present as rhinorrhea via the eustachian tube. Otorrhea is often unrecognized, especially if the tympanic membrane is intact, as in the case reported by Kramer and colleagues in which a congenital defect in the temporal bone led to occult otorrhea that simulated serous otitis media.[35] Tomography showed the bony defect clearly.

Treatment of Nontraumatic Leaks

The treatment of nontraumatic CSF leaks is primarily surgical, although nonsurgical measures have resulted in successful management of such patients on rare occasions. The principles of treatment of both traumatic and nontraumatic leaks is summarized in Table 274-6.

Remission of leakage, rarely permanent, may follow lumbar puncture, meningitis, or dye injection. It has been reported that long-term medical management with antibiotics is possible,[4] but with the increasing number of resistant organisms, this conservative therapy becomes hard to justify. Repeated lumbar punctures have been tried and recommended, but this may now be considered an obsolete method and, as indicated above, liable to precipitate meningitis. Instillation of substances such as silver nitrate nasally to promote closure of the fistula from below has not been routinely successful, but the cure of a case of CSF rhinorrhea has been reported after the application of methyl 2-cyanoacrylate to the roof of the ethmoid sinus.[25] It is often recommended that, following the identification of CSF in a rhinorrhea, expectant treatment—including nursing in a semi-Fowler position and discouragement of nose blowing, sneezing, and straining—and antibiotic administration be tried for 6 to 8 weeks before surgery is considered. While it is true that most cases of CSF rhinorrhea, particularly the traumatic variety, will stop leaking, it would be risky to suggest that this conservative therapy be adopted routinely. Indeed, the occurrence of repeated attacks of meningitis after spontaneous closure of such fistulas, even in the absence of obvious leakage of fluid,[59] would support a more active approach to some of these patients. Thus, in nontraumatic CSF rhinorrhea, a conservative attitude is probably justifiable only in those patients with high-pressure leaks in whom the causal lesion cannot be removed. This was the initial management of our case 16 in Table 274-5. However, after apparently complete regression of this patient's adenocarcinoma following deep x-ray therapy, her fistula was closed intracranially to prevent recurrent meningitis.

TABLE 274-6 Summary of Principles of Treatment of CSF Leaks

Traumatic Rhinorrhea[37]

1. Intradural surgical repair of the dural laceration is recommended for *all* cases of proven CSF rhinorrhea as prophylaxis against infection.
2. Surgery should be performed 10–14 days after trauma for *acute* leaks and as soon as possible after the onset of delayed CSF rhinorrhea.
3. Conservative management is reserved for older and poor risk patients only.

Nontraumatic Rhinorrhea[53]

1. *High-pressure leaks* Treat the cause, e.g., remove a tumor or perform CSF shunt surgery for hydrocephalus. Only if the leak persists after the cause is treated should the fistula be localized and surgically closed.
2. *Normal-pressure leaks* The fistula will be found either in the anterior fossa (usually via the cribriform area) or in the middle fossa (usually via the sellar or parasellar area and sphenoid sinus). Localize and close either by an intradural or transsphenoidal method.

In normal-pressure leaks, surgical repair of the fistula is usually easy and is to be recommended as soon as the diagnosis is established. A cautionary note should be made regarding anesthesia for such surgery. Positive pressure respiration at induction must be carefully avoided to protect against the risk of infection. Thus, tracheal intubation while the patient is awake is recommended.

The use of synthetic adhesives has been reviewed by VanderArk and colleagues, and this option should be considered in difficult cases not responding to the more routine methods described above.[64] Nystrom[48] and Probst and Rahn[55] have used a combination of an adhesive (Biobond) and fascia to achieve good results.

Surgical Techniques for Fistula Closure

The techniques for fistula closure may be considered briefly under two headings: first, the extracranial, usually transnasal, approach, and, second, the intracranial approach. An extracranial, extranasal approach to fistulas through the frontal and ethmoidal sinuses has been recommended by Aboulker et al.[1] Mennig has described a transethmoidal trans-sphenoidal approach that was used to repair a fistula through the floor of the sella turcica and was successful after an intracranial attempt at closing the leak had failed.[44] A review of such extracranial techniques may be found in a paper by Vrabec and Hallberg.[67] In my opinion, such extracranial techniques should be reserved for sellar and parasellar leaks in carefully selected patients in whom the etiology of the leak has been clearly understood and the fistula tract demonstrated and in whom the intracranial methods cannot be undertaken for definite reasons. The rationale for this opinion is that treating CSF rhinorrhea is not simply a matter of closing the bony defect but, more importantly, necessitates repair of the meningeal defects. Such meningeal repairs are best conducted after adequate inspection intradurally, and rhinologic procedures seldom provide an adequate view within the dura mater except for the lower part of the sella turcica as exposed through the sphenoid sinus. Therefore, leaks through the sella turcica and sphenoid sinus are best approached via the microneurosurgical trans-sphenoidal route. In one case we were able to stop a trans-sphenoidal leak using tantalum-impregnated methacrylate after three prior craniotomies had failed to stop the flow. Use of intraoperative fluoroscopy while injecting the opacified semiliquid methacrylate transnasally made possible complete and solid filling of the sphenoid sinus after polymerization had occurred.

More recently, McCormack and coworkers have recommended the extracranial approach, carried out with the help of an otorhinolargyngologist, as their preferred method for repairing CSF leaks.[42] They claim that this procedure gives a success rate equal or superior to that achieved by the intracranial approach while avoiding the morbidity of craniotomy. In reviewing the early results of Lewin and coworkers[37] along with our own experiences, and excluding the trans-sphenoidal leaks as indicated above, we find no significant morbidity from craniotomy and a success rate equal or superior to that of extracranial procedures. When the help of an otorhinolaryngologist skilled in the extracranial approach is not available, we recommend the intracranial approach.

Intracranial procedures have been adequately described by Dandy,[14] and only a few comments are necessary. The crucial factor in adequate surgical treatment is closure of the meningeal defect. This is often quite small in nontraumatic leaks and easy to overlook. Some neurosurgeons have resorted to filling the craniotomy site with saline, and with the help of the anesthesiologist they obtain a visual demonstration of the hole by forcing air from the nasopharynx into the exposure area, where the escape of bubbles may be seen.[57] However, with accurate preoperative diagnosis, this maneuver with its attendant risk of sepsis may be avoided. After demonstration of the meningeal defect, the patient's own fascia lata, pericranium, muscle, or strips of fat may be used to provide the intradural repair, with fascia lata plus fat grafts being most satisfactory. It is not essential to strip the dura and to seal bony defects exposed with bone wax, acrylic cements, or other substances. This is necessary only where the bony defect is large enough to necessitate support of the intradural graft. In such cases, methyl methacrylate is a satisfactory caulking material.

The intracranial, intradural approach is recommended for most traumatic and nontraumatic cerebrospinal fistulas, with careful "patching" of the fistula site, preferably using the patient's own fat with or without fascia lata as free grafts. Sealing of subjacent bony defects is required only when the hole is of significant size—for example, greater than 2 mm in diameter. In high-pressure leaks, removal or bypass of the tumor or obstruction should always precede repair of the fistula, which should be carried out only where it is positively established that the "safety valve" function of the CSF leakage is no longer required. In normal-pressure leaks, obliteration of the arachnoid hernia should accompany careful intradural repair of the fistula.

Pneumocephalus

Air in the subarachnoid pathways, ventricles, or brain substance is usually a post-traumatic phenomenon. However, iatrogenic pneumocephalus should also be kept in mind. The most common cause of the latter condition is the placement of a CSF drain for the treatment of CSF leaks via the nose or ear. Certainly such drains should not be placed in the presence of a CSF leak associated with a pneumocephalus. Most cases with pneumocephalus are traumatic. When the vault or base of the skull is fractured, and particularly when such fractures involve the paranasal sinuses, mastoid air cells, or petrous temporal regions, air can enter the cranium. Lacerations of the dura enable the air to pass into the subarachnoid space or even the ventricles without direct brain laceration via an "upstream" flow of air along the normal CSF pathways and, of course, directly into the brain substance and/or the ventricles in the presence of tears in the brain tissues. Plain x-ray films are the best way to follow the presence of the air, and CT scans can provide further detail as needed. Typical sulcal patterns are seen when air is in the subarachnoid space over the convexities. If the pneumocephalus is confined to the subdural compartment, it tends to collect in the frontal polar region when films are taken with the patient in the supine position. If x-ray films do not reveal the associated skull fracture, thin section CT scans usually succeed in doing so. Occasionally, small "bubbles" of air may be seen in the scalp tissues in association with scalp lacerations. When the air is associated with depressed skull fractures, tangential views will be required to differentiate intracranial and extracranial subcutaneous pneumocephalus.

Tension pneumocephalus is the term used to describe the trapping of air intracranially. Usually, it occurs in patients whose brains do not expand after removal of a chronic subdural hematoma, but it can also occur as part of a traumatic pneumocephalus without overt CSF leakage. It is a serious complication if coupled with clinical deterioration and requires separate drainage using a subdural needle tap. The management of pneumocephalus in general means *closing the causative breech in the cerebral integuments* and has the same implications as for CSF leaks. In our previous publications, we have discussed the significance of pneumocephalus associated with CSF leaks relative to the indications for timing of surgical intervention.[52–54] The recommendation for immediate surgical treatment that we made has not been well clarified and has often been misquoted, for example, in a monograph on complications and sequelae of head injury.[11] We recommend such intervention only for CSF leaks that have persisted for more than 6 to 8 days.[52]

References

1. Aboulker P, Le Beau J, Sterkers JM, Elbaz P. Traitement des fistules méningées ethmoïdo-frontales: a propos de 15 cas opérés avec succès par voie exocrânienne. *Ann Otolaryngol Chir Cervicofac* 1966; 83:27–32.
2. Alazraki NP, Halpern SE, Ashburn WL, Coel M. Hyberbaric cisternography: experience in humans. *J Nucl Med* 1973; 14:226–229.
3. Allen MB Jr, El Gammal T, Ihnen M, Cowan MA. Fistula detection in cerebrospinal fluid leakage. *J Neurol Neurosurg Psychiatry* 1972; 35:664–668.
4. Anderson WM, Schwarz GA, Gammon GD. Chronic spontaneous cerebrospinal rhinorrhea. *Arch Intern Med* 1961; 107:723–731.
5. Bergstrand G, Bergstrom M, Eriksson L, et al. Positron emission tomography with ^{68}Ga-EDTA in the diagnosis and localization of CSF fistulas. *J Comput Assist Tomogr* 1982; 6:320–324.
6. Bernasconi V, Giovanelli MA, Papo I. Primary empty sella. *J Neurosurg* 1972; 36:157–161.
7. Busch W. Die Morphologie der Sella turcica und ihre Beziehungen zur Hypophyse. *Virchows Arch [Pathol Anat]* 1951; 320:437–458.

8. Cairns H. Injuries of the frontal and ethmoidal sinuses with special reference to cerebrospinal fluid rhinorrhoea and aeroceles. *J Laryngol Otol* 1937; 52:589–623.
9. Cairns H. Discussion on injuries of the frontal and ethmoidal sinuses. *Proc R Soc Med* 1942; 35:809–810.
10. Ciric IS, Tarkington J. Transsphenoidal microsurgery. *Surg Neurol* 1974; 2:207–212.
11. Cooper PR. Cerebrospinal fluid fistulas and pneumocephalus. In Barrow DL (ed): *Complications and Sequelae of Head Injury*. Park Ridge, IL: American Association of Neurological Surgeons, 1992, pp 1–12.
12. Crow HJ, Keogh C, Northfield DWC. The localisation of cerebrospinal-fluid fistulae. *Lancet* 1956; 2:325–327.
13. Cushing H. Experiences with orbito-ethmoidal osteomata having intracranial complications. *Surg Gynecol Obstet* 1927; 44:721–742.
14. Dandy WE. Pneumocephalus (intracranial pneumatocele or aerocele). *Arch Surg* 1926; 12:949–982.
15. Di Chiro G, Grove AS Jr. Evaluation of surgical and spontaneous cerebrospinal fluid shunts by isotope scanning. *J Neurosurg* 1966; 24:743–748.
16. Di Chiro G, Ommaya AK, Ashburn W, Briner WH. Isotope cisternography in the diagnosis and follow-up of cerebrospinal fluid rhinorrhea. *J Neurosurg* 1968; 28:522–529.
17. Di Chiro G, Reames PM, Matthews WB Jr. RISA-ventriculography and RISA-cisternography. *Neurology (Minneap)* 1964; 14:185–191.
18. Dohlman G. Spontaneous cerebrospinal rhinorrhea: case operated by rhinologic methods. *Acta Otolaryngol (Stockh) [Suppl]* 1948; 67:20–23.
19. Doron Y, Simon J, Peyser E. Positive contrast myeloencephalography for visualization of cerebrospinal fluid fistula. *Neuroradiology* 1972; 3:228–230.
20. Drolet M, Bouche B, Bélanger C. Syndrome de la grosse selle turcique vide et de la rhinorrhée du liquide céphalo-rachidien. *Can Med Assoc J* 1972; 107:1199–1202.
21. Eden K. Traumatic cerebrospinal rhinorrhoea: repair of the fistula by a transfrontal intradural operation. *Br J Surg* 1941; 29:299–303.
22. Engels EP. Roentgenographic demonstration of a hypophysial subarachnoid space. *Am J Roentgenol* 1958; 80:1001–1004.
23. Front D, Penning L. Occult spontaneous cerebrospinal fluid rhinorrhea diagnosed by isotope cisternography. *Neuroradiology* 1971; 2:167–169.
24. Gadeholt H. The reaction of glucose-oxidase test paper in normal nasal secretion. *Acta Otolaryngol (Stockh)* 1964; 58:271–272.
25. Gotham JE, Meyer JS, Gilroy J, Bauer RB. Observations on cerebrospinal fluid rhinorrhea and pneumocephalus. *Ann Otol Rhinol Laryngol* 1965; 74:215–233.
26. Grant FC. Intracranial aerocele following fracture of the skull: report of a case with review of the literature. *Surg Gynecol Obstet* 1923; 36:251–255.
27. Hodgson SF, Randall RV, Holman CB, MacCarty CS. Empty sella syndrome. *Med Clin North Am* 1972; 56:897–907.
28. Holman BL, Davis DO. Radioisotopic assessment of cerebrospinal fluid pathways. *Prog Nucl Med* 1972; 1:359–375.
29. Hooper AC. Sphenoidal defects—a possible cause of cerebrospinal fluid rhinorrhoea. *J Neurol Neurosurg Psychiatry* 1971; 34:739–742.
30. House WF, Hitselberger WE. Surgical complications of acoustic tumor surgery. *Arch Otolaryngol* 1968; 88:659–667.
31. Jacobson I, Maran AG. Localization of cerebrospinal fluid rhinorrhea. *Arch Otolaryngol* 1971; 93:79–80.
32. Jones HM. The problem of recurrent meningitis. *J R Soc Med* 1974; 67:1141–1147.
33. Keravel Y. Contribution au diagnostic et au traitement chirurgical de la selle turcique ''vide.'' Thesis. Paris, 1973.
34. King D. Report to Westminster Medical Society. *Lond Med Surg J* 1834; 4:823–825.
35. Kramer SA, Yanagisawa E, Smith HW. Spontaneous cerebrospinal fluid otorrhea simulating serous otitis media. *Laryngoscope* 1971; 81:1083–1089.
36. Leclercq TA, Hardy J, Vezina JL, Mercky F. Intrasellar arachnoidocele and the so-called empty sella syndrome. *Surg Neurol* 1974; 2:295–299.
37. Lewin W. Cerebrospinal fluid rhinorrhea in nonmissile head injuries. *Clin Neurosurg* 1966; 12:237–252.
38. Linell EA, Robinson WL. Head injuries and meningitis. *J Neurol Neurosurg Psychiatry* 1941; 4:23–31.
39. MacGee EE, Cauthen JC, Brackett CE. Meningitis following acute traumatic cerebrospinal fluid fistula. *J Neurosurg* 1970; 33:312–316.
40. Manelfe C, Cellerier P, Sobel D, et al. Cerebrospinal fluid rhinorrhea: evaluation with metrizamide cisternography. *Am J Roentgenol* 1982; 138:471–476.
41. Marc JA, Schecter MD. The significance of fluid-gas displacement in the sphenoid sinus in post-traumatic cerebrospinal fluid rhinorrhea. *Radiology* 1973; 108:603–606.
42. McCormack B, Cooper PR, Persky, M, et al. Extracranial repair of cerebrospinal fluid fistulas: techniques and results in 37 patients. *Neurosurgery* 1990; 27:412–417.
43. McKusick KA, Malmud LS, Lordela PA, et al. Radionuclide cisternography: normal values for nasal secretion of intrathecally injected ^{111}In-DTPA. *J Nucl Med* 1973; 14:933–934.
44. Mennig H. Heilung einer schwierigen Liquorfistel durch rhinochirugisches Vorgehen. *Laryngol Rhinol Otol (Stuttg)* 1964; 43:412–419.
45. Metzger J, Helias A, Messimy R, et al. Nouveaux cas de selles turciques dites vides avec signes neuro-ophtalmologiques ou rhinorrhée. *Rev Neurol (Paris)* 1970; 123:435–442.
46. Miller C. Case of hydrocephalus chronicus, with some unusual symptoms and appearances on dissection. *Trans Med Chir Soc Edinb* 1826; 2:243–248.
47. Nori A, Carteri A. Rinoliquorrea: trattamento e risultati a distanza. *Chir Ital* 1964; 16:161–165.
48. Nystrom SHM. On the use of Biobond in the treatment of cerebrospinal rhinorrhea and frontobasal fistula. *Int Surg* 1970; 54:332–340.
49. Oberson R. Radioisotopic diagnosis of rhinorrhea. *Radiol Clin Biol* 1972; 41:28–35.
50. Obrador S. Primary non-traumatic spontaneous cerebro-spinal fluid rhinorrhea with normal cerebro-spinal fluid pressure. *Schweiz Arch Neurol Neurochir Psychiatr* 1972; 111:369–376.
51. O'Connell JEA. Primary spontaneous cerebrospinal fluid rhinorrhea. *J Neurol Neurosurg Psychiatry* 1964; 27:241–246.
52. Ommaya AK. Spinal fluid fistulae. *Clin Neurosurg* 1976; 23:363–392.
53. Ommaya AK, Di Chiro G, Baldwin M, Pennybacker JB. Non-traumatic cerebrospinal fluid rhinorrhea. *J Neurol Neurosurg Psychiatry* 1968; 31:214–225.
54. Ommaya AK, O'Tuama LA, Lorenzo AV. CSF dynamics, hydrocephalus and leaks. In Wagner H (ed): *Principles of Nuclear Medicine*, 2d ed. Philadelphia: Saunders, 1995.
55. Probst C, Rahn BA. La fermeture plastique des fistules frontobasales au moyen de Biobond-Tabotamp: expériences cliniques et expérimentales. *Neurochirurgie* 1972; 18:203–212.
56. Raskin R. Cerebrospinal fluid rhinorrhea and otorrhea: diagnosis and treatment in 35 cases. *Int Surg* 1965; 43:141–154.
57. Ray BS, Bergland R. Cerebrospinal fluid fistula: clinical aspects, techniques of localization, and methods of closure. *J Neurosurg* 1969; 30:399–405.
58. Rockett FX, Wittenborg MH, Shillito J Jr, Matson DD. Pantopaque visualization of a congenital dural defect of the internal auditory meatus causing rhinorrhea: report of a case. *Am J Roentgenol* 1964; 91:640–646.
59. Schneider RC, Thompson JM. Chronic and delayed traumatic cerebrospinal rhinorrhea as a source of recurrent attacks of meningitis. *Ann Surg* 1957; 145:517–529.
60. Spetzler RF, Wilson CB. Dural fistulae and their repair. In Youmans JR (ed): *Neurological Surgery*, 2d ed. Philadelphia: Saunders, 1982, pp 2209–2227.
61. Teng P, Edalatpour N. Cerebrospinal fluid rhinorrhea with demonstration of cranionasal fistula with Pantopaque. *Radiology* 1963; 81:802–806.

62. Teng P, Papatheodorou C. Cerebrospinal rhinorrhea and otorrhea. *Arch Otolaryngol* 1965; 82:56–61.
63. Thomson St C. *The Cerebrospinal Fluid; Its Spontaneous Escape from the Nose.* London: Cassell, 1899.
64. VanderArk GD, Pitkethly DT, Ducker TB, Kempe LG. Repair of cerebrospinal fluid fistulas using a tissue adhesive. *J Neurosurg* 1970; 33:151–155.
65. VanGilder JC, Goldenberg IS. Hypophysectomy in metastatic breast cancer. *Arch Surg* 1975; 110:293–295.
66. Voena G. Considerazioni su un caso di grave cranio-rino-liquorrea da persistenza del canale basi-occipitale. *Arch Ital Otol* 1959; 70:212–222.
67. Vrabec DP, Hallberg OE. Cerebrospinal fluid rhinorrhea. *Arch Otolaryngol* 1964; 80:218–229.
68. Wehrle PF, Mathies AW Jr, Leedom JM. Management of bacterial meningitis. *Clin Neurosurg* 1967; 14:72–85.
69. Wocjan J, Klisiewicz R, Krolicki L. Overpressure radionuclide cisternography and metrizamide computed tomographic cisternography in the detection of intermittent rhinoliquorrheas in children. *Childs Nerv Syst* 1989; 5:238–240.
70. Wolman L. The neuropathological effects resulting from the intrathecal injection of chemical substances. *Paraplegia* 1966; 4:97–115.
71. Yasargil MG, Fox JL. The microsurgical approach to acoustic neurinomas. *Surg Neurol* 1974; 2:393–398.

275 Cranial Defects and Cranioplasty

Donald J. Prolo

The cranium is the province of the neurosurgeon, who must respect and understand its unique biological nature no less than that of the brain itself. Craniotomy for various cerebral lesions requires safe passage to and from cephalic areas with eventual restoration of conformity of the head. The temporary exteriorization of sections of the skull, either free or hinged on a muscle pedicle, in every craniotomy is followed by a form of fresh autogeneic (formerly called "autogenous") cranioplasty. Discontinuity defects of the cranium for which there is no replaceable skull section have engaged the ingenuity of surgeons from antiquity to the present. The problem of reconstructing the smooth symmetrical and rounded contours of the skull is complex, the moment for accomplishing this is often fleeting, and the diversity of methods advanced through the years testifies to the unsolved nature of this Sisyphean task.

Brief Historical Review

Trepanation is the oldest operation known and dates from prehistoric neolithic time (10,000–7,000 BC). Stone Age Celts of France and Incas of Peru performed such cranial operations with an apparent 70 percent survival rate for patients. Repair of skull defects (cranioplasty) paralleled the practice of trepanation among these ancient cultures. Gold and silver pieces corresponding to the size and shape of defects have been discovered in graves in Peru, and skull allografts ("rondells," round discs) in neolithic Celt remains.[72,73,83] Primitive races trepanned by scraping away bone until dura was exposed. Coconut shells were used by South Sea Islanders to repair the defect. Petronius in 1565 used a gold plate to repair cleft palates—the first use of an alloplastic material to repair a defect.

J. van Meekren is credited with the first bone graft in history when in 1670 he used canine bone to repair a skull defect in a Russian; however, he removed the implant under threat of excommunication by the church. Merrem in 1810 transplanted bone in dogs, and in 1821 P. von Walther performed the first human autogeneic bone graft. The work of Ollier in 1859 established the importance of periosteum in bone regeneration. Macewen in 1873 reimplanted calvarial bone fragments after treating them with bichloride of mercury, and in 1878 he was the first to transplant a human bone allograft.[8]

In 1889 Senn wrote on the repair of cranial defects with antiseptic decalcified bone. In that same year Seydel transplanted an autograft of tibia with attached periosteum to repair a parietal defect. Müller and König in 1890 independently advocated a flap of scalp periosteum and outer skull table to be swung over a skull defect. Bunge (1903) first used fresh osteoperiosteal homograft (allograft) skull. The work of Sicard, Dambrin, and Roger from 1917 to 1919 introduced cadaver skull in cranioplasty. The transplantation of fresh autogeneic bone in cranioplasty followed the initial work of Kappis (1915) with whole ribs, Brown (1917) with split ribs, and Mauclaire (1914) with ilium.[17,72,97] The histologic sequence of autogeneic bone transplant repair was first fully documented in 1907 by Axhausen, who described the process of invasion of blood vessels along preexisting channels followed by dynamic reconstructive processes of resorption and appositional new bone formation (*schleichender Ersatz,* translated "creeping substitution").[8]

Alloplastic repair of cranial defects has followed the availability of various plastics and metals throughout this past century. Celluloid, used by Fraenkel in 1890, had an extensive trial but later was abandoned because of cellular reactions and biodegradative processes in tissue.[17,72,97] Aluminum, one of the first metals used by Booth and Curtis in 1893, was soon followed by gold, utilized successfully by Gersten (1895) and more extensively tried by Estor (1916). Subsequently many metals have had clinical trials, including vitallium alloy (cobalt, chromium, and molybdenum), used by Geib (1941); tantalum, used by Pudenz and Odom (1942) and Fulcher (1943); stainless steel mesh, used by Boldrey (1944); stainless steel, used by Scott, Wycis, and Murtagh (1956); and titanium, used by Simpson (1965) and Gordon and Blair (1974).[5,87] Seven decades after its introduction, Black (1978) returned to the use of aluminum because of its malleability, radiolucency, and low tissue reactivity.[4]

Acrylic resins became available as industrial materials in 1937. Under trade names of Vitacrilic, Lucite, Plexiglas, Crystallite, and Cranioplastic, methyl methacrylate was introduced to human cranioplasty by Zander in October 1940.[97] A one-stage acrylic method described by Spence (1954) is now the most widely used method.[82] Galicich and Hovind in 1967 found that incorporating stainless steel mesh within the methyl methacrylate rendered it less brittle.[15] More recently Habal and colleagues have reconstructed cranial defects with an alloplastic tray of polyurethane terephthalate (cured Dacron-urethane composite) filled with autogeneic cancellous bone.[22]

Polyethylene, introduced by Alexander and Dillard in 1950 and initially not available in pure form, has had resurgent use in the form of a high density porous implant.[10,33,87,94] The softness of silicon rubber, along with its tendency to encapsulate, accumulate fluid, and erode adjacent bone (as an onlay), has militated against its use in cranioplasty since it was first used by Courtemanche and Thompson in 1968.[11,21] Plaster of Paris (calcium sulfate hemihydrate, CaO_4S) has been used as a bone substitute to fill extracranial defects since 1892.[58,70] It is easily heat sterilized, can be used in areas of infection, is absorbable, and can be used as a filler that resorbs as bone grows into a defect and as a binder for the ceramic hydroxylapatite. Hydroxylapatite, $Ca_{10}(PO_4)_6(OH)_2$, the mineral of bone and teeth, is variably resorbable, is osteoconductive, and bonds to adjacent bone.[28,76] However, it is brittle, with low impact resistance and tensile strength.[35] The combination of hydroxylapatite and plaster of Paris has been used successfully in cats to close surgically created defects in the skull (12-mm parietal defects and frontal sinus defects).[70] The variable resorption and limited mechanical strength of hydroxlapatite, whether alone or in combination with autogeneic or allogeneic bone in the human, make this ceramic a less reliable biomaterial in human cranioplasty.[28,48,76,78,79]

Over this century, the plethora of methods tried and later abandoned for various reasons has paralleled the increasing need for a suitable implant. The incidence of trauma through wars and vehicular accidents and multiplying neurosurgical procedures have provided an experimental base upon which principles of cranioplasty have evolved.

Causes of Skull Defects; Indications for and Timing of Cranioplasty

Skull defects most commonly result from trauma. Contaminated compound depressed skull fractures among civilians and penetrating head injuries among military personnel are the most frequent types. In addition, a defect resulting from a growing skull fracture has been found in children, usually under 3 years of age, which develops within 4 to 6 months after a skull fracture (usually parietal) and is associated with a dural tear, cerebral herniation, and ventricular dilatation and porencephaly.[19,36]

Skull defects also arise from excision of tumors (osteomas, hemangiomas, meningiomas, eosinophilic granulomas, epidermoids, metastatic tumors, fibrous dysplasia), from infections (osteomyelitis, infected skull flaps), from aseptic necrosis of skull flaps, from radionecrosis and electrical burns of the skull, and from congenital absence of portions of the skull (encephaloceles, large parietal foramina, and other anomalies of the obelion). Cerebral swelling from brain tumors, trauma, infections, and lead intoxication at times requires external decompression, which results in a skull defect.

Defects larger than 2 to 3 cm over the cerebral convexity and defects of any size in the glabrous frontal areas are universally repaired. Exceptions to this rule include cases where there is deficient skull under temporal or occipital muscles or cases of calvarial discontinuity in the elderly or mentally impaired. If cerebral seizures occur among these latter patients, a cranioplasty should be done to protect the brain.

Among the possible indications for cranioplasty, the two commonly accepted ones address issues of cerebral protection and appearance. These two indications also partially delimit the materials used to restore the integrity of the cranium. Although cranioplasty was once thought to be able to relieve wound discomfort and seizures, that does not often seem to be the case. Neither is the "syndrome of the trephined," consisting of headaches, dizziness, intolerance of vibration and noise, irritability, fatigability, loss of motivation and concentration, depression, and anxiety, universally accepted as an indication to reconstruct the skull.[18,93] However, this last constellation of symptoms is regaining some credibility from reports that describe the effects of direct atmospheric pressure on the brain.[14,83,85] Both ventricular migration toward a small defect with a corresponding ipsilateral midline shift and contralateral shift of central structures under a large defect (the "sinking skull flap syndrome") have been reported.[36,83–85] Associated with this anatomic displacement of brain has been contralateral hemiplegia,[85] increased intracranial pressure, hemispheric collapse,[84] and cerebrospinal hydrodynamic changes[14] in patients with large cranial defects. In these large defects with anatomic displacement of cerebral structures, the return of the patient to normal after cranioplasty was noted in each of the above reports.

Four persuasive indications for cranioplasty, therefore, are restoration of cerebral protection, physical appearance, and intracranial pressure relationships and the provision of an intact vault for the normal growth and development of cephalic structures in the young. Evidence supporting the organic basis of the syndrome of the trephined is the improvement in symptoms following cranioplasty with the reversion of intracranial pressure relationships to normal. Improvement in electroencephalographic abnormalities, seizures, and neurological dysfunction (motor, speech) has been reported.[18,83,85]

Contraindications to cranioplasty include the presence of hydrocephalus, cerebral swelling, infection, a compound wound, contiguous functional paranasal sinuses (as indicated by air in a sinus on x-ray), and thin, scarred, or devitalized scalp. Children under 4 years of age will frequently regenerate skull, provided that the dura is intact and not grafted. At least 1 year should be allowed to elapse after craniectomy before a cranioplasty is considered in children.

The timing of cranioplasty is critical for avoiding the development of infection in devitalized autografts or around alloplastic materials. It is generally accepted that cranioplasty should be delayed 3 to 6 months after compound wounds and at least 1 year after a wound infection. The report of Rish and colleagues in 1979 based on 491 cranioplasties performed by numerous neurosurgeons clearly established the desirability of waiting 1 year after penetrating or compound cranial injuries.[75] The use of stainless steel mesh and antibiotics by Koslow and Ransohoff suggests an alternative method in rare and exceptional circumstances.[38]

Attributes of Ideal Cranioplastic Material

Most will agree that no alloplastic plate will ever exceed in quality the properties of viable full-thickness autogeneic skull. That such tissue is quantitatively unavailable explains the search for an acceptable, albeit imperfect, substitute. An ideal material would be (1) viable and thereby capable of growth and resistant to infection, (2) radiolucent, (3) thermally nonconductive and with a coefficient of expansion identical to that of the surrounding skull, (4) nonionizing and noncorrosive, (5) stable (durable, nonbiodegradable), (6) inert (nonreactive, nonantigenic, nonsensitizing, noncarcinogenic), (7) esthetically pleasing, (8) protective and having biomechanical properties equal to those of skull, (9) malleable and easily contoured, (10) inexpensive, (11) readily available, and (12) sterilizable.[13] For various reasons no present material satisfies all of these criteria.

Autogeneic bone (cranium, rib, ilium) removed from its blood supply slowly becomes viable (capable of growth and resistant to infection). However, the frequently unsatisfactory esthetic result (up to 50 percent),[37] the necessity of harvesting from and thereby violating another area of the body, and the tendency for the cranioplasty to resorb with compromise of biomechanical properties and cosmetic results, are all disadvantages in the use of autogeneic cranium, rib, or ilium.

Metals are strong, can be sterilized, and do not require a second operation. However, they more often become infected, and they erode the scalp, indent, conduct cold and heat, ionize and corrode, are difficult to shape, and usually are radiopaque. They are no longer used.

Acrylic resins provide favorable properties, including stability, strength, esthetic qualities, inertness, availability, thermal nonconductivity, and ease of application. The plate remains a foreign body, however, with attendant risks of infection, brittleness, and stationary size. With a pore size of 50 μm, bacteria may colonize within the plate.[20] Methyl methacrylate is well tolerated for both cranioplasty and aneuroplasty,[6,7,23] but macrophages aggregate around such implants; methyl methacrylate particles have been found in the liver,[20] and there is concern over potential release of toxic monomer. No carcinoma or sarcoma has been reported following the use of any plastic, including polyethylene, in humans, despite the reports of such developments in rats.[56]

Technique of Cranioplasty with Methyl Methacrylate

The use of methyl methacrylate has been widespread since Spence described the one-stage method in 1954.[82] The brittleness of this material resulted in reports of fractures,[27,31] leading Galicich and Hovind to recommend embedding wire mesh in the plate during the autopolymerization process.[15] Lake and colleagues confirmed the better mechanical properties of methyl methacrylate strengthened by coarse wire mesh.[40] Whereas stainless steel mesh was originally used to increase the tensile and impact strength of the acrylic, Malis reported the far more desirable properties of titanium mesh: it is lightweight, malleable, comparable in strength to stainless steel (in terms of ductility, elastic modulus, and tensile strength), nearly radiolucent, neither magnetic nor paramagnetic (hence eliminating the risk of plate movement and artifacts on magnetic resonance imaging), stable, with no tendency to diffuse into surrounding tissue or corrode, and biocompatible (causing no toxicity or inflammation).[44] The plate should be at least 5 mm thick, except over the temporal region or in a child's skull (Figs. 275-1 and 275-2).

Preparation of the Patient

Because acrylic is a foreign body, some neurosurgeons deliver preoperative antibiotics active against *Staphylococcus* species and continue them for 48 h postoperatively. All the hair over the scalp is clipped on the ward, and the scalp is scrubbed with disinfectant soap several times. After the induction of general anesthesia, the entire head is shaved and then positioned with the plane of the skull defect horizontal in order to facilitate molding of the congealing plastic later (Fig. 275-1).

Preparation of the Wound

Scalp incisions must be designed to lie outside of the defect, behind the hairline, never parallel to previous wounds or scars, and with a broad flap base to accommodate the vascular supply to the area of skin within the flap. If an incision is made through the old scar, one must exercise great care to avoid incising the dura. The entire scalp flap is elevated cautiously to avoid penetrating the dura in areas where it is adherent to the scalp. It is important to maintain the full thickness of the scalp, especially where it will overlie the acrylic plate. The temporalis muscle is reflected off the dura. The pericranium surrounding the cranial defect should be incised and the margins of the defect demarcated by removing soft tissue down to the dura with a curet. After all cottonoids (but not Gelfoam) are removed from the field, a 3- to 5-mm ledge is then drilled around the entire circumference of the defect to the diploe with a high-speed burr. This ledge allows the edges of the acrylic plate to be recessed and provides a smooth contour and firm fixation. All bone dust is irrigated off the field. At least four drill holes are placed through the skull around the circumference of the defect for securing the plate.

Preparation and Positioning of the Acrylic Plate

Strips of saline-soaked bulk cotton of various thicknesses are laid over the dura within the defect to establish the desired contour over which the plate will be molded. This material also further protects the brain from thermal or chemical injury from the acrylic plate.[2,16,49] Methylene blue or another marker is used to outline the edges of the defect along the ledge. A sheet of paper is then placed over the defect, thus transferring the outline of the defect to the paper, which is then cut to the shape of the defect. This pattern is then superimposed onto titanium mesh, and an appropriate configuration of wire mesh is prepared. The wire mesh is then contoured over the bulk cotton in the defect. Thin radial sections may be cut into the mesh to help in bending and contouring the titanium mesh. The mesh has 1-mm spacing (24 $\times$ 24 mesh) and permits penetration by the methyl methacrylate. A clamp is used to open up holes in the wire at 2-cm intervals.

A folded sheet of polyethylene is laid over the defect, and the contoured wire mesh is positioned between the two layers of the sheet. Liquid monomer (the catalyst) is then added to the powdered methacrylate polymer. This mixture is continuously stirred until its consistency is doughy (like a soft putty), at which point it is poured over the wire mesh between the layers of polyethylene sheet. Enough methyl methacrylate is mixed to form a plate at least 5 mm thick for the adult skull. The surgeon, assistant surgeon, and nurse then firmly press with their fingers along the edges of the defect to establish the boundaries of the plate. Intermittent molding of the plate will smooth out irregularities and promote equal thickness. Because this autopolymerization process is exothermic, the plate should be irrigated with cold saline while it hardens.[16,49] Studies have shown that the subdural temperatures rise very little.

When the plate has solidified enough to hold its shape (at a point when the exothermic process peaks), it is removed from its position over the defect. It is then trimmed, and irregularities are removed with a drill. In the areas of the previously placed holes in the wire mesh, the drill is used to create 3- to 5-mm openings in the plate. This allows egress of epidural fluid and also allows fibrosis to occur through the plate, with the scalp eventually becoming adherent to it. Smaller drill holes are placed at four points along the edges of the plate opposite the holes in the skull, and the plate is secured in position either with wire pulled from the edge of the discarded titanium mesh or with 2-0 Nurolon (Ethicon, Inc, Somerville, NJ) sutures.[44] The high-speed drill is then further used to remove any excrescences over the plate. The bulk cotton overlying the dura is removed, and copious saline irrigation is used to purge the wound of debris. The temporalis muscle, galea, and skin are closed in layers.

The postoperative roentgenographic appearance of such a plate shows the wire mesh separated by a margin of acrylic from the edge of the skull defect (Fig. 275-2*A* and *B*). (The plate in this figure is reinforced with stainless steel mesh; titanium mesh is

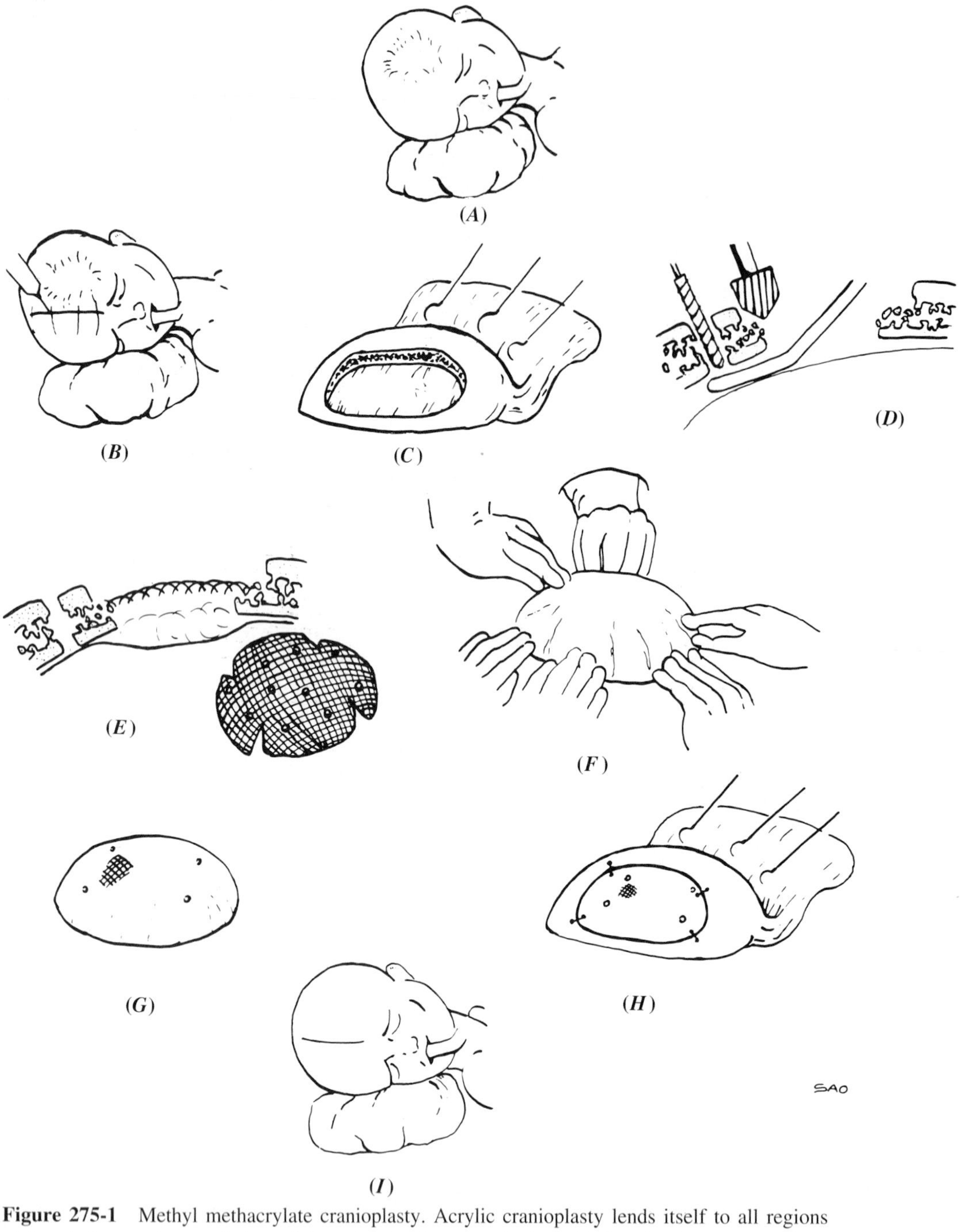

Figure 275-1 Methyl methacrylate cranioplasty. Acrylic cranioplasty lends itself to all regions of the skull except areas that are infected or in direct contiguity with functional paranasal sinuses. *A*. At operation, the head is positioned with the plane of the defect horizontal to facilitate later molding of the hardening plastic. *B*. The scalp incision is outlined on the skin outside the area of the defect and is infiltrated with a local anesthetic containing adrenalin. *C*. The margins of the defect are defined with removal of soft tissue down to the dura; penetration of this protective membrane is avoided. *D*. With a drill, a 5-mm ledge is carved around the defect. At least four holes are placed around the defect. *E*. Bulk cotton is placed over the dura to approximate the normal cranial contour. Methylene blue is traced over the ledge. This outline is then transferred onto paper spread over the defect. A paper pattern of the defect is then placed over titanium wire mesh, and the wire mesh is cut in the shape of the defect. If necessary, sectors are cut out of the wire mesh to facilitate bending it, and 5-mm holes are opened up in the mesh with a small clamp. *F*. Enough acrylic monomer and polymer are mixed to provide for a 5-mm thick plate. The wire mesh and acrylic of doughy consistency are placed within a folded plastic sheet that is positioned over the defect. At least three pairs of hands are positioned around the defect to fashion a plate of the desired shape and thickness. *G*. Excrescences are removed with a burr, and holes are drilled around the edges of the plate to secure it to the skull and through the interior of the plate to allow for the escape of extradural fluid and penetration of binding fibroblasts. *H*. The plate is secured with 2-0 Nurolon or titanium wire separated from the edge of the mesh, and the wound is closed (*I*).

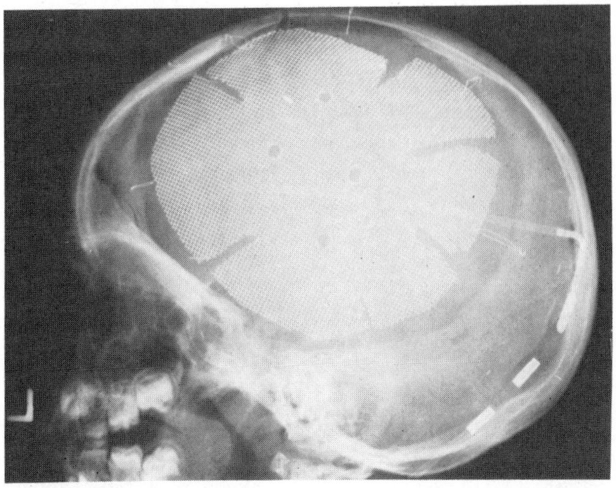

(*A*)

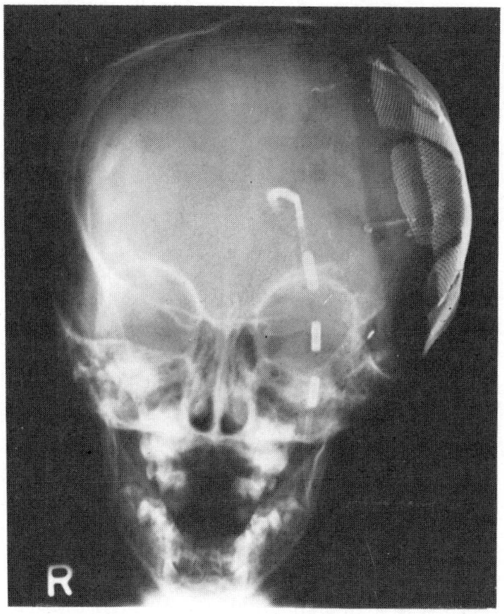

(*B*)

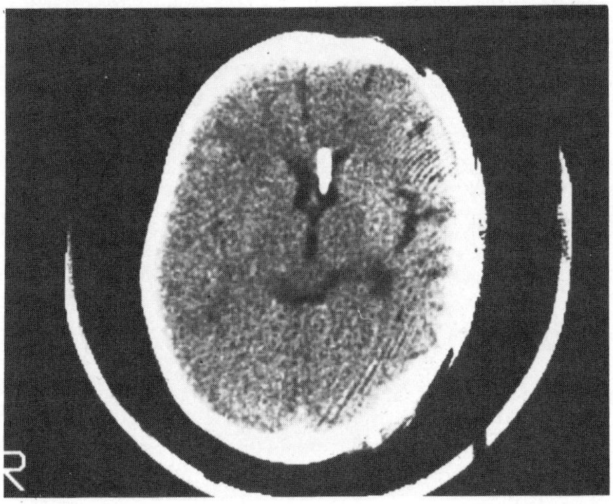

(*C*)

Figure 275-2 A 2-year-old patient with a cranioplasty. *A*. A lateral skull film shows the methyl methacrylate–wire mesh plate. The wire mesh does not reach the margins of the defect and is surrounded by and embedded within a 5-mm-thick acrylic plate. A diversionary shunt installed 9 months previously for communicating hydrocephalus is seen. *B*. An anteroposterior skull film also shows the acrylic-mesh cranioplasty. A rim of acrylic surrounds the mesh. The child's head is asymmetric as a result of hydrocephalus and disturbed cranial growth after a severe injury with cerebral swelling and an acute subdural hematoma. *C*. A CT scan shows brain reaching the inner portion of the acrylic-mesh plate, some artifact from the wire mesh, and evidence of treated communicating hydrocephalus.

considerably more radiolucent.) The contour of such a plate should follow that of the brain. Otherwise, in striving for perfect skull symmetry, one risks compressing the brain. The stainless steel or titanium wire mesh embedded within the acrylic plate imposes little artifact on computed tomograms (Fig. 275-2*C*).

As an alternative to direct formation of an acrylic plate, some neurosurgeons prefer to prefabricate an implant of this type by impression techniques to ensure a good cosmetic result and reduce operating time. Maniscalco and Garcia-Bengochea,[45] Jordan et al.,[32] Cooper et al.,[9] and Van Gool[92] have described such procedures, which require the services of a dental prosthetics laboratory. If the patient's own bone flap or that of another patient of identical cranial contour is available for use as a model, a plate may be prefabricated without estimating the margins of the defect through the intact scalp.[3] Asimacopoulos and colleagues reported forming an impression and thereafter a plate of methyl methacrylate during the operative procedure to improve the cosmetic appearance and strength of the implant.[2] The prefabrication techniques are most applicable to very large hemicraniectomy defects, where they make it possible to avoid irregularities and low stress points in the plate.[9,32,33,45]

Methyl methacrylate and titanium mesh are available commercially (Cranioplastic and Malis titanium mesh; Codman & Shurtleff, Inc., Randolph, MA).

Technique of Cranioplasty with Porous Polyethylene

High-density polyethylene, sintered to create a framework of interconnecting pores, has been available for use in humans since 1985. The large surface negative charge of polyethylene is thought to favor osteogenesis through pores that are larger than the 100-μm minimum size required for bone ingrowth.[94] The material is nontoxic, inert, and stable. It is used as a standard for biocompatibility testing and has had over 30 years of human application.[29,77] Ingrowth of soft tissue and bone occurs rapidly. Porous polyethylene is available as Flexblock (Medpor Surgical Implant; Porex Surgical, College Park, GA), with dimensions of 56 mm × 91 mm × 4 mm thick (that is, having a 1-mm thick smooth external surface and 3-mm descending cones; Fig. 275-3). It is easily cut, shaped,

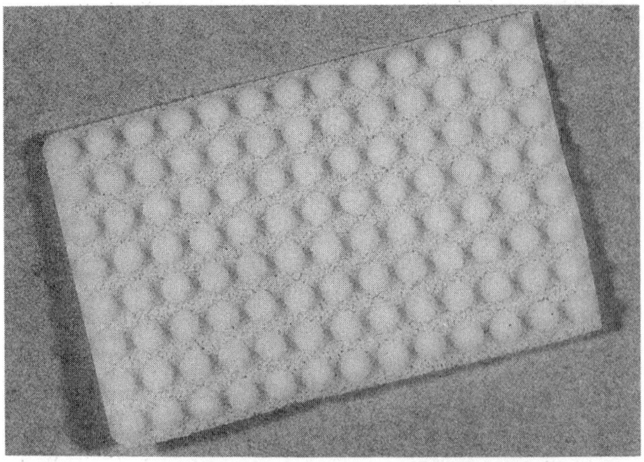

Figure 275-3 Porous, flexible high-density polyethylene may be used to fill small and medium sized defects. The Flexblock measures 91 mm × 56 mm × 4 mm thick; it has a 1-mm thick smooth external surface and an undersurface of cones 3 mm long. The flexibility of this alloimplant allows it to be contoured. After the size of the defect is transferred to a paper template and the outline traced onto the Flexblock, scissors or a scalpel are used to cut the alloimplant to size and to ''feather'' the perimeter of the Flexblock by removing peripheral cones. The 1-mm thick sheet can then be secured to the adjacent cranium with sutures. Fibrous tissue and bone grow into the pores of the polyethylene and strengthen it.

and sutured to adjacent skull. Small and medium-sized defects can quickly be filled with this product.[10] For larger defects, Flexblock does not provide adequate cerebral protection. Porous polyethylene blocks are available measuring up to 38 mm × 63 mm with thicknesses of 3 mm, 6 mm, and 9.5 mm. Soaking a block in sterile saline at 180°F will relax its memory and allow its shape to be modified. Alternatively, an implant can be fitted preoperatively to a defect from data based on computed tomographic imaging. The degree of cerebral protection these solid blocks offer for larger defects is not presently known. However, even a successful cranioplasty with autogeneic cranium has only 50 percent of the mechanical strength of adjacent skull.[20,96]

Preparation of the Patient and Wound

The patient and wound preparation is identical with that described for acrylic cranioplasty.

Preparation and Positioning of the Flexblock or Solid Block

The cones on the undersurface of the Flexblock allow the material to be flexed in any direction within the range permitted by the spacing and size of the cone tips (Fig. 275-3). A low-speed drill is used to create a 5-mm shelf around the margin of the bony defect on which to seat the implant. A pattern of the defect is drawn on paper or plastic and then transferred to the smooth surface of the Flexblock. The implant is cut with scissors or a knife on a nylon carving block. The underside of the implant is cut with a scalpel to feather the edges that will overlie the shelf. Titanium microscrews or sutures are used to secure the implant onto the adjacent bone.

A survey of 200 human skulls showed that the skull thickness over the parietal convexity averaged 6.80 mm to 7.72 mm, with a minimum of 3 mm and maximum of 12 mm.[59] Although the Flexblock allows flexibility, a solid porous polyethylene block of 6 to 9.5 mm thickness provides greater biomechanical protection. To shape such a block, the operating surgeon puts it in sterile saline heated to at least 180°F, molds it to the appropriate form, and then cuts and implants it as described above.

Wellisz and coworkers and Couldwell and coworkers have described their use of Flexblock in human cranioplasty.[10,94]

Technique of Autogeneic Bone Cranioplasty

Despite the universal popularity of cranioplasty with alloplastic materials, most surgeons acknowledge that the viability, potential for growth, and resistance to infection of fresh autogeneic bone are compelling advantages in grafting skull defects.[12,21,37,42,43,53,61,63,65,67,69] In children whose brain and skull are actively growing, autogeneic bone grafting is obviously advantageous because of the capacity of the bone to respond to developmental forces in step with the surrounding skull. It has been shown, further, that viable bone is more resistant to infection. When an alloplastic plate must be removed in an adult because of infection, fracture, or hypersensitivity, then consideration must be given to the use of autogeneic bone.

Cranioplasty with Split Calvaria

Since the early 1980s, there has been renewed use of cranium in grafting skull defects. Split-thickness calvarial grafts of optimal curvature and form are recoverable through a coronal scalp opening, which allows total exposure of the skull and visual comparison of both sides, and avoids a second, more painful wound at the ilium or thorax.[47] Müller and König independently initiated partial thickness skull cranioplasty in 1890. Over the past century, the technique has flourished, with Woolf and Walker listing 94 references to autogeneic cranioplasty up to 1945.[34,97] Santoni-Rugiu advocated a large outer table graft in 1969,[80] and this report has been followed by numerous other publications by plastic surgeons who have ''discovered'' this technique.[47,62,86] Smith and Abramson in 1974 and Zins and Whitaker in 1983 demonstrated that grafts from the membranous calvaria are less likely to resorb than grafts from bone of endochondral origin.[81,101] Split-thickness calvaria is today the autograft of choice.

Thin, motorized oscillating blades and fine curved osteotomes have been used to implement a variety of cranial splitting techniques. Either a section of donor skull is totally removed and then split, or the outer table is removed *in situ* (Fig. 275-4).[47] Intravenous infusion of antibiotics is started with the induction of anesthesia and is continued for 24 h after the operation.

The patient's head is prepared and positioned on the headrest to allow exposure of the defect and planned donor cranium. A coronal incision is made unless existing scars dictate a more prudent choice. The scalp is elevated in a subperiosteal plane, great care being exercised where the deeper levels of scalp adhere to the dura mater. The edges of the carniectomy defect are denuded of fibrous tissue to bleeding bone, preferably with a curet, or else with a burr

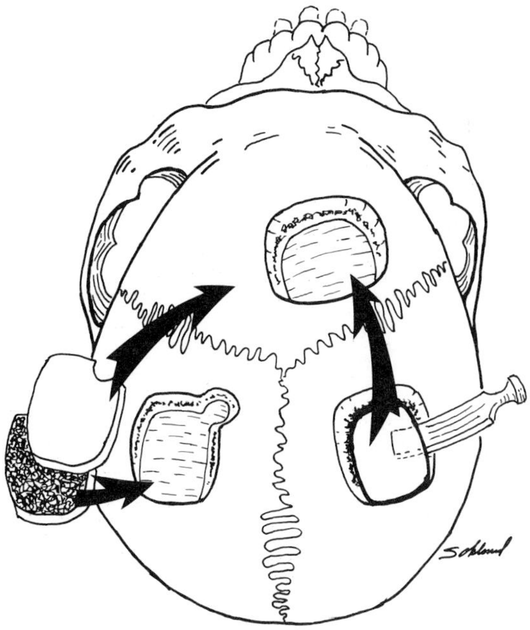

Figure 275-4 Autogeneic cranioplasty with split calvaria. Skull defects may be closed with split-thickness cranium. A 5-mm shelf is created around the outer edge of the defect by removing the external table. A pen is used to mark the outer limit of the shelf, and an imprint of this area is transposed to paper laid over it. The paper is cut along this line to form a template, which is then placed over a donor area of skull of appropriate contour. The pattern is traced on the donor skull with pen and marks the external boundary of the graft. On the *left* of this figure one burr hole is placed; then a craniotome is directed around the line to elevate a plate, which is split with thin curved osteotomes or an oscillating saw. The inner table is returned to the donor defect and the outer is transferred to the skull defect to be closed. On the *right* an outer table graft is elevated with a thin curved osteotome. The groove around the perimeter of the donor graft site is cut with a power burr, beveled outward to allow for angling the osteotome between tables of the skull with avoidance of dural penetration. The groove is of the right depth when bleeding signals the level of diploe. The autograft is secured to the recipient site over the shelf with no. 28 stainless steel wire.

using saline irrigation to limit heat-induced cell necrosis. Along the margin of the defect, the outer bone table is removed to create a 5-mm shelf. A marking pen is used to delimit the outer edge of this shelf, and this line is transferred to paper placed over the defect. Bone wax is avoided over bleeding bone.

A suitable graft donor region is identified, which will match the contour of the recipient site and avoid cranial sutures. The area of the donor graft is outlined around the paper pattern, and the full thickness of the skull is excised with the Gigli saw or craniotome (Fig. 275-4, left side). The calvaria is thickest over the parietal area, averaging about 7.5 mm thick with a range from 3 mm to 12 mm. The exteriorized cranium is then split into inner and outer tables with an oscillating saw and thin flexible osteotomes. The inner table is returned to the graft donor site and secured with wire. The outer table is stabilized over the bone shelf with at least four no. 28 or no. 30 stainless steel wires or with the more expensive titanium mini- or microplates and screws. If the donor bone contour is unsatisfactory, the skull section can be cut into strips, remodeled, and wired together, according to the method of Tessier.[86]

The outer skull table is removed in the *in situ* technique, with great care taken to avoid deep penetration and injury of the underlying dura and brain (Fig. 275-4, right side). A drill is used to create a beveled, partial-thickness groove to bleeding diploic bone around the area marked for donor bone. The outer ridge of the groove is flattened to allow introduction of thin osteotomes between the two tables, and this diploic plane is followed over the area of the donor graft. This outer-table graft is then secured over the recipient site. Some bone dust can be placed over the donor site, or even some demineralized allogeneic bone. The wound is closed in two layers over a drain.

Although this technique usually gives a good cosmetic result, both the donor and recipient areas are less biomechanically protective than adjacent skull. Resorption of 25 to 50 percent of the bone mass can occur, although resorption is usually less than with bone of endochondral origin.[46]

Titanium mini- and microplates and screws for fixation should be avoided in infants and children, as they can penetrate through the dura. In patients younger than 2 years, the cranium cannot be split into tables.[61]

Cranioplasty with Split Rib and Ilium

Although Kappis in 1915 used whole rib, it was Brown in 1917 who suggested splitting the rib to increase its area and make the autograft easier to contour. Credit must be given to Longacre for emphasizing the clinical utility of autogeneic rib and providing a scientific base through studies in the monkey.[43] He emphasized the unique osteogenic proliferative capacity of transplanted rib, the large reservoir of autogeneic ribs in the body, and the regenerative character of these bones. If its thoracic periosteal bed is preserved, a rib will regenerate within 5 weeks in the young child, and if necessary may be used again for transplantation. McClintock and Dingman reported the successful use of iliac bone for cranioplasty in 1951 even before the studies of Longacre.[87]

Two operative fields are necessary for autogeneic rib and ilium cranioplasty (Fig. 275-5). The source of autogeneic bone for smaller defects may be the iliac crest. For larger defects, rib grafts should be employed. Incisions for rib grafts are made to take some combination of alternate ribs (e.g., ribs 4 and 6). The thoracic incision is curved posteriorly to allow exposure of more ribs. An incision is made through the periosteum overlying the rib, and as much rib as possible is removed from the transverse process to the costal cartilage.

The total length of rib needed is estimated by the formula $L = A/W \times 2$, where L is the required rib length in centimeters, A is the surface area of the defect in square centimeters, and W is the average width of the rib in centimeters.[53] Ribs are cut 4 mm longer than the defect. The costal periosteum is then closed with no. 000 catgut suture. If the pleural cavity is entered, closure should be effected at the time of a Valsalva maneuver. The chest wall is then closed.

The cranial wound is prepared in the manner described above for alloplastic cranioplasty. In this case, however, the eburnated margins of the defect must be curetted and rid of fibrous tissue back to bleeding bone. The high-speed drill may destroy cells by heat production. It and the use of bone wax should be avoided. Either a 1-cm ledge is created along the edge of the defect on which to inlay the rib graft, or a groove is tunneled between the inner and outer tables of the skull to hold the tapered ends of the

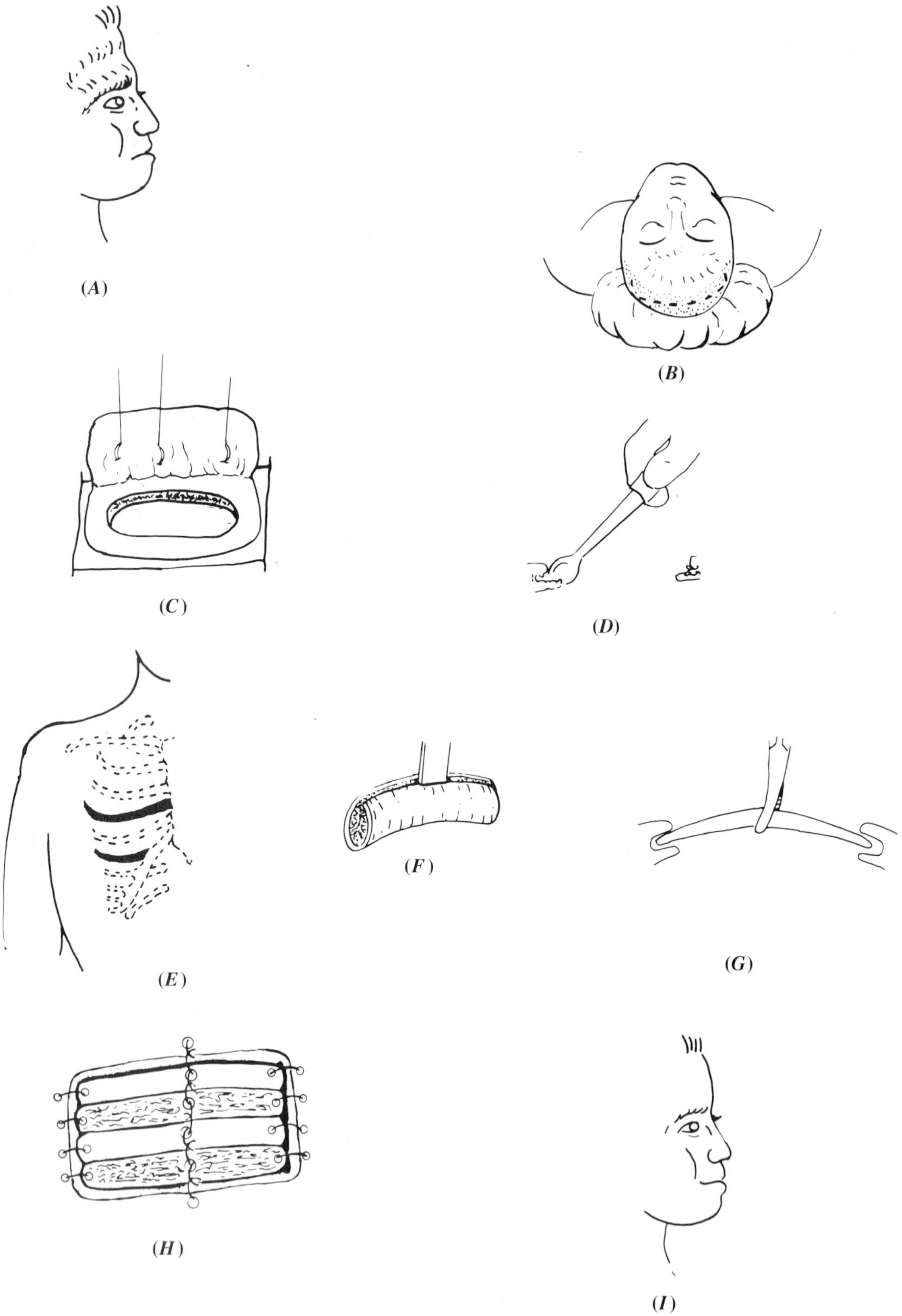

Figure 275-5 Autogeneic rib cranioplasty. *A*. This cranioplasty is indicated in defects previously infected or contiguous with paranasal sinuses and is used by some neurosurgeons in children. *B*. The scalp incision is made behind the hairline and never directly over the defect. *C*. The skull defect is exposed, with removal of all soft tissue from the margins of the defect to the dura. A curet is used to fashion a ledge (*D*) or a groove (*G*) for inlaying the tapered ends of the rib. *E*. Alternate ribs are removed and are split with an osteotome (*F*) after a groove is made along one edge. *H*. Split-thickness ribs are placed across the defect, with medullary and cortical surfaces facing the dura in alternation. The ribs are stabilized in position with 28-gauge stainless steel wire at each end and also across the middle with interlocking wire to hold them together in tight contact and thus to stimulate bony union.

ribs. The ribs are split with osteotomes and contoured with strong clamps or bone benders to provide a suitable cosmetic result. It is extremely important that the sections of rib be firmly secured to the exposed corticocancellous bone at the margins of the defect. Contact compression forces at the junction between autograft and host skull determine whether the grafts will become viable or will ultimately resorb. The inlaid ribs are then secured at either end with 28-gauge stainless steel wire. The ribs are alternated in terms of whether the cortical or the medullary surface faces the dura. Adjacent ribs must be closely approximated to one another to stimulate osseous rather than fibrous union. Wiring adjacent ribs together in the manner of a chain-linked fence has even been suggested.[53] The wound is closed in layers as described above, and a mildly compressive dressing is applied.

Cranioplasty with Allogeneic Skull and Particulate Demineralized Bone Matrix

Since the reports of Sicard, Dambrin, and Roger in 1917–1919, allogeneic human skull plates or extracranial bone have been periodically used for filling cranial defects. Contemporary papers on the use of skull allografts are sparse and are incompletely documented, with imprecise methodology and unsatisfactory follow-up.[50,78]

In the early 1980s, a spate of reports from one group seemed to herald the successful use of demineralized allogeneic bone powder as an osteoinductive matrix in craniofacial surgery.[51,52] However, while demineralized bone powders are osteoinductive in mice, rats, and rabbits, bone defects in dogs, monkeys, and humans will regenerate consistently only with a composite transplant of bone or bone morphogenetic protein and autogeneic bone marrow.[91] Subsequent clinical reports emphasized the unpredictability of demineralized human allografts in inducing osteogenesis.[51] Ousterhout reported up to 60 percent resorption in forehead cranioplasties.[57] Toriumi and colleagues found an average rate of resorption of demineralized allografts used for facial applications of 49 percent; this rate reached 82.5 percent when follow-up was longer than 2 years.[88]

Successful, reproducible repair of large and medium-sized skull defects with allogeneic powders and plates has not been demonstrated in humans. However, surface demineralized allogeneic skull discs do provide a suitable matrix for osteogenesis in small defects in the baboon and human.[64,67,74] Over the past 14 years, demineralized and undemineralized skull discs have been used successfully in hundreds of patients to fill in burr hole defects (Fig. 275-6).[64] These allografts become revitalized and incorporated into the adjacent skull and the replaced exteriorized skull plate through osteoconductive ''creeping substitution.''

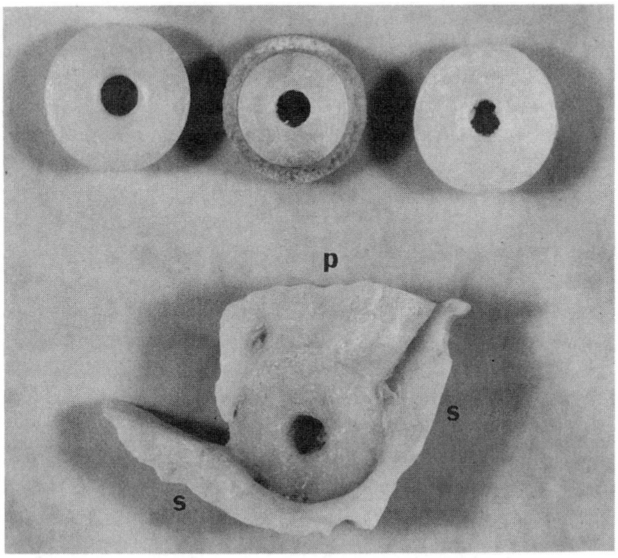

Figure 275-6 Allogeneic mineralized or demineralized skull discs have been successfully used to fill skull defects. Outer and inner surfaces of three skull discs are shown. The lower specimen, from a 42-year-old patient, was removed 4 years after a craniotomy for astrocytoma. The allograft was incorporated and remodeled despite radiotherapy with 5500 cGy. s, adjacent skull; p, section of devitalized free skull plate exteriorized at the time of the original craniotomy. The skull, the free plate, and the allogeneic skull discs are all remodeled and viable.

Complications and Results

Complications from cranioplasty may be divided between those characteristic of the operative procedure in general and those related more to the type of implant used. The risk of death in a patient who has marginal cardiopulmonary reserve who is bedridden or sedentary is extraordinary in relation to the fact that the aims of the procedure are cerebral protection and appearance. If a large prefabricated plate does not follow the cranial contours, compression of the underlying brain and internal herniation may result and cause death. Infection in a plate with subsequent meningitis or cerebral abscess formation may lead to permanent morbidity or even death. A frequent instructive comment by all authors is the need to obliterate contiguous paranasal sinuses months before implanting any plate. Otherwise the alloplastic material or devitalized autogeneic bone are subject to external microbial colonization.[23]

Metallic and plastic plates are foreign bodies that become encapsulated by host tissue. Sinus tracts between plate and skin, granulomas, and pneumatoceles have been reported.[87] Plates may loosen and erode the skin. Acrylic plates, which are especially brittle unless fortified with titanium wire mesh, may fracture and injure the underlying brain or protrude through the skin. Infection remains the predominant concern for all foreign bodies, and, if infection does occur, the foreign body must be removed. Autogeneic bone grafts are initially nonviable and therefore are subject to infection. These grafts later may resorb or produce cosmetically undesirable ridges.

The mortality rate for cranioplasty is very low. Even before the modern era, Grant and Norcross reported a mortality rate of 0.73 percent among 1385 reported cases.[17] Whereas complications were relatively frequent for cranioplasty with tantalum,[95] the experience with methyl methacrylate has been much better. Infection rates usually range between 1 and 8 percent,[23,75,89,102] with an inexplicably high rate of 12 percent in one report.[60] Hammon and Kempe reported 1 percent infection, 2 percent morbidity, and no mortality among 417 cranioplasties.[23] The most comprehensive survey involved 491 cranioplasties performed by many surgeons and was published by Rish and colleagues in 1979.[75] Their mortality rate of 0.2 percent with a total morbidity of 5.5 percent (infection rate of 3.7 percent, plate loss 3.1 percent) is likely representative of the results achievable in the community practice of neurosurgery. Manson and colleagues tabulated 45 different series of cranioplasties over all areas of the skull and found an average infection rate of 5 percent.[46]

Over the past 40 years of use, there have been no reports of malignancy associated with acrylic resin implants, and the plastic is well tolerated by the adjoining tissue.[6,7] In general the cosmetic result with methyl methacrylate is good, although large plates may give the head a flattened appearance, and wire mesh must be imbedded to prevent these brittle prostheses from fracturing.

Autogeneic bone is preferred by many, especially for children and in areas of previous infection or adjacent to sinuses.[17,37,42,43,57,60,61,80] Among 55 cranioplasties with autogeneic bone (46 rib cranioplasties, 9 ilium cranioplasties), Körloff and colleagues in 1973 reported one infection.[37] The cosmetic result was satisfactory in only 50 percent of these cases, however. Petty (1974) reported no infections in 19 rib cranioplasties and only one case of resorption.[60] Leivy and Tovi (1970) reported no complications among nine patients (seven cranioplasties with rib, two with ilium).[42] Including the use of osteoperiosteal grafts of skull, Grant and Norcross (1939) reported an infection rate of 5.1 percent among 89 cases (75 osteoperiosteal grafts, 7 rib grafts, etc.). They recommended using the seventh and ninth ribs for defects larger than 6 × 6 cm.[17] Santoni-Rugiu (1969) transplanted 12 osteoperiosteal grafts from adjacent cranium without complications.[80]

Complications related to the use of split-thickness cranial grafts include intracerebral hematoma,[9] subarachnoid hemorrhage, and dural tears.[30,100] Some authors warn against using titanium screws and plates in young patients because of the possibility that they may penetrate the dura into the underlying brain.

The general disinclination of many neurosurgeons to use autogeneic bone results from the need for two operative fields when donor sites are the ribs or ilium, the longer operative time, the difficulty of sculpturing the autograft, some tendency for the grafts to resorb, the occurrence of donor wound complications (pain, pneumothorax), and the frequently unacceptable cosmetic result.

Preservation and Delayed Reimplantation of Skull Flaps

Sections of cranium are often exteriorized for various periods with the prospect of delayed reimplantation. The treatment of this skull bone after its removal largely determines its natural history after replacement. Odom and colleagues (1952)[54] and Abbott (1953)[1] reported success with delayed cranioplasty after freezing the autograft. Hancock (1963) cautioned against autoclaving exteriorized skull because of the high rate of aseptic necrosis and infection with these replaced frozen autografts.[24] Fresh bone separated from its blood supply dies, with the exception of some periosteal, endosteal, and medullary cells and osteocytes within 0.2 mm of cortical bone surfaces. Frozen bone is entirely devitalized. The reorganization of a dead bone plate requires revascularization followed by resorption of dead bone trabeculae and cortex, then finally appositional new bone formation.[55,63] After bone is frozen, there is impaired coupling of new bone formation to follow the initial resorptive phase.

At this time the only generally accepted method of preserving cranium is by freezing to −70°C or freeze-drying after aseptic removal from the skull. The extent of resorption within these frozen plates is considerable in many cases and is not reduced even by augmentation with fresh corticocancellous bone.[65,66,83] Some of these frozen plates must be removed later and an acrylic cranioplasty performed if resorptive processes leave a thin, unprotective, and cosmetically undesirable plate.[66] The length of time the cranial flap is frozen has no bearing on the outcome; neither does sterilization with ethylene oxide adversely affect the biological events in the replaced plate.[67] Despite this tendency toward resorption, restoration of skull with frozen autogeneic skull is generally successful, except in individuals under 13.[24] In younger people with a very thin cranium, resorption reduces the replaced plate to only a small remnant.

In an effort to prevent resorption of an externalized plate, many clinicians have tried novel approaches for cranial bone preservation. Kreider (1920) and more recently Häuptli and Segantini (1980) and Stula (1984) have implanted the skull section subcutaneously in the abdomen.[25,72,83] This technique would likely maintain viability of some superficial cells and perhaps some matrix proteins. Yamada and colleagues advocated coating the exteriorized bone graft with acrylic resin to reduce resorption, but report an infection rate of 11 percent.[99]

Contaminated skull must not be boiled or autoclaved, because these procedures denature the essential bone proteins and result in nearly universal resorption. Cold-cycle ethylene oxide may be used to sterilize skull bone, provided the residues are desorbed by lyophilization or prolonged aeration over at least 5 days at room temperature.[68]

Fresh skull autografts remain the best kind of graft. No preservative method for bone yet equals the osteogenic capacity of a fresh autograft.[67,69] That such a graft is often unavailable accounts for the search for a suitable alternative.

Prospects for the Future

Calvarial bone has the lowest regenerative capacity of any bone in the body. This characteristic led Barth (1893–1898) to conclude in error that all fresh transplanted bone dies and must be replaced by surrounding tissues.[8] It is known that fractures of the cranial base (of chondral origin) heal faster than those over the convexity (of membranous origin).[43] This limited regenerative capacity of calvaria provides the ultimate test for effectiveness of grafts and biological bone substitutes. Paradoxical, therefore, are reports that autogeneic transplants of membranous bone resorb less and vascularize more rapidly as onlay grafts than do those of endochondral origin.[39,81,101] These observations in animals have induced maxillofacial surgeons to use cranium as the preferred source for autogeneic bone grafts.[21,47]

The biology of repair of skull autografts and allografts is complex and incompletely understood. In contrast to fracture repair, bone graft remodeling occurs after revascularization without intermediary cartilage formation. The successful revitalization of a graft requires a coupled sequence of resorption of the necrotic bone of the graft followed by appositional new bone formation. In contrast to extracranial bone healing, osteoclasts within resorption cavities uniquely are not seen in skull repair.[66]

It is possible that in the adult skull, the diminished functional demands and stresses (Wolff's law) result in the predominance of resorption over appositional new bone formation in the implant. There are further biological differences in the proliferative capacities of living periosteum derived from bone of cartilaginous as compared to membranous origin (the pericranium and dura mater). Physical and chemical treatments (boiling, freezing, irradiation, etc.) further alter the bone by denaturing collagen and other structural proteins and interrupt chemical bonds and polypeptide growth factors. These substances ordinarily enhance new bone formation at the recipient site in the fresh autograft.

A human cranium reconstituted with bone identical in esthetic, viability, and mechanical properties represents the consummate cranioplasty. Alloplastic materials will always fall short of the goal of viability, though they may be inert, nontoxic, cosmetically desirable, and protective. The fresh autograft, long regarded as the "gold standard," usually becomes viable, but it tends to resorb and to lose desired cosmetic and mechanical properties. Allografts suffer the same fate to a greater extent.

Over the past decade revolutionary progress has unraveled some mysteries of the molecular biology of bone healing. Since Urist's seminal discovery of an osteogenic protein in 1965, he and others have pursued the identification of the bone morphogenetic protein and of a panoply of polypeptide growth factors.[71,90,98] Soft and hard tissue healing is now known to involve interactions between a multitude of cellular species and autocrine, paracrine, and endocrine factors. Preeminent among these are the bone morphogenetic proteins (BMPs) responsible for osteoinduction—that is, the phenotypic conversion of pluripotential stem cells into osteoblasts as a consequence of interaction with a bioactive molecule. BMPs are glycoproteins and are extractable from bone matrix with chaotropic agents such as 4 M guanidine hydrochloride, 6 M urea in 0.5 M $CaCl_2$, or ethylene glycol. They are insoluble in aqueous solution because of their close association with noncollagenous matrix proteins and are present in quantities of less than 1 μg per kilogram of cortical bone. The arrival of biochemical purification and recombinant DNA techniques has made possible the identification of a series of BMPs with a relative migration rate of 30 kD. Using tryptic peptide sequence from the 30 kD region, seven cDNAs have been cloned and named BMP-1, 2, 3, 4, 5, 6, and 7. All but BMP-1 are members of the transforming growth factor-β (TGF-β) superfamily of molecules. Recombinant human BMP-2 (rhBMP-2), manufactured by Genetics Institute, is now undergoing field trials for augmenting the repair of traumatic limb fractures.

A cascade for graft healing is triggered by BMP and then further promoted by complex cytokine interactions, which cause mesenchymally derived cells such as fibroblasts and monocytes to migrate (by chemotaxis), proliferate, and differentiate. These polypeptide growth factors are released from platelets, macrophages, and fibroblasts. They include platelet-derived growth factor (PDGF), epidermal growth factor (EGF), basic fibroblast growth factor (bFGF), TGF-β, insulin-like growth factor (IGF), and platelet-derived endothelial cell growth factor (PD-ECGF).

TGF-β, PDGF, and bFGF are central to bone repair. Studies by Urist and Landesman and Reddi show that osteogenic factors have to be delivered within a 3 to 5 day window after transplantation.[41,91] Simultaneous activation of cell populations by these growth factors is essential. Responding cell populations decrease with age. The ratio of mesenchymal stem cells to bone marrow cells is 1/10,000 in the newborn, 1/100,000 in the adolescent, 1/250,000 at 35 years, 1/400,000 at 50 years, and 1/2,000,000 at 80 years.[26] The greater osteogenic capacity in the young reflects this dynamic interplay between cells and growth and differentiation factors.

Senn in 1889 reported demineralized bovine bone to have some osteogenic capacity. Urist in 1965 and Reddi and Huggins in 1972 demonstrated osteoinduction resulting from the placement of demineralized bone in extraskeletal sites.[71,90] Contemporary neurosurgery now stands on the threshold of revolutionary contributions to bone healing from the findings and applications of molecular biology. Bioactive molecules sequentially released from biodegradable delivery systems to interact with responding cells will transform surgical efforts at regeneration of the cranium.

References

1. Abbott KH. Use of frozen cranial bone flaps for autogenous and homologous grafts in cranioplasty and spinal interbody fusion. *J Neurosurg* 1953; 10:380–388.
2. Asimacopoulos TJ, Papadakis N, Mark VH. A new method of cranioplasty: technical note. *J Neurosurg* 1977; 47:790–792.
3. Bernstein TW, Stewart WA, Andrews EE. Cranioplasty: utilization of bank bone flaps to prepare acrylic cranioplasties: a technical note. *J Trauma* 1972; 12:133–134.
4. Black SPW. Reconstruction of the supraorbital ridge using aluminum. *Surg Neurol* 1978; 9:121–128.
5. Blair GAS, Fannin TF, Gordon DS. Titanium-strip cranioplasty. *Br Med J* 1976; 2:907–908.
6. Cabanela ME, Coventry MB, MacCarty CS, Miller WE. The fate of patients with methyl methacrylate cranioplasty. *J Bone Joint Surg [Am]* 1972; 54-A:278–281.
7. Charnley J. The reaction of bone to self-curing acrylic cement: a long-term histological study in man. *J Bone Joint Surg [Br]* 1970; 52-B:340–353.
8. Chase SW, Herndon CH. The fate of autogenous and homogenous bone grafts: a historical review. *J Bone Joint Surg [Am]* 1955; 37-A:809–841.
9. Cooper PR, Schechter B, Jacobs GB, et al. A pre-formed methyl methacrylate cranioplasty. *Surg Neurol* 1977; 8:219–221.
10. Couldwell WT, Chen TC, Weiss MH, et al. Cranioplasty with the Medpor porous polyethylene Flexblock implant: technical note. *J Neurosurg* 1994; 81:483–486.
11. Courtemanche AD, Thompson GB. Silastic cranioplasty following craniofacial injuries. *Plast Reconstr Surg* 1968; 41:165–170.
12. Edwards MSB, Ousterhout DK. Autogeneic skull bone grafts to reconstruct large or complex skull defects in children and adolescents. *Neurosurgery* 1987; 20:273–280.
13. Firtell DN, Grisius RJ. Cranioplasty of the difficult frontal region. *J Prosthet Dent* 1981; 46:425–429.
14. Fodstad H, Ekstedt J, Fridén H. CSF hydrodynamic studies before and after cranioplasty. *Acta Neurochir (Wien) [Suppl]* 1979; 28:514–518.
15. Galicich JH, Hovind KH. Stainless steel mesh-acrylic cranioplasty: technical note. *J Neurosurg* 1967; 27:376–378.
16. Genest AS. Cranioplasty made easier. *Surg Neurol* 1978; 10:255–257.
17. Grant FC, Norcross NC. Repair of cranial defects by cranioplasty. *Ann Surg* 1939; 110:488–512.
18. Grantham EG, Landis HP. Cranioplasty and the post-traumatic syndrome. *J Neurosurg* 1948; 5:19–22.
19. Haar FL. Complication of linear skull fracture in young children. *Am J Dis Child* 1975; 129:1197–1200.
20. Habal MB. Current status of biomaterial's clinical applications in plastic and reconstructive surgery. *Biomater Med Devices Artif Organs* 1979; 7:229–241.
21. Habal MB. Craniofacial surgery. In Habal MB, Reddi AH (eds): *Bone Grafts and Bone Substitutes.* Philadelphia: Saunders, 1992, pp 316–365.
22. Habal MB, Leake DL, Maniscalco JE. A new method for reconstruction of major defects in the cranial vault. *Surg Neurol* 1976; 6:137–138.
23. Hammon WM, Kempe LG. Methyl methacrylate cranioplasty: 13 years experience with 417 patients. *Acta Neurochir (Wien)* 1971; 25:69–77.
24. Hancock DO. The fate of replaced bone flaps. *J Neurosurg* 1963; 20:983–984.

25. Häuptli J, Segantini P. Neue Aufbewahrungsart von Schädelkalottenstücken nach dekompressiver Kraniotomie. *Helv Chir Acta* 1980; 47:121–124.
26. Haynesworth SE, Goldberg VM, Caplan AI. Diminution of the number of mesenchymal stem cells as a cause of skeletal aging. In Buckwalter JA, Goldberg VM. Woo S L-Y (eds): *Musculoskeletal Soft Tissue Aging: Impact on Mobility.* American Association of Orthopaedic Surgeons, 1994, pp 80–86.
27. Henry HM, Guerrero C, Moody RA. Cerebrospinal fluid fistula from fractured acrylic cranioplasty plate. *J Neurosurg* 1976; 45:227–228.
28. Holmes RE, Hagler HK. Porous hydroxyapatite as a bone graft substitute in cranial reconstruction: a histometric study. *Plast Reconstr Surg* 1988; 81:662–671.
29. Homsy CA. Bio-compatibility in selection of materials for implantation. *J Biomed Mater Res* 1970; 4:341–356.
30. Jackson IT, Helden G, Marx R. Skull bone grafts in maxillofacial and craniofacial surgery. *J Oral Maxillofac Surg* 1986; 44:949–955.
31. Jackson IJ, Hoffmann GT. Depressed comminuted fracture of a plastic cranioplasty. *J Neurosurg* 1956; 13:116–117.
32. Jordan RD, White JT, Schupper N. Technique for cranioplasty prosthesis fabrication. *J Prosthet Dent* 1978; 40:230–233.
33. Karvounis PC, Chiu J, Sabin H. The use of prefabricated polyethylene plate for cranioplasty. *J Trauma* 1970; 10:249–254.
34. Keen WW. *Surgery: Its Principles and Practice.* Philadelphia: Saunders, 1909.
35. Kent JN, Zide MF. Wound healing: bone and biomaterials. *Otolaryngol Clin North Am* 1984; 17:273–319.
36. Kingsley D, Till K, Hoare R. Growing fractures of the skull. *J Neurol Neurosurg Psychiatry* 1978; 41:312–318.
37. Körloff B, Nylén B, Rietz K. Bone grafting of skull defects: a report on 55 cases. *Plast Reconstr Surg* 1973; 52:378–383.
38. Koslow M, Ransohoff J. Primary wire mesh cranioplasty in flap infections. *Neurosurgery* 1979; 4:290–291.
39. Kusiak JF, Zins JE, Whitaker LA. The early revascularization of membranous bone. *Plast Reconstr Surg* 1985; 76:510–516.
40. Lake PA, Morin MA, Pitts FW. Radiolucent prosthesis of mesh-reinforced acrylic: technical note. *J Neurosurg* 1970; 32:597–602.
41. Landesman R, Reddi AH. *In vivo* analysis of the half-life of the osteoinductive potential of demineralized bone matrix using diffusion chambers. *Calcif Tissue Int* 1989; 45:348–353.
42. Leivy DM, Tovi D. Autogenous bone cranioplasty. *Acta Chir Scand* 1970; 136:385–387.
43. Longacre JJ. Deformities of the forehead, scalp and cranium. In Converse JM (ed): *Reconstructive Plastic Surgery,* vol 2. Philadelphia: Saunders, 1964, pp 564–597.
44. Malis LI. Titanium mesh and acrylic cranioplasty. *Neurosurgery* 1989; 25:351–355.
45. Maniscalco JE, Garcia-Bengochea F. Cranioplasty: a method of prefabricating alloplastic plates. *Surg Neurol* 1974; 2:339–341.
46. Manson PN, Crawley WA, Hoopes JE. Frontal cranioplasty: risk factors and choice of cranial vault reconstructive material. *Plast Reconstr Surg* 1986; 77:888–904.
47. Marchac D. Deformities of the forehead, scalp, and cranial vault. In McCarthy JG (ed): *Plastic Surgery,* vol 2. Philadelphia: Saunders, 1990, pp 1538–1573.
48. Matukas VJ, Clanton JT, Langford KH, Aronin PA. Hydroxylapatite: an adjunct to cranial bone grafting. *J Neurosurg* 1988; 69:514–517.
49. McComb JG, Heiden J, Weiss MH. Cortical damage from methyl methacrylate cranioplasty. *Neurosurgery* 1978; 3:233 (abstr).
50. Merville L, Brunet C, Derome P. Reconstruction frontale et des sinus frontaux. *Ann Chir Plast* 1982; 27:205–210.
51. Mulliken JB. Induced osteogenesis and craniofacial surgery. In Caronni EP (ed): *Craniofacial Surgery.* Boston: Little, Brown, 1985, pp 42–53.
52. Mulliken JB, Glowacki J, Kaban LB, et al. Use of demineralized allogeneic bone implants for the correction of maxillocraniofacial deformities. *Ann Surg* 1981; 3:366–372.
53. Munro IR, Guyuron B. Split-rib cranioplasty. *Ann Plast Surg* 1981; 7:341–346.
54. Odom GL, Woodhall B, Wrenn FR Jr. The use of refrigerated autogenous bone flaps for cranioplasty. *J Neurosurg* 1952; 9:606–610.
55. Oklund SA, Prolo DJ, Gutierrez RV, King SE. Quantitative comparisons of healing in cranial fresh autografts, frozen autografts and processed autografts and allografts in canine skull defects. *Clin Orthop* 1986; 205:269–291.
56. Olson NR, Newman MH. Acrylic frontal cranioplasty. *Arch Otolaryngol* 1969; 89:774–777.
57. Ousterhout DK. Clinical experience in cranial and facial reconstruction with demineralized bone. *Ann Plast Surg* 1985; 15:367–373.
58. Peltier LF, Speer DP. Calcium sulfate. In Habal MB, Reddi AH (eds): *Bone Grafts and Bone Substitutes.* Philadelphia: Saunders, 1992, pp 243–246.
59. Pensler J, McCarthy JG. Anatomical study of calvarial thickness. *Plast Reconstr Surg* 1985; 75:648–651.
60. Petty PG. Cranioplasty: a follow-up study. *Med J Aust* 1974; 2:806–808.
61. Posnick JC, Goldstein JA, Armstrong D, Rutka JT. Reconstruction of skull defects in children and adolescents by the use of fixed cranial bone grafts: long-term results. *Neurosurgery* 1993; 32:785–791.
62. Powell NB, Riley RW. Cranial bone grafting in facial aesthetic and reconstructive contouring. *Arch Otolaryngol Head Neck Surg* 1987; 113:713–719.
63. Prolo DJ, Burres KP, McLaughlin WT, Christensen AH. Autogenous skull cranioplasty: fresh and preserved (frozen), with consideration of the cellular response. *Neurosurgery* 1979; 4:18–29.
64. Prolo DJ, Gutierrez RV, DeVine JS, Oklund SA. Clinical utility of allogeneic skull discs in human craniotomy. *Neurosurgery* 1984; 14:183–186.
65. Prolo DJ, Oklund SA. Composite autogeneic human cranioplasty: frozen skull supplemented with fresh iliac corticocancellous bone. *Neurosurgery* 1984; 15:846–851.
66. Prolo DJ, Oklund SA. The use of bone grafts and alloplastic materials in cranioplasty. *Clin Orthop* 1991; 268:270–278.
67. Prolo DJ, Pedrotti PW, Burres KP, Oklund S. Superior osteogenesis in transplanted allogeneic canine skull following chemical sterilization. *Clin Orthop* 1982; 168:230–242.
68. Prolo DJ, Pedrotti PW, White DH. Ethylene oxide sterilization of bone, dura mater, and fascia lata for human transplantation. *Neurosurgery* 1980; 6:529–539.
69. Prolo DJ, Rodrigo JJ. Contemporary bone graft physiology and surgery. *Clin Orthop* 1985; 200:322–342.
70. Rawlings CE III, Wilklins RH, Hanker JS, et al. Evaluation in cats of a new material for cranioplasty: a composite of plaster of Paris and hydroxylapatite. *J Neurosurg* 1988; 69:269–275.
71. Reddi AH, Huggins C. Biochemical sequences in the transformation of normal fibroblasts in adolescent rats. *Proc Natl Acad Sci USA* 1972; 69:1601–1605.
72. Reeves DL. *Cranioplasty.* Springfield, IL: Charles C Thomas, 1950.
73. Rifkinson-Mann S. Cranial surgery in ancient Peru. *Neurosurgery* 1988; 23:411–416.
74. Ripamonti U. Calvarial regeneration in primates with autolyzed antigen-extracted allogeneic bone. *Clin Orthop* 1992; 282:293–303.
75. Rish BL, Dillon JD, Meirowsky AM, et al. Cranioplasty: a review of 1030 cases of penetrating head injury. *Neurosurgery* 1979; 4:381–385.
76. Roux FX, Brasnu D, Loty B, et al. Madreporic coral: a new bone graft substitute for cranial surgery. *J Neurosurg* 1988; 69:510–513.
77. Rubin LR. Polyethylene as a bone and cartilage substitute: a 32-year retrospective. In Rubin LR (ed): *Biomaterials in Reconstructive Surgery.* St. Louis: Mosby, 1983, pp 474–493.
78. Salyer KE, Gendler E, Menendez JL, et al. Demineralized perforated bone implants in craniofacial surgery. *J Craniofac Surg* 1992; 3:55–62.
79. Salyer KE, Hall CD. Porous hydroxylapatite as an onlay bone-graft substitute for maxillary surgery. *Plast Reconstr Surg* 1989; 84:236–244.
80. Santoni-Rugiu P. Repair of skull defects by outer table osteoperiosteal free grafts. *Plast Reconstr Surg* 1969; 43:157–161.

81. Smith JD, Abramson M. Membranous vs. endochondral bone autografts. *Arch Otolaryngol* 1974; 99:203–205.
82. Spence WT: Form-fitting plastic cranioplasty. *J Neurosurg* 1954; 11:219–225.
83. Stula D. *Cranioplasty: Indications, Techniques, and Results.* New York: Springer, 1984, pp 1–112.
84. Stula D, Müller HR. Schädeldachplastic nach grossen dekompressiven Kraniotonien mit Massenverschieburg; CT Analyse. *Neurochirurgia (Stuttg)* 1980; 23:41–46.
85. Tabaddor K, LaMorgese J. Complication of a large cranial defect: case report. *J Neurosurg* 1976; 44:506–508.
86. Tessier P. Autogenous bone grafts taken from the calvarium for facial and cranial applications. *Clin Plast Surg* 1982; 9:531–538.
87. Timmons RL. Cranial defects and their repair. In Youmans JR (ed): *Neurological Surgery: A Comprehensive Reference Guide to the Diagnosis and Management of Neurosurgical Problems,* 2d ed. Philadelphia: Saunders, 1982, pp 2228–2250.
88. Toriumi DM, Larrabee WF Jr, Walike JW, et al. Demineralized bone. Implant resorption with long-term follow-up. *Arch Otolaryngol Head Neck Surg* 1990; 116:676–680.
89. Tysvaer AT, Hovind KH. Stainless steel mesh-acrylic cranioplasty. *J Trauma* 1977; 17:231–233.
90. Urist MR. Bone: formation by autoinduction. *Science* 1965; 150:893–899.
91. Urist MR. Bone morphogenetic protein, bone regeneration, heterotopic ossification and bone-bone marrow consortium. *Bone Mineral Res* 1989; 6:57–112.
92. Van Gool AV. Preformed polymethylmethacrylate cranioplasties: report of 45 cases. *J Maxillofac Surg* 1985; 13:2–8.
93. Walker AE, Erculei F. The late results of cranioplasty. *Arch Neurol* 1963; 9:105–110.
94. Wellisz T, Dougherty W, Gross J. Craniofacial applications for the Medpor porous polyethylene flexblock implant. *J Craniofac Surg* 1992; 3:101–107.
95. White JC. Late complications following cranioplasty with alloplastic plates. *Ann Surg* 1948; 128:743–755.
96. Wilkinson HA. Autogeneic skull bone grafts. *Neurosurgery* 1987; 21:760. Letter.
97. Woolf JI, Walker AE. Cranioplasty: collective review. *Int Abst Surg* 1945; 81:1-23.
98. Wozney JM. Bone morphogenetic proteins. *Prog Growth Factor Res* 1989; 1:267–280.
99. Yamada H, Sakai N, Takada M, et al. Cranioplasty utilizing a preserved autogenous bone flap coated with acrylic resin. *Acta Neurochir (Wien)* 1980; 52:273–280.
100. Young VL, Schuster RH, Harris LW. Intracerebral hematoma complicating split calvarial bone-graft harvesting. *Plast Reconstr Surg* 1990; 86:763–765.
101. Zins JE, Whitaker LA. Membranous versus endochondral bone: implications for craniofacial reconstruction. *Plast Reconstr Surg* 1983; 72:778–785.
102. Zotti G, De Vito R. Cranioplastica con resina acrilica: considerazioni su 139 casi. *Minerva Med* 1971; 62:3760–3769.

276

Traumatic Intracranial Hematomas

Srinath Samudrala
Paul R. Cooper

It is convenient to classify subdural hematomas (SDHs) into acute lesions, which present within 48 to 72 h of injury, subacute lesions, which become manifest at 3 to 20 days, and chronic lesions, which do not produce symptoms until from 3 weeks to several months after injury.

Acute Subdural Hematoma

Epidemiology

Acute SDH occurs in approximately 5 to 22 percent of patients with severe head injury.[31,56,75] Males predominate in most series in a ratio of 3:1. Older people have a greater risk of developing acute SDH, and the average age of patients with acute SDH is greater than for other types of head injury.[20,72] Head trauma from a fall is more apt to produce an acute SDH than are head injuries from vehicle accidents, assaults, or other common causes.[20]

Pathogenesis

Acute SDH is caused by a high-speed impact that accelerates the brain relative to the fixed dural structures, tearing bridging veins that traverse the space between the cortical surface and the venous sinuses. Subdural hemorrhages can also result from injury to the surface of the brain with bleeding from cortical vessels into the subdural space. The impact that produces an acute SDH may also cause diffuse parenchymal injury, which can be graded as to severity and correlates strongly with outcome.[39] This diffuse injury, which is manifested by brain shifting and obliteration of the basal cisterns on computed tomography (CT) scans, can have a greater influence on the patient's outcome and prognosis than the presence of a hematoma in the subdural space.[75]

Clinical Findings and Diagnosis

The clinical findings are related to the size and rapidity of growth of the SDH and the severity of diffuse injury to the brain. Patients who are rendered immediately unconscious with decerebrate posturing at the time of injury may be assumed to have sustained diffuse (and perhaps irreversible) injury to the cerebral parenchyma. Recovery often does not take place regardless of how rapidly the hematoma is removed or intracranial pressure (ICP) controlled.

In patients with less severe injuries, the sequence of changes in the level of consciousness is determined by the magnitude of the impact injury and the rapidity of hematoma accumulation. Patients with minor injuries may lose consciousness only briefly or not at all at the time of impact, and thus have a lucid interval. As the hematoma expands in the early post-trauma period, however, consciousness is gradually lost.

An altered level of consciousness, pupillary inequality, and motor deficit are common signs in patients with acute SDH (Table 276-1). These signs are seen with other expanding mass lesions and are not pathognomonic for SDH. However, regardless of the type of mass, they may provide information as to the side of the lesion: mass lesions are usually ipsilateral to the dilated pupil and contralateral to the motor deficit. Contralateral (false localizing) pupillary dilation may be seen as a result of direct trauma to the globe, oculomotor or optic nerve injury, or direct midbrain trauma. Ipsilateral (false localizing) motor deficit is not uncommon and results from cerebral parenchymal injury on the side opposite the SDH or from compression of the contralateral cerebral peduncle against the edge of the tentorium (Kernohan's notch).[35]

Specialized Diagnostic Evaluation

Skull roentgenograms are commonly obtained in head-injured patients who have a focal neurological deficit or depressed level of consciousness, in a search for a linear skull fracture. However, the presence of a skull fracture does not reliably predict the presence or site of an intracranial hematoma. Although skull films may be used to assess a pineal shift, emergency room skull films are often of poor quality, and they reveal a pineal shift in less than 20 percent of patients with an acute SDH.[40,41] For the obtunded patient suspected of having an SDH or other intracranial hematoma, skull films delay the diagnostic evaluation, provide little information that will help the neurosurgeon to make therapeutic decisions, and are unnecessary except to evaluate a depressed skull fracture or localize the site of a cerebrospinal fluid fistula.

In most institutions, CT scanners are readily available and should be used as the first diagnostic procedure for patients suspected of having an acute SDH. CT scanning is rapid, visualizes the entire intracranial compartment, and can reliably distinguish the density and thus the nature of intra- and extra-axial mass lesions. Acute SDHs appear as hyperdense crescentic areas over the cerebral hemispheres (Fig. 276-1). They may be localized to one or more lobes or may be holohemispheric, extending over the entire convexity. Acute SDHs are sometimes isointense to brain when patients have a low hemoglobin level or when cerebrospinal fluid

TABLE 276-1 Frequency of Various Signs in Patients with Acute Subdural Hematoma*

Sign	Patients, %
Anisocoria	51
Papilledema	16
Cranial nerve VI palsy	5
Hemiparesis	49

*As compiled from a number of large series in the literature.

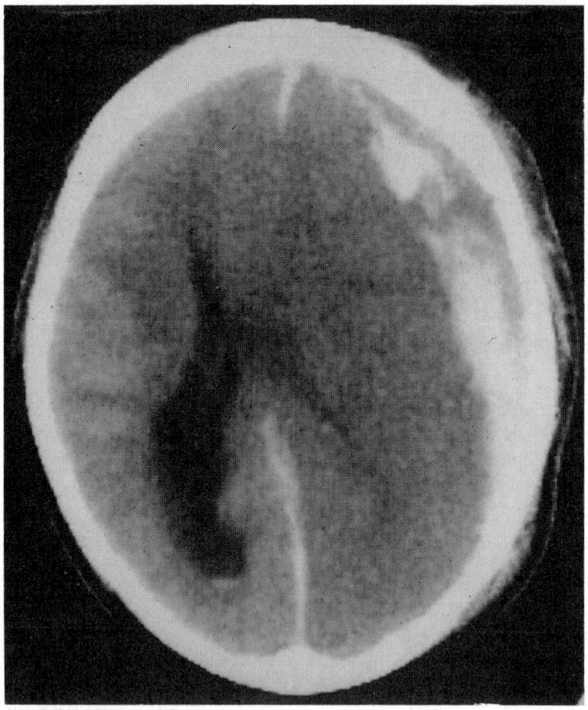

Figure 276-1 A CT scan of a patient with an acute subdural hematoma. There is a significant mass effect and shift, causing compression of the ipsilateral lateral ventricle.

from torn arachnoid dilutes the extravasated blood. The volume of the hematoma (as found at operation) may be underestimated by the CT scan because the intensity of blood is similar to that of the inner skull table, and this fact should be considered when debating evacuation. Prior to the widespread use of CT scanners, carotid angiography was used as an alternative means of diagnosis. Now it is of historical interest only.

Although magnetic resonance imaging (MRI) is more sensitive than CT at detecting intraparenchymal lesions caused by head trauma, it has been of limited value in the radiographic diagnosis of acute SDH.[78] MRI takes too long and involves too many restrictions on patient monitoring to be practical for the evaluation of severely injured patients. Moreover, its great sensitivity is not of immediate value for the diagnosis of surgical lesions that are readily demonstrated by CT. MRI is useful in assessing the intraparenchymal injury associated with an SDH and may be performed in the stabilized patient.

Treatment

Patients who are admitted with a depressed level of consciousness and a suspected intracranial mass should be assumed to have an increase in ICP. Medical treatment to lower elevated ICP should begin after the initial evaluation and is discussed elsewhere in this textbook. In determining whether surgical evacuation will benefit the patient, one must evaluate the contribution of the SDH to the neurological deficit, ICP, and overall condition of the patient. In general, all SDHs that are more than 5 mm thick and that contribute significantly to the mass effect and shift should be considered for evacuation. Patients who are in good neurological condition and harbor a small SDH may not need surgery. Adult patients who are still flaccid with absent brain stem reflexes after aggressive resuscitative efforts will almost certainly have a poor result and are not candidates for operation. Some patients who have exhausted their reserves of intracranial compliance may benefit from the evacuation of even small hematomas. We believe that if an operation is to be done, it should be done as early as possible.

The definitive treatment of an acute SDH consists of operative removal using a large craniotomy centered over the maximum thickness of the hematoma.[16] The wide exposure provided by the craniotomy allows complete removal of solid clot and visualization and control of the source of the hemorrhage. When present, contused brain is resected and intraparenchymal hematomas are evacuated. Real-time ultrasound should be used before dural closure to rule out newly developed intraparenchymal lesions and to assess the adequacy of hematoma removal. We leave a drain in the subdural space, close the dura around the drain, and wire the bone flap in place. In the postoperative period the ICP is monitored; a CT scan is obtained within 24 h of operation and again 2 days after, even if the patient is apparently doing well, to rule out the presence of recurrent extra-axial hematoma formation or delayed parenchymal bleeding. Prophylactic antibiotics are given for the first 24 h.

Burr holes have been used in the past for the treatment of acute SDH. For rapidly deteriorating patients with clear signs of focality, emergency burr holes may be useful to diagnose the presence of an acute SDH and to evacuate enough of it to stabilize the patient's neurological condition or reverse signs of herniation.[63] However, burr holes or small trephine openings are not adequate for the definitive treatment of acute SDH, because visualization of the hematoma is limited and total evacuation of a solid hematoma cannot be accomplished through small openings.[31] Real-time ultrasound can improve the diagnostic accuracy of burr holes and can be used if CT scanning is not available.[1,2] In most institutions, rapid CT scanning and emergent craniotomy can obviate the need for emergency burr holes, which may delay definitive decompression.

Large decompressive craniectomies have been proposed as a means of reducing mortality from acute SDH by providing external decompression of a swollen brain.[52] Decompression does reduce ICP and improve compliance, but outcome has not been improved by the procedure. This failure probably reflects the fact that many patients with acute SDH have severe parenchymal injury that cannot be reversed by decompression. Moreover, there is experimental evidence that decompression may increase edema formation and result in strangulation of cortical vessels at the edges of the craniectomy, producing cerebral infarction.[14]

Complications

As many as one-half of patients will have elevations of ICP after the operation.[38,43] Postoperative ICP greater than 45 mmHg has been shown to correlate with poor outcome.[74] CT scanning will clarify the cause of these elevations and distinguish the patients who need reoperation from the patients whose ICP should be managed medically. The most common cause of elevated ICP in the postoperative period is cerebral swelling, which results from compression of the brain by the SDH and from direct parenchymal injury sustained at the time of trauma. The edema is often diffuse and generally is not amenable to operative treatment. Therapy consists of controlling the ICP by medical means.

Recurrent or residual hematoma is not an uncommon complication. If the hematoma is small and the ICP not elevated, operative removal may not be necessary, although the patient must be followed with appropriate imaging studies to detect the formation of a chronic SDH. Large hematomas or those associated with elevated ICP should be removed. Delayed intracerebral hemorrhage may occur into areas of the brain that have undergone shearing or in loci that show minor contusions on the initial CT scan. This complication is more frequent than was suspected in the past but is readily identified by frequent CT scanning in the postoperative period. Post-traumatic seizures occur in up to one-third of patients with severe head injury. Phenytoin has been shown to decrease their incidence in the first week after trauma but has no antiepileptic effect after this period.[70]

Outcome

The outcome from acute SDH has been generally unsatisfactory. Most series in the literature report a mortality of over 50 percent, and none records a mortality of less than 35 percent. Of the patients who do survive, most do not return to normal functioning, and a significant number have disabilities that render them dependent.[10,39,53,74,75]

For the individual patient, however, there are factors that affect outcome in either a beneficial or detrimental way. McKissock et al. found that mortality was 20 percent for patients under age 40 and 65 percent for patients over age 40.[40] Others have found that mortality changes after age 50 or 60.[27,33] Elderly patients—those older than 80 years—have a mortality of 88 percent from acute SDH.[10] The initial and postresuscitative Glasgow Coma Scale (GCS) score has been shown to correlate reliably with outcome.[53,75] Patients who are conscious at the time of operation have a mortality of 9 percent, whereas unconscious patients have a 40 to 65 percent mortality.[31] While Seelig et al. and Haselberger et al. have shown that prompt operation has an important bearing on outcome, other studies have shown no statistical difference.[23,56,74,75] Patients who are alcohol abusers have a higher incidence of morbidity and mortality after acute SDH than nonalcoholics.[62] Associated brain injury also influences outcome; acute SDH without evidence of parenchymal injury is associated with a mortality of 22 percent, but patients with a concurrent brain injury have a mortality between 30 and 64 percent.[23] Elevations in postoperative ICP, especially when refractory to medical management, indicate a poor prognosis.[43,75]

Chronic Subdural Hematoma

As mentioned above, SDHs that develop from 3 days to 3 weeks after head injury are called subacute, and those that appear later than 3 weeks after injury are called chronic. Little has been written about subacute SDH, and for all practical purposes hematomas that produce symptoms within the first week clinically resemble acute SDH, and those that appear 1 to 3 weeks after injury are much like chronic SDH.

The incidence of chronic SDH is 1 to 2 per 100,000 people per year.[18] Most patients are 50 years of age or older. Between one-quarter and one-half have no history of head injury, and in those with a history of trauma the injury was often a mild one. A significant proportion of patients are predisposed to SDH by chronic alcoholism, epilepsy, or coagulopathies.

Pathogenesis

Small amounts of hemorrhage into the subdural space or larger hematomas in patients with brain atrophy may fail to produce symptoms. Within 1 week, the hematoma is covered by another membrane beneath the dura, and by 3 weeks an inner membrane forms between the hematoma and the arachnoid surface over the brain, thus completely enclosing the hematoma. During this period the hematoma liquefies and becomes progressively more hypodense on the CT scan. In some patients the hematoma gradually enlarges over the next weeks, whereas in others there is gradual resorption of the liquefied blood.

It has been postulated that a chronic SDH enlarges because the capsule acts as an osmotic membrane, with cerebrospinal fluid diffusing into the hematoma and increasing its volume. Zollinger and Gross suggested that the flow across the membrane occurs as a result of an increase in osmotic pressure from a breakdown of hemoglobin molecules.[79] This theory has now been discredited, because it has been shown that the osmolality of the hematoma does not change with time.[73] Moreover, the ratios of albumin to gamma globulin and of albumin to total protein are higher in the hematoma than in serum. It is likely that albumin diffuses across the hematoma membrane, and that the hematoma also enlarges from recurrent hemorrhage into its surrounding membranes.[29]

There is considerable angiographic and CT evidence that some hematomas regress in size and do not need surgical treatment. It is likely that there is a balance between hematoma formation and resorption; when the rate of resorption exceeds the rate of formation, the hematoma will shrink, and, conversely, when formation exceeds resorption, the hematoma will enlarge.

Symptoms and Signs

The symptoms and signs of chronic SDH are variable and are not pathognomonic. In the elderly patient the insidious onset of symptoms is sometimes interpreted as dementia. In other patients the onset of a motor deficit is confused with a cerebrovascular accident, transient ischemic attacks, or a brain tumor.[28] Common signs are listed in Table 276-2.

Diagnostic Evaluation

The diagnostic procedure of choice for the evaluation of a chronic SDH is CT. In the first week after injury, a chronic SDH appears hyperdense in relation to brain, and in the next 2 weeks most hematomas will appear isodense (although some will appear hyperdense or hypodense). After 3 weeks, the vast majority will be hypodense and will assume a lenticular appearance. Nevertheless, because recurrent bleeding frequently occurs from the vascular hematoma membranes, a chronic SDH can appear as a mixture of hypo- and hyperdense material.

Older, less sophisticated CT scanners could not always readily distinguish isodense hematomas from cerebral parenchyma, and the shift of midline structures was often mistakenly attributed to

TABLE 276-2 Frequency of Various Signs in Patients with Chronic Subdural Hematoma*

Sign	Patients, %
Hemiparesis	45
Papilledema	24
Hemianopsia	7
Cranial nerve III abnormality	11
Impaired consciousness	53

*Mean calculated from several large series in the literature.

cerebral swelling or even to a tumor. Bilateral isodense SDHs were even more likely to result in misdiagnosis, because they produce no midline shift. Most of the newer CT scanners show the interface between cortical gray matter and the underlying white matter quite well. When the interface is seen to be well away from the inner table, a chronic SDH should be suspected. If there is remaining uncertainty, contrast material (300 ml of 30% diatrizoate meglumine) injected intravenously will cause the membranes of an otherwise isodense hematoma to opacify.

MRI reliably identifies and characterizes chronic SDHs.[17,59,71] For the most part, short-TR and long-TR images both show the hematoma to be hyperintense relative to brain and CSF (Fig. 276-2). The change of signal intensity correlates with the length of time the hematoma has been present and with the breakdown of blood in the hematoma capsule.[17] MRI can also demonstrate acute hemorrhages within chronic SDHs and can differentiate chronic SDHs from subdural hygroma.[17] This modality is more sensitive and specific than contrast CT in identifying isodense SDHs and obviates the risks of an intravenous contrast agent.

Although cerebral angiography was formerly the primary modality for the diagnosis of chronic SDH, it is now rarely used for this purpose. The hematoma appears as an avascular space between the brain and skull at the frontal or occipital poles. Between 15 and 20 percent of chronic SDHs are bilateral, so bilateral carotid injections must be performed in all patients.

Treatment

Chronic SDH has been managed by both medical and surgical means. Proponents of medical management have used combinations of bed rest, osmotic diuretics, and corticosteroids in selected patients who had minimal neurological signs.[5,67] Unfortunately, medical treatment is unsuccessful in a considerable number of patients[5] and entails the risks of prolonged immobilization and the administration of corticosteroids and potent diuretics; sudden neurological deterioration is not uncommon.

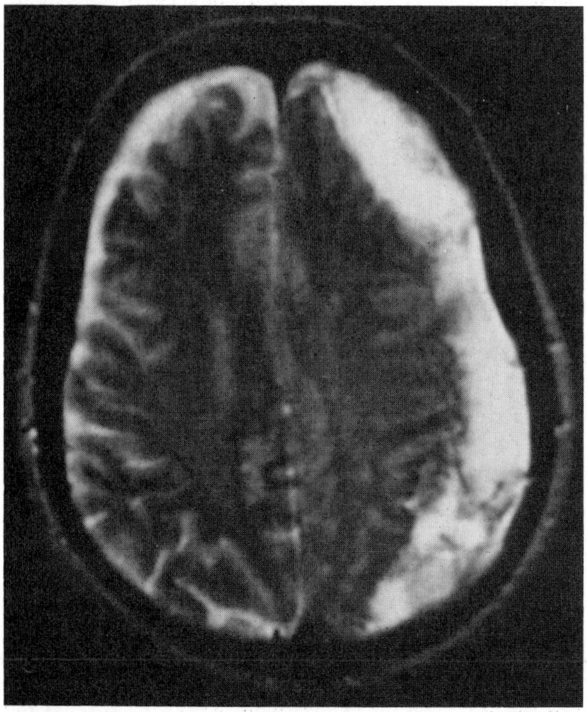

Figure 276-2 A T2-weighted MR image of a patient with a chronic SDH, showing an area of hyperintensity along the left hemisphere that causes compression and effacement of the sulci.

Opinion today overwhelmingly supports the operative treatment of symptomatic chronic SDH. Evacuation of chronic SDHs has been achieved with the use of craniotomy, burr holes, or twist-drill aspiration. Putnam and Cushing advocated craniotomy because of the exposure it provides for treatment of the solid components of the SDH.[51] Others have employed craniotomy to permit removal of the membranes surrounding the hematoma. There is no evidence that craniotomy is necessary for the adequate treatment of chronic SDH. These hematomas are liquid, and removal may be accomplished without a craniotomy. Similarly, removal of membranes is unnecessary and has no advantage over simple hematoma evacuation.

The most common treatment for chronic SDH has been evacuation using burr holes at the site of maximum hematoma thickness. A single burr hole is usually sufficient, although two are sometimes helpful. A catheter is left in the subdural space for 24 h after the operation to allow any residual hematoma to be removed using gravity drainage or gentle suction.

Twist-drill craniostomy performed at the bedside using local anesthesia is also an effective treatment for most hypodense or isodense chronic SDHs.[68] A twist-drill hole is made at a 45 degree angle to the skull, and a plastic ventricular catheter or small pediatric feeding tube is passed into the subdural space and connected to a closed sterile collection system. Because rapid evacuation of a chronic SDH by craniotomy or other means can cause brain shift, neurological deterioration, or brain stem hemorrhages,[40] we initially place the drainage bag at or slightly below the patient's head and gradually lower it over a period of hours to facilitate slow drainage. After 24 h, the subdural drain is removed and the patient is allowed out of bed.

Occasionally, when the CT scan shows a loculated hematoma, two twist-drill drains must be inserted. Twist-drill drainage will not work if the hematoma has a significant solid component. When the CT scan shows a hyperdense collection, the solid hematoma should be evacuated using a burr hole or a small trephine opening.

Complications

The use of CT scanning to follow the postoperative progress of patients with a chronic SDH has shown that residual hematoma is quite common regardless of the operative technique used. In spite of this, removal of most of the hematoma will generally result in alleviation of symptoms, and the residual hematoma will gradually resorb over a period of weeks.

True reaccumulation of the hematoma is reported to occur as often as 45 percent of the time in some series and probably results from bleeding from the vascular outer membrane. The possibility that reaccumulation has occurred should be considered in all patients who deteriorate or do not improve after operation. When reaccumulation is suspected, a CT scan should be obtained; if reaccumulation has occurred, the CT scan will show a hematoma that is hyperdense or of mixed density.

When bilateral hematomas exist, it is essential that both be evacuated. If only one is removed, the remaining hematoma can cause a rapid shift of midline structures with resultant neurological deterioration.

Infectious complications include subdural empyema, brain abscess, and meningitis. These complications are uncommon, occurring in less than 1 percent of patients. Seizures are reported in about 10 percent of cases, and all patients with a chronic SDH should be treated prophylactically with anticonvulsant medication prior to operation. Medication may be discontinued 1 month postoperatively if seizures have not occurred.

Results of Treatment

The mortality following treatment of a chronic SDH is less than 10 percent in most large series, and about 80 percent of patients are able to resume normal functioning.[64] The outcome correlates most closely with the patient's neurological state at the time of treatment; McKissock and colleagues reported a 13 percent mortality in patients who were comatose or stuporous at the time of operation, and a 5 percent mortality in patients who were alert or drowsy.[40]

Subdural Hygroma

Collections of clear, xanthochromic, or slightly bloody fluid in the subdural space following head injury are termed subdural hygromas. Hygromas probably form as a result of a tear in the arachnoid, which allows cerebrospinal fluid to escape into the subdural space.[22,24,66] Enlargement occurs as cerebrospinal fluid becomes trapped in the subdural space.

Subdural hygromas represent about 10 percent of all traumatic intracranial mass lesions. The severity of the precipitating head injury varies from very minor to severe, and the reported age of patients ranges from infancy to the seventies. Subdural hygromas are frequently seen in association with other injuries to the cerebral parenchyma, and the interval between the injury and the discovery of the hygroma depends, in large part, on the nature of the underlying brain injury. Many patients are asymptomatic, but depression of consciousness and focal motor deficit are common manifestations.

The CT scan shows a crescentic extra-axial collection with a density similar to that of cerebrospinal fluid (Fig. 276-3). The collections are bilateral in more than half of patients, but even when unilateral the midline shift is often small or absent, which serves to distinguish hygromas from chronic SDHs. Unlike the chronic SDH, there are no membranes and there is no enhancement with intravenous contrast injection. In patients who are asymptomatic, treatment is not necessary. In symptomatic patients, therapy consists of burr hole or twist-drill drainage. In patients with coexisting parenchymal lesions, a craniotomy may be necessary. Because of the nature of the lesion, recurrence is frequent. Recurrent symptomatic hygromas may be treated with a shunt placed from the subdural space to the peritoneal cavity. Mortality has been reported to range from 12 to 25 percent but the morbidity and mortality of patients with this lesion are most likely associated with the severity of intraparenchymal injuries.[66]

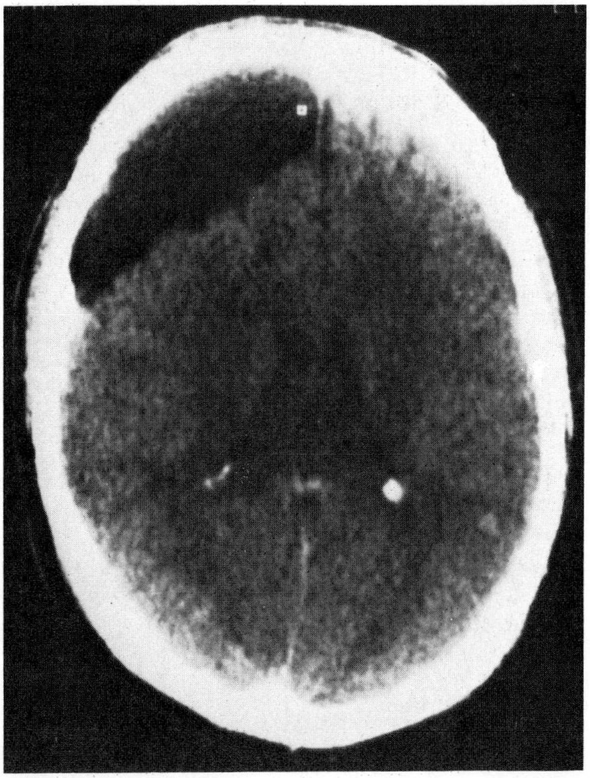

Figure 276-3 A CT scan showing a frontal subdural hygroma. The lesion density is the same as that of cerebrospinal fluid. There is no ventricular shift and only slight effacement of the frontal horn of the lateral ventricle. At operation (performed for severe headache), clear colorless fluid not enclosed by membranes was removed.

Extradural Hematoma

Epidemiology

Extradural hematoma (EDH), a collection of blood between the inner table of the skull and the dura, is an infrequent sequel of head injury, occurring in less than 2 percent of patients admitted with craniocerebral trauma.[30] The age distribution of patients with EDH is generally similar to that seen in patients with other types of head injury. However, it is rare in those over age 60 (probably because of the increased adherence of the dura to the inner skull table in the elderly) and in children in the first 2 years of life. The types of trauma that cause EDH are the same as those that cause other types of head injuries and include falls, vehicular accidents, and assault.[3,20,46,58]

Pathogenesis

Impact to the skull can cause inbending and stripping of the dura mater from the inner table. The skull is usually (although not invariably) fractured, and meningeal vessels are torn. Bleeding occurs into the region where the dura has been separated from the inner skull table, and the dura is further stripped by a confluent hematoma.

EDH results from injury to the middle meningeal artery or vein, the diploic veins, or the dural venous sinuses. The hematoma arises from the middle meningeal artery in over one-half of patients, from the middle meningeal vein in one-third, and from diploic veins or a torn dural venous sinus in the remainder. The hematoma is almost always unilateral, and most are found in the temporal region, although extension to adjacent frontal, parietal, and occipital areas is common. In adults a fracture is present 90 percent of the time, although in children fractures are less common.

Associated intracranial injury occurs in a minority of patients, and in this sense EDH is quite different from acute SDH, where associated parenchymal injury is usual and has such a detrimental influence on outcome.

Clinical Manifestations

Patients with EDH follow one of the following five clinical courses:

1. Conscious throughout
2. Unconscious throughout
3. Initially conscious and subsequently unconscious
4. Initially unconscious and subsequently lucid
5. Initially unconscious followed by a lucid interval and then unconsciousness again

The concept of a "lucid interval" has come to be associated with EDH; a transient loss of consciousness results from a concussive blow and is followed by a return of consciousness until the growing EDH results in unconsciousness once again. Although a lucid interval is seen in patients with EDH, it is less frequent than commonly imagined and was the mode of presentation in less than one-third of patients reported in the literature. Moreover, a lucid interval is not pathognomonic for EDH; other post-traumatic mass lesions can present in similar fashion.

Patients with acute EDH may present with only minimal complaints such as headache, nausea, and vomiting.[44] The rapidity of the appearance and progression of symptoms and signs is variable. In a series described by Bricolo and Pasut, 57 percent of patients with acute EDH had an operation within 6 h of injury, and most underwent operation within 24 h.[7] Other series report a longer interval from trauma to the development of symptoms, with some patients presenting days to weeks after injury.[30,47] The clinical signs associated with EDH depend on the location and speed of growth of the hematoma and on the presence of associated intradural lesions. Temporal hematomas can cause early deterioration because of their proximity to the brain stem. Hematomas originating from a laceration of the middle meningeal vein or dural sinus extravasate at low pressure, accumulate slowly, and may be associated with a long interval from trauma to the time of clinical presentation. Patients with intradural lesions will have more severe neurological impairment and present earlier than if they had EDH alone.[23,55] In some patients, the EDH may decompress through the skull fracture and scalp laceration and cause less severe neurological impairment. Depressed consciousness, hemiparesis, and pupillary dilation are frequently seen with EDH but are not pathognomonic and are of little use in distinguishing EDH from other post-traumatic intracranial mass lesions. The incidence of delayed EDH following an initially negative CT scan has been reported to range from 10 to 30 percent, possibly because CT scanning is usually done within 60 min of injury and the EDH may enlarge later.[48,60]

Diagnosis

When an EDH is suspected, a CT scan should be performed; the hematoma will appear as a hyperdense, biconvex area between the skull and the brain (Fig. 276-4). Hematomas over the vertex and at the floor of the temporal fossa may be difficult to visualize owing to the similar intensity of adjacent bone. A mass effect, shift, and compression of the basal cisterns may be present.

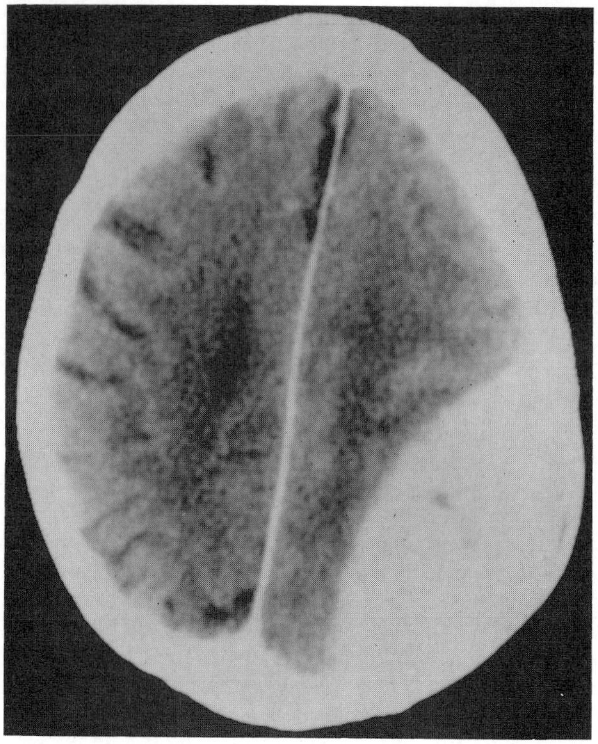

Figure 276-4 A CT scan showing a large hyperdense parietal epidural hematoma.

Treatment

The condition of most patients can be stabilized initially with diuretics and hyperventilation so that a CT scan can be obtained to confirm the diagnosis. Following the CT scan, an immediate craniotomy with evacuation of the hematoma is the treatment of choice. In rapidly deteriorating patients with a suspected EDH, a CT scan is inappropriate, and a burr hole is placed ipsilateral to the side of pupillary dilatation and contralateral to the side of motor signs.[63] After emergency hematoma evacuation, there is usually a rapid improvement in neurological signs, and the patient is taken to the operating room, where a craniotomy is made that is large enough to expose the site of bleeding and to visualize and permit removal of the entire hematoma. Dural tacking sutures should be placed to prevent hematoma reaccumulation. In patients who have not had a preoperative CT scan, intraoperative real-time ultrasonography may be used to identify coexisting intradural lesions. If this is not available, the dura should be opened to rule out an underlying acute SDH, and a postoperative CT scan should be obtained to identify any other occult intradural lesions.

Although most patients with acute EDH will require operative evacuation, a few selected patients with small hematomas may be managed without surgery.[21,36,57] This approach requires prolonged hospitalization, careful observation, and serial CT scans. The costs and risks of nonsurgical management must be weighed against the minimal morbidity and mortality of prompt operative treatment.

Complications

Delay in diagnosis and treatment is the most common preventable cause of morbidity and mortality. In one study the mean delay in evacuation of the hematoma in patients who made a good recovery was 2 h, whereas in those who died it was over 15 h.[42]

Although the placement of burr holes is an acceptable lifesaving emergency procedure, burr holes are inadequate for the definitive treatment of EDH. Recurrent or residual hematoma may result from failure to gain full access to the hematoma and to the lacerated meningeal vessel or multiple small bleeders on the dura where it has been stripped off the inner table of the skull.

Outcome

Mortality following treatment of EDH varies from 5 to 43 percent.[7,13,30,33,47,58] Mortality is low (5 to 10 percent) in children and increases sharply in those over age 40 (35 to 50 percent). Associated intracranial lesions such as SDH, intracerebral hematoma, and cerebral contusion have a detrimental effect on outcome and result in a mortality rate four times greater than in patients without such lesions.[23] Increased age, poor neurological condition, large hematoma volume, delay in operative evacuation, large midline shift, and postoperative elevation in ICP are all associated with poor outcome.[10,13,33,37] Patients who are alert or slightly lethargic at the time of operation should have virtually no mortality, while those who are unconscious with brain stem signs will have a mortality of well over 50 percent.

Cerebral Contusion

Cerebral contusions consist of heterogeneous areas of hemorrhage, brain necrosis, and infarction. It is the most common lesion seen after head injury at autopsy or on CT scans. Cerebral contusions are usually multiple and are commonly associated with other intracranial hemorrhagic lesions.

Contusions occur in the brain underlying the site of impact (coup lesions), but the largest and most serious contusions are generally located far from the site of impact (contrecoup contusions), at the frontal and temporal poles, as a result of injury against the bony floor of the frontal and middle fossa as the brain accelerates within the skull. Contusion of the medial cerebral hemispheres or corpus callosum may occur as a result of acceleration of the brain against the falx cerebri. Small hemorrhagic lesions are also found in the deep white and gray matter and result from the shearing that occurs with rapid acceleration and deceleration of the brain.

Symptoms and Signs

The symptoms and signs produced by cerebral contusion will vary according to the size and location of the contusion and the type of associated lesions. Small contusions pose no threat to the patient's life, but when they occur in speech areas of the dominant hemisphere or in the motor cortex, permanent deficits can result. Large contusions or multiple contusions involving both frontal and temporal lobes (the so-called tetrapolar injury) may produce elevations of ICP, shift, and concomitant coma.

In the period following the injury, the contused areas become necrotic and heterogeneously hemorrhagic. Although the hemorrhage is eventually resorbed, the total mass effect may initially increase as a result of edema around the contused brain, with a rise in ICP, depression of the patient's level of consciousness, and the appearance or exacerbation of focal neurological deficits.

Diagnosis

The diagnosis of cerebral contusion is established by the CT scan; hemorrhagic contusions appear as small areas of increased density mixed with areas of decreased density characteristic of edema and necrotic brain (Fig. 276-5). These lesions are usually located superficially near the cortex and extend into the white matter. Some superficial contusions may not be visible on CT scans because of the high density of adjacent bone. Serial CT scans may show the contused areas coalescing to form larger hematomas with surrounding edema and a mass effect.

Treatment

The optimal management of patients with cerebral contusions is often not clear-cut. Patients with small or deep lesions are managed nonoperatively. Patients with larger contusions and a mass effect should have a craniotomy and resection of contused brain at the time of presentation. The clinical course of patients who are initially in satisfactory neurological condition and have moderate-sized contusions is variable. Some patients will show continuous improvement, while in others with an apparent stable neurological status, the brain may suddenly herniate as late as 7 to 9 days after injury. It is sometimes difficult to identify the patients who have a high risk of deterioration and in whom early operation is justified.

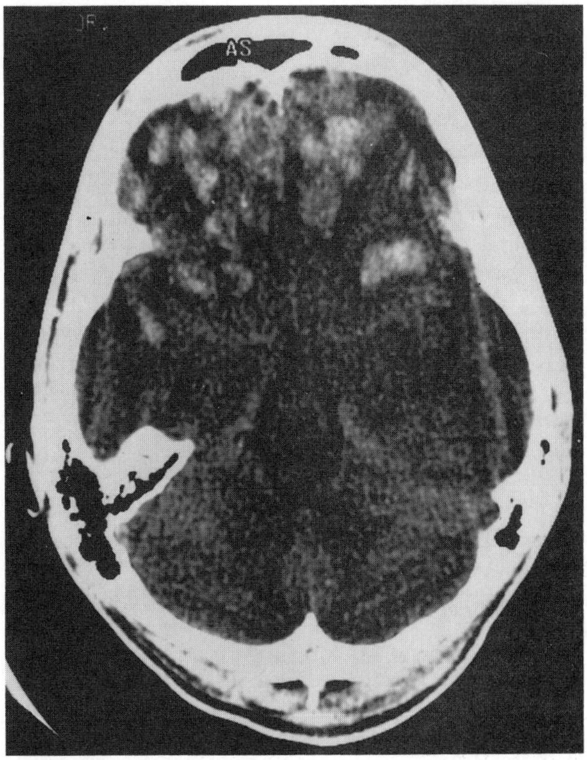

Figure 276-5 A CT scan showing multiple contusions. The superficial location in the frontal area is common. This scan was performed shortly after injury, and subsequent scans showed areas of edema around the lesions.

Medical therapy may be attempted initially. However, if the ICP becomes difficult to control or the neurological status deteriorates, prompt operative evacuation is recommended. Large contusions should be resected shortly after injury to minimize the chance of subsequent neurological deterioration. Temporal lobe contusions, because of their proximity to the brain stem, are especially dangerous. The importance of post-traumatic masses in the temporal lobe will be discussed in the next section.

Outcome

The mortality from cerebral contusion has been reported to be from 25 to 60 percent.[34] Outcome is influenced by the same factors that are important for other mass lesions, which have been discussed in previous sections of this chapter.

Intracerebral Hematoma

Traumatic intracerebral hematomas are well-defined, homogeneous areas of hemorrhage that appear hyperdense on the CT scan. Before CT came into use, the incidence of traumatic intracerebral hematoma was reported as 0.6 percent.[30] However, CT scanning shows that it occurs in as many as 23 percent of head trauma patients.[61,77]

Pathogenesis

Intracerebral hematomas are produced by a mechanism similar to the one that produces contrecoup contusions when the brain is propelled forward in the cranium. Confluent hemorrhages resulting from trauma are found in the same locations as cerebral contusions; the frontal and temporal lobes account for 80 to 90 percent of total hemorrhages. Hemorrhages may also occur in the corpus callosum, brain stem, and deep gray matter as a result of shearing injury. Multiple hemorrhages are seen in 20 percent of patients, and 30 to 60 percent of intracerebral hemorrhages are associated with extracerebral hematomas.[8,15,61] CT evaluation of patients with acute head injury has revealed that intraventricular hemorrhages are not uncommon and can be seen in the absence of CT-demonstrable parenchymal injury.

Symptoms and Signs

Injuries that result in intracerebral hemorrhage are generally severe, and over one-half of all patients lose consciousness as a direct result of the impact. The subsequent level of consciousness is determined by the severity of the impact injury and the growth of the intracerebral hematoma or of coexisting extracerebral hematomas. In up to 46 percent of patients, an intracerebral hematoma appears after a delay of 24 h or more.[61]

The symptoms and signs of intracerebral hematoma are not pathognomonic, and this entity cannot be reliably distinguished from other intracranial mass lesions on clinical grounds alone. The fact that these lesions so frequently coexist with extracerebral collections makes their diagnosis even more difficult. The neurological findings depend on the location and size of the hematoma. Enlargement of the hematoma or increase in the edema adjacent to it in the days following injury may produce additional mass effect with deterioration of consciousness and an increase in neurological deficit.

Diagnosis

CT is the favored diagnostic procedure for detecting intracerebral hematomas and will reliably distinguish the mass effect caused by parenchymal hematomas from edema or cerebral contusions (Fig. 276-6).

Treatment

Patients who have a large intracerebral hematoma with a midline shift, altered consciousness, and a focal deficit require operative evacuation of the hematoma. We create a large craniotomy centered over the site of the hematoma (which facilitates complete hematoma removal), resect adjacent injured brain, and evacuate extraparenchymal hematomas. Patients whose hematomas are small (whether or not a neurological deficit is present) usually do not need an operation. Similarly, patients with hemorrhages involving the deep white matter or basal ganglia are not candidates for operation.

The clinical course of patients who do not have an early operation and are managed with medical therapy is variable. Some show continuous improvement, while others deteriorate rapidly and often unexpectedly. Patients who are not initially considered candidates for operation should have ICP monitoring and serial CT scans every 2 to 4 days for the first week or 10 days after injury. The initial ICP may be predictive of patients likely to deteriorate.

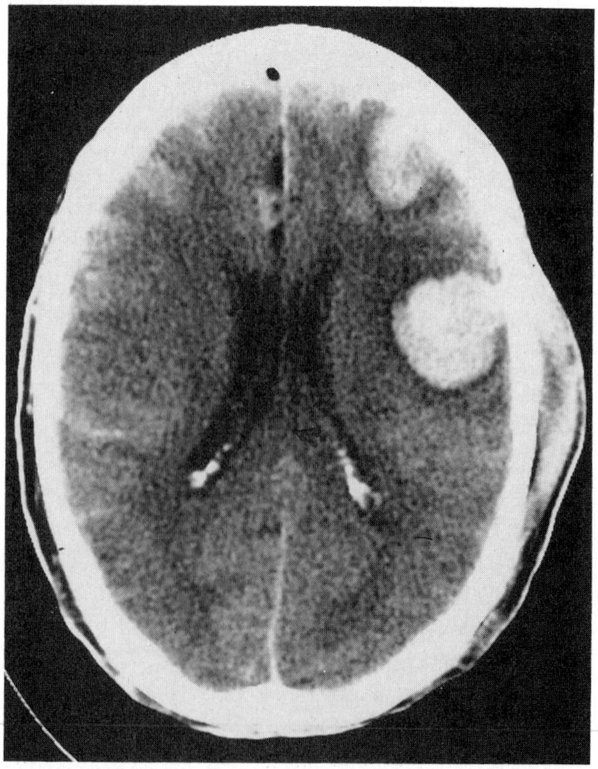

Figure 276-6 A CT scan showing post-traumatic frontal and temporal intracerebral hematomas. The superficial location in the frontal or temporal area is characteristic of a traumatic hematoma.

Teasdale and colleagues report that most patients with an initial ICP greater than 20 mmHg will need an operation.[69] Surgery is indicated if the ICP cannot be controlled by medical means, if there is neurological deterioration, or if CT scans show an increasing mass effect from hematoma growth or edema. Single photon emission computed tomography (SPECT) scanning using technetium 99m has been advocated as a way to assess which patients will deteriorate. Patients in whom the SPECT scan shows large perfusion defects are more likely to develop edema in this region and subsequently deteriorate.[11] Temporal lobe hematomas are an especially dangerous entity because of their proximity to the incisura and midbrain. In spite of an ICP that is often surprisingly low, and minimal midline shift on a CT scan, rapid neurological deterioration with little or no warning is a frequent occurrence. For this reason, we have been aggressive in treating these lesions with early operation and hematoma removal.

Outcome

Mortality rates of 25 to 72 percent have been reported; mortality depends to a large degree on the patient's neurological status at the time of operation.[8,9,32,61] Patients who are conscious at operation have a mortality of 6 percent, whereas those who are unconscious have a mortality of 45 percent. Advanced age and temporal lobe hematomas are associated with poor prognosis.[32,34,61]

Mass Lesions of the Posterior Fossa

Posterior fossa structures are remarkably well protected from injury; trauma-induced hemorrhagic lesions are unusual and represent less than 5 percent of all intracranial traumatic lesions. EDH is the most common lesion seen, followed by SDH and intracerebellar hematoma.

Epidural Hematoma of the Posterior Fossa

EDHs of the posterior fossa are invariably associated with occipital trauma and skull fracture.[65] The time of onset of neurological signs in patients with an EDH of the posterior fossa is variable: about 40 percent of patients become symptomatic in the first 24 h; just over 50 percent become symptomatic in the next 6 days, and in a small percentage symptoms appear after 1 week.

Headache and stiff neck are common.[25,26,50,76] Cranial nerve deficits are sometimes present. Cerebellar signs are seen in less than one-half of all patients and are uncommon in those with a rapid course. Corticospinal tract findings may result from coexisting supratentorial injury or extension of the hematoma superiorly to overlie the occipital lobe. Later in the patient's course, corticospinal tract signs result from medullary compression and are associated with depressed consciousness.

Because EDH of the posterior fossa is rare and coexisting supratentorial injury is often present, the diagnosis is often not suspected. A posterior fossa EDH or some other infratentorial mass should be considered when a depressed level of consciousness without localizing signs appears after occipital trauma.

The CT scan will rapidly and accurately establish the diagnosis of posterior fossa EDH (Fig. 276-7). In all head-injured patients, and particularly those with altered consciousness and few localizing signs, the posterior fossa should be scanned. In the past, ventriculography and angiography were used to evaluate suspected lesions. They have been superseded by CT and are indicated only where it is unavailable.

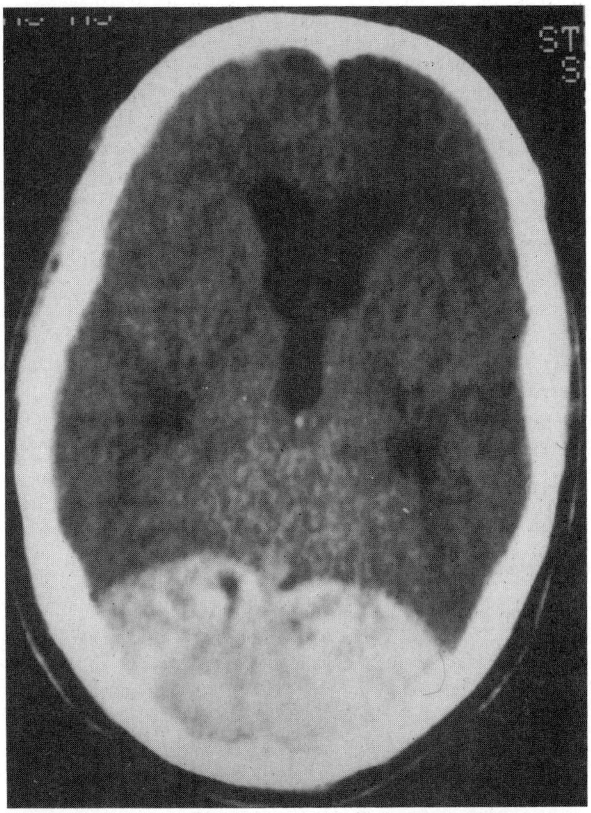

Figure 276-7 A CT scan showing an EDH of the posterior fossa and occipital area. The hematoma extended both above and below this cut. Acute hydrocephalus is also present.

Treatment of these lesions is operative. Posterior fossa epidural hematomas usually arise from a tear in the dural venous sinuses underlying a skull fracture. Therefore a craniectomy is performed where the skull fracture crosses the torcular, transverse sinus, or sigmoid sinus. The craniectomy is enlarged superiorly, if necessary, for the visualization of a hematoma above the transverse sinus compressing the occipital lobe. The outcome is most closely related to the patient's level of consciousness at the time of operation. Although earlier series reported a mortality of 37 to 69 percent, some recent studies in the CT era have shown no mortality.[4,6,19,25,45,54]

Subdural Hematoma of the Posterior Fossa

Posterior fossa SDHs represent less than 1 percent of the total number of SDHs reported. Bleeding from torn bridging veins over the cerebellum, injury to the dural venous sinuses, or hemorrhage from cerebellar contusions is the usual source of SDHs.

Disturbance of consciousness, headache, and vomiting are common. Cranial nerve palsies, nuchal rigidity, and cerebellar signs are each seen in less than one-half of patients. The clinical course is variable, and symptoms and signs may appear immediately after injury or after an interval of over 24 h.

Treatment is similar to that described for posterior fossa EDH. After an SDH has been removed, a careful search must be made for the injured vessels that gave rise to it, and hemostasis achieved to prevent recurrence. Mortality is reported to be in the range of 50 percent.[12]

Traumatic Intracerebellar Hematoma

Traumatic intracerebellar hematomas are unusual lesions that originate from direct blows to the suboccipital area. A fracture is frequently present.[76] Posterior fossa SDH is a frequent co-existing lesion. Symptoms and signs are indistinguishable from those produced by extra-axial posterior fossa lesions. Operative treatment consists of removal of the hematoma and adjacent contused cerebellum. Associated supratentorial contrecoup contusions and hematomas are frequently found, and attention is directed first to the lesion that is considered the most clinically significant. Mortality is high, and survivors are often left with significant neurological impairment.[49]

References

1. Andrews BT, Bederson JB, Pitts LH. Use of intraoperative ultrasonography to improve the diagnostic accuracy of exploratory burr holes in patients with traumatic tentorial herniation. *Neurosurgery* 1979; 24:345–347.
2. Andrews BT, Pitts LH, Lovely MP, Bartkowski H. Is computed tomographic scanning necessary in patients with tentorial herniation? Results of immediate surgical exploration without computed tomography in 100 patients. *Neurosurgery* 1986; 19:408–414.
3. Baykaner K, Alp H, Ceviker N, et al. Observation of 95 patients with extradural hematoma and review of the literature. *Surg Neurol* 1988; 30:339–341.
4. Beller AJ, Peyser E. Extradural cerebellar hematoma: report of three cases with review of the literature. *J Neurosurg* 1952; 9:291–298.
5. Bender MB, Christoff N. Nonsurgical treatment of subdural hematomas. *Arch Neurol* 1974; 31:73–79.
6. Brambilla G, Rainoldi F, Gipponi D, Paolatte P. Extradural haematoma of the posterior fossa: a report of eight cases and a review of the literature. *Acta Neurochir (Wien)* 1986; 80:24–29.
7. Bricolo AP, Pasut LM. Extradural hematoma: toward zero mortality. A prospective study. *Neurosurgery* 1984; 14:8–12.
8. Browder J, Turney MF. Intracerebral hemorrhage of traumatic origin: its surgical treatment. *NY State J Med* 1942; 42:2230–2235.
9. Bullock R, Golek J, Blake G. Traumatic intracerebral hematoma—which patients should undergo surgical evacuation? CT scan features and ICP monitoring as a basis for decision making. *Surg Neurol* 1989; 32:181–187.
10. Cagetti B, Cossu M, Pau A, et al. The outcome from acute subdural and epidural intracranial haematomas in very elderly patients. *Br J Neurosurg* 1992;6:227–231.
11. Choksey MS, Costa DC, Ianotti F, et al. ^{99m}TC-HMPAO SPECT studies in traumatic intracerebral haematoma. *J Neurol Neurosurg Psychiatry* 1991; 54:6–11.
12. Ciembroniewicz JE. Subdural hematoma of the posterior fossa: review of the literature with addition of 3 cases. *J Neurosurg* 1965; 22:465–473.
13. Cook RJ, Dorsch NWC, Fearnside MR, Chaseling R. Outcome prediction in extradural haematomas. *Acta Neurochir (Wien)* 1988; 95:90–94.
14. Cooper PR, Hagler H, Clark WK, Barnett P. Enhancement of experimental cerebral edema after decompressive craniectomy: implications for the management of severe head injuries. *Neurosurgery* 1979; 4:296–300.
15. Dublin AB, Fench BN, Rennick JM. Computed tomography in head trauma. *Radiology* 1977; 122:365–369.
16. Fell DA, Fitzgerald S, Moiel RH, Caram P. Acute subdural hematomas: review of 144 cases. *J Neurosurg* 1975; 42:37–42.
17. Fobben ES, Grossmand RI, Atlas SW, et al. MR characteristics of subdural hematomas and hygromas at 1.5 T. *Am J Neuroradiol* 1989; 153:589–595.
18. Fogelholm R, Waltimo O. Epidemiology of chronic subdural haematoma. *Acta Neurochir (Wien)* 1975; 32:247–250.
19. Garza-Mercado R. Extradural hematoma of the posterior cranial fossa. Report of seven cases with survival. *J Neurosurg* 1983; 59:664–672.
20. Gutman MB, Moulton RJ, Sullivan I, et al. Risk factors predicting operable intracranial hematomas in head injury. *J Neurosurg* 1992; 77:9–14.
21. Hamilton M, Wallace C. Nonoperative management of acute epidural hematoma diagnosed by CT: the neuroradiologist's role. *Am J Neuroradiol* 1992; 13:853–862.
22. Hasegawa M, Yamashima T, Yamashita J, et al. Traumatic subdural hygroma: pathology and meningeal enhancement on magnetic resonance imaging. *Neurosurgery* 1992; 31:580–585.
23. Haselberger K, Pucher R, Auer LM. Prognosis after acute subdural or epidural haemorrhage. *Acta Neurochir (Wien)* 1988; 90:111–116.
24. Hoff J, Bates E, Barnes B, et al. Traumatic subdural hygroma. *J Trauma* 1973; 13:870–876.
25. Holzschuh M, Schuknecht B. Traumatic epidural haematomas of the posterior fossa: 20 new cases and a review of the literature since 1961. *Br J Neurosurg* 1989; 3:171–180.
26. Hooper RS. Extradural haemorrhages of the posterior fossa. *Br J Surg* 1954; 42:19–26.
27. Howard MA III, Gross AS, Dacey RG Jr, Winn HR. Acute subdural hematomas: an age-dependent clinical entity. *J Neurol* 1989; 71:858–863.
28. Ikeda K, Ito H, Yamashita J. Relation of regional cerebral blood flow to hemiparesis in chronic subdural hematoma. *Surg Neurol* 1990; 33:87–95.
29. Ito H, Komai T, Yamamoto S. Fibrinolytic enzyme in the lining walls of chronic subdural hematoma. *J Neurosurg* 1978; 48:197–200.
30. Jamieson KG, Yelland JDN. Extradural hematoma: report of 167 cases. *J Neurosurg* 1968; 29:13–23.
31. Jamieson KG, Yelland JDN. Surgically treated traumatic subdural hematomas. *J Neurosurg* 1972; 37:137–149.
32. Jamieson KG, Yelland JDN. Traumatic intracerebral hematoma: report of 63 surgically treated cases. *J Neurosurg* 1972; 37:528–532.
33. Jamjoom A. The influence of concomitant intradural pathology on the presentation and outcome of patients with acute traumatic extradural haematoma. *Acta Neurochir (Wien)* 1992; 115:86–89.
34. Jayakumar PN, Sastry Kolluri VR, Basavakumar DG, et al. Prognosis in contre-coup intracranial haematomas—a clinical and radiological study of 63 patients. *Acta Neurochir (Wien)* 1991; 108:30–33.
35. Kernohan JW, Woltman HW. Incisura of the crus due to contralateral brain tumor. *Arch Neurol Psychiatry* 1929; 21:274–287.
36. Knuckey NW, Gelbard S, Epstein MH. The management of "asymptomatic" epidural hematomas: a prospective study. *J Neurosurg* 1989; 70:392–396.
37. Lobato RD, Rivas JJ, Cordobes F, et al. Acute epidural hematoma: an analysis of factors influencing the outcome of patients undergoing surgery in coma. *J Neurosurg* 1988; 68:48–57.
38. Marmarou A, Anderson RL, Ward JD, et al. Impact of ICP instability and hypotension on outcome in patients with severe head trauma. *J Neurosurg* 1991; 75(Suppl):S59–S66.
39. Marshall LF, Gautille T, Klauber MR, et al. The outcome of severe closed head injury. *J Neurosurg* 1991; 75(Suppl):S28–S36.
40. McKissock W, Richardson A, Bloom WH. Subdural haematoma: a review of 389 cases. *Lancet* 1960; 1:1365–1369.
41. McLaurin RL, Tutor FH. Acute subdural hematoma: review of 90 cases. *J Neurosurg* 1961; 18:61–67.
42. Mendelow AD, Karmi MZ, Paul KS, et al. Extradural haematoma: effect of delayed treatment. *Br Med J* 1979; 1:1240–1242.
43. Miller JD, Becker DP, Ward JD, et al. Significance of intracranial hypertension in severe head injury. *J Neurosurg* 1977; 47:503–516.
44. Miller JD, Murray LS, Teasdale GM. Development of a traumatic

intracranial hematoma after a ''minor'' head injury. *Neurosurgery* 1990; 27:669–673.
45. Neubauer UJ. Extradural haematoma of the posterior fossa. Twelve years experience with CT-scan. *Acta Neurochir (Wien)* 1987; 87:105–111.
46. O'Sullivan MGJ, Gray WP, Buckley TF. Extradural haematoma in the Irish Republic: an analysis of 82 cases with emphasis on 'delay.' *Br J Surg* 1990; 77:1391–1394.
47. Phonprasert C, Suwanwela C, Hongsaprabhas C, et al. Extradural hematoma: analysis of 138 cases. *J Trauma* 1980; 20:679–683.
48. Poon WS, Rehamn SU, Poon CYF, Li AKC. Traumatic extradural hematoma of delayed onset is not a rarity. *Neurosurgery* 1992; 30:681–686.
49. Pozzati E, Grossi C, Padovani R. Traumatic intracerebellar hematomas. *J Neurosurg* 1982; 56:691–694.
50. Pozzati E, Tognetti F, Cavallo M, Acciarri N. Extradural hematomas of the posterior cranial fossa: observations on a series of 32 consecutive cases treated after the introduction of computed tomography scanning. *Surg Neurol* 1989; 32:300–303.
51. Putnam TJ, Cushing H. Chronic subdural hematoma: its pathology, its relation to pachymeningitis hemorrhagica and its surgical treatment. *Arch Surg* 1925; 11:329–393.
52. Ransohoff J, Benjamin MV, Gage L Jr, Epstein F. Hemicraniectomy in the management of acute subdural hematoma. *J Neurosurg* 1971; 34:70–76.
53. Richardson NS III, Paysinger BD. Outcome of acute subdural and epidural hematomas in a level I trauma center in South Carolina. *J SC Med Assoc* 1990; 86:573–576.
54. Rivano C, Borzone M, Altamonte M, Capuzzo T. Traumatic posterior fossa extradural hematomas. *Neurochirurgia (Stuttg)* 1992; 35:43–47.
55. Rivas JJ, Lobato RD, Sarabia R, et al. Extradural hematoma: analysis of factors influencing the courses of 161 patients. *Neurosurgery* 1988; 23:44–51.
56. Seelig JM, Becker DP, Miller JD, et al. Traumatic acute subdural hematoma: major mortality reduction in comatose patients treated within four hours. *N Engl J Med* 1981; 304:1511–1518.
57. Servadei F, Faccani G, Roccella P, et al. Asymptomatic extradural haematomas. Results of a multicenter study of 158 cases in minor head injury. *Acta Neurochir (Wien)* 1989; 96:39–45.
58. Servadei F, Piazza G, Seracchioli A, et al. Extradural haematomas: an analysis of the changing characteristics of patients admitted from 1980 to 1986. Diagnostic and therapeutic implications in 158 cases. *Brain Inj* 1988; 2:87–100.
59. Sipponen JT, Sepponen RE, Sivula A. Chronic subdural hematoma: demonstration by magnetic resonance. *Radiology* 1984; 150:79–85.
60. Smith HK, Miller JD. The danger of an ultra-early computed tomographic scan in a patient with an evolving acute epidural hematoma. *Neurosurgery* 1991; 29:258–260.
61. Soloniuk D, Pitts LH, Lovely M, Bartkowski H. Traumatic intracerebral hematomas: timing of appearance and indications for operative removal. *J Trauma* 1986; 26:787–794.
62. Sonne NM, Tonnesen H. The influence of alcoholism on outcome after evacuation of subdural haematoma. *Br J Neurosurg* 1992; 6:125–130.
63. Springer MF, Baker FJ. Cranial burr hole decompression in the emergency department. *Am J Emerg Med* 1988; 6:640–646.
64. Steimle R, Jacquet G, Godard J, et al. Hématome sous-dural chronique des personnes agées et scanner: étude de 80 cas. *Chirurgie* 1990; 116:160–167.
65. St. John JN, French BN. Traumatic hematomas of the posterior fossa: a clinicopathological spectrum. *Surg Neurol* 1986; 25:457–466.
66. Stone JL, Lang RGR, Sugar O, Moody RA. Traumatic subdural hygroma. *Neurosurgery* 1981; 8:542–550.
67. Suzuki J, Takaku A. Nonsurgical treatment of chronic subdural hematoma. *J Neurosurg* 1970; 33:548–553.
68. Tabaddor K, Shulman K. Definitive treatment of chronic subdural hematoma by twist-drill craniostomy and closed-system drainage. *J Neurosurg* 1977; 46:220–226.
69. Teasdale G, Galbraith S, Jennett B. Operate or observe? ICP and the management of the ''silent'' traumatic intracranial haematoma. In Shulman K, Marmarou A, Miller JD, et al (eds): *Intracranial Pressure IV.* Berlin: Springer-Verlag, 1980, pp 36–38.
70. Temkin NR, Dikmen SS, Wilensky AJ, et al. A randomized, double-blind study of phenytoin for the prevention of post-traumatic seizures. *N Engl J Med* 1990; 323:497–502.
71. Thulborn KR, Atlas SW. Intracranial hemmorrhage. In Atlas SW (ed): *Magnetic Resonance Imaging of the Brain and Spine.* New York: Raven Press, 1991 pp 175–222.
72. Vollmer DG, Torner JC, Jane JA, et al. Age and oucome following traumatic coma: why do older patients fare worse? *J Neurosurg* 1991; 75(Suppl):S37–S49.
73. Weir BKA. The osmolality of subdural hematoma fluid. *J Neurosurg* 1971; 34:528–533.
74. Wilberger JE Jr, Harris M, Diamond DL. Acute subdural haematoma: morbidity and mortality related to timing of operative intervention. *J Trauma* 1990; 30:733–736.
75. Wilberger JE Jr, Harris M, Diamond DL. Acute subdural hematoma: morbidity, mortality, and operative timing. *J Neurosurg* 1991; 74:212–218.
76. Wright RL. Traumatic hematomas of the posterior cranial fossa. *J Neurosurg* 1966; 25:402–409.
77. Zimmerman RA, Bilaniuk LT, Gennarelli T, et al. Cranial computed tomography in diagnosis and management of acute head trauma. *Am J Roentgenol* 1978; 131:27–34.
78. Zimmerman RA, Bilaniuk LT, Hackney DB, et al. Head injury: early results of comparing CT and high-field MR. *Am J Neuroradiol* 1986; 7:757–764.
79. Zollinger R, Gross RE. Traumatic subdural hematoma: an explanation of the late onset of pressure symptoms. *JAMA* 1934; 103:245–249.

277

Delayed and Recurrent Intracranial Hematomas and Post-Traumatic Coagulopathies

Michael E. Miner

Patients with acute traumatic intracranial hematomas require prompt decisions and treatment.[1] The incidence of traumatic intracranial hematomas that are visible on the initial computed tomography (CT) scans of the brain is probably between 4 and 15 percent in patients with severe brain injuries, although an incidence as high as 30 percent has been reported.[12,13,22,34] Delayed hematomas—those first seen on a later scan—have been reported by Gudeman and colleagues and Sweet and colleagues to occur in 7 to 9 percent of head-injured patients.[11,28] On the other hand, Gentleman and colleagues found that only 3 percent of patients with traumatic intracranial hematomas developed a delayed intracerebral hematoma after hospital admission.[9] The differences between these reports seem to reflect differences in the time after injury at which the patient is first seen and in the frequency of brain imaging after hospitalization. Clearly, delayed traumatic intracerebral hematomas are more often identified in patients who have early and frequent brain CT scans. A smaller but significant number of patients who have had early emergency craniotomy for evacuation of an extracerebral hematoma develop recurrent intracranial hematomas within the first 10 days after the operation. Thus, the incidence of delayed or recurrent traumatic intracerebral hematomas is significant; fortunately, both types of hematoma are relatively easily diagnosed by CT. However, the diagnosis of delayed and recurrent post-traumatic intracranial hematomas does require a high index of clinical suspicion, an understanding of the clinical features and CT findings, and, most important, an understanding of the pathophysiology of these lesions.

Clinical Features and CT Findings

The neurological abnormalities associated with delayed or recurrent intracranial hematomas occurring in the first week after severe head injury may be difficult to distinguish from those due to brain edema.[13] A deteriorating state of consciousness, a newly developed third nerve palsy, or a rise in intracranial pressure does not indicate which intracranial component has increased in volume. Laboratory evaluations also do not distinguish the cause, even though blood clotting abnormalities are more often due to new brain destruction with hematoma formation than to brain swelling. Certainly a sudden deterioration in neurological status should prompt another brain CT scan, which will allow a diagnosis to be made. However, in many situations, a new intracerebral hematoma may be relatively silent with regard to the patient's neurological status. For example, the hemorrhage may be small or may occur in a relatively silent area of the brain; the patient may be in such desperate condition that further deterioration is difficult to identify; or the treatment regimen may interfere with neurological evaluation. Thus, we routinely perform brain CT twice a week for the first two or three weeks in injured patients who remain unable to follow commands, even if they do not deteriorate neurologically. Because the clinical signs are frequently insidious, we obtain a second brain scan in less severely injured patients if they are not clearly improving and certainly if they deteriorate neurologically. Delayed epidural and subdural hematomas occur about as often as delayed intracerebral hematomas. Poon and colleagues observed that fully 30 percent of epidural hematomas requiring surgery were delayed in onset, which emphasizes the need for repeated brain CT scanning.[24]

CT is the test of choice for diagnosing delayed or recurrent intracranial hematomas.[6,7] Delayed intracerebral hematomas are nearly always lobar, are occasionally multiple, and often occur in areas of previously demonstrated cerebral contusion. However, delayed intracerebral hematomas can occur even after a normal initial CT scan.[11] Small areas of contusion, best appreciated on the contrast-enhanced CT scans, frequently evolve into delayed parenchymal hemorrhages.

Over the past decade, it has become increasingly apparent that severe brain injury results in pathological changes in multiple organ systems. Accordingly, the best treatment for the head-injured person addresses these other organ systems as well as the brain. A number of reports have noted that brain injury can result in abnormalities of blood coagulation.[5,7,8,10,14–17,20,23,25–27,31] These coagulation changes may in turn cause cerebral hemorrhage or infarction, resulting in a self-perpetuating, ever-worsening course with a predictable outcome. Neurosurgeons must be aware that head trauma can result in coagulopathies that can be treated successfully and must be able to recognize when and how to initiate treatment. To do this, a basic understanding of normal hemostasis and the required screening coagulation studies is essential.

Normal and Abnormal Blood Coagulation

Normal hemostasis results from a complex series of reactions that are still incompletely understood. Platelets aggregate at the site of hemorrhage and serve to mechanically occlude the vessel. Serotonin and other vasoactive peptides are released by platelets, resulting in a local vasoconstriction. Two fundamental clotting pathways are well described: the tissue-activated, or extrinsic, pathway and the plasma-originated, or intrinsic, pathway. The extrinsic pathway, initiated by tissue thromboplastin, requires calcium ions and plasma factor VII. There are high concentrations of thromboplastin in the intima of small vessels throughout the body, but the brain has exceedingly high thromboplastin activity.[2,29,32] The intrinsic pathway does not require thromboplastin, but rather coagulation factors normally present in plasma (factors IX and VIII), calcium ions, and platelet phospholipid. This pathway results from a cascade of clotting enzymes, converts a precursor to an activated form that catalyzes the next reaction.[17] Ultimately, both the intrinsic and extrinsic pathways generate activated factor X, the Stuart factor. Although both pathways are complex, it is striking that a fibrin clot can be produced in a matter of seconds by the extrinsic pathway but requires several minutes to form by the intrinsic pathway. This time difference may be related to the normal functions of the two pathways. The final common pathway, originating from activated Stuart factor, catalyzes the conversion of prothrombin to thrombin, which in turn catalyzes the conversion of fibrinogen to fibrin. Fibrin monomers can self-polymerize to yield a durable plug and thus hemostasis.

Intravascular coagulation is a normal process that is constantly occurring throughout all organs. Similarly, fibrinolysis is a constantly occurring normal process. Control of this homeostatic mechanism, although incompletely understood, is amazingly accurate. Plasminogen activator substance, present in blood and many body tissues, converts plasminogen to plasmin, which dissolves fibrin clots. Fibrin clots are thus split or degraded to smaller molecules (fibrin split products or degradation products), which are themselves antihemostatic in that they inhibit the polymerization of fibrin monomers.

Although the foregoing overview of normal hemostasis is brief and simplified, it is sufficient to explain the screening tests used for blood clotting and fibrinolysis. Platelet quantification is important because platelet aggregation is the first step in hemostasis and because platelets are critical to the intrinsic clotting pathway. The prothrombin time screens primarily for abnormalities in the extrinsic pathway, whereas a normal activated partial thromboplastin time (APTT) reflects the integrity of the intrinsic clotting pathway. Even minor abnormalities of these clotting tests may indicate major hemostatic abnormalities. The prothrombin time and the APTT do not become prolonged until one or more of the clotting factors have decreased to 20 to 30 percent of normal. Fibrinogen quantification provides information about the integrity of the final common pathway to hemostasis. The level of fibrin split products reflects the magnitude of fibrinolytic activity. However, even though this assay is highly sensitive, it is not highly specific for the syndrome of disseminated intravascular coagulation and fibrinolysis (DICF). The presence of cross-linked fibrin, D-dimer, in the plasma confirms that thrombin and plasmin generation are actively occurring.[4] One definition of DICF that is not dependent on clinical findings is the presence of abnormal levels of both fibrin degradation products and D-dimers in the plasma.

There is justification for using a wide variety of screening tests to determine the integrity of the clotting and fibrinolytic systems. Autopsy studies have shown that brain injury results in microthrombi in multiple organs, including the brain, lungs, and kidneys.[5,23,25,33] The contribution of DICF to intraoperative bleeding is a very real phenomenon to the trauma surgeon.[18] Abnormalities of the coagulation system may have profound effects on the outcome ot patients with brain injuries. DICF may be important in such diverse secondary problems as intracranial intravascular clotting, particularly in the venous system, and the adult respiratory distress syndrome that frequently follows severe brain injury.

Although the screening tests for clotting function indicate that abnormalities of the thromboplastin-activated extrinsic clotting system are more common than abnormalities of the intrinsic system, abnormalities of both systems are common, and both systems can be abnormal at the same time in a single patient. Abnormal platelet counts are relatively uncommon, but the count is abnormally low in up to 5 percent of severely head-injured patients. Our experience indicates that the frequency of hemostatic abnormalities is directly related to the severity of the neurological deficits. Patients who can be presumed to have more brain cell destruction (e.g., patients with gunshot wounds and depressed skull fractures) have a greater incidence of hemostatic abnormalities than patients with less brain tissue destruction.[21] It is also apparent that severe abnormalities of hemostasis are likelier to be discovered the sooner patients are evaluated after brain injury. It may be that patients with the most severe abnormalities die early enough that the abnormalities are not identified in some centers.[9]

Because, as mentioned above, relatively minor abnormalities in clotting test results may indicate major hemostatic abnormalities, the laboratory diagnosis of DICF can be rather liberal, requiring only the demonstration of fibrin split products in the serum or decreased levels of fibrinogen or platelets. On the other hand, some workers require a fibrinogen level below 130 μg/dl and fibrin split products greater than 40 μg/ml for a diagnosis of DICF. Either of these criteria will identify 70 to 85 percent of severely brain-injured patients as having DICF. We have developed a somewhat more restrictive criterion, which requires abnormalities in three or more major hemostatic screening studies for a diagnosis of DICF, to ensure that a clotting disorder exists unequivocally and is severe. Even so, nearly half of our severely injured patients have had DICF when initially evaluated.[20]

The fact that both abnormalities of individual clotting tests and "full-blown" DICF correlate with the severity and pathology of the brain injury implies not only that the incidence of clotting abnormalities is related to the amount of brain tissue destruction but also that the severity of the coagulopathy is related to the severity of the injury. However, it is equally clear that absence of demonstrable brain tissue destruction does not rule out DICF,[30] because the latter can likewise result from injury to other organs, most notably the liver.

Given that over 40 percent of our severely brain-injured patients had DICF when first evaluated, it is surprising that this condition has not been a generally recognized phenomenon. The reason may be because DICF after brain injury either is a transient phenomenon or causes such high mortality that most patients with severe head injuries and DICF do not survive to reach a medical facility. Case reports of DICF after head injury generally involve patients evaluated very soon after their injury, and all of our patients were initially evaluated less than 2 h after their injury. The relationship between DICF and morbidity and mortality after head injury is impressive. van der Sande and colleagues compared CT scans, neurological status, and coagulation studies on hospital admission and found that coagulations studies were more sensitive than CT at demonstrating brain contusion.[31] In our studies, the presence of DICF increased mortality by a factor of three to six times.[20] However, the cause of death is not obvious in all cases. Many patients died after their clotting studies had returned to normal, and the autopsy generally did not reveal massive hemorrhage or intravascular clots. It is likely that the influence on mortality is due to diffuse microvascular fibrin deposits that plug small vessels and result in increased brain damage and multiple organ failure. Thus, DICF after brain injury may be life-threatening, may occur without overwhelming brain injury, may affect multiple organs, and may affect long-term recovery.

A Treatment Regimen for Delayed and Recurrent Intracerebral Hematomas and Post-Traumatic Coagulopathies

Currently, we obtain coagulation screening tests on admission for all patients with diffuse brain injuries who are not following commands, as well as for all of those who have brain-penetrating injuries or intracranial hematomas. Fresh frozen plasma is used as an initial resuscitation fluid if the prothrombin time or the activated partial thromboplastin time is increased or if the fibrinogen level is less than 130 mg/dl. Platelet packs are given if the platelet count is less than 100,000 per cubic millimeter. If possible, we delay operation until the coagulation studies normalize. However, abnormal levels of fibrin split products or fibrinogen are not regarded as a contraindication to surgery but are treated with fresh frozen plasma while preparation is made for surgery. If the clotting study results are abnormal, we use a hollow screw in the subarachnoid space to monitor intracranial pressure rather than a ventriculostomy or intraparenchymal monitor. If D-dimer levels are elevated, we consider the abnormal clotting process to be ongoing and continue therapy.

An increase in intracranial pressure, a decrease in the state of consciousness, or the development of a focal or lateralizing finding prompts repeat CT scanning. Also, patients in whom cerebral contusion or hematomas are seen on the initial CT scan are routinely re-scanned on the third to fifth day after injury. If a recurrent or delayed intracerebral hematoma is identified, repeat coagulation studies are performed, and the same hematologic resuscitation is used as on admission. Surgical decisions and timing are based on the patient's clinical status and the results of the CT scan and the coagulation studies. We operate to remove intraparenchymal clots of approximately 35 cc volume or greater if they are in a surgically accessible location. Deeper clots are stereotactically aspirated on a more elective basis. Of course, we do not delay operating on life-threatening surgical lesions in order to correct abnormal laboratory values.[3] However, the correction of hemostatic abnormalities is just as important as the correction of a low hemoglobin level or arterial oxygen tension. We have found that this policy decreases blood loss during operation, decreases morbidity, and ultimately saves lives.

References

1. Aldrich EF. Surgical management of traumatic intracerebral hematomas. *Neurosurg Clin North Am* 1991; 2:373–385.
2. Astrup T. Assay and content of tissue thromboplastin in different organs. *Thromb Haemost* 1965; 14:401–416.
3. Becker DP, Miller JD, Ward JD, et al. The outcome from severe head injury with early diagnosis and intensive management. *J Neurosurg* 1977; 47:491–502.
4. Bick RL, Baker WF. Diagnostic efficiency of the D-dimer assay in disseminated intravascular coagulation (DIC). *Thromb Res* 1992; 65:785–790.
5. Clark JA, Finelli RE, Netsky MG. Disseminated intravascular coagulation following cranial trauma: case report. *J Neurosurg* 1980; 52:266–269.
6. Clifton GL, Grossman RG, Makela ME, et al. Neurological course and correlated computerized tomography findings after severe closed head injury. *J Neurosurg* 1980; 52:611–624.
7. Diaz FG, Yock DH Jr, Larson D, Rockwald GL. Early diagnosis of delayed posttraumatic intracerebral hematomas. *J Neurosurg* 1979; 50:217–223.
8. Drayer BP, Poser CM. Disseminated intravascular coagulation and head trauma—two case studies. *JAMA* 1975; 231:174–175.
9. Gentleman D, Nath F, MacPherson P. Diagnosis and management of delayed traumatic intracerebral haematomas. *Br J Neurosurg* 1989; 3:367–372.
10. Goodnight SH, Kenoyer G, Rapaport SI, et al. Defibrination after brain tissue destruction: a serious complication of head injury. *N Engl J Med* 1974; 290:1043–1047.
11. Gudeman SK, Kishore PRS, Miller JD, et al. The genesis and significance of delayed traumatic intracerebral hematoma. *Neurosurgery* 1979; 5:309–313.
12. Gurdjian ES, Thomas LM. Traumatic intracranial hemorrhage. In Feiring EH (ed): *Brock's Injuries of the Brain and Spinal Cord and Their Coverings.* New York: Springer Verlag, 1974, pp 203–282.
13. Jennett B, Teasdale G. *Management of Head Injuries.* Philadelphia: Davis, 1981.
14. Kaufman HH, Moake JL, Olson JD, et al. Delayed and recurrent intracranial hematomas related to disseminated intravascular clotting and fibrinolysis in head injury. *Neurosurgery* 1980; 7:445–449.
15. Keimowitz RM, Annis BL. Disseminated intravascular coagulation associated with massive brain injury. *J Neurosurg* 1973; 39:178–180.
16. Kim H, Suzuki M, Lie JT, Titus JL. Clinically unsuspected disseminated intravascular coagulation (DIC): an autopsy survey. *Am J Clin Pathol* 1976; 66:31–39.
17. Macfarlane RG. An enzyme cascade in the blood clotting mechanism and its function as a biochemical amplifier. *Nature* 1964; 202:498–499.
18. McGauley JL, Miller CA, Penner JA. Diagnosis and treatment of diffuse intravascular coagulation following cerebral trauma: case report. *J Neurosurg* 1975; 43:374–376.
19. McKay DG, Latour JG, Parrish MH. Activation of Hageman factor by α-adrenergic stimulation. *Thromb Haemost* 1970; 23:417–422.
20. Miner ME, Kaufman HK, Graham SH, et al. Disseminated intravascular coagulation, a fibrinolytic syndrome following head injury in children: frequency and prognostic implications. *J Pediatr* 1982; 100:687–691.
21. Peck SD. Disseminated intravascular coagulation. How often have you missed it? *Rocky Mt Med J* 1970; 67:25–31.
22. Piepmeier J, Wagner FC Jr. Delayed post traumatic extracerebral hematomas. *J Trauma* 1982; 22:455–460.
23. Pondaag W. Disseminated intravascular coagulation related to outcome in head injury. *Acta Neurochir (Wien) [Suppl]* 1979; 28:98–102.
24. Poon WS, Rehman SU, Poon CY, Li AKC. Traumatic extradural hematoma of delayed onset is not a rarity. *Neurosurgery* 1992; 30:681–686.
25. Preston FE, Malia RG, Sworn MJ, et al. Disseminated intravascular coagulation as a consequence of cerebral damage. *J Neurol Neurosurg Psychiatry* 1974; 37:241–248.
26. Pretorius ME, Kaufman HH. Rapid onset of delayed traumatic intracerebral haematoma with diffuse intravascular coagulation and fibrinolysis. *Acta Neurochir (Wien)* 1982; 65:103–109.
27. Strinchini A, Baudo F, Nosari AM, et al. Defibrination and head injury. *Lancet* 1974; 2:957.
28. Sweet RC, Miller JD, Lipper M, et al. Significance of bilateral abnormalities on the CT scan in patients with severe head injury. *Neurosurgery* 1978; 3:16–21.
29. Tovi D. Fibrinolytic activity of human brain: a histochemical study. *Acta Neurol Scand* 1973; 49:152–162.
30. van der Sande JJ, Emeis JJ, Lindeman J. Intravascular coagulation: a common phenomenon in minor experimental head injury. *J Neurosurg* 1981; 54:21–25.
31. van der Sande JJ, Veltkamp JJ, Boekhout-Mussert RJ, Vielvoye GJ. Hemostasis and computerized tomography in head injury: their relationship to clinical features. *J Neurosurg* 1981; 55:718–724.
32. Vecht CJ, Sibinga CTS, Minderhoud JM. Disseminated intravascular

coagulation and head injury. *J Neurol Neurosurg Psychiatry* 1975; 38:567–571.

33. Watts C. Disseminated intravascular coagulation. *Surg Neurol* 1977; 8:258–262.
34. Zimmerman RA, Bilaniuk LT, Gennarelli T, et al. Cranial computed tomography in diagnosis and management of acute head trauma. *Am J Roentgenol* 1978; 131:27–34.

278 Penetrating Wounds of the Head

William S. Rosenberg
Griffith R. Harsh IV

Missile injuries to the head account for the majority of penetrating wounds of the brain and are responsible for a significant number of deaths. With over 250,000,000 firearms in the United States, approximately 150,000 people are shot each year and more than 30,000 of them will die.[35] According to data obtained in San Francisco, 50 percent of trauma deaths resulted from brain injury and 35 percent of these were caused by a gunshot wound to the head.[8] Recent data from Harris County, Texas, showed that gunshot wound to the head was present in 2.5 percent of all deaths, 16 percent of deaths from traumatic causes, and 45 percent of all fatal gunshot wounds.[36] There are several types of injuries, with urban conflict, terrorism, hunting accidents, and industrial explosions creating wounds similar to those seen in combat. Violence involving firearms, and therefore penetrating head injury, is increasing, and the management of these injuries will need to concern all neurosurgeons.

Physicians have been challenged by penetrating wounds to the head since antiquity.[13] Within a few hundred years of the Mongols' bringing gunpowder to Europe from China in the 1300s, a firearm (the Spanish musket) was invented that could propel a projectile at 1000 ft/s,[56] and could inflict previously unimaginable wounds. The modern management of these injuries began with the application of antiseptic technique to combat neurosurgery in the Anglo-Boer War (1899 to 1902)[23] and was further advanced and codified by Harvey Cushing during his tour of duty with the United States Expeditionary Force in France during World War I.[21,22] Cushing clearly delineated the principles of treatment for gunshot wounds to the head that resulted in a decrease in mortality from 54 to 28 percent.

The neurosurgical management of all penetrating head wounds derives from the same fundamental concepts, whether the penetration involves the scalp alone or the skull, dura, and the brain. The intent of treatment is to increase the incidence and quality of survival by preventing early and late infection, by controlling and relieving increased intracranial pressure, and by reducing secondary damage to the affected brain tissue.

This chapter will focus on wounds penetrating the dura and brain produced by power-driven missiles (bullets or shrapnel). Other piercing injuries may be caused by such sharp objects as nails, sticks, pencils, pens, screwdrivers, hatchets, pointed toys, and rocks. Injuries caused by these objects evoke similar therapeutic considerations but are modified primarily by a general absence of significant impact force and its deleterious secondary consequences.

Ballistics

Following ignition of the propellant, a projectile interacts with the firing chamber and barrel (internal ballistics) and is then propelled from the weapon on its flight toward the target (external ballistics). Once it strikes its target, the projectile interacts with the encountered material in complicated and variable ways.[9] An understanding of the effect of the missile on the target (terminal ballistics), and specifically on living tissue (wound ballistics), is of utmost importance in the treatment of gunshot wounds.

Using 10 percent ordnance gelatin as tissue simulant, Fackler and colleagues studied the ''wounding profiles'' of various projectiles,[24,25,27] and defined three fundamental biomechanical effects of missile passage.[11] The first is a direct crush injury produced by the projectile, which results in a permanent cylindrical cavity. The second, temporary cavitation, is produced by the cyclical radial expansion and contraction of the walls of the permanent cavity with pressures ranging from subatmospheric to 4 atm.[24] This pressure wave causes a stretch injury in both the region of the missile track and distant from it. In addition, the subatmospheric phases of the cycle can draw contaminated surface material into the wound. Of least clinical significance is the third effect, the sonic pressure wave, generated when the missile strikes the surface of the target. While pressures in this wave can reach 100 atm, tissue is spared injury by the brevity of the wave (approximately 2 μs).[11]

The major determinant of injury is the behavior of the missile within the tissue, which in turn depends on deformation, yaw (rotation about the long axis), and fragmentation of the projectile. Prior clinical literature on wound ballistics has excessively emphasized the velocity of the projectile, differentiating wounds on the basis of ''low-velocity'' versus ''high-velocity'' weapons. Velocity is not, however, a primary, independent determinant of wounding potential[24]; increased velocity is not always correlated with increased tissue disruption. The Vetterli 10.4 mm round used by the Swiss and Italian armies during the late 1800s, caused significant temporary cavitation at a ''low velocity'' because of its deformation[11]; its contemporary, the 6.5 mm round of the Mannlicher-Carcano rifle used in Holland, Romania, and Italy, caused virtually no temporary cavitation, even at velocities characteristic of the modern assault rifle.[26] Furthermore, cavitation may be delayed in certain nondeforming rounds. The 7.62 mm full metal jacketed projectile of the AK-47 assault rifle, for instance, can traverse 25 cm of tissue prior to cavitating, which coincides with its beginning to yaw.[27] This delayed cavitation may be important in certain neurosurgical injuries, as missile paths may be short enough to exit the head prior to temporary cavitation. Since deforming rounds were banned from military conflict by the Hague Convention of 1899, but are still used for nonmilitary purposes, civilian wounds may be more serious than those incurred in military combat.

Some clinical publications equated a missile's kinetic energy to its wounding potential. Kinetic energy [$\frac{1}{2} m(V^2_{entry} - V^2_{exit})$; where m is bullet mass, V_{entry} is the velocity of the bullet on entry, and V_{exit} is the velocity of the bullet on exit] is a useful first approximation, but it represents only the energy available to a projectile, not the energy actually delivered to the target. The energy delivered is related more to the deformation and/or fragmentation of the missile, its motion in flight and on impact, and aspects of the tissue it encounters. Ryan et al.[45] proposed the useful concept of "high and low energy-transfer wounding" to encompass these various factors.

Penetrating wounds can also arise from explosions during conventional warfare, terrorist operations, or industrial accidents. The irregular shape of the resulting fragments alters their ballistic behavior and wounding profile.[45] Initial velocities may be extremely high, and, in combination with blast effects, can result in a near 100 percent mortality rate for people close to the explosion. However, the nonaerodynamic nature of the fragments causes a rapid decline in velocity with distance, typically producing low energy-transfer injuries in those who survive the initial blast.

Explosive rounds, such as the projectiles used in the assassination attempt on President Reagan, result in even more complicated wounds (see Sykes et al.[51] for review). These missiles have a high failure rate when striking at less than a 90 degree angle. The unexploded round is a potential danger to both patient and health care providers. Evidence of their use includes explosive ammunition in the weapon or at the scene, a single lead shot on x-ray examination or within the wound, a large amount of black powder residue within the wound, and/or percussion caps on x-ray examination or within the wound. If an explosive round is suspected, all personnel should take precautions, such as wearing metal-proof goggles and using long, rubber-tipped forceps for handling the bullet. Unexploded missiles should be removed because the dangers of tissue injury from toxicity and delayed detonation are unknown.

Neurosurgically, the important ballistic concepts are as follows: (1) wounds can be divided into high and low energy-transfer injuries, but all wounds need to be evaluated individually, regardless of ammunition or weapon used; (2) many nondeforming rounds can traverse substantial amounts of tissue before initiating temporary cavitation, which may cause tissue damage distant from the missile track; (3) the brain, a high density/low elasticity organ, is very susceptible to temporary cavitation. Temporary cavitation represents a stretch injury, and probably mandates no more debridement than other such stretch injuries; (4) bone fragments from the skull can be secondary missiles (Fig. 278-1*B*), which exacerbate the primary injury.[6] Moreover, the bullet can ricochet from the inner table (Fig. 278-1*C*), resulting in complicated missile tracts; and (5) special ammunition, such as an explosive bullet, needs to be sought and handled appropriately.

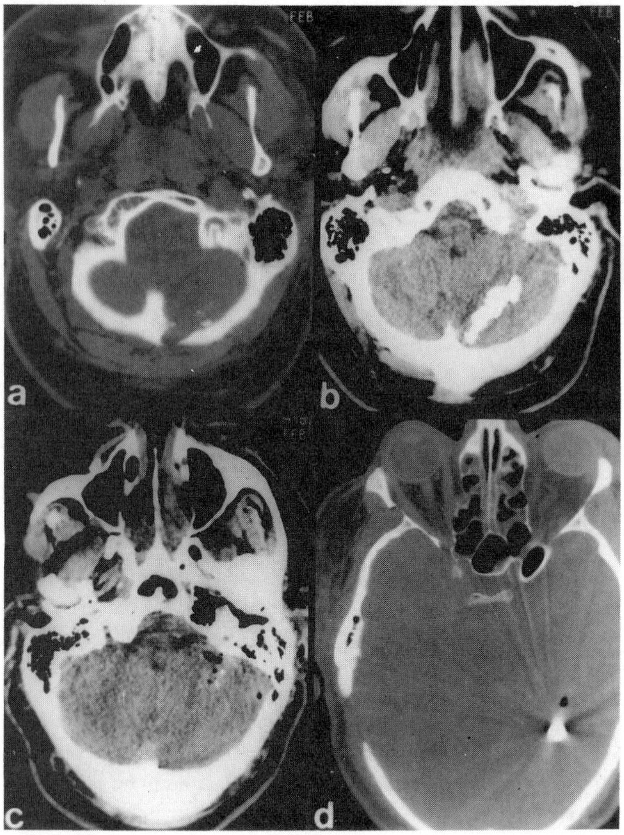

Figure 278-1 The patient is a 60-year-old man who was shot in the back of the neck. The bullet entered the posterior fossa (*A*), produced indriven bone fragments (*B*), ricocheted off the petrous apex (*C*), and lodged above the tentorium (*D*). The patient's only deficit was a transient trigeminal neuropathy. He was managed conservatively and made a full recovery.

Pathophysiology

Impact of the missile on the head is followed by a variety of primary and secondary pathophysiologic alterations within the cranium. As the projectile travels through the brain, it crushes neural tissue, producing a permanent cavity. Direct laceration of significant vascular structures may lead to intracranial hemorrhage, the incidence of which, in civilian series using computed tomography (CT), is approximately 50 percent.[19,38,47] Although typically thought of as a phenomenon of temporary cavitation, distant vascular injury can also result from missile passage directly. Nichols and Sens,[42] using modern cytologic techniques, examined the residue adherent to the projectiles in 38 consecutive gunshot wound deaths. Bullets passing through the brain were the only ones found to carry long, arborizing fragments of capillaries and blood vessels. The authors hypothesized that this resulted from biomechanical attributes of the Virchow-Robin space and/or the blood-brain barrier and may explain some of the distant cerebrovascular effects of missile passage. Temporary cavitation, the second pressure wave caused by the projectile, induces a stretch injury extending radially from the missile track that can also affect cerebral vasculature. Although many believe the sonic pressure wave, the third pressure wave of missile passage, has no adverse effects on living tissue, one group of investigators[50] has attributed the myelin invaginations, axoplasmic shrinkage, decrease in microtubule number, and chromatolysis found in cerebellar Purkinje cells following peripheral wounding in the thighs of young pigs to the distant effects of these waves.

Damage created instantaneously by the missile is soon compounded by a series of secondary changes that occur over minutes to hours. These changes were initially studied in monkeys with a trephined skull opening by Crockard et al.,[20] and later by Carey et al. in a closed-skull cat model.[14] In the cat, the mean arterial blood pressure (MAP) rose within seconds of injury and gradually returned to baseline over the next several minutes. The intracranial pressure (ICP) also demonstrated a large initial rise, followed by a gradual fall over the next several minutes to a level still elevated above baseline. In the most severely wounded cats, the ICP then increased over the 2 to 3 h following injury. Both initial and delayed increases in ICP were proportional to the energy delivered via the missile. The cerebral perfusion pressure (CPP) increased for the first hour after wounding secondary to the increase in MAP, and then gradually decreased as the effect of increasing ICP became predominant and the MAP returned to baseline. Respiratory variations also occurred; the duration of apnea following injury correlated with the wounding energy. Immediate ventilatory support for apneic animals improved outcome, a finding corroborated by subsequent human data.[28] The hypothesized mechanism for these cardiopulmonary changes is the rostrocaudal displacement or distortion of the brain stem induced by the pressure differential created across the foramen magnum.[14,20] This hypothesis is supported, but not proved, by changes found in epinephrine- and serotonin-containing brain stem nuclei following experimental craniocerebral missile injury,[49] by the absence of postinjury apnea in cats wounded through a skull trephination,[14] and by differences in the cardiopulmonary changes of cats injured without a trephination as compared to monkeys injured through a trephination.[20]

The edema that develops following penetrating cerebral injury has also been studied in the cat model.[16] Animals were examined for up to 7 days following injury. Edema occurred only adjacent to the missile track. First evident at 6 h, it peaked at 48 h and spontaneously resolved within 1 week of wounding. At its peak, the edema was relatively mild when compared to that of cold-induced injury. In addition, electrolyte composition and intravascular Evans blue dye studies[15] showed the edema to be vasogenic, secondary to disruption of the blood-brain barrier along the missile track.

Craniocerebral missile wounds also induce systemic changes in coagulation. Following experimental missile injury in cats, disseminated intravascular coagulopathy was detectable within 2 h and persisted until the end of the study at 6 h.[7] The pattern of coagulation factor depletion was consistent with activation of the extrinsic coagulation system, possibly by brain thromboplastin. Platelet number and aggregability decreased by 2 h after injury, but normalized within the 6 h of the experiment. These findings have been confirmed in human victims of gunshot wounds to the head with 71 percent of survivors, and 94 percent of nonsurvivors displaying at least one abnormal test suggestive of disseminated intravascular coagulopathy.[36]

To summarize, the pathophysiology of craniocerebral missile passage has primary and secondary aspects. During the primary injury, the bullet causes direct trauma, as well as distant stretch injury, and may have more potential for cerebrovascular injury than previously appreciated. Second, severe derangements of cardiopulmonary regulation occur, possibly because of brain stem dysfunction. These are often transient and, if appropriate hemodynamic and ventilatory support are provided, secondary injury can be prevented. Coagulopathy is a common accompaniment of penetrating missile injury and may contribute to secondary intracranial hemorrhage.

Initial Assessment and Resuscitation

Presentation of a patient following missile injury to the brain is highly variable due to the combinations of external signs of trauma and neurological deficit that occur. External wounds may or may not involve extensive soft tissue disruption (e.g., the difficult to find orbital-facial entry wound). Significant external hemorrhage and hypovolemic shock may occur from discrete, as well as extensive wounds. Skull fractures may be almost linear, but usually are comminuted, displaced, and accompanied by the inward carriage of fragments and debris. Simultaneous infracranial injuries are common.

Any combination of alteration in consciousness and focal neurological deficit may be seen. Some degree of agitation or depression of awareness is usually found. Consciousness may or may not be lost in penetrating brain injury; its presence does not preclude sudden, severe neurological deterioration. Focal deficits may be absent if a missile traverses only noneloquent brain, or they may be multiple and profound if eloquent cortex is damaged at the sites of entry, ricochet, and/or exit. Loss of brain stem reflexes may be transient. An enlarging intracranial mass lesion should be suspected when there is progressive loss of brain stem function in a pattern consistent with herniation, or if the brain stem examination is dramatically better than the overall Glasgow Coma Scale (GCS) score.[28]

Proper initial treatment of a patient with a gunshot wound to the head involves prompt cardiopulmonary resuscitation as needed. Endotracheal intubation is indicated in any patient whose current or future ability to maintain an adequate airway is questionable. Aggressive resuscitation, both before and during transport to the hospital, improves the outcome of patients who initially appear moribund.[28,48] Definitive treatment decisions based on the neurological status should be deferred until adequate hemodynamic resuscitation and oxygenation are achieved.[28] Significant bleeding from the scalp or other wounds should be controlled immediately. Cardiovascular compromise from blood loss or arrhythmia should be corrected as rapidly as possible. The usual precautions for spinal instability must be observed, as some patients will have fallen and sustained spine injuries following the gunshot wound. A careful inspection of the entire patient for other injuries should be performed, and appropriate treatment instituted. In the case of multiple injury, first priority is given to the most life-threatening injuries, and occasionally simultaneous laparotomy or thoracotomy and craniotomy are necessary.

CT may demonstrate the bullet track, as well as intracranial hemorrhage, indriven radiopaque material, and diffuse cerebral edema. Most of the recent civilian series[10,28,36,38,41,48] and some of the modern wartime studies[12,53] have relied heavily on CT for the initial and continued evaluation of the patient. Only the most life-threatening circumstances should delay or prevent its use. An adequate lateral skull film can be obtained from the scout film of the CT scan. Arteriography is indicated if the bullet track passes near major intracranial vessels and the clinical status of the patient allows it (Fig. 278-2*D*). The role of arteriography in other cases, and its timing remain controversial (see Post-Traumatic Cerebrovascular Lesions below).

Complete shaving of the head facilitates the search for small wounds of entrance or exit. Open wounds exuding cerebrum or cerebrospinal fluid (CSF) should be bandaged until definitive treatment is possible. Neurological assessment should be as thorough as time permits; the appearance of rapid deterioration with signs of progressive herniation requires immediate surgical intervention.

Definitive Management

Medical Therapy

Preoperative and intraoperative medical therapy attempts to control intracranial pressure and to prevent secondary neural injury, seizures, infection, and gastrointestinal hemorrhage. Elevated ICP should be assumed in all patients who present with a depressed level of consciousness, and these patients should be treated empirically with hyperventilation and mannitol. The efficacy of corticosteroids in penetrating head injury is unsubstantiated, and consequently their use is not recommended.

The problem of post-traumatic epilepsy has been reviewed recently (see Temkin et al.[54]). Victims of penetrating brain injury are

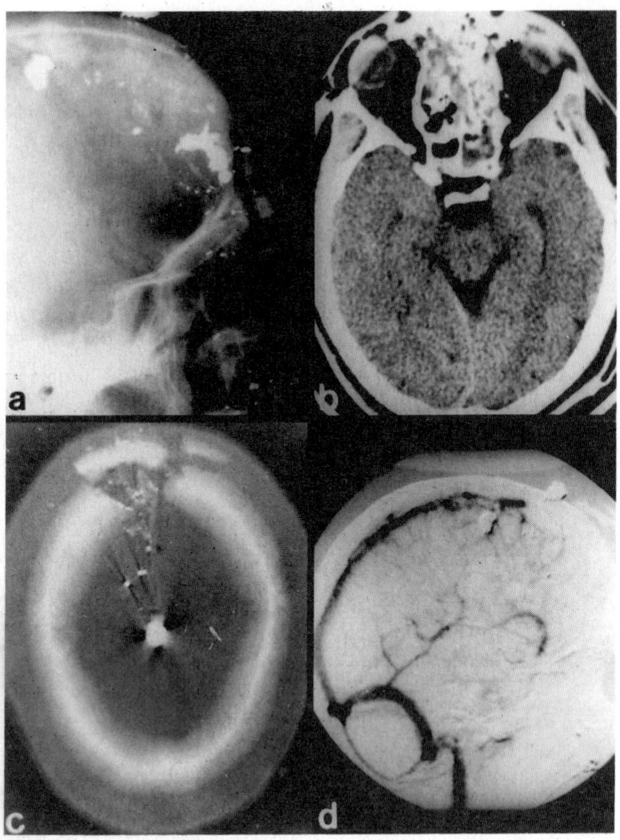

Figure 278-2 The patient is a 38-year-old police officer who attempted suicide by shooting himself through the palate with his service revolver (*A*). The bullet fragmented the ethmoid sinuses (*B*), and traversed the midline of the anterior cranial fossa (*C*). Arteriography demonstrated compromise of flow through the anterior aspect of the superior sagittal sinus, and adjacent bullet fragments (*D*). Initially, he was neurologically intact, but acute deterioration secondary to bifrontal swelling necessitated an emergency craniotomy. He recovered fully.

at high risk for both post-traumatic seizures and delayed epilepsy. Seizure rates following these injuries approach 50 percent in some long-term studies. The use of prophylactic anticonvulsants in Vietnam did not reduce the rate of delayed epilepsy below that in previous conflicts, in which they were not used.[39] Nonetheless, given the high rate of post-traumatic epilepsy following penetrating head injury, it seems reasonable to use prophylactic antiepileptics until well-designed, prospective studies are available. The duration of antiepileptic treatment is also controversial. Ninety-five percent of patients with blunt head injury who will develop seizures within 15 years of their injury will have their first seizure within 3 years of the injury.[54] Status epilepticus is a medical emergency, and should be treated with intravenous benzodiazepines (while ensuring adequate ventilation), followed by longer acting antiepileptics.

In Vietnam, 11 percent of cultures from craniocerebral missile tracks yielded bacterial growth.[17] Bullets fired into experimental animals carry bacteria with them, although the colony counts do not become clinically significant until 24 h after wounding.[55] Culture data from the Iran-Iraq War[1,3] and the Lebanese Civil War[52] show approximately equal numbers of gram-positive and gram-negative bacterial infections. The high incidence of gram-negative bacterial contamination may reflect a change in skin colonization secondary to the suboptimal living conditions encountered in combat. However, Taha et al.[53] showed gram-positive antibiotic coverage to be sufficient for the prevention of infection. Incomplete initial dural closure, wound dehiscence, CSF leakage, and violation of an air sinus are the most important risk factors for infection.[52] Cultures obtained from a dehisced scalp wound correlate well with those obtained from brain abscesses and can be used to guide the therapy of deep infections.[52] Prophylactic antibiotic coverage, initially broad spectrum and directed toward non-nosocomial wound flora, is warranted. The exact choice of antibiotics, as well as the duration of administration, should be dictated by the circumstances of the injury and the characteristics of the individual wound. Antibiotic coverage for normal skin flora, particularly staphylococcus and streptococcus, remains the mainstay of prophylaxis. If there is gross contamination of the wound, or there is a question of suboptimal hygiene and therefore changes in skin flora, antibiotics directed toward gram-negative bacteria should be added. All antibiotics chosen should adequately penetrate the CSF.

A nasogastric tube, or an orogastric tube when injury to the paranasal sinuses mandates it (Fig. 278-2*B*), should be inserted in all patients. The gastric mucosa should be protected during the period of postinjury stress by an H2-blocker and/or an antacid.

Surgical Selection—Overall Morbidity and Mortality

The selection of patients for surgical intervention should be guided by morbidity and mortality data. Preoperative identification of patients who will recover without intervention and those who will succumb despite all treatment would be particularly helpful. Wartime series[4,12,18,32] have a much lower mortality rate than civilian series. This difference reflects the higher proportion of low energy-transfer injuries (long-range bullets and shrapnel), and the longer evacuation time that selects for the less critically injured patients. In modern civilian studies that rely extensively on CT scans, the overall morbidity and mortality of patients with craniocerebral gunshot wounds who survive until hospitalization has been remarkably stable (Fig. 278-3).[10,28,36,38,41,48] The retrospective nature of most of these studies makes them susceptible to selection bias: patients presenting in poor neurological condition were not operated on because of the surgeon's perception that they will not have a satisfactory outcome. However, there is a general concordance that the most important prognosticator of outcome is the presenting GCS score. Other risk factors for poor outcome are age, suicide attempt, delay in effective resuscitation, bihemispheric or multilobar injury (Fig. 278-4), and intraventricular hemorrhage.

Grahm et al.,[28] using a prospectively designed protocol to treat 100 consecutive craniocerebral gunshot wound victims, confirmed the above findings and proposed the following algorithm. All patients exhibiting neurological function are aggressively resuscitated and receive a CT scan. Surgery is reserved for patients with: (1) a GCS score of 3 to 5 and a large extra-axial hematoma, (2) a GCS score of 6 to 8 without transventricular, bihemispheric, or multilobar dominant hemisphere injury, or (3) a GCS score of 9 to 15. No treatment is given to those patients with a GCS score of 3 to 5 without hematoma, or a GCS score of 6 to 8 with intraventricular, bihemispheric, or multilobar dominant hemisphere injury. The value of this treatment plan is well supported by scientific data. However, the surgical debridement used was perhaps more aggressive than necessary (see Operative Technique below). In general, patients either do well or die; very few are left in a persistent vegetative state.

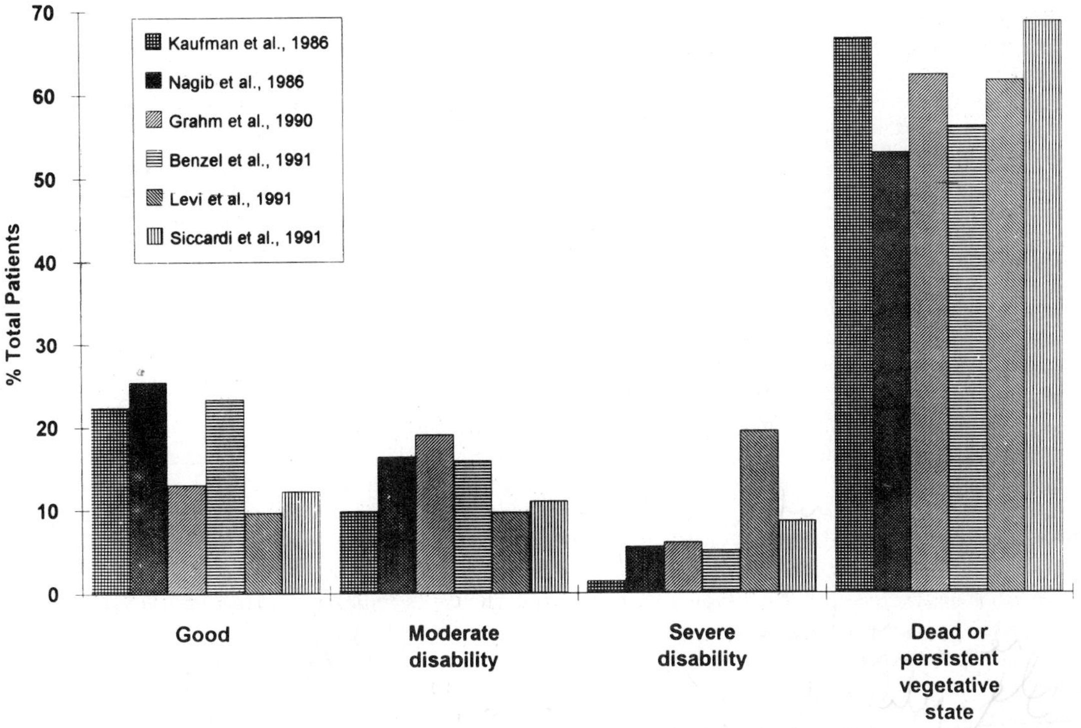

Figure 278-3 Morbidity and mortality of patients arriving at the hospital with a craniocerebral gunshot wound in civilian series using CT.

Several reports emphasize individual cases of patients appearing to be fatally wounded who make a meaningful neurological recovery.[10,28,36] Such cases suggest the value of aggressively treating patients with poor neurological presentation, and further studies are necessary. Until these are available, categorical or protocol decisions would seem inappropriate.

Evidence from the Lebanese Civil War indicates that there may be a subset of highly functional patients who do not need surgery. Taha and colleagues[53] initiated a prospective protocol in which patients were selected if they met the following criteria: (1) initial GCS score over 10, (2) examination within 6 h of injury, (3) diameter of entrance wound less than 2 cm, (3) no exit wound, (4) proximal Sylvian fissure not traversed, (4) no extra-axial hematoma, and (5) no intracerebral hematoma that was enlarging or measured more than 4 cm in diameter. These patients were treated with simple wound debridement and closure (one layer nylon) in the emergency room and given intravenous methicillin for 14 days and antiepileptics. Only one of 32 patients developed complications (seizure and abscess), and they were treated successfully.

Operative Technique

The goals of modern neurosurgical therapy, as first outlined by Cushing,[21] include the removal of clinically significant intracranial mass lesions, control of hemorrhage, prevention of further loss of functioning neural tissue, and the deterrence of infection and seizures. Surgery consists of removal of extra-axial hematomas, evacuation of intracerebral hematomas large enough to cause neurological deficit, careful hemostasis, and meticulous wound closure

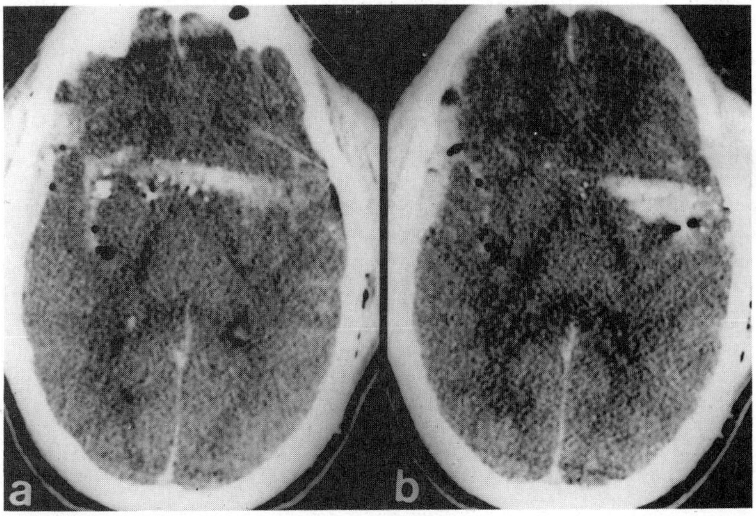

Figure 278-4 The patient was a 15-year-old high school student who shot himself while at school. There is a through-and-through missile track filled with blood, debris, and bone (*A, B*). The patient met brain death criteria shortly after admission to the Emergency Ward.

resulting in a watertight dura and a tension-free wound. The entire head is shaved and a thorough search for entrance and exit wounds is made. The head is positioned to allow access first to the entrance wound, and then to the exit wound, unless a distal intracranial hematoma evident on the preoperative CT scan mandates initial exit wound exploration. The scalp wound is excised and incorporated into the incision, if possible. Using either a craniectomy or a craniotomy, structurally sound dura is exposed on all sides of the penetration site to facilitate watertight dural closure. The subdural space is inspected, and any hematoma evacuated. Any debris, whether comminuted bone fragments, missile remnants, or necrotic brain, that presents itself easily to the surface should be removed. This protocol is a departure from the previous teaching of aggressive surgical debridement of the wound track. Removal of ''a surrounding margin of 0.5 to 1 cm of normal brain''[18] was advocated during the Vietnam War. Aggressive debridement for removal of indriven bone or bullet fragments was thought to reduce the risk of infection and seizure. Secondary and even tertiary operations were undertaken to remove such retained debris. Recent military data,[12,53] as well as some civilian studies,[10,41,48] indicate that such an aggressive approach is unnecessary, and that acceptable rates of morbidity and mortality can be achieved while preserving as much neural tissue as possible. There has been no evidence from the era of antibiotics, modern neurosurgical techniques, and CT that retained fragments, of either bone or metal, result in increased rates of infection or epilepsy. In patients with retained bone fragments who develop in intracranial infection, other important risk factors such as CSF leakage and wound dehiscence are almost always present.[1,52]

After gentle debridement of easily accessible debris and necrotic brain, the subdural space is again inspected and the dura closed. Watertight dural closure is crucial for prevention of postoperative infection, and dural grafting with pericranium, temporal or occipital fascia, or fascia lata should be performed as necessary. Intracranial pressure should be monitored if there is evidence of brain swelling, and/or difficulty evaluating the neurological condition of the patient is expected. If the wound is more than 36 h old, soft tissue should be closed with a single layer of stainless steel wire. A tension-free skin closure completes the operation.

Special Surgical Considerations

Post-Traumatic Cerebrovascular Lesions

As state-of-the-art angiographic services are becoming available to both military and civilian neurosurgeons, cerebrovascular damage is increasingly recognized as a component of penetrating brain injury. There are numerous reports of post-traumatic aneurysms, vascular occlusions, dural sinus injuries, and arteriovenous fistulae following gunshot wound to the head.[2,5,10,30,33,34,37,43,46] One prospective angiographic study[34] found a 50 percent incidence of such cerebrovascular injuries in a civilian population. Aneurysms have an incidence as high as 42 percent following gunshot wound to the head.[34] They usually result from injury to the vessel wall from close passage of the projectile, and typically occur on the distal branches of major vessels. If the missile track is near major intracranial vessels or dural venous sinuses, angiography should be performed (Fig. 278-2*D*) unless precluded by the need for other emergency treatment.[10] Whether arteriography should be done acutely or be delayed has not been resolved by a well-controlled trial.

Perforation of Air Sinuses

Passage of the missile through an air sinus or mastoid air cell prior to its entry into the cranium is associated with a high incidence of CSF leakage, infection, and mortality.[3,52] If the wounding site is accessible, the same principles of management as for uncomplicated wounds apply. Special attention should be given to dural repair at sites of possible CSF leakage. If the entrance or exit wounds are not easily accessible, surgery can be deferred until mandated by the presence of a CSF leak. Any leakage that develops should be treated with standard techniques.

Tangential Wounds

Termed ''gutter wounds'' by Cushing,[21] tangential wounds are those in which the missile delivers a glancing, nonpenetrating blow to the cranium. Such an injury may be associated with significant brain damage, with or without visible bone involvement. Even if there is no disruption of the skull, or only a nondisplaced, linear skull fracture, significant neurological injury may result from brain hematoma, laceration, or contusion underlying the point of tangential impact.[29] Computed tomography has made a dramatic impact on the treatment of these injuries. Therapy is the same as that for other types of penetrating injuries to the head.

Opening of Intact Dura

Dura left intact by the injury should be opened at the time of operation, if it is tense, protuberant, and darkened in appearance, or if the neurological examination and CT scan suggest an underlying mass lesion.

Migratory Projectiles

Bullets can migrate within the cranium under several conditions.[44] Migratory projectiles can be located within the ventricular system, within a cavity of liquefied necrotic brain, pus, or hematoma or, if heavy enough, within the white matter of the brain. Intraventricular missiles can cause acute obstructive hydrocephalus, and missiles within a cavity may induce an abscess. Continued movement of a missile through the white matter can damage critical white matter tracts, such as the internal capsule. Although no statistical studies of such cases exist, it seems prudent to remove the potentially migratory projectile whenever possible.

Pediatric Injuries

The one study published on pediatric craniocerebral gunshot wounds[40] suggests that these are similar to adult injuries. The mortality rate is similar, but morbidity is lower because of the ability of children to recover more fully.

Postoperative Care

Prevention of further injury to the brain during the postoperative period is crucial to outcome. Close neurological monitoring for signs of increased ICP or infection is essential. An ICP monitor may be used if problems with pressure control or evaluation of the patient are anticipated. Intracranial hypertension should be investigated by emergency CT scan and treated aggressively with mild sedation, hyperventilation, mannitol, barbiturates, and reoperation, as necessary. Prophylactic antibiotics and antiepileptics are continued. Rigorous medical intensive care monitoring is essential for the prevention of cardiac, pulmonary, or metabolic derangement that might jeopardize brain recovery.

Complications encountered in the early postoperative period include recurrent bleeding, uncontrollable intracranial hypertension, infection, and CSF leakage.[31] Recurrent bleeding mandates a repeat craniotomy. Infection requires treatment directed at the source (e.g., repair of a continuing CSF fistula, removal of an abscess) and appropriate antibiotics.

Conclusions

The principles of management of penetrating brain injuries are the same for wounds sustained in military combat and in civilian life. The ballistics of wounding range, projectile deformation and cavitation, and skull-missile interactions provide pathophysiologic insight. Aggressive resuscitation in both the field and the hospital, and prompt correction of physiologic abnormalities are of paramount importance to clinical outcome. Computed tomography and, when appropriate, arteriography are cornerstones of the diagnostic evaluation of these patients. The surgical principles of aggressive treatment of mass lesions, limited brain debridement, watertight dural closure, and tension-free skin closure should be applied in all situations with accessible entrance and/or exit wounds. Intensive postoperative monitoring and control of ICP, cardiorespiratory function, and metabolic status, are required for optimizing the outcome of victims of penetrating craniocerebral injuries.

References

1. Aarabi B. Comparative study of bacteriological contamination between primary and secondary exploration of missile head wounds. *Neurosurgery* 1987; 20:610–616.
2. Aarabi B. Traumatic aneurysms of brain due to high velocity missile head wounds. *Neurosurgery* 1988; 22:1056–1063.
3. Aarabi B. Causes of infections in penetrating head wounds in the Iran-Iraq war. *Neurosurgery* 1989; 25:923–926.
4. Aarabi B. Surgical outcome in 435 patients who sustained missile head wounds during the Iran-Iraq war. *Neurosurgery* 1990; 27:692–695.
5. Achram M, 'Rizk G, Haddad FS. Angiographic aspects of traumatic intracranial aneurysms following war injuries. *Br J Radiol* 1980; 53:1144–1149.
6. Amato JJ, Syracuse D, Seaver PR Jr, et al. Bone as a secondary missile: an experimental study in the fragmenting of bone by high-velocity missiles. *J Trauma* 1989; 29:609–612.
7. Awasthi D, Rock WA, Carey ME, et al. Coagulation changes after an experimental missile wound to the brain in the cat. *Surg Neurol* 1991; 36:441–446.
8. Baker CC, Oppenheimer L, Stephens B, et al. Epidemiology of trauma deaths. *Am J Surg* 1980; 140:144–148.
9. Barach E, Tomlanovich M, Nowak R. Ballistics: a pathophysiologic examination of the wounding mechanisms of firearms: Part I. *J Trauma* 1986; 26:225–235.
10. Benzel EC, Day WT, Kesterson L, et al. Civilian craniocerebral gunshot wounds. *Neurosurgery* 1991; 29:67–72.
11. Bowen TE, Bellamy RF (eds) *Emergency War Surgery,* 2d ed. Washington, DC: United States Government Printing Office, 1988, pp 13–34.
12. Brandvold B, Levi L, Feinsod M, et al. Penetrating craniocerebral injuries in the Israeli involvement in the Lebanese conflict, 1982–1985: analysis of a less aggressive surgical approach. *J Neurosurg* 1990; 72:15–21.
13. Breasted JH. *The Edwin Smith Surgical Papyrus.* Chicago: University of Chicago Press, 1930.
14. Carey ME, Sarna GS, Farrell JB, et al. Experimental missile wound to the brain. *J Neurosurg* 1989; 71:754–764.
15. Carey ME, Sarna GS, Farrell JB. Brain edema after an experimental missile wound. *Adv Neurol* 1990; 52:301–305.
16. Carey ME, Sarna GS, Farrell JB. Brain edema following an experimental missile wound to the brain. *J Neurotrauma* 1990; 7:13–20.
17. Carey ME, Young H, Mathis JL, et al. A bacteriological study of craniocerebral missile wounds from Vietnam. *J Neurosurg* 1971; 34:145–154.
18. Carey ME, Young HF, Mathis JL. The neurosurgical treatment of craniocerebral missile wounds in Vietnam. *Surg Gynecol Obstet* 1972; 135:386–389.
19. Clark WC, Muhlbauer MS, Watridge CB, et al. Analysis of 76 civilian craniocerebral gunshot wounds. *J Neurosurg* 1986; 65:9–14.
20. Crockard HA, Brown FD, Calica AB, et al. Physiological consequences of experimental cerebral missile injury and use of data analysis to predict survival. *J Neurosurg* 1977; 46:784–794.
21. Cushing H. A study of a series of wounds involving the brain and its enveloping structures. *Br J Surg* 1918; 5:558–684.
22. Cushing H. Notes on penetrating wounds of the brain. *Br Med J* 1918; 1:221–226.
23. De Villiers JC. The management of missile injuries of the head during the Anglo-Boer War. *Br J Neurosurg* 1987; 1:53–61.
24. Fackler ML. Wound ballistics. A review of common misconceptions. *JAMA* 1988; 259:2730–2736.
25. Fackler ML. Wound ballistics: the management of assault rifle injuries. *Mil Med* 1990; 155:222–225.
26. Fackler ML, Dougherty PJ. Theodor Kocher and the scientific foundation of wound ballistics. *Surg Gynecol Obstet* 1991; 172:153–160.
27. Fackler ML, Malinowski JA, Hoxie SW, et al. Wounding effects of the AK-47 rifle used by Patrick Purdy in the Stockton, California, schoolyard shooting of January 17, 1989. *Am J Forensic Med Pathol* 1990; 11:185–189.
28. Grahm TW, Williams FC Jr, Harrington T, et al. Civilian gunshot wounds to the head: a prospective study. *Neurosurgery* 1990; 27:696–700.
29. Hadas N, Schiffer J, Rogev M, et al. Tangential low-velocity missile wound of the head with acute subdural hematoma: case report. *J Trauma* 1990; 30:358–359.
30. Haddad FS, Haddad GF, Taha J. Traumatic intracranial aneurysms caused by missiles: their presentation and management. *Neurosurgery* 1991; 28:1–7.
31. Hagan D. Early complications following penetrating wounds of the brain. *J Neurosurg* 1971; 34:132–141.
32. Hammon WM. Analysis of 2187 consecutive penetrating wounds to the brain from Vietnam. *J Neurosurg* 1971; 34:127–131.
33. Hanigan WC, Wright RM, Berkman WA, et al. MR imaging of a false carotid aneurysm. *Stroke* 1986; 17:1317–1319.
34. Jinkins JR, Dadsetan MR, Sener RN, et al. Value of acute-phase angiography in the detection of vascular injuries caused by gunshot wounds to the head: analysis of 12 cases. *Am J Roentgenol* 1992; 159:365–368.
35. Kaufman HH. Treatment of civilian gunshot wounds to the head. *Neurosurg Clin North Am* 1991; 2:387–397.
36. Kaufman HH, Makela ME, Lee KF, et al. Gunshot wounds to the head: a perspective. *Neurosurgery* 1986; 18:689–695.
37. Kaufman HH, Sadhu VK, Clifton GL, et al. Delayed intracerebral hematoma due to traumatic aneurysm caused by a shotgun wound: a problem in prophylaxis. *Neurosurgery* 1980; 6:181–184.

38. Levi L, Linn S, Feinsod M. Penetrating craniocerebral injuries in civilians. *Br J Neurosurg* 1991; 5:241–247.
39. Meirowsky AM. Notes on posttraumatic epilepsy in missile wounds of the brain. *Mil Med* 1982; 147:632–634.
40. Miner ME, Ewing-Cobbs L, Kopaniky DR, et al. The results of treatment of gunshot wounds to the brain in children. *Neurosurgery* 1990; 26:20–25.
41. Nagib MG, Rockswold GL, Sherman RS, et al. Civilian gunshot wounds to the brain: prognosis and management. *Neurosurgery* 1986; 18:533–537.
42. Nichols CA, Sens MA. Cytologic manifestations of ballistic injury. *Am J Clin Pathol* 1991; 95:660–669.
43. Rahimizadeh A, Abtahi H, Daylami MS, et al. Traumatic cerebral aneurysms caused by shell fragments. Report of four cases and review of the literature. *Acta Neurochir (Wien)* 1987; 84:93–98.
44. Rengachary SS, Carey M, Templer J. The sinking bullet. *Neurosurgery* 1992; 30:291–295.
45. Ryan JM, Cooper GJ, Haywood IR, et al. Field surgery on a future conventional battlefield: strategy and wound management. *Ann R Coll Surg Engl* 1991; 73:13–20.
46. Salar G, Mingrino S. Traumatic intracranial internal carotid aneurysm due to gunshot wound. *J Neurosurg* 1978; 49:100–102.
47. Sherman WD, Apuzzo MLJ, Heiden JS, et al. Gunshot wounds to the brain—a civilian experience. *West J Med* 1980; 132:99–105.
48. Siccardi D, Cavaliere R, Pau A, et al. Penetrating craniocerebral missile injuries in civilians: a retrospective analysis of 314 cases. *Surg Neurol* 1991; 35:455–460.
49. Soblosky JS, Rogers NL, Adams JA, et al. Central and peripheral biogenic amine effects of brain missile wounding and increased intracranial pressure. *J Neurosurg* 1992; 76:119–126.
50. Suneson A, Hansson HA, Seeman T. Pressure wave injuries to the nervous system caused by high-energy missile extremity impact: Part II. Distant effects on the central nervous system—a light and electron microscopic study on pigs. *J Trauma* 1990; 30:295–306.
51. Sykes LN Jr, Champion HR, Fouty WJ. Dum-dums, hollow-points, and devastators: techniques designed to increase wounding potential of bullets. *J Trauma* 1988; 28:618–623.
52. Taha JM, Haddad FS, Brown JA. Intracranial infection after missile injuries to the brain: report of 30 cases from the Lebanese conflict. *Neurosurgery* 1991; 29:864–868.
53. Taha JM, Saba MI, Brown JA. Missile injuries to the brain treated by simple wound closure: results of a protocol during the Lebanese conflict. *Neurosurgery* 1991; 29:380–384.
54. Temkin NR, Dikmen SS, Winn HR. Management of head injury: posttraumatic seizures. *Neurosurg Clin North Am* 1991; 2:425–435.
55. Tian HM, Deng GG, Huang MJ, et al. Quantitative bacteriological study of the wound track. *J Trauma* 1988; 28(Suppl):S215–S216.
56. West CGH. A short history of the management of penetrating missile injuries of the head. *Surg Neurol* 1981; 16:145–149.

279

Vascular Lesions Resulting from Head Injury

Jamshid Ahmadi
Michael L. Levy
Bizhan Aarabi
Steven L. Giannotta

Cerebrovascular trauma can result from a broad array of injuries—both direct and indirect. Epidural hematoma and carotid-cavernous sinus fistula are two examples of the better recognized sequelae of intracranial vascular disruption. Unfortunately, not all vascular injuries associated with head trauma are as readily identifiable nor are they associated with definite treatment guidelines. Symptoms and signs of major extra- or intracranial cerebrovascular injuries such as aneurysm formation, carotid thrombosis, or dissection may be delayed in onset or remain unrecognized because of superimposed brain injury. Such patients are at risk for further irreversible deterioration due to ischemia or emboli. Thus, the recognition of clinical and/or radiologic findings can result in the early diagnosis and treatment of traumatic injuries to major intra- or extracranial cerebrovascular structures.

From its inception, computed tomography (CT) has essentially supplanted cerebral arteriography in the initial evaluation of head-injured patients. Despite the numerous benefits of CT, arteriography still remains the definitive examination for the subsequent evaluation of patients potentially harboring cerebrovascular lesions. More recently, magnetic resonance imaging (MRI), with its high level of sensitivity, has also become an integral tool both in the initial and subsequent evaluation of patients presenting with traumatic craniocerebral injuries.

Since the majority of traumatic vascular injuries associated with head injury are not suspected prior to imaging, a high index of suspicion and a firm concept of the pathophysiology and presenting symptoms of vascular insufficiency associated with head trauma are needed. Our reliance on CT for the initial evaluation of patients with head injuries may potentially decrease the number of occult vascular injuries identified. At our medical center, the number of cerebral angiographic examinations in patients with traumatic head injuries has decreased from approximately 900 per year to just over 100 per year since CT scanning has been available. The incidence of documented intracranial traumatic aneurysms over that period has fallen proportionally.[113] It is for this reason that MRI is now the imaging modality of choice in the evaluation of these patients for traumatic cerebrovascular injuries. While angiography remains the ''gold-standard'' for documenting the vast majority of traumatic vascular lesions, the technologic progression with regard to the sensitivity of MRI should result in its becoming the imaging modality of choice in the future diagnosis of these injuries.

In this chapter we will discuss a number of cerebrovascular lesions known to occur in association with head trauma. Although the list will by no means be exhaustive, a discussion of the presenting symptoms and signs, natural history, radiographic evaluation, pathology, and management may serve to emphasize the importance of early diagnosis and a high index of suspicion in the prevention of the ''stroke after head injury'' syndrome.

Extracranial Traumatic Arterial Lesions

Injury to the extracranial carotid and vertebral arteries is uncommon but certainly by no means rare. Other injuries have also been reported to result in neurological compromise including injuries to the subclavian artery[56] and superficial temporal artery.[264] A thorough physical exam and consideration of the etiology of the injury will usually result in the diagnosis of such injuries. For example, a 15-year-old boy presented with left visual loss and a left upper extremity monoparesis which resolved within 15 min. His neurological examination on admission was normal. The right arm radial pulse was weak and the blood pressures of the right and left arms were significantly different. Doppler sonography and subsequent angiography documented a right subclavian artery aneurysm containing several clots.[56]

More than 90 percent of the major arterial trauma in the neck is caused by penetrating wounds, especially from firearms.[190,282,291] Historically, our knowledge of the management of extracranial cerebrovascular injuries has come from reports of military actions in which the majority of injuries were penetrating. With the current and progressive increase in penetrating injuries suffered by civilian populations, we have accumulated a more thorough understanding of these injuries in both populations.

In the setting of civilian head trauma, nonpenetrating traumatic lesions of the extracranial cerebral vasculature provide the most difficult diagnostic and management problems. We will discuss these in this chapter.

Carotid Arterial Injuries

The incidence of extracranial carotid artery injuries in association with head trauma is generally unknown. In one series of 2000 head injuries, the carotid artery was found to be injured in 0.5 percent.[89] When one considers that more than 1.5 million head injuries occur in the United States each year, the problem assumes greater magnitude. The mortality rate for a traumatic lesion of the carotid artery in the neck is between 20 and 40 percent.[145,180,266,345,365] This combined with the fact that the incidence of neurological deficit can be up to 80 percent in those who survive further underscores the importance of this entity.[291]

Because of the relatively low incidence of carotid artery injuries, a typical patient profile is difficult to construct. The majority of cases are subjects of isolated case presentations in the literature. Yamada et al., in a review of the literature, put together a series of 52 cases of blunt trauma to the carotid artery.[365] They found that 75 percent of the patients had some history of head injury prior to their presentation, 23 percent of which were severe. An important feature of this study was the fact that there was a significant delay in recognizing the vascular injury in 94 percent of the cases. A number of clinical features peculiar to traumatic lesions of the carotid artery may explain the reasons for this delay.

Following an injury that results in disruption of the arterial intima, subsequent hemodynamic and thrombogenic events will determine the ultimate pathologic injury. The fractured intima initially serves as a substrate for platelet deposition and thrombus formation. As this process proceeds, several different sequelae may occur. A concomitant mural hematoma may constrict the vessel lumen and predispose it to complete thrombosis; an ischemic infarction of the brain is the usual result. Prior to, or in the absence of, complete vessel occlusion, distal embolization of fragments from the growing thrombus may occur causing transient ischemic attacks (TIAs), seizures, or cerebral infarction.

The most important symptoms of carotid arterial injury are those of cerebral ischemia. Following a traumatic incident, the patient may develop a hemiparesis or a hemisensory deficit with or without associated hemianopsia, suggesting ischemia in the internal carotid territory.[253] Symptoms may be fleeting, as in TIAs, or more prolonged in their presentation, as in reversible ischemic neurological deficit (RIND). With severe ischemia, the neurological deficit worsens and eventually becomes permanent. Also, the level of consciousness may be affected, but frequently the neurological deficit is disproportional to any reduction in the level of consciousness, in contradistinction to what would be expected solely as a result of the head injury.

Several factors may have a negative impact on the examiner's index of suspicion of an associated extracranial traumatic arterial lesion. Less than half of the patients in the series of Yamada et al. showed any sign of injury to the neck.[365] Those who did had only a bruise on the neck or at most an abrasion on the neck or forehead. Second, symptoms and signs of carotid territory insufficiency were delayed in their appearance. Less than 10 percent of the patients developed ischemic symptoms within 1 h of the time of the injury. Half of the patients remained asymptomatic for up to 10 h. Indeed, 17 percent of their cases were still asymptomatic with respect to the arterial injury at 24 h following the injury. The presence of associated injuries, especially traumatic brain injuries, can mask symptoms related to the arterial trauma. This scenario is especially true in those cases where severe head injury accompanies the vascular lesions.

Other physical findings may herald the presence of an associated carotid injury in the setting of a traumatic brain injury. A number of patients will manifest a Horner's syndrome caused by injury to the sympathetic nerves surrounding the internal carotid artery. Also, the presence of a carotid bruit due to turbulence at the site of an unsuspected injury should cause one to further consider the possibility of an internal carotid lesion. The association of a fractured mandible with that of traumatic carotid injury has been underscored by a number of authors.[25,160,330] Although the mechanism is unclear, the presence of facial fractures, especially a mandible fracture, should alert one to the possibility of an underlying carotid injury.[25,327,332,341]

Delayed visual loss following head trauma as a result of indirect trauma to the internal carotid artery has also been reported.[356] Visual loss occurred from 1 day to 13 years after the initial injury and was related to the formation of either an aneurysm or pseudoaneurysm or a carotid-cavernous fistula. The diagnosis in all patients was established by CT, MRI, and angiography. Different pathophysiologic mechanisms could be correlated with the delayed visual loss produced by the two types of lesions. The pathologic changes included direct compression of optic nerves and/or chiasm and intracranial hematoma formation. The delayed onset of decreased vision following head trauma should alert the physician to the possibility of a traumatic aneurysm/pseudoaneurysm or a carotid-cavernous fistula. Neurosurgical or interventional neuroradiologic procedures resulted in significant visual improvement in five of six patients. In a recent series of 133 patients with penetrating cerebrovascular injuries, the frequency of preoperative neurological deficit was 20 percent (27 patients). Neurological deficits were related to injuries of the common carotid (29 percent) and internal carotid (15 percent) artery most frequently.[284]

Successful management of trauma-induced extracranial carotid lesions will be influenced by three major factors: (1) the type of injury as depicted by carotid angiography, (2) the location of the injury along the course of the internal carotid artery, and (3) the preexisting severity of the neurological deficit. The rapidity with which the diagnosis is made will influence two of these factors, namely the type of angiographic injury (stenosis vs. occlusion), and the amount of neurological deficit. Therefore, the key to successful management of these injuries is early diagnosis. Richardson et al. reviewed a series of 133 patients with penetrating cerebrovascular injuries. Carotid repair was performed in nine patients with a preoperative deficit limited to weakness or paralysis with improvement in seven patients but no change in two. Four patients improved and four patients worsened or died following carotid repair in patients with preoperative obtundation. Carotid ligation resulted in improvement in one patient, no change in one patient, and worsening or death in three patients.[284]

Carotid Dissection

While many cases of carotid dissection occur in association with cervical trauma, they can also occur in association with underlying vasculopathy, mild head trauma, or spontaneously without any history of trauma. Dissections can be bilateral[119,214] or associated with dissection of the vertebral artery. Dissections occur equally in males and females and predominantly in the young or middle-aged. The dissection is thought to result from bleeding into the arterial wall. As in thrombosis, the critical element is disruption of the intima. The rapid pulsatile blood column further elevates the intima and subintimal layers, occasionally over long stretches of the vessel. This may proceed up to the carotid canal at the base of the skull. A long segment of severe stenosis may result in restriction of flow or serve as the site for the origination of cerebral emboli.[29,331]

The cervical portion of the carotid artery can be injured in association with head trauma in several ways. The most common mechanism is direct blunt trauma to the neck. Among the cervical cephalic arteries, the extracranial segment of the internal carotid artery is the vessel most commonly involved; intracranial carotid dissections are much rarer.[214] In this situation, the internal carotid artery just above the bifurcation seems to be the most vulnerable in the section of the artery adjacent to the C1 and C2 vertebrae. It is theorized that the artery is rapidly compressed against the vertebral column, resulting in injury to the medial or to the intima. As mentioned, mandibular fractures may in some way be responsible for injuring the internal carotid artery above the bifurcation. A fracture fragment or bony spicule may compress the artery, causing disruption of one or more layers of the arterial wall. More likely, the fracture simply identifies the patient most likely to have arterial trauma, much like a first rib fracture suggests a major injury to branches of the aortic arch.[283,330]

The internal carotid artery in its cervical portion can also be injured by stretching.[25] Boldrey et al. directed attention to this particular mechanism of injury.[36] Because the carotid is firmly rooted in the carotid canal at the base of the skull, a blow to the head or face that results in hyperextension and rotation can pull the internal carotid artery tightly against the lateral mass of either the C1 or C2 vertebra. Subsequent stretching or compression of the artery against the bony prominence causes intimal disruption and possibly hematoma formation in the media. This mechanism has been invoked to explain injuries that result in internal carotid artery dissections in the upper cervical portion. A number of young patients with high internal carotid dissections have been reported, suggesting that older people with more redundant elongated arteries may somehow be protected from this type of injury.[25,29,199,327]

Clinical Manifestations

The clinical manifestations resulting from dissections can range from an isolated headache to stroke. Most commonly, the patients present with localized findings including head or neck pain, Horner's syndrome, pulsatile tinnitus, or lower cranial nerves palsy. Neurological compromise following these injuries can also be gradual in presentation. A recent study reported a patient who, 16 h after a closed head injury, developed an alteration in his level of consciousness and infarction of the left hemisphere followed by death 4 days postinjury. Autopsy demonstrated multiple dissections of the inner wall of the left internal carotid artery and the left middle cerebral artery. Thus, a small temporarily sealed tear of the extracranial vessel resulted in a large intramural hemorrhage between the media and adventitia with associated compression of the lumen.[218]

Another study described five patients with carotid dissection following blunt injury and delayed clinical presentation (from 2 weeks to 6 months). Cerebrovascular symptoms developed in four patients while a fifth suffered loss of vision as a result of a giant intracranial dissecting aneurysm. Arteriography demonstrated a "string sign" in two patients and a cervical carotid aneurysm in three. Two of the latter also had siphon occlusion, and one had a superimposed supraclinoid dissection aneurysm.[273]

The delay following the traumatic event (nonpenetrating) until the documentation of a carotid dissection is 0 to 1 h in 10 percent, 1 to 24 h in 73 percent, and after 24 h in 17 percent.[357] Specific guidelines for the treatment of traumatic carotid dissection are still a matter of anecdote because the natural history of this entity has not been defined. Although a number of these cases have presented with neurological deficits presumably due to emboli, some have remained asymptomatic during follow-up. New and Momose[246] and Sullivan et al.[330] have reported cases in which the dissection has eventually resolved completely; however, other cases have been documented to result in pseudoaneurysm formation, complete thrombosis, or further embolization.[25,246,330]

Radiologic Evaluation

Angiography has long been considered the gold standard for the diagnosis of dissections. An irregular narrowing of the contrast column over several centimeters is the typical angiographic picture indicative of these injuries. An intramural hematoma may almost totally occlude the artery, and thrombus formation may be apparent. The artery usually assumes its normal caliber in the region of the carotid canal at the base of the skull. Branch occlusions or evidence of distal emboli may be seen in the intracranial vasculature. An intimal flap along the cervical segment of the internal carotid artery is another important angiographic sign of dissection (Fig. 279-1). Given the invasive nature of angiography and its inherent risks, noninvasive diagnostic approaches [including MRI, single photon emission computed tomography (SPECT), and transcranial Doppler sonography] are being used more frequently.[214,288] Currently, extracranial and transcranial ultrasound findings can suggest the presence of dissecting injuries subsequently substantiated by intra-arterial digital subtraction angiography.[240]

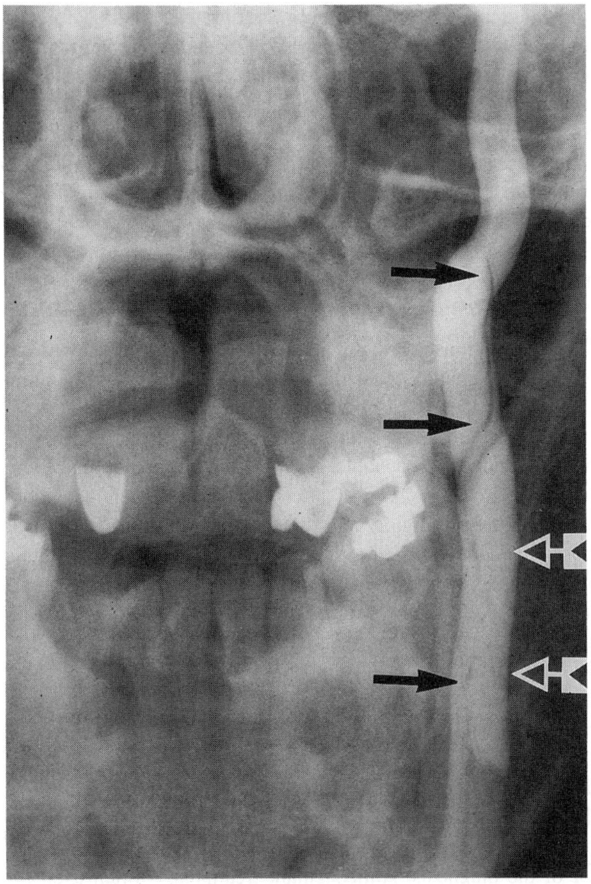

Figure 279-1 Traumatic dissection of the internal carotid artery. This angiogram demonstrates a long intimal flap (*arrows*) and false lumen (*crossed arrows*). Despite adequate anticoagulant therapy, the patient continued to have TIAs. The involved internal carotid artery was successfully trapped by detachable balloons. (Courtesy of Dr. Mehringer, Harbor General Hospital, Los Angeles, CA.)

In a recent retrospective correlation of MRI and angiography in nine patients with cervical dissections, MRI documented vascular abnormalities in eight patients, seven of whom had dissections. One MRI false negative was reported.[329] In this and a number of other studies, MRI was able to demonstrate the presence of an intramural hematoma and false lumen in the dissected artery. MRI demonstration of mural hematomas is specific for the diagnosis and follow-up of dissections.[183,200,273,373] These techniques also have been used for serial follow-up examinations.

MRI findings suggestive of dissection include (1) increased signal from the entire vessel; (2) increased periluminal signal; (3) luminal narrowing; (4) decreased or absent visualization of the vessel; and (5) vessel compromise resulting from adjacent tissue with an abnormal, increased signal.[329] While the combined use of extra- and transcranial Doppler and duplex sonography can increase the diagnostic yield in the evaluation of these patients, there

To date, only 16 dissecting injuries of the vertebral artery have been reported.[196] Dissecting aneurysms of the vertebral artery have also been described.[147,235,312,318] In addition, injury to the subclavian artery with aneurysm formation and thrombosis has been reported. In one case, the aneurysm was surgically removed and the right vertebral artery reimplanted.[56]

Meiser et al. have reported that the liberal use of four-vessel angiography in patients suspected of having major vascular injury in the neck will increase the yield in documenting vertebral artery injuries.[227] Therefore, a discussion of the circumstances surrounding vertebral artery trauma as well as the related symptoms and signs is in order.

Symptoms and Signs

Most patients with vertebral artery injuries associated with head and neck trauma will present with the delayed onset of symptoms and signs of brain stem or cerebellar ischemia. Vertigo, blurred vision, ataxia, and dysarthria are common. In the setting of cervical vertebral artery trauma, neck ache, suboccipital pain, and headache are also frequent concomitants. The classical Wallenberg syndrome as a result of trauma to the vertebral artery is also known to occur following minor head and neck injury.[51,80,104,195] This results in Horner's syndrome plus decreased sensation to pain and temperature on the ipsilateral face and contralateral arm and leg, and ipsilateral ataxia. These symptoms may follow any traumatic incident that causes acute hyperextension or rotation of the cervical spine. Frequently the head injury is minor, and usually the patient will be unable to recall a period of unconsciousness. Neurological symptoms may be delayed as long as a month after the trauma but usually occur within 24 h. In some cases associated neck movements serve to exacerbate the symptoms of ischemia.[321] This situation should alert the treating physician to a potential vertebral artery injury.

Schneider and Schemm brought to our attention the occurrence of spinal cord ischemia from vertebral arterial insufficiency due to cervical trauma.[305] They theorized that traumatic vertebral artery occlusion may compromise blood flow to the anterior spinal artery, producing ischemia to the cervical portion of the spinal cord. The manifestations would include a typical central cord lesion with disproportionately more motor impairment of the upper than the lower extremities, bladder dysfunction, and varying degrees of sensory loss below the level of the lesion.

Outward signs of trauma to the head or neck may be lacking or may simply exist in the form of bruises or abrasions. Neck pain, as noted in some patients with vertebral artery injuries, may be simply ascribed to bony or ligamentous injury to the spine. Therefore, one must maintain a very high index of suspicion when dealing with patients who have minor head and neck injury.

Mechanism of Injury

Injuries to the extracranial vertebral artery commonly occur in three places: at or below the C6 level, at the atlantoaxial level, and at the atlanto-occipital level. The artery is susceptible to blunt or penetrating injury below or at its entrance into the foramen transversarium at C6. It is here that the artery, relatively free in the base of the neck, becomes fixed to the bony orifice of the foramen. This combined with the fact that the mobility of the cervical spine is greatest at the C6 joint makes the vertebral artery particularly vulnerable to hyperextension injuries. The vessel can be stretched at its entrance into the foramen, causing a mural hemorrhage or possibly an intimal disruption and culminating ultimately in thrombosis or distal embolization. The artery is also susceptible to injuries at the atlantoaxial joint and the atlanto-occipital joint. The spine has its greatest rotational mobility in this region. Stretch injuries are liable to occur during rotation and extension because of the relative fixation of the artery at the atlanto-occipital membrane.[48]

Cadaver studies have shown that the vertebral artery can be occluded or narrowed when the head is rotated toward the opposite side.[340] This may occur even when movement is within physiologic limits. Therefore it is not surprising that traumatically induced extension and rotation injure the vessel. The presence of congenital spinal abnormalities such as congenital subluxations or fusions tends to increase the mobility of the adjacent cervical spinal segments and increases the possibility of stretch injury to the vertebral artery.[321] Patients with these anomalies should be closely scrutinized for any delayed symptoms of cerebrovascular insufficiency.

Injuries to the cervical vertebral arteries most commonly result in thrombosis. However, intimal disruption, dissection, aneurysm formation, and fistula formation are also known to occur (Fig. 279-3). Ischemia usually results from distal embolization but also may result from flow-restrictive lesions in dominant vertebral arteries.

Treatment

Little has been written about the management of acute vertebral artery injury because the diagnosis is frequently delayed or

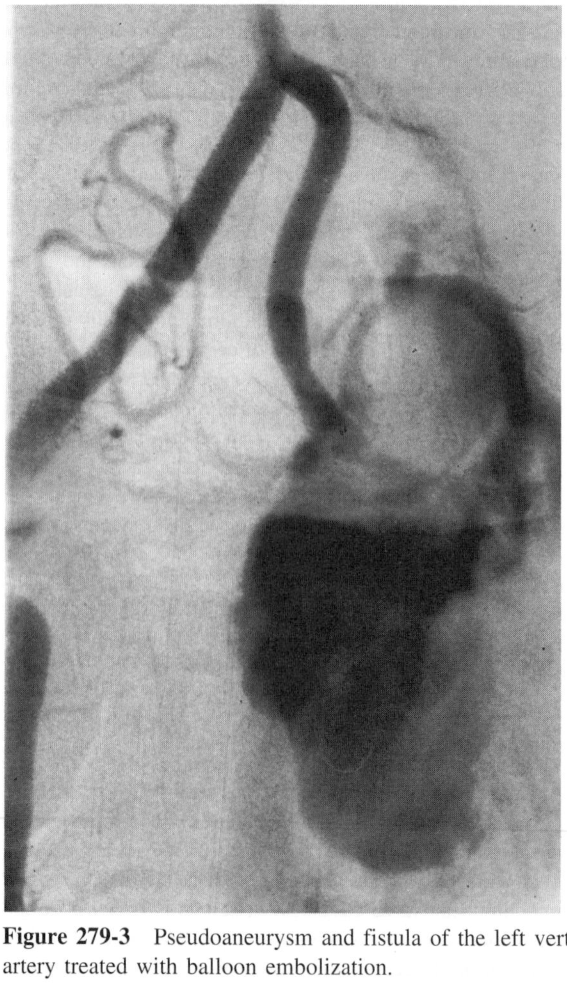

Figure 279-3 Pseudoaneurysm and fistula of the left vertebral artery treated with balloon embolization.

is only made at the time of autopsy. Scrutiny of the few cases that exist in the literature suggests that it is not unusual for a lucid interval to occur before episodes of vertebrobasilar ischemia. Thus a high index of suspicion and early and liberal use of angiography in suspected arterial lesions might provide for management alternatives.

As with carotid arterial injuries, treatment will depend on the location and nature of the lesion as well as any existing neurological deficit. Total occlusion of the vertebral artery may not lead to ischemic symptoms because of a patent vertebral artery on the other side. In this instance no further therapy is warranted. In those cases where vertebral thrombosis results in significant neurological symptoms, attempts at thrombus removal or thromboendarterectomy of the vertebral artery have usually been unsuccessful.[321] Supportive therapy with a trial of increased intravascular volume or mild hypertension may obviate some of the ischemic manifestations. Other injuries, including traumatic narrowing, dissection, and mural hemorrhage with pseudoaneurysm formation, are potential sources for distal embolization. In documented cases of embolization with mild or transient neurological deficits, anticoagulation with heparin is recommended with consideration given to repair of the vessel.

As with dissections of the carotid artery, medical therapy with anticoagulants should be initiated immediately and continued for up to 6 months. Evidence of progression of a lesion on serial angiography or the persistence of symptoms despite medical treatment are indications for surgery. Surgical intervention is based on proximal clip ligation of the vertebral artery if the contralateral vertebral is not hypoplastic or absent.[106,318,364] Trapping or trapping with resection of the vessel is rarely necessary.

If angiography documents that the injured vessel is the dominant vertebral, reconstruction or repair using suitable graft material or, more likely, ligation or balloon occlusion with concomitant EC-IC bypass grafting might be contemplated. In a situation where the nondominant vertebral artery is injured and is considered to be nonrepairable, a successful trial of balloon occlusion under local anesthesia may be followed by permanent occlusion. In the presence of a major cerebral infarction, revascularization or anticoagulation should only be attempted as a last resort.

In those patients in whom cervical subluxation or cervical spondylosis has caused or exacerbated vertebral arterial stenosis, decompression or fusion may be all that is necessary to avoid further trauma to the artery and obviate further ischemic episodes.[321] Follow-up angiography is strongly recommended in vertebral dissection and traumatic aneurysm formation. Evidence of increasing stenosis or enlargement of the aneurysm in those patients initially treated with conservative measures should prompt surgical intervention to avoid the potential for emboli or vertebrobasilar ischemia.

Halbach et al. recently reported on a series of 16 patients with dissecting aneurysms or pseudoaneurysms of the vertebral artery who underwent endovascular occlusion. They concluded that symptomatic vertebral artery dissections involving the intradural and extradural segments can be managed effectively by endovascular techniques.[125]

Intracranial Vascular Injuries

Disruption of intracranial vasculature is the rule rather than the exception with severe head injury. Subarachnoid hemorrhage due to loss of integrity of small pial vessels can be documented in most fatal brain injuries. However, documentation of traumatic lesions to major branches of the circle of Willis or to dural venous sinuses is relatively uncommon in blunt head trauma. In a series of over 2000 head injuries from Scandinavia, injury to a major intracranial vessel as proved by angiography or at autopsy occurred in just over 3 percent of the cases.[89] A report from Canada surveyed 431 industrial head injuries; nine cases were found that demonstrated evidence of trauma-induced cerebral arterial occlusion.[35] A review of these types of injuries with discussion of presenting symptoms, mechanisms, and outcome should help emphasize the difficulty in identifying and treating these patients.

Occlusion

The most common intracranial arterial structure to be occluded in blunt head injury is the internal carotid artery. Although the majority of injuries to the internal carotid occur in its cervical portion, injury at the base of the skull, within the carotid canal, or at its cavernous segment has been reported with some regularity.[3,7,52,178,222,368] Injuries to the carotid artery at the skull base occur usually in the setting of major head trauma. The patient is typically admitted comatose following an auto accident. Within 24 h the neurological condition deteriorates further, during which time evidence of a hemiparesis may emerge. In slightly less than one-third of intracranial carotid injuries, head trauma may be relatively mild.[3,368] In this situation the clinical syndrome mimics that of traumatically induced carotid occlusion in the neck.[179]

Mechanism of Injury

Several important mechanisms are thought to be responsible for intracranial carotid thrombosis secondary to head trauma. Autopsies frequently demonstrate a fracture at the base of the skull that narrows the carotid canal. Fracture fragments may compress the vessel, causing irreversible injury and subsequent thrombosis. Pathologic examination may reveal an intimal dissection, mural hematoma, aneurysm formation, or total disruption. In the absence of a fracture, stretching or torsion of the carotid artery as it exists from the carotid canal or the cavernous sinus is thought to be another cause of occlusion. Differential motion between the brain and skull during acute acceleration and deceleration can injure the arterial wall, setting in motion the thrombotic process. An equally important mechanism for intracranial thrombosis of the carotid artery involves emboli originating more proximally in the vessel secondary to an arterial injury in the neck. In a small number of cases, usually older individuals, traumatic disruption of atherosclerotic plaques may also cause distal embolization and possibly internal carotid occlusion.[29,143,214]

Radiologic Findings

Angiographically, an abrupt, usually smooth obstruction or stenosis is noted near the skull base. Frequently the occlusion will propagate to the next patent branch, namely the ophthalmic artery. Occlusion may, however, extend to the internal carotid bifurcation, resulting in cerebral infarction. Evidence of distal embolization including the absence of small branches of the middle cerebral artery or intraluminal filling defects may also be appreciated.[3,368]

Management and Outcome

Eighty-five percent of patients with traumatic internal carotid artery occlusion at the base of the skull or intracranially can be expected to die or suffer a severe neurological deficit.[3,216,368] The severity of head injury also governs the outcome. Aarabi and McQueen, reviewing reports of 21 cases, found that of 15 patients who suffered major brain trauma, 12 died.[3] There was only one death among the six patients who suffered minor head trauma. Management of intracranial thrombosis of the internal carotid artery remains a frustrating exercise. In those patients who have suffered a major ischemic neurological deficit, steroid administration and attempts to control the intracranial pressure may be of some potential benefit. Barbiturate-induced coma has also been utilized in this setting with unspectacular results. Acute revascularization also seems an unlikely adjunct to the management of these cases since the diagnosis is usually delayed and cerebral infarction has already occurred. In those few instances where emboli are found to occur in the absence of a major infarction, anticoagulation may be attempted in order to obviate further neurological deficit.

Occlusion of the Middle Cerebral Artery

Occlusion of other major intracranial vessels has also been documented subsequent to head trauma. Evidence of injury to cerebral cortical branches may be seen, especially in relation to calvarial fractures. Findings may include branch occlusion, segmental narrowing, traumatic aneurysm formation, or slow flow in the cortical surface veins. A sharp angulation of a damaged cortical branch (Z deformity) suggests entrapment of the vessel within the fracture line.[292]

Dujovny et al. catalogued eight cases of traumatically induced middle cerebral artery thrombosis.[82] Five were caused by motor vehicle accidents, and the remaining three were caused by falls. Five of their patients demonstrated a lucid interval, which varied from 9 to 15 days. Either after the lucid interval or from the outset of the traumatic event, a contralateral hemiparesis or hemiplegia occurred. Four patients also demonstrated a homonymous hemianopsia. No obvious injury to the head was present on physical examination, and x-ray films of the skull revealed a linear skull fracture in only two patients. All of the patients had occlusion of the middle cerebral artery at its origin from the internal carotid bifurcation. One patient in their series died, and although the remainder suffered severe cerebral infarctions, four eventually became ambulatory. This report is in sharp distinction to others that suggest a 38 percent mortality rate for traumatically induced middle cerebral artery thrombosis.[143,155,202,287]

The mechanisms of middle cerebral artery thrombosis secondary to trauma are incompletely explained. The middle cerebral artery may become occluded indirectly secondary to injury to the internal carotid artery. In a report of three cases and a review of the literature, Hollin and colleagues suggested that one-third of the cases of traumatic middle cerebral artery occlusion were caused by emboli from injury to the internal carotid.[143] Alternatively, the middle cerebral artery may be compressed by extra- or intracerebral hematomas. A more likely mechanism for thrombosis of the middle cerebral artery is stretching due to acceleration or deceleration of the brain resulting from blunt head trauma. Others have theorized that the artery may directly impact against the sphenoid bone causing intimal dissection or a mural hematoma resulting in eventual occlusion.[202]

The management of traumatically induced middle cerebral occlusion remains empirical and supportive only. In the majority of those patients who survive and have follow-up angiography, the middle cerebral artery is again patent.[202]

Occlusion of the Basilar Artery

Basilar artery occlusion has also been noted secondary to head trauma.[307,320] These patients invariably present with ischemic brain stem symptoms, and most do not survive. Basilar artery occlusion or stenosis can often be inferred from a carotid arteriogram that shows filling of the distal basilar artery through a posterior communicating artery. This observation should prompt complete examination of the vertebrobasilar circulation. Frequently, the basilar artery may be occluded due to associated injury to one or both vertebral arteries, which then acts as a source of emboli. Basilar occlusion may also be related to a fracture at the base of the skull across the clivus, which in some instances may serve to trap the artery within the fracture.[320] The majority of cases of basilar artery occlusion are documented at the time of autopsy; thus, no satisfactory treatment regimen has yet evolved.

Traumatic Aneurysms

Trauma has been implicated as a significant factor in the genesis of less than 1 percent of intracranial aneurysms.[27,101,326,369,371] The proportion of traumatic intracranial aneurysms (TICAs) that are "true" as opposed to "false" has not been determined.[45,229,370] None of the intracranial aneurysms catalogued in the Cooperative Aneurysm Study was of traumatic origin.

From the first report of a traumatic infraclinoid carotid artery aneurysm by Guibert in 1895, close to 435 cases with traumatic aneurysms have been reported in the world literature.[1,2,4,5, 8–16, 18, 20, 21, 23, 26–28, 30–33, 37–42, 44–47, 49, 50, 53, 54, 57–59, 61–63, 65–68, 71, 72, 74–79, 83, 84, 87, 90–94, 97, 99–103, 106–111, 114, 115, 120–123, 131–138, 140–142, 144, 149–154, 156–159, 161–168, 171, 172, 174, 175, 178, 181, 184, 185, 187–189, 191, 192, 194, 198, 201, 203–206, 208–210, 213, 215, 217, 219, 221, 223–226, 228–231, 233, 234, 236–243, 245, 247, 250–252, 254–256, 258, 259, 261–263, 265, 267–269, 271, 272, 275–280, 286, 290, 293–299, 301–304, 308, 310, 311, 313–317, 319, 322–324, 326, 333–337, 339, 342–344, 346, 350–356,360,363,366–372] Two hundred and seventy-five (63 percent) of these aneurysms resulted from closed head injuries and 126 (29 percent) from penetrating head injuries. Thirty-four (8 percent) were iatrogenic (following craniotomy, trans-sphenoidal hypophysectomy, or ENT procedures).

They occur in 2 to 8 percent of projectile injuries (shell and missile fragments), if an angiogram is performed on an average of 20 days after injury.[1,2,5,135,276] There is a sharp increase in the incidence, however, if diagnostic studies are performed within 48 h of hospitalization.[161] Often, the initial angiogram may be normal.[1,2,49,153,236,295,324] Our own experience consists of 36 patients who presented with traumatic aneurysms following closed or penetrating head injury from 1967 until the advent of CT in 1976. We also reviewed a series of 16 patients who presented with traumatic aneurysms following closed or penetrating head injury from 1977 until 1985. Of these 52 patients, 10 had traumatic aneurysms that resulted from penetrating injuries.[349]

Traumatic aneurysms can occur at the level of major skull base arteries,[1,2,49,66,77,153,208,236,267,295,298,301,303] or arterial bifurcations[2,81] and at times are seen distant from the missile track.[2] These aneurysms have also been found to enlarge over time,[1,2,20,78,122,153,295,298,301] spontaneously rupture, or heal.[1,2] It is important to remember that traumatic aneurysms can occur following projectile (tangential) injuries without violation of dura or skull.[2]

Location

Most traumatic cerebral aneurysms are located on branches of the middle cerebral artery. The next most common site is the internal carotid artery as it enters the skull. The pericallosal artery is another important site for the occurrence of traumatically induced aneurysms (most likely because of its proximity to the falx). The internal carotid artery is primarily involved following closed head injuries whereas the middle cerebral artery is involved following penetrating injuries. The anterior cerebral, ophthalmic, basilar, vertebral, superior cerebellar, and anterior inferior cerebellar arteries are also involved, though less often.

Etiology

Theories regarding the mechanism of traumatic cerebral aneurysm formation abound. Blunt trauma can produce the vascular injury as a result of differential velocity of the brain and skull. The brain and its vessels impact against bony or connective tissue protuberances such as the falx, tentorium, or sphenoid wing. Traction injuries thought to be due to adhesions between cortical vessels and the underlying dura as described by Drake are also believed to be operative in producing traumatic tears of cortical arteries with subsequent aneurysm formation.[81] Trapping of the cortical vessel in a fracture site has also been reported as a mechanism for traumatic cerebral aneurysm formation.[292]

Angiography

Angiographic hallmarks of traumatic aneurysms include delayed filling and emptying of the aneurysm, irregular contour, and the absence of a neck. A peripheral location, other than at a branching point, will also help distinguish the traumatically induced aneurysm from the congenital or atherosclerotic form.

With the obvious and highly important exception of risk, MRA still has not replaced catheter angiography in the evaluation of patients with potentially ruptured intracranial aneurysms, traumatic or otherwise. Currently, MRA has a true-positive diagnostic rate of 86 percent using time-of-flight MRA[306] alone or combined with standard spin-echo imaging rate[116,289] in the diagnosis of spontaneous intracranial aneurysms. No studies detailing the efficacy of MRA in the evaluation of patients with traumatic aneurysms have been published. Recently, a review of 16 patients harboring 27 aneurysms failed to replicate this detection rate.[148] The true-positive diagnostic rate reported was 26 percent for T1-weighted MRI, 48 percent for T2-weighted MRI, 56 percent for time-of-flight MRA, and 44 percent for phase-contrast MRA.

Despite the technologic advances that have resulted in a high level of sensitivity in the detection of aneurysms, certain inherent technical limitations remain that need to be circumvented before MRA can serve as the definitive diagnostic modality for the assessment of traumatic aneurysms.[289] While the false-positive rate among control subjects remains negligible, the documentation of aneurysms smaller than 5 mm remains adequate at best.[289] In addition, certain information is required in the evaluation of patients with traumatic aneurysms, namely, the actual presence of an aneurysm; the determination of rupture; the location and configuration of the aneurysm; the presence of arteriovenous associated sister aneurysms or malformations (AVMs); and the presence of atherosclerotic changes in the proximal vessels.[361] Currently, MRA cannot sufficiently answer all of these questions but it can contribute on a secondary level.

In conclusion, MRI and MRA remain valuable screening techniques in the evaluation of patients who may harbor traumatic aneurysms. A combination of these studies is required in addition to the evaluation of the individual MRA partitions and the "cine" loop in order to maximize the diagnostic yield of these lesions. At the present time, MRA cannot be relied on to detect all vascular lesions. Thus, in patients with a high probability of a traumatic vascular lesion, catheter angiography remains the procedure of choice. Once a vascular lesion is documented by catheter angiography, MRA may be used as a follow-up modality. In patients with a low clinical suspicion, and particularly in children with a high Glasgow Coma Scale (GCS) score, MRA may be utilized as a noninvasive screening test. With future technologic advances, it is likely that MRA will reach a high level of sensitivity in the detection of aneurysms and replace catheter angiography as the diagnostic modality of choice.

Following Closed and Penetrating Head Trauma

Blunt head trauma is responsible for the majority of these lesions; up to 40 percent may be seen in the absence of a fracture on skull films.[45] In aneurysms resulting from penetrating injuries, 70 of 126 were secondary to gunshot wounds whereas 56 were secondary to low-velocity (mainly knife) injuries. The majority of the reported traumatic aneurysms due to projectile injuries are caused by schrapnel,[1,2,122,153,276,277] shotgun pellets,[6,16,23,66,278,295,324] or missile fragments of low caliber or energy.[6,122,161,268,295,298] The proximity of the missile track to the location of the aneurysm, in the majority of the cases, indicates that direct contact of the missile, schrapnel, or secondary bone fragments with the vessel is required for aneurysm formation.[6,276] This could result in a partial laceration of the related artery or the avulsion of a perforating branch, or produce enough shearing force to cause a rent in the arterial wall.[1,2,78,122]

The reported pathologic studies on the excised aneurysmal wall indicate that all traumatic aneurysms due to projectile injuries are indeed false.[1,2,6,66,97,122,276,295] There is a clear tendency for the penetrating fragments around the face or pterion to damage basal or cortical arteries. Close to 65 percent of the aneurysms reported in the literature have had facio-orbito-craniocerebral (35.5 percent), frontal (18.8 percent), or pterional injury (10 percent).[2,6,20,66,77,78,97,122,153,165,208,233,267,276,277,295,298,304,324]

Most traumatic aneurysms will manifest themselves within 2 to 3 weeks following penetrating missile injuries. The initial positive angiogram in 41 patients reported in the literature was noted after a mean of 20 days following their injury (S.D. = 13 days).[1,2,6,20,49,66,78,153,161,208,236,267,278,295,324] Symptomatic aneurysmal rupture can be varied in presentation following these injuries. Courville presented the case of a patient who bled 10 years after shotgun wound to the head.[66] Careful attention to the neurodiagnostic examination in addition to the recognition and consideration of certain variables should allow for the rapid recognition of a traumatic aneurysm. Only with rapid diagnosis can one exclude these arterial injuries from the cerebral circulation in due time before rupture occurs.[1,2]

Principles of Diagnosis

Parkinson and West collected five cases of traumatically induced intracranial aneurysm, adding to them six cases of traumatically induced fistula, and emphasized the fact that since angiography has been replaced by CT scanning in the evaluation of head injuries, these aneurysms are even more likely to escape attention.[259] Over 60 percent of the traumatic aneurysms reported in the literature have been diagnosed by angiography before their overt clinical presentation.[1,2,6,20,78,97,122,161,276,280,295,301,324] Since CT has become the first line of approach in imaging patients with penetrating and closed head injuries, it is all the more significant to perform angiography in patients who are at high risk to develop a traumatic aneurysm. With the technologic progression of neuroimaging we are beginning to determine those variables which may enable us to predict the occurrence of traumatic aneurysms, especially following penetrating injuries, and the associated outcome.[1,2,122] Most important is the development of imaging techniques which will allow for the accurate localization followed by the rapid management of these lesions.[166,194]

Our own experience tends to confirm this. Since 1977, when we began to use the CT scanner in our department, the number of traumatic intracranial aneurysms documented by angiography has dropped dramatically.[113] Our experience with traumatic intracranial aneurysms is based on over 40 cases since 1968. The majority of these were unsuspected and were found in conjunction with angiographic evaluation usually in an unconscious head trauma victim. The most common mode of presentation in symptomatic patients is a delayed subarachnoid hemorrhage (SAH) following a head injury. Typically, a decrease in the level of consciousness to the point of coma heralds the subarachnoid hemorrhage. Further evaluation may reveal nuchal rigidity or complaints of a severe headache. Unless a high index of suspicion is maintained, the symptoms may be ascribed to an intracranial expanding process such as a hematoma or edema or possibly post-traumatic hydrocephalus. Other presenting symptoms include progressive deterioration following head trauma, most likely due to vasospasm following rupture of the aneurysm. Epistaxis or a delayed cranial nerve palsy following trauma may also give evidence of the presence of an internal carotid aneurysm near the skull base. Extracerebral hematomas following trivial head trauma and unexplained arterial bleeding during hematoma removal have all been reported as evidence of traumatically induced cerebral aneurysms.[6,45,101,113,259,292]

In conclusion, with the emphasis placed on CT as the first line of approach in managing missile injuries of the head,[193] it is all the more significant to perform angiography in patients with the following findings: (1) Facio-orbito-pterional injuries; (2) penetrating fragments, especially if they cross the midline or traverse into another dural compartment; and (3) severe subarachnoid hemorrhage, and intracerebral or subdural hematomas.[1,2,122,194] In this regard, facio-orbito-pterional injuries by penetrating fragments which have caused intracranial hemorrhage are highly suspicious. Intracranial hematomas, either at the time of admission or occurring in the hospital course, are significant.[2,6,66,122,166,276,308] A small number of the aneurysms could present with epistaxis if they involve the infraclinoid portion of the internal carotid artery,[77,130,153,208,236,267,295,303] or present with progressive neurological compromise associated with mass effect.[49,277,298]

Treatment

A review of the literature shows that in those cases where no immediate surgical treatment was rendered, 40 percent of the aneurysms bled at some point after the diagnosis was made. Further, 21 percent were found to enlarge with follow-up cerebral angiography. This often occurred within 3 weeks of the trauma. A small number of aneurysms were noted to become either smaller or totally thrombosed on follow-up angiography.[6,45,101,113] As with other types of intracranial aneurysm, management is directed toward avoiding recurrent hemorrhage.[105] Fleischer et al. reported increased survival rates in those patients treated surgically.[101] Unfortunately, the amount of underlying brain injury may negatively affect the outcome in selected cases. Operative mortality is now around 16 percent. Conservative therapy in these lesions has produced a mortality of 41 percent.[113]

A plethora of surgical procedures have been applied to the treatment of projectile-induced traumatic aneurysms. In a few cases, clip application alone has been successful.[78] Most often simple excision with or without an arterial bypass graft seems to be the procedure of choice.[1,2,122,276] Other approaches include clipping the parent artery with or without an arterial bypass.[1,2,6,20,97,287] Wrapping, cauterizing, or the endovascular introduction of thrombogenic wire inside the aneurysmal sac has also been tried.[77,91,165] Trapping has been widely used for carotid artery aneurysms.[1,49,97,153,236,267] Intraluminal occlusion of traumatic aneurysms at the base of skull with preservation of carotid flow has been tried in nonmissile traumatic aneurysms and is the treatment of choice if preoperative angiographic studies reveal insufficient cross-flow from the opposite hemisphere.[139,226,313] In selected patients a direct approach to the cavernous sinus has been tried with variable success.[79,346]

Arteriovenous Fistulas

Arteriovenous fistulas secondary to head injury are not rare lesions. The most dramatic and therefore most well recognized is the carotid-cavernous sinus fistula[178] which occurs in 0.2 percent of patients. This lesion is discussed in more detail in another section of this text and will only be reviewed briefly here.

Carotid-cavernous fistulas are classified as direct or indirect. Indirect fistulas are located within the dural leaves surrounding the cavernous sinus whereas direct fistulas involve a direct connection between the internal carotid artery and cavernous sinus and are usually traumatic in origin. Direct fistulas most often result from injuries involving the sphenoid bone[124,196] and are more common in males. Indirect fistulas can also be traumatic in origin following injuries to the intracavernous branches of the internal carotid artery.[257] The clinical presentation of carotid-cavernous fistulas is based on venous drainage.[17,186,211] Clinical signs include headache, progressive proptosis, chemosis, orbital bruits, progressive ophthalmoplegia, and visual loss. Visual loss is usually related to ischemia and is usually irreversible if treatment is delayed.[300]

The remainder of traumatic fistulas usually involve dural vessels and are found incidentally at the time of angiography. An arteriovenous fistula fed by the middle meningeal artery can be found in 2 percent of head trauma victims.[96,98] Typically a fistulous communication develops between the meningeal artery and the accompanying veins, producing the so-called train track sign. However, fistulas between the meningeal artery and diploic veins may also occur, usually in association with lacerations of the dura. These fistulas are almost always found in association with a fracture line. The fistula itself does not usually cause symptoms over and above those that result from the head injury. Thus they represent more of an arteriographic curiosity than a threat to the well-being of the patient. Spontaneous closure has been reported, but the natural history of these lesions remains unknown.

Traumatic dural AV fistulas usually do not produce symptoms. As with carotid-cavernous fistulas, the clinical presentation is based on the pattern of venous drainage. The few cases in the literature of symptomatic AV fistulas described headache, ophthalmologic complaints, and bruit developing in a delayed fashion from 30 days to 1 year following the head injury.[73,98] In contradistinction, spontaneous dural AV fistulas have been known to present with subarachnoid hemorrhage increased intracranial pressure, progressive neurological deficit, or hydrocephalus.[24,248]

An unusual case of traumatic AV fistula fed by cortical arteries was reported by Feldman et al.[96] Their case was unique in that cortical branches of the middle cerebral artery directly fed branches of the superior sagittal sinus. Eventually the sagittal sinus became completely arterialized and no longer served as a conduit for venous return. Treatment was eventually completed by totally excising the fistula, including most of the superior sagittal sinus.

Indications for the Treatment of Carotid-Cavernous Fistulas

Indications for treatment are based on the natural history of these lesions. Spontaneous thrombosis of indirect fistulas is more common than in direct fistulas though the actual incidence remains unknown.[309] Poor outcome has been found to correlate significantly with epistaxis or cortical venous drainage in a series of 155 patients.[124] The presence of increased intracranial pressure, progressing proptosis, and visual loss were also related to poor outcome. Rapid treatment should be considered in patients with progressive proptosis, visual loss, or ophthalmoplegia.[70,348]

Management of Carotid-Cavernous Fistulas

Embolization of carotid-cavernous fistulas can be accomplished via a transarterial,[69,140,169] or (more recently) a transvenous approach.[126] Transarterial approaches are preferred and allow for the delivery and passage of an embolic substrate via a microcatheter, through the defect in the cavernous carotid into the cavernous sinus. Embolic substrates include detachable balloons, platinum coils, glues, and silk sutures. These substrates can become lodged within the cavernous sinus or stick to the dural walls, resulting in occlusion and avoiding distal loss. The goal of the procedure, occluding the fistula with a balloon or coil while maintaining the patency of the parent artery, is realized in 60 to 88 percent of patients as reported in the larger series of 54 and 234 patients. Complications include the formation of a false aneurysm (44 percent), transient third nerve palsy, and stroke in 2 to 4 percent.[69,140,169]

With the development of steerable microcatheters, transvenous approaches are now being reported.[24,69,126,212] These approaches are usually reserved when transarterial approaches are impossible or have failed. Transvenous approaches allow for the delivery of an embolic substrate via a microcatheter through the draining veins into the cavernous sinus, resulting in occlusion of the fistula.[69,126,140,212,239] As with the transarterial approaches, embolic substrates include platinum coils (most common), detachable balloons, glues, and silk sutures. In a series of 14 patients treated via the transvenous approach, 12 had successful occlusion of the fistula. Complications included rupture of the inferior petrosal sinus and a fatal hemorrhage following diversion of the blood flow to the cortical draining veins.[126]

Indications for the Treatment of Arteriovenous Fistulas

In addition to the symptomatology noted above, indications for intervention include intracranial hemorrhage, progressive neurological deficits, tinnitus, and progressive visual loss. Given the lack of knowledge regarding the natural history of arteriovenous fistulas, it is unclear as to whether treatment is indicated in asymptomatic individuals.

Management of Arteriovenous Fistulas

Early therapeutic interventions based on the proximal ligation of the external carotid feeding vessels often resulted in recurrence of the fistula secondary to the recruitment of collateral vessels. To circumvent such recurrences, direct approaches with attempts at isolating the fistula itself were developed but they were associated with large amounts of blood loss.[182,331] Advances in digital subtraction angiography techniques and catheter design and development of novel embolic agents have resulted in endovascular intervention becoming the primary therapeutic modality. The endovascular approach itself is based on the anatomic location of the fistula. Transfemoral-transarterial approaches are preferred in the treatment of fistulas of the transverse sinus. As noted, transarterial approaches are also preferred in the management of cavernous sinus fistulas although a transvenous approach may be indicated if branches of the internal carotid artery are involved.[128,338,348] In addition, complex fistulas of the transverse sinus, cavernous sinus, or tentorium may require combined surgical and endovascular approaches.[118,129,270] Benefits of combined approaches include preoperative embolization which can significantly decrease the blood loss associated with surgical approaches to these lesions.[22] Given the potential for embolization of the ophthalmic artery, surgery is preferred in the treatment of fistulas in the anterior cranial fossa.[177] Indications for stereotactic radiosurgical ablation of smaller (<2.5 cm) fistulas remains unclear.[55,177]

Transverse, sigmoid, and cavernous sinus fistulas are usually approached using a coaxial microcatheter and microguidewire system via a transfemoral-transarterial route. *N*-butyl-cyanoacrylate (NBCA, Histoacryl; Yocan Medical, Thornhill, Ontario) is the embolic agent of choice for transarterial approaches given its permanent nature and adjustable polymerization period. Polyvinyl alcohol is an attractive alternative given its ability to embolize smaller fistulas, although the incidence of recanalization is higher than with NBCA.[170,249] Embolization of the external carotid feeders is generally sufficient. Patients with intracranial hemorrhage or progressive neurological deficits may require obliteration of the fistula itself. Embolization of cavernous internal carotid artery feeders or transvenous approaches are indicated in the setting of progressive ocular signs.

In fistulas that cannot be approached via a transarterial route (i.e., internal carotid artery) or in which a transarterial approach has failed to result in complete obliteration of the fistula, a transvenous approach is preferred.[127] Methods of cannulating the superior ophthalmic vein or inferior petrosal sinus have been described.[128,338] Finally, technologies used in obliterating carotid-cavernous fistulas such as balloon occlusion or embolization with or without the use of bilateral simultaneous velocity recordings of the middle cerebral arteries with Doppler ultrasonography[244] are also used to obliterate fistulas in other areas.

Vasospasm

Cerebral vasospasm, a common cause of ischemic symptoms following the rupture of a cerebral aneurysm, has also been implicated in the pathophysiology of head injury. Angiographically evident spasm following severe closed head trauma has been reported to range from 5 to 58 percent.[60,95,117,146,197,207,347,358,359]

Suwanwela and Suwanwela reviewed angiograms in a series of 350 patients. Moderate head injury was associated with narrowing of the internal carotid, middle cerebral, or anterior cerebral arteries in 5.1 percent of all patients.[332] Data from human as well as experimental cases suggest that the accumulation of blood in the subarachnoid space is in part responsible for vascular narrowing,[86,197] and spasm angiographically.[222] Vasospasm has been implicated in the pathophysiology of head injury.[88,113,194] Despite these findings there is no satisfactory hypothesis relating angiographic vasospasm and neurological compromise.

Transcranial Doppler ultrasonography has been found to reproducibly document a number of vascular phenomena which can occur following head injury.[325] These include increased intracranial vascular flow resistance due to raised intracranial pressure, hypeaemia due to transient ischemia, decreased perfusion, and increased flow velocities in AV fistulas or vasospasm. Traumatic AV fistulas and injuries to the circle of Willis are manifested by high mean flow velocities with increased end-diastolic flow values.[43] In a study of 86 patients with head injuries with admission GCS scores between 3 and 12, the amount of subarachnoid hemorrhage on the initial CT scan correlated with the average middle cerebral artery/ICA flow velocity ratio ($r = 0.5$). Subarachnoid hemorrhage on CT was correlated with poor outcome. Vasospasm remained subcritical, and no negative relationship to outcome could be identified. Hyperperfusion, as based on ICA flow velocities, and vasospasm were correlated with diminished vasoreactivity, although abnormal vasoreactivity, particularly during the first days, was common and did not always predict a poor outcome.[288]

McCullough et al. found a direct correlation between the magnitude of hemorrhage in the basal cisterns and the degree of narrowing on angiography.[222] Other mechanisms, such as associated brain or vascular damage, certainly contribute to this phenomenon. Evidence linking angiographic constriction with neurological deficit is lacking. Miller and Gudeman studied the CT scans of 162 patients with severe head injury and found a 14 percent incidence of low-density lesions unassociated with hematomas or contusions.[232] Autopsy data on some of the fatal cases confirmed the suspicion that these were areas of ischemic damage. Unfortunately, because of the relative lack of angiographic data in these cases, vasospasm remains a possible but unverified explanation for their findings. Until further research into this phenomenon is available, the contribution of vasospasm to cerebral ischemia following head injury will remain conjectural.

Kistler et al., in a prospective study of 41 patients with aneurysmal SAH, predicted the absence or development of severe vasospasm on angiography based on the appearance of subarachnoid blood on CT.[176] Vasospasm was present in 20 of 22 patients with thick blood in the basilar cisterns and was absent in 14 of 19 patients with diffuse SAH. Pasqualin et al. also reported on a significant correlation between radiographic evidence of SAH on CT and the development of vasospasm.[260] Blood in the interhemispheric region carried the lowest risk of associated vasospasm. Blood in the insular and sylvian cisterns was associated with medium risk. The involvement of multiple cisterns had the highest correlation with the onset of vasospasm. Black reported that large amounts of SAH evident on CT were associated with the occurrence of vasospasm and hydrocephalus.[34]

The use of transcranial Doppler ultrasonography suggests that vasospasm is present in approximately 40 percent of patients with severe head injury. This was closely correlated with the amount of cisternal blood documented on CT.[119] Eisenberg et al., in a prospective multicenter study, examined data derived from admission CT scans of 753 patients with severe closed head injury.[88] The presence of subarachnoid blood was found to be significantly related to abnormal intracranial pressure and death. This represents the first significant association between SAH following closed head trauma and outcome. To our knowledge there have been no prior associations between SAH and outcome following penetrating injury other than our initial report in 1986. It was reported at that time that outcome was a function of the severity of the initial head injury whereas the role of TICAs and their potential for hemorrhage could contribute to additional morbidity. Angiographic spasm has not been found to be a salient feature in TICA.[122]

It remains unclear why the presence of SAH would contribute to poor outcome. It is likely that SAH may not only reflect the extent of the injury (SAH was significantly associated with increased morbidity (Chi Square, $p < 0.01$) and mortality (Chi Square, $p < 0.005$), in our series but also contribute to secondary vasospasm. It may also reflect a combination of both. The presence of multiple injuries (a combination of intracerebral hemorrhage, intraventricular hemorrhage, fragmentation, or bihemispheric injury) was always indicative of poor outcome (Chi Square, $p < 0.005$). Regardless of the presence or absence of these other variables, SAH was found to be significantly correlated with poor outcome (Chi Square hierarchical classification, $p < 0.05$).

As CT scanning continues to supplant cerebral angiography as the sole method of evaluating head trauma patients, information about the exact frequency and influence on prognosis of major vascular injuries will remain scarce. Increasing vigilance on the part of the physician, with liberal use of angiography in high-risk patients or those who deteriorate inexplicably, may allow for better management alternatives. MRA is a fairly sensitive technique, but lacking in specificity. A normal MR angiogram is very helpful in ruling out intracranial vascular lesions. However, if an MR angiogram is abnormal, conventional angiography is needed to work up the details. The need for patient cooperation (or heavy sedation) and the difficulty in evaluating acutely sick patients (such as a patient on a respirator) limits the use of MRI and MRA in the acute setting.

References

1. Aarabi B. Traumatic aneurysms of brain due to high velocity missile head wounds. *Neurosurgery* 1988; 22:1056–1063.
2. Aarabi B, Koleini MK. Traumatic aneurysms due to missile head wounds: report of twenty cases. *Iranian J Med. Sci.* 1989; 14:26–32.
3. Aarabi B, McQueen JD. Traumatic internal carotid occlusion at the base of the skull. *Surg Neurol* 1978; 10:233–236.
4. Abad JM, Alvarez F, Blazquez MG. An unrecognized neurological syndrome: sixth-nerve palsy and Horner's syndrome due to traumatic intracavernous carotid aneurysm. *Surg Neurol* 1981; 16:140–144.
5. Achram M, Rizk G, Haddad FS. Angiographic aspects of traumatic intracranial aneurysms following war injuries. *Br J Radiol* 1980; 53:1144–1149.
6. Acosta C, Williams PE Jr, Clark K. Traumatic aneurysms of the cerebral vessels. *J Neurosurg* 1972; 36:531–536.
7. Ajir F, Tibbeus JC. Post-traumatic occlusion of the supraclinoid internal carotid artery. *Neurosurgery* 1981; 9:173–176.
8. Alexander E Jr, Adams JE, Davis CH Jr. Complications in the use of temporary intracranial arterial clip. *J Neurosurg* 1963; 20:810–811.
9. Ali S, Bihari J. Intracranial traumatic aneurysm following hypophysectomy. *J Laryngol Otol* 1981; 95:749–755.
10. Aliquo-Mazzei A. Contributo alla conoscenza della sindromi oculari da aneurisma della carotide interna. *Boll d'Oculo* 1929; 8:1187–1211.

11. Allen GW. Angiography in otolaryngology. *Laryngoscope* 1967; 77:1909–1961.
12. Almeida GM, Pindaro J, Plese P, et al. Intracranial arterial aneurysms in infancy and childhood. *Child Brain* 1977; 3:193–199.
13. Andrew J, Nathan PW, Spanos NC. Disturbances of micturition and defecation due to aneurysms of the anterior communicating or anterior cerebral arteries. *J Neurosurg* 1966; 24:1–10.
14. Araki C, Handa H, Handa J, et al. Traumatic aneurysm of the intracranial extradural portion of the internal carotid artery. Report of a case. *J Neurosurg* 1965; 23:64–67.
15. Arseni C, Ionesco S. Hemorragie nasale grave provoquee par la rupture d'un anevrysme carotidien intracranien posttraumatique. *Rev Otoneuroophtalmol* 1969; 41:149–154.
16. Asari S, Nakamura S, Yamada O, et al. Traumatic aneurysm of peripheral cerebral arteries: report of two cases. *J Neurosurg* 1977; 46:795–803.
17. Awad IA, Little JR, Akarawi WP, et al. Intracranial dural arteriovenous malformations: factors predisposing to an aggressive neurological course. *J Neurosurg* 1990; 72:839–850.
18. Awad I, Sawhny B, Little JR. Traumatic post-surgical aneurysm of the intracavernous carotid artery: a delayed presentation. *Surg Neurol* 1982; 18:54–57.
19. Ballard JL, Bunt TJ, Fitzpatrick B, Malone JM. Bilateral traumatic internal carotid artery dissections: case report. *J Vasc Surg* 1992; 15:431–435.
20. Bank WO, Nelson PB, Drayer BP, et al. Traumatic aneurysm of the basilar artery. *Am J Roentgenol* 1978; 130:975–977.
21. Barcia-Marino C, Katramiz H, Tormo FF. Aneurisma carotideo infraclinoideo de origen traumatico. Presentacion de un caso y revision de la literature. *Rev Esp Otoneurooftalmol Neurochir* 1976; 34:165–176.
22. Barnwell SL, Halbach VV, Higashida RT, et al. Complex dural arteriovenous fistulas: results of combined endovascular and neurosurgical treatment in 16 patients. *J Neurosurg* 1989; 71:352–358.
23. Barrett JH, Lawrence VL. Aneurysm of the internal carotid artery as a complication of mastoidectomy. *Arch Otolaryngol* 1960; 72:366–368.
24. Barrow DL, Spector RH, Braun IF, et al. Classification and treatment of spontaneous carotid-cavernous sinus fistulas. *J Neurosurg* 1985; 62:248–256.
25. Batzdorf U, Bentson JR, Machleder HL. Blunt trauma to the high cervical carotid artery. *Neurosurgery* 1979; 5:195–201.
26. Becker DH, Newton TH. Distal anterior cerebral artery aneurysm. *Neurosurgery* 1979; 4:495–503.
27. Benoit BG, Wortzman G. Traumatic cerebral aneurysms. Clinical features and natural history. *J Neurol Neurosurg Psychiatry* 1973; 36:127–138.
28. Berger PE, Harwood-Nash DC, Fitz CR. Computerized tomography: abnormal intracerebral collections of blood in children. *Neuroradiology* 1976; 11:29–33.
29. Bergquist BJ, Boone SC, Whaley RA. Traumatic dissection of the internal carotid artery treated by ECIC anastomosis. *Stroke* 1981; 12:73–76.
30. Bergstrom K, Hemmingsson A. False cortical aneurysm in subdural hematoma following head injury without fracture. *Acta Radiol* 1973; 14:657–661.
31. Bernard MH, Rosseaux P, Scherpereel B, et al. Traumatic aneurysms of cerebral convexity. Report of 4 cases. *Neurochirurgie* 1978; 24:343–346.
32. Bingas B, Vogt U. The traumatic aneurysm of intracranial vessels. *Neurosurg Rev* 1980; 3:197–199.
33. Birley JL. Traumatic aneurysm of the intracranial portion of the internal carotid artery. *Brain* 1928; 51:184–208.
34. Black P McL. Hydrocephalus and vasospasm after subarachnoid hemorrhage from ruptured intracranial aneurysms. *Neurosurgery* 1986; 18:12–16.
35. Blau, A, Richardson JC. Strokes and head injury. *Can J Neurol Sci* 1978; 5:263–266.
36. Boldrey E, Maass L, Miller E. The role of atlantoid compression in the etiology of internal carotid thrombosis. *J Neurosurg* 1956; 13:127–139.
37. Bonnal J, Stevenaert A, Beaujean M, et al. Epistaxis repetees graves, parfois mortelles, secondares a des lesions de la carotide interne. Rupture traumatique ou rupture d'un anevrysme infraclinoidien. *Neurochirurgie* 1967; 13:417–430.
38. Bonnet P. Epistaxis mortelle, par rupture traumatique de la carotide interne dans le sinus sphenoidal. *Rev Otoneuroophtalmol* 1955; 27:25–27.
39. Brenner H. Fontale Schadelspaltung mit traumatischem Aneurysma der Arteria pericallosa. *Acta Neurochir (Wien)* 1962; 10:145–152.
40. Brihaye J, Mage J, Verriest G. Anevrysme traumatique de la carotide interne dans sa portion supraclinoidienne. *Acta Neurol Psychiatr Belg* 1954; 54:411–438.
41. Brunon J, Duquesnel J, Fischer G. Embolisation libre percutanee avec conservation de flux carotidien d'une fistule carotido- caverneuse traumatique. *Neurochirurgie* 1977; 23:453–462.
42. Buckingham MJ, Crone KR, Ball WS, et al. Traumatic intracranial aneurysms in childhood: two cases and a review of the literature. *Neurosurgery* 1988; 22:398–408.
43. Burger R, Hassler W. Transkranielle Dopplersonographie beim Schadel-Hirn-Trauma: Wertvolle Methode in der traumatologischen Notfallsituation. *Aktuel Traumatol* 1993; 23:14–19.
44. Burton C, Velasco F, Dorman J. Traumatic aneurysm of a peripheral cerebral artery. Review and case report. *J Neurosurg* 1968; 28:468–474.
45. Burton R. Massive epistaxis from a ruptured traumatic internal carotid artery aneurysm. *Med J Aust* 1973; 1:692–694.
46. Busby DR, Slemmons DH, Miller TF Jr. Fatal epistaxis via carotid aneurysm and eustachian tube. *Arch Otolaryngol* 1968; 87:295–298.
47. Cairns HL. The vascular aspects of head injuries. *Lisboa Med* 1942; 19:375–410.
48. Cantu-R-C. Cerebral stroke in a semi-pro football player: a case report. *Med Sci Sports Exerc* 1991; 23:1119–1121 (see comments).
49. Capanna AH. Traumatic intracranial aneurysm and Gradenigo's syndrome secondary to gunshot wound. *Surg Neurol* 1984; 22:263–266.
50. Carothers A. Orbitofacial wounds and cerebral artery injuries caused by umbrella tips. *JAMA* 1978; 239:1151–1152.
51. Carpenter S. Injury of neck as cause of vertebral artery thrombosis. *J Neurosurg* 1961; 18:849–853.
52. Caveness WF. Incidence of craniocerebral trauma in the United States in 1976 with trends from 1970 to 1975. *Adv neurol* 1979; 22:1–3.
53. Chadduck WM. Intracavernous compression of the third nerve by an extracavernous carotid aneurysm: case report. *J Neurosurg* 1969; 30:501–503.
54. Chambers EF, Rosenbaum AE, Norman D, Newton TH. Traumatic aneurysms of cavernous internal carotid artery with secondary epistaxis. *Am J Neuroradiol* 1981; 2:405–409.
55. Chandler HC Jr, Friedman WA. Successful radiosurgical treatment of a dural arteriovenous malformation: case report. *Neurosurgery* 1993; 33:139–142.
56. Chevallier B, Renaud C, Parat S, et al. Revelation par des signes neurologique d'un anevrysme de la sous-claviere droite. *Arch Fr Pediatr* 1993; 50:235–238.
57. Christensen JC. Epistaxis por aneurismas carotideos infraclinoideos. *Acta Neurol Latinoam* 1955; 1:60–70.
58. Clark P, Whittaker M. Traumatic aneurysms of the internal carotid artery and rupture of the duodenum following seatbelt injury. *Injury* 1980; 12:158–160.
59. Cockrill HH Jr, Jimenez JP, Goree JA. Traumatic false aneurysm of the superior cerebellar artery simulating posterior fossa tumor. *J Neurosurg* 1977; 46:377–380.
60. Columella F, Delzanno GB, Gaist G, et al. Angiography in traumatic cerebral lacerations with special regard to some less common aspects. *Acta Radiol (Diagn)* 1963; 1:239–247.
61. Connaughton PN, Williams JP. Iatrogenic intracranial aneurysms. *Acta Radiol [Suppl]* 1976; 347:59–62.
62. Cooper PR, Maravilla K, Cone J. Computerized tomographic scan

and gunshot wounds of the head: indications and radiographic findings. *Neurosurgery* 1979; 4:373–380.
63. Cosgrove GR, Villemure JG, Melancon D. Traumatic intracranial aneurysm due to arterial injury at surgery. Case report. *J Neurosurg* 1983; 58:291–294.
64. Countee RW, Vijayanathan T, Barrese C. Cervical carotid aneurysm presenting as recurrent cerebral ischemia with head turning. *Stroke* 1979; 10:144–147.
65. Courson B, Dumas M, Collomb H. Les anevrysmes arteriels distaux ou des branches peripheriques de l'artere cerebrale moyenne. *Neurochirurgie* 1970; 16:15–24.
66. Courville CB. Traumatic aneurysms of an intracranial artery: description of a lesion incident to a shotgun wound of the skull and brain. *Bull Los Angeles Neurol Soc* 1960; 25:48–54.
67. Cressman MR, Hayes GJ. Traumatic aneurysm of the anterior choroidal artery. Case report. *J Neurosurg* 1966; 24:102–104.
68. Davis EDD. Severe epistaxis difficult to control. *Br Med J* 1939; 1:721–723.
69. Debrun G, Lacour P, Vinuela F, et al. Treatment of 54 traumatic carotid-cavernous fistulas. *J Neurosurg* 1981; 55:678–692.
70. Debrun GM, Vinuela F, Fox AJ, et al. Indications for treatment and classification of 132 carotid-cavernous fistulas. *Neurosurgery* 1988; 22:285–289.
71. Dechaume JP, Cuche M, Requin JL. Les raports des traumatismes craniens et des anevrysmes arteriels intracraniens. (A propos de huit observations). *Med Leg Dommage Corpor* 1969; 2:3–20.
72. Denecke HJ, Hartert H. Carotis interna-Verletzung unt unstillbarem Nasenbluten, geheilt durch intraarterielle Thrombininjektion. Mit einem experimentellen Beitrag. *Chirurgie* 1954; 25:470–472.
73. Dennery JM, Ignacio BS. Post-traumatic arteriovenous fistula between the external carotid arteries and the superior longitudinal sinus: report of a case. *Can J Surg* 1967; 10:333–336.
74. De-Trevou MD, van Dellen JR. Penetrating stab wounds to the brain: the timing of angiography in patients presenting with the weapon already removed. *Neurosurgery* 1992; 31:905–912.
75. Dharker SR, Chandy MJ, Chandy SM, et al. Giant traumatic aneurysm of the intracranial carotid artery (case report). *Neurol India* 1975; 23:207–209.
76. Dial DL, Maurer GB. Intracranial aneurysms. Report of 13 cases. *Am J Surg* 1937; 35:2–21.
77. Ding MX. Traumatic aneurysm of the intracavernous part of the internal carotid artery presenting with epistaxis. Case report. *Surg Neurol* 1988; 30:65–67.
78. Ditmore QM, Samson DS, Beyer CW. Traumatic middle cerebral artery aneurysm. Case report. *Neurosurgery* 1980; 6:293–296.
79. Dolenc V. Direct microsurgical repair of intracavernous vascular lesions. *J Neurosurg* 1983; 58:824–831.
80. Dragon R, Saranchak H, Lakin P, Strauch G. Blunt injuries to the carotid and vertebral arteries. *Am J Surg* 1981; 141:497–500.
81. Drake CG. Subdural hematoma from arterial rupture. *J Neurosurg* 1961; 8:597–601.
82. Dujovny M, Laha RK, Decastro S, Briani S. Post-traumatic middle cerebral artery thrombosis. *J Trauma* 1979; 19:775–779.
83. Dupuy JP, Ravon R, Bokor J, et al. Post-traumatic pseudo-aneurysm of the anterior cerebral artery. *J Radiol Electrol Med Nucl* 1975; 56:715–716.
84. Duthel R, Brunon J, Deruty R, et al. Giant traumatic aneurysms of the internal carotid developing in the sphenoid sinus. Apropos of 2 cases. *Neurochirurgie* 1985; 31:309–315.
85. Easton JD, Sherman DG. Cervical manipulation and stroke. *Stroke* 1977; 8:594–597.
86. Echlin F. Spasm of basilar and vertebral arteries caused by experimental subarachnoid hemorrhage. *J Neurosurg* 1965; 23:1–11.
87. Eichler A, Story JL, Bennett DE, et al. Traumatic aneurysm of a cerebral artery. Case report. *J Neurosurg* 1969; 31:72–76.
88. Eisenberg HM, Gary HE Jr, Aldrich EF, et al. Initial CT findings in 753 patients with severe head injury: a report from the NIH Traumatic Coma Data Bank. *J Neurosurg* 1990; 73:688–698.
89. El Gindi S, Salama M, Tawfik E, et al. A review of 2,000 patients with craniocerebral injuries with regard to intracranial haematomas and other vascular complications. *Acta Neurochir (Wien)* 1979; 48:237–244.
90. Endo S, Sato S, Uneoka K, et al. Traumatic aneurysm of the callosomarginal artery. Case report. *Neurol Surg (Tokyo)* 1974; 2:329–336.
91. Endo S, Takaku A, Aihara H, Suzuki J. Traumatic cerebral aneurysm associated with widening skull fracture. Report of two infancy cases. *Childs Brain* 1980; 6:131–139.
92. Enomoto H, Shibata T, Ito A, Harada T. Traumatic aneurysm of supraclinoid internal carotid artery: report of a case. *Neurosurgery* 1984; 15:700–702.
93. Fabian G. Traumatisches Aneurysma der Carotis interna in der Keilbeinhohle. *HNO* 1952; 3:346–349.
94. Fabian G. Traumatisches Aneurysma der Carotis interna in der Keilbeinhohle. *HNO* 1956; 6:42–45.
95. Falsetti HL, Moody RA. Electrocardiographic changes in head injuries. *Dis Chest* 1966; 49:420–424.
96. Feldman RA, Hieshima G, Giannotta SL, Gade GF. Traumatic dural arteriovenous fistula supplied by scalp, meningeal, and cortical arteries: case report. *Neurosurgery* 1980; 6:670–674.
97. Ferry DJ Jr, Kempe LG. False aneurysm secondary to penetration of the brain through orbitofacial wounds: report of two cases. *J Neurosurg* 1972; 36:503–506.
98. Fincher EF. Arteriovenous fistula between the middle meningeal artery and the greater petrosal sinus: case report. *Ann Surg* 1951; 133:886–888.
99. Finkemeyer H. Verletzungen der A. carotis interna in ihrem intrakraniellen extraduralen Abschnitt. *Zentralbl* 1955; 15:65–73.
100. Finkemeyer H. Ein säckchenförmiges Aneurysma der A. cerebri media als postoperativ Komplikation. *Zentralbl* 1955; 15:302–305.
101. Fleischer AS, Patton JM, Tindall GT. Cerebral aneurysms of traumatic origin. *Surg Neurol* 1975; 4:233–239.
102. Ford FR. *Diseases of the Nervous System in Infancy, Childhood and Adolescence,* 6th ed. Springfield, IL: Charles C Thomas, 1973, pp 1023–1034.
103. Fox JL. *Intracranial Aneurysms.* New York: Springer-Verlag, 1983, vol 1, pp 423–431; vol 3, pp 1453–1463.
104. Fraser RAR, Zimbler SM. Hindbrain stroke in children caused by extracranial vertebral artery trauma. *Stroke* 1975; 6:153–159.
105. Freytag E. Fatal rupture of intracranial aneurysms. Survey of 250 medicolegal cases. *Arch Pathol* 1966; 81:418–424.
106. Friedman AH, Drake CG. Subarachnoid hemorrhage from intracranial dissecting aneurysm. *J Neurosurg* 1984; 60:325–334.
107. Funahashi K, Mishima T, Hayashi S, et al. Traumatic aneurysm of intracranial portion of the internal carotid artery. Report of a case in which the development of aneurysm was documented by several carotid angiographies. *No Shinkei Geka* 1977; 5:619–625.
108. Funakoshi T, Tsuchiya J, Sakai N, et al. Peripheral arterial aneurysm of the brain occurring after brain abscess extirpation and healing spontaneously. Report of a case and review of the literature. *Neurol Surg (Tokyo)* 1976; 4:405–410.
109. Gallina E, Gallo O, Boccuzzi S, Galeotti T. Intracranial post-traumatic aneurysm of the internal carotid artery as cause of epistaxis: considerations of 2 cases. *Acta Otorhinolaryngol Ital* 1990; 10:607–613.
110. Garcia-Bengochea F, Revuelta R, Fernandez Carrera JC. Aneurisma sacular traumatico de le carotida internal en el seno aereo esfenoidal tratado con ligadura de ambas carotidas externas y de la carotida interna homolateral. *Acta Neurol Latinoam* 1957; 3:395–399.
111. Gerlach J, Kley W. Fronto-basal skull and brain injuries involving the sphenoid sinus. In de Vet AC (ed): Proceedings of the Third International Congress of Neurological Surgery. (Excerpta Medica International Congress Series, No. 110). Amsterdam: Excerpta Medica, 1966, pp 292–298.
112. Giannotta SL, McGillicuddy JE, Kindt GW. Gradual carotid artery occlusion in the treatment of inaccessible internal carotid artery aneurysms. *Neurosurgery* 1979; 5:417–421.
113. Giannotta SL, Weiss MH. Pitfalls in the diagnosis of head injury. *Clin Neurosurg* 1982; 29:288–299.

114. Glickman MG. Angiography in head trauma. In Newton TH, Potts DG (eds): *Radiology of the Skull and Brain,* vol 2, book 4, *Angiography.* St. Louis: Mosby, 1974, pp 2598–2658.
115. Go KG, Penning L, Oen TS. Acute subdural hematoma in connection with angiographically demonstrated traumatic rupture of a cortical cerebral artery (presenting as false aneurysm). A report of 2 cases. *Neuroradiology* 1971; 2:107–110.
116. Gouliamos A, Gotsis E, Vlahos L, Samara C. Magnetic resonance angiography compared to intra-arterial digital subtraction angiography in patients with subarachnoid hemorrhage. *J Neuroradiol* 1992; 35:46–49.
117. Greitz T, Lindgren E. Intracranial traumatic changes. In Abrams HL (ed): *Angiography.* Boston: Little, Brown, 1961, pp 95–100.
118. Grisoli F, Vincentelli F, Fuchs S, et al. Surgical treatment of tentorial arteriovenous malformations draining into the subarachnoid space. *J Neurosurg* 1984; 60:1059–1066.
119. Grolimund P, Weber M, Seiler RW, et al. Time course of cerebral vasospasm after severe head injury. *Lancet* 1988; 2:1173. (letter)
120. Guest PG, Schnetler J. Traumatic cavernous carotid aneurysm resulting in blindness. *Br J Oral Maxillofac Surg* 1992; 30:395–397.
121. Guibert. Anévrysme artériel de la carotide interne au niveau du sinus caverneux gauche: communication avec le sinus sphénoidal droit, hémorrhagies nasales, mort, autopsie. *Ann d'Oculist* 1895; 113:314–318.
122. Haddad FS, Haddad GF, Taha J. Traumatic intracranial aneurysms caused by missiles: their presentation and management. *Neurosurgery* 1991; 28:1–7.
123. Hahn YS, Welling B, Rechman OH, Azar Kia B. Traumatic intracavernous aneurysm in children: massive epistaxis without ophthalmic signs. *Childs Nerv Syst* 1990; 6:360–364.
124. Halbach VV, Hieshima GB, Higashida RT, et al. Carotid cavernous fistulae: indications for urgent treatment. *Am J Neuroradiol* 1987; 8:627–633.
125. Halbach VV, Higashida RT, Dowd CF, et al. Endovascular treatment of vertebral artery dissections and pseudoaneurysms. *J Neurosurg* 1993; 79:183–191.
126. Halbach VV, Higashida RT, Hieshima GB, et al. Transvenous embolization of direct carotid-cavernous fistulas. *Am J Neuroradiol* 1988; 9:741–747.
127. Halbach VV, Higashida RT, Hieshima GB, et al. Transvenous embolization of dural fistulas involving the transverse and sigmoid sinuses. *Am J Neuroradiol* 1988; 10:385–392.
128. Halbach VV, Higashida RT, Hieshima GB, et al. Transvenous embolization of dural fistulas involving the cavernous sinus. *Am J Neuroradiol* 1989; 10:377–383.
129. Halbach VV, Higashida RT, Hieshima GB, et al. Treatment of dural fistulas involving the deep cerebral venous system. *Am J Neuroradiol* 1989; 10:393–399.
130. Hamilton JG. Massive epistaxis following closed head injury. *Guy's Hosp Rep* 1953; 102:360–367.
131. Handa J, Handa H. Severe epistaxis caused by traumatic aneurysm of cavernous carotid artery. *Surg Neurol* 1976; 5:241–243.
132. Handa J, Kamijyo Y, Handa H. Posttraumatisches Aneurysma der leptomeningealen Arterien (Bericht uber einen Fall). *Arch Psychiatr Nervenkr* 1968; 211:357–364.
133. Handa J, Kikuchi H, Iwayama K, et al. Traumatic aneurysm of the internal carotid artery. *Acta Neurochir (Wien)* 1967; 17:161–177.
134. Handa J, Shimizu Y, Matsuda M, et al. Traumatic aneurysms of the middle cerebral artery. *Am J Roetgenol* 1970; 109:127–129.
135. Hatashita S, Nitta T, Koga N, et al. Traumatic aneurysm of the intracavernous carotid artery. A case report. *Neurol Med Chir (Tokyo)* 1983; 23:885–890.
136. Hayakawa I, Sugiyama H, Yanagihashi K. Zur Entstehung eines traumatischen Karotisaneurysmas nach Behandlung einer Karotis-Sinus Kavernosus-Fistel durch Muskelembolisierung. *Acta Neurochir (Wien)* 1972; 27:45–51.
137. Heidrich R. Hirntrauma und Aneurysma. *Psychiatr Neurol Med Psychol (Leipz)* 1969; 21:121–124.
138. Herrmann HD, Fischer D, Loew F. Experiences with intraluminal occlusion with the Fogarty catheter in the treatment of carotid-cavernous sinus fistula and other lesions at the base of the skull. *Acta Neurochirur (Wien)* 1975; 32:35–54.
139. Heyn K, Noetzel H. Über verschiedene Formen der Rupturblutungen intercranieller Aneurysmen. *Beitr Pathol Anat* 1956; 116:61–70.
140. Higashida RT, Halbach VV, Tsai FY, et al. Interventional neurovascular treatment of traumatic carotid and vertebral artery lesions: results in 234 cases. *Am J Roentgenol* 1989; 153:577–582.
141. Hirsh LF. Intracranial aneurysm and hemorrhage following skull caliper traction. Review of skull traction complications. *Spine* 1979; 4:206–208.
142. Hirsch JF, David M, Sachs M. Les anévrysmes artériels traumatiques intracraniens. *Neurochirurgie* 1962; 8:189–201.
143. Hollin SA, Sukoff MH, Silverstein A, Gross SW. Post-traumatic middle cerebral artery occlusion. *J Neurosurg* 1966; 25:526–535.
144. Holmes B, Harbaugh RE. Traumatic intracranial aneurysms: a contemporary review. *J Trauma* 1993; 35:855–860.
145. Houck WS, Jackson JR, Odom GL, Young WG. Occlusion of the internal carotid artery in the neck secondary to closed trauma to the head and neck. *Ann Surg* 1964; 159:219–221.
146. Huber P. Posttraumatische Kaliberschwankungen der Hirngefässe im Angiogramm. *Fortschr Geb Rontgenstr Nuklearmed* 1963; 98:292–302.
147. Hugenholtz H, Pokrupa P, Montpetit VJA, et al. Spontaneous dissecting aneurysms of the extracranial vertebral artery. *Neurosurgery* 1982; 10:96–100.
148. Huston J, Nichols DA, Luetmer PH, et al. Blinded prospective evaluation of sensitivity of MR angiography to known intracranial aneurysms: importance of aneurysm size. *Am J Neuroradiol* 1994; 15:1607–1614.
149. Iob I, Scanarini M, Salar G, Ori C. Traumatic cerebral aneurysm in pediatric age. Case report. *J Neurosurg Sci* 1983; 27:187–190.
150. Isfort A. Traumatisches Hirnrindenaneurysma. *Monatsschr Unfallheilkd* 1961; 64:14–20.
151. Ishikawa S, Kajikawa H, Hibino H, et al. Massive epistaxis from intracranial extradural aneurysm of the internal carotid artery associated with head injury. *Neurol Surg (Tokyo)* 1976; 4:953–961.
152. Ito H, Hanyu T, Fujii H, et al. Traumatic aneurysm of the anterior cerebral artery, in reference to the role of cerebral falx. *Brain Nerve (Tokyo)* 1975; 27:787–793.
153. Jackson FE, Augusta FA, Sazima HJ, et al. Head injury and delayed epistaxis: report of a case of rupture of traumatic aneurysm of internal carotid artery due to grenade fragment wound received in Vietnam conflict. *J Trauma* 1970; 10:1158–1167.
154. Jackson FE, Gleave JRW, Janon E. Traumatic aneurysms, cranial and intracranial. *US Navy Med* 1974; 63:34–40.
155. Jacques S, Shelden CH, Rogers DT Jr, Trippi AC. Posttraumatic bilateral middle cerebral artery occlusion: case report. *J Neurosurg* 1975; 42:217–221.
156. Jakobsson KE, Carlsson C, Elfverson J, von-Essen C. Traumatic aneurysms of cerebral arteries. A study of five cases. *Acta Neurochir (Wien)* 1984; 71:91–98.
157. Jamart P, Stevenaert A, Thibaut A, et al. Epistaxis cataclysmique par rupture d'un anevrisme de la carotide interne dans le sinus sphenoidal. *Acta Otorhinolaryngol Belg* 1967; 21:21–30.
158. Jeanmart L, Noterman J, Brihaye J, et al. Les anevrysmes de la carotide intra-caverneuse. *Neurochirurgie* 1973; 19:61–73.
159. Jenewein K, Pirker E, Furtschegger A, et al. Verletzungen intrakranieller Arterien im Angiogramm. *Rofo Fortschr Geb Rontgenstr Neuen Bildgeb Verfahr* 1989; 151:706–712.
160. Jernigan WR, Gardner WC. Carotid artery injuries due to closed cervical trauma. *J Trauma* 1971; 11:429–435.
161. Jinkins JR, Dadsetan MR, Sener RN, et al. Value of acute-phase angiography in the detection of vascular injuries caused by gunshot wounds to the head: analysis of 12 cases. *Am J Roentgenol* 1992; 159:365–368.
162. Jungmichel G. Aneurysma einer basalen Gehirnarterie nach Trauma. *Dtsch Z Gesamte Gerichtl Med* 1932; 19:197–223.

163. Kahlau G. Uber die traumatische Entstehung von Aneurysmen der Hirnbasisarterien. *Frankf Z Pathol* 1937; 51:319–343.
164. Kamijo Y, Namba A, Handa J, et al. Posttraumatic pial artery aneurysm with special reference to a case with surgical treatment and histological examination following carotid artery angiography. *Brain Nerve (Tokyo)* 1968; 20:965–970.
165. Kaufman HH. Civilian gunshot wounds to the head. *Neurosurgery* 1993; 32:962–964.
166. Kaufman HH, Sadhu VK, Clifton GL, Handel SF. Delayed intracerebral hematoma due to traumatic aneurysm caused by a shotgun wound: a problem in prophylaxis. *Neurosurgery* 1980; 6:181–184.
167. Keane JR. Automobile accidents caused by unsuspected neurological disease. *J Neurosurg* 1973; 38:581–583.
168. Keane JR, Talalla A. Posttraumatic intracavernous aneurysm. Epistaxis with monocular blindness preceded by chromatopsia. *Arch Ophthalmol* 1972; 87:701–705.
169. Kendall B. Results of treatment of arteriovenous fistulae with the Debrun technique. *Am J Neuroradiol* 1983; 4:405–408.
170. Kerber CW, Newton TH. The macro and microvasculature of the dura mater. *Neuroradiology* 1973; 6:175–179.
171. Kieck CF, de Villiers JC. Vascular lesions due to transcranial stab wounds. *J Neurosurg* 1984; 60:42–46.
172. Kimbell FD Jr, Llewellyn RC, Kirgis HD. Surgical treatment of ruptured aneurysm with intracerebral and subarachnoid hemorrhage in a 16-month-old infant. *J Neurosurg* 1960; 17:331–332.
173. Kindt G, McGillicuddy J, Giannotta S, Pritz M. The reversal of neurologic deficit in patients with acute cerebral ischemia by profound increases in intravascular volume. *Acta Neurol Scand Suppl* 1979; 72:468–469.
174. Kinley GJ, Leighninger DS. Aneurysm of anomalous ophthalmic artery presenting in the sphenoid sinus and simulating an aneurysm of the internal carotid artery on routine arteriography. *J Neurosurg* 1952; 9:544–547.
175. Kintzel D. Traumatisches Karotisaneurysma im Bereich der Schadelbasis mit lebensbed-rohlicher Blutung in den Nasen-Rachen-Raum. *Zentralbl Neurochir* 1978; 39:65–72.
176. Kistler JP, Crowell RM, Davis KR, et al. The relation of cerebral vasospasm to the extent and location of subarachnoid blood visualized by CT scan: a prospective study. *Neurology* 1983; 33:424–436.
177. Kobayashi H, Hayashi M, Noguchi Y, et al. Dural arteriovenous malformations in the anterior cranial fossa. *Surg Neurol* 1988; 30:396–401.
178. Kojima T, Waga S, Furuno M. Fracture of the sella turcica. *Neurosurgery* 1985; 16:225–229.
179. Kojimahara M, Ikeda N, Tsuji A, et al. An autopsy case of traumatic middle cerebral artery occlusion. *Nippon Hoigaku Zasshi* 1993; 47:134–136.
180. Krajewski LP, Hertzer NR. Blunt carotid artery trauma: report of two cases and review of the literature. *Ann Surg* 1980; 191:341–346.
181. Krauland W. Zur Entstehung traumatischer Aneurysmen der Schlagadern am Hirngrund. *Schweiz Z Pathol Bakteriol* 1949; 12:113–127.
182. Kuhner A, Krastel A, Stoll W. Arteriovenous malformations of the transverse dural sinus. *J Neurosurg* 1976; 45:12–19.
183. Kuroda S, Abumiya T, Takahashi A, et al. Magnetic resonance findings in spontaneous dissection of the cervical internal carotid artery—case report. *Neurol Med Chir (Tokyo)* 1992; 32:773–777.
184. Kurozumi S, Harada Y, Okazaki H, et al. [Severe recurrent epistaxis caused by traumatic aneurysm of the internal carotid artery]. *Jibiinkoka* 1971; 43:685–690.
185. Laitinen L. Arterial aneurysm with subarachnoid hemorrhage in children. *Nord Med* 1964; 71:329–333.
186. Lasjaunias P, Chiu M, Ter Brugge K, et al. Neurological manifestations of dural arteriovenous malformations. *J Neurosurg* 1986; 64:724–730.
187. Lassman LP, Ramani PS, Sengupta RP. Aneurysms of peripheral cerebral arteries due to surgical trauma. *Vasc Surg* 1974; 8:1–5.
188. Laun A. Traumatische zerebrale Aneurysmen. *Unfallheilkunde* 1978; 81:482–491.
189. Laurent JP, Cheek WR, Mims T, McCluggage CW. Traumatic intracranial aneurysm in an infant: case report and review of the literature. *Neurosurgery* 1981; 9:303–306.
190. Ledgerwood AM, Mullins RJ, Lucas CE. Primary repair vs ligation for carotid artery injuries. *Arch Surg* 1980; 115:488–493.
191. Lee JP, Wang AD. Epistaxis due to traumatic intracavernous aneurysm: case report. *J Trauma* 1990; 30:619–622.
192. Levy A, Kellerhals B, Nawaz AW. Foudroyante Epistaxis aus carotis interna. *Acta Neurochir (Wien)* 1971; 24:37–53.
193. Levy ML, Masri LS, Levy KM, et al. Penetrating craniocerebral injury resultant from gunshot wounds: gang-related injury in children and adolescents. *Neurosurgery* 1993; 33:1018–1025.
194. Levy ML, Rezai A, Masri LS, et al. The significance of subarachnoid hemorrhage following penetrating craniocerebral injury: correlations with angiography and outcome in a civilian population. *Neurosurgery* 1993; 32:532–540.
195. Levy RL, Dugan TM, Bernat JL, Keating J. Lateral medullary syndrome after neck injury. *Neurology* 1980; 30:788–790.
196. Leys D, Lesoin F, Pruvo JP et al. Bilateral spontaneous dissection of extracranial vertebral arteries. *J Neurol* 1987; 234:237–240.
197. Lin JP, Chase NE, Kricheff II, et al. Microangiographic changes in the traumatized brain. *Acta Radiol (Diagn)* 1966; 5:341–351.
198. Lister JR, Sypert GW. Traumatic false aneurysms and carotid-cavernous fistula: a complication of sphenoidotomy. *Neurosurgery* 1979; 5:473–475.
199. Little JM, May J, Vanderfield GK, Lamond S. Traumatic thrombosis of the internal carotid artery. *Lancet* 1969; 2:926–930.
200. Liu JS, Tsai TC, Chang YY. Extracranial internal carotid artery dissection secondary to neck massage: visualization of mural hematoma by MRI. *Kao Hsiung I Hsueh Ko Hsueh Tsa Chih* 1993; 9:322–327.
201. Liu MY, Shih CJ, Wang YC, Tsai SH. Traumatic intracavernous carotid aneurysm with massive epistaxis. *Neurosurgery* 1985; 17:569–573.
202. Loar CR, Chadduck WM, Nugent GR. Traumatic occlusion of the middle cerebral artery: case report. *J Neurosurg* 1973; 39:753–756.
203. Loiseau G, Marchand J, Moncade J, et al. Epistaxis grave par infraclinoidien. *Ann Otolaryngol Chir Cervicofac* 1967; 84:472–475.
204. Lombardi G, Passerini A, Migliavacca F. Intracavernous aneurysms of the internal carotid artery. *Am J Roentgenol* 1963; 89:361–371.
205. Lukin R, Chambers A. Traumatic aneurysm of peripheral cerebral artery. *Neuroradiology* 1974; 8:1–3.
206. Mackenzie I. The intracranial bruit. *Brain* 1955; 78:350–368.
207. Macpherson P, Graham DL. Arterial spasm and slowing of the cerebral circulation in the ischaemia of head injury. *J Neurol Neurosurg Psychiatry* 1973; 36:1069–1072.
208. Mahmoud NA. Traumatic aneurysm of the internal carotid artery and epistaxis: review of literature and report of a case. *J Laryngol Otol* 1979; 93:629–656.
209. Majchrzak H, Wencel T, Gajos L, Bazowski P. [Traumatic aneurysm of the cortical branch of the middle cerebral artery]. *Neurol Neurochir Pol* 1983; 17:153–155.
210. Maki Y, Kono M. Posttraumatic pial artery aneurysm. *Saiga Igaku* 1971; 14:92–95.
211. Malik GM, Pearce JE, Ausman JI, et al. Dural arteriovenous malformations and intracranial hemorrhage. *Neurosurgery* 1984; 15:332–339.
212. Manelfe C, Berenstein A. treatment of carotid-cavernous fistulas by venous approach: report of one case. *J Neuroradiol* 1980; 7:13–19
213. Marubayashi T, Kaku M, Yoshida A, et al. Traumatic aneurysm of the frontopolar artery developing after evacuation of the subdural effusion in a 6-month-old girl. *Neurol Surg (Tokyo)* 1975; 3:177–183.
214. Mas JL. Internal carotid artery dissection. *Rev Prat* 1993; 43:2509–2514.
215. Masana Y, Taneda M. Direct approach to a traumatic giant internal carotid artery aneurysm associated with a carotid cavernous fistula. Case report. *J Neurosurg* 1992; 76:524–527.
216. Mastaglia FL, Savas S, Kakulas BA. Intracranial thrombosis of the

internal carotid artery after closed head injury. *J Neurol Neurosurg Psychiatry* 1969; 32:383–388.
217. Maurer JJ, Mills M, German WJ. Triad of unilateral blindness, orbital fractures and massive epistaxis after head injury. *J Neurosurg* 1961; 18:837–840.
218. Maxeiner H, Finck GA. Traumatischer Hirninfarkt bei mehrzeitig verlaufender Dissektion der extrakraniellen Arteria carotis interna. Unfallchirurgie 1989; 92:321–327.
219. Mayo F, Benjamin V. Aneurisma traumatico del sifon carotideo derecho. *Acta Neurol Latinoam* 1971; 17:365–373.
220. McCollum CH, Wheeler WG, Noon GP, DeBdcey ME. Aneurysms of the extracranial carotid artery: twenty-one years' experience. *Am J Surg* 1979; 137:196–200.
221. McCormick WF, Beals JD. Severe epistaxis caused by ruptured aneurysm of the internal carotid artery. *J Neurosurg* 1964; 21:678–686.
222. McCullough D, Nelson KM, Ommaya AK. The acute effects of experimental head injury on the vertebrobasilar circulation: angiographic observations. *J Trauma* 1971; 11:422–428.
223. McDonald EJ, Winestock DP, Hoff JT. The value of repeat cerebral arteriography in the evaluation of trauma. *Am J Roentgenol* 1976; 126:792–797.
224. McGrail KM, Heros RC, Debrun G, Beyerl D. Aneurysm of the ICA petrous segment treated by balloon entrapment after EC-IC bypass. Case report. *J Neurosurg* 1986; 65:249–252.
225. Meder JF, Gaston A, Merienne L, et al. Traumatic aneurysm of the internal and external carotid arteries. One case and a review of the literature. *J Neuroradiol* 1992; 19:248–255.
226. Meguro K, Rowed DW. Traumatic aneurysm of the posterior inferior cerebellar artery caused by fracture of the clivus. *Neurosurgery* 1985; 16:666–668.
227. Meier DE, Brink BE, Fry WJ. Vertebral artery trauma: acute recognition and treatment. *Arch Surg* 1981; 116:236–239.
228. Melvill RL, de Villiers JC. Peripheral cerebral arterial aneurysms caused by stabbing. *S Afr Med J* 1977; 51:471–473.
229. Menezes AH, Graf CJ. True traumatic aneurysm of anterior cerebral artery. Case report. *J Neurosurg* 1974; 40:544–548.
230. Menschel H. Uber einen Fall von Aneurysma der Arteria vertebralis dextra nach einem Trauma. *Aerztl Sachverst Ztg* 1922; 28:13–17.
231. Meyer-Horstgen H, Bettag W. Uber eintraumatisches Aneurysma der Arteria pericallosa bei einem elfjahrigen Jungen. *Neurochirurgia (Stuttg)* 1980; 23:239–244.
232. Miller JD, Gudeman SK. Cerebral vasospasm after head injury. In Wilkins RH (ed): *Cerebral Arterial Spasm: Proceedings of The Second International Workshop, Amsterdam, The Netherlands.* Baltimore: Williams & Wilkins, 1980, pp 476–479.
233. Miyahara S, Cheng CL, Kitamura K. Intracranial aneurysm due to arterial injury during surgery. Case report. *No Shinkei Geka* 1977; 5:991–994.
234. Miyazaki S, Ohmori H, Munekata K, et al. [Spontaneous healing of traumatic aneurysm occurring after brain tumor removal]. *No Shinkei Geka* 1981; 9:531–537.
235. Miyazaki S, Yamaura A, Kamata K, et al. A dissecting aneurysm of the vertebral artery. *Surg Neurol* 1984; 21:171–174.
236. Moore D, Budde RB, Hunter CR, et al. Massive epistaxis from aneurysm of the carotid artery. *Surg Neurol* 1979; 11:115–117.
237. Morley TP, Barr HWK. Giant intracranial aneurysms: diagnosis, course, and management. *Clin Neurosurg* 1969; 16:73–94.
238. Mounier-Kuhn P, Gaillard J, Fontvieille J, et al. Epistaxis par rupture d'un anévrisme traumatique de la carotide interne 33 dans la sinus sphénoidal. *J Fr Otorhinolaryngol Chir Maxillofac* 1960; 9:631–637.
239. Mullan S. Experiences with surgical thrombosis of intracranial berry aneurysms and carotid cavernous fistulas. *J Neurosurg* 1974; 41:657–670.
240. Mullges W, Ringelstein E-B, Leibold M. Non-invasive diagnosis of internal carotid artery dissections. *J Neurol Neurosurg Psychiatry* 1992; 55:98–104.
241. Nagpal RD, Kirtane M, Parikh VR. Traumatic intracranial aneurysm. A case report with a suggested definitive line of treatment. *Neurol India* 1978; 26:31–33.
242. Nakamura N, Sato O. A case of ruptured intracranial aneurysm within the subdural space. *Brain Nerve (Tokyo)* 1965; 17:41–45.
243. Nakamura T, Matsuoka Y, Nishimura S. Traumatic cerebral aneurysm showing remarkable extravasation into the lateral ventricle: report of a case in an infant. *Neurol Surg (Tokyo)* 1977; 5:371–378.
244. Nakstad PH, Hald JK, Sorteberg W. Carotid-cavernous fistula treated with detachable balloon during bilateral transcranial Doppler monitoring of middle cerebral arteries. A case report. *Acta Radiol* 1992; 33:145–148.
245. Negoro N, Kageyama N, Ishiguchi T. Cerebrovascular occlusion by catheterization and embolization: clinical experience. *Am J Neuroradiol* 1983; 4:362–365.
246. New PFJ, Momose KJ. Traumatic dissection of the internal carotid artery at the atlantoaxial level, secondary to nonpenetrating injury. *Radiology* 1969; 93:41–49.
247. Newbarr FD, Courville CB. Trauma as the possible significant factor in the rupture of congenital intracranial aneurysms. *J Forensic Sci* 1958; 3:174–200.
248. Newton TH, Hoyt WF. Dural arteriovenous shunts in the region of the cavernous sinus. *Neuroradiology* 1970; 1:71–81.
249. Nishijima M, Takaku A, Endo S, et al. Etiological evaluation of dural arteriovenous malformations of the lateral and sigmoid sinuses based upon histopathological examinations. *J Neurosurg* 1992; 76:600–606.
250. Nishimoto A, Matsumoto K, Ueda S, et al. Traumatic aneurysm of middle cerebral artery. *Nippon Acta Neuroradiol* 1967; 8:4–9.
251. Noterman J, Flament-Durand J, Hermanus N, Brotchi J. Traumatic aneurysm of the anterior cerebral artery associated with a contralateral carotid-cavernous fistula: a case report. *Neurosurgery* 1985; 17:807–810.
252. Nov AA, Cromwell LD. Traumatic pericallosal artery aneurysm. *J Neuroradiol* 1984; 11:3–8.
253. Olafson RA, Christoferson LA. The syndrome of carotid occlusion following minor craniocerebral trauma. *J Neurosurg* 1970; 33:636–639.
254. Overton MC III, Calvin TH Jr. Iatrogenic cerebral cortical aneurysm. Case report. *J Neurosurg* 1966; 24:672–675.
255. Papo I, Caruselli G, Salvolini U. Epistaxis posttraumatique massive par rupture d'anevrisme infraclinoidien. *Neurochirurgie* 1969; 15:283–290.
256. Parent AD, Smith RR. Traumatic aneurysm complications EC-IC bypass: successful surgical clipping. *Surg Neurol* 1981; 15:229–231.
257. Parkinson D. Carotid-cavernous fistula: direct repair with preservation of the carotid artery: technical note. *J Neurosurg* 1973; 38:99–106.
258. Parkinson D, Jain KK, Johnston JB. Saccular aneurysm of the ophthalmic artery. Report of an unusual case. *Can J Surg* 1961; 4:229–232.
259. Parkinson D, West M. Traumatic intracranial aneurysms. *J Neurosurg* 1980; 52:11–20.
260. Pasqualin A, Rosta L, Da Pian R, et al. Role of computed tomography in the management of vasospasm after subarachnoid hemorrhage. *Neurosurgery* 1984; 15:344–353.
261. Paul GA, Shaw CM, Wray LM. True traumatic aneurysm of the vertebral artery: case report. *J Neurosurg* 1980; 53:101–105.
262. Paullus WS, Norwood CW, Morgan HW. False aneurysm of the cavernous carotid artery and progressive external ophthalmoplegia after transsphenoidal hypophysectomy. Case report. *J Neurosurg* 1979; 51:707–709.
263. Pecker J, Hoel J, Javaleta A, et al. Volumineux anevrisme motor oculaire externe. *Bull Soc Ophtalmol Fr* 1960; 5:283–290.
264. Peick AL, Nichols WK, Curtis JJ, Silver D. Aneurysms and pseudoaneurysms of the superficial temporal artery caused by trauma. *J Vasc Surg* 1988; 8:606–610.
265. Perneczky A, Wruhs O, Matras H. Traumatisches intrakranielles Aneurysma der Arteria carotis interna bei longitudinaler Frakturdes Orbitadaches. *Unfallchirurgie* 1982; 8:195–199.

266. Perry MO, Snyder WH, Thal ER. Carotid artery injuries caused by blunt trauma. *Ann Surg* 1980; 192:74–77.
267. Petty JM. Epistaxis from aneurysm of the internal carotid artery due to a gunshot wound. Case report. *J Neurosurg* 1969; 30:741–743.
268. Philippides D, Buchheit F, Roth A, et al. Anevrysme post-traumatique de la carotide intra-caverneuse. *Rev Otoneuroophtalmol* 1969; 41:345–349.
269. Philippides D, Steimle R. Anevrysme posttraumatique du siphon de la carotide interne. *Rev Otoneuroophtalmol* 1956; 28:144–147.
270. Pierot L, Chiras J, Meder JF, et al. Dural arteriovenous fistulas of the posterior fossa draining into subarachnoid veins. *Am J Neuroradiol* 1992; 13:315–323.
271. Pool JL, Potts DG. *Aneurysms and Arteriovenous Anomalies of the Brain. Diagnosis and Treatment.* New York: Harper & Row, 1965.
272. Pozzati E, Gaist G, Servadei F. Traumatic aneurysms of the supraclinoid internal carotid artery. *J Neurosurg* 1982; 57:418–422.
273. Pozzati E, Giuliani G, Poppi M, Faenza A. Blunt traumatic carotid dissection with delayed symptoms. *Stroke* 1989; 20:412–416.
274. Pritz MB, Giannotta SL, Kindt GW, et al. Treatment of patients with neurological deficits associated with cerebral vasospasm by intravascular volume expansion. *Neurosurgery* 1978; 3:364–368.
275. Quattrocchi KB, Nielsen SL, Poirier V, Wagner FC Jr. Traumatic aneurysm of the superior cerebellar artery: case report and review of the literature. *Neurosurgery* 1990; 27:476–479.
276. Rahimizadeh A, Abtahi H, Daylami MS, et al. Traumatic cerebral aneurysms caused by shell fragments. Report of four cases and review of the literature. *Acta Neurochir (Wien)* 1987; 84:93–98.
277. Rahmat H, Abbassioun K, Amirjamshidi A. Pulsating unilateral exophthalmos due to traumatic aneurysm of the intraorbital ophthalmic artery: case report. *J Neurosurg* 1984; 60:630–632.
278. Raimondi AJ, Yashon D, Reyes C, et al. Intracranial false aneurysms. *Neurochirurgia (Stutt)* 1968; 11:219–233.
279. Reddy SV, Sundt TM Jr. Giant traumatic false aneurysm of the internal carotid artery associated with a carotid-cavernous fistula. Case report. *J Neurosurg* 1981; 55:813–818.
280. Reichel J, Intrau H. Traumatisches intrakranielles Aneurysma *Zentralbl Neurochir* 1975; 36:199–202.
281. Rhodes EL, Stanley JC, Hoffman GL, et al. Aneurysms of extracranial carotid arteries. *Arch Surg* 1976; 111:339–343.
282. Rich NM, Spencer FC. *Vascular Trauma.* Philadelphia: Saunders, 1978.
283. Richardson JD, McElvein RB, Trinkle JK. First rib fracture: a hallmark of severe trauma. *Ann Surg* 1975; 181:251–254.
284. Richardson R, Obeid FN, Richardson JD, et al. Neurologic consequences of cerebrovascular injury. *J Trauma* 1992; 32:755–760.
285. Rittenhouse EA, Radke HM, Sumner DS. Carotid artery aneurysms: review of the literature and report of a case with rupture into the oropharynx. *Arch Surg* 1972; 105:786–789.
286. Robbins JB, Fitz-Hugh GS, Jane JA. Intracranial carotid catastrophies encountered by the otolaryngologist. *Laryngoscope* 1976; 86:893–902.
287. Roessmann U, Miller RT. Thrombosis of the middle cerebral artery associated with birth trauma. *Neurology* 1980; 30:889–892.
288. Romner B, Sjoholm H, Brandt L. Transcranial Doppler sonography, angiography and SPECT measurements in traumatic carotid artery dissection. *Acta Neurochir (Wien)* 1994; 126:185–191.
289. Ross JS, Masaryk TJ, Modic MT, et al. Intracranial aneurysms: evaluation by MR angiography *Am J Neuroradiol* 1994; 11:449–455.
290. Rousseau F, Spillman J. Deux cas d'epistaxis incoersibles avec cecite homolaterale par lésion de la carotide interne intracranienne après chut sur la tete. *Ann Otolaryngol* 1951; 68:461–465.
291. Rubio PA, Reul GA Jr, Beall AC Jr, et al. Acute carotid artery injury: 25 years' experience. *J Trauma* 1974; 14:967–973.
292. Rumbaugh CL, Bergeron RT, Kurze T. Intracranial vascular damage associated with skull fractures: radiographic aspects. *Radiology* 1972; 104:81–87.
293. Rumbaugh CL, Bergeron RT, Talalla A, et al. Traumatic aneurysms of the cortical cerebral arteries. Radiographic aspects. *Radiology* 1970; 96:49–54.
294. Sachdev VP, Drapkin AJ, Hollin SA, et al. Subarachnoid hemorrhage following intranasal procedures. *Surg Neurol* 1977; 8:122–125.
295. Sadar ES, Jane JA, Lewis LW, et al. Traumatic aneurysms of the intracranial circulation. *Surg Gynecol Obstet* 1973; 137:59–67.
296. Sadik AR, Adachi M, Ranshoff J. Rupture of an intracranial aneurysm within the subdural space—in association with trauma. A case report. *J Neurosurg* 1963; 20:609–612.
297. Saito R, Yazaki T, Kawase T, Toya S. [Traumatic intracranial aneurysms after removal of tuberculum sellae meningioma: case report]. *No Shinkei Geka* 1992; 20:973–977.
298. Salar G, Mingrino S. Traumatic intracranial internal carotid aneurysm due to gunshot wound: case report. *J Neurosurg* 1978; 49:100–102.
299. Salmon JH, Blatt ES. Aneurysm of the internal carotid artery due to closed trauma. *J Thorac Cardiovasc Surg* 1968; 56:28–32.
300. Sanders MD, Hoyt WF. Hypoxic ocular sequelae of carotid-cavernous fistulae: study of the causes of visual failure before and after neurosurgical treatment in a series of 25 cases. *Br J Ophthalmol* 1969; 53:82–97.
301. Sarwar M, Batnitzky S, Schechter MM, et al. Growing intracranial aneurysms. *Radiology* 1976; 120:603–607.
302. Scharfetter F, Fodisch HJ, Menardi G, et al. Falsches Aneurysma der Arteria gyri angularis durch Gefassverletzung bei einer Ventrikelpunktion. *Acta Neurochir (Wien)* 1976; 33:123–132.
303. Schlosshauer B, Vosteen KH. Zur Diagnostik und Therapie der Carotisblutung nach Keilbeinhohlenfrakturen. *Arch Ohren Nasen Kehlkopfheilkd* 1954; 165:270–277.
304. Schmidt-Vanderheyden W, Backmund H. Angiographische Verlaufsbeobachtung eines traumatischen, intracerebralen Aneurysmas. *Arch Psychiatr Nervenkr* 1971; 214:10–16.
305. Schneider RC, Schemm GW. Vertebral artery insufficiency in acute and chronic spinal trauma: with special reference to the syndrome of acute central cervical spinal cord injury. *J Neurosurg* 1961; 18:348–360.
306. Schuierer G, Huk WJ, Laub G. Magnetic resonance angiography of intracranial aneurysms: comparison with intra-arterial digital subtraction angiography. *Neuroradiology* 1992; 35:50–54.
307. Scott GE, Neubuerger KT, Denst J. Dissecting aneurysms of intracranial arteries. *Neurology* 1960; 10:22–27.
308. Sedzimir CB, Occleshaw JV, Buxton PH. False cerebral aneurysm. Case report. *J Neurosurg* 1968; 29:636–639.
309. Seeger JF, Gabrielsen T, Giannotta SL, et al. Carotid-cavernous sinus fistulas and venous thrombosis. *Am J Neuroradiol* 1980; 1:141–148.
310. Seftel DM, Kolson H, Gordon BS. Ruptured intracranial carotid aneurysm with fatal epistaxis. *Arch Otolaryngol* 1959; 70:52–60.
311. Sekino H, Katoh Y, Kanki T, Nakamura N. [Iatrogenic traumatic intracranial aneurysm. Case report]. *Neurol Med Chir (Tokyo)* 1985; 25:945–951.
312. Senter HJ, Sarwar M. Nontraumatic dissecting aneurysm of the vertebral artery: case report. *J Neurosurg* 1982; 56:128–130.
313. Serbinenko FA, Lazarev VA. [Use of balloon catheter in cases of traumatic pseudoaneurysm of the carotid artery complicated by profuse nosebleed]. *Zh Vopr Neirokhir* 1981; 6:9–16.
314. Shallat RF, Taekman MS, Nagle RC. Delayed complications of craniocerebral trauma: case report. *Neurosurgery* 1981; 8:569–573.
315. Shaw C-M, Alvord EC Jr. Injury of the basilar artery associated with closed head trauma. *J Neurol Neurosurg Psychiatry* 1972; 35:247–257.
316. Shigemori M, Shirahama M, Hara K, et al. [Traumatic aneurysms of intracranial internal carotid arteries. Case reports]. *Neurol Med Chir (Tokyo)* 1982; 22:241–247.
317. Shima T, Uozumi T, Nishimura S, et al. [False traumatic aneurysm secondary to penetration of the brain through supraorbital wound: report of a case]. *No Shinkei Geka* 1978; 6:1025–1030.
318. Shimoji T, Bando K, Nakajima K, et al. Dissecting aneurysm of the vertebral artery: report of seven cases and angiographic findings. *J Neurosurg* 1984; 61:1038–1046.
319. Shirai S, Tomono Y, Owada T, et al. Traumatic aneurysm of the

internal carotid artery. Report of a case with late epistaxis. *Eur Neurol* 1977; 15:212–216.
320. Sights WP Jr. Incarceration of the basilar artery in a fracture of the clivus: case report. *J Neurosurg* 1968; 28:588–591.
321. Simeone FA, Goldberg HL. Thrombosis of the vertebral artery from hyperextension injury to the neck: case report. *J Neurosurg* 1968; 29:540–544.
322. Smith DR, Kempe LG. Cerebral false aneurysm formation in closed head trauma. Case report. *J Neurosurg* 1970; 32:357–359.
323. Smith KR Jr, Bardenheier JA III. Aneurysm of the pericallosal artery caused by closed cranial trauma. Case report. *J Neurosurg* 1968; 29:551–554.
324. Spetzler RF, Owen MP. Extracranial-intracranial arterial bypass to a single branch of the middle cerebral artery in the management of traumatic aneurysm. *Neurosurgery* 1979; 4:334–337.
325. Steiger HJ, Aaslid R, Stooss R, Seiler RW. Transcranial Doppler monitoring in head injury: relations between type of injury, flow velocities, vasoreactivity, and outcome. *Neurosurgery* 1994; 34:79–86.
326. Steinmetz H, Heiss E, Mironov A. Traumatic giant aneurysms of the intracranial carotid artery presenting long after head injury. *Surg Neurol* 1988; 30:305–310.
327. Stringer WL, Kelly DL Jr. Traumatic dissection of the extra-cranial internal carotid artery. *Neurosurgery* 1980; 6:123–130.
328. Sturzenegger M, Mattle HP, Rivoir A, et al. Ultrasound findings in spontaneous extracranial vertebral artery dissection. *Stroke* 1993; 24:1910–1921.
329. Sue DE, Brant-Zawadzki MN, Chance J. Dissection of cranial arteries in the neck: correlation of MRI and arteriography. *Neuroradiology* 1992; 34:273–278.
330. Sullivan HG, Vines FS, Becker DP. Sequelae of indirect internal carotid injury. *Radiology* 1973; 109:91–98.
331. Sundt TM Jr, Piepgras DG. The surgical approach to arteriovenous malformations of the lateral and sigmoid dural sinuses. *J Neurosurg* 1983; 59:32–39.
332. Suwanwela C, Suwanwela N. Intracranial arterial narrowing and spasm in acute head injury. *J Neurosurg* 1972; 36:314–323.
333. Symonds CP. Delayed traumatic intracerebral haemorrhage. *Br Med J* 1940; 1:1048–1051.
334. Takahashi A, Kamiyama H, Imamura H, et al. "True" posterior communicating artery aneurysm: report of two cases. *Neurol Med Chir (Tokyo)* 1992; 32:338–341.
335. Tani S, Funahashi K, Hashimoto T, et al. [Traumatic aneurysm of the posterior inferior cerebellar artery]. *No Shinkei Geka* 1982; 10:423–427.
336. Taylor PE. Delayed postoperative hemorrhage from intracranial aneurysm after craniotomy for tumor. *Neurology* 1961; 11:225–231.
337. Teal JS, Bergeron RT, Rumbaugh CL, et al. Aneurysms of the petrous or cavernous portion of the internal carotid artery associated with non-penetrating head trauma. *J Neurosurg* 1973; 38:568–574.
338. Teng MMH, Guo WY, Huang CI, et al. Occlusion of arteriovenous malformations of the cavernous sinus via the superior ophthalmic vein. *Am J Neuroradiol* 1988; 9:539–546.
339. Thompson JR, Harwood-Nash DC, Fitz CR. Cerebral aneurysms in children. *Am J Roentgenol* 1973; 118:163–175.
340. Toole JF, Tucker SH. Influence of head position upon cerebral circulation. *Arch Neurol* 1960; 2:616–623.
341. Towne JB, Neis DD, Smith JW. Thrombosis of the internal carotid artery following blunt cervical trauma. *Arch Surg* 1972; 104:565–568.
342. Tranmer BI, Humphreys RP, Chuang SH. Microsurgical recovery of a migrated balloon from the internal carotid artery of a child. *Neurosurgery* 1985; 16:381–386.
343. Tsubokawa T, Kotani A, Sugawara T, et al. Treatment for traumatic aneurysm of the cerebral artery: identification between deteriorating type and spontaneously disappearing type. *Neurol Surg (Tokyo)* 1975; 3:663–672.
344. Umebayashi Y, Kuwayama M, Handa J, et al. Traumatic aneurysm of a peripheral cerebral artery. Case report. *Clin Radiol* 1970; 21:36–38.
345. Unger SW, Tucker WS Jr, Mrdeza MA, et al. Carotid arterial trauma. *Surgery* 1980; 87:477–487.
346. Van-Dellen JR. Intracavernous traumatic aneurysms. *Surg Neurol* 1980; 13:203–207.
347. Vilato RJ, LeBeau J. Le spasme des artères du cercle de Willis au cours des hémorragies traumatiques ou anévrismales. *Neurochirurgie* 1962; 8:217–221.
348. Vinuela F, Fox AJ, Debrun GM, et al. Spontaneous carotid-cavernous fistulas: clinical, radiological, and therapeutic considerations: experience with 20 cases. *J Neurosurg* 1984; 60:976–984.
349. Von Hanwehr RI, Giannotta SL, Weiss MH. The impact of traumatic cerebral aneurysms and their sequelae on selective morbidity following head trauma. In Kikuchi H, Fukushima T, Watanabe K (eds): *Intracranial Aneurysms: Surgical Timing and Techniques: Proceedings of the First International Workshop on Intracranial Aneurysms.* Tokyo, Japan: Nishimura Co Ltd, 1986, pp 96–104.
350. Voris HC, Basile JXR. Recurrent epistaxis from aneurysm of the internal carotid artery. Case report with cure by operation *J Neurosurg* 1961; 18:841–842.
351. Waga S, Morikawa A, Fujimoto K. Carotid-cavernous fistula associated with traumatic aneurysm of the internal carotid artery. *Surg Neurol* 1978; 9:367–369.
352. Wakai S, Yoshimasu N, Eguchi T, Ashikawa R. Traumatic intracavernous aneurysm of the internal carotid artery following surgery for chronic sinusitis. *Surg Neurol* 1980; 13:391–394.
353. Wang AN, Winfield JA, Gucer G. Traumatic internal carotid artery aneurysm with rupture into the sphenoid sinus. *Surg Neurol* 1986; 25:77–81.
354. Weaver DF, Gates EM, Neilsen AE. Traumatic intracranial vascular lesions producing late massive nasal hemorrhage. *Trans Am Acad Ophthalmol Otolaryngol* 1961; 65:759–774.
355. Weiler G, Reinhardt V, Nau HE, Gerhard L. Beitrag zum intracraniellen "traumatischen Aneurysma". *Z Rechtsmed* 1980; 85:225–233.
356. Weinstein JM, Rufenacht DA, Partington CR, et al. Delayed visual loss due to trauma of the internal carotid artery. *Arch Neurol* 1991; 48:490–497.
357. Welling RE, Taha A, Goel T, et al. Extracranial carotid artery aneurysms. *Surgery* 1983; 93:319–323.
358. Wilkins RH. Trauma-induced cerebral vasospasm. In Wilkins RH (ed): *Cerebral Arterial Spasm: Proceedings of the Second International Workshop, Amsterdam, The Netherlands.* Baltimore: Williams & Wilkins, 1980, pp 472–475.
359. Wilkins RH, Odom GL. Intracranial arterial spasm associated with craniocerebral trauma. *J Neurosurg* 1970; 32:626–633.
360. Wilson CB, Christensen FK, Subrahmanian MV. Intracranial aneurysms at the pericallosal artery bifurcation. *Am Surg* 1965; 31:386–393.
361. Winn HR. Intracranial aneurysms and MR angiography: questions and answers. *Am J Neuroradiol* 1994; 15:1617 (commentary).
362. Wolpert SM, Caplan LR. Current role of cerebral angiography in the diagnosis of cerebrovascular diseases. *Am J Roentgenol* 1992; 159:191–197.
363. Wortzman D, Tucker WS, Gershater R. Traumatic aneurysm in the posterior fossa. *Surg Neurol* 1980; 13:329–332.
364. Yamada K, Hayakawa T, Ushio Y, et al. Therapeutic occlusion of the vertebral artery for unclippable vertebral aneurysm: relationship between site of occlusion and clinical outcome. *Neurosurgery* 1984; 15:834–838.
365. Yamada S, Kindt GW, Youmans JR. Carotid artery occlusion due to nonpenetrating injury. *J Trauma* 1967; 7:333–342.
366. Yamaura A, Makino H, Hachisu H, et al. Secondary aneurysm due to arterial injury during surgical procedures. *Surg Neurol* 1978; 10:327–333.
367. Yarborough WL, Harrill JA, Alexander E Jr. Traumatic internal carotid aneurysm rupture into sphenoid sinus with angiographic demonstration. *Laryngoscope* 1963; 73:1313–1325.
368. Yashon D, Johnson AB II, Jane JA. Bilateral internal carotid artery occlusion secondary to closed head injuries. *J Neurol Neurosurg Psychiatry* 1964; 27:547–552.

369. Yokota H, Tazaki H, Murayama K, et al. [Traumatic cerebral aneurysm: 94 cases from the literature and 5 cases observed by the authors]. *No Shinkei Geka* 1983; 11:521–528.
370. Yonas H, Dujovny M. ''True'' traumatic aneurysm of the intracranial internal carotid artery: case report. *Neurosurgery* 1980; 7:499–502.
371. Yuge T, Shigemori M, Tokutomi T, et al. Diffuse axonal injury associated with multiple traumatic aneurysms of the distal anterior cerebral artery—case report. *Neurol Med Chir (Tokyo)* 1990; 30:412–416.
372. Zakrzewski A, Konopacki K, Kwaskowski A, et al. Rupture of the internal carotid artery during fracture of the cranial base. *Otolaryngol Pol* 1969; 23:685–692.
373. Zipp F, Herdt P, Goetz GF, et al. Isolierte einseitige Hypoglossvsparese bei Karotisdissektion. *Nervenarzt* 1993; 64:535–538.

280 Sequelae of Head Injury

Byron Young

Post-Traumatic Epilepsy

Post-traumatic epilepsy is divided into two types: early and late. Early post-traumatic epilepsy is characterized by one or more seizures occurring within 1 week of head injury without any other obvious causes. Seizures occurring more than 1 week after head injury are referred to as late post-traumatic epilepsy. Temkin et al. subdivided the category of early epilepsy to distinguish seizures occurring within the first 24 h from those occurring from day 2 to day 7.[42] Those occurring during the first 24 h are called immediate seizures. The most common classification, however, is that used by Jennett and adopted by most other authors (i.e., seizures are divided simply into early and late epilepsy).

Post-traumatic epilepsy is not an infrequent occurrence. An estimated 422,000 people are hospitalized for head injury each year in the United States.[20] The incidence of early epilepsy in large head injury studies ranges from 2.5 to 7 percent.[1,19] In the retrospective study by Annegers et al.[1] of a civilian population during the first year after head injury, late seizures occurred in 7.1 percent of patients. Five percent of the patients admitted to the hospital in Jennett's series of unselected head injuries developed late epilepsy.[19] On the basis of these data, between 8000 and 30,000 people in the United States each year have an early or late post-traumatic seizure.

Early Post-Traumatic Epilepsy

Risk and Characteristics of Early Epilepsy

The risk of early post-traumatic seizures is related to the type and severity of brain injury. Subdural and intracerebral hematomas are associated with a 30 to 36 percent incidence of early seizures.[18] Epidural hematomas, frontal and parietal depressed skull fractures, and brain injuries causing focal neurological signs or post-traumatic amnesia longer than 24 h are associated with an early seizure incidence of 9 to 13 percent.[9,18,19] Patients with combat missile wounds have an early seizure incidence of about 2 to 6 percent.[2,37] The incidence of early seizures in civilians who have suffered missile wounds has not been established in any large series. Only 1 to 2 percent of patients with minor head injuries and no neurological signs have an early seizure.[19]

Age also seems to be a factor in determining the susceptibility to early seizures. In Jennett's series,[19] early seizures occurred more frequently in children under 5 years of age. Early seizures more often began in the first hour and by 24 h in children than in adults.

Slightly less than one-third of early seizures occur within 1 hour of injury, one-third occur during the next 24 h, and slightly more than one-third occur during the remaining days of the first week after injury.[19] Rish and Caveness also reported that early post-traumatic seizures occur most frequently during the first 5 days after a combat head injury, with a peak incidence on the first day.[34]

Focal seizures account for approximately half of all early seizures. Most early focal seizures are focal motor seizures. Focal seizures occur more frequently after missile injuries than after blunt injuries.[19]

A generalized seizure occurring within a few moments of injury is termed *immediate epilepsy* and is distinguished by most investigators from the *early seizures* that occur more than a few seconds after injury. An immediate seizure follows a mild injury, is an infrequent occurrence, and, unlike early seizures, does not predispose to subsequent seizures.[19]

Significance of Early Epilepsy

The primary significance of early epilepsy is as an indicator of an increased risk of developing late post-traumatic seizures. Approximately 25 percent of patients with an early seizure have late seizures. This high frequency includes even mild injuries that would, in the absence of an early seizure, have only a slight risk for late seizures. The risk for late seizures is unaffected by the number or type of early seizures, except that early focal seizures in children do not increase the risk of late seizures.[19]

The occurrence of an early seizure complicates the treatment of head-injured patients. Depression of consciousness after a seizure hinders the evaluation of the patient's neurological condition. Computed tomography (CT) scans may have to be repeated to rule out the possibility of a newly developed intracranial mass lesion. Occasionally, secondary complications, such as aspiration pneumonitis, are caused by post-traumatic seizures. Eleven percent of all patients, and 22 percent of children under the age of 5, develop status epilepticus.[19] A series of 116 patients who were able to talk after a head injury but who subsequently died included two children (only mildly injured), whose sole cause of death was poorly controlled epilepsy.[35]

Late Post-Traumatic Epilepsy

Risk and Characteristics of Late Epilepsy

Although researchers have developed many experimental animal models for post-traumatic epilepsy,[29] no animal model exactly reproduces the human brain injury milieu leading to post-traumatic epilepsy. Thus, the mechanisms responsible for the development of late post-traumatic epilepsy have not yet been well elucidated. Because very few late seizures occur during the first 2 months after head injury,[19] a period of approximately 8 weeks seems to be necessary for the development of the epileptogenic focus. Some of the elements that have been suggested as causes for the development of the epileptogenic focus include (1) biochemical, electrical, and structural changes; (2) the development of pacemaker neurons; (3) decreased inhibitory controlling mechanisms; (4) biochemical deficits in acetylcholine, glutamic acid, and potassium; (5) postsynaptic hypersensitivity; (6) impairment of acid-base balance; (7) the deposition of iron salts from the hemorrhage; (8) lipid peroxidation; and (9) genetic factors.[8,13,17,25,26,28,40,43–45,47–49,51]

The severity of the head injury plays an important role in the development of late epilepsy. The incidence of post-traumatic seizures after traumatic intracranial hematoma is very high; one-fifth of patients who have suffered epidural hematomas and almost one-half of patients with subdural or intracerebral hematomas will develop late seizures.[18] The incidence of late epilepsy after depressed skull fractures depends on a wide range of factors and ranges from only 4 percent to more than 60 percent. Other associated factors, such as focal signs, dural laceration, post-traumatic amnesia longer than 24 h, or an early seizure, greatly increase the incidence of late seizures in patients with depressed fractures. In the absence of these factors, the incidence of late epilepsy is below 10 percent.[19] Approximately one-third of patients with combat missile wounds develop post-traumatic seizures.[10] Certain characteristics of the injury are important risk factors for subsequent seizures. The extent of focal damage, the association of focal damage and prolonged coma, and injuries adjacent to the central sulcus increase the incidence of late seizures. In the Vietnam War head injury series,[10,38] one-half of the patients having early seizures had late seizures.

Severe head injuries are not the only injuries that have a high association with late epilepsy. A patient with a mild injury, but having an early seizure, has a 25 percent chance of having late seizures. A mild injury alone, without significant loss of consciousness and no early epilepsy, is associated with only a 1 to 2 percent chance of late seizures. Jennett's series provides considerable data based on the features of the injury for the accurate calculation of the exact risk of the individual patient for late epilepsy.[19]

Caveness et al. and Potter have suggested that the individual's personal or constitutional make-up, such as genetic traits, may play an important role in his or her susceptibility to post-traumatic epilepsy.[10,28] The significance of these factors remains unestablished. Electroencephalography performed soon after head injury provides few reliable data to predict the risk of late seizures.[11] However, after a late seizure has occurred, focal EEG abnormalities suggest an increased risk of additional seizures.

The frequency of late seizures varies within a wide range. There may be only a single seizure, or so many that no effort is made to keep count. According to Caveness et al., once post-traumatic epilepsy is established, there is little change in the frequency of attacks.[10] Caveness et al. divided the patients in their Korean War series into three frequency patterns: those who had experienced 1 to 3, 4 to 30, or more than 30 seizures. Each of these groups comprised approximately one-third of the seizure patients. In this series, which was based on a 10-year follow-up, one-half of those patients having early seizures developed late seizures. A highly significant relationship exists between the frequency and duration of seizures. The greater the frequency of seizures, the greater the probability of persistence.

Mechanisms of Late Post-Traumatic Epilepsy

Surgical specimens removed to control post-traumatic epilepsy show neuronal and oligodendroglial loss, gliosis, and hemosiderosis. The epileptogenic focus is adjacent to the injury site. The hyperirritable epileptogenic focus may be caused by mechanical stress or by long-standing localized ischemia.[17] Tower and Elliot demonstrated that an epileptogenic focus has biochemical defects in acetylcholine, glutamic acid, and potassium metabolism.[43,44] Schmidt et al. attributed the burst of autonomous electrical activity in the epileptogenic focus to a dendritic depolarization and the difference in potential between the cell body and the dendritic network.[40] Westrum et al. proposed that the decreased synaptic endings or dendrites within the epileptogenic focus permit post-synaptic hypersensitivity.[45] Gliotic changes may also impair the glial control of acid-base balance and allow an excessive excitability of adjacent neurons.[26]

Post-traumatic epilepsy is characterized by a latency period between the time of the trauma and the appearance of the first seizure. The brain injury presumably sets into motion a series of biochemical, electrical, and structural changes that lead to the development of an epileptogenic focus.[30] The time for development of the epileptogenic focus in humans is about 8 weeks. Late seizures make their appearance after this incubation phase. In Jennett's series, the seizure incidence during the first week after head injury is 30 times the incidence in any one of the seven subsequent weeks.[19]

Post-Traumatic Epilepsy: Prophylaxis Clinical Trials

Many clinical and laboratory investigations suggest that administering antiepileptics as a prophylactic measure will reduce the incidence of post-traumatic epilepsy. Young[52] and Temkin et al.[42] provide reviews of these reports. Some early clinical trials indicated that administering a prophylactic antiepileptic drug reduced the incidence of late seizures, but these trials were not well designed. More recent and better controlled studies do not support this conclusion.

Prophylaxis must be distinguished from treatment or suppression of an established epileptogenic focus. To be considered successful as *prophylaxis*, the antiepileptic regimen must prevent the development of the epileptogenic focus and consequent seizures. Once this has been accomplished, the administration of the prophylactic agent can cease after 2 or 3 months with significantly less risk of seizure occurrence. By contrast, successful *treatment* suppresses the electrical activity of the developed epileptogenic focus so that seizures do not occur. Seizures are still likely in this setting, however, if the antiepileptic drug is withdrawn.

Prophylaxis of Early Post-Traumatic Epilepsy

Young et al.[54] performed a randomized, double-blinded, placebo-controlled study to determine whether administering phenytoin soon after injury decreased the incidence of epilepsy in the first week after severe head injury. Two hundred forty-four patients were randomized into two groups and were given either phenytoin or a placebo. The patients in the phenytoin group were given the drug within 24 h of being admitted to the hospital. At 1, 3, and 7 days after injury, plasma concentrations of at least 10 μg/ml had been achieved in more than 78 percent of the phenytoin patients. No significant difference was found in the percentage of patients in either group who had early seizures ($p = 0.99$), nor was there a significant difference between the treated and placebo groups in the interval from injury to first seizure ($p = 0.41$). The early administration of phenytoin was not effective as prophylaxis in reducing the occurrence of seizures in the first week after head injury. The authors therefore recommended that antiepileptic drugs be administered as prophylaxis only after an early seizure has occurred.

Temkin et al.[41] performed a double-blinded, placebo-controlled study of 404 severely head-injured patients who were determined to be at high risk for the development of post-traumatic seizures. Patients were randomly assigned to receive either phenytoin or a placebo. The intent of the study was to obtain and maintain high therapeutic levels of serum phenytoin in the treated patients. These patients received an initial loading dose of phenytoin within the first 24 h after injury. Results demonstrated that the phenytoin group had a cumulative early seizure rate of 3.6 ± 1.3 percent, whereas 14.2 ± 2.6 percent of the placebo group had seizures. The authors found a significant difference between the placebo and the prophylactic phenytoin groups and concluded that phenytoin reduced the risk of early seizures by 73 percent. The authors did not, however, make specific recommendations as to whether phenytoin should be administered prophylactically to prevent early seizures.

Prophylaxis of Late Post-Traumatic Epilepsy

Many patients make an excellent recovery from head injuries but retain a significant disability because of post-traumatic seizures. Late post-traumatic epilepsy has considerably more severe medical, economic, social, and psychological consequences than early post-traumatic epilepsy. Late post-traumatic seizures greatly lessen the chance for gainful employment after rehabilitation.

A large body of experimental evidence suggests that antiepileptic prophylaxis tends to prevent epilepsy induced by a variety of epileptogenic causes.[31,55] However, the evidence from older clinical studies testing the efficacy of prophylaxis for late post-traumatic seizures is conflicting and, by modern standards, is fraught with methodologic deficiencies.[4,10,16,27,50,53,56] The rationale for prophylactic administration of antiepileptic drugs is to prevent or to arrest the progression of the development of the epileptogenic focus.

Of the patients in the series reported by Temkin et al.[41] (followed for up to 2 years), no significant difference in the seizure rates could be demonstrated between the phenytoin and the placebo patients. Twenty-seven percent of the patients treated with phenytoin and 21 percent of the patients given a placebo developed late post-traumatic seizures. Temkin et al. could not demonstrate that phenytoin is effective as a prophylaxis against late post-traumatic epilepsy. Of the patients who could be followed, 70 percent had therapeutic phenytoin levels at their subsequent clinic visits. By the end of the first year, 21 percent of the phenytoin group and 15 percent of the control group had experienced late seizures. At the end of 2 years, 27 percent of the phenytoin group and 21 percent of the control group had suffered seizures.

Young et al.[55] performed a randomized, double-blinded, placebo-controlled study of 179 patients to determine whether administering phenytoin soon after head injury would decrease the incidence of late post-traumatic epilepsy. Patients in the study were followed for 18 months to detect the occurrence of seizures and to serially measure concentrations of plasma phenytoin. No significant difference in the percentage of late seizures was found between the treated and placebo groups ($p = 0.75$), nor was there a significant difference between the two groups in the amount of time between injury and seizures. The results of this study demonstrated that low therapeutic ranges of phenytoin provided no prophylaxis against late post-traumatic seizures.

Because Young et al. found that no patients with phenytoin plasma concentrations of 12 μg/ml or higher had a seizure, they could not conclude that higher therapeutic plasma concentrations of phenytoin and higher compliance rates would not have significantly decreased the occurrence of post-traumatic epilepsy.[55] In the study by Temkin et al.,[41] 7 of 9 patients receiving phenytoin had therapeutic levels on the day of their first seizure, which provides even stronger evidence that phenytoin does not prevent the development of late post-traumatic seizures.

Combined Analysis

Temkin et al.[42] reviewed four studies of prophylactic administration of antiepileptics to prevent early and late post-traumatic epilepsy. The authors concluded that the studies by Young et al.[55] and Temkin et al.[41] were compatible and, when combined, showed an estimated decrease in early seizures of 64 percent. This analysis of late-seizure studies estimated that phenytoin contributed to a 10 percent increase in late-seizure incidence.

Recommendations for Prophylaxis and Treatment

Considering the available data, we cannot recommend the prophylactic administration of phenytoin to prevent either early or late seizures. If an early seizure occurs, however, phenytoin should be administered intravenously in an attempt to prevent subsequent seizures. Phenytoin should be given for approximately 10 days and then discontinued. No prophylaxis should be given to prevent late post-traumatic seizures; such prophylaxis is not justified on the basis of the evidence obtained in well-controlled studies of late-seizure prophylaxis. If a late seizure occurs, an antiepileptic drug (e.g., phenytoin, valproate, or carbamazepine) should be administered. Treatment should be initiated after the first seizure, because late post-traumatic seizures are likely to be multiple. The duration of treatment for patients with late post-traumatic seizures should follow the principles for treatment of all late seizures, regardless of their cause.

Other drugs, such as phenobarbital or valproate, have not been adequately tested to justify their prophylactic administration. A trial being conducted at the National Institute of Neurological Disorders and Stroke (NINDS) is testing whether prophylactically administered valproate reduces the incidence of late post-traumatic epilepsy.

Resection of the epileptogenic focus is rarely required to control post-traumatic seizures intractable to medical management. Late post-traumatic seizures tend to diminish with time, and surgery should not be performed for at least 2 years after the injury. The general principles of the surgical treatment of post-traumatic epilepsy are the same as those for surgical treatment of other focal seizures. Rasmussen's classic report indicated that 40 percent of patients become seizure-free after surgery, 26 percent have a significant reduction in seizure frequency, and 35 percent have no or only a moderate reduction in seizure frequency.[31]

Postconcussion Syndrome

The term ''postconcussion syndrome'' refers to a variety of symptoms including headache, dizziness, forgetfulness, anxiety, irritability, and impaired concentration, which occur after minor head injury.[6,12,21] Minor head injury is generally defined as a Glasgow Coma Scale (GCS) score of 13 to 15. Patients within this range, however, may have a normal CT scan or skull films, or may have associated lesions such as skull fracture or brain hemorrhage or contusion. Patients with such associated lesions perform significantly worse on tests of verbal fluency and speed of information processing.[46] The duration of the postconcussion syndrome is usually 1 to 6 months.[14] Middle-aged patients appear to have more postconcussion symptoms and longer duration of the syndrome than young patients.[15] Levin et al.[22] found that one-fourth of moderately and severely injured patients had long-term memory impairments, although intelligence test scores were in the normal range. These authors demonstrated that the GCS score, duration of disturbed consciousness, nonreactive pupils, and oculocephalic/oculovestibular disturbance were significant predictors of prolonged memory impairment.

There are widely differing opinions about the cause of the postconcussion syndrome. This etiologic controversy and the dilemma for the physician faced with the treatment of an individual patient focuses on whether the symptoms are a psychological consequence of a seemingly trivial head injury, whether they are caused by structural damage associated with a minor head injury, or whether they are caused by a combination of both factors.

Post-traumatic headaches are characterized by their variability.[6] The headaches range from mild to excruciatingly severe, steady to intermittent, throbbing to dull, burning to pressure-like, and generalized to localized. Common causative factors are change in posture, stress, fatigue, or effort. Temporary respite can usually be obtained by rest or simple analgesics. The characteristics of the headache do not seem to be related to the length of persistence of the headache after the injury. However, headaches lasting longer than 2 months are commonly accompanied by dizziness, anxiety, fatigability, and impaired concentration.

Post-traumatic dizziness is intermittent, with each episode usually lasting a few minutes.[12] A change in posture commonly initiates the attack, but stress is occasionally also a precipitating factor. The severity and frequency of attacks are highly variable. The symptoms usually subside with recumbency with the eyes closed.

Brenner et al. studied 200 patients who were hospitalized for a minor head injury and who were followed for 6 months or more.[6] Sixty-nine percent of their patients complained of headache at some time after injury. Thirty-two percent of the patients (slightly less than one-half of those with headaches) had headaches for more than 2 months. Prolonged headaches occurred more often in patients with neurotic symptoms before injury, occupational difficulties, pending litigation, immediate emotional reaction to the injury, and scalp laceration. Prolonged headaches occurred infrequently after very mild injury or recreational accidents.

Fifty-one percent of these patients had dizziness at some time after injury. Thirty-four percent of the total group (70 percent of the patients with dizziness) had dizziness persisting after discharge from the hospital. Twenty-three percent of the total group had dizziness lasting for more than 2 months. About three-fourths of patients having dizziness also had headaches; likewise, a similar proportion of those with headaches had dizziness. Dizziness persisting longer than 2 months was associated with neurosis or nervousness before the injury, anxiety, fatigability, impaired memory after hospitalization, occupational difficulties, pending litigation, retrograde amnesia, postoperative amnesia, disorientation, and definite loss of consciousness. True vertigo was much less common than dizziness. Only 6 percent of the patients in this series had true vertigo at some time after injury, but vertigo tended to be more persistent than dizziness.

In a study by Rimel et al.,[32] minor head injury was defined as cranial trauma with loss of consciousness for 20 min or less and an admission GCS score of 13 or higher. Three months after injury, 78 percent of their patients complained of persistent headache. A change in memory was noted by 59 percent of the patients. Fourteen percent reported difficulties with the activities of daily life. Only one-sixth of the patients had no complaints. Mild neuropsychological impairment was detected in most patients tested 3 months after injury. One-third of the patients who were employed before the injury were not employed 3 months after injury.

Brenner et al.[6] and Friedman et al.[12] concluded that both physical and psychological factors are important in persistent post-traumatic headache and dizziness. The symptoms lasting only a few days or weeks are often due to local scalp injury or subtle structural brain injury or dysfunction.

The treatment of most patients with symptoms after mild injury depends on the duration, severity, and type of symptoms. Most patients need no treatment other than encouragement and the passage of a little time to resume work and the normal activities of daily life. When disabling symptoms persist for more than 2 or 3 months, continued encouragement by the treating neurosurgeon often must be supplemented by psychiatric evaluation and occupational rehabilitative programs. Evoked sensory potential testing, electroencephalography, CT scanning of the brain, and neuropsychological testing may be helpful in separating psychiatric and structural factors contributing to persistent symptoms. Mild analgesics, medication for vertigo and dizziness, and antidepressant or antianxiety drugs may be helpful. Fortunately, the postconcussion syndrome almost always resolves with the passage of time. In some cases, cessation of symptoms occurs only after the settlement of litigation.

Intellectual Impairment

The Glasgow outcome scale is widely used to grade overall recovery and adjustment to daily life after head injury. Only a few studies have been published, however, that precisely quantify intellectual and psychological recovery after severe closed head injury. Levin et al. evaluated the neuropsychological recovery of patients with severe head injuries.[23] They classified the injury as severe when the initial GCS score was 8 or less. Of the 27 patients selected for their study, 10 made a good recovery, 12 were moderately disabled, and 5 were severely disabled. The study included only patients who could be tested, that is, those who improved beyond a persistent vegetative state. The median follow-up exceeded a year, and the minimum follow-up was 6 months. This study showed that patients attaining a good recovery level on the Glasgow outcome scale ''recovered to within one standard deviation of the population mean (100) on both the Verbal and Performance Scales of the WAIS, that is, no patient had an IQ below 85.'' Patients with a good recovery had median verbal IQ scores of 94 and performance scores of 100; moderately disabled patients had a median verbal IQ of 90 and a median performance IQ of 88; severely disabled patients had a median verbal IQ of 66 and a median performance IQ of 60. The verbal IQ was not statistically different between patients achieving a good outcome and those having a moderately disabled outcome, but the performance IQ was significantly lower in the latter patients.

In the study by Levin et al.,[23] long-term memory storage was impaired in 10 percent of patients with a good recovery (only 1 patient of 10), in one-third of moderately disabled patients, and in all severely disabled patients. Approximately one-third of the patients had a deficit in memory storage or retrieval. Speech deficits were confined to moderate and severely disabled patients. Writing impairment was confined to severely disabled patients.

The study of neuropsychiatric symptoms and signs by Levin et al.[23] tested for disordered thinking, hostility-suspicion, withdrawal-retardation, and anxietal depression. Disorders in these areas were infrequent in patients with a good recovery, but behavioral disturbances were very common in moderately and severely disabled patients. Two-thirds of the patients had chronic disability.

Only one-fifth returned to full-time employment. Levin et al. suggested that a characteristic pattern of neuropsychological and psychiatric deficits are responsible for the chronic disability seen after severe closed head injury. The characteristic pattern includes impairment in performance IQ, memory, and retrieval of names, as well as behavioral changes such as thinking disturbance and withdrawal-retardation. These sequelae were minimal in patients with a good recovery. Moderately disabled patients varied widely in neuropsychological impairments, and severely disabled patients uniformly had marked neurobehavioral disturbances.

Scherzer et al.[39] showed that severe brain injury causes deficits in abstract thinking when the individual is questioned so that preexisting overlearned or automatic knowledge is not tested. Additionally, this group detected no differences in abstract thinking between patients with predominantly left or right hemisphere damage.

In the study by Rimel et al.[33] of moderate head injury, which was defined as a GCS score of 9 to 12 at 6 h after admission to the hospital, 93 percent of the patients had headaches and 90 percent had memory impairment at 3 months after injury. Forty-two percent had multiple subjective problems. Although 38 percent were categorized as having a good recovery at 3 months, only 4 percent were asymptomatic and only 31 percent were employed. Only 69 percent of those employed before injury were working 3 months after injury. The significant predictor of employment was not a premorbid factor, such as age, education, and socioeconomic status, but was the severity of injury. Twenty-one percent of the patients in this study were chronically unemployed, and 21 percent were unskilled laborers. Some alcohol was present in the blood of 73 percent of the patients, and 53 percent were intoxicated. Forty-two percent had had a previous head injury. Definite neuropsychological impairment was shown by the Halstead-Reitan neuropsychological test battery in these patients. The proportion of patients scoring beyond the standard cutoff scores for the normal range ranged from 34 to 66 percent.

The minimum time from injury to full recovery depends on the severity of injury. In Becker's study of mild head injury, substantial recovery occurred by 11 weeks.[3] The study by Bond and Brooks of severe closed head injuries suggests that the largest part of recovery occurs within 6 months.[5] Considerable individual variations in recovery rate occur and are dependent on age, neurological findings, and preinjury ability.[21] Rosenbaum et al. indicate that significant improvement in motor function, overall functional state, and (to a lesser extent) intellectual function can occur in some cases for as long as 3 years.[36]

Rehabilitation

Although the efficacy of rehabilitation services has been difficult to demonstrate,[7,24] rehabilitation efforts are generally accepted as the standard of care. Current efforts at rehabilitation are more extensively employed, more intense, more sophisticated, and more comprehensive than just a few years ago. A large amount of information is now available, however, about the cognitive and behavioral sequelae of head injury and the patterns and extent of recovery.

Rehabilitation efforts should commence as soon as practical after head injury. The rehabilitation team should consist of a physiatrist, clinical psychologist, physical therapist, speech therapist, occupational therapist, and social worker. The neurosurgeon usually serves as a consultant but ideally should be an active participant in a rehabilitation program. The neurosurgeon's attendance at rounds and conferences, even if only once a month, can improve the rehabilitation effort and provide an important educational service to other members of the rehabilitation team. A psychiatrist is also an essential consultant.

The importance of counseling for the family cannot be overemphasized. Misunderstanding and outright refusal to accept the effects of the head injury on a loved one are frequent. Carefully informing the family about realistic recovery rates and probable eventual outcome enhances the relationship between the family and the injured individual and fosters confidence and respect for the personnel attempting rehabilitation.

Some programs do accept for rehabilitation those patients who are still unconscious, but most allow entry into their program only after a potential for retraining is established, such as verbal or performance IQ test scores of at least 80. Programs accepting comatose patients can aid the family in tracheostomy care, nasogastric tube feeding, bladder care, and coping with the emotional and economic effects of the head injury. Individuals with potential for retraining are entered into programs that are designed to permit reemployment, or at least an independent daily life. Cognitive retraining, vocational rehabilitation, and management of behavioral or family problems form the mainstay of the rehabilitation program.

The study by Bond and Brooks[5] shows that verbal skills recover more rapidly than nonverbal skills, that the severity of injury is the significant determinant of outcome, that severely injured individuals reach their final level of outcome sooner than less injured persons, that older patients are left with greater disability than younger patients, and that psychosocial factors have an important influence on recovery.

References

1. Annegers JF, Grabow JD, Groover RV, et al. Seizures after head trauma: a population study. *Neurology* 1980; 30:683–689.
2. Ascroft PB. Traumatic epilepsy after gunshot wounds of the head. *Br Med J* 1941; 1:739–744.
3. Becker B. Intellectual changes after closed head injury. *J Clin Psychol* 1975; 31:307–309.
4. Birkmayer von W. Die Behandlung der traumatischen Epilepsie. *Wien Klin Wochenschr* 1951; 63:606–609.
5. Bond MR, Brooks DN. Understanding the process of recovery as a basis for the investigation of rehabilitation for the brain injured. *Scand J Rehabil Med* 1976; 8:127–133.
6. Brenner C, Friedman AP, Merritt HH, Denny-Brown DE. Post-traumatic headache. *J Neurosurg* 1944; 1:379–391.
7. Brooks N, McKinlay W, Symington C, et al. Return to work within the first seven years of severe head injury. *Brain Inj* 1987; 1:5–19.
8. Caveness WF. Epilepsy, a product of trauma in our time. *Epilepsia* 1976; 17:207–215.
9. Caveness WF, Liss HR. Incidence of post-traumatic epilepsy. *Epilepsia* 1961; 2:123–129.
10. Caveness WF, Meirowsky AM, Rish BL, et al. The nature of posttraumatic epilepsy. *J Neurosurg* 1979; 50:545–553.
11. Courjon J. A longitudinal electro-clinical study of 80 cases of post-traumatic epilepsy observed from the time of the original trauma. *Epilepsia* 1970; 11:29–36.
12. Friedman AP, Brenner C, Denny-Brown D. Post-traumatic vertigo and dizziness. *J Neurosurg* 1945; 2:36–46.
13. Goldensohn ES, Ward AA Jr. Pathogenesis of epileptic seizures. In Tower DB (ed): *The Nervous System,* vol 2, *The Clinical Neurosciences.* New York: Raven Press, 1975, pp 249–260.

14. Goldstein FC, Levin HS. Postconcussion syndrome and neurobehavioral disorders. In Barrow DL (ed): *Complications and Sequelae of Head Injury.* Park Ridge, IL: American Association of Neurological Surgeons, 1992, pp 133–148.
15. Gronwall D. Cumulative and persisting effects of concussion on attention and cognition. In Levin HS, Eisenberg HM, Benton AL (eds): *Mild Head Injury.* New York: Oxford University Press, 1989, pp 153–162.
16. Hoff von H, Hoff H. Fortschritte in der Behandlung der Epilepsie. *Monatschr Psychiat Neurol* 1947; 114:105–118.
17. Jasper HH. Physiopathological mechanisms of post-traumatic epilepsy. *Epilepsia* 1970; 11:73–80.
18. Jennett B. Epilepsy and acute traumatic intracranial haematoma. *J Neurol Neurosurg Psychiatry* 1975; 38:378–381.
19. Jennett B. *Epilepsy after Non-Missile Head Injuries,* 2d ed. Chicago: Year Book, 1975.
20. Kalsbeck WD, McLaurin RL, Harris BSH III, Miller JD. The National Head and Spinal Cord Injury Survey: major findings. *J Neurosurg* 1980; 53 (11 Suppl):519–531.
21. Levin HS, Benton AL, Grossman RG. *Neurobehavioral Consequences of Closed Head Injury.* New York: Oxford University Press, 1982.
22. Levin HS, Goldstein FC, High WM Jr, Eisenberg HM. Disproportionately severe memory deficit in relation to normal intellectual functioning after closed head injury. *J Neurol Neurosurg Psychiatry* 1988; 51:1294–1301.
23. Levin HS, Grossman RG, Rose JE, Teasdale G. Long-term neuropsychological outcome of closed head injury. *J Neurosurg* 1979; 50:412–422.
24. Malec JF. Ethics in brain injury rehabilitation: existential choices among western cultural beliefs. *Brain Inj* 1993; 7:383–400.
25. Penfield W, Erickson TC. *Epilepsy and Cerebral Localization.* Springfield, IL: Charles C Thomas, 1941, pp 3–7.
26. Pollen DA, Trachtenberg MC. Neuroglia: gliosis and focal epilepsy. *Science* 1970; 167:1252–1253 (abstr).
27. Popek K. Preventive treatment of post-traumatic epilepsy following severe brain injury. *Cesk Neurol* 1972; 35:169–174.
28. Potter JM. The personal factor in the maturation of epileptogenic brain scars: review and hypothesis. *J Neurol Neurosurg Psychiatry* 1978; 41:265–271.
29. Purpura DP, Penry JK, Woodbury DM, et al. *Experimental Models of Epilepsy: A Manual for the Laboratory Worker.* New York: Raven Press, 1972.
30. Rapport RL II, Ojemann GA. Prophylactically administered phenytoin: effects on the development of chronic cobalt-induced epilepsy in the cat. *Arch Neurol* 1975; 32:539–548.
31. Rasmussen T. Surgical therapy of post-traumatic epilepsy. In Walker AE, Caveness WF, Critchley M (eds): *The Late Effects of Head Injury.* Springfield, IL: Charles C Thomas, 1969, pp 277–305.
32. Rimel RW, Giordani B, Barth JT, et al. Disability caused by minor head injury. *Neurosurgery* 1981; 9:221–228.
33. Rimel RW, Giordani B, Barth JT, Jane JA. Moderate head injury: completing the clinical spectrum of brain trauma. *Neurosurgery* 1982; 11:344–351.
34. Rish BL, Caveness WF. Relation of prophylactic medication to the occurrence of early seizures following craniocerebral trauma. *J Neurosurg* 1973; 38:155–158.
35. Rose J, Valtonen S, Jennett B. Avoidable factors contributing to death after head injury. *Br Med J* 1977; 2:615–617.
36. Rosenbaum M, Lipsitz N, Abraham J, Najenson T. A description of an intensive treatment project for the rehabilitation of severely brain-injured soldiers. *Scand J Rehabil Med* 1978; 10:1–6.
37. Russell WR, Whitty CWM. Studies in traumatic epilepsy: I. Factors influencing the incidence of epilepsy after brain wounds. *J Neurol Neurosurg Psychiatry* 1952; 15:93–98.
38. Salazar AM, Jabbari B, Vance SC, et al. Epilepsy after penetrating head injury. I. Clinical correlates: a report of the Vietnam Head Injury Study. *Neurology* 1985; 35:1406–1414.
39. Scherzer BP, Charbonneau S, Solomon CR, Lepore F. Abstract thinking following severe traumatic brain injury. *Brain Inj* 1993; 7:411–423.
40. Schmidt RP, Thomas LB, Ward AA Jr. The hyper-excitable neurone: micro-electrode studies of chronic epileptic foci in the monkey. *J Neurophysiol* 1959; 22:285–296.
41. Temkin NR, Dikmen SS, Wilensky AJ, et al: A randomized, double-blind study of phenytoin for the prevention of post-traumatic seizures. *N Engl J Med* 1990; 323:497–502.
42. Temkin NR, Dikmen SS, Winn HR. Management of head injury: post-traumatic seizures. *Neurosurg Clin North Am* 1991; 2:425–435.
43. Tower DB. *Neurochemistry of Epilepsy: Seizure Mechanisms and Their Management.* Springfield, IL: Charles C Thomas, 1960.
44. Tower DB, Elliott KAC. Activity of acetylcholine system in human epileptogenic focus. *J Appl Physiol* 1952; 4:669–676.
45. Westrum LE, White LE, Ward AA Jr. Morphology of the experimental epileptic focus. *J Neurosurg* 1964; 21:1033–1046.
46. Williams DH, Levin HS, Eisenberg HM. Mild head injury classification. *Neurosurgery* 1990; 27:422–428.
47. Willmore LJ, Rubin JJ. The effect of tocopherol and dimethyl sulfoxide on focal edema and lipid peroxidation induced by isocortical injection of ferrous chloride. *Brain Res* 1984; 296:389–392.
48. Willmore LJ, Sypert GW, Munson JB. Recurrent seizures induced by cortical iron injection: a model of posttraumatic epilepsy. *Ann Neurol* 1978; 4:329–336.
49. Willmore LJ, Triggs WJ. Effect of phenytoin and corticosteroids on seizures and lipid peroxidation in experimental posttraumatic epilepsy. *J Neurosurg* 1984; 60:467–472.
50. Wohns RNW, Wyler AR. Prophylactic phenytoin in severe head injuries. *J Neurosurg* 1979; 51:507–509.
51. Wyler AR, Ray MW. Anticonvulsant prophylaxis against posttraumatic seizures. *Contemp Neurosurg* 1985; 7:1–6.
52. Young B. Post-traumatic epilepsy. In Youmans JR (ed): *Neurological Surgery: A Comprehensive Reference Guide to the Diagnosis and Management of Neurosurgical Problems,* 3d ed. Philadelphia: Saunders, 1990, pp 2243–2249.
53. Young B, Rapp R, Brooks WH, et al. Posttraumatic epilepsy prophylaxis. *Epilepsia* 1979; 20:671–681.
54. Young B, Rapp RP, Norton JA, et al. Failure of prophylactically administered phenytoin to prevent early posttraumatic seizures. *J Neurosurg* 1983; 58:231–235.
55. Young B, Rapp RP, Norton JA, et al. Failure of prophylactically administered phenytoin to prevent late posttraumatic seizures. *J Neurosurg* 1983; 58:236–241.
56. Zervit Z, Musil F. Prophylactic treatment of posttraumatic epilepsy: results of a long-term follow-up in Czechoslovakia. *Epilepsia* 1981; 22:315–320.

SECTION C

Spinal Trauma

281

Pathophysiology and Pathology of Spinal Cord Injury

Charles H. Tator

Recently, there has been a great expansion of knowledge of the pathophysiology of acute spinal cord injury due to a large number of basic investigations of the injury process in experimental models. The knowledge gained from experimentation supplements many excellent pathologic descriptions of human spinal cord injuries[31,58] which have been shown to occur in a variety of circumstances involving diverse injury mechanisms including compression, concussion, stretch, and others. Thus, there is merit in having available a wide variety of experimental models to simulate the human condition. One of the most remarkable findings based on the models has been the similarity among the models regarding the acute pathophysiology which suggests that there are similar basic processes underlying all types of acute spinal cord injury. There are also similarities in the pathologic findings among the various experimental models and also between the models and human spinal cord injury, highlighting the rule that there are fundamental injury processes. It is important to note that many, if not all, of these fundamental processes are also common to brain injury, cerebral ischemia, subarachnoid hemorrhage, and spinal cord injury. A knowledge of these common and fundamental pathophysiologic processes is helpful for understanding the pathology. This chapter will emphasize the fundamental injury processes and will synthesize the results from clinical and experimental studies.

Pathophysiology of Acute Spinal Cord Injury

Primary and Secondary Injury Mechanisms

One of the most important experimental and clinical observations of spinal cord injury is that the pathologic appearance of the lesion changes dramatically during the first few days after injury. To explain this evolution, investigators have provided strong evidence that the injury process includes primary and secondary mechanisms of injury. Human spinal cord injury can result from a variety of primary injury mechanisms as shown in Table 281-1. The most common mechanism is the combination of impact plus persisting compression. This combination of mechanical forces occurs in a variety of mechanisms of injury including burst fractures, fracture-dislocations, missile injuries, and ruptured discs. Impact alone, without persisting compression, occurs with injuries such as hyperextension of the spine in cervical spondylosis which momentarily compresses the cord between a bulging disc or osteocartilaginous bar anteriorly and an infolded ligamentum flavum posteriorly. Spinal column dislocation can occur during hyperflexion especially in children with lax ligaments and underdeveloped paraspinal musculature. This type of injury is one of the mechanisms of spinal cord injury without radiologic abnormality (SCIWORA) that occurs more frequently in children and adolescents,[42] but also occurs in adults. More common in adults, especially those with cervical spondylosis, is the syndrome of spinal cord injury without radiologic evidence of trauma (SCIWORET).[52] Laceration of the cord, with or without dural laceration, can occur from sharp bone fragments or severe distraction. Missile injuries can produce a combination of laceration, compression, and concussion.[31] Cord lacerations can occur to varying degrees up to total transection.

TABLE 281-1 Primary Mechanisms of Human Spinal Cord Injury

Mechanical Force	Mechanism of Injury
Impact plus persisting compression	Burst fracture
	Fracture-dislocation
	Disc rupture
Impact alone (temporary compression)	Hyperextension
Distraction	Hyperflexion
Laceration, transection	Burst fracture
	Laminar fracture
	Fracture-dislocation
	Missile

Experimental models of acute cord injury have been developed which simulate almost all of these mechanisms of human cord injury. The most popular model has been the weight-drop model introduced in 1911 by Allen[1] that causes impact alone without significant persisting compression since the weight is usually removed quickly. Several models of impact plus persisting compression have been developed including the author's acute extradural clip compression technique.[44] There are several comprehensive reviews of experimental models of spinal cord injury.[26,51]

The concept of the secondary mechanism of injury was first postulated by Allen[1] in 1911 when he found that myelotomy and removal of the post-traumatic hematomyelia in the central aspect of the injured dog cord resulted in improvement of neurological function after weight-drop injury. He theorized that there was a noxious agent present in the hemorrhagic necrotic material which caused further damage to the cord. He concluded that

> The physiology of the beneficial action of this means was ascribed to a draining of the cord at this point of blood and serum and thereby not only preventing the pressure of this exudate on the nerve elements but also removing what would in time, through chemical change, give rise to a biochemical irritation with destruction of tissue.[2]

This process, which was later termed autodestruction by Nemecek,[41] has been the subject of much experimental work, but has still not been fully elucidated. Since 1911, numerous injurious pathophysiologic processes have been discovered[3] as listed in Table 281-2 and illustrated diagrammatically in Fig. 281-1. Similar theories have been postulated to explain the progressive damage in head injury, cerebral ischemia, and subarachnoid hemorrhage.

TABLE 281-2 Secondary Injury Mechanisms Involved in the Pathophysiology of Spinal Cord Injury

Systemic Effects (Neurogenic Shock)
Heart rate—brief increase, then prolonged bradycardia
Blood pressure—brief hypertension, then prolonged hypotension
Peripheral resistance—decreased
Cardiac output—decreased
Catecholamines—increased, then decreased
Local Vascular Damage of the Cord Microcirculation—Initial and Progressive
Mechanical disruption of capillaries and venules
Hemorrhage—especially gray matter
Loss of microcirculation—mechanical, thrombosis, vasospasm
Reduction of spinal cord blood flow—thrombosis, vasospasm
Loss of autoregulation
Biochemical Changes
Excitotoxicity—glutamate
Neurotransmitter accumulation
Catecholamines—noradrenaline, dopamine
Arachidonic acid release
Free radical production
Eicosanoid production
Prostaglandins
Lipid peroxidation
Endogenous opioids
Cytokines
Electrolyte Shifts
Increased intracellular calcium
Increased extracellular potassium
Increased intracellular sodium
Edema
Loss of Energy Metabolism
Decreased adenosine triphosphate production

Systemic Effects of Acute Spinal Cord Injury—Neurogenic Shock

Spinal cord injury is one of the causes of neurogenic shock—the magnitude of which is directly related to the level and severity of the injury. Complete cervical injuries cause the greatest systemic changes including bradycardia and hypotension which may be profound initially and prolonged for days to months after the injury. Peripheral resistance and cardiac output may also remain depressed for long periods. Neurogenic shock in spinal cord injury (see Kiss and Tator[36] for a recent review) is due to a combination of decreased sympathetic tone, unopposed cardiac vagotonia, and possible secondary changes in the heart.[29] During the acute management of patients with spinal cord injury it is important to be aware of these systemic effects, because failure to treat neurogenic shock may worsen the other pathophysiologic effects described below.

Local Vascular Damage to the Cord Microcirculation

One of the strikingly common and dramatic effects of spinal cord injury in all experimental models and in human cord injury is the early and often progressive development of hemorrhages in the central region of the injured cord, especially in the gray matter (Figs. 281-2 and 281-3). Certainly, there is direct mechanical disruption of capillaries and venules and some arterioles due to the initial mechanical force of injury and distortion of tissue by impact, compression, stretching, or laceration.[19] However, the hemorrhagic effects may be progressive as seen in experimental studies which have shown in severe cases that hemorrhaging can continue for hours. One of the remarkable findings is the usual sparing of the large vessels such as the anterior spinal artery and the anterior sulcal arteries from direct mechanical damage. Angiographic studies in humans and microangiographic studies experimentally have consistently shown patency of the large arterioles and arteries.[37–39,51] The major loss of the microcirculation involves the capillaries and venules not only at the injury site, but spreading for a considerable distance rostrally and caudally (Figs. 281-4 and 281-5). Also of great importance is the progressive nature of these changes over time as demonstrated by serial measurements of spinal cord blood flow. Progressive post-traumatic ischemia has been shown in a variety of injury models with several different blood flow techniques and in several species ranging from rats to primates (see Tator[51] and Tator and Fehlings[53]). Another interesting feature of these studies has been the spatial relationship between the hemorrhagic and ischemic zones which highlights the early views of Allen that there may be an injurious "biochemical irritation" unleashed by the hemorrhagic necrotic zone.[2] In addition to a direct mechanical cause of vasospasm, a number of potential biochemical factors have been investigated as the possible noxious agent on the microcirculation including catecholamines, glutamate, and prostaglandins.[51,53] Vasospasm has recently been conclusively demonstrated after experimental spinal

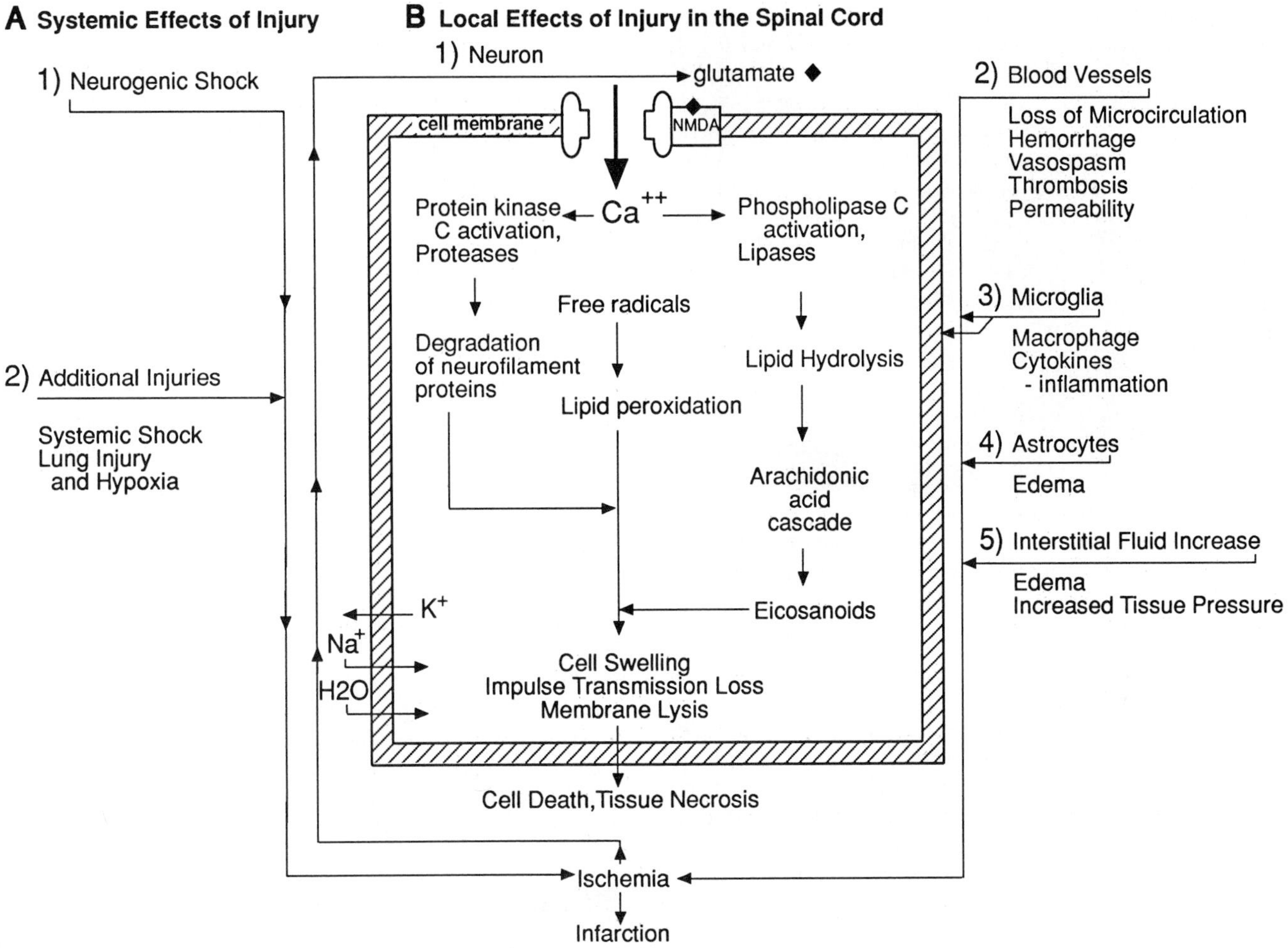

Figure 281-1 Schema of pathophysiologic events after acute spinal cord injury. Physical trauma directly affects the individual components of the spinal cord (B 1–5) including neurons, blood vessels, microglial cells, and astrocytes and also has systemic (A 1 and 2) or general effects due to any accompanying neurogenic or systemic shock, hypoxia, or other complication. The secondary neuronal effects are emphasized in this diagram and in the center a single neuron is depicted bounded by its cell membrane. Although there are numerous types of receptors on the surface of neurons, axons, astrocytes, and other cells in the spinal cord and its blood vessels, for simplicity, only the NMDA receptor is shown. The excitotoxic series of events begins with an increase in extracellular glutamate with subsequent glutamate activation of the NMDA receptor in the neuronal cell membrane which in turn opens the receptor-dependent NMDA channel resulting in a marked influx of calcium ions (sodium also). Increased intracellular calcium in turn activates calcium-dependent enzymes such as phospholipase C and protein kinase C with subsequent cellular events which ultimately produce cell lysis and tissue necrosis. The interrelationships between the systemic, neuronal, and vascular events are stressed with the final results being cell death, tissue necrosis, and post-traumatic infarction. For example, vasoactive prostaglandins produced as a result of the arachidonic acid cascade may in turn affect the adjacent blood vessels to produce infarction. In addition, ischemia of neuronal tissue may produce elevations of extracellular glutamate which can in turn trigger further neuronal damage.

cord injury in our laboratory both by scanning[37,38] and transmission electron microscopy.[4] Other studies suggest that intravascular thrombosis is a cause of post-traumatic ischemia, perhaps due to an agent such as thromboxane A2.[17] Indeed, Nemecek[41] observed intravascular thrombosis with the light microscope and in our laboratory we have seen excellent examples with the electron microscope[4] after experimental spinal cord injury. Thrombosed vessels have also been present in some human cases of spinal cord injury as discussed below.

Several investigators have found loss of autoregulation after trauma (i.e., the ability of the spinal cord to maintain relatively constant blood flow over a wide range of levels of systemic blood pressure). Thus, systemic hypotension or neurogenic shock after severe spinal cord injury may worsen post-traumatic ischemia of

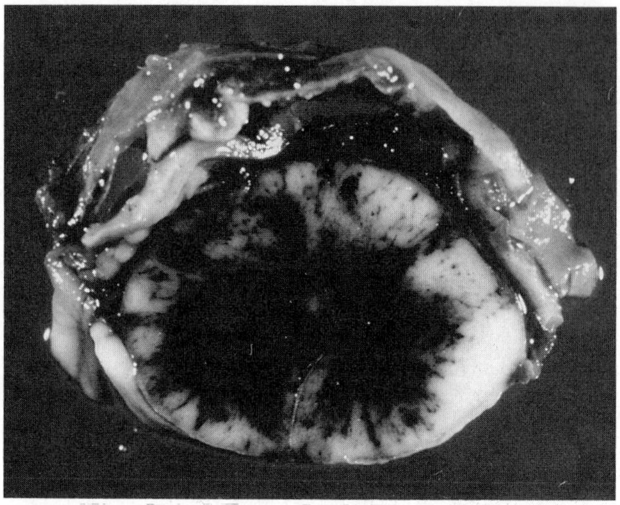

Figure 281-2 Human cervical spinal cord at site of injury. The patient died on the day of injury. The ventral dura was removed at autopsy. Almost the entire gray matter is hemorrhagic, including the dorsal and ventral horns. The hemorrhages have also extended into the white matter.

the injured cord due to the concomitant loss of autoregulatory homeostasis. Conversely, gross elevations of systemic pressure may lead to increased blood flow in adjacent segments of the injured cord (sometimes found to be hyperemic) and lead to further hemorrhage.

Biochemical Changes

Numerous theories of biochemical damage have been postulated regarding direct damage to neural tissue and indirect damage exerted via the microcirculation and subsequent ischemic effects. One of the most compelling biochemical derangements in the injured spinal cord is the accumulation and subsequent damage exerted by the excitatory amino acid neurotransmitter, glutamate.[24,43] Also, it has been hypothesized that cell membrane receptor activation by glutamate may play a key role in the development of ischemic damage,[45] the mechanism of which is an early intracellular accumulation of sodium, producing cytotoxic edema and a concomitant elevation of intracellular calcium. Raised levels of intracellular calcium can in turn activate calcium-dependent proteases or lipases that cause further damage due to breakdown of cytoskeletal components including neurofilaments, and dissolution of cell membranes. There are several types of excitatory amino acid receptors, although the *N*-methyl-D-aspartate (NMDA) receptor seems to be the principal receptor involved in glutamate-induced excitotoxicity. Indeed, blockage of this receptor with MK-801, a specific NMDA receptor antagonist, has had a protective effect on experimental spinal cord injury.[24]

The successful use of steroids in human spinal cord injury[12] is strong evidence for the beneficial interruption or prevention of secondary mechanisms of injury, especially those related to lipid peroxidation and the production of oxygen-free radicals. Indeed, it has been postulated that the inhibition of lipid peroxidation is the main cytoprotective mechanism of action of steroids.[13,30] The excess production of arachidonic acid and eicosanoids such as prostaglandins may be related to lipid peroxidation and oxygen-free radicals and may in turn cause tissue damage. For example, the release of vasoactive eicosanoids from damaged neuronal membranes may cause progressive post-traumatic ischemia by inducing vasospasm. Endogenous opioids may also be involved in the secondary injury process,[23] by either their effects on the local or systemic circulation or by direct effects on the injured cord.

Electrolyte Shifts

There is considerable evidence that there are major electrolyte shifts between the extracellular and intracellular compartments and vice versa after spinal cord injury. One of the best defined electrolyte changes is the marked increase of intracellular calcium.[50,59] An excess of free intracellular calcium ions plays a fundamental role in mediating the pathogenesis of all neural injuries, but especially ischemia and traumatic injuries. Indeed, intracellular influx

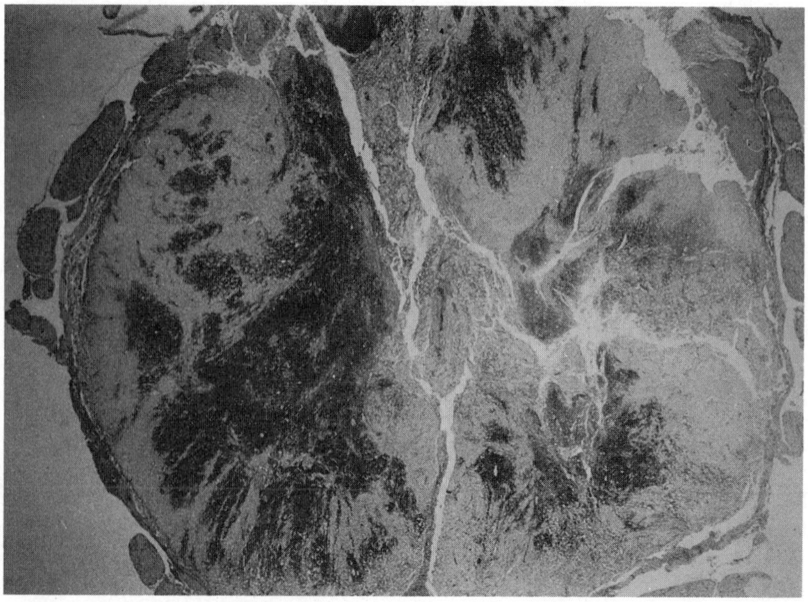

Figure 281-3 Human cervical cord at the injury site (C4-C5), 3 days after injury (stained with hematoxylin and eosin). The fissures are artifacts produced when this softened spinal cord was removed at autopsy. The gray matter on the left side is much more hemorrhagic than on the right. Hemorrhages are also seen in the white matter. Most of the cord centrally is necrotic, while there is some preservation of nervous tissue peripherally. The anterior spinal artery (not seen) was patent.

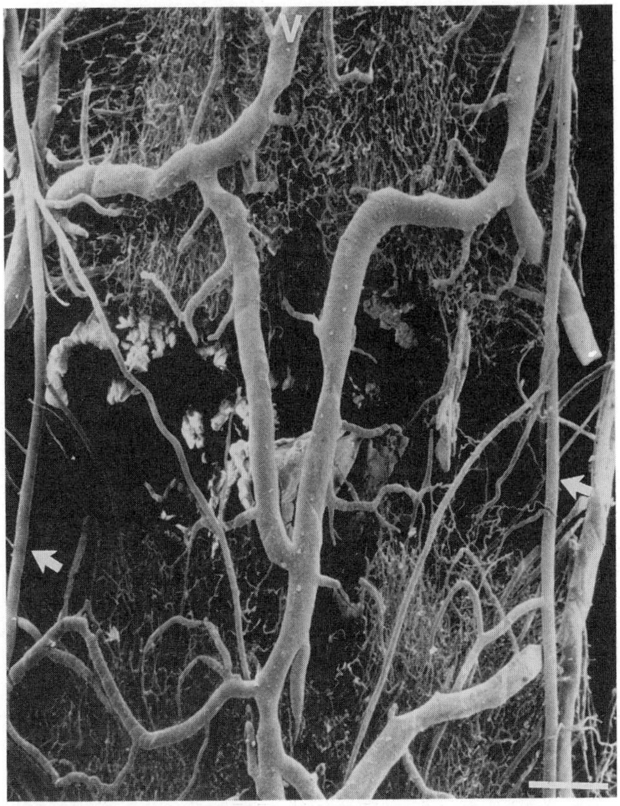

Figure 281-4 Dorsal view of the rat spinal cord 15 min after clip compression injury as demonstrated by the vascular corrosion cast technique and the scanning electron microscope. The capillary network in the central segment of the cord fails to fill, indicating severe damage. The irregular masses are extravasations of the resin due to continuing bleeding. The dorsal vein (V) and other large veins are patent. The paired posterior spinal arteries (*arrows*) are also patent. Scale bar = 1 mm.

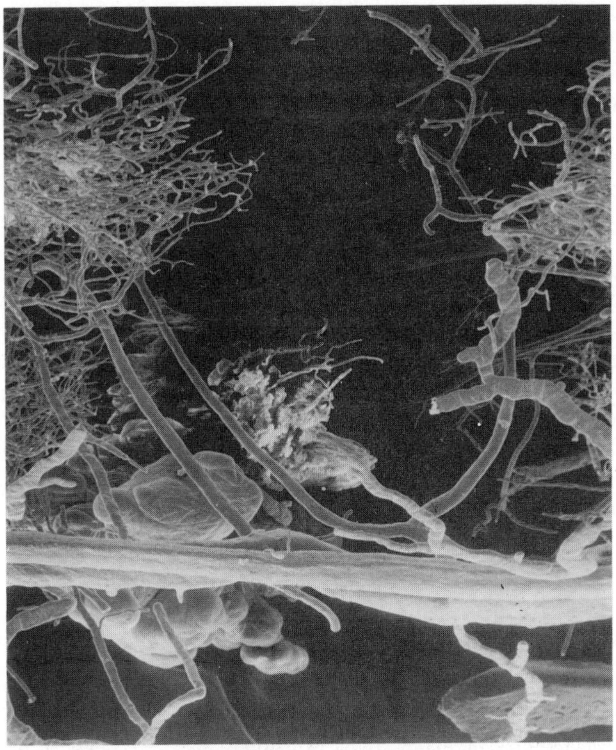

Figure 281-5 Parasagittal view of the rat spinal cord 15 min after acute clip compression injury as demonstrated by the vascular corrosion cast technique and the scanning electron microscope. The ventral aspect of the spinal cord is toward the bottom and shows the patent anterior spinal artery and vein. The anterior sulcal arteries extend almost vertically upward from the anterior spinal artery and are displaced away from the site of the injury which is the large avascular zone in the center. The ''mushroom'' appearing object is an extravasation of the resin.

of calcium has been termed the ''final common pathway of toxic cell death'' in the nervous system.[16,47] After trauma, calcium can shift into neurons in a variety of ways including through disrupted cell membranes, or by depolarization and entry through voltage-sensitive calcium channels, or through receptor-mediated calcium channels activated by glutamate. Ischemia can also increase intracellular calcium through glutamate release. In turn, increased intracellular calcium appears to trigger neurotoxicity in a variety of ways including activation of proteases such as protein kinase C which disrupt microtubules and neurofilaments and lipases such as phospholipase C which disrupt cell membranes as indicated above. There is also the possibility that spinal cord trauma increases intracellular calcium in vascular smooth muscle in the microcirculation at the site of spinal cord injury which results in vasospasm and post-traumatic ischemia. Support for this mechanism is the successful use of calcium-channel blockers such as nimodipine to reverse post-traumatic ischemia of the spinal cord.[27] Recent studies of intracellular calcium in an in vitro model of spinal cord injury in our laboratory confirm the damaging effects of glutamate and its relationship to levels of intracellular calcium in cultured spinal cord neurons.[54] Also, we confirmed the importance of the NMDA channel for triggering neurotoxicity, and that the calcium overload and resulting damage were only minimally reduced by N-type calcium-channel blockers such as nimodipine.

Edema

It is well known that significant and progressive edema can follow spinal cord injury,[55] but it is not known whether the edema is injurious in itself or whether it is an epiphenomenon of another injury mechanism such as ischemia or glutamate toxicity. For example, as noted above, the latter causes sodium to enter neurons with resulting cytotoxic edema. Edema can spread in the cord from the site of injury for a considerable distance rostrally and caudally in both experimental models[57] and clinical cases.[31,58]

Conduction Block in Spinal Cord Injury

Of special importance are the temporary or persistent failure of axonal conduction in acute spinal cord injury and the later conduction defects in the chronic stage. In the acute phase conduction block may be due to biochemical changes, especially electrolyte shifts. For example, increased extracellular potassium may cause excessive depolarization and account for spinal shock.[22] More severe mechanical axonal injuries with membrane disruption would account for persisting failure of conduction. The recent demonstration that conduction can be restored in clinically complete human injuries by the potassium channel antagonist, 4-amino-pyridine, emphasizes the role of increased extracellular potassium on the demyelinated axons present in the chronic phase of cord injury.[9] In addition, a direct relationship exists between the severity of post-traumatic ischemia and conduction block after spinal cord injury.[28]

Pathology of Acute Spinal Cord Injury

Our knowledge of the pathologic features of acute spinal cord injury (Table 281-3) is based on a relatively small number of clinical studies supplemented by a much larger number of experimental studies of the pathologic features of several different injury models. As noted, there are obvious similarities in the clinical and experimental pathologic findings which suggests that several of the models accurately simulate the human lesion, and that there are common pathologic processes underlying different mechanisms of injury.

The Central Zone of Injury

The central region of the cord at the injury site comprising the gray matter and the immediately adjacent white matter is more severely affected than the more peripheral white matter, especially in the acute compression injuries such as those due to burst fracture or fracture-dislocation (Figs. 281-2 and 281-3). The reasons given for the gray matter predilection include its softer consistency and greater vascularity.[58] In the initial stages, severe injuries usually produce numerous petechial hemorrhages due to diapedesis from smaller vessels with an admixture of some larger coalescent hemorrhages, especially in the gray matter. Bleeding usually results from capillaries, venules, and arterioles, but almost never from arteries such as the anterior spinal artery. Bleeding can continue at the injury site for about 2 h.[2] Central hematomyelia, which can be defined as a large space-occupying hemorrhage with distension of the cord, is very rare.[31,35,58] Remote hemorrhages can occur at considerable distances rostral and caudal to the injury site, especially at the base of the dorsal columns at the junction of the dorsal while commissure and gray matter immediately dorsal to the central canal.[31,58] Many of these remote hemorrhages have been shown experimentally to be venous in origin.[39]

At 12 to 24 h after trauma, structures in the central region of the cord begin to lose their definition and the picture begins to resemble central hemorrhagic necrosis with the hemorrhagic zones becoming more confluent. The definition of gray and white matter becomes blurred (Fig. 281-6). Several authors have noted the worsening of the pathologic changes over time.[21,58] In our autoradiographic studies of spinal cord blood flow in the monkey, we were able to show major ischemic zones at the injury site with extremely low or absent blood flow persisting for 24 h after trauma; the corresponding histologic sections at 24 h showed the features of infarction,[46] and thus we have termed this phenomenon post-traumatic infarction (Fig. 281-7).

Subarachnoid hemorrhage is very common with lesions producing contusions or lacerations, but subdural or extradural hematomas are very rare[38,58]; the latter occurs in a small number of patients with ankylosing spondylitis who sustain spinal fractures. During the first 24 h, there is gross swelling and softening of the spinal cord at the injury site which spreads rostrally and caudally for a considerable distance depending on the severity of the injury.[31,57,58]

TABLE 281-3 Pathology of Acute Spinal Cord Injury

Central hemorrhages—especially into gray matter from capillaries, venules, and arterioles
Hematomyelia (rarely large)
Remote hemorrhages—especially venous
Central hemorrhagic necrosis
Post-traumatic infarction
Subarachnoid hemorrhage
Subdural or extradural hematomas—rare
Edema
Local
Spreading
Axonal injuries
Transection
Axolemma rupture
Swelling
Giant axons
Granular dissolution
Organelle accumulation
Myelin sheath injuries
Rupture
Vesicular disruption
Periaxonal spaces
Inflammation
Macrophages
Microglia

Degree of Transection

It has been generally accepted that even after severe injury a portion of the spinal cord at the injury site usually remains in continuity. However, Bunge et al.[15] recently examined the pathology of 22 cases of human spinal cord injuries, 14 of whom had injury-to-death intervals of 6 months or less, and made a number of important observations with regard to the incidence and degree of intactness of the spinal cord. They found that only 62 percent of the cases had "central neural tissue continuity through the epicentre of the lesion." They specifically excluded cases in which the continuity consisted of only noncentral nervous tissue such as nerve roots or meninges. Indeed, only eight (50 percent) of the 16 cases with complete injuries on clinical examination showed "some parenchymal continuity across the epicentre of the lesion" including "nerve fibers transversing the lesion site." Thus, the incidence of neural continuity in clinically complete cases is lower than previously thought. These findings also provide some pathologic confirmation of Dimitrijevic's[18] concept of the "discomplete" injury, a term used to describe those clinically complete cases in whom sensory or motor evoked potentials or other neurophysiologic tests show signals traversing the injury site. Bunge et al.[15] classified the human lesions into four pathologic types: (1) The contusion/cyst was present in 23 percent of their cases and was believed to be due to moderate contusive forces which leave the continuity of the cord intact but result in a centrally located hematomyelia which evolves to become a stable cyst; (2) Cord maceration due to massive compression was present in 32 percent and was characterized by severe destruction of most or all nervous tissue, breaching of the pia, and subsequent connective tissue scarring. Surprisingly, in a minority of cases there was a "fragment of remaining CNS parenchyma"; (3) Cord laceration due to open injuries such as gunshot wounds was present in 27 percent and was characterized by torn cord parenchyma and ingrowth of dense scar tissue; and (4) Solid cord injury in which the overall form of the cord was retained without central hematomyelia or cyst was found in 18 percent of cases. In these cases, the damage was largely confined to the white matter,

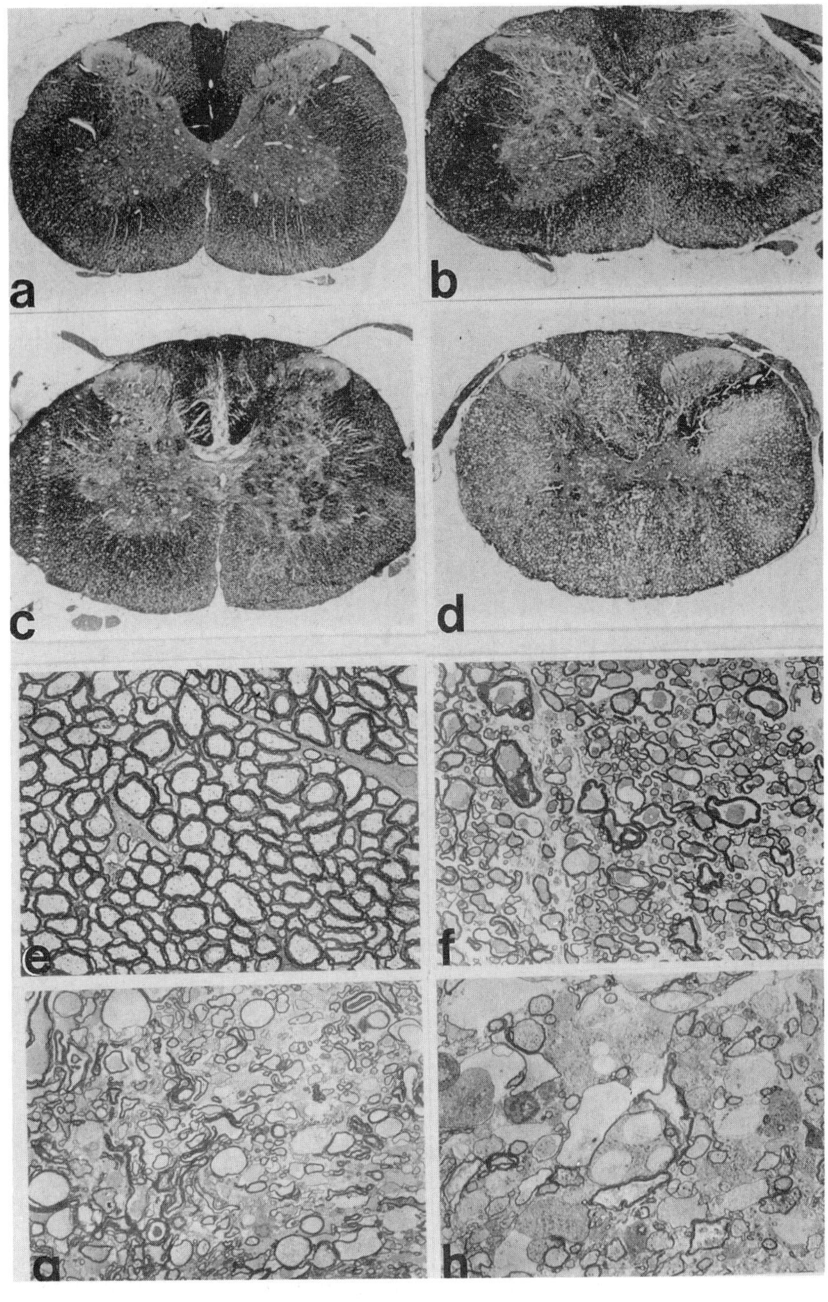

Figure 281-6 Pathologic changes during the first 24 h after acute cord compression injury in the rat showing the progression of changes. *a, e* = normal cord; *b, f* = 15 min after injury; *c, g* = 2 h after injury; and *d, h* = 24 h after injury. There is gradual worsening of the gross and microscopic changes. *e* to *h* are from the dorsolateral white matter and show progressive damage to the myelinated axons. There is a marked decline in the number of intact axons with increasing time. The myelin sheaths become very thin, and some giant axons appear at 24 h.

especially the dorsal part of the lateral funiculus in the region of the corticospinal tract where there was diffuse axonal disruption, especially of the large diameter axons. Surprisingly, the gray matter was not affected in this type. All four patients in this group had been diagnosed clinically as cases of the central cord syndrome which previously was thought to involve primarily central hematomyelia with spreading edema.[49] Thus, the pathophysiology of the central cord syndrome may have to be reexamined. Only types 2 and 3 where the pia was breached showed connective tissue scarring. Thus, connective tissue scarring cannot be an important impediment to axonal recovery or regeneration in a significant number of cases. Indeed, even in cases with extensive scarring, its role in preventing recovery by blocking axonal regeneration is not firmly established. In this author's view, scarring is a minor factor preventing axonal recovery or regeneration in most spinal cord injury cases.

Cord Injury in Cervical Spondylosis

The common mechanism of acute cord injury in the elderly associated with cervical spondylosis and hyperextension was well described pathologically by Hughes and Brownell[32] in three severe cases. They found evidence of direct compression damage to the cord as seen by contusion and indentation of the cord immediately opposite a large spondylotic bulge. In all three cases the bulge was associated with a torn intervertebral disc, which suggested that this was the point where the spine was abnormally hinged at the time of the injury. No spinal fracture or dislocation was present in any of these three cases. The site of the injuries was marked by a well-demonstrated area of necrosis which did not correspond to an arterial territory. Adjacent to the sites of maximum destruction were areas of central hemorrhagic infarction with the tissue in the adjacent surviving anterior horns showing ischemic changes con-

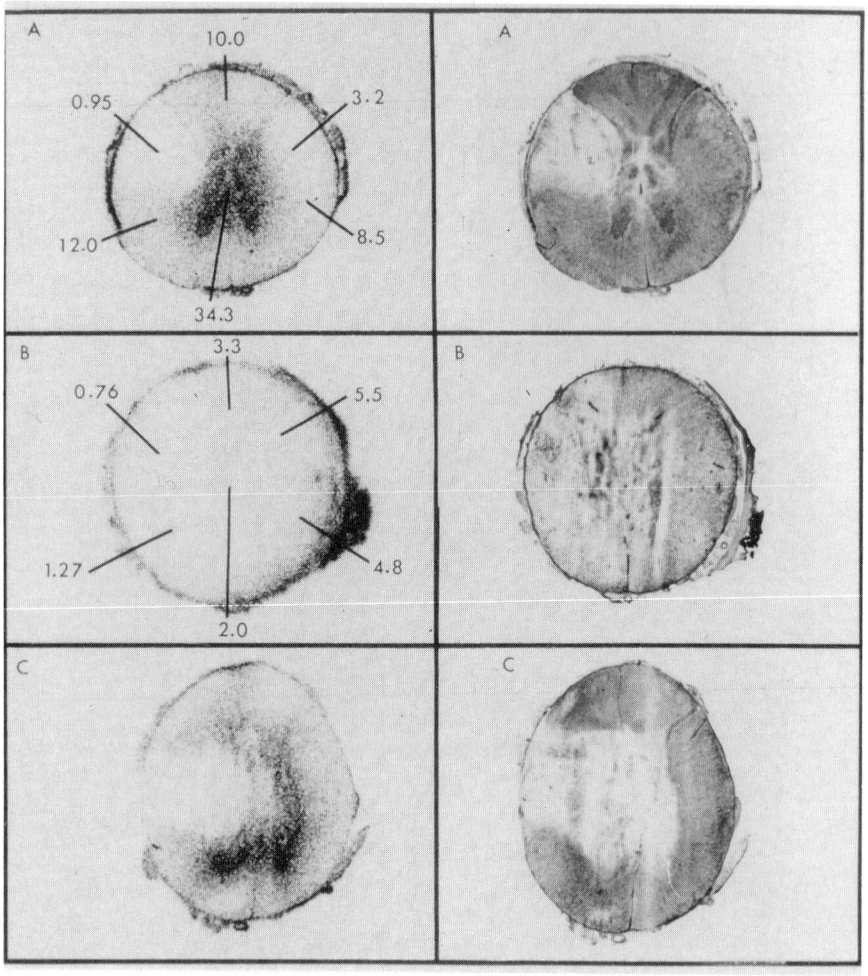

Figure 281-7 The three images *A, B, C* on the left are autoradiographs and the three images on the right *A, B, C* are the corresponding histologic sections of primate spinal cord 24 h after acute cuff compression injury. *B* is at the injury site and shows almost total cessation of blood flow in the gray matter with marked ischemia in the white matter. *A* and *C* are 1 cm caudal and rostral to the injury site, respectively, and show marked general ischemia with focal areas of major ischemia on the autoradiograph, and the corresponding infarcted zones in the histologic sections.

sisting of depletion of neurons and shrinkage and pyknosis of surviving neurons. This is the classical picture of the complete cord injury consisting of central hemorrhagic necrosis or infarction and ischemic changes in adjacent sites, as compared with the much less severe changes described above for the central cord syndrome found by Bunge et al.,[15] some of which were also due to falls in elderly patients with cervical spondylosis. These findings suggest that a wide spectrum of injuries exist in this patient population which vary in severity depending on the degree of mechanical compression. Perhaps the more severe forces cause not only more direct compression, but also induce more severe secondary mechanisms such as ischemia.

The Question of Large Vessel Occlusion

Schneider[48] suggested that some spinal cord injuries, especially those with the anterior cervical cord syndrome, were due to thrombosis or at least impaired circulation in the anterior spinal artery, and that some cases of thoracic cord injuries especially in the T4 ''watershed'' zone may have been due to a more remote traumatic or compressive interruption of a major radicular vessel or of the anterior spinal artery itself.[49] Wolman's series of 95 fatal spinal cord injuries contained three cases of thrombosis of the anterior spinal artery in the thoracic cord but none in the cervical cord.[58] However, he frequently found thrombosis of small pial arteries and intramedullary vessels. Holmes[31] had also observed thrombosis of vessels at the injury site in his early study. Yet other authors of clinical studies found no evidence of traumatic occlusion of the major arteries such as the anterior spinal artery.[11,34] Experimental studies have supported the latter findings. Indeed, even after extremely severe cord injury in the rat, the anterior spinal artery always remained patent[37–39] (Fig. 281-5).

Axonal and Myelin Sheath Injuries

Many types of axonal injuries have been described in clinical and experimental studies of acute spinal cord injury. The electron microscopic studies by Dohrmann et al.,[20] Bresnahan,[14] Balentine,[6] and Anthes et al.[4,5] have shown significant axonal changes within 15 min of injury which then progress markedly during the next 24 h (Figs. 281-6 and 281-8). The axonal changes include rupture of the axolemma with spillage of organelles into the extracellular space, granular degeneration of the axoplasm, axonal swelling and the development of giant axons, and excess accumulation of organelles such as mitochondria within the axoplasm around a neurofilamentous core. Our laboratory studies regarding acute clip compression injury have also documented axonal transection.[5]

The changes in the myelin sheaths also progress rapidly during the first few hours. The changes include rupture of the myelin sheaths, separation of the myelin from the axons with the development of large periaxonal spaces, and vesicular myelin[5] (Figs.

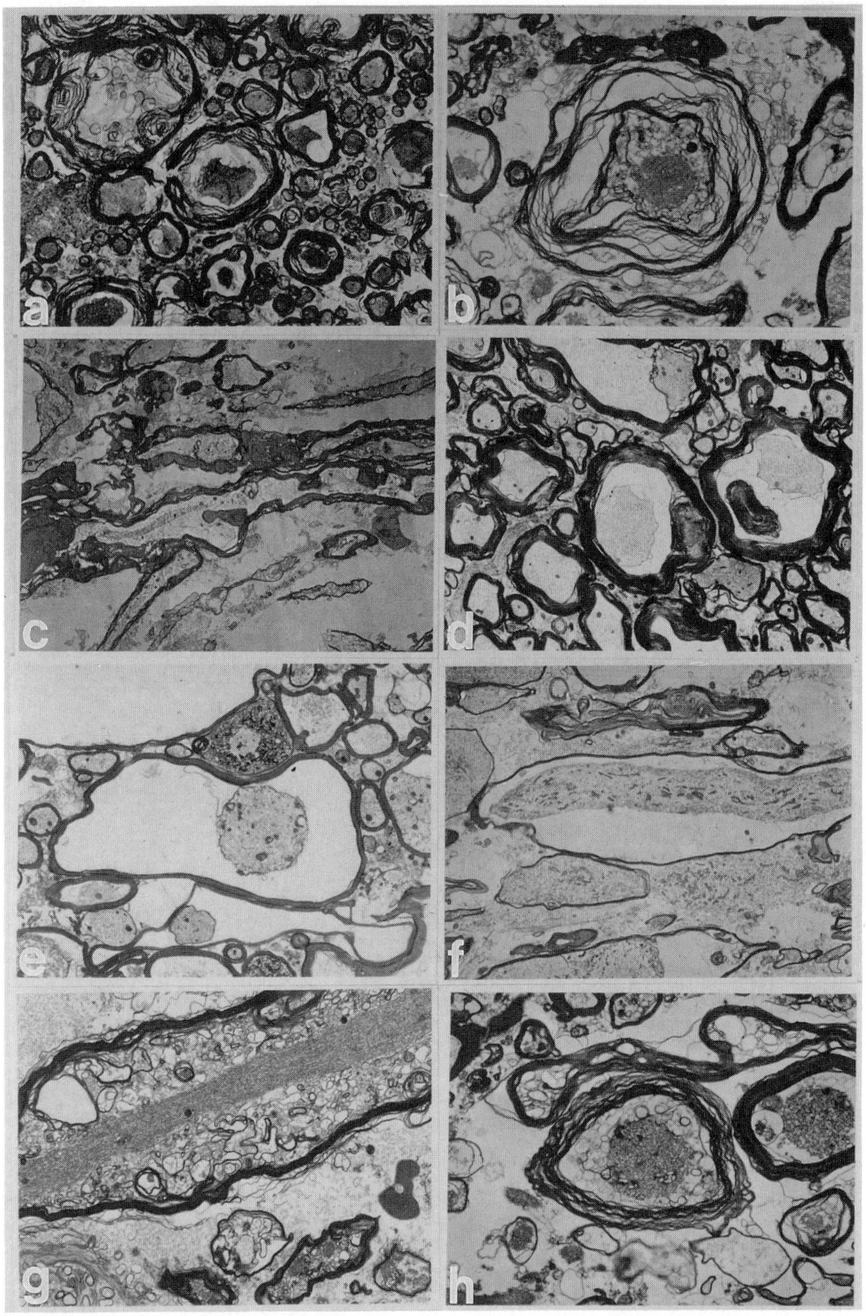

Figure 281-8 Pathologic changes in the axons after acute clip compression injury in the rat. In *a* there is rupture of the myelin sheaths around two axons in the center; *b* shows vesicular myelin change with separation of the myelin lamellae; *c* and *d* show examples of myelin invagination within the periaxonal space in a longitudinal section (*c*) and a transverse section (*d*); *e* and *f* show marked enlargement of the periaxonal space between the axon and myelin sheath; *g* and *h* show central accumulation of axoplasmic organelles around a neurofilamentous core.

281-6 and 281-8). Some of these early axonal and myelin changes have also been observed at the light microscopic level in human cases.[31,58]

Pathology of Spinal Cord Injury in the Chronic Phase

Within days of the acute injury, a large number of reparative, degenerative, and regenerative processes begin to occur at the injury site as well as rostrally and caudally, and then continue even for several years in severe cases (Table 281-4). The polymorphonuclear leukocytes diminish in number and there is then a marked increase in macrophages derived from resident microglial cells and from the circulating blood. The macrophages phagocytose debris, especially myelin and red blood cells, and have been given a

TABLE 281-4 Pathology of Spinal Cord Injury in the Chronic Phase

Central cavitation
Persisting subpial rim of axons
Post-traumatic infarction
Injury site
Remote
Post-traumatic syringomyelia
Cystic myelomalacia
Remote necrotic foci
Demyelination and the discomplete syndrome
Inflammation—macrophages
Wallerian degeneration
Scarring and gliosis
Arachnoiditis
Atrophy
Regenerative processes
Axons
Schwann cells
Ependyma

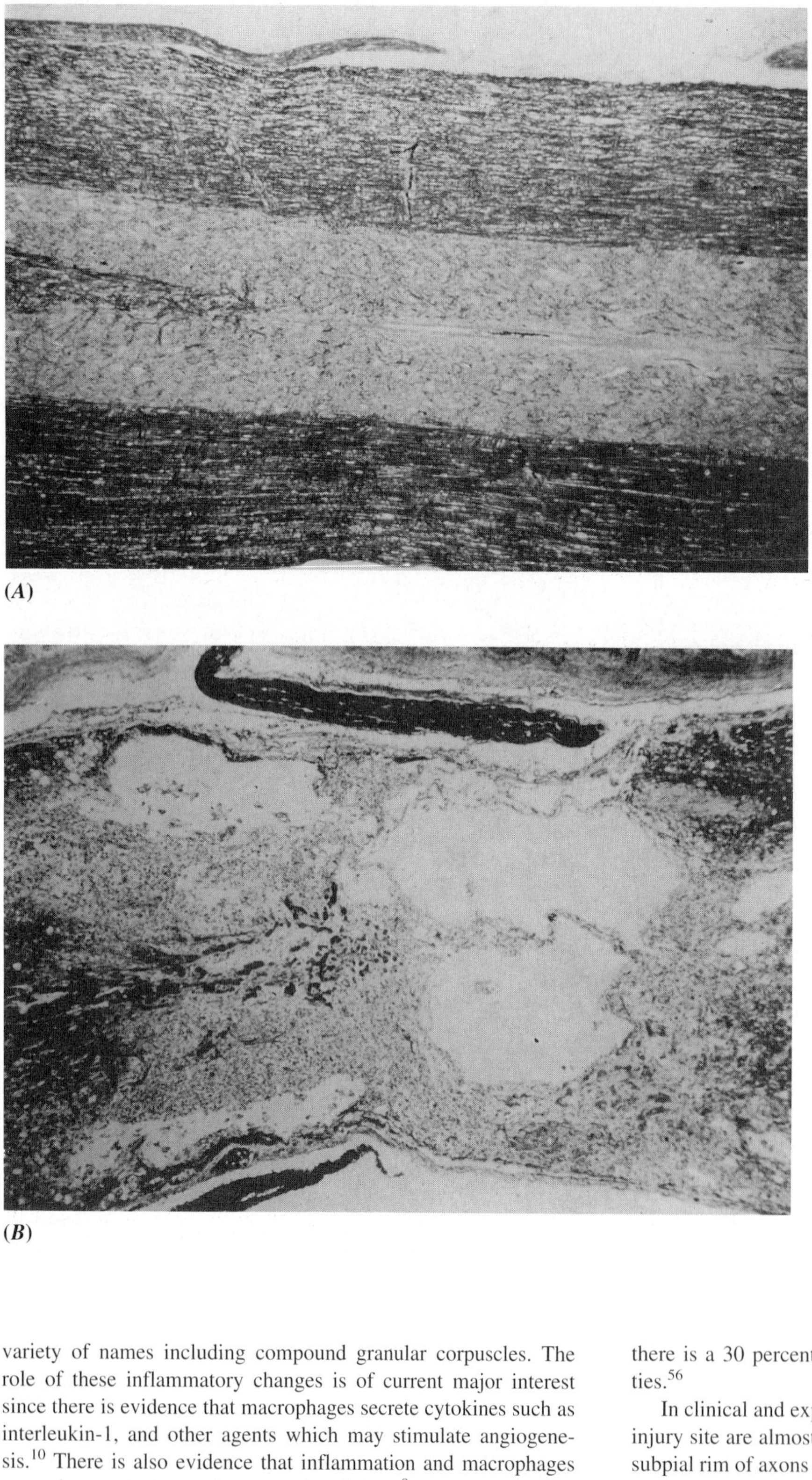

Figure 281-9 *A*. Coronal section of a normal rat thoracic cord stained with luxol fast blue (a myelin stain), hematoxylin, and eosin, demonstrating the normal white matter tracts of the lateral columns above and below and the gray matter centrally. *B*. Coronal section of a rat thoracic spinal cord stained with luxol fast blue, hematoxylin, and eosin 8 weeks after clip compression injury showing marked cavitation at the injury site with major necrosis and demyelination. In this rat there was ascending post-traumatic syringomyelia which extended for several segments above the injury site. There was also extensive arachnoiditis and ependymal cell proliferation centrally (seen in the center of the section as small islands of darkly staining cells). It is of major interest that the nerve root at the top of the section survived the injury reasonably well in comparison with the cord, although both the root and the cord were compressed by the clip.

variety of names including compound granular corpuscles. The role of these inflammatory changes is of current major interest since there is evidence that macrophages secrete cytokines such as interleukin-1, and other agents which may stimulate angiogenesis.[10] There is also evidence that inflammation and macrophages may play a role in causing secondary injury.[8]

In the more severe injuries, small and large cavities routinely develop at the injury site (Fig. 281-9), only some of which communicate with the ependymal-lined central canal. In about 10 percent of cord injuries, the small cavities at the injury site coalesce to form a larger cavity which can increase in size and extend for a considerable distance rostrally and caudally, producing the syndrome of post-traumatic syringomyelia. In some animal models there is a 30 percent incidence of ascending or descending cavities.[56]

In clinical and experimental studies, any persisting axons at the injury site are almost always located subpially (Fig. 281-10). This subpial rim of axons may extend around the entire perimeter of the cord or may exist along one side only.[7] These axons are often demyelinated or have thinner myelin sheaths than normal axons, and also show a shift in caliber toward smaller size as compared with uninjured axons.[25]

Sharply circumscribed areas of necrosis with the appearance of infarcts are more readily identified in the chronic stage (Fig. 281-7). These necrotic foci may occur at a considerable distance from the injury site, and have been identified in both experimental[46] and

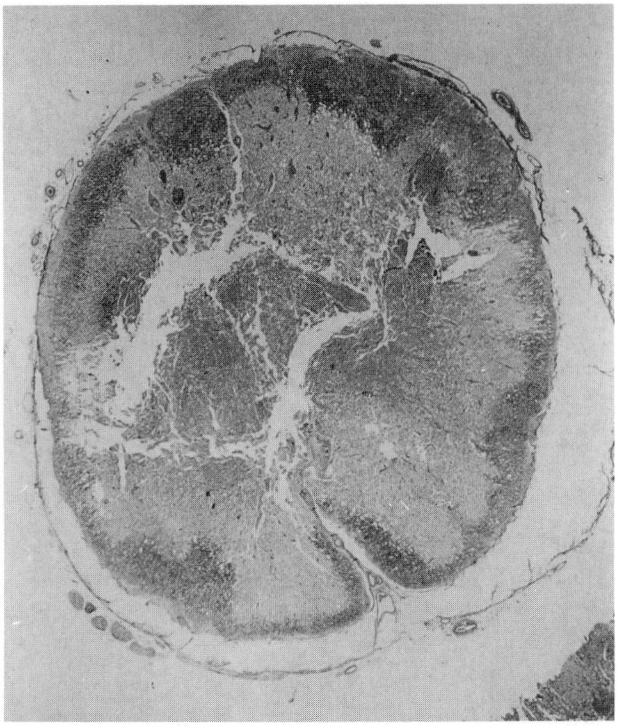

Figure 281-10 Human spinal cord at C1-C2 18 days after injury stained with luxol fast blue, hematoxylin, and eosin. The central portion of the cord is entirely necrotic but there is a preserved peripheral rim of myelinated axons. The anterior spinal artery at the ventral aspect of the anterior median sulcus is patent.

clinical material.[31,58] Some of these lesions conform to the distribution of anterior sulcal arteries,[37–39] while others do not conform to arterial zones and may be venous in origin. The exact pathophysiology of these lesions is unknown. They are clinically important because they help explain why some of the clinical deficits are remote from the principal site of injury.

There is another form of post-traumatic central degeneration without frank syringomyelia which has been described as a microcystic myelomalacia or ''marshy cord syndrome.''[40] Arachnoiditis has been associated with this condition as well as with post-traumatic syringomyelia. Indeed, arachnoiditis may play an etiologic role in the progression of both post-traumatic syringomyelia and cystic myelomalacia. Intramedullary fibrosis or scarring occurs to a variable extent, even in major injuries. Extensive scarring with collagen in the cord, or bridging to the arachnoid and dura frequently occurs as a sequela to lacerations of the dura. In the absence of a dural laceration, intramedullary collagenous scarring is usually minimal. Similarly, the degree of astrocytic scarring or gliosis is variable.

Wallerian degeneration involving axonal degeneration and demyelination can be detected in the afferent tracts such as the dorsal columns and spinothalamic tracts rostral to the lesion, and in the efferent tracts such as the lateral corticospinal tract caudal to the lesion. As a result, the spinal cord in the chronic stage is not only atrophic at the injury site, but also rostrally and caudally.

A range of regenerative changes can also be seen in the chronic stage; the most marked change is ingrowth of Schwann cells and associated peripheral axons and peripheral myelin from both the dorsal and ventral roots (Fig. 281-11). The proliferation of Schwann cells may be so extensive in some patients that they produce the appearance of an intramedullary neuroma.[33] There may also be a proliferation of small blood vessels,[10] and ependymal cells can also proliferate and migrate for a considerable distance from the central canal.[56]

Conclusions

Although much has been learned about the pathophysiology of spinal cord injury, there are still many unanswered questions. The experimental studies have revealed a large variety of secondary injury mechanisms which cause progressive damage to the cord and contribute to the rich variety of pathologic changes in the acute and chronic stages. The evidence is strong for the damaging effects

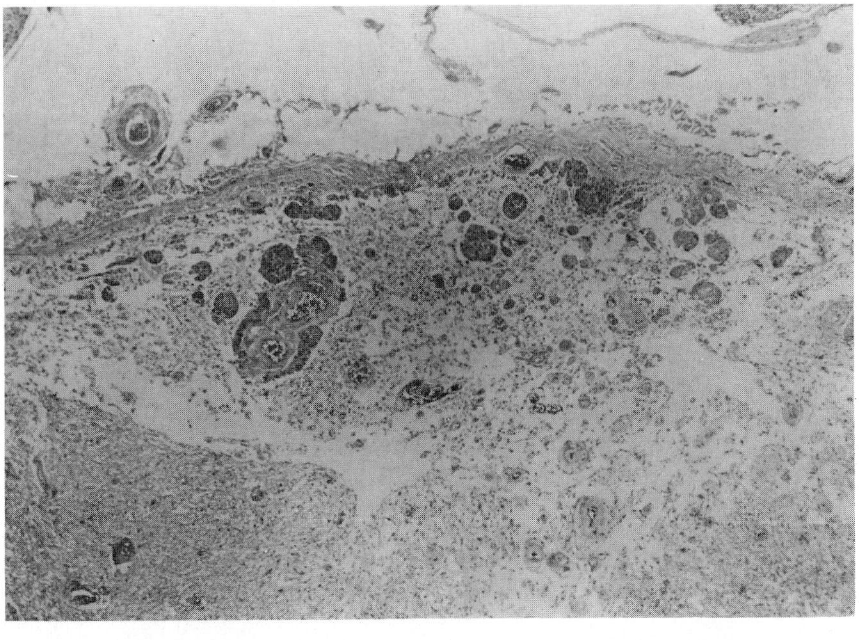

Figure 281-11 The dorsal columns of the human spinal cord near the injury site at C1-C2 9 months after an acute spinal cord injury show infiltration of the necrotic white matter by proliferating Schwann cells forming small neuromatous knots. There is also severe arachnoiditis surrounding the cord with virtually complete obliteration of the subarachnoid space.

of ischemia, excitotoxicity, lipid peroxidation, and elevation of intracellular calcium. The counteracting of each of these processes has led to very promising therapeutic studies. A knowledge of the pathology in the various stages of injury assists the clinician in the interpretation of the clinical and imaging findings, and thus is beneficial for the management of patients with spinal cord injury.

References

1. Allen AR. Surgery of experimental lesions of the spinal cord equivalent to crush injury of fracture dislocation of the spinal column. A preliminary report. *JAMA* 1991; 57:878–880.
2. Allen AR. Remarks on the histopathological changes in the spinal cord due to impact. An experimental study. *J Nerv Ment Dis* 1914; 41:141–147.
3. Anderson DK, Hall ED. Pathophysiology of spinal cord trauma. *Ann Emerg Med* 1993; 22:987–992.
4. Anthes DL, Theriault E, Tator CH. An ultrastructural assessment of microcirculatory pathophysiology following spinal cord trauma. Manuscript submitted, 1995.
5. Anthes DL, Theriault E, Tator CH. Characterization of ultrastructural pathology following experimental spinal cord compression injury. Manuscript submitted, 1995.
6. Balentine JD. Pathology of experimental spinal cord trauma. II. Ultrastructure of axons and myelin. *Lab Invest* 1978; 39:254–266.
7. Blight AR. Cellular morphology of chronic spinal cord injury in the cat: analysis of myelinated axons by line-sampling. *Neuroscience* 1983; 10:521–543.
8. Blight AR. Delayed demyelination and macrophage invasion: a candidate for secondary cell damage in spinal cord injury. *Cent Nerv Syst Trauma* 1985; 2:299–315.
9. Blight AR. Effect of 4-aminopyridine on axonal conduction-block in chronic spinal cord injury. *Brain Res Bull* 1989; 22:47–52.
10. Blight AR. Remyelination, revascularization, and recovery of function in experimental spinal cord injury. *Adv Neurol* 1993; 59:91–104.
11. Braakman R, Penning L. Injuries of the cervical spine. In Vinken PJ, Bruyn GW (eds): *Handbook of Clinical Neurology,* vol 25. Amsterdam: North-Holland Publishing Co., 1976, pp 227–380.
12. Bracken MB, Shepard MJ, Collins WF, et al. A randomized, controlled trial of methylprednisolone or naloxone in the treatment of acute spinal cord injury. Results of the Second National Acute Spinal Cord Injury Study. *N Engl J Med* 1990; 322:1405–1411.
13. Braughler JM, Pregenzer JF, Chase RL, et al. Novel 21-amino steroids as potent inhibitors of iron-dependent lipid peroxidation. *J Biol Chem* 1987; 262:10438–10440.
14. Bresnahan JC. An electron-microscopic analysis of axonal alterations following blunt contusion of the spinal cord of the rhesus monkey (macaca mulatta). *J Neurol Sci* 1978; 37:59–82.
15. Bunge RP, Puckett WR, Becerra JL, et al. Observations on the pathology of human spinal cord injury. A review and classification of 22 new cases with details from a case of chronic cord compression with extensive focal demyelination. *Adv Neurol* 1993; 59:75–89.
16. Cheung JY, Bonventre JV, Malis CD, et al. Calcium and ischemic injury. *N Engl J Med* 1986; 314:1670–1676.
17. De La Torre JC. Spinal cord injury: review of basic and applied research. *Spine* 1981; 6:315–335.
18. Dimitrijevic MR. Residual motor functions in spinal cord injury. *Adv Neurol* 1988; 47:138–155.
19. Dohrmann GJ, Wagner FC Jr, Bucy PC. The microvasculature in transitory traumatic paraplegia. An electron microscopic study in the monkey. *J Neurosurg* 1971; 35:263–271.
20. Dohrmann GJ, Wagner FC Jr, Bucy PC. Transitory traumatic paraplegia: electron microscopy of early alterations in myelinated nerve fibers. *J Neurosurg* 1972; 36:407–415.
21. Ducker TB, Kindt GW, Kempf LG. Pathological findings in acute experimental spinal cord trauma. *J Neurosurg* 1971; 35:700–708.
22. Eidelberg E, Sullivan J, Brigham A. Immediate consequences of spinal cord injury: possible role of potassium in axonal conduction block. *Surg Neurol* 1975; 3:317–321.
23. Faden AI, Jacobs TP, Mougey E, et al. Endorphins in experimental spinal injury: therapeutic effect of naloxone. *Ann Neurol* 1981; 10:326–332.
24. Faden AI, Simon RP. A potential role for excitotoxins in the pathophysiology of spinal cord injury. *Ann Neurol* 1988; 23:623–626.
25. Fehlings MG, Lewicki M, Tator CH. The relationship between axon counts and neurological function after experimental spinal cord injury. *J Neurotrauma* 1989; 6:218 (abstr).
26. Fehlings MG, Tator CH. A review of experimental models of acute spinal cord injury. In Illis LS (ed): *Spinal Cord Dysfunction: Assessment.* Oxford: Oxford University, 1988, pp 3–43.
27. Fehlings MG, Tator CH, Linden RD. The effect of nimodipine and dextran on axonal function and blood flow following experimental spinal cord injury. *J Neurosurg* 1989; 71:403–416.
28. Fehlings MG, Tator CH, Linden RD. The relationships among the severity of spinal cord injury, motor and somatosensory evoked potentials and spinal cord blood flow. *Electroencephalogr Clin Neurophysiol* 1989; 74:241–259.
29. Guha A, Tator CH. Acute cardiovascular effects of experimental spinal cord injury. *J Trauma* 1988; 28:481–490.
30. Hall ED. Effects of the 21-aminosteroid U74006F on post-traumatic spinal cord ischemia in cats. *J Neurosurg* 1988; 68:462–465.
31. Holmes G. The Goulstonian lectures on spinal injuries of warfare. 1. The pathology of acute spinal injuries. *Br Med J* 1915; 2:769–774.
32. Hughes JT, Brownell B. Spinal cord damage from hyperextension injury in cervical spondylosis. *Lancet* 1963; 1:687–690.
33. Hughes JT, Brownell B. Aberrant nerve fibers within the spinal cord. *J Neurol Neurosurg Psychiatry* 1963; 26:528–534.
34. Jellinger K. Neuropathology of cord injuries. In Vinken PJ, Bruyn GW (eds): *Handbook of Clinical Neurology,* vol 25. Amsterdam: North-Holland Publishing, 1976, pp 43–121.
35. Kakulas BA. Pathology of spinal injuries. *Cent Nerv Syst Trauma* 1984; 1:117–129.
36. Kiss ZHT, Tator CH. Neurogenic shock. In Geller ER (ed): *Shock and Resuscitation.* New York: McGraw-Hill, 1993, pp 421–440.
37. Koyanagi I, Tator CH, Lea PJ. Three-dimensional analysis of the vascular system in the rat spinal cord with scanning electron microscopy of vascular corrosion casts. Part 1: Normal spinal cord. *Neurosurgery* 1993; 33:277–284.
38. Koyanagi I, Tator CH, Lea PJ. Three-dimensional analysis of the vascular system in the rat spinal cord with scanning electron microscopy of vascular corrosion casts. Part 2: Acute spinal cord injury. *Neurosurgery* 1993; 33:285–292.
39. Koyanagi I, Tator CH, Theriault E. Silicone rubber microangiography of acute spinal cord injury in the rat. *Neurosurgery* 1993; 32:260–268.
40. MacDonald RL, Schwartz ML, Mirich D, et al. Diagnosis of cervical spine injury in motor vehicle crash victims: how many x-rays are enough. *J Trauma* 1990; 30:392–397.
41. Nemecek S. Morphological evidence of microcirculatory disturbances in experimental spinal cord trauma. *Adv Neurol* 1978; 20:395–405.
42. Pang D, Wilberger JE Jr. Spinal cord injury without radiographic abnormalities in children. *J Neurosurg* 1982; 57:114–129.
43. Panter SS, Yum SW, Faden AI. Alteration in extracellular amino acids after traumatic spinal cord injury. *Ann Neurol* 1990; 27:96–99.
44. Rivlin AS, Tator CH. Effect of duration of acute spinal cord compression in a new acute cord injury model in the rat. *Surg Neurol* 1978; 10:38–43.
45. Rothman SM, Olney JW. Glutamate and the pathophysiology of hypoxic-ischemic brain damage. *Ann Neurol* 1986; 19:105–111.
46. Sandler AN, Tator CH. Effect of acute spinal cord compression injury on regional spinal cord blood flow in primates. *J Neurosurg* 1976; 45:660–676.
47. Schanne FAX, Kane AB, Young EE, et al. Calcium dependence of toxic cell death: a final common pathway. *Science* 1979; 206:700–702.

48. Schneider RC. The syndrome of acute anterior spinal cord injury. *J Neurosurg* 1955; 12:95–122.
49. Schneider RC, Crosby EC, Russo RH, et al. Traumatic spinal cord syndromes and their management. *Clin Neurosurg* 1973; 20:424–492.
50. Stokes BT, Fox P, Hollinden G. Extracellular calcium activity in the injured spinal cord. *Exp Neurol* 1983; 80:561–572.
51. Tator CH. Review of experimental spinal cord injury with emphasis on the local and systemic circulatory effects. *Neurochirurgie* 1991; 37:291–302.
52. Tator CH. Spinal cord syndromes with physiological and anatomic correlations. In Menezes AH, Sonntag VKH (eds): *Principles of Spinal Surgery.* New York: McGraw-Hill, 1996 (in press).
53. Tator CH, Fehlings MG. Review of the secondary injury theory of acute spinal cord trauma with special emphasis on vascular mechanisms. *J Neurosurg* 1991; 75:15–26.
54. Tymianski M, Charlton MP, Carlen PL, et al. Secondary Ca^{2+} overload indicates early neuronal injury which precedes staining with viability indicators. *Brain Res* 1993; 607:319–323.
55. Wagner FC Jr, Stewart WB. Effect of trauma dose on spinal cord edema. *J Neurosurg* 1981; 54:802–806.
56. Wallace MC, Tator CH, Lewis AJ. Chronic regenerative changes in the spinal cord after cord compression injury in rats. *Surg Neurol* 1987; 27:209–219.
57. Wang R, Ehara K, Tamaki N. Spinal cord edema following freezing injury in the rat: relationship between tissue water content and spinal cord blood flow. *Surg Neurol* 1993; 39:348–354.
58. Wolman L. The disturbance of circulation in traumatic paraplegia in acute and late stages: a pathological study. *Paraplegia* 1965; 2:213–226.
59. Young W, Yen V, Blight A. Extracellular calcium ionic activity in experimental spinal cord contusion. *Brain Res* 1982; 253:105–113.

282

Management of Acute Spinal Cord Injury

Edward C. Benzel

Prognostication

Historically, the prognosis for neurological recovery after spinal cord injury (SCI) has been dismal. The prognosis, however, has improved remarkably over the past several decades. Many factors have played a role in this improvement. They are, for the most part, founded on an increased understanding of the processes involved with the medical care of the SCI patient.

Prognosis for Neurological Recovery

The prognosis for neurological recovery following SCI has been well outlined by multiple authors.[7,9,19,27,31,46,54,73,79] It is affected predominantly by the patient's neurological grade at admission to the hospital. Patients with motor and sensory complete myelopathies have a minimal chance for recovery. Patients with motor complete myelopathies have an improved, but nevertheless, relatively poor recovery potential. The presence of motor function at the time of admission allows for recovery of function that is proportional to the extent of function initially present.

Similarly, mobility gains can be predicted by using a mobility index. In patients with cervical spine injuries, important predictive variables have been observed. These include the patient's gender, rectal tone status, reflexes, medical and surgical management, motor and sensory neurological history since injury, neurological status, and initial mobility score.[54]

Time Course of Recovery

Late or delayed neurological improvement or deterioration often occurs following incomplete SCI. Piepmeier and Jenkins[68] observed that the majority of neurological improvement occurs within the first year after injury; however, changes in neurological status continue for many years. In their patients, at 3 years postinjury nearly 23.3 percent of the patients continued to improve, whereas 7.1 percent had deteriorated. At 5 or more years, 12.5 percent had improved and 5 percent had deteriorated.[68] Tominaga, however, reported that the chance for recovery exists only for about 6 months.[84]

Approximately 5 percent of SCI patients deteriorate in the early postinjury period.[52] These cases are predominantly cervical injuries and most are associated with specific management events that include early surgery and ineffective or inappropriate immobilization. Therefore, one must question the wisdom of early or emergency decompression surgery for SCI patients.

Grading Scales

The "chance" for neurological recovery after SCI is particularly affected by admission neurological grade.[7,9] This has also been documented following both aggressive surgical and medical management.[17,33] Multiple grading schemes have been used.[7,9,22,31,49,54,56,83] The Frankel grading scheme is the most popular.[31] A recent revision has enhanced the clarity of this scale.[56] It does not offer the ability to sort out motor useful function, however. The Benzel/Larson scale offers this ability by expanding the motor useful aspect of the Frankel scale and the walking aspect of the Maynard modification of the Frankel scale[56]; thus establishing a 7 rather than a 5 grade scale.[7,9] This scheme more accurately assesses function and functional levels by expanding a motor useful function grade into three separate grades. This allows for a more "fine-tuned" recovery assessment, particularly when combined with a motor strength assessment scheme, such as the ASIA scale.[33]

Complete Myelopathy

Many have observed that long tract recovery does not ensue, or rarely ensues, after a complete post-traumatic myelopathy.[7,9,16] Others have observed recovery to occur in this patient population.[4,17] This discrepancy requires further consideration. The definition of complete myelopathy may vary from surgeon to surgeon. Its definition is often inadequately outlined in the literature. Because the term complete myelopathy implies the absence of long tract neural transmission past the injured site, and because this determination may be difficult in the early postinjury period, the establishment of this diagnosis requires meticulous serial neurological examinations.[76]

Perhaps this issue can be clarified by assessing autonomic function preservation. Patients with complete motor and sensory myelopathies have been observed (in a carefully performed study), to have a 26 percent incidence of distal sensory function return. This was correlated with admission blood pressure (normotensive) and pulse (absence of bradycardia); perhaps indicating the preservation of some autonomic long tract function. This long tract preservation, however minimal, reflects the perseveration of the potential for additional long tract function recovery.[47] The medical and surgical implications of this potential are profound. Other diagnostic techniques may be useful in the future in this regard.[74]

Medical versus Combined Medical and Surgical Management

Outcome after SCI depends, to some extent, on therapy. The original and traditional therapy designed to improve neurological outcome after SCI is surgical decompression. Although not proved in randomized prospective studies, surgical therapy does appear to offer a clear advantage.[5,7,9,46,54,73] This is despite the fact that the degree of neural encroachment does not directly correlate with extent of neurological injury.[44] Frankel et al. established baseline data for neurological recovery after nonoperative management of SCI.[31] Several reports have documented better neurological recovery than that reported by Frankel et al. for patients with thoracolumbar fractures who had undergone neural element decompression operations.[7–9,46,73] Mason and Gunst also reported that the best treatment regimen regarding neurological recovery included immobilization, medication, surgical stabilization, and surgical decompression.[54]

The type of surgical procedure appears to affect the extent of neurological recovery. In fact, some reports demonstrate no neurological advantage to surgical decompression. Burke and Murray confirmed the recovery rate observed by Frankel et al. They also demonstrated that posterior surgical approaches failed to offer a neurological advantage over nonoperative approaches.[19] Dickson et al. also compared their results regarding posterior spinal surgery to those of Frankel et al. and found that surgery did not provide a neurological advantage.[27] The correlation of the information regarding anterior and posterior surgical approaches implies that appropriate decompressive procedures (usually involving an anterior decompression of the spine) provide a neurological advantage over simple stabilization procedures alone.

Burke and Murray[19] and Dickson et al.[27] observed no significant difference between the neurological outcome of surgically and nonsurgically treated patients and thus illustrates that the neurological outcome may reflect the effects of many different variables. These variables include distraction, which results in a varying degree of deformity reduction and, thus, neural element decompression (Fig. 282-1*A, B*). It may be of significance that stabilization procedures commonly involve the application of distraction forces to the spinal column. On the other hand, distraction, in the face of a persistent ventral mass, may result in the stretching of the spinal cord over the ventral mass. This, in turn, may worsen neurological function or minimize the chance for neurological recovery (Fig. 282-1*C*). These factors may, indeed, counteract each other, thus potentially negating any neurological advantage or the decompression associated with posterior stabilization procedures.

The neurological recovery advantage associated with spinal cord decompression is also evident after cervical spine trauma.[9] Furthermore, there appears to be an advantage to recovery of nerve root function after surgical decompression of neural foramina following cervical spine trauma.[8] Finally, although conus medullaris lesions complicate the neurological evaluation, they appear to be associated with a better prognosis than higher injuries.[85]

Medical management schemes are assuming a greater and greater role in the management of patients with neural trauma. Laboratory investigations regarding the secondary injury phenomenon have been instrumental in the establishment of the foundation for this clinical work. Several very promising medical interventions are currently under investigation.

Acute Treatment Strategies

Surgical Decompression and Fusion

Treatment strategies for SCI usually include a surgical management component.[3] The rationale for this is outlined above. From this information, appropriate goals for the surgical component of the management scheme include a dural sac decompression, the prevention of dural sac tethering, and spinal stabilization to prevent further injury.

The selection of the most appropriate time for surgery is complicated by a lack of meaningful prospective information to correlate outcome with timing of surgery. From an emotional point of view, one could easily conclude that early surgery (emergency surgery) is a rational approach. It is intuitive that the quicker a compressive mass is removed, the greater the chance for permanent neurological improvement. Anecdotal information has

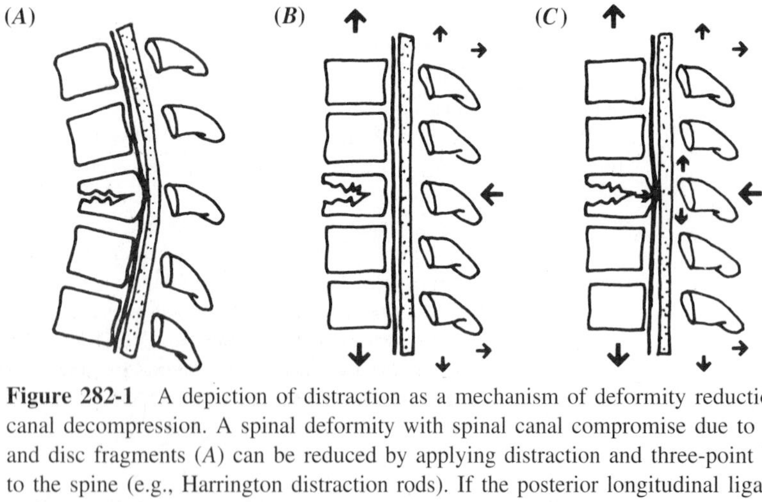

Figure 282-1 A depiction of distraction as a mechanism of deformity reduction and spinal canal decompression. A spinal deformity with spinal canal compromise due to retropulsed bone and disc fragments (*A*) can be reduced by applying distraction and three-point bending forces to the spine (e.g., Harrington distraction rods). If the posterior longitudinal ligament is intact **and** the unstable segment is mobile, a reduction of the retropulsed bone and disc fragments, with a relative restoration of the normal anatomic arrangement, will occur. This results in a decompression of the spinal canal (*B*). This may occur, however, at the expense of the stretching of the dural sac over the ventral mass during the reduction process (which may result in neural compromise). A more obvious problem arises if either the posterior longitudinal ligament is incompetent or the unstable segment is not mobile. In either case, the retropulsed fragments cannot be reduced by the distraction plus three-point bending mechanism. If this occurs, distraction can result in dural sac distortion (*C*). This may explain the reported lack of neurological efficacy of posterior stabilization procedures.

supported this. However, neurological deterioration after spinal cord injury has been shown to be greatest in those patients who had undergone early (emergency) surgery.[52] In addition, others have shown that neurological recovery does not appear to depend on the timing of surgery.[7–9] Indeed, early surgery has been associated with a poorer neurological outcome.[52] Finally, decompressive surgery that was delayed for a significant time (greater than 6 months) was associated with neurological recovery in a large portion of the neurologically incomplete patients.[50]

Secondary Injury and Neural Regeneration

Secondary injury has been defined as ''an injury to a neuron and its supporting cells which is delayed and follows a primary neurologic insult by a finite period of time. This injury results in a cell dropout (death) which is greater than that observed with the primary injury alone.''[11] It is now generally accepted that the phenomenon of secondary injury does indeed exist. Its nature is extremely complex, thus offering multiple potential avenues for intervention. These address the secondary injury scheme (as it is understood at this time) at a variety of points.

Although controversial, the second National Acute Spinal Cord Injury Study (NASCIS-II) has played a seminal role in establishing (1) that there is clinical significance to the secondary injury phenomenon noted in the laboratory, and (2) that the timing of intervention is critical.[17] Steroids and narcotic antagonists have garnered the majority of the initial clinical interest regarding the prevention of the ''secondary injury'' response to neural injury. The majority of experimental evidence suggests that massive doses of steroids will decrease the delayed neural injury response (secondary injury). This has been clinically demonstrated by the NASCIS-II study.[17] This report presented the first clinical evaluation that clearly demonstrated the efficacy of a treatment that theoretically alters the secondary injury response following trauma.

The importance of the relationship between the timing of treatment and neurological outcome was also documented by the NASCIS-II study. Patients whose treatment was initiated within 8 h of injury received benefit from treatment, whereas those who were treated after 8 h received no significant benefit. Others have observed a similar temporal relationship with manipulations of the secondary injury response.[6] These temporal relationships underscore the necessity for evaluating the timing of administration of a treatment, in addition to the dose administered. The 8 h therapeutic window observed in the NASCIS-II study may be pertinent only to methylprednisolone therapy in the particular clinical situation evaluated, however. Because the secondary injury response is very complex, it most likely takes place over a much wider time frame than 8 h and involves many more potential points of intervention than the inhibition of lipid peroxidation and free radical scavenging (the hypothesized mechanism of action of methylprednisolone in the NASCIS-II study).

The Methylprednisolone Treatment Regimen

The recommended methylprednisolone treatment regimen involves the intravenous administration of a 30 mg/kg bolus (administered over 15 min), followed by a 45 min pause. This is followed over the next 23 h by a maintenance intravenous infusion of methylprednisolone (5.4 mg/kg per h). Thus, the total administration time is 24 h. Treatment must be initiated within 8 h of the injury. The efficacy of this regimen was only established for closed injuries of the spinal cord. The efficacy of methylprednisolone administration for penetrating injuries and for closed injuries below the conus medullaris has not been established. Therefore, it seems prudent not to administer methylprednisolone to these patients; particularly because this methylprednisolone scheme doubles the wound infection rate and increases the chance of gastrointestinal hemorrhage.[17]

Other pharmacologic regimens also may be clinically effective. However, to date, only GM_1 ganglioside has been shown to be effective.[33] In this study, GM_1 ganglioside enhanced the recovery of neurological function at the 1-year follow-up. Further investigations regarding the efficacy of GM_1 ganglioside are currently proceeding.

Physiologic Parameter Management

The optimization of spinal cord blood flow or, more important spinal cord perfusion pressure, offers a theoretical advantage regarding outcome.[28,29,32,37] Therefore, it appears prudent to manage spinal cord injury patients aggressively with intravascular volume expansion. The etiology of hypotension in this patient population is multifactorial. Hypovolemia and vasodilation (secondary to the loss of sympathetic nervous system output) may both be involved. If sympathetic nervous system dysfunction secondary to cervical or high thoracic spinal cord injury exists, relative hypovolemia can be caused by the vasodilation. Therefore, even in cases where blood loss does not contribute to hypovolemia, significant volume expansion may be required to compensate for this phenomenon. The management scheme should essentially be identical to standard protocols for the management of hypovolemic shock.

Intravascular volume loss should be replaced rapidly, while intravascular volume status is monitored by maintaining the pulmonary artery wedge pressure between 12 and 16 mmHg, in most cases. Following the rapid acquisition of euvolemia, normotension should be achieved with pressors (in the range of 110 to 140 mmHg systolic). This scheme should optimize perfusion of the spinal cord.

Turning Techniques

The advantages of minimizing tissue pressure to critical cutaneous regions in spinal cord injury patients have been clearly documented. The time-honored treatment is an aggressive nursing program. Turning beds have been advocated.[18,35,58,75] However, proponents of these beds have not provided convincing supportive clinical information regarding them. There is no substitute for aggressive skilled nursing care. Treatment modalities that detract from this, such as complicated adjuncts to patient care, require close scrutiny.

Early Mobilization

Early mobilization of the patient may provide significant advantages regarding pulmonary care, decubitus ulcer prevention, and deep venous thrombosis and pulmonary embolus prevention. The advantages provided by early and aggressive orthotic management may assist in this process.[5,10,80] Early aggressive surgical stabilization, however, may provide more of an advantage regarding the extent of stability acquired in the severely impaired spinal cord injury patient by decreasing the need for confining and mobility limiting orthotics. Thus, early stabilization surgery provides significant advantages, if indicated.

Deep Vein Thrombosis Prophylaxis

Deep vein thrombosis prophylaxis may decrease the incidence of fatal complications of SCI. Therefore, a management scheme that includes either passive lower extremity motion, intermittent pressure boots or stockings, or low-dose heparin may be of benefit.[72] Each of these therapeutic regimens seems to be as effective as the others. Their risks are minimal. The most significant risk regarding passive motion or intermittent compression boot therapy is the potential for suboptimal compliance on the part of both the patient and the hospital personnel. Ineffective or inadequate placement or inconsistent utilization may negate their advantages.

Management of Orthostatic Hypotension

The effective management of orthostatic hypotension after spinal cord injury can allow the patient with a complete or high-grade myelopathy to ambulate earlier and, thus, optimize the rehabilitation process.[40] Pharmacologic management with pressors (i.e., oral ephedrine), with or without abdominal binders, are useful for this problem. Conditioning also plays a role. Many clinically significant problems diminish with time. Similarly, tolerance to orthostatism improves with time.

Pulmonary Complication Prophylaxis

Aggressive patient mobilization and early ambulation play a major role in avoiding pulmonary complications. This is obviously enhanced further by minimizing the time spent with ventilator support.[18,51,61]

Nutrition

The nutritional management of the spinal cord injury patient is more complex than one might expect.[2,70] An obligatory negative nitrogen balance ensues for weeks after spinal cord injury. An awareness of this phenomenon should alter traditional nutritional supplementation regimens.[70] Traditional caloric utilization calculation techniques overestimate nutritional requirements. Furthermore, they lack predictability. Therefore, the serial use of indirect calorimetry to assess nutritional requirements may be useful in difficult cases, particularly when ventilator dependence persists.

Rehabilitation

Physical Restoration Techniques

The purpose of the rehabilitation process is primarily related to the strengthening of existing motor groups and patient education. Physical restoration techniques do not augment neuronal recovery. They, therefore, do not augment neurological recovery. They do, however, take advantage of function recovered spontaneously by allowing strengthening of reinnervated and nonimpaired muscle groups and the education of the patient regarding his or her motor and sensory recovery.[41,45,77]

Functional Restoration

The enhancement of the quality of outcome by functional restoration modalities includes the improvement of quality of life-enhancing techniques,[41] instruction regarding ambulation and transfer skills,[45,77] biofeedback,[34] wheelchair considerations, and structural support and function augmentation. The latter can be accomplished by functional electrical stimulation,[25,53,62–67,87] reconstructive surgery,[43,60] and braces and orthotics.[5,10,80]

Education and psychological stabilization[55] also play a role in this process. The goal obviously is independence and community reentrance, when feasible.

The management of depression in this patient population may play a significant role in enhancing the rehabilitation process. Tricyclic antidepressant medication, if not contraindicated, should be considered early in the postinjury course in selected patients.

Medical Follow-Up

The medical follow-up of spinal cord injury patients should include the assessment and management of pain, decubitus ulcers,[78] urologic and bowel complications,[1,14,26,48,78,86] orthostatic hypotension,[40] respiratory complications,[51] muscle spasm, autonomic dysreflexia,[15] heterotopic ossification, sexual dysfunction (i.e., pregnancy, erection, orgasm, etc.),[12,13,20,21,23,36,69,71,81,82] spinal neuropathy,[24] burns,[30] alcoholism,[38] limb fractures,[42,59] exercise intolerance,[57] and post-traumatic syringomyelia. Cost should obviously be taken into account. Outpatient follow-up plans and schedules assist in the organization of long-term care.

The Comprehensive Rehabilitation Program

Where should I send my patients for SCI rehabilitation? This is, perhaps, the most pertinent question facing the spine surgeon today. Questions regarding family convenience, the quality of the rehabilitation program, and the capabilities for medical management, psychological management, postrehabilitation follow-up, and patient and family education must be answered by the referring physician prior to transferring the patient to a rehabilitation facility.[39]

The Future

What does the SCI victim of the future have to look forward to? Are there reasonable expectations regarding improvements in the anticipated quality of life of SCI patients? These questions are obviously rhetorical. Their answer, however, essentially depends on five factors: (1) SCI prevention, (2) medical management and secondary injury prevention techniques, (3) surgical management techniques, (4) augmented ambulation techniques, and (5) the improvement of the tolerance of the environment regarding the ''disabled.'' The research and medical community's investment into these areas will play a major role in dictating their success.

References

1. Achong MR. Urinary tract infections in the patient with a neurogenic bladder. In Bloch RF, Basbaum M (eds): *Management of Spinal Cord Injuries.* Baltimore: Williams & Wilkins, 1986, pp 164–179.
2. Agarwal N, Lee BY. Nutrition in spinal cord injured patients. In Lee BY, Ostrander LE, Cochran GVB, Shaw W (eds): *The Spinal Cord Injured Patient: Comprehensive Management.* Philadelphia: Saunders, 1991, pp 330–335.
3. Albin MS. Resuscitation of the spinal cord. *Crit Care Med* 1978; 6:270–276.
4. Bedbrook GM, Prince HG. A study of the influence of posterior column sensory sparing on initial presentation of cervical injuries on the ultimate prognosis. *Paraplegia* 1987; 25:441–445.
5. Benzel EC, Hadden TA, Saulsbery CM. A comparison of the Minerva and halo jackets for stabilization of the cervical spine. *J Neurosurg* 1989; 70:411–414.
6. Benzel EC, Lancon JA, Bairnsfather S, et al. Effect of dosage and timing of administration of naloxone on outcome in the rat ventral compression model of spinal cord injury. *Neurosurgery* 1990; 27:597–601.
7. Benzel EC, Larson SJ. Functional recovery after decompressive operation for thoracic and lumbar spine fractures. *Neurosurgery* 1986; 19:772–778.
8. Benzel EC, Larson SJ. Recovery of nerve root function after complete quadriplegia from cervical spine fractures. *Neurosurgery* 1986; 19:809–812.
9. Benzel EC, Larson SJ. Functional recovery after decompressive operation for cervical spine fractures. *Neurosurgery* 1987; 20:742–746.
10. Benzel EC, Larson SJ. Postoperative stabilization of the posttraumatic thoracic and lumbar spine: a review of concepts and orthotic techniques. *J Spinal Disord* 1989; 2:47–51.
11. Benzel EC, Wild GC. Biochemical mechanisms of posttraumatic neural injury. *Perspect Neurol Surg* 1991; 2:95–126.
12. Berard EJJ. The sexuality of spinal cord injured women: physiology and pathophysiology. A review. *Paraplegia* 1989; 27:99–112.
13. Beretta G, Chelo E, Zanollo A. Reproductive aspects in spinal cord injured males. *Paraplegia* 1989; 27:113–118.
14. Binnie NR, Creasey GH, Edmond P, et al. The action of cisapride on the chronic constipation of paraplegia. *Paraplegia* 1988; 26:151–158.
15. Bloch RF. Autonomic dysfunction. In Bloch RF, Basbaum M (eds): *Management of Spinal Cord Injuries.* Baltimore: Williams & Wilkins, 1986, pp 149–163.
16. Bohlman HH, Freehafer A, Dejak J. The results of treatment of acute injuries of the upper thoracic spine with paralysis. *J Bone Joint Surg [Am]* 1985; 67-A:360–369.
17. Bracken MB, Shepard MJ, Collins WF, et al. A randomized, controlled trial of methylprednisolone or naloxone in the treatment of acute spinal cord injury: results of the second National Acute Spinal Cord Injury Study. *N Engl J Med* 1990; 322:1405–1411.
18. Brackett TO, Condon N. Comparison of the wedge turning frame and kinetic treatment table in the acute care of spinal cord injury patients. *Surg Neurol* 1984; 22:53–56.
19. Burke DC, Murray DD. The management of thoracic and thoracolumbar injuries of the spine with neurologic involvement. *J Bone Joint Surg [Br]* 1976; 58-B:72–78.
20. Chapelle PA, Durand J, Lacert P. Penile erection following complete spinal cord injury in man. *Br J Urol* 1980; 52:216–219.
21. Chapelle PA, Roby-Brami A, Yakovleff A, et al. Neurological correlations of ejaculation and testicular size in men with a complete spinal cord section. *J Neurol Neurosurg Psychiatry* 1988; 51:197–202.
22. Chehrazi B, Wagner FC Jr, Collins WF Jr, et al. A scale for evaluation of spinal cord injury. *J Neurosurg* 1981; 54:310–315.
23. Comarr AE. Sexual concepts in traumatic cord and cauda equina lesions. *J Urol* 1971; 106:375–378.
24. Crim JR, Bassett LW, Gold RH, et al. Spinal neuroarthropathy after traumatic paraplegia. *Am J Neuroradiol* 1988; 9:359–362.
25. Dan BB. One small step for paraplegics, a giant leap for bioengineering. *JAMA* 1983; 249:1113–1114.
26. de Groot GH, de Pagter GF. Effects of cisapride on constipation due to a neurological lesion. *Paraplegia* 1988; 26:159–161.
27. Dickson JH, Harrington PR, Erwin WD. Results of reduction and stabilization of the severely fractured thoracic and lumbar spine. *J Bone Joint Surg [Am]* 1978; 60-A:799–805.
28. Dolan EJ, Tator CH. The treatment of hypotension due to acute experimental spinal cord compression injury. *Surg Neurol* 1980; 13:380–384.
29. Dolan EJ, Tator CH. The effect of blood transfusion, dopamine, and gamma hydroxybutyrate on posttraumatic ischemia of the spinal cord. *J Neurosurg* 1982; 56:350–358.
30. Formal C, Goodman C, Jacobs B, et al. Burns after spinal cord injury. *Arch Phys Med Rehabil* 1989; 70:380–381.
31. Frankel HL, Hancock DO, Hyslop G, et al. The value of postural reduction in the initial management of closed injuries of the spine with paraplegia and tetraplegia—Part I. *Paraplegia* 1969; 7:179–192.
32. Frankel HL, Mathias CJ. The cardiovascular system in tetraplegia and paraplegia. In Vinken PJ, Bruyn GW (eds): *Handbook of Clinical Neurology,* vol 26. Amsterdam: North Holland, 1976, pp 313–333.
33. Geisler FH, Dorsey FC, Coleman WP. Recovery of motor function after spinal cord injury; a randomized placebo-controlled trial with GM-1 ganglioside. *N Engl J Med* 1991; 324:1829–1838.
34. Goldsmith MF. Computerized biofeedback training aids in spinal injury rehabilitation. *JAMA* 1985; 253:1097–1099.
35. Gonzalez-Arias SM, Goldberg ML, Baumgartner R, et al. Analysis of the effect of kinetic therapy on intracranial pressure in comatose neurosurgical patients. *Neurosurgery* 1983; 13:654–656.
36. Guttmann L, Frankel HL, Paeslack V. Cardiac irregularities during labour in paraplegic women. *Paraplegia* 1965; 3:144–151.
37. Haghighi SS, Chehrazi BB, Wagner FC Jr. Effect of nimodipine-associated hypotension on recovery from acute spinal cord injury in cats. *Surg Neurol* 1988; 29:293–297.
38. Heinemann AW, Keen M, Donohue R, Schnoll S. Alcohol use by persons with recent spinal cord injury. *Arch Phys Med Rehabil* 1988; 69:619–624,
39. Heinemann AW, Yarkony GM, Roth EJ, et al. Functional outcome following spinal cord injury. A comparison of specialized spinal cord injury center vs general hospital short-term care. *Arch Neurol* 1989; 46:1098–1102.
40. Hoeldtke RD, Cavanaugh ST, Huges JD. Treatment of orthostatic hypotension: interaction of pressor drugs and tilt table conditioning. *Arch Phys Med Rehabil* 1988; 69:895–898.
41. Hussey RW, Stauffer ES. Spinal cord injury: requirements for ambulation. *Arch Phys Med Rehabil* 1973; 54:544–547.
42. Ingram RR, Suman RK, Freeman PA. Lower limb fractures in the chronic spinal cord injured patient. *Paraplegia* 1989; 27:133–139.
43. Johnstone BR, Jordan CJ, Buntine JA. A review of surgical rehabilitation of the upper limb in quadriplegia. *Paraplegia* 1988; 26:317–339.
44. Keene JS, Fischer SP, Vanderby R Jr, et al. Significance of acute posttraumatic bony encroachment of the neural canal. *Spine* 1989; 14:799–802.
45. Kostuik JP, Stauffer ES. The rehabilitation of the patient with neurologic dysfunction as a result of injuries to the thoracolumbar spine. In Frymoyer JW (ed): *The Adult Spine: Principles and Practice.* New York: Raven Press, 1991, pp 1353–1366.
46. Larson SJ, Holst RA, Hemmy DC, et al. Lateral extracavitary approach to traumatic lesions of the thoracic and lumbar spine. *J Neurosurg* 1976; 45:628–637.
47. LeDoux MS, Rosner MJ. Importance of cardiopulmonary function in prognosis after spinal cord injury. Presented at the 59th Annual Meeting of the American Association of Neurological Surgeons, New Orleans, April 24, 1991.
48. Lloyd LK, Kuhlemeier KV, Fine PR, et al. Initial bladder management in spinal cord injury: does it make a difference? *J Urol* 1986; 135:523–527.

49. Lucas JT, Ducker TB. Motor classification of spinal cord injuries with mobility, morbidity and recovery indices. *Am Surg* 1979; 45:151–158.
50. Maiman DJ, Larson SJ, Benzel EC. Neurological improvement associated with late decompression of the thoracolumbar spinal cord. *Neurosurgery* 1984; 14:302–307.
51. Mansel JK, Norman JR. Respiratory complications and management of spinal cord injuries. *Chest* 1990; 97:1446–1452.
52. Marshall LF, Knowlton S, Garfin SR, et al. Deterioration following spinal cord injury: a multicenter study. *J Neurosurg* 1987; 66:400–404.
53. Marsolais EB, Kobetic R. Functional walking in paralyzed patients by means of electrical stimulation. *Clin Orthop* 1983; 175:30–36.
54. Mason RL, Gunst RF. Prediction of mobility gains in patients with cervical spinal cord injuries. *J Neurosurg* 1976; 45:677–682.
55. Mawson AR, Jacobs KW, Winchester Y, et al. Sensation-seeking and traumatic spinal cord injury: case-control study. *Arch Phys Med Rehabil* 1988; 69:1039–1043.
56. Maynard FM, Reynolds GG, Fountain S, et al. Neurological prognosis after traumatic quadriplegia. Three-year experience of California Regional Spinal Cord Injury Care System. *J Neurosurg* 1979; 50:611–616.
57. McAdam R, Natvig H. Stairclimbing and ability to work for paraplegics with complete lesions—a sixteen-year follow-up. *Paraplegia* 1980; 18:197–203.
58. McGuire RA, Green BA, Eismont FJ, et al. Comparison of stability provided to the unstable spine by the kinetic therapy table and the Stryker frame. *Neurosurgery* 1988; 22:842–845.
59. McMaster WC, Stauffer ES. The management of long bone fracture in the spinal cord injured patient. *Clin Orthop* 1975; 112:44–52.
60. Moberg E. The present state of surgical rehabilitation of the upper limb in tetraplegia. *Paraplegia* 1987; 25:351–356.
61. Morgan MDL, Silver JR, Williams SJ. The respiratory system of the spinal cord patient. In Bloch RF, Basbaum M (eds): *Management of Spinal Cord Injuries.* Baltimore: Williams & Wilkins, 1986, pp 78–116.
62. Nene AV, Jennings SJ. Hybrid paraplegia locomotion with the ParaWalker using intramuscular stimulation: a single subject study. *Paraplegia* 1989; 27:125–132.
63. Peckham PH, Marsolais EB, Mortimer JT. Restoration of key grip and release in the C6 tetraplegic patient through functional electrical stimulation. *J Hand Surg [Am]* 1980; 5:462–469.
64. Peckham PH, Mortimer JT, Marsolais EB. Alternation in the force and fatigability of skeletal muscle in quadriplegic humans following exercise induced by chronic electrical stimulation. *Clin Orthop* 1976; 114:326–333.
65. Peckham PH, Mortimer JT, Marsolais EB. Upper and lower motor neuron lesions in the upper extremity muscles of tetraplegics. *Paraplegia* 1976; 14:115–121.
66. Peckham PH, Mortimer JT, Marsolais EB. Controlled prehension and release in the C5 quadriplegic elicited by functional electrical stimulation of the paralyzed forearm musculature. *Ann Biomed Eng* 1980; 8:369–388.
67. Peckham PH, Poon CW, Ko WH, et al. Multichannel implantable stimulator for control of paralyzed muscle. *IEEE Trans Biomed Eng* 1981; 28:530–536.
68. Piepmeier JM, Jenkins NR. Late neurological changes following traumatic spinal cord injury. *J Neurosurg* 1988; 69:399–402.
69. Robertson DNS. Pregnancy and labour in the paraplegic. *Paraplegia* 1972; 10:209–212.
70. Rodriguez DJ, Clevenger FW, Osler TM, et al. Obligatory negative nitrogen balance following spinal cord injury. *J Parenter Enteral Nutr* 1991; 15:319–322.
71. Rossier AB, Ruffieux M, Ziegler WH. Pregnancy and labour in high traumatic spinal cord lesions. *Paraplegia* 1969; 7:210–216.
72. Sachs BL, Bargar WL, Rechtine GR, et al. An improvised passive motion apparatus. *Clin Orthop* 1985; 194:205–206.
73. Schmidek HH, Gomes FB, Seligson D, et al. Management of acute unstable thoracolumbar (T-11–L-1) fractures with and without neurological deficit. *Neurosurgery* 1980; 7:30–35.
74. Schrader SC, Sloan TB, Toleikis JR. Detection of sacral sparing in acute spinal cord injury. *Spine* 1987; 12:533–535.
75. Stauffer ES. Complications associated with the use of the circular electrical turning frame. *J Bone Joint Surg [Am]* 1975; 57-A:711–713.
76. Stauffer ES. Diagnosis and prognosis of acute cervical spinal cord injury. *Clin Orthop* 1975; 112:9–15.
77. Stauffer ES. The rehabilitation of the patient with neurologic dysfunction as a result of cervical trauma. In Frymoyer TW (ed): *The Adult Spine: Principles and Practice.* New York: Raven Press, 1991, pp 1131–1141.
78. Sugarman B, Brown D, Musher D. Fever and infection in spinal cord injury patients. *JAMA* 1982; 248:66–70.
79. Suwanwela C, Alexander E Jr, Davis CH Jr. Prognosis in spinal cord injury, with special reference to patients with motor paralysis and sensory preservation. *J Neurosurg* 1962; 19:220–227.
80. Sypert GW. External spinal orthotics. *Neurosurgery* 1987; 20:642–649.
81. Szasz G. Sexual health care. In Zejdlik CM (ed): *Management of Spinal Cord Injury.* Belmont, CA: Wadsworth, 1983, pp 125–151.
82. Tarabulcy E. Sexual function in the normal and in paraplegia. *Paraplegia* 1972; 10:201–208.
83. Tator CH, Rowed DW, Schwartz ML. Sunnybrook cord injury scales for assessing neurological injury and neurological recovery. In Tator CH (ed): *Early Management of Acute Spinal Cord Injury.* New York: Raven Press, 1982, pp 7–24.
84. Tominaga S. Periodical, neurological-functional assessment for cervical cord injury. *Paraplegia* 1989; 27:227–236.
85. Toscano J. Prevention of neurological deterioration before admission to a spinal cord injury unit. *Paraplegia* 1988; 26:143–150.
86. Verkuyl A. Sexual function in paraplegia and tetraplegia. In Vinken PJ, Bruyn GW (eds): *Handbook of Clinical Neurology,* vol 26. Amsterdam: North Holland, 1976, pp 437–461.
87. Woltring HJ, Marsolais EB. Optoelectric (Selspot) gait measurement in two- and three-dimensional space—a preliminary report: technical note. *Bull Prosthet Res* 1980; 17:46–52.

283 Spinal Cord Injury without Radiographic Abnormality in Children

Paul A. Grabb
A. Leland Albright

For almost a century, it has been known that spinal cord injury can occur without vertebral fracture or deformation.[12] Burke in the early 1970s was the first to report a substantial series in which 12 children with spinal cord injury showed "no evidence of bony injury on x-ray."[3] Three of the 12 children underwent laminectomy, and a grossly contused or "pulped" spinal cord was discovered in all cases, but no soft tissue damage or bony injury was apparent. These findings highlighted the severe injury that the pediatric spinal cord can incur without any associated spine or soft tissue injury.

Children sustain fewer spine and spinal cord injuries than do adults. In reports by Hamilton and Myles, and by Osenbach and Menezes, pediatric spinal cord injury accounted for only 5.4 and 9 percent of all patients hospitalized with spine or spinal cord injuries, respectively.[7,9] Some spinal cord injuries in children have characteristics which suggest important differences in the mechanism of injury as compared to adults. One of these characteristics is spinal cord injury without radiographic abnormality (SCIWORA).

SCIWORA was defined by Pang and Wilberger in 1982 as the "objective signs of myelopathy as a result of trauma" in which no evidence of fracture, subluxation, or instability on plain radiographs, or computed tomography (CT) is demonstrable.[12] They reported on 24 children with SCIWORA and outlined the clinical spinal cord injury syndromes and injury levels according to age.[12] Their initial findings of age-related injury severity and injury level have been reinforced by subsequent reports.[9,11] Computed tomography is now used instead of plain tomography when excluding occult fractures. The above definition of SCIWORA has been adopted by most authors but should be expanded to include patients with symptoms, as well as signs, indicative of SCIWORA.

Epidemiology

The proportion of SCIWORA cases among all pediatric spinal cord injuries varies from 28[7] to 67 percent.[12] In two large series, 33 to 35 percent of pediatric spinal cord injuries were SCIWORA injuries.[6,9] The different percentages reflect different criteria: some studies included only children who were admitted to the hospital.[7] It is possible that children with lesser degrees of SCIWORA were not hospitalized at some institutions. The practice at the Children's Hospital of Pittsburgh has been to admit all children diagnosed with SCIWORA, no matter how mild—for reasons to be discussed.

The frequency of SCIWORA is higher in children younger than 8 or 9 years.[7,12] In one series, 42 percent of all spinal column or cord injuries in children younger than 9 years were diagnosed as SCIWORA.[7] Of the 31 children with SCIWORA reported by Osenbach and Menezes, 22 were younger than 9 years, and 18 were younger than 3 years.[9] This disproportionate representation of younger children (<9 years old) suggests a predisposition of the immature spine to SCIWORA. In addition, younger children are much more likely to have complete or severe SCIWORA injuries than older children. In three large series, 49 of 60 children younger than 9 years had severe or complete injuries.[7,9,11]

All levels of the spinal cord are susceptible to SCIWORA; the cervical cord is most often affected, followed by the thoracic and lumbosacral cord, respectively.[4,9,11] Upper cervical (C1-C4) SCIWORA occurs more often in children younger than 9 years.[9] Pang and Pollack reported upper cervical (C1-4) SCIWORA in nine of 21 children younger than 9 years, but in only one of 22 children ages 9 to 16 years.[11] This differential distribution of injury levels is explained by differences in the sites of maximum flexion. In the young child, maximum flexion occurs at C2-C3 and C3-C4, but as the child matures the point of maximal flexion migrates caudally to the adult level of maximum flexion, C5-C6, around age 8.[12]

The causes of SCIWORA vary with age. In young children, birth trauma, falls, and motor vehicle versus pedestrian accidents account for most cases, whereas in older children motor vehicle accidents and athletic injuries predominate.[7,11]

Proposed Mechanisms

Characteristics of the pediatric spine that make it more susceptible to SCIWORA than the adult spine are (1) more horizontal orientation of facet joints, (2) anterior wedging of the superior aspect of the vertebral bodies, and (3) more elastic ligaments and joint capsules. These characteristics allow for excess intersegmental motion to occur in flexion, extension, or distraction, resulting in neural injury without bony or overt ligamentous injury. The relatively large head and immature neck musculature in young children predispose to intersegmental motion when flexion or extension forces are applied. SCIWORA secondary to birth trauma can often be ascribed to longitudinal distractive forces. In a cadaver study of the neonatal spine, it was demonstrated that the spinal *column* could be stretched 2 in. without overt ligamentous disruption whereas the spinal *cord* could tolerate no more than ¼ in. before neural tissue disruption.[8]

There currently is no definitive evidence for any of the proposed mechanisms of SCIWORA. Information obtained from clinical observations, cadaver studies, and magnetic resonance imaging (MRI) of these children supports a mechanism involving abnormal intersegmental motion and neural compression. Although ischemia was initially thought to be a possible mechanism of SCIWORA, because of the ease with which the vertebral arteries can be occluded between the occiput and C1 during extension and rotation, there is no convincing evidence that it plays a significant primary role. MRI of childhood SCIWORA has documented ligamentous and disc injury but not compressive or vascular injuries, thus supporting excessive intersegmental motion and transient neural compression or distraction as the prominent mechanisms.[5] The high proportion (27 percent) of children with delayed onset SCIWORA and the occurrence of recurrent SCIWORA further implicate intersegmental motion in the pathogenesis. Interestingly, in half the children with recurrent SCIWORA, the second injury occurred after a force notably less in magnitude than in the first injury.[13]

Clinical Presentation and Diagnosis

SCIWORA can present with a spectrum of symptoms and neurological deficits, from a history of transient parasthesias or weakness to a permanent complete spinal cord syndrome. The presenting neurological syndromes can be grouped into three categories: complete, partial, and Brown-Sequard. The latter two can be further subdivided into severe and mild injuries. Some authors have divided incomplete injuries further into central and anterior cord syndromes, but for this review we will consider all incomplete injuries as partial with the exception of the Brown-Sequard syndrome.

Younger children are more likely to present with severe neurological injuries. Sensory changes (other than the ability to sense pinprick) are difficult to detect in a young child. In older children, subtle sensory deficits are frequently present at the time of admission, and usually persist longer than any accompanying motor deficit before complete resolution. Given the often subtle findings of a mild traumatic myelopathy in the older age group, it is possible that similar injuries go undiagnosed in the young child who is more difficult to examine and less able to articulate specific complaints.

As with any disease process, the key to diagnosis is a careful history and examination. We will not concentrate on the features of obvious traumatic myelopathies, but instead will concentrate on the subsets of the SCIWORA population which offer specific diagnostic challenges. The three subsets to be discussed are (1) children with transient symptoms that have abated before neurological evaluation, (2) children with a head injury and a mechanism of injury compatible with spinal cord injury, and (3) children with crush injuries of the torso, when general surgical problems may overshadow an accompanying thoracic SCIWORA.

For children who describe transient neurological symptoms or who are witnessed to have transient paresis that completely abates before neurological evaluation, great caution must be exercised before discharging them from the office or emergency room. A careful neurological examination may reveal subtle sensory, motor, or reflex changes consistent with a traumatic myelopathy. When such evidence is present, it is imperative to proceed with imaging studies and admission for appropriate observation and treatment. When a careful neurological examination is normal, however, one may be inclined to end the evaluation. This may not be appropriate given the high frequency of delayed neurological deterioration in childhood with SCIWORA often after minor transient neurological symptoms. Hamilton and Myles, and Pang and Pollack reported a 23 and 27 percent incidence of such delayed neurological deterioration in childhood SCIWORA, respectively.[7,11] Because of this evidence, if the mechanism of injury and the history are consistent with transient neurological symptoms from spinal cord trauma, we proceed with immobilization and further evaluation as an inpatient. The history cannot be discounted, even in the presence of a normal neurological examination, if the mechanism of injury and complaints make neuroanatomic sense. Although the original definition of SCIWORA put forth by Pang and Wilberger stated "objective *signs* of myelopathy . . . ," given the well-documented occurrence of delayed deterioration, a diagnosis of SCIWORA is also appropriate for children with transient neurological *symptoms* but a normal examination.

Severe head injuries are occasionally accompanied by spinal injury, which is traditionally diagnosed by spine radiographs since the head-injured patient cannot cooperate for a thorough neurological examination. In children, however, SCIWORA accounts for roughly one-third of all pediatric spinal cord injuries[6,7,9] and normal plain radiographs (including normal flexion/extension radiographs), therefore, cannot exclude SCIWORA. For severely head-injured children whose mechanism of injury is likely to have caused a spinal cord injury, we apply cervical immobilization until somatosensory evoked potentials (SSEPs) can be obtained. Although SSEPs only evaluate the posterior columns of the cord, they are currently the only practical means of assessing cord function when the appropriate neurological examination is not possible.

Lower thoracic cord injury may occur with crush injuries of the torso, such as those that occur when a vehicle runs over a prone child and hyperextends the thoracic spine. In one report of seven children with thoracic SCIWORA, all had "significant non-neural injuries."[11] The presence of life-threatening general surgical injuries may result in the overlooking of a thoracic cord injury. Tire marks were present on the torsos of all these seven children and thus should serve as a clue to the possibility of a thoracic SCIWORA.

Diagnostic Studies

Radiographs and CT are the crux of obtaining a diagnosis of SCIWORA. The neurological level indicated by symptoms and signs indicates the specific region to be studied. Initially, standard anterior-posterior and lateral spine radiographs are obtained. If these are normal, CT will exclude occult fractures. If the child is cooperative and comfortable enough to perform flexion and extension views of the involved spinal segment, dynamic plain radiographs are obtained to rule out overt ligamentous instability, although the reliability of acute flexion-extension films may be diminished by paravertebral muscle spasm. The finding of fracture, subluxation, or abnormal intersegmental motion at the level of neurological injury excludes SCIWORA as a diagnosis.

The role of SSEPs in the evaluation of possible childhood SCIWORA is unclear. Pang and Pollack noted SSEP abnormalities in 17 or 22 children with SCIWORA[11]; of the five with normal SSEPs, the cord injury was considered mild, with no clinical posterior column dysfunction. SSEPs are unlikely to detect mild cord injuries, especially those without overt posterior column dysfunction. We utilize SSEPs most often to try to detect subclinical spinal cord dysfunction when the history suggests SCIWORA but the examination is equivocal, and when a severe head injury prevents an adequate neurological examination and the mechanism of injury could be associated with a spinal cord injury.

MRI does have a role in the evaluation of childhood SCIWORA, but not in its diagnosis (since MRI is not a radiograph). SCIWORA is diagnosed by history, examination, plain radiographs, CT, and, rarely, SSEPs. MRI is able to exclude compressive lesions (e.g., herniated disc, hematoma), to detect ligamentous damage, and to assess the cord parenchyma for hemorrhage, transection, or edema. The greatest use of MRI in SCIWORA is for *prognostic* information: there is a close correlation between the status of the cord parenchyma and outcome. In a series of seven children with SCIWORA who had an MRI evaluation because of persisting or worsening neurological status, four had signal abnormalities of the cord, and four had disc or ligament abnormalities.[5] The cord signal abnormalities consisted of transection, edema only, and minor and major parenchymal hemorrhage. MRI evidence of major hemorrhage (>50 percent of the transverse diameter of the cord) or cord transection was associated with permanent complete injuries (Fig. 283-1). MRI evidence of minor hemorrhage or edema only was associated with severe cord syndromes at presentation but with substantial recovery to near normal (Fig. 283-2). Those children with normal MRI of the cord, including one with an acute complete T11 cord syndrome, made complete neurological recoveries independent of the presenting neurological picture. The ligamentous and disc abnormalities corresponded to the neurological level of injury as well as to the mechanism of injury (e.g., anterior longitudinal ligament disruption with hyperextension injury). The finding of ligamentous and disc injury on MRI strongly supports the proposed pathogenesis of incipient instability and potentially injurious intersegmental motion in SCIWORA, but does not predict overt instability.

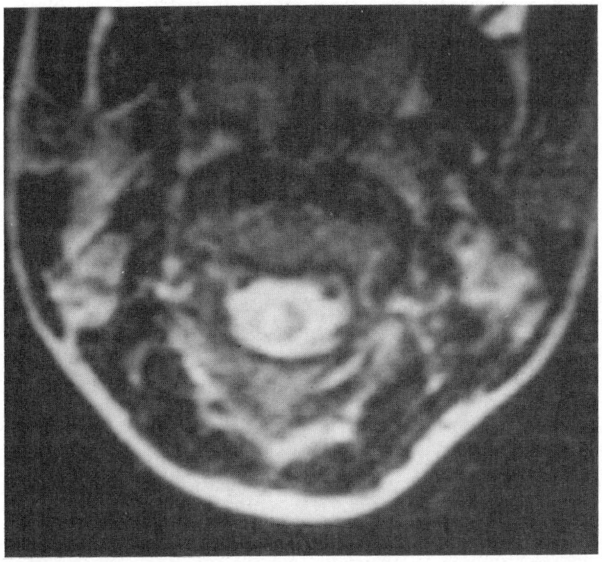

Figure 283-2 Long TR (TR = 4000, TE = 144) axial MRI of a 9-year-old boy with Brown-Sequard's syndrome after sustaining a lateral flexion injury shows a right hemicord hyperintensity consistent with edema.

Treatment

The mainstay of SCIWORA treatment is spinal immobilization. The duration and method of immobilization vary, however. Pang has championed 12 weeks of external immobilization because of the risk of recurrent injury if immobilization is discontinued earlier.[11,13] No other center has reported recurrent SCIWORA, however, and many pediatric neurosurgeons remain skeptical of the need to maintain 12 weeks of immobilization.[2] MRI evidence of ligament and disc injury may influence the duration of immobilization.

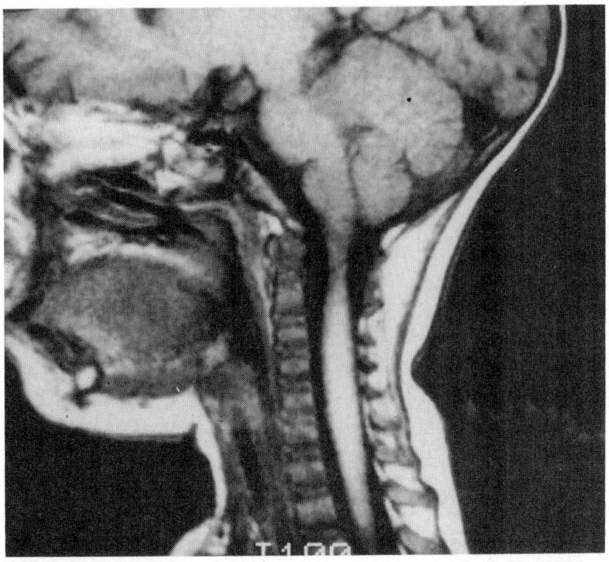

Figure 283-1 Short TR (TR = 600, TE = 20) sagittal MRI of a quadriplegic 21-month-old infant after physical abuse shows intraparenchymal hyperintensity expanding and replacing the cord. The hyperintensity is consistent with methemoglobin.

Methods of immobilization vary depending on the level of injury, age of the child, and physician preference. For cervical injuries, we employ a Guilford cervicothoracic brace (Guilford Inc., Cleveland, OH), which is more difficult for children to remove than a Philadelphia collar. Unless the parents perform daily skin care, skin (chin) breakdown is likely to be a problem. For thoracic injuries we employ a molded thoracolumbosacral orthosis (TLSO). Immobilization of infants is difficult. In fact, in cases of birth trauma associated with SCIWORA, a ventilated posterior thermoplastic shell contoured to the infant's occiput, torso, and buttocks is strapped to the infant with Velcro bands. A platform handle can be added to the back so that the neonate can be held, nursed, and turned with ease while maintaining immobilization.

Almost as important as immobilization in the treatment of SCIWORA is the emphasis to the parents and the child of the severity and potential consequences of SCIWORA. Especially in older children, when the injuries seem to be minor, the temptation to discard immobilization and return to normal activity can be great. In a review by Pollack et al. of recurrent SCIWORA, seven of eight children with recurrent injury engaged in activities which were clearly against medical advice.[13] The recurrent injuries were induced by mechanisms of relatively less force than the initial trauma, but the neurological deficits were more severe than with the initial injuries. Because of this experience and MRI documentation of ligamentous injury, emphasis must be placed on the lowered threshold a child with SCIWORA may have for recurrent spinal cord injury.

High dose methylprednisone is given intravenously to children presenting with severe or complete SCIWORA within 24 h of their injury in accord with the National Acute Spinal Cord Injury

Study.[1] We thus far have experienced no morbidity with this protocol, but cannot comment on the effectiveness of the steroids in these children.

Children with SCIWORA treated at the Children's Hospital of Pittsburgh are advised to maintain external immobilization for 4 to 12 weeks and advised against any physical activity which would put them at risk for reinjury. If the initial flexion/extension radiographs show no abnormality other than straightening of the cervical lordosis, the likelihood of later instability is approximately 2 percent.[11] If high quality flexion/extension radiographs are obtained initially, then repeat studies before discontinuing immobilization may not be necessary unless persistent neck pain or progressive neurological deficits occur.

Prognosis and Outcome

The single most important predictor of SCIWORA, as with other spinal cord injuries, is the initial neurological status.[9,11,12] Other important variables are the level of injury, age of the child, and MRI appearance of the spinal cord.

Many authors note that the presenting neurological status correlates closely with outcome.[9,11,12] In one report, 12 of 14 children with complete or severe cord syndrome at presentation are now dead or totally disabled.[12] In another report, none of the children with initial severe cord injury ''regained useful neurological function.''[9] Mild cord injuries are associated with much better outcomes. Of 33 children with mild to moderate injuries, 26 are neurologically normal, and five have mild residual deficits ''that did not preclude a full psychosocial lifestyle.''[11]

The level of injury is associated with the severity of the injury. The higher the level of injury in the cervical and thoracic cord, respectively, the more severe the injury. The majority of patients with SCIWORA at C1-4 in one report had complete or severe deficits.[11] Children with upper cervical SCIWORA are more likely to die, or to require long-term mechanical ventilatory support, tracheostomy, and gastrostomy. Likewise, upper thoracic SCIWORA is associated with a complete or severe syndrome much more often than lower thoracic SCIWORA.[11] Those children with severe or complete thoracic injuries are often able to achieve some independence through intensive rehabilitation and the use of orthoses. Severe or complete lower cervical cord injuries, while less frequent, carry a prognosis intermediate to that of upper cervical and thoracic injuries.

The age of the child is important because of the correlation between age and severity of injury. Of 104 reported cases of SCIWORA reviewed by Dickman et al., children age 0 to 8 years had a 75 percent incidence of complete injuries, whereas children age 9 to 16 years had only a 27 percent incidence of complete injuries.[4] As mentioned, young age confers not only a greater risk for complete SCIWORA but also a higher level of injury, both of which negatively impact on prognosis.

Finally, as noted earlier, MRI provides prognostic information by demonstrating transection, hemorrhage, and edema, and by allowing the evaluation of adjacent soft tissues, intervertebral discs, and ligaments, which may be injured despite normal radiographs. While it is neither practical nor advisable to obtain MR images in all children with SCIWORA, it is useful in evaluating children with severe or complete cord syndromes, or progressive neurological deficits. MRI provides valuable prognostic information and excludes the unlikely possibility of a significant compressive lesion.

At the Children's Hospital of Pittsburgh there have been no cases of SCIWORA complicated by an extradural or intradural-extramedullary compressive lesion. Reports in the literature lack any case of SCIWORA that required operative intervention to remove a cord-compressing disc or hematoma. While MRI has documented herniated disc material and extra-axial hematomas in childhood SCIWORA, none of these abnormalities has been substantial enough to warrant operative intervention.[5,10]

Conclusion

SCIWORA is a diagnosis practically limited to children because of the unique biomechanics of the immature spine, ligaments, and soft tissues. The definitive diagnosis of SCIWORA can only be made after normal flexion and extension radiographs and the exclusion of occult fractures. MRI almost never reveals surgically treatable abnormalities. The most important means of improving outcome in children with SCIWORA is early recognition and immobilization. No cases of recurrent SCIWORA or neurological deterioration have been reported after adequate immobilization. Patient and family education of the potential seriousness of the injury is an important aspect of management. While outcome has been most closely linked to presenting neurological status, MRI may be at least an equally accurate predictor of outcome.

References

1. Bracken MB, Shepard MJ, Collins WF, et al. A randomized, controlled trial of methylprednisolone or naloxone in the treatment of acute spinal-cord injury. Results of the Second National Acute Spinal Cord Injury Study. *N Engl J Med* 1990; 322:1405–1411.
2. Bruce D. Spinal cord injury without radiographic abnormality in children. *Pediatr Neurosci* 1989; 15:175, (editorial comment).
3. Burke DC. Traumatic spinal paralysis in children. *Paraplegia* 1974; 11:268–276.
4. Dickman CA, Rekate HL, Sonntag VKH, Zabramski JM. Pediatric spinal trauma: vertebral column and spinal cord injuries in children. *Pediatr Neurosci* 1989; 15:237–256.
5. Grabb PA, Pang D. Magnetic resonance imaging in the evaluation of spinal cord injury without radiographic abnormality in children. *Neurosurgery* 1994; 35:406–414.
6. Hadley MN, Zabramski JM, Browner CM, et al. Pediatric spinal trauma. Review of 122 cases of spinal cord and vertebral column injuries. *J Neurosurg* 1988; 68:18–24.
7. Hamilton MG, Myles ST. Pediatric spinal injury: review of 174 hospital admissions. *J Neurosurg* 1992; 77:700–704.
8. Leventhal HR. Birth injuries of the spinal cord. *J Pediatr* 1960; 56:447–453.
9. Osenbach RK, Menezes AH. Spinal cord injury without radiographic abnormality in children. *Pediatr Neurosci* 1989; 15:168–175.
10. Pan G, Kulkarni MV, MacDougall DJ, Miner ME. Traumatic epidural hematoma of the cervical spine: diagnosis with magnetic resonance imaging. Case report. *J Neurosurg* 1988; 68:798–801.
11. Pang D, Pollack IF. Spinal cord injury without radiographic abnormality in children—the SCIWORA syndrome. *J Trauma* 1989; 29:654–664.
12. Pang D, Wilberger JE Jr. Spinal cord injury without radiographic abnormalities in children. *J Neurosurg* 1982; 57:114–129.
13. Pollack IF, Pang D, Sclabassi R. Recurrent spinal cord injury without radiographic abnormalities in children. *J Neurosurg* 1988; 69:177–182.

284 Atlanto-Occipital Dislocation

Vincent C. Traynelis
Howard H. Kaufman

Traumatic atlanto-occipital dislocation appears to be a more common problem than previously appreciated. Well over 80 percent of the reported clinical cases of atlanto-occipital dislocation have been published since 1975, a fact most likely linked to increased sophistication in on-scene resuscitation and rapid transportation by emergency medical service units.[9] In 1979, Powers et al. reported that this usually fatal injury was detected in 1 percent of patients with cervical spine injuries presenting to the emergency room at their institution.[8] Neurosurgeons can expect to see a number of such cases in the future.

Mechanism of Injury

Most survivors of atlanto-occipital dislocation have been either passengers in automobiles or pedestrians involved in automobile accidents. These individuals have been subjected to forces significant enough to cause severe ligamentous disruption at the craniocervical junction.

The craniocervical articulation contains two separate groups of ligaments (Fig. 284-1).[10] The skull is attached to the first cervical vertebra (C1) by the articular capsule ligaments, the anterior and posterior atlanto-occipital membrane ligaments, and the two lateral atlanto-occipital ligaments. The cruciate ligament (a longitudinally oriented structure associated with the transverse ligament of the atlas) provides additional stability to this articulation. It should be noted, however, that a second set of ligaments coursing from the occiput to the second cervical vertebra (C2) provides the major structural support for the craniocervical junction. These ligaments, which include the apical dental ligament, the paired alar ligaments, and the tectorial membrane, also restrict extreme motion at the craniovertebral articulation. Specifically, hyperextension is limited by the tectorial membrane and lateral flexion by the alar ligaments. Excessive flexion is restricted by contact of the odontoid process with the basion.

Although forward dislocation of the cranium with respect to the cervical spine occurs after sectioning the alar ligaments and tectorial membrane, traumatic atlanto-occipital dislocation probably involves more extensive ligamentous injury.[9,10] Hyperextension can lead to tearing the tectorial membrane, and extreme lateral flexion can produce injury to the alar ligaments. Separation of the posterior elements of the axis and atlas, presumably a result of hyperflexion, is also present in many patients.

Atlanto-occipital dislocation appears to have its highest incidence in the pediatric age group which may be related to a relatively high incidence of automobile-pedestrian accidents, to specific features of the craniovertebral articulation in the young, or to both.[9] The craniocervical junction in children seems to be inherently less stable than that of the adult because of two factors. Early in life, the plane of articulation between the cranium and the atlas is almost horizontal.[4] Development of the occipital condyles occurs with maturation and allows the craniocervical articulation to function in a more stable vertically oriented plane. Furthermore, the occipital condyles of infants and children are not deeply seated into the fossa of the superior facet of the atlas. With maturation, condylar mass increases and the fossa of the superior facet of C1 develops more fully, thereby increasing the stability of this articulation.

Clinical Presentation

Neurological dysfunction related to atlanto-occipital dislocation may be categorized into lesions involving the brain stem, cranial nerves, upper spinal cord, and cervical nerve roots.[9] Many patients also have head injuries which can complicate the neurological picture.

Pang and Wilberger believe that brain stem injury, although common in atlanto-occipital dislocation, is not always fully appreciated.[7] Decerebrate posturing or complete lack of brain stem function may be seen, although it is difficult to ascribe such findings totally to atlanto-occipital dislocation in patients who also suffer head injuries. Discrete pyramidal involvement may result in paraparesis. Cardiopulmonary instability leading to bradycardia, irregular respirations, or even apnea can occur following a brain stem injury. It is severe brain stem damage which most likely accounts for the high mortality of this lesion.

Craniocervical dislocation may result in avulsion or stretching of the lower cranial nerves. The sixth nerve as well as the ninth through twelfth nerves are at particular risk. The true etiology of a sixth nerve dysfunction is difficult to ascertain in patients with concomitant head injuries. Severe hypertension may develop if both carotid sinuses are denervated following ninth nerve injuries.

Impairment of upper spinal cord function may result in quadriplegia, although hemiparesis appears to be a more common finding in patients with atlanto-occipital dislocation. Such motor dysfunction may also indicate brain stem injury. Some patients may present with a Brown-Sequard syndrome.

Traumatic atlanto-occipital dislocation may be associated with injury of the cervical roots. Unilateral dysfunction of multiple cervical roots may mimic a brachial plexus lesion.

Atlanto-occipital dislocation has been associated with compression, intimal tearing, spasm, and thrombosis of the vertebral arteries.[7,8] Such vascular injuries may produce brain stem or cerebellar infarctions.

Patients with atlanto-occipital dislocation may experience progression of their deficits. This may be due to additional trauma to the nervous system (secondary to movement of the unstable spine) or to other problems such as ischemia from emboli or thrombosis of damaged vessels. Patients suffering atlanto-occipital dislocation are often victims of multiple trauma and as such they must be fully evaluated for other injuries.

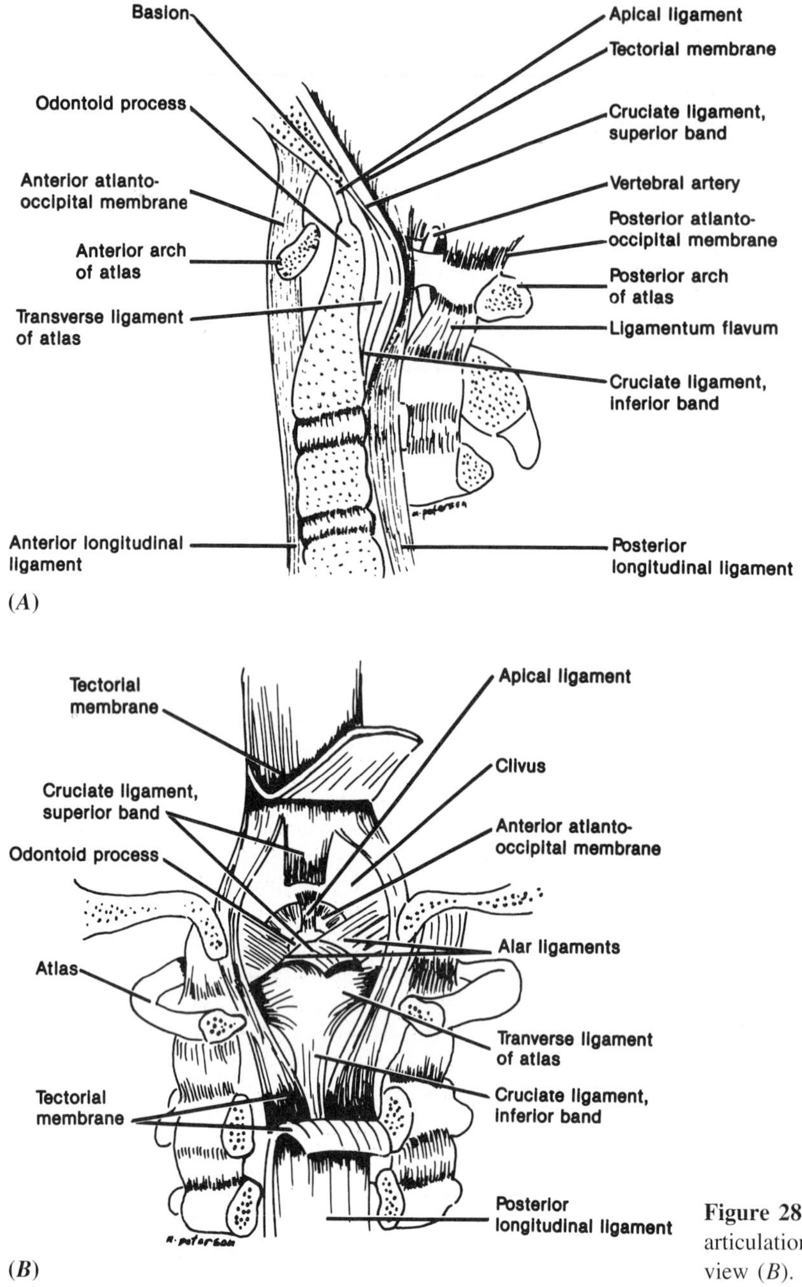

Figure 284-1 Anatomy of the craniocervical articulation, lateral view (*A*) and posteroanterior view (*B*).

Radiographic Features

The diagnosis of atlanto-occipital dislocation is made radiographically. Although the findings on plain radiographs may be subtle, the recognition of a retropharyngeal hematoma, which is invariably present, should alert the clinician to the possibility of serious spinal injury.

The diagnosis of atlanto-occipital dislocation may be confirmed by one of several radiographic criteria. Powers et al. proposed that the relation between the base of the skull and C1 could be defined by the ratio of the lengths of two lines (Fig. 284-2*A*).[8] One line is the distance between the basion (B) and the posterior arch of C1 (C), and the other is the distance between the opisthion (O) and the anterior arch of the atlas (A). The mean BC/OA ratio in normal individuals is 0.77. Any value greater than 1 may indicate atlanto-occipital dislocation. The BC/OA ratio is dimensionless and therefore not influenced by magnification which may be introduced with nonstandard film positioning. The BC/OA ratio is unreliable, however, in patients with congenital anomalies of the foramen magnum or fractures of the atlas. It may be less than 1 in some cases of longitudinal or posterior atlanto-occipital dislocation.

Lee et al. evaluated the craniovertebral junction with a pair of lines (*x*-lines): one from the basion to the midpoint of the C2 spinolaminar line (BC2S1) and the other from the opisthion to the posteroinferior corner of the dens (C2O).[6] The BC2S1 line intersects tangentially with the posterosuperior aspect of the dens and

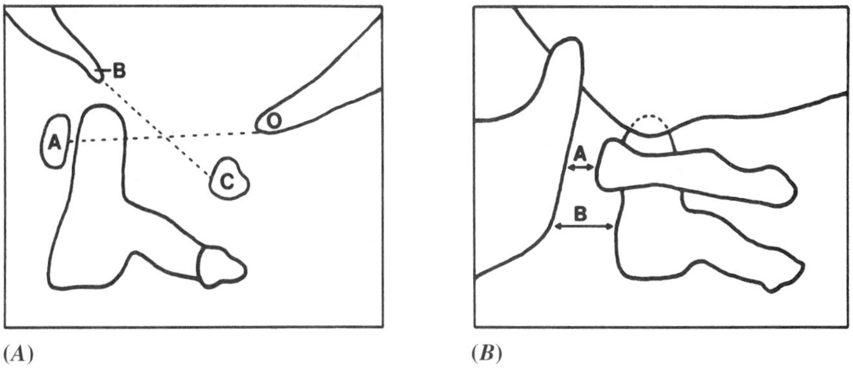

Figure 284-2 *A*. The diagram depicts the relation of the basion (B) and the posterior arch of C1 (C) to the opisthion (O) and the anterior arch of the atlas (A). *B*. Distances (in the neutral position) between the mandible and the anterior arch of the atlas (A) and the odontoid (B) average 2 and 10 mm, respectively.

the C2O line intersects tangentially with the highest point on the C1 spinolaminar line in normal patients over the age of 5 years. These relationships are altered by atlanto-occipital dislocation.

The *x*-line method may be more sensitive than the ratio proposed by Powers et al. Its validity is dependent on a normal C1-C2 relationship, however, and in over 50 percent of patients with atlanto-occipital dislocation, there is abnormal separation of the posterior elements of C1 and C2.[9]

Atlanto-occipital dislocation may be diagnosed by determining an increase in the distances from the most posteriorly located mandibular cortex to the anterior arch of C1 and to the odontoid process (Fig. 284-2*B*).[3] Precise radiographic positioning, utilizing well-oriented 72-cm films, is necessary to obtain valid measurements but this is not always feasible in the emergency room setting. This method is unreliable in patients with posterior atlanto-occipital dislocation, and furthermore, a displaced mandibular fracture can invalidate these measurements.

Kaufman et al. studied the radiographic separation between the occipital condyle and the superior facet of C1 in children and found the actual distance is never more than 5 mm.[5] They proposed that any displacement greater than 5 mm indicates atlanto-occipital dislocation. This measurement may be obtained from the anteroposterior or lateral radiograph, and it seems to be particularly useful in determining the presence of longitudinal dislocation. This distance has not been fully evaluated in adults.

Gross abnormalities of the craniovertebral junction are relatively easy to diagnose with plain radiographs. When atlanto-occipital dislocation is suspected, but the lateral cervical radiographic findings are inconclusive, thin-section computed tomography (CT) scanning of the craniovertebral junction should be performed. Two- and three-dimensional CT reconstructions may be very useful for evaluating the relationship of the occipital condyle to the atlas.

Hematomas, ligamentous injury or avulsion, bone fractures, and spinal alignment can be assessed with magnetic resonance imaging (MRI). MRI scans can provide visual confirmation of traumatic cord lesions. In addition, they can detect vertebral artery injury and/or thrombosis. Rarely, the diagnosis of atlanto-occipital dislocation is made solely by MRI scan.[2]

Traynelis et al. have suggested that there are three specific types of atlanto-occipital dislocation: (1) type I atlanto-occipital dislocation consists of anterior displacement of the occiput with respect to C1; (2) type II is primarily a longitudinal distraction with separation of the occiput from the atlas; and (3) type III atlanto-occipital dislocation exists when the occiput is posteriorly dislocated from C1 (Fig. 284-3).[9] Recently, Dickman et al. have described rotatory occipital-cervical dislocation.[2]

Management and Outcome

All trauma victims, particularly those with head and neck injuries, must be suspected of having atlanto-occipital dislocation. The initial management entails maintenance of adequate ventilation while the cervical spine is immobilized in the neutral position. Nasotracheal intubation should be attempted in patients requiring airway protection or suffering from respiratory distress. If this is unsuccessful or difficult, a tracheostomy should be performed promptly. Patients with spinal cord deficits should receive methylprednisolone as recommended by Bracken et al.[1]

The safety and usefulness of traction in the initial management of patients is controversial. Although there is concern that neural structures may be stretched and injured by traction, this has not been clearly reported to occur. The subdivision of atlanto-occipital dislocation into three types may be utilized to guide initial therapy.[9] In patients with type II atlanto-occipital dislocation, the primary problem is longitudinal distraction; therefore, traction, which may result in further distraction, is contraindicated. However, in patients with type I (anterior) or type III (posterior) atlanto-occipital dislocation and neurological deficit, traction may be indicated to realign the bony structures and thereby decompress the neural

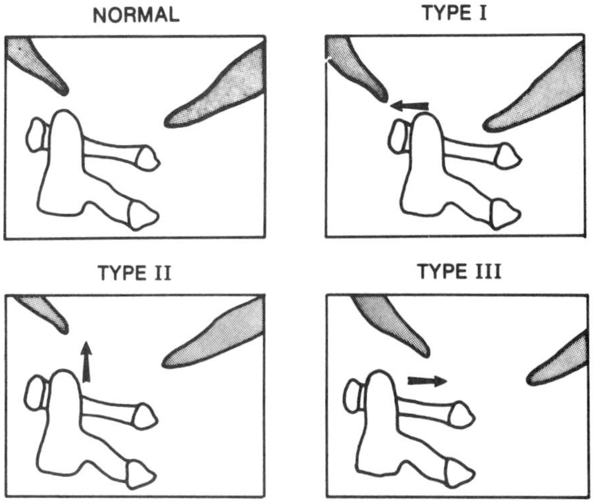

Figure 284-3 Diagrams illustrate the normal craniocervical relationship and the three types of atlanto-occipital dislocation: type I (anterior dislocation), type II (longitudinal separation), and type III (posterior dislocation).

elements. Rapid resolution of major neurological deficits has been noted in both type I and type III patients treated in this manner.[9]

The sole presence of a type I or type III atlanto-occipital dislocation does not absolutely mandate the use of traction. If there is only a minimal amount of malalignment and/or slight deficit, it may be reasonable to attempt realignment by careful positioning under fluoroscopy. Traction should be considered only in cases of gross misalignment or major neurological deficit.

Treatment with traction should be gentle (5 lb or less). Excessive weight must be avoided, and close clinical and radiographic monitoring is necessary. Following resolution of the deficit or radiographic realignment of the spine, the traction may be reduced to 1 or 2 lb, or it may even be discontinued and the patient immobilized in a halo vest.

Traction may be applied with Gardner-Wells tongs or a halo ring. Children require special consideration. By the age of 4 years (and perhaps as early as 2 years) there is sufficient development of the calvarium for safe tong application. Halo pins should only be tightened to 4 lb torque in patients 2 to 4 years old.

Although some patients have been successfully treated with traction and prolonged immobilization, most have remained unstable and required open fusion.[2,9] Injuries which are primarily ligamentous, such as atlanto-occipital dislocation, frequently fail to heal with conservative therapy, and therefore we recommend definitive treatment with posterior fusion as soon as medically feasible. Fusion of the occiput with C1 and C2 (and perhaps C3) is required despite the fact that this may reduce cervical spine mobility by as much as 50 percent.[9] Rigid internal fixation should be performed in conjunction with the fusion.[2]

Patients surviving atlanto-occipital dislocation for the first 48 h may have a good outcome. Up to one-quarter may survive neurologically intact, and another 25 percent are left with only minor deficits.[9]

References

1. Bracken MB, Shepard MJ, Collins WF, et al. A randomized, controlled trial of methylprednisolone or naloxone in the treatment of acute spinal-cord injury. Results of the Second National Acute Spinal-Cord Injury Study. *N Engl J Med* 1990; 322:1405–1411.
2. Dickman CA, Papadopoulos SM, Sonntag VKH, et al. Traumatic occipitoatlantal dislocations. *J Spinal Discord* 1993; 6:300–313.
3. Dublin AB, Marks WM, Weinstock D, et al. Traumatic dislocation of the atlanto-occipital articulation (AOA) with short-term survival: with a radiographic method of measuring the AOA. *J Neurosurg* 1980; 52:541–546.
4. Englander O. Non-traumatic occipito-atlanto-axial dislocation: a contribution to the radiology of the atlas. *Br J Radiol* 1942; 15:341–345.
5. Kaufman RA, Carroll CD, Buncher CR. Atlantooccipital junction: standards for measurement in normal children. *Am J Neuroradiol* 1987; 8:995–999.
6. Lee C, Woodring JH, Goldstein SJ, et al. Evaluation of traumatic atlantooccipital dislocations. *Am J Neuroradiol* 1987; 8:19–26.
7. Pang D, Wilberger JE Jr. Traumatic atlanto-occipital dislocation with survival: case report and review. *Neurosurgery* 1980; 7:503–508.
8. Powers B, Miller MD, Kramer RS, et al. Traumatic anterior atlanto-occipital dislocation. *Neurosurgery* 1979; 4:12–17.
9. Traynelis VC, Marano GD, Dunker RO, et al. Traumatic atlanto-occipital dislocation: case report. *J Neurosurg* 1986; 65:863–870.
10. Werne S. Studies in spontaneous atlas dislocation. *Acta Orthop Scand [Suppl]* 1957; 23:1–150.

285 Cervical Spine Injuries: Diagnosis and Management

Charles B. Stillerman
Ranjan S. Roy
Martin H. Weiss

Serious injury to the cervical spine resulting in spinal column structural damage or injury to the spinal cord is a problem of major public health proportions in the United States. The sequelae of such injuries may be devastating with respect to long-term disability for the patient and the demands on public resources. Our primary objective as physicians responsible for caring for such individuals is to minimize the extent of spinal cord injury subsequent to cervical trauma while providing an environment for the spinal cord to recover maximally. Spinal decompression, stabilization, and fusion procedures are often required to achieve recovery, as well as to promote fracture healing, to circumvent problems associated with prolonged bedrest, and in many instances to avoid the use of prolonged cervical fixation.

Epidemiology

The yearly incidence of spinal cord trauma in the United States ranges from 28 to 50 patients per million people. There are approximately 10,000 new cases occurring each year, with an estimated prevalence of 300,000 to 500,000 living victims.[32] An increase in prevalence during the past decade has been attributed mainly to enhanced longevity of spine-injured patients. Increased survivorship as well as improvements in neurological outcome have been attributed to enhanced medical, surgical, and prehospital care. In the spinal cord injured population the incidence of paraplegia and quadriplegia is roughly equal. Twenty percent of traumatic cervical instabilities will result in quadriplegia; however, there is a growing percentage of incomplete injuries. Approximately 25 percent of these patients will not have any associated neurological dysfunction. The remaining 55 percent will have incomplete spinal cord injuries or radiculopathies.[1]

Spinal cord trauma is most frequently a problem of the young adult male. It is estimated that 63 percent of new traumatic injuries occur in individuals between the ages of 16 and 30 with a 4:1 male to female ratio.[75] Most injuries occur as a result of motor vehicle accidents (50 percent), followed by falls (21 percent), acts of violence [mostly gunshot wounds (14 percent)], and sports-related activities (14 percent).[21] A large number of injuries occur in the early morning and are often associated with alcohol or drug ingestion. Multisystem trauma commonly accompanies spinal cord injury, the most frequent being long bone fractures. Visceral injuries to the chest and abdomen, fractures of the pelvis, and severe head injuries are common. Although patients with spinal cord injury are usually young, certain etiologies account for more injuries in some age groups than others. Motor vehicle accidents are the leading cause in the young, with a significant decrease in frequency with increasing age. The proportion of injuries occurring due to falls increases with age whereas sports-related injury is relatively rare in older patients. Acts of violence are fairly evenly distributed up to age 60, after which the frequency declines greatly. In the older group, traffic-related injuries and falls are responsible for almost 90 percent of spinal cord injury.[75]

Other contributing factors depend on environmental and geographic considerations relative to the region of study. Interest has long focused on the significance of athletics as a cause of spinal injury. Much focus has been directed toward contact sports as a precipitating cause; however, the occurrence of spinal cord injury from participation in football in the United States is rather insignificant when compared with other athletic activities. Certainly, in California, the greatest percentage of spinal cord injuries is related to water sports (i.e., diving, surfing, and water skiing) and snow skiing. These activities account for more than 80 percent of the athletically related spinal cord injuries seen in that state.

While 60 percent of spinal cord injuries occur in individuals under 30 years of age, occurrence in childhood and adolescence is uncommon. The incidence is believed to be between 1 and 3 percent in individuals under the age of 15.[31,63] When a cervical spine injury occurs in childhood, anatomic and developmental factors predispose the upper cervical spine. Because of this, childhood cervical traumatic instability that results in quadriplegia is not uncommon. The male to female ratio in spinal injured children is 2:1 with peak of injury being in summer. Traffic-related injuries account for 40 percent of the incidence followed closely by diving and other sports-related accidents (27 percent). Surprisingly, acts of violence are responsible for a larger proportion of injuries in this age group (20 percent) than for any other age groups but it is not clear whether these children are just innocent victims or active participants.[75]

Although the overall use of seat belts in automobiles has significantly reduced mortality secondary to automobile accidents, the lap-shoulder type of seat belts has actually resulted in a small increase in the overall number of spinal cord injured patients. Certainly, this occurrence does not compare to the protective effects.

Approximately 20 percent of all fatal victims of traffic accidents have an associated severe cervical spinal cord injury that contributes significantly, if not primarily, to the mortality. Eighty percent of these lesions involve the articulations between the occiput, C1, and C2. Studies have shown that in auto injuries which require towing from the scene of the accident, cervical spine injuries occur with a frequency of 1 in 300 victims. If an occupant is ejected from the vehicle, the frequency increases to 1 in 9.[47] Interestingly, severe neck injuries are associated predominantly with impacts occurring at the front end or side; such injuries occur much less frequently with impacts at the rear end.

The most common site of cervical vertebral body fracture is C5. Neurological injury at this level is estimated to be about 30 percent which is greater than at any other level in the cervical spine. When a cervical spine injury is associated with a fracture of the vertebral body and posterior elements, a 61 percent incidence of neurological deficit secondary to the injury is observed. Noncontiguous multiple spinal fractures occur in approximately 5 percent of cases; failure to recognize these injuries may result in devastating spinal cord damage.

Predisposing Factors

The most important factor associated with the genesis of significant cervical spine injury is the concomitant occurrence of a serious head or trunk injury. Transmission of forces through the cranial vault to the cervical spine has been readily demonstrated. Our general program of head-injury management requires that all patients rendered unconscious from a blow to the head be considered a victim of an associated cervical spinal cord injury until proved otherwise. The high frequency of alcoholic intoxication associated with craniocerebral trauma is also witnessed in cervical spinal cord injuries associated with traffic accidents. Not only does alcoholic intoxication contribute to the likelihood of becoming involved in such an accident but the potential chemical toxicity of ethanol on the traumatized spinal cord may increase the severity of the cord injury.

A number of underlying medical diseases may also predispose to the development of spinal cord injury. Although infrequent, people with a generalized seizure disorder have been reported to develop significant cervical spine injuries. Certainly, unrecognized metastatic disease renders an individual vulnerable to spinal cord injury subsequent to even trivial trauma. Of greatest consequence, however, is the existence of other underlying cervical spine disease—congenital or developmental. Three disorders that potentiate the occurrence of cervical spinal cord injury relate to the preexistence of (1) ankylosing spondylitis, (2) degenerative spondylosis, or (3) congenital fusion of cervical vertebrae. The first two are associated with a particularly high incidence of severe spinal cord injury related to trauma to the cervical spine; such injury most commonly occurs at the level of C5-C7.[76,89]

Imaging

Optimal treatment of patients with cervical spine injury relies on an accurate radiologic assessment of the traumatic lesions both with respect to existing abnormalities and the underlying mechanism of injury. Failure to recognize a cervical fracture or cervical instability may result in the subsequent development of severe neurological sequelae.

A lateral plain x-ray film encompassing the area between C1 and T1 is probably the single most important film for the initial evaluation of patients with a suspected or demonstrated cervical spine injury. However, it is important to remember that only 75 to 85 percent of cervical spine injuries are detected by such a single view. This accuracy increases to nearly 100 percent when anteroposterior, open-mouth odontoid, and flexion-extension radiographs are also obtained.[52,53] Inadequate visualization of the cervicothoracic junction due to overlapping shoulders is a common cause of a suboptimal x-ray evaluation. This problem is greatly magnified in obese patients or in those with a muscular body habitus. Downward pull on the arms is often necessary to adequately visualize the C7-T1 area. If this is technically inadequate, a swimmer's view may be needed. If both methods fail, tomography, computed tomography (CT), or magnetic resonance imaging (MRI) will be required for adequate visualization.

When the lateral cervical spine film is being reviewed, a number of areas must be addressed. The anterior prevertebral soft tissue width should be measured at the inferior aspect of C3. The normal width of the soft tissue at this level is less than 5 mm; any increase in soft tissue size should make one suspect prevertebral hemorrhage secondary to cervical spine injury. This sign must be interpreted with caution because crying, talking, or a film taken during inspiration may give a false positive result. The presence of an endotracheal or nasogastric tube invalidates this measurement. Loss of the normal lordotic curve frequently accompanies injury to the cervical spine. Although this finding may be an indication of a severe cervical injury, it must be noted that the lordotic curve is absent in 20 percent of normal patients. Careful inspection of the relationship of the posterior aspect of the vertebral bodies on the lateral x-ray films provides good evidence for anterior or posterior displacement. Likewise, close inspection for angular deformity or changes in the bony configuration of the vertebral bodies is essential. Abnormal separation anteriorly at the level of the intervertebral disc that may or may not be associated with an avulsion fracture of the adjacent vertebral body, or increased separation between the spinous processes posteriorly provide evidence of injury to the ligamentous structures supporting the vertebral column.

Anteroposterior (AP) views of the mid- and lower cervical spine are helpful in defining the presence of a unilateral facet dislocation that may not be evident on the lateral projection. In such circumstances one must carefully view the spinous processes as they appear on the AP view, looking for rotation of the spines toward the side of the dislocation above the level of the injury. One may also detect a widening of the uncovertebral joints as well as fractures of articular processes, vertebral bodies, and transverse and uncinate processes on the AP view. In the event that the clinical picture suggests a facet dislocation but x-rays are not definitive, oblique views of the cervical spine taken with the physician in attendance may lend further support in establishing a diagnosis. Open-mouth views, in conjunction with lateral films, are necessary to evaluate the atlantoaxial articulations and different patterns of odontoid fractures. One should inspect the integrity of the lateral masses of C1, and note the alignment relative to C2. Abnormal alignment may reflect damage to the transverse ligament. This view is particularly helpful in looking for a Jefferson's fracture and rotatory instability secondary to bony or ligamentous disruption.

Between 15 and 20 percent of patients who have cervical spinal cord injuries will have no overt radiographic findings on plain films. Of these patients, approximately two-thirds will demonstrate abnormalities when thin-section CT of the spine is subsequently added to the radiographic evaluation. Of particular importance is the capacity of the studies to demonstrate the projection of bone and/or disc material into the spinal canal and the presence of nondisplaced fractures of the laminae, pedicles, facets, and vertebral body.[13,30] CT offers the added advantage of reformatting images to give a three-dimensional configuration of fractures thereby permitting increased visualization of the extent of injury. A drawback of reformatting, however, is that it may give rise to "pseudofractures." Limitation of CT is evidenced by the evaluation of certain types of odontoid, atlantal, or subaxial fractures in which the plane of the fracture parallels the plane of the CT scan. In such cases, lateral x-ray films or tomography may be more useful.

With the intrathecal administration of a water-soluble contrast agent, CT myelography has essentially replaced conventional cervical myelography for assessing intraspinal contents. The contrast agent may be administered via a lateral C1-2 puncture or through the lumbar route, with subsequent CT evaluation, giving a precise assessment of the bony structures around the spinal canal as well as the contents of the spinal canal. Intrathecal contrast provides an outline of the spinal cord. This is extremely helpful in assessing the degree of spinal cord and/or neural foraminal compression. Spinal cord parenchymal injury is inferred by cord widening and a corresponding decrease in the size of the subarachnoid space at the level of injury. The CT scan is also helpful in defining the presence of spinal stenosis, regardless of the underlying etiology. It is important to remember, however, that such a static study may not reflect the relationship between the spinal column and the neural elements that occur during weight bearing.

X-ray films demonstrate a static situation with respect to the pathology of the cervical spine. Even though major disruptions of ligamentous structures may strongly argue that a given fracture is unstable, demonstrations or proof of instability may require dynamic assessment. Flexion-extension views are recommended only in conscious patients and preferably when one has direct visualization of the cervical spine. These maneuvers are only done under direct supervision of a physician in those situations in which there is no evidence of gross instability and an absence of neurological deficit and/or significant intracanalicular bone or disc material. Dynamic studies are especially valuable in the absence of subluxation when one suspects ligamentous instability.[52] It should be emphasized that, in patients with major spinal injury, any radiographic evaluation of the patient, especially any involving transportation to an x-ray table, should be under the direction of a physician; cervical immobilization with a head holder, cervical collar, or sandbag should be used to reduce neck motion prior to and during x-ray evaluation. In a patient with major muscular spasm, frequently observed after cervical spine injury, it may be impossible to adequately assess instability of the spine. We place such patients in traction or a restrictive cervical orthosis until such spasm abates in order to more adequately assess spinal stability, with the physician once again in attendance during this assessment. Occult ligamentous injury should be considered when displacement is greater than 5 mm or angulation of 5 degrees or more is noted on lateral or flexion-extension films.

MRI has recently been used to evaluate patients with acute cervical spine injury.[19,30] Despite its relatively short existence, MRI has already demonstrated significant advantages over that offered by CT or CT-myelography. A major advance of MRI is its ability to provide superior soft-tissue contrast resolution using combinations of T1-weighted, proton-density, and T2-weighted images. Exquisite detail of soft tissue injury including the disc herniation, ligamentous rupture, and intrinsic cord injury can now be provided by MRI.

Among the noninvasive modalities available to determine the presence of a traumatic cervical disc herniation, MRI is now being used more frequently. In a series of patients with traumatic cervical disc herniations, Flanders et al. reported that CT without contrast detected only 44 percent of disc protrusions when compared to MRI.[30] Others have reported similar findings. No comparisons were reported between CT-myelography and MRI regarding evaluation of disc herniation.

Another advantage of MRI is its ability to assess spinal column ligaments, which offers additional information regarding the stability of the cervical spine. Ligamentous abnormalities, once only inferred through other studies, can now be imaged directly.[60] Evaluation is best performed using sagittal T2-weighted images. Damage to the anterior and posterior longitudinal ligaments is suggested by the discontinuity of the signal void on either side of the vertebral body at the level of injury. Massive prevertebral swelling, seen as a hyperintense signal on T2-weighted images, accompanies damage to the anterior longitudinal ligament. In a similar fashion, flexion-distraction injuries reveal a hyperintense T2-weighted signal, demonstrating edema and/or hemorrhage in the region of the posterior ligamentous complex.

Direct nonreformatted multiplanar imaging is easily acquired by MRI and serves to enhance lesion detection. Sagittal imaging of the spine by MRI is at least equal to, and usually superior to, reformatted CT images. Reconstructed CT scans may not be as anatomically correct as direct MR images.

MRI has the inherent ability to create "myelographic-equivalent" images using T2-weighted signal sequences.[30,33,81] In the past, only the invasive technique of myelography with subsequent CT provided an outline of the spinal cord and hence information regarding thecal sac or spinal cord compression. T2-weighted MR images can be used to assess the extent of compressive cord pathology. MRI sequences can further delineate the exact underlying cause (i.e., bony osteophyte, disc herniation, and/or epidural hematoma).

Another unique capability of MRI is its ability to directly image intrinsic cord injury ranging from mild contusion and intramedullary hemorrhage to complete cord transection.[30] Earlier studies with the midfield strength unit (0.5 T) did not easily distinguish between edema and cord hemorrhage. Increasing the magnet size to 1.5 T solved this problem. The value of imaging spinal cord parenchymal injury is obvious considering that a direct correlation is not always found between neurological deficits and the degree of spinal canal compromise. Intrinsic cord injury may be responsible, at least in part, for some of the neurological deficits.

A relative disadvantage of MRI is that it does not image cortical bone well.[45] Thus, bony fractures may not be as well defined on MRI as on bone windows of CT scans, tomograms, or plain films. Nevertheless, the contrast discrimination between the hypointense cortical bone and the hyperintense marrow on T1-weighted images permits adequate visualization of fractures. Acute fractures through the cortex appear mildly hyperintense whereas fractures through the bone marrow are usually hypointense on T1-weighted images; cortical fractures are usually more obvious and well defined than fractures through the marrow. CT is the better test for demonstrating anterior and posterior element fractures with retropulsed bone fragments in the spinal canal, and bony anatomy in general. The degree of thecal sac compression by these fragments is most precisely depicted by contrast CT scans.

Because the spinal cord can be imaged directly with MRI, recent studies have focused on attempts to correlate specific MRI findings with the degree of neurological injury at admission. In a series of 78 patients with acute cervical spinal cord injuries, MRI revealed abnormal cord parenchymal signals in all patients with a neurological deficit.[30] There was also a direct relationship between the severity of injury and cord swelling as visualized on T2-weighted images. The presence of intramedullary hemorrhage signified severe trauma and was predictive of a complete and possibly permanent lesion. As expected, the degree of bony and soft tissue injury did not correlate with the extent of spinal cord trauma or neurological deficit. The prognostic significance of initial MR images in patients with acute cervical injuries and associated neurological deficits has been reported.[51] Patients with a large parenchymal hemorrhage had a poor prognosis; a somewhat better outcome occurred in those patients with a small, focal hematoma. Patients with intramedullary edema over multiple segments but no hemorrhage had a much higher rate of recovery but not as much as those with edema involving one spinal segment or less.

From a practical standpoint, MRI for acute cervical spine

trauma may not always be feasible as a first method of evaluation for several reasons.[61] An MRI unit may not be accessible or it may be housed in a separate facility, thus making examination of hemodynamically unstable patients impossible. The long image acquisition time (relative to CT) and the requirement that the patient be absolutely still during the entire imaging procedure is impractical for patients with severe neck pain or for those with impaired cognition. Critically ill patients requiring life support systems may be difficult to image with MRI. Electrical devices can interfere with image acquisition and may not function properly within the magnetic field. Some patients require, as part of their initial treatment based on plain films, cervical immobilization and traction. Not all MRI suites are equipped with in-line cervical traction devices. Moreover, these devices may cause local magnetic field changes and image distortion. Progress has been made in handling some of these obstacles. Ventilatory support systems have been designed to be within close proximity to the magnet without interfering with the quality of the images. MRI-compatible graphite traction tongs and nonferrous pulleys and waterbags can be used during imaging of the acutely injured patient requiring cervical traction. Preliminary studies have also reported the use of ultrafast imaging techniques and motion suppression techniques to obtain higher quality MR images.

Anatomy

Fundamental to the discussion of cervical spine injuries is an understanding of the normal anatomic relationships of the cervical spine. Complete familiarity of this region is essential for treating traumatic injuries.

Upper Cervical Spine

The upper cervical spine serves as a transition zone between the rigid calvarium and the mobile spine. It consists of the foramen magnum, paired occipital condyles, atlas, and axis, and is often referred to as the cervicocranium (Fig. 285-1). The craniocervical articulation houses the lower medulla and the upper cervical spinal cord and also provides protection for the paired vertebral arteries. This region is distinct in morphology and physiology when compared to the middle and lower cervical spine, which extends from the third to the seventh cervical vertebrae. The effects of a traumatic event on the cervicocranium are greatly modified largely due to its unique structural and biomechanical characteristics.

The posterior skull base is formed predominantly by the occipital bone (Fig. 285-2). At the floor of the fossa is the foramen magnum through which the lower medulla and upper cervical cord and their surrounding meninges become continuous. The opening also transmits the vertebral arteries, a few small veins, and the spinal roots of the accessory nerve. The anterior rim of the foramen magnum is the basion and is normally within 5 mm and directly above the tip of the dens. The opisthion refers to the posterior aspect of the foramen. The occipital condyles lie on the inferior surface of the occipital bone and along the anterolateral edges of the foramen magnum. These paired structures are convex and semilunar in shape, and articulate with the reciprocally concave superior aspect of the lateral masses of the first cervical vertebra (Fig. 285-3).

The first cervical vertebra, the atlas, is ring-like and consists of a shorter anterior and longer posterior arch and a lateral mass on each side (Fig. 285-4). Unlike the other six cervical vertebrae, the atlas does not have a vertebral body, pedicles, laminae, or a true spinous process. Although the anterior and posterior arches are relatively thin, the lateral masses are heavy and thick and correspond to the pedicles and articular pillars of the lower cervical vertebrae. The ventral surface of the anterior arch is the anterior tubercle upon which the longus colli muscles insert. The dorsal surface of the anterior arch has a depression for articulation with the dens. A prominent tubercle of bone on the anteromedial aspect of each lateral mass permits attachment of the transverse ligament that confines the dens and maintains stable articulation with the axis.

Extending laterally from each lateral mass is a rudimentary transverse process containing the transverse foramen through which runs the vertebral artery. The artery passes upward and then loops dorsally and medially around the lateral mass prior to entering the foramen magnum. The superior facet of the atlas, ovoid and concave in configuration, articulates with the convex occipital condyles and forms the atlanto-occipital joints. This allows for flexion and extension of the head. The inferior facet, almost circular in shape and gently concave, articulates with the superior facet of the axis, or second cervical vertebra forming the atlantoaxial joints and permitting rotation of the atlas on the axis (Figs. 285-1 and 285-3).

The axis is the largest and heaviest cervical vertebra, consisting

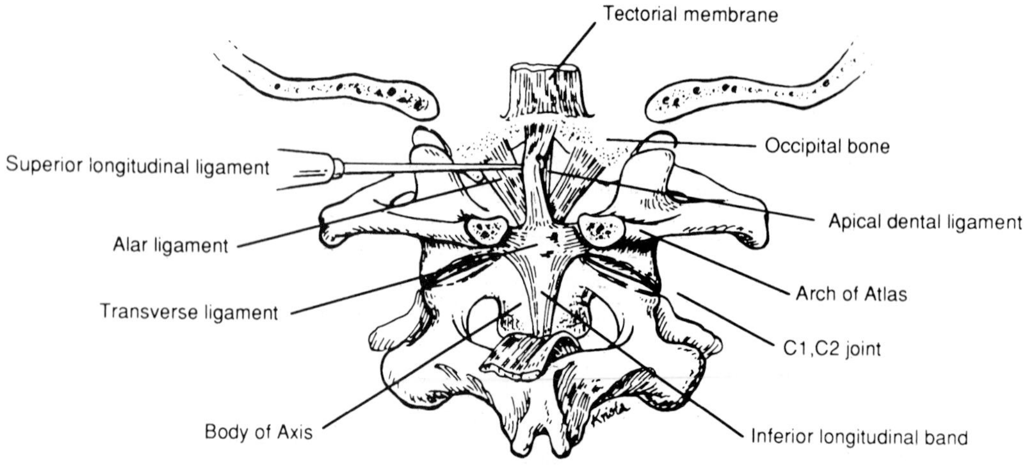

Figure 285-1 Diagram of the craniocervical junction (posterior view).

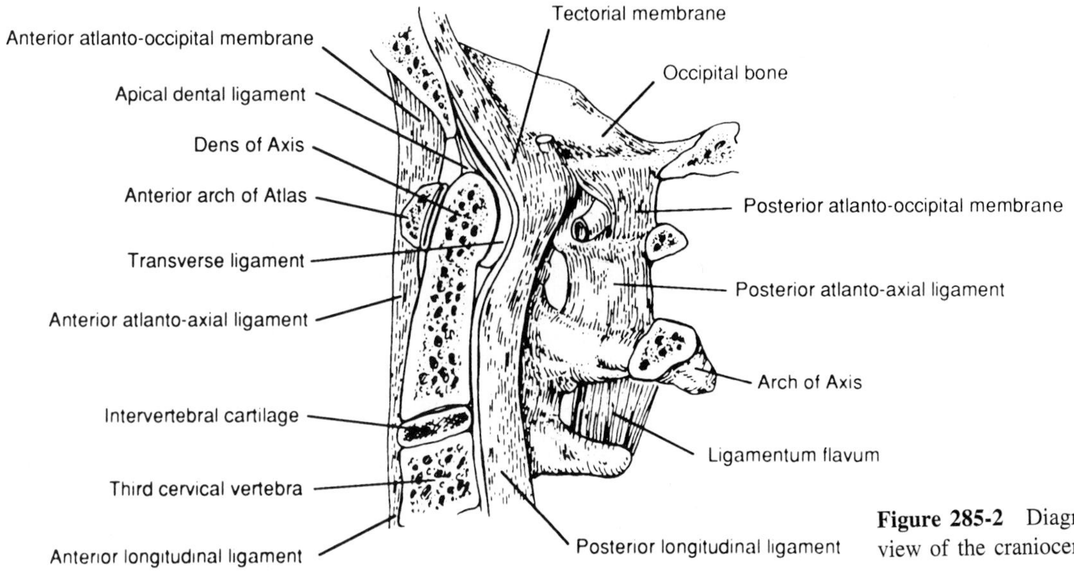

Figure 285-2 Diagram illustrating a lateral view of the craniocervical junction.

of a body, bilateral masses, laminae, and a prominent, bifid spinous process (Fig. 285-5). The lateral masses with their superior and inferior articulating facets and transverse processes lie on each side of the body. Of note is the ''offsetting'' of the articular processes with the superior pair being more anterior than the inferior pair. In addition, the superior facet of the axis is convex and faces upward and outward to articulate with the atlas while the inferior facet faces obliquely forward and downward articulating with the third cervical vertebra. Unique to the axis is the dens (odontoid process) projecting upward from the axis body; it serves as a pivot for articulation with the atlas and provides rotational mobility.

The transverse process of the axis contains the foramen transversarium for the vertebral artery and serves as an attachment site for muscles involved in head rotation. Three joints comprise the atlantoaxial articulation (Figs. 285-4 and 285-5). The articulation between the anterior arch of the atlas and the anterior surface of the dens and that between the posterior surface of the dens and the transverse ligament of the atlas together constitute the medial atlantoaxial joint. The two lateral atlantoaxial joints are formed by the articulating surfaces of the lateral masses of the atlas and axis.

Ligamentous structures are vitally important in allowing for large ranges of motion of the cervical spine while maintaining stability. This is no exception in the region of the cervicocranium. The ligaments of the craniocervical articulation appear to bypass the atlas and extend from the occiput to the axis. In essence, the atlas serves only as a spacer.

The major cranial cervical ligaments are classified as either internal or external depending on their location inside or outside the vertebral canal (Fig. 285-1). The principal internal ligaments are (1) the thin and flat tectorial membrane, which is a cranial extension of the posterior longitudinal ligament that passes posterior to the body, odontoid process, and transverse ligament and attaches to the anterior margin of the foramen magnum; (2) the transverse atlantal ligament, passing horizontally behind the dens and maintaining a normal relationship between the dens and the atlas; and (3) the paired alar ligaments which extend from the posterolateral tip of the dens to the medial surface of the occipital condyles thereby limiting rotation of the head with respect to the atlas. Ligaments of lesser importance in this region include the apical dental ligament extending from the apex of the dens to the anterior midpoint of the foramen magnum and the accessory ligament that connects the body of the dens near its base to the lateral mass of the atlas. The accessory ligament, in conjunction with the alar ligament, restricts atlantoaxial rotation.

The major external craniocervical ligaments are (1) the anterior atlanto-occipital membrane, a structural extension of the anterior

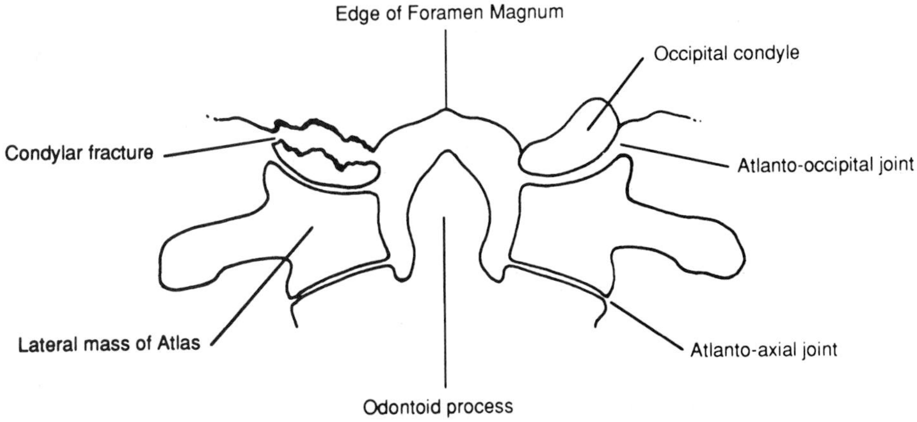

Figure 285-3 Illustration of a type III occipital condyle fracture.

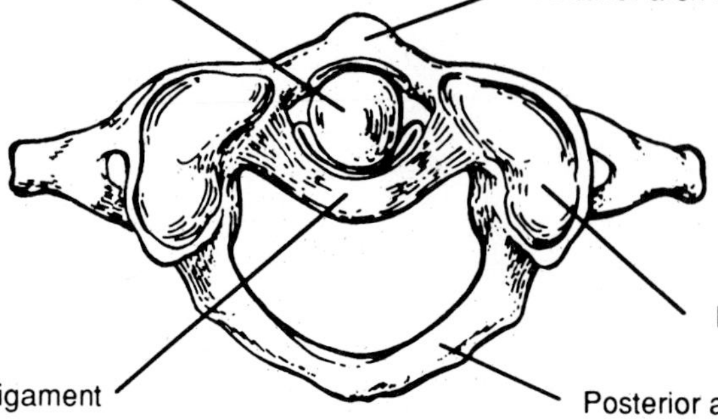

Figure 285-4 Axial diagram of the atlas. Note that the anterior arch of C1 is shorter than the posterior arch.

longitudinal ligament, that extends from the anterior arch of the atlas to the basion; (2) the posterior atlanto-occipital membrane located between the posterior rim of the foramen magnum and superior surface of the posterior arch of the atlas and believed to be homologous to the ligamenta flava; (3) the anterior and posterior atlantoaxial membranes; and (4) the articular capsules and ligamentum nuchae (Fig. 285-2).

Subaxial Cervical Spine

The third through the seventh cervical vertebrae are similar in most respects (Fig. 285-6*A*). Although they are uniform in configuration, there is a gradual increase in size with the seventh vertebra being the largest (Fig. 285-6*B*). The vertebral body is oval shaped with the transverse diameter greater than the anteroposterior diameter (Fig. 286-6*C*). The superior surface of the vertebral body is concave with a raised projection on either side called the uncinate process, while the inferior surface is reciprocally convex. The joint of Luschka is formed by the uncinate process of the vertebra below and the lateral margin of the vertebra above (Fig. 285-6*B*). Superiorly and inferiorly, the vertebral body is bounded by intervertebral discs.

Pedicles project posterolaterally from the body whereas the laminae are medially directed to join the spinous processes. Lateral to the junction of the pedicles and laminae are the lateral pillars with obliquely directed superior and inferior articular facets. Each vertebra has a transverse process pierced by a foramen through which passes the vertebral artery and vein as well as sympathetic fibers (Fig. 285-6*C*).

The seventh cervical vertebra is sometimes called the vertebra prominens because of its long and prominent spinous process. Because it protrudes beyond the other processes, it is easily palpable under the skin. The transverse process of this vertebra may lack a foramen; when present, the foramen may or may not transmit the vertebral artery.

Soft tissue structures (intervertebral discs and ligaments) are present throughout the cervical spine. Major ligaments include the anterior and posterior longitudinal ligaments, articular capsule of each interfacetal joint, ligamentum flavum, and the interspinous and supraspinous ligaments (Fig. 285-6*A*).

The anterior longitudinal ligament extends from the anterior surface of the axis to the sacrum (Figs. 285-2 and 285-6*A*). The fibers are ''ribbon like'' and are adherent to the discs and end plates but not to the anterior surface of the vertebral bodies; it maintains stability during cervical extension. Cranially, the fibers are continuous with the atlantoaxial ligament and atlanto-occipital membrane.

The posterior longitudinal ligament courses along the dorsal surface of the vertebral bodies and discs within the spinal canal along its entire length (Fig. 285-6*A*). The ligament is closely adherent to the intervertebral discs, broad over the disc space, and narrower over the vertebral body. The tectorial membrane is the cephalad extension of this ligament (Fig. 285-2). The articular capsule of the facet joints are thin, loose structures which attach to the margins of the adjacent facets. The ligamenta flava are thick, dense structures which connect the laminae of adjacent vertebrae, forming the posterior ligamentous margin of the spinal canal. The supraspinous and interspinous ligaments connect the spinous processes from the external occipital protuberance to the seventh cervical vertebra. They provide stability during flexion movements.

The intervertebral disc is a fibrocartilagenous complex interposed between two adjacent vertebrae. It is attached to the vertebral end plates through dense Sharpey's fibers, a component of the anulus fibrosus. Discs are closely adherent to both anterior and

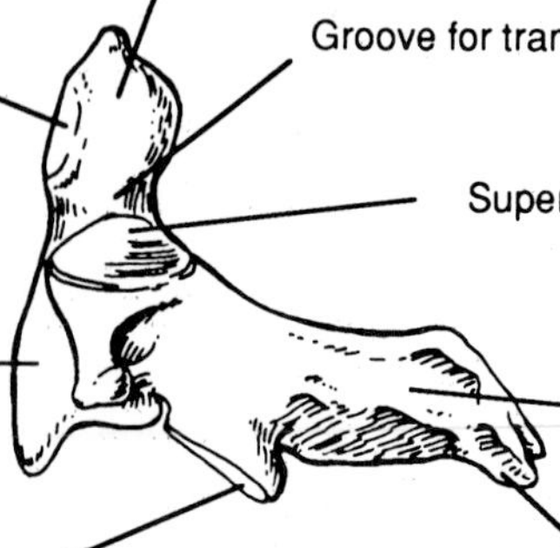

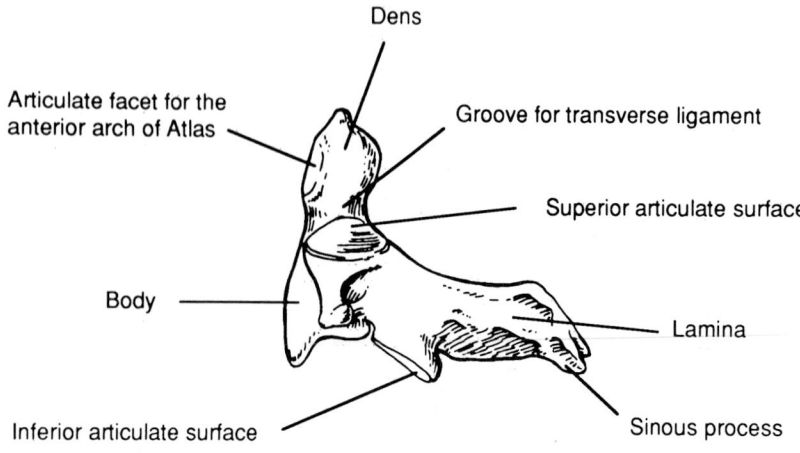

Figure 285-5 Lateral diagram of the axis.

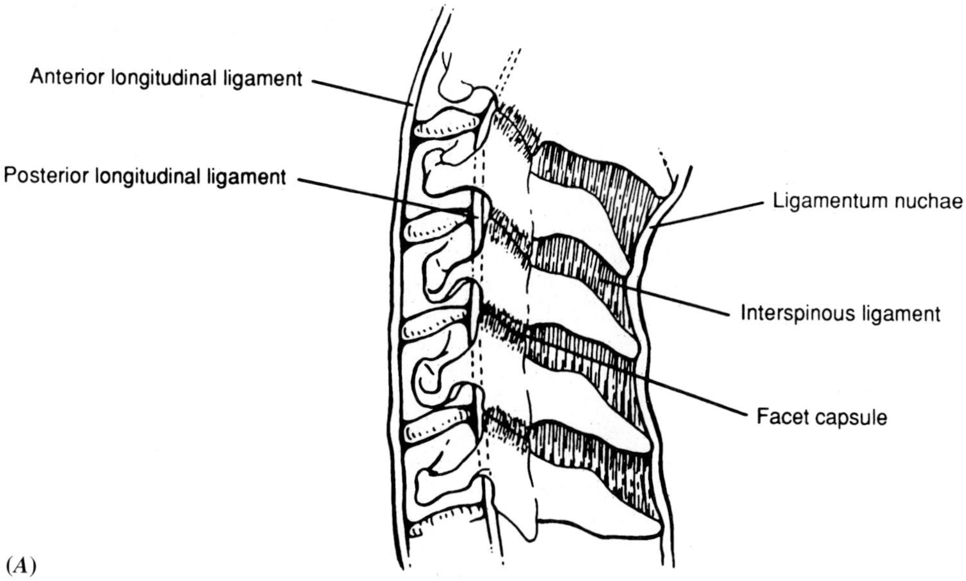

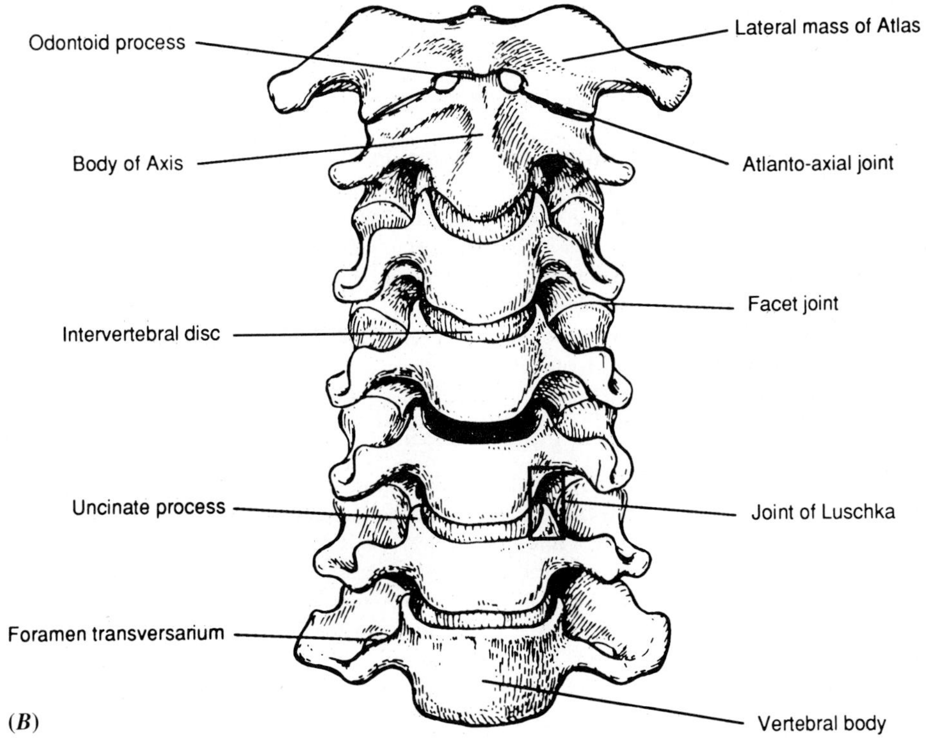

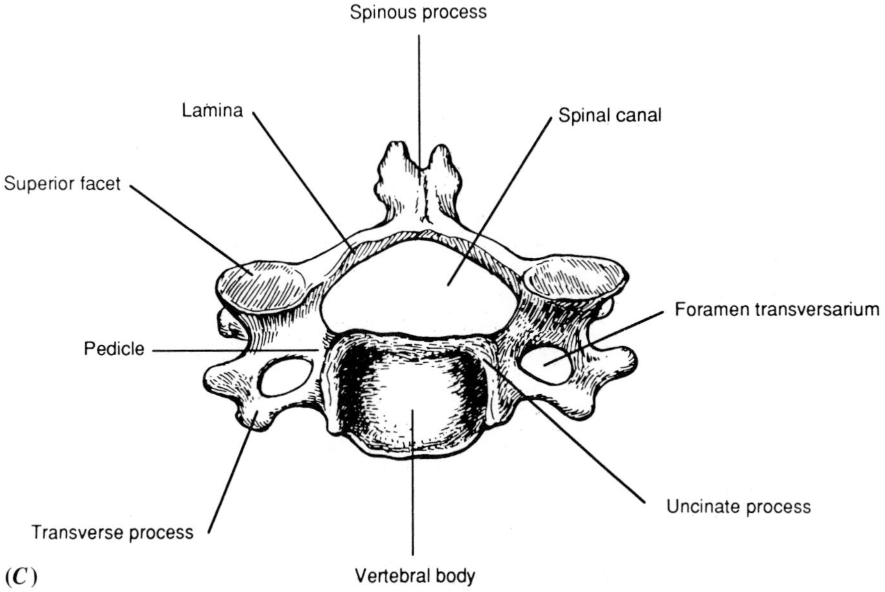

Figure 285-6 *A*. Lateral illustration of the mid- and lower cervical spine, C3-C7. *B*. Frontal view. Note how the uncinate process from the level below and the lateral margin of the vertebral body above form the joint of Luschka. The vertebral bodies increase in size moving down the cervical spine. *C*. Axial view.

posterior longitudinal ligaments. An important function of discs is to distribute weight over the entire vertebral body surface during bending motion instead of concentrating the weight toward the side the spine is bent. In addition, discs function as ''shock-absorbers'' during direct axial loading. The inner nucleus pulposus contains a macromolecular proteoglycan which serves to imbibe water molecules and thereby increase the disc's ability to resist axial loads. With aging, the water content of the discs significantly diminishes and may result in loss of disc space height. Subsequently more of the load-bearing responsibilities are subjected to the posterior elements, particularly the facet joints, which results in hypertrophic degenerative changes. This degenerative process may serve to potentiate the neurological deficit resulting from a cervical injury.

Biomechanics

Biomechanical analysis of the ligaments of the upper cervical spine has shown that hyperflexion is prevented by contact of the basion with the anterior arch of the atlas, while hyperextension and vertical translation are checked by the tectorial membrane. The alar ligaments limit lateral bending and rotation. Distraction between the occiput and atlas or atlas and axis is checked by both the tectorial membrane and the alar ligaments.

From his extensive studies, Werne concluded that the tectorial membrane and alar ligaments were most important for stability.[82] Sectioning of these ligaments resulted in atlanto-occipital dislocation. This was confirmed by Bucholz and Burkhead's postmortem examinations of patients with known atlanto-occipital dislocations that showed disruption of most, if not all, the atlanto-occipital ligaments.[17] The craniocervical articulations derive minimal stability from the apical ligaments, atlanto-occipital membranes, and articular facet capsules. Stability at the atlantoaxial articulation is largely dependent on the transverse ligament which limits anterior translation. Hyperflexion is limited by the tectorial membrane, while hyperextension is checked by impingement of the anterior arch of the atlas on the odontoid. Excessive rotation is checked by the paired alar ligaments.

White and Panjabi[83] have studied cervical spine mobility at different levels and in the various planes of motion. The representative values for rotation are indicated in Table 285-1. In the upper cervical spine, ligaments allowed 13 degrees of flexion-extension, 8 degrees of lateral bending, and zero degrees of rotation between the occiput and the atlas; and 47 degrees of axial rotation, 10 degrees of flexion-extension, and zero degrees of lateral bending between the atlas and axis. In the subaxial spine, the range of motion is greatest in the central region with the C4-C5 and C5-C6 interspaces being the most mobile. Flexion in the subaxial spine is limited largely by the chin touching the chest, although the posterior neck ligaments and musculature also play a significant role. Anterior neck muscles and fascia as well as the anterior longitudinal ligament restrict hyperextension. Lateral bending and axial rotation are also most prominent in the midcervical region and decline as one approaches the lower cervical and upper thoracic segments. Lateral motion is held in check by the articular pillars and the intertransverse ligaments.

Spinal Column Injuries

Upper Cervical Spine

It has been reported that up to 25 percent of cervical trauma occurs in the upper cervical spine, defined as the occiput to C3.[11,44,70] In the skeletally immature patient, the upper cervical spine is involved in the majority of injuries. Of lesions occurring in this region, the axis is involved the most, comprising up to 20 percent of cervical spine injuries.[4,8,24,26,38,56] Atlas fractures occur in between 3 to 13 percent[10,23,39] and C3 fractures occur in less than 5 percent.[70]

Occipital-Atlantal Dislocations

Occipital-atlantal dislocation is considered to be rare; however, the frequency may be underestimated as a result of the high fatality rate.[12] Recent literature reveals an increasing number of these injuries in survivors. The mechanism of injury is thought to be distraction with the neck hyperflexed. These injuries are associated with rupture of the anterior occipitoatlantal ligament, tectorial membrane, and alar ligaments. The occipital-atlantal joints are disrupted with dislocation of the occipital condyles on the lateral masses of the atlas.[78] These injuries may also occur in combination with atlantoaxial instability. The occipital-atlantal region is stabi-

TABLE 285-1 Representative Angles (Degrees) of Rotation of the Cervical Spine

	Type of Motion		
Interspace	**Combined Flexion/Extension (x-Axis Rotation)**	**One Side Lateral Bending (z-Axis Rotation)**	**One Side Axial Rotation (y-Axis Rotation)**
Upper			
Ocp-C1	13	8	0
C1-C2	10	0	47
C2-C3	10	10	3
Middle			
C3-C4	15	11	7
C4-C5	20	11	7
C5-C6	20	8	7
Lower			
C6-C7	17	7	6
C7-T1	9	4	2

Source: From White and Panjabi,[83] with permission.

lized by the inner and outer sets of ligaments. These inner ligaments include the apical ligament, the paired alar ligaments, the cruciate ligament, and the tectorial membrane. The outer ligaments are the articular capsules, the anterior and posterior atlanto-occipital membranes, and the ligamentum nuchae.[12,17,25,27,46]

Three subgroups of occipital-atlantal dislocations have been described by Traynelis et al.[77]

Type I. Figure 285-7. This type involves anterior translation of the cranium relative to the cervical spine and is thought to be the most common variety. When the ratio of the distance between the basion and posterior arch of the atlas, and the opisthion and the anterior arch of C1 is greater than 1 (with normal being 0.77), suspicion of an anterior dislocation should be entertained.

Type II. Type IIA consists of longitudinal distraction between the occiput and the atlas. The IIB group involves vertical distraction between the occiput and atlas as well as between the atlas and axis.

Type III. These injuries consist of posterior displacement of the skull relative to the cervical spine.

Although patients surviving these injuries may not have any neurological deficits, a variety of presentation patterns have been reported. These include upper cervical and lower cranial nerve injuries, vertebral artery abnormalities, and brain stem and spinal cord dysfunction.[59]

Although treatment is generally considered to be reduction with the judicious application of skeletal traction followed by posterior fusion, it needs to be emphasized that the application of traction may prove devastating to the patient. In our practice, we closely monitor this process either by measuring evoked potentials or by keeping the patient awake for serial neurological testing. We have observed the loss of sensory evoked potentials with the application of 4 lb of traction followed by immediate improvement in potentials after removing the weight. We have subsequently abandoned the use of traction in these patients and have chosen controlled posterior reduction across the occipital-atlantal-axial segment followed by posterior fusion and stabilization (Fig. 285-8*A, B*).

Occipital Condylar Fractures

Bell first described fractures of the occipital condyle in 1817. These injuries are considered to be rare and at this time there are

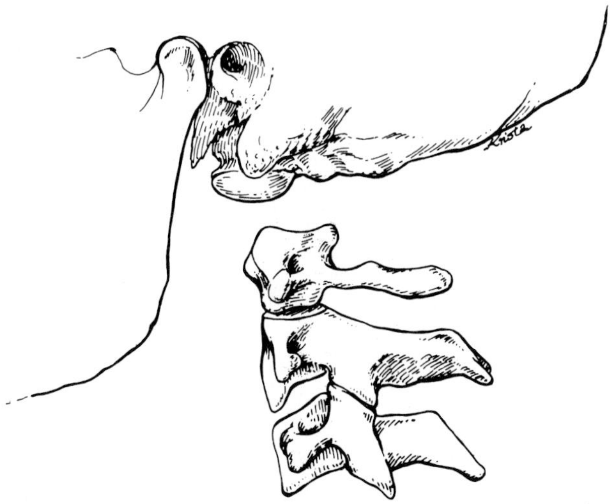

Figure 285-7 Type I occipital-atlantal dislocation. There is anterior translation of the cranium relative to the cervical spine.

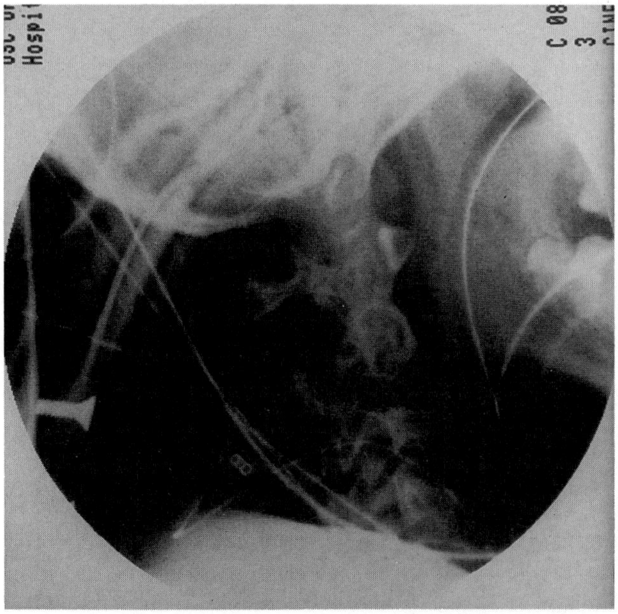

(*A*)

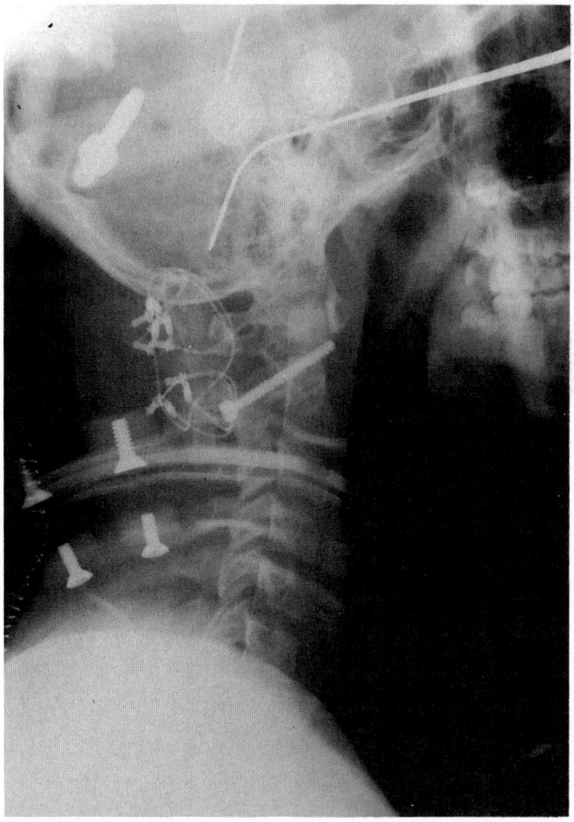

(*B*)

Figure 285-8 *A*. Lateral x-ray film of type IIB occipital-atlantal-axial dislocation. Note that in addition to the longitudinal distraction of the occiput relative to the atlas there is also a distractive injury at the atlantoaxial segment. *B*. Postoperative lateral x-ray film demonstrates the screw-cable-rib construct used to stabilize this occipital-atlantal-axial instability. Posterior C1-C2 transarticular screw fixation was used to provide rigid fixation across the atlantoaxial level, thereby blocking rotational movement at this level. Multiple titanium cables were also placed to achieve occiput to C2 fixation. Rib was used because it conforms to the occipital-atlantal-axial contour.

only 35 reported survivors in the literature. This probably reflects the high frequency of associated fatal head injuries. These fractures may be difficult to detect on plain radiographs and may require CT scanning for definitive diagnosis. The index of suspicion should be raised in patients sustaining closed head injuries with lower cranial nerve deficits and neck pain.[94] Three types of injury patterns have been described.[6,94]

Type I. This group involves a nondisplaced comminuted condylar fracture which is believed to occur from an axial load impacting the occipital condyle into the lateral mass of C1. These are stable injuries that are treated with a semirigid cervical collar.

Type II. This type involves a fracture through the skull base extending into the occipital condyle. The supporting ligamentous structures are thought to remain intact, preserving stability. Treatment consists of a semirigid collar.

Type III. Figure 285-3. This group consists of an avulsion fracture of the condyle by the ipsilateral alar ligament. Although these injuries are generally considered to be stable, dynamic imaging may be required prior to and following cervical immobilization. Bracing in most series consists of either a halo, Minerva, or comparable orthosis.

C1 Arch Fractures—Jefferson Fracture

The "Jefferson's fracture" was described in 1920 by Sir Geoffrey Jefferson and consisted of a fracture of the ring of C1 in four locations[49,68] (Fig. 285-9*A*, *B*). The mechanism of injury appears to be an axial load applied to the cranial vertex which drives the occipital condyles downward into the lateral masses of C1. This downward load serves to fracture the ring of C1. Fractures of the atlas are thought to comprise between 3 and 13 percent of cervical spine injuries.[39] The open mouth plain x-ray view is helpful to look for lateral displacement of the lateral masses of C1 on C2. If the combined distance is greater than 6.9 mm there is likely a loss of competence of the transverse ligament. In the absence of transverse ligament injuries this fracture generally can be treated with rigid external fixation. Transverse ligament disruption requires surgical fusion.

Atlantoaxial Instability

Both bone and ligamentous structures help stabilize the atlantoaxial region. The transverse ligament is most important and inserts onto the medial tubercles of the lateral masses of the atlas, passing behind the odontoid process. Other structures involved in the stability at this level include the alar ligaments, accessory atlantoaxial ligaments, and tectorial membrane. The odontoid and the anterior arch of C1 also are stabilizing structures.

The degree of motion at this level is about 47.5 degrees of rotation and 10 degrees of flexion-extension. Lateral bending does not occur here.[83] Flexion is limited by the tectorial membrane, extension by the anterior arch of C1 contacting the odontoid process, anterior translation by the transverse ligament, and rotation by the alar ligaments. A distance of greater than 3 mm in an adult and 4.5 mm in a child between the posterior surface of the anterior arch of C1 and the anterior surface of the dens is thought to represent incompetence of the transverse ligament with associated instability.

A variety of pathologic processes lead to atlantoaxial instability with the potential for damage to the cervical spinal cord. These include trauma, rheumatoid arthritis, neoplastic disease, basilar invagination, occipitalization of the atlas, os odontoideum, aplasia or dysplasia of the dens, Down's syndrome, ankylosing spondylitis, and retropharyngeal infections.[59,78]

Treatment of this disorder must take into consideration the patient's neurological status, the degree of spinal deformity and the ability to achieve reduction, the presence of spinal cord compression, and the patient's age and overall medical condition. For reducible instabilities, we generally perform a posterior fusion and stabilization via C1-C2 transarticular screw fixation. Our initial experience using this technique without associated wiring suggests that this can be a safe procedure with a high rate of osseous fusion. Additionally, patients did not require postoperative stabilization with a halo or Minerva brace.[74] The experience of others using posterior C1-C2 screw fixation adds further support for this technique in the management of atlantoaxial instability[37,54,57] (Fig. 285-10). C1-C2 transarticular screws can also be used in conjunction with occipital stabilization techniques to enhance construct

Figure 285-9 Axial (*A*) and frontal (*B*) diagrams of a classic Jefferson's fracture.

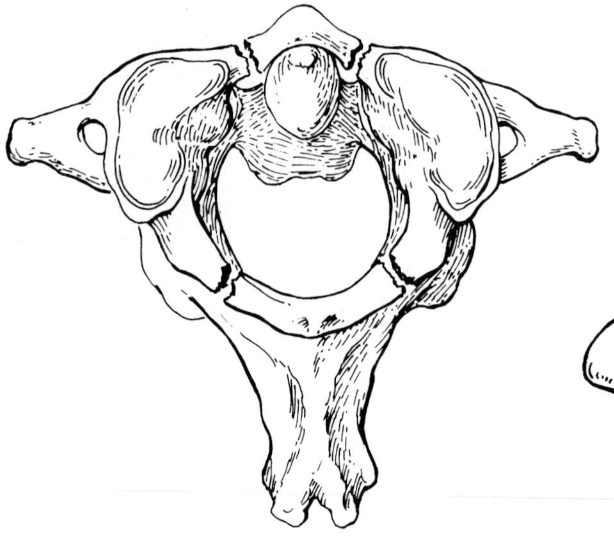

(*A*)

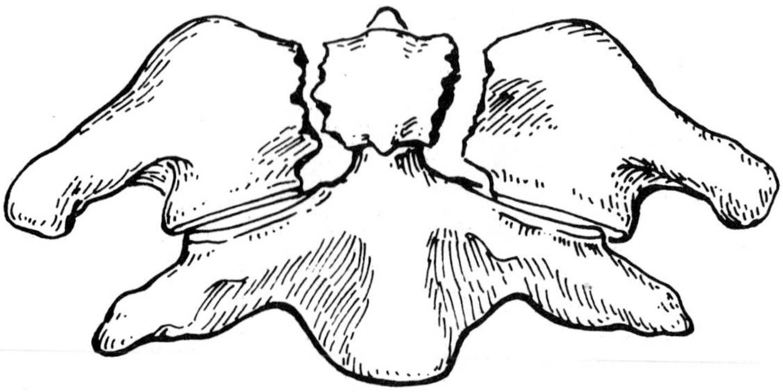

(*B*)

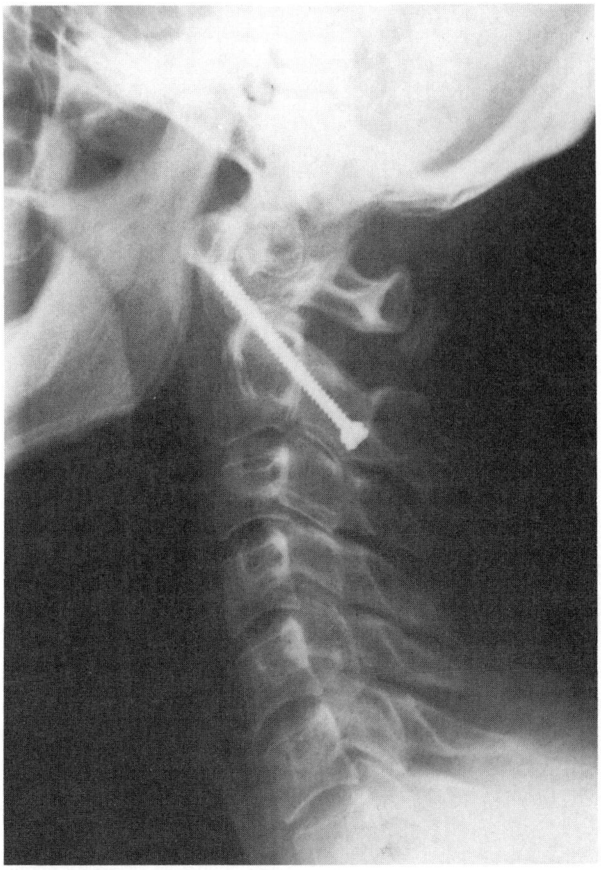

Figure 285-10 Unstable atlantoaxial region in a patient with os odontoideum. This was stabilized using posterior C1-C2 transarticular screw fixation.

fixation strength in the presence of occipital-atlanto-axial instability (Figs. 285-8*A*, *B* and 285-11*A–C*).

Rotatory Subluxations

Rotatory subluxations are far more common in children than in adults. These injuries have been subgrouped into types I to IV,[12,18,29,78] based on whether there is integrity of the transverse ligament.

Type I. These types are the most common. The transverse ligament is intact, and there is no anterior displacement of the atlas. These are initially treatable with bracing after reduction.

Type II. There is rupture of the transverse ligament with anterior translation of the anterior arch of the atlas up to 5 mm from the dens. The atlas rotation exceeds 35 degrees. Treatment in part is influenced by the duration of rotation. Reduction and subsequent external stabilization for 12 weeks is frequently successful. If the duration of rotational deformity is greater than 2 to 4 weeks, or if there is also incompetence of the occipitoatlantal level a posterior fusion procedure is required.

Type III. There is rupture of both the transverse and alar ligaments with rotation of greater than 40 degrees, and anterior translation of the atlas relative to the dens of more than 5 mm. This requires surgical fusion after reduction.

Type IV. This is a rare lesion with retrodisplacement of the atlas relative to the axis. Reduction followed by surgical fusion is required.

When the transverse ligament is intact, bilateral dislocation does not occur until the head rotates approximately 65 degrees. When there is rupture of this ligament, bilateral dislocation can occur at 45 degrees.[11,12,18] With a competent ligament the dens acts as a pivot, preventing rotation of more than 35 degrees. This deformity is generally thought to be reducible. Examination of the patient may reveal the abnormal head tilt or "cockrobin" posture. Plain AP open mouth x-ray films reveal an asymmetrical overhang of the atlas relative to the axis. The lateral projections may show the lateral mass of C1 anterior to the dens. Although the neurological examination is usually normal, devastating brain stem and spinal cord injury can occur (Fig. 285-12*A*, *B*).

Odontoid Fractures

Injuries of the axis are thought to comprise up to 17 percent of cervical spine injuries.[4,9,24,26,38,56] Most of these are odontoid fractures. The most widely accepted classification for these fractures was proposed by Anderson and D'Alonzo in 1974.[5] Their scheme divides these fractures into three subtypes based on the location of the fracture.

Type I. Figure 285-13*A*. These are the rarest of the odontoid fractures and involve the tip of the odontoid process above the synchondrosis. Although these may occur in association with injury to the apical ligaments, they are generally stable and can be managed by using a cervical collar. They have a very low incidence of osseous nonunion.

Type II. Figure 285-13*B*. The majority of odontoid fractures involve the synchondrosis where the dens fuses with the body of C2. This fracture pattern is thought to disrupt the blood supply to the dens and leaves a small surface area for fracture healing. Nonunion rates for this injury range from 9 to 100 percent.[5,74] The management of these injuries is controversial. Advanced age and significant translational changes are thought to predispose to nonunion. Subluxation of greater than 4 to 6 mm is believed to significantly enhance the likelihood of nonosseous union.[9]

Surgical treatment of these injuries consists of either C1-C2 fusion or transodontoid screw fixation. When there is rupture of the transverse ligament we perform a posterior C1-C2 fusion. Our preferred technique is generally a percutaneous posterior transarticular screw fixation and fusion[7,57,74,85] (Fig. 285-14*A–D*). Comparative mechanical testing suggests that this technique of fixation is superior to other posterior methods. Transarticular screwing is particularly effective in blocking rotational movement.[36,62] The inability to prevent rotational movement using nonscrew techniques may account for their high rate of nonunion.

When the transverse ligament is intact there is growing enthusiasm for anterior transodontoid screw fixation. This technique has recently been popularized and refined in North America by Apfelbaum.[7] The biggest advantage of this procedure appears to be preservation of atlantoaxial motion, which accounts for approximately 50 percent of cervical rotation. The procedure requires the ability to perform biplanar, realtime fluoroscopic imaging. It appears ideally suited for small-chested patients with acute fractures (Fig. 285-15*A–C*).

Type III. Figure 285-13*C*. These include fractures that extend into the body of the axis. They generally will heal with 3 months of halo or Minerva external bracing.

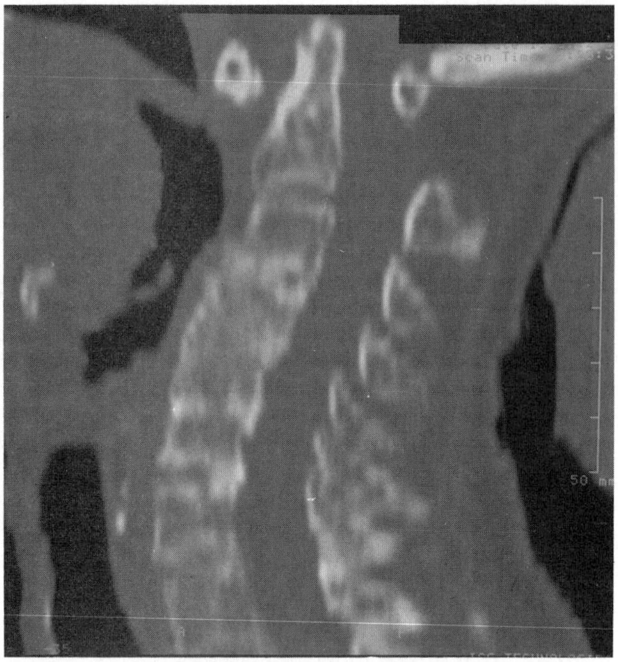

(*A*)

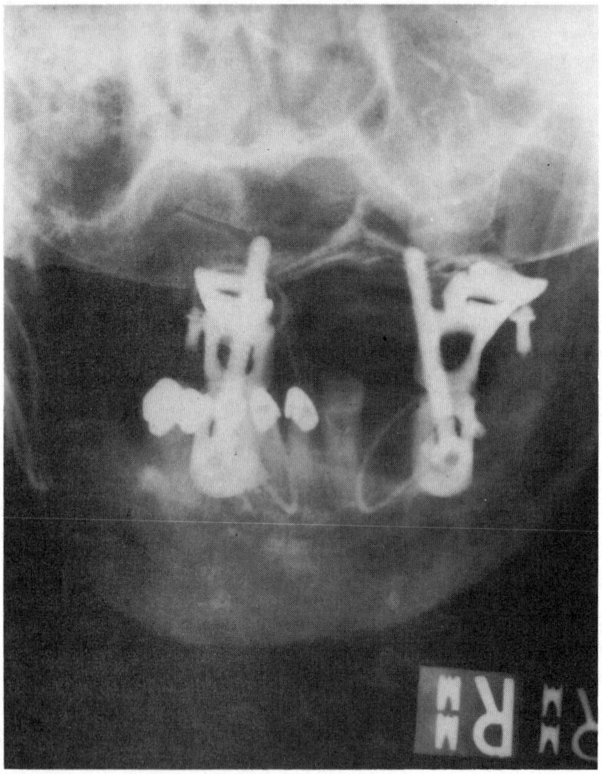

(*B*)

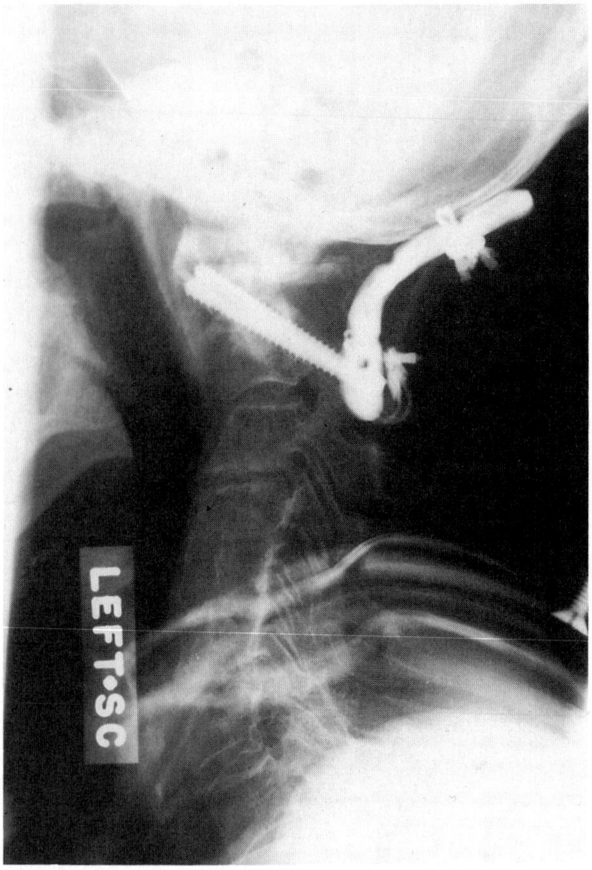

(*C*)

Figure 285-11 *A*. C1-C2 subluxation and cranial settling causing neck pain and myelopathy in a patient with rheumatoid arthritis. *B*, *C*. Occipital-atlantal-axial fixation was performed following skeletal traction reduction using C1-C2 screw-plate-cable fixation. The myelopathy and neck pain significantly improved following surgery.

C2 Traumatic Spondylolisthesis— "Hangman's Fracture"

Fractures of the neural arch of C2 may result in a traumatic spondylolisthesis, or the so-called "Hangman's Fracture" (Fig. 285-16). This injury pattern was first reported by Wood-Jones in 1913, as the characteristic injury resulting from a judicial hanging.[87] In 1965 Schneider et al. reported eight such injuries resulting from motor vehicular accidents suggesting a hyperextension mechanism.[69] Specifically, the anatomic disruption is commonly thought to involve bilateral pars interarticularis fractures. Unlike hangings that produce irreversible injury to the vertebral arteries and cervicomedullary junction, most of these injuries are not associated with neurological injury. The majority of these injuries are stable and heal in a cervical collar.

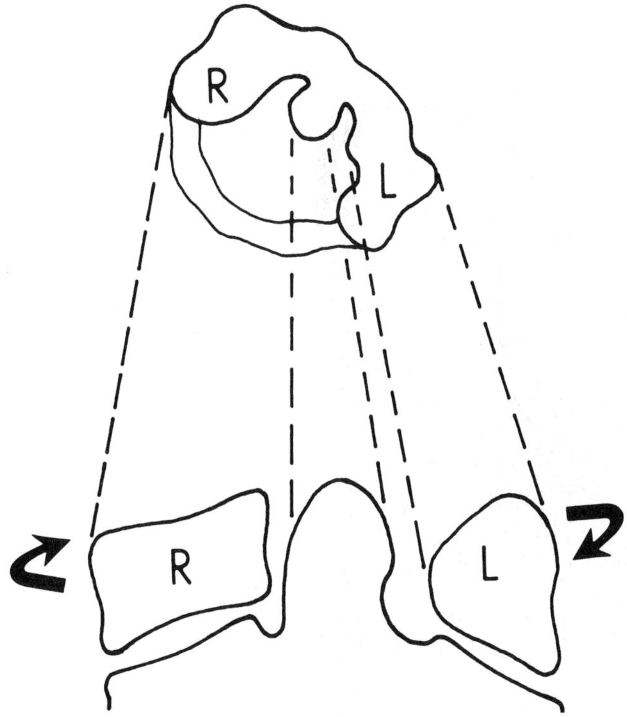

(*A*)

Figure 285-12 *A*. Illustration of a rotatory subluxation. *B*. Lateral x-ray film of a rotatory subluxation. Note the significant volume of bone (the lateral mass of C1; *arrow*) anterior to the odontoid process.

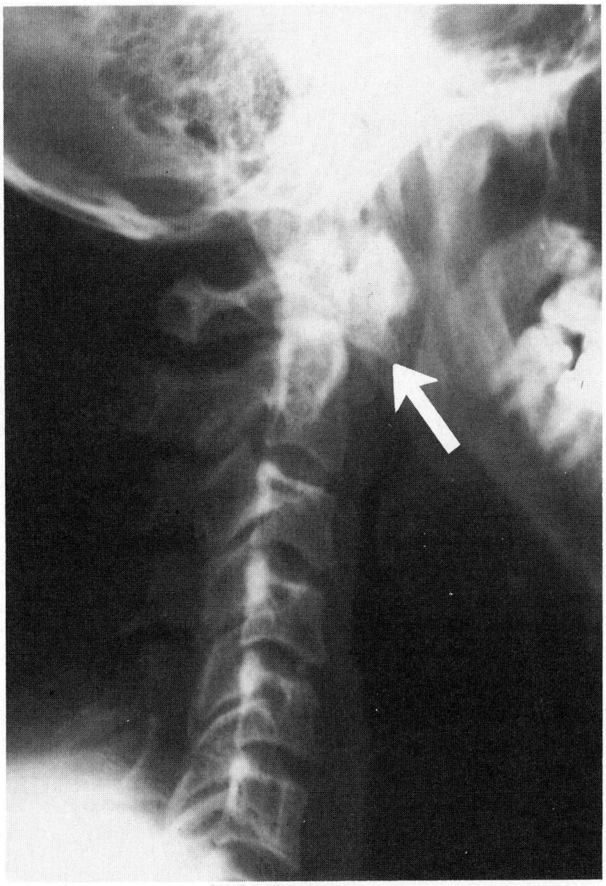

(*B*)

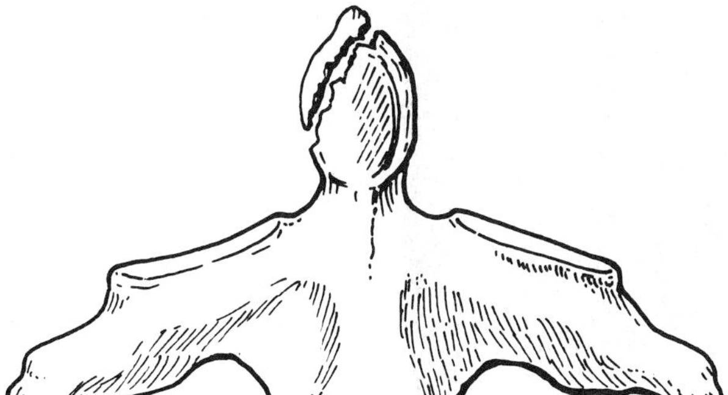

(*A*)

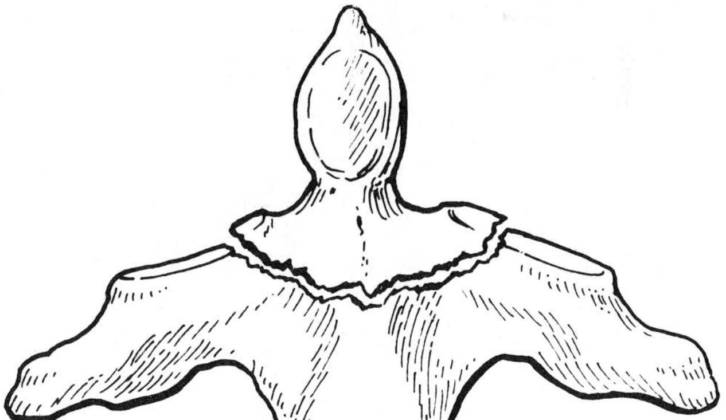

(*C*)

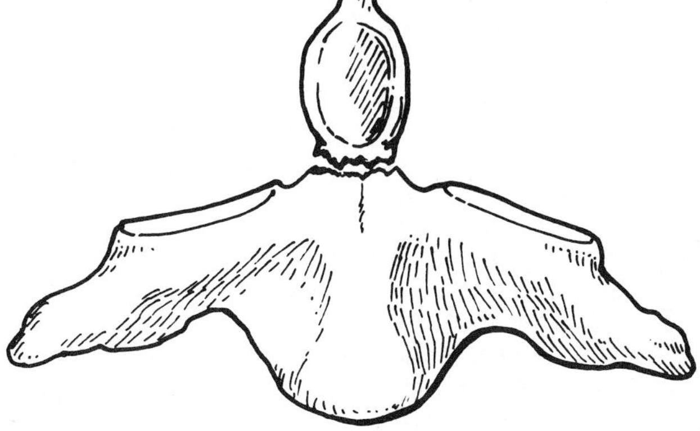

(*B*)

Figure 285-13 *A*. Type I odontoid fracture. The rarest type. Low incidence of nonunion when treated in hard collar. *B*. Type II odontoid fracture. The most common variety of axis fractures. The fracture line involves the synchondrosis where the dens fuses with the body of C2. Management of these fractures often requires surgery for fusion, especially if there is more than 4 mm of subluxation associated with the fracture. *C*. Type III odontoid fracture. The fracture extends into the body of C2. These generally heal with an osseous union when treated with an external brace for 3 months.

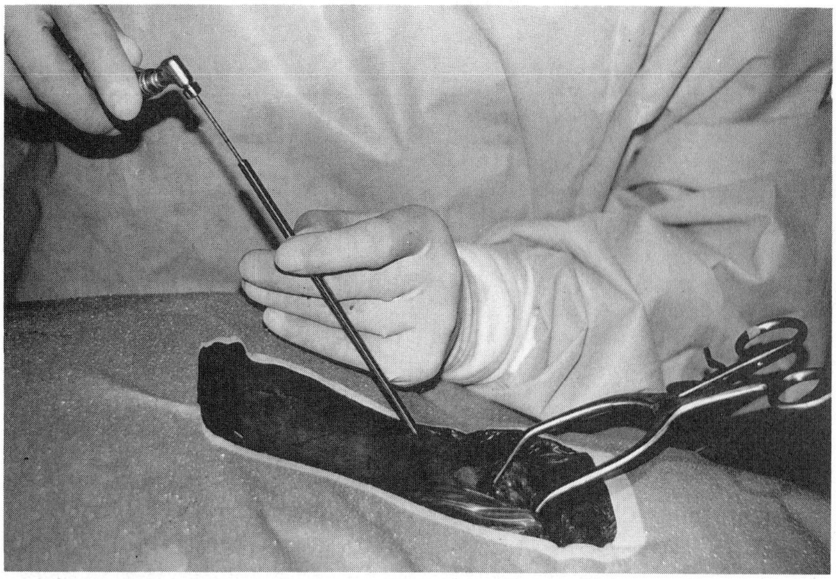

(*A*)

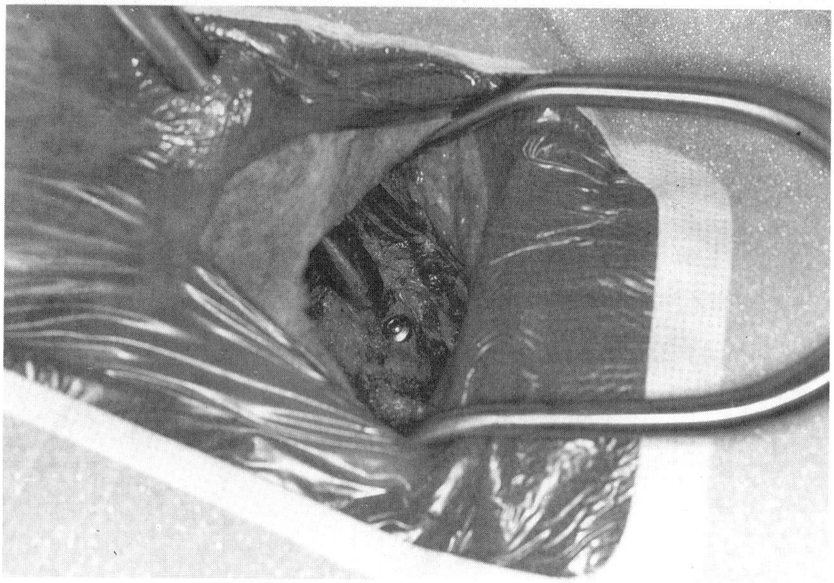

(*B*)

Figure 285-14 Percutaneous posterior C1-C2 transarticular screw fixation. *A*. A small midline incision is used to expose from the posterior arch of C1 down to the C2-C3 facet joint only. Cannulated trocars are introduced through stab wounds. Drilling is performed using extended instruments. *B*. The permanent screw is introduced through the cannula and threaded into place. Prior to screw placement an extended tap is used to prepare the pilot hole for a nontapping permanent screw. The procedure is repeated on the opposite side. Biplanar real-time fluoroscopic imaging is used during hole preparation and screw placement.

Subaxial Spine

The work of Allen et al. led to the development of a mechanically oriented classification scheme for cervical spine injuries.[2,3] Although there is presently no universally accepted classification for cervical fractures, there are a few important reasons why we routinely use this mechanistic scheme in our practice: (1) it requires a systematic evaluation of x-rays looking for evidence of disruption; (2) it facilitates interobserver consistency regarding injury type; and (3) by forcing the managing physician to postulate the forces leading to the instability, a stabilization procedure that counteracts these forces can be thoughtfully planned.

The scheme is based on the hypothesis that injuries can consistently be grouped based on x-ray evidence of anatomic disruption. Major and minor forces, or "injury vectors," are thought to work in tandem to create these fractures. The severity of the spinal disruption is a function of the magnitude of the vectors, and similar vectors will produce similar injury patterns.

Although controversy surrounds the mechanical precision of this scheme, it does, however, provide a standardized format for mid- and lower cervical spine injuries. Shortening of an area results from compression, whereas lengthening arises from distraction or tension; translational failure is inferred if there is spondylolisthesis, retrodisplacement, or lateral displacement. According to this system there are six patterns seen in indirect, mid- to low cervical (subaxial) failure. Compression flexion, compression extension, and distraction flexion are the most commonly occurring injury patterns. Lateral flexion and distractive extension are the least likely to occur. Vertical compression is intermediate in frequency.[2,3] Each group is subsequently subdivided into subgroups based on the magnitude of the injury. Treatment is instituted based on the group (mechanism of injury) and severity (magnitude of the injury vectors) of the injury.

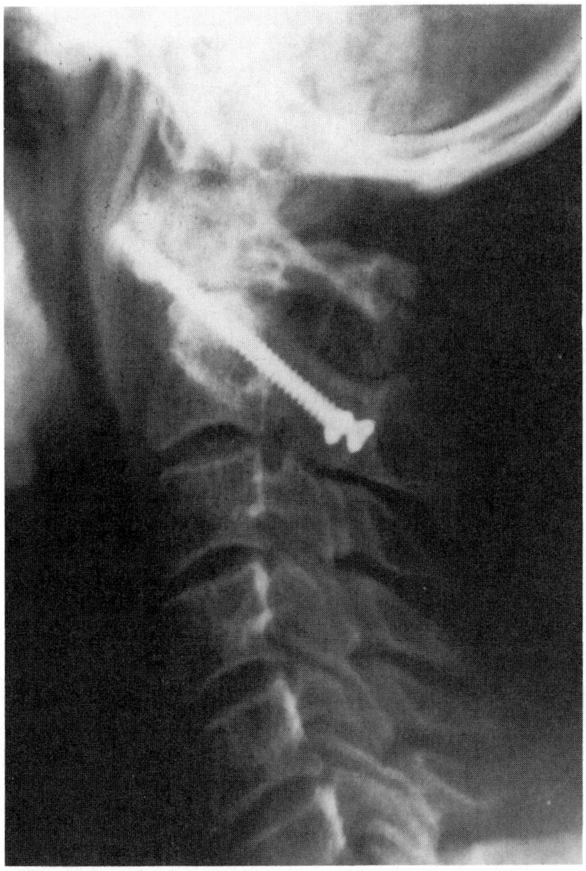

(*C*)

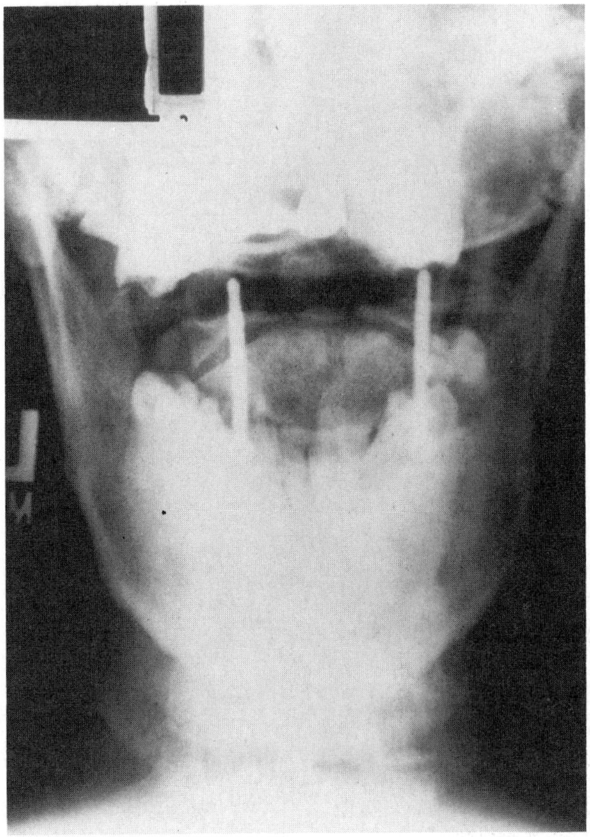

(*D*)

Figure 285-14 (*Continued*) *C, D*. Postoperative x-ray films with the permanent screws in place. On the lateral radiograph (*C*), the screw is generally advanced to the posterior cortical surface of the anterior arch of C1. The open mouth view (*D*) is especially helpful at determining the number of screw threads capturing the C1 lateral mass. Additionally, this view provides valuable information regarding screw position and the lateral margins of the C2 pars interarticularis and the lateral mass of C1. Lateral penetration may result in catastrophic vertebral artery injury. Preoperative CT scans and/or MRI must be evaluated to avoid missing an anomalous vertebral artery.

Compression Injuries

The following injuries may be grouped together because they all have an axial load contributing to their failure. These axial forces result in shortening of a portion of the injured segment. This group includes flexion compression, vertical compression, and compression extension injuries.

Flexion-Compression Injuries (Fig. 285-17*A*) Termed the compressive flexion (CF) group, this category is subdivided into five subgroups. CF injuries are thought to result from forces directed inferiorly and anteriorly. They range from isolated compressive failure involving the anterior-superior vertebral body to significant vertebral body collapse with associated retropulsion of the posterior porticn into the canal. Additionally, the most severe type (CF5) has posterior column disruption which may be associated with distraction of the facet joints, widening of the interspinous distance suggesting injury to the supraspinous and interspinous ligaments, and incompetence of the posterior longitudinal ligament. The most severe injuries are thought to result from compressive loading of a flexed spine. The entire group is thought to comprise up to 20 percent of subaxial cervical spine injuries. There is a predilection for the midcervical spine with a peak incidence occurring at the C4-C5 and C5-C6 levels.

The treatment of flexion compression injuries is influenced by several factors including the neurological status of the patient, the presence of intracanalicular bone or disc, the degree and reducibility of the flexion deformity, the quality of the patient's bone, and the age and medical condition of the patient. Type I and II injuries (CF1 and CF2) can generally be treated with rigid external support. The probability for neurological injury appears to increase proportionally with the severity of radiographic disruption. Higher grade injuries without complete cord deficit frequently require anterior decompression combined with circumferential fusion because of the presence of ventral intracanalicular bone and/or disc in association with pancolumn spinal disruption. When this approach is indicated, we combine anterior cervical screw-plate fixation with the decompression and fusion procedure. There are presently several anterior cervical fixators that may be used in this situation. We use the ''Manny Stillerman'' fixator device which was designed and developed to improve anterior column fixation. Following cadaveric comparative mechanical testing this device has been used in 34 consecutive patients who required anterior cervical stabilization with encouraging results (Fig. 285-17*B*–*E*).[71,72]

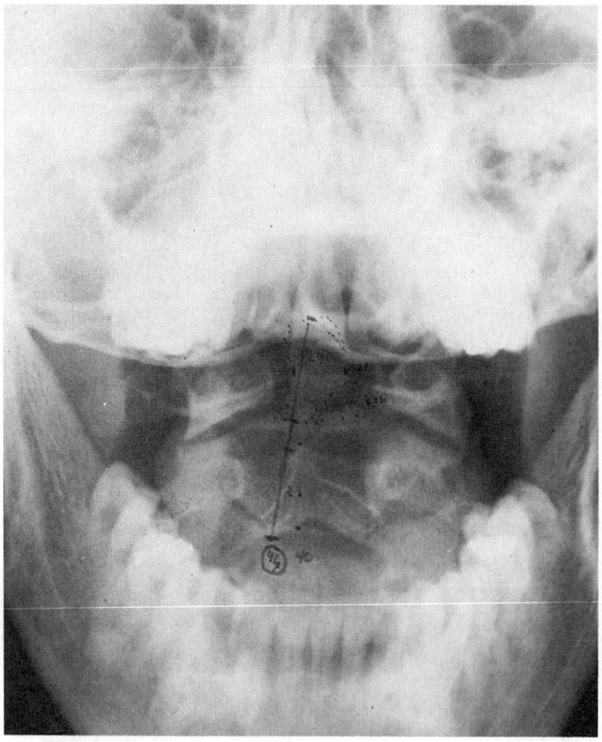

(*A*)

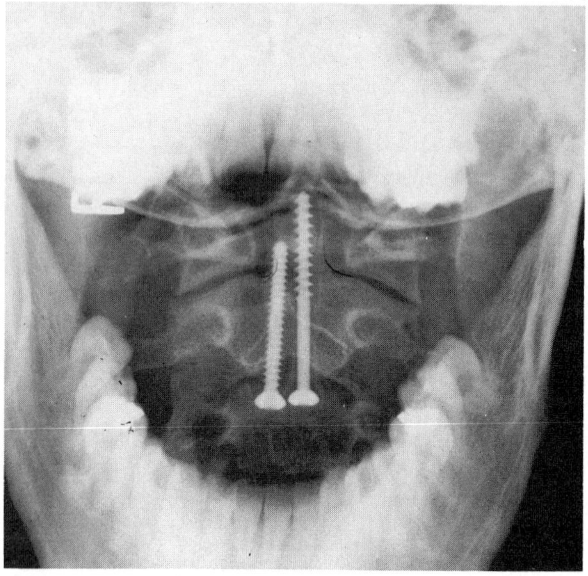

(*B*)

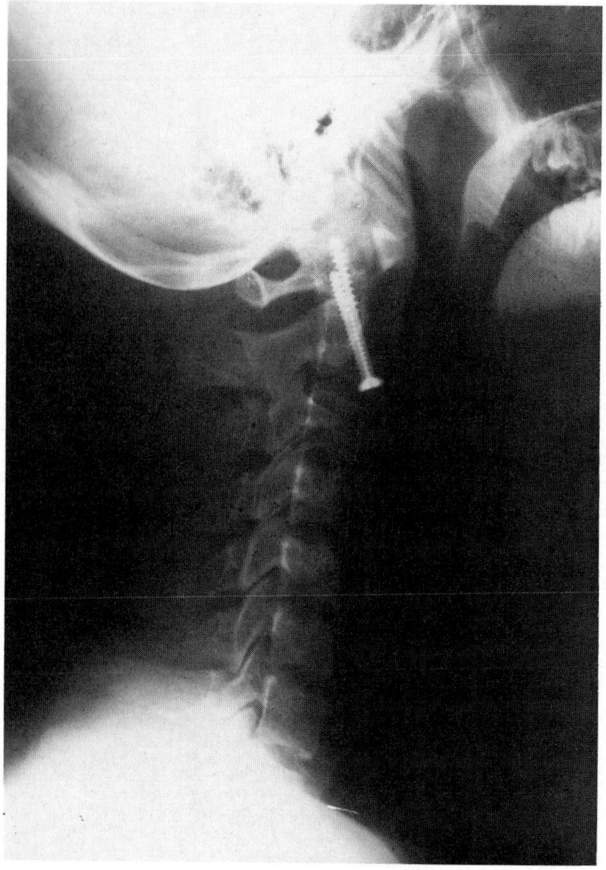

(*C*)

Figure 285-15 Transodontoid screw fixation. *A*. Preoperative open mouth x-ray film showing a large defect in the odontoid 4 months after the patient was placed in a halo for a type II odontoid fracture (this 16-year-old patient had been involved in an auto vs. pedestrian accident). The transverse ligament was assessed as intact based on MRI scans and dynamic lateral x-ray films. Because of the age of the patient it was deemed desirable to preserve motion at the C1-C2 segment. Pen marks outline the odontoid process as well as the large cortical defect. Preoperative markings are placed to help determine screw trajectory and permanent screw size. *B*, *C*. Permanent screws are in place. Note that a curette was used to refracture the fibrous union repair of the odontoid fracture prior to screw placement. A lag screw (with distal threads) was passed first down the center of C2. The threaded portion of the screw was passed across the fracture so that compression across the fracture site could be facilitated. A second fully threaded screw was then passed to enhance fixation strength. No brace was worn postoperatively.

Vertical Compression A compressive load delivered to the center of the vertebrae distinguishes this group from the CF group where the axial loading is oblique. Additionally, the neck is thought to be in neutral position at the time of impact loading. These injuries are also referred to as ''burst'' fractures and may be associated with retropulsion of vertebral fragments into the spinal canal (Fig. 285-18*A*) and severe neurological dysfunction. There are three subgroups, VC1-3. These injuries occur most commonly in the lower cervical spine, involving C6-C7, and C7-T1 with greatest frequency. They are generally considered to be stable injuries in the absence of injury to the posterior ligamentous structures and can be treated initially with either halo or Minerva external fixation.[11,44] The severity of neurological injury parallels the degree of compression failure. The VC3 subgroup with severely comminuted and retropulsed fragments may require surgery for decompression and fusion of the anterior column (Fig. 285-18*B*, *C*).

Compression-Extension Injuries In this group, the major compressive force is delivered to the posterior elements with the neck in extension (Fig. 285-19). There are five subgroups and interestingly the magnitude of spinal disruption does not seem to correlate

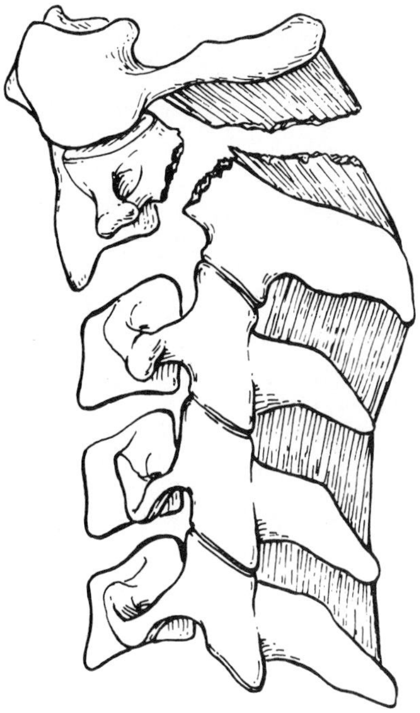

Figure 285-16 C2 traumatic spondylolisthesis. ''Hangman's'' fracture. Fractures of the C2 pars interarticularis may result in anterior translation and/or angulation of C2 relative to C3.

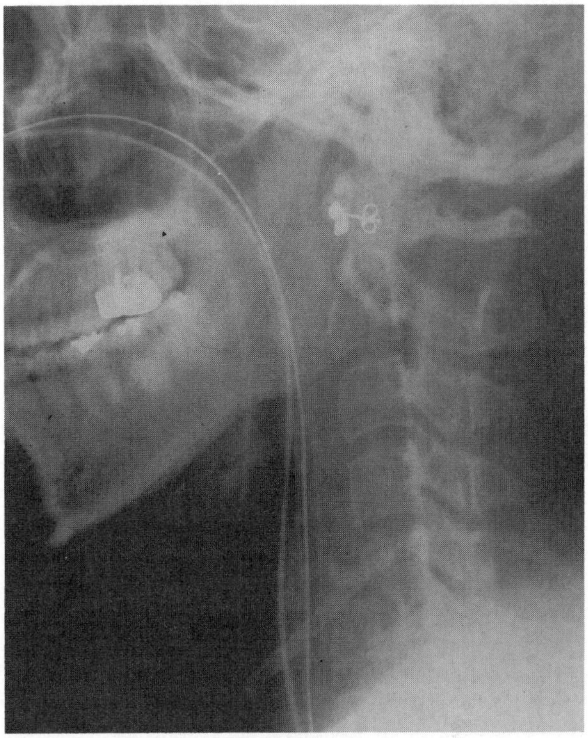

(*B*)

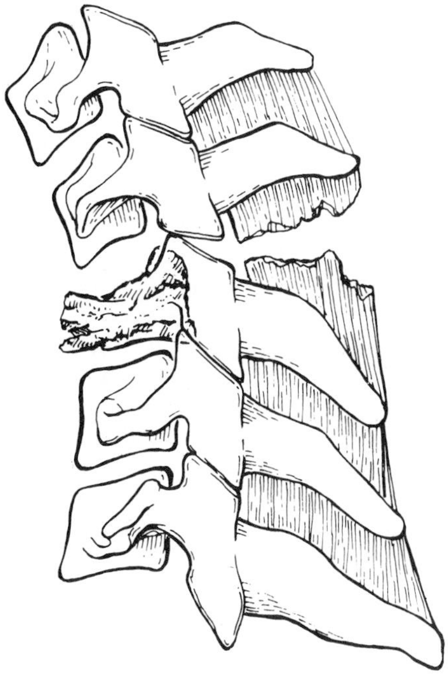

(*A*)

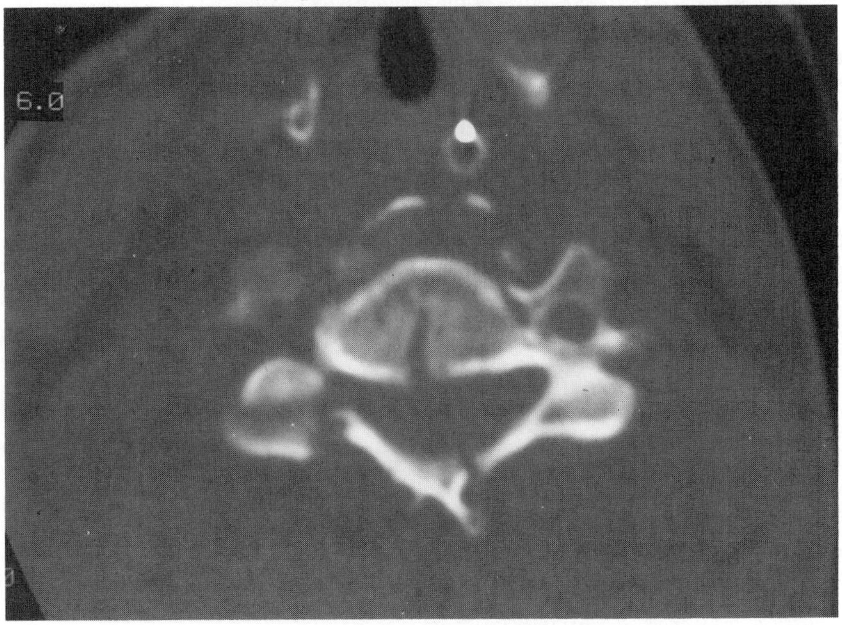

(*C*)

Figure 285-17 *A*. Diagram of a flexion-compression injury. Lateral x-ray film (*B*) and CT bone window axial view (*C*) of CF injury. Patient with axial loading to the anterior column sustained compression fractures of both C5 and C6, and significant posterior element disruption and flexion deformity.

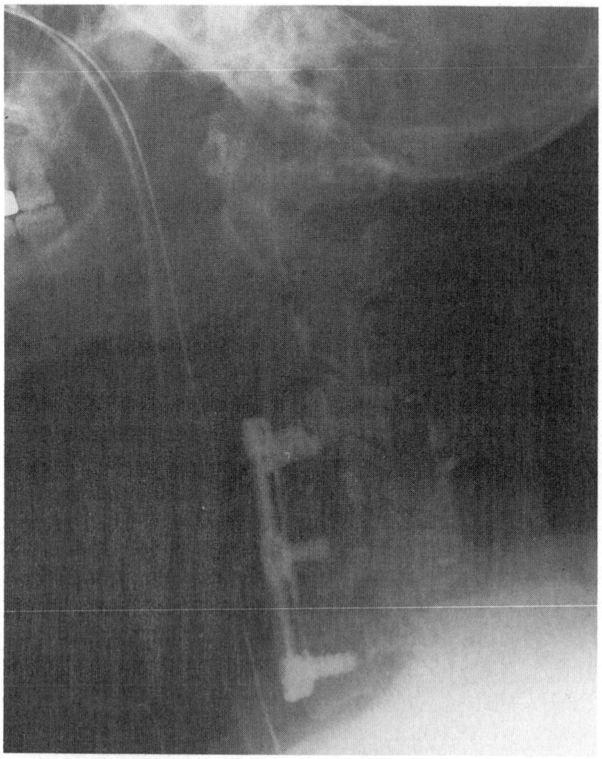

(*D*)

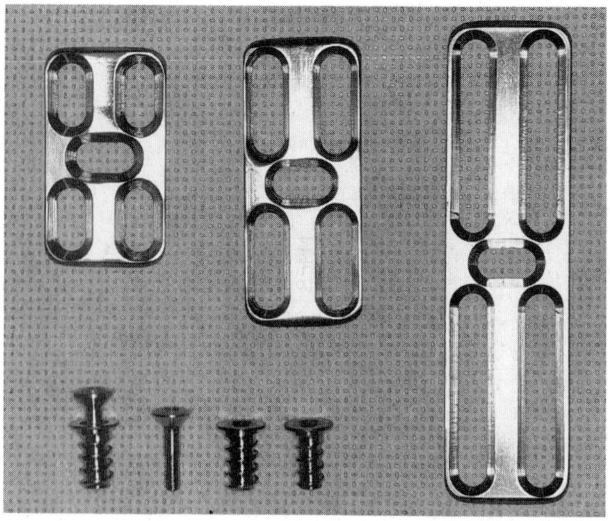

(*E*)

Figure 285-17 (*Continued*) *D*. Postoperative lateral x-ray film. Following anterior column reconstruction and interbody grafting using iliac crest bone, anterior column fixation was implemented using one of several presently available devices, the "Manny" fixator. Because of the pancolumn disruption, posterior stabilization and fusion was performed with cable and iliac crest grafts. Posterior fusion and stabilization was not extended down to C7 because of significant neural arch disruption at this level. *E*. Photograph shows the "Manny Stillerman" fixator for stabilizing the anterior cervical spine. Assembly of the implant consists of initially placing short, large diameter anchor screws into the vertebral bodies. Three different screws varying in major and minor diameters are shown. These include 4.5, 5.5, and 6.5 mm major diameters as shown in the photograph. Following drilling and tapping, permanent screws are threaded into the vertebral body. A plate is selected, contoured, and then placed over the anchor screws. The plate is secured to the anchor screws by inserting the "universal" locking screw through the plate.

with the severity of neurological dysfunction. This is a common injury type, comprising approximately 25 percent in the large series of Allen et al.[3]

The type I lesion consists of a unilateral vertebral arch fracture and is the most commonly occurring subtype. This may involve any portion of the laminar-facet-pedicle complex. Although this type of injury occurs throughout the cervical spine, level C6-C7 is the most common.

Distraction Injuries

These injuries result in part from supraphysiologic distractive forces which cause tension failure or lengthening of the involved spinal segment. These include the commonly occurring distractive flexion injuries as well as the distractive extension group.

Distractive Flexion Distractive flexion injuries (Fig. 285-20*A*) account for almost 40 percent of the cervical injuries in the series of Allen et al.,[3] making it the most commonly occurring injury pattern. There are four subgroups seen.

1. Type I is characterized by widening of the space between the spinous processes and facet subluxation in flexion (Fig. 285-20*B–D*).
2. Type II has an associated unilateral facet dislocation.
3. Type III has bilateral facet dislocation, with 50 percent vertebral body translation.
4. Type IV has bilateral facet dislocations with translational changes of up to a full vertebral width. Loading to the occiput with the neck in flexion is known to result in this type of injury pattern. The major injury vector is tension which acts on the posterior elements. Additionally, a compressive force is thought to be a minor contributor involving the vertebral bodies. These injuries involve early failure of the posterior ligamentous complex.

The higher grade injuries may be difficult to distinguish from the compression flexion injuries because both types exhibit pancolumn failure.[3] The more advanced subgroups occur with greater frequency in the lower cervical spine.

Management of patients with these injuries is controversial.[55,86] Factors influencing treatment include the subgroup of lesion, the presence of myelopathy or radiculopathy, the age and overall medical condition of the patient, and the presence of intracanalicular

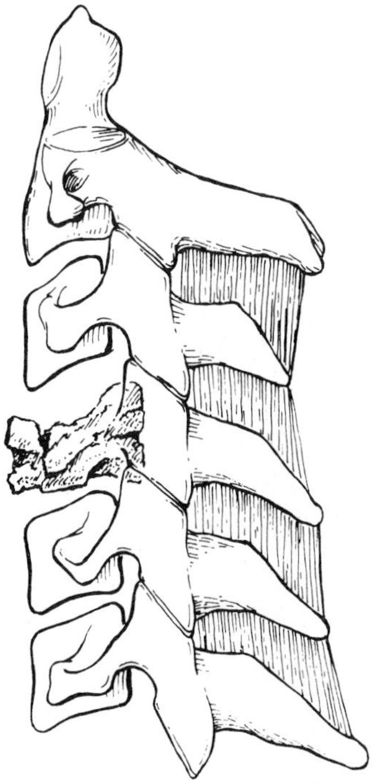

(*A*)

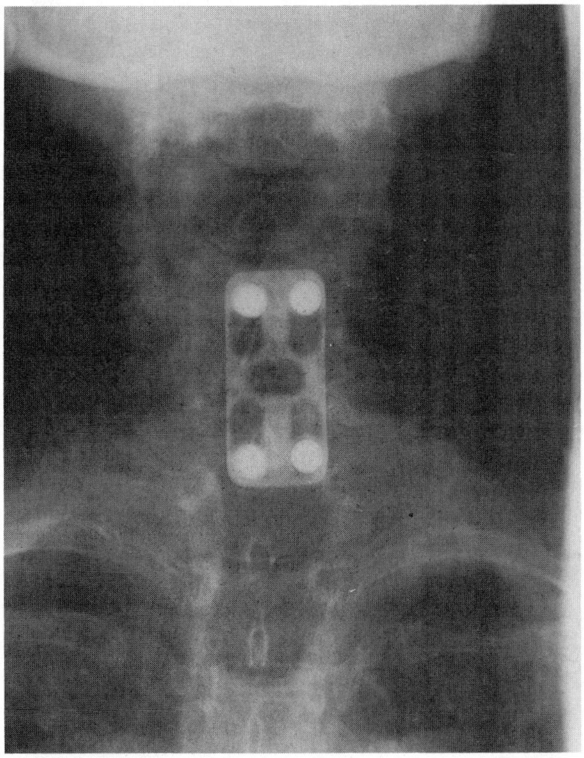

(*C*)

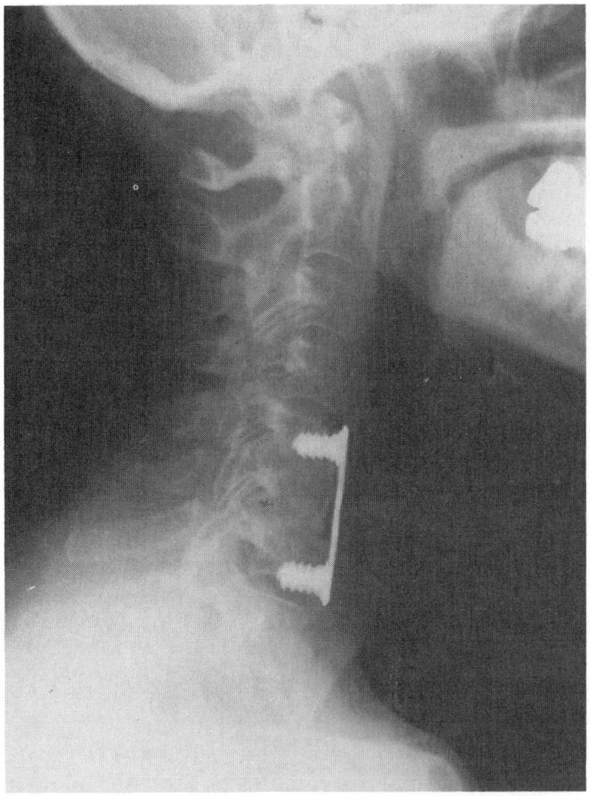

(*B*)

Figure 285-18 *A*. Illustration of a vertical compression injury. *B*, *C*. Following a C6 corpectomy and interbody graft placement, anterior cervical screw-plate fixation was performed. No posterior stabilization and fusion was required because the spinal column failure was confined to the anterior column.

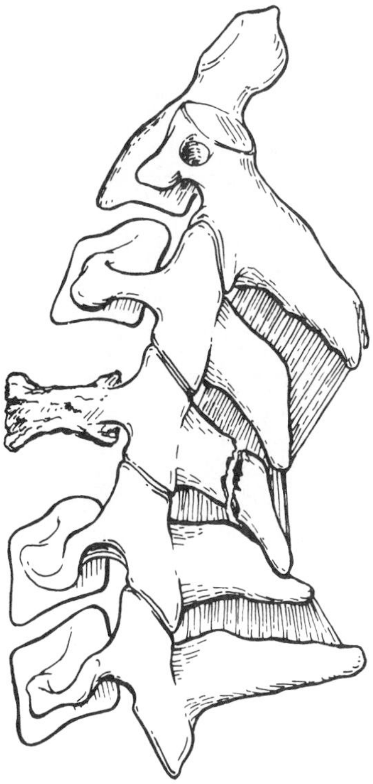

Figure 285-19 Diagram of a compression extension injury.

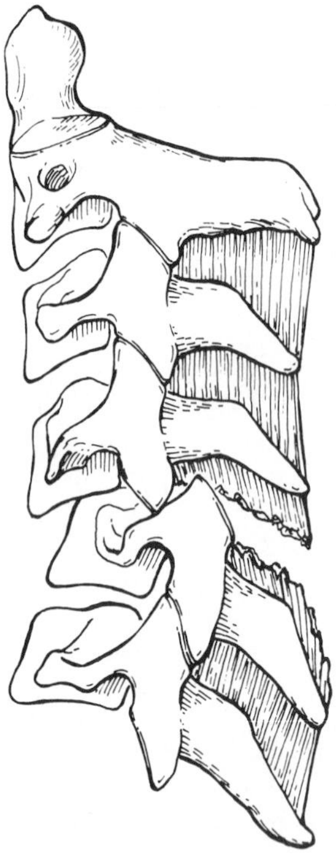

(*A*)

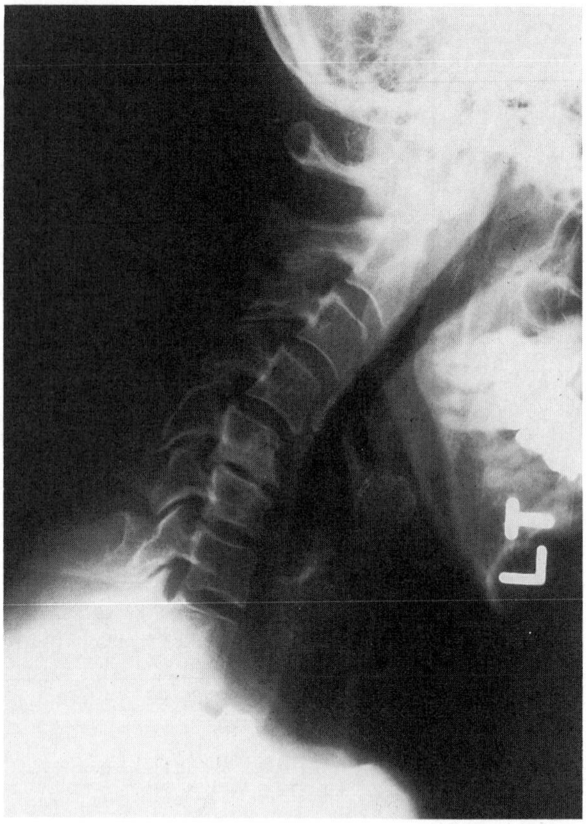

(*B*)

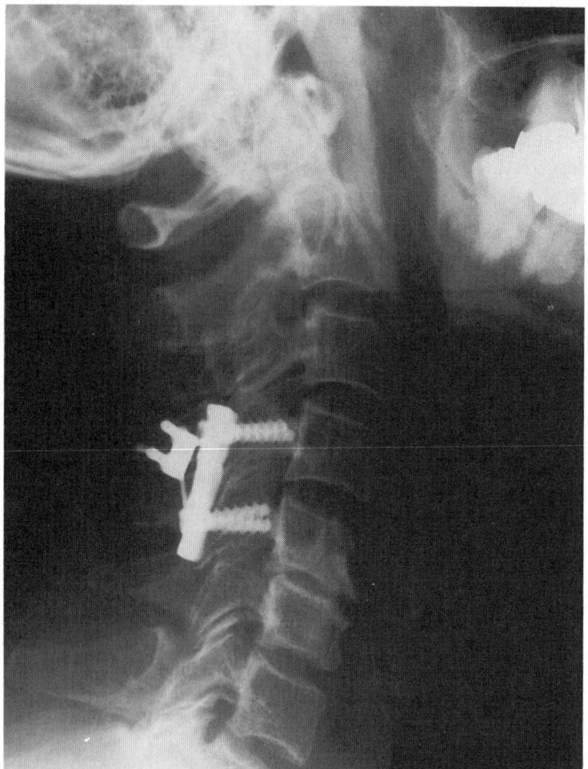

(*C*)

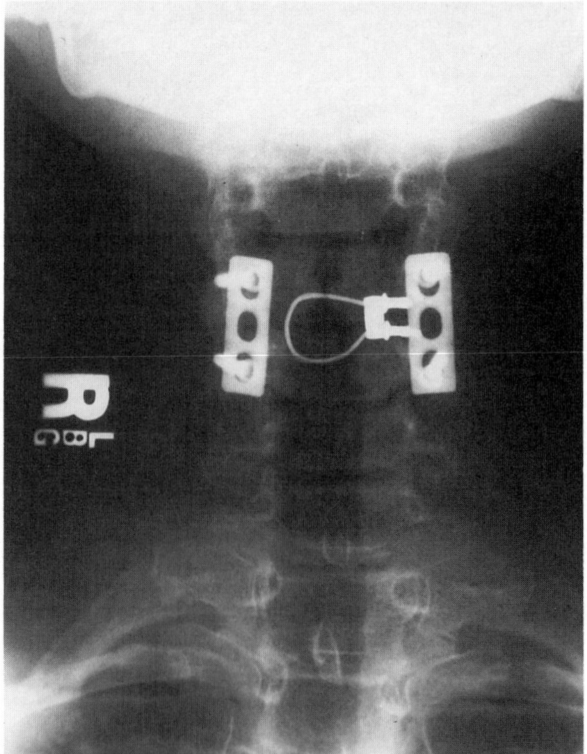

(*D*)

Figure 285-20 Distractive flexion injuries. *A*. Illustration of a type III distractive flexion injury with more than 50 percent vertebral body translation. *B*. Type I distractive flexion injury with posterior ligamentous instability causing C4-C5 hypermobility. There is no associated facet subluxation. *C*, *D*. Posterior stabilization and fusion was performed using C4-C5 lateral mass plates, spinous process cable, and iliac crest en lay fusion.

disc and/or end plate. Although the highest grades of this type of injury are frequently associated with devastating neurological deficits, this is not always true. Because of the frequency with which these injuries occur, the lack of consensus in the literature regarding optimal treatment, and our dissatisfaction with "conventional" management schemes (Fig. 285-21), we have developed treatment algorithms for these injuries (Figs. 285-22, 285-23).[73] The most important of these algorithms are for the management of all unilateral facet dislocations as well as the problematic subgroup of patients with bilateral dislocations who are neurologically intact, or have only a radiculopathy or incomplete neurological dysfunction. The impetus for this latter scheme was the exceptionally disappointing results experienced in three patients while strictly following conventional methods. It must be emphasized that these treatment algorithms were developed based on our observations. Although we have used them in our practice to safely treat both unilateral and bilateral facet dislocations, future evaluation will require a nonrandomized cohort study.

The key to treating these patients is to prevent deterioration of neurological status, and, when possible, to safely restore normal spinal alignment. Prior to attempting reduction, all patients with unilateral facet dislocation should initially undergo imaging in the form of either MRI or CT scans with low dose intrathecal contrast. Patients found not to have disc and/or significant end plate herniations undergo traction for reduction, regardless of neurological status. Of these patients, those with neck pain only are braced for 8 to 12 weeks regardless of whether the traction provides reduction. Patients with a neurological deficit whose facet dislocation does not reduce undergo surgery for facetectomy and posterior stabilization and fusion. The duration and degree of postoperative bracing is determined by the construct. Those patients with a neurological deficit whose dislocation reduces with traction are braced for up to 12 weeks. If the neurological status does not improve with the reestablishment of physiologic alignment, a repeat MRI scan is obtained.

No patient with unilateral dislocation and a scan positive for significant intracanalicular disc material is treated with traction (Fig. 285-22). Our concern is that these patients will develop irreversible neurological symptoms from spinal cord compression with closed reduction. Despite immediate detection of symptomatic spinal cord compression, there is no guarantee that emergency decompression will restore cord function. These patients are managed based on their neurological status. Patients with only neck pain are placed in a semirigid brace like a Philadelphia collar for up to 12 weeks.

All patients with unilateral dislocation with disc herniation on MRI and myelopathy and/or radiculopathy, or with bilateral facet dislocations with normal or incomplete neurological dysfunction, undergo anterior cervical microdiscectomy without attempting closed reduction (Figs. 285-22, 285-23). We have found MRI unreliable for predicting who will develop symptoms of spinal cord compression from disc herniation once bilateral facet dislocations are reduced.[73] Following disc removal (or vertebrectomy if significant angular deformity accompanies the bilateral dislocations),

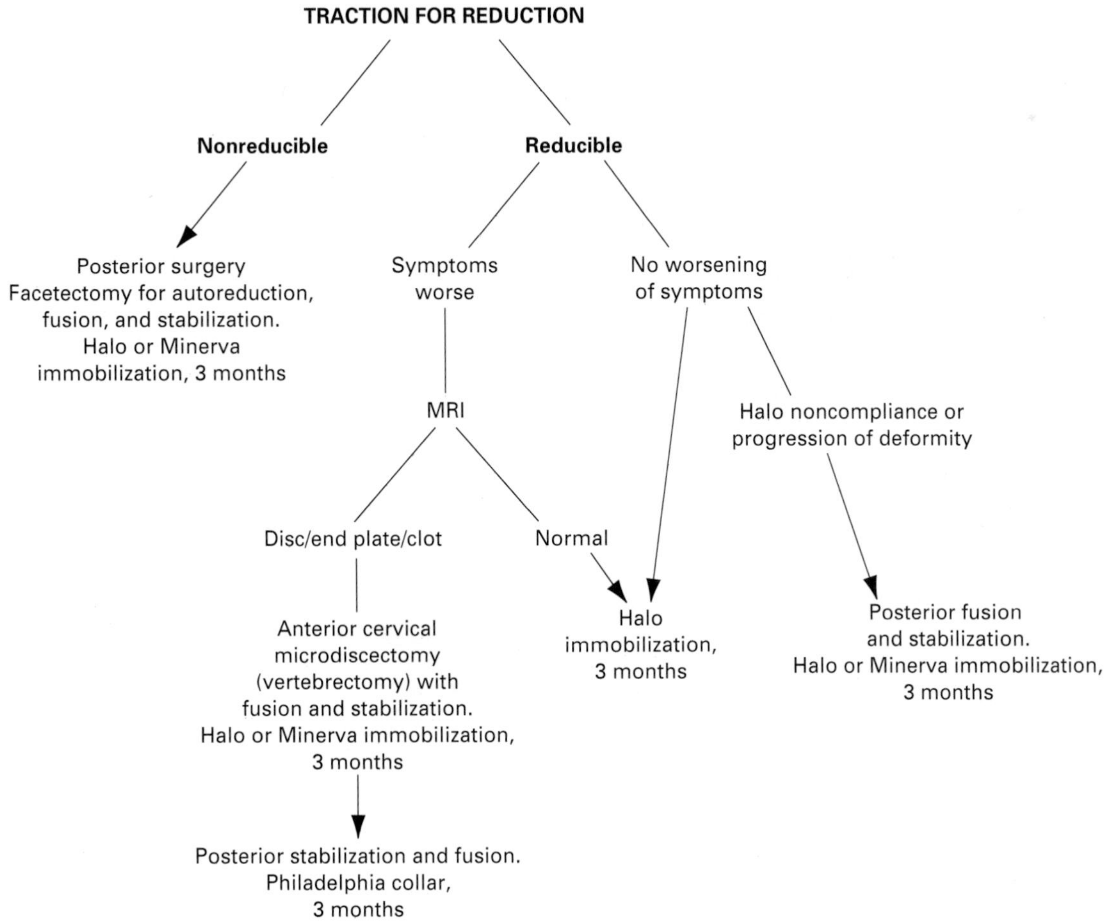

Figure 285-21 Conventional management of bilateral facet dislocation in intact patients or those with incomplete neurological deficits.

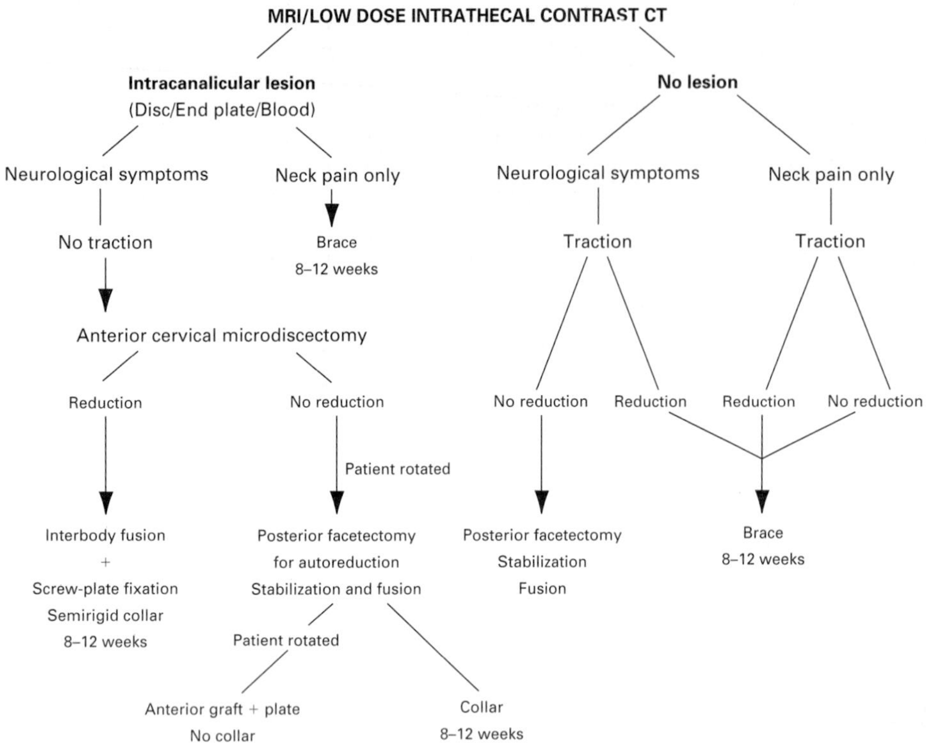

Figure 285-22 Unilateral facet dislocation.

gentle distraction is applied to try to reduce the dislocated facet joint(s). If reduction is achieved, an interbody graft and screw-plate fixator are placed; a Philadelphia collar is worn for 12 weeks. If reduction is not possible, the patient is rotated to a prone position on the Stryker bed and a facetectomy is performed for autoreduction. Posterior stabilization and fusion is carried out. Finally, the patient may be returned to the supine position for placement of an interbody bone graft. The type of bracing is determined by the type of construct established (Fig. 285-24*A–D*).

Bilateral facet dislocations in patients with complete spinal cord injuries are treated with traction. Surgery can be avoided if the deformity can be corrected and then can be maintained in a halo brace. Patients who do not experience reduction undergo a posterior operation for reduction, stabilization, and fusion.

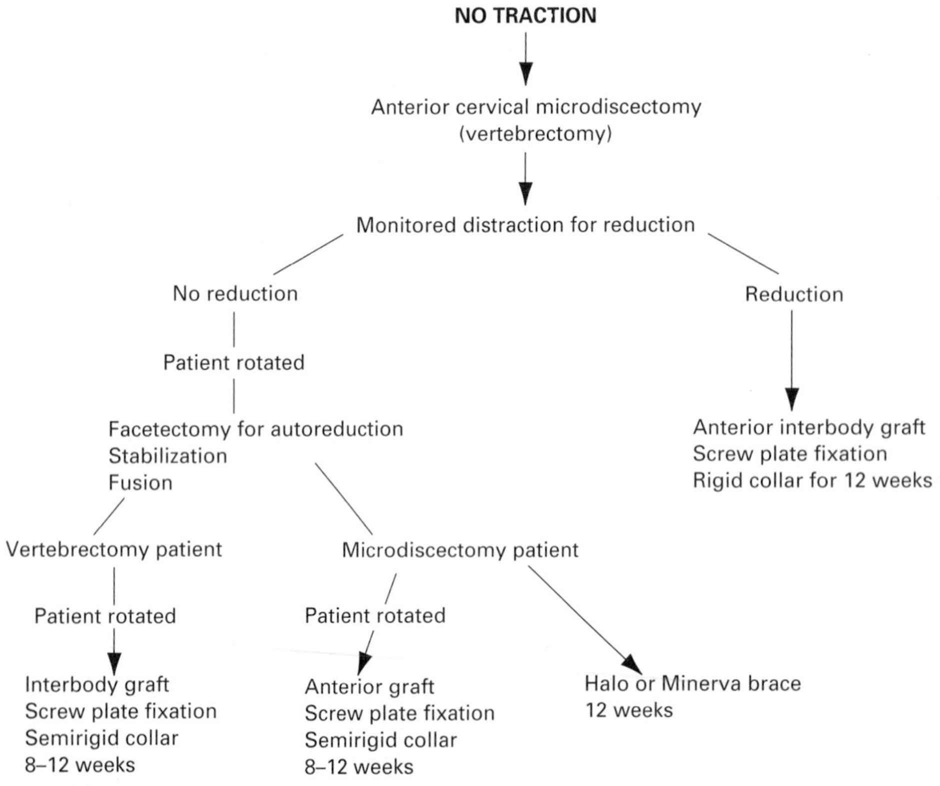

Figure 285-23 Bilateral facet dislocation in intact patients or those with incomplete neurological deficits.

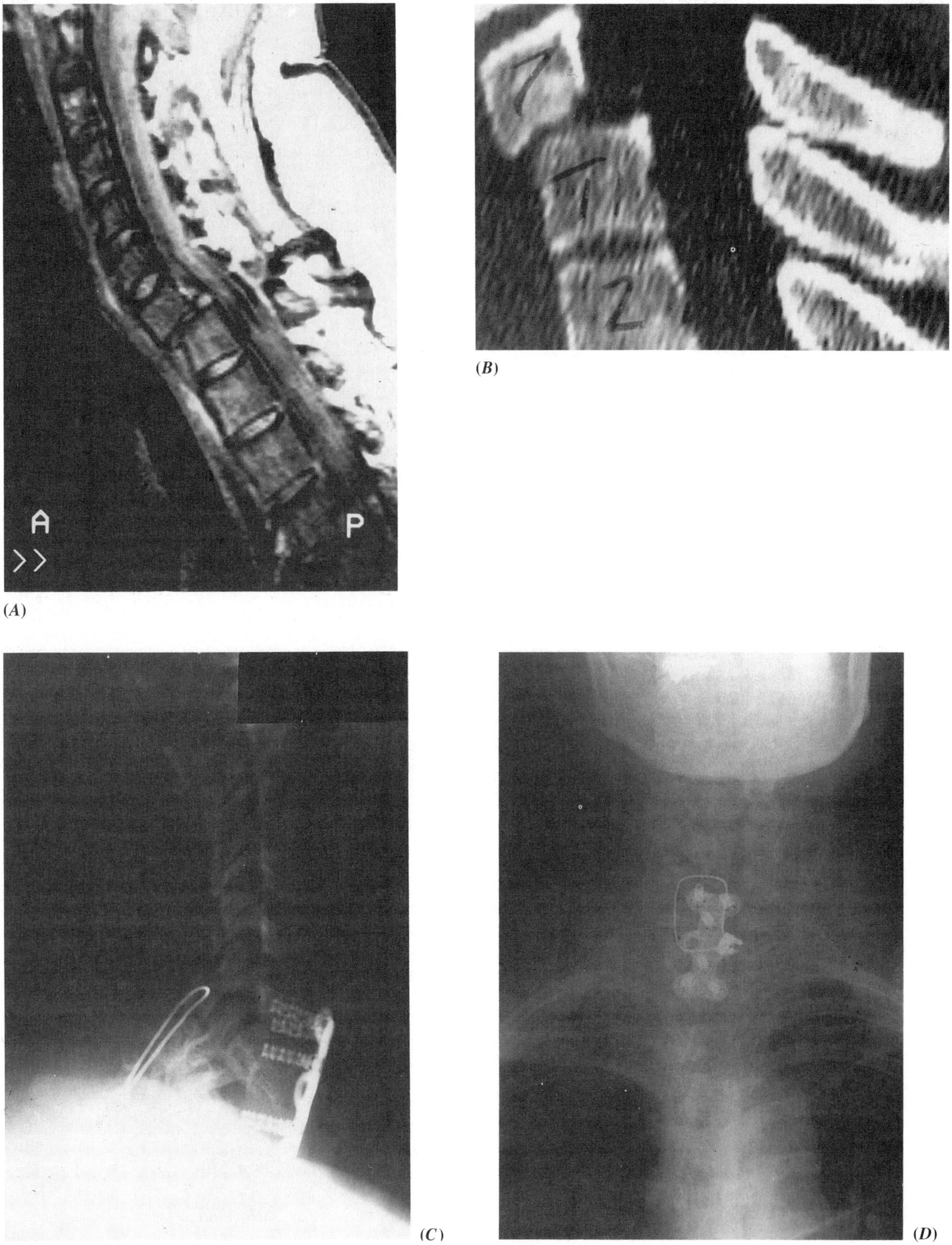

Figure 285-24 Bilateral facet dislocations in a patient with an incomplete neurological deficit. *A*. MRI scan showing C7-T1 bilateral facet dislocations in a patient with no myelopathy and only radicular symptoms. Note the extensive disc disruption. *B*. Sagittal reformatted CT scan of the same injury. *C, D*. Postoperative x-ray films. Based on our dissatisfaction with "conventional" management strategies, a treatment algorithm was designed for intact and incomplete patients with bilateral facet dislocations (see Fig. 285-23). The algorithm was followed in this patient. No traction was attempted. The patient underwent an anterior cervical vertebrectomy. Reduction could not be achieved. The patient was rotated on the Stryker bed and C7-T1 facetectomies and a C6-T1 stabilization and fusion were performed. The patient was turned supine again and a C6-T1 interbody graft and screw-plate fixator were placed. The patient had an excellent postoperative course with total resolution of radiculopathy and no development of myelopathy.

Distractive Extension There are two subgroups of distractive extension injuries (Fig. 285-25). In type I injuries there is widening of the disc space. The major injury vector is tension along the anterior elements. In type II injuries there is associated failure of the posterior elements which occurs as the tension forces are transmitted posteriorly. Falls onto the face with the neck in extension are known to result in these types of injuries. These injuries occur throughout the cervical spine, with the greatest number reported between C5-C6. This injury pattern is usually seen in older patients. Neurological injury is thought to occur as a result of posterior displacement of the cephalad vertebral segment with ''pinching'' of the adjacent spinal cord between the vertebral body and neural arch of the level below. These types of injuries may reduce spontaneously and therefore may not be detected on static plain x-ray films. Significant panligamentous disruption associated with the type II distraction-extension injuries generally requires surgical stabilization and fusion.

Lateral Flexion Injuries

These injuries are rare and consist of an asymmetrically applied lateral bending or flexion force that results in spinal column disruption (Fig. 285-26). The major force vector is thought to be compression along the side of the spine that is flexed laterally. The minor injury force is tension or distraction along the opposite side. There are two types of lateral flexion injuries. Both reveal asymmetrical compression of the vertebrae on anteroposterior views. Type I has ipsilateral vertebral and neural arch compression failure without any displacement of the neural arches. Type II lesions have vertebral body and ipsilateral neural arch compression fractures with either ipsilateral displacement of the neural arch or ligamentous injury manifested by separation of the contralateral facet joints. The lateral flexion injuries have a high incidence of associated brachial plexus injuries. They tend to involve the lower segments of the cervical spine. Some series report a high incidence of complete neurological deficit with the type II injuries. The rarity of these lesions and the wide spectrum of injury patterns make it difficult to generalize regarding appropriate treatment. Optimal treatment must be individualized based on a precise evaluation of the injury pattern.

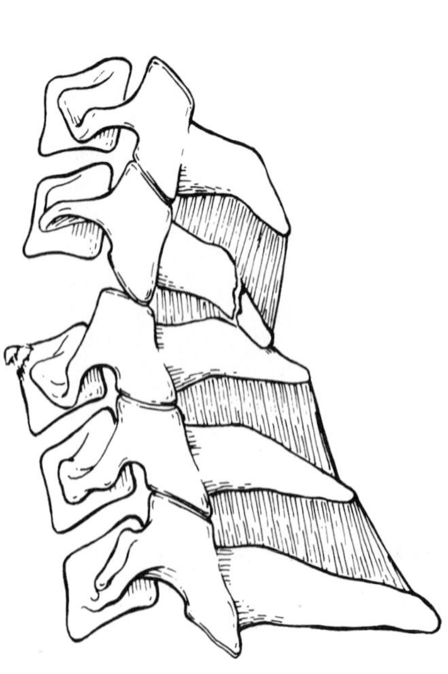

Figure 285-25 Diagram of a distractive extension injury.

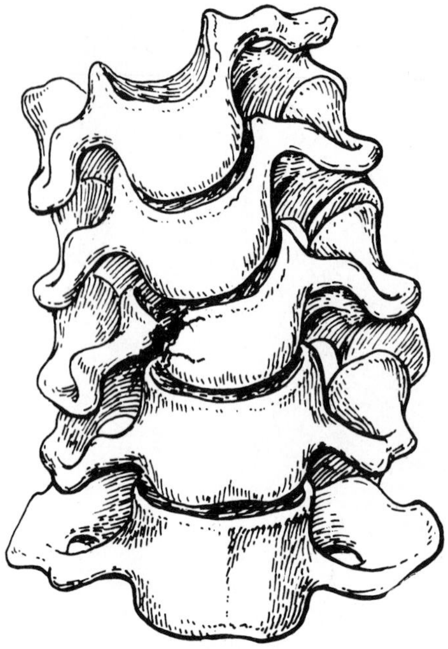

Figure 285-26 Illustration of a lateral flexion injury.

Management of Cervical Spine Injuries

Care of the patient who has sustained an injury to the cervical spine is designed to minimize the potential for further injury and to provide an environment that will maximize recovery of spinal cord dysfunction. Such a program demands that one be alert to the possibility of a cervical spine injury so as to take measures radiographically and clinically to evaluate this potential. The presence of a complete transverse myelopathy involving the cervical spinal cord poses a major medical challenge to the physician charged with the care of such patients; such challenges may also occur in patients with a partial or incomplete cord lesion.

One of the major causes contributing to the worsening of a patient with a mechanical spinal cord injury is a superimposed ischemic injury to the spinal cord. The finding of neurogenic shock, characterized by systemic hypotension and bradycardia, must be attended to immediately. Adequate volume expansion supplemented with judicious use of pressor agents to maintain normotension may avoid conversion of an incomplete or reversible lesion to one that is complete or fails to respond to therapy. Interruption of the corticospinal fibers may impede pulmonary function as a result of intercostal muscle denervation with a subsequent decrease in pulmonary excursion. Frequent pulmonary function tests and arterial blood gas determinations may alert the physician to an impending hypoxic insult.

Sympathetic denervation will result in the loss of thermal regulation, allowing for the development of hypothermia with potentially disastrous cardiovascular consequences. Loss of bladder control after such injuries requires meticulous attention to a bladder drainage system. A massively distended bladder may never recover sufficient tone to function adequately even in the face of spinal cord recovery. Intermittent catheterization every 6 h even in the acute phase helps to avoid complications of bladder overdistension and urinary stasis. This technique is preferred over an indwelling catheter for drainage since it is considered to be associated with a lower incidence of urinary tract infections. Finally, careful attention to skin care in the spinal cord injured patient is paramount. With the loss of skin sensation, and perhaps of motor function preventing voluntary changes in position, the patient is prone to develop pressure sores and decubitus ulcers. Precautions must be taken to prevent skin damage. Mechanical kinetic therapy beds have been used in an effort to minimize skin compression with possible necrosis. Log-rolling the patient every 2 to 3 h and padding bony prominences are also effective for preventing skin necrosis.

One additional potential catastrophic complication of immobilization in the spinal cord injured patient is development of deep vein thrombosis and subsequent pulmonary embolization. Pulmonary embolism is a common cause of sudden death in the spinal cord injured patient. Various measures have been used to reduce this potential including compression stockings, subcutaneous heparin injections, and kinetic therapy beds.

Once stabilization of systemic parameters has been achieved, attention should be directed to the need for alignment and immobilization of the spine. The use of skeletal traction to restore and/or maintain the normal alignment of the spinal column is a long practiced and effective approach for treating many patients with cervical spine fractures. Exceptions to this may include the dislocations and other distractive injuries discussed above. Throughout the years, a number of different cervical traction devices have evolved with the Gardner-Wells tongs being popular because of its ease of application and maintenance. The device has several advantages including that it may be applied directly in the emergency room, it does not require any surgical manipulation, and it can even be used in the face of a suspicious injury to help stabilize the spine while an evaluation is in progress. Application is simple and generally poses minimal risk to the patient, particularly when compared with the potential for excess motion of the unprotected cervical spine. We often prefer the immediate application of the halo ring for traction in those patients in whom halo immobilization is anticipated for maintaining reduction of the cervical injury. With a defined lesion of the cervical spine, we apply weight to the traction device with a maximum of 5 lb for each level below the occiput based on the guidelines promulgated by Crutchfield many years ago in the evaluation of vigorous male patients. Under these circumstances, reduction of highly unstable cervical fractures is usually readily accomplished. Because of the potential for overdistraction at the fracture site, however, we begin with 10 lb (for lesions at C4 or below) and then, under x-ray or fluoroscopic control, add weights up to the maximum weight if necessary. Patients with highly unstable injuries, and particularly when there is associated spondylosis, may be vulnerable to overdistraction and thus weights less than those recommended by Crutchfield should be used initially.

Once reduction has been accomplished, the question arises regarding the best mode of therapy to ensure healing with permanent stability at the fracture site. Application of a halo or rigid brace to the cervical spine may be satisfactory. This technique may be effective when there is adequate reduction of the cervical spine without persistent angulation due to extensive ligamentous disruption. We use the halo device or an effective rigid cervical brace to immobilize and treat patients who are neurologically intact with reduced yet unstable cervical spine fractures and fracture-dislocations.

Contraindications to the use of the halo include preexisting infection of the scalp, severe restrictive respiratory expansion of the chest, and severe chronic pulmonary disease. The patient with a complete transverse myelopathy who has an anesthetic shoulder and chest may develop pressure necrosis under a halo vest, which is, in our view, a relative although not absolute contraindication for using the halo apparatus.

Controversy surrounds the issue pertaining to optimal timing of spinal decompression. The major indication for early or acute surgical intervention in acute spinal cord injury is the avoidance of non-neurological complications such as pneumonia, urinary tract infection, deep vein thrombosis, pulmonary embolus, and skin necrosis that are shown to develop in patients not mobilized quickly following their injury.[84] There appears to be an 8 to 12 h window of opportunity for surgery; if passed, surgery does not lower these non-neurological complications. Another indication for surgery is preservation or restoration of neurological function if this is deemed possible. Numerous studies have evaluated the impact of decompression of the spinal cord acutely after cervical trauma on eventual outcome of spinal cord injury. These studies have failed to demonstrate any evidence of improved neurological function from acute operative decompression of the cervical spine in the face of spinal cord injury.

Although there have been reports of small series of patients with complete motor dysfunction demonstrating functional motor improvement following decompression, those patients generally considered candidates for surgical decompression have preservation of at least some distal neurological function but either fail to improve under observation or demonstrate evidence of a progressive neurological deficit. Progression of a neurological deficit demands emergency intervention if a compressive lesion is demonstrated. It should be stressed that an attempt at definitive stabilization of the cervical spine should be made at the same time that any indicated operative decompression is carried out. Our approach has been to assess by radiologic and clinical criteria the underlying mechanism responsible for the spinal injury and to direct our operative intervention at that particular site, via either an anterior or posterior approach or a combination of both. We no longer undertake ''decompression'' in the face of an unimproved complete transverse cervical myelopathy.

Treatment of Spinal Cord Injury

A critical hypothesis of acute spinal cord injury research is that preservation of surviving axons from further damage provides the best chance for recovery from injury. An acutely injured spinal cord undergoes progressive pathologic changes. This constitutes a common feature regardless of whether the initial mechanism of injury was trauma or ischemia. The primary injury (i.e., mechanical disruption of axons), triggers a cascade of events which produce secondary and irreversible structural damage to the spinal cord. Many mechanisms have been posited to explain secondary injury including (1) post-traumatic fall in spinal cord blood flow,[50] (2) release of neurotransmitters and toxic by-products,[64] (3) extracellular ionic and metabolic derangements,[90] (4) calcium influx into traumatized axons with subsequent activation of proteases and phospholipases,[16,43] and (5) generation of oxygen free radicals.[22] These mechanisms most probably act in concert to enhance cellular autodestruction after spinal cord injury.

The recognition that acute injury to the spinal cord is naturally progressive led investigators to design therapeutic interventions to prevent or reduce the extent of secondary damage. In the past 30 years, many treatment modalities have been attempted. One which has had some success is the use of pharmacologic agents given shortly after injury.

Two promising drugs that were found to alter the injury response and improve neurological outcome in animal models were the glucocorticoid hormone, methylprednisolone, and the opiate antagonist, naloxone. Many investigators have reported the positive effects that methylprednisolone has on functional recovery and histological appearance of injured spinal cords. Others, however, have not found steroids to be effective in spinal cord injury. This may be due in part to differences in methodology, treatment protocols, steroid preparations, and doses. Studies with dexamethasone (a relatively weak inhibitor of lipid peroxidation), or relatively low levels of methylprednisolone (<15 mg/kg) showed minimal protection against experimental spinal injury. On the other hand, methylprednisolone at doses of 30 mg/kg was neuroprotective.[93] The beneficial effects of methylprednisolone at such high doses has been attributed largely to its ability to scavenge free radicals and maximally inhibit lipid peroxidation and, less likely, to its anti-inflammatory or antiedema properties.[41] In light of this, a new class of steroids, the lazaroids, have been developed. These compounds, an example of which is tirilazad mesylate, are even more potent inhibitors of lipid peroxidation and have been shown to be efficacious in spinal trauma, but without the glucocorticoid effect of methylprednisolone.[40] No report has documented the use of tirilazad in human spinal cord injury.

High doses of naloxone (>2 mg/kg) have been reported to improve post-traumatic spinal cord blood flow and functional outcome after spinal cord injury. Other opiate antagonists, namely nalmefene and thyrotropin releasing hormone (TRH), are even more effective than naloxone. The mechanism by which naloxone has its effects is not entirely understood. Faden et al. demonstrated release of opiate-like substances in the blood of cats subjected to spinal cord injury. Because of their peripheral vasodilatory effect, opiates were held responsible for the systemic hypotension and decreased spinal cord perfusion that accompany spinal cord injury.[28] Based on these observations, Faden et al. proposed that naloxone, by blocking opiate receptors, improved mean systemic pressure and ameliorated the hypotension associated with trauma. Others have proposed that naloxone increases cardiac output without significantly increasing systemic pressure. More recently, Wallace and Tator challenged the positive results obtained with naloxone.[79,80] They reported no improvement in cardiac output, spinal cord blood flow, or functional outcome after spinal cord injury. However, spinal cord blood flow improved by simply raising the blood pressure and cardiac output with fluids and pressors.

Based on the observation that methylprednisolone improved recovery in spinal injured animals, the National Acute Spinal Cord Injury Study (NASCIS) group conducted a multicenter double-blind randomized trial with high dose methylprednisolone in human spinal cord injury.[14,15] Between 1979 and 1984, the first NASCIS investigation (NASCIS 1) randomized 330 patients and compared the effects of high dose (1000 mg bolus followed by 1000 mg/day for 10 days) versus low dose (100 mg bolus followed by 100 mg/day for 10 days) methylprednisolone started within 48 h after spinal cord injury. Admission and follow-up examinations at 6 weeks, 6 months, and 1 year after injury were performed. Recovery was defined as the difference between admission and follow-up motor and sensory scores. At 6 months and 1 year after injury, there were no significant differences in motor or sensory recovery between the two groups. In addition, a higher rate of wound infection accompanied the high dose group, perhaps due to immunosuppression from the prolonged steroid treatment.

NASCIS 1 was criticized for three reasons[91]: (1) the treatment groups were not compared against placebo, therefore, it is difficult to state with certainty that steroid at low doses had no effect on functional recovery; (2) the high dose of methylprednisolone used in the study was suboptimal. A 70 kg person receiving 1000 mg of the drug per day, as in the NASCIS 1 investigation is equivalent to a dose of 15 mg/kg. Later evidence from animal studies suggested an optimal dose of 30 mg/kg for methylprednisolone to effectively inhibit lipid peroxidation, increase post-traumatic blood flow, and improve motor function: and (3) experimental studies indicated that the drug needed to be administered within a few hours after injury to have maximal effect. In contrast, the treatment protocol for NASCIS 1 allowed for drug delivery as late as 48 h after injury by which time much damage had already occurred.

Important lessons learned from NASCIS 1 including earlier treatment with a higher dose and comparison of the results with a placebo group were incorporated into NASCIS 2. The study was started in 1985 and randomized 487 patients to treatment with methylprednisolone (30 mg/kg bolus followed by 5.4 mg/kg per h for 23 h), naloxone (5.4 mg/kg bolus followed by 4.0 mg/kg per h for 23 h), and placebo.[92] Bolus and maintenance doses of drugs were largely based on dose-response testing in animals. To avoid the complication of prolonged steroid therapy, the study chose a treatment duration of 24 h. The conclusion of the study was that methylprednisolone, if given within 8 h after injury, significantly improved motor and sensory recovery at 6 weeks, 6 months, and 1 year postinjury. Improvement in motor scores was consistent with up to two Frankel grade category changes for both "plegic" and "paretic" patients. Patients receiving naloxone or methylprednisolone more than 8 h after injury did not differ in their scores from the placebo group. This study does suggest that high dose methylprednisolone does provide a neuroprotective effect when administered within 8 h of injury. It is not certain whether this is clinically relevant.

Generation of oxygen free radicals by injured cells is now thought to be a primary secondary injury mechanism in spinal cord injury.[42] Superoxide free radicals are produced by the univalent reduction of molecular oxygen. This free radical and subsequent derived oxygen species are highly reactive and attack lipids and proteins. Superoxide dismutase, catalase, and other antioxidants effectively reduce post-traumatic changes and promote function and survival in experimental studies on various organ systems. Among the potential sources of free radicals which may contribute to post-traumatic myelopathy (i.e., arachidonic acid metabolism, polymorphonuclear cell infiltration, and mitochondrial dysfunction), one that is becoming increasingly popular is xanthine oxidase. The in vivo form of the enzyme, xanthine dehydrogenase, is unable to produce superoxide.[58] Under ischemic conditions, it converts to xanthine oxidase which can produce free radicals in the presence of oxygen and xanthine derived from adenosine triphosphate (ATP) catabolism.[65] Such conversion has been documented in human head injury and acutely injured spinal cords.[88] Endothelial cells are a rich source of xanthine oxidase.[48] The high concentration in endothelial cells correlates with the microvasculature as being the trigger for post-traumatic hypoperfusion and subsequent secondary damage. A recent study evaluated the role of xanthine oxidase in rat spinal cord injury using allopurinol to specifically inhibit the enzyme. The results revealed a strong neuroprotective effect with allopurinol, suggesting that xanthine oxidase-derived free radicals contribute significantly to secondary damage.[66,67]

Many other drugs have reportedly produced beneficial effects in animal impact injury models. These include a number of antioxidants, neurotransmitter receptor blockers, cyclo-oxygenase inhibitors, protease inhibitors, calcium channel blockers, modulators of intracellular messengers, and others.[91] The demonstration of post-injury treatment being neuroprotective by such diverse drugs confirms the fact that primary injury initiates a cascade of endogenous mechanisms which can be manipulated at many levels. Thus far, methylprednisolone has been the only drug to have an impact on the treatment of human spinal cord injury. Other promising drugs have yet to be evaluated in a clinical setting.

A novel treatment for the acutely traumatized spinal cord is the use of a pedicled omental on-lay graft at the site of the injury.[34,35] The rationale for this procedure is based on the sequelae of spinal cord trauma, i.e., cord swelling and local ischemia, and the omentum's ability to absorb extraordinary amounts of vasogenic edema fluid and to revascularize traumatized spinal cords. In previous studies, Goldsmith had shown the formation of vascular connections between omentum and the cerebral surface with a consequent increase in blood flow, sufficient to prevent infarction following occlusion of the middle cerebral artery. Revascularization was also confirmed at the omental-spinal cord interface and in deep spinal cord tissue in normal and traumatized spinal cords. The omentum also prevents formation of scar tissue at the site of injury. The hypothesis is that omentum decreases fibroblastic proliferation by reducing the level of fibrinogen in vasogenic edema fluid, which is believed to initiate scar formation. Alternatively, omental tissue may possess antifibrotic activity. Despite such convincing evidence provided by animal studies and limited human studies, the use of the omentum in acute spinal cord injury remains experimental.

Syndromes of Spinal Cord Trauma

The extent of spinal cord injury relates, of course, most directly to the amount of force applied to the spinal cord at the time of impact, although vascular consequences, both hemorrhagic and ischemic, secondary to the injury may contribute significantly to the ultimate clinical picture. The most severe consequence of spinal cord trauma is complete transverse myelopathy in which all functional activity below the level of the lesion is lost. This entity is frequently, if not always, associated with spinal shock in which there is impairment of sensation and absence of motor modalities and monosynaptic reflexes below the level of the lesion at the initial evaluation. Complete spinal shock rarely persists longer than 24 h after injury. If no recovery is noted within this time frame, there is usually permanent paralysis and sensory deficit below the lesion. Complete cord injury may occur as a result of true anatomic disruption of the spinal cord, physiologic disruption of neural function because of compression or ischemia, or a combination of both. One may rarely witness an extensive injury to the spinal cord, including even the clinical picture of a complete transverse myelopathy, that spontaneously resolves within 24 to 72 h after the injury. Such an occurrence relates to transient physiological dysfunction secondary to trauma and may be considered a concussion of the spinal cord.

The patient with preservation of some neurological function below the level of injury is classified as having incomplete or partial cord injury. Such injuries have a much better prognosis for neurological recovery than do complete injuries. Progressive deterioration of partial injury to total neurological deficit is rare but can happen in the presence of cord compression by bone fragments, extruded disc material, or hematoma, or by spinal instability causing further cord damage. Specific syndromes of incomplete injury may occur, depending on the degree and location of the injury.

In the anterior spinal cord syndrome, one observes dysfunction of those substrates of spinal cord function subserved by the anterior two-thirds of the spinal cord embracing the corticospinal tracts and the anterolateral spinothalamic systems. Under such circumstances one observes a loss of all voluntary motor activity along with absence of sensation to pain and temperature below the level of the lesion. On the other hand, posterior column function, as evaluated by proprioceptive responses, is generally preserved. Reflex activity below the level of such lesions is generally absent acutely, although one may see extensor plantar responses. The degree of the motor deficit in both the upper and lower extremities below the level of the lesion is generally equal. The pathophysiologic process underlying the genesis of this syndrome has not been precisely defined. Direct trauma to the anterior and lateral aspect of the cord is the usual cause. It may also relate to stretch applied by the attachment of the dentate ligaments at the equatorial plane of the cord or ischemic injury due to compromise of the anterior spinal artery which supplies the anterior two-thirds of the cord. Based on autopsy studies, thrombosis of the anterior spinal artery is not the cause, although it may occur and may add to the pathology of anterior cord syndrome. Recovery is variable and, in general is poor with only a 10 to 20 percent chance of recovering functional motor control.

Another syndrome of partial injury is the central cord syndrome. The focus of trauma lies within the centrum of the cervical spinal cord, therein involving those structures traversing this area. Underlying pathologic substrates include edema and hemorrhagic contusion to the centrum of the cord, mechanical disruption, ischemia, or a combination of these. Clinically, one observes disproportionate weakness in the upper extremities below the level of the lesion when compared with the lower extremities. The anatomic position of the lower extremity fibers laterally in the corticospinal and spinothalamic tracts provides an explanation for the relative preservation of leg function. Sensory loss is usually minimal, although it varies and frequently occurs in no specific pattern. The extent of the motor deficit may vary, with the key clinical observation being that the motor deficit in the upper extremities is greater than that in the lower extremities. Deep tendon reflexes in the lower extremities are generally preserved and may show signs of an upper motor neuron pattern; deep tendon reflexes in the upper extremities at the level of the lesion will generally be absent.

Characteristically, the central cord syndrome is associated with hyperextension injury in elderly patients with cervical spondylosis and a stenotic spinal canal. This may be the result of a forward fall or of inadvertent hyperextension during endotracheal intubation. An entity which mimics the central cord syndrome is cruciate paralysis secondary to a fractured odontoid. Paresis of both upper extremities with relative sparing of the lower limbs occurs due to injury involving the midline and upper portion of the anterior cervicomedullary junction where arm fibers decussate. Fibers to the legs, traversing through the lower decussation, are less affected.

Different opinions exist regarding the management of central cord injury. This is in large part due to variable recovery patterns, ranging from complete recovery to profound and permanent residual deficits. Some authors prefer conservative treatment while others favor surgery for patients with cord deformation who have plateaued neurologically. On occasion, removal of the offending abnormality has led to significant improvement.

The Brown-Sequard syndrome or hemisection of the spinal cord is yet another example of partial cord injury. Classic features of the syndrome include ipsilateral loss of lower motor neurons at the level of injury, ipsilateral loss of strength and proprioception, and contralateral loss of pain and temperature sensation below the injury level. The syndrome is most commonly observed secondary to penetrating injuries such as stab wounds, although blunt spinal cord trauma causing lateral cord compression can produce some of the findings. Functional recovery has a more favorable prognosis in patients with cord hemisection than in those with the anterior cord or central cord injury.

Prognosis

Critical review of the literature shows that neurological improvement occurs in patients with spinal cord injuries and that the eventual outcome depends greatly on the initial degree of sparing from the trauma. Information released by the National Spinal Cord Injury Statistical Center (NSCISC) data base in 1991 confirmed this finding.[20] To assess the severity of deficits and to evaluate functional changes following acute care and rehabilitation, the authors utilized the Frankel Classification system. Spinal cord injured patients were segregated into five functional categories: "A" when they had no motor or sensory function below the lesion level, "B" when they had sensory but no motor function below the lesion, "C" when motor function was present but not useful, "D" when useful motor function was present in the lower limbs, or "E" if normal. Complete injuries were thus differentiated from incomplete injuries and patients with partial function were further subdivided into different categories based on their motor capabilities. Of the 4934 persons enrolled in the study, initial evaluation revealed 51.9 percent to have complete loss, that is, Frankel grade A. The others were classified as Frankel grade B (13.1 percent), Frankel grade C (13.1 percent), and Frankel grade D (21.9 percent). Only 10.3 percent of patients in the grade A category showed improvement significant enough to be placed into a higher functional category. In contrast, 45.2 percent and 55.9 percent of patients in Frankel grades B and C, respectively, experienced improved function, by at least one Frankel grade, prior to discharge. Patients with Frankel grade D also improved, with 7.3 percent showing complete neurological recovery; most, however, left the hospital with some degree of residual motor impairment.

In terms of long-term outcome, neurological recovery continues for some patients for up to 18 months, after which further improvement is rare. Outcome and follow-up data from a population of 186 persons reported by Gerhart showed a similar positive outlook following traumatic injury to the cervical spinal cord.[32] Thirty-six percent of patients improved neurologically by at least one Frankel grade before hospital discharge, regardless of their initial Frankel classification. Approximately 10 percent continued to improve 2 years postdischarge by an additional grade.

Conclusion

The study of cervical spine injury has evolved dramatically during the past several decades. A greater understanding of the anatomic and mechanical considerations has enabled a more accurate classification of these injuries. Refinements in the medical and surgical treatment of these unfortunate individuals have significantly improved both short-term and long-term outcome. Future developments in the area of neural protection and axonal regeneration will undoubtedly provide the important key to the management puzzle of the spinal cord injured patient.

References

1. Acton PA, Farley T, Freni LW, et al. Traumatic spinal cord injury in Arkansas, 1980 to 1989. *Arch Phys Med Rehabil* 1993; 74:1035–1040.
2. Allen BL Jr. Recognition of injuries to the lower cervical spine. In Sherk HH, Dunn EJ, Eismont FJ, Fielding JW, Long DM, Ono K, Penning L, Raynor R (eds): *The Cervical Spine,* 2d ed. Philadelphia: Lippincott, 1989, pp 286–298.
3. Allen BL Jr, Ferguson RL, Lehmann TR, et al. A mechanistic classification of closed, indirect fractures and dislocations of the lower cervical spine. *Spine* 1982; 7:1–27.
4. Anderson LD, Clark CR. Fractures of the odontoid process of the axis. In Sherk HH, Dunn EJ, Eismont FJ, Fielding JW, Long DM, Ono K, Penning L, Raynor R (eds): *The Cervical Spine,* 2d ed. Philadelphia: Lippincott, 1989, pp 325–343.
5. Anderson LD, D'Alonzo RT. Fractures of the odontoid process of the axis. *J Bone Joint Surg [Am]* 1974; 56-A:1663–1674.
6. Anderson PA, Montesano PX. Traumatic injuries of the occipital-cervical articulation. In Camins MB, O'Leary PF (eds): *Disorders of the Cervical Spine.* Baltimore: Williams & Wilkins, 1992, pp 273–283.
7. Apfelbaum RI. Anterior screw fixation of odontoid fractures. In Camins MB, O'Leary PF (eds): *Disorders of the Cervical Spine.* Baltimore: Williams & Wilkins, 1992, pp 603–608.
8. Apfelbaum RI. Posterior transarticular C1-2 screw fixation for atlantoaxial instability. In *Aesculap Scientific Information.* South San Francisco: Aesculap, 1993, vol 25, pp 1–12.
9. Apuzzo MLF, Heiden JS, Weiss MH, et al. Acute fractures of the odontoid process. An analysis of 45 cases. *J Neurosurg* 1978; 48:85–91.
10. Bauer RD, Errico TJ. Cervical spine injuries. In Errico TJ, Bauer RD, Waugh T (eds): *Spinal Trauma.* Philadelphia: Lippincott, 1991, pp 71–121.
11. Bohlman HH. Acute fractures and dislocations of the cervical spine: an analysis of three hundred hospitalized patients and review of the literature. *J Bone Joint Surg [Am]* 1979; 61-A:1119–1142.
12. Borges LF. Clinical assessment of posttraumatic spinal instability. In Cooper PC (ed): *Management of Posttraumatic Spinal Instability.* Park Ridge, IL: American Association of Neurological Surgeons, 1990, pp 37–49.
13. Borock EC, Gabram SG, Jacobs LM, Murphy MA. A prospective analysis of a two-year experience with computed tomography as an adjunct for cervical spine clearance. *J Trauma* 1991; 31:1001–1006.
14. Bracken MB, Collins WF, Freeman DF, et al. Efficacy of methylprednisolone in acute spinal cord injury. *JAMA* 1984; 251:45–52.
15. Bracken MB, Shepard MJ, Hellenbrand KG, et al. Methylprednisolone and neurological function one year after spinal cord injury: results of the National Acute Spinal Cord Injury Study. *J Neurosurg* 1985; 63:704–713.
16. Braughler JM, Duncan LA, Chase RL. Interaction of lipid peroxidation and calcium in the pathogenesis of neuronal injury. *Cent Nerv Syst Trauma* 1985; 2:269–283.
17. Bucholz RW, Burkhead WZ. The pathological anatomy of fatal atlanto-occipital dislocations. *J Bone Joint Surg [Am]* 1979; 61-A:248–250.
18. Coutts MB. Atlanto-epistropheal subluxations. *Arch Surg* 1934; 29:297–311.
19. Davis SJ, Teresi LM, Bradley WG Jr, et al. Cervical spine hyperextension injuries: MR findings. *Radiology* 1991; 180:245–251.

20. De Vivo MJ, Richards JS, Stover SL, Go BK. Spinal cord injury: rehabilitation adds life to years. *West J Med* 1991; 154:602–606.
21. De Vivo MJ, Rutt RD, Black KJ, et al. Trends in spinal cord injury demographics and treatment outcomes between 1973 and 1986. *Arch Phys Med Rehabil* 1992; 73:424–430.
22. Demopoulos HB, Flamm ES, Pietronigro DD, et al. The free radical pathology and the microcirculation in the major central nervous system disorders. *Acta Physiol Scand* 1980; 492:91–119.
23. Dickman CA, Hadley MN, Browner C, Sonntag VKH. Neurosurgical management of acute atlas-axis combination fractures: a review of 25 cases. *J Neurosurg* 1989; 70:45–49.
24. Dreyzin V, Esses SI. Trauma of the cervical spine. *Curr Opin Orthop* 1993; 4(II):78–88.
25. Eismont FJ, Bohlman HH. Posterior atlanto-occipital dislocation with fractures of the atlas and odontoid process. *J Bone Joint Surg [Am]* 1978; 60-A:397–399.
26. Errico TJ. Techniques and management of cervical spine fractures. *Spine: State Art Rev* 1993; 7:157–180.
27. Evarts CM. Traumatic occipito-atlantal dislocation: report of a case with survival. *J Bone Joint Surg [Am]* 1970; 52-A:1653–1660.
28. Faden AI, Jacobs TP, Holaday JW. Opiate antagonist improves neurologic recovery after spinal injury. *Science* 1981; 211:493–494.
29. Fielding JW, Hawkins RJ, Hensinger RN, et al. Atlantoaxial rotatory deformities. *Orthop Clin North Am* 1978; 9:955–967.
30. Flanders AE, Schaeffer DM, Doan HT, et al. Acute cervical spine trauma: correlation of MR imaging findings with degree of neurologic deficit. *Radiology* 1990; 177:25–33.
31. Gaufin LM, Goodman SJ. Cervical spine injuries in infants: problems in management. *J Neurosurg* 1975; 42:179–184.
32. Gerhart KA. Spinal cord injury outcomes in a population-based sample. *J Trauma* 1991; 31:1529–1535.
33. Goldberg AL, Deeb ZL, Rothfus WE, Daffner RH. Magnetic resonance imaging in evaluation of acute spinal trauma. *Spine State Art Rev* 1989; 3:339–348.
34. Goldsmith HS, Duckett S, Chen WF. Spinal cord vascularization by intact omentum. *Am J Surg* 1975; 129:262–265.
35. Goldsmith HS, Steward E, Duckett S. Early application of pedicled omentum to the acutely traumatised spinal cord. *Paraplegia* 1985; 23:100–112.
36. Grob D, Crisco JJ III, Panjabi MM, et al. Biomechanical evaluation of four different posterior atlantoaxial fixation techniques. *Spine* 1992; 17:480–490.
37. Grob D, Jeanneret B, Aebi M, et al. Atlanto-axial fusion with transarticular screw fixation. *J Bone Joint Surg [Br]* 1991; 73-B:972–976.
38. Hadley MN, Browner C, Sonntag VKH. Axis fractures: a comprehensive review of management and treatment in 107 cases. *Neurosurgery* 1985; 17:281–290.
39. Hadley MN, Dickman CA, Browner CM, Sonntag VKH. Acute traumatic atlas fractures: management and long term outcome. *Neurosurgery* 1988; 23:31–35.
40. Hall ED. Effects of the 21-aminosteroid U74006F on posttraumatic spinal cord ischemia in cats. *J Neurosurg* 1988; 68:462–465.
41. Hall ED, Braughler JM. Glucocorticoid mechanisms in acute spinal injury: a review and therapeutic rationale. *Surg Neurol* 1982; 18:320–327.
42. Hall ED, Braughler JM, McCall JM. Antioxidant effects in brain and spinal cord injury. *J Neurotrauma* 1992; 9:S165–S172.
43. Happel RD, Smith KP, Powers JM, et al. Ca^{2+} accumulation in experimental spinal cord trauma. *Brain Res* 1983; 211:476–479.
44. Heiden JS, Weiss MH, Rosenberg AW, et al. Management of cervical spinal cord trauma in Southern California. *J Neurosurg* 1975; 43:732–736.
45. Heier LA, Johnson CE. Efficacy of magnetic resonance imaging in the diagnosis of spinal cord trauma. In Lee BY, Ostrander LE, Cochran GVB, Shaw W (eds): *The Spinal Cord Injured Patient.* Philadelphia: Saunders, 1991, pp 90–114.
46. Hohl M. Normal motions in the upper portion of the cervical spine. *J Bone Joint Surg [Am]* 1964; 46-A:1777–1779.
47. Huelke DF, O'Day J, Mendelsohn RA. Cervical injuries suffered in automobile crashes. *J Neurosurg* 1981; 54:316–322.
48. Jarasch ED, Grund C, Bruder G, et al. Localization of xanthine oxidase in mammary-gland epithelium and capillary endothelium. *Cell* 1981; 25:67–82.
49. Jefferson G. Remarks on fractures of the first cervical vertebra: founded on a portion of a Hunterian Lecture delivered at the Royal College of Surgeons of England, Feb 1924. In *Selected Papers, Geoffrey Jefferson.* Springfield, IL: Charles C Thomas, 1960, pp 213–231.
50. Kobrine AI, Doyle TF, Martins AN. Local spinal cord blood flow in experimental traumatic myelopathy. *J Neurosurg* 1975; 42:144–149.
51. Kulkarni MV, McArdle CB, Kopanicky D, et al. Acute spinal cord injury: MR imaging at 1.5T. *Neuroradiology* 1987; 164:837–843.
52. Lewis LM, Docherty M, Ruoff BE, et al. Flexion-extension views in the evaluation of cervical spine injuries. *Ann Emerg Med* 1991; 20:117–121.
53. MacDonald RL, Schwartz ML, Mirich D, et al. Diagnosis of cervical spine injury in motor vehicle crash victims: how many x-rays are enough? *J Trauma* 1991; 30:392–397.
54. Magerl F, Seemann PS. Stable posterior fusion of the atlas and axis by transarticular screw fixation. In Kehr P, Weidner A (eds): *Cervical Spine,* vol I. New York: Springer Verlag, 1987, pp 322–327.
55. Maiman DJ, Barolat G, Larson SJ. Management of bilateral locked facets of the cervical spine. *Neurosurgery* 1986; 18:542–547.
56. Maiman DJ, Larson SJ. Management of odontoid fractures. *Neurosurgery* 1982; 11:471–476.
57. Marcotte P, Dickman CA, Sonntag VKH, et al. Posterior atlantoaxial facet screw fixation. *J Neurosurg* 1993; 79:234–237.
58. McCord JM, Roy RS. The pathophysiology of superoxide: roles in inflammation and ischemia. *Can J Physiol Pharmacol* 1982; 60:1346–1352.
59. Menezes AH, Muhonen M. Management of occipito-cervical instability. In Cooper PC (ed): *Management of Posttraumatic Spinal Instability.* Park Ridge, IL: American Association of Neurological Surgeons, 1990, pp 65–76.
60. Mirvis SE, Geisler FH, Jelinek JJ, et al. Acute cervical spine trauma: evaluation with 1.5 T MR imaging. *Radiology* 1988; 166:807–816.
61. Mirvis SE, Rothman M. Magnetic resonance imaging of the cervical spine. In Camins MB, O'Leary PF (eds): *Disorders of the Cervical Spine.* Baltimore: Williams & Wilkins, 1992, pp 69–103.
62. Montesano PX, Juach EC, Anderson PA, et al. Biomechanics of cervical spine internal fixation. *Spine* 1991; 16(Suppl 3): S10–S16.
63. Ogden JA (ed). *Skeletal Injury in the Child.* Philadelphia: Lea & Febiger, 1982, pp 385–422.
64. Osterholm JL. The pathophysiological response in spinal cord injury: the current status of related research. *J Neurosurg* 1974; 40:5–33.
65. Roy RS, McCord JM. Superoxide and ischemia: conversion of xanthine dehydrogenase to xanthine oxidase. In Greenwald RA, Cohen G (eds): *Oxy Radicals and Their Scavenger Systems: Vol II. Cellular and Medical Aspects.* New York: Elsevier, 1983, pp 145–153.
66. Roy RS, Young W. Allopurinol reduces lesion volumes in injured rat spinal cords. *J Neurotrauma* 1994; submitted.
67. Roy R, Zagzag D, Miller DC, et al. Allopurinol minimizes histological changes in spinal cord injury. *J Neurosurg* 1994; 80:388A (abstr).
68. Schneider RC. High cervical spine injuries. In Wilkins RH, Rengachary SS (eds), *Neurosurgery.* New York: McGraw-Hill, 1985, pp 1701–1708.
69. Schneider RC, Livingston KE, Cave AJE, et al. ''Hangman's fracture'' of the cervical spine. *J Neurosurg* 1965; 22:141–154.
70. Sonntag VKH, Hadley MN. Management of nonodontoid upper cervical spine injuries. In Cooper PC (ed): *Management of Posttraumatic Spinal Instability.* Park Ridge, IL: American Association of Neurological Surgeons, 1990, pp 99–110.
71. Stillerman CB, Chen TC, Gruen JP, et al. Anterior cervical fixation using the Manny fixator: clinical experience and follow-up on 32 patients. Presented at the 62nd Annual Meeting of the American Association of Neurological Surgeons, San Diego, April 9–14, 1994 (poster).
72. Stillerman CB, Mueller W, Baker G. Clinical and biomechanical characteristics of a new anterior cervical screw-plate fixation device: the

Manny fixator. Presented at the 61st Annual Meeting of the American Association of Neurological Surgeons, Boston, April 24–29, 1993 (poster).
73. Stillerman CB, Mueller W, Tung H. The management of bilateral facet dislocations in patients with incomplete neurologic deficits. Presented at a meeting of the Joint Section on Disorders of the Spine and Peripheral Nerves, Miami, 1992.
74. Stillerman CB, Wilson JA. Atlanto-axial stabilization with posterior transarticular screw fixation: technical description and report of 22 cases. *Neurosurgery* 1993; 32:948–955.
75. Stover SL, Fine PR. *Spinal Cord Injury: The Facts and Figures.* Birmingham, AL: University of Alabama, 1986.
76. Survin VV. Fractures of the cervical spine in patients with ankylosing spondylitis. *Acta Orthop Scand* 1980; 51:79–84.
77. Traynelis VC, Marano GD, Dunker RO, Kaufman HH. Traumatic atlanto-occipital dislocation: case report. *J Neurosurg* 1986; 65:863–870.
78. VanGilder JC, Menezes AH, Dolan KD. *The Craniovertebral Junction and Its Abnormalities.* New York: Futura Publishing, 1987, pp 195–215.
79. Wallace MC, Tator CH. Failure of naloxone to improve spinal cord blood flow and cardiac output after spinal cord injury. *Neurosurgery* 1986; 18:428–432.
80. Wallace MC, Tator CH. Failure of blood transfusion or naloxone to improve clinical recovery after experimental spinal cord injury. *Neurosurgery* 1986; 19:489–494.
81. Wehner JM. Magnetic resonance imaging in spinal trauma. *Spine State Art Rev* 1993; 7:181–186.
82. Werne S. Studies in spontaneous atlas dislocation. *Acta Orthop Scand [Suppl]* 1957; 23:1–150.
83. White AA III, Panjabi M. *Clinical Biomechanics of the Spine,* 2d ed. Philadelphia: Lippincott, 1990.
84. Wilberger JE. Diagnosis and management of spinal cord trauma. *J Neurotrauma* 1991; 8(Suppl 1):21–30.
85. Wilson JA, Stillerman CB. Percutaneous posterior transarticular screw fixation for atlanto-axial instability. In preparation.
86. Wolf A, Levi L, Mirvis S, et al. Operative management of bilateral facet dislocation. *J Neurosurg* 1991; 75:883–890.
87. Wood-Jones F. The ideal lesion produced by judicial hanging. *Lancet* 1913; 1:53.
88. Xu J, Beckman JS, Hogan EL, Hsu GY. Xanthine oxidase in experimental spinal cord injury. *J Neurotrauma* 1991; 8:11–18.
89. Young JS, Chesire JE, Pierce JA, Vivian JM. Cervical ankylosis with acute spinal cord injury. *Paraplegia* 1977; 15:133–146.
90. Young W. Blood flow, metabolic and neurophysiologic mechanisms in spinal cord injury. In Becker D, Povlishock JT (eds): *Central Nervous System Trauma Status Report.* Bethesda, MD: NIH, NINCDS, 1985, pp 463–473.
91. Young W. Medical treatments of acute spinal cord injury. *J Neurol Neurosurg Psychiatry* 1992; 55:635–639.
92. Young W, Bracken MB. The Second National Acute Spinal Cord Injury Study. *J Neurotrauma* 1992; 9(Suppl 1):S397–S405.
93. Young W, Ransohoff J. Acute spinal cord injuries: experimental therapy, pathophysiological mechanisms, and recovery of function. In Sherk HH, Dunn EJ, Eismont FJ, Fielding JW, Long DM, Ono K, Penning L, Raynor R (eds): *The Cervical Spine,* 2d ed. Philadelphia: Lippincott, 1989, pp 464–495.
94. Young WF, Rosenwasser RH, Getch C, Jallo J. Diagnosis and management of occipital condyle fractures. *Neurosurgery* 1994; 34:257–261.

286 Cervical Traction

John C. Stevenson

Cervical traction creates a longitudinal pull along the cervical spine that reduces deformity, restores normal anatomic alignment, and provides stabilization. This form of traction is most commonly used for treating injuries from the atlantooccipital joint to T1. There are essentially three methods of applying cervical traction: the head halter, cranial tongs, and the halo head ring. The head halter is easy to apply and is useful for soft tissue injuries to reduce muscle spasm, but it has no place in the treatment of dislocations or fractures. Tongs are more invasive because they are embedded in the outer table of the cranium; however, more traction can be applied to the cervical spine to reduce a subluxation or fracture-dislocation. The disadvantages of tongs are that they do not provide rigid immobilization and they confine the patient to bed. The halo ring is often preferable to tongs because a rigid vest jacket can be aplied that allows the patient to become ambulatory following successful traction and reduction of a fracture-dislocation.

History

Spinal traction was described as a form of treatment by Hippocrates over 2000 years ago. Hippocrates suggested a method for treating posterior dislocations of the vertebrae; the patient was placed face down, and pressure was applied to the protruding vertebrae while traction was maintained simultaneously at both ends of the body.[3] According to Schneider,[13] Glisson in 1650 introduced the use of the sling for overcoming deformities of the spine due to rickets, and Sayre in 1877 used the Glisson sling in his overhead suspension technique for reducing spinal deformity. In 1929, Taylor described a method of physician-controlled manual head halter traction for the reduction of fracture-dislocation of the cervical spine.[14]

The introduction of tongs for skeletal traction to treat a cervical fracture-dislocation (reported in 1933) is attributed to Crutchfield.[1] His original patient had a mandibular fracture that prevented Crutchfield from using head halter traction; he removed the sharp points from Edmonton extension tongs, and placed each tip into a surgical perforation in the ipsilateral parietal eminence. Crutchfield later designed his own tongs, which are placed in the parietal region of the calvaria, above the widest diameter of the cranium. They have blunted tips that require bone holes for placement. Their unique position and small size allow the patient to be turned in bed with relative ease. The main disadvantages are the time required for tong placement and their vertex position, which makes them relatively easy to dislodge. Crutchfield tongs were widely used until the early 1970s, when the Gardner-Wells tongs were introduced.

In 1936, Hoen described a technique in which, on each side of the skull, a wire was passed between two cranial burr holes; traction was then applied to the cranium via the two wires.[4] Complications associated with this technique included loss of traction caused by the wire cutting through the overlying bone and scalp, laceration of the dura, and the development of meningitis.

In 1973, Gardner introduced the easily applied tongs that are the most commonly used type of tongs today. Each of the two tips of these tongs is placed below the greatest diameter of the skull; there is a spring-loaded pin that only allows 30 lb of compressive force. Gardner-Wells tongs do not require shaving or incising of the scalp or drilling into the skull.[8] The main advantage over previous tongs is the relative ease with which they can be applied. However, the most effective immobilizing device today is the halo system. This was first described by Nickel and coworkers in 1968.[12]

Head Halter Traction

Indications

The indications for head halter traction include cervical radiculopathy caused by a herniated disc or spondylosis and cervical muscle spasm. Head halter traction is also used for distraction purposes during anterior cervical discectomy and fusion. This type of simple cervical traction is most commonly used for the conservative management of neck pain both in the hospital and as a form of outpatient therapy. Inpatient head halter traction is usually applied with the patient lying supine in bed; the patient's body supplies the countertraction. The direction of the traction should be that which is most comfortable for the patient. Ordinarily a neutral or slightly flexed neck position is the most comfortable, whereas neck extension tends to accentuate the pain. The amount of traction is usually limited to a maximum of 3 to 7 lb, and even this may be too much for some patients. Cervical traction by head halter is generally applied intermittently to avoid prolonged pressure on the chin and occiput (the sites of pull by the halter system). Head halter traction is usually not applied for cervical spine stabilization. The patient may be allowed to ambulate between sessions of traction.

Application

Head halter systems vary in design, but generally they consist of two pads, one placed under the chin and the other under the occiput. (The Crile head halter is an exception: it has a pad beneath the occiput and a padded forehead piece so that the chin is free.) These pads are fitted so that relatively even pressure is applied on the chin and occiput. A metal spreader can be hooked to the side pieces so that compression of lateral soft tissues can be avoided when traction is applied.

The application of cervical traction using the head halter device in the supine position is performed with the patient in the semi-flexed position (flexed at the waist). The head of the bed is usually elevated to 30 or 40 degrees, with the patient's hips and knees flexed to about 45 degrees.[10] This position will provide a straight line of pull from the buttocks to the pulley. If the pull is completely straight, there will be equal pressure on the chin and occiput. The patient may complain of a tender chin or occiput, in which case the pressure may be changed by altering the direction of pull. This is usually accomplished by raising or lowering the head of the bed, provided that the pulley remains in the same position. Lowering the head of the bed will place more traction on the occiput in the case of a tender chin. Conversely, raising the head of the bed will create more pull on the chin. These positional points are important for patients who may require more prolonged head halter traction.

Cervical traction is often prescribed as an outpatient treatment for patients with cervical spondylosis and muscle spasm. Halter traction in this circumstance may be applied in the sitting position. The device for this maneuver consists of a pulley system that is attached to the door by a bracket. Many different devices have been manufactured and are on the market for home cervical traction. They usually consist of the head halter device plus the necessary attachments for the door. The amount of traction in these patients can be greater (up to 15 lb) because the period of traction is less than with patients who are in the supine position. This much weight is often necessary because the weight of the head is 7 to 10 lb. The initial starting weight is usually 5 lb, increasing by 5-lb increments to a maximum of 15 lb. Most physicians will prescribe a period of 10 to 15 min in traction twice a day. If the patient feels that too much pressure is being place on the chin or occiput, then the head should be tilted either forward to put more pull on the chin strap or backward to put more pull on the occiput strap. Most patients who require cervical traction do not need cervical stabilization; therefore, head halter traction is a very useful method for applying a noninvasive form of traction.

Risks

Skin problems caused by pressure are the main adverse effects of this type of traction. Inpatient head halter traction should not be used for more than 6 to 8 h during the day. Outpatient head halter traction has few complications if the patient is instructed carefully in its use. The most common complaint is that the traction increases pain. If this occurs, the patient should be instructed to discontinue the traction and contact the physician.

LaBan and colleagues reported 12 patients who had been treated with intermittent cervical traction for complaints of cervical radicular pain who subsequently developed lumbar radicular discomfort. They suggested that axial tension induced in the dural coverings of the spinal cord can be transmitted to lumbar nerve roots.[9]

Skeletal Traction

Indications

In situations in which the potential for instability of the cervical spine exists (e.g., cervical fractures, dislocations, or fracture-dislocations), a more efficient type of cervical traction will be required. Cervical skeletal traction must be applied in these circumstances. Skeletal traction is used commonly in the management of serious injuries to the cervical spine to reduce a dislocation or fracture-dislocation. This form of traction is also used to maintain the position of the cervical spine before and after operative fusion and occasionally for the treatment of cervical spondylosis with a severe nerve root compression syndrome. Herman and Sonntag have reported the successful use of external skeletal traction in reducing kyphosis which has developed following cervical laminectomy.[2] Cervical skeletal traction has also been used to reduce spinomedullary compression from cranial settling secondary to rheumatoid arthritis, infection, neoplastic processes, or trauma.[11]

Pull is exerted along the axis of the spine; the traction forces preserve alignment and thus the volume of the vertebral bony canal, protecting the spinal cord. The advantages of skeletal traction include the following: (1) such traction is very efficient and can be regulated closely by the amount of weight applied; (2) the traction can be much greater in amount than that tolerated with the halter; and (3) the traction can be applied continuously, 24 h a day, over protracted periods of time.

Traction should be commenced at 10 to 15 lb. Marked distraction may occur if weights of more than 15 lb are used initially in the presence of ligamentous injury. Analgesics and muscle relaxants are often required to help overcome the forces generated by the cervical musculature. Traction weights are usually increased every 30 to 60 min in 5- to 10-lb increments following radiographic evaluation.

Debate exists in the literature over the amount of weight required for reduction of a fracture-dislocation and the maximum weight that should be used. Crutchfield developed a rule of 5 lb per cervical level, starting with 10 lb for the head. A C1–C2 injury would therefore be allowed a maximum of 15 lb and a C5–C6 injury would be allowed up to 35 lb. It is generally accepted practice to add weight in 5-lb increments until reduction is achieved, or to a maximum of 70 lb. Once reduction is achieved, the spine is extended and the weight reduced to 5 or 10 lb. If a halo vest is being used, the jacket can be applied at this time to maintain the reduction.

Gardner-Wells Tongs

Gardner-Wells tongs are currently being used with good results and have largely replaced the Crutchfield tongs because they are easier to apply. Their ease of application and their self-contained tension devices are definite advantages. They are less likely to dislodge than Crutchfield tongs.

Application

Gardner-Wells tongs come with application instructions on a metal tag attached to the tongs. These tongs are readily applied using local anesthesia. Pin location is just below the equator of the skull and just above the ears (2 to 3 cm) in line with the external auditory meatus and the mastoid process. This site places the pins in the longitudinal axis of the spine, thus balancing the extension and flexion forces. The hair in this region is usually not shaved, and the area is prepared with an aerosol antiseptic solution. Infiltration of the skin with a local anesthetic (1% lidocaine without epinephrine) down to the galea is required. The physician must ensure that the pins are sharp and have been wiped with an antiseptic. The tong pins are then placed over the appropriate scalp position and held by an assistant. The pins are then tightened simultaneously by hand until the tension indicator on the spring-loaded pin protrudes 1 mm. The tongs should be tilted back and forth to set the points.

After the tongs are set, traction is applied by attaching a traction line through the eye at the top of the tongs. This line is taken through a pulley situated at the top of the bed and then attached to weights. The amount of traction applied is determined by the level of the injury. To prevent the patient from sliding up the bed, countertraction is applied by elevating the head of the bed (20 to 30 degrees) before adding the weights for traction. Elevation must be increased as the traction weight is increased. The final step in application is obtaining x-ray films of the skull and cervical spine to ascertain the position of the tongs and the alignment of the spine. Additional lateral films of the cervical spine will be required after each application of additional weight. The pins are normally retightened 24 h after the initial application. Further retightening is not required. Pin site care is essential to avoid local skin infection. One successful routine is the frequent (twice a day) application of hydrogen peroxide using soaked cotton swabs. The metal pins can be wiped with alcohol to keep them free of debris.

Risks

Great care must be taken when applying the tongs so that excessive manipulation of the cervical spine does not occur. Neurological assessment must be carried out after each increase in traction weight to avoid neurological worsening. Improper positioning can lead to the tongs pulling out. The risk of dislodgement is much less with the Gardner-Wells tongs than with the Crutchfield tongs. The mean pull-off strength for Gardner-Wells tongs is 137 lb when the indicator stem is protruding 1 mm (manufacturer's recommendations).[8] Infection may occur at the pin sites with prolonged traction or poor pin site care. Underlying osteomyelitis has been reported. Loosening of the tongs can occur, especially when low-grade infection is present or small tong movements are occurring. A more serious complication is penetration of the inner bony table of the skull if the pin sites are too low (with possible later meningitis or brain abscess). An occipital decubitus ulcer can occur where the occiput comes into contact with the bed. Awareness of this potential problem and careful nursing will help to avoid this complication.

Cranial Halo Traction

The introduction of the halo by Nickel and associates represented a real advancement in the management of cervical spine fractures and subluxations. The cranial halo provides a more efficient skeletal fixation to the skull. The direction of the traction force, both lateral and rotatory, can be controlled better than with the Gardner-Wells tongs. There is no movement between the skull and the pins with the halo ring. The main advantage of the halo traction system is that it allows early ambulation of the patient while traction is being maintained. After the fracture has been reduced and stabilized with the patient in the supine position, the halo may be fitted to an MRI-compatible metal frame attached to a plastic body jacket. Different styles of halo vests are now available from a number of manufacturers.

Indications

Halo traction has been used to stabilize fractures and reduce fracture-dislocations and dislocations of the upper and lower cervical spine following trauma, infection, inflammation, and tumor invasion. The halo vest provides good immobilization in the upper cervical spine for fractures of C1 and C2. Biomechanical studies performed on patients wearing halo vests have shown that as little as 4 percent or as much as 30 percent of cervical spine movement occurs as the patient moves from the supine to the sitting position.[5–7] Higher redislocation rates have been seen at the lower cervical levels in patients wearing the halo vest. Even with careful patient selection, at least 10 to 15 percent of patients fail halo vest therapy and require operative stabilization. Patients who do poorly in the halo vest include those with unstable pure cervical ligamentous injuries (especially injuries involving the posterior ligamentous complex securing the facet joints). Redislocation is common in this group.

Application

The halo ring comes in different sizes, which depend on the manufacturer. The initial step is to measure the circumference of the patient's skull at the equator. The tape is pulled tight to ensure that the measurement does not include the hair. The appropriate size of halo ring can then be selected with the help of the manufacturer's instructions. The pin sites on the scalp are prepared by shaving the hair and then sterilizing the region with a surgical antiseptic. The safe area for the anterior pin sites is over the lateral eyebrow areas, avoiding the nerves (supraorbital nerves) and frontal sinus medially, and the thin temporal bone and temporalis muscle laterally. The posterior pin sites are located just behind the superior half of each pinna over the temporal bone. Many manufacturers provide a device to slightly elevate the patient's head for halo placement. The halo ring is then placed over the patient's head.

Some rings have positioning pads to ensure a 1-cm separation between the halo ring and the head at the pin sites. Correct alignment of the halo ring is assured if the following criteria are met: (1) the ring lies 1 cm above the eyebrows, (2) there is a 1-cm separation between the scalp and the ring at each of the pin sites, (3) the ring does not touch the ears, (4) the posterior pin sites are below the equator of the skull, and (5) the arch of the ring does not touch the top of the head.

The skin and periosteum are now anesthetized at each pin site using 1% lidocaine without epinephrine (3 to 4 ml). Epinephrine together with pressure from the pins may cause a skin slough. With the patient's eyes closed and the halo ring position maintained, the skull pins are inserted into the selected holes. Opposing pins are tightened with the fingers until the skin is penetrated. Some manufacturers provide torque-limiting caps that are placed on the pins and will usually allow 8 lb of torque to be applied (at which time the cap will automatically break off). Opposing pins are tightened simultaneously, two turns apiece until the caps break. Alternatively, the four pins are each tightened separately until the torque force at each pin site is 8 in./lb. At this stage the patient is ready for either halo vest placement or traction hoop placement. Prior to traction, the four pin sites should be retorqued to 8 lb. The traction hoop is attached and bolted at the junction of the halo ring and the arch of the ring.

Pins should be retorqued at 24 and 48 h after the initial application (8 in./lb). Every 2 to 3 weeks or on patient complaint of pain at pin sites, the pins should be retorqued (2 to 3 in./lb). Pin care is similar to that for the Gardner-Wells tongs.

Risks

Several different types of complications have been described with the halo ring and vest. Infection of the pin sites has been reported in as many as 20 percent of patients. Loosening of pins usually occurs as a result of infection. A loose pin site is usually heralded by a complaint of pain. Pins that become loose or infected need to be replaced by a new pin at a different site. Perhaps the most serious complication of halo ring placement is penetration of the inner table of the skull by the pins. This could lead to bleeding or infection (meningitis or cerebral abscess). Improper placement of the anterior pins could lead to damage of the supraorbital nerves and hypalgesia over the frontal area of the scalp. Once the halo jacket is fitted, close inspection of the thorax and back is required to avoid the development of pressure sores. Loss of reduction of a fracture or subluxation is possible with the halo jacket in place.

Conclusions

Cervical traction has been readily available as a treatment for various disorders of the cervical spine for many years. The development of a wide variety of devices has made it easier for the physician to select the most appropriate therapy for the patient. The head halter is useful as a conservative measure for managing soft tissue injury and painful cervical radiculopathy. However, it has no place in the management of dislocations or fractures. In circumstances where long-term halo bracing is not required, tongs are easy to apply and will provide excellent traction. A halo ring will provide traction and stabilization which, when combined with a vest, translates into early ambulation for the patient.

References

1. Crutchfield WG. Skeletal traction for dislocation of the cervical spine: report of a case. *South Surgeon* 1933; 2:156–159.
2. Herman JM, Sonntag VKH. Cervical corpectomy and plate fixation for postlaminectomy kyphosis. *J Neurosurg* 1994; 80:963–970.
3. Hippocrates. On the articulations. In Adams F (ed): *The Genuine Works of Hippocrates. Translated from the Greek with a Preliminary Discourse and Annotations,* vol II. New York: William Wood, 1886, pp 75–156 (see pp 114–124).
4. Hoen TLI. A method of skeletal traction for treatment of fracture dislocation of cervical vertebrae. *Arch Neurol Psychiatry* 1936; 36:158–161.
5. Johnson RM, Hart DL, Simmons EF, et al. Cervical orthoses: a study comparing their effectiveness in restricting cervical motion in normal subjects. *J Bone Joint Surg [Am]* 1977; 59-A: 332–339.
6. Johnson RM, Owen JR, Hart DL, et al. Cervical orthoses: a guide to their selection and use. *Clin Orthop* 1981; 154:34–45.
7. Koch RA, Nickel VL. The halo vest: an evaluation of motion and forces across the neck. *Spine* 1978; 3:103–107.
8. Krag MH, Byrt W, Pope M. Pull-off strength of Gardner-Wells tongs from cadaveric crania. *Spine* 1989; 14:247–250.
9. LaBan MM, Macy JA, Meerschaert JR. Intermittent cervical traction: a progenitor of lumbar radicular pain. *Arch Phys Med Rehabil* 1992; 73:295–296.
10. Lewis RC Jr. *Handbook of Traction, Casting and Splitting Techniques.* Philadelphia: Lippincott, 1977, pp 20–26.
11. McAfee PC, Cassidy JR, Davis RF, et al. Fusion of the occiput to the upper cervical spine: a review of 37 cases. *Spine* 1991; 16:S490–S494.
12. Nickel VL, Perry J, Garrett A, et al. The halo: a spinal skeletal traction fixation device. *J Bone Joint Surg [Am]* 1968; 50-A:1400–1409.
13. Schneider RC. Cervical traction, with evaluation of methods, and treatment of complications. *Int Abstr Surg* 1957; 104:521–530.
14. Taylor AS. Fracture dislocation of the cervical spine. *Ann Surg* 1929; 90:321–341.

287 Halo Immobilization of Cervical Spine Injuries

William T. Hardaker, Jr.

The halo was first introduced as a traction apparatus in 1959 by Perry and Nickel in the management of severe cervical instability secondary to poliomyelitis.[12] Over the ensuing years, its advantages over previous traction systems have been well recognized. The early halo systems have undergone significant modifications to expand their role in the management of a variety of spinal disorders, including traumatic instability.[4,5,7–13,18] Cervical stability can be achieved by attaching the halo to a body jacket by means of metal uprights. The halo-jacket system offers distinct advantages over previous traction and stabilization systems.

Crutchfield, Vinke, Barton, and Gardner-Wells tongs are effective in applying traction in only one axis. This limits these devices primarily to longitudinal traction. Complex cervical fractures and fracture-dislocations often require multiplanar forces to achieve satisfactory realignment of the spine and decompression of the neural tube. Some of the tong systems require skin incisions as well as cranial drill holes to achieve fixation. Motion occurs at the tong-skull junction, thus increasing the possibility for infection. In addition, calipers alone do not provide rigid external fixation for the unstable spine, necessitating prolonged bed rest until stabilization is achieved. This form of treatment increases the likelihood of thrombophlebitis, muscle atrophy, and demineralization, as well as renal and pulmonary complications. Hospitalization and rehabilitation time can be lengthy.

The plaster of paris Minerva jacket has been the traditional method of obtaining external fixation of the unstable cervical spine. However, even the most expertly applied Minerva jacket allows movement of the cervical spine. The jacket is heavy, hot, and uncomfortable, and adjustment of head or neck position is impossible once the jacket is applied. Radiologic evaluation of the spine is difficult through the plaster of paris jacket. If surgery were to be performed, a small window could be cut in the cast. These windows provide only adequate exposure, at best, for the surgeon.

The halo–plastic jacket system is better than tongs as a traction device, and better than the Minerva jacket as a stabilization device. The halo pins are applied directly to the skull without the need for a skin incision or predrilling. No motion occurs at the pin penetration site, thus allowing the patient less discomfort and providing a decreased potential for infection. The halo-vest system can be applied quickly and, once in place, allows precise three-dimensional positioning of the cervical spine.

To allow rigid external fixation of the cervical spine, the halo can be mounted on a plastic vest. The halo-vest allows the patient to sit, stand, and walk, thus decreasing the time of recumbency and its potential complications. The time and cost of rehabilitation can be reduced significantly. Adjustable aluminum uprights allow radiologic examination of the spine, and surgical access is very satisfactory. In case of cardiac arrest, the anterior portion of the vest can be removed quickly to provide access for closed chest message.

Indications

Over the past 20 years, the indications for halo traction and halo-vest stabilization have expanded to include a variety of unstable cervical spinal lesions, including traumatic, congenital, neoplastic, and arthritic conditions.[4,5,7–13,16,18] The indications for the halo include:

A. Reduction of cervical
   1. Fractures
   2. Fracture-dislocations
   3. Subluxations
B. Realignment of thoracic kyphosis and scoliosis using
   1. Halo-femoral traction
   2. Halo-pelvic traction
C. External fixation of the unstable cervical spine in
   1. Severe muscle paralysis
   2. Fracture-dislocation
   3. Rheumatoid arthritis
   4. Primary or metastatic neoplastic disease
   5. Extensive laminectomy
   6. Following arthrodesis
   7. Osteomyelitis

Description

Stabilization of the cervical spine is achieved in the halo-jacket system by externally fixing the skull in reference to the chest. The system consists of three major components: the halo ring and pins, the plastic vest, and adjustable uprights that connect the halo ring to the jacket.

The halo ring is available in various sizes, configurations, and materials to allow for magnetic resonance imaging (MRI) compatibility. Conventional halo rings usually contain an occipital offset to allow clearance for high cervical fusions (Fig. 287-1). The halo is attached to the skull above the eyes and ears in four quadrants using pins that penetrate the skin and outer table (Fig. 287-2). The pins have sharp points and require no skin incision on introduction. The pins rapidly flare into broad shoulders, thus minimizing penetration and increasing the contact area (Fig. 287-3). The pins and the channels within the halo ring are threaded to firmly fix the halo-pin assembly to the skull. Additional pin channels are available in each of the four quadrants to allow for alternate pin placement if the pins should migrate or loosen or induce inflammation.

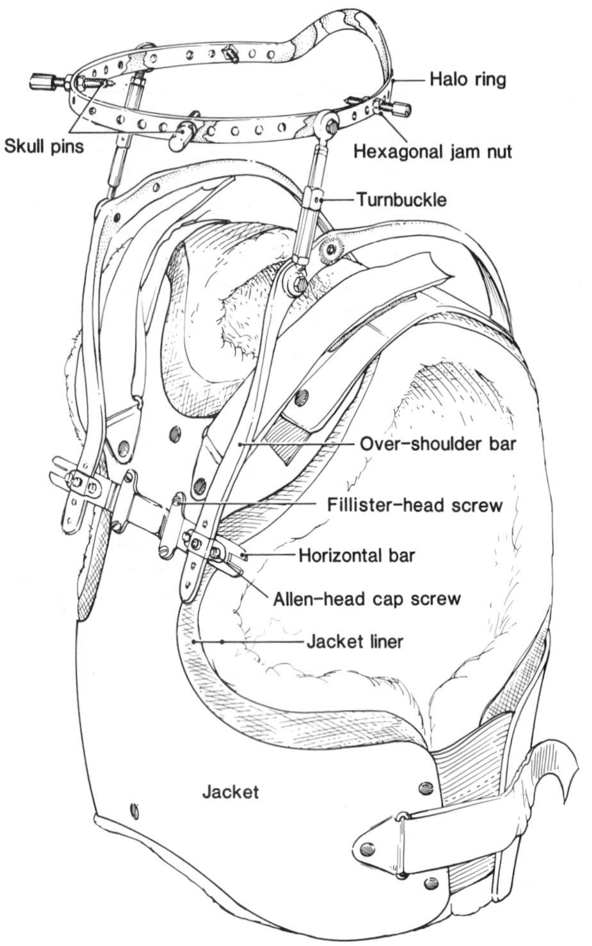

Figure 287-1 Components of the halo-jacket system.

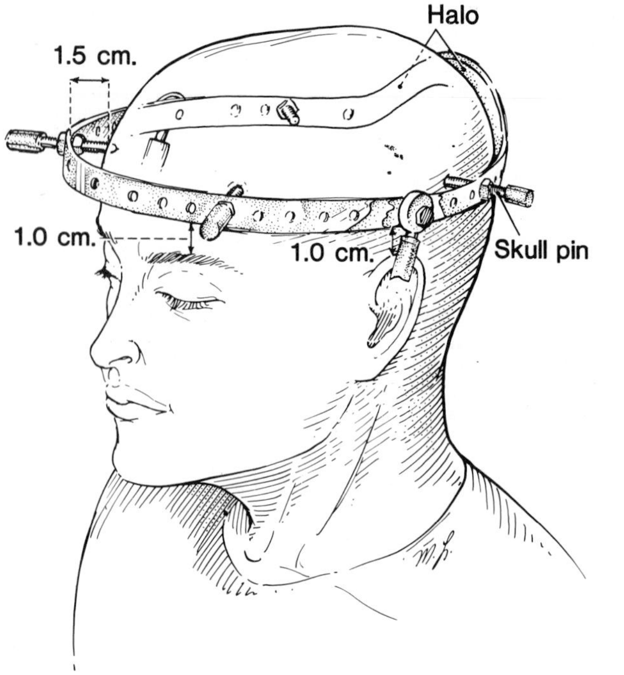

Figure 287-2 An assembled halo ring demonstrating correct pin placement.

The pins are firmly locked to the halo by hexagonal nuts on either side of the halo ring (Fig. 287-1).

The halo ring and the jacket are connected to one another by uprights on each side. The uprights are adjustable to provide variable traction, flexion, extension, or cervical translation (Fig. 287-1).

The polyethylene body jacket is available in multiple sizes to permit optimum fit for the dissipation of forces and thus minimize pressure on the soft tissues. To further reduce the pressure on the soft tissues, the jacket is lined with synthetic lamb's wool (Fig. 287-1). The jacket allows full use of the arms, and the anterior compartment can be rapidly removed to gain direct access to the chest in case of cardiac arrest. Once in place, the system firmly fixes the cervical spine, allowing less than 4 percent of normal motion in flexion-extension and lateral bending, and less than 1 percent of normal rotation.[6]

Magnetic resonance imaging has become an invaluable technique in the evaluation of patients with cervical and cerebral trauma. Conventional halo systems with components of ferromagnetic materials can produce artifacts which may distort or obscure the imaging of anatomic structures. Halo rings and jacket systems composed of graphite-carbon and other nonferrous materials are capable of producing distortion-free MR images.[1,2,15] These systems are recommended in those patients in whom MRI may be anticipated.

Materials and Methods

The materials necessary for application of the halo-jacket system include:

1. Halo ring, available in multiple sizes.
2. Skull pins, available in two sizes.
3. Hexagonal nuts, to fix and lock the skull pins to the halo ring.
4. Uprights, to connect the halo ring to the jacket. They are radiolucent and adjustable to provide varying amounts of traction, and are available in various lengths.
5. Shoulder bars, to allow the upright assembly to be fixed to the jacket. They are radiolucent and are available in multiple sizes to correspond with varying jacket sizes.
6. Jacket bars, to mount the shoulder bars to the jacket. Horizontal slots within the jacket bars allow for multiple adjustments.
7. Allen head screws, to hold the jacket bars to the shoulder bars.
8. Polyethylene jacket, lined with synthetic lamb's wool.
9. Tools necessary for halo-jacket application (Fig. 287-4): two torque screwdrivers, two open-ended wrenches, and one Allen wrench.

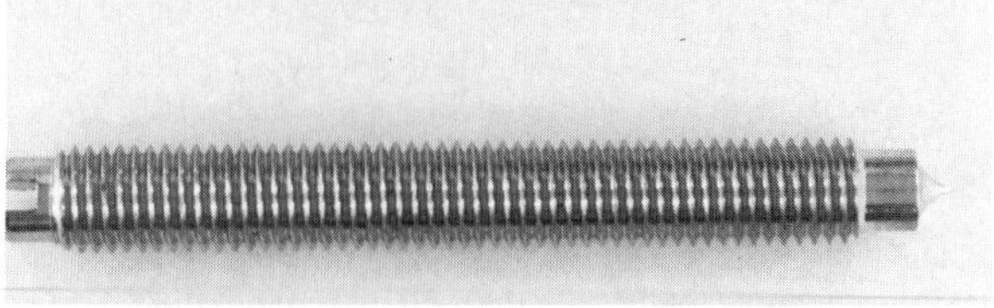

Figure 287-3 The halo pin with its sharp point and broad shoulder.

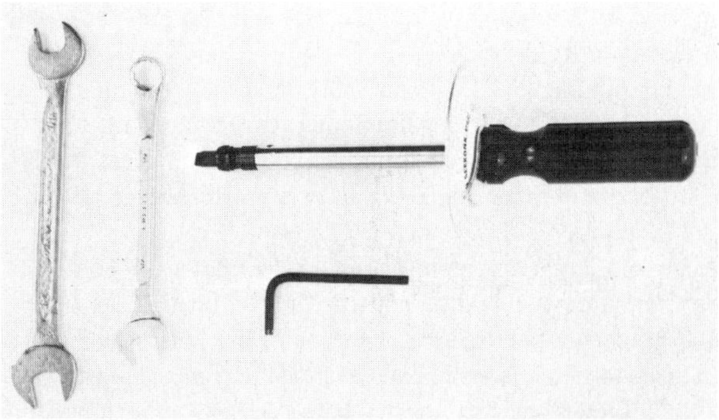

Figure 287-4 Tools required for the application of the halo-jacket system.

Application

Patient Premedication and Positioning

On most occasions, a mild sedative and an analgesic are helpful in relieving the anxiety and pain associated with halo application. In addition, the physician should thoroughly explain the procedure to the patient so that he or she will know what to expect.

The patient is positioned on a stretcher or bed with the head beyond the edge. The head is supported on a thin wooden board. Traditionally, the halo is held in position by the first assistant and the second assistant assists the surgeon with the materials. However, with a specially designed positioning fixture (Fig. 287-5), the entire procedure can be performed more effectively and with less assistance.[3] The positioning fixture not only supports the head but also securely holds the halo in the correct position during application. Such a device obviates the need for positioning pins and the wooden board and allows the surgeon to apply the halo with only one assistant.

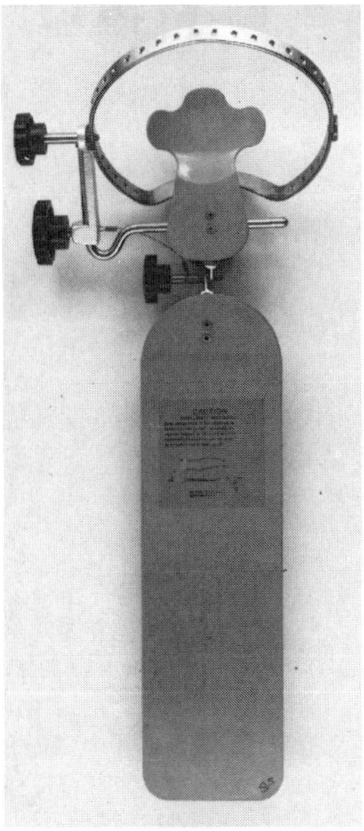

Figure 287-5 The halo positioning fixture.

Halo and Jacket Selection

Halo rings are generally available in different sizes. Approximately 1 to 1½ cm of halo-to-skull circumferential clearance should be present, with the halo positioned just below the maximum diameter of the skull. When correctly placed, the halo is 1 cm above the eyebrows anteriorly and 1 cm above the pinnae of the ears laterally (Fig. 287-2). The polyethylene jacket is available in several sizes, based on chest circumference. Intermediate chest sizes are accommodated by adjustment of the Velcro straps or plastic buckles connecting the anterior and posterior shells.

Skin Preparation and Local Anesthesia

The hair is clipped and shaved in a bandlike pattern just above and posterior to each ear in preparation for the posterior pins. Some surgeons have, in the past, placed the anterior pins within the hairline. This is not routinely recommended, however. These areas are characterized by relatively thinner and less supportive bone. In addition, the temporalis muscle must be penetrated, leading to patient discomfort while chewing and also a greater chance for skin and muscle necrosis and infection. Finally, if these sites are selected, there is a danger of directly injuring the superficial temporal artery.

The skin is thoroughly scrubbed, and the skin and underlying periosteum at the four pin sites are infiltrated with a 1% lidocaine solution. A trial positioning of the halo is recommended to ensure that the exact sites are well prepared and infiltrated.

Fixation of the Halo Ring

The autoclaved halo ring is held in correct position by the assistant, by positioning plates, or by the halo positioning fixture (Fig. 287-5). If the positioning fixture is employed, the positioning plates and screws and the second assistant will not be needed. With the halo properly centered on the head, the anterior pins are placed in channels overlying sites 1 cm above the lateral third of the eyebrows (Fig. 287-2). The posterior pins are diagonally opposite the anterior pins in channels approximately 1.5 cm posterior to the ears. Hexagonal lock nuts should be loosely placed on each pin between the ring and the skull prior to advancing the pin.

The skull pins are advanced by hand until just above the skin. The anterior and the diagonally opposite posterior pins are simultaneously tightened by hand. The surgeon and the assistant then simultaneously tighten each diametrically opposite pin using the torque screwdriver to a maximum torque of 6 kg. Alternate tightening of the halo pins is necessary to prevent displacement of the halo into an asymmetric position. The pins with their sharp points and broad shoulders are designed to penetrate the periosteum and impact into the outer table but not to penetrate into the inner surface. When the halo is in place, at or near the maximum diameter of the skull, the pins impact at 90 degrees to the skull surface, thus providing maximum fixation in order to prevent superior migration of the halo when traction is applied.

Once the pins have been placed, the inner hexagonal nuts are tightened using the open-ended wrench. An additional outer hexagonal nut is placed on each pin. These are tightened to further lock the halo firmly to the pins. Plastic caps are then placed on each pin to prevent impalement in sheets or bed clothing.

Attachment of Traction or Jacket

The cervical spine may be placed in longitudinal traction using a traction hoop attached to a rope, weight, and pulley system. Alternatively, the surgeon may proceed immediately to fixation of the cervical spine by connecting the halo superstructure to a polyethylene jacket. When this is the case, the posterior half of the jacket is first gently placed under the patient. With the head supported, the anterior portion of the jacket is placed and secured to the posterior shell using Velcro straps. The uprights are then adjusted to achieve the desired cervical translation and flexion or extension. The hexagonal open-ended screws are then placed to securely fix the uprights to both the halo and the shoulder bars. The hexagonal open-end wrenches and the Allen wrenches should then be securely taped to the anterior aspect of the jacket. This ensures their immediate availability should the anterior shell need to be removed in case of cardiac arrest.

X-Ray Views

Supine anteroposterior and lateral x-ray films of the cervical spine are then taken to ensure that the desired cervical alignment has been achieved.

After Care

The hexagonal lock nuts should be loosened and the pins tightened using the torque screwdriver the day after the initial application. Continued tightening after 72 h is not recommended. The pin sites should be cleansed with peroxide several times daily to remove any coagulum at the pin-skin interface. Following pin irrigation, povidone-iodine solution should be applied with a cotton-tipped applicator to each pin site. The pins are left undisturbed otherwise. No surgical dressings or paste antiseptic solutions should be applied at the pin sites.

A pin may need to be replaced because of loosening or significant inflammation or actual infection of the pin site. Patients often detect a loose pin because of a "clicking" sensation at that site. Loosening can occur secondary to pressure osteonecrosis or from infection itself. Regardless, the involved pins should not be advanced further. To replace a loose pin, the new sterile pin is first placed in an adjacent channel in the halo and tightened before removal of the loose pin.

Complications

Complications associated with the halo apparatus relate primarily to the skull pins. In most cases, these potential complications can be prevented by strict adherence to the correct techniques of halo application and meticulous daily care of the pin sites.

Superior migration of the halo can occur if the halo is not placed below the maximum diameter of the skull. When properly placed, the pins impact the skull at right angles in thick cortical bone. Traction forces are then directed into a thickening bony mass rather than into a thinning, obliquely sloped cortical margin.

Skin necrosis can occur if the halo ring is allowed to contact the scalp or the ears. A circumferential clearance of 1 cm will provide room for edema following pin placement and will prevent contact with the scalp by the ring.

Infection of the pin sites is probably the most common problem associated with the halo device. Some pin drainage and mild inflammation is to be expected, but active infection requires early recognition and proper management or premature removal of the halo may be required.

Many pin problems can be avoided by correct application techniques. Great care should be taken to prevent tension on the skin and surrounding soft tissues at the time of pin insertion. Tension often leads to tissue ischemia and eventual necrosis. Tissue necrosis then provides the medium for bacterial infection. Loose pins similarly promote inflammation of surrounding tissues and should be replaced promptly. Properly placed pins still require meticulous daily care to prevent later infection. Peroxide debridement is routinely necessary to remove coagulum around the pins and to prevent the tracks from sealing and trapping bacteria within.

Soft tissue infection that does not respond to local care and antibiotics requires removal of the involved pin after first inserting a sterile fifth pin in a nearby channel. Local wound care will usually clear the infection from the involved pin track. Deep infection, involving bone, requires soft tissue debridement as well as removal of the underlying bony sequestrum. Following adequate debridement, these wounds can likewise be expected to heal. Brain abscesses, involving pins that have penetrated the inner table, have been described.[17] This is indeed a more serious complication and requires early diagnosis and aggressive management.

Other complications encountered with the halo apparatus relate to its use as a traction device. The halo is a powerful traction instrument capable of causing serious neurological damage.[9,14] Excessive traction can lead to cranial nerve, spinal nerve root, and spinal cord injury. The sixth cranial nerve is quite sensitive to traction and is frequently affected early in the setting of improper traction.[7] Accordingly, lateral rectus function should be assessed periodically in all patients in halo traction.

References

1. Ballock RT, Hajek PC, Byrne TP, Garfin SR. The quality of magnetic resonance imaging, as affected by the composition of the halo orthosis: a brief note. *J Bone Joint Surg [Am]* 1989; 71-A:431–434.
2. Clayman DA, Murakami ME, Vines FS. Compatibility of cervical spine braces with MR imaging: a study of nine nonferrous devices. *Am J Neuradiol* 1990; 11:385–390.
3. Hardaker WT Jr, Reed WO, Vaughn DW, Clippinger FW. Duke halo-positioner, improved technique for halo application. *Orthop Rev* 1984; 13:37–43.
4. Houtkin S, Levine DB. The halo yoke: a simplified device for attachment of the halo to a body cast. *J Bone Joint Surg [Am]* 1972; 54-A:881–883.
5. James JIP. Fracture dislocation of cervical spine. *J R Coll Surg Edinb* 1960; 5:232–233.
6. Johnson RM, Hart DL, Simmons EF, et al. Cervical orthoses: a study comparing their effectiveness in restricting cervical motion in normal subjects. *J Bone Joint Surg [Am]* 1977; 59-A:332–339.
7. Keim HA. Spinal stabilization following trauma. *Clin Orthop* 1971; 81:53–55.
8. Kopits SE, Steingass MH. Experience with the "halo-cast" in small children. *Surg Clin North Am* 1970; 50:935–943.
9. Nickel VL, Perry J, Garrett A, Heppenstall M. The halo: a spinal skeletal traction fixation device. *J Bone Joint Surg [Am]* 1968; 50-A:1400–1409.

10. O'Brien JP, Yau ACMC, Smith TK, Hodgson AR. Halo pelvic traction. *J Bone Joint Surg [Br]* 1971; 53-B:217–229.
11. Perry J. The halo in spinal abnormalities: practical factors and avoidance of complications. *Orthop Clin North Am* 1972; 3:69–80.
12. Perry J, Nickel VL. Total cervical-spine fusion for neck paralysis. *J Bone Joint Surg [Am]* 1959; 41-A:37–60.
13. Prolo DJ, Runnels JB, Jameson RM. The injured cervical spine: immediate and long-term immobilization with the halo. *JAMA* 1973; 224:591–594.
14. Ransford AO, Manning CWSF. Complications of halo-pelvic distraction for scoliosis. *J Bone Joint Surg [Br]* 1975; 57-B:131–137.
15. Shellock FG, Slimp G. Halo vest for cervical spine fixation during MR imaging. *Am J Radiol* 1990; 154:631–632.
16. Thompson H. The ''halo'' traction apparatus: a method of external splinting of the cervical spine after injury. *J Bone Joint Surg [Br]* 1962; 44-B:655–661.
17. Victor DI, Bresnan MJ, Keller RB. Brain abscess complicating the use of halo traction. *J Bone Joint Surg [Am]* 1973; 55-A:635–639.
18. Zwerling MT, Riggins RS. Use of the halo apparatus in acute injuries of the cervical spine. *Surg Gynecol Obstet* 1974; 138:189–193.

288

Management of Upper Cervical Spinal Instability

Volker K. H. Sonntag
Mark N. Hadley

Instability of the Upper Cervical Spine

Instability of the vertebral column may be defined as excessive motion (hypermobility), beyond physiologic limits, of one vertebra upon another in at least one of three motion planes: the *x* axis (flexion-extension), the *y* axis (rotation), and the *z* axis (lateral bending).[4,26,34] The most common cause of instability of the superior cervical spine (the atlas, axis, and cervical vertebra 3) is traumatic injury. Degenerative, metabolic, neoplastic, and congenital disorders may also contribute to spinal instability; however, only traumatic spinal instability will be addressed in this chapter. Traumatic instability of the vertebral column may be due to vertebral fracture or fracture-dislocation, ligamentous injury, and/or facet complex disruption-dislocation.

The anatomy and biomechanics of the superior three cervical vertebrae are complex and are unique to the human vertebral column. These superior cervical spinal segments are predisposed to instability following traumatic injury due to the thin but broad, flat ring of the atlas, the large, stout second cervical vertebra with its vulnerable odontoid process, the biconvex articular interfaces between C1 and C2, and the marked degrees of physiologic rotation at C1-C2 and flexion at C2-C3.[4,15,18,31,32,34]

Several investigators have attempted to identify injury criteria that would help predict instability of the superior cervical spine after trauma (Table 288-1).[1,4,6,7,10,12,18,30,32] Atlanto-axial instability, typically reflecting excessive rotation (*y* axis) of C1 on C2, or *x* axis translation (flexion-extension) can be suggested on radiographs of the cervical spine.[4,12,30,32] An open mouth, anterior-posterior (AP) radiograph of the C1-C2 articulations and a lateral radiograph, which will allow determination of the predental space at C1-C2, may be quite helpful. Displacement of the articular surfaces of C1 over the superior articular surfaces of C2 on the AP C1-C2 radiograph provides data about the integrity of the ring of the atlas and the transverse atlantal ligament. A predental space greater than 3.0 mm in adults and 4.0 mm in children in any lateral view (flexion, neutral, or extension) indicates C1-C2 instability.[4,12] Precise fracture anatomy and ligamentous injury are best determined with computed tomography (CT) and magnetic resonance imaging (MRI), respectively.

Several useful radiographic criteria have been offered to assist in the determination of stability of the cervical spine following an axis fracture.[1,6,9,16,18,29] The most common C2 fracture, an odontoid type II fracture, is considered unstable if the dens fracture/dislocation is 6.0 mm or greater. Hangman's fractures of the axis may be unstable if a significant axial load is applied to the axis in addition to the marked extension forces compromising the superior cervical spine.[4,10,33] The combination of these forces may compromise the anterior longitudinal ligament and annulus at C2-C3, leading to C2-C3 subluxation and instability. C2-C3 *x* axis translation greater than 3.0 mm is considered unstable.

TABLE 288-1 Factors Suggestive of Upper Cervical Spinal Instability

Predental space >3.0 mm
Overlap of C1 on C2 on AP x-ray film >6.9 mm
Rupture of transverse ligament (MRI)
Dens type II fracture-dislocation >6.0 mm
C2-C3 *x* axis translation >3.0 mm
Flexion-extension range >11 degrees (C1-C3)
Loss of facet contact >50%
Loss of facet parallelism
Interspinous widening

Injuries of the Upper Cervical Spine

Incidence

There are an estimated 200,000 traumatic spinal column injuries per year in the United States. Most of these injuries involve the cervical spine and have a high incidence of paralysis and death. The neurological morbidity after cervical spine trauma is reportedly between 45 and 60 percent and the mortality rate has been cited as high as 17 percent.[2,27,31]

Males are much more likely to sustain vertebral column trauma than females, and individuals between 15 and 30 years old remain the most likely population to sustain injury. Accordingly, the most common cause of cervical spine injury in the United States is a motor vehicle accident, followed by falls, and diving and recreational-athletic accidents.[2,16,21,27,31]

Approximately 25 percent of all cervical spine fractures involve the superior cervical vertebrae, C1, C2, and C3 (Table 288-2).[6,16–18,31] The unique anatomy, orientation, articulations, and biomechanics of these vertebrae (the atlas, axis, and cervical vertebra 3) predispose them to several specific types of injury. The incidence of neurological injury is relatively low after C1-C2-C3 fracture-dislocation.[1,2,6,9,11,16–18,29,31] This incidence is probably artificially low and describes the incidence of neurological injury of patients with C1-C2 or C3 trauma who survive transport to the hospital. A neurological injury at the superior cervical spine level may compromise respiration, leading to rapid death at the scene of the accident before medical attention can be rendered. Investigators estimate that 25 to 40 percent of patients with high cervical spine fracture-dislocations after automobile accidents die at the scene from their neurological injuries.[15,20]

Evaluation

A high index of suspicion of spinal injury must be maintained until a cervical fracture or cervical instability can be ruled out by radiography. Immobilization of the head and neck with respect to the

TABLE 288-2 Distributions of 304 Acute C1, C2, and C3 Fractures from a Total of 1280 Acute Cervical Spine Fractures (1976–1988)

Fracture Type	Number of Patients	Percent of Total
Atlas fractures		
Isolated	32	2.5
Combination	25	2.0
	57	4.5
Axis fractures		
Odontoid I	0	0
Odontoid II	87	6.8
Odontoid III	49	3.8
Hangman's	46	3.6
Miscellaneous	47	3.7
	229	17.9
Third cervical vertebral fractures		
Isolated	10	0.8
Combination	8	0.6
	18	1.4

torso is essential during the initial resuscitation, triage, and evaluation of the patient. Nearly half of the patients who sustain cervical spine trauma will present without evidence of neurological injury.[2,27,31] The fact that 10 percent of patients in one review[28] developed new symptoms or signs of cervical spinal cord compromise during evaluation in the emergency department or during some later phase of their early hospital course (radiographic workup or initial treatment) underscores the importance of proper cervical spine immobilization and external stabilization until a careful and compulsive examination has provided a definitive diagnosis.

Sixty percent of patients with cervical spine fractures will have other organ system trauma, a fact which highlights the significance of basic life support and resuscitation to avoid the potentially deleterious effects of hypoxia and hypotension on spinal cord function.[27,31] Persistent immobilization and serial neurological examinations during the resuscitation period are important to document (and preserve) the patients' functional ability and to serve as a reference for further determinations of recovery (or loss) of neurological function.

The radiographic examination of the cervical spine includes anteroposterior and lateral roentgenograms from the skull base through the first thoracic vertebra. Lateral and swimmer's view x-ray films of the cervical spine will depict most of the traumatic injuries to the cervical spine. To assess the superior cervical spine adequately, particularly if the patient has skull base or superior cervical spine pain or if the initial lateral roentgenograms are suspicious for injury, the open-mouth view of the odontoid process and the C1-C2 articulations should be obtained. The pillar view of the odontoid process (oblique view) will reveal the integrity of the dens in patients who will not (or cannot) cooperate with the open-mouth view. Approximately 15 percent of patients with a high cervical fracture will have a second associated vertebral column fracture, an incidence that warrants a complete spinal column radiographic survey in such patients.[16,27,31]

Areas of suspected injury identified on the plain roentgenograms should be studied with thin section CT.[5,31] This is particularly true for C1 and C2 fractures because the precise fracture subtype is often difficult to discern on the plain x-ray films.[6,17–19] In addition, there is a high frequency of combination fractures involving *both* the atlas and the axis, which are difficult to identify without CT images.[6,17] The CT evaluation precedes dynamic flexion and extension roentgenograms (when indicated), myelography, angiography, and magnetic resonance studies (depending on individual patient circumstances).

The exception to proceeding to CT following the initial cervical spine films is the patient with a fracture-dislocation. Every attempt should be made to reduce the fracture-subluxation to restore the anatomic alignment of the spinal column early in the patient's hospital course.[2,31] Traction with a halo ring or with Gardner-Wells tongs (GWT) is usually effective for reduction but requires monitoring the patient closely. We treat patients with cervical spine injuries that require traction reduction in the intensive care unit (ICU) on a Stokes bed. The ICU setting also allows for prompt treatment of respiratory insufficiency (common with upper cervical spine injuries) and spinal shock when present, and facilitates treatment of other associated injuries. Immobilization of the head and neck with respect to the torso can be a problem despite traction when treating a fracture-dislocation of the upper cervical spine where only a small amount of weight is needed for reduction. This is particularly true for the combative or uncooperative patient.

Difficult patients with upper cervical spinal instability may be further immobilized in a rigid collar with sandbags placed at both sides of the patient's head and neck (in addition to traction). These are the patients we attempt to immobilize with rigid external stabilization (halo vest) early in the hospital course to prevent subluxation and potential neurological injury (even if they are surgical candidates waiting for surgery). The early application of an MRI-compatible halo ring allows both the early application of traction forces and the early application of the halo immobilization device, without having to remove the traction device (GWT) when halo application is necessary.

Patient Distribution

Atlas Fractures

The atlas, uniquely positioned between the skull and the remainder of the vertebral column, is predisposed to a variety of acute traumatic injuries. The incidence of acute C1 fractures ranges between 3 and 13 percent in most cervical spine series.[2,17,24,30–32] We have experience with 57 acute atlas fractures. This represents 4.5 percent of the patients treated for acute cervical vertebral column injuries in a 12-year period.

Thirty-two patients had isolated C1 fractures, and 25 sustained combination C1-C2 fractures. That 44 percent of patients with a C1 fracture also had a fracture of the axis is important with respect to treatment and will be discussed under combination C1-C2 fractures. Five patients (9 percent) sustained an additional noncontiguous cervical spine fracture, and 12 patients (21 percent) had associated head injuries. Motor vehicle accidents were the most common cause of injury (68 percent of fractures) followed by falls (13 percent) and motorcycle accidents (7 percent). Twelve percent of the patients sustained an atlas fractures from miscellaneous causes including diving, hang gliding, skateboarding, and other sports-related injuries. Not one of the 32 patients with an isolated C1 fracture sustained neurological injury (0 percent), although several complained of dysesthesias at the base of the skull and neck at the time of presentation.

The majority of isolated C1 fractures [18 of 32 (56 percent)] were acute bilateral or multiple fractures of the ring of the atlas

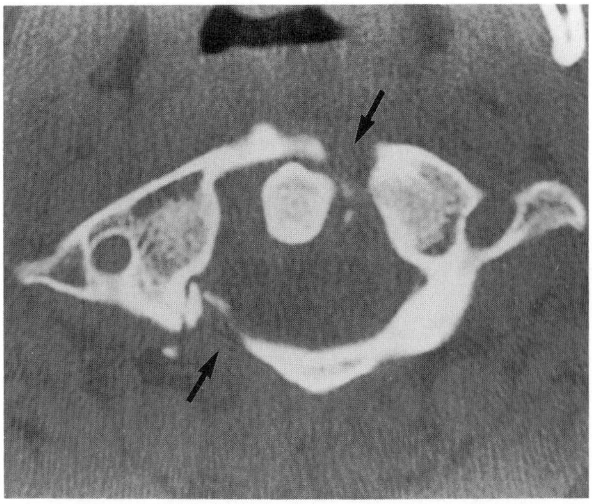

Figure 288-1 CT scan depicting multiple ring fractures of the atlas. (From Sonntag and Hadley,[31] with permission.)

(Fig. 288-1). There were 10 unilateral ring fractures (31 percent) and 4 isolated lateral mass fractures (13 percent). Twelve of the isolated atlas fractures were without C1-C2 dislocation as determined by anteroposterior (AP), open-mouth view roentgenograms. Fifteen of the fractures had less than 6.9 mm of displacement of C1 and C2 (determined by measuring and summing the spread of the lateral masses on the AP x-ray film), and five fractures were displaced by greater than 6.9 mm. These radiographic features are important when determining the appropriate treatment of isolated atlas fractures.[17,31,32] We do not solely rely on AP or lateral x-ray films to determine the extent of C1 fracture of ligamentous injury. Thin-section CT may reveal an atlas lateral mass fracture implying disruption of the inferior site of the transverse ligament. MRI is an excellent diagnostic tool for the assessment of the integrity of the transverse ligament and potential C1-C2 instability.[7]

Axis Fractures

The unique anatomy and articulations of the second cervical vertebra predispose it to a wide variety of fractures and fracture-dislocations.[14,31] We treated 229 acute axis fractures between 1976 and 1988. Axis fractures represented 18 percent of the total acute cervical spine injuries during this period.

Odontoid fractures were the most common fracture types encountered (n = 136, 60 percent of total). There were no odontoid type I fractures in this series. Eighty-seven patients had odontoid type II fractures; 49 had odontoid type III fractures. Hangman's fractures (n = 46) and miscellaneous axis fractures (nonodontoid-nonhangman's fractures, n = 47) each represented 20 percent of the axis fracture population. Males outnumbered females 2:1, and the median age by sex was 37 years for males (range, 10 to 94 years) and 41 years for females (range, 2 months to 90 years). The most common causes of injury were motor vehicle accidents (65 percent), followed by falls (15 percent), diving injuries (6 percent), and miscellaneous accidents (14 percent).

Thirteen patients with axis fractures sustained neurological injury from their C2 level injury (5.7 percent). Three patients had odontoid type II fractures, 4 had type III fractures, 2 had hangman's fractures, and 4 patients had miscellaneous axis fractures. Fifteen patients died in this series (6.5 percent), most as a result of severe cardiopulmonary compromise or severe head injury.

Atlas-Axis Combination Fractures

Twenty-five patients presented with acute atlas-axis combination fractures. These patients represented 2 percent of the total population of acute cervical spine injured patients treated over a period of 12 years. Sixteen patients were male, with a median age of 40 years (range, 14 to 82 years), and 9 patients were female, with a median age of 51 years (range, 21 to 86 years). Combination C1-C2 injuries accounted for 44 percent of all acute atlas fractures (n = 57) during this time period and 11 percent of all axis fractures (n = 229). The causes of traumatic combination C1-C2 injury are similar to those described for isolated C1 or C2 fractures.

The classification of combination atlas-axis injuries is based on the type of *axis* fracture present.[6] The most common type of C1-C2 combination fractures in our review was C1–odontoid type II injury (40 percent), followed by C1–miscellaneous C2 fractures (nonodontoid, nonhangman's fractures), C1–odontoid type III fractures, and C1–hangman's fractures. C1–odontoid type II fractures were present twice as frequently as C1–odontoid type III fractures.

Each of the three patients with C1–hangman's fracture combinations had associated multiple fractures of the posterior arch of the *atlas*. The C1 fractures in the remaining atlas-axis fracture combinations were divided among multiple ring fractures, unilateral C1 ring fractures, or lateral mass fractures.

Three patients (12 percent) with acute combination C1-C2 fractures had neurological deficits on admission. Two of these patients had central cord findings due to C1-C2 body fractures (combination C1–miscellaneous C2 fractures). The third patient had a complete neurological injury at the C2 level from a combination C1–odontoid type II fracture. The latter patient sustained severe thoracic and abdominal injuries and died from cardiopulmonary complications on his fourth postinjury day. He represents the only death in the combination C1-C2 fracture population.

Third Cervical Vertebral Fractures

Isolated fractures of the third cervical vertebra are rare.[2,31] We identified 10 isolated C3 fractures among 1280 acute cervical fractures (0.8 percent). These were primarily chip fractures of the body or isolated lamina or spinous process fractures. We treated another 8 patients who sustained C3 fractures in addition to axis fractures. The third cervical vertebra appears to be provided partial protection from injury due to its unique position between the more vulnerable axis and that portion of the spine where the greatest flexion occurs (i.e., the C5 level).

Treatment

Atlas Fractures

The treatment of most atlas fractures and lesser forms of C1-C2 dislocation is almost exclusively nonsurgical and depends on the type of atlas fracture and the presence of associated axis or other cervical vertebral body injuries.[17,31] Thin-section CT is the radiographic diagnostic study of choice to accurately define the extent of a C1 (and/or C2) fracture injury.[5,17,23,31] MRI is the study of choice to identify the integrity of the transverse atlantal ligament.[7]

For isolated C1 fractures, uncomplicated by an axis fracture or other associated cervical spine fracture (for which more rigid external immobilization or even surgery may be required), Spence et al. have provided criteria which help determine appropriate therapy.[32] They documented that if the sum of the spread of the lateral masses of C1 over C2 as determined on the AP C1-C2 x-ray film exceeded 6.9 mm, then the likelihood of transverse ligament disruption was great. In cadaver studies, this degree of dislocation was associated with transverse ligament disruption and C1-C2 instability. The authors concluded that injuries of this magnitude require a more aggressive approach to treatment and advocated surgical stabilization of C1 and C2.[32] Dickman et al. have demonstrated that MRI can accurately identify transverse ligament injuries following C1 fracture or C1-C2 dislocation.[7] Disruption of the transverse ligament implies C1-C2 instability and usually requires surgical stabilization and fusion of the atlas and axis.

Experience has demonstrated that isolated acute C1 fractures rarely require early surgical intervention (in the absence of bone compromising the spinal cord or disruption of the transverse ligament). Isolated atlas fractures without rupture of the transverse ligament can be treated effectively with less rigid cervical support (typically a Philadelphia collar) for a duration of 8 to 12 weeks. We advocate more rigid external immobilization and/or surgical stabilization for atlas fractures with a 6.9-mm (or greater) dislocation of the lateral masses and those with transverse ligament disruption.[17,31] In our experience, rigid external immobilization is most effectively accomplished with the halo-vest immobilization device for a duration of 10 to 14 weeks. Periodic clinical and radiologic follow-up of these patients is essential to document patient compliance and adequate alignment and fusion. Dynamic flexion and extension films are required to confirm bony union without instability. Patients with marked C1-C2 instability with ligamentous disruption and those who fail rigid external immobilization are offered operative reduction, internal fixation, and fusion, typically a C1-C2 posterior wiring and fusion procedure (Figs. 288-2 and 288-3). We now favor bilateral C1-C2 transarticular screw fixation/fusion in addition to C1-C2 interspinous fixation and fusion (Fig. 288-4).[13,25]

The treatment administered for the 32 isolated C1 fractures in our series is depicted in Table 288-3. The form of external immobilization employed depended on the degree of C1-C2 lateral mass dislocation (Fig. 288-5). None of these 32 patients required surgical stabilization or fusion. The median length of treatment for the group was 12 weeks, with a range of 8 to 16 weeks. Three of 32 patients were lost to follow-up. The remaining 29 patients had no evidence of nonunion or instability on follow-up roentgenograms (including dynamic studies). No patients developed a late neurological injury. Three patients complained of intermittent neck pain (median follow-up, 40 months).

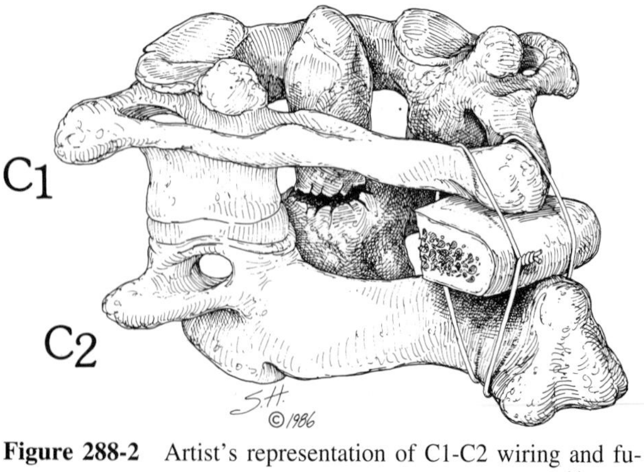

Figure 288-2 Artist's representation of C1-C2 wiring and fusion with an iliac crest bone plug. (From Hadley et al.,[14] with permission.)

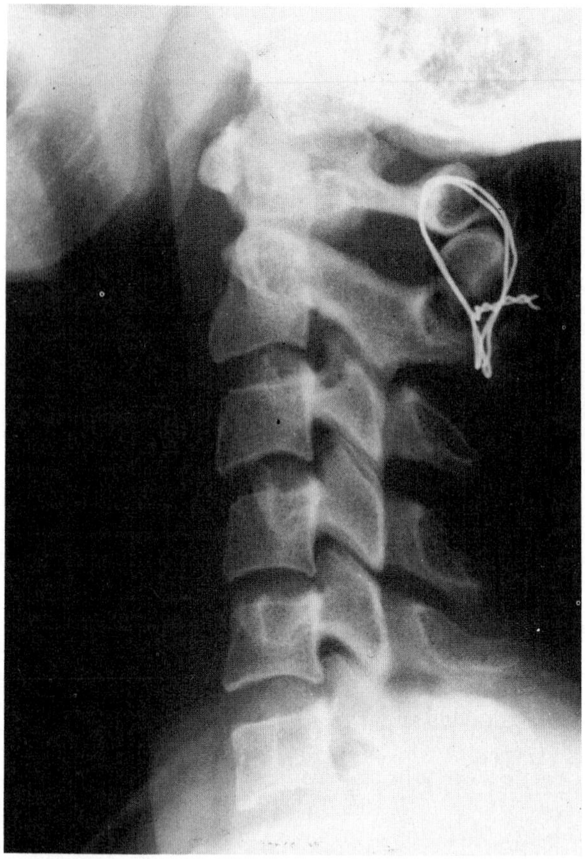

Figure 288-3 Postoperative lateral x-ray film reveals realignment of C1, the odontoid, and C2 with a C1-C2 wiring and fusion procedure. Note the bone plug secured between C1 and C2 with wires.

Axis Fractures

Several types of axis fractures are best treated by nonoperative means.[18,19,31] These include hangman's fractures, odontoid type III fractures, and miscellaneous axis fractures (Fig. 288-6).

Hangman's fractures (Fig. 288-7) are fractures through the pars interarticularis (bilateral) of the axis.[3,19,29,31] Of 46 patients with hangman's fractures we have treated, 4 patients died early in their hospital course due to severe head injury or multiple trauma. The remaining 44 patients were treated with rigid external immobilization (39, halo vest; 5, SOMI brace) for periods of 10 to 16 weeks (median duration, 11 weeks).

TABLE 288-3 Treatment of 32 Patients with Isolated Atlas Fractures

Fracture Displacement	Number of Patients	Method of Treatment*
Nondisplaced	1	Soft collar
	10	Rigid collar
	1	SOMI brace
	12	
Displaced <6.9 mm	8	Rigid collar
	3	SOMI brace
	4	Halo vest
	15	
Displaced ≥6.9 mm	5	Halo vest

*The duration of treatment ranged from 8 to 16 weeks (median, 12 weeks).

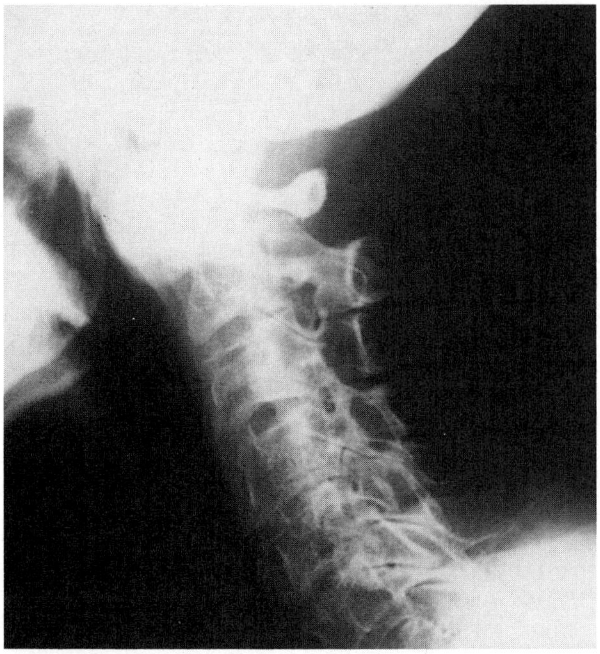

(*A*)

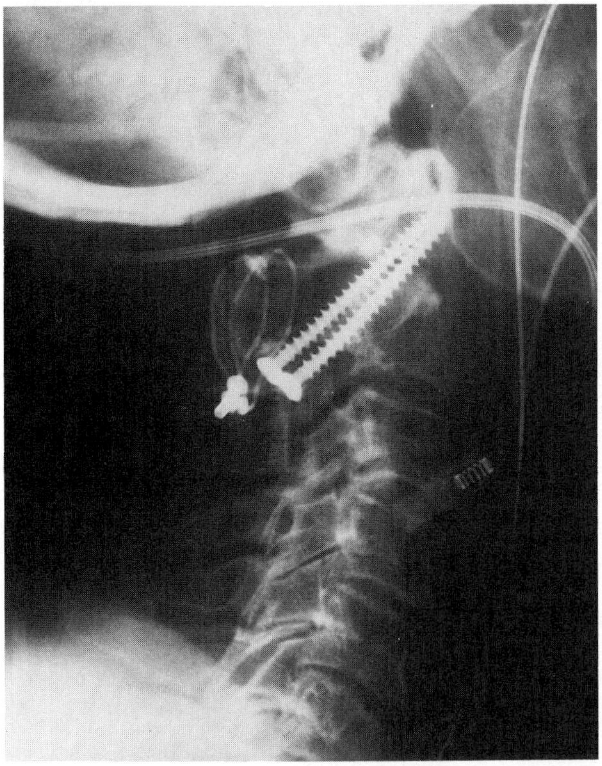

(*B*)

Figure 288-4 *A*. Lateral cervical spine radiograph documenting C1-C2 instability. *B*. Lateral postoperative x-ray film revealing bilateral C1-C2 transarticular screw fixation supplemented with a C1-C2 dorsal wiring and fusion procedure.

Two patients (4.5 percent) failed nonoperative therapy and required surgical stabilization. Both were initially treated with a halo vest and both had marked C2-C3 instability. One patient underwent a posterior wiring and fusion procedure of C1-C2-C3. The second patient had a C1 ring fracture, a C2 hangman's fracture,

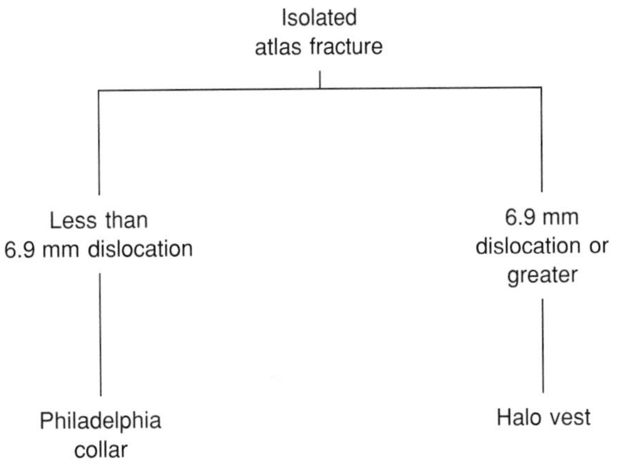

Figure 288-5 Treatment algorithm for patients with isolated atlas fractures.

and a C3 posterior arch fracture in addition to 4-mm C2-C3 subluxation (Fig. 288-8). He was treated with an anterior C2-C3 discectomy and anterior autologous iliac crestbone graft fusion, secured with C2-C3 Caspar plating (Fig. 288-9). No other patient treated nonoperatively for a hangman's fracture had post-treatment instability. The two surgical patients had no evidence of nonunion or instability at last follow-up.

Odontoid type III fractures (fractures through the base of the odontoid process that extend into the body of the axis), occur half as frequently as odontoid type II fractures.[16,18,19,31] Type III fractures rarely lead to nonunion or long-term instability if adequately immobilized with an external brace. Forty-eight of the 49 patients we treated with odontoid type III fractures responded to nonoperative immobilization (47, halo vest; 2, SOMI brace) for a period of 10 to 20 weeks (median, 11 weeks). One patient with a marked C2-C3 subluxation required operative reduction and fusion. All patients with type III fractures were stable with good bony union at last evaluation.

Miscellaneous fractures of the axis are all axis fracture subtypes which are not encompassed by hangman's and odontoid fractures.[15,19,31] These include C2 body, lateral mass, lamina, and spinous process fractures. The treatment of patients with miscellaneous fractures must be individualized and depends on the severity of the fracture and the presence of associated C2-C3 subluxation.[15,31] Clearly, an isolated spinous process or lamina fracture will not require the same type of immobilization or duration of therapy required to treat a C2 body or lateral mass fracture with a 3-mm C2-C3 subluxation.

Of 47 patients with miscellaneous axis fractures in our series, 3 died. The remaining 44 patients were treated in a halo vest (n = 36), a SOMI brace (n = 4), a rigid Philadelphia collar (n = 3), or with early surgery (n = 1). The patient who underwent early surgery was treated with a posterior wiring and fusion of C1-C3 for a C2 lateral mass fracture and 5-mm subluxation of C2 on C3. Only one patient treated nonoperatively (15 weeks, halo vest) had instability with nonunion. She had a C2 body fracture with a 4-mm C2-C3 subluxation. She was ultimately treated with a C2-C3 wiring and fusion procedure. No other patient had evidence of nonunion or instability at last follow-up.

Of 135 patients with hangman's, odontoid type III, or miscellaneous fractures of the axis who were treated nonoperatively on whom follow-up was obtained, 4 had persistent instability with nonunion after treatment (3 percent nonunion rate). Common to all 4 patients (2 hangman's, 1 type III, and 1 miscellaneous fracture)

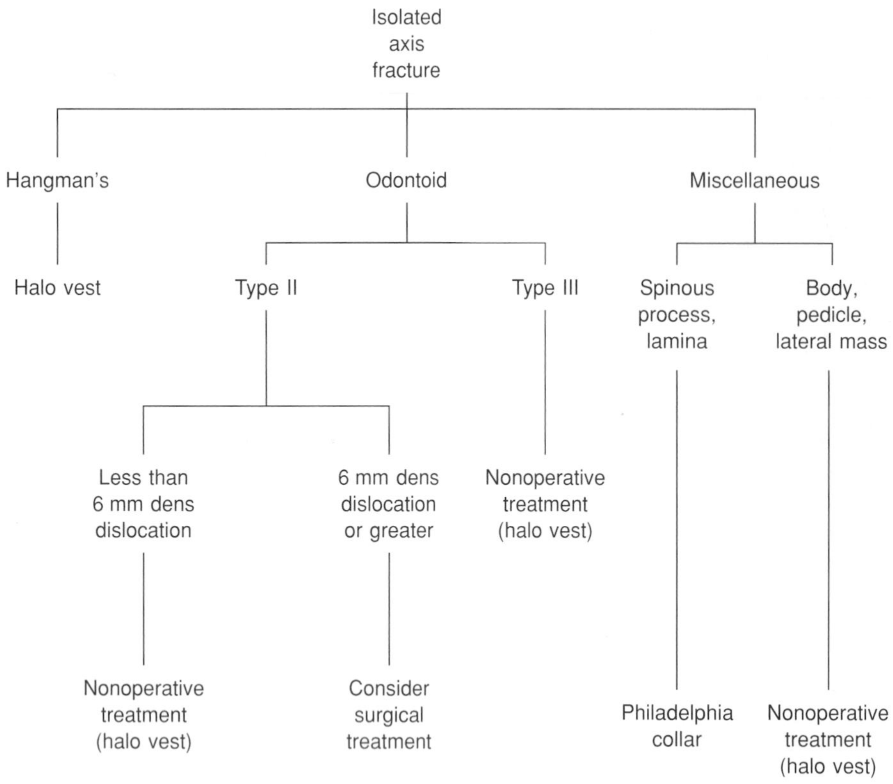

Figure 288-6 Treatment algorithm for patients with axis fractures.

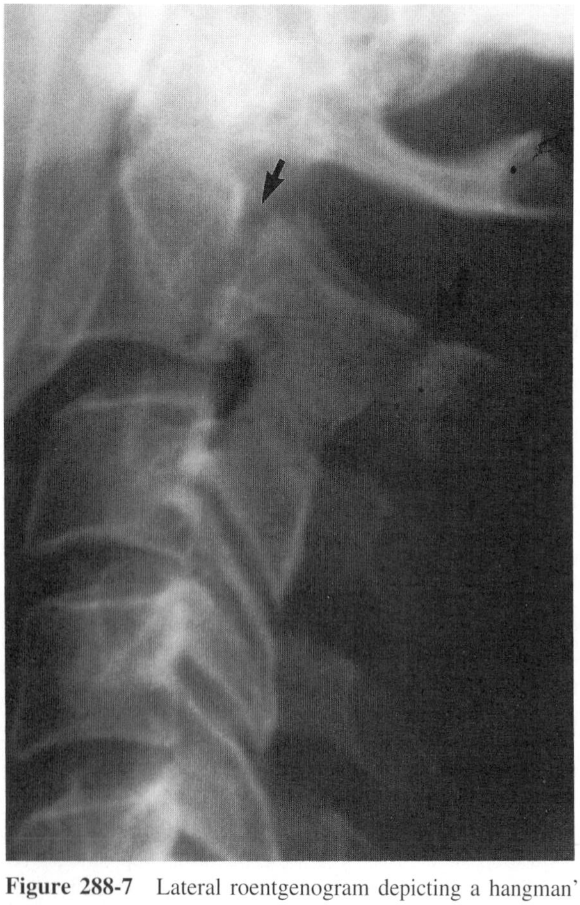

Figure 288-7 Lateral roentgenogram depicting a hangman's fracture (*small arrow*) with an additional C2 spinous process fracture (*large arrow*).

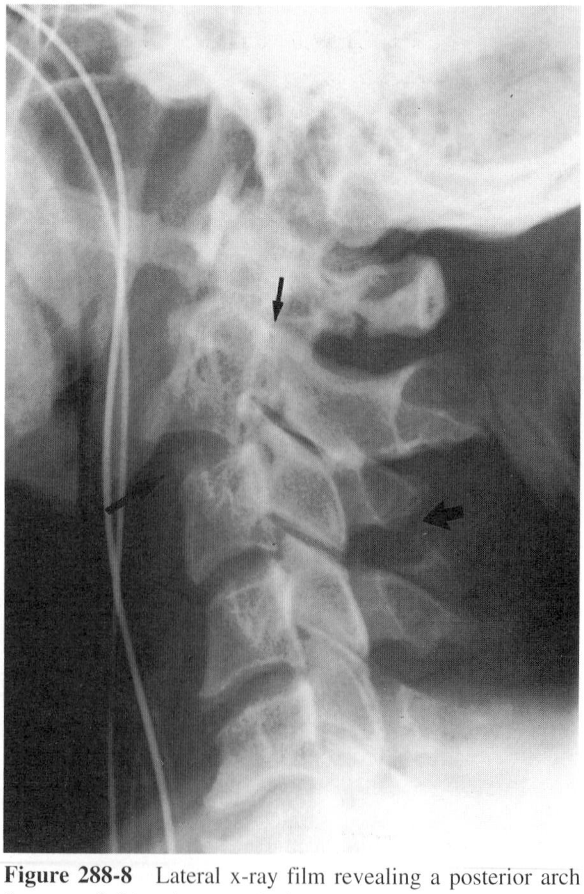

Figure 288-8 Lateral x-ray film revealing a posterior arch fracture of C1, a hangman's fracture of C2 (*small arrow*), and a spinous process fracture of C3 (*broad arrow*). Note the marked C2-C3 subluxation (*long arrow*).

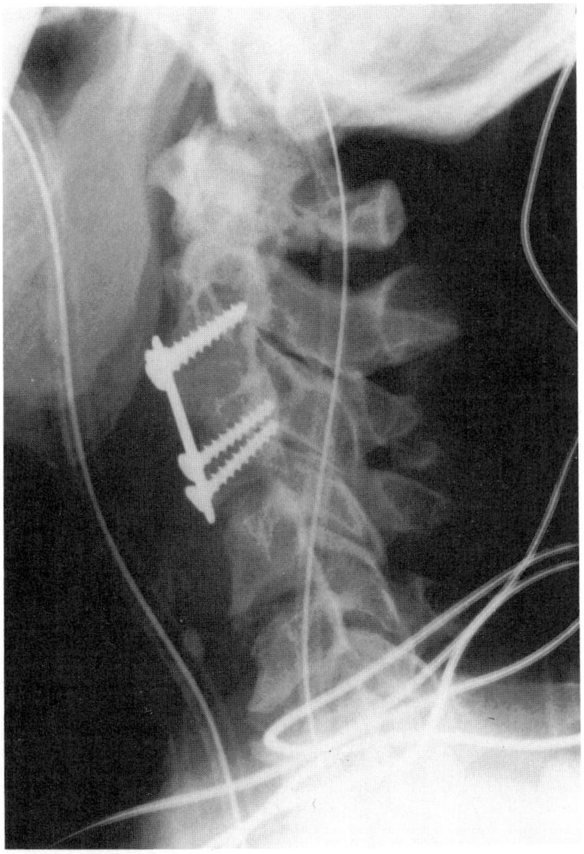

Figure 288-9 Postoperative roentgenogram of the same patient (Fig. 288-8) after C2-C3 discectomy, fusion, and anterior plating.

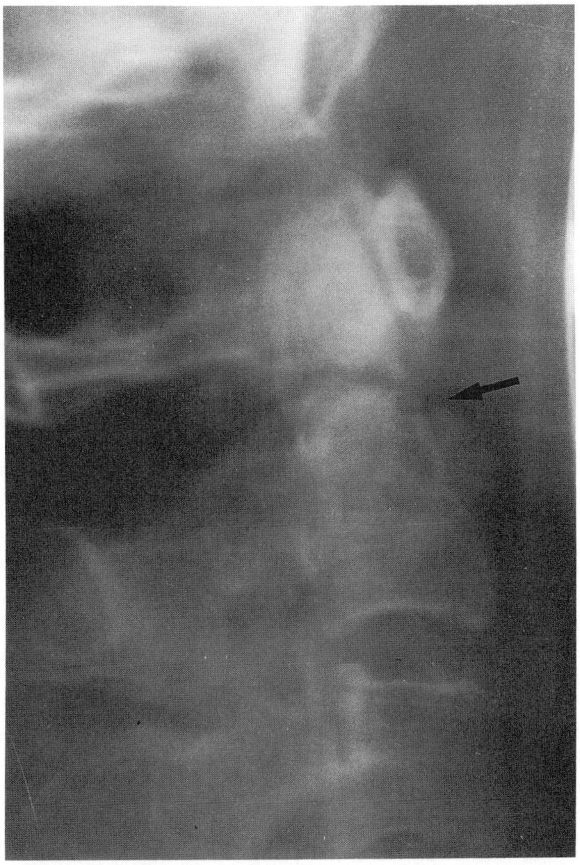

Figure 288-10 Lateral roentgenogram reveals a nondisplaced type II odontoid fracture (*arrow*).

was pronounced subluxation and instability at C2-C3. The presence of instability and subluxation (greater than 3.0 mm) at the C2-C3 level is an indication for consideration of early surgical therapy in patients with acute axis fractures.

The treatment of the most common type of axis fracture, type II odontoid fractures (Fig. 288-10), remains controversial.[1,9,11,16,18,19,31] Investigators have attempted to identify specific patient (age, neurological examination) or fracture (direction, degree of dens dislocation) characteristics that might help guide appropriate therapy.[1,9,11,16,19,31] The degree of dens dislocation has been cited as the single most important factor that determines the success or failure of nonoperative treatment of type II odontoid fractures.[16,18,19,31] Several authors have suggested that patient age is an important consideration when deciding between operative and nonoperative therapy.[1,9,11]

We reviewed our experience with 87 patients who had acute traumatic type II fractures. Three patients died early in their hospital course from associated injuries; nine patients were treated with early surgery. These nine patients had type II fractures with dens dislocation of 6 mm or greater ($n = 6$) or were patients with type IIA fractures ($n = 3$).[14] They were treated with posterior wiring and fusion procedures.

Seventy-five patients with type II fractures were initially treated with nonoperative external immobilization (65, halo vest; 8, SOMI brace; 2, Philadelphia collar) for durations of 10 to 23 weeks (median, 12 weeks). Excluding early surgery cases, deaths, and patients lost to follow-up, 68 patients were available for long-term evaluation and review (median follow-up, 4 years, 9 months).

The nonunion rate for type II fractures initially treated with nonoperative immobilization-stabilization was 28 percent. This rate corresponds with that of other reported series.[1,9,11,16,18,19] Of these 19 patients, 5 developed long-term union and stability after a *further* period of immobilization in a halo vest (the initial treatment being: 2, Philadelphia collar; 2, halo vest; 1, SOMI brace). The remaining 14 patients required surgical stabilization and fusion.

Individuals with odontoid type II fractures with the dens dislocated less than 6 mm had only a 10 percent nonunion rate compared with a 78 percent nonunion rate for patients with a dens location of 6 mm or greater, irrespective of the patient's neurological condition or the direction of the dens dislocation ($P < 0.001$, $\chi^2 = 30.20$) (Fig. 288-11).

The age of the patient with a type II fracture has been cited as a factor used to determine optimal therapy. Patients in our series aged 60 years or older had three times the nonunion rate (39 percent) as did patients under the age of 60 (15 percent) ($P < 0.05$, $\chi^2 = 6.06$). These figures are altered somewhat by our previous bias to perform early surgical therapy on younger patients with a 6-mm or greater dens dislocation ($n = 9$) and a relative reluctance to proceed with early surgical treatment in the older-age group patients. Although patients 60 years of age and older had a slightly higher incidence of nonunion if the dens was dislocated 6 mm or greater than did patients under 60 years of age (85 percent vs. 75 percent; $P < 0.6$, $\chi^2 = 0.19$) and a higher incidence of nonunion for dens dislocation less than 6 mm (13 percent vs. 7 percent), these differences were not statistically significant. If one examines

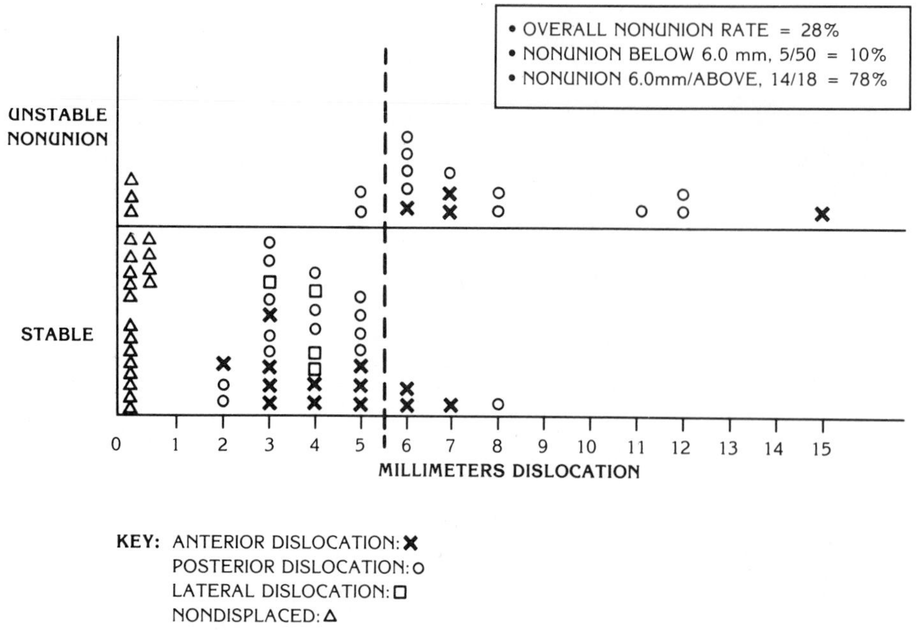

Figure 288-11 Graphic representation of the relationship between nonunion and the degree of dens dislocation for type II odontoid fractures. (From Hadley et al.,[18] with permission.)

the nonunion rate for a dens dislocation of 6 mm or greater compared with a dislocation less than 6 mm among the two age groups, the message is clear: patients in either age group have a statistically significantly higher incidence of nonunion if the initial dens dislocation is 6.0 mm or greater (Fig. 288-12; Table 288-4).

Based on these data, we advocate 10 to 12 weeks of halo-vest immobilization for patients with type II odontoid fractures with less than 6 mm dislocation. Individuals with a 6 mm (or greater) type II odontoid dislocation (regardless of patient age) or those with traumatic injuries that preclude the application of the halo device should be offered early surgical therapy.

Three percent of patients with acute odontoid type II fractures will have additional bone fragments at the base of the odontoid fracture identified by plain roentgenograms and CT studies (Figs. 288-13 and 288-14). We believe that these represent a unique subtype of type II odontoid fracture and have labeled them type IIA fractures.[14,18,19] These fractures are extremely unstable and are probably associated with significant ligamentous disruption. The additional bone fragments hinder anatomic realignment and inhibit proper bony union with external immobilization. Patients with this fracture subtype should be offered early surgical therapy.

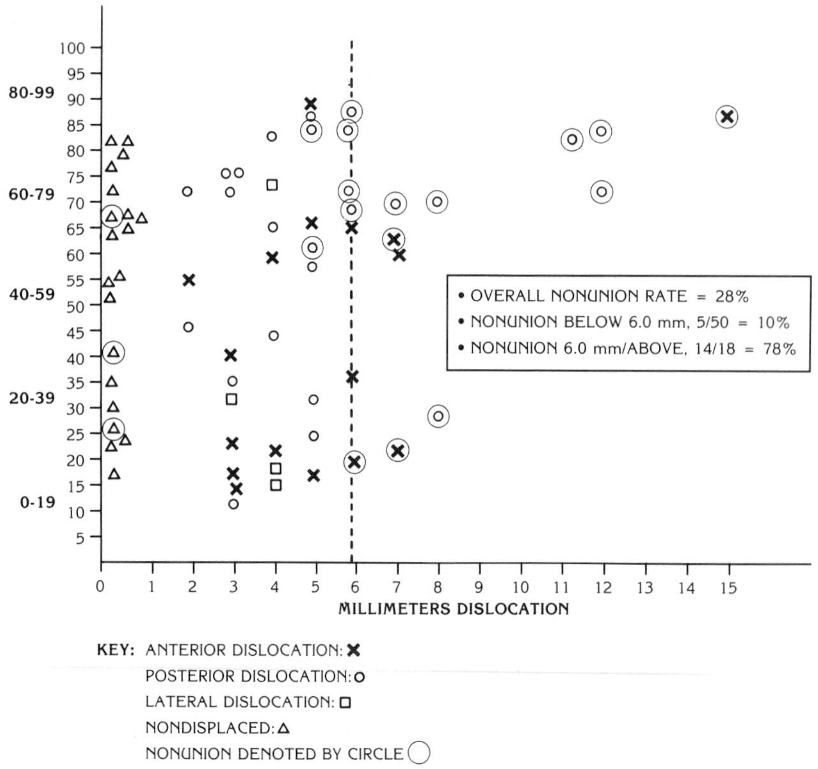

Figure 288-12 Comparison of the degree of dens dislocation and patient age with respect to nonunion for type II fractures of the odontoid. (From Hadley et al.,[18] with permission.)

TABLE 288-4 Odontoid Type II Fracture: Rate of Nonunion following Nonoperative Immobilization-Stabilization in Relation to Amount of Dens Dislocation*

	Dens Dislocation		
Patient Age	**<6 mm**	**≥6 mm**	**Statistical Significance**
60 years or older	13%*	85%*	$P < 0.001$; $\chi^2 = 17.0$
Less than 60 years	7%*	75%*	$P < 0.001$; $\chi^2 = 16.3$

*Percent of patients with nonunion.
Source: Adapted from Hadley et al.,[18] with permission.

Combination Atlas-Axis Fractures

Although much has been written about the treatment of isolated C1 and isolated C2 fractures, little attention has been directed toward the combination C1-C2 fracture injury.[6] Do these combination fractures have special characteristics which require specific therapy? Is there a rational means of classifying and treating these traumatic injuries?

Lipson, in one of the few papers specifically addressing the treatment of C1-C2 combination fractures, proposed a lengthy treatment course which incorporated both nonoperative and operative strategies.[24] He advocated external immobilization in a halo vest for 6 to 8 weeks to allow the *atlas* fracture to heal, followed

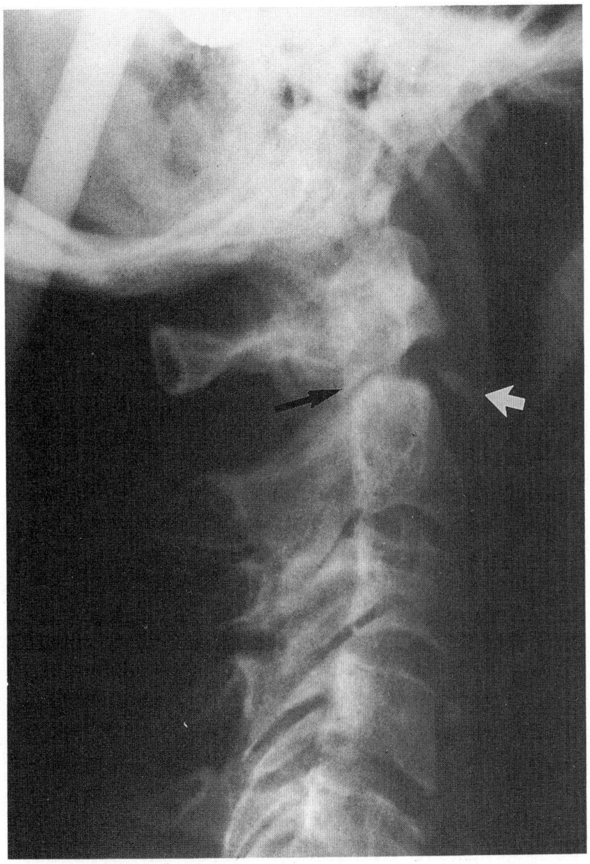

Figure 288-13 Lateral roentgenogram of a patient with a type IIA odontoid fracture. Note the bone chip (*white arrow*) anterior to the odontoid fracture (*black arrow*). This patient could not be effectively immobilized despite this degree of realignment in a halo vest.

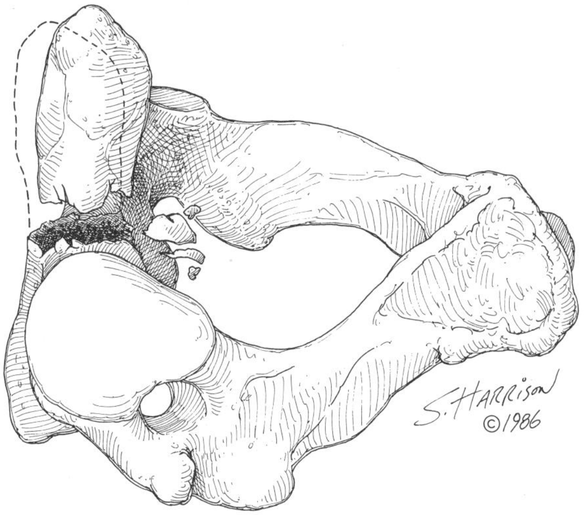

Figure 288-14 Artist's representation of a type IIA odontoid fracture.

by surgical wiring and fusion as definitive treatment of the *axis* fracture-dislocation. More recent experience with the management of patients with *axis* fractures, improved radiographic diagnostic studies, and the knowledge that not all *atlas* fractures are unstable has led us to conclude that a more refined approach to combination C1-C2 fractures is necessary.[6,17–19,31] A unilateral arch fracture of the atlas or an isolated C1 lateral mass fracture does not preclude early surgical wiring of C1 to C2 in the treatment of combination C1-C2 fracture injuries. If the atlas fracture is a bursting type (bilateral or multiple arch fractures), then C1 cannot be incorporated in the wiring and a bilateral C1-C2 transarticular screw fixation/fusion procedure or an occiput to C2 wiring and fusion procedure should be considered. The additional immobilization of patients for 6 to 8 weeks *prior* to definitive surgical therapy of their combination C1-C2 injury as advocated by Lipson can thus be obviated.

We base the decision to perform early surgery (within 3 to 12 days after injury) on patients with combination C1-C2 fractures upon the type of *axis* fracture present (Fig. 288-15). Several reviews of patients with isolated axis fractures have demonstrated that odontoid type III fractures, hangman's fractures, miscellaneous C2 fractures, and many odontoid type II fractures heal with external immobilization alone, when treated for 8 to 14 weeks.[16,18,19,31] Odontoid type II fractures with a dens dislocation of 6 mm or greater have a high incidence of nonunion with rigid external immobilization (regardless of the patient's age, the direction of dens dislocation, or the degree of neurological impairment).[16,18,19,31] As emphasized earlier, early surgical stabilization and fusion has been recommended for these patients.[16,18,31] Applying these principles to the atlas-axis combination fractures, if the axis fracture component of the C1-C2 combination injury is an odontoid type II fracture with a 6 mm or greater dens dislocation, then early operative intervention should be considered. All other axis fractures encountered in combination with a C1 fracture should be managed initially with rigid external immobilization. We favor the halo vest for its superior immobilization characteristics[22,31,35]; however, the SOMI brace was effective in the treatment of two patients in this series.

The treatment of the 25 combination C1-C2 fracture patients in our series was determined by the type of C2 fracture present. Nonoperative therapy was the initial treatment in 84 percent of patients; 18 patients had immobilization with a halo vest and 2 with a

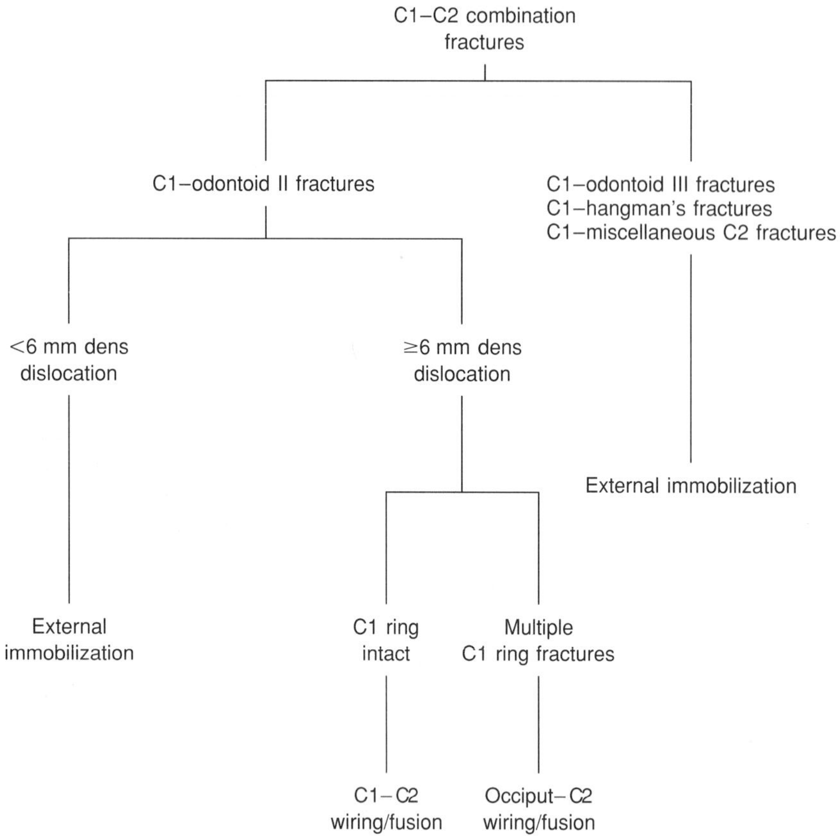

Figure 288-15 Treatment algorithm for C1-C2 combination fractures.

SOMI brace (Table 288-5). The median duration of external immobilization was 12 weeks, with a range of 10 to 22 weeks. Early operative reduction and internal fixation (ORIF) was performed in four patients (16 percent of the series). These patients had combination C1–odontoid type II fractures with a dens dislocation of 6 mm or greater. In the group treated with early ORIF, the integrity of the ring of the atlas was considered when determining the extent of the wiring and fusion procedure. Three patients had unilateral C1 arch or lateral mass fractures. These patients underwent wiring and fusion of C1 and C2. The one patient with a multiple ring fracture of the atlas underwent an occiput to C2 wiring and fusion procedure.

TABLE 288-5 Treatment of Combination C1-C2 Fractures

Fracture Combinations	Number of Patients	Method of Treatment*
C1–hangman's fractures	3	Halo vest
C1–odontoid II fractures	5	Halo vest†
	4	ORIF
	9	
C1–odontoid III fractures	1	SOMI brace
	4	Halo vest
	5	
C1–miscellaneous C2 fractures	1	SOMI brace
	6	Halo vest
	7	

*The duration of treatment ranged from 10 to 22 weeks (median, 12 weeks).
†One patient with nonunion required a late surgical fusion.
ORIF, operative reduction and internal fixation.
Source: Adapted from Hadley et al.,[17] with permission.

Follow-up was achieved in 23 of 25 patients (92 percent) with a median follow-up of 41 months (range, 2 to 101 months). One patient with a C1–odontoid type II combination fracture with an initial dens dislocation of 5 mm had nonunion with recurrent dens dislocation despite good alignment in the halo immobilization vest. He underwent C1-C2 wiring and fusion with an autologous iliac crest bone graft at 12 weeks after injury. All other patients treated solely with external immobilization healed without evidence of nonunion or instability on follow-up flexion and extension roentgenograms. All five patients treated with ORIF (4 early, 1 delayed) had a good bony fusion without evidence of subluxation on follow-up radiographic studies.

Third Cervical Vertebral Fractures

The treatment of C3 fractures must be individualized according to the type of fracture and the presence of associated fractures or fracture-dislocations. We have treated 10 isolated C3 fractures. All were treated nonoperatively with external immobilization (1, halo vest; 1, SOMI brace; 8, Philadelphia collar). The majority of the isolated C3 fractures were spinous process or isolated lamina fractures. There were two C3 body fractures. One was a stable chip fracture of the inferior aspect of the body. The second was a body fracture with 3-mm C3-C4 subluxation that was effectively treated with a halo vest.

Eight patients in our series of 1280 cervical fractures had C3 fractures in combination with C2 fractures. The treatment of these patients requires consideration of all of the fracture injuries. Six of eight patients were satisfactorily treated with halo-vest immobilization. One patient with a type II odontoid fracture with 6 mm dislocation and a C3 lateral mass fracture was treated with early posterior wiring and fusion of C1-C2-C3. The other patient had

C1, C2 (hangman's), and C3 posterior arch fractures with 4 mm of C2-C3 subluxation and was treated anteriorly with a C2-C3 discectomy and fusion procedure (Figs. 288-8 and 288-9).

Surgical Options

When surgery is indicated for axis fractures or combination C1-C2 fractures, we traditionally have performed a posterior atlas-axis wiring and autologous iliac crest bone graft fusion procedure[8] (Figs. 288-2 and 288-3). If an unstable atlas fracture (multiple ring fractures) complicates the axis fracture-dislocation, then the occiput is included in the C1-C2 wiring and fusion or a dorsal C1-C2 (bilateral) transarticular screw fixation procedure is added to the C1-C2 wiring and fusion procedure (Fig. 288-4). If the axis fracture is associated with significant C2-C3 subluxation, C3 is incorporated in the stabilization procedure. Each patient and each fracture combination must be individualized. In the patient who presented with a C1 ring fracture, C2 hangman's fracture, and C3 posterior arch fracture with 4 mm of C2-C3 subluxation, we elected to go anteriorly to repair the C2-C3 subluxation rather than proceed posteriorly and attempt to fuse and stabilize already disrupted posterior elements. We utilized a Caspar plate internal fixation device to provide additional support[33] (Fig. 288-9). More recently we have been performing C1-C2 transarticular screw fixation and fusion in addition to dorsal atlas-axis wiring and fusion procedures for C1-C2 instability or fracture-dislocations. This combination of internal fixation techniques provides the most rigid stabilization and fusion construct and usually precludes the use of an external immobilization device.[13,25] The specifics of the surgical techniques for each of these procedures is recorded elsewhere in this volume.

Cervical Orthoses

Except for the mildest injuries (either cervical sprain or an isolated, stable spinous process fracture), foam collars should not be used as an orthotic device for the cervical spine.[19,31] The Philadelphia collar, which provides significantly better immobilization of the neck than the foam collar ($P < 0.001$), has application in the treatment of atlas fractures displaced less than 6.9 mm, less severe miscellaneous axis fractures, and minor C3 fractures.[22,31,35]

More significant fracture-dislocations of C1, C2, or C3 require rigid immobilization of the head and neck with respect to the torso to maintain anatomic alignment and to ensure bony union.[6,16–18,30–32] Several cervicothoracic braces have been designed to serve this purpose. The SOMI brace provides fair immobilization with respect to flexion but allows considerable extension, rotation, and lateral bending of the cervical spine.[19,22,35] The rigid cervicothoracic orthosis and the Yale brace are slightly better at head and spine immobilization than the SOMI; however, both allow a significant range of neck flexion, rotation, and lateral bending compared with the halo immobilization brace. While not absolute in its ability to restrict head and neck movements, the halo ring attached to the plastic body vest represents the best form of external cervical spine immobilization currently available.[19,22,31,35] We rely extensively on the halo vest for nonoperative management of atlas fractures with less than 6.9 mm lateral dislocations, combination C1-C2 fractures, odontoid type II fractures (with less than 6 mm dens dislocation), odontoid type III fractures, hangmans' fractures, and the more severe miscellaneous axis fractures. Our results have been good, with few complications.[6,16–19,31] We recommend the rigid cervicothoracic brace as an alternative for patients who will not tolerate halo-vest immobilization, particularly those with flexion injuries.

Summary

A significant number of traumatic spine injuries involve the upper cervical spine. The incidence of neurological injury among patients who survive transport to the emergency department is relatively low after a C1, C2, or C3 fracture when compared with lower cervical levels and can be explained by the larger subarachnoid space at these superior levels. A wide variety of fractures and fracture-dislocations may occur between the occiput and C3. The treatment of these injuries begins with immobilization and rapid evaluation. Standard roentgenograms and CT studies, and occasionally MRI studies, are essential in determining the precise nature and stability of each fracture injury and guiding subsequent therapy. The optimal treatment of each high cervical injury must be individualized. Specific guidelines have been proposed to help determine whether operative or nonoperative management is the most efficacious. Regardless of the form of treatment used, compulsive follow-up is necessary to monitor therapy and to optimize patient outcome.

References

1. Apuzzo MLJ, Heiden JS, Weiss MH, et al. Acute fractures of the odontoid process: an analysis of 45 cases. *J Neurosurg* 1978; 48:85–91.
2. Bohlman HH. Acute fractures and dislocations of the cervical spine: an analysis of three hundred hospitalized patients and review of the literature. *J Bone Joint Surg [Am]* 1979; 61:1119–1142.
3. Bohlman HH, Boada E. Fractures and dislocations of the lower cervical spine. In The Cervical Spine Research Society (ed): *The Cervical Spine*. Philadelphia: Lippincott, 1983, pp 232–267.
4. Borges LF. Clinical assessment of posttraumatic spinal instability. In Cooper PR (ed): *Management of Posttraumatic Spinal Instability*. Park Ridge, IL: American Association of Neurological Surgeons, 1990, pp 37–49.
5. Brant-Zawadzki M, Miller EM, Federle MP. CT in the evaluation of spine trauma. *Am J Radiol* 1981; 136:369–375.
6. Dickman CA, Hadley MN, Browner C, et al. Neurosurgical management of acute atlas-axis combination fractures: a review of 25 cases. *J Neurosurg* 1989; 70:45–49.
7. Dickman CA, Mamourian A, Sonntag VKH, Drayer BP. Magnetic resonance imaging of the transverse atlantal ligament for the evaluation of atlantoaxial instability. *J Neurosurg* 1991; 75:221–227.
8. Dickman CA, Sonntag VKH, Papadopoulos SM, Hadley MN. The interspinous method of posterior atlantoaxial arthrodesis. *J Neurosurg* 1991; 74:190–198.
9. Dunn ME, Seljeskog EL. Experience in the management of odontoid process injuries: an analysis of 128 cases. *Neurosurgery* 1986; 18:306–310.
10. Effendi B, Roy D, Cornish B, et al. Fractures of the ring of the axis. A classification based on the analysis of 131 cases. *J Bone Joint Surg [Br]* 1981; 63-B:319–327.
11. Ekong CEU, Schwartz ML, Tator CH, et al. Odontoid fracture: management with early mobilization using the halo device. *Neurosurgery* 1981; 9:631–637.

12. Fielding JW, Cochran GVB, Lawsing JF III, et al. Tears of the transverse ligament of the atlas: a clinical and biomechanical study. *J Bone Joint Surg [Am]* 1974; 56-A:1683–1691.
13. Grob D, Crisco JJ III, Panjabi MM, et al. Biomechanical evaluation of four different posterior atlantoaxial fixation techniques. *Spine* 1992; 17:480–490.
14. Hadley MN, Browner CM, Liu SS, et al. New subtype of acute odontoid fractures (Type IIA). *Neurosurgery* 1988; 22:67–71.
15. Hadley MN, Browner C, Sonntag VKH. Miscellaneous fractures of the second cervical vertebra. *BNI Q* 1985; 1(4):34–39.
16. Hadley MN, Browner C, Sonntag VKH. Axis fractures: a comprehensive review of management and treatment in 107 cases. *Neurosurgery* 1985; 17:281–290.
17. Hadley MN, Dickman CA, Browner CM, et al. Acute traumatic atlas fractures: management and long term outcome. *Neurosurgery* 1988; 23:31–35.
18. Hadley MN, Dickman CA, Browner CM, et al. Acute axis fractures: a review of 229 cases. *J Neurosurg* 1989; 71:642–647.
19. Hadley MN, Sonntag VKH. Acute axis fractures. *Contemp Neurosurg* 1987; 9(2):1–6.
20. Hadley MN, Sonntag VKH, Grahm TW, et al. Axis fractures resulting from motor vehicle accidents: the need for occupant restraints. *Spine* 1986; 11:861–864.
21. Heiden JS, Weiss MH, Rosenberg AW, et al. Management of cervical spine cord trauma in Southern California. *J Neurosurg* 1975; 43:732–736.
22. Johnson RM, Owen JR, Hart DL, et al. Cervical orthoses: a guide to their selection and use. *Clin Orthop* 1981: 154:34–45.
23. Keene GCR, Hone MR, Sage MR. Atlas fracture: demonstration using computerized tomography. *J Bone Joint Surg [Am]* 1978; 60:1106–1107.
24. Lipson SJ. Fractures of the atlas associated with fractures of the odontoid process and transverse ligament ruptures. *J Bone Joint Surg [Am]* 1977; 59:940–943.
25. Magerl F, Seemann P-S. Stable posterior fusion of the atlas and axis by transarticular screw fixation. In Kehr P, Weidner A (eds): *Cervical Spine,* vol 1. New York: Springer Verlag, 1987, pp 322–327.
26. Panjabi MM, White AA III, Brand RA Jr. A note on defining body parts configurations. *J Biomech* 1974; 7:385–387.
27. Reiss SJ, Raque GH Jr, Shields CB, et al. Cervical spine fractures with major associated trauma. *Neurosurgery* 1986; 18:327–330.
28. Rogers WA. Fractures and dislocations of the cervical spine: an end-result study. *J Bone Joint Surg [Am]* 1957; 39:341–376.
29. Seljeskog EL, Chou SN. Spectrum of the hangman's fracture. *J Neurosurg* 1976; 45:3–8.
30. Sherk HH, Nicholson JT. Fractures of the atlas. *J Bone Joint Surg [Am]* 1970; 52:1017–1024.
31. Sonntag VKH, Hadley MN. Nonoperative management of cervical spine injuries. *Clin Neurosurg* 1986; 34:630–649.
32. Spence KF Jr, Decker S, Sell KW. Bursting atlantal fracture associated with rupture of the transverse ligament. *J Bone Joint Surg [Am]* 1970; 52:543–549.
33. Tuite GF, Papadopoulos SM, Sonntag VKH. Caspar plate fixation for the treatment of complex hangman's fractures. *Neurosurgery* 1992; 30:761–765.
34. White AA III, Panjabi MM. The basic kinematics of the human spine: a review of past and current knowledge. *Spine* 1978; 3:12–20.
35. Wolf JW Jr, Johnson RM. Cervical orthoses. In The Cervical Spine Research Society (ed): *The Cervical Spine.* Philadelphia: Lippincott, 1983, pp 54–61.

289 Management of Lower Cervical Spinal Instability

George W. Sypert
E. Joy Arpin

Lower cervical spinal (C3-C7) instability is most commonly the result of traumatic injuries. The vast majority of civilian lower cervical spine injuries are closed-type injuries with forces indirectly acting on the cervical spine. Injuries to the cervical spine range in consequence from simple myofascial stretch injuries and neck pain (sprains, strains) to quadriplegia and death. Traumatic instability of the lower cervical spine may result in serious injury to the cervical spinal cord which may be devastating to the patient with respect to long-term disability and suffering. The principal objective of the physicians responsible for the care of such patients is to prevent or minimize the extent of spinal cord injury subsequent to cervical spine trauma and instability. A corollary of this objective is to provide the optimal environment for the cervical spinal cord to recover maximally from any damage suffered at the time of the traumatic event.

In spite of continuing notable attempts by physicians to identify therapies that improve the spinal cord injured patient's chances of neurological recovery, no specific treatment or combination of therapeutic modalities has come forth that offers significant improvement over a variety of conventional approaches. It is clear, however, that inappropriate management can prevent expected recovery or cause further loss of neurological function. In one of the largest reported series of lower cervical spine injuries, approximately one-third of such patients suffered permanent additional injuries related to either errors in judgment or lack of suspicion on the part of the initial treating physician.[4] Current management methods must be designed to prevent post-traumatic complications, particularly those related to instability, that may lead to further disability and inhibit spontaneous recovery of neurological function.

Classification

The medical literature is replete with numerous attempts at the classification of acute cervical spine injuries and instability. The fact that none has gained general acceptance is indicative of the complexity of cervical spine injuries and/or failure of these classification systems to satisfy the requirements of clinicians working in this field. Most investigators concur that the mechanism of injury should be a major basis for segregation of these injuries into classes. Such an approach should contribute substantially to an understanding of the pathophysiology of cervical spine injuries and instability as well as offer a framework for clinical application and research.

Biomechanical[43] and cadaver model[1] experiments have established the basic relationship between the mechanisms of injury (vector forces) and the acute osseomusculoligamentous injuries of the lower cervical spine. In these controlled laboratory experiments, "pure" vector forces such as flexion, extension, vertical compression (axial loading), vertical distraction, lateral flexion (lateral bending), rotation, shear, or a combination of these forces have been demonstrated to produce cervical spine osseoligamentous injuries specific to each vector force or combination of forces.

Lower cervical spine injuries usually result from trauma to the head or trunk or a combination of both such that vector forces are transmitted to the cervical spine with injury to the osseomusculoligamentous, neural, and vascular structures. In fact, approximately 90 percent of serious lower cervical spine injuries appear to occur by the accelerating head or body striking a stationary object.[14] Clinically, the causative force(s) responsible for acute cervical spine instability can only be inferred retrospectively in most cases by correlating the available historical, physical examination, and neurodiagnostic imaging data because the conditions of injury are not controlled and rarely directly observed. It is reasonable, however, to apply knowledge regarding the mechanisms of cervical spine osseoligamentous injury obtained in controlled laboratory experiments to clinical injuries as there appears to be sufficient pathologic and radiographic similarity between the experimental and clinical injuries.

A clinically useful lower cervical spine osseoligamentous injury classification based on certain assumptions regarding the mechanisms of injury is presented in Table 289-1.[23] These acute cervical spine injuries are assumed to result from either predominant (pure) vector forces (flexion, extension, axial loading) or combinations of such forces (flexion-rotation, extension-rotation) and are grouped accordingly. Because the majority of serious lower cervical spine injuries are caused by being accelerated headfirst against a nonyielding object, excessive axial loading probably

TABLE 289-1 Mechanistic Classification of Osseomusculoligamentous Injuries of the Lower Cervical Spine

I. Flexion
   A. Anterior dislocation (hyperflexion sprain)
   B. Bilateral facet dislocation (locked facets)
   C. Simple wedge compression fracture
   D. Clay-shoveler fracture (spinous process avulsion)
   E. Flexion teardrop fracture
II. Flexion-rotation
   A. Unilateral facet dislocation
III. Vertical compression (axial loading)
   A. Burst fracture
IV. Extension
   A. Hyperextension dislocation (hyperextension sprain)
   B. Laminar fracture
   C. Hyperextension fracture-dislocation
V. Extension-rotation
   A. Lateral mass (pillar) fracture
VI. Lateral flexion
   A. Uncinate process fracture

Source: Adapted from Harris et al.,[23] with permission.

occurs in most injuries classified as flexion and extension injuries. Predominant distraction (atlanto-occipital and/or atlanto-axial dislocation), lateral flexion (uncinate process fracture), and shear vector forces appear to be infrequent in the clinical setting and often do not produce characteristic cervical spine injuries in the laboratory. This classification scheme is dependent on the additional reasonable assumptions that different injuries may be caused by a single predominant vector force and that there is a direct relationship between the magnitude of the force(s) and the type of injury.[43]

The principal clinical goal of the management of lower cervical spine instability is to prevent or minimize neurological injury subsequent to the injury and to provide an optimal environment for the spinal cord and nerve roots to maximally recover from any damage sustained at the time of the injury. An objective essential to achieving this goal is to obtain a stable healed cervical spine osseomusculoligamentous complex. A stable cervical spine will prevent further or future injury of the neural elements and offer the best opportunity for future pain-free function.

In order to make rational management plans regarding spinal instability, it is essential that the treating physician understand the osseomusculoligamentous pathology, the nature of any neural tissue injury or compression, and the healing processes that can be expected for any given injury. Moreover, it is necessary to consider the risks inherent in the various treatment methods available. Without such knowledge, the treating physician will not likely be able to obtain the greatest benefit for the individual patient with the least risks.

Clinical cervical spine stability has been defined using three parameters: (1) the motion segment will not further displace or deform under physiologic loads; (2) there is no progressive displacement or deformity during the healing process; and (3) there is no progressive compression or injury to the neural element.[36,43] In the clinical situation of an acute lower cervical spine injury, it is frequently difficult for the managing physician to definitely determine stability. As a general rule, it is safest to assume that all cervical spine injuries are unstable and to initially treat them as such until it is determined that the lesion is stable.

Based on experiments using fresh human cadaver models, White et al. defined lower cervical spine instability biomechanically.[42,43] These investigators suggested that cervical spine instability is imminent or exists if there is more than 3.5 mm of horizontal displacement of one vertebra on the adjacent vertebra, or if there is more than 11 degrees of angulation between adjacent vertebrae. Although specific measurements of traumatic injuries and subsequent clinical instability have not been established, these measurements may offer reasonable guidelines to indicate that instability is quite likely. However, values of less displacement or absence of angulation in the lateral neurodiagnostic image do not ensure clinical stability. Severe posterior ligamentous rupture with transient facet subluxation and spontaneous reduction does occur and is generally not evident on conventional lateral cervical spine roentgenograms. Even erect lateral dynamic flexion-extension films may not demonstrate acute instability due to reflex muscle contraction and spasm. Therefore, it is important to initially treat the acute cervical spine injured patient as if he or she is unstable using some external orthotic device until the acute response to the trauma has subsided and follow-up dynamic imaging assures stability.

Although the two-column concept of the spine[24] has been invaluable in understanding the mechanisms of injuries occurring as a result of predominant flexion or extension vector forces, the more recent redefinition of the spinal columns to include a middle column has substantial biomechanical and clinical merit.[15] The *three-column concept* that was originally applied to the thoracic and lumbar spine appears to have substantial applicability for the lower cervical spine as well. The posterior column is formed by the posterior neural arch, spinous process, facetal articular processes, and their corresponding posterior ligamentous complex. The middle column consists of the posterior one-third of the vertebral body and annulus fibrosus and the posterior longitudinal ligament. The anterior column comprises the anterior longitudinal ligament and the anterior two-thirds of the vertebral body and annulus fibrosus. As a first approximation, if two or more columns are disrupted, then acute spinal instability exists and predicts the possibility of late instability. Injuries that involve a single column generally do not lead to instability.

Lower Cervical Spinal Injuries

The treatment of lower cervical spinal injuries and instability remains controversial. Disagreement exists regarding the roles of external orthotic immobilization, surgical decompression, and surgical stabilization, both generally and specifically. Moreover, the type of appropriate external stabilizing device for specific injuries as well as the optimal type of surgical stabilization for specific injuries remain topics of debate. The following discussion will attempt to cover specific management methods for the common injuries of the lower cervical spine. The classification scheme presented in Table 289-1 will be followed.

Flexion Injuries

Anterior Dislocation

Anterior dislocation (subluxation) is the result of severe limited disruption of the posterior ligamentous complex.[12,19,41] This injury is characterized on the lateral radiographic view by a hyperkyphotic angulation of the cervical spine localized to the motion segment involved (Fig. 289-1). It is associated with a 20 to 30 percent incidence of delayed instability due to failure of ligamentous healing.[12,20]

Anterior subluxation (hyperflexion sprain) of the lower cervical spine is infrequently associated with a cervical spinal cord injury. The most common presenting complaint is post-traumatic neck pain and muscle spasm. The conventional lateral x-ray film is often diagnostic. These lesions may be missed, however, if the patient is supine or in extension when the lateral film is taken. Therefore, voluntary dynamic flexion-extension films may be necessary to make the diagnosis.

The management of anterior dislocation is initially nonoperative. If anterior subluxation is present, the patient should be reduced with extension or skeletal traction. The application of a halo-vest orthosis, which will maintain optimal spinal alignment for a time period of 10 to 12 weeks, provides the greatest opportunity for ligamentous healing. If instability persists despite external immobilization, then posterior internal fixation and fusion of the involved motion segments are appropriate. For patients who cannot tolerate rigid external immobilization, early posterior operative therapy may be considered.

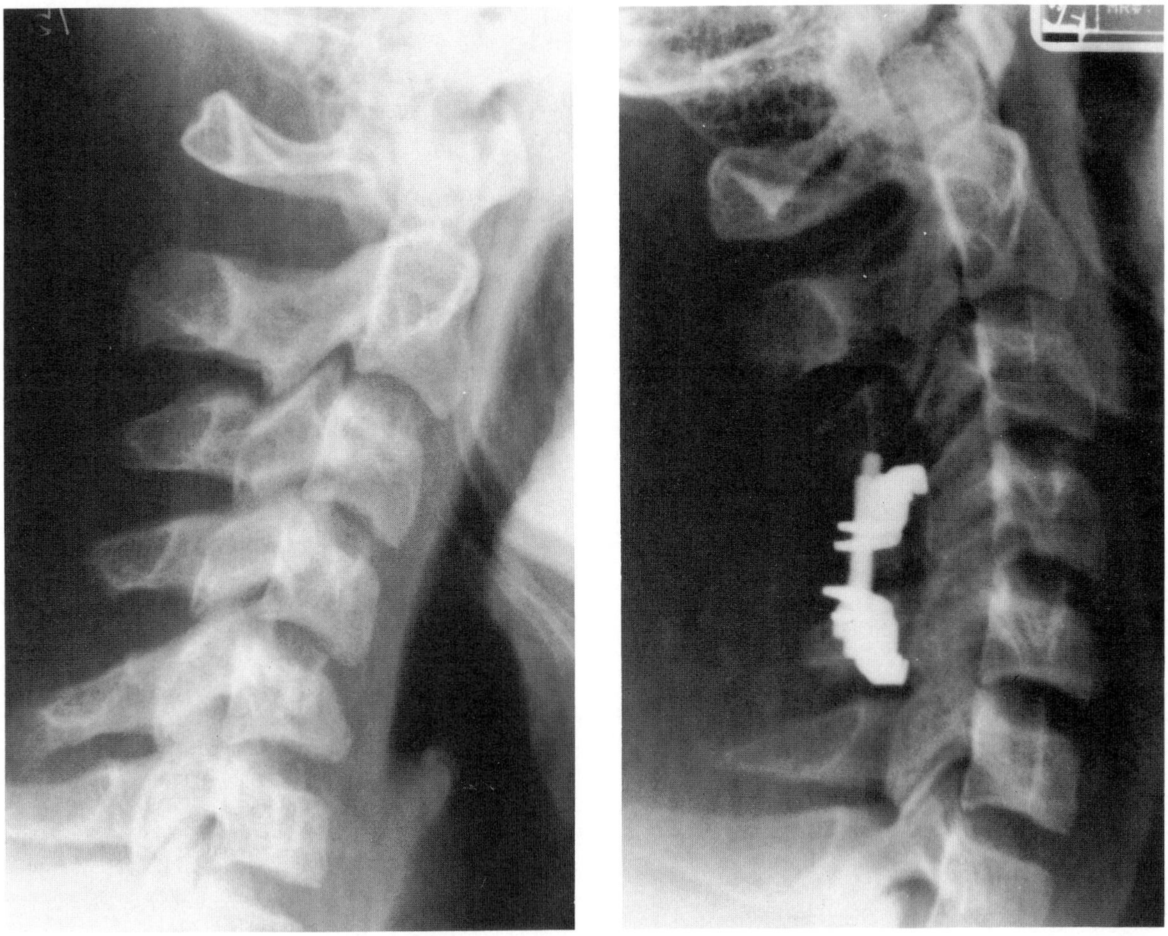

(*A*) (*B*)

Figure 289-1 Anterior dislocation (subluxation) at C4-C5 in a 17-year-old male who was treated initially with a SOMI orthosis and presented 3 months later complaining of intractable neck pain when weight bearing. After posterior internal fixation and fusion, the patient was pain-free and returned to competitive athletics. *A.* A lateral roentgenogram 3 months following injury (dynamic flexion-extension films revealed persistent instability). *B.* A postoperative lateral roentgenogram demonstrating internal fixation and autogenous fusion.

Bilateral Facet Dislocation

Anterior subluxation of lower cervical spine with bilateral facet dislocation is usually the result of a severe hyperflexion-shear injury.[21,26,35,44] Bilateral interlocking occurs when the inferior articular facets of the upper dislocated vertebra slide forward over the superior facets of the vertebra below. These injuries are serious three-column ligamentous injuries; they include rupture of the posterior ligamentous complex, the joint capsules, the intervertebral disc, and, usually, the posterior and anterior longitudinal ligaments.[8,21,26,35,44] Therefore, these dislocations are very unstable and great caution must be exercised when closed reduction is attempted. Excessive cervical skeletal traction can cause distraction injuries of the cervical spinal cord.[8,30]

Bilateral facet dislocation occurs in as many as 5 percent of major cervical spine injuries.[26] In most instances (about 80 percent), irreversible complete transverse myelopathy is present at the time of the insult due to spinal cord crush from the vertebral dislocation.[21,26,35,44] Similarly, nerve root function at the level of the dislocation is lost due to traction, compression, or avulsion.

The lateral roentgenogram demonstrates an anterior subluxation of the rostral vertebra of about 50 percent or more of the vertebral body surface. On the anteroposterior film, there is little or no displacement of the spinous processes.

The optimal management of bilateral facet dislocation with locking is controversial. In many spinal injury centers, a high priority is given to the urgent closed reduction of the dislocation using skeletal traction and manipulation or early surgical reduction via a posterior approach if closed methods are unsuccessful.[8,21,26,35,44] Maiman et al. reported that early reduction failed to promote significant neurological recovery.[26] They suggested that immediate reduction may not be justified. Similarly, nerve root recovery does not appear to be affected by early or late reduction.[36]

Approximately 60 percent of bilateral facet dislocations heal with spontaneous interbody ankylosis using halo-vest stabilization for a time period of 12 weeks.[11,20,36] If the vertebral body is compressed in association with facet dislocation, the incidence of chronic instability reportedly exceeds 66 percent.[36] Therefore, early posterior internal fixation and fusion seem to be reasonable alternatives to prolonged halo-vest immobilization. In patients who develop delayed instability during or after treatment with closed stabilization, appropriate anterior or posterior surgical arthrodesis is indicated. Internal fixation may be achieved safely with posterior interspinous process tension band wiring or interlaminar clamps. Reported attempts at surgical fusion using an anterior approach alone in the absence of posterior ligamentous support have documented a high failure rate.[30,38] However, the application of an anterior plate-screw fixation system in combination with anterior bone arthrodesis has been shown to be successful in achieving a high rate of stability.[32,44]

Although most clinicians are of the opinion that decompressive operations are rarely indicated in patients sustaining bilateral facet dislocations, recent evidence indicates that significant anterior neurocompressive mass lesions including herniated intervertebral discs are not infrequent in these patients.[22,26] Maiman et al. performed anterior decompression to reconstruct the normal anatomy of the spinal canal in 13 patients (28 cases total) who demonstrated a persistent ventral mass effect despite optimal reduction with skeletal traction.[26] Improvement in nerve root and spinal cord function seemed to be related to the surgery. Single-stage anterior decompression combined with posterior arthrodesis is preferred by Maiman et al. when an anterior decompression is performed. Other authors have successfully achieved stability following anterior microsurgical decompression using anterior plate-screw fixation with bone auto- or allograft reconstruction.[25,32,44]

Simple Wedge Compression Fracture

Simple compression fracture is the result of hyperflexion injury of sufficient force to cause impaction of one vertebra against the subjacent vertebra. This fracture is typically characterized by impaction of the superior endplate and impaction and kyphotic angulation of the anterior superior margin of the involved vertebral body, which are readily verified on a lateral roentgenogram. Although some patients with this injury escape neurological injury, many unfortunately suffer spinal cord damage.

The initial management of this injury is closed realignment. Optimal alignment for the wedge compression fracture is usually achieved with the patient supine using skeletal traction. Slightly elevating the patient's shoulders to induce some mild extension of the cervical spine is often helpful. Some clinicians recommend using large weights (50 to 60 lb) in an attempt to optimize alignment and reconstitute the vertebral body height.[17] They further advocate prolonged traction using these weights for several days followed by a slow reduction in weight over the next 2 to 3 weeks in order to maintain the reduction. Skeletal traction is maintained for 3 to 4 weeks to allow the anterior vertebral body to reconstitute itself in its normal configuration, followed by halo-vest application for an additional 8 weeks. If the initial x-ray films indicate posterior ligamentous disruption, some clinicians further advocate early halo-vest application after reduction and stabilization of the patient, with surgical treatment reserved for those patients with delayed instability manifested during or after the period of rigid external immobilization.[11–13,20]

In patients sustaining a neurological deficit that is persistent after optimal realignment and stabilization, appropriate neurodiagnostic imaging [computed tomography (CT) myelography or magnetic resonance imaging (MRI)] is recommended to determine whether a neurocompressive lesion is present. Generally, no such lesion will be found. When a neurocompressive lesion is present, it is usually located anterior to the neural elements. If the neurocompressive lesion is a herniated intervertebral disc, it is often one level above the compressed vertebra. Surgical decompression with reconstruction of the spinal canal for ventrally located mass lesions requires an anterior approach.[3,4] Appropriate anterior strut grafting, posterior arthrodesis if the posterior ligamentous complex is disrupted, and rigid external immobilization postoperatively are required when an anterior decompression is performed.

The optimal management of these lesions remains in dispute. In simple wedge compression fractures without posterior ligamentous damage, the incidence of delayed instability (progressive kyphotic deformity) is about 10 to 15 percent of patients treated with halo-vest immobilization.[11,20] Hence, patients sustaining such osseous lesions associated with posterior ligamentous damage should be told that surgical stabilization may be necessary to achieve spinal stability in spite of 12 weeks of external immobilization. For patients with both anterior and posterior column injuries who cannot tolerate rigid immobilization, early surgical stabilization should be considered.

Clay-Shoveler Fracture

The clay-shoveler fracture is an avulsion fracture of the spinous process(es) of lower cervical vertebra(e). The C7 spinous process is the most commonly affected, followed by C6 and T1. The clay-shoveler fracture occurs when head and upper cervical spinal segments are forced into flexion against the opposing action of the posterior musculoligamentous complex. On lateral radiographic views, this fracture is characterized by an oblique fracture limited to the spinous process of the involved vertebra. Because the spine is stable, the treatment consists of immobilization in an external orthosis such as a Philadelphia collar for 8 weeks.

Flexion Teardrop Fracture

The teardrop fracture is a consequence of severe hyperflexion with complete disruption of the intervertebral disc and all of the ligaments of all three columns associated with an oblique fracture of the anterior inferior body of the involved vertebra.[34] The lateral roentgenogram reveals a triangular fracture of the anteroinferior vertebral body or, more commonly, a larger triangular or quadrilateral fracture of the anterior vertebral body. The vertebral body is displaced posteriorly and the anterior fragment is displaced anteriorly. The involved vertebra is compressed, with narrowing of the intervertebral disc and kyphotic deformity of the cervical spine.

The teardrop fracture is highly unstable and is generally a devastating injury. It is usually associated with a complete transverse myelopathy or severe anterior cervical spinal cord syndrome.

The initial management is stabilization and realignment using skeletal traction. If optimal alignment can be achieved, the spinal canal will be reconstituted in most cases. The subsequent management remains controversial. Some authors recommend maintaining skeletal traction for 4 weeks followed by 8 weeks in a halo vest.[17] Most authors prefer early application of the halo vest and its continuation for 10 to 12 weeks.[11,12,20] The incidence of delayed instability ranges from 10 to 15 percent for such injuries.[11,20] If an anterior surgical decompression is performed for persistent anterior neurological compression, anterior plate-screw fixation or posterior arthrodesis followed by the application of a rigid external orthosis is probably indicated.[3]

Flexion-Rotation Injuries

Unilateral Facet Dislocation

Unilateral facet dislocation seems to be the result of simultaneous flexion and rotation vector forces.[30] In this injury, there is a unilateral facet dislocation at one level on the side opposite that of the direction of rotation. Usually the dislocated rostral facet is displaced anterior to the caudal facet and becomes wedged or locked in the intervertebral neural foramen anterior to the rostral edge of the caudal facet. The facet capsule and posterior ligamentous complex are disrupted. The posterior and anterior longitudinal ligaments and the intervertebral disc are also injured. An impaction fracture of either of the facet masses of the affected joint may also occur. Such fractures may make closed reduction difficult. An ipsilateral nerve root injury is frequently associated with this injury. Spinal cord injury occurs in about 25 percent of cases.[30]

The lateral roentgenogram typically shows forward displacement (30 percent or less) of the rostral dislocated vertebra on the caudal vertebra. The rotated vertebra demonstrates a narrow double posterior margin and the paired articular masses do not line up (double facet configuration). On the anteroposterior roentgenogram, the spinous processes at and above the level of dislocation are rotated (i.e., displaced toward the side of the dislocated facet complex).

Although the unilateral facet dislocation with locking is a stable injury and will heal without instability if treated with external immobilization, this injury causes chronic pain and has a high incidence of nerve root injury. Therefore, the dislocated facet should be reduced with closed skeletal traction if possible. Careful manipulation while undergoing skeletal traction may be required to achieve closed reduction. If closed reduction is unsuccessful, posterior open surgical reduction is readily accomplished when performed during the first 2 weeks after injury. Most patients who undergo successful closed reduction may then be treated effectively with halo-vest immobilization for 12 weeks.[21] The incidence of delayed instability after halo-vest immobilization is about 15 percent. Some authors advocate posterior internal fixation with wires or interlaminar clamps and fusion to prevent redislocation and chronic instability.[37]

Vertical Compression (Axial Loading) Injuries

Burst Fracture

The burst fracture is a result of vertical compressive forces acting on the longitudinal axis of the lower cervical spine. This axial loading leads to comminuted fracture of the vertebral body with retropulsion of posterior body fragments into the spinal canal. Posterior element fractures, particularly laminar fractures, are almost invariably present. Serious spinal cord injury is frequently present in these patients.

The lateral x-ray film will reveal loss of vertebral body height with comminution of the body resulting in variable retropulsion of posterior body bone fragments into the spinal canal. There is an absence of distraction of the posterior elements. The anteroposterior film will frequently demonstrate a vertical fracture line through the vertebral body. Axial CT imaging will demonstrate the vertebral body fractures and generally a posterior element fracture.

The management of this fracture remains controversial. The same issues exist for this lesion as for the teardrop fracture (see prior discussion).

Extension Injuries

Hyperextension injuries of the lower cervical spine are the result of posteriorly directed vector forces that cause posterior rotation and/or translocation of the cervical vertebrae.[27] These forces result in a family of spinal column injuries as listed in Table 289-1. Such injuries often leave little radiographic evidence of acute spinal column damage. In the *hyperextension dislocation or sprain,* the spinous processes and lateral masses act as a fulcrum, causing the anterior longitudinal ligament and anterior disc to rupture. The radiographic examination may be normal. Radiographic evidence of this injury includes prevertebral soft tissue swelling, a widened intervertebral disc space, a small anterior avulsion fracture, and normal alignment of the cervical vertebrae. An isolated *laminar fracture* may also occur related to compression of the posterior elements. These injuries are relatively stable. Spinal cord injury, usually a central cord syndrome, is a common consequence of these injuries in patients with cervical spinal stenosis (the younger patient with congenital stenosis and/or block vertebrae and the older patient with degenerative cervical spondylosis and/or ossification of the posterior longitudinal ligament).

The management of hyperextension dislocation without a neurological deficit is usually symptomatic. In those patients presenting with an acute spinal cord injury, the initial management generally involves the application of skeletal traction although a cervical collar may be just as effective for immobilization. If skeletal traction is applied, usually 10 lb is all that is required to maintain optimal alignment. Those patients who show an early improvement in their neurological deficit (during the first 48 h after injury) have the greatest probability of excellent neurological function.[18] After the patient's neurological deficit has stabilized, neurodiagnostic imaging (CT myelography) is generally necessary to determine whether persistent neural compression is present. If myelography is performed early, a widened swollen spinal cord is frequently demonstrated.[18] Appropriate surgical decompression may require either an anterior or posterior approach depending on the location of the neurocompressive lesion.[18]

Hyperextension fracture-dislocation is usually the result of a severe rotatory hyperextension vector force causing compression injury of the posterior elements, including the articular masses, pedicles, laminae, and spinous processes. The vertebral body is frequently subluxed forward. The intervertebral disc is disrupted and the anterior longitudinal ligament may rupture causing a small avulsion fracture of either the anteroinferior corner or the vertebral body above the involved disc or the anterosuperior corner of the vertebral body below the involved disc. Patients sustaining this injury may or may not sustain a serious neurological injury. This injury is, however, very unstable and carries the risk of new or additional spinal cord injury if not managed appropriately.

The lateral roentgenogram may demonstrate mild to moderate anterior or posterior subluxation of the vertebral body. Compression fractures of the lateral masses or spinous processes may be evident on either the lateral or anteroposterior projections. Thin-section CT imaging with sagittal and coronal reconstructions clearly delineates the extent of bony injury.

The management of this injury initially requires the application of skeletal traction to achieve optimal alignment. Generally, excessive weight should be avoided to prevent overdistraction with the risk of inducing a neurological injury. Those patients without a neurological deficit and with no neurocompressive lesion may be managed with halo-vest immobilization for 12 weeks. The incidence of delayed instability seems to be very low in such patients. The optimal management for those patients with a persistent neurological deficit and a neurocompressive lesion is complex and highly individualized, and remains controversial.

Surgical Management

The indications for surgical management of lower cervical spine injuries and instability are two: (1) *neural decompression* and (2) *reduction-stabilization.* In spite of substantial recent advances in our knowledge of the biomechanics of spinal instability and our understanding of adequate neural decompression, the indications for surgical decompression and stabilization remain controversial. However, recent advances and contributions have brought about a more rational application of modern surgical techniques to the management of cervical traumatic neural compression and instability. The present goals of surgical therapy are to prevent injury to the neural elements, to decompress the neural elements, to maximize neurological recovery, to prevent delayed instability and spine deformity with their corresponding risks of delayed loss of neurological function, and to permit early mobilization and rehabilitation of patients with a corresponding reduction in the morbidity and mortality associated with prolonged recumbency and hospitalization.

A careful, comprehensive neurodiagnostic evaluation is essential for the proper assessment of lower cervical spine injuries and instability in order to adequately define the pathologic anatomy and biomechanics of the injury if operative therapy is contemplated. In patients with persistent incomplete neurological recovery or transient neurological deficits after appropriate external reduction and immobilization, it is appropriate to further assess the need for operative decompression, looking specifically for evidence of spinal canal encroachment by bone fragments, disc material, or hematoma which may prevent additional recovery or lead to delayed loss of neurological function. Presently, CT myelography (CT scanning with CSF contrast enhancement) seems to be the neurodiagnostic imaging procedure of choice for accurately delineating the location and degree of neurological compressive lesions. Modern high quality MRI of the cervical spine can also be used to visualize traumatic neurocompressive lesions, thus obviating the need for dural puncture. Depending on the location of the mass lesion compressing the neural elements, an appropriate surgical approach can be logically selected which will adequately decompress the neural elements. Similarly, an appropriate stabilizing procedure must be planned to achieve correction of spinal instability if one is to minimize treatment complications. In each case presenting with cervical spine instability, sufficient neurodiagnostic imaging is essential to obtaining an understanding of the predominant biomechanical vector forces responsible for the given injury. The treatment selected must be designed to counteract the forces producing the spinal instability/deformity if a stable cervical spine is to be achieved and maintained. If those forces are not adequately counteracted, then mechanical failure of the cervical spine is the likely consequence.

The timing of surgical management in patients with lower cervical spine injuries is continually evolving with the advances in our understanding of the nature of cervical spine neurological and osseomusculoligamentous injuries and the rational application of improved surgical techniques and approaches.[25] The spinal surgeon must always take into account those factors relating to coexisting conditions or injuries. Approximately 60 percent of patients with severe cervical spine injuries suffer other major organ system trauma. Therefore, the surgeon should not risk aggravating these life-threatening conditions by performing additional surgery. Cervical operative decompression and/or stabilization should be delayed until the patient's condition permits its accomplishment without additional risk. Of major importance is the problem of respiratory insufficiency, particularly in those patients with cervical spinal cord injuries whose pulmonary insufficiency is compounded by neurogenic paralysis of the intercostal muscles. Preoperative assessment of respiratory function is useful in determining the timing of nonemergent surgery. It has been suggested that nonemergent surgery should be postponed if the patient's total vital capacity is less than 700 to 800 ml in order to avoid postoperative respiratory failure.

In patients with lower cervical spine injuries without neurological deficit, surgical management should be performed only after all major medical problems have been resolved and the cervical spinal column has been reduced and immobilized by external methods. This recommendation includes those patients with injuries that cannot be safely realigned using external methods. Open reduction should be postponed and the spinal column immobilized externally until all life-threatening conditions have been controlled.

Timing of surgical management continues to remain controversial regarding patients with neurological deficits, both complete and incomplete, who have neurodiagnostic evidence of continued compression of the neural elements after closed reduction. Although various authors have recommended early operative decompression of the neural elements,[10,40] there are no statistically significant data to indicate that early operative decompression within the first few hours or days after cervical spinal injury results in any greater recovery of neurological function than surgery performed days or weeks later.[25] In fact, Benzel and Larson were not able to demonstrate a correlation between the timing of surgery and the degree of neurological return in a study of 99 patients with lower cervical spine injuries treated surgically.[2,3] Furthermore, early surgical management has been shown to be associated with a much higher rate of serious postoperative complications than delayed surgery.[6] Therefore, available evidence is consistent with the concept that the only indication for early or emergency operation is neurological deterioration in the presence of neurological element compression by bone, soft tissues, or hematoma.

In the preparation of the patient for operation, protection of the neural elements is paramount and requires considerable attention on the part of the surgeon and anesthesiologist. If there is any question regarding the stability of the cervical spine, it is essential that an exceedingly careful awake endotracheal intubation be performed so that the neurological status can be constantly monitored. This can be accomplished via the nasotracheal route. In difficult cases, it may be necessary to use the fiber-optic bronchoscope to achieve a safe intubation. Positioning as well as turning of the patient should also be accomplished with the patient awake, maintaining the preoperative cervical spine alignment. Manipulation of the cervical spine must be kept to a minimum with induction of anesthesia and positioning of the patient. A lateral cervical spine film should be used to verify optimal position of the cervical spinal column prior to beginning the operation. As a general principle, if reduction and alignment were achieved preoperatively using skeletal traction, the traction should be maintained during the preparation and surgical procedure until adequate intraoperative stabilization has been accomplished and verified radiographically.

In cervical spine injured patients with persistent neurological compression who are candidates for surgical decompression, the majority will have the neurocompressive mass lesion located ventral to the neural elements.[3–5,29] Under these circumstances, the appropriate procedure is an anterior approach (Fig. 289-2). When an anterior approach is used to decompress the spinal cord and nerve roots, the posterior longitudinal ligament should be excised and adequate decompression of the dura should be directly verified visually. We believe that the operative microscope is an important element for ensuring the success and safety of this surgical procedure. All disc, soft tissue, and bone compressing the dura must be removed. In some cases, an appropriate decompression may require partial or complete wide mesial corpectomy with discectomies rostral and caudal to the involved vertebral body.

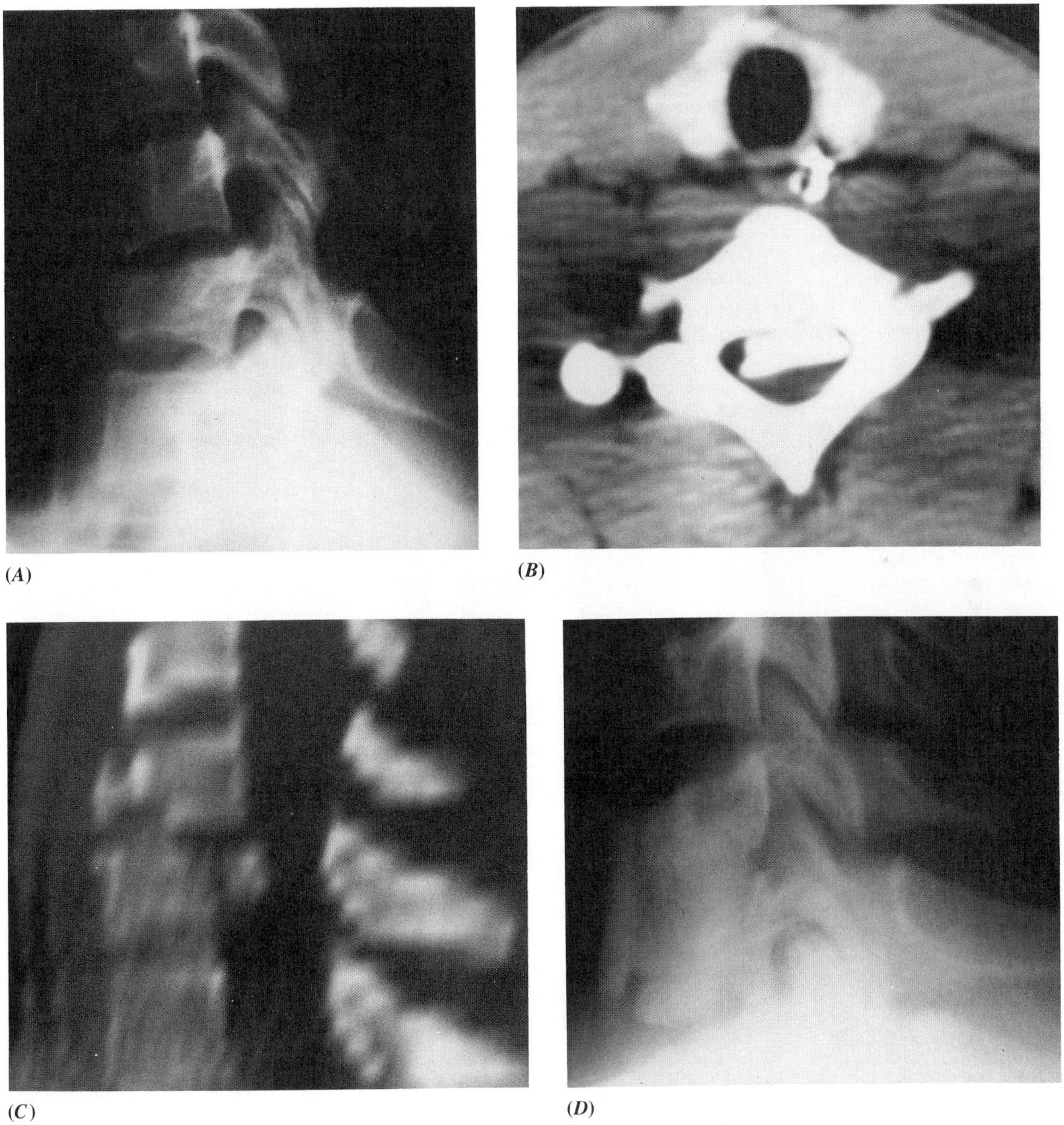

Figure 289-2 Neurodiagnostic studies of an 18-year-old male who sustained a burst fracture of C5 and an incomplete myelopathy that did not improve with adequate closed reduction and alignment using skeletal tong traction. After an anterior decompressive partial corpectomy and fibula allograft reconstruction, the patient's spinal cord function recovered fully. *A.* Lateral roentgenogram; *B.* axial CT scan; *C.* sagittal CT reconstruction; and *D.* postoperative lateral roentgenogram.

After achieving an adequate neural decompression, an appropriate cervical fusion is carried out using a bone graft. Although we advocate using a fibular strut allograft, many surgeons prefer the block graft technique using a tricortical iliac crest autograft. Tibial bone may also be used. However, Verbiest reported two tibial fractures in a series of 47 tibial autografts.[39] When a bone strut is used, both the bone graft and the vertebral bodies should be notched (tongue and groove configuration) to decrease the chance of dislodgment of the graft. Recent retrospective analyses of relatively large numbers of patients with cervical spine injuries strongly indicate that adequate surgical restoration of the normal relationships between the neural and structural spinal elements can result in improvement in spinal cord neurological function.[3,4] Moreover, appropriate surgical decompression in patients suffering irreversible complete transverse myelopathy seems to be followed by better recovery of nerve root function than does nonsurgical management.[3,4]

In those infrequent patients who present with isolated anterior column instability, anterior cervical arthrodesis using a bone graft after decompression may yield sufficient stability that a well-fitted Philadelphia collar or similar orthosis may be adequate for postoperative immobilization until fusion occurs. However, the majority of patients present with coexisting posterior element instability (two- or three-column instability). In the latter, more common, situation, anterior cervical decompression, particularly with removal of the destroyed vertebral body and posterior longitudinal ligament, will aggravate the instability. In some patients, the surgeon may elect to use a halo-vest orthosis postoperatively. However, the instability after anterior decompression and reconstruction may be of such a degree that graft dislodgment may occur despite the use of the halo vest. In the latter circumstance, the surgeon may perform a posterior cervical internal fixation and fusion (Fig. 289-3). The other way to manage such patients is to lock the bone graft in place with anterior plates and vertebral body bone screws (Caspar or Synthes anterior cervical instrumentation) (Fig. 289-4).

Attempted decompression of the spinal cord compressed by a ventrally located mass lesion such as retropulsed bone fragments or intervertebral disc material using a posterior approach or posterolateral approach (laminectomy) is difficult and hazardous with an unacceptably high risk of inducing additional spinal cord injury. This is the most likely explanation for the neurological deterioration frequently reported in earlier studies of patients with cervical spinal cord injuries treated by so-called decompressive laminectomies. In such series, a permanent increase in neurological deficit after a conventional decompressive laminectomy was a relatively common complication, with a reported incidence of 22 percent in one series.[7,28] These data do not imply that posterior decompression is contraindicated in all cases. On rare occasions, when neurodiagnostic imaging demonstrates posterior neural compression by

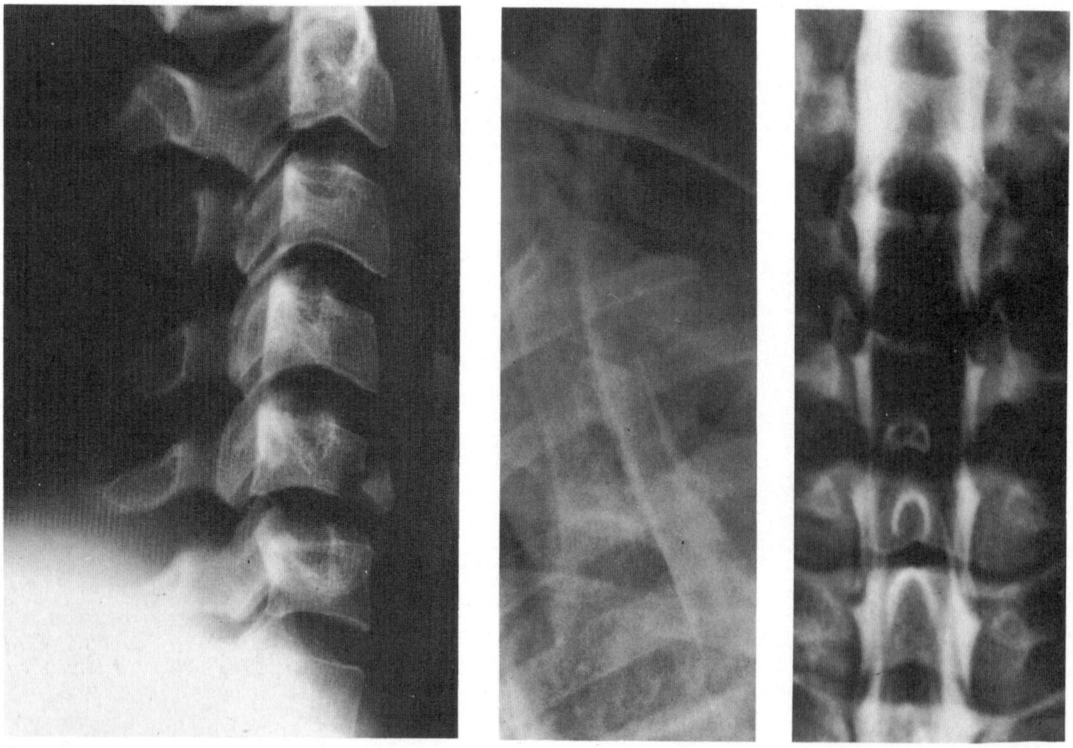

(*A*) (*B*) (*C*)

Figure 289-3 Neurodiagnostic studies of a 20-year-old male who sustained a teardrop fracture of C5 and an incomplete cervical myelopathy (anterior cord syndrome). Adequate reduction and immobilization using skeletal tong traction failed to yield any recovery of spinal cord function. After a single-stage anterior microsurgical decompressive mesial corpectomy and fibula allograft reconstruction and posterior internal fixation and autogenous bone fusion, the patient's spinal cord function returned to normal. The posterior internal fixation and arthrodesis was performed because posterior ligamentous disruption was demonstrated during closed skeletal traction (overdistraction at C5-C6). *A.* Lateral roentgenogram; *B, C,* myelogram (note the widened spinal cord);

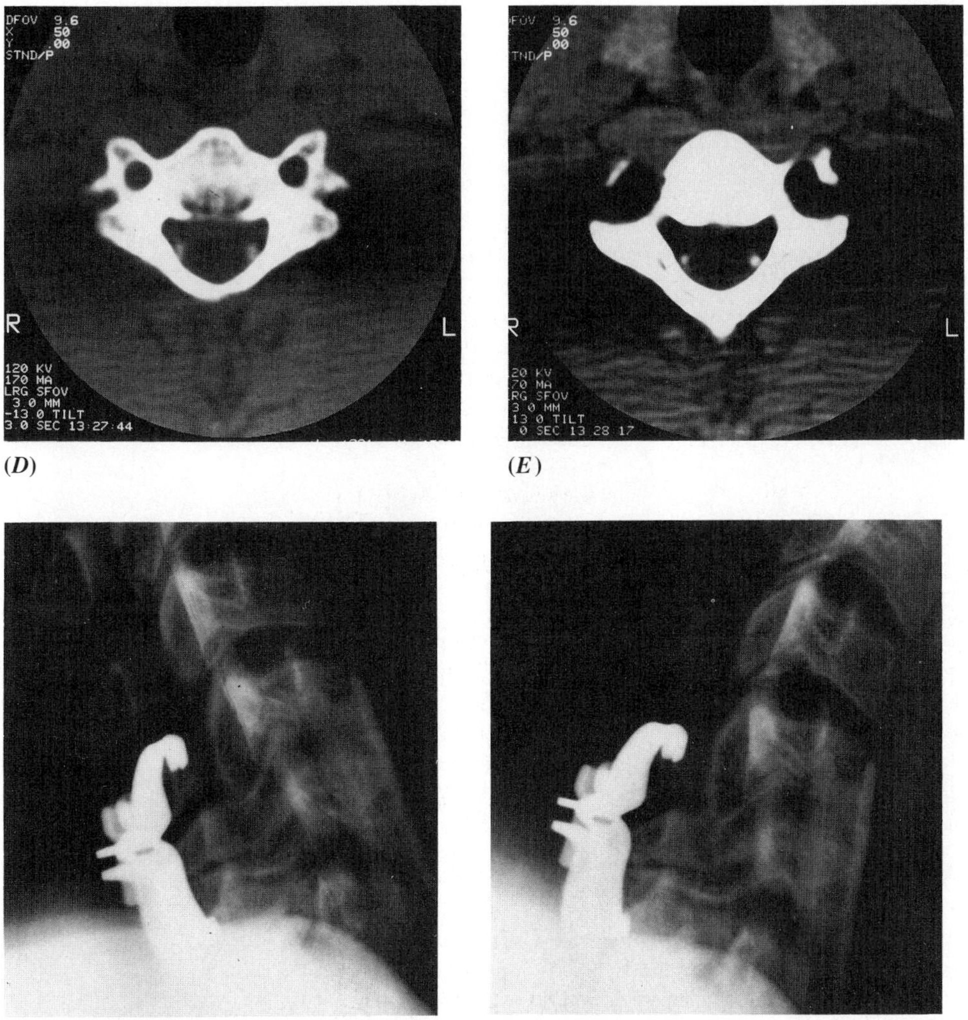

(*D*) (*E*)

(*F*) (*G*)

Figure 289-3 (*Continued*) *D, E,* axial CT myelogram [note the large retrovertebral mass compressing the spinal cord (a ventral epidural hematoma and a swollen posterior longitudinal ligament)]; and *F, G,* postoperative lateral extension and flexion films.

fractured laminar elements or a hematoma, a traditional decompressive laminectomy may be the preferred surgical procedure. Another circumstance in which the posterior approach for decompression of the injured spinal cord may be indicated is when neurodiagnostic imaging clearly demonstrates focal enlargement of the spinal cord consistent with an intramedullary hematoma. It has been suggested that some of the latter patients may benefit from myelotomy and evacuation of the intramedullary hematoma and necrotic debris. However, no data are available in the literature to clearly support such an aggressive approach over conventional nonsurgical management of this situation.

In most circumstances, acute lower cervical spine instability requiring surgical management may be accomplished electively after the patient has been medically stable and the spinal column reduced and immobilized by external methods. Operative reduction, fixation, and fusion are indicated if the patient's cervical spinal instability is such that external devices (e.g., halo orthosis) are not likely to adequately immobilize the injured segments, to result in a healed stable spine, or to prevent fracture collapse and late deformity. Examples of such injuries include major subluxations associated with severe ligamentous disruption and major traumatic kyphotic deformities. As a general principle, we prefer posterior internal reduction and/or fixation and bony fusion as the procedure of choice for ligamentous injuries with minimal or no osseous injury. Fewer complications seem to be associated with this approach than with attempts at stabilization of such injuries using an anterior operation.[9,31,38,39]

The type of internal fixation and the material used for operative stabilization of the unstable lower cervical spine varies widely among spinal surgeons. Posterior interspinous wiring, sublaminar wiring, facet to spinous process wiring, facet to bone graft wiring, interlaminar clamps, and plates with bone screws have been used with varying success. Anterior fixation has been achieved using interbody bone grafts alone or supplemented with wire fixation or plates and screws. Late perforation of the esophagus has been reported with anterior wire fixation. At present, an adequate series of long-term follow-up using the anterior screw-plate technique is lacking in the literature.

In general, we advocate using autograft bone for posterior cervical fusion whereas allograft fibula is advocated for anterior cervical arthrodesis. The patient's own bone yields the most rapid union and the highest incidence of satisfactory fusion when used in

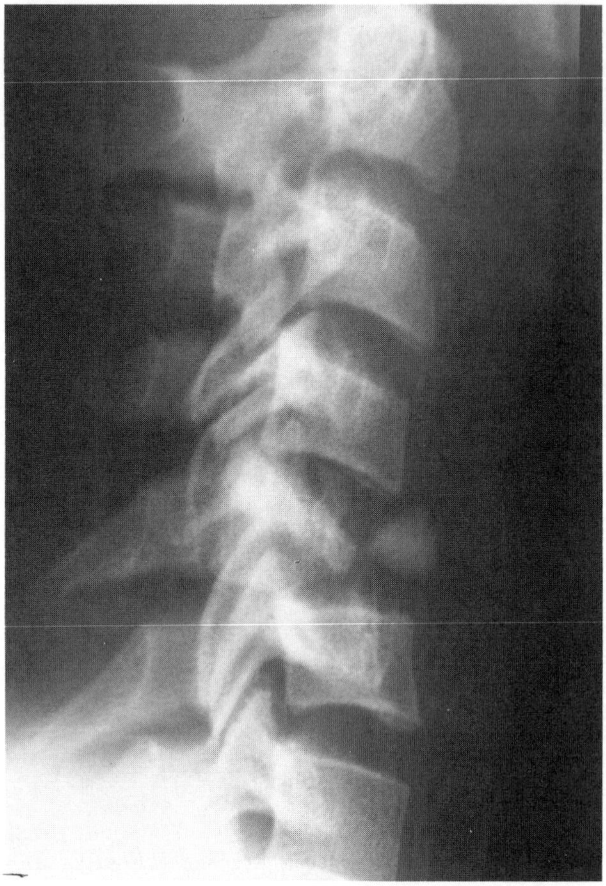

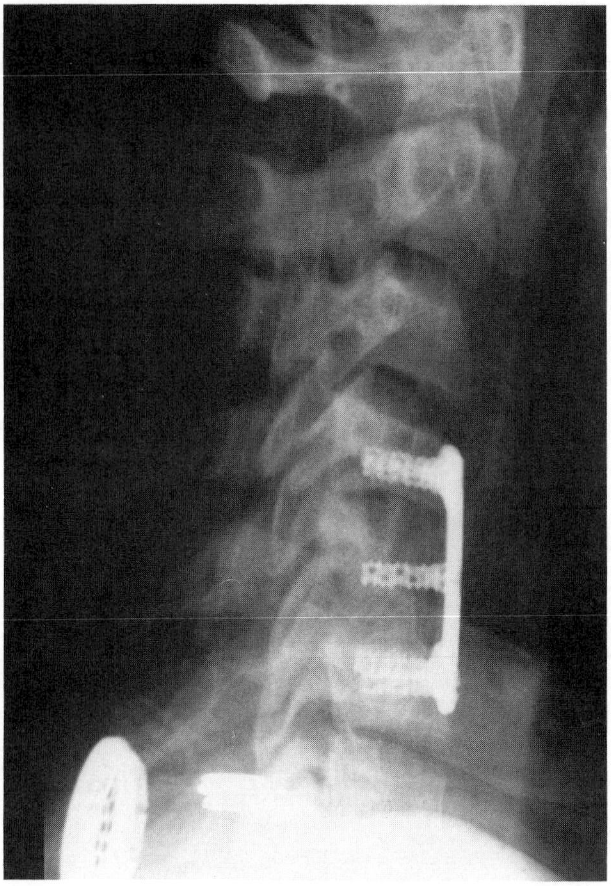

(*A*) (*B*)

Figure 289-4 Preoperative lateral roentgenogram (*A*) and postoperative lateral roentgenogram (*B*) of a 20-year-old male who sustained a severe unstable burst fracture of C5 and a complete transverse cervical myelopathy. The patient underwent anterior microsurgical decompressive corpectomy, fibula allograft reconstruction, and Synthes anterior plate-vertebral body screw fixation that provided improved patient care and facilitated earlier transfer to a spinal cord rehabilitation center. Postoperatively, the patient regained bilateral C6 nerve root function but not spinal cord function.

an onlay mode as when performing a posterior spine fusion. Review of the literature fails to reveal any substantial difference between the bony union rate of allograft bone compared with autograft bone when used for anterior interbody cervical fusion. Hence, we prefer to avoid donor site complications whenever possible.

One additional comment merits consideration; that is, intraoperative radiographic assessment should always be obtained immediately after any bone grafting or internal spinal fixation procedure to verify the satisfactory location and position of the graft and implant(s) as well as the adequacy of the spinal column reconstruction and realignment.

Finally, management of lower cervical spine injuries in patients with ankylosing spondylitis needs to be addressed. Lower cervical spine injuries are the most common spinal injuries suffered by these patients and are often secondary to rather minor trauma. The most common injuries consist of fracture-subluxations secondary to disruption of all three columns. Spinal cord injury is very frequent in these extremely unstable injuries. These patients may be managed by either the initial application of axial traction to carefully reduce the patient to their original deformity followed by early surgical decompression-stabilization,[33] or the initial application of a halo-vest orthosis with careful incremental correction of the deformity followed by halo-vest immobilization for 3 months.[16] Operative decompression-stabilization is required for patients with neurocompressive lesions and operative stabilization-arthrodesis for recurrent or persistent instability.

Conclusion

The optimal management of lower cervical spinal instability requires an extensive knowledge of the anatomy, physiology, biomechanics, pathology, and natural history of injuries of the cervical spinal column, spinal cord, and nerve roots as well as the benefits and limitations of the treatment methods available. Our most important goal should be to prevent these injuries. Short of prevention, recent advances in our understanding of spinal disorders coupled with improved surgical approaches and techniques have substantially increased our ability to optimize the treatment of patients who suffer such spinal instability.

References

1. Beatson R. Fractures and dislocation of the cervical spine. *J Bone Joint Surg [Br]* 1963; 45-B:21–35.
2. Benzel EC, Larson SJ. Recovery of nerve root function after complete quadriplegia from cervical spine fractures. *Neurosurgery* 1986; 19:809–812.
3. Benzel EC, Larson SJ. Functional recovery after decompressive spine operation for cervical spine fractures. *Neurosurgery* 1987; 20:742–746.
4. Bohlman HH. Acute fractures and dislocations of the cervical spine. *J Bone Joint Surg [Am]* 1979; 61-A:1119–1142.
5. Bohlman HH. Later anterior decompression for spinal cord injury: review of 100 cases with long term results. *Orthop Trans* 1980; 4:42–43 (abstr).
6. Braakman R. Some neurological and neurosurgical aspects of injuries of the lower cervical spine. *Acta Neurochir (Wien)* 1970; 22:245–260.
7. Breig A. *Adverse Mechanical Tension in the Central Nervous System.* Stockholm: Almqvist and Wiksell, 1978.
8. Burke CD, Berryman D. The place of closed manipulation in the management of flexion-rotation dislocations of the cervical spine. *J Bone Joint Surg [Br]* 1971; 53-B:165–182.
9. Capen DA, Garland DE, Waters RL. Surgical stabilization of the cervical spine: a comparative analysis of anterior and posterior spine fusions. *Clin Orthop* 1985; 196:229–237.
10. Carol M, Ducker TB, Byrnes DP. Minimyelogram in cervical spinal cord trauma. *Neurosurgery* 1980; 7:219–224.
11. Chan RC, Schweigel JF, Thompson GB. Halo-thoracic brace immobilization in 188 patients with acute cervical spine injuries. *J Neurosurg* 1983; 58:508–515.
12. Cheshire DJ. The stability of the cervical spine following the conservative treatment of fractures and fracture-dislocations. *Paraplegia* 1969; 7:193–203.
13. Cooper PR, Maravilla KR, Sklar FH, et al. Halo immobilization of cervical spine fractures: indications and results. *J Neurosurg* 1979; 50:603–610.
14. Davis D, Bohlman H, Walker EA, et al. The pathological findings in fatal craniospinal injuries. *J Neurosurg* 1971; 34:603–613.
15. Denis F. The three column spine and its significance in the classification of acute thoracolumbar spinal injuries. *Spine* 1983; 8:817–831.
16. Detwiler KN, Loftus CM, Godersky JC, et al. Management of cervical spine injuries in patients with ankylosing spondylitis. *J Neurosurg* 1990; 72:210–215.
17. Ducker TB, Bellegarrique R. Management of the fractured cervical spine. *Contemp Neurosurg* 1982; 4(16):1–8.
18. Epstein N, Epstein JA, Benjamin V, et al. Traumatic myelopathy in patients with cervical spinal stenosis without fracture or dislocation: methods of diagnosis, management, and prognosis. *Spine* 1980; 5:489–496.
19. Evans DK. Anterior cervical subluxation. *J Bone Joint Surg [Br]* 1976; 58-B:318–321.
20. Glaser JA, Whitehill R, Stamp WG, et al. Complications associated with the halo-vest: a review of 245 cases. *J Neurosurg* 1986; 65:762–769.
21. Hadley MN, Fitzpatrick BC, Sonntag VKH, et al. Facet fracture-dislocation injuries of the cervical spine. *Neurosurgery* 1992; 31:661–666.
22. Harrington JF, Likavec MJ, Smith AS. Disc herniation in cervical fracture subluxation. *Neurosurgery* 1991; 29:374–379.
23. Harris JH Jr, Edeiken-Monroe B, Kopaniky DR. A practical classification of acute cervical spine injuries. *Orthop Clin North Am* 1986; 17:15–30.
24. Holdsworth FW. Fractures, dislocations, and fracture-dislocations of the spine. *J Bone Joint Surg [Br]* 1963; 45-B:6–20.
25. Levi L, Wolf A, Rigamonti D, et al. Anterior decompression in cervical spine trauma: does the timing of surgery affect the outcome? *Neurosurgery* 1991; 29:216–222.
26. Maiman DJ, Barolat G, Larson SJ. Management of bilateral locked facets of the cervical spine. *Neurosurgery* 1986; 18:542–547.
27. Marar BC. Hyperextension injuries of the cervical spine: the pathogenesis of damage to the spinal cord. *J Bone Joint Surg [Am]* 1974; 56-A:1655–1662.
28. Morgan TH, Wharton GW, Austin GN. The results of laminectomy in patients with incomplete spinal cord injuries. *Paraplegia* 1971; 9:14–23.
29. Norrell H, Wilson CB. Early antetior fusion for injuries of the cervical portion of the spine. *JAMA* 1970; 214:525–530.
30. O'Brien PJ, Schweigel JF, Thompson WJ. Dislocations of the lower cervical spine. *J Trauma* 1982; 22:710–714.
31. Pierce DS. Spinal cord injury with anterior decompression, fusion, stabilization and early rehabilitiation. *J Bone Joint Surg [Am]* 1969; 51-A:1675 (abstr).
32. Randle MJ, Wolf A, Levi L, et al. The use of anterior Caspar plate fixation in acute cervical spine injury. *Surg Neurol* 1991; 36:181–189.
33. Rowed DW. Management of cervical spinal cord injury in ankylosing spondylitis: the intervertebral disc as a cause of cord compression. *J Neurosurg* 1992; 77:241–246.
34. Schneider RC, Kahn EA. Chronic neurological sequelae of acute trauma to the spine and spinal cord: Part 1. The significance of the acute flexion or "tear drop" fracture-dislocation of the cervical spine. *J Bone Joint Surg [Am]* 1956; 38-A:985–997.
35. Sonntag VKH. Management of bilateral locked facets of the cervical spine. *Neurosurgery* 1981; 8:150–152.
36. Stauffer ES. Neurologic recovery following injuries to the cervical spinal cord and nerve roots. *Spine* 1984; 9:532–534.
37. Stauffer ES. Management of spine fractures C3 to C7. *Orthop Clin North Am* 1986; 17:45–53.
38. Stauffer ES, Kelly EG. Fracture-dislocations of the cervical spine: instability and recurrent deformity following treatment by anterior interbody fusion. *J Bone Joint Surg [Am]* 1977; 59-A:45–48.
39. Verbiest H. Anterolateral operations for fractures and dislocations in the middle and lower parts of the cervical spine. *J Bone Joint Surg [Am]* 1969; 51-A:1489–1530.
40. Wagner FC Jr, Chehrazi B. Early decompression and neurological outcome in acute cervical spinal cord injuries. *J Neurosurg* 1982; 56:699–705.
41. Webb JK, Broughton RBJ, McSweeney T, et al. Hidden flexion injury of the cervical spine. *J Bone Joint Surg [Br]* 1976; 58-B:322–327.
42. White AA III, Johnson RM, Panjabi MM, et al. Biomechanical analysis of clinical stability in the cervical spine. *Clin Orthop* 1975; 109:85–96.
43. White AA III, Panjabi MM. *Clinical Biomechanics of the Spine.* Philadelphia: Lippincott, 1978.
44. Wolf A, Levi L, Mirvis S, et al. Operative management of bilateral facet dislocation. *J Neurosurg* 1991; 75:883–890.

290 Occipitocervical and High Cervical Fusion

Volker K.H. Sonntag
Curtis A. Dickman

Indications for Surgery

Atlantoaxial or occipitocervical fusion is required for a wide spectrum of problems that result in upper cervical instability. Tumors, rheumatoid arthritis, fractures, ligament avulsions, surgery, congenital malformations, infections, and other pathologic conditions can cause instability of the craniovertebral junction. Atlantoaxial instability is manifested by movement beyond the normal range. No anterior or posterior translation of C1 normally occurs; however, there are 40 degrees of unilateral axial rotation, 20 degrees of combined flexion and extension, and 5 degrees of lateral bending.[12,15,61] Clinically, instability appears as subluxation or spinal deformity accompanied by severe pain or neurological deficits.

Translational or rotational instability of C1 can develop. Translational anterior atlantoaxial instability is detected on lateral cervical radiographs as a widened, mobile atlantodental interval (>3 mm). This occurs from laxity or disruption of the transverse atlantal ligament, or from an odontoid fracture.[8,27,61] Posterior translation of C1 can occur if the dens or anterior C1 arch is fractured or incompetent (i.e., os odontoideum). Rotational atlantoaxial instability appears as asymmetric rotation of the C1 lateral masses on plain radiographs. CT shows C1 rotated more than 40 degrees in relation to C2. Rotational subluxations that are irreducible, recurrent, or associated with transverse ligament disruption require surgery.[8,15,16,61]

Steele's "rule of thirds" was formulated to estimate the space available for the spinal cord at the craniovertebral junction.[57] The spinal canal at the C1 level is occupied equally by three components: the odontoid process, the spinal cord, and the subarachnoid space. Each component occupies approximately 1 cm of space. Atlantoaxial subluxations can compress the spinal cord. In instances of acute or chronic instability, even minor trauma can cause permanent paralysis or sudden death.[8,9,15,16,47]

Occipitoatlantal instability is often more difficult to diagnose radiographically than atlantoaxial instability because of the difficulty in identifying landmarks of the skull base.[5] Occipitoatlantal instability is demonstrated radiographically by movement between the dens and basion (i.e., increased dens-basion distance), by distraction or translation of the occipital condyles, or by vertical migration.[5,43]

The normal atlas is relatively rigidly fixed to the occipital condyles and skull base. Twenty-five degrees of flexion plus extension, 5 degrees of axial rotation, and 5 degrees of lateral bending occur between the occiput and C1.[61] C1 tends to move in conjunction with the occiput.[12,15,17] C1 acts as a transition zone, like a "washer," entrapped between the skull base and C2. The transverse ligament and alar ligaments allow C1 and the skull base to rotate around the dens. These ligaments are very strong; they allow a wide range of rotation, yet restrict excessive movement.[12,15,17]

Surgical stabilization is required to correct instability when nonoperative therapy has failed or when spontaneous healing with an orthosis is unlikely. Pure ligamentous injuries, such as transverse ligament disruption or occipitoatlantal dislocations, cannot heal well enough to restore structural support to the craniovertebral junction.[8,9,14–17,48] In contrast, most upper cervical fractures heal satisfactorily with an orthosis, such as a halo brace.[6,16,26,27,35,54,55] Surgery for internal fixation is required for irreducible fractures, fractures that cannot be kept aligned with a rigid cervical orthosis, fractures that have failed to heal (nonunions), or fractures that are at very high risk for nonunion (i.e., widely displaced odontoid type II fractures[27]). Surgery may also be considered for patients who either prefer surgery to a rigid orthosis, or cannot tolerate a rigid orthosis (i.e., because of multiple skull fractures).

Tumors, rheumatoid arthritis, infections, or surgery can cause irreversible instability due to destruction of the bone and ligaments of the craniovertebral junction. In rheumatoid arthritis, atlantoaxial subluxations exceeding 6 mm are at high risk for neurological injury and sudden death, and should be considered for fusion.[47] Patients with rheumatoid arthritis are also at high risk for instability after a transoral decompression, with more than 90 percent of these patients needing fusion.[7]

Selection of an Approach

Several issues must be considered when contemplating surgery for upper cervical instability. Is there just spinal instability, or is there also neural compression? Is neural compression reducible with traction or head positioning, or is decompressive surgery also required? Can decompression and fusion be achieved with one operative approach, or are staged approaches needed? Is there extensive destruction of bone architecture that requires reconstruction? Should the fusion extend to the occiput or just involve the cervical spine? These questions need to be addressed for each patient.

The selection of an operative approach must reflect the patient's medical condition, the specific spinal levels involved, the extent of neurological involvement, the radiologic abnormalities, and the individual pathology. The extent of spinal deformity, the ligament integrity, the bone strength, and the bone architecture influence how extensive a fusion is needed and which techniques can be applied safely.

Anterior or posterior operative approaches can be used to access the craniovertebral junction (Table 290-1). Occipitocervical or atlantoaxial stabilization is best achieved using posterior approaches. Anterior approaches have serious limitations. Transoral bone grafts resist compression but do not provide satisfactory immediate fixation and are at risk for infection.[4,43,56] Anterior C1-C2 facet screw fixation is difficult to perform and bone grafts cannot be added to promote fusion.[10] Odontoid screw fixation is an excellent method to fixate odontoid fractures; this procedure is discussed elsewhere in this textbook. Our chapter focuses on

TABLE 290-1 Surgical Techniques for Fixation of the Craniovertebral Junction

- I. Atlantoaxial Stabilization
  - A. Anterior Approaches
    1. Transoral bone graft
    2. Anterior C1-C2 facet screw fixation
    3. Odontoid screw fixation
  - B. Posterior Approaches
    1. C1-C2 wiring and bone graft
       - a. Interspinous fusion
       - b. Brooks fusion
       - c. Gallie fusion
    2. Posterior C1-C2 facet screws
    3. C1-C2 Halifax clamps
- II. Occipitocervical Stabilization
    1. Wire and bone grafts
    2. Steinmann pin, metal rods
    3. Occipitocervical screw plate

techniques for posterior stabilization of the craniovertebral junction and upper cervical spine.

Neural decompression, spinal reconstruction, and spinal stabilization may all need to be performed. Posterior operative approaches can often achieve these goals in a single operative session. However, when there is instability accompanying irreducible ventral compression of the cervicomedullary junction, then we recommend staged approaches; an anterior approach for neural decompression and a posterior approach for stabilization. Compression of the cervicomedullary junction should be treated first. Instrumenting a stenotic spinal canal can cause neurological injury. When compression is reducible with traction or with head positioning, then only a fusion is needed.

The goals of surgery are to achieve anatomic alignment, to protect the neural elements, and to stabilize the spine, yet preserve the motion of normal spinal segments. Fusions should be confined only to the unstable segments whenever possible. The occiput should not routinely be incorporated into a fusion without a good reason. Increasing the length of a fusion increases the pseudarthrosis rate and causes a loss of normal motion.[14,21,28,31,46,61] Atlantoaxial instability is best treated with a C1-C2 fusion. Adjacent segments are fused only if C1 or C2 cannot be directly fixed and incorporated into a fusion, or if the adjacent segments are unstable.

Rigid external cervical immobilization (i.e., a halo brace) may be required as an adjunct to some forms of internal fixation.[36] Extensive fractures, osteoporotic bone, tumors, long segment fusions, or inadequate internal fixation purchase require supplemental external immobilization to guarantee osseous union. The spine must be temporarily shielded from excessive stress while the fusion becomes mature.

Onlay fusion techniques should only be performed when there is inadequate bone structure for fixation with instrumentation or wires. After onlay grafting, a halo brace is mandatory to provide immobilization while the bone fuses.

Surgical Techniques

Posterior Cervical Exposure and Preparation of the Fusion Site

The posterior craniovertebral junction is accessed with the patient in a prone position on the operating table. The head is fixated with a Mayfield head clamp. If a halo brace was applied preoperatively, a Mayfield head holder adaptor for the halo brace is used (Fig. 290-1). The back plate of the halo vest may be removed if needed to access the iliac crest or posterior occipitocervical region. The surgery is usually performed with the head and neck in a slightly flexed position. Flexing the head facilitates exposure; however, this should be performed carefully, under fluoroscopic monitoring to avoid complications.

A linear posterior cervical incision is extended from the inion to the spinous process of C7. The incision is deepened, with sharp division of the nuchal fascia and posterior cervical muscles in the midline sagittal plane. The posterior arches of C1 and C2 and other segments to be fused are exposed. The occipital squamosa and foramen magnum are exposed if the occiput is to be fused. Gentle dissection technique is used to avoid translocation or displacement of the unstable vertebral segments. Broad-surfaced, lightweight periosteal elevators are used to dissect the suboccipital and paraspinous muscles subperiosteally from the bone surfaces. The muscles are detached from the midline and are swept laterally. The posterior arches of C1 and C2 are exposed widely, but the laterally positioned vertebral arteries are avoided. The soft tissues are meticulously removed from the bone surfaces to facilitate fusion. The ligamentum flavum and posterior occipitoatlantal membrane are removed with sharp curettes to allow safe sublaminar wire passage. The bone surfaces for fusion are segmentally decorticated with a high-speed drill. The decortication exposes bleeding cancellous bone surfaces; however, the bone must not be weakened with excessive drilling. The bone grafts and fusion surfaces must be prepared to maximize the fitting of the grafts. Tight apposition of cancellous bone surfaces promotes fusion.

Proper preparation of the bone surfaces is critical for successful fusion.[14,37] Instrumentation is susceptible to fatigue and can break, even after a fusion has formed. Only a solid osseous union ensures long-term spinal stability. The surgeon must meticulously remove all soft tissue from the fusion site. Soft tissue can form a fibrous tissue interface which creates a pseudarthrosis. All periosteum, fascia, and ligaments are stripped from the surfaces of the bone grafts and from the fusion bed. The articular cartilage should be

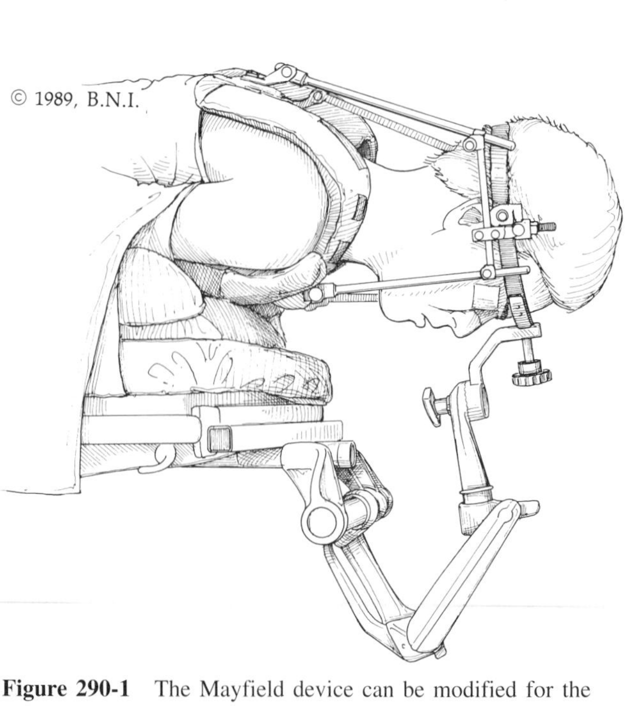

Figure 290-1 The Mayfield device can be modified for the halo brace to stabilize the patient to the operating table.

removed from the articular surfaces whenever possible. Atraumatic dissection technique is used to avoid devascularizing the bone. The segments to be fused are roughened with a high-speed drill to create bleeding bone surfaces. Bone grafts are placed under compression and are fitted precisely. The unstable vertebrae are rigidly and segmentally instrumented.

Autogenous bone grafts are preferred for cervical arthrodesis. Live bone contains active cellular and structural components for bone remodeling, new bone formation, and fusion. Cervical fusions with autograft have a higher union rate than similar procedures using allograft.[13,62] Tricortical or bicortical iliac crest strut grafts provide a mixture of cortical and cancellous bone which provides excellent structural support.[5,11,60,61] Cortical bone is stronger than cancellous bone in resisting tension and compression.[61] Cancellous bone is important because it becomes vascularized rapidly and is better than cortical bone for promoting fusion.[14,37,61] We use autograft struts for reconstruction and cancellous bone fragments to promote fusion. Allograft bone is used only when the patient's bone stock is inadequate.

Methyl methacrylate should be considered only for the patient with a neoplasm who has a short life expectancy.[41] Methacrylate provides only temporary fixation; a pseudocapsule forms around it and it can loosen. It is not incorporated in the bone healing process. It covers the surfaces that could be used for bone fusion. Osseous union should be pursued in all patients capable of long-term survival.

Atlantoaxial Stabilization Methods

Wire and Bone Grafts

Interspinous Fusion

For interspinous fusion,[11] a routine posterior exposure of the atlas and axis is performed. The inferior surface of the ring of C1 and the superior surfaces of the spinous process and laminae of C2 are cleaned of soft tissue and decorticated with a drill or Kerrison rongeur. To seat the wire, notches are made bilaterally in the inferior surfaces of the C2 laminae, where they join the C2 spinous process (Fig. 290-2*A*).

An autologous, curved, tricortical bone graft is obtained from the posterior iliac crest. The rounded upper cortical edge of the graft is removed with a Lexsell rongeur to create a bicortical, curvilinear strut graft (Fig. 290-2*B*). The strut graft is fitted between C1 and C2. A precise fit restores the normal relationship between C1 and C2 posteriorly. This allows reduction and restoration of normal atlantoaxial alignment. The curve of the graft should approximate the curve of the ring of C1. The inferior margin of the bone graft is notched in the midline to match the contour of the spinous process of C2. The graft is temporarily removed to allow wire placement. A braided cable[33,53] or double-stranded, 24-gauge twisted surgical wire, with 2 to 3 turns per centimeter[58] is halved, looped, and passed superiorly beneath the posterior arch of C1 in the midline (Fig. 290-2*C*). The wire must be simultaneously fed and pulled using a two-handed process to avoid traction or manipulation of the atlas and to avoid displacing the wire anteriorly. Next, the graft is repositioned between the atlas and axis. The loop of wire is passed over the ring of C1, behind the graft, and is secured beneath the base of the C2 spinous process. The free ends of the wire are positioned anterior to the graft and passed beneath the spinous process of C2. The wires are tightened, compressing the bone graft between the posterior arches of C1 and C2. The wire is twisted while applying upwardly directed tension. If a braided cable is used, a tensioner is used to tighten the cable and a crimp is used to fixate the cable into its final position (Fig. 290-2*D*).[33,53] The graft is fixed by wire anteriorly and posteriorly and compressed between C1 and C2. The posterior surfaces of C1, C2, and the bone graft are roughened with a drill. Any additional fragments of cancellous bone are packed into the fusion bed. The wound is closed routinely.

Brooks Fusion

In 1978, Brooks and Jenkins described a wedge compression technique of C1-C2 fixation.[2] A modification of this technique has become popular.[22] The atlas and axis are exposed and prepared using routine techniques. The ligamentum flavum adjacent to the C2 laminae is removed completely and the dura is visualized to prevent injury during wire passage. Bilaterally, wires are halved, looped, and passed sublaminar beneath C1 and then beneath C2 (Fig. 290-3*A*). Two rectangular corticocancellous wedges of autologous iliac crest bone are fitted bilaterally between the C1 ring and C2 laminae. The bone grafts are positioned into the interlaminar space on each side. The wires on each side are tightened dorsal to the grafts thereby compressing and fixing the grafts (Fig. 290-3*B*). The fusion site is decorticated with a drill. The wounds are closed routinely.

Gallie Fusion

In 1937, Gallie referred to the principle of performing a cervical fusion using wires and bone grafts; however, he did not publish the details of his wiring technique.[18,19] Several authors have referred to a midline wiring technique for C1-C2 and have named this the "Gallie fusion."[16,23,42,50] A 5- to 8-mm thick unicortical bone graft is harvested from the iliac crest and shaped into a modified "H." The graft is positioned dorsal to the C1 arch. The inferior notch of the "H" is fitted to straddle the C2 spinous process. The graft is removed and the wiring is performed.

Wire or braided cable is halved, looped, and passed sublaminar at C1, directed superiorly (Fig. 290-4*A*). The loop is fixed beneath the C2 spinous process. Next, the graft is positioned behind the wire loop (Fig. 290-4*B*). The free ends of the wire at C1 are wrapped behind the graft to hold the graft in position (Fig. 290-4*C*). A routine wound closure is performed.

Results of Posterior Wire and Bone Grafts

Traditionally, wire and bone grafts have been the most popular methods for atlantoaxial internal fixation and arthrodesis. These techniques are relatively safe and reasonably reliable. Wire, without grafts, should not be used because (1) overreduction can occur, (2) fusion is not promoted, and (3) the wire can fatigue and break.

Clinically, the different C1-C2 wiring techniques have fusion rates ranging from 75 to 95 percent.[2,11,16,22,42,46,47] The pathologic process causing the atlantoaxial instability influences the fusion rate. Patients with rheumatoid arthritis have a high nonunion rate with any technique.[2,47] The different distributions of pathology in each series account for the variability in fusion rates.

Biomechanically, wire and bone grafts provide semirigid fixation of C1-C2. Moderate translation and rotation can occur in

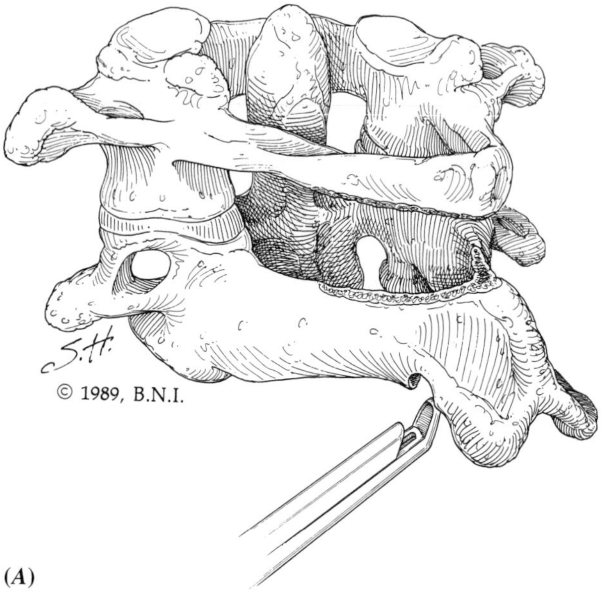

(*A*)

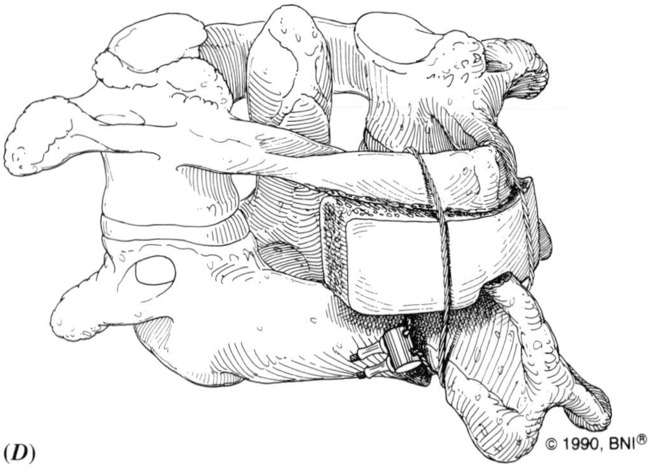

(*D*)

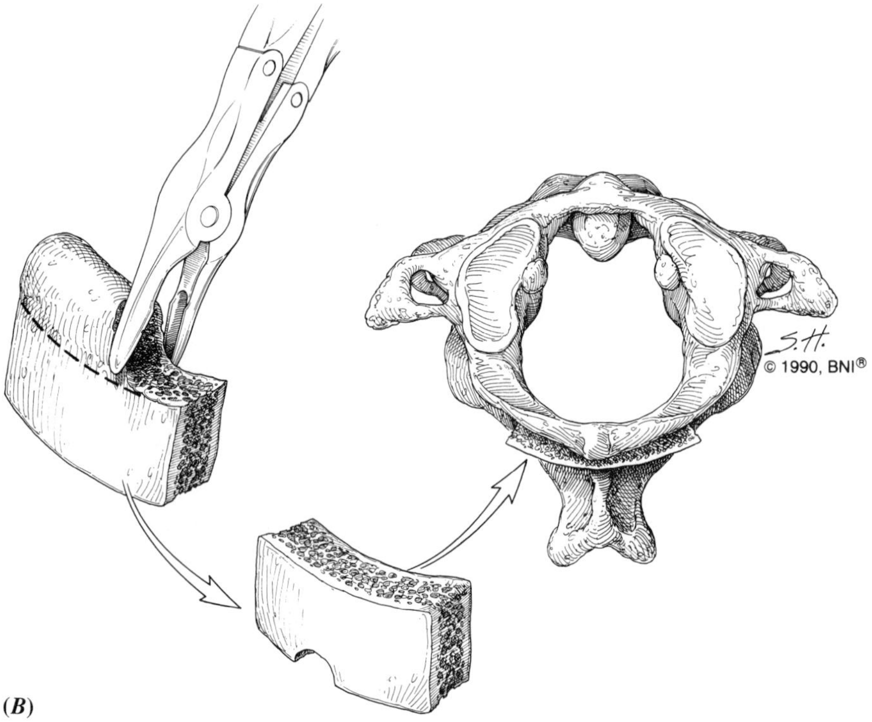

(*B*)

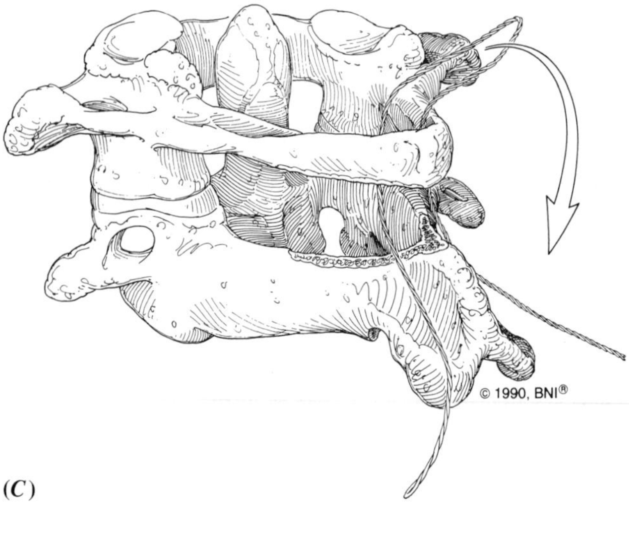

(*C*)

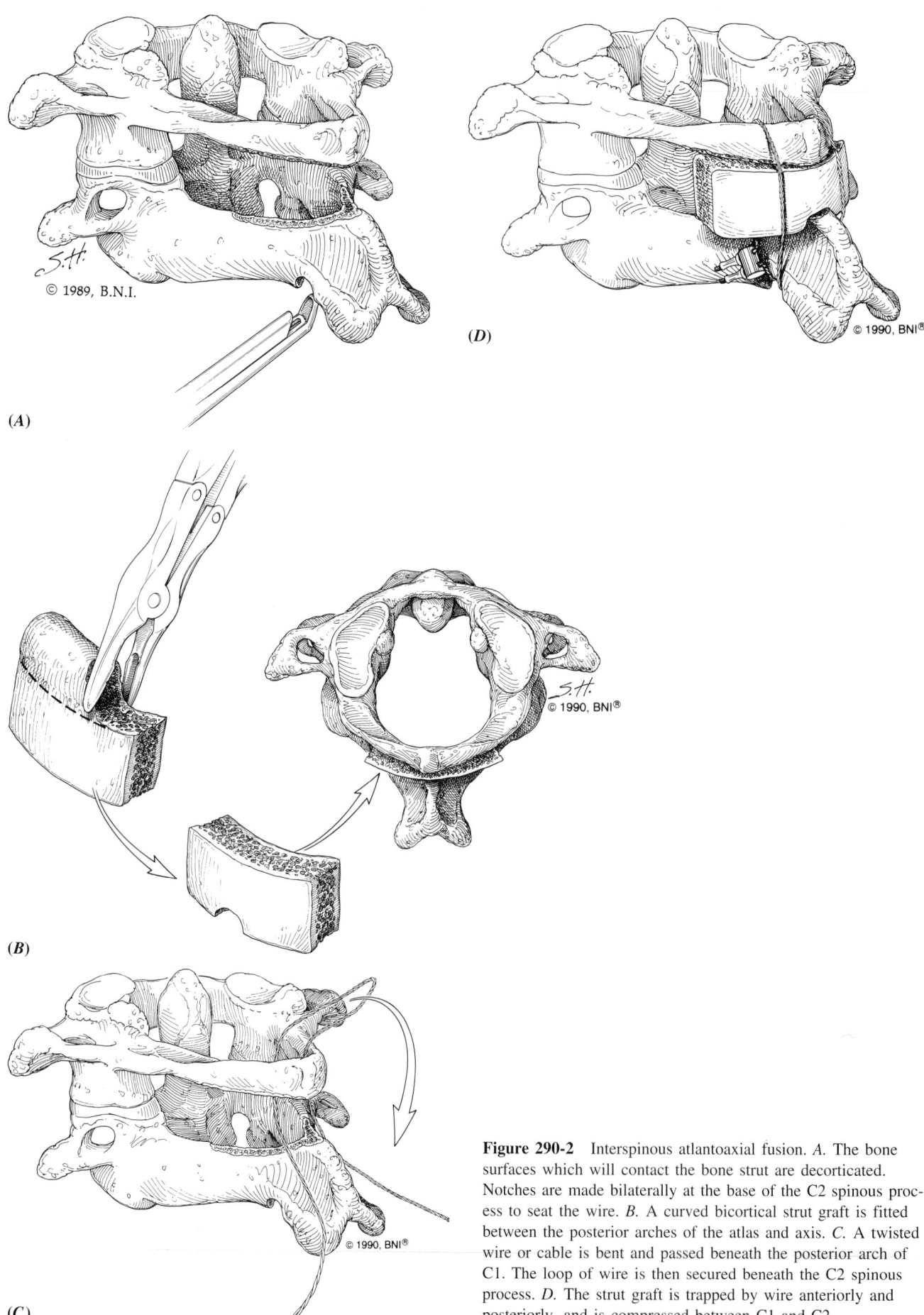

Figure 290-2 Interspinous atlantoaxial fusion. *A.* The bone surfaces which will contact the bone strut are decorticated. Notches are made bilaterally at the base of the C2 spinous process to seat the wire. *B.* A curved bicortical strut graft is fitted between the posterior arches of the atlas and axis. *C.* A twisted wire or cable is bent and passed beneath the posterior arch of C1. The loop of wire is then secured beneath the C2 spinous process. *D.* The strut graft is trapped by wire anteriorly and posteriorly, and is compressed between C1 and C2.

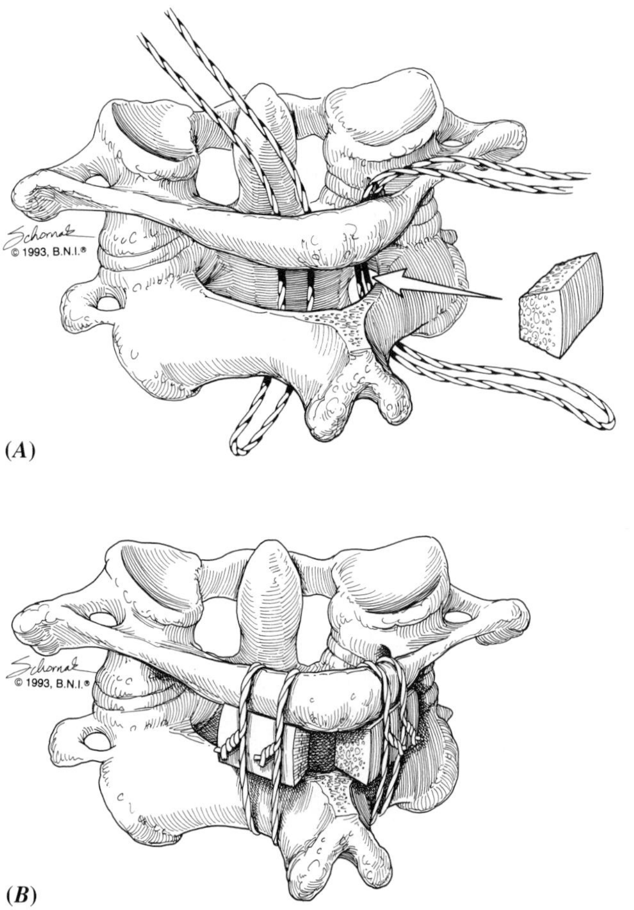

(*A*)

(*B*)

Figure 290-3 Brooks wedge compression technique. *A.* Wires are halved and passed sublaminar beneath C1 and C2. Bilaterally, wedges of bone are compressed between C1 and C2. *B.* The wires are twisted to fixate C1, C2, and the grafts. Two wires fixate each graft.

wired specimens.[23,29,44] In vitro biomechanical studies have demonstrated that the Gallie technique allows significantly more rotation than the Brooks technique for C1-C2 fixation.[23,29] However, both techniques provided stiffness that exceeded the normal and pathologic movement of C1.[23,29] Because the fixation with wire at C1-C2 is moderate, the fusion rate with wiring techniques can be improved by supplementing the internal fixation with a halo brace.[11]

The interspinous method of atlantoaxial fusion was developed to overcome the disadvantages of the Brooks and Gallie methods.[11] The bicortical strut graft and wiring construct provides translational and rotational stability. The graft is compressed between the arches of C1 and C2 to prevent overreduction and to promote fusion. This technique, unlike the Brooks or Gallie method, can be used when C1 is posteriorly dislocated, and requires only one sublaminar wire passage at C1, thus minimizing the risk of neurological injury. Among 74 cases treated with the interspinous method, an 86 percent fusion rate was obtained (Table 290-2).

Posterior Atlantoaxial Facet Screw Fixation

This technique, developed by Friedrich Magerl, achieves rigid C1-C2 fixation by placing a bone screw through each C2 pedicle,

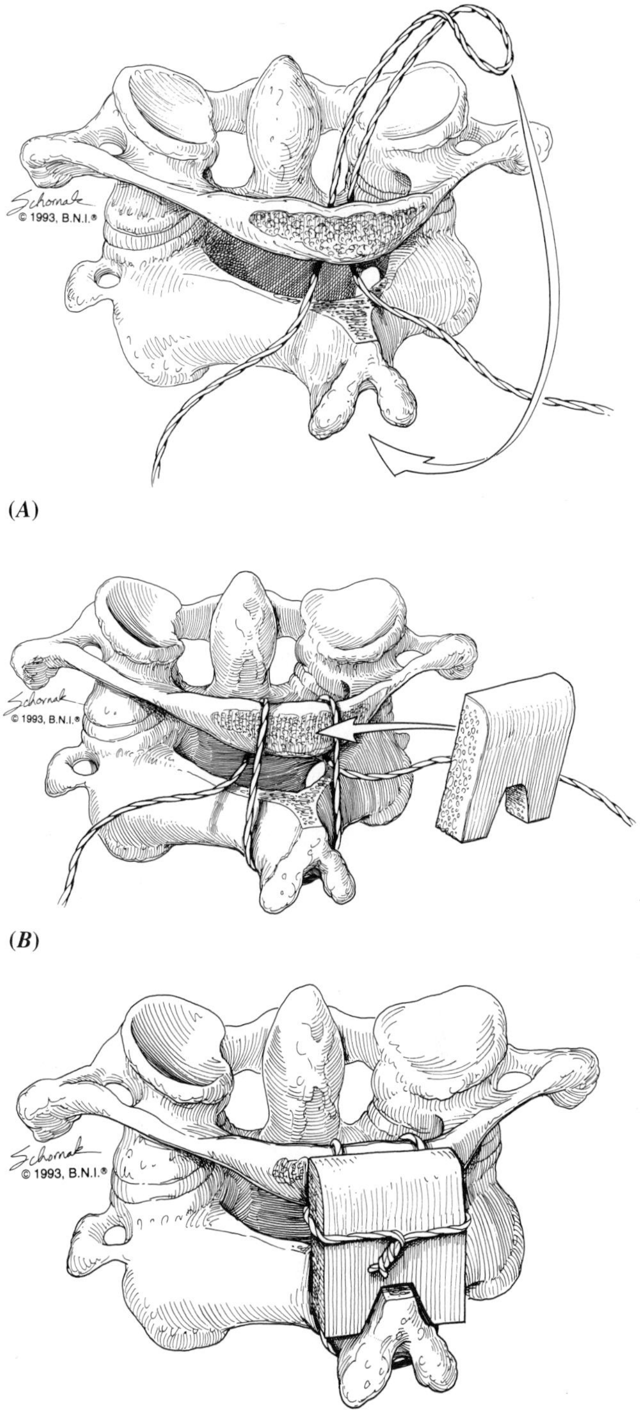

(*A*)

(*B*)

(*C*)

Figure 290-4 Gallie technique. *A.* A wire is halved and passed beneath C1. The loop of wire is secured beneath the C2 spinous process. *B.* An unicortical graft is notched to fit over the C2 spinous process, behind the C1 ring. *C.* The free ends of the wire are wrapped behind the graft for fixation.

across the C1-C2 facet, and into the C1 lateral mass.[25,34,40] Before posterior atlantoaxial screw fixation is attempted, the morphology of the atlas and axis must be studied carefully with CT. Comminuted fractures of C1 or C2 or an anomalous course of the vertebral artery contraindicate screw fixation. Subluxations should be reducible with positioning. Atlantoaxial alignment must be restored to be able to perform C1-C2 screw fixation satisfactorily.

TABLE 290-2 Pathology and Results of 74 Patients Treated with Interspinous Atlantoaxial Fusion*

Etiology of Instability	Total	Osseous Union	Fibrous Union	Non-union	Periop-erative Deaths
Unstable C2 fractures	16	16	—	—	—
Unstable C1-C2 combination fractures	12	12	—	—	—
Rheumatoid arthritis	28	18	4	4	2
Os odontoideum	8	7	—	1	—
Transverse ligament disruption	6	6	—	—	—
Tumor	4	3	—	1	—
Total	74	62	4	6	2

*Mean follow-up 31 months, range 12 to 57 months.

The superior facets of C2 and lateral masses of C1 must be properly aligned to provide an adequate screw purchase.

Intraoperatively, controlled flexion of the patient's neck facilitates the proper drill trajectory (Fig. 290-5). The patient's head is affixed with a Mayfield skull clamp and the patient is placed in the prone position. Lateral fluoroscopic visualization with a C-arm is used to avoid increasing the atlantoaxial dislocation during positioning and to monitor the drilling and screw placement. If a long incision or percutaneous access is required for drilling, the skin preparation should extend to the upper thoracic levels. A routine posterior cervical incision is made to expose the atlas and axis. The atlas and axis are realigned by manual reduction. With anterior atlantoaxial subluxations, C2 is gently displaced anteriorly and C1 is pulled posteriorly. Opposite forces are applied for posterior C1 subluxations. A wire is placed around the ring of C1 for traction and for subsequent bone graft fixation. Traction can be applied to C2 with an Allis clamp attached to the C2 spinous process. The C2 spinous process can be retracted toward the occiput to improve the drill trajectory.

The ligamentum flavum adjacent to the C2 laminae and pedicles must be removed to visualize each C2 pedicle and the C1-C2 articular surfaces. A number four Penfield dissector or a thin Kirschner wire (K-wire) is placed directly along the surface of the C2 pedicle into the atlantoaxial facet joint. The K-wire or dissector is used to retract the C2 nerve root upward to allow direct visualization of the C2 pedicle and the atlantoaxial facet joint.

The drill enters the posterior C2 cortex 2 to 3 mm above the C2-C3 facet, and 2 to 3 mm lateral to the medial edge of the C2-C3 facet. The cortical bone is first penetrated using a high-speed drill or bone awl to precisely direct the drill for the pilot hole. Lateral fluoroscopic monitoring is used while the pilot hole is made. The drill trajectory is aimed toward the dorsal cortex of the anterior arch of C1 (Fig. 290-6*A*). The drill is directed through the central axis of the C2 pedicle. An axial trajectory of 0 to 10 degrees medially is required (Fig. 290-6*B*). A 3.5-mm diameter Synthes cortical screw system (Synthes Maxillofacial/Spine, Paoli, PA) is used. The pilot hole is prepared using a 2.5-mm diameter drill. If percutaneous drilling is needed, a 9-in. long, calibrated, 2.4-mm diameter guide pin is used. The pin is threaded along the distal 1 cm of the shaft for drilling. The smooth shaft of the guide pin will not entangle the soft tissues (Fig. 290-6*C*).

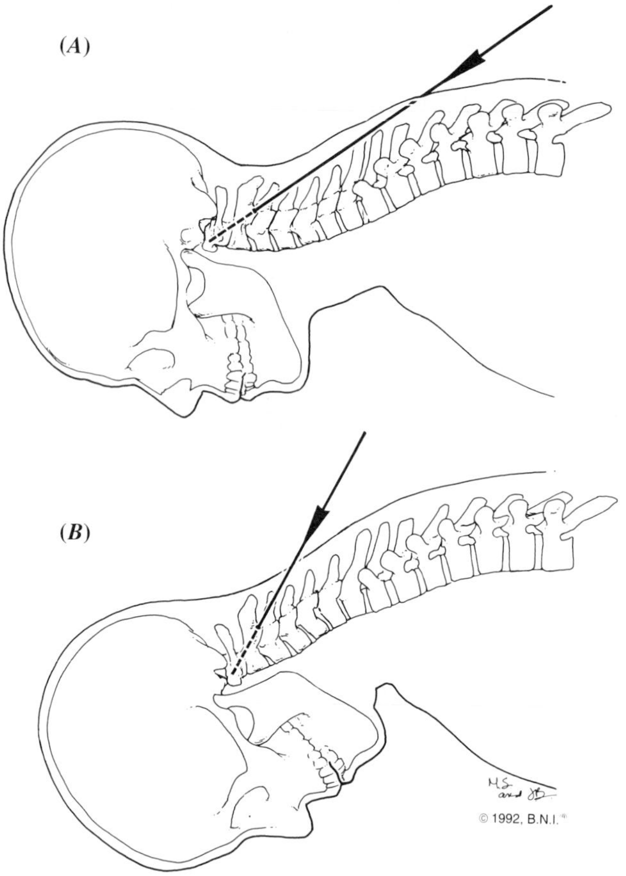

Figure 290-5 The intraoperative position of the neck determines the method needed for drilling the posterior atlantoaxial facet screws. *A.* Percutaneous drilling is performed when the neck cannot be flexed. *B.* Neck flexion permits drilling directly through the neck incision used to expose C1 and C2.

A 3.5-mm diameter cortical bone screw is inserted into the pilot hole. A screw length between 35 and 45 mm is required, depending on the size of the vertebrae. As the screws cross the joint space into C1, the atlas and axis become rigidly coupled. The hole can be tapped to cut the screw thread pattern into the bone if desired. Satisfactory fixation can be achieved using a minimum number of operative steps by inserting the screw directly into the hole without tapping the hole. Tapping does not improve the pullout strength of screws for spinal fixation.[38]

Figure 290-6 (*Opposite*) Posterior atlantoaxial facet screw fixation. *A.* Lateral fluoroscopic imaging is used to direct the drill and screw trajectories toward the dorsal cortex of the anterior arch of C1. *B.* A trajectory of 0 to 10 degrees medially is required to place the screws through the central axis of the C2 pedicle. The vertebral artery is preserved by avoiding a lateral drill trajectory. *C.* A 3.5-mm diameter cortical bone screw is used for fixation. The pilot hole is drilled with a 2.5-mm diameter cylindrical bit. A partially threaded, calibrated, 9-in. long guide pin (*center*) can be used for percutaneous drilling.
D. The screws enter the C2 inferior facet, just above the C2-C3 facet joint. The C2 nerve root and venous plexus are retracted superiorly during drilling. *E.* Lateral radiograph. *F.* A wired bone strut provides three-point mechanical stabilization and facilitates fusion.

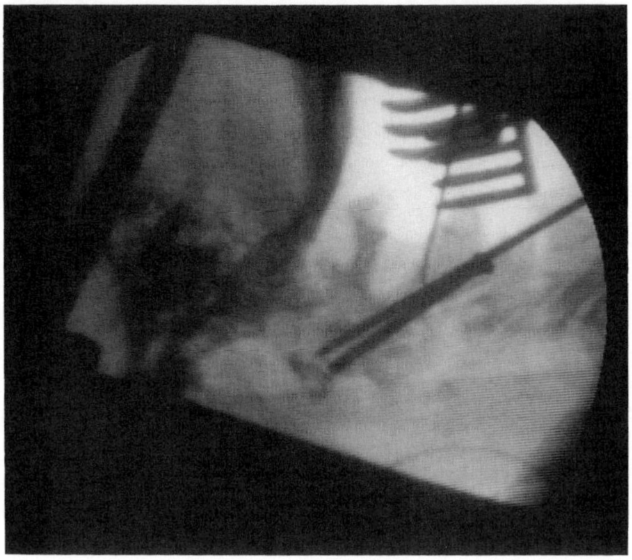

(*A*)

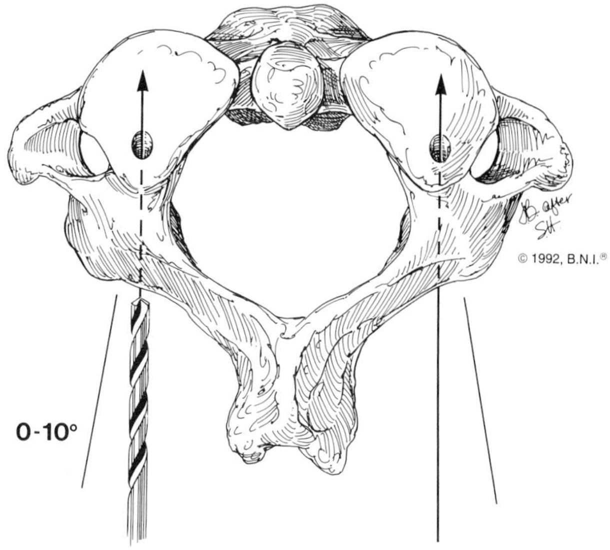

(*B*)

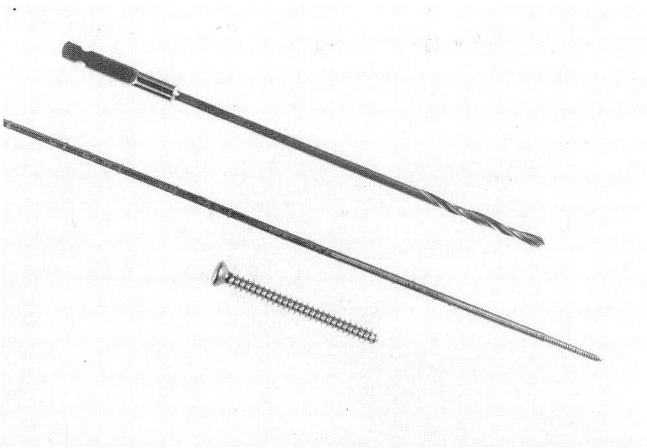

(*C*)

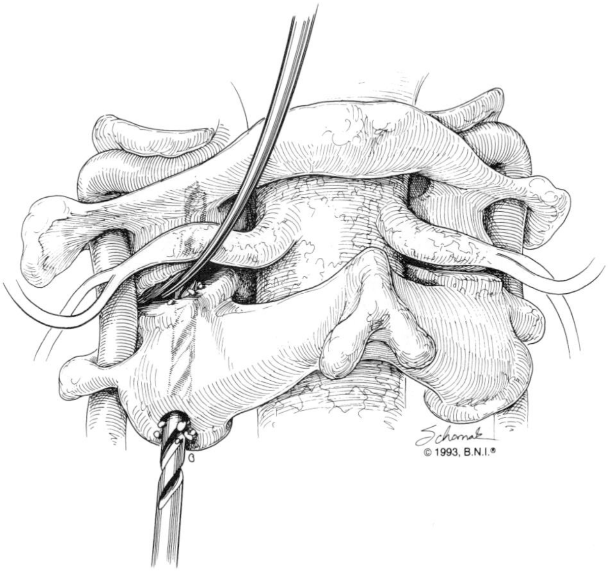

(*D*)

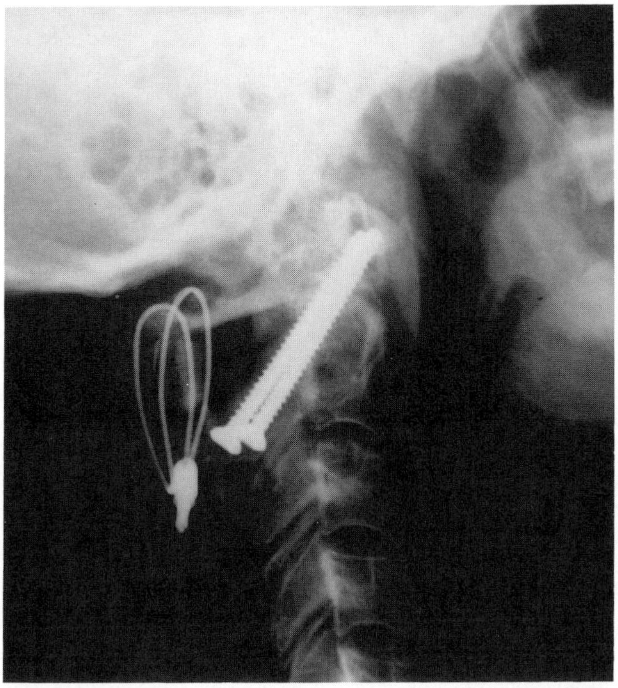

(*E*)

Figure 290-6

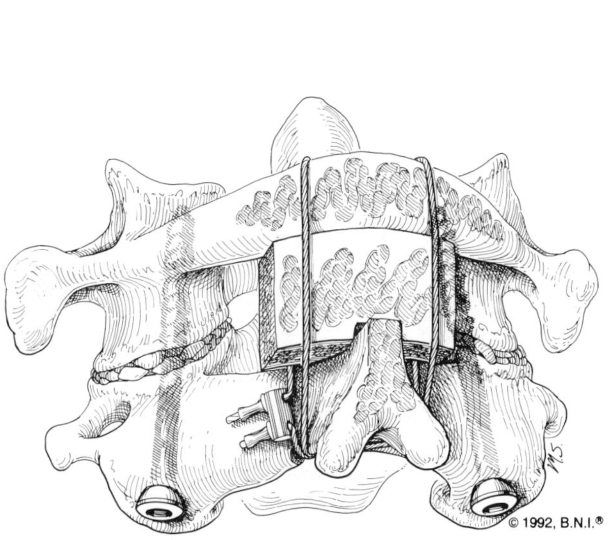

(*F*)

If a lag effect is desired to compress the C1-C2 facet joint, it can be achieved by overdrilling the proximal bone of C2, or by using a partially threaded 4.0-mm diameter cancellous bone screw. The screw threads should not cross the joint space.

The C1-C2 facet screws are supplemented with a wired interspinous bone strut to promote fusion (Fig. 290-6*F*). The bone graft, which is compressed between the posterior arches of C1 and C2, facilitates the formation of a solid fusion and provides additional fixation. Three-point fixation of C1-C2 (with the two screws and the wired graft) provides greater mechanical stability than either technique used alone.[10,23,30] If the posterior arches of C1 or C2 are fractured, wiring is not performed but bone grafts are still added. Posterior atlantoaxial facet screws rigidly couple the facets of the atlas and axis and provide immediate segmental fixation. Because of the rigid coupling of C1 and C2, a postoperative halo

TABLE 290-3 Results Among 18 Patients Treated with Posterior Atlantoaxial Facet Screw Fixation

Etiology of Instability*	Osseous Union†	Complications‡
Unstable C2 fractures	6	—
Unstable C1-C2 combination fractures	1	—
Rheumatoid arthritis	6	—
Os odontoideum	2	—
Transverse ligament disruption	1	—
Tumor	2	1

*Four patients had nonunions of prior C1-C2 graft procedures.
†Mean follow-up 12 months, range 6–16 months.
‡Died 3 months postoperatively from metastatic tumor with an intact spinal fixation.

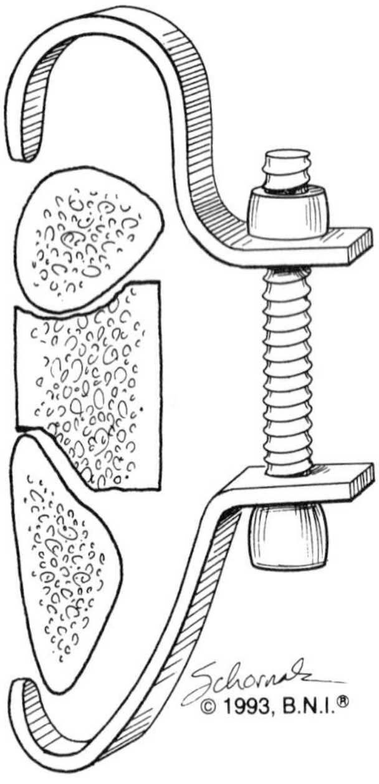

(*A*)

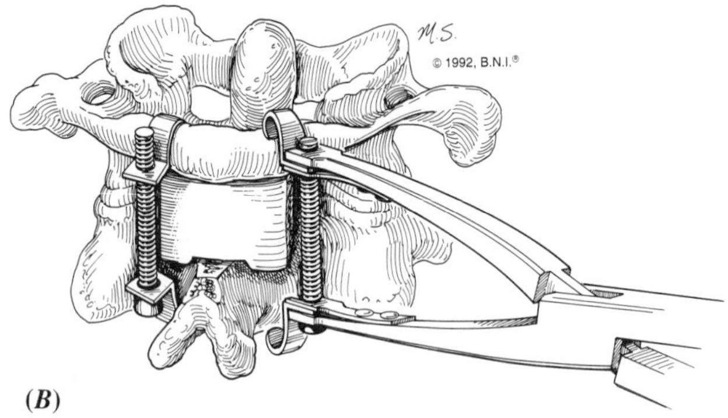

(*B*)

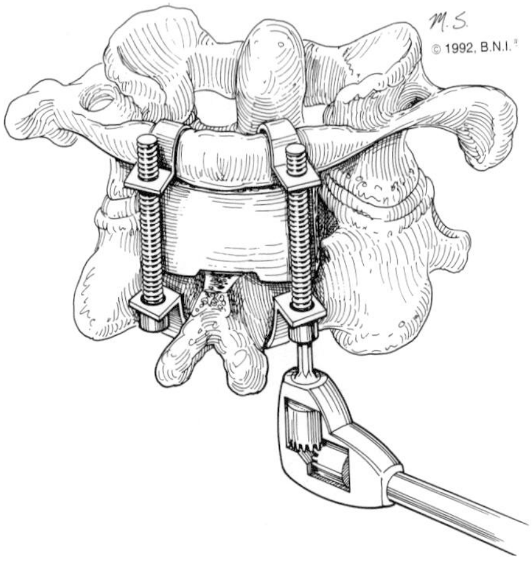

(*C*)

Figure 290-7 Halifax clamps. *A*. The clamps for C1 and subaxial levels have different profiles to conform to the shape of the bone surfaces. *B*. A bone strut is used to prevent hyperextension and inhibit rotation. Clamp applicator forceps are used to hold and position the clamps. *C*. A 90 degree-angled wrench is used to tighten the screws.

brace is unnecessary. Facet screws are biomechanically superior to wire or Halifax clamps for prohibiting atlantoaxial rotation and translation.[23,30,44]

This is an excellent method of fixation but requires meticulous technique to avoid complications. We have had no major complications and no failures of treatment among 18 patients (Table 290-3). Experience with screw fixation techniques is a prerequisite. Careful preoperative planning and precise screw trajectories are mandatory to avoid injury to the vertebral artery or neural structures. Facet screws are especially useful after a laminectomy has been performed, after a C1-C2 wiring procedure has failed, or when a maximally rigid fixation of C1-C2 is required.

Halifax Interlaminar Clamp Fixation

Halifax interlaminar clamps were designed by Tucker, and subsequently reported by Holness et al. in 1984.[1,32,45] They are used for posterior atlantoaxial fixation using a standard posterior cervical exposure. Several hook sizes and shapes are available. The clamps for C1 have a semicircular profile. The clamps for subaxial levels are hook-shaped to fit beneath the lamina (Fig. 290-7*A*). An upper clamp is sized to fit around the posterior ring of C1. The lower clamp is fitted beneath the lamina of C2. The clamp is preassembled with a screw and mounted on a clamp applicator forceps. Laminotomies are performed so that the clamps fit the bone surfaces precisely. Since the hooks extend along the undersurface of the laminae, the ligamentum flavum is removed to prevent neural compression. An interspinous strut graft or two wedges of bone are positioned between the posterior arches of C1 and C2 to prevent hyperextension and limit rotation (Fig. 290-7*B*).[45] The clamps are tightened using a 90 degree-angled wrench (Fig. 290-7*C*). The site should be inspected to ensure that the clamps engage the laminae securely and that the hooks are seated properly.

Halifax clamps are easy to apply. They provide mechanical stability comparable to the Brooks wiring technique. They are not as rigid as C1-C2 facet screws.[45] Unilateral clamps have reduced rotational stability and should not be used. Clamps should also be used with bone struts to prevent excessive rotation and extension of C1. Screw loosening and clamp displacement have been reported.[1,32,45] Subsequently, the clamp design was modified to alleviate this problem. Care must be used to avoid neural compression since hooks are placed beneath the C2 laminae and C1 ring.

Occipitocervical Fusion Techniques

Occipitocervical fusion is performed using a posterior cervical exposure. The patient positioning, preparation, and incisions are identical to the techniques for atlantoaxial fusion. In contrast, however, the osseous exposure is more extensive and involves subperiosteal dissection of the squamous portion of the occipital bone, the rim of the foramen magnum, and the cervical vertebrae to be fused.

Wiring Techniques

Wire is best fixed where the occipital bone is thick since the occipital squamous is thin laterally and wire can easily pull through the bone. The midline crest, the bone near the nuchal line, or the bone adjacent to the foramen magnum provides an excellent site for wire fixation. To prepare the occiput adjacent to the foramen magnum for wiring, the posterior rim of the foramen magnum is enlarged with a Kerrison rongeur. Two burr holes are placed into the occipital bone, 0.5 cm superior to the rim of the foramen magnum (Fig. 290-8). The burr holes are waxed for hemostasis and the dura is separated from the inner table of the skull using dural elevators. Several alternative techniques can be used for wiring the cervical levels. The C1 ring can be wired or the posterior elements of C2 to C7 can be fixated with wire attached to the spinous processes, the laminae, or the facets.

Spinous process wiring is a versatile technique.[28,31,33,50,60] A drill hole is made in the base of the spinous processes. The hole is completed with a towel clip. Twenty-gauge wire is looped through the hole and around the base of the adjacent spinous process. Segmental fixation is achieved by wiring two bone graft struts to the spinous processes (Fig. 290-9).

Sublaminar wires can be used to fixate rod constructs or bone struts.[5,39,46,49,52,53] Laminotomies must be performed and the ligamentum flavum must be completely removed to safely pass

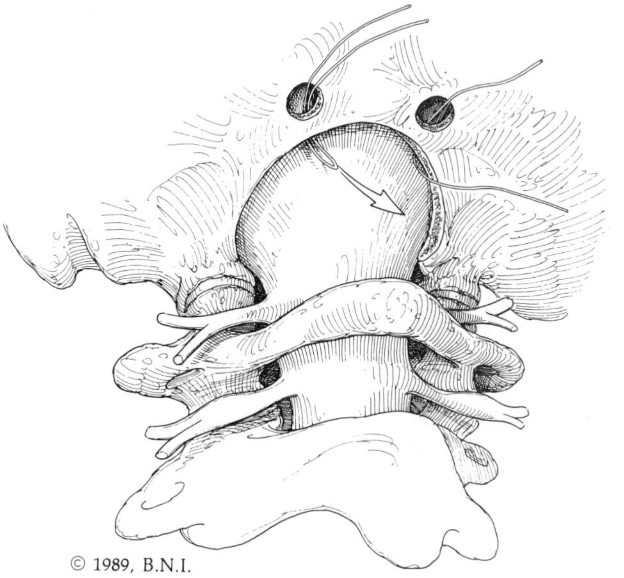

Figure 290-8 The occiput can be wired after enlarging the dorsal rim of the foramen magnum. Two burr holes are placed in the occiput adjacent to the foramen magnum. The dura is elevated prior to wire passage.

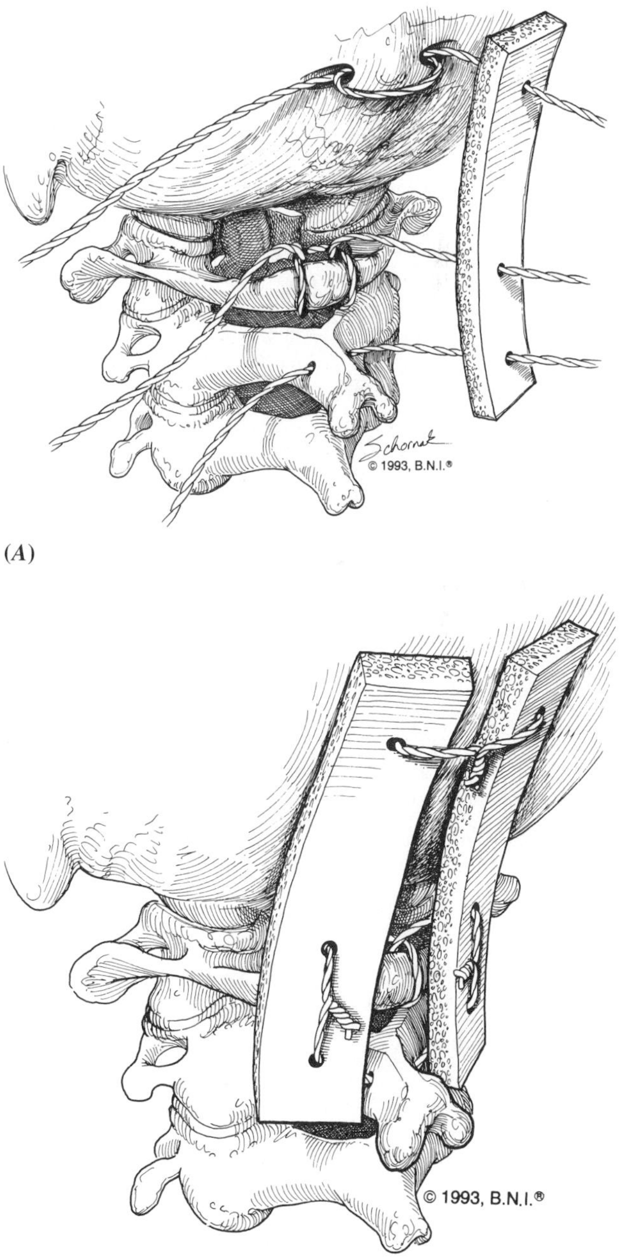

(*B*)

Figure 290-9 Occipitocervical fusion. *A*. Bone struts are wired to the occiput and cervical vertebrae. *B*. The wire is threaded through holes in the grafts, and tightened to compress the grafts against the fusion surfaces.

sublaminar wires. There is a risk of neurological injury with sublaminar wire passage, especially in the middle and lower cervical spine. Notches are made in the lamina where the wire is to be passed (Fig. 290-10*A*). The dura is directly visualized during wire passage. The distal end of the wire is contoured so that it can hug the undersurface of the lamina. The wire is passed using a two-handed process, simultaneously feeding and pulling the wire (Fig. 290-10*B*). The wire is positioned laterally against cortical bone for a strong purchase.

Facet wires are useful after a laminectomy has been performed.[3,20] Since the cervical facets are thin, facet wires are weaker than sublaminar wires. However, facet wires avoid the risk of neurological injury associated with sublaminar wires. The articular surface of the facet joint is opened and roughened with a small curette. The joint is held open with a Penfield instrument. A drill hole is made at a 90-degree angle to the inferior facet, entering the joint. Twenty-gauge monofilament wire or double-stranded 24-gauge twisted wire is passed through the hole (Fig. 290-11).

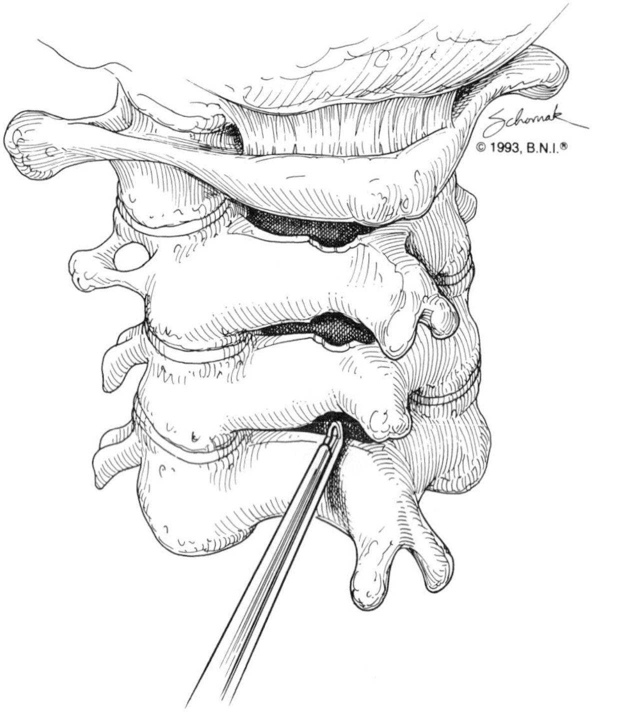

(*A*)

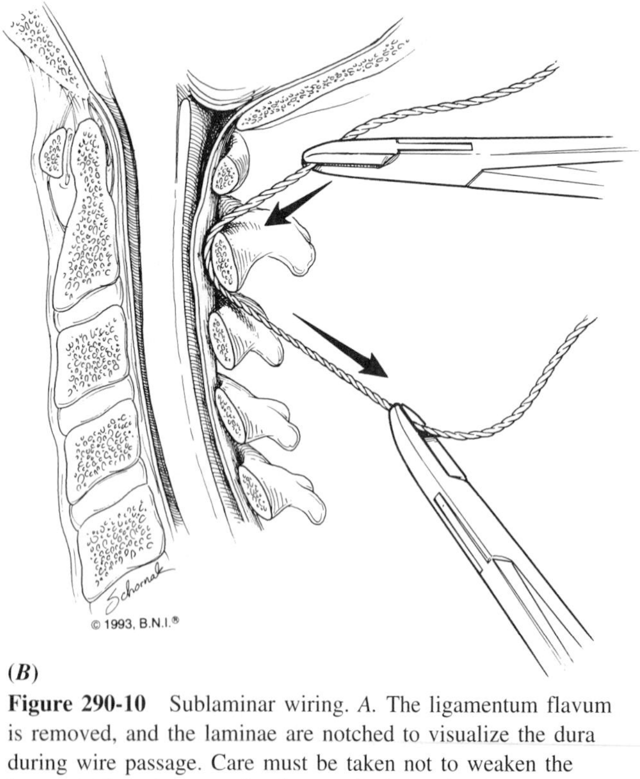

(*B*)

Figure 290-10 Sublaminar wiring. *A*. The ligamentum flavum is removed, and the laminae are notched to visualize the dura during wire passage. Care must be taken not to weaken the bone. *B*. The wires are simultaneously fed and pulled during passage to prevent neural compression.

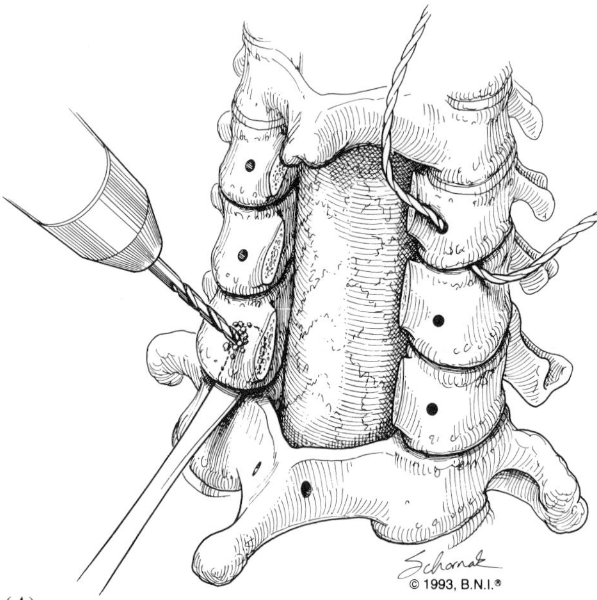

(*A*)

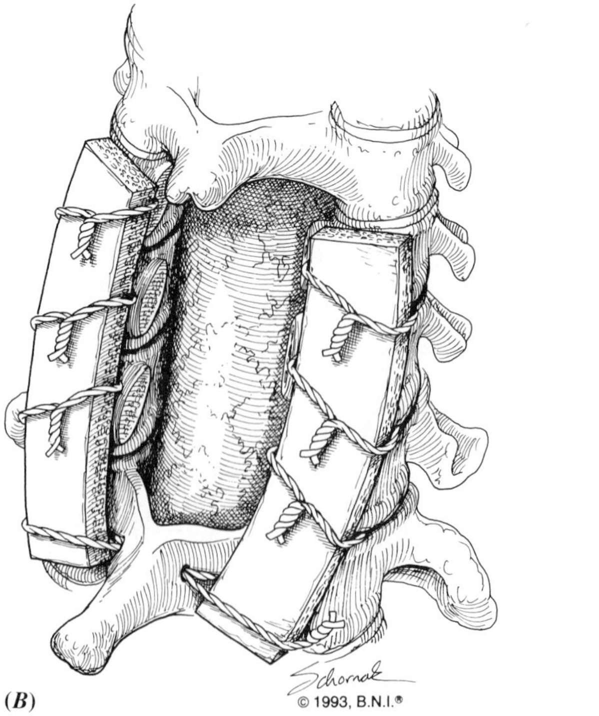

(*B*)

Figure 290-11 Facet wiring. *A*. The facet joints are opened and the articular cartilage is removed. A drill hole is made into the facet joint. Wires are passed through the hole. *B*. Bone grafts are wired to the facets.

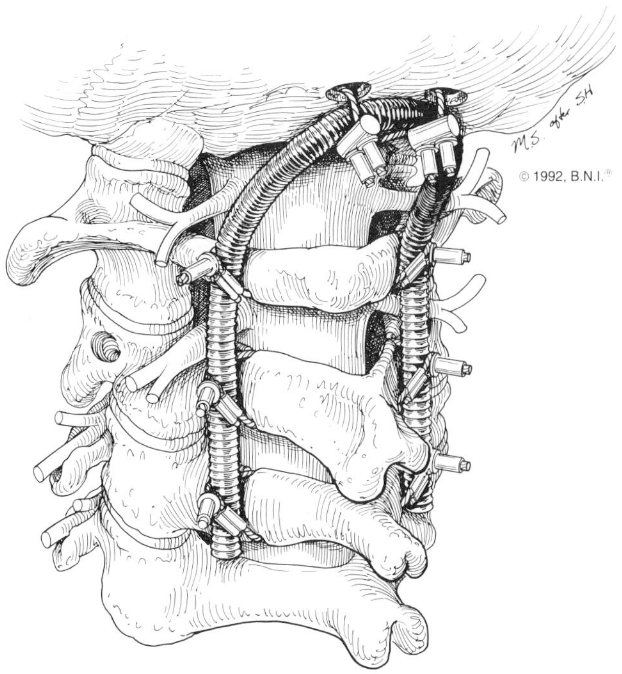

(*A*)

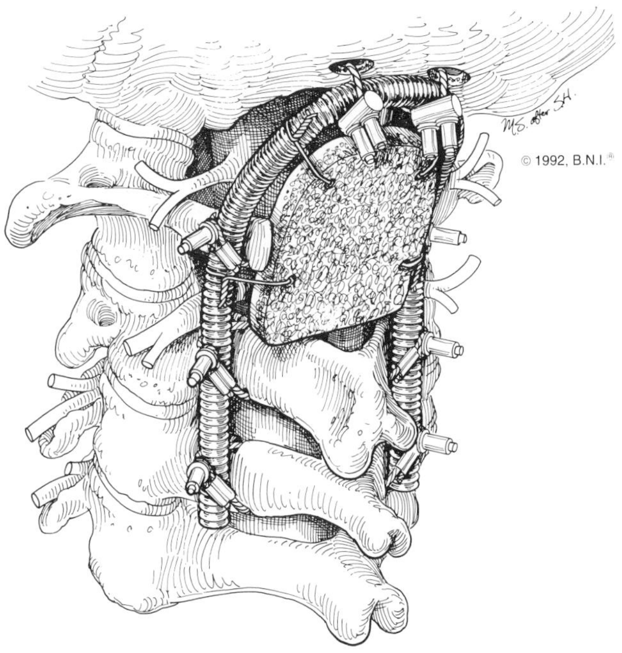

(*B*)

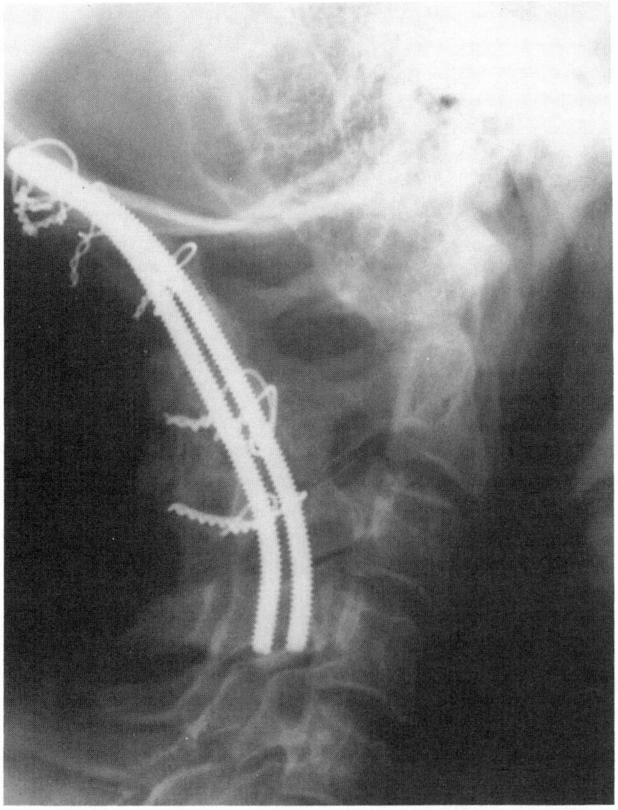

(*C*)

Figure 290-12 Occipitocervical fixation with a threaded Steinmann pin ($\frac{5}{32}$ in. diameter). *A.* The pin is smoothly contoured to avoid stress risers. The threads of the pin prevent settling of the fixation. *B.* When a suboccipital decompression or cervical laminectomy has been performed, a bone plate is wired to the pin to preserve the decompression site. *C.* Lateral cervical radiograph demonstrates a well-formed osseous union, 3 months postoperatively.

Bone struts or contoured metal rods can be fixed with wire for occipitocervical stabilization. Iliac crest or rib struts provide initial stabilization and subsequently promote fusion. The fixation of bone struts, however, is semirigid. The bone grafts can fracture if excessive force is applied prior to healing. Therefore, a halo brace or some other cervical orthosis is needed until a fusion occurs. Metal rods or screw plates have been used to provide immediate rigid fixation for occipitocervical fusion.[4,5,24,39,49,51,52] Metal implants must be supplemented with bone grafts to ensure fusion.

Steinmann Pin Fusion

A wide diameter ($\frac{5}{32}$ in.), *threaded* Steinmann pin is bent into a ''U'' shape. Secondary curves are fashioned with bending irons so that the pin fits the lordotic contour of the occipitocervical region. The bends of the pin should be smooth. Sharp angles create stress risers where the pin may fatigue and fracture. The pin is cut so that the ends do not extend beyond the fused segments. After the Steinmann pin is contoured to the desired curvature and length, it is wired against the occiput and against the cervical lamina or facets (Fig. 290-12*A*).[5,54] The pin should contact all bone surfaces. Gaps between the pin and lamina will result in inadequate fixation of the vertebra.

Cortical and cancellous bone grafts for fusion are obtained from the iliac crest. The occiput and posterior surfaces of the cervical levels to be fused are decorticated with a high-speed air drill. Cancellous bone grafts are compressed against the levels to be fused. When a suboccipital craniotomy or cervical laminectomy has been performed, a plate of cortical iliac crest bone is wired to the central portion of the Steinmann pin (Fig. 290-12*B*). This bone plate provides a template for the fusion to develop and preserve the dural decompression. A routine multilayered wound closure is performed.

TABLE 290-4 Results of Occipitocervical Fusion with a Threaded Steinmann Pin*

Pathology	No.	Osseous Unions	Fibrous Unions	Non-unions†	Postoperative Deaths	Instrument Complications‡
Rheumatoid arthritis	11	9	2	—	—	2
Congenital anomalies	8	7	—	—	1	—
Occipitoatlantal dislocations	3	3	—	—	—	—
Fractures	4	4	—	—	—	—
Tumor	2	1	—	1	—	—
Total	28	24	2	1	1	2

*Mean follow-up 29.6 months (range, 6 to 62 months). Five patients had nonunion of prior fusions.
†The nonunion occurred in a 10-year-old boy with progressive bone destruction from tumor.
‡Instrument complications included delayed pin breakage (n = 1) and facet wire pullout (n = 1). Both occurred in patients with osseous unions.
Source: Adapted from Sonntag VKH, Dickman CA. Craniocervical stabilization. *Clin Neurosurg* 1993; 40:243–272.

An 89 percent rate of fusion (Table 290-4) has been achieved using the threaded Steinmann pin for occipitocervical fusion (Fig. 290-12*C*). A wide diameter Steinmann pin provides rigid fixation and minimizes implant failure. The threads of the pin prevent vertical translocation or settling of the construct. This technique was developed as an alternative to metal fixtures with smooth rod surfaces, because they can allow settling.[39,49,52]

Screw Plates

A screw-plate technique can be used for occipitocervical stabilization.[24,31,51,59] An inverted "Y" shaped steel plate is contoured and affixed with bilateral posterior atlantoaxial facet screws and midline screws placed into the occiput near the nuchal line (Fig. 290-13). Posterior cervical lateral mass screws can be added to fixate the plate to the C3 to C7 levels if needed. Autologous bone grafts are used and the fusion bed is decorticated to promote fusion. The thickness of the occipital bone should be measured individually with CT prior to screw insertion. The occiput has an average midline thickness of 14 mm (range, 10 to 18 mm) at the nuchal line.[24]

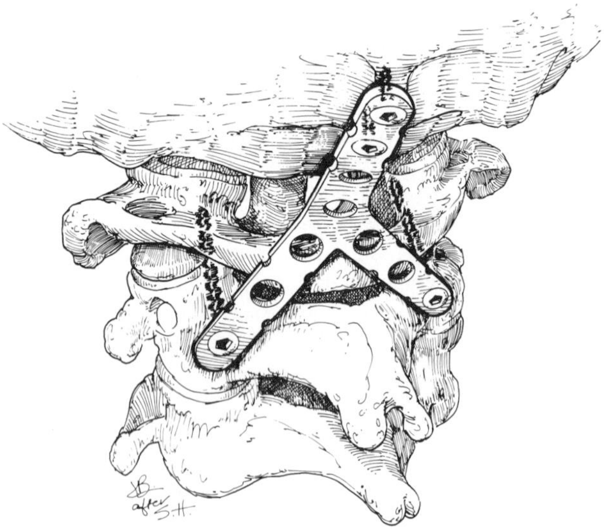

© 1992, B.N.I.®

Figure 290-13 An inverted "Y" shaped screw plate for occipitocervical fixation. The plate is secured to the occiput with midline screws near the nuchal crest. The plate is fixed to the cervical spine with posterior atlantoaxial facet screws.

Short screws must be placed in the occiput to avoid intradural penetration and cerebellar injury. Short screws have relatively limited pullout strength.

Occipitocervical screw plates are particularly useful if a multilevel cervical laminectomy has been performed or if the lamina cannot be fixated; however, it is technically demanding. The posterior atlantoaxial facet screws obliterate motion at C1-C2. Screw plates can avoid overlap of instruments with nonfused segments and can provide immediate rigid segmental fixation.

Surgical Outcome

The type of pathology causing the spinal instability affects the likelihood of success of an operative procedure for internal fixation. Rheumatoid arthritis causes progressive ligamentous weakening, bone softening, and poor healing—all of which contribute to a high risk for failure of fusion. Osteoporosis, arthritis, primary and metastatic neoplasms of the spine, widespread bone destruction, and osteomyelitis cause a high risk of failure of internal fixation. In soft, weak bone, instrumentation (e.g., screws, wires, clamps) may pull out and fail easily. Diseased bone tissue heals slowly or inadequately and tolerates instrumentation poorly. In contrast, patients who have fractures or congenital malformations usually have good bone quality and thus have an excellent capacity to heal.

A fibrous union or pseudarthrosis is a manifestation of inadequate bone healing. A fibrous union is a well-aligned, nonmobile fusion that has failed to form bone trabeculae or that is associated with bone resorption. There is a risk of delayed instrument breakage or failure in these cases. Long-term follow-up is necessary to detect late complications. A nonunion (pseudarthrosis) is a failed fusion and is characterized by subluxation, pathologic movement, and fibrous interfaces between the bone surfaces.

Conclusions

Several methods have evolved for surgical stabilization of the craniovertebral junction and upper cervical spine. Rigid internal fixation is desirable since it promotes fusion and minimizes the need for adjunctive external immobilization. The specific operative approach should be individualized and depends on the patient's pathology, a thorough understanding of the anatomy, the sites of instability, and the architecture of the osseous and ligamentous injuries. Wiring and autogenous bone grafts provide simple, safe, and effective methods for stabilization. Screw fixation techniques are useful when wiring is impossible, when wiring is inadequate to stabilize the spine, or when a highly rigid implant is needed. A rigid cervical orthosis should be considered to supplement the internal fixation when the bone is weak or diseased, when there are three-column spine injuries, or when semirigid fixation methods are used.

References

1. Aldrich EF, Crow WN, Weber PB, et al. Use of MR imaging-compatible Halifax interlaminar clamps for posterior cervical fusion. *J Neurosurg* 1991; 74:185–189.
2. Brooks AL, Jenkins EB. Atlanto-axial arthrodesis by the wedge compression method. *J Bone Joint Surg [Am]* 1978; 60-A:279–284.
3. Callahan RA, Johnson RM, Margolis RN, et al. Cervical facet fusion for control of instability following laminectomy. *J Bone Joint Surg [Am]* 1977; 59-A:991–1002.
4. Crockard HA, Pozo JL, Ransford AO, et al. Transoral decompression and posterior fusion for rheumatoid atlanto-axial subluxation. *J Bone Joint Surg [Br]* 1986; 68-B:350–356.
5. Dickman CA, Douglas RA, Sonntag VKH. Occipitocervical fusion: posterior stabilization of the craniovertebral junction and upper cervical spine. *BNI Q* 1990; 6:(2)2–14.
6. Dickman CA, Hadley MN, Browner C, et al. Neurosurgical management of acute atlas-axis combination fractures: a review of 25 cases. *J Neurosurg* 1989; 70:45–49.
7. Dickman CA, Locantro J, Fessler RG. The influence of transoral odontoid resection on stability of the craniovertebral junction. *J Neurosurg* 1992; 77:525–530.
8. Dickman CA, Mamourian A, Sonntag VKH, et al. Magnetic resonance imaging of the transverse atlantal ligament for the evaluation of atlantoaxial instability. *J Neurosurg* 1991; 75:221–227.
9. Dickman CA, Papadopoulos SM, Sonntag VKH, et al. Traumatic occipitoatlantal dislocations. *J Spinal Disord* 1993; 6:300–313.
10. Dickman CA, Sonntag VKH, Marcotte PJ. Techniques of screw fixation of the cervical spine. *BNI Q* 1992; 8(2):9–26.
11. Dickman CA, Sonntag VKH, Papadopoulos SM, et al. The interspinous method of posterior atlantoaxial arthrodesis. *J Neurosurg* 1991; 74:190–198.
12. Dvorak J, Schneider E, Saldinger P, et al. Biomechanics of the craniocervical region: the alar and transverse ligaments. *J Orthop Res* 1988; 6:452–461.
13. Fernyhough JC, White JI, LaRocca H. Fusion rates in multilevel cervical spondylosis comparing allograft fibula with autograft fibula in 126 patients. *Spine* 1991; 16(10) (Suppl):S561–S564.
14. Fielding JW. The status of arthrodesis of the cervical spine. *J Bone Joint Surg [Am]* 1988; 70-A:1571–1574.
15. Fielding JW, Cochran Gvan B, Lawsing JF III, et al. Tears of the transverse ligament of the atlas. A clinical and biomechanical study. *J Bone Joint Surg [Am]* 1974; 56-A:1683–1691.
16. Fielding JW, Hawkins RJ, Ratzan SA. Spine fusion for atlanto-axial instability. *J Bone Joint Surg [Am]* 1976; 58-A:400–407.
17. Frank C, Amiel D, Woo SL-Y, et al. Normal ligament properties and ligament healing. *Clin Orthop* 1985; 196:15–25.
18. Gallie WE. Skeletal traction in the treatment of fractures and dislocations of the cervical spine. *Ann Surg* 1937; 106:770–776.
19. Gallie WE. Fractures and dislocations of the cervical spine. *Am J Surg* 1939; 46:495–499.
20. Garfin SR, Moore MR, Marshall LF. A modified technique for cervical facet fusions. *Clin Orthop* 1988; 230:149–153.
21. Grantham SA, Dick HM, Thompson RC Jr, et al. Occipitocervical arthrodesis. Indications, technic and results. *Clin Orthop* 1969; 65:118–129.
22. Griswold DM, Albright JA, Schiffman E, et al. Atlanto-axial fusion for instability. *J Bone Joint Surg [Am]* 1978; 60-A:285–292.
23. Grob D, Crisco JJ III, Panjabi MM, et al. Biomechanical evaluation of four different posterior atlantoaxial fixation techniques. *Spine* 1992; 17:480–490.
24. Grob D, Dvorak J, Panjabi M, et al. Posterior occipitocervical fusion. A preliminary report of a new technique. *Spine* 1991; 16(3) (Suppl):S17–S24.
25. Grob D, Jeanneret B, Aebi M, et al. Atlanto-axial fusion with transarticular screw fixation. *J Bone Joint Surg [Br]* 1991; 73-B:972–976.
26. Hadley MN, Dickman CA, Browner CM, et al. Acute traumatic atlas fractures: management and long term outcome. *Neurosurgery* 1988; 23:31–35.
27. Hadley MN, Dickman CA, Browner CM, et al. Acute axis fractures. A review of 229 cases. *J Neurosurg* 1989; 71:642–647.
28. Hamblen DL. Occipito-cervical fusion. Indications, technique and results. *J Bone Joint Surg [Br]* 1967; 49-B:33–45.
29. Hanley EN Jr, Harvell JC Jr. Immediate postoperative stability of the atlantoaxial articulation: a biomechanical study comparing simple midline wiring, and the Gallie and Brooks procedures. *J Spinal Disord* 1992; 5:306–310.
30. Hanson PB, Montesano PX, Sharkey NA, et al. Anatomic and biomechanical assessment of transarticular screw fixation for atlantoaxial instability. *Spine* 1991; 16:1141–1145.
31. Heywood AW, Learmonth ID, Thomas M. Internal fixation for occipitocervical fusion. *J Bone Joint Surg [Br]* 1988; 70-B:708–711.
32. Holness RO, Huestis WS, Howes WJ, et al. Posterior stabilization with an interlaminar clamp in cervical injuries: technical note and review of the long term experience with the method. *Neurosurgery* 1984; 14:318–322.
33. Huhn SL, Wolf AL, Ecklund J. Posterior spinal osteosynthesis for cervical fracture/dislocation using a flexible multistrand cable system: technical note. *Neurosurgery* 1991; 29:943–946.
34. Jeanneret B, Magerl F. Primary posterior fusion C1/2 in odontoid fractures: indications, technique, and results of transarticular screw fixation. *J Spinal Disord* 1992; 5:464–475.
35. Jefferson G. Fracture of the atlas vertebra. Report of four cases, and a review of those previously recorded. *Br J Surg* 1920; 7:407–422.
36. Johnson RM, Hart DL, Simmons EF, et al. Cervical orthoses. A study comparing their effectiveness in restricting cervical motion in normal subjects. *J Bone Joint Surg [Am]* 1977; 59-A:332–339.
37. Kaufman HH, Jones E. The principles of bony spinal fusion. *Neurosurgery* 1989; 24:264–270.
38. Krag MH. Biomechanics of thoracolumbar spinal fixation. A review. *Spine* 1991; 16(3)(Suppl):S84–S99.
39. MacKenzie AI, Uttley D, Marsh HT, et al. Craniocervical stabilization using Luque/Hartshill rectangles. *Neurosurgery* 1990; 26:32–36.
40. Magerl F, Seemann P-S. Stable posterior fusion of the atlas and axis by transarticular screw fixation. In Kehr P, Weidner PA (eds): *Cervical Spine I.* New York: Springer-Verlag, 1987, pp 322–327.
41. McAfee PC, Bohlman HH, Ducker TB, et al. Failure of methylmethacrylate stabilization of the spine. A retrospective analysis of 24 cases. In Cervical Spine Research Society Editorial Committee (ed): *The Cervical Spine,* 2d ed. Philadelphia: Lippincott, 1989, pp 838–849.
42. McGraw RW, Rusch RM. Atlanto-axial arthrodesis. *J Bone Joint Surg [Br]* 1973; 55-B:482–489.
43. Menezes AH, VanGilder JC, Graf CJ, et al. Craniocervical abnormalities. A comprehensive surgical approach. *J Neurosurg* 1980; 53:444–455.
44. Montesano PX, Juach EC, Anderson PA, et al. Biomechanics of cervical spine internal fixation. *Spine* 1991; 16(3)(Suppl):S10–S16.
45. Moskovich R, Crockard HA. Atlantoaxial arthrodesis using interlaminar clamps. An improved technique. *Spine* 1992; 17:261–267.
46. Murphy MJ, Southwick WO. Posterior approaches and fusions. In Cervical Spine Research Society Editorial Committee (ed): *The Cervical Spine,* 2d ed Philadelphia: Lippincott, 1989, pp 775–791.
47. Papadopoulos SM, Dickman CA, Sonntag VKH. Atlantoaxial stabilization in rheumatoid arthritis. *J Neurosurg* 1991; 74:1–7.
48. Papadopoulos SM, Dickman CA, Sonntag VKH, et al. Traumatic atlantooccipital dislocation with survival. *Neurosurgery* 1991; 28:574–579.

49. Ransford AO, Crockard HA, Pozo JL, et al. Craniocervical instability treated by contoured loop fixation. *J Bone Joint Surg [Br]* 1986; 68-B:173–177.
50. Robinson RA, Southwick WO. Surgical approaches to the cervical spine. *Instr Course Lect* 1960; 17:229–230.
51. Roy-Camille R, Saillant G, Mazel C. Internal fixation of the unstable cervical spine by a posterior osteosynthesis with plates and screws. In Cervical Spine Research Society Editorial Committee (ed): *The Cervical Spine,* 2d ed. Philadelphia: Lippincott, 1989, pp 390–403.
52. Sakou T, Kawaida H, Morizono Y, et al. Occipitoatlantoaxial fusion utilizing a rectangular rod. *Clin Orthop* 1989; 239:136–144.
53. Songer MN, Spencer DL, Meyer PR Jr, et al. The use of sublaminar cables to replace Luque wires. *Spine* 1991; 16(8)(Suppl):S418–S421.
54. Sonntag VKH, Dickman CA. Operative management of occipitocervical and atlantoaxial instability. In Holtzman RNN, Farcy J-PC, McCormick PC, (eds): *Spinal Instability.* Berlin: Springer-Verlag, 1993, pp 255–292.
55. Spence KF Jr, Decker S, Sell KW. Bursting atlantal fracture associated with rupture of the transverse ligament. *J Bone Joint Surg [Am]* 1970; 52-A:543–549.
56. Spetzler RF, Dickman CA, Sonntag VKH. The transoral approach to the anterior cervical spine. *Contemp Neurosurg* 1991; 13(9):1–6.
57. Steel HH. Anatomical and mechanical considerations of the atlanto-axial articulations. *J Bone Joint Surg [Am]* 1968; 50-A:1481–1482.
58. Taitsman JP, Saha S. Tensile strength of wire-reinforced bone cement and twisted stainless-steel wire. *J Bone Joint Surg [Am]* 1977; 59-A:419–425.
59. Weidner A. Internal fixation with metal plates and screws. In Cervical Spine Research Society Editorial Committee (ed): *The Cervical Spine,* 2d ed. Philadelphia: Lippincott, 1989, pp 404–421.
60. Wertheim SB, Bohlman HH. Occipitocervical fusion. Indications, technique, and long-term results in thirteen patients. *J Bone Joint Surg [Am]* 1987; 69-A:833–836.
61. White AA III, Panjabi MM. *Clinical Biomechanics of the Spine.* Philadelphia: Lippincott, 1978.
62. Zdeblick TA, Ducker TB. The use of freeze-dried allograft bone for anterior cervical fusion. *Spine* 1991; 16:726–729.

291 Stabilization of the Spine Using Flexible Multistrand Cables

Setti S. Rengachary
Abhay Sanan

Stabilization of the cervical spine with the use of wire was first described by Hadra in 1891.[3] Heavy-gauge wire continues to see considerable use in the stabilization of the cervical spine. Wires can be used as the primary stabilization method or as adjuncts to other spinal implants. The ultimate strength of the wire–bone construct depends on several factors, most notably the geometry of the construct and the mechanical properties of the wire itself. Historically, the wire of choice has been a thick (16- or 18-gauge) monofilament wire. However, several disadvantages of monofilament wire have been noted.[1,4,5] First, the wires tend to break over time. They usually fracture just below the twisted ends, and it is hypothesized that a stress riser occurs just below the twist and reduces the fatigue strength of the wire. If the wire breaks prematurely, the clinical result is a higher pseudoarthrosis rate. Second, the stiffness of the wire poses a danger to the dura and spinal cord with sublaminar passage. Direct dural contusions during wire passage have been reported. Perioperative rates of neural injury have been reported to be as high as 17 percent. Even when the wire passage is successful, the unyielding nature of monofilament wire can result in a loop that protrudes into the canal and causes pressure necrosis of the dura or chronic spinal cord compression. Removal of broken wires or spinal implants held by wires can pose a risk to both the patient and the surgeon. The broken ends tend to be sharp and can cut the dura or a surgeon's glove during removal.

A cable system offers several advantages over monofilament wire. The most important advantage is a higher fatigue strength. Stainless steel monofilaments and cables of equal diameters have roughly equal static strength, but the cable has six times the fatigue strength as measured by cycles to failure. When the wire and cable systems are tested in a loop configuration, the differences become more dramatic. For example, the Songer cable has 2.85 times the static strength of wire and 6 to 22 times the fatigue strength.[7] Similar results have been obtained with other cable systems. Since an implant is subjected to repeated loading and unloading, the fatigue strength is likely to be a very important indicator of its resistance to fracture. Another advantage is the possibility of using a cinch or crimp system for fixation, in place of twisting with its accompanying stress risers. In fact, during biomechanical testing, the cable fails before the cinch or crimp. In addition to avoiding stress risers, the fixation system has another benefit, in that it allows the tension produced in the cable to be controlled and reliably reproduced. This feature allows for adjustments based on the local anatomy, bone quality, and type of construct. The flexibility of the cable system is also highly desirable. Sublaminar passage is safer, and there is less risk of acute injury to the canal structures. Furthermore, the cable hugs the contour of the laminar surface. This has two advantages. First, chronic pressure injury to canal structures is reduced. Second, the zone of contact between bone and cable is increased, thereby distributing the stress more uniformly over the length of cable. Minor disadvantages of the multistrand cable are the requirement for a special instrument to secure the cable and the additional cost. On the whole, the flexible multistrand cable system represents a significant advance in posterior wire fusion constructs.

Instrumentation

Currently three companies offer cable systems for stabilization of the spine. These systems are The Danek Cable (Danek, Memphis, TN), The Songer Cable (AcroMed, Cleveland, OH), and The Sof'Wire (Codman, Randolph, MA). The products differ in the weave of the cable, and there are minor differences in cable instrumentation. Table 291-1 summarizes the salient differences among the three products.

Cables

The cables consist of braided strands made of either stainless steel or titanium alloy (Fig. 291-1). Titanium creates less artifact on magnetic resonance imaging. The number of strands in the cable ranges from 49 to 133, depending on the manufacturer. The cables

TABLE 291-1 Comparison of Three Cable Systems

Feature	Songer Cable	Danek Cable	Sof'Wire
Number of wires per cable	75	49	133
Cable diameter	0.041 in.	0.041 in.	0.034 in.
Equivalent diameter of wire	18 G	18 G	20 G
Provision for measuring cable tension	Yes	Yes	No
Fixation device	Crimp	Crimp	Cinch
Disposability	No	No	Yes
Provisional crimp	No	Yes	No

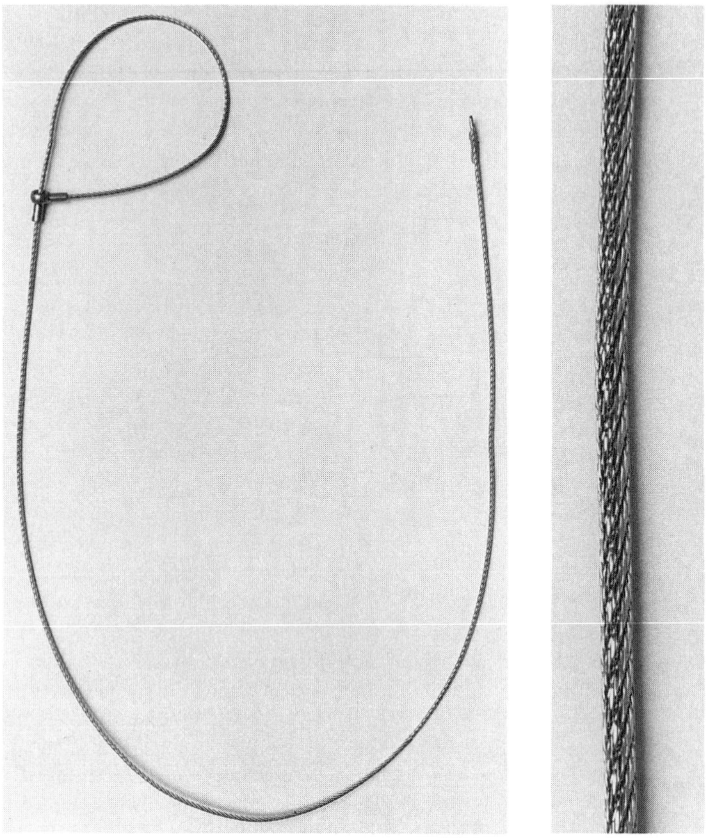

Figure 291-1 *A.* The cable is pliable and can easily be looped. *B.* A magnified view shows the braided nature of the cable.

come in diameters approximating those of 18 or 20 gauge monofilament wires. Because of the weaker biomechanical properties of titanium, the diameter of the titanium alloy cable is slightly greater than that of the steel cable. One end of the cable has a leader, and the other has either an eyelet or some other device that can connect with the leader end. Cables are sold as double or single cables. The double cable consists of two single cables welded to a single, looped monofilament leader. It is designed primarily for sublaminar constructs. After passing the double cable under the lamina, the leader loop can be cut, creating two single cables that can be used in the construct.

Tensioner and Fixator

The tensioner device tightens the cable loop. For the Danek and Songer cables, tension can be adjusted as necessary by a ratchet mechanism. The Danek and Songer cable systems have a worm gear with a 5-to-1 ratio, so the tension read from the instrument should be multiplied by 5 to arrive at the true cable tension. In general, for the cervical spine, 40 to 60 lb of tension is required for stainless steel cable and 30 to 40 lb is adequate for the thicker titanium cable. Cable tensions should be lower in patients with osteopenia. The Sof'Wire system does not allow for measurement of tension; instead it relies on palpation by the surgeon. The Songer and Danek cables use a crimp for fixation. A crimp is a small device that fits over the cable and is crimped (compressed) around it to hold it fast. The Sof'Wire cable uses a tubular cinch that operates in a similar way. A typical set of basic instruments is shown in Fig. 291-2.

Other Differences

The Sof'Wire system is the only one that is entirely disposable. The Danek system is the only one that offers a provisional crimp. A provisional crimp allows for the temporary maintenance of tension in the cable and is useful when staged tightening and crimping is desired, as in multisegmented constructs for correction of scoliosis or kyphosis. The Danek and Songer cables are approved by the Food and Drug Administration for use in the entire spine, whereas the Sof'Wire cable is approved for use only in the cervical spine.

Internal Fixation

In general, a cable system can be used in place of monofilament wire as the situation requires. Regardless of the manufacturer, the general principles of cable fixation remain the same. The cable is first wrapped around the items to be immobilized, then secured to itself using any of a number of devices, and then tightened using a tensioner device. Once the desired tension has been achieved, the cable ends are fixed using a fixation device. Finally, the excess

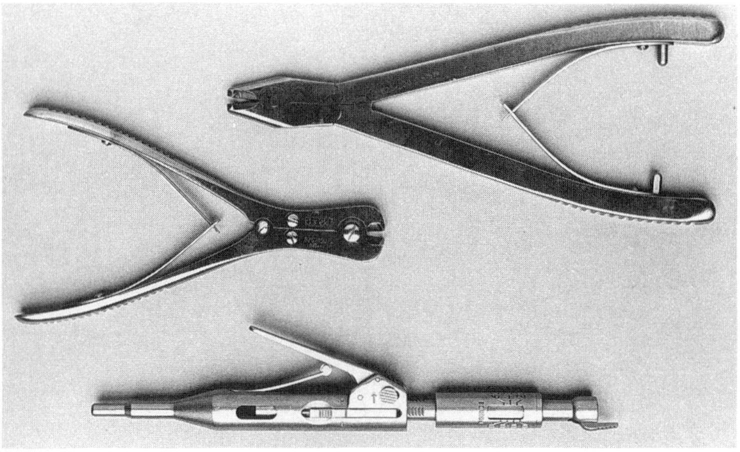

Figure 291-2 The basic set of instruments includes a crimp applier (top), wire cutter (middle), and tensioner device (bottom).

wire is cut off and discarded. The cable should be cut flush so that sharp strands do not protrude. Some common constructs are described, to highlight the safety and versatility of the cable system.

Upper Cervical Spine (Occiput, C1, C2)

The indications for posterior atlantoaxial stabilization include traumatic disorders such as unstable type II odontoid fractures and degenerative disorders such as rheumatoid arthritis. Achieving a successful result in the upper cervical spine with the cable system requires adherence to certain basic principles. The incision should expose the occipitocervical area from the inion to C3 to allow room for the required instruments. The passage of sublaminar wires, even flexible cables, can be hazardous. The following technique minimizes this risk. A large blunt needle (e.g., an aneurysm needle with the point cut off) is threaded with no. 1 silk suture. The needle is then carefully passed under the lamina in an inferior-to-superior direction. The silk suture is then tied to the cable. Both the suture and the cable are held taut so the lamina will be hugged, and the suture is used to pull the cable under the lamina.

The modified Gallie technique offers the classic construct for fusion of the posterior atlantoaxial joint (Fig. 291-3). Decortication of the inferior lamina of C1 and superior lamina of C2 is performed with a high-speed burr. A looped single cable is passed under the arch of C1 in an inferior-to-superior direction and then hooked under the spinous process of C2. A contoured corticocancellous graft is inserted between the C1 and C2 arches. By applying tension to the cable, a noose is formed around the C2 spinous process. After fixation, the free ends of the wire are cut, and then additional bone can be packed into any defects as desired.

The Brooks technique is an alternative method for accomplishing a C1-to-C2 posterior arthrodesis that involves the sublaminar passage of wire at both levels (Fig. 291-4).[2] While this construct offers better biomechanical stability than the Gallie construct, it also carries higher risks from sublaminar wire placement. A double cable is used, and the leader end is passed in an inferior-to-superior direction under the lamina of C2 and then C1. It is important to pass the cable in two steps to avoid injury to the dura and spinal cord. Once the cable is recovered from the top of C1, the tip of the leader is cut. This converts the double cable into two individual cables. Decortication of the inferior lamina of C1 and superior lamina of C2 is then performed, and two tricortical wedge grafts are placed between the laminae of C1 and C2. The free end of each cable is pulled through its respective eyelet and then tightened and fixed, and the excess cable is cut and discarded.

Incorporation of the occiput can be accomplished by using the cables as anchors for any rectangular metal construct (Fig. 291-5).[6] The construct can be anchored to the laminae of the upper cervical spine in the manner described. Anchoring the construct to the occiput can be achieved by drilling two holes on either side of the external occipital protuberance. A double cable can be passed through each set of holes, and the construct can be fixed to the occiput in a figure-of-eight fashion.

Lower Cervical Spine

Posterior arthrodesis of the lower cervical spine has been used in patients with instability of the posterior column caused by trauma, extensive laminectomies, or destruction of bony elements by

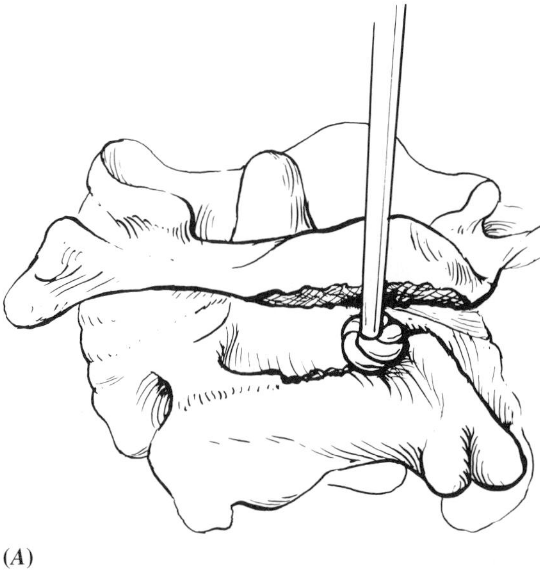

(*A*)

Figure 291-3 The modified Gallie construct for C1-to-C2 fusion. *A*. The opposing laminar surfaces of C1 and C2 are decorticated with a high-speed burr.

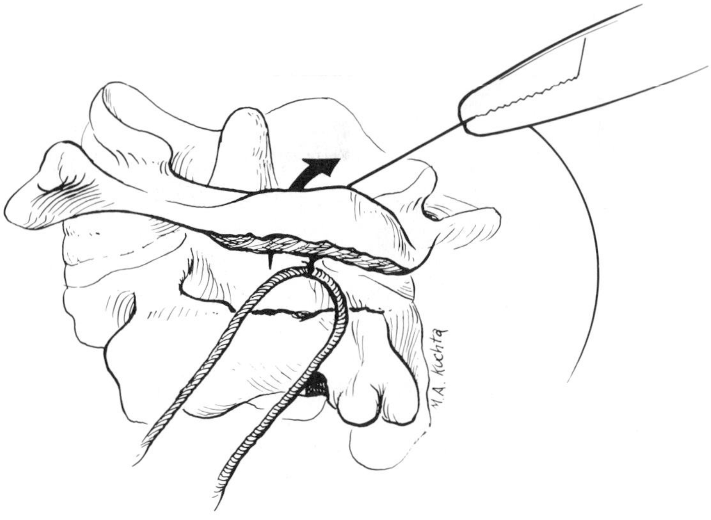

(*B*)

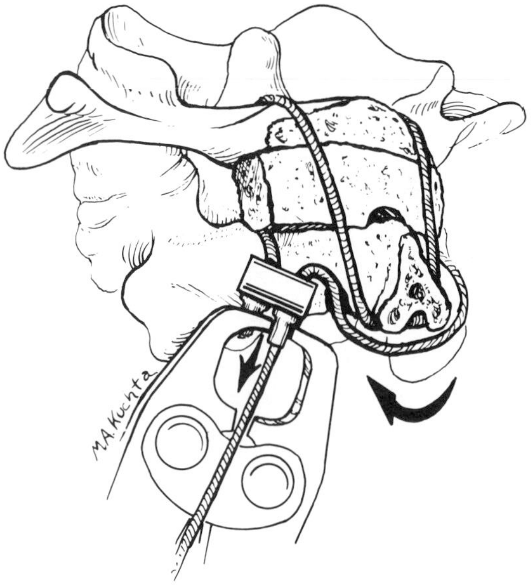

(*D*)

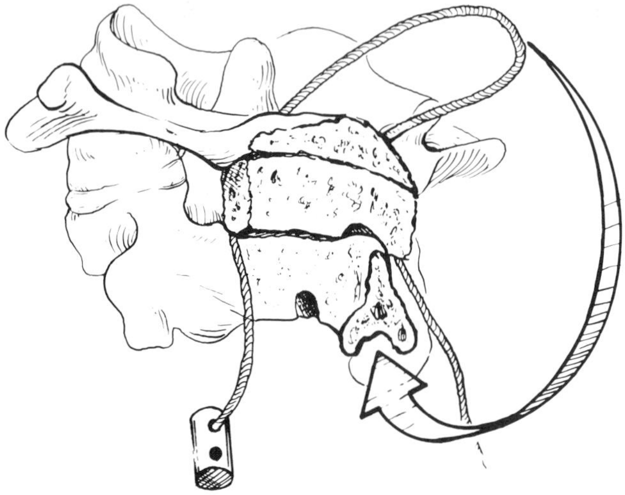

(*C*)

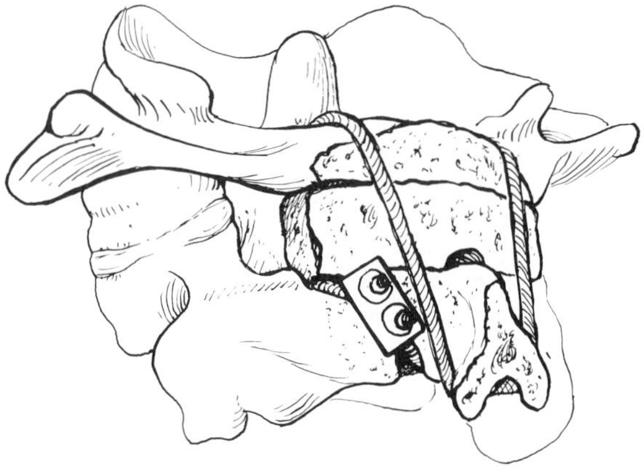

(*E*)

Figure 291-3 *(Continued) B.* A looped single cable is passed under the arch of C1. *C.* The bone graft is placed, and the cable is looped under the spinous process of C2. *D.* The cable is tightened and crimped. *E.* The final construct.

infectious or neoplastic processes. There are many techniques for cervical wiring and fusion, but a popular and biomechanically sound technique of fusion is the triple-wire technique (Fig. 291-6). This construct compresses bone grafts to the underlying laminae. For fusion of two adjacent vertebrae, the technique involves drilling a 3-mm hole at the base of both spinous processes. One double cable and one single cable are required. A single cable is passed through the cephalad spinous process, and both ends are looped underneath the caudad spinous process. The ends are then attached to each other, tightened, and fixed in place, thus immobilizing the two vertebrae. The remainder of the technique is aimed at promoting arthrodesis. The laminae and facets of both vertebrae are decorticated. Two pieces of corticocancellous bone of an appropriate size are obtained, and a hole is drilled on each end. The second and third cables are obtained by cutting the tip of the double cable leader. A cable is passed through the bone graft, then the spinous process, then the bone graft again at each level. The cables are introduced in opposite directions at each level so that the free end of one cable will be ipsilateral to the leader of the other. The cables are then tightened and fixed. If there is a fracture of the spinous process or lamina, wiring should be avoided at that level. Instead, wiring is anchored to levels above and below in a fashion similar to that described.

Total Cervical Constructs

There is a growing consensus that the appropriate treatment for multilevel cervical spondylitic myelopathy should include a multilevel decompressive laminectomy followed by fusion of the involved levels. Other indications for total cervical fusion might include correction of deformity from ankylosing spondylitis. This

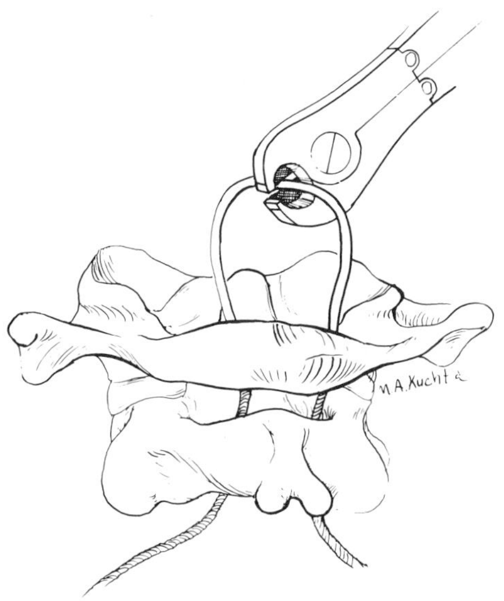

(*A*)

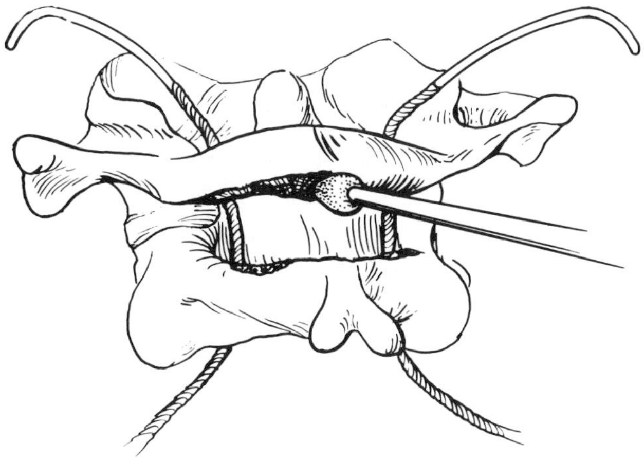

(*B*)

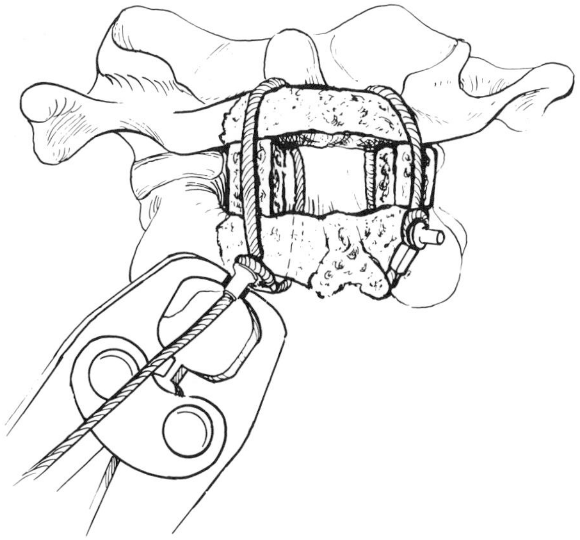

(*C*)

Figure 291-4 The Brooks technique is an alternative to the Gallie technique for C1-to-C2 fusion. *A.* A double cable is passed under the arches of C1 and C2. The leader is cut to yield two single cables. *B.* The opposing laminar surfaces of C1 and C2 are decorticated with a high-speed burr. *C.* Two bone grafts are placed between C1 and C2. The cables are tightened and crimped.

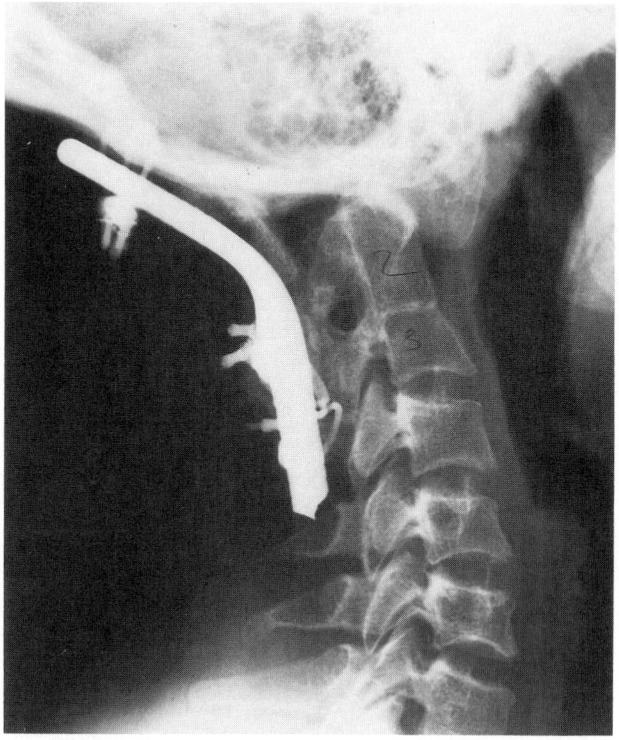

Figure 291-5 A bent metal rectangle can be used to incorporate the occiput into a high cervical fusion.

stabilization procedure can be performed using a cable system and any suitable metal construct, such as the Luque loop. After the laminectomy is completed, the metal rectangle is placed so that it covers one intact level cranially and two intact levels caudally. The cable system is then used in a sublaminar fashion to rigidly fix the construct to the spine. An example of such an approach is shown in Fig. 291-7, in which a C3-to-C7 decompressive laminectomy has been performed and the cervical spine has been immobilized from C2 to T2.

Thoracic and Lumbar Constructs

The cable system can also be used for segmental fixation in the thoracic and lumbar regions. Its use is primarily restricted to the

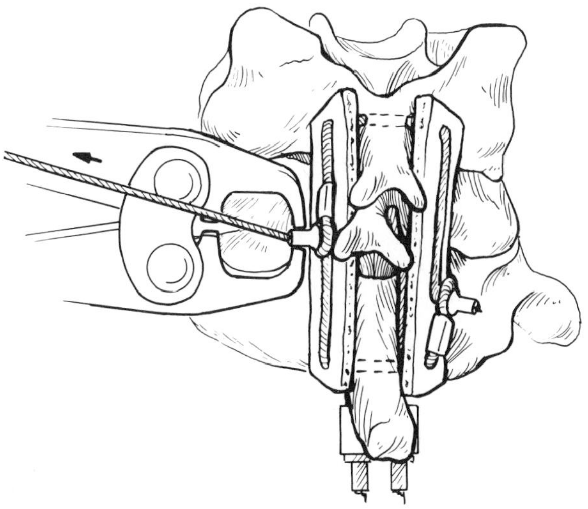

Figure 291-6 A C5-to-C7 fusion using the triple cable technique.

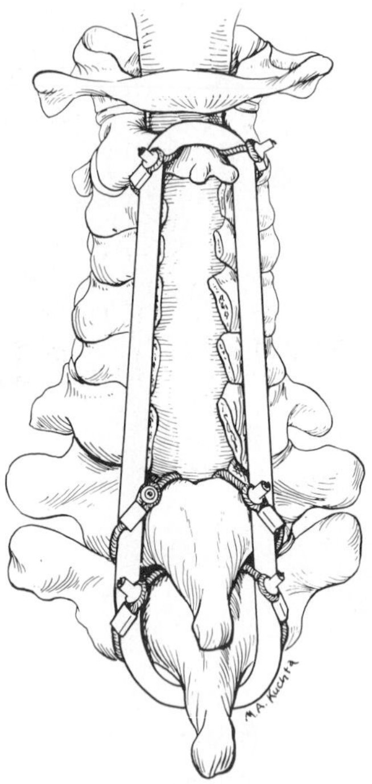

Figure 291-7 Extensive cervical stabilization using a Luque loop and sublaminar cables.

correction of scoliotic deformities. The cables are used to augment the segmental universal fixation devices by applying tension to malpositioned vertebrae.

Precautions

Although the cable system is quite safe, several precautions should be taken. The passage of cables under C1 and C2 should be well controlled. The tension in the cable should be balanced in relation to a number of factors. Too high a tension can fracture or cut through the bone. Excessively aggressive tightening of two adjacent levels should be avoided to prevent foraminal narrowing and root compression. Sharp bends should be avoided, as they will produce stress risers. The leader wire should not be used as part of the construct. The tension should be reduced in patients with osteopenic bone. In the Songer and Danek systems, the crimp should be applied before the leader wire is cut off; otherwise, application of the crimp becomes difficult. Because the Sof'Wire system does not give a measurement of the tension, the surgeon should check the tautness of the cable frequently to prevent fractures.

References

1. Bernard TN Jr, Johnston CE II, Roberts JM, et al. Late complications due to wire breakage in segmental spinal instrumentation. Report of two cases. *J Bone Joint Surg [Am]* 1983; 65:1339–1345.
2. Brooks AL, Jenkins EB. Atlanto-axial arthrodesis by the wedge compression method. *J Bone Joint Surg [Am]* 1978; 60:279–284.
3. Hadra BE. The classic. Wiring of the vertebrae as a means of immobilization in fracture and Potts' disease: Berthold E. Hadra. Med Times and Register, vol 22, May 23, 1891. *Clin Orthop* 1975; 112:4–8.
4. Johnston CE II, Happel LT Jr, Norris R, et al. Delayed paraplegia complicating sublaminar segmental spinal instrumentation. *J Bone Joint Surg [Am]* 1986; 68:556–563.
5. Schrader WC, Bethem D, Scerbin V. The chronic local effects of sublaminar wires. An animal model. *Spine* 1988; 13:499–502.
6. Seifert V, Stolke D, Stürz H. Cranio-cervical stabilization using contoured Luque rectangles. *Acta Neurochir (Wien)* 1991; 109:20–25.
7. Songer MN, Spencer DL, Meyer PR Jr, et al. The use of sublaminar cables to replace Luque wires. *Spine* 1991; 16:S418–S421.

292

Luque Loop Stabilization after Extensive Cervical Laminectomy

Paul Kurt Maurer

Advances in technology have enhanced the surgeon's ability to combine the benefits of posterior decompression with those of stabilization.[5,10,13,15,16] Surgical history is replete with procedures that were cast aside as "outdated," only to be "reborn" as advances allowed their reapplication. Posterior decompression of the cervical spinal cord was the standard in neurosurgery for decades, but fell from prominence in the 1970s and 1980s with the expansion of anterior cervical approaches.[6,9,12] It is now possible to combine the excellent decompression achieved from a posterior approach with the benefits of immobilization and stabilization. Luque instrumentation combined with sublaminar/facet cable techniques allows extensive immobilization in a relatively "low friction" manner.[16]

Indications

The indications for posterior cervical laminectomy are numerous, and include laminectomy for purposes of exposure of an intramedullary lesion (e.g., cervical spinal cord tumor, vascular malformation, syrinx) and decompression of the spinal cord affected by extra-axial pathology (e.g., extramedullary tumor, cervical spondylosis, ossification of the posterior longitudinal ligament). While it has long been theorized that simple multilevel cervical laminectomy causes instability of the spine, there is ample evidence to the contrary.[6,15] A standard laminectomy that preserves the facets may cause some angulation deformity but frank instability is unusual. In spite of advances in instrumentation technique, there is clearly some increase in the morbidity of a procedure when instrumentation is included and its use should be restricted to two basic settings: instability of the cervical spine, and pathologic processes in which the inherent dynamic motion of the cervical spine may aggravate the underlying disease process.

Luque rod instrumentation with sublaminar cable techniques allows fixation and bone fusion over long segments of the cervical spine.[15,16] Its applicability is, therefore, greatest in processes that require immobilization from C2 to approximately C7 or T1. As will be discussed below, sublaminar cable techniques allow very strong and rigid fixation, but are most safely used in regions with an ample subarachnoid space (i.e., C2 or T1). Instability of the cervical spine or pathologic lesions requiring less extensive immobilization are better addressed with posterior lateral mass plates over 2 or 3 segments, Hartshill/Ti-Frame rectangle with cable, or anterior approaches without or with plating techniques. In those disease processes that do require an extensive laminectomy and immobilization, we have found the Luque loop-sublaminar cable procedure to be very effective and safe.[15,16] Preformed Hartshill/Ti-Frame rectangles are applied with the same technique as will be discussed below.

Instability of the Cervical Spine

As noted above, one of the two broad indications for extensive stabilization is frank cervical instability after an extensive laminectomy. In that a standard cervical laminectomy without facetectomy does not cause true instability, the vast majority of extensive cervical procedures do not require any associated fusion.[5] This basic tenet is violated, however, when any of the posterior or anterior elements are degraded by trauma or disease. A common example is a patient with metastatic involvement of the vertebral bodies and multiple pathologic compression fractures.[5,14] The posterior elements (pedicles, laminae, facets, and associated ligaments) are often compromised as well. An extensive cervical laminectomy in this setting can lead to frank instability. If multilevel decompression is needed, it is appropriate to consider Luque instrumentation. Less extensive involvement (e.g., one vertebral body with an epidural tumor mass) could be dealt with by an anterior corpectomy and fusion, or by a laminectomy over 2 or 3 segments with lateral mass plates or preformed Ti-Frame rectangle with cable application and fusion. Trauma may also require treatment by a laminectomy and fusion. It is relatively uncommon for the laminectomy to span greater than 3 segments, however, and techniques requiring lesser degrees of immobilization are often more applicable (anterior plates, lateral mass plates, etc.).

Detrimental Effects of Spinal Motion

We have used Luque instrumentation extensively in the treatment of cervical spondylotic myelopathy (CSM).[15,16] Cervical spondylosis is a degenerative disease that is the most common cause of myelopathy in patients over 55 years of age.[3] It was initially described in detail in the 1950s, but its natural history and exact pathophysiologic nature remain controversial.[3,15] CSM is, in part, caused by a progressive decrease in the anterior-posterior (AP) dimension of the cervical spinal canal that results in compression of the spinal cord. It has long been thought that a spinal canal with an AP dimension of less than 10 to 12 mm was sufficiently constricted to place the patient at risk for a slow, stuttering, progressive loss of spinal cord function, or even an abrupt central cord syndrome. Although the AP dimension of the cervical canal clearly determines the potential for compression, it has been amply demonstrated over several decades that the dynamic, inherent motion of the cervical spine greatly exacerbates the progression of myelopathy in CSM.[1–4,8,15]

The disc/spur complexes that cause encroachment of the spinal canal are located anterior to the cord. This led to the logical (but not necessarily correct) assumption that removal of the offending pathology must be done from an anterior approach. It is noteworthy that autopsy studies have consistently demonstrated that the spinal cord in CSM is most heavily damaged not in its anterior aspects but rather in its lateral and posterolateral portions.[3] If the pathophysiology were a simple anterior compressive issue, one would have expected different findings. It was noted in the United Kingdom more than 20 years ago that CSM patients who were immobilized prior to surgery often improved dramatically in spite of the lack of a decompression.[1,2] Several reviews of cervical laminectomy found improved results in patients with a limited range of motion of the neck.[1,2] An extensive review of surgical techniques for CSM and their results in Europe in the 1970s demonstrated that patients had a better outcome if they were immobilized over 3 or more segments of the cervical spine, regardless of whether the approach was anterior or posterior.[8] All of the aforementioned data suggest that it is not the simple act of compression that leads to spinal cord dysfunction in CSM, but rather it is the compression associated with the inherent dynamic motion of the cervical spine causing traction and compression insults.[1–3,15]

Treatment of CSM requires addressing both components of its pathophysiology: the compressive forces (i.e., the reduction in the AP diameter of the spinal canal) and the dynamic forces (i.e., the inherent motion of the cervical spine).[1,3,4,15,16,18] Interestingly, the success of anterior cervical procedures may be as much related to the fusion that accompanies anterior cervical procedures as to the fact that it removes the osteophytes. When the encroachment on the canal is limited to 1 or 2 levels, simple anterior cervical discectomy with fusion can address the problems of both compression and reduction of motion, with a fairly low morbidity. The advent of lateral mass plates should also allow decompression with reduction of motion from a posterior approach over two segments, although no outcome data are available at the time of this writing.

Often, the CSM patient has disease at C4-5, C5-6, and C6-7. A three-level corpectomy requires a more extensive anterior grafting technique.[9,12,18] Although a three-level anterior approach (with a fibular strut graft or plate technique) can certainly address both the compressive and dynamic aspects of CSM, there has been a fairly notable complication rate with such procedures even in experienced hands.[12,18]

The somewhat mixed results obtained with posterior approaches in CSM and ossification of the posterior longitudinal ligament in the past may have been due to the failure to address the dynamic aspects of the disease, not because there was continued compression. Multilevel cervical laminectomy provides the extensive decompression required in CSM, and Luque-sublaminar cable techniques now allow a relatively ''low friction'' manner in which to address the dynamic aspects of the disease when three or more levels are involved.[16] Sublaminar fixation techniques allow very solid construct formation.[7,15–17] When wire was the sole means of sublaminar fixation, concern was raised about the safety of passing such wires in the sublaminar compartment.[7] The newer cable materials are a major advance because they are soft, pliable, and easily passed in the sublaminar space.[10,16,17] Additionally, the cables are 6 to 10 times stronger than wire of similar gauge.[17] Assuming the passage of the sublaminar cables at a level with an adequate subarachnoid space (C2, T1, or T2) and attention to proper technique, the sublaminar methods of instrument (Luque rod, loop, Hartshill rectangle, Ti-Frame rectangle, etc.) fixation are a reasonable option.

Operative Technique

The technique of extensive posterior cervical laminectomy and Luque loop instrumentation may be performed consistently with low morbidity if attention is paid to the details of each step.

Decompression

The first portion of the procedure involves a standard multilevel cervical laminectomy from C3 to C7. Although a cervical laminectomy can be accomplished in either the sitting or the prone position, the extent of the dissection needed for instrumentation (C2-T2) favors using the prone position. It is important to have the patient's neck placed in a neutral position and the head fixed with a Mayfield head holder. Flexion or extension can cause spinal cord compression during the operation. Additionally, because the head will be limited in its range of motion after fusion, instrumenting the patient in flexion or extension makes for an uncomfortable head position postoperatively. As noted above, passage of sublaminar cables requires a reasonable ''safe space'' under the lamina. For this reason, the decompression should include all bone and associated ligaments to the inferior lip of C2 and to the superior lip of T1. We have generally utilized spinous process/facet cable techniques in regions of less ample subarachnoid space such as C_3–C_5.

An equator-to-equator decompression of the spinal cord from C2 to C7 is achieved easily with standard cervical techniques. The author generally prefers a high speed drill, using cutting and diamond bits to form a trough at the laminar-facet groove. This method eliminates the risk of placing the foot plate of an instrument in the already compromised spinal canal. At each spinal level, after the laminae are freed at both lateral limits, the spinous process is grasped, the bony arch is gently lifted off the dura, and the ligamentum flavum on each side is sectioned with an angled arachnoid knife or a number 11 scalpel blade. Posterolateral foraminotomies can be added if necessary in the patient with combined myeloradiculopathy. The completed decompression is depicted in Fig. 292-1.

Instrumentation and Fusion

The second part of the procedure involves placement of the Luque loop and the sublaminar cables to fix the loop to the spine. This portion of the procedure is performed in steps, as follows.

Clearing Passage for the Sublaminar Cables

It is very important to have a ''clean'' dura over which to pass the cables. Any retained soft tissue such as ligamentum flavum or epidural venous plexus can prevent a smooth passage under the lamina and cause the cable to bunch and compress the subarachnoid space. Note in Fig. 292-2 that dissection has provided a clear zone between C1 and C2 so that the cable can be visualized entering the epidural compartment at the inferior lip of the posterior arch of C2, and the dura visualized throughout the passage of the cable into the C1-C2 space. A similar clear area of dura is prepared at the C7-T1 and T1-T2 zones. Sublaminar fixation is recommended at both the T1 and T2 levels to further strengthen the construct.

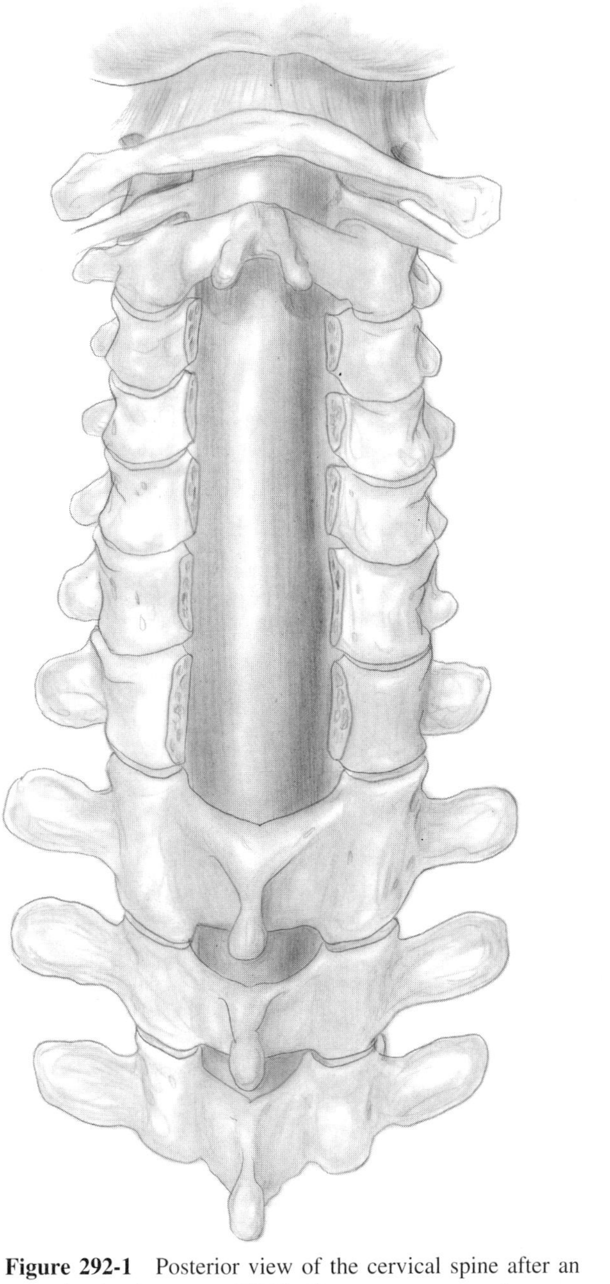

Figure 292-1 Posterior view of the cervical spine after an extensive laminectomy (C3-7). Equator to equator decompression is achieved; foraminotomies can be included if necessary. Note that for subsequent sublaminar cable placement and Luque instrumentation the interlaminar spaces at C7-T1 and T1-T2 must be cleared of ligament and epidural soft tissue.

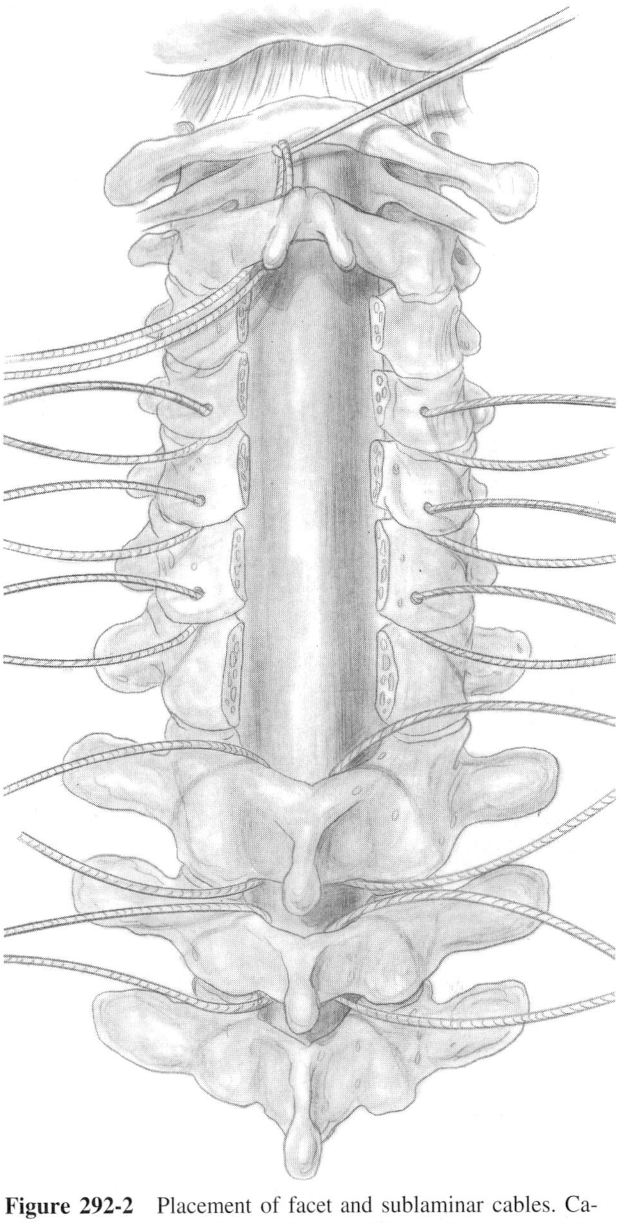

Figure 292-2 Placement of facet and sublaminar cables. Cables are passed through facet holes drilled with a small cutting bit. The articular surface of the facet is "roughened" with a curette or diamond bit prior to passage of the cable in anticipation of bone graft placement. Six additional sublaminar cables are used. It is critical to clear the sublaminar zone of all soft tissue prior to passage of the cables so that the dura can be visualized both superior and inferior to the lamina at the time of passage. As shown, a nerve hook is used to pull the cable under the lamina (the cable should never be pushed).

Drilling Holes for the Facet Cables

This portion of the procedure uses techniques employed in standard trauma care. A Penfield #3 dissector is wedged into the space between the inferior and superior articular facets. A gentle amount of traction is applied which spreads the facet joint. A high speed drill with a 2 mm cutting burr is then angled medially and inferiorly to form a hole in the inferior articular facet. It is not necessary to place a cable through each facet, but the use of three facet cables per side is desirable.

Forming the Luque Loop

Luque rods are made of stainless steel in both 3/16 in. and 1/4 in. sizes. The 3/16 in. rod is selected for the cervical spine. The rod is marketed in a straight configuration, and is fashioned into a loop (or rectangle) of appropriate size with Isola rod benders (Fig. 292-3). It has been our experience that the use of the Isola benders eliminates the need for other bending instruments because they

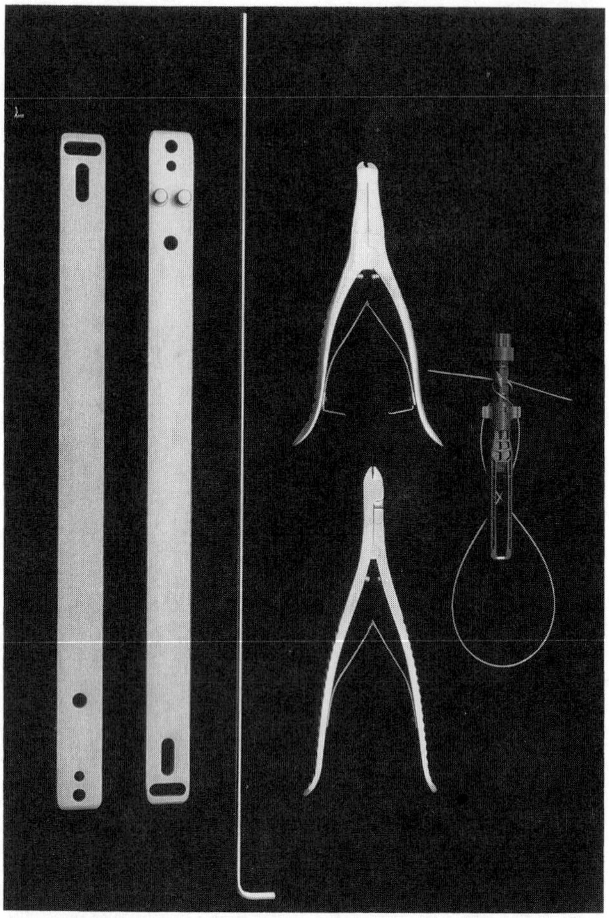

Figure 292-3 Instrumentation for Luque stabilization (left to right): Two flat Isola rod benders allow the Luque rod to be bent to appropriate size and shape based on an 18 gauge wire template fashioned for the individual patient at the time of surgery. The Luque rod is a straight 3/16 in. metal rod. The Codman "Sof-Wire" sublaminar cable kit includes the "crimper" pliers to lock the cable in position, the cable cutting pliers, and the tension ratchet device (depicted with a cable loaded) used to tighten the cable around the lamina and rod. Preformed titanium rectangles may reduce the requirement to form an individual loop. Titanium cables are available for Ti-Frame application.

allow fashioning of the acute angles at the top and bottom of the loop as well as the gentle lordotic curve needed.

The final configuration of the rod is based on a template (model) made of 18 gauge wire. A piece of 18 gauge wire is bent into a shape that will fit over the C2 spinous process and under the T2 spinous process. This loop is placed gently into the wound, and is fashioned for the specific patient. The wire loop is removed to serve as a model; the actual Luque rod is then bent accordingly to provide a custom fit for a given patient. It is helpful for the surgeon to practice bending such rods in advance to gain experience before performing this maneuver during an operation. Preformed Hartshill rectangles or Ti-Frame rectangles may eliminate the need to form an individual loop for each patient. They are applied with the same cable technique as described below.

Placement of the Cables

Cables are now placed (Fig. 292-2); these eventually will be tightened around the Luque loop to fix it in position (Fig. 292-4). The cables [the author currently prefers the Codman Sof' Wire (Codman/Johnson & Johnson Professional, Inc., Randolph, MA) type because of their flexibility and ease of placement] are supplied as a double strand, with a so-called leader loop which facilitates passage under the lamina (Fig. 292-2). Sublaminar passage can be very safe and simple. The leader loop is gently slid in a superior direction over the dura from the inferior laminar lip. The leader loop is passed until it is visualized emerging from under the lamina. Then a nerve hook is placed in the loop, and the cable is pulled through. It is important to emphasize that the cable should only be pulled through; never pushed through. Attempting to push the cable under the lamina (rather than pull it through as above) can lead to "bunching" of the cable with compression of the subjacent neural elements. The leader loop is cut and one passage under the lamina has therefore produced two cables (one on each side) for fixation of the rod. Similar passage is made under the T1 and T2 laminae, thereby affording a total of six sublaminar cables for fixation (Fig. 292-2).

A single stranded cable is passed through each facet hole. If the facet holes have been drilled with a gentle inferior and medial angle, the cable can be grasped with a fine needle holder after the facet is spread with a Penfield #3 dissector. Four to six facet cables are placed, giving a total of 10 to 12 cables for fixation (Figs. 292-2 and 292-5).

Fixation of the Luque Loop

The Luque loop which was fashioned previously is now delivered over the cables and slid into position, with one end over the C2 spinous process and the other under the T2 spinous process. One end of each cable is passed inside the loop so that each cable will act as a noose around the Luque loop (Fig. 292-4). The "tensioner-crimper" portion of the cable system (Figs. 292-3 and 292-4) is now used to tighten each cable over the loop. Alternate cables are tightened, such as one would tighten lug nuts on an automobile wheel. Unlike wire, the cables tighten in a consistent manner. A small metal clasp is crimped over each cable, fixing it in position (Fig. 292-4).

Bone Grafting

Although some authors have used various types of instrumentation without bone grafts, bone grafting forms a permanent fusion, thereby eliminating the requirement for long-term resistance of instrument fatigue. Although our initial protocol used standard iliac crest graft harvesting, we currently use the bone from the resected laminae and spinous processes for the fusion. A recent review validates the effectiveness of this technique.[11] The advantages include eliminating the need for a second incision at the iliac crest. The bone is crushed into a pâte after the soft tissues are removed, and the pâte is wedged between the articular surfaces of the facets at each level. Prior to placement of the graft material, the articular surfaces of each facet should be scraped with a small curette or a diamond burr to encourage effective fusion. However, the facets should not be overpacked. The remainder of the pâte is placed over the lateral masses that have been gently buffed with the diamond burr.

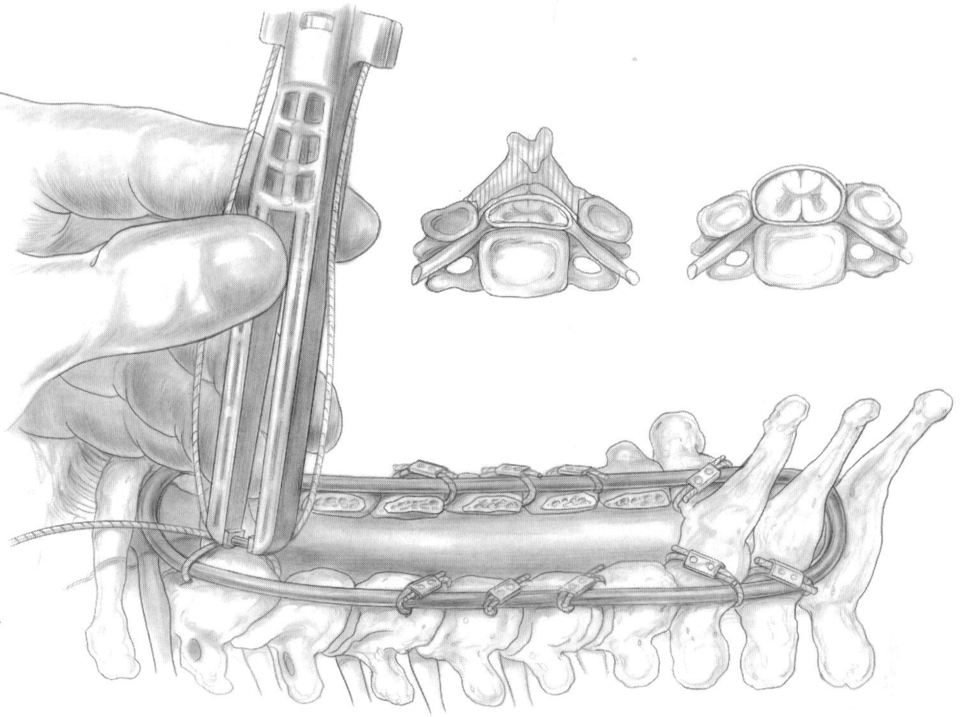

Figure 292-4 The Luque loop has been placed, and the cables are shown holding it in position. Each cable is tightened with the "tensioner-crimper" and fixed in position with a metal clasp which is closed with a crimping pliers. The *inset diagrams* depict preoperative (*left*) and postoperative (*right*) axial views of the cervical spinal canal.

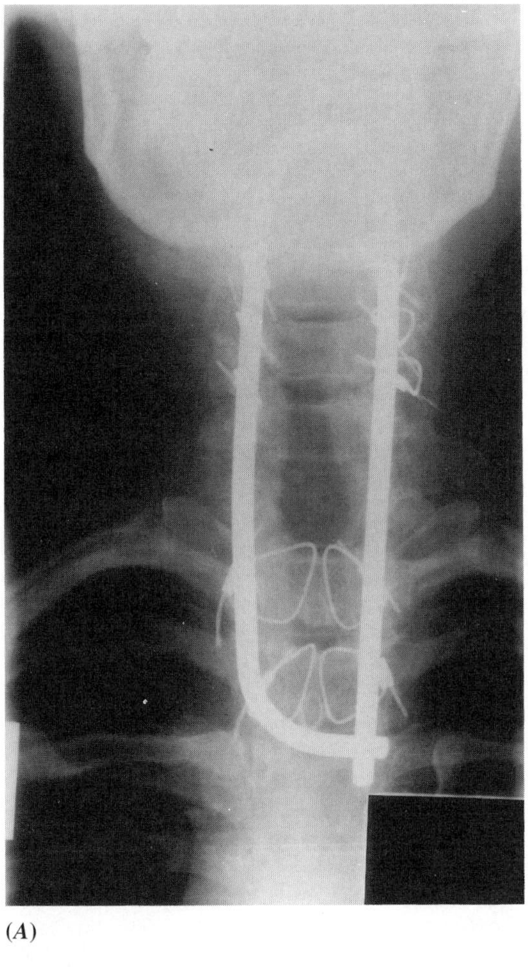

(*A*)

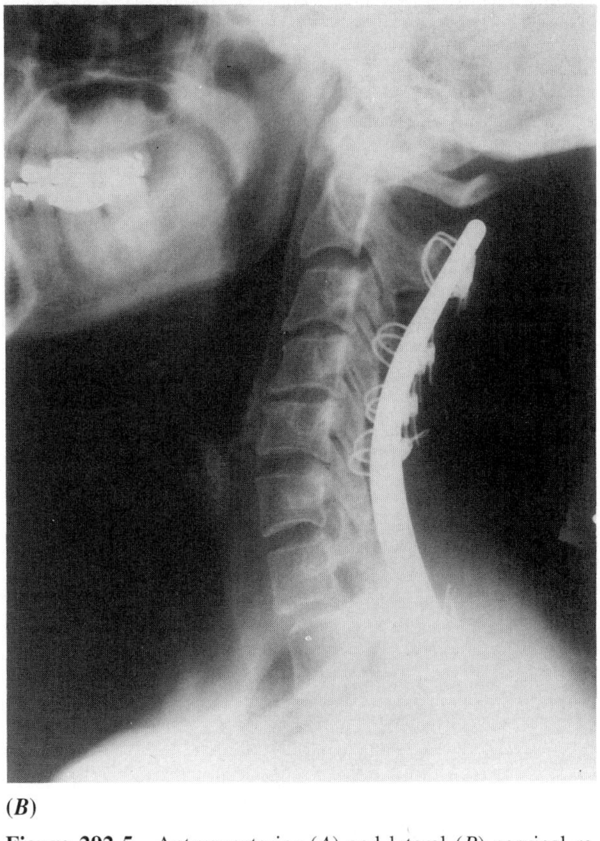

(*B*)

Figure 292-5 Anteroposterior (*A*) and lateral (*B*) cervical radiographs after placement of a Luque loop in a 46-year-old woman with cervical spondylotic myelopathy. Note the six sublaminar and six facet cables fixing the Luque loop in position.

Closure

The closure is similar to that of a standard cervical laminectomy. The dissection is somewhat more extensive because of the length of the wound as well as the need to expose most of each facet to its lateral margin. A tight closure with interrupted 2-0 Vicryl (polyglactin 910; Ethicon, Inc., Somerville, NJ) sutures in the muscles and fascia and a subsequent subcutaneous closure is recommended. Staples are used in the skin. Attention is paid to hemostasis prior to closure and no drains are used.

Postoperative Care

The patient is placed in a Philadelphia collar prior to being rolled from the prone position. The Philadelphia collar is worn at all times for the next 8 to 10 weeks. A single postoperative dose of an antibiotic is given. The patient may ambulate on the day after surgery and a regular diet is resumed. The patient is generally discharged between the fourth and fifth postoperative day.

Results

Luque instrumentation has been used extensively for stabilization of the thoracic and lumbar spinal regions.[5,13,14] Surgical decompression and resection for metastatic disease has been a common indication for its use.[5,14] Sublaminar wire was used initially to fix the rods in position, but concern was raised about the safety of the sublaminar method.[13] The advent of soft cable technology has enhanced the use of safe sublaminar techniques.[10] It is now possible to safely immobilize an extensive portion of the cervical spine with sublaminar cables and Luque loop instrumentation.

Our initial review of the use of Luque loop immobilization after extensive laminectomy was published in 1991.[15] Ten patients underwent a laminectomy and immobilization for cervical spondylotic myelopathy. Nine of the ten patients had significant improvement and the tenth had no progression. Since that time, 41 additional patients have been treated in similar fashion. The results have been encouraging. No patient has incurred a neurological deficit. Three of the initial ten patients developed seromas, two of the remaining group have done so as well. One patient has required removal of the instrumentation because of chronic drainage. Luque instrumentation with sublaminar cable techniques seems to offer a safe and effective method of cervical spine stabilization after an extensive laminectomy.

References

1. Adams CB, Logue V. Studies in cervical spondylotic myelopathy. II: The movement and contour of the spine in relation to the neural complications of cervical spondylosis. *Brain* 1971; 94:569–586.
2. Barnes M, Saunders M. The effect of cervical mobility on the natural history of cervical spondylotic myelopathy. *J Neurol Neurosurg Psychiatry* 1984; 47:17–20.
3. Bernhardt M, Hynes RA, Blume HW, et al. Cervical spondylotic myelopathy. *J Bone Joint Surg [Am]* 1993; 75-A:119–128.
4. Cusick JF, Steiner RE, Berns T. Total stabilization of the cervical spine in patients with cervical spondylotic myelopathy. *Neurosurgery* 1986; 18:491–495.
5. Cybulski GR. Methods of surgical stabilization for metastatic disease of the spine. *Neurosurgery* 1989; 25:240–252.
6. Fager CA. Results of adequate decompression in the relief of spondylotic myelopathy. *J Neurosurg* 1973; 38:684–692.
7. Fielding JW. The status of arthrodesis of the cervical spine. *J Bone Joint Surg [Am]* 1988; 70-A:1571–1574.
8. Gonzalez-Feria L. The effect of surgical immobilization after laminectomy in the treatment of advanced cases of cervical spondylotic myelopathy. *Acta Neurochir (Wien)* 1975; 31:185–193.
9. Harsh GR IV, Sypert GW, Weinstein PR, et al. Cervical spine stenosis secondary to ossification of the posterior longitudinal ligament. *J Neurosurg* 1987; 67:349–357.
10. Huhn SL, Wolf AL, Ecklund J. Posterior spinal osteosynthesis for cervical fracture/dislocation using a flexible multistrand cable system: technical note. *Neurosurgery* 1991; 29:943–946.
11. Keene JS, McKinley NE. Iliac crest versus spinous process grafts in post-traumatic spinal fusions. *Spine* 1992; 17:790–794.
12. Lunsford LD, Bissonette DJ, Zorub DS. Anterior surgery for cervical disc disease. Part 2: Treatment of cervical spondylotic myelopathy in 32 cases. *J Neurosurg* 1980; 53:12–19.
13. Luque ER. The anatomic basis and development of segmental spinal instrumentation. *Spine* 1982; 7:256–259.
14. MacKenzie AI, Uttley D, Marsh HT, et al. Craniocervical stabilization using Luque Hartshill rectangles. *Neurosurgery* 1990; 26:32–36.
15. Maurer PK, Ellenbogen RG, Ecklund J, et al. Cervical spondylotic myelopathy: treatment with posterior decompression and Luque rectangle bone fusion. *Neurosurgery* 1991; 28:680–684.
16. Maurer PK, Nussbaum C. Posterior decompression and fusion for cervical spondylotic myelopathy. In Rengachary SS, Wilkins RH (eds): *Neurosurgical Operative Atlas,* vol 2. Park Ridge, IL: American Association of Neurological Surgeons, 1992, pp 465–474.
17. Songer MN, Spencer DL, Meyer PR Jr, et al. The use of sublaminar cables to replace Luque wires. *Spine* 1991; 16:418–421.
18. Sypert GW. Anterior decompression and fusion for cervical myelopathy. In Camins MB, O'Leary PF (eds): *Disorders of the Cervical Spine.* Baltimore: Williams & Wilkins, 1992, pp 407–416.

293 Screw Fixation of Odontoid Fractures

Ronald I. Apfelbaum

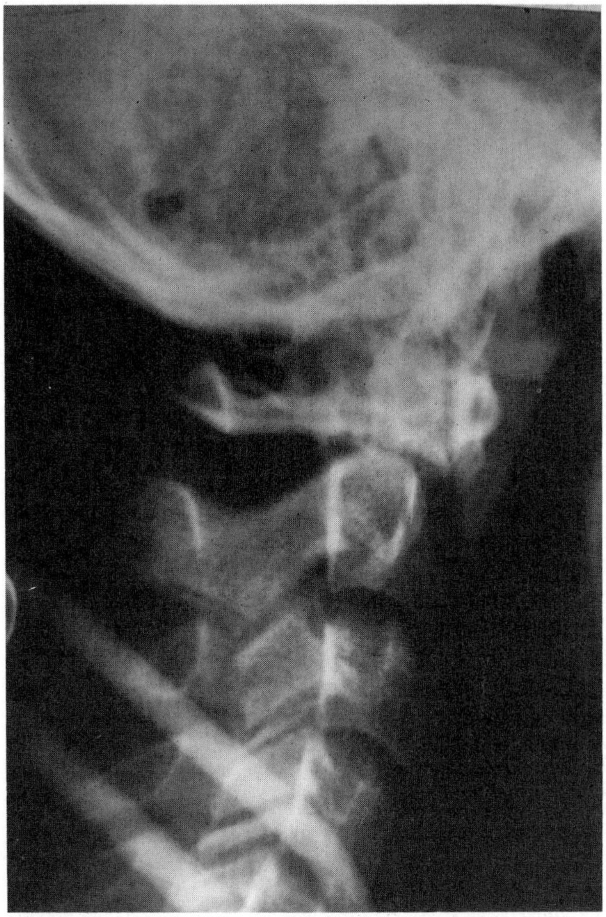

(*A*)

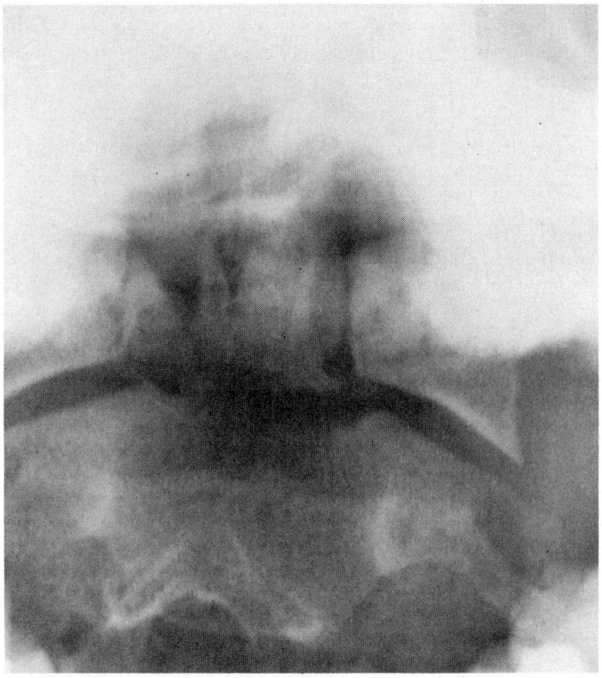

(*B*)

Figure 293-1 *A, B.* Typical type II odontoid fracture across the neck of the odontoid with anterolisthesis of C1 on C2. (From Apfelbaum,[4] with permission.)

The dens or odontoid process of the second cervical vertebra serves as a pivot point around which the skull and first cervical vertebra rotate. The anatomy of this region is well designed to allow this rotation. The lateral articulations at C1-C2 lie in a flat coronal plane. This, combined with the absence of an intervertebral disc and constraining annulus, loose capsular ligaments, and absence of a restraining elastic ligamentum flavum at C1-C2 posteriorly all facilitate such motion.[38] While the diameter of the spinal canal is widest at this level to accommodate such rotation,[40] it would be compromised to a potentially disastrous degree if anterior-posterior translation at C1-C2 were to occur. To prevent this, the strongest and thickest ligament in the cervical spine, the transverse ligament, with an average diameter of 10 mm,[29] constrains the odontoid into the anterior portion of the C1-C2 ring.

A fracture of the odontoid process, chronically nonunited odontoid (including os odontoideum), or disruption of the transverse ligament results in atlantoaxial instability and mandates efforts to restabilize this critical region. If not achieved, catastrophic neurological compromise can follow even minor trauma. I will discuss management of odontoid fractures in this chapter; the subject of ligamentous incompetence will be discussed elsewhere.

Odontoid Fractures

Odontoid fractures have been classified by Anderson and DeAlonzo[2] as type I, involving the apex of the odontoid, type II, across its neck, and type III, involving the body of C2. Type I fractures are quite rare and are thought to be stable, although some authors question that assumption.[36] Type II fractures are the most common (Fig. 293-1). These can result in either anterolisthesis or retrolisthesis of the odontoid relative to C2. Type III fractures, into the body of C2, are not infrequent. These have a good record of successful healing and fusion (greater than 80 percent) with immobilization, usually in a rigid external orthosis such as a halo vest.[12,15,16,18,22,27,32,37] They rarely require surgical intervention.

Type II fractures of the odontoid, on the other hand, are much less successfully managed by such immobilization. Various published series report widely discrepant results from external immobilization,[1,6,7,12,15,16,18,22,24,26,27,32,34,37] ranging from 0 percent[27] to 93 percent[26] success. An approximate average of reported cases suggests only a 40 to 50 percent chance of successful healing of a type II odontoid fracture by external immobilization.

Various authors have tried to define predictors of success or failure by retrospective review of their series. Such analyses have not yielded any unanimity of opinion, however. Apuzzo et al.[6] reported that greater than 4 mm of offset and age above 40 years correlated with increased chance of nonunion with immobilization (88 percent nonunion versus 16 percent). Dunn and Selgeskog[15] found that age above 65 years and retrolisthesis predicted nonunion with immobilization (70 to 78 percent). However, Hadley et al.[23] could correlate only 6 mm of offset in any direction with a higher nonunion rate (67 versus 26 percent). They also have identified a subtype they have called a type IIA odontoid fracture.[21] This type has comminuted fracture fragments at the base of the odontoid and is thought to be markedly unstable.

Quite likely the discrepancies noted by the various authors may represent a sampling problem, since the degree of offset is determined by that seen on what is essentially a random x-ray study. Any patient may indeed have significantly more offset if dynamic studies were obtained, but no one would advocate obtaining flexion and extension films in these unstable patients.

These discrepancies have led some authors to recommend that type II odontoid fractures be treated by a trial of immobilization in a rigid external orthosis (halo vest or Minerva jacket),[1,7,8,11,26,30,32,37] while others have recommended early surgical stabilization, either in all patients[24,27,34,35,39] or in those who meet specific criteria.[6,12,13,15,16,18,22,31]

External immobilization may be likened to trying to hold a snake at both ends in order to prevent movement between those ends. Indeed, we have seen patients move from significant anterolisthesis to significant retrolisthesis on fluoroscopy with each respiratory excursion, despite their being immobilized in a halo. Owing to the high degree of mobility of the cervical spine and the increased motion conferred by the fracture, immobilization will not be successful in many instances.

Posterior Fusion

The conventional surgical approach to atlantoaxial stabilization after a type II odontoid fracture has been a posterior C1-C2 fusion. This may be applied either as an initial treatment or after a failed trial of immobilization. Commonly used techniques involve placing a bone graft between or over the posterior arches of C1 and C2 and securing it with an encircling wire. Such techniques require an intact C1 posterior arch, which may not always be present with concomitant injury or prior surgery. The Gallie,[19] Brooks,[10] and Sonntag-Dickman[14] approaches have all been used with success for C1-C2 posterior fusion. Most also require external immobilization as well, since they offer little or no protection from translation until the fusion is solid. Although not uniformly successful,[17] posterior fusions, when successful, restore C1-C2 stability and protect the neural elements, but in so doing eliminate all normal C1-C2 motion. This is unfortunate because one-half of the axial rotation possible in the cervical spine occurs at the C1-C2 joint.[38] Nevertheless, this result is certainly preferable to the potentially disastrous complications associated with persistent C1-C2 instability.

Anterior Screw Fixation

Fortunately, an alternative technique has evolved: direct screw fixation of the odontoid fracture. This has proved quite successful in stabilizing the C1-C2 complex immediately, preserving normal C1-C2 motion. It has a high likelihood of long-term success.

The procedure was first reported by Nakanishi[28] in 1980 and Böhler[9] in 1982. Subsequently, Lesoin et al.[25] described an approach that required an extensive neck dissection. Geisler et al.[20] in 1989 reported on nine patients treated by a low cervical anterior approach. We have subsequently developed a set of instruments that greatly facilitate this procedure using a similar approach[3–5] (Aesculap Instrument Corporation, South San Francisco, CA, and Aesculap AG, Tuttlingen, Germany). The approach I recommend utilizes a small, transverse, low cervical incision in a natural skin crease at about the C5 level with a standard (Cloward type) approach to the vertebral column at that level. This is identical to that employed for an anterior cervical discectomy. Special retractors, a guide tube system, and fluoroscopic guidance in both the anteroposterior (AP) and lateral planes facilitate this procedure.

Surgical Technique

The reader is referred to two publications[4,5] for further details and illustrations of this procedure. Under lateral fluoroscopic control, the patient is positioned supine and the neck is extended as far as possible without displacing the odontoid process posteriorly into the spinal canal. Even with a retrolisthesed odontoid, anterior translation of the head while extending the rest of the neck may be possible as long as careful fluoroscopic control is maintained.

Halter traction holds the head in position. A radiolucent mouth gag (wine bottle cork or plastic padded tongue blade) keeps the mouth open for transoral AP fluoroscopy. If available, two C-arm fluoroscopes are used for AP and lateral imaging, respectively. Placing the lateral unit with its arc at or somewhat above the level of the head of the table allows the AP unit to be brought in over it (Fig. 293-2). One can then image frequently in either plane by

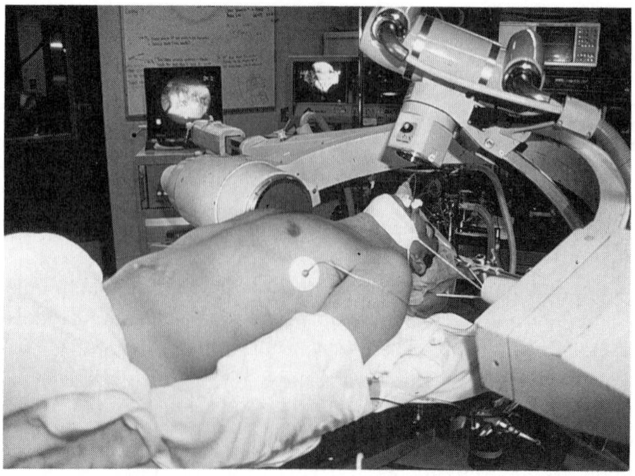

Figure 293-2 Patient positioned with two C-arm fluoroscopic units for transoral AP and lateral imaging. The folded sheet under the shoulders increases neck extension and facilitates exposure in this patient, whose fracture reduced in extension.

stepping on the appropriate foot control pedal. If only one fluoroscope is available, it should be positioned to allow frequent rotation into either the AP or lateral plane. In such a case, draping the patient in such a way as to make a tent of sheets to keep the fluoroscope out of the sterile field facilitates frequent change of fluoroscope position without the need for redraping.

In either case, only high-quality fluoroscopic units with digital processing should be used to allow precise screw placement. The OEC units (OEC Medical Systems, Inc, Salt Lake City, UT) are our preference, although others also meet these requirements. Having an image storage and display capability allows the surgeon to hold an image on one screen while matching the image on the other. This makes possible, for example, placing the screw into a previously prepared track by realigning the vertebrae precisely at each step when there is instability.

After routine prepping and draping, the incision site is determined by placing a straight object such as a K-wire alongside the neck and aligning it fluoroscopically with the desired trajectory to the inferior edge of C2. Routine dissection in natural tissue planes allows access to the prevertebral space at the selected level, usually about C5-C6, (Fig. 293-3), where the anterior longitudinal ligament is incised in the midline over one and a half vertebral bodies. Periosteal elevators allow elevation of the longus coli muscle bellies bilaterally at this level. Sharp-toothed Caspar retracting blades are securely placed beneath this muscle to anchor a specially modified retractor (Fig. 293-3). Blunt dissection in the loose areolar prevertebral space *anterior* to the longus coli muscles with a "peanut dissector" held in a tonsil clamp and swept from side to side quickly allows access to the C1-C2 region. An angled titanium (for radiolucency) retractor blade placed in this space is attached to a retractor that mates with the lateral retractor. In this manner a working tunnel is created from the incision to the C2 region. No inferior retraction is needed, and its absence improves the low trajectory required to place the screw into the body of C2 and then into the odontoid process across the fracture site.

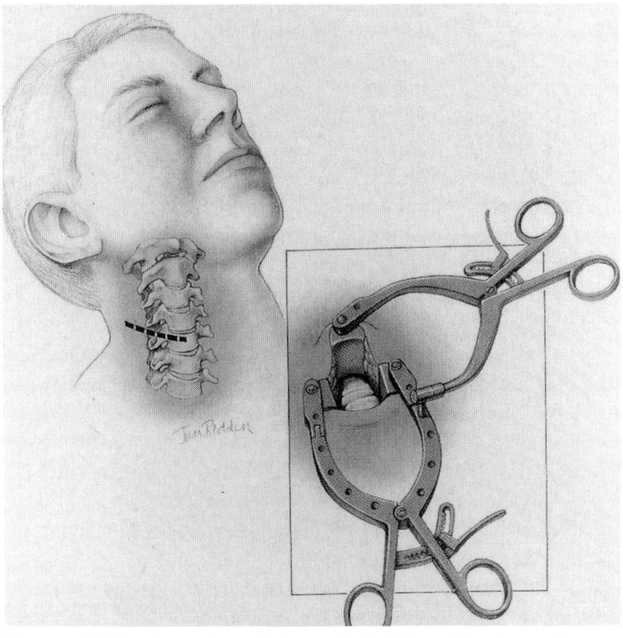

Figure 293-3 Location of the neck incision. The *inset* shows the retractor in place.

This screw placement is achieved as follows. First a K-wire is impacted into the anterior inferior edge of C2 (Fig. 293-4*A*). The entry site is carefully chosen under biplane fluoroscopy. A paramedian location about 2 mm off the midline and aimed toward the odontoid tip is chosen if two odontoid screws are to be placed (see later discussion). A midline site is chosen if only one screw will be placed.

A 7-mm hollow overdrill is then placed over the K-wire and rotated by hand (Fig. 293-4*C*) to create a shallow trough (Fig. 293-4*B, D*) in the anterior face of C3 and the C2-C3 annulus. This trough will accommodate the inner guide tube. The guide tube system (Fig. 293-5) consists of an inner and outer guide tube, which mate together and then are placed over the K-wire. The outer guide tube has fixation spikes which are placed into C3 once the tube has been manipulated over the K-wire to that level. Once so secured the inner guide tube is advanced through the aforementioned trough to the inferior edge of C2. The K-wire is then withdrawn and a pilot hole is drilled through the body of C2 and up to the tip of the odontoid (Fig. 293-6). It is possible and desirable to complete the realignment of the odontoid to the body of C2 before crossing the fracture site with the drill. This usually can be done by moving the C2-C3 complex relevant to the C1-odontoid complex with the drill guide. The odontoid is quite constrained by its investing periosteum to which are attached the restraining alar and apical ligaments. It will not be displaced by the drill or screw placement, as one might fear.

The drilling must be monitored fluoroscopically in both planes. It is possible, using the guide tube system, to aim the drill in the desired direction, but it is hard to correct the trajectory once a hole has been drilled. Proceeding slowly and with frequent monitoring in both planes is therefore essential for optimal positioning.

The drill should pierce the full thickness of the odontoid apical cortex (Fig. 293-7). Note that the direction of drilling is such that penetration beyond the odontoid carries the drill into the apical ligaments and toward the clivus, providing a generous safety margin for the neural elements. Once the pilot hole is drilled through the apex of the odontoid, the depth of penetration of the drill may be read on the calibrated shaft of the drill bit (Fig. 293-6). This requires that the inner drill guide be extended to abut the inferior edge of C2. The drill is then withdrawn and the inner drill guide removed. A tap is placed through the outer drill guide and used to cut threads in the bone to and through the odontoid apical cortex. This ensures proper screw-thread–bone interface and prevents splitting of the dense odontoid cortical bone.

A partially threaded lag screw is then placed through the guide tube. It should firmly engage the distal odontoid cortex (Fig. 293-8). In fresh fractures it will draw the odontoid back to the body of C2. This lag effect is achieved even if some of the threads cross the fracture line, since the softer, cancellous bone in that area will readily yield.

A second screw, if one is used, is then placed by means of an identical series of steps using an entry site 3 to 4 mm away from the first, toward the contralateral side. If a second screw is placed it may be fully threaded, since no further lag effect is anticipated (Fig. 293-8).

If screw fixation is attempted in chronically nonunited fractures (see discussion below), the screw may be placed into the body of C2, stopping short of crossing the fracture line, and the guide tube assembly removed (Fig. 293-9*A*). Bifaced angled curettes are available to curette out the fracture site to remove fibrous tissue and "freshen" the bone edges in the hope of promoting fusion.

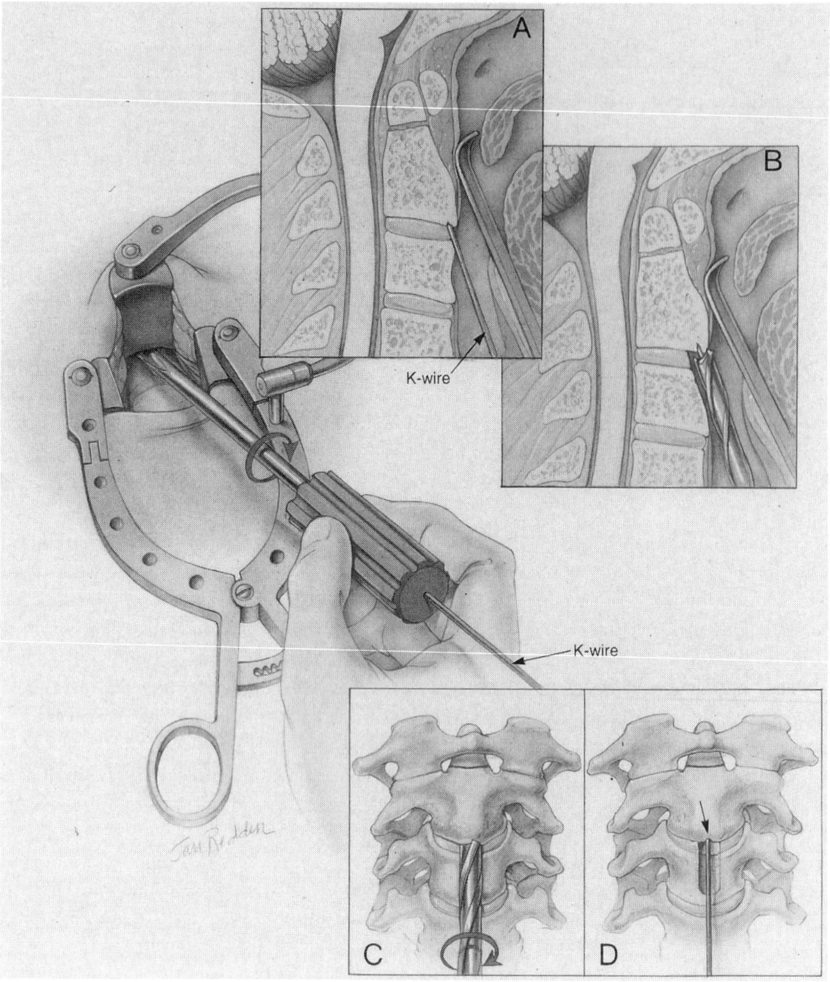

Figure 293-4 *A*. A K-wire in place in the anterior inferior edge of C2. *B–D*. A hollow hand-drill placed over the K-wire is used to create a trough in the face of C3 and in the C2-C3 annulus. (From Apfelbaum,[4] with permission.)

These are angled such that rotation of the handle simultaneously curettes both upper and lower surfaces(Fig. 293-9*B*). A ball-tipped screwdriver then facilitates reengaging the screw head to fully seat the screw (Fig. 293-9*C*). In chronic nonunions, usually no significant lag effect can be seen because scar tissue and shortening of the ligaments will prevent full approximation of the odontoid to the body of C2.

After assuring hemostasis, the retractor system is removed and stability is confirmed by flexing the patient's neck under lateral fluoroscopic monitoring. While combined disruption of both the transverse ligament and odontoid is unlikely, this must be tested for by the maneuver described above to ensure that stabilization has been achieved. Closure is then effected in standard fashion with interrupted absorbable sutures in layers and sterile skin tapes. No drain is placed. Unless bone quality is poor, a cervical collar is not routinely used, but one may be used if required for comfort or external protection. Hospital stay is usually quite brief, often only 1 to 3 days; patients may resume normal activities including nonjarring or strenuous work within a few days. Acute fractures normally will demonstrate good bone healing on serial radiographs within 3 months. Chronic nonunions, however, may take considerably longer, and some will only achieve fibrous union, defined as persistent long-term stabilization with intact hardware despite absence of demonstrable bony union.

Results

We have employed this technique in 44 patients operated upon over a 7.5-year period. Two-thirds of these procedures were for fractures incurred within the six months prior to repair, termed ''acute fractures.'' The remaining one-third were all fractures of over 18 months' duration and are referred to as ''chronic nonunions.'' The average patient age was 46 years, with a range of 15 to 83 years.

Of the 29 patients with acute fractures, more than 3 months have elapsed since surgery for 27, and, hence, data are available for analysis. One patient in this group died of unrelated pulmonary problems 1 month after surgery; another out-of-state patient has been lost to follow-up. The remaining 25 patients have all gone on to bony union, although one fracture healed in an anterolisthesed position when the screws failed to hold well in the fractured C2 body. This patient failed to return for scheduled follow-up. Had she done so, fusion in proper position might have been obtained by manipulating her back into position and using an external orthosis, as was done in another patient when such failure to hold in C2 was recognized promptly.

Patients with chronic, nonunited fractures of the odontoid process (which may include some patients with os odontoideum) fared less well. Of the 15 patients in this category we have been unable

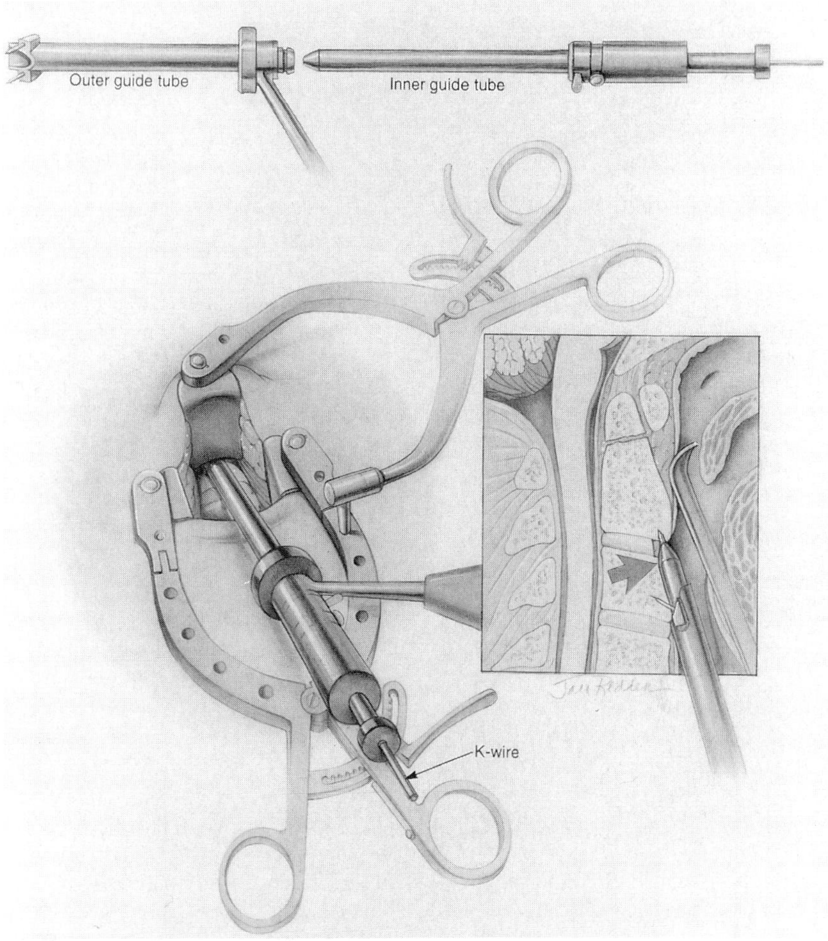

Figure 293-5 The guide tube system. The inner and outer guide tubes mate together. They are placed over the K-wire, and the fixation spikes are set into C3 *(right inset)*. The inner drill guide is then advanced to the inferior edge of C2 over the K-wire (*arrow*). (From Apfelbaum,[4] with permission.)

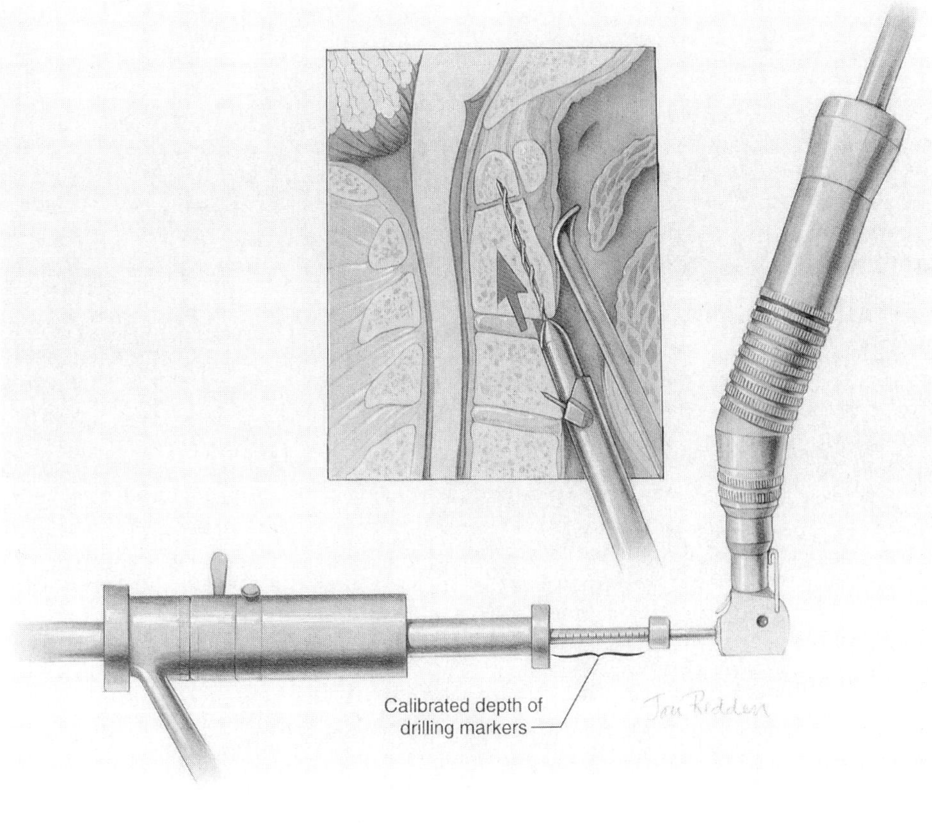

Figure 293-6 A pilot hole is being drilled (under biplane fluoroscopic control) through the body of C2 and to the apex of the odontoid. The drill should pierce the distal odontoid cortex (Fig. 293-7). The depth of penetration is then measured on the calibrated drill shaft. (From Apfelbaum,[4] with permission.)

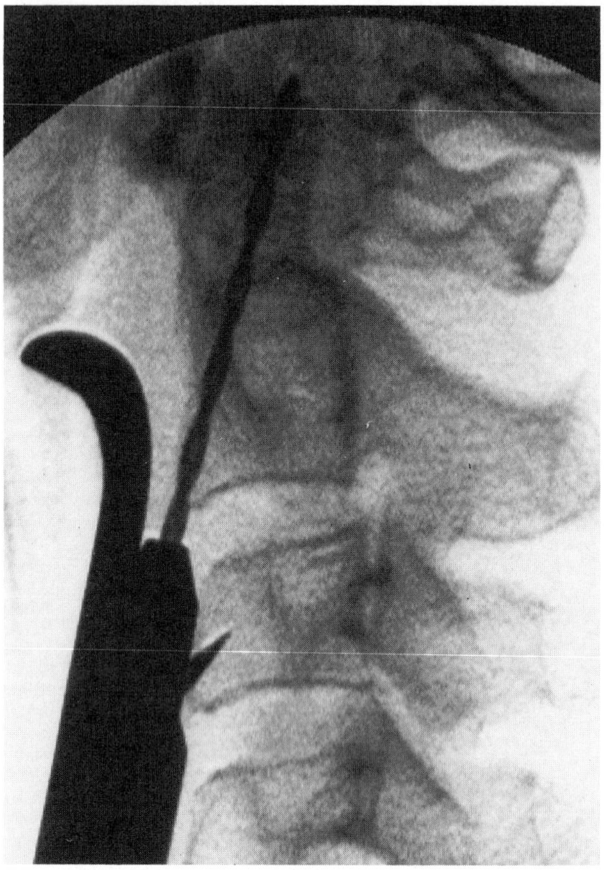

Figure 293-7 Lateral fluoroscopic view of drill bit to and through the distal odontoid cortex.

to obtain follow-up in two. Of the remaining 13, four have achieved bony union, and five have fibrous union, defined as intact hardware and stability on flexion/extension films, but without definite bony bridging. In the remaining four patients, screw fractures occurred in three and a small os odontoideum failed to hold the screws in one. Only one of these was a late occurrence, several years after apparent satisfactory fibrous union. All of these patients who failed odontoid screw fixation were treated successfully with atlantoaxial fusion.

There were no neurological complications. In no instance was there any dural penetration, CSF leakage, or neurological worsening. One patient had a minor esophageal leak at the site of the lateral retractors (C5-C6), and this quickly resolved. There were no other significant complications.

Technical Considerations

Biomechanical studies have suggested that the addition of a second screw may not augment structural strength very much.[33] Two screws, however, can prevent rotation of the odontoid on the body of C2. This may be less important with acute fractures, where the irregular bone surfaces seem to lock together well when drawn together by the lag screw, than with chronic nonunions, where smooth sclerotic edges exist that often cannot be fully approximated. Since anatomic studies have suggested that the dens often can accept two screws, and this adds very little to the operative time, we have therefore tried to use two screws whenever possible and have been able to do so in 21 of our last 22 patients.

The screws in current use are made of titanium or titanium alloy. These are fully MRI compatible. They do not produce any significant artifact on MRI, so the atlantoaxial region can be well imaged if there is need in the future.

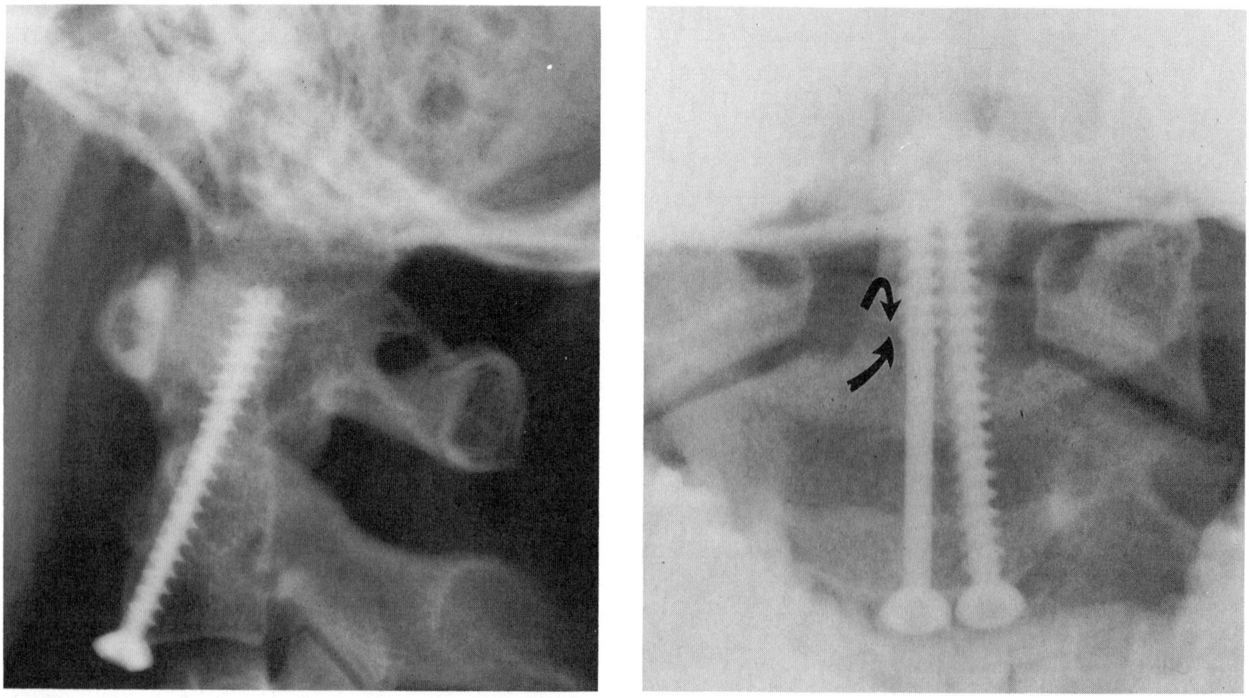

(A) *(B)*

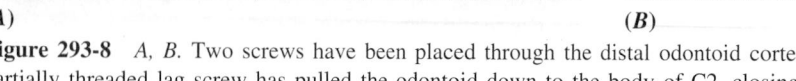

Figure 293-8 *A, B.* Two screws have been placed through the distal odontoid cortex. The first partially threaded lag screw has pulled the odontoid down to the body of C2, closing the fracture gap (*arrows*).

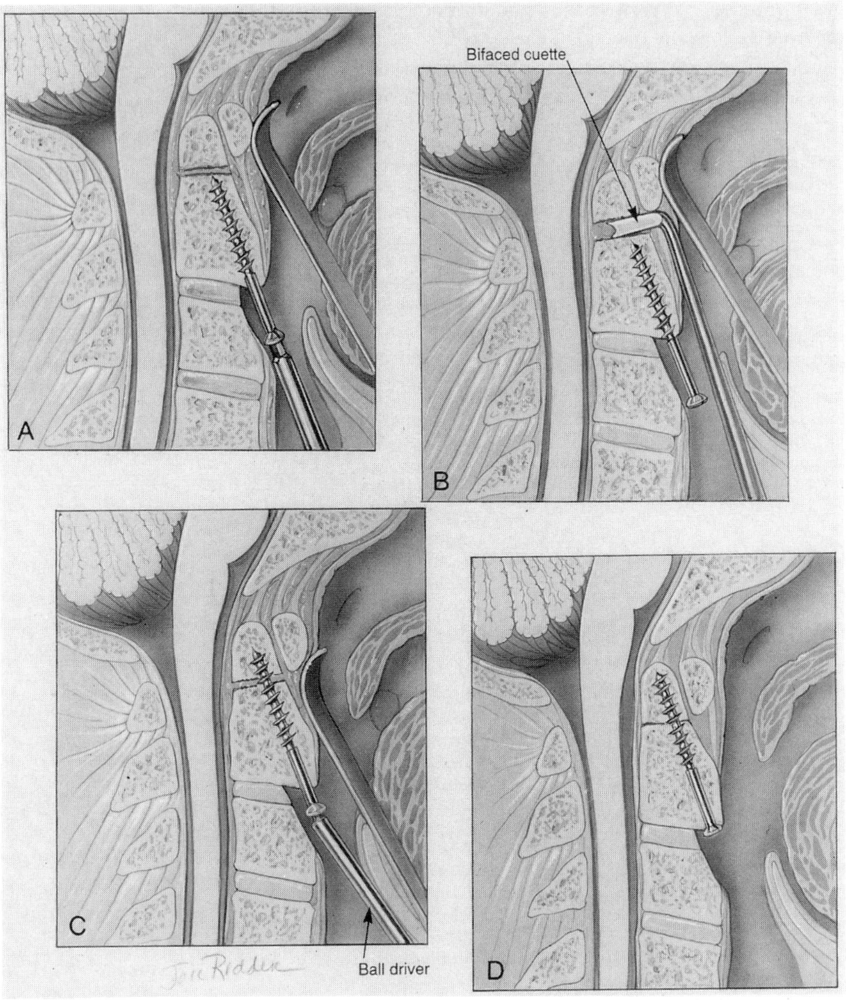

Figure 293-9 *A*. The screw is inserted through the guide tube (omitted in artist's drawing) and advanced through the threaded pilot hole. *B*. In chronic nonunion, special bifaced curettes are used to freshen the fracture site. *C*. The screw is then advanced using the ball driver. *D*. The final screw position. (From Apfelbaum,[4] with permission.)

Discussion

Halo vest immobilization, as noted earlier, has an uncertain success rate, which may be no greater than 50 to 60 percent overall for type II odontoid fractures. Fractures in patients at either end of the age spectrum may be less likely to fuse when immobilized—the elderly owing to poor or slow healing capability and the young who are more flexible and, hence, harder to immobilize successfully.

Immobilization in a halo vest is not inexpensive. When one considers the cost of the device and the cost of daily pin site care, there may be little economic advantage over direct screw fixation with its brief 1- to 3-day hospital stay. Complications of halo vest treatment such as pin site infections further add to its cost. Factoring in the loss of income if the patient is unable to work in the halo and the nontangible but very real issues of patient comfort (or discomfort) and social morbidity appear to give direct screw fixation a significant advantage.

The use of screw fixation in acute odontoid fractures has proved to be a very satisfactory treatment. All the patients we have been able to follow adequately have fused successfully. Ten of these had failed prior halo vest immobilization; eight had been immobilized in a rigid collar prior to surgery. As noted, the cost of halo vest immobilization and its associated social morbidity makes screw fixation appear to be quite cost-effective. We therefore feel justified in recommending this as a primary treatment for odontoid fractures of less than 6 months duration.

The chronically nonunited fracture, and os odontoideum as well, present a more difficult problem. Successful bony union was achieved in 27 percent, and successful stabilization (bony plus fibrous union) in 60 percent. Some of the patients with fibrous union may fail in the future, although to date only one has done so (all other failures have occurred within a few months of surgery). When successful, however, odontoid screw fixation preserves normal C1-C2 rotation, which as noted earlier accounts for 50 to 60 percent of the capacity for axial rotation of the cervical spine. For this reason the procedure probably should be considered as an option and discussed with patients. If the patient is willing to accept the lower success rate (60 percent) versus almost assured fusion (if C1-C2 posterior fusion is augmented with C1-C2 transarticular screw fixation) to try to avoid the C1-C2 fusion, it should be offered as long as the patient understands that failure means a second operation. In our experience, however, most patients, when approached in this manner, have elected to have an atlantoaxial fusion; therefore, we infrequently employ odontoid screw fixation for chronic nonunions.

If, in preoperative evaluation, the odontoid is found to have spontaneously fused to the anterior arch of C1 or clivus, anterior screw fixation is not indicated. Such fusion will likely place much more stress on the screw fixation and likely will lead to hardware failure. Also, even if the odontoid can be successfully fused to C2 in such a situation, the patient would still lose C1-C2 rotation.

Careful preoperative evaluation of the integrity of C2 is also necessary to assure its ability to hold the fixation screws. Concomitant body fractures, as noted above, led to screws pulling out of the body of C2 when these secondary injuries were not fully appreciated or respected.

A final relative contraindication is an anteriorly sloping oblique odontoid fracture. In such cases the fixation screw will tend to pull the fractured odontoid down the slope and increase anterolisthesis.

An occasional type III odontoid fracture involving only the upper one quarter of the body of C2 may also be amenable to screw fixation if the patient is unwilling to accept halo vest immobilization. The high success rate of that latter treatment, however, must be factored into such a decision.

Conclusions

Direct anterior screw fixation of type II odontoid fractures has proved to be a very successful treatment. With the development of specialized instrumentation, the procedure can be performed quickly and safely under biplane fluoroscopic control. The ability to immediately stabilize the C1-C2 complex and achieve bony union of the odontoid for long-term stability while avoiding the cost, discomfort, and medical and social morbidity of halo vest immobilization on one hand and the loss of normal C1-C2 rotatory motion on the other makes this both the treatment of choice and the surgical procedure of choice for acute (less than 6 months old) odontoid fractures.

It is also a treatment option for chronically nonunited odontoid processes when, on balance, the patient is willing to accept its lower long-term success rate to try to avoid loss of normal atlanto-axial motion.

References

1. Althoff B, Bardholm P. Fracture of the odontoid process. A clinical and radiographic study. *Acta Orthop Scand (Suppl)* 1979; 177:61–95.
2. Anderson LD, D'Alonzo RT. Fractures of the odontoid process of the axis. *J Bone Joint Surg [Am]* 1974; 56-A:1663–1674.
3. Apfelbaum RI. Anterior screw fixation of odontoid fractures. In Camins MD, O'Leary PF (eds): *Disorders of the Cervical Spine.* Baltimore: Williams & Wilkins, 1992, pp 603–608.
4. Apfelbaum RI. Anterior screw fixation of odontoid fractures. In Rengachary SS, Wilkins RH (eds): *Neurosurgical Operative Atlas,* vol 2. Baltimore: Williams & Wilkins, 1992, pp 189–199.
5. Apfelbaum RI. Anterior screw fixation of odontoid fractures. Aesculap Scientific Information #24, Tuttlingen, Germany: Aesculap AG, 1993.
6. Apuzzo MLJ, Heiden JS, Weiss MH, et al. Acute fractures of the odontoid process: an analysis of 45 cases. *J Neurosurg* 1978; 48:85–91.
7. Blockey NJ, Purser DW. Fractures of the odontoid process of the axis. *J Bone Joint Surg [Br]* 1956; 38-B:794–817.
8. Böhler J. Fractures of the odontoid process. *J Trauma* 1965; 5:386–391.
9. Böhler J. Anterior stabilization for acute fractures and non-unions of the dens. *J Bone Joint Surg [Am]* 1982; 64-A:18–27.
10. Brooks AL, Jenkins EB. Atlanto-axial arthrodesis by the wedge compression method. *J Bone Joint Surg [Am]* 1978; 60-A:279–284.
11. Chan RC, Schweigel JF, Thompson GB. Halo-thoracic brace immobilization in 188 patients with acute cervical spine injuries. *J Neurosurg* 1983; 58:508–515.
12. Clark CR, White AA III. Fractures of the dens. A multicenter study. *J Bone Joint Surg [Am]* 1985; 67-A:1340–1348.
13. Cooper PR, Maravilla KR, Sklar FH, et al. Halo immobilization of cervical spine fractures: indications and results. *J Neurosurg* 1979; 50:603–610.
14. Dickman CA, Sonntag VKH, Papadopoulos SM, et al. The interspinous method of posterior atlantoaxial arthodesis. *J Neurosurg* 1991; 74:190–198.
15. Dunn ME, Seljeskog EL. Experience in the management of odontoid process injuries: an analysis of 128 cases. *Neurosurgery* 1986; 18:306–310.
16. Ekong CEU, Schwartz ML, Tator CH, et al. Odontoid fracture: management with early mobilization using the halo device. *Neurosurgery* 1981; 9:631–637.
17. Fried LC. Atlanto-axial fracture-dislocations. Failure of posterior C1 to C2 fusion. *J Bone Joint Surg [Br]* 1973; 55-B:490–496.
18. Fujii E, Kobayashi K, Hirabayashi K. Treatment in fractures of the odontoid process. *Spine* 1988; 13:604–609.
19. Gallie WE. Fractures and dislocations of the cervical spine. *Am J Surg* 1939; 46:495–499.
20. Geisler FH, Cheng C, Poka A, et al. Anterior screw fixation of posteriorly displaced type II odontoid fractures. *Neurosurgery* 1989; 25:30–38.
21. Hadley MN, Browner CM, Liu SS, et al. New subtype of acute odontoid fractures (type IIA). *Neurosurgery* 1988; 22:67–71.
22. Hadley MN, Browner CM, Sonntag VKH. Axis fractures: a comprehensive review of management and treatment in 107 cases. *Neurosurgery* 1985; 17:281–290.
23. Hadley MN, Dickman CA, Browner CM, et al. Acute axis fractures: a review of 229 cases. *J Neurosurg* 1989; 71:642–647.
24. Hentzer L, Schalimtzek M. Fractures and subluxations of the atlas and axis. A follow-up study of 20 patients. *Acta Orthop Scand* 1971; 42:251–258.
25. Lesoin F, Autricque A, Franz K, et al. Transcervical approach and screw fixation for upper cervical spine pathology. *Surg Neurol* 1987; 27:459–465.
26. Lind B, Nordwall A, Sihlbom H. Odontoid fractures treated with halo-vest. *Spine* 1987; 12:173–177.
27. Maiman DJ, Larson SJ. Management of odontoid fractures. *Neurosurgery* 1982; 11:471–476.
28. Nakanishi T. Internal fixation of the odontoid fracture (in Japanese). *Cent Jpn J Orthop Traumatic Surg* 1980; 23:399–406.
29. Panjabi MM, Oxland TR, Parks EH. Quantitative anatomy of cervical spine ligaments. Part II. Middle and lower cervical spine. *J Spinal Disord* 1991; 4:277–285.
30. Paradis GR, Janes JM. Posttraumatic atlantoaxial instability: the fate of the odontoid process fracture in 46 cases. *J Trauma* 1973; 13:359–367.
31. Pepin JW, Bourne RB, Hawkins RJ. Odontoid fractures with special reference to the elderly patient. *Clin Orthop* 1985; 193:178–183.
32. Ryan MD, Taylor TKF. Odontoid fractures: a rational approach to treatment. *J Bone Joint Surg [Br]* 1982; 64-B:416–421.
33. Sasso RC, Heggeness MH, Doherty BJ. Biomechanics of odontoid fracture fixation: a comparison of one and two screw technique. Presented at the 20th Annual Meeting of the Cervical Spine Research Society, Palm Desert, CA, December 1992.

34. Schatzker J, Rorabeck CH, Waddell JP. Fracture of the dens (odontoid process). An analysis of thirty-seven cases. *J Bone Joint Surg [Br]* 1971; 53-B:392–405.
35. Schiess RJ, DeSaussure RL, Robertson JT. Choice of treatment of odontoid fractures. *J Neurosurg* 1982; 57:496–499.
36. Scott EW, Haid RW, Peace D. Type I fractures of the odontoid process: implications for atlanto-occipital instability. Case report. *J Neurosurg* 1990; 72:488–492.
37. Wang GJ, Mabie KN, Whitehill R, et al. The nonsurgical management of odontoid fractures in adults. *Spine* 1984; 9:229–230.
38. White AA, Panjabi MM. *Clinical Biomechanics of the Spine,* 2d ed. Philadelphia: Lippincott, 1990, pp 92–97.
39. Wilson TAS Jr, McWhorter JM. Atlantoaxial injuries. In Camins MB, O'Leary PF (eds): *Disorders of the Cervical Spine.* Baltimore: Williams & Wilkins, 1992, pp 285–291.
40. Wolf BS, Khilnani M, Malis L. The sagittal diameter of the bony cervical spinal canal and its significance in cervical spondylosis. *J Mt Sinai Hosp NY* 1956; 23:283–292.

294

Caspar Plating for Stabilization of the Cervical Spine

H. Louis Harkey

The complexion of spinal neurosurgery has changed dramatically over the past decade as neurosurgeons have embraced orthopedic concepts of stabilization. The traditional neurosurgical charge, decompression of the spinal cord and nerve roots, is now recognized as only one therapeutic component in the surgical treatment of many spinal disorders. The importance of preservation, reconstruction, or stabilization of motion segments is increasingly appreciated. Granted, neurosurgeons have been stabilizing cervical spine fractures for many years, but the use of sophisticated implantable devices is relatively new.

The expanding horizons of spinal surgery mandate new emphasis within the framework of traditional neurosurgical education. Basic science training must include concepts of spinal biomechanics and bone healing. The surgical skills for adequate but minimally destructive decompression and internal instrumentation techniques should be taught. Finally, the spinal neurosurgeon must know the proper indications for each decompressive and reconstructive procedure.

European surgeons were the first to report the use of bone plates to stabilize the traumatized cervical spine. Orozco and others designed plates specifically for the cervical spine,[9] but the Caspar plate was the first plate to attain widespread usage.[1] The success of this plate can be attributed to an overall system concept. Caspar developed instrumentation in accordance with a procedural concept of enhanced exposure, crafted interbody reconstruction, and individually adaptable implants. The Caspar technique and instrumentation continue to be refined and have stimulated other novel techniques of anterior cervical spine stabilization.

Indications and Patient Selection

The most biomechanically sound indication for anterior cervical plating is the hyperextension injury, including those with a component of distraction or compression.[2,11] The destabilizing forces of hyperextension disrupt the anterior longitudinal ligament and anulus fibrosus of the disc space. The stabilizing forces of an anterior plate are in the opposite direction of the destabilizing forces. The plate acts as a tension band, restoring integrity to the anterior column.

Compression and flexion/compression injuries resulting in vertebral burst fractures or anterior wedge fractures are also good indications for anterior cervical plating. Many of these fractures require anterior decompression of the cord and nerve roots followed by either internal or external immobilization. The Caspar osteosynthetic stabilization technique allows for decompression and stabilization in a one-stage procedure. Flexion injuries resulting in cervical fracture dislocation can also be treated with anterior grafting and plating. Although biomechanical theory would predict anterior plating to be a less desirable stabilization technique for fractures with posterior instability, laboratory studies and clinical experience have proved otherwise.[1,3,4,13,14]

Caspar plate stabilization is useful in other types of cervical trauma as well. Some highly unstable hangman's fractures with C2-C3 and posterior longitudinal ligament disruption cannot be treated adequately by external immobilization.[15] These fractures can be reduced and stabilized with a Caspar plate because it can be bent acutely to follow the contour of the axis body and screws can be placed at various angles if necessary (Fig. 294-1).

It has become apparent from recent use of magnetic resonance imaging (MRI) in cervical trauma that disc herniation associated with simple fracture subluxation is more common than previously thought.[6] Following the removal of displaced disc fragments, anterior plating provides immediate internal stabilization, obviating the need for a second posterior stabilization procedure or halo immobilization. The decreased risk of supine positioning and the ease of operative exposure afforded by the anterior approach make anterior cervical plate stabilization an increasingly popular alternative to posterior stabilization techniques even when decompression is not necessary.

Most locked facets can be reduced after anterior decompression with a combination of distraction and gentle manipulation and therefore do not constitute an absolute contraindication to anterior

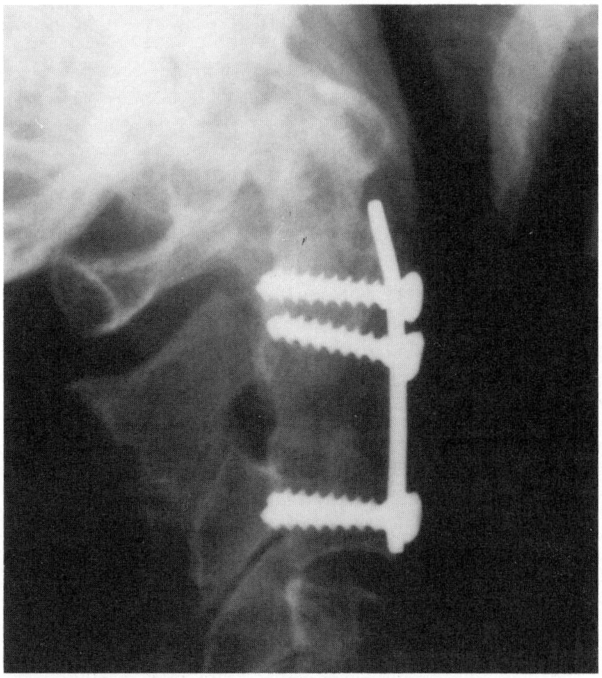

Figure 294-1 This 71-year-old woman had an unstable hangman's fracture that failed halo stabilization. She was treated successfully with an intervertebral graft and a contoured anterior cervical plate.

cervical plating. However, if a locked facet is disassociated from the vertebral body by a fracture through the pedicle, reduction via an anterior approach may not be possible. Locked facets not requiring anterior decompression are still best treated by posterior reduction and stabilization.

The indications for Caspar plating are not limited to traumatic lesions of the cervical spine but also include the treatment of degenerative diseases, tumors, and other processes requiring stabilization.[5,7] Degenerative subluxation with associated osteophytic root or cord compression can be decompressed, reduced, and stabilized with the Caspar plate. Ossification of the posterior longitudinal ligament, severe multilevel cervical spondylosis, and tumors of the vertebral body or anterior spinal canal increasingly are being treated with cervical corpectomy followed by strut graft reconstruction. The major complication associated with cervical corpectomy is graft extrusion. The addition of a Caspar plate provides an anterior tension band that deters graft extrusion and enhances fusion. Likewise, the risk of pseudarthrosis increases following multilevel discectomies for cervical spondylosis as the number of levels of decompression increases. Caspar plating with fixation at each intervening vertebral body will decrease the chance of malunion.

A stabilizing bone plate merely acts as an internal splint while bony remodeling occurs. If bony union is not ultimately achieved, repeated stress on the instrumentation will eventually lead to treatment failure. Young healthy bone, most common in traumatic cervical spine injuries, is ideally suited for anterior cervical stabilization. It provides excellent screw purchase and rapid bone healing. On the other hand, osteoporotic bone has decreased density and heals more slowly; therefore, the risk of screw-loosening is greater and the stresses on the plate are prolonged. The surgeon should recognize the increased risk of instrumentation failure and malunion in patients with osteoporotic bone and should augment the stabilization with external bracing in accordance with the quality of the patient's bone.

General Principles of Anterior Cervical Stabilization

Most neurosurgeons are comfortable with the anterior approach to the cervical spine and recognize the advantages it offers in treatment of some cervical lesions. Likewise, most are familiar with interbody arthrodesis techniques which, when successful, result in a highly stable block fusion that maintains normal cervical lordosis and intervertebral distances. Anterior internal instrumentation is easily adopted if certain basic rules for successful anterior cervical stabilization are followed.

The overall effectiveness of any anterior plating procedure depends on the quality of the reconstruction. The plate acts simply to stabilize the vertebral segment(s) *temporarily*, and any compromise in technique undermines its effectiveness. The interbody graft plays an even more important role than plating itself since the graft provides the foundation for postoperative stability and subsequent bony arthrodesis. Most axial load and bending moment forces should be borne by the intervertebral strut. Without a substantial intervertebral spacer, the plate will become overwhelmed and will fail. Attention to detail and careful craftsmanship during reconstruction are exceedingly important if any plating procedure is to be effective.

Within reason, every attempt should be made to restore the normal anatomic alignment of the vertebrae when stabilizing the spine. Malalignment of the spinal elements results in excessive forces on the healing segment and potentially can result in failure. Even if healing occurs, a nonanatomic center of gravity can result in accelerated degeneration of adjacent levels. The plate should conform to the curve of the spine (preferably lordotic) and fit flush with the surface of the vertebral body.

A plate should never be placed across an intact disc space. The motion allowed by an intact disc will result in screw-loosening and ultimate failure of the construct. An interbody graft should always be utilized underneath a Caspar plate.

The Caspar system relies on bicortical purchase of the screws. Although some recent laboratory data questioned the validity of this concept, clinical experience has demonstrated that screws that fail to purchase the posterior cortex are more likely to back out.[8] To engage the posterior cortex safely, a true lateral fluoroscopic view during drilling and screw placement is mandatory.

Operative Procedure

Preparation and Positioning

When dealing with cervical spine trauma, an attempt should be made to restore alignment with skeletal traction. The traction apparatus can be left in place to maintain alignment and prevent rotation of the spine during the procedure. Because of the increased risk of infection associated with foreign body implantation, prophylactic antibiotics are recommended to cover the common offending organisms including gram-negative organisms if a Foley catheter is used.

As with any cervical spine surgery, care should be taken during intubation to avoid movement of an unstable spine or excessive hyperextension of a stable spine. Nasal intubation with the assistance of a bronchoscope is often preferable, particularly when the spine is unstable. When available, somatosensory and/or motor evoked potentials are recommended.

The patient is positioned supine with the head of the table elevated 10 to 15 degrees relative to the feet, providing a direct line of vision through the plane of the disc space. The head should rest on a narrow support, such as a horseshoe head-holder, in order to facilitate fluoroscopy. The addition of an adjustable neck support assists in restoring and maintaining the proper cervical lordosis throughout the procedure. The shoulders must be retracted with tape, or traction applied to the arms, to allow radiographic imaging of the lower cervical segments. The fluoroscopic unit is positioned to provide a true lateral view with the x-ray tube on the operative side (Fig. 294-2). The surgeon and assistant stand on either side of the x-ray tube, which is draped into the sterile field. The cervical spine is adjusted with the head-rest, neck support, and traction to restore normal lordotic curvature and to remove any rotation. The hip should be slightly elevated with padding to facilitate exposure of the iliac crest if a graft is to be harvested.

Skin Incision and Exposure

The standard anterior cervical approach is modified to provide the additional exposure required for cervical plating. A wide transverse neck incision is placed obliquely within a skin fold and extended 1 or 2 cm beyond the midline. Generous myocutaneous

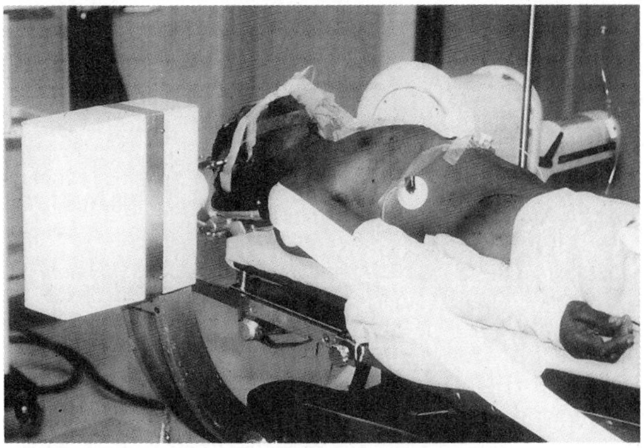

Figure 294-2 Surgical positioning includes placing a C-arm fluoroscope for lateral imaging during the anterior plating procedure. The patient's head is supported in a horseshoe holder, and the shoulders are retracted toward the feet with tape.

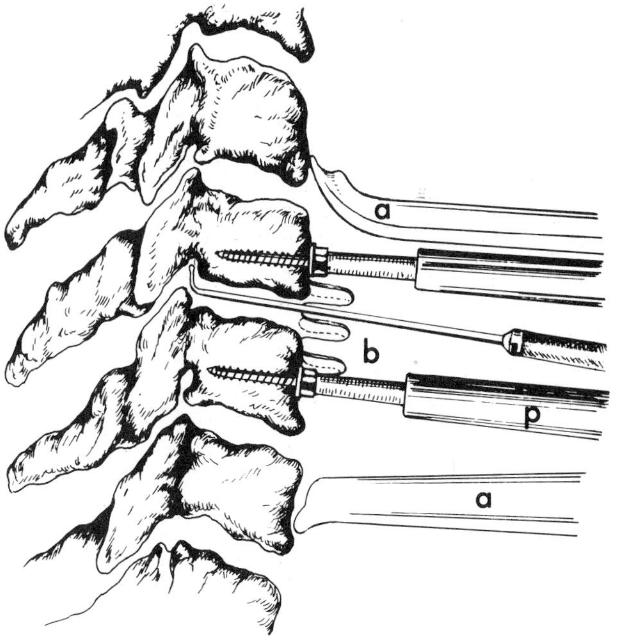

Figure 294-3 This illustration demonstrates the intraoperative positioning of the longitudinal (a) and lateral (b) retractor blades. The distraction pins (p) are inserted into the center of the vertebral body so that the baseplate is flush with the anterior cortex.

flaps, incorporating skin and platysma muscle, are developed superiorly and inferiorly in the fascial plane below the platysma. The cervical fascia is opened along the medial border of the sternocleidomastoid muscle, and the anterior aspect of the vertebral column is exposed with blunt dissection. The exposure required for plating is much greater than that required for a simple anterior discectomy and interbody arthrodesis. It is exceedingly important to adequately dissect the soft tissues of the neck in order to provide ample exposure without injuring the fine neurovascular structures of the neck. Inadequate exposure leads to excessive swelling, dysphagia, and hoarseness in the postoperative period.

Dissection of the longus coli muscles is the key to holding the self-retaining retractors. They are elevated bilaterally from the disc space above to the disc space below the level of fusion. They should be dissected widely while avoiding maceration of the muscle belly since it must sustain powerful lateral retraction. Serrated blades readily retain their position beneath the longus coli muscles and are much less likely to become dislodged than the toothless blades. Toothless blades are used for longitudinal countertraction. For extensive exposure, lateral retractor systems placed in tandem can be used. Radiolucent blades for lateral retraction are preferable because they do not interfere with the fluoroscopic view during screw placement.

Decompression and Graft Site Preparation

The anterior portion of the disc is removed as far as the uncovertebral junction on either side so that the midline can be readily identified. Holes are drilled into the center of the vertebral body for the distraction pins. They are directed parallel to the vertebral endplate using the drill guide and fluoroscopy. The pins are inserted until the baseplate is flush with the anterior surface of the vertebral body. The base plate rather than the depth of pin insertion is responsible for transmitting distraction forces to the vertebral body. Under typical circumstances, it is not necessary for the pin tip to engage or penetrate the posterior cortical surface.

Distraction pins are inserted into the vertebral bodies on either side of the disc space(s) to be fused (Fig. 294-3). Each pin can be inserted freehanded or with the immobile distractor arm–drill guide assembly to insure that the pins are parallel. The vertebral body distractor is placed over the shafts of the distraction pins and distraction forces are applied gradually. In the presence of a kyphotic deformity, individual distraction pins may be placed parallel to the endplates of the vertebral bodies, allowing the distractor to restore the normal curvature.

With the vertebral bodies gently distracted, the discectomy is completed, taking care to remove the cartilaginous endplates. The overhanging anterior vertebral body lip can be removed with a high-speed drill to facilitate the discectomy. This maneuver will be necessary for graft site preparation anyway. If a total or partial corpectomy is planned, the disc above and the disc below the vertebral body are removed. The anterior portion of the corpectomy can then be performed using a rongeur and the bony fragments can be saved as augmentation for the strut graft. After the decompression is completed, any persistent abnormal cervical curvature or locked facets can be corrected by manipulating the distractors and the neck-rest.

Reconstruction begins at this point and, as mentioned earlier, the success of stabilization depends largely on the quality of reconstruction. The endplates provide the foundation for the graft and, therefore, should be level but should have substantial cortical bone remaining. During preparation of the graft site, cortical bone is removed from adjacent endplates. Owing to the different shape of the superior and inferior endplates, production of parallel surfaces for grafting requires selective drilling of the anterior third and posterior third of the caudal endplate and the posterior third or half of the rostral endplate (Fig. 294-4). The surgeon should avoid exposing excessive amounts of underlying cancellous bone because this will decrease the intrinsic supporting capacity of the vertebral body and will predispose a sturdy graft to penetrate the weakened vertebral bodies. A common error is failure to remove enough anterior and posterior bony lip, thus leaving a central gap between

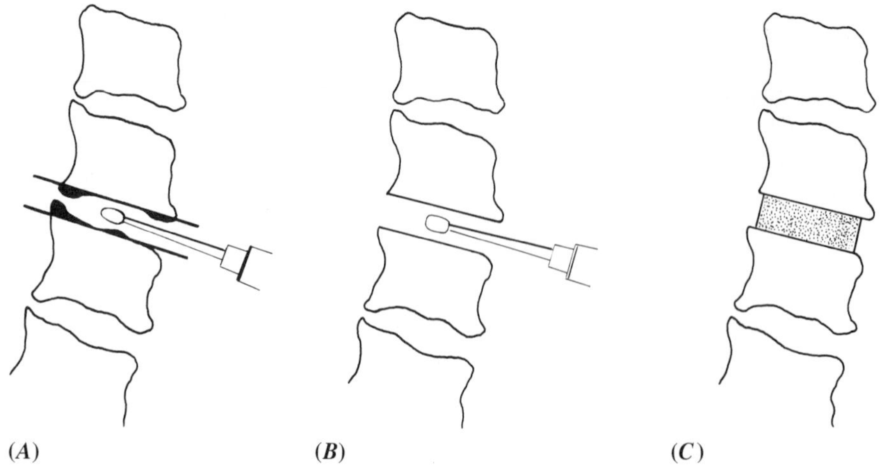

Figure 294-4 Creating parallel vertebral surfaces makes intervertebral grafting easier and enhances the graft-to-vertebral endplate contact. Cortical bone is judiciously removed from the vertebral endplates, as illustrated by the shaded area in (*A*). This results in parallel intervertebral surfaces (*B*) for a ''gapless'' fit between the graft and the adjacent vertebrae (*C*). (From Harkey et al.,[5] with permission.)

the bone graft and vertebral endplate. Maximizing the area of contact between the graft and the vertebral body produces a more stable construct and enhances bony union.

Grafting

The selection of graft material depends on the degree of decompression and the indications for stabilization. The objective in trauma surgery is to restore long-lasting stability; this is best achieved with an autogenous graft, which heals faster and more reliably than other types of graft. An allograft may be preferable in surgery for degenerative disease when the spine is generally not as unstable as it is following trauma. Acrylic or other inert spacers are suitable following decompressions for malignant tumor. A tricortical iliac crest bone graft is ideal for interbody arthrodesis up to a two-level corpectomy. Larger decompressions may require a fibular graft.

A tight-fitting ''gapless'' graft requires an appropriately sized, well formed bone plug in addition to a meticulously prepared graft site. The exact dimensions of the bone plug are determined by measuring the maximally distracted disc space with a micrometer and depth gauge. The average graft should measure 7 to 8 mm in height, but should not be more than 10 mm to avoid overdistraction when there is severe ligamentous disruption.

The graft should be rectangular so that the end surfaces are parallel. It is not necessary to create mortises in the graft or vertebral body. A properly shaped graft should fit snugly with ample surface contact to prevent it from becoming dislodged. A double-bladed oscillating saw cuts a perfect iliac crest graft for a single level fusion. Strut grafts used for subtotal or total body replacement should be cut several millimeters longer than measured to allow for reshaping.

The depth of the graft should measure 3 mm less than the anteroposterior diameter of the prepared interspace—generally about 15 mm in depth. This allows a sufficient margin of safety anterior to the spinal cord once the bone plug is seated into place. Contrary to standard anterior fusion techniques, the bone plug is not countersunk for plating but is left flush with the anterior surface of the spine. A slight bevel on the leading edges of the graft facilitates insertion.

Without using excessive force or hammering, the fabricated graft is tamped into position with the vertebral bodies in the distracted position. The graft should fit snugly and remain secure after the distraction is released. Cancellous bone chips can be laid alongside the graft to enhance the fusion, but care must be taken to avoid compression of the neural structures with these smaller bits of bone.

At this point, the distraction pins can be removed and a small piece of Gelfoam (absorbable gelatin sponge; The Upjohn Company, Kalamazoo, MI) or bone wax used to stop the hemorrhage from the hole. Any remaining bony irregularities of the anterior vertebral bodies can be removed with a drill to ensure that the plate fits flush. This is an important step that maximizes plate-to-bone contact, enhancing the structural stability of the construct.

Plating

Two very important points regarding Caspar anterior cervical plating cannot be overstated. First, plate stabilization cannot be properly or safely performed without fluoroscopy. Dispensing with x-ray guidance will very likely lead to faulty plate fixation and possibly to disastrous complications. Second, a plate should never be placed across an unfused disc space. One should keep in mind that plate stabilization is merely a temporary internal splint which enhances the fusion process. It is the ossification of the graft placed in the cleared disc space that provides the long-term stability. If the plate crosses an intact disc space, screw-loosening or fracture will eventually occur because of the micromotions that remain.

The plate selected will bind the intact vertebral bodies above and below the level(s) of instability. The plate should span the fusion site and all but 2 mm of the adjacent vertebral bodies. After selecting the appropriate length of plate by inspecting its fit with the C-arm, the plate is bent in a convex fashion to reapproximate a normal lordotic posture after fixing the plate to the spine. Generally speaking, the curve should be smoothly distributed along the length of the plate except when C2-C3 instability is being treated. In this instance, the upper edge of the plate should be more sharply bent in order to conform to the ventral shape of the C2 vertebral body (Fig. 294-1).

The plate should be positioned carefully prior to drilling the screw holes. Since the exposure is not truly midline, there is a tendency to position the plate slightly toward the side of the incision. The uncovertebral joints and longus coli muscle insertions are useful landmarks for identifying the midline. Longitudinal positioning is verified by direct vision and fluoroscopy.

The ideal screw position should maximize bone contact and engage both the anterior cortex and the posterior cortex of the vertebral body (Fig. 294-5). There is ample room between the spinal cord and the posterior cortex of the midvertebral body to accommodate slight penetration of the screw tip. The intact posterior longitudinal ligament protects the dura. The screws are preferably placed within the central third of the vertebral body in the sagittal plane, but can be placed outside this region as long as they do not violate the vertebral endplate. The optimal screw trajectory is a slightly oblique, medially directed angle of approximately 15 degrees, parallel to the vertebral endplates. At least two screws should be placed into each vertebral body, not only for the added holding power but to prevent rotation. A distraction pin hole should not be used as a screw hole, as it may have been widened during the distraction process.

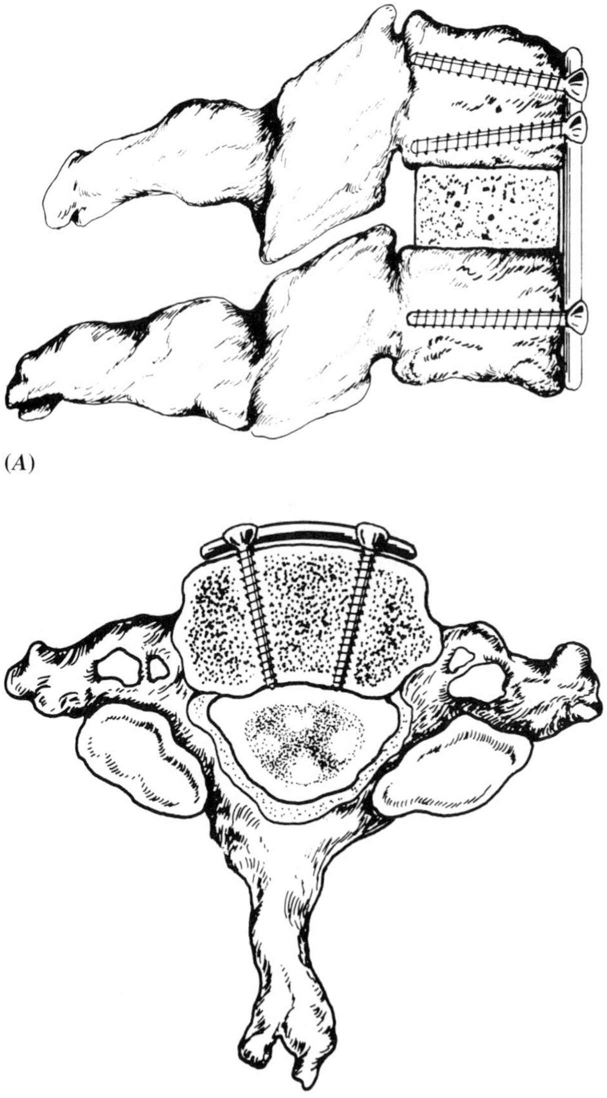

(*A*)

(*B*)

Figure 294-5 Screws should be inserted into the middle third of the vertebral body and should penetrate the posterior cortex (*A*). It is acceptable for the screws to angle cephalad or caudad, but they should not penetrate the disc space. The dual drill guide assists in achieving the optimal transverse screw trajectory, an oblique, converging angle (*B*). (From Harkey et al.,[5] with permission.)

The drili-guides are adjustable for depth and direct the screw holes in a converging course toward the posterior cortex of the vertebral body. The appropriate depth can be estimated from the previously measured depth of the interspace and adjustments made in the guide to safeguard against overpenetration with the drill bit. Generally, the most easily accessible level is drilled first so the plate can be loosely fixed with two screws. With the plate in position over the vertebral bodies, the drill-guide tips are inserted into the holes of the plate. The drill is inserted into the guide and the final trajectory is verified with fluoroscopy. Holes should be drilled deliberately and carefully, relying on the feel of the drill and frequent fluoroscopic visualization. A blunt K-wire is inserted into the freshly drilled hole under fluoroscopic vision. The K-wire is useful for palpating the posterior cortex and posterior longitudinal ligament at the depth of the drill hole and it temporarily stabilizes the plate and drill guide.

The screw holes are measured using the depth gauge with the plate in position. The appropriate screw is selected and inserted but not fully tightened. Once all the screws are in position they can be sequentially tightened "two-fingers" tight. Ideally, the screw tips should completely penetrate the posterior cortex without extending into the spinal canal. Some penetration beyond the posterior cortex is allowable, but no more than the width of one thread. Screws manufactured with a flat tip can fully engage the posterior cortex without penetrating the canal.

Stripped screws should be removed and one of several salvage techniques applied. These include using an oversized rescue screw, redirecting and drilling a new hole with the single drill guide, or filling the stripped hole with acrylic.

Subtotal and Total Body Replacement

When teardrop fractures or anterior body compression fractures accompany an unstable spine, the bone fragments can be removed along with the discs above and below the fractured body. A "U-shaped" block graft is constructed to span the distance between the adjacent intact vertebral bodies and envelop the intervening partially resected body (Fig. 294-6*A*). A plate is then applied with screws through both the anterior and posterior cortices of the intact vertebral bodies. Screws are also placed at the center of the plate through the strut graft and the posterior cortex of the partially resected vertebral body. As the screws are tightened, any residual subluxation is usually reduced and the normal lordotic curvature can be restored.

Following complete corpectomy to decompress the spinal canal, a strut graft can be utilized for reconstruction (Figs. 294-6*B*, 294-7). The plate and screws are applied in the same fashion; however, screws should penetrate only the anterior two-thirds of the graft, thereby preventing posterior displacement of the graft. Locking the graft to the plate eliminates an intercalated segment and produces a more stable construct.

At completion, a closed system drain is placed at the depth of the wound to reduce retropharyngeal swelling, which can be more problematic than occurs following simple anterior cervical discectomy procedures. Postoperative bracing should be tailored to the individual based on the quality and complexity of the reconstruction.

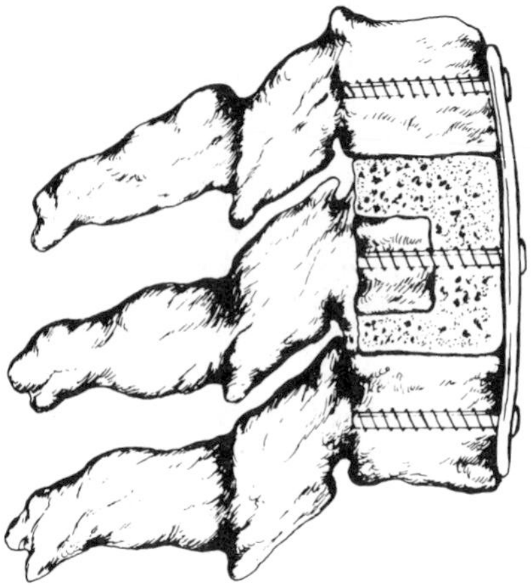
(A)

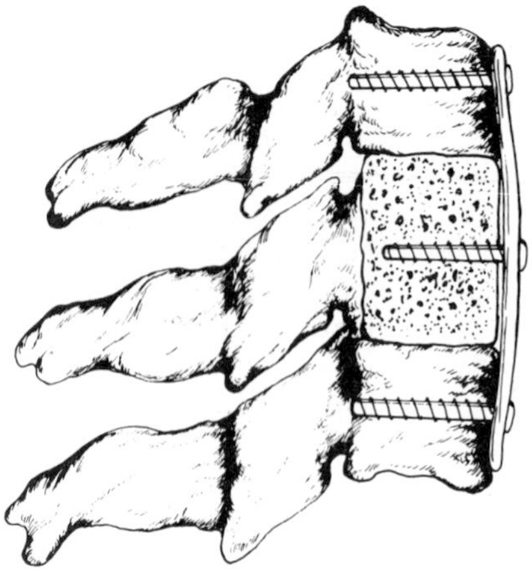
(B)

Figure 294-6 Two of the reconstruction techniques available with the Caspar system are shown. *A*. Subtotal body replacement; *B*. total body replacement.

Outcome

The experience with Caspar plating is compiled from five published reports that each reviewed 25 or more patients in order to determine outcome.[1,4,10,12,13] A total of 220 patients undergoing Caspar plating were reported by these authors. All but nine of these patients were treated for traumatic instability. Four patients (1.8 percent) developed instability in the early postoperative period and required additional intervention. Three underwent reoperation and one had a halo brace applied. In each case, failure was attributed to technical faults of grafting and/or plating. Apparently all 220 patients have ultimately formed a stable fusion, recognizing the limitations of x-ray filming to confirm bony fusion. In the author's personal experience of 50 cases, two patients required later additional intervention owing to early postoperative instability. In one case, the graft, which was not secured to the plate, dislocated posteriorly but did not significantly compromise the spinal canal. This patient was treated successfully with the addition of a halo brace. One other osteoporotic patient, who was treated for a longstanding kyphotic deformity, required posterior stabilization when the screws began to back out.

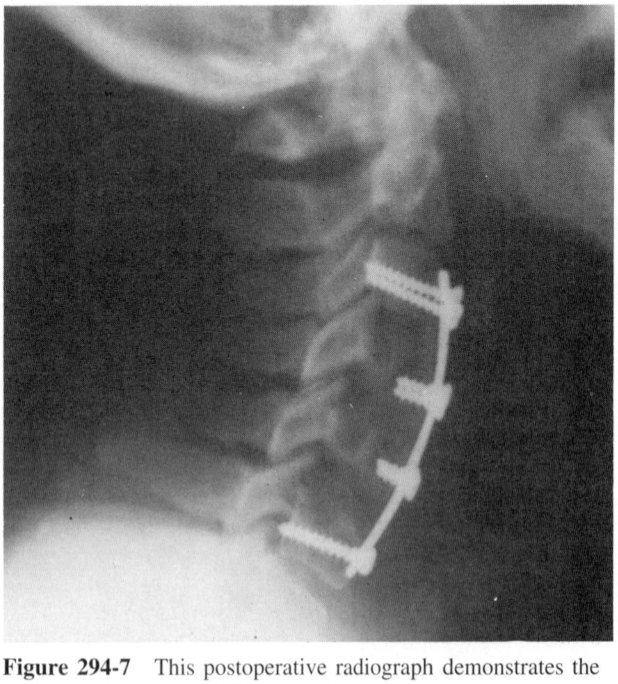

Figure 294-7 This postoperative radiograph demonstrates the reconstruction and stabilization following a two-level anterior decompression for ossification of the posterior longitudinal ligament.

Complications associated with Caspar plating can be divided into clinical complications, such as infection or neurological injury, and technical complications, such as screw-loosening and plate failure. In the compiled series of 220 patients, there were no perioperative deaths or major neurological deficits attributable to the plating procedure. Three patients were reported to have transient vocal cord paralysis. In the author's experience, temporary vocal cord paralysis is somewhat more common, but occurs only in longer fusions requiring exposure of four or more vertebral segments or in cervicothoracic fusions. Dysphagia lasting more than 10 days was reported in three patients when it was mentioned at all. Again, the author's experience indicates that dysphagia is more of a problem than the literature suggests. Fortunately, it is usually short-lived, lasting less than 5 days. Dysphagia can be minimized by developing adequate tissue planes during surgical exposure and by leaving a $\frac{3}{16}$-in. suction drain in the wound for 24 to 48 h following surgery. Infections were reported in only four cases, which is within the expected rate for any surgical procedure.

The Caspar plating technique is clearly a reliable method for stabilizing the cervical spine. Although there is a theoretical risk of injury to the spinal cord during screw placement, practical experience has not established this to be a problem. There is a relatively steep learning curve, particularly for the surgeon not experienced in other plate/screw stabilization techniques. However, any surgeon interested in learning this technique may gain invaluable experience by attending hands-on practical courses and by assisting seasoned surgeons. By paying meticulous attention to detail during the reconstruction and following the guidelines for successful plating described in this chapter, the surgeon should find this technique very satisfying and effective.

References

1. Caspar W, Barbier DD, Klara PM. Anterior cervical fusion and Caspar plate stabilization for cervical trauma. *Neurosurgery* 1989; 25:491–502.
2. de Oliveira JC. Anterior plate fixation of traumatic lesions of the lower cervical spine. *Spine* 1987; 12:324–329.
3. Garvey TA, Eismont FJ, Roberti LJ. Anterior decompression, structural bone grafting, and Caspar plate stabilization for unstable cervical spine fractures and/or dislocations. *Spine* 1992; 17 (Suppl 10):S431–S435.
4. Goffin J, Plets C, Van den Bergh R. Anterior cervical fusion and osteosynthetic stabilization according to Caspar; a prospective study of 41 patients with fractures and/or dislocations of the cervical spine. *Neurosurgery* 1989; 25:865–871.
5. Harkey HL, Caspar W, Tarassoli Y. Caspar plating of the cervical spine. In Rengachary SS, Wilkins RH (eds): *Neurosurgical Operative Atlas,* vol 2. Baltimore: Williams & Wilkins, 1992, pp 261–271.
6. Harrington JF, Likavec MJ, Smith AS. Disc herniation in cervical fracture subluxation. *Neurosurgery* 1991; 29:374–379.
7. Kalfas I, Papadopoulos SM, Sonntag VKH. Anterior cervical fusion and Caspar plate stabilization for degenerative disorders of the cervical spine. *J Spinal Disord* 1991; 4:385–386 (abstr).
8. Maiman DJ, Pintar FA, Yoganandan N, et al. Pull-out strength of Caspar cervical screws. *Neurosurgery* 1992; 31:1097–1101.
9. Orozco R, Llovet TJ. Osteosintesis en las fractures de requis cervical. *Rev Ortop Traumatol* 1970; 14:285–288.
10. Randle MJ, Wolf A, Levi L, et al. The use of anterior Caspar plate fixation in acute cervical spine injury. *Surg Neurol* 1991; 36:181–189.
11. Ripa DR, Kowall MG, Meyer PR Jr, et al. Series of ninety-two traumatic cervical spine injuries stabilized with ASIF plate fusion technique. *Spine* 1991; 16(Suppl 3):S46–S55.
12. Shoung HM, Lee LS. Anterior metal plate fixation in the treatment of unstable lower cervical spine injuries. *Acta Neurochir (Wien)* 1989; 98:55–59.
13. Tippets RH, Apfelbaum RI. Anterior cervical fusion with the Caspar instrumentation system. *Neurosurgery* 1988; 22:1008–1013.
14. Traynelis VC, Donaher PA, Roach RM, et al. Biomechanical comparison of anterior Caspar plate and three-level posterior fixation techniques in a human cadaveric model. *J Neurosurg* 1993; 79:96–103.
15. Tuite CF, Papadopoulos SM, Sonntag VKH. Caspar plate fixation for the treatment of complex hangman's fractures. *Neurosurgery* 1992; 30:761–765.

295

Anterior Stabilization of the Cervical Spine Using Locking Plate Systems

Setti S. Rengachary
Abhay Sanan

Anterior cervical fusion has become the standard of care for a wide variety of disorders of the cervical spine. Simple discectomy and fusion is adequate in spondylotic disc disease at a single level; however, the rate of graft extrusion, kyphosis, and pseudarthrosis have been demonstrated to be quite high with multilevel fusions or with anterior fusion for traumatic lesions with posterior instability. The introduction of locking plate systems represents a significant advance and has substantially increased the stability of the initial fusion. This result has reduced the need for postoperative immobilization in a rigid external orthosis or the requirement for later posterior stabilization. The plate systems offer immediate stability with the use of multiple fixation points and a rigid plate-screw interface. They are safe to use and do not require bicortical purchase, thus avoiding injury to the spinal cord, nerve roots, or vascular structures. The operative approach is very similar to that for standard anterior fusions, and in general the locking plates are easy to implant. All of these advantages have made the locking plate systems the state of the art for complicated anterior cervical fusions.

Historical Perspective

Anterior cervical fusion was first performed in 1952 at the University of Michigan by Dr. Bailey and Dr. Badgley.[1] Cloward, Robinson and Smith, Dereymaeker and Mulier, and Verbiest stressed the importance of decompression of the spinal canal in addition to fusion. The initial indications were single-level degenerative disc disease and spondylosis. When the technique was used for multilevel disease, the rate of pseudarthrosis approached one-third, and late kyphotic deformities were common.[6] The technique was even less successful in treating traumatic injuries in which posterior instability was also present. Despite the use of external orthoses, the success rate was not satisfactory, and many patients were subjected to a posterior stabilization procedure. Furthermore, orthotic devices are associated with a significant amount of patient inconvenience and complications. Dissatisfaction with the traditional methods available served as an impetus for the development of a rigid internal stabilization device that would allow for a one-step anterior decompression and immediate stability.

Internal stabilization of the cervical spine was first performed posteriorly over a century ago. Anterior internal stabilization is a more recent advance, having been developed in the last three decades. Bohler, in 1964, was the first to fixate the cervical spine anteriorly using a plate and screw system.[2] Orozco and Tapies, in 1970, were the first to report the use of a plate produced by the Association for the Study of Internal Fixation (ASIF), a nonprofit European physician group. They and others subsequently began to use H-shaped ASIF plates that were the forerunners of the current Synthes plate (Synthes Spine, Paoli, PA). Caspar popularized anterior cervical plating in the 1980s by developing a standardized technique and, in collaboration with the Aesculap company (Aesculap, South San Francisco, CA), a set of instruments.[3] The Caspar/Aesculap system gained widespread use in the late 1980s, but several major disadvantages were soon noted. The technique demanded bicortical screw purchase, which was often technically demanding. Overpenetration could result in neurological injury, whereas underpenetration could result in construct failure and eventual screw pullout with erosion into the esophagus. Fluoroscopy was necessary, and was cumbersome and involved a radiation risk to both the surgeon and patient. Almost simultaneously with the development of the Caspar system, Raveh developed the titanium-coated hollow screw reconstruction plate at the University of Berne.[4] By inserting an expansion bolt into the screw, the screw was rigidly fixed to the plate; this feature avoided the need for bicortical screw purchase. Morscher, also from Switzerland, modified the Orozco plate for use with Raveh's hollow, unicortical, locking screws and reported his results in 1986. The system was introduced in the United States by Synthes in 1991 and seems to have solved many of the problems of the Caspar plate. Other locking plate systems have now entered the marketplace: the Orion system (Sofamor Danek, Memphis, TN) and the Codman system (Codman/Johnson & Johnson Professional, Inc, Randolph, MA), have been recently introduced.

Indications for the Use of Locking Plates

In general, the locking plate is indicated for the treatment of anterior cervical instability. It should be emphasized that instrumentation is unnecessary in the overwhelming majority of routine single-level anterior discectomies and fusions. The rate of successful fusion without instrumentation in these cases is greater than 95 percent. The locking plates should be reserved for conditions in which a bone graft alone will not suffice. Multilevel cervical spondylosis treated by discectomy or corpectomy is perhaps the most common indication, followed by cervical trauma. Other indications include destructive malignant neoplasms, degenerative conditions such as rhematoid arthritis, and kyphotic deformities following infectious conditions such as osteomyelitis.

Operative Technique

The technique is fundamentally the same irrespective of the system used. The patient is placed in a stable supine position with a roll beneath the shoulders to provide physiologic lordosis. A standard transverse incision is sufficient for most one- or two-level constructs. An oblique vertical incision, similar to the one used for carotid endarterectomy, may be required for longer constructs. The cervical spine is then exposed in the usual fashion as outlined elsewhere in this book. Once the discectomy or corpectomy has been performed, distraction should be applied, and a bone graft impacted so that it will fit firmly. The distraction should then be released, and the stability of the impacted bone assessed. A strong and appropriate bony construct is essential for a successful fusion; the locking plate will not compensate for a poorly designed bony construct. Plating should never be performed across an unfused segment, because the hardware will ultimately fail.

The vertebral bodies must be properly prepared for the plate. Any soft tissue adhering to the bone should be removed using a curet or Leksel rongeur. Typically, the cervical spine is not smooth, and there is a natural concavity at the midvertebral level and a convexity from osteophytes at the superior and inferior borders. In addition, the edges of the graft may protrude slightly above the vertebral body. These irregularities must be gently smoothed with a high-speed drill, bearing in mind that over-aggressive drilling may thin the cortical bone and reduce the strength of screw purchase. The plate should encompass the vertebral bodies both above and below the bone graft. Once the appropriate plate has been chosen, it should be gently bent in the sagittal plane to conform to the natural lordosis of the spine. The Orion and Codman systems supply a prebent plate. In the Synthes system, the bend should not go through any of the screw holes because that will weaken the screw-plate fixation.

The next step is the placement of the screws. Ideally, two screws should be placed close to the cortical endplate of each vertebral body that is spanned. Placing a screw into the graft is helpful but not necessary in short constructs. A power or hand drill is used to define a tract, which is then tapped. The foundation screw is then placed. The other screws are placed using the same sequence (drilling, tapping, and placing a foundation screw). Once all the screws have been placed, they are retightened. If a screw strips, one can attempt to pack the hole with crushed cancellous bone and apply the screw again. True rescue screws (larger diameter) are not available at present with any system. With the Orion or Codman system one can place a longer-length screw and partially salvage an entry hole. Once all the screws are in place, the locking screws can be applied. The procedure is complete at this point. It is advisable to obtain anteroposterior and lateral radiographs prior to wound closure. Figure 295-1 shows radiographs of a completed construct.

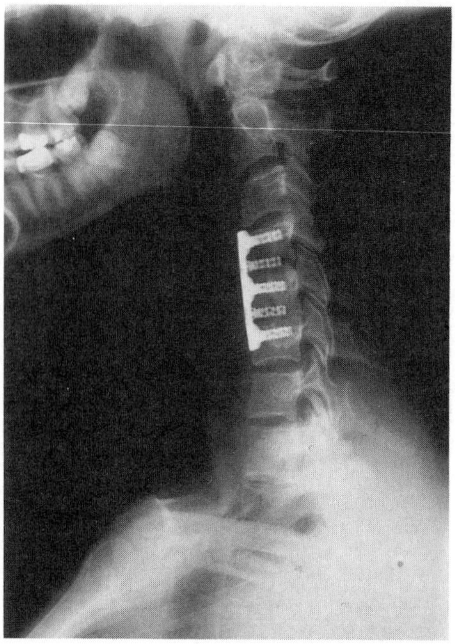

(A)

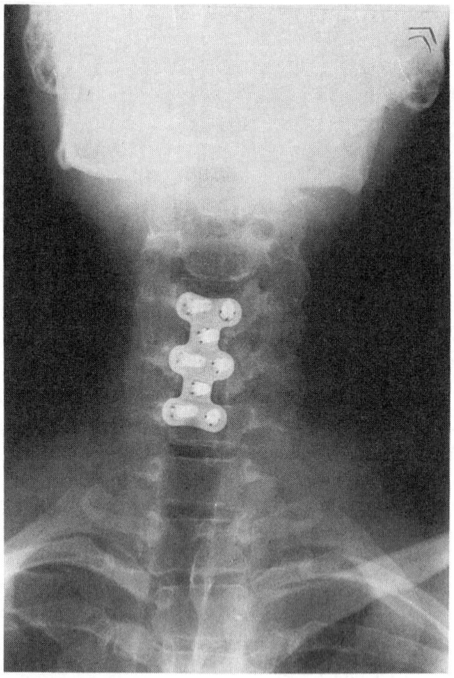

(B)

Figure 295-1 (*A*) Lateral and anteroposterior (*B*) radiographs of a completed Synthes construct. Note that the plate is flush with the lordotic curve of the spine. The screws are placed near the cortical end plate of the vertebrae. Two screws have also been placed into the graft.

Comparison between Locking Plate Systems and Nonlocking Plate Systems Using Bicortical Screws

The most striking feature of the locking plate systems is their ease of use. Because bicortical purchase is not required, fluoroscopy is not necessary, which decreases the operative time. Biomechanically, the nonlocking bicortical screw system is at a distinct disadvantage. Screw migration continues to occur in bicortical systems, a problem that is almost never seen in locking plate systems. If the bicortical screw loses one cortical purchase, the plate and screw can move independently; this produces a claw-hammer effect and results in screw backout. When the screw is fixed rigidly to the plate, neither can move independent of the other, and they function as a single metal unit. Since the rate of fusion produced by locking systems and bicortical systems is virtually the same, namely 99

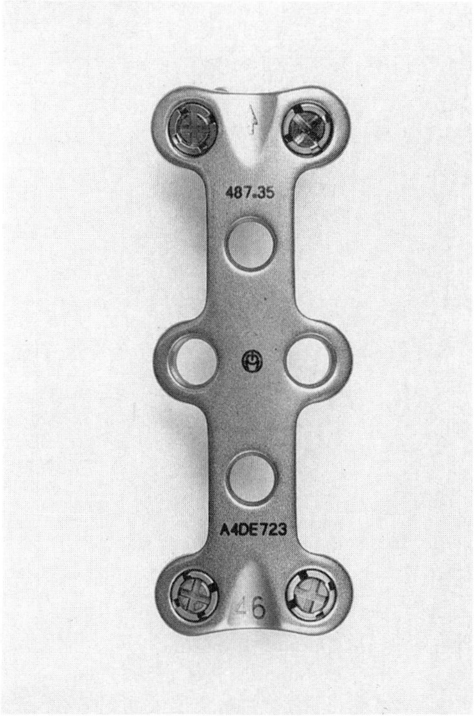

(*A*)

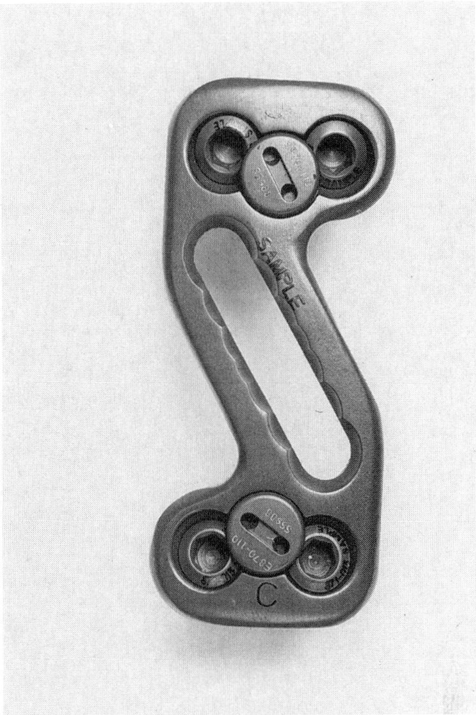

(*C*)

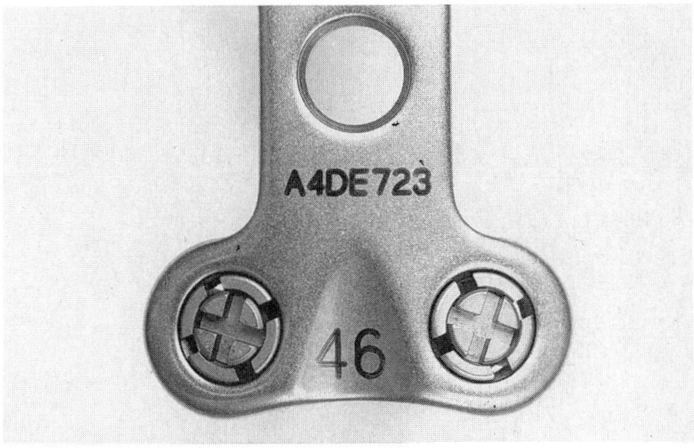

(*B*)

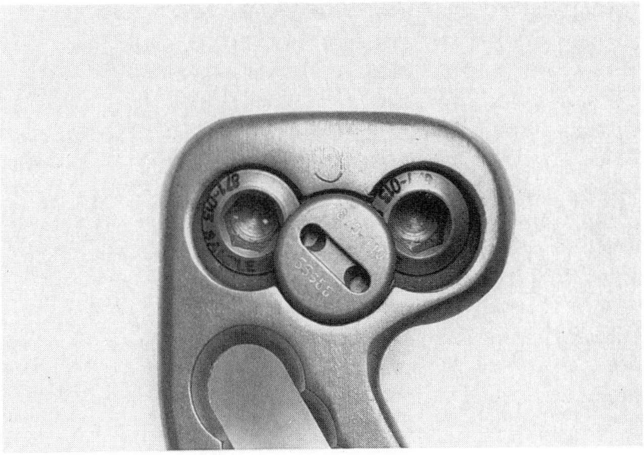

(*D*)

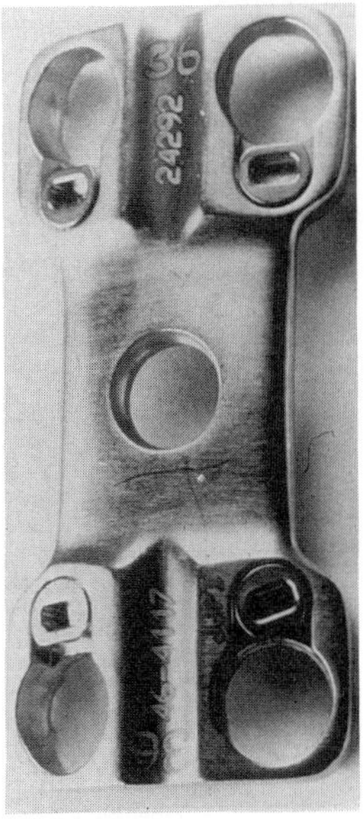

(*E*)

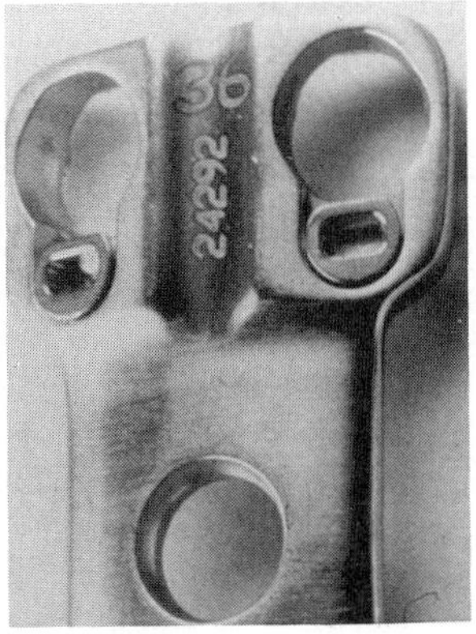

(*F*)

Figure 295-2 The systems are quite similar in design and concept. The locking mechanism is different in each system: Synthes plate (*A*) and expansion screw (*B*); Orion plate (*C*) and covering screw (*D*); Codman plate (*E*) and cam lock (*F*).

TABLE 295-1 Comparison Among the Three Locking Plate Systems

Technical Features	System		
	Synthes	Orion	Codman
Material	Titanium	Titanium	Titanium
Locking mechanism	Internal expansion screw	External covering screw	Cam lock
Screw diameter			
Core	3.0 mm	2.4 mm	2.5 mm
Thread	4.35 mm	4.0 mm	4.5 mm
Rescue screws	No	No*	No*
Screw length	Fixed (14 mm)	Variable (10–26 mm)	12 or 15 mm
Plate shape	Flat	Lordotic	Lordotic
Medial entry angle	12°	6°	Variable
Cephalad/caudal angle	12°/0°	15°/15°	Variable
Screw construct	Convergent (fixed angle)	Convergent (fixed angle)	Variable

*Larger diameter screws are not available (true rescue screw). However, application of a longer screw may partially salvage an entry hole.

percent, and the locking plate system is easier to use and has less complications, we believe that the locking systems are now the gold standard for anterior cervical fusions. The rapid popularity and success of the locking systems attests to this statement.

Comparison Among the Three Locking Plate Systems

The three systems (Synthes, Orion, and Codman) are basically similar in design and concept. Figure 295-2 shows the plate and screw designs of the three manufacturers. Table 295-1 reviews some of the differences among the three systems. All are made of titanium to minimize magnetic resonance imaging (MRI) artifact. The Synthes system uses an internal expansion screw to lock the screw to the plate; the Orion system uses an external covering screw; and the Codman system uses a cam lock. The Synthes system is the oldest and most standardized.[5] All of the Synthes screws are 14 mm long and have a fixed angle of entry with respect to the plate. Since the average diameter of an adult vertebral body is 21 to 22 mm, it is virtually impossible to inadvertently penetrate the posterior cortex. However, the Synthes screws are too long for use in children. The Orion system is more versatile and has a variety of screw lengths; this allows for either unicortical or bicortical purchase in both adults and children. The Codman system is the most recent arrival into the locking plate market. Like the Synthes system, the screw length is restricted. The standard screw is 12 mm; a 15-mm length is also produced. The Codman system allows for an infinitely variable screw entry angle, whereas the angle of convergence is fixed at 12 degrees for the Synthes screws and 6 degrees for the Orion screws. The Synthes plate is flat and has a predetermined cephalad angle of 12 degrees on the superior two screws and 0 degrees on the inferior ones. The Orion plate has a preshaped lordotic curve and has a cephalad and caudal angle of 15 degrees for the superior and inferior screws, respectively. The Codman plate is also lordotic but allows for a variable screw entry angle.

Precautions and Complications

The anterior cervical approach has a number of complications, including wound hematoma, vascular injury, esophageal injury, superior or recurrent laryngeal nerve injury, and infection. This section will focus only on the complications specific to plate application. Although the locking plate system can provide a good deal of load sharing to a destabilized spine, it has limitations. Long fusions are particularly prone to screw breakage or pullout because of the long lever arm created. Severe trauma may disrupt both the anterior and posterior elements, and anterior plating may be insufficient. In these two situations, either the patient should be placed in a halo vest, or a posterior stabilization procedure should be performed.

References

1. Bailey R, Badgley C. Stabilization of the cervical spine by anterior fusion. *J Bone Joint Surg [Am]* 1960; 42-A:565–594.
2. Bohler J, Gaudernak T. Anterior plate stabilization for fracture-dislocations of the lower cervical spine. *J Trauma* 1980; 20:203–205.
3. Caspar W, Barbier DD, Klara PM. Anterior cervical fusion and Caspar plate stabilization for cervical trauma. *Neurosurgery* 1989; 25:491–502.
4. Raveh J, Stich H, Sutter F, Greiner R. Use of the titanium-coated hollow screw and reconstruction plate system in bridging of lower jaw defects. *J Oral Maxillofac Surg* 1984; 42:281–294.
5. Rechtine GR, Cahill DW, Gruenberg M, et al. The Synthes cervical spine locking plate and screw system in anterior cervical fusion. *Tech Orthop* 1994; 9:86–91.
6. White AA III, Southwick WO, DePonte RJ, et al. Relief of pain by anterior cervical-spine fusion for spondylosis. A report of sixty-five patients. *J Bone Joint Surg* 1973; 55A:525–534.

296

Injuries to the Thoracic and Lumbar Spine

Wesley A. Cook, Jr.
William T. Hardaker, Jr.

Seventy percent of the injuries to the spinal cord result from trauma, whereas disease (neoplastic, neurological, or congenital) accounts for only 30 percent.[31,32] Trauma secondary to motor vehicle accidents is responsible for more than one-half of the total number of spinal cord injuries, which approaches 10,000 cases per year. The death toll from motor vehicle accidents in the United States has been about 50,000 per year, and slightly more than one-half of those accidents have been related to alcohol. In perspective, the loss of life during a single year from motor vehicle accidents nearly equals the number of Americans lost during the entire Vietnam War.

The significance of these tragic numbers is that the majority of deaths and major injuries from motor vehicle accidents are preventable. To diminish this highway tragedy, society must learn to dissociate drinking and driving. Furthermore, greater utilization must be made of existing restraint systems while driving. It has been demonstrated that serious and fatal injuries can be reduced 65 to 80 percent by employing restraint systems.[9,47] In those states with mandatory seat belt legislation, usage of restraints is usually above 50 percent. The combination of increased usage of restraints and the increasingly severe penalties for driving under the influence has resulted in a steady decline in fatalities since 1988.

Types of Thoracolumbar Injuries

The mobility of the thoracolumbar spine (T10-L5) is considerably greater than that of the thoracic spine (T1-T9) because of the stability imparted to the latter by the rib cage and sternum. This mobility contributes to the more frequent occurrence of injury at the thoracolumbar junction.

Fractures of the thoracolumbar spine are divided into three groups: wedge fractures, burst fractures, and fracture-dislocations.[25,28] The wedge fracture results primarily from severe flexion forces applied to the spine (Fig. 296-1). Mild wedge fractures are generally stable, particularly in the thoracic spine. Chronic instability may result from multiple contiguous wedge fractures or from single fractures with greater than 50 percent anterior vertebral body deformation. Instability in this case refers to the progressive flexion-angulation of the spine that may occur with the passage of time. Severe wedge fractures are often associated with fractures of the laminae, pedicles, or facets.

Burst fractures result from axial compression, frequently associated with varying degrees of flexion. These forces result in failure of both the anterior and posterior cortices of the vertebral body (Fig. 296-2). Severe burst fractures are often associated with posterior element fractures, and the anteroposterior roentgenogram will demonstrate widening of the interpedicular distance (Fig. 296-3). Miller et al. have noted that dural lacerations are commonly associated with severe burst fractures.[39]

Varying degrees of retropulsion of bone into the neural canal characterize the radiographic appearance of burst fractures. In our series of patients, computed tomography (CT) has consistently demonstrated that the bone fragments compressing the dural contents arise from the upper portion of the vertebral body (Fig. 296-4). Similar findings have also been noted by Jelsma and associates.[28] This pattern should be recognized and considered when planning surgical decompression for these lesions.

When rotation is added to the force producing a fracture-dislocation, a so-called slice fracture often results. In this injury a "slice" of the lower vertebra remains attached to the upper displaced vertebra. The slice may be composed of a single bone fragment or multiple fragments attached to the annulus.[30]

A distinctive distraction injury of the thoracolumbar spine results from extreme flexion and is often associated with lap belt injuries.[21,44,51] This type of injury is most likely to occur when the lap belt is worn above the iliac crests or when the belt slides up during the accident. The characteristics of this injury are listed in Table 296-1 and are shown in Fig. 296-5. A clinical analysis of this injury by Smith and Kaufer suggests that the axis for flexion is shifted from the center of the nucleus pulposus in the normal situation to a point between the seat belt and the abdominal wall.[44]

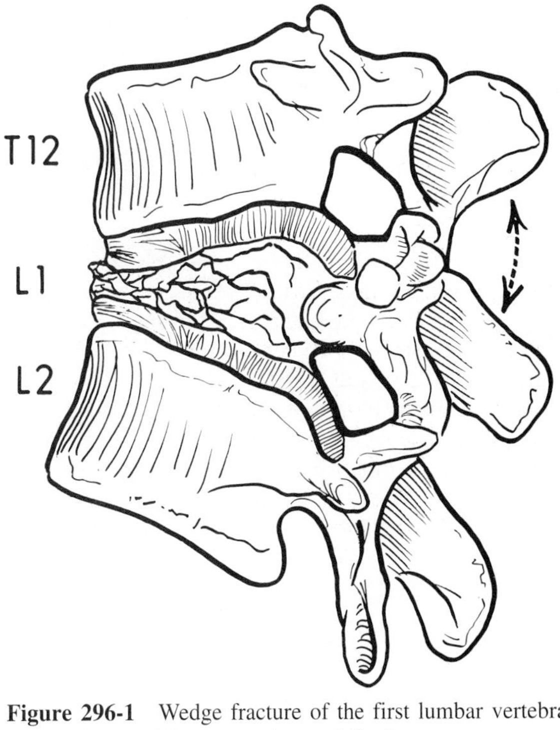

Figure 296-1 Wedge fracture of the first lumbar vertebra resulting from axial compression and flexion.

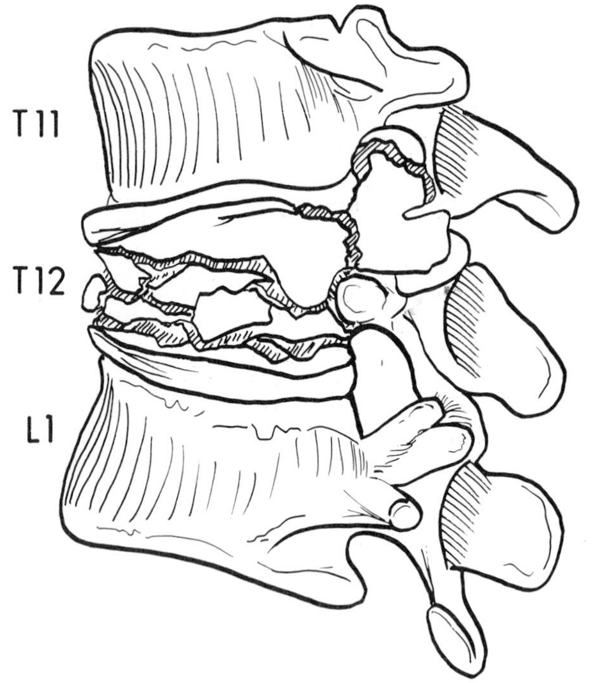

Figure 296-2 Burst fracture of the twelfth thoracic vertebra resulting from axial compression.

With the axis for flexion at the latter point, the spine is then subjected to a distractive force. It would also appear that an extreme degree of flexion is required to produce this type of injury, since only 1 in 24 cases involved the driver of the vehicle, the remaining cases being passengers. Presumably, the steering wheel prevented the required amount of flexion.

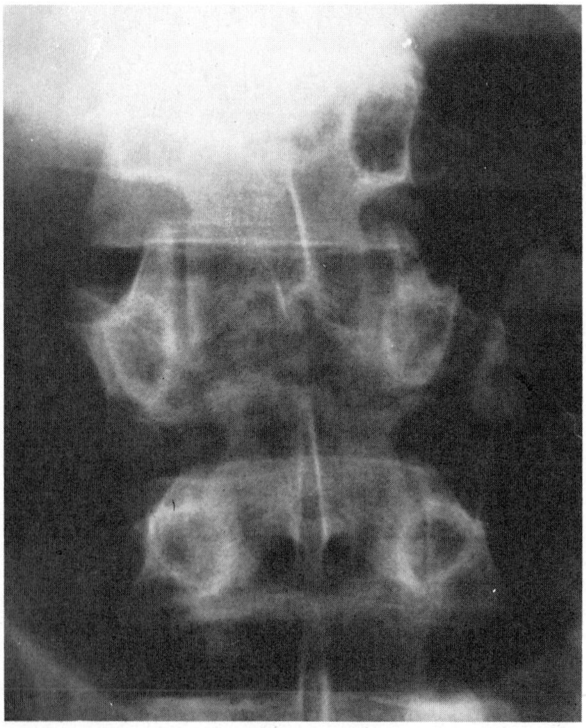

Figure 296-3 Anteroposterior roentgenogram of an L2 burst fracture showing widening of the interpedicular distance.

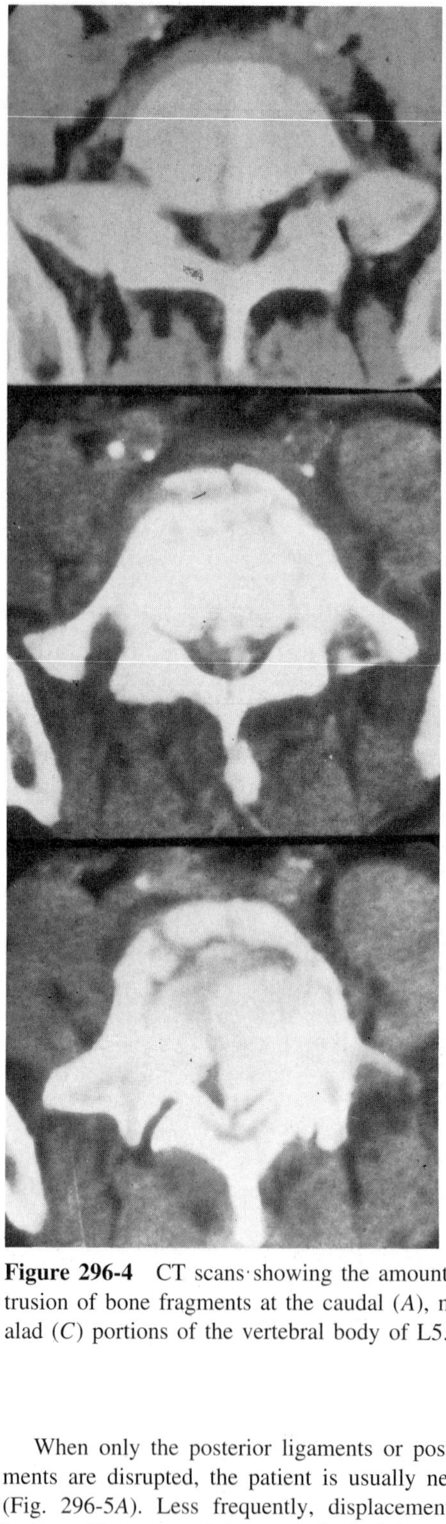

(*A*)

(*B*)

(*C*)

Figure 296-4 CT scans showing the amount of posterior protrusion of bone fragments at the caudal (*A*), mid (*B*), and cephalad (*C*) portions of the vertebral body of L5.

When only the posterior ligaments or posterior osseous elements are disrupted, the patient is usually neurologically intact (Fig. 296-5*A*). Less frequently, displacement of the vertebral bodies will occur, and then neurological damage can be expected (Fig. 296-5*B*). Incomplete neurological deficits are unusual with this lesion. Patients are either intact or demonstrate a complete neurological deficit.

When fracture does occur, it is of the variety described by Chance, that is, a horizontal splitting of the spinous process and neural arch with extension of the fracture into the vertebral body (Fig. 296-5*C*).[6] Not all of these fractures are grossly unstable, and many will heal satisfactorily with a hyperextension brace. The more severe examples require posterior fusion augmented by compression instrumentation.

TABLE 296-1 Characteristics of Distraction Injuries

Disruption and separation of posterior elements, either ligamentous or osseous
Little, if any, anterior wedging of the vertebral body
Little, if any, anterior or lateral displacement
L1, L2, and L3 most commonly involved
Patient usually neurologically intact unless displacement occurs
Intra-abdominal injuries common

Abdominal wall ecchymoses will be noted in many patients with lap belt injuries, although their absence does not exclude this type of injury. Intra-abdominal injuries are common with lap belt injuries and should not be overlooked.

Radiology of Thoracolumbar Injuries

The radiologic evaluation of spine fractures has been revolutionized by the advent of CT, water-soluble intrathecal contrast agents, and magnetic resonance imaging (MRI). Following initial plain films, computed tomography of the injured spine will provide the necessary information in most clinical situations. The CT scan provides a more accurate picture of the degree of spinal canal compromise and is of less risk to the patient than conventional polytomography. The radiation dose is greater with polytomography; and with most tomographic units the patient must be shifted to a lateral position for the lateral tomography, which entails a certain risk if the spine fracture is unstable. A comparative study suggests that conventional polytomography is the procedure of choice only for suspected fractures of the pars interarticularis.[30]

CT myelography or an MRI scan is indicated in those patients whose neural deficit is not consistent with the level or extent of vertebral involvement. CT myelography is not necessary in cases of marked fracture-dislocation with an appropriate neurological level. On the other hand, a minimal burst fracture or dislocation with severe neurological damage is an indication for CT myelography or an MRI scan, as is the situation in which the neurological level is not consistent with the radiologic level of injury.

Therapy of Thoracolumbar Injuries

The question as to whether the final neurological outcome following spinal cord injury reflects the form of treatment or the extent of damage to the spinal cord at the time of injury remains controversial. While it would appear reasonable to assume that both factors are operative, the small number of complete spinal cord injuries that improve, irrespective of treatment modality, is considered to prove the importance of the initial injury by many investigators. However, there is rationale for treating acute spinal cord injuries with high-dose steroid therapy,[23] and interest and optimism have been stimulated by the results of a multicenter study of high dose methylprednisolone.[5] Neurological improvement was noted at 6 weeks, 6 months and 12 months when the high dose steroid protocol was initiated within 8 h of injury.

The goals of therapy are listed in Table 296-2. Irrespective of the treatment modality employed, a team approach to the spinal patient is essential if these goals are to be achieved. Each patient should receive input from neurosurgical, orthopedic, urologic, nursing, physical therapy, rehabilitation, and social service specialists.

Essential to the initial management of the spinal cord injured patient is an accurate recorded neurological examination against

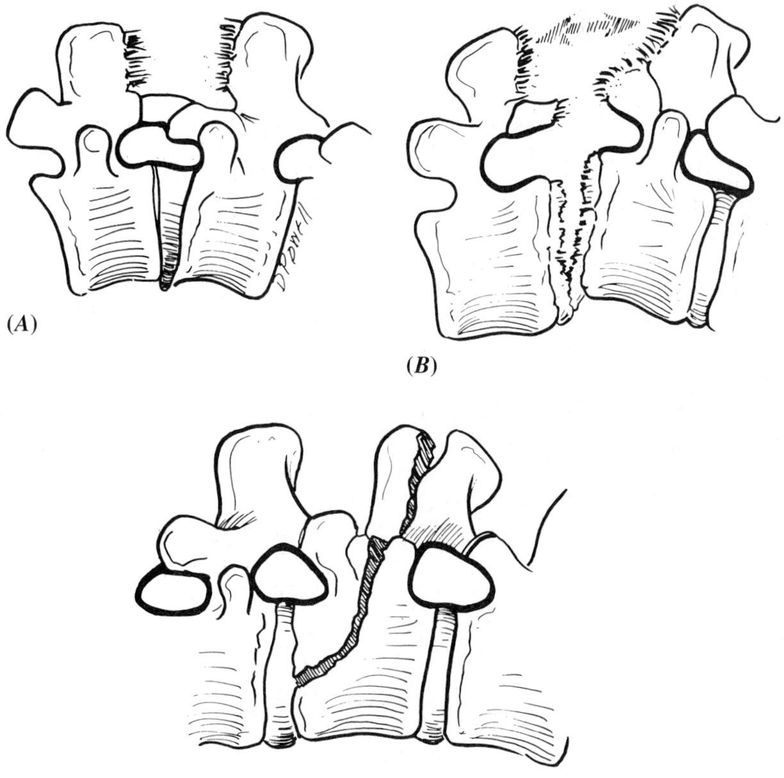

Figure 296-5 Distraction fracture-dislocations. *A, B.* Primarily ligamentous injury. *C.* Chance fracture.

TABLE 296-2 Goals of Therapy

Preservation of remaining spinal cord function
Maximization of the degree of neurological recovery
Restoration of spinal alignment
Achievement of a stable and pain-free fracture site
Prevention of pulmonary, gastrointestinal, genitourinary, and cutaneous complications
Prevention of delayed neurological complications
Rapid mobilization and early rehabilitation
Cost containment

which future examinations can be compared. Improper movement of the patient, hypoxia, and hypotension must be avoided to prevent further damage to the spinal cord. Associated injuries must be recognized and treated. In thoracic fractures, injury to the lungs and cardiovascular structures is not uncommon. Thoracolumbar fractures may be associated with retroperitoneal or visceral injuries. It should be emphasized that the characteristic signs of peritoneal irritation may be abolished by spinal shock. Finally, the care of the bladder and anesthetic skin should begin immediately to avoid the debilitating complications of urinary tract infections and decubitus ulcers. The latter remain the single most important complication in terms of hospital stay and cost.

Nonsurgical Therapy

Postural reduction is a nonsurgical means of treating spinal fractures that was developed by Guttman in 1944.[22] Although this form of therapy has not gained widespread acceptance in this country, the contributions of Guttman and his colleagues to the care of the spine-injured patient have been considerable, and the degree of initial neurological improvement achieved by postural reduction is similar to that reported in many surgical series. For example, in patients with thoracolumbar fractures and partial neurological involvement, Guttman in 1963[22] and Frankel in 1969[15] reported that 60 percent and 63 percent of the patients, respectively, improved one or more neurological grades (Frankel classification). Patients undergoing surgery (laminectomy with or without fusion) during the same period did not improve neurologically to any greater extent.[52] A more recent study reported improvement in 95 percent of patients treated by postural reduction.[8] In comparison, two surgical series (posterolateral decompression and Harrington instrumentation) documented 90 percent or more improvement in a similar group of patients.[14,27]

For this form of therapy to be successful, a team approach is required, and the nursing staff must be both talented and dedicated. Disadvantages of postural reduction include a prolonged immobilization period (9 to 13 weeks) and the complications associated with prolonged bed rest. Although the displacement of the fracture-dislocation can usually be corrected by postural reduction, the abnormal angulation of the spine will frequently recur. In the series of patients reported by Davies et al. the prereduction angulation of the spine measured 16 degrees.[8] This was reduced to 6 degrees by postural reduction but then increased to 18 degrees at follow-up.

Surgical Therapy

The primary indications for surgical intervention with thoracolumbar fractures are to relieve actual or anticipated neural compression and to stabilize the spine (Table 296-3). The universally accepted indication is progressive neurological deterioration due to a compressive lesion; however, this situation is not commonly encountered. The remaining indications continue to be controversial. It is our opinion that the spinal canal should be decompressed with removal of all bone and disc fragments to provide an optimum environment for spinal cord recovery. The compression of the spinal cord or cauda equina may be actual or anticipated. In the latter case, the lumen of the spinal canal is reduced, and with healing of the fracture and further angulation of the spine, neural compression and deficit occur with time. Dural lacerations should be identified and repaired.[12] Frequently, portions of the cauda equina will herniate through the laceration, and if the dura is not repaired, scarring and a chronic pain syndrome may result. Although many believe that the spinal canal should be decompressed and experimental evidence suggests that spinal cord recovery is related to both the force and duration of the compressing agent,[29] it must be recalled that, in terms of neural recovery, the results of operative and nonoperative therapy appear to be approximately the same.

Controversy also exists as to which fractures are stable and which are unstable (Table 296-3). This reflects, in part, the different definitions of the term *stability*. For example, some authors do not consider progressive angulation of the spine as a sign of instability, yet late progressive kyphosis may be accompanied by loss of neurological function.

When surgical intervention is indicated, timing is the next important consideration. Initially we attempted to operate within the first few hours following injury with the expectation that immediate decompression and stabilization would improve the degree of neurological recovery. This has not proved to be the case, either in our series or in those of others.[14,27] We now believe a more orderly and complete diagnostic workup, stabilization of the patient, and therapy for associated injuries should be completed first. With this approach the majority of our spine fractures are operated on within 3 to 4 days following injury. The result has been fewer complications and no detectable loss in the degree of neurological recovery.

A variety of intraoperative aids are available to improve the technical aspects of the surgery and to diminish potential complications. These include improved lighting, magnification, high-speed drills of different configurations, and the monitoring of evoked potentials. The intraoperative monitoring of spinal somatosensory evoked potentials (SSEPs) is a useful, but not absolute, method of minimizing spinal cord injury during spine fracture surgery.[19,20] With stimulus intensities three times the motor threshold, the evoked potentials primarily reflect activity in the dorsal columns[19,35] and thus do not provide precise information regarding the status of the more ventrally placed motor tracts. Varying degrees of motor paralysis have been reported to occur without significant change in SSEPs. Several reports of animal models suggest that this limitation of SSEPs may be overcome in the future.[34,42]

TABLE 296-3 Indications for Surgical Treatment

Progressive neurological deficit
Spinal cord compression
Dural laceration
Unstable spine
Fracture-dislocation
Anteroposterior or lateral translocation
Severe wedge or burst fracture
Progressive angulation

Surgical procedures designed to decompress and stabilize thoracolumbar fractures are primarily anterior or posterior approaches. The anterior approach involves resection of the fractured vertebral body followed by strut grafting using autogenous iliac or fibular strut grafts. Posterior operative approaches include laminectomy, lateral extracavitary decompression (modified costotransversectomy), and posterolateral decompression via the pedicle combined with posterior instrumentation.

Anterior Vertebral Body Resection

Anterior exposure of the vertebral body is gained by either a transthoracic, a transabdominal, or a combined approach.[49] Since the portion of the vertebral body compromising the dural contents invariably involves the cephalad portion of the vertebral body, the resection should begin at the lower interspace where the anatomy is relatively normal. A high speed drill and thin upbiting curettes are useful for this. Once the posterior longitudinal ligament and dura have been exposed, the resection is carried cephalad through the fractured vertebral body to the interspace above. The dura should be exposed completely from below to above and from one lateral gutter to the other. Iliac crest or fibular strut grafts are utilized for the fusion. Simple anterior fusion alone is often inadequate to prevent graft collapse and progressive angulation of the spine with weight bearing. Anterior implants are bulky and are ineffective in securing vertebral bodies. Therefore, these procedures are often combined with posterior stabilization.

Laminectomy

Laminectomy as primary therapy for thoracolumbar fractures is being viewed with increasing disfavor in this country, and, although late in coming, this is a welcome trend. There are very few reasons to recommend laminectomy for this condition, and many reasons to condemn it. For example, the abnormality in the majority of thoracolumbar fractures is anterior to the spinal cord (Fig. 296-4), and laminectomy does little to relieve the traction of the spinal cord over an anterior lesion. Furthermore, laminectomy increases the instability of the damaged spinal column. Removal of the interspinous and yellow ligaments increases the possibility of a progressive flexion deformity. There is also a risk of further damaging the spinal cord when a laminectomy is carried out for thoracic fractures. The diameter relationships of the thoracic spinal column and spinal cord are such that there may be insufficient space to safely insert the jaw of a rongeur between the lamina and the posteriorly displaced spinal cord. If there is any doubt regarding this point, the history of surgery for thoracic disc disease should be recalled. In our opinion, there is little justification for the routine use of laminectomy. The procedure should be reserved for those few specific situations where laminectomy will benefit the patient.

Posterior compression of the spinal cord resulting from bone fragments or epidural hematoma formation may be an indication for laminectomy. Preoperative utilization of CT myelography will indicate whether the main lesion is anterior or posterior to the spinal cord. Another indication for laminectomy is the severe burst (impaction) fracture with associated dural lacerations.[24,39] This diagnosis is suspected by noting the widened interpedicular distance on the plain film. In this case laminectomy may be required to reduce herniated nerve roots and repair the dura.

The following technical points should be considered when laminectomy is utilized for fractures of the spine. The exposure for the laminectomy must be accomplished by sharp dissection and not by use of a periosteal elevator, which may drive bone fragments into the spinal canal. In some cases it is possible to remove the lamina with rongeurs, but in other cases, when the spinal cord has been displaced posteriorly, there is insufficient space to insert an instrument between the lamina and the dura. To prevent further damage to the spinal cord in this situation, removal of the lamina with a drill is advisable. In addition, lateral and central dural tack-up sutures should be employed to prevent postoperative epidural bleeding from compressing the spinal cord.

Lateral Extracavitary Approach

Another posterior approach to the spinal column is the lateral extrapleural or extraperitoneal approach.[33] This involves resection of the posterior portion of the ribs and the transverse processes to gain exposure to the lateral aspect of the spinal column. It will be recognized that this is a modification of the costotransversectomy originally developed to deal with tuberculous involvement of the spine. Once the lateral aspect of the vertebral body is exposed, the posteriorly protruded fragments may be removed as described below.

Posterolateral Decompression

A posterolateral approach to the spinal canal through the pedicle provides direct access to the cephalad portion of the vertebral body while avoiding the disadvantages of laminectomy.[13,24,27,29,37,43] Furthermore, following decompression of the spinal canal, posterior instrumentation can be accomplished, thus eliminating the need for a second procedure that is often required when the fractured vertebral body is removed by an anterior approach. However, from the technical standpoint, the procedure is tedious, and meticulous attention to detail is required to achieve adequate decompression without further neural injury.[24]

In this procedure, the patient is placed prone and is carefully positioned to avoid abdominal compression and brachial plexus stretch injuries. A midline incision of sufficient length to encompass the posterior implant is selected. Over the fracture site only sharp dissection should be employed to avoid driving bone fragments into the spinal canal with a periosteal elevator. The fracture is identified visually, and the level is confirmed by a lateral x-ray film. The pedicle is entered with a high speed drill. Whether the right or left pedicle is removed is based on the configuration of the fracture as determined by the preoperative CT scan. The crucial step is leaving a thin rim of bone to protect the dural contents. The posterior portion of the vertebral body is then removed with the drill, again leaving a rim of bone. The remaining rim of bone is then fractured into the cavity with a thin impactor and is removed with pituitary rongeurs. If complete decompression is not obtained, the procedure is repeated from the contralateral side (Fig. 296-6*A–E*). The decompression is confirmed by visual inspection and palpation, or, alternatively, with intraoperative ultrasonography. Following posterior instrumentation and bone grafting drains are placed and the wound is closed.

The following points regarding this operative procedure are worth emphasizing. During inspection of the fracture site, CSF leaks must be recognized, and if present, the dural lacerations must be repaired. With many of these fractures, the ligamentum flavum is torn, and if this is so, the ligamentum should be removed. If it is not resected, spinal realignment may buckle the torn ligamentum inward and produce posterior spinal cord compression. A final point to recall is the relationship of the neurovascular bundle to the

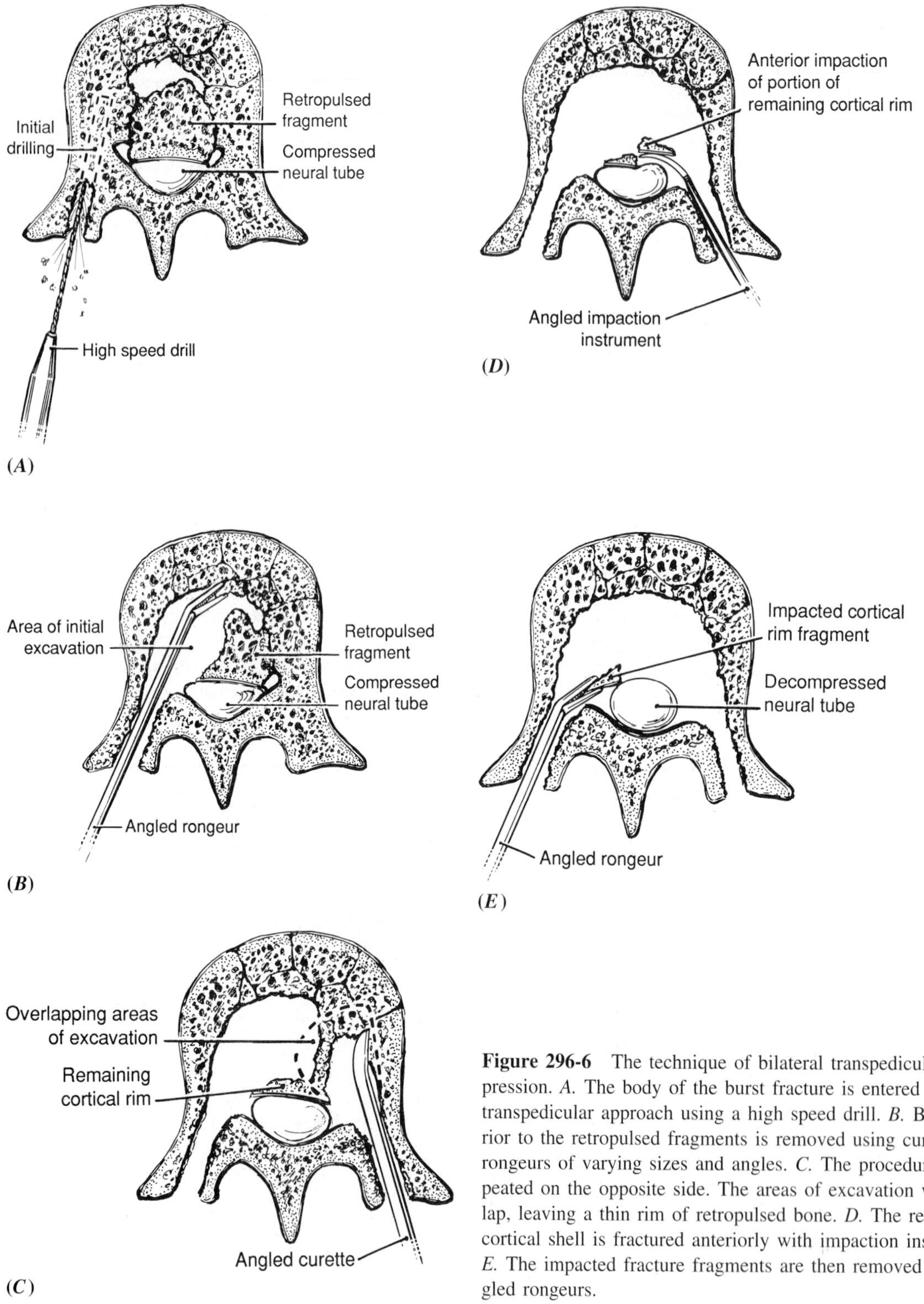

Figure 296-6 The technique of bilateral transpedicular decompression. *A.* The body of the burst fracture is entered through a transpedicular approach using a high speed drill. *B.* Bone anterior to the retropulsed fragments is removed using curettes and rongeurs of varying sizes and angles. *C.* The procedure is repeated on the opposite side. The areas of excavation will overlap, leaving a thin rim of retropulsed bone. *D.* The remaining cortical shell is fractured anteriorly with impaction instruments. *E.* The impacted fracture fragments are then removed with angled rongeurs.

pedicle, so that the vessels and nerves are not damaged when the pedicle is drilled out.

Posterior Instrumentation

Posterior instrumentation systems have made a major contribution to the operative management of fractures and fracture-dislocations of the thoracolumbar spine. Initial reports suggested that realignment of the spinal column using distraction instrumentation might effectively decompress the neural tube. Experience has demonstrated, however, that satisfactory decompression in most cases requires direct removal of bony and disc elements from the spinal canal and that distraction instrumentation alone cannot be relied on to achieve consistent and effective decompression.[2–4,10,18,36,38,46,48,50] The primary role of spinal instrumentation, therefore, is the realignment and stabilization of the spinal column.

Restoration of height and alignment of the spinal column with distraction implants utilizes both the principles of distraction and three-point bending.[1,16,17,24,26,40,45] These considerable mechanical forces, if not controlled, can be transmitted through the bony and soft tissue elements of the spinal column to the neural structures. Direct observation of the neural tube at the fracture site must be maintained to ensure that displacement of bone fragments into the spinal canal or overdistraction does not occur. In this manner, a safe, controlled realignment can be accomplished. Operative roentgenograms are employed to confirm satisfactory reduction. Somatosensory evoked potentials are closely monitored during the following realignment.

In some cases, the rods may require prebending prior to distraction in order to achieve satisfactory restoration of the normal kyphotic and lordotic contours of the thoracolumbar junction. During the following spinal alignment with the initial distraction rod, the injury site is inspected to ensure that complete decompression has been maintained. The second rod is then placed in conjunction with the standard posterior decortication and fusion using autogenous iliac bone grafts. The grafting is bilateral from the level of the superior hooks to the level of the inferior hooks of the distraction system. Graft material is placed medially between the rods and the borders of the spinous processes and laterally within the facet joints and spanning the transverse processes.

Suction drains are placed in the graft donor site and in the fusion site, and these are routinely removed within 36 to 48 h. Postoperatively, the patient is placed in a prefabricated plaster splint. At 5 days, the dressings are removed and the surgical wounds are inspected. The patient is then placed in a plaster body jacket awaiting fabrication of a polypropylene thoracolumbar spinal orthosis. Patients with insensitive skin are fitted with a bivalved polypropylene jacket held with Velcro straps. This facilitates periodic removal for skin inspection to prevent pressure skin necrosis. Neurologically intact patients are maintained in a riveted body jacket until satisfactory fusion can be demonstrated on x-ray films.

The results of posterolateral decompression and instrumentation for thoracolumbar injuries can be considered in light of the goals of therapy (Table 296-2). The immediate stabilization of the fracture permits rapid weight bearing and early rehabilitation. This has reduced the acute hospital stay to approximately 10 days, with a corresponding reduction in cost and in the complications related to prolonged bed rest. The stabilization and fusion have eliminated the problem of progressive angulation of the spine and have diminished, but not abolished, pain at the fracture sites. Whether or not decompression of the spinal canal and repair of the dural lacerations will diminish the late complications of chronic pain, spinal stenosis, tethering, and intra- or extradural scarring[41] remains to be proved. Our early results suggest a significant reduction of the number of patients with chronic pain. The amount of neurological recovery that can be achieved by posterolateral decompression and instrumentation is greater than that obtained by postural reduction if the comparison is made with the earlier reports by Guttman[22] and Frankel et al.[15] A more recent report indicates an equal degree of improvement.[8]

Thoracic Injuries

The thoracic spine is stabilized by the rib cage, and a much greater force is required to produce fracture-dislocation here than for the more mobile cervical and thoracolumbar areas of the spine. Thus, thoracic fracture-dislocations are less common, but when they do occur, the spinal cord injury is usually complete. In addition to the force required to overcome the stability imparted by the rib cage, two other factors contribute to the high percentage of complete

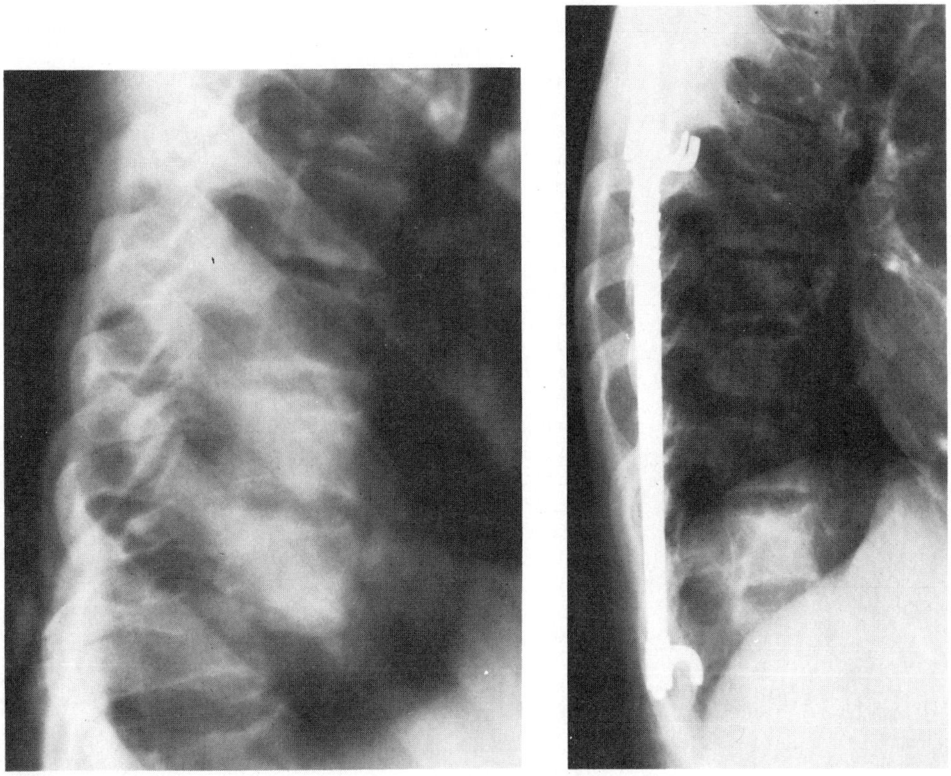

(*A*) (*B*)

Figure 296-7 Thoracic fracture-dislocation before (*A*) and after (*B*) posterolateral decompression and Harrington instrumentation.

thoracic spinal cord injuries. The first is that the diameters of the thoracic spinal canal and thoracic spinal cord are nearly equal, so that minimal displacement results in cord compression. Secondly, the blood supply to the thoracic cord is such that watershed zones are present and thus ischemic as well as compressive damage may occur. Guttman has pointed out that complete thoracic spinal cord injuries have the least chance of any neurological return but that incomplete lesions have a greater degree of return than do incomplete cervical or lumbar spinal cord injuries.[22] The inherent stability of the thoracic spine may explain the better recovery rate for the incomplete injuries.

Similar to thoracolumbar injuries, the mechanisms of injury include flexion, extension, compression, and rotation. Most commonly, the major force is flexion, with the upper vertebra shearing forward on the lower vertebra. Because of the magnitude of the force, associated injuries are common and include damage to the lungs, great vessels, and myocardium.

Traumatic or nontraumatic compression fractures of thoracic vertebrae are frequently encountered in elderly patients. These fractures are generally not associated with neurological deficit and will respond to symptomatic therapy, which may vary from simple analgesics to a hyperextension brace.

In contrast to thoracolumbar fractures, thoracic (T1-9) fracture-dislocations are generally stable, and significant progressive angulation of the spine is an infrequent problem. Thus, many of these fractures can be managed by postural reduction and external stabilization with an appropriate orthosis. When faced with a major unstable dislocation, operative reduction followed by instrumentation and fusion is the procedure of choice (Fig. 296-7).

Surgical decompression of the thoracic spinal cord in the face of complete neurological deficit is an unrewarding procedure. If the neurological deficit is incomplete, then posterolateral or anterior decompression may be indicated. As noted earlier, decompression by laminectomy is to be avoided.

Lumbar Injuries

Fractures of the lower lumbar spine and lumbosacral junction are encountered infrequently.[7] These fractures usually result from flexion and compression. A rotational component to the injury may also be present. With these injuries only the cauda equina is involved; thus the potential for neurological recovery is high. Our current practice includes decompression of the cauda equina, either by a posterolateral or transdural approach, and fusion. Stabilization is usually achieved by employing a transpedicular screw-plate system or a rod system combined with posterolateral bone grafting.

References

1. Aebi M, Etter C, Kehl T, et al. Stabilization of the lower thoracic and lumbar spine with the internal spinal skeletal fixation system: indications, techniques, and first results of treatment. *Spine* 1987; 12:544–551.
2. Akbarnia BA, Fogarty JP, Tayob AA. Contoured Harrington instrumentation in the treatment of unstable spinal fractures: the effect of supplementary sublaminar wires. *Clin Orthop* 1984; 189:186–194.
3. Benson DR. Unstable thoracolumbar fractures, with emphasis on the burst fracture. *Clin Orthop* 1988; 230:14–29.
4. Bohlman HH. Treatment of fractures and dislocations of the thoracic and lumbar spine. *J Bone Joint Surg [Am]* 1985; 67-A:165–169.
5. Bracken MB, Shepard MJ, Collins WF, et al. A randomized, controlled trial of methylprednisolone or naloxone in the treatment of acute spinal cord injury: results of the Second National Acute Spinal Cord Injury Study. *N Engl J Med* 1990; 322:1405–1411.
6. Chance GO. Note on a type of flexion fracture of the spine. *Br J Radiol* 1948; 21:452–453.
7. Das De S, McCreath SW. Lumbosacral fracture-dislocations: a report of four cases. *J Bone Joint Surg [Br]* 1981; 63-B:58–60.
8. Davies WE, Morris JH, Hill V. An analysis of conservative (non-surgical) management of thoracolumbar fractures and fracture-dislocations with neural damage. *J Bone Joint Surg [Am]* 1980; 62-A:1324–1328.
9. Dooley BJ. The role of seat-belts in reducing the road toll. *J Bone Joint Surg [Br]* 1982; 64-B:518–519.
10. Durward QJ, Schweigel JF, Harrison P. Management of fractures of the thoracolumbar and lumbar spine. *Neurosurgery* 1981; 8:555–561.
11. Eismont FJ, Green BA, Berkowitz BM. The role of intra-operative ultrasonography in the treatment of thoracic and lumbar spine fractures. *Spine* 1984; 9:782–787.
12. Eismont FJ, Wiesel SW, Rothman RH. Treatment of dural tears associated with spinal surgery. *J Bone Joint Surg [Am]* 1981; 63-A:1132–1136.
13. Erickson DL, Leider LL, Brown WE. One-stage decompression-stabilization for thoracolumbar fractures. *Spine* 1977; 2:53–56.
14. Flesch JR, Leider LL, Erickson DL, et al. Harrington instrumentation and spine fusion for unstable fractures and fracture-dislocations of the thoracic and lumbar spine. *J Bone Joint Surg [Am]* 1977; 59-A:143–153.
15. Frankel HL, Hancock DO, Hyslop G, et al. The value of postural reduction in the initial management of closed injuries of the spine with paraplegia and tetraplegia. *Paraplegia* 1969; 7:179–192.
16. Gepstein R, Latta L, Shufflebarger HL. Cotrel-Dubousset instrumentation for lumbar burst fractures: a biomechanical study. *Orthop Trans* 1987; 11:452 (abstr).
17. Gepstein R, Shufflebarger HL, Hallel T. Cotrel-Dubousset (C-D) instrumentation: technical notes and our experience in trauma, tumors, and scoliosis cases, *Orthop Trans* 1987; 11:531 (abstr).
18. Golimbu C, Firooznia H, Rafii M, et al. Computed tomography of thoracic and lumbar spine fractures that have been treated with Harrington instrumentation. *Radiology* 1984; 151:731–733.
19. Grundy BL. Monitoring of sensory evoked potentials during neurosurgical operations: Methods and applications. *Neurosurgery* 1982; 11:556–575.
20. Grundy BL. Intraoperative applications of evoked responses. In Owen JH, Davis H (eds): *Evoked Potential Testing: Clinical Applications.* New York: Grune & Stratton, 1985, pp 159–212.
21. Gumley G, Taylor TKF, Ryan MD. Distraction fractures of the lumbar spine. *J Bone Joint Surg [Br]* 1982; 64-B:520–525.
22. Guttman L. The conservative management of closed injuries of the vertebral column resulting in damage to the spinal cord and spinal roots. In Vinken PJ, Bruyn GW (eds): *Handbook of Clinical Neurology,* Vol 26. New York: American Elsevier, 1976, pp 285–306.
23. Hall ED, Braughler JM. Glucocorticoid mechanisms in acute spinal cord injury: a review and therapeutic rationale. *Surg Neurol* 1982; 18:320–327.
24. Hardaker WT Jr, Friedman AH, Fitch RD. Bilateral transpedicular decompression and Harrington rod stabilization in the management of severe thoracolumbar burst fractures. *Spine* 1992; 17:162–171.
25. Holdsworth F. Fractures, dislocations, and fracture-dislocations of the spine. *J Bone Joint Surg [Am]* 1970; 52-A:1534–1551.
26. Jacobs RR, Asher MM, Snider RK. Thoracolumbar spinal injuries: a comparative study of recumbent and operative treatment in 100 patients. *Spine* 1980; 5:463–477.
27. Jelsma RK, Kirsch PT, Jelsma LF, et al. Surgical treatment of thoracolumbar fractures. *Surg Neurol* 1982; 18:156–166.
28. Jelsma RK, Kirsch PT, Rice JF, Jelsma LF. The radiographic description of thoracolumbar fractures. *Surg Neurol* 1982; 18:230–236.

29. Jelsma RK, Rice JF, Jelsma LF, Kirsch PT. The demonstration and significance of neural compression after spinal injury. *Surg Neurol* 1982; 18:79–92.
30. Keene JS, Goletz TH, Lilleas F, et al. Diagnosis of vertebral fractures: a comparison of conventional radiography, conventional tomography, and computed axial tomography. *J Bone Joint Surg [Am]* 1982; 64-A:586–595.
31. Kraus JF, Franti CE, Riggins RS, et al. Incidence of traumatic spinal cord lesions. *J Chronic Dis* 1975; 28:471–492.
32. Kurtzke JF. Epidemiology of spinal cord injury. *Exp Neurol* 1975; 48 (Part 2):163–236.
33. Larson SJ, Holst RA, Hemmy DC, Sances A Jr. Lateral extracavitary approach to traumatic lesions of the thoracic and lumbar spine. *J Neurosurg* 1976; 45:628–637.
34. Levy WJ. Spinal evoked potentials from the motor tracts. *J Neurosurg* 1983; 58:38–44.
35. Macon JB, Poletti CE, Sweet WH, et al. Conducted somatosensory evoked potentials during spinal surgery: Part 2. Clinical applications. *J Neurosurg* 1982; 57:354–359.
36. Maiman DJ, Larson SJ, Benzel EC. Neurological improvement associated with late decompression of the thoracolumbar spinal cord. *Neurosurgery* 1984; 14:302–307.
37. McAfee PC, Yuan HA, Lasda NA. The unstable burst fracture. *Spine* 1982; 7:365–373.
38. McEvoy RD, Bradford DS. The management of burst fractures of the thoracic and lumbar spine: experience in 53 patients. *Spine* 1985; 10:631–637.
39. Miller CA, Dewey RC, Hunt WE. Impaction fracture of the lumbar vertebrae with dural tear. *J Neurosurg* 1980; 53:765–771.
40. Olerud S, Karstrom G, Sjostrom L. Transpedicular fixation of thoracolumbar vertebral fractures. *Clin Orthop* 1988; 227:44–51.
41. Osborne DRS, Vavoulis G, Nashold BS Jr, et al. Late sequelae of spinal cord trauma: myelographic and surgical correlation. *J Neurosurg* 1982; 57:18–23.
42. Powers SK, Bolger CA, Edwards MSB. Spinal cord pathways mediating somatosensory evoked potentials. *J Neurosurg* 1982; 57:472–482
43. Schmidek HH, Gomes FB, Seligson D, McSherry JW. Management of acute unstable thoracolumbar (T11–L1) fractures with and without neurological deficit. *Neurosurgery* 1980; 7:30–35.
44. Smith WS, Kaufer H. Patterns and mechanisms of lumbar injuries associated with lap seat belts. *J Bone Joint Surg [Am]* 1969; 51-A:239–254.
45. Steffee AD, Biscup RS, Sitkowski DJ. Segmental spine plates with pedicle screw fixation: a new internal fixation device for disorders of the lumbar and thoracolumbar spine. *Clin Orthop* 1986; 203:45–53.
46. Trafton PG, Boyd CA Jr. Computed tomography of thoracic and lumbar spine injuries. *J Trauma* 1984; 24:506–515.
47. Watson N. Road traffic accidents, spinal injuries and seat belts. *Paraplegia* 1983; 21:63–64.
48. White RR, Newberg A, Seligson D. Computerized tomographic assessment of the traumatized dorsolumbar spine before and after Harrington instrumentation. *Clin Orthop* 1980; 146:150–156.
49. Whitesides TE Jr, Shah SGA. On the management of unstable fractures of the thoracolumbar spine. *Spine* 1976; 1:99–107.
50. Willen J, Lindahl S, Irstam L, et al. Unstable thoracolumbar fractures: a study by CT and conventional roentgenology of the reduction effect of Harrington instrumentation. *Spine* 1984; 9:214–219.
51. Williams JS, Kirkpatrick JR. The nature of seat belt injuries. *J Trauma* 1971; 11:207–218.
52. Young JS, Dexter WR. Neurological recovery distal to the zone of injury in 172 cases of closed, traumatic spinal cord injury. *Paraplegia* 1978; 16:39–49.

297

Management of Thoracic and Lumbar Spinal Instability

William J. Richardson
William T. Hardaker, Jr.

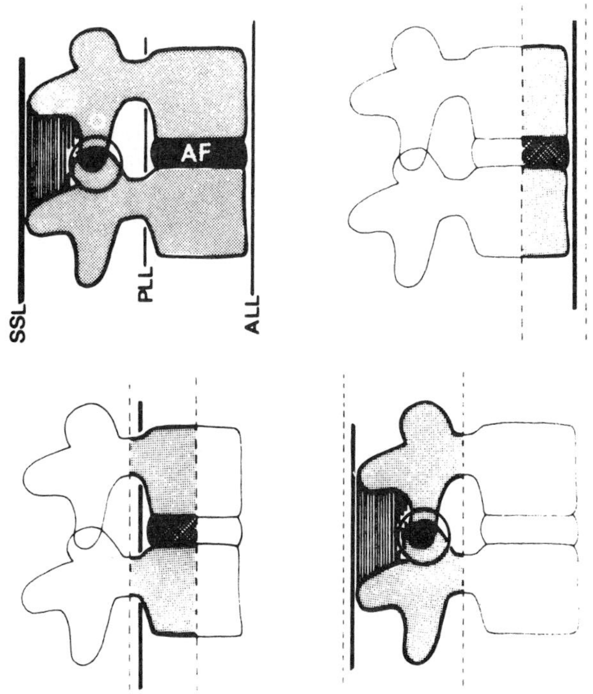

Figure 297-1 The anterior, middle, and posterior spinal columns are illustrated. (From Denis,[1] with permission.)

Clinical spinal instability has been defined by White and Panjabi as the "loss of the ability of the spine under physiologic loads to maintain relationships between vertebrae in such a way that there is neither damage nor subsequent irritation to the spinal cord or nerve roots, and, in addition, there is no development of incapacitating deformity or pain due to structural changes."[23] The task of identifying when instability exists in the clinical situation is difficult and requires careful evaluation of all data available; incorrect decisions may lead to progression of neurological deficits, deformity, or death. Commonly used information which is available to help make this decision includes the radiographic appearance, the anatomic location, the neurological status, the etiologic agent (trauma, tumor, infection, etc.), and an analysis of forces involved. Authors have offered a variety of approaches to help make the diagnosis of clinical instability and to develop a treatment plan. Most interest has been in the study of fractures secondary to major trauma and, thus, our clearest understanding of instability exists in this area.

Identification and Classification of Instability in the Thoracic and Lumbar Spine

Holdsworth in reviewing thoracic and lumbar fractures divided them into two major groups[8]: stable fractures (simple wedge compression fractures, burst fractures, and extension injuries) and unstable fractures (dislocations, rotational fracture-dislocations, and shear fractures). This did not account for the clinically observed instability seen with some burst fractures. Thus, Whitesides proposed a classification based on a two-column system.[24] The anterior column was visualized as resisting compressive forces with the posterior column resisting tension forces. Denis[1] and McAfee et al.[16] added a third or middle column to the classification system (Fig. 297-1).

Denis recommends the subdivision of instability into three categories (first, second, and third degree).[1] Instability of the first degree, or mechanical instability, includes severe compression fractures with failure of the posterior column as seen in distraction and seatbelt injuries. With these fractures the neural elements are not at great risk in the acute period, but the spine can buckle, leading to further deformity or chronic mechanical instability. External support is usually adequate. Instability of the second degree, or neurological instability, would include burst fractures without neurological involvement. The middle column, having failed in compression, may further compromise the neural elements unless protected from further axial load. Stabilization operatively might be considered for this category. Instability of the third degree, or mechanical and neurological instability, would include fracture-dislocations and burst fractures with acute neurological involvement. These are at significant risk of developing progressive neurological loss and deformity; they may require reduction, decompression, and stabilization. Denis' system becomes cumbersome clinically with over 20 subcategories, although it does allow us to classify almost all fractures which are observed in the thoracolumbar spine and thus may be valuable in research studies (Table 297-1).

TABLE 297-1 Basic Modes of Failure of the Three Columns in the Four Major Types of Spinal Injuries

Type of Fracture	Column		
	Anterior	**Middle**	**Posterior**
Compression	Compression	None	None or distraction (severe)
Burst	Compression	Compression	None
Seatbelt type	None or compression	Distraction	Distraction
Fracture-dislocation	Compression, rotation, shear	Distraction, rotation, shear	Distraction, rotation, shear

Source: Adapted from Denis.[1]

McAfee et al., based on an analysis of 100 thoracolumbar fractures with CT scans and based on the three-column concept, offered a simplified classification system.[16] It divides the forces acting on the middle column into axial compression, axial distraction, and translation or shear which would include rotational forces. Based on this system, they suggest six types of injuries: (1) wedge compression fracture, (2) stable burst fracture, (3) unstable burst fracture,[17] (4) Chance fracture, (5) flexion-distraction injury, and (6) translational (shear) injuries to include slice and rotational fracture-dislocations. This system is useful because the method of treatment is suggested by the mechanism by which the middle column fails. If the middle column fails in compression, distraction instrumentation is used posteriorly; for failure in distraction, compression instrumentation should be used; for failure in translation or shear, segmental instrumentation should be used. Thus, this is a relatively simple classification system that is clinically useful.

The three-column concept has been developed and used to evaluate spinal fractures. Clinical instability may also be caused by infection, inflammation, neoplasia, or degeneration, or may be iatrogenically induced. Each etiologic agent is associated with unique circumstances which make a universal classification system somewhat impractical.

In addition, the anatomic area in which the lesion occurs provides unique biomechanical characteristics. In the thoracic area, the spine tends to be stiffer and less mobile due to the ribs; there is less room for the spinal cord; and the blood supply to the cord is more precarious. These characteristics differ from those of the lumbar spine that is more mobile and has relatively more space for the neural elements in the canal. The thoracolumbar junction is frequently subjected to higher stresses because it links the stiff thoracic spine to the mobile lumbar spine.

White and Panjabi, using biomechanical studies of cervical, thoracic, and lumbar spine cadaveric specimens, made observations that are helpful in the evaluation of clinical instability.[23] They have incorporated these data along with information from a review of the clinical literature to develop checklists for each spinal area. Relative point values are given to different criteria. If the relative points from the checklist total more than five, then clinical instability is considered to exist. This system can be used to determine instability caused by infection, tumor, or surgery.

The checklist for clinical instability in the thoracic and thoracolumbar spine is presented in Table 297-2. Because of the overlying shoulder girdle in the upper thoracic spine and ribs, radiographic evaluation is frequently difficult and planar tomograms and/or computed tomography (CT) scanning may be necessary to adequately evaluate this area. The checklist can be valuable in assessing patients preoperatively as a guide to a surgical approach. For example, if the anterior elements are destroyed (as frequently occurs with infection or tumor), and there is any gibbus or listhesis, it would be ill-advised to remove the posterior elements without performing some type of stabilization procedure because that would further destabilize the spine. Depending on the circumstances, one might then direct attention to the anterior approach if practical.

A similar checklist is provided for the lumbar spine (Table 297-3).[18] Neurological deficits are relatively less common in this area and may have a greater propensity for recovery if decompressed. The values for sagittal plane translation in this checklist are percentages to eliminate the problem of x-ray magnification.

Degenerative and/or iatrogenic instability of the lumbar spine is controversial. Several techniques and criteria have been suggested to identify the problem.[23] Most frequently the symptom is chronic low back pain, with neurological compromise being less common. Most criteria are derived from static or stress roentgenograms. When evaluating this area, it is important to have standing anteroposterior and lateral x-ray films of the lumbar spine because there is more likely to be sagittal plane translation in these views than with supine films. Currently suggested criteria include greater than 3 mm of sagittal plane translation on standing or bending x-ray films, retrolisthesis, traction spurs, and asymmetric disc collapse with flexion/extension. Unfortunately, no well-controlled studies exist that document the reliability of these criteria in predicting a successful outcome if a solid fusion is obtained. Most frequently these patients are difficult to evaluate clinically with a long clinical history and many psychosocial issues. Prior to embarking on a stabilization procedure, a multidiscipline evaluation, including a psychosocial assessment, should be completed.

TABLE 297-2 Checklist for the Diagnosis of Clinical Instability in the Lumbar (L1-L5) Spine

Element	Point Value*
Cauda equina damage	3
Relative flexion sagittal plane translation >8% or extension sagittal plane translation >9%	2
Relative flexion sagittal plane rotation <−9 degrees	2
Anterior elements destroyed	2
Posterior elements destroyed	2
Dangerous loading anticipated	1

*Total of 5 or more = clinically unstable.
Source: Data from White and Panjabi.[23]

Once a lesion is identified and fully evaluated, a treatment plan is made. The plan is based on its relative value to the patient's overall well-being versus the risks involved. This must consider the natural history of the disease process (if known), the general medical condition of the patient, the patient's goals, and the experience of the treating physician. Options include nonoperative treatment (bed rest or external support) and operative treatment, to include stabilization and/or decompression.[9] This chapter will not deal extensively with techniques of decompression but will offer limited recommendations or options available to be used depending on the stabilization technique chosen. It will not deal with nonoperative techniques. A variety of commonly used operative techniques to provide stabilization are described with their indications, contraindications, advantages, and disadvantages.

Techniques of Posterior Surgical Stabilization

Harrington Distraction Instrumentation

Background

Originally used by Harrington in 1958 for thoracolumbar fractures, there are numerous reports of the use of Harrington distraction instrumentation, with and without sublaminar wires, to treat spinal fractures.[3,4,9,19,21] It is ideally suited for the treatment of burst fractures where the middle column fails in compression. It can be used whenever the anterior longitudinal ligament is intact. If the anterior ligament is destroyed or disrupted in tension, distraction instrumentation can lead to further neurological compromise by overdistraction. If used early (within 48 to 72 h) with burst fractures, the deformity can be reduced and there is some evidence suggesting that the compromise of the canal can be cleared through ligamentotaxis. However, there have been reports of neurological

TABLE 297-3 Checklist for the Diagnosis of Clinical Instability in the Thoracic and Thoracolumbar Spine

Element	Point Value*
Anterior elements destroyed or unable to function	2
Posterior elements destroyed or unable to function	2
Relative sagittal-plane translation >2.5 mm	2
Relative sagittal-plane rotation >5 degrees	2
Spinal cord or cauda equina damage	2
Disruption of costovertebral articulations	1
Dangerous loading anticipated	2

*Total of 5 or more = clinically unstable.
Source: Data from Posner et al.[18]

deterioration after using distraction instrumentation with failure of reduction of the bony fragments within the canal. In addition, the adequacy of reduction must be evaluated by intraoperative myelography or ultrasonography or a postoperative myelogram and CT scan. If reduction is incomplete, a second-stage anterior decompressive procedure may be indicated.

We prefer to accomplish decompression using a posterolateral approach[5] through the pedicle prior to attempts at reduction of the deformity and stabilization. In our experience this is a safer approach because the canal is cleared of bone fragments that decrease the risk of further neurological compromise. This is imperative if surgery is delayed more than 48 to 72 h.

Dawson has shown in a cadaveric biomechanical study that with burst fractures, placement of the hooks, three levels above the fractured segment and two below, tends to maximize stability.[12] This can be a problem in the lower lumbar spine because instrumentation below L3 leads to an increased incidence of lower back pain. In addition, the use of distraction instrumentation in the lower lumbar spine can create an iatrogenic lumbar kyphosis or flat back syndrome, which is quite disabling.[13] For these reasons, distraction instrumentation should not be used below L4. When instrumenting to L3 or L4, all attempts should be made to maintain a sagittal curve. To aid in this, the following should be done: (1) the hip should be hyperextended to help maintain lumbar lordosis, (2) the spinous processes of the lower segments can be wired together to prevent distraction at these levels, and (3) a square-ended rod should be utilized to allow sagittal plane contouring.

Some authors have popularized the concept of instrumenting long and fusing short. With this approach, the spine is instrumented three segments above and two below, but the fusion is limited to one segment above and one below. The rods are then removed between 1 and 2 years postoperatively with the hope that the nonfused segments will regain mobility. The physiologic effect of enforced immobility of the facets and discs for a year or longer is not known, but there are some laboratory studies suggesting that it may be detrimental. This technique is not necessary at the thoracolumbar junction and newer methods are available lower; thus, this technique is seldom indicated.[4,10,15]

Segmental wiring results in increased stability and can be provided by sublaminar wires or interspinous process (Wisconsin) wires.[4,15,21,22] Both techniques increase the operative time, the use of sublaminar wires also increases blood loss and has a greater inherent risk of iatrogenic neurological injury. Spinous process wires provide improved stability without the risk of neurological loss.

Surgical Technique

The patient is placed prone with the abdomen free from compression using chest and iliac crest rolls. The area of the spine is draped to include the iliac crest. A midline exposure is made with subperiosteal dissection, three levels above and two below the injured level. Typically, spinal cord evoked potential monitoring is used and, if this is done, four spaces above are exposed to allow the introduction of an epidural electrode which does not interfere with the hook sites. The normal laminae above and below are exposed first and then exposure at the fracture site is accomplished with sharp dissection. The upper hook sites are prepared to accept a 1262 or a 1253 hook. This is accomplished by removing a small portion of the inferior facet, lamina, and ligamentum flavum (Fig. 297-2). The lower hook sites are prepared by excising the ligamentum flavum, a small portion of the inferior facet, and the adjacent laminal edges. The lower hooks are the 1254 (round hole) or 1201 (square hole) hook.

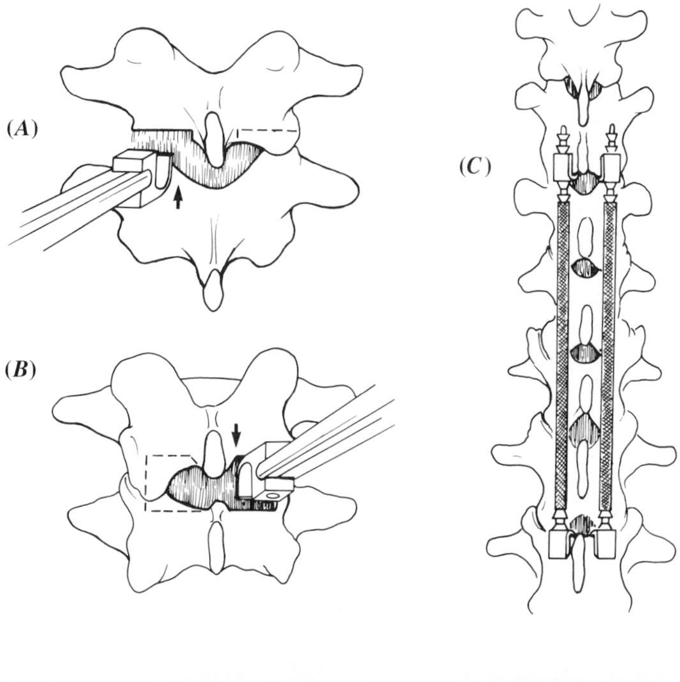

Figure 297-2 Insertion of Harrington distraction rods. *A.* Insertion of the upper hook after removal of a small portion of the inferior facet, lamina, and ligamentum flavum. *B.* Insertion of the lower hook after removal of a small portion of the inferior facet, upper and lower laminae, and ligamentum flavum. *C.* Completed insertion of the dual Harrington distraction rods with upper and lower hooks and distraction applied.

In most instances, the square-ended rods and hooks should be used to maintain sagittal contouring. If using the rods to obtain reduction, the distractor may be helpful. After inserting the hooks on one side, the distractor is applied and axial length is restored, taking care not to overdistract. Translational or rotational deformity can then be corrected by manipulating the spinous processes of the intact levels above and below with Kocher clamps. This reduction can be maintained by placing wires through the base of the spinous process at the level above and likewise at the level below. Care should be taken to remove the ligamentum flavum and joint capsule at the injured level to be sure that these do not impinge on the neural elements at the time of reduction.

If sublaminar wires are to be used, they are passed at this time as described below. Likewise, spinous process wires (Fig. 297-3) are prepared at this time. For their use, a hole is made at the base of each spinous process which is intact over the instrumented segment with a curved awl or bone tenaculum. Beaded Wisconsin wires with attached buttons are then inserted through the hole from each side and the wire threaded through the button and pulled tight until the button is flush against the side of the spinous processes.

After the hook sites are prepared and the sublaminar or spinous process wires are passed, the distraction rods are selected and inserted (Fig. 297-2*C*). Rod length is selected such that a single ratchet will be exposed beneath the upper hook. The rods are contoured to allow correction of kyphosis if it exists and to attempt to maintain lumbar lordosis. If distraction is being utilized in the lumbar spine, the lower spinous processes are wired together in an attempt to maintain lumbar lordosis. If contouring of the rods is required, the square-ended hooks and rods are utilized. One rod is inserted and distraction is applied to correct the deformity. The second rod is then inserted and distraction is likewise applied.

If decompression has not been accomplished through a transpedicular approach, the canal is inspected using either the ultrasound or an intraoperative myelogram at this time. If adequate decompression has been accomplished, the sublaminar or spinous process wires are secured to the rods using a wire twister in a clockwise fashion (Fig. 297-4). Segmental wires are then cut and bent toward the midline. C clamps are applied to the ratchet below the hook to avoid loss of distraction. The spine is decorticated and an autogenous iliac crest bone graft is placed posteriorly and posterolaterally. The wound is closed in layers over drains that are deep to the fascia.

The patient is kept at bed rest until the drains are removed and then is fitted with a thoracolumbar orthosis and mobilized. The rods are usually left in place unless they become symptomatic because of limited soft tissue coverage or if a limited fusion is done because of the involvement of the lower lumbar spine. The rods then are typically removed between 12 and 24 months, postoperatively.

Luque Instrumentation

Luque segmental instrumentation provides better stability against translational and rotational stresses. It is weaker in resisting flexion-extension and provides no axial protection.[15,22] Therefore, it is typically used in the treatment of fracture-dislocations where the middle column fails in shear.[13,22] It may also be used in patients with metastatic tumor involving multiple levels anteriorly where anterior resection and grafting is not feasible. The operative time is typically longer, blood loss greater, and risk of neurological damage greater from sublaminar passage of wires as well as handling of the wires. Sublaminar wires should not be passed at a level where the canal is narrowed.

The positioning, prepping, draping, and exposure are accomplished as for the Harrington instrumentation. Instrumentation generally extends from three levels above to two to three levels below the level of injury. If reduction is necessary, this can frequently be accomplished as with the Harrington instrumentation. Hook sites are prepared at the upper level and the Harrington distractor is utilized to carefully apply distraction under direct vision (to avoid overdistraction) while the translational or rotational component is corrected by manipulating the intact spinous processes above and below the injured level with Kocher clamps. The

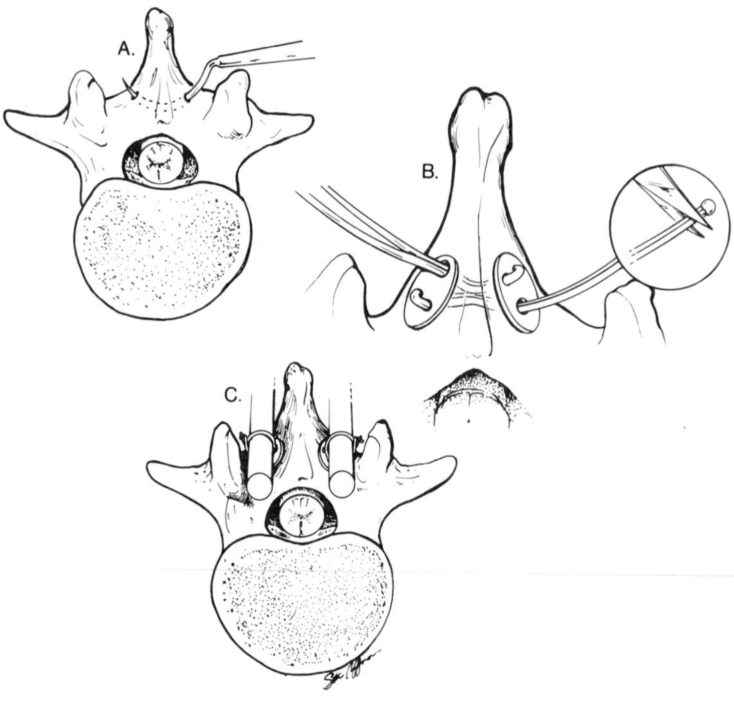

Figure 297-3 Use of Wisconsin wires. *A.* A hole is made at the base of the spinous process with a bone awl and enlarged with a bone tenaculum. *B.* The interspinous process wires are threaded from each side of the spinous process until the metal button is flush with the base of the spinous process. (*Inset*) The wires are separated after the ball tip is removed. *C.* After the rods are inserted, the wires are twisted about the rods and the ends cut.

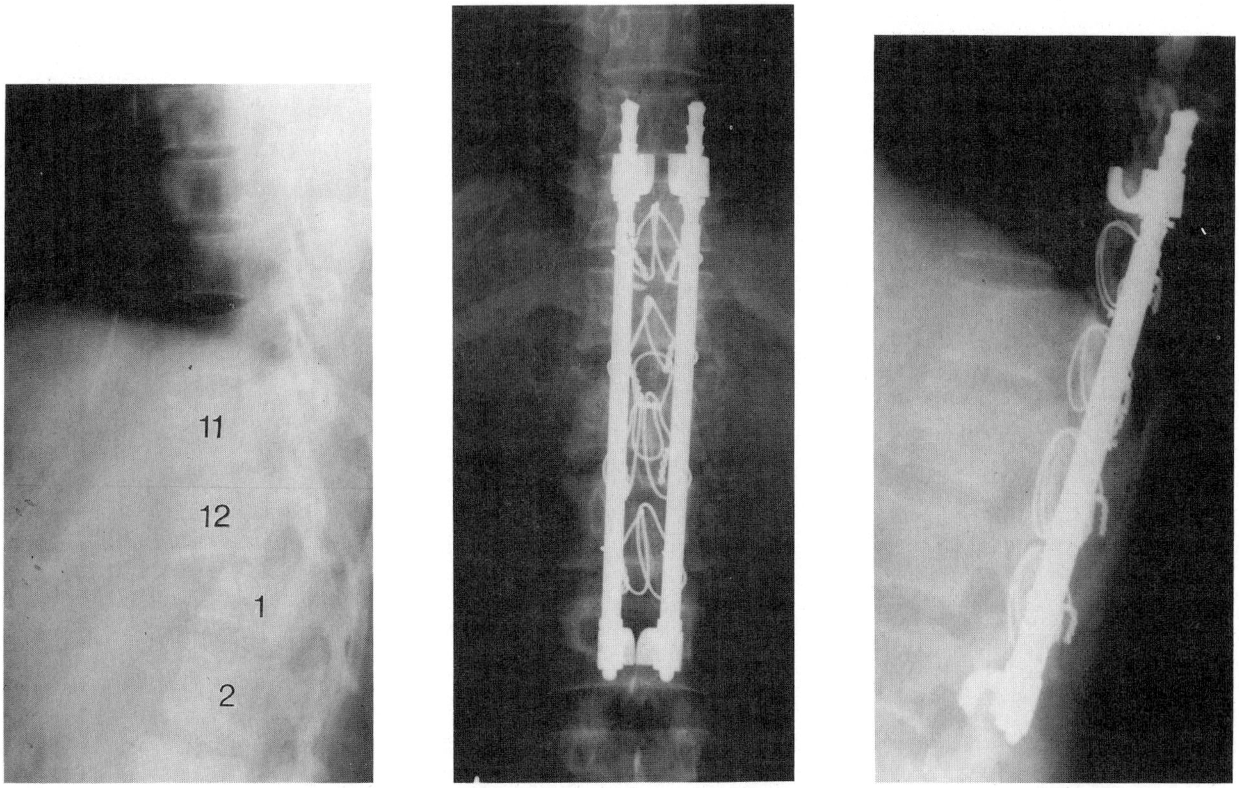

(*A*) (*B*) (*C*)

Figure 297-4 Patient with a fracture-dislocation at T12-L1 (*A*). Care must be taken with distraction instrumentation to avoid overdistraction intraoperatively. *B.* Postoperative anteroposterior film after reduction using a distractor and Kocher clamps to obtain reduction, and an interspinous wire posteriorly to maintain reduction and prevent overdistraction. *C.* Postoperative lateral film showing maintained reduction with dual Harrington distraction rods and sublaminar wires (with an interspinous process wire at the level of injury).

spinous processes are wired together to maintain temporary reduction while the remaining sites are prepared for wire passage. The distractor and hooks are then removed.

Sites are prepared for passage of the wires by removing the interspinous process ligaments in the midline with a rongeur and removing the ligamentum flavum in the midline to expose epidural fat or dura. Kerrison rongeurs are then used to remove the remaining ligamentum flavum and a limited amount of lamina to allow easy passage to the wires. A stainless-steel wire of 18 gauge (0.040 mm) or 16 gauge (0.048 mm) is used. The wire is doubled and bent into an S shape, the diameter of the first bend being slightly larger than the width of the lamina. The tip of the wire is placed in the neural canal at the inferior edge of the lamina in the midline and the wire is advanced along the inner cortex of the lamina parallel to the floor. Once it has passed half the width of the lamina, it is rotated to present the tip above the lamina, maintaining slight constant pressure upward to keep the wire against the undersurface of the lamina and to minimize compromise of the spinal canal. The tip of the wire is grasped with a small Kocher clamp and advanced by pulling up with the clamp (Fig. 297-5*A*). The hand holding the opposite end of the wire should not advance the wire by pushing it, but should apply a slight upward force to keep the wire from plunging into the canal. Depending on preference, the wire may be cut and one half used for each side at the middle levels. Some prefer to use a double wire at each level, requiring passage of a second doubled wire at each level. If single wires are used, they should only be at the midlevels. Doubled wires should be used at the cephalad and caudad extremes.

It is imperative that care be taken and attention continue to be given to the wires once they have been passed beneath the lamina. It is still easy to damage the cord by plunging the wires into the canal while performing other tasks once the wires have been passed. The wires should carefully be bent so that they lie flat over the posterior surface of the lamina (Fig. 297-5*B*) and then bent at right angles over the extensor muscles (Fig. 297-5*C*). These can be held in place with rubber-shod clamps or covered with a towel to minimize manipulation.

Two standard $\frac{3}{16}$-in. (4.8-mm diameter) stainless-steel L rods are selected and cut to the appropriate length. The rods are contoured to preserve or restore sagittal alignment. The rods can be used to obtain correction of the kyphosis by wiring them securely to the lamina above or below the fracture and then levering the attached spine into the proper frontal and sagittal plane alignment (Fig. 297-5*D*).[22] The sublaminar wires at the extreme cephalad and caudad laminae are bent with the superior portion of the wire lateral to the rod and the inferior portion exiting medially. The center wires are all bent with the superior portion medial to the rod and the inferior portion lateral to it. It is important that a rod pusher be used to approximate the rod to the lamina before the wire is tightened. Tightening the wire should never be used to pull the rod to the lamina, as this will frequently result in failure of the wire and/ or lamina. Two additional double 16-gauge wires are used to

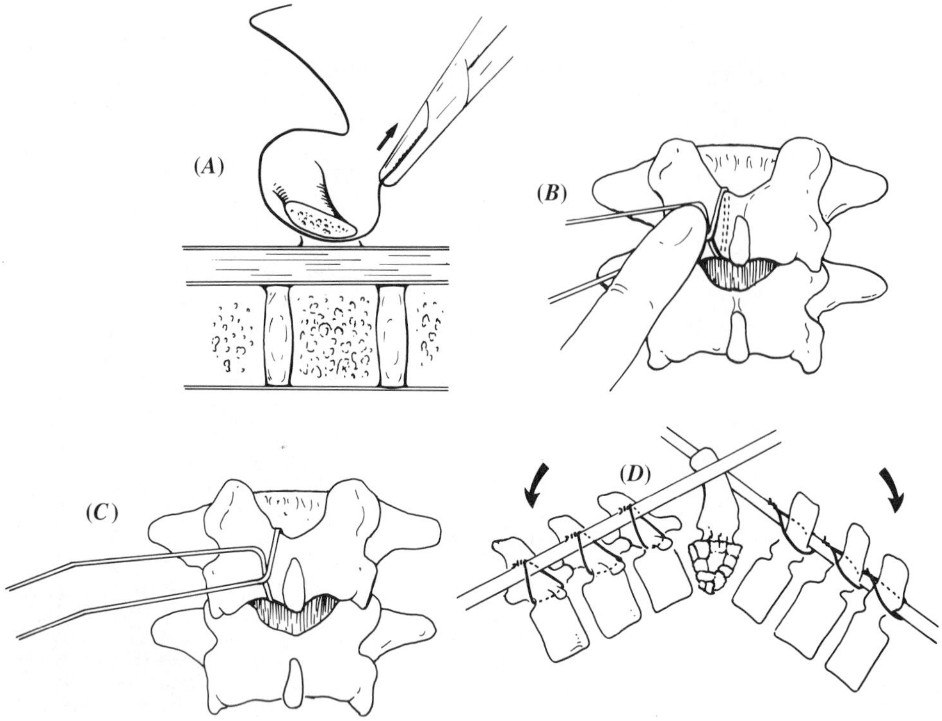

Figure 297-5 Insertion of Luque wires and rods. *A.* Passage of a sublaminar wire with care by constant upward pressure to maintain the wire along the undersurface of the lamina. *B.* Bending the wire along the upper surface of the lamina to prevent it from plunging into the canal. *C.* Bending the wire over the posterior extensor musculature to prevent it from plunging into the canal. *D.* Use of rods and sublaminar wires to reduce kyphosis.

transversely approximate the two L rods at the cephalad and caudad extremes (Fig. 297-6). Decortication is then accomplished and bone is placed posteriorly and posterolaterally for the fusion. Closure and postoperative care are the same as for Harrington distraction instrumentation.

Cotrel-Dubouset (CD) Instrumentation

We prefer the CD instrumentation system over the Harrington distraction and compression systems. The CD system has a solid rod with a knurled surface. There are a variety of closed- and open-ended hooks which allow either compression or distraction to occur. Utilizing closed hooks at the cephalad and caudad extremes and open hooks centrally allows segmental fixation. Depending on the direction of the hooks, both distraction and compression can be used on the same rod in different locations. Typically the cephalad and caudad laminae are secured using two hooks in opposite directions in a claw technique (Fig. 297-7). The rods may be contoured in the frontal and sagittal planes to obtain correction as well as to preserve the sagittal contour. Finally, the two rods are coupled with two transverse traction rods, creating a rectangular structure with improved stability. Generally, instrumentation and fusion can be limited to two levels above and one or two levels below the injured segment.

The disadvantages of the system are that it is somewhat more cumbersome and complex to use as well as being more expensive. Thus, the operative time tends to be slightly longer and blood loss slightly greater. The system is somewhat bulkier and may be more prominent in the thin patient. It occupies more area which otherwise would be utilized for the bone graft. Its advantages are the flexibility that the system provides as well as increased stability. The system is used to provide a posterior compressive force for Chance fractures and flexion distraction injuries (Fig. 297-8). It is utilized to provide a distractive force for unstable burst fractures (Fig. 297-9). It is quite effective in neutralizing the shear forces with translational injuries such as a slice, and rotational fracture-dislocations. It can also be used for patients with multilevel metastatic disease for which anterior decompression is not feasible because of multilevel involvement. However, in severely osteoporotic patients, we have continued to use Luque segmental instrumentation, thinking that it provides more support.

The patient is positioned, prepped, draped, and approached in the same fashion as for the Harrington distraction instrumentation. The spine is exposed two levels above and one to two levels below the level of injury. Hook sites are prepared, as with the Harrington system, to accept closed lamina hooks with narrow (4-mm) blades in claw configuration both cephalad and caudad to the fracture. A total of four hooks are used for each side. The spine is then decorticated and some bone graft is inserted prior to placement of the rods. The rod is threaded through the hooks on one side, using the sagittal contour to correct any kyphosis. Distraction or compression is applied depending on the mode of failure of the middle column. The locking screws of the hooks are then tightened to maintain the distraction or compression. The second rod is threaded through the hooks, with locking screws being tightened as the appropriate corrective force is applied. Once all screws are tightened, two transverse loaders are applied near the end of the rod to form a rigid stable system. All locking screws are twisted until broken. Remaining bone graft is added around the implants and the wounds are closed in layers over drains deep to the fascia. Postoperatively the patient frequently does not require external support.

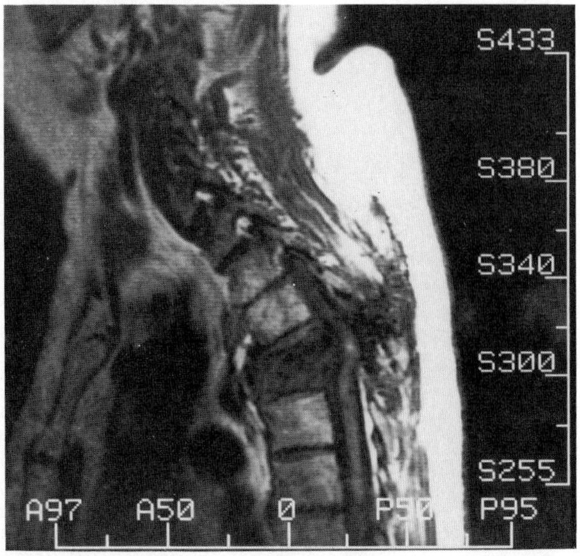

(*A*)

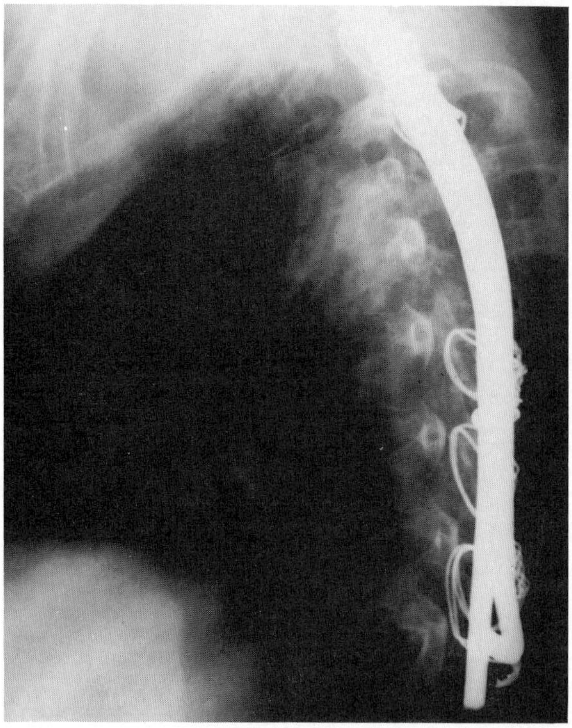

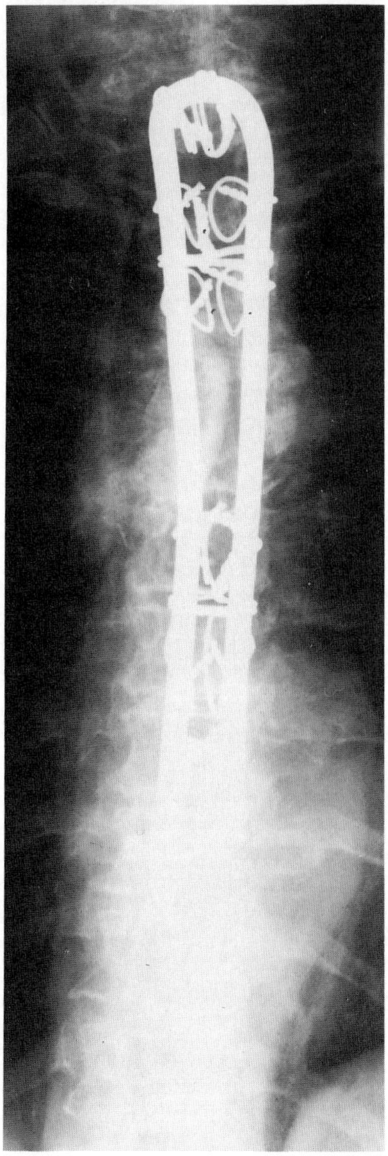

(*C*)

Figure 297-6 *A.* Magnetic resonance image of a patient with vertebral osteomyelitis who had undergone a laminectomy with worsening of kyphosis and neurological status. *B.* Postoperative lateral x-ray film after an anterior decompression with tricortical iliac crest strut grafting and a second-stage posterior stabilization and bone grafting with Luque instrumentation. *C.* Postoperative anteroposterior film showing a rectangular Luque rod with sublaminar wires.

(*A*)

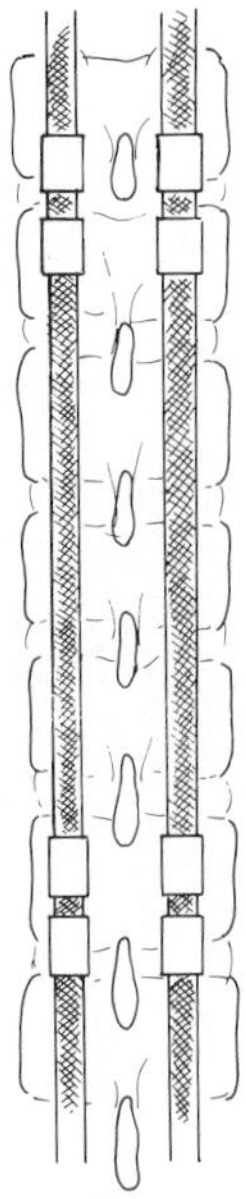

(*B*)

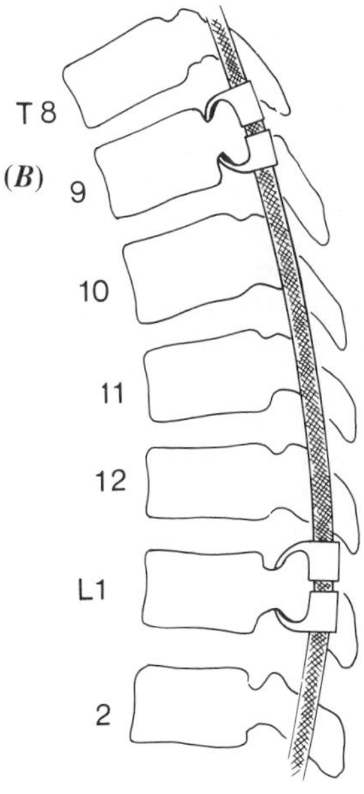

Figure 297-7 Cotrel-Dubouset instrumentation in the coronal plane (*A*) and sagittal plane (*B*). Two hooks are used to form a claw around the upper and lower laminae.

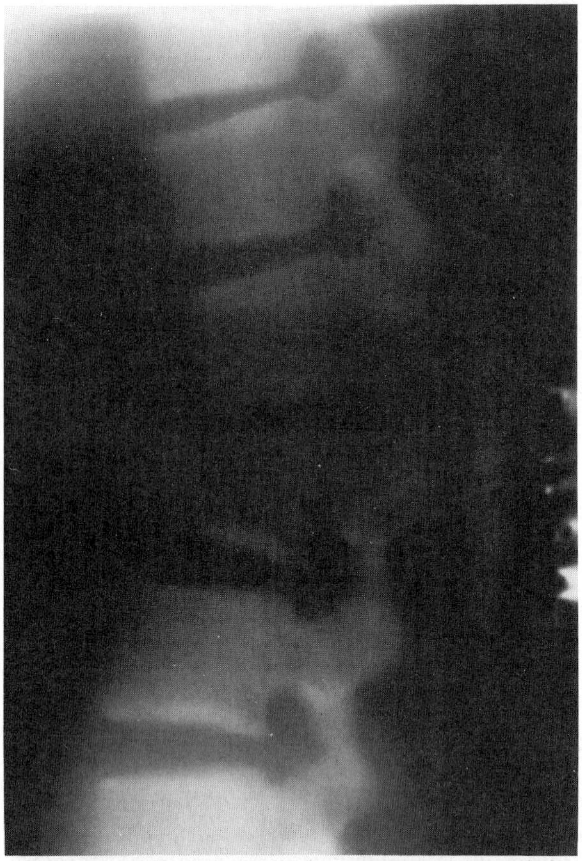

(*A*)

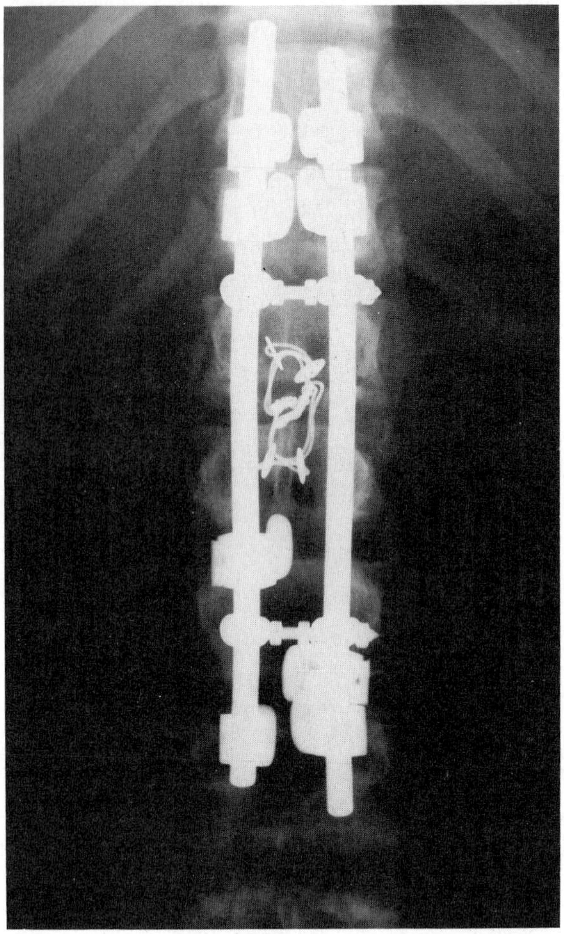

(*B*)

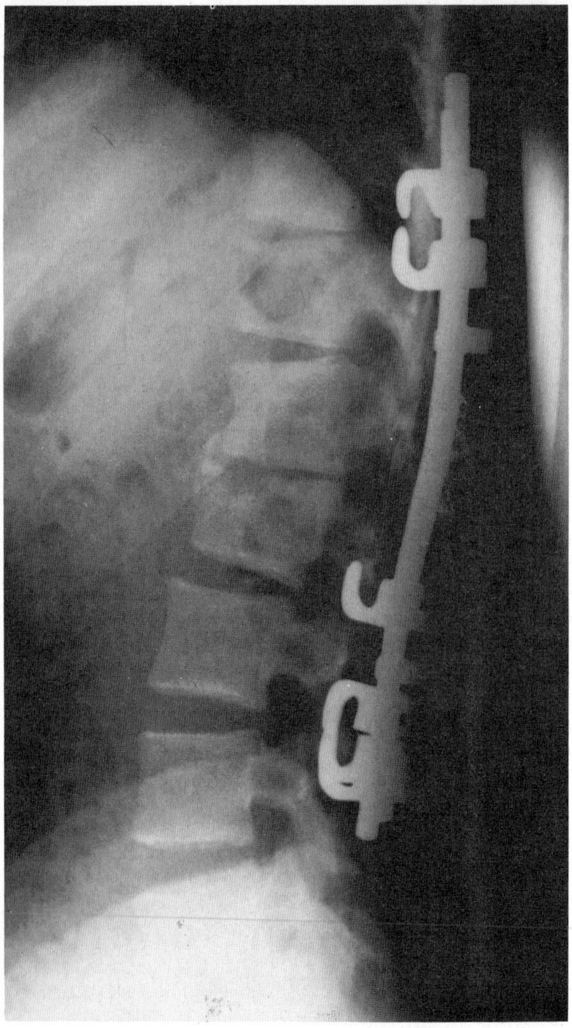

(*C*)

Figure 297-8 *A.* Seatbelt injury with distraction through the posterior elements. *B.* Postoperative anteroposterior film showing interspinous process wiring to supplement the reduction and CD instrumentation applying compression. *C.* Postoperative lateral film showing reduction with CD instrumentation.

The Anterior Surgical Approach

The anterior approach was first popularized by Hodgson and associates in the treatment of tuberculous spondylitis.[7] The major advantage of the anterior approach is that it allows a direct attack on anterior compressive lesions. This is particularly important with infections and metastatic tumors because more than 90 percent of such lesions occur anteriorly. In addition, it can be invaluable for treating burst fractures, particularly those addressed after 72 h. Its disadvantages have been the inability to provide stable fixation in the past and the relative inexperience of orthopaedic surgeons and neurosurgeons with these approaches.

A variety of anterior fixation devices have been developed with the major disadvantage being the risk of vascular compromise. Because of its bulk, the Dunn device[2] has been associated with vascular injury both early and late and is thus no longer available. The Kostuik-Harrington device[11] has been used for several years with no reported intraoperative or postoperative vascular complications. Methyl methacrylate spacers reinforced with metallic rods have been used anteriorly for metastatic disease,[6,20] providing immediate stabilization and improved quality of life for patients with a shortened life expectancy.

Anterior internal fixation devices and methyl methacrylate are contraindicated in the face of infection. Likewise, internal fixation

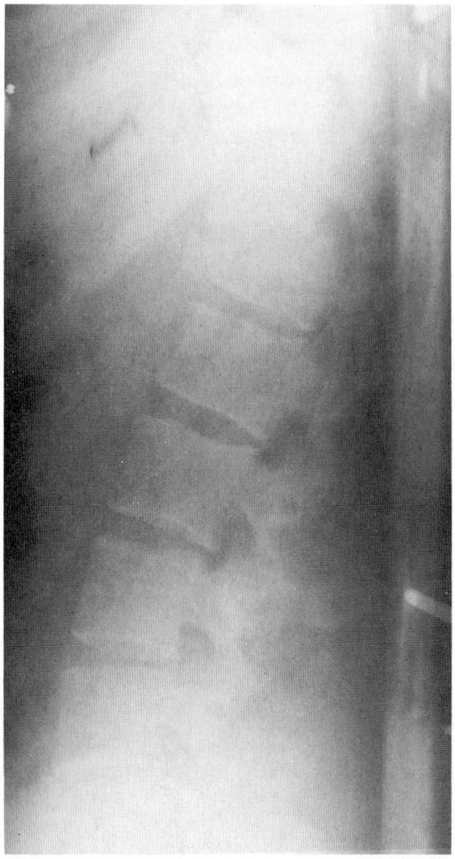

(*A*)

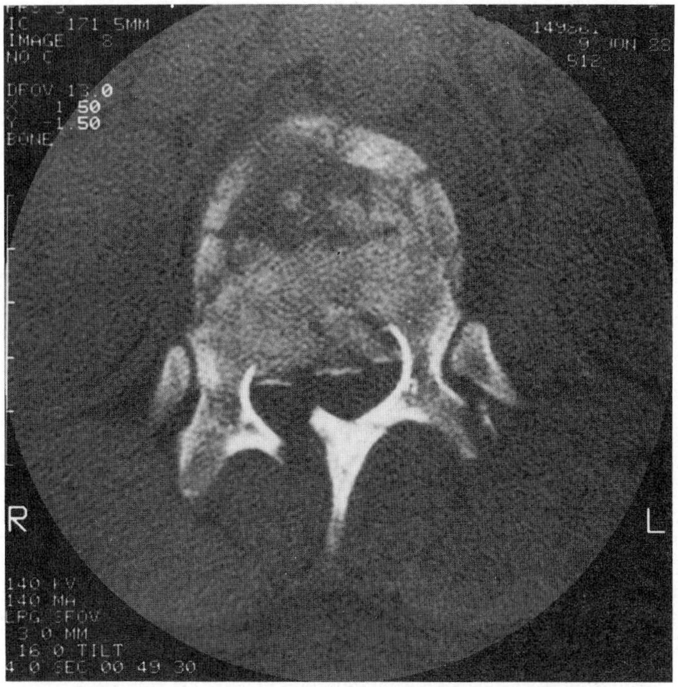

(*B*)

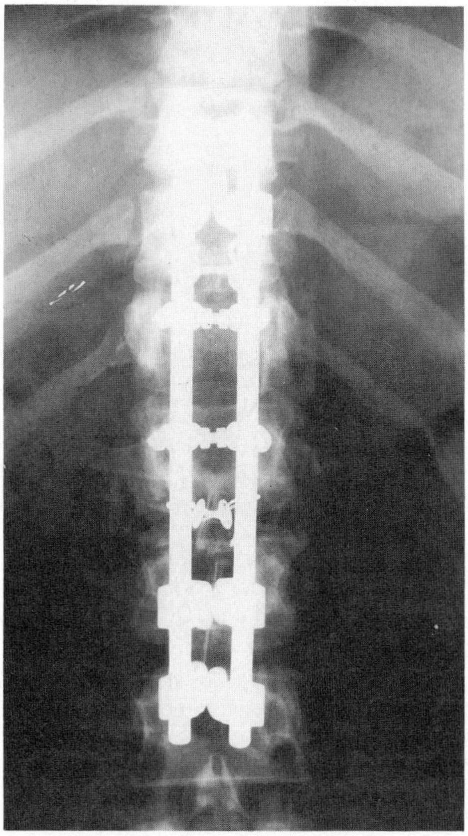

(*C*)

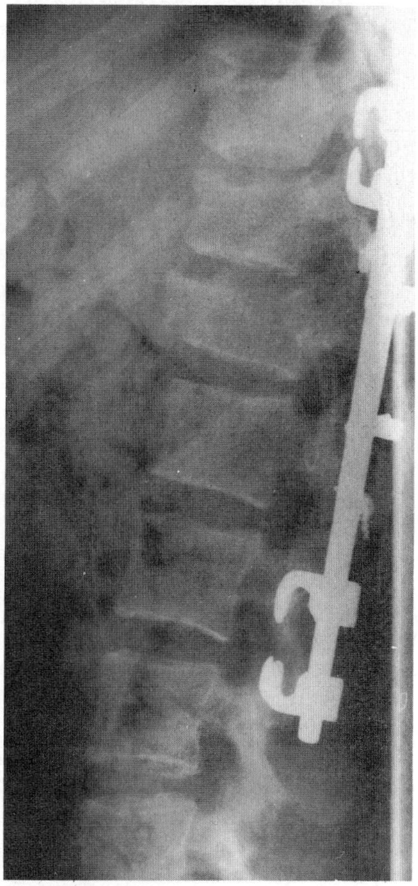

(*D*)

Figure 297-9 *A.* Patient with an L1 burst fracture with retropulsion of bone into the canal. *B.* CT scan showing bony retropulsion and lamina fractures. *C.* Postoperative anteroposterior film showing CD instrumentation supplemented with interspinous process wires. *D.* Postoperative lateral film. Decompression was performed through a posterolateral transpedicular approach and some correction of kyphosis was achieved with distraction.

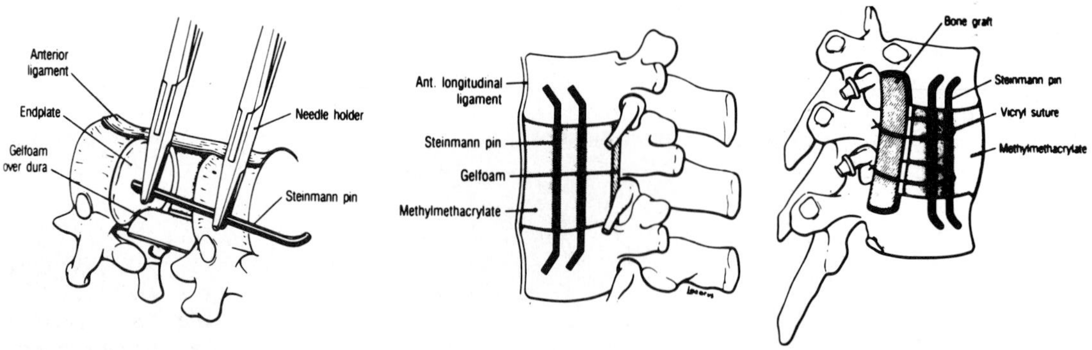

Figure 297-10 Reconstruction after vertebral resection for malignant tumor. (From Sundaresan N, Galicich JH, Lane JM, et al. Treatment of neoplastic epidural cord compression by vertebral body resection and stabilization. *J Neurosurg* 1985; 63:676–684, with permission.)

should not be used for the lumbosacral junction because it requires placing the instrumentation beneath the iliac vessels (nor should it be used at the cervicothoracic junction). If the posterior elements are intact with burst fractures at the thoracolumbar junction and with thoracic fractures or tumors, a simple tricortical iliac crest strut graft supplemented with external support post-operatively may be adequate.[14] If there is posterior element involvement, a strut graft can be placed anteriorly, followed by a second-stage posterior instrumentation and fusion procedure. Similarly, the anterior procedure can be done as a second stage if an attempt at reduction through ligamentotaxis fails in the acute burst fracture.

The thoracic and lumbar spine can be approached anteriorly through a variety of approaches that are well described in a number of texts. The L5 vertebra and lumbosacral junction can be approached either transperitoneally or retroperitoneally. The L1 to L5 vertebrae can be reached through a retroperitoneal approach. The T11 to L1 vertebrae can be reached through a thoracoabdominal approach by removing the tenth rib and then extending retroperitoneally and taking down the diaphragm. The T6 through T11 vertebrae can be reached through a thoracotomy that usually involves removing the rib two levels above the level of the major spinal lesion. The T3 to T5 vertebrae can be approached through a third rib thoracotomy.

The segmental vessels at the involved level and usually the level above and below are ligated and divided. Ligation is carried out near the midline to avoid interference with a major radicular artery. Bleeding around an intervertebral foramen should be controlled with absorbable gelatin sponge (Gelfoam; The Upjohn Company, Kalamazoo, MI) or oxidized regenerated cellulose (Surgicel; Johnson & Johnson, New Brunswick, NJ) and gentle compression; cauterization should be avoided in this area to minimize the possibility of a vascular insult to the cord. In the thoracic spine, the intercostal nerve is identified and traced to the foramen and the pedicle exposed cephalad and caudad with subperiosteal dissection. The pedicle is then removed with a Kerrison rongeur and the dura exposed. The anterior portion of the vertebral body is removed with a rongeur as is the disc above and below. The remaining posterior third of the body is removed with a burr and Kerrison rongeurs. Decompression is complete once the opposite pedicle is exposed.

If decompression is accomplished for a metastatic tumor with postoperative radiation planned and with a life expectancy of less than 2 years, stabilization can be provided with methyl methacrylate (Fig. 297-10). This is accomplished by creating a hole in the end plates of the cephalad and caudad vertebrae and removing enough bone to allow the insertion of the tip of the finger into each vertebral body through these holes. Next, a Harrington compression rod or a Cotrel-Dubouset rod is cut to fit within the hole. The rod is removed and methyl methacrylate which has been cooled is packed by finger into the vertebral bodies and then the rod is reinserted. The dura is protected with a malleable retractor or rubber dam and methacrylate is placed between the bodies surrounding the rod. Copious irrigation prevents thermal damage to the dura or cord as the methacrylate cures. The malleable retractor or rubber dam is removed and the wound is closed. Usually the patient can be mobilized as soon as the drains are removed, without the need for external support.

If Kostuik-Harrington instrumentation (Fig. 297-11) is selected, the large Kostuik screws for the ratcheted rod are inserted anterolaterally in the vertebral body above and vertebral the body below, aiming to penetrate the opposite cortex at the base of the

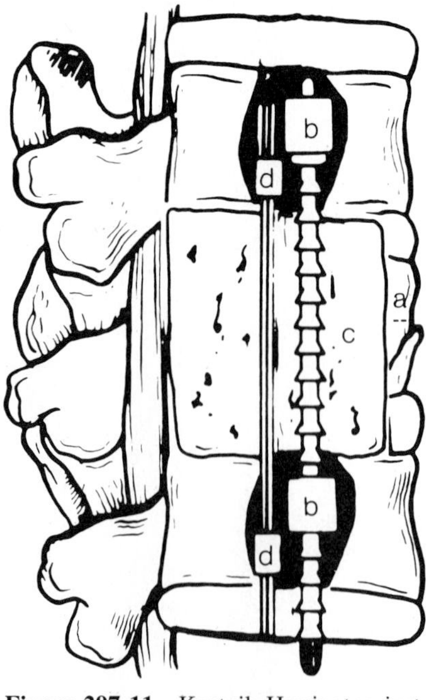

Figure 297-11 Kostuik-Harrington instrumentation. The anterior portion of the body (*a*) is preserved as a viable graft, but the dura is decompressed by removing the posterior third of the body. Kyphosis is reduced with an anterior Kostuik-Harrington distraction apparatus (*b*). An iliac crest graft (*c*) is inserted. Kostuik screws with a Harrington compression rod (*d*) are inserted for neutralization. (From Kostuik,[11] with permission.)

pedicle on the far side. A Harrington distraction rod is then inserted and distraction is applied to correct the deformity. An appropriate size tricortical iliac crest bone graft is harvested and inserted to act as a strut. The collar-ended Kostuik screws are then inserted posterolaterally in the bodies above and below and a Harrington compression rod is threaded through these; the screws are crimped to act as a neutralization rod. A C clamp is placed around the ratcheted rod to prevent loss of fixation. The wound is closed and the patient is mobilized, once the drains are removed, in a TLSO brace for 6 to 12 weeks.

If the patient has already had a posterior procedure with stabilization or if the posterior elements are intact, a tricortical iliac crest strut graft can be keyed into the vertebral bodies above and below after they are prepared as for the methyl methacrylate. The tricortical graft is fashioned into a T shape and locked into place by inserting the upper limbs of the T through the holes of the end plates of the cephalad and caudad vertebrae, with the rounded cortical edge of the iliac crest directed toward the patient's opposite side. The wounds are closed and the patient is mobilized, once the drains are removed, in a TLSO brace. A brace is usually required for 6 to 12 weeks.

References

1. Denis F. The three column spine and its significance in the classification of acute thoracolumbar spinal injuries. *Spine* 1983; 8:817–831.
2. Dunn HK. Anterior stabilization of thoracolumbar injuries. *Clin Orthop* 1984; 189:116–124.
3. Flesch JR, Leider LL, Erickson DL, et al. Harrington instrumentation and spine fusion for unstable fractures and fracture-dislocations of the thoracic and lumbar spine. *J Bone Joint Surg* [*Am*] 1977; 59-A:143–153.
4. Gaines RW, Breedlove RF, Munson G. Stabilization of thoracic and thoracolumbar fracture-dislocations with Harrington rods and sublaminar wires. *Clin Orthop* 1984; 189:195–203.
5. Garfin SR, Mowery CA, Guerra J Jr, et al. Confirmation of the posterolateral technique to decompress and fuse thoracolumbar spine burst fractures. *Spine* 185; 10:218–223.
6. Harrington KD. Metastatic disease of the spine. Current concepts review. *J Bone Joint Surg* [*Am*] 1986; 68-A:1110–1115.
7. Hodgson AR, Stock FE. Anterior spinal fusion: a preliminary communication on the radical treatment of Pott's disease and Pott's paraplegia. *Br J Surg* 1956; 44:266–275.
8. Holdsworth F. Fractures, dislocations, and fracture-dislocations of the spine. *J Bone Joint Surg* [*Am*] 1970; 52A:1534–1551.
9. Jacobs RR, Asher MA, Snider RK. Thoracolumbar spinal injuries: a comparative study of recumbent and operative treatment in 100 patients. *Spine* 1980; 5:463–477.
10. Kahanovitz N, Arnoczky SP, Levine DB, et al. The effects of internal fixation of the articular cartilage of unfused canine facet joint cartilage. *Spine* 1984; 9:268–272.
11. Kostuik JP. Anterior fixation for fractures of the thoracic and lumbar spine with or without neurologic involvement. *Clin Orthop* 1984; 189:103–115.
12. Kostuik JP, Maurais GR, Richardson WJ, et al. Combined single stage anterior and posterior osteotomy for correction of iatrogenic lumbar kyphosis. *Spine* 1988; 14:257–266.
13. Luque ER, Cassis N, Ramirez-Wiella G. Segmental spinal instrumentation in the treatment of fractures of the thoracolumbar spine. *Spine* 1982; 7:312–317.
14. McAfee PC, Bohlman HH, Yuan HA. Anterior decompression of traumatic thoracolumbar fractures with incomplete neurological deficit using a retroperitoneal approach. *J Bone Joint Surg* [*Am*] 1985; 67A:89–104.
15. McAfee PC, Werner FW, Glisson RR. A biomechanical analysis of spinal instrumentation systems in thoracolumbar fractures. *Spine* 1988; 10:204–217.
16. McAfee PC, Yuan HA, Fredrickson BE, et al. The value of computed tomography in thoracolumbar fractures. *J Bone Joint Surg* [*Am*] 1983; 65-A:461–473.
17. McAfee PC, Yuan HA, Lasda NA. The unstable burst fracture. *Spine* 1982; 7:365–373.
18. Posner I, White AA III, Edwards TW, et al. A biomechanical analysis of the clinical stability of the lumbar and lumbosacral spine. *Spine* 1982; 7:374–389.
19. Purcell GA, Markolf KL, Dawson EG. Twelfth thoracic-first lumbar vertebral mechanical stability of fractures after Harrington-rod instrumentation. *J Bone Joint Surg* [*Am*] 1981; 63-A:71–78.
20. Siegal T, Tiqva P, Seigal T. Vertebral body resection for epidural compression by malignant tumors: results of forty-seven consecutive operative procedures. *J Bone Joint Surg* [*Am*] 1985; 67-A:375–382.
21. Sullivan JA. Sublaminar wiring of Harrington distraction rods for unstable thoracolumbar spine fractures. *Clin Orthop* 1984; 189:178–185.
22. Wenger DR, Carollo JJ. The mechanics of thoracolumbar fractures stabilized by segmental fixation. *Clin Orthop* 1984; 189:89–96.
23. White AA III, Panjabi MM. *Clinical Biomechanics of the Spine.* Philadelphia: Lippincott, 1978.
24. Whitesides TE Jr. Traumatic kyphosis of the thoracolumbar spine. *Clin Orthop* 1977; 128:78–92.

298 Texas Scottish Rite Hospital Universal System for Stabilization of the Thoracic or Lumbar Spine

Richard G. Fessler
Michael Sturgill

The Texas Scottish Rite Hospital (TSRH) Universal Instrumentation system was developed out of attempts to resolve the problem of rod migration, which is noted particularly during attempted corrections of scoliosis of neuromuscular etiology and cases with pelvis obliquity. Biomechanical testing demonstrated that "locking" the rods together would prevent rod migration; thus the crosslink, which has become one of the trademarks of the TSRH system, was developed for use with the Luque "L" rod/sublaminar wire system.

In 1986, the Cotrel Dubousset (CD) system was introduced to the United States. Many of the CD innovations were similar to concepts incorporated into prior experiments performed at the Texas Scottish Rite Hospital, and solved several of the problems noted with Harrington and/or Luque systems (e.g., straight back syndrome from two-point fixation). Therefore, the surgeons at the Texas Scottish Rite Hospital began using the CD system for corrective spinal surgery, but requested the crosslink system as an addition to the CD instrumentation. This request, as well as requests directed toward different hook and screw designs, led to the development of a complete, independent, TSRH spinal instrumentation system.

The TSRH system has several benefits. First, as with all "universal" systems, it allows for immediate "segmental" stabilization of the spine. This can be accomplished even in the absence of laminae, by using a combination of pedicle screws, pedicle hooks, and transverse process hooks. Second, because it is a "rod" and not a "plate" system, it provides a larger posterolateral surface area for bony fusion. Third, the side bolt locking assembly, and the top loading system, are relatively easy to use. Finally, since all components of the system are fully removable without destroying any component of the system, revision surgery is easier than with previous systems.

In this chapter we will emphasize the TSRH universal instrumentation system. In discussing its use, we will first consider indications for instrumentation of the thoracolumbar spine. Thereafter, the specific techniques used with this system will be discussed. Finally, the results and complications of the University of Florida series will be presented.

Indications

The general indications for fusion and instrumentation of the spine are (1) to provide stability to the unstable spine, (2) to prevent injury to neurological structures, (3) to decrease malalignment and deformity, (4) to improve the probability of fusion, and (5) to decrease long-term pain. The efficacy of spinal instrumentation systems in providing the first four of these benefits has previously been reviewed.[6] Furthermore, the influence of spinal fusion on back vs. radicular pain has also been discussed previously.[4] These topics, therefore, will not be considered here. Instead, we will focus on the indications for stabilization of specific pathologic conditions.

Spinal instability can result from various pathologic lesions, such as trauma, tumor, infection, spondylolisthesis associated with spondylolysis, degenerative spine disease, iatrogenic spinal instability, pseudarthrosis, and deformity. The indications for rigid fixation using TSRH are clear in certain pathologic conditions but less clear, or even controversial, in other situations. The controversy results from a relative lack of prospective, randomized evaluations, specifically addressing each pathologic condition. Although many of these studies are currently under way, or in the planning stages, data from them are not yet available. Therefore, the following indications represent those generally accepted based on the available retrospective data.

Trauma

Table 298-1 compares the classification schemes of spinal instability proposed by Denis[3] and McAfee et al.[13] and indicates recommended treatments. Trauma that results in injury to two (or three) of three columns (McAfee et al.[13]) or the posterior ligamentous complex (Denis[3]) produces a spinal injury that is sufficiently unstable to require surgical stabilization.

The use of TSRH spinal instrumentation techniques to treat thoracic and lumbar fractures has been described by Benzel et al.[2] Twenty-eight patients underwent decompression and fusion procedures with the placement of TSRH rods. Each patient underwent either lateral extracavitary decompression and fusion or posterolateral-transpedicular dural sac decompression and fusion. The posterolateral-transpedicular decompression was used in the patients whose examination demonstrated complete functional spinal cord disruption and whose magnetic resonance imaging (MRI) studies demonstrated complete anatomic neural transection. In the early part of the series, sublaminar hooks were used below the level of the conus and transverse process hooks and/or pedicle hooks were used above the level of the conus with a longer rod segment above the fracture than below. The longer rod was used above because it was thought that the transverse process hook "purchase" was less secure than the pedicle or laminar hook. However, patients entered later in the study received a "short-rod two-claw" (SRTC) system. This system utilized upward and downward facing hooks on

TABLE 298-1 Comparison of Spinal Fracture Classification Schemes of Denis[3] and McAfee et al.[13]

Fracture Types		Spinal Column Failure			Assessment of Stability	
Denis	**McAfee et al.**	**Anterior**	**Middle**	**Posterior**	**McAfee et al.**	**Denis**
Wedge compression	Wedge compression	F			Generally stable[a]	Stable[b]
Seatbelt type injury	Chance fracture		F	F	Generally stable[f]	Unstable[c]
	Flexion distraction injury	F	F	F	Generally unstable	
Burst fracture	Stable burst	F	F		Stable	Unstable[d]
	Unstable burst	F	F	F	Unstable	
Fracture dislocation	Translational injury	F	F	F	Unstable	Unstable[e]

[a] Multilevel wedge compression fractures may require surgical therapy.
[b] Potential mechanical instability is seen with severe wedge fractures. This instability does not acutely threaten the neural elements.
[c] Potential mechanical instability.
[d] Burst fractures are either neurologically unstable, or both mechanically and neurologically unstable.
[e] Fracture dislocations are both mechanically and neurologically unstable.
[f] Unstable if there is facet dislocation or subluxation or facet fractures.
F = failure.

the same lamina applied to the laminae above and below the fractured level. The results of Benzel and his associates revealed no cases of instability or pseudarthrosis observed during an average follow-up of 9 months. There were no cases of instrumentation failure, regardless of the number of spinal levels fused or the number of levels instrumented. The authors argued that the SRTC system resulted in a lower incidence of delayed instability and discomfort from loosening at the hook/bone interface compared to that observed with long-rod systems.

Tumors

Primary and metastatic tumors of the spinal column cause pain, instability, deformity, and neurological deficits. The goals of surgery are to relieve pain, to decompress the neural elements, and to provide immediate mechanical stability. The approach and fusion technique may be anterior, posterior, or a combination of both. Since the vertebral body is involved in 85 percent of spinal metastases, the benefit of the anterior approach for adequate decompression and fusion is clear.

The definition of instability for tumors of the spinal column follows the three-column theory of Denis.[3] Currently, no study has been published which specifically evaluates the use of TSRH instrumentation for spinal tumors. Several reports have included such patients within their series, with good results. The authors of one study that is relevant to the use of TSRH instrumentation in spinal tumors performed an in vitro biomechanical analysis of the ability of various spinal instrumentation techniques to restore stability after destruction of the anterior and middle columns in a calf corpectomy model.[9] The results of this study indicated that, compared to posterior constructs using sublaminar wire with and without crosslinks and constructs embedded in polymethyl-methacrylate, axial stability and torsional stiffness were best restored by a cross-linked, rectangular, anterior TSRH construct.[10] Construct adequacy had previously been reported by Gurr et al. for posterior transpedicular instrumentation two levels above and two levels below the corpectomy site.[8,9]

Infection

Spinal stabilization may be necessary in cases of osteomyelitis in which more than 50 percent of the vertebral body is eroded, or in which aggressive surgical debridement is expected to produce an unstable spine. Progressive angulation and new or increasing neurological deficit are additional indications for instrumentation in spinal infections.

Traditionally, debridement and stabilization were performed as separate procedures, with a long delay between the two to minimize the possibility of infecting the rods. A recent analysis by Dietze and Haid[5] has demonstrated that primary reconstruction with TSRH instrumentation for spinal infections can be performed safely, in conjunction with the administration of parenteral and oral antibiotics, without infection of the inserted bone graft or instrumentation material.[5] This surgical series represents an aggressive management of advanced infections of the spine. The series by Dietze and Haid included 20 surgical cases (6 cervical, 8 thoracic, and 6 lumbar). All were nontuberculous bacterial infections, except two tuberculous infections, involving 18 interbody grafts and 14 posterolateral onlay grafts with spinal instrumentation used in 15 cases. Five TSRH hook/rod constructs and six screw/rod constructs were used. Parenteral antibiotics were used for an average of 6 weeks followed by a 3-month course of oral antibiotics. Patients with tuberculosis were treated with oral antibiotics for 1 year. Seventeen of the 20 patients had an improved clinical status postoperatively and 15 of 18 had radiographic evidence of bony fusion. Successful outcomes were a function of aggressive debridgment of infectious foci and prolonged parenteral administration of antibiotics.

Spondylolisthesis Associated with Spondylolysis

The indications for surgery and fusion in spondylolisthesis are persistent pain unresponsive to conservative therapy and progressive subluxation. The indications for reduction are slippage of more than 75 percent, and a slip angle greater than 45 degrees.

Degenerative Disease

Segmental instability secondary to spinal degeneration is a controversial topic. Although several classification schemes exist, Frymoyer and Selby[7] have done extensive work to develop a classification scheme which clearly defines the different types of degenerative disease processes and provides criteria for fusion and stabilization. They define segmental instability as a loss of motion segment stiffness such that force applied to that motion segment produces greater displacement than would occur in a normal segment. They divide degenerative disease into two major categories: primary degenerative instability and fixed deformity. Based on clinical, radiographic, and biomechanical data, they further divide primary degenerative instability into translational instability, retrolisthetic instability, torsional instability, disc disruption, and scoliotic degeneration. They subdivide fixed deformity into degenerative spondylolisthesis, fixed retrolisthesis, disc space collapse, and fixed scoliotic deformity.

Table 298-2 lists the guidelines recommended by Frymoyer and Selby for stabilizing each primary degenerative process. Indications for fusion in translational instability include (1) forward displacement on plain standing x-ray films, (2) persistent or recurrent low back pain or claudication, (3) relatively preserved disc space, (4) minimal bridging osteophytes, and (5) greater than 8 degrees of motion on flexion and extension roentgenograms. Indications for fusion of retrolisthetic instability include (1) posterior displacement on plain standing x-ray films, (2) an increase and decrease in deformity during flexion and extension roentgenograms, and (3) lateral recess symptoms. In addition to the same indications as for translational instability, fusion for torsional instability is also recommended for spinous process malalignment, and a myelographic ''pedicle-to-pedicle'' defect. Fusion should be considered for disc degeneration in the presence of recurrent disc herniations and discographic disc disruption with symptom reproduction. Finally, for degenerative scoliosis, indications for fusion include (1) progression of the curve over time on standing x-ray films, (2) increasing symptoms of stenosis, (3) translation on lateral standing x-ray films, (4) rotational deformity, and (5) potentially destabilizing surgery.

Table 298-3 lists the indications for fusion and stabilization for ''secondary'' instability. Secondary instability can be divided into four general categories: (1) instability after disc excision; (2) instability after decompressive laminectomy; (3) instability after spinal fusion (at adjacent levels); and (4) postfusion pseudarthrosis. Indications for stabilization following disc excision include increasing deformity over time and recurrent disc herniation. Following decompressive laminectomy, indications for stabilization include accentuation of preexisting deformity and multilevel decompression in the presence of scoliotic deformity. Indications for stabilization following a previous fusion are (1) progressive degenerative spondylolisthesis, (2) symptoms of stenosis, and (3) pseudarthrosis. Pseudarthrosis is suggested when there is (1) a visible defect on x-ray films, (2) relief of symptoms by local anesthetic injection into the defect, (3) greater than 4 degrees of motion on flexion and extension roentgenograms, and (4) recurrent disc herniation.

Specific fusions have been suggested for several of these specific instabilities. Antitorsion facet fusion is suggested for axial rotational instabilities. Anterior or posterior interbody fusion is recommended for translational instabilities, and fusion in flexion is recommended for retrolisthetic instabilities. Postsurgical instability syndromes require special approaches, based on the overall pathology and remaining osseous elements.[7] TSRH, being a universal system, would be useful for any of these fusions.

Since the ultimate objective in bony fusion is the rigidity of the fusion mass, rigid fixation must be demonstrated to enhance such fusion to justify its additional time, expense, and risk. To date the only prospective randomized study which addresses this question is that by Zdeblick.[14] This study examined the efficacy of several instrumentation techniques to improve fusion rates in lumbar fusion for degenerative conditions in 124 patients divided into three groups: (1) group 1 had a bone graft only, (2) group 2 had a semirigid screw-plate fixation system (Luque II) with bone grafting, and (3) group 3 had combined rigid fixation with pedicle screws and rods (TSRH) with bone grafting. The overall fusion rate was best for group 3, 95 percent, compared to 77 percent in group 2, and 65 percent in group 1. Group 3 also had good (i.e., mild back

TABLE 298-2 Indications for Fusion and Stabilization of the Spine in Degenerative Disease*

Transitional Instability
- Forward displacement on plain standing x-ray films
- Persistent or recurrent low back pain or claudication
- Relatively preserved disc space
- Minimal bridging osteophytes
- Greater than 8 degrees of motion on flexion and extension roentgenograms

Retrolisthetic Instability
- Posterior displacement on plain standing x-ray films
- Increase and decrease in deformity during flexion and extension roentgenograms
- Lateral recess symptoms

Torsional Instability
- Same as for translational instability
- Spinous process malalignment
- ''Pedicle-to-pedicle'' defect

Disc Degeneration
- Recurrent disc disruption
- Discographic disc disruption with reproduction of symptoms

Degenerative Scoliosis
- Progression of curve over time on standing x-ray films
- Increasing symptoms of stenosis
- Translation on lateral standing x-ray films
- Rotational deformity
- Potentially destabilizing surgery

*Guidelines proposed by Frymoyer and Selby.[7]

TABLE 298-3 Indications for Fusion and Stabilization for ''Secondary'' Instability

Instability Following

Disc Excision
- Increasing deformity over time
- Recurrent disc herniation

Decompressive Laminectomy
- Accentuation of preexisting deformity
- Multilevel decompression in the presence of scoliotic deformity

Previous Fusion
- Progressive degenerative spondylolisthesis
- Symptoms of stenosis
- Pseudarthrosis

ache but returning to work) to excellent (i.e., pain free; returning to work) functional results 95 percent of the time. This was statistically significant when compared to groups 2 and 1. These results support animal studies that have shown that spinal instrumentation increases the fusion rate in a destabilized canine lumbar spine, and that as the rigidity of the instrumentation increases so does the rigidity of the fusion mass.[11,12]

Instrumentation

The TSRH system consists of a series of rods, screws, hooks, and crosslinks, with the application devices described below. All TSRH screws, hooks, and crosslink plates use a ''three-point shear clamp'' locking mechanism to attach to the spinal rods. Axial and torsional strength in static strength testing has been superior or equal to that of similar systems.[1]

Rods

Rod strength and fatigue resistance have been enhanced by ''shot peening'' surface treatment. All rods have hexagonal ends to facilitate rod rotation with a small wrench. Three rod stiffnesses are available: 3⁄16 TSRH, 1⁄4 flex TSRH, and 1⁄4 rigid. The rigid 1⁄4 in. rod is similar in stiffness to the Harrington rod. The type of rod selected is based on an assessment of the stiffness of the deformity, the weight and size of the patient, and the length of time until fusion is anticipated.

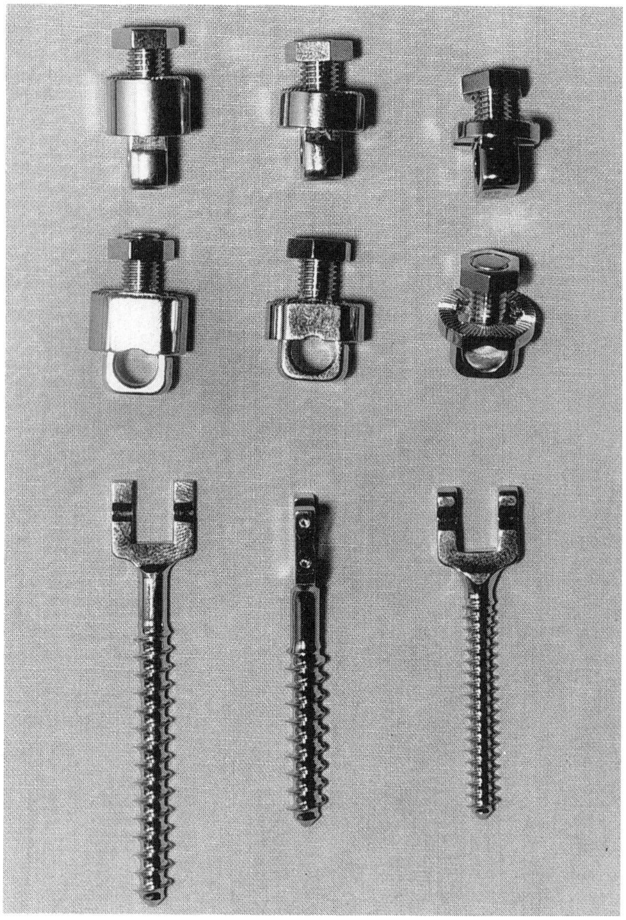

Figure 298-1 TSRH fixed angle screw examples of 5.5 and 6.5 mm diameters *(bottom).* TSRH variable angle eyebolts of 0, 3, and 6 mm offset for use with variable angle screws *(top).*

Screws

TSRH screws come in two head styles: fixed angle (Fig. 298-1) and variable angle (Fig. 298-2). Outer diameters are 5.5, 6.5, 7.5, and 8.5 mm. Three locking assemblies are available: (1) shear clamp locking eyebolt and nut assembly for the fixed and variable angle screws (see Fig. 298-5), (2) a serrated spacer attachment unique to TSRH for the variable angle screw (Fig. 298-1), and (3) a top tightening variable angle screw (Fig. 298-3). Serrations allow angle changes in 6-degree increments, thus offering many degrees of angulation. Three offset sizes in the eyebolt minimize necessary rod bending by accepting a variable amount of displacement between the rod and the screw. To minimize pullout, all threads have the standard cancellous thread pattern. Because biomechanical data indicate that the shank of the screw is the most prone to fatigue and breakage, TSRH has increased the diameter of this location and tapered the upper threads.

Hooks

TSRH hooks (Fig. 298-4) come in various sizes and shapes (i.e., large, small, and pediatric), using a central post configuration. Hooks are designed to anatomically mirror specific vertebral structures. Thus, the laminar, pedicle, and transverse process hooks contour to the laminae, pedicles, and transverse processes, respectively. Finally, lumbar laminar hooks come in standard and elevated sizes. Standard (round) laminar hooks are perhaps the most versatile, fitting many aspects of the posterior elements without infringing significantly into the canal. Round elevated hooks allow closer placement to the midline. Cranial and caudal angled hooks are used to attach to lumbar laminae in lumbar claw constructs.

Crosslinks

Axial and torsional forces are more significant than transverse forces between rods. Crosslinks (Fig. 298-5) prevent rod migration and enhance the rigidity of the system. The crosslink uses the same eyebolt locking mechanism as do the hooks and screws. One-half inch nuts are used with crosslink plates. This provides a broad, smooth surface, which minimizes sharp edges on areas of skin prominence. Care must be taken to ensure that eyebolts for crosslink plates are preplaced on the rod in the desired position prior to setting all hooks and/or screws. Split eyebolts can be used with crosslink plates if all other hooks and screws are already in place. The strength of the split eyebolt is comparable to that of the regular eyebolts. Mechanical testing has demonstrated that two crosslink plates create a construct as rigid as one with three crosslink plates. One crosslink plate should be located at the superior end of the construct, caudal to the top hook while the other crosslink is placed at the lower end of the construct above the bottom hook or pelvic fixation instrumentation. Crosslinks should not be applied at the

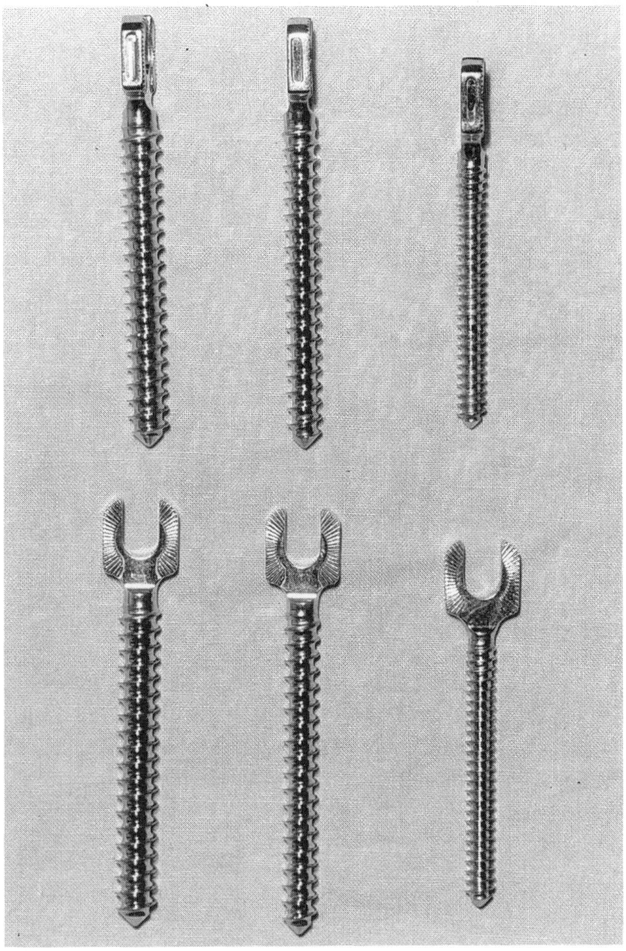

Figure 298-2 TSRH variable angle screw examples of 5.5, 6.5, and 7.5 mm diameters.

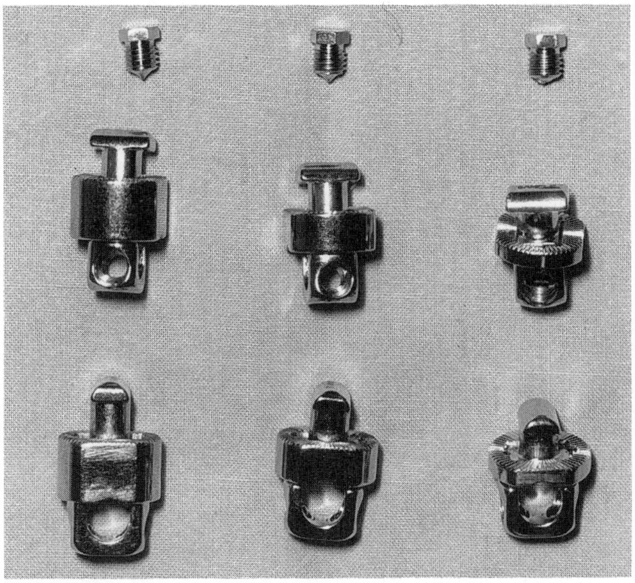

Figure 298-3 TSRH variable angle, top loading eyebolts of 0, 3, and 6 mm offset.

point of maximum curve on the rods (due to stress and skin prominence). In short constructs, a single crosslink is adequate. Crosslink plates can be bent or torqued about their axis with the crosslink benders.

Application Instrumentation

Instruments used to apply the above hooks, screws, and rods are important adjuncts, and a familiarity with their use can be both time saving and important in the quality of the ultimate construct. The TSRH Spinal Implant System is specific for TSRH implants. Hook holders are designed to ensure a positive attachment to the hooks and screws, and are color coded by size (Fig. 298-6). Eyebolts and rods can be inserted with the hook holders in place. Trial hook holders can be used for site preparation. All, except the transverse process hook trial, are angled at 30 degrees. The trials can serve as laminar elevators and pedicle finders, but because they are shaped like hooks they are less likely to invade the spinal canal. The mini-corkscrew can be used with hooks and screws to reduce the rod downward so that the eyebolt aligns properly with the top of the hook or screw. Excessive force usually means that the rod has been poorly contoured. In situ benders are provided but the entire rod can also be easily removed, recontoured, and reapplied.

The three-point shear clamp mechanism provides significant resistance to axial, torsional, and shear forces, as long as the nut is torqued down to 150 in./lb. Top tightening screws should be torqued to 100 in./lb. Several wrenches, (i.e., open and closed face, 10 in. long) are provided to facilitate tightening the nuts. Applying a force of 150 in./lb can cause the patient to move on the table if the construct is not stabilized. An in situ bender, rod pusher, or vice clamp can be used to secure the rods during final tightening. It is better to overtighten the rod then to undertighten it.

The instrumentation system developed at the Texas Scottish Rite Hospital has been demonstrated to be highly versatile in many pathologic conditions. Versatility of the TSRH system can be noted by its ability to build hybrid constructs such as lumbar screws with thoracic or laminar hooks all attached to the same rod. Revision screws and variable angle screws also add to its versatility. One can also add a preexisting rod construct to a revision construct by using crosslink offset plates or crosslink axial plates. Differing hook sizes, angle screws, and different rod sizes allow for several different positions in which the rods can be applied.

Surgical Technique

Techniques for placement of the TSRH system follow general guidelines but vary in the design of the construct depending on the location of the pathologic lesion. For example, pedicle screws are thought to be stronger in the lumbar spine and lower thoracic spine. The pedicles of the midthoracic spine are thought to be too small to safely accommodate the screws. Consequently, hooks are usually used in the mid to upper thoracic spine.

Patient Positioning and Exposure

All patients receive general endotracheal anesthesia, pneumatic compression stockings, and appropriate arterial and venous lines,

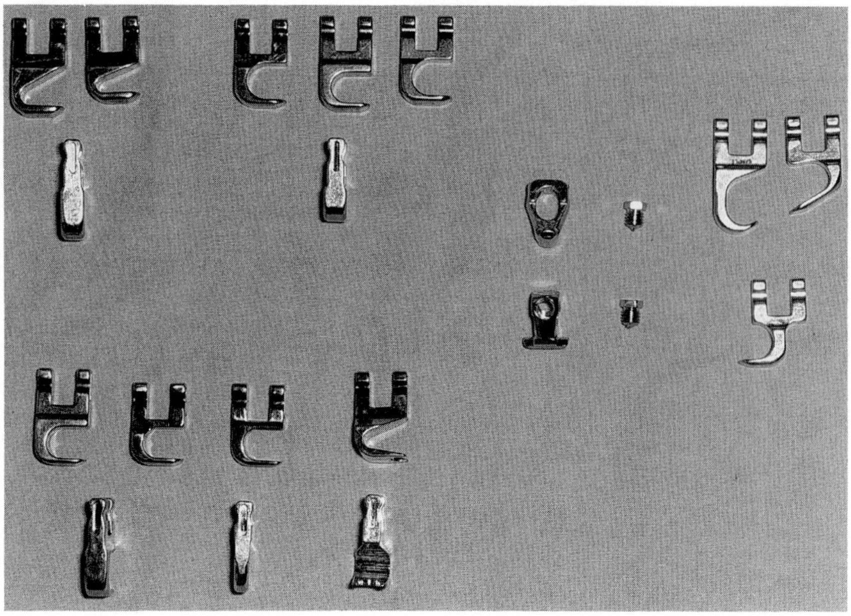

Figure 298-4 TSRH hook alternatives. Hooks demonstrated are thoracic laminar and small thoracic laminar hooks *(top left),* large and elevated laminar hooks *(top middle),* small and small elevated, wide and narrow laminar hooks *(bottom left),* pedicle hooks *(bottom center),* eyebolts and screws *(center left),* caudal and cranial angle lumbar laminar hooks *(center right, top),* and transverse process hook *(center right, bottom).*

prior to being turned prone onto the radiolucent operating table. Prophylactic antibiotics are begun before surgery and continued for 48 h after surgery. Whenever possible, autologous blood is donated in advance, and a cell saver is used in all cases, unless contraindicated. An adjustable fluoroscopic image intensifier and patient frames or chest rolls are used to permit intraoperative anteroposterior, oblique, and lateral fluoroscopy of the spine. Patients are positioned prone on the operating table, with the thorax supported laterally to avoid epidural venous distention from abdominal compression. An appropriate midline thoracic or lumbar incision is made, extending 2 to 3 in. above and below the segments to be instrumented. Subperiosteal dissection to the lateral tips of the transverse processes of the segments to be fused is performed to maximize available bone surface for fusion. Prior to posterior instrumentation, neural decompression and/or vertebral body reconstruction are performed as indicated.

Pedicle Preparation and Screw Placement

After exposure and decompression of the spine, the external landmarks over the pedicles are identified. Pedicle identification, hole preparation, and screw placement are performed under fluoroscopic guidance.

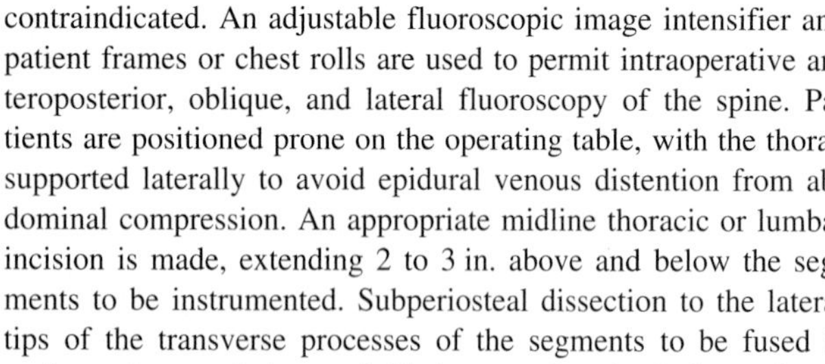

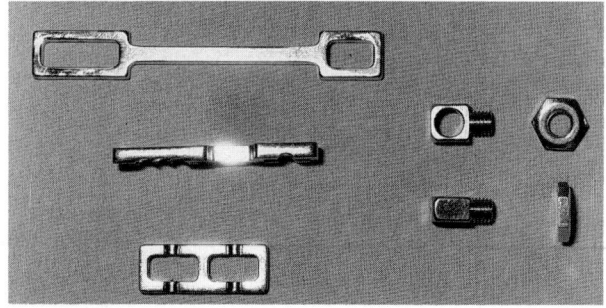

Figure 298-5 TSRH crosslink assembly.

In the thoracic and lumbar spine, the external landmark for the pedicle is the intersection of the axial plane through the middle of the transverse process and the sagittal plane through the superior facet. Identification of the facet complex is facilitated by moving the spinous process with a Kocher clamp and then removing the soft tissue from the surface of the superior facet.

A Steinmann pin is then placed over this point of intersection and the correct entry position is verified radiographically by orienting the pin along the axis of the central portion of the pedicle. On anteroposterior (or slightly oblique) fluoroscopic images, the pedicle and aligned pin appear as a "bull's eye" or "target sign" within an oval pedicle. The cortical point of intersection can then be entered with either a high-speed drill or Leksell rongeur, and the pin twisted down into the cancellous bone of the pedicle to the desired depth in the vertebral body in preparation for the screw placement. A Steinmann pin with a diameter corresponding to the minor diameter of the screw is used (for example, a $\frac{9}{64}$-in. pin for a 5.5-mm screw or a $\frac{5}{32}$-in. pin for a 6.5-mm screw), and the placement is facilitated by holding the pin with a Jacob's chuck. This procedure is repeated at each pedicle, and the final anteroposterior orientation of each pin is assessed fluoroscopically. The progress of pin and screw penetration into the vertebral body is monitored using lateral imaging. This procedure minimizes the possibility of malpositioning any screw.

Sacral screw sites are prepared in a similar manner. The external anatomic landmarks differ from those in the thoracic and lumbar regions since the sacrum has no transverse processes. Manipulating the L5 spinous process helps to identify the L5-S1 facet. Soft tissue dissection delineates the first dorsal sacral foramina and the osseous recession caudal to the L5-S1 facets. The external landmark for the first sacral pedicle is located at the inferolateral portion of the superior S1 facet. The correct entry sites into the S1 pedicles are verified fluoroscopically.

Each pin is manually positioned parallel to the end plate of the vertebra; however, penetration into the adjacent disc space is avoided. This maneuver requires a vertical orientation for the thoracic and lumbar spine and a 30-degree caudal angle for the sacrum. The medial trajectory corresponds to the angle of the pedicles

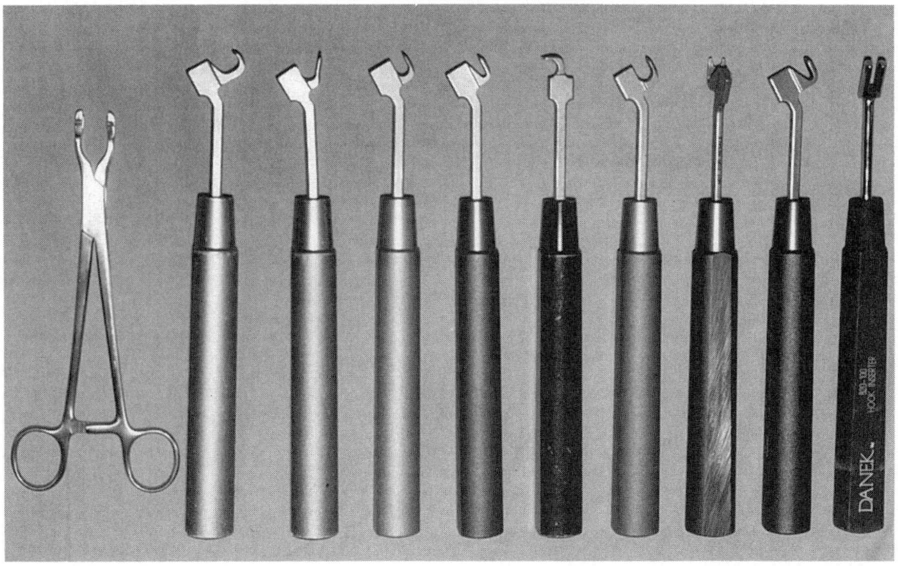

Figure 298-6 TSRH hook holder and trial hook inserters. These are *(left to right)* cranial angle hook trial, caudal angle hook trial, small laminar hook trial, small thoracic laminar hook trial, transverse process hook trial, large laminar hook trial, pedicle hook trial, large thoracic laminar hook trial, and hook inserter.

at each level. Penetration of the pin through the hard pedicle into the soft cancellous bone of the vertebral body provides a distinct feel, with a reduction in resistance.

After all pins have been placed into the vertebral bodies to create tracks for the screws, the Steinmann pins are removed, and the superficial 5- to 10-mm area of each track is enlarged with a drill or bone awl. This allowed the threads of the pedicle screw to engage a purchase upon the bone.

Pedicle screw sizes are preselected on the basis of the CT characteristics of the particular vertebra. The screws are placed into the prepared holes with a trajectory identical to that of the Steinmann pins. Screw purchase is obtained by advancing the screw with a screwdriver, penetrating 70 to 80 percent of the vertebral body. To avoid injuring the vascular and visceral structures anterior to the vertebral column, the anterior portion of the vertebral body is not penetrated. Throughout the procedure, the progress, depth, and position of the screws is monitored.

Construct Assembly

After hook site preparation and hook placement have been accomplished, the construct is assembled. A malleable wire or sterile endothracheal tube stylet is used as a template to approximate the desired rod curvature. The rods are selected, cut to the desired length, and bent to match the contour of the template. An S-shaped curve is used for thoracolumbar rods and a lordotic curve for lumbar or lumbosacral rods. The rods are then connected to the pedicle screws by attaching the eyebolts to the rods and tightening the nut assemblies.

Final adjustments in rod contour are achieved with in situ rod benders. Hook holders, corkscrew devices, wrenches, and a variety of other tools help the surgeons connect the rods, screws, and hooks. Spinal reductions are performed and instruments can be placed under compression, distraction, or in a neutral position as indicated. Crosslinks can then be used to connect the right and left rods as described above. All connections of the screws, hooks, rods, and crosslinks are then tightened securely for final fixation.

Fusion Site Preparation and Wound Closure

The fusion site, which extends over the entire length of the instrumentation system, is usually prepared prior to rod placement. After all soft tissue is removed from the surface of the fusion bed, the transverse processes, facet joints, and other bone fusion surfaces are decorticated using a high-speed drill. The articular surfaces of the facet joints are curetted or drilled to remove the cartilage, and cancellous bone grafts are packed into the facets. The rods are then placed and the wound is thoroughly irrigated with a bacitracin solution. Cancellous bone and/or cortical matchstick grafts are then placed over the transverse processes and facets for a posterolateral fusion. Autogenous iliac bone is the preferred grafting material. Closed suction drainage systems are then placed and the wound is closed in multiple layers.

Postoperatively, patients with a thoracic or lumbar fusion wear an appropriate thoracic or thoracolumbar orthosis for 3 to 6 months. Patients with a lumbosacral fusion wear an orthosis with one thigh immobilized. Ambulation is begun within the first few postoperative days, after which progressive rehabilitative therapy is administered.

Results

Patient Population

The results of pedicle screw instrumentation in 104 patients operated on at the University of Florida between 1987 and 1991 have been reported.[4] Details of the patient population were discussed elsewhere, and will not be repeated here. The pathologic conditions responsible for their instability were (1) fractures in 28 patients; (2) isthmic or degenerative spondylolisthesis in 29; (3) primary or metastatic neoplasms in four; (4) vertebral osteomyelitis in two; and (5) postsurgical instability after operations for spinal stenosis in 26.

Neurological Function and Back Pain

Neurological improvement occurred in 85 of 96 patients presenting with deficits. In 73 patients with nerve root or cauda equina compression, 66 experienced improved motor function or resolution of radicular pain; 49 of these patients recovered normal function. Improved motor function or sensation (average recovery, 1.6 Frankel grades) was experienced by 19 of 23 patients with spinal cord or conus medullaris compression; five of these patients recovered normal function.

The resolution of back pain varied more than neurological recovery. The criterion for evaluation was based on the patient's subjective responses regarding limitations due to back symptoms. Severe, incapacitating back pain was present preoperatively in the entire patient population. Postoperatively, 20 patients had excellent relief of back pain, 57 had moderate back pain, and 19 had severe, persistent pain.

Fusion Rate

At long-term follow-up examination (10 to 50 months postoperatively), 96 percent of the patients developed osseous union. These patients demonstrated solid, continuous radiographic fusion masses on plain radiographic studies or tomography and had no clinical or radiographic evidence of instability.

Pseudarthrosis occurred in four patients, three of whom underwent additional surgery for reinstrumentation and fusion with successful results. The fourth patient refused another operation, and continues to have severe back pain. Factors contributing to nonunion included the use of fresh frozen allograft bone in two patients, prior pseudarthrosis in three, osteoporosis in two, obesity in two, and cigarette smoking in two. Obviously, each patient had multiple factors contributing to his or her pseudarthrosis. Although patients with a prior pseudarthrosis had a higher risk of failure, the 92 percent fusion rate for this group of patients was excellent after pedicle screw instrumentation.

Correction of Deformity

In the patients with spondylolisthesis, the vertebrae were fused in situ without attempting to correct the spinal deformity. Reduction of spinal deformity was attempted in all other patients, achieving a mean reduction of 14 degrees. Nineteen patients underwent major reductions, which were defined as a correction of 1 cm or more of vertebral body height or a reduction of 30 degrees or more of sagittal angulation. Ten patients developed a minor reversal of correction during long-term follow-up, with a mean loss of reduction of 2.4 degrees.

Complications

Four patients experienced neurological complications. Three of these developed new postoperative radiculopathy. One patient had spontaneous resolution of the radiculopathy, with no radiographic evidence of root impingement. This transient radiculopathy was attributed to intraoperative root manipulation during foraminotomy. Two cases of radicular deficits occurred secondary to pedicle screw malpositioning and were treated by removing the offending screw and by foraminal decompression. One patient recovered completely; the other had persistent unilateral L5 weakness and numbness at 21 months after surgery. The fourth patient with neurological complications developed a cauda equina syndrome from a spinal epidural hematoma due to a postoperative coagulopathy. Although this complication was treated with urgent operative decompression, the patient had residual neurological dysfunction.

Three would infections (one superficial and two deep) developed postoperatively. The superficial infection cleared with local wound debridement, packing, and oral antibiotic therapy. The two deep wound infections cleared after open debridement, irrigation, primary closure, and parenteral antibiotic treatment. The instrumentation was not removed in any of these cases and no recurrent infections developed. Subsequently, all three patients attained a successful arthrodesis.

Other perioperative complications included pneumonia in six patients, urinary tract infection in nine, deep venous thrombosis in three, and a decubitus ulcer in one. Four intraoperative dural tears occurred unrelated to instrument placement; these tears were satisfactorily treated with primary closure of the dural defect. There were no postoperative deaths.

Instrument Failure

Instrument failure eventually developed in 18 cases. Nine patients were asymptomatic with solid fusions, and required no therapy. In the other nine patients, however, the instrument failure was symptomatic or associated with a pseudarthrosis and required operative revision.

Trauma was responsible for two early cases of instrument failure. Both patients fell and dislodged the instrumentation constructs within the first 8 weeks postoperatively. These patients required immediate operative revision.

The rods became uncoupled from the screw systems in six patients. Four of these required operative revision, two for instrument prominence and two for pseudarthrosis. No rods bent or broke.

Screws failed in 10 patients, three of whom required reoperation. Among these patients there were nine bent screws, six broken screws, and 10 loose screws, representing an overall 4.8 percent screw failure rate (25 of 516 screws). Five of the six screws that broke had a narrow diameter (4.5 or 5.0 mm); the other was 7 mm in diameter. Screw breakage was eliminated after discontinuing the use of narrow-diameter screws. No TSRH screws had broken at the termination of follow-up in this group of patients. A variety of screw sizes (5 to 7 mm) bent or loosened. Although the TSRH screws had a lower breakage rate, no significant difference existed in the overall instrument failure rate between the CD and the TSRH systems.

References

1. Ashman RB, Birch JG, Bone LB, et al. Mechanical testing of spinal instrumentation. *Clin Orthop* 1988; 227:113–125.
2. Benzel EC, Kesterson L, Marchand EP. Texas Scottish Rite Hospital rod instrumentation for thoracic and lumbar spine trauma. *J Neurosurg* 1991; 75:382–387.
3. Denis F. The three column spine and its significance in the classification of acute thoracolumbar spinal injuries. *Spine* 1983; 8:817–831.

4. Dickman CA, Fessler RG, MacMillan M, Haid RW. Transpedicular screw-rod fixation of the lumbar spine: operative technique and outcome in 104 cases. *J Neurosurg* 1992; 77:860–870.
5. Dietze DD Jr, Haid RW Jr. Antibiotic-impregnated methylmethacrylate in treatment of infections with spinal instrumentation. *Spine* 1992; 17:981–987.
6. Fessler RG. Decision making in spinal instrumentation. *Clin Neurosurg* 1993; 40:227–242.
7. Frymoyer JW, Selby DK. Segmental instability: rationale for treatment. *Spine* 1985; 10:280–286.
8. Gurr KR, McAfee PC. Cotrel-Dubousset instrumentation in adults: a preliminary report. *Spine* 1988; 13:510–520.
9. Gurr KR, McAfee PC, Shih C. Biomechanical analysis of posterior instrumentation systems after decompressive laminectomy: an unstable calf-spine model. *J Bone Joint Surg [Am]* 1988; 70-A:680–691.
10. Heller JG, Zdeblick TA, Kunz DA, McCabe R. Spinal instrumentation for metastatic disease: in vitro biomechanical analysis. *J Spinal Disord* 1993; 6:17–22.
11. Johnston CE II, Ashman RB, Baird AM, Allard RN. Effect of spinal construct stiffness on early fusion mass incorporation. Experimental study. *Spine* 1990; 15:908–912.
12. Johnston CE II, Ashman RB, Corin JD. Mechanical effects of crosslinking rods in Cotrel-Dubousset instrumentation. *Orthop Trans* 1987; 11:96–97 (abstr).
13. McAfee PC, Yuan HA, Fredrickson BE, Lubicky JP. The value of computed tomography in thoracolumbar fractures. An analysis of one hundred consecutive cases and a new classification. *J Bone Joint Surg [Am]* 1983; 65-A:461–473.
14. Zdeblick TA. A prospective, randomized study of lumbar fusion: preliminary results. *Spine* 1993; 18:983–991.

299 Isola Instrumentation for Stabilization of the Thoracic and Lumbar Spine

Setti S. Rengachary
Abhay Sanan

The Isola spinal system is one of a number of universal spinal instrumentation systems currently available. Originally developed for the correction of scoliosis, universal instruments are also able to correct virtually any type of instability of the thoracic or lumbar spine. The Isola and other similar systems have gained popularity because of several key advantages, including versatility, the ability to achieve multisegment fixation, the preservation of motion segments if pedicle screws are used, the reduced need for external bracing, and the achievement of a high rate of bony fusion.

Historical Perspective

Hadra, in 1891, was the first to attempt spinal fusion by using interspinous wiring for the treatment of cervical Potts' disease.[2] However, the pioneers of spinal fusion are generally considered to be Hibbs and Albee, who, in 1911, independently reported techniques for posterior bony fusion. The initial indications were restricted to spinal infection, scoliosis, and trauma. Fusions for degenerative conditions did not appear in the literature until 1929, when Hibbs and Swift published the first cases. The overwhelming majority of early lumbosacral fusions used bone autografts and were not augmented with metal constructs.

Harrington's development of a rod and hook system in the 1950s represented a major advance in the history of spinal surgery.[3] The hooks were placed in a sublaminar position and attached to rods. By using various combinations of compression and distraction forces, the system could instantly bring the spine into better alignment. The system proved to be a boon for correcting the scoliosis secondary to poliomyelitis (which was reaching epidemic proportions in the 1950s) and was later also used for idiopathic scoliosis and degenerative spondylolisthesis. The initial enthusiasm for the system was later tempered by a growing number of failures. After prolonged periods, the rods would break or the hooks would break the lamina. Numerous modifications were made to the system, including strengthening the rods and redesigning the hooks, but none was very effective in improving the longevity of the implant. The lesson learned from the Harrington experience was that spinal fusion was a necessary adjunct to dynamic correction if a permanent reduction of deformity was desired.

The concept of segmental fixation was first proposed by Lange, who, in 1910, conceived of a system of steel rods that could be attached to the spinous processes for the correction of kyphosis. The concept of segmental fixation using multiple fixation points proved attractive. Corrective forces were more evenly distributed, and the rate of construct failure was low. Luque used these principles to his advantage and in 1982 described a technique of spinal fixation using L-shaped rods anchored to the spine with multiple sublaminar wires. When tested biomechanically, the Luque system proved superior to the Harrington system in all axes of movement. The major drawback of the system was the use of sublaminar wires. Significant neurological complications (including paraplegia) have been reported with the improper sublaminar passage of wire, particularly in the already compromised scoliotic spine.

Interest in the pedicle as an anchor for posterior constructs began with Boucher who, in 1959, placed pedicle screws for fusions and achieved excellent results. Advantages of pedicle fixation soon became evident, and a complete plating system that was anchored by pedicle screws was developed by Roy-Camille in the 1960s. His work set the foundation for subsequent pedicle screw instrumentation, including the AO dynamic compression plate and the variable screw placement (Steffee) plate.

The introduction of a screw and rod system (instead of a plate system) by Cortrel and Dobousset in 1984 allowed for greater versatility in construct design. The rods were better suited for the longer constructs required for the correction of scoliosis, because the rods could be bent in any plane to accommodate a change in pedicle direction. The system was soon designated a *universal spinal instrumentation system* because of its ability to stabilize the entire thoracic and lumbar spine for virtually any type of instability. Other universal systems soon emerged, including the Texas Scottish Rite Hospital (TSRH) system and the Isola system.

The Isola System

Developed by Asher and associates,[1] the Isola system (Acromed Corporation, Cleveland, OH) draws its name from a North American butterfly species, *Hemiargus isola* (Fig. 299-1), because the initial sacral implant resembled outstretched butterfly wings. Originally a sacral fixation device, the Isola system quickly evolved into a universal spinal system. It is a posterior thoracolumbosacral instrumentation system that consists of spinal anchors (screws, hooks, and wires) that can be attached to smooth rods by a versatile connector system. Isola implants are fully compatible with the variable screw placement (VSP) plate.

The implant design is based on Harrington's emphasis on precisely defining the anatomy of the deformity and then maintaining spinal balance with whatever correction is undertaken. Toward this end, the approach emphasizes understanding the three-dimensional

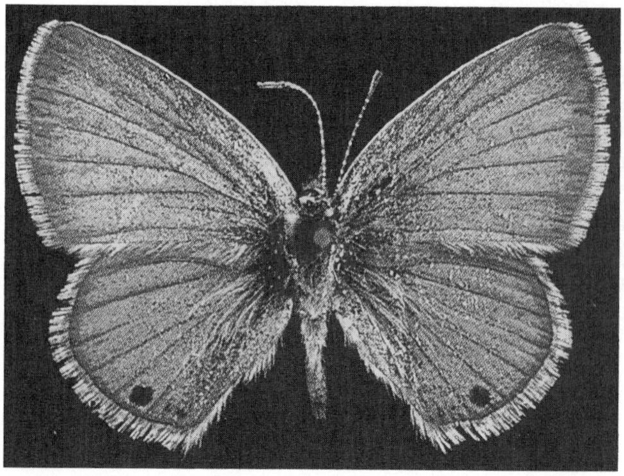

Figure 299-1 The *Hemiargus isola* species of butterfly, indigenous to the Americas. The shape of the first sacral implant developed by Asher was reminiscent of the wings of this species of butterfly.

nature of the six degrees of freedom of motion when analysis of spinal angulation is performed. The system's goals have been defined as the following: (1) correcting spinal deformity of any type; (2) improving access to the anchor sites of the spine with a wide variety of devices; (3) minimizing the requirement for external support; and (4) preserving the number of motion segments.[1] The indications for using the Isola implant are no different from those for other universal systems and include the correction of congenital, degenerative, or traumatic deformity and the stabilization of traumatic, degenerative, or iatrogenic mechanical insufficiency.

Implants

The implants can be divided into four basic categories: anchors, longitudinal members, connectors, and accessories. Each category will be discussed separately.

Anchors

Anchors for the system include bone screws, hooks, and wires.

Bone screws The Food and Drug Administration has approved the implantation of bone screws in the sacrum and ilium. Although approval for transpedicular placement is under review, many surgeons will use them if it is thought to be in the best interest of the patient. The Isola screws have the same design as the VSP screws. A portion of the screw (cancellous threaded) acquires anchoring purchase and another portion (machine threaded) is used to attach connectors. The screw has an integral hex nut over which the connector is placed. The connector is secured in place using a hex nut. Through the use of straight or angled washers placed over the machine-threaded portion, variabilities in the sagittal displacement of the rod can be corrected (Fig. 299-2). This basic design is biomechanically engineered to eliminate the claw-hammer pullout effect on the screw, and it decreases shearing of the threads on the bone.

The pedicle screws are available in diameters of 5.5, 6.25, 7.0, and 7.75 mm. The cancellous-threaded portion ranges in length from 25 to 50 mm in 5-mm increments, while the machine-threaded portion is available in 16, 19, and 30-mm sizes. The sacral screws are thicker, with a fixed diameter of 8.5 mm, and also longer—30 to 50 mm in 5-mm increments. The machine-threaded sacral screw length is 24 mm. Because of their large diameter, a special 8.5 mm tap is made for sacral screws, and this tap should not be used in the pedicles. Iliac screws are designed for placement between the iliac cortices and are available in diameters of 6.25 and 7.0 mm and lengths of 80 and 100 mm. Special rods with eyes can be attached to the screws, thus allowing a longitudinal member to gain pelvic anchoring.

Hooks Drop-entry (closed-body) and top-entry (open-body) hooks are available for anchoring to the laminae or transverse processes. The hooks have a low profile to minimize any canal impingement. The drop-entry hook may be slid onto the rod first, and the rod-hook combination can then be placed in the spine. Alternatively, the drop-entry hook can be placed first and the rod threaded through it. On the other hand, the top-entry hook easily allows for the hook to be secured to the spine prior to placement of the rod (Fig. 299-3).

The hook and rod are fixed together using a V-groove hollow-ground design patented by the Isola developers. It is different from the conventional hole and set screw connection in that the rod is driven into a smaller-diameter hole on tightening of the set screw, thus generating a stronger circumferential gripping force on the rod (Fig. 299-4). Set screw torques of 6.8 Nm (60 in./lb) are recommended. It is important to remember that the rod size must correspond to the hook hole size; otherwise, the benefit of the V-groove design is lost. For similar reasons, the hook should not be applied to a highly curved portion of the rod. A unique feature of the Isola drop-entry hooks is that the angle between the hook and rod changes on tightening of the set screw. When the hook is loose on the rod, it can rotate 15 degrees satittally with respect to the rod. As the set screw is tightened, the hook is forced to be nearly parallel with the rod, this design provides better fixation against the bone anchor site (Fig. 299-5). This feature is not present on the top-entry hooks.

The hooks are available in two hole sizes and four throat sizes. One hole size is designed for the 6.35 mm (¼ in.) rod and is available in throat sizes of 6.5, 8, 9.5, and 11 mm. The other hole size is designed for the 4.76 mm (3⁄16 in.) rod and is available in throat sizes of 5, 6.5, 8.0, 9.5, and 11 mm. The smaller throat sizes are designed for the laminae and the larger for the transverse processes.

Cables Because of the danger of sublaminar passage with monofilament wire, the use of multistranded cable is preferred. However, wires are available for providing a sublaminar anchor to the rod and are usually used in correction of scoliosis by providing a posterolateral force at the apex of the scoliotic curve. The wires provided are a 16-gauge single-strand wire with beaded ends, a 16-gauge preformed double-stranded wire, and a 18-gauge wire with button.

Longitudinal Members

Longitudinal members are used to interconnect anchor points. The Isola longitudinal members include smooth rods, eyelet rods, and plate-rod combinations. The VSP plates can be incorporated into the construct as well. Rods are preferred over plates for longer constructs because of their length and superior bending capability in both the sagittal and coronal planes. The Isola rod surface is designed to be smooth, because smooth rods have better strength

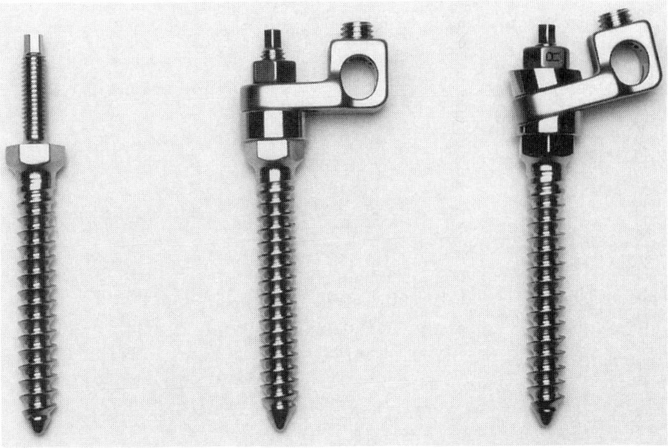

Figure 299-2 *Left:* A typical bone screw. The integral hex nut lies between the cancellous-threaded portion and the machine-threaded portion. *Middle.* A straight washer and slotted connector have been locked onto the screw with a hex nut. *Right.* Angled washers have been used to alter the angulation between the screw and connector.

and resistance to fatigue than rods with knurls, threads, or ratchets. Rod diameters are 4.76 mm ($\frac{3}{16}$ in.) and 6.35 mm ($\frac{1}{4}$ in.). The standard length is 46 mm (18 in.), but a 61 cm (24 in.) rod is available by special request. The eyelet rod has a hole at one end to allow it to be secured to an iliac screw. The plate-rod combination has a 16-mm-wide VSP plate attached to a 6.35-mm-diameter rod and a 12.7-mm-wide VSP plate attached to a 4.76-mm-diameter rod. The rods are 203 mm (12 in.) long, and the plates come with a variety of slot arrangements. Six rod and plate benders, including two in-situ benders, are part of the basic set.

Connectors

Connectors are used to fix the longitudinal member to the anchor point or to another longitudinal member. As in the hooks, the V-groove hollow ground design is used in all of the connectors.

Longitudinal connectors The slotted connectors fix the rod to a screw anchor. The connector is composed of a 16-mm plate portion and a body. The plate portion with a slot attaches to the machine-threaded portion of the screw using a hex and locking nut system, and the body contains the V-groove passage for the rod. Connector sizes correspond to the rod diameter (4.76 and 6.35 mm) and secure the rod using a set screw. Connectors are of six types: straight, angled, offset left, offset right, extended, and open (Fig. 299-6). The extended connector offers a 24-mm-long plate. Open connectors offer the advantage of placement even after the rod has been placed in the spine; this feature is not present on the closed connectors, which must be slipped on the rod prior to placement. What the open connectors gain in convenience, they lose in biomechanical stability, and they should be avoided whenever possible. The open connectors use the V-groove design but do not have a set screw. Instead, two pieces grip the rod and can be tightened using an 8-mm hex nut torqued to 7.3 Nm (65 lb/in.).

Transverse connectors Transverse connectors join two longitudinal elements together and increase the torsional strength of a construct. They also provide resistance to axial loads and, when placed adjacent to hooks, prevent hook migration. The standard transverse connectors are composed of two sets of split connector jaws with passages corresponding to either the 4.76-mm or 6.35-mm-diameter rod (Fig. 299-7). Each set of jaws are connected with a 4.76-mm-diameter, 10-cm-long threaded rod. The jaws can be made to grasp a rod by tightening a 8.0-mm hex nut. Recently, a transverse connector that uses a J clamp has been introduced. The advantage of this connector is that it is easier to use and has a low profile.

A dual (bypass) connector is also made, but it is designed for rod splicing and not for increased stability. It consists of a three-unit piece that can tighly hold two rods in place by the use of a 8.0-mm hex nut. Different sizes are available, such that any combination of 4.76-mm and 6.35-mm rods can be connected.

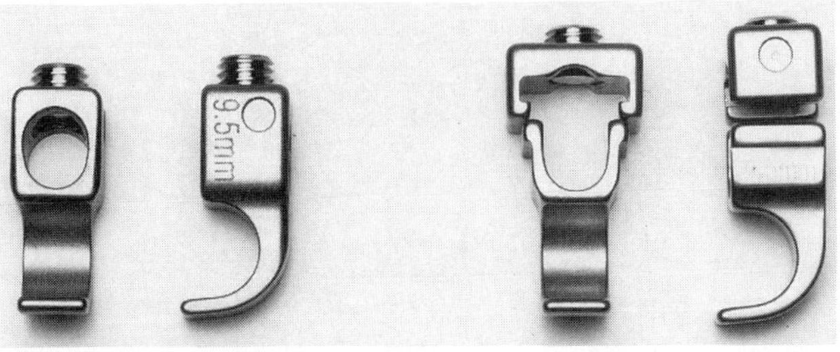

Figure 299-3 *Left.* The drop-entry (closed-body) hook. *Right.* The top-entry (open-body) hooks, which allows for placement on the bone prior to assembly with the rod.

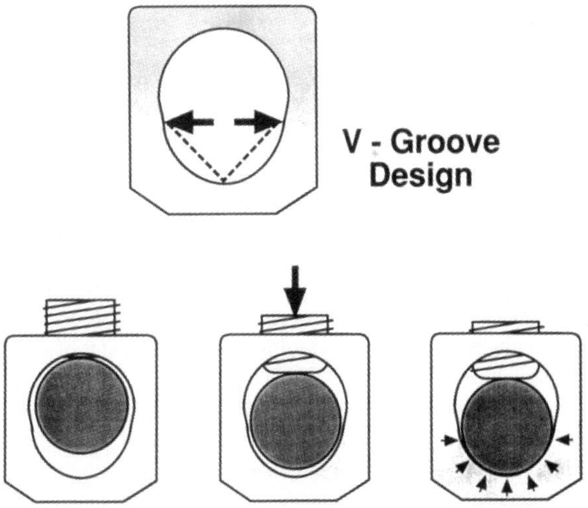

Figure 299-4 The V-groove hollow design is a unique feature of the Isola system. Lateral gripping forces are produced by driving the rod into a smaller-diameter hole.

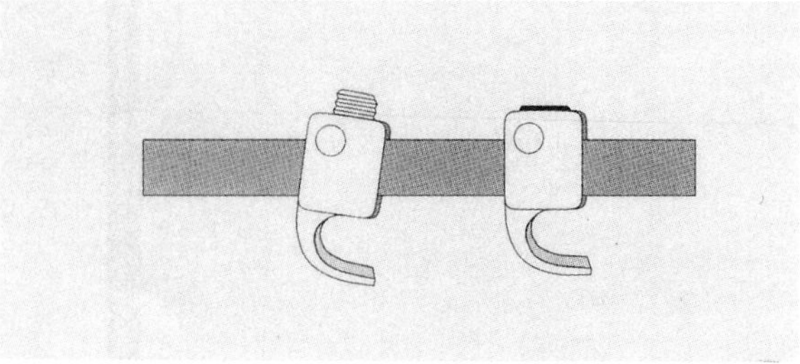

Figure 299-5 The drop-entry hook rotates 15 degrees on tightening of the set screw and provides superior fixation against the bone.

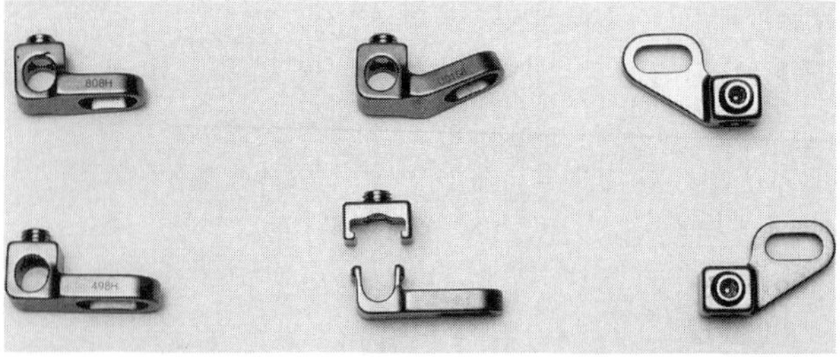

Figure 299-6 Extreme versatility can be achieved with the slotted connectors. *Clockwise from top:* straight, angled, offset left, offset right, open, and extended connectors.

Tandem connectors Tandem connectors are used to connect rods end to end. They come in various sizes, so any combination of 4.76-mm rods and 6.35-mm rods can be connected.

Accessories

Washers can be placed on the machine-threaded portion of a bone screw to allow for elevation of the connector plate. The elevation produces less interference with underlying bony structures and allows additional bone to be placed underneath the construct. Angled washers are also available to allow for rotation of the connector (Fig. 299-2). The use of washers is biomechanically sound, and they increase the construct strength when plates are used. The washers are 11 mm in diameter and are available in heights of 3 or 5 mm. The angled washers are 12.7 mm in diameter and offer a 15 degree angulation.

Implantation Technique

Preoperative Considerations

The procedure is carried out under general anesthesia. Nonparalyzing muscle relaxation is preferred so that detection of nerve root irritation is preserved. Special requirements such as a wake-up test should be discussed with the anesthesiology team. If a large blood loss is anticipated, preparation for autologous blood units or a cell saver should be made. Hypotensive anesthesia techniques to minimize blood loss should be used with caution because of the risk of end-organ failure, particularly myocardial infarction.

Positioning of the patient can be done with rolls, posts, or a spine frame. Because the operations are often long, special attention should be paid to the neck, brachial plexuses, and ulnar nerves. The ability to take radiographs should not be compromised, and good-quality films should be taken after positioning to inspect preoperative spinal alignment. Prophylactic broad-spectrum antibiotics should be administered prior to incision and should be repeated later if the procedure is lengthy. Meticulous attention to the handling of tissue and judicious placement of self-retaining retractors will prevent devascularization, which can act as a nidus for bacterial growth. Any devitalized tissue should be removed at the conclusion of the procedure, and the wound should be irrigated copiously. The neurological status can be monitored by somatosensory evoked potentials, motor evoked potentials, wake-up tests, or testing for clonus. Particular attention should be paid to muscle activity during pedicle screw placement, because it may represent nerve root irritation.

Operative Technique

A generous midline incision is required to allow for sufficient lateral retraction to expose the transverse processes. The muscle layer is dissected off the bone with attention to hemostasis. Some adherent soft tissue and ligament may need to be scraped off using curettes or rongeurs. In order to preserve stability, facet capsules and joints that will not be fused should not be violated, nor should motion segments avove and below the instrumented levels be unduly disturbed. Decompression can be done before or after the instrumentation is implanted, but it is technically more difficult to do it afterward.

The choice of the Isola construct depends on a number of factors, the most important of which is the level of the spine. In the upper and middle thoracic regions, hooks are used as the spinal anchors. Open hooks are easier to couple to a rod but are weaker than closed hooks. It is better to use closed hooks at each end of the construct, reserving the open hooks for the middle. The 11-mm throat size hook can be placed on the superior border of the transverse process, and a second, 8-mm hook can be placed under the lamina and facet. A part of the inferior articular facet needs to be removed with a ¼ in. osteotome for proper placement of the laminar hook. Both the lamina and the transverse process should be cleaned of ligament and soft tissue to maximize the metal-bone contact area. In this fashion, the two hooks face each other and form a "claw." The claw construct (Fig. 299-8) can be used with the transverse process and lamina of the same vertebra (intrasegmental claw) or adjacent ones (intersegmental claw). The intersegmental claw avoids excessive stress on a single level. Claw constructs are required a few segments (generally three) above and

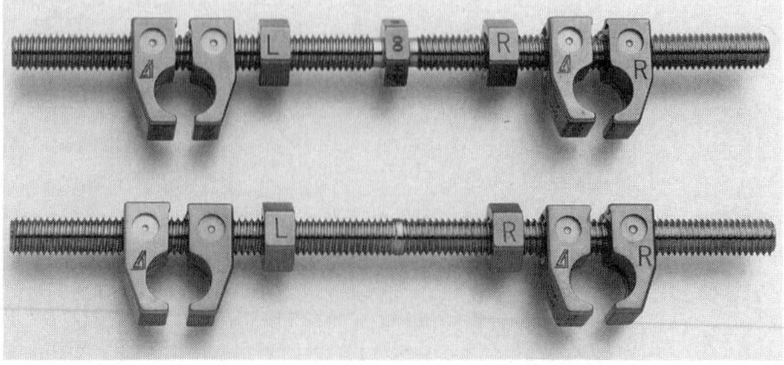

Figure 299-7 The torsional strength of the construct is increased with the transverse connector.

below the area of instability, and then an appropriate-sized rod is cut and contoured. It is important to remember that the rod shape needs to do more than match the hook placement; it must provide a corrective force when secured. The rod can be threaded through the closed hooks or placed on the top of the open hooks. The caps for the open hooks can then be lightly applied. One end of the rod can be secured to the hooks using the set screws. Each set of claws can then be secured by compression and tightening of the set screw. An important step is the application of compressive or distractive forces to the level of instability as the clinical situation requires. Cross-links can then be placed at the cranial and caudal ends, but a single midportion cross-link may suffice in a small construct (Fig. 299-9). Once the implant is secure, the spinous processes, laminae, and transverse processes are decorticated using a high-speed air drill, and autologous cortical and cancellous bone is packed to create a fusion mass. It is critical to remember that the hardware alone will eventually fail and it is imperative to assure a bony fusion.

The use of sublaminar cable is occasionally worthwhile, particularly in the treatment of scoliosis. Sublaminar cables provide superior dorsal rigidity and resist flexion better than hooks; however, they do not provide axial rigidity. Cable passage can have serious neurological complications when performed in the thoracic area, so extreme attention should be paid to detail. If possible, cables should be passed prior to rod placement. The lamina must be cleared of soft tissue, and the ligamentum flavum should be excised. A small portion of the lamina may be removed to allow unobstructed passage. Only when the anatomic boundaries are well defined is passage performed. An arc is made in the cable so that it will hug the undersurface of the lamina at all times. It is usually passed in a caudal-to-cranial direction. Once the cable is seen at the superior edge of the lamina, it is grasped with a hemostat and pulled; upward tension is maintained on it constantly. The cable can then be secured to a longitudinal member.

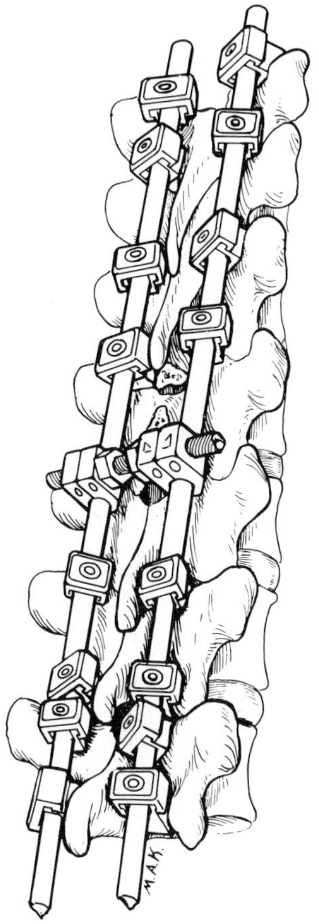

Figure 299-9 A completed thoracic construct using multiple claws. A transverse connector is present in the middle.

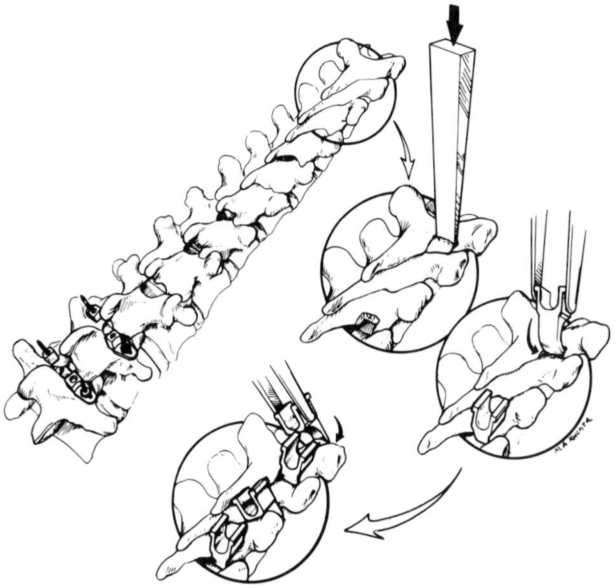

Figure 299-8 Preparation for a claw construct. A ¼ in. osteotome is used to remove a portion of the inferior articular facet, and a laminar hook is placed. Placement of an opposing hook on the transverse process constitutes the claw.

Lumbar stabilization can be accomplished with the use of pedicle screws. The most critical portion of this technique is pedicle localization. The pedicle can be located with the help of external landmarks, with radiographic confirmation, and, if there is a laminotomy, by direct inspection. The junction of the superior facet, transverse process, and lamina is the conventional site of entry (Fig. 299-10). The mamillary process often lies in this exact spot and is a useful bony landmark. Evaluating the plain roentgenograms and computed tomography scans is helpful in determining the axial and sagittal entry angles.

The entry site is decorticated with a rongeur or drill. A pedicle probe is used to create a tract down the pedicle and to confirm the proposed trajectory. If there is sufficient concern, this may be done under C-arm radiography, but this precaution usually becomes unnecessary with experience. The probe is advanced into the vertebral body under proprioceptive control. Typically, little downward pressure is required, and the probe will pass through cancellous bone with the help of a moderate side-to-side rocking motion. Cortical bone is unyielding to these maneuvers, and excessive pressure followed by a sudden ''give'' may represent penetration of the pedicle's cortical rim. The probe should be inserted as far as the proposed screw depth, which should gain purchase on 50 to 80% of the vertebral body. Penetration beyond the anterior vertebral cortex may risk injury to the great vessels. Removal of the probe is often followed by slow cancellous bone bleeding, and some fat globules may even drip out. The sides of the tract are then explored with a feeler to assure that no breaks in the cortex have occurred.

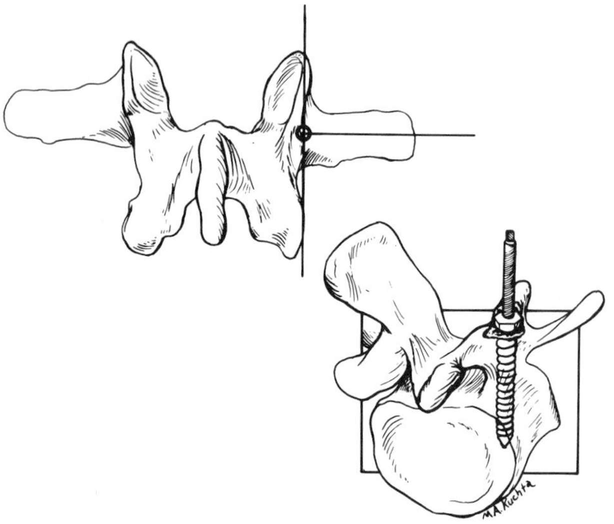

Figure 299-10 The pedicle is located at the junction of the superior facet, the lamina, and the transverse process.

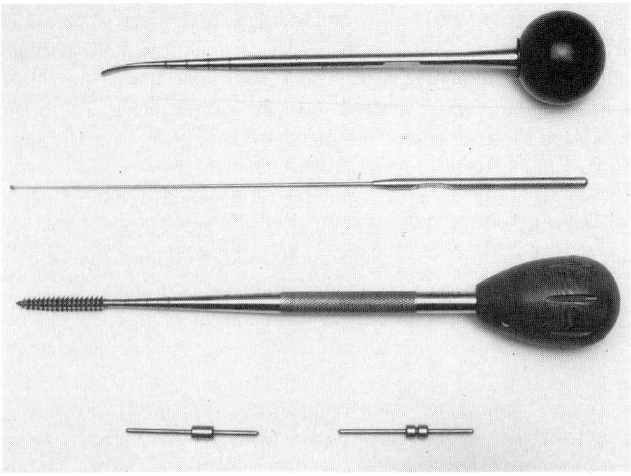

Figure 299-11 Instruments required in preparation for screw placement. *Top to bottom:* bone probe, bone feeler, tap, and marker pins.

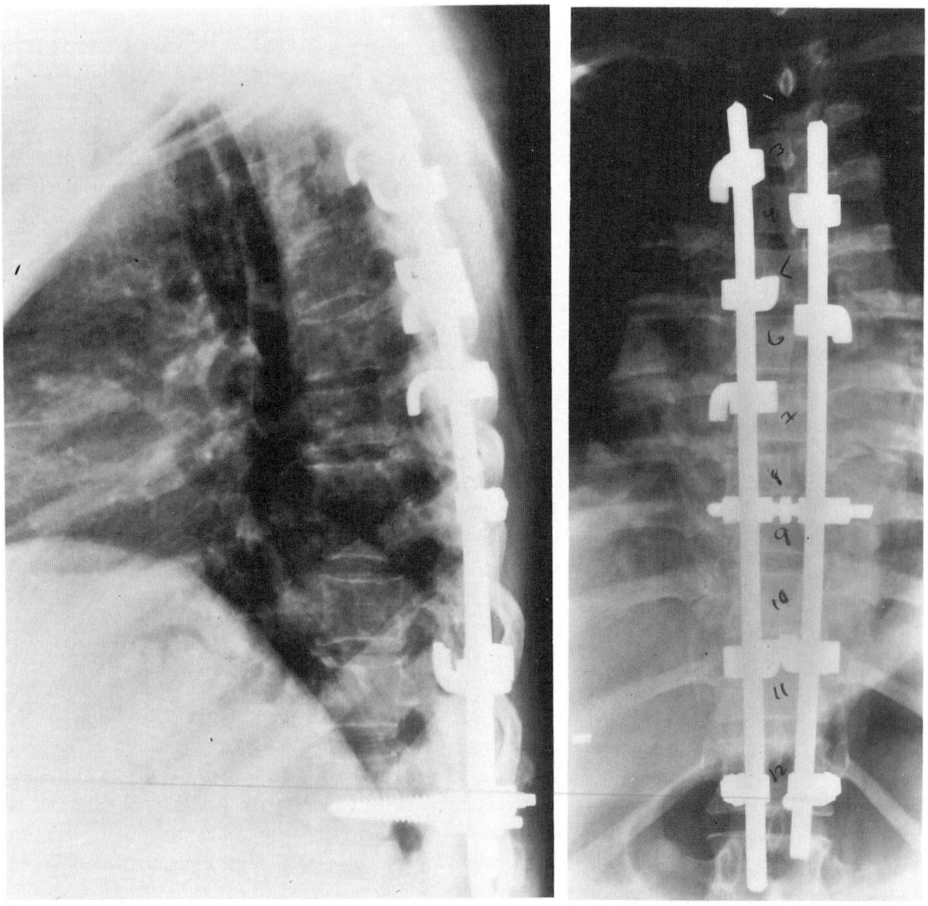

Figure 299-12 A hybrid construct for stabilization of thoracolumbar instability. Claw constructs have been placed in the thoracic spine, and pedicle screws have been placed in the lumbar spine. A transverse connector is present in the middle.

Blunt-tipped pins can be introduced into the tracts and a radiograph taken to preview the proposed screw trajectories. A guiding principle of screw choice is that the largest diameter that will not cause pedicale fracture should be chosen.[4] A tap is used to cut threads into the cortical bone of the pedicle, and then the screw is placed (Fig. 299-11). The connectors are then used to join the screws to the rods.

Instrumentation of thoracolumbar regions may require a hybrid construct, with claws used as anchors in the thoracic spine and pedicle screws used as the lumbar spine anchors.

An example of the Isola system applied to a clinical problem is shown in Fig. 299-12.

Complications

Each aspect of the instrumentation process has its attendant risks and complications. None is unique to the Isola system. The hook with the smallest throat size should be used to minimize any canal compromise. Sublaminar passage of wire or cable can result in neurological compromise, so considerable attention should be paid during this step. Placement of a pedicle screw can cause neural injury with inadvertent entry into the canal or foramen. Dural tears can result in cerebrospinal fluid leaks. Injury to the great vesels can occur with too deep a screw. Infection rates have been reported to be higher with instrumentation, but this is most likely secondary to the longer procedure time.

References

1. Asher MA, Strippgen WE, Heinig CF, et al. Isola spinal implant system: principles, design, and applications. In An HS, Cotler JM (eds): *Spinal Instrumentation*. Baltimore: Williams & Wilkins, 1992, pp 325–351.
2. Hadra BE. The classic. Wiring of the vertebrae as a means of immobilization in fracture and Potts' disease: Berthold E. Hadra. Med Times and Register, Vol 22, May 23, 1891. *Clin Orthop* 1975; 112:4–8.
3. Harrington PR. The history and development of Harrington instrumentation by Paul R. Harrington, 1973. *Clin Orthop* 1988; 227:3–5.
4. Stillerman CB, Gruen JP. Universal spinal instrumentation. In Benzel EC (ed): *Spinal Instrumentation*. Park Ridge, IL: American Association of Neurological Surgeons, 1994, pp 147–174.

300 Lumbosacral Stabilization Using Screw Fixation Techniques

Gregory J. Bennett

Screw fixation techniques have dramatically changed surgical capabilities in the lumbar spine. Since their early description as a supplement to posterior fusions,[3] the design configuration and biomechanical properties of pedicle fixation systems have steadily evolved.[1,4,5,12,25,29,32] Current lumbar screw fixation techniques include posterior transpedicular systems and anterior screw-plate systems. Their relative advantages and disadvantages, surgical indications, techniques, and results of surgery are discussed in this chapter.

Indications for Surgery

Spondylolysis and Spondylolisthesis

Posterior transpedicular stabilization techniques are very useful for patients with spondylolysis and spondylolisthesis.[7,9,13,16] These patients frequently develop severe leg and back pain that is consistent with both a radiculopathy and an instability syndrome. Laminectomy and foraminotomy without stabilization may result in progression of the instability syndrome.

The lumbosacral stabilization procedure should only include one disc level if the adjacent disc is normal. For example, the adjacent disc at L4-L5 is typically normal, so the minimal stabilization procedure should only include L5-S1. Since the posterior elements at L5 are lacking after the decompressive laminectomy, the only stabilization technique available is pedicle fixation (Fig. 300-1). At these levels, the pedicles are quite large and easily accommodate screws.

In the mid- and upper lumbar spine, the pedicles vary considerably in size and can be quite small relative to the size of the currently available screws. This increases the risk of surgical damage to both the pedicle and adjacent nerves during screw insertion.[2,6,14,15,18,26] Spondylolysis is very rare at these levels, unless there has been a previous laminectomy or fusion.

Degenerative spondylolisthesis is most commonly seen at L4-L5 and occasionally at L3-L4 or above. Surgery for spondylo-

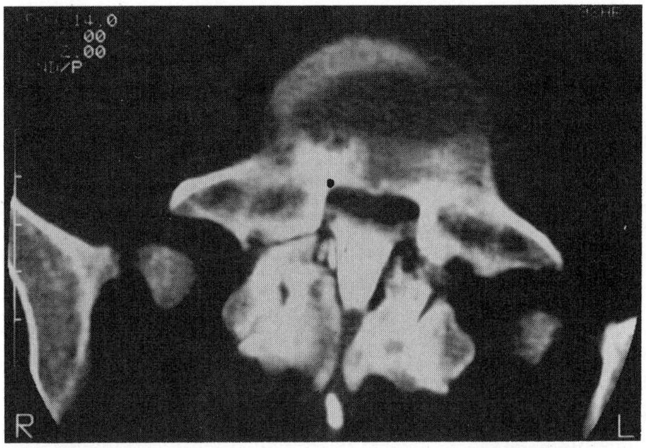

(*A*)

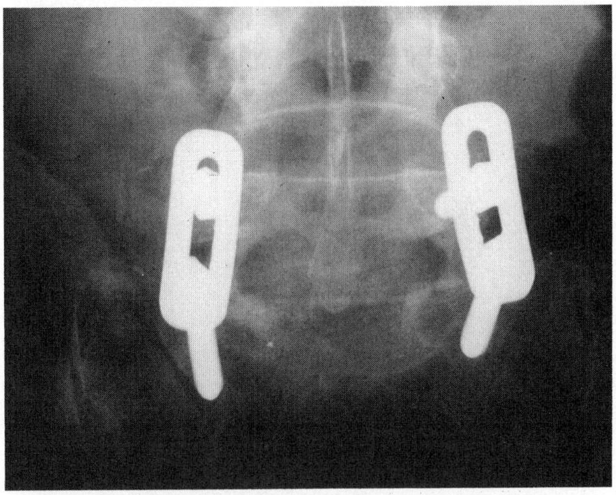

(*B*)

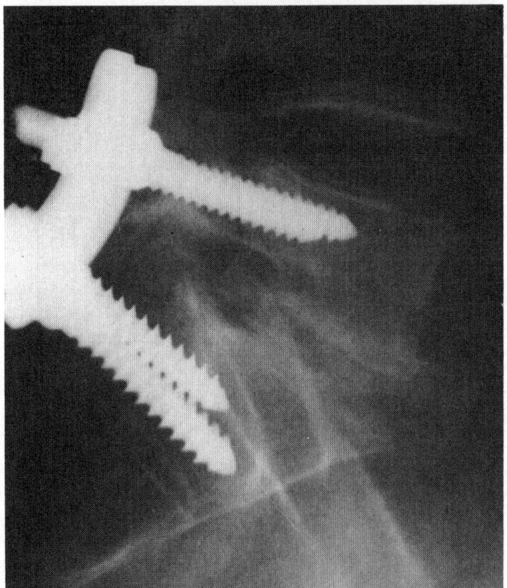

(*C*)

Figure 300-1 A 42-year-old woman with severe back and leg pain. Note the defect at the pars interarticularis of L5 adjacent to the pedicle. (*A*). Decompression involves *partial* removal of the lamina and pars (*B*), which leaves only the pedicles for stabilization (*C*).

listhesis usually involves a laminectomy or extensive laminotomy and partial or complete facetectomy for decompression. (Fig. 300-2). Since the posterior elements have been removed, pedicle screw fixation is the only posterior technique that can stabilize the motion segment.

Central and Recurrent Disc Herniation

Patients with central disc herniation and recurrent disc herniation can be treated with lumbar stabilization procedures. Those patients with a central disc herniation may experience a predominance of back pain that is worse with prolonged upright postures, such as when driving a motor vehicle or working in a standing position. Microdiscectomy may remove enough disc to decompress the nerves and adjacent structures. If the patient is able to rest, exercise, and rehabilitate carefully, the spine usually heals with good function and satisfactory relief of symptoms. Unfortunately, in some patients, the discectomy further destabilizes the spine which settles at that segment, resulting in increased back pain and occasionally foraminal stenosis. At L5-S1, retrolisthesis may occur, further exacerbating the foraminal stenosis.

The lumbar instability syndrome consists of severe back pain which occurs with upright postures and axial loading of the spine. It can be difficult to diagnose but, in my experience, exists in some patients. Surgical candidates for stabilization procedures are those patients who have good function of the paraspinal muscles and a normal range of motion in the lumbar spine, but who have severe pain despite conservative measures. These patients can greatly benefit from discectomy and fusion using a variety of stabilizing implants (Fig. 300-3).

Spinal stabilization surgery for central disc herniation can incorporate a variety of approaches. Discectomy can be performed unilaterally or bilaterally, depending on the surgeon's ability to adequately remove the disc and scar tissue from previous surgery and on the type of fusion to be done after discectomy. Unilateral discectomy may not create enough space for an adequate interbody fusion and should probably be used only in patients in whom an intertransverse fusion is planned. By comparison, bilateral discectomy permits an excellent neural decompression and provides

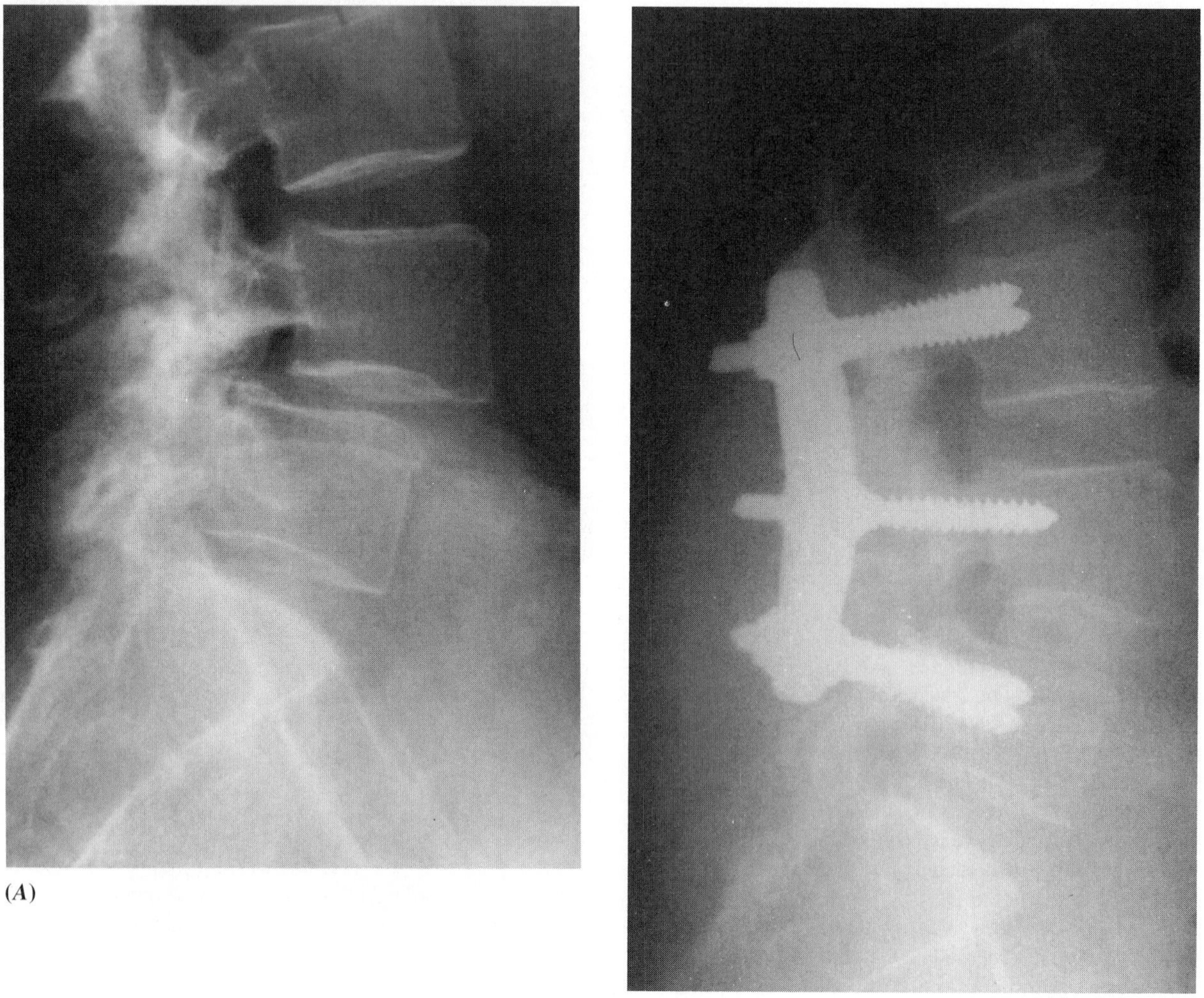

(*A*)

Figure 300-2 A 66-year-old woman with degenerative spondylolisthesis at L4-L5 (*A*). The laminotomy at L4-L5 with discectomy was followed by fusion from L3 to L5 with pedicle fixation (*B*).

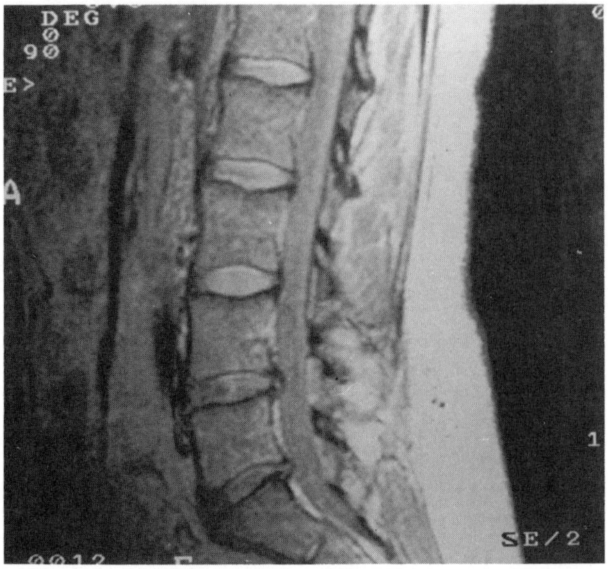

(*A*)

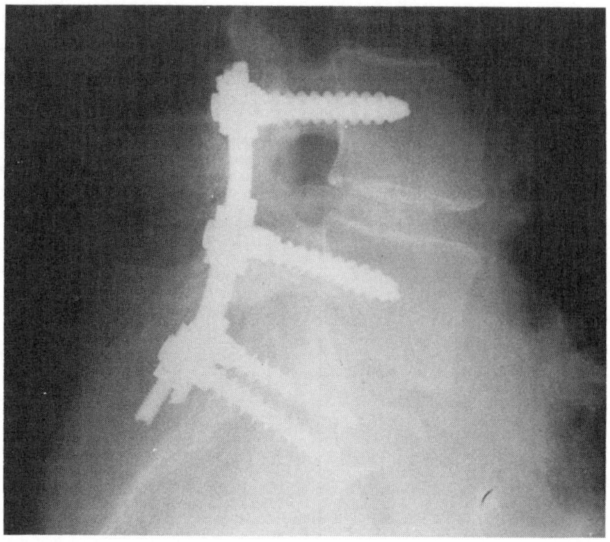

(*B*)

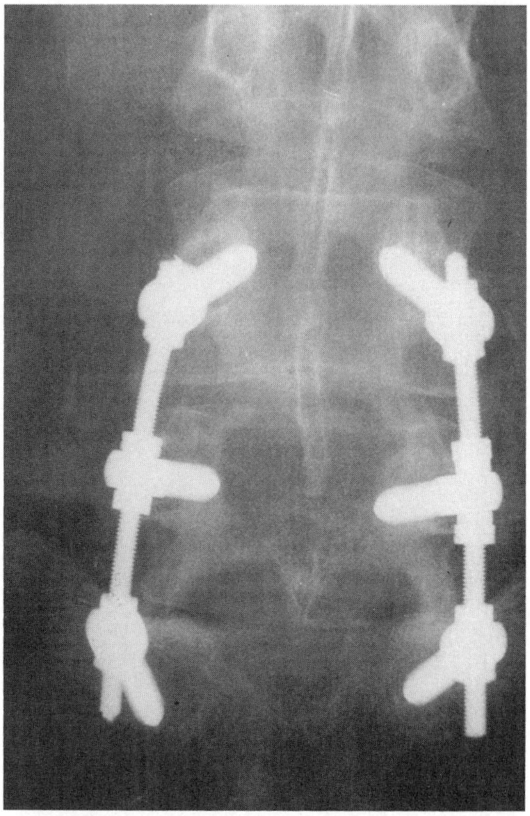

(*C*)

Figure 300-3 A 40-year-old man with severe back pain and minimal leg pain with central disc herniations (*A*). Pedicle fixation (*B, C*) can be used to increase the stiffness of the surgical construct, to permit more extensive facetectomy for insertion of bone grafts without retracting nerve roots, and to decrease the risk of graft displacement.

abundant space for subsequent interbody fusion but is destabilizing and may result in excessive axial loads on pedicle screws if the fusion is only intertransverse.

Pedicle fixation with intertransverse fusion is usually adequate for patients of moderate body size and for those in whom excessive loads on the implant from postoperative activities are not anticipated. Occasionally pedicle screws will fracture several weeks after surgery. The presumed mechanism of screw failure is micromotion, abrasion of the screw surface, and excessive bending moment which creates a weak point at the outermost 2 to 3 screw threads and eventually a fatigue fracture of the metal. In patients in whom high axial loads are anticipated, an interbody fusion can lessen the strain on pedicle screws and may permit the use of smaller screws with less risk of pedicle fracture and neural damage.[19,20,30]

Recurrent disc herniation may indicate that the spinal motion segment has failed to function and will progressively deteriorate. For these patients, a fusion may reduce the severity of back pain and other instability symptoms. The scar tissue from previous surgery can complicate a direct epidural dissection of the nerve root and increase the risk of damage to the dura and root. Wide facetectomy and additional laminotomy will usually expose fresh dural margins and greatly facilitate discectomy. The biomechanical function of the facet joints can be largely recreated by pedicle fixation.[10,21,23,31] For patients with extensive epidural scar tissue, facetectomy and stabilization with pedicle fixation is advantageous and may be safer than more limited approaches which spare the facet. Fusion technique, either intertransverse or interbody, can be selected by considering the anticipated loads from patient size and activity and the availability of autograft or allograft.

Degenerative Scoliosis

Lumbar scoliosis with spinal stenosis is best considered an instability syndrome with stenosis similar to degenerative spondylolisthesis.[22] The nerve roots may be adequately decompressed using conventional laminectomy, but progressive spinal deformity can cause recurrent symptoms. Lateral foraminal stenosis can be present on the concavity of the caudal curve and typically affects the L5 root. Removal of the disc bulge and facetectomy may be necessary to decompress the root, resulting in an instability syndrome. Pedicle fixation with a rod-based system (Fig. 300-4) is essential for stabilization. The posterior elements are largely removed by the decompressive surgery, and the deformity requires that screws be connected by a curved implant which precludes the use of a plate.[17,24,27]

Interbody fusions can be used in patients with degenerative scoliosis; in my experience, however, the deformity is quite stiff and cannot easily be corrected. If fused in situ, there is usually very little space on the concavity for interbody grafts, even after thorough discectomy. For most patients, an intertransverse fusion is sufficient, and attempted interbody grafting may be needlessly traumatic to nerves.

Previous Failed Fusion

Patients who have had a previous fusion with failure at fused or adjacent levels can be very challenging for the surgeon. Some of the difficulties they present include (1) the lack of anatomic landmarks for identifying pedicles, facets, and nerve roots; (2) the lack of available autograft bone; and (3) high localized stresses on bone and implants due to the lack of motion at adjacent segments. Spinal fusion in such patients should include rigid fixation and optimal bone grafting, such as interbody grafts with pedicle fixation (Fig. 300-5). As in surgery for recurrent disc herniation, wide exposure with foraminotomy, facetectomy, and thorough discectomy reduces the risk of nerve root damage. These measures also facilitate positioning of interbody grafts and insertion of pedicle screws under direct visualization of the pedicle margins and adjacent roots.

Lumbar Tumors

Palliative surgery for metastatic spinal tumors and definitive resection for primary tumors are well described and increasingly facili-

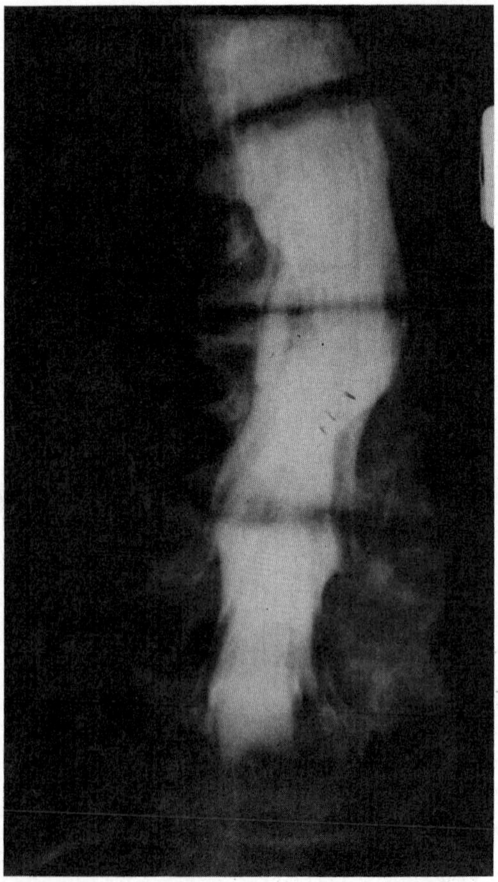

(*A*)

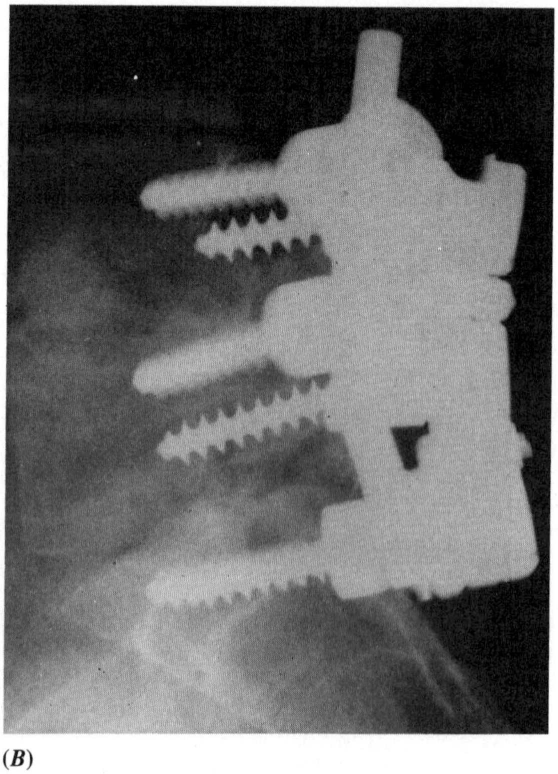

(*B*)

Figure 300-4 A 73-year-old woman with back pain and severe left L5 radiculopathy (*A*), underwent partial L5-S1 facetectomy and fusion (*B*) to decompress the L5 root. The screws appear offset on the lateral view because of the scoliotic deformity.

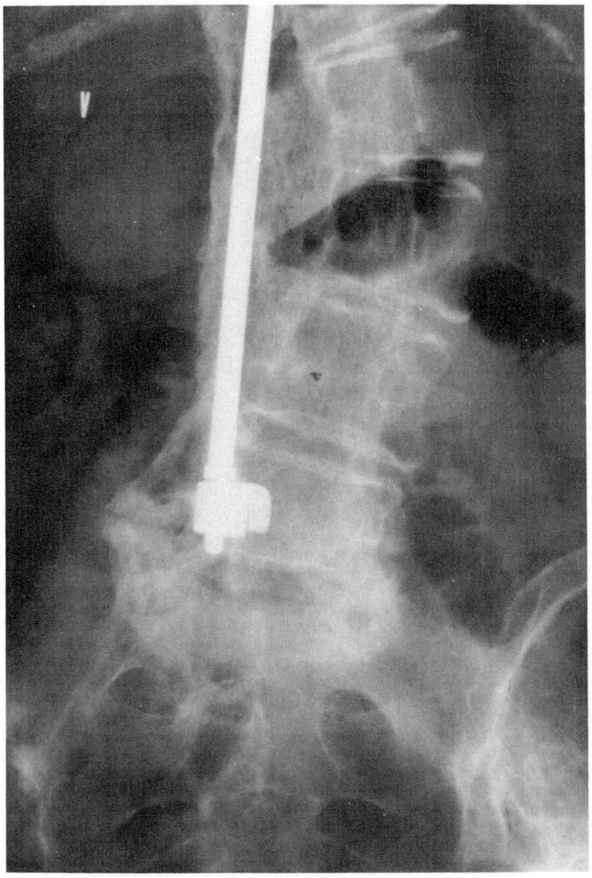

(*A*)

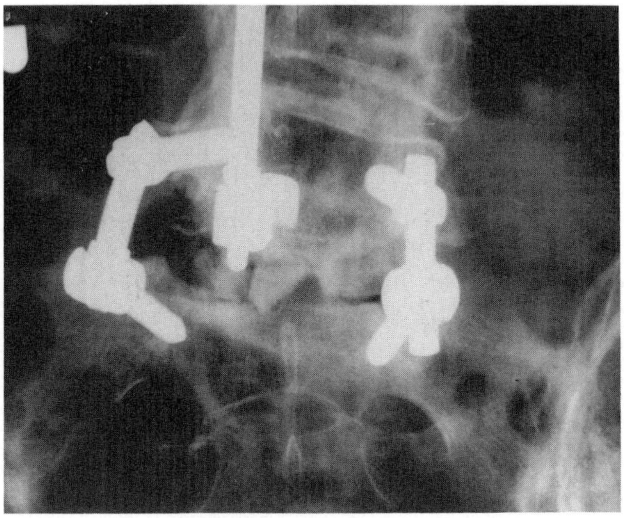

(*B*)

Figure 300-5 A 49-year-old man who had undergone a thoracolumbar fusion to the sacrum (*A*) for idiopathic scoliosis at age 11 and presented with severe back and moderate leg pain. Surgical exploration revealed a pseudarthrosis and L5 foraminal compression. An interbody fusion at L5-S1 with pedicle fixation was performed (*B*).

tated by the use of stabilizing implants.[11] A destructive lesion can be removed and the patient can be quickly mobilized with added safety and effectiveness using pedicle fixation (Fig. 300-6).

Anterior Screw-Plate Stabilization

The role of anterior stabilization implants for lumbar spine disorders remains somewhat undefined. The best indications for anterior stabilization include the presence of previously radiated or otherwise damaged soft tissues which preclude a posterior approach. Severely damaged pedicles from previous failed posterior fusion may also require the anterior approach and screw-plate stabilization.

The hazards of anterior implants include the proximity to the aortic and iliac vessels and the possibility of delayed implant loosening with migration of the implant into veins and arteries. A transabdominal surgical approach may be difficult at L5-S1 because of a prominent lumbosacral lordosis and at L3-4 and L4-5 because of the proximity of the aortic bifurcation and iliac vessels.

A lateral retroperitoneal approach can be used at L2-L4, and the lateral extracavitary approach provides adequate exposure for screw-plate fixation at T11-L2 (Fig. 300-7). Screws that lock to the plate with internal expansion screws or other external locking devices may be used as a monocortical screw which reduces the risk of vascular injury from direct screw trauma or delayed loosening of the implant.

Lumbosacral Stabilization with Screws: Surgical Technique

Transpedicular stabilization techniques are heavily dependent on lateral soft tissue exposure for medial screw orientation and lateral bony landmarks for identification of the screw entry site. The most common and easily preventable cause of poor screw placement is a skin incision that is too short. A variety of approaches can be used to facilitate the spinal exposure. Large patients need a very long incision, frequently from L1-S2. Very obese patients may be impossible to expose in a conventional manner. These patients require the use of a wide transverse incision with undermining of all skin and soft tissue to the lumbodorsal fascia, after which the skin and fat are rostrally and caudally retracted to reduce the bulk of laterally retracted tissues. A midline fascia incision, muscle dissection, and laminectomy can then be performed in the usual manner. Alternatively, separate paramedian incisions with muscle splitting techniques may be used to spare the midline structures if the bony exposure consists only of bilateral laminotomy, facetectomy, and pedicle screw fixation.

Once the paraspinal muscles have been dissected to the lateral tips of the transverse processes, the superior articular process of the vertebral levels to be fused should be identified. This process is located at the facet joint, one level above the facet commonly encountered during laminotomy for discectomy. The surgical orientation to posterior approaches to the lamina is somewhat misleading, since the lamina is positioned at the caudal end of the

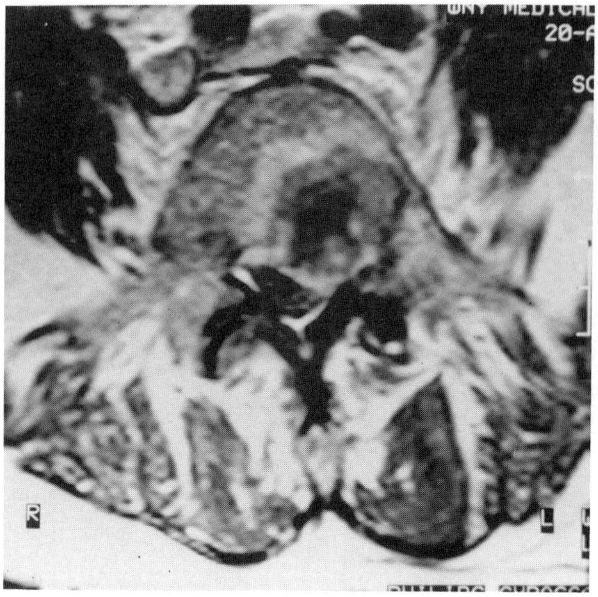

(*A*)

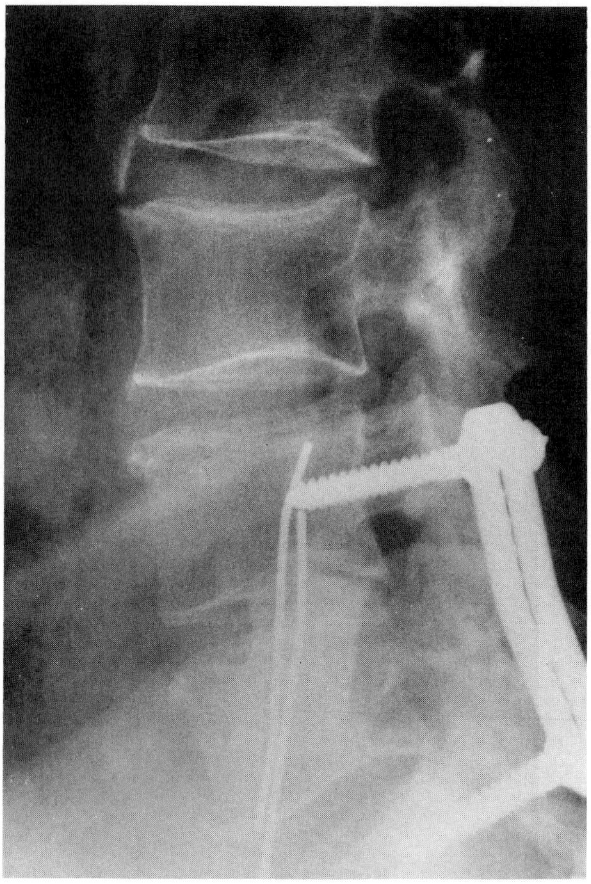

(*B*)

Figure 300-6 A 64-year-old healthy and active man with apical adenocarcinoma of the lung, a solitary metastasis at L5, and a short history of severe back pain, leg pain, and a left foot drop (*A*). The tumor was removed using a paraspinal approach. The spine was stabilized with polymethyl methacrylate bone cement, Steinmann pins, and pedicle fixation (*B*). The lung tumor was also removed, and the spine was radiated.

vertebra, and the pedicle and vertebral body are rostral relative to the lamina. The screw entry site is created by drilling medially into the lateral cortical margin of the superior process approximately 3 to 4 mm and then down into the pedicle.

The orientation of the screw in the sagittal plane, relative to the lumbar lordosis, and in the axial plane, relative to the transverse diameter of the pedicle, is then carefully considered from radiographs and computed tomography (CT) scans. Pedicle morphometry progressively varies between L1 and S1, with the upper lumbar pedicles being narrow in the transverse dimension and the L5 and S1 pedicles being short and wide. The pedicle orientation in the axial plane also varies, with the upper pedicles being straight anterior-posterior and the lower pedicles progressively more angled medially.[15] Screw orientation should attempt to maximally utilize the medial orientation of the pedicles to create the longest trajectory for the screw in bone and to direct the tip of the screw toward the midline of the vertebral body. This ''ideal'' axial plane screw orientation (Fig. 300-8) also adds intrinsic stability by triangulating the implant and protects the iliac vessels and lumbar plexus from accidental displacement of the screw. When positioning pedicle screws, it is important to remember that although the least anatomic tolerance and the greatest potential for serious nerve damage are at the caudal and medial margins of the pedicle, the screw must also avoid the spinal nerve from the level above that travels immediately lateral to the pedicle.

Before the screw is inserted, the pedicle is probed with an object, such as a curette. A gradual increase in resistance should be identified until the probe enters the vertebral body and a drop in resistance is noted. Then, the probe is removed, and a Steinmann pin is inserted. Bleeding around the pin commonly occurs, which confirms that the vertebral body has been entered. The position of the probe or pins should be monitored with fluoroscopy or plain radiographs in both lateral and anterior-posterior views. A sudden drop in pedicle stiffness indicates that the probe has fractured through the cortical margins of the pedicle and may be displaced. This requires radiographic confirmation of the location of the probe followed by repositioning.

Once the pins have been confirmed to be in satisfactory position, the pedicle screws can be selected. At L4 and above, the narrowest available screw (usually with an outside diameter of 5.5 to 6.0 mm) should be selected for all but the largest individuals. Larger screws (up to 7.0 mm) can be used at L5 and S1. Screw lengths will vary, but may be as long as 45 to 50 mm in large patients, particularly if medially oriented. In general, shorter screws (averaging 30 to 35 mm) are used at L5 and S1.

Sacral fixation can be problematic, since the pedicles consist primarily of cancellous bone and the sacral entry site may be soft. To avoid inadequate fixation, the surgeon should do the following: (1) use screws with wide deep threads, (2) make a tiny puncture site at the lateral aspect of the sacral superior articular process, and (3) avoid tapping the bone prior to screw entry. At other levels, bone taps can be very helpful for reducing the expansion stress in the pedicle created by screw insertion, thereby decreasing the risk of pedicle fracture. If the pedicle seems hard and the screw does not draw itself in, bone taps can be used to prepare the path for the screw.

Once the screws are in good position, they are connected by plates or rods. If one motion segment is being fused, plates can

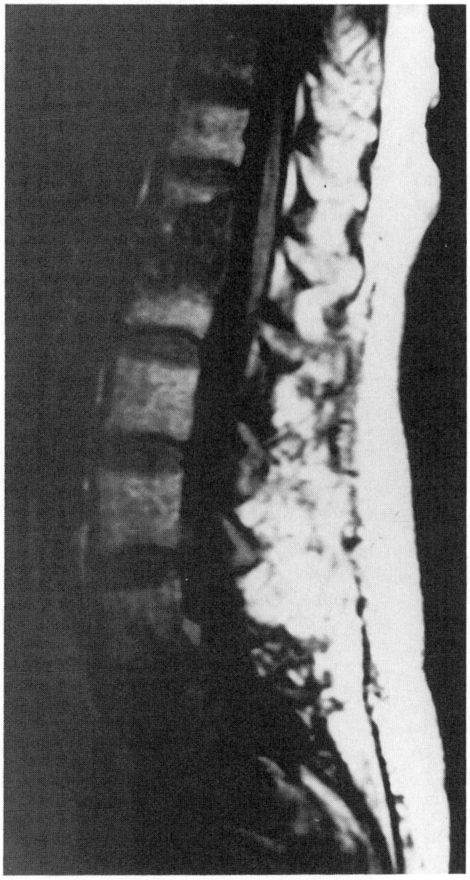

(*A*)

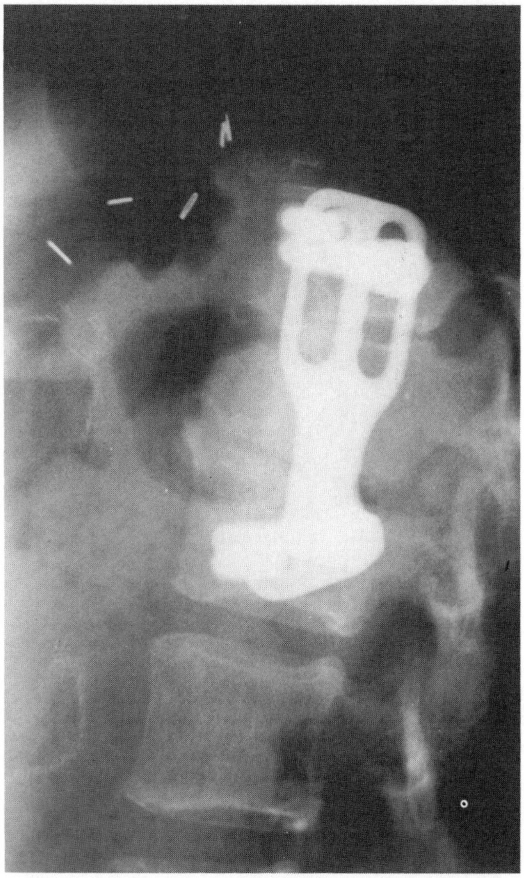

(*B*)

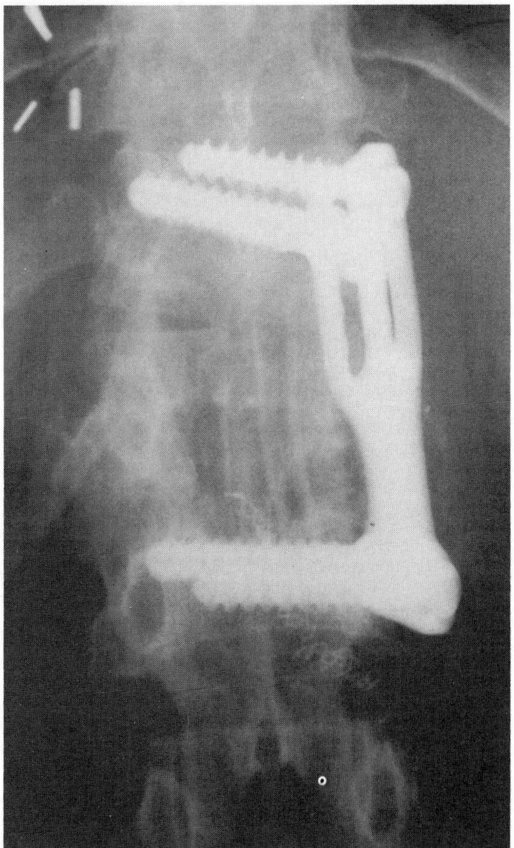

(*C*)

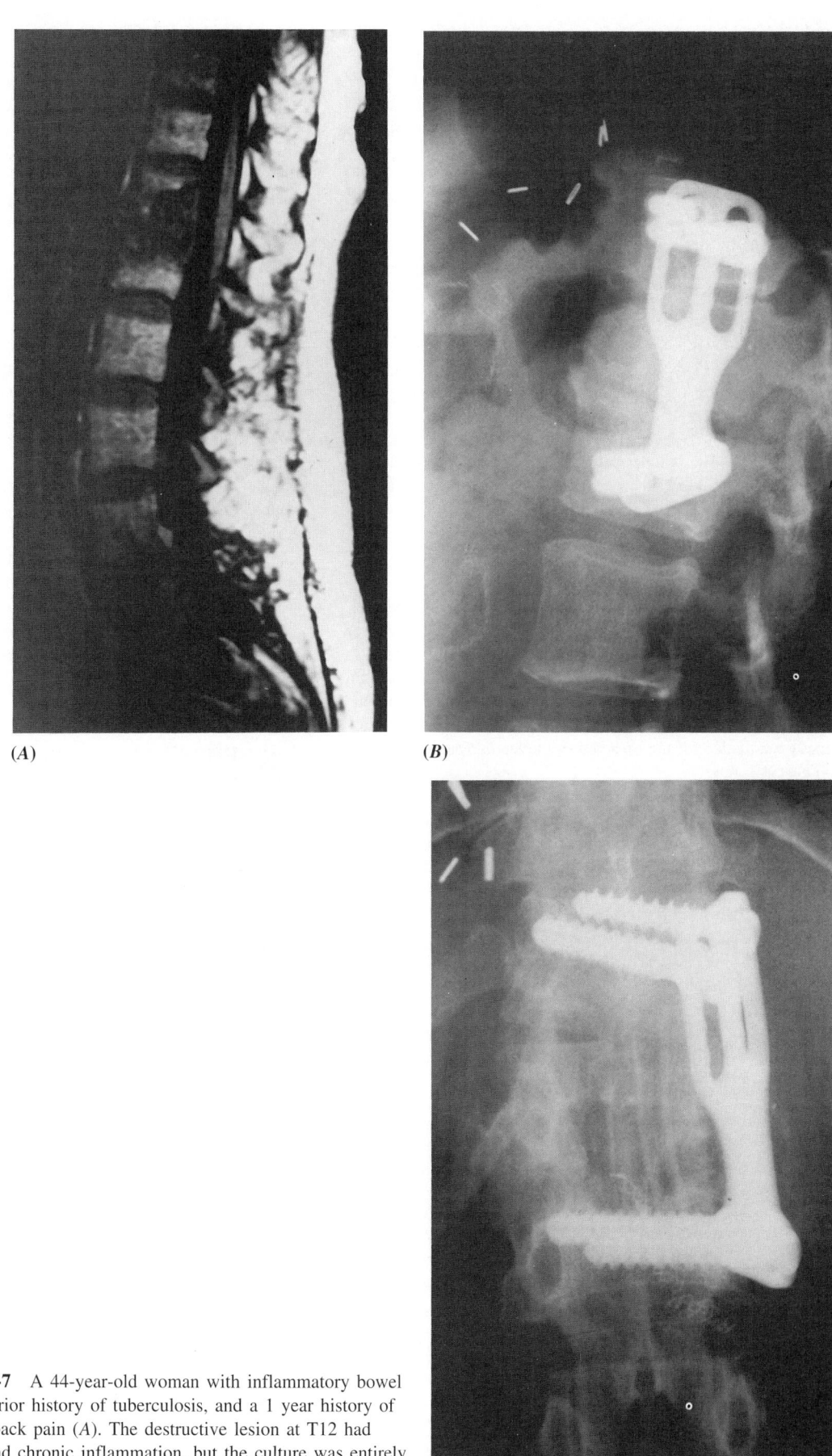

Figure 300-7 A 44-year-old woman with inflammatory bowel disease, a prior history of tuberculosis, and a 1 year history of increasing back pain (*A*). The destructive lesion at T12 had caseation and chronic inflammation, but the culture was entirely negative. A plate and screws were applied from a lateral approach after vertebral body debridement and grafting (*B, C*).

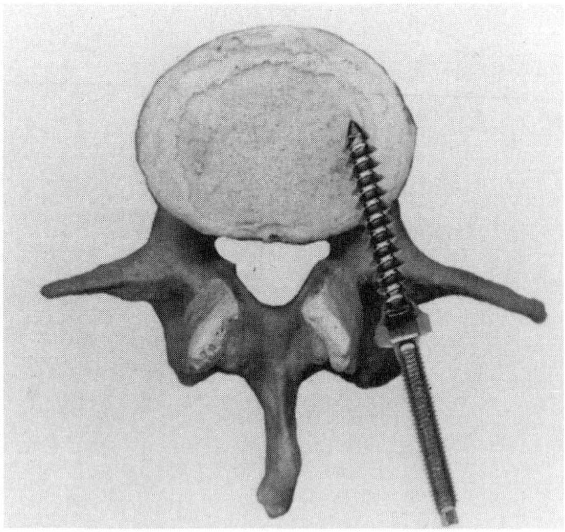

Figure 300-8 The optimal pedicle screw orientation is along the predominant axis of the pedicle to maximize the available bone for screw contact and to minimize the risk of nerve damage.

usually be oriented between the screws to provide very rigid fixation. For spondylolisthesis, the double-threaded screws for rods or plates can be used to correct some of the displacement by securing the caudal level first and slowly tightening the rostral level. Two motion segment fusions incorporating three screws can make the use of plates technically difficult if the screws are offset transversely, particularly if the L5 screw is too lateral in relation to the L4 and S1 screws.

Lateral spinal deformities and degenerative scoliosis can also require rods to connect the screws. Acute spinal instability, such as caused by an acute unstable fracture, can sometimes be corrected with pedicle screw implants using in situ rod contouring, distraction, and eventually compression of anterior grafts. Extensive trauma with associated ligamentous injury is easy to realign. When treating degenerative deformities, attempting partial correction is better than risking pedicle fracture by trying to correct rigid, longstanding misalignments.

Results of Pedicle Screw Stabilization

The anatomic results of pedicle screw stabilization are well documented.[25,29] Pedicle screw fixation is quite rigid by comparison with other implants and greatly reduces but does not entirely eliminate intervertebral movement.[31] Reduced movement is known to be associated with increased rates of successful fusion from both clinical and experimental studies.[8] Additionally, pedicle screw fixation can greatly facilitate interbody fusion, thereby permitting the successful use of allograft bone, which does not fuse at the intertransverse location, and avoiding postoperative iliac crest pain. Relief of symptoms and improvement in statistical measures of quality of life and functional status have been associated with lumbar stabilization surgery for degenerative disease. Rigid stabilization for fractures and tumors makes excellent clinical sense and can significantly benefit patients by reducing the rate of stabilization failure and permitting more extensive posterior exposure for decompression.

The dilemmas associated with clinical decisions concerning the use of pedicle screws for degenerative disease are largely caused by our limited understanding of many aspects of back pain and lumbar instability and the low but definite risk of serious additional damage to nerves from surgical treatment. Back pain may be disabling but is essentially a benign disorder that should be treated accordingly. Although surgery can be very helpful, the treatment of back pain can also be influenced by several different exercise, behavioral, and psychosocial interventions.

Patients with chronic pain become depressed and desperate for relief as their physiologic, social, and psychological compensatory mechanisms become exhausted. Physicians can easily misjudge a patient's prospects for recovery and eventual rehabilitation to a socially healthy and functional lifestyle if this decompensated state is not also considered during treatment, preferably before surgery. A good anatomic result can be easily obscured by persistent social and psychological disability and dependency. Recognizing the severity of these associated problems, a surgeon must individualize treatment decisions and insist on full patient responsibility for lifestyle changes, remembering that all rehabilitative resources should be utilized before a patient is considered a treatment failure.

Standardized outcome measures in the form of short questionnaires can be quite helpful for monitoring symptoms and functional status. When the records of 246 patients undergoing 251 lumbar fusions for degenerative disease were reviewed retrospectively, significant improvements in symptoms and functional status were noted.[28]

Complications of Lumbosacral Stabilization

The complications of pedicle screw stabilization have been well described[6,19,20] and include (1) nerve damage resulting from displaced screws, (2) immediate or delayed pedicle fracture with nerve damage caused by bone fragments or screws, (3) loss of fixation resulting from screw fracture or delayed screw loosening, (4) failed fusion caused by inadequate preparation of bone surfaces, (5) insufficient autografting or allografting, and (6) insufficient stabilization.

Between 1988 and 1993, 124 lumbar stabilization procedures using pedicle screw fixation were performed at our institution. Table 300-1 lists the indications for, and the complications and their eventual outcomes from these procedures. The complication rate was 14/124 or 11 percent.

Preventing complications requires careful attention to surgical details. Excellent muscle and soft tissue exposure permits medial orientation during screw insertion. Optimal axial and sagittal plane screw orientation adds intrinsic stability and protects the great vessels from accidental screw displacement. Atraumatic insertion of guidance pins allows radiographic confirmation of the screw trajectory before atraumatic screw insertion along a constant path within the pedicle. Direct inspection of pedicle margins if screw penetration is suspected allows for repositioning before complete insertion. Postoperative CT scans with intravenous contrast should be used if anterior cortex penetration is suspected. Avoidance of excessive off-axis loads on screws by precise alignment and contouring of longitudinal connectors, such as plates and rods, will decrease the risk of delayed screw fracture through the pedicle.

TABLE 300-1 Lumbar Stabilizations Using Pedicle Screw Fixation 1988–1993

Indication for Procedure	**No. of Patients**
Spondylolysis and spondylolisthesis	54
Central disc herniation	46
Failed previous fusion	7
Fracture	5
Recurrent disc herniation	4
Degenerative scoliosis	3
Retrolisthesis	1
Discitis	1
Tumor	2
Lumbar osteotomy for ankylosing spondylitis	1
No. of Procedures	124
Complications and Eventual Outcome	**No. of Patients**
Displaced screw not resulting in symptoms	1
Displaced screw causing symptoms, requiring screw removal with partial or complete relief of pain and no deficit	3
Displaced allograft from interbody fusion causing leg pain, revised with implant removal	1
Screw fracture, no revision	2
Rod fracture requiring revision	1
Displaced screw through anterior cortex adjacent to iliac vessels, removed electively	2
Failed fusion requiring reoperation	1
Deep infection with osteomyelitis in diabetic patient, no implant removal, resolved with antibiotic therapy	1
Inflammatory response from nickel allergy requiring implant removal, resolved	2
No. of Complications	14

Summary

Lumbar pedicle screw fixation is now an established technique in spine surgery. Screw fixation provides excellent stability and greatly increases the surgeon's options in decompression and fusion techniques. Nevertheless, many questions remain including safety issues, implant bulk and the need for extensive exposures for accurate insertion, and the ultimate patient benefits of stabilization procedures for lumbar degenerative disease with instability.

References

1. Aebi M, Etter C, Kehl T, et al. The internal skeletal fixation system: a new treatment of thoracolumbar fractures and other spinal disorders. *Clin Orthop* 1988; 227:30–43.
2. Bernard TN Jr, Seibert CE. Pedicle diameter determined by computed tomography: its relevance to pedicle screw fixation in the lumbar spine. *Spine* 1992; 17(6)(Suppl):S160–S163.
3. Boucher HH. A method of spinal fusion. *J Bone Joint Surg [Br]* 1959; 41-B:248–259.
4. Carl AL, Tromanhauser SG, Roger DJ. Pedicle screw instrumentation for thoracolumbar burst fractures and fracture-dislocations. *Spine* 1992; 17(8)(Suppl):S317–S324.
5. Dick W. The "fixateur interne" as a versatile implant for spine surgery. *Spine* 1987; 12:882–900.
6. Gertzbein SD, Robbins SE. Accuracy of pedicular screw placement in vivo. *Spine* 1990; 15:11–14.
7. Gurr KR, McAfee PC. Cotrel-Dubousset instrumentation in adults. A preliminary report. *Spine* 1988; 13:510–520.
8. Gurr KR, McAfee PC, Warden KE, Shih CM. Roentgenographic and biomechanical analysis of lumbar fusions: a canine model. *J Orthop Res* 1989; 7:838–848.
9. Guyer DW, Wiltse LL, Peek RD. The Wiltse pedicle screw fixation system. *Orthopedics* 1988; 11:1455–1460.
10. Gwon JK, Chen J, Lim TH, et al. In vitro comparative biomechanical analysis of transpedicular screw instrumentations in the lumbar region of the human spine. *J Spinal Disord* 1991; 4:437–443.
11. Hammerberg KW. Surgical treatment of metastatic spine disease. *Spine* 1992; 17:1148–1153.
12. Herrmann HD. Transarticular (transpedicular) metal plate fixation for stabilization of the lumbar and thoracic spine. *Acta Neurochir (Wien)* 1979; 48:101–110.
13. Kamioka Y, Yamamoto H. Lumbar trapezoid plate for lumbar spondylolisthesis. A clinical study on preoperative and postoperative instability. *Spine* 1990; 15:1198–1203.
14. Krag MH, Beynnon BD, Pope MH, et al. An internal fixator for posterior application to short segments of the thoracic, lumbar, or lumbosacral spine. Design and testing. *Clin Orthop* 1986; 203:75–98.
15. Krag MH, Weaver DL, Beynnon BD, et al. Morphometry of the thoracic and lumbar spine related to transpedicular screw placement for surgical spinal fixation. *Spine* 1988; 13:27–32.
16. Louis R. Fusion of the lumbar and sacral spine by internal fixation with screw plates. *Clin Orthop* 1986; 203:18–33.
17. Marchesi DG, Aebi M. Pedicle fixation devices in the treatment of adult lumbar scoliosis. *Spine* 1992; 17(8)(Suppl):S304–S309.
18. Marchesi D, Schneider E, Glauser P, et al. Morphometric analysis of the thoracolumbar and lumbar pedicles, anatomoradiologic study. *Surg Radiol Anat* 1988; 10:317–322.
19. Matsuzaki H, Tokuhashi Y, Matsumoto F, et al. Problems and solutions of pedicle screw plate fixation of lumbar spine. *Spine* 1990; 15:1159–1165.
20. Misenhimer GR, Peek RD, Wiltse LL, et al. Anatomic analysis of pedicle cortical and cancellous diameter as related to screw size. *Spine* 1989; 14:367–372.
21. Pintar FA, Cusick JF, Yoganandan N, et al. The biomechanics of lumbar facetectomy under compression-flexion. *Spine* 1992; 17:804–810.
22. Pritchett JW, Bortel DT. Degenerative symptomatic lumbar scoliosis. *Spine* 1993; 18:700–703.
23. Rahmatalla AT, Hastings GW, Dove J, et al. A pedicle screw bridging device for posterior segmental fixation of the spine: preliminary mechanical testing results. *J Biomed Eng* 1991; 13:97–102.
24. Robin GC, Span Y, Steinberg R, et al. Scoliosis in the elderly: a follow-up study. *Spine* 1982; 7:355–359.
25. Roy-Camille R, Saillant G, Mazel C. Internal fixation of the lumbar spine with pedicle screw plating. *Clin Orthop* 1986; 203:7–17.
26. Scoles PV, Linton AE, Latimer B, et al. Vertebral body and posterior element morphology: the normal spine in middle life. *Spine* 1988; 13:1082–1086.
27. Simmons ED Jr, Kowalski JM, Simmons EH. The results of surgical treatment for adult scoliosis. *Spine* 1993; 18:718–724.
28. Sorini P, Bennett GJ, Egnatchik J. Clinical and functional outcomes following lumbar fusion: a retrospective analysis. Presented at the 60th Annual Meeting of The American Association of Neurological Surgeons, San Francisco, April 15, 1992.
29. Steffee AD, Biscup RS, Sitkowski DJ. Segmental spine plates with pedicle screw fixation: a new internal fixation device for disorders of the lumbar and thoracolumbar spine. *Clin Orthop* 1986; 203:45–53.
30. Steffee AD, Sitkowski DJ. Posterior lumbar interbody fusion and plates. *Clin Orthop* 1988; 227:99–102.
31. Yoganandan N, Larson SJ, Pintar F, et al. Biomechanics of lumbar pedicle screw/plate fixation in trauma. *Neurosurgery* 1990; 27:873–881.
32. Zucherman J, Hsu K, White A, et al. Early results of spinal fusion using variable spine plating system. *Spine* 1988; 13:570–579.

301

Anterior Fixation Devices for the Thoracic and Lumbar Spine

Peter M. Klara

Early attempts at internal fixation of the thoracic and lumbar spine date back to Humphries et al.[13] They were discouraged by the results of posterior fusion and used a transperitoneal approach to perform an anterior lumbar interbody arthrodesis. Immobilization was accomplished by insertion of an internal metallic device.

The modern era of internal fixation began with Dwyer,[6] who used staples and flexible cable to provide corrective forces after anterior discectomy in the treatment of scoliosis. The Dwyer construct did not, however, provide rigid fixation. Zielke connected a threaded rod to screws placed in the vertebral body. This allowed him to apply forces to correct coronal plane deformities as well as rotational deformities. Kostuik reported his results with anterior decompression and internal fixation using plates and screws, Dwyer cables, rods, and screws, as well as an anterior Harrington rod construct. The latter construct was the forerunner of the Kostuik-Harrington device.[16] Dunn developed a similar device for anterior distraction and fixation of the thoracolumbar spine. Two threaded rods were connected to vertebral bodies by staples and bone screws. Although bony fusions were obtained, the high profile of this device was responsible for vascular complications.

Anterior internal fixation was slow to achieve widespread acceptance and use. This was partially due to the lack of familiarity with the anterior surgical approach on the part of many spine surgeons. Another factor was the lack of standardized techniques and devices for internal fixation. The ability to achieve excellent neural decompression under direct visualization, fusion, and internal fixation in a single procedure gradually attracted much attention and is now widely accepted.

With the exception of the Dunn device, all the devices mentioned above remain commercially available and in use. In this chapter, I will describe commonly used and presently available anterior fixation devices, their indications, installation, advantages, disadvantages, and complications.

Indications

Anterior surgical decompression of the thoracic and lumbar spine became a widely utilized technique in response to the prevalence of tuberculous lesions of the spine in the mid-1900s.[11] It was reasoned that anterior neural compression could best be treated with anterior decompression. Since that time anterior decompression for pyogenic osteomyelitis, rigid kyphotic deformities, tumors (both primary and metastatic), and trauma has been widely accepted. Humphries et al. thought that anterior grafting favored fusion because of better blood supply and bone contact; also, the graft is under compression.[13] Internal fixation devices are indicated when spinal stability has been compromised either iatrogenically by surgery or by the disease process.[21] Evidence exists that internal fixation may improve fusion rates[1] as well as accelerate rehabilitation. The untoward effects of decreased activity are minimized, as is hospitalization. It is therefore useful in the treatment of failed posterior fusion or if posterior internal fixation is impossible.

Surgical Approaches

Access to the thoracic and lumbar spine for placement of anterior instrumentation may be gained through several standard approaches. Each has its advantages and limitations. These have been described in this textbook and elsewhere. The details of the surgical approaches lie beyond the scope of this chapter. The thoracic and lumbar spine can be separated into regions which assist surgical planning.

Approaches to the upper thoracic spine (T1-T3) include the (1) lateral parascapular extrapleural, (2) supraclavicular, (3) transmanubrial, (4) trans-sternal (C4-T4), and (5) transthoracic (3d rib) approaches. Those to the lower thoracic spine (T3-T10) include the (1) lateral extracavitary, (2) transthoracic, and (3) costotransversectomy approaches. Those to the thoracolumbar area (T11-L1) include the (1) transthoracic and (2) 10th rib resection approaches, with or without the step of taking down the diaphragm. Approaches to the lumbar spine (L2-L5) include the (1) retroperitoneal and (2) transperitoneal approaches.

Anterior Fixation Devices

Various anterior fixation devices are available for use, as listed in Table 301-1 and discussed below.

Cable Devices

Dwyer Device

This titanium device (Fig. 301-1) was designed to treat scoliosis and has been in use since 1964. Through an anterior approach, discectomy and fusion are performed. Screws are placed through a staple-plate that hooks over and under the vertebral body and centers the screw. A ⅛-in. titanium cable is then passed through the head of each screw, and tension is applied sequentially. The cable is then secured at each screw head. In this manner significant correction can be gained. Successful results have been reported by Dwyer and others.[6,7,24] This device remains useful in the treatment of scoliosis, but cannot be used in the presence of posterior element disruption. Although vascular and urologic complications have been reported, this system remains useful today.

TABLE 301-1 Anterior Fixation Devices

Device	Type	Uses	Compress	Distract	Neutral
Dwyer	Cable	Scoliosis	X		
Zielke	Rod (single)	Scoliosis	X		
Kostuik-Harrington	Rod (double)	Kyphotic deformities,	X	X	
Slot-Zielke	Rod (single, double)	fractures, tumors,			
Kaneda	Rod (double)	degenerative disease,	X	X	
		latrogenic instability			
DCP plate	Plate	Fractures, tumors,	+/−		X
ALPS	Plate	adjunct to posterior			X
CASP	Plate	instrumentation,			X
I plate	Plate	degenerative			X
Z plate	Plate	disease	X	X	
Rezaian	Interbody device	Interbody distractor			
Moss cage	Interbody device	Interbody spacer/graft			

Rod Devices

Zielke Device

This device, developed in 1975 and made of stainless steel, substitutes a threaded rod for the cable of the Dwyer device (Fig. 301-2). The rigidity of the rod allows for restoration of lumbar lordosis (with the use of an outrigger device) as well as for correction of scoliosis. The threaded rod allows gradual, controlled application of the compressive force. The ability to correct kyphosis makes this device useful in the treatment of failed posterior fusions.[18] Excellent results also have been reported in the treatment of degenerative lumbar scoliosis.[20] However, complications and pseudarthrosis rates as high as 30 percent have been reported.[25] Increased rates of pseudarthrosis have been reported when this device is used for stabilization alone. More favorable results are obtained when the device is applied under tension and the graft is compressed.[16]

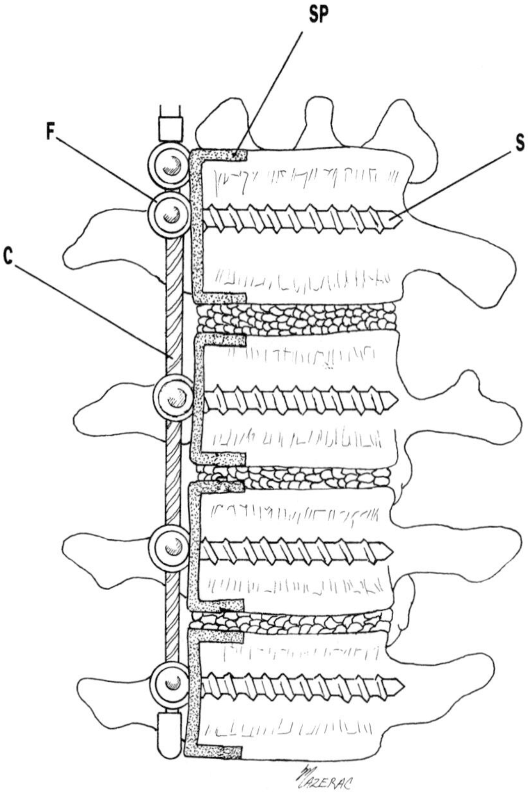

Figure 301-1 Dwyer device. First of the modern anterior thoracolumbar devices, this construct uses a flexible cable *(C)* threaded through screws. The screws *(S)* pass through a staple-like plate *(SP)* that fits over and under the vertebral body for added stability. The cable is fastened to the screws *(F)* after tension is applied.

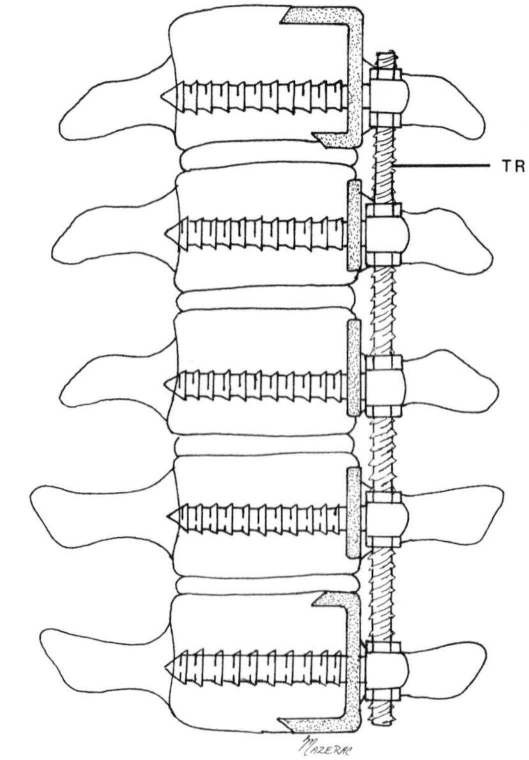

Figure 301-2 Zielke device. A rigid threaded rod *(TR)* is substituted for the flexible cable of the Dwyer device. This provides an adjustable compressive force and controlled application of lordosis. Correction of a coronal plane deformity as well as rotational deformity can be accomplished. This device is still in use for the treatment of scoliosis.

Slot-Zielke Device

Originally this was a single rod device used for correcting kyphotic deformities. Zielke screws are placed through staple plates into the vertebral body. Following discectomy or corpectomy, correction of kyphosis is accomplished with an outrigger. An appropriate Slot rod with antirotation notches is then connected to the screws. In the treatment of burst fractures, this system achieved 41 percent fusion rates and an average loss of reduction of greater than 5 percent. Hardware failure occurred, but no vascular or neurological complications were reported.[2] The device is now available as a two-rod system with cross connectors (Fig. 301-3). This design change increases rotational stability and axial support. Little clinical data are presently available on the two rod design.

Kostuik-Harrington Device

In an attempt to develop a device that provided distraction, compression, and stabilization as needed, Kostuik combined a Harrington distraction rod with a compression rod. The posteriorly placed rod is connected to screws in the vertebral body. A parallel rod is placed anteriorly and is similarly fixed with screws to the vertebral body. This arrangement allows for distraction and correction of a kyphotic deformity and facilitates insertion of the bone graft, which is then seated under compression. This enables the construct to share the load with the graft and prevents graft failure. Tricortical iliac struts have been shown to fail under loads applied to this area of the spine. Alternative grafts (e.g., allograft fibula) are structurally stronger but are slow to become vascularized.

The Kostuik-Harrington device (Fig. 301-4) has been used extensively, and excellent results have been reported in the treatment of kyphotic and flat-back deformities, symptomatic pseudarthrosis, and burst fractures.[17] Complications have been reported but appear to be within acceptable limits without reported vascular or neurological complications.[18]

Dunn Device

Dunn's clinical experience with thoracolumbar trauma demonstrated that anterior decompression and internal fixation could produce superior neurological recovery. In the early 1980s he produced a series (Dunn type I, type II, and type III) of anterior internal fixation devices. Vascular complications, thought to be related to the devices' high profile, resulted in their recall from the commercial market.

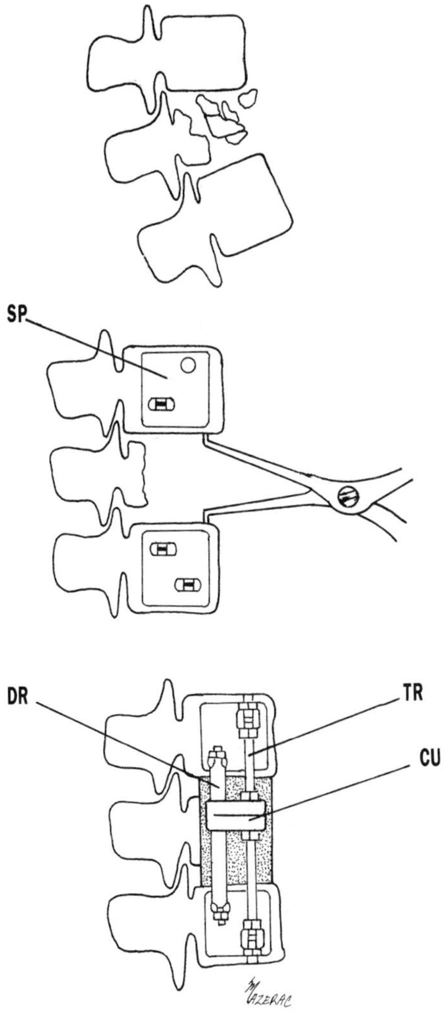

Figure 301-3 Slot-Zielke device. While the dual-rod construct is illustrated, the device may be used with only a single rod. Used mainly for the correction of kyphotic deformities, the device resembles both the Kostuik-Harrington device and the Kaneda device. *SP,* staple plate; *TR,* threaded rod; *DR,* dual rod; *CU,* cross connector.

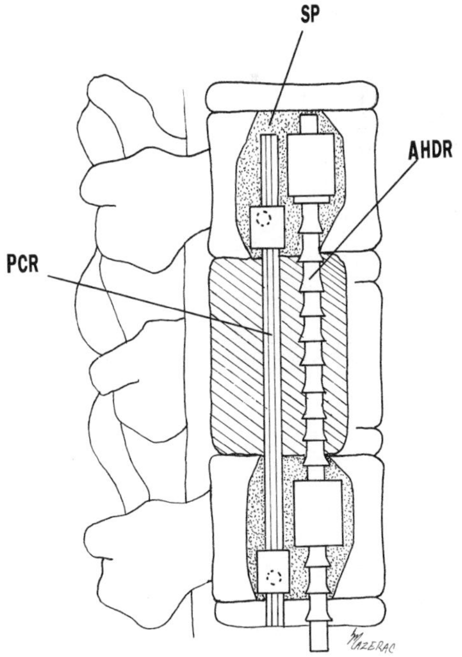

Figure 301-4 Kostuik-Harrington device. An anterior Harrington distraction rod *(AHDR)* is installed and used to reduce kyphosis after corpectomy or discectomy. Graft insertion is facilitated. A posterior Harrington compression rod *(PCR)* is added to the construct to increase stability. The rods are connected to screws which pass through staple-plates *(SP)* and into the vertebral body. Use of the device from T2 to L5 and an extensive clinical experience in the treatment of burst fractures and various kyphotic deformities has been reported.

Kaneda Device

Posterior distraction has been used to treat burst fractures. However, reduction of canal fragments is not always achieved by ligamentataxis. In 1988, Gertzbein et al. reported success with combined anterior decompression and grafting followed by posterior stabilization with Harrington rods (three levels above and two levels below).[9] While efficacious, this technique involves two surgical incisions and fusion over at least five motion segments. Kaneda reasoned that anterior decompression and anterior internal fixation could insure neural decompression under direct visualization, involve less surgery, and require fusion over fewer levels. Encouraged by his success with the Kostuik-Harrington construct, he developed the Kaneda device (Fig. 301-5). This device provides distractive and compressive capabilities as well as anterior internal fixation and load-sharing with an anterior graft.[14]

The device consists of two tetra spikes that are applied to the vertebral body after decompression has been accomplished. Two screws are placed through each plate, and bicortical purchase is obtained. A distractive force can then be applied with a spreader to correct kyphosis. Insertion of a tricortical iliac graft is facilitated. The screw heads accept threaded rods, which are secured with nuts. Two rods form a trapezoid with the anterior base longer than the posterior base. Tightening the nuts applies compression to the graft and promotes fusion. The rods are coupled with a transverse fixator forming a construct which biomechanically compares favorably to the stability imparted by posterior instrumentation systems.[10] Excellent results have been reported in the treatment of burst fractures.[15]

In the hands of experienced surgeons, complications are few and consist mainly of pseudarthrosis and breakage of screws and rods. No vascular or neurological complications have been reported in over 300 cases.[14]

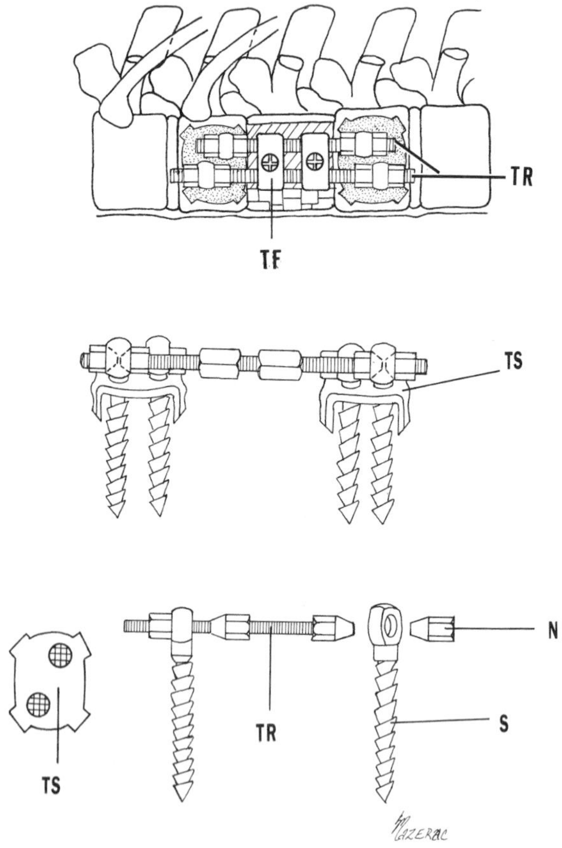

Figure 301-5 Kaneda device. The dual threaded rod *(TR)* design allows for distraction and compression while the transverse fixators *(TF)* couple the rods and increase stability. Bicortical screw *(S)* penetration is required. The device has been used extensively and has been recommended for anterior reconstruction following corpectomy or discectomy. A standardized technique and array of instruments facilitate surgery. *TS,* tetra spike; *N,* nut.

Plate Devices

DCP Plate

The principles of long bone internal fixation have been adapted to spinal surgery. Anterior plate fixation with large DCP plates (Fig. 301-6) has been used to impart stability to the anterior spinal column following trauma or surgical decompression. The plate functions as a tension band in extension and a buttress plate in flexion. Plates are applied through standard surgical approaches to the thoracic or lumbar spine. Bicortical penetration is required because screw back-out is the primary mechanism of failure. Early reports of this technique were favorable, and the development of numerous anterior plating systems followed.[23]

Synthes I Plate

In 1988, Yuan et al. developed a plate that afforded more resistance to rotation than did the standard AO/ASIF DC plate (Fig. 301-7).[26] The 3-mm thick plates are of variable length, have a curvature of 60 degrees and accept four 6.5-mm cancellous screws of varying lengths. The necks of the screws are smooth at the plate interface, fit flush, and provide a friction slip fit. This design minimizes screw back-out as well as providing a low plate and screw profile. This low profile and decreased risk of vascular injury are

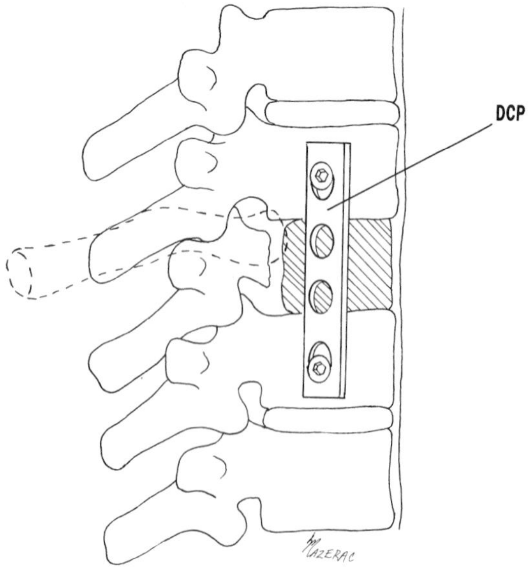

Figure 301-6 DCP plate. This long bone plate can be applied to the thoracolumbar spine anteriorly following corpectomy and grafting. The plate serves as a tension band, and bicortical screw purchase is desirable. Poor rotational stability is achieved and a strong cortical graft is required to prevent late kyphosis. This construct was the forerunner of all plate devices.

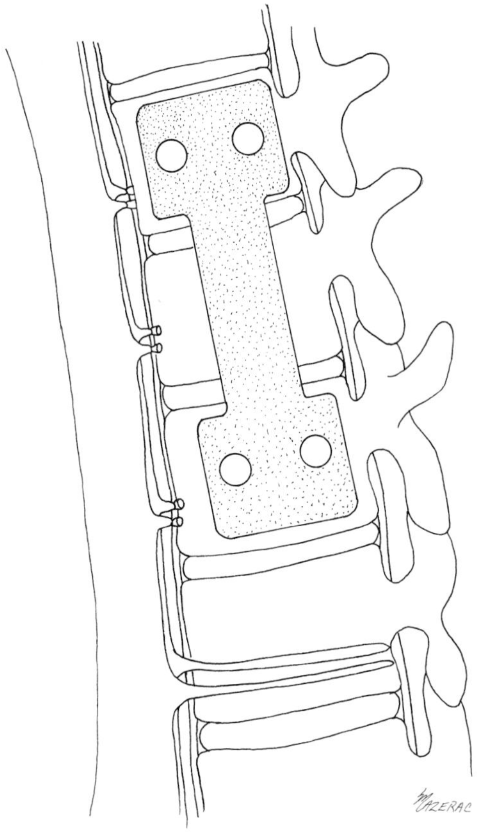

Figure 301-7 I plate. Essentially a modified DCP plate, the portion of the plate overlying intact vertebral bodies was enlarged to accept additional screws and increase stability. Bicortical screw purchase is required and this device, like most plate constructs, serves as a neutralization plate. Screws are not truly fixed to the plate, but are coupled by a friction-slip fit.

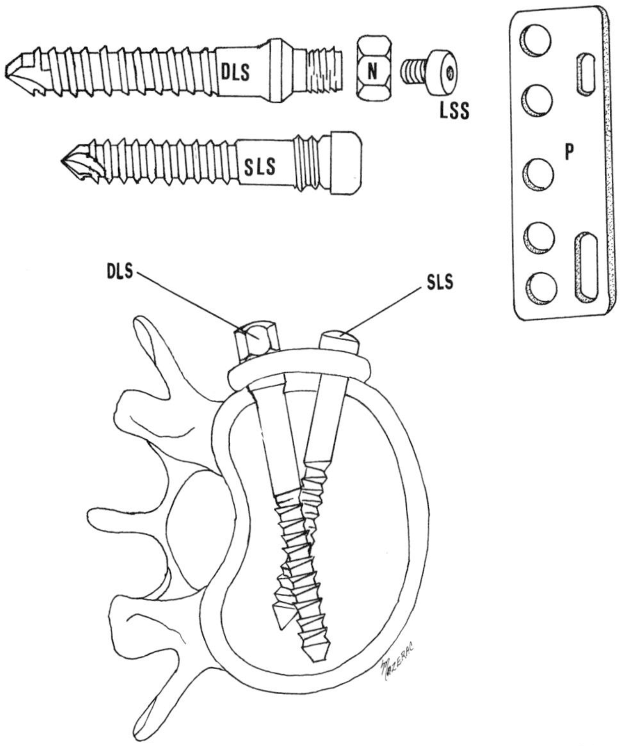

Figure 301-8 ALPS plate. Unlike other plate constructs, this device does not require bicortical screw placement. Two different screw types are used to secure the plates. The double-locking screws *(DLS)* have a metal-metal interface and are secured with a nut *(N)* and locking set-screw *(LSS)* through the elliptical holes in the plate *(P)*. The self-locking screws *(SLS)* pass through the round hole in the plate, and threads on the screw neck secure it to the plate. As with most plates, correction of kyphosis must be obtained with vertebral body spreaders following corpectomy.

the main advantage of the I plate as compared to rod systems. Biomechanical studies in a burst fracture model showed the I plate to be as stable as the intact spine in axial rotation.[19] Increased stability was seen in flexion, extension, and lateral bending. The developers of this device recommend its use from T11 to L5. Thoracolumbar neoplasms (both primary and metastatic) with anterior column involvement and unstable burst injuries are the main indication for this device.

Anterior Locking Plate Systems (ALPS)

This plate system differs from those previously described in that bicortical screw penetration is not required (Fig. 301-8). Seven-mm double-locking screws are placed posteriorly, and a constrained screw and plate interface is formed. A nut and set-screw secure this construct and help prevent screw back-out. Smaller 6-mm self-locking screws are then placed anteriorly and are affixed to the plate by threads just below the screw head. These screws do not require additional securing nuts or set-screws. The plates are available in straight and contoured designs to allow for vertebral malalignment. Also available are notched plates that prevent sacral impingement when used at the L5 level. Few biomechanical data are presently available on the system, and published results of clinical studies are not currently available.

The Contoured Anterior Spinal Plate (CASP)

This device has its origin in the AO femoral plate. Armstrong[1] believed that additional points of fixation and a stronger plate were needed (Fig. 301-9). He contoured the end of the plate to prevent impingement on iliac vessels when the plate is used at lower levels. The present device is 0.5 cm thick and 2.5 cm wide. Various lengths are available. The plate is fixed to the vertebral bodies using 6.5-mm cancellous screws and bicortical penetration.

Biomechanical testing in a burst fracture model has been conducted, and the CASP device performed similarly to the AO/ASIF plates in axial and torsional stiffness. The CASP device was superior in axial stiffness when compared with the Zielke and Kostuik devices.[3] Clinical results are limited but appear to be favorable for this device.[4]

Z Plate

This system shares characteristics with the ALPS system in that bolts and screws are used to secure the plate to the vertebral bodies (Fig. 301-10). Advantageous design features include (1) distraction instruments that assist in the reduction of kyphosis; (2) titanium construction and improved postoperative imaging with both computed tomography (CT) and magnetic resonance imaging (MRI); (3) compression capability for seating the graft and

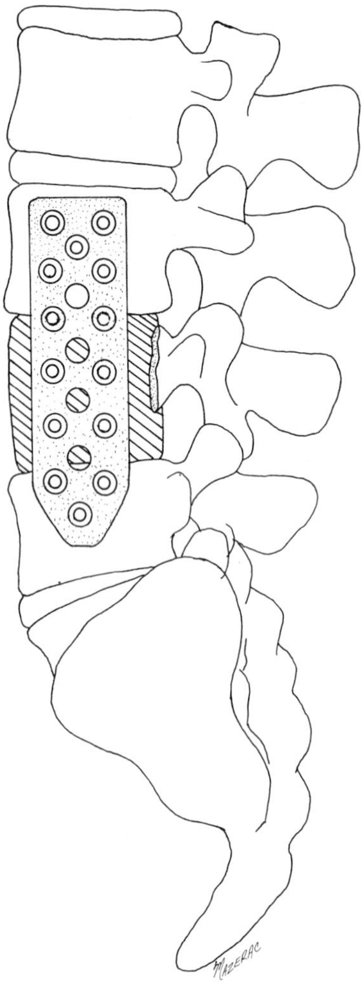

Figure 301-9 CASP plate. A low flush profile of plate and screws is the hallmark of this device. Bicortical screw purchase is required, and placement of more than two screws per level is desirable. A modified plate with a tapered end is available for use at L5.

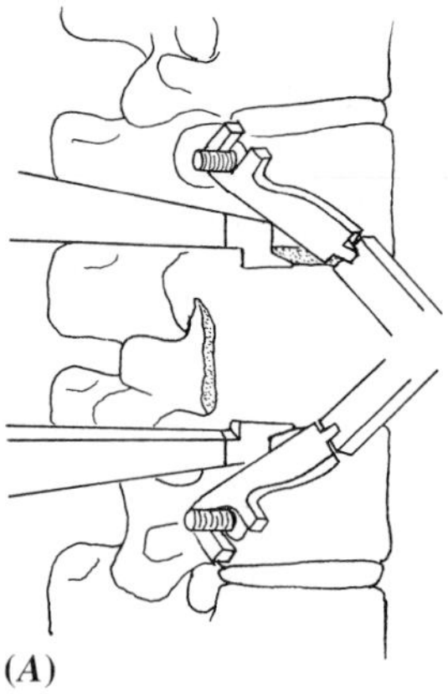

(*A*)

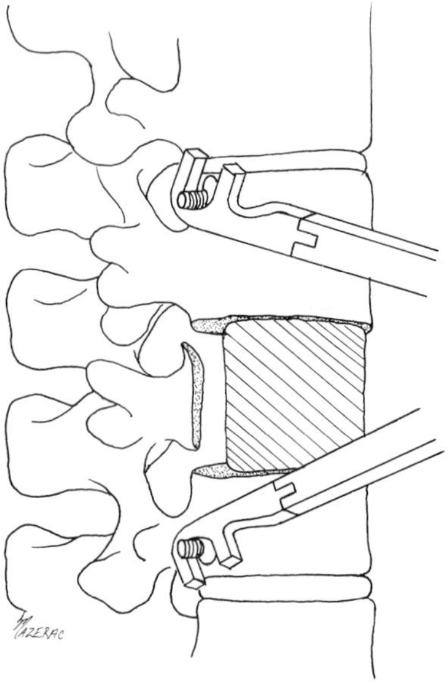

(*B*)

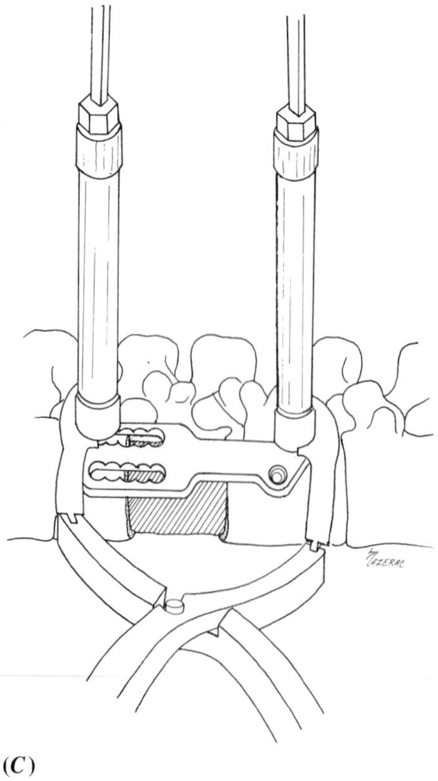

(*C*)

Figure 301-10 Z plate. Unlike other plate devices, this system provides distraction and compression. *A, B.* Posteriorly, plate bolts accept a distractor that corrects kyphosis and facilitates graft placement. The metal-metal interface is similar to the ALPS design. *C.* Scalloped slots allow for application of compression prior to final tightening of the nuts. Anterior screws are then placed; as with the posterior bolts, bicortical purchase is achieved. The system is made of titanium and provides improved postoperative CT and MRI visualization. The device is easily applied from T9 to L5 and maintains a low profile. It is currently my system of choice.

enhancing fusion; (4) low-profile smooth surface to minimize risks of vascular injury.

The various-sized plates can accommodate multiple level decompression. After decompression, posterior bolts (7 mm) are placed in the superior and inferior vertebra using a template. Bolts are angled anteriorly (10 degrees) to avoid any possible canal impingement. Bicortical purchase is desirable, and a constrained construct between the bolt and plate is formed. Correction of kyphosis can be obtained using a distractor. Insertion of the graft is facilitated. The appropriate plate is applied (5 to 13 cm) and hex nuts are used to secure the plate and bolt assembly. Compression is then applied to seat the graft; final tightening of the hex nuts secures the construct. Anterior screws (6 mm) are implanted with up to 10 degrees of posterior angulation, and again bicortical penetration is required.

Although this system holds promise, few clinical data are currently available. These plates are difficult to use above T9. Z plates for use above T9 will have to be made smaller and given a greater radius of curvature.

Interbody Devices

Rezaian Device

This device is basically an interbody distractor (Fig. 301-11). It is impaled into the endplates of the vertebral body above and below by the distractive force generated by a cellar-jack mechanism. It is available in three sizes, is made of surgical stainless steel, and serves as a vertebral body replacement. The size of the device limits room for graft material.

Limited biomechanical or clinical data are available.[22] The device is advocated as a vertebral body replacement in the treatment of burst fractures or metastatic disease of the spine.

Titanium (Moss) Cage

Constructed of titanium mesh formed into a cylinder, this device is available in variable diameters and lengths and serves as a support following decompression (Fig. 301-12). While not actually an interbody distractor, this device is packed with autologous bone, serving both as a graft and as an interbody support. Favorable clinical results in over 100 cases of tumor resection have been reported. Personal clinical experience suggests that results with this construct are at least comparable to those of a tricortical iliac autograft. Decreased donor site complications, improved availability, and indefinite shelf-life make it desirable compared with allograft. MRI and CT after surgery are excellent owing to the titanium construction.

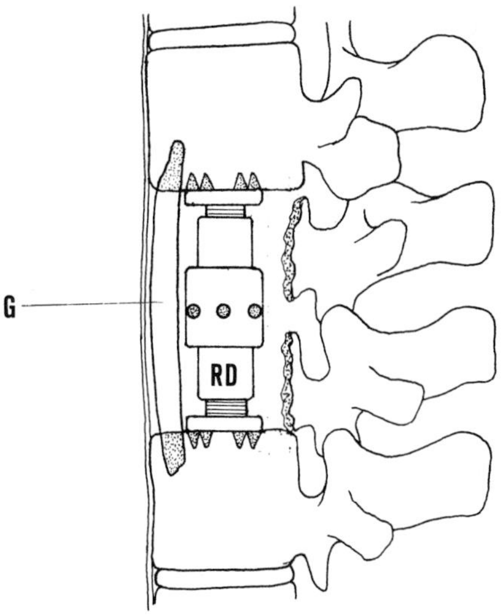

Figure 301-11 Rezaian device. This expanding device *(RD)* operates like a cellar-jack and serves as an interbody distractor. Its size leaves little room for graft *(G)* material and its stainless steel construction interferes with CT and MRI.

Complications

Complications encountered in the implantation of anterior and anterolateral fixation devices of the thoracic and lumbar spine may be separated into categories, as shown in Table 301-2. The reader is referred to texts that discuss the subject of complications in detail.[8,12]

In addition to the complications listed in Table 301-2, several other issues deserve special attention. These include (1) the role of preoperative angiography; (2) hardware breakage (early vs. late); and (3) infection.

TABLE 301-2 Complications of Anterior Fixation Devices

Surgical Approach (General)	
	Inadequate exposure
	Wrong level
	Vascular injury/hemorrhage
	Secondary ischemic injury
	Direct neural injury
	Associated structural injury
	Iatrogenic instability
	Infection
Regional Specific Complications	
Cervicothoracic	
	Recurrent laryngeal/superior laryngeal nerve injury
	Tracheoesophageal injury
	Thoracic duct injury
	Carotid artery injury
Thoracic	
	Intercostal neuralgia
	Dural laceration
	CSF pleural effusion
	Pulmonary injury
	Direct spinal cord injury
	Secondary ischemic injury
Lumbar	
	Lumbar plexopathy
	Left iliac vein injury
	Sympathetic injury—retrograde ejaculation
	Injury to intraperitoneal structures
Graft Complications	
	Fracture
	Extrusion
	Pseudarthrosis
Instrumentation	
	Loosening
	Breakage

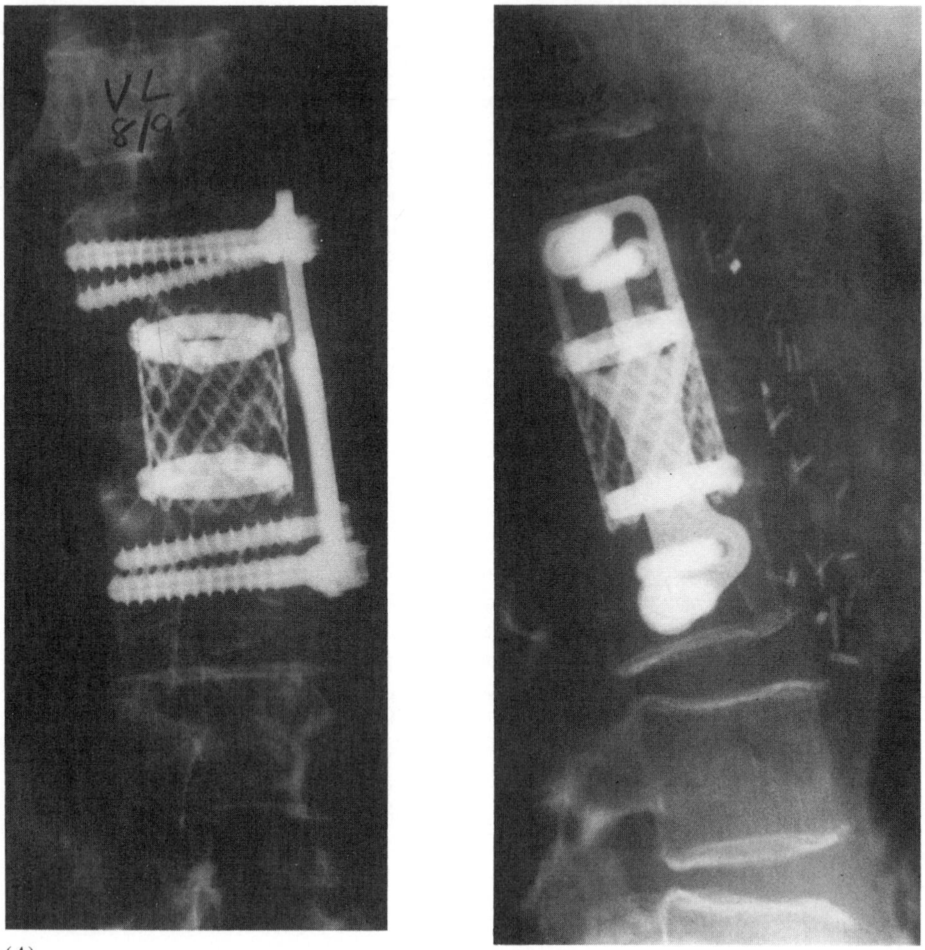

(*A*) (*B*)

Figure 301-12 Moss cage. Not technically an anterior fixation device, the cage serves as an interbody distractor. When packed with cancellous bone, it provides structural support for the graft material. Personal experience shows that this device can support applied loads in the thoracolumbar area when it is supplemented with anterior plates. Titanium construction allows for good postoperative imaging *(A, B)*.

Preoperative Angiography

Arterial arcades provide significant anastomosis for segmental arteries, including the artery of Adamkiewicz. Preservation of this vessel does not completely prevent ischemic injury, nor does sacrifice of this vessel routinely result in ischemic injury.[5] Routine angiography is not performed in patients undergoing anterior decompression and internal fixation. Of course, complicated cases still may benefit from angiography.

Hardware Breakage

While early dislodgement or breakage usually is an indication for revision surgery, late breakage does not always mandate revision. Because of the differences in the modulus of elasticity between bone and metal implants, breakage secondary to micromotion may occur within a solid fusion mass. Only patients with symptomatology that can be explained by hardware failure should be considered for revision.

Infection

Implantation of a foreign body always carries an increased risk of infection. This holds true with anterior thoracic and lumbar instrumentation. Meticulous surgical technique and keeping operating time as short as possible should result in minimizing infection rates. Prophylactic antibiotics, while commonly used, are no substitute for good surgical technique. It should also be recognized that infection does not necessarily mandate removal of hardware. Closed irrigation and appropriate antibiotic therapy can prove adequate. Careful postoperative patient assessment is necessary because early diagnosis of infection is important.

Summary

Anterior decompression of the thoracic and lumbar spine may be accomplished via several surgical approaches. Anterior decompression can be accomplished under direct visualization, thus insuring adequacy of decompression. Internal fixation offers the possibility of immediate postoperative stability, restoration of normal alignment, improved fusion rates, early patient mobilization with decreased pain, and fewer complications associated with prolonged inactivity. The combination of anterior decompression with anterior internal fixation offers the additional benefit of a single surgical procedure and a potentially shorter hospital stay.

Although attractive, these potential benefits must be weighed against inherent surgical risks. Furthermore, prospective well-controlled studies must be undertaken to prove the efficacy of these techniques compared with alternatives. It should be remembered that most presently available data are anecdotal and retrospective. Certainly, a given patient's treatment should be individualized, and surgeons should be reluctant to abandon time-tested techniques with proven results. In the final analysis there is no substitute for good clinical judgment. Unfortunately, this comes only after making bad clinical judgments and learning from them.

References

1. Armstrong GWD, Chow D. The contoured anterior spinal plate. In An HS, Cotler JM (eds): *Spinal Instrumentation.* Baltimore: Williams & Wilkins, 1992, pp 379–396.
2. Been HD. Anterior decompression and stabilization of thoracolumbar burst fractures by the use of the Slot-Zielke device. *Spine* 1991; 16:70–77.
3. Bone LB, Johnson CE II, Ashman RB, et al. Mechanical comparison of anterior spinal instrumentation in a burst fracture model. *J Orthop Trauma* 1988; 2:195–201.
4. Chow DM, Armstrong GWD, Feibel R, et al. The contoured anterior spinal plate: design, rationale and results of the first 25 cases. Presented at the Scoliosis Research Society Meeting, Honolulu, 1990.
5. Crock HV, Yoshizawa H. *The Blood Supply of the Vertebral Column and Spinal Cord in Man.* New York: Springer-Verlag, 1977.
6. Dwyer AF. Anterior instrumentation for scoliosis. *J Bone Joint Surg [Br]* 1970; 52-B:782 (abstr).
7. Dwyer AF, Schafer MF. Anterior approach to scoliosis: results of treatment in fifty-one cases. *J Bone Joint Surg [Br]* 1974; 56-B:218–224.
8. Garfin SR (ed). *Complications of Spine Surgery.* Baltimore: Williams & Wilkins, 1989.
9. Gertzbein SD, Court-Brown CM, Jacobs RR, et al. Decompression and circumferential stabilization of unstable spinal fractures. *Spine* 1988; 13:892–895.
10. Gurr KR, McAfee PC, Shih CM. Biomechanical analysis of anterior and posterior instrumentation systems after corpectomy. A calf-spine model. *J Bone Joint Surg [Am]* 1988; 70-A:1182–1191.
11. Hodgson AR, Stock FE. Anterior spinal fusion: a preliminary communication on the radical treatment of Pott's disease and Pott's paraplegia. *Br J Surg* 1956; 44:266–275.
12. Horowitz NH, Rizzoli HV (eds). *Postoperative Complications of Extracranial Neurological Surgery.* Baltimore: Williams & Wilkins, 1987.
13. Humphries AW, Hawk WA, Berndt AL. Anterior interbody fusion of lumbar vertebrae: a surgical technique. *Surg Clin North Am* 1961; 41:1685–1700.
14. Kaneda K. Kaneda anterior spinal instrumentation for the thoracic and lumbar spine. In An HS, Cotter JM (eds): *Spinal Instrumentation.* Baltimore: Williams & Wilkins, 1992, pp 413–433.
15. Kaneda K, Abumi K, Fujiya K. Burst fractures with neurologic deficits of the thoracolumbar-lumbar spine. Results of anterior decompression and stabilization with anterior instrumentation. *Spine* 1984; 9:788–795.
16. Kostuik JP. Anterior spinal cord decompression for lesions of the thoracic and lumbar spine: techniques, new methods of internal fixation, results. *Spine* 1983; 8:512–531.
17. Kostuik JP. Anterior Kostuik-Harrington distraction system for the treatment of kyphotic deformities. *Iowa Orthop J* 1988; 8:68–77.
18. Kostuik JP. Anterior Kostuik-Harrington distraction systems. In An HS, Cotler JM (eds): *Spinal Instrumentation.* Baltimore: Williams & Wilkins, 1992, pp 359–377.
19. Mann KA, McGowan AP, Fredrickson BR, et al. A biomechanical investigation of short segment spinal fixation for burst fractures with varying degrees of posterior disruption. *Spine* 1990; 15:470–478.
20. Moe JH, Purcell GA, Bradford DS. Zielke instrumentation (VDS) for the correction of spinal curvature: analysis of results in 66 patients. *Clin Orthop* 1983; 80:133–153.
21. Müller ME, Allgower M, Schneider R, Willenegger (eds): *Manual of Internal Fixation,* 3d ed. New York: Springer-Verlag, 1991.
22. Rezaian SM, Dombrowski ET, Ghista DN. Spinal fixator for the management of spinal injury (the mechanical rationale). *Eng Med* 1983; 12:95–97.
23. Ryan MD, Taylor TKF, Sherwood AA. Bolt-plate fixation for anterior spinal fusion. *Clin Orthop* 1986; 203:196–202.
24. Simmons EH, Sue A, Quan EA, et al. An analysis of Dwyer instrumentation of the spine with assessment of its place in spinal surgery. *J Bone Joint Surg [Br]* 1977; 59-B:117 (abstr).
25. Trammell TR, Benedict F, Reed D. Anterior spine fusion using Zielke instrumentation for adult thoracolumbar and lumbar scoliosis. *Orthop Trans* 1989; 13:506 (abstr).
26. Yuan HA, Mann KA, Found EM, et al. Early clinical experience with the Syracuse I-plate: an anterior spinal fixation device. *Spine* 1988; 13:278–285.

302

Injuries to the Sacrum and Pelvis

Carlos A. David
Barth A. Green

The first reported case of a fracture of the sacral spine is attributed to Malgaigne in 1847,[15] and the first series and classification system was presented by Bonnin in 1945.[2] Despite these historical reports, injuries of the sacrum and its neural elements have been considered an unusual medical rarity. These significant injuries and their commonly associated neurological deficits have until now received relatively little attention. However, with the recent publication of several large series,[4,24] sacral fractures have emerged as a significant and important clinical problem.

Sacral fractures are frequently associated with significant pelvic and visceral injury and are commonly seen in the multiply injured trauma patient. These patients often have acute injuries so severe that the early diagnosis of a sacral injury is precluded. In the past many of these patients have succumbed to their massive injuries; however, with the advent of modern trauma networks and advances in the care of the acutely injured patient, the prognosis is now more favorable. Consequently, there has been a relative increase in the number of sacral injuries brought to treatment. Increased awareness and knowledge of sacral injuries on the part of the neurological surgeon is therefore necessary if we are to meet the challenge of these relatively uncommon but complex injuries.

Epidemiology

Most of the available information on sacral fractures is based on small series and case reports, hence the true incidence is unknown. However, it is generally accepted that sacral fractures compromise somewhere around 1 percent of all spine fractures.[7] These fractures, as already stated, are commonly associated with pelvic fractures.[21] Studies report that the incidence of sacral fractures associated with pelvic fractures lies somewhere between 4 and 74 percent.[2,4,20,28] However, one must recall that many of these fractures are missed during the treatment of the severely injured patient. Denis et al.[4] reported in their series of 236 cases that the diagnosis of sacral fracture on admission was made in only 50 percent of the patients with sacral fracture. Other studies have reported as many as 61 percent of sacral fractures missed on admission.[14,19]

The incidence of neurological deficit associated with sacral fractures also has yielded a wide range of statistics. Gibbons et al.[8] reported an incidence of 34 percent; others have reported rates of 22 to 60 percent.[4,24,25] A neurological deficit associated with injury to the pelvis is less common. Reported ranges in the literature vary from 0.75 to 11 percent,[3,9,29] with the occurrence of deficit being more prevalent in pelvic fractures that involve the sacrum.

Most sacral fractures are due to indirect trauma as the result of motor vehicle accidents. These indirect injuries occur when biomechanical forces are exerted on the sacrum through the pelvis or lumbar spine.[25] However, direct trauma to the sacral area also can result in injury. The most common cause of direct injury is gunshot wounds, although hard falls and blows to the sacral region also have been cited.[25]

Classification

Since the publication of Bonnin's scheme for the classification of sacral fractures in 1945,[2] a variety of other systems have been proposed and used. Of the many systems, the classifications of Schmidek et al.[25] and, more recently, Denis et al.[4] have been the most useful and most widely used.

Schmidek Classification of Sacral Fractures

The classification of Schmidek et al.[25] subdivides sacral injuries according to direct and indirect trauma (Table 302-1).

Direct Trauma

Under the heading of direct trauma, gunshot wounds account for the majority. These injuries result in various degrees of tissue and sacral damage. The majority are considered structurally stable, depending on the integrity of the sacrum and sacroiliac joints above the level of the S1 foramina.[25] Direct blunt trauma to the sacrum such as that occurring during falls or blows to the area comprise the remainder of the direct injuries. This mechanism usually results in a low transverse fracture of the sacrum (Fig. 302-1). Low transverse fractures occur when the distal sacrum acts as a lever arm below the level of fixation by the sacroiliac joints.[2,7,22,29] The fracture typically occurs below S3, most commonly through the foramina of S4.[25] Low transverse fractures are generally considered stable since the fracture segment is not involved in weight-bearing. Neurological injury occurs rarely with this type of fracture; however, since the fractured segment is usually displaced anteriorly, rectal perforation and cerebrospinal fluid leakage may occur.[22,29]

TABLE 302-1 Classification of Sacral Fractures

Direct Trauma	Indirect Trauma
Penetrating	Vertical
Low transverse	Lateral mass
	Juxta-articular
	Cleaving
	Avulsion
	High Transverse
	Type I
	Type II
	Type III

Source: Adapted from Schmidek et al.[25] and Roy-Camille et al.[23]

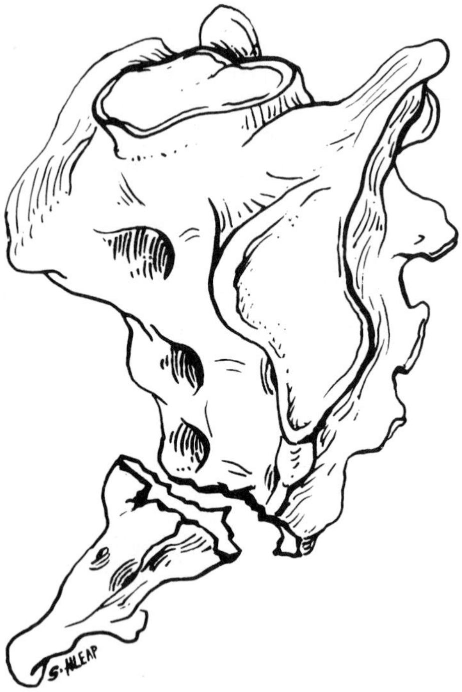

Figure 302-1 Low transverse sacral fracture.

Indirect Trauma

Indirect injuries represent by far the majority of sacral fractures. They are commonly associated with a neurological deficit arising from compression, avulsion, or stretching of sacral nerve roots.[2] Indirect injuries are the result of forces placed on the sacrum through the pelvis or lumbar spine; as such, they result in a wide variety of fracture types. These can be subclassified into two groups: *vertical fractures* and *high transverse fractures.*[25]

Vertical Fractures Vertical fractures are the largest group of fractures resulting from indirect trauma, and they always occur in association with a pelvic fracture. They are named to emphasize the general vertical orientation of the fracture lines. Vertical fractures have been further subdivided into four different patterns: lateral mass fractures, juxta-articular fractures, cleaving fractures, and avulsion fractures (Fig. 302-2).[25] The lateral mass fracture typically begins in the superior sacral notch (site of S1 fusion with the sacral ala) and extends through the sacral foramina of that side. Juxta-articular fractures occur in the lateral mass adjacent to the sacroiliac joint. Cleaving fractures arise in the superior sacral notch and extend inferiorly to the area of the coccyx. This fracture type may or may not involve one or more neural foramina. Avulsion type fractures occur at the site of insertion of the sacrotuberous and sacrospinous ligaments.

These vertical fractures are not uncommonly associated with a neurological deficit. Schmidek et al.[25] reported a 54 percent incidence of neurological deficit with vertical type fractures. This is most likely to be an L5 or S1 radiculopathy; however, plexopathies have been noted to occur. The stability of vertical sacral fractures is variable and is a function of the pattern and stability of the associated pelvic fracture. Three general patterns of pelvic fracture have been recognized. These include *anteroposterior compression, lateral compression,* and *vertical shear.* Essentially, all of these involve dual sites of pelvic ring discontinuity.

Anteroposterior compression injuries are the result of separation of the symphysis pubis in conjunction with disruption of the sacroiliac ligaments.[25] This pattern is most commonly associated with the cleaving or avulsion type of vertical fracture and is generally considered unstable.

The lateral compression pattern is the most common pattern of injury to the pelvic ring. This pattern is characterized by disruption of the symphysis pubis and inward rotation of the anterior hemipelvis.[25] This inward rotation creates tension on the posterior sacroiliac ligaments and a compressive force on the anterior sacroiliac joint and lateral mass of the sacrum. The resulting associated sacral fracture is the lateral mass or juxta-articular type of vertical fracture. This pattern is usually stable.

Vertical shear injuries usually occur when sudden deceleration forces applied to the lower extremities are transmitted to the pelvis. The injury commonly occurs with falls and motor vehicle accidents. This pattern is characterized by disruption of the pubic rami or symphysis pubis in conjunction with disruption of the posterior pelvic ring via injury to the sacrum, sacroiliac joint, or ilium.[25] This pelvic fracture pattern can be associated with any type of vertical sacral fracture, but is most commonly associated with the juxta-articular type. Owing to the complete disruption of the posterior pelvic ring, all vertical shear injuries are unstable.[25]

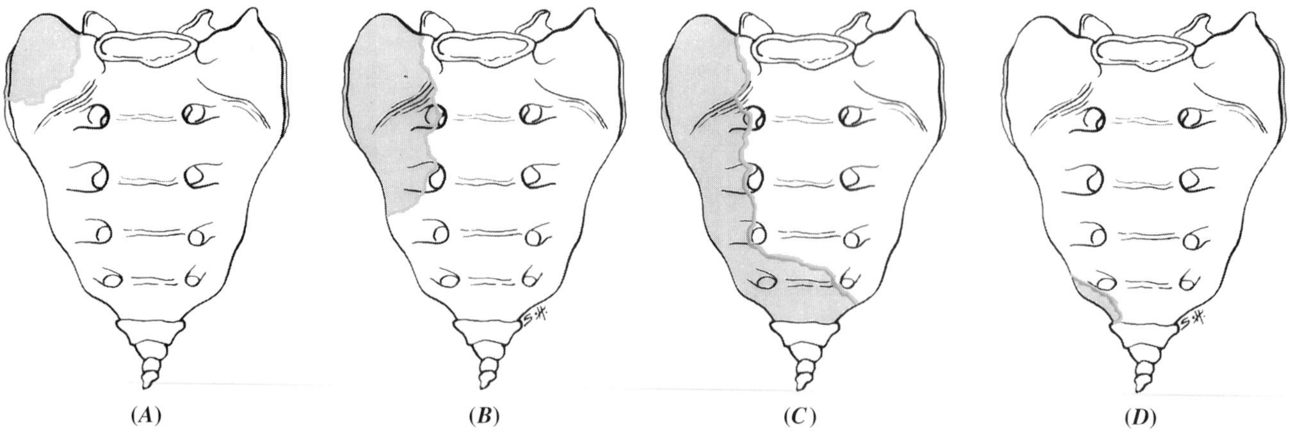

Figure 302-2 Four vertical fracture subtypes: (*A*) juxta-articular fracture, (*B*) lateral mass fracture, (*C*) cleaving fracture, (*D*) avulsion fracture.

High Transverse Fractures High transverse fractures make up a second group of indirect injuries. The mechanism for this type of fracture is the result of a flexion force being applied to a flexed lumbosacral spine (hip flexion) with the knees locked in extension.[18] The resultant fracture is characterized by a traumatic spondylolisthesis, most commonly at the level of the S1-S2 foramina (Fig. 302-3). High transverse fractures are extremely rare, comprising only 5 percent of all sacral fractures.[2,7,17,28] These fractures are considered unstable and are invariably associated with a neurological deficit.[25]

Roy-Camille et al.[23] have further subdivided high transverse fractures into three types (Fig. 302-3). Type I results when there is an anterior bend to the upper sacral fragment. Type II occurs when the upper sacral fragment is horizontally and posteriorly displaced relative to the lower segment, resulting in a lumbar kyphosis. Type III is characterized by anterior displacement of the upper fragment in front of the lower segment, resulting in a lumbar lordosis.

Denis Classification of Sacral Fractures

Denis et al.[4] devised a classification system based on the involvement of the sacral foramina and sacral canal. This modest classification scheme which allows prediction of neurological injury has gained in popularity, and is presently the most useful classification system available. This system divides the sacrum into three anatomic zones of injury (Fig. 302-4):

Zone I

Zone I injuries are fractures through the sacral ala and do not involve the sacral foramina or sacral canal. Injuries to this zone are generally due to lateral compression type forces on the pelvis with preservation of the posterior sacroiliac ligaments. They are typically stable injuries, and neurological injury is uncommon. Denis et al.[4] reported a 5.9 percent incidence of neurological deficit with injuries to Zone I. However, in a smaller series an incidence as high as 24 percent has been reported.[8]

Zone II

Zone II fractures involve one or more sacral foramina but do not involve the sacral canal. This type of fracture is analogous to the lateral mass fracture and cleaving fracture of Schmidek. As such, the stability of Zone II fractures is similarly dependent on the pattern of pelvic injury. Neurological injury associated with this type of fracture is not uncommon, as would be expected in view of the involvement of neural foramina. In one study, Zone II injuries were associated with a 28 percent incidence of neurological injury.[4]

Zone III

Zone III injuries comprise both vertical and transverse fractures that involve the sacral canal. The vertical subtype usually is associated with significant pelvic injury, and invariably there is a high degree of neurological injury. Denis et al.[4] reported an 87 percent incidence of neurological injury associated with a Zone III injury. A recent study by Gibbons et al.[8] looked at the incidence of neurological injury specifically with vertical and transverse Zone III injuries and found a 60 and 57 percent incidence, respectively.

Pattern of Neurological Injury

Depending on the specific type of sacral fracture and degree of pelvic involvement, different patterns of neurological injury may occur. These neurological deficits may be radiculopathic or may take the form of cauda equina or lumbar-sacral plexopathy syndromes. A review by Schmidek et al.[25] identified three patterns of neural lesions associated with sacral fractures. This study reported

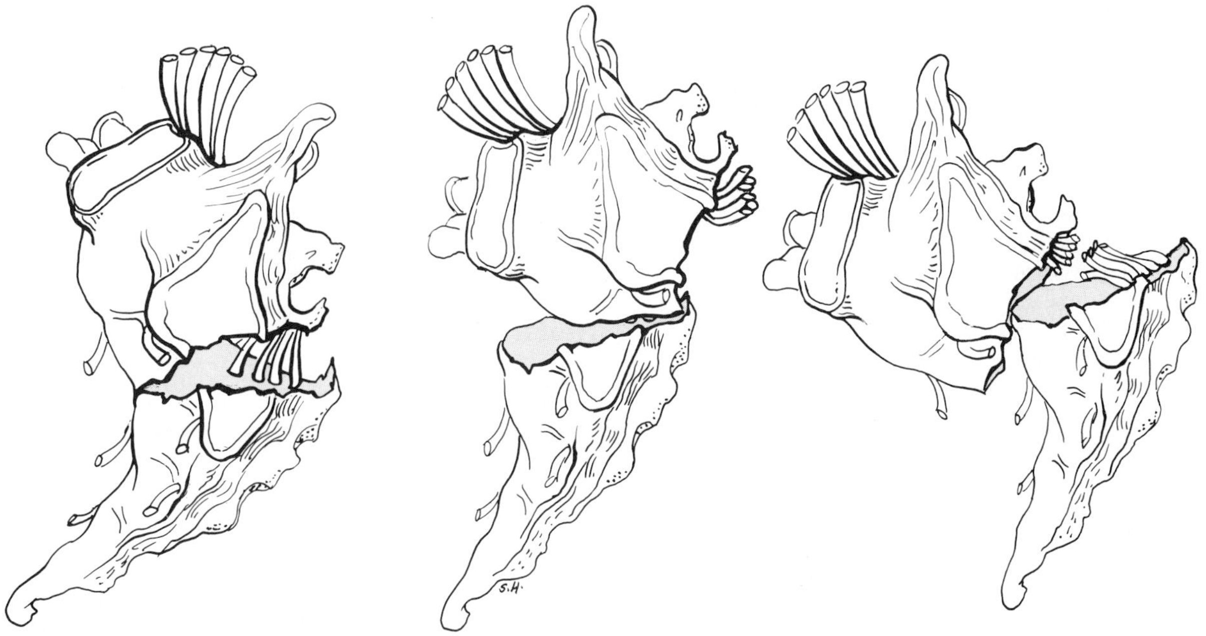

Figure 302-3 High transverse sacral fractures.

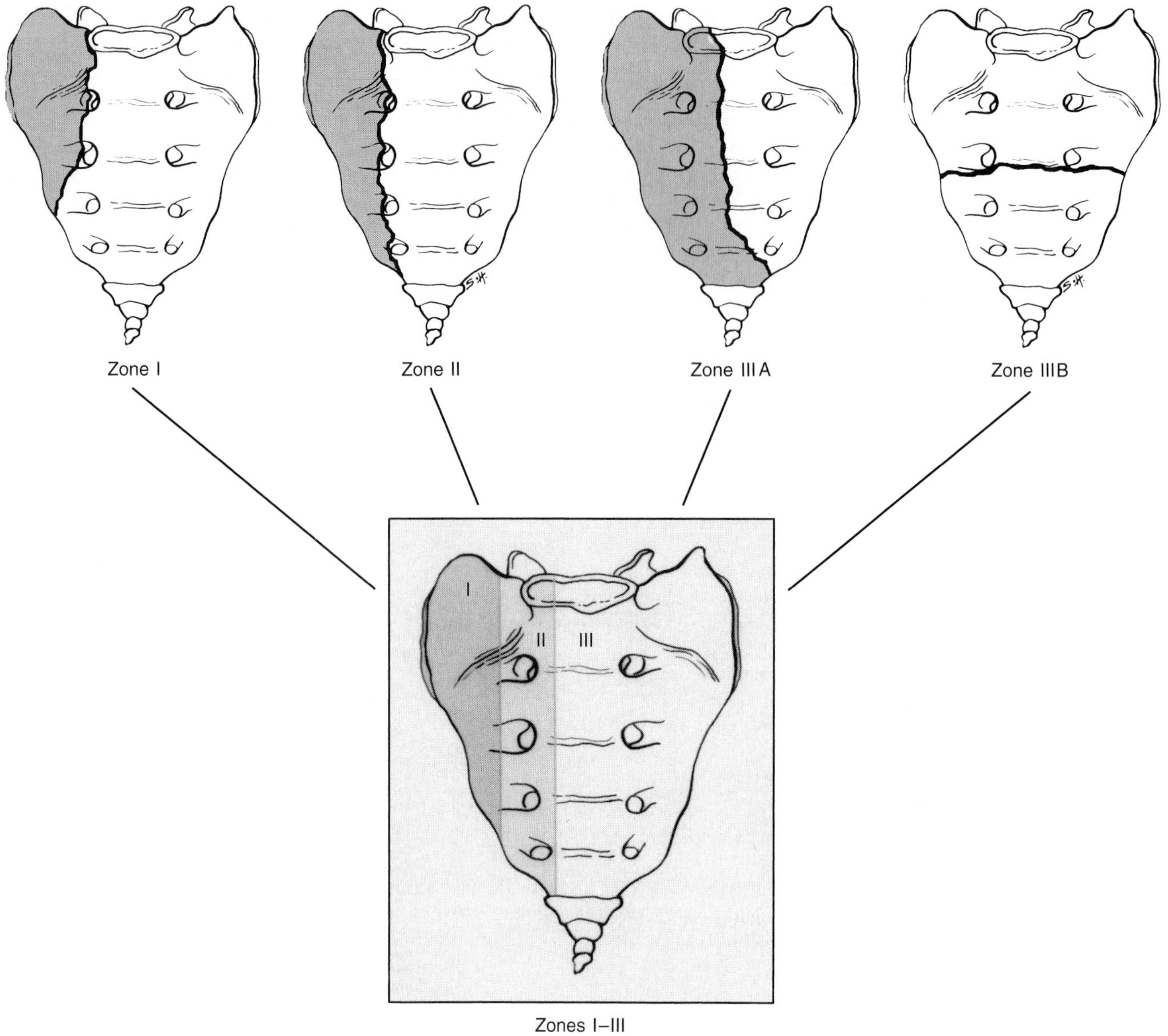

Figure 302-4 Classification of sacral fractures according to zones as defined by Denis et al.[4] (*inset*), and examples of different fracture patterns classified by zones.

a 50 percent incidence of nerve traction injuries, occurring most commonly at the lumbosacral trunk and superior gluteal nerves as they crossed the sacroiliac joints. Avulsions were the second most common pattern of injury, comprising 40 percent of the lesions in this study. The avulsions most commonly involved the cauda equina, the superior gluteal nerve, the obturator nerve, and the fifth lumbar nerve. Compression injuries accounted for 10 percent of this series and were observed at the ventral rami of S1 through S3.

Despite these patterns, it remains difficult to predict neurological deficits with specific patterns of sacral fracture. The popularity of the classification system brought forth by Denis et al.[4] is that it allows better prediction of the pattern of neurological injury with the specific sacral fracture zone. According to this system, Zone I injuries are rarely associated with neurological injury. However, when a Zone I fracture results in a significantly displaced sacral ala, an L5 root injury may occur. According to Denis, Zone II injuries resulted in a 28 percent incidence of neurological deficit; these comprised various patterns of L5, S1, and S2 nerve root injuries and cauda equina syndromes. Zone III injuries are commonly associated with a neurological injury. Depending on whether this is a high or low transverse fracture or a vertical fracture upper sacral or lower sacral root injury with significant bowel and bladder dysfunction will result.

Evaluation of Sacral Spine Injuries

Emergency Room Assessment

The initial management of the patient sustaining a possible pelvic or sacral injury should follow the fundamentals of trauma resuscitation. The first priority of treatment in the emergency room is stabilization of physiologic parameters and immobilization and stabilization of the spinal column in order to prevent and minimize secondary injury. The highest priority is the establishment of a secure airway to maintain oxygenation.

Of equal importance is the systemic circulatory status of the victim. Decreased perfusion to all critical organs, not just the central nervous system, must be avoided. Hypotension from a massive retroperitoneal hematoma is a well-known entity associated with pelvic fractures and must always be considered.

Once a reasonable degree of systemic stabilization is achieved, attention can be directed toward a thorough physical and spinal nervous system examination. If the patient requires emergency surgery for associated injuries, as complete a neurological assessment as possible in the time available should be performed. The definitions recommended by the American Spinal Injury Association (ASIA) should be followed.[1] The level and character of the injury should be ascertained. Accurate differentiation between complete and incomplete injuries is vital. Special attention should be given to any ecchymosis over the buttock, complaints of severe low back pain, deformity, rectal bleeding from perforation, and sacral pain on rectal examination. The neurological examination should include careful scrutiny of motor strength in the foot and ankle, sphincter strength and tone, and, if possible, assessment of sensory loss, particularly in the perineal region. Bulbocavernosus and anal wink reflexes also should be tested and the results recorded.

Although difficult in this setting, a history (as complete as possible) should be obtained. The mechanism of injury sometimes can be ascertained by noting the position and actual method of injury, and such information can be extremely helpful in raising clinical suspicion for a particular fracture type. Premorbid history, such as other medical problems, medication, allergies, and preexisting spinal problems should be obtained.

Neurological Assessment

The neurological sequelae of sacral-pelvic injuries can be quite varied, as delineated above. Careful neurological evaluation combined with a thorough knowledge of the expected deficits associated with a neural injury are prerequisites to accurate and timely diagnosis.

Injury to the L5, S1, and S2 nerve roots usually results in dermatomal sensory loss according to the particular nerve root(s) involved and various degrees of lower extremity weakness. If the injury occurs distally in the superior gluteal nerve, weakness of hip abduction and internal rotation will be found. A more proximal injury at the L5 nerve root results in weakness of the anterior tibial muscles and sensory changes over the medial dorsum of the foot and the anterolateral aspect of the calf. S1 nerve root injuries result in weakness of plantar flexion and sensory changes along the lateral aspect of the foot, as well as a diminished ankle jerk. The S2 nerve, although involved in the innervation of the leg muscles by way of the inferior gluteal and sciatic nerves, plays a minor role when compared to the S1 input to these same levels. Therefore, injury to the S2 nerve root usually does not manifest as sensorimotor changes to the extremity; but rather results in disorders of sexual and bowel and bladder function, for which S2 plays a major role. The S3 and S4 nerve roots also are involved in these functions. These roots, together with the S2 nerve root, form a major constituent of the pudendal nerve, subserving innervation to the external urethral and anal sphincters as well as sensation from the penis, labia majora, urethra, perianal region, and anal canal.

Bowel and bladder emptying, sexual potency, and ejaculation are coordinated by integrated input from the autonomic nervous system. Parasympathetic input arises from the ventral rami of S2–S4 and is distributed via the inferior hypogastric plexus. The sympathetic input to the inferior hypogastric plexus derives from the sacral splanchnic nerves of the S2 and S3 sympathetic ganglia located medial to the ventral foramina. Injury to these roots manifests as varying degrees of bowel, bladder, and sexual dysfunction. There is also resultant perianal hypesthesia, as well as loss of the anal wink reflex. Often this part of the examination is not performed, resulting in delayed diagnosis. The diagnosis is usually made days to weeks later when the patient complains of perineal numbness and difficulty with urination after removal of an indwelling catheter.

The S5 and Co1 nerve roots subserve minor functions, innervating the coccygeus muscle and supplying the skin over the coccyx with sensory innervation. Injury to these roots is easily overlooked owing to the minor resulting deficit.

Radiographic Evaluation

Because of the curve of the sacrum and the lordosis at the lumbosacral junction, the sacrum is poorly visualized on the standard anteroposterior pelvic radiograph used as the screening test when evaluating trauma victims. In addition, fecal material and intestinal gas further obscure anatomic details on the plain radiograph. Despite this, specific findings on a standard anteroposterior pelvic radiograph may suggest possible sacral injury and the need for further investigation.[2,5,12,14,19] These include: (1) fracture of a lower lumbar transverse process; (2) significant anterior pelvic fractures without evident posterior pelvic injury; (3) discontinuity or asymmetry of the sacral notch; (4) clouding of the trabecular pattern in the lateral sacral mass; and (5) irregularity in the arcuate lines (the thin horizontal arches that outline the sacral foramina) of the upper three sacral foramina.

More detailed visualization of the sacrum can be achieved with the x-ray beam projected 50 degrees cephalad; however, no single view on plain radiography will delineate all the anatomic features of the sacrum. Therefore, a lateral view that includes the coccyx, and anteroposterior as well as lateral pelvic tomograms are suggested when suspicion is high for a sacral fracture.

Computed tomography (CT) offers much better anatomic detail of the sacral canal and foramina and thus will provide much clearer delineation of most fracture patterns. Thin cuts and sagittal reconstructions should be obtained in order not to miss transverse fractures.[4,6,26,30] In these instances, plain lateral tomograms may be more conclusive.

The utility of sacral myelography is limited to the evaluation of neural injuries of S1 associated with transverse fractures at this level. This is due to the termination of the thecal sac at the level of S2. Despite these limitations, findings of meningeal diverticula or rupture of the subarachnoid space may suggest nerve root avulsions. Furthermore, foraminal compromise with nerve root impingement and the extent of sacral canal compromise can be ascertained. Experience with magnetic resonance imaging (MRI) has been limited, but this modality may prove very useful in evaluating soft tissues as well as neural involvement below S1.

Neurophysiologic Evaluation

A variety of neurophysiologic tests such as evoked potentials, electromyography, and urodynamics have become powerful adjuncts in the evaluation of sacral injuries. These studies can aid in localizing and determining the degree of injury to nerves, nerve plexi, and nerve roots.

Electromyography (EMG) and evoked potentials can be vital in localizing the area of injury and determining the long-term outlook for recovery. Areas of abnormality may reveal denervation changes such as positive sharp waves and fibrillation potentials. Because the paraspinal muscles are innervated by early branches off the primary rami, they provide important information when one attempts to determine the location of injury. If EMG reveals abnormalities in these muscles, the nerve injury must be located within the spinal canal, whereas normal EMG recordings from the paraspinal muscles suggest a peripheral nerve or plexus injury.[25] A good prognostic indicator is the concurrence of sacral root paralysis with normal EMG and normal nerve conduction studies. This pattern suggests a neuropraxic injury, which has a good prognosis for functional recovery. EMG has no diagnostic value during the acute phase of injury, and several weeks usually must pass before there is evidence of abnormality on EMG recordings. Furthermore, owing to its lack of motor representation for roots below S2, EMG is not useful in evaluating root injuries below that level.

Urodynamics in the form of cystometrography has provided a good way to assess damage to the conus medullaris and lower sacral roots, as made evident by detrusor paralysis, areflexia, and uninhibited sphincter relaxation.[25] Furthermore, this technique provides a means for monitoring neurological improvement and the status of a neurogenic bladder. Therefore, we advocate establishing a baseline and making subsequent serial measurements.

Treatment of Sacral Fractures

The definitive treatment of sacral fractures is based primarily on determining the pattern and stability of the associated pelvic fracture(s). Second, one must take into account the presence and extent of nerve injury. Both operative and nonoperative treatments have been proposed and used successfully in treating these injuries. Despite this, no large series comparing operative and nonoperative treatment strategies has been published to date, and the optimal method of treatment has yet to be determined.

Using the classification system of Denis et al.[4], basic recommendations for the logical evaluation and treatment of sacral fractures can be made, as follows.

Vertical Fractures of Zones I-III

Vertical fractures are always associated with pelvic ring fractures; therefore, treatment strategies are dictated by the extent of pelvic ring disruption, fragment displacement, and pelvic stability. Zone I fractures are usually associated with *lateral compression* type pelvic stability. These Zone I fractures are usually stable and have no associated neurological deficit. As long as the posterior sacroiliac ligaments are intact, the pattern is stable. These patients can be treated symptomatically, with early mobilization and weight-bearing on the uninjured side. If disruption of the posterior sacroiliac ligaments is present, the fracture must be considered unstable, and treatment consists of either internal fixation, external fixation, or bedrest.

If the associated pelvic fracture is of the *anteroposterior compression* pattern, stability is determined by the intactness of the sacrum and ileum and the integrity of the posterior sacroiliac ligaments. However, in practical terms, these fractures should be considered unstable; they require reduction and either external or internal fixation, which in turn will indirectly stabilize the sacrum.

When the *vertical-shear* pattern of pelvic fracture is present, the situation is life-threatening. This fracture pattern is usually associated with severe trauma and massive retroperitoneal hemorrhage, and as such necessitates emergent external stabilization of the pelvis. Definitive stabilization of the pelvis and the sacral injury is delayed until the patient is stable.

Definitive stabilization of the above described sacropelvic injuries consists of stabilizing the posterior pelvis, which will indirectly stabilize the sacral injury. With relatively undisplaced sacroiliac joint disruption, stability may be achieved by an anterior external fixation frame in conjunction with plating of the symphysis pubis when an associated symphysis diastasis is present.[27] This method requires bedrest while the injuries heal because it does not provide enough stabilization for weight-bearing.

Various operative methods are available for stabilization of sacropelvic injuries. These include anterior or posterior plating, Harrington's sacral bars, sacral screws placed through the ilium posteriorly into the sacral promontory, and fixation of the posterior iliac crests posterior to the sacrum, thus creating the "posterior tension band."[10,13,16] The incidence of nerve injury with these fracture patterns varies, as already described; however, these neurological injuries usually recover with fracture reduction.

Transverse Fractures of Zone III

Clinical experience with transverse Zone III fractures is limited and the optimal method of treatment remains controversial. These fractures comprise the low transverse and high transverse fractures already described. Low transverse fractures, which most commonly occur through S4, are considered stable. Such fractures are best treated symptomatically. Digital reduction through the rectum combined with 4 to 6 weeks of bedrest has been advocated.[11,29] The importance of bedrest must be stressed to allow adequate osseous healing and to prevent the development of a pseudarthrosis at the fracture site.[29]

High transverse fractures are uncommon and treatment options vary. These injuries are invariably associated with severe neurological deficits, many of which improve without surgical intervention.[24] However, when significant displacement exists in addition to a neurological deficit (as in type II and type III transverse fractures), surgical decompression and reduction should be contemplated. The surgical options include sacral laminectomy and foraminotomy to decompress the canal, or laminectomy with reduction and fixation. Roy-Camille et al.[23] recommend wide laminectomies over the sacrum and L5 level, followed by opening and reducing the fracture line, and finally fixation by a variety of methods—lumboiliac plates, lumbosacral plates with pedicle screws, or Harrington rod fixation. In addition, a posterolateral bony fusion is also recommended.

The neurological prognosis for high transverse fractures is variable. Schmidek et al.[25] described 15 patients with transverse fractures and neurological deficits, of whom 11 underwent operative decompression. All operated patients experienced neurological improvement; however, the four nonoperated patients showed improvement as well. Denis et al.[4] also reported eight cases, of whom five underwent surgical decompression with improvement when compared to the lack of improvement noted for the three treated nonoperatively.

The role and benefit of surgery in these fractures cannot be determined conclusively at the present time. Although the literature supports surgical decompression and reduction in a large number of cases, the information is sparse. More definitive recommendations will be forthcoming as experience with these rare fractures continues to accumulate.

References

1. American Spinal Injury Association. *Standards for Neurological Classification of Spinal Injury Patients*, 1989.
2. Bonnin JG. Sacral fractures and injuries to the cauda equina. *J Bone Joint Surg* 1945; 27:113–127.
3. Byrnes DP, Russo GL, Ducker TB, Cowley RA. Sacrum fractures and neurologic damage. *J Neurosurg* 1977; 47:459–462.
4. Denis F, Davis S, Comfort T. Sacral fractures: an important problem. Retrospective analysis of 236 cases. *Clin Orthop* 1988; 227:67–81.
5. Fardon D. Sacral fractures. *J Neurosurg* 1978; 48:316 (letter).
6. Fishman EK, Magid D, Brooker AF, Siegelman SS. Fractures of the sacrum and sacroiliac joint: evaluation by computerized tomography with multiplanar reconstruction. *South Med J* 1988; 81:171–177.
7. Fountain SS, Hamilton RD, Jameson RM. Transverse fractures of the sacrum: a report of six cases. *J Bone Joint Surg [Am]* 1977; 59-A:486–489.
8. Gibbons KJ, Soloniuk DS, Razack N. Neurological injury and patterns of sacral fractures. *J Neurosurg* 1990; 72:889–893.
9. Goodell CL. Neurological deficits associated with pelvic fracture. *J Neurosurg* 1966; 24:837–842.
10. Gunterberg B. Effects of major resection of the sacrum: clinical studies on urogenital and anorectal function and a biomechanical study on pelvic strength. *Acta Orthop Scand Suppl* 1976; 162:1–38.
11. Heckman JD, Keats PK. Fracture of the sacrum in a child. *J Bone Joint Surg [Am]* 1978; 60-A:404–405.
12. Jackson H, Kam J, Harris JH Jr, Harle TS. The sacral arcuate lines in upper sacral fractures. *Radiology* 1982; 145:35–39.
13. Kellam JF, McMurtry RY, Paley D, Tile M. The unstable pelvic fracture. Operative treatment. *Orthop Clin North Am* 1987; 18:25–41.
14. Laasonen EM. Missed sacral fractures. *Ann Clin Res* 1977; 9:84–87.
15. Malgaigne JF. *A Treatise on Fractures*. Philadelphia: Lippincott, 1859.
16. Mears DC, Fu FH. Modern concepts of external skeletal fixation of the pelvis. *Clin Orthop* 1980; 151:65–72.
17. Mendelman JP. Fractures of the sacrum: their incidence in fracture of the pelvis. *Am J Roentgenol* 1939; 42:100–103.
18. Nicoll EA. Fractures of the dorso-lumbar spine. *J Bone Joint Surg [Br]* 1949; 31-B:376–394.
19. Northrop CH, Eto RT, Loop JW. Vertical fracture of the sacral ala: significance of non-continuity of the anterior superior sacral foraminal line. *Am J Roentgenol* 1975; 124:102–106.
20. Patterson FP, Morton KS. Neurologic complications of fractures and dislocations of the pelvis. *Surg Gynecol Obstet* 1961; 112:702–706.
21. Pennal GF, Tile M, Waddell JP, Garside H. Pelvic disruption: assessment and classification. *Clin Orthop* 1980; 151:12–21.
22. Rowell CE. Fracture of the sacrum with hemisaddle anaesthesia and cerebro-spinal fluid leak. *Med J Aust* 1965; 1:16–19.
23. Roy-Camille R, Saillant G, Gagna G, Mazel C. Transverse fracture of the upper sacrum. Suicidal jumper's fracture. *Spine* 1985; 10:838–845.
24. Sabiston CP, Wing PC. Sacral fractures: classification and neurologic implications. *J Trauma* 1986; 26:1113–1115.
25. Schmidek HH, Smith DA, Kristiansen TK. Sacral fractures. *Neurosurgery* 1984; 15:735–746.
26. Soye I, Levine E, Batnitzky S, et al. Computed tomography of sacral and presacral lesions. *Neuroradiology* 1982; 24:71–76.
27. Tile M. *Fractures of the Pelvis and Acetabulum.* Baltimore: Williams & Wilkins, 1984.
28. Wakeley CPG. Fracture of the pelvis: an analysis of 100 cases. *Br J Surg* 1929; 17:22–29.
29. Weaver EN, England GD, Richardson DE. Sacral fracture: case presentation and review. *Neurosurgery* 1981; 9:725–728.
30. Whelan MA, Hilal SK, Gold RP, et al. Computed tomography of the sacrum: 2. Pathology. *Am J Neuroradiol* 1982; 3:555–559.

303 Penetrating Wounds of the Spine

Carlos A. David
Howard J. Landy
Barth A. Green

History

Much of the contemporary literature regarding penetrating spinal wounds (mostly gunshot injuries) presents analyses of neurosurgical and orthopedic military experience. The early literature concerning spinal missile injuries described poor outcomes and very high mortality rates. Cushing reported an overall mortality of 71.8 percent during World War I, with only patients with incomplete injuries surviving. Operative treatment consisted of debridement and decompressive laminectomy. However, the high operative mortality (62.2 percent) during World War I gave rise to much controversy regarding the optimal management of these injuries. Generally, it was thought that complete injuries should undergo only debridement of entrance and exit wounds, and that laminectomy should be reserved for those incomplete injuries displaying further neurological deterioration.[50]

This controversy persisted into World War II, leading Matson[35] to conclude that spinal cord injuries received less uniform treatment than any other type of injury during that war. Despite this lack of treatment uniformity, advances in resuscitation, antibiotics, and long-term care decreased the overall mortality rates to 7.4 to 14.5 percent.[21,23,25] Most surgeons, however, remained pessimistic regarding the prospects for neurological improvement with surgical treatment. Despite this bleak outlook, some surgeons began reporting improvement with surgical exploration and decompression.[35,37,50] Slowly, these views became more widespread, with the small chance of improvement in "some" patients justifying surgical treatment of "all" patients.

Operative exploration became the policy for all penetrating spinal injuries during the Korean conflict. Patients were reported to show significant neurological improvement and an operative mortality of 1 percent.[52] During the conflict in Vietnam, further advances in triage, rapid evacuation of casualties, and resuscitation allowed patients access to trauma and neurosurgical medical care quickly and efficiently.[27,28] Despite these advances, there were no reports of neurological improvement with surgical treatment of penetrating spinal injuries.

In the past three decades, there has been a steady increase in the incidence of penetrating spinal injuries in civilians. Most are gunshot injuries; stabbings and other penetrating injuries occur much less frequently in the United States. Civilian experience with these injuries has generated even less optimism than previous military reports.[24,31,46,47,57] However, with the advent of modern trauma networks, interdisciplinary trauma teams, and helicopter ambulances, more patients are receiving better treatment much sooner. This has improved the outlook for survival for severe trauma victims; however, the prognosis for significant neurological recovery remains uncertain. Consequently, it has become very important for neurosurgeons to familiarize themselves with the mechanisms of injury and the pathophysiology and current management of penetrating wounds of the spine.

Epidemiology

The incidence of penetrating spinal cord injuries has risen steadily over the past three decades. Data from the National Spinal Cord Injury Data Research Center, which compiled data from various regional spinal cord injury units, indicated that of 6014 cases of spinal cord injury between 1973 and 1981, 14 percent were penetrating injuries.[58] Seven hundred eighty-two (13 percent) were caused by gunshot wounds. In this series gunshot wounds were the third leading cause of spinal cord injury. Since most of these injuries are due to acts of violence, it is not surprising that they tend to occur in large metropolitan areas with high crime rates. In a series of 148 penetrating spinal injuries from Los Angeles, 135 were attributable to gunshot, 12 were due to stab wounds, and 1 was secondary to impalement after a fall.[58] Other less commonly reported mechanisms include penetrating glass injuries and acupuncture needles.[4,26] Therefore, in the United States gunshot wounds predominate, whereas stab wounds occur far more frequently outside the United States, with the largest number reported from South Africa.[32,39]

Ballistics

A basic understanding of firearms and ballistics is needed to appreciate the wounding capacity of gunshot wounds. Firearms exist with different sizes, muzzle velocities, and general uses. Light firearms, including handguns, rifles, and shotguns, are most commonly seen in civilian use. There is also a variety of bullets, some used exclusively by the military and others found commonly in civilian settings.

Bullets behave in different ways depending on their size, shape, composition, and velocity. With regard to size, bullets can be classified into three groups: large (45 caliber), medium (32 and 38 caliber, including 9 mm), and small (22 and 25 caliber). Caliber refers to the diameter in hundredths of an inch. One must understand the shape and composition of bullets to understand their behavior in air and tissue. The shape can vary from pointed to rounded, flat, or hollow. Sharp-pointed bullets are aerodynamically more efficient, enabling them to travel greater distances.[12] Bullets commonly are composed of lead and are ensheathed or jacketed with such materials as copper, nickel, or steel. The purpose of this jacketing is to maintain the shape of the bullet and to decrease the deformation that occurs when lead is exposed to heat and friction. This allows for further tissue penetration. The jacket may be left incomplete, allowing some deformation and mushrooming of the tip upon tissue impact and resulting in more tissue destruction.[11] To further this deformation, some bullets are hollowed at the tip. This adds the secondary advantage of rapid deceleration, ensuring that the bullet remains in the target and does not pass through, injuring bystanders.

Unlike military gunshot injuries, civilian gunshot wounds are produced by low-velocity weapons. Low-velocity bullets travel at speeds <1000 ft/s, whereas medium- and high-velocity bullets travel between 1000 and 2000 ft/s and >2000 ft/s, respectively.[11] This speed depends on the acceleration through the muzzle, which is limited by the size and powder charge of the bullet. The ratio of weight/charge is critical. For a given charge, a lighter bullet can be accelerated to higher velocities. Magnum shells have larger powder charges than standard bullets of the same caliber, thus increasing their velocity.

Once in flight, multiple destabilizing forces come to bear on the projectile.[25] These include: *yaw,* which is deviation from the longitudinal axis of motion, *tumble,* the rotation of the projectile around the center of mass, and *wobbling,* which is circular motion or spiraling around the center of mass. *Spin,* which is imparted to the projectile as it travels through the gun barrel, helps to stabilize its flight. This spin, however, is usually insufficient once the bullet enters tissue, resulting in tumbling of bullets within tissues.[25]

Pathophysiology

Owing to the complex bony structure of the spinal canal, the spinal cord is generally protected from injury. Except in the cervical spine, a significant amount of force is needed to damage the spinal cord. However, in penetrating injuries the protection afforded by the spinal column is breached by the sharp penetrating object. Furthermore, depending on the nature of the penetrating object, direct and indirect damage can occur. Generally, direct injuries are the result of stabs or impalements with sharp objects, whereas indirect injuries result from missiles passing through or near the spinal column.

Stab wounds cause more damage to the spinal cord than to the spinal column. The spinal cord is usually directly damaged by the stabbing instrument, resulting in localized severe damage. The entrance is generally a small inconspicuous puncture wound; however, the underlying spinal cord damage may vary from small contusions and dural tears to total cord transection. Hemisection tends to predominate, owing to the protective effect of the spinal laminae, spinous processes, and associated ligaments. These structures are believed to force the penetrating object to enter slightly off the midline, resulting in asymmetric cord injury. This results in the classically described Brown-Séquard syndrome, although most cases do not completely fit the syndrome definition. There can also exist associated injury to vascular structures such as major spinal radicular arteries or even the aorta; resulting in ischemic vascular injury as well as epidural, subdural, and even intramedullary hemorrhage.

The pathophysiology of gunshot wounds is complex. The main factor in the degree of damage sustained from a bullet is the amount of energy delivered to the affected tissues. This energy can be approximated by the kinetic energy of the projectile.[11–13] Kinetic energy can be calculated from the following expression:

$$E_k = \frac{1}{2} mv^2$$

where m = mass, and v = velocity. Inspecting this expression, one can see the importance of bullet weight, size, composition, and velocity to its wounding capacity. Doubling the mass of a bullet doubles its kinetic energy, whereas doubling the velocity quadruples the kinetic energy, resulting in much greater tissue damage.

Missile injuries cause damage to the spinal cord and nerve roots by (1) direct injury, (2) concussive injury secondary to shock waves, and (3) temporary cavitation.

Direct injury by the penetrating projectile and associated bone and disc fragments is the main mechanism involved in civilian gunshot wound injuries. The missile can pass through the spinal canal and cord, causing total or subtotal transection over several segments. The cord can also be damaged by bone and disc fragments, even though the missile itself did not come in contact with the spinal cord. The cord may sustain a *concussive injury,* resulting in a partial or complete loss of function that may recover completely in time. This type of injury is related to the *shock wave* created by the projectile.[5,33,35] This shock wave is due to the compressive effect which occurs when a missile impacts on tissue. The area compressed initially moves away, but then reverberates back to its original position, generating a pulsation or pressure wave which then travels through the tissue. *Temporary cavitation* occurs when the penetrating missile's kinetic energy is transferred to the wound tract, resulting in outward movement of the surrounding tissues. The creation of this temporary cavity results in a negative pressure gradient which may even suck in air and debris. The temporary cavity then collapses, leaving behind a smaller permanent wound tract.[1,8,25]

Pathologically, these mechanisms may result in significant intramedullary hemorrhage, particularly in the more susceptible gray matter. Significant hematoma formation in the epidural or subdural space is seen infrequently. Central chromatolysis, neuronal death, and axonal degeneration may be seen for variable distances on either side of the lesion. Chronically, cystic change with resultant syrinx formation or myelomalacia may be seen.

Evaluation of Penetrating Spinal Injuries

Emergency Room Assessment

The initial management of the patient sustaining a penetrating spinal injury should follow the fundamentals of trauma resuscitation. The first priority of treatment in the emergency room is stabilization of physiologic parameters and immobilization and stabilization of the spinal column in order to prevent and minimize secondary injury. The highest priority is the establishment of a secure airway to maintain oxygenation.

Of equal importance is the systemic circulatory status of the victim. Decreased perfusion to all critical organs, not just the central nervous system, must be avoided. The usual etiology of hypotension is acute blood loss from the penetrating injury; however, this may be unclear in cases of cervical and upper thoracic level injuries owing to the frequent compromise of autonomic nervous system function (i.e., neurogenic shock). These patients usually present with hypotension and bradycardia; however, some cases have coexistent hypovolemic shock, making the distinction quite difficult. The mainstay in the management of these patients is judicious intravascular volume replacement; however, some may require a combination of a vagolytic, such as atropine, and pressors, such as dopamine or dobutamine. In extreme cases of refractory bradycardia, temporary cardiac pacing may be instituted.

Once a reasonable degree of systemic stabilization is achieved, attention can be directed to the spinal nervous system. A careful neurological examination is performed. If the patient requires emergency surgery for associated injuries, as complete a neurological assessment as possible in the time available should be performed. The definitions recommended by the American Spinal Injury Association (ASIA) should be followed.[2] The level and character of the injury should be ascertained. An accurate differentiation between complete and incomplete injuries is vital. Entrance and exit wounds need to be inspected carefully with attention to the possible presence of CSF leakage and to weapon fragments, which should never be removed in the emergency department. These partially penetrating fragments are often tamponading major vascular structures, and their removal can precipitate uncontrollable hemorrhage. Removal should be undertaken only in the controlled environment of the operating room.

Although difficult in this setting, a complete as possible history should be obtained. Mechanism of injury, caliber of weapon, trajectory, and the like provide valuable information to the treating physician. Furthermore, photographs or even a brief sketch of the entrance and exit wounds can be quite helpful in dealing with the ever-present medical-legal issues surrounding these cases. Premorbid history, such as other medical problems, medications, allergies, and preexisting spinal problems should be obtained.

Diagnostic Imaging

Routine multiplanar spinal radiographs should be obtained in the emergency room and analyzed for the presence of fractures and metal fragments. Note should be made of any bullet fragments in the canal or neural foramina (Fig. 303-1). Spinal column alignment and stability are assessed, despite the common belief that most gunshot wounds are stable. Computed tomography (CT) is an important adjunct in the assessment of penetrating wounds of the spine. Precise delineation of fractures, location of bone and disc fragments, and visualization of bullet fragments can be made (Fig. 303-2). Significant cord contusion and hematoma also may be visualized. Magnetic resonance imaging (MRI), although the preferred modality for most spinal disorders, is less useful and may be hazardous in this setting; at least theoretically, movement of retained bullet fragments may lead to further neurological deterioration. In selected cases, particularly if there is persistent CSF drainage, CT-myelography may be quite helpful.

Stability Determination

Spinal instability occurs only rarely after gunshot wounds to the spine. In a series of 1300 gunshot wound cases, Meyer et al.[38] reported no case of spinal instability. However, in this center we have seen the occasional gunshot wound with spinal instability. These cases are usually high-velocity injuries that disrupt the major columns of stability in the spine. Children, especially, may have a higher incidence of instability, owing to their smaller and more fragile spinal column. This leads to greater tissue destruction from the penetrating missile; hence, unstable spinal injuries in children are not infrequent.

Despite the common belief that gunshot injuries to the spine are inherently stable, the bullet trajectory and the involved structures need to be considered carefully in each case before reaching any conclusions. If spinal instability is possible, then such further studies as controlled flexion-extension radiographs should be obtained.

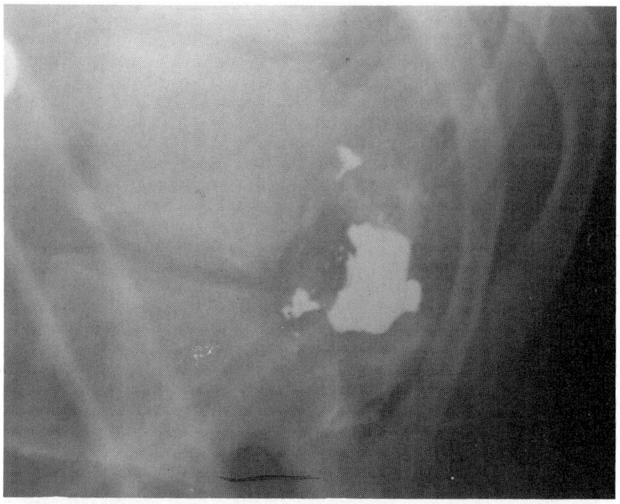

(*A*)

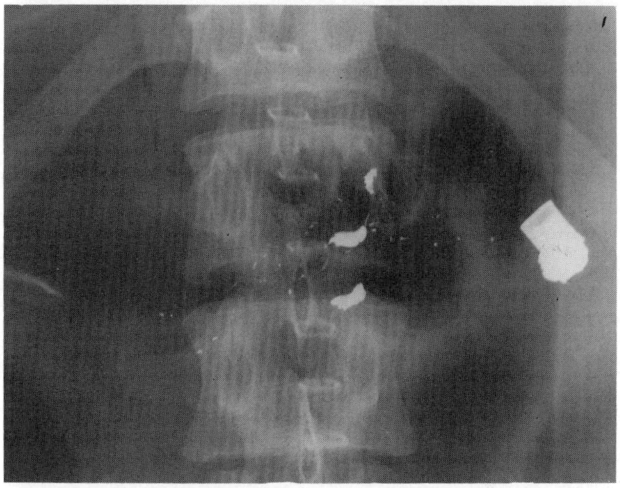

(*B*)

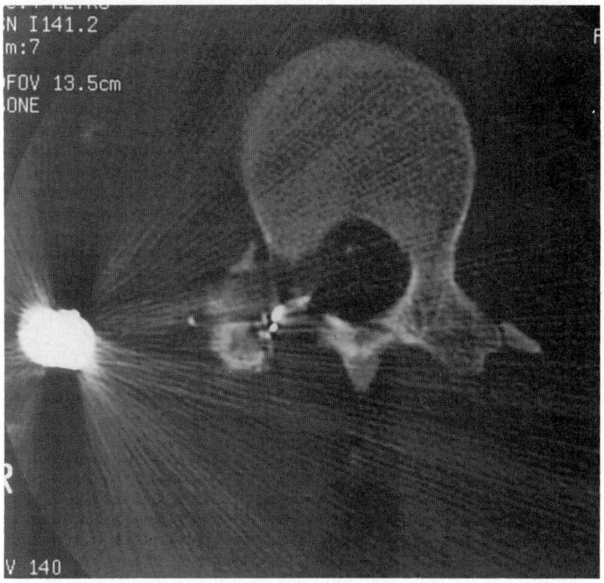

(*C*)

Figure 303-1 Lateral (*A*) and anteroposterior (*B*) radiographs showing bullet fragments in the neural foramina and canal. CT scan (*C*), illustrating the bullet path through the posterior vertebral elements and the associated fractures of the lamina, pedicle, and transverse process.

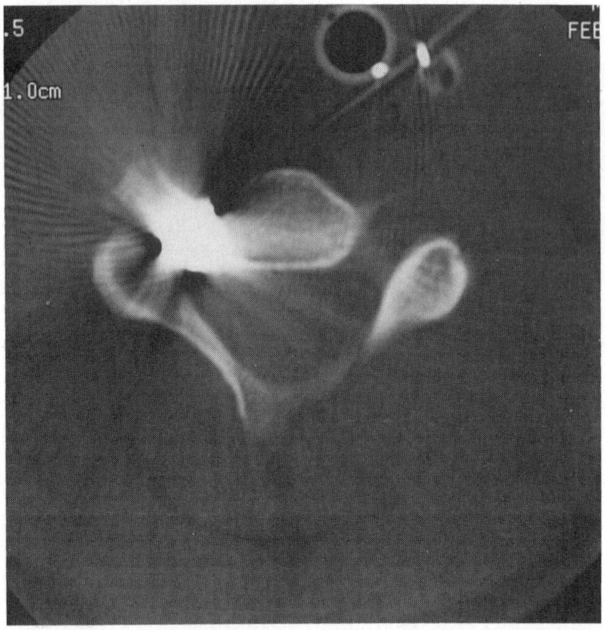

Figure 303-2 CT of a bullet lodged in neural foramen of C5. This patient had evidence of an appropriate nerve root injury as well as radicular pain in that distribution.

Management of Penetrating Spinal Injuries

Role of Surgery

There exists considerable debate as to the role of surgery in the management of penetrating wounds of the spine. Reports from wartime experience favor laminectomy and removal of bullet fragments. In contrast, the civilian literature favors nonsurgical management unless there is evidence of incomplete injury with progressive neurological decline. Those who favor surgical intervention, base their decision on the results of wartime experience. They argue that surgery prevents complications such as infection, CSF leakage, lead toxicity, pain, and late deterioration, and that it also improves the patient's chances for neurological improvement. The disparity between military and civilian reports, however, may be due to the higher incidence of spinal cord concussion from higher velocity missiles in military injuries, which in turn leads to a higher false incidence of improvement after uniformly applied surgical exploration.[56,57]

Reports based on civilian experience generally do not support surgical exploration unless there is evidence of neurological deterioration. This is based on the results of surgical experience with spinal gunshot wounds that revealed no benefit. In a series of 65 patients, 24 had a laminectomy for initially complete lesions, but none showed significant neurological recovery.[57] In a group of 38 civilian cervical injuries, operative treatment did not improve the outcome for complete or incomplete injuries.[24] In a report of 185 civilian injuries, laminectomy had no effect on either complete or incomplete injuries, and surgical treatment led to an increase in morbidity from wound infections, CSF fistulae, and spinal instability.[47]

To add further controversy, some surgeons consider laminectomy alone to be adequate; others believe that bullet removal is critical. A report by Waters and Adkins[55] concluded that removal of bullets from the thoracolumbar region allowed highly significant neurological improvement in patients with both complete and incomplete injury. Removal of bullets from the thoracic region produced no neurological improvement. This author attributed this difference to the regional anatomy of the spinal cord and nerve roots. In bullet removal from the thoracolumbar region more nerve roots with a greater recovery potential were decompressed than when bullets were removed from the thoracic region.

With regard to the management of stab wounds, there is considerably more agreement. Generally, stab wounds and penetrating injuries from sharp objects have a significantly more favorable prognosis for functional recovery.[36] Surgical exploration in these cases is performed for persistent CSF leakage and for retained weapon fragments.[10,16] There is no controversy with regard to removal of retained knife fragments; it is accepted that these fragments have a higher potential for late complications and neurological decline. In fact, a recent report on nonmissile penetrating injuries documented neurological improvement in seven of nine patients who underwent surgical exploration and a 100 percent mortality with conservative management.[49]

General agreement exists that patients with progressive neurological deterioration and incomplete lesions should be afforded surgical treatment. At our institution, complete penetrating injuries of the spinal cord usually are not explored operatively. We believe that the surgical risks of infection, CSF fistula formation, and anesthetic complications far outweigh the minimal chances of significant neurological recovery. In contrast, incomplete spinal cord injuries with a significant persistent compressive effect undergo exploration, laminectomy, debridement, and removal of the foreign body.

Furthermore, with complete injuries in the cervical region, we may on occasion surgically explore such a lesion if the radiologic studies suggest that operative decompression may carry significant potential for improvement in function of one or more nerve roots. We think that in this region, recovery of even a single nerve root may enhance functional and rehabilitative outcome.

Complete and incomplete lesions of the cauda equina region carry a better functional prognosis due to the predominant involvement of nerve roots and not spinal cord. Removal of bullet or bone fragments decompresses the nerve roots, allowing for better recovery of function and less scarring. Therefore, our policy is to remove fragments that occupy the spinal canal at this level. In addition we believe that fragments in the cauda equina are more likely to cause chronic pain if not removed.

Timing of Surgery and Surgical Technique

The exact timing of surgery depends on associated injuries. We consider these cases as elective and perform them at the first convenient opportunity after systemic stability is achieved. After positioning the patient for surgery and prior to incision, intraoperative radiographs should be obtained to recheck the position of the foreign body, which may be mobile if it is in the epidural or subarachnoid space. Exploration is then usually performed via laminectomy with the assistance of intraoperative ultrasound. Bone and bullet fragments are located and removed. However, not all fragments need be removed. Some fragments, especially those that are intramedullary, may lead to further neurological injury if removal is attempted. After the removal of fragments is completed, any necrotic tissue is debrided and the wound cleaned with antibiotic irrigation. Dural repair, if needed, is achieved with lyophilized cadaver dura or fascial grafts, and the wound is closed in a meticulous fashion in multiple layers using interrupted sutures. If there is spinal instability, the appropriate fusion and/or instrumentation is performed. Intraoperative monitoring of somatosensory evoked potentials and real-time electromyography are performed when appropriate (e.g., incomplete lesions, cauda equina injuries).

Peri- and Postoperative Management

Upon reversal of anesthesia, a baseline assessment should be performed, again according to the definitions of the ASIA.[2] Patients at our institution are nursed pre- and postoperatively on a kinetic therapy treatment table. The constant rotation of the bed promotes drainage of pulmonary secretions, promotes venous drainage from the lower extremities, and protects skin integrity.[19] The patient should receive a 14-day course of broad spectrum antibiotics—especially if there has been transpleural or a transperitoneal trajectory with bowel injury. Rapid mobilization is essential, and multidisciplinary rehabilitation is instituted within 24 to 48 hours after surgery. This allows for a smooth transition from the acute care setting to the transitional and rehabilitation phases, thereby optimizing the chances for functional recovery.[18]

Complications

Infection

Spinal infections were once the major argument for bullet removal and debridement, particularly if the bullet perforated the alimentary tract before injuring the spine. Meningitis, epidural abscess, intramedullary abscess, and osteomyelitis have all been reported.[9,22,40,45] Romanick et al.[45] reported 20 patients with transperitoneal gunshot wounds of the spine. Eight had associated colonic perforation, and seven of these developed infection. However, one must consider that most of these patients received little antibiotic therapy. Roffi et al.[44] reviewed 42 such patients, but all received a 1- to 2-week course of broad spectrum antibiotics. No patient in this series developed septic complications. A recent review[51] found no increase in septic complications with transperitoneal gunshot wounds of the spine treated with broad spectrum antibiotics. Therefore, it appears that antibiotic therapy without laminectomy and removal of fragments yields good results without increasing infectious complications.

Migration of Bullet Fragments

There have been multiple reports of spontaneous migration of fragments within the central nervous system.[3,30,48,54] These migrations may result in variable neurological deficits ranging from radicular pain and paresthesia to motor weakness. The fragments usually are located in the subarachnoid space, and excision usually results in resolution of the symptoms.

Fistula Formation

Fistula formation may occur between the subarachnoid space and the bowel, bladder, or even the pleural cavity.[7,14,53] Although these complications are rare, they should be considered in the differential diagnosis of a paralyzed patient with persistent diarrhea, excessive urine output, or persistent pleural effusion. These fistulae are created when there is simultaneous perforation of the dura and an adjacent body cavity. More common, however, are CSF fistulae from the subarachnoid space to the entrance or exit wound. The diagnosis of such a fistula can be confirmed with myelography or noninvasively with CINE-MRI. Initial management should be conservative and consist of continuous lumbar drainage and concurrent use of acetazolamide to reduce CSF production. A persistent or recurrent fistula may require exploration and surgical repair.

Spinal Cord Cysts

Progressive post-traumatic cystic myelopathy (PPCM), i.e., post-traumatic syringomyelia, may be the cause of late deterioration in these patients. Historically, it was thought that these cysts develop either from ischemic necrosis of neural tissue or possibly from lysosomal destruction of the spinal cord.[6,29] Contemporary opinion holds that tethering of the spinal cord results in altered CSF flow dynamics, which in turn creates a progressive cystic degeneration of the cord which may advance both rostrally and caudally. The presence of a syrinx should be suspected in a patient who develops new progressive motor weakness, sensory loss, local or radicular pain, changes in bladder function, hyperhidrosis, dysreflexia, or increased spasticity. MRI, which by this time is safe, is usually diagnostic. Alternatively, delayed CT following myelography may reveal the cyst. Shunting of the cyst to the pleural space or peritoneum may significantly improve the symptoms.[15,34,41]

Recently, we have described a syndrome of progressive post-traumatic myelomalacic myelopathy (PPMM). In this case the spinal cord develops microcystic or malacic changes and not a confluent cyst. The etiology of this syndrome is unclear, but as in the case of PPCM, we believe it is the result of spinal cord tethering occurring after prolonged supine positioning in the immediate post-injury period when the cord is contused and inflamed. This sequence of events allows scar tissue to form dorsolaterally between the cord and surrounding dura. Surgical untethering has shown promising results preliminarily.[15,34]

Lead Intoxication

Lead intoxication from retained bullet fragments, although reported,[20] is relatively rare. Lead projectiles in nervous tissue produce relatively little tissue reaction. Generally, bullet fragments become encapsulated by fibrous tissue scar. Lead intoxication is a risk if bullet fragments are located in disc spaces or joint regions where there is prolonged bathing by body fluids. Symptoms may occur years later. Elevated serum and urine lead levels support the diagnosis. Therapy should consist of the administration of a chelating agent and removal of the lead source.

Pain

A distressing problem in this population is the development of late pain of spinal deafferentation. The pain is usually dysesthetic in nature and quite intractable to treatment.[17] Removal of bullets in this setting has not been helpful,[42,43,55] the exception being the radicular type of pain associated with retained fragments in the cauda equina and cervical area. Carbamazepine, phenytoin, and amitriptyline have been used alone or in combination with limited success. However, for penetrating injuries in the thoracic region, the dorsal root entry zone (DREZ) lesioning procedure and spinal cord stimulation have shown promising results.

Conclusion

Missile injuries and penetrating wounds of the spine and spinal cord are encountered increasingly by neurosurgeons, who must familiarize themselves with the mechanisms and management of these injuries. As a rule, complete injuries do not require surgery unless the bullet fragment is in the cauda equina region, and incomplete injuries should be explored if there is evidence of compression and neurological deterioration. Retained bullet fragments rarely lead to infection or lead intoxication; therefore, prophylactic removal is not necessary. However, retained glass or knife fragments have been known to cause delayed neurological deterioration or infection, thus justifying operative removal.

Despite the advances made in trauma resuscitation, neurological evaluation, surgical technique, and intraoperative monitoring, the prognosis for complete spinal cord injuries remains poor. The national cooperative study unfortunately did not address penetrating injuries, and there are few scientific data available with regard to medical therapy in this population. The GM ganglioside investigation, which addressed these patients, is currently being analyzed, and conclusions are forthcoming. Future advances in medical therapy will most likely attempt to limit secondary injury rather than to reverse the paralysis. Ultimately there are hopes of implementing cellular regeneration and of neural tissue transplantation. However, the most effective treatment of a disease is to prevent it; effective gun control and violence prevention programs would be more likely to have a significant impact on penetrating spinal injuries than will future advances in therapy.

References

1. Amato JL, Billy LJ, Lawson NS, et al. High velocity missile injury: an experimental study of the retentive forces of tissue. *Am J Surg* 1974; 127:454–459.
2. American Spinal Injury Association. *Standards for Neurological Classification of Spinal Injury Patients,* 1989.
3. Arasil E, Tascioglu AO. Spontaneous migration of an intracranial bullet to the cervical spinal canal causing Lhermitte's sign: case report. *J Neurosurg* 1982; 56:158–159.
4. Baghai P, Sheptak PE. Penetrating spinal injury by a glass fragment: case report and review. *Neurosurgery* 1982; 11:419–422.
5. Baker GS, Daniels F Jr. Concussion of the spinal cord in battle casualties. *J Neurosurg* 1946; 3:206–211.
6. Barnett HJM, Jousse AT, Ball MJ. Pathology and pathogenesis of progressive cystic myelopathy as a late sequel to spinal cord injury. In Barnett HJM, Foster JB, Hudgson P (eds): *Syringomyelia.* Philadelphia: Saunders, 1973, pp 179–219.
7. Beutel EW, Roberts JD, Langston HT, Barker WL. Subarachnoid-pleural fistula. *J Thorac Cardiovasc Surg* 1980; 80:21–24.
8. Charters AC III, Charters AC. Wounding mechanism of very high velocity projectiles. *J Trauma* 1976; 16:464–470.
9. Craig JB. Cervical spine osteomyelitis with delayed onset tetraparesis after penetrating wounds of the neck. *S Afr Med J* 1986; 69:197–199.
10. Criado E, Oller D, Fulghum J. Delayed diagnosis of a foreign body in the spinal canal. *South Med J* 1990; 83:332–333.
11. Demuth WE Jr. Bullet velocity and design as determinants of wounding capability: an experimental study. *J Trauma* 1966; 6:222–232.
12. Demuth WE. Bullet velocity as applied to military rifle wounding capacity. *J Trauma* 1969; 9:27–38.
13. Dillman RO, Crumb CK, Lidsky MJ. Lead poisoning from a gunshot wound: report of a case and review of the literature. *Am J Med* 1979; 66:509–514.
14. Djergaian RS, Roberts JD, Ditunno JF Jr, et al. Subarachnoid-pleural fistula in traumatic paraplegia. *Arch Phys Med Rehabil* 1982; 63:488–489.
15. Falcone S, Quencer RM, Green BA, et al. Progressive posttraumatic myelomalacic myelopathy: imaging and clinical features. *Am J Neuroradiol* 1994; 15:747–754.
16. Fung CF, Ng TH. Delayed myelopathy after a stab wound with a retained intraspinal foreign body: case report. *J Trauma* 1992; 32:539–541.
17. Green BA, Edgar R. Spinal injury pain. In Long DM (ed): *Current Therapy in Neurological Surgery.* Toronto: Decker, 1987, pp 294–297.
18. Green BA, Eismont FJ. Acute spinal cord injury: a systems approach. *Cent Nerv Sys Trauma* 1984; 1:173–195.
19. Green BA, Green KL, Klose KJ. Kinetic therapy for spinal cord injury. *Spine* 1983; 8:722–728.
20. Grogan DP, Bucholz RW. Acute lead intoxication from a bullet in an intervertebral disc space: a case report. *J Bone Joint Surg [Am]* 1981; 63-A:1180–1182.
21. Guttman L. *Spinal Cord Injuries: Comprehensive Management and Research.* Oxford: Blackwell Scientific Publications, 1976.
22. Hales DD, Duffy K, Dawson EG, Delamarter R. Lumbar osteomyelitis and epidural and paraspinous abscesses. Case report of an unusual source of contamination from a gunshot wound to the abdomen. *Spine* 1991; 16:380–383.
23. Haynes WG. Acute war wounds of the spinal cord. Analysis of 184 cases. *Am J Surg* 1946; 72:424–433.
24. Heiden JS, Weiss MH, Rosenberg AW, et al. Penetrating gunshot wounds of the cervical spine in civilians. Review of 38 cases. *J Neurosurg* 1975; 42:575–579.
25. Hopkinson DA, Marshall TK. Firearm injuries. *Br J Surg* 1967; 54:344–353.
26. Isu T, Iwasaki Y, Sasaki H, Abe H. Spinal cord and root injuries due to glass fragments and acupuncture needles. *Surg Neurol* 1985; 23:255–260.
27. Jacobs GB, Berg RA. The treatment of acute spinal cord injuries in a war zone. *J Neurosurg* 1971; 34:164–167.
28. Jacobson SA, Bors E. Spinal cord injury in Vietnamese combat. *Paraplegia* 1970; 7:263–281.
29. Kao CC, Chang LW. The mechanism of spinal cord cavitation following spinal cord transection: Part I. *J Neurosurg* 1977; 46:197–209.
30. Karim NO, Nabors MW, Golocovsky M, Cooney FD. Spontaneous migration of a bullet in the spinal subarachnoid space causing delayed radicular symptoms. *Neurosurgery* 1986; 18:97–100.
31. Kupcha PC, An HS, Cotler JM. Gunshot wounds to the cervical spine. *Spine* 1990; 15:1058–1063.
32. Lipschitz R. Stab wounds of the spinal cord. In Vinken PJ, Bruyn GW (eds): *Handbook of Clinical Neurology,* vol 25. Amsterdam: North-Holland, 1976, pp 197–207.
33. Livingston WK, Newman HW. Spinal cord ''concussion'' in war wounds. *West J Med* 1946; 54:131–139.
34. Madsen PW III, Green BA, Bowen BC. Syringomyelia. In Rothman RH, Simeone FA (eds): *The Spine,* 3d ed. Philadelphia: Saunders, 1992, pp 1575–1604.
35. Matson DD. *The Treatment of Acute Compound Injuries of the Spinal Cord due to Missiles.* Springfield, IL: Charles C Thomas, 1948.
36. Maynard FM, Reynolds GG, Fountain S, et al. Neurological prognosis after traumatic quadriplegia: three-year experience of California Regional Spinal Cord Injury Care System. *J Neurosurg* 1979; 50:611–616.
37. McCravey A. A plea for exploration of spinal cord and cauda equina injuries. *JAMA* 1945; 129:152–154.

38. Meyer PR, Apple DF, Bohlman HH, et al. Symposium: management of fractures of the thoracolumbar spine. *Contemp Orthop* 1988; 16:57–86.
39. Peacock WJ, Shrosbree RD, Key AG. A review of 450 stabwounds of the spinal cord. *South Afr Med J* 1977; 51:961–964.
40. Pool JL. Gunshot wounds of the spine. Observations from an evacuation hospital. *Surg Gynecol Obstet* 1945; 81:617–622.
41. Quencer RM, Green BA, Eismont FJ. Posttraumatic spinal cord cysts: clinical features and characterization with metrizamide computed tomography. *Radiology* 1983; 146:415–423.
42. Richards JS. Pain secondary to gunshot wound during the initial rehabilitation process in spinal cord injury patients. *J Rehabil Res Dev* 1988; 25:75.
43. Richards JS, Meredith RL, Nepomuceno C, et al. Psycho-social aspects of chronic pain in spinal cord injury. *Pain* 1980; 8:355–366.
44. Roffi RP, Waters RL, Adkins RH. Gunshot wounds to the spine associated with a perforated viscus. *Spine* 1989; 14:808–811.
45. Romanick PC, Smith TK, Kopaniky DR, Oldfield D. Infection about the spine associated with low-velocity missile injury to the abdomen. *J Bone Joint Surg [Am]* 1985; 67-A:1195–1201.
46. Six E, Alexander E Jr, Kelly DL Jr, et al. Gunshot wounds to the spinal cord. *South Med J* 1979; 72:699–702.
47. Stauffer ES, Wood RW, Kelly EG. Gunshot wounds of the spine: the effects of laminectomy. *J Bone Joint Surg [Am]* 1979; 61-A:389–392.
48. Tanguy A, Chabannes J, Deubelle A, et al. Intraspinal migration of a bullet with subsequent meningitis: a case report. *J Bone Joint Surg [Am]* 1982; 64-A:1244–1245.
49. Thakur RC, Khosla VK, Kak VK. Non-missile penetrating injuries of the spine. *Acta Neurochir (Wien)* 1991; 113:144–148.
50. Tinsley M. Compound injuries of the spinal cord. *J Neurosurg* 1946; 3:306–309.
51. Velmahos G, Demetriades D. Gunshot wounds of the spine: should retained bullet fragments be removed to prevent infection. *Ann R Coll Surg Engl* 1994; 76:85–87.
52. Wannamaker GT. Spinal cord injuries: a review of the early treatment in 300 consecutive cases during the Korean conflict. *J Neurosurg* 1954; 11:517–524.
53. Ward WC, Maltby GL. Associated complications in war wounds of the spine. *JAMA* 1945; 129:155–157.
54. Wasserman SM, Cohen JA. Spontaneous migration of an intracranial bullet fragment. *Mt Sinai J Med* 1979; 46:512–515.
55. Waters RL, Adkins RH. The effects of removal of bullet fragments retained in the spinal canal. A collaborative study by the National Spinal Cord Injury Model Systems. *Spine* 1991; 16:934–939.
56. Yashon D. Missile injuries of the spinal cord. In Vinken PJ, Bruyn GW (eds): *Handbook of Clinical Neurology,* vol 25. Amsterdam: North-Holland, 1976, pp 209–220.
57. Yashon D, Jane JA, White RJ. Prognosis and management of spinal cord and cauda equina bullet injuries in sixty-five civilians. *J Neurosurg* 1970; 32:163–170.
58. Young JS, Burns PE, Bowen AM, McCutchen R. *Spinal Cord Injury Statistics: Experience of the Regional Spinal Cord Injury Systems.* Phoenix, AZ: Good Samaritan Medical Center, 1982.

304

Post-Traumatic Syringomyelia

Joseph H. Piatt, Jr.

In 1898 in one of his very earliest literary efforts, Harvey Cushing reported a nonprogressive syringomyelic syndrome in a young woman who had suffered a cervical gunshot wound.[11] He viewed hematomyelia as the pathologic substrate of both acute and delayed post-traumatic syringomyelia. Reporting his observations of battlefield injuries in 1915, Gordon Holmes described "curious cavities" in the segments of the spinal cord adjoining traumatic lesions, and he speculated that such secondary changes might be responsible for late progression of neurological deficits.[12] Improved understanding of the clinical and pathologic features of delayed post-traumatic syringomyelia did not occur until the antibiotic era and the prolonged survival of large numbers of paraplegic and quadriplegic patients. In 1966, Barnett and colleagues drew on their experiences at a major center for the rehabilitation of patients with spinal cord injuries to report eight cases of late, progressive neurological deficit referable to the cervical cord,[6] and the subsequent monograph by Barnett, Foster, and Hudgson[7] led to wide recognition of and interest in this syndrome. Our current understanding of post-traumatic syringomyelia continues to evolve as heightened clinical awareness and sophisticated neuroimaging techniques augment our experience with this devastating but treatable complication of spinal cord injury.

Post-traumatic syringomyelia is a clinical syndrome characterized by delayed progressive myelopathy often corresponding to spinal cord segments distant from the level of a preceding injury. The prevalence of this syndrome among spinal cord–injured patients has been reported between 1.3 and 51 percent, but such figures are artificial products of particular institutional referral patterns and varying periods of follow-up.[2,6,26] Although the probability of developing this complication seems to be proportional to the completeness of the original lesion, [2,6] post-traumatic syringomyelia has been described after spinal fractures without apparent spinal cord injury.[8] The mean latency from injury to the development of new symptoms has been reported to be between 4 and 9 years, and although there may be a subgroup of patients who deteriorate slowly but continuously after the original injury, a prolonged static hiatus between the initial trauma and subsequent progression is the rule.[7,23,26,28,32]

The most common initial complaint is pain at or above the level of the original spinal cord injury, usually localized to the chest wall or upper extremity. It may be acute in onset and is frequently related by the patient to coughing or straining. In the presence of spinal cord tethering by arachnoiditis at the site of injury, movements of the head and neck or spinal motion during transfer from a bed to a wheelchair may activate the pain. Other symptoms include paresthesias, numbness, weakness, hyperhidrosis, and orthostatic hypotension. Examination reveals hypesthesia, especially to pain and temperature, extending cephalad from the old spinal level, although clinically normal segments may be interposed. Depressed reflexes accompany the sensory changes cephalad and precede weakness and atrophy. Bulbar involvement may be heralded by facial hypesthesia and may progress to dysphonia, dysphagia, and atrophy of the tongue. Less frequently noted are Horner's syndrome, neurogenic arthropathy of the joints of the upper extremity and autonomic dysreflexia.[26] If the original spinal injury was incomplete, progression of spasticity in the lower extremities and loss of retained bowel, bladder, and sexual function may occur. Like the pathologic changes, the symptoms and signs of post-traumatic syringomyelia are usually unilateral in onset and remain asymmetric with the passage of time and the progression of the neurological deficits.

The natural history of this condition is not well documented in the literature, but the trend is gradual progression over months to years. In one large series, no patient was followed longer than 3 years without development of new deficits or more severe symptoms.[26] Remissions are mentioned infrequently.[7,18] Clinical or neuroimaging features predicting the rate of progression have not been identified.[31]

Well-studied autopsy cases of post-traumatic spinal cord cavitation remote from the site of injury are few. Holmes described cylindrical cavities adjoining the injured segment, extending as many as four or five segments cephalad or caudad, and situated posteriorly and laterally.[12] He believed these cavities were under pressure. The age of these changes was not explicitly stated but was probably a matter of weeks. A more recent case studied 2 months after injury exhibited an angular cavity in the posterolateral quadrant extending cephalad and caudad from the level of the trauma.[14] The walls of the cavity were lined with macrophages and incipient glial proliferation; there was no iron pigment. Autopsy material further removed in time from the initial injury demonstrates long tubular cavities adjoining the injured segment and extending through the cervical enlargement, where they attain their greatest dimensions.[7,25] At levels where the anatomy of the cord is not totally obliterated, syrinxes tend to be situated posterolaterally, separate from the central canal and generally without an ependymal lining. Gliosis with or without collagen constitutes the walls, small portions of which may have an ependymal lining.[25] The ends of the cavities are blunted and capped by thick fibroglial scar, and similar glial scar tissue forms internal septations. More than one channel may develop.[7] The pathologic changes are nonspecific, the wall of the post-traumatic syrinx is not readily distinguishable from the walls of other syrinx cavities or from the wall of the hydrocephalic ventricle.[25,29]

The pathogenesis of post-traumatic syringomyelia remains obscure, but it is expedient to consider three aspects of syrinx development separately: initiation, extension, and maintenance.

Clearance of necrotic debris after spinal cord injury leads in some cases to a cystic myelomalacia that may be a precursor to post-traumatic syringomyelia.[19] Holmes believed that the cavities he observed probably not long after injury were created by transuded fluid and degeneration products tracking away from the site of injury under pressure along paths of least resistance.[12] He alluded to a possible role for vascular factors, and subsequent work has confirmed that the ventral posterior columns and posterior horns are an arterial end field.[30] This anatomic arrangement may be responsible for the "en crayon" pattern of central cord infarction and may have a role in the initiation of syrinxes.[33] Venous infarction of the cord assumes a similar central pattern,[13] as does traumatic hematomyelia. On a subcellular level, autolysis of neural tissue by lysosomal enzymes transported to the site of injury along traumatized axons appears to have a role in cord cavitation.[15] The relative importance of these pathologic processes in the initiation of post-traumatic syrinxes is unclear. The pathophysiology of acute spinal cord injury is reviewed in another chapter.

Mechanical considerations best explain the extension of syrinxes into segments remote from the original injury. Fluid injected into a cadaver spinal cord under pressure tracks preferentially through the gray matter of the posterior horns, which as a region of terminal capillary beds lacks the mechanical support provided by larger vessels.[17] Williams has proposed that coughing and straining cause transmission of pressure from the abdomen to the thoracolumbar epidural venous plexus and thence to the cyst fluid, which ''sloshes'' cephalad through the tissue planes that offer the least resistance.[32] Tethering of the cord at the level of injury by a meningeal cicatrix may also play a role[20,24]; movement of the head and neck may stretch the tethered cord, narrowing it and, like Chinese handcuffs, many transmit pressure to its cystic contents (Fig. 304-1). Circumferential tethering may transform flexion and extension of the spine into destructive shearing forces in the central portion of the cord.[32] Furthermore, tension in a spinal cord segment harboring an intramedullary mass inflicts a compressive injury on the tissue surrounding the mass and may, if that mass is a syrinx, cause progressive tissue loss and cavitation.[9]

The origin and maintenance of the syrinx fluid have been investigated as well. Ball and Dayan injected India ink at low pressure into a cervical syrinx at necropsy and observed percolation of the dye particles centrifugally along dilated perivascular Virchow-Robin spaces.[3] Perivascular centripetal passage of dye particles has been demonstrated in animal experimentation.[10] Thus, even in the absence of gross cyst-subarachnoid fistulas, cyst fluid may be in relatively free communication with the cerebrospinal fluid (CSF) and would be expected to contain normal or only moderately elevated amounts of protein, as is true of samples obtained at surgery and during endomyelography.[26]

Advances in neuroimaging have simplified the diagnosis of post-traumatic syringomyelia and have offered insights into its pathogenesis. Myelography with gas or with oil-based iodinated contrast material detects syringomyelia only if the spinal cord is grossly enlarged; however, spinal cord enlargement may be present in only a minority of cases.[7,23] In 1981, Seibert and associates first reported uptake of metrizamide into traumatic spinal cord cysts, producing in transaxial computed tomography (CT) images what has come to be called the *target sign* (Fig. 304-2).[27] This seepage of contrast from the subarachnoid space across spinal cord tissue into the syrinx cavity illustrates the ''porosity'' of the spinal

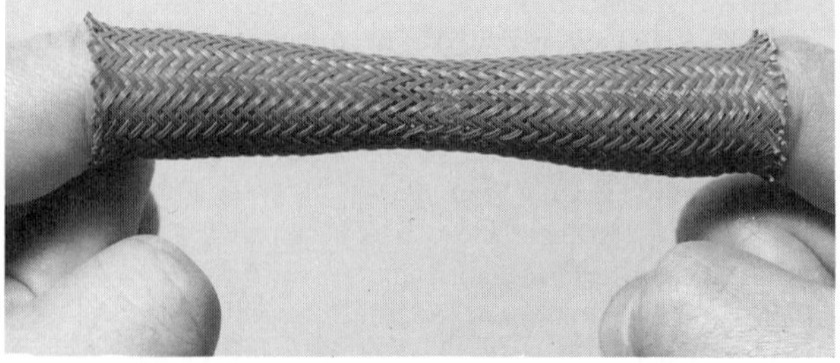

Figure 304-1 Chinese handcuffs illustrate a mechanism for transformation of longitudinal tension into circumferential compression. Such a mechanism may be operative in the cross-sectional enlargement and segmental extension of post-traumatic syrinxes.

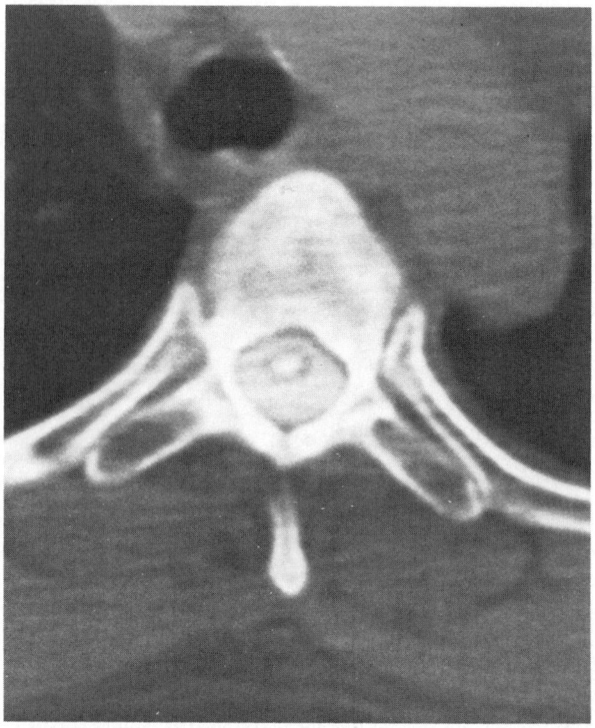

Figure 304-2 A transaxial CT scan 4 h after subarachnoid instillation of metrizamide displays the target sign; contrast has penetrated the substance of the spinal cord and collected in the syrinx cavity. This patient was rendered paraplegic 30 years before by a midthoracic fracture. (Courtesy of Dr. Dennis R. S. Osborne.)

cord, a concept that figures prominently in theories of the pathogenesis of syringomyelia.[32] CT myelography with water soluble iodinated contrast material has demonstrated a surprisingly high prevalence of post-traumatic cavitation in atrophic spinal cord segments,[23] and has also proved useful in the definition of related spinal lesions, such as cord tethering, arachnoid adhesions and cysts, and extradural fibrosis.[21]

Despite its enormous advantages over preceding techniques, CT myelography has been almost entirely displaced in the diagnosis of post-traumatic syringomyelia by magnetic resonance imaging (MRI).[2,5,22,29] On T1-weighted images, syringomyelia appears as a low signal lesion within the substance of the spinal cord (Fig. 304-3), and this sequence is most useful for demonstrating anatomic detail. T2-weighted spin echo images offer additional information regarding pathology and pathophysiology; gliosis appears as areas of high signal intensity in the wall of the syrinx cavity.[29] Foci of low signal intensity within the syrinx cavity are flow voids caused by pulsatile movement of CSF. Disappearance of flow voids has been correlated with collapse of the syrinx cavity after treatment, and, because of the role of CSF pulsation in the pathophysiology of syrinx extension, it is reasonable to view elimination of flow voids as a therapeutic goal.[5] Because of the rapid rate of technologic progress, it is difficult to estimate the sensitivity and specificity of MRI, but both false-negatives and false-positives have been reported.[19,22]

The simplicity of MRI has stood the clinical problem of post-traumatic syringomyelia on its head. In the past, patients presented with clearly progressive neurological syndromes, and the difficulty was to demonstrate subtle radiographic correlates. Now patients present with subtle symptoms, and the difficulty is to interpret the

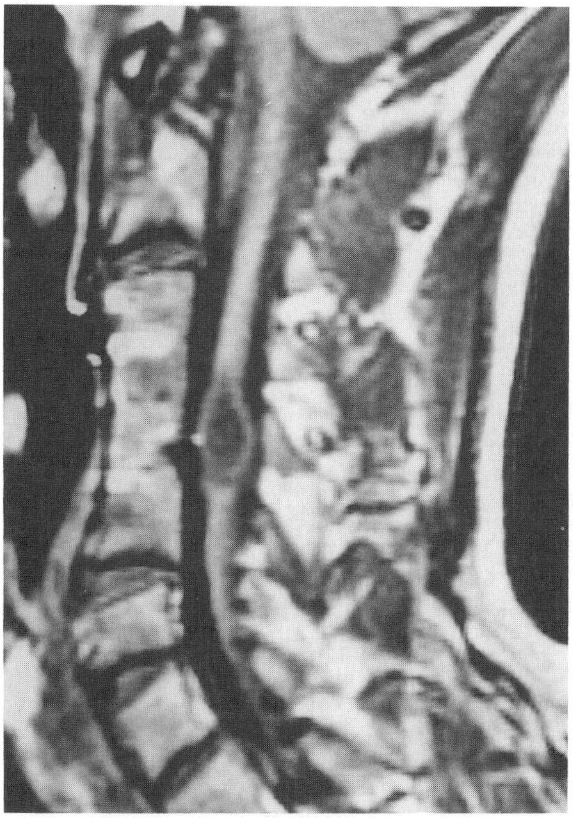

Figure 304-3 A sagittal T1-weighted MR image of the cervical spine demonstrates an expansile, low signal lesion of the spinal cord adjacent to an old anterior cervical fusion. This patient sought neurosurgical consultation because of progressive spasticity; he had suffered a partial spinal cord injury 10 years before. (Courtesy of Dr. Edmund H. Frank.)

relevance of the findings demonstrated so clearly by MRI. Backe and associates recently reported a series of 88 spinal cord injury patients who underwent MRI ''as a baseline study'' on admission to a rehabilitation unit; 45 patients (51 percent) had post-traumatic spinal cord cysts![2] Post-traumatic spinal cord cysts are thus much more common among spinal cord injured patients than is the clinical syndrome of post-traumatic syringomyelia, and judgment must be exercised in recommending treatment on the basis of neuroimaging. Pain is particularly problematic. It is the most common presenting complaint in post-traumatic syringomyelia, but patients with spinal cord injury may have pain of many other etiologies. (Pain following spinal cord injury is discussed in detail in another chapter.)

The surgical treatment of post-traumatic syringomyelia has not yet coalesced around a single technique, and it is not possible to present scientific conclusions about the relative merits of the various operations that have been described. Perhaps the most commonly recommended procedure is drainage of the syrinx into the subarachnoid space by means of a syringosubarachnoid shunt.[1,4,18,26,32] The apparent simplicity of this operation may be offset by the practical difficulty of finding unscarred subarachnoid space into which to insert the shunt; syringocisternal shunting has been promoted as a solution to this problem.[18] Another common technique is syringopleural or syringoperitoneal shunting.[1,4,16,18,32] Cordectomy, either by itself or combined with a shunt, has been effective for patients with physiologically complete spinal cord injuries.[4,18,28,32] Terminal ventriculostomy has been proposed for syrinxes of the conus.[32] Williams has recently described creation of an artificial meningocele, a maneuver which corrects the underlying abnormalities of CSF flow that may be responsible for the development of the syrinx.[32] Whichever the technique, there is consensus that surgical treatment is effective in properly selected patients in the control of syringomyelic pain.[1,4,16,18,26] Motor abnormalities are more likely to improve after surgical treatment than sensory deficits.[1,4,16,26] Unfortunately, treatment seldom leads to significant functional recovery,[1,32] and the question of preemptive intervention to prevent functional loss deserves consideration, particularly for syrinxes in the cervical cord.[18] Although little is known about the long-term course of patients who have been treated surgically, argument by analogy with the treatment of syringomyelia of other causes and with the treatment of hydrocephalus suggests that patients require indefinitely prolonged follow-up, ideally with periodic MRI, in order to detect syrinx reaccumulation and neurological progression at an early stage before functional loss can occur.

References

1. Anton HA, Schweigel JF. Posttraumatic syringomyelia: the British Columbia experience. *Spine* 1986; 11:865–868.
2. Backe HA, Betz RR, Mesgarzadeh M, et al. Post-traumatic spinal cord cysts evaluated by magnetic resonance imaging. *Paraplegia* 1991; 29:607–612.
3. Ball MJ, Dayan AD. Pathogenesis of syringomyelia. *Lancet* 1972; 2:799–801.
4. Barbaro NM, Wilson CB, Gutin PH, Edwards MSB. Surgical treatment of syringomyelia. Favorable results with syringoperitoneal shunting. *J Neurosurg* 1984; 61:531–538.
5. Barkovich AJ, Sherman JL, Citrin CM, Wippold FJ II. MR of postoperative syringomyelia. *Am J Neuroradiol* 1987; 8:319–327.
6. Barnett HJM, Botterell EH, Jousse AT, Wynne Jones M. Progressive myelopathy as a sequel to traumatic paraplegia. *Med Serv J Can* 1966; 22:631–650.
7. Barnett HJM, Foster JB, Hudgson P. *Syringomyelia.* Toronto: WB Saunders Company Ltd, 1973.
8. Bleasel A, Clouston P, Dorsch N. Post-traumatic syringomyelia following uncomplicated spinal fracture. *J Neurol Neurosurg Psychiatry* 1991; 54:551–553.
9. Breig A. Overstretching of and circumscribed pathological tension in the spinal cord—a basic cause of symptoms in cord disorders. *J Biomech* 1970; 3:7–9.
10. Brierley JB. The penetration of particulate matter from the cerebrospinal fluid into the spinal ganglia, peripheral nerves, and perivascular spaces of the central nervous system. *J Neurol Neurosurg Psychiatry* 1950; 13:203–215.
11. Cushing HW. Haematomyelia from gunshot wounds of the spine: a report of two cases, with recovery following symptoms of hemilesion of the cord. *Am J Med Sci* 1898; 115:654–683.
12. Holmes G. The Goulstonian Lectures on spinal injuries of warfare. *Br Med J* 1915; 2:769–774.
13. Hughes JT. Venous infarction of the spinal cord. *Neurology* 1971; 21:794–800.
14. Jensen F, Reske-Nielsen E. Post-traumatic syringomyelia: review of the literature and two new autopsy cases. *Scand J Rehabil Med* 1977; 9:35–43.
15. Kao CC, Chang LW. The mechanism of spinal cord cavitation following spinal cord transection: Part 1. A correlated histochemical study. *J Neurosurg* 1977; 46:197–209.
16. La Haye PA, Batzdorf U. Posttraumatic syringomyelia. *West J Med* 1988; 148:657–663.

17. Leyden-Goldscheider. Die Erkrankungen des Rückenmarkes und der Medulla Oblongata. Wien, 1895, cited in Cushing HW.[11]
18. Lyons BM, Brown DJ, Calvert JM, et al. The diagnosis and management of post traumatic syringomyelia. *Paraplegia* 1987; 25:340–350.
19. Macdonald RL, Findlay JM, Tator CH. Microcystic spinal cord degeneration causing posttraumatic myelopathy. Report of two cases. *J Neurosurg* 1988; 68:466–471.
20. McLean DR, Miller JDR, Allen PBR, Ezzeddin SA. Posttraumatic syringomyelia. *J Neurosurg* 1973; 39:485–492.
21. Osborne DRS, Vavoulis G, Nashold BS Jr, et al. Late sequelae of spinal cord trauma: myelographic and surgical correlation. *J Neurosurg* 1982; 57:18–23.
22. Pojunas K, Williams AL, Daniels DL, Haughton VM. Syringomyelia and hydromyelia: magnetic resonance evaluation. *Radiology* 1984; 153:679–683.
23. Quencer RM, Green BA, Eismont FJ. Posttraumatic spinal cord cysts: clinical features and characterization with metrizamide computed tomography. *Radiology* 1983; 146:415–423.
24. Ragnarsson TS, Durward QJ, Nordgren RE. Spinal cord tethering after traumatic paraplegia with late neurological deterioration. *J Neurosurg* 1986; 64:397–401.
25. Reddy KKV, Del Bigio MR, Sutherland GR. Ultastructure of the human posttraumatic syrinx. *J Neurosurg* 1989; 71:239–243.
26. Rossier AB, Foo D, Shillito J, Dyro FM. Posttraumatic cervical syringomyelia. Incidence, clinical presentation, electrophysiological studies, syrinx protein and results of conservative and operative treatment. *Brain* 1985; 108:439–461.
27. Seibert CE, Dreisbach JN, Swanson WB, et al. Progressive posttraumatic cystic myelopathy: neuroradiologic evaluation. *Am J Neuroradiol* 1981; 2:115–119.
28. Shannon N, Symon L, Logue V, et al. Clinical features, investigation and treatment of post-traumatic syringomyelia. *J Neurol Neurosurg Psychiatry* 1981; 44:35–42.
29. Sherman JL, Barkovich AJ, Citrin CM. The MR appearance of syringomyelia: new observations. *Am J Roentgenol* 1987; 148:381–391.
30. Turnbull IM, Breig A, Hassler O. Blood supply of the cervical spinal cord in man: a microangiographic cadaver study. *J Neurosurg* 1966; 24:951–965.
31. Vernon JD, Silver JR, Ohry A. Post-traumatic syringomyelia. *Paraplegia* 1982; 20:339–364.
32. Williams B. Post-traumatic syringomyelia, an update. *Paraplegia* 1990; 28:296–313.
33. Zülch KJ. Réflexions sur la physiopathologie des troubles vasculaires médullaires. *Rev Neurol (Paris)* 1962; 106:632–645.

INDEX

Note: Pages in italic indicate figures; pages followed by t indicate tables.

ISBN 0-07-079991-1
90000>
9 780070 799912

ISBN 0-07-070313-2
90000>
9 780070 703131

ISBN 0-07-070314-0
90000>
9 780070 703148

ISBN 0-07-070315-9
90000>
9 780070 703155